Creating a Floor-Ready Nurse

Instructor Resources—Redefined!

INTRODUCING
Pearson Nursing Class Preparation Resources

- **New and Unique!** Correlation to Today's Nursing Standards!
  - Correlation guides link book and supplement content to nursing standards such as the *2010 ANA Scope and Standards of Practice, QSEN, National Patient Safety Goals, AACN Essentials of Baccalaureate Education* and more!

- **New and Unique!** Pearson Nursing Lecture Series
  - Highly visual, fully narrated and animated, these short lectures focus on topics that are traditionally difficult to teach and difficult for students to grasp
  - All lectures accompanied by case studies and classroom response questions for greater interactivity within even the largest classroom
  - Useful as lecture tools, remediation material, homework assignments and more!

- **Additional instructor resources!**
  - Find assets such as **videos, animations, lecture starters, classroom and clinical activities** and more!
  - **Add selected resources** to presentations that can be shown online or exported to PowerPoint™ or HTML pages
  - Organized by topic and **fully searchable** by type and keyword
  - **Upload your own resources** to keep everything in one place
  - **Rate resources** and view other instructor ratings!

- **Pearson** Nursing Question Bank
  - Even **more** accessible with both pencil and paper and online delivery options
  - **All NCLEX®-style** questions
  - **All New!** Approximately 30% of questions now in alternate-item format!
  - **Complete rationales** for both correct and incorrect answers mapped to learning outcomes

Book-specific resources also available to instructors including:

- Instructor's Manual and Resource Guide organized by learning outcome
- Comprehensive PowerPoint™ presentations integrating lecture notes and images
- Image library
- Classroom Response Questions
- Online course management systems complete with instructor tools and student activities

mynursinglab

- Saves instructor time by providing quality feedback, ongoing formative assessments, and customized remediation for students
- **New and Unique!** *ECG: The Art and Science of Interpretation.* A special ECG module prepares students for the important skill of interpreting ECGs. Includes:
  - Mini-lectures, quizzes, animations, and hundreds of practice strips
- **New!** Select *Real Nursing Simulation* scenarios
- Includes select set of *Real Nursing Skill 2.0* videos
- Available with *Pearson's Interactive e-Text*
  - Integrated media and website links
  - Full search capability and note-taking functionality
  - Customizable organization

REAL NURSING SIMULATIONS

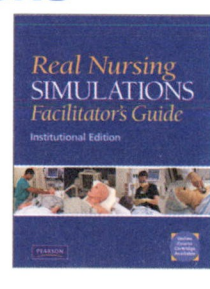

- 25 simulation scenarios that span the nursing curriculum
- Consistent format includes learning objectives, case flow, set-up instructions, debriefing questions and more!
- Companion online course cartridge with student pre- and post-simulation activities, videos, skill checklists and reflective discussion questions

Brief Contents

Medical-Surgical NURSING

Critical Thinking in Patient Care

FIFTH EDITION

Priscilla LeMone, RN, DSN, FAAN
Associate Professor Emeritus
Sinclair School of Nursing
University of Missouri
Columbia, Missouri

Karen Burke, RN, MS
Education Consultant
Astoria, Oregon

Gerene Bauldoff, RN, PhD, FAAN
Associate Professor of Clinical Nursing
The Ohio State University
Columbus, Ohio

Pearson
Boston   Columbus   Indianapolis   New York   San Francisco   Upper Saddle River
Amsterdam   Cape Town   Dubai   London   Madrid   Milan   Munich   Paris   Montreal   Toronto
Delhi   Mexico City   Sao Paulo   Sydney   Hong Kong   Seoul   Singapore   Taipei   Tokyo

Library of Congress Cataloging-in-Publication Data

LeMone, Priscilla.
  Medical-surgical nursing : critical thinking in client care / Priscilla LeMone, Karen Burke, Gerene
Bauldoff. -- 5th ed.
    p. ; cm.
  Rev. ed. of: Medical-surgical nursing. 4th ed. c2008.
  Includes bibliographical references and index.
  ISBN-13: 978-0-13-507594-4
  ISBN-10: 0-13-507594-7
  1. Nursing. 2. Surgical nursing. 3. Critical thinking. I. Burke, Karen M. II. Bauldoff, Gerene. III.
Medical-surgical nursing. IV. Title.
  [DNLM: 1. Nursing Process. 2. Nursing Care. 3. Patient Care Planning. 4. Perioperative Nursing.
WY 100.1]
  RT41.M493 2011
  617'.0231--dc22
                        2010042914

Publisher: Julie Levin Alexander
Assistant to Publisher: Regina Bruno
Executive Acquisitions Editor: Pamela Fuller
Editorial Assistant: Lisa Pierce/Cynthia Gates
Development Editor: Barbara Price
Director of Marketing: David Gesell
Marketing Manager: Phoenix Harvey
Marketing Specialist: Michael Sirinides
Managing Editor, Production: Patrick Walsh
Production Editor: GEX Publishing Services
Production Liaison: Cathy O'Connell
Digital Media Product Manager: Travis Moses-Westphal
Media Project Manager: Rachel Collett
Manufacturing Manager: Ilene Sanford
Senior Art Director: Mary Siener
Art Editor: Patricia Gutierrez
Assistant Editor for Media: Sarah Wrocklage
Interior Design: GEX Publishing Services
Cover and Interior Design: Mary Siener
Manager, Image Rights and Permissions: Annette Linder
Composition: GEX Publishing Services
Printer/Binder: Courier Kendallville
Cover Printer: Lehigh-Phoenix Color/Hagerstown
Cover Photograph: Rick Brady

Notice: Care has been taken to confirm the accuracy of information presented in this book. The authors, editors, and the pub-lisher, however, cannot accept any responsibility for errors or omissions or for consequences from application of the informa-tion in this book and make no warranty, express or implied, with respect to its contents.

  The authors and publisher have exerted every effort to ensure that drug selections and dosages set forth in this text are in accord with current recommendations and practice at time of publication. However, in view of ongoing research, changes in government regulations, and the constant flow of information relating to drug therapy and reactions, the reader is urged to check the package inserts of all drugs for any change in indications or dosage and for added warning and precautions. This is particularly important when the recommended agent is a new and/or infrequently employed drug.

---

10 9 8 7 6 5 4 3 2 1

ISBN-13: 978-0-13-507594-4
ISBN-10: 0-13-507594-7

www.pearsonhighered.com

About the Authors

Priscilla LeMone, RN, DSN, FAAN

Associate Professor Emeritus, Sinclair School of Nursing, University of Missouri; Adjunct Associate Professor of Nursing, College of Nursing, The Ohio State University

Priscilla LeMone spent most of her career as a nurse educator, teaching medical-surgical nursing and pathophysiology at all levels from diploma to doctoral students. She has a diploma in nursing from Deaconess College of Nursing (St. Louis, Missouri), baccalaureate and master's degrees from Southeast Missouri State University, and a doctorate in nursing from the University of Alabama–Birmingham. She is retired as an Associate Professor Emeritus, Sinclair School of Nursing, University of Missouri, but continues to keep up to date in nursing both as an Adjunct Associate Professor at The Ohio State University, College of Nursing and as an author of nursing textbooks.

Dr. LeMone had numerous awards for scholarship and teaching during her more than 30 years as a nurse educator. She is most honored for receiving the Kemper Fellowship for Teaching Excellence from the University of Missouri, the Unique Contribution Award from the North American Nursing Diagnosis Association, and for being selected as a Fellow in the American Academy of Nursing

Dr. LeMone currently lives in Ohio. She enjoys traveling, gardening, knitting, and reading fiction.

She believes that her education gave her solid and everlasting roots in nursing. Her work with students has given her the wings that have allowed her love of nursing and teaching to continue through the years.

I dedicate this book to all the students who will become the caregivers. The following quote provides a solid base for your professional future:

How far you go in life depends on your being tender with the young, compassionate with the aged, sympathetic with the striving and tolerant of the weak and the strong, because someday in your life you will have been all of these. (George Washington Carver)

Priscilla LeMone

Karen M. Burke, RN, MS

Karen Burke has been a nurse educator for much of her career, teaching basic and advanced medical-surgical nursing and pathophysiology. She retired as director of the nursing and health occupations programs at Clatsop Community College in Astoria, Oregon, subsequently serving as nursing education consultant and program manager for the Oregon State Board of Nursing. She currently provides consulting services for nursing and higher education.

Ms. Burke earned her diploma in nursing from Emanuel Hospital School of Nursing in Portland, Oregon, later completing baccalaureate studies at Oregon Health & Science University, and a master's degree in nursing at the University of Portland. She has been actively involved in nursing education and clinical nursing education reform, as well as in initiatives to address the nursing faculty shortage. Ms. Burke is coauthor of another text, *Medical-Surgical Nursing Care* (3rd edition) with Elaine Mohn-Brown and Linda Eby.

Ms. Burke strongly values the nursing profession and the importance of providing a strong education in the art and science of nursing for students preparing to enter the profession, no matter which educational path is being pursued.

I dedicate this book to Brad, Faith, Max, and Aliya – who will carry our family into the future – and to all the nursing students who carry our profession into the future.

Karen Burke

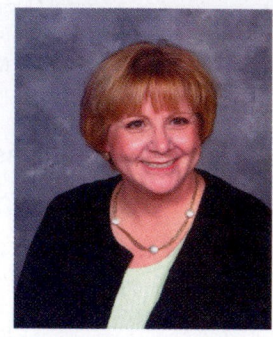

Gerene Bauldoff, RN, PhD, FAAN

Gerene Bauldoff is an Associate Professor of Clinical Nursing at The Ohio State University College of Nursing in Columbus, Ohio. She has been a nurse educator for ten years, teaching medical-surgical nursing, clinical specialist role and translational science courses at the baccalaureate, master's and doctoral levels. Prior to her nursing educator role, her clinical background includes home health nurse, lung transplant coordinator and pulmonary rehabilitation coordinator. Dr. Bauldoff has a diploma from the Western Pennsylvania Hospital School of Nursing, Pittsburgh, PA, and a BSN from LaRoche College in Pittsburgh. Her graduate education is from the University of Pittsburgh, with a MSN in medical-surgical nursing (Cardiopulmonary clinical nurse specialist) and PhD in nursing in 2001, training under Leslie Hoffman, PhD, RN, FAAN.

Dr. Bauldoff is an active member in multiple professional organizations including Sigma Theta Tau International Honor Society of Nursing, the American Association of Cardiovascular and Pulmonary Rehabilitation (AACVPR), the American Thoracic Society Nursing Assembly and the American College of Chest Physicians (ACCP). She is a recognized expert in medical-surgical nursing, focusing on the care of the patient with chronic pulmonary disease and served as the nursing representative on the ACCP/AACVPR Evidence-based Guidelines for Pulmonary Rehabilitation published in 2007. She has been honored with fellowship in AACVPR and ACCP. She currently serves on the Board of Directors of the American Association of Cardiovascular and Pulmonary Rehabilitation and has been appointed to the Community-Based Care board of the Ohio Council of Home Care and Hospice.

Dr. Bauldoff feels nursing is the best profession, using scientific evidence to provide the highest quality of care while maintaining the personal relationship with the patient and their family. Her experiences provide her with insights and lessons learned that she shares with her students.

Dr. Bauldoff resides in central Ohio. She enjoys reading, walking, bicycling, golf, and spending time with her family and friends. She is learning the intricacies of social networking and keeps up to date with technology to be able to interface with her students, family, and friends.

I dedicate this book to my parents, Melvin and the late Frieda Bauldoff, who taught me and my sisters that education is the springboard to a life of great joy and adventure. I also dedicate this book to Dr. Leslie Hoffman, my mentor and role model—she remains who I would like to be when I grow up!

Gerene Bauldoff

Thank You

Contributors

We extend a heartfelt thanks to our contributors, who gave their time, effort, and expertise so tirelessly to the development and writing of chapters and resources that helped foster our goal of preparing student nurses for evidence-based practice.

Textbook Contributors

Jane E. Bostick, PhD, RN, PMHCNS-BC

Associate Teaching Professor, University of Missouri Sinclair School of Nursing, Columbia, Missouri
Chapters 3 and 6

Renae L. Dougal, MSN, RN, CLNC, CCRP

Nurse Educator Specialist, Clinical Education & Research Department , Saint Alphonsus Regional Medical Center, Boise, Idaho, *Research Feature*

Mei R. Fu, PhD, RN, ACNS-BC

Assistant Professor, College of Nursing, New York University, New York, New York
Chapter 14

Gina Dahlby, MSN, RN

Assistant Professor, MedCentral College of Nursing, Mansfield, Ohio, *Chapter 7*

Bonnie L. Kirkpatrick RN, MS, CNS, CNL

Clinical Instructor, The Ohio State University College of Nursing, Columbus, Ohio
Chapter 10

Kimberly R. Regis, RN, MS, CPNP

Nurse Practitioner, Section of Molecular and Human Genetics, Nationwide Children's Hospital, Columbus, Ohio, *Chapter 8*

Mary Ann Towle, BSN, MSN, MEd

Senior Instructor, Boise State University, Boise, Idaho, *Clinical competencies/End of unit features*

Marjorie Whitman RN, MSN, AOCN

Nursing Consultant, University of Missouri Hospital & Clinics (retired), Columbia, Missouri, *Chapters 4, 12, 13, 19, 20*

Janice Wilcox, MSN, RN

Nursing Educator, The Ohio State Medical Center, Columbus, Ohio
Chapters 48 and 49

Student and Instructional Resource Contributors

Tracy Blanc, RN, BSN

Nursing Instructor, Ivy Tech Community College, Terre Haute, Indiana

Wanda Bonnel, PhD, RN, ANEF

Associate Professor, University of Kansas, Kansas City, Kansas

Jane Bostick, PhD, RN, PMHCNS-BC

Associate Teaching Professor, University of Missouri-Columbia, Columbia, Missouri

Donna Bowles, RN, EdD, CNE

Associate Professor, Indiana University Southeast, New Albany, Indiana

Janet Brown, PhD, RN, CNE

Associate Professor, The University of Tennessee, Knoxville, Knoxville, Tennessee

Janet E. Burton, MSN, RN, CMSRN

Medical-Surgical Nursing Instructor, Ivy Tech Community College, Columbus, Indiana

Emily Cannon, RN, MSN

Associate Professor, Ivy Tech Community College, Terre Haute, Indiana

Kathleen A. Clark, BSN, MSN

Assistant Professor, College of Saint Mary, Omaha, Nebraska

Kim D. Cooper, RN, MSN

Nursing Department Chair, Ivy Tech Community College, Terre Haute, Indiana

Renae L. Dougal, MSN, RN, CLNC, CCRP

Nurse Educator Specialist, Clinical Education & Research Department , Saint Alphonsus Regional Medical Center, Boise, Idaho

Daniel B. Flores Jr., MSN, RN

Faculty, Baptist Health System School of Health Professions, San Antonio, Texas

Pam Fowler, MS, RN

Retired, Rogers State University, Claremore, Oklahoma

Kathy Garza, MS, BSN, RN

Associate Professor, Hocking College, Nelsonville, Ohio

Caushauana Harvey, MSN, RN

Nursing Faculty, Fortis College-Columbus, Westerville, Ohio

Tiffany Johnson, MSN, RN

Instructor, West Georgia Technical College, Waco, Georgia

Christina D. Keller, RN, MSN

Assistant Professor, Virginia Western Community College, Roanoke, Virginia

Cynthia J. Larsen, MSN, RN, CNE

Nursing Instructor, Southwest Wisconsin Technical College, Fennimore, Wisconsin

Anne M Larson PhD, RN, CNE, BC

Professor, Midland Lutheran College, Fremont, Nebraska

Wanda Lawrence, PhD, RNC, MSN

Assistant Professor, Winston-Salem State University, Winston-Salem, North Carolina

Dawna Martich, RN, MSN

Nursing Education Consultant, Pittsburgh, Pennsylvania

Joni Meeker, RN, MSN, FNP-BC

Professor, Hondros College, Westerville, Ohio

Dona Molyneaux, PhD

Associate Professor, Gwynedd Mercy College, Gwynedd Valley, Pennsylvania

Leigh Moore, MSN, RN, CNOR, CNE

Associate Professor, Southside Virginia Community College, Alberta, Virginia

Traci Moxley, RN, MSN

Nursing Faculty, Harrisburg Area Community College, Lancaster, Pennsylvania

Christina C. Olson, RN, MSN

Program Coordinator of Nursing, San Antonio College, San Antonio, Texas

Felicia Vergara Omick, MSN, RN, CNE

Assistant Professor, Southside Virginia Community College, Alberta, Virginia

Jill Price, MSN, RN, CCRN

Online Services, DeVry Inc., Faculty Manager, Chamberlain College of Nursing, Senior Faculty, Chamberlain College of Nursing, US Virgin Islands

Sharon R. Redding, MN, RN, CNE

Associate Professor of Nursing, College of Saint Mary, Omaha, Nebraska

Margaret Reneau, RN, MSN

Online Faculty Manager and Operations Liaison, Chamberlain College of Nursing, Jacksonville, Florida

Elizabeth Schneider, RN, MSN, CNS

Program Director, Keiser University, Ft. Lauderdale Campus, Florida

Caryn A. Sheehan, DNP, ARNP, RN

Associate Professor, Saint Anselm College, Manchester, New Hampshire

Judy K. Smith, MSN, RN, BC

Assistant Professor, Lamar University, Beaumont, Texas

Betsy Swinny, MSN, RN, CCRN

Faculty II, BHS School of Health Professions, San Antonio, Texas

Jeri Taylor, BS, RN

Associate Professor, Ivy Tech Community College, Terre Haute, Indiana

Charlotte A. Wisnewski, PhD, RN, BC, CDE, CNE

Associate Professor, University of Texas Medical Branch, Galveston, Texas

Reviewers

Our heartfelt thanks go out to our colleagues from schools of nursing across the country who have given their time generously to help create this exciting new edition of our medical–surgical nursing textbook. These individuals helped us plan and shape our book and resources by reviewing chapters, art, design, and more. *Medical–Surgical Nursing: Critical Thinking in Patient Care* has reaped the benefits of your collective knowledge and experience as nurses and teachers, and we have improved the materials due to your efforts, suggestions, objections, endorsements, and inspiration. Among those who gave their time generously to help us are the following:

Academic Reviewers

Julie Baldwin, RN, MSN, BC

Assistant Professor, Missouri Western State University, St. Joseph, Missouri

Michael Beach DNP, ACNP-BC, PNP

Assistant Professor, University of Pittsburgh, Pittsburgh, Pennsylvania

Sophia Beydoun RN MSN

Nursing Instructor, Henry Ford Community College, Dearborn, Michigan

Tracy Blanc, RN, BSN

Nursing Instructor, Ivy Tech Community College, Terre Haute, Indiana

Jill Brennan-Cook, DNP, RN, CEN

Associate Professor of Nursing, Mount Saint Mary College, Newburgh, New York

Janet E. Burton, MSN, RN, CMSRN

Medical-Surgical Nursing Instructor, Ivy Tech Community College, Columbus, Indiana

Theresa Delahoyde, EdD, RN

Associate Professor, BryanLGH College of Health Sciences, Waverly, Nebraska

Deborah Ellis RN, MSN, NP-C

Assistant Professor, Missouri Western State University, St. Joseph, Missouri

Maria Farber, MSN, RN, BC,OCN

Instructor, Middlesex County College, Edison, New Jersey

Karlynne Galczyk MPH, MSN, RN

Lecturer, Widener University, Chester, Pennsylvania

Carman Godfrey, MSN, RN

Nursing Instructor, Faulkner State Community College, Bay Minette, Alabama

Janet Riga Goeldner, RN, MSN, AOCN

Professor, University of Cincinnati, Cincinnati, Ohio

Claudia Haile, RN, MSN

Instructor, Corning Community College, Corning, New York

Jackie Harris, MNSc, RN

Assistant Professor, Harding University, Searcy, Arkansas

Caushauana Harvey, MSN, RN

Nursing Faculty, Fortis College-Columbus, Westerville, Ohio

Roseann Kaminsky, RN, BSN, BSEd, MSN

Associate Professor, Lorain County Community College, Elyria, Ohio

Cheryl Lantz, RN, MS, PhDc

Assistant Professor, Dickinson State University, Dickinson, North Dakota

Anne M Larson PhD, RN, CNE, BC

Professor, Midland Lutheran College, Fremont, Nebraska

Karla Larson, MSN, RN, GNP

Assistant Professor, Indiana Wesleyan University, Marion, Indiana

Virginia Lester, RN MSN

Assistant Professor, Department of Nursing, Angelo State University, San Angelo, Texas

Margie Lovett-Scott, FNP

Associate Professor, The College at Brockport, Brockport, New York

Ann Marie E. McSwain, RN, MSN, CCNS, CCRN, APRN, BC

Assistant Professor, Lincoln University, Jefferson City, Missouri

Dianne Murphy, DNP, RN, CCRN

Associate Professor, Mount Saint Mary College, Newburgh, New York

Donna Molyneaux, PhD

Associate Professor, Gwynedd-Mercy College, Gwynedd Valley, Pennsylvania

Karen Sheffield O'Brien, RN PhD, ACNP-BC

Assistant Professor, University of Texas Medical Branch, Galveston, Texas

Stefani O'Connor, MS, RN, CCM

Clinical Instructor, The Ohio State University, Columbus, Ohio

Mia Toles-Pickard, MSN, MHA

Instructor, University of Phoenix/Axia College, Phoenix, Arizona

Sharon R. Redding, MN, RN, CNE

Associate Professor of Nursing, College of Saint Mary, Omaha, Nebraska

Stacy Rose, MSN, RN, CRNP

Assistant Professor, Kent State University, Ashtabula, Ohio

Sonia Rudolph, RN, MSN, ARNP, FNP-BC

Associate Professor, Jefferson Community & Technical College, Louisville, Kentucky

Joanne Farley Serembus, EdD, RN, CCRN, CNE

Clinical Associate Professor, Drexel University, Philadelphia, Pennsylvania

Marianne F. Swihart, RN, BSN, MEd, MSN

Associate Professor, Pasco Hernando Community College, New Port Richey, Florida

Shirley Van Zandt, MS, MPH, CRNP

Instructor, Johns Hopkins University, Baltimore, Maryland

Denyce Watties-Daniels, RN, MSN

Assistant Professor, Coppin State University, Baltimore, Maryland

Charlotte A. Wisnewski, PhD, RN, BC, CDE, CNE

Associate Professor, University of Texas Medical Branch, Galveston, Texas

Denise York, RNC, CNS, MS, MEd

Professor, Columbus State Community College, Columbus, Ohio

Preface

Why We Wrote this Book

Medical-Surgical Nursing: Critical Thinking in Patient Care is based on our philosophy that nursing care is provided for the whole person, and not just for a malfunction of one or more body systems. Therefore, our text is structured by functional health patterns. Functional health patterns, as defined by Dr. Marjorie Gordon, include several important components: patterns of behavior, nursing assessment, and nursing diagnoses. Patterns indicate a sequence of recurring behavior and are interrelated, interactive, and interdependent. Health behaviors may be functional or dysfunctional. Dysfunctional patterns of health are indicated by manifestations of an illness or trauma, or may be risk factors for illness or injury. Both functional and dysfunctional patterns of health are identified by assessment and are given labels (nursing diagnoses) to direct care within the nursing process.

We revised and updated the fifth edition of *Medical-Surgical Nursing: Critical Thinking in Patient Care* to provide the knowledge and skills needed to care for adult patients to promote health, facilitate recovery from illness and injury, and provide support when coping with disability or loss. Throughout the text, we make every effort to communicate that both nurses and patients may be male or female; and that patients require holistic, individualized care regardless of their age, gender, or racial, cultural, or socioeconomic background. Our goal is to provide the knowledge and resources that ensure a solid base for critical thinking and clinical judgment and that can be applied to provide safe, individualized, and competent clinical nursing care. We use understandable language and a consistent format, and students overwhelmingly report that they actually like reading our text. We have developed multiple learning strategies to facilitate success—audio, illustrations, teaching tips, and video and animation media.

Starting with the first edition, we have held fast to our vision that this textbook

- maintains a strong focus on nursing care as the essential element in learning and doing nursing, regardless of the gender, age, race, culture, or socioeconomic background of the patient or the setting for care.

- provides a balance of pathophysiology, pharmacology, and interdisciplinary care to support dependent, interdependent, and independent nursing interventions.

- emphasizes the nurse's role as a caregiver, educator, advocate, leader and manager, and as an essential member of the interdisciplinary healthcare team.

- uses functional health patterns and the nursing process as the structure for providing nursing care in today's world by prioritizing nursing diagnoses and interventions specific to altered responses to illness.

- fosters critical thinking and decision-making skills as the basis for safe, knowledgeable, individualized clinical practice.

ORGANIZATION

The book is organized into 50 chapters in six major parts, organized by functional health patterns. Each part opens with a concept map illustrating the relationship of a specific functional health pattern to possible nursing diagnoses. The parts are then divided into units based on alterations in human structure and function. Each unit with a focus on altered health states opens with an assessment chapter. This chapter draws upon the student's prerequisite knowledge, and serves to reinforce basic principles of anatomy and physiology as applied to assessment in both health and illness. To increase student learning, each chapter in the book includes key terms, learning outcomes and clinical competencies, chapter highlights (not included in the assessment chapters), test yourself NCLEX-type questions, and a bibliography that provides additional reading.

Following the assessment chapter in each unit, the nursing care chapters provide information about major illnesses and traumatic injuries. Each of the nursing care chapters follows a consistent format, including three key components:

PATHOPHYSIOLOGY The discussion of each *major* illness or injury begins with incidence and prevalence, risk factors, and an overview of pathophysiology, followed by manifestations (signs and symptoms) and complications. Selected *Focus on Cultural Diversity* boxes demonstrate how race, age, and gender affect differences in incidence, prevalence, and mortality. *Pathophysiology Linkage* tables provide the pathophysiologic basis for manifestations. Throughout, *Pathophysiology Illustrated* and *Multisystem Effects of Illness* art brings changes in physiologic processes to life. *Manifestation* boxes summarize specific subjective and objective manifestations.

INTERDISCIPLINARY CARE Interdisciplinary care considers diagnosis and treatment by the healthcare team. The section includes information, as appropriate, about specific tests necessary for diagnosis, medications, surgery and other treatments, fluid management, dietary management, and complementary and alternative therapies. Specific information with related nursing care is highlighted in *Medication Administration* boxes, *Nursing Care of Patients (such as those having a specific treatment or surgery)* boxes, and Procedure boxes describing care for advanced procedures.

NURSING CARE Because illness prevention is critical in health care today, health promotion information introduces the nursing care discussion of major illnesses or injuries. Selected major illnesses also include *Evidence for Nursing Care* boxes with resources for additional review in applying evidence to practice. We discuss nursing assessment and care within a context of priority nursing diagnoses and interventions, with rationales provided for each intervention. Boxes throughout each illness discussion section present information essential to patient care. These features include *Nursing Care, Nursing Care of the Older Adult, Meeting Individualized Needs, Practice Alerts, Safety Alerts, Moving Evidence into Action* (a summary of a nursing study with critical thinking questions), and *NANDA, NIC, and NOC Linkages*. Last, for 80 major disorders or trauma, we provide a narrative *Case Study & Nursing Care Plan*. Critical thinking questions specific to the care plan conclude with a section called *Evaluate Your Response* that provides additional guidance for critical thinking (with suggestions for decisions provided in the appendix). The nursing care section ends with information about community-based care with suggestions for referrals and additional patient resources.

CHAPTER REVIEW This end-of-chapter section concludes with ten or more multiple-choice NCLEX-type review questions to reinforce comprehension of the chapter content. (The correct answers with rationales are found in Appendix C.) Students can log on to the student resources website to apply what they have learned from the textbook through critical thinking and interactive exercises.

What's New in the Fifth Edition

- We are delighted to welcome Gerene Bauldoff as a co-author of this book. Information about Dr. Bauldoff is included in a separate section.

  All the chapters of the fifth edition of this book were extensively reviewed, and reviewer comments were used to make this revision. New features of the fifth edition include the following:

- Using the term *patient* to describe the recipient of nursing care; this change reflects current language used by major nursing organizations.

- A reorganization of some units as follows:

  - *Responses to Altered Nutrition* (unit 6) includes chapters on assessment and care of patients with nutritional disorders, upper gastrointestinal disorders, bowel disorders, and disorders of the gallbladder, liver, and pancreas.

  - *Responses to Altered Cardiovascular Function* (unit 8) includes chapters on assessment and care of patients with coronary heart disease, cardiac disorders, vascular and lymphatic disorders, and hematologic disorders.

  - *Responses to Altered Neurologic Function* includes chapters on assessment and care of patients with intracranial disorders, spinal cord disorders, and neurologic disorders.

- The diagnostic tables in each assessment chapter have been expanded and are listed alphabetically, and a question about spirituality was added to the functional health pattern interview guide.

- Memory cues provide methods of remembering important information.

- Pathophysiology Linkage tables illustrate the way in which a specific disease pathophysiology results in patient manifestations.

Features

PATHOPHYSIOLOGY ILLUSTRATED

The 3-D art brings the content to life—visual illustrations of disease processes make processes easy to visualize.

PATHOPHYSIOLOGY LINKAGE

Pathophysiology linkages are tables that show the relationships between specific disease pathophysiologies and resulting clinical manifestations.

PATHOPHYSIOLOGY ILLUSTRATED
Acute Renal Failure

The initial kidney injury is usually associated with an acute condition such as sepsis, trauma, and hypotension, or the result of treatment for an acute condition with a nephrotoxic medication. Injury to the kidney can occur because of glomerular injury, vasoconstriction of capillaries, or tubular injury. All consequences of injury lead to decreased glomerular filtration and oliguria.

PATHOPHYSIOLOGY LINKAGE	Fluid Volume Excess
MANIFESTATIONS	**RELATED PATHOPHYSIOLOGY**
Peripheral edema, or if severe, anasarca (severe, generalized edema)	Excess fluid in the interstitial spaces, usually resulting from conditions that cause retention of both sodium and water (heart failure, cirrhosis of the liver, renal failure, adrenal gland disorders, corticosteroid administration, and stress conditions causing the release of ADH and aldosterone, such as surgery)
Full bounding pulse, distended neck and peripheral veins, increased central venous pressure (>11–12 cm of water), cough, dyspnea (labored or difficult breathing), **orthopnea** (difficult breathing when supine)	Circulatory overload from increased water and sodium retention
Dyspnea at rest	Impaired gas exchange from pulmonary interstitial edema
Tachycardia and hypertension	Increased circulatory fluid volume
Reduced oxygen saturation	As fluid increases in the interstitial spaces and alveoli, gas exchange is impaired, leading to hypoxia and hypercapnia
Moist crackles on auscultation of the lungs, pulmonary edema	Excess fluid in pulmonary interstitial spaces and alveoli
Increased urine output (polyuria)	Increased sodium and water retention resulting in increased circulatory volume and increased perfusion of the renal arteries
Ascites (excess fluid in the peritoneal cavity)	Sodium and water retention
Decreased hematocrit and BUN	Dilutional effect of increased circulatory volume
Altered mental status and anxiety	Pressure on the cerebral cortex from an increase in cerebral contents and cerebral hypertension causes decreased oxygenation (hypoxia) of neurons
Pulmonary edema	Elevation of left-sided filling pressures resulting from increased circulatory volume and heart failure

Features

DIAGNOSTIC TESTS

The three-column tables summarize information about key diagnostic tests for each body system.

MOVING EVIDENCE INTO ACTION

These boxes focus on research into specific topics and how the research relates to current nursing care. Critical-thinking questions help students understand the material.

MOVING EVIDENCE INTO ACTION   Preventing Pressure Ulcers in Acute Care and Home Care Settings

Despite advances in health care to extend life and improve functional status, older adults with chronic illnesses are at increased risk of developing pressure ulcers. The older adult, with age-related compromised cellular activity is especially vulnerable to impaired healing of injured tissue such as pressure ulcers. This article (Frantz, 2004) describes an evidence-based protocol designed to enhance the healing of pressure ulcers in older patients by using evidence-based interventions. The following interventions are recommended:

- Assess all individuals admitted to a healthcare facility with a pressure ulcer for the risk of developing additional pressure ulcers by using a standardized risk assessment scale.
- Perform a complete history and physical examination, combined with a detailed assessment of the ulcer characteristics (location, stage, type of tissue, presence of tunneling or tracts, exudate, odor, and condition of skin around the ulcer).
- Remove necrotic tissue and debris from the ulcer to decrease the growth of bacteria and remove foreign materials, such as exudates and metabolic wastes.
- Provide a moist wound environment to promote reepithelialization and healing.
- Control bacterial levels in the wound by using cleansing and debridment, as well as systemic and topical antibiotics.
- Supply essential substrates for tissue repair, including protein, calories, vitamins, and minerals. Maintain a positive nitrogen balance.
- Manage tissue loads by positioning to avoid external force on the ulcer.

IMPLICATIONS FOR NURSING

The design and implementation of a pressure ulcer prevention and treatment plan is essential for any person at risk, including older adults, those with debilitating or multiple illnesses, and those with health problems limiting mobility. To effectively implement a plan, it is important to prepare providers to use a standard protocol through educational programs, and to monitor indicators of improvement or deterioration in the ulcer and presence or absence of new ulcers. These outcomes should be assessed and recorded on a weekly basis.

CRITICAL THINKING IN PATIENT CARE

1. Describe the differences and similarities in a pressure ulcer prevention plan of care you would develop for two patients: a 76-year-old man in a nursing home who has had a stroke that paralyzed his left side, and a 36-year-old man with a spinal cord injury from a motorcycle accident who cannot walk and lives at home.
2. Consider the activities to treat pressure ulcers, and answer the following:
   a. What level of healthcare provider would you delegate to care for the patient?
   b. How much time in an 8-hour period would be needed for nursing care?
3. What would you teach family caregivers about providing care at home?

DIAGNOSTIC TESTS of the Integumentary System

NAME OF TEST	PURPOSE & DESCRIPTION	RELATED NURSING INTERVENTIONS
Biopsy	A punch biopsy is done to differentiate benign lesions from skin cancers. An instrument is used to remove a small section of dermis and subcutaneous fat. Depending on size, the incision may be sutured with a single suture. An incisional biopsy is done to differentiate benign lesions from skin cancers. An incision is made and the skin lesion or tumor is removed for analysis. The incision is closed with sutures.	Apply dressing and provide information about self-care and when to return for suture removal.
Culture	A culture of scrapings from a lesion, from drainage, or of exudate is done to identify fungal, bacterial, or viral skin infections.	Obtain the culture with a sterile Culturette swab and culture tubes. Maintain strict asepsis while obtaining the culture.
Immunofluorescent Slides	Immunofluorescent studies of samples from skin and/or serum may be done to identify IgG antibodies (present in pemphigus vulgaris) and to identify varicella in skin cells (for herpes zoster). Skin or blood samples are placed on a slide and examined microscopically.	No special preparation is necessary.
Oil Slides	Oil slides are used to determine the type of skin infestation present. Scrapings of the lesion are placed on a slide with mineral oil and examined microscopically.	No special preparation is necessary.
	These tests are used to determine a specific allergen. In a patch test, a small amount of the suspected material is placed on the skin under an occlusive bandage. In a scratch test, a needle is used to "scratch" small amounts of potentially allergic materials on the skin surface.	Explain to the patient the need to return in 48 hours to have the patched area or scratched areas evaluated.
	A specimen from hair or nails is examined for a fungal infection. The specimen is obtained by placing material from a scraping on a slide, adding a potassium hydroxide solution, and examining it microscopically.	No special preparation is necessary.
	This test is used to diagnose herpes infections, but it does not differentiate herpes simplex from herpes zoster. Fluid and cells from the vesicles are obtained, put on a slide, stained, and examined microscopically.	
	This test uses an ultraviolet light that causes certain organisms to fluoresce (such as *Pseudomonas* organisms and fungi). The skin is examined under a special lamp.	

GENETIC CONSIDERATIONS

For each unit, this feature lists genetic issues related to the body system.

GENETIC CONSIDERATIONS
Examples of Integumentary Disorders

- Oculocutaneous albinism, an autosomal recessive inheritance disorder, causes hypopigmentation (albinism or absence of color) of the skin, hair, and eyes as a result of an inability to synthesize melanin.
- Keloids, which are elevated scars, have a familial tendency and are more commonly found in Blacks.
- Vitiligo, the sudden appearance of white patches on the skin, has a familial tendency.
- Male pattern baldness (the most common cause of baldness in men) is genetically predetermined.
- Hirsutism (excessive hair in women) may be genetically predetermined.
- Blacks may have very dry scalps and dry, fragile hair of genetic origin.
- A family history of skin cancer is a risk factor for skin cancer

EVIDENCE FOR NURSING CARE   The Patient with Bacterial Infection of the Skin

Selected resources that nurses may find helpful when planning evidence-based nursing care follow.

- Casey, M. L., & Chasens, E. R. (2009). Community-associated methicillin-resistant staphylococcus aureus: Implications for emergency department nursing. *Journal of Emergency Nursing, 35*(3), 224–229.
- Haas, J. P., & Larson, E. L. (2008). Compliance with hand hygiene. *The American Journal of Nursing, 108*(8), 40–44.
- Hodgkinson, B., Agnew, J., Godfrey, C., Goldie, B., Kenner, C., González, R. L., Ramirez, B. A., Maria, E. G., McInerney, P., & Robertson-Malt, S. (2007). Topical skin care in aged care facilities. *Best Practice, The Joanna Briggs Institute, 11*(3), 1–4. Retrieved from, http://www.joannabriggs.edu.au/pdf/BPISEng_11_3.pdf
- Johnson, D., Lineweaver, L., & Maze, L. M. (2009). Patients' bath basins as potential sources of infection: A multicenter sampling study. *American Journal of Critical Care, 18*(1), 31–38.

EVIDENCE FOR NURSING CARE

Evidence for Nursing Care boxes provide resources for additional review in applying evidence to practice.

FUNCTIONAL HEALTH PATTERN ASSESSMENT

Health history questions are described for the functional health patterns related to each unit.

FUNCTIONAL HEALTH PATTERN INTERVIEW   Integumentary System

Functional Health Pattern	Interview Questions and Leading Statements
Health Perception-Health Management	■ Describe any health problems, injuries, or surgeries you have had. How were these treated? ■ Describe medications, herbs, and vitamins you currently are taking. ■ Describe your current problem. How long has it lasted? What have you done to treat it? ■ Do you have allergies to foods, plants, pets? Explain how the allergy affects you. ■ Describe what you do each day to care for your skin, hair, and nails.
Nutritional-Metabolic	■ Describe what you eat and how much and type of fluids you drink in a 24-hour period. ■ Do you have a history of food allergies? If so, describe what you are allergic to and how you respond. ■ Have you recently eaten any new foods? ■ Do you take any nutritional supplements, herbs, or vitamins? If so, what are they? ■ How well do your cuts and scratches heal?
Elimination	■ Is your skin and scalp dry or oily? ■ Have you noticed swelling around your eyes or ankles? ■ Do you perspire a lot?
Activity-Exercise	■ Describe your physical activities in a typical day. ■ Do you bruise easily? ■ Do you use a sunscreen when you are outside? If so, what SPF? ■ Do you visit tanning salons?
Sleep-Rest	■ How many hours do you sleep each night? ■ Do you have trouble sleeping because of itching or sweating?
Cognitive-Perceptual	■ Do you have any of the following: pain, discomfort, itching, tingling, burning, tenderness, or numbness? If so, where?
Self-Perception-Self-Concept	■ How does this condition make you feel about yourself?
Role-Relationships	■ How does this condition affect your relationships with others? ■ Is there anything in your work environment that may have caused this condition?
Sexuality-Reproductive	■ Has this condition interfered with your usual sexual activities?
Coping-Stress-Tolerance	■ Have you experienced any type of stress that may have worsened this condition? ■ Has this condition created stress for you? ■ Describe what you do when you feel stressed.
Value-Belief	■ Tell me how specific relationships or activities help you cope with this condition. ■ Describe specific cultural beliefs or practices that affect how you care for and feel about this condition. ■ Is there anything interfering with your spiritual beliefs, needs, or practices as a result of this condition? What can I or another caregiver do to help you with your spiritual needs? ■ Are there any specific treatments that you would not use to treat this condition?

MEDICATION ADMINISTRATION

Drugs appropriate for the chapter disorders are featured, as well as the related nursing responsibilities and patient/family teaching.

MEDICATION ADMINISTRATION **Therapeutic Baths**

AGENTS USED IN THERAPEUTIC BATHS

Saline or tap water

Antibacterial agents: potassium permanganate, acetic acid, hexachlorophene

Colloid substances: oatmeal (Aveeno), cornstarch, sodium bicarbonate

Coal tar derivatives: Balnetar, Zetar, Polytar

Emollients: Alpha Keri, Lubath, mineral oil

Therapeutic baths have a variety of uses in treating skin disorders. Depending on the agent used, therapeutic baths soothe the skin, lower the skin bacteria count, clean and hydrate the skin, loosen scales, and relieve itching.

Nursing Responsibilities

■ Ensure that the bath water is at a comfortable temperature that is neither too hot nor too cool, usually 110°F to 115°F (45°C to 46°C).
■ Fill the tub one-third to one-half full.
■ Mix the agent well with the water.

■ Assist the patient into and out of the tub to prevent falls.
■ Dry the patient's skin by blotting with the towel.

Health Education for the Patient and Family

■ Use a bath mat in the tub because the medications may cause the tub to become slippery.
■ Keep the bathroom warm but adequately ventilated.
■ Follow directions carefully for the amount of medication to use in the bath.
■ Fill the bath one-third to o[...] comfortable temperature.
■ Stay in the bath for 20 to [...] areas to be treated.
■ Do not get the bathwater [...]
■ Dry by blotting (not rubbing [...]
■ If the medications cause s[...]
■ If the itching is not relieve[...] dry, call your healthcare p[...]

NURSING CARE OF THE OLDER ADULT

This feature provides essential guidelines for caring for older adults.

NURSING CARE OF THE OLDER ADULT **Age-Related Skin Changes**

AGE-RELATED CHANGE	SIGNIFICANCE
Epidermis: ← thickness and miotic activity	■ Skin is more fragile and at greater risk for tears or injury ■ Delayed wound healing ■ Hyperkeratoses and skin cancers in sun-exposed areas are more evident
Epidermis: ← permeability, ← Langerhans cells	■ Increased risk of reactions to irritants ■ Decreased inflammatory response
Epidermis: ← number of active melanocytes	■ Increased susceptibility to sun exposure
Epidermis: hyperplasia of melanocytes, especially in sun-exposed areas	■ Small areas of hyperpigmentation ("liver spots") and hypopigmentation ("age spots"), especially on the hands
Epidermis: ← vitamin D production	■ Increased risk of osteomalacia, osteoporosis
[...]on flattens	■ Increased risk of skin tears, purpura, and pressure ulcers
	■ More susceptible to dry skin ■ Decreased sensation (pain, touch, temperature, and peripheral vibration) ■ Increased risk of injury
	■ Greater risk of hyperthermia and hypothermia
	■ Decreased tone and elasticity, with wrinkle formation
	■ Cherry hemangiomas are common
	■ Greater risk of hypothermia ■ Increased risk of pressure ulcers
[...]tissue is redistributed	■ Cellulite forms ■ Bags over and under the eyes ■ Double chin forms ■ Abdominal fat increases ■ Breasts sag ■ Skin returns to normal more slowly when pinched (also called tenting)
[...]tivity	■ Dry skin is common ■ Absent perspiration

CASE STUDY & NURSING CARE PLAN A Patient with Herpes Zoster

Jesus Rivera is a 34-year-old migrant farm worker who currently lives in temporary housing in a rural area of the southwestern United States. His family includes his wife, Marta, who is 3 months pregnant, and two children, ages 3 and 5. He takes his wife to a medical clinic staffed by volunteer nurses, physicians, and students from a nearby university for a prenatal checkup. The clinic is open only on Saturday and provides care on a sliding fee scale or for free if the family is unable to pay. While Mrs. Rivera is being examined, Mr. Rivera asks the nurse to have someone look at some very painful blisters on his chest that developed about a week ago. He is afraid that exposure to pesticides has caused the sores.

ASSESSMENT

Mr. Rivera speaks Spanish and is able to communicate only slightly in English. The initial assessment of Mr. Rivera is performed by Anita Mendez, a student nurse fluent in Spanish. Mr. Rivera's history reveals problems with lower back pain but no significant past medical illnesses. He is not aware of any allergies and cannot remember having had chickenpox as a child. Two years ago, both children were sick and had blisters on their bodies, and a friend told them it was chickenpox. Mrs. Rivera thinks she had chickenpox as a child.

Because Mr. Rivera has not had any medical care for several years, baseline laboratory tests are ordered to screen for any other illnesses. The complete blood count (CBC), blood chemistry, and urinalysis are all within normal limits.

Mr. Rivera says that he did not feel well for several days before the blisters appeared, having experienced chills and general achiness. He had not taken his temperature because the family does not own a thermometer. Current vital signs are as follows: T 99°F (37.2°C), P 74, R 22, and BP 148/88.

Physical examination of the trunk reveals a bandlike pattern of lesions across the left thorax. Some of the lesions are vesicles filled with serous fluid; others are darker in color and are oozing a light yellow drainage. The skin around the lesions is red and inflamed. Mr. Rivera complains of a severe, burning pain with itching across his chest. He is diagnosed with herpes zoster.

DIAGNOSES

■ *Risk for Infection* related to open oozing areas on the left thorax
■ *Acute Pain* related to the presence of lesions and pruritus
■ *Deficient Knowledge* of the cause of the skin disorder and recommended treatment
■ *Anxiety* related to need to work in areas of pesticide application
■ *Ineffective Health Maintenance* related to limited access to health care due to transitory work conditions and cultural and language barriers

EXPECTED OUTCOMES

■ Skin lesions will heal without evidence of a secondary infection.
■ Limit exposure (as much as possible) to his wife and children and to persons with debilitating illnesses to prevent the spread of the virus.
■ Obtain relief of pain and pruritus with the proper use of medications.

■ Verbalize an understanding of the disease process and participate in the treatment plan.
■ Obtain follow-up care.
■ Make an appointment for a referral for information about occupational hazards.

PLANNING AND IMPLEMENTATION

■ Provide verbal and written instructions (in Spanish) for self-care:
  ■ Wear a clean cotton undershirt each day.
  ■ Trim the fingernails short, and keep the nails clean.
  ■ Wash the hands each time the infected area is touched.
  ■ Wash any soiled clothes or linens in hot water and soap.
  ■ Do not allow other family members to use your towels.
  ■ Take medications as prescribed for itching and pain.
  ■ Take the medicine for your sores every 4 hours, even during nighttime hours, for 7 days.
  ■ As much as possible, do not touch your wife and children until the sores are covered with scabs. Do not have sex with your wife while you have these sores.
■ Teach how to take care of skin lesions:
  ■ Wear disposable gloves every time you do this treatment.
  ■ Wash the sores and the skin around them very gently with a soft washcloth and a mild soap.
  ■ Using your fingers, carefully rub the cream on the sores. Do this once every morning after breakfast and once every evening after supper.
  ■ Wash your hands carefully before and after each treatment.
■ Make a follow-up appointment for the next week.
■ Provide Mr. Rivera with the name and phone number of the Occupational Safety and Health Administration (OSHA) and recommend he call for an appointment to discuss his concerns about pesticides.

EVALUATION

Mrs. Rivera explains how she has taken care of her husband, and Mr. Rivera is careful to describe how he has followed the nurse's instructions. The skin lesions are dry and crusty, with no new blister formation. Mr. Rivera says he has not called OSHA and is not sure that he will, but he thanks Miss Mendez for the phone number. The nurses make an appointment in 1 month for a prenatal checkup for Mrs. Rivera and for follow-up of Mr. Rivera's herpes zoster. Mr. Rivera promises to return if they are still living close enough to keep the appointment.

CRITICAL THINKING IN THE NURSING PROCESS

1. Identify barriers to care present in this case study. How may nursing interventions promote healthcare delivery to disadvantaged populations?
2. Although most cases of herpes zoster are self-limiting, what further assessments and interventions might have been indicated had the lesions shown little improvement over time and/or the pain remained severe?
3. If Mr. Rivera is advised not to work until his lesions heal, the family may face economic and sociocultural hardships. Develop a plan of care for Mr. Rivera for the nursing diagnosis *Ineffective Role Performance*.

See Evaluating Your Response in Appendix C.

NURSING CARE OF THE PATIENT
Receiving Intraspinal Analgesia

Intraspinal analgesia is used to manage chronic intractable malignant pain and postoperative pain, particularly after orthopedic and abdominal surgeries. The intraspinal route may be either intrathecal (into the subarachnoid space) or epidural (into the epidural space). Infusion of an opioid into these spaces provides for a direct effect on the opiate receptors in the dorsal horn of the spinal cord. The opioid analgesic is also absorbed systemically, affecting pain responses in the brain. This method can provide complete pain relief but has some potentially dangerous adverse effects.

PROCEDURE

The physician places a catheter into the epidural space. The catheter is connected to infusion tubing and an infusion pump, and the prescribed medication is administered. A portable or implantable pump may be used for longer term opioid analgesic administration.

NURSING CARE

■ Monitor vital signs every 15 minutes for the first 2–3 hours and every hour for the first 24 hours; the patient is at risk for respiratory depression and hypotension. These adverse responses may not develop immediately, becoming evident only after several hours.

CASE STUDY & NURSING CARE PLAN

The two-column Case Study & Nursing Care Plan includes Assessment, Diagnoses, Expected Outcomes, Planning and Implementation, Evaluation, and Critical Thinking in the Nursing Process.

NURSING CARE OF THE PATIENT

Essential information needed for nursing care of various disorders is described—detailed illustrations help students understand the steps of the nursing process.

Features

END OF CHAPTER TEST YOURSELF NCLEX-RN® REVIEW

At the end of each chapter, NCLEX-style review questions reinforce comprehension of the chapter content.

UNIT 3

Building Clinical Competence
Pathophysiology and Patterns of Health

Functional Health Pattern: Health Perception/Health Management

Think about patients with altered health perception or health management for whom you have cared in your clinical experiences.

- What were their major medical diagnoses? Had they been injured in an accident? Had they or will they be experiencing a loss of body function, loss of an important object, or loss of a family member? Had they had surgery? Did they have a genetic disorder?
- What manifestations did each of these patients have? Were these manifestations similar or different?
- How did the patients' healthcare behaviors interfere with their health status? Did the patient have a genetic disorder? Was there a family history of genetic disorders? Did the patient have genetic studies done? Did the patient complain of pain? If so, what type of pain? In what region of the body was the pain? Did the pain radiate? What was the quality and quantity of pain? What was the severity of the pain? What did the patient do to relieve pain? Did the patient have a significant body fluid loss? If so, what was the loss: vomiting, diarrhea, or hemorrhage? Did the patient have excess body fluid such as edema? Did the patient complain of cardiac dysrhythmias? Did the patient complain of muscle weakness or muscle spasms? Did the patient complain of numbness or tingling around the mouth or of the fingers and toes? Did the patient exhibit changes in respiratory patterns? Did the patient exhibit personality changes or confusion? Did the patient have any seizure activity? Did the patient have any traumatic injuries: multiple trauma injuries, abuse? Did the patient have a blood transfusion? Was the patient treated for shock? Was the patient treated for an infection? Did the patient have a problem with wound healing? Was the patient up-to-date with immunizations? Did the patient have allergies? Did the patient have any autoimmune disorders? Had the patient had an organ or tissue transplant? Had the patient been tested for HIV? Did the patient have HIV or AIDS?

The Health Perception/Health Management Functional Health Pattern includes healthcare behaviors such as health promotion and illness prevention activities, medical treatments, and follow-up care. Early intervention and health-promotion-focused care can result in a longer life and a better quality of life. Health perception and health maintenance are affected by perceived health status in two primary ways:

- Factors that change or disrupt genes are genetic alterations (e.g., Down's syndrome, Turner syndrome, chronic myelogenous leukemia, Alzheimer's disease), autosomal dominant inheritance patterns (e.g., breast and ovarian cancer, neurofibromatosis, Huntington disease), autosomal recessive inheritance patterns (e.g., cystic fibrosis, sickle cell anemia), X-linked recessive inheritance (e.g., hemophilia), and monogenic inheritance (e.g., Prader-W...

- Factors that change or disrupt cells are altered immune response (e.g., hypersensitivity, rheumatoid arthritis, systemic lupus erythematosus, HIV/AIDS), inflammation (e.g., osteoarthritis, *mycobacterium tuberculosis*, infection (e.g., influenza, meningitis), cancer (e.g., leukemia, lymphoma, sarcomal, trauma (e.g., rape, burns, fractures, gunshot wound), shock (e.g., hypovolemic, septic, anaphylactic), fluid volume (e.g., dehydration, edema), electrolyte imbalance (e.g., hyponatremia, hyperkalemia, hypocalcemia), and acid-base imbalance (e.g., respiratory acidosis, metabolic alkalosis).

The human body is continually threatened by foreign substances, infectious agents, and abnormal cells, resulting in alterations that cause abnormalities or disease processes. A patient's perceived pattern of health and well-being affects how health is managed, leading to manifestations such as the following:

- **Rapid weight loss** (neoplastic cells divert nutrition for own use causes increase in serum glucose and increased metabolic rate resulting in reduced appetite)
- **Tachycardia** (shock or trauma causes vasoconstriction and decreased blood volume resulting in rapid, weak, and thready pulse to increase cardiac output)
- **Tachypnea** (decreased perfusion of alveoli causes impaired gas exchange resulting in increased carbon dioxide and respiratory acidosis)

Priority nursing diagnoses within the health perception and health management functional health pattern that may be appropriate for patients include the following:

- **Risk for Infection** as evidenced by traumatized tissue, malnutrition, stasis of body tissue, leucopenia, and decreased hemoglobin
- **Acute pain** as evidenced by guarding, facial grimacing, crying, diaphoresis, restlessness, and pupillary dilation
- **Disturbed Body Image** as evidenced by verbalization of feelings, fear of rejection, preoccupation with loss, feelings of helplessness, and hiding body part
- **Risk for Violence** as evidenced by verbal threats, physical injury to others, refusal to take medications, impulsivity, and clenching fists and jaw

Two nursing diagnoses from other functional health patterns often are of high priority for the patient with deficits in health perception or health maintenance:

- **Impaired Tissue Integrity** (nutritional-metabolic functional health pattern)
- **Risk for Post-trauma Syndrome** (cognitive-perceptual functional health pattern)

1. Besides administration of medication, what did you do to help your patients manage their health related to pain, fever, inflammation, tachycardia, and tachypnea?

TEST YOURSELF NCLEX-RN® REVIEW

1. Following a burn involving several layers of skin, the healed burn area does not grow hair or sweat. Which layer of the skin was a part of the burn?
   1. epidermis
   2. dermis
   3. stratum basale
   4. stratum spinosum
2. What pigment is responsible for skin tanning?
   1. carotene
   2. red blood cells
   3. melanin
   4. sebum
3. Which of the four assessment techniques are used during assessment of the integumentary system? Select all that apply.
   1. inspection
   2. palpation
   3. percussion
   4. auscultation
4. A nurse takes a patient's body temperature orally and finds it elevated by 3 degrees. What other assessment would also be commonly found?
   1. erythema
   2. jaundice
   3. pallor
   4. cyanosis
5. A nurse is assessing a patient who is complaining of severe itching. What would be an appropriate interview question?
   1. "Tell me how this itch feels."
   2. "Why do you keep scratching it?"
   3. "Have you used a new soap?"
   4. "Describe your daily fluid intake."
6. A nurse is assessing the skin of an older adult patient for dehydration. What finding would indicate this condition?
   1. decreased turgor
   2. increased moisture
   3. presence of lesions
   4. pallor or cyanosis
7. A nurse is assessing for edema. What part of the body would he or she palpate?
   1. scalp
   2. fingers
   3. clavicle
   4. ankle/foot
8. A nurse documents that a patient with chronic dermatitis has rough, thickened areas of skin. What term would he or she use?
   1. ulcers
   2. papules
   3. atrophy
   4. lichenification
9. While making a home visit to an older woman, a nurse notices multiple angiomas on her arms and body. What might these indicate?
   1. high intake of vitamin A
   2. poor hygiene
   3. caregiver strain
   4. aging skin
10. While assessing the hair of a family, a nurse notices small white eggs on the hair shaft. What type of infestation is being assessed?
    1. bacterial
    2. viral
    3. head lice
    4. head lichens

See Test Yourself answers in Appendix C.

BUILDING CLINICAL COMPETENCE

Appearing at the end of each unit, this feature integrates information from the unit chapters and gives readers opportunities to apply what they have learned to simulated clinical situations. "Building Clinical Competence" is made up of three separate assignments, which focus on the essential skills of critical thinking, prioritization, and delegation.

FUNCTIONAL HEALTH PATTERN ACTIVITY

This feature provides more detail about how the disorders discussed in the unit impact patients' functional health status. The Functional Health Patterns are described in further detail. Priority nursing diagnoses are described and critical thinking questions focus on applying the most important content.

CLINICAL SCENARIO

This activity presents the reader with multiple patients, and the associated questions focus on setting priorities while managing multiple patients. This activity is particularly good preparation for NCLEX questions that test prioritization, delegation, and safe nursing care.

CLINICAL SCENARIO

Directions: Read the following clinical scenarios and answer the questions that follow. To complete this exercise successfully, you will utilize not only knowledge of the content in this unit but also principles related to priority setting and maintaining patient safety.

You have been assigned to work with the following four patients for the 0700 shift on a medical-surgical unit. Significant data obtained during report is as follows:

- Allen Barber is a 55-year-old patient with diabetes mellitus who is 4 days postoperative abdominal surgery with an inflammation of the incision site. Temperature is 101°F, pulse 94, respirations 24, blood pressure 138/82. The abdominal incision appears red with warmth and edema around the incision. The patient states his pain level is 8 on a pain scale of 0 to 10. Labs and wound cultures have been ordered.

- Tamra Sanders is a 22-year-old patient with Down syndrome. She is admitted in sickle cell crisis with a temperature of 102°F, pulse 90, respirations 30 and shallow, and blood pressure of 110/84. She is complaining of severe chest pain with shortness of breath. She states her pain scale level is 10 of 10. She has an order to begin morphine PCA.
- Mia Windham is a 26-year-old who was admitted yesterday with a maculopapular rash on her hands and feet that is spreading to her arms and legs. This morning she is complaining of abdominal pain, nausea, and bloody diarrhea. The patient has a history of having a bone marrow transplant 3 months ago as treatment for leukemia.
- Harry Anderson is a 40-year-old in late stages of AIDS. He is confused, incontinent, and is very spastic. He is on seizure precautions. He needs to be turned every 2 hours to prevent pressure sores. He is currently yelling that he needs help.

CASE STUDY WITH CONCEPT MAP

This activity offers readers opportunities to apply specific patient information to the process of concept mapping. Critical-thinking questions prepare the groundwork for creating the concept map, and readers have the opportunity to create a concept map of their own in the Student Resources section of the student website.

CASE STUDY: Mr. Blount

Mr. Blount is a 60-year-old African American construction worker who is seen in the physician's office with complaints of dull chest pain, shortness of breath, swelling of his hands and feet, weight loss, fatigue, and weakness. Upon physical assessment, vital signs are temperature 99.8°F, pulse 84, respirations 24, blood pressure 168/92. His height is 5' 11" and weight is 175 pounds. Mr. Blount states this is a loss of 35 pounds over the past 3 months. Wheezing is heard when breath sounds are auscultated. Coughing is noted with deep breathing. Remainder of the physical assessment is unremarkable. He has a medical history of high blood pressure for which he takes diltiazem and ramipril. He has a history of smoking 1 to 2 packs of cigarettes per day since he was 15 years old. He states he has been exposed to asbestos in his employment. Mr. Blount's nutrition assessment indicates that his diet consists of fried meats (especially chicken), green vegetables cooked in fatback, eggs, and bacon for breakfast, and at break time he eats doughnuts or cookies. His fluid intake consists of coffee for breakfast and break time, soda at lunch, and 3 to 4 beers at night.

Blood is drawn for a complete blood count, electrolytes, blood glucose, calcetonin, CEA, haptoglobulin, GGT, and creatinine. A sputum specimen is sent to the laboratory. A chest x-ray and CT scan are done. Based on the results of the chest x-ray, bronchoscopy and needle aspiration biopsies are performed to confirm the diagnosis of lung cancer. The pathophysiology of lung cancer is formation of tumors that begin as mucosal lesions that grow to form masses that obstruct the bronchi and invade adjacent lung tissue. The lung tumor can hemorrhage, causing hemoptysis. The cancer cells can spread via the lymph system to lymph nodes and other organs. Manifestations of lung cancer are chronic cough, hemoptysis, wheezing, shortness of breath, dull and aching chest pain, hoarseness, dysphagia, weight loss, anorexia, fatigue, weakness, bone pain, and clubbing of the fingers and toes. Complications of lung cancer are metastasis to other organs, superior vena cava syndrome, anemia, Cushing's syndrome, syndrome of inappropriate antidiuretic syndrome (SIADH), thrombophlebitis, osteoarthropathy, peripheral neuropathy, and cerebellar degeneration.

Due to Mr. Blount's symptoms, a nursing diagnosis of Ineffective Breathing Pattern is appropriate for guiding nursing care on this patient.

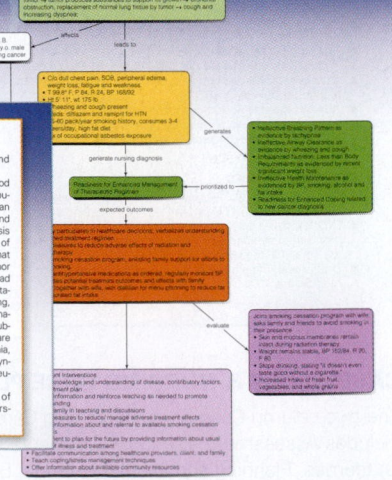

Contents

Medical-Surgical Nursing Practice

PART

1

Functional Health Patterns with Related Nursing Diagnoses

HEALTH PERCEPTION HEALTH MANAGEMENT

- Perceived health status
- Perceived health management
- Health care behaviors: health promotion and illness prevention activities, medical treatments, follow-up care

VALUE-BELIEF

- Values, goals, or beliefs (including spirituality) that guide choices or decisions
- Perceived conflicts in values, beliefs, or expectations that are health related

COPING-STRESS-TOLERANCE

- Capacity to resist challenges to self-integrity
- Methods of handling stress
- Support systems
- Perceived ability to control and manage situations

NUTRITIONAL-METABOLIC

- Daily consumption of food and fluids
- Favorite foods
- Use of dietary supplements
- Skin lesions and ability to heal
- Condition of the integument
- Weight, height, temperature

PART I

Medical Surgical Nursing Practice: Practical Examples Related NANDA Nursing Diagnoses

- Anxiety
- Caregiver Role Strain
- Chronic Pain
- Compromised Family Coping
- Death Anxiety
- Decisional Conflict
- Deficient Knowledge
- Fatigue
- Fear
- Fluid Volume Excess
- Health Promoting Behavior
- Infection
- Latex Allergy Response
- Nausea
- Powerlessness
- Risk for Bleeding
- Risk for Electrolyte Imbalance
- Risk for Injury
- Risk for Shock
- Risk Prone Health Behavior
- Self-Care Deficit
- Situational Low Self-Esteem

Functional Health Patterns with Related Nursing Diagnoses
Adapted from Gordon, M., (1994). *Nursing diagnosis: Process and application* (3rd ed.). St. Louis: Mosby-Year Book, pp. 80–96.
Copyright © 1994, with permission from Elsevier Science.

SEXUALITY-REPRODUCTIVE

- Satisfaction with sexuality or sexual relationships
- Reproductive pattern
- Female menstrual and perimenopausal history

ELIMINATION

- Patterns of bowel and urinary excretion
- Perceived regularity or irregularity of elimination
- Use of laxatives or routines
- Changes in time, modes, quality or quantity of excretions
- Use of devices for control

ROLE-RELATIONSHIP

- Perception of major roles, relationships, and responsibilities in current life situation
- Satisfaction with or disturbances in roles and relationships

ACTIVITY-EXERCISE

- Patterns of personally relevant exercise, activity, leisure, and recreation
- ADLs which require energy expenditure
- Factors that interfere with the desired pattern (e.g., illness or injury)

SELF-PERCEPTION– SELF-CONCEPT

- Attitudes about self
- Perceived abilities, worth, self-image, emotions
- Body posture and movement, eye contact, voice and speech patterns

SLEEP-REST

- Patterns of sleep and rest/relaxation in a 24-hr period
- Perceptions of quality and quantity of sleep and rest
- Use of sleep aids and routines

COGNITIVE-PERCEPTUAL

- Adequacy of vision, hearing, taste, touch, smell
- Pain perception and management
- Language, judgment, memory, decisions

Dimensions of

Medical-Surgical Nursing

UNIT 1

1 Medical-Surgical Nursing in the Twenty-first Century

LEARNING OUTCOMES

1. Describe the core competencies for healthcare professionals: patient-centered care, interdisciplinary teams, evidence-based practice, quality improvement, safety, and informatics.
2. Apply the attitudes, mental habits, and skills necessary for critical thinking when using the nursing process in patient care.
3. Explain the importance of nursing codes and standards as guidelines for clinical nursing practice.
4. Explain the activities and characteristics of the nurse as caregiver, educator, advocate, leader and manager, and researcher.

CLINICAL COMPETENCIES

1. Demonstrate critical thinking when using the nursing process to provide knowledgeable, safe, and patient-centered care.
2. Provide clinical care within a framework that integrates, as appropriate, the medical-surgical nursing roles of caregiver, educator, advocate, leader/manager, and researcher.

KEY TERMS

code of ethics, *11*	delegation, *14*	nursing process, *6*
core competencies, *5*	dilemma, *12*	patient, *4*
critical pathway, *9*	ethics, *11*	professional boundaries, *11*
critical thinking, *5*	medical-surgical nursing, *4*	standard, *11*

Nursing, as defined by the American Nurses Association (ANA) (2004a), "is the protection, promotion, and optimization of health and abilities, prevention of illness and injury, alleviation of suffering through the diagnosis and treatment of human response, and advocacy in the care of individuals, families, communities, and populations" (p. 7). **Medical-surgical nursing** is the health promotion, health care, and illness care of adults based on knowledge derived from the arts and sciences and shaped by knowledge (the science) of nursing. The adult **patient**—the person with whom and for whom nursing care is designed and implemented—ranges in age from the late teens to the early 100s. Medical-surgical nursing focuses on the adult patient's response to actual or potential alterations in health. Medical-surgical nurses must be knowledgeable about all body systems, the disorders that affect them, and the interrelatedness of body systems and health problems. Medical-surgical nurses need to be strong communicators, able to effectively communicate with other members of the healthcare team, patients, and their families. Medical-surgical nurses need to be able to safely perform often complex nursing care skills and tasks. Delegation to and management and supervision of nursing assistive personnel is an ever-increasing component of effective medical-surgical nursing care.

The wide range of ages and the variety of healthcare needs specific to individual patients make medical-surgical nursing an ever-changing and challenging area of nursing practice. It also is important to remember that individual patients are part of families and live in communities. In some instances, nursing care is directed toward the family (for example, supporting the family of a dying person) or even the community (for example, immunizing people to prevent an outbreak of hepatitis A).

In this textbook, discussions of the human responses are structured within the framework of functional health patterns, and nursing care is presented within the context of nursing diagnoses. Throughout the text, nursing care planning is based on a philosophy that individuals, their families, and communities are active participants in health and illness as well as consumers of healthcare services.

No matter the type of healthcare service or setting, medical-surgical nurses must use knowledge and skills to provide competent and safe patient care. The ability to effectively prioritize activities and patient care needs is critical. Nursing care is structured by the activities planned and carried out through clinical reasoning and critical thinking within the nursing process, is based on ethics and standards established by nursing organizations, and is focused on returning the patient to a state of functional health. This chapter provides a broad overview of the clinical practice of medical-surgical nursing, including core competencies, framework and guidelines for care delivery, and the roles of the nurse in medical-surgical care.

Core Competencies for Safe and Effective Health Care

The healthcare system in North America faces numerous challenges, including an increasingly older patient population, changing consumer desires and expectations, rapidly expanding information and technologies, and a focus on improving quality and safety of care. After examining a number of studies about these challenges, the Institute of Medicine (IOM) (2001) found that although misuse of services and injuries resulting from errors are becoming more common, the safety and quality problems exist largely because of problems within the system and not through fault of highly dedicated healthcare professionals.

To meet the challenges, the National Academy of Sciences (2003) proposed a set of five **core competencies** that all healthcare professionals should possess, regardless of their discipline, to meet the needs of the twenty-first-century health system. The competencies are based on using communication, knowledge, technical skills, clinical reasoning, critical thinking, and values in clinical practice. The Quality and Safety Education for Nurses (QSEN) initiative (Cronenwett et al., 2007) followed, with a major goal of preparing nurses with the necessary knowledge, skills, and attitudes to continuously improve the quality and safety of care in healthcare systems (Sullivan, 2010, p. 37). The core competencies with a description of related activities are outlined in Table 1–1.

Framework for Practice: Critical Thinking in the Nursing Process

As nurses care for patients, they use nursing knowledge, critical thinking, clinical reasoning, and the nursing process as they care for patients. It is these mental activities and their application that differentiate nursing from other helping professions.

Critical Thinking

Critical thinking is goal-oriented, purposeful, and reflective thinking. It is self-directed thinking that is focused on what to believe or do in a specific situation. It involves attitudes and skills. The nurse uses critical thinking to collect and interpret information, consider the patient's needs, and determine appropriate interventions.

As you practice critical thinking, you will use the following:

- Knowledge gained though classroom studies, textbooks and current resources, and by interacting with experienced nurses
- Experience gained by working with patients experiencing similar problems or disorders
- An understanding of the patient as an individual who presents with both current and previous illness experiences
- Personal values and beliefs, including recognition of prejudices that may influence thinking (e.g., believing that all homeless people are dirty, or that aged people cannot learn to care for themselves)

TABLE 1–1 Core Competencies for Healthcare Professionals

COMPETENCY	DESCRIPTION OF ACTIVITIES
Provide patient-centered care	<ul><li>Identify, respect, and communicate patient's differences, values, preferences, and expressed needs.</li><li>Relieve pain and suffering, considering patient values, preferences, and needs.</li><li>Coordinate care, promoting active patient and family involvement in health care.</li><li>Listen to, communicate with, and educate patients.</li><li>Facilitate informed patient consent for care.</li><li>Communicate care needs and provide them at each transition in care.</li></ul>
Work in interdisciplinary teams	<ul><li>Effectively communicate with team members to develop and achieve patient goals.</li><li>Clarify roles and responsibilities of team members, collaborating and integrating care.</li><li>Use communication practices that minimize risks associated with care transitions.</li></ul>
Use evidence-based practice	<ul><li>Integrate research and evidence with clinical expertise and patient values for optimum care.</li><li>Participate in learning and research activities to the extent possible.</li></ul>
Apply quality improvement	<ul><li>Identify actual and potential errors and hazards in care.</li><li>Understand and implement basic safety principles and tools.</li><li>Understand and measure quality of care in terms of structure, process, and outcomes in relation to patient and community needs.</li><li>Design and test interventions to change processes and systems of care, with the objective of improving quality.</li></ul>
Promote safety	<ul><li>Effectively use technology and practices that support safety and quality.</li><li>Effectively use strategies to reduce the risk of harm to self or others.</li><li>Communicate recognized hazards or concerns to patients, families, and the healthcare team.</li><li>Use organizational systems to report near misses and errors.</li><li>Participate in root cause analysis of errors and near misses to identify and design system improvements.</li></ul>
Use informatics	<ul><li>Communicate, manage knowledge, decrease error, and support decision making [critical thinking] using information technology.</li></ul>

Source: Data from National Academy of Sciences. (2003). Health professions education: A bridge to quality, pp. 1–15. Available at http://www.nap.edu, and from Quality and safety education for nurses (2007). Nursing Outlook, 55(3), pp. 122–131.

■ An ability to identify other possible options, evaluate the alternatives, and reach a conclusion

It takes practice to make critical thinking an integral component of a nurse's clinical reasoning. The beginning nurse uses a deliberate process of assessing, considering possible alternative causes and action options, and choosing the most appropriate of the alternatives considered. With knowledge and experience, the nurse recognizes expected patterns of response, deviations from the expected, and the probable meaning of the deviation. Clinical reasoning and critical thinking gradually become more internalized; the nurse begins "thinking like a nurse." Critical-thinking exercises are included throughout this book to provide practice in clinical reasoning.

Attitudes and Mental Habits Necessary for Critical Thinking

Thinking critically involves more than just cognitive (knowledge) skills. It is strongly influenced by one's attitudes and mental habits. To think critically, you must be aware of your attitudes and how they affect your thinking. These attitudes and mental habits are the following:

■ Being able to think independently so that you make clinical decisions based on sound thinking and judgment. This means, for example, that you are not influenced by negative comments from other healthcare providers about a patient.

■ Being willing to listen to and be fair in your evaluation of others' ideas and beliefs. This involves listening carefully to other ideas and thoughts, and making a decision based on what you learn instead of how you feel.

■ Having empathy by being able to put yourself in the place of another to better understand that other person. For example, if you put yourself in the place of the person with severe pain, you are better able to understand why he or she is so upset when pain medications are late.

■ Being fair-minded and considering all viewpoints before making a decision through a sense of justice and being humble. This means you consider the viewpoints of others that may be different from yours before reaching a conclusion. You also realize that you are constantly learning from others. You are not afraid to say, "I don't know the answer to that question, but I will find out and let you know."

■ Being disciplined so that you do not stop at easy answers, but continue to consider alternatives.

■ Being creative and self-confident. Nurses often need to consider different ways of providing care and constantly look for better, more cost-effective methods. Confidence in one's decisions is gained through critical thinking.

Critical Thinking Skills

The major critical thinking skills used by nurses are divergent thinking, reasoning, clarifying, and reflection. A description of each follows:

Divergent thinking is the ability to weigh the importance of information. This means that when you collect data from a patient, you can sort out the data that are relevant for care from the data that are not relevant, and explore alternatives to draw a conclusion. Abnormal data are usually considered relevant; normal data are helpful but may not change the care you provide.

Reasoning is the ability to discriminate between facts and guesses. By using known facts, problems are solved and decisions are made in a systematic, logical way. For example, when you take a pulse you must know the facts of normal pulse rate for a person of this age, types of medications the patient is taking that may alter the pulse rate, and the emotional and physical state of the patient. Based on these facts, you are able to decide if the pulse rate is normal or abnormal.

Clarifying involves noting similarities and differences to sort information to help focus on the present situation. For example, when caring for a patient with chronic pain, you must know the definition of chronic pain and the similarities and differences between acute pain and chronic pain.

Reflection occurs when you take time to think about something, comparing different situations with similar solutions. It cannot take place in an emergency situation. As you reflect on your experiences in nursing, many of those experiences may in turn become alternatives when caring for a different patient.

All nurses are expected to think critically, making reasoned clinical judgments. Using critical thinking to provide care that is structured by the nursing process allows the nurse to provide safe, effective, holistic, and individualized care.

The Nursing Process

The **nursing process** is the series of critical-thinking and clinical-reasoning activities nurses use as they provide care to patients. As nurses gain increasing autonomy in their practice, the nursing process helps them identify their independent practice domain. The nursing process provides a common reference system and a common terminology to serve as a base for improving clinical practice through research. In addition, the nursing process can serve as a framework for the evaluation of quality care.

The nursing process can be used in any setting. The purpose of care may be to promote wellness, maintain health, restore health, or provide comfort and facilitate coping with disability or death. Regardless of the purpose of care, the planned process of nursing allows for the inclusion of specific, individualized, and holistic activities.

The nursing process also benefits the patient receiving care and the agency or institution providing that care. The patient receives planned, individualized interventions; participates in all steps of the process; and is assured continuity of care through the written care plan. The nursing process benefits the healthcare institution through better resource utilization, increased patient satisfaction, and improved documentation of care.

The five phases in the nursing process are assessment, diagnosis, planning, implementation, and evaluation. These phases are interrelated and interdependent. They are often used cyclically, with the patient central to all phases, as illustrated in Figure 1–1 ■. The steps have been legitimized by the ANA Standards of Practice, state nursing practice acts, and licensing examinations that are structured on a nursing model of care based on the nursing process.

This textbook assumes that the student already has a basic understanding of the nursing process and is now ready to expand and apply that knowledge to adult patients with medical-surgical health problems. The following discussion is intended to serve only as a review; for more information, consult books specifically

Figure 1–1 ■ Steps of the nursing process. Notice that the steps are interrelated and interdependent. For example, evaluation of the patient might reveal the need for further assessment, additional nursing diagnoses, and/or a revision of the plan of care.

focused on the use of the nursing process, and read the case studies in the nursing care chapters throughout this textbook.

In addition to nursing care plans based on a patient care situation that describe each step of the process, charts are included throughout the text that illustrate the relationship of nursing diagnoses (NANDA), nursing interventions (NIC), and nursing outcomes (NOC). Categorized as the NNN Alliance, the links between and among NANDA, NIC, and NOC represent the collaborative relationship between the North American Nursing Diagnosis Association (NANDA) and the Center for Nursing Classification and Clinical Effectiveness (Nursing Interventions Classification [NIC] and Nursing Outcomes Classification [NOC]) at the University of Iowa.

Assessment

Assessment is a critical element in each phase of the nursing process. It begins with the patient's first encounter with the healthcare system and continues as long as the patient requires care. During assessment, data (pieces of information) about health status are collected, validated, organized, clustered into patterns, and communicated either verbally or in written form. Assessment serves as the basis for deriving accurate nursing diagnoses, for planning and implementing both initial and ongoing individualized care, and for evaluating care.

The nurse collects holistic assessment data, considering all dimensions of the patient. The data collected are both objective and subjective. Information that the nurse perceives by the senses is *objective data*; it is seen, heard, touched, or smelled, and can be verified by another person (e.g., blood pressure, temperature, pulse, or the presence of infected drainage). Information that is perceived only by the person experiencing it (e.g., pain, dizziness, or anxiety) is *subjective data*.

Nurses conduct both initial and ongoing assessments. The initial assessment, conducted through a nursing history and physical assessment, is obtained to provide a comprehensive

picture of the patient's health status. It is necessary to provide comprehensive data about the individual's health responses, identify specific factors that contribute to these responses, and facilitate mutually established goals and outcomes of care.

Focused assessments are ongoing and continuous, occurring whenever the nurse interacts with the patient. In a focused assessment, data is gathered about an identified or potential problem. This data is used to evaluate nursing actions and make decisions about whether to continue or change interventions to meet outcomes. Assessments also provide structure for documenting nursing care. In addition, focused assessments enable the nurse to identify responses to a disease process or treatment modality not present during the initial assessment, and to identify new problems (Alfaro-LeFevre, 2009).

To make accurate and holistic assessments, nurses must have and use a wide variety of knowledge and skills. The ability to assess the physical status of the patient is essential, as is the ability to communicate effectively. Nurses must know and understand pathophysiology and pharmacology and be able to identify abnormal laboratory and diagnostic test data. Finally, nurses need a solid foundation of nursing knowledge and skill to interpret assessment data and to use that interpretation as the basis for individualized care.

Nurses use a number of critical thinking skills when assessing. An attitude of inquiry is used during data gathering. The nurse must distinguish data that is relevant from that which is irrelevant, as well as important data from unimportant data. In addition, the nurse identifies missing data and seeks additional information to fill in gaps (Wilkinson, 2007).

MEMORY CUE

Remember that assessment is collecting and interpreting the meaning of data; it is *not* forming judgments. "Patient is angry and out-of-control" is a judgment; "Pacing, talking loudly and with a rapid cadence" is an assessment.

Diagnosis

The ANA defines nursing as "the protection, promotion, and optimization of health and abilities, prevention of illness and injury alleviation of suffering through the diagnosis and treatment of human response" (2004a, p. 7). In the diagnosis phase of the nursing process, the nurse uses assessed data, knowledge of expected responses, intuition, and prior experience to analyze data and draw conclusions about its meaning. The nurse then labels each identified health problem with a nursing diagnosis, a statement that describes the patient's current health status. Nursing diagnoses describe actual or potential health problems that can legally be diagnosed by the nurse, for which the nurse can prescribe the primary interventions, and for which the nurse is accountable (Wilkinson, 2007).

The nurse analyzes assessment data to support appropriate nursing diagnoses. During analysis, the nurse organizes or categorizes data so that it can be used to identify actual or potential health problems. Data can be organized within a variety of frameworks. Methods commonly used are basic human needs (Maslow, 1970), body systems, human response patterns, and functional health patterns (Gordon, 1982). The broad organizational structure used to categorize information in this book is based on functional health patterns, outlined in Box 1–1.

Identifying health problems or needs and making a diagnosis is a complex process that always involves uncertainty. Therefore, the nurse uses diagnostic reasoning to choose nursing diagnoses that best define the individual patient's health problems. Diagnostic reasoning is a form of clinical judgment used to make decisions about which label (or diagnosis) best describes the patterns of data. Box 1–2 outlines the steps and processes the nurse uses in diagnostic reasoning.

Diagnoses made by nurses generally fall within three categories:

1. Actual nursing diagnoses: A health problem identified during assessment that can be relieved or resolved through nursing interventions
2. Potential (or risk) nursing diagnoses: A health problem that is likely to develop unless the nurse intervenes
3. Collaborative problems: A health problem that requires both medical and nursing interventions; nurses monitor for and intervene to reduce complications (Wilkinson, 2007)

NANDA   Although there is no universal list of diagnoses used in nursing, the ongoing work of NANDA is widely accepted. The diagnoses are classified by a taxonomy; that is, they are grouped into classes and subclasses based on patterns and relationships. The NANDA system was accepted in 1988 by the ANA as the official system of nursing diagnosis for the United States. Nursing diagnoses within the NANDA taxonomy are used in this book. Where appropriate, collaborative problems also are identified. A complete list of current NANDA nursing diagnoses can be found in ∞ Appendix B.

BOX 1–1 Functional Health Patterns

1. *Health perception–health management pattern.* Describes client's perceived pattern of health and well-being and how health is managed.
2. *Nutritional-metabolic pattern.* Describes pattern of food and fluid consumption relative to metabolic need and pattern indicators of local nutrient supply.
3. *Elimination pattern.* Describes pattern of excretory function (bowel, bladder, and skin).
4. *Activity-exercise pattern.* Describes pattern of exercise, activity, leisure, and recreation.
5. *Cognitive-perceptual pattern.* Describes sensory-perceptual and cognitive patterns.
6. *Sleep-rest pattern.* Describes patterns of sleep, rest, and relaxation.
7. *Self-perception–self-concept pattern.* Describes self-concept pattern and perceptions of self (e.g., body comfort, body image, feeling state).
8. *Role-relationship pattern.* Describes patterns of role engagements and relationships.
9. *Sexuality-reproductive pattern.* Describes client's patterns of satisfaction and dissatisfaction with sexuality; describes reproductive patterns.
10. *Coping–stress tolerance pattern.* Describes general coping pattern and effectiveness of the pattern in terms of stress tolerance.
11. *Value-belief pattern.* Describes patterns of values, beliefs (including spiritual), or goals that guide choices or decisions.

Source: Adapted from Gordon, M., (1994). *Nursing diagnosis: Process and application* (3rd ed.), St. Louis: Mosby-Year Book. Used with permission.

BOX 1–2 Overview of Diagnostic Reasoning

Interpret the Data

Level I—Identify significant cues
1. *Organize data* in a concise format, using nursing framework
2. *Compare individual data to standards and norms* to identify significant cures

Level II—Cluster cures and identify data gaps
3. *Cluster significant cues*; look for patterns and relationships
4. *Categorize clusters* according to your framework
5. *Identify data gaps and inconsistencies*

Level III—Draw conclusions about the present health status
6. *Think of as many explanations as possible for each cue cluster. Then decide which hypothesis best explains it.* (Note: You can sometimes identify both the problem and etiology in this step.)
7. *Identify problem* (wellness diagnoses; actual, potential, and possible nursing diagnoses; collaborative problems; and medical problems)
8. *Identify patient and family strengths.*

Level IV—Determine etiologies and categorize problems
9. *Determine the etiologies of the problems*
10. *Categorize problems* according to your framework

Verify the Diagnoses
11. *Verify the diagnoses and strengths* with the patient, family, other professionals, and references

Label the Diagnoses
12. *Choose standardized problem label.* Write formal health status statements: nursing and wellness diagnoses, collaborative problems, and strengths
13. *Prioritize the problems*

Record the Data
14. *Record the problem statements* on the appropriate documents: patent care plan, chart, etc.

Source: From Wilkinson, Judith M., *Nursing Process and Critical Thinking*, 4th, © 2007. Reproduced by permission of Pearson Education, Inc., Upper Saddle River, New Jersey.

WRITING DIAGNOSES   A diagnosis is written in two parts joined by the phrase "related to." The first part of the statement describes the patient's health status. It identifies what needs to change in a specific patient as a result of nursing interventions, and suggests the patient outcomes that measure the change. The part of the statement that follows the "related to" phrase identifies the physical, psychosocial, cultural, spiritual, and/or environmental factors (etiologies) that cause or contribute to the occurrence of the response.

Many nurses write nursing diagnoses using a method known as PES (Gordon, 1994). Diagnoses written with this method have three components:

1. The problem (P), which is the NANDA label.
2. The etiology (E) of the problem, which names the related factors and is indicated by the phrase "related to."
3. The signs and symptoms (S), which are the defining characteristics and are indicated by the phrase "as manifested by."

Examples of nursing diagnoses written with the PES method are as follows:

- *Anxiety* related to hospitalization as manifested by statements of nervousness and by crying
- *Bowel incontinence* related to loss of sphincter control as manifested by involuntary passage of stool

■ *Fatigue* related to the side effects of chemotherapy as manifested by the inability to carry out normal daily routines and statements of overwhelming exhaustion

Planning

During the planning step, the nurse identifies the desired patient outcomes of care and nursing interventions to achieve those outcomes. *Outcomes*, which are mutually established by the patient and nurse, describe the expected patient responses that will occur as a result of the nursing interventions. Nursing interventions (actions) are specifically planned to achieve the desired outcomes. Both outcomes and nursing interventions are documented in a written plan of care that directs nursing activities and documentation and provides a tool for evaluation (Alfaro-LeFevre, 2009).

Nurses plan interventions for problems that require nursing management (stated as nursing diagnoses) and for collaborative or clinical problems. Nursing diagnoses provide the basis for selecting nurse-initiated interventions to achieve outcomes for which the nurse is accountable. Collaborative problems are often based on medical diagnoses (such as hemorrhage) that nurses monitor to detect onset or changes in status.

Outcome criteria for nursing diagnoses are patient centered, time specific, and measurable. They are classified into three domains: cognitive (knowing), affective (feeling), and psychomotor (doing). The nurse considers all three domains to ensure holistic care.

The Nursing Outcomes Classification (NOC) provides standardized outcome labels and measurable indicators that can be used to evaluate patient status and nursing care.

Outcome criteria for collaborative problems follow the same pattern. For example, "Respiratory complications will not occur as evidenced by clear lung sounds, pulse, respiratory rate, and temperature in normal range for patient throughout recovery period."

Planned nursing interventions must be specific and individualized. If, for example, the nurse identifies that a patient is at risk for fluid volume deficit, it is not enough that the nurse simply encourage the patient to drink increased amounts of fluid. The nurse and the patient together must identify those liquids the patient prefers, the times that will be best for drinking them, and the amount of fluid (in ounces or milliliters); this information is documented as a nursing order on the written care plan. Only then does care truly become a part of the plan of care.

EVIDENCE-BASED PRACTICE GUIDELINES Whenever possible, planned nursing interventions are based on evidence, that is, nursing research and nursing practice guidelines. Currently, significant work is being done to develop evidence-based nursing practice guidelines. Guidelines are collections of practical information used to help guide decisions related to specific circumstances (Hanson et al., 2008). Nurses use guidelines to help identify appropriate interventions for a given nursing care problem or diagnosis. Evidence-based nursing care guidelines also show the strength of the evidence (research) used, allowing nurses to evaluate the appropriateness of a given guideline for the individual circumstance. Evidence-based nursing guidelines are available through specialty nursing organizations, healthcare systems, on the web, and in published resources. See the accompanying Moving Evidence into Action feature for more information about nurses' use of evidence for nursing practice.

Using research and evidence for planning nursing care is a relatively new skill for many nurses. Brief features such as the accompanying box will be found throughout this book. These boxes identify potential resources for planning evidence-based nursing care.

NURSING INTERVENTIONS CLASSIFICATION Just as NANDA has provided standardized language for nursing diagnoses and NOC provides standardized outcome labels and criteria, the NIC provides standardized nursing intervention labels and nursing activities to carry out the intervention.

CRITICAL PATHWAYS A **critical pathway** (also called a clinical path or pathway) is a healthcare plan designed to provide care with a multidisciplinary, managed action focus. Such pathways are generally developed for specific diagnoses—usually

---

MOVING EVIDENCE INTO ACTION **Nursing Practice**

Recognition of the need to base nursing practice on the best available evidence has significantly increased in recent years. Despite this recognition and the increased availability of published nursing research, current nursing practice often is based on experience, tradition and intuition—not on science. Koehn & Lehman (2008) surveyed registered nurses in a large medical center to identify their knowledge and skills, attitudes, and current use of evidence-based practice (EBP). Overall, nurses rated their knowledge and skills lower than their attitudes and use of EBP. Lack of time was identified by nurses as the major barrier to implementing EBP; nurses identified limited knowledge of research as a significant barrier as well.

IMPLICATIONS FOR NURSING

With increasing emphasis on and recognition of the importance of EBP, it is clear that practicing nurses need support to effectively implement it. Many nurses in the current workforce were educated at a time when EBP was not taught or emphasized. In addition to administrative leadership and support for implementing

evidence-based nursing practice, nurses need support for developing the knowledge and skills to find and critically evaluate the research to support EBP.

CRITICAL THINKING IN PATIENT CARE
1. In this study, less than half of the nurses responding to the survey reported reading or subscribing to a professional journal. What implications do you think this finding has for the use of evidence-based nursing practice? What do you think nurse managers and administrators could do to encourage more nurses to stay up-to-date on current nursing practice?
2. Lack of time was identified in this study as a major barrier to implementing EBP. How could you, as a staff nurse, support your peers in developing and implementing EBP?
3. Nurses are responsible for not only using evidence in their nursing practice, but also for contributing to nursing research and the evidence for nursing practice. What steps might you take to identify a research question that could provide evidence for practicing nurses to use?

EVIDENCE FOR NURSING CARE — Planning Nursing Care

Selected resources that nurses may find helpful when planning evidence-based nursing care follow.

- Carlson, C. (2009, December). Use of three evidence-based postoperative pain assessment practices by registered nurses. *Pain Management Nursing, 10*(4), 174–187.
- D'Arcy, Y. (2009). Putting pain research into practice. *Nursing 2009, 39*(8), 58.
- Rauen, C. A., Makic, M. B. F., & Bridges, E. (2009). Evidence-based practice habits: Transforming research into bedside practice. *Critical Care Nurse, 29*(2), 46–59.
- Scott, K., & McSherry, R. (2009). Evidence-based nursing: Clarifying the concepts for nurses in practice. *Journal of Clinical Nursing, 18*(8), 1085–1095.
- Sund-Levander, M., & Grodzinsky, E. (2010, January 12–18). What is the evidence base for the assessment and evaluation of body temperature? *Nursing Times, 106*(1), 10–13.

high volume, high risk, and high cost case types—with the collaboration of members of the healthcare team. Critical pathways are outcome driven and provide a time line to achieve specified goals. They also establish the sequence of multidisciplinary interventions, including education, discharge planning, consultations, medication administration, diagnostics, therapeutics, and treatments.

The overall goal is to design pathways that facilitate a reproducible standard of care for specific patient populations and improve the quality and proficiency of that care.

When patients do not achieve expected outcomes, variances (deviations from the established plan) from the critical pathways are recorded and studied by the multidisciplinary team. In many agencies, critical pathways are designed so that interventions and variances can be easily documented. Most documentation systems require a check off when interventions are performed or variances occur.

Implementation

The implementation step is the action or "doing" phase of the nursing process, during which the nurse carries out planned interventions. In some instances, the nurse assigns and supervises nursing assistive personnel in carrying out planned interventions. Ongoing assessment of the patient before, during, and after the intervention is an essential component of implementation in either case. Although the plan may be appropriate, many variables can modify or negate any planned intervention, making a change in the plan necessary. For example, the nurse would not be able to force fluids if the patient were nauseated or vomiting.

When implementing the planned interventions, the nurse follows several important principles:

- Set daily priorities, based on initial assessments and on the patient's condition as reported during the change of shift report and/or documented in the patient's chart. Ensure that critical assessments (such as status of invasive lines, fluids infusing, or changes in health status during the preceding shift) take first priority.
- Be aware of the interrelated nature of nursing interventions. For example, while giving a bath the nurse can also assess

physical and psychologic status, use therapeutic communication, teach the patient, do range-of-motion exercises, and provide skin care.

- Determine the most appropriate interventions for each patient, based on health status and illness treatment. Examples of appropriate interventions include the following:
  - Directly performing the activity for the patient.
  - Assisting the patient to perform the activity.
  - Supervising the patient/family while they are performing the activity.
  - Assigning and supervising nursing assistive personnel to perform the activity.
  - Teaching the patient/family about health care.
  - Monitoring the patient at risk for potential complications or problems.
- Use available resources to provide interventions that are realistic for the situation and practical in terms of equipment available, financial status of the patient, and resources available (including staff, agency, family, and community resources).

Documenting interventions is the final component of implementation, and it is a legal requirement. There are many different ways of documenting care. Narrative source-oriented and problem-oriented charting methods are used, as are focused charting, charting by exception, and computer-assisted documentation.

Evaluation

The evaluation step allows the nurse to determine whether the plan was effective and either to continue the plan, to revise the plan, or to terminate the plan. The outcome criteria that were established during the planning step provide the basis for evaluation. Evaluation takes place continuously throughout patient care, as illustrated in Figure 1–1.

To evaluate a plan, the nurse collects data from the patient and the patient's chart. The nurse then compares the status of the patient with the written outcomes. If the outcomes have been accomplished, the nurse may either continue or terminate the plan. If the outcomes have not been accomplished, the nurse must modify the nursing diagnoses, outcomes, or plan.

The Nursing Process in Clinical Practice

With experience, the nurse does not consciously stop and consider each step. Rather, using the process as a framework, care is based on the patient's specific, individualized needs. For example, when caring for a patient who is hemorrhaging, the nurse uses all five steps simultaneously to meet critical, life-threatening needs. In contrast, when considering long-term needs for a patient with a chronic illness or disability, the nurse makes in-depth assessments, mutually determines goals with the patient, and documents a written plan of care that is developed and revised as necessary by all nurses providing care. As a nurse becomes an expert practitioner, the nursing process becomes so much a part of the nurse that he or she may not even consciously consider it while providing care; the practice is the process (Benner, 1984).

Guidelines for Nursing Practice

Nursing practice is structured by codes of ethics and standards that guide nursing practice and protect the public. Individual nursing practice is held to these standards in a court of law. The guidelines are especially important because nurses encounter legal and ethical problems almost daily.

Codes for Nurses

An established **code of ethics** is one criterion that defines a profession. **Ethics** are principles of conduct. Ethical behavior is concerned with moral duty, values, obligations, and the distinction between right and wrong. Codes of ethics for nurses provide a frame of reference for "professionally valued and ideal nursing behaviors that are congruent with the principles expressed in the Code for Nurses" (Ketefian, 1987, p. 13).

The large number of ethical issues facing nurses in clinical practice makes the established codes for nurses critical to moral and ethical decision making. The codes also help to define the roles of nurses. The codes of ethics presented here were developed by and for members of the International Council of Nurses (ICN) and the ANA.

The ICN Code

The ICN Code of Ethics for Nurses (2006) helps guide nurses in setting priorities, making judgments, and taking action when they face ethical dilemmas in clinical practice. The ICN Code specifies what nurses are accountable for in terms of people, practice, society, coworkers, and the profession. The philosophical base for the ICN code is that nurses are responsible to promote health, to prevent illness, and to alleviate suffering.

The ANA Code

The ANA Code for Nurses (2001) states principles of ethical concern, guiding the behavior of nurses and also defining nursing for the general public (Box 1–3).

Standards of Nursing Practice

A **standard** is a statement or criterion that can be used by a profession and by the general public to measure quality of practice. Established standards of nursing practice make each individual nurse accountable for practice. This means that each nurse providing care has the responsibility or obligation to account for his or her own behaviors within that role. Professional nursing organizations develop and implement standards of practice to identify clearly the nurse's responsibilities to society.

The ANA standards of nursing practice (2004) are outlined in Box 1–4. These standards allow objective evaluation of nursing licensure and certification, institutional accreditation, quality assurance, and public policy.

Health Information Privacy Rules

Although the right to privacy of health and other personal information is an accepted ethical principle of nurses and other healthcare providers, federal rules also govern what can be shared and with whom. The Health Insurance Portability and Accountability Act and the Standards for Privacy of Individually Identifiable Health Information, commonly referred to together as HIPAA, are designed to protect individuals' health information while allowing such information to be shared as needed for effective care. The rules apply to those who transmit health information electronically—including nurses and others employed in hospitals, clinics, and other settings.

While often misinterpreted, HIPAA rules allow disclosure of health information for treatment purposes, even without the

BOX 1–3 The American Nurses Association Code of Ethics for Nurses

- The nurse, in all professional relationships, practices with compassion and respect for the inherent dignity, worth, and uniqueness of every individual, unrestricted by considerations of social or economic status, personal attributes, or the nature of health problems.
- The nurse's primary commitment is to the patient, whether an individual, family, group, or community.
- The nurse promotes, advocates for, and strives to protect the health, safety, and rights of the patient.
- The nurse is responsible and accountable for individual nursing practice and determines the appropriate delegation of tasks consistent with the nurse's obligation to provide optimum patient care.
- The nurse owes the same duties to self as to others, including the responsibility to preserve integrity and safety, to maintain competence, and to continue personal and professional growth.
- The nurse participates in establishing, maintaining, and improving health care environments and conditions of employment conducive to the provision of quality health care and consistent with the values of the profession through individual and collective action.
- The nurse participates in the advancement of the profession through contributions in practice, education, administration, and knowledge development.
- The nurse collaborates with other health professionals and the public in promoting community, national, and international efforts to meet health needs.
- The profession of nursing, as represented by associations and their members, is responsible for articulating nursing values, for maintaining the integrity of the profession and its practice, and for shaping social policy.

Source: ©2001 From *Code of Ethics for Nurses with Interpretive Statements.* By American Nurses Association. Reprinted with permission. All Rights Reserved.

patient's explicit consent. Although the patient's privacy is to be protected, safety protections such as posting the patient's name outside his or her room are allowed to help ensure that care is provided to the correct patient (Anderson, 2007). Unless the patient specifically objects, health information also can be shared with family members who are involved in the patient's care. Other state or federal laws may override the patient's right to privacy of health information, for example, laws that require nurses and other healthcare providers to report evidence of child, elder, or spousal abuse.

Professional Boundaries

Nurses are expected to act in the best interests of the patient, avoiding use of their position for personal gain or to become involved in the patient's personal relationships. **Professional boundaries** are the borders between the vulnerability of the patient and the power of the nurse. The nurse's position as care provider and knowledge of private information about the patient places the nurse in a position of power. It is vital that nurses recognize this relationship, and establish boundaries to safely and effectively meet the patient's needs. Confusion between the needs of the nurse and those of the patient can result in boundary violations (National Council of State Boards of Nursing, 1996). It is the nurse's responsibility to establish and maintain professional boundaries, maintaining an appropriate level of involvement for effective care.

BOX 1–4 ANA Standards of Practice

Standards of Practice	Standards of Professional Practice
■ Assessment: The registered nurse collects comprehensive data pertinent to the patient's health or the situation. ■ Diagnosis: The registered nurse analyzes the assessment data to determine the diagnoses or issues. ■ Outcomes Identification: The registered nurse identifies expected outcomes for a plan individualized to the patient or the situation. ■ Planning: The registered nurse develops a plan that prescribes strategies and alternatives to attain expected outcomes. ■ Implementation: The registered nurse implements the identified plan, coordinates care delivery, and employs strategies to promote health and a safe environment. The advanced practice registered nurse also provides consultation and uses prescriptive authority, procedures, referrals, treatments and therapies. ■ Evaluation: The registered nurse evaluates progress toward attainment of outcomes.	■ Quality of Practice: The registered nurse systematically enhances the quality and effectiveness of nursing practice. ■ Education: The registered nurse attains knowledge and competency that reflects current nursing practice. ■ Professional Practice Evaluation: The registered nurse evaluates one's own nursing practice in relation to professional practice standards and guidelines, relevant statutes, rules, and regulations. ■ Collegiality: The registered nurse interacts with and contributes to the professional development of peers and colleagues. ■ Collaboration: The registered nurse collaborates with patient, family, and others in the conduct of nursing practice. ■ Ethics: The registered nurse integrates ethical provisions in all areas of practice. ■ Research: The registered nurse integrates research findings into practice. ■ Resource Utilization: The registered nurse considers factors related to safety, effectiveness, cost, and impact on practice in the planning and delivery of nursing services. ■ Leadership: The registered nurse provides leadership in the professional practice setting and the profession.

Source: ©2004 From *Nursing Scope and Standards of Practice.* By American Nurses Association. Reprinted with permission. All Rights Reserved.

Legal and Ethical Dilemmas in Nursing

A **dilemma** is a choice between two unpleasant, ethically troubling alternatives. Nurses who provide medical-surgical nursing care face dilemmas almost daily. Many commonly experienced dilemmas involve confidentiality, patient rights, and issues of dying and death. The nurse must use ethical and legal guidelines to make decisions about moral actions when providing care in these and in many other situations.

Nurses respect the right to confidentiality of patient information found in the patient's record or secured during interviews. However, an individual's right to privacy and confidentiality creates a dilemma when it conflicts with the nurse's right to information that may affect personal safety. The law in most states mandates that HIV test results can be given to another person only with the patient's written consent. Many healthcare providers believe that this law violates their own right to personal safety.

The right to refuse treatment (including surgery, medication, medical therapy, and nourishment) also raises nursing dilemmas. The situation, the alternatives, and the potential harm from refusal must be carefully explained. The nurse is faced with the dilemma of respecting the patient's autonomy or following the ethical principle of beneficence, doing what is best for the patient.

Issues surrounding dying and death have become increasingly pressing as advances in technology extend the lives of people with chronic, debilitating illness and major trauma. These changes have altered concepts of living and dying, resulting in ethical conflicts regarding quality of life and death with dignity versus technologic methods of preserving life in any form.

Even if the patient is competent and requests that no heroic measures be used to maintain life, many questions arise in nursing care. What constitutes a heroic measure? Should nursing interventions to provide comfort include administering narcotics at a level known to depress respirations? These and other questions are being debated not only within the healthcare system but also in the courts.

Roles of the Nurse in Medical-Surgical Nursing Practice

Health care today is a vast and complex system. It reflects changes in society, changes in the populations requiring nursing care, and a philosophical shift toward health promotion rather than illness care. Roles of the medical-surgical nurse have broadened and expanded in response to these changes. Medical-surgical nurses are increasingly expected to be care managers, educators, advocates, leaders, and researchers. The nurse assumes these various roles to promote and maintain health, to prevent illness, and to facilitate coping with disability or death for the adult patient (a person requiring healthcare services) in any setting.

The Nurse as Caregiver

Nurses have always been caregivers. However, the activities carried out within the caregiver role have changed tremendously in the twenty-first century. From 1900 to the 1960s, the nurse was regarded primarily as the person who gave personal care and carried out physicians' orders. This dependent role has changed as a result of the increased education of nurses, research in and the development of nursing knowledge, and the recognition that nurses are autonomous and informed professionals.

The caregiver role for the nurse today is both independent and collaborative. Nurses independently make assessments and plan and implement patient care based on nursing knowledge and skills. Nurses also collaborate with other members of the healthcare team to implement and evaluate care (Figure 1–2 ■).

Figure 1–2 ■ The healthcare team discusses the individualized plan of care and outcomes.

As a caregiver, the nurse practices both the science and the art of nursing. In medical-surgical nursing, the science requires a deep understanding of normal physiology and the pathophysiology underlying disease processes commonly affecting adults. Just as the pediatric nurse must understand the physical and psychosocial development of children, the medical-surgical nurse must understand the physical, psychosocial, economic and developmental differences among adults spanning a range of more than 60 years. Using critical

thinking in the nursing process as the framework for care, the nurse provides interventions to meet not only the physical needs but also the psychosocial, cultural, spiritual, and environmental needs of patients and families. See Box 1–5 for a discussion of culturally sensitive nursing care. Considering all aspects of the patient ensures a holistic approach to nursing. Holistic nursing care is based on a philosophical view that interacting wholes are greater than the sum of their parts. A holistic approach also emphasizes the uniqueness of the individual.

In providing comprehensive, individualized care, the nurse uses critical thinking skills to analyze and synthesize knowledge from the arts, the sciences, and nursing research and theory. The science (knowledge base) of nursing is translated into the art of nursing through caring. Caring is the means by which the nurse is connected with and concerned for the patient (Benner & Wrubel, 1989). Thus, the nurse as caregiver is knowledgeable, skilled, empathic, and caring.

The Nurse as Educator

The nurse's role as educator is increasingly important for several reasons. Healthcare providers and consumers as well as local, state, and federal governments are placing greater emphasis on health promotion and illness prevention, hospital stays are shorter, and the number of chronically ill in our society is increasing. Early discharge of patients from the hospital setting or rehabilitation facility to home care means that family

BOX 1–5 Culturally Sensitive Nursing

The primary focus of nursing care is the patient, as the patient relates to the environment and experiences events or situations related to health or illness. These experiences are given shape and personal meaning by culture—the socially inherited characteristics of a human group. These characteristics include the beliefs, practices, habits, likes, dislikes, customs, and rituals people learn from their families and pass on to their children. Cultural background is an essential component of a person's ethnic identity. A person's ethnic identity includes belonging to a social group within a culture and a social system and sharing a common religion, language, ancestry, and physical characteristics.

The healthcare system encompasses patients who are culturally diverse. This diversity includes differences in country of origin, health beliefs, sexual orientation, race, socioeconomic level, and age. Despite increasing diversity, nursing has been slow to address the need for culturally sensitive care. Many different factors account for this inattention, including ethnocentrism (people's belief that their own cultural group's beliefs and values are the only acceptable ones) and prejudice. The healthcare system is itself a culture, composed primarily of white middle-class people, and it often serves as a barrier to culturally sensitive care.

The 1992 American Academy of Nursing Expert Panel on Culturally Competent Nursing Care identified several reasons why it has become increasingly important that nurses plan culturally sensitive care:

■ The demographic and ethnic composition of the population of the world in general, and the United States in particular, has changed markedly, and there is a lack of ethnic representation in healthcare professionals in the healthcare system. Information on and knowledge about values, beliefs, experiences, and healthcare needs of various populations is limited.

■ There is a growing awareness and acceptance of diversity and an increased willingness to maintain and support ethnic and cultural heritage.

■ People of color and immigrants are facing increasing unemployment, decreasing opportunity, and limited access to health care. These conditions may contribute to the establishment of new minorities, such as the homeless.

■ The international focus on providing health care for all people (within the context of inequity, barriers, and lack of access) may have raised the consciousness of healthcare professionals to some of the inequities inherent in healthcare systems in both developing countries and developed countries.

■ Nurses comprise the largest force in the delivery of health care and therefore have the potential to contribute to the changing inequities in and inaccessibility to health care.

■ Consumers are becoming increasingly aware of what is competent and sensitive health care.

This same panel of experts proposed general principles for nurses for becoming sensitive to cultural diversity and providing culturally sensitive care. For example,

■ nurses must learn to appreciate intergroup and intragroup cultural diversity and commonalties in racial/ethnic minority populations.

■ nurses must understand how social structure factors shape health behaviors and practices among members of racial/ethnic minorities.

■ nurses must confront their own ethnocentrism and racism.

■ nurses must begin rehearsing, practicing, and evaluating services provided to cross-cultural populations.

People of every culture have the right to have their cultural values known, respected, and addressed appropriately in nursing and other healthcare services (Leininger, 1991). To provide nursing care that is culturally sensitive, nurses must develop a sensitivity to personal fundamental values about health and illness; must accept the existence of differing values; and must be respectful of, interested in, and understanding of other cultures without being judgmental.

caregivers must learn how to perform complex skills. All these factors make the educator role essential to maintaining the health and well-being of patients.

The framework for the role of educator is the teaching–learning process. Within this framework, the nurse assesses learning needs, plans and implements teaching methods to meet those needs, and evaluates the effectiveness of the teaching. To be an effective educator, the nurse must have effective interpersonal skills and be familiar with adult learning principles (Figure 1–3 ■).

A major component of the educator role today is discharge planning. Discharge planning, which begins on admission to a healthcare setting, is a systematic method of preparing the patient and family for exit from the healthcare agency and for maintaining continuity of care after the patient leaves the setting. Discharge planning also involves making referrals, identifying community and personal resources, and arranging for necessary equipment and supplies for home care.

The Nurse as Advocate

The patient entering the healthcare system may be unprepared to make independent decisions. However, today's healthcare consumer is better educated about options for care, and may have very definite opinions. The nurse as patient advocate actively promotes the patient's rights to autonomy and free choice. The nurse as advocate speaks for the patient, mediates between the patient and other persons, and/or protects the patient's right to self-determination (Ellis & Hartley, 2007). The goals of the nurse as advocate are to do the following:

- Assess the need for advocacy.
- Communicate with other healthcare team members.
- Provide patient and family teaching.
- Assist and support patient decision making.
- Serve as a change agent in the healthcare system.
- Participate in health policy formulation.

The nurse must practice advocacy based on the belief that patients have the right to choose treatment options, based on information about the results of accepting or rejecting the treatment, without coercion. The nurse must also accept and

Figure 1–3 ■ The nurse's role as educator is an essential component of care. As part of the discharge planning process, the nurse is responsible for teaching for self-care at home.

respect the decision of the patient, even though it may differ from the decision the nurse would make.

The Nurse as Leader and Manager

All nurses are leaders and managers. They practice leadership and they manage time, people, resources, and the environment in which they provide care. Nurses carry out these roles by directing, delegating, supervising and coordinating nursing activities. Nurses must be knowledgeable of how and when to delegate, as well as the legal requirements of delegation. Nurses also evaluate the quality of care provided.

Models of Care Delivery

Nurses are leaders and managers of patient care within a variety of models of care delivery. Examples are primary nursing, team nursing, and case management. The nursing shortage made the combination of primary and team nursing more economically feasible.

PRIMARY NURSING   Primary nursing allows the nurse to provide individualized direct care to a small number of patients during their entire inpatient stay. This model was developed to reduce the fragmentation of care experienced by the patient and to facilitate family-centered continuity of care. In primary nursing, the nurse provides and coordinates care; communicates with patients, families, and other healthcare providers; and carries out discharge planning.

TEAM NURSING   Team nursing is practiced by teams of variously educated healthcare providers. For example, a team may consist of a registered nurse, a licensed practical nurse, and two unlicensed assistive personnel (UAPs). The registered nurse is the team leader. The team leader is responsible for making assignments and has overall responsibility for patient care by team members. All team members work together, each performing the activities for which he or she is best prepared.

CASE MANAGEMENT   Case management focuses on management of a caseload (group) of patients and the members of the healthcare team caring for those patients. The purpose of case management is to maximize positive outcomes and contain costs. The nurse who is case manager is usually a clinical specialist, and the caseload consists of patients with similar healthcare needs. As case manager, the nurse makes appropriate referrals to other healthcare providers and manages the quality of care provided, including accuracy, timeliness, and cost. The case manager also is in contact with patients after discharge, ensuring continuity of care and health maintenance.

Delegation

Delegation is carried out when the nurse assigns appropriate and effective work activities to other members of the healthcare team. When the nurse delegates nursing care activities to another person, that person is authorized to act in the place of the nurse, while the nurse retains the accountability for the activities performed. Delegation skills are becoming increasingly important in healthcare as agencies restructure and implement cost containment measures. More categories of healthcare workers with often minimal nursing education and experience are being hired to assist the registered nurse as *nurse extenders,* or *UAPs.* Guidelines for delegation include the following:

- Consider the training, experience, and competence of each member of the healthcare team, the complexity of the task to be assigned, and the amount of time available to supervise the tasks.
- Determine the level of nursing judgment and evaluation required for the task.
- Consider the patient's condition and the potential harm and difficulty of performing the task.
- Know the state's nurse practice act and any practice limitations that may exist.
- Delegate only tasks that are within the scope of practice or authorized duties for each category of worker.
- Assign the right job to the right person. Tasks that are routine and standard are the best to assign to others.
- Know when it is appropriate to retain direct responsibility for care activities. Tasks that are complex or require a high level of nursing judgment should be performed by the nurse.
- Give clear and complete directions for assignments. Ask questions to be sure directions have been understood.
- Give the team member the authority to complete the task while remaining accountable for the outcomes of care.
- Monitor the care provided and give constructive evaluation if necessary.

Quality and Safety

As a major sector within the healthcare workforce, nurses have a significant responsibility for ensuring the quality and safety of care patients receive. This responsibility goes beyond ensuring that individual patients receive safe and effective patient-centered nursing care to recognizing healthcare system issues that impact quality of care. The current focus of safety initiatives is on minimizing the risk of harm to patients and providers by improving the performance and effectiveness of both individuals and healthcare systems (Cronenwett et al., 2007). All nurses must be prepared to understand, take seriously, and participate in quality and safety improvement strategies.

As a leader and manager, the nurse encourages the use of strategies such as standardized practices, checklists, and technology to improve safety and quality. When an error or near miss occurs, the nurse's focus is on reporting the incident to promote analysis of the factors and systems leading up to it, not on blaming the individuals involved.

In the role of leader and manager, the nurse is responsible for the quality of patient care through a process of quality improvement. Quality improvement uses data to monitor the outcomes of care and the processes used to deliver that care. Changes to improve the quality and safety of healthcare systems are continuously designed and tested through quality improvement strategies and initiatives (Cronenwett et al., 2007).

Quality improvement methods also are used to evaluate patient care. They commonly evaluate actual care against an established set of standards of care. Nurses and other healthcare providers make this evaluation by reviewing documentation, by conducting patient surveys and nurse interviews, and/or by direct observation of nurse or patient performance. The data are then used to identify differences between actual practice and established standards and to develop a plan of action to resolve the differences. The actions are then assessed through internal peer review or by an external medical review organization, called a utilization and quality control peer review organization (PRO), to determine whether they were effective in improving practice.

The Nurse as Researcher

Nurses have always identified problems in patient care. Early nurse researchers showed the link between effective preoperative patient education and shorter postoperative hospital stays with fewer complications. Today, nurse researchers are studying a broad variety of questions and issues. To develop the science of nursing, nursing knowledge must be established through clinical research and then published so that the findings can be used by all nurses to provide evidence-based patient care.

To be relevant, nursing research must have a goal to improve the care that nurses provide patients. This means that all nurses must consider the researcher role to be integral to nursing practice. Summaries of relevant nursing research are included in almost all the nursing care chapters of this textbook. After the summary and discussion of each study, a critical-thinking section specifically related to the findings of the study encourages the student to apply the findings to the clinical setting.

CHAPTER HIGHLIGHTS

- Recommended core competencies for all healthcare professionals include providing patient-centered care, working in interdisciplinary teams, using evidence-based practice, applying quality improvement, promoting safe healthcare systems, and using informatics.
- The nursing process is the cyclical series of critical-thinking activities used by nurses to provide patient care to promote wellness, maintain health, restore health, or facilitate coping with disability or death. The five inter-related phases of the nursing process are assessment, diagnosis, planning, implementation, and evaluation.
- The clinical practice of nursing is guided by codes for nurses and standards of practice.
- The human responses that nurses must consider when planning and implementing care result from changes in the structure and/or function of all body systems, as well as the effects of those changes on the psychosocial, cultural, spiritual, economic, and personal life of the patient.
- Nurses function as caregivers, educators, advocates, leaders and managers, and researchers to promote and maintain health, prevent illness, improve health care delivery and systems, and facilitate coping with disability or death for the adult patient.

TEST YOURSELF NCLEX-RN® REVIEW

1. The National Academy of Sciences has proposed a set of core competencies for healthcare professionals. What is the primary purpose of these competencies?
   1. to make all healthcare professionals equal
   2. to improve safety and quality of care
   3. to reduce the number of medical law suits
   4. to maintain public faith in physicians

2. What does the nurse use in the practice setting to make clinical judgments and decisions?
   1. nursing process
   2. standards of care
   3. nursing ethics
   4. critical thinking

3. Which of the following statements is true of outcomes developed during the planning phase of the nursing process?
   1. Outcomes are mutually established by the patient and the nurse.
   2. Outcomes are mutually established by the nurse and the physician.
   3. Outcomes are mandated by institutional policies and standards.
   4. Outcomes are written by patients and family members.

4. The phases of the nursing process are used when providing care to patients. From the following list, choose the order in which these phases are most often used.
   1. outcomes
   2. assessment
   3. evaluation
   4. implementation
   5. planning

5. When nurses discuss the "science of nursing," what does this phrase mean?
   1. clinical competency
   2. holistic care
   3. knowledge base
   4. practice component

6. What role does the nurse demonstrate when developing and providing health information?
   1. advocate
   2. caregiver
   3. researcher
   4. educator

7. What goal is a component of the nurse's role as advocate?
   1. assisting and supporting patient decision making
   2. conducting research about the effects of exercise
   3. delegating responsibilities for patient care to others
   4. performing range-of-motion exercises

8. A nurse assigns appropriate work activities to other members of his or her team. What role is being illustrated?
   1. advocate
   2. leader/manager
   3. researcher
   4. caregiver

9. A method of establishing a standard of care and evaluating outcomes of that standard involves which of the following?
   1. writing a dress code policy for a healthcare agency
   2. creating a critical pathway for a specific type of patient
   3. establishing quality assurance regulations
   4. implementing a new procedure to change dressings

10. A nurse delegates vital sign assessment to a UAP. Who is accountable for the assessment findings?
    1. the UAP
    2. the patient
    3. the nurse
    4. the physician

See Test Yourself answers in Appendix C.

Pearson Nursing Student Resources
Find additional review materials at
www.nursing.pearsonhighered.com
Prepare for success with additional NCLEX®-style practice questions, interactive assignments and activities, Web links, animations and videos, and more!

BIBLIOGRAPHY

Alfaro-LeFevre, R. (2009). *Applying nursing process: A tool for critical thinking* (7th ed.). Philadelphia: Lippincott.

American Nurses Association. (2001). *Code of ethics for nurses.* Silver Spring, MD: Author.

American Nurses Association. (2003). *Nursing's social policy statement* (2nd ed.). Washington, DC: Author.

American Nurses Association. (2004a). Managed care: Challenges & opportunities for nursing. Retrieved from http://nursingworld.org/readroom/fsmgdcar.htm

American Nurses Association. (2004b). *Nursing: Scope and standards of practice.* Silver Spring, MD: Author.

American Nurses Association. (2005). *ANA's health care agenda 2005.* Washington, DC: Author.

Anderson, F. (2007). Finding HIPAA in your soup: Decoding the privacy rule. *American Journal of Nursing, 107*(2), 66–71.

Andrews, M. M., & Boyle, J. S. (2008). *Transcultural concepts in nursing care* (5th ed.). Philadelphia, PA: Lippincott.

Banning, M. (2008, May). Clinical reasoning and its application to nursing: concepts and research studies. *Nurse Education in Practice, 8*(3), 177–183.

Benner, P. (1984). *From novice to expert: Excellence and power in clinical nursing practice.* Redwood City, CA: Addison-Wesley Nursing.

Benner, P., & Wrubel, J. (1989). The primacy of caring: Stress and coping in clinical nursing practice. Redwood City, CA: Addison-Wesley Nursing.

Bulechek, G. M., Butcher, H. K., & Dochterman, J. M. (2008). *Nursing Interventions Classification (NIC)* (5th ed.). St. Louis: Mosby.

Chitty, K., & Black, B. P. (2007). *Professional nursing: Concepts & challenges* (5th ed.). Philadelphia: Saunders.

Cronenwett, L., Sherwood, G., Barnsteiner, J., Disch, J., Johnson, J., Mitchell, P., et al. (2007). Quality and safety education for nurses. *Nursing Outlook, 55*(3), 122–131.

Ellis, J., & Hartley, C. (2008). *Managing and coordinating nursing care* (5th ed.). Philadelphia: Lippincott.

Esterhuizen, P. (2006). Is the professional code still the cornerstone of clinical nursing practice? *Journal of Advanced Nursing, 53*(1), 104–110.

Foust, J. (2007, May). Discharge planning as part of daily nursing practice. *Applied Nursing Research, 20*(2), 72–77.

Giger, J. N., & Davidhizar, R. E. (2008). *Transcultural nursing: Assessment and intervention* (5th ed.). St. Louis, MO: Mosby.

Greggs-McQuilkin, D. (2003). The specialty of medical-surgical nursing: The solid rock, not the stepping stone. *MEDSURG Nursing, 12*(1), 5, 26.

Hanks, R. (2008, July). The lived experience of nursing advocacy. *Nursing Ethics, 15*(4), 468–477.

Hanson, D., Hoss, B., & Wesorick, B. (2008, August). Evaluating the evidence: Guidelines. *AORN Journal, 88*(2), 184, 186, 188–196.

International Council of Nurses. (2006). *The ICN Code of ethics for nurses.* Geneva: Imprimerie Fornara.

Institute of Medicine. Committee on Quality of Health Care in America. (2001). *Crossing the quality chasm: A new health system for the 21st century.* Washington, DC: National Academy Press.

Johnson, K., Hallsey, D., Meredith, R., & Warden, E. (2006, April). A nurse-driven system for improving patient quality outcomes. *Journal of Nursing Care Quality, 21*(2), 168–175.

Klenner, S. (2000). Mapping out a clinical pathway. *RN, 63*(6), 33–36.

Koehn, M., & Lehman, K. (2008). Nurses' perceptions of evidence-based nursing practice. *Journal of Advanced Nursing, 62*(2), 209–215.

Lachman, V. D. (2007). Ethics, law, and policy. Moral courage in action: Case studies. *Medsurg Nursing, 16*(4), 275–277.

Lachman, V. (2008, October). Making ethical choices: weighing obligations & virtues. *Nursing, 38*(10), 42–46.

Leininger, M. (1991). Transcultural care principles, human rights, and ethical considerations. *Journal of Transcultural Nursing, 3*(1), 21–23.

Mathes, M. (2005). Ethics, law, and policy. On nursing, moral autonomy, and moral responsibility. *Medsurg Nursing, 14*(6), 395–398.

Matter, S. (2006, December). Empower nurses with evidence-based knowledge. *Nursing Management.* Retrieved from www.nursingmanagement.com

National Academy of Sciences. (2003). Executive summary. *Health professions education: A bridge to quality,* pp. 1–10. Retrieved from http://www.nap.edu

National Council of State Boards of Nursing, Inc. (1996). Professional boundaries: A nurse's guide to the importance of appropriate professional boundaries. Chicago, IL: National Council of State Boards of Nursing, Inc.

Olson, D. P. (2007). Ethical issues. Unwanted treatment: What are the ethical implications? *American Journal of Nursing, 107*(9), 51–53.

Radwin, L. (1990). Research on diagnostic reasoning in nursing. *Nursing Diagnosis, 1*(2), 70–77.

Riddell, T. (2007, March). Critical assumptions: thinking critically about critical thinking. *Journal of Nursing Education, 46*(3), 121–126.

Spector, R. (2009). *Cultural diversity in health and illness* (7th ed.). Upper Saddle River, NJ: Prentice Hall.

Spotlight on medical-surgical nursing. (2003). *Nursing, 33*(4), 88–R2.

Sullivan, D. (2010). Connecting nursing education and practice: A focus on shared goals for quality and safety. *Creative Nursing, 16*(1), 37–43.

Tanner, C. A. (2006). Thinking like a nurse: A research-based model of clinical judgment in nursing. *Journal of Nursing Education, 45*(6), 204–211.

Uhrenfeldt, L., & Hall, E. (2007, May). Clinical wisdom among proficient nurses. *Nursing Ethics, 14*(3), 387–398.

Wallace, C., Bigelow, S., Xu, X., & Elstein, L. (2007, January–February). Collaborative practice: usability of text-based, electronic patient care guidelines. *CIN: Computers, Informatics, Nursing, 25*(1), 39–44.

Wilkinson, J. M. (2007). *Nursing process and critical thinking* (4th ed.). Upper Saddle River, NJ: Prentice Hall.

World Health Organization. (1974). *Constitution of the World Health Organization: Chronicle of the World Health Organization.* Geneva: World Health Organization.

Health and Illness in Adults

KEY TERMS

acute illness, *22*	family, *31*	illness, *22*
chronic illness, *23*	health, *18*	manifestations, *22*
disease, *22*	health–illness continuum, *18*	remission, *23*
exacerbation, *23*	holistic health care, *19*	wellness, *18*

The human responses that nurses must consider when planning and implementing care result from changes in the structure and/or function of all body systems, as well as the interrelated effects of those changes on the psychosocial, cultural, spiritual, economic, and personal life of the patient.

In 1948, the World Health Organization (WHO) defined **health** as "a state of complete physical, mental, and social well-being, and not merely the absence of disease or infirmity." This definition, which WHO maintains to date, addresses the importance of physical, mental, emotional, and social components of health, but fails to take into account the various levels of health a person may experience. Health is

not just a state of being, but the resources (e.g., physical, personal, social) used by each person in dealing with the challenges of living. These factors, which greatly influence nursing care, include the health–illness continuum and high-level wellness.

The Health–Illness Continuum and High-Level Wellness

The **health–illness continuum** represents health as a dynamic process, with high-level **wellness** at one extreme of the continuum and death at the opposite extreme (Figure 2–1 ■).

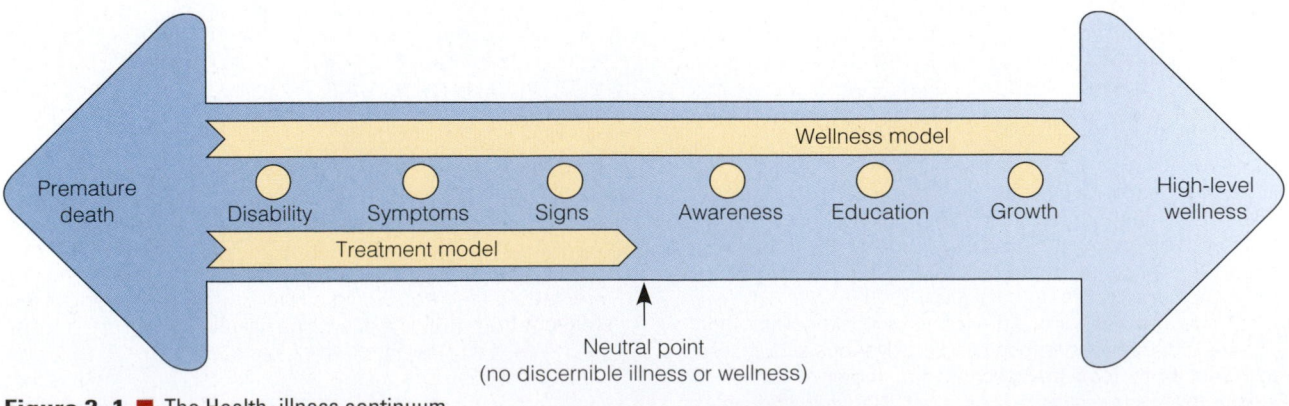

Figure 2–1 ■ The Health–illness continuum.

Source: From Travis, J. W., & Ryan, R. S. (1998). *Wellness Workbook.* Berkeley, CA: Ten Speed Press. Used with permission.

Individuals place themselves at different locations on the continuum at specific points in time.

Dunn (1959) expanded the concept of a continuum of health and illness in his description of high-level wellness. Dunn conceptualized wellness as an active process influenced by the environment. He differentiated good health from wellness:

> Good health can exist as a relatively passive state. . . . Wellness is an integrated method of functioning. . . oriented toward maximizing the potential of which the individual is capable, within the environment where he is functioning. (1959, p. 4)

A variety of factors influence wellness, including self-concept, environment, culture, and spiritual values. Providing care based on a framework of wellness facilitates active involvement by both the nurse and the patient in promoting, maintaining, or restoring health. It also supports the philosophy of **holistic health care**, in which all aspects of a person (physical, psychosocial, cultural, spiritual, and intellectual) are considered as essential components of individualized care.

Factors Affecting Health

Many different factors affect a person's health or level of wellness. These factors often interact to promote health or to become risk factors for alterations in health.

Genetic Makeup

Each person's genetic makeup influences health status throughout life. Genetic makeup affects personality, temperament, body structure, intellectual potential, and susceptibility to the development of hereditary alterations in health. Examples of chronic illnesses that are associated with genetic makeup include sickle cell disease, hemophilia, diabetes mellitus, and cancer.

Cognitive Abilities and Educational Level

Although cognitive abilities are determined prior to adulthood, cognitive development affects whether people view themselves as healthy or ill; cognitive levels also may affect health practices. Injuries to and illnesses affecting the brain may alter cognitive abilities. Educational level affects the ability to understand and follow guidelines for health. For example, if an individual is functionally illiterate, written information about healthy behaviors and health resources is worthless.

Race, Ethnicity, and Cultural Background

Certain diseases occur at a higher rate of incidence in some races and ethnic groups than in others. For example, in the United States hypertension is more common in African Americans, diabetes mellitus and chronic liver disease are among the leading causes of illness in Native Americans, and eye disorders are more prevalent in Chinese Americans. See the accompanying Cultural Diversity feature. The ethnic and cultural background of an individual also influences health values and behaviors, lifestyle, and illness behaviors. Every culture defines health and illness in a way that is unique; in addition, each culture has its own health beliefs and illness treatment practices.

Age, Gender, and Developmental Level

Age, gender, and developmental level are factors in health and illness. Cardiovascular disorders are uncommon in young adults, but the incidence increases after the age of 40. Myocardial infarctions are more common in men than women until women are postmenopausal. Some diseases occur only in one gender or the other (e.g., prostate cancer in men and cervical cancer in women). The older adult often has increased incidence of chronic illness and increased potential for serious illness or death from infectious illnesses such as influenza and pneumonia.

Lifestyle and Environment

The components of a person's lifestyle that affect health status include patterns of eating, use of chemical substances (alcohol, nicotine, caffeine, legal and illegal drugs), exercise and rest patterns, and coping methods. Examples of altered responses are the relationship of obesity to hypertension, cigarette smoking to chronic obstructive pulmonary disease, a sedentary lifestyle to heart disease, and a high-stress career to alcoholism. The environment has a major influence on health. Occupational exposure to toxic substances (such as asbestos and coal dust) increases the risk of pulmonary disorders. Air, water, and food pollution increase the risk of respiratory disorders, infectious diseases, and cancer. Environmental temperature variations can result in hypothermia or hyperthermia, especially in the older adult.

FOCUS ON CULTURAL DIVERSITY
Biologic Variations Among Cultures

As genetic science and our understanding of disease causes and pathology have advanced, there is increasing recognition that differences between peoples of the world are more than skin deep. Certain diseases and conditions are much more likely to develop in some groups than in others; for example, sickle cell anemia occurs more frequently in people whose ancestors are from central Africa, the Near East, the Mediterranean region, and parts of India; Caucasian women of small stature and of Scandinavian heritage have a higher risk of developing osteoporosis. Biological variations also may affect the way the body metabolizes drugs, leading to an effect that is either less than or greater than anticipated. In other cases, selected drugs may be found to be effective for people of one race but not another.

Biologic differences among people of various cultural groups also affect both food preferences and food tolerance. Most Mexican Americans, African Americans, Native Americans, and Asians are lactose intolerant; that is, they do not produce enough lactose to tolerate large amounts of milk and milk products. If too much milk (or yogurt or milk chocolate) is eaten, undigested lactose in the intestine causes manifestations such as cramping, flatulence, abdominal bloating, and diarrhea (Giger & Davidhizar, 2008).

Although known biologic variables among people of different races and cultures can be helpful in providing individualized health education, it is important to avoid stereotyping based on racial and cultural differences. For example, a person who appears to be African American may actually identify with Native American culture as a result of having a Native American parent; a recent emigrant from Ethiopia has a significantly different cultural background than a black person who is a descendent of U.S. slaves. Making assumptions about health risk factors and preferences could lead to inappropriate care planning for these individuals.

Socioeconomic Background

Both lifestyle and environmental influences are affected by one's income level. The culture of poverty, which crosses all racial and ethnic boundaries, negatively influences health status. Living at or below the poverty level may result in crowded, unsanitary living conditions or homelessness. Housing often is overcrowded, lacks adequate heating or cooling, and is infested with insects and rats. Crowded living conditions increase the risk of transferring communicable diseases. Other problems include lack of infant and child care, lack of medical care for injuries or illness, inadequate nutrition, use of addictive substances, and violence.

Geographic Area

The geographic area in which one lives influences health status. Such illnesses as malaria are more common in tropical areas of North America, whereas multiple sclerosis occurs with greater frequency in the northern United States and Canada. Other geographic influences are seen in the number of skin cancers in people living in sunny, hot areas and sinus infections in people living in areas of high humidity.

Health Promotion and Maintenance

For many years, the emphasis in nursing was on care of the acutely ill patient in the hospital setting. With changes in society and in health care, this emphasis is shifting toward preventive, community-based care, including managing chronic illness. Although the focus of this textbook is not community health nursing, the importance of teaching health-promoting behaviors is an essential component of medical-surgical nursing.

Healthy Living

Practices that are known to promote health and wellness include the following:

- Eat three balanced meals a day, following the guidelines developed jointly by the U.S. Department of Agriculture

(sidebar, left margin, rotated) Health Promotion for Young Adults Video

BOX 2–1 Dietary Guidelines for Health

- Eat a variety of foods to get the energy, proteins, vitamins, minerals, and fiber needed for good health.
- Balance intake of food with physical activity. Maintain or improve body weight to reduce the risks of high blood pressure, heart disease, stroke, certain cancers, and type 2 diabetes mellitus.
- Choose a diet with plenty of grain products, vegetables, and fruits, which provide needed fiber and complex carbohydrates and can help lower intake of fat.
- Choose a diet low in fat, saturated fat, and cholesterol to reduce the risk of heart attack and certain types of cancer, and to help maintain a healthy weight.
- Choose a diet moderate in sugars. Increased sugar intake can increase weight, decrease nutrient intake, and contribute to tooth decay.
- Choose a diet moderate in salt and sodium to help reduce the risk of high blood pressure.
- Drink alcoholic beverages, if at all, in moderation. Alcohol provides non-nutrient calories, may be addicting, and causes many health problems.

(USDA) and the U.S. Department of Health and Human Services (HHS) (Box 2–1). It is also helpful to follow a general guideline of what to eat each day, such as with the Food Guide Pyramid illustrated in Figure 2–2 ■. The food pyramid was revised in 2005, with recommendations for a greater emphasis on monounsaturated and polyunsaturated fats, the inclusion of whole-grain foods with each meal, and increased intake of fish and vegetables. The goal of the revision is to reduce obesity and cardiovascular disease. A website is available to individualize the plan by helping consumers choose foods and amounts. After entering their age, gender, and activity level, consumers get their own plan at an appropriate calorie level, and can print out a miniposter and worksheet to track progress.

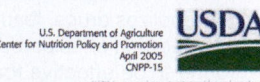

Figure 2–2 ■ The USDA Food Guide Pyramid is designed to be used as a method of helping Americans make healthy food choices and be active every day.

Source: U.S. Department of Agriculture and U.S. Department of Health and Human Services. (2005). Retrieved from http://www.mypyramid.gov/downloads/miniposter.pdf

- Exercise moderately and regularly, engaging in at least 20 minutes of continuous activity (such as walking) five or more days per week.
- Sleep 7 to 8 hours each day.
- Limit alcohol consumption to a moderate amount (no more than two drinks per day for men or one drink daily for women), and favor red wine.
- Eliminate smoking and use of other tobacco products such as smokeless tobacco.
- Keep sun exposure to a minimum.
- Maintain recommended immunizations (Table 2–1).

The nurse promotes health by teaching the activities that maintain wellness, by providing information about the characteristics and consequences of diseases when risk factors have been identified, and by supplying specific information about decreasing risk factors (Pender, Parsons, & Murdaugh, 2006). The nurse also promotes health by following healthy practices and serving as a role model.

NATIONAL HEALTH PROMOTION The U.S. Department of Health and Human Services (HHS) has published national public health objectives each decade since 1980. Overarching goals for the current decade are described in Box 2–2.

BOX 2–2 *Healthy People 2020:* **Overarching Goals**

With the overall mission of improving the nation's health, *Healthy People 2020* has four overarching major goals. These goals address factors that contribute to the health status of individuals or populations, and include social and physical determinants of health.

Overarching Goals
- Eliminate preventable disease, disability, injury, and premature death.
- Achieve health equity, eliminate disparities, and improve the health of all groups.
- Create social and physical environments that promote good health for all.
- Promote healthy development and healthy behaviors across every stage of life.

Objectives to achieve these overarching goals fall under such diverse topics as the following:
- Access to health services
- Chronic disease conditions
- Educational and community-based programs
- Food safety
- Global health
- Injury and violence prevention
- Nutrition and weight status, and
- Social determinants of health

Source: U.S. Department of Health and Human Services. (2010). *Healthy People 2020.* Washington, DC: Author.

TABLE 2–1 Recommended Immunizations for Adults

VACCINE	INDICATIONS	DO NOT GIVE TO
Measles-mumps-rubella	Anyone born after 1956 and never infected, or those likely to be exposed, such as those entering college or the military and healthcare personnel.	Pregnant women, immunocompromised people, or anyone with a history of anaphylactic reaction to egg protein or neomycin.
Tetanus, diphtheria, pertussis (Td, Tdap)	Anyone who has never been vaccinated should have the primary tetanus and diphtheria toxoid series, followed by booster every 10 years. Adults younger than 65 years should receive one dose of Tdap.	People with a history of anaphylactic reaction to the vaccine. People with a history of encephalopathy following pertussis vaccine should not receive Tdap.
Hepatitis A	Anyone who wishes protection and those traveling to countries in which hepatitis A infection is endemic.	People with a history of hypersensitivity to aluminum hydroxide or phenoxyethanol.
Hepatitis B	Anyone likely to have repeated exposure (such as healthcare providers or sex partners of a known carrier) or who have had exposure (such as a needle-stick injury to a healthcare worker).	People with a history of anaphylactic reaction to common baker's yeast.
Human papillomavirus (HPV)	All previously unvaccinated women through age 26 years.	People with a history of anaphylactic reaction to the vaccine or its components.
Influenza	Anyone at high risk for complications, healthcare providers, and those wanting immunity.	Those with a high fever, or a history of anaphylactic reaction to egg protein.
Pneumococcal pneumonia	Anyone at high risk for pneumococcal disease, those over 65 years of age.	Pregnant women.
Varicella	Anyone never infected, especially healthcare providers and child care workers.	Pregnant women, immunocompromised people, those who have received an immune globulin or a blood transfusion within 5 months, or those with a history of anaphylactic reactions to neomycin or gelatin.
Zoster (shingles)	Persons age 60 years and older.	Pregnant women, immunocompromised people, and those with a history of anaphylactic reactions to neomycin or gelatin.

Disease and Illness

Disease and *illness* are terms that are often used interchangeably, but in fact they have different meanings. In general, nursing is concerned with illness, whereas medicine is concerned with disease.

Disease

Disease (literally meaning "without ease") is a medical term describing alterations in structure and function of the body or mind. Diseases may have mechanical, biologic, or normative causes. Mechanical causes of disease result in damage to the structure of the body and are the result of trauma or extremes of temperature. Biologic causes of disease affect body function and are the result of genetic defects, the effects of aging, infestation and infection, alterations in the immune system, and alterations in normal organ secretions. Normative causes are psychologic but involve a mind–body interaction, so that physical manifestations occur in response to the psychologic disturbance.

The cause of many diseases is still unknown. The following are generally accepted as common causes of disease:

- Genetic defects
- Developmental defects resulting from exposure to viruses, chemicals, or drugs that affect the developing fetus
- Biologic agents or toxins (including viruses, bacteria, rickettsia, fungi, protozoa, and helminths)
- Physical agents such as temperature extremes, radiation, and electricity
- Chemical agents such as alcohol, drugs, strong acids or bases, and heavy metals
- Generalized response of tissues to injury or irritation
- Alterations in the production of antibodies, resulting in allergies or hypersensitivities
- Faulty metabolic processes (e.g., a production of hormones or enzymes above or below normal)
- Continued, unabated stress

Diseases may be classified as acute or chronic, communicable, congenital, degenerative, functional, malignant, psychosomatic, idiopathic, or iatrogenic. These classifications are defined in Table 2–2. In all types of disease, alterations in structure or function cause signs and symptoms (**manifestations**) that prompt a person to seek treatment from a physician or traditional healer. Although both subjective symptoms and objective signs commonly appear with disease, objective signs often predominate. Subjective symptoms may include such manifestations as nausea, general malaise, or fatigue. Examples of objective signs include bleeding, vomiting, diarrhea, limitation of movement, swelling, visual disturbances, and changes in elimination. However, pain (a subjective symptom) is often the primary reason that prompts a person to seek health care.

Illness

Illness is the response a person has to a disease. This response is highly individualized because the person responds not only to his or her own perceptions of the disease but also to the perceptions of others. Illness integrates pathophysiologic alterations; psychologic effects of those alterations; effects on roles, relationships, and values; and cultural and spiritual beliefs. A person may have a disease and not categorize him- or herself as ill, or may validate feelings of illness through the comments of others ("You don't look as though you feel well today").

ACUTE ILLNESS An **acute illness** occurs rapidly, lasts for a relatively short time, and is self-limiting. The condition responds to self-treatment or to medical-surgical intervention. Patients with uncomplicated acute illnesses usually have full recovery and return to normal pre-illness functioning.

Illness behaviors are the way people cope with the alterations in health and function caused by a disease. Illness behaviors are highly individualized and are influenced by age, gender, family values, socioeconomic status, culture, educational level, and mental status. The commonly recognized sequence of illness behaviors follows:

1. *Experiencing symptoms.* In the first stage of an acute illness, a person experiences one or more manifestations that prompt awareness of a change in normal health. Examples of symptoms that signal an illness are pain, bleeding, swelling, fever, or difficulty with breathing. If the manifestations are mild or are familiar (such as symptoms of the common cold or influenza), the person usually uses over-the-counter medications or a traditional remedy for self-treatment. If the symptoms are relieved, no further action is taken; however, if the symptoms are severe or become worse, the person moves to the next stage.

2. *Assuming the sick role.* In the second stage of illness behavior, the person assumes the sick role. This signals acceptance of the symptoms as indicative of an illness. The person usually validates this belief with others and seeks support for seeking professional treatment or remaining

TABLE 2–2 Disease Classifications and Definitions

CLASSIFICATION	DEFINITION
Acute	A disease that has a rapid onset, lasts a relatively short time, and is self-limiting
Chronic	A disease that requires continuing management over a long period—years or even decades
Communicable	A disease that can spread from one person to another
Congenital	A disease or disorder that exists at or before birth
Degenerative	A disease that results from deterioration or impairment of organs or tissues
Functional	A disease that affects function or performance but does not have manifestations of organic illness
Malignant	A disease that tends to become worse and cause death
Psychosomatic	A psychologic disease that is manifested by physiologic symptoms
Idiopathic	A disease that has an unknown cause
Iatrogenic	A disease that is caused by medical therapy

home from school or work. Self-preoccupation is characteristic of this stage, and the person focuses on alterations in function resulting from the illness. If the illness is resolved, the person validates a return to health with others and resumes normal activities; however, if manifestations remain or increase in severity and others agree that no improvement has occurred, the person moves to the next stage by seeking medical care.

3. *Seeking medical care.* In our society, a physician or other healthcare provider usually provides validation of illness. People who believe themselves to be ill (and who are encouraged by others to contact a healthcare provider) make the medical contact for diagnosis, prognosis, and treatment of the illness. If the medical diagnosis is of an illness, the person moves to the next stage. If the medical diagnosis does not support illness, the patient may return to normal functioning or may seek validation from a different healthcare provider.

4. *Assuming a dependent role.* The stage of assuming a dependent role begins when a person accepts the diagnosis and planned treatment of the illness. As the severity of the illness increases, so does the dependent role. It is during this stage that the person may enter the hospital for treatment and care. The responses of the person to care depend on many different variables: the severity of the illness, the degree of anxiety or fear about the outcome, the loss of roles, the support systems available, individualized reactions to stress, and previous experiences with illness care. The severity of the illness and the individual's resources affect whether the person moves to the next stage, recovery and rehabilitation, or to chronic illness or even death.

5. *Achieving recovery and rehabilitation.* The final stage of an acute illness is recovery and rehabilitation. The person now gives up the dependent role and resumes normal roles and responsibilities. As a result of education during treatment and care, the person may be at a higher level of wellness after recovery is complete. There is no set timetable for recovery from an illness. The severity of the illness and the method of treatment affect the length of time required, as does the person's compliance with treatment plans and motivation to return to normal health.

CHRONIC ILLNESS **Chronic illness** is a term that encompasses many different long-term pathologic and psychologic alterations in health. It is the leading health problem in the world today, accounting for 70% of all deaths in the United States (CDC, 2009). The incidence and prevalence of chronic illness is increasing, a trend that is predicted to continue. Current trends contributing to an increased incidence of chronic illnesses include an aging population, diseases of lifestyle and behavior (e.g., obesity, smoking), and environmental factors.

Chronic illness is defined as a condition that requires continuing management over a long period—years or even decades. Chronic conditions may be caused by noncommunicable disease (e.g. cancer, heart disease); persistent illnesses such as asthma or diabetes; long-term mental health disorders such as schizophrenia; or physical, sensory, or structural impairments (e.g. arthritis, visual impairment).

Chronic illness is often also characterized by impaired function in more than one body system; responses to this impaired function may occur in sensory perception, self-care abilities, mobility, cognition, and social skills. The demands on the individual and family as a result of these responses are often lifelong (Crumbie et al., 2004; Lee, 2009).

The intensity of a chronic illness and its related manifestations range from mild to severe. Chronic illness may be characterized by periods of remission and exacerbation. During periods of **remission**, the person does not experience symptoms, even though the disease is still clinically present. During periods of **exacerbation**, the symptoms reappear. These periods of change in symptoms do not appear in all chronic diseases.

Each person with a chronic illness has a unique set of responses and needs. The response of the person to the illness is influenced by the following factors:

- The point in the life cycle at which the illness develops
- The type and degree of limitations imposed by the illness
- The visibility of impairment or disfigurement
- The pathophysiology causing the illness
- The relationship between the impairment and functioning in social roles
- Pain and fear

These factors are highly complex. They are interrelated within each person, resulting in individualized illness behaviors and needs. Because there are so many different chronic diseases and because the experience of each person with the illness is a composite of individualized responses, it is difficult to generalize about needs. However, almost all people with a chronic illness will need to do the following:

- Live as normally as possible, despite symptoms and treatment that may make the person with a chronic illness feel alienated, lonely, and different from others without the illness.
- Learn to adapt activities of daily living and self-care activities.
- Grieve the loss of physical function and, in some cases, life roles, structure, income, status, and dignity.
- Learn to manage an ongoing treatment plan.
- Maintain a positive self-concept and a sense of hope.
- Maintain a feeling of being in control.
- Confront the inevitability of death (Miller, 2000).

Many people with chronic illness successfully meet health-related needs, whereas others do not. Research indicates that adaptation is influenced by variables such as anger, depression, denial, self-concept, locus of control, hardiness, and disability. Nursing interventions for the person with a chronic illness focus on education to promote independent functioning, reduce healthcare costs, and improve well-being and quality of life.

ILLNESS PREVENTION Activities to prevent illness include any measures that limit the progression of an illness at any point of its course. Three levels of illness prevention have been defined (Leavell & Clark, 1965). Each level of prevention occurs at a distinct point in the development of a disease process and requires specific nursing interventions (Edelman & Mandle, 2006). The levels are as follows:

1. *Primary level of prevention.* This level includes generalized health promotion activities as well as specific actions

that prevent or delay the occurrence of a disease. Following are examples of primary prevention activities:

- Reducing exposure to environmental risks, such as air and water pollution
- Eating nutritious foods
- Protecting oneself against industrial hazards
- Obeying seat belt and helmet laws
- Obtaining sex counseling and practicing safer sex
- Obtaining immunizations
- Undergoing genetic screenings
- Eliminating the use of alcohol and cigarettes

2. *Secondary level of prevention.* This level involves activities that emphasize early diagnosis and treatment of an illness to stop the pathologic process and enable the person to return to his or her former state of health as soon as possible. Following are examples of secondary prevention activities:

- Being screened for diseases such as hypertension, diabetes mellitus, and glaucoma
- Obtaining physical examinations and diagnostic tests for cancer
- Performing self-examination for breast and/or testicular cancer
- Obtaining tuberculosis skin tests
- Obtaining specific treatment for illness (e.g., treatment of streptococcal infections of the throat helps prevent secondary disorders involving the heart and/or kidneys)

3. *Tertiary level of prevention.* This level focuses on stopping the disease process and returning the affected individual to a useful place in society within the constraints of any disability. The activities primarily revolve around rehabilitation. Following are examples of tertiary prevention measures:

- Obtaining medical or surgical treatment for an illness
- Enrolling in specific rehabilitation programs for cardiovascular problems, head injuries, and strokes
- Joining work training programs following illness or injury
- Educating the public to employ rehabilitated people to the fullest possible extent

Meeting Health Needs of Adults

The adult years commonly are divided into three stages: the young adult (ages 18 to 40), the middle adult (ages 40 to 65), and the older adult (over age 65). Although developmental markers are not as clearly delineated in the adult as in the infant or child, specific changes do occur with aging in intellectual, psychosocial, and spiritual development, as well as in physical structures and functions.

The developmental theories specific to the adult, with related stages and tasks, are listed in Table 2–3. Applying a variety of developmental theories is important to the holistic care of the adult as nurses assess, plan and implement care, and provide teaching.

The Young Adult

From ages 18 to 25, the healthy young adult is at the peak of physical development (Figure 2–3 ■). All body systems are functioning at maximum efficiency. Then, during the 30s, some

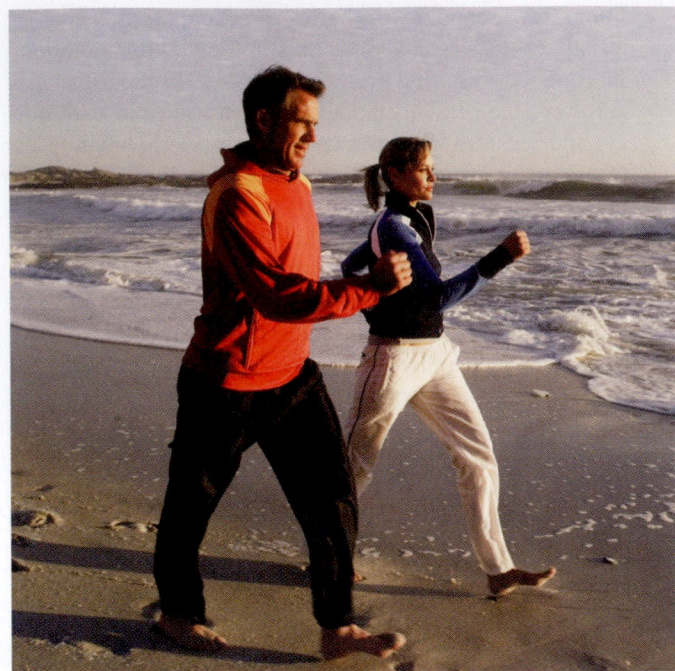

Figure 2–3 ■ Regular exercise is a key healthy behavior for the young adult.

normal physiologic changes begin to occur. A comparison of physical status for young adults during their 20s and 30s is shown in Table 2–4.

Risks for Alterations in Health

The young adult is at risk for alterations in health from accidents, sexually transmitted infections, substance abuse, and physical or psychosocial stressors. These risk factors may be interrelated (see the Moving Evidence into Action Moving Evidence into Action).

INJURIES Unintentional injuries are the leading cause of injury and death in people between ages 15 and 24 (National Center for Health Statistics [NCHS], 2007). Most injuries and fatalities occur as the result of motor vehicle crashes, but injuries and death also result from assaults (homicide), drowning, fire, guns, occupational accidents, and exposure to environmental hazards. Accidental injury or death is often associated with the use of alcohol or other chemical substances, or with psychologic stress. Intentional self-harm (suicide) is the third leading cause of death in young adults of both genders.

SEXUALLY TRANSMITTED INFECTIONS Sexually transmitted infections include genital herpes, chlamydia, gonorrhea, syphilis, and HIV/AIDS. The young adult who is sexually active with a variety of partners and who does not use condoms is at greatest risk for development of these diseases. Nursing care of patients with sexually transmitted infections is discussed in ∞ Chapter 50.

SUBSTANCE ABUSE Substance abuse is a major cause for concern in the young adult population. Although alcohol abuse occurs at all ages, it is greater in the 20s than during any other decade of the life span. Alcohol contributes to motor vehicle crashes and physical violence, and it is damaging to the developing fetus in pregnant women. It can also cause liver disease and nutritional deficits.

TABLE 2–3 Theories of Adult Development

	THEORIST	AGE	TASK
Psychosocial Development	Erikson	18–25	Identity versus role confusion
			■ Establishing an intimate relationship with another person
			■ Committing oneself to work and to relationships
		25–65	Generativity versus stagnation
			■ Accepting one's own life as creative and productive
			■ Having concern for others
		65–death	Integrity versus despair
			■ Accepting worth of one's own life
			■ Accepting inevitability of death
Spiritual Development	Fowler	After 18	■ Having a high degree of self-consciousness
			■ Constructing one's own spiritual system
		After 30	■ Being aware of truth from a variety of viewpoints
	Westerhoff	Young adult	Searching faith
			■ Acquiring a cognitive and an affective faith through questioning one's own faith
		Middle–older adult	Owned faith
			■ Putting faith into action and standing up for beliefs
Moral Development	Kohlberg	Adult	Postconventional level
			Social contract/legalistic orientation
			■ Defining morality in terms of personal principles
			■ Adhering to laws that protect the welfare and rights of others
			Universal-ethical principles
			■ Internalizing universal moral principles
			■ Respecting others; believing that relationships are based on mutual trust
Developmental Tasks	Havighurst	18–35	■ Selecting and learning to live with a mate
			■ Starting a family and rearing children
			■ Managing a home
			■ Starting an occupation
			■ Taking on civic responsibility
			■ Finding a congenial social group
		35–60	■ Achieving civic and social responsibility
			■ Establishing and maintaining an economic standard of living
			■ Assisting teenage children in becoming responsible and happy adults
			■ Developing leisure-time activities
			■ Relating to one's spouse as a person
			■ Accepting and adjusting to the physiologic changes of middle age
			■ Adjusting to aging parents
		60 and over	■ Meeting civic and social obligations
			■ Establishing an affiliation with one's own age group
			■ Establishing satisfactory physical living arrangements
			■ Adjusting to decreasing physical strength, health, retirement, reduced income, death of spouse

Source: Data from Erickson, E. (1963). *Childhood and Society* (2nd ed.). New York: Norton; Fowler, W. (1981). *Stages of Faith: The Psychology of Human Development and the Quest for Meaning.* New York: Harper & Row; Havighurst, R. J. (1972). *Human Development and Education* (3rd ed.). New York: Longman; Kohlberg, L. (1979). *The Meaning and Measurement of Moral Development.* New York: Clark University; and Westerhoff, J. (1976). *Will Our Children Have Faith?* New York: Seabury Press.

Other substances that are commonly abused include nicotine, marijuana, amphetamines (including methamphetamine), cocaine, and crack. Smoking increases the risk of respiratory and cardiovascular diseases. Marijuana can affect memory and learning for days to weeks after its use. Methamphetamine, a highly addictive substance, can lead to structural and functional changes in the areas of the brain associated with emotion and memory. Cocaine and crack can cause death from cardiovascular effects (increased heart rate and ventricular dysrhythmias), and can lead to addiction and health problems in the baby born to an addicted mother. Nursing care of patients with problems of substance abuse is discussed in ∞ Chapter 6.

TABLE 2–4 Physical Status and Changes in the Young Adult Years

ASSESSMENT	STATUS DURING THE 20S	STATUS DURING THE 30S
Skin	Smooth, even temperature	Wrinkles begin to appear
Hair	Slightly oily, shiny	Graying may begin
	Balding may begin	Balding may begin
Vision	Snellen 20/20	Some loss of visual acuity and accommodation
Musculoskeletal	Strong, coordinated	Some loss of strength and muscle mass
Cardiovascular	Maximum cardiac output	Slight decline in cardiac output
	60–90 beats/minute	60–90 beats/minute
	Mean BP: 120/80	Mean BP: 120/80
Respiratory	Rate: 12–20	Rate: 12–20
	Full vital capacity	Slight decline in vital capacity

PHYSICAL AND PSYCHOSOCIAL STRESSORS Physical stressors that increase the risk of illness include environmental pollutants and work-related risks (e.g., electrical hazards, mechanical injuries, or exposure to toxins or infectious agents). Other physical stressors include exposure to the sun, participation in high-risk activities (e.g., contact sports, driving too fast), ingestion of chemical substances (e.g., caffeine, alcohol, nicotine), and pregnancy. Young adults have the highest rate of injury-related visits to emergency departments (NCHS, 2009).

Many different and individualized psychosocial stressors may affect the young adult. Choices must be made about education, occupation, relationships, independence, and lifestyle. These choices indirectly affect future health. The young adult without adequate education or job skills may face unemployment, poverty, homelessness, and limited access to health care. Nearly half of all marriages end in divorce, usually within the first 10 years. People who are divorced have more health problems than those who remain married (NCHS, 2002). Divorce often results in loneliness, feelings of failure, financial difficulties, domestic violence, and child abuse. The inability of the young adult to cope with these stressors may result in suicide, which ranks close to accidents as a major cause of death in this age group. Although difficult to prove, it is believed that some accidental deaths, especially when associated with substance abuse, are actually suicides.

Assessment Guidelines

The following guidelines are useful in assessing the achievement of significant developmental tasks in the young adult. Does the young adult

- feel independent from parents?
- have a realistic self-concept?
- like oneself and the direction in which life is going?
- interact well with family?
- cope with the stresses of constant change and growth?
- have well-established bonds with significant others, such as marriage partners or close friends?
- have a meaningful social life?
- have a career or occupation?
- demonstrate emotional, social, and economic responsibility for his or her own life?
- have a set of values that guide behavior?
- have a healthy lifestyle?

Physical assessment of the young adult includes height and weight, blood pressure, and vision. During the health history, the nurse should ask specific questions about substance use, sexual activity and concerns, exercise, eating habits, menstrual history and patterns, coping mechanisms, any familial chronic illnesses, and family changes. See Table 2–5 for health screening recommendations for young and middle adults.

MOVING EVIDENCE INTO ACTION Health Promotion for Young Adults

Traditional college students who fall into the young adult age group (ages 18 to 24) often engage in risky behaviors that increase their health risks. Students responding to a 2008 survey by the American College Health Association reported the following:

- stress that interfered with academic performance (34%)
- sleep difficulties (26%)
- consuming one to four drinks while partying (38%)
- engaging in behaviors they regretted after drinking (36%)
- feeling depressed (18.4%)
- being in an emotionally abusive relationship (13.6%)

These behaviors have major implications for the health of this segment of young adults. This survey also found that students identify health educators and health center staff as credible sources of health-related information.

IMPLICATIONS FOR NURSING

Nurses in college-based health centers and primary care settings are in position to provide resources and education for college-age students. Interventions that focus on wellness, health promotion, and coping strategies can have a positive impact on student outcomes (Ahern, 2009). Nurses should reach out to young, college-age adults to provide support and education to promote healthy behaviors.

CRITICAL THINKING IN PATIENT CARE

1. Considering the current preferred methods of communicating among adolescents and young adults, develop potential strategies for outreach to and health and wellness education for students on a traditional, residential college campus.
2. How might you modify these planned strategies to reach students enrolled in a college where the primary student population is commuters?
3. Would your strategies and focus change if your goal was health promotion for nontraditional college students (ages 25 and older)?

TABLE 2–5 Recommended Health Screening for Healthy Adults (without specific risk factors)

EXAMINATION	RECOMMENDED FREQUENCY		
	YOUNG ADULTS (18–40)	MIDDLE ADULTS (40–65)	OLDER ADULTS (65 AND OLDER)
Health maintenance examination: ■ Height, weight, body mass index ■ Risk evaluation & counseling ■ Safety ■ Behavioral assessment	Every 1 to 5 years	Every 1 to 3 years	Every 1 to 2 years
Blood pressure	Every 2 years; more frequently if 120/80 or higher	Every 2 years; more frequently if 120/80 or higher	Every 2 years; more frequently if 120/80 or higher
Breast cancer: ■ Clinical breast exam ■ Mammography	Every 3 years	Annually Annually	Annually Annually to age 75
Cervical cancer (Pap test)	Annually until age 30, then every 2 to 3 years after three normal results	Every 2 to 3 years if normal	May discontinue; resume if has new sexual partner
Cholesterol and lipid profile	Every 5 years	Every 5 years	Every 5 years
Chlamydia	All sexually active women under age 26		
Colorectal cancer: ■ Fecal occult blood test (FOBT) or fecal immunochemical test (FIT) ■ Flexible sigmoidoscopy or double contrast barium enema ■ Colonoscopy		Annually beginning at age 50 Every 5 years beginning at age 50 Every 10 years beginning at age 50	Annually Every 5 years Every 10 years to age 80
Diabetes mellitus		Fasting plasma glucose every 3 years	Fasting plasma glucose every 3 years
Glaucoma			Every 2 years
Osteoporosis			Bone mineral density; repeat every 2 years for those at risk
Prostate cancer		Digital rectal exam (DRE) and prostate-specific antigen (PSA) annually beginning at age 50 (age 45 for black males and men with strong family history of prostate cancer)	DRE and PSA annually

Sources: Cokkinides, V., Bandi, P., Siegel, R., Ward, E. M., & Thun, M. J. (2007). *Cancer prevention & early detection facts & figures 2008.* Atlanta, GA: American Cancer Society; National Guideline Clearinghouse. (2006). Adult preventive services (ages 18–49). Southfield, MI: Michigan Quality Improvement Consortium; National Guideline Clearinghouse. (2006). Adult preventive services (ages 50–65+). Southfield, MI: Michigan Quality Improvement Consortium.

Promoting Healthy Behaviors in the Young Adult

The nurse promotes health in the young adult by teaching the behaviors listed in Box 2–3. Health information for the young adult is primarily provided in community settings. Examples are as follows:

■ Health-related courses and seminars at colleges and universities include information on the use of sports and exercise facilities, alcohol and drug abuse, smoking cessation, mental health, and sexual health.
■ Workplace programs include blood pressure monitoring, exercise, smoking cessation, cafeteria nutrition guidelines, and stress reduction activities.
■ Community programs include media information, health fairs, support groups, and information about risk factors for disease and injury.

The Middle Adult

The middle adult, ages 40 to 65, has physical status and function similar to that of the young adult. However, many changes take place between ages 40 and 65. Table 2–6 lists the physical changes that normally occur in the middle years.

Risks for Alterations in Health

The middle adult is at risk for alterations in health from obesity, cardiovascular disease, cancer, substance abuse, and physical and psychosocial stressors. These factors may be interrelated.

OBESITY   The middle adult often has a problem maintaining a healthy weight. Weight gain in middle adulthood is usually the result of continuing to consume the same number of calories while decreasing physical activity and experiencing a

BOX 2–3 Healthy Behaviors in the Young Adult

- Choose foods from all food groups, and eat a variety of foods.
- Choose a diet low in fat (30% or less of total calories), saturated fat (less than 10% of calories), and cholesterol (less than 300 mg daily).
- Choose a diet that each day includes at least seven servings of fruits and vegetables, and six servings of grains.
- Use sugar, salt, and sodium in moderation.
- For females, increase to or maintain 18 mg of iron daily in the diet, 1000 mg of calcium, and 400 mg of folic acid per day through diet or supplements.
- Have regular dental examinations and cleanings.
- Make exercise a regular part of life, carrying out activities that increase the heart rate to a set target, and maintain that rate for 30–60 minutes five or more days a week.
- Include exercise as part of any weight reduction program.
- Maintain immunizations.

decrease in basal metabolic rate. Obesity affects all of the major organ systems of the body, increasing the risk of atherosclerosis, hypertension, elevated cholesterol and triglyceride levels, and diabetes. Obesity is also associated with heart disease, cancer, osteoarthritis, and gallbladder disease.

TABLE 2–6 Physical Changes in the Middle Adult Years

ASSESSMENT	CHANGES
Skin	■ Decreased turgor, moisture, and subcutaneous fat result in wrinkles. ■ Fat is deposited in the abdominal and hip areas.
Hair	■ Loss of melanin in hair shaft causes graying. ■ Hairline recedes in males.
Sensory	■ Visual acuity for near vision decreases (presbyopia) during the 40s. ■ Auditory acuity for high-frequency sounds decreases (presbycusis); more common in men. ■ Sense of taste diminishes.
Musculoskeletal	■ Skeletal muscle mass decreases by about age 60. ■ Thinning of intervertebral discs results in loss of height (about 2.5 cm [1 inch]). ■ Postmenopausal women may develop low bone density or osteoporosis.
Cardiovascular	■ Blood vessels lose elasticity. ■ Systolic blood pressure may increase.
Respiratory	■ Loss of vital capacity (about 1 L from age 20 to 60) occurs.
Gastrointestinal	■ Large intestine gradually loses muscle tone; constipation may result. ■ Gastric secretions are decreased.
Genitourinary	■ Hormonal changes occur: menopause, women (↓ estrogen); andropause, men (↓ testosterone).
Endocrine	■ Gradual decrease in glucose tolerance occurs.

CARDIOVASCULAR DISEASE   The major risk factors, especially for coronary heart disease, include age, male gender, family history, physical inactivity, cigarette smoking, hypertension, elevated blood cholesterol levels, and diabetes. Other contributing factors include obesity, stress, and lack of exercise. The middle adult is at risk for peripheral vascular, cerebrovascular, and cardiovascular disease.

CANCER   Cancer is the third leading cause of death in adults between ages 25 and 64 in the United States, with one-third of cases occurring between ages 35 and 64. Cancers of the breast, colon, lung, and reproductive system are common in the middle years. Prolonged exposure to environmental carcinogens and use of alcohol and nicotine are significant cancer risk factors for the middle adult. Nursing care of the patient with cancer is discussed in ∞ Chapter 14.

SUBSTANCE ABUSE   Although the middle adult may abuse a variety of substances, the most commonly abused are alcohol, nicotine, and prescription drugs. Excess alcohol use in the middle adult contributes to an increased risk of liver cancer, cirrhosis, pancreatitis, hyperlipidemia, and anemia. Alcoholism also increases the risk of accidental injury or death and disrupts careers and relationships. Cigarette smoking increases the risk of cancer of the larynx, lung, mouth, pharynx, bladder, pancreas, esophagus, and kidney; of chronic obstructive pulmonary disorders; and of cardiovascular disease.

PHYSICAL AND PSYCHOSOCIAL STRESSORS   The middle adult years are ones of change and transition, frequently resulting in stress. Both men and women must adapt to changes in physical appearance and function and accept their own mortality. Children may leave home or choose to remain at home longer than they are welcome. Parents are aging, with illness probable and death inevitable. The middle adult thus becomes part of what has been called "the sandwich generation," caught between the need to care for both children and aging parents. Both men and women may make career changes, and approaching retirement becomes a reality. Divorce in the middle years is a major emotional, social, and financial stressor.

Assessment Guidelines

The following guidelines are useful in assessing the achievement of significant developmental tasks in the middle adult. Does the middle adult

- accept the aging body?
- feel comfortable with and respect him- or herself?
- enjoy some new freedom to be independent?
- accept changes in family roles?
- enjoy success and satisfaction from work and/or family roles?
- interact well and share companionable activities with a partner?
- expand or renew previous interests?
- pursue charitable and altruistic activities?
- consider plans for retirement?
- have a meaningful philosophy of life?
- follow preventive healthcare practices?

EVIDENCE FOR NURSING CARE	Health Promotion for Middle Adults

Selected resources that nurses may find helpful when planning evidence-based nursing care follow.

- O'Rourke, J. (2009). Blazing the trail into boomer wellness and prevention. *Rehab Management, 22*(6), 10, 12–13.
- Zender, R., & Olshansky, E. (2009). Promoting wellness in women across the life span. *The Nursing Clinics of North America, 44*(3), 281–291.

Physical assessment of the middle adult includes all body systems, including blood pressure, vision, and hearing. Monitoring for risks and onset of cancer symptoms is essential (see Table 2–5). During the health history, the nurse should ask specific questions about food intake and exercise habits, substance abuse, sexual concerns, changes in the reproductive system, coping mechanisms, and family history of chronic illnesses.

Promoting Healthy Behaviors in the Middle Adult

The nurse promotes health in the middle adult by teaching the behaviors listed in Box 2–4. Information about health for the middle adult may be provided in a variety of community settings, including outpatient clinics, occupational health clinics, and private practice. Examples are as follows:

- Specific programs emphasize accepting responsibility for one's own health. This type of teaching can be in a seminar or on a one-to-one basis, and includes information specific to a group of individuals with an identified need, such as smokers, women who have just entered the workforce, or men nearing retirement.
- The community and industries provide information about safety hazards in the home and workplace, as well as during leisure activities.
- Literature about community resources is available for health promotion, including programs offered at alcohol/drug abuse treatment centers, clinics and health centers, counseling services, crisis intervention centers, spouse abuse programs, and health education and promotion agencies (e.g., American Red Cross, American Cancer Society, American Heart Association, YWCA, YMCA).

BOX 2–4 Healthy Behaviors in the Middle Adult

- Choose foods from all food groups, and eat a variety of foods.
- Choose a diet low in fat (30% or less of total calories), saturated fat (less than 10% of calories), and cholesterol (less than 300 mg daily). Adjust daily calorie intake to maintain healthy weight.
- Choose a diet that each day includes at least seven servings of fruits and vegetables, and six servings of grains.
- Use sugar, salt, and sodium in moderation.
- Increase calcium intake (in perimenopausal women) to 1200 mg daily.
- Consume high-fiber foods.
- Have regular dental examinations and cleanings.
- Make exercise a part of life, carrying out regular exercise that is moderately strenuous, is consistent, and avoids overexertion; exercise for 30 minutes five or more days a week.
- Include exercise as part of any weight reduction program.

The Older Adult

The older adult period begins at age 65, but it can be further divided into three periods: the young-old (ages 65 to 74), the middle-old (ages 75 to 84), and the old-old (age 85 and over). With increasing age, a number of normal physiologic changes occur, as listed in Table 2–7.

The older adult population is increasing more rapidly than any other age group. In the last century, the number of adults in the United States living to age 65 or older increased from 4% in 1900 to 12.4% in 2006. There will be 71.5 million older adults by the year 2030, almost twice the number in 2005. The average life expectancy in the United States is 75.2 years for men and 80.4 years for women (Administration on Aging, 2007; NCHS, 2009).

FAST FACTS

Diversity in Older Adults

- Currently, minority older adults comprise over 19% of all older Americans.
- By 2030, the minority older adult population is projected to increase by 183%, compared with 74% for the older adult white population.
- Minority elders will increase as follows: African Americans = 147%, Asians = 208%, Hispanic Americans = 254%, American Indians and Alaska Natives = 143%.

Source: Data from Administration on Aging. (2007). *A profile of older Americans: 2007.* Retrieved from www.aoa.gov/prof/Statistics/profile/profiles.aspx

The increasing numbers of older adults have important implications for nursing. Patients in all healthcare settings will be older, with nursing care and teaching needs that differ from those of young and middle adults. Although gerontologic nursing (care of the older adult) is a nursing specialty area, it is also an integral component of medical-surgical nursing (Figure 2–4 ■).

Risks for Alterations in Health

The older adult is at risk for alterations in health from a variety of causes. Most older adults have one or more chronic health problems; many have multiple illnesses. The most frequently

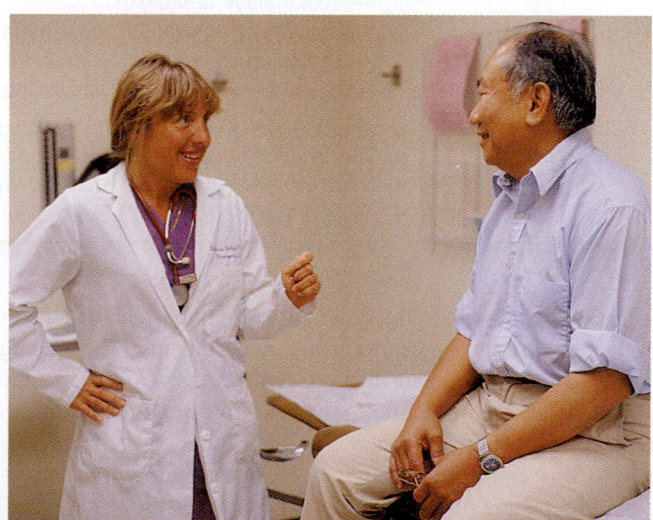

Figure 2–4 ■ The older adult population is increasing more rapidly than any other age group, making gerontologic nursing an integral component of medical-surgical nursing practice.

TABLE 2–7 Physical Changes in the Older Adult Years

ASSESSMENT	CHANGES
Skin	■ Decreased turgor and sebaceous gland activity result in dry, wrinkled skin. Melanocytes cluster, causing "age spots" or "liver spots."
Hair and nails	■ Scalp, axillary, and pubic hair thins; nose and ear hair thickens. Women may develop facial hair. ■ Nails grow more slowly; may become thick and brittle.
Sensory	■ Visual field narrows, and depth perception is distorted. ■ Pupils are smaller, reducing night vision. ■ Lenses yellow and become opaque, resulting in distortion of green, blue, and violet tones and increased sensitivity to glare. ■ Production of tears decreases. ■ Sense of smell decreases. ■ Age-related hearing loss progresses, involving middle- and low-frequency sounds. ■ Threshold for pain and touch increases. ■ Proprioception (sense of physical position) may be altered, increasing risk for falls.
Musculoskeletal	■ Loss of overall mass, strength, and movement of muscles occurs; tremors may occur. ■ Loss of bone structure and deterioration of joint cartilage results in kyphosis, increased risk of fractures, and restricted range of motion.
Cardiovascular	■ Systolic blood pressure rises. ■ Cardiac output decreases. ■ Peripheral resistance increases, and capillary walls thicken.
Respiratory	■ Continued loss of vital capacity occurs as the lungs become less elastic and more rigid. ■ Anteroposterior chest diameter and residual volume increase. ■ Although blood carbon dioxide levels remain relatively constant, blood oxygen levels decrease by 10%–15%.
Gastrointestinal	■ Decreased saliva production and loss of taste buds decrease ability to taste salt and sweet. ■ Gag reflex is decreased, stomach motility reduced, and gastric emptying is delayed. ■ Both large and small intestines have some atrophy, with decreased peristalsis. ■ The liver decreases in weight and storage capacity; gallstones increase; pancreatic enzymes decrease.
Genitourinary	■ Kidneys lose mass, and the glomerular filtration rate is reduced (by nearly 50% from young adulthood to old age). ■ Bladder capacity decreases, and the micturition reflex is delayed. Urinary retention is more common. ■ Women may have stress incontinence; men may have an enlarged prostate gland. ■ Reproductive changes in men occur: —Testosterone decreases. —Sperm count decreases. —Testes become smaller. —Length of time to achieve an erection increases; erection is less full. ■ Reproductive changes in women occur: —Estrogen levels decrease. —Breast tissue decreases. —Vagina, uterus, ovaries, and urethra atrophy. —Vaginal lubrication decreases. —Vaginal secretions become alkaline.
Endocrine	■ Pituitary gland loses weight and vascularity. ■ Thyroid gland becomes more fibrous, and plasma T_3 levels decrease. ■ Pancreas releases insulin more slowly; increased blood glucose levels are common. ■ Adrenal glands produce less cortisol.

occurring conditions in the older adult are hypertension, arthritis, heart diseases, cancer, sinusitis, and diabetes. The leading causes of death are heart disease, cancer, and stroke. Like the middle adult, the older adult is at risk for alterations in health from obesity and a sedentary lifestyle. Other risk factors specific to this age group include accidental injuries, pharmacologic effects, and physical and psychosocial stress.

INJURIES Injuries in the older adult cause many different problems: illness, financial burdens, hospitalization, self-care deficits, loss of independence, and even death. The risk of injury is increased by normal physiologic changes that accompany aging, pathophysiologic alterations in health, environmental hazards, and lack of support systems. The three major causes of injury in the older adult are falls, fires, and motor vehicle crashes. Of these, falls with resultant hip fractures are the most significant in terms of long-term disability and death.

PHARMACOLOGIC EFFECTS A number of risk factors predispose the older adult to toxic drug effects. Age-related changes in tissue and organ structure and function alter the absorption of both oral and parenteral medications. Low nutritional levels and decreased liver function may alter drug metabolism. The aging kidney may not excrete drugs at the normal clearance rate. Self-administration of both prescribed and over-the-counter medications presents risks for error resulting from confusion, forgetfulness, or misreading the directions. The older adult may take several drugs at once, increasing the risk for adverse drug interactions. In addition, the older adult living on a fixed income may have to make a choice between buying medications or food, resulting in undermedication and ineffective treatment of an illness.

PHYSICAL AND PSYCHOSOCIAL STRESSORS The older adult is exposed to the same environmental hazards as the young and middle adult, but the effects of an accumulation of years of exposure may now appear. For example, exposure to the sun in earlier years may be manifested by skin cancer, and the long-term effects of exposure to noise pollution can result in impaired hearing. The older adult is at increased risk for respiratory disorders as a result of years of smoking, or from such pollutants as coal or asbestos dust. Living conditions and economic constraints may prevent the older adult from having necessary heating and cooling, contributing to thermal-related illnesses and even death. Elder abuse and neglect further increase the risk of injury or illness.

Psychosocial stressors for the older adult include the illness or death of a spouse, decreased or limited income, retirement, isolation from friends and family because of lack of transportation or distance, return to the home of a child, or relocation to a long-term healthcare facility. A further stressor may be role loss or reversal—for example, when the wife becomes the caretaker of her chronically ill husband.

Assessment Guidelines

The following guidelines are useful in assessing the achievement of significant developmental tasks in the older adult. Does the older adult

- adjust to the physiologic changes related to aging?
- manage retirement years in a satisfying manner?
- have satisfactory living arrangements and income to meet changing needs?
- participate in social and leisure activities?
- have a social network of friends and support persons?
- view life as worthwhile?
- have high self-esteem?
- have the abilities to care for self or to secure appropriate help?
- gain support from a value system or spiritual philosophy?
- adapt lifestyle to diminishing energy and ability?
- accept and adjust to the death of significant others?

Physical assessment of the older adult includes a careful examination of all body systems. During the health history, the nurse should ask specific questions about usual dietary patterns; elimination; exercise and rest; use of alcohol, nicotine, over-the-counter medications and prescription drugs; sexual concerns; financial concerns; and support systems.

Promoting Healthy Behaviors in the Older Adult

The nurse promotes health in the older adult by teaching the behaviors listed in Box 2–5 and encouraging screening examinations as outlined in Table 2–5. Medicare covers the cost of

EVIDENCE FOR NURSING CARE | **Health Promotion for Older Adults**

Selected resources that nurses may find helpful when planning evidence-based nursing care follow.

- Kennedy, R. D., & Cullamar, K. (2007). Try this: Best practices in nursing care to older adults. Immunizations for older adults. The Hartford Institute for Geriatric Nursing, Division of Nursing, New York University. Available at www.hartfordign.org.
- Lee, C. (2009). A comparison of health promotion behaviors in rural and urban community-dwelling spousal caregivers. *Journal of Gerontological Nursing, 35*(5), 34–40.

most regular screening examinations, based on recommended frequency of the exam. Older adults may be concerned about the cost of undergoing health promotion and screening exams; providing information about Medicare coverage can relieve concerns and promote compliance with recommended schedules.

Older adults get the same benefits from health teaching as young adults and middle adults; they should never be viewed as being "too old" for healthy living practices. However, nurses should structure teaching activities to meet age-related physiologic changes, such as using charts and literature with large print. Health education for the older adult is provided in hospitals, long-term care facilities, retirement centers, outpatient clinics, senior citizen centers, and other community settings. Examples are as follows:

- Educational seminars teach about accident prevention in the home, in automobiles, and when taking public transportation.
- Health screenings and information from health fairs can specifically aid the older adult.
- Community programs provide immunization for influenza and pneumonia.
- Literature is available about financial assistance for health care, crisis hot lines, community services and resources (as described earlier for the middle adult), transportation, and nutrition (such as the Meals on Wheels program).

The Family of the Adult Patient

Although some patients are totally alone in the world, most have one or more people who are significant in their lives. These significant others may be related or bonded to the patient by birth, adoption, marriage, or friendship. Although not always meeting traditional definitions, people (or even pets) significant to the patient are the patient's family. The nurse includes the family as an integral component of care in all healthcare settings.

Definitions and Functions of the Family

What is a **family**? The definitions of family vary by culture and change as society changes. According to one definition, a family is a unit of people related by marriage, birth, or adoption (Duvall, 1977). A more comprehensive definition is that a family is a social unit composed of two or more people who are emotionally involved with each other.

Although every family is unique, all families have certain structural and functional features in common. Family structure (family roles and relationships) and family function

BOX 2–5 Healthy Behaviors in the Older Adult

- Eat a variety of nutrient-dense foods and beverages within and among the basic food groups while choosing foods that limit the intake of saturated and trans fats, cholesterol, added sugars, salt, and alcohol.
- Choose a diet low in fat (30% or less of total calories), saturated fat (less than 10% of calories), and cholesterol (less than 300 mg daily). Choose foods high in fiber, low in sodium, and high in potassium.
- People with dark skin and those with little sunlight exposure should consume extra vitamin D from fortified foods or supplements.
- Individuals with hypertension and African Americans should consume no more than 1500 mg of sodium each day.
- If weight loss is needed, aim for a slow, steady loss by decreasing caloric intake while maintaining an adequate nutrient intake and increasing physical activity.
- Increase calcium intake to 1200 mg daily.
- Make exercise a part of life, carrying out regular exercise that is moderately strenuous, is consistent, and avoids overexertion; exercise for 30 to 60 minutes every day, if possible.
- Practice good oral hygiene with teeth brushing and flossing and have a dental checkup one to two times a year.
- Use sunscreen and avoid sunburn.
- Obtain an annual influenza immunization and have the pneumonia vaccine at age 65. *(Medicare pays for an annual influenza immunization once a year in the fall or winter and covers the cost of the pneumococcal vaccine, which most people only need once.)*

(interactions among family members and with the community) provide the following:

- *Interdependence.* The behaviors and developmental level of individual family members constantly influence and are influenced by the behaviors and developmental level of all other members of the family.
- *Maintaining boundaries.* The family creates boundaries that guide its members, providing a distinct and unique family culture. This culture, in turn, provides values.
- *Adapting to change.* The family changes as new members are added, current members leave, and the development of each member progresses.
- *Performing family tasks.* Essential tasks maintain the stability and continuity of the family. These tasks include physical maintenance of the home and the people in the home, the production and socialization of family members, and the maintenance of the psychologic well-being of members.

Family Developmental Stages and Tasks

The family, like the individual, has developmental stages and tasks. Each stage brings change, requiring adaptation; each new stage also brings family-related risk factors for alterations in health. The nurse must consider the needs of the patient both at a specific developmental stage and within a family with specific developmental tasks. Family developmental stages and developmental tasks are described next; related risk factors and health problems for each stage are listed in Table 2–8.

Couple

Two people living together with or without being married are in a period of establishing themselves as a couple. The developmental tasks of the couple include adjusting to living together as a couple, establishing a mutually satisfying relationship, relating to kin, and deciding whether to have children (in those of child-bearing age).

Family with Infants and Preschoolers

The family with infants or preschoolers must adjust to having and supporting the needs of more than two members. Other developmental tasks of the family at this stage are developing an attachment between parents and children, adjusting to the economic costs of having more members, coping with energy depletion and lack of privacy, and carrying out activities that enhance growth and development of the children.

Family with School-Age Children

The family with school-age children has the developmental tasks of adjusting to the expanded world of children in school and encouraging educational achievement. A further task is promoting joint decision making between children and parents.

Family with Adolescents and Young Adults

The developmental tasks of the family with adolescents and young adults focus on transition. While providing a supportive home base and maintaining open communications, parents must balance freedom with responsibility and release adult children as they seek independence.

Family with Middle Adults

The family with middle adults (in which the parents are middle aged and children are no longer at home) has the developmental tasks of maintaining ties with older and younger generations and planning for retirement. If the family consists of just the middle-aged couple, they have the developmental task of reestablishing the relationship and (if necessary) acquiring the role of grandparents.

Family with Older Adults

The older adult family has the developmental tasks of adjusting to retirement, adjusting to aging, and coping with the loss of a spouse. If a spouse dies, further tasks include adjusting to living alone or closing the family home.

The Family of the Patient with a Chronic Illness

The patient with a chronic illness may be hospitalized for diagnosis and treatment of acute exacerbations, but the care of the patient is primarily provided at home. Chronic illness in a family member is a major stressor that may cause changes in family structure and function, as well as changes in performing family developmental tasks.

Many different factors affect family responses to chronic illness; family responses in turn affect the patient's response to and perception of the illness. Factors influencing response to chronic illness include personal, social, and economic resources; the nature and course of the disease; and demands of the illness as perceived by family members.

Support for the family is essential. The following information should be considered when performing any family assessment and developing a patient's plan of care:

- Cohesiveness and communication patterns within the family
- Family interactions that support self-care

TABLE 2–8 Family-Related Risk Factors for Alterations in Health

STAGE	RISK FACTORS	HEALTH PROBLEMS
Couple or Family with Infants and Preschoolers	■ Lack of knowledge about family planning, contraception, sexual and marital roles ■ Inadequate prenatal care ■ Altered nutrition: inadequate nutrition, overweight, underweight ■ Smoking, alcohol/drug abuse ■ First pregnancy before age 16 or after age 35 ■ Low socioeconomic status ■ Lack of knowledge about child health and safety	Sexually transmitted infection Premature pregnancy Infertility Low-birth-weight infant Birth defects Poisoning Injury to infant or child Accidents Psychologic stress Family violence (child or spousal abuse)
Family with School-Age Children	■ Unsafe home environment ■ Working parents with inappropriate or inadequate resources for child care ■ Low socioeconomic status ■ Child abuse or neglect ■ Multiple, closely spaced children ■ Repeated infections, accidents, and hospitalizations ■ Unrecognized and unattended health problems ■ Poor or inappropriate nutrition ■ Toxic substances in the home	Behavior problems Speech and vision problems Learning disabilities Communicable diseases Physical abuse Cancer Developmental delay Obesity, underweight
Family with Adolescents and Young Adults	■ Family values of aggressiveness and competition ■ Lifestyle and behavior leading to chronic illness (substance abuse, inadequate diet) ■ Lack of problem-solving skills ■ Conflicts between parent and children	Violent death and injury Alcohol/drug abuse Unwanted pregnancy Suicide Sexually transmitted infections Domestic abuse
Family with Middle Adults	■ High-fat, high-cholesterol diet ■ Overweight ■ Hypertension ■ Smoking, alcohol abuse ■ Physical inactivity ■ Personality patterns related to stress ■ Exposure to environment: sunlight, radiation, asbestos, water or air pollution ■ Depression	Cardiovascular disease (coronary heart disease and cerebral vascular disease) Cancer Diabetes mellitus Accidents Suicide Mental illness
Family with Older Adults	■ Depression ■ Drug interactions ■ Chronic illness ■ Death of spouse ■ Reduced income ■ Poor nutrition ■ Lack of exercise ■ Past environment and lifestyle	Impaired vision and hearing Hypertension Acute illness Chronic illness Infectious diseases (influenza, pneumonia) Injuries from burns and falls Depression, suicide Alcohol abuse

■ Number of friends, relatives, and social support systems (e.g., church members) available
■ Family values and beliefs about health and illness
■ Cultural and spiritual beliefs
■ Developmental level of the patient and family

It is important to remember that standardized teaching plans may not be effective. Rather, patients with chronic illnesses and their families should be given the freedom to choose appropriate literature, self-help or support groups, and interactions with others who have the same illness.

CHAPTER HIGHLIGHTS

- Health, an ever-changing state, is affected by genetic makeup; cognitive abilities and educational level; race, ethnicity, and cultural background; age, gender, and developmental level; lifestyle and environment; socioeconomic background; and geographic area.
- The emphasis of nursing has shifted from acute illness care in the hospital setting to preventive community-based care. An essential component of medical-surgical nursing is teaching health-promoting behaviors to promote and maintain functional health status.
- Illnesses may be acute or chronic, with behaviors of illness individualized within a fairly predictable sequence of experiencing symptoms, assuming the sick role, seeking medical help, assuming a dependent role, and achieving recovery and rehabilitation.

- Young adults are at risk for alterations in health from injuries, sexually transmitted infections, substance abuse, workplace exposure to pollutants, sun exposure, and psychologic stressors.
- Middle adults are at risk for alterations in health from obesity, cardiovascular disease, cancer, substance abuse, and the stresses of change and transition.
- Older adults are at risk for alterations in health from chronic illnesses (including hypertension, heart disease, cancer, and stroke), injuries, drug toxicities, and changes in income and marital status.
- The family is an integral component in planning and implementing nursing care for the adult patient.

TEST YOURSELF NCLEX-RN® REVIEW

1. Which definition best describes wellness?
   1. a complete absence of disease
   2. presence of no more than one chronic illness
   3. never having to take medications
   4. actively practicing healthy behaviors
2. Many different factors affect the health of an individual. Which of the following are included? **Select all that apply.**
   1. genetic makeup
   2. cognitive abilities
   3. height
   4. age
   5. race
3. Which of the following diseases has a genetic basis?
   1. tuberculosis
   2. sickle cell disease
   3. appendicitis
   4. indigestion
4. Primary levels of prevention are general health promotion actions that prevent or delay the occurrence of a disease. Which of the following is a primary preventive activity?
   1. practicing safer sex
   2. having a screening for hypertension
   3. doing a self-breast examination
   4. having surgery
5. You call your instructor to say you have the "flu" and will not be in class. What level of illness behavior are you demonstrating?
   1. experiencing symptoms
   2. assuming the sick role
   3. seeking medical care
   4. assuming a dependent role

6. Your nephew was born with a heart defect. How would this disorder be classified?
   1. an acute illness
   2. a malignant illness
   3. an iatrogenic illness
   4. a congenital illness
7. Of the following descriptors, which is specific to a chronic illness?
   1. occurs rapidly
   2. lasts for a lifetime
   3. self-limiting
   4. lasts for a short time
8. Mr. Jones, aged 50, is 30 pounds overweight, smokes, and rarely exercises. As a middle adult, these factors increase his risk for disorders of which body system?
   1. cardiovascular
   2. renal
   3. gastrointestinal
   4. nervous
9. You have been asked to present a health-related program at the local senior center. What would be an appropriate topic?
   1. the hazards of substance abuse
   2. accident prevention in the home
   3. family roles and tasks
   4. treating acute illness
10. Which of the following developmental tasks are a part of the life of a family with older adults if a spouse dies? **Select all that apply.**
    1. coping with lack of privacy
    2. planning for retirement
    3. adjusting to aging
    4. coping with loss
    5. relating to kin

See Test Yourself answers in Appendix C.

BIBLIOGRAPHY

Administration on Aging, U.S. Department of Health and Human Services. (2007). *A profile of older Americans: 2007.* Retrieved from www.aoa.gov/prof/Statistics/profile/profiles.aspx

Administration on Aging, U.S. Department of Health and Human Services. (2008). *A statistical profile of older Americans aged 65+.* Retrieved from www.aoa.gov

Amella, E. J. (2004). Presentation of illness in older adults. *American Journal of Nursing, 104*(10), 40–51.

Brooks, Y., Black, D., Coster, D., Blue, C., Abood, D., & Gretebeck, R. (2007, November). Body mass index and percentage body fat as health indicators for young adults. *American Journal of Health Behavior, 31*(6), 687–700. Retrieved from Health Source: Nursing/Academic Edition database.

Byrne, S. (2008, September). Healthcare avoidance: a critical review. *Holistic Nursing Practice, 22*(5), 280–292. Retrieved from CINAHL database.

Centers for Disease Control and Prevention. (2007). Recommended adult immunization schedule—United States, October 2007–September 2008. Atlanta, GA: MMWR.

Centers for Disease Control and Prevention and The Merck Company Foundation. (2007). The state of aging and health in America 2007. Retrieved from www.cdc.gov/aging

Cokkinides, V., Bandi, P., Siegel, R., Ward, E. M., & Thun, M. J. (2007). *Cancer prevention & early detection facts & figures 2008.* Atlanta, GA: American Cancer Society.

Cumbie, S., Conley, V., & Burman, M. (2004 January–March). Advanced practice nursing model for comprehensive care with chronic illness. *Advances in Nursing Science, 27*(1), 70–80.

D'Cruz, P. (2003). Family-focused interventions in health and illness. *Journal of Health Management, 5*(1), 37–56.

Dunn, H. (1959). High-level wellness for man and society. *American Journal of Public Health, 49,* 786–972.

Duvall, E. (1977). *Marriage and family development.* Philadelphia: Lippincott.

Edelman, C., & Mandle, C. (2006). *Health promotion throughout the lifespan* (6th ed.). St. Louis, MO: Mosby.

Erikson, E. (1963). *Childhood and society* (2nd ed.). New York: Norton.

Federal Citizen Information Center. (2004). *The food guide pyramid.* Retrieved from http://www.pueblo.gsa.gov/cic_text/food/food-pyramid/main.htm

Fowler, J. (1981). *Stages of faith: The psychology of human development and the quest for meaning.* New York: Harper & Row.

Freidman, M., Bowden, V., & Jones, E. (2003). *Family nursing: Research, theory and practice.* Upper Saddle River, NJ: Prentice Hall.

Grossman, S. & Lange, J. (2006). Theories of aging as a basis for assessment. *MEDSURG Nursing, 15*(2), 77–83.

Havighurst, R. (1972). *Human development and education* (3rd ed.). New York: Longman.

Kennedy, R. D., & Cullamar, K. (2007). Try this: Best practices in nursing care to older adults. Immunizations for older adults. The Hartford Institute for Geriatric Nursing, Division of Nursing, New York University. Retrieved from www.hartfordign.org

Kohlberg, L. (1979). *The meaning and measurement of moral development.* New York: clark University.

Langer, N. (2008, May). Integrating Compliance, communication, and culture: Delivering health care to an aging population. *Educational Gerontology, 34*(5), 385–396.

Leavell, H., & Clark, A. (1965). *Preventive medicine for doctors in the community.* New York: McGraw-Hill.

Lee, C. (2009). A comparison of health promotion behaviors in rural and urban community-dwelling spousal caregivers. *Journal of Gerontological Nursing, 35*(5), 34–40.

Lubkin, I., & Larsen, P. (2006). *Chronic illness: Impact and interventions* (6th ed.). Boston: Jones & Bartlett.

Miller, C. (2003). Safe medication practices: Nursing assessment of medications in older adults. *Geriatric Nursing, 24*(5), 314–315, 317.

Miller, C. (2008). *Nursing for wellness in older adults: Theory and practice* (5th ed.). Philadelphia: Lippincott.

Miller, J. (2000). *Coping with chronic illness: Overcoming powerlessness* (3rd ed.). Philadelphia: F. A. Davis.

National Center for Health Statistics. (2009). *Health, United States, 2008.* Hyattsville, MD: U. S. Department of Health and Human Services, Centers for Disease Control and Prevention.

National Guideline Clearinghouse. (2006). Adult preventive services (ages 18–49). Southfield, MI: Michigan Quality Improvement Consortium. Retrieved from www.guideline.gov

National Guideline Clearinghouse. (2006). Adult preventive services (ages 50–65+). Southfield, MI: Michigan Quality Improvement Consortium. Retrieved from www.guideline.gov

Pender, N., Parsons, M., & Murdaugh, C. (2006). *Health promotion in nursing practice* (5th ed.). Upper Saddle River, NJ: Prentice Hall.

Senior Site. (2004). *Learning to cope with chronic illness.* Retrieved from http://seniors-site.com/coping/chronic.html

Strandberg, T., & Pitkälä, K. (2007, April 21). Frailty in elderly people. *Lancet,* pp. 1328, 1329. Retrieved from Health Source: Nursing/Academic Edition database.

Strauss, A., et al. (1984). *Chronic illness and the quality of life.* St. Louis, MO: Mosby.

Suchman, E. (1972). Stages of illness and medical care. In E. Jaco (Ed.), *Patients, physicians and illness.* New York: Free Press.

Tabloski, P. A. (2006). *Gerontological nursing.* Upper Saddle River, NJ: Pearson/Prentice Hall.

U.S. Department of Health and Human Services. (2010). *Healthy people 2020.* Washington, DC: Author.

Westerhoff, J. (1976). *Will our children have faith?* New York: Seabury Press.

World Health Organization. (1974). *Constitution of the World Health Organization: Chronicle of the World Health Organization.* Geneva: Author.

3 Community and Home Care of Adults

LEARNING OUTCOMES

1. Differentiate community-based care from community health care.
2. Discuss selected factors affecting health in the community.
3. Describe services and settings for healthcare consumers receiving community-based and home care.
4. Describe the components of the home healthcare system, including agencies, patients, referrals, nursing care, physicians, reimbursement, and legal considerations.

5. Compare and contrast the roles of the nurse providing home care with the roles of the nurse in medical-surgical nursing discussed in ∞ Chapter 1.
6. Discuss nursing interventions to deliver safe and competent care to patients in their homes.
7. Explain the purpose of rehabilitation in health care.

CLINICAL COMPETENCIES

1. Assess factors affecting the health of individuals in the community.
2. Provide patient care in community-based settings and the home.

3. Apply the nursing process to care of the patient in the home.

KEY TERMS

community-based care, *36*
contracting, *42*
disability, *47*
faith community nursing, *38*

handicap, *47*
home care, *38*
hospice care, *39*
impairment, *47*

referral source, *39*
rehabilitation, *47*
respite care, *39*

Healthcare is provided by medical-surgical nurses in a variety of settings. Currently, only patients requiring complex surgery, who are acutely ill or seriously injured, or who are having babies are hospitalized and then only for a minimum period of time. As a result, most healthcare services are provided in settings outside the hospital. Those settings include clinics, schools, prisons, day-care centers for children and seniors, offices, and homes. The discussion in this chapter focuses on selected community services and settings and home care.

People requiring healthcare services may access and use the system through a variety of providers and settings, including hospital-based outpatient care, community-based offices and clinics, and home care. In the healthcare system of the twenty-first century, hospitals are primarily acute care providers with services focused on high-technology care for severely ill or injured people or for people having major surgery. Even those patients rarely remain in the hospital for long. They are moved as rapidly as possible to less acute care settings within the hospital and then to community-based and home care. Health care has become a managed care, community-based system. Although many nurses are still employed in hospitals, they are increasingly providing nursing care outside of the acute care, in-hospital setting.

Community-Based Nursing Care

A community may be a small neighborhood in a major urban city or a large area of rural residents. Communities are formed by the characteristics of people, area, social interaction, and common ties. Each community, however, is unique. People who live in a community may share a culture, history, or heritage. Although a community is where people live, have homes, raise families, and carry on daily activities, its members often cross community boundaries to work or to seek health care. Nurses who provide care within a community must know the composition and characteristics of the patients with whom they will work.

In contrast to community health nursing, which focuses on the health of the community, **community-based care** centers on individual and family healthcare needs. The nurse practicing community-based care provides direct services to individuals to manage acute or chronic health problems and to promote self-care. The care is provided in the local community, is culturally competent, and is family centered. The philosophy of community-based nursing directs nursing care for patients wherever they are, including where they live, work, play, worship, and go to school.

Nurses provide community-based care in many different ways and locations, ranging from leading support groups in a hospital (for individuals and family members diagnosed with such illnesses as cancer or diabetes) to managing a freestanding clinic to providing care at the patient's home. Box 3–1 illustrates the varied settings within the community in which a nurse may provide care.

Factors Affecting Health in the Community

Many factors can affect the health of individuals in a community. These factors include social support systems, the community healthcare structure, environmental factors, and economic resources.

Social Support Systems

A person's social support system consists of the people who lend assistance to meet financial, personal, physical, or emotional needs. In most instances, family, friends, and neighbors provide the best social support within the community. To understand the community social structure, the nurse needs to know what support is available for health care for the patient and family, including neighbors, friends, their church, organizations, self-help groups, and professional providers. The nurse also must know and respect the cultural and ethnic background of the community.

Community Healthcare Structure

The healthcare structure of a community has a direct effect on the health of the people living and working within it. The size of the community often determines the type of services provided as well as the access to the services. For example, urban residents have various means of transportation to a variety of community healthcare providers, whereas rural residents must often travel long distances for any type of care. The financial base of the community is also important, in many cases determining state and county funding of services.

Nurses who provide community-based care must know about public health services, the number and kind of health screenings offered, the location and specialty of healthcare professionals within the community, and the availability and accessibility of services and supplies. Other factors to consider include facilities (e.g., day care and long-term care), housing, and the number and kind of support agencies providing assistance (e.g., for housing, shelter, and food).

Environmental Factors

The environment within which a person lives and works may have both helpful and harmful effects on health. Air and water quality differ across communities. Air pollution may occur across a large area, or may be limited to the home. Within the home, pollution may occur from such sources as molds, pesticides, and fumes from new carpet. The water source also varies, with water supplies coming from rivers, lakes, reservoirs, or wells. No matter the source, chemical runoff or bacteria may contaminate water. It is critical to determine whether patients have a safe supply of running water.

Household and community safety and health resource accessibility are also important. Nurses must consider lighting, street and sidewalk or road upkeep and conditions, effects of ice and snow, condition of stairs and floors, and usefulness and availability of bathroom facilities. Physical barriers to residents accessing community resources include lack of transportation, distance to services, and location of services.

Economic Resources

Economic resources encompass the financial and insurance coverage necessary to provide the means for health care within the community. As private medical insurance becomes more and more expensive, fewer citizens have it, and many U.S. citizens have no insurance at all. Most unskilled and semi-skilled jobs do not provide healthcare benefits, resulting in a substantial percentage of what might be labeled "the working poor," those who have no financial assistance for illness care or healthcare screenings from an employer. However, the healthcare bill of 2010 mandates healthcare insurance for all citizens, with provisions made requiring employers to provide insurance and Medicaid expanded to assist low-income people. Older adults with fixed or limited incomes often find their monthly income consumed by medicines and medical supplies.

Medicare and Medicaid are health assistance programs created by 1965 Social Security amendments. Medicare is a federal health insurance plan for acute care needs of the disabled and those over 65 years. This plan covers some services provided in hospitals, long-term facilities, and the home; however, many necessary healthcare components are not covered fully or at all, including prescribed and over-the-counter medications and adaptive equipment for safety, such as shower seats or raised toilet seats. Coverage for care at home continues only as long as skilled providers are needed, and the person is not considered homebound even if he or she needs a wheelchair and assistance from others to leave the home. Medicaid is a state-run health insurance program for people with limited incomes. Each state has different benefits and criteria for coverage.

Community-Based Healthcare Services

Community-based healthcare services have many forms. Selected examples are discussed in the following sections.

Community Centers and Clinics

Community centers and clinics may be directed by physicians, advanced practice nurses in collaboration with physicians, or advanced practice nurses working independently (depending on state regulations). These healthcare settings may be located within a hospital, be part of a hospital but located in another area, or be independent of a hospital base. Healthcare centers and clinics provide a wide range of services and often meet the health needs of patients who are unable to access care elsewhere. This group includes the homeless, the poor, those with substance abuse problems, those with sexually transmitted diseases, and the victims of violent or abusive behavior.

Day Care Programs

Day care programs, such as senior centers, are usually located where people gather for social, nutritional, and recreational purposes. They may provide care for older adults with physical

BOX 3–1 Community-Based Nursing Care Settings

- Hospitals
  - Outpatient (ambulatory) surgery
  - Outpatient diagnostics and treatments
  - Cardiac rehabilitation
  - Support groups
  - Education groups
- County health departments
- Senior centers
- Long-term care
- Parish nursing
- Adult day care centers
- Homeless shelters
- Mobile vans
- Mental health centers
- Schools
- Crisis intervention centers
- Ambulatory surgery centers
- Alcohol/drug rehabilitation
- Healthcare provider offices
- Healthcare clinics
- Free clinics
- Urgent care centers
- Rural health centers
- Home care
- Hospice care
- Industry
- Jails and prisons

disabilities or mild Alzheimer's disease while family care-givers are at work. These programs vary among communities. Meals may be provided at low cost.

Faith Community Nursing

Faith community nursing, also known as parish nursing, is a nontraditional, community-based way of providing health promotion and health restoration nursing interventions to specific groups of people. It meets the needs of people who are often underserved by the traditional healthcare system.

A nurse who practices faith community nursing works with the pastor and staff of a faith community to promote health and healing through counseling, referrals, teaching, and assessment of healthcare needs. A faith community nurse may be employed by a hospital and contracted by a church, be employed directly by a church, or work as a volunteer with the congregation of a church. The faith community nurse helps bridge gaps between members of the church and the healthcare system (American Nurses Association [ANA], 2005).

Meals on Wheels

Many communities have a food service, usually called Meals on Wheels, for older people who do not have assistance in the home for food preparation. A hot, nutritionally balanced meal is delivered once a day, usually at noon. Volunteers often deliver the meals, providing not only nutrition but also a friendly, caring visit each day.

Home Care

Home care is not easily defined. It is not simply illness care at home, nor is it the act of setting up a hospital room in someone's house. The National Association for Home Care and Hospice (NAHC) (2009) defines **home care** as services for recovering, disabled, or chronically ill people who are in need of treatment or support to function effectively in the home environment. The U.S. Department of Health and Human Services places home care along a continuum of health care. Home care is provided in the patient's place of residence for the purpose of promoting, maintaining, or restoring health or of maximizing the level of independence while minimizing the effects of disability and illness, including terminal illness.

Home care encompasses both health and social services provided to the chronically ill, disabled, or recovering person in his or her own home. Home care is usually provided when a person needs help that cannot be provided by a family member or friend. Among patients who benefit from home care services are those who

- cannot live independently at home because of age, illness, or disability.
- have chronic, debilitating illnesses such as congestive heart failure, heart disease, kidney disease, respiratory diseases, diabetes mellitus, or muscle-nerve disorders.
- are terminally ill and want to die with comfort and dignity at home.
- do not need in-patient hospital or nursing home care but require additional assistance.
- need short-term help at home for postoperative care.

The services provided in the home may include professional nursing care, care provided by home care aides, physical therapy, speech therapy, occupational therapy, medical social worker services, and nutritional services. Patients receiving home care services are usually under the care of a physician, with the focus of care being treatment or rehabilitation. Registered nurses or licensed practical nurses provide nursing care based on physician orders. These nurses give direct care, supervise other care providers, coordinate patient care with the physician, advocate for the patient and family, and teach family members and friends how to care for the patient when professional services are no longer necessary.

Home care is both professional and technical. Professional home care is provided by people who are practice driven, licensed, certified, and/or have special qualifications. Nurses, therapists, social workers, and home aides are considered professional providers. Durable medical equipment companies (businesses that deliver medical equipment to homes) are technical providers. Technical home care providers are business and product driven. Customer satisfaction, field service, reimbursement, and profits are their primary concerns.

Brief History of Home Care

Many milestones marked the growth and development of home care in the United States. The passage of Medicare in 1965, Medicaid in 1970, the addition of hospice benefits in 1973, and the introduction of diagnosis-related groups (DRGs) in 1983 dramatically affected home care. Medicare legislation entitled the nation's older adult to home care services, primarily skilled nursing, and other curative or restorative therapies. This same benefit was extended to certain disabled younger Americans in 1973.

The introduction of DRGs to help control healthcare costs greatly increased home care. DRGs are categories for reimbursement of inpatient services. The DRG system pays the same predetermined amount of money for the care of different persons with the same medical diagnosis. Many changes in the healthcare system have been attributed to the introduction of DRGs, including earlier discharge from hospitals and the increased need for home care services.

Hospice and Respite Care

Hospice care is a special component of home care, designed to provide medical, nursing, social, psychological, and spiritual care for terminally ill patients and their families. Hospice care relies on a philosophy of relieving pain and suffering and allowing the patient to die with dignity in a comfortable environment. Licensed nurses, medical social workers, physicians, occupational and physical therapists, and volunteers provide care. Hospice care is discussed in ∞ Chapter 5.

Respite care provides short-term or intermittent home care, often using volunteers. These services exist primarily to give the family member or friend who is the primary caregiver some time away from care. Respite care does much to relieve the burden of full-time caregiving.

The Home Care System

Nurses who practice home care do so within a system that includes home healthcare agencies, patients, referral sources, physicians, reimbursement sources, and legal considerations. The system is interactive and functions best when its members communicate, cooperate, and collaborate with one another.

Types of Home Health Agencies

Home care agencies are either public or private organizations engaged in providing skilled nursing and other therapeutic services in the patient's home. The several different types of home care agencies differ only in the way their programs are organized and administered. All home care agencies are similar in that they must meet uniform standards for licensing, certification, and accreditation. Home care agencies include the following:

- *Official or public agencies.*   State or local governments operate these agencies, which are financed primarily by tax funds. Most official agencies offer home care, health education, and disease-prevention programs in the community.
- *Voluntary or private not-for-profit agencies.*   Donations, endowments, charities such as the United Way, and third-party (insurance company) reimbursement support these agencies. They are governed by a volunteer board of directors, which usually represents the community they serve.
- *Private, proprietary agencies.*   Most of these agencies are for-profit organizations governed by either individual owners or national corporations. Although some participate in third-party reimbursement, others rely on patients paying their own bills (often called out-of-pocket expenses).
- *Institution-based agencies.*   These agencies operate under a parent organization, such as a hospital. The home care agency is governed by the sponsoring organization, and the mission of both is similar. Often, the majority of home care referrals come from the parent organization.

Home care agency personnel typically include administrators, managers, care providers (these may be experienced in areas such as social work, medical-surgical care, mental health care, or infusion services) and business office staff. Depending on the agency and geographic location, professional providers may include registered nurses, practical nurses, nurse practitioners, enterostomal therapists, physical therapists, occupational therapists, speech therapists, respiratory therapists, social workers, a chaplain or pastoral minister, dietitians, and home care aides. It is not unusual for patients to require the services of several professionals simultaneously. No matter how many providers are in the home, the responsibility for case coordination (also called case management) remains with the registered nurse.

Patients

The patients in home care are the person receiving care and the person's family. The recognition that the family is also a patient acknowledges the powerful influence that families exert on health. A patient's family is not limited to persons related by birth, adoption, or marriage. In the home, family members may include partners, friends, colleagues, other significant people, and even animals that hold the potential of greatly affecting the health care environment.

Age and functional disability are the primary predictors of need for home care services. Information from a national survey conducted by the Agency for Health Care Policy and Research found that about half of all home care patients are over the age of 65 and that the number of home care services that patients need seems to increase with age.

The old adage that discharge plans begin at admission makes more sense today than ever before. With shortened lengths of hospital stay, it is imperative for nurses to evaluate all patients for their ability to manage at home. Nurses preparing to send patients home must consider many of the questions outlined in the Meeting Individualized Needs box on page 40.

Referrals

A **referral source** is a person recommending home care services and supplying the agency with details about the patient's needs. The source may be a physician, nurse, social worker, therapist, or discharge planner. Families sometimes generate their own referrals, either by approaching one of the sources already mentioned or by calling a home care agency directly to make an inquiry. When the family seeks a referral and the agency believes that the patient qualifies for services, usually the agency contacts the patient's physician and requests a referral on the patient's behalf.

The nurse may make a referral to a home care agency, a hospice, or a community resource if the patient seems to need formal follow-up beyond the present clinical setting. Hospital discharge planners, social workers, organizations for older adults, and local nonprofit agencies usually have a good command of the services and support groups available in their communities.

The nurse must talk to patients and their caregivers about concerns related to home management. It is not unusual for one family member to think that no additional help is necessary and

QUESTIONS FOR CONSIDERATION

- Does the patient need follow-up therapy, treatments, or additional education?
- What equipment, supplies, or information about community resources is necessary?
- What teaching materials can be sent home? Are they written at an acceptable reading level? Do they come in other languages?
- What cognitive abilities do the patient and the caregiver seem to have? Are there any sensory deprivations that impede learning?
- Who will be the principal caregiver in the home? Is there one? Are all caregivers comfortable in doing what needs to be done? If not, what support do they need to become comfortable?
- Was the caregiver present during and included in instruction? How have the patient and caregiver responded to health teaching thus far? Have they comprehended what has been taught? Was their stress level such that they could not listen?
- Has a devastating diagnosis and/or prognosis just been determined?
- Is high-technology intervention necessary?

for another to feel differently. The nurse can facilitate an informal family meeting in which everyone shares concerns and can make inquiries about the family's insurance coverage for home care. Suggesting services that families cannot afford only adds to the problem. For patients with limited means, the nurse can consult with staff in the institution who are most knowledgeable about funding. In every instance, it is important that the nurse avoid making assumptions: Well-educated and financially secure patients can be just as overwhelmed by illness as patients who are poor and less learned. Everyone is a referral candidate.

If the family believes that no help is necessary and the nurse believes otherwise, then the nurse may ask the family to consider an evaluation visit, explaining how the situation may look different once the patient is home. If family members continue to refuse, the nurse can let them know that the door is never closed and give them contacts in the community that they can access independently should their needs change.

Physicians

Home care cannot begin without a physician's order, nor can it proceed without a physician-approved treatment plan. This is a legal and reimbursement requirement. Only after a referral is made and an initial set of physician orders is obtained can a nursing assessment visit be scheduled to identify the patient's needs. If the input of another provider, such as a physical therapist, is necessary to complete the initial assessment, then the nurse arranges for this visit.

At the nursing assessment visit, the nurse begins to formulate the plan of care. Box 3–2 lists Medicare's required data for the nursing plan of care. Once formulated, the nurse sends the plan of care back to the physician for review and approval. The physician's signature on the plan of care authorizes the home care agency's providers to continue with services and also serves as a contract indicating agreement to participate in the care of the patient on an ongoing basis. The plan is reviewed as necessary, but at least once every 60 days.

Reimbursement for Services

A reimbursement source pays for home care services. Medicare is home care's largest single reimbursement source, although other sources exist (Medicaid, other public funding, private insurance, and public donation). The reimbursement source evaluates each treatment plan to determine if the goals and plans set forth by the professional providers match the needs assessed. Only interventions identified on the treatment plan

are covered. Periodically the reimbursement source may ask for the home care provider's notes to substantiate what is being done in the home. This is one reason why accurate documentation is critical.

Medicare does not reimburse visits made to support general health maintenance, health promotion, or patients' emotional or socioeconomic needs. Both patient and nurse must meet specific criteria to secure Medicare reimbursement. The patient must meet all of the following criteria:

- The physician must decide that the patient needs care at home and make a plan for home care.
- The patient must need at least one of the following: intermittent (not full time) skilled nursing care, physical therapy, speech language pathology services, or occupational therapy.
- The patient must be homebound. This means leaving the home is a major effort. When leaving the home, it must be infrequent, for a short time, to get medical care, or to attend religious services.
- The home care agency must be Medicare approved.

Medicare will reimburse only when the skilled provider performs at least one of the following tasks:

- Teaching about a new or acute situation.
- Assessing an acute process or a change in the patient's condition.
- Performing a skilled procedure or a hands-on service requiring the professional skill, knowledge, ability, and judgment of a licensed nurse (Figure 3–1 ■).

BOX 3–2 Medicare's Required Data for the Plan of Care

1. All pertinent diagnoses
2. A notation of the beneficiary's mental status
3. Types of services, supplies, and equipment ordered
4. Frequency of visits to be made
5. Patient's prognosis
6. Patient's rehabilitation potential
7. Patient's functional limitations
8. Activities permitted
9. Patient's nutritional requirements
10. Patient's medications and treatments
11. Safety measures to protect against injuries
12. Discharge plans
13. Any other items the home health agency or physician wishes to include

Source: Data from Medicare Health Insurance Manual-11, Section 204.2.

Figure 3–1 ■ The nurse is arriving for a home visit.

The reimbursement guidelines present problems because they are not sensitive to the full scope of nursing practice. Many of the patient and family needs that nurses encounter during home visits are complex and time consuming, reflecting both intense psychosocial and economic concerns. This situation presents a profound dilemma. How are nurses to reconcile spending time on issues for which their agency will receive no payment? How are they to meet agency home visit productivity standards when each home they enter requires more and more from them? How are they to document activities and interventions that are not considered "skilled"? There are no easy answers to these questions.

Legal Considerations

The legal considerations in home care center around issues of privacy and confidentiality, the patient's access to health information, the patient's freedom from unreasonable restraint, witnessing of documents, informed consent, and matters of negligence and/or malpractice. Numerous sources suggest that nurses can best avoid lawsuits by familiarizing themselves with the standards of practice, providing care that is consistent with both the standards and their agency's policies, and documenting all care fully and accurately according to agency guidelines.

Home care nurses are responsible for adhering to the same codes and standards that guide all other nurses. These codes and standards guide nursing practice and protect the public. In addition to these guidelines, other codes and statements give specific guidance on issues that affect care in the home.

The ANA Scope and Standards of Practice for Home Health Nursing (2007a) and Public Health Nursing (2007b) are used in conjunction as a basis for the practice of nursing in the home. These standards address the nursing process, interdisciplinary collaboration, quality assurance, professional development, and research. The standards speak to two levels of practitioners (generalist, who is prepared on the baccalaureate level, and specialist, who is prepared on the graduate level) and outline what achievements are expected of the professional nurse in the home.

Another source of guidance regarding home care is the National Association of Home Care (NAHC) Bill of Rights. Its use is a federal requirement for all home care agencies. Although they are permitted to make additions to the NAHC's original bill of rights, home care agencies are required by law to address the concepts in the NAHC Bill of Rights with all home care patients on the initial visit. The bill of rights is listed in Box 3–3.

The Nursing Process in Home Care

The nursing process used in home care is no different from that practiced in any other setting. The unique challenges of home care present themselves chiefly in the implementation step. Generally, the differences lie in assessing how the home's unique environment affects the need or problem and using outcome criteria and mutual participation to plan goals and interventions.

Assessment

In home care, nursing assessment and data collection center chiefly around the first home visit. This is not to say that nurses do not collect information on an ongoing basis, but because most agencies require the submission of a plan of care within 48 hours of the initial evaluation, the first visit carries tremendous weight. Under ideal circumstances, a preliminary review of background information initiates the assessment process; the reality in home care, however, is that few patients are referred with copies of either their medical records or their discharge summaries. If the patient has received home care services in the past, records may be available, but often all the nurse has prior to initiating care is the referral form describing the present problem, some notations about past medical history, and a projection of the skilled interventions needed. Therefore, it falls to the nurse to try to obtain as complete a clinical picture as possible when meeting the patient.

Assessment begins when the nurse calls the patient to arrange a visit. This initial telephone call can yield much information to the nurse who pays close attention. For example,

- How alert, oriented, and stressed does the patient (and/or family) seem to be?
- Does the patient know the reason for the home care referral?
- How open to intervention do the patient and family seem to be?
- Have they encountered any difficulties since discharge from the prior setting?
- Do they need any supplies on the first visit?

During the visit, much of the assessment process centers on collecting the information requested on the tools and forms contained in the agency's admission packet. These packets usually include a physical and psychosocial database; a medication sheet; forms for pain assessment, spiritual assessment, financial assessment; and a family roster. It is extremely important that the data collected be as complete and accurate as possible and reflect subjective, objective, current, and historical information. Through interviewing, direct observation, and physical assessment, the nurse can achieve the goal of the initial visit, namely, to gain as clear and accurate a clinical picture of the patient as possible.

Diagnosis

After completing the initial assessment, the nurse identifies the real and/or potential patient problems that emerge from the data. Nursing diagnoses describing the patient's health problems and needs, based on data collection, must be part of the home care record both to organize care and to justify reimbursement.

In almost all home care situations, *Deficient Knowledge* is an appropriate nursing diagnosis. Nursing interventions for this diagnosis specific to a patient with Alzheimer's disease and the patient's family can be found in the Meeting Individualized Needs box on page 43.

BOX 3–3 Example of a Home Health Agency's Bill of Rights

The agency acknowledges the patient's rights and encourages the patient and family to participate in their plan of care through informed decision making. In accordance with this belief, each patient/family member will receive, prior to admission, the following bill of rights and responsibilities.

1. The patient and the patient's property will be treated with respect by the program's staff.
2. The patient will receive care without regard to race, color, creed, age, sex, religion, national origin, or mental or physical handicap.
3. The patient has the right to be free from mental and physical abuse.
4. The patient's medical record and related information is maintained in a confidential manner by the program.
5. The patient will receive a written statement of the program's objectives, scope of services, and grievance process prior to admission.
6. The patient, family, or guardian has the right to file a complaint regarding the services provided by the program without fear of disruption of service, coercion, or discrimination.
7. The patient will be advised of the following in advance of service:
   a. Description of services and proposed visit frequency
   b. Overview of the anticipated plan of care and its likely outcome
   c. Options that may be available
8. The patient/family is encouraged to participate in the plan of care. The patient will receive the necessary information concerning the patient's condition and will be encouraged to participate in changes that may arise in care.
9. The program shall provide for the right of the patient to refuse any portion of planned treatment to the extent permitted by law without relinquishing other portions of the treatment plan, except where medical contraindications exist. The patient will be informed of the expected consequences of such action.

10. The patient has a right to continuity of care:
    a. Services provided within a reasonable time frame
    b. A program that is capable of providing the level of care required by the patient
    c. Timely referral to alternative services, as needed
    d. Information regarding impending discharge, continuing care requirements, and other services, as needed
11. The patient will be informed of the extent to which payment will be expected for items or services to be furnished to patients by Medicare, Medicaid, and any other program that is funded partially or fully with federal funds. Upon admission, the patient will be informed orally and in writing of any charges for items and services that the program expects will not be covered upon admission. The patient will be informed of any change in this amount as soon as possible, but no later than within 25 days after the program is made aware of the change.
12. Upon request, the patient may obtain:
    a. An itemized bill
    b. The program's policy for uncompensated care
    c. The program's policy for disclosure of the medical record
    d. Identity of healthcare providers with which the program has contractual agreements, insofar as the patient's care is concerned
    e. The name of the responsible person supervising the patient's care and how to contact this person during regular business hours
13. The patient has the right to obtain medical equipment and other health-related items from the company of the patient's choice and assumes financial responsibility for such. The program's staff will assist in obtaining supplies and physician approvals as needed.
14. The patient/family is responsible for:
    a. Giving the program accurate, necessary information
    b. Being available and cooperative during scheduled visits
    c. Assisting, as much as possible, in the plan of care
    d. Alerting the staff to any problems as soon as possible

Planning

Planning in home care includes setting priorities, establishing goals, and deciding on interventions designed to meet the needs of the patient. The greatest level of success is achieved when patients feel an ownership of the suggested plan. For this reason, planned interventions and outcome criteria should be patient centered, realistic, achievable, and mutually accepted. The nurse works with the patient to do the following:

- Identify significant issues and needs.
- Set mutually agreed-upon goals (outcome criteria).
- Make and initiate acceptable plans to meet the goals.

Outcome criteria should be verbally stated to patients and documented clearly and concisely, in timed, measurable, and observable terms. These measures help patients and care providers better focus their work together and evaluate the effectiveness of care. In addition, outcome criteria provide the reimbursement source a measurable standard from which to judge the appropriateness of the plan of care.

Implementation

The home care nurse implements most of the planned interventions, although some may be carried out by another agency provider, a paraprofessional introduced into the setting by the nurse case manager, or the patient.

Nurses and patients reach an agreement about the implementation of care through a process called **contracting**, the negotiation of a cooperative working agreement between the nurse and patient that is continuously renegotiated. Contracting is a concept used often in, but not exclusive to, many home and community health settings. Contracting can occur both formally and informally. It involves exploring a need, establishing goals, evaluating resources, developing a plan, assigning responsibilities, agreeing on a time frame, and evaluating or terminating. Contracting requires the nurse to relinquish control as the expert and consider the patient as an equal partner in the process.

Contracting is not appropriate with all patients. It is certainly inadvisable if the nurse–patient relationship is to be no more than two visits or if the patient has limited cognitive abilities. However, contracting is useful for patients who demonstrate a willingness to be active participants in their health care. It is empowering, can save time, and keeps the nursing goals directed and focused.

Evaluation

Evaluation in home care is both formative and summative. Formative evaluation is the systematic, ongoing comparison of the plan of care with the goals actually being achieved from visit to

MEETING INDIVIDUALIZED NEEDS   Family Home Care for the Older Adult with a Dementing Disorder

NURSING DIAGNOSIS
Deficient Knowledge related to lack of information about Alzheimer's disease process and care

OUTCOME CRITERIA
Short term: Adequate knowledge, as evidenced by family's stating of disease progression and treatment (expected within 1 week)
Long term: Adequate knowledge, as evidenced by family's following of the recommended interventions throughout illness course (within 1 month) or by discharge from home health

INTERVENTIONS
- Alert the family to both environmental hazards and patient habits that could threaten safety. (first visit)
- Provide the family with specific recommendations for keeping the patient safe, for example, serving foods warm, not hot; allowing the patient to eat with fingers; cutting food in small pieces; wearing an ID bracelet; discouraging daytime sleep. (first visit)
- Discuss the disease course (degenerative), the prognosis (incurable), typical issues of concern (promoting adequate nutrition, activity, rest, safety, and independence); supporting cognitive function; communication, socialization, and family caregiving; the supportive care available; and the ultimate need for long-term placement with disease progression. (first visit)
- Discuss local resources, including adult day care, support groups, and Alzheimer's Disease Association. Give family a list of these resources. (first visit)
- Include all family members or significant persons in teaching and planning care. (each visit)
- Prepare the family for typical types of Alzheimer's disease behaviors: forgetfulness, disorientation, agitation, screaming, crying, physical or verbal abuse, accusations of infidelity. (subsequent visits)
- Teach the family specific interventions for dealing with these behaviors: calm, unhurried manner, music, stroking, rocking, structuring the environment, distracting the patient. (subsequent visits)
- Stress the importance of both exercise and recreation in terms of quality of life and decreasing nighttime restlessness. (subsequent visits)
- Reinforce the patient's continued needs for socialization and intimacy. (subsequent visits)
- Suggest specific interventions for meeting socialization needs: limiting visitors to one or two at a time, pet therapy, use of the phone. (subsequent visits)
- Suggest useful interventions that are described in the literature and/or that are utilized in more formal Alzheimer's disease settings and may also be helpful in the home. (subsequent visits)
- Keep the environment safe for the patient.
- Use reality orientation with patient several times a day, and post clocks, calendars, and telephone numbers within easy sight of the patient.
- Give patient simple directions, using simple sentences and a quiet, monotone voice so as not to excite the patient.
- Allow the use of the telephone, because calls will help orient the patient.

visit. In summative evaluation, the nurse reviews the total plan of care and the patient's progress toward goals to determine the patient's eligibility for discharge.

Reimbursement guidelines may be helpful in driving the evaluation process. Because reimbursement sources require that all skilled services be justified, many home care agencies have designed their clinical notes to include areas for evaluation of the patient's response to the visit's interventions and documentation of a plan of care for the next scheduled visit.

Roles of the Home Care Nurse
The role expectations of the home care nurse are similar to those of the professional nurse in any setting. On behalf of patients in the home, the nurse serves as an advocate, a provider of direct care, an educator, and a coordinator of services.

Advocate
As patient advocate, the nurse explores, informs, supports, and affirms the choices of patients. Advocacy begins on the first visit, when the nurse discusses advanced directives, living wills, and durable power of attorney for health care. The home care agency's bill of rights also needs to be discussed. During the course of care, patients may need help negotiating the complex medical system (especially in regard to healthcare insurance), accessing community resources, recognizing and coping with required changes in lifestyle, and making informed decisions. When the family's desires differ from the patient's, advocacy

can be a challenge. If a conflict arises, the nurse must remain the patient's primary advocate.

In the home there are no colleagues present to consult, to assist, or to rely on for support. The home is a practice setting where nurses learn to trust their theoretical and intuitive knowledge and to be totally accountable.

Provider of Direct Care
Home care nurses usually are not involved in providing personal care for patients (such as bathing and changing linens). The families often provide routine personal care, or the nurse may arrange for a home care aide. If a personal care need arises during the course of the skilled visit (e.g., if a patient has an incontinent episode), the nurse typically either bathes and changes the patient or assists the caregiver to do so before moving on to the skilled activities planned for the visit.

As a provider of direct care, the nurse uses the nursing process to assess, diagnose, plan care, intervene, and evaluate patient needs. During the course of this process, home care nurses frequently are involved in performing specific procedures and treatments such as physical assessments, care of intravenous lines, ostomy care, wound care, and pain management.

Personal health habits, living conditions, resources, and support systems may leave much to be desired. It is not unusual for home care nurses to face unchanged dressings, undertreated infections, off-and-on self-medication, poor nutrition, filthy conditions, and unreliable caregivers. No matter how vigilant nurses may be, practice settings like these work against their best efforts. If the conditions cannot be changed, the nurse may withdraw from the situation, or continue to practice within the environment and report substandard care by caregivers.

Educator

Most of the home care nurse's time is spent teaching. Many nurses believe that their role as teacher is the crux of their nursing practice and that nurses in the home are always teaching (Figure 3–2 ■). For this reason, it is important that home care nurses develop expertise in the theory and principles of patient education.

The greatest educational challenge may be motivating the patient. Discovering what it takes to make the patient want to learn and focusing the patient on what is most important can tax the ingenuity of even the most dedicated nurse. Despite the work involved, nurses are rewarded by the knowledge that through their efforts, patients have learned to manage independently. Because the nurse's role as educator is becoming increasingly important, guidelines for community-based care are included in the discussion of each major disorder addressed in this textbook.

Figure 3–2 ■ Home visits offer opportunities to carry out health promotion activities. This nurse takes a patient's blood pressure while visiting for an unrelated condition.

SAFETY ALERT

Promoting Safety in Home Care

When preparing patients for discharge to home, the nurse focuses on safety and survival first. Even if health education is to continue with home care, a day or two may elapse before the nurse arrives, and patients must be able to manage by themselves until then. The nurse must not discharge patients without giving them the correct information and supplies to get them through the first few days at home. Additionally, patients should not be discharged without phone numbers and complete written information about their medications and the manifestations of complications they should report to their doctor or the nurse that discharged them. Finally, all patients should be able to at least minimally manage any necessary treatments. Management includes not only performing procedures safely but also knowing how to obtain necessary supplies in the community.

Patients need help understanding their situations, making healthcare decisions, and changing health behaviors. It is unrealistic, however, to believe that patients can be taught everything they need to know during today's shortened hospital stays. The nurse should therefore recommend a home care referral for anyone in need of follow-up teaching. Prioritized teaching is essential: Even under the best of circumstances, patients generally forget about one-third of what is said to them and their recall of specific instructions and advice is less than 50%. Comprehensive information related to patient and family teaching is included in most of the following chapters in this textbook. This can be used as a guide in planning teaching.

Coordinator of Services

As coordinator of services, the home care nurse is the main contact with the patient's physician and all other providers involved in the treatment plan. It is the responsibility of the registered nurse case coordinator (or clinical case manager) to report patient changes, discuss responses, and develop and secure treatment plan revisions on an ongoing basis. This is accomplished formally, through scheduled case and team conferences, and informally (often over the phone) with concerned providers. Documentation of all coordination activities is legally required.

Special Considerations in Home Care Nursing

Nursing practice in the home is a unique experience that differs in many ways from nursing practice in a hospital setting. The word "home" generates strong feelings of ownership, control, security, family history, independence, comfort, protection, and conflict. Family members perceive a sharing of self when they consistently allow entry to a stranger. Because patients and nurses most often meet during periods of vulnerability and crisis, and because socializing is such an integral part of the home visit process, nurse providers are often perceived as friends or extended family members, blurring the boundaries of practice.

Nurses are invited into homes, meaning they are guests and cannot assume entry as they do in formal clinical settings. The environment belongs to the patient, who retains control. Every nursing action must communicate respect for these boundaries. To negotiate both repeated entry and a share of power in the patient's domain, the nurse must establish trust and rapport quickly. This is often difficult because most home care nurses are with each patient for only 1 hour a few times a week.

During the course of establishing rapport and getting to know each other as people, the nurse–patient relationship often becomes something more. Nurses and patients end up giving to each other and learning from each other. By connecting as human beings, they touch each other's spirits in profound ways (Taylor, 2008). In home health, it is not unusual for nurses to realize suddenly not only that they do things to create a healing environment but also that their very presence has become the healing environment. Over time, as the nurse becomes a familiar presence and the family's behavior relaxes, the nurse can gain a clearer and more complete picture of family relationships, dynamics, lifestyle choices, and coping patterns.

Caregiver burden is not easily hidden in the home. In nearly one out of four American households (23%), people are taking care of disabled relatives and friends (USDHHS, 2008). Many

Special Needs of Older Adults Living Alone

Many older adults live alone. Some may have current or potential caregivers nearby, whereas others, for various reasons, have no one. These people often require considerable nursing support to remain strong, independent, and resourceful. Caring for "families of one" can take a toll on even the strongest home care nurse. Some nurses have reported calling between visits, keeping in touch after discharge, and driving by on days off because they have such difficulty "letting go" their concerns about these

patients. Transitioning between healthcare settings is especially problematic for those with chronic illness or long-term health problems. Older adults are at high risk for "falling through the gap" and frequently need assistance to navigate the complex healthcare system. High quality transitional care can reduce adverse events and re-hospitalization rates while improving patient satisfaction with care (Naylor & Keating, 2008).

of these caregivers are themselves older adults. Healthcare planners visualize the home as a place where all kinds of medical services can occur but may give little thought to how people manage. Few ever ask whether families can cope with the level of care they are expected to assume. Caregiving has only recently been acknowledged as a complex activity, requiring adjustment in family living patterns, relationships, and finances. Early hospital discharge of family members with chronic conditions places enormous emotional, physical, and financial burdens on family caregivers (Toofany, 2008). For some families, the crisis of caregiving is short lived, but for others it lasts for years. As a result, caregivers are at great risk for both physical and emotional illness. Because the success of home care heavily depends on the supports in place, addressing the needs of the support network is imperative.

Nursing Interventions to Ensure Competent Home Care

Despite differences in the setting, nursing care for patients in their homes is a highly rewarding clinical practice. The following discussion provides practical information for competent care with successful outcomes.

Establish Trust and Rapport

To establish trust and rapport in the patient's home, nurses must try to find common ground and let go of ethnocentric ("my culture's way is the best way") views. Nurses must be sure everything they say and do communicates an understanding that they are guests—offering suggestions in a way that acknowledges the patient's right to say no, sensing and honoring "where people are in their situation," maintaining a respectful distance, and noticing and honoring family customs ("I see that no one wears shoes in your house; I'll take mine off, too."). Nurses should try to negotiate their schedules around the family's needs; nursing should enhance family coping, not complicate it. Above all, nurses should validate patients' illness experiences, remembering that everyone needs someone who is willing to listen and say, "I hear what you are saying, and I think I have a sense of how you feel."

Proceed Slowly

The nurse must enter the home with awareness that the first contact is important. On the first nursing visit, the nurse can suggest to patients that they have someone else present "to help them listen." To avoid overwhelming patients with too much information, the nurse stresses the essential information and

repeats it on subsequent visits. When making suggestions, the nurse offers patients the pluses and minuses of each alternative. Informed decisions are difficult to make if people are too overwhelmed to think of their options. The nurse speaks slowly, directly, and within the patient's range of vision (the patient may have to lip-read) and refrains from shouting at patients who are hearing-impaired. The nurse must also allow time for families to process new information.

Set Goals and Boundaries

The nurse explores patients' expectations of home care. In particular, the nurse explains the primary goal (to achieve self-care), defines nurse and patient roles within this framework, and discusses limitations. The nurse may make statements such as, "No, a home care nurse is not the same as a private duty nurse" and "Home care nurses do not routinely do that, but today I will make an exception." It is important that the nurse stresses mutual accountability, choice, and negotiation as part of the process.

Assess the Home Environment

The nurse surveys the overall home environment, using common sense, intuition, and imagination. Among the variables to note are sights, sounds, smells, dress, tone of voice, body language, and the use of touch; visiting patterns among family members; significant relationships; what is sacred and what is not; the appearance of the house, yard, sidewalk, and neighborhood; and the effect of illness on the family. The nurse asks questions and listens carefully to stories and offhand remarks.

Set Priorities

It is important that nurses are flexible and realize they cannot tackle everything. Although it is necessary to enter the home with a plan in mind, nurses must be prepared to modify the plan according to conditions they encounter once inside. Safety, issues that are of concern to patients, and those problems that can most easily be solved should be addressed first. Alternatively, the nurse can focus on safety first, then short-term and long-term goals. If the priorities that are set are primarily the nurse's and not the patient's, then they may not be met.

Promote Learning

Instead of just teaching the patient, the nurse tries actively to promote the patient's ability to learn by, for example, identifying what is most important to the patient and teaching that. Survival takes first priority; the nurse teaches the information people need to ensure their safety until the next visit. The nurse prioritizes material on a needs-to-know, wants-to-know, ought-to-know basis, assessing and responding to learner readiness.

Timing is important; people who are not ready to listen cannot be taught. In addition, the nurse must allow a sufficient amount of time to teach, ask patients how and when they learn best, use appropriate methods and materials when possible, and capitalize on patients' frustrations and desires to regain control of self-care. When possible, the nurse teaches while providing care.

The nurse can empower patients to learn by talking them through learning tasks, encouraging them to listen to their own bodies and to ask questions, and urging them to write thoughts and questions about their care and bring them to the next visit or doctor's appointment.

Limit Distractions

Homes are full of events or circumstances that may divert attention from the job at hand. Such distractions as children, animals, noise, clutter, and mannerisms that are controlling, manipulative, or aggressive can try even the most experienced nurse. However, environmental and behavioral distractions can yield useful information about people, their relationships, and their values. For example, a dirty house could indicate a lack of interest in housekeeping, outright neglect and abuse, depression, or increased disability.

Distractions should be limited as much as possible. For example, the nurse might ask a patient, "May I please turn off your television while we visit?" or "I would like to schedule my next visit for a time when the children are in school. Is that all right with you?" The nurse must be truthful about allergies, fear of a patient's pet, or difficulty hearing in a particular room, but should not debate the priority of the visit over the distraction (such as a favorite television show). The nurse may not change the patient's views and may also risk losing the patient's trust and rapport. If all efforts at limiting distractions fail, the nurse should leave the home and return on another day: "I can see this is not going to work for us today. I will need to leave."

If any distraction originates with the nurse, such as fear of harm, reaction to the patient's lifestyle, preoccupation with role or a feeling of being overwhelmed by the situation in the home, the nurse should seek out a colleague to discuss the problem. Often, another perspective helps when dealing with the issue.

Put Safety First

Safety assessment in the home is a nursing responsibility and a legal requirement. Nurses cannot close their eyes to an unsafe environment. Upon entering the home and on a continuing basis, it is imperative that the nurse alert the family to unsafe and hazardous conditions, suggest remedies, and document in the clinical record the family's response to the nurse's suggestions. See Box 3–4 for a sample home safety assessment list. In particular, nurses must remain alert to the following:

- How patients handle stairs.
- How patients manage their own care if they are alone.
- The presence of a smoke detector in the home.
- The presence of bathroom safety equipment.
- Electrical hazards.
- Slippery throw rugs, clutter, or a furniture arrangement that may cause a fall.
- A supply of expired medications.
- Inappropriate clothing or shoes.
- Cooking habits that may precipitate a fire.

BOX 3–4 Home Safety Assessment Checklist

General Household Safety
1. Do stairwells and halls have good lighting?
2. Do staircases have handrails on both sides?
3. Are rugs securely tacked down?
4. Is the telephone readily accessible? Is the dial easy to read?
5. Are electrical cords in good condition and out of the way?
6. Is furniture sturdy?
7. Is the temperature of the home comfortable?
8. Are protective screens in front of fireplaces or heating devices?
9. Are smoke detectors and carbon monoxide detectors present and working?

Bathroom
1. Are grab bars present in the tub and/or shower? Around the toilet?
2. Are toilet seats high enough?
3. Are nonskid materials (rugs, mats) on the floor, tub/shower?
4. Are medications stored safely? Out of the reach of children?
5. Is the water temperature safe?
6. Are electrical outlets and appliances a safe distance from the tub?

Kitchen
1. Are floors slippery? Are nonskid rugs used?
2. Is the stove in good working order?
3. Is the refrigerator in good working order? Clean?
4. Are electrical outlets overloaded with appliance cords?
5. Are sharp objects kept in a special container or safe area?
6. Is food storage adequate? Clean?
7. Are cleaning materials stored safely?

- An inadequate food supply.
- Poorly functioning utilities.
- Chipping paint.
- Signs of abusive behavior.

Nurses cannot go into homes and change the family's living space and lifestyle, but they can register their concern and react appropriately if the situation suggests that an injury is about to occur or if they suspect abuse or neglect. In the home and community setting, ignoring an unsafe environment is considered nursing negligence.

The disposal of toxic medications and sharp objects (such as needles used for injections) is also a safety issue in the home, especially if young children are present. Once again, it is imperative that the nurse address this with the patient, demonstrate safe disposal, and provide the necessary equipment to accomplish that end. Documentation should address what information the nurse has covered, the family's response to the teaching, and assessment of the family's ongoing practice of safety precautions.

Nurses must focus on safety and survival first, for themselves as well as their patients, in all that they do. When traveling in the community, the nurse takes such precautions as keeping car doors locked, having a cellular phone, keeping supplies out of sight, and staying inside the car in potentially dangerous situations. Colleagues, families, and community members can offer useful guidelines for maintaining safety and self-protection.

It is important to avoid overwhelming families with numerous healthcare providers in the home. Most people dislike having strangers in their home, no matter how helpful they may seem to be. The nurse can help families manage moments of crisis by staying as close as possible. If abuse is suspected, the nurse must notify authorities and/or remove patients from potentially dangerous situations.

Make Do

Nurses must learn to be resourceful and cost conscious with equipment, supplies, and services in the home. When needing to make do or improvise, they should do so in a low-key manner to avoid causing the family additional anxiety. The nurse must make every effort to convey the message that the situation is under control; after leaving the home, the nurse can react as necessary.

Control Infection

Infection control in the home centers on protecting patients, caregivers, and the community from the spread of disease. Within the home, nurses may encounter patients with infectious or communicable diseases, patients who are immuno-compromised, and/or patients having multiple access devices, drainage tubes, or draining wounds. The home presents a challenging environment in which to practice infection control for several reasons: Families typically are set in their own ways of doing things; caregivers often lack any formal education on the subject; the setting itself may not be conducive; and the facilities for even the most basic of aseptic practices (hand hygiene) may be lacking. Without a doubt, the single most important nursing intervention in controlling infection is health teaching. Patients and caregivers need to know the importance of effective hand hygiene, the use of gloves, the disposal of wastes and soiled dressings, the handling of linens, and the practice of standard precautions. Unfortunately, the imparting of important information does not always bring about a change in behavior. Trying to change a family's values frequently demands a great deal of ingenuity from the nurse.

Rehabilitation

Rehabilitation is the process of learning to live to one's maximum potential with a chronic impairment and its resultant functional disability. Rehabilitation nursing is based on a philosophy that each person has a unique set of strengths and abilities that can enable that person to live with dignity, self-worth, and independence. Nursing care to promote rehabilitation primarily focuses on patients with chronic illnesses or impairments. Rehabilitation most often begins in the acute phase of an illness or injury.

The terms *impairment*, *disability*, and *handicap* are often used as synonyms, but they have different meanings. **Impairment** is a disturbance in structure or function resulting from physiologic or psychologic abnormalities. A **disability** is the degree of observable and measurable impairment. A **handicap** is the total adjustment to disability that limits functioning at a normal level (Stanhope & Lancaster, 2006). For example, following a motorcycle accident, a patient had damage to her left leg that led to impairment in the ability to flex her knee. This resulted in a 50% disability of that leg and caused a handicap because the patient was a school bus driver and could no longer operate the bus safely.

Rehabilitation promotes reintegration into the patient's family and community through a team approach. Many different aspects of the patient's life are included in the plan of care, including physical function, mental health, interpersonal relationships, social interactions, family support, and vocational status. This comprehensive consideration of the patient requires the expertise of a team of healthcare providers who usually meet weekly to discuss the achievement of patient goals.

Assessment of the patient and family includes functional health level and self-care abilities, educational needs, psychosocial needs, and the home environment. It is critical to determine the priorities of needs from the patient and family perspective before establishing any plan of care. The nurse assesses the patient's level of physical function, goals, concerns, stage of loss, home environment, and available resources.

Interventions to facilitate rehabilitation are revised to meet patient and family needs as the patient progresses toward reintegration. In general, interventions are planned and implemented to prevent complications, assist in achieving a realistic level of independence, educate the patient and family about home care, and make referrals to community agencies (for nursing care, special equipment or supplies, support groups, counseling, physical therapy, occupational therapy, respiratory therapy, vocational guidance, house cleaning, and meals).

CHAPTER HIGHLIGHTS

- In contrast to community health, which focuses on health of a population, community-based care focuses on individual and family healthcare needs. Services are provided in many different settings, including community centers and clinics, day care programs, faith community nursing, and Meals on Wheels.
- Factors affecting health in the community include social support systems, community healthcare structures, environment, and economic resources.
- Home care is defined as services for recovering, disabled, or chronically ill people who are in need of treatment or support to function effectively in the home environment.
- Two special components of home care are hospice care and respite care.

- The home care system includes agencies, patients, referral sources, physicians, reimbursement sources, and legal considerations.
- The roles of the home care nurse include advocate, provider of direct care, educator, and coordinator of services.
- Nursing interventions to ensure competent care include those used to establish trust and rapport, proceed slowly, set goals and boundaries, assess the home environment, set priorities, promote learning, limit distractions, put safety first, and control infection.
- Rehabilitation is the process of learning to live to one's maximum potential with a chronic health impairment and its resultant disability.

TEST YOURSELF NCLEX-RN® REVIEW

1. What is the focus of community-based nursing care?
 1. the function of the community
 2. the health of the community
 3. individual and family health
 4. older adult needs and services
2. What is one way in which urban and rural residents may differ?
 1. access to healthcare services
 2. age and gender of residents
 3. family tasks and values
 4. ability to follow directions
3. As part of the initial assessment of a disabled older adult receiving community-based care, the nurse asks, "Who takes you to your doctor's appointments and picks up your prescriptions or groceries for you?" Which of the following factors is the nurse assessing?
 1. social support systems
 2. community healthcare structure
 3. environmental factors
 4. economic resources
4. Which of the following services helps relieve the stress of full-time caregiving?
 1. faith community nursing
 2. block nursing
 3. day care
 4. respite care
5. Home health nurses provide care to patients with a wide variety of healthcare needs. Which of the following patients would benefit from home care? **Select all that apply.**
 1. an older adult recently discharged from the hospital after a total hip replacement
 2. a teenager recently discharged from the hospital following an appendectomy
 3. a middle-aged patient with a terminal illness who wants to die at home
 4. a single mother of toddlers recently discharged following major abdominal surgery
 5. a frail older adult experiencing weakness and impaired mobility from osteoarthritis

6. While making the first home health visit, the nurse discusses advance directives, living wills, and durable power of attorney for health care. These topics are part of which nursing role?
 1. provider of direct care
 2. coordinator of services
 3. educator
 4. advocate
7. The nurse is assessing the safety of a patient's home environment. Which of the following outcomes indicate an unsafe environment? **Select all that apply.**
 1. the presence of overloaded extension cords
 2. the presence of a smoke detector in the home
 3. the presence of several throw rugs and a cluttered floor space
 4. a supply of expired medications
 5. a supply of frozen dinners and canned goods
8. Which of the following factors should have the highest priority when planning rehabilitative care for the patient?
 1. physician and nurse perspective of needs
 2. patient and family perspective of needs
 3. patient and family insurance coverage
 4. physician and nurse goals and concerns
9. Nurses practicing in the home provide teaching for a variety of topics. Which of the following areas is essential to maintaining infection control?
 1. fire and smoke detectors
 2. hand hygiene
 3. uncluttered floors and stairs
 4. medications
10. What element of home care is a requirement for reimbursement?
 1. family member approval
 2. completion of agency forms
 3. physician's order
 4. treatment plan

See Test Yourself answers in Appendix C.

Pearson Nursing Student Resources

Find additional review materials at
www.nursing.pearsonhighered.com

Prepare for success with additional NCLEX®-style practice questions, interactive assignments and activities, Web links, animations and videos, and more!

BIBLIOGRAPHY

American Nurses Association. (2005). *Faith community nursing scope and standards of practice.* Washington, DC: Author.

American Nurses Association. (2007a). *Home health nursing scope and standards of practice.* Washington, DC: Author.

American Nurses Association. (2007b). *Public health nursing scope and standards of practice.* Washington, DC: Author.

Carter, A. (2009). Home healthcare nurses and clinicians can bring significant savings to the table. *Home Healthcare Nurse, 27*(1), 64–65.

Eddy, T., Kilburn, E., Chang, C., Bullock, L., & Sharps, B. (2008). Facilitators and barriers for implementing home visit interventions to address intimate partner violence. *Nursing Clinics of North America, 43*(3), 419–435.

Grafova, I., Freedman, V., Kumar, K., & Ropgowski, J. (2008). Neighborhoods and obesity in later life. *American Journal of Public Health, 98*(11), 2065–2071.

Hoare, K. (2004). Care home placement: Can admission direct from acute hospital be justified? *Nursing Older People, 16*(6), 14–17.

Medicare. (2007). Types of long-term care. Retrieved from http://www.medicare.gov/LongTermCare/Static/TypesOverview.asp

National Association for Home Care and Hospice. (2009). *What are my rights as a patient?* Retrieved from http://www.nahc.org/consumer/rights.html

Naylor, M., & Keating, S. (2008). Transitional care. *American Journal of Nursing, 108*(9 supplement), 58–63.

North American Nursing Diagnosis Association International. (2009). *Nursing diagnoses: Definitions & classification 2009–2011.* Oxford, UK: Wiley-Blackwell.

Schneider, J., Barkauskas, V., & Keenan, G. (2008). Evaluating home health care nursing outcomes with OASIS and NOC. *Journal of Nursing Scholarship, 40*(1), 76–42.

Spotlight on home health nursing. (2007). *Nursing, 37*(12), 56–R2.

Stanhope, M., & Lancaster, J. (2006). Foundations of nursing in the community (2nd ed.). St. Louis: Mosby.

Taylor, E. J. (2008). Promoting spiritual health in home healthcare. *Home Healthcare Nurse 26*(6), 367–374.

Toofany, S. (2008). Hospital at home: A resurgence. *Primary Health Care, 18*(7), 20–23.

US Department of Health and Human Services (USDHHS), Administration on Aging (AOA). (2007). *Hospice care: A guide for families*. Retrieved from http://www.aoa.gov/press/prodsmats/fact/pdf/fs_hospice.pdf

US Department of Health and Human Services (USDHHS), Administration on Aging (AOA). (2008). *National family caregiver support program*. Retrieved from http://www.aoa.gov/prof/aoaprog/caregiver/caregiver.aspx

US Department of Health and Human Services (USDHHS), Centers for Medicare & Medicaid Services (CMS). (2007). *Medicare and home health care*. (Pub. No. CMS-10969). Baltimore, MD: CMS. Retrieved from http://www.medicare.gov/Publications/Pubs/pdf/10969.pdf

US Department of Health and Human Services (USDHHS), Centers for Medicare & Medicaid Services (CMS). (2008). *Medicare & You 2009*. (Pub. No. CMS-10050). Baltimore, MD: CMS. Retrieved from http://www.medicare.gov/Publications/Pubs/pdf/10050.pdf

Wilkinson, J. & Ahern, N. (2008). *Prentice Hall nursing diagnosis handbook with NIC interventions and NOC outcomes*, (9th ed.). Upper Saddle River, NJ: Prentice Hall.

Building Clinical Competence
Dimensions of Medical-Surgical Nursing

Functional Health Pattern: Health Perception-Health Management

Think about patients with altered health perception or health management for whom you have cared in your clinical experiences.

- What were the patient's major medical diagnoses (e.g. hypertension, diabetes mellitus, cancer, chronic obstructive pulmonary disease, stroke and alcoholism)?

- What kinds of manifestations did each of these patients have? Were these manifestations similar or very different?

- How did the patients' healthcare behaviors interfere with their health status? Did they have yearly physical examinations and routine eye examinations? Did they obtain recommended immunizations? Did they use preventative measures, such as breast self-examinations or testicular examinations, sunscreen, dietary changes, decreasing alcohol intake, stopping smoking, beginning exercising regularly, practicing safe sex, and using stress reduction activities? Did they achieve developmental tasks appropriate for their age? Did they interact well with family, friends, and coworkers?

The Health Perception-Health Management Functional Health Pattern include healthcare behaviors, such as health promotion and illness prevention activities, medical treatments, and follow-up care. Individuals are at different locations on the illness-wellness continuum at specific points in time. Health perception and health maintenance are affected by factors that influence the individual's health status or level of wellness in two primary ways:

- Factors affecting health that can be altered to possibly prevent disease processes are diet (e.g., osteoporosis), substance abuse (e.g., alcoholism), smoking (e.g., chronic obstructive pulmonary disease, lung cancer), socioeconomic status (e.g., communicable disease, violence or abuse) or occupational exposure (e.g., pulmonary disease due to asbestos, tuberculosis).

- Factors affecting health that cannot be altered and that may result in disease processes are genetics (e.g., sickle cell disease, hemophilia), age (e.g., type II diabetes mellitus, myocardial infarction), or race (e.g., hypertension).

A patient's perceived pattern of health and well-being affects how health is managed. Improper health management affects the body's ability to maintain itself, leading to manifestations such as the following:

- **Vomiting** (*unpleasant, wave-like sensations in the stomach with sweating and pulse rate changes result in sudden, forceful expulsion of stomach contents through the mouth*)

- **Bleeding** (*trauma, decreased platelets or deficient clotting factors result in the delay of or inability of the activation of the clotting pathway cause leakage of blood*)

- **Pain** (*swollen tissue, changes in pH and inflammatory changes cause tissue damage stimulate pain receptors transmit pain impulses to the brain*)

Priority nursing diagnoses within the health perception and health management functional health pattern that may be appropriate for patients include the following:

- *Health-Seeking Behaviors* as evidenced by dietary changes as prescribed, decreasing alcohol intake, stopping smoking, and joining a health club to participate in an exercise program.

- *Deficient Knowledge* as evidenced by lack of interest in learning about health care, inability to understand healthcare teaching (developmental level), and misinterpretation of healthcare teaching completed.

- *Ineffective Health Maintenance* as evidenced by smoking, drinking alcohol or other substance abuse, sedentary lifestyle, and not seeking routine health care.

- *Risk for Injury* as evidenced by poor hygiene habits, self treatment of illnesses, not taking prescribed medications, and participation in risk-seeking behaviors.

Two nursing diagnoses from other functional health patterns often are of high priority for the patient with deficits in health perception or health management:

- *Self-Care Deficit* (Activity-Exercise Functional Health Pattern)

- *Low Self-Esteem* (Self-Perception–Self-concept Functional health pattern)

Question

1. What questions will you ask your patients to determine his or her perceived pattern of health and well-being?

CLINICAL SCENARIO

Directions: *Read the following clinical scenario and answer the related questions. To complete this exercise successfully you will not only use knowledge of the content in this unit, but also principles related to setting priorities and maintaining patient safety.*

You have been assigned to work with the following home health care patients on the day shift. You receive a report at 0800. Significant data obtained during report is as follows:

- Mrs. Cora Swank, a 76-year-old female, had surgery 10 days ago for an obstructed colon that resulted in a permanent transverse colostomy. She was discharged from the acute care hospital yesterday. She lives with her 78-year-old husband. You need to evaluate her care of the colostomy and how well she can care for herself at home.
- Tom Smith is a 24-year-old who is at home due to osteomyelitis in the left leg from a previous leg fracture obtained when the motorcycle he was riding was involved in an accident. You need to change his left leg dressing and administer IV vancomycin (Vancocin) that is to be given every 12 hours. The next dose is due at 0930.
- Marguerite Garcia is an 86-year-old Hispanic who lives alone. She has hypertension, type II diabetes mellitus, and congestive heart failure. She is to have her blood pressure taken and a glucometer check for her blood sugar level. You will need to make sure she is taking her prescribed medications and set up her medications for the week.
- Sebastian Huian is a 56-year-old Asian who had a stroke which left him with left-sided weakness and some speech difficulties in addition to speaking little English. He smokes a half a pack of cigarettes daily. He is being discharged from the rehabilitation unit this morning. You will be doing an intake as the first home health visit to determine what his needs will be and how much assistance he will need from home health.

Questions

Priority Setting

1. What factors will you consider when deciding in which order you will visit these patients after report?
   A. _____
   B. _____
   C. _____

Health Promotion

1. An important part of primary prevention is to provide patient teaching related to the primary diagnosis. What primary prevention interventions will you talk to each patient about?
   A. _____
   B. _____
   C. _____
   D. _____

2. Tertiary level of prevention focuses on stopping the disease process and returning the affected patient to a useful place in society. Which is an example of a tertiary level of prevention for Mr. Huian?
   A. Eating a nutritious diet to promote healing and gain more strength.
   B. Having screenings for other disease processes, such as hypertension.
   C. Enrolling in a work training program for individuals with extremity weakness.
   D. Eliminating the use of smoking and alcohol.

Nursing Process

1. Besides obtaining vital signs, what diagnosis-specific assessment data should be collected for each patient?
   A. _____
   B. _____
   C. _____
   D. _____

2. Identify one nursing diagnoses for each of the patients presented earlier. What is the rationale for your choices?

	Nursing Diagnosis	Rationale
Cora Swank		
Tom Smith		
Marguerite Garcia		
Sebastian Huian		

3. Nursing interventions to ensure competent home care for Mr. Huian include which of the following? Select all that apply.
   A. Establish trust and rapport.
   B. Have his 14-year-old son translate for him.
   C. Assess the home environment for safety.
   D. Discuss having family members feed him due to his left arm weakness.
   E. Set goals for home health care and rehabilitation.

4. The nurse explains a diet of low sodium foods to Mrs. Garcia. What is the best way to evaluate Mrs. Garcia's understanding of the low sodium diet?

Communication

1. What information will you report to the next home health nurse who will be caring for Mr. Huian?

Delegation

1. What care or data collection for each patient can be delegated to a home health certified nursing assistant?

Nursing Ethics

1. During your initial visit to Tom Smith, he states, "When my leg is better, let's go dancing." How will you respond?

CASE STUDY: Betty Jo Moore

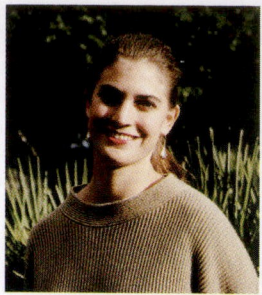

Betty Jo Moore is a 20-year-old who is admitted to the women's health unit for treatment of lower abdominal pain and tenderness, chills, and foul-smelling vaginal discharge. During the admission assessment she states that she is unmarried and has been sexually active for the past three years with multiple sexual partners. Vital signs are as follows: temperature 100.4°F, pulse 92, respirations 22, blood pressure 118/76. Lab studies drawn in the emergency department indicate a WBC count of 25,000 mm³, an erythrocyte sedimentation rate of 22mm/h, and a positive c-reactive protein. She is to begin IV antibiotic therapy and is in need of being educated about safe sex practices.

Ms. Moore is diagnosed with pelvic inflammatory disease. The pathophysiology of pelvic inflammatory disease (PID) is that pathogenic microorganisms enter the vagina during intercourse or other sexual activity and alter the cervical mucosa, allowing the microorganisms to travel to the uterus. The microorganisms can travel to the fallopian tubes and ovaries also. Multiplication of the microorganisms results in infection and possibly abscess formation. Manifestations of pelvic inflammatory disease include fever, chills, purulent vaginal discharge, vaginal bleeding, severe lower abdominal pain, pain on movement of the cervix, and dysuria. Complications that can occur from pelvic inflammatory disease are pelvic abscess, infertility, ectopic pregnancy, chronic pelvic pain, pelvic adhesions, and dyspareunia. Due to her medical diagnosis and history of unsafe sexual practices, the nursing diagnosis of Deficient Knowledge is appropriate for guiding nursing care.

BJM 20 y.o. female PID — affects →

- Pathogenic organisms enter the vagina through sexual activity
- Changes occur in the cervical mucosa, decreasing protection
- Microorganisms travel to the uterus, fallopian tubes, and ovaries
- Microorganisms multiply and invade mucous membranes, causing infection and abscesses

leads to

assess →

- States she has had unprotected sexual activity with multiple partners
- T 100.4 F
- Lower abdominal pain (8 on a scale of 1 to 10) on abdominal palpation
- Thick, odorous, green vaginal discharge

generates →

- Acute Pain related to inflammation as evidenced by statements of pain on abdominal palpation
- Ineffective Health Maintenance related to unprotected sexual activity with multiple partners as evidenced by pelvic infection
- Risk for Injury related to pelvic infection

generate nursing diagnosis

prioritized to

Deficient Knowledge: Safer Sex

expected outcomes

- Normal oral temperature
- Lab values within normal limits
- Takes total prescribed antibiotic dose
- Verbalize understanding of STIs
- Verbalize need for male partner to wear condom during sexual intercourse

evaluate →

- Temperature within normal range
- Lab values within normal ranges
- Completes entire dose of prescribed medications
- Verbalizes understanding of cause, effects, and treatment of STIs
- Demonstrates correct application of male condom

Interdisciplinary Interventions
- Monitor lab values on return to clinic.

Independent Interventions
- Instruct to call clinic if oral temperature is over 100° F.
- Explain rationale for taking all of prescribed antibiotic even when manifestations are gone.
- Teach cause, manifestations, complications, and treatment for PID caused by a sexually transmitted organism.
- Provide information about safer sex, including how to apply a male condom.

Activity:

1. After reviewing the concept map, go to the Pearson Nursing Student Resources for this book at www.nursing.pearsonhighered.com to write a concept map based on the nursing diagnosis *Risk-Prone Health Behavior* as evidenced by multiple sexual partners. See answers and hints in Appendix C.

Alterations in Patterns of Health

UNIT 2

Nursing Care of Patients Having Surgery

LEARNING OUTCOMES

1. Compare the differences and similarities between outpatient and inpatient surgery.
2. Identify the three phases of perioperative care.
3. Interpret the significance of diagnostic tests used in the perioperative period.
4. Explain nursing implications for medications prescribed for the surgical patient.
5. Identify variations in perioperative care for the older adult.
6. Describe principles of pain management specific to acute postoperative pain control.

CLINICAL COMPETENCIES

1. Assess the physiologic and psychosocial health status of patients for surgery to determine their ability to tolerate surgery and identify risks for complications.
2. Participate in patient and family teaching prior to anesthesia, during postoperative care, and prior to discharge from the facility.
3. Use appropriate communication techniques to minimize risks associated with handoffs among healthcare team members during transitions between phases of the perioperative experience.
4. Observe and participate as appropriate with nursing responsibilities and interventions to promote patient safety and integrity and to prevent hazards in the operating room.
5. Use the nursing process to provide safe and effective nursing care for the patient in the preoperative, intraoperative, and postoperative phases of surgery.

KEY TERMS

anesthesia, *64*
circulating nurse, *67*
conscious sedation, *65*
dehiscence, *79*
equianalgesia, *80*

evisceration, *79*
general anesthesia, *64*
informed consent, *55*
intraoperative phase, *54*
perioperative nursing, *54*

postoperative phase, *54*
preoperative phase, *54*
regional anesthesia, *64*
scrub person, *67*
surgery, *54*

Perioperative nursing is a specialized area of practice. It incorporates the three phases of the surgical experience: preoperative, intraoperative, and postoperative. The **preoperative phase** begins when the decision for surgery is made and ends when the patient is transferred to the operating room. The **intraoperative phase** begins with the patient's entry into the operating room and ends with admittance to the postanesthesia care unit (PACU), or recovery room. The **postoperative phase** begins with the patient's admittance to the PACU and ends with the patient's complete recovery from the surgical intervention. Although the perioperative nurse works in collaboration with other healthcare professionals to identify and meet the patient's needs, the perioperative nurse has the primary responsibility and accountability for nursing care of the patient undergoing surgery.

Surgery

Surgery is an invasive medical procedure performed to diagnose or treat illness, injury, or deformity. Although surgery is a medical treatment, the nurse assumes an active role in caring for the patient before, during, and after surgery. Interdisciplinary care and independent nursing care together prevent complications and promote the surgical patient's optimal recovery

Classification of Surgical Procedures

Surgical procedures can be classified according to purpose, risk, and urgency (see Table 4–1). Based on this information, nursing care can be individualized to best meet patient needs.

Settings for Surgery

Surgical patients may be inpatients or outpatients. The complexity of the surgery and recovery and the expected level of care needed upon completion of the surgery are the major differences. Cataract removal with or without lens implants, hernia repairs, tubal ligations, vasectomies, dilation and curettage (D&C), hemorrhoidectomies, diagnostic procedures, and biopsies are commonly performed as outpatient (same-day) surgeries.

Inpatient and outpatient surgeries are performed in the same operating suites in most hospitals. Outpatient surgery is also performed in freestanding surgical facilities and in physician's

TABLE 4–1 Classification of Surgical Procedures

	CLASSIFICATION	FUNCTION	EXAMPLES
Purpose	Diagnostic	Determine or confirm a diagnosis	Breast biopsy, bronchoscopy
	Ablative	Remove diseased tissue, organ, or extremity	Appendectomy, amputation
	Constructive	Build tissue/organs that are absent (congenital anomalies)	Repair of cleft palate
	Reconstructive	Rebuild tissue/organ that has been damaged	Skin graft after a burn, total joint replacement
	Palliative	Alleviate symptoms of a disease (not curative)	Bowel resection in patient with terminal cancer
	Transplant	Replace organs/tissue to restore function	Heart, lung, liver, kidney transplant
Risk	Minor	Minimal physical assault with minimal risk	Removal of skin lesions, dilation and curettage (D&C), cataract extraction
	Major	Extensive physical assault and/or serious risk	Transplant, total joint replacement, thoracotomy, colostomy, nephrectomy
Urgency	Elective	Suggested, though no foreseen ill effects if postponed	Cosmetic surgery, cataract surgery, bunionectomy
	Urgent	Necessary to be performed within 1 to 2 days	Heart bypass surgery, amputation resulting from gangrene, fractured hip
	Emergency	Performed immediately	Obstetric emergencies, bowel obstruction, ruptured aneurysm, life-threatening trauma

offices. The number of outpatient surgeries has grown rapidly in the past decade as part of the effort to contain the high costs of surgery. Moreover, increasingly complex surgeries on patients with complicated medical problems are now commonly performed on an outpatient basis. This increase in number of procedures and acuity level of the patients has presented a challenge to the perioperative nurse, the patient, and the family.

Outpatient surgery potentially offers several advantages:

- Decreased cost to the patient, hospital, and insuring agency
- Reduced risk of hospital-acquired infection
- Less interruption in the patient's and family's routine
- Possible reduction in time lost from work and/or other responsibilities
- Less physiologic stress to the patient and family

Many similarities exist between nursing care of inpatient and outpatient surgical patients. Physical care is provided in much the same manner in the preoperative, intraoperative, and postoperative phases of surgery. The major differences lie in the degree of teaching and emotional support that are necessary for outpatient surgical patients and their families. In addition to the physiologic insult of surgery, the outpatient surgical patient must cope with the additional stress of needing to learn a great deal of information in a short span of time. The nurse teaches the patient and family in both the preoperative and postoperative periods to enable the patient to perform self-care following discharge. More extensive teaching and emotional support is essential as patients requiring more complex surgical procedures and experiencing more complicated health problems undergo outpatient surgery.

PRACTICE ALERT

Patients having outpatient surgery should wear or bring clothing that will be easy to put on after surgery and will accommodate any dressings or appliances. Patients must also bring any medications, including herbal preparations, they regularly use.

Following outpatient surgery, the patient is discharged after meeting the institution's criteria, which are typically as follows:

- Vital signs are stable.
- Patient is able to stand and begin to walk without dizziness or nausea.
- Pain is controlled or alleviated.
- Patient is able to urinate.
- Patient is oriented.
- Patient and/or significant other demonstrates understanding of postoperative instructions.

Legal Requirements

It is the responsibility of the surgeon who performs the procedure to obtain the patient's consent for care. The surgeon should discuss the procedure with the patient and family in language they can understand. **Informed consent** is disclosure of risks associated with the intended procedure or operation to the patient, and is usually obtained by means of a legal document required for certain diagnostic procedures or therapeutic measures, including surgery. The language of the document varies according to statutory and common law of each state. This legal document protects the patient, nurse, physician, and healthcare facility. Informed consent includes the following information:

- Need for the procedure in relation to the diagnoses
- Description and purpose of the proposed procedure
- Possible benefits and potential risks
- Likelihood of a successful outcome
- Alternative treatments or procedures available
- Anticipated risks should the procedure not be performed
- Physician's advice as to what is needed
- Right to refuse treatment or withdraw consent

Ideally, the nurse should be present when the preceding information is provided. Later, the nurse can discuss the information with the patient and family, if necessary. If the patient has questions or concerns that were not discussed or made clear, or if the nurse questions the patient's understanding, the surgeon is responsible for supplying further information. If these situations arise, the nurse should contact the surgeon before having the patient sign a consent for the operation or special procedures. Following a thorough discussion of the consent, the nurse witnesses the patient's voluntary signature on the form (Figure 4–1 ■). The nurse also signs the form, indicating that the correct patient (or legal designee) is signing the form and that the patient was alert and aware of what was being signed.

Risk Factors

An independent national organization called the Institute for Healthcare Improvement (IHI) launched a campaign in 2004 to prevent an alleged 100,000 avoidable deaths in U.S. hospitals by 2006. Guided by these goals, hospitals implemented changes that spared more than 122,000 lives (Daniels, 2007). A 2006 initiative by IHI to further reduce medical harm was joined by a coalition of healthcare organizations called the Surgical Care Improve Project (SCIP). SCIP focuses on evidence-based interventions to reduce surgical complications including surgical site infections (SSIs), adverse cardiac events, and blood clots. Perioperative nursing should support and follow guidelines that will achieve these goals.

Prior to planning and implementing care for the surgical patient, the nurse must first assess the patient's needs and the factors that may increase the risks associated with surgery. The type of surgical procedure determines the assessment and interventions planned by the nurse. However, a complete assessment is also necessary to identify *risk factors* and to determine the patient's overall health status. Table 4–2 lists common risk factors for the patient undergoing surgery, and the related nursing interventions and implications. For example, when a patient is admitted for surgery on the right knee, it should be of concern to the nurse if this patient has diabetes, smokes 1.5 packs of cigarettes per day, has numbness in the right foot, and takes insulin. This information should be incorporated into a care plan, using appropriate nursing diagnoses and interventions to meet the patient's needs and assist the patient toward full postoperative recovery.

Risks are associated with all phases of surgery. For example, transporting the patient to and from the operating room (OR) requires assessment of the needs of the patient for supplemental oxygen, intravenous therapy, cardiac monitoring, and safety issues pertaining to the means of transport. Many patients enter the operating suite highly anxious and may benefit from medication to help them relax prior to administration of anesthesia. This can be discussed with the anesthetist. Chemicals, electrical equipment, and environmental hazards in the surgical area have the potential for harm and must be monitored and maintained carefully. Also read about risks for the older patient in the Nursing Care of the Older Adult box on page 69.

Patient and Procedure Identification

The 2009 Patient Safety Goals issued by the Joint Commission specifically address patient and procedure identification prior to any treatment or procedure. The patient must be actively involved in identification procedures, and if the patient is not able to participate or reliability is questioned, the family or designated caregiver is responsible for verifying identification. Hence any patient whose reliability is questionable must be accompanied by the caregiver into the surgical area for the "time out" procedure (AORN, 2010).

Unfortunately, there is a risk of performing the wrong surgery on the wrong patient: wrong site, wrong procedure, wrong person (Gibbs, 2005). In 2004, the Joint Commission issued the Universal Protocol (Box 4–1) mandating preoperatively (1) verifying the procedure, (2) physically marking and initialing the site, and (3) taking a "time out" before starting any procedure. A time out is an intentional stoppage of the preparation for the operation in the operating suite before the patient is anesthetized. The goal of the time out is to ensure the right procedure will be performed on the right patient on the correct site with the necessary and correct healthcare providers in attendance. All participants are introduced, including the patient, and encouraged to ask any questions or express any concerns before the surgery is commenced.

BOX 4–1 The Universal Protocol

The Universal Protocol to reduce surgical errors calls for three specific actions by the healthcare team:

1. *Conduct a pre-procedure verification process* when the procedure is scheduled, during pre-admission testing, on admission to the facility, before entering the procedure room, and whenever the patient is transferred to another caregiver during the procedure. This process includes verifying the availability of the following:
   - ✓ Relevant documents such as the history and physical, pre-anesthesia assessment
   - ✓ Accurate, complete, and signed procedure consent form
   - ✓ Correct and accurately labeled diagnostic test results including x-rays
   - ✓ Any required blood products, implants, devices, or special equipment
2. *Mark the procedure site* for any procedure that involves incisions, punctures, or insertion of instruments. The site is to be marked by the healthcare provider performing the procedure or by an individual who will be directly involved and present during the procedure and while the patient is awake.
3. *"Time out" before starting the procedure* to conduct a final verification that the correct patient, site, positioning, and procedure are identified, and that all relevant documents, information, and equipment are available.

M.R. # _____

Informed Consent to Operation, Administration of Anesthetics, and to the Rendering of Other Medical Services

Saint
Francis
Medical
Center

1. I do hereby authorize and direct _____ M.D./D.O./D.D.S., my physician, and/or such associates or assistants of his choice, to perform the following operation or procedure:

_____

_____

upon _____ (patient's name). I understand that the above named physician and his associates or assistants are employed by me and will be occupied solely with performing such operation or procedure.

2. The nature of the operation or procedure has been explained to me and no warranty or guarantee has been made as to result or cure. I have been advised that additional surgical and/or medical procedures or treatment may be deemed necessary during the course of the operation or procedure consented hereto, and I fully consent to such additional procedures and treatment which, in the opinion of my physician, are deemed necessary or desirable for the well-being of the patient. The possible risks and complications of the operation or procedure have been explained to me. The physician has explained to me the above medical terminology and I satisfactorily understand the type of operation/procedure.

3. I hereby authorize and direct the above named physician and/or his associates or assistants or those working under his direction to provide for _____ (patient's name) such additional services as he or they may deem reasonable and necessary, including, but not limited to, the administration and maintenance of anesthesia, blood or blood derivatives, and the performance of services involving pathology and radiology and I hereby consent thereto. The possible risks and complications of blood transfusions and the administration of anesthetics have also been explained to me.

4. I understand also that the persons in attendance at such operation or procedure for the purpose of administering anesthesia, and the radiologists in attendance at such operation or procedure for the purpose of performing radiological (X-ray) service are not the agents, servants, or employees of St. Francis Medical Center nor of any physician, but are independent healthcare providers who are employed by me in the same way that my surgeon and physician are employed by me.

5. I hereby authorize the Medical Center pathologist or personnel to use their discretion in the disposal of any severed tissue or member.

6. I hereby grant permission for St. Francis Medical Center to obtain clinical photographs for educational purposes or for my patient record as deemed necessary by my physician.

7. The **exception to this consent:** (If none, write "none".) _____
_____ and I assume full responsibility for these exceptions.

_____   _____
            PATIENT'S SIGNATURE   **DATE**

If the patient is a minor or incompetent or is unable to sign, the following must be completed:

I hereby certify that I am the (relationship) _____ of the above named patient

who is unable to sign because _____ ,

and I am fully authorized to give the consent herein granted.

_____   _____
            SIGNATURE   DATE

_____   _____
      WITNESSED BY/date   **WITNESSED BY/date**

If signed in the physician's office, the following   **MUST be completed by the Medical Center.**

_____   _____
  REVIEWED BY (patient name) **/date**   **WITNESSED BY /date**

Figure 4–1 ■ Informed consent form.

TABLE 4–2 Nursing Implications for Surgical Risk Factors

FACTOR	ASSOCIATED RISK	NURSING IMPLICATIONS
Adolescence	Diversity in age and physical, cognitive, and psychologic maturation makes preparation for surgery vary in content and inclusion of significant others. Increased need for control, privacy, and peer interaction poses special challenges in the acute care setting.	Adapt assessment and interventions to the development level of individual patients, involving them in preparation and care to the extent possible. Allow for regressive and independent behavior including rejection of adult support.
Advanced age	Older adults have age-related changes that affect physiologic, cognitive, and psychosocial responses to the stress of surgery; decreased tolerance of general anesthesia and postoperative medications; and delayed wound healing.	Selected nursing interventions are summarized in Table 4–6.
Malnutrition	Reserves may not be sufficient to allow the body to respond satisfactorily to the physical assault of surgery; organ failure and shock may result. Increased metabolic demands may result in poor wound healing and infection.	With the physician and dietitian, promote weight gain by providing a well-balanced diet high in calories, protein, and vitamin C. Administer parenteral nutrition, nutritional supplements, and enteral feedings as prescribed. Daily weights and calorie counts also may be ordered.
Obesity	The obese patient is at increased risk for delayed wound healing, wound dehiscence, infection, pneumonia, atelectasis, thrombophlebitis, dysrhythmias, and heart failure.	Promote weight reduction if time permits. Monitor closely for wound, pulmonary, and cardiovascular complications postoperatively. Encourage coughing, turning, and diaphragmatic breathing exercises and early ambulation.
Poverty	Because of limited access to health care, pathology may be more advanced at diagnosis. Greater risk of exposure to hazardous waste and emotional stress, poor nutrition, lack of exercise, and poor social support systems.	Assess for undiagnosed chronic conditions, assess nutritional status, and involve a social worker for help with resources. Unattended children may accompany the patient and need assistance.
Chronic Conditions		
Alcoholism	The patient may be malnourished and experience delirium tremens (acute withdrawal symptoms). More general anesthesia may be required. Hemorrhage and delayed wound healing can result from liver damage and poor nutritional status.	Monitor closely for signs of delirium tremens. Encourage well-balanced diet. Monitor for wound complications. Administer supplemental nutrients parenterally as ordered.
Arthritis	Inflammation or degenerative changes in joints limits mobility and comfort.	Position and pad arthritic joints including the spine. Handle joints gently to avoid strain on ligaments and tendons.
Cardiovascular disorders	Presence of cardiovascular disease increases the risk of heart failure, hemorrhage and shock, hypotension, venous thrombosis, pulmonary embolism, stroke (especially in the older patient), and fluid volume overload.	Diligently monitor vital signs, especially pulse rate, regularity, and rhythm, and general condition of the patient. Closely monitor fluid intake (oral and parenteral) to prevent circulatory overload. Assess skin color. Assess for chest pain, lung congestion, and peripheral edema. Observe for signs of hypoxia, and administer oxygen as ordered. Early postoperative ambulation and leg exercises reduce the risk of vascular problems, such as venous thrombosis and pulmonary embolism. Determine that prescribed beta-blockers are given preoperatively.
Diabetes mellitus	Diabetes causes an increased risk for fluctuating blood glucose levels, which can lead to life-threatening hypoglycemia or ketoacidosis. Diabetes also increases the risk for cardiovascular disease, delayed wound healing, and wound infection.	Monitor the patient closely for manifestations of hypoglycemia and hyperglycemia. Monitor blood glucose levels every 4 hours or as ordered. Administer insulin as prescribed. Encourage intake of food at the designated meal and snack times.
Immune suppression	Suppressed immunity impairs ability to resist infection and promote tissue repair. Advanced age, HIV, autoimmune diseases, chronic pain, immune deficiency diseases, malnutrition, splenectomy, and alcohol abuse compromise immunity.	Prevent hypothermia, maintain sterile fields, consistently prevent infection. Nourishment and normoglycemia promote wound healing.

TABLE 4–2 Nursing Implications for Surgical Risk Factors (continued)

FACTOR	ASSOCIATED RISK	NURSING IMPLICATIONS
Nicotine use	Cigarette smokers are at increased risk for respiratory complications such as pneumonia, atelectasis, and bronchitis because of increased mucous secretions and a decreased ability to expel them.	Ideally, the patient should quit smoking. Be supportive of the patient, and monitor closely for respiratory difficulties. Coughing, turning, and diaphragmatic breathing exercises with early ambulation are very important. Increase daily fluid intake to 2500–3000 mL (unless contraindicated) to help liquefy respiratory secretions to aid expectoration. A nicotine patch may help the patient tolerate withdrawal during the postoperative period.
Renal and liver disorders	The patient with renal or liver dysfunction may poorly tolerate general anesthesia, have fluid/electrolyte and acid–base imbalances, decreased metabolism and excretion of drugs, increased risk for hemorrhage, and delayed wound healing.	Monitor for fluid volume overload, intake and output (I&O), and response to medication. Evaluate closely for drug side effects and evidence of acidosis or alkalosis.
Respiratory disorders	Respiratory complications such as bronchitis, atelectasis, and pneumonia are some of the most common and serious postoperative complications. Respiratory depression from general anesthesia and acid–base imbalance may also occur. Patients with pulmonary disease are more at risk for developing these complications.	Closely monitor respirations, pulse, and breath sounds. Also assess for hypoxia, dyspnea, lung congestion, and chest pain. Encourage coughing, turning, and diaphragmatic breathing exercises and early postoperative ambulation. Encourage the patient to quit smoking or at least to reduce the number of cigarettes smoked.
Medical Therapies		
Medications	Anesthesia interaction with some medications can cause respiratory difficulties, hypotension, and circulatory collapse. Other medications can produce side effects that may increase surgical risk.	Inform the anesthesiologist of all prescribed and over-the-counter medications, as well as any herbal preparations.
Anticoagulants	May cause intraoperative and postoperative hemorrhage.	Monitor for bleeding. Assess PT/PTT values.
Antidepressants (particularly monoamine oxidase inhibitors)	Increase the hypotensive effects of anesthesia.	Closely monitor blood pressure.
Antihypertensives	Increase the hypotensive effects of anesthesia.	Closely monitor blood pressure.
Antibiotics (particularly the "mycin" group)	May cause apnea and respiratory paralysis.	Monitor respirations.
Diuretics	May lead to fluid and electrolyte imbalances, producing altered cardiovascular response and respiratory depression.	Monitor I&O and electrolytes. Assess cardiovascular and respiratory status.
Herbal supplements	Some may prolong the effects of anesthesia. Others may increase the risks of bleeding or raise blood pressure.	Inquire about the use of herbs or other dietary supplements. These should be discontinued at least 2 weeks before surgery.
Immunosuppressants	Steroids, drugs to treat cancer, and transplant rejection drugs suppress the immune system and increase the risk of infection and hypothermia (Neil, 2007).	Monitor CBC with differential for leukopenia. Document current dosage of medications and time of last dose. Administer prescribed steroids in the perioperative period to prevent adrenal crisis. Prevent hypothermia and maintain sterile fields. Monitor wound and protect from infection.
Treatments	Radiation therapy	Tissue integrity may be compromised in targeted fields.
In the OR		
Fluid/electrolyte imbalance	Depending on the degree of dehydration and/or the type of electrolyte imbalance, cardiac dysrhythmias or heart failure may occur. Liver and renal failure may also result.	Administer intravenous fluids as ordered. Monitor I&O. Monitor patient for evidence of electrolyte imbalance (∞ see Chapter 10).
Hypothermia/hyperthermia	Deviations from normothermia, either hypothermia or hyperthermia, may cause infection, cardiac morbidity, myocardial ischemia, surgical bleeding, skin damage, or patient discomfort.	Monitor core temperatures and prevent chilling or overheating. Remove wet drapes and test the temperature of fluids used.

(continued)

TABLE 4–2 Nursing Implications for Surgical Risk Factors (continued)

FACTOR	ASSOCIATED RISK	NURSING IMPLICATIONS
Surgical site infections	Contamination of sterile fields as well as opening body organs containing pathogens leads to infection.	Administer antibiotics prior to incision as ordered. Carefully maintain sterile fields. Monitor and sustain core body temperature between 36°C and 38°C.
Venous stasis	Lower limbs, especially when tourniquets are applied, are susceptible to blood clotting. Patients with cancer have higher risks of blood clots.	Promote venous circulation with intermittent pneumatic compression devices as ordered. Monitor circulation in arms and legs during surgery.

SAFETY ALERT

It is very important to establish the right and duty of all members of the surgical team to advocate for the safety of the patient. Important processes such as counting of sponges and equipment are time-consuming and may seem less important when urged by team members with less "power" (Jackson & Brady, 2008).

Retainment of Foreign Objects

Another potential error is retained foreign bodies such as instruments, needles, or sponges. To prevent accidental retention the American College of Surgeons recommends

- consistent application and adherence to standardized procedures for the counting of objects used in the surgery,
- methodical wound exploration before closing the site,
- using x-ray detectable materials in the wound,
- maintenance of optimal OR environments to allow focused surgical performance (minimizing distractions such as change of personnel, telephone calls, beepers, and pages),
- employing technological methods to ensure no unintended item remains, and
- suspension of these measures as needed in life-threatening situations (Gibbs, 2005; Jackson & Brady, 2008).

While not all surgeries have equal risk for retainment of items, those that do must include a careful count procedure with appropriate action if the count is incorrect. Stopping a closing procedure to recount and search for missing items increases anesthesia and wound exposure, but leaving items contributes to serious infections and other potential liabilities (Jackson & Brady, 2008).

Medication Reconciliation

A complete history of medications the patient has been taking regularly is vital information at every transition point in the care continuum. Over-the-counter medicines and herbal preparations as well as prescription medications may interact with drugs given during surgery, putting a patient at increased risk (Saber, 2006). As part of the preoperative planning and teaching, early consideration of all medications including complementary and alternative medicine is important. This information should be obtained in a matter-of-fact and nonjudgmental manner, because a judgmental attitude could cause the patient to withhold information. This process needs to be repeated at every transition: admission to the hospital, preoperatively, in postoperative reports, and at discharge.

Medications may interact with anesthesia drugs during surgery, augmenting hemodynamic effects such as hypertension or hypotension. Some categories of medication require special consideration in regard to surgery (Saber, 2006). These include drugs that alter blood clotting, replace adrenal hormones, prevent seizures, antiparkinsonian drugs, antipsychotics, anxiolytics, bronchodilators, cardiovascular drugs, glaucoma drugs, immunosuppressants, and thyroid or antithyroid drugs. Patients with diabetes or HIV infection who are being treated with antivirals require expert advice (Rahman & Beattie, 2008).

Anticoagulant medications should be discontinued prior to surgery to prevent excessive blood loss during surgery. These include aspirin and nonsteroidal anti-inflammatory drugs. If laboratory tests of bleeding time, prothrombin time (PT), partial thromboplastin time (PTT), and international normalized ratio (INR) are elevated, the surgery may be cancelled. Guidelines for discontinuing use vary according to the particular medication; it is generally recommended that aspirin or products containing aspirin be discontinued 5 days or longer before surgery. Similarly, herbs or nutritional supplements that impair clotting should be discontinued 2 weeks prior to surgery (Saper, 2005). The most common self-prescribed medicines that may inhibit coagulation are vitamin E, garlic, ginkgo, ginseng, fish oil, and chamomile. Many plants contain coumarins with the potential to interact with warfarin and inhibit coagulation. Others inhibit platelet aggregation or prevent the conversion of fibrinogen to fibrin. Patients taking warfarin for the risk of blood clots due to atrial fibrillation will be counseled about the appropriate time to withdraw warfarin. If surgery is urgent due to trauma or sudden onset of morbidity, the impact of anticoagulants needs to be evaluated with PT, PTT, and INR before the operation and appropriate support for clotting administered.

In addition to clotting impairment, excessive consumption of herbal medicines or dietary supplements can produce levels of chemicals that interact with conventional medications, exacerbating or impairing the intended effect. Anesthesia drugs often decrease hepatic blood flow and interfere with metabolism and elimination of medications (Bressler, 2005). This increases the risk of adverse drug–herbal supplement interactions during surgery. Cardiovascular instability, impaired glucose control, increased metabolism of perioperative medication, and unpredictable response to anesthesia are categories of adverse reactions of perioperative herbal use (Saper, 2005).

Thromboembolism

The risk of bleeding has to be balanced against the risk of postoperative deep venous thrombosis (DVT) and thromboembolism. Prophylactic anticoagulation with low-dose unfractionated heparin, low-molecular-weight heparin, factor Xa, or warfarin may be used for this purpose. Aspirin-only therapy is not considered adequate protection from DVT formation (Daniels, 2007). In addition, use of intermittent pneumatic compression devices (IPCDs) and graduated compression stockings is recommended. DVTs can lead to pulmonary embolism (PE) and to significant patient morbidity, mortality, and increased healthcare cost. Each patient's risk for developing DVT and PE needs to be assessed and appropriate prophylaxis initiated when indicated.

Hypothermia

Hypothermia is a risk in the perioperative period. The anesthetized patient loses heat intraoperatively and is unable to restore temperature through the normal mechanisms of shivering or muscle contractions. Typically, surgical suites are maintained quite cold for the comfort of the personnel gowned in several layers of protective clothing and wearing masks. Lowering environmental temperature is common in surgical suites, but research shows that normothermia (core body temperature in the range of 36.0°C to 37.5°C [Porth, 2007]) in the patient provides less risk to the patient for infection, cardiac morbidity, myocardial ischemia, surgical bleeding, and patient discomfort. Methods to minimize the risk of hypothermia include applying warm blankets, limiting the amount of skin exposed, warming intravenous fluids, and monitoring the patient's temperature.

Hyperthermia should also be avoided. Heating of fluids or use of heating units necessitates accurate measurement of the temperature and assessment of the patient's skin integrity. Body temperature is best evaluated through core temperature monitoring, which includes esophageal or tympanic assessment (AORN, 2010; Weirich, 2008).

Surgical Site Infections (SSIs)

Despite the carefully clean OR environment and use of sterile equipment, gloves, and gowns, a significant percentage of patients develop wound infections. Patients suffer increased morbidity and mortality, and healthcare costs increase dramatically as a result of SSIs. Four strategies are recommended by SCIP guidelines: prophylactic antibiotics in select procedures, appropriate hair removal, glucose control in patients having major cardiac surgery, and normothermia in patients undergoing colon surgery. Prophylactic antibiotic administration immediately before the surgical incision is indicated for hip and knee arthroplasty, cardiac surgery including coronary artery bypass graft, hysterectomy, and some colon and vascular procedures (Daniels, 2007).

Adverse Cardiac Events

Myocardial infarction is a risk following major surgery, especially among elderly patients. The circulatory system is stressed during surgery, increasing the risk for cardiac ischemia. Beta-blocker medications slow nerve conduction to the myocardium and reduce oxygen demand, thereby reducing the risk for infarction. Any patient who is taking beta-blocker medication regularly needs to take the usual dose prior to any type of surgery.

Interpreting and responding to identified risk factors require nursing judgment. It is important to bring information to the attention of the surgeons and anesthesiologists prior to surgery so necessary modifications can be made for the patient.

Interdisciplinary Care

The patient undergoing surgery receives care from a number of healthcare providers. Surgeons, nurses, scrub technicians, anesthetists, phlebotomists, x-ray technicians, registration clerks, and transporters are often involved in securing the safety and health of patients. Case managers, social workers, and spiritual care providers are available based on patient need and desire. This interdisciplinary approach focuses on placing the patient in the best possible health status before, during, and after surgery.

Diagnostic Tests

Diagnostic tests performed prior to surgery provide baseline data or reveal problems that may place the patient at additional risk during and after surgery. Because of the trend toward shortened hospital stays, many diagnostic studies and procedures are performed in a preadmission clinic within a week prior to elective surgery.

Complete blood counts, electrolyte studies, coagulation studies, and urinalysis are the most commonly performed preoperative laboratory tests. Table 4–3 discusses the significance and nursing implications of abnormal findings for these common tests. Additional diagnostic tests may be performed as the history and physical findings indicate. For example, if the patient has a low hemoglobin and hematocrit, and significant blood loss during surgery is anticipated, the surgeon may order a type and crossmatch of the patient's blood for a possible transfusion.

In addition to laboratory tests, older patients or those with risk factors related to heart and lung function typically have a chest x-ray. This radiologic procedure provides baseline information about the size, shape, and condition of the heart and lungs. Pulmonary complications such as lung disease, tuberculosis, calcification, infiltration, or pneumonia may require that surgery be postponed to allow the patient to undergo further evaluation or treatment. If findings are abnormal and the surgery cannot be postponed, information from the chest x-ray study can be used to determine the safest form of anesthesia.

Another commonly performed preoperative diagnostic procedure is the electrocardiogram (ECG). This test is ordered routinely on patients undergoing general anesthesia when they are over 40 years of age or have cardiovascular disease. The ECG provides data for evaluation about either new or preexisting cardiac conditions. The patient's surgery may be cancelled or postponed if a life-threatening cardiac condition is discovered.

In addition to the chest x-ray study and ECG, other diagnostic tests may be performed preoperatively to gather further assessment data. For example, for patients who have chronic

TABLE 4–3 Laboratory Tests for Perioperative Assessment

TEST	SIGNIFICANCE OF INCREASED VALUES	SIGNIFICANCE OF DECREASED VALUES	NURSING IMPLICATIONS
Hemoglobin (Hgb) and hematocrit (Hct)	Dehydration, excessive fluid plasma loss, polycythemia vera	Fluid overload, excessive blood loss, anemia	Monitor oxygenation, and vital signs; assess for bleeding.
Glucose and hemoglobin-A1c	Impaired glucose metabolism, stress, or infection	Inadequate glucose intake in relation to insulin	If decreased, monitor for manifestations of hypoglycemia. Notify surgeon of glucose <70 mg/dL or >180 mg/dL.
White blood cell (WBC) count	Infectious/inflammatory processes, leukemia	Immune deficiencies	Monitor for manifestations of inflammation; monitor drainage, temperature, and pulse. Use strict standard precautions.
Platelet count	Malignancies, polycythemia vera	Clotting deficiency disorders, chemotherapy	If decreased, assess for bleeding at incision sites and drainage tubes, and assess for hematomas.
Carbon dioxide (CO_2)	Emphysema, chronic bronchitis, asthma, pneumonia, respiratory acidosis, vomiting, nasogastric suctioning	Metabolic acidosis, hyperventilation	Monitor respiratory status and arterial blood gases (ABGs).
Electrolytes			
Potassium (K^+)	Kidney dysfunction, dehydration, suctioning	Side effects of diuretics, vomiting, NG suctioning	Monitor K^+ level, cardiac and neurologic function, and preoperative diuretic therapy.
Sodium (Na^+)	Kidney dysfunction, dehydration, normal saline-containing intravenous fluids	Side effects of diuretics, vomiting, NG suctioning, fluid volume excess	Monitor Na^+ level and I&O; assess for peripheral edema and effects of perioperative diuretic therapy.
Chloride (Cl^-)	Kidney dysfunction, dehydration, alkalosis	Side effects of diuretics, vomiting, NG suctioning	Monitor Cl^- level and I&O; assess for peripheral edema and perioperative diuretic therapy.
Prothrombin time (protime, or PT) and partial thromboplastin time (PTT)	Defect in mechanism for blood clotting, anticoagulant therapy (aspirin, heparin, warfarin), side effect of other drugs affecting clotting time	Hypercoagulability of the blood may lead to thrombus formation in the veins	If clotting time is elevated, monitor PT/PTT values. Assess for bleeding at incision site and drainage tubes and for hematomas. If clotting time is decreased, monitor for thrombus formation (pulmonary emboli, venous thrombosis), and evaluate PT and PTT values.
Urinalysis	Varied	Varied	Used to detect abnormal substances (e.g., protein, glucose, red blood cells, or bacteria) in the urine. Notify surgeon if abnormalities are detected.
Serum creatinine, BUN	Renal dysfunction	Malnutrition, musculoskeletal wasting	Monitor urinary output, wound healing.

obstructive pulmonary disease, pulmonary function studies often are performed to determine the extent of respiratory dysfunction. This information guides the anesthesiologist before and during surgery in choosing the type of anesthetic to be used, and it guides the surgeon and nursing staff in the recovery phase.

Renal function is evaluated on the basis of glomerular filtration rate (GFR) which is estimated by using serum creatinine (reported as the eGFR) or by measuring urinary creatine. Creatinine is a stable product of muscle mass; it is filtered by the kidneys or secreted by the kidney tubules. In kidney failure, serum creatinine rises and the GFR is low. The best indicator of GFR is the creatinine clearance, a comparison of both serum and urinary creatinine levels. In older adults with decreased

muscle mass and low dietary meat intake, serum creatinine may be falsely low. Older adults are especially susceptible to renal insufficiency, which puts them at risk for fluid volume overload in the perioperative period and for accumulation of metabolic by-products and medications dependent on renal clearance (Loran et al., 2005; Giannelli, 2007).

Medications

The patient having surgery receives medications before, during, and after surgery to achieve specific therapeutic outcomes. Traditionally, all medication orders are cancelled when the patient goes to surgery and must be rewritten by the physician when the patient returns to the postsurgical care unit. Following surgery it

CHAPTER 4 / Nursing Care of Patients Having Surgery **63**

is very important that medications are re-ordered so that chronic as well as acute conditions will be treated.

PREOPERATIVE MEDICATIONS A combination of preoperative drugs may be ordered to achieve a multitude of desired outcomes with minimal side effects. Such outcomes include sedation, reducing anxiety, inducing amnesia to minimize unpleasant surgical memories, increasing comfort during preoperative procedures, reducing gastric acidity and volume, increasing gastric emptying, decreasing nausea and vomiting, and reducing the incidence of aspiration by drying oral and respiratory secretions.

The surgical patient usually is given preoperative medications 45 to 70 minutes before the scheduled surgery. Any delay in administration should be reported promptly to the surgical department. Preoperative medications are often given in the surgical holding area.

TABLE 4–4 Examples of Commonly Used Preoperative Medications

GENERIC	TRADE	ACTION BY CATEGORY	NURSING IMPLICATIONS
Antibiotics			
Cefazolin	Ancef	Prevents surgical site infections in orthopedic and general surgeries and is associated with lower risk of mortality in elderly patients	Patients with beta-lactam allergies receive vancomycin or clindamycin.
Benzodiazepines			
Midazolam	Versed	Decreases anxiety and produces sedation to some extent	Monitor for respiratory depression, hypotension, drowsiness, and lack of coordination.
Diazepam	Valium	Induces amnesia	
Lorazepam	Ativan	May induce substantial amnesia	
Opioid Analgesics			
Morphine	Morphine	Decreases anxiety, provides analgesia	Monitor for respiratory depression and safety if ambulating. ∞ See Chapter 9 for nursing implications of specific opioid analgesics.
Fentanyl	Sublimaze	Allows reduced anesthetic dose	
Oxycodone	Roxicodone		
Hydrocodone	Vicodin		
Tramadol	Ultram		
Codeine	Tylenol with Codeine		
Antacids			
Sodium citrate	Bicitra	Increases the pH and reduces volume of gastric fluid; used in patients with GERD and/or trauma	No significant factors in this setting.
H$_2$ Receptor Antagonists			
Cimetidine	Tagamet	Reduces gastric acid volume and concentration	Monitor for confusion and dizziness in older adults.
Famotidine	Pepcid		
Nizatidine	Axid		
Ranitidine	Zantac		
Gastric Acid (Proton) Pump Inhibitors			
Lansoprazole	Prevacid	Suppresses gastric acid secretion	Monitor for dizziness and headache, rash, or thirst.
Omeprazole	Prilosec		
Pantoprazole	Protonix		
Antiemetics			
Metoclopramide	Reglan	Enhances gastric emptying	Monitor for sedation and extrapyramidal symptoms (involuntary movement, muscle tone changes, and abnormal posture).
Droperidol	Inapsine	Tranquilizer	
Anticholinergics			
Atropine sulfate	Atropine sulfate	Reduces oral and respiratory secretions to decrease risk of aspiration; decreases vomiting and laryngospasm	Monitor for confusion, restlessness, and tachycardia. Prepare patient to expect a dry mouth.
Glycopyrrolate	Robinul		
Scopolamine	Scopolamine		

Preoperative antibiotic prophylaxis is effective in the prevention of postoperative complications in many surgeries (Andersen et al., 2005; Daniels, 2007). Table 4–4 outlines commonly prescribed preoperative medications.

An increasingly common and controversial strategy to prevent intense or lingering pain is the use of *preemptive analgesia* (D'Arcy, 2008). The goal of preemptive analgesia is to prevent sensitization of the central and peripheral nervous system from painful stimuli by blocking the pain pathways with local, regional, or epidural analgesia prior to incision. Sensitization to pain is believed to prolong the painful experience; blocking the sensitization throughout the perioperative period should result in decreased pain in the postoperative period, shortened hospital stay, quicker return to self-care, and decreased residual pain (Polomano et al., 2008; Ong et al., 2005). To date, the best combination of methods and medications for the great variety of surgical interventions has not been identified. The best method to improve postoperative pain scores, reduce total analgesic consumption, and extend the time to first rescue dose following anesthesia seems to be a combination of epidural, local wound infiltration, and nonsteroidal anti-inflammatory drugs (NSAIDs). Opioids given preoperatively do not enhance comfort in the postoperative period (Ong et al, 2005).

Decisions about which of the patient's routine medications to administer prior to surgery when the patient is NPO require careful analysis. The best guideline is to confer with the surgeon and anesthetist about specific medications. The reason for caution has to do with potential interactions between anesthesia and medications and the effect on the patient if drugs such as steroids, antiseizure medications, and tranquilizers are discontinued abruptly. Generally, insulin is withheld when the patient is NPO, but depending on the anticipated length of the surgery, the dosage may be adjusted for the previous evening as well as the morning of surgery. Under anesthesia the manifestations of hypoglycemia (insulin reaction) are absent, so withholding insulin the morning of surgery when the patient is NPO is advisable. Plasma glucose is monitored intermittently during surgery with the goal of maintaining normal blood sugar level (see Table 4–2). Patients who ordinarily manage their diabetes mellitus with oral medications often are placed on sliding scale insulin to manage blood glucose during the perioperative experience. Evidence-based practice supports subcutaneous basal insulin administration for hyperglycemic patients to maintain glycemia below 180 mg/dL throughout the perioperative period. This practice is associated with better healing, fewer infections, and shorter hospital stays (Odom-Forren, 2006).

INTRAOPERATIVE MEDICATIONS **Anesthesia** is used to produce unconsciousness, analgesia, reflex loss, and muscle relaxation during a surgical procedure. **General anesthesia** produces all of these effects, whereas **regional anesthesia** results in analgesia, reflex loss, and muscle relaxation but does not cause the patient to lose consciousness. An anesthesiologist (physician) or certified registered nurse anesthetist (CRNA) administers anesthetics during the intraoperative phase of surgery.

General Anesthesia General anesthesia is most commonly administered by inhalation and, to a lesser extent, by the intravenous route. It produces central nervous system depression. As a result, the patient loses consciousness and does not perceive pain, the skeletal muscles relax, and reflexes diminish.

Advantages to general anesthesia include rapid excretion of the anesthetic agent and prompt reversal of its effects when desired. Additionally, general anesthesia can be used with all age groups and any type of surgical procedure. It produces amnesia.

Disadvantages of general anesthesia include risks associated with circulatory, respiratory, hepatic, and renal side effects. Patients with serious respiratory or circulatory diseases, such as emphysema or congestive heart failure, are at greater risk for complications. Patients with renal or hepatic disease cannot metabolize and eliminate anesthetics safely. Inhalation agents are avoided in patients with a history of malignant hyperthermia (MH) because they can trigger MH (Box 4–1). With the increase in ambulatory and minimally invasive surgeries, anesthetics are used that enable shorter recovery phases. Drugs with a very short half-life have a rapid recovery phase, allowing *fast-tracking*, often bypassing the post anesthesia care unit (PACU) (Hassan & Fahy, 2005).

The phases of general anesthesia are divided into three distinct categories: induction, maintenance, and emergence. During the induction phase, the patient receives the anesthetic agent intravenously or by inhalation. During this phase, airway

BOX 4–2 Malignant Hyperthermia (MH)

Malignant hyperthermia (MH) is a rare autosomal dominant disorder that can be triggered by inhalational anesthetic gases and succinylcholine, a depolarizing neuromuscular blocker. The initial manifestations are an unexplained rise in end-tidal carbon dioxide that does not respond to ventilation and sustained skeletal muscle contraction (Carter-Templeton, 2005). The temperature rises rapidly to as high as 43°C as result of sustained hypermetabolism. Cardiac dysrhythmias develop and oxygen and ATP are rapidly consumed. Lactate and carbon dioxide, byproducts of metabolism, are produced in excess (Porth & Matfin, 2009). If unchecked the condition will progress to hyperkalemia, myoglobinuria, disseminated intravascular coagulation, congestive heart failure, bowel ischemia, and compartment syndrome in the limbs.

MH can develop during surgery or when the patient returns to the PACU. If the early symptoms of MH (e.g., escalating temperature, increased carbon dioxide production) are identified, suspected triggering agents are immediately discontinued. Oxygen is immediately administered with a nonrebreather mask. The patient should not be unattended, good IV access should be maintained, and the anesthesia provider should be summoned. Dantrolene, a muscle relaxant, is administered and measures to decrease core body temperature should be started at once and continued until core temperature is 36.0°C. A urinary catheter should be placed to monitor urine output and blood drawn for testing. Blood gases should be drawn to measure pH; sodium bicarbonate is given to correct metabolic acidosis. Insulin may be ordered to decrease serum potassium. This patient may be transferred to the ICU for continued monitoring and doses of dantrolene every 4–6 hours.

patency is achieved and maintained with either endotracheal intubation or newer devices including the laryngeal mask airway (LMA) esophageal-tracheal Combitube, or lighted stylet or wand (Hassan & Fahy, 2005). These newer methods of airway maintenance do not require direct visualization of the vocal cords for placement. They allow effective ventilation and can prevent the need for surgical tracheostomy in patients who are difficult to intubate.

The next phase of general anesthesia is maintenance. During this period, the patient is positioned, the skin is prepared, and surgery is performed. The anesthesiologist maintains the proper depth of anesthesia while constantly monitoring physiologic parameters such as heart rate, blood pressure, respiratory rate, temperature, and oxygen and carbon dioxide levels.

The final phase of anesthesia is the patient's emergence from this altered physiologic state. As the anesthetic agents are withdrawn or the effects reversed pharmacologically, the patient begins to awaken. The endotracheal tube or laryngeal mask is removed (extubated) once the patient is able to reestablish voluntary breathing. It is critical to ensure airway patency during this period, because extubation may cause bronchospasm or laryngospasm.

Regional Anesthesia   Regional anesthesia is a type of anesthesia in which medication instilled around the nerves blocks transmission of nerve impulses in a particular area. Regional anesthesia produces analgesia, relaxation, and reduced reflexes. The patient is awake and conscious during the surgical procedure but does not perceive pain. Regional anesthesia may be classified in several ways:

- Local nerve infiltration is achieved by injecting lidocaine, bupivacaine, or tetracaine around a local nerve to suppress sensation over a limited area of the body. This technique may be used when a skin or muscle biopsy is obtained or when a small wound is sutured.
- Nerve blocks are accomplished by injecting an anesthetic agent at the nerve trunk to produce a lack of sensation over a specific larger area, such as an extremity.
- Epidural blocks are local anesthetic agents injected into the epidural space, outside the dura mater of the spinal cord. This type of intraspinal anesthesia provides safe and effective pain relief for patients of all ages with less risk of adverse effects than general anesthesia. It is indicated for surgeries of the arms and shoulders, thorax, abdomen, pelvis, and lower extremities (Schwartz, 2006). The epidural catheter is often left in place for pain relief in the postoperative period; it can also be used for chronic pain management.

Spinal anesthesia is administered similarly to epidural except the anesthetic medication is infused in a single injection. Spinal anesthesia is effective for approximately 90 minutes. Surgeries of the lower abdomen, perineum, and lower extremities are likely to use this type of regional anesthesia. Leakage of cerebrospinal fluid (CSF) into the epidural space can cause reduced CSF pressure and postoperative headaches. Treatment may include hydration, caffeine, analgesics, or administration of an epidural blood patch (Schwartz, 2006). Hypotension is common with epidural and spinal anesthesia. Blood pressure should be monitored and, if critical hypotension occurs, the anesthesia provider should be alerted and expected to increase intravenous fluids and administer vasoactive medications.

Conscious Sedation   An increasing number of surgical and diagnostic procedures are being performed using **conscious sedation**. This type of anesthesia provides analgesia, amnesia, and moderate sedation. The pharmacologic effects are produced by administering a combination of intravenous medications with opioids (such as morphine sulfate or fentanyl [Sublimaze]) or sedatives (such as diazepam [Valium] and midazolam [Versed]). During conscious sedation the patient is able to independently maintain an open airway. This allows the patient to respond to verbal and physical stimulation. Physician supervision is always required and a registered nurse must be prepared to initiate rescue if sedation becomes too deep. Institutions base their policies defining the qualifications of those who care for patients undergoing conscious sedation on professional organization guidelines, regulatory agency requirements, and state law.

Assessment prior to conscious sedation includes evaluating the appropriateness of the patient based on physical status. Patients with compromised circulation or airway, a history of sleep apnea or snoring, a history of problems with anesthesia or analgesia, or medications that would potentially interact with conscious analgesia medications may require the anesthesiologist to manage conscious sedation procedures. Patients need to be appropriately fasting, and baseline vital signs must be taken prior to giving the sedative. A consent form must be signed by the patient, and a patent IV line must be in place. Equipment to rescue the patient should be available if sedation becomes too deep. Oxygen saturation, pulse, breathing, and level of consciousness must be monitored throughout the procedure.

Common adverse side effects include venous thrombosis, phlebitis, local irritation, confusion, drowsiness, hypotension, and apnea. Reversal agents (naloxone hydrochloride [Narcan] and flumazenil [Romazicon]) are used as needed to enhance the safety of conscious sedation.

POSTOPERATIVE MEDICATIONS   Management of acute postoperative pain by medication improves with greater understanding of pain physiology and the development of better methods to deliver adequate pain medication. For more information on pain management, ∞ see Chapter 9.

Established, persistent, severe pain is more difficult to treat than pain that is at its onset. Therefore, postoperative analgesics should be administered at regular intervals around the clock (ATC) to maintain a therapeutic blood level. Administering analgesics as needed (prn) lowers this therapeutic level; delays in medication administration further increase pain intensity. Therefore, prn administration of analgesics is not recommended in the first 36 to 48 hours postoperatively. Patients using patient-controlled analgesia (PCA) or patient-controlled epidural analgesia (PCEA) in the postoperative period need to be taught the importance of using the allowed dosages regularly to prevent increasing pain levels.

In the immediate postoperative period, older adult patients benefit from the same protocol for morphine titration as do younger patients. Intravenous morphine may be initiated at a slightly reduced dose and then titrated to the same protocol as for younger patients. Morphine-related adverse effects such as nausea, vomiting, respiratory depression, constipation, urinary retention, pruritus, and allergy or sedation are similar among varying age groups. However, older adult patients require fewer opioids than younger patients in the later postoperative period. PCEA may be more effective for older adult patients and is associated with earlier improved mental status and bowel activity (Loran et al., 2005).

> **PRACTICE ALERT**
> Nurses are responsible for assessing patients' pain level and administering pain medication. They must work collaboratively with surgeons to schedule postoperative analgesics rather than rely on prn administration orders.

NSAIDs treat mild to moderate postoperative pain. This category of drugs should be given soon after surgery (orally, parenterally, or rectally) along with opioids unless contraindicated. Although NSAIDs may not be sufficient to control pain completely, they allow lower doses of opioid analgesics and therefore fewer side effects. NSAIDs can be given safely to older patients, but they should be observed closely for side effects, particularly gastric and renal toxicity.

Opioid analgesics, such as morphine, are considered the foundation for managing moderate to severe postoperative pain. Opioid dosage requirements vary greatly from one patient to another, so the dosage must be individually tailored. Later in the postoperative recovery period, opioid analgesics (oral or parenteral) may be given prn. In this way, pain relief can be maintained, while the potential for drug side effects is decreased.

Contrary to the belief of many healthcare providers (including nurses), physical dependence and tolerance to opioid analgesics is extremely uncommon in short-term postoperative use. Additionally, opioid analgesics, when used to treat acute pain, rarely lead to psychologic dependence and addiction. According to the World Health Organization pain ladder, acute pain is appropriately treated with opioids, tapering to acetaminophen as healing progresses. Chronic pain, in contrast, is treated with analgesics that increase from acetaminophen to opioids as tolerance develops or the condition worsens.

Analgesic options continue to develop, especially methods of delivery. Relatively new is the Q-ball, which provides wound infiltration with analgesia. Using combinations of analgesics and simultaneous methods of delivery, the patient can appreciate better pain control and experience fewer analgesic gaps (periods of ineffective pain control). Among the newest methods to achieve control are transdermal fentanyl by iontophoresis and extended-release epidural morphine. Iontophoresis is the delivery of "charged molecules across intact skin using a small electric current" (Polomano et al., 2008, p. S48). By providing combinations of opioids via multiple routes preemptively as well as intraopertively and postoperatively, the doses of each can be reduced and pain control enhanced.

Older patients tend to be more sensitive to the analgesic effects of opioids, experiencing a higher peak effect with a longer duration of pain control. The Moving Evidence into Action box on page 67 provides additional information.

> **PRACTICE ALERT**
> Oral analgesia requires a significantly greater dose than parenteral for most analgesics. Teach patients who are being discharged and their caregivers the relative strength of oral analgesics. (Caution them to not rely on trade names to gauge effectiveness.) Two acetaminophen with codeine (30 mg) is *equianalgesia* to 10 mg parenteral morphine; however, oral meperidine 100 mg does not provide equianalgesia with 10 mg parenteral morphine. (∞ See Chapter 9 for details about equianalgesia.)

Surgical Environment

MEMBERS OF THE SURGICAL TEAM Because of the complexity of the intraoperative environment, members of the surgical team must function as a coordinated unit. The surgeon, surgical assistant(s), anesthesiologist or CRNA, circulating nurse, and scrub person or operating room technician (Figure 4–2 ■) constitute the surgical team. Each member provides specialized skills and is essential to the successful outcome of the surgery. Risks to members of the surgical team

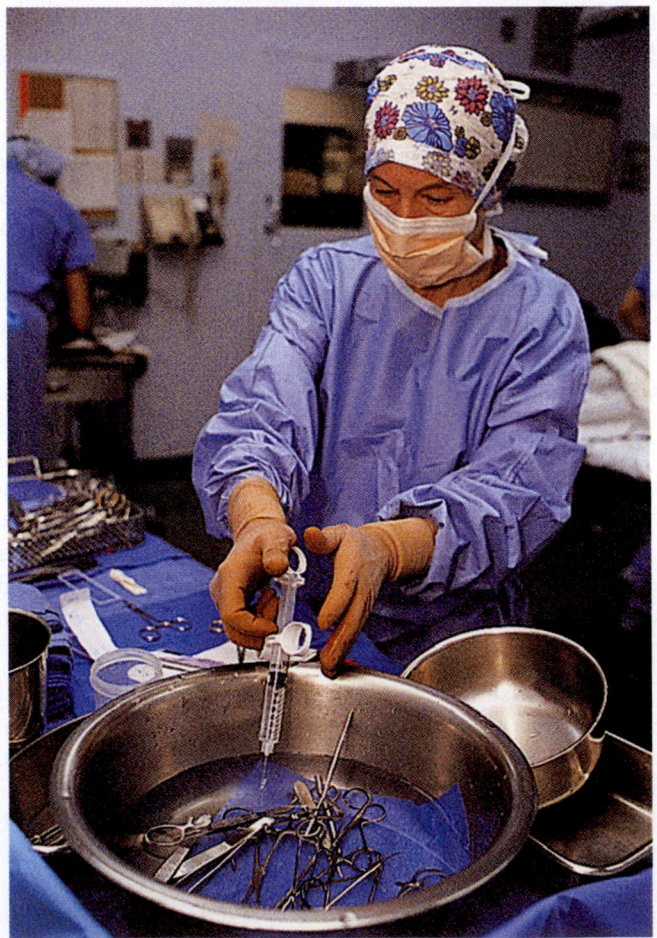

Figure 4–2 ■ A scrub nurse in the operating room.

Assisting Older Adults to Communicate Postoperative Pain

Pain is a subjective experience. Nurses rely heavily on patients' assessments of the pain they are experiencing. Rating of pain intensity by the patient is the gold standard for knowing when to provide an intervention to decrease pain, and it is considered more accurate than nurses' evaluations of behavioral manifestations of pain. Older patients who believe that healthcare providers know best how to manage their pain are at risk for inadequately treated pain.

McDonald and colleagues (2005) used a program for coaching older adults about postoperative pain communication and management. In this study, older adults preparing for single-knee replacement surgery attended a preoperative joint replacement class where they learned about recovering from the surgery and pain management. Forty subjects greater than age 65 were randomly assigned either to the regular class, which included pain management information, or an intervention class, which included both information on pain management and skills to effectively communicate about pain. Pain severity scores were similar for both groups on postoperative days 1 and 2. There was no significant difference between the two groups in the postdischarge measures (day 7) of any pain dimension.

IMPLICATIONS FOR NURSING

Findings from this study highlight the importance of coaching older adults to report their pain experience candidly, particularly in the immediate postoperative period. Establishing trust within the nurse–patient relationship is critical to relieving pain. Coaching older patients to describe their pain location, intensity, and sensation gives them permission to communicate in a manner with which they may feel uncomfortable at first. Coaching is necessary to dispel myths about professional expertise and to allow patients control and independence so that they are willing to ask for pain medications. Exploring with older patients their perception of pain, as well as the significance it has for recovery from illness, are necessary elements in providing adequate pain relief and restoring health.

CRITICAL THINKING IN PATIENT CARE

1. Your older patient says, "I deserved this pain, so I don't want to take anything to make it better." What would be your response and why?
2. A man of Native American descent, aged 76, replies that "something doesn't feel right" when asked to rate his pain on a scale of 0 to 10. His pulse is increased and he is protective of his abdominal incision. What could you ask or do to accurately assess his pain?
3. An independent, 85-year-old woman has a PCA pump for analgesia following major surgery. She continuously presses the pump button, but continues to complain of severe pain. What do you do now?

---

from bloodborne pathogens or injury are minimized when the surgical team is well organized and prepared.

The surgeon is the physician performing the procedure. As head of the surgical team, the surgeon is responsible for all medical actions and judgments.

The surgical assistant works closely with the surgeon in performing the operation. The number of assistants varies according to the complexity of the procedure. The assistant may be another physician, a nurse, a physician assistant, or other trained person. The assistant performs such duties as exposing the operative site, retracting nearby tissue, sponging and/or suctioning the wound, ligating bleeding vessels, and suturing or helping suture the surgical wound.

The anesthesiologist (medical doctor) or CRNA relieves the surgeon of the responsibility for the patient's general well-being, thus allowing the surgeon to focus on the technical aspects of the procedure. The anesthesiologist or CRNA evaluates the patient preoperatively, administers the anesthesia and other required medications, transfuses blood or other blood products, infuses intravenous fluids, continuously monitors the patient's physiologic status, alerts the surgeon to developing problems and treats them as they arise, and supervises the patient's recovery in the PACU.

The **circulating nurse** is a highly experienced registered nurse who coordinates and manages a wide range of activities before, during, and after the surgical procedure. The circulating nurse oversees the physical aspects of the operating room itself, including the equipment, assists with transferring and positioning the patient, prepares the patient's skin, ensures that no break in aseptic technique occurs, and counts all sponges and instruments. The circulating nurse assists all other team members, including the anesthesiologist or CRNA. Thorough documentation of the case in the surgical area is essential, and the circulating nurse is responsible for documenting intraoperative nursing activities, medications, blood administration, placement of drains and catheters, and length of the procedure. The circulating nurse also formulates a care plan based on physiologic and psychosocial assessments of the patient. Finally, the circulating nurse is at all times an advocate for the safety and well-being of the patient.

The role of the **scrub person** primarily involves technical skills, manual dexterity, and in-depth knowledge of the anatomic and mechanical aspects of a particular surgery. The scrub person handles sutures, instruments, and other equipment immediately adjacent to the sterile field. The role of the scrub person may be assumed by a registered nurse or an operating room technician (ORT), depending on hospital policy and the complexity of the surgery. Registered nurses are responsible for patient outcomes including the performance of the person functioning in the role of scrub person. The Association of Operating Room Nurses (AORN) believes that registered nurses should maintain an active presence in the role of scrub person to ensure appropriate delegation and supervision of scrub duties and to maintain an integral link between scrub and circulating responsibilities (AORN, 2010).

The role of nurses in surgery continues to evolve to improve patient care. Although not participating in the surgical procedure, PACU nurses are part of the surgical team. In recent years, nurses have begun to specialize within the already specialized field of perioperative nursing. Specialty surgical teams are developing in response to the demands of increasingly complex technical surgeries. For example, a designated open heart surgical team may be responsible for all open heart cases and ordinarily not be involved with other procedures. The use of specialty surgical teams allows nurses to become highly skilled in a particular range of procedures.

Safety in the surgical environment is important for surgical team members as well as patients. Team members need to be aware of and strictly comply with guidelines to prevent exposure to scatter radiation when fluoroscopy is used in surgical procedures. Fluoroscopy is a real time continuous image of the internal structures of a patient. This technique is used in many types of surgeries including cardiac catheterization, orthopedic placement of metalwork, urologic cases, cardiovascular cases, and digestive system cases. The facility's radiation safety officer assures that protective equipment such as lead aprons, protective eye-glasses, and thyroid shields are available to all personnel at risk for exposure. In the surgical setting, the risk of scatter radiation is small with each event, but the cumulative dose may exceed safe limits. Therefore, personnel need to be informed about protection and limit their exposure (AORN, 2010).

SURGICAL METHODS   Open invasive surgical procedures have traditionally been the gold standard for successful outcomes. This approach was necessary in order to see and protect vital structures surrounding a target organ. Today, miniaturization and technology allow minimally invasive surgeries carried out through small incisions with the aid of cameras and remotely controlled tools and instruments for incising and suturing. While laparoscopic surgeries have been available since 1985, a newer method of minimally invasive surgery is robot-assisted surgery. Robotic technology offers three-dimensional views, while laparoscopic technology offers only two-dimensional views. Instruments are easier for the surgeon to manipulate with the robotic systems. Robotic, computer-aided surgical systems are not independent, preprogrammed systems. Two surgeons perform the procedures—the primary surgeon at the robotic controls and the other at the patient's side to exchange sterile instruments, retract patient tissues, and manipulate nonrobotic sterile instruments used to assist the procedure (Francis & Winifield, 2006). Nurses must be familiar with the equipment and the procedures and ready to assist at all times.

Minimally invasive surgery, whether performed robotically or laparoscopically, has advantages for patients. There is less operative trauma, leading to improved postoperative comfort and decreased pain. While these procedures may take longer than similar open surgeries, they result in decreased hospital stays and fewer complications such as adhesions. General anesthesia is required for most minimally invasive surgeries and the risk for some complications similar to open surgeries remains.

SURGICAL ATTIRE   Strict dress codes are necessary in the surgical department to provide infection control within the operating room suites, reduce cross-contamination between the surgery department and other hospital units or departments, and promote both personnel and patient health and safety. While based on research and recommendations by hospital infection control authorities, guidelines for attire differ among surgical facilities. Following institutional guidelines, all personnel in the surgical department must be in proper surgical attire. The design and composition of the surgical attire minimize bacterial shedding, thus reducing wound contamination. The area in the surgical department is divided into *unrestricted*, *semirestricted*, and *restricted* zones. The unrestricted zones permit access by those in hospital uniforms or street clothes. These areas facilitate communication with operating room personnel.

The semirestricted zones require scrub attire, including a scrub suit, shoe covers, and a cap or hood (Figure 4–3 ■). Hallways, work areas, and storage areas are considered semirestricted. New guidelines exist for attire in the semirestricted and restricted areas of the OR. Previously, each person had to disrobe and don hospital-laundered scrubs. Today, home-laundered scrubs are accepted by many institutions based on data comparing hospital and home-laundered apparel. Only woven or disposable fabrics that will not harbor bacteria are allowed, and all items of apparel must be covered by appropriate fabric. No fabric other than the approved scrub uniform fabric can be exposed to the environment. AORN guidelines (2010) suggest that home-laundered scrubs be brought to the OR in a clean covering and donned at the facility, not worn into the hospital from home. Institutions vary in their interpretation of these guidelines. Artificial nails are discouraged in surgery and anywhere the nurse will have direct contact with high-risk patients. These nails are associated with glove tears and even after careful hand hygiene can harbor potential pathogens (Ogg & Peterson, 2007).

Restricted zones are within operating rooms. Personnel wear masks, sterile gowns, and gloves in addition to appropriate scrub attire if they are participating at the operating table.

A   B

Figure 4–3 ■ Surgical attire. *A*, Scrub attire includes scrub suit, shoe covers, and cap or hood to cover hair. *B*, Sterile attire includes scrub suit, shoe covers, and cap or hood, plus gown, gloves, and mask.

Because of cardiovascular and tissue changes that result from aging, long, complicated surgeries (especially of the thorax and abdomen) place the older adult at increased risk for complications The older adult is more prone to hypotension, hypothermia, and hypoxemia resulting from anesthesia and the cool temperature in the operating room

Positioning may cause complications in the older adult. Intraoperative positioning of arthritic joints can cause postoperative joint pain unrelated to the operative site. Also, the longer the surgery, the greater the chance of decubitus ulcer formation. The older patient is at increased risk for developing decubitus ulcers because of decreased subcutaneous fat tissue and reduced peripheral circulation.

Infections are a particular problem in the older adult because of increased susceptibility from potential immune system decline and unusual manifestations such as confusion, lethargy, and anorexia. The classic signs of infection, fever, redness, pain, and swelling may be diminished in the elderly patient especially if there is immune system decline. The focus of care needs to be strongly on prevention.

Finally, the older adult often has some degree of hearing and/or visual impairment. These impairments coupled with a strange environment can make the operating room a frightening, disorienting place. By effectively communicating with the patient, the nurse can provide support and reassurance to minimize these factors. To decrease confusion and assist in communication, hearing aids and glasses should be used when appropriate and possible.

Factors that contribute to successful surgical outcomes for older adults include stabilizing nutrition and hydration, controlling concurrent chronic conditions with appropriate medication reconciliation, and providing information for realistic expectations about the surgery and the recovery (Clayton, 2008). Advanced age alone is not a contra-indication for surgery.

The outer sterile covering is changed between procedures and when it becomes soiled or wet. These practices are designed to protect the patient and the practitioner, especially from blood-borne pathogens. Continual evaluation by the hospital's infection control team is the source for guiding these practices. Strict adherence to proper usage of gowns, gloves, and masks is vital for protection (Belkin, 2006).

THE SURGICAL SCRUB   The surgical scrub is performed to render hands and arms as clean as possible in preparation for a procedure. All personnel who participate directly in the procedure must perform a surgical scrub with a brush and antimicrobial soap. Skin cannot be rendered sterile, but it can be considered "surgically clean" following the scrub. The purposes of the surgical scrub are to do the following:

- Remove dirt, skin oils, and transient microorganisms from hands and forearms.
- Increase patient safety by reducing microorganisms on surgical personnel.
- Leave an antimicrobial residue on the skin to inhibit growth of microbes for several hours.

Following the 5- to 10-minute surgical scrub, hands and arms are dried with sterile towels.

Patient Preparation

Although much preparation has taken place prior to the patient's transfer to the surgical department, additional activities such as hair removal and positioning may be performed there. The skin preparation, which usually includes cleansing the area with a prescribed antimicrobial agent, may have been performed either by the patient or by nursing personnel before the transfer to the surgical department. Additional skin cleansing is performed in the surgical department to further decrease microorganisms on the skin and thereby reduce the possibility of wound infection.

Shaving as part of skin preparation is associated with increased risk for infection secondary to nicks in the skin. Hair removal by clippers or by depilatory solutions is preferable (Daniels, 2007). The surgeon may order hair removed in and around the proposed incision area. This is more often performed in the holding area of the surgical department. Generally, the prepared area is wider than the planned incision because of the possibility of unexpected extension of the incision. Hospital policy and surgeon preference should be followed.

Preparing the patient for surgery also includes positioning the patient on the operating table. Table 4–5 shows frequently used positions and describes corresponding surgical procedures and possible adverse effects. Positioning exposes the operative site and provides access for anesthesia administration.

> **SAFETY ALERT**
> Proper positioning is imperative to prevent injury to the patient. Pressure, rubbing, and/or shearing forces can cause injury to the tissue over bony prominences. If positioning causes normal joint range of motion to be exceeded, injury to muscles and joints can occur.

Improper positioning also can lead to sensory and motor dysfunction, resulting in nerve damage. Pressure on peripheral blood vessels can decrease venous return to the heart and negatively affect the patient's blood pressure. Additionally, oxygenation of the blood can be decreased if the patient is not properly positioned to promote lung expansion.

Because the anesthetized patient cannot respond to discomfort, it is the surgical team's responsibility to position the patient not only for the best surgical advantage but also for patient safety and comfort. The circulating nurse refers to hospital policy, the surgeon's preference, and the patient's history to ensure optimal positioning, and continuously assesses the patient. Be aware that tendons and ligaments can be overstretched by improper positioning (Clayton, 2008).

INTRAOPERATIVE AWARENESS   Prior to induction of anesthesia, the circulating nurse establishes rapport with the patient to assess the patient's psychologic status. This assessment is continued throughout the surgical procedure. After anesthetic medications have been given, the patient may appear oblivious to the surroundings; however, anesthesiologists are concerned

TABLE 4–5 Common Surgical Positions

POSITION AND USE	POSSIBLE ADVERSE EFFECTS AND NURSING INTERVENTIONS
(a) The *dorsal recumbent* (or *supine*) *position* is used for many abdominal surgeries (e.g., colostomy and herniorrhaphy) as well as for some thoracic surgeries (e.g., open heart surgery) and some surgeries on the extremities.	This position may cause excessive pressure on posterior bony prominences, such as the back of the head, scapulae, sacrum, and heels. Pad these areas with soft materials. To avoid compression of blood vessels and sluggish circulation, ensure that the knees are not flexed. Use trochanter rolls or other padding to avoid internal or external rotation of the hips and shoulders.
(b) The *semisitting position* is used for surgeries on the thyroid and neck areas.	This position can lead to postural hypotension and venous pooling in the legs. It may promote skin breakdown on the buttocks. Sciatic nerve injury is possible. Assess for hypotension. Ensure that knees are not sharply flexed. Use soft padding to prevent nerve compression.
(c) The *prone position* is used for spinal fusions and removal of hemorrhoids.	This position causes pressure on the face, knees, thighs, anterior ankles, and toes. Pad bony prominences, and support the feet under the ankles. To promote optimum respiratory function, raise the patient's chest and abdomen, and support with padding. Corneal abrasion could occur if the eyes are not closed or are insufficiently padded.
(d) The *lateral chest position* is used for some thoracic surgeries, as well as hip replacements.	This may cause excessive pressure on the bony prominences on the side on which the patient is positioned. Ensure adequate padding and support, especially of the downside arm. The weight of the upper leg may cause peroneal nerve injury on the downside leg. Both legs must therefore be padded.
(e) The *lithotomy position* is used for gynecologic, perineal, or rectal surgeries.	This position causes an 18% decrease (from a standing position) in vital capacity of the lungs. Monitor respirations, and assess for hypoxia and dyspnea. The lithotomy position can lead to joint damage, peroneal nerve damage, and damage to peripheral blood vessels. To avoid injury, ensure adequate padding, and manipulate both legs into the stirrups simultaneously.
(f) The *jackknife position* is used for proctologic surgeries, such as removal of hemorrhoids, and for some spinal surgeries.	This position causes a 12% decrease (from a standing position) in vital capacity of the lungs. Monitor respirations, and assess for hypoxia and dyspnea. In this position, the greatest pressure is felt at the bends in the table. Therefore, the patient is supported with pads at the groin and knees, as well as at the ankles. Padding of the chest and knees helps prevent skin breakdown. Padding and proper positioning help prevent pressure on the ear, the neck, and the nerves of the upper arm.

about patient awareness with recall of intraoperative events (Hassan & Fahy, 2005). Intraoperative awareness is the patient's subconscious awareness of what is being said and done during surgery. Although most patients do not consciously remember what happened or what was said, psychologic trauma can result. Because loss of consciousness is gradual, conversations during surgery should be professional.

> **PRACTICE ALERT**
> Do not say anything while the patient is unconscious that would be inappropriate if the patient were awake. Maintain a respectful, professional demeanor throughout the operative period.

Nutrition

Wound healing after surgery depends on adequate nutritional intake. During the immediate postoperative phase, dietary intake is withheld until evidence of peristalsis (either audible bowel sounds or passage of flatus) is found and the patient can tolerate liquids without nausea and vomiting. While intravenous fluids maintain hydration and electrolyte balance, they do not provide nutrition. Unless balanced nutrition through gastrointestinal intake can be reestablished within 3 to 4 days, parenteral nutrition is critical for homeostasis and wound healing.

- Protein, calories, and vitamins are needed for wound healing and recovery from surgery.
- Low-fat, high-fiber diets are important for chronic cardiovascular fitness, but are contraindicated in the wound healing phase following surgery.
- Failure to use the gastrointestinal tract for more than 4 or 5 days allows the intestinal mucosa to atrophy, putting the patient at risk for infection.

Fluid administered through peripheral veins must be isotonic or only moderately hypertonic to prevent injury to the small peripheral veins. Solutions of 10% dextrose are tolerable peripherally for a short time but do not provide adequate calories for healing and maintenance. To provide adequate nutrition, central vein access must be established and solutions must be prepared with protein, carbohydrates, lipids, vitamins, and minerals. This is important for patients who have extended recovery periods without eating after surgery.

Parenteral nutrition has serious risks. Central vein access may cause infection and sepsis. Normal stimulation to the intestinal tract is lost when the parenteral approach is used alone. Using the gut is better than using the vein because it (1) prevents intestinal atrophy, which results in a very thin bowel wall poorly suited to absorb nutrients; (2) prevents bacteria and inert particles from translocating across the bowel lining into the bloodstream; (3) introduces fats and other large particles into the lymphatic circulation and stimulates the immune system; and (4) is safer and far less expensive than parenteral nutritional support (Heimburger & Weinsier, 1997; Lindgren & Ames, 2005). Education and counseling to support adequate nutritional intake should be ongoing throughout the preoperative and postoperative period.

Nursing Care

The following section discusses nursing care in each of the three phases of surgery. The Case Study & Nursing Care Plan at the end of the section follows one patient through the postoperative experience, bringing this information together.

Preoperative Nursing Care

The patient's response to planned surgery varies greatly. When planning and implementing nursing care, consider individual psychologic and physical differences, the type of surgery, and the circumstances surrounding the need for surgery. A thorough nursing assessment is needed to determine the most appropriate care for each patient undergoing surgery.

Before planning and implementing care for the surgical patient, gather assessment information by taking a nursing history and performing a physical examination. Use this information to establish baseline data, identify physical needs, determine teaching needs and psychologic support for the patient and family, and prioritize nursing care. The type of surgical procedure directs the assessment and intervention planned by the nurse.

> **PRACTICE ALERT**
> Be sure to assess information about use of over-the-counter medications including herbal supplements. These drugs can interact with medications administered in the perioperative period.

Surgery is a significant and stressful event. Regardless of the nature of the surgery (whether major or minor), the patient and family will be anxious. Some patients and their families seek care from a spiritual provider during this time. The degree of anxiety they will feel is not necessarily proportional to the magnitude of the surgical procedure. For example, a patient scheduled to have a biopsy to rule out cancer, which is considered minor surgery, may be more anxious than a patient undergoing gallbladder removal, which is considered major surgery.

The nurse's ability to listen actively to both verbal and nonverbal messages is imperative to establishing a trusting relationship with the patient and family (Majasaari et al., 2005). Therapeutic communication can help the patient and family identify fears and concerns. The nurse can then plan nursing interventions and supportive care to reduce the patient's anxiety level and assist the patient to cope successfully with the stressors encountered during the perioperative period.

Preoperative Patient and Family Teaching

Patient teaching is an essential nursing responsibility in the preoperative period. Patient education and emotional support have a positive effect on the patient's physical and psychologic well-being, and on family members, both before and after surgery. Majasaari et al. (2005) surveyed 100 patients who underwent general, orthopedic, or gynecologic surgery as outpatients and their family members. Results of the survey showed the greatest dissatisfaction with outpatient surgery was lack or inadequacy of information. Because outpatient surgical stays are

BOX 4–3 Preoperative Patient Teaching

Diaphragmatic Breathing Exercise

Diaphragmatic (abdominal) breathing exercises are taught to the patient who is at risk for developing pulmonary complications, such as atelectasis or pneumonia. Risk factors for pulmonary complications include general anesthesia, abdominal or thoracic surgery, history of smoking, chronic lung disease, obesity, and advanced age.

In diaphragmatic breathing, the patient inspires deeply while allowing the abdomen to expand outward. On expiration, the abdomen contracts inward as air from the lungs is expelled.

1. Explain to the patient that the diaphragm is a muscle that makes up the floor of the abdominal cavity and assists in breathing. The purpose of diaphragmatic breathing is to promote lung expansion and ventilation and enhance blood oxygenation.
2. Position the patient in a high or semi-Fowler's position.
3. Ask the patient to place the hands lightly on the abdomen (see the following figure).
4. Instruct the patient to breathe in deeply through the nose, allowing the chest and abdomen to expand.
5. Have the patient hold the breath for a count of 5.
6. Tell the patient to exhale completely through pursed (puckered) lips, allowing the chest and abdomen to deflate.
7. Have the patient repeat the exercise five times consecutively.

Encourage the patient to perform diaphragmatic breathing exercises every 1 to 2 waking hours, depending on the patient's needs and institutional protocol.

Diaphragmatic breathing exercise.

Coughing Exercise

Coughing exercises are also taught to the patient who is at risk for developing pulmonary complications. The purpose of coughing is to loosen, mobilize, and remove pulmonary secretions. Splinting the incision decreases the physical and psychologic discomfort associated with coughing.

1. Assist the patient in following steps 1 through 4 for diaphragmatic breathing.
2. Ask the patient to splint the incision with interlocked hands or a pillow (see the following figure).
3. Tell the patient to take three deep breaths and then cough while contracting abdominal muscles.
4. Have the patient repeat the exercise five times consecutively every 2 hours while awake, taking short rest periods between coughs if necessary.

Splinting abdomen while coughing.

Leg, Ankle, and Foot Exercises

Leg exercises are taught to the patient who is at risk for developing venous thrombosis (formation of blood clots in a vein, often accompanied by inflammation). Risk factors for developing venous thrombosis include decreased mobility preoperatively and/or postoperatively; a history of difficulties with peripheral circulation; and cardiovascular, pelvic, or lower extremity surgeries.

The purpose of leg exercises is to promote venous blood return from the extremities. As the leg muscles contract and relax, blood is pumped back to the heart, promoting cardiac output and reducing venous stasis. These exercises also maintain muscle tone and range of motion, which facilitate early ambulation.

Teach the patient to perform the following exercises while lying in bed:

1. Muscle pumping exercise: Contract and relax calf and thigh muscles at least 10 times consecutively.
2. Leg exercises:
   a. Bend the knee and raise it toward the chest (see the following figure).
   b. Straighten out leg and hold for a few seconds before lowering the leg back to the bed.
   c. Repeat exercise five times consecutively prior to alternating to the other foot.

1 Flexed **2** Straight out **3** Then down

Leg exercises.

3. Ankle and foot exercises:
   a. Rotate both ankles by making complete circles, first to the right and then to the left (see the following figure).
   b. Repeat five times and then relax.
   c. With feet together, point toes toward the head and then to the foot of the bed (see the following figure).
   d. Repeat this pumping action 10 times, and then relax.

(continued)

BOX 4–3 Preoperative Patient Teaching (continued)

Encourage the patient to perform leg, ankle, and foot exercises every 1 to 2 hours while awake, depending on the patient's needs and ambulatory status, the physician's preference, and institutional protocol.

Ankle and foot exercises.

Turning in Bed

The patient who is at risk for circulatory, respiratory, or gastrointestinal dysfunction following surgery is taught to turn in bed. Although this may be a simple task prior to surgery, after surgery (particularly after abdominal surgery) the patient may find it a difficult procedure. To make the procedure more comfortable, the patient may need to splint the incision by using the hand placed on a small pillow or blanket. Additionally, the patient should be taught that analgesics can be given to ease postoperative discomfort involved with turning. Encourage the patient to turn every 2 hours while awake.

1. Tell the patient to grasp the side rail toward the direction to be turned, to rest the opposite foot on the mattress, and to bend the knee.
2. Instruct the patient to roll over in one smooth motion by pulling on the side rail while pushing off with the bent knee.
3. Pillows may need to be positioned behind the patient's back to help the patient maintain a side-lying position. The older patient may also need padding over pressure points between the knees and ankles to decrease the chance of decubitus ulcer formation from pressure.

---

brief, it is valuable for nurses to be sensitive, perceptive, and able to listen to and identify the patient as an individual within a unique family.

Patient teaching should begin as soon as the patient learns of the upcoming surgery. Teaching may begin as early as in the physician's office or at the time of preadmission testing. Although education continues during postoperative care, most teaching is done before surgery because pain and the effects of anesthesia can greatly diminish the patient's ability to learn.

The amount of information desired varies from patient to patient. Therefore, assess the patient's need for and readiness to accept information. The teaching will be directed in part by the particular surgical procedure that is being performed and by the type of anesthesia. The information in Box 4–3 is relevant to most patients undergoing major surgery.

In addition to teaching the patient and family about measures that will decrease the risk of complications, provide other preoperative information to prepare the patient and family for surgery. This information should include the following:

- Diagnostic tests—reasons and preparations
- Arrival time if surgery is scheduled the day of admission
- Preparations for surgery, including fasting prior to surgery, skin preparation, indwelling catheter or bladder elimination, start of intravenous infusion, preoperative medication, handling of valuables (rings, watch, money)
- Sedative/hypnotic medication to be taken the night before surgery to promote rest and sleep
- Counseling on whether to take significant medications the morning of surgery
- Informed consent
- Expected timetable for surgery and the recovery room
- Method to inform family of progress throughout surgery
- Transfer to the surgery department
- Location of the surgical waiting room
- Transfer to recovery room

- Anticipated postoperative routine and devices or equipment (drains, tubes, equipment for IV infusions, oxygen or humidifying mask, dressings, splints, casts)
- Plans for postoperative pain control
- Appropriate clothing for dressing prior to discharge from outpatient surgery

The American Society of Anesthesiologists provides guidelines for preoperative fasting in healthy patients undergoing elective procedures; they are available online. Withdrawal from caffeine in beverages such as coffee or colas may cause headaches and irritability. Dehydration, hypovolemia, and hypoglycemia are other recognized side effects. Thirst, worry, and hunger are reported by patients to be related to fasting. Fasting does not ensure that the stomach will be empty or that the gastric contents will be less acidic.

Preoperative Patient Preparation

A preoperative surgical checklist (Figure 4–4 ■) serves as an outline for finalizing preparation of the patient for surgery in most institutions. Complete the checklist before the patient is transported to surgery. Nursing responsibilities the day of surgery are as follows:

- Assist with bathing, grooming, and changing into operating room gown.
- Ensure that the patient takes nothing by mouth (NPO). Provide additional teaching, and reinforce prior teaching.
- Remove nail polish, lipstick, and makeup to facilitate circulatory assessment during and after surgery. Artificial nails worn by the patient should not be altered.
- Ensure that identification, blood, and allergy bands are correct, legible, and secure.
- Remove hair pins and jewelry; a wedding ring may be worn if it is removed from the finger, covered with gauze, replaced, and then taped to the finger.
- Complete skin or bowel preparation as ordered.

To be completed 24 hours prior to surgery

DATE: _____

* CALL REPORT AT 4474 (6 AM - 6 PM)
CALL REPORT AT 6171 (6 PM - 6 AM & weekends & holidays)

INSTRUCTIONS: Indicate that the task has been completed or the proper form is on the chart by initializing the item. Place NA in the column if item does not apply. Sign full name and title at bottom of page. Complete new form for each surgery procedure date.

REVIEW MEDICAL RECORD AND PHYSICIAN'S ORDER:	INITIALS

1. History and Physical completed and in chart .... 1. _____
2. Laboratory studies/Reports in chart .... 2. _____
3. EKG report in chart .... 3. _____
4. Chest X-ray report in chart .... 4. _____
5. Operative Permit completed, signed, & witnessed in chart .... 5. _____
   ☐ Patient Affirmation ☐ Witness Affirmation ☐ Physician Attestation
6. Anesthesia Permit completed, signed, & witnessed in chart .... 6. _____
   ☐ Patient Affirmation ☐ Witness Affirmation ☐ Physician Attestation
7. Consent for blood transfusion completed, signed, & witnessed in chart .... 7. _____
   ☐ Patient Affirmation ☐ Witness Affirmation ☐ Physician Attestation
8. Medication Reconciliation Form Completed & Signed .... 8. _____
9. 4 pages of labels .... 9. _____

PREOPERATIVE PREPARATION:	INITIALS

1. Identification bracelet accurate and affixed to wrist or ankle prior to transport ...... 1. _____
2. Allergies checked, allergies bracelet on and allergy sticker on chart .... 2. _____
3. Isolation label on chart .... 3. _____
4. Jewelry, hairpieces, hairpins, contact lenses, glasses, prosthesis, underwear, money removed .. 4. _____
5. Vital signs taken and recorded .... 5. _____
   Time taken_____ BP_____ Temp_____ HR_____ Resp_____ FS_____ 6. _____
6. Dentures: ☐ Full: ☐ Upper ☐ Lower   ☐ Partial: ☐ Upper ☐ Lower
   ☐ Other:_____
   ☐ **Removed:** ☐ Sent Home ☐ Left at bedside
   ☐ **Left in place as requested by:** ☐ Anesthesiologist ☐ Patient
7. Patient NPO ☐ yes since _____ ☐ no .... 7. _____
   If no: O.R. notified (Time) _____ (Whom)..
8. Medication sheets on chart.. 8. _____
9. Most recent nursing assessment attached.. 9. _____
10. Report called to _____ at_____(time) .... 10. _____

INITIALS	SIGNATURE AND TITLE	INITIALS	SIGNATURE AND TITLE

THE GEORGE WASHINGTON UNIVERSITY HOSPITAL

UHS
Universal Health

Patient Label

NURSING PREOPERATIVE CHECKLIST

OP0070

75-041 (12/06)

Figure 4–4 ■ The preoperative checklist helps ensure consistent completion of preoperative care activities.

- Insert an indwelling catheter, intravenous line, or nasogastric tube as ordered.
- Remove dentures, artificial eye, and contact lenses, and store them in a safe place.
- Leave a hearing aid in place if the patient cannot hear without it, and notify the operating room nurse.
- Verify that the informed consent has been signed prior to administering preoperative medications.
- Weigh the patient and record height and weight in the chart (for dosage of anesthesia).
- Verify that all ordered diagnostic test reports are in the chart.
- Have the patient empty the bladder immediately before the preoperative medication is administered (unless an indwelling catheter is in place).
- Administer preoperative medication as scheduled (refer to the Medications section earlier in the chapter and Table 4–4).
- Ensure the safety of the patient once the medication has been given by placing the patient on bed rest with raised side rails and by placing the call light within reach.
- Obtain and record vital signs.
- Provide ongoing supportive care to the patient and the patient's family.
- Document all preoperative care in the appropriate location, such as the preoperative surgical checklist, the medication record, and the narrative preoperative nursing notes.
- Verify with the surgical personnel the patient's identity, and verify that all patient information is documented appropriately.
- Help the surgical personnel transfer the patient from the bed to the stretcher.
- Prepare the patient's room for postoperative care, including making the surgical bed and ensuring that the anticipated supplies and equipment are in the room.

Having completed the preoperative check list and upon "call" from the OR, the patient enters the operating suite via stretcher and resides in a "holding area" prior to entry into the designated operating room. Additional preparations are made here and may include hair removal and intravenous access. Surgery nurses rotate their staffing assignments among holding areas, operating room, and postanesthesia care units. Preoperative care is completed in this setting. Some hospitals allow a family member or significant other to accompany the patient in the holding area while awaiting transfer to the operating room.

Intraoperative Nursing Care

The intraoperative phase of surgery begins when the patient enters the operating room and ends when the patient is transferred to the postanesthesia care unit. Nursing care in this phase focuses on keeping the patient and the environment safe and providing physiologic monitoring and psychologic support. Circulating nurses and scrub nurses, according to specific role definitions, support and care for the patient and assist the surgeons.

On entry into the surgical suite, the nurse verifies the patient's identity, the type and site of surgery, and previously obtained assessment data. The nurse participates in the Universal Protocol, calling for a "time out" before the procedure to conduct final verification of the correct patient, site,

positioning, and procedure, and that all relevant documents, information, and equipment are available.

The patient is appropriately positioned, using safety belts to secure him or her while assuring distal circulation remains unimpaired. Bone prominences are padded to reduce the risk of tissue breakdown. During surgery, the nurse observes for and informs the team if any breaks or potential breaks in sterile technique are noted.

> ### PRACTICE ALERT
> Objects on the sterile drape are considered sterile. Remain a minimum of 12 inches away from draped tables and sterile fields to avoid contamination if you are not attired in sterile gown and gloves.

Postoperative Nursing Care

Immediate Postoperative Care

Immediate postoperative care begins when the patient has been transferred from the operating room to the PACU. The PACU nurse immediately assesses the patient's airway and breathing and monitors vital signs and the surgical site to determine the response to the surgical procedure and to detect significant changes. Assessing mental status and level of consciousness is another ongoing nursing responsibility, and the patient may require repeated orientation to time, place, and person. Emotional support also is essential, because the patient is in a vulnerable and dependent position. Assessing and evaluating hydration status by monitoring intake and output is crucial to detecting cardiovascular or renal complications. In addition, the PACU nurse assesses the patient's pain level. Careful administration of analgesics provides comfort without compounding the potential side effects from the anesthesia.

Care When the Patient Is Stable

When awake and after being stabilized, the patient is transferred to his or her room. The PACU nurse communicates information about the patient's condition and postoperative orders to the floor nurse prior to the patient's arrival. This prepares the floor nurse for additional problems or needed equipment.

Immediate and continuing assessment is essential to detect and/or prevent complications. In documenting assessment findings, the nurse completes a flow record of the individual patient's situation. Baseline data are obtained and compared with preoperative data. A postoperative head-to-toe assessment includes but may not be limited to the following:

- General appearance
- Vital signs
- Level of consciousness
- Emotional status
- Quantity of respirations
- Skin color and temperature
- Discomfort/pain
- Nausea/vomiting
- Type of intravenous fluids and flow rate
- Dressing site

- Drainage on the dressing and/or bed linen
- Urinary output (catheter or ability to urinate)
- Ability to move all extremities

The hospital policy or physician's orders dictate the frequency of follow-up assessments. After major surgery, the nurse generally assesses the patient every 15 minutes during the first hour and, if the patient is stable, every 30 minutes for the next 2 hours, and then every hour during the subsequent 4 hours. Assessments are then carried out every 4 hours, subject to change according to the patient's condition and protocol for the particular surgical procedure. It is critically important to inform the surgeon immediately if the assessment reveals any signs of impending shock or other life-threatening changes.

After carrying out the initial assessment and ensuring the patient's safety by lowering the bed, raising the side rails, and placing the call light within reach, the nurse notes the physician's postoperative orders. These orders guide the nurse in the care of the postoperative patient. For example, the orders specify activity level, diet, medications for pain and nausea, antibiotics, continuation of preoperative medications, frequency of vital sign assessments, administration of intravenous fluids, and laboratory tests such as hemoglobin and potassium level. In most institutions, orders written prior to surgery must be reordered following surgery because the patient's condition is presumed to have changed.

Nursing Care of Common Postoperative Complications

Several factors place the patient at risk for postoperative complications. Nursing care before, during, and after surgery is aimed at preventing and/or minimizing the effects of these complications.

Preoperative care and teaching to decrease postoperative complications have been discussed. The following section addresses postoperative cardiovascular, respiratory, and wound complications, and problems associated with elimination.

Cardiovascular Complications

Common postoperative cardiovascular complications include shock, hemorrhage, deep venous thrombosis, and pulmonary embolism.

SHOCK   Shock is a life-threatening postoperative complication. It results from an insufficient blood flow to vital organs, an inability to use oxygen and nutrients, or the inability to rid tissues of waste material. Hypovolemic shock, the most common type in the postoperative patient, results from a decrease in circulating fluid volume. Decreased fluid volume develops with blood or plasma loss or, less commonly, from severe prolonged vomiting or diarrhea. Symptoms vary according to the severity of the shock; the greater the loss of fluid volume, the more severe the symptoms. ∞ Chapter 11 provides a detailed discussion of nursing care of the patient with various types of shock.

HEMORRHAGE   Hemorrhage is an excessive loss of blood. A concealed hemorrhage occurs internally from a blood vessel that is no longer sutured or cauterized or from a drainage tube that has eroded a blood vessel. An obvious hemorrhage occurs externally from a dislodged or ill-formed clot at the wound. Hemorrhage also may result from abnormalities in the blood's ability to clot; these abnormalities may result from a pathologic condition, or they may be a side effect of medications.

Hemorrhage from a venous source oozes out quickly and is dark red, whereas an arterial hemorrhage is characterized by bright red spurts of blood pulsating with each heartbeat. Whether the hemorrhage is from a venous or an arterial source, hypovolemic shock will occur if sufficient blood is lost from the circulation.

Assessment findings with hemorrhage depend on the amount and rate of blood loss. Restlessness and anxiety are observed in the early stage of hemorrhage. Frank bleeding will be present if the hemorrhage is external. The patient will have symptoms characteristic of shock.

Care of the patient who is hemorrhaging centers around stopping the bleeding and replenishing the circulating blood volume. Nursing care includes providing care for shock and one or more of the following:

- Applying one or more sterile gauze pads and a snug pressure dressing to the area
- Applying pressure with gloved hands (may be necessary for severe external bleeding)
- Preparing patient and family for emergency surgery (in severe situations when bleeding cannot be stopped)

DEEP VENOUS THROMBOSIS   Deep venous thrombosis (DVT) is the formation of a thrombus (blood clot) in association with inflammation in deep veins. This complication most often occurs in the lower extremities of the postoperative patient. It may result from the combination of several factors, including trauma during surgery, pressure applied under the knees, and sluggish blood flow during and after surgery. Patients particularly at risk for developing DVT include those who are over age 40 and who

- have experienced trauma or undergone orthopedic surgery to lower extremities; urologic, gynecologic, or obstetric surgeries; or neurosurgery.
- are pregnant or have recently given birth, have varicose veins, are undergoing hormone replacement therapy, or are using birth control pills.
- have a history of venous thrombosis, pulmonary emboli, or atrial fibrillation.
- are obese, smoke, have prolonged travel time in plane or car, or are immobilized.
- have an infection or sepsis.
- have a malignancy.

Prevention of venous stasis is an important nursing responsibility; it reduces adverse patient outcomes and decreases healthcare costs. Early ambulation is the key to preventing venous stasis but when patients are immobilized there is risk for blood clots. Anticoagulant medications such as low molecular weight heparin are used in high risk populations. Use of mechanical prophylactic devices (intermittent pneumatic compression devices [IPCDs]) on the foot, entire leg, or calf only is documented as effective prevention. Given the frequency and seriousness of the development of DVT and pulmonary embolism, attention to prevention is very important.

Common assessment findings reveal pain or cramping in the involved calf or thigh. Redness and edema of the entire extremity may occur along with a slightly elevated temperature. The patient may have a positive Homans' sign (pain in the calf on dorsiflexion of the affected foot).

Nursing care of the patient with DVT focuses on preventing a portion of the clot from dislodging and becoming an embolus (traveling blood clot) circulating to the heart, brain, or lungs; preventing other clots from forming; and supporting the patient's own physiologic mechanism for dissolving clots. Nursing care includes the following measures:

- Administer anticoagulants and analgesics as prescribed.
- Monitor laboratory values for clotting times.
- Maintain bed rest and keep affected extremity at or above heart level.
- Apply thigh-high antiemboli stockings or IPCDs to stimulate venous return.
- Ensure that the affected area is not rubbed or massaged.
- Apply heat as prescribed.
- Record bilateral calf or thigh circumferences every shift.
- Teach and support the patient and family.
- Assess color and temperature of involved extremity every shift.

PULMONARY EMBOLISM A pulmonary embolism is a dislodged blood clot or other substance that lodges in a pulmonary artery. For the postoperative patient with DVT, the threat that a portion of the thrombus may break off or dislodge from the vein wall and travel to the lung is a constant concern. Early detection of this potentially life-threatening complication depends on the nurse's astute, continuing assessment of the postoperative patient.

Common assessment findings of the patient experiencing a pulmonary embolism include mild to moderate dyspnea, chest pain, diaphoresis, anxiety, restlessness, rapid respirations and pulse, dysrhythmias, cough, and cyanosis. The severity of the symptoms is determined by the degree of pulmonary vascular blockage. Sudden death can occur if a major pulmonary artery becomes completely blocked.

Stabilizing respiratory and cardiovascular functioning while preventing the formation of additional emboli is of utmost importance in the care of the patient with a pulmonary embolism. Nursing care includes the following measures:

- Immediately notify the physician and nursing supervisor.
- Frequently assess and record general condition and vital signs.
- Maintain the patient on bed rest, and keep the head of the bed elevated.
- Provide oxygen as ordered and monitor pulse oximetry.
- Administer prescribed intravenous fluids to maintain fluid balance while preventing fluid overload.
- Administer prescribed anticoagulants.
- Maintain comfort by administering analgesics and sedatives (use caution to prevent respiratory depression).
- Provide supportive measures for the patient and family.

Refer to ∞ Chapter 37 for a detailed discussion of pulmonary embolism.

Respiratory Complications
Common postoperative respiratory complications include pneumonia and atelectasis.

PNEUMONIA Pneumonia is an inflammation of lung tissue. Inflammation is caused either by a microbial infection or by a foreign substance in the lung, which leads to inflammation. Numerous factors may be involved in the development of pneumonia, including aspiration of gastric contents, retained pulmonary secretions, failure to cough deeply, and impaired cough reflex and decreased mobility.

Common assessment findings of the postoperative patient with pneumonia are as follows:

- High fever
- Rapid pulse and respirations
- Chills (may be present initially)
- Productive cough (may be present depending on the type of pneumonia)
- Dyspnea
- Chest pain
- Crackles and wheezes

Treating the pulmonary infection, supporting the patient's respiratory efforts, promoting lung expansion, and preventing the organisms' spread are the goals in the care of the patient with pneumonia. Nursing care includes the following measures:

- Obtain sputum specimens for culture and sensitivity testing.
- Position patient with the head of the bed elevated.
- Encourage the patient to turn, cough, and perform deep-breathing exercises at least every 2 hours.
- Assist with incentive spirometry, intermittent positive pressure breathing (IPPB), and/or nebulizer treatments as ordered.
- Ambulate patient as condition permits and as prescribed.
- Administer oxygen as ordered.
- Assess vital signs, breath sounds, oxygen saturation, and general condition.
- Maintain hydration to help liquefy pulmonary secretions.
- Administer antibiotics, expectorants, antipyretics, and analgesics as ordered.
- Provide or assist with frequent oral hygiene.
- Prevent the spread of microorganisms by teaching proper disposal of tissues, covering mouth when coughing, and good hand hygiene technique.
- Provide supportive measures for the patient and family. ∞ Chapter 36 provides a detailed discussion of pneumonia.

ATELECTASIS Atelectasis is an incomplete expansion or collapse of lung tissue resulting in inadequate ventilation and retention of pulmonary secretions. Common assessment findings include dyspnea, diminished breath sounds over the affected area, anxiety, restlessness, crackles, and cyanosis.

Promoting lung expansion and systemic oxygenation of tissues is a goal in the care of the patient with atelectasis. Nursing care includes these tasks:

- Position the patient with the head of the bed elevated.

- Administer oxygen as prescribed.
- Encourage coughing, turning, and deep breathing every 2 hours.
- Ambulate the patient as condition permits and as prescribed.
- Assist with incentive spirometry or other pulmonary exercises, such as inflating a balloon, as ordered.
- Administer analgesics as prescribed.
- Promote hydration.
- Provide supportive measures to the patient and family.

Wound Complications

Discussion of the complications associated with surgical wounds follows an overview of wound healing, wound drainage, and nursing care of wounds.

Wounds heal by either *primary*, *secondary*, or *tertiary intention* (Figure 4–5 ■). Healing by primary intention takes place when the wound is uncomplicated and clean and has sustained little tissue loss. The edges of the incision are well approximated (have come together well) with sutures, staples, or superglue for drain holes or superficial wounds (Zide, 2005). This type of surgical incision heals quickly, and very little scarring is expected.

Secondary intention refers to the healing that occurs when the wound is large, gaping, and irregular. Tissue loss prevents wound edges from approximating; therefore, granulation tissue fills in the wound. This type of wound takes longer to heal, is more prone to infection, and develops more scar tissue.

Primary intention

Clean incision   Early suture   "Hairline" scar

Secondary intention

Gaping wound with blood clot   Granulation tissue fills in wound   Large scar

Tertiary intention

Contaminated wound   Granulation tissue   Closure with wide scar

Figure 4–5 ■ Wound healing by primary, secondary, and tertiary intention.

If enough time passes before a wound is sutured, healing by tertiary intention occurs. Infection is more likely to take place. Because the wound edges are not approximated, tissue is regenerated by the granulation process. Closure of the wound results in a wide scar.

From the time the surgical incision is made until the wound is completely healed, all wounds progress through four stages of healing. However, healing time varies according to many factors, such as age, nutritional status, general health, and the type and location of the wound. Figure 4–5 provides a summary of the stages of wound healing.

Wound drainage (exudate) results from the inflammatory process in the first two stages of wound healing. The drainage is from the rich blood supply that surrounds the wound tissue and is composed of escaped fluid and cells. The drainage is described as serous, sanguineous, or purulent.

- Serous drainage contains mostly the clear serous portion of the blood. The drainage appears clear or slightly yellow and is thin in consistency.
- Sanguineous drainage contains a combination of serum and red blood cells and has a thick, reddish appearance. This is the most common type of drainage from a noncomplicated surgical wound.
- Purulent drainage is composed of white blood cells, tissue debris, and bacteria. Purulent drainage is the result of infection and tends to be of a thicker consistency, with various colors specific to the type of organism. It also may have an unpleasant odor.

Box 4–4 describes and illustrates various types of wound drainage devices. These devices decrease pressure in the wound area by removing excess fluid, which promotes healing and decreases complications.

Nursing care of the postoperative patient with a surgical wound focuses on preventing and monitoring for wound complications. The nurse assumes a leading role in supporting the wound healing process, providing emotional support to the patient and teaching wound care to the patient.

Common assessment findings of an infected wound include pain; purulent, odorous discharge and redness; warmth; tenderness; and edema around the edges of the incision. Additionally, the patient may have a fever, chills, and increased respiratory and pulse rates. Nursing care includes the following measures:

- Maintain medical asepsis (e.g., by using good hand hygiene technique).
- Follow Centers for Disease Control and Prevention guidelines for wound care.
- Observe aseptic technique during dressing changes and handling of tubes and drains.
- Assess vital signs, especially temperature.
- Evaluate the characteristics of wound discharge (color, odor, and amount).
- Assess the condition of the incision (approximation of the edges, sutures, staples, or drains).
- Clean, irrigate, and pack the wound in the prescribed manner. Sterile normal saline is often prescribed; povidone-iodine (Betadine) is no longer recommended for wound care.

BOX 4–4 **Wound Drainage Devices**

A Penrose drain, used for passive wound drainage, promotes healing from the inside to the outside (see figure A). The use of the drain decreases the chance of abscess formation. The safety pin in the Penrose drain prevents the exposed end from slipping down into the wound. Wound care focuses on cleaning around the drain with a prescribed solution, such as sterile normal saline, and replacing the precut gauze dressing as necessary to keep the surrounding skin dry and encourage further drainage. An absorbent dressing is placed over the drain and gauze (not shown).

Wound suction devices promote drainage of fluid from the incision site, decreasing pressure on healing tissues and reducing abscess formation. Shown are the Jackson-Pratt and Hemovac wound suction devices (see figures B and C).

The frequency with which the nurse empties the device depends on the time elapsed since surgery, type of surgery, amount of drainage, and hospital policy. For example, immediately after surgery the nurse may empty the device every 15 to 60 minutes. With time, as drainage decreases, the device is emptied every 2 to 4 hours (per hospital policy). Care is taken to maintain asepsis when emptying suction devices, avoiding contamination of the drain or the drain plug. Amount, color, consistency, and odor of drainage are documented. Usually, the drain is removed on the second to fourth day after surgery. Removal causes minor patient discomfort. The drain site is cleaned, superglue may be applied to the hole, and a sterile dressing is applied.

Wound drainage devices. *A,* Penrose passive wound drainage device. *B,* Jackson-Pratt wound suction device. *C,* Hemovac wound suction device.

- Maintain the patient's hydration and nutritional status.
- Culture the wound prior to beginning antibiotic therapy.
- Administer antibiotics and antipyretics as prescribed.
- Provide supportive measures to patient and family.

Dehiscence is a separation in the layers of the incisional wound (Figure 4–6A ■). Treatment depends on the extent of wound disruption. If the dehiscence is extensive, the incision must be resutured in surgery. **Evisceration** is the protrusion of body organs from a wound dehiscence (Figure 4–6B). These serious complications may result from delayed wound healing or may occur immediately following surgery. They also may occur after forceful straining (coughing, sneezing, or vomiting). When dehiscence occurs, immediately cover the wound with a sterile dressing moistened with normal saline. Emergency surgery is performed to repair these conditions.

Either the nurse, physician, physician assistant (PA), or nurse practitioner (NP) removes sutures or staples after the wound has healed sufficiently (usually 5 to 10 days after surgery). Removal is performed using medical aseptic technique. Additional support may be provided to the incision by applying strips of tape (or Steri-Strips) as directed by institutional policy or by the physician.

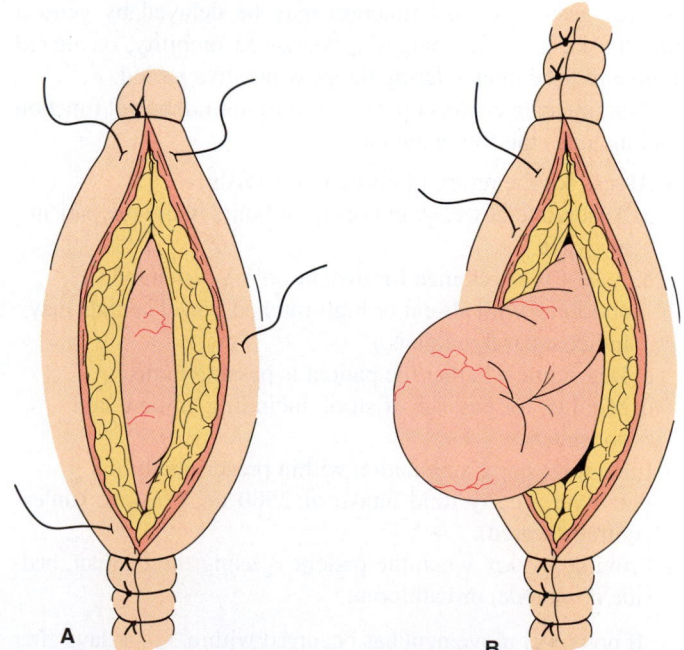

Figure 4–6 ■ Wound complications. *A,* Dehiscence is a disruption in the incision resulting in a separation of the layers of the wound. *B,* Evisceration is a protrusion of a body organ through a surgical incision.

Complications Associated with Elimination

Common postoperative complications associated with elimination include urinary retention and altered bowel elimination. The inability to urinate with urinary retention may occur postoperatively as a result of the recumbent position, effects of anesthesia and narcotics, inactivity, altered fluid balance, nervous tension, or surgical manipulation in the pelvic area. Nursing care centers on promoting normal urinary elimination and includes the following measures:

- Assess for bladder distention if the patient has not voided within 7 to 8 hours after surgery or if the patient is urinating small amounts frequently.
- Assess the amount of urine in the bladder with a portable ultrasound scanner. This noninvasive procedure provides information to prevent unnecessary catheterization and decreases the potential for urinary tract infections and urethral trauma from repeated catheterizations.
- Monitor intake and output.
- Maintain intravenous infusion if fluids are prescribed.
- Increase daily oral fluid intake to 2500 to 3000 mL if the patient's condition permits.
- Insert a straight or indwelling catheter if ordered.
- Promote normal urinary elimination by
  a. assisting and providing privacy when the patient uses a bedpan.
  b. helping the patient use the bedside commode or walk to the bathroom.
  c. assisting male patients to stand to void.
  d. pouring a measured amount of warm water over the perineal area. (If urination occurs, subtract the amount of water from the total amount for an accurate output measurement.)

Bowel elimination frequently is altered after abdominal or pelvic surgery and sometimes after other surgeries. Return to normal gastrointestinal function may be delayed by general anesthesia, narcotic analgesia, decreased mobility, or altered fluid and food intake during the perioperative period.

Nursing care centers on the return of normal bowel function and includes the following measures:

- Assess for the return of normal peristalsis:
  a. Auscultate bowel sounds every 4 hours while the patient is awake.
  b. Assess the abdomen for distention. (A distended abdomen with absent or high-pitched bowel sounds may indicate paralytic ileus.)
  c. Determine whether the patient is passing flatus.
  d. Monitor for passage of stool, including amount and consistency.
- Encourage early ambulation within prescribed limits.
- Facilitate a daily fluid intake of 2500 to 3000 mL (unless contraindicated).
- Provide privacy when the patient is using the bedpan, bedside commode, or bathroom.

If no bowel movement has occurred within 3 to 4 days after surgery, a suppository or an enema may be ordered.

Special Considerations for Older Adults

Physiologic, cognitive, and psychosocial changes associated with the aging process place the older adult at increased risk for postoperative complications. These age-related changes with selected nursing interventions are summarized in Table 4–6. With an ever-increasing population of older adults, particularly the very old, the nurse must be aware of these normal changes and modify nursing care accordingly in an effort to provide safe, supportive care.

Managing Acute Postoperative Pain

Pain is expected after surgery. It is neither realistic nor practical to eliminate postoperative pain completely. Nevertheless, the patient should receive substantial relief from and control of this discomfort and experience minimal "analgesic gaps: periods of ineffective pain relief" (Polomano et al., 2008, p. S44). Controlling postoperative pain not only promotes comfort but also facilitates coughing, turning, deep-breathing exercises, earlier ambulation, and decreased length of hospitalization, resulting in fewer postoperative complications, and therefore reducing healthcare costs. Despite the apparent benefits and methods of effective pain control and improved understanding of pain physiology, many postoperative patients do not receive adequate pain relief or control (MacLellan, 2004).

Managing acute postoperative pain is an important nursing role before, during, and after surgery. Successful pain management involves the cooperative efforts of the patient, physician, and nurse. The American Society of Anesthesiologists suggests six specific guidelines for perioperative pain management. These include education and training for healthcare providers, monitoring of patient outcomes, 24-hour availability of anesthesiologists providing perioperative pain management, and use of a dedicated acute pain service. Preoperatively, the patient should learn how much pain to anticipate and what methods are available to control pain. After discussing options with the patient, healthcare providers must respect the patient's personal preferences.

Postoperative medications were discussed earlier in the chapter. Various nonpharmacologic approaches to pain management are used alone or in combination to control acute postoperative pain. Relaxation, music, distraction, and imagery techniques can decrease mild pain and anxiety. Massage and the application of heat or cold can also relieve postoperative pain. Transcutaneous electrical nerve stimulation (TENS) has been used successfully to decrease postoperative incisional pain. Other approaches include acupuncture, acupressure, and therapeutic touch. Additional information on pain management techniques is found in ∞ Chapter 9.

Opioid dosage requirements vary greatly from one patient to another and by the route they are taken. Remember that oral doses of analgesics are not equal to parenteral doses. Oral doses need to be higher to provide **equianalgesia**. (See Table 9–3 for equianalgesic doses.)

The patient's input and participation in assessing pain and pain relief is essential to a successful pain control regime. For example, the patient can rate the pain on a scale of 0 to 10

TABLE 4–6 Nursing Interventions for Older Surgical Patients

SYSTEM	AGE-RELATED CHANGES	NURSING INTERVENTIONS
General appearance	Change in height, weight, and fat distribution	Assess physical parameters. Provide for warmth. Turn frequently.
Integument	Diminished integrity secondary to loss of subcutaneous fat and decreased oil production, elasticity, and hydration	Provide careful preoperative preparation to avoid trauma. Avoid shaving. Assess oxygenation and hydration by evaluation of mucous membranes, laboratory studies, and urine output.
Sensory-perceptual	Decline in vision and hearing ability; dryness of mouth	Compensate for sensory deficits: speak low, not loud; minimize noise in environment; provide adequate room light; stay within patient's field of vision when speaking; encourage patient to wear hearing aid to the operating room. Whenever possible, do not remove dentures or glasses. Provide comfort measures when NPO.
Respiratory	Decreased efficiency of cough reflex and decreased aeration of lung fields	Teach and encourage coughing and diaphragmatic breathing exercises. Assess baseline parameters. Constantly monitor lung sounds and respiratory status.
Cardiovascular	Less efficient, decreased adaptation to stress	Monitor for hypotension and shock. Assess for thrombus formation, cardiac dysrhythmias, peripheral pulses, and edema.
Gastrointestinal	Decline in gastric motility	Encourage intake of adequate fluids, nutritious meals, soft diet. Assist with feeding; monitor bowel function.
Genitourinary	Decreased efficiency of kidney; loss of bladder control	Monitor I&O and electrolyte levels. Assess for drug side effects. Assist with voiding as needed.
Musculoskeletal	Stiffness of joints; decrease in strength; brittleness of bones	Carefully position on OR table. Move carefully and gently. Prevent pressure sores.
Cognitive-psychosocial	Decreased reaction time; stable intellectual ability; proneness to delirium and altered mental status while in hospital	Provide ample time for making decisions. Implement safety measures. Talk to patient as adult, not as child. Unique to older adults, fear of increasing dependency on others. Orient frequently.

Reprinted from *AORN Journal*, Vol. 83, No. 3, Judith L. Clayton, "Special Needs of Older Adults Undergoing Surgery," p 557–574, © 2008, Association of periOperative Registered Nurses, with permission from Elsevier.

(where 0 signifies no pain and 10 signifies unbearable pain). Assess and document pain at scheduled intervals to determine the degree of pain control, to observe for drug side effects, and to assess the need for changes in the dosage and/or frequency of medication administration. When a range of dosage is ordered, carefully titrate opioid dosages based on individual assessments of need and response to therapy.

Using NANDA, NIC, and NOC

Linkages between a selected NANDA nursing diagnosis, NIC, and NOC for the postoperative patient are shown in the chart that follows.

Community-Based Care

Because the postoperative phase does not end until the patient has recovered completely from the surgical intervention, the nurse plays a vital role as the patient nears discharge. As the patient prepares to recuperate at home, provide information and support to help the patient successfully meet self-care demands. All aspects of teaching should be accompanied by written guidelines, directions, and information. This is

NANDA, NIC, AND NOC LINKAGES
The Postoperative Patient

NANDA — Acute Pain

NIC — Medication Administration
Patient-Controlled Analgesia
(PCA) Assistance
Pain Management
Postanesthesia Care

NOC — Pain Level
Pain Control
Symptom Control

Data from NANDA International. (2009). *Nursing diagnoses: Definitions & classification 2009–2011.* Oxford, UK: Wiley-Blackwell; Bulechek, G. M., Butcher, H. K., & Dochterman, J. M. (Eds.). (2008). *Nursing Interventions Classification (NIC)* (5th ed.). St. Louis, MO: Mosby; and Moorhead, S., Johnson, M., Maas, M., & Swanson, E. (Eds.). (2008). *Nursing Outcomes Classification (NOC)* (4th ed.). St. Louis, MO: Mosby.

CASE STUDY & NURSING CARE PLAN   A Patient Having Surgery

Martha Overbeck is a 74-year-old widow of German descent who lives alone in a senior citizens' housing complex. She is active there, as well as in the Lutheran Church. She has been in good health and is independent, but she has become progressively less active as a result of arthritic pain and stiffness. Mrs. Overbeck has degenerative joint changes that have particularly affected her right hip. On the recommendation of her physician and following a discussion with her friends, Mrs. Overbeck has been admitted to the hospital for an elective right total hip replacement. Her surgery has been scheduled for 8:00 AM the following day.

Mrs. Eva Jackson, a close friend and neighbor, accompanies Mrs. Overbeck to the hospital. Mrs. Overbeck explains that her friend will help in her home and assist her with the wound care and prescribed exercises.

ASSESSMENT

Gloria Nobis, RN, is assigned to Mrs. Overbeck's care on return to her room. Ms. Nobis performs a complete head-to-toe assessment and determines that Mrs. Overbeck is drowsy but oriented. Her skin is pale and slightly cool. Mrs. Overbeck states she is cold and requests additional covers. Ms. Nobis places a warmed cotton blanket next to Mrs. Overbeck's body, adds another blanket to her covers, and adjusts the room's thermostat to increase the room temperature. Mrs. Overbeck states that she is in no pain and would like to sleep. She has even, unlabored respirations and stable vital signs as compared to preoperative readings.

Mrs. Overbeck is NPO. An intravenous solution of dextrose and water is infusing at 100 mL/h per infusion pump. No redness or edema is noted at the infusion site. Ms. Nobis notes that the antibiotic ciprofloxacin hydrochloride (Cipro) is to be administered by mouth when the patient is able to tolerate fluids. Mrs. Overbeck has a large gauze dressing over her right upper lateral thigh and hip with no indications of drainage from the wound. Tubing protrudes from the distal end of the dressing and is attached to a passive suctioning device (Hemovac). Ms. Nobis empties 50 mL of dark red drainage from the suctioning device and records the amount and characteristics on a flow record. Mrs. Overbeck has a Foley catheter in place with 250 mL of clear, light amber urine in the dependent gravity drainage bag.

When assessing Mrs. Overbeck's lower extremities, Ms. Nobis finds her feet slightly cool and pale with rapid capillary refill time bilaterally. Dorsalis pedis and posterior tibial pulses are strong and equal bilaterally. Ms. Nobis notes slight pitting edema in the right foot and ankle as compared with the left extremity. She also notes sensation and ability to move both feet and toes, without numbness or tingling (paresthesia).

Ms. Nobis records these findings on a postoperative flowsheet. After ensuring that Mrs. Overbeck is safely positioned and can reach her call light, Ms. Nobis gives Mrs. Overbeck's friend, Mrs. Jackson, a progress report. They then go into Mrs. Overbeck's room.

DIAGNOSES

Ms. Nobis makes the following postoperative nursing diagnoses for Mrs. Overbeck:

- *Risk for Infection* of right hip wound related to disruption of normal skin integrity by the surgical incision
- *Risk for Injury* related to potential dislocation of right hip prosthesis secondary to total hip replacement
- *Pain* related to right hip incision and positioning of arthritic joints during surgery
- *Risk for Impaired Physical Mobility* related to right hip wound

EXPECTED OUTCOMES

The expected outcomes established in the plan of care specify that Mrs. Overbeck will

- regain skin integrity of the right hip incision without experiencing signs or symptoms of infection.

- demonstrate (along with Mrs. Jackson) proper aseptic technique while performing the dressing change.
- verbalize signs and symptoms of infection to be reported to her physician.
- describe measures to be taken to prevent dislocation of right hip prosthesis.
- report control of pain at incision and in arthritic joints.
- remain afebrile.
- remain free of complications related to immobility such as respiratory obstruction, muscle weakness, urinary retention, constipation, and disorientation.

PLANNING AND IMPLEMENTATION

Ms. Nobis develops a care plan that includes the following interventions to assist Mrs. Overbeck during her postoperative recovery:

- Use aseptic technique while changing dressing.
- Monitor temperature and pulse every 4 hours to assess for elevation.
- Assist to change positions frequently (q2h) and cough and deep breathe. Assist with early ambulation.
- Assess wound every 8 hours for purulent drainage and odor. Assess edges of wound for approximation, edema, redness, or inflammation in excess of expected inflammatory response.
- Teach Mrs. Overbeck and Mrs. Jackson how to use aseptic technique while assessing the wound and performing the dressing change.
- Teach Mrs. Overbeck and Mrs. Jackson the signs and symptoms of infection and when to report findings to the physician.
- Review and discuss with Mrs. Overbeck the written materials on total hip replacement.
- Convey empathetic understanding of Mrs. Overbeck's incisional and arthritic joint pain.
- Medicate Mrs. Overbeck every 4 hours (or as ordered) to maintain a therapeutic analgesic blood level.

EVALUATION

Throughout Mrs. Overbeck's hospitalization, Ms. Nobis works with Mrs. Overbeck and Mrs. Jackson to ensure that Mrs. Overbeck can care for herself after discharge from the hospital. Five days after her surgery, Mrs. Overbeck is discharged with a well-approximated incision with no indications of an infection. Prior to discharge, Ms. Nobis is confident that with Mrs. Jackson's help Mrs. Overbeck can properly assess the incision. With minimal help, Mrs. Overbeck is able to replace the dressing using aseptic technique. She can cite the signs and symptoms of an infection, take her own oral temperature, and describe preventive measures to decrease the chances of dislocating her prosthetic hip. Because of her reduced mobility the past 5 days, Mrs. Overbeck says she can tell the arthritis in her "old bones" is "acting up." She reports less pain in her right hip than before the surgery. Mrs. Overbeck tells Ms. Nobis she will be back the following winter to have her left hip replaced.

CRITICAL THINKING IN THE NURSING PROCESS

1. Describe risk factors for Mrs. Overbeck's safety. What changes in her home environment would you suggest to promote safety until she recovers more fully?
2. Why is Mrs. Overbeck placed on the antibiotic Cipro although she has no indications of an infection? What teaching would you do?
3. Mrs. Overbeck's clotting time is slightly elevated as a result of an ordered anticoagulant. Why would this medication be ordered? Consider the patient's age and the area of surgery.
4. Mrs. Overbeck is 30 pounds above her ideal weight and has osteoarthritis. Develop a care plan for the nursing diagnosis *Ineffective Health Maintenance* related to intake in excess of metabolic requirements.

See Evaluating Your Response in Appendix C.

particularly helpful when a large amount of unfamiliar, detailed information is presented. Because the hospital stay is often brief, make an organized, coordinated effort to educate the patient and family. Teaching needs vary, but the most common needs include the following:

- How to perform wound care. Teaching is more effective if the nurse first demonstrates and explains the procedure for the patient and family or other caregiver. The patient and family should then participate in the care. To evaluate the effectiveness of the teaching, ask the patient or caregiver to demonstrate the procedure in return. Ideally, teaching is carried out over several days, evaluated, and periodically reinforced.

- Signs and symptoms of a wound infection. The patient should be able to determine what is normal and what should be reported to the physician.
- Method and the frequency of taking one's temperature.
- Limitations or restrictions that may be imposed on such activities as lifting, driving, bathing, sexual activity, and other physical activities.
- Control of pain. If analgesics are prescribed, instruct the patient in the dosage, frequency, purpose, common side effects, and other side effects to report to the physician. Reinforce the use of relaxation, distraction, imagery, or other pain control techniques that the patient has found useful in controlling postoperative pain.

CHAPTER HIGHLIGHTS

- Surgeries take place in traditional and nontraditional settings with increasing use of minimally invasive procedures that expedite discharge, facilitate healing, and increase patient satisfaction.
- Surgery is an invasive procedure and legal guidelines must be followed to protect the patient and the healthcare providers. The surgical team includes surgeons, anesthetists, nurses, and technicians; all are responsible for the safety of the patient and the progression of the surgery.
- The focus on safety during surgery continues to increase with attention directed to preventing wrong site and wrong patient surgeries (using the Universal Protocol), surgical site infections, DVT and PE, and adverse cardiac events. A team approach to safety works best; each member of the team must feel accountable for the results of the surgery and entitled to share observations and concerns as the procedure progresses.
- Inpatients have relatively short stays. Providing information for self-care is challenging with the shortened stays and rate of admissions and discharges. From the time of entry to the surgical setting, the patient's discharge must be planned and prepared.
- Patient teaching prior to and following surgery empowers patients to achieve successful recovery, discharge, and rehabilitation. Most of the care patients receive during healing is either provided by self or a caregiver outside the healthcare environment. Patients and their families need to know appropriate

assessments and interventions to monitor the healing process and contact information for additional help.
- Pain management is offered prior to, during, and after surgery with methods designed to give the best therapeutic response. While acute pain occurs related to the surgery, many patients also experience chronic pain that affects their response to pain management therapies.
- Behaviors characteristic of older adult patients and ethnically diverse populations increase the need for individualized care. Assessment of physical and emotional status can be more difficult when patients have hearing or visual impairments or when individuals speak and understand a foreign language. Surgery can be frightening to patients and their families and they need reassurance and interventions to decrease pain, relieve anxiety, and promote healing.
- Operating room and postanesthesia care nursing are professional specialties that require unique orientation and education. These professionals make careful assessments of the risks each patient faces and make plans to ensure safe, successful surgical outcomes. Special attention is focused on early recognition and treatment of postoperative complications associated with cardiopulmonary function, respiratory function, wound healing, elimination, and pain.

TEST YOURSELF NCLEX-RN® REVIEW

1. The nurse's primary responsibility related to informed consent is which of the following?
   1. defining the risks and benefits of the surgery
   2. witnessing the patient's signature on the consent form
   3. explaining the right to refuse treatment or withdraw consent
   4. advising the patient and family about what is needed for the diagnosis
2. Given shorter hospital stays for outpatient surgery, patients require which of the following?
   1. increased opioid doses
   2. increased information about complications
   3. increased attention to nutrition
   4. increased parenteral hydration

3. Nonsteroidal anti-inflammatory drugs are given in the postoperative period to do which of the following?
   1. stimulate appetite
   2. increase amnesia
   3. potentiate analgesia
   4. improve renal function
4. When reviewing a preoperative patient's chart, the nurse notes some abnormal findings. Which abnormal finding may indicate renal impairment?
   1. decreased hemoglobin
   2. increased chloride
   3. decreased glucose
   4. increased creatinine

5. In the immediate postoperative period for knee surgery, neurovascular concern is raised if which of the following is found distal to the site?
   1. bounding pedal pulse
   2. muscle cramps in the foot
   3. redness or swelling in the calf
   4. skin that is cool to the touch

6. What would the nurse do postoperatively about medications prescribed prior to surgery?
   1. continue after surgery
   2. decrease by half for 36 hours
   3. order anew prior to administration
   4. withhold until evidence of anesthesia is absent

7. A nurse is preparing a patient with diabetes mellitus for surgery. The patient is NPO prior to surgery. What would the nurse consider about this patient?
   1. has no risk for hyperglycemia
   2. should receive sliding-scale insulin prescriptions
   3. will benefit from hypoglycemia during anesthesia
   4. will fail to manifest signs of hypoglycemia under anesthesia

8. Acute pain management medications in the immediate postoperative period generally do which of the following?
   1. progress from NSAIDs to opioids
   2. progress from oral to parenteral routes
   3. are scheduled rather than prn to promote control
   4. induce a strong sedative effect to decrease the risk of nausea

9. What risks for the older adult patient are posed from lengthy operative procedures?
   1. memory loss due to blood loss
   2. hearing loss due to extended anesthesia
   3. weight loss due to lack of nutritional intake
   4. pressure sores and joint pain from operative positioning

10. A nurse working in the PACU would know that hypothermia in the perioperative period has what effect?
    1. decreases cardiac ischemia
    2. reduces the risk for wound infection
    3. increases patient comfort and analgesia
    4. is associated with cardiac morbidity and surgical bleeding

See Test Yourself answers in Appendix C.

Pearson Nursing Student Resources

Find additional review materials at
www.nursing.pearsonhighered.com
Prepare for success with additional NCLEX®-style practice questions, interactive assignments and activities, Web links, animations and videos, and more!

BIBLIOGRAPHY

American Society for Pain Management Nursing and the American Pain Society. (2010). Consensus statement: The use of "as needed" range orders for opioid analgesics in the management of acute pain. Retrieved from http://www.ampainsoc.org/advocacy/opiods2.htm

Andersen, B. R., Kallehave, F. L., & Andersen, H. K. (2005). Antibiotics versus placebo for prevention of postoperative infection after appendectomy (Review). *The Cochrane Database of Systematic Reviews, 4.*

AORN. (2010). *Perioperative standards and recommended practices.* Denver, CO: AORN, Inc.

AORN Journal. (2007). AORN Guidelines for prevention of venous stasis. *AORN Journal, 85,* 607–614; 616–624.

Asher, M. E. (2004). Surgical considerations in the elderly. *Journal of Perianesthesia Nursing, 19*(6), 406–414.

Belkin, N. L. (2006). Masks, barriers, laundering, and gloving: Where is the evidence? *AORN, 84*(4), 655–657; 660–664.

Berry, D., Wick, C., & Magons, P. (2008). A Clinical Evaluation of the cost and time effectiveness of the ASPAN Hypothermia Guideline. *Journal of PeriAnesthesia Nursing 23*(1), 24–35.

Bhattacharyya, T., Yeon, H., & Harris, M. B. (2005). The medical-legal aspects of informed consent in orthopaedic surgery. *The Journal of Bone and Joint Surgery, 87A*(11), 2395–2400.

Brandom, B. W. (2005). The genetics of malignant hyperthermia. *Anesthesiology Clinics of North America, 23,* 615–619.

Bratzler, D. W., & Houck, P. M. (2005). Surgical Infection Prevention Guideline Writers Workgroup. Antimicrobial prophylaxis for surgery: An advisory statement from the National Surgical Infection Prevention Project. *American Journal of Surgery, 189*(4), 395–404.

Brendle, T. A. (2007). Surgical Care Improvement Project and the perioperative nurse's role. *AORN Journal, 86*(1), 94–95; 97–101.

Bressler, R. (2005). Herb-drug interactions: Interactions between Kava and prescription medications. *Geriatrics, 60*(9), 24–25.

Byme, M. (2006). Special needs populations: Patients in poverty. *AORN, 84*(5), 837–839.

Carter-Templeton, H. (2005). Malignant hyperthermia. *Nursing, 35*(6), 88.

Cawley, Y. (2008). Mechanical thromboprophylaxis in the perioperative setting. *MedSurg Nursing 17*(3), 177–182.

Clayton, J. L. (2008). Special needs of older adults undergoing surgery. *AORN, 87*(3), 557–570.

Cohen, M. J., & Schecter, W. P. (2005). Perioperative pain control: A strategy for management. *Surgical Clinics of North America, 85,* 1243–1257.

Daniels, S. M. (2007). Protecting patients from harm: Improving hospital care for surgical patients. *Nursing 2007, 37*(8), 36–42.

D'Arcy, Y. (2008). First strike: Does preemptive analgesia work? *Nursing, 38*(4), 52–55.

Fanning, J., Fenton, B, & Purohit, M. (2008). Robotic radical hysterectomy. *American Journal of Obstetrics & Gynecology, 198,* 649.e1–649e1.

Francis, P. & Winifield, H.N. Medical robotics: The impact on perioperative nursing practice. *Urology Nursing, 26*(2), 99–108.

Giannelli, S. V., Patel, K. V., Windham, B. G., Pizzarelli, F., Ferrucci, L., & Guralnik, J. M. (2007). Magnitude of underascertainment of impaired kidney function in older adults with normal serum creatinine. *Journal of the American Geriatrics Society, 55*(6), 816–823.

Gibbs, V. C. (2005). Patient safety practices in the operating room: Correct-site surgery and nothing left behind. *Surgical Clinics of North America, 85,* 1207–1319.

Hassan, Z., & Fahy, B. G. (2005). Anesthetic choices in surgery. *Surgical Clinics of North America, 85,* 1075–1089.

Jackson, S., & Brady, S. (2008). Counting difficulties: Retained instruments, sponges, and needles. *AORN, 87*(2), 315–321.

Lindgren, V. A., & Ames, N. (2005). Caring for patients on mechanical ventilation: What research indicates is best practice. *American Journal of Nursing, 105*(5), 50–60.

Loran, D. B., Hyde, B. R., & Zwischenberger, J. B. (2005). Perioperative management of special populations: The geriatric patient. *Surgical Clinics of North America, 85,* 1259–1266.

MacLellan, K. (2004). Postoperative pain: Strategy for improving patient experiences. *Journal of Advanced Nursing, 46*(2), 179–193.

Majasaari, H., Sarajärvi, A., Koskinen, H., Autere, S., & Paavilainen, E. (2005). Patients' perceptions of emotional support and information provided to family members. *AORN Journal, 81*(5), 1030–1039.

McDonald, D. D., Thomas, G. J., Livingston, K. E., & Severson, J. S. (2005). Assisting older adults to communicate their postoperative pain. *Clinical Nursing Research, 14*(2), 109–126.

Neil, J. A. (2007). Perioperative care of the immunocompromised patient. *AORN Journal, 85*(3), 544–560.

Odom-Forren, J. (2006). Preventing surgical site infections. *Nursing, 36*(6), 58–63.

Ogg, M., & Petersen, C. (2007). Clinical issues: surgical hand antisepsis; hand lotions and creams, gel overlays as artificial nails; benchmarking. *AORN Journal, 85*(4), 815–818.

Pagana, K. D., & Pagana, T. J. (2009). *Mosby's manual of diagnostic and laboratory tests* (9th. ed.). St. Louis, MO: Mosby.

Phillips, N. (2007). *Berry & Kohn's operating room technique* (11th ed.). St. Louis, MO: Mosby.

Polomano, R. C., Rathmell, J. P., Krenzischek, D. A., & Dunwoody, C. J. (2008). Emerging trends and new approaches to acute pain management. *Journal of PeriAnesthesia Nursing (23)*1a, 843–853.

Porth, C. M. (2007). *Essentials of Pathophysiology: Concepts of altered health states* (2nd ed.). Philadelphia: Lippincott Williams & Wilkins.

Porth, C. M., & Matfin, G. (2009). *Pathophysiology: Concepts of altered health states.* (8th ed.). Philadelphia: Lippincott Williams & Wilkins.

Rahman, M. H., & Beattie, J. (2004). Medication in the perioperative period. *The Pharmaceutical Journal, 272,* 287–289.

Saber, W. (2006). Perioperative medication management: a case-based review of general principles. *Cleveland Clinic Journal of Medicine, 73,* S1, S82–S87.

Saper, R. B. (2005). *Overview of herbal medicine.* UpToDate online. Retrieved January 9, 2006, from http://www.uptodate.com

Schwartz, A. J. (2006). Learning the essentials of epidural anesthesia. *Nursing, 36*(1), 44–50.

Silber, J. H., Rosenbaum, P. R., Trudeau, M. E., Chen, W., Zhang, X., Lorch, S. A., et al. (2005). Preoperative antibiotics and mortality in the elderly. *Annals of Surgery, 242*(1), 107–114.

The Joint Commission (2009). The Universal Protocol. Retrieved from www.jointcommission.org/PatientSafety/UniversalProtocol/

The Joint Commission. (2008). 2009 National Patient Safety Goals. Accreditation Program: Hospital, 01.01.01. Retrieved September, 6 2008, from http://www.jointcommission.org/NR/rdonlyres/31666E86-E7F4-423E-9BE8-F05BD1CB0AA8/0/HAP_NPSG.pdf

Washington, G. T., & Matney, J. L. (2007). Comparison of temperature measurement devices in post anesthesia patients. *Journal of PeriAnesthesia Nursing, 23*(1), 36–348.

Weirich, T. L. (2008). Hypothermia/warming protocols: Why are they not widely used in the OR? *AORN, 87*(2), 333–344.

Zide, B. M. (2005). Seven more tips for the operating room. *Plastic & Reconstructive Surgery, 115*(3), 973–975.

Nursing Care of Patients Experiencing Loss, Grief, and Death

LEARNING OUTCOMES

1. Compare and contrast theories of loss and grief.
2. Explain factors affecting responses to loss.
3. Explain the physiologic basis for manifestations associated with the end of life.
4. Discuss legal and ethical issues in end-of-life care.
5. Describe the philosophy and activities of hospice and palliative care.

CLINICAL COMPETENCIES

1. Identify physiological changes in the dying patient.
2. Use assessments, patient values, and evidence to provide nursing interventions to promote a comfortable and dignified death.
3. Effectively communicate with and function within the interdisciplinary team to plan and provide individualized care for patients and families experiencing loss, grief, or death.
4. Adapt individual and cultural values and variations, as well as expressed needs and preferences, into the plan of care for patients and families experiencing loss, grief, or death.

KEY TERMS

advance directives, *92*
bereavement, *93*
chronic sorrow, *98*
death, *87*
death anxiety, *98*
do-not-resuscitate order, *92*

durable power of attorney, *92*
end-of-life, *91*
euthanasia, *92*
grief, *86*
grieving, *86*
healthcare surrogate, *92*

hospice, *92*
living will, *92*
loss, *86*
mourning, *86*
palliative care, *93*

Loss may be defined as an actual or potential situation in which a valued object, person, body part, or emotion that was formerly present is lost or changed and can no longer be seen, felt, heard, known, or experienced. A loss may be temporary or permanent, complete or partial, objectively verifiable or perceived, physical or symbolic. Only the person who experiences the loss can determine the meaning of the loss. Although the order of importance varies with the person, people most commonly fear the losses listed in Box 5–1.

Loss always results in change. The stress associated with the loss may be the precipitating factor leading to physiologic or psychologic change in the person or family. The effective or ineffective resolution of feelings surrounding the loss determines the person's ability to deal with the resulting changes.

BOX 5–1 Types of Losses

- Death
- Health
- Body part
- Social status
- Lifestyle
- Marital relationship (i.e., through divorce)
- Reproductive function
- Sexual function

There are many different types of loss, with responses to the loss individualized within each person. This chapter considers loss from both a general and from a specific focus. There is, within the chapter, a greater emphasis on loss from death, as this is often a difficult situation because nurses care for the person who is dying and also for the people who are left to experience the loss. Some of the terms that are used throughout the chapter are introduced in the following paragraphs.

Grief is the emotional response to loss and its accompanying changes. Grief as a response to loss is an inevitable dimension of the human experience. The loss of a job, a role (e.g., the loss of the role of spouse, as occurs in divorce), a goal, body integrity, a loved one, or the impending loss of one's own life or a loved one's life may trigger grief. Although death is the ultimate loss, losses that occur in any phase of the life cycle may produce grief responses as intensely painful as those observed in the death experience.

Grieving may be thought of as the internal process the person uses to work through the response to loss. **Mourning** describes the actions or expressions of the bereaved, including the symbols, clothing, and ceremonies that make up the outward manifestations of grief. Both grieving and mourning are healthy responses to loss because they ultimately lead the person to invest energy in new relationships and to develop positive self-regard.

Death is defined in many ways. One commonly used definition of death is an irreversible cessation of circulatory and respiratory functions or irreversible cessation of all functions of the entire brain, including the brainstem. With the current life-support systems available, the most often used criterion for determining death is whole-brain death (permanent irreversible cessation of the functioning of all areas of the brain). The criteria for whole-brain death are listed in ∞ Chapter 11.

Although death is an inevitable part of life, it is often an immensely difficult loss for the person who is dying and for his or her loved ones. Death may be accidental (for example, from trauma), purposeful (from suicide), occur suddenly or at the end of a long and painful struggle with a terminal illness such as cancer or AIDS, or be the natural end of the aging process.

Theories of Loss, Grief, and Dying

Medical-surgical nurses often care for patients exhibiting responses typical of various stages of the grieving process. Highly individual in quality and duration, the grief process may range from discomforting to debilitating, and it may last a day or a lifetime, depending on what the loss means to the person experiencing it. Although each person experiences loss in a different manner, knowledge of some of the major theories of loss, grief, and dying can give the nurse a framework for holistic care of the patient and family anticipating or experiencing a loss. Table 5–1 summarizes these theories.

Freud: Psychoanalytic Theory

Freud (1917, 1957) wrote about grief and mourning as reactions to loss. Freud described the process of mourning as one in which the person gradually withdraws attachment from the lost object or person. He observed that with normal grieving, this withdrawal of attachment is followed by a readiness to make new attachments. In comparing melancholia (prolonged gloominess, depression) with the "normal" emotions of grief and its expression in mourning, Freud observed that the "work of mourning" is a nonpathologic condition that reaches a state of completion after a period of inner labor.

Bowlby: Attachment Theory

Bowlby (1973, 1980) believed that the grieving process initiated by a loss or separation from a loved object or person successfully ends when the grieving person experiences feelings of emancipation from the lost object or person. He divided the grieving process into three phases and identified behaviors characteristic of each phase.

- *Protest.* The protest phase is marked by a lack of acceptance of the loss. All energy is directed toward protesting the loss. The person experiences feelings of anger toward self and others, and feelings of ambivalence toward the lost object or person. Crying and angry behaviors characterize this phase.
- *Despair.* The person's behavior becomes disorganized. Despair mounts as efforts to deny the loss compete with acceptance of permanent loss. Crying and sadness, coupled with a desire for the lost object or person to return, result in disorganized thoughts as the patient recognizes the reality of the loss.
- *Detachment.* As the person realizes the permanence of the loss and gradually relinquishes attachment to the lost object, a reinvestment of energy occurs. Both the positive and negative aspects of the relationship are remembered. Expressions of hopefulness and readiness to move forward are characteristic of this phase.

Bolby's theory was used as a base for a "continuing bonds" theory, developed by Field, Gao, and Paderna (2005). This theory poses the belief that mourners of loved ones lost by death continue to have memories of the deceased, feel their presence, and save meaningful belongings. These actions bring comfort to the bereaved, and allow a new relationship to form with those lost by death. As a result the mourners resolve their grief and accept the loss.

Engel: Acute Grief, Restitution, and Long-Term Grief

Engel (1964) related the grief process to other methods of coping with stress: After the person perceives and evaluates the loss (the stressful event), the person adapts to it. Engel's recognition of the effect of cognitive factors on the grieving process was an important contribution to the understanding of grieving. The acute stage is initiated by shock and disbelief and may be manifested by denial, which in turn may help the person to cope with the overwhelming pain. As the shock and disbelief begin to fade the loss becomes a reality, and pain, anguish, anger, guilt, and blame surface. Culturally patterned behaviors, such as maintaining a stoic pose in public or weeping openly, characterize this phase. During restitution friends and family gather to support the grieving person through rituals dictated by their culture. The mourner continues to feel a painful void and is preoccupied with thoughts of the loss. The mourner may join

TABLE 5–1 Summary of Selected Theories of Loss

THEORIST	DYNAMICS
Freud	Grief and mourning are reactions to loss. Grieving is the inner labor of mourning a loss. Inability to grieve a loss results in depression.
Bowlby	The successful grieving process initiated by a loss or separation during childhood ends with feelings of emancipation from the lost person or object.
Engel	After the person perceives and evaluates the loss, the person adapts to it. Shock and disbelief, developing awareness, and restitution occur during the first year following the loss; in the months following, the person puts the lost relationship into perspective.
Lindemann	A sequence of responses is experienced following a catastrophic event; concepts of anticipatory grieving and morbid grief reactions are defined.
Caplan	Periods of psychologic crisis are precipitated by hazardous circumstances; successful resolution of grief involves feelings of hope and engaging in activities of ordinary living.
Kübler-Ross	Five stages define the response to loss: denial, anger, bargaining, depression, and acceptance. Stages are not necessarily sequential.

a support group or seek other social support for coping with the loss. This stage lasts about one year, after which the mourner begins to come to terms with the loss and interests in people and activities are renewed.

Lindemann: Categories of Symptoms

Lindemann (1944) interviewed people who had lost a loved one during the course of medical treatment, disaster victims, and relatives of members of the armed forces who had died. Lindemann's research led him to describe normal grief, anticipatory grieving, and morbid grief reactions. He described symptoms characteristic of normal grief into categories of somatic (physical symptoms without an organic cause) distress, preoccupation with the image of the deceased, feelings of guilt, hostile reactions, and loss of patterns of conduct.

Anticipatory grieving was defined as a cluster of predictable responses to an anticipated loss. These responses include the range of feelings experienced by the person or family preoccupied with an anticipated loss. The term *morbid grief reaction* described delayed and dysfunctional reactions to loss; a variety of debilitating health problems were seen in people who displayed excessive or delayed responses to loss.

Caplan: Stress and Loss

Caplan's (1990) theory of stress and its relationship to loss is useful in understanding the grief process. He expanded the focus of the grief process to include not only bereavement but also other episodes of stress that people experience, such as may result from surgery or childbirth. Caplan described three factors that influence the person's ability to deal with a loss. He believed these factors might cause distress for a year or more following the loss.

- The psychic pain of the broken bond and the agony of coming to terms with the loss
- Living without the assets and guidance of the lost person or resource
- The reduced cognitive and problem-solving effectiveness associated with the distressing emotional arousal

Caplan described the process of building new attachments to replace those that have been lost as involving two elements: a feeling of hope and the assumption of regular activity as a form of participating in ordinary living.

Kübler-Ross: Stages of Coping with Loss

Kübler-Ross's (1969, 1978) research on death and dying provided a framework for gaining insight about the stages of coping with an impending or actual loss. According to Kübler-Ross, not all people dealing with a loss go through these stages, and those who do may not experience the stages in the sequence described. In identifying the stages of death and dying, Kübler-Ross stressed the danger of prematurely labeling a "stage" and emphasized that her goal was to describe her observations of how people come to terms with situations of loss.

Some or all of the following reactions may occur during the grieving process and may reappear as the person experiences the loss:

- *Denial.* A person may react with shock and disbelief after receiving word of an actual or potential loss. After receiving a terminal diagnosis, notification of a death, or other serious loss, people may make such statements as "This can't be happening to me" or "This can't be true."
- *Anger.* In the anger stage, the person resists the loss. The anger is often directed toward family and healthcare providers.
- *Bargaining.* The bargaining stage serves as an attempt to postpone the reality of the loss. The person makes a secret bargain with God, expressing a willingness to do anything to postpone the loss or change the prognosis.
- *Depression.* The person enters a stage of depression as the full impact of the actual or perceived loss is realized. The person prepares for the impending loss by working through the struggle of separation. While grieving over "what cannot be," the person may either talk freely about the loss or withdraw from others.
- *Acceptance.* The person begins to come to terms with the loss and resumes activities with hopefulness for the future. Some dying people reach a stage of acceptance in which they may appear to be almost devoid of emotion. The struggle is past, and the emotional pain is gone.

Factors Affecting Responses to Loss

A variety of factors affect a person's responses to loss. These include age, social support, families, culture and spiritual practices, and rituals of mourning.

Age

The understanding of and reaction to loss is influenced by the age of the person experiencing the loss. In general, as people experience life transitions, their ability to understand and accept the losses associated with the transitions increases. From the age of 3 years, the development of the concept of death as a loss proceeds rapidly. Table 5–2 outlines the development of the concept of death throughout the life span.

Social Support

Grieving is painful and lonely. One's social support system is important because of its potentially positive influence on the successful resolution of grief. Some losses may lead to social isolation, placing affected people at high risk for dysfunctional grief reactions. For example, partners of people who die with AIDS often report feeling excluded by the deceased person's family and by healthcare providers. Characteristic factors that can interfere with successful grieving include the following:

- Perceived inability to share the loss
- Lack of social recognition of the loss
- Ambivalent relationships prior to the loss
- Traumatic circumstances of the loss

A move, a divorce, or even the death of a pet can cause a person to feel extremely isolated, yet the person experiencing these types of loss does not ordinarily receive the same social support offered to the person mourning the death of a loved one. A woman having an abortion or giving up a child for adoption seldom receives the same social support as the mother of a child who died at birth. It is therefore especially important that

TABLE 5–2 Development of the Concept of Death

AGE	BELIEFS/ATTITUDES ABOUT DEATH
3	Fears separation; lacks comprehension of permanent separation.
3 to 5	Believes death is like sleeping and is reversible.
	Expresses curiosity about what happens to the body.
6 to 10	Understands finality of death.
	Views own death as avoidable.
	Associates death with violence.
	Believes wishes can be responsible for death.
11 to 12	Reflects views of death expressed by parents. Expresses interest in afterlife as an understanding of mortality develops. Recognizes death as irreversible and inevitable.
13 to 21	Usually has a religious and philosophic view of death but seldom thinks about it.
	Views own death as distant or a challenge, acting out defiance through reckless behavior.
	Previously held developmental awareness of death may still be present.
22 to 45	Does not think about death unless confronted with it.
	Emotionally distances self from death.
	Attitude toward death influenced by religious and cultural beliefs.
46 to 65	Experiences the death of parents or friends.
	Accepts own mortality.
	Experiences waves of death anxiety.
	Puts life in order to prepare for death and decrease anxiety.
66 and older	Fears lingering, incapacitating illness. Views death as inevitable but from a philosophical viewpoint, that is, as freedom from pain and illness or as a spiritual reunion with deceased friends and loved ones.

the nurse does not place a value on the patient's loss when assessing the need for support.

The painful nature of grief can cause the patient to withdraw from a previously established social support system, thereby increasing the feelings of loneliness caused by the loss. A recently widowed woman, for example, may refuse invitations involving married couples with whom she had socialized while her husband was alive, even though her needs for social interaction remain similar to those established before the loss.

Families

A well-functioning family usually rallies after the initial shock and disbelief and provides support for each other during all phases of the grieving process. After a loss, the functional family is able to shift roles, levels of responsibility, and ways of communicating. See the Moving Evidence into Action box for research about factors that affect a family member's ability to care for a dying family member at home.

The family may have negative as well as positive effects. For example, the dying patient may request that someone the family perceives as an outsider be near, and the family may respond with anger to the perceived "intrusion." Similarly, certain family members may express hurt feelings or anger if the patient is unresponsive to other family members. Well-meaning family members also may try to shield the patient from the pain of grieving. It is rare for the family and the patient to experience anger, denial, and acceptance in unison. While one member is in denial, another may be angry because "not enough is being done."

Culture and Spiritual Practices

The influence of culture and ethnic identity on communication, family values, and beliefs about and practices related to illness and death are important considerations when providing nursing care. There are countless ethnocultural and religious differences in the way people observe dying, death, and mourning. For example, differences in the way death is expressed in the United States include "passed away," "died peacefully," "departed this life," "went home to be with God," and "passed from this life." Objects, too, express death and death rituals, such as masks, statues, and candles. Examples of religious traditions in mourning and end-of-life rituals (Spector, 2009) include the following:

- *Catholicism:* An obligation to take ordinary, not extraordinary, measures to prolong life. Autopsy and organ donation are acceptable.
- *Islam:* Euthanasia is prohibited. Medical help to prolong life is not sought. The body is washed only by Muslims of the same gender.
- *Judaism:* Neither autopsy nor organ donation is acceptable. The body is ritually washed and burial is as soon as possible. There is a 7-day mourning period.
- *Protestantism:* Organ donation, autopsy, burial, or cremation are individual decisions. Prolonging life many have restrictions.

Spiritual Beliefs

Patients who are dying often ask questions of themselves and others as to what their life has meant, why this illness has affected them, and what will happen to them when they die. They may feel abandoned by God, or worry that their behavior caused the illness resulting in death. These questions and concerns lead to spiritual distress, which if unresolved may lead to hopelessness, anxiety, and depression. When spiritual distress is resolved, the patient can die more peacefully.

The principles, values, personal philosophy, and meaning of life by which the patient has pursued goals and self-actualization may be called into question when the patient responds to an actual or perceived loss. Because of a fear of intruding on the personal spiritual beliefs and practices of the patient, the nurse often feels uncertain about implementing interventions that would be helpful to the patient responding to a loss. The following questions (using the mnemonic device FICA) may be used to assess a patient's spiritual or religious practices (AACN, 2002):

- *Faith:* What is your faith or belief? Do you consider yourself a spiritual or a religious person? Does religious faith or spirituality play an important part in your life? What do you believe gives your life meaning?

MOVING EVIDENCE INTO ACTION   **End-of-Life Care at Home**

Patients who are terminally ill often choose to die at home and are supported in this choice by many healthcare providers as a way to enhance the dying experience for the patient and for his or her family members. This shift to the setting for healthcare as a patient nears the end of life is contingent upon the availability and readiness of members of the family to assume care of the patient at home. Family caregivers become responsible for providing most of the physical and emotional care of the patient, for managing complex care in the home, and for organizing and coordinating health services on behalf of the dying person. Stajduhar, Martin, Barwidh, & Fykes (2008) collected data from family caregivers of home-care patients who were diagnosed with advanced cancer and had a life expectancy of 6 months or less. The themes identified were (1) the caregiver's approach to life (having a "just do it" positive attitude), (2) the patient's illness experience (caregivers coped best when the patient was "doing well"), (3) the patient's recognition of the caregivers' contribution to his or her care (coping was facilitated by patient's recognition and appreciation of caregiving efforts), (4) the quality of the relationship between the caregiver and dying person (caregiving was easier when the relationship was based on mutual love and respect), and (5) the caregiver's sense of security (security in the caregiving role was enhanced by having family and friends to listen and provide hands-on help, access to relevant and timely information, and support from the healthcare system when it was needed).

IMPLICATIONS FOR NURSING

Although this study focused on patients with terminal cancer, the findings are applicable to family caregivers of all patients who require end-of-life care at home. As the population of older

adults increases, so too will the number of people who wish to die at home. Nurses must be able to teach the skills of physical care and the importance of maintaining comfort. It is also important for nurses to know how to help family members learn to talk with the patient about dying and what the patient wants to facilitate a good death. The family caregiver must know that other family members and friends support what is being done and that it is often a difficult and lonely responsibility. Nurses can provide emotional support through referrals for hospice care and spiritual support, and by being available to provide information throughout end-of-life care. Caring for the caregiver of a dying patient is an important nursing role.

CRITICAL THINKING IN PATIENT CARE

1. An older man, dying of advanced lung caner, says, "I just want to go home to die." He has no family living near him. How would you respond?
2. Make a list of teaching topics needed by the daughter of an 83-year-old woman who has had three major strokes and also has Alzheimer's disease. The daughter wants to care for her mother at home during the last days of her life.
3. The wife of a man dying of kidney failure says, "I just can't leave him. I don't need time for myself." What could you say to convince her that she does need time for herself?

Data from Stajduhar, K., Martin, W., Barwidh, D., & Fyles, G. (2008). Factors influencing family caregivers' ability to cope with providing end-of-life cancer care at home. *Cancer Nursing, 31*(1), 77–85.

■ *Influence:* How does your religious faith or spirituality influence your thoughts about health? How does it affect the way that you take care of yourself?

■ *Community:* Do you consider yourself part of a spiritual or religious community or congregation? How is that community or congregation a source of support for you?

■ *Address:* Do you have any special religious or spiritual issues or concerns that you would like me to address with you? Is there someone else you would like to speak to about these matters?

It is often difficult for patients with an incurable illness to maintain hope and a sense that their lives have had meaning. To meet spiritual needs, nurses can help patients accept the uncertainty that comes with their illness and future death, and respect the spiritual beliefs and practices of patients and their families. Patients who are religious need opportunities for prayer, devotions, and religious rituals. Other resources for spirituality include meditation, guided imagery, music, and art. Privacy and space for these activities should be provided without question.

Rituals of Mourning

Through participation in religious ceremonies such as baptism, confirmation, and bat or bar mitzvah, people joyously celebrate progression to a new stage of life and loss of a former way of being. The funeral ceremony serves many of the same purposes in meeting the needs of the bereaved as people gather to share loss. Through the ceremony, people symbolically express

triumph over death and deny the fear of death. Culture is the primary factor that dictates the rituals of mourning. See the Focus on Cultural Diversity feature on page 91, which provides examples of values and rituals for death in selected groups of people.

Nurses' Response to Patients' Loss

Nurses care for patients and families at various stages of the grief process and may feel that crisis situations are not the time for self-reflection. However, because the nurse's conscious or unconscious reactions to the patient's responses to the loss will influence the outcome of any intervention, nurses need to take time to analyze their own feelings and values related to loss and the expression of grief. The nurse can promote self-awareness by reflecting on the following questions:

■ What are my personal feelings about how grief should be expressed?

■ Am I making judgments about the meaning of this loss to the patient?

■ Are unresolved losses in my own life preventing me from relating therapeutically to the patient?

The following Internet resources may be useful in helping nurses provide care to dying patients:

■ Dying Well
■ National Hospice and Palliative Care Organization
■ AARP Grief and Loss Program
■ GriefNet
■ National Resource Center on Diversity at End-of-Life Care

FOCUS ON CULTURAL DIVERSITY
Cultural Aspects of Terminal Illness Care

Culture/Ethnicity	Nursing Considerations
American Indian	Some tribes prefer not to openly discuss terminal prognosis and do-not-resuscitate (DNR) decisions, because negative thoughts may make inevitable loss occur sooner. Suggest a family meeting to discuss care and end-of-life issues. If the family feels comfortable, all members of the family and close friends may remain 24 hours a day (eating, joking, singing). Mourning is done in private, away from the dying person. After death, the family may hug, touch, sing, and stay close to the deceased.
Black/African American	Suggest that the family have a family meeting or talk with a minister or family elder. Patients may decide to have older family member disclose a poor prognosis. Care for the dying family member is often done at home until death is imminent.
Chinese American	Ensure the head of the family is present when terminal illness is discussed. The patient may not want to discuss approaching death. Special amulets or cloths may be brought from home. Family members may prefer to bathe the body after death.
Iranian	Information about a terminal illness should be presented by a trusted member of the healthcare team to the family, and never to the patient when he or she is alone. Most Iranians believe in tagdir (will of God) in life and death as a predestined journey. When death occurs, notify the head of the family first. DNR decisions are often made by the family. The family may want to bathe the body.
Mexican American	Based on the belief that worry may make health worse, the family may want to protect the patient from the seriousness of illness. The information is often handled by an older daughter or son. Extended family members are obligated to pay respects to the sick and dying, although pregnant women do not care for dying persons or attend funerals. The family may prefer the patient die at home. Prayers, amulets, and rosary beads are used, and the priest should be notified. Death is seen as an important spiritual event. The family may bathe the body and spend time with the body.
Vietnamese	Consult head of family before telling patient about a terminal illness. The entire family will make DNR decision, often with assistance from a priest or monk. Patients often prefer to die at home. Family should have extra time with the body, and may cry loudly and uncontrollably. Spiritual/religious rites are often conducted in the room.

Source: Adapted from Lipson, J. G., Dibble, S. L., & Minarik, P. A. (Eds.). (1996). *Culture & nursing care: A pocket guide.* San Francisco: UCSF Nursing Press; Spector, R. E. (2009). *Cultural diversity in health & illness* (7th ed.). Upper Saddle River, N.J.: Prentice Hall Health.

End-of-Life Care

End-of-life (the final weeks of life when death is imminent) nursing care that ensures a peaceful death was mandated by the International Council of Nurses (1997) and further supported by the American Association of Colleges of Nursing (AACN) (1999). Following are selected competencies necessary for nurses to provide high-quality end-of-life care as defined by the AACN (2004).

- Promote the provision of comfort care to the dying as an active, desirable, and important skill, and an integral component of nursing care (Figure 5–1 ■).
- Communicate effectively and compassionately with the patient, family, and healthcare team members about end-of-life issues.
- Recognize one's own attitudes, feelings, values, and expectations about death and the individual, cultural, and spiritual diversity existing in those beliefs and customs.
- Demonstrate respect for the patient's views and wishes during end-of-life care.
- Use scientifically based standardized tools to assess manifestations (e.g., pain, dyspnea, constipation, anxiety, fatigue, nausea/vomiting, and altered cognition) experienced by patients at the end of life.
- Use data from assessment to plan and intervene in symptom management using state-of-the-art traditional and complementary approaches.
- Assist the patient, family, colleagues, and one's self to cope with suffering, grief, loss, and bereavement in end-of-life care.

Figure 5–1 ■ The nurse helps the patient visualize the hospital room as a safe, comfortable place to die by surrounding the patient with familiar pictures and objects.

End of Life Care or Grieving Video

Nursing Considerations for End-of-Life Care

Nurses care for the dying patient in critical care units, emergency rooms, hospital units, long-term care facilities, and the home. Regardless of the setting, the patient's wishes about death should be respected. The Dying Person's Bill of Rights states that each person has "the right to be cared for by caring, sensitive, knowledgeable people who will attempt to understand my needs and will be able to gain some satisfaction in helping me face my death" (Barbus, 1975).

Legal and Ethical Issues

Issues such as those involved in advance directives and living wills, euthanasia, and quality of life are especially important to nurses in upholding the specific care requests of their patients.

Advance Directives

Advance directives are legal documents that allow a person to plan for health care and/or financial affairs in the event of incapacity. They include living wills, healthcare surrogates, and durable power of attorney.

FAST FACTS

Types of Advance Directives

- **Living will**:   A document that provides written directions about life-prolonging procedures to provide instructions when a person can no longer communicate in a life-threatening situation.
- **Healthcare surrogate**:   An individual selected to make medical decisions when a person is no longer able to make them for him- or herself.
- **Durable power of attorney**:   A document that can delegate the authority to make health, financial, and/or legal decisions on a person's behalf. It must be in writing and must state that the designated person is authorized to make healthcare decisions.

A living will is a legal document that formally expresses a person's wishes regarding life-sustaining treatment in the event of terminal illness or permanent unconsciousness. It is not a type of durable power of attorney and usually does not designate a substitute decision maker. It is the responsibility of the nurse as patient advocate to request and record the patient's preference for care and include it in the plan of care. The nurse's documentation helps communicate these preferences to the other members of the healthcare team.

Facilities that receive Medicare and Medicaid funds are required to provide all patients with written information and counseling about advance directives and the institution's policies governing them. The specific terms of this requirement are found in the Patient Self-Determination Act (PSDA). A copy of the signed advance directive must be kept in the patient's medical record, but patients do not have to sign it in order to be treated. Nurses are the ones in close contact with patients, so they are often left with unresolved feelings about the moral, ethical, and legal aspects of their actions. Although advance directives do not ease the pain of seeing patients die, they do help nurses provide patients with the care that the patients have chosen.

Do-Not-Resuscitate Orders

A **do-not-resuscitate order** (DNR, or "no-code") is written by the physician for the patient who has a terminal illness or is near death. This order is based on the wishes of the patient and family that no cardiopulmonary resuscitation be performed for respiratory or cardiac arrest. A "comfort measures only" order indicates that no further life-sustaining interventions are necessary and that the goal of care is a comfortable, dignified death. Agency protocols should be established defining "comfort care" for consistency in nursing care. Confusing or conflicting DNR orders create dilemmas because nurses are involved in resuscitation and either begin CPR or ensure that unwanted attempts do not occur. The American Nurses' Association (ANA) (2004) recommends that the DNR order should be directed by what the informed patient wants or wanted. The ANA further recommends that guidelines and policies be developed to help resolve conflicts between patients and their families, between patients and healthcare professionals, and among healthcare professionals.

Euthanasia

Euthanasia (from the Greek for "painless," "easy," "gentle," or "good death") is now commonly used to signify a killing prompted by some humanitarian motive. There are many arguments for and against euthanasia, and nurses have often found themselves at the center of the debate. As a result, nurses have pushed for the development of appropriate guidelines and procedures for DNR orders. When no such orders exist, the nurse faces a dilemma. Certainly, there are situations in which the nurse's role is clear. For example, it is considered malpractice to participate in "slow codes" (in which the nurse does not hurry to alert the emergency team when a terminally ill patient who does not have a DNR order stops breathing).

The natural death laws seek to preserve the notion of voluntary versus involuntary euthanasia. In voluntary euthanasia, the competent adult patient and a physician, nurse, or adult friend or relative make the decision to terminate life. Involuntary euthanasia ("mercy killing") is performed without the patient's consent. Because care settings offer many complex and technologic interventions, it is not likely that the ethical aspects of euthanasia will soon be resolved. However, advance directives do give patients a much more active role in decisions about their own care.

Settings and Services for End-of-Life Care

Settings and services for end-of-life care range from the critical care unit in a hospital to the patient's own home. Two methods of providing end-of-life care—hospice and palliative care—are described in this section.

Hospice

Hospice is a philosophy of care rather than a program of care. It is comprehensive and coordinated care for patients with limited life expectancy, provided at home, hospitals, and long-term care facilities, that reaffirms the right of every patient and family to fully participate in the final stages of life. Provided by hospice agency nurses and other members of a healthcare team (including social workers, ministers, home health aides, and volunteers), it is based on a philosophy of death with comfort and dignity, encompassing biomedical, psychosocial, and spiritual aspects of the dying experience. Although most hospice care is provided in the home, it may also be provided in hospitals, long-term care facilities, or other community-based settings.

There are more than 3250 hospice agencies in the United States, with services and care reimbursed by private insurance or a Medicare hospice benefit. Services are reimbursed by Medicare for an initial 90-day period, followed by a subsequent 90-day period, and an unlimited number of 60-day periods as long as the patient continues to meet eligibility requirements. The average length of service is 71 days (Hospice Association of America, 2008). Hospice services usually begin when the patient has 6 months or less to live and ends with the family 1 year after the death of the patient. This continuation of care for the family is called bereavement care (**bereavement** is the time of mourning experienced after a loss).

To be eligible for hospice benefits from Medicare or Medicaid, the patient must have a serious, progressive illness with a limited life expectancy. In most cases, a family (or other) caregiver must be continuously in the home with the patient. The patient must have Medicare, waive traditional Medicare benefits for the terminal illness, have physician certification of a terminal illness with a life expectancy of 6 months or less, and care must be provided by a Medicare-certified hospice agency or program. Hospice care under Medicare includes home care, inpatient care when needed, and a variety of services not otherwise covered by Medicare (US Department of Health & Human Services, 2008). The focus is on care, not cure.

Palliative Care

Palliative care is an area of care that has evolved out of the hospice experience, but exists outside of hospice programs, is not restricted to the end of life, and is used earlier in the disease experience. Palliative care, which can be used in all types of healthcare settings, is focused on the relief of physical, mental, and spiritual distress for individuals who have an incurable illness. The goal of palliative care is to prevent and relieve suffering by early assessment and treatment of pain and other physical, psychosocial, and spiritual needs to improve the patient's quality of life.

Although palliative care may be provided by a single person, it usually involves the combined efforts of an interdisciplinary team, including physicians, nurses, social workers, chaplains, home health aides, and volunteers. Care is provided in the patient's home (or long-term care facility, senior living facility, or hospital). The expected outcomes of care are directed by interventions to manage current manifestations of the illness and to prevent new manifestations from occurring.

Physiological Changes in the Dying Patient

Death is a highly individualized process, and may occur rapidly or slowly. Physiological changes are a part of the dying process. These changes result in any or all of the manifestations listed in the accompanying box as death nears. Although each person responds differently, there are certain manifestations common in the dying process, regardless of the trauma or disease process that is causing death. The discussion that follows includes treatments and related nursing care.

MANIFESTATIONS of Impending Death

- Difficulty talking or swallowing
- Nausea, flatus, abdominal distention
- Urinary and/or bowel incontinence, constipation
- Decreased sensation, taste, and smell
- Weak, slow, and/or irregular pulse
- Decreasing blood pressure
- Decreased, irregular, or Cheyne-Stokes respirations
- Changes in level of consciousness
- Restlessness, agitation
- Coolness, mottling, and cyanosis of the extremities

Pain

A common problem for patients at the end of life, pain is what people often say they fear the most. Pain, a subjective experience, is influenced by the patient's emotions, previous experiences with pain, and family and culture. Unfortunately, pain is often undertreated at the end of life because physicians and nurses fear they will cause addiction or cause harm from the high does of opioids necessary to control pain. However, nearly all pain at the end of life can be managed without causing addiction or hastening death through respiratory depression. It is of utmost importance to keep the patient comfortable through general comfort measures (Box 5–2) and by administering ordered medications for pain, neuropathic pain (which is rarely relieved by opioids), seizures, and/or anxiety. The pathophysiology, treatment, and nursing care of patients experiencing pain are fully described in ∞ Chapter 9.

PRACTICE ALERT
There is no maximum allowable dose for full agonist opioids such as morphine sulfate; the dose should be increased to whatever is necessary to relieve pain. Meperidine (Demerol) is not useful for chronic pain as it has a short half-life and a toxic metabolite that can caused irritability and seizures (McPhee, Papadakis, & Tierney, 2008, p. 69).

Dyspnea

Respiratory changes, including dyspnea, are normal as death nears. Dyspnea is a subjective experience, and the patient often reports having a feeling of suffocation, shortness of breath, or

BOX 5–2 Providing Comfort for the Patient Nearing Death

- Maintain clean skin and bed linens.
- Use a draw sheet to turn the patient as often as possible so the patient is comfortable.
- Position the patient to promote comfort and protect bony areas with padding. Reposition the patient and raise the head of the bed if fluids accumulate in the upper airways and back of the throat.
- Use bed pads or insert a Foley catheter (if ordered) for urinary incontinence.
- Use gentle massage to improve circulation and shift edema.
- Provide small, frequent sips of fluids, ice chips, or Popsicles.
- Provide oral care, using a soft moist brush or glycerin swab.
- Clean secretions from the eyes and nose.
- Administer ordered pain medications as needed to maintain comfort.
- Administer oxygen as prescribed to relieve dyspnea.

tightness in the chest. Up to 50% of dying patients have severe dyspnea, especially those with lung tumors (primary or metastatic), restrictive lung disease, or pleural effusion (Tierney et al. 2008). Regardless of the terminal illness or fatal injury, the final cause of death is a lack of oxygen to the brain.

As death nears, respirations often become fast or slow, shallow, and labored. The patient may have apnea or Cheyne-Stokes respirations (regular periods of deep, rapid breathing following by no breaths for 5 to 30 seconds). Fluid may accumulate in the lungs, causing crackles, especially in patients who are well hydrated, and in those who are having difficulty swallowing or coughing. These sounds are not painful for the patient, but they may be treated with oxygen, opioids (to improve respirations and decrease anxiety), and medications to decrease secretions (atropine, scopolamine, hyoscyamine, or glycopyrrolate). It should be noted that oxygen and suctioning are only temporary measures, and (especially with suctioning) may even be traumatic for the patient. Nursing care to improve respirations include keeping the head of the bed elevated. Keeping the room cool and providing a breeze from a fan often makes the patient more comfortable.

PRACTICE ALERT
Morphine is the medication of choice for palliative treatment of dyspnea. Nebulized morphine may be used, and is often more effective than that given by other routes, but it increases the risk of bronchospasm. Nebulized morphine is contraindicated in patients with chronic obstructive pulmonary disease because of the risk of respiratory depression and increasing hypercapnia.

Anorexia, Nausea, and Dehydration

Although anorexia and a decrease in food and fluid intake are normal in the dying patient, the family often views this as "giving up." Anorexia may be a protective mechanism; the breakdown of body fats results in ketosis, which leads to a sense of well-being and helps decrease pain. Parenteral or enteral feedings do not improve manifestations or prolong life and may actually cause discomfort. As weakness and difficulty swallowing progress, the gag reflex is decreased and patients are at increased risk for aspiration if oral foods are given.

Nausea, with or without vomiting, is a common problem in dying patients. Nausea and vomiting may be caused by reduced gastric emptying, constipation, bowel obstruction (a side effect of morphine), uremia, or hypercalcemia. If the patient is conscious and complains of nausea, antiemetics such as prochlorperazine (Compazine) or ondansetron (Zofran) should be administered.

Dehydration is less of a problem than overhydration. Forcing fluids or initiating intravenous fluids for hydration may in turn increase fluid in the lungs, peripheral edema, ascites, and vomiting. Dehydration in the patient nearing death primarily causes discomfort from dry mouth and thirst. The patient should be given small sips of water or an atomizer can be used to spray the inside of the mouth. Oral care should be given at least every 2 hours, and more often if the patient is breathing through his or her mouth. Glycerine swabs may be used to moisten the lips.

Altered Levels of Consciousness

Neurologic dysfunction results from any or all of the following: decreased cerebral perfusion, hypoxemia, metabolic acidosis, sepsis, an accumulation of toxins from liver and renal failure, the effects of medications, and disease-related factors. These changes may result in decreased level of consciousness or agitated delirium. Patients with terminal delirium may be confused, restless, or agitated. Moaning, groaning, and grimacing often accompany the agitation and may be misinterpreted as pain. Level of consciousness often decreases to the point where the patient cannot be aroused. Although decreased consciousness and agitation are both normal states at the end of life, they are very distressing to the patient's family.

If possible, confusion or agitation is treated based on its cause, for example, by relieving pain or dyspnea. Other medications include low doses of neuroleptics, tranquilizers, or anti-anxiety medications. A patient near death often has altered cerebral function, so the nurse must stand near the bedside and speak clearly. Hearing is thought to be the last sense a dying patient loses; the nurse should never whisper or engage in conversation with the family as if the patient were not there. Nursing care for the comatose patient includes the following:

- Using artificial tears if the patient does not blink
- Keeping lights at a low level
- Keeping skin clean and dry
- Covering the patient only with a light blanket
- Using adult incontinence pads or pants for incontinence
- Turning every 2 hours and maintaining joints in position of comfort

Hypotension

As death nears, the cardiac output decreases, as does intravascular blood volume. As a result, blood pressure gradually decreases and the pulse is often rapid and irregular. The extremities are cooler, and cyanosis is present in nailbeds, skin, and lips. The skin on the legs and in dependent areas may become mottled in color. Renal perfusion decreases and the kidneys cease to function. Urinary output is scanty. The patient will have tachycardia, hypotension, cool extremities, and cyanosis with skin mottling.

Support for the Patient and Family

As the patient's condition deteriorates, the nurse's knowledge of the patient and family guides the care provided. It may be necessary to provide opportunities for patients to express personal preferences about where they want to die and about funeral and burial arrangements. If the family feels that this is morbid, the nurse explains that it helps patients to keep a sense of control as they approach death.

The patient needs the opportunity to say goodbye to others. The nurse encourages and supports the patient and family as they terminate relationships as a necessary part of the grief process. The nurse acknowledges that termination is painful and, if the patient or family desires, stays with them during this time. Family members are often afraid to be present at the moment of death, yet dying alone is the greatest fear expressed by patients.

Death

The manifestations listed below are seen after death occurs, and are the basis for pronouncing death. They appear gradually and not in any special order. Pronouncement of death is legally required by a physician or other healthcare provider to confirm death. The time of death, with any related data, is documented in the patient's chart.

The nurse may also fear being present at the moment of the patient's death. In fact, Kübler-Ross (1969) noted that the nurse's fear of death frequently interferes with the ability to provide support for the dying patient and family. Thoughts such as, "Please, God, don't let him die on my shift," are common, and they express the nurse's emotional turmoil in dealing with the task. Nurses who have worked through their own feelings about death and dying are more at ease in assisting the dying patient toward a peaceful death.

After the death, the family is encouraged to acknowledge the pain of loss. The nurse's presence and support as the bereaved express their sorrow, anger, or guilt can help them resolve their grief. It is important for the bereaved not to suppress the pain of grieving with drugs. By accepting variations in the expression of grief, the nurse supports the family's grief reactions.

Resolution of grief begins with acceptance of the loss. The nurse can encourage this acceptance by maintaining open, honest dialogue and by providing the family with the opportunity to view, touch, hold, and kiss the person's body. As family members realize the finality of the death, they are often comforted by the presence of the nurse who cared for the patient during the final days.

Postmortem Care

The nurse documents the time of death (required for the death certificate and all official records), notifies the physician, and assists the family (if needed) in choice of a funeral home. If the patient dies at home, death must be pronounced before the body is removed. In some states and in some situations, nurses can pronounce death; for specifics, consult state practice acts, laws, and agency policy. All jewelry is removed and given to the family unless the request is made that it be left on. The body is kept in place until the family is ready and gives permission for it to be moved. If an autopsy is required or requested, the body must be left undisturbed (e.g., do not remove any tubes) for transportation to the medical examiner.

Documentation of the death is completed by sending a completed death certificate to the funeral home (for a death in the home), or by completing the required paperwork and sending the body to the morgue or funeral home (for a death in the hospital or long-term care setting).

MANIFESTATIONS of Death

- Absence of respirations, pulse, and heartbeat
- Fixed and dilated pupils; eyes may stay open
- Release of stool and urine
- Waxen color (pallor) as blood settles to dependent areas
- Body temperature drops
- Lack of reflexes
- Flat encephalogram

Nurses' Grief

The nurse who has developed a close relationship with the patient who has died may experience strong feelings of grief. Sharing grief with the family after the death of a loved one helps both the nurse and family to cope with their feelings about the loss. Taking time to grieve after the death of a patient provides a release that can help prevent "blunting" of feelings, a problem often experienced by nurses who care for patients who are terminally ill.

> **PRACTICE ALERT**
> Crying with families, at one time considered unprofessional, is now recognized as an expression of empathy and caring.

Nurses working with critically or terminally ill patients should be aware that witnessing a patient's death and the family's grief may reactivate feelings about some unresolved grief in their own lives. In these cases, nurses may need to reflect on their responses to their own losses. Also, nurses who work with dying patients need support from peers and other professionals to work through the often overwhelming feelings that result from dealing with death, grief, and loss (Figure 5–2 ■).

Interdisciplinary Care

Interventions for loss and grief may be planned and implemented by any or all members of the healthcare team. Nurses and social workers provide interventions to help patients or families adapt to a loss. They also make referrals to mental health professionals (grief counselors, social services), support groups, chaplains, or legal or financial assistance agencies.

Grieving patients frequently enter the healthcare system with significant somatic symptoms. In some cases, the symptoms of

Figure 5–2 ■ Nurses who work with dying patients need support from their colleagues to work through their often overwhelming feelings of grief.

grief and loss are overlooked until the patient reaches a crisis state requiring psychiatric medical intervention. Collaborative care by the physician and the nurse early in the normal grieving process can help the patient achieve an early and effective resolution of grief and avoid physical or psychiatric health problems.

Nursing Care

Nurses practicing in all types of settings care for patients who are in various stages of the grieving process. Grief is highly individual. The grief process may range from uncomfortable to debilitating, and it may last for a day or a lifetime, depending on what the loss means to the person experiencing it. A case study and care plan for a patient who is grieving is included at the end of this section.

Health Promotion

In planning and implementing nursing care for the patient experiencing a loss, the nurse considers the individual responses, which may vary greatly. In an era of short acute care stays for patients, nurses may feel that an elaborate grief assessment is impossible or, at the least, impractical. But research and clinical experience suggest that patients who delay the grieving process after a loss are prone to have health problems that may last a lifetime. See below for an end-of-life checklist for older adults.

Assessment

Knowledge of the expected physical reactions to loss provides the nurse with a basis for identifying reactions requiring further assessment. To assess the extent of physical distress, the nurse observes for changes in sensory processes and asks questions about the patient's sleeping and eating patterns, activities of daily living, general health status, and pain.

Physical Assessment

People who experience a loss may experience one or more predictable somatic (physical) symptoms. Gastrointestinal manifestations such as indigestion, nausea or vomiting, anorexia, weight gain or loss, constipation, or diarrhea occur frequently.

The shock and disbelief that accompany a loss may cause shortness of breath, a choking sensation, hyperventilation, or weakness. Some people also report insomnia, preoccupation with sleep, fatigue, and decreased or increased activity level.

Crying and sadness are observed during normal grief states. Crying may make the individual feel exhausted and interfere with carrying out activities of daily living. However, a person who is unable to cry may have difficulty completing the mourning process. If the person does not express feelings of grief, somatic symptoms may increase.

Reactions to loss are not always obvious. For example, in patients who experience an illness following a serious loss, assessment may reveal somatic complaints related to the grief state as well as the illness. When a person who has been healthy begins to develop patterns of increased illness, the nurse should be aware that this may signal dysfunctional grieving. This is especially common in the loss and grieving associated with a change in body image. In addition to making a physical assessment, assess the patient's perception of the alteration in body image. The loss of a body part, weight gain or loss, and scars from surgery or trauma can be difficult for the patient to accept. Some patients may grieve hair loss that accompanies chemotherapy used in cancer treatment.

It is imperative that the dying patient's concerns about pain be assessed, especially if the patient has cancer or another painful illness. Knowledge of pain theories and pain assessment can help the nurse assess the need for pain medication (∞ see Chapter 9). During the last stages of dying, the patient usually becomes very weak, and sensations and reflexes decrease; these changes call for careful assessment of the patient's physical needs.

Spiritual Assessment

Because spiritual beliefs and practices greatly influence people's reaction to loss, it is important to explore them with the patient when assessing a loss. The spiritually healthy patient has inner resources that help work through the grief process. Faith, prayer, trust in God or a superior being, perception of a purpose in life, or belief in immortality are examples of the inner resources that may sustain the patient during an actual or

---

NURSING CARE OF THE OLDER ADULT — End-of-Life Checklist

- Take time a day or so before appointments with your healthcare provider to think about the questions you need answered and concerns you want to discuss. It is often a good idea to keep a pad of paper and a pen handy so you can write down things as they come to you.
- Do not hesitate to have your doctor explain your diagnosis again if you didn't understand the explanation the first time or if you missed some key points. The same goes for details about using medications and possible side effects.
- You may wish to have a friend or family member go with you to medical appointments.
- When you visit the doctor, take an up-to-date list of all the medications (prescribed and over-the-counter) you are currently taking.
- If you have physical pain, tell your healthcare provider. You will probably be asked to rate your pain on a scale of 1 (no pain) to 10 (severe pain). Your rating helps determine what pain relief measures are appropriate.

- It is a good idea to ask your healthcare provider about hospice services well before you are likely to need them.
- Your family and close friends should be aware of your treatment preferences (such as the existence of a DNR order). You might consider documenting your wishes in a living will.
- Think about asking and appointing someone you trust to make your healthcare decisions in case the moment comes when you can no longer make them yourself.
- If you are feeling depressed or anxious or need emotional support, consider talking to a pastor, chaplain, rabbi, or other trusted person in your faith community. If necessary, ask your healthcare provider to recommend someone to help you sort out your feelings.
- Avoid withdrawing from social activities. Keep communicating with your family, friends, and the people who help care for you. If you are open with them you are more likely to get the care you need.

perceived loss. Patients who had not considered themselves religious before the actual or perceived loss often turn to religion to seek comfort or to cope with feelings of despair, helplessness, hopelessness, or guilt.

Assessing the dying patient's spiritual life and its significance to the patient and family helps identify spiritual support systems. Some nurses are uncomfortable with assessing the patient's spiritual needs; the following questions may be helpful.

- What are the spiritual aspects of the patient's philosophy about life? Death?
- Are the values and beliefs about life and death congruent with those of people who are important to the patient?
- Which spiritual resources and rituals have significance for the patient?

Belief systems that are incompatible with those of family members can be an additional source of stress for patients dealing with a loss. The anger and resentment often observed among families faced with decisions concerning dying members may be avoided if the nurse assesses the potential effect of differing beliefs.

Patients coping with a loss often perceive that it is a punishment from God for their wrongdoing or for their failure to remain faithful to their religious practices. Therefore, it is important to assess the level of guilt the patient or family expresses. Assessing the patient's comments regarding feelings of responsibility for the loss helps determine whether these feelings are an expected phase of grieving or indicate dysfunctional grieving.

Psychosocial Assessment

When working through the grief process, patients can be overwhelmed by the fears associated with the loss and the changes it will produce. The patient responding to an actual or perceived loss commonly expresses anxiety (fear of the unknown). An extreme level of anxiety can threaten the patient's wellbeing. Assessment includes helping patients openly acknowledge their fears. Some patients may fear the feelings they experience while proceeding through the grief process more than the loss itself. The most common fear expressed by patients facing a loss is that of losing self-control.

Talking with dying patients is often difficult. The following suggestions by Roncour (personal communication) provide assistance.

- Often, when patients initiate conversations about dying, you may feel unprepared for their questions. They can take you by surprise, and can often lead you to believe that the patient expects a crystal ball response. Remember that the purpose of all such discussions is to keep the lines of communication open with the patient. The idea is to make the subject of dying discussible, and to communicate to the patient that it does not make you afraid to do so. An open-ended statement, such as "Tell me what concerns you the most" provide a means of encouraging communication.
- Some patients may be too fearful to ask physicians such questions. They often approach staff who they perceive as less intimidating or more approachable. The question often comes in the middle of the night, when there are no distractions, when anxiety or pain may keep the patient awake, and when the patient may feel most alone with psycho-spiritual

distress. In any case, it is often on the nurse's watch when questions about dying may arise.

- Because of the surprising nature of such questions, you may feel tempted to escape ("I've got to go take that patient's vital signs right now"), or pass the buck ("That sounds like a question for your doctor"). Be vigilant about such impulsive behavior and realize that it only serves your own need to reduce your anxiety, but does nothing to assist the patient with his or her own. It is well within the scope of your professional practice as a competent nurse to provide counseling and death education, especially when the patient asks you for it or indicates an unmet need for such information and support. *When in doubt, ask a question in response, such as "Tell me how you feel about that" or "What have you been told already?"* This will accomplish several things. First, it will help you to regain your composure. The second point of asking a question is that it will give you more information about what is on the patient's mind so that your intervention can be as specific and responsive to that patient as possible.
- Do not provide false reassurance. It is important to remember that avoiding discussions about death robs the patient of precious time to accomplish goals that produce hope. Dying people hope for many things even when they cannot hope for a cure, such as hope for freedom from pain, to be surrounded by loved ones, and for the rest of their allotted time to be spent in meaningful pursuits.

Awareness of the altered sensorium observed during the stage of shock and disbelief provides parameters for assessment. The nurse may note in the patient feelings of numbness, unreality, emotional distance, intense preoccupation with the lost object, helplessness, loneliness, and disorganization. As awareness of the loss begins to develop, preoccupation with the lost person or object may increase, and self-accusation and ambivalence toward the lost person or object may follow.

Nursing Diagnoses and Interventions

A variety of nursing diagnoses may be appropriate for the patient experiencing loss and grief, as well as for the patient who is nearing death. Nurses practicing medical-surgical nursing will most often provide interventions for grieving, chronic sorrow, and death anxiety.

Grieving

Grieving is a combination of intellectual and emotional responses and behaviors by which people adjust their selfconcept in the face of an actual or potential loss. Grieving may be a response to one's own future death; to loss of body parts or functions; to loss of a significant person, animal, or possession; or to loss of a social role. Nursing interventions are designed to assist with grief resolution.

- Assess for factors causing or contributing to the grief. Ask about support systems, how many losses have occurred, relationship with the lost person, significance of the body part, and previous experiences with loss and grief. *Grief and mourning occur when a person experiences any type of loss.*
- Use open-ended questions to encourage the person to share concerns and the possible effect on the family. *Grief resolution cannot occur until the patient acknowledges the loss.*

■ Promote a trusting nurse–patient relationship: Allow enough time for communications; speak clearly, simply, and concisely; listen; be honest in responses to questions; do not give unrealistic hope; offer support; and demonstrate respect for the person's age, culture, religion, race, and values. *An effective nurse–patient relationship begins with acceptance of the patient's feelings, attitudes, and values related to the loss. If the patient is ready to talk, listening and being present are the most appropriate interventions.*

■ Ask about strengths and weakness in coping with the other losses. *Current responses are influenced by past experiences with loss, illness, and death. Socioeconomic and cultural background, as well as cultural and spiritual beliefs and values, affect a person's ability to adapt to loss.*

■ Teach the patient and family the stages of grief. *This helps them to be aware of their emotions in each stage and reassures them that their reactions are normal.*

■ Provide time for decision making. *In periods of stress, people may need extra time to make informed decisions.*

■ Provide information about appropriate resources, including support from family, friends, support groups, community resources, and legal/financial aides. *Support from others decreases feelings of loneliness and isolation and facilitates grief work.*

Chronic Sorrow

Chronic sorrow is a "cyclical, recurring, and potentially progressive pattern of pervasive sadness experienced in response to continual loss, throughout the trajectory of an illness or disability" (Nanda International, 2009, p. 276). It is triggered by situations that bring to mind the person's losses, disappointments, or fears. It may be experienced by a patient, parent or caregiver, or person with chronic illness or disability.

■ Explain the difference between chronic sorrow and chronic grieving. *Grieving is time-limited and ends in adaptation to the loss. Chronic sorrow may vary in intensity, but it persists as long as the person with the disability or chronic sorrow condition lives.*

■ Encourage verbalization of feelings about the loss, and about the personal relevance of the changes to hopes for the future. *Expressing feelings is normal and necessary to decrease the emotional pain.*

■ Help identify triggers that intensify the sorrow, such as birthdays, anniversaries, and holidays. *When triggers have been identified, role-playing may make the events less painful.*

■ Refer to appropriate community support groups. *Participating in support groups with others experiencing grief is helpful in coping with loss.*

■ Encourage use of personal, family, significant other, and spiritual support systems *to facilitate coping with loss.*

Death Anxiety

Death anxiety is worry or fear related to death or dying. It may be present in patients who have an acute life-threatening illness, who have a terminal illness, who have experienced the death of a family member or friend, or who have experienced multiple deaths in the same family.

■ Explore the patient's knowledge of the situation. For example, ask, "What has your doctor told you about your condition?" *This provides information about the patient's*

knowledge base about the condition and about his or her ability to make informed decisions.

■ Ask the patient to identify specific fears about death. *This provides data about any unrealistic expectations or misperceptions.*

■ Determine the patient's perceptions of strengths and weakness in coping with death. *Identifying past strengths can help the patient cope with loss, illness, and death.*

■ Ask the patient to identify needed help. *This determines whether available resources are adequate.*

■ Encourage independence and control in decisions about treatment and care. *This promotes self-esteem, decreases feelings of powerlessness, and allows the patient to retain dignity in dying.*

■ Facilitate access to culturally appropriate spiritual rituals and practices. *This provides spiritual comfort.*

■ Explain advance directives and assist with them if necessary. *Advance directives help ensure that the patient's wishes for end-of-life care are carried out.*

■ Encourage life review and reminiscence. *Life review is self-affirming.*

■ Encourage activities such as listening to music, aromatherapy, massage, or relaxation exercises. *These activities decrease anxiety.*

■ Suggest keeping a journal or leaving a written legacy. *A written document provides continuing support to others after death.*

Using NANDA, NIC, and NOC

Linkages between a selected NANDA nursing diagnosis, NIC, and NOC for the patient experiencing death anxiety are shown in the chart that follows.

Community-Based Care

In addition to teaching patients and families to carry out the physical skills that are necessary to the patient's care, nurses also provide information on identifying signs of deterioration

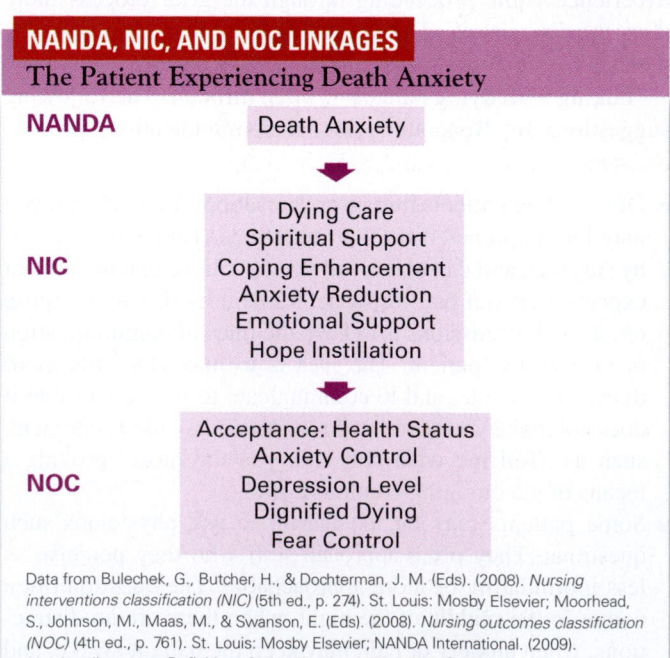

NANDA, NIC, AND NOC LINKAGES
The Patient Experiencing Death Anxiety

NANDA Death Anxiety

NIC
Dying Care
Spiritual Support
Coping Enhancement
Anxiety Reduction
Emotional Support
Hope Instillation

NOC
Acceptance: Health Status
Anxiety Control
Depression Level
Dignified Dying
Fear Control

Data from Bulechek, G., Butcher, H., & Dochterman, J. M. (Eds). (2008). *Nursing interventions classification (NIC)* (5th ed., p. 274). St. Louis: Mosby Elsevier; Moorhead, S., Johnson, M., Maas, M., & Swanson, E. (Eds). (2008). *Nursing outcomes classification (NOC)* (4th ed., p. 761). St. Louis: Mosby Elsevier; NANDA International. (2009). *Nursing diagnoses: Definitions & classification 2009–20011.* Oxford, UK: Wiley-Blackwell.

Pearl Rogers is a 79-year-old woman who is admitted to the Methodist Home Nursing Center. Mrs. Rogers lived with her husband of 58 years until his death 9 months ago. She had one son who died in an auto crash 2 years ago, and she has one daughter who lives nearby. After her husband's death, Mrs. Rogers lived with her daughter until her admission to the nursing center. Mrs. Rogers has become increasingly agitated and helpless, complaining constantly of pain. Her daughter states that Mrs. Rogers is chronically constipated, has difficulty sleeping, and has stopped engaging in all social activities, including weekly church services. She cries frequently. Extensive medical testing prior to her admission to the nursing center revealed Mrs. Rogers has arthritis but no other pathologic disorder.

ASSESSMENT

On admission to the nursing center, Mrs. Rogers says, "I'm a sick woman, and no one will listen to me! I can't walk, I'm so weak. My head hurts, and I'm always sick at my stomach. I haven't had a bowel movement in a week, and I never sleep more than 3 hours a night." Physical assessment findings include swollen knees and ankles, with limited mobility of the lower extremities.

DIAGNOSES

- Grieving related to stress of husband's death
- Disturbed Sleep Pattern related to grieving
- Constipation related to inactivity

EXPECTED OUTCOMES

- Engage in normal grief work: Work through grief process, discuss reality of losses, use nondestructive coping mechanisms, and discuss positive and negative aspects of the loss.
- Experience adequate and restful sleep: Fall asleep 20 to 30 minutes after retiring and awaken feeling rested after 7 to 8 hours of sleep.
- Have a bowel movement with soft, formed stools at least every other day.

PLANNING AND IMPLEMENTATION

- Promote trust: Show empathy and caring, demonstrate respect for Mrs. Roger's culture and values, offer support and reassurance, be honest, engage in active listening.

- Assist in labeling Mrs. Roger's feelings: anger, fear, loneliness, guilt, isolation.
- Explore previous losses and the ways in which the patient has coped.
- Encourage review of Mrs. Roger's relationship with her dead husband.
- Reinforce expressions of behaviors associated with normal grieving.
- Encourage participation in usual spiritual practices.
- Encourage participation in a grief group that meets at the facility.
- Consult with the physical and recreational therapist to help the nursing staff provide afternoon activities.
- Provide measures that assist in bowel evacuation: Encourage exercise as tolerated, including walks and rocking in a rocking chair. Offer foods that stimulate bowel movements. Offer privacy: Close the door, ensuring that the emergency call bell is within reach, and do not interrupt.
- Administer a mild laxative and/or stool softener, if necessary, but discontinue as soon as possible.

EVALUATION

After 4 weeks at the nursing center, Mrs. Rogers states, "I don't feel any better, but I know I have to accept my situation." Although Mrs. Rogers states that she doesn't feel better, she is walking the length of the hall, sleeping better, and having regular bowel movements. Mrs. Rogers is also less withdrawn and has openly discussed her feelings related to her husband's death, including her anger at the loss of her son and her husband less than 2 years apart. She has attended the grief group once and has attended chapel services on Sunday for the past 2 weeks. Her daughter visits her each Saturday and takes her in a wheelchair to the shopping mall.

CRITICAL THINKING IN THE NURSING PROCESS

1. What common physical manifestations of grief did Mrs. Rogers experience?
2. How might Mrs. Rogers's daughter be more involved in developing and implementing her mother's plan of care?
3. Suppose Mrs. Rogers says that she does not want any help, that she just wants to be left alone to die. How would you respond?

See Evaluating Your Response in Appendix C.

and additional sources of support. General guidelines for teaching patients and families about grief include those suggested in the accompanying Meeting Individualized Needs feature that appears below. In addition, suggest the following resources:

- Hospice
- Home healthcare agencies
- Support groups
- Public health departments
- Church, synagogue, or mosque
- Pastoral counseling centers
- Mental health agencies

- Encourage both children and adults to discuss expected or impending loss and to express feelings.
- Teach problem-solving skills: Define what the possible changes and problems are related to the predicted loss, develop potential strategies for dealing with problems, list pros and cons of each strategy, and decide which strategies might be most useful to try first to solve potential problems associated with loss.
- Teach individuals and families how to support a person who is dealing with an impending loss.

- Explain what to expect with a loss: sadness, fear, rejection, anger, guilt, loneliness.
- Teach signs of grief resolution:
  - No longer living in the past, becoming future oriented
  - Breaking ties with the lost object or person (acute stage often shows signs of resolving in 6 to 12 months)
  - The possibility of having painful "waves" of grief years after the loss, especially on the anniversary of the loss and in response to "triggers" such as pictures, events, songs, or memories

CHAPTER HIGHLIGHTS

■ Grief is the emotional response to a loss, experienced by a person as grieving. Bereavement, a form of depression accompanied by anxiety, is a common response to loss of a loved one by death. Death, although inevitable, is an immensely difficult loss.

■ There are many different theories of how people respond to loss, grief, and death. These theories are useful when providing nursing care to patients and families.

■ A person's response to loss is influenced by age, culture, social support, family members, spiritual beliefs, and rituals of mourning. Nurses need to assess the way in which they respond to loss to better care for patients.

■ Legal and ethical issues involved in end-of-life care include advance directives (living wills, healthcare surrogate, and durable power of attorney), do-not-resuscitate orders, and euthanasia.

■ Hospice, a model of care for patients and their families when faced with limited life expectancy, supports a dignified and peaceful death. Palliative care is focused on the relief of physical, mental, and spiritual distress for people with an incurable illness.

■ To provide knowledgeable and compassionate care at the end of life, nurses must recognize physiological changes as the patient nears death, support the patient and family, provide postmortem care, and resolve their own grief.

■ Nursing care of patients experiencing an actual or potential loss includes accurate physical, spiritual, and psychosocial assessment, and interventions for the human responses of grieving, chronic sorrow, and/or death anxiety.

TEST YOURSELF NCLEX-RN® REVIEW

1. Which of the following statements best describes loss?
   1. It is determined by one's cultural values.
   2. It is largely dependent on support of family and friends.
   3. It can be determined only by the person who experiences it.
   4. It is the same as grief and mourning.

2. A newly diagnosed patient states, "I hate this cancer." According to Kübler-Ross, what stage of loss is being verbalized?
   1. anger
   2. bargaining
   3. depression
   4. denial

3. What is an important factor in the successful resolution of grief?
   1. social isolation
   2. support systems
   3. triggers of grief
   4. loss acknowledgement

4. What element is the primary factor that dictates the rituals of mourning?
   1. culture
   2. age
   3. gender
   4. religion

5. A patient says, "I don't want anything heroic done if I die. Just let me go." What document expresses a person's wishes for life-sustaining treatment in the event of terminal illness or permanent unconsciousness?
   1. durable power of attorney
   2. living will
   3. no-code order
   4. healthcare surrogate

6. A patient has been referred to hospice and asks what it means. The nurse's response is based on what knowledge about hospice?
   1. Hospice is a special place of care.
   2. Hospice care is a life-long type of care.
   3. Hospice is a model of care rather than a place of care.
   4. Hospice is designed for patients with serious chronic illness.

7. A patient nearing death requests that no medication be given that would cause a loss of consciousness, including pain medication. What would a nurse do to provide the best end-of-life care in this situation?
   1. Give the medication; comfort is the highest priority.
   2. Give half the ordered dose to provide compassionate care.
   3. Discuss this with family members and follow their wishes.
   4. Respect the patient's wishes and withhold pain medications.

8. Which of the senses is believed to be the last one lost as a person nears death?
   1. hearing
   2. vision
   3. touch
   4. smell

9. Which of the following statements best describes the treatment of pain at the end of life?
   1. As patient nears death, no pain is perceived and no medications are necessary.
   2. It is important to withhold pain medications if the patient has respiratory changes.
   3. There is no maximum allowable dose for opioids during end-of-life care.
   4. Nurses should not administer opioids to the dying patient.

10. A woman, recently widowed, tells the nurse, "I just can't even get out of bed in the mornings anymore." What response by the nurse would be most helpful in resolving the patient's grief?
   1. "I don't know why you feel that way."
   2. "This must be a difficult time for you."
   3. "Why do you think you feel this way?"
   4. "After you get up, you will feel better."

See Test Yourself answers in Appendix C.

Pearson Nursing Student Resources
Find additional review materials at
www.nursing.pearsonhighered.com
Prepare for success with additional NCLEX®-style practice questions, interactive assignments and activities, Web links, animations and videos, and more!

BIBLIOGRAPHY

American Association of Colleges of Nursing (AACN). (2004). *Peaceful death: Recommended competencies and curricular guidelines for end-of-life nursing care.* Washington, DC: AACN.

American Association of Retired Persons (AARP). (2010). *End of life: Beginning the conversation.* Retrieved from http://www.aarp.org

American Geriatrics Society. (2007). *Position statement: The care of dying patients.* Retrieved from http://americangeriatrics.org/products/positionpapers/careofd

American Nurses Association. (2003). *Position statements: Pain management and control of distressing symptoms in dying patients.* Retrieved from http://www.nursingworld.org/readroom/position/ethics/etpain.htm

Bialk, J. (2004). Ethical guidelines for assisting patients with end-of-life decision making. *MEDSURG Nursing, 13*(2), 87–90.

Bowlby, J. (1973). *Attachment and loss, Separation, anxiety, and anger* (Vol. 2). New York: Basic Books.

Bowlby, J. (1980). *Attachment and loss, loss, sadness, and depression* (Vol. 3). New York: Basic Books.

Bulechek, G., Butcher, H., & Dochterman, J. M. (Eds.). (2008). *Nursing interventions classification (NIC)* (5th ed). St. Louis: Mosby Elsevier.

Caplan, G. (1990). Loss, stress, and mental health. *Community Mental Health Journal, 26*(1), 27–48.

Chart Smart: Documenting a patient's death. (2008). *Nursing, 38* (7), 19.

Emanuel, L., Ferris, F., von Guten, C., & Von Rooenn, J. (2006). *The last hours of living: Practical advice for clinicians.* Medscape. Retrieved from http://cme.medscape.com/viewprogram/5808?src=top10

Engel, G. (1964). Grief and grieving. *American Journal of Nursing, 64,* 93.

Field, N., Gao, B., & Paderna, L. (2005). Continued bonds in bereavement: An attachment theory based perspective. *Death Studies, 29*(4), 277–299.

Fields, L. (2007). DNR does not mean no care. *Journal of Neuroscience Nursing, 39*(5), 294–296

Florida Department of Elder Affairs and the Florida Partnership for End-of-life Care. (2005). *Making choices: A guide to plan for end-of-life planning.* Retrieved from http://elderaffairs.state.fl.us

Freud, S. (1917/1957). Mourning and melancholia. In J. Strachey & A. Tyson (Eds.), *The complete psychological works of Sigmund Freud* (Vol. 14). London: Hogarth Press.

Henneman, E., & Karras, G. (2004). Determining brain death in adults: A guideline for use in critical care. *Critical Care Nurse, 24,* 50–56. Retrieved from http://ccn.aacnjournals.org/cgi/contents/full/24/5/50

Holtslander, L. (2008). Ways of knowing hope: Carper's fundamental patterns as a guide for hope research with bereaved palliative caregivers. *Nursing Outlook, 56*(1), 25–30.

Hospice Foundation of America. (2005). *The dying process: A guide for caregivers.* Washington, DC: Hospice Foundation of America.

Hospice Foundation of America. (2008). *HFA grief resource page. What is grief?* Retrieved from http://www.hospicefoundation.org/griefAndLoss/

Huggins, M., & Brooks, L. (2007). Discussing end-of-life care with older patients: What are you waiting for? *Geriatrics Aging, 10*(7), 461–464.

International Council of Nurses. (2005). *The ICN definition of nursing.* Geneva: The International Council of Nurses.

Jonhson, J., & Johnson, M. (1995). *Grief. What it is and what you can do.* Omaha, NE: Centering Corporation.

Kantor, D. (2008). Caring for the dying patient. *American Journal of Nursing, 108*(11), 72CCC.

Kübler-Ross, E. (1969). *On death and dying.* New York: Macmillan.

Kübler-Ross, E. (1978). *To live until we say goodbye.* Englewood Cliffs, NJ: Prentice Hall.

Kübler-Ross, E. (1997). *On death and dying: What the dying have to teach doctors, nurses, clergy, and their own families.* New York: Simon & Schuster.

Living wills and health care proxies. (2004). *Harvard Women's Health Watch, 11*(5), 6–7.

Mananec, P., & Tyler, M. (2003). Cultural considerations in end-of-life care. *American Journal of Nursing, 103*(3), 50–58.

McPhee, S. J., Papadakis, M. A., & Tierney, L. M. (2008). *Current medical diagnosis & treatment* (47th ed.). New York: McGraw Hill.

Moorhead, S., Johnson, M., Maas, M., & Swanson, E. (Eds.). (2008). *Nursing outcomes classification (NOC)* (4th ed.). St. Louis: Mosby Elsevier.

NANDA International. (2009). *Nursing diagnoses: Definitions & classification 2009–2011.* Oxford, UK: Wiley-Blackwell.

National Association for Home Care & Hospice. (2008). *Hospice facts & statistics.* Washington, DC: National Association for Home Care & Hospice.

Norlander, L. (2008). *To comfort always: A nurse's guide to end-of-life care.* Indianapolis: Sigma Theta Tau International.

Pomeranz, J., & Brustman, M. (2005). When's the time right to enter hospice care? *Nursing, 55*(8), 43.

Rancour, P. (2008). *Personal communications.* Columbus, OH.

Rancour, P. (2008). *Tales from the pager chronicles.* Indianapolis: Sigma Theta Tau International.

Rushton, C., Roshi, J., & Dossey, B. (2007). Being with dying: Contemporary practices for compassionate end-of-life care. *American Nurse Today, 2*(9), 16–18.

Spector, R. (2009). *Cultural diversity in health and illness* (7th ed.). Upper Saddle River, NJ: Pearson Prentice Hall.

Springhouse (Eds.). (2006). *End of life: A nurse's guide to compassionate care.* Philadelphia: Lippincott Williams & Wilkins.

Stajduhar, K., Martin, W., Barwich, D., & Fyles, G. (2008). Factors influencing family caregivers' ability to cope with providing end-of-life cancer care at home. *Cancer Nursing, 31*(1), 77–85.

Ufema, J. (2007). *Insights on death & dying.* Philadelphia: Lippincott Williams & Wilkins.

U.S. Department of Health & Human Services. (2008). *Medicare hospice benefits.* Baltimore: Centers for Medicare & Medicaid Services.

Wilkinson, J., & Ahern, N. (2009). *Prentice Hall nursing diagnosis handbook* (9th ed.). Upper Saddle River, NJ: Pearson Prentice Hall.

6 Nursing Care of Patients with Problems of Substance Abuse

LEARNING OUTCOMES

1. Discuss risk factors associated with substance abuse.
2. Recognize the manifestations of potential substance abuse in coworkers.
3. Describe common characteristics of substance abusers.

4. Explain the effects of addictive substances on physiological, cognitive, psychological, and social well-being.
5. Support interdisciplinary care for the patient with substance abuse problems, including diagnostic tests, emergency care for overdose, and treatment of withdrawal.

CLINICAL COMPETENCIES

1. Assess functional health status of patients with substance abuse or dependence.
2. Monitor for signs of withdrawal and life-threatening conditions.
3. Provide skilled nursing care during the detoxification period.
4. Collaborate with other disciplines when caring for patients with substance abuse problems.

5. Educate patients about stress management, coping skills, nutrition, relapse prevention, and healthy lifestyle choices.
6. Use the nursing process to provide individualized nursing care for patients experiencing problems with substance abuse.
7. Revise plan of care as needed to promote, maintain, or restore functional health status to patients with substance abuse problems.

KEY TERMS

alcohol, 107
amphetamine, 108
caffeine, 105
cannabis sativa, 106
central nervous system depressants, 108
cocaine, 108
co-occurring disorders, 103
delirium tremens (DT), 108

hallucinogens, 109
inhalants, 110
kindling, 103
Korsakoff's psychosis, 108
nicotine, 106
opiates, 109
polysubstance abuse, 115

psychostimulants, 108
substance abuse, 102
substance dependence, 102
tolerance, 102
Wernicke's encephalopathy, 108
withdrawal, 102
withdrawal symptoms, 102

Disease Process: The Patient with Substance Abuse Problems

Substance abuse refers to the use of any chemical in a fashion inconsistent with medical or culturally defined social norms despite physical, psychological, or social adverse effects. Anxiety and depressive disorders frequently occur with substance abuse. More than 90% of people who commit suicide have a depressive or substance abuse disorder (National Institute of Mental Health [NIMH], 2008). In 2007, over 22 million Americans, or 9% of the population, were classified with substance dependence or abuse (Substance Abuse and Mental Health Services Administration [SAMHSA], 2008a).

The *Diagnostic and Statistical Manual of Mental Disorders* (*DSM-IV-TR*) (American Psychiatric Association [APA], 2000) includes a classification scheme for distinguishing between substance abuse and substance dependence. **Substance dependence** refers to a severe condition occurring when the use of the chemical substance is no longer under an individual's control for at least 3 months. Continued use of the substance usually persists despite adverse effects on the

person's physical condition, psychological health, and interpersonal relationships. The *DSM-IV-TR* criteria deal with the behavioral aspects and the maladaptive patterns of substance use, emphasizing the physical symptoms of **tolerance** and **withdrawal**. Tolerance is a cumulative state in which a particular dose of the chemical elicits a smaller response than before. With increased tolerance, the individual needs higher and higher doses to obtain the desired effect. When a person is physically addicted to the drug and stops taking it, **withdrawal symptoms** can occur within hours. Withdrawal is an uncomfortable state lasting several days, manifested by tremors, diaphoresis, anxiety, high blood pressure, tachycardia, and possibly convulsions. An overview of the *DSM-IV-TR* diagnostic criteria for substance abuse and substance dependence is shown in Box 6–1.

Pathophysiology and Manifestations

The human tendency to seek pleasure and avoid stress and pain is partially responsible for substance abuse. Although far from definite, evidence implicates the endogenous opioid system in

BOX 6–1 Substance Abuse versus Substance Dependence

Substance Abuse

Maladaptive pattern of substance use leading to clinically significant impairment or distress, manifested by **one or more** of the following within a 12 month period:

1. Failure to fulfill major role obligations at work, school, and home.
2. Involvement in physically hazardous situations while impaired (driving while intoxicated, operating a machine, exacerbation of physical symptoms such as ulcers).
3. Recurrent legal or interpersonal problems.
4. Continued use despite recurrent social and interpersonal problems.

Substance Dependence

Maladaptive pattern of substance use leading to clinically significant impairment or distress, manifested by **three or more** of the following within a 12-month period:

1. Presence of tolerance to the drug.
2. Presence of withdrawal symptoms.
3. Substance is taken in larger amounts or for longer periods than is intended.
4. Unsuccessful or persistent desire to cut down or control substance use.
5. More time spent in getting, taking, and recovering from the substance. May withdraw from family or friends and spend more time using substance in private.
6. Decline in or absence of important social, occupational, or recreational activities.
7. Continued use of substance despite knowledge of adverse effects.

Adapted from American Psychiatric Association. (2000). *Diagnostic and Statistical Manual of Mental Disorders* (4th ed., text rev.). Washington, DC: APA.

---

the development and maintenance of addictive behaviors. Current data suggest that alcohol increases opioid neurotransmission and that this activation is partly responsible for its reinforcing effect. Dopamine has been identified as the primary neurotransmitter responsible for sustaining the addictive quality of drugs as well as increasing drug-seeking behavior. The reinforcing properties of drugs can create a pleasurable experience and reduce the intensity of unpleasant experiences.

The craving one has for a particular substance may also be heightened by a phenomenon known as the "kindling" effect. **Kindling** refers to long-term changes in brain neurotransmission that occur after repeated detoxifications. Recurrent detoxifications increase neuron sensitivity and are thought to intensify obsessive thoughts or cravings for a substance. Eventually the brain responds spontaneously in a dysfunctional manner even when the substance is no longer being used (Stuart, 2009). This phenomenon may explain why subsequent episodes of withdrawal from a substance tend to progressively worsen.

Although there is no greater prevalence of psychiatric illness in substance abusers than in the general population, co-occurring disorders are often present. **Co-occurring disorders** (previously called dual diagnosis and dual disorders) refer to the coexistence of substance abuse or dependence and a psychiatric disorder in one individual. One disorder can be an indication of another, such as the relationship between alcoholism and depression. Alcohol dependence and major depression commonly occur together, posing a significant risk for the development of the other disorder. A depressed person may use self-medication in the form of alcohol to treat the depression, or the alcoholic person may become depressed. The most commonly co-occurring mental disorders in adults are alcohol abuse or alcohol dependence with depression or psychoses. Patients with co-occurring disorders are more likely to be unemployed younger males living in unstable conditions with more than one psychiatric diagnosis and a personality disorder. The combination of these factors results in more crises and a greater risk to the person and others. Box 6–2 lists terminology associated with substance abuse.

Risk Factors

Various risk factors help explain why one person becomes addicted while another does not. Genetic, biological, psychological, and sociocultural factors shed light on how a person may abuse or become dependent on a substance.

- *Genetic factors* include an apparent hereditary factor, especially with alcohol use and dependence. Most of the related genetic research has focused on alcoholism. Evidence supports the D2 dopamine receptor gene (DRD2 A1 allele) as a genetic marker in adolescent males with increased risk for developing substance use problems (Conner et al., 2005). The discovery that the DRD2 A1 allele gene appeared to be associated with alcoholism has led to a growing body of genetic research into substance abuse disorders (Stuart, 2009).

GENETIC CONSIDERATIONS
Alcoholic Fathers and Their Sons

Genetic research has also identified that children of alcoholics (COAs) are at higher risk for developing substance use problems (Conner et al., 2005). This is primarily true with male relatives. One type of alcoholism seen mostly in the sons of alcoholic fathers is associated with an early onset, inability to abstain, and an antisocial personality (Stuart, 2009). Results of one study revealed that adolescent boys of alcoholics with the D2 dopamine receptor gene (DRD2 A1 allele) tried and got intoxicated on alcohol more often than boys without this genetic marker. In addition, they tried more, and used more substances overall. Boys with the allele developed a tobacco habit more and experienced a marijuana high at an earlier age than boys without the allele (Conner et al., 2005).

Critical Thinking in Patient Care

1. Why is it important to ask your patients if they have a family history of substance abuse?
2. What questions should you ask when assessing for increased risk of substance abuse?
3. Does having a positive family history of substance abuse indicate that a person will develop a substance abuse problem? Why or why not?

BOX 6–2 Terminology Associated with Substance Abuse

Term	Definition
Abstinence	Voluntarily going without drugs or alcohol.
Addiction	A disease process characterized by the continued use of a specific chemical substance despite physical, psychological, or social harm (used interchangeably with substance dependence).
Codependence	A cluster of maladaptive behaviors exhibited by significant others of a substance abusing individual that serves to enable and protect the abuse at the expense of living a full and satisfying life.
Co-occurring disorders	Concurrent diagnosis of a substance use disorder and a psychiatric disorder. One disorder can precede and cause the other, such as the relationship between alcoholism and depression.
Cross-tolerance	Tolerance to one drug confers tolerance to another.
Delirium tremens	A medical emergency usually occurring 3 to 5 days following alcohol withdrawal and lasting 2 to 3 days. Characterized by paranoia, disorientation, delusions, visual hallucinations, elevated vital signs, vomiting, diarrhea, and diaphoresis.
Detoxification	The process of helping an addicted individual safely through withdrawal.
Dual diagnosis	The coexistence of substance abuse/dependence and a psychiatric disorder in one individual (used interchangeably with dual disorder and co-occurring disorders).
Kindling	Brain sensitization to events such as stress, trauma, or the effects of substance use.
Korsakoff's psychosis	Secondary dementia caused by thiamine (B_1) deficiency that may be associated with chronic alcoholism; characterized by progressive cognitive deterioration, confabulation, peripheral neuropathy, and myopathy.
Physical dependence	A state in which withdrawal syndrome will occur if drug use is discontinued.
Polysubstance abuse	The simultaneous use of many substances.
Psychologic dependence	An intensive subjective need for a particular psychoactive drug.
Substance abuse	Continued use of a chemical substance in a fashion inconsistent with medical or social norms, for at least 1 month, despite related problems.
Substance dependence	A severe condition occurring when the use of the chemical substance is no longer under control, for at least 3 months; continued use persists despite adverse effects (used interchangeably with addiction).
Tolerance	State in which a particular dose elicits a smaller response than it formerly did. With increased tolerance the individual needs higher and higher doses to obtain the desired response.
Wernicke's encephalopathy	Caused by thiamine (B_1) deficiency, characterized by nystagmus, ptosis, ataxia, confusion, coma, and possible death. Thiamine deficiency is common in chronic alcoholism.
Withdrawal syndrome	Constellation of signs and symptoms that occurs in physically dependent individuals when they discontinue drug use.

Women drink less alcohol and have fewer alcohol-related problems than men. In addition, women are less likely to have characteristics associated with heavy drinking including aggressiveness, drinking to reduce distress, and antisocial tendencies. See the Genetics Consideration box on page 103.

- *Biological factors* were first identified by Jellinek in his Disease Model of Alcoholism. He hypothesized that addiction to alcohol may have a biochemical basis and identified specific phases of the disease (Jellinek, 1946). Expanding on Jellinek's early work, researchers have implicated low levels of dopamine and serotonin in the development of alcohol dependence. Dopamine and dopamine receptor sites are intricately involved in the complex workings between the nervous system and abusive substances. Any drug's ability to have an impact on the biochemical mechanism of the brain must be able to do so at a receptor site or at a number of receptor sites (Figure 6–1 ■). Most abused substances either mimic or block the brain's most important neurotransmitters at their respective receptor sites. For example, heroin and other opiates mimic natural opiate-like neurotransmitters such as endorphin, enkephalin, and dynorphin. In contrast, cocaine

and other stimulants block the reuptake of dopamine, serotonin, and norepinephrine (Stuart, 2009).

- *Psychological factors* attempt to explain substance abuse through a combination of psychoanalytic, behavioral, and family system theories. Psychoanalytic theorists view substance abuse as a fixation at the oral stage of development, while behavioral theorists see addiction as a learned, maladaptive behavior. Family system theory focuses on the pattern of family relationships throughout several generations. No addictive personality type has been identified; however, several common factors seem to exist among alcoholics and drug users. Another type of alcoholism may be more environmentally influenced and is linked with onset after the age of 25, inability to stop after one drink, and a passive-dependent personality (Stuart, 2009). Many substance abusers have experienced sexual or physical abuse in their childhood and as a result have low self-esteem and difficulty expressing emotions. A link also exists between substance abuse and psychiatric disorders such as depression, anxiety, and antisocial and dependent personalities. The habit of using a substance becomes a form of self-medication to cope with day-to-day problems, and over time develops into an addiction.

Agonistic effects

Drug induces increase in synthesis of neurotransmitter

Drug increases release of transmitter

Drug activates receptors that normally respond to neurotransmitter

Drug

Receptor site

Antagonistic effects

Synaptic vesicle

Drug

Receptor site

Drug interferes with release of neurotransmitter

Drug acts as a false transmitter, occupying receptor sites normally sensitive to neurotransmitter

Drug causes leakage of neurotransmitter from synaptic vesicles

Figure 6–1 ■ Action of abusive substances at brain receptor sites.

■ *Sociocultural factors* often influence individuals' decisions as to when, what, and how they use substances. Ethnic differences in the way alcohol is metabolized may explain why some individuals choose not to drink. Compared to other ethnic groups, Asian Americans report the lowest prevalence of family history of alcoholism. It is hypothesized that the Asian population has a deficiency of aldehyde dehydrogenase (ADH), the chemical in the brain that breaks down alcohol acetaldehyde (Cook et al., 2005). A buildup of acetaldehyde in the brain causes toxic symptoms characterized by vomiting, flushing and tachycardia. Caucasians, Hispanics, and African Americans, on the other hand, have sufficient ADH for metabolizing alcohol and report higher alcoholism rates (Bersamin, Paschall, & Flewelling, 2005).

Religious background may also correlate with the likelihood that a person will abuse alcohol. Among major religions, people of Jewish faith have the lowest rate of alcoholism while Roman Catholics have the highest rate. See the accompanying Focus on Diversity feature.

Many factors place a person at risk for substance use, abuse, and dependence. No single cause can explain why one individual develops a pattern of drug use and another person does not. Thorough assessment of these factors is necessary to understand the whole person and plan appropriate interventions.

Characteristics of Abusers

As mentioned, no addictive personality type exists; however, many abusers have several characteristics in common. Addictive behavior associated with alcoholism and other substances is characterized by compulsive preoccupation with obtaining the substance, loss of control over consumption, and development of tolerance and dependence as well as impaired social and occupational functioning. There is a tendency for drug users to indulge in impulsive, risk-taking behaviors. Abusers often have a low tolerance for frustration and pain. Often, drug users are rebellious against social norms and engage in various antisocial and risky behaviors such as stealing, promiscuity, driving while intoxicated, and violence against others. There is also a tendency toward anxiety, anger, and low self-esteem in substance abusers. Many people have a desire for social acceptance and initiate drug use to "fit in" with a peer group. Others may suffer from social anxiety and need drugs or alcohol to feel less inhibited while interacting with others.

Addictive Substances and Their Effects
Caffeine

Caffeine is a stimulant that increases the heart rate and acts as a diuretic. Although commonly consumed daily in soft drinks, coffee, tea, chocolate, and some pain relievers, an excessive amount of caffeine can cause negative physiologic effects, especially cardiac related risks. Approximately 300 mg per day

Ethnic identity plays a unique role in drug use behavior. Patterns of substance use are influenced by cultural norms and practices, in addition to other environmental and biological factors. Adolescents in particular are influenced by ethnic and cultural practices. Positive ethnic identity (i.e., strong ethnic affiliation, attachment, and pride) may "protect" adolescents against drug use and help them form resistant behaviors to substance abuse (Marsiglia, Kulis, Hecht, & Sills, 2004). A higher number of Black and Hispanic children are exposed to alcohol problems in the home than white children (Ramisetty-Mikler & Caetano, 2004). Use of tobacco, alcohol, and illicit drugs are reportedly different in racial and ethnic groups. American Indians and Alaska Natives have higher levels of tobacco, alcohol, and illicit drug use when compared to other racial groups (SAMHSA, 2008a). Substance abuse and Type 2 diabetes are serious health problems among

American Indians (Leonardson et al., 2005). Asian Americans have the lowest rates of tobacco, alcohol, and illicit drug usage (SAMHSA).

CRITICAL THINKING IN PATIENT CARE

1. You are a school nurse with a large population of American Indians, Latin Americans, and African Americans in the community. An increasing problem with alcohol use and binge drinking among the high school students has become evident. The school superintendent has asked you for ideas to address this problem. How would you respond?

2. You are caring for a 23-year-old Asian American female brought to the emergency room by her boyfriend who tells you they were at a college party where she had alcohol for the first time. She is weak, her face is flushed, and she is vomiting violently. What would you do?

is safe for most people, but over 600 mg is considered excessive and not recommended (Kneisl & Trigoboff, 2009). Individuals with a history of cardiac disease are advised to cut down or eliminate caffeine intake altogether. Caffeine, if consumed in large quantities, can also cause higher total cholesterol levels and insomnia.

Many people in today's society recognize the adverse effects of too much caffeine in the system and voluntarily cut down on caffeine by drinking decaffeinated beverages. A caffeine-addicted person who abruptly withdraws from caffeine often experiences headaches and irritability. A rising number of adolescents are developing caffeine dependence by consuming sizeable quantities of soft drinks and coffee.

Nicotine

Nicotine is found in tobacco and enters the system via the lungs (cigarettes and cigars) and oral mucous membranes (chewing tobacco as well as smoking). In low doses, nicotine stimulates nicotinic receptors in the brain to release norepinephrine and epinephrine, causing vasoconstriction. As a result, the heart rate accelerates and the force of ventricular contractions increases. Gastrointestinal (GI) effects include an increase in gastric acid secretion, tone and motility of GI smooth muscle, and promotion of vomiting. Nicotine acts on the central nervous system (CNS) as a stimulant, binding to acetylcholine receptors in the brain and causing the release of dopamine and norepinephrine. Quitting smoking is thought to be more difficult because of dopamine release, which in turn reinforces the addictive craving for more. Smoking cessation can pose a problem for hospitalized patients. See Moving Evidence into Action: Smoking Cessation in Hospitalized Patients.

Initially, nicotine increases respiration, mental alertness, and cognitive ability, but eventually depresses these responses (Kneisl & Trigoboff, 2009). Moderate doses of nicotine can cause tremors. High doses of nicotine, found in some insecticides, can cause acute poisoning, resulting in convulsions and death.

Tolerance can develop to nausea and dizziness, but not to the cardiovascular effects. Nicotine dependence results from chronic use with withdrawal seen as craving, nervousness, restlessness, irritability, impatience, increased hostility, insomnia, impaired concentration, increased appetite, and weight gain. Gradual reduction in nicotine use seems to prolong suffering. Chronic health problems from smoking have been well established in the form of cancer, heart disease, emphysema, hypertension, and death (Kneisl & Trigoboff, 2009).

Since the 1990s, smoking rates among American women have steadily increased. Smoking is now the number one cause of preventable death and disease among women. An estimated 22.4% (about one in five) women in the United States are current smokers (SAMHSA, 2008a). Far more women are dying of lung cancer than of breast cancer. An estimated 178,000 women die annually from smoking-related diseases such as cancer, stroke, and heart disease (U.S. Department of Health and Human Services [USDHHS], 2006). Women are also confronted with unique health concerns from smoking during pregnancy. Smoking during pregnancy leads to increased risks for infants such as low birth weight, stillbirth, preterm delivery, perinatal mortality, and sudden infant death syndrome (USDHHS). Secondhand effects from smoking have been demonstrated, especially to fetuses during pregnancy. Smoking also increases the risk for infertility. Postmenopausal women who smoke have lower bone density and increased risk for hip fracture than women who have never smoked (USDHHS).

Cannabis

Cannabis sativa is the source of marijuana. According to 2007 NSDUH data, marijuana is the most commonly used illicit drug (14.4 million users) (SAMHSA, 2008a). A majority of illicit drug users (56.2%) reported that their first drug was marijuana,

---

MOVING EVIDENCE INTO ACTION   **Smoking Cessation in Hospitalized Patients**

Despite the well-publicized deleterious health effects posed by cigarette smoking and the legally restricted access to cigarettes, it still remains a persistent problem. Smoking has been banned in stores, malls, hospitals, office buildings, and even a number of restaurants. Admission to the hospital provides an excellent opportunity for nurses to assist patients to quit smoking. Patients in hospitals may find it easier to quit in an environment where smoking is restricted or prohibited. In addition, individuals may be more open to cessation efforts when faced with the risks associated with surgery. In a review of the literature, researchers found that high intensity behavioral interventions that include at least 1 month of follow-up contact were effective in helping hospitalized patients quit smoking (Rigotti, Munafo, Murphy, & Stead, 2005). Healthcare professionals, especially nurses, can be very instrumental in smoking cessation efforts. Another literature review provided evidence that nursing interventions for smoking cessation has potential benefits (Rice & Stead, 2005). Nicotine replacement therapy (NRT) also increases quit rates with or without additional counseling (Rice & Stead, 2005; Silagy et al., 2005). NRT aims to reduce withdrawal from tobacco products by replacing nicotine in the blood. All forms of NRT, available as chewing gum, skin patches, nose spray, inhalers, and tablets, increases the likelihood that a person will succeed in quitting smoking (Silagy et al., 2005). Effective nursing strategies include asking patients about their tobacco use, counseling those who want to quit, reinforcing cessation efforts, and early follow-up with those who quit smoking. This evidence points to the important role nurses possess to encourage their patients to quit smoking and the need for nurses to incorporate smoking cessation interventions as part of their standard practice.

CRITICAL THINKING IN PATIENT CARE

1. You are caring for a 55-year-old man recently hospitalized for acute angina who asks you what is the best way to stop smoking. What would you do?
2. Why do you think nurses and other healthcare professionals should (or should not) quit smoking?
3. You are caring for a 12-year-old girl who tells you she has smoked cigarettes occasionally and believes it makes her more popular with her older friends. She admits that she knows that smoking is supposed to be bad for you but doesn't see the harm in smoking a few cigarettes every day. How would you respond?

CHAPTER 6 / Nursing Care of Patients with Problems of Substance Abuse **107**

supporting the notion that marijuana is a "gateway" drug. The greatest psychoactive substances are in the flowering tops of the cannabis plant. Marijuana (also know as grass, weed, pot, dope, joint, and reefer) and hashish are the most common derivatives. The psychoactive component of marijuana is an oily chemical known as delta-9-tetrahydrocannabinol (THC). THC activates specific cannabinoid receptors in the brain. Evidence suggests that marijuana may act like opioids and cocaine in producing a pleasurable sensation, probably by causing release of endogenous opioids and then dopamine (Kneisl & Trigoboff, 2009). Marijuana use can trigger psychosis in schizophrenic patients and according to recent research cannabis use may be a risk factor in developing future psychotic symptoms (Ferdinand et al., 2005).

Physiologic effects of cannabis are dose related and can cause an increase in heart rate and bronchodilation in short-term use. Chronic long-term use can lead to airway constriction, bronchitis, sinusitis, asthma, and increased risk for respiratory cancer. The reproductive system is also affected by marijuana; it causes decreased spermatogenesis and testosterone levels in males and suppresses follicle-stimulating, luteinizing, and prolactin hormones in females, making breast feeding for new mothers impossible. Birth defects may also be associated with cannabis use. Marijuana crosses the placental barrier and is spread to fetal tissues. When a pregnant woman smokes marijuana she increases the risk of abnormalities in the fetus such as CNS disturbances, low birth weight, decreased length, smaller head circumference, and fetal death (Kneisl & Trigoboff, 2009). Subjective effects of marijuana include euphoria, sedation, and hallucinations. In addition, chronic use of marijuana can result in amotivational behaviors such as apathy, dullness, poor grooming, reduced interest in achievement, and disinterest. At extremely high doses, tolerance and physical dependence result.

Alcohol

Alcohol is the most commonly used and abused legal substance in the United States. Alcohol and other CNS depressants act on other neurotransmitters in the brain such as gamma-aminobutyric acid (GABA). GABA is the most prevalent inhibitory neurotransmitter in the brain and has a major role in decreasing neuronal excitability. Alcohol creates an additive effect with GABA, further inhibiting arousal and depressing the autonomic nervous system. This may explain why cross-tolerance effects occur when alcohol and other CNS depressants are used in combination. When taken together, alcohol and other CNS depressants such as benzodiazepines and barbiturates can lead to respiratory depression and death.

Slightly more than half, or 126.8 million, of the nation's population over age 12 report current alcohol use (SAMHSA, 2008a). Of this number, an estimated 17 million, or 1 in every 7, report heavy drinking (defined as binge drinking on at least 5 days in the past 30 days) (SAMHSA). Although the legal drinking age in all 50 states is 21, many underage people use alcohol. Of the 14 million adults in America who abuse alcohol, 95% report drinking before the age of 21 (SAMHSA, 2008b). Alcohol use increases with increasing age among underage persons and, unfortunately, this pattern has remained stable since 2002. In 2007, slightly more

than half (50.7%) of 18 to 20 year olds drank alcohol during the month before they were surveyed (SAMHSA, 2008a). Alcohol is considered a "gateway" drug, leading to the use of "harder" substances like cocaine, heroin, or methamphetamine. During 2006, over 130,000 alcohol-related emergency department (ED) visits were made by patients under the age of 21 (SAMSHA, 2008b). Almost one-third (31%) of those alcohol-related ED visits for minors involved other substances as well. Table 6–1 lists the drugs most frequently reported with alcohol in ED visits.

> **FAST FACTS**
> **Underage Drinking**
> - The rate of underage drinking remains consistently high. In 2007, approximately 10.7 million persons aged 12 to 20 reported drinking alcohol in the past month (27.9% of this age group).
> - Of these, nearly 18.6% were binge drinkers, and 6% were heavy drinkers.
> - Among persons aged 12 to 20 in 2007, past month alcohol use rates were lowest among Asians (16.8%) and highest among whites (32%).
> - The highest prevalence of binge and heavy drinking in 2007 was for young adults aged 18 to 20 (50.7%).
> - In 2007, over 26% of teens (16 to 20 years) reported driving under the influence at least once in the past year.
>
> *Source: SAMHSA, 2008a NSDUH.*

Alcohol is absorbed in the mouth, stomach, and digestive tract. The liver metabolizes approximately 95% of the ingested alcohol and the rest is excreted via the skin, kidney, and lungs. Generally, an individual can break down approximately 1 ounce of whiskey every 90 minutes. Factors such as body mass, food intake, and liver function can affect the rate of alcohol absorption.

When used in moderation, certain types of alcohol can have positive physiological effects by decreasing coronary artery disease and protecting against stroke. However, when consumed in excess, alcohol can severely diminish one's ability to function and will ultimately lead to life-threatening conditions. Chronic use of alcohol can cause severe neurological and psychiatric disorders. Severe damage to the liver occurs with chronic alcohol abuse, and can progress from fatty liver to other

TABLE 6–1 Drugs Most Frequently Reported with Alcohol-Related ED Visits

RANK	DRUG	ESTIMATED VISITS
1	No other drug	126,704
2	Cocaine only	101,588
3	Marijuana only	41,653
4	Cocaine and marijuana	21,241
5	Heroin only	14,958
6	Stimulants only	7,895
7	Alprazolam only	8,007
8	Cocaine and heroin	10,628

Source: SAMHSA, Office of Applied Studies, Drug Abuse Warning Network, 2008b.

liver diseases such as hepatitis or cirrhosis. Chronic alcoholism is the major cause of fatal cirrhosis. Alcohol causes damaging effects to many other systems; its effects include myocardial disease, erosive gastritis, acute and chronic pancreatitis, sexual dysfunction, and an increased risk of breast cancer.

Malnutrition is another serious complication of chronic alcoholism, especially thiamine (B_1) deficiency that can result in neurological impairments. Thiamine depletion is thought to cause the Wernicke-Korsakoff syndrome observed in chronic alcoholics (Stuart, 2009). Severe cognitive impairment is a principal feature of **Wernicke's encephalopathy** and **Korsakoff's psychosis**. Although these are sometimes considered to be two distinctive disorders, they are actually different phases of the same disease, commonly called Wernicke-Korsakoff syndrome. Wernicke's encephalopathy indicates the acute stage of the illness, and Korsakoff's psychosis indicates the chronic stage.

Although alcohol is a CNS depressant, it actually disrupts sleep, thus altering the sleep cycle, decreasing the quality of sleep, intensifying obstructive sleep apnea, and reducing total sleeping time. Heavy drinkers have a higher mortality rate and many fatalities occur from alcohol-related accidents. Blood alcohol levels (BALs) are highly predictive of CNS effects. Euphoria, reduced inhibitions, impaired judgment, and increased confidence are seen at 0.05% (Kneisl & Trigoboff, 2009). The legal level of intoxication in many states is 0.08%. Toxic levels in excess of 0.5% can cause coma, respiratory depression, peripheral collapse, and death (Kneisl & Trigoboff, 2009). Chronic consumption of alcohol produces tolerance and creates cross-tolerance to general anesthetics, barbiturates, benzodiazepines, and other CNS depressants. If alcohol is withdrawn abruptly, the brain becomes overly excited because receptors previously inhibited are no longer inhibited. This hyperexcitability manifests clinically as anxiety, tachycardia, hypertension, diaphoresis, nausea, vomiting, tremors, sleeplessness, and irritability (Llussier et al., 2007). Severe manifestations of alcohol withdrawal include seizures, convulsions, and **delirium tremens (DT)**. Episodes of delirium tremens have a mortality rate of 1% to 5%.

CNS Depressants

Central nervous system depressants, including barbiturates, benzodiazepines, paraldehyde, meprobamate, and chloral hydrate are also subject to abuse. Cross dependence exists among all CNS depressants and cross-tolerance can develop to alcohol and general anesthetics. Chronic users of barbiturates require progressively higher doses to achieve subjective effects as tolerance develops, but they develop little tolerance to respiratory depression. The depressant effects related to barbiturates are dose dependent and range from mild sedation to sleep to coma to death. With larger doses over time and a combination of alcohol and barbiturates, the risk of death increases greatly. The risk of accidental overdose and death resulting from barbiturates has resulted in decreased use, yet barbiturates are still clinically useful for seizure disorders and alcohol withdrawal. Benzodiazepines have replaced barbiturates as the drugs of choice for anxiety-related disorders. Benzodiazepines alone are safer than barbiturates, because an overdose of oral benzodiazepines rarely results in death. However, CNS depressants when taken together (for example alcohol and benzodiazepines) can result in death.

Psychostimulants

Psychostimulants such as cocaine and amphetamines have a high potential for abuse. Euphoria is the main subjective effect associated with cocaine and amphetamines, leading to addiction. **Cocaine** powder has been "snorted" (inhaled through the nostrils) for thousands of years, but a more dangerous method now is called freebasing. Cocaine base (freebased cocaine, or "crack") is heat stable and is usually "cooked" in a baking soda solution and smoked (freebasing). Cocaine hydrochloride (HCl) is diluted or cut before sale and the pure form ("rocks") is administered intranasally (snorted) or injected intravenously. "Skin popping," a subcutaneous method many substance abusers are using to administer drugs, may lead to the formation of abscesses under the skin. Mild overdose of cocaine produces agitation, dizziness, tremor, and blurred vision. Severe overdose produces anxiety, hyperpyrexia, convulsions, ventricular dysrhythmias, severe hypertension, and hemorrhagic stroke with possible angina or myocardial infarction (MI). The use of cocaine during pregnancy is especially problematic because the drug crosses the placenta and enters the fetal bloodstream. Spontaneous abortion, premature delivery, retardation of intrauterine growth, congenital abnormalities, and fetal addiction can result. Long-term intranasal use of cocaine can cause atrophy of the nasal mucosa, necrosis and perforation of the nasal septum, and lung damage. The growing practice of crack cocaine injection requires serious attention, as this new drug use behavior is associated with increased rates of high risk behaviors. Recent research indicates that injection drug users (IDUs) exhibit significantly higher rates of risky health behaviors. High risk sexual behaviors were especially prevalent among female crack cocaine injectors. Higher self-reported rates of adverse health outcomes, such as sexually transmitted infections (STIs), Hepatitis C, and abscesses among crack injectors were found, although no differences in rates of HIV infection were self-reported (Buchanan et al., 2006).

Amphetamine use is on the rise and poses a severe health risk to society due to its devastating physical and neurological consequences, including amphetamine-induced mental disorders. Methamphetamine is illegally manufactured, distributed, and abused and is currently the most widespread amphetamine used in the United States (SAMHSA, 2008a). In 2007, there were an estimated 529,000 current users of methamphetamine aged 12 or older (SAMHSA). Methamphetamine is a powerful stimulant drug commonly referred to as "speed," "crystal," "crank," "go," and, most recently, "ice," a smokable form of methamphetamine. The manufacture of methamphetamine is a relatively simple process and can be carried out by individuals without special knowledge or expertise in chemistry. Methamphetamine is often taken in combination with other drugs such as cocaine and marijuana and, like heroin and cocaine, can be inhaled, injected, ingested, or smoked.

It appears that methamphetamine is an "equal-opportunity" drug for addiction without regard to gender, age, race, or sexual preferences. In regard to race or ethnicity, the highest percentage rates of methamphetamine use were found among Native Hawaiians or other Pacific Islanders and the lowest rates of methamphetamine use were among Caucasians, Hispanics, Asians, and African Americans (SAMHSA, 2008a).

Methamphetamine use has been linked with human immunodeficiency virus (HIV) infection and high rates of sexually transmitted infections (STIs) in homosexual, heterosexual, and bisexual men and women all over the United States (Brown, Domier, & Rawson, 2005; Semple Grant, & Patterson, 2004; Shoptaw et al., 2005). Heterosexual men and women displayed severe to moderate depressive symptoms due to perceived stigma associated with methamphetamine use, emphasizing the importance of identifying and treating depression in this population (Semple, Patterson, & Rant, 2005).

Amphetamines cause arousal and an elevation of mood with a sense of increased strength, mental capacity, self-confidence, and a decreased need for food and sleep. Methamphetamine users experience numerous physical symptoms including weight loss, tachycardia, tachypnea, hyperthermia, insomnia, and muscular tremors. The behavioral and psychiatric symptoms reported most often include violent behavior, repetitive activity, memory loss, paranoia, delusions of reference, auditory hallucinations, and confusion or fright. A psychotic state with hallucinations and paranoia is common with long-term use, requiring treatment similar to other psychotic disorders. The cardiovascular effects of amphetamines are comparable to those of cocaine, including vasoconstriction, tachycardia, hypertension, angina, and dysrhythmias. Tolerance to mood elevation, appetite suppression, and cardiovascular effects develops with amphetamines; however, dependence is more psychological than physical.

Withdrawal from amphetamines produces dysphoria and craving with fatigue, prolonged sleep, excessive eating, and depression. Although a large number of people cope with amphetamine dependence worldwide, limited evidence exists for effective treatment (Srisuraponont, Jarusuraisin, & Kittirattanapalboon, 2005). In a systematic review of treatment measures for amphetamine dependence and abuse, antidepressants provided little benefit concerning amphetamine use. Both biological and psychosocial treatments should be further investigated (Srisuraponont, Jarusuraisin, & Kitirattanapalboon, 2005).

Opiates

Opiates such as morphine, meperidine, codeine, hydrocodone, and oxycodone are narcotic analgesics. Examples of some common brand names include Vicodin®, Percocet®, OxyContin®, and Darvon®. Narcotic analgesics are a type of pain reliever derived from natural or synthetic opiates. A small percentage of individuals are originally exposed to opiates in the context of prescription pain management; however, most people use opiates under social or illicit circumstances. The urban poor constitute the majority of abusers, although opiates are used and abused by people of all socioeconomic statuses. The problem of abuse of and addiction to prescribed narcotics has resurfaced as a major issue for the United States in the past decade and has worsened over the past few years (Compton & Volkow, 2006). Approximately 6.9 million Americans over the age of 12 reported nonmedical use of prescription pain relievers (SAMHSA, 2008a). According to the 2007 NSDUH, the number of new nonmedical users of OxyContin® was 554,000, with an average age at first use of 24 years (SAMHSA). A steady increase in opiate abuse seems to reflect, in part, changes in

medication prescribing practices, changes in drug formulations, and fairly easy access via the Internet or from family and friends. Over 56% of persons abusing pain relievers reported that the source of the drug was from a friend or relative for free.

Although the use of narcotic analgesics for acute pain management looks benign, long-term use has been associated with significant rates of abuse or addiction. OxyContin® is a controlled-released form of oxycodone prescribed for the management of moderate to severe pain. OxyContin® diversion and abuse has become a major problem in certain areas of the United States, particularly rural areas and Appalachia. A retrospective review of 534 medical records revealed that 27% of patients admitted and discharged from an addiction detoxification unit were dependent on prescription opiate medications (Miller & Greenfeld, 2004). The most frequently mentioned medication was Vicodin® (hydrocodone) followed by OxyContin® (oxycodone). Almost 0.75 million ED visits in 2006 involved illicit use of prescription or over-the-counter (OTC) pharmaceuticals (SAMHSA, 2008b). The most frequent opiates included methadone, oxycodone, and combination forms (e.g., hydrocodone with acetaminophen).

Heroin has been abused for many centuries and is usually administered intravenously. It induces a "rush" or "kick" that lasts less than a minute, followed by a sense of euphoria lasting several hours. Tolerance develops to the euphoria, respiratory depression, and nausea but not to constipation and miosis. Physical dependence occurs with long-term use of opiates. Initial withdrawal symptoms such as drug craving, lacrimation, rhinorrhea, yawning, and diaphoresis usually take 10 days to run their course, with the second phase of opiate withdrawal lasting for months with insomnia, irritability, fatigue, and potential GI hyperactivity and premature ejaculation as problems. Methadone is a synthetic opiate used to treat chronic pain and addiction to other opiates. Methadone does not hinder one's ability to function productively as other narcotics do and is a viable support for withdrawal (Stuart, 2009).

Hallucinogens

Hallucinogens are also called psychedelics and include phencyclidine (PCP), 3,4-methylenediosy-methamphetamine (MDMA), d-lysergic acid diethylamide (LSD), mescaline, dimethyltryptamine (DMT), and psilocin. Psychedelics bring on the same types of thoughts, perceptions, and feelings that occur in dreams. PCP (also called angel dust and peace pill) was developed in the 1950s as an anesthetic similar to ketamine, but due to its severe side effects its development for human use was discontinued. PCP is known for inducing violent behavior and for inducing negative physical reactions such as seizures, coma, and death. The most common route of administration is smoking tobacco, marijuana, or herbal cigarettes laced with PCP powder or the liquid form of PCP.

MDMA, commonly known as Ecstasy, had high use in the 1980s as a popular recreational "club drug" associated with dance clubs or "raves" and has reappeared in recent years as a date or rape drug. According to 2007 NSDUH data, approximately 0.5 million persons aged 12 or older (0.2%) used Ecstasy during the past year (SAMHSA, 2008a). Ecstasy use peaked in 2002, but has shown a steady decline in recent years, possibly due to a heightened awareness and vigilance. Parties where other drugs such as marijuana or alcohol are present may lead to easier access or availability of Ecstasy, thereby increasing the chances for first-time Ecstasy use. One study suggests that cannabis use is a powerful risk factor for subsequent first onset of Ecstasy use (Zimmerman et al., 2005). Another study reported approximately 20% of youths aged 16 to 23 admitted to using one or more of the following drugs: methamphetamine, MDMA (Ecstasy), LSD, ketamine, GHB (gamma-hydroxybutyrate), and flunitrazepam (Rohypnol) (Wu, Schlenger, & Galvin, 2006). Females were more likely than males to report using multiple club drugs. Staying in school and getting married were associated with decreased odds of club drug use. On the other hand, use of club drugs was increased by criminal behaviors and recent alcohol abuse or dependence.

LSD was first used to simulate psychosis. It affects serotonin receptors at multiple sites in the brain and spinal cord. LSD is usually taken orally but can be injected or smoked, as in tobacco- or marijuana-laced cigarettes. The individual's response to a "trip," the experience of being high on LSD, cannot be predicted and psychological effects and "flashbacks" are common. Serotonin imbalance is thought to affect impulse control and may be responsible for uninhibited sexual responses in women who have been given the drug without their knowledge. Other hallucinogens are similar to LSD but with different potency and course of action. Because physical dependence to hallucinogens does not appear to occur, withdrawal symptoms are not present.

Inhalants

Inhalants are categorized into three types: anesthetics, volatile nitrites, and organic solvents. Nitrous oxide (laughing gas) and ether are the most abused anesthetics. Amyl nitrite, butyl nitrite, and isobutyl nitrite are volatile nitrites used especially by homosexual males to induce venodilation and anal sphincter relaxation. Amyl nitrite is manufactured for medical use, but butyl and isobutyl nitrites are sold for recreational use. Other names for butyl and isobutyl nitrites are climax, rush, and locker room. Street names for amyl nitrite are "poppers" or "snappers" (Box 6–3). Brain damage or sudden death can occur the first, tenth, or hundredth time an individual uses an inhalant, resulting in "sudden sniffing death." This danger makes the use of inhalants more hazardous than some other substances.

Another danger is the wide assortment of organic solvents that are available to and inhaled by young children. Organic solvents are ingested in three different methods: bagging, huffing, or sniffing. *Bagging* involves pouring the solvent in a plastic bag and inhaling the vapor. *Huffing* refers to pouring the solvent on a rag and inhaling. *Sniffing* refers to inhaling the solvent directly from the container. Common organic solvents are toluene, gasoline, lighter fluid, paint thinner, nail polish remover, benzene, acetone, chloroform, and model airplane glue. The effects from inhaling organic solvents are similar to alcohol, with prolonged use leading to multiple toxicities and an increased risk for abusing other substances. Children who used inhalants before the age of 14 were twice as likely to initiate opiate use, as compared to those who had never tried opiates (Storr, Westergaard, & Anthony, 2005). There are no antidotes for these inhalants; therefore, management of overdose is supportive.

BOX 6–3 Common Street Names for Abused Substances

Substance	Street Name
Alcohol	Booze, brew, spirits, juice, hootch
Amphetamines	Bennies, crystal, crystal meth, crank, dexies, diet pills, dolls, eye-openers, ice, lid poppers, pep pills, purple hearts, speed, uppers
Barbiturates	Barbs, beans, black beauties, blue angels, candy, downers, goof balls, ludes, nebbies, reds, sleepers, tranks, yellow jackets, yellows
Benzodiazepines	Bennies, blues, rainbows, reds, sopors, yellows
Cocaine	Bernice, bernies, big C, blow, Charlie, coke, dust, girl, heaven, jay, lady, nose candy, nose powder, snow, sugar, white lady
	Crack: conan, freebase, rock, toke, white cloud, white tornado
Heroin, morphine	H, horse, harry, boy, M, Miss Emma, scag, "shit," smack, stuff, white junk, white stuff
Opiates	Meperidine (Demerol), hydrocodone (Vicodin®), Percocet®, oxycodone (OxyContin®), and Darvon®
Marijuana	Acapulco gold, Aunt Mary, broccoli, dope, grass, grunt, hay, hemp, herb, J, joint, joy stick, killer weed, Mary Jane, pot, ragweed, reefer, smoke, weed, "shit"
Hallucinogens	Acid, big D, blotter, blue heaven, cap D, deeda, flash, L, mellow yellows, microdots, paper acid, sugar, ticket, yello, Ecstasy

Interdisciplinary Care

Effective treatment of substance abuse and dependence results from the efforts of an interdisciplinary team specializing in the treatment of psychiatric and substance abuse disorders. Therapies may include detoxification, aversion therapy to maintain abstinence, group and/or individual psychotherapy, psychotropic medications, cognitive-behavioral strategies, family counseling, and self-help groups. Patients suffering from substance abuse can be treated in either inpatient or outpatient settings. A substance overdose is a life-threatening condition that requires emergency hospitalization to stabilize the patient medically before implementing any of these interventions. Several diagnostic tests can provide valuable information about the patient's physical condition and set the course for treatment.

Diagnostic Tests

The body fluids most often tested for drug content are blood and urine, although saliva, perspiration, and even hair can be tested. The simplest method of detecting blood alcohol content is by using a Breathalyzer. More invasive procedures such as serum drug levels are useful in the ED and other hospital settings to treat drug overdoses or complications. Urine drug screens (UDS) and/or blood alcohol levels (BAL) are the main biological measures for assessment purposes. Urine drug screening is noninvasive and the preferred method for detecting substances in the body. Companies often require a UDS of prospective employees before hiring them. In addition, professional and college athletes are now required to submit to random drug testing. Results of UDS are also used within the court system to determine drug use in relation to criminal activity. The length of time that drugs can be found in blood and urine varies according to dosage and metabolic properties of the drug. All traces of the drug may disappear within 24 hours or may still be detectable 30 days later. The psychoactive substance found in marijuana, delta 6-3, 4-tetrahydrocannabinol (THC) is stored in fatty tissues (especially the brain and reproductive system) and can be detected in the body for up to 6 weeks (Kneisl & Trigoboff, 2009).

Knowledge of the BAL is helpful in ascertaining the level of intoxication, the level of tolerance, and whether the person accurately reported recent drinking. At 0.10% (after 5 to 6 drinks in 1 to 2 hours), voluntary motor action becomes clumsy and reaction time is impaired. The degree of impairment varies with gender, weight, and food ingestion. Small women who drink alcohol on an empty stomach will experience intoxication more rapidly than large males who have eaten a full meal. At 0.20% (after 10 to 12 drinks in 2 to 4 hours), function of the motor area in the brain is depressed, causing staggering and ataxia (Kneisl & Trigoboff, 2009). A level above 0.10% without associated behavioral symptoms indicates the presence of tolerance. A BAL greater than 0.08% is considered legal intoxication in most states. High tolerance is a sign of physical dependence. Assessing for withdrawal symptoms is important when the BAL is high.

PRACTICE ALERT
Medications given for treatment of withdrawal from alcohol are usually not started until the BAL is below a set norm (usually below 0.10%) unless withdrawal symptoms become severe. The BAL may be repeated several times, several hours apart, to determine the body's metabolism of alcohol and when it is safe to give the patient medication to minimize the withdrawal symptoms.

High Acuity Care

Emergency Care for Overdose

The care of a patient who has overdosed on any substance is a serious medical emergency. Respiratory depression may require mechanical ventilation. The patient may become severely sedated and difficult to arouse. Every effort must be made to keep the patient awake; however, stupor and coma may often result. A seizure is another serious complication that requires emergency treatment. If the overdose was intentional, the patient must be constantly monitored for further signs of suicidal ideation. Never leave an actively suicidal patient alone. Signs of overdose and withdrawal from major substances are summarized in Table 6–2 along with recommended treatments.

Treatment of Withdrawal

All CNS depressants, including alcohol, benzodiazepines, and barbiturates, have a potentially dangerous progression of withdrawal. Alcohol and the entire class of CNS depressants share the same withdrawal syndrome. Early signs of withdrawal appear within a few hours following cessation of the drug, peak after 24 to 48 hours, and then rapidly disappear unless the withdrawal progresses to delirium tremens. Severe withdrawal or delirium tremens is a medical emergency that usually occurs 2 to 5 days following alcohol withdrawal and persists 2 to

3 days. The symptoms of severe withdrawal include disorientation, paranoid delusions, visual hallucinations, and marked withdrawal symptoms. Seizures may also occur, requiring the use of emergency equipment. Treatment of severe withdrawal during detoxification is mostly symptomatic through acetaminophen, vitamins, and medications to minimize discomfort.

In managing alcohol withdrawal, the goal is to minimize adverse outcomes, such as patient discomfort, seizures, delirium and mortality, and to avoid the adverse effects of withdrawal medications, such as excess sedation. Close monitoring is essential to assure protection of the patient. Critical care monitoring may be indicated to manage alcohol withdrawal delirium, particularly when very high doses of benzodiazepines are needed, or when there are significant concurrent medical conditions. Medications such as benzodiazepines are effectively used to minimize the discomfort associated with alcohol withdrawal and prevent serious adverse effects, in particular seizures. A symptom-triggered approach to the administration of benzodiazepines during alcohol withdrawal results in less total medication use and requires a shorter duration of treatment.

PRACTICE ALERT
The Clinical Institute Withdrawal Assessment for Alcohol (CIWA-Ar) is recommended to manage the symptoms of acute alcohol withdrawal. Benzodiazepines such as lorazepam (Ativan) are commonly administered according to a sliding scale based on the CIWA-Ar score. Medication is given only when the CIWA-Ar score is higher than 8 points.

Medications used to treat alcoholism are disulfiram (Antabuse), naltrexone (ReVia, Depade), and acamprosate (Campral). Disulfiram is a form of aversion therapy that prevents the breakdown of alcohol, causing physical illness (intense vomiting) if taken while drinking alcohol. All forms of alcohol, including OTC cough and cold preparations, must be avoided.

Naltrexone can help reduce the craving for alcohol by blocking the pathways to the brain that trigger a feeling of pleasure when alcohol and other narcotics are used. Because naltrexone blocks opiate receptors, patients should avoid taking any narcotics, such as codeine, morphine, or heroin, while on naltrexone. Patients should also discontinue all narcotics 7 to 10 days before starting on naltrexone. It is also recommended that patients wear a medical alert bracelet stating they are on naltrexone, in case of emergency medical treatment. While on disulfiram or naltrexone, psychosocial treatments such as Alcoholics Anonymous meetings, individual counseling, or group therapy are important, as the desire to "take a break" from treatment can overcome the patient's motivation to continue taking the medication.

Acamprosate is another medication prescribed for patients wanting to abstain from alcohol. The chemical structure of acamprosate is similar to gamma amino butyric acid (GABA) and glutamate neurotransmitters. Acamprosate is thought to block glutamate receptors while simultaneously activating GABA receptors in the brain; thus stabilizing the chemical imbalance that is disrupted by alcoholism. Evidence suggests that acamprosate is fairly effective in reducing cravings of alcohol-dependent patients when used in combination with psychosocial interventions (Snyder & Bowers, 2008).

TABLE 6–2 Signs and Treatment of Overdose and Withdrawal

	OVERDOSE		WITHDRAWAL	
DRUG	**SIGNS**	**TREATMENT**	**SIGNS**	**TREATMENT**
CNS Depressants: Alcohol Barbiturates Benzodiazepines	Cardiovascular or respiratory depression or arrest (mostly with barbiturates) Coma Shock Convulsions Death	*If awake:* Keep awake Induce vomiting Activated charcoal to absorb drug VS q 15 minutes *Coma:* Clear airway, intubate IV fluids Gastric lavage Seizure precautions Possible hemo or peritoneal dialysis Frequent VS Assess for shock and cardiac arrest	Nausea and vomiting Tachycardia Diaphoresis Anxiety or agitation Tremors Marked insomnia Grand mal seizures Delirium (after 5–15 years of heavy use)	Carefully titrated detoxification with similar drug *NOTE:* Abrupt withdrawal can lead to death.
Stimulants: Cocaine-crack Amphetamines	Respiratory distress Ataxia Hyperpyrexia Convulsions Coma Stroke Myocardial infarction (MI) Death	Antipsychotics Management for 1. Hyperpyrexia 2. Convulsions 3. Respiratory distress 4. Cardiovascular shock 5. Acidify urine (ammonium Cl for amphetamine)	Fatigue Depression Agitation Apathy Anxiety Sleepiness Disorientation Lethargy Craving	Antidepressants (desipramine) Dopamine agonist Bromocriptine
Opiates: Heroin Meperidine Morphine Methadone	Pupil dilation due to anoxia Respiratory depression-arrest Coma Shock Convulsions Death	Narcotic antagonist, (Narcan) quickly reverses CNS depression	Yawning, insomnia Irritability Rhinorrhea Panic Diaphoresis Cramps Nausea and vomiting Muscle aches Chills and fever Lacrimation Diarrhea	Methadone tapering Clonidine-naltrexone detoxification Buprenorphine substitution
Hallucinogens:		Low stimuli with minimal light, sound, activity	No pattern of withdrawal	
Lysergic acid diethylamide (LSD)	Psychosis Brain damage Death	Have one person "talk down patient," reassure Speak slowly and clearly Diazepam or chloral hydrate for anxiety		
Phencyclidine piperidine (PCP)	Possible hypertensive crisis Respiratory arrest Hyperthermia Seizures	Acidify urine to help excrete drug (cranberry juice, ascorbic acid); in acute stage use ammonium chloride Minimal stimulus Do NOT attempt to talk down, speak slowly in low voice Diazepam or Haldol		

TABLE 6–2 Signs and Treatment of Overdose and Withdrawal (continued)

DRUG	OVERDOSE SIGNS	TREATMENT	WITHDRAWAL SIGNS	TREATMENT
Inhalants: Volatile solvents such as butane, paint thinner, airplane glue, or nail polish remover	Intoxication: Excitation Drowsiness Disinhibition Staggering Lightheadedness Agitation Side Effects: Damage to nervous system Death	Support affected systems	No pattern of withdrawal	
Nitrates	Enhance sexual pleasure	Neurological symptoms may respond to vitamin B$_{12}$ and folate		
Anesthetics such as nitrous oxide	Giggling, laughter Euphoria	Chronic users may experience polyneuropathy and myelopathy		

MEMORY CUE

Alcohol abuse is a disease with definite genetic propensity, passed down from generation to generation through family members' DNA. The three main medications currently available to help alcohol-dependent patients maintain sobriety can be easily remembered by using the acronym DNA: Disulfiram, Naltrexone, and Acamprosate. Disulfiram interacts with alcohol to cause adverse effects, while naltrexone and acamprosate help to reduce the craving for alcohol.

Withdrawal symptoms from opiates and stimulants can be very unpleasant but are generally not life threatening. The patient experiencing an acute phase of cocaine withdrawal may become suicidal. Common drugs used in the treatment of substance abuse and withdrawal are presented in Table 6–3.

TABLE 6–3 Drugs Used in the Treatment of Substance Withdrawal/Abuse

DRUG	DOSE	PURPOSE
Benzodiazepines		
Clordiazepoxide (Librium)	15–100 mg	Diminishes anxiety and has anticonvulsant qualities to provide safe withdrawal. May be ordered q4h or prn to manage adverse effects from withdrawal; then dose is tapered to zero.
Diazepam (Valium)	4–40 mg	
Oxazepam (Serax)	30–120 mg	
Lorazepam (Ativan)	2–6 mg	
Vitamins		
Thiamine (Vitamin B$_1$)	100 mg/day	Prevents Wernicke's encephalopathy.
Folic acid	1 mg/day	Corrects vitamin deficiency caused by heavy long-term alcohol abuse.
Multivitamins	1 tab/cap daily	
Anticonvulsants		
Phenobarbital	30–320 mg	For seizure control and sedation.
Magnesium sulfate	1 g q6h	Reduces postwithdrawal seizures.
Abstinence medications		
Disulfiram (Antabuse)	250 mg/day	Prevents breakdown of alcohol.
Naltrexone (ReVia)	50 mg/day	Diminishes cravings for alcohol and opioids.
Acamprosate (Campral)	300 mg/TID	Diminishes cravings for alcohol.
Methadone	40 mg/day	Blocks craving for heroin.
Antidepressants		
Fluoxetine (Prozac)	20–80 mg/day	Enhances and stabilizes mood and diminishes anxiety.
Sertraline (Zoloft)	50–200 mg/day	

NURSING CARE OF THE OLDER ADULT   **Substance Abuse in the Older Adult**

Substance abuse in older adults is likely to increase over subsequent decades as baby boomers reach retirement age. People of any age can have substance abuse problems, but the consequences in older adults can be more critical (Lewis, 2008). Falls and accidents can rob older adults of their independence, and substance abuse increases the risk of falls by affecting alertness, judgment, coordination, and reaction time. In addition, older adults (especially older women) are more likely than younger people to use prescription or OTC medicines, which can be harmful when mixed with alcohol and/or illicit drugs (Lantz, 2005). Alcohol and drug abuse can also make certain medical problems hard to diagnose, for example, by dulling a pain sensation that might warn of a heart attack.

While substance abuse and dependence is not as common in older adults, it is less likely to be recognized. Unfortunately, a substance abuse problem in an older adult can be difficult to detect because many of the symptoms of abuse (e.g., insomnia, depression, loss of memory, anxiety, musculoskeletal pain) may be confused with conditions commonly seen in older patients (Lantz, 2005). Healthcare professionals frequently attribute these symptoms to the aging process and fail to address the misuse and abuse of substances in the elderly. Often, the *symptoms* of substance abuse are treated rather than confronting the abuse itself. Older adults are also at greater risk for numerous physical problems and premature death because alcohol negatively interacts with the natural aging process to increase risks for injuries, hypertension, cardiac dysrhythmias, cancers, gastrointestinal problems, cognitive deficits, bone loss, and emotional challenges, most notably depression (Stevenson, 2005). Because depression and alcohol abuse are the most frequently found disorders in completed suicides, nurses should routinely screen older adults for both substance abuse and mental disorders.

✑ Nursing Care

(margin: Substance Abuse Video)

Nurses may interact with patients experiencing substance abuse or substance dependence in a variety of settings. The most common setting is an alcohol and drug abuse (ADA) treatment program where patients are hospitalized for 20 to 30 days for detoxification and in-patient therapy. These patients may be voluntarily admitted but most are court-ordered to undergo treatment after charges of driving under the influence (DUI) or driving while intoxicated (DWI). Patients with substance abuse or dependence have impaired senses and risk-taking behaviors that lead to injuries from falls and accidents requiring medical attention. Therefore, hospital EDs as well as medical and surgical units are places where nurses will frequently encounter these patients. Box 6–4 summarizes key safety considerations for hospitalized patients with substance abuse problems. Occupational nurses and community health nurses will also interact with substance abusing patients in employee assistance programs and community health departments. Urgent care, pain clinics, and ambulatory care centers are other settings in which patients with substance abuse disorders will frequently appear for minor health problems associated with chronic disorders related to substance abuse or dependence.

Health Promotion

Nursing care of the patient with substance abuse or dependence is challenging and requires a nonjudgmental atmosphere promoting trust and respect. Health promotion efforts are aimed at preventing drug use among children and adolescents and reducing the risks among adults. Adolescence is the most common phase for the first experience with drugs (Stuart, 2009); therefore, teenagers are a vulnerable population, often succumbing to peer pressure. Healthy lifestyles, parental support, stress management, good nutrition, and information about ways to steer clear of peer pressure are important topics for the nurse to provide in school programs.

Nurses should provide adults with information on healthy coping mechanisms, relaxation, and stress reduction techniques to decrease the risks of substance abuse. Nurses have a responsibility to educate their patients about the physiological effects of substances on the body as well as ways to manage stress and anxiety. Nurses must encourage and support periods of abstinence while assisting patients to make major changes in lifestyles, habits, relationships, and coping methods. See Nursing Care of the Older Adult for meeting the individualized needs of older patients with substance abuse problems.

Assessment

A comprehensive approach to the assessment of substance use is essential to ensure adequate and appropriate intervention. Three important areas to assess are a history of the patient's past substance use, medical and psychiatric history, and the presence of psychosocial concerns. Questions should be asked in a nonthreatening, matter-of-fact manner, phrased as to not imply wrongdoing (Savage, 2008). For instance, a nonthreatening question such as "How much alcohol do you drink?" is preferable to the judgmental question "You don't drink too much alcohol, do you?" Open-ended questions that elicit more than a simple yes or no answer help to determine the direction of future counseling. Examples of open-ended questions are

---

BOX 6–4 **Safety Considerations for Hospitalized Patients with Substance Abuse**

- Closely monitor patients admitted for a drug overdose for signs of suicidal ideation.
- Never leave an actively suicidal patient alone.
- During acute alcohol withdrawal (first 72 hours), assess for withdrawal symptoms and administer benzodiazepines as ordered.
- Monitor unconscious patients closely for possibility of aspiration. Never place an intoxicated, unconscious patient in a supine position.
- Seizure precautions are indicated for patients experiencing acute withdrawal symptoms.
- Expect signs of delirium tremens to occur after 72 hours of abstinence from alcohol.
- Monitor patient for signs of hallucinations, delusions, or altered sensory perceptions that may lead to injuries.
- Assess for fall and choking risk. Provide one-to-one assistance as needed.
- Maintain fluid and electrolyte balance.

provided in Box 6–5. Use therapeutic communication techniques to establish trust prior to the assessment process.

History of Past Substance Use

A thorough history of the patient's past substance use is important to ascertain the possibility of tolerance, physical dependence, or withdrawal syndrome. The following questions are helpful in eliciting a pattern of substance use behavior.

- How many substances has the patient used simultaneously (**polysubstance abuse** or simultaneous use of many substances) in the past?
- How often, how much, and when did the patient first use the substance(s)?
- Is there a history of blackouts, delirium, or seizures?
- Is there a history of withdrawal syndrome, overdoses, and complications from previous substance use?
- Has the patient ever been treated in an alcohol or drug abuse clinic?
- Has the patient ever been arrested for DUI or charged with any criminal offense while using drugs or alcohol?
- Is there a family history of drug or alcohol use?

Medical and Psychiatric History

The patient's medical history is another important area for assessment and should include the existence of any concomitant physical or mental condition (e.g., HIV, hepatitis, cirrhosis, esophageal varices, pancreatitis, gastritis, Wernicke-Korsakoff syndrome, depression, schizophrenia, anxiety, or personality disorder). Ask about prescribed and OTC medications as well as any allergies or sensitivity to drugs. A brief overview of the patient's current mental status is also significant.

- Is there a history of abuse (physical or sexual) or family violence?
- Has the patient ever tried to commit suicide?
- Is the patient currently having suicidal or homicidal ideation?

Psychosocial Issues

Information about the patient's level of stress and other psychosocial concerns can help in the assessment of substance use problems.

- Has the patient's substance use affected his or her ability to hold a job?
- Has the patient's substance use affected relationships with spouse, family, friends, or coworkers?
- How does the patient usually cope with stress?

BOX 6–5 Examples of Open-Ended Questions for Assessment

- On average, how many days per week do you drink alcohol or use drugs?
- On a typical day when you use drugs or alcohol, how many hits or drinks do you have?
- What is the greatest number of drinks you have had at any one time during the past month?
- What drug(s) did you take before coming to the hospital or clinic?
- How long have you been using the substances?
- How often and how much do you usually use?
- What kinds of problems has substance use caused for you, your family, friends, finances, and health?

- Does the patient have a support system that helps in times of need?
- How does the patient spend his or her leisure time?

Screening Tools

Several screening tools such as the Michigan Alcohol Screening Test (MAST) (Pokorny, Miller, & Kaplan, 1972), Brief Drug Abuse Screening Test (B-DAST) (Skinner, 1982), and the CAGE questionnaire (Ewing, 1984) may help the nurse determine the degree of severity of substance abuse or dependence (Figure 6–2 ■). These screening tools provide a nonjudgmental, brief, and easy method to ascertain patterns of substance abuse behaviors.

- *Michigan Alcohol Screening Test (MAST) Brief Version* is a 10-question, dichotomous, self-administered questionnaire that takes 10 to 15 minutes to complete. An answer of yes to 3 or more questions indicates a potentially dangerous pattern of alcohol abuse.
- *CAGE questionnaire* is more useful when the patient may not recognize he or she has an alcohol problem or is uncomfortable acknowledging it. This questionnaire is designed to be a self-report of drinking behavior or may be administered by a professional. One affirmative response indicates the need for further discussion and follow-up. Two or more yes answers signify a problem with alcohol that may require treatment.
  - Have you ever felt you should *Cut* down on your drinking?
  - Have people *Annoyed* you by criticizing your drinking?
  - Have you ever felt bad or *Guilty* about your drinking?
  - Have you ever had a drink first thing in the morning (an *"Eye-opener"*) to steady your nerves or to get rid of a hangover?
- *Brief Drug Abuse Screening Test (B-DAST)* is a yes/no self-administered questionnaire that is useful in identifying people who are possibly addicted to drugs other than alcohol. A positive response to one or more questions suggests significant drug abuse problems and warrants further evaluation. Because self-report tools are not always answered truthfully, all patients who screen positive for drug addiction should be evaluated according to other diagnostic criteria.

Withdrawal Assessment Tools

Nurses working in medical-surgical units, psychiatric units, and special substance abuse units routinely care for patients experiencing acute alcohol or opiate withdrawal. Several assessment tools are available to determine the severity of withdrawal symptoms and indicate the need for pharmacological treatment to manage withdrawal symptoms. Examples of withdrawal assessment tools are the revised *Clinical Institute Withdrawal Assessment (CIWA-Ar)* (Sullivan et al., 1989) and the *Clinical Opiate Withdrawal Scale (COWS)* (Wesson & Ling, 2003).

- The *Clinical Institute Withdrawal Assessment of Alcohol-Revised (CIWA-Ar)* (Sullivan et al., 1989) (Figure 6–3 ■) is used widely in clinical and research settings for initial assessment and ongoing monitoring of alcohol withdrawal signs and symptoms. The CIWA-Ar scale is a validated 10-item assessment tool that can be used to monitor and medicate patients going through alcohol withdrawal. The CIWA-Ar assesses for several alcohol withdrawal symptoms (e.g. high blood pressure, rapid pulse

Brief MAST   Scoring Yes to 3 or more indicates alcoholism

1. Do you feel you are a normal drinker?
2. Do friends or relatives think you are a normal drinker?
3. Have you ever attended a meeting of Alcoholics Anonymous?
4. Have you ever gotten in trouble at work because of drinking?
5. Have you ever lost friends or girlfriends/boyfriends because of drinking?
6. Have you ever neglected your obligations, your family, or your work for 2 or more days in a row because of your drinking?
7. Have you ever had delirium tremens (DTs), severe shaking, or heard voices or seen things that were not there after heavy drinking?
8. Have you ever gone to anyone for help about your drinking?
9. Have you ever been in a hospital because of your drinking?
10. Have you ever been arrested for drunken driving or other drunken behavior?

B-DAST   The following questions concern information about your involvement with drugs *not including alcoholic beverages* during the past 12 months.

In the statements, "drug abuse" refers to (1) the use of prescribed or OTC drugs in excess of the directions and (2) any nonmedical use of drugs. The various classes of drugs may include cannabis, solvents, antianxiety drugs, sedative-hypnotics, cocaine, stimulants, hallucinogens, and narcotics. Remember *do not include alcoholic beverages*.

Have you used drugs other than those required for medical purposes?	Yes ___	No ___
Do you abuse more than one drug at a time?	Yes ___	No ___
Are you always able to stop using drugs when you want to?	Yes ___	No ___
Have you had "blackouts" or "flashbacks" as a result of drug use?	Yes ___	No ___
Do you ever feel bad about your drug abuse?	Yes ___	No ___
Does your spouse (or parents) ever complain about your involvement with drugs?	Yes ___	No ___
Have you neglected your family because of your use of drugs?	Yes ___	No ___
Have you engaged in illegal activities in order to obtain drugs?	Yes ___	No ___
Have you ever experienced withdrawal symptoms (felt sick) when you stopped taking drugs?	Yes ___	No ___
Have you had medical problems as a result of your drug use (e.g., memory loss, hepatitis, convulsions, bleeding, etc.)?	Yes ___	No ___

Scoring: one positive response warrants further evaluation

Figure 6–2 ■ Screening Tools for Alcohol and Drug Abuse.

Source: Brief MAST adapted from "The Brief MAST: A Shortened Version of the Michigan Alcohol Screening Test" by A. D. Porkorny, B. A. Miller, and H. B. Kaplan, 1972, *American Journal of Psychiatry,* September 1972, Vol. 129, pp. 342–345, Table 3. Used with permission from the American Journal of Psychiatry, © 1972 American Psychiatric Association. *Source:* Reprinted from Addictive Behaviors, Vol. 7, No. 4, H. A. Skinner, "Brief Drug Abuse Screening Test (B-DAST)", p. 363, © 1982, with permission from Elsevier.

and respirations, tremors, insomnia, irritability, sweating, and convulsions) and results in a score that is used to direct the administration of benzodiazepines or other drugs to relieve associated symptoms of withdrawal and prevent seizures. A score of 8 points or fewer corresponds to mild withdrawal symptoms. Scores of 9–15 points indicate moderate withdrawal, while a score of 15 or greater denotes severe withdrawal and an increased risk of delirium tremens and seizures.

■ *Clinical Opiate Withdrawal Scale (COWS)* (Wesson & Ling, 2003) rates eleven common signs or symptoms of opiate withdrawal. The summed total score of the 11 items can be used to assess the intensity of opiate withdrawal and determine the extent of a patient's physical dependence on opioids. A score of less than 12 on the COWS indicates mild or no opiate withdrawal symptoms while a score of 13 or more indicates moderate to severe withdrawal symptoms (Figure 6–4 ■).

Nursing Diagnoses and Interventions

The primary nursing diagnoses and interventions for patients with substance abuse problems are listed in this section. Implications for nursing care in acute and home care settings are combined in this discussion. See the Case Study & Nursing Care Plan on page 119 for the patient experiencing withdrawal from alcohol.

Injury, Risk for; Violence, Risk for

■ Assess patient's level of disorientation to determine specific risks to safety. *Knowledge of the patient's level of cognitive functioning is essential to the development of an appropriate plan of care.*

■ Obtain a drug history as well as urine and blood samples for laboratory analysis of substance content. *Subjective history is often not accurate and knowledge regarding substance use is important for accurate assessment.*

■ Place patient in a quiet, private room to decrease excessive stimuli, but do not leave patient alone if excessive hyperactivity or suicidal ideation is present. *Excessive stimuli increase patient's agitation.*

■ Frequently orient patient to reality and the environment, ensuring that potentially harmful objects are stored outside the patient's access. *Patient may harm self or others if disoriented and confused.*

■ Monitor vital signs every 15 minutes until stable and assess for signs of intoxication or withdrawal. *The most reliable information about withdrawal symptoms are vital signs; they provide information about the need for medication during detoxification.*

Clinical Institute Withdrawal Assessment of Alcohol Scale, Revised (CIWA-Ar)

Patient:_____ Date: _____ Time: _____ (24 hour clock, midnight = 00:00)

Pulse or heart rate, taken for one minute:_____ Blood pressure:_____

NAUSEA AND VOMITING -- Ask "Do you feel sick to your stomach? Have you vomited?" Observation.
0 no nausea and no vomiting
1 mild nausea with no vomiting
2
3
4 intermittent nausea with dry heaves
5
6
7 constant nausea, frequent dry heaves and vomiting

TREMOR -- Arms extended and fingers spread apart. Observation.
0 no tremor
1 not visible, but can be felt fingertip to fingertip
2
3
4 moderate, with patient's arms extended
5
6
7 severe, even with arms not extended

PAROXYSMAL SWEATS -- Observation.
0 no sweat visible
1 barely perceptible sweating, palms moist
2
3
4 beads of sweat obvious on forehead
5
6
7 drenching sweats

ANXIETY -- Ask "Do you feel nervous?" Observation.
0 no anxiety, at ease
1 mild anxious
2
3
4 moderately anxious, or guarded, so anxiety is inferred
5
6
7 equivalent to acute panic states as seen in severe delirium or acute schizophrenic reactions

AGITATION -- Observation.
0 normal activity
1 somewhat more than normal activity
2
3
4 moderately fidgety and restless
5
6
7 paces back and forth during most of the interview, or constantly thrashes about

TACTILE DISTURBANCES -- Ask "Have you any itching, pins and needles sensations, any burning, any numbness, or do you feel bugs crawling on or under your skin?" Observation.
0 none
1 very mild itching, pins and needles, burning or numbness
2 mild itching, pins and needles, burning or numbness
3 moderate itching, pins and needles, burning or numbness
4 moderately severe hallucinations
5 severe hallucinations
6 extremely severe hallucinations
7 continuous hallucinations

AUDITORY DISTURBANCES -- Ask "Are you more aware of sounds around you? Are they harsh? Do they frighten you? Are you hearing anything that is disturbing to you? Are you hearing things you know are not there?" Observation.
0 not present
1 very mild harshness or ability to frighten
2 mild harshness or ability to frighten
3 moderate harshness or ability to frighten
4 moderately severe hallucinations
5 severe hallucinations
6 extremely severe hallucinations
7 continuous hallucinations

VISUAL DISTURBANCES -- Ask "Does the light appear to be too bright? Is its color different? Does it hurt your eyes? Are you seeing anything that is disturbing to you? Are you seeing things you know are not there?" Observation.
0 not present
1 very mild sensitivity
2 mild sensitivity
3 moderate sensitivity
4 moderately severe hallucinations
5 severe hallucinations
6 extremely severe hallucinations
7 continuous hallucinations

HEADACHE, FULLNESS IN HEAD -- Ask "Does your head feel different? Does it feel like there is a band around your head?" Do not rate for dizziness or lightheadedness. Otherwise, rate severity.
0 not present
1 very mild
2 mild
3 moderate
4 moderately severe
5 severe
6 very severe
7 extremely severe

ORIENTATION AND CLOUDING OF SENSORIUM -- Ask "What day is this? Where are you? Who am I?"
0 oriented and can do serial additions
1 cannot do serial additions or is uncertain about date
2 disoriented for date by no more than 2 calendar days
3 disoriented for date by more than 2 calendar days
4 disoriented for place/or person

Total **CIWA-Ar** Score _____
Rater's Initials _____
Maximum Possible Score 67

The **CIWA-Ar** is not copyrighted and may be reproduced freely. This assessment for monitoring withdrawal symptoms requires approximately 5 minutes to administer. The maximum score is 67 (see instrument). Patients scoring less than 10 do not usually need additional medication for withdrawal.

Sullivan, J.T.; Sykora, K.; Schneiderman, J.; Naranjo, C.A.; and Sellers, E.M. Assessment of alcohol withdrawal: The revised Clinical Institute Withdrawal Assessment for Alcohol scale (**CIWA-Ar**). *British Journal of Addiction* 84:1353-1357, 1989.

Figure 6–3 ■ Assessment Tool for Alcohol Withdrawal.

Clinical Opiate Withdrawal Scale

For each item, circle the number that best describes the patient's signs or symptom. Rate on just the apparent relationship to opiate withdrawal. For example, if heart rate is increased because the patient was jogging just prior to assessment, the increase pulse rate would not add to the score.

Patient's Name:_____   Date and Time ____/____/____:_____

Reason for this assessment:_____

Resting Pulse Rate: _____ beats/minute *Measured after patient is sitting or lying for one minute* 0 pulse rate 80 or below 1 pulse rate 81-100 2 pulse rate 101-120 4 pulse rate greater than 120	**GI Upset**: *over last ½ hour* 0 no GI symptoms 1 stomach cramps 2 nausea or loose stool 3 vomiting or diarrhea 5 Multiple episodes of diarrhea or vomiting
Sweating: *over past ½ hour not accounted for by room temperature or patient activity.* 0 no report of chills or flushing 1 subjective report of chills or flushing 2 flushed or observable moistness on face 3 beads of sweat on brow or face 4 sweat streaming off face	**Tremor** *observation of outstretched hands* 0 No tremor 1 tremor can be felt, but not observed 2 slight tremor observable 4 gross tremor or muscle twitching
Restlessness *Observation during assessment* 0 able to sit still 1 reports difficulty sitting still, but is able to do so 3 frequent shifting or extraneous movements of legs/arms 5 Unable to sit still for more than a few seconds	**Yawning** *Observation during assessment* 0 no yawning 1 yawning once or twice during assessment 2 yawning three or more times during assessment 4 yawning several times/minute
Pupil size 0 pupils pinned or normal size for room light 1 pupils possibly larger than normal for room light 2 pupils moderately dilated 5 pupils so dilated that only the rim of the iris is visible	**Anxiety or Irritability** 0 none 1 patient reports increasing irritability or anxiousness 2 patient obviously irritable anxious 4 patient so irritable or anxious that participation in the assessment is difficult
Bone or Joint aches *If patient was having pain previously, only the additional component attributed to opiates withdrawal is scored* 0 not present 1 mild diffuse discomfort 2 patient reports severe diffuse aching of joints/ muscles 4 patient is rubbing joints or muscles and is unable to sit still because of discomfort	**Gooseflesh skin** 0 skin is smooth 3 piloerrection of skin can be felt or hairs standing up on arms 5 prominent piloerrection
Runny nose or tearing *Not accounted for by cold symptoms or allergies* 0 not present 1 nasal stuffiness or unusually moist eyes 2 nose running or tearing 4 nose constantly running or tears streaming down cheeks	Total Score _____ The total score is the sum of all 11 items Initials of person completing Assessment: _____

Score: 5-12 = mild; 13-24 = moderate; 25-36 = moderately severe; more than 36 = severe withdrawal

Provided by: Physician Clinical Support System, (877) 630-8812; PCSSproject@asam.org; www.PCSSmentor.org

Figure 6–4 ■ Assessment Tool for Opiate Withdrawal.

Source: Excerpted from Wesson & Ling "The Clinical Opiate Withdrawal Scale (COWS)," Vol. 35, No. 2, of the Journal of Psychoactive Drugs. Reprinted with permission of Haight Ashbury Publications (www.hajpd.com).

George Russell, aged 58, fell at home and broke his arm. His wife took him to the ER and an open reduction internal fixation (ORIF) of his right wrist was performed under general anesthesia in the operating room. He was admitted to the postoperative unit for observation following surgery because he required large amounts of anesthesia during the procedure.

Mr. Russell has a ruddy complexion and looks older than his stated age. He discloses that he was laid off from his factory job 2 years ago and has been working odd jobs until last week when he was hired by a local assembly plant. His father was a recovering alcoholic and his 30-year-old son has been treated for alcohol abuse in the past. Mr. Russell states that he knows alcoholism runs in the family, but he feels that he has his drinking under control. However, he cannot remember the events that led up to his fall and how he might have broken his arm.

ASSESSMENT

During the nursing assessment, Mr. Russell is hesitant to provide information and refuses to make eye contact. Prior to his operation, a BAL was drawn because the ER nurse detected alcohol on his breath. His BAL was 0.40 %, which is 5 times the legal limit for intoxication in many states. His vital signs are within the upper limits of normal, but he is confused and disoriented with slurred speech and a slight tremor of the hands. He is 6 feet tall and weighs 140 pounds. His total albumin is 2.9 mg and he has elevated liver enzymes. His wife states that he rarely eats the meals she prepares because he is usually drinking and has no appetite for food.

DIAGNOSES

- *Ineffective Coping* related to possible hereditary factor and personal vulnerability
- *Risk for Injury* related to aggressive behavior, unsteady gait and impaired motor responses
- *Ineffective Denial* related to inability to recognize maladaptive behaviors caused by substance use
- *Imbalanced Nutrition: Less than Body Requirements* related to anorexia manifested by decreased weight and low serum protein levels

EXPECTED OUTCOMES

- Patient will express his true feelings associated with using alcohol as a method of coping with stressful situations.
- Patient will identify three adaptive coping mechanisms he can use as alternatives to alcohol in response to stress.
- Patient will verbalize the negative effects of alcohol and agree to seek professional help with his drinking.

- Patient will be free of injury as evidenced by steady gait and absence of subsequent falls.
- Patient will gain 1 lb (0.45 kg) per week without evidence of increased fluid retention. Serum albumin levels will return to normal range.

PLANNING AND IMPLEMENTATION

- Establish trusting relationship with patient and spend time with him discussing his feelings, fears, and anxieties.
- Consult with a physician regarding a schedule for medications during detoxification and observe for signs of withdrawal syndrome.
- Explain the effects of alcohol abuse on the body and emphasize that prognosis is closely associated with abstinence.
- Teach a relaxation technique that is useful in the patient's opinion.
- Provide community resource information about self-help groups and, if patient is receptive, a list of meeting times and phone numbers.
- Consult with a dietitian to determine number of calories needed to provide adequate nutrition and realistic weight gain. Document intake, output, and calorie count.
- Consult with physician to begin vitamin B_1 (Thiamine) and dietary supplements.

EVALUATION

Mr. Russell was discharged from the postoperative unit without complications. He successfully underwent detoxification and contacted the Employee Assistance Program (EAP) at his new place of employment. He was on medical leave while his arm completely healed and now attends Alcoholics Anonymous meetings 5 days a week. He reports that he enjoys taking long walks with his wife in the warm weather and that his appetite has returned. He has gained 10 pounds in the past 6 weeks and feels physically better than he has in many years.

CRITICAL THINKING IN THE NURSING PROCESS

1. Explain why it would be important to include questions about Mr. Russell's medication history and his use of other medications during the initial nursing assessment.
2. Mr. Russell asks you to explain the risks of taking disulfiram (Antabuse). What should you tell him?
3. Develop a care plan for Mr. Russell for the nursing diagnosis of *Alteration in Nutrition: Less than Body Requirements*. Why is this necessary?

See Evaluating Your Response in Appendix C.

Denial, Ineffective

- Be genuine, honest, and respectful of the patient. Keep all promises and convey an attitude of acceptance of the patient. *The development of a nonjudgmental, therapeutic nurse–patient relationship is essential to gain the patient's trust.*
- Identify maladaptive behaviors or situations that have occurred in the patient's life and discuss how the use of substances may have been a contributing factor. *The first step in combating denial is for the patient to recognize the relationship between substance use and personal problems.*
- Do not accept the use of defense mechanisms such as rationalization or projection as the patient attempts to blame others or make excuses for his or her behavior. Use confrontation with caring to avoid placing the patient on the defensive. *Confrontation interferes with the patient's ability to use denial.*

- Encourage patient participation in therapeutic group activities such as co-occurring disorder or Alcoholics Anonymous (AA) meetings with other people who are experiencing or have experienced similar problems. *Peer feedback is often more accepted than feedback from authority figures.*

Coping, Ineffective

- Establish trusting relationship. *Trust is essential to the nurse–patient relationship.*
- Set limits on manipulative behavior and maintain consistency in responses. *Patient is unable to set own limits and must begin to accept responsibility without being manipulative.*
- Encourage patient to verbalize feelings, fears, or anxieties. Use attentive listening and validate patient's feelings with observations or statements that acknowledge feelings.

Verbalization of feelings helps patient to develop insight into behaviors and long-standing problems.

■ Explore methods of dealing with stressful situations other than resorting to substance use. Provide encouragement for changing to a healthier lifestyle. Teach healthy coping mechanisms (e.g., physical exercise, progressive muscle relaxation, deep breathing exercises, meditation, and imagery). *Patient needs knowledge about how to adapt to stress without resorting to drug use.*

Nutrition, Imbalanced: Less than Body Requirements

■ Administer vitamins and dietary supplements as ordered by physician. *Vitamin B₁ is necessary to prevent complications from chronic alcoholism such as Wernicke's syndrome.*

■ Monitor lab work (e.g., total albumin, complete blood count, urinalysis, electrolytes, and liver enzymes) and report significant changes to physician. *Objective laboratory tests provide necessary information to determine the extent of malnourishment.*

■ Collaborate with dietitian to determine number of calories needed to provide adequate nutrition and realistic weight gain. Document intake, output, and calorie count. Weigh daily if condition warrants. *Weight loss or gain is important assessment information so that an appropriate plan of care can be developed.*

■ Teach the importance of adequate nutrition by explaining the food guide pyramid and relating the physical effects of malnutrition on body systems. *Patient may have inadequate knowledge of proper nutritional habits.*

Self-Esteem, Chronic or Situational Low

■ Spend time with the patient and convey an attitude of acceptance. Encourage the patient to accept responsibility for his or her own behaviors and feelings. *An attitude of acceptance enhances self-worth.*

■ Encourage the patient to focus on strengths and accomplishments rather than weaknesses and failures. *Minimize attention to negative ruminations.*

■ Encourage participation in therapeutic group activities. Offer recognition and positive feedback for actual achievements. *Success and recognition increase self-esteem.*

■ Teach assertiveness techniques and effective communication techniques such as the use of "I feel" rather than "You make me feel" statements. *Previous patterns of communication may have been aggressive and accusatory, causing barriers to interpersonal relationships.*

Deficient Knowledge

■ Assess the patient's level of knowledge and readiness to learn the effects of drugs and alcohol on the body. *Baseline assessment is required to develop appropriate teaching material.*

■ Develop a teaching plan that includes measurable objectives. Include significant others, if possible. *Lifestyle changes often affect all family members.*

■ Begin with simple concepts and progress to more complex issues. Use interactive teaching strategies and written materials appropriate to the patient's educational level. Include information on physiological effects of substances, the propensity for physical and psychological dependence, and the risks to a

fetus if the patient is pregnant. *Active participation and handouts enhance retention of important concepts.*

Sensory Perception, Disturbed

■ Observe for withdrawal symptoms. Monitor vital signs. Provide adequate nutrition and hydration. Place on seizure precautions. *These actions provide supportive physical care during detoxification.*

■ Assess level of orientation frequently. Orient and reassure the patient of safety in presence of hallucinations, delusions, or illusions. *Patient may be frightened.*

■ Explain all interventions before approaching the patient. Avoid loud noises and talk softly to the patient. Decrease external stimuli by dimming lights. *Excessive stimuli increase agitation.*

■ Administer prn medications according to detoxification schedule. *Benzodiazepines help to minimize the discomfort of withdrawal symptoms.*

Thought Processes, Disturbed

■ Give positive reinforcement when thinking and behavior are appropriate or when the patient recognizes that delusions are not based in reality. *Drugs and alcohol can interfere with the patient's perception of reality.*

■ Use simple, step-by-step instructions and face-to-face interaction when communicating with the patient. *Patient may be confused or disoriented.*

■ Express reasonable doubt if the patient relays suspicious or paranoid beliefs. Reinforce accurate perception of people or situations. *It is important to communicate that you do not share that false belief as reality.*

■ Do not argue with delusions or hallucinations. Convey acceptance that the patient believes a situation to be true, but that the nurse does not see or hear what is not there. *Arguing with the patient or denying the belief serves no useful purpose, because delusions are not eliminated.*

■ Talk to the patient about real events and real people. Respond to feelings and reassure the patient that he or she is safe from harm. *Discussions that focus on the delusions may aggravate the condition. Verbalization of feelings in a nonthreatening environment may help the patient develop insight.*

Using NANDA, NIC, and NOC

Linkages between a selected NANDA nursing diagnosis, NIC, and NOC for the patient with a substance abuse problem are shown in the chart that follows.

Community-Based Care

The community provides many options for treating substance abuse including a mixture of individual, group, and family therapy. Medical detoxification can occur in hospitals, psychiatric units, special substance abuse units, methadone clinics, or outpatient settings. Less restrictive environments include residential rehabilitation programs, halfway houses, and partial hospitalization programs. These programs provide structured environments for the recovering substance abuser while maintaining a viable presence in the community. In addition, patients can obtain vocational counseling, become involved in self-help groups such as Alcoholics Anonymous or Narcotics Anonymous, and receive drug and health education.

NANDA, NIC, AND NOC LINKAGES
The Patient with a Substance Abuse Problem

Nursing Diagnoses	Nursing Interventions	Nursing Outcomes
■ Defensive Coping	■ Patient Contracting ■ Anxiety Reduction ■ Coping Enhancement ■ Counseling ■ Decision-Making Support ■ Self-Awareness Enhancement	■ Risk Control: Alcohol Use, Drug Use, Tobacco Use ■ Anxiety Control ■ Coping ■ Symptom Control Behavior ■ Self-Esteem

Note: Data from Moorhead, S., Johnson, M., Maas, M., & Swanson, E. (Eds.). (2008). *Nursing outcomes classification (NOC)* (4th ed.). St. Louis: Mosby; North American Nursing Diagnosis Association. (2009). *Nursing diagnoses: Definitions & classification 2009–2011.* Philadelphia: Wiley-Blackwell; Bulechek, G. M., Butcher, H. K., & Dochterman, J. (2008). *Nursing interventions classification (NIC)* (4th ed.). St. Louis: Mosby. Reprinted by permission.

Teaching the patient and family includes the following:

- The negative effects of substance abuse, including physical and psychological complications of substance abuse
- The signs of relapse and the importance of after care programs and self-help groups to prevent relapse
- Information about specific medications that help to reduce the craving for alcohol (naltrexone [ReVia] and acamprosate [Campral]) and maintain abstinence (disulfiram [Antabuse]), including the potential side effects, possible drug interactions, and any special precautions to be taken (e.g., avoiding OTC medications such as cough syrup that may have alcohol content)
- Ways to manage stress including techniques such as progressive muscle relaxation, abdominal breathing techniques, imagery, meditation, and effective coping skills

In addition, suggest the following resources:

- Alcoholics Anonymous, Narcotics Anonymous, and other self-help groups
- Employee assistance programs
- Individual, group, and/or family counseling
- Community rehabilitation programs
- National Alliance for the Mentally Ill

MEMORY CUE
Patients are at highest risk for relapse within the first few months after stopping the abused substance. An acronym that can assist the patient in recognizing behaviors that lead to relapse is **HALT**: **h**ungry, **a**ngry, **l**onely, and **t**ired. Nurses should emphasize the importance of a balanced diet, adequate sleep, healthy recreation activities, and a caring support system to prevent relapse.

Impaired Nurses

Healthcare providers are as susceptible as anyone else for developing substance abuse. By nature of their roles, dentists, pharmacists, physicians, and nurses are in frequent contact with drugs and are at high risk for substance abuse problems. One study exploring family history of alcohol and drug use in healthcare professionals found that nurses reported a higher

prevalence of alcoholism in their families than dentists and physicians (Kenna & Wood, 2005). However, no significant differences were found in healthcare professionals' drinking levels. As a rule, nurses experience many pressures in the workplace and have easy access to drugs. This temptation may result in greater vulnerability for substance abuse and dependence and can lead to impaired professional practice. Nurses must act responsibly when coworkers display signs of substance use. Healthcare professionals have a higher risk for opiate abuse than other professionals due to the high accessibility of opiates in their line of work. If colleagues are showing signs of a substance abuse problem, information about impaired nurse programs is available through most state boards of nursing to help individual nurses. Nurses convicted of working or driving under the influence of alcohol, illegal substances, or nonmedical use of prescription drugs are subject to disciplinary action by their state board of nursing. A disciplinary hearing is held and may result in censure, probation, or suspension of a professional license. The loss of professional licensure is the most severe form of disciplinary action and may prevent an individual from ever practicing nursing again. Warning signs of impaired nurses in the workplace are listed in Table 6–4.

TABLE 6–4 Warning Signs of Impaired Nurses in the Workplace

AT-RISK SITUATIONS	OBSERVABLE WARNING SIGNS
Easy access to prescription drugs	Inaccurate narcotic counts or frequent missing drugs Patients complain of ineffective pain control, deny receiving pain meds Excessive "wasting" of drugs Volunteering to give medications to patients Frequent trips to the bathroom
Role strain	Frequent tardiness or absenteeism, especially before and after scheduled days off Haphazard, shoddy charting Patient care judgment errors Unorganized, erratic behavior, unkempt appearance
Depression	Irritability, unable to focus or concentrate Abrupt mood swings Isolating self, taking long breaks Apathetic, depressed, lethargic Unexplained absences from assigned unit
Signs of alcohol or drug use	Smell of alcohol on breath Excessive use of perfumes, mouthwash, or mints Slurred speech, flushed face, reddened eyes, unsteady gait Wearing long sleeves in hot weather to cover up arms
Signs of withdrawal	Tremors, restlessness, sweating Watery eyes, runny nose, stomach aches

CHAPTER HIGHLIGHTS

- Substance abuse is the unsanctioned use of any chemical despite adverse effects on the individual's physical, psychological, interpersonal, or social health.
- Substance dependence occurs when control over the chemical substance is lost and the individual must use increasing amounts to produce the desired effect (tolerance) and must use the substance to avoid or relieve uncomfortable symptoms (withdrawal).
- Combinations of genetic, biologic, psychological, and sociocultural factors contribute to substance abuse or dependence. Addictive behavior has been linked to biochemical changes in dopamine and serotonin brain levels as well as heredity, ethnic differences, and peer pressure. Thorough assessment of individual risk factors is necessary to plan and deliver appropriate nursing interventions.
- Adolescents are particularly influenced by society and peers to use substances, predominantly tobacco, alcohol, and illicit drugs. A positive ethnic identity and family environment act as "protective" deterrents for substance use.
- Substance abusers have common characteristics including risk-taking behavior, low tolerance for frustration or pain, compulsive preoccupation with the substance, anxiety, anger, and low self-esteem. Stress management, anger control, social support, and counseling are helpful strategies to avoid substance abuse and dependence.
- Alcohol is the most commonly used and abused legal substance in America; however, polysubstance abuse is frequent in many

individuals. Marijuana is the most commonly used illicit drug. Both alcohol and marijuana are considered "gateway" drugs to harder substance abuse. Substances such as cocaine and methamphetamine are often used in conjunction with alcohol. Prescription anti-anxiety agents have been abused in the past, and there is a growing trend in prescription narcotic analgesic abuse.
- Nursing care of patients experiencing substance abuse problems includes health promotion efforts to prevent substance abuse; comprehensive physical, spiritual, and psychosocial assessment; and interventions for the human responses of ineffective coping and denial, imbalanced nutrition, low self-esteem, disturbed thought processes, disturbed sensory perception, and risk for injury or violence.
- Severe alcohol withdrawal or delirium tremens is a medical emergency that usually occurs 2 to 5 days following cessation of use. A symptom-triggered approach to the administration of benzodiazepines during alcohol withdrawal results in less total medication use and requires a shorter duration of treatment.
- The community provides many options for treating substance abuse including a mixture of individual, group, and family therapy. A successful after-care program includes resources to help manage stress and prevent relapse.
- Nurses are susceptible to substance abuse due to pressures in the workplace and easy access to drugs. Nurses need to assess their response to stress and seek early treatment for depressive symptoms to avoid impaired professional practice.

TEST YOURSELF NCLEX-RN® REVIEW

1. What is the minimum level of alcohol in the blood for an individual to be considered intoxicated?
   1. 0.05%
   2. 0.08%
   3. 0.50%
   4. 1.00%
2. Which of the following questions is *most* appropriate when interviewing the patient who is suspected of alcohol abuse problems?
   1. "Typically, how many days per week do you drink alcoholic beverages?"
   2. "Have you been drinking lately?"
   3. "You don't drink much alcohol, do you?"
   4. "Has your drinking caused a lot of problems between you and your spouse?"
3. What is the rationale behind ordering thiamine (vitamin B_1) for a person with a history of chronic alcoholism?
   1. to prevent acute pancreatitis
   2. to prevent cirrhosis of the liver
   3. to prevent hepatic encephalopathy
   4. to prevent Wernicke's encephalopathy
4. Which of the following substances present the highest medical danger during withdrawal?
   1. CNS stimulants and amphetamines
   2. opiates and marijuana
   3. alcohol and CNS depressants
   4. amphetamines and hallucinogens
5. What is the rationale for prescribing disulfiram (Anatabuse) for a person who suffers from alcohol abuse?
   1. to decrease the discomfort of withdrawal symptoms

   2. to decrease the pleasant, reinforcing effects of alcohol
   3. to prevent the breakdown of alcohol, thereby inhibiting impulsive drinking
   4. to block the signs and symptoms of alcohol withdrawal
6. Which is NOT a warning sign of substance abuse in the nurse?
   1. impaired motor coordination, slurred speech, bloodshot eyes
   2. unkempt appearance, disorganized, erratic behavior
   3. patients consistently report effective pain control
   4. frequent absenteeism or tardiness, unexplained absences from the unit
7. Which of the following statements is false?
   1. Smoking is the leading known cause of preventable death and disease among women.
   2. The smoking rates for women have steadily declined since the 1950s.
   3. Women who smoke during pregnancy have a higher risk for spontaneous abortions.
   4. Women who smoke have an increased risk for stroke and heart disease.
8. Which statement by the patient illustrates an understanding of your teaching regarding naltrexone (ReVia)?
   1. "I should read labels of OTC cold medicines to make sure they don't have alcohol."
   2. "I should stop taking all pain medications before starting on naltrexone."
   3. "I should go to my Narcotics Anonymous meetings for 1 month, then I can stop going."
   4. "I should wear a medical alert bracelet that states I'm taking naltrexone."

9. Which of the following is a realistic goal for a patient with substance abuse?
1. The patient will identify ways to deal with stressful situations instead of resorting to substance use.
2. The patient will refrain from using substances until craving for the substance has been eliminated.
3. The patient will focus on negative aspects of past behaviors and interpersonal relationships.
4. The patient will be able to use alcohol or drugs in moderation.

10. An appropriate nursing diagnosis for a patient with substance abuse problems is which of the following.
1. *Imbalanced Nutrition: Greater than Body Requirements* related to food intake in excess of energy expenditure
2. *Excess Fluid Volume* related to increased intake of vitamins and dietary supplements
3. *Ineffective Denial* related to inability to recognize maladaptive behaviors related to substance use
4. *Disturbed Thought Processes* related to infectious process and pain

See Test Yourself answers in Appendix C.

Pearson Nursing Student Resources

Find additional review materials at
www.nursing.pearsonhighered.com
Prepare for success with additional NCLEX®-style practice questions, interactive assignments and activities, Web links, animations and videos, and more!

BIBLIOGRAPHY

American Psychiatric Association (2000). *Diagnostic and statistical manual of mental disorders (DSM-IV-TR)* (4th ed., text revision). Washington, DC: Author.

Bersamin, M., Paschall, M. F., & Flewelling, R. L. (2005). Ethnic differences in relationships between risk factors and adolescent binge drinking: A national study. *Prevention Science, 6*(2), 127–137.

Brown, A. H., Domier, C. P., & Rawson, R. A. (2005). Stimulants, sex, and gender. *Sexual Addiction & Compulsivity, 12*(2-3), 169–180.

Buchanan, D., Tooze, J. A., Shaw, S., Kinzly, M., Heimer, R., & Singer, M. (2006). Demographic, HIV risk behavior, and health status characteristics of "crack" cocaine injectors compared to other injection drug users in three New England cities. *Drug and Alcohol Dependence, 81*(3), 221–229.

Bulechek, G. M., Butcher, H. K. & Dochterman, J. M. (Eds.). (2008). *Nursing interventions classification (NIC)* (5th ed.). St. Louis: Mosby.

Compton, W. M. & Volkow, N. D. (2006). Major increases in opioid analgesic abuse in the United States: Concerns and strategies. *Drug and Alcohol Dependence, 81*(2), 103–107.

Conner, B. T., Noble, E. P., Berman, S. M., Ozkaragoz, T., Ritchie, T., Antolin, T., & Sheen, C. (2005). DRD2 genotypes and substance use in adolescent children of alcoholics. *Drug and Alcohol Dependence, 79*(3), 379–387.

Cook, T. A., Luczak, S. E., Shea, S. H., Ehlers, C. L., Carr, L. G., & Wall, T. L. (2005). Associations of ALDH2 and ADH1B genotypes with response to alcohol in Asian Americans. *Journal of Studies on Alcohol, 66*(2), 196–204.

Ewing, J. A. (1984). Detecting alcoholism: The CAGE questionnaire. *Journal of the American Medical Association, 252*(14), 1905–1907.

Ferdinand, R. F., Sondeijker, F., van der Ende, J., Selten, J., Huizink, A., & Verhulst, F. C. (2005). Cannabis use predicts future psychotic symptoms, and vice versa. *Addiction, 100*(5), 612–618.

Jellinek, E. (1946). *Phases in the drinking history of alcoholics.* New Haven, CT: Hillhouse Press.

Kenna, G. A., & Wood, M. D. (2005). Family history of alcohol and drug use in healthcare professionals. *Journal of Substance Use, 10*(4), 225–238.

Kneisl, C. R., & Trigoboff, E. (2009). *Contemporary psychiatric–mental health nursing* (2nd ed.). Upper Saddle River, NJ: Prentice Hall.

Lantz, M. S. (2005). Prescription drug and alcohol abuse in an older woman. *Clinical Geriatrics, 12*(1), 39–43.

Leonardson, G. R., Kemper, E., Ness, F. K., Koplin, B. A., Daniels, M. C., & Leonardson, G. A. (2005). Validity and reliability of the audit and CAGE-AID in Northern Plains American Indians. *Psychological Reports, 97*(1), 161–166.

Lewis, T. (2008). Assessing an older adult for alcohol use disorders. *Nursing, 32*(8), 60–61.

Llussier-Cushing, M., Repper-DeLisi, J., Mitchell, M., Lakatos, B., Mahmoud, F., & Lipkos-Orlando. (2007). Is your medical-surgical patient withdrawing from alcohol? *Nursing2007, 37*(10), 50–55.

Miller, N. S., & Greenfeld, A. (2004). Patient characteristics and risk factors for development of dependence on hydrocodone and oxycodone. *American Journal of Therapeutics, 11*(1), 26–32.

Moorhead, S., Johnson, M., & Maas, M. & Swanson, E. (Eds.). (2008). *Nursing outcomes classification (NOC)* (4th ed.). St. Louis: Mosby.

National Institute of Mental Health. (2008). *The numbers count: Mental disorders in America.* NIH Publication No. 01-4584. Bethesda, MD: NIMH. Retrieved from http://www.nimh.nih.gov/publicat/numbers.cfm

North American Nursing Diagnosis Association International. (2009). *Nursing diagnoses: Definitions & classification 2009–2011.* Philadelphia: Wiley-Blackwell.

Pokorny, A. D., Miller, B. A., & Kaplan, H. B. (1972). The brief MAST: A shortened version of the Michigan Alcohol Screening Test. *American Journal of Psychiatry, 129,* 342–345.

Rice, V. H., & Stead, L. F. (2005). Nursing interventions for smoking cessation. *The Cochrane Database of Systematic Reviews,* Issue 4, The Cochrane Collaboration: John Wiley & Sons.

Rigotti, N. A., Munafo, M. R., Murphy, M. F. G., Stead, L. F. (2005). Interventions for smoking cessation in hospitalized patients. *The Cochrane Database of Systematic Reviews,* Issue 4, The Cochrane Collaboration: John Wiley & Sons.

Savage, C. (2008). How to screen patients for alcohol use disorders. *American Nurse Today, 3*(12), 7–9.

Semple, S. J., Patterson, T. L., & Rant, I. (2005). Methamphetamine use and depressive symptoms among heterosexual men and women. *Journal of Substance Use, 10*(1), 31–47.

Shoptaw, S., Reback, C. J., Peck, J. A., Yang, X., Rotheram-Fuller, E., Larkins, S., Veniegas, R. C., Freese, T. E., & Hucks-Ortiz, C. (2005). Behavioral treatment approaches for methamphetamine dependence and HIV-related sexual risk behaviors among urban gay and bisexual men. *Drug and Alcohol Dependence, 78*(2), 125–134.

Silagy, C. Lancaster, T., Stead, M., & Fowler, G. (2005). Nicotine replacement therapy for smoking cessation. *The Cochrane Database of Systematic Reviews,* Issue 4, The Cochrane Collaboration: John Wiley & Sons.

Skinner, H. A. (1982). *Drug Abuse Screening Test (DAST)* (p. 363). Langford Lance, England: Elsevier Science Ltd.

Snyder, J. L., & Bowers, T. G. (2008). The efficacy of acamprosate and naltrexone in the treatment of alcohol dependence: a relative benefits analysis of randomized controlled trials. *Journal of Drug and Alcohol Abuse, 34*(4), 449–461.

Srisurapanont, M., Jarusuraisin, N., & Kittirattanapalboon, P. (2005). Treatment for amphetamine dependence and abuse. *The Cochrane Database of Systematic Reviews,* (4): ID #CD003022.

Stevenson, J. S. (2005). Alcohol use, misuse, abuse, and dependence in later adulthood. *Annual Review of Nursing Research, 23,* 245–280.

Storr, C. L., Westergaard, R., & Anthony, J. C. (2005). Early onset inhalant use and risk for opiate initiation by young adulthood. *Drug and Alcohol Dependence, 78*(3), 253–261.

Stuart, G. W. (2009). *Principles and practice of psychiatric nursing* (9th ed.). St. Louis: Mosby.

Substance Abuse and Mental Health Services Administration (SAMHSA), Office of Applied Studies. (2008a). *Results from the 2007 National Survey on Drug Use and Health: National findings* (NSDUH Series H-34, DHHS Publication No. SMA 08-4343). Rockville, MD.

Substance Abuse and Mental Health Services Administration (SAMHSA), Office of Applied Studies. (2008b). *Drug abuse warning network, 2006: National estimates of drug-related emergency department visits* (DAWN Series D-30, DHHS Publication No. (SMA) 08-4339). Rockville, MD: Author.

Sullivan, J. T., Sykora, K., Schneiderman, J., Naranjo, C. A., & Sellers, E. M. (1989). Assessment of alcohol withdrawal: the revised Clinical Institute Withdrawal Assessment for Alcohol scale (CIWA-Ar). *British Journal of Addictions, 84,* 1353–1357.

U.S. Department of Health and Human Services (USDHHS), Centers for Disease Control and Prevention. (2007). *Fact sheet: Women and tobacco.* National Center for Chronic Disease Prevention and Health Promotion, Office on Smoking and Health. Retrieved January 12, 2009, from http://www.cdc.gov/tobacco/data_statistics/fact_sheets/populations/women_tobacco.htm

Wesson, D. R., & Ling, W. (2003). The clinical opiate withdrawal scale (COWS). *Journal of Psychoactive Drugs, 35*(2), 253–259.

Wu, L. T., Schlenger, W. E. & Gavin, D. M. (2006). Concurrent use of methamphetamine, MDMA, LSD, ketamine, GHB, and flunitrazepam among American youths. *Drug and Alcohol Dependence, 84*(1), 102–113.

Zimmerman, P., Wittchen, H., Waszak, F., Nocon, A., Hofler, M., & Lieb, R. (2005). Pathways into Ecstasy use: the role of prior cannabis use and Ecstasy availability. *Drug and Alcohol Dependence, 79*(3), 331–341.

7 Nursing Care of Patients Experiencing Disasters

LEARNING OUTCOMES

1. Distinguish the difference between an emergency and a disaster.
2. Describe the types of injuries and manifestations associated with biologic, chemical, or radiologic terrorism.
3. Discuss nursing interventions for the treatment of injuries related to biologic, chemical, or radiologic terrorism.
4. Explain the rationale for reverse triage in disasters versus conventional triage in emergencies.
5. Discuss situations requiring the need for patient isolation or patient decontamination.
6. Discuss the role of the nurse in disaster planning, response, and mitigation.

CLINICAL COMPETENCIES

1. Assess health status of patients who have experienced a disaster and monitor, document, and triage to the appropriate level of care.
2. Use evidence-based interventions to plan and implement nursing care for patients with injuries suffered as a result of a disaster.
3. Using assessment skills, implement and evaluate individualized nursing interventions for patients who are victims of disasters.
4. Provide safe and knowledgeable nursing care to treat disaster-related injuries.
5. Evaluate and revise plan of care to restore functional health status to patients who have sustained injuries due to a disaster.
6. Provide education to promote prevention of disaster-related injuries.

KEY TERMS

bioterrorism, *126*
cold zone, *133*
conventional weapons, *125*
disasters, *124*
emergency, *125*
hot zone, *133*
man-made disasters, *125*
mass casualty incidents, *125*

mitigation, *131*
multiple casualty incidents, *125*
natural disasters, *124*
nonconventional terrorist
   weapons, *125*
personal protective equipment (PPE), *133*
preparedness, *131*

radiation sickness, *129*
recovery, *131*
reverse triage, *132*
surge capacity, *131*
terrorism, *125*
triage, *132*
warm zone, *133*

All nurses will be expected to know how to provide care for victims of disasters whether they work in acute care settings, ambulatory sites, long-term care facilities, or at home in their communities. There is no way to know where or when disasters may strike. Because of this, nurses must be prepared to assist patients, families, friends, healthcare workers, first responders, and communities in their recovery from disastrous events. There are a number of basic competencies that nurses should be cognizant of related to disaster preparedness. The International Nursing Coalition for Mass Casualty Education (INCMCE) was founded to ensure a competent nurse workforce to respond to mass casualty incidents (MCIs) by facilitating the development of policies related to mass casualty events as they influence the public health infrastructure and affect nursing practice, education, research, and regulation (International Nursing Coalition for Mass Casualty Education [INCMCE], 2003).

The purpose of the *Educational Competencies for Registered Nurses Responding to Mass Casualty Incidents* publication (2003) is to provide registered nurses with the awareness of critical competencies necessary to respond effectively to mass casualty events (Box 7–1). Nurses are expected to have sufficient knowledge to recognize the potential for a disaster event; when such an event has occurred; and what nurses can do to protect themselves, family members, and community members from harm or from potential exacerbation of conditions. Nurses must be aware of their role in disaster planning, response, and mitigation. Equally important, nurses must be aware of professional limitations and be able to respond to MCIs appropriately within the scope of nursing practice.

Disasters and Emergencies

Noji (1997) defined disasters as "events that require extraordinary efforts beyond those needed to respond to everyday emergencies." **Disasters** may be natural or man-made. **Natural disasters** are caused by acts of nature or emerging diseases. They may be predictable through advanced meteorologic technologies or unexpected. For example, Hurricane Katrina hit landfall on August 29, 2005, along the Central Gulf Coast. The hurricane caused vast devastation as its storm surge breached the levee system that protected New Orleans from Lake Ponchartrain and the Mississippi River. Most of the New Orleans area was flooded, and heavy damage was also inflicted on the coasts of Mississippi and Alabama. Katrina is considered one of the most destructive and costliest natural disasters in the history of the United States (U.S. Department of Homeland Security, 2008). **Man-made disasters** are either accidental or intentional. They include complex emergencies, technologic disasters, material shortages, and other disasters not caused by natural hazards. Examples of man-made or human-generated disasters include war; chemical, biologic, radiologic, and nuclear terrorism; transportation accidents; group violence; food or water contamination; deforestation; and building collapses. Contamination of large amounts of vegetables at a grocery store is an example of a deliberate or *intentional* man-made disaster. A campfire that has been left unattended such that the embers are carried by high winds to the dry trees and brush nearby, creating a massive forest fire is an example of a man-made *accidental* disaster.

An **emergency** is distinguished from a disaster in that an emergency encompasses an unforeseen combination of circumstances calling for immediate action for a range of victims from one to many. For example, a motor vehicle crash may call for emergency assistance for a small number of individuals whose injuries are minor to very severe or fatal. Emergencies are generally accommodated within the emergency management system. Disasters seldom involve a single victim. Instead, disasters are complex emergencies that significantly overwhelm available hospitals, emergency medical services, facilities, and resources. Disasters are typically labeled as **multiple casualty incidents** with more than 2 but fewer than 100 persons injured or **mass casualty incidents** in which 100 or more casualties are involved (Beachley, 2005). An example of a mass casualty incident is that of an entire community affected by the release of a hazardous material such as a chemical as a result of a train derailment. With human fatalities of approximately 200,000 and 1,300 in Banda Aceh and the Gulf

Coast, respectively, the tsunami in Indonesia and Hurricane Katrina are prime examples of mass casualty incidents (American Red Cross, 2006). In summary, the key difference between an emergency and a disaster is that an emergency can be handled by the usual emergency management systems already in place, while a disaster overwhelms general emergency systems and requires additional resources.

Causes of Disasters

Disasters may result from a variety of causes, including hazardous materials and terrorism.

Hazardous Materials

Hazardous materials pose a potential risk to life, health, or property if they are released because of their chemical, biologic, or physical nature. The hazard exists during any stage of use, from the production and storage of these substances to their transportation, use, or disposal. Hazardous materials accidents range from the unintentional release of household hazardous materials, to chemical spills on highways, to groundwater contamination by naturally occurring methane gas (Langan & James, 2005).

Terrorism

Terrorism is defined by the U.S. Department of Defense as the "calculated use of violence or the threat of violence to inculcate fear; intended to coerce or to intimidate governments or societies in the pursuit of goals that are generally political, religious or ideological." One of the goals of terrorism is to cause psychologic effects that reach a much wider audience than the immediate victims or object of an attack. High-profile acts draw attention to the terrorists and their cause. It is thought that terrorists seek to obtain leverage, influence, and power through the publicity generated by their violence (Hoffman, 2008).

The weapons terrorists use are often described as conventional and nonconventional. **Conventional weapons** include bombs and guns. Car and truck bombs have become powerful weapons in suicide attacks such as the Oklahoma City bombing of the Alfred P. Murrah Federal Building on April 19, 1995. Terrorists use explosive bombs such as letter, parcel, pipe, barometric, and fertilizer truckbombs, as well as incendiary bombs such as Molotov cocktails. Other types of conventional terrorist weapons include handguns, rifles, semiautomatic weapons, hand grenades, rocket-propelled devices, and even surface-to-air, shoulder-fired missiles that can bring down helicopters, fighter aircraft, and civilian airliners (Through The Eyes of Terror, n.d.).

Nonconventional terrorist weapons include those in the chemical, biologic, and nuclear categories. Chemical terrorism attacks may manifest as the release of a toxin into highly populated areas, bodies of water, and unventilated areas. Another type of chemical terrorism is a specific attack on a particular product, especially a food product. This is accomplished by introducing a toxic chemical substance directly into the product. The anthrax attacks against U.S. public officials after 9/11 illustrate how these small amounts of "white powder" can encourage mass panic and hysteria in the public (Simonsen & Spindlove, 2007) (See Box 7–2).

BOX 7–1 Educational Competencies for Registered Nurses Responding to Mass Casualty Incidents

Core Competencies
1. Critical thinking
2. Assessment
3. Technical skills
4. Communication

Core Knowledge Areas
1. Health promotion, risk reduction, and disease prevention
2. Healthcare systems and policy
3. Illness and disease management
4. Information and healthcare technologies
5. Ethics
6. Human diversity

Professional Role Development
1. A description of nursing roles in MCIs
2. Identification of the most appropriate or most likely healthcare role for oneself during an MCI

Source: INCMCE (2003).

Bioterrorism

Another name for biologic terrorism is **bioterrorism**. Biologic terrorism is the "use of etiological agents (disease) to cause harm or kill a population, food, and/or livestock. Biological terrorism includes the use of organisms such as bacteria, viruses, and rickettsia and the use of products of organisms—toxins. The main purpose of biologic weapon use is mass devastation. Unfortunately, it is not uncommon for the results of a biologic attack not to be known for several hours or days after the attack because aerosolized biologic particles are odorless, colorless, and tasteless. Unless the terrorists announce the biologic attack, it may remain unknown until patients begin to present at emergency departments or physicians' offices a few days or weeks after the release of the agent. Detection is difficult because of the numerous different healthcare facilities available for patient treatment. Surveillance is essential to detect such an event. The goal of the surveillance system is to determine the status of the public's health and detect any sudden change in that status. Fortunately, biologic weapons are not as common, accessible, or available as chemical weapons.

Healthcare providers must be alert to the recognition, reporting, and treatment of high-priority biologic agents. A disaster preparedness plan should be established in every healthcare facility that outlines the protocol and procedures to be taken with a suspected bioterrorism attack. Hospital staff will alert the infection control nurse when subtle changes or trends in symptoms among patients are seen. The public health department is also given this data. When an unusual disease pattern presents itself, laboratories perform tests on cultures that would normally be discarded as contaminants. Laboratory personnel report unusual clusters of laboratory results. Special laboratories have been established to perform a battery of tests on suspicious specimens of rarely seen bacteria, toxins, viruses, or increased numbers of a particular strain or specimen. The Centers for Disease Control and Prevention (CDC) have created detailed "Fact Sheets" about bioterrorism agents and diseases for healthcare providers.

Nuclear/Radiologic Terrorism

The nuclear category of nonconventional terrorist weapons encompasses the use of a nuclear device to cause mass murder and devastation. This category of terrorism includes the use or threat of the use of fissionable radioactive materials in an attack. An explosion at a nuclear power plant is an example of this type of terrorism. Using conventional weapons against one of the many nuclear reactors in the world could cause an explosion that would cause extensive and possibly irreversible environmental damage. Damage to the reactors could cause radioactive matter to be released into the atmosphere, potentially endangering large population centers (U.S. Department of State, 2009).

The radiologic dispersion bomb is probably the most accessible nuclear device to be used by terrorists. Another name for this device is dirty bomb because it consists of a conventional explosive and radioactive waste by-products from nuclear reactors. The dirty bomb discharges deadly radioactive particles into the environment. It is cheaper to make than a nuclear bomb

BOX 7–2 Biologic Threat Infections

Following the terrorist attacks on September 11, 2001, and the development of anthrax cases in the United States, concern has arisen about the possible use of biologic weapons. The most likely pathogens to be used for this purpose include anthrax, smallpox, botulism, pneumonic plague, and viral hemorrhagic fevers.

Anthrax is an acute bacterial infection caused by *Bacillus anthracis*, a gram-positive, spore-producing organism that occurs in inhaled, cutaneous, and gastrointestinal forms. The spores are impervious to temperature and sunlight, and remain viable for years.

Inhalation anthrax carries the highest mortality rate because spores of one to five microns are easily inhaled and deposited in the alveoli. The patient initially exhibits influenza-like symptoms such as fever, nonproductive cough, headache, and malaise that advances to respiratory distress, mediastinal widening, and hemodynamic collapse in 3 to 5 days. Death may occur shortly thereafter. Untreated patients die in 2 to 3 days. The characteristic lesion of cutaneous anthrax progresses from an itching papule to a painless, serosanguineous-filled vesicle that forms a black necrotic center. Patients who ingest the anthrax bacillus develop nausea, vomiting, severe abdominal pain, and bloody diarrhea. Diagnosis is confirmed by a positive blood culture, polymerase chain reaction, and serology. On confirmation of anthrax exposure, prophylaxis is initiated with oral ciprofloxacin (Cipro) or doxycycline (Doxycin) for 60 days; people with confirmed systemic anthrax cases must receive anti-infectives intravenously (CDC, 2006).

Healthcare workers risk exposure to anthrax through direct contact with a contaminated surface, exposed persons' contaminated clothes, or direct unprotected contact with the open lesions of cutaneous anthrax. Guidelines for decontamination of extensively exposed persons include removal of clothing and storage in a sealed plastic bag, and showering with soap and water. If gross contamination with the agent occurs and soap and water decontamination is ineffective, use a bleach solution (1:10 dilution of household bleach/final hypochlorite concentration 0.5%) and rinse after 10 to 15 minutes (Heymann, 2004).

In 1980, the World Health Organization certified that *smallpox* was eradicated. Routine smallpox vaccination was discontinued in 1972, leaving people under the age of 39 at risk for this disease if it reappears or is used as a weapon. Smallpox spreads by direct contact or by inhalation of respiratory droplets. Symptoms include a high fever, headache, and malaise, followed by a vesicular/pustular rash appearing simultaneously on the face and extremities. Once the lesions break open and spread large amounts of the virus into the mouth and throat, people are highly contagious and should be placed in negative-pressure rooms. Anyone exposed to the patient should be vaccinated and monitored closely. Vaccination up to 4 days after exposure and before a rash appears provides almost complete protection (World Health Organization (WHO), 2009). Healthcare providers should be alert to illness patterns that could indicate an unusual infectious disease outbreak. Indicators of a biologic agent release include increased disease incidence among people in the same geographic area (e.g., people who attended the same event); the disease pattern is inconsistent with patient age, such as chickenpox among adults; and a patient presents with symptoms of a rare disease. The presence of one or more of these indicators should be reported to public health authorities to determine the infectious disease source and to prevent further exposure (WHO, 2009).

and radioactive waste material is relatively easy to obtain. Radioactive waste is found throughout the world and is typically not as well guarded as nuclear weapons.

Types of Disasters with Common Injuries

This section describes a variety of disasters with the injuries that are common to each specific disaster. Table 7–1 outlines types of disasters with related injuries and nursing implications.

Hurricanes, Tornados, and Tsunamis

A hurricane is a type of tropical cyclone. It is a low-pressure system that generally forms in the tropics. Hurricanes can wreak havoc on coastlines as well as several hundred miles inland. Hurricanes and tropical storms can also spawn tornadoes, create storm surges along the coast, and cause extensive damage from heavy rainfall. Floods are deadly and destructive. Excessive rain can trigger landslides or mudslides, especially in mountainous regions. Flooding on rivers and streams may persist for several days or more after the storm (Federal Emergency Management Agency, 2008).

Common physical effects include asphyxia due to drowning; wounds; bone, joint, and muscle injuries; aggravation of chronic illnesses; stress-related symptoms; upper respiratory infections; gastrointestinal illnesses; clean-up injuries; animal, snake, and insect bites; skin irritations and infections; obstetrical complications; and waterborne and insect-borne diseases from contaminated water supplies and insect breeding grounds (Clark, 2008; Smith & Maurer, 2005).

As a result of Hurricane Katrina, many people lost their homes, family members, friends, and the environment that supported their daily routines. Many basic physical needs in the aftermath of the hurricane could not be met, which put survivors at risk of dehydration, starvation or malnutrition, heat-related illnesses, and diseases and injuries related to lack of sanitation and safe housing (Myers-Walls, 2005). The CDC offers a number of specific strategies to promote health and safety after a hurricane.

A tsunami, a seismic sea wave, is a series of ocean waves characterized by having a long period and wavelength and the ability to travel at speeds greater than 500 miles per hour. As the tsunami encounters shallow water, its height increases drastically, resulting in a sudden increase in sea level, thereby flooding low-lying coastal areas. Injuries are similar to those seen with hurricanes.

Thunderstorms

Risk of a lightning strike is possible during a thunderstorm. The short duration of a lightning strike results in a very short flow of current internally, despite the high voltage of lightning. Additionally, the almost immediate flashover of current around the body usually results in very little, if any, skin breakdown or burning of tissues (Daley et al., 2008).

High electrolyte and water content in the body conduct the greatest electrical current. Hence, the greatest conductors of

electrical current in the body are the nerves, muscle, and blood vessels. High resistors to electric current are bone, tendon, and fat, due to their tendency to heat up and coagulate instead of transmitting current. Much of the energy current may be dissipated at the skin surface. This results in significant surface burns, especially in calloused areas (Daley et al., 2008).

Tornados

Flying debris causes most fatalities and injuries in tornadoes. The physical effects include bone, muscle, and joint injuries; fractures; aggravation of chronic illnesses, obstetrical complications, stress-related symptoms; upper respiratory infections and those associated with fiberglass; eye injuries (see Box 7–3 for first aid); clean-up wounds; and gastrointestinal illnesses (Smith & Maurer, 2005).

Earthquakes

Earthquakes have a high incidence of mortality and morbidity. The most common health effects experienced by victims of earthquakes include stress-related symptoms; wounds; bone, joint, and muscle injuries; burns from explosions; clean-up injuries; gastrointestinal and respiratory problems; aggravation of chronic illnesses; obstetrical complications; and death (Smith & Maurer, 2005).

Snowstorms

Overexertion and exhaustion are major problems during the snow shoveling that is done following a snowstorm. The exertion required to shovel heavy snow in the extreme cold may cause a myocardial infarction.

BOX 7–3 First Aid for Eye Injuries

Specks in the Eye
- Do not rub the eye.
- Flush the eye with large amounts of water.
- Seek medical attention if the speck does not wash out.

Cuts, Punctures, and Foreign Objects in the Eye
- Do NOT wash out the eye.
- Do NOT try to remove a foreign object stuck in the eye.
- Seek immediate medical attention.

Chemical Burns
- Immediately flush the eye with water or any drinkable fluid. Open the eye as wide as possible. Continue flushing for at least 15 minutes. For caustic or basic solutions, continue flushing while on the way to medical care.
- If a contact lens is in the eye, begin flushing over the lens immediately. Flushing may dislodge the lens.
- Seek immediate medical attention.

Blows to the Eye
- Apply a cold compress without pressure, or tape crushed iced in a plastic bag to the forehead and allow it to rest gently on the injured eye.
- Seek immediate medical attention if pain continues, if vision is reduced, or if blood or discoloration appears in the eye.

Source: National Institute for Occupational Safety and Health (NIOSH). (2009). Available at http://www.cdd.gov/niosh/topics/eye/eyesafe.html

TABLE 7–1 Types of Disasters and Common Injuries

TYPE OF DISASTER	COMMON INJURIES	NURSING IMPLICATIONS
Hurricane-Related Injuries	Drowning; clean-up injuries; aggravation of chronic illnesses; stress-related symptoms; upper respiratory infections; gastrointestinal illnesses; animal, snake, and insect bites; obstetrical complications; contaminated water supplies and insect-breeding grounds; heat-related illnesses; lack of sanitation and safe housing	Asphyxia; wounds; bone, joint, and muscle injuries; infections; skin irritations; waterborne and insect-borne diseases; dehydration; starvation or malnutrition; diseases.
Tsunami-Related Injuries	"Tsunami lung," a severe infection caused by swallowing muddy, bacteria-laden water	Requires aggressive respiratory and ventilator management, blood transfusions, antibiotics, and other medical support.
Thunderstorm-Related Injuries	Resistance of body tissues to electrical current *Least resistance:* nerves, blood, mucous membranes, muscle *Intermediate resistance:* dry skin *Most resistance:* tendon, fat, bone	Potential for tissue destruction with longer duration of contact with high-voltage current; if energy current is dissipated at the skin surface, significant surface burns result, especially in calloused areas.
Tornado-Related Injuries	Flying debris; injuries similar to hurricane-related injuries	Injuries and fatalities can occur.
Earthquake-Related Injuries	High incidence of mortality and morbidity; explosions	May result in stress-related symptoms; wounds; bone, joint, and muscle injuries; clean-up injuries; gastrointestinal and respiratory problems; aggravation of chronic illnesses; obstetrical complications; burns.
Snowstorm-Related Injuries	Overexertion and exhaustion	Myocardial infarction can occur.
Disaster-Related Eye Injuries	"Specks" of dust or debris; cuts, punctures, or stuck objects; blows to the eye	Administer eyewash or flushing versus rubbing; stabilize eye with rigid shield. Apply cold compress, no pressure; patient should visit healthcare professional to rule out serious injury or internal eye damage.
Blast Injuries	Auditory	Tympanic membrane rupture, ossicular disruption, and cochlear damage occur; damage from foreign body can occur.
	Eye, orbit, face	Perforated globe, air embolisms, fractures are common; damage from foreign body can occur.
	Respiratory	May result in blast lung, hemothorax, pneumothorax, pulmonary contusion and hemorrhage, atrioventricular fistulas (source of air embolism), airway epithelial damage, aspiration pneumonitis, sepsis.
	Digestive	May result in bowel perforation, hemorrhage, ruptured liver or spleen, sepsis, mesenteric ischemia from air embolism.
	Circulatory	Cardiac contusion, myocardial infarction from air embolism, shock, vasovagal hypotension, peripheral vascular injury, and air embolism-induced injury can occur.
	Central nervous system injury	Concussion, closed and open brain injury, stroke, spinal cord injury, air embolism-induced injury can occur.
	Renal injury	May result in renal contusion, laceration, acute renal failure due to rhabdomyolysis, hypotension, and hypovolemia.
	Extremity injury	Traumatic amputation, fractures, crush injuries, compartment syndrome, burns, cuts, lacerations, acute arterial occlusion, air embolism-induced injury can occur.
Blunt Trauma	Head and torso blunt trauma, penetrating trauma	Fractured limbs and spinal injury can occur.
Pressure Trauma	Lungs	Tearing of the alveoli cause swelling, fluid accumulation, possible pulmonary emboli, eventual hypoxia.
	Ear injury: ear pain, hearing loss	Keep auditory canal clean.

TABLE 7–1 Types of Disasters and Common Injuries (continued)

TYPE OF DISASTER	COMMON INJURIES	NURSING IMPLICATIONS
	Bowel injury	Make the patient comfortable.
Radiological Dispersion Bomb (Dirty Bomb) Blast	Radiation sickness	Get rid of contaminated clothes, shower, and evacuate the area within a day of a small or medium blast. Those close to the blast could suffer radiation sickness and require hospital care.
Nuclear Detonation	Thermal burns	May involve only the epidermis and upper layers of dermis with short duration of heat exposure.
Bright Light Flash of Nuclear Detonation	Eye burn injuries	May blind the patient momentarily, effects will disappear with time, can impair a patient's ability to perform self-care and other ADLs.
Radiation Exposure Injury	Bone marrow and blood cell damage	A reduction in the blood's oxygen-carrying capacity results in nausea, fatigue, and a general feeling of malaise. Reduced platelet production causes clotting disorders and possibly hemorrhage. When the body's white blood cells are destroyed, it is important to reduce the patient's exposure to infection. Infection at the time of reduced WBC production can be severe and even fatal.
	Bowel	Cells that reproduce the bowel lining are damaged, resulting in nausea, loss of appetite, vomiting, diarrhea, fluid loss, and malaise in the acute stage; later, dehydration, malnutrition, bowel hemorrhage, and perforation may occur; if radiation exposure is not exacerbated by other injury or pathology, patients will generally survive.
	Integument	Erythema or generalized reddening of the skin occurs when skin cells are damaged, with the appearance of a sunburn; more serious burns may occur with persistent exposure or extremely high radiation doses.
	Nervous and cardiovascular systems	With acute radiation exposure, blood vessel and nerve cells are damaged and the patient is incapacitated and experiences cardiovascular collapse, confusion, and even an "on fire" sensation throughout the body; symptoms this severe generally do not permit survival.
Chemical Burns	Range from minor to life-threatening injuries	Remove clothing from injury site as well as any jewelry; flush chemical from skin with thorough decontamination; cover wounds loosely with a dry, sterile, or clean cloth.

Source: Adapted from *Centers for Disease Control and Prevention* (2003a), Daley, Aycinena, & Mallat (2008), DeLorenzo & Porter (2000), and Harris (2002).

Explosives

Blast injuries are the result of explosive munitions, often involving car or package bombs. Care for persons injured by blast injuries typically focuses on abdominal and lung injuries, penetrating wounds, traumatic amputations, and burns (Scott, Vanderploeg, Belanger & Scholten, 2005).

Radiologic Dispersion Bomb (Dirty Bomb) Blast

A dirty bomb consists of a conventional explosive such as trinitrotoluene (TNT) packed with radioactive waste by-products from nuclear reactors. When the dirty bomb explodes, the radioactive material spreads in the wind like a dust cloud. In this way, it reaches far wider areas than the initial explosion (Harris, 2005). The long-term destructive force of the dirty bomb is caused by the ionizing radiation from the radioactive material. In a person's body, an ion's electrical charge may lead

to unnatural chemical reactions inside the cells. The charge can break DNA chains. Cells with broken DNA strands either die or the DNA develops a mutation. Diseases develop as the result of widespread cell death. If the DNA mutates, a cell may become cancerous. The cancer may spread and the cells may malfunction. This series of events may result in a wide variety of symptoms collectively referred to as **radiation sickness**. While this condition can be deadly, it is survivable with bone marrow transplantation.

People are exposed to ionizing radiation frequently, but in small doses, with little if any ill effects. Some of the sources of this everyday exposure are outer space, the stars, sun, natural radioactive isotopes, and x-ray machines. The risk of cancer and radiation sickness is increased by exposure to a dirty bomb and the subsequent rise in radiation levels above normal. The fatal effects of the dirty bomb may not be apparent in the short term after exposure, but could kill people years later.

Nuclear Detonations

A thermal burn is the most common mechanism resulting in injury and death associated with nuclear detonation. A tremendous amount of thermal energy is created by a nuclear reaction. This energy travels unimpeded through the air. The energy is absorbed by the contact surface. It may create burns or ignite combustibles. The burns may involve only the epidermis and upper layers of dermis because of the short duration of heat exposure. Thermal burn injuries can be severe and are treated as any other burn. Radiation exposure results in injury from ionizing radiation altering some cell structures. Cells are damaged from the changes in DNA in bone marrow, blood, bowel, skin, and nervous and cardiovascular systems. Radiation suppresses the immune system, so special care must be taken to reduce the potential infection often associated with full-thickness burns. More information on burn care can be found in ∞ Chapter 17.

The major activities performed for patients who have suffered a nuclear casualty are triage, evacuation or sheltering, search and rescue, radioactive monitoring, decontamination, and direct patient care. The patient will be assessed for injuries such as burns or blunt trauma. Pressure injuries such as lung injury, difficult breathing, or minor stroke-like symptoms (air emboli) must be assessed quickly. There may be some early complaints of radiation exposure such as nausea or fatigue. The manifestations of serious radiation exposure may not occur for several hours and do not suggest imminent death. Since radiation has a cumulative danger, shorter exposure times are less damaging. Flash blindness to the eyes caused by a detonation blast lasts only a few minutes during daylight and up to 30 minutes at night. Reassure patients that their eyesight will return and have someone remain with them until their sight is restored.

The victim should be evacuated from the exposure area, along with the healthcare provider and first responders. Wind shifts are monitored continuously to minimize exposure. Triage is done to classify the patients into categories of immediate, delayed, and minimal. Comfort measures, such as psychologic support and empathy, are given to patients.

Disaster Planning, Response, and Mitigation

In the United States, disaster preparedness has been a priority issue for government and military agencies. These efforts have been expanded to public and private healthcare sectors. Healthcare professionals are among the essential personnel in addressing disaster preparations and in dealing with the consequences of a disaster. Nurses comprise the largest group of healthcare professionals, and will play key roles in disaster relief whether they work in hospitals, residential facilities, ambulatory care, schools, or simply at home in their communities. The general public looks to nurses for information and trusts that what nurses advise is true and accurate. Nurses have a responsibility to be educated and to assimilate the new skills and demands necessary to assist patients, families, and communities in preparing for and responding to disastrous situations effectively.

Numerous disaster agencies are involved in disaster planning, response, and mitigation depending on the severity of the disaster and the resultant necessary response:

- A Level I disaster is dealt with effectively by local emergency response personnel and organizations.
- A Level II disaster requires mutual aid from surrounding communities and regional efforts.
- A Level III disaster overwhelms local and regional assets and statewide or federal assistance is required (Goolsby & Mothershead, 2008).

Agencies that may become involved include the Federal Emergency Management Agency (FEMA), the U.S. Army Corps of Engineers, the U.S. Department of Health and Human Services (DHHS), the American Red Cross (an international disaster relief agency), United Nations Headquarters of the Disaster Relief Organization, Pan American Health Organization (PAHO), International Reserve Committee, and local volunteer organizations such as the Boy Scouts of America, Goodwill Industries, and Volunteers of America. National agencies have state and local offices that respond to disasters. However, the most immediate response is from the local groups and organizations. Individual states may request aid from neighboring states or the federal government if the disaster exceeds local and state resources. The local disaster response organizations include fire departments, police departments, public health departments, public works, emergency services, and the local branch of the American Red Cross.

Local disaster response plans include action plans for various types of disaster situations, designation of the overall incident commander, and identification of community resources. The local emergency management agency is also represented in the state management planning efforts.

Hospitals and other healthcare agencies develop their own disaster plans. However, it is very important that each agency understands its role within the larger community disaster plan. When disasters occur, competing healthcare systems must put the competition aside and work collaboratively in the response effort to ensure favorable outcomes following the impact of the disaster.

Stages of Disaster Preparedness

The five stages of disaster preparedness are the *nondisaster* or *interdisaster* stage, the *predisaster* stage, the *impact* stage, the *emergency* stage, and the *reconstruction* or *rehabilitation* stage (see Figure 7–1 ■). The nondisaster stage is the time for planning and preparation as the threat of a disaster is still in the future. It is a time for prevention, preparedness, and mitigation activities. The predisaster stage occurs when there is knowledge about an impending disaster that has not yet occurred. Activities during this stage include warning, preimpact mobilization, and evacuation if appropriate. The impact stage is a time when the disaster event has occurred and the community experiences the immediate effects. The emergency stage involves the immediate response to the effects of the disaster. The community relies on local assistance or aid because outside sources of aid have not yet arrived. In the reconstruction or recovery stage, restoration, reconstitution, and mitigation take

STAGES AND PHASES OF A DISASTER

V. Reconstruction Stage
(Recovery phase)

I. Nondisaster Stage
(Interdisaster phase)

IV. Emergency Stage
(Postimpact phase)

II. Predisaster Stage
(Preimpact phase)

III. Impact Stage
(Impact phase)

Figure 7–1 ■ The stages of a disaster are cyclical. After a disaster, the planning cycle begins again, with evaluation of the current disaster plan and community response, debriefing with all disaster response agencies and personnel, and modifying disaster plans based on lessons learned.

Source: From Langan, Joanne C.; James, Dotti C., *Preparing Nurses for Disasters Management*, 1st, © 2005. Reproduced by permission of Pearson Education, Inc., Upper Saddle River, New Jersey.

place. This stage involves rebuilding and returning to some semblance of "normalcy" but also includes mitigation activities or planning to prevent subsequent disasters or to minimize the effects of future disasters (Langan & James, 2005b).

The key to effective disaster management is predisaster planning and preparation. Clark (2008) stated that the two purposes of disaster planning are to reduce the community's vulnerability to the disaster and to prevent it, if possible, and to ensure that resources are available for effective response in the event of a disaster. A comprehensive emergency management plan addresses four major areas: mitigation, preparedness, response, and recovery.

Mitigation is the action taken to prevent or reduce the harmful effects of a disaster on human health or property. It involves future-oriented activities to prevent subsequent disasters or to minimize their effects. Mitigation may take the form of reinforcing highway over-passes and levees, sandbagging, developing communication strategies as backup systems to what is currently in place, and educating professionals and the public regarding preparation and response to disasters. A key nursing activity related to mitigation is the active participation in learning about the major aspects of disasters to remain current in their knowledge base and be able to teach the general public. Another mitigation activity is the anticipation of needed resources and policies to assist nurses and other professionals in implementing an effective disaster response.

Preparedness is having a comprehensive disaster plan in place that coordinates efforts among many people, agencies, and levels of government. The plan will be based on familiarity with possible disaster agents based on previous experiences, as well as experiences of others from various regions and countries. It is

imperative that all persons and agencies who may be involved in the disaster response be involved in the planning. In this way, information is shared and representatives from each agency explain and offer their respective resources and expertise and note deficiencies in the plan. Planning committees will exist on all levels—federal, regional, state, local, and individual agency. Nurses participate in this facet of disaster planning by having a nurse representative on the planning committee at least at the agency level.

Response to disasters happens in the emergency stage, after the disaster event has occurred. The community has been rapidly assessed for damage, and the types and extent of injuries suffered as well as the immediate needs of the community have been determined. Hospital disaster planners must plan for the possibility that the next disaster may involve the hospital. The hospital's response may include the evacuation of patients as well as relocating and operating from an independent facility. **Surge capacity** is the healthcare system's ability to rapidly expand beyond normal services to meet the increased demand for qualified personnel, medical care, and public health in the event of a large-scale disaster. The Agency for Healthcare Research and Quality (2005) has published a report discussing the use of former "shuttered" hospitals to expand surge capacity during mass casualty events. Hospitals must be constantly aware of the number of beds available, which patients may be discharged, staffing, equipment, other resources, and their overall ability to manage casualties quickly.

The local community provides assistance or aid initially, because outside sources of aid have not yet arrived. Assistance from outside of the affected area arrives later and search and rescue operations commence as well as first aid, emergency medical assistance, establishment or restoration of communication and transportation, assessment of infectious diseases and mental health problems, and evacuation of residents, if necessary. Nurses should follow the disaster plan of their agencies, communities, and the local emergency management agency. This includes having a disaster plan for the nurse's immediate family. In this way, the nurse will feel secure in the fact that the immediate family is situated safely and the nurse can respond to the staging area to await instructions. Nurses use their expertise in infectious disease control and in assessing physical as well as psychosocial needs. In a disaster, mental health issues are extremely significant for victims, families, friends, first responders, and all healthcare workers. Nurses will ensure that patients receive follow-up care for both physical wounds and mental health concerns. Advanced practice nurses may take on significantly greater responsibilities especially if they are competent and prepared in emergency and trauma care. Protocols and standards of care are in place to guide the practice of all nurses. It is imperative that nurses determine the boundaries of their practice in times of emergencies when mass numbers of victims must be treated without the luxury of an on-site physician.

The **recovery** aspect of disaster response is also called *reconstruction*. During this stage, restoration, reconstitution, and mitigation take place. Restoration includes rebuilding, replacing lost or damaged property, returning to school and work, and continuing life without those who were killed in the disaster. Reconstitution occurs when the life of the community returns to a new normal. The final stage of recovery is mitigation, which is also an activity in the preparation and planning aspects of the nondisaster stage. This illustrates the cyclical nature of planning and disaster response. The work is never complete. Future-oriented activities take place to prevent subsequent disasters or to minimize their effects. Some of these activities may include increased security and surveillance measures. Nurses may suggest ideas for responding to the victims of disasters more effectively and efficiently. For example, nurses may communicate the need for carts stocked with specific items that will assist them in treating patients faster. They may also suggest a more efficient method of tracking patients as they enter the healthcare system and move from area to area based on the patients' acuity and condition. Nurses will participate in mock disasters, read updated protocols, and practice their skills repeatedly to maintain competence. Mock disasters or disaster drills can take the form of tabletop exercises/discussions or simulated drills with mock victims. Mock disaster drills allow the participants to become familiar with the plan, and the areas that need strengthening in the plan will become evident (Langan & James, 2005b).

Casualty Management

During a disaster, nurses may be expected to perform triage. Nurses perform triage every day in every emergency department. **Triage** means sorting. A very basic triage system is to categorize or label victims needing the most support and emergency care as "red." Those less critical but still in need of transport to emergency centers for care are classified as "yellow." Victims who have minor injuries and do not warrant transport to an emergency center are categorized as "green." Victims who are least likely to survive or are already deceased are color coded as "black" (see Table 7–2). These are the triage levels given to patients under normal circumstances or when there are only a few victims. However, when there is a mass casualty event with greater than 100 victims, **reverse triage** may be instituted. Reverse triage works on the principle of the greatest good for the greatest number. For example, if there were a collision between a train full of railroad cars filled with toxic chemicals and a full tour bus in a highly populated area, this disaster would likely be called a mass casualty event. In this case, those persons who were the most ambulatory and

least injured would be transported or instructed to move quickly to the warm zone, away from the immediate accident site to get decontaminated and processed first (see Box 7–4). Those with minor injuries would be decontaminated next. Those with more severe to most severe injuries would be treated in that order. In this way, the most victims with the greatest chance of survival could be saved most efficiently with limited resources. Many emergency personnel will share the difficulty of making these decisions at disaster sites when the first inclination might be to rescue the most severely injured.

Triage is a continuous process in which priorities are reassigned as needed treatments, time, and the condition of the victims change. This process must balance human lives with the realities of the situation, such as supplies and personnel (see Box 7–5). The triage role requires a person who is able to rapidly assess patients' conditions under stressful, often adverse conditions and assign a category. Those assigned to triage are expected to function independently, yet as part of a coordinated team effort (James et al., 2005). It has been suggested that emergency personnel should triage/categorize the victims so that physicians and nurses can be best utilized in the treatment area, performing patient care. Advanced practice personnel will continue to triage and perform more complete assessments.

Isolation and Personal Protective Equipment

Persons suspected of having smallpox or some other highly contagious disease will need to be isolated from other patients, visitors, or healthcare personnel. For example, persons with pulmonary tuberculosis and a severe illness requiring hospitalization should be placed in a private room with negative-pressure ventilation. Patients are taught to cover their nose and mouth when coughing or sneezing. All persons entering the room should wear personal respiratory protective devices capable of filtering submicron particles. Decontamination of the air may be achieved through ventilation and supplemented by ultraviolet light.

Gas masks are used in a broad range of military, industrial, and emergency situations to protect the user from hazardous dust, gas, or other aerosols. Biologic contaminants that are spread through aerosolized droplets create a threat to those not wearing PPE. A gas mask may be considered a high-performance respirator and is

---

TABLE 7–2 Simple Triage and Rapid Transport (START) System

Red (Immediate)	Critically injured, with problems that will require immediate intervention to correct. (Patients with a respiratory rate above 30 are tagged "red." If their respirations are below 30, assess their circulatory status. If capillary refill takes more than 2 seconds, tag them "red." If it is below 2 seconds, assess mental status.)
Yellow (Delayed)	Injured, and will require some medical attention, but they will not die if care is delayed while you care for other patients; not ambulatory and will require a stretcher for transportation. (Patients who can follow simple commands such as hand grips are tagged as "yellow." Patients who cannot follow simple commands are tagged "red.")
Green (Ambulatory)	Not critically injured, and can walk and care for themselves. (Have them walk to a safe place, but do not lose track of them; every patient triaged at an incident is tracked to the best of the responder's ability.)
Black (Expectant)	Deceased, or have such catastrophic injuries that they are not expected to survive to be transported. (If the patient is not breathing, open the airway manually. If they remain apneic, tag them "black"; if they begin breathing, they are tagged "red.")

Source: Start.(n.d.) Managing the scene. Retrieved January 10, 2009, from http://www.citmt.org/start/rpm.htm

BOX 7–4 Hot, Warm, and Cold Zones

The site of the disaster where a weapon was released or where the contamination occurred is called the **hot zone**. It is considered contaminated and only those persons in the appropriate **personal protective equipment (PPE)** may enter it. PPE is equipment used for the protection of personnel and includes gloves, masks, goggles, gowns, and biologic disposal bags. Typically, fire, police, and military personnel will collect evidence and begin their investigation in this zone. The **warm zone** is adjacent to the hot zone. Another name for this area is the *control zone*. This area is where decontamination of victims or triage and emergency treatment take place. The level of PPE required is based on the dynamic risk assessment of the threat and agent involved. The **cold zone** is considered to be the safe zone. It is adjacent to the warm zone and is the area where a more in-depth triage of victims would occur. Survivors may find shelter in this area, and the command and control vehicles would be found here as well as the emergency transport vehicles.

usually equipped with both eye protection and air supply protection or treatment. A hood, helmet, or headgear is generally worn to protect the skin, eyes, airways, and respiratory systems. Protective clothing is made to guard against mild irritants and even serious lethal materials. Some protective suits are disposable, intended for one use only. Others are durable, multilayered fabrics that are completely impermeable and are reusable. The Occupational Safety and Health Administration (OSHA) (2005) has issued guidelines to inform healthcare workers and first responders about the correct level of PPE for various situations. The Chemical, Biological, Radiological, and Nuclear (CBRN) Personal Protection Equipment Selection Matrix for Emergency Responders and other information specific to PPE can be located online at the OSHA website. In addition to the isolation of patients, special air handling systems are used in the isolation

BOX 7–5 Key Triage Points to Remember

1. Use a triage system that is easy to learn, easy to implement in stressful conditions, and does not require advanced diagnostic skills yet allows for basic patient interventions.
2. Use the Incident Management System (defined by each facility, and based on the area's civilian and military authorities) for every incident and wear personnel identification vests. Incident management systems use logical management structure, defined responsibilities, clear reporting channels, and a common language (Langan & James, 2005).
3. Get accurate preliminary and final patient counts and relay this information to the incident commander.
4. Use some type of visual color-coded identification system to indicate patient priority.
5. Do not fall into the trap of using your time providing one-to-one patient care.
6. Retriage patients frequently, at the incident, on arrival at the treatment area, and periodically thereafter.
7. Make certain the walking-wounded are gathered and treated.
8. Preplan for potential incidents that may occur.
9. Be aware that emergency responders may be potential targets.
10. Practice, practice, practice.

rooms to prevent the spread of the contaminated droplets into the general hospital air vents. Many hospitals also have the capability to shut off airflow in contaminated areas to prevent the spread of contaminants to other "clean" areas of the hospital. The heating, ventilation, air conditioning, and refrigeration (HVAC) systems are closely monitored and can be shut down in designated areas to avoid air intake from the outside as well, especially in cases of outdoor environmental contamination.

Recording Victim Data

The CDC has created a Mass Trauma Data Instrument (available on the CDC website: Mass Casualty Event Preparedness and Response) to record data about victims of disasters. The categories on the data sheet include demographics, circumstances of the injury, injury conditions, and disposition and details of the conditions. The completion of this form is initiated by the triage nurse and completed by the nurse who implements the treatment or transfers the patient to another unit/department.

Crowd Control

When a disaster occurs, many people converge on the site. Those who come are the curious and those who truly mean to assist in the rescue and recovery of victims. However, this crowd of people needs to be controlled by authorities in charge of the site and rescue and recovery. Similarly, crowds may arrive at the hospital or healthcare delivery sites when injured or even when they just think they may be injured or contaminated in some way. The job of crowd control is not under the auspices of nurses or other healthcare personnel. The agency's security personnel and/or the local police force must control these crowds. If control is not maintained, chaos ensues and those in greatest need of medical assistance may be unable to reach healthcare providers in order to avoid further declines in their health status. In fact, nurses, physicians, and other healthcare workers should not enter an area that has not been secured. To put one's safety at risk jeopardizes the potential treatment of many. Additionally, social services personnel or psychiatric service providers should be available to assist the "worried well" cope with the trauma they have experienced or witnessed or simply heard about through the news media.

Psychosocial Needs

The importance of mental health services for victims, the public, first responders, and healthcare workers cannot be overstated. Both those persons directly affected by the disaster as well as those indirectly affected will seek medical care and advice. Many who seek medical attention are simply anxious about the threat of injury. At times, reassurance is all that is necessary. However, with large numbers of people seeking health care, the system is quickly overwhelmed. Mental health experts may quickly assess individual needs, offer immediate advice, and refer for follow-up care if deemed appropriate.

People react to disasters in a variety of ways, both physically and behaviorally. Their reactions depend on the severity of the threat and their proximity to the area of direct impact. The closer the person is to the area of impact and the longer the exposure, the greater the likelihood of a more severe reaction to the event. Table 7–3 summarizes the normal initial responses aimed at survival (Ganong, 2005; Murray, Zentner & Yakimo, 2009; Selye, 1965, 1980).

Most people exhibit great coping mechanisms and resilience in the aftermath of a disaster. However, mechanisms should be developed for identifying and referring those who need psychologic counseling. After the September 2001 terrorist attacks on the World Trade Center and the Pentagon, it was reported that 71% of the persons surveyed felt depressed, 49% had difficulty concentrating, and 33% had trouble sleeping at night. Most (92%) felt sad when watching news coverage of the event, yet 63% stated a compulsion to continue to watch the news (Pew Research Center for the People and the Press, 2001). Reactions to terrorist events and disasters in general are influenced by developmental level and maturity, prior experiences with disasters, and cultural background (McLaughlin et al., 2005).

∞ Nursing Care

The Role of the Nurse in Disaster Relief

Because nurses have an obligation to keep current in new and emerging trends in health care and threats to society, learning about the prevention and mitigation of disasters is essential. Nurses must be aware of the roles they play in all aspects of disaster preparedness and response (Box 7–6.) It is imperative that nurses first know how to take care of themselves in order to assist others. By educating oneself and being proactive in regular drills and practice of skills, nurses take an active role in helping others to save lives and fulfill an important obligation to society.

Applying basic first aid skills can be very helpful in immediate disaster relief efforts until emergency help can be obtained. The American Red Cross invites nurse volunteers and will provide the necessary training. Many nurses have taken advantage of online disaster certificate programs, and efforts are being made to integrate disaster preparedness content into nursing courses.

BOX 7–6 Roles of Nurses in Disasters

1. Prepare selves, families, friends, and communities for disasters in conjunction with the local disaster preparedness plan.
2. Continue educating self on various types of disasters and appropriate response.
3. Provide emergency services with consideration of victims' abilities, deficits, culture, language, or special needs.
4. Assist in the mobilization of healthcare personnel, food, water, shelter, medication, clothing, and other assistive devices.
5. Collaborate with agencies in authority including local, state, and federal representatives to deploy resources based on the greatest good for the greatest number.
6. Consider needs of victims including shelter both temporary and permanent, as well as psychologic, economic, legal, and spiritual factors.
7. Become involved with local, state, and national disaster planning agencies to schedule regular meetings to continually review and modify disaster plans.

In many different practice settings, nurses serve on disaster preparedness and response planning committees. Nurses are receiving in-service education on biologic, chemical, and radiologic threats to patient health as well as surveillance and reporting of suspicious activities. Although nursing professionals may not be asked to don decontamination gear to decontaminate victims, nurses should be aware of decontamination basics so that they will remain safe from exposure and be able to direct others when threatened with contamination. Some nurses choose to be actively involved with disaster medical assistance teams as part of the National Disaster Medical System (NDMS). The NDMS is a program, coordinated by the federal government, that supplements an integrated national medical response to assisting states and local authorities in dealing with the medical aspects of peacetime disasters.

In a true mass casualty event, it is impossible to have physicians present at every station where they are needed. Nurses may have to assume expanded roles in making decisions for the most appropriate treatment of casualties. Discussions should

---

TABLE 7–3 Responses to Stress: General Adaptation Syndrome (GAS) and Levels of Anxiety

GAS STAGE	PHYSICAL RESPONSE	BEHAVIORS RELATED TO ANXIETY
Alarm Stage	Pupils dilate; blurred vision. Hearing sharper or diminished.	Misinterpretation of stimuli. Confusion. Poor concentration. Selective inattention. Need for assistance.
Severe Anxiety or Panic	Stronger, faster heart rate and respirations. Palpitations, arrhythmias, elevated blood pressure.	Feeling of impending doom. Terror. Fear. Agitation. Irritability. Increased demands. Impulsivity. Paresthesias.
	Muscle tone increased. Headaches.	Muscle tension. Excitability, restless movements. Tremors. Rigidity. Weakness.
	Basal metabolism rate increased. Body temperature. Perspiration. Altered glucose, protein, and lipid metabolism. Increased startle response.	Insomnia. Urgency of speech and movement. Fatigue. Dehydration. Weight loss. Appetite changes. Smooth muscle of gastrointestinal and urinary tracts less motile, interfering with digestion and elimination of wastes.
	Hypoglycemia from glycogenolysis due to high energy demands.	Blood glucose increase. Appetite changes. Dehydration. Fatigue. Poor concentration.
	Increased blood clotting and suppressed immune response if stage persists.	Blood stasis; thrombus formation. Resistance to infection and disease reduced.

take place among physicians, nurses, and policy makers regarding the necessity of the nurses' expanded roles in crisis situations. As noted earlier in the chapter, these agency policies must be documented in the agency-wide plan. Additionally, all healthcare personnel must receive any specialized training required to be safe and competent practitioners of the expanded duties. This training must be practiced and updated and those participating in the training must be tracked and notified of additional requirements as necessary. See the Moving Evidence into Action box on page 135.

Roles of Nurses Working with Victims of Disasters

The role of the nurse in a disaster depends greatly on a number of variables including the nature of the disaster, the number of victims and severity of injuries, the location of the disaster as well as the location of the nurse, the availability of supplies, rescue and command personnel, and other necessary resources. The nurse must be able to perform under stressful conditions but will not be expected to endanger self, other nurses, or other rescuers.

If it is safe to do so, the nurse begins by triaging and assessing the victims for the best care and best use of available resources. Very quick, direct treatment may be given, or the nurse may be involved in extended periods of time with a mobile surgical unit. Local authorities such as the police, fire, and emergency medical services will guide the nurse in securing the area and determining the safe zone for the nurse and others to work. The National Disaster Medical System is the agency responsible for coordinating disaster relief with local fire, police, and emergency medical services to provide overall disaster assistance. Victim assistance may be offered in the field in mobile shelters, in local clinics, in hospitals, or in makeshift buildings.

Nurses take on a variety of roles based on their expertise and the needs of the victims. Nurses will be expected to follow the emergency preparedness plans outlined in their communities and in their agencies of employment. When a disaster occurs, it is not a time for individual creativity. However, individual nurses should be the leaders in their communities in discussing emergency preparedness and contingency plans.

Considerations for Patients with Special Needs

Older Adults

It is not appropriate to generalize needs to all older adults. Many are quite independent and active into their 90s. However, some older persons lack the physical stamina to recover quickly from disastrous events. The nurse must assess the individual's ability to cope with and recover from unexpected events, socioeconomic factors, support systems, potential healthcare needs, and resources. See the accompanying Case Study & Nursing Care Plan.

Teaching about disaster preparedness is important in all communities. Older adults need to determine the appropriateness of "sheltering in place" should there be an environmental event outside of their homes, or of being evacuated if they are unable to care for themselves for extended periods of time. This becomes a very real issue when roads become impassable or usual modes of transportation and communication are disrupted.

MOVING EVIDENCE INTO ACTION · Disaster Education

The nursing profession has recognized the need to develop resources to teach practicing and future nurses to improve their response to victims of radiologic, biologic, and chemical terrorism. However, nursing students may have different perceptions about working with disaster victims. The purpose of this descriptive study (Young & Persell, 2004) was to identify student nurses' major concerns and learning needs in working with victims of terrorism. Ninety-five junior and senior baccalaureate nursing students participated in the study by completing an anonymous questionnaire regarding their concerns about terrorism and how their lives had changed following September 11, 2001 ("9/11"). The students' main concern was for the safety of themselves and their families. The students indicated they would not be willing to care for victims if there was a lack of protection for all types of terrorist agents for themselves and their families. The students did not demonstrate an accurate understanding of the pathogenic nature of many terrorist agents even though the nursing faculty members had provided self-education articles for the students. The students' concerns for specific infectious agents appeared to be based on unnecessary fear or inappropriate confidence.

IMPLICATIONS FOR NURSING

If nurses do not believe that a terrorist event is a real threat in their communities, they may not be motivated to become more prepared for terrorist events. The nation's emergency healthcare planners and trauma nurses will have a major challenge preparing more nurses for disasters, especially mass casualty events. During a terrorist attack, the general public will seek information about the event from all healthcare providers. The public will also expect nurses to deliver safe and competent care to the victims of terrorism. Disaster care information should be a part of the curriculum in all basic nursing education schools. Continuing education and elective courses should continue to be planned. Basic disaster preparedness competencies should be required for all new graduate nurses so that they have a solid foundation on which to build.

CRITICAL THINKING IN PATIENT CARE

1. Make a list of all the barriers that nurses might express as reasons they do not need or value disaster/terrorism education and preparation.
2. Discuss the rationale for including basic disaster preparedness content in all basic nursing education programs.
3. Consider the results of this study. What could have been done differently to assist nursing students in learning facts and the pathogenic nature of the terrorist agents presented in the articles?

Source: Young, C. F., & Persell, D. (2004). Biological, chemical, and nuclear terrorism readiness: Major concerns and preparedness of future nurses. *Disaster Management & Response, 2*(4), 109–114.

A current list of medications, doses, and times of administration should be kept in an easily accessible, secure place. The names and phone numbers of significant persons, relatives, those with power of attorney, healthcare providers, or any others to be notified in case of emergency should also be kept in an easily accessible place. Additionally, the following materials should be considered essential in keeping with the person should evacuation to a shelter be necessary: eyeglasses and eyeglass prescriptions, style and serial numbers of medical devices such as pacemakers, healthcare policies and numbers, identification, list of allergies, blood type, checkbook, credit cards, insurance agent's name and number, driver's license, 72-hour supply of medications, dentures, list of special dietary needs, sturdy shoes, warm clothing, blankets, incontinence briefs, prostheses, hearing aids, hearing aid batteries, extra wheelchair batteries, oxygen, and other assistive devices.

Immunocompromised Patients

Patients who are immunocompromised pose special problems to the healthcare community especially if these persons are unable to access health care quickly in a disaster situation. A compromised immune system may be due to treatments such as chemotherapy or immunosuppressants or from an underlying disease such as HIV. The immunocompromised population would be at greater risk for complications and death than the general population should a bioterrorist attack occur. For example, a potential complication following smallpox vaccination is generalized vaccinia. It is believed to result from a vaccinia viremia with skin manifestations. In noncompromised persons, generalized vaccinia consists of vesicles or pustules appearing on normal skin distant from the vaccination site. The rash is generally self-limited and usually requires only supportive therapy. However, immunocompromised patients may have a toxic course and require vaccinia immune globulin (VIG), available only from the CDC (Center for Disease Control (CDC), 2008).

An additional issue the nurse should discuss with this population is the patients' preparation for disaster events related to infection control. Patients should carry treatment calendars with them at all times so that any healthcare provider can determine where they are in their treatment program and disease process. Patients should plan a backup location to visit for chemotherapy if their usual office is inaccessible. Nurses should also assess their patients' knowledge level regarding the avoidance of raw seafood or possibly contaminated water. Bottled water should be ready so the patient can avoid drinking water of questionable purity. Bone marrow transplant patients are instructed not to eat fresh fruits and vegetables due to the risk of contamination and subsequent infection. It is safest for this population of patients to consume processed or canned foods if they can be heated to the proper temperatures.

Patients with Sensory, Speech, or Literacy Deficits

Persons who have sensory deficits, speech or language impairments, or who are illiterate must be assessed for the most effective means of communicating steps to be taken in the case of a disaster. One cannot generalize that all people with hearing impairments or speech impairments will choose a particular means of communication. This may be an individual preference. A multitude of communication means are available through technological support systems as well as written and visual cue boards. Public service announcements may inform the general public about impending natural disasters and about proper steps to be taken to be safely rescued or sheltered. Nurses are in the position of alerting community leaders about special needs of members of their communities. Public service personnel, including fire, police, and emergency services, should be alerted to extenuating circumstances and needs of specific individuals in the community. The collaborative planning efforts of the individual, family members, caregivers, and emergency service personnel will help alleviate any undue pain and suffering caused by the lack of understanding of emergency messages and directives.

Patients with Mobility and Sensory Deficits

The U.S. Department of Health and Human Services (2005) has estimated that 13% of the U.S. population experiences some form of activity limitation due to a chronic condition. Many persons require the use of assistive technology devices (ATDs) to accommodate mobility and other impairments. Careful planning must be in place in order to provide necessary support during and after a disaster. Arrangements must be made in advance to provide adequate numbers of volunteers or staff to assist when this group must be relocated or regrouped in a safe room or shelter. These individuals or their caregivers must provide input to service personnel to determine what kind of support services would be necessary in an emergency or disaster. Emergency personnel or rescue teams may need to learn a few basic phrases in American Sign Language. Something as simple as carrying a notepad and pencil or directions in large print may be just what is necessary to share information with people who have hearing impairments or visual impairments, respectively.

Non-English-Speaking Patients

The literacy of non-English-speaking patients should be assessed in both their own language and in English. One cannot assume that individuals are literate in their own language. It is ideal to obtain the assistance of an interpreter, preferably an interpreter with whom the patient is familiar, to assist in translating information for the patient. Communication aids can be prepared in advance of disasters to be used during emergencies. The communication aids or disaster preparedness and response procedures should be practiced on a regular basis prior to an emergency. The use of visual aids is very helpful. Do not use children as interpreters if adults are available. The stress of interpretation can be overwhelming to the children and place an unnecessary burden on them.

Spiritual Considerations

Religion tends to be a source of comfort for those who are experiencing the threat of loss of life, property, or way of living. Churches, synagogues, and clergy become active in supporting

CASE STUDY & NURSING CARE PLAN   A Patient with Injuries from a Natural Disaster

Mr. Ed Jones, a 84-year-old widower, is retired from his job as a cabinet-maker. He continues to work with wood as a hobby in the basement of his home located on the banks of the Deep River. He sells small toys at craft fairs and flea markets in nearby communities. His daughter lives approximately 20 minutes away and checks in on him at least every weekend. Mr. Jones is independent and sees his primary care physician occasionally for monitoring of his blood pressure, which is controlled with antihypertensive medications. Following a week of heavy rainstorms, flash flooding occurred in the area and Mr. Jones's basement sustained much water damage and ruined most of his stored wood, wooden toy products, and the woodworking machinery. Mr. Jones waded through the waist-deep water to get to the rescue boat rather than wait for the boat to get to him. He is subsequently admitted to the medical/surgical unit due to concerns from the EMTs who triaged him at the fire station 5 miles inland from Mr. Jones's neighborhood.

ASSESSMENT

Lisa Smith, RN, obtains a nursing assessment. Mr. Jones states that he has been on antihypertensive medications for "a few years" but only takes his medication "once in awhile" since it has been some time since his last office visit and he wants his remaining pills "to last" until he can get back to the doctor. He has had numerous cuts to his hands from his woodworking and has had a big ulcer on his right foot "for a few weeks" caused by a tool that fell on his foot. He did not seek medical care because he believed it would get better on its own. "It looks worse than it is. It really doesn't even hurt."

When asked about his home he stated, "Everything is gone. My wife is gone, my wood, my tools...it's all over."

Physical assessment findings include T 100.7°F PO, P 96, R 20, and BP 178/100. Skin cool and dry with multiple lesions on both hands and a Stage II ulcer on his right dorsal foot with yellow-green exudate. Pain rated at a 2 on a 10 scale with 10 being the worst pain there could be. Lungs are clear, heart rate regular. No edema noted. Abdominal assessment is normal. Neurologically intact. Weight is normal for height and frame. A culture is ordered and taken of the yellow-green exudate of the right foot.

Preliminary blood work results show WBCs at 15,000/mm³. A peripheral IV is initiated with continuous fluids and IV antibiotics are ordered every 6 hours. An antihypertensive medication is ordered on a regular schedule plus a prn antihypertensive for systolic >180 and diastolic >90.

DIAGNOSES

- *Impaired Skin Integrity* of the right foot and hands related to lesions (cuts) on the hands and Stage II ulcer with exudates on the right foot
- *Powerlessness* related to perceived loss of control over life situation
- *Ineffective Thermoregulation* related to trauma
- *Acute Pain* related to expression of pain secondary to skin lesions

EXPECTED OUTCOMES

- Regain skin integrity—ulcer on right foot and lesions on hands will heal.
- Identify aspects of his life still under his control.
- Maintain body temperature at normothermic levels.
- Express feeling of comfort and relief from pain.

PLANNING AND IMPLEMENTATION

- Assess skin every shift; describe and document skin condition; report changes.
- Clean lesions on hands and right foot every 8 hours and assess healing.
- Administer prescribed antibiotics and assess for effectiveness in treating infection.
- Arrange psychosocial consult(s).
- Guide Mr. Jones through a life review. Encourage reflection on past achievements.
- Help Mr. Jones identify the aspects of his life that are still under his control.
- Monitor temperature every 4 hours, more often if indicated.
- Monitor and record patient's heart rate and rhythm, blood pressure, and respiratory rate every 4 hours.
- Administer analgesics, antipyretics, and medications as indicated.
- Maintain hydration; monitor intake and output.
- Assess level of pain and administer pain medication as prescribed.

EVALUATION

Mr. Jones was hospitalized for 3 days, receiving intravenous antibiotic therapy, analgesics, an antidepressant, monitoring of his cardiac response to a new antihypertensive medication, wound care, and sessions with the social services representative and his daughter. His hand lesions are healed, the foot ulcer has developed new granulation tissue with no signs of infection, he is afebrile, and his blood pressure is maintained within normal limits. He will be discharged to his daughter's home until his home can be assessed for the extent of the water damage and feasibility of repair. He has agreed to visit a therapist to work through his feelings of grief and loss. He has expressed an interest in attending monthly support group meetings with his neighbors who also experienced losses in this disaster.

CRITICAL THINKING IN THE NURSING PROCESS

1. What action did Mr. Jones take that probably exacerbated his skin lesions?
2. What other testing might you anticipate related to Mr. Jones's delayed healing?
3. What were the contributing factors to Mr. Jones's fever?
4. What life situations contributed to Mr. Jones's attitude about life?

See Evaluating Your Response in Appendix C.

---

their congregations in times of disaster. Religious leaders should be actively involved in community planning for disaster preparedness especially if certain religious considerations should be strictly followed. For example, in some religions, the human body and all of its parts are considered sacred. To be sensitive to this religious belief, all tissues and blood would be collected at the site of a disaster by those trained to collect such material versus washing this matter away from the scene. In general, rescue personnel would need to be informed of specific religious obligations or rights to be able to be sensitive to the individual's religious beliefs and practices.

CHAPTER HIGHLIGHTS

■ Disasters require extraordinary efforts beyond those needed to respond to everyday emergencies.

■ Nurses have an obligation to keep current in new and emerging trends in health care and threats to society.

■ Learning about the prevention and mitigation of bioterrorism and disasters in general is essential.

■ Reverse triage is used in mass casualty events instead of traditional triage in order to do the greatest good for the greatest number.

■ Nurses will be actively engaged in assessing the physical as well as the mental needs of victims, their families, first responders, and other healthcare personnel.

■ Nurses need to have their own family disaster plans in place to be able to assist others in times of disasters.

■ Nurses are actively involved in disaster mitigation, planning, and response efforts by learning and practicing their communities' and agencies' disaster preparedness systems.

TEST YOURSELF NCLEX-RN® REVIEW

1. What is the key difference between emergencies and disasters?
   1. Emergencies are controlled.
   2. Disasters result from man-made errors.
   3. Emergencies can typically be handled by available emergency services.
   4. Disasters typically involve the local emergency services and no other agencies.

2. Which of the following is NOT true regarding nurses' responsibilities in disaster preparedness?
   1. Nurses have a responsibility to the public to be knowledgeable about disaster preparedness and response.
   2. Nurses must have a personal and family plan as a part of their disaster preparedness and response plan.
   3. Nurses will be the leaders in the incident command structure set up at the site of the disaster.
   4. Nurses who are prepared for disasters will be better able to help themselves, their families, and their communities in a disaster situation.

3. What is the purpose of reverse triage?
   1. Save scarce resources for future use.
   2. Test first responders on their triage classification categories.
   3. Save those persons who are in the most critical condition.
   4. Do the greatest good for the greatest number with limited resources.

4. Why is important for nurses to assess patients' literacy in their primary language?
   1. They are most comfortable speaking in their primary language.
   2. They are most comfortable reading in their primary language.
   3. They may not be able to read and comprehend in their primary language.
   4. They may be too shy to communicate in English if it is not their primary language.

5. Which of the following is true about personal protective equipment (PPE)?
   1. PPE protects by creating a barrier against hazards.
   2. Eye, face, head, foot, and hand protection are addressed in PPE programs.
   3. PPE should reduce the likelihood of occupational injury and/or illness.
   4. Healthcare workers do not need to wear PPE if they follow strict hand hygiene protocol and universal precautions.

6. Which of the following is NOT true about decontamination?
   1. Decontamination corridors should be set up in an area downwind from the hospital entrance.
   2. Decontamination begins in the hot zone, closest to the site of the disaster.
   3. Decontamination must take place before the patient enters the hospital.
   4. Decontaminating a person should be done by sweeping strokes away from you and the patient.

7. What is another name for a radiological dispersion bomb?
   1. a dirty bomb
   2. an ionization radiation bomb
   3. a nonfiltered bomb
   4. a radio-controlled remote bomb

8. One of the results of DNA mutation inside cells exposed to ionizing radiation that can be deadly, but is survivable with bone marrow transplantation, is a description of which of the following?
   1. ionizing sickness
   2. radiation sickness
   3. TNT sickness
   4. compromised immune sickness

9. Why should a nurses assess the special needs of older adults as part of the emergency preparedness plan?
   1. All older adults will need some kind of special support.
   2. Some older adults will take the lead in evacuation efforts in nursing homes.
   3. Not all older adults need the same level of support in emergencies and disasters.
   4. Some older adults will be unable to evacuate even with multiple support agencies.

10. Why would nurses need the assistance of a mental health worker following a disaster?
   1. All nurses need the help of a mental health worker at one point or another in their nursing careers.
   2. Nurses are trained to provide care, regardless of the situation encountered.
   3. Nurses maintain good mental health and rarely require mental health assistance.
   4. The nurse may feel as overwhelmed and traumatized as the population for whom he or she is caring.

See Test Yourself answers in Appendix C.

Pearson Nursing Student Resources
Find additional review materials at
www.nursing.pearsonhighered.com
Prepare for success with additional NCLEX®-style practice questions, interactive assignments and activities, Web links, animations and videos, and more!

BIBLIOGRAPHY

Agency for Healthcare Research and Quality. (2005, September). *Use of former ("shuttered") hospitals to expand surge capacity.* Retrieved from http://www.ahrq.gov/research/shuttered/American Red Cross

American Red Cross. (n.d.). *Disaster preparedness for seniors.* Retrieved from http://www.redcross.org/services/disaster/beprepared/seniors.html

American Red Cross. (n.d.). *Your evacuation plan.* Retrieved from http://www.redcross.org/services/disaster/0,1082,0_6_,00.html

American Red Cross and IOM open new homes in Indonesia. (2006). Retrieved from http://www.redcross.org/article/0,1072,0_332_5110,00.html

Beachley, M. (2005). Nursing in a disaster. In C. M. Smith & F. A. Maurer (Eds.), *Community public/health nursing practice* (pp. 496–514). Philadelphia: Elsevier Health Sciences.

Centers for Disease Control and Prevention. (2006a). *Explosions and blast injuries: A primer for clinicians.* Retrieved from http://www.bt.cdc.gov/masstrauma/explosions.asp

Centers for Disease Control and Prevention. (2006b). *Fact sheet: Anthrax information for health care providers.* Retrieved from http://www.bt.cdc.gov/agent/anthrax/anthrax-hcp-factsheet.asp#cutaneous

Centers for Disease Control and Prevention. (2008a). *Key facts about hurricane recovery: Protect your health and safety after a hurricane.* Retrieved from http://www.bt.cdc.gov/disasters/hurricanes/pdf/recovery.pdf

Centers for Disease Control and Prevention. (2008b) *Blast injuries: Fact sheets for professionals.* Retrieved from http://www.bt.cdc.gov/masscasualties/blastinjuryfacts.asp

Centers for Disease Control and Prevention. (2008c). *Smallpox fact sheet—Adverse reactions following smallpox vaccination.* Retrieved from http://www.bt.cdc.gov/agent/smallpox/vaccination/reactions-vacc-clinic.asp

Clark, M. J. (2008). Care of client patients in disaster settings. In M. J. Clark, *Community health nursing: Advocacy for population health* (5th ed.) (Chapter 27). Upper Saddle River, NJ: Pearson/Prentice Hall.

Clark, M. J. (2008). Communicable diseases. In M. J. Clark, *Community health nursing: Advocacy for population health* (5th ed.) (Chapter 28). Upper Saddle River, NJ: Pearson/Prentice Hall.

County of Henrico (n.d.). *Community disaster preparedness manual.* Retrieved from http://www.co.henrico.va.us/fire/pdfs/cpm_man.pdf

Daley, B. J., Aycinena, J. F., & Mallat, A. F. (2008). *Electrical Injuries.* Retrieved from http://emedicine.medscape.com/article/433682-overview

Federal Emergency Management Agency. (2008). *Are you ready? Hurricanes.* Retrieved from http://www.fema.gov/areyouready/hurricanes.shtm

Ganong, W. (2005). *Review of medical physiology* (22nd ed.). New York: McGraw-Hill.

Goolsby, C., & Mothershead, J. L. (2008). *Disaster planning.* Retrieved from http://www.emedicine.com/emerg/topic718.htm

Hoffman, B. (2008). Terrorism. *In Microsoft Encarta Online Encyclopedia 2008.* Retrieved from http://encarta.msn.com/encyclopedia_761564344/Terrorism.html#s3

International Nursing Coalition for Mass Casualty Education. (2003). *Educational competencies for registered nurses related to mass casualty incidents.* Retrieved from http://www.aacn.nche.edu/Education/pdf/INCMCECompetencies.pdf

James, D. C., Langan, J. C., Sandkuhl, H., & Benbenishty, J. (2005). Preparing staff and inactive registered nurses to manage casualties. In J. C. Langan & D. C. James (Eds.), *Preparing nurses for disaster management* (pp. 95–123). Upper Saddle River, NJ: Pearson/Prentice Hall.

Laditka, S., Laditka, J., Zirasagar, S., Cornman, C., Davis, C., & Richter, J. (2008). Providing shelter to nursing home evacuees in disasters: Lessons learned from hurricane Katrina. *American Journal of Public Health, 98*(7), 1288–1293.

Langan, J. C. & James, D. C. (2005). *Preparing nurses for disaster management.* Upper Saddle River, NJ: Pearson/Prentice Hall.

McLaughlin, D. E., Murray, R. B., & Benbenishty, J. (2005). Promoting mental health: Predisaster and postdisaster. In J. C. Langan & D. C. James (Eds.), *Preparing nurses for disaster management* (pp. 55–77). Upper Saddle River, NJ: Pearson/Prentice Hall.

Murray, R. B., Zentner, J., & Yakimo, R. (2009). *Health promotion strategies through the life span* (8th ed.). Upper Saddle River, NJ: Pearson/Prentice Hall.

National Institute of Mental Health. (2002). *Mental health and mass violence: Evidence-based early psychological interventions for victims/survivors of mass violence. A workshop to reach consensus on best practices* (NIH Publication No. 02-5138). Washington, DC: U.S. Government Printing Office.

National Institute for Occupational Safety and Health. (2009). *Eye safety for emergency response and disaster recovery.* Retrieved from http://www.cdc.gov/niosh/topics/eye/eyesafe.html

Noji, E. K. (1997). The nature of disaster: General characteristics and public health effects. In E. K. Noji (Ed.), *The public health consequences of disasters* (pp. 3–20). New York: Oxford University Press.

North Carolina Department of Health and Human Services. (2007). *After the storm: Injury prevention.* Retrieved from http://www.dhhs.state.nc.us/docs/hurricanepreventinjury.htm

Occupational Safety and Health Administration. (2005). *CBRN personal protective equipment selection matrix for emergency responders.* Retrieved from http://www.osha.gov/SLTC/emergencypreparedness/cbrnmatrix/index.html

Pacific Tsunami Museum. (2007). *Tsunami glossary.* Retrieved from http://www.tsunami.org/definitions.html

Pew Research Center for the People and the Press. (2001). *American psyche reeling from terror attacks.* Retrieved from http://people-press.org/reports/display.php3?ReportID=3

Pryor, T. (2005). Remembering the tsunami: Story of hope. *Reflections on Nursing Leadership,* 4th Quarter, pp. 26–27.

Scott, S. G., Vanderploeg, R. D., Belanger, H. G., & Scholten, J. D. (2005). Blast injuries: Evaluating and treating the postacute sequelace. *Federal Practitioner,* 67–75.

Selye, H. (1965). Stress syndrome. *American Journal of Nursing, 65*(3), 97–99.

Simonsen, C. E., & Spindlove, J. R. (2007). *Terrorism today: The past, the players, the future* (3rd ed.). Upper Saddle River, NJ: Pearson/Prentice Hall.

Smith, C. M., & Maurer, F. A. (2005). *Community/public health nursing practice: Health for families and populations* (3rd ed.). Philadelphia: Saunders.

Start. (n.d.). Managing the scene. Retrieved from http://www.citmt.org/start/rpm.htm

Stevens, S., & Slone, L. (2005). *Tsunami and mental health: What can we expect?* Retrieved from http://www.ncptsd.va.gov/ncmain/ncdocs/fact_shts/fs_tsunami_mental_health.html

Through The Eyes of Terrorism. (n.d.). *Weapons.* Retrieved from http://library.thinkquest.org/CR0212088/terweap.htm

U. S. Department of Homeland Security. (2008, October 16). *The first year after Hurricane Katrina: What the federal government did.* Retrieved from http://www.dhs.gov/xprepresp/programs/gc_1157649340100.shtm

U.S. Department of State. (2009). *Fact sheet: Guidance for responding to radiological and nuclear incidents.* Retrieved from http://travel.state.gov/travel/tips/health/health_1184.html

World Health Organization. (2009). *Smallpox.* Retrieved from http://www.who.int/mediacentre/factsheets/smallpox/en/index.html

Functional Health Pattern: Health Perception-Health Management

Think about patients with altered health perception or health management for whom you have cared in your clinical experiences.

■ What were their major medical diagnoses (e.g., surgery, terminal illness, impending death, alcoholism or other substance abuse, or victim of multiple or mass casualty incident)?

■ What kinds of manifestations did each of these patients have? Were these manifestations similar or different?

■ How did the each patient's healthcare behaviors interfere with his or her health status? Had the patient had surgery before? Did the patient experience any complications due to having surgery? Did the patient have any problems with anesthesia? What medications was the patient taking? Did the patient take medications as prescribed? Did the patient use any substances other than prescribed medications and over-the-counter medications? If so, what substances and how much were used? How much alcohol did the patient drink? What kind of problems had substance abuse caused for the patient, family, friends, finances, and health? Was the patient exposed to environmental hazards? Did the patient have sensory deficits or sight or speech impairments? Did the patient speak English? What religious considerations did the patient verbalize? Did the patient have a living will, do-not-resuscitate orders, or power of attorney? Had end-of-life issues been discussed with the family?

The Health Perception-Health Management Functional Health Pattern includes healthcare behaviors such as health promotion and illness prevention activities, medical treatments, and follow-up care. Individuals may or may not have the ability to change their healthcare practices. Health perception and health maintenance are affected by perceived health status in two primary ways:

■ Factors that interfere with health care are lack of understanding basic health practices (e.g., altered cognition, altered coping), inability to take responsibility for meeting health needs (e.g., alcoholism, substance abuse), or lack of communication skills (e.g., non-English-speaking, illiterate).

■ Factors that interfere with the desire to seek higher level of wellness are inability to change declining health status (e.g., cancer, kidney failure, impending death), need for treatment (e.g., surgery), catastrophic events (e.g., motor vehicle accidents injuries, weather-related event injuries, thermal or chemical burns).

A patient's perceived pattern of health and well-being affects how health is managed. Unexpected events can alter the patient's health status, leading to manifestations such as the following:

■ **Anxiety** (*uneasy feeling of the unknown* → *resulting in sympathetic nervous system responses*)

■ **Grief** (*physical and emotional responses* → *due to loss or impending loss* → *resulting in withdrawal of attachment*)

■ **Death** (*irreversible condition* → *resulting from cessation of circulatory and respiratory functions or irreversible cessation of all functions of the brain*)

Priority nursing diagnoses within the health perception and health management functional health pattern that may be appropriate for patients include the following:

■ *Impaired Skin Integrity* as evidenced by surgical incisions, injuries due to accidents or falls, physical immobility, and skin changes in the elderly

■ *Risk for Injury* as evidenced by misuse of drugs and alcohol, environmental hazards, intraoperative complications, and inadequate postoperative care

■ *Ineffective Therapeutic Regimen Management* as evidenced by ineffective patterns of health care, lack of knowledge of health care, and mistrust of healthcare personnel

■ *Powerlessness* as evidenced by loss of privacy, loss of control due to chronic or debilitating conditions, and dependency on others

Two nursing diagnoses from other functional health patterns often are of high priority for the patient with alterations in patterns of health perception or health maintenance:

■ *Impaired Verbal Communication* (Cognitive-Perceptual Functional Health Pattern)

■ *Ineffective Individual Coping* (Coping-Stress-Tolerance Functional Health Pattern)

Question

1. How did you decrease your patient's anxiety, thus altering his or her health status?

Questions

Refer to the Clinical Scenario on the next page in order to answer the following questions.

Priority Setting

1. In what order would you visit these patients after report? What is your rationale for your choice?
   A. _____
   B. _____
   C. _____
   D. _____

Health Promotion

1. Diet is important for wound healing. What nutrients will you encourage Mary Black to eat in order to ensure proper healing of her fractured ankle?

2. Mary Black understands her diet when she picks which meal plan?
   A. hamburger, french fries, and a cola beverage
   B. tossed salad, chocolate pudding, and iced tea
   C. baked chicken, broccoli and cheese, and lemonade
   D. salmon patty, baked potato, and milk

CLINICAL SCENARIO

Directions: *Read the following clinical scenario and answer the questions that follow. To complete this exercise successfully you will not only use knowledge of the content in this unit, but also principles related to setting priorities and maintaining patient safety.*

You have been assigned to work with the following four patients for the 0700 shift on a medical-surgical unit. Significant data obtained during report is as follows:

- Peter Black is a 46-year-old who was admitted from the emergency room 2 hours ago for observation after being thrown 50 yards during a tornado. His vital signs on admission were stable: T 99.8°F, P 86, R 24, and BP 140/86. He had multiple abrasions and lacerations that were sutured in the emergency room. He is now complaining of numbness in both legs.

- Mary Black is a 44-year-old wife of Peter Black who was admitted 1 hour ago with multiple abrasions and ecchymotic areas. She is scheduled to go to surgery at 0900 for an open reduction of a left ankle fracture. Current vital signs are T 99°F, P 90, R 26, BP 134/88. She is requesting pain medication and wants to see her children, who were admitted to the pediatric unit, before going to surgery.

- John Linzer, aged 67, was admitted one week ago in the terminal stages of colon cancer. Vital signs are T 96.8°F, P 54, R 10, BP 88/68. The family is requesting that a nurse check on Mr. Linzer as they feel that death is imminent. There is a do-not-resuscitate order.

- Paul Goetz, aged 47, was admitted three days ago due to being found unconscious in his car. On admission his alcohol level was 0.45. Current vital signs are T 100°F, P 110, R 30, BP 168/94. He is diaphoretic, disoriented, and complaining of nausea and seeing spiders on the wall.

Nursing Process

1. Besides obtaining vital signs, what diagnosis-specific assessment data should be collected for each patient?

   A. _____

   B. _____

   C. _____

   D. _____

2. Identify one priority nursing diagnosis for each patient presented earlier. What is the rationale for your choices?

	Nursing Diagnosis	Rationale
Peter Black		
Mary Black		
John Linzer		
Paul Goetz		

3. Identify five nursing interventions for John Linzer as he progresses through the dying process.

4. With history of alcoholism for 5 years, which is a priority nursing intervention in the plan of care for Mr. Goetz?

   A. Identify maladaptive behaviors that may contribute to the alcoholism.

   B. Encourage patient participation in therapeutic group activities.

   C. Teach the patient the effects of alcohol use on his body.

   D. Use a respectful, nonjudgmental approach to gain the patient's trust.

5. Paul Goetz is given Ativan (lorazepam) to prevent symptoms of alcohol withdrawal. How would you evaluate the effectiveness of this medication?

6. Mrs. Black understands the postoperative teaching done by the nurse when she states which of the following?

   A. "Since my surgery is on my ankle, I will need to stay still in the bed to prevent pain."

   B. "I will need to cough frequently to remove fluids from my lungs."

   C. "Since I will have a PCA machine for pain medication, I will not have to ask for pain medication."

   D. "I will be able to eat and drink as soon as I return from surgery."

Communication

1. What information will you report to Peter Black's doctor regarding his new symptom of numbness in both legs?

2. What information should be communicated with the pediatric unit nurses prior to Mary Black's being allowed to visit her children before she has surgery on her ankle?

Delegation

1. What nursing interventions for each patient can be delegated to a certified nursing assistant (CNA)?

   A. _____

   B. _____

   C. _____

   D. _____

Nursing Ethics

1. Paul Goetz asks you to bring him some beer. He says, "You can smuggle it in and no one will know." How will you respond?

2. When preparing for the role the nurse will play in disaster relief, the nurse must first do which of the following?

   A. Be able to apply basic first aid skills.

   B. Be aware of decontamination procedures.

   C. Serve on disaster preparedness committees.

   D. Know how to take care of him- or herself.

CASE STUDY: Maria Rodriguez

Mrs. Maria Rodriguez is admitted to the emergency room with an open left leg fracture, left upper quadrant pain, and reddened areas across the left shoulder, neck, and chest. According to the paramedics, she was involved in a multiple car accident on an icy highway. Upon assessment she is found to be a non-English-speaking Hispanic, 28 years of age, 5' 4'' in height, and weighing 115 pounds. Her vital signs are T 100°F, P 100, R 28 and shallow, BP 150/86. She indicates that her pain scale level is at 9 out of 10, even after being medicated with Morphine in the ambulance.

After chest, abdominal, and leg x-rays, Mrs. Rodriguez is diagnosed with a severe comminuted left leg fracture; a lacerated spleen; and bruising across the shoulder, neck, and chest due to the seat belt. With the use of a translator, the physician explains to the patient that due to the seriousness of the left leg fracture, the left leg may need to be amputated during surgery. Mrs. Rodriguez begins crying and wringing her hands after speaking with the physician.

Blood is drawn for the following laboratory studies: complete blood count with differential, electrolytes, prothrombin time (PT),

partial thromboplastin time (PTT), and blood gases. A urine specimen is sent to the laboratory for a urinalysis. Preoperative preparation is completed. Through the use of a translator, the nurse explains postoperative teaching to the patient to prevent the following complications of surgery: shock, hemorrhage, deep vein thrombosis, pulmonary embolism, pneumonia, infection, urinary retention, and delayed bowel elimination. The nurse tries to calm the patient and answer any questions she has regarding the surgery and what will happen in the postoperative period. The nurse attempts to contact family members and a priest to see the patient before she goes to surgery. At the ordered time, the nurse administers preoperative medication as ordered and the patient is sent to the operating room.

Due to difficulty understanding the English language, the need for surgery, and the possibility of leg amputation, the patient is very anxious. The nursing diagnosis of Anxiety is appropriate for guiding nursing care. Anxiety is an uneasy feeling of not knowing what is going to happen. The pathophysiology of anxiety is anticipation of danger or a threat to health status that leads to a "fight or flight" response from the sympathetic nervous system. Manifestations of anxiety are restlessness, tachycardia, rapid breathing, facial flushing, increased perspiration, weakness, tremors, and impaired attention and concentration. Complications of anxiety are nausea, vomiting, diarrhea, loss of appetite, insomnia, immobility, and powerlessness that can lead to panic or phobias.

Activity:

1. After reviewing the concept map, go to the Pearson Nursing Student Resources for this book at www.nursing. pearsonhighered.com to write a concept map based on the nursing diagnosis Grieving related to potential amputation of

left leg. In your concept map, be sure to include consideration of Mrs. Rodriguez's communication barriers and culture. See answers and hints in Appendix C.

2. Write another concept map using another appropriate nursing diagnosis.

Pathophysiology and Patterns of Health

UNIT 3

CHAPTER 8

Genetic Implications of Adult Health Nursing

LEARNING OUTCOMES

1. Discuss the role of genetic concepts in health promotion and health maintenance.
2. Apply knowledge of the principles of genetic transmission and risk factors for genetic disorders.
3. Describe the significance of delivering genetic education and counseling follow-up in a professional manner.
4. Explain the implications of genetic advances on the role of nurses with particular attention to spiritual, cultural, ethical, legal, and social issues.
5. Identify the significance of recent advances in human genetics and the effect on healthcare delivery.

CLINICAL COMPETENCIES

1. Integrate genetic physical assessment and the use of a pedigree family history into delivery of nursing care.
2. Identify patients or families with actual or potential genetic conditions and initiate referrals to a genetics professional.
3. Prepare patients and their families for a genetic evaluation and facilitate the genetic counseling process.
4. Integrate basic genetic concepts into patient and family education and the reinforcement of information provided to patients by genetic professionals.

KEY TERMS

alleles, *147*
autosomes, *145*
biological markers, *148*
chromosomes, *145*
gene, *147*
genotype, *147*
heterozygous, *147*

homozygous, *147*
human genome, *144*
meiosis, *146*
mitosis, *146*
penetrance, *149*
phenotype, *147*
polymorphisms, *148*

sex chromosomes, *146*
somatic cell, *146*
translocation, *147*
trisomy 21, *146*
X-linked dominant, *148*
X-linked recessive, *148*

Ongoing research in genetics has enhanced our understanding of the causes and natural course for disease, and our understanding of the factors that increase risk for the development of many diseases. Genetics research is not only focused on traditional genetic disorders, but also common complex diseases such as heart disease, stroke, diabetes, and several kinds of cancer. The knowledge gained from the Human Genome Project (Box 8–1) and the continued efforts of scientists and clinicians has and will continue to have a profound impact on the prevention, diagnosis, and treatment of genetic disorders and complex diseases (Figure 8–1 ■).

Integrating Genetics into Nursing Practice

Genetic knowledge will continue to revolutionize how persons perceive themselves, their health status, and their health potential. Therefore, it is expected that nurses must integrate genetics into nursing practice. The *Statement on the Scope and Standards of Genetics Clinical Nursing Practice* from the American Nurses Association and the International Society of Nurses in Genetics (ANA/ISONG) defines the role of all nurses regardless of practice setting (Box 8–2), thus emphasizing the importance of genetics in every arena of health care.

Nurses must have basic genetic knowledge to care for the needs of patients and their families with known or suspected genetic disease. Basic interventions that meet the standard of genetic nursing include the following:

- Identifying simple risk factors by completing genetics-focused family history
- Performing an accurate and thorough physical assessment

BOX 8–1 Human Genome Project

In 1986, the U.S. Department of Energy (USDOE) announced the Human Genome initiative, and in 1990 the USDOE joined with the National Institutes of Health (NIH) to develop the Human Genome Project (HGP). The ultimate goal was to sequence the **human genome** and to identify all human genes. The completion of a high-quality reference sequence was announced in April 2003. Information obtained through the sequencing of the human genome has had a tremendous impact on finding the genes associated with human disease. Future research will now be directed toward understanding the complex functions of cellular regulation, human variation, and the interplay of genes and environment and how all the cell organelles, genes, and proteins work together in life's functions (USDOE Genome Programs, 2008).

Source: From Ball, Jane W.; Bindler, Ruth McGillis W.; Cowen, Kay J., Child Health Nursing: Partnering with Children and Families, 2nd, © 2010. Reproduced by permission of Pearson Education, Inc., Upper Saddle River, New Jersey.

Nursing Role in Genetic Testing Video

Trillions of cells

Each cell:
- 46 human chromosomes
- 2 meters of DNA
- 3 billion DNA subunits (the bases: A, T, C, G)
- 25,000 genes code for proteins that perform all life functions

DNA
the molecule of life

Cell

Chromosomes

DNA

Protein

Gene

Figure 8–1 ■ Each cell nucleus throughout the body contains the genes, DNA, and chromosomes that make up the majority of an individual's genome. The remaining portion of the human genome is in the mitochondria.

Source: From Ball, Jane W., Bindler, Ruth McGillis W., and Cowen, Kay J., Child Health Nursing: Partnering with Children and Families, 2nd, p. 89, © 2009 Pearson Prentice Hall. Reproduced by permission of Pearson Education, Inc., Upper Saddle River, New Jersey.

- Applying concepts of health promotion and health maintenance to assist the patient and family in making informed decisions about their health and lifestyle choices while facilitating autonomy
- Being a patient advocate and providing patients with information about available resources and services
- Providing patient education and making referrals when appropriate
- Completing an evaluation of the plan of care for the patient
- Applying knowledge of the ethical, legal, and social implications of genetic information

Nurses can improve the nursing care provided to patients by applying fundamental genetic concepts to their practice.

Genetic Basics

Life starts as a single cell, but the developed human body is made up of many cells. These cells share common features such as a nucleus that contains 46 chromosomes, and organelles such as mitochondria. There are many different types of specialized cells that function differently depending on their location. For example, pancreatic cells have a very different function than that of nerve cells.

All human cells, except mature red blood cells, contain a complete set of deoxyribonucleic acid (DNA) molecules. DNA molecules consist of long sequences of nucleotides or bases represented by the letters A, T, G, and C. The order of these bases gives the exact instructions for the functioning of that particular cell. Writing the correct order of the bases using the abbreviations represents the sequence of the bases in DNA. Together, the total sum of DNA in a human cell is referred to as the human *genome*, or the complete set of inheritance for an individual. The human genome includes the DNA in the cell nucleus as well as the DNA found in the mitochondria, which will be discussed later in this section. Each person's genome is unique. Identical (monozygotic) twins are the exception because they develop from only one fertilized ovum and share identical DNA.

The cell nucleus contains about 6 feet of DNA that is tightly wound and packaged into 23 pairs of chromosomes, making a complete set of 46 **chromosomes**. The structure and number of chromosomes can be shown by a karyotype, or picture, of an individual's chromosomes (Figure 8–2 ■) There are two copies of each chromosome. One copy, or half of the complete set of these 46 chromosomes, is inherited from the mother and the other copy, or the other half of the 46 chromosomes, is inherited from the father. For example, an individual will have two copies of chromosome 1, one inherited from his or her mother and one inherited from his or her father. These two copies or pairs of inherited chromosomes are called homologous (the same) chromosomes. Chromosomes are numbered according to size (largest to smallest), with chromosome 1 being the largest. The first 22 pairs of chromosomes, known as **autosomes**, are alike

Nursing Role in Genetic Testing Animation

Figure 8–2 ■ A karyotype is a picture of an individual's chromosomes. It shows the chromosomal structure and number of the 22 pairs of autosomes and the sex chromosomes.

in males and females. The 23rd pair, the **sex chromosomes**, determines an individual's gender. A female has two copies of the X chromosome (one copy inherited from each parent) and a male has one X chromosome (inherited from his mother) and a Y chromosome (inherited from his father).

Cell Division

Mitosis and meiosis are the two types of cell division in human cells. **Mitosis** is the process of making new cells and it takes place in the **somatic**, or tissue, **cells** of the body. Cell division through mitosis heals wounds and replaces cells lost daily on skin surfaces and in the lining of gastrointestinal and respiratory tracts. In addition, mitosis is responsible for human development. The mitotic activity of the zygote and its daughter cells is the foundation for a human's growth and development. The zygote undergoes mitosis to form a multicellular embryo, then fetus, then infant. Cell division through mitosis results in two cells called *daughter cells* that are genetically identical to the original cell, or *mother cell*, and each other.

Meiosis is also known as the reduction division of the cell. Meiosis occurs only in the sex cells of the testes and ovaries and results in the formation of the sperm and oocyte (gametes). Meiosis is very similar to mitosis in that it is a form of cell division; however, through a series of complex mechanisms, the amount of genetic material is reduced in half (23 chromosomes). This is very important because when the two sex cells combine during fertilization, the total number of chromosomes (46) is present in the offspring's cells. There are three purposes of meiosis: (1) to produce gametes, (2) to reduce the number of chromosomes by half, and (3) to make new combinations of genetic material from crossing over and independent assortment processes, which allows diversity in the human population.

Chromosomal Alterations

Alterations in chromosomes often occur during cell division and are classified as either alterations in the number of chromosomes or structural alterations. They involve either part of or the whole chromosome. The clinical consequences of number and structural changes in the chromosomes in an individual vary depending on the amount and type of DNA affected by the alterations.

Alterations in Chromosome Number

An increase or decrease in chromosomal numbers can occur during meiosis or mitosis (Box 8–3). Alterations occur often during meiosis because meiosis is a highly specific and complex process and each new daughter cell must contain exactly one chromosome from each homologous pair of chromosomes. During meiosis, the paired chromosomes may fail to separate, resulting in an egg or sperm cell with either two copies or no copies of a particular chromosome. This is known as *nondisjunction*. When these egg or sperm cells are fertilized by a normal gamete that contains 23 copies of all of the chromosomes, a zygote that is monosomic (one member of the chromosome pair is missing) or trisomic (having three chromosomes instead of the usual two) results. These circumstances produce such conditions as *monosomy* of the sex chromosomes in a female (Turner syndrome) or *trisomy* of autosomes, of which **trisomy 21** (Down syndrome) is one of the more commonly known.

Alterations in Chromosome Structure

Alterations in chromosome structure include inversions, deletions, duplications, and translocations. In a chromosomal inversion a segment of a chromosome is reversed, changing the DNA sequence for that portion of the chromosome. It occurs when a chromosome breaks in two places and the piece between the breaks turns upside down and reattaches within the same chromosome. The clinical consequences of an inversion

---

BOX 8–3 Variations in Chromosomal Number

Aneuploidy—the condition when extra or missing chromosomes exist; in affected living individuals, physical abnormalities and/or mental retardation are common

Monosomy—the loss of a single chromosome from a pair, i.e., Turner syndrome (45,XO)

Trisomy—the gain of a single chromosome, making a total of three copies of a certain chromosome, i.e., trisomy 21 or Down syndrome

Euploidy—the presence of the normal number of 46 chromosomes

Polyploidy—the condition when more than two pairs of all the chromosomes are present depend on how much chromosomal material is involved, where the inversion occurs, and what type of inversion is present.

A chromosomal alteration that includes a missing (deletion) or additional (duplication) whole chromosome or segment of a chromosome is an unbalanced rearrangement. An unbalanced rearrangement can result in missing genes, confusing directions from the genes, or too much gene product, which often results in a condition that is not compatible with life or altered physical and/or mental development. An example is *cri du chat* syndrome (mental retardation, crying that sounds like a cat mewing, and low-set ears), which results from a large deletion on 5p (the short arm of chromosome 5).

Translocation (chromosomal reshuffling) occurs when a segment of a chromosome transfers or moves and attaches itself to another chromosome. An example is the reciprocal translocation that is found in 95% of patients with chronic myelogenous leukemia (CML) (Wang et al., 2006). The contributing translocation occurs between chromosomes 9 and 22 and is known as the Philadelphia chromosome. The translocation that occurs between chromosomes 9 and 22 is not inheritable. However, this is not true for all translocations. About 4% of trisomy 21 cases are caused by a translocation; of these, half can be attributed to a translocation inherited from a parent (Mayo Clinic, 2008). The parent remains unaffected because although he or she has extra material his or hers is a balanced chromosomal rearrangement.

Genes

A **gene** is a small portion (segment) of the nucleotide (base) sequence of a chromosome DNA molecule that can be identified as having specific directions for a particular function or characteristic. The specific sequence of nucleotides (the genes and the variations therein) is referred to as the individual's **genotype**. Each chromosome contains numerous genes arranged in a linear order. Researchers currently believe there are about 20,000 to 25,000 genes in the human genome (USDOE Human Genome Programs, 2008).

All genes come in pairs because chromosomes come in pairs. The only exception to all genes being paired are the genes on the sex chromosomes (X and Y) present in males. All genes have a specific location on a specific chromosome. This is known as the *genetic locus*. For example, one of the many genes located on chromosome 19 is a gene for eye color. There may be slight variations or different forms of a gene, for instance, green versus blue eye color, and these different forms or versions of genes are called **alleles**. When an individual has two identical forms (alleles) of a gene they are said to be **homozygous** (homo = same). If an individual has two different forms (alleles) of the gene, they are said to be **heterozygous** (hetero = different). Genes can be described as *altered* or *mutated* when a change has taken place, or *expressed* when the gene has an impact on the outward appearance of an individual and/or the functioning of cells. The observable, outward expression of an individual's entire physical, biochemical, and physiologic makeup, as determined by his or her genotype (alleles) and environmental factors, is referred to as **phenotype**.

Function and Distribution of Genes

One function of genes is to provide directions for how to make proteins. These protein-directing genes are very important to life and functioning as a human and are responsible for transmitting messages between cells, fighting infection, directing genes to turn "on" or "off," forming structures, as well as sensing light, taste, and smell (U.S. National Library of Medicine, 2008). Some gene activities change from moment to moment in response to tens of thousands of intra- and extracellular environmental signals (USDOE Genome Programs, 2008). An example of this is the feedback mechanism that stimulates a cell to produce insulin after eating a candy bar. After eating, a gene on chromosome 11 directs pancreatic cells to produce, modify, and secrete insulin. Although the gene for producing insulin is present in all nucleated cells of the body, it is only functional in insulin-secreting pancreatic cells.

Mitochondrial Genes

Chromosomes in the cell nucleus are not the only site where genes reside. Several dozen that are involved in energy metabolism are located in the cell mitochondria (the "powerhouse" of the cell). *Mitochondria* are concerned with energy production and metabolism. Some cells contain more mitochondria than others, but each mitochondrion contains its own copies of DNA identified as mitochondrial DNA (mtDNA). Because ova have many mitochondria and sperm do not (most mitochondria are located in the tail of the sperm that detaches after fertilization), mtDNA is primarily inherited from the mother. Therefore, mitochondrial genes and any diseases due to DNA alterations on those genes are transmitted through the mother in a matrilineal pattern. This pattern of inheritance is very different from the pattern of inheritance of genes found in the nucleus of the cell. Thus, an affected female will pass the mtDNA mutation to all of her children; however, an affected male will not pass the mtDNA mutation to any of his children (Nussbaum et al., 2007). Manifestations of conditions as a result of mitochondrial gene alterations are primarily involved in high-energy tissues and organs such as skeletal muscle, heart muscle, the liver, kidney, brain, and nerve cells. The ears, eyes, and endocrine system are also affected. Symptoms develop over years as unhealthy or dying cells are not replaced. Hypertrophic cardiomyopathy, heart block, seizures, and deafness are also associated with mtDNA gene alterations (Nussbaum et al., 2007).

Gene Alterations and Disease

Today, we know that gene alterations are responsible for approximately 6000 hereditary diseases (Winkleman, 2004). However, different gene alterations within a particular gene can result in a wide variety of signs and symptoms. For example, the *CFTR* gene for cystic fibrosis is a very large gene located on chromosome 7. More than 1100 different mutations of the CFTR gene have been reported to be associated with disease (Giusti et al., 2007). The area of the *CFTR* gene that controls mucous production can have more than 300 different gene alterations resulting in a variety of symptoms ranging from mild, to severe, or no symptoms at all (U.S. National Library of Medicine, 2008). Gene alterations, not the genes themselves, cause genetic diseases and conditions.

Gene Alterations That Decrease Risk of Disease

Although it is common to associate gene mutations with disease, it is important to remember that gene mutations can also be helpful to decrease the risk of disease. Gene alterations and genetic variations may also have a protective role in the expression of diseases. A common example is the protective value of the gene alteration that causes sickle cell disease. Those individuals with this gene alteration have protection against malaria. Another example is the APOE gene. The APOE gene provides instructions for making a protein called apolipoprotein E. This protein combines with fats (lipids) in the body to form molecules called lipoproteins that are responsible for packaging cholesterol and other fats and carrying them through the bloodstream. There are at least three slightly different versions (alleles) of the APOE gene. The major alleles are called e2, e3, and e4. Research has shown that a person who inherits at least one e4 allele will have a greater chance of developing Alzheimer's disease. However, inheriting the e2 allele seems to indicate that a person is less likely to develop Alzheimer's (Genetics Home Reference, 2008).

Single Nucleotide Polymorphisms

Greater than 99% of human DNA sequences are the same (HGP, 2008c). **Polymorphisms** are DNA sequences that are natural variations in a gene in which each possible sequence is present in at least 1% of people, but usually have no adverse effect on the individual. *Single nucleotide polymorphisms* (SNPs, or "snips") are the most common type of genetic variation among humans and are one-letter (base pair) variations in the DNA sequence and serve as biological markers. **Biological markers** are important for the construction of chromosome maps and are easily tracked, stable segments of DNA. Scientists are hopeful that information gained from SNPs will provide information on how subtle differences in humans impact their response to drugs and the environment, thus making medical treatment and pharmacologic management more individualized.

Principles of Inheritance

Knowledge of inheritance allows the nurse to provide genetic information to patients and their families to assist them in managing their care and in making reproductive decisions. The basic underlying principles of inheritance that nurses can apply to inheritance risk assessment and teaching include (1) all genes are paired, (2) only one gene of each pair is transmitted (passed on) to an offspring, and (3) one copy of each gene in the offspring comes from the mother and the other copy comes from the father. Understanding the Mendelian patterns of inheritance is made easier by relating these principles.

Mendelian Pattern of Inheritance

Conditions that are caused by a mutation or alteration of a single gene are known as *monogenic* or *single-gene disorders*. The most common gene alterations that result in genetic disorders are categorized into Mendelian inheritance patterns because they are predictably passed on from generation to generation following Mendel's laws of inheritance. These single-gene mutations follow an autosomal dominant, autosomal recessive, **X-linked recessive**, or **X-linked dominant** inheritance pattern. The first three of these patterns are the most common. Modes of transmission or inheritance for thousands of conditions resulting from monogenic alterations have been identified (U.S. National Library of Medicine, 2008).

Autosomal Dominant

Autosomal dominant (AD) conditions are the result of an altered gene on any of the 22 autosomes or non–sex chromosomes (Figure 8–3 ■). More than half of the known Mendelian

Figure 8–3 ■ This Punnett square shows potential gene combinations (genotypes) and resulting phenotypes of children from parent genotypes with an autosomal dominant altered gene. Phenotypes are expressed (affected) when a male *or* female has one copy of the gene alteration.

Source: From Ball, Jane W.; Bindler, Ruth McGillis W.; Cowen, Kay J., Child Health Nursing: Partnering with Children and Families, 2nd, © 2010. Reproduced by permission of Pearson Education, Inc., Upper Saddle River, New Jersey.

conditions are autosomal dominant. In AD conditions, disease occurs in spite of the fact that there exists one unaltered or normal gene. Also, homozygous dominant conditions are generally much more severe than heterozygous dominant conditions and are often lethal. Because homozygous dominant conditions are usually lethal and would result from both parents being affected, the nurse should consider an individual exhibiting an autosomal dominant condition as heterozygous. See Box 8–4 for characteristics of an AD pattern of inheritance.

Autosomal Recessive

A gene or genetic condition is considered recessive when two copies of altered genes are needed to express the condition. Autosomal recessive (AR) conditions are the result of an

---

BOX 8–4 Autosomal Dominant Mendelian Inheritance Characteristics

(Examples: neurofibromatosis, breast and ovarian cancer, autosomal dominant polycystic kidney disease, Marfan syndrome, Huntington disease, familial hypercholesterolemia)

When the nurse gathers a family history, the nurse should assess for any of the following characteristics of autosomal dominant inheritance:

1. Both males and females are affected.
2. Males and females are usually affected in equal numbers.
3. An affected child will have an affected parent and/or all generations will have an affected individual (appearing as a vertical pattern of affected individuals on the family pedigree).
4. Unaffected children of an affected parent will have unaffected offspring.
5. A significant proportion of isolated cases are due to a new mutation.

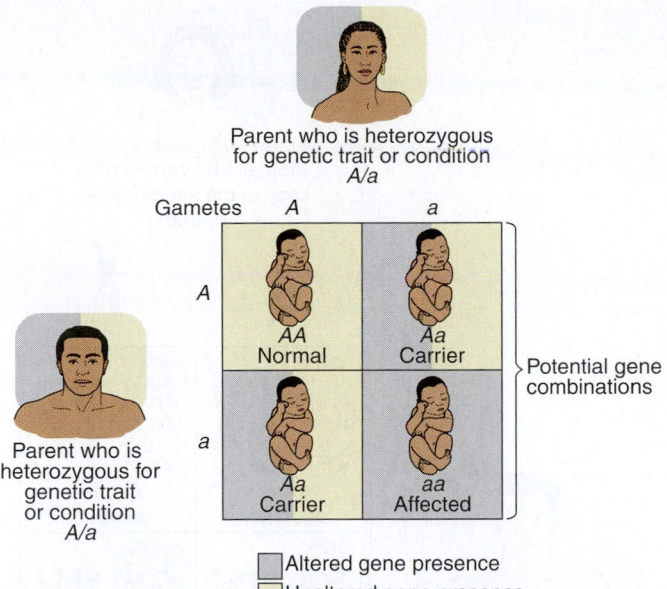

Parent who is heterozygous
for genetic trait or condition
A/a

Parent who is
heterozygous for
genetic trait
or condition
A/a

Potential gene
combinations

☐ Altered gene presence
☐ Unaltered gene presence

Figure 8–4 ■ This Punnett square shows potential gene combinations (genotypes) and resulting phenotypes of children from parent genotypes with an autosomal recessive altered gene. Phenotypes are expressed (affected) when a male *or* female has two copies of the gene alteration.

Source: From Ball, Jane W.; Bindler, Ruth McGillis W.; Cowen, Kay J., Child Health Nursing: Partnering with Children and Families, 2nd, © 2010. Reproduced by permission of Pearson Education, Inc., Upper Saddle River, New Jersey.

altered gene on any of the 22 autosomes or non–sex chromosomes (Figure 8–4 ■). An individual with a recessive condition has inherited one altered gene from his mother and one from his father. In most cases, neither of the parents is affected and, therefore, each of the parents must have a single gene alteration on one chromosome of a pair and the normal, wild-type or unaltered form of the gene on the other chromosome. These parents would be known as *carriers* of the condition and they do not usually exhibit any signs and symptoms of the condition. Because the gene alteration occurs on a non–sex chromosome, both males and females have an equal chance of inheriting the altered gene from their parent. See Box 8–5 for characteristics of an AR pattern of inheritance.

X-Linked Recessive

X-linked conditions are the result of an altered gene on the X chromosome. Unlike the autosomes, the sex chromosome, X, is unevenly distributed to males and females. The female has two X chromosomes and the male has only one. Thus, the family history and pattern of inheritance has a characteristic distribution pattern among the males and females in the family (Figure 8–5 ■). Because the male has only one copy of any gene on the X chromosome, it becomes the only copy available to give direction for those particular functions of these genes regardless of whether it is considered dominant or recessive in the female. Thus, if any of these genes are altered, an unaltered counterpart is not present to "override" the altered functioning gene.

The consequences of the altered gene on an X chromosome will be expressed in all males. Females, on the other hand, will have two copies and the unaltered gene generally compensates for the altered gene, making the female a carrier. The male

BOX 8–5 Autosomal Recessive Mendelian Inheritance Characteristics

(Examples: hemochromatosis type 1, cystic fibrosis, phenylketonuria, sickle cell anemia)

When the nurse gathers a family history, the nurse should assess for any of the following characteristics of autosomal recessive inheritance:

1. Both males and females are affected.
2. Males and females are usually affected in equal numbers.
3. An affected child will have an unaffected parent but may have affected siblings (appearing as a horizontal pattern of affected individuals on the family pedigree).
4. The condition may appear to skip a generation.
5. The parents of the affected child may be consanguineous (close blood relatives).
6. The family may be descendants of a certain ethnic group that is known to have a more frequent occurrence of a certain genetic condition.

receives his X chromosome from his mother and his Y chromosome from his father. The female offspring receives an X chromosome from each of her parents. Thus, all affected males will pass on the altered X chromosome to all of his daughters who will be carriers of the altered gene. A male can never transmit an altered gene on the X chromosome to his sons because the male will transmit only the Y chromosome to his sons. Because of these transmission patterns, the most commonly occurring transmission of an X-linked condition is through a female who is a carrier of an altered gene. See Box 8–6 for characteristics of an X-linked recessive pattern of inheritance.

X-Linked Dominant

X-linked dominant conditions also exist but these conditions are very rare. If a male is affected, the condition is severe and often lethal. A family history of multiple male miscarriages may be a sign of an X-linked dominant condition. An example of a viable X-linked dominant condition is vitamin-D resistant rickets, also known as hypophosphatemic rickets.

Variability in Classic Mendelian Patterns of Inheritance

Along with understanding the classic Mendelian inheritance patterns, several other concepts are also important for families to understand when the nurse is assisting patients with or at risk for inheriting a genetic disorder. These include the following exceptions or variations to the traditional Mendelian patterns of inheritance.

Penetrance

Penetrance is the probability that a gene will be expressed phenotypically. It is an "all or none" concept in that either the gene will be expressed (even if mildly expressed) or it will not be expressed at all. Penetrance can be measured in the following way. In a certain group of individuals with the same genotype, what percentage of them will exhibit at least some signs and/or symptoms of the condition? If the number is less than 100%, then that condition is said to show reduced penetrance. For example, the gene alterations that cause achondroplasia (dwarfism) exhibit 100% penetrance and all individuals with

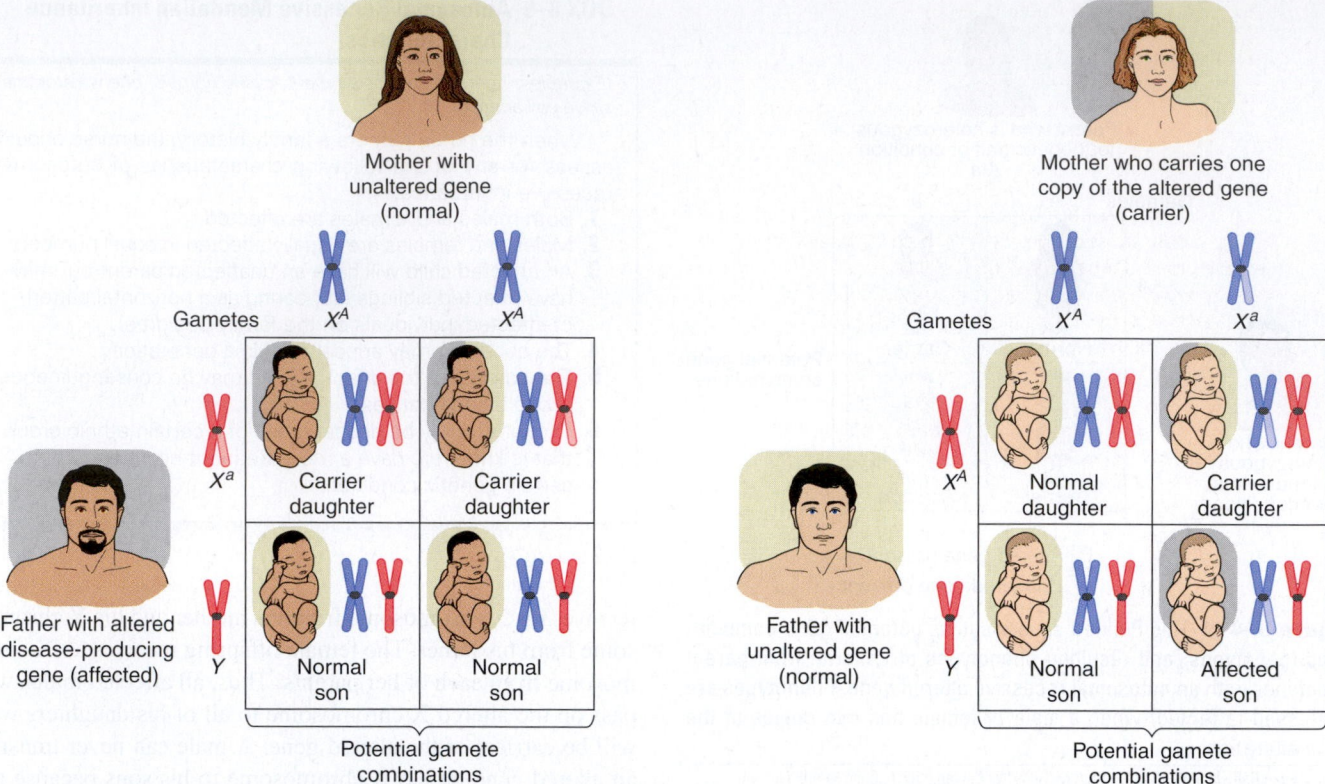

Figure 8–5 ■ These Punnett squares show potential gene combinations (genotypes) and resulting phenotypes of children from different parent genotypes with an X-linked recessive altered gene. Phenotypes are expressed (affected) in a male with only one copy of the gene alteration and in a female with two copies of the altered gene.

Source: From Ball, Jane W.; Bindler, Ruth McGillis W.; Cowen, Kay J., Child Health Nursing: Partnering with Children and Families, 2nd, © 2010. Reproduced by permission of Pearson Education, Inc., Upper Saddle River, New Jersey.

one copy of the gene alteration will exhibit signs and symptoms of the disease (Nussbaum et al., 2007).

New Mutation

When there is no previous history of a condition including even subtle signs and symptoms of the disease in any other immediate or distant family member, the disease may be caused by a spontaneous new mutation. This case is usually called a *de novo* mutation. New mutations of a gene are most frequently seen in autosomal dominant conditions because one copy of an altered gene is all that is necessary to elicit a state of altered health. Autosomal dominant diseases known to have high mutation rates include neurofibromatosis, achondroplasia, and

BOX 8–6 X-Linked Recessive Mendelian Inheritance Characteristics

(Examples: hemophilia A; Duchenne muscular dystrophy)

When the nurse gathers a family history, he or she should assess for any of the following characteristics of X-linked recessive inheritance:

1. More males will be affected than females; rarely seen in females.
2. An affected male will have all carrier daughters.
3. There is no male-to-male inheritance.
4. Affected males are related by carrier females.
5. Females may report varying milder symptoms of the condition.
6. A new sporadic case could be due to a new mutation.

Marfan syndrome. New mutations are also possible in autosomal recessive diseases although rarely expressed because two altered genes are necessary for signs and symptoms to appear. Finally, new mutations are often seen in X-linked recessive disorders, such as hemophilia A, as the male with just one altered gene will express the disease phenotype.

Anticipation

Anticipation occurs when successive generations of a family exhibit more severe signs and symptoms of certain diseases and the disease often has an earlier onset. An example of a condition where this occurs is fragile X. Fragile X is the most common cause of inherited mental impairment, caused by a mutation in a gene known as FMR-1, which is located on the X chromosome. The mutation is a "genetic stutter" in which a small section within the gene is repeated too many times. A person who does not have fragile X has between 6 and 45 repeats (trinucleotide repeats). Individuals with 55 to 200 repeats have a pre-mutation that can possibly expand when passed on to offspring. When this mutation is greater than 200 repeats an individual has a full mutation. See Box 8–7 for more information about fragile X.

Variable Expressivity

Expressivity is used to describe the severity of the *gene expression* of the phenotype. When people with the same genetic makeup (genotype) exhibit signs and/or symptoms with varying degrees of severity the phenotype is described as

BOX 8–7 Fragile X and Anticipation

- **Normal number of repeats.** Individuals with a normal number of repeats (6 to 45) cannot pass fragile X syndrome on to their offspring. The number of repeats in the offspring generally does not change.
- **Intermediate number of repeats or "gray zone":** When an individual has more than about 45 repeats but fewer than 55 repeats, the number of repeats can sometimes expand slightly when passed from parent to child. Individuals who have between about 45 and 55 repeats are considered in a "gray zone." These individuals have not been found to have a child with fragile X syndrome. However, the number of repeats can grow with each generation, so their grandchildren could be at risk.
- **Pre-mutation.** Individuals with between about 55 and 200 repeats have what is called a pre-mutation. Both men and women can be carriers of the pre-mutation. About 1 in 250 women and 1 in 800 men carries the pre-mutation. However, only women who carry the pre-mutation are at risk for having a child with fragile X syndrome.

    A pre-mutation carrier mother has a 50 percent chance of passing along the abnormal gene to her baby during each pregnancy. Some children who inherit the abnormal gene have a pre-mutation and no symptoms of fragile X syndrome. However, the number of repeats is likely to expand when the gene is passed from mother to child. As a result, some children of carrier mothers inherit the full mutation (more than 200 repeats) and show symptoms of fragile X syndrome.

    A male pre-mutation carrier passes on the pre-mutation to all of his daughters but to none of his sons. The daughters generally have no symptoms of fragile X syndrome, but they are carriers of a pre-mutation that may be passed on to their children. Unlike in females, in males the pre-mutation does not usually expand in size when passed on to their daughters. Sons of men with the pre-mutation do not inherit it because they do not get an X chromosome from their father.
- **Full mutation.** Individuals with more than 200 repeats have the full mutation. A woman with a full fragile X mutation has a 50 percent chance of passing along the full mutation in each pregnancy. If a man with a full mutation has children, he will pass the pre-mutation on to all of his daughters. For reasons that are not understood, the full mutation shrinks back to a pre-mutation in sperm. His sons are not at risk because they do not inherit the X chromosome from their father.

Source: Copyright 2007 March of Dimes. Used by permission.

variable expression (Nussbaum et al., 2007). Variable expression is common in the autosomal dominant condition, neurofibromatosis. Although neurofibromatosis has 100% penetrance, variable expressivity can occur within family members with each family member exhibiting a variety of signs and/or symptoms.

Multifactorial (Polygenic or Complex) Disorders

Many birth defects such as cleft lip and palate, as well as many adult-onset conditions such as cancer, mental illness, asthma, diabetes, obesity, heart disease, and Alzheimer's disease have a multifactorial cause. *Multifactorial conditions* occur as a result of several gene (polygenic) variations, lifestyle, and environmental influences that work together. The polygenic concept is illustrated with the multiple genes involved in an individual's susceptibility for breast cancer. These genes have been identified on chromosomes 6, 11, 13, 14, 15, 17, and 22. Exactly which genes interrelate and how many environmental influences are enough to cause the presentation of many of the common complex diseases or conditions is not known. However, it is believed that by 2010, the major contributing genes for many common complex conditions will be identified (HGP, 2008a).

Multifactorial conditions accumulate in families but these conditions do not follow the characteristic Mendelian pattern of inheritance seen with single-gene conditions. Inheritable recurrence risks vary in multifactorial conditions. Scheuner et al. (1997) developed a method of risk stratification that allows risk to be quantified for common adult diseases. For example, premature death in a first-degree relative, two affected first-degree relatives, and two second-degree maternal or paternal relatives with at least one individual having premature onset of the disease are all considered high inheritance risks. A patient considered as high risk for an inheritable condition should be referred for genetics consultation.

Interdisciplinary Care

Many health professionals work together in screening, diagnosis, identification, and treatment of genetic disorders. The goals of interdisciplinary care are early diagnosis through testing and assessment and development of an effective treatment plan, combined with psychosocial support to enhance coping and referral to a genetic specialist when needed.

Genetic Testing

Genetic testing involves the analysis of DNA, RNA, chromosomes, and serum levels of specific enzymes or metabolites. Genetic tests can be classified into two categories: screening and diagnostic. A positive screening genetic test result indicates an increased risk or probability but must always be confirmed by diagnostic testing. Screening genetic tests are most commonly completed in prenatal, newborn, and carrier circumstances. In contrast, a diagnostic test can definitively validate or eliminate a genetic disorder in the symptomatic patient and then guide clinical management. Box 8–8 lists some of the benefits and negative outcomes of genetic testing. Several categories of genetic tests follow:

- *Newborn screening* provides a means to identify children who have an increased risk for having a genetic disease such as phenylketonuria, sickle cell disease, or maple syrup urine disease. Several states now screen for more than 30 conditions (expanded newborn screen) as part of routine newborn care.
- *Carrier testing* is completed on asymptomatic individuals who may be carriers of one copy of a gene alteration that can be transmitted to future children in an autosomal recessive or X-linked pattern of inheritance. This may be part of a couple's premarriage or preconception planning if they belong to a particular ethnic group with known incidence to genetic disorders such as sickle cell anemia and Tay-Sachs disease.

BOX 8–8 Outcomes Related to Genetic Testing

Benefits of Genetic Testing

Provide for:

- Early screening and preventive measures
- Future planning and life preparation
- Lifestyle adaptations
- Decreased confusion and anxiety
- Psychologic stress relief
- Reproductive choices
- Informed immediate/extended family members
- Early medical and/or surgical intervention
- Cost of medical follow-up reduced (if negative result)

Possible Negative Outcomes of Genetic Testing

- Survivor guilt
- Loss of identity
- No treatment may exist
- Employability and insurability affected
- Confusion about accessing health care and resources
- Risk for invasion of confidentiality and privacy
- Social stigmatization

Source: Data from Secretary's Advisory Committee on Genetic Testing (SACGT), National Institutes of Health, 2000.

It may be necessary to determine the exact gene mutation from an affected family member prior to carrier testing. This is often completed through lineage analysis.

- *Preimplantation genetic diagnosis (PGD)* involves the detection of disease-causing gene alterations in human embryos just after *in vitro* fertilization and before implantation in the uterus, thus providing an opportunity for preselection of unaffected embryos for implantation. This type of genetic testing is most often used by parents who are both carriers of a single-gene recessive disorder and who wish to implant into the uterus only the embryo(s) without the disease-causing gene alteration. It has also been used to determine tissue type for donation of tissue such as bone marrow to a sibling or parent PGD is usually not covered by insurance, is very costly, and is available at only a small number of centers and for only a small number of disorders (U.S. National Library of Medicine, 2008).

- *Predictive genetic testing* is usually made available to the asymptomatic individual and includes both predispositional and presymptomatic testing. A positive predispositional testing result will indicate there is an increased risk that the individual might eventually develop the disease. Common examples include breast cancer and hereditary nonpolyposis colorectal cancer. A presymptomatic test is performed when development of the disease is certain if the gene alteration is present. These tests are medically indicated when the seriousness and mortality of the disease can be reduced with knowledge of the gene alteration. An example of this would be hereditary hemochromatosis or familial hypercholesterolemia. Life planning and lifestyle choices can be influenced by predictive testing.

- Other uses of genetic testing include organ transplantation tissue typing and pharmacogenetic testing, which involves predicting or studying the patient's response to particular medications. For example, pharmacogenetic testing has shown that 20% of Caucasians have a polymorphism on the cytochrome P450 CYP2C9 gene and consequently metabolize Warfarin more slowly and take longer to achieve therapeutic dosing (Ryan, Byrne, & O'Shea, 2008). These patients require significantly less Warfarin and are two to three times more likely to have a hemorrhagic adverse event. Controversy remains as to whether genetic testing should be undertaken for every patient prior to initiating Warfarin therapy; however, the United States Food and Drug Administration has revised the product label for Warfarin to include information on the benefits of genetic testing to guide Warfarin treatment (2008).

DIAGNOSING CHROMOSOMAL ALTERATIONS Chromosomal diagnostic examination can be accomplished with a blood, skin, or buccal cell sampling. A karyotype is completed in a cytogenetics laboratory. Chromosomes can be identified by their size and unique light and dark banding patterns. The pairs of autosomal chromosomes are arranged from 1 to 22 according to each chromosome's size, unique banding patterns, and *centromere* position. The sex chromosomes complete the picture, with the X chromosome(s) first, then the Y chromosome (if present). The karyotype shows all of the chromosome pairs lined up and positioned on a piece of paper allowing for visual chromosomal analysis. (See Figure 8–2 earlier in this chapter.) The final report contains numerical data that includes the total number of chromosomes present. Guidelines for writing results of karyotyping are determined by the International System of Human Cytogenetic Nomenclature (ISCN). The guidelines established by this organization allow for a standardized universal language that is utilized by cytogenetic laboratories and in medical publications. For example, a normal female karyotype is written as 46, XX, whereas a karyotype of a female with trisomy 21 is written as 47, XX, +21. In the second example, the (+) symbol signifies an additional copy of chromosome 21, whereas a (−) would signify a deletion (ISCN, 2005).

DIAGNOSING GENE ALTERATIONS More than 1000 tests are available from several laboratories, with some tests only available by a small number of sites. *DNA-based tests* involve sophisticated technology that permits the examination of the DNA itself. Genetic testing that is DNA based can be obtained from blood, bone marrow, amniotic fluid, fibroblast cells of the skin, or buccal cells from the mouth. These tests can be focused looking for common mutation(s) for a specific disorder or a mutation already identified in a previous family member. Several of the conditions screened for on newborn screening such as galactosemia are biochemical tests that look at enzyme levels. Genotyping must be done to confirm the diagnosis and specific type of galactosemia the patient has and to provide more accurate genetic counseling for family planning. A third type of DNA-based test is a complete gene sequence that may be utilized when only one mutation can be found in a symptomatic patient or when none of the common mutations were found (U.S. National Library of Medicine, 2008).

Nursing Care

The Role of the Nurse in Genetic Testing

Although confidentiality and privacy are integral parts of delivery of care for all nurses, this issue is of even more concern as it relates to genetic information. Results of genetic tests can affect employment and insurance options. Will the results affect the patient's ability to obtain and/or maintain insurance coverage? Can an employer refuse to hire or promote an individual because of genetic testing results? Can genetic information be released to the courts, military, schools, or adoption agencies? Would a patient with a known gene alteration for Huntington disease be offered a college scholarship to the best law school? There is debate over whether genetic privacy is different from medical privacy. The nurse should inform patients of their rights and responsibility to know who will have access to the genetic test results. Those providing the genetic tests must provide the patient with assurance that the results will be handled confidentially, and that there will be no access to the genetic information by a third party without written permission of the individual being tested. All genetic testing should be voluntary and it is the nurse's responsibility to ensure that the informed consent process includes discussion of the risks and benefits of the test, including any physical harm as well as potential psychologic and societal injury by stigmatization, discrimination, and emotional stress. Healthcare providers are legally liable to maintain that confidence. Exceptions to the individual's privacy may be made only when the individual refuses to inform extended family members when a very high probability of irreversible harm exists for an extended family member and informing the family member can prevent harm from occurring (National Human Genome Research Institute, 2005).

Psychosocial Issues

Although family and individual anxiety may be decreased with a negative test result, potential problems do exist and the nurse must be prepared to address them. Concerns about carrier status may interfere with development of intimacy and interpersonal relationships. Nonpaternity may be revealed through genetic testing. For example, the parents of a child born with an autosomal recessive condition will be considered carriers of the altered gene the majority of the time. To counsel the parents about future pregnancies, the parents would be tested to confirm their genotype, and nonpaternity may become an issue. A positive test result may lead to feelings of unworthiness, confusion, anger, depression, and self-image disturbance. Survivor guilt may affect adults with negative results if their siblings are positive. The individual carrying a gene alteration for a late-onset disease may have an increased tendency for risky behaviors and may choose not to be a positive member of society. Relatives of an individual affected with a genetic disorder may be very frightened when they realize what their own future might be. The individual who has inherited an altered disease-producing gene may foster deep resentment toward the parent who carries the altered gene. Parents and older generations may feel tremendous guilt for passing the altered gene to their children and grandchildren.

Economic Issues

The nurse should consider the cost of genetic tests, which can range from hundreds to thousands of dollars, depending on the size of the gene being tested. Most insurance companies do not cover genetic tests, but if there is insurance coverage the individual must weigh the cost of allowing the insurance company to have access to the genetic information (HGPb, 2008). Additionally, depending on the information that will be gained from obtaining the test, the family may wish to defer testing if it does not provide better outcomes or change in treatment strategy for the patient.

Assessment

Health Promotion and Health Maintenance

Health promotion and health maintenance of the patient are viewed as goals of nursing care.

With knowledge of genetic conditions, the nurse can ensure health teaching and early detection of complications from genetic conditions with emphasis on primary and secondary care interventions. For example,

- a woman with a strong family history and/or mutations in the *BRCA1* and *BRCA2* tumor suppressor genes should have screening clinical breast exams and mammographies at an earlier age than the general population.
- a man with a strong family history and/or mutations in the *BRCA1* and *BRCA2* tumor suppressor genes should report any mass, tenderness, or swelling in the breast tissue and maintain early screening for prostate cancer.
- colonoscopy screening every 1 to 2 years beginning at age 25 is important for the individual with a positive family history and/or mutations in the *MLH1/MSH2* gene, which increases the risk for hereditary nonpolyposis colorectal cancer.

Patients receiving early intervention and health-promotion-focused care can live longer and with a much better quality of life that those who do not. The nurse must be able to identify both community-based and genetic-based resources that are available to assist the patient in strategies to support both health promotion and health maintenance activities.

Patient Intake and History

Family history has long been a part of nursing assessment, but the relative importance of obtaining a family history has recently increased as our knowledge of the interaction of genes and the environment has expanded. In fact, it is an inexpensive first "genetic screen," often underused by healthcare professionals. Yet, with the number of genetics professionals being less than the projected need, professionals in primary care and other specialties will have to share some of the responsibility in obtaining this information and making appropriate referrals.

Pedigrees

A pedigree is a pictorial representation or diagram of the medical history of a family (typically three generations). Multiple symbols are utilized to present this picture (Figure 8–6 ■) and the finished pedigree presents a family's medical data and biologic

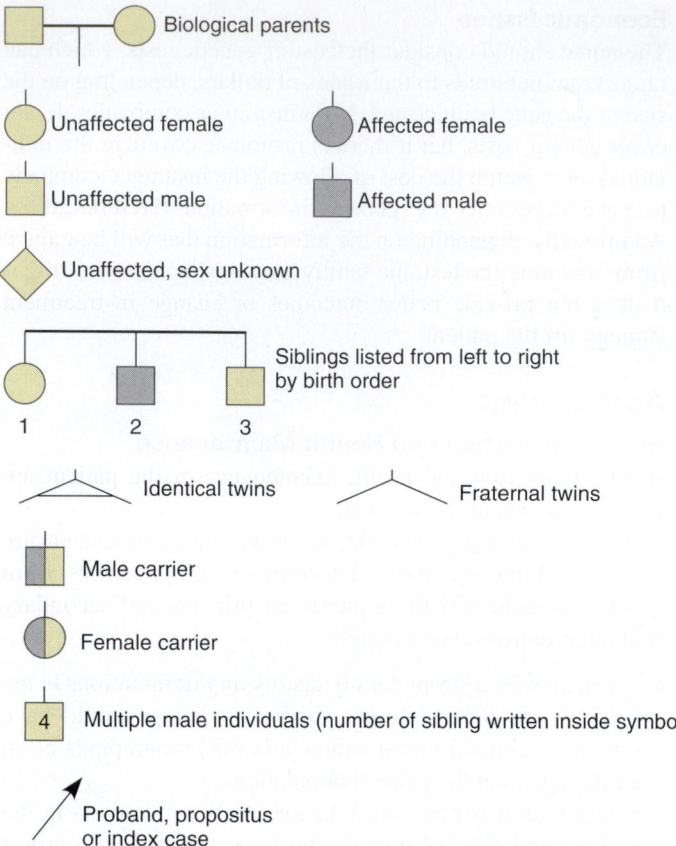

Biological parents

Unaffected female

Affected female

Unaffected male

Affected male

Unaffected, sex unknown

Siblings listed from left to right by birth order

1 2 3

Identical twins

Fraternal twins

Male carrier

Female carrier

4 Multiple male individuals (number of sibling written inside symbol)

Proband, propositus or index case

Figure 8–6 ■ Selected standardized symbols for use in drawing a pedigree.

Source: From Ball, Jane W.; Bindler, Ruth McGillis W.; Cowen, Kay J., *Child Health Nursing: Partnering with Children and Families*, 2nd, © 2010. Reproduced by permission of Pearson Education, Inc., Upper Saddle River, New Jersey.

relationship information at a glance (Figure 8–7 ■). A pedigree provides the nurse, genetic counselor, or geneticist with a clear, visual representation of relationships of affected individuals to the immediate and extended family. It can identify other individuals in the family who might benefit from a genetic consultation. It also can identify a single-gene alteration pattern of inheritance or a cluster of multifactorial conditions, and a referral and/or reproductive risk teaching for the individual and family can result. A family's learning can be enhanced by the visual teaching contribution a pedigree can provide and also clarify any inheritance misunderstandings or misconceptions.

By simply integrating into practice the genetic aspects of assessment, observation, and history gathering, the nurse can improve the standard of care delivered and have a positive effect on the patient. The nurse does not need to be a genetic expert, but with heightened awareness, appropriate inquiries and referrals to genetic specialists can be completed.

Nursing Diagnosis and Interventions

Nurses are responsible for comprehensively delivering the correct standard of care to patients, but at the same time being aware of the limitations of their own knowledge and expertise. In addition to the continuous integration of genetic aspects into nurses' assessments of family history and physical assessment, nurses are also responsible for carrying out interventions that include initiating referrals to genetic specialists and delivering

care to the individual or family in any of the following ways. Nursing diagnoses to consider include the following:

- *Grieving*
- *Anxiety*
- *Disturbed Body Image*
- *Ineffective Coping*
- *Decisional Conflict*
- *Interrupted Family Processes*
- *Ineffective Health Maintenance*
- *Deficient Knowledge*
- *Powerlessness*
- *Spiritual Distress*

Genetic Referrals and Counseling

Referral of a patient with a suspected genetic problem to a geneticist, genetic clinical nurse specialist, or genetic clinic is an expected nursing responsibility in the same way as referrals to a dietitian or a social worker. After gathering assessment data that incorporates genetic concepts, the nurse is able to initiate a referral to genetic specialists if there are indicators for a genetic referral (Box 8–9). The nurse should provide the patient with information about the advantages of a referral to genetic specialists, the disadvantages of not following through with the referral, and provide anticipatory guidance as to what to expect from his or her visit (Box 8–10).

Usually before the first genetic evaluation visit, the patient will be contacted to provide a detailed medical and family history and to make an appointment for genetic consultation. The patient should be prepared to give as exact a family history as possible so that a detailed three-generation pedigree can be constructed. The patient should be informed that a genetic consultation usually lasts several hours. During the appointment, a genetic clinical nurse, genetic counselor, and/or a physician will perform an initial interview with the patient. A geneticist will examine the patient in order to establish an accurate diagnosis. Tests may be ordered. These may include chromosome (cytogenetic) analysis, DNA-based testing, x-rays, biopsy, biochemical tests, and linkage studies (Lashley, 2005). After the exam and the completion of any applicable testing, the geneticist and/or genetic counselor will discuss the findings with the patient and make recommendations. The discussion will include the natural history of the condition, the inheritance patterns, the current preventive or treatment options, and the risks to the patient and/or family. The visit will also include opportunities for questions and answers as well as the assessment and evaluation of the patients' understanding. It is typical for the retention of information for a patient facing a new genetic diagnosis to be very low. This makes it imperative for the nurse to take advantage of opportunities to reinforce genetic concepts at a later time when the patient is ready.

As the visit concludes, the patient can expect appropriate referrals to be made, discussion of available services or research studies, and possible scheduling of a follow-up visit. A summary of the information is usually sent to the patient and the patient's healthcare provider will receive a report if requested by the patient.

Genetic healthcare providers present the patient with information to promote informed decisions. They are also sensitive to the importance of protecting the individual's autonomy. A challenge during any visit to a genetic specialist is providing

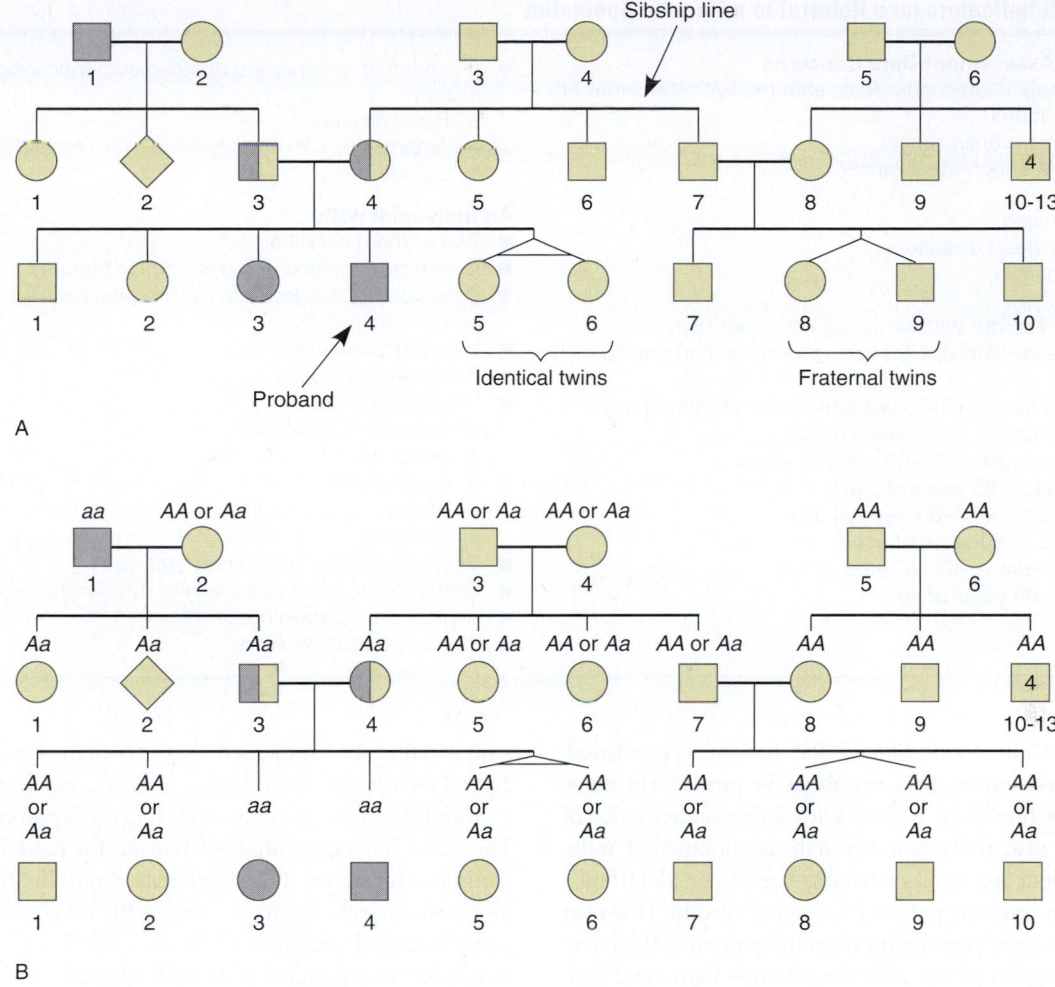

(A) A representative pedigree for a single character or genetic condition through three generations.
(B) The most probable genotypes of each individual in the pedigree for an autosomal recessive condition, represented by AA, Aa, or aa.

Figure 8–7 ■ Sample three-generation pedigree.

Source: Fig. 3.13, p. 63 from *Concepts of Genetics*, 7th ed. by William S. Klug and Michael R. Cummings. Copyright © 2003 by William S. Klug and Michael R. Cummings. Reproduced by permission of Pearson Education, Inc..

nondirective counseling. Patients should be permitted to make decisions that are not influenced by any biases or values from the nurse, counselor, or geneticist. Many patients are accustomed to practitioners and nurses providing direction and guidance in their decision making, and patients may be very uncomfortable with the nondirectional approach of the nurse. They may believe that the nurse or healthcare provider is withholding very bad news. The nurse should discuss the positives and negatives of each decision and present as many options as possible through the use of therapeutic listening and communication skills.

Patient Teaching and Support

The nurse must be aware of available genetic resources and participate in the education of genetic disorders as well as health promotion and prevention. The cultural and religious beliefs and values of the patient must be assessed prior to teaching. Are the gene alterations viewed as uncontrollable and believed to be occurring secondary to cultural belief such as a stranger looking at the patient? Or, are the gene alterations considered a "punishment"? Obtaining educational materials in the native language of the patient will also help facilitate the

teaching–learning experience. Also, identifying and dealing with barriers to learning, such as denial, anxiety, or guilt, will enable teaching to be more useful and effective for the patient and family.

Nurses should encourage open discussions and the expression of fears and concerns. Reinforce to patients that genetic alterations are caused by changes within a gene and not by superstitions related to sin or other cultural beliefs. However, it is important to remember that everyone has superstitions or beliefs and the nurse must remain nonjudgmental. The nurse is responsible for assessing the patient's coping mechanisms as well as available family, spiritual, cultural, and community support systems. Genetic conditions can cause a permanent strain on family dynamics and relationships. The nurse may need to help the patient reaffirm his or her self-worth and value (Lashley, 2005).

Growth and development and meeting adult developmental milestones can be altered by actual or potential genetic disorders. Especially unique is the potential or actual inheritance of a late-onset condition such as Huntington disease. The patient with this altered gene may not meet any of the developmental tasks in

BOX 8–9 Adult Indicators for a Referral to a Genetic Specialist

Adult History Assessment Data Concerns

- Several closely related individuals affected with the same or related conditions:
  - Breast and ovarian cancer
  - Colon and endometrial cancer
  - Diabetes
  - Hypertension
  - Coronary heart disease
  - Thyroid cancer
  - Colon polyps
- A common disorder with earlier age of onset than typical (increase concern if it occurs in more than one family member):
  - Breast cancer: < 45–50 years of age or premenopausal
  - Colon cancer: < 45–50 years of age
  - Prostate cancer: < 45–60 years of age
  - Vision loss: < 55 years of age
  - Hearing loss: < 50–60 years of age
  - Dementia: < 60 years of age
  - Heart disease: < 40–60 years of age
  - Stroke: < 60 years of age

- A sudden or unexpected death in someone who seemed healthy:
  - Renal disease
  - Asthma
  - Suicide

An Individual with:
- Two or more conditions
- A medical condition and dysmorphic features
- Developmental delay with dysmorphic features and/or physical birth anomalies
- Learning disabilities
- Behavioral problems
- Unexplained:
  - Movement disorders
  - Seizures
  - Hypotonia
  - Ataxia
  - Infertility
- Disproportionate tall or short stature
- Proportionate short stature with dysmorphic features
- Atypical sexual development
- Premature ovarian failure

---

moving through adulthood. Should the patient get married, attend college, save money, or worry about the future? The nurse must identify the impact of genetic knowledge on activities of daily living but also movement through developmental milestones. Both patient and family strengths need to be identified.

The nurse can refer the patient to a support group. However it is important to have permission from the patient if the nurse is providing a support group with the patient's name and contact information.

Another key role for the nurse is to help patients with the often difficult task of communicating genetic information such as inheritance patterns to extended family members. Cultural values of autonomy and privacy are affected when a patient must consider whether to communicate genetic information to extended family members who may also carry the altered gene. The history of a genetic alteration that may or may not cause disease can be extensive within a family, affecting multiple family members. Family members often have difficulty understanding that some genetic conditions have variable expressivity. Members of the extended family often are shocked and feel a profound sense of

guilt that they are the one who has carried the gene alteration that caused their loved one to have a genetic condition.

Careful self-assessment of feelings is essential for the nurse. The nurse must continually advocate for patients and support their decisions even if the decisions contradict the nurse's own ideals and morals. Coping with genetic revelations and making genetic-related treatment decisions are difficult. The nurse must remember that patients will need resources and support, and also help in gathering information about reproductive options.

Evaluation

Expected outcomes of delivering nursing care with a genetic focus include the following:

- The patient will make informed and voluntary decisions related to genetic health issues.
- The patient will accurately identify the following:
  - Basic genetic concepts and simple inheritance risk probabilities
  - What to expect from a genetic referral
  - The influence of genetic factors in health promotion and health maintenance
  - Differences between medical and genetic tests
  - Social, legal, and ethical issues related to genetic testing

Visions for the Future

Nurses are often the primary caregivers to whom patients turn for information, guidance, and clarification of ideas. This nursing role is essential not only in providing direct nursing care but as a member of the community. As more information about the genetic revolution becomes available to consumers—in areas such as pharmacogenomics, gene transfer, ethics, genetic engineering, and stem cell research—the role of nurses remains not only vital but grows enormously. Nurses should remain educated, informed, knowledgeable, and ready to discuss trends and changes with patients and their families.

BOX 8–10 Genetic Information Nondiscrimination Act of 2008 (GINA)

After 13 years of debate, on May 21, 2008, President George W. Bush signed into law the Genetic Information Nondiscrimination Act of 2008 (GINA). The purpose of this federal law is to protect consumers from discrimination by employers and health insurance companies based on genetic information. Examples of protected tests are BRCA1/BRCA2 (breast cancer); Huntington's disease; and carrier screening for cystic fibrosis, sickle cell anemia, and cystic fibrosis. The health insurance regulations will take place 1 year after legislation was signed, while employment regulations are effective 6 months after signing. Some of the things not covered under GINA are life, disability, or long-term care insurance, and members of the military.

CHAPTER HIGHLIGHTS

- Nurses are responsible for basic genetic knowledge and delivering the expected standard of genetic nursing care. The nurse must be aware of the social, ethical, cultural, and spiritual issues related to the delivery of genetic nursing care.
- When cell division does not occur as expected, chromosomal alterations on the autosomes or sex chromosomes can result. Chromosomal alterations can be seen in a human karyotype.
- An individual may be identified as heterozygous or homozygous for a single gene. Some gene alterations cause disease and some are protective from disease. Multifactorial inheritance does not follow Mendelian inheritance patterns.
- Many types of genetic tests are available. All genetic tests have special considerations related to social, financial, ethical, and

legal implications. Genetic healthcare providers are obligated to present the individual and his or her family with information to promote informed decisions.
- Basic genetic nursing care involves family risk assessment through a detailed family history, integrating genetic concepts into a physical assessment, and initiating a referral to a genetic specialist.
- Genetic concepts can be applied to health promotion and health maintenance. Knowledge of the principles of inheritance allows the nurse to not only offer and reinforce genetic information to patients and their families but also to assist them in managing their care and in making reproductive decisions.

TEST YOURSELF NCLEX-RN® REVIEW

1. The patient is discussing the inheritance of an autosomal dominant trait. The patient has the condition and the patient's wife does not. They have one child without the condition. The nurse would be correct in explaining to the patient that he is most likely which genotype?
   1. FF
   2. Ff
   3. ff
   4. X_fY

2. A male patient diagnosed with Fabry disease is admitted to the unit. Which statement made by the patient would indicate to the nurse that the patient understands Mendelian inheritance concepts? "I have the disease because...
   Select all that apply.
   1. my mother had Fabry and my father did not."
   2. my father's mother had Fabry disease."
   3. my grandmother's brother had Fabry disease."
   4. my father has Fabry disease."

3. The nurse is providing information regarding genetic testing to a couple who believe they are carriers of an autosomal recessive gene alteration. Which statement by the nurse is appropriate?
   1. "If both of you are carriers, all of your sons will be affected and all of your daughters will be carriers."
   2. "Chromosomal studies will reveal if you are actually a carrier."
   3. "Newborn screening will reveal if your child is affected."
   4. "During the genetic evaluation, you will be asked to provide at least a three-generation family history."

4. When analyzing a family pedigree, the nurse notes the pedigree demonstrates that successive generations contain affected individuals, both males and females are affected, and there is no father-to-offspring inheritance. What is the most likely pattern of inheritance?
   1. autosomal dominant
   2. autosomal recessive
   3. x-linked recessive
   4. mitochondrial

5. When the nurse is developing a teaching plan, which statement is a correct rationale regarding the health promotion and health maintenance benefits from an assessment of family history?
   1. Clinical treatment options can be more focused.
   2. Prophylactic treatments can be started early.
   3. Specific diet, exercise regimen, and genotype can be determined.
   4. Single-gene alteration can be diagnosed.

6. When developing a teaching plan for a patient with a newly diagnosed genetic disorder, what is the rationale for including time for questions and answers?
   1. genetic disorders frequently are accompanied by learning difficulty
   2. retention of information is typically low at this time
   3. the information is complex and high-level
   4. many patients do not want to know this information

7. The patient asks the nurse if a genetic referral is necessary. Which information would be appropriate for the nurse to provide? Most likely genetic specialists will do which of the following? **Select all that apply.**
   1. Provide direction for important decision making.
   2. Complete chromosomal studies.
   3. Ask to see photographs of relatives.
   4. Provide information about the natural history of the condition.

8. The nurse would consider which assessment finding(s) as minor anomalies? **Select all that apply.**
   1. café au lait spots
   2. ear pits
   3. atrial septal defect (ASD)
   4. hypertelorism

9. A young man has a positive family history for mutations of the MLH/MLH2 gene. What would the nurse recommend?
   1. clinical breast examinations annually
   2. self-testing of blood glucose daily
   3. colonoscopy screening every 1 to 2 years
   4. hematocrit levels every 3 months

10. What was one purpose of the Genetic Information Nondiscrimination Act (GINA), signed into law in 2008?
    1. protection against gender bias in the workplace
    2. guidelines for specific sexual harassment activities
    3. mandated genetic testing for all government employees and their children
    4. protection against discrimination by employers based on genetic information

See Test Yourself answers in Appendix C.

Pearson Nursing Student Resources

Find additional review materials at
www.nursing.pearsonhighered.com
Prepare for success with additional NCLEX®-style practice questions, interactive assignments and activities, Web links, animations and videos, and more!

BIBLIOGRAPHY

American Nurses Association and International Society of Nurses in Genetics, Inc. (2007). *Statement on the scope and standards of genetics clinical nursing practice.* Washington, DC: American Nurses Publishing.

Bradley, A. (2005). Utility and limitations of genetic testing information. *Nursing Standard, 20*(5), 52–55.

Burke, W. (2004). Genetic testing in primary care. *Annual Review Genomics: Human Genetics, 5,* 1–14.

Chinnery, P. F. (2005, April 12). Leber hereditary optic neuropathy. In *GeneReviews at GeneTests: Medical Genetics Information Resource* [Online database]. University of Washington, Seattle, 1997–2005. Retrieved from http://www.genetests.org

Dietz, H. C. (2005, October 26). Marfan syndrome. In *GeneReviews at GeneTests: Medical Genetics Information Resource* [Online database]. University of Washington, Seattle, 1997–2005. Retrieved from http://www.genetests.org

Duncan, R., Savulescu, J., & Gillam, L. et al., (2005). An international survey of predictive genetic testing in children for adult onset conditions. *Genetics in Medicine, 7*(6), 390–396.

Gene reviews. In *GeneTests: Medical Genetics Information Resource* [Online database]. University of Washington, Seattle, 1993–2005. Retrieved from http://www.genetests.org

Genetics Home Reference (2008). *Genes: APOE.* Retrieved from http://ghr.nlm.nih.gov/gene=apoe

Giusti, R., Badgwell, A., Iglesias, A. D., & New York State Cystic Fibrosis Newborn Screening Consortium. (2007). New York State Cystic Fibrosis Consortium: The first 2.5 years of experience with cystic fibrosis newborn screening in an ethnically diverse population. *Pediatrics, 119,* e460–e467.

Guttmacher, A. E., Collins, F. S., & Carmona, R. H. (2004). The family history—more important than ever. *New England Journal of Medicine, 35*(22), 2333–2336.

Hudson, K., Holohan, M., & Collins, F. (2008). Keeping pace with the times – the genetic information nondiscrimination act of 2008. *The New England Journal of Medicine, 358*(25), 2661–2663.

Human Genome Project. (2008a). *From genome to the proteome.* Retrieved from http://www.ornl.gov/sci/techresources/Human_Genome/project/info.shtml

Human Genome Project. (2008b). *Gene testing.* Retrieved from http://www.ornl.gov/sci/techresources/Human_Genome/medicine/genetest.shtml

Human Genome Project. (2008c). *SNP fact sheet.* Retrieved from http://www.ornl.gov/techresources/Human_Genome/faq/snps.shtml

International Society of Nurses in Genetics. (2005). *Position statement: Informed decision-making consent: The role of the nurse.* Retrieved from http://www.isong.org/about/position_statements/index.html

Jones, K. L. (2005). *Smith's recognizable patterns of human malformations* (6th ed.). Philadelphia: Saunders.

Klug, W. S., Cummings, M. R., Spencer, C., & Palladino, M. A. (2009). *Concepts of genetics* (8th ed.). Upper Saddle River, NJ: Pearson/Prentice Hall.

Klug, W. S., Cummings, M. R., Spencer, C., & Palladino, M. A. (2010). *Essentials of genetics.* (7th ed.). Upper Saddle River, NJ: Pearson/Prentice Hall.

Lashley, F. R. (2005). *Clinical genetics in nursing practice.* (3rd ed.). New York: Springer.

Lea, D. (2008, January). Genetic and genomic healthcare: Ethical issues of importance to nurses. *The Online Journal of Issues in Nursing,* Vol. 13, No. 1.

Levy, H. P. (2007, May 1). Ehlers-Danlos Syndrome, Hypermoblity Type I. *Gene reviews.* In *GeneTests: Medical Genetics Information Resource.* Retrieved from http://www.ncbi.nlm.nih.gov/sites/GeneTests/?db=GeneTests [Online database].

Mayo Clinic. (2008). *Children's Health: Down Syndrome.* Retrieved from www.mayoclinic.com

National Cancer Institute. (2009). *Chronic myelogenous leukemia.* Retrieved from http://www.cancer.gov

National Coalition for Health Professional Education in Genetics. (2005). *Core competencies in genetics essential for all health-care professionals.* Retrieved from http://www.nchpeg.org

National Human Genome Research Institute. (2008). *FISH Fact Sheet.* Retrieved from http://www.genome.gov/10000206

Nussbaum, R. L., McInnes, R. R., Willard, H. F., & Boerkoel, C. F. (2007). *Thompson & Thompson genetics in medicine* (6th ed.). Philadelphia: Saunders.

Online Mendelian Inheritance in Man. (2003). McKusick-Nathans Institute for Genetics Medicine, Johns Hopkins University (Baltimore, MD) and National Center for Biotechnology Information Library of Medicine (Bethesda, MD). Retrieved from http://www.ncbi.nlm.nih.gov/omim/

Ryan, F., Byrne, S., & O'Shea, S. (2008). Managing oral anticoagulation therapy: Improving clinical outcomes: A review. *Journal of Clinical Pharmacy and Therapeautics. 33,* 581–590.

Theos, A., &, Korf, B. (2006). Pathophysiology of neurofibromatosis type 1. *Annals of Internal Medicine, 144*(11), 842–849.

U.S. Department of Energy Biological and Environmental Research Source. (2008). *Gene gateway—Exploring genes and genetic disorders.* Retrieved from http://www.ornl.gov/TechResources/Human_Genome/posters/chromosome/

U.S. Department of Energy Genome Programs. (2008). *Genomics and its impact on science and society: The human genome project and beyond.* Retrieved from http://www.ornl.gov/hgmis/publicat/primer/

U.S. National Library of Medicine (2008). *Genetics home reference.* Retrieved from http://ghr.nlm.nih.gov/

Winkleman, C. (2004). Genomics: What every critical care nurse needs to know about the genetic contribution to critical illness. *Critical Care Nurse, 24*(3), 34–35.

Nursing Care of Patients in **Pain**

9 CHAPTER

LEARNING OUTCOMES

1. Describe the neurophysiology of pain.
2. Compare and contrast definitions and characteristics of acute, chronic, central, malignant, phantom, and psychogenic pain.
3. Discuss factors affecting individualized responses to pain.
4. Discuss interdisciplinary care for the patient in pain, including medications, surgery, transcutaneous electrical nerve stimulation, and complementary therapies.
5. Use the nursing process as a framework for providing individualized nursing care for patients experiencing pain.

CLINICAL COMPETENCIES

1. Assess patients' pain intensity, quality, location, pattern, intensifiers, relievers; side effects of analgesics; and effect on function and mood.
2. Determine patient's expressed desire, values, preference, and support for pain management.
3. In collaboration with the healthcare team, intervene with appropriate evidence-based pharmacologic and nonpharmacologic methodologies. Revise plan of care according to patient's response to interventions and need for control.
4. Use equianalgesia tables to select and transition between opioid analgesics.
5. Teach patients about safe and effective self-management of pain.
6. Evaluate effectiveness of interventions to relieve pain and promote comfort; re-treat or adjust doses of medication and interventions as necessary.

KEY TERMS

acute pain, *163*
addiction, *166*
analgesic, *167*
breakthrough pain, *165*

chronic pain, *164*
equianalgesic, *168*
neuropathic pain, *165*
nociceptive pain, *165*

nociceptors, *161*
pain, *159*
titrate, *172*

Pain is a subjective response to both physical and psychologic stressors. All people experience pain at some point during their lives. An estimated 50 million Americans live with chronic pain; low back pain is one of the most common types of chronic pain, along with migraine or severe headache and joint pain. Another 25 million experience acute pain related to surgery or trauma (American Academy of Pain Management, 2009; Centers for Disease Control and Prevention [CDC], 2006). Although pain as a health condition falls within the cognitive-perceptual health pattern, its effects have the potential to cause dysfunction in all functional health patterns, whether the pain is acute, chronic, severe, or mild to moderate.

Although pain usually is experienced as uncomfortable and unwelcome, it also serves a protective role, warning of potentially health-threatening conditions. For this reason, pain is increasingly referred to as the *fifth vital sign*, with recommendations to assess pain with each vital sign assessment. The Joint Commission (2001) established pain standards that identify the relief of pain as a patient right. Joint Commission standards require healthcare facilities to implement specific procedures for, and provider education on, pain assessment and management.

Pain is a distinct and personal experience influenced by physiologic, psychologic, cognitive, sociocultural, and spiritual factors. It is the symptom most associated with describing oneself as ill, and it is the most common reason for seeking health care. The International Association for the Study of Pain (IASP) defines pain as an unpleasant sensory and emotional experience associated with actual or potential tissue damage, or described in terms of such damage. Although there are many definitions and descriptors of pain, the one most relevant for nurses is that pain is "whatever the person experiencing it says it is, and existing whenever the person says it does" (McCaffery, 1979, p. 11). This definition acknowledges the

FAST FACTS

- More than 25% of adults report low back pain within the past 3 months.
- Approximately 15% of adults, most between age 18 and 44, experience recurrent migraine or severe headache.
- Pain is common among older adults, with 20% reporting pain lasting more than 24 hours within the past month (CDC, 2006).

patient as the only person who can accurately define and describe his or her own pain and serves as the basis for nursing assessment and care of patients in pain. It also supports the values and beliefs about pain necessary for holistic nursing care, including the following:

■ Only the person affected can experience pain; that is, pain has a personal meaning.
■ If the patient says he or she has pain, the patient is in pain. All pain is real.
■ Pain has physical, emotional, cognitive, sociocultural, and spiritual dimensions.
■ Pain affects the whole body, usually negatively.
■ Pain may serve as both a response to and a warning of actual or potential trauma.

Myths and Misconceptions about Pain

Myths and misconceptions about pain and its management are common in both healthcare providers and patients. Some of the most common of these myths are included here.

■ *Pain is a result, not a cause.*   According to the traditional view of pain, pain is a symptom, not a condition. Pain is now recognized to have both immediate and long-term effects, such as immobility, anger, and anxiety; pain may also delay healing and rehabilitation.
■ *Chronic pain is really a masked form of depression.* Serotonin plays a chemical role in pain transmission and is also the major modulator of depression. Therefore, pain and depression are chemically related, not mutually exclusive. It is common to find them coexisting.
■ *Narcotic medication is too risky to be used in chronic pain.*   This common misconception often deprives patients of the most effective source of pain relief. Opioid (narcotic) analgesics are now recognized as an appropriate strategy for managing chronic pain unrelieved by other strategies.
■ *It is best to wait until a patient has pain before giving medication.*   Relieving pain before it escalates is widely accepted as having a noticeable effect on the amount of pain a patient experiences.
■ *Many patients lie about the existence or severity of their pain.*   Very few patients lie about their pain.
■ *Pain relief interferes with diagnosis.*   Effective pain management with analgesics in the emergency department (ED) has been shown to have no impact on physical assessment findings or diagnosis (Pasero, 2003).

Neurophysiology of Pain

The peripheral nervous system has two types of neurons: sensory and motor. The pain experience involves both sensory stimulation and perception. Pain stimuli are generated and transmitted through the sensory neurons, perceived within the central nervous system, and responded to through the motor neurons. Connections or synapses occur within the spinal cord and again within the brain, where interpretation of the painful stimulus leads to a response. A pain stimulus may prompt an immediate reflex response that precedes awareness of the pain.

Pain Theories

Several theories explain the response to pain and the diversity of human experiences with pain. The meaning or perception of pain can be modified by past experiences, motivation, attention, suggestion, personality, and culture. *Specificity* and *pattern* theories describe nerve impulses of varying intensity terminating in pain centers in the forebrain. These theories provide explanations of the neurophysiologic basis of pain. Later, in 1965, Melzack and Wall postulated the *gate-control theory* (Helms & Barone, 2008). According to this theory, activation of large-diameter, faster-propagating fibers by a tactile stimulus (e.g., massaging the elbow after hitting it on a sharp object) activates a gating mechanism that then blocks impulses from smaller pain fibers (Porth & Matfin, 2009). This mechanism was thought to exist at the segmental spinal cord level (Figure 9–1 ■).

Ongoing research demonstrates that the control and modulation of pain is much more complex than the description in the gate-control theory, which served as a base for further research about pain-modulating systems Tactile information is now known to be transmitted by both large- and small-diameter fibers, and interaction between sensory neurons is known to occur at multiple levels of the central nervous system. Melzack subsequently developed the *neuromatrix* theory of pain to integrate cultural and genetic factors with basic neurophysiologic function. This theory is consistent with but more complex than the gate-control theory. According to the neuromatrix theory, the brain contains a *body-self neuromatrix*, a widely distributed network of neurons that is affected by both genetic factors and sensory experiences. The neuromatrix integrates multiple sources of input in addition to the stimuli of pain and touch. The pain experience for the individual is affected by inputs from other sensory systems that help interpret the stimuli (e.g., seeing

Theoretical gate (open)

Dorsal horn

Large-diameter fiber

Small-diameter fiber carrying pain impulses to brain

Spinal cord

Theoretical gate (closed)

Large-diameter fiber carrying nonpain impulses to brain

Small-diameter fiber carrying pain impulses

Figure 9–1 ■ The spinal cord component of the gate-control theory. Pain transmission by small-diameter fibers is blocked when large-diameter fibers carrying touch impulses dominate, closing the gate in the dorsal horn of the spinal cord.

a wound); factors such as attention, expectation, personality, and culture; innate pain modulation systems; and components of stress-regulation systems (Porth & Matfin, 2009).

One pain theory that is quite significant in clinical terms describes the effect of sensitizing the central and peripheral nervous system to painful stimuli. According to this theory, painful signals create a cascade of changes in the nervous system that increase the responsiveness of the peripheral and central neurons. These changes, in turn, increase the response to future signals and amplify pain. Studies of infants undergoing painful procedures show that those who received analgesia experienced reduced sensitivity to future painful events, while those who did not receive analgesia experienced greater sensitivity (Taddio & Katz, 2005). Sensitization occurs from nociceptive barrage as well as inflammation that follows the injury or incision. In adults this theory indicates the value of preventing sensitization as well as treating perceived pain with multimodal pain therapy. Local and regional anesthesia used in combination with central anesthesia prior to incision to diminish sensitization of these pathways results in significantly reduced consumption of intravenous morphine by PCA in the 5 days following surgery (Hartrick, 2004).

Physiology

Nerve receptors for pain are called **nociceptors** (Figure 9–2 ■). These free nerve endings are woven throughout all the tissues of the body except the brain. Nociceptors are especially numerous in the skin and muscles. Pain occurs when the tissue containing nociceptors is subjected to a noxious insult. The intensity and duration of the stimuli determine the sensation. Long-lasting, intense stimulation produces greater pain than brief, mild stimulation.

Nociceptors respond to several different types of noxious stimuli: mechanical, chemical, or thermal. Some nociceptors respond to only a single type of stimulus, whereas others respond to all three types of stimuli (Table 9–1). The perception of pain in different parts of the body is affected by this variation in sensitivity to type of stimulus and the distribution of nociceptors in various tissues.

Tissue trauma, inflammation, and ischemia prompt the release of a number of biochemicals. These biochemicals have several effects. Chemicals such as bradykinin, histamine, serotonin, and potassium ion directly stimulate nociceptors, producing pain. These chemicals and others (such as ATP and prostaglandins) also sensitize nociceptors, intensifying the pain response and causing normally innocuous stimuli (such as touch) to be perceived as pain. Chemical mediators also act to perpetuate inflammation, which, in turn, causes release of additional chemicals that stimulate pain receptors. Furthermore, so-called *silent nociceptors* (e.g., sensory receptors in the gut that normally do not respond to mechanical or thermal stimuli) can become sensitive to mechanical stimuli in the presence of inflammatory mediators, leading to severe and debilitating pain and tenderness (Fauci et al., 2008).

Figure 9–2 ■ *A,* Touching the hot lid activates nociceptors in the skin, generating pain impulses that travel via fast Aδ and slower C fibers to the spinal cord. *B,* Secondary neurons in the dorsal horn pass impulses across the spinal cord to the anterior spinothalamic tract. *C,* Pain impulses ascend to the thalamus and, from there, to the cerebral cortex and the reticular and limbic systems in the brainstem, which integrate the emotional, cognitive, and autonomic responses to pain.

TABLE 9–1 Painful Stimuli

STIMULUS	EXAMPLES
Chemical	■ Ischemia (e.g., angina, bowel infarct) ■ Tissue trauma ■ Inflammation, inflammatory mediators such as histamine, prostaglandins
Mechanical	■ Spasm (ureteral colic, gallstones) ■ Compression (e.g., mechanical or by a tumor, carpal tunnel syndrome, or compartment syndrome) ■ Extreme muscle stretch or contraction (e.g., following a fracture)
Thermal	■ Contact with extreme heat or cold

Pain Pathways

The neural pathways of pain are illustrated in Figure 9–1 and can be summarized as follows:

1. A noxious stimulus is translated by nociceptors into an action potential that then is transmitted through small A-delta (Aδ) and even smaller C nerve fibers to the spinal cord. Aδ fibers are myelinated and transmit impulses rapidly. They produce what is called *fast pain* or first pain—sharp, well-defined pain sensations, such as those that result from cuts, electric shocks, or the impact of a blow. Aδ fibers are associated with acute pain from mechanical or thermal injury. C fibers are not myelinated and thus transmit pain impulses more slowly. Pain transmitted by C fibers may be described as *slow-wave pain* or second pain because it is slower to develop and lasts longer. This pain is more often prompted by chemical stimuli or persistent mechanical or thermal stimuli (Porth & Matfin, 2009). The pain from deep body structures (such as muscles and viscera) is primarily transmitted by C fibers, producing diffuse burning or aching sensations. C fibers are associated with chronic pain. Both Aδ and C fibers are involved in most injuries. For example, if a person bangs an elbow, Aδ fibers transmit this pain stimulus within 0.1 second, and can actually prompt reflex withdrawal from the stimulus before pain is perceived. The person feels this pain as a sharp, localized, smarting sensation. One or more seconds after the blow, the person experiences a duller, aching, diffuse sensation of pain impulses carried by the C fibers.

2. The sensory neuron enters the spinal cord via the dorsal root and terminates in the dorsal horn of the spinal cord. Here it synapses with spinal (or *second-order*) neurons that transmit the pain signal to the brain. Several chemical neurotransmitters, including glutamate, norepinephrine, and substance P, carry the pain signal from the sensory neuron to the spinal neurons. Each neuron contacts many spinal neurons, and each spinal neuron receives input from many peripheral neurons. This accounts for the phenomenon of referred pain (discussed under types of pain). Spinal neurons transmit the impulses via axons that cross over to the spinothalamic tract.

3. The impulses ascend the spinothalamic tracts and pass through the medulla and midbrain to the thalamus.

4. From the thalamus, the pain signal is distributed via third-order neurons to several areas of the cerebral cortex. The

somatosensory area of the cerebral cortex localizes the pain and interprets its intensity and quality. Other thalamic neurons reach areas of the frontal lobe, generating an emotional or affective response to pain. Connections to the reticular and limbic systems of the brain also are involved in the emotional and autonomic responses to painful stimuli. Pain signals to these areas can activate the "fight or flight" response, stress responses, and cardiovascular changes. A noxious impulse becomes pain when the sensation reaches conscious levels and is perceived and evaluated by the person experiencing the sensation.

Pain Modulation

No two people experience pain from an identical stimulus in the same way or at the same intensity; furthermore, the same person may perceive pain from the same stimulus differently on different occasions. A number of neural and chemical responses explain some of these differences.

Neural circuits that are thought to arise in the cerebral cortex link with the hypothalamus, midbrain, and medulla. These circuits interact with peripheral sensory axon terminals in the dorsal horn of the spinal cord to selectively control neurons that transmit pain signals. As a result, that pain response can be modified, that is, changed, increased, or dampened. Neurons within this circuit produce *endogenous opioids*, naturally occurring morphine-like neuropeptides. They also contain opioid receptors sensitive to endorphins and opioid drugs. Four types of endogenous opioids have been identified: enkephalins, endorphins, dynorphins, and endomorphins. They are hormones that act like neurotransmitters, binding with opioid receptors to block transmission of painful stimuli (Figure 9–3 ■). These

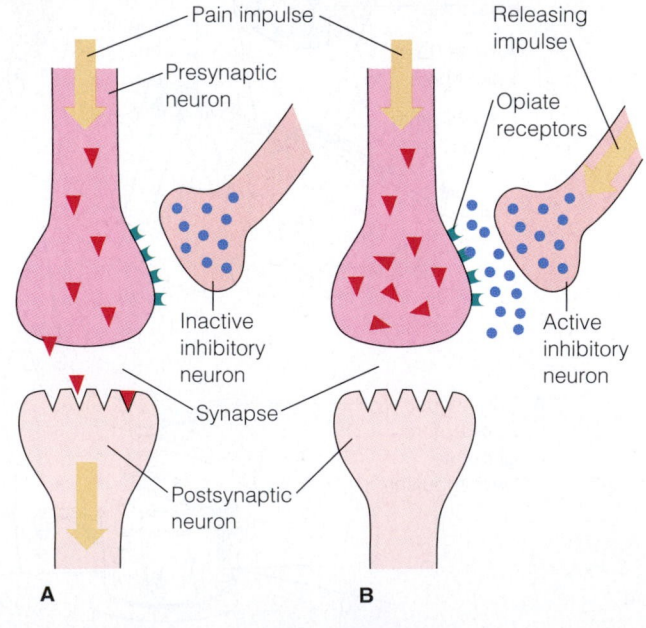

■ = Neurotransmitters   ● = Endorphins

Figure 9–3 ■ *A,* Pain impulse causes presynaptic neuron to release burst of neurotransmitters across synapse. These bind to postsynaptic neuron and propagate impulse. *B,* Inhibitory neuron releases endorphins, which bind to presynaptic opiate receptors. Neurotransmitter release is inhibited, and pain impulse interrupted.

substances also have been linked to a general sense of well-being (McCance & Huether, 2010).

Chemicals such as peptides and neurotransmitters also affect responses to pain stimuli. Locally, inflammatory mediators (e.g., prostaglandins, nitric oxide, histamine) lower the threshold for pain perception and tend to augment pain. ATP, substance P, and other peptides promote the local spread of pain and contribute to vasodilation and vascular permeability, increasing discomfort (McCance & Huether, 2010). In contrast, substances such as serotonin, norepinephrine, and others inhibit pain impulse transmission in the spinal cord and brain.

Types and Characteristics of Pain

Pain typically is described and characterized in several ways: by its duration (acute or chronic), its source or location, and referral.

Acute Pain

Acute pain has a sudden onset, is usually self-limited, and is localized. The cause of acute pain generally can be identified ("I tripped and twisted my ankle; now it really hurts"). The onset is usually sudden, most often resulting from tissue injury from trauma, surgery, or inflammation. The pain is usually sharp and localized, although it may radiate. Tissue healing relieves the pain. The three major types of acute pain are the following:

■ *Cutaneous and deep somatic pain*, which arises from nerve receptors originating in the skin (e.g., from a laceration), subcutaneous tissues, or deep body structures such as periosteum, muscles, tendons, joints, and blood vessels (acute pain from a fracture or sprain, for example). Somatic pain may be either sharp and well localized, or dull and diffuse.

■ *Visceral pain*, which arises from body organs. Visceral pain is dull and poorly localized because of the low number of nociceptors. The viscera are sensitive to stretching, inflammation, and ischemia but relatively insensitive to cutting and temperature extremes. Visceral pain often radiates or is referred. It may be described as deep cramping, splitting or stabbing pain, intermittent pain, or colicky pain. A kidney stone passing through the ureter to the bladder causes severe, acute visceral pain.

■ *Referred pain* is pain that is perceived in an area distant from the site of the stimuli. It commonly occurs with pain that originates in thoracic or abdominal viscera. Visceral sensory fibers synapse at the level of the spinal cord, close to fibers innervating other subcutaneous tissue areas of the body (Figure 9–4 ■). For example, the phrenic nerve, which innervates the central part of the diaphragm enters the spinal cord at the C3 to C5 level; pain originating in the diaphragm or the parietal peritoneum lining it (e.g., peritonitis) may be perceived as shoulder pain. Sites of referred pain are determined during embryologic development.

Acute pain warns of actual or potential injury to tissues. As a stressor, it initiates the fight-or-flight autonomic stress response. Characteristic physical responses include tachycardia, rapid and shallow respirations, increased blood pressure, dilated pupils, sweating, and pallor. The pain may be accompanied by nausea and vomiting. Secondary reflex muscle spasms may develop, intensifying the pain. The person experiencing acute pain responds to this threat with anxiety and fear. This psychologic

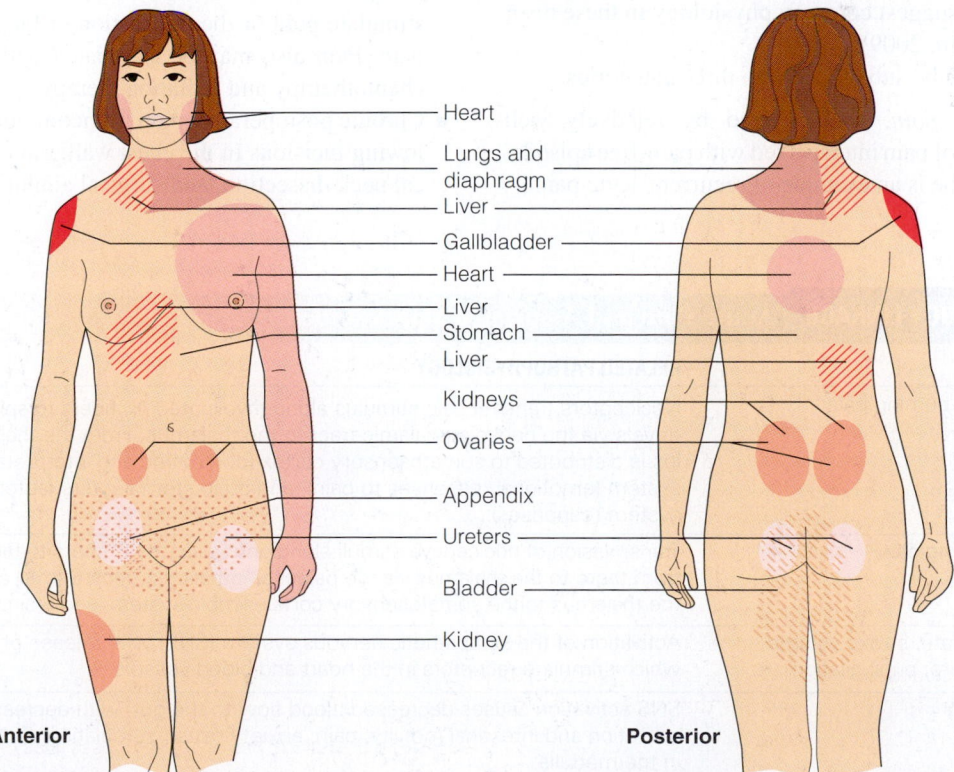

Figure 9–4 ■ Referred pain results of the convergence of sensory nerves from certain areas of the body within the spinal cord. For example, a toothache may be felt in the ear, pain from inflammation of the diaphragm may be felt in the shoulder, and pain from ischemia of the heart muscle (angina) may be felt in the left arm.

response may further increase the physical responses to acute pain. The accompanying Pathophysiology Linkage box describes manifestations of pain with an abbreviated explanation of the pathophysiology underlying the manifestation.

Chronic Pain

Chronic pain is prolonged pain, or pain that persists after the condition causing it has resolved. Although the cause may be identifiable (e.g., arthritis, cancer, migraine headache, diabetic neuropathy), chronic pain does not always have an identifiable cause. In some cases, pain may be perpetuated by disease-caused damage that persists after the disease has resolved (e.g., sensory nerve damage or reflex muscle contraction). In others, an imbalance of pain modulation mechanisms is thought to cause the persistent pain. This imbalance may relate to changes in the peripheral nervous system such as increased neuronal sensitivity to stimuli (a lower pain threshold) or spontaneous impulse generation by damaged neurons. Changes in the dorsal root, spinal cord, and brain also affect pain modulation. Repeated stimulation of peripheral nerves leads to a progressive buildup of electrical response in the central nervous system (CNS), leading to more intense and prolonged pain.

Unlike acute pain, chronic pain has much more complex and poorly understood neurophysiology and purpose. Persistent chronic pain often serves no useful function. The pain itself becomes the problem, creating physical, psychosocial, and economic stresses on the affected individual and his or her family. Furthermore, emotional and psychologic factors can cause the pain itself or make it worse. There is a clear association between chronic pain and depression. Depletion of serotonin (a neurotransmitter) and endorphins, found in both chronic pain and in depression, suggest common physiology in these disorders (Porth & Matlin, 2009).

Chronic pain can be subdivided into three categories:

- *Recurrent acute pain*, characterized by relatively well-defined episodes of pain interspersed with pain-free episodes. Migraine headache is an example of recurrent acute pain.

- *Chronic malignant pain*, caused by advance of a life-threatening disease or associated with treatment. Cancer pain is a type of chronic malignant pain.
- *Chronic nonmalignant pain*, non-life-threatening pain that nevertheless persists beyond the expected time for healing. Chronic lower back pain, a major cause of suffering and lost work time, falls into this category.

Patients with chronic pain often do not have the same physiologic responses to pain as are seen in acute pain. The heart and respiratory rates and blood pressure may remain within the normal range. Other autonomic nervous system responses such as nausea, vomiting, pallor, or sweating may not occur with persistent pain. The patient with chronic pain often is depressed, may have difficulty sleeping, and may be preoccupied with the pain. Table 9–2 compares acute and chronic pain.

The most common chronic pain condition is lower back pain. Other common chronic pain conditions include the following (McCance & Huether, 2010):

- *Myofascial pain syndromes* are marked by injury to or disease of muscle and fascia. They include myositis, fibrositis, myofibrositis, myalgia, and muscle strain. Pain results from muscle spasm, stiffness, and collection of lactic acid in the muscle. The pain leads to *guarding* (a defensive tensing of the muscle) and limited motion, which, in turn, leads to weakness, stiffness, and spasm—and more pain.
- Cancer often produces chronic pain, usually due to factors such as tumor growth that presses on nerves or other structures, stretching of viscera, obstruction of ducts, or metastasis to bones. The malignant tumor also may mechanically stimulate pain or the production of biochemicals that cause pain. Pain also may be associated with treatments such as chemotherapy and radiation therapy.
- Chronic postoperative pain is uncommon, but may occur following incisions in the chest wall, radical mastectomy, radical neck dissection, and surgical amputation.

PATHOPHYSIOLOGY LINKAGE Acute Pain and Associated Manifestations

MANIFESTATION	RELATED PATHOPHYSIOLOGY
Localized, sharp, burning pain	Nociceptors transmit pain stimulus along myelinated Aδ fibers to spinal cord, where it travels via the neospinothalamic tract to the thalamus. From the thalamus, the stimulus is distributed to somatosensory cortex (perception and interpretation), the limbic system (emotional responses to pain), and brain stem centers (autonomic nervous system responses).
Diffuse, dull, aching pain	Transmission of nociceptive stimuli along unmyelinated C fibers to the spinal cord, and from there to the thalamus via the paleospinothalamic tract. Stimuli are distributed from the thalamus to the somatosensory cortex, limbic system, and brain stem centers.
Increased heart rate, stroke volume, and blood pressure; pupil dilation	Activation of the sympathetic nervous system (SNS) with release of catecholamines, which stimulate receptors in the heart and blood vessels.
Nausea, vomiting	SNS activation causes decreased blood flow to the gut, with decreased gastric acid secretion and intestinal motility; pain, anxiety cause stimulation of the vomiting center in the medulla.
Muscle tension	Protective responses initiated by higher brain centers to reduce nociceptive stimuli.
Anxiety, fear	Emotional responses to pain stimuli generated by limbic system.

TABLE 9–2 Characteristics of Acute and Chronic Pain

CHARACTERISTIC	ACUTE PAIN	CHRONIC PAIN
Purpose	Signals actual or potential tissue damage	May serve no useful function
Onset and duration	Sudden; relieved by healing	Persists after acute problem is resolved
Cause	Actual or potential tissue damage	May not be readily identifiable May result from nerve damage or pain modulation mechanism imbalance
Associated symptoms	Sympathetic nervous system responses (increased pulse and respiratory rates, increased blood pressure, sweating, nausea) Muscle spasms Anxiety, fear	Depression common Insomnia Possible preoccupation with pain

Breakthrough Pain

Breakthrough pain is pain that exceeds baseline chronic or persistent pain. It is often described as a sudden flare that exceeds the analgesic effect of long-acting pain medications. Whether the pain is malignant or non-malignant in origin, treated or untreated, breakthrough pain is temporary and can be debilitating. The onset and intensity of breakthrough pain vary; its unpredictability and inconsistency are distressing to the patient and can make it difficult to manage.

Incident pain is a subtype of breakthrough pain. Incident or *episodic pain* is predictable, precipitated by an event or activity such as coughing, changing position, or being touched. Pain associated with a fractured bone is a good example of incident pain. When the patient remains still and the fracture is aligned and supported, little pain is experienced. Movement of the affected part, however, can precipitate sharp, intense pain.

Nociceptive Pain

Nociceptive pain is pain caused by stimulation of peripheral or visceral pain receptors. It generally is localized and responsive to treatment. Nociceptive pain may be either acute or chronic, resulting from disease processes (e.g., arthritis), tissue trauma, and medical treatment (e.g., surgery).

Neuropathic Pain

Neuropathic pain results from injury to the peripheral nerves that leads to abnormal impulse processing by the peripheral and central nervous systems. Although neuropathic pain may be acute (e.g., the pain associated with shingles [herpes zoster]), usually it is chronic, associated with conditions such as diabetic neuropathy or postherpetic neuralgia. Neuropathic pain is thought to result from hyperactivity of neurons in the spinal cord and thalamus. The hyperactive neurons generate *ectopic* (arising from an abnormal site) impulses, leading to spontaneous paresthesias, numbness, pain, and tenderness, despite peripheral nerve damage. The pain may be described as gnawing, electric shock-like, burning, shooting, or tingling. Pain may occur with a stimulus such as touch that normally does not produce pain (*allodynia*), or its intensity may be disproportionate to the stimulus (*hyperalgesia*) (Helms & Barone, 2008; McCance & Huether, 2010).

Central Pain

Central pain is caused by a lesion or damage in the brain or spinal cord. This damage leads to spontaneous generation of impulses that are perceived as pain. An infarction, tumor, trauma, or disorder such as multiple sclerosis or epilepsy may cause central pain. Central pain is constant, of moderate to severe intensity, and difficult to treat. The location of the pain depends on the area of the CNS affected. The pain may be described as burning, pressing, lacerating, or aching. "Pins and needles" sensations may be experienced along with the underlying pain. Affected areas may have decreased sensation (numbness). Thalamic pain, a type of central pain, may cause hyperesthesia (an abnormal sensitivity to touch, pain, or other sensory stimuli) on the side of the body opposite to the thalamic lesion.

Complex Regional Pain Syndromes

Complex regional pain syndromes (CRPS) cause extremity pain that is severe, diffuse, and burning. The pain is accompanied by vasomotor changes that affect skin color and temperature. Initially the affected extremity has typical inflammatory symptoms, with redness, warmth, and swelling. Later, it is cool, cyanotic, and edematous; skin and nail changes may be seen (McCance & Huether, 2010). The cause of CRPS is unclear; there may, in fact, be several causes, including damage to the central or peripheral nervous system, or a disrupted healing or immune process. In CRPS, pain receptors in the affected part of the body become sensitized to catecholamines, neurotransmitters associated with sympathetic nervous system activity.

Phantom Limb Pain

Phantom limb pain is a pain syndrome that occurs following amputation of a body part. The patient experiences pain in the missing body part that may be described as burning, cramping, or shooting. Phantom limb pain more frequently affects people who had pain in the amputated limb prior to its removal than those who did not. Several theories for phantom limb pain have been developed. These include regeneration of severed peripheral nerves and abnormal impulses generated by spinal cord neurons that no longer receive normal sensory input from the body (Porth & Matfin, 2009).

Adverse Effects of Pain

Acute pain has a defined purpose: to warn of injury to body tissues. Although often attributable to a defined disorder (such as arthritis, migraine, or cancer), chronic pain often serves no useful purpose, becoming instead part of the problem. Physiologic responses to pain extend beyond the muscle spasm and fight-or-flight response (increased blood pressure, heart rate, and cardiac output, decreased gastric and intestinal motility), and can have adverse effects on the patient's health. Pain interferes with sleep quantity and quality, leading to exhaustion and possible disorientation. Metabolism and myocardial oxygen demand are increased. Catabolism (breakdown of body tissues) increases, and healing is impaired. Immune function is suppressed, increasing the risk for infection. Research shows a clear link between chronic pain and depression.

Factors Affecting Responses to Pain

Responses to pain stimuli are as individualized as the person experiencing the stimulus. The previous discussion focused on types of pain and physiologic responses to pain stimuli. The individualized response to pain is shaped not only by physiologic responses, but by multiple and interacting factors, including age, gender, sociocultural influences, emotional state, past experiences with pain, the source and meaning of the pain, and knowledge base.

The *pain threshold* is the point at which a stimulus elicits a response. Although the pain threshold is relatively consistent, meaning that a given pain stimulus will elicit pain perception among most people, it can be affected by factors such as the presence of chronic pain (which tends to lower the threshold) or more intense pain at another site (which tends to raise the threshold).

Pain tolerance is the amount (duration, intensity) of pain a person can endure before outwardly responding to it (McCance & Huether, 2010). Pain tolerance varies significantly among individuals and within an individual over time. It is influenced by culture, expectations, emotions, and psychosocial factors. The ability to tolerate pain may be decreased by repeated episodes of pain, fatigue, anger, anxiety, and sleep deprivation. Medications, alcohol, hypnosis, warmth, distraction, and spiritual practices may increase pain tolerance.

Age

Age influences a person's perception and expression of pain. There is, however, no evidence that nociception is altered by age. When compared with younger adults, pain stimulus transmission relies more on C fibers in older adults than on Aδ fibers. As a result, pain stimulus transmission is slower, and pain more frequently may be described as burning, dull, or aching. Central processing often is slowed, resulting in a slower response time

to pain. Referred pain is less typical in older adults, and visceral pain may present as less severe than in younger adults. The older adult may report vague complaints of pain, or may present with manifestations such as delirium rather than subjective reports of pain (Helms & Barone, 2008; Tabloski, 2006).

Many older adults experience both acute and chronic pain related to disorders such as arthritis or peripheral neuropathy. While peripheral vascular disease or diabetes may lead to neuropathy and interfere with normal nerve impulse transmission, neuropathy can manifest as hyperesthesias as well as hypoesthesias. Both of these manifestations cause discomfort. Pain tolerance decreases with aging, perhaps related to the prevalence of chronic pain in this population. Studies of elderly nursing home residents found daily, persistent pain among them, with 40% of those who reported pain on the first assessment still in pain 60 to 180 days later (Teno, 2002).

Effective assessment and management of pain in the elderly can be challenging. Patients and healthcare professionals (including nurses) may believe that pain and discomfort are unavoidable aspects of aging. Individuals in this age group may fail to acknowledge pain, believing that pain is inevitable or fearing dependency if they alarm their loved ones. Patients and healthcare professionals may have misconceptions about the use of analgesics, including opioid medications, fearing adverse effects (such as respiratory depression) or **addiction**. Sensory impairments (e.g., impaired hearing) or cognitive impairments can interfere with the patient's ability to report pain and the healthcare professional's ability to assess pain. The Nursing Care of the Older Adult table lists some age-related changes and their effects on pain.

Gender

Clinical and animal studies show that women have a lower pain threshold and experience higher intensity of pain than men (Toomey, 2008; Wilson, 2006). It has long been held that sociocultural factors account for these recognized differences in the pain experience. Research has recently provided evidence of physiologic differences in pain responses and the analgesic effect of opioid medications. Positron emission tomography (PET) demonstrates greater activation of areas of the brain associated with emotions in women experiencing a painful stimulus than in men (Toomey, 2008). These physiologic responses appear to be genetically encoded, involving the sex

NURSING CARE OF THE OLDER ADULT — **Age-Related Changes in Pain Perception and Response**

AGE-RELATED FACTOR	EFFECTS
Decreased Aδ fiber transmission, greater reliance on C fiber transmission	Pain perceived as dull, aching, more diffuse rather than sharp, localized
Slowed central processing	Slower motor or avoidance responses
Reduced norepinephrine levels	Reduced sympathetic nervous system responses to pain (pulse, blood pressure, papillary dilation)
Decreased referred pain	May not exhibit "classic" manifestations of such disorders as myocardial infarction, acute abdomen
Reduced neurotransmitter levels	Increased risk of depression related to chronic pain

hormones and the activity of opioid receptors in the brain. Fluctuating estrogen levels associated with the menstrual cycle affect perceived pain intensity. The circuits that mediate the pain response differ in men and women, the opioid pain modulatory system in particular. Because of these differences, women and men may respond differently to opioid analgesics such as morphine (Wilson, 2006).

Sociocultural Influences

Each person's response to pain is strongly influenced by the family, community, and culture. Sociocultural influences affect pain behavior, dictating appropriate and inappropriate expressions of pain. In general, cultural responses to pain fall into two categories: stoic and emotive (Andrews & Boyle, 2008). For example, if the patient's culture teaches that people should tolerate pain stoically, the patient may appear withdrawn and refuse (or not request) pain medication. If the cultural norm encourages open and intense emotional expression, the patient may cry freely and appear comfortable requesting pain medication.

Cultural standards also teach an individual how much pain to tolerate, what types of pain to report, to whom to report the pain, and what kind of treatment to seek. For example, patients of northern European ancestry may value "being a good patient," which may cause them to avoid "complaining" about their pain, whereas patients of Jewish ancestry may value seeking information about their pain, which may cause them to discuss their pain often and in detail. Note, however, that behaviors vary greatly within a culture and from generation to generation. The nurse should approach each patient as an individual, observing the patient carefully, taking the time to ask questions, and avoiding assumptions.

The nurse also has a set of sociocultural values and beliefs about pain. If these values and beliefs differ from those of the patient, the assessment and management of pain may be based on the values of the nurse rather than on the needs of the patient. The nurse must be familiar with ethnic and cultural diversity in pain expression and management and respect cultural differences. It is particularly important to remember that pain behaviors are not an objective indicator of the amount of pain present for any individual. Finally, most experts agree that cultural differences in the expression of, response to, and interpretation of the meaning of pain need further research.

Psychological Influences

The intensity of perceived pain has been shown to be affected by psychological variables such as attention, expectation, and suggestion. The sensation of pain may be blocked by intense concentration (during sports activities, for example) or may be increased by anxiety or fear. Pain often is increased when it occurs in conjunction with other illnesses or physical discomforts such as nausea or vomiting. The presence or absence of support people or caregivers that genuinely care about pain management also may alter emotional status and the perception of pain. The placebo effect, a positive patient response to an inactive substance, has been demonstrated through both observational studies and brain MRI studies (Fauci et al., 2008).

Anxiety may increase the perception of pain, and pain in turn may cause anxiety. In addition, the muscle tension common with anxiety can create its own source of pain. This association explains why nonpharmacologic interventions such as relaxation or guided imagery are helpful in relieving or decreasing pain.

Fatigue, lack of sleep, and depression also are related to pain experiences. Pain interferes with a person's ability to fall asleep and stay asleep and thus induces fatigue. In turn, fatigue can lower pain tolerance. Depression is clearly linked to pain: Serotonin, a neurotransmitter, is involved in the modulation of pain in the CNS. In clinically depressed people, serotonin is decreased, leading to an increase in pain sensations. The reverse is also true: In the presence of pain, depression is common.

The meaning associated with the pain influences the experience of pain. For example, the pain of labor to deliver a baby is experienced differently from the pain following removal of a major organ for cancer. Because pain is the major signal for health problems, it is strongly linked to all associated meanings of health problems, such as disability, loss of role, and death. A lack of understanding of the source, outcome, and meaning of the pain can contribute negatively to the pain experience. For this reason, it is important to explain to patients the etiology and prognosis for the pain assessed.

If the patient perceives the pain as deserved (e.g., "just punishment for sins"), the patient may actually feel relief that the "punishment" has commenced. If the patient believes that the pain will relieve him or her from an unrewarding job, dangerous military service, or even stressful social obligations, there may similarly be a feeling of relief. In contrast, pain that is perceived as meaningless—for example, chronic low back pain or the unrelieved pain of arthritis—can cause anxiety and depression.

Interdisciplinary Care

Effective pain relief results from collaboration among patient and all members of the healthcare team. Acute pain management may be straightforward, accomplished though short-term analgesia and management of the underlying problem. Chronic pain, on the other hand, frequently requires a multidisciplinary approach. Pain clinics are centers staffed by a team of healthcare professionals who use traditional pharmacologic agents as well as herbs, vitamins, and other dietary supplements; nutritional counseling; psychotherapy; biofeedback; hypnosis; acupuncture; massage; and other treatments. Hospices for dying patients also provide a multifaceted approach to pain management. Chapter 5 provides information about pain management during end-of-life care.

Medications

Medication is the most common approach to pain management. Management of acute pain often is relatively straightforward, relying on **analgesic** (pain-relieving) drugs such as acetaminophen, nonsteroidal anti-inflammatory drugs (NSAIDs), and opioid analgesics. Chronic pain presents additional challenges; a broader range of drug classes may be employed, including antidepressant medications, anticonvulsants, and chronic opioid medication use.

In addition to administering the prescribed medications, the nurse may act interdependently in selecting the appropriate dosage and timing. The nurse is also responsible for assessing the side effects of the medications, evaluating the medication's effectiveness, and providing patient teaching. The nurse's role in pain relief is patient advocate as well as direct caregiver.

The World Health Organization (WHO) "ladder of analgesia" effectively guides the use of medications for patients with malignant pain (WHO, 2009) (Figure 9–5 ■). Aspirin and NSAIDs are initially used, followed by the addition of mild opioid analgesics and then strong opioids until pain is relieved, reflecting the interactive nature of these two types of analgesics. Adjuvant drugs are used to manage fear and anxiety. This approach also emphasizes administering analgesics by the clock, rather than on-demand, to maintain comfort.

ASPIRIN, ACETAMINOPHEN, AND NSAIDS Nonopioid analgesics such as acetaminophen (Tylenol), aspirin and NSAIDs produce analgesia and reduce fever. They are used to treat mild to moderate pain, and are particularly effective for treating headache and musculoskeletal pain.

Acetaminophen appears to act on the CNS to relieve pain. Its exact mechanism of action is unknown, but it is believed to raise the pain threshold by acting on receptors in pain pathways. Acetaminophen is considered to be a very safe drug, and often is combined with opioid analgesics to allow effective pain relief with a lower opioid dose (e.g., Percocet, Tylenol #3, Vicodin). It is important to remember, however, that acetaminophen is toxic to the liver. Hepatotoxicity is a particular risk in patients who are malnourished or who have a history of alcohol abuse (DiPiro et al., 2008). It also is a consideration when given in combination with an opioid analgesic. As the patient develops tolerance to the opioid, increasing doses may be required to achieve effective analgesia, resulting in acetaminophen doses that increase the risk for hepatotoxicity.

Aspirin and NSAIDs act on peripheral nerve endings and minimize pain by interfering with two enzymes necessary for prostaglandin synthesis, cyclooxygenase type 1 (COX-1) and cyclooxygenase type 2 (COX-2). Examples include ibuprofen, indomethacin (Indocin), and ketorolac (Toradol). The NSAIDs have anti-inflammatory, analgesic, and antipyretic actions. NSAIDs are the treatment of choice for mild to moderate pain and continue to be effective when combined with narcotics for moderate to severe pain. NSAIDs are increasingly used in a *multimodal* approach to analgesic therapy; that is, in combination with opioid and adjunctive pain relief measures.

As a class, aspirin and NSAIDs are associated with gastric irritation. As cyclooxygenase (COX) inhibitors, they interfere with prostaglandin production. While this accounts for their anti-inflammatory effects, prostaglandins are necessary to maintain the gastric mucosal barrier. The gastric mucosal barrier (composed of mucus and bicarbonate) protects gastric mucosa from the irritating effects of ingested substances. NSAIDS, therefore, are not only irritating to gastric mucosa, they interfere with its protection as well. The risk for resultant gastrointestinal bleeding is greatest with aspirin, because it also interferes with platelets and blood clotting (Lehne, 2007).

NSAIDs also increase blood pressure in many patients, and, with long-term use, may be toxic to the kidneys. With the exception of aspirin, NSAIDs have been shown to have an associated increased cardiovascular risk (DiPiro, 2008). They are not recommended for use in people with kidney or liver disease, bleeding disorders, peptic ulcer disease, pregnancy, or a history of hypersensitivity to aspirin or other NSAIDs. Nursing implications for NSAIDs are found in the Medication Administration box on page 169. For more information about doses and precautions for specific NSAIDs, see Table 40–5 on page 1368.

OPIOID ANALGESICS *Opioid* (also called *narcotic*) analgesics are derivatives of the opium plant. These drugs (and their synthetic forms) are the most potent pain relieving drugs available, and are the treatment of choice for acute moderate-to-severe pain. Examples are morphine, codeine, and fentanyl (Duragesic, Actiq). Opioid analgesics produce analgesia by binding to opioid receptors both within and outside the CNS. They differ from one another in potency, speed of onset, duration of action, and preferred route of administration. Opioid *agonists* such as morphine produce their effect by stimulating the receptor they bind with. Drugs with a mixed *agonist-antagonist* effect block the activity of some receptors (mu receptors), while activating others (kappa receptors). This mixed agonist-antagonist activity can actually intensify pain responses in some patients. Buprenorphine (Buprenex), butorphanol (Stadol), nalbuphine (Nubain), and pentazocine (Talwin) are examples of opioids with mixed agonist-antagonist effects.

A summary of **equianalgesic** or approximate equivalent doses of selected opioid analgesics used to treat moderate to severe pain, their peak effect and duration, and nursing implications is provided in Table 9–3.

Opioid analgesics tend to have similar unintended effects. They are CNS and respiratory depressants. They commonly produce sedation, drowsiness, and dizziness. All should be

Freedom from cancer pain

Opioid for moderate to severe pain
± Nonopioid analgesic
± Adjuvant therapy

Pain persisting or increasing

Opioid for mild to moderate pain
+ Nonopioid analgesic
± Adjuvant therapy

Pain persisting or increasing

Nonopioid analgesic
± Adjuvant therapy

Pain

Figure 9–5 ■ The WHO analgesic ladder illustrates the process for selection of analgesic medications for pain management.

Source: The WHO Analgesic Ladder from Cancer Pain Relief and Palliative Care, Technical Report Series, No. 804, The World Health Organization, Geneva, Switzerland. Reprinted by permission.

MEDICATION ADMINISTRATION Nonsteroidal Anti-Inflammatory Drugs

EXAMPLES OF NSAIDS ARE THE FOLLOWING:

aspirin (acetylsalicylic acid)

celecoxib (Celebrex)

diflunisal (Dolobid)

fenoprofen calcium (Nalfon)

ibuprofen (Advil, Motrin)

indomethacin (Indocin)

ketoprofen (Actron, Orudis)

ketorolac tromethamine (Toradol)

nabumetone (Relafen)

naproxen (Aleve, Naprosyn)

piroxicam (Feldene)

sulindac (Clinoril)

tolmetin (Tolectin)

The NSAIDs have anti-inflammatory, analgesic, and antipyretic effects. It is believed that they inhibit the enzyme COX, thereby decreasing synthesis of prostaglandins. These drugs provide analgesic effects by reducing inflammation and by perhaps blocking the generation of noxious impulses.

Nursing Responsibilities

- Do not administer aspirin with other NSAIDs.
- Assess and document if the patient is taking a hypoglycemic agent or insulin; the NSAIDs may increase the hypoglycemic effect.
- Administer with meals, milk, or a full glass of water to decrease gastric irritation.
- Assess patients who are also taking anticoagulants for bleeding; the NSAIDs increase this risk.

Health Education for the Patient and Family

- Drugs may cause gastrointestinal bleeding (report nausea, vomiting of blood, dark stools), visual disturbances (report blurred or diminished vision), increased blood pressure, hearing problems, dizziness, skin rash, and kidney problems (report weight gain or edema).
- Take medications with meals to decrease gastric irritation.
- Avoid drinking alcohol or taking any over-the-counter drug unless approved by the healthcare provider.
- The desired effects may not appear for 3–5 days, and the full effects may not appear for 2–4 weeks.
- Maintain regular healthcare appointments.

avoided or used with caution in patients with chronic obstructive lung disease (COPD) or who are experiencing an acute asthma attack because they can suppress respirations. Nausea and vomiting are common adverse effects, as is constipation. All opioid analgesics have the potential to cause physical and psychologic dependence, particularly when taken at high doses for an extended time (Adams, Holland, & Bostwick, 2008).

A common myth among healthcare professionals is that using opioids for pain treatment poses a real threat of addiction.

Actually, when the medications are used as recommended, there is little to no risk of addiction. Rather, if pain is not adequately treated, the patient may seek more and more analgesic relief, thus increasing the risk of an adversarial relationship with the provider and a weakening of the trust relationship between patient and provider (Trame, 2002) (Box 9–1).

Opioid analgesics commonly are used to treat chronic malignant pain (see Figure 9–5). Because of their potency and efficacy, they also may be used to treat chronic nonmalignant

BOX 9–1 Pain Management, Addiction, and Regulation

The goals of pain control are to minimize discomfort and promote normal functioning. While these goals often can be achieved through use of nonpharmacologic strategies and nonnarcotic analgesics, opioid medications currently provide the only effective option for pain associated with acute trauma, surgery, cancer, and some chronic conditions.

Crude opium has been available for thousands of years. Abuse of opium and its derivatives (e.g., heroin, morphine) increased dramatically with development of the hypodermic syringe. International efforts to control narcotic trafficking and abuse while ensuring availability for medical and scientific purposes began in the early twentieth century. And yet today, while much of the world's population still lacks access to these effective and inexpensive analgesics, illicit narcotic trafficking accounts for $400–$500 billion per year; nearly 10% of world trade (Taylor, 2007).

The WHO estimates than 80% of people with severe pain are inadequately treated (Taylor, 2007). Despite significant data showing very little *addiction* as the result of treating pain with adequate analgesia, prescribers still tend to undertreat chronic nonmalignant pain (American Pain Society, 2009). Cook et al. (2004) found that physicians prescribe significantly more nonopioid analgesics for a patient addicted to heroin than for a non-addicted patient with identical injuries. The authors observe that analgesics may be rationed to addicted persons in an effort to wean them from their addiction. Addiction is a neurophysiologic disease, separate and distinct from *physical dependence* and tolerance. See the following list for definitions of relevant terms.

The development of highly effective oral opioid analgesics such as oxycodone (OxyContin) and hydrocodone (Vicodin) has resulted in increased illegal trafficking of legally manufactured opioids. This has led to calls for legislation to limit the use and availability of these drugs, an option that concerns palliative care specialists.

Opioid analgesics are among the most effective, highly regulated, and significantly abused drugs available today. Clearly, there are no simple answers to the problems associated with drug trafficking, abuse, and addiction.

- *Addiction:* A primary, chronic neurobiologic disease characterized by compulsive use of a substance despite negative consequences, such as health threats or legal problems.
- *Drug abuse:* The use of any chemical substance for other than a medical purpose.
- *Physical drug dependence:* A biologic need for a substance. If the substance is not supplied, physical withdrawal symptoms occur.
- *Psychologic drug dependence:* A psychologic need for a substance. If the substance is not supplied, psychologic withdrawal symptoms occur.
- *Drug tolerance:* Physical adaptation to the drug resulting in its diminished effects over time.
- *Equianalgesic:* Having the same pain-killing effect when administered to the same individual. Drug dosages are equianalgesic if they have the same effect as morphine sulfate 10 mg administered parenterally.
- *Pseudoaddiction:* Behavior involving drug seeking; a result of receiving inadequate pain relief.

TABLE 9–3 Equianalgesic Drug Chart

ANALGESIC	DOSAGE(MG)	PEAK(MIN)	DURATION(H)	NURSING CONSIDERATIONS
Morphine sulfate	10 SC, IV	30–60 min	4–5 h	PO dose is 3–6 times the IM dose. A lower dose may be appropriate for older patients with chronic pain.
	30–60 PO	60–120 min	4–5 h	Smaller doses (e.g., 2 to 5 mg) may be administered more frequently when using IV route.
Codeine	130 IM, SC	30–60 min	4 h	PO dose is about 1.5 times the parenteral dose. IM absorption unpredictable.
	200 PO	60–120 min	4 h	Analgesic potency about one-sixth that of morphine.
				Often given in combination with aspirin or acetaminophen for mild to moderate pain.
				Also used for its antitussive (cough suppressant) effect.
Fentanyl (Duragesic, Sublimaze)	0.1(100 mcg)/h IV or transdermal	1 min	5–7 min IV	100 mcg/hr parenteral or transdermal is equivalent to 4 mg/hr of parenteral morphine.
				Rapid onset and short half-life; tissue storage can prolong half-life and effect with longer-term use.
				Transdermal fentanyl not recommended for acute pain management.
				Available by oral transmucosal route (lozenge on a stick).
Hydromorphone HCl (Dilaudid)	1.5 IM, SC, IV	15–30 min	4 h	PO dose is 5 times IM dose. Shorter acting than morphine.
	7.5 PO	30 min	4 h	
Levorphanol (Levo-Dromoran)	2 IM, SC, IV	60 min	4–5 h	Longer acting than morphine when given in repeated, regular doses. Accumulates, so analgesic effect may increase over time.
	4 PO	90–120 min	4–5 h	
Meperidine (Demerol)	75 IM, SC, IV	30–50 min	2–4 h	Not recommended as first-line opioid for acute or chronic pain. Metabolized to normeperidine, which is toxic to the CNS.
	300 PO	60–90 min	2–4 h	
				Not recommended for older adults, patients with impaired kidney function, or for administration by continuous IV infusion.
Methadone HCl (Dolophine)	10 IM, SC, IV	60–120 min	4–6 h	Initial PO dose is twice IM dose. Accumulates, so analgesic effect may increase over time.
	20 PO	90–120 min	4–6 h	Initial doses lower in opioid-tolerant patients.
				Also used for heroin detoxification and temporary maintenance.
Oxycodone (Percocet, OxyContin)	30 PO (NA parenteral)	60 min	3–6 h	Used in combination with nonopioid analgesic (Percocet, Tylox) for moderate pain.
				Available as a single-entity product in immediate- or controlled-release forms (OxyContin) for severe pain. Has faster onset and higher peak effect than most PO narcotics, equivalent to oral morphine.
Oxymorphone (Numorphan)	1–1.5 IM, SC, IV	30–60 min	3–6 h	Also available as rectal suppository (10 mg equianalgesic).
	10 PO or PR	30–60 min	4–6 h	Used for moderate to severe pain.
Tramadol (Ultram, Zydol)	100 PO	120–180 min	3–6 h	Used for moderate to moderately severe pain. Causes less respiratory depression than morphine.

Note: Morphine sulfate 10 mg IM is the analgesic dose to which all other parenteral and PO doses in this table are considered equianalgesic.

pain. Oral preparations of a fixed combination of an opioid and acetaminophen are used with caution. Tolerance can lead to higher required doses of the opioid, increasing the risk for hepatoxicity due to the increasing dose of acetaminophen. Nursing implications for opioid analgesics are found in the Medication Administration box on page 171.

Certain opioid analgesics, while still available, are not recommended for use because of toxic effects or their potential for abuse. As previously noted, the metabolite of meperidine (Demerol) is toxic to the CNS. While a single dose of meperidine may be used to relieve acute pain (e.g., migraine), it is not recommended for continued use (DiPiro, 2008). Propoxyphene (Darvon, Darvocet, Balacet), a synthetic opioid analgesic for mild to moderate pain has a high potential for abuse, with significant risk for psychologic dependence. The risk of fatal overdose is significant with propoxyphene (FDA, 2009), and it

MEDICATION ADMINISTRATION Opioid Analgesics

EXAMPLES OF OPIOID ANALGESICS ARE THE FOLLOWING:

buprenorphine HCl (Buprenex)

codeine

fentanyl (Duragesic)

hydrocodone (Hycodan, Vicodin)

hydromorphone HCl (Dilaudid)

levorphanol (Levo-Dromoran)

morphine sulfate

nalbuphine HCl (Nubain)

oxycodone (OxyContin)

oxymorphone HCl (Numorphan)

pentazocine (Talwin)

Opioid analgesics are used to treat severe pain. The drugs in this category include morphine, codeine, opium derivatives, and synthetic substances with activity similar to natural opioids. Morphine and codeine are pure chemical substances isolated from opium. These drugs decrease the awareness of the sensation of pain by binding to opiate receptors in the brain and spinal cord. It is also believed that they diminish the transmission of pain impulses by altering cell membrane permeability to sodium and by affecting the release of neurotransmitters for efferent nerves sensitive to noxious stimuli. Opioid analgesics affect the central nervous system, causing analgesia, euphoria, drowsiness, mental clouding, and lethargy. They also have various other effects: Depending on the drug used, they can depress respirations, stimulate the vomiting center, suppress the cough reflex, induce peripheral vasodilatation (resulting in hypotension), constrict the pupils, and decrease intestinal peristalsis (DiPiro, 2008). Opioid analgesics have the potential to cause tolerance and psychologic and physical dependence.

Nursing Responsibilities

- Opioids are regulated by federal law; the nurse must record the date, time, patient name, type and amount of the drug used, and sign the entry in a narcotic inventory sheet. If the drug must be wasted after it is signed out, the act must be witnessed and the narcotic sheet signed by the nurse and the witness. Computerized narcotic documentation methods are also available.
- Keep an opioid antagonist, such as naloxone, immediately available to treat respiratory depression.
- Assess allergies or adverse effects from opioids previously experienced by the patient.

- Assess for respiratory disorders (e.g., asthma or COPD), neuromuscular disorders (e.g. multiple sclerosis), and other conditions that might increase the risk associated with respiratory depression.
- Assess the characteristics of the pain and the effectiveness of drugs that have been previously used to treat the pain.
- Take and record baseline vital signs before administering the drug.
- Administer the drugs, following established guidelines.
- Monitor vital signs and respiratory status, level of consciousness, papillary response, nausea, bowel function, urinary function, and effectiveness of pain management at regular intervals and as indicated.
- Provide for patient safety.
- Report adverse effects such as continued nausea, vomiting, or itching.
- Employ protocols or prn orders as needed to promote bowel function and prevent constipation.
- Meperidine (Demerol) is associated with CNS toxicity and thus involves significant patient risk (DiPiro, 2008). Monitor any patient who is receiving more than one dose for nervousness, restlessness, tremors, twitching, shakiness, myoclonic jerks, diaphoresis, changes in level of awareness, agitation, disorientation, confusion, delirium, hallucinations, violent shivering, and/or seizures. Toxicity can occur with any route of administration or any dosing regimen. The risk is increased in patients with decreased renal function (including normal changes with aging). Report these manifestations to the physician. Oral administration is not recommended.
- Teach noninvasive methods of pain management for use in conjunction with opioid analgesics.

Health Education for the Patient and Family

- The use of opioid analgesics to treat severe pain is unlikely to cause addiction (American Pain Society, 2009).
- Do not drink alcohol while taking these drugs.
- Do not take over-the-counter medications unless approved by the healthcare provider.
- Increase intake of fluids and fiber in the diet to prevent constipation. Contact your provider if additional measures (such as laxatives) are needed to manage constipation.
- The drugs often cause dizziness, drowsiness, and impaired thinking; use caution when driving or making decisions.
- Report adverse effects or decreasing effectiveness to the physician.

should not be taken concurrently with any other CNS depressant such as alcohol. Furthermore, clinical studies have shown propoxyphene to be no more effective as an analgesic than acetaminophen.

ANTIDEPRESSANTS Antidepressants, particularly those within the tricyclic and related chemical groups, are useful for treating chronic pain. Tricyclic antidepressants act on the production and retention of serotonin in the CNS, thus inhibiting pain sensation. The dose to provide analgesia is lower than that required to treat depression. These drugs also potentiate the effects of opioid analgesics, and may be used to help manage severe persistent or malignant pain. They also promote normal sleeping patterns, further alleviating the suffering of the patient in pain. They are particularly useful in treating neuropathic pain. Tricyclic antidepressants are not without adverse

effects, however. They may cause orthostatic hypotension, drowsiness, urinary retention, constipation, and impaired memory. These effects can limit their usefulness in older adults in particular. Antidepressants from other classes such as serotonin norepinephrine reuptake inhibitors (venlafaxine [Effexor], duloxetine [Cymbalta]) appear to have an analgesic effect similar to that of tricyclic antidepressants with fewer adverse effects (Fauci et al., 2008).

ANTICONVULSANTS Similar to antidepressants, some seizure medications such as gabapentin (Neurontin), pregabalin (Lyrica), and carbamazepine (Tegretol) are useful with neuropathic pain, including shingles (herpes zoster), migraine headaches, and diabetic neuropathy. These drugs reduce pain and sleep disruption. Drugs that are primarily used to treat epilepsy (seizures) have been used to treat nerve pain conditions and migraine headache for several decades. Many anticonvulsant drugs have been shown in clinical studies to be effective in managing chronic pain (DiPiro, 2008).

LOCAL ANESTHETICS Drugs such as benzocaine and lidocaine are part of a large group of substances that block the initiation and transmission of nerve impulses in a local area, thus blocking pain as well. Local anesthetics can be delivered by a variety of methods, including via transdermal patch to treat focal neuropathic pain (DiPiro, 2008). They are sometimes used to enable a patient to begin moving and using a painful area to diminish long-term pain.

Local anesthetics can be delivered directly to the sheath of a nerve through a peripheral nerve catheter. During surgery, a soaker type catheter can be inserted along a surgical incision to deliver local relief; this method may decrease the need for opioids and allow the patient to resume activity sooner (D'Arcy, 2005).

Analgesic Administration

The ideal drug, route of administration, and dosing schedule to provide optimal pain relief varies, depending on such factors as the type of pain, its intensity and duration, and the individual patient. Each drug has a unique absorption and duration of action. The nurse must understand that no drug will have a totally predictable effect, because each person absorbs, metabolizes, and excretes medications at different dosage levels. The only way to obtain reliable data about the effectiveness of the medication for the individual is to assess how that patient responds. Therefore, the best choice is to individualize the drug, route, and schedule.

Giving analgesics before the pain occurs or increases prevents some of the untoward effects of pain. This holds true for both acute and chronic pain: Poorly managed acute pain is one of the leading causes of persistent pain syndrome. Additional benefits of a preventive approach to pain can be summarized as follows:

- The patient may spend less time in pain. Pain has been shown to have a negative effect on healing; poorly relieved pain is associated with longer hospital stays.
- Inadequate relief of acute pain has been shown to be a significant contributing factor to chronic pain (Barclay, Lee, & Martin, 2008).
- Frequent analgesic administration may allow for smaller doses and less analgesic administration.
- Smaller doses will in turn mean fewer side effects.
- The patient's fear and anxiety about the return of pain will decrease.
- Pain relief allows the patient to be more physically active and avoid complications of immobility.

Analgesics may be given either around-the-clock (ATC) or as necessary (PRN, meaning *pro re nata*, Latin for "as circumstances may require"). ATC administration is recommended for the first 48 hours for acute pain related to surgery or traumatic injury. It also is appropriate for pain that has a predictable intensity and pattern. PRN administration is appropriate for pain that is not predictable or constant. PRN medication should be given as soon as the pain begins. Breakthrough pain occurs to patients receiving long-acting analgesics for chronic pain. It

is a transitory experience of moderate to severe pain often precipitated by coughing or movement but that may occur spontaneously. Breakthrough pain is managed using short-acting opioid analgesics in addition to ATC medications.

Maintaining effective pain relief while minimizing adverse effects of the medication can be challenging. Within a prescribed range, the nurse can choose the correct dose according to the patient's response. It is also the role of the nurse to notify the physician if the prescribed dosage does not meet the patient's needs or causes excessive drowsiness, unsteadiness, or significant adverse effects.

Routes of Administration

The route of administration significantly affects how much of the medication is needed to relieve pain. For example, because of differences in absorption and distribution, oral doses of some opioids must be up to five times greater than parenteral doses to achieve the same degree of pain relief. In addition, the potency of opioid analgesics vary. Consulting an equianalgesic chart when converting from one route of administration to another or from one drug to another helps ensure an equivalent effect for the patient. The analgesic effect of 10 mg of parenteral morphine is used as the base to which other opioids and routes of administration are compared. Table 9–3 is an example of an equianalgesic chart.

ORAL The simplest route for both patient and nurse is the oral (PO) route. Unless contraindicated, the oral route is preferred for most patients. Special nursing care is still required, because some medications must be given with food, some are irritating to the gastrointestinal system, and some patients have trouble swallowing pills. Liquid and timed-release forms are available for special applications.

Some analgesics, such as fentanyl, are available in alternative forms, including a buccal tablet, a lozenge, or a lollipop. The buccal route provides a rapid onset of action, as the medication is absorbed directly into the circulation, bypassing the gastrointestinal tract and first-pass liver metabolism. These delivery systems are particularly helpful for managing breakthrough pain. Special precautions must be taken in storing the lozenge and lollipop, as these may be mistaken for candy by children and pets (Cranwell-Bruce, 2007).

RECTAL The rectal route is helpful for patients who are unable to swallow or who are experiencing nausea and vomiting. Acetaminophen, aspirin, and some NSAIDs and opioid analgesics are available in this form. The rectal route is effective and simple, but the patient and family may not accept it. To be effective, any rectal medication must be placed above the rectal sphincter.

TRANSDERMAL The transdermal, or "patch," form of medication is increasingly being used because it is simple, painless, and delivers a continuous level of medication (Figure 9–6 ■). Transdermal medications are easy to store and apply. Reapplication every 72 hours enhances compliance. Additional short-acting medication may be needed for breakthrough pain. As with any route of administration, overdosage can occur. It is important to start with a low dose and **titrate** (which means to increase or decrease dose in small increments) to the effective

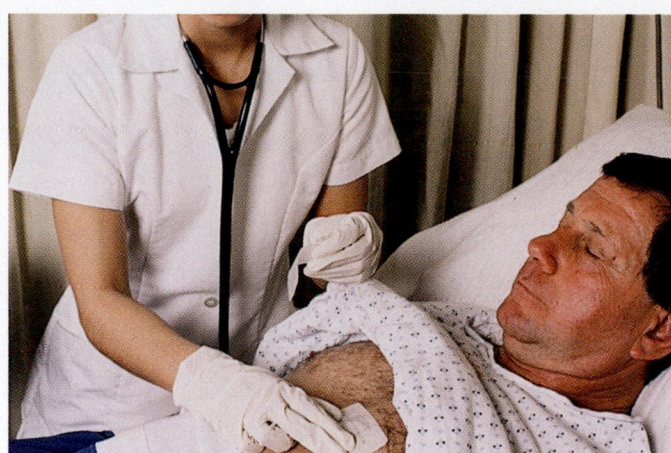

Figure 9–6 ■ The transdermal patch administers medication in predictable doses.

Figure 9–7 ■ PCA units allow the patient to self-manage acute pain. The units may be portable or mounted on intravenous poles.

level. Medication administered transdermally is in a lipid-soluble form, and may be stored in fat cells longer than expected. Monitor level of sedation and respiratory effort.

A transdermal patch is applied to a clean, dry area on the upper torso. If hair is present, it should be clipped before applying the patch. Apply the patch immediately after opening the package, ensuring complete contact with the skin, especially around the edges. The patch is effective for about 72 hours. When replaced, the new patch should be applied on a different site. When transdermal therapy is initiated, approximately 12–24 hours is necessary until therapeutic level is absorbed; similarly, when discontinuing, expect a gradual decline in level because of medication reservoir in the skin. Absorption is enhanced by fever or inflammation of the skin, exercise, and use of electric blankets or heating pads.

PARENTERAL   Once the most popular route for pain medication administration, the intramuscular (IM) route is no longer preferred. Its disadvantages include uneven absorption from the muscle, discomfort on administration, and time consumed to prepare and administer the medication. Subcutaneous administration may be used, primarily when continuous analgesic administration via a parenteral route is required.

INTRAVENOUS   The intravenous (IV) route provides the most rapid onset of effect, usually ranging from 1 to 15 minutes. Medication can be given by drip, bolus, or patient-controlled analgesia (PCA). PCA uses a pump with a control mechanism that allows the patient to self-manage pain (Figure 9–7 ■).The advantages of PCA are dose precision, timeliness, and convenience. The patient does not have to wait for a nurse to assess the need for pain medication, then procure and deliver the analgesia. Respiratory depression and sedation is minimized when plasma levels of opioids are steady. PCA, especially with basal dosing (continuous infusion of a very small dose), facilitates frequent small dosing. Several drugs can be administered by this route. The disadvantages are the nursing care needed for any intravenous line, the potential for infection, and the cost of disposable supplies. In addition, the risk for serious medication error requiring interventions in response has been shown to be greater with PCA than when other methods of analgesic delivery are used. Adverse events associated with PCA errors include

depressed respirations, inadequate pain relief, and even patient death (Sheehan, 2008). This increased risk is attributed to the complexity of the systems involved when PCA is used to provide analgesia. The PCA method of administration requires close attention by the physician, pharmacist, and nurse, as well as careful patient teaching and monitoring.

INTRASPINAL   The intraspinal (intrathecal or epidural) route is invasive and requires more extensive nursing care but may provide better analgesia and postoperative recovery than intravenous delivery for some patients. When a combination of local anesthetics and opioids are infused by the epidural route, many patients experience better pain relief, earlier bowel recovery, and earlier mobility. The risk for respiratory depression and failure is lower with epidural analgesia than with administration by other parenteral routes. Other complications can occur, however, including hypotension, development of an epidural hematoma or abscess, and neurologic damage. Some patients achieve little or no pain relief with epidural analgesia, another potential complication (Gendall, Kennedy, Watson, & Frizell, 2007). See page 174 for nursing implications for patients receiving epidural analgesia.

NERVE BLOCKS   In a nerve block, a local anesthetic, sometimes in combination with steroidal anti-inflammatory drugs, is injected by a physician or nurse anesthetist into or near a nerve, usually in an area between the nociceptor and the dorsal root. The procedure may be performed to determine the precise location of the source of the pain: Pain relief indicates that the injection site is the site of the source of the pain.

Temporary (local) nerve blocks may give the patient enough relief to (1) develop a more hopeful attitude that pain relief is possible, (2) allow local procedures to be performed without causing discomfort, or (3) exercise and move the affected part. A temporary nerve block may be particularly useful for such painful conditions as fractured ribs, allowing the patient to deep breathe, cough, and move with more ease during healing. Nerve blocks may also be performed to predict the results of neurosurgery. For long-term pain relief, a permanent neurolytic agent is used. Neurolytic blocks usually are reserved for terminally ill patients because of the risks of weakness, paralysis, and bowel and bladder dysfunction.

NURSING CARE OF THE PATIENT
Receiving Intraspinal Analgesia

Intraspinal analgesia is used to manage chronic intractable malignant pain and postoperative pain, particularly after orthopedic and abdominal surgeries. The intraspinal route may be either intrathecal (into the subarachnoid space) or epidural (into the epidural space). Infusion of an opioid into these spaces provides for a direct effect on the opiate receptors in the dorsal horn of the spinal cord. The opioid analgesic is also absorbed systemically, affecting pain responses in the brain. This method can provide complete pain relief but has some potentially dangerous adverse effects.

PROCEDURE
The physician places a catheter into the epidural space. The catheter is connected to infusion tubing and an infusion pump, and the prescribed medication is administered. A portable or implantable pump may be used for longer term opioid analgesic administration.

NURSING CARE
- Monitor vital signs every 15 minutes for the first 2–3 hours and every hour for the first 24 hours; the patient is at risk for respiratory depression and hypotension. These adverse responses may not develop immediately, becoming evident only after several hours.

SAFETY ALERT
Ensure that naloxone, an opioid antagonist, is immediately available to reverse respiratory depression if necessary.
- Monitor the effectiveness of the pain management. Administer supplemental analgesics as ordered, and notify the physician if analgesia is inadequate (patient rates pain at 4 or higher on a scale of 0 to 10).
- Monitor intake and output. Intraspinal narcotics may block the micturition reflex, causing urinary retention and necessitating intermittent catheterization or placement of an indwelling urinary catheter.
- Use sterile technique to care for the intraspinal catheter.

Surgery

As a pain-relief measure, surgery usually is considered only after all other methods have failed. Surgical intervention typically is reserved for patients experiencing nerve pain, for example, the pain of trigeminal neuralgia, complex regional pain syndrome, or pain associated with spinal nerve or spinal cord injury. Patients need thorough knowledge of the implications of the use of surgery for pain relief. For example, motor function loss is an unwelcome side effect of some surgeries. Surgical procedures used to relieve pain are shown in Figure 9–8 ■. Some surgical procedures can be accomplished through minimally invasive techniques (e.g., percutaneously); others require an open surgical procedure. Surgical approaches to pain relief may include the following:

CORDOTOMY   A *cordotomy* is an incision into the anterolateral tracts of the spinal cord to interrupt the transmission of pain. Because it is difficult to isolate the nerves responsible for upper body pain, this surgery is most often performed for pain in the abdominal region and legs, including severe pain from terminal cancer. A percutaneous cordotomy produces lesions of the anterolateral surface of the spinal cord by means of a radio frequency current.

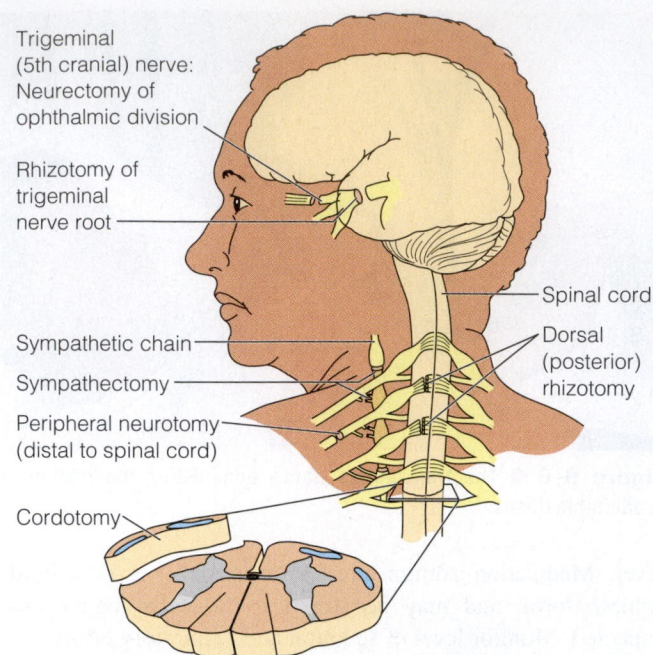

Figure 9–8 ■ Surgical procedures may be used to treat severe pain that does not respond to other types of management. They include cordotomy, neurectomy, sympathectomy, and rhizotomy.

NEURECTOMY   A *neurectomy* is the removal or destruction of a nerve. It is sometimes used for pain relief, for example, to relieve the pain of trigeminal neuralgia. The nerve may be destroyed through several different methods, including injection of glycerol into the nerve, using radiofrequency-generated heat, or by compressing the nerve using a balloon. When an open approach is used, the nerve is exposed and severed. A peripheral neurectomy is the severing of a nerve at any point distal to the spinal cord.

SYMPATHECTOMY   The sympathetic nerves play an important role in producing and transmitting the sensation of pain. A *sympathectomy* involves destruction by injection or incision of the ganglia of sympathetic nerves, usually in the lumbar region or the cervicodorsal region at the base of the neck.

RHIZOTOMY   *Rhizotomy* is surgical severing of the dorsal spinal roots. It is most often performed to relieve the pain of cancer of the head, neck, or lungs. A rhizotomy may be performed by surgically cutting the nerve fibers, by injecting a chemical such as alcohol or phenol into the subarachnoid space, or by using a radio frequency current to selectively destroy pain fibers.

Transcutaneous Electrical Nerve Stimulation (TENS)

Transcutaneous electrical nerve stimulation (TENS) is the application of electrical current through the skin to control acute or chronic pain. A TENS unit consists of a battery-operated low-voltage transmitter connected to the skin using two or more electrodes (Figure 9–9 ■). Electrodes may be placed by the patient or by the physical therapist. The TENS unit generates a high-frequency or a low-frequency electrical pulse. With high-frequency application, pulse intensity is low and does not cause muscle contraction; low-frequency applications produce an intensity that does produce muscle contraction. The patient experiences a gentle tapping or vibrating sensation over the electrodes. He or she can adjust the voltage to achieve maximum pain relief.

Figure 9–9 ■ The TENS unit is used to assist in acute and chronic in pain management. Electrodes deliver low-voltage electrical stimuli through the skin to block transmission of pain stimuli.

TENS controls pain in several ways. It activates opioid receptors in the spinal cord and medulla. It also affects release of both excitatory and inhibitory neurotransmitters, reducing the transmission of pain signals within the CNS. Furthermore, TENS stimulates large-diameter A-beta touch fibers to close the gate controlling pain transmission within the spinal cord. Low frequency TENS stimulates serotonin release and activates serotonin receptors, as well as prompting endorphin release.

A TENS unit is most commonly used to relieve chronic benign pain, neuropathic pain, and acute postoperative pain. Their use during obstetric care (labor in particular) is increasing, as is their use in treating orthopedic conditions. In any case, thorough patient teaching is essential, including an explanation of manufacturer's directions, instructions on where to place the electrodes, and the importance of placing the electrodes on clean, unbroken skin. The patient should assess the skin daily for signs of irritation. Patients who have a cardiac pacemaker or implanted cardioverter-defibrillator should not use TENS.

TENS offers several advantages: avoidance of drug side effects, patient control, and good interaction with other therapies. Disadvantages are its cost and the need for expert training for initiation. It also should be noted that TENS is not effective in relieving all types of pain or for all patients.

Complementary Therapies

The benefit of complementary and adjunctive therapies (or *CAM*—complementary and alternative medicine) as part of a comprehensive pain management strategy is increasingly recognized. According to a report issued in December 2008 by the National Center for Complementary and Alternative Medicine (NCCAM) and National Center for Health Statistics (part of the Centers for Disease Control and Prevention), about 38% of adults in the United States are using some form of CAM. See the accompanying Focus on Cultural Diversity box for the prevalence of CAM use among people of various cultures.

Pain—back, neck, or joint pain—and arthritis are the most common conditions that prompt adults to use CAM. A number of CAM therapies are used to treat pain, including acupuncture, chiropractic and osteopathic medicine, massage, and relaxation. Some of the more commonly used therapies follow.

ACUPUNCTURE Acupuncture is an ancient Chinese system involving the stimulation of certain specific points on the body to enhance the flow of vital energy (chi) along pathways called meridians. Acupuncture points can be stimulated by inserting and withdrawing needles, applying heat, massage, laser, electrical stimulation, or a combination of these methods. Only care providers with training in acupuncture techniques can use this method. Acupuncture is becoming a more widely accepted therapy, although evidence of its effectiveness in treating pain is mixed. Acupuncture has been shown to enhance traditional analgesia when used after abdominal surgery. The effectiveness of acupuncture in relieving chronic musculoskeletal pain has been extensively studied, with a beneficial effect shown in relieving chronic pain in the neck, lower back, or shoulder. Numerous studies also have shown that acupuncture may increase the pain threshold and promote well-being in patients with fibromyalgia (Spencer & Jacobs, 2003).

BIOFEEDBACK Biofeedback is method for learning to control physiologic responses of the body. Physiologic responses such as brain waves, muscle contraction, and skin temperature are measured electronically, "feeding" this information back to the patient. Biofeedback units use electrodes placed on the skin to transform data into visual cues, such as colored lights. The patient thus learns to recognize stress-related responses and to replace them with relaxation responses. Eventually, the patient learns to repeat independently those actions that produce the desired brain wave effect.

Biofeedback gives the patient a measure of control over the response to pain. It has been studied as a CAM therapy for migraine, fibromyalgia, traumatic brain injury, and temporomandibular disorder (TMD). In all studies, a beneficial effect was found, for example, reduced frequency of migraine headache or reduced intensity of pain associated with fibromyalgia and TMD (Fontaine, 2005; Spencer & Jacobs, 2003).

CHIROPRACTIC Chiropractic uses on hands-on therapy, focusing on the relationship between body structure and function. This relationship between structure (primarily that of the spine) and function and its affect on health is a key concept of chiropractic medicine. Chiropractic therapy is directed at normalizing the relationship between structure and function to promote the body's innate ability to self-heal (NCCAM, 2008). The practice of chiropractic in the United States is limited to those who earn a doctor of chiropractic degree from an accredited college. Chiropractic is among the 10 most commonly used CAM procedures, with an estimated 20% of Americans receiving chiropractic care at some point during their lives. Most often, it is used in conjunction with conventional medical services.

Spinal manipulation has been demonstrated to be as effective for relieving mild-to-moderate low back pain as conventional treatments (NCCAM, 2008). Chiropractic generally is safe, with discomfort of the treated area, headache, and fatigue the most common adverse effects. Chiropractors may combine treatments such as application of heat or ice, electrical stimulation, exercise prescriptions, counseling, and dietary supplements with spinal manipulation.

DISTRACTION Distraction involves redirecting attention away from the pain and onto something that the patient finds more pleasant. Examples of distracting activities are practicing focused breathing, listening to music, or doing some form of rhythmic activity to music. For example, the patient using recorded music for distraction may sing along with the song, tap out the rhythm with the fingers or foot, clap to the music, conduct the music, or add harmony.

Participating in an activity that promotes laughter, such as reading a joke book or viewing a comedy, has been found to be highly effective in pain relief. Laughing for 20 minutes or more is known to produce an increase in endorphins that may continue pain relief even after the patient stops laughing.

HYPNOTHERAPY AND GUIDED IMAGERY Hypnotherapy is the use of hypnosis, a trance state in which the mind becomes extremely responsive to suggestion, to address a specific problem such as pain. Guided imagery is similar, helping patients achieve a state of focused attention. During hypnotherapy or guided imagery, the patient enters a trance state in which he or she is aware of the surroundings without focusing on them. The patient may go through three trance levels: superficial trance, in which awareness of the surroundings is maintained; alpha trance, a deeper trance state during which the heart rate, blood pressure, and respirations fall; and somnambulism, the level believed to be most beneficial. The patient's muscles relax, alpha brain waves predominate, and the patient experiences a sense of well-being and the ability to accept new ideas. During this state, the therapist may make suggestions to encourage pain relief. It is possible to achieve complete anesthesia or to modify pain in a variety of ways through hypnotism. For the technique to work, however, the patient must be fully relaxed and must want to be hypnotized.

Guided imagery, also called creative visualization, is use of the mind to create a scene or sensory experience that relaxes the muscles and moves the attention of the mind away from the pain experience. Images may be created by the therapist to help the patient modify physical responses to stressors such as pain. To use guided imagery, the patient must be able to concentrate,

use the imagination, and follow directions. The nurse can facilitate this technique by asking the patient for some descriptions of what the patient finds most relaxing. The nurse then speaks to the patient in a calm, soothing voice about those places or situations. Imagery can cause changes in vital signs, brain wave patterns, blood flow, and hormone and neurotransmitter levels (Fontaine, 2005).

Advantages hypnotherapy and guided imagery include patient control and lack of side effects. Disadvantages include the need for a skilled practitioner and a willing patient. However, some patients can learn to enter into a trance state without assistance by a practitioner to achieve pain relief.

MASSAGE Massage therapy often is employed as a CAM therapy to relieve pain and promote relaxation. In massage therapy, muscles and soft tissues of the body are manipulated with the intent of relaxing soft tissues; increasing warmth, blood flow, and oxygen delivery to the area; and decreasing pain. There are over 80 different types of massage therapy. Among the most common are Swedish massage, deep tissue massage, trigger point massage, and shiatsu massage. Massage therapy carries very little risk, but should be used appropriately and performed by a licensed or certified massage professional.

NATURAL PRODUCTS Natural products are the most frequently employed CAM therapy overall, used by nearly 20% of adults. A number of products, including herbals, natural oils, and other natural substances are available. Glucosamine, a natural substance that is found in cartilage, is among the most commonly used natural products. When combined with chondroitin, another natural substance found in cartilage, glucosamine has been found to have a beneficial effect on moderate to severe pain associated with osteoarthritis of the knee (NCCAM, 2006). Other natural products have been studied for the relief of pain associated with migraine and other musculoskeletal conditions such as fibromyalgia and rheumatoid arthritis with mixed results (Spencer & Jacobs, 2003).

RELAXATION Relaxation involves learning activities that deeply relax the body and mind. Relaxation distracts the patient's focus from the pain, lessens the effects of stress from pain, increases pain tolerance, increases the effectiveness of other pain relief measures, and increases perception of pain control. Some examples of relaxation activities are the following:

- *Diaphragmatic breathing* can relax muscles, improve oxygen levels, and provide a feeling of release from tension. This technique is more effective when the patient either lies down or sits comfortably, remains in a quiet environment, and keeps the eyelids closed. Inhaling and exhaling slowly and regularly is also helpful. The technique for diaphragmatic breathing is described and illustrated in ∞ Chapter 4.
- *Progressive muscle relaxation* may be used alone or in conjunction with deep breathing to help manage pain. The patient is taught to tighten one group of muscles (such as those of the face), hold the tension for a few seconds, and then relax the muscle group completely, repeating these actions for all parts of the body. This method is also more effective when the patient lies or sits comfortably, is in a quiet environment, and

keeps the eyelids closed. There are tapes available to help the patient with this relaxation process.

- *Meditation* is a process whereby the patient empties the mind of all sensory data and, typically, concentrates on a single object, word, or idea. This activity produces a deeply relaxed state in which oxygen consumption decreases, muscles relax, and endorphins are produced. At its deepest level, the meditative state may resemble a trance state. A variety of exercises can induce the meditative state, and all are relatively easy to learn. Many books and tapes are available commercially.

- *Music therapy* uses music and the therapeutic relationship to reduce pain, anxiety, and depression. Music provides a familiar sensory stimulus that can provoke favorable responses such as muscle relaxation and reduced heart rate and blood pressure. Studies on the efficacy of music therapy to reduce pain perception in an acute care setting have been mixed; however, patients rated music therapy as a positive experience even when its effect on pain perception was statistically insignificant (Richards, Johnson, Sparks, & Emerson, 2007).

ᴂ Nursing Care

Nursing care of the patient with pain presents perhaps more of a challenge than almost any other type of illness or injury. Regardless of the type of pain, the goal of nursing care is to assist the patient to achieve optimal control of the pain. See the accompanying Case Study & Nursing Care Plan: A Patient Experiencing Chronic Pain.

Health Promotion

Health promotion activities related to pain focus on providing effective relief of acute pain to avoid the negative consequences of inadequately managed pain. Evidence points to the existence of pain circuits established when acute pain is inadequately treated that perpetuate pain and contribute to chronic pain. Furthermore, pain has a negative effect on quality of life, resulting in decreased job performance, exercise, socialization, and activity-of-daily-living (ADL) performance. Longerterm effects include depression, isolation, and loss of self-esteem (American Academy of Pain Management, 2009).

CASE STUDY & NURSING CARE PLAN   **A Patient Experiencing Chronic Pain**

Susan Akers, aged 37, is currently being seen at an outpatient clinic for chronic nonmalignant pain. She works at a local paper factory. She has a 3-year history of neck and shoulder pain that usually is accompanied by headaches. She believes the pain is related to lifting objects at work, but it is now precipitated by activities of daily living. Susan is absent from work approximately three times a month and states that the absences are due to her pain and headaches. She has been seeking care in the local emergency department on the average of twice monthly for injections for pain. She does not regularly use medications but does take Percocet-5 as needed (usually two to three times a day). Ms. Akers is divorced and has two children. She states that she has several friends in the area, but her parents and siblings live in another part of the United States.

ASSESSMENT

During the nursing history, Ms. Akers rates her pain during an acute episode as a 7 on a scale of 1 to 10. She states that lifting objects and moving her hands and arms above shoulder level precipitate sharp pain. The pain never really goes away, but it does decrease with upper extremity rest. She says that when she lifts a lot at work, she has difficulty sleeping that night. She takes two Percocet-5 tablets every 6 hours when the pain is severe, but does not get complete relief.

DIAGNOSIS

- *Chronic Pain* related to muscle inflammation

EXPECTED OUTCOMES

Ms. Akers will:

- Return for follow-up visits with a journal of activities and pain experiences.
- After 3 to 5 days on regularly scheduled doses of pain medication, report a decrease in the level of pain from 7 to 3 or 4 on a scale of 1 to 10.
- Decrease number of absences from work.
- Modify activities at work and at home, especially when pain is intense.

PLANNING AND IMPLEMENTATION

- Encourage discussion of pain, and acknowledge belief in Ms. Akers's report of pain.
- Consult with a physician for an appropriate nonsteroidal anti-inflammatory analgesic with a minimum of side effects, and instruct in maintaining regular dosing schedules.
- For episodes of acute pain, take opioid analgesic as soon as the pain begins and every 6 hours while continuing the dosage of NSAID analgesic.
- Teach one relaxation technique that is personally useful.
- Explore distraction techniques such as listening to music, watching comedies, or reading.
- Provide clinic phone number and instruct to call if pain is unrelieved with opioid and NSAID analgesics.

EVALUATION

Ms. Akers returns for scheduled follow-up visits with a completed journal of her activities and associated pain. She reports that taking oral opioid analgesics has relieved her pain and that within 3 weeks regular use, NSAID analgesics brought her pain under control. She also reports that her supervisor has reassigned her to a position that requires no lifting. She now rates her pain at 2 or 3 on a scale of 1 to 10. She has missed only 1 day of work in the last 3 months and reports that her children and friends have helped with her household tasks when she has requested they do so.

CRITICAL THINKING IN THE NURSING PROCESS

1. Describe three factors that support the statement "Pain is a personal experience."
2. Ms. Akers asks you how often she should take her pain medications. You tell her to (a) take them on a regular basis or (b) wait until she experiences pain. Which action would you choose, and why?
3. Develop a care plan for Ms. Akers for the nursing diagnosis of *Risk for Constipation*. Why is this necessary?

See Evaluating Your Response in Appendix C.

Assessment

Pain assessment varies by the acuity of the pain and circumstances surrounding the patient's entry into the healthcare setting. Identifying the location, intensity, and triggering event may be the most appropriate initial assessment for a patient experiencing acute pain related to trauma. The approach to a patient experiencing acute pain without known trauma (e.g., acute chest, flank, or abdominal pain) may still be very focused due to the acuity of the situation. Additional information regarding the quality and timing of the pain, as well as the patient's health history often provide valuable clues about the underlying cause. When pain is chronic, a comprehensive approach to pain assessment is essential to ensure adequate and appropriate interventions. The four essential areas to assess are patient perceptions, physiologic responses, behavioral responses, the patient's attempts to manage the pain, and the effectiveness of these pain-management strategies.

Patient Perceptions

The most reliable indicator of the presence and degree of pain is the patient's own statement about the pain.

> **MEMORY CUE**
>
> The PQRST mnemonic provides a useful tool for conducting a focused pain assessment:
>
> P = What precipitated (triggered, stimulated) the pain? Has anything relieved the pain? What is the pattern of the pain (constant, episodic)?
>
> Q = What are the qualities of the pain? How would you describe the pain (sharp, stabbing, aching, burning, stinging, deep, crushing, viselike, gnawing)?
>
> R = What is the region (location) of the pain? Can you put your finger on where the pain is? Does the pain radiate to other areas of the body?
>
> S = What is the severity or intensity of the pain?
>
> T = What is the timing of the pain? When does it begin, how long does it last, and how is it related to other events in the patient's life?

The McGill Pain Questionnaire is a useful tool in assessing the subjective pain experience. It asks the patient to locate the pain and to describe its quality and intensity using terms to describe its sensory, affective, evaluative, and miscellaneous

Figure 9–10 ■ The McGill Pain Questionnaire. The descriptors fall into four major groups: sensory (1–10), affective (11–15), evaluative (16), and miscellaneous (17–20). The rank value for each descriptor is based on its position in the word set; the sum of the rank values is the pain rating index (PRI). The present pain intensity (PPI) is based on a scale of 0 to 5.

components. Additional components of the questionnaire address the pattern and timing of the pain (Figure 9–10 ■).

The most common method to assess the severity of pain is a pain rating scale. Pain rating scales can be used even in the most emergent situations. Several scales are illustrated in Figure 9–11 ■. For patients who do not understand English or numerals, a scale using colors (e.g., light blue for no pain through bright red for worst possible pain) or the Faces Pain Scale-Revised (FPS-R) may be helpful. The following guidelines will help the nurse effectively use a pain rating scale:

■ To ensure consistent communication, explain the specific pain rating scale being used. If a word descriptor scale is used, verify that the patient can read the language being used. If a numerical scale is used, be sure the patient can count to 10. Discuss the definition of the word "pain" to ensure that the patient and the provider are communicating on the same level. It is often helpful to use the patient's own words when describing the pain.

■ Explain that the report of pain is important for promoting recovery, not just for achieving temporary comfort.

■ Ask the patient to establish a comfort-function goal. This is a level of pain that does not interfere with or prevent the performance of essential activities of recovery or living. Often, pain assessment is made while a patient is sedentary. In this state the patient may experience less pain than when active and falsely estimate tolerable pain ratings. Provide guidelines for setting goals. Researchers found that pain ratings higher than 3 (scale of 0–10) interfered significantly with patients' activities, and scores of 6 and 7 decrease quality of life (Slaughter, Pasero, & Manworren, 2002).

Figure 9–11 ■ Examples of commonly used pain scales.

Research has shown the numeric rating, verbal descriptor, and faces rating scales to be effective with young, middle, and older adults. These scales also are effective in cognitively impaired older adults, although the faces scale was the preferred tool. Additionally, the faces scale was preferred by African Americans and Hispanics (Flaherty, 2007).

Physiologic Responses

Predictable physiologic changes occur in the presence of acute pain. These may include muscle tension; tachycardia; rapid, shallow respirations; increased blood pressure; dilated pupils; sweating; and pallor. Over time, however, the pain stimulus triggers less of a sympathetic nervous system response, and these physiologic changes may be extinguished in patients with chronic pain.

Behavioral Responses

Some behaviors are so typical of people in pain that the behaviors are referred to as *pain behaviors*. They include bracing or guarding the painful part, taking medication, crying, moaning, grimacing, withdrawing from activity and socialization, becoming immobile, talking about pain, holding the painful area, breathing with increased effort, exhibiting a sad facial expression, and being restless.

Behavioral responses to pain may or may not coincide with the patient's report of pain and are not always reliable cues to the pain experience. Discrepancies between the patient's report of pain and behavioral responses may be the result of cultural factors, coping skills, fear, denial, or the utilization of relaxation or distraction techniques.

Patients may deny pain for a variety of reasons, including fear of injections, fear of drug/narcotic addiction, misinterpretation of terms (the patient may not think that aching, soreness, or discomfort qualify as pain), or the misconception that healthcare providers know when patients experience pain. Some patients may deny pain as part of an attempt to deny that there is something wrong with them. Other patients, by contrast, may think that "as needed" medications will be given only if their pain rating is high. Patients may also use pain as a mechanism to gain attention from family and healthcare providers.

Patients with Advanced Dementia

Behavior cues are critical for assessing pain intensity in patients with advanced dementia (unable to respond to simple yes or no questions) or who are nonverbal. The Pain Assessment in Advanced Dementia (PAINAD) scale uses five behavioral indicators of pain. Once trained, the nurse can use the scale by observing patient behaviors related to breathing (normal, labored, hyperventilation), vocalization (moaning, calling out, crying), facial expression (smiling or without expression, sad, frowning, grimacing), body language (relaxed, tense, rigid or striking out), and consolability (distractible, reassured, or unable to console) (Horgas & Miller, 2008).

Self-Management of Pain

The patient's attempts to manage pain are useful additions to the assessment database. This information is individualized and patient specific, including many factors such as culture, age, and patient knowledge. Get detailed descriptions of actions the patient or significant others took, when and how these measures were applied, and how well they worked.

Nursing Diagnoses and Interventions

The primary nursing diagnoses for patients in pain are acute pain and chronic pain.

Acute Pain

Assess the characteristics of the pain by asking the patient to do the following:

- Point to the pain location or mark the pain location on a figure drawing. *Pain location provides information about the etiology of the pain and the type of pain being experienced.*
- Rate the intensity of the pain by using an evidence-based pain scale (see Figure 9–11). Use the same scale with each assessment. *Pain and its intensity is a subjective experience. Consistently using the same scale to rate pain intensity allows evaluation of intervention effectiveness.*

PRACTICE ALERT

Do not assume that the older patient or the cognitively-impaired patient is not having pain or is unable to identify its intensity. Many cognitively impaired patients are able to use a pain scale such as faces, numeric rating, or verbal descriptor (Flaherty, 2007).

- Describe the quality of the pain, saying, for example, "Describe what your pain feels like." If necessary, suggest word descriptors for the patient to select. *Descriptive terms provide insight into the nature and cause of the pain.*
- Describe the pattern of the pain, including time of onset, duration, persistence, and times without pain. Ask whether the pain is worse at regular times of the day and about its relationship to activity. *The pattern of pain provides clues about cause and location.*
- Describe any precipitating or relieving factors. *Precipitating factors provide clues to any underlying pathophysiology of the pain; relieving factors provide information that can be used when planning nursing interventions for pain management.*
- Monitor manifestations of pain by taking vital signs; assessing skin temperature and moisture; observing pupils; observing facial expressions, position in bed, guarding of body parts; and noting restlessness. *Autonomic responses to pain may result in an increased blood pressure, tachycardia, rapid respirations, perspiration, and dilated pupils. Other responses to pain include grimacing, clenching the hands, muscle rigidity, guarding, restlessness, and nausea.*

PRACTICE ALERT

Consider pain the fifth vital sign and assess patients for pain every time you check temperature, pulse, respirations, and blood pressure.

- Communicate belief in the patient's pain. *Verbally acknowledge the presence of the pain, listen carefully to the description of pain, and act to help the patient manage the pain. Because pain is a personal, subjective experience, the nurse must convey belief in the patient's pain. By conveying belief in the patient's pain, the nurse reduces anxiety and thereby lessens pain.* See the accompanying Moving Evidence into Action box.
- Administer prescribed analgesics, determining the preferred route of administration. Provide pain-relieving measures for

MOVING EVIDENCE INTO ACTION — The Patient Experiencing Pain

Pain that is not adequately managed is the focus of regulatory agencies, professional healthcare organizations, and consumer groups. Despite well-defined guidelines for pain management, there is a gap between guideline standards of care and implementation of care. A number of studies have compared nurses' perceptions of pain management with the experience related by patients. In a study by Manias et al. (2005) nurses were observed for 2-hour periods of high environmental, patient, and nursing activity, revealing varied responses to patients' pain. The pain was (1) responded to effectively; (2) prioritized as less important than other nursing tasks; (3) ignored because cues were missed; (4) treated as part of the medication administration regimen, with medication given or withheld according to schedule; (5) prevented through comfort measures, pre-medicating, and teaching the importance of early communication about pain; and (6) only addressed reactively, after the painful experience. A later study by Gunningberg and Idvall (2007) compared patient and nurse assessments of the pain management of postoperative patients on two surgery units. This study found areas for improvements in pain management related to communication, action, trust, and environment. Patients who experienced more pain than expected were less satisfied with their care and reported higher levels of pain intensity. The study also pointed to the importance of considering patients' previous pain experience and goals for pain relief in accurately assessing pain.

IMPLICATIONS FOR NURSING

Appropriate pain management is increasingly recognized as a critical component of care, with increasing attention given to patients' self-reported pain scores. These studies provide valuable information to guide nursing practice. Communication among nurses, physicians, and patients is key to pain relief. Developing and maintaining caregiver competence in the effective use of pharmacologic and nonpharmacologic pain management is critical. Although few conditions have higher priority for the patient than pain relief, these studies reveal that nurses accept pain as a normal component of the postoperative experience. Pain management is an important component of professional nursing; nurses should be supported in their efforts to address pain with compassion and efficiency.

CRITICAL THINKING IN PATIENT CARE

1. Reflect on your own experiences with pain. How will those experiences facilitate or hinder your assessments and interventions for patients in pain?
2. You are caring for a young man who has multiple injuries from a motorcycle accident. He tells you his pain is so bad that "he just wants to die." How would you respond?
3. You are caring for an 80-year-old man with diabetes who has had his left foot amputated for gangrene. He is restless and moaning. Another nurse tells you to only give one-half of the ordered dose of narcotics because "he is old and there is a danger of respiratory depression." What would you do?
4. Why do you think nurses tend to underestimate and under-medicate pain?

severe pain on a regular around-the-clock basis or by self-administration (such as with a PCA pump). *The patient is a part of the decision-making process and can exert some control over the situation by choosing the administration route. Analgesics are usually most effective when they are administered before pain occurs or becomes severe. Around-the-clock administration has been proven to provide better pain management for both acute and chronic pain.*

> **SAFETY ALERT**
> Use extreme care to ensure the correct patient, medication, and dose when setting up and monitoring PCA for analgesia. Patient harm resulting from medication errors with PCA often is greater than harm resulting from other types of medication errors.

- To reduce the risk of medication error associated with PCA, work with administration to develop the following strategies:
  - Use a single brand or type of pump within a facility to reduce programming and use complexity for caregivers.
  - Use bar codes and electronic medical records to reduce errors that involve the wrong medication.
  - Develop and use easily understood and standardized forms for PCA.
    The complexity of activities required to safely program PCA pumps, the use of different medications and concentrations, confusion of medical orders, and variations in documentation related to PCA are identified as contributing factors to PCA medication errors (Sheehan, 2008).
- Evaluate and monitor the effects of analgesics and other pain-relieving measures. Teach family members or significant others to be alert for adverse reactions to pain medications. Sedation, constipation, nausea and dizziness are common side effects of opioid analgesics. *Opioid analgesics stimulate mu receptors, leading to common adverse effects such as respiratory depression, nausea, and constipation.*
- Provide for safety of the patient receiving opioid analgesics:
  - Check respiratory rate and oxygen saturation every 2 hours at the beginning of opioid therapy and after increasing dosage. Reduce the dose and notify the physician if the respiratory rate falls to eight per minute or lower or if the oxygen saturation falls. *Excessive sedation can progress to significant respiratory depression.*

- Prevent falls that may result from sedation or dizziness. *Opioid analgesics can affect balance and judgment, increasing the risk for falls, particularly in the elderly.*
- Administer an opioid antagonist such as naloxone (Narcan) if the patient develops symptoms of excessive opioid dosage. Administer prescribed dose (0.4–2 mg) by direct intravenous push over 10 to 15 seconds or by intravenous infusion. Titrate infusion or repeat direct IV push every 2–3 minutes (up to a total of 10 mg) to reverse respiratory depression or excessive sedation. Continue to monitor respiratory status and sedation, repeating naloxone as necessary. *The opioid agonist causing excessive sedation and respiratory depression may have a longer half-life than naloxone, leading to a fall in respiratory rate and decreased LOC after the initial dose of naloxone has been substantially eliminated. Administration of excessive naloxone may cause acute withdrawal and failure of pain relief. It may take considerable time to re-establish a therapeutic comfort level.*
- Teach the patient and family nonpharmacologic methods of pain management, such as relaxation, distraction, and cutaneous stimulation. *These techniques are especially useful when used in conjunction with pain medications. They can be beneficial for patients experiencing either acute or chronic pain.*
- Provide comfort measures, such as changing positions, back massage, oral care, skin care, and changing bed linens. *Basic comfort measures for personal cleanliness, skin care, and mobility promote physical and psychosocial well-being, lessening the perception of pain.*
- Provide patient and family teaching, and make referrals if necessary to assist with coping, financial resources, and home care. *The patient (and family) with pain requires information about medications, noninvasive techniques for pain management, and sources of assistance with home-based care. The patient with acute pain requires information about the expected course of pain resolution.*

Chronic Pain

The patient who has chronic pain may not demonstrate the same physiologic and behavioral responses to pain as are seen in the patient with acute pain. The intensity of the pain, however, may be as high or even higher than acute pain. Furthermore, chronic pain, whether of malignant or nonmalignant origin, has a negative

Chronic Pain Video

NURSING CARE OF THE OLDER ADULT — Pain Management for the Older Adult

Older adults often have medical conditions associated with pain, such as arthritis, peripheral vascular disease, and diabetes. Many older adults have multiple health disorders causing them to experience both acute and chronic pain.

The nursing standard of care calls for older adults to be pain free or have their pain controlled to an acceptable level that allows the highest possible level of functioning (Horgas & Yoon, 2008). Achieving this standard requires comprehensive assessment of the patient, including the patient's history, subjective reports of pain, nonverbal and behavioral responses, and information from family members about the patient's pain experiences.

In addition to frequent and ongoing assessment, nursing care guidelines call for the nurse to anticipate and treat pain before, during, and after painful procedures and treatments. The nurse should educate the patient, family, and other clinicians about prophylactic analgesic use, using analgesics on a regular basis, and how to avoid allowing pain to escalate. Teaching must include information about the medications themselves, their side and adverse effects, and issues about addiction, dependence, and tolerance. Finally, the nurse teaches the patient, family, and other healthcare providers about nonpharmacologic pain management strategies such as relaxation, massage, and application of heat or cold (Horgas & Yoon, 2008).

EVIDENCE FOR NURSING CARE — The Patient with Acute Pain

Selected resources that nurses may find helpful when planning evidence-based nursing care follow.

- Herr, K., Bjoro, K., Steffensmeier, J., & Rakel, B. (2006, July). *Acute pain management in older adults.* Iowa City, IA: University of Iowa Gerontological Nursing Interventions Research Center, Research Translation and Dissemination Core.
- Institute for Clinical Systems Improvement. (2008). *Health care guideline: Assessment and management of acute pain* (6th ed., pp. 1–58). Retrieved from http://www.icsi .org/pain_acute/pain__acute__assessment_and_ management_of__3.html
- Registered Nurses Association of Ontario (RNAO). (2007 February 27). *Assessment and management of pain: supplement.* Toronto, ON: Author.

effect on the patient's physical, psychosocial, emotional, and functional status. In addition to the nursing assessments and interventions identified for acute pain, consider the following interventions for the patient experiencing chronic pain.

- Ask the patient to describe the pain and its meaning, including its effects on life style, self-concept, roles, and relationships. *Pain is a stressor that may affect the patient's coping ability. Chronic pain often interferes with sleep quality, job performance, personal relationships, and social interactions. The patient may have concerns about addiction to pain medication and costs as well.*
- Assess for depression using an accepted depression screening tool. *Chronic pain and depression commonly occur concurrently (Fauci et al., 2008).*
- If the underlying cause of chronic pain has not been identified, advocate for consultations, diagnostic testing, or other means of establishing an accurate diagnosis. *Guidelines for chronic pain management call for treatment of the underlying cause whenever it can be identified (WHO, 2008).*

EVIDENCE FOR NURSING CARE — The Patient with Chronic Pain

Selected resources that nurses may find helpful when planning evidence-based nursing care follow.

- D'Arcy, Y. (2009). Chronic opioid therapy clinical guidelines. *The Nurse Practitioner: The American Journal of Primary Health Care, 34*(10), 13–15. Retrieved from http:// www.nursingcenter.com/library/JournalArticle.asp?Article _ID=935533
- D'Arcy, Y. (2009). Overturning barriers to pain relief in older adults. *Nursing2009, 39*(10), 32–39. Retrieved from www .nursing2009.com
- Institute for Clinical Systems Improvement (ICSI). (2008, July). *Assessment and management of chronic pain.* Bloomington, MN: Institute for Clinical Systems Improvement.
- University of Michigan Health System. (2009, March). *Managing chronic non-terminal pain including prescribing controlled substances.* Ann Arbor, MI: University of Michigan Health System.

- Administer prescribed NSAIDs, opioid and nonopioid analgesics, and other medications around the clock and as ordered. Whenever possible, the oral or transdermal routes should be used. *Around-the-clock analgesic administration helps maintain pain within an acceptable range within which the patient remains comfortable and functional. As needed medications may be required for breakthrough pain.*
- Do not crush or break or allow patients to chew controlled-release oral preparations. *Crushing, breaking or chewing controlled release oral preparations may lead to overdose. Capsules containing controlled-release pellets can be opened and sprinkled over soft food. See the accompanying box for more information about standards of pain management in the older adult.*
- Teach the patient, family, and caregivers how to manage side and adverse effects of prescribed medications. Advise about the importance of taking NSAIDs with food to reduce the risk of gastrointestinal irritation and bleeding. Provide information about appropriate laxatives for the patient taking opioid analgesics. Instruct when to contact the prescribing care provider should adverse effects become problematic. *Many analgesics, while effective, have adverse effects that may limit the patient's willingness to continue therapy. In most cases, appropriate management of these effects allows continued use of the medication.*
- Encourage and advocate for a multimodal approach to pain management, teaching about the use of heat, cold, and CAM therapies, providing for referrals to healthcare providers (e.g. physical therapists, chiropractic physicians, massage therapists, acupuncturists) and chronic pain clinics as appropriate. *Using a multimodal approach to management of chronic pain improves the patient's perception of control over the pain and its effect on lifestyle. This also may allow less dependence on opioid and nonopioid analgesics.*

Using NANDA, NIC, and NOC

Linkages between a selected NANDA nursing diagnosis, NIC, and NOC for the patient with chronic pain are shown in the chart that follows.

NANDA, NIC, AND NOC LINKAGES
The Patient with Chronic Pain

NANDA — Chronic Pain

NIC — Pain Management / Teaching: Prescribed Medication / Meditation Facilitation / Cutaneous Stimulation

NOC — Discomfort Level / Pain: Disruptive Effects / Knowledge: Pain Management / Depression Level

Data from NANDA International. (2009). *Nursing diagnoses: Definitions and classification 2009–2011.* Oxford, UK: Wiley-Blackwell; Bulecheck, G., Butcher, H., Dochterman, J. (Eds.). (2008). *Nursing interventions classification (NIC)* (5th ed.). St. Louis, MO: Mosby; and Moorhead, M., Johnson, M., Maas, M., Swanson, M. (Eds.). (2008). *Nursing outcomes classification (NOC)* (4th ed.). St. Louis, MO: Mosby.

Community-Based Care

Teaching the patient and family includes the following:

- Specific drugs to be taken, including the frequency, potential side effects, possible drug interactions, and any special precautions to be taken (such as taking with food or avoiding alcohol).
- How to take or administer the drugs ordered for managing chronic malignant or nonmalignant pain (Box 9–2).
- The importance of taking pain medications before the pain becomes severe.
- An explanation that the risk of addiction to pain medications is very small when they are used for pain relief and management.
- Discussion about physical tolerance and the importance of contacting the prescriber should medications become less effective.
- The importance of scheduling periods of rest and sleep.
- Use of CAM therapies to supplement or enhance traditional approaches to pain management.
- In addition, suggest the following resources:
  - Pain clinics
  - Community support groups
  - American Cancer Society
  - American Pain Society

BOX 9–2 Opioids for Long-Term Analgesia for Chronic Pain

Drug	Route	Nursing Implications
Oxycodone (OxyContin)	Oral	Available in a timed-release formulation for 12-hour dosing and as fast-acting formulations (OxyIR, OxyFAST) for breakthrough pain.
Morphine (Kadian)	Oral	Formulated of timed-release particles in a capsule. If patient can't swallow the capsule, may be sprinkled over food or given by nasogastric or gastric tube.
Fentanyl (Duragesic)	Transdermal	Absorbed slowly through the skin; allows 72-hour dose schedule. Up to 14 ours to achieve therapeutic level; when discontinued therapeutic effect will decay slowly.
Fentanyl citrate (Actiq)	Transmucosal	A lozenge formulation used to treat breakthrough cancer pain in opioid-tolerant patients.

CHAPTER HIGHLIGHTS

- Pain is transmitted by the peripheral and central nervous systems and perceived in the CNS. Opioids and other analgesics block the perception of pain; NSAIDs and most nonpharmacological interventions block or decrease the transmission of pain from the periphery to the CNS. Measures to block the sensitization of pain-transmitting fibers can help prevent chronic pain.

- There are many types of pain and treatment varies according to the type and combination of types. Acute pain, which may be cutaneous or deep somatic, visceral, or referred, usually decreases as healing progresses. Chronic pain may be episodic, experienced as recurrent acute pain, or may be persistent pain of either malignant or nonmalignant origin. Breakthrough pain is that which exceeds the baseline or persistent level of pain. Phantom limb pain is a type of neuropathic pain that occurs after amputations. Central pain and complex regional pain syndrome also are types of neuropathic pain.

- Culture and gender impact pain perception and behavior. A patient's emotional state, past experiences with pain, and the underlying cause and meaning of the painful experience also affect responses to pain. A mnemonic such as PQRST or a tool such as the McGill Pain Questionnaire may be used when assessing pain. Important components of the assessment include the location, intensity, and character (quality) of the pain; its onset, duration, and timing; factors that aggravate or relieve the pain; associated symptoms; and measures taken to treat the pain or its cause. When rating pain intensity, one pain scale should be consistently used with the individual patient.

- Behavioral assessment of pain intensity is less accurate than a patient's report of pain intensity, particularly when pain is chronic. Behavioral responses may be used to assess pain in patients who are significantly cognitively impaired, however. Older adults perceive pain as intensely as younger adults, but may hesitate to report pain for fear of losing independence or being considered a bother. Physical tolerance develops with long-term opioid use, necessitating dose increases to achieve the same effect. Although patients who are addicted to opioids need greater doses of opioid analgesics to control pain because of tolerance, treating physicians and nurses providing care often withhold or use lower doses of opioid analgesics, leading to inadequate pain relief.

- Pain management includes assessment, intervention, and evaluation. It is important to verify that interventions have been effective. If not, interventions must be identified that bring pain down to a level of intensity with which the patient feels satisfied.

TEST YOURSELF NCLEX-RN® REVIEW

1. During your assessment, a patient tells you he has had lower back pain for 9 months. When planning nursing care, you recognize this type of pain as which of the following?
   1. neuropathic pain
   2. chronic pain
   3. visceral pain
   4. somatic pain

2. A patient presents to the ED after smashing her finger in the car door. She relates that her pain initially was sharp and so intense she thought she would faint, but now it is dull and throbbing. The nurse appropriately recognizes this as which of the following?
   1. indicative that the injury is less severe than initially perceived
   2. the result of interpretation of the pain stimulus by the thalamus
   3. an example of the gate theory of pain transmission
   4. transmission of pain stimuli via unmyelinated C fibers

3. You are taking a health history for a patient who has taken an NSAID for several years. Which of the following questions should you ask? **Select all that apply.**
   1. "Tell me how and when you take this drug."
   2. "Have you ever vomited blood or had very dark stools?"
   3. "Do you know that you may become addicted to this drug?"
   4. "Have you noticed any problems with your breathing?"
   5. "Do you have your blood pressure checked regularly?"

4. Which of the following would you include when teaching a patient about a transdermal pain medication?
   1. Contact your physician if this medication makes you excessively sleepy.
   2. Replace this patch every 24 hours, applying it to clean, dry skin.
   3. When reapplying the patch, place it on the anterior thigh.
   4. This medication should be effective within 2 to 4 hours; contact your physician if your pain is not at an acceptable level after that.

5. Which of the following statements would be most useful in determining the quality of a patient's pain?
   1. "Tell me where you hurt."
   2. "Rate your pain on a scale of 0–10."
   3. "Describe what your pain feels like."
   4. "Tell me how this pain affects your sleep."

6. When assessing a postoperative patient's pain, you note that he is relaxed, smiling, and visiting with friends. He rates his pain as a 7 on a scale of 0–10. The most appropriate response is to do which of the following?
   1. Reassess the patient's pain after his friends have left.
   2. Document your assessment but take no further action.
   3. Administer the prescribed analgesic dose.
   4. Note that the patient is developing tolerance to the prescribed opioid analgesic.

7. When teaching a patient with chronic malignant pain about using opioid analgesics, you would include which of the following instructions?
   1. "This drug may interfere with urination; contact your physician if that becomes a problem."
   2. "Increase fluid and fiber intake; you may need a stool softener or laxative to prevent constipation."
   3. "This drug may cause itching and rash; take Benadryl (diphenhydramine) as needed."
   4. "There is a risk of addiction with this drug; stop the drug if you find that it no longer provides the degree of pain relief necessary."

8. When assessing pain in a patient who is moderately cognitively impaired due to dementia, the nurse should do which of the following?
   1. Ask the patient to rate his pain using the faces pain scale.
   2. Use only behavioral cues such as grimacing, pacing, or agitation.
   3. Have the family evaluate the intensity of the patient's pain.
   4. Administer the prescribed analgesic on an around-the-clock basis.

9. A patient asks the nurse if she should take glucosamine for her knee pain. The nurse bases her response on the knowledge of which of the following?
   1. There is no evidence that natural products such as glucosamine are effective for treating any type of pain.
   2. Chronic pain such as that associated with osteoarthritis is best treated with NSAIDs and acetaminophen.
   3. When combined with chondroitin, glucosamine has been effective in relieving moderate to severe knee pain in some patients.
   4. Although no studies have shown a benefit from taking glucosamine, other CAM therapies such as acupuncture are effective for treating pain.

10. A patient who recently took up running to lose weight asks why she feels better after running when she should be tired and sore. The most accurate response would be which of the following?
    1. Natural narcotic-like substances are released during physical activities like running.
    2. Activities such as running activate a natural "gate" in the spinal cord, blocking pain signals.
    3. Engaging in activities that actively use large muscle groups changes pain circuits in the brain, reducing the perception of pain.
    4. With repeated stimulation through activities such as running, nociceptors in deep tissues become less sensitive to stimuli.

BIBLIOGRAPHY

Adams, M., P., Holland, L. N., Jr., & Bostwick, P. M. (2008). *Pharmacology for nurses: A pathophysiologic approach* (2nd ed.). Upper Saddle River, NJ: Pearson Prentice Hall.

American Academy of Pain Management. (2009). Pain is an epidemic – A message from the director. Retrieved from www.aapainmanage.org

American Music Therapy Association, Inc. Music therapy in the treatment and management of pain. Retrieved from www.musictherapy.org

Andrews, M. M., & Boyle, J. S. (2008). *Transcultural concepts in nursing care* (5th ed.). Philadelphia, PA: Lippincott Williams & Wilkins.

Ashley, J. L. (2008). Pain management: Nurses in jeopardy. *Oncology Nursing Forum, 35*(5), E70–E75.

ASPAN pain and comfort clinical guideline. (2008). Retrieved from www.guideline.gov

Barclay, L., Lee, D., & Martin, B., N. (2008). Patients may need better pain interventions after traumatic injury. *Medscape Medical News, 2008 March 25.*

Barnes, P. M., Bloom, B., Nahin, R. (2008 December). Complementary and alternative medicine use among adults and children: United States, 2007. *CDC National Health Statistics Report #12.* Retrieved from www .nccam.nih.gov

Breivik, H., Borchgrevink, P. C., Allen, S. M., Rosseland, L. A., Romundstad, L., Breivik Hals, E. K., et al. (2008). Assessment of pain. *British Journal of Anaesthesia, 101*(1), 17–24. Retrieved from www.medscape.com

Centers for Disease Control and Prevention (CDC). (2006). New report finds pain affects millions of Americans. Retrieved from www.cdc.gov

Comptom, P., & Athanasos, P. (2003). Chronic pain, substance abuse and addiction. *The Nursing Clinics of North America, 38*; 525–537.

Cranwell-Bruce, L. (2007 October). Update on pain management: New methods of opiate delivery. *Medsurg Nursing, 16*(5), 333–335.

DiPiro, J., Talbert, R., Yee, G., Matzke, G., Wells, B., & Posey, L. (2008). *Pharmacotherapy: A pathophysiologic approach* (7th ed.). New York, NY: McGraw Hill.

Doyle, S. (2008). Fentanyl buccal tablets safe, well tolerated in cancer patients. *Medscape Medical News, 2008.* Retrieved from www.medscape.com

Fauci, A. S., Braunwald, E., Kasper, D. L., Hauser, S. L., Longo, D. L., Jameson, J. L., et al. (2008). *Harrison's principles of internal medicine* (17th ed.). New York, NY: McGraw Hill.

Flaherty, E. (2007). Pain assessment for older adults. *Try This: Best Practices in Nursing Care to Older Adults.* New York, NY: The Hartford Institute for Geriatric Nursing, College of Nursing, New York University.

Flaherty, E. (2008). How to try this. Using pain-rating scales with older adults. *American Journal of Nursing, 108*(6), 40–47.

Fontaine, K. L. (2005). *Complementary & alternative therapies for nursing practice* (2nd ed.). Upper Saddle River, NJ: Pearson Prentice Hall.

Galvagno, S. M., Jr., Correll, D. J., & Narang, S. (2007 April). Safe oral equianalgesic opioid dosing for patients with moderate-to-severe pain. *Resident & Staff Physician, 2007-04.* Retrieved from www.residentandstaff.com

Gendall, K. A., Kennedy, R. R., Watson, A. J. M., & Frizelle, F. A. (2007 March). The effect of epidural analgesia on postoperative outcome after colorectal surgery. *Colorectal Disease, 9,* 584–600.

Gunningberb, L., & Idvall, E. (2007). The quality of postoperative pain management from the perspectives of patients, nurses and patient records. *Journal of Nursing Management, 15,* 756–766.

Hartrick, C. T. (2004). Multimodal postoperative pain management. *American Journal of Health-System Pharmacology, 61,* S1, S4–S10.

Helms, J. E., & Barone, C. P. (2008 December). Physiology and treatment of pain. *Critical Care Nurse, 28*(6), 38–49.

Horgas, A., & Miller, L. (2008 July). How to try this. Pain assessment in people with dementia. *American Journal of Nursing, 108*(7), 62–70.

Horgas, A. L., & Yoon, S. L. (2008 January). Want to know more: Pain. Nursing Standard of Practice Protocol: Pain management in older adults. New York, NY: The Harford Institute for Geriatric Nursing, New York University. Retrieved from www.consultgerirn.org

International Association for the Study of Pain (IASP). (2008). What's new: IASP pain terminology. Retrieved from www.iasp-pain.org

Joint Commission on Accreditation of Healthcare Organizations. (2004). *Joint Commission on Accreditation of Healthcare Organizations pain standards for 2004.* Retrieved from www.jcaho.org

Lehne, R. A. (2007). *Pharmacology for Nursing Care* (6th ed.). St. Louis, MO: W.B. Saunders.

Low, J., Johnston, N., & Morris, C. (2008). Editorial. Epidural analgesia: First do no harm. *Anaesthesia, 63,* 1–3.

McCaffery, M. (1979). *Nursing management of the patient with pain.* Philadelphia: Lippincott.

McCaffery, M., Pasero, C., & Ferrell, B. R. (2007 December). Pain control. Nurses' decisions about opioid dose. *American Journal of Nursing, 107*(12), 35–39.

McCance, K., & Huether, S. (2010). *Pathophysiology: The biologic basis for disease in adults and children* (6th ed.). St. Louis: Mosby.

McCarberg, B. H. (2008). What are we afraid of? Barriers to providing adequate pain relief. *Medscape Neurology & Neurosurgery, 2008.* Retrieved from www.medscape.com

McCarberg, B., & D'Arcy, Y. (2007 July). Target pain with topical peripheral analgesics. *The Nurse Practitioner, 32*(7), 44–49.

Melzack, R. (1975). The McGill Pain Questionnaire: Major properties and scoring methods. Pain, 1, 277.

Miaskowski, C., Cleary, J., Burney, R., Coyne, P., Finley, R., Foster, R., et al. (2008). Guideline for the treatment of cancer pain in adults and children. Glenview, IL: American Pain Society (APS). Retrieved from www.guideline.gov

NANDA International. (2009). *Nursing diagnoses: Definitions and classification 2009–2011.* Oxford, UK: Wiley-Blackwell.

National Center for Complementary and Alternative Medicine (NCCAM). (2008). CAM use by race/ethnicity among adults—2007. Retrieved from www.nccam.nih.gov

NCCAM. (2006). Efficacy of glucosamine and chondroitin sulfate may depend on level of osteoarthritis pain. Retrieved from www.nccam.nih.gov

NCCAM. (2008). Spinal manipulation for low-back pain. Retrieved from www.nccam.nih.gov

National Comprehensive Cancer Network. (2008). NCCN practice guidelines in oncology: Adult cancer pain. Retrieved from www.nccn.org

National Institute of Neurological Disorders and Stroke. (2008). NINDS central pain syndrome information page. Retrieved from www.ninds.nih.gov

National Institute of Neurological Disorders and Stroke. (2009). Complex regional pain syndrome fact sheet. Retrieved from www.ninds.nih.gov

Pasero, C. (2003). Pain in the emergency department. Withholding pain medication is not justified. *American Journal of Nursing, 103*(7), 73–74.

Porth, C., & Matfin, G. (2009). Pathophysiology: Concepts of altered health states (8th ed.). Philadelphia: Lippincott.

Richards, T., Johnson, J., Sparks, A., & Emerson, H. (2007 February). The effect of music therapy on patients' perception and manifestation of pain, anxiety, and patient satisfaction. *MEDSURG Nursing, 16*(1), 7–14.

Sheehan, S. (2008). Study: Patient harm more common with patient-controlled pain medication. Joint Commission Resources. Retrieved from www.jcrinc.com

Slatkin, N. E., & Rhiner, M. I. (2008). Breakthrough pain: Improving recognition and management to enhance quality of life. Retrieved from www.medscape.com

Spencer, J. W., & Jacobs, J. J. (2003). *Complementary and alternative medicine: An evidence-based approach* (2nd ed.). St. Louis, MO: Mosby.

Tabloski, P. (2006). *Gerontological Nursing.* Upper Saddle River, NJ: Pearson Prentice Hall.

Taddio, A., & Katz, J. (2005). The effects of early pain experience in neonates on pain responses in infancy and childhood. *Pediatric Drugs, 7*(4), 245–257.

Taylor, A. (2007 Winter). Addressing the global tragedy of needless pain: Rethinking the United Nations Single Convention on Narcotic Drugs. *Journal of Law, Medicine & Ethics, Winter 2007,* 556–570.

Toomey, M. (2008, October). Gender differences in pain: Does X = Y? *AANA Journal, 76*(5), 355–359.

World Health Organization (WHO). (2008). *Scoping document for WHO treatment guidelines on chronic non-malignant pain in adults.* Geneva: WHO.

WHO. (2008). S*coping document for WHO treatment guidelines on pain related to cancer, HIV and other progressive life-threatening illnesses in adults.* Geneva: WHO.

WHO. (2009). *WHO's pain ladder.* Geneva: WHO.

Wilkinson, J. M., & Ahern, N. R. (2009). *Nursing diagnosis handbook* (9th ed.). Upper Saddle River, NJ: Pearson Prentice Hall.

Wilson, B. A., Shannon, M. T., Shields, K. M., & Stang, C. L. (2008). *Nurse's drug guide 2008.* Upper Saddle River, NJ: Pearson Prentice Hall.

CHAPTER 10

Nursing Care of Patients with Altered Fluid, Electrolyte, and Acid–Base Balance

LEARNING OUTCOMES

1. Describe the functions and regulatory mechanisms that maintain water and electrolyte balance in the body.
2. Compare and contrast the causes, effects, and care of the patient with fluid volume or electrolyte imbalance.
3. Explain the pathophysiology and manifestations of imbalances of sodium, potassium, calcium, magnesium, and phosphorus.
4. Describe the causes and effects of acid–base imbalances.

CLINICAL COMPETENCIES

1. Assess and monitor fluid, electrolyte, and acid–base balance.
2. Administer fluids and medications knowledgeably and safely.
3. Determine priority nursing diagnoses, based on assessment data, to select and implement individualized nursing interventions.
4. Use assessed data, patient values, and evidence to provide patient and family teaching about diet and medications used to promote, restore, and maintain fluid, electrolyte, and acid–base balance.
5. Effectively communicate and function within the interdisciplinary team to plan and provide care to patients with altered fluid, electrolyte, and acid–base balance.
6. Adapt individual cultural values and variations and expressed needs and preferences into the plan of care to provide knowledgeable and safe care to patients with fluid and electrolyte imbalances.

KEY TERMS

acidosis, 222
alkalis, 222
alkalosis, 222
arterial blood gases (ABGs), 201
atrial natriuretic peptide (ANP), 192

base excess (BE), 223
dehydration, 193
fluid volume deficit (FVD), 193
fluid volume excess, 198
homeostasis, 186

Kussmaul's respirations, 227
orthopnea, 198
serum bicarbonate, 223
tetany, 214
third spacing, 193

Normal physiologic processes depend on **homeostasis** (the ability to maintain internal equilibrium by adjusting physiological processes) in the internal environment of the body. The fluid volume, electrolyte composition, and pH of both intracellular and extracellular spaces must remain constant within a relatively narrow range to maintain health and life. Changes in the normal distribution and composition of body fluids often occur in response to illness and trauma. These changes affect fluid balance of the intracellular and extracellular compartments of the body, the concentration of electrolytes within fluid compartments, and the body's hydrogen ion concentration (pH). Fluid and electrolyte imbalances occur in all adult age groups, and in all healthcare settings.

Changes in the normal volume of fluids, their composition, distribution, and relative acidity or alkalinity have the potential to disrupt most functional health patterns. Imbalances of fluids, electrolytes, and pH affect the ability to maintain activities of daily living (activity-exercise), think clearly (cognitive-perceptual), and engage in self-care (health perception-health management). Conversely, alterations in a number of health patterns affect the ability to maintain homeostasis. Alterations in the nutritional-metabolic pattern affect the ability to consume adequate food and fluids. Disruptions of the elimination pattern may lead to retention or loss of excess amounts of fluids and electrolytes. Disrupted heart or respiratory function, which falls within the activity-exercise pattern, has the potential to affect fluid, electrolyte, and acid–base balance.

The goal in managing fluid, electrolyte, and acid–base imbalances is to reestablish and maintain homeostasis. Nursing care includes identifying and assessing patients who are likely to develop imbalances, monitoring patients for early manifestations, and implementing interdisciplinary and nursing interventions to prevent or correct imbalances. Effective nursing interventions require an understanding of the multiple processes that maintain fluid, electrolyte, and acid–base balance and an understanding of the causes and treatment of imbalances that occur. This chapter contains many references to disease processes that are discussed throughout the book and is most useful as a reference when learning about those disorders.

Overview of Fluid and Electrolyte Balance

Fluid and electrolyte balance in the body involves regulatory mechanisms that maintain the composition, distribution, and movement of fluids and electrolytes.

Body Fluid Composition

Body fluid is composed of water and various dissolved substances (solutes).

Water

Water is the primary component of body fluids and functions in several ways to maintain normal cellular function. Water provides a medium for the transport and exchange of nutrients and other substances such as oxygen, carbon dioxide, and metabolic wastes to and from cells; provides a medium for metabolic reactions within cells; and assists in regulating body temperature through the evaporation of perspiration.

Total body water constitutes about 60% of the total body weight, but this amount varies with age, gender, and the amount of body fat. Total body water decreases from 45% to 50% of total body weight with obesity and with aging (Porth & Matfin, 2009). Fat cells contain comparatively little water: In the person who is obese, the proportion of water to total body weight is less than in the person of average weight; in a person who is very thin, the proportion of water to total body weight is greater than in the person of average weight. Adult females have a greater ratio of fat to lean tissue mass than adult males; therefore, they have a lower percentage of total body water.

To maintain normal fluid balance, body water intake and output should be approximately equal. The average fluid intake and output is about 2500 mL over a 24-hour period. Most water gain is from the intake of foods and fluids; carbohydrate metabolism and other metabolic processes produce an additional small amount. Urine production and excretion account for most water loss. The average daily urine output is 1500 mL in adults. About 300 mL to 400 mL of urine per day is required to excrete metabolic wastes produced by the body (Porth & Matfin, 2009). Insensible water loss occurs through the skin, lungs, and feces. These losses, while normally small, can increase significantly during exercise, when environmental temperatures are high, and during illness that increases the respiratory rate, perspiration, or gastrointestinal (GI) losses (particularly diarrhea). Table 10–1 shows the sources of fluid gain and loss (Porth & Matfin, 2009).

Electrolytes

Body fluids contain both water molecules and chemical compounds. These chemical compounds can either remain intact in solution or dissociate into discrete particles. Electrolytes are substances that dissociate in solution to form charged particles called ions. Cations are positively charged electrolytes; anions are negatively charged electrolytes. Electrolytes have many functions, including assisting with the regulation of water balance, regulating and maintaining acid–base balance, and contributing to enzyme reactions. They are also essential for neuromuscular activity.

Body Fluid Distribution

Body fluid is classified by its location inside or outside of cells. Intracellular fluid (ICF) is found within cells (Figure 10–1 ■). ICF is essential for normal cell function, providing a medium for metabolic processes. Extracellular fluid (ECF) is located outside of cells and is further classified by location:

- Interstitial fluid is located in the spaces between most of the cells of the body.
- Intravascular fluid, called *plasma*, is contained within the arteries, veins, and capillaries.
- Transcellular fluid includes urine; digestive secretions; perspiration; and cerebrospinal, pleural, synovial, intraocular, gonadal, and pericardial fluids.

Solutes. Although the overall concentration of solutes in ICF and ECF is nearly identical, the concentration of specific electrolytes differs significantly between these compartments, as shown in Figure 10–2 ■. ICF contains high concentrations of

TABLE 10–1 24-Hour Fluid Gain and Loss for an Adult

	SOURCE	AMOUNT (mL)
Gain	Fluids taken orally	1000
	Water in food	1300
	Water as by-product of food metabolism	200
		↓
	Total	2500
		↑
Loss	Urine	1500
	Feces	200
	Perspiration	500
	Respiration	300

Figure 10–1 ■ The major fluid compartments of the body.

Intracellular fluid
40% of total
body weight

Total body fluid
60% of total
body weight

Plasma
5% of total
body weight

Interstitial and
transcellular fluid
15% of total
body weight

Extracellular
fluid
20% of total
body weight

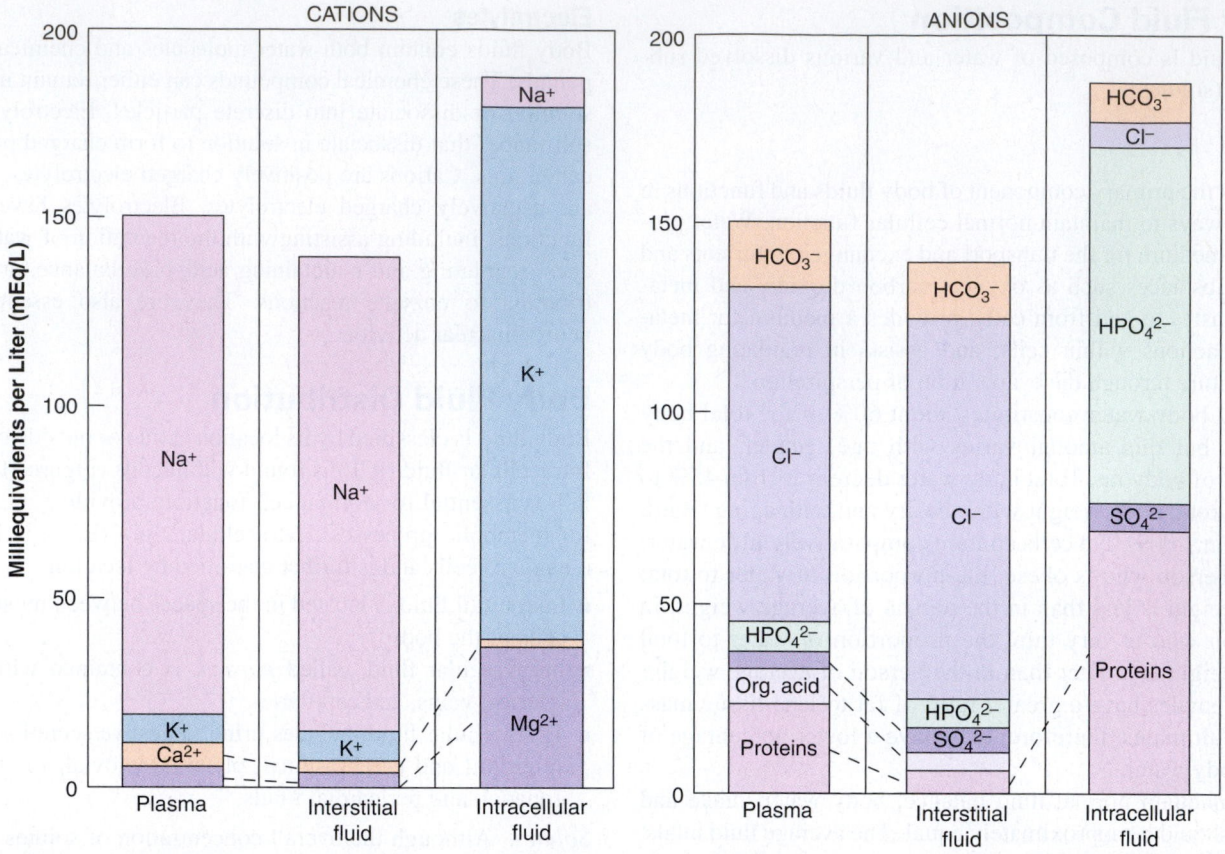

Figure 10–2 ■ Electrolyte composition (cations and anions) of body fluid compartments.

Source: Fig. 27.2, p. 1009 from *Fundamentals of Anatomy and Physiology*, 4th ed. by Frederic H. Martini. Copyright © 1998 by Frederic H. Martini, Inc. Reproduced by permission of Pearson Education, Inc.

potassium (K^+), magnesium (Mg^{2+}), and phosphate (PO_4^{2-}), as well as other solutes such as glucose and oxygen. Sodium (Na^+), chloride (Cl^-), and bicarbonate (HCO_3^-) are the principal extracellular electrolytes. The high sodium concentration in ECF is essential to regulating body fluid volume. The concentration of potassium in ECF is low. There is a minimal difference in electrolyte concentration between plasma and interstitial fluid. Normal values for electrolytes in plasma are shown in Table 10–2.

The body fluid compartments are separated by cell membranes and epithelial membranes. The cell membrane is selectively permeable; that is, it allows the passage of water, oxygen, carbon dioxide, and small water-soluble molecules, but bars proteins and other intracellular colloids. Capillary membranes separate plasma from interstitial fluid. The capillary membrane separating the plasma from the interstitial space is made of squamous epithelial cells. Pores in the membrane allow solute molecules (such as glucose and sodium), dissolved gases, and

TABLE 10–2 Normal Values for Electrolytes and Serum Osmolality

SERUM COMPONENT	VALUES	
	CONVENTIONAL	SI
Electrolytes		
Sodium (Na^+)	135–145 mEq/L	135–145 mmol/L
Chloride (Cl^-)	98–106 mEq/L	98–106 mmol/L
Bicarbonate (HCO_3^-)	22–26 mEq/L	22–26 mmol/L
Calcium (Ca^{2+}) (total)	8.5–10.0 mg/dL	2.1–2.6 mmol/L
Potassium (K^+)	3.5–5.0 mEq/L	3.5–5.0 mmol/L
Phosphate/inorganic phosphorus (PO_4^{-2})	1.7–2.6 mEq/L (2.5–4.5 mg/dL)	0.8–1.5 mmol/L
Magnesium (Mg^{2+})	1.6–2.6 mg/dL (1.3–2.1 mEq/L)	0.8–1.3 mmol/L
Serum osmolality	275–295 mOsm/kg	275–295 mmol/kg

water to cross the membrane. Epithelial membranes separate transcellular fluid from interstitial fluid and plasma. These membranes include the mucosa of the stomach, intestines, and gallbladder; the pleural, peritoneal, and synovial membranes; and the tubules of the kidney.

Body Fluid Movement

Four chemical and physiologic processes control the movement of fluid, electrolytes, and other molecules across membranes between the intracellular and interstitial space and the interstitial space and plasma. These processes are osmosis, diffusion, filtration, and active transport.

OSMOSIS Osmosis is the process by which water moves across a selectively permeable membrane from an area of lower solute concentration to an area of higher solute concentration (Figure 10–3 ■). A selectively permeable membrane allows water molecules to cross but is relatively impermeable to dissolved substances (solutes). Osmosis continues until the solute concentration on both sides of the membrane is equal. For example, if pure water and a sodium chloride solution are separated by a selectively permeable membrane, then water molecules will move across the membrane to the sodium chloride solution. Osmosis is the primary process that controls body fluid movement between the ICF and ECF compartments.

Osmolality Osmolality, or concentration of a solution, refers to the number of solutes per kilogram of water (by weight); it is reported in milliosmoles per kilogram (mOsm/kg). The osmolality of the ECF depends chiefly on sodium concentration. Serum osmolality may be estimated by doubling the serum sodium concentration (approximately 142 mEq/L). Glucose and urea contribute to the osmolality of ECF, although to a lesser extent than sodium.

Osmotic Pressure and Tonicity The power of a solution to draw water across a membrane is known as the osmotic pressure of the solution. The composition of interstitial fluid and intravascular plasma is essentially the same except for a higher concentration of proteins in the plasma. These proteins (especially albumin) exert colloid osmotic pressure (also called oncotic pressure), pulling fluid from the interstitial space into the intravascular compartment. Because the osmolality of intravascular and interstitial fluid is essentially identical, the osmotic activity of plasma proteins is important in maintaining fluid balance between the interstitial and intravascular spaces, helping hold water within the vascular system.

Tonicity refers to the effect a solution's osmotic pressure has on water movement across the cell membrane of cells within that solution. Isotonic solutions have the same concentration of solutes as plasma. Cells placed in an isotonic solution will neither shrink nor swell because there is no net gain or loss of water within the cell, and no change in cell volume (Figure 10–4A ■). Normal saline (0.9% sodium chloride solution) is an example of an isotonic solution.

Hypertonic solutions have a greater concentration of solutes than plasma. In their presence, water is drawn out of a cell, causing it to shrink (Figure 10–4B). A 3% sodium chloride solution is hypertonic. Hypotonic solutions (such as 0.45% sodium chloride) have a lower solute concentration than plasma (Figure 10–4C). When red blood cells are placed in a hypotonic solution, water moves into the cells, causing them to swell; rupture (hemolysis) of cells may occur with extremely hypotonic solutions.

The concepts of osmotic draw and tonicity are important in understanding the pathophysiologic changes that occur with fluid and electrolyte imbalances, as well as treatment measures. For example, an increased sodium concentration of extracellular fluid pulls water from the ICF compartment into the ECF compartment, causing cells to shrink. In this case, administering a hypotonic IV solution to reduce the sodium concentration and osmolality of ECF will facilitate water movement back into the cells.

DIFFUSION Diffusion is the process by which solute molecules move from an area of high solute concentration to an area of low solute concentration to become evenly distributed (Figure 10–5 ■). The two types of diffusion are simple and facilitated diffusion. Simple diffusion occurs by the random movement of particles through a solution. Water, carbon dioxide, oxygen, and solutes move between plasma and the interstitial space by simple diffusion through the capillary membrane. Water and solutes move into the cell by passing through protein channels or by dissolving in the lipid cell membrane. Facilitated diffusion, also called carrier-mediated diffusion, allows large water-soluble molecules, such as glucose and amino acids, to diffuse across cell membranes. Proteins embedded in the cell membrane function as carriers, helping large molecules cross the membrane. The rate of diffusion is influenced by a number of factors, such as the concentration of solute and the availability of carrier proteins in the cell membrane. The effect of both simple and facilitated diffusion is to establish equal concentrations of the molecules on both sides of a membrane.

FILTRATION Filtration is the process by which water and dissolved substances (solutes) move from an area of high hydrostatic pressure to an area of low hydrostatic pressure. This usually occurs across capillary membranes. Hydrostatic pressure

Higher solute concentration   Lower solute concentration

Dissolved substances   Selectively permeable membrane   Water molecules

Figure 10–3 ■ Osmosis. Water molecules move through a selectively permeable membrane from an area of low solute concentration to an area of high solute concentration.

Fluid Volume Deficit Animation

A Isotonic solution

B Hypertonic solution

C Hypotonic solution

Figure 10–4 ■ The effect of tonicity on red blood cells. *A,* In an isotonic solution, RBCs neither gain nor lose water, retaining their normal biconcave shape. *B,* In a hypertonic solution, cells lose water and shrink in size. *C,* In a hypotonic solution, cells absorb water and may burst (hemolysis).

is created by the pumping action of the heart and gravity against the capillary wall. Filtration occurs in the glomerulus of the kidneys, as well as at the arterial end of capillaries.

A balance of hydrostatic (filtration) pressure and osmotic pressure regulates the movement of water between the intravascular and interstitial spaces in the capillary beds of the body. Hydrostatic pressure within the arterial end of the capillary pushes water into the interstitial space. At the venous end of the capillary, the osmotic force of plasma proteins draws fluid back into the capillary (Figure 10–6 ■).

ACTIVE TRANSPORT Active transport allows molecules to move across cell membranes and epithelial membranes against a concentration gradient. This movement requires energy (adenosine triphosphate [ATP]) and a carrier mechanism to maintain a higher concentration of a substance on one side of the membrane than on the other. The sodium-potassium pump is an important example of active transport (Figure 10–7 ■). High concentrations of potassium in intracellular fluids and of sodium in extracellular fluids are maintained because cells actively transport potassium from interstitial fluid into intracellular fluid.

Figure 10–5 ■ Diffusion. Solute molecules move through a semipermeable membrane from an area of high solute concentration to an area of low solute concentration.

Body Fluid Regulation

Homeostasis requires several regulatory mechanisms and processes to maintain the balance between fluid intake and excretion. These include thirst, the kidneys, the renin–angiotensin–aldosterone mechanism, antidiuretic hormone, and atrial natriuretic peptide. These mechanisms affect the volume, distribution, and composition of body fluids.

Thirst

Thirst is the primary regulator of water intake. Thirst plays an important role in maintaining fluid balance and preventing dehydration. The thirst center, located in the hypothalamus, is stimulated when the blood volume drops because of water losses or when serum osmolality increases. The thirst mechanism is highly effective in regulating extracellular sodium levels. Increased sodium in ECF increases serum osmolality, stimulating the thirst center. Fluid intake in turn reduces the sodium concentration of ECF and lowers serum osmolality. Conversely, a drop in serum sodium and low serum osmolality inhibit the thirst center.

> ### PRACTICE ALERT
> The thirst mechanism declines with aging, making older adults more vulnerable to dehydration and hyperosmolality. Patients with an altered level of consciousness or who are unable to respond to thirst, such as intubated patients and artificially fed patients, are also at risk.

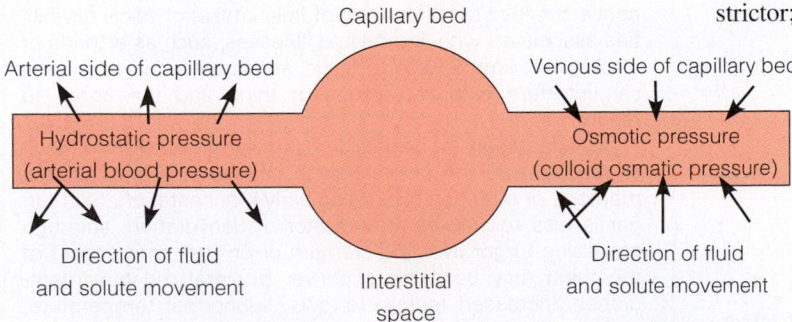

Figure 10–6 ■ Fluid balance between the intravascular and interstitial spaces is maintained in the capillary beds by a balance of filtration at the arterial end and osmotic draw at the venous end.

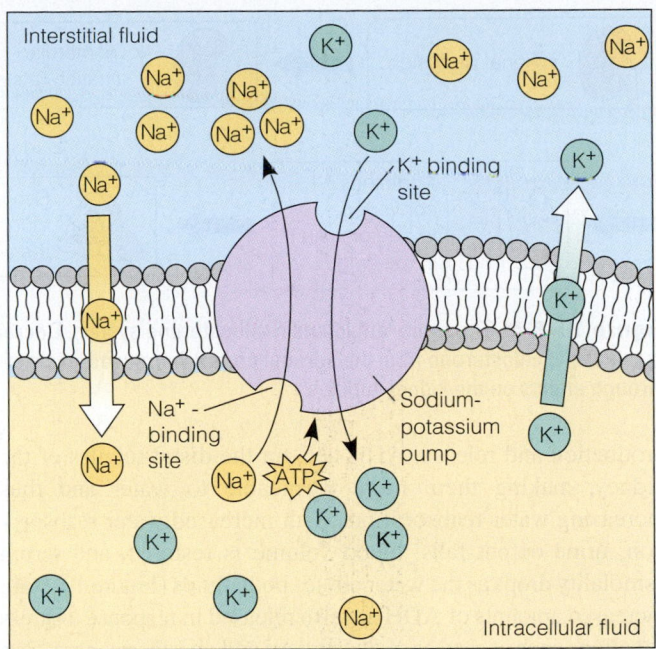

Figure 10–7 ■ The sodium-potassium pump. Sodium and potassium ions are moved across the cell membranes against their concentration gradients. This active transport process is fueled by energy from ATP.

Kidneys

The kidneys are primarily responsible for regulating fluid volume and electrolyte balance in the body. They regulate the volume and osmolality of body fluids by controlling the excretion of water and electrolytes. In adults, about 170 L of plasma are filtered through the glomeruli every day. By selectively reabsorbing water and electrolytes, the kidneys maintain the volume and osmolality of body fluids. About 99% of the glomerular filtrate is reabsorbed, and only about 1500 mL of urine is produced over a 24-hour period (Porth & Matfin, 2009).

Renin–Angiotensin–Aldosterone System

The renin–angiotensin–aldosterone system helps to maintain intravascular fluid balance and blood pressure. A decrease in blood flow or blood pressure to the kidneys stimulates specialized receptors in the juxtaglomerular cells of the nephrons to produce renin, an enzyme. Renin converts angiotensinogen (a plasma protein) in the circulating blood into angiotensin I. Angiotensin I travels through the bloodstream to the lungs where it is converted to angiotensin II by angiotensin-converting enzyme (ACE). Angiotensin II is a potent vasoconstrictor; it raises the blood pressure. It also stimulates the thirst mechanism to promote fluid intake and acts directly on the kidneys, causing them to retain sodium and water. Angiotensin II stimulates the adrenal cortex to release aldosterone. Aldosterone promotes sodium and water retention in the distal nephron of the kidney, restoring blood volume (Figure 10–8 ■).

Antidiuretic Hormone

Antidiuretic hormone (ADH), released by the posterior pituitary gland, regulates water excretion from the kidneys. Osmoreceptors in the hypothalamus respond to increases in serum osmolality and decreases in blood volume, stimulating ADH

Respiratory Acidosis Animation

Figure 10–8 ■ The renin–angiotensin–aldosterone system. Decreased blood volume and renal perfusion set off a chain of reactions leading to release of aldosterone from the adrenal cortex. Increased levels of aldosterone regulate serum K⁺ and Na⁺, blood pressure, and water balance through effects on the kidney tubules.

production and release. ADH acts on the distal tubules of the kidney, making them more permeable to water and thus increasing water reabsorption. With increased water reabsorption, urine output falls, blood volume is restored, and serum osmolality drops as the water dilutes body fluids (Figure 10–9 ■). Increased amounts of ADH are also released in response to stress situations such as nausea, pain, surgery and anesthesia, narcotics, and nicotine. Its release is inhibited by alcohol and medications such as phenytoin, as well as by increased blood volume and decreased serum osmolality (Porth, 2007).

Atrial Natriuretic Peptide

Atrial natriuretic peptide (ANP) is a hormone released by atrial muscle cells in response to distention from fluid overload. ANP affects several body systems, including the cardiovascular, renal, neural, GI, and endocrine systems, but it primarily opposes the renin–angiotensin–aldosterone system by inhibiting renin secretion and blocking the secretion and sodium-retaining effects of aldosterone. As a result, ANP promotes sodium wasting and increased urine output.

Figure 10–9 ■ Antidiuretic hormone (ADH) release and effect. Increased serum osmolality or a fall in blood volume stimulates the release of ADH from the posterior pituitary. ADH increases the permeability of distal tubules, promoting water reabsorption.

NURSING CARE OF THE OLDER ADULT **Fluid Volume Deficit**

Changes in the normal aging process affect homeostasis in several ways. In older adults, the percentage of total body water is about 10% lower than in younger or middle-aged adults, and thus they have less body reserve. Lean muscle mass is lower in older adults, and the percentage of body fat is higher; as a result water accounts for about 50% of the total body weight (TBW) of an older man and about 45% TBW of an older woman (Porth & Matfin, 2009). Sodium and water regulation become less efficient with aging. Renal blood flow and glomerular filtration decline with aging; the kidneys are less able to effectively concentrate the urine and conserve sodium and water. The perception of thirst decreases, interfering with the thirst mechanism. Consequently, the older adult may become dehydrated without being aware of the need to increase fluid intake.

Undetected fever in older adults can increase the total body need for water with every degree of temperature. Dehydration can cause a fever and further compound dehydration in the older adult. Older adults who have self-care deficits, or who are confused, depressed, tube fed, on bed rest, or taking medications (such as sedatives, tranquilizers, diuretics, and laxatives) are at greatest risk for fluid volume imbalance. Older adults without air conditioning are at risk during extremely hot weather. In addition, functional changes and illnesses can affect fluid balance. For example, fear of incontinence can lead to self-limiting of fluid intake; physical disabilities associated with age-related illnesses, such as arthritis or stroke, may limit access to fluids; and cognitive impairments can interfere with recognition of thirst and the ability to respond to it.

Manifestations of fluid volume deficit may be more difficult to recognize in the older adult. A change in mental status, memory, or attention may be an early manifestation. Skin turgor is less reliable as an indicator of dehydration, although assessing turgor over the sternum or on the inner aspect of the thigh may be more effective. Dry oral mucous membranes, increased tongue furrows, subnormal temperature, tachycardia, and a pinched facial expression are also indicative of dehydration. Orthostatic vital signs may not demonstrate typical changes in the dehydrated older adult.

Fluid and Electrolyte Imbalances

Fluid Imbalance

The Patient with a Fluid Volume Deficit

Fluid volume deficit (FVD) is a decrease in intravascular, interstitial, and/or intracellular fluid in the body. Fluid volume deficits may be the result of excessive fluid losses, insufficient fluid intake, or failure of regulatory mechanisms and fluid shifts within the body. FVD is a relatively common problem that may exist alone or in combination with other electrolyte or acid–base imbalances. The term **dehydration** refers to loss of water alone, even though it often is used interchangeably with fluid volume deficit.

Pathophysiology

The most common cause of fluid volume deficit is excessive loss of GI fluids from vomiting, diarrhea, GI suctioning, intestinal fistulas, and intestinal drainage. Other causes of fluid losses include diuretics, renal disorders, endocrine disorders, excessive exercise, hot environment, hemorrhage, and chronic abuse of laxatives and/or enemas. Other factors involved in inadequate fluid intake include inability to access fluids, inability to request or to swallow fluids, oral trauma, or altered thirst mechanisms. Older adults are at particular risk for fluid volume deficit (see the Nursing Care of the Older Adult box on page 192).

Fluid volume deficit can develop slowly or rapidly, depending on the type of fluid loss. Loss of extracellular fluid volume can lead to hypovolemia, decreased circulating blood volume. Electrolytes often are lost along with fluid, resulting in an isotonic fluid volume deficit. When both water and electrolytes are lost, the serum sodium level remains normal, although levels of other electrolytes such as potassium may fall. Fluid is drawn into the vascular compartment from the interstitial spaces as the body attempts to maintain tissue perfusion. This eventually depletes fluid in the intracellular compartment as well.

Hypovolemia stimulates regulatory mechanisms to maintain circulation. The sympathetic nervous system is stimulated, as is the thirst mechanism. ADH and aldosterone are released, prompting sodium and water retention by the kidneys. Severe fluid loss, as in hemorrhage, can lead to shock and cardiovascular collapse.

THIRD SPACING   **Third spacing** is a shift of fluid from the vascular space into an area where it is not available to support normal physiologic processes. Fluid may be sequestered in the abdomen or bowel, or in other actual or potential body spaces as the pleural or peritoneal space. Fluid may also become trapped within soft tissues following trauma or burns. The trapped fluid represents a volume loss and is unavailable for normal physiologic processes.

In many cases, fluid is sequestered in interstitial tissues and is unavailable to support cardiovascular function. As an example, surgery triggers adaptive stress responses and the release of stress hormones (ACTH, cortisol, and catecholamines). These hormones increase blood glucose levels to provide increased fuel for metabolic processes and promote vasoconstriction that redistributes blood to vital organs (the heart and brain). Renal blood flow falls, stimulating the renin–angiotensin–aldosterone system. This promotes sodium and water retention to maintain intravascular volume. The blood vessel and tissue damage caused by surgery stimulate the release of inflammatory mediators such as histamine and prostaglandins. These substances lead to local vasodilation and increased capillary permeability, allowing fluid to accumulate in interstitial tissues.

Assessing the extent of FVD resulting from third spacing is difficult. It may not be reflected in weight or intake and output records, and it may not become apparent until after organ malfunction occurs. Daily weights may be helpful in uncovering third spaced fluids; however, due to fluid or weight loss due to disease processes, these gains may be obscured. Delays in recognition and treatment can lead to irreversible shock and multiorgan system failure (Perrin, 2009).

Manifestations

With a rapid fluid loss (such as hemorrhage or uncontrolled vomiting), manifestations of hypovolemia develop rapidly. When the loss of fluid occurs more gradually, the patient's fluid volume may be very low before manifestations develop. See the Multisystem Effects of Fluid Volume Deficit feature on page 194.

Rapid weight loss is a good indicator of fluid volume deficit. Each liter of body fluid weighs about 1 kg (2.2 lb). The severity of the fluid volume deficit can be estimated by the percentage of rapid weight loss: A loss of 2% of body weight represents a mild FVD; 5%, moderate FVD; and 8% or greater, severe FVD (Metheny, 2000). Loss of interstitial fluid causes skin turgor to diminish. When pinched, the skin of a patient with FVD remains elevated. Postural or orthostatic hypotension is a sign of hypovolemia. A drop of more than 15 mmHg in systolic blood pressure when changing from a lying to standing position often indicates loss of intravascular volume. Venous pressure falls as well, causing flat neck veins, even when the patient is recumbent. Compensatory mechanisms to conserve water and sodium and maintain circulation account for many of the manifestations of fluid volume deficit, such as tachycardia; pale, cool skin (vasoconstriction); and decreased urine output. The specific gravity of urine increases as water is reabsorbed in the tubules. Table 10–3 compares manifestations of fluid imbalances.

Interdisciplinary Care

The primary goals of care are to prevent deficits in patients at risk and to correct deficits and their underlying causes. Depending on the acuity of the imbalance, treatment may include replacement of fluids and electrolytes by the IV, oral, or enteral route. When possible, the oral or enteral route is preferred for administering fluids. In acute situations, however, IV fluid administration is necessary.

Diagnosis

Laboratory and diagnostic tests may be ordered when fluid volume deficit is suspected. Such tests measure the following:

■ *Serum electrolytes.* In an isotonic fluid deficit, sodium levels are within normal limits; when the loss is water only, sodium levels are high. Decreases in potassium are common.

MULTISYSTEM EFFECTS OF
Fluid Volume Deficit

Neurologic
- Altered mental status
- Anxiety, restlessness
- Diminished alertness/cognition
- Possible coma (severe FVD)

Mucous Membranes
- Dry; may be sticky
- ↓ tongue size, longitudinal furrows ↑

Integumentary
- Diminished skin turgor
- Dry skin
- Pale, cool extremities

Urinary
- ↓ urine output
- Oliguria (severe FVD)
- ↑ urine specific gravity

Cardiovascular
- Tachycardia
- Orthostatic hypotension (moderate FVD)
- Falling systolic/diastolic pressure (severe FVD)
- Flat neck veins
- ↓ venous filling
- ↓ pulse volume
- ↓ capillary refill
- ↑ hematocrit

Potential Complication
- Hypovolemic shock

Musculoskeletal
- Fatigue

Metabolic Processes
- ↓ body temperature (isotonic FVD)
- ↑ body temperature (dehydration)
- Thirst
- Weight loss
  2–5% mild FVD
  6–9% moderate FVD
  >10% severe FVD

TABLE 10–3 Comparison of the Manifestations of Fluid Imbalance

ASSESSMENT	FLUID DEFICIT	FLUID EXCESS
Blood pressure	Decreased systolic	Increased
	Postural hypotension	
Heart rate	Increased	Increased
Pulse amplitude	Decreased	Increased
Respirations	Normal	Moist crackles
		Wheezes
Jugular vein	Flat	Distended
Edema	Rare	Dependent
Skin turgor	Loose, poor turgor	Taut
Output	Low, concentrated	May be low or normal
Urine specific gravity	High	Low
Weight	Loss	Gain

- *Serum osmolality.* Measurement of serum osmolality helps to differentiate isotonic fluid loss from water loss. With water loss, osmolality is high; it may be within normal limits with an isotonic fluid loss.
- *Hemoglobin and hematocrit.* The hematocrit often is elevated due to loss of intravascular volume and hemoconcentration.
- *Urine specific gravity and osmolality.* As the kidneys conserve water, both the specific gravity and osmolality of urine increase.
- *Central venous pressure (CVP).* The CVP measures the mean pressure in the superior vena cava or right atrium, providing an accurate assessment of fluid volume status. The technique for measuring CVP is described in ∞ Chapter 31.

Fluid Management

Oral rehydration is the safest and most effective treatment for fluid volume deficit in alert patients who are able to take oral fluids. Adults require a minimum of 1500 mL of fluid per day or approximately 30 mL per kg of body weight (ideal body weight is used to calculate fluid requirements for obese patients) for maintenance. Fluids are replaced gradually, particularly in older adults, to prevent rapid rehydration of the cells.

For mild fluid deficits in which a loss of electrolytes has been minimal (e.g., moderate exercise in warm weather), water alone may be used for fluid replacement. When the fluid deficit is more severe and when electrolytes have also been lost (e.g., FVD due to vomiting and/or diarrhea, strenuous exercise for longer than an hour or two), a carbohydrate/electrolyte solution such as a sports drink, ginger ale, or a rehydrating solution (e.g., Pedialyte or Rehydralyte) is more appropriate. These solutions provide sodium, potassium, chloride, and calories to help meet metabolic needs.

IV THERAPY When the fluid deficit is severe or the patient is unable to ingest fluids, the IV route is used to administer replacement fluids. Table 10–4 describes commonly administered IV fluids with nursing implications. Isotonic electrolyte solutions (0.9% NaCl or Ringer's solution) are used to expand plasma volume in hypotensive patients or to replace abnormal losses, which are usually isotonic in nature. Normal saline (0.9% NaCl) tends to remain in the vascular compartment, increasing blood volume. When administered rapidly, however, this solution can precipitate acid–base imbalances, so balanced electrolyte solutions such as Lactated Ringer's solution are preferred to expand plasma volume.

Five percent dextrose in 0.45% saline (D_5 1/2; NS) or 0.45% NaCl (one-half normal saline or 1/2 NS) are given to provide water to treat total body water deficits. D_5W, although isotonic in the bag, is not used for fluid resuscitation as the dextrose is rapidly metabolized and the subsequent fluid is hypotonic (David, 2007). Saline solution (0.45% NaCl with or without added electrolytes) or 5% dextrose in 0.45% sodium chloride (D_5 1/2 NS) are used as maintenance solutions. These solutions provide additional electrolytes such as potassium, a buffer (lactate or acetate) as needed, and water. When dextrose is added, they also provide a minimal number of calories.

∞ Nursing Care

Nurses are responsible for identifying patients at risk for fluid volume deficit, initiating and carrying out interventions to prevent and treat fluid volume deficit, and monitoring the effects of therapy.

Health Promotion

Health promotion activities focus on teaching to prevent fluid volume deficit. Discuss the importance of maintaining adequate fluid intake, particularly when exercising and during hot weather. Advise patients to use commercial sports drinks to replace both water and electrolytes when exercising during warm weather. Instruct patients to maintain fluid intake when ill, particularly during periods of fever or when diarrhea is a problem.

Carefully monitor the intake and output of patients at risk for abnormal fluid losses through vomiting, diarrhea, nasogastric suction, increased urine output, fever, or draining wounds. Monitor

TABLE 10–4 Commonly Administered IV Fluids with Nursing Implications

I. Isotonic Solutions

0.9% Saline
Lactated Ringer's solution

- Monitor for fluid overload; if manifestations occur, discontinue fluids and notify the healthcare provider.
- Do not administer lactated Ringer's solution to patients with severe liver disease as the liver may be unable to convert the lactate to bicarbonate and the patient may become acidotic. Do not administer if the patient has a blood pH of > 7.50.
- If administering lactated Ringer's solution, monitor potassium levels and cardiac rhythm; if abnormals are present, notify the healthcare provider.

II. Hypotonic Solutions

0.45% saline or 0.25% saline
D_5W

- Monitor for inflammation and infiltration at IV insertion site as hypotonic solutions may cause cells to swell and burst, including those at the insertions site; this narrows the lumen of the vein.
- Monitor blood sodium levels.
- Do not administer to patients at risk for increased intracranial pressure (e.g., head trauma, stroke, neurosurgery).
- Do not administer to patients at risk for third-space shifts (burns, trauma, liver disease, malnutrition).

III. Hypertonic Solutions

Hypertonic fluids have a tonicity > 350 mEq/L and include the following:
Fluids containing medications
D_5W sodium chloride
D_5W in lactated Ringer's solution
Total parenteral solutions

- Monitor for inflammation and infiltration at IV insertion site as hypertonic solutions cause cells to shrink, exposing the basement membrane of the vein.
- Monitor blood sodium levels.
- Monitor for circulatory overload.
- Do not administer to patients with diabetic ketoacidosis or impaired cardiac or kidney function.

Clinical alert: The Infusion Nurses Society mandates that all fluids with a tonicity exceeding 500 mEq/L be infused through a central venous access device; this includes $D_{10}W$, 5% protein hydrolysate, or a high electrolyte solution.

Adapted from David, K. (2007). *IV fluids: Do you know what's hanging and why?* RN Web and AHA Media LLC; Hogan, M., Gringrich, M., Overby, P., & Ricci, M. (2007). *Fluids, electrolytes, & acid–base balance* (2nd ed). Upper Saddle River, NJ: Pearson Prentice Hall; and Rosenthal, K., (2009). *Tonicity and IV fluids.* Resource Nurse.com.

fluid intake in patients with decreased level of consciousness, disorientation, nausea, anorexia, and physical limitations.

Assessment

Collect assessment data through the health history interview and physical examination.

- *Health history:* Risk factors such as medications, acute or chronic renal or endocrine disease; precipitating factors such as hot weather, extensive exercise, lack of access to fluids, recent illness (especially if accompanied by fever, vomiting, and/or diarrhea); onset and duration of manifestations.
- *Physical assessment:* Weight; vital signs including orthostatic blood pressure and pulse; peripheral pulses and capillary refill; jugular neck vein distention; skin color, temperature, turgor; level of consciousness and mentation; urine output. Allow the older adult to stand quietly for a full minute before rechecking blood pressure and pulse when measuring orthostatic vital signs.

Nursing Diagnoses and Interventions

Nursing diagnoses and interventions for the patient with fluid volume deficit focus on managing the effects of the deficit and preventing complications.

Deficient Fluid Volume

Patients with a fluid volume deficit due to abnormal losses, inadequate intake, or impaired fluid regulation require close monitoring as well as immediate and ongoing fluid replacement.

- Assess intake and output accurately, monitoring fluid balance. In acute situations, hourly intake and output may be indicated. *Urine output should normally be 30 to 60 mL per hour. Urine output of less than 30 mL per hour in adults indicates inadequate renal perfusion and an increased risk for acute renal failure and inadequate tissue perfusion (Perrin, 2009).*

> **PRACTICE ALERT**
> Report a urine output of less than 30 mL per hour to the patient's healthcare provider.

- Assess vital signs, CVP, and peripheral pulse volume at least every 4 hours. *Hypotension, tachycardia, low CVP, and weak, easily obliterated peripheral pulses indicate hypovolemia.*
- Weigh daily under standard conditions (time of day, clothing, and scale). *In most instances (except third spacing), changes in weight accurately reflect fluid balance.*

- Administer and monitor the intake of oral fluids as prescribed. Identify beverage preferences and provide these on a schedule. *Oral fluid replacement is preferred when the patient is able to drink and retain fluids.*
- Administer IV fluids as prescribed using an infusion pump. Monitor for indicators of fluid overload if rapid fluid replacement is ordered: dyspnea, tachypnea, tachycardia, increased CVP, jugular vein distention, and edema. *Rapid fluid replacement may lead to hypervolemia, resulting in pulmonary edema and cardiac failure, particularly in patients with compromised cardiac and renal function.*
- Monitor laboratory values: electrolytes, serum osmolality, blood urea nitrogen (BUN), and hematocrit. *Rehydration may lead to changes in serum electrolytes, osmolality, BUN, and hematocrit. In some cases, electrolyte replacement may be necessary during rehydration.*

Ineffective Tissue Perfusion

A fluid volume deficit can lead to decreased perfusion of renal, cerebral, and peripheral tissues. Inadequate renal perfusion can lead to acute renal failure. Decreased cerebral perfusion leads to changes in mental status and cognitive function, causing restlessness, anxiety, agitation, excitability, confusion, vertigo, fainting, and weakness.

- Monitor for changes in level of consciousness and mental status. *Restlessness, anxiety, confusion, and agitation may indicate inadequate cerebral blood flow and circulatory collapse.*
- Monitor serum creatinine, BUN, and cardiac enzymes, reporting elevated levels to the physician. *Elevated levels may indicate impaired renal function or cardiac perfusion related to circulatory failure.*
- Turn at least every 2 hours. Provide good skin care and monitor for evidence of skin or tissue breakdown. *Impaired circulation to peripheral tissues increases the risk of skin breakdown. Turn frequently to relieve pressure over bony prominences. Keep skin clean, dry, and moisturized to help maintain integrity.*

Risk for Injury

The patient with fluid volume deficit is at risk for injury because of dizziness and loss of balance resulting from decreased cerebral perfusion secondary to hypovolemia.

- Institute safety precautions, including keeping the bed in a low position, using side rails as needed, and slowly raising the patient from supine to sitting or sitting to standing position. *Using safety precautions and allowing time for the blood pressure to adjust to position changes reduce the risk of injury.*
- Teach patient and family members how to reduce orthostatic hypotension:
  a. Move from one position to another in stages; for example, raise the head of the bed before sitting up, and sit for a few minutes before standing.
  b. Avoid prolonged standing.
  c. Rest in a recliner rather than in bed during the day.
  d. Use assistive devices to pick up objects from the floor rather than stooping.

Teaching measures to reduce orthostatic hypotension reduces the patient's risk for injury. Prolonged bed rest increases skeletal muscle weakness and decreases venous tone, contributing to postural hypotension. Prolonged standing allows blood to pool in the legs, reducing venous return and cardiac output.

Using NANDA, NIC, and NOC

Linkages between a selected NANDA nursing diagnosis, NIC, and NOC for the patient with fluid volume deficit are shown in the chart that follows.

Community-Based Care

Depending on the severity of the fluid volume deficit, the patient may be managed in the home or long-term care facility, or may be admitted as a hospital inpatient. Assess the patient's understanding of the cause of the deficit and the fluids necessary for providing replacement. Address the following topics when preparing the patient and family for home care:

- The importance of maintaining adequate fluid intake (at least 1500 mL per day; more if extra fluid is being lost through perspiration, fever, or diarrhea)
- Manifestations of fluid imbalance, and how to monitor fluid balance
- How to prevent fluid deficit:
  - Avoid exercising during extreme heat.
  - Increase fluid intake during hot weather.
  - If vomiting, take small frequent amounts of ice chips or clear liquids, such as weak tea, flat cola, or ginger ale.
  - Reduce intake of coffee, tea, and alcohol, which increase urine output and can cause fluid loss.
- Replacement of fluids lost through diarrhea with fruit juices or bouillon, rather than large amounts of tap water
- Alternate sources of fluid (such as gelatin, frozen juices, or ice cream) for effective replacement of lost fluids.

NANDA, NIC, AND NOC LINKAGES
The Patient with Fluid Volume Deficit

NANDA Deficient Fluid Volume

NIC
Fluid Management
Fluid Monitoring
Hypovolemia Management
IV (IV) Therapy
Shock Management: Volume

NOC
Vital Signs
Fluid Balance
Hydration

Data from NANDA International. (2009). *Nursing diagnoses: Definitions & classification 2009–2011.* Oxford, UK: Wiley-Blackwell; Bulechek, G., Butcher, H., Dochterman, K. (Eds.). (2008). *Nursing interventions classification (NIC)* (5th ed.). (pp. 370–371, 372, 420–421, 441, 655), St. Louis: Elsevier Mosby; and Moorhead, M., Johnson, M., Maas, M., and Swanson, E. (Eds.). (2008). *Nursing outcomes classification (NOC)* (4th ed.) (p. 771). St. Louis: Elsevier Mosby.

The Patient with Fluid Volume Excess

Fluid volume excess results when both water and sodium are retained in the body. Fluid volume excess may be caused by fluid overload (excess water and sodium intake) or by impairment of the mechanisms that maintain homeostasis. The excess fluid can lead to excess intravascular fluid (hypervolemia) and excess interstitial fluid (edema).

Pathophysiology

Fluid volume excess usually results from conditions that cause retention of both sodium and water. These conditions include heart failure, cirrhosis of the liver, renal failure, adrenal gland disorders, corticosteroid administration, and stress conditions causing the release of ADH and aldosterone. Other causes include an excessive intake of sodium-containing foods, drugs that cause sodium retention, and the administration of excess amounts of sodium-containing IV fluids (such as 0.9% NaCl or Ringer's solution). This *iatrogenic* (induced by the effects of treatment) cause of fluid volume excess primarily affects patients with impaired regulatory mechanisms.

In fluid volume excess, both water and sodium are gained in about the same proportions as normally exists in extracellular fluid. The total body sodium content is increased, which in turn causes an increase in total body water. Because the increase in sodium and water is isotonic, the serum sodium and osmolality remain normal, and the excess fluid remains in the extracellular space.

Stress responses activated before, during, and immediately after surgery commonly lead to increased ADH and aldosterone levels, leading to sodium and water retention. In the immediate postoperative period, however, this additional fluid tends to be sequestered in interstitial tissues and unavailable to support cardiovascular and renal function (see the earlier Third Spacing section in this chapter). This sequestered fluid is reabsorbed into the circulation within about 48 to 72 hours after surgery. Although it is then normally eliminated through a process of diuresis, patients with heart or kidney failure are at risk for developing fluid overload.

Manifestations

Excess extracellular fluid leads to hypervolemia and circulatory overload. Excess fluid in the interstitial space causes peripheral or generalized edema. The manifestations of fluid volume excess relate to both the excess fluid and its effects on circulation. Manifestations of fluid volume excess with related pathophysiology are described in the table below.

Complications

Congestive heart failure (CHF) is not only a potential cause of fluid volume excess, but it is also a potential complication of the condition if the heart is unable to increase its workload to handle the excess blood volume. Severe fluid overload and CHF can lead to pulmonary edema, a medical emergency. ∞ See Chapter 31 for information about CHF and pulmonary edema.

Interdisciplinary Care

Managing fluid volume excess focuses on prevention in patients at risk, treating its manifestations, and correcting the underlying cause. Management includes limiting sodium and water intake and administering diuretics.

PATHOPHYSIOLOGY LINKAGE   Fluid Volume Excess

MANIFESTATIONS	RELATED PATHOPHYSIOLOGY
Peripheral edema, or if severe, anasarca (severe, generalized edema)	Excess fluid in the interstitial spaces, usually resulting from conditions that cause retention of both sodium and water (heart failure, cirrhosis of the liver, renal failure, adrenal gland disorders, corticosteroid administration, and stress conditions causing the release of ADH and aldosterone, such as surgery)
Full bounding pulse, distended neck and peripheral veins, increased central venous pressure (>11–12 cm of water), cough, dyspnea (labored or difficult breathing), **orthopnea** (difficult breathing when supine)	Circulatory overload from increased water and sodium retention
Dyspnea at rest	Impaired gas exchange from pulmonary interstitial edema
Tachycardia and hypertension	Increased circulatory fluid volume
Reduced oxygen saturation	As fluid increases in the interstitial spaces and alveoli, gas exchange is impaired, leading to hypoxia and hypercapnia
Moist crackles on auscultation of the lungs, pulmonary edema	Excess fluid in pulmonary interstitial spaces and alveoli
Increased urine output (polyuria)	Increased sodium and water retention resulting in increased circulatory volume and increased perfusion of the renal arteries
Ascites (excess fluid in the peritoneal cavity)	Sodium and water retention
Decreased hematocrit and BUN	Dilutional effect of increased circulatory volume
Altered mental status and anxiety	Pressure on the cerebral cortex from an increase in cerebral contents and cerebral hypertension causes decreased oxygenation (hypoxia) of neurons
Pulmonary edema	Elevation of left-sided filling pressures resulting from increased circulatory volume and heart failure

Diagnosis

The following laboratory tests may be ordered.

- *Serum electrolytes* and *serum osmolality* are measured, but usually remain within normal limits.
- *Serum hematocrit* and *hemoglobin* often are decreased due to plasma dilution from excess extracellular fluid.

Additional tests of *renal* and *liver function* (such as serum creatinine, BUN, and liver enzymes) may be ordered to help determine the cause of fluid volume excess.

Medications

Diuretics are commonly used to treat fluid volume excess. They inhibit sodium and water reabsorption, increasing urine output. The three major classes of diuretics, each of which acts on a different part of the kidney tubule, are as follows:

- Loop diuretics act in the ascending loop of Henle.
- Thiazide-type diuretics act on the distal convoluted tubule.
- Potassium-sparing diuretics affect the distal nephron.

The nursing implications for diuretics are outlined in the following Medication Administration box.

Treatments

FLUID MANAGEMENT Fluid intake may be restricted in patients who have fluid volume excess. The amount of fluid allowed per day is prescribed by the primary care provider. All fluid intake must be calculated, including meals and that used to administer medications orally or IV. Box 10–1 provides guidelines for hospitalized patients with a fluid restriction.

PRACTICE ALERT

Recommendations for oral care in the critically ill:
- Brush teeth, gums and tongue at least twice a day using a soft pediatric or adult toothbrush.
- Provide oral moisturizing to oral mucosa and lips every 2–4 hours.
- Use an oral chlorhexidine gluconate (0.12%) rinse twice a day during the perioperative period for adult patients who undergo cardiac surgery (American Association of Critical Care Nurses, 2007).

DIETARY MANAGEMENT Because sodium retention is a primary cause of fluid volume excess, a sodium-restricted diet often is prescribed. The primary dietary sources of sodium are the salt shaker, processed foods, and foods themselves.

A mild sodium restriction can be achieved by instructing the patient and primary food preparer in the household to reduce the amount of salt in recipes by half, avoid using the salt shaker during meals, and avoid foods that contain high levels of sodium (either naturally or because of processing). In moderate and severely sodium-restricted diets, salt is avoided altogether, as are all foods containing significant amounts of sodium.

MEDICATION ADMINISTRATION — Diuretics for Fluid Volume Excess

Diuretics increase urinary excretion of water and sodium. They are categorized into three major groups: loop diuretics, thiazide and thiazide-like diuretics, and potassium-sparing diuretics. Diuretics are used to enhance renal function and to treat vascular fluid overload and edema. Common side effects include orthostatic hypotension, dehydration, electrolyte imbalance, and possible hyperglycemia. Diuretics should be used with caution in the older adult. Examples of each major type follow.

LOOP DIURETICS

Furosemide (Lasix)

Ethacrynic Acid (Edecrin)

Bumetanide (Bumex)

Torsemide (Demadex)

Loop diuretics inhibit sodium and chloride reabsorption in the ascending loop of Henle (∞ see Chapter 26 for the anatomy of the kidneys). As a result, loop diuretics promote the excretion of sodium, chloride, potassium, and water.

THIAZIDE AND THIAZIDE-LIKE DIURETICS

Bendroflumethiazide (Naturetin)

Chlorothiazide (Diuril)

Hydrochlorothiazide (HydroDIURIL, Oretic)

Metolazone (Zaroxolyn)

Polythiazide (Renese)

Chlorthalidone (Hygroton)

Trichlormethiazide (Naqua)

Indapamide (Lozol)

xipamid (Xipamide)

Thiazide and thiazide-like diuretics promote the excretion of sodium, chloride, potassium, and water by decreasing absorption in the distal tubule.

POTASSIUM-SPARING DIURETICS

Spironolactone (Aldactone)

Amiloride HCl (Midamor)

Triamterene (Dyrenium)

Potassium-sparing diuretics promote excretion of sodium and water by inhibiting sodium-potassium exchange in the distal tubule.

NATRIURETIC PEPTIDE FAMILY

The natriuretic peptide family consists of atrial natriuretic peptide, brain natriuretic peptide, and C-type natriuretic peptide. Although the primary action of the natriuretic peptides is vasodilation, it has multiple effects on the kidneys including diuresis from renal hemodynamics and direct renal tubular effects.

Health Education for the Patient and Family

- The drug will increase the amount and frequency of urination.
- The drugs must be taken even when you feel well.
- Take the drugs in the morning and afternoon to avoid having to get up at night to urinate.
- Change position slowly to avoid dizziness.
- Report the following to your primary healthcare provider: dizziness; trouble breathing; or swelling of face, hands, or feet.
- Weigh yourself every day, and report sudden gains or losses.
- Avoid using the salt shaker when eating.
- If the drug increases potassium loss, consume foods high in potassium, such as orange juice and bananas.
- Do not use salt substitute if you are taking a potassium sparing diuretic.

BOX 10–1 Fluid Restriction Guidelines

- Subtract required fluids (e.g., ordered IV fluids, fluid used to dilute IV medications) from total daily allowance.
- Divide remaining fluid allowance—Day shift: 50% of total; Evening shift: 25% to 33% of total; Night shift: Remainder.
- Explain the fluid restriction to the patient and family members.
- Identify preferred fluids and intake pattern of patient.
- Place allowed amounts of fluid in small glasses (gives perception of a full glass).
- Offer ice chips (when melted, ice chips are approximately half the frozen volume).
- Provide frequent oral care.
- Provide sugarless chewing gum (if allowed) to reduce thirst sensation.

Examples of food high in sodium include lunch meat, bacon, cheese, dry cereal, canned soup, popcorn, ketchup, pickles, and seafood.

Nursing Care

Nursing care focuses on preventing fluid volume excess in patients at risk and on managing problems resulting from its effects.

Health Promotion

Health promotion related to fluid volume excess focuses on teaching preventive measures to patients who are at risk (e.g., patients who have heart disease or kidney failure). Discuss the relationship between sodium intake and water retention. Provide guidelines for a low-sodium diet, and teach patients to carefully read food labels to identify sodium in processed foods. Instruct patients at risk to weigh themselves on a regular basis, using the same scale, and to notify their primary care provider if they gain more than 5 lb in a week or less.

Assessment

Collect assessment data through the health history interview and physical examination.

- *Health history:* Risk factors such as medications, heart failure, acute or chronic renal or endocrine disease; precipitating factors such as a recent illness, change in diet, or change in medications. Recent weight gain; complaints of persistent cough, shortness of breath, swelling of feet and ankles, or difficulty sleeping when lying down.
- *Physical assessment:* Weight; vital signs; peripheral pulses and capillary refill; jugular neck vein distention; edema; lung sounds (crackles or wheezes), dyspnea, cough, and sputum; urine output; mental status.

Nursing Diagnoses and Interventions

Nursing diagnoses and interventions for the patient with fluid volume excess focus on the multisystem effects of the fluid overload.

Fluid Volume Excess

Nursing care for the patient with excess fluid volume includes collaborative interventions such as administering diuretics and maintaining a fluid restriction, as well as monitoring the status

and effects of the excess fluid volume. This is particularly critical in older patients because of the age-related decline in cardiac and renal compensatory responses.

- Assess vital signs, heart sounds, and volume of peripheral arteries. *Hypervolemia can cause hypertension, bounding peripheral pulses, and a third heart sound (S_3) due to the volume of blood flow through the hearts.*
- Assess for the presence and extent of edema, particularly in the lower extremities and the back, sacral, and periorbital areas. *Initially, edema affects the dependent portions of the body—the lower extremities of ambulatory patients and the sacrum in bedridden patients. Periorbital edema indicates more generalized edema.*

PRACTICE ALERT

Assess urine output hourly. Maintain accurate intake and output records. Note urine output of less than 30 mL per hour or a positive fluid balance on 24-hour total intake and output calculations. Congestive heart failure and inadequate renal perfusion may result in decreased urine output and fluid retention.

- Obtain daily weights at the same time of day, using approximately the same clothing and a balanced scale. *Daily weights are one of the most important gauges of fluid balance. Acute weight gain or loss represents fluid gain or loss. Weight gain of 2.2 lbs is equivalent to 1 L of fluid gain.*
- Administer oral fluids cautiously, adhering to any prescribed fluid restriction. Discuss the restriction with the patient and significant others, including the total volume allowed, the rationale, and the importance of reporting all fluid taken. *All sources of fluid intake, including ice chips, are recorded to avoid excess fluid intake.*
- Provide oral hygiene at least every 2 hours. *Oral hygiene contributes to patient comfort and keeps mucous membranes intact; it also helps relieve thirst if fluids are restricted.*
- Teach patient and significant others about the sodium-restricted diet (see Box 10–2), and emphasize the importance of checking before bringing foods to the patient. *Excess sodium promotes water retention; a sodium-restricted diet is ordered to reduce water gain.*
- Administer prescribed diuretics as ordered, monitoring the patient's response to therapy. *Loop or high-ceiling diuretics such as furosemide can lead to rapid fluid loss and manifestations of hypovolemia and electrolyte imbalance.*
- Promptly report significant changes in serum electrolytes or osmolality or abnormal results of tests done to determine contributing factors to the fluid volume excess. *Gradual correction of serum electrolytes and osmolality is expected; however, aggressive diuretic therapy can lead to overcorrection.*

Risk for Impaired Skin Integrity

Tissue edema decreases oxygen and nutrient delivery to the skin and subcutaneous tissues, increasing the risk of injury.

- Frequently assess skin, particularly in pressure areas and over bony prominences. *Skin breakdown can progress rapidly when circulation is impaired.*
- Reposition the patient at least every 2 hours. Provide skin care with each position change. *Frequent position changes minimize tissue pressure and promote blood flow to tissues.*

- Provide an egg-crate mattress or alternating pressure mattress, foot cradle, heel protectors, and other devices to reduce pressure on tissues. *These devices, which distribute pressure away from bony prominences, reduce the risk of skin breakdown.*

Impaired Gas Exchange

With fluid volume excess, gas exchange may be impaired by edema of pulmonary interstitial tissues. Acute pulmonary edema is a serious and potentially life-threatening complication of pulmonary congestion.

- Auscultate lungs for presence or worsening of crackles and wheezes; auscultate heart for extra heart sounds. *Crackles and wheezes indicate pulmonary congestion and edema. A gallop rhythm (S_3) may indicate diastolic overloading of the ventricles secondary to fluid volume excess.*
- Place in Fowler's position if dyspnea or orthopnea is present. *Fowler's position improves lung expansion by decreasing the pressure of abdominal contents on the diaphragm.*
- Monitor oxygen saturation levels and **arterial blood gases (ABGs)** for evidence of impaired gas exchange ($SaO_2 < 92\%$ to 95%; $PaO_2 < 80$ mmHg). Administer oxygen as indicated. *Edema of interstitial lung tissues can interfere with gas exchange and delivery to body tissues. Supplemental oxygen promotes gas exchange across the alveolar-capillary membrane, improving tissue oxygenation.*

Community-Based Care

Teaching for home care focuses on managing the underlying cause of fluid volume excess and preventing future episodes of excess fluid volume. Address the following topics when preparing the patient and family for home care:

- Manifestations of excess fluid and when to contact the care provider
- Prescribed medications: when and how to take, intended and adverse effects, what to report to care provider

BOX 10–2 Patient Teaching: Low-Sodium Diet

Low-Sodium Diet
- Reducing sodium intake will help the body excrete excess sodium and water.
- The body needs less than one-tenth of a teaspoon of salt per day.
- Approximately one-third of sodium intake comes from salt added to foods during cooking and at the table; one-fourth to one-third comes from processed foods; and the rest comes from food and water naturally high in sodium.
- Sodium compounds are used in foods as preservatives, leavening agents, and flavor enhancers.
- Many nonprescription drugs (such as analgesics, cough medicine, laxatives, and antacids) as well as toothpastes and mouthwashes contain high amounts of sodium.
- Low-sodium salt substitutes are not really sodium free and may contain half as much sodium as regular salt.
- Use salt substitutes sparingly; larger amounts often taste bitter instead of salty.
- The preference for salt will eventually diminish.
- Salt, monosodium glutamate, baking soda, and baking powder contain substantial amounts of sodium.
- Read labels.
- In place of salt or salt substitutes, use herbs, spices, lemon juice, vinegar, and wine as flavoring when cooking.

- Recommended or prescribed diet; ways to reduce sodium intake; how to read food labels for salt and sodium content; use of salt substitutes, if allowed
- If restricted, the amount and type of fluids to take each day; how to balance intake over 24 hours
- Monitoring weight; changes reported to care provider
- Ways to decrease dependent edema:
  a. Change position frequently.
  b. Avoid restrictive clothing.
  c. Avoid crossing the legs when sitting.
  d. Wear support stockings or hose.
  e. Elevate feet and legs when sitting.
- How to protect edematous skin from injury:
  a. Do not walk barefoot.
  b. Buy good-fitting shoes; shop in the afternoon when feet are more likely to be swollen.
- Using additional pillows or a recliner to sleep, to relieve orthopnea

Sodium Imbalance

Sodium is the most plentiful electrolyte in ECF, with normal serum sodium levels ranging from 135 to 145 mEq/L. Sodium is the primary regulator of the volume, osmolality, and distribution of ECF. It also is important in maintaining neuromuscular activity. Because of the close interrelationship between sodium and water balance, disorders of fluid volume and sodium balance often occur together. Sodium imbalances affect the osmolality of ECF and water distribution between the fluid compartments. When sodium levels are low (hyponatremia), water is drawn into the cells of the body, causing them to swell. In contrast, high levels of sodium in ECF (hypernatremia) draw water out of body cells, causing them to shrink.

Most of the body's sodium comes from dietary intake. Although a sodium intake of 500 mg per day is usually sufficient to meet the body's needs, and the CDC suggests that two-thirds of Americans should limit their intake to 1500 mg per day (about 3/4 teaspoon), the average intake of sodium by adults in the United States is about 3500 mg per day (CDC, 2009). Other sources of sodium include prescription drugs and some self-prescribed remedies.

The kidney is the primary regulator of sodium balance in the body. The kidney excretes or conserves sodium in response to changes in vascular volume. A fall in blood volume prompts several mechanisms that lead to sodium and water retention:

- The renin–angiotensin–aldosterone system (see Figure 10–8) is stimulated. Angiotensin II prompts the renal tubules to reabsorb sodium. It also causes vasoconstriction, slowing blood flow through the kidney and reducing glomerular filtration. This further reduces the amount of sodium excreted. Angiotensin II promotes the release of aldosterone from the adrenal cortex. In the presence of aldosterone, more sodium is reabsorbed in the cortical collecting tubules of the kidney, and more potassium is eliminated in the urine.
- ADH is released from the posterior pituitary (see Figure 10–9). ADH promotes sodium and water reabsorption in the distal tubules of the kidney, reducing urine output and expanding blood volume.

In contrast, when blood volume expands, sodium and water elimination by the kidneys increases.

- The glomerular filtration rate increases, allowing more water and sodium to be filtered and excreted.
- The hormone ANP is released by cells in the atria of the heart. ANP increases renal blood flow and glomerular filtration rate and also inhibits the aldosterone secretion to increase sodium excretion by the kidneys.
- ADH release from the pituitary gland is inhibited by ANP. In the absence of ADH, the distal tubule is relatively impermeable to water, allowing more to be excreted in the urine. Table 10–5 summarizes the manifestations of sodium imbalances.

The Patient with Hyponatremia

Hyponatremia is a serum sodium of less than 135 mEq/L. Hyponatremia usually results from a loss of sodium from the body, but it may also be caused by water gains that dilute ECF.

Pathophysiology

Excess sodium loss can occur through the kidneys, GI tract, or skin. Diuretics, kidney diseases, or adrenal insufficiency with impaired aldosterone and cortisol production can lead to excessive sodium excretion in urine. Vomiting, diarrhea, and GI suction are common causes of excess sodium loss through the GI tract. Sodium may also be lost when GI tubes are irrigated with water instead of saline, or when repeated tap water enemas are administered (Porth & Matfin, 2009). Excessive sweating, loss of skin surface (as with an extensive burn), and third spacing can also cause excessive sodium loss.

Hyponatremia causes a decrease in serum osmolality. Water shifts from ECF into the intracellular space, causing cells to swell and reducing the osmolality of intracellular fluid. Many of the manifestations of hyponatremia can be attributed to cellular edema and hypo-osmolality. Water gains that can lead to hyponatremia may occur with systemic diseases such as heart failure, renal failure, or cirrhosis of the liver; syndrome of inappropriate secretion of antidiuretic hormone (SIADH); excessive administration of hypotonic IV fluids; and self-induced water intoxication.

TABLE 10–5 Manifestations of Sodium Imbalances

HYPONATREMIA	HYPERNATREMIA
■ Plasma sodium <135 mEq/L	■ Plasma sodium >145 mEq/L
■ Decreased serum osmolality	■ Increased serum osmolality
■ Decreased hematocrit and BUN	■ Increased hematocrit and BUN
■ Weight loss	■ Weight gain
■ Muscle cramps, weakness	■ Increased thirst, oliguria, increased urine output and specific gravity
■ Headache	■ Dry skin and mucous membranes, decreased skin turgor, furrowed tongue, dry mouth
■ Anxiety	
■ Lethargy, stupor, coma	
■ Anorexia, nausea, vomiting, diarrhea	■ Headache, restlessness
■ Hypotension, shock	■ Seizures, coma
	■ Tachycardia, hypotension, vascular collapse

Manifestations

The manifestations of hyponatremia depend on the rapidity of onset, the severity, and the cause of the imbalance. If the condition develops slowly, manifestations are usually not experienced until the serum sodium levels reach 125 mEq/L. In addition, the manifestations of hyponatremia vary, depending on extracellular fluid volume. Early manifestations of hyponatremia include muscle cramps, weakness, and fatigue from its effects on muscle cells. Gastrointestinal function is affected, causing anorexia, nausea and vomiting, abdominal cramping, and diarrhea.

As sodium levels continue to decrease, the brain and nervous system are affected by cellular edema. Neurologic manifestations progress rapidly when the serum sodium level falls below 120 mEq/L and include headache, depression, dulled sensorium, personality changes, irritability, lethargy, hyperreflexia, muscle twitching, and tremors. If serum sodium falls to very low levels, coma is likely to occur. When hyponatremia is associated with decreased ECF volume, the manifestations are those of hypovolemia (*hypotonic dehydration*). In hyponatremia associated with fluid volume excess, manifestations include those of hypervolemia.

Interdisciplinary Care

Interdisciplinary management of hyponatremia focuses on restoring normal blood volume and serum sodium levels.

Diagnosis

The following laboratory tests may be ordered.

- *Serum sodium* and *osmolality* are decreased in hyponatremia.
- A *24-hour urine specimen* is obtained to evaluate sodium excretion. In conditions associated with normal or increased extracellular volume (such as SIADH), urinary sodium is increased; in conditions resulting from losses of isotonic fluids (e.g., sweating, diarrhea, vomiting, and third-space fluid accumulation), by contrast, urinary sodium is decreased.

Medications

When both sodium and water have been lost (hyponatremia with hypovolemia), sodium-containing fluids are given to replace both water and sodium. Isotonic Ringer's solution or isotonic saline (0.9% NaCl) solution may be administered. Cautious administration of IV 3% or 5% NaCl solution may be necessary in patients who have very low plasma sodium levels (110 to 115 mEq/L).

Loop diuretics are administered to patients who have hyponatremia with normal or excess ECF volume. Loop diuretics promote an isotonic diuresis and fluid volume loss without hyponatremia. Thiazide diuretics are avoided because they cause a relatively greater sodium loss in relation to water loss. In addition, drugs to treat the underlying cause of hyponatremia may be administered.

Fluid and Dietary Management

If hyponatremia is mild, increasing the intake of foods high in sodium may restore normal sodium balance. Fluids often are restricted to help reduce ECF volume and correct hyponatremia (see Box 10–1 for fluid restriction guidelines).

Nursing Care

Nursing care of the patient with hyponatremia focuses on identifying patients at risk and managing problems resulting from the systemic effects of the disorder.

Health Promotion

People at risk for mild hyponatremia include those who participate in activities that increase fluid loss through excessive perspiration (diaphoresis) and then replace those losses by drinking large amounts of water or drinks with high sugar content. This includes athletes, people who do heavy labor in high environmental temperatures, and older adults living in non-air-conditioned settings during hot weather. Teach the following to patients who are at risk:

- Manifestations of mild hyponatremia, including nausea, abdominal cramps, and muscle weakness
- The importance of drinking liquids containing sodium and other electrolytes at frequent intervals when perspiring heavily, when environmental temperatures are high, and/or if watery diarrhea persists for several days

Assessment

Assessment data related to hyponatremia include the following:
- *Health history:* Current manifestations, including nausea and vomiting, abdominal discomfort, muscle weakness, headache, other manifestations; duration of manifestations and any precipitating factors such as heavy perspiration, vomiting, or diarrhea; chronic diseases such as heart or renal failure, cirrhosis of the liver, or endocrine disorders; current medications.
- *Physical assessment:* Mental status and level of consciousness; vital signs including orthostatic vital signs and peripheral pulses; presence of edema or weight gain.

Nursing Diagnoses and Interventions

Risk for Imbalanced Fluid Volume

Because of its role in maintaining fluid balance, sodium imbalances often are accompanied by water imbalances. In addition, treatment of hyponatremia can affect the patient's fluid balance.

- Monitor intake and output, weigh daily, and calculate 24-hour fluid balance. *Fluid excess or deficit may occur with hyponatremia.*

> **PRACTICE ALERT**
> Carefully monitor patients receiving sodium-containing IV solutions for manifestations of hypervolemia (increased blood pressure and CVP, tachypnea, tachycardia, gallop rhythm [S_3 and/or S_4 heart sounds], shortness of breath, crackles). Hypertonic saline solutions can lead to hypervolemia, particularly in patients with cardiovascular or renal disease.

- Use an infusion pump to administer hypertonic saline (3% and 5% NaCl) solutions; carefully monitor flow rate and response. *Hypertonic solutions can increase the risk of pulmonary and cerebral edema due to water retention. Careful monitoring is vital to prevent these complications and possible permanent damage.*

- If fluids are restricted, explain the reason for the restriction, the amount of fluid allowed, and how to calculate fluid intake. *Teaching increases the patient's sense of control and compliance.*

For additional nursing interventions that may apply to the patient with hyponatremia, review the discussions of fluid volume deficit and fluid volume excess.

Risk for Ineffective Cerebral Tissue Perfusion

The patient with severe hyponatremia experiences fluid shifts that cause an increase in intracellular fluid volume. This can cause brain cells to swell, increasing pressure within the cranial vault.

- Monitor serum electrolytes and serum osmolality. Report abnormal results to the healthcare provider. *As serum sodium and osmolality levels fall, the manifestations and neurologic effects of hyponatremia become increasingly severe.*
- Assess for neurologic changes, such as lethargy, altered level of consciousness, confusion, and convulsions. Monitor mental status and orientation. Compare baseline data with continuing assessments. *If serum sodium levels continue to fall, the patient may become increasingly less responsive.*
- Assess muscle strength and tone, and deep tendon reflexes. *Increasing muscle weakness and decreased deep tendon reflexes are manifestations of increasing hyponatremia.*

Community-Based Care

Teaching for home care focuses on the underlying cause of the sodium deficit and prevention. Teach patients about the following:

- Manifestations of mild and more severe hyponatremia to report to the primary care provider
- The importance of regular serum electrolyte monitoring if taking a potent diuretic or on a low-sodium diet
- Types of foods and fluids to replace sodium orally if dietary sodium is not restricted
- Older adults' increased risk for hyponatremia from the effects of medications and potential fluid imbalances

The Patient with Hypernatremia

Hypernatremia is a serum sodium level greater than 145 mEq/L. It may develop when sodium is gained in excess of water, or when water is lost in excess of sodium. Either fluid volume deficit or fluid volume excess often accompany hypernatremia.

Pathophysiology

Two regulatory mechanisms protect the body from hypernatremia: Excess sodium in ECF stimulates the release of ADH so more water is retained by the kidneys, and the thirst mechanism is stimulated to increase the intake of water. These two factors increase extracellular water, diluting the excess sodium and restoring normal levels.

Hypernatremia (also known as *hypertonic dehydration*) causes hyperosmolality of the ECF. As a result, water is drawn out of cells, leading to cellular dehydration. The most serious effects of cellular dehydration are seen in the brain. As brain cells contract, neurologic manifestations develop. The brain itself shrinks, causing mechanical traction on cerebral vessels. These vessels may tear and bleed. Although the brain rapidly adapts to hyperosmolality to minimize the water loss, acute hypernatremia can cause coma and seizures (Porth & Matfin, 2009).

Water deprivation is a cause of hypernatremia in patients who are unable to respond to thirst due to altered mental status or physical disability. Excess water loss may also occur with watery diarrhea or increased water losses from fever, hyperventilation, excessive perspiration, or massive burns. Unless water is adequately replaced, patients with diabetes insipidus (∞ see Chapter 19) also may develop hypernatremia. Excess sodium intake can result from ingestion of excess salt or hypertonic IV solutions. Patients who experience near-drowning in seawater are at risk for hypernatremia, as are patients with heatstroke.

Manifestations

Thirst is the first manifestation of hypernatremia. If thirst is not relieved, the primary manifestations relate to altered neuro-logic function (see Table 10–5). Initial lethargy, weakness, and irritability can progress to seizures, coma, and death in severe hypernatremia. Both the severity of the sodium excess and the rapidity of its onset affect the manifestations of hypernatremia.

Interdisciplinary Care

Treatment of hypernatremia depends on its cause. Hypernatremia is corrected slowly (over a 48-hour period) to avoid development of cerebral edema secondary to a shift of water into the brain cells.

Diagnosis

The following laboratory and diagnostic tests may be ordered:

- *Serum sodium levels* are greater than 145 mEq/L in hypernatremia.
- *Serum osmolality* is greater than 295 mOsm/kg in hypernatremia.

Medications

The principal treatment for hypernatremia is oral or IV water replacement. Hypotonic IV fluids such as 0.45% NaCl solution or 5% dextrose in water (which is isotonic when administered, but becomes hypotonic and provides pure water when the glu-cose is metabolized) may be administered to correct the water deficit. Diuretics may also be given to increase sodium excretion.

ᏯᎧ Nursing Care

The primary focus of nursing care related to hypernatremia is prevention. Measures to prevent hypernatremia include identi-fying risk factors, teaching patients and caregivers, monitoring laboratory test results, and collaborating with the interdiscipli-nary team to reduce the potential for hypernatremia.

Health Promotion

Patients at risk for hypernatremia, as well as their caregivers, need teaching to prevent this electrolyte disorder. Instruct care-givers of debilitated patients who are unable to perceive thirst or unable to respond to it to offer fluids at regular intervals. If the patient is unable to maintain adequate fluid intake, contact the healthcare provider about an alternate route for fluid intake (e.g., a feeding tube). Teach caregivers the importance of providing adequate water for patients receiving tube feedings (many of which are hypertonic).

Assessment

Assessment data related to hypernatremia include the following:

- *Health history:* Duration of manifestations and any pre-cipitating factors such as water deprivation, increased water loss due to heavy perspiration, temperature or rapid breath-ing, diarrhea, excess salt intake, or diabetes insipidus; cur-rent medications; perception of thirst.
- *Physical assessment:* Vital signs, mucous membranes; mental status or level of consciousness; manifestations of fluid volume excess or fluid volume deficit.

Nursing Diagnoses and Interventions

Risk for Injury

Mental status and brain function may be affected by hypernatremia itself or by rapid correction of the condition that leads to cerebral edema. In either case, closely monitor the patient and take precautions to reduce risk of injury.

- Monitor and maintain fluid replacement to within the prescribed limits. Monitor serum sodium levels and osmo-lality; report rapid changes to the care provider. *Rapid water replacement or rapid changes in serum sodium or osmolality can increase the risk of bleeding or cerebral edema.*
- Monitor neurologic function, including mental status, level of consciousness, and other manifestations such as headache, nausea, vomiting, hypertension, and bradycardia. *Both hypernatremia and rapid correction of hypernatremia affect cerebral function. Careful monitoring is vital to detect changes in mental status that may indicate cerebral bleeding or edema.*
- Institute safety precautions as necessary: Keep the bed in its lowest position, side rails up and padded, and an airway at bedside. *Patients with sodium disorders are at risk for injury due to seizure activity and changes in mental status.*
- Keep clocks, calendars, and familiar objects at bedside. Orient to time, place, and circumstances as needed. Allow significant others to remain with the patient as much as possible. *An unfamiliar environment and altered thought processes can further increase the patient's risk for injury. Significant others provide a sense of security and reduce the patient's anxiety.*

Community-Based Care

When preparing the patient who has experienced hypernatremia for home care, discuss the following topics:

- The importance of responding to thirst and consuming ade-quate fluids (If the patient is dependent on a caregiver, stress to the caregiver the importance of regularly offering fluids.)
- If prescribed, guidelines for following a low-sodium diet (see Box 10–2)
- Use and effects of any prescribed diuretic
- The importance of following a schedule for regular monitor-ing of serum electrolyte levels and reporting manifestations of imbalance to healthcare provider

Potassium Imbalance

Potassium, the primary intracellular cation, plays a vital role in cell metabolism and cardiac and neuromuscular function. The normal serum (ECF) potassium level is 3.5 to 5.0 mEq/L. To maintain balance, potassium must be replaced daily through diet. Virtually all foods contain potassium, although some foods and fluids are richer sources of this element than others.

Most potassium in the body is found within the ICF, which has a concentration of 140 to 150 mEq/L. This significant difference in the potassium concentrations of ICF and ECF helps maintain the resting membrane potential of nerve and muscle cells. Potassium imbalances affect transmission and conduction of nerve impulses, maintenance of normal cardiac rhythms, and contraction of skeletal and smooth muscle. The higher intracellular potassium concentration is maintained by the sodium-potassium pump. Potassium constantly shifts into and out of the cells. This movement between ICF and ECF can significantly affect the serum potassium level. For example, potassium shifts into or out of the cells in response to changes in hydrogen ion concentration (pH, discussed later in this chapter) as the body strives to maintain a stable acid–base balance.

Aldosterone helps regulate potassium elimination by the kidneys. An increased potassium concentration in ECF stimulates aldosterone production by the adrenal gland. The kidneys respond to aldosterone by increasing potassium excretion. Changes in aldosterone secretion can profoundly affect the serum potassium level.

The Patient with Hypokalemia

Hypokalemia is an abnormally low serum potassium level (less than 3.5 mEq/L). It usually results from excess potassium loss, although hospitalized patients may be at risk for hypokalemia because of inadequate potassium intake.

Pathophysiology

Hypokalemia may result from inadequate intake of potassium; excessive renal, intestinal, or skin losses; or redistribution between the ICF and ECF. An intake of a minimum of 40 to 50 mEq/day is needed to compensate for urinary losses (Porth & Matfin, 2009). The kidneys are the main source of potassium loss. Normally only small amounts of potassium are lost in the feces, but substantial amounts may be lost from the GI tract with diarrhea or through drainage from an ileostomy (a permanent opening into the small bowel). Excessive sweating may also cause potassium loss.

These losses deplete total potassium stores in the body.

- Excess potassium loss through the kidneys often is secondary to drugs such as potassium-wasting diuretics, corticosteroids, amphotericin B, and large doses of some antibiotics. Hyperaldosteronism, a condition in which the adrenal glands secrete excess aldosterone, also causes excess elimination of potassium through the kidneys. Renal losses of potassium also occur from stress, trauma, metabolic acidosis, and a magnesium deficit.
- Gastrointestinal losses of potassium result from severe vomiting, gastric suction, or loss of intestinal fluids through diarrhea or ileostomy drainage.
- Transcellular shifts (from the ECF to the ICF) occur in conditions such as treatment of diabetic ketoacidosis with insulin (insulin increases the movement of potassium into the cells) and the use of beta2-adrenergic decongestants and bronchodilators (these drugs have the same effect as insulin).

Potassium intake may be inadequate in patients who are unable or unwilling to eat for prolonged periods. Hospitalized patients are at risk, especially those on extended parenteral fluid therapy with solutions that do not contain potassium. Patients with anorexia nervosa or alcoholism may develop hypokalemia due to both inadequate intake and loss of potassium through vomiting, diarrhea, or laxative or diuretic use.

PATHOPHYSIOLOGY LINKAGE Hypokalemia

MANIFESTATIONS	RELATED PATHOPHYSIOLOGY
Characteristic electrocardiogram (ECG) changes of hypokalemia include flattened or inverted T waves, the development of U waves, and a depressed ST segment (Figure 10–10).	Low levels of potassium interfere with the contractility of cardiac muscle and the regulation and transmission of cardiac impulses, which maintain normal cardiac rhythms.
Nausea and vomiting, anorexia, decreased bowel sounds, ileus	Loss of potassium from severe vomiting, gastric suctioning, diarrhea, or ileostomy drainage affects the resting membrane potential and intracellular enzymes in smooth muscle cells, slowing peristalsis of the GI tract.
Decreased cardiac output, dysrhythmias (abnormal rhythms)	Decreased strength of cardiac contractions and dysrhythmias in turn cause a decrease in cardiac output. The most serious cardiac effect is an increased risk of atrial and ventricular dysrhythmias. Hypokalemia increases the risk for digitalis toxicity in patients receiving this drug used to treat heart failure (∞ see Chapter 31).
Muscle weakness and leg cramps	Low potassium levels affect the resting membrane potential and intracellular enzymes in skeletal muscle cells. Muscles of the lower extremities are affected first, then the trunk and upper extremities. This effect of hypokalemia is magnified when serum calcium levels are above normal. Severe hypokalemia can lead to rhabdomyolysis, a condition in which muscle fibers disintegrate, releasing myoglobin to be excreted in the urine.
Altered kidney function	Inability to concentrate urine due to decreased collecting tubule responsiveness to antidiuretic hormone.

Manifestations

Hypokalemia affects the transmission of nerve impulses, interfering with the contractility of smooth, skeletal, and cardiac muscle, as well as the regulation and transmission of cardiac impulses. Carbohydrate metabolism is affected by hypokalemia. Insulin secretion is suppressed, as is the synthesis of glycogen in skeletal muscle and the liver.

See the Pathophysiology Linkages box for manifestations of hypokalemia.

Manifestations of hypokalemia are more pronounced when potassium losses occur acutely. When hypokalemia develops gradually, potassium shifts out of the cells, helping maintain the ratio of intracellular to extracellular potassium. As a result, the neuromuscular manifestations of hypokalemia are less severe. See the Multisystem Effects of Hypokalemia feature on the following page.

Interdisciplinary Care

The management of hypokalemia focuses on prevention and treatment of a deficiency.

Diagnosis

The following laboratory and diagnostic tests may be ordered:

- *Serum potassium* (K^+) is used to monitor potassium levels in patients who are at risk for or who are being treated for hypokalemia.
- *Arterial blood gases (ABGs)* are measured to determine acid–base status. An increased pH (alkalosis) often is associated with hypokalemia. (See Table 10–10 later in this chapter for normal ABG values.)
- *Renal function studies*, such as *serum creatinine* and *blood urea nitrogen (BUN)*, may be ordered to evaluate for potential causes or effects of hypokalemia.

- *ECG recordings* are obtained to evaluate the effects of hypokalemia on the cardiac conduction system.

Medications

Oral and/or parenteral potassium supplements are given to prevent and, as needed, treat hypokalemia. To prevent hypokalemia in the patient taking nothing by mouth, potassium chloride is added to IV fluids. The dose used to treat hypokalemia includes the daily maintenance requirement, replacement of ongoing losses (e.g., gastric suction), and additional potassium to correct the existing deficit. Several days of therapy may be required. Commonly prescribed potassium supplements, their actions, and nursing implications are described in the following Medication Administration box.

Nutrition

A diet high in potassium-rich foods is recommended for patients at risk for developing hypokalemia or to supplement drug therapy. Examples of foods high in potassium include bananas, oranges, avocados, spinach, potatoes, tomatoes, meat, seafood, milk, and yogurt.

Nursing Care

See the Case Study & Nursing Care Plan on page 209.

Health Promotion

When providing general health education, discuss using balanced electrolyte solutions (e.g., Pedialyte or sports drinks) to replace abnormal fluid losses (excess perspiration, vomiting, or severe diarrhea). Discuss the necessity of preventing hypokalemia with patients at risk. Provide diet teaching and refer patients with anorexia nervosa for counseling. Stress the potassium-losing effects of diuretics. Encourage a diet rich in high-potassium foods, as well as regular monitoring of serum potassium levels.

MEDICATION ADMINISTRATION Hypokalemia

POTASSIUM SOURCES

Potassium acetate (Tri-K)

Potassium bicarbonate (K + Care ET)

Potassium citrate (K-Lyte)

Potassium chloride (K-Lease, Micro-K 10, Apo-K)

Potassium gluconate (Kaon Elixir, Royonate)

Potassium is rapidly absorbed from the GI tract; potassium chloride is the agent of choice, because low chloride often accompanies low potassium. Potassium is used to prevent and/or treat hypokalemia (e.g., with parenteral nutrition and potassium-wasting diuretics, and prophylactically after major surgery).

Nursing Responsibilities

- When giving oral forms of potassium
  a. dilute or dissolve effervescent, soluble, or liquid potassium in fruit or vegetable juice or cold water.
  b. chill to increase palatability.
  c. give with food to minimize GI effects.
- When giving parenteral forms of potassium (KCl)
  a. do not administer IV push, do not add to fluids already hanging, and infuse at rate not to exceed 10 mEq/hour.
  b. do **NOT** administer undiluted.

  c. assess injection site frequently for manifestations of pain and inflammation. Discontinue and restart in another vein at first sign of infiltration.
  d. use an infusion pump.
  e. use cardiac monitoring if high or rapid doses are administered.
- Assess for abdominal pain, distention, GI bleeding; if present, do not administer medication. Notify healthcare provider.
- Monitor fluid intake and output.
- Assess for manifestations of hyperkalemia: weakness, feeling of heaviness in legs, mental confusion, hypotension, cardiac dysrhythmias, changes in ECG, increased serum potassium levels.

Health Education for the Patient and Family

- Do not take potassium supplements if you are also taking a potassium-sparing diuretic.
- When parenteral potassium is discontinued, eat potassium-rich foods.
- Do not chew enteric-coated tablets or allow them to dissolve in the mouth; this may affect the potency and action of the medications.
- Take potassium supplements with meals.
- Do not use salt substitutes when taking potassium (most salt substitutes are potassium based).

MULTISYSTEM EFFECTS OF
Hypokalemia

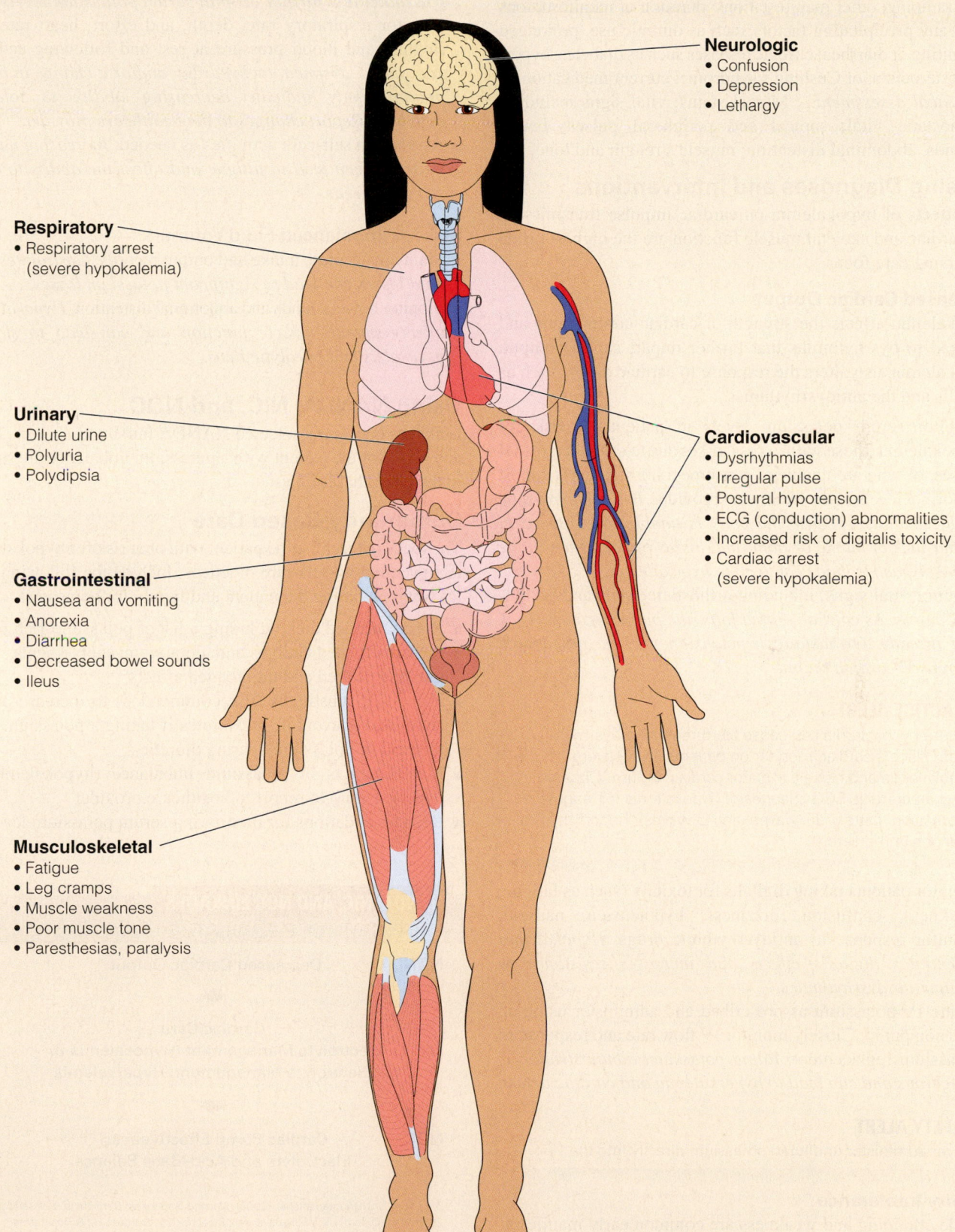

Neurologic
- Confusion
- Depression
- Lethargy

Respiratory
- Respiratory arrest
  (severe hypokalemia)

Urinary
- Dilute urine
- Polyuria
- Polydipsia

Cardiovascular
- Dysrhythmias
- Irregular pulse
- Postural hypotension
- ECG (conduction) abnormalities
- Increased risk of digitalis toxicity
- Cardiac arrest
  (severe hypokalemia)

Gastrointestinal
- Nausea and vomiting
- Anorexia
- Diarrhea
- Decreased bowel sounds
- Ileus

Musculoskeletal
- Fatigue
- Leg cramps
- Muscle weakness
- Poor muscle tone
- Paresthesias, paralysis

Assessment

Assessment data related to hypokalemia include the following:

- *Health history:*   Current manifestations, including anorexia, nausea and vomiting, abdominal discomfort, muscle weakness or cramping, other manifestations; duration of manifestations and any precipitating factors such as diuretic use, prolonged vomiting or diarrhea; chronic diseases such as diabetes, hyperaldosteronism, or Cushing's syndrome; current medications.
- *Physical assessment:*   Mental status; vital signs including orthostatic vitals, apical and peripheral pulses; bowel sounds, abdominal distention; muscle strength and tone.

Nursing Diagnoses and Interventions

The effects of hypokalemia on cardiac impulse transmission and cardiac and skeletal muscle function are the highest priority nursing care focus.

Decreased Cardiac Output

Hypokalemia affects the strength of cardiac contractions and can lead to dysrhythmias that further impair cardiac output. Hypokalemia also alters the response to cardiac drugs, such as digitalis and the antidysrhythmics.

- Monitor serum potassium levels in patients at risk for hypokalemia (those with excess losses due to drug therapy, GI losses, or who are unable to consume a normal diet). Report abnormal levels to the healthcare provider. *Potassium must be replaced daily because the body is unable to conserve it. Either lack of intake or abnormal losses of potassium in the urine or gastric fluids can lead to hypokalemia.*
- Monitor vital signs, including orthostatic vitals and peripheral pulses. *As cardiac output falls, the pulse becomes weak and thready. Orthostatic hypotension may be noted with decreased cardiac output.*

> **PRACTICE ALERT**
> Severe hypokalemia can cause life-threatening dysrhythmias. Place a cardiac monitor on patients with severe hypokalemia and closely monitor cardiac rhythm. Observe for characteristic ECG changes of hypokalemia (ST segment depression, flattened T waves, and U waves). Report rhythm changes immediately.

- Monitor patients taking digitalis for toxicity (such as fatigue, weakness, confusion, dizziness, hypotension, nausea). Monitor response to antidysrhythmic drugs. *Hypokalemia potentiates digitalis effects and increases resistance to certain antidysrhythmics.*
- Dilute IV potassium as prescribed and administer using an infusion pump. Closely monitor IV flow rate and response to potassium replacement. *Rapid potassium administration is dangerous and can lead to hyperkalemia and cardiac arrest.*

> **SAFETY ALERT**
> Never administer undiluted potassium directly into the vein.

Activity Intolerance

Muscle cramping and weakness are common early manifestations of hypokalemia. The lower extremities are usually affected first. This muscle weakness can cause the patient to fatigue easily, particularly with activity.

- Monitor skeletal muscle strength and tone, which are affected by moderate hypokalemia. *Increasing weakness, paresthesias, or paralysis of muscles or progression of affected muscles to include the upper extremities or trunk can indicate a further drop in serum potassium levels.*
- Monitor respiratory rate, depth, and effort; heart rate and rhythm; and blood pressure at rest and following activity. *Tachypnea, dyspnea, tachycardia, and/or a change in blood pressure may indicate decreasing ability to tolerate activities. Report changes to the healthcare provider.*
- Assist with self-care activities as needed. *Increasing muscle weakness can lead to fatigue and affect the ability to meet self-care needs.*

Risk for Imbalanced Fluid Volume

- Maintain accurate intake and output records. *Gastrointestinal fluid losses can lead to significant potassium losses.*
- Monitor bowel sounds and abdominal distention. *Hypokalemia affects smooth muscle function and can lead to slowed peristalsis and paralytic ileus.*

Using NANDA, NIC, and NOC

Linkages between a selected NANDA nursing diagnosis, NIC, and NOC for the patient with a potassium imbalance are shown in the chart that follows.

Community-Based Care

The focus in teaching the patient with or at risk for hypokalemia is prevention by self-care practices. Include the following topics when preparing the patient and family for home care.

- Recommended diet, including a list of potassium-rich foods
- Prescribed medications and potassium supplements, their use, and desired and unintended effects
- Using salt substitutes (if recommended) to increase potassium intake; avoiding substitutes if taking a potassium supplement or potassium-sparing diuretic
- Manifestations of potassium imbalance (hypokalemia or hyperkalemia) to report to healthcare provider
- Recommendations for monitoring serum potassium levels

NANDA, NIC, AND NOC LINKAGES
The Patient with Potassium Imbalance

NANDA	Decreased Cardiac Output
NIC	Cardiac Care Electrolyte Management: Hypokalemia *or* Electrolyte Management: Hyperkalemia
NOC	Cardiac Pump Effectiveness Electrolyte and Acid–Base Balance

Data from NANDA International. (2009). *Nursing diagnoses: Definitions & classification 2009–2011.* Oxford, UK: Wiley-Blackwell; Bulechek, G., Butcher, H., & Dochterman, K. (Eds.). (2008). *Nursing interventions classification (NIC)* (5th ed.) (pp. 195–196, 286–287, 294–295). St. Louis, Elsevier Mosby; and Moorhead, S., Johnson, M., Maas, M., & Swanson, E. (Eds.). (2008). *Nursing outcomes classification (NOC)* (4th ed.) (pp.211–212, 340–341). St. Louis: Elsevier Mosby.

CASE STUDY & NURSING CARE PLAN Hypokalemia

Rose Ortiz is a 72-year-old widow who lives alone, although close to her daughter's home. Ms. Ortiz has mild heart failure and is being treated with digoxin (Lanoxin) 0.125 mg, furosemide (Lasix) 40 mg PO daily, and a mildly restricted sodium diet (2 g daily). For the last several weeks, Ms. Ortiz has complained that she feels weak and sometimes faint, light-headed, and dizzy. Serum electrolyte tests ordered by her physician reveal a potassium level of 2.4 mEq/L. Potassium chloride solution (Kaochlor 10%, 20 mEq/15 mL) PO twice daily is prescribed, and Ms. Ortiz is referred to Nancy Walters, RN, for follow-up care.

ASSESSMENT

Ms. Ortiz's health history reveals that she has adhered to her sodium-restricted diet and has been compliant in taking her prescribed medications, with the exception of occasionally taking an additional "water pill" when her ankles swell. She takes a laxative every evening to ensure a daily bowel movement. She states that she is reluctant to take the potassium chloride the doctor has ordered because her neighbor complains that his potassium supplement upsets his stomach. Physical assessment findings included T 98.4, P 70, R 20, and BP 138/84. Muscle strength in her upper extremities is normal and equal; lower extremity strength is weak but equal. Sensation is normal.

DIAGNOSES

- *Risk for Injury* related to muscle weakness
- *Risk for Ineffective Health Maintenance* related to lack of knowledge about how diuretic therapy and laxative use affect potassium levels

EXPECTED OUTCOMES

- Maintain potassium level within normal limits (3.5 to 5.0 mEq/L).
- Regain normal muscle strength.
- Remain free of injury.
- Verbalize understanding of the effects of diuretic therapy and laxatives on potassium levels.

- Identify measures to avoid GI irritation when taking oral potassium.
- Identify potassium-rich foods.

PLANNING AND IMPLEMENTATION

- Explain need to use caution when ambulating, particularly when going up and down stairs.
- Discuss side effects of furosemide, and explain how taking additional tablets may have contributed to hypokalemia.
- Discuss alternative measures to prevent constipation without using laxatives on a regular basis (e.g., high-fiber diet, adequate fluid intake).
- Explain purpose of the prescribed potassium and its role in reversing muscle weakness.
- Teach to take potassium supplement after breakfast and supper, diluted in 4 oz of juice or water, and to sip it slowly over a 5- to 10-minute period. Advise to call if gastric irritation occurs.
- Discuss dietary sources of potassium; provide a list of potassium-rich foods.

EVALUATION

On a follow-up visit 1 week later, Ms. Ortiz states that her muscle weakness, dizziness, and other manifestations have resolved. She is taking the prescribed drugs as directed and is using laxatives only two or three times a week. Ms. Ortiz reports that she has increased her intake of potassium-rich foods and fluids and of high-fiber foods. Her potassium level is within normal limits.

CRITICAL THINKING IN THE NURSING PROCESS

1. What is the pathophysiologic basis for Ms. Ortiz's muscle weakness and dizziness?
2. How might the chronic overuse of laxatives contribute to hypokalemia?
3. Describe the interaction of digitalis, diuretics, and potassium.
4. Develop a plan of care for Ms. Ortiz for the nursing diagnosis of *Perceived Constipation*.

See Evaluating Your Response in Appendix C.

- If taking digitalis, manifestations of digitalis toxicity to report to healthcare provider
- Managing GI disorders that cause potassium loss (vomiting, diarrhea, ileostomy drainage) to prevent hypokalemia

The Patient with Hyperkalemia

Hyperkalemia is an abnormally high serum potassium (greater than 5 mEq/L). Hyperkalemia can result from inadequate excretion of potassium, excessively high intake of potassium, or a shift of potassium from the ICF to the ECF. Hyperkalemia affects neuromuscular and cardiac function.

Pathophysiology

Impaired renal excretion of potassium is a primary cause of hyperkalemia. Untreated renal failure, adrenal insufficiency (e.g., Addison's disease or inadequate aldosterone production), and medications (such as potassium-sparing diuretics, the antimicrobial drug trimethoprim [Trimpex], and some NSAIDs) impair potassium excretion by the kidneys.

Rapid IV administration of potassium or transfusion of aged blood can lead to hyperkalemia. A shift of potassium ions from the ICF can occur in acidosis, with severe tissue trauma, during

chemotherapy, and due to starvation. In acidosis, excess hydrogen ions enter the cells, displacing potassium and causing it to shift into the extracellular space. The extent of this shift is greater with metabolic acidosis than with respiratory acidosis (see the Acid–Base Disorders section later in this chapter).

Hyperkalemia alters the cell membrane potential, affecting the heart, skeletal muscle function, and the GI tract. The most harmful consequence of hyperkalemia is its effect on cardiac function. The cardiac conduction system is affected first, with slowing of the heart rate, possible heart blocks, and prolonged depolarization. ECG changes include peaked T waves, a prolonged PR interval, and widening of the QRS complex (see Figure 10–10 ■). Ventricular dysrhythmias develop, and cardiac arrest may occur. Severe hyperkalemia decreases the strength of myocardial contractions.

Manifestations

The manifestations of hyperkalemia result from its effects on the heart, skeletal, and smooth muscles. Early manifestations include diarrhea, colic (abdominal cramping), anxiety, paresthesias, irritability, and muscle tremors and twitching. As serum potassium levels increase, muscle weakness develops,

A Normal ECG

B ECG in hypokalemia

C ECG in hyperkalemia

Figure 10–10 ■ The effects of changes in potassium levels on the electrocardiogram (ECG). *A,* Normal ECG; *B,* ECG in hypokalemia; *C,* ECG in hyperkalemia.

progressing to flaccid paralysis. The lower extremities are affected first, progressing to the trunk and upper extremities. The heart rate may be slow (bradycardia) and irregular. Table 10–6 summarizes the pathophysiologic indicators and manifestations of hyperkalemia.

TABLE 10–6 Pathophysiologic Indicators and Manifestations of Hyperkalemia	
PATHOPHYSIOLOGIC INDICATOR	**MANIFESTATIONS**
Changes in laboratory values	■ Serum sodium level >145 mEq/L ■ Increased serum osmolality ■ Increased hematocrit and BUN
Increased ADH	■ Thirst ■ Decreased urine output ■ Increased urine specific gravity
Intracellular dehydration	■ Dry skin, dry mucous membranes ■ Increased tongue furrows ■ Decreased salivation
Hyperosmolality of ECF = Dehydration of brain neurons	■ Headache ■ Restlessness ■ Seizures ■ Coma
Decreased vascular volume	■ Tachycardia ■ Pulse weak and thready ■ Decreased blood pressure ■ Vascular collapse ■ ECG changes (see Figure 10–10)

Interdisciplinary Care

The management of hyperkalemia focuses on returning the serum potassium level to normal by treating the underlying cause and avoiding additional potassium intake. The choice of therapy for existing hyperkalemia is based on the severity of the hyperkalemia.

Diagnosis

The following laboratory and diagnostic tests may be ordered:

■ *Serum electrolytes* show a serum potassium level greater than 5.0 mEq/L. Low calcium and sodium levels may increase the effects of hyperkalemia; therefore, these electrolytes are usually measured as well.

■ *ABGs* are measured to determine if acidosis is present.

■ An *ECG* is obtained and *continuous ECG monitoring* is instituted to evaluate the effects of hyperkalemia on cardiac conduction and rhythm.

Medications

Medications are administered to lower the serum potassium and to stabilize the conduction system of the heart. For moderate to severe hyperkalemia, calcium gluconate is given IV to counter the effects of hyperkalemia on the cardiac conduction system. While the effect of calcium gluconate lasts only for 1 hour, it allows time to initiate measures to lower serum potassium levels. To rapidly lower these levels, regular insulin and 50 g of glucose are administered. Insulin and glucose promote potassium uptake by the cells, shifting potassium out of ECF. In some cases, a ß$_2$-agonist such as albuterol may be given by nebulizer to temporarily push potassium into the cells. Sodium bicarbonate may be given to treat acidosis. As the pH returns toward normal, hydrogen ions are released from the cells and potassium returns into the cells.

To remove potassium from the body, sodium polystyrene sulfonate (Kayexalate), a resin that binds potassium in the GI tract, may be administered orally or rectally. If renal function is normal, diuretics such as furosemide are given to promote potassium excretion. Commonly prescribed drugs, their actions, and nursing implications are listed in the accompanying Medication Administration box.

Dialysis

When renal function is severely limited, either peritoneal dialysis or hemodialysis may be implemented to remove excess potassium. These measures are invasive and typically used only when other measures are ineffective. ∞ See Chapter 28 for more information about dialysis.

℘ Nursing Care

Nursing care interventions related to hyperkalemia include identifying patients at risk, preventing hyperkalemia, and addressing problems resulting from the systemic effects of hyperkalemia. A Case Study & Nursing Care Plan for a patient with hyperkalemia is found on page 212.

Health Promotion

Patients at the greatest risk for developing hyperkalemia include those taking potassium supplements (prescribed or over-the-counter), using potassium-sparing diuretics or salt substitutes, and experiencing renal failure. Athletes participating in competition sports such as body building and those using anabolic steroids, muscle-building compounds, or "energy drinks" also may be at risk for hyperkalemia.

Teach all patients to carefully read food and dietary supplement labels. Discuss the importance of taking prescribed potassium supplements as ordered, and not increasing the dose unless prescribed by the care provider. Advise patients taking a potassium supplement or potassium-sparing diuretic to avoid salt substitutes, which usually contain potassium. Discuss the importance of maintaining an adequate fluid intake (unless a fluid restriction has been prescribed) to maintain renal function to eliminate potassium from the body.

Assessment

Assessment data related to hyperkalemia include the following:

- *Health history:* Current manifestations, including numbness and tingling, nausea and vomiting, abdominal cramping, muscle weakness, palpitations; duration of manifestations and any precipitating factors such as use of salt substitutes, potassium supplements, or reduced urine output; chronic diseases such as renal failure or endocrine disorders; current medications.
- *Physical assessment:* Apical and peripheral pulses; bowel sounds; muscle strength in upper and lower extremities; ECG pattern.

MEDICATION ADMINISTRATION   Hyperkalemia

DIURETICS
Potassium-wasting diuretics, such as furosemide (Lasix), may be used to enhance renal excretion of potassium.

Nursing Responsibilities
- Monitor serum electrolytes.
- Monitor and record weight at regular intervals under standard conditions (same time of day, balanced scale, same clothing).
- Monitor intake and output.

INSULIN, HYPERTONIC DEXTROSE, AND SODIUM BICARBONATE
Insulin, hypertonic dextrose (10% to 50%), and sodium bicarbonate are used in the emergency treatment of moderate to severe hyperkalemia. Insulin promotes the movement of potassium into the cell, and glucose prevents hypoglycemia. The onset of action of insulin and hypertonic dextrose occurs within 30 minutes and is effective for approximately 4 to 6 hours.

Sodium bicarbonate elevates the serum pH; potassium is moved into the cell in exchange for hydrogen ion. Sodium bicarbonate is particularly useful in the patient with metabolic acidosis (Perrin, 2009). Onset of effects occurs within 15 to 30 minutes and is effective for approximately 2 hours.

Nursing Responsibilities
- Administer IV insulin and dextrose over prescribed interval of time using an infusion pump.
- Administer sodium bicarbonate as prescribed. It may be administered as an IV bolus or added to a dextrose-in-water solution and given by infusion.
- In patients receiving sodium bicarbonate, monitor for sodium overload, particularly in patients with hypernatremia, heart failure, and renal failure.

- Monitor the ECG pattern closely.
- Monitor serum electrolytes (K^+, Na^+, Ca^{2+}, Mg^{2+}) frequently during treatment.

CALCIUM GLUCONATE AND CALCIUM CHLORIDE
IV calcium gluconate or calcium chloride is used as a temporary emergency measure to counteract the toxic effects of potassium on myocardial conduction and function.

Nursing Responsibilities
- Closely monitor the ECG of the patient receiving IV calcium, particularly for bradycardia.
- Calcium should be used cautiously in patients receiving digitalis, because calcium increases the cardiotonic effects of digitalis and may precipitate digitalis toxicity, leading to dysrhythmias.

SODIUM POLYSTYRENE SULFONATE (KAYEXALATE) AND SORBITOL
Sodium polystyrene sulfonate (Kayexalate) is used to treat moderate or severe hyperkalemia. Categorized as a cation exchange resin, Kayexalate exchanges sodium or calcium for potassium in the large intestine. Sorbitol is given with Kayexalate to promote bowel elimination. Kayexalate and sorbitol may be administered orally, through a nasogastric tube, or rectally as a retention enema.

Nursing Responsibilities
- Because Kayexalate contains sodium, monitor patients with heart failure and edema closely for water retention.
- Monitor serum electrolytes (K^+, Na^+, Ca^{2+}, Mg^{2+}) frequently during therapy.
- Restrict sodium intake in patients who are unable to tolerate increased sodium load (e.g., those with CHF or hypertension).

CASE STUDY & NURSING CARE PLAN   Hyperkalemia

Montigue Longacre, a 51-year-old African American male, has end-stage renal failure. He arrives at the emergency clinic complaining of shortness of breath on exertion and extreme weakness.

ASSESSMENT

Mr. Longacre tells the nurse, Janet Allen, RN, that he normally receives dialysis three times a week. He missed his last treatment, however, to attend his father's funeral. During the last several days, he has eaten a number of fresh oranges he received as a gift. Physical assessment findings include T 99.2, P 100, R 28, BP 168/96, 2+ pretibial edema, and a 6-lb (3.6-kg) weight gain since his last hemodialysis treatment 4 days ago. Laboratory and diagnostic tests show the following abnormal results:

- K^+ 6.5 mEq/L (normal 3.5 to 5 mEq/L)
- BUN 118 mg/dL (normal 7 to 18 mg/dL)
- Creatinine 14 mg/dL (normal 0.7 to 1.3 mg/dL)
- HCO_3^- 17 mEq/L (normal 22 to 26 mEq/L)
- Peaked T wave noted on ECG

Mr. Longacre is placed on continuous ECG monitoring, and the physician prescribes hemodialysis. As an interim measure to lower the serum potassium, the physician prescribes D50W (25 g of dextrose), one ampule, to be administered IV with 10 units of regular insulin over 30 minutes.

DIAGNOSES

- *Activity Intolerance* related to skeletal muscle weakness
- *Risk for Decreased Cardiac Output* related to hyperkalemia
- *Risk for Ineffective Health Maintenance* related to inadequate knowledge of recommended diet
- *Fluid Volume Excess* related to renal failure

EXPECTED OUTCOMES

- Gradually resume usual physical activities.
- Maintain serum potassium level within normal range.

- Verbalize causes of hyperkalemia, the importance of hemodialysis treatments as scheduled, and the role of diet in preventing hyperkalemia.

PLANNING AND IMPLEMENTATION

- Monitor intake and output.
- Monitor serum potassium and ECG closely during treatment.
- Teach causes of hyperkalemia and the relationship between hemodialysis and hyperkalemia.
- Discuss the importance of avoiding foods high in potassium to prevent or control hyperkalemia.

EVALUATION

Following emergency treatment and hemodialysis, Mr. Longacre's ECG and serum potassium level have returned to normal. His muscle strength has returned to near normal, and he verbalizes an understanding of his prescribed hemodialysis regimen. Janet Allen provides verbal and written information about hyperkalemia, the importance of complying with the hemodialysis regimen, and the importance of limiting intake of dietary sources of potassium in renal failure. She also furnishes a list of foods high in potassium and cautions against using potassium-containing salt substitutes and nonprescription drugs.

CRITICAL THINKING IN THE NURSING PROCESS

1. What information given by Mr. Longacre indicated that he might be experiencing hyperkalemia?
2. Why was continuous ECG monitoring instituted as an emergency measure?
3. What additional emergency measures might have been instituted if Mr. Longacre's serum potassium level had been 8.5 mEq/L and his ECG had showed changes in impulse conduction?
4. Develop a care plan for Mr. Longacre for the nursing diagnosis of *Anxiety*.

See Evaluating Your Response in Appendix C.

Nursing Diagnoses and Interventions

The effects of excess potassium on the electrical conduction and contractility of the heart are the highest priority for nursing care, particularly when the serum potassium level is 6.5 mEq/L or higher.

Risk for Decreased Cardiac Output

Hyperkalemia affects depolarization of the atria and ventricles of the heart. Severe hyperkalemia can cause dysrhythmias with ventricular fibrillation and cardiac arrest. The cardiac effects of hyperkalemia are more pronounced when the serum potassium level rises rapidly. Low serum sodium and calcium levels, high serum magnesium levels, and acidosis contribute to the adverse effects of hyperkalemia on the heart muscle.

PRACTICE ALERT

Monitor the ECG pattern for development of peaked, narrow T waves, prolongation of the PR interval, depression of the ST segment, widened QRS interval, and loss of the P wave (see Figure 10–10). Notify the physician of changes. Progressive ECG changes from a peaked T wave to loss of the P wave and widening of the QRS complex indicate an increasing risk of dysrhythmias and cardiac arrest.

- Closely monitor the response to IV calcium gluconate, particularly in patients taking digitalis. *Calcium increases the risk of digitalis toxicity.*

Risk for Activity Intolerance

Both hypokalemia (low serum potassium levels) and hyperkalemia (high serum potassium levels) affect neuromuscular activity and the function of cardiac, smooth, and skeletal muscles. Hyperkalemia can cause muscle weakness and even paralysis.

- Monitor skeletal muscle strength and tone. *Increasing weakness, muscle paralysis, or progression of affected muscles to affect the upper extremities or trunk can indicate increasing serum potassium levels.*
- Monitor respiratory rate and depth. Regularly assess lung sounds. *Muscle weakness due to hyperkalemia can impair ventilation. In addition, medications such as sodium bicarbonate or sodium polystyrene sulfonate can cause fluid retention and pulmonary edema in patients with preexisting cardiovascular disease.*
- Assist with self-care activities as needed. *Increasing muscle weakness can lead to fatigue and affect the ability to meet self-care needs.*

Community-Based Care

Preventing future episodes of hyperkalemia is the focus when preparing the patient for home care. Include the family, a significant other, or a caregiver when teaching the following topics:

- Recommended diet and any restrictions including salt substitutes and foods high in potassium
- Medications to be avoided, including over-the-counter and fitness supplements

Calcium Imbalance

Calcium is one of the most abundant ions in the body. The normal adult total serum calcium concentration is 8.5 to 10.0 mg/dL. Calcium is obtained from dietary sources, although only about 20% of the calcium ingested is absorbed into the blood. The remainder is excreted in feces. Extracellular calcium is excreted by the kidneys. Approximately 99% of the total calcium in the body is bound to phosphorus to form the minerals in bones and teeth. The remaining 1% is in extracellular fluid. About half of this extracellular calcium is ionized (free); it is this ionized calcium that is physiologically active. The remaining extracellular calcium is bound to protein or other ions. Ionized calcium is essential to a number of processes: stabilizing cell membranes, regulating muscle contraction and relaxation, maintaining cardiac function, and blood clotting.

Serum calcium levels are regulated by the interaction of three hormones: parathyroid hormone (PTH), calcitonin, and calcitriol (a metabolite of vitamin D). When serum calcium levels fall, the parathyroid glands secrete PTH, which mobilizes skeletal calcium stores, increases calcium absorption in the intestines, and promotes calcium reabsorption by the kidneys (Figure 10–11 ■). Calcitriol facilitates this process by stimulating calcium release from the bones, absorption in the intestines, and reabsorption by the kidneys. Calcitonin is secreted by the thyroid gland in response to high serum calcium levels. Its effect on serum calcium levels is the opposite of PTH: It inhibits the movement of calcium out of bone, reduces intestinal absorption of calcium, and promotes calcium excretion by the kidneys.

Serum calcium levels are also affected by acid–base balance. When hydrogen ion concentration falls and the pH rises (alkalosis), more calcium is bound to protein. While the total serum calcium remains unchanged, less calcium is available in the ionized, active form. Conversely, when hydrogen ion concentration increases and the pH falls (acidosis), calcium is released from protein, making more ionized calcium available.

Finally, the total amount of calcium in blood plasma fluctuates with plasma protein levels, particularly the albumin level. As the albumin level falls, the total amount of plasma calcium declines. Table 10–7 summarizes the manifestations of calcium imbalances.

The Patient with Hypocalcemia

Hypocalcemia is a total serum calcium level of less than 8.5 mg/dL. Hypocalcemia can result from decreased total body calcium stores or low levels of extracellular calcium with normal amounts of calcium stored in bone. The systemic effects of hypocalcemia are caused by decreased levels of ionized calcium in extracellular fluid.

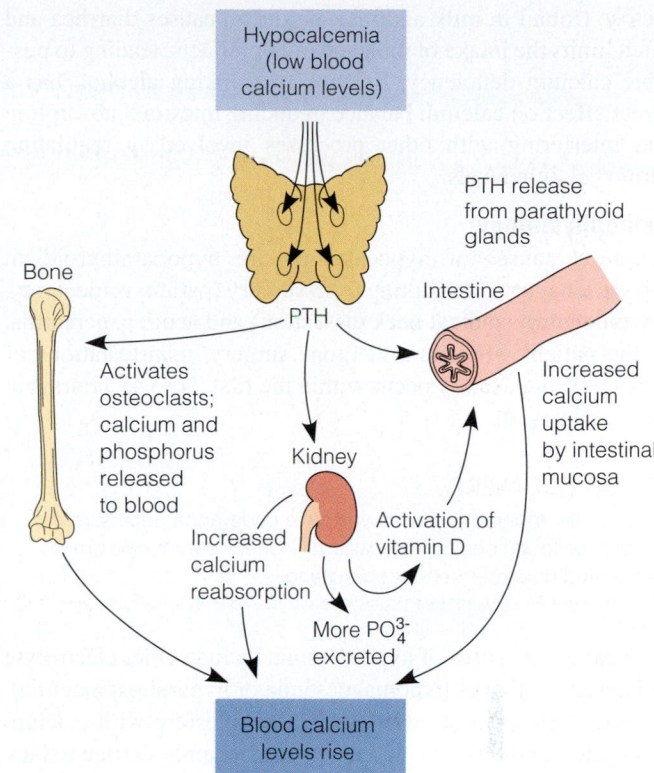

Figure 10–11 ■ Low calcium levels (hypocalcemia) trigger the release of parathyroid hormone (PTH), increasing calcium ion levels through stimulation of bones, kidneys, and intestines.

Risk Factors

Certain people are at greater risk for hypocalcemia: those who have had a parathyroidectomy (removal of the parathyroid glands), older adults (especially women), people with lactose intolerance, and those who have alcoholism. Older adults often consume less milk and milk products (good sources of calcium) and may have decreased exposure to the sun (a source of vitamin D). Older adults also may be less active, promoting calcium loss from bones. They are more likely to be taking drugs that interfere with calcium absorption or promote calcium excretion (e.g., furosemide). Older women are at particular risk after menopause because of reduced estrogen levels. Intolerance to

TABLE 10–7 Manifestations of Calcium Imbalances

HYPOCALCEMIA	HYPERCALCEMIA
■ Serum calcium level <8.5 mg/dL	■ Serum calcium level >10.0 mg/dL
■ Numbness and tingling	■ Increased thirst and urine output
■ Muscle cramping	■ Anorexia
■ Hyperactive reflexes	■ Nausea, vomiting
■ Tetany	■ Constipation
■ Carpopedal and laryngeal spasms	■ Muscle weakness
■ Positive Chvostek and Trousseau signs (see Figure 10–12)	■ Increased blood pressure
■ Decreased blood pressure	■ AV block
■ Ventricular dysrhythmias	■ Lethargy
■ Bone pain, fractures (chronic form)	■ Coma

lactose (found in milk and milk products) causes diarrhea and often limits the intake of milk and milk products, leading to possible calcium deficiency. Ethanol, or drinking alcohol, has a direct effect on calcium balance, reducing intestinal absorption and interfering with other processes involved in regulating serum calcium levels.

Pathophysiology

Common causes of hypocalcemia are hypoparathyroidism (∞ see Chapter 19) resulting from surgery (parathyroidectomy, thyroidectomy, radical neck dissection) and acute pancreatitis. In the patient who has undergone surgery, manifestations of hypocalcemia usually occur within the first 24 to 48 hours, but may be delayed.

PRACTICE ALERT
Carefully monitor patients who have undergone neck surgery for manifestations of hypocalcemia. Check serum calcium levels, and document and report changes.

Additional causes of hypocalcemia include other electrolyte imbalances (such as hypomagnesemia or hyperphosphatemia), alkalosis, malabsorption disorders that interfere with calcium absorption in the bowel, and inadequate vitamin D (due to lack of sun exposure or malabsorption). Hyperphosphatemia often occurs in acute renal failure, with reciprocal hypocalcemia. Massive transfusion of banked blood can lead to hypocalcemia. Citrate is added to blood to prevent clotting and as a preservative. When blood is administered faster than the liver can metabolize the citrate, it can bind with calcium, temporarily removing ionized calcium from circulation. Many drugs increase the risk for hypocalcemia, including loop diuretics (such as furosemide [Lasix]), anticonvulsants (such as phenytoin [Dilantin] and phenobarbital), phosphates (including phosphate enemas), and drugs that lower serum magnesium levels (such as cisplatin [Platinol]).

Extracellular calcium acts to stabilize neuromuscular cell membranes. This effect is reduced in hypocalcemia, increasing neuromuscular irritability. The threshold of excitation of sensory nerve fibers is lowered as well, leading to paresthesias (altered sensation). The nervous system becomes more excitable, and muscle spasms develop. In the heart, this change in cell membranes can lead to dysrhythmias such as ventricular tachycardia and cardiac arrest. Hypocalcemia decreases the contractility of cardiac muscle fibers, leading to decreased cardiac output.

Manifestations and Complications

The most serious manifestations of hypocalcemia are **tetany** (tonic muscular spasms) and convulsions. Numbness and tingling around the mouth (circumoral) and in the hands and feet develop. Muscle spasms of the face and extremities occur, and deep tendon reflexes become hyperactive. Chvostek's sign, contraction of the facial muscles produced by tapping the facial nerve in front of the ear (Figure 10–12A ■), and Trousseau's sign, carpal spasm induced by inflating a blood pressure cuff on the upper arm to above systolic blood pressure for 2 to 5 minutes (Figure 10–12B), indicate increased neuromuscular excitability in patients without obvious manifestations. Tetany can also cause bronchial muscle spasms, simulating an asthma attack,

Figure   10–12 ■ A, Positive Chvostek's sign. B, Positive Trousseau's sign.

and visceral muscle spasms, producing acute abdominal pain. Cardiovascular manifestations include hypotension, possible bradycardia (slow heart rate), and ventricular dysrhythmias.

Serious complications of hypocalcemia include airway obstruction and possible respiratory arrest from laryngospasm, ventricular dysrhythmias, prolonged QT intervals, cardiac arrest, heart failure, and convulsions.

Interdisciplinary Care

Management of hypocalcemia is directed toward restoring normal calcium balance and correcting the underlying cause.

Diagnosis

The following laboratory and diagnostic tests may be ordered when hypocalcemia is known or suspected:

■ *Total serum calcium*, the amount of ionized (active) calcium available, usually is estimated. In critically ill patients, however, *ionized calcium* may be directly measured using ion-selective electrodes. Direct measurement of ionized calcium requires special handling of the blood specimen, including placing the specimen on ice and analyzing it immediately.

- *Serum albumin*, because the albumin level affects serum calcium results. When the albumin level is low (hypoalbuminemia), the amount of ionized calcium may remain normal even though the total calcium level is low.
- *Serum magnesium*, because hypocalcemia is often associated with hypomagnesemia (serum magnesium < 1.6 mg/dL). In this case, normal magnesium levels must be restored to correct the hypocalcemia.
- *Serum phosphate*, because hyperphosphatemia (serum phosphate > 4.5 mg/dL) can lead to hypocalcemia due to the inverse relationship between phosphorus and calcium (as phosphate levels rise, calcium levels fall).
- *Parathyroid hormone (PTH)*, to identify the possible diagnoses of hyperparathyroidism.
- An *ECG*, to evaluate the effects of hypocalcemia on the heart, such as a prolonged ST segment.

Medications

Hypocalcemia is treated with oral or IV calcium. The patient with severe hypocalcemia is treated with IV calcium to prevent life-threatening problems such as airway obstruction. The most common IV calcium preparations include calcium chloride and calcium gluconate. Although calcium chloride contains more elemental calcium than calcium gluconate, it also is more irritating to the veins and may cause venous sclerosis (hardening of the vein walls) if given into a peripheral vein. IV calcium preparations can cause necrosis and sloughing of tissue if they infiltrate into subcutaneous tissue. Rapid drug administration can lead to bradycardia and possible cardiac arrest due to over-correction of hypocalcemia with resulting hypercalcemia. See the accompanying Medication Administration box for further information about calcium administration.

Oral calcium preparations (calcium carbonate, calcium gluconate, or calcium lactate) are used to treat chronic, asymptomatic hypocalcemia. Calcium supplements may be combined with vitamin D, or vitamin D may be given alone to increase GI absorption of calcium.

Nutrition

A diet high in calcium-rich foods may be recommended for patients with chronic hypocalcemia or with low total body stores of calcium. Foods high in calcium include dairy products, canned salmon, broccoli, spinach, and tofu.

Nursing Care

Health Promotion

Because of the large stores of calcium in bones, most healthy adults have a very low risk of developing hypocalcemia. However, a deficit of total body calcium is often associated with aging, increasing the risk of osteoporosis, fractures, and disability. Women have a higher risk for developing osteoporosis than men due to lower bone density and hormonal influences. Teach women of all ages the importance of maintaining adequate calcium intake through diet and, as needed, calcium supplements. Stress the relationship between weight-bearing exercise and bone density, and encourage women to engage in a regular aerobic and weight-training exercise regime. Recommend screening for bone density in older women. See Chapter 40 for more information about osteoporosis.

Assessment

Assessment data related to hypocalcemia include the following:
- *Health history:* Current manifestations, including numbness and tingling around mouth and of hands and feet, abdominal pain, shortness of breath; acute or chronic diseases such as pancreatitis, liver or kidney disease; current medications.

MEDICATION ADMINISTRATION Calcium Salts

CALCIUM SALTS
Calcium carbonate (BioCal, Calsam, Caltrate, OsCal, Tums, others)
Calcium chloride
Calcium citrate (Citracal)
Calcium glubionate
Calcium gluceptate
Calcium gluconate (Kalcinate)
Calcium lactate

Calcium salts are given to increase calcium levels when there is a deficit (a total body deficit or inadequate levels of extracellular calcium). Calcium is necessary to maintain bone structure and for multiple physiologic processes including neuromuscular and cardiac function as well as blood coagulation. In the presence of vitamin D, calcium is well absorbed from the GI tract. Severe hypocalcemia is treated with IV calcium preparations.

Nursing Responsibilities
Oral calcium salts:
- Administer 1 to 1.5 hours after meals and at bedtime.
- Give calcium tablets with a full glass of water.
IV calcium salts:
- Assess IV site for patency. Do not administer calcium if there is a risk of leakage into the tissues.

- May be given by slow IV push (dilute with sterile normal saline for injection prior to administering) or added to compatible parenteral fluids such as NS, lactated Ringer's solution, or D_5W.
- Administer into the largest available vein; use a central line if available.
- Do not administer with bicarbonate or phosphate.
- Continuously monitor ECG when administering IV calcium to patients taking digitalis due to increased risk of digitalis toxicity.
- Frequently monitor serum calcium levels and response to therapy.

Health Education for the Patient and Family
- Take calcium tablets with a full glass of water 1 to 2 hours after meals. Do not take with food or milk. If possible, do not take within 1 to 2 hours of other medications.
- Maintain adequate vitamin D intake through diet or exposure to the sun to promote calcium absorption.
- Calcium carbonate can cause constipation. Eat a high-fiber diet and maintain a generous fluid intake to prevent constipation.

■ *Physical assessment:* Muscle spasms; deep tendon reflexes; Chvostek's sign and Trousseau's sign; vital signs and apical pulse; presence of convulsions.

Nursing Diagnoses and Interventions

The effect of hypocalcemia on neuromuscular irritability, with the risk for muscle spasm and convulsions, is the highest priority for nursing care of the patient.

Risk for Injury

The patient with hypocalcemia is at risk for injury from possible laryngospasm, cardiac dysrhythmias, or convulsions. In addition, too rapid administration of IV calcium or infiltration of the medication into subcutaneous tissues can lead to injury.

■ Frequently monitor airway and respiratory status. Report changes such as respiratory stridor (a high-pitched, harsh inspiratory sound indicative of upper airway obstruction) or increased respiratory rate or effort to the physician. *These changes may indicate laryngeal spasm due to tetany.*

> **PRACTICE ALERT**
> Laryngeal spasm is a respiratory emergency, requiring immediate intervention to maintain ventilation and gas exchange.

■ Monitor cardiovascular status including heart rate and rhythm, blood pressure, and peripheral pulses. *Hypocalcemia decreases myocardial contractility, causing reduced cardiac output and hypotension. It also can cause bradycardia or ventricular dysrhythmias. Cardiac arrest may occur in severe hypocalcemia.*

■ Continuously monitor ECG in patients receiving IV calcium preparations, especially if the patient also is taking digitalis. *Rapid administration of calcium salts can lead to hypercalcemia and cardiac dysrhythmias. Calcium administration increases the risk of digitalis toxicity and resultant dysrhythmias.*

■ If the patient has tetany, provide a quiet environment and institute seizure precautions such as raising the side rails and keeping an airway at bedside. *A quiet environment reduces central nervous system stimuli and the risk of convulsions in the patient with tetany.*

Community-Based Care

In preparing the patient with hypocalcemia for home care, consider the circumstances leading to low serum calcium levels. Discuss risk factors for hypocalcemia specific to the patient, and provide information about managing these risk factors to avoid future episodes of hypocalcemia. Teach about prescribed medications, including calcium supplements. Provide a list of foods high in calcium, as well as sources of vitamin D if recommended. Discuss manifestations to report to the healthcare provider, and stress the importance of follow-up care as scheduled.

The Patient with Hypercalcemia

Hypercalcemia is a serum calcium value greater than 10.0 mg/dL. Excess ionized calcium in ECF can have serious widespread effects.

Pathophysiology

Hypercalcemia usually results from increased resorption of calcium from the bones. The two most common causes of bone resorption are hyperparathyroidism and malignancies. In hyperparathyroidism, excess PTH is produced. This causes calcium to be released from bones, as well as increased calcium absorption in the intestines and retention of calcium by the kidneys. Hypercalcemia is a common complication of malignancies. It may develop as a result of bone destruction by the tumor or due to hormone-like substances produced by the tumor itself. Prolonged immobility and lack of weight bearing also cause increased resorption of bone with calcium release into extracellular fluids. Self-limiting hypercalcemia may follow successful kidney transplant. Levels of parathyroid hormone may be altered in chronic renal failure, leading to increased serum calcium levels.

Increased intestinal absorption of calcium also can lead to hypercalcemia. This may result from excess vitamin D, overuse of calcium-containing antacids, or excessive milk ingestion. Renal failure and some drugs such as thiazide diuretics and lithium can interfere with elimination of calcium by the kidneys, causing high serum calcium levels.

The effects of hypercalcemia largely depend on the degree of serum calcium elevation and the length of time over which it develops. In general, higher serum calcium levels are associated with more serious effects. Calcium has a stabilizing effect on the neuromuscular junction; hypercalcemia decreases neuromuscular excitability, leading to muscle weakness and depressed deep tendon reflexes. Gastrointestinal motility is reduced as well. In the heart, calcium exerts an effect similar to digitalis (∞ see Chapter 30), strengthening contractions and reducing the heart rate. Hypercalcemia affects the conduction system of the heart, leading to bradycardia and heart blocks. The ability of the kidneys to concentrate urine is impaired by hypercalcemia, causing excess sodium and water loss and increased thirst.

Extremely high serum calcium levels affect mental status. This is thought to be due to increased calcium in cerebrospinal fluid. Behavioral effects range from personality changes to confusion, impaired memory, and acute psychoses.

Manifestations and Complications

Manifestations of hypercalcemia relate to its effects on neuromuscular activity, the central nervous system, the cardiovascular system, and the kidneys. Decreased neuromuscular excitability causes muscle weakness and fatigue, as well as GI manifestations such as anorexia, nausea, vomiting, and constipation. Central nervous system (CNS) effects may include confusion, lethargy, behavior or personality changes, and coma. Cardiovascular effects include dysrhythmias, ECG changes, and possible hypertension. Hypercalcemia causes polyuria and, as a result, increased thirst (see Table 10–7).

Complications of hypercalcemia can affect several different organ systems. Peptic ulcer disease may develop due to increased gastric acid secretion. Pancreatitis can occur as a result of calcium deposits in pancreatic ducts. Excess calcium can precipitate out of urine to form kidney stones. Hypercalcemic crisis, an acute increase in the serum calcium level, can lead to cardiac arrest.

Interdisciplinary Care

The management of hypercalcemia focuses on correcting the underlying cause and reducing the serum calcium level. Treatment is particularly important in patients who have one or more of the following: serum calcium levels greater than 12 mg/dL, overt manifestations of hypercalcemia, compromised renal function, and inability to maintain an adequate fluid intake.

Diagnosis

The laboratory and diagnostic tests that may be ordered are as follows:

- *Serum electrolytes* show a total serum calcium greater than 10.0 mg/dL.
- *Serum PTH levels* are measured to identify or rule out hyperparathyroidism as the cause of hypercalcemia.
- *ECG* changes in hypercalcemia include a shortened QT interval, shortened and depressed ST segment, and widened T wave. Bradycardia or heart block may be identified on the ECG.
- *Bone density scans* may be done to monitor bone resorption and the effects of treatment measures on mineralization of bone.

Medications

Measures to promote calcium elimination by the kidneys and reduce calcium resorption from bone are used to treat hypercalcemia. In acute hypercalcemia, IV fluids are given with a loop diuretic such as furosemide [Lasix] to promote elimination of excess calcium. Calcitonin, which promotes the uptake of calcium into bones, also may be used to rapidly lower serum calcium levels.

A number of drugs that inhibit bone resorption are available. The bisphosphonates (pamidronate and etidronate) are commonly used to treat hypercalcemia associated with malignancies. These drugs also are used to prevent and treat osteoporosis. Nursing implications for calcitonin and bisphosphonate drugs are presented in the Medication Administration boxes in ∞ Chapter 40. When a bisphosphonate drug is ineffective to correct hypercalcemia, mithramycin, a chemotherapeutic agent, may be used.

Rapid reversal of hypercalcemia in emergency situations may be accomplished by IV administration of sodium phosphate or potassium phosphate. Calcium binds to phosphate, thus decreasing serum calcium levels. Paradoxically, complications of this therapy can include fatal hypocalcemia resulting from binding of the ionized calcium and soft tissue calcifications.

Other drug therapies include the use of IV plicamycin (Mithramycin) to inhibit bone resorption. Glucocorticoids (cortisone), which compete with vitamin D, and a low-calcium diet may be prescribed to decrease GI absorption of calcium, inhibit bone resorption, and to increase urinary calcium excretion. Also, calcitonin may be prescribed to decrease skeletal mobilization of calcium and phosphorus and to increase renal output of calcium and phosphorus. ∞ See Chapter 19 for more information about and nursing implications of glucocorticoid therapy.

Fluid Management

IV fluids, usually isotonic saline, are administered to patients with severe hypercalcemia to restore vascular volume and promote renal excretion of calcium. Isotonic saline is used because sodium excretion is accompanied by calcium excretion. Careful assessment of cardiovascular and renal function is done prior to fluid therapy; the patient is carefully monitored for evidence of fluid overload during treatment.

∞ Nursing Care

Health Promotion

Identify and monitor patients at risk for hypercalcemia. Promote mobility in patients when possible. Assist hospitalized patients to ambulate as soon as possible. In the home setting, discuss the benefits of regular weight-bearing activity with patients, families, and caregivers. Encourage a generous fluid intake of up to 3 to 4 quarts per day. Encourage patients at risk to limit their intake of milk and milk products, as well as calcium-containing antacids and supplements. In addition, patients with prolonged immobility or hypercalcemia are encouraged to consume fluids that increase the acidity of urine (which inhibits calcium stone formation), such as cranberry or prune juice.

Assessment

Assessment data related to hypercalcemia include the following:
- *Health history:* Current manifestations, including weakness or fatigue, abdominal discomfort, nausea or vomiting, increased urination and thirst; changes in memory or thinking; duration of manifestations and any risk factors such as excess intake of milk or calcium products, prolonged immobility, malignancy, renal failure, or endocrine disorders; current medications.
- *Physical assessment:* Mental status and level of consciousness; vital signs including apical pulse; bowel sounds; muscle strength of upper and lower extremities; deep tendon reflexes.

> **MEMORY CUE**
> Remember, calcium has a stabilizing or sedative effect on neuromuscular transmission. Therefore,
> Hypocalcemia → Increased neuromuscular excitability, muscle twitching, spasms, and possible tetany
> Hypercalcemia → Decreased neuromuscular excitability, muscle weakness, and fatigue

Nursing Diagnoses and Interventions
Risk for Injury

Patients with hypercalcemia are at risk for injury due to changes in mental status, the effects of hypercalcemia on muscle strength, and loss of calcium from bones.

- Institute safety precautions if confusion or other changes in mental status are noted. *Changes in mental status may impair judgment and the patient's ability to maintain his or her own safety.*

- Observe for manifestations of digitalis toxicity (if administered), including vision changes, anorexia, and changes in heart rate and rhythm. Monitor serum digitalis levels. *Hypercalcemia increases the risk of digitalis toxicity.*
- Promote fluid intake to keep the patient well hydrated and maintain dilute urine. Encourage fluids such as prune or cranberry juice to help maintain acidic urine. *Acidic, dilute urine reduces the risk of calcium salts precipitating out to form kidney stones.*
- If excess bone reabsorption has occurred, use caution when turning, positioning, transferring, or ambulating. *Bones that have lost excess calcium may fracture with minimal stress or trauma (pathologic fractures).*

Risk for Fluid Volume Excess

Large amounts of isotonic IV fluid often are administered to help correct acute hypercalcemia, leading to a risk for hypervolemia. Patients with preexisting cardiac or renal disease are at particular risk. Loop diuretics may be prescribed to help eliminate excess fluid and calcium.

- Closely monitor intake and output. *A loop diuretic such as furosemide may be necessary if urinary output does not keep up with fluid administration.*
- Frequently assess vital signs, respiratory status, and heart sounds. *Increasing pulse rate, dyspnea, adventitious lung sounds, and an S_3 on auscultation of the heart may indicate excess fluid volume and potential heart failure.*
- Place in semi-Fowler's to Fowler's position. *Elevating the head of the bed improves lung expansion and reduces the work of breathing.*

Community-Based Care

Discuss the following topics when preparing the patient for discharge:

- Avoid excess intake of calcium-rich foods and antacids.
- Use prescribed drugs to prevent excess calcium resorption. Discuss their dose, use, and desired and possible adverse effects.
- Increase fluid intake to 3 to 4 quarts per day; increase the intake of acid ash foods (meats, fish, poultry, eggs, cranberries, plums, prunes); increase dietary fiber and fluid intake to prevent constipation.
- Maintain weight-bearing physical activity to prevent hypercalcemia.

Magnesium Imbalance

Only about 1% of the magnesium in the body is in extracellular fluid; the rest is found within the cells and in bone. The normal serum concentration of magnesium ranges from 1.6 to 2.6 mg/dL (1.3 to 2.1 mEq/L).

Magnesium is obtained through the diet (it is plentiful in green vegetables, grains, nuts, meats, and seafood) and excreted by the kidneys. Magnesium is vital to many intracellular processes, including enzyme reactions and synthesis of proteins and nucleic acids. Magnesium exerts a sedative effect on the neuromuscular junction, decreasing acetylcholine release. It is an essential ion for neuromuscular transmission and cardiovascular function. The physiologic effects of magnesium are affected by both potassium and calcium levels.

The Patient with Hypomagnesemia

Hypomagnesemia is a magnesium level of less than 1.6 mg/dL. It is a common problem in critically ill patients. Hypomagnesemia may be caused by deficient magnesium intake, excessive losses, or a shift between the intracellular and extracellular compartments.

Risk Factors

Loss of GI fluids, particularly from diarrhea, an ileostomy, or intestinal fistula is a major risk factor for hypomagnesemia. Disruption of nutrient absorption in the small intestine also increases the risk. Multiple factors associated with alcoholism contribute to hypomagnesemia: deficient nutrient intake, increased GI losses, impaired absorption, and increased renal excretion. Other risk factors for hypomagnesemia include protein-calorie malnutrition or starvation; diabetic ketoacidosis; kidney disease; drugs such as loop or thiazide diuretics, aminoglycoside antibiotics, amphotericin B, and cyclosporine; and rapid administration of citrated blood.

Pathophysiology

Magnesium deficiency usually occurs along with low serum potassium and calcium levels. The effects of hypomagnesemia relate not only to the magnesium deficiency but also to hypokalemia and hypocalcemia.

Hypomagnesemia causes increased neuromuscular excitability, with muscle weakness and tremors. The accompanying hypocalcemia contributes to this effect. In the central nervous system, this increased neural excitability can lead to seizures and changes in mental status. Deficient intracellular magnesium in the myocardium increases the risk of cardiac dysrhythmias and sudden death. Hypokalemia increases this risk. Hypomagnesemia also increases the risk of digitalis toxicity. Chronic hypomagnesemia may contribute to hypertension, probably due to increased vasoconstriction. Severe hypomagnesia is strongly linked to low serum calcium levels because both are associated with renal and GI losses.

Manifestations and Complications

Neuromuscular manifestations of hypomagnesemia include tremors, hyperreactive reflexes, positive Chvostek's and Trousseau's signs (see Figure 10–12), tetany, paresthesias, and seizures. CNS effects include confusion, mood changes (apathy, depression, agitation), hallucinations, and possible psychoses. An increased heart rate and ventricular dysrhythmias are common, especially when hypokalemia is present or the patient is taking digitalis. Cardiac arrest and sudden death may occur. Table 10–8 summarizes manifestations of magnesium imbalances.

TABLE 10–8 Manifestations of Magnesium Disorders

HYPOMAGNESEMIA	HYPERMAGNESEMIA
■ Serum magnesium level < 1.6 mg/dL	■ Serum magnesium level > 2.6 mg/dL
■ Changes in personality	■ Confusion and lethargy
■ Nystagmus (lateral twitching of eyeballs)	■ Hypotension
■ Positive Babinski, Chvostek, and Trousseau signs	■ Cardiac dysrhythmias
■ Hypertension	■ Coma
■ Tachycardia	■ Cardiac arrest
■ Cardiac dysrhythmias	

Interdisciplinary Care

Hypomagnesemia is diagnosed by measuring serum electrolyte levels. The ECG shows a prolonged PR interval, widened QRS complex, and depression of the ST segment with T-wave inversion. Treatment is directed toward prevention and identification of an existing deficiency. Magnesium is added to IV total parenteral nutrition solutions to prevent hypomagnesemia.

In patients able to eat, a mild deficiency may be corrected by increasing the intake of foods rich in magnesium (such as green leafy vegetables, seafood, milk, bananas, citrus fruits, and chocolate), or with oral magnesium supplements. Oral magnesium supplements may cause diarrhea, however, limiting their use.

Patients with manifestations of hypomagnesemia are treated with parenteral magnesium sulfate. Treatment is continued for several days to restore intracellular magnesium levels. Magnesium may be given IV or by deep IM injection. Renal function is evaluated prior to administration, and serum magnesium levels are monitored during treatment. The IV route is used for severe magnesium deficiency or if neurologic changes or cardiac dysrhythmias are present. See the Medication Administration box below for the nursing implications of parenteral magnesium sulfate.

✑ Nursing Care

Health Promotion

Discuss the importance of maintaining adequate magnesium intake through a well-balanced diet, particularly with patients at risk (people with alcoholism, malabsorption, or bowel surgery). Many hospitalized patients are at risk for hypomagnesemia due to protein-calorie malnutrition and other disorders.

Monitor serum magnesium levels, reporting changes to the healthcare provider.

Assessment

In addition to asking questions related to risk factors for hypomagnesemia, assess for manifestations of hypokalemia and hypocalcemia. Monitor diagnostic studies such as serum electrolytes, serum albumin levels, and the ECG.

Nursing Diagnoses and Interventions

Nursing care for patients with hypomagnesemia focuses on careful monitoring of manifestations and responses to treatment, promoting safety, patient and family teaching, and administering prescribed medications.

Risk for Injury

- Monitor serum electrolytes, including magnesium, potassium, and calcium. *Magnesium deficiency often is accompanied by deficiencies of potassium and calcium.*
- Monitor GI function, including bowel sounds and abdominal distention. *Hypomagnesemia reduces GI motility.*
- Initiate cardiac monitoring, reporting and treating (as prescribed) ECG changes and dysrhythmias. In patients receiving digitalis, monitor for digitalis toxicity. *Low magnesium levels can precipitate ventricular dysrhythmias, including lethal dysrhythmias such as ventricular fibrillation.*
- Assess deep tendon reflexes frequently during IV magnesium infusions and prior to each IM dose. *Depressed tendon reflexes indicate a high serum magnesium level.*
- Maintain a quiet, darkened environment. Institute seizure precautions. *Increased neuromuscular and CNS irritability can lead to seizures. A quiet, dark environment reduces stimuli.*

Community-Based Care

Prior to discharge, instruct the patient to increase dietary intake of foods high in magnesium and provide information about magnesium supplements. In addition, if alcohol abuse has precipitated a magnesium deficit, discuss alcohol treatment options, including support groups such as Alcoholics Anonymous, Al-Anon, and/or Alateen.

The Patient with Hypermagnesemia

Hypermagnesemia is a serum magnesium level greater than 2.6 mg/dL. It is much less common than hypomagnesemia. Hypermagnesemia can develop in renal failure, particularly if

---

MEDICATION ADMINISTRATION   **Magnesium Sulfate**

Magnesium sulfate is used to prevent or treat hypomagnesemia. It may be given IV or by IM injection.

Nursing Responsibilities
- Assess serum magnesium levels and renal function tests (BUN and serum creatinine) prior to administering. Notify the care provider if magnesium levels are above normal limits or renal function is impaired.
- Frequently monitor neurologic status and deep tendon reflexes during therapy. Withhold magnesium and notify the care provider if deep tendon reflexes are hypoactive or absent.

- Monitor intake and output.
- Administer IM doses deep into the ventral or dorsal gluteal sites.
- IV magnesium sulfate may be given by direct IV push or by continuous infusion.

Health Education for the Patient and Family
Explain purpose and duration of treatment. Discuss reason for frequent neurologic and reflex assessments.

magnesium is administered parenterally or orally (e.g., magnesium-containing antacids or laxatives). Older adults are at risk for hypermagnesemia as renal function declines with aging and they may be more likely to use over-the-counter laxatives and other preparations that contain magnesium.

Pathophysiology and Manifestations

Elevated serum magnesium levels interfere with neuromuscular transmission and depress the central nervous system. Hypermagnesemia also affects the cardiovascular system, potentially causing hypotension, flushing, sweating, and bradydysrhythmias.

Predictable manifestations occur with increasing serum magnesium levels. With lower levels, nausea and vomiting, hypotension, facial flushing, sweating, and a feeling of warmth occur. As levels increase, manifestations of CNS depression appear (weakness, lethargy, drowsiness, weak or absent deep tendon reflexes). Marked elevations cause respiratory depression, coma, and compromised cardiac function (ECG changes, bradycardia, heart block, and cardiac arrest).

Interdisciplinary Care

The management of hypermagnesemia focuses on identifying and treating the underlying cause. All medications or compounds containing magnesium (such as antacids, IV solutions, or enemas) are withheld. In the patient with renal failure, hemodialysis or peritoneal dialysis is instituted to remove the excess magnesium.

Calcium gluconate is administered IV to reverse the neuromuscular and cardiac effects of hypermagnesemia. The patient may require mechanical ventilation to support respiratory function, and a pacemaker to maintain adequate cardiac output.

Nursing Care

Nursing care includes instituting measures to prevent and identify hypermagnesemia in patients at risk, monitoring for critical effects of hypermagnesemia, and providing measures to ensure the patient's safety. Consider the following nursing diagnoses for the patient with hypermagnesemia:

- *Decreased Cardiac Output* related to altered myocardial conduction
- *Ineffective Breathing Pattern* related to respiratory depression
- *Risk for Injury* related to muscle weakness and altered level of consciousness
- *Risk for Ineffective Health Maintenance* related to lack of knowledge about use of magnesium-containing supplements, antacids, laxatives, and enemas.

Phosphate Imbalance

Although most phosphate (85%) is found in bones, it is the primary intracellular anion. About 14% is in intracellular fluid, and the remainder (1%) is in extracellular fluid. The normal serum phosphate (or phosphorus) level in adults is 2.5 to 4.5 mg/dL. Phosphorus levels vary with age, gender, and diet.

Overview of Normal Phosphate Balance

Phosphate is essential to intracellular processes such as the production of ATP, the fuel that supports muscle contraction, nerve cell transmission, and electrolyte transport. Phosphate is vital for red blood cell function and oxygen delivery to tissues; nervous system and muscle function; and the metabolism of fats, carbohydrates, and protein. It also assists in maintaining acid–base balance.

Phosphorus is ingested in the diet, absorbed in the jejunum, and primarily excreted by the kidneys. When phosphate intake is low, the kidneys conserve phosphorus, excreting less. An inverse relationship exists between phosphate and calcium levels: When one increases, the other decreases. Regulatory mechanisms for calcium levels (parathyroid hormone, calcitonin, and vitamin D) also influence phosphate levels. The manifestations of phosphate imbalances are summarized in Table 10–9.

The Patient with Hypophosphatemia

Hypophosphatemia is a serum phosphorus of less than 2.5 mg/dL. Low serum phosphate levels may indicate a total body deficit of phosphate or a shift of phosphate into the intracellular space, the most common cause of hypophosphatemia. Decreased GI absorption of phosphate or increased renal excretion of phosphate also can cause low phosphate levels. Hypophosphatemia often is iatrogenic (related to treatment). Selected causes of hypophosphatemia include the following:

- Refeeding syndrome can develop when malnourished patients are started on enteral or total parenteral nutrition. Glucose in the formula or solution stimulates insulin release, which promotes the entry of glucose and phosphate into the cells, depleting extracellular phosphate levels.
- Medications frequently contribute to hypophosphatemia, including IV glucose solutions, antacids (aluminum- or magnesium-based antacids bind with phosphate), anabolic steroids, and diuretics.
- Alcoholism affects both the intake and absorption of phosphate.
- Hyperventilation and respiratory alkalosis cause phosphate to shift out of extracellular fluids into the intracellular space.
- Other causes include diabetic ketoacidosis with excess phosphate loss in the urine, stress responses, and extensive burns.

TABLE 10–9 Manifestations of Phosphate Imbalances

HYPOPHOSPHATEMIA	HYPERPHOSPHATEMIA
■ Serum phosphate level < 2.5 mg/dL	■ Serum phosphate level > 4.5 mg/dL
■ Intention tremor, paresthesias	■ Paresthesias
■ Confusion, stuporous	■ Muscle weakness
■ Bone pain	■ Nausea and vomiting
■ Joint stiffness	■ Dysphagia
■ Bleeding disorders (platelet dysfunction)	■ Tetany
■ Impaired white blood cell function	■ Decreased blood pressure
■ Seizures	■ Cardiac dysrhythmias

Pathophysiology and Manifestations

Most effects of hypophosphatemia result from depletion of ATP and impaired oxygen delivery to the cells due to a deficiency of the red blood cell enzyme 2,3-DPG. Severe hypophosphatemia affects virtually every major organ system:

- *Central nervous system:* Reduced oxygen and ATP synthesis in the brain causes neurologic manifestations such as irritability, apprehension, weakness, paresthesias, lack of coordination, confusion, seizures, and coma.
- *Hematologic:* Oxygen delivery to the cells is reduced. Hemolytic anemia (excessive RBC destruction) may develop due to lack of ATP in red blood cells.
- *Musculoskeletal:* Decreased ATP causes muscle weakness and release of creatinine phosphokinase (CPK, a muscle enzyme); acute rhabdomyolysis (muscle cell breakdown) can develop. Muscle cell destruction, in turn, can lead to acute renal failure as myoglobin, a muscle cell protein, exerts a toxic effect on the kidney tubule.
- *Cardiovascular:* Hypophosphatemia decreases myocardial contractility; decreased oxygenation of the heart muscle can cause chest pain and dysrhythmias.
- *Gastrointestinal:* Anorexia can occur, as well as dysphagia (difficulty swallowing), nausea and vomiting, decreased bowel sounds, and possible ileus due to reduced GI motility.

Interdisciplinary Care

Treatment for hypophosphatemia is directed at prevention, treating the underlying cause of the disorder, and replacing phosphate. An improved diet and oral phosphate supplement (such as Neutra-Phos or Neutra-Phos K capsules) may restore normal phosphate levels in patients with a mild to moderate deficiency. IV phosphate (sodium phosphate or potassium phosphate) is given when serum phosphate levels are less than 1 mg/dL.

Nursing Care

Nurses can be instrumental in identifying patients at risk for phosphate deficiency and preventing it from developing. Nurses should closely monitor serum electrolyte values in patients at risk, including those who are malnourished, receiving IV glucose solutions or total parenteral nutrition, or being treated with diuretic therapy or antacids that bind with phosphate. Nursing diagnoses that may be appropriate for the patient with hypophosphatemia include the following:

- *Impaired Physical Mobility* related to muscle weakness and poor coordination
- *Decreased Cardiac Output* related to reduced myocardial contractility
- *Risk for Injury* related to muscle weakness and altered mental status

Community-Based Care

In preparing for discharge, teach the patient and family about the causes and manifestations of hypophosphatemia. Discuss the importance of avoiding phosphorus-binding antacids, unless prescribed. Stress a well-balanced diet to maintain an adequate intake of phosphate.

The Patient with Hyperphosphatemia

Hyperphosphatemia is a serum phosphate level greater than 4.5 mg/dL. As with other electrolyte imbalances, it may be the result of impaired phosphate excretion, excess intake, or a shift of phosphate from the intracellular space into extracellular fluids.

- Acute or chronic renal failure is the primary cause of impaired phosphate excretion.
- Rapid administration of phosphate-containing solutions, including phosphate enemas, can increase serum phosphate levels. In addition, excess vitamin D increases phosphate absorption and can lead to hyperphosphatemia in patients with impaired renal function.
- A shift of phosphate from the intracellular to extracellular space can occur during chemotherapy, from sepsis or hypothermia, or because of extensive trauma or heat stroke.
- Because phosphate levels are affected by serum calcium concentrations, disruption of the mechanisms that regulate calcium levels (e.g., hypoparathyroidism, hyperthyroidism, or vitamin D intoxication) can lead to hyperphosphatemia.

Pathophysiology and Manifestations

Excessive serum phosphate levels cause few specific manifestations. The effects of high serum phosphate levels on nerves and muscles (muscle cramps and pain, paresthesias, tingling around the mouth, muscle spasms, tetany) are more the result of hypocalcemia that develops secondary to an elevated serum phosphorus level. The phosphate in the serum combines with ionized calcium, and the ionized serum calcium level falls.

Interdisciplinary Care

Treatment of the underlying disorder often corrects hyperphosphatemia. When this is not feasible, phosphate-containing drugs are eliminated and intake of phosphate-rich foods such as organ meats and milk and milk products is restricted. Agents that bind with phosphate in the GI tract (such as calcium-containing antacids) may be prescribed. If renal function is adequate, IV normal saline may be given to promote renal excretion of phosphate. Dialysis may be necessary to reduce phosphate levels in patients with renal failure.

Nursing Care

When providing nursing care for the patient with hyperphosphatemia, monitor the laboratory data for an excess of phosphorus and a deficit of calcium, as well as the manifestations of hypocalcemia.

Community-Based Care

Discuss the risk of hyperphosphatemia related to using phosphate preparations as laxatives or enemas, particularly with patients who have other risk factors for the disorder. When preparing the patient for discharge, teach about the use of phosphate-binding preparations as ordered and dietary phosphate restrictions.

Acid–Base Disorders

Homeostasis and optimal cellular function require maintenance of the hydrogen ion (H^+) concentration of body fluids within a relatively narrow range. Hydrogen ions determine the relative acidity of body fluids. Acids release hydrogen ions in solution; bases (or **alkalis**) accept hydrogen ions in solution. The hydrogen ion concentration of a solution is measured as its pH. The relationship between hydrogen ion concentration and pH is inverse; that is, as hydrogen ion concentration increases, the pH falls, and the solution becomes more acidic. As hydrogen ion concentration falls, the pH rises, and the solution becomes more alkaline or basic. The pH of body fluids is slightly basic, with the normal pH ranging from 7.35 to 7.45 (a pH of 7 is neutral).

Regulation of Acid–Base Balance

A number of mechanisms work together to maintain the pH of the body within normal range. Metabolic processes in the body continuously produce acids, which fall into two categories: volatile acids and nonvolatile acids. Volatile acids can be eliminated from the body as a gas. Carbonic acid (H_2CO_3) is the only volatile acid produced in the body. It dissociates into carbon dioxide (CO_2) and water (H_2O); the carbon dioxide is then eliminated from the body through the lungs. All other acids produced in the body are nonvolatile acids that must be metabolized or excreted from the body in fluid. Lactic acid, hydrochloric acid, phosphoric acid, and sulfuric acid are examples of nonvolatile acids. Most acids and bases in the body are weak; that is, they neither release nor accept a significant amount of hydrogen ion.

Three systems work together in the body to maintain the pH despite continuous acid production: buffers, the respiratory system, and the renal system.

Buffer Systems

Buffers are substances that prevent major changes in pH by removing or releasing hydrogen ions. When excess acid is present in body fluid, buffers bind with hydrogen ions to minimize the change in pH. If body fluids become too basic or alkaline, buffers release hydrogen ions, restoring the pH. Although buffers act within a fraction of a second, their capacity to maintain pH is limited. The major buffer systems of the body are the bicarbonate-carbonic acid buffer system, phosphate buffer system, and protein buffers.

The bicarbonate-carbonic acid buffer system can be illustrated by the following equation:

$$CO_2 + H_2O \; 4 \; H_2CO_3 \; 4 \; H^+ + HCO_3^-$$

Bicarbonate (HCO_3^-) is a weak base; when an acid is added to the system, the hydrogen ion in the acid combines with bicarbonate, and the pH changes only slightly. Carbonic acid (H_2CO_3) is a weak acid produced when carbon dioxide dissolves in water. If a base is added to the system, it combines with carbonic acid, and the pH remains within the normal range. Although the amounts of bicarbonate and carbonic acid in the body vary to a certain extent, as long as a ratio of 20 parts

bicarbonate (HCO_3^-) to 1 part carbonic acid (H_2CO_3) is maintained, the pH remains within the 7.35 to 7.45 range (Figure 10–13 ■).

The normal serum bicarbonate level is 24 mEq/L, and that of carbonic acid is 1.2 mEq/L. Thus, the ratio of bicarbonate to carbonic acid is 20:1. It is this ratio that maintains the pH within the normal range. Adding a strong acid to extracellular fluid depletes bicarbonate, changing the 20:1 ratio and causing the pH to drop below 7.35. This is known as **acidosis**. Addition of a strong base depletes carbonic acid as it combines with the base. The 20:1 ratio again is disrupted and the pH rises above 7.45, a condition known as **alkalosis**.

Intracellular and plasma proteins also serve as buffers. Plasma proteins contribute to buffering of extracellular fluids. Proteins in intracellular fluid provide extensive buffering for organic acids produced by cellular metabolism. In red blood cells, hemoglobin acts as a buffer for hydrogen ion when carbonic acid dissociates. Inorganic phosphates also serve as extracellular buffers, although their roles are not as important as the bicarbonate-carbonic acid buffer system. Phosphates are, however, important intracellular buffers, helping to maintain a stable pH within the cells.

Respiratory System

The respiratory system (and the cerebral respiratory center) regulates carbonic acid in the body by eliminating or retaining carbon dioxide. Carbon dioxide is a potential acid; when combined with water, it forms carbonic acid (see the previous equation), a volatile acid. Acute increases in either carbon dioxide or hydrogen ions in the blood stimulate the respiratory center in the brain. As a result, both the rate and depth of respiration increase. The increased rate and depth of lung ventilation eliminate carbon dioxide from the body, and carbonic acid levels fall, bringing the pH to a more normal range. Although this compensation for increased hydrogen ion concentration occurs

Figure 10–13 ■ The normal ratio of bicarbonate to carbonic acid is 20:1. As long as this ratio is maintained, the pH remains within the normal range of 7.35 to 7.45.

within minutes, it becomes less effective over time. Patients with chronic lung disease may have consistently high carbon dioxide levels in their blood.

Alkalosis, by contrast, depresses the respiratory center. Both the rate and depth of respiration decrease, and carbon dioxide is retained. The retained carbon dioxide then combines with water to restore carbonic acid levels and bring the pH back within the normal range.

Renal System

The renal system is responsible for the long-term regulation of acid–base balance in the body. Excess nonvolatile acids produced during metabolism normally are eliminated by the kidneys. The kidneys also regulate bicarbonate levels in extracellular fluid by regenerating bicarbonate ions as well as reabsorbing them in the renal tubules. Although the kidneys respond more slowly to changes in pH (over hours to days), they can generate bicarbonate and selectively excrete or retain hydrogen ions as needed. In acidosis, when excess hydrogen ion is present and the pH falls, the kidneys excrete hydrogen ions and retain bicarbonate. In alkalosis, the kidneys retain hydrogen ions and excrete bicarbonate to restore acid–base balance.

Assessing Acid–Base Balance

Acid–base balance is evaluated primarily by measuring arterial blood gases. Arterial blood is used because it reflects acid–base balance throughout the entire body better than venous blood. Arterial blood also provides information about the effectiveness of the lungs in oxygenating blood. The elements measured are pH, the $PaCO_2$, the PaO_2, and bicarbonate level.

The abbreviations $PaCO_2$ and PaO_2 are used interchangeably with PCO_2 and PO_2. The P stands for partial pressure, the pressure exerted by the gas dissolved in the blood. The *a* indicates that the sample is arterial blood. Because these measurements rarely are done on venous blood, the *a* often is deleted from the abbreviation.

The $PaCO_2$ measures the pressure exerted by dissolved carbon dioxide in the blood. It reflects the respiratory component of acid–base regulation and balance, and is regulated by the lungs. The normal value is 35–45 mmHg. A $PaCO_2$ of less than

35 mmHg is known as *hypocapnia*; a $PaCO_2$ greater than 45 mmHg is *hypercapnia*.

The PaO_2 is a measure of the pressure exerted by oxygen that is dissolved in the plasma. Only about 3% of oxygen in the blood is transported in solution; most is combined with hemoglobin. However, it is the dissolved oxygen that is available to the cells for metabolism. As dissolved oxygen diffuses out of plasma into the tissues, more is released from hemoglobin. The normal value for PaO_2 is 80 to 100 mmHg. A PaO_2 of less than 80 mmHg is indicative of hypoxemia. The PaO_2 is valuable for evaluating respiratory function, but is not used as a primary measurement in determining acid–base status.

The **serum bicarbonate** (HCO_3^-) reflects the renal regulation of acid–base balance. It is often called the metabolic component of arterial blood gases. The normal HCO_3^- value is 22 to 26 mEq/L.

The **base excess (BE)** is a calculated value also known as *buffer base capacity*. The base excess measures substances that can accept or combine with hydrogen ion. It reflects the degree of acid–base imbalance by indicating the status of the body's total buffering capacity. It represents the amount of acid or base that must be added to a blood sample to achieve a pH of 7.4. This is essentially a measure of increased or decreased bicarbonate. The normal value for base excess for arterial blood is –3.0 to +3.0. Normal ABG values are summarized in Table 10–10.

ABGs are analyzed to identify acid–base disorders and their probable cause, to determine the extent of the imbalance, and to monitor treatment. When analyzing ABG results, it is important to use a systematic approach. First evaluate each individual measurement, then look at the interrelationships to determine the patient's acid–base status (see Box 10–3).

Acid–Base Imbalance

Acid–base imbalances fall into two major categories: acidosis and alkalosis. Acidosis occurs when the hydrogen ion concentration increases above normal (pH below 7.35). Alkalosis occurs when the hydrogen ion concentration falls below normal (pH above 7.45).

Acid–base imbalances are further classified as metabolic or respiratory disorders. In metabolic disorders, the primary

TABLE 10–10 Normal Arterial Blood Gas Values

VALUE	NORMAL RANGE	SIGNIFICANCE
pH	7.35 to 7.45	Reflects hydrogen ion (H+) concentration
		■ < 7.35 = acidosis ■ > 7.45 = alkalosis
$PaCO_2$	35 to 45 mmHg	Partial pressure of carbon dioxide (CO_2) in arterial blood
		■ < 35 mmHg = hypocapnia ■ > 45 mmHg = hypercapnia
PaO_2	80 to 100 mmHg	Partial pressure of oxygen (O_2) in arterial blood
		■ < 80 mmHg = hypoxemia
HCO_3^-	22 to 26 mEq/L	Bicarbonate concentration in plasma
BE	–3 to +3	Base excess; a measure of buffering capacity

BOX 10–3 Interpreting Arterial Blood Gases

1. Look at the pH.
   - pH < 7.35 = acidosis
   - pH > 7.45 = alkalosis
2. Look at the $PaCO_2$.
   - $PaCO_2$ < 35 mmHg = hypocapnia; more carbon dioxide is being exhaled than normal
   - $PaCO_2$ > 45 mmHg = hypercapnia; carbon dioxide is being retained
3. Evaluate the pH–$PaCO_2$ relationship for a possible respiratory problem.
   - If the pH is < 7.35 (acidosis) and the $PaCO_2$ is > 45 mmHg (hypercapnia), retained carbon dioxide is causing increased H^+ concentration and *respiratory acidosis*.
   - If the pH is > 7.45 (alkalosis) and the $PaCO_2$ is < 35 mmHg (hypocapnia), low carbon dioxide levels and decreased H^+ concentration are causing *respiratory alkalosis*.
4. Look at the bicarbonate.
   - If the HCO_3^- is < 22 mEq/L, bicarbonate levels are lower than normal.
   - If the HCO_3^- is > 26 mEq/L, bicarbonate levels are higher than normal.
5. Evaluate the pH, HCO_3^-, and BE for a possible metabolic problem.
   - If the pH is < 7.35 (acidosis), the HCO_3^- is < 22 mEq/L, and the BE is < –3 mEq/L, then low bicarbonate levels and high H^+ concentrations are causing *metabolic acidosis*.
   - If the pH is > 7.45 (alkalosis), the HCO_3^- is > 26 mEq/L, and the BE is > +3 mEq/L, then high bicarbonate levels are causing *metabolic alkalosis*.
6. Look for compensation.
   - *Renal compensation:*
     - In respiratory acidosis (pH < 7.35, $PaCO_2$ > 45 mmHg), the kidneys retain HCO_3^- to buffer the excess acid, so the HCO_3^- is > 26 mEq/L.
     - In respiratory alkalosis (pH > 7.45, $PaCO_2$ < 35 mmHg), the kidneys excrete HO_3^- to minimize the alkalosis, so the HCO_3^- is < 22 mEq/L.
   - *Respiratory compensation*
     - In metabolic acidosis (pH < 7.35, HCO_3^- < 22 mEq/L), the rate and depth of respirations increase, increasing carbon dioxide elimination, so the $PaCO_2$ is < 35 mmHg.
     - In metabolic alkalosis (pH > 7.45, HCO_3^- > 26 mEq/L), respirations slow, carbon dioxide is retained, so the $PaCO_2$ is > 45 mmHg.
7. Evaluate oxygenation.
   - PaO_2 < 80 mmHg = hypoxemia; possible hypoventilation
   - PaO_2 > 100 mmHg = hyperventilation

change is in the concentration of bicarbonate. In metabolic acidosis, the amount of bicarbonate is decreased in relation to the amount of acid in the body (Figure 10–14A ■). It can develop as a result of abnormal bicarbonate losses or because of excess nonvolatile acids in the body. The pH falls below 7.35 and the bicarbonate concentration is less than 22 mEq/L. Metabolic alkalosis, by contrast, occurs when there is an excess of bicarbonate in relation to the amount of hydrogen ion (Figure 10–14B). The pH is above 7.45 and the bicarbonate concentration is greater than 26 mEq/L.

In respiratory disorders, the primary change is in the concentration of carbonic acid. Respiratory acidosis occurs when carbon dioxide is retained, increasing the amount of carbonic acid in the body (Figure 10–15A ■). As a result, the pH falls to less than 7.35, and the $PaCO_2$ is greater than 45 mmHg. When too much carbon dioxide is "blown off," carbonic acid levels fall and respiratory alkalosis develops (Figure 10–15B). The pH rises to above 7.45 and the $PaCO_2$ is less than 35 mmHg.

Acid–base disorders are further defined as *primary* (simple) and *mixed*. Primary disorders usually are due to one cause. For example, respiratory failure often causes respiratory acidosis due to retained carbon dioxide; renal failure usually causes metabolic acidosis due to retained hydrogen ion

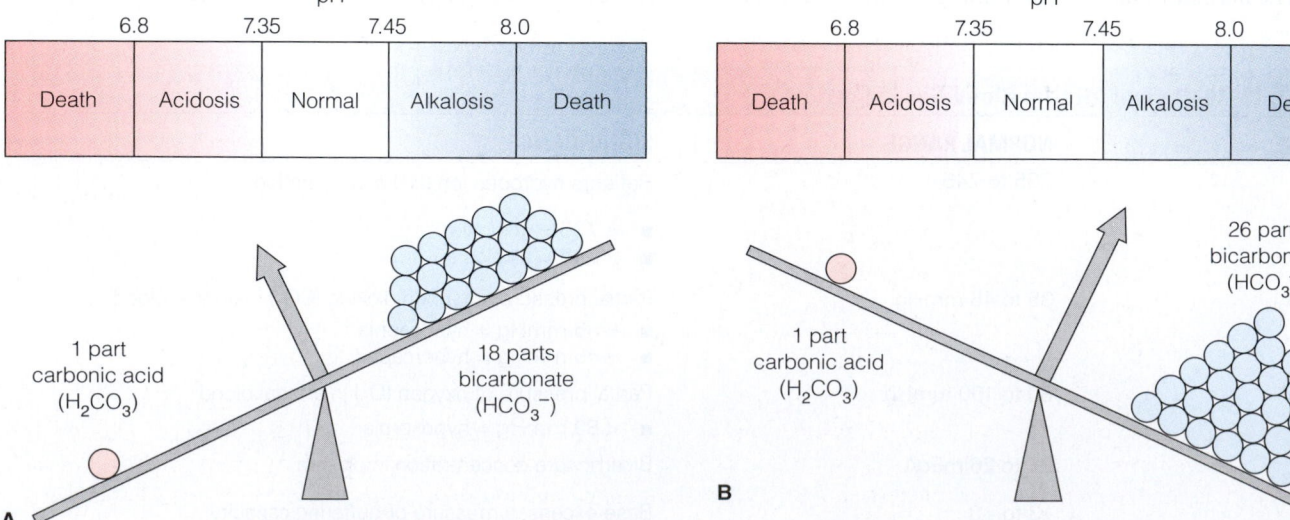

Figure 10–14 ■ Metabolic acid–base imbalances. *A*, Metabolic acidosis. *B*, Metabolic alkalosis.

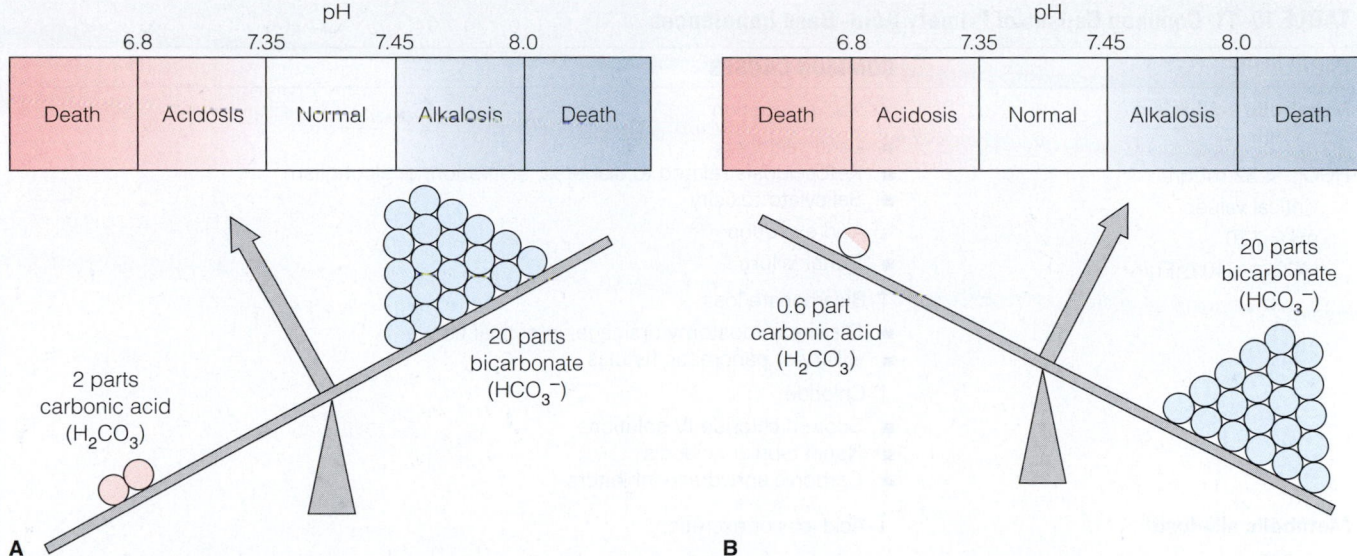

Figure 10–15 ■ Respiratory acid–base imbalances. *A,* Respiratory acidosis. *B,* Respiratory alkalosis.

and impaired bicarbonate production. Table 10–11 summarizes primary acid–base imbalances with common causes of each. Mixed disorders occur from combinations of respiratory and metabolic disturbances. For example, a patient in cardiac arrest develops a mixed respiratory and metabolic acidosis due to lack of ventilation (and retained CO_2) and hypoxia of body tissues that leads to anaerobic metabolism and acid by-products (excess nonvolatile acids).

Compensation

With primary acid–base disorders, compensatory changes in the other part of the regulatory system occur to restore a normal pH and homeostasis. In metabolic acid–base disorders, the change in pH affects the rate and depth of respirations. This, in turn, affects carbon dioxide elimination and the $PaCO_2$, helping restore the carbonic acid to bicarbonate ratio. The kidneys compensate for simple respiratory imbalances. The change in pH affects both bicarbonate conservation and hydrogen ion elimination (Table 10–12).

Compensatory changes in respirations occur within minutes of a change in pH. These changes, however, become less effective over time. The renal response takes longer to restore the pH, but is a more effective long-term mechanism. If the pH is restored to within normal limits, the disorder is said to be fully compensated. When these changes are reflected in ABG values but the pH remains outside normal limits, the disorder is said to be partially compensated.

The Patient with Metabolic Acidosis

Metabolic acidosis (bicarbonate deficit) is characterized by a low pH (< 7.35) and a low bicarbonate (< 22 mEq/L). It may be caused by excess acid in the body or loss of bicarbonate from the body. When metabolic acidosis develops, the respiratory system attempts to return the pH to normal by increasing the rate and depth of respirations. Carbon dioxide elimination increases, and the $PaCO_2$ falls (< 35 mmHg).

Risk Factors

Metabolic acidosis rarely is a primary disorder; it usually develops during the course of another disease:

- Acute lactic acidosis usually results from tissue hypoxia due to shock or cardiac arrest.
- Patients with type 1 diabetes mellitus are at risk for developing diabetic ketoacidosis. (∞ See Chapter 20 for more information about diabetes and its complications.)
- Acute or chronic renal failure impairs the excretion of metabolic acids.
- Diarrhea, intestinal suction, or abdominal fistulas increase the risk for excess bicarbonate loss.

Other common causes of metabolic acidosis are listed in Table 10–11.

Pathophysiology

Three basic mechanisms that can cause metabolic acidosis are the following:

- Accumulation of metabolic acids
- Excess loss of bicarbonate
- An increase in chloride levels

An accumulation of metabolic acids can result from excess acid production or impaired elimination of metabolic acids by the kidney. Lactic acidosis develops due to tissue hypoxia and a shift to anaerobic metabolism by the cells. Lactate and hydrogen ions are produced, forming lactic acid. Both oxygen and glucose are necessary for normal cell metabolism. When intracellular glucose is inadequate due to

TABLE 10–11 Common Causes of Primary Acid–Base Imbalances

IMBALANCE	COMMON CAUSES

Metabolic acidosis
 	
pH < 7.35
HCO_3^- < 22 mEq/L
  Critical values
  pH < 7.20
  HCO_3^- < 10 mEq/L
	↑ Acid production
	  ■ Lactic acidosis
	  ■ Ketoacidosis related to diabetes, starvation, or alcoholism
	  ■ Salicylate toxicity
	↓ Acid excretion
	  ■ Renal failure
	↑ Bicarbonate loss
	  ■ Diarrhea, ileostomy drainage, intestinal fistula
	  ■ Biliary or pancreatic fistulas
	↑ Chloride
	  ■ Sodium chloride IV solutions
	  ■ Renal tubular acidosis
	  ■ Carbonic anhydrase inhibitors

Metabolic alkalosis
 	
pH > 7.45
HCO_3^- > 26 mEq/L
  Critical values
  pH > 7.60
  HCO_3^- > 40 mEq/L
	↑ Acid loss or excretion
	  ■ Vomiting, gastric suction
	  ■ Hypokalemia
	↑ Bicarbonate
	  ■ Alkali ingestion (bicarbonate of soda)
	  ■ Excess bicarbonate administration

Respiratory acidosis
 	
pH < 7.35
$PaCO_2$ >45 mm Hg
  Critical values
  pH < 7.2
  $PaCO_2$ > 77 mmHg
	Acute respiratory acidosis
	  ■ Acute respiratory conditions (pulmonary edema, pneumonia, acute asthma)
	  ■ Opiate overdose
	  ■ Foreign body aspiration
	  ■ Chest trauma
	Chronic respiratory acidosis
	  ■ Chronic respiratory conditions (COPD, cystic fibrosis)
	  ■ Multiple sclerosis, other neuromuscular diseases
	  ■ Stroke

Respiratory alkalosis
 	
pH > 7.45
$PaCO_2$ < 35 mm Hg
 	
  Critical values
  pH > 7.60
  $PaCO_2$ < 20 mmHg
	■ Anxiety-induced hyperventilation (e.g., anxiety)
	  ■ Fever
	  ■ Early salicylate intoxication
	  ■ Hyperventilation with mechanical ventilator

starvation or a lack of insulin to move it into cells, the body breaks down fatty tissue to meet its metabolic needs. In this process, fatty acids are released, which are converted to ketones; ketoacidosis develops. Substances such as aspirin, methanol (wood alcohol), and ethylene (contained in antifreeze and solvents) cause a toxic increase in body acids by either breaking down into acid products (salicylic acid) or stimulating metabolic acid production (Porth & Matfin, 2009). Renal failure impairs the body's ability to excrete excess hydrogen ions and form bicarbonate.

Excess metabolic acids increase the hydrogen ion concentration of body fluids. The excess acid is buffered by bicarbonate, leading to what is known as a high anion gap acidosis (see Box 10–4).

The pancreas secretes bicarbonate-rich fluid into the small intestine. Intestinal suction, severe diarrhea, ileostomy drainage,

or fistulas can lead to excess losses of bicarbonate. Hyperchloremic acidosis can develop when excess chloride solutions (such as NaCl or ammonium chloride) are infused, causing a rise in chloride concentrations. It also may be related to renal disease or administration of carbonic anhydrate inhibitor diuretics. The anion gap remains normal in metabolic acidosis due to bicarbonate loss or excess chloride.

Acidosis depresses cell membrane excitability, affecting neuromuscular function. It also increases the amount of free calcium in ECF by interfering with protein binding. Severe acidosis (pH of 7.0 or less) depresses myocardial contractility, leading to a fall in cardiac output. If kidney function is normal, acid excretion and ammonia production increase to eliminate excess hydrogen ions.

Acid–base imbalances also affect electrolyte balance. In acidosis, potassium is retained as the kidney excretes excess

TABLE 10–12 Compensation for Simple Acid–Base Imbalances

PRIMARY DISORDER	CAUSE	COMPENSATION	EFFECT ON ABGS
Metabolic acidosis	Excess nonvolatile acids; bicarbonate deficiency	Rate and depth of respirations increase, eliminating additional CO_2.	↓ pH ↓ HCO_3 ↓ $PaCO_2$
Metabolic alkalosis	Bicarbonate excess	Rate and depth of respirations decrease, retaining CO_2.	↑ pH ↑ HCO_3^- ↑ $PaCO_2$
Respiratory acidosis	Retained CO_2 and excess carbonic acid	Kidneys conserve bicarbonate to restore carbonic acid: bicarbonate ratio of 1:20.	↓ pH ↑ $PaCO_2$ ↑ HCO_3^-
Respiratory alkalosis	Loss of CO_2 and deficient carbonic acid	Kidneys excrete bicarbonate and conserve H^+ to restore carbonic acid:bicarbonate ratio.	↑ pH ↓ $PaCO_2$ ↓ HCO_3^-

hydrogen ions. Excess hydrogen ions also enter the cells, displacing potassium from the intracellular space to maintain the balance of cations and anions within the cells. The effect of both processes is to increase serum potassium levels. Also in acidosis, calcium is released from its bonds with plasma proteins, increasing the amount of ionized (free) calcium in the blood. Magnesium levels may fall in acidosis.

Manifestations

Metabolic acidosis affects the function of many body systems. Its general manifestations include weakness and fatigue, headache, and general malaise. Gastrointestinal function is affected, causing anorexia, nausea, vomiting, and abdominal pain. The level of consciousness declines, leading to stupor and coma. Cardiac dysrhythmias develop, and cardiac arrest may occur. The skin is often warm and flushed. Skeletal problems may develop in chronic acidosis, as calcium and phosphate are released from the bones.

Manifestations of compensatory mechanisms are seen. The respirations are labored, deep and rapid, known as **Kussmaul's respirations**. The patient may complain of shortness of breath or dyspnea. See the Manifestations box on page 228.

Interdisciplinary Care

Management of metabolic acidosis focuses on treating the underlying cause of the disorder and correcting the acid–base imbalance.

Diagnosis

The following laboratory and diagnostic tests may be ordered.

- *ABGs* generally show a pH of less than 7.35 and a bicarbonate level of less than 22 mEq/L. A compensatory decrease in $PaCO_2$ to less than 35 mmHg is usually present.

BOX 10–4 Unraveling the Anion Gap

Calculation of the anion gap can help identify the underlying mechanism in metabolic acidosis if it is unclear.

The number of cations (positively charged ions) and anions (negatively charged ions) in ECF normally is equal (refer to Figure 10–2). Not all of these ions, however, are measured in laboratory testing (e.g., organic acids and proteins). The anion gap is calculated by subtracting the sum of two measured anions, chloride and bicarbonate, from the concentration of the major cation, sodium (see the following figure). The normal anion gap is 8 to 12 mEq/L.

Excess acids in ECF are buffered by bicarbonate, reducing serum bicarbonate levels and the total measured concentration of anions. This increases the anion gap (B in figure). When bicarbonate is lost from the body or chloride levels increase, however, the anion gap remains within normal limits (C in figure). This occurs because an increase or decrease in one of these negatively charged ions causes a corresponding change in the other to maintain balance (e.g., $\downarrow HCO_3^- \leftrightarrow \uparrow Cl^-$), and there is no change in the amount of unmeasured anions.

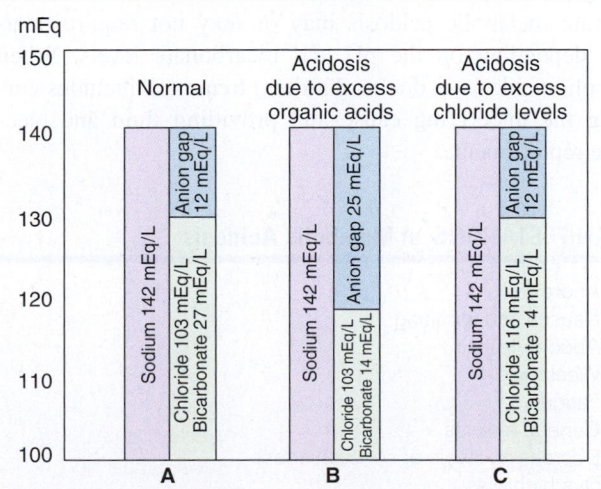

Illustration of the anion gap in metabolic acidosis. *A*, Normal anion gap. *B*, High anion gap caused by excess acids. *C*, Normal anion gap with hyperchloremia.

- *Serum electrolytes* demonstrate elevated serum potassium levels and possible low magnesium levels. The total calcium may remain unchanged, although more physiologically active ionized calcium is available. Sodium, chloride, and bicarbonate levels are used to calculate the anion gap.
- The *ECG* may show changes that reflect both the acidosis (particularly when severe) and the accompanying hyperkalemia.
- Other diagnostic studies such as the blood glucose and renal function studies may be ordered to identify the underlying cause of metabolic acidosis.

Medications

An alkalinizing solution such as bicarbonate may be given if the pH is less than 7.2 to reduce the effects of the acidosis on cardiac function. Sodium bicarbonate is the most commonly used alkalinizing solution; others include lactate, citrate, and acetate solutions (which are metabolized to bicarbonate). Alkalinizing solutions are given IV for severe acute metabolic acidosis. In chronic metabolic acidosis, the oral route is used.

The patient treated with bicarbonate must be carefully monitored. Rapid correction of the acidosis may lead to metabolic alkalosis and hypokalemia. Hypernatremia and hyperosmolality may develop as well, leading to water retention and fluid overload.

> **PRACTICE ALERT**
> As metabolic acidosis is corrected, potassium shifts back into the intracellular space. This can lead to hypokalemia and cardiac dysrhythmias. Carefully monitor serum potassium levels during treatment.

Treatment for diabetic ketoacidosis includes IV insulin and fluid replacement (∞ see Chapter 20 for the treatment of diabetic ketoacidosis). Alcoholic ketoacidosis is treated with saline solutions and glucose. Treatment for lactic acidosis from decreased tissue perfusion (e.g., shock or cardiac arrest) focuses on correcting the underlying problem and improving tissue perfusion. Patients with chronic renal failure and mild or moderate metabolic acidosis may or may not require treatment, depending on the pH and bicarbonate levels. When metabolic acidosis is due to diarrhea, treatment includes correcting the underlying cause and providing fluid and electrolyte replacement.

MANIFESTATIONS of Metabolic Acidosis

- Anorexia
- Nausea and vomiting
- Abdominal pain
- Weakness
- Fatigue
- General malaise
- Decreasing levels of consciousness
- Dysrhythmias
- Bradycardia
- Warm, flushed skin
- Hyperventilation (Kussmaul's respirations)

✍ Nursing Care

Nurses frequently provide care for patients with metabolic acidosis, although the focus of care often is the disorder underlying the acidosis (e.g., diabetes mellitus, renal failure) rather than the acidosis itself. For this reason, it is vital for the nurse to be aware of the effects of the acidosis and its implications for nursing care.

Health Promotion

To promote health in patients at risk for metabolic acidosis, discuss management of their underlying disease process (e.g., type 1 diabetes or renal failure) to prevent complications such as diabetic ketoacidosis and metabolic acidosis. Because early manifestations of metabolic acidosis (e.g., fatigue, general malaise, anorexia, nausea, abdominal pain) resemble those of common viral disorders such as "the flu," stress the importance of promptly seeking treatment if these manifestations develop.

Assessment

Assessment data related to metabolic acidosis include the following:

- *Health history:* Current manifestations, including anorexia, nausea, vomiting, abdominal discomfort, fatigue, lethargy, other manifestations; duration of manifestations and any precipitating factors such as diarrhea, ingestion of a toxin such as aspirin, methanol, or ethylene; chronic diseases such as diabetes or renal failure, cirrhosis of the liver, or endocrine disorders; current medications.
- *Physical assessment:* Mental status and level of consciousness; vital signs; apical and peripheral pulses; skin color and temperature; abdominal contour and distention; bowel sounds; urine output.

> **PRACTICE ALERT**
> Apply firm pressure to the puncture site for 2–5 minutes after the needle is withdrawn following aspiration of arterial blood to measure ABGs to prevent bleeding into the surrounding tissues. Pressure may need to be applied longer for patients receiving anticoagulation medications.

Nursing Diagnoses and Interventions

Nursing management of patients with metabolic acidosis often focuses on the primary disorder (e.g., diabetic ketoacidosis or renal failure); however, the acidosis itself has effects that must be attended to when providing care.

Decreased Cardiac Output

Metabolic acidosis affects cardiac output by decreasing myocardial contractility, slowing the heart rate, and increasing the risk for dysrhythmias. The accompanying hyperkalemia increases the risk for decreased cardiac output as well (see the earlier discussion about hyperkalemia).

- Monitor vital signs, including peripheral pulses and capillary refill. *Hypotension, diminished pulse strength, and slowed capillary refill may indicate decreased cardiac output and impaired tissue perfusion. Poor tissue perfusion can increase the risk for lactic acidosis.*

- Monitor the ECG pattern for dysrhythmias and changes characteristic of hyperkalemia. Notify the physician of changes. *Progressive ECG changes such as widening of the QRS complex indicate an increasing risk of dysrhythmias and cardiac arrest. Dysrhythmias further decrease cardiac output, possibly intensifying the degree of acidosis.*
- Monitor laboratory values, including ABGs, serum electrolytes, and renal function studies (serum creatinine and BUN). *Frequent monitoring of laboratory values allows evaluation of the effectiveness of treatment as well as early identification of potential problems.*

Risk for Fluid Volume Excess

Administering bicarbonate to correct acidosis increases the risk for hypernatremia, hyperosmolality, and fluid volume excess.

- Monitor and maintain fluid replacement as ordered. Monitor serum sodium levels and osmolality. *Bicarbonate administration can cause hypernatremia and hyperosmolality, leading to water retention.*
- Monitor heart and lung sounds, CVP, and respiratory status. *Increasing dyspnea, adventitious lung sounds and a high CVP reading, and a third heart sound (S_3) due to the volume of blood flow through the heart are indicative of hypervolemia and should be reported to the healthcare provider.*
- Assess for edema, particularly in the back, sacral, and periorbital areas. *Initially, edema affects dependent tissues—the back and sacrum in patients who are bedridden. Periorbital edema indicates more generalized edema.*
- Assess urine output hourly. Maintain accurate intake and output records. Note urine output less than 30 mL/hour or a positive fluid balance on 24-hour total intake and output calculations. *Heart failure and inadequate renal perfusion may lead to decreased urine output.*
- Obtain daily weights using consistent conditions. *Daily weights are an accurate indicator of fluid balance.*
- Administer prescribed diuretics as ordered, monitoring the patient's response to therapy. *Loop or high-ceiling diuretics such as furosemide [Lasix] can lead to further electrolyte imbalances, especially hypokalemia. This is a significant risk like that seen during correction of metabolic acidosis.*

Risk for Injury

Mental status and brain function are affected by acidosis, increasing the risk for injury.

- Monitor neurologic function, including mental status, level of consciousness, and muscle strength. *As the pH falls, mental functioning declines, leading to confusion, stupor, and a decreasing level of consciousness.*
- Institute safety precautions as necessary: Keep the bed in its lowest position, side rails raised. *These measures help protect the patient from injury resulting from confusion or disorientation.*
- Keep clocks, calendars, and familiar objects at bedside. Orient to time, place, and circumstances as needed. Allow significant others to remain with the patient as much as possible. *An unfamiliar environment and altered thought processes can further increase the risk for injury. Significant others provide a sense of security and reduce anxiety.*

Nursing care also includes measures to treat the underlying disorder, such as diabetic ketoacidosis. Refer to the chapters on diabetes (∞ Chapter 20) and renal failure (∞ Chapter 28) for specific interventions.

Community-Based Care

Discharge planning and teaching focus on the underlying cause of the imbalance. The patient who has developed ketoacidosis as a result of diabetes mellitus, starvation, or alcoholism needs interventions and teaching to prevent future episodes of acidosis. Diet, medication management, and alcohol dependency treatment are vital teaching areas. When metabolic acidosis is related to renal failure, the patient should be referred for management of the renal failure itself. Patients who have experienced diarrhea or excess ileostomy drainage leading to bicarbonate loss need information about appropriate diarrhea treatment strategies and when to call their primary care provider.

The Patient with Metabolic Alkalosis

Metabolic alkalosis (bicarbonate excess) is characterized by a high pH (> 7.45) and a high bicarbonate (> 26 mEq/L). It may be caused by loss of acid or excess bicarbonate in the body. When metabolic alkalosis develops, the respiratory system attempts to return the pH to normal by slowing the respiratory rate. Carbon dioxide is retained, and the $PaCO_2$ increases (> 45 mmHg).

Risk Factors

As is the case with other acid–base imbalances, metabolic alkalosis rarely occurs as a primary disorder. Risk factors include hospitalization, hypokalemia, and treatment with alkalinizing solutions (e.g., bicarbonate).

Pathophysiology

Hydrogen ions may be lost via gastric secretions through the kidneys, or because of a shift of H^+ into the cells. Metabolic alkalosis due to loss of hydrogen ions usually occurs because of vomiting or gastric suction. Gastric secretions are highly acidic (pH 1 to 3). When these are lost through vomiting or gastric suction, the alkalinity of body fluids increases. This increased alkalinity results both from the loss of acid and selective retention of bicarbonate by the kidneys as chloride is depleted. (Chloride is the major anion in ECF; when it is lost, bicarbonate is retained as a replacement anion.)

Increased renal excretion of hydrogen ions can be prompted by hypokalemia as the kidneys try to conserve potassium, excreting hydrogen ion instead. Hypokalemia contributes to metabolic alkalosis in another way as well. When potassium shifts out of cells to maintain extracellular potassium levels, hydrogen ions shift into the cells to maintain the balance between cations and anions within the cell.

Excess bicarbonate usually occurs as a result of ingesting antacids that contain bicarbonate (such as soda bicarbonate or Alka-Seltzer) or overzealous administration of bicarbonate to treat metabolic acidosis. Common causes of metabolic alkalosis are summarized in Table 10–11.

In alkalosis, more calcium combines with serum proteins, reducing the amount of ionized (physiologically active) calcium in the blood. This accounts for many of the common manifestations of metabolic alkalosis. Alkalosis also affects potassium balance: Hypokalemia not only can cause metabolic alkalosis (see the earlier discussion), but it also can result from metabolic alkalosis. Hydrogen ions shift out of the intracellular space to help restore the pH, prompting more potassium to enter the cells and depleting ECF potassium. The high pH depresses the respiratory system as the body retains carbon dioxide to restore the carbonic acid to bicarbonate ratio.

Manifestations and Complications

Manifestations of metabolic alkalosis (see the following box) occur as a result of decreased calcium ionization and are similar to those of hypocalcemia, including numbness and tingling around the mouth, fingers, and toes; dizziness; Trousseau's sign; and muscle spasm. As the respiratory system compensates for metabolic alkalosis, respirations are depressed and respiratory failure with hypoxemia and respiratory acidosis may develop.

Interdisciplinary Care

Interdisciplinary management of metabolic alkalosis focuses on diagnosing and correcting the underlying cause.

Diagnosis

The following laboratory and diagnostic tests may be ordered.

- *ABGs* show a pH greater than 7.45 and bicarbonate level greater than 26 mEq/L. With compensatory hypoventilation, carbon dioxide is retained, and the $PaCO_2$ is greater than 45 mmHg.
- *Serum electrolytes* often demonstrate decreased serum potassium (< 3.5 mEq/L) and decreased chloride (< 95 mEq/L) levels. The serum bicarbonate level is high. Although the total serum calcium may be normal, the ionized fraction of calcium is low.
- *Urine pH* may be low (pH 1 to 3) if metabolic acidosis is caused by hypokalemia. The kidneys selectively retain potassium and excrete hydrogen ion to restore ECF potassium levels. Urinary chloride levels may be normal or greater than 250 mEq/24 hours.
- The *ECG pattern* shows changes similar to those seen with hypokalemia. These changes may be due to hypokalemia or to the alkalosis.

MANIFESTATIONS of Metabolic Alkalosis

- Confusion
- Decreasing level of consciousness
- Hyperreflexia
- Tetany
- Dysrhythmias
- Hypotension
- Seizures
- Respiratory failure

Medications

Treatment of metabolic alkalosis includes restoring normal fluid volume and administering potassium chloride and sodium chloride solution. The potassium restores serum and intracellular potassium levels, allowing the kidneys to more effectively conserve hydrogen ions. Chloride promotes renal excretion of bicarbonate. Sodium chloride solutions restore fluid volume deficits that can contribute to metabolic alkalosis. In severe alkalosis, an acidifying solution such as dilute hydrochloric acid or ammonium chloride may be administered. In addition, drugs may be used to treat the underlying cause of the alkalosis.

Nursing Care

Health Promotion

Health promotion activities focus on teaching patients the risks of using sodium bicarbonate as an antacid to relieve heartburn or gastric distress. Stress the availability of other effective antacid preparations and the need to seek medical evaluation for persistent gastric manifestations. In the hospital setting, carefully monitor laboratory values for patients at risk for developing metabolic alkalosis, particularly patients undergoing continuous gastric suction.

Assessment

Focused assessment data related to metabolic alkalosis include the following:

- *Health history:* Current manifestations, such as numbness and tingling, muscle spasms, dizziness, other manifestations; duration of manifestations and any precipitating factors such as bicarbonate ingestion, vomiting, diuretic therapy, or endocrine disorders; current medications.
- *Physical assessment:* Vital signs including apical pulse and rate and depth of respirations; muscle strength; deep tendon reflexes.

Nursing Diagnoses and Interventions

As with metabolic acidosis, nursing care of the patient with metabolic alkalosis often focuses on intervening for patient responses to the primary problem, rather than the alkalosis itself. However, the risk for impaired gas exchange is a priority problem, especially with severe metabolic alkalosis.

Risk for Impaired Gas Exchange

Respiratory compensation for metabolic alkalosis depresses the respiratory rate and reduces the depth of breathing to promote carbon dioxide retention. As a result, the patient is at risk for impaired gas exchange, especially in the presence of underlying lung disease.

- Monitor respiratory rate, depth, and effort. Monitor oxygen saturation continuously, reporting an oxygen saturation level of less than 95% (or as ordered). *The depressed respiratory drive associated with metabolic alkalosis can lead to hypoxemia and impaired oxygenation of tissues. Oxygen saturation levels of less than 90% indicate significant oxygenation problems.*
- Assess skin color; note and report cyanosis around the mouth. *Central cyanosis, seen around the mouth and oral mucous membranes, indicates significant hypoxia.*

- Monitor mental status and level of consciousness (LOC). Report decreasing LOC or behavior changes such as restlessness, agitation, or confusion. *Changes in mental status or behavior may be early manifestations of hypoxia.*
- Place in semi-Fowler's or Fowler's position as tolerated. *Elevating the head of the bed facilitates alveolar ventilation and gas exchange.*
- Schedule nursing care activities to allow rest periods. *The patient who is hypoxemic has limited energy reserves, necessitating frequent rest and limited activities.*
- Administer oxygen as ordered or necessary to maintain oxygen saturation levels. *Supplemental oxygen can help maintain blood and tissue oxygenation despite depressed respirations.*

Fluid Volume Deficit

Patients with metabolic alkalosis often have an accompanying fluid volume deficit.

- Assess vital signs, CVP, and peripheral pulse volume at least every 4 hours. *Hypotension, tachycardia, a low CVP, and weak, easily obliterated peripheral pulses indicate hypovolemia.*
- Weigh daily under standard conditions (time of day, clothing, and scale). *Rapid weight changes accurately reflect fluid balance.*
- Administer IV fluids as prescribed using an infusion pump. Monitor for indicators of fluid overload if rapid fluid replacement is ordered: dyspnea, tachypnea, tachycardia, increased CVP, jugular vein distension, and edema. *Rapid fluid replacement may lead to hypervolemia, resulting in pulmonary edema and cardiac failure, particularly in patients with compromised cardiac and renal function.*
- Monitor serum electrolytes, osmolality, and ABG values. *Rehydration and administration of potassium chloride will affect both acid–base and fluid and electrolyte balance. Careful monitoring is important to identify changes.*

Community-Based Care

When preparing the patient with metabolic alkalosis for discharge, consider the cause of the alkalosis and any underlying factors. For example, provide teaching about the following:

- Using appropriate antacids for heartburn and gastric distress
- Using potassium supplements as ordered or eating high-potassium foods to avoid hypokalemia if taking a potassium-wasting diuretic or if aldosterone production is impaired
- Contacting the primary care provider if uncontrolled or extended vomiting develops

The Patient with Respiratory Acidosis

Respiratory acidosis is caused by an excess of dissolved carbon dioxide, or carbonic acid. It is characterized by a pH less than 7.35 and a $PaCO_2$ greater than 45 mmHg. Respiratory acidosis may be either acute or chronic. In chronic respiratory acidosis, the bicarbonate is higher than 26 mEq/L as the kidneys compensate by retaining bicarbonate.

Risk Factors

Acute or chronic lung disease (e.g., pneumonia or chronic obstructive pulmonary disease [COPD]) is the primary risk factor for respiratory acidosis. Other conditions that depress or interfere with ventilation, such as excess narcotic analgesics, airway obstruction, or neuromuscular disease, also are risk factors for respiratory acidosis. Selected causes of respiratory acidosis are listed in Table 10–11.

Pathophysiology

Both acute and chronic respiratory acidosis result from carbon dioxide retention caused by alveolar hypoventilation. Hypoxemia (low oxygen in the arterial blood) frequently accompanies respiratory acidosis.

ACUTE RESPIRATORY ACIDOSIS Acute respiratory acidosis occurs as the result of a sudden failure of ventilation. Chest trauma, aspiration of a foreign body, acute pneumonia, and overdoses of narcotic or sedative medications can lead to this condition. Because acute respiratory acidosis occurs with the sudden onset of hypoventilation—for example, with cardiac arrest—the $PaCO_2$ rises rapidly and the pH falls markedly. A pH of 7 or lower can occur within minutes (Metheny, 2000). The serum bicarbonate level initially is unchanged because the compensatory response of the kidneys occurs over hours to days.

Hypercapnia (increased carbon dioxide levels) affects neurologic function and the cardiovascular system. Carbon dioxide rapidly crosses the blood–brain barrier. Cerebral blood vessels dilate and, if the condition continues, intracranial pressure increases and papilledema (swelling and inflammation of the optic nerve where it enters the retina) develops (Porth & Matfin, 2009). Peripheral vasodilation also occurs, and the pulse rate increases to maintain cardiac output.

CHRONIC RESPIRATORY ACIDOSIS Chronic respiratory acidosis is associated with chronic respiratory or neuromuscular conditions such as COPD, asthma, cystic fibrosis, or multiple sclerosis. These conditions affect alveolar ventilation because of airway obstruction, structural changes in the lung, or limited chest wall expansion. Most patients with chronic respiratory acidosis have COPD with chronic bronchitis and emphysema. (∞ See Chapter 37 for more information about COPD.) In chronic respiratory acidosis, the $PaCO_2$ increases over time and remains elevated. The kidneys retain bicarbonate, increasing bicarbonate levels, and the pH often remains close to the normal range.

The acute effects of hypercapnia may not develop because carbon dioxide levels rise gradually, allowing compensatory changes to occur. When carbon dioxide levels are chronically elevated, the respiratory center becomes less sensitive to the gas as a stimulant of the respiratory drive. The PaO_2 provides the primary stimulus for respirations. Patients with chronic respiratory acidosis are at risk for developing carbon dioxide narcosis, with manifestations of acute respiratory acidosis, if the respiratory center is suppressed by administering excess supplemental oxygen.

> **PRACTICE ALERT**
> Carefully monitor neurologic and respiratory status in patients with chronic respiratory acidosis who are receiving oxygen therapy. Immediately report a decreasing LOC or depressed respirations.

Manifestations

The manifestations of acute and chronic respiratory acidosis differ. In acute respiratory acidosis, the rapid rise in $PaCO_2$ levels causes manifestations of hypercapnia. Cerebral vasodilation causes manifestations such as headache, blurred vision, irritability, and mental cloudiness. If the condition continues, the level of consciousness progressively decreases. Rapid and dramatic changes in ABGs can lead to unconsciousness and ventricular fibrillation, a potentially lethal cardiac dysrhythmia. The skin of the patient with acute respiratory acidosis may be warm and flushed, and the pulse rate is elevated.

The manifestations of chronic respiratory acidosis include weakness and a dull headache. Sleep disturbances, daytime sleepiness, impaired memory, and personality changes also may be manifestations of chronic respiratory acidosis (see the following box).

Interdisciplinary Care

Patients with acute respiratory failure usually require treatment in the emergency department or intensive care unit. The focus is on restoring adequate ventilation and gas exchange. Hypoxemia often accompanies acute respiratory acidosis, so oxygen is administered as well. Supplemental oxygen is administered with caution to patients with chronic respiratory acidosis.

Diagnosis

The following laboratory and diagnostic tests may be ordered.

- *ABGs* show a pH of less than 7.35 and a $PaCO_2$ of more than 45 mmHg. In acute respiratory acidosis, the bicarbonate level is initially within normal range but increases to greater than 26 mEq/L if the condition persists. In chronic respiratory acidosis, both the $PaCO_2$ and the HCO_3^- may be significantly elevated.
- *Serum electrolytes* may show hypochloremia (chloride level < 98 mEq/L) in chronic respiratory acidosis.
- *Pulmonary function tests* may be done to determine if chronic lung disease is the cause of the respiratory acidosis. These studies would not be done during the acute period, however.

Additional diagnostic tests may be done to identify the underlying cause of the respiratory acidosis. *Chest x-ray* and *sputum studies* (cytology and culture) may be ordered to identify an acute or chronic lung disorder. If drug overdose is suspected, serum levels of the drug may be obtained.

Medications

Bronchodilator drugs may be administered to open the airways and antibiotics prescribed to treat respiratory infections. If excess narcotics or anesthetic has caused acute respiratory acidosis, drugs to reverse their effects (such as naloxone) may be given.

Respiratory Support

Treatment of respiratory acidosis, either acute or chronic, focuses on improving alveolar ventilation and gas exchange. Patients with severe respiratory acidosis and hypoxemia may require intubation and mechanical ventilation (∞ see Chapter 37 for more information about these procedures). The $PaCO_2$ level is lowered slowly to avoid complications such as cardiac dysrhythmias and decreased cerebral perfusion. In patients with chronic respiratory acidosis, oxygen is administered cautiously to avoid carbon dioxide narcosis.

Pulmonary hygiene measures, such as breathing treatments or percussion and drainage, may be instituted. Adequate hydration is important to promote removal of respiratory secretions.

∾ Nursing Care

See the Case Study & Nursing Care Plan: Acute Respiratory Acidosis on page 234.

Health Promotion

Health promotion activities related to respiratory acidosis focus on identifying, monitoring, and teaching patients at risk. Carefully monitor patients receiving anesthesia, narcotic analgesics, or sedatives for manifestations of respiratory depression. Monitor the response of patients with a history of chronic lung disease to oxygen therapy. Teach patients who have an identified risk for respiratory acidosis (such as people using narcotic analgesia for cancer pain and people with chronic lung disease) and their families about early manifestations of respiratory depression and acidosis, and instruct them to immediately contact their care provider if manifestations develop.

Assessment

Assessment data related to respiratory acidosis include the following:

- *Health history:* Current manifestations, including headache, irritability or lethargy, difficulty thinking, blurred vision, and other manifestations; duration of manifestations and any precipitating factors such as drug use or respiratory infection; chronic diseases such as cystic fibrosis or COPD; current medications.
- *Physical assessment:* Mental status and level of consciousness; vital signs; skin color and temperature; rate and depth of respirations, pulmonary excursion, lung sounds; examination of optic fundus for possible papilledema.

Nursing Diagnoses and Interventions

Restoring effective alveolar ventilation and gas exchange is the priority of interdisciplinary and nursing care for patients with respiratory acidosis.

MANIFESTATIONS of Respiratory Acidosis

ACUTE RESPIRATORY ACIDOSIS
- Headache
- Warm, flushed skin
- Blurred vision
- Irritability, altered mental status
- Decreasing level of consciousness
- Cardiac arrest

CHRONIC RESPIRATORY ACIDOSIS
- Weakness
- Dull headache
- Sleep disturbances with daytime sleepiness
- Impaired memory
- Personality changes

Impaired Gas Exchange

- Frequently assess respiratory status, including rate, depth, effort, and oxygen saturation levels. *Decreasing respiratory rate and effort along with decreasing oxygen saturation levels may signal worsening respiratory failure and respiratory acidosis.*
- Frequently assess level of consciousness. *A decline in LOC may indicate increasing hypercapnia and the need for increasing ventilatory support (such as intubation and mechanical ventilation).*
- Promptly evaluate and report ABG results to the physician and respiratory therapist. *Rapid changes in carbon dioxide or oxygen levels may necessitate modification of the treatment plan to prevent complications of overcorrection of respiratory acidosis.*
- Place in semi-Fowler's to Fowler's position as tolerated. *Elevating the head of the bed promotes lung expansion and gas exchange.*
- Administer oxygen as ordered. Carefully monitor response. Reduce the oxygen flow rate or percentage and immediately report increasing somnolence. *Supplemental oxygen can suppress the respiratory drive in patients with chronic respiratory acidosis.*

Ineffective Airway Clearance

- Frequently auscultate breath sounds (whether on or off a mechanical ventilator). *Increasing adventitious sounds or decreasing breath sounds (faint or absent) may indicate worsening airway clearance due to obstruction or fatigue.*
- Encourage the patient with chronic respiratory acidosis to use pursed-lip breathing. *Pursed-lip breathing helps maintain open airways throughout exhalation, promoting carbon dioxide elimination.*
- Frequently reposition and encourage ambulation as tolerated. *Repositioning, sitting at the bedside, and ambulation promote airway clearance and lung expansion.*
- Encourage fluid intake of up to 3000 mL per day as tolerated or allowed. *Fluids help liquefy secretions and hydrate respiratory mucous membranes, promoting airway clearance.*
- Administer medications such as inhaled bronchodilators as ordered. *Inhaled bronchodilators help relieve bronchial spasm, dilating airways.*
- Provide percussion, vibration, and postural drainage as ordered. *Pulmonary hygiene measures such as these help loosen respiratory secretions so they can be coughed out of airways.*

Using NANDA, NIC, and NOC

Linkages between a selected NANDA nursing diagnosis, NIC, and NOC for the patient with respiratory acidosis are shown in the chart that follows.

Community-Based Care

Planning and teaching for home care focuses on the health problem that caused the patient to develop respiratory acidosis. The patient who developed acute respiratory acidosis as a result of acute pneumonia or chest trauma may only require teaching to prevent future problems. If acute respiratory acidosis occurred secondarily to a narcotic overdose, determine if the drug was prescribed for pain or if it was an illicit street drug.

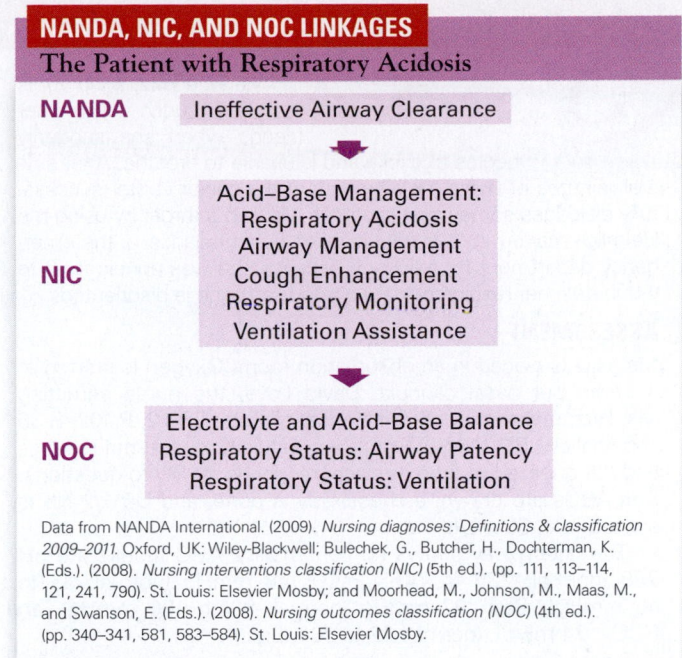

NANDA, NIC, AND NOC LINKAGES
The Patient with Respiratory Acidosis

NANDA — Ineffective Airway Clearance

NIC — Acid–Base Management: Respiratory Acidosis
Airway Management
Cough Enhancement
Respiratory Monitoring
Ventilation Assistance

NOC — Electrolyte and Acid–Base Balance
Respiratory Status: Airway Patency
Respiratory Status: Ventilation

Data from NANDA International. (2009). *Nursing diagnoses: Definitions & classification 2009–2011*. Oxford, UK: Wiley-Blackwell; Bulechek, G., Butcher, H., Dochterman, K. (Eds.). (2008). *Nursing interventions classification (NIC)* (5th ed.). (pp. 111, 113–114, 121, 241, 790). St. Louis: Elsevier Mosby; and Moorhead, M., Johnson, M., Maas, M., and Swanson, E. (Eds.). (2008). *Nursing outcomes classification (NOC)* (4th ed.). (pp. 340–341, 581, 583–584). St. Louis: Elsevier Mosby.

Provide teaching to the patient who requires narcotic medication on a continuing basis. Refer the patient using illicit drugs to a substance abuse counselor, treatment center, or Narcotics Anonymous as appropriate.

For patients with chronic lung disease, discuss ways to avoid future episodes of acute respiratory failure. Encourage the patient to be immunized against pneumococcal pneumonia and influenza. Discuss ways to avoid acute respiratory infections and measures to take when respiratory status is further compromised.

The Patient with Respiratory Alkalosis

Respiratory alkalosis is characterized by a pH greater than 7.45 and a $PaCO_2$ of less than 35 mmHg. It is always caused by hyperventilation leading to a carbon dioxide deficit.

Risk Factors

Anxiety with hyperventilation is the most common cause of respiratory alkalosis; therefore, anxiety disorders increase the risk for this acid–base imbalance. In the patient who is critically ill, mechanical ventilation is a risk factor for respiratory alkalosis.

Pathophysiology

In acute respiratory alkalosis, the pH rises rapidly as the $PaCO_2$ falls. Because the kidneys are unable to rapidly adapt to the change in pH, the bicarbonate level remains within normal limits. Anxiety-based hyperventilation is the most common cause of acute respiratory alkalosis. Other physiologic causes of hyperventilation include high fever, hypoxia, gram-negative bacteremia, and thyrotoxicosis. Early salicylate intoxication (aspirin overdose), encephalitis, and high progesterone levels in pregnancy directly stimulate the respiratory center, potentially leading to hyperventilation and respiratory alkalosis. Hyperventilation also can occur during anesthesia or mechanical ventilation if the rate and tidal volume (depth) of ventilations is excessive.

If hyperventilation continues, the kidneys compensate by eliminating bicarbonate to restore the bicarbonate to carbonic

Marlene Hitz, aged 76, is eating lunch with her friends when she suddenly begins to choke and is unable to breathe. After several minutes of trying, an attendant at the senior center successfully dislodges some meat caught in Ms. Hitz's throat by using the Heimlich maneuver. Ms. Hitz is taken by ambulance to the emergency department for follow-up because she was apneic for 3 to 4 minutes, her respirations are shallow, and she is disoriented.

ASSESSMENT

Ms. Hitz is placed in an observation room. Oxygen is started at 4 L/min per nasal cannula. David Love, the nurse admitting Ms. Hitz, makes the following assessments: T 98.2, P 102, R 36 and shallow, BP 146/92. Skin is warm and dry. Alert but restless and not oriented to time or place; responds slowly to questions. Stat ABGs are drawn, a chest x-ray is done, and D5 1/2 NS is started IV at 50 mL/h.

The chest x-ray shows no abnormality. ABG results are pH 7.38 (normal: 7.35 to 7.45), $PaCO_2$ 48 mmHg (normal: 35 to 45 mmHg), PaO_2 92 mmHg (normal: 80 to 100 mmHg), and HCO_3^- 24 mEq/L (normal: 22 to 26 mEq/L).

DIAGNOSES

- *Impaired Gas Exchange* related to temporary airway obstruction
- *Anxiety* related to emergency hospital admission
- *Risk for Injury* related to confusion

EXPECTED OUTCOMES

- Regain normal gas exchange and ABG values.
- Be oriented to time, place, and person.
- Regain appropriate mental status.
- Remain free of injury.

PLANNING AND IMPLEMENTATION

- Monitor ABGs, to be redrawn in 2 hours.
- Monitor vital signs and respiratory status (including oxygen saturation) every 15 minutes for the first hour, then every hour.
- Assess color of skin, nail beds, and oral mucous membranes every hour.
- Assess mental status and orientation every hour.
- Monitor anxiety level as evidenced by restlessness and agitation.
- Maintain a calm, quiet environment.
- Provide reorientation and explain all activities.
- Keep side rails in place, and place call bell within reach.

EVALUATION

Ms. Hitz remains in the emergency department for 6 hours. Her ABGs are still abnormal, and David now notes the presence of respiratory crackles and wheezes. She is less anxious and responds appropriately when asked who and where she is. Because she has not regained normal gas exchange, Ms. Hitz is admitted to the hospital for continued observation and treatment.

CRITICAL THINKING IN THE NURSING PROCESS

1. Describe the pathophysiologic process that leads to acute respiratory acidosis in Ms. Hitz.
2. Describe the effect of acidosis on mental function.
3. What teaching would you provide to Ms. Hitz to prevent future episodes of choking?

See Evaluating Your Response in Appendix C.

---

acid ratio. The bicarbonate level is lower than normal in chronic respiratory alkalosis, and the pH may be close to the normal range.

Alkalosis increases binding of extracellular calcium to albumin, reducing ionized calcium levels. As a result, neuromuscular excitability increases and manifestations similar to hypocalcemia develop. Low carbon dioxide levels in the blood cause vasoconstriction of cerebral vessels, increasing the neurologic manifestations of the disorder.

Manifestations

The manifestations of respiratory alkalosis include lightheadedness, a feeling of panic and difficulty concentrating, circumoral and distal extremity paresthesias, tremors, and positive Chvostek's and Trousseau's signs. The patient also may experience tinnitus, a sensation of chest tightness, and palpitations (cardiac dysrhythmias). Seizures and loss of consciousness may occur. (See the following Manifestations box.)

Interdisciplinary Care

Management of respiratory alkalosis focuses on correcting the imbalance and treating the underlying cause.

Diagnosis

ABGs generally show a pH greater than 7.45 and a $PaCO_2$ of less than 35 mmHg. In chronic hyperventilation, there is a compensatory decrease in serum bicarbonate to less than 22 mEq/L and the pH may be near normal.

Medications

A sedative or antianxiety agent may be necessary to relieve anxiety and restore a normal breathing pattern. Additional drugs to correct underlying problems other than anxiety-induced hyperventilation may be ordered.

Respiratory Therapy

The usual treatment for anxiety-related respiratory alkalosis involves instructing the patient to breathe more slowly and having the patient breathe into a paper bag or rebreather mask. This allows rebreathing of exhaled carbon dioxide, increasing $PaCO_2$ levels, and reducing the pH. If excessive ventilation by a mechanical ventilator is the cause of respiratory alkalosis, ventilator settings are adjusted to reduce the respiratory rate and tidal volume as indicated. When hypoxia is the underlying cause of hyperventilation, oxygen is administered.

MANIFESTATIONS of Respiratory Alkalosis

- Dizziness
- Numbness and tingling around mouth, hands, and feet
- Palpitations
- Dyspnea
- Chest tightness
- Anxiety/panic
- Tremors
- Tetany
- Seizures, loss of consciousness

✐ Nursing Care

Health Promotion

Identify patients at risk in the hospital (e.g., patients on mechanical ventilation or who have a fever or infection), and monitor assessment data and ABGs to identify early manifestations of hyperventilation and respiratory alkalosis.

Assessment, Diagnoses, and Interventions

Ineffective Breathing Pattern

The usual cause of hyperventilation and respiratory alkalosis is psychologic, although physiologic disorders also can lead to hyperventilation. It is important to not only address the hyperventilation, but also to identify the underlying cause.

- Assess respiratory rate, depth, and ease. Monitor vital signs (including temperature) and skin color. *Assessment data can help identify the underlying cause, such as a fever or hypoxia.*
- Obtain subjective assessment data such as circumstances leading up to the current situation, current health and recent illnesses or medication use, and current manifestations. *Subjective data provide cues to the cause and circumstances of the hyperventilation response.*
- Reassure the patient that he or she is not experiencing a heart attack and that manifestations will resolve when breathing returns to normal. *Manifestations of hyperventilation and respiratory alkalosis such as dyspnea, chest tightness or pain, and palpitations can mimic those of a heart attack.*
- Instruct the patient to maintain eye contact and breathe with you to slow the respiratory rate. *These measures help to make the patient aware of respirations and provide a sense of support and control (Ackley & Ladwig, 2006).*
- Have the patient breathe into a paper bag. *This allows the patient to rebreathe exhaled carbon dioxide, increasing the $PaCO_2$ and decreasing the pH.*
- Protect the patient from injury. *If hyperventilation continues to the point at which the patient loses consciousness, respirations will return to normal, as will acid–base balance.*
- If the patient has experienced repeated episodes of hyperventilation or has a chronic anxiety disorder, refer for counseling. *Counseling can help the patient develop alternative strategies for dealing with anxiety.*

Community-Based Care

Planning and teaching for home care is directed toward the underlying cause of hyperventilation. If anxiety precipitated the episode, discuss anxiety management strategies with the patient. Refer the patient and family to a counselor if appropriate. Teach the patient to identify a hyperventilation reaction, and how to breathe into a paper bag to manage it at home.

CHAPTER HIGHLIGHTS

- The volume and composition of body fluid is normally maintained by a balance of fluid and electrolyte intake; elimination of water, electrolytes, and acids by the kidneys; and hormonal influences. Change in any of these factors can lead to a fluid, electrolyte, or acid–base imbalance that adversely affects health.
- Fluid, electrolyte, and acid–base imbalances can affect all body systems, especially the cardiovascular system, the central nervous system, and the transmission of nerve impulses. Conversely, primary disorders of the respiratory, renal, cardiovascular, endocrine, or other body systems can lead to an imbalance of fluids, electrolytes, or acid–base status.
- Fluid and sodium imbalances are related; both affect serum osmolality.
- Potassium imbalances are commonly seen in patients with acute or chronic illnesses. Both hypokalemia and hyperkalemia affect cardiac conduction and function. Carefully monitor cardiac rhythm and status in patients with very low or very high potassium levels.
- Calcium imbalances primarily affect neuromuscular transmission: Hypocalcemia increases neuromuscular irritability; hypercalcemia depresses neuromuscular transmission. Magnesium imbalances have a similar effect.
- Acid–base imbalances may be caused by either metabolic or respiratory health problems. Simple acid–base imbalances (respiratory or metabolic acidosis or alkalosis) are more commonly seen than mixed imbalances.
- Buffers, lungs, and kidneys work together to maintain acid–base balance in the body. Buffers respond to changes almost immediately; the lungs respond within minutes; the kidneys, require hours to days to restore normal acid–base balance.
- The lungs compensate for metabolic acid–base imbalances by excreting or retaining carbon dioxide. This is accomplished by increasing or decreasing the rate and depth of respirations.
- The kidneys compensate for respiratory acid–base imbalances by producing and retaining or excreting bicarbonate, and by retaining or excreting hydrogen ions.
- Careful monitoring of respiratory and cardiovascular status, mental status, neuromuscular function, and laboratory values is an important nursing responsibility for all patients with fluid, electrolyte, or acid–base imbalances.

TEST YOURSELF NCLEX-RN® REVIEW

1. A patient is admitted to the emergency department with hypovolemia. Which IV solution would the nurse anticipate administering?
   1. lactated Ringer's solution
   2. 10% dextrose in water
   3. 3% sodium chloride
   4. 0.45% sodium chloride

2. When assessing a patient with fluid volume deficit, what would the nurse expect to find?
   1. increased pulse rate and blood pressure
   2. dyspnea and respiratory crackles
   3. headache and muscle cramps
   4. orthostatic hypotension and flat neck veins

3. The nurse caring for a patient with acute hypernatremia includes which of the following in the plan of care? **Select all that apply.**
   1. Conduct frequent neurologic checks.
   2. Restrict fluids to 1500 mL per day.
   3. Orient to time, place, and person frequently.
   4. Maintain IV access.
   5. Limit length of visits.

4. Laboratory results for a patient show a serum potassium level of 2.2 mEq/L. Which of the following nursing actions is of highest priority for this patient?
   1. Keep the patient on bed rest.
   2. Initiate cardiac monitoring.
   3. Start oxygen at 2 L/min.
   4. Initiate seizure precautions.

5. The nurse evaluates teaching about calcium supplement therapy as effective when the patient states that she will take her calcium tablets how?
   1. all at one time in the morning
   2. with meals
   3. as needed for tremulousness
   4. with a full glass of water

6. A patient who is known to be an alcoholic presents with confusion, hallucinations, and a positive Chvostek's sign. Which medication(s) should the nurse anticipate administering?
   1. magnesium sulfate
   2. calcium chloride
   3. insulin and glucose
   4. sodium bicarbonate

7. Arterial blood gas results for a patient show pH 7.21, PaO_2 98 mmHg, $PaCO_2$ 32 mmHg, and HCO_3^- 17 mEq/L. The nurse correctly interprets these values as indicative of which of the following acid–base imbalances?
   1. metabolic acidosis
   2. metabolic alkalosis
   3. respiratory acidosis
   4. respiratory alkalosis

8. A patient is admitted with a suspected heroin overdose and a respiratory rate of 5 to 6 per minute. Which of the following assessment data would the nurse anticipate? **Select all that apply.**
   1. pH 7.29
   2. alert and oriented
   3. $PaCO_2$ 54 mmHg
   4. HCO_3^- 32 mEq/L
   5. skin warm and flushed

9. The nurse caring for a patient undergoing several days of gastric decompression recognizes that the patient is at risk for which of the following acid–base imbalances?
   1. metabolic acidosis
   2. metabolic alkalosis
   3. respiratory acidosis
   4. respiratory alkalosis

10. A patient undergoing mechanical ventilation following a severe chest wall injury and flail chest complains of chest tightness, anxiety, and feeling as though she cannot get enough air. She is afraid she is having a heart attack. The nurse should first do which of the following?
    1. Administer prescribed analgesic.
    2. Contact respiratory therapy to evaluate ventilator settings.
    3. Obtain arterial blood gases.
    4. Notify the physician.

See Test Yourself answers in Appendix C.

Pearson Nursing Student Resources

Find additional review materials at
www.nursing.pearsonhighered.com

Prepare for success with additional NCLEX®-style practice questions, interactive assignments and activities, Web links, animations and videos, and more!

BIBLIOGRAPHY

American Association of Critical Care Nurses. (2007). Practice alert: Oral care in the critically ill. Retrieved from http://www.aacn.org

Astle, S. M. (2005). Restoring electrolyte balance. *RN, 68*(5), 34–40.

Beer, M. H., Porter, R., & Jones, T. V. (Eds.). (2008). *The Merck manual of diagnosis and therapy* (18th ed.). Merck & Co., Inc. Internet edition provided by Medical Services, USMEDSA, USHH.

Blackmer, S. (2010). Cerebral salt wasting: An overlooked cause of hyponatremia. *American Nurse Today, 5*(3), 34, 36.

Bulechek, G., Butcher, H., & Dochterman, J. (Eds.). (2008). *Nursing interventions classification (NIC)* (5th ed.). Mosby Elsevier.

Centers for Disease Control. (2009). Application of lower sodium intake recommendations to adults—United States, 1999–2006. *MMWR Weekly,* March 27, 2009/ *58*(11), 291–283.

David, K. (2007). *IV fluids: Do you know what's hanging and why?* RN Web. Available RN/AHC Home Study Program.

Dougherty, L. (2008). Back to basics in IV therapy: An unfortunate necessity. *British Journal of Nursing, 17*(19), S3.

Edwards, S. L. (2005). Maintaining calcium balance: Physiology and implications. *Nursing Times, 101*(19), 58–61.

Fauci, A. S., Braunwald, E., Kasper, D., Hauser, S. L., Longo, D. L., Jameson, J. L., & Loscalzo (Eds.). (2008). *Harrison's principles of internal medicine* (17th ed.). New York: McGraw-Hill.

Fournier, M. (2009). Perfecting your acid-base balancing act. How to detect and correct acid-base disorders. *American Nurse Today, 4*(1), 17–22.

Gobbi, M., Cowen, M., & Ugboma, D. (2006). Fluid and electrolyte balance. In M. Alexander, J. Fawcett, & P. Runciman (Eds.) *Nursing practice: Hospital and home: The adult* (3rd ed., pp. 763–785). Philadelphia: Churchill Livingstone.

Hayes, D. (2007). How to respond to abnormal serum sodium levels. *Nursing, 37*(12), 56hn1–2, 56hn4.

Hogan, M., Gingrich, M., Overby, P., & Ricci, M. (2007). *Fluids, electrolytes, & acid-base balance* (2nd ed.) Pearson Prentice Hall.

Holman, C., Roberts, S., & Nicol, M. (2005). Promoting adequate hydration in older people. *Nursing Older People, 17*(4), 31–32.

Kee, J. L. (2008). *Prentice Hall handbook of laboratory and diagnostic tests with nursing implications* (6th ed). Pearson Prentice Hall.

Lawes, R. (2009). Body out of balance: Understanding metabolic acidosis and alkalosis. *Nursing, 39*(11), 50–54.

Macafee, D., Allison, S., & Lobo, D. (2005). Some interactions between GI function and fluid and electrolyte homeostasis. *Current Opinion in Clinical Nutrition and Metabolic Care, 8*(2), 197–203.

McPhee, S., Papadakis, M., & Tierney, L. (2008). *Current medical diagnosis and treatment* (47th ed.). New York: Lange /McGraw-Hill.

Mentes, J. (2008). *Hydration management: Nursing standard of practice protocol: Oral hydration management.* Hartford Institute for Geriatric Nursing. Retrieved from http://www.consultgerirn.org/topics

Metheny, N. M. (2000). *Fluid and electrolyte balance: Nursing considerations* (4th ed.). Philadelphia: Lippincott.

Moorhead, S., Johnson, M., Maas, M., & Swanson, E. (Eds.). (2008). *Nursing outcomes classification (NOC)* (4th ed.). St. Louis: Mosby Elsevier.

NANDA International. (2009). *Nursing diagnoses: Definitions and classification 2009–2011.* Oxford, UK: Wiley-Blackwell.

Nemec, K., Kopelent-Frank, H., & Greif, R. (2008). Standardization of infusion solutions to reduce the risk of incompatibility. *American Journal of Health-System Pharmacy, 65*(17), 1648–1654.

Oh, H., & Seo, W. (2007). Alterations in fluid, electrolytes and other serum chemistry values and their relations with enteral tube feeding in acute brain infarction patients. *Journal of Clinical Nursing, 16*(2), 298–307.

Oh, H., Suh, Y., Hwang, S., & Seo, W. (2005). Effects of nasogastric tube feeding on serum sodium, potassium and glucose levels. *Journal of Nursing Scholarship, 37*(2), 141–147.

O'Keeffe, S. (2005). Clinician's guide to interpreting arterial blood gases (ABG's). *Clinical Times, 2*(3), 3.

O'Neill, P. (2007). Helping your patient to restrict potassium: Teach him how to modify his diet to maintain optimum levels of this vital electrolyte. *Nursing, 37*(4), 64hn6, 64hn8.

Perrin, K. O. (2009). *Understanding the essentials of critical care nursing.* Upper Saddle River: Pearson Prentice Hall.

Porth, C. M. (2007). *Essentials of pathophysiology: Concepts of altered health states* (2nd ed.). Philadelphia: Lippincott Williams & Wilkins.

Porth, C. M., & Matfin, G. (2009). *Pathophysiology: Concepts of altered health states.* (8th ed.). Philadelphia: Lippincott Williams & Wilkins.

Pruitt, W. C., & Jacobs, M. (2004). Interpreting arterial blood gases: Easy as ABC. *Nursing, 34*(8), 50–53.

Rosenthal, K. (2009). *Tonicity and IV fluids.* Resource Nurse. Retrieved from http://www.resourcenurse.com/feature_tonicity_fluids.html

Scroggs, J. (2008). Improving patient safety using clinical needs assessment in IV therapy. *British Journal of Nursing, 17*(19), S22–S28.

Stanner, S. (2005). Preventing undernutrition and dehydration in older people. *Nursing & Residential Care, 7*(1), 17–19.

Sweeney, J. (2005a). What causes hyponatremia? *Nursing, 35*(6), 18.

Sweeney, J. (2005b). What causes sudden hypokalemia? *Nursing, 35*(4), 12.

Ulrich, S., & McCutcheon, H. (2008). Nursing practice and oral fluid intake of older people with dementia. *Journal of Clinical Nursing, 17*(21), 2910–2919.

Urden, L. D., Stacy, K. M., & Lough, M. E. (2006). *Thelan's critical care nursing: Diagnosis and management* (5th ed.). St. Louis, MO: Mosby.

Wilson, B., Shannon, M., & Shields, K. (2009). *Prentice Hall Nurses Drug Guide 2009.* Pearson Prentice Hall.

Young, E., Shrrard-Jacob, A., Knapp, K., et al., (2009). Perioperative fluid management. *AORN Journal, 39*(1), 167–182.

CHAPTER

11

Nursing Care of Patients
Experiencing Trauma and Shock

LEARNING OUTCOMES

1. Define the word *trauma*.
2. Define the components and types of trauma.
3. Describe the result of energy transfer to the human body.
4. Discuss causes, effects, and initial management of trauma.
5. Discuss diagnostic tests used in assessing patients experiencing trauma and shock.
6. Describe collaborative interventions for patients experiencing trauma and shock, including medications, blood transfusion, and intravenous fluids.
7. Discuss organ donation and forensic implications of traumatic injury or death.
8. Discuss cellular homeostasis and basic hemodynamics.
9. Discuss the risk factors, etiologies, and pathophysiologies of hypovolemic shock, cardiogenic shock, obstructive shock, and distributive shock.
10. Use the nursing process as a framework for providing individualized care to patients experiencing trauma and shock.

CLINICAL COMPETENCIES

1. Describe steps of the primary survey to diagnose and manage life-threatening injuries.
2. Obtain initial subjective and objective data of the trauma patient to include history taking, assessment, review of past medical history, and communication with pre-hospital and other healthcare providers and family members.
3. Evaluate patient response to medical and surgical interventions for patients sustaining multiple trauma and shock.
4. Provide essential ongoing written communication for patient care and continuity of the trauma patient.
5. Describe the role of the nurse in trauma prevention education and develop a plan of care to restore the functional health status of trauma patients.
6. Communicate significant data and changes in the condition of the patient who has sustained trauma.
7. Identify nursing diagnoses based on signs and symptoms recognized during the nursing assessment.
8. Develop a plan of care for the trauma patient based on scientific knowledge and patient diversity that addresses the nursing diagnosis.
9. Document quality of care issues associated with the trauma patient.
10. Advocate for the patient's rights as indicated by documents that address end-of-life issues.
11. Comply with guidelines related to the Uniform Anatomical Gift Act.

KEY TERMS

abrasion, *242*
brain death criteria, *248*
contusion, *242*
laceration, *242*

pneumothorax, *241*
puncture wound, *242*
shock, *253*

tension pneumothorax, *241*
transfusion, *245*
trauma, *238*

The Patient Experiencing Trauma

Trauma is defined as injury to human tissues and organs resulting from the transfer of energy from the environment. In the past the term *trauma* has been associated with the word *accident*. *Accident* means that the injury occurred without intent, a result of random chance. We now know that a considerable number of injuries are preventable and not of random chance. Intentional and nonintentional trauma encompasses a variety of injuries resulting from motor vehicle crashes, pedestrian injuries, gunshot wounds, falls, violence toward others, or self-inflicted violence. The injuries, disabilities, and deaths resulting from these acts constitute a major healthcare challenge.

FAST FACTS
- Trauma kills more people between the ages of 1 and 44 than any other disease or illness.
- Forty-three percent of all deaths from ages 1 to 4 are due to trauma.
- Forty-eight percent of all deaths from ages 5 to 14 are due to trauma.
- Sixty-two percent of all deaths from ages 15 to 24 are due to trauma.

Trauma usually occurs suddenly, leaving the patient and family with little time to prepare for its consequences. Nurses provide a vital link in both the physical and psychosocial care for the injured patient and family. In caring for the patient who has experienced trauma, nurses must consider not only the initial physical injury, but also its long-term consequences, including rehabilitation. Trauma may alter the patient's previous way of life, potentially effecting independence, mobility, cognitive thinking, and appearance.

Components of Trauma

Trauma results from an abnormal exchange of energy between a host and a mechanism in a predisposing environment. The *host* is the person or group at risk of injury. Multiple factors influence the host's potential for injury: age, sex, race, economic status, preexisting illnesses, and use of substances such as street drugs and alcohol.

The *mechanism* is the source of the energy transmitted to the host. The energy exchanged can be mechanical, gravitational, thermal, electrical, physical, or chemical. Table 11–1 lists the most common mechanisms for each type of energy. Mechanical energy is the most common type of energy transferred to a host in trauma. The most common mechanical source of injury in all adult age groups is the motor vehicle.

Guns are another common mechanical source of injury. Trauma from gunshot wounds has steadily increased over the past 20 years and remains a major reason for emergency department and trauma center admissions, especially in large cities.

When describing a traumatic injury, *intention* is included as a component. Most gunshot and stab wounds are examples of intentional injuries. It is important to remember, however, that some gunshot wounds are unintentional, such as those that occur when children play with their parents' guns. Other common unintentional injuries result from motor vehicle crashes, falls, drowning, fires, and hunting accidents.

The final component of trauma is the *environment*. For example, a road that has become slippery after a snowstorm is a physical environment that may contribute to an injury.

TABLE 11–1 Common Mechanisms of Injury by Energy Source

ENERGY SOURCE	COMMON MECHANISMS OF INJURY
Mechanical	Motor vehicles
	Firearms
	Machines
Gravitational	Falls
Thermal	Heating appliances
	Fire
	Freezing temperatures
Electrical	Wires, sockets, and other electrical objects
	Lightning
Physical	Fists, feet, and other body parts (as in physical assault)
	Sharp objects, such as knives
	Ultraviolet radiation
	Ionizing radiation
	Water (drowning)
	Other submersion agents (e.g., grain)
	Explosions
Chemical	Drugs
	Poisons
	Industrial chemicals

Occupation is an important environmental factor to consider. Those in certain occupations face a high risk of trauma; examples include police officers, firefighters, professional athletes, racecar drivers, and taxi cab drivers. One's social environment also influences risk for injury, such as the presence of gangs and neighborhood violence. (See the following box for one example, intimate partner violence.)

Assessing Intimate Partner Violence (IPV)

Most IPV incidents are not reported, thus it is believed that the available data greatly underestimates the true magnitude of the problem. It is estimated that more than 5.3 million women are beaten by male partners every year, resulting in 1300 deaths annually. Among men, 3.2 million IPV episodes occur annually, accounting for approximately 800,000 men raped or physically assaulted by an intimate partner. IPV is the single largest cause of injury to women in the United States. This is a widespread problem that occurs regardless of age, sex, race, socioeconomic status, or education. IPV is also referred to as partner abuse or spousal abuse (CDC, 2003). In 2001, intimate partner violence made up 20% of violent crime against women. The same year, intimate partners committed 3% of all violent crimes against men.

Note: From Bureau of Justice Statistics Crime Data. *Intimate Partner Violence, 1993–2001.* February 2003.

VIOLENCE IN THE ELDERLY

Elder abuse is defined as anything that endangers the life of an elderly person. This can range from physical or emotional assault to intimidation, neglect, or financial exploitation. In addition, willful deprivation of food or medical care is included. The National Elder Abuse Incidence study found that approximately 551,000 persons aged 60 or older were abused or neglected in a 1-year period. Persons 80 years of age and older experienced abuse and neglect two to three times their proportion of the older population. The perpetrator is a family member in 90% of the cases.

The general approach to diagnosis in abuse situations is challenging and many times hidden. As with spousal, elder, or child abuse, the task of identification is complex. The following are clues to identify violence-related injuries:

- Injuries that do not correlate with the history
- Injuries that suggest a defensive posture
- Injuries during pregnancy
- Pattern injuries
- Pattern burns
- Sexual abuse/rape
- Unusual or unexplained fractures
- Signs of confinement
- Unusual interaction between patient and caregiver
- Lack of medical attention; immunizations not up to date, poor dental health
- Unexplained dehydration or malnutrition

Types of Trauma

Minor trauma causes injury to a single part or system of the body and is usually treated in a physician's office or in the hospital emergency department. A fracture of the clavicle, a small second-degree burn, and a laceration requiring sutures are examples of minor trauma. Major or multiple trauma involves serious single-system injury (such as the traumatic amputation of a leg) or multiple-system injuries. Multiple trauma is most often the result of a motor vehicle crash.

Trauma is further classified as either blunt or penetrating. Blunt trauma occurs when there is no communication between the damaged tissues and the outside environment. It is caused by various forces including *deceleration* (a decrease in the speed of a moving object), *acceleration* (an increase in the speed of a moving object), *shearing* (forces occurring across a plane, with structures slipping across each other), *compression* (acute tissue pressure resulting in increased density), and *crushing* (high force that results in tissue destruction). Blunt forces often cause multiple injuries that may affect the head, spinal cord, bones, thorax, and abdomen. Blunt trauma is frequently caused by motor vehicle crashes, falls, assaults, and sports activities.

Penetrating trauma occurs when a foreign object enters the body, causing damage to body structures. Structures commonly affected include the brain, lungs, heart, liver, spleen, the intestines, and the vascular system. Examples of penetrating trauma are gunshot or stab wounds and impalement.

Other types of trauma include inhalation injuries from gases, smoke, or steam, burn or freezing injuries, and blast injuries from explosions. Blast injuries result from the temperature and velocity of air movement and the force of projectiles from the explosion. Blast injuries are more severe in water than in air since blast waves travel farther and faster in water. Trauma from blast injuries includes pulmonary edema and hemorrhage, damage to abdominal organs, burns, penetrating injuries, and ruptured tympanic membranes.

Outcome studies show a correlation between survival rates of multiple trauma victims and rapid response times by pre-hospital providers, coupled with appropriate decision making with regards to transporting victims to a facility capable of treating their injuries. As a result, a system was devised to assist pre-hospital providers to make the appropriate decisions. Trauma patients are classified as Class 1, 2, or 3 based on factors including mechanism of injury, vehicle speed, height of falls, and location of penetrating injuries. Class 3 trauma is the least severe. An example would be a same level fall without loss of consciousness or significant injury. Class 1 trauma involves life-threatening injuries likely to require medical specialists or immediate surgical intervention. While any hospital emergency department should be capable of caring for Class 3 trauma patients, patients meeting Class 1 or 2 criteria should be transported to a designated trauma center when possible. Facilities designated as trauma centers have medical specialists and surgical coverage available or on call 24 hours a day.

Effects of Traumatic Injury

Death is a common result of serious traumatic injury, and may be immediate, early, or late. Immediate death happens within minutes at the scene from such injuries as a torn thoracic aorta or decapitation. Early death occurs during the "golden hour" (the first hour following the injury) from major abdominal or thoracic injuries or progression of intracranial hemorrhage. Appropriate care during this time has been shown to improve survival. Late death generally occurs days or weeks after the injury and results from multiple organ failure, sepsis, and coagulopathies.

Because of the serious consequences of trauma, it is important to rapidly identify the patient's injuries and institute appropriate interventions quickly. Following are common results of trauma and interventions necessary for good outcomes.

Head and Neck Effects—Airway Obstruction

Maintenance of the airway and cervical spine are the highest priority in the trauma patient. Other distracting injuries may take the inexperienced practitioner away from the airway, but if the airway is not patent and the patient is unable to deliver oxygen to vital organs, all other interventions are futile.

Assessment includes determining airway patency. If the patient is unresponsive, manual opening of the airway using a jaw thrust maneuver is necessary. The jaw thrust is recommended in patients with actual and potential C-spine injury. Once the airway is opened, the practitioner must identify any potential obstruction from the tongue, loose teeth, foreign bodies, bleeding, secretions, vomitus, or edema. If the patient is responsive and can vocalize, that is a good indication that the airway is clear.

Any time the nurse performs an intervention it is important that you reassess the effectiveness of the intervention. For example, if you suction the airway to remove vomitus, you would reassess the airway after suctioning to determine if that intervention was successful or if you have to re-suction the airway a second time.

All trauma patients should receive high flow oxygen until stabilized. Assessment of breathing effectiveness is paramount. Assessment should include if the patient has spontaneous breathing, good rise and fall of the chest, determination of skin color, general rate and depth of respirations, abdominal or accessory muscle use, position of the trachea, observation of chest wall integrity and presence of jugular vein distention, bilateral breath sounds, as well as the presence of any surface trauma.

In addition to suctioning, other airway adjuncts available include oral or nasal pharyngeal airways, oxygen delivery devices, laryngeal mask airway, Combitube, and endotracheal intubation (Figure 11–1 ■). Intubation is the preferred method of airway management if the patient is unable to maintain oxygenation or an open airway.

Trauma patients may exhibit several aspects of airway management that are unique and require special preparation and precautions, as discussed next.

CLOSED HEAD INJURY Changes in hemodynamics, oxygenation, and ventilation should be minimized in order to maintain adequate cerebral perfusion pressure. Laryngoscopy causes a marked increase in intracranial pressure (ICP).

The goal is to maintain a $PaCO_2$ of 30–35 mmHg. Lidocaine administered 3–5 minutes prior to intubation can blunt an increase in ICP that is secondary to laryngeal stimulation. In a normotensive patient, beta blockers are given 2–3 minutes prior to intubation to attenuate the sympathetic response. Effective induction agents such as Etomidate or thiopental have not been shown to increase ICP.

Figure 11–1 ■ Placement of an oral endotracheal tube (ETT) for intubation. When the ETT is in place, air or oxygen can be blown into the external opening of the tube and enter the trachea.

MAXILLOFACIAL TRAUMA   Significant distortion of normal anatomy in facial trauma and respiratory compromise is not uncommon. Even in patients who present with mild respiratory compromise rapid deterioration from edema or hemorrhage can occur. A surgical airway may be the only alternative.

DIRECT AIRWAY TRAUMA   Penetrating trauma to the neck is associated with a high degree of morbidity and mortality. Airway involvement includes dyspnea, cyanosis, subcutaneous emphysema, hoarseness, or air bubbling from the wound. Orotracheal intubation with rapid sequence intubation is the technique of choice. The key is early identification of the need for intubation before the patient has no airway at all. Tracheobronchial injury occurs in approximately 10%–20% of patients with penetrating neck injuries.

CERVICAL SPINE INJURY   Precautions for securing an airway in the presence of a presumed C-spine injury is not unusual. Approximately 3%–6% of major trauma victims have clinically significant C-spine injuries. Oral intubation with manual in-line axial head and neck stabilization (MIAS) is a safe method. There is a decreased probability of C-spine injury if the following criteria are met:

- Absence of midline cervical spine tenderness
- Normal alertness
- Absence of intoxication
- Absence of a painful distracting injury
- No focal neurological defects

BURNS   Burn patients with airway compromise require aggressive management. Upper airway edema associated with inhalation or enclosed space fires can progress during the post burn phase. Securing an airway sooner than later is the goal. ∞ See Chapter 17 for nursing care of the patient with burns.

Thoracic Effects

TENSION PNEUMOTHORAX   A **pneumothorax** results when air enters the potential space between the parietal and visceral pleura. The thorax is completely filled by the lungs. Surface tension between the pleural surfaces hold the lungs to the chest wall. Air present in the pleural space will eventually collapse the lungs. A **tension pneumothorax** is life threatening and requires immediate intervention. On inspiration air enters the pleural space, does not escape on expiration, and increases the intrapleural pressure. This pressure collapses the injured lung, shifts the mediastinal contents, compressing the heart, great vessels, trachea, and eventually the uninjured lung. In turn, this causes the following signs and symptoms:

- Severe respiratory distress
- Hypotension
- Jugular vein distension
- Tracheal deviation toward the uninjured side
- Cyanosis

The immediate short-term life-saving intervention is a needle thoracostomy, inserting a large bore over the needle catheter into the second intercostal space at the mid-clavicular line (MCL). See Figure 11–2 ■.

FLAIL CHEST   Flail chest is the fracture of two or more ribs in two or more separate locations, leading to an unstable thoracic wall segment. Paradoxical movement of the chest wall is

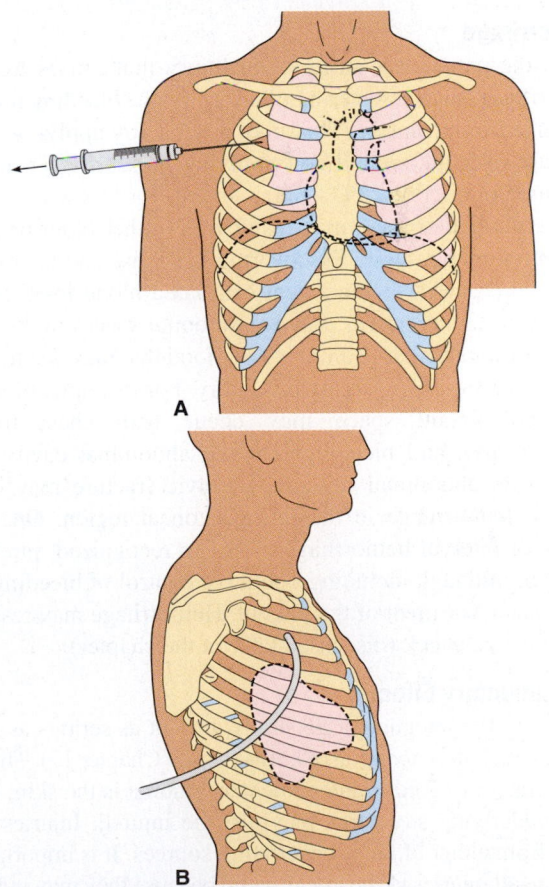

Figure 11–2 ■ A needle thoracostomy may be used in the emergency treatment of a tension pneumothorax. *A,* A large-gauge needle is introduced, and air and fluid are aspirated. *B,* Alternatively, a chest tube may be inserted and connected to a chest drainage system.

Hemo/Pneumothorax Animation

seen with the area sinking into the chest cavity with inspiration and protrusion with expiration. The area must be supported quickly to re-establish the thoracic bellows effect.

THORACIC CONTUSION AND RUPTURE Bruising of thoracic tissue is referred to as contusion. Pulmonary contusion is the most common traumatic chest injury. As a shock wave of force travels through the parenchyma, diffuse hemorrhage and alveolar edema develops, impairing gas exchange. Motor vehicle accidents are the most common cause of pulmonary contusions. Diaphragmatic rupture is a rare traumatic injury but can result in herniation of abdominal contents into the thoracic cavity, causing respiratory compromise.

Myocardial contusion results in extravasation of red blood cells into myocardial fibers. As myocardial cells are injured, it is believed that cardiac output diminishes due to reductions in contractile strength. Myocardial rupture is an acute traumatic tear of any structures of the heart. While rare, myocardial rupture is usually fatal with atrial rupture having the best chance for survival.

Cardiac tamponade occurs when blood or fluid collects in the pericardial sac. Resulting in myocardial compression, this condition is potentially life threatening and should be addressed immediately with pericardiocentesis.

Aortic rupture (transection) can result in acceleration-deceleration injury or blunt chest trauma. This injury is commonly fatal due to profuse bleeding. Aortic rupture is the second most common cause of trauma death after traumatic brain injury.

Hemorrhage

When the patient has suffered an injury that causes external hemorrhage, such as severing of an artery, the bleeding must be controlled immediately. This may be done by applying direct pressure over the wound and applying pressure over arterial pressure points (Figure 11–3 ■).

Internal hemorrhage may result from either blunt or penetrating traumatic injury. Discovering the cause and location of the injury, as well as the extent of related blood loss, are the most important concerns. Several potential spaces in the body can accommodate large amounts of blood that may accumulate (called *third spacing*) following injury. For example, bleeding into the pleural space may occur with chest trauma (*hemothorax*), and bleeding into the abdominal cavity may occur with abdominal trauma. A pelvic fracture may cause massive hemorrhage in the retroperitoneal region. Once the source of internal hemorrhage has been recognized, interventions are initiated, including operative control of bleeding and continual assessment of the patient. Hemorrhage may result in hypovolemic shock (discussed later in the chapter).

Integumentary Effects

Injuries to the integument generally are not as serious as other injuries, with the exception of burns (∞ see Chapter 17). The primary organ involved in integumentary trauma is the skin; however, underlying structures may also be injured. Injuries may result from either blunt or penetrating sources. It is important to evaluate all injuries to the integument, because they may indicate a more serious injury such as an open fracture. Additionally, large wounds may contribute to significant blood loss.

Five specific injuries to the integument are contusions, abrasions, puncture wounds, lacerations, and full thickness avulsion

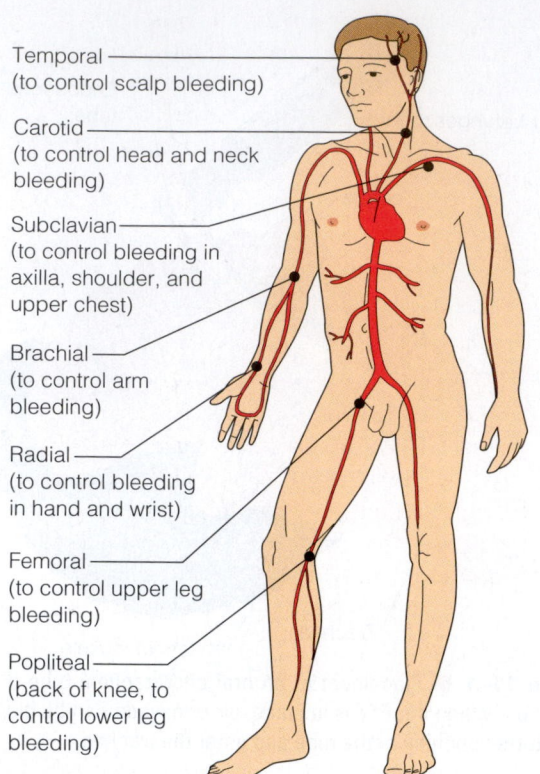

Temporal (to control scalp bleeding)

Carotid (to control head and neck bleeding)

Subclavian (to control bleeding in axilla, shoulder, and upper chest)

Brachial (to control arm bleeding)

Radial (to control bleeding in hand and wrist)

Femoral (to control upper leg bleeding)

Popliteal (back of knee, to control lower leg bleeding)

Figure 11–3 ■ The major pressure points used for the control of bleeding.

injuries (Figure 11–4 ■). **Contusions**, or superficial tissue injuries, result from blunt trauma that causes the breakage of small blood vessels and bleeding into the surrounding tissue. **Abrasions**, or partial-thickness denudations of an area of integument, generally result from falls or scrapes. **Puncture wounds** occur when a sharp or blunt object penetrates the integument. **Lacerations** are

A   B

C   D

Figure 11–4 ■ Traumatic injuries to the skin include *A*, contusion; *B*, abrasion; *C*, puncture wound; and *D*, laceration.

open wounds that result from sharp cutting or tearing. Injuries to the integument are at risk for contamination from dirt, debris, or foreign objects. Infection may cause further physical stress to the patient with multiple injuries. Full thickness avulsion injuries are injuries that result in loss of all of the layers of the skin, causing fat and muscle to be exposed. The size of the wound impacts both the length of time necessary for healing to take place as well as the risk for infection. These types of injuries are treated by allowing new skin to grow from the edges, stitching the wound together, reattaching avulsed skin, or by skin grafting.

Abdominal Effects

The abdomen contains both solid organs (liver, spleen, and pancreas) and hollow organs (stomach and intestines). Direct trauma to the abdomen can lacerate and compress the solid organs and cause burst injuries to the hollow organs. Blood vessels may be torn and organs may be displaced from their blood supply, producing life-threatening hemorrhage. Damage to the mesenteric vessels supplying the bowel can result in bowel ischemia and infarction. Injury to the stomach, pancreas, and small bowel may allow digestive enzymes to leak out into the abdominal cavity. Rupture of the large bowel results in escape of feces, which causes peritonitis. The immediate threat following abdominal trauma is hemorrhage; the later threat is peritonitis.

Musculoskeletal Effects

Musculoskeletal injuries may occur alone or with multiple injuries as the result of blunt or penetrating trauma. Musculoskeletal injuries usually are not considered a high priority in the care of the patient with multiple injuries. Exceptions are the life- or limb-threatening musculoskeletal injury, such as a dislocated hip, pulseless extremity, or significant blood loss such as from a femur or pelvic fracture. Other exceptions include fractures or dislocations with neurovascular compromise, open fractures, or compartment syndromes. Musculoskeletal injuries may provide clues to the presence of other serious injuries; for example, a fractured clavicle may indicate an associated thoracic injury. Care of the patient who has suffered a musculoskeletal injury is discussed in ∞ Chapter 38.

Neurologic Effects

Head injuries are a common type of injury sustained as the result of trauma. Injuries to the spinal cord, resulting in loss of neurologic function, are devastating outcomes of trauma, but they are much less common than head injuries. Most head and spinal cord injuries result from blunt trauma and are sustained in motor vehicle crashes. Falls, sports injuries, and assault are other sources of neurologic injury. Care of the patient with a neurologic injury is discussed in ∞ Chapters 41 and 42.

Multiple Organ Dysfunction Syndromes (MODS)

Multiple organ dysfunction syndrome (MODS) is a common complication of severe injury and a frequent cause of death in intensive care units. It is a progressive impairment of two or more organ systems. This is the result of an uncontrolled inflammatory response to severe injury or illness.

Patients at risk for MODS are those with a disturbance in homeostasis resulting from one or a combination of the following conditions:

- infection
- injury

- inflammation
- ischemia
- immune response
- intoxication of substances
- iatrogenic factors

The primary organ systems involved in MODS are the respiratory, renal, hepatic, hematologic, cardiovascular, gastrointestinal, and neurological. Supportive therapy depends on the identification of correctable causes. It may be one or a combination of several therapies. Surgical intervention, antibiotic administration, corticosteroid administration, or correction coagulopathies are some therapies used for this condition. MODS following injuries produces more than half of the late mortality following trauma.

Effects on the Family

Trauma usually occurs suddenly and with little warning. It may result in death or cause injury serious enough to alter both the patient's and the family's lives. The suddenness and seriousness of the event are precipitating factors in the development of a psychologic crisis. Over the past decade, some emergency departments have instituted care plans that allow families to be present during resuscitation. This type of care is not without controversy, but it should be considered when appropriate.

Interdisciplinary Care

Interdisciplinary care of the trauma patient depends on a team approach. Providing trauma care with a team focus helps each team member know his or her role. Prompt delegation of tasks and responsibilities improves the patient's chances for survival and decreases the morbidity that may result from traumatic injuries.

Pre-hospital Care

The major functions of pre-hospital care include injury identification, critical interventions, and rapid transport.

INJURY IDENTIFICATION   Emergency care of the patient experiencing trauma is based on rapid assessment to identify injuries and begin appropriate interventions. Injuries that indicate the need for trauma center care include the following:

- Penetrating injuries to the abdomen, pelvis, chest, neck, or head
- Spinal cord injuries with deficit
- Crushing injuries to the abdomen, chest, or head
- Major burns
- Injuries leading to airway compromise or obstruction

Many methods help healthcare providers determine the seriousness of the patient's injuries and the potential for survival. Scoring systems such as the Champion Revised Trauma Scoring System can be helpful (Table 11–2). A primary trauma assessment follows an alphabet mnemonic:

- **A** is airway assessment (with C-spine immobilization) to determine if the airway is patent, maintainable, or nonmaintainable.
- **B** is breathing evaluation for spontaneous respirations or ventilatory impedance such as by rib fractures or a collapsed lung.
- **C** is circulatory assessment to palpate peripheral and central pulses; to assess capillary refill, skin color, and temperature; and to identify any external sources of bleeding.
- **D** is disability and refers to the neurovascular status. Assessment includes level of consciousness, pupillary function, and response to verbal or painful stimuli.

TABLE 11–2 Champion Revised Trauma Scoring System

TEST	SCORE	CODED VALUE
Glasgow Coma Scale*	13 to 15	4
	9 to 12	3
	6 to 8	2
	4 to 5	1
	3	0
Systolic blood pressure	> 89	4
	76 to 89	3
	50 to 75	2
	1 to 49	1
	0	0
Respiratory rate	10 to 29	4
	> 29	3
	6 to 9	2
	1 to 5	1
	0	0
	Total score:	_____

The highest possible total score is 12. The lowest possible score is 0. The higher the total score, the greater the chance of survival.

*∞ See Chapter 41 for instructions for using the Glasgow Coma Scale.

Note: From "A Revision of the Trauma Score" by H. Champion et al., 1989, *Journal of Trauma*, Vol 29, No 5, p. 624, with permission from Wolters Kluwer Health.

- **E** is expose/environment where a whole body assessment is completed while assuring that hypothermia doesn't occur (i.e., heated blankets, warmed intravenous fluids).

Secondary assessment usually begins while the primary assessment is underway. This assessment extends the alphabetical mnemonic:

- **F** is "full set of vital signs." F can also stand for having family members present during treatment.
- **G** is giving comfort measures for both physical and emotional comfort for the patient and family.
- **H** is head-to-toe assessment and medical history that includes visual and manual assessment as well as appropriate auscultation.
- **I** is inspection of posterior surfaces for any injuries.

The Glasgow Coma Scale is another scoring system that is used to quantify the level of consciousness following traumatic brain injury. ∞ See Chapters 41 and 45.

CRITICAL INTERVENTIONS As life-threatening problems are identified during the primary assessment, appropriate on-the-scene interventions must be performed immediately. These include providing life support, immobilizing the cervical spine, managing the airway, and treating hemorrhage and shock.

Immobilization of the patient's cervical spine is a primary intervention. The patient is placed on a spine board, and a cervical collar and a head immobilizer are applied (Figure 11–5 ■). The cervical spine may also be immobilized by logrolling the patient onto a board, placing towel rolls or a head immobilizer along the sides of the patient's head, and securing the patient to the board. If

Figure 11–5 ■ Immobilization of the cervical spine at the scene of the accident is essential to preventing further injury to the spinal cord. The combined use of a hard cervical collar, head blocks, and tape best restricts flexion, extension, rotation, and lateral bending of the neck.
Source: Spencer Grant/Photo Researchers, Inc.

the patient was wearing a helmet at the time of injury, the helmet should remain on until the patient arrives at the hospital, unless the patient's airway is at risk. If necessary, healthcare personnel at the scene will remove the helmet by manipulating it over the patient's nose and ears while holding the patient's head and neck immobile; safe removal requires at least two people. Improper removal risks injury or additional injury to the spinal cord.

If the patient's airway is patent, oxygen is administered. Ventilations may be assisted with a bag-valve-mask resuscitator until airway management is achieved. Active external bleeding is controlled by direct pressure. Measures to reverse shock (discussed later in the chapter) are initiated.

RAPID TRANSPORT Patients who have multiple injuries must be transported as soon as possible to a regional trauma center. The most common modes of rapid transport are ground ambulance and air ambulance, which includes helicopters specially staffed and equipped to care for trauma victims. Figure 11–6 ■ shows a flight nurse assessing a patient. Stable patients within access of a ground ambulance are best transported by ground. Unstable patients and those injured in the wilderness or other areas in which ground access is difficult may best be transported by air. When these transport systems are unavailable, the patient is transported by any possible means.

Emergency Department Care

DIAGNOSIS The diagnostic tests ordered once the patient reaches the hospital depend on the type of injury the patient has sustained. Tests that may be ordered for victims of trauma include the following:

- *Blood type and crossmatch* involves typing the patient's blood for ABO antigens and Rh factor, screening the blood for antibodies, and crossmatching the patient's serum and donor red blood cells.
- *Complete blood count* evaluates the components of blood including red blood cell count and white blood cell count.
- *Arterial blood gas* evaluates oxygenation, acid–base balance, presence of metabolic or respiratory compensatory mechanisms.

Figure 11–6 ■ Flight nurses provide initial assessment, stabilization, and support for patients with trauma.
Courtesy of University Air Care/University of Cincinnati Hospital.

- *Blood alcohol level* measures the amount of alcohol in a patient's blood. It has been found that between 20% and 50% of people who are injured may be intoxicated. Alcohol alters the patient's level of consciousness and response to pain.
- *Urine drug screen* may also be ordered. Like alcohol, such drugs as cocaine alter the patient's level of consciousness and overall response to the primary survey.
- *Pregnancy test* for any woman of childbearing age rules out the potential for pregnancy and fetal injury.
- *Focused assessment by sonography in trauma (FAST)* primarily focuses on evaluating the identification of blood in body cavities where it is not supposed to be. Primary focus is on the peritoneum. It is also helpful in identification of blood in the pleura and pericardium.
- *Diagnostic peritoneal lavage* determines the presence of blood in the peritoneal cavity, which may indicate abdominal injury. The test is generally done in the emergency department. A local anesthetic (such as lidocaine) is injected subcutaneously, and a small incision is made in the lower abdomen. A catheter is placed into the peritoneal cavity, and any free blood is aspirated. If 10 mL of blood is found, the patient is taken to the operating room for exploratory surgery. If no free blood is aspirated, 1 L of a warm isotonic solution (Ringer's solution or normal saline) is rapidly infused into

the peritoneal cavity and then allowed to drain by gravity. If the solution returns pink and is found to have a red blood cell count of 100,000 mm^3; a white blood cell count of $\geq$ 500; or bile, food, or feces, the test is considered positive and the patient is taken to the operating room for exploratory surgery. This procedure is used less with the inception of the FAST exam. This test does not detect retroperitoneal injuries (injuries of the kidneys, pancreas, great vessels, duodenum, or portions of the ascending or descending colon).

- *Computerized tomography (CT) scans* can discover injuries to the brain, skull, spine, spinal cord, chest, and abdomen.
- *Magnetic resonance imaging (MRI) scans* can discover injuries to the brain and spinal cord.

Medications

Medications used to treat the patient who has experienced trauma depend on the type and severity of the injuries, as well as the degree of traumatic shock that is present. The following general categories of medications may be used. (Fluid administration and the drugs listed are covered later in the chapter in discussion of the collaborative care of the patient in shock.)

- Blood components and crystalloids are administered intravenously in the initial treatment of traumatic shock to replace intravascular volume.
- Inotropic drugs (drugs that increase myocardial contractility) are given to increase cardiac output and improve tissue perfusion. These drugs, administered only after fluid volume restoration, include dopamine (Dopastat, Intropin), dobutamine (Dobutrex), and isoproterenol (Isuprel).
- Vasopressors may be administered in conjunction with fluid replacement to treat neurogenic, septic, or anaphylactic shock. Examples of vasopressors include dopamine (Dopastat), epinephrine (Adrenalin), norepinephrine (Levophed), and phenylephrine (Neo-synephrine).
- Opioids, administered by bolus or continuous infusion, are used to treat pain as soon as possible. However, the effects of the pain medications may alter patient responses to injury, cause hypotension and respiratory depression, and mask potential injuries. If pain medications are administered, they must be carefully regulated, and the patient must be closely monitored.
- Immunization: If the patient has penetrating and open wounds, tetanus immunization status must be determined. If the patient is unable to remember when the last tetanus immunization was given, is unable to answer, or has not received a tetanus immunization within the past 5 years, then tetanus prophylaxis is given.

Blood Transfusions

Blood and blood components are initially produced in the body and then donated for use by another person through a **transfusion** (an infusion of blood or blood components). A patient may be given whole blood, packed red blood cells (RBCs), platelets, plasma, albumin, clotting factors, prothrombin, or cryoprecipitate (Table 11–3). Blood and blood components increase the amount of hemoglobin available to carry oxygen to the cells, improve hemoglobin and hematocrit levels during active bleeding, increase intravascular volume, and replace deficient substances such as platelets and clotting factors.

TABLE 11–3 Volume Resuscitation Therapies

COMPONENT	INDICATIONS	ADVANTAGES	DISADVANTAGES
Ringer's lactate	■ Restoration of circulating volume ■ Replacement of electrolyte deficits	■ Good availability ■ Safe to use ■ Low cost ■ Aids in buffering acidosis	■ Rapid movement from the intravascular to the extravascular space, leading to three or more times requirement for replacement
Normal saline	■ Restoration of circulating volume ■ Vehicle compatible with administration of blood	■ Good availability ■ Low cost ■ Safe to use	■ Hyperchloremic acidosis associated with prolonged use of sodium solutions
Whole blood	■ Replaces blood volume and oxygen carrying capacity in hemorrhage and shock	■ Contains RBCs, plasma proteins, clotting factors, and plasma	■ Contains few platelets or granulocytes; deficient in clotting factors V and VII ■ Greatest risks are for incompatibility or circulatory overload ■ Risk of transmitting blood-borne pathogens
Packed red blood cells (RBCs)	■ Restoration of intravascular volume ■ Replacement of oxygen carrying capacity	■ One unit of RBCs should increase the hemoglobin of a 70 kg adult by approximately 1 gm/dl in the absence of volume overload or continuing blood loss.	■ Red cells require compatibility testing ■ Risk of transmitting blood borne pathogens ■ Should be warmed to prevent hypothermia ■ Contains little or no clotting factors
Platelets	■ Significant thrombocytopenia (platelet count less than 20,000–50,000 per mm^3) ■ Continued hemorrhage	■ Compatibility testing is not required ■ Typical platelet transfusion should raise the platelets of a 70 kg adult approximately 30,000–50,000/UL	■ Post exposure prophylaxis with anti-Rh immune globulin should be considered following Rh+ platelet transfusion to an Rh− woman ■ Risk of transmitting blood-borne pathogens
Albumin	■ Expends blood volume in shock and trauma	■ Good availability	■ Is not a substitute for whole blood ■ Risk of hypersensitivity reactions ■ Risk of transmitting blood-borne pathogens
Fresh frozen plasma (FFP)	■ Documented coagulopathy ■ Restoration of clotting factors ■ Supplies plasma proteins	■ Cross matching and Rh compatibility is not required	■ Must be thawed in a 37°C water bath for approximately 30 minutes ■ Should be ABO compatible ■ Risk of transmitting blood-borne pathogens
Cryoprecipitate	■ Coagulopathy with low fibrinogen ■ Restoration of fibrinogen	■ Rh type not important	■ Risk of transmitting blood-borne pathogens ■ Contains hemagglutinins ■ If large volume of ABO incompatible cryoprecipitate are administered intravascular hemolysis can occur

Each person has one of four blood types: A, B, AB, or O. The blood group antigens A and B, present on RBC membranes, form the basis for the ABO blood categorization. The presence or absence of these inherited antigens determines one's blood type. People with blood type A have A antigens, those with type B have B antigens, those with type AB have both antigens, and those with neither antigen have blood type O (called a universal donor).

FAST FACTS
■ Type AB blood is the "universal receiver."
■ Type O blood is the "universal donor."

ABO antibodies develop in the serum of people whose RBCs lack the corresponding antigen; these antibodies are called anti-A and anti-B. The person with blood type B has A antibodies, the person with type A has B antibodies, the person with type O has both types of antibodies, and the person with blood type AB has no antibodies (called a universal recipient).

A third antigen on the RBC membrane is D. People who are Rh positive have the D antigen, whereas people who are Rh negative do not. These antigens and antibodies may cause ABO and Rh incompatibilities.

A transfusion of incompatible blood causes hemolysis (breakdown) of the RBCs and agglutination of erythrocytes. (Agglutination is the clumping of cells that results from their interaction with specific antibodies.) The ABO blood group names and compatibilities are listed in Table 11–4.

TABLE 11–4 Blood Group Types and Compatibilities

BLOOD GROUP	RBC AGGLUTINOGENS	SERUM AGGLUTINOGENS	COMPATIBLE DONOR BLOOD GROUPS	INCOMPATIBLE DONOR BLOOD GROUPS
A	A	Anti-B	A, O	B, AB
B	B	Anti-A	B, O	A, AB
AB	A, B	None	A, B, AB, O	None
O	None	Anti-A, Anti-B	O	A, B, AB

Before RBCs or whole blood can be administered, a series of procedures determine donor and recipient ABO types and Rh groups. These procedures, called a type and crossmatch, are performed by mixing the donor cells with the recipient's serum and watching for agglutination. If none occurs, the blood is considered compatible.

Despite meticulous procedures for matching blood types and antigens, blood transfusion reactions may still occur. The most common is a *febrile reaction*. Antibodies within the patient receiving the blood are directed against the donor's white blood cells, causing fever and chills. Febrile reactions typically begin during the first 15 minutes of the transfusion. Using leukocyte-poor blood avoids future febrile reactions.

Hypersensitivity reactions result when antibodies in the patient's blood react against proteins, such as immunoglobulin A, in the donor blood. Hypersensitivity reactions may appear during or after the transfusion. The manifestations of hypersensitivity reaction include *urticaria* (the appearance of reddened wheals of various sizes on the skin) and itching.

Hemolytic reactions, the most dangerous transfusion reactions, usually result from an ABO incompatibility. Clumping RBCs block capillaries, decreasing blood flow to vital organs. In addition, macrophages engulf the clumped RBCs, releasing free hemoglobin into the circulating blood; the hemoglobin is then filtered by the kidneys and may block the renal tubules, causing renal failure. Hemolytic reactions usually begin after infusion of 100 to 200 mL of the incompatible blood. Manifestations of a hemolytic reaction include flushing of the face, a burning sensation along the vein, headache, urticaria, chills, fever, lumbar pain, abdominal pain, chest pain, nausea and vomiting, tachycardia, hypotension, and dyspnea. If any of these manifestations appear, the blood transfusion must be immediately discontinued.

Other risks to patients receiving blood include circulatory overload, electrolyte imbalances, and infectious diseases such as hepatitis or cytomegalovirus.

Patients who have experienced trauma of any severity have had substantial blood loss and are usually in hypovolemic shock. Blood replacement is the treatment of choice to restore oxygen-carrying capacity. Patients in severe shock with active bleeding are given universal, type O red blood cells immediately. Patients with less severe injuries or bleeding may be stabilized with other types of fluids until type-specific or crossmatched blood is available.

Some emergency departments and trauma centers use autotransfusion to provide blood for transfusions for the patient with multiple injuries and/or severe shock. Autotransfusion is a method of blood administration in which special equipment collects and returns the patient's own blood. The chest cavity is the typical source of blood to be autotransfused.

Nursing considerations for blood transfusion therapy are described in the following Medication Administration box.

Emergency Surgery

Immediate surgical intervention is indicated when the patient remains in shock despite resuscitation and there is no obvious external sign of blood loss. Abdominal and chest x-rays, ultrasound studies, diagnostic peritoneal lavage, or CT scan may be performed to help identify the potential source of the blood loss. It is important that the emergency or trauma nurse speak with the family as soon as possible and keep everyone informed about what is happening to his or her family member. Unfortunately, the need for emergency surgery may not allow time for family members or significant others to see their loved one before transfer to the operating room.

Organ Donation

The Uniform Anatomical Gift Act (1968, 1987) requires that people be informed about their options for organ donation. Under this act, consent for organ donation may be given not only by the donor but also by a spouse, adult children, parents, adult siblings, guardian, or any adult authorized to do so. The act also encourages people to carry donor cards.

The increased success of organ transplant has made it a more common and valuable method of prolonging and improving life; however, many people are still waiting for organs, and many people who may be suitable organ donors die each year from trauma. Organs and tissues that may be transplanted include bones, eyes, liver, lungs, skin, muscles and tendons, pancreas, intestines, kidneys, heart, and heart valves.

The organ donation process begins with identification of the potential organ donor. Most people are potential organ donors. Exceptions include those who

- currently abuse intravenous drugs.
- have preexisting untreated infections, such as septicemia.
- have any malignancy other than a primary brain tumor.
- have active tuberculosis.

In the past HIV positive patients were excluded as donors. A recent legislative change now allows HIV positive patients to donate to HIV positive recipients.

The family needs to be made aware of the patient's prognosis and presented with the option of donating the patient's organs. Both the family's and the patient's feelings about

MEDICATION ADMINISTRATION   Blood Transfusion

The risk for and seriousness of blood transfusion reactions require that extreme caution be taken when blood is administered. Most fatal transfusion reactions are the result of human error. Although general guidelines are provided here, each institution has specific policies and procedures that must be followed. Prior to beginning the transfusion, the nurse must determine that typed and crossmatched blood is available and collect the needed equipment: a Y-tubing blood administration set with a filter, a large-bore intravenous catheter (usually 18 or 19 gauge), and normal saline solution. Only normal saline is used with a blood transfusion. Dextrose causes clumping of RBCs, and distilled water causes hemolysis.

Nursing Responsibilities

- Obtain patient consent.
- Assess for any previous reactions to blood.
- Explain the procedure to the patient, and answer any questions.
- Prepare the intravenous equipment. Shut off one side of the Y tubing, and attach the other side to the saline solution. Flush the tubing and filter with the saline.
- If venous access is not already in place, insert the intravenous needle (following body substance precautions), and begin administering the saline.
- Using institutional procedure, obtain the blood from the blood bank or laboratory. Administer the blood immediately; if this is not possible, return it to the blood bank or laboratory.
- Check and document that the donor and recipient blood have been tested and are compatible. This usually involves two nurses, each verifying the following:
  a. an order for blood has been written
  b. type and crossmatch have been done
  c. the name of the patient and the name on the blood bag are identical
  d. the number assigned to the unit of blood is identical to the one on the requisition for the blood
  e. blood type and Rh factor are compatible
  f. the blood has not exceeded its expiration date
  g. the unit of blood is intact and has no bubbles or discoloration
- Identify the patient by reading the arm band and asking the patient to tell you his or her name. Check the arm band against the unit of blood.
- Gently invert the blood bag several times to mix the plasma and RBCs.
- Take and record vital signs as a baseline.
- Attach the open side of the Y tubing to the blood unit, and begin the transfusion at a slow rate of about 2 mL per minute. (Some trauma patients may have blood infused at a rapid rate. If blood is infused rapidly, it may need to be warmed prior to administration to prevent hypothermia.)

- Stay with the patient for at least the first 15 minutes of the transfusion, monitoring for manifestations of a reaction and taking the patient's vital signs.
- Continue to monitor the patient during the transfusion, assessing for manifestations of hypersensitivity or hemolytic reactions and taking and recording vital signs as directed by institutional policy.
- After the first 15 minutes, the rate of infusion is increased. If there is no danger of fluid volume overload, most patients can tolerate an infusion of a unit of blood (ranging from 250 to 500 mL, depending on the blood component administered) in 2 hours. The unit of blood should be administered in 3 to 4 hours; after this time, it has warmed and begins to deteriorate.
- Take the following actions if manifestations of a reaction occur:
  a. Stop the infusion of blood immediately, and notify the physician. Continue to infuse the saline.
  b. Take vital signs and assess manifestations.
  c. Compare the blood slip with the unit of blood to ensure that an identification error was not made.
  d. Save the blood bag and any remaining blood for return to the laboratory for further tests to determine the cause of the reaction.
  e. Follow institutional policy for collecting urine and venous blood samples.
  f. Continue to monitor the patient and provide prescribed interventions to treat hypersensitivity or hemolytic manifestations.

Health Education for the Patient and Family

- The possible risks of blood transfusions include infectious diseases and acquired immune deficiency syndrome (AIDS). However, because of careful handling and storage of blood, bacterial contamination is rare. Although hepatitis may be transmitted by contaminated blood, new tests for hepatitis antibodies in the donor blood are reducing this risk. Many people are afraid of contracting AIDS from blood; however, donor screening and HIV-antibody testing of donor blood has virtually eliminated the transmission of HIV by blood transfusion. A new risk that has been identified is the transmission of West Nile Virus through blood transfusions. Screening for this risk is asking potential donors about the presence of symptoms indicative of West Nile Virus.
- During the transfusion, immediately report any warm feelings, chills, itching, feelings of weakness or fainting, or difficulty breathing.
- Report any signs of a delayed transfusion reaction: chills, fever, cough, difficulty breathing, hives, itching, or changes in circulation, and seek medical care immediately.
- Discuss any religious or cultural considerations related to blood transfusions.

---

organ donation must be explored. Even if the patient carries an organ donation card, many institutions will not remove any organs without a signature from a family member or other authorized person. The nurse must always respect the family's concerns and feelings in this process. Organ procurement agencies employ specially trained personnel who oversee organ donor identification and procurement. These professionals are trained to approach families regarding potential organ donation. Box 11–1 lists **brain death criteria**. Once brain death has been confirmed, the family must also

understand the diagnosis and be allowed time to accept the patient's death.

When caring for an adult patient who is an organ donor, the nurse carries out the following:

- Maintain systolic blood pressure of 90 mmHg to keep the patient's organs perfused until removal.
- Maintain urine output at more than 30 mL per hour. This is usually accomplished by administering fluids and/or inotropic agents such as dopamine.
- Maintain oxygen saturation at 90% or greater.

BOX 11–1 Brain Death Criteria

Clinical Signs
- Irreversible condition
- Apnea with a $PaCO_2$ greater than 60 mmHg
- No response to deep stimuli
- No spontaneous movement (some spinal cord reflexes may be present)
- No gag or corneal reflex
- No oculocephalic or oculovestibular reflex
- Absence of toxic or metabolic disorders

Confirmatory Tests
- Cerebral blood flow study
- Electroencephalogram

Forensic Considerations

Injuries often happen under circumstances that require legal investigation. Many injuries, particularly penetrating trauma, may involve criminal activity. Therefore, the nurse must recognize the need to identify, store, and properly transfer potential evidence for medical–legal investigations.

Each item of clothing removed from the patient must be placed in a breathable container, such as a paper bag, and documented appropriately. Bullets or knives should be labeled, with their source specified, and given to the proper authorities. Holes found in clothing should not be disturbed. When it is necessary to cut off clothing, these areas should be avoided and never cut through if at all possible.

The patient's hands may yield important evidence, such as powder burns or residue on the skin, or tissue or hair samples beneath the fingernails. In the case of death, it is recommended that paper bags be placed over the patient's hands if the presence of evidence is suspected; otherwise, the evidence should be collected by nail clippings.

Identify all wounds and document these findings with pictures, diagrams, or written descriptions. Once the evidence has been collected, identified, and properly stored, ensure that it is given to the appropriate authorities. A chain of custody needs to be maintained throughout the entire process. All evidence must be identified and labeled, and documentation procedures must chronicle where and in whose possession the evidence has been. For the chain of custody to remain intact, the evidence must remain in the continuous possession of identified people and be marked and sealed in tamper-proof containers.

✑ Nursing Care

Nursing care of the patient who has been injured begins with a primary assessment and the initiation of collaborative interventions for any life-threatening injuries. Nursing care is directed toward the patient's specific responses to trauma.

Health Promotion

Prevention efforts can reduce the incidence and severity of trauma. Areas of health promotion and trauma prevention interventions for individuals and communities include the following:

- Motor vehicle safety: seatbelts, airbags, helmets, driving under the influence of alcohol or drugs, reckless driving,

visual or cognitive deficits in the older adult, cell phone use, driver fatigue
- Home safety: snow and ice removal, electrical wiring, falls, burns, drowning
- Farm safety: operating heavy equipment, safe storage of chemicals such as fertilizers
- Work safety: operating work equipment, wearing safety equipment, removal of jewelry
- Relationships: domestic violence, child abuse, elder abuse, or neglect
- Communities: gun control, gangs, condition of streets, neighborhood safety

(In providing information about trauma prevention to members of the community, the nurse serves as a healthcare educator, political activist, and safety advocate.)

Assessment

See Interdisciplinary Care for assessment of the patient experiencing trauma.

Nursing Diagnoses and Interventions

The trauma patient has many complex and interrelated actual or potential alterations in health. The nursing care in this section focuses on patient and family problems with respirations, infection, immobility, and spirituality. Nursing interventions for decreased cardiac output and altered perfusion are discussed in the section of the chapter on nursing care of the patient in shock. See the accompanying Case Study & Nursing Care Plan on page 252.

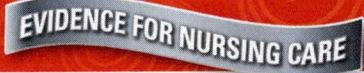

EVIDENCE FOR NURSING CARE — **The Patient with Brain Death**

Selected resources that nurses may find helpful when planning evidence-based nursing care follow.

- Arbour, R. (2009). Cardiogenic oscillation and ventilator autotriggering in brain-dead patients: A case series. *American Journal of Critical Care, 18*(5), 496, 488–495.
- Catlin, A. J. & Volat, D. (2009). When the fetus is alive but the mother is not: Critical care somatic support as an accepted model of care in the twenty-first century? *Critical Care Nursing Clinics of North America, 21*(2), 267–276.
- Greer, D. M., Varelas, P. N., Haque, S., & Wijdicks, E. F. M. (2008). Variability of brain death determination guidelines in leading US neurologic institutions. *Neurology, 70*(4), 284–289.
- Linde, E. B. (2009). Speaking up for organ donors. *Nursing2009, 39*(1), 29–31.
- Recommendations for end-of-life care in the intensive care unit: A consensus statement by the American Academy of Critical Care Medicine. (2008). National Guideline Clearinghouse. Retrieved from http://www.guideline.gov/summary/summary.aspx?doc_id=12655&nbr=006550&string=brain+AND+death
- Wijdicks, E. F. M., Rabinstein, A. A., Manno, E. M. & Atkinson, J. D. (2008). Pronouncing brain death: Contemporary practice and safety of the apnea test. *Neurology, 71*(16), 1240–1244.

MOVING EVIDENCE INTO ACTION   The Care of ICU Patients

SUSTAINING MULTIPLE TRAUMA

Ventilator-associated pneumonia (VAP) is an important patient safety issue in critically injured patients. The purpose of this study (Dodek, 2004) was to develop an evidenced-based guideline for prevention of ventilator-assisted pneumonia.

Data extraction consisted of gathering physical, positional, and pharmacologic interventions that may influence the development of VAP. The authors searched for pertinent randomized trails and case reviews that involved patients on mechanical ventilation. The study was isolated to include only adults and only studies published before 1 April 2003 were considered.

Physical strategies included the following:
- Route of endotracheal intubations
- Systematic search for maxillary sinusitis
- Frequency of ventilator circuit changes
- Airway humidification
- Endotracheal suctioning system
- Sublette secretion drainage
- Chest physiology
- Timing of tracheotomy

Positional strategies included the following:
- Kinetic bed therapy
- Semi-recumbent positioning
- Prone positioning

Pharmacologic strategies include the following:
- Stress ulcer prophylaxis
- Prophylactic antibiotics, including selective decontamination of the digestive track

IMPLICATIONS FOR NURSING

The following section identifies pertinent findings to support the conclusion that effectively implemented guidelines may decrease the morbidity, mortality, and costs of VAP in mechanically ventilated patients.

Based on direct evidence the following recommendations are encouraged:
- Alternatively, orotracheal intubations should be used when intubation is necessary.
- Recommend that new circuits for each patient be instituted and changed if the circuits become soiled.
- Recommend weekly changes of heat and moisture exchangers on equipment providing mechanical ventilation.
- Recommend the use of closed endotracheal suction systems that are changed for each new patient and as clinically indicated.
- Recommend that clinicians consider the use of subglottic secretion drainage.
- Recommend that clinicians consider the use of kinetic beds.
- Recommend the use of semi-recumbent positioning, with a goal of 45 degrees, in patients without contraindications.

The pharmacologic strategies that were studied were unfounded and not recommended for the VAP guideline.

CRITICAL THINKING IN PATIENT CARE

1. Considering the information from this study, how would you communicate the recommendations to the medical staff for the patient with mechanical ventilation?
2. What is the rationale behind the preceding recommendations?

Ineffective Airway Clearance

The patient with multiple injuries is at great risk for developing airway obstruction and apnea. Facial injuries, loose teeth, blood, and vomitus increase the risk for aspiration and obstruction. Neurologic injuries and cerebral edema alter the patient's respiratory drive and ability to keep the airway clear.

- Assess if airway is patent, maintainable, or nonmaintainable. Assess for manifestations of airway obstruction: stridor, tachypnea, bradypnea, cough, cyanosis, dyspnea, decreased or absent breath sounds, changes in oxygen levels, and changes in level of consciousness. *Assessing the airway and initiating interventions are the first steps in managing the patient with multiple injuries.*
- Monitor oxygen saturation by applying a pulse oximeter. Adjust oxygen flow to maintain oxygen saturation from 94% to 100%. *Changes in oxygen saturation as measured by the pulse oximeter indicate the effectiveness of the patient's airway. Pulse oximetry in patients who have been exposed to carbon monoxide (i.e., house fires) is unreliable since it cannot differentiate carboxyhemoglobin from oxyhemoglobin.*
- Monitor level of consciousness. *An early sign of an ineffective airway is change in the patient's behavior. If the patient becomes restless, anxious, combative, or unresponsive, the effectiveness of the airway needs to be immediately evaluated and appropriate interventions initiated.*

Risk for Infection

Traumatic injuries are considered dirty wounds. Projectiles enter the body through dirty surfaces and clothing, carrying dirt and debris into the wound. Open fractures provide a portal for the entry of bacteria and dirt. Even with surgical intervention, the wounds often remain contaminated.

- Use careful hand hygiene practices. *Hand hygiene remains the single most important factor in preventing the spread of infection.*
- Use strict standard precautions and aseptic technique when caring for wounds. *Standard precautions are essential to protect the patient and the nurse from infection.* In addition,
  - monitor wounds for odor, redness, heat, swelling, and copious or purulent drainage.
  - monitor hidden wounds, such as those under casts, by asking the patient whether the pain has increased and observing for increased drainage and heat over the area of the wound.
  - ensure that cross-contamination between wounds does not occur. Collect drainage in ostomy bags if it is copious. *The skin is the first line of defense against infection. Wounds provide a portal of entry for organisms. Risk factors for wound infection include contamination, inadequate wound care, and the condition of the wound at the time of closure. Aseptic techniques used in applying and changing dressings reduce the entry of organisms.*

- Take and record vital signs, including temperature, every 2 to 4 hours. *Vital signs, particularly an elevated body temperature, indicate the presence of an infection.*
- Provide adequate fluids and nutrition. *Adequate fluids, calories, and protein are essential to wound healing.*
- Assess for manifestations of gas gangrene: fever, pain, and swelling in traumatized tissues; drainage with a foul odor. *Gas gangrene is usually caused by the organism* Clostridium perfringens. *This bacterium is found in the soil and can be introduced into the body during a traumatic injury. The organism grows in the tissues, causing necrosis; hydrogen and carbon dioxide are released, with resultant swelling of tissues. If the infection continues, tissues are progressively destroyed, and sepsis and death may result.*
- Assess for development of potentially life-threatening conditions such as necrotizing fasciitis where flesh-eating bacteria infect subcutaneous and dermal layers, spreading to the fascial plane. Many types of bacteria can cause necrotizing fasciitis; however, the methicillin-resistant *Staphylococcus aureus* is occurring with increasing frequency.
- Assess the status of tetanus immunization and administer tetanus toxoid or human toxin-antitoxin (TAT) as prescribed. *Tetanus is caused by an exotoxin produced by* Clostridium tetani, *usually introduced through an open wound. The organism is commonly found in the soil.*
- Use strict aseptic technique when inserting catheters, suctioning, administering parenteral medications, or performing any other invasive procedure. *Using aseptic technique during invasive procedures reduces the risk of entry of organisms.*

Impaired Physical Mobility

The patient with trauma injuries is often unable to change positions independently and is at risk for complications of the integumentary, cardiovascular, gastrointestinal, respiratory, musculoskeletal, and renal systems. Patients at greatest risk are those who have had multiple injuries, spinal cord injuries, peripheral nerve injuries, and traumatic amputations. Collaborate with the physical therapist and occupational therapist (if available) to determine the most effective types and schedule of exercises and assistive devices.

- If active bleeding or edema is not present, provide active or passive exercises to affected and unaffected extremities at least once every 8 hours. *Exercise improves muscle tone, maintains joint mobility, improves circulation, and prevents contractures.*
- Help the patient turn, cough, and deep breathe and use the incentive spirometer at least every 2 hours. *Changing positions, coughing, deep breathing, and incentive spirometry reduce the risk of integumentary and respiratory complications.*
- If the patient is unable to be moved and positioned, consider a specialty bed, such as the kinetic continuous rotation bed (Figure 11–7 ■). *The kinetic continuous rotation bed allows continuous turning of the patient; the motion decreases pulmonary complications, venous stasis, postural hypotension, urinary stasis, muscle wasting, and bone demineralization.*
- Monitor the lower extremities each day for manifestations of deep vein thrombosis: heat, swelling, and pain. Measure and record the circumference of the thigh and calf each day. If antiemboli stockings or intermittent compression stockings

Figure 11–7 ■ A kinetic continuous rotation bed provides a means of turning the patient with multiple injuries to decrease the hazards of immobility.
Courtesy of Kinetic Concepts, Inc.

are used, remove them for 1 hour during each shift and assess the skin. *Venous stasis results when surrounding muscles are unable to contract and help move the blood through the veins. Thrombus (clot) formation in deep veins is a major risk for pulmonary embolism.*

Spiritual Distress

Trauma generally strikes without warning and carries potentially devastating consequences, including severe alterations in the lives of the victim and family, and death. The traumatic death of a loved one may be the most difficult event a family may ever experience. The decision to cease life support systems or to donate organs challenges the family's belief systems and psychologic stability. Nursing care of the family (or patient) experiencing spiritual distress includes the following:

- Offer referral to spiritual advisor if needed. *Most hospitals have chaplain programs.*
- Give the family information about the option to donate the patient's organs. *The decision to donate organs needs to be based on information about the patient's condition, prognosis, and criteria by which brain death is determined. It is important to convey to family members that organ donation is only an option and that they should not feel they are obligated to consent or are doing something wrong if they do not consent.*
- Encourage the family to ask questions and express any feelings about the traumatic event and/or organ donation. *Allowing families to express their feelings may help prevent long-term consequences such as guilt.*

CASE STUDY & NURSING CARE PLAN   A Patient with Multiple Injuries

Jane Souza is a 25-year-old married woman with two children who provides day care for preschool children in her home. As she is driving the interstate at 65 miles per hour, a car crosses the median and strikes her vehicle head-on. Mrs. Souza, who is not wearing a seat belt, is thrown forward against the steering wheel. The front of her car is pushed up against her by the car that struck her, entrapping her lower extremities.

After extensive efforts to extricate her from the car, Jane is transported to the local trauma center. She is still conscious, is receiving high-flow oxygen by mask, and has one intravenous line in place. Her vital signs are a palpable systolic blood pressure of 80, a pulse rate of 120, and a respiratory rate of 36. On arrival, she states that she is having difficulty breathing.

ASSESSMENT

- Airway: Maintainable with high-flow oxygen in place.
- Breathing: Respiratory rate of 36, multiple bruising and abrasions on right side of her chest, decreased breath sounds on the right side.
- Circulation: No palpable radial pulses; palpable brachial pulses. Monitor shows sinus tachycardia. No active external bleeding noted. Skin color pale, cool to the touch, and diaphoretic. One intravenous line already established.
- Neurologic: Moved her fingers when asked; complains of difficulty breathing; denies that she is hurt. Pupils 4 mm, equal, and react to light. Has a broken right arm and an open fracture of the left ankle; because of these injuries, extremity movement is limited.

Because of Mrs. Souza's respiratory distress, she is intubated and ventilated with 100% oxygen. Another intravenous line is inserted and O-negative blood administered. It is determined that Jane has sustained a pneumothorax in the right side and a chest tube is inserted.

DIAGNOSES

- *Ineffective Breathing Pattern* related to multiple bruises and abrasions on the right side of the chest, and respiratory difficulty

- *Deficient Fluid Volume* related to acute internal blood loss (presumed because no active bleeding can be found)
- *Risk for Injury* related to trauma resuscitation

EXPECTED OUTCOMES

- Maintain adequate oxygenation.
- Maintain adequate circulating blood volume.

PLANNING AND IMPLEMENTATION

- Monitor airway and assist in any needed airway management.
- Explain all procedures.
- Monitor the effects of fluid and blood administration, including any changes in blood pressure and pulse.
- Prepare for transfer to the operating room for emergency surgery.
- Keep family informed about her condition.

EVALUATION

Mrs. Souza is transferred to the operating room, where it is determined that she has a ruptured spleen and a serious pelvic fracture. Her treatment continues in the operating room.

CRITICAL THINKING IN THE NURSING PROCESS

1. Is the nursing diagnosis Deficient Fluid Volume appropriate for Jane Souza? Why or why not?
2. The assessment of a patient who has experienced trauma is, in order, A = airway, B = breathing, and C = circulation. What is the rationale for this sequence?
3. Following surgery, Mrs. Souza is moved to the surgical intensive care unit. She is very anxious and restless. What methods of assessments would help you identify the cause of her restlessness?
4. Infection is a common complication for the trauma patient. Describe five risks for infection that are present from the time of injury to the time of hospital discharge.

See Evaluating Your Response in Appendix C.

- Refer the family for follow-up care. Long-term follow-up is important for the family facing the sudden death of a loved one. *Grieving is not an overnight process, and providing the family with resources that may be used in the future may help prevent future crises and dysfunction.* (For more information, ∞ see Chapter 5.)

Post-traumatic Stress Disorder

Post-traumatic stress disorder is an intense, sustained emotional response to a disastrous event. It is also referred to as post-trauma syndrome. It is characterized by emotions that range from anger to fear and by flashbacks or psychic numbing. In the initial stage, the patient may be calm or may express feelings of anger, disbelief, terror, and shock. In the long-term phase, which begins anywhere from a few days to several months after the event, the patient often experiences flashbacks and nightmares of the traumatic event. The patient may call on ineffective coping mechanisms, such as alcohol or drugs, and withdraw from relationships.

- Assess emotional responses while providing physical care. Observe for crying, sleep problems, suspiciousness, and fear

during the initial phase of treatment. If the patient is unconscious, encourage family members and friends to express their feelings. *These assessments provide valuable information about the patient's ability to cope with the trauma.*

- Be available if the patient wishes to talk about the trauma, and encourage expression of feelings. *The patient may initially deny negative feelings; this denial is a coping mechanism in the initial phase of recovery.*
- Teach relaxation techniques, such as deep breathing, progressive muscle relaxation, or imagery (∞ see Chapter 4). *These techniques are often useful in coping when thoughts of the trauma recur.*
- Refer the patient and family members for counseling, psychotherapy, or support groups as appropriate. *Continued therapy may be necessary in assisting the patient and family to resolve the acute and long-term effects of trauma.*

Using NANDA, NIC, and NOC

Linkages between a selected NANDA nursing diagnosis, NIC, and NOC for the patient experiencing trauma are shown in the chart that follows.

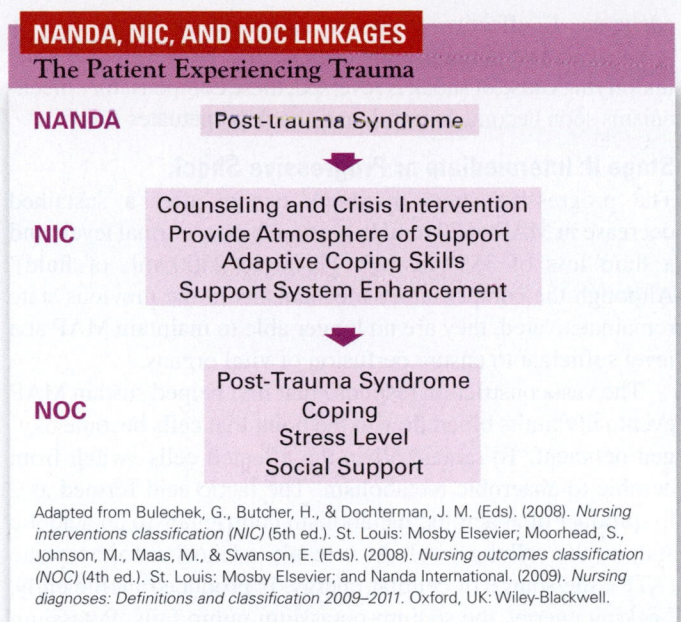

Adapted from Bulechek, G., Butcher, H., & Dochterman, J. M. (Eds). (2008). *Nursing interventions classification (NIC)* (5th ed.). St. Louis: Mosby Elsevier; Moorhead, S., Johnson, M., Maas, M., & Swanson, E. (Eds). (2008). *Nursing outcomes classification (NOC)* (4th ed.). St. Louis: Mosby Elsevier; and Nanda International. (2009). *Nursing diagnoses: Definitions and classification 2009–2011*. Oxford, UK: Wiley-Blackwell.

Community-based Care

Address the following topics to prepare the patient and family for home care:

- The type of home environment to which the patient will be returning, including any changes that will be required to let the patient function in that environment
- Medications, dressings, wound care, equipment, and supplies
- Special diet, if needed
- Rehabilitation plan and its effect on the patient's family
- Follow-up appointments with the physician or at the trauma clinic
- Emotional changes that the patient may undergo as a result of the trauma
- Helpful resources:
  - Home health care
  - Community support groups
  - National Institute of Neurological Disorders and Stroke

The Patient Experiencing Shock

Shock is a clinical syndrome characterized by a systemic imbalance between oxygen supply and demand. This imbalance results in a state of inadequate blood flow to body organs and tissues, causing life-threatening cellular dysfunction.

Overview of Cellular Homeostasis and Hemodynamics

To maintain cellular metabolism, cells of all body organs and tissues require a regular and consistent supply of oxygen and the removal of metabolic wastes. This homeostatic regulation is maintained primarily by the cardiovascular system and depends on four physiologic components.

1. A cardiac output sufficient to meet bodily requirements
2. An uncompromised vascular system, in which the vessels have a diameter sufficient to allow unimpeded blood flow and have good tone (the ability to constrict or dilate to maintain normal pressure)

3. A volume of blood sufficient to fill the circulatory system, and a blood pressure adequate to maintain blood flow
4. Tissues that are able to extract and use the oxygen delivered through the capillaries

In a healthy person, these components function as a system to maintain tissue perfusion.

During shock, however, one or more of these components are disrupted. An understanding of basic hemodynamics is necessary to understand the pathophysiology of shock.

- Stroke volume (SV) is the amount of blood pumped into the aorta with each contraction of the left ventricle.
- Cardiac output (CO) is the amount of blood pumped per minute into the aorta by the left ventricle. CO is determined by multiplying the SV by the heart rate (HR): $CO = SV \times HR$.
- Systemic vascular resistance (SVR) is the resistance offered by the peripheral circulation.

> **PRACTICE ALERT**
> Cardiac Output (CO) = Stroke Volume (SV) × Heart Rate (HR).

- Mean arterial pressure (MAP) is the product of cardiac output and SVR: $MAP = CO \times SVR$. It can also be calculated as MAP = [(2x diastolic BP) + systolic BP] / 3. When CO, SVR, or total blood volume rises, MAP and tissue perfusion increase. Conversely, when CO, SVR, or total blood volume falls, MAP and tissue perfusion decrease. A MAP of 70 to 110 is normal. A MAP of 60 mmHg is required to maintain adequate perfusion to the brain, heart, and kidneys.
- The sympathetic nervous system maintains the smooth muscle surrounding the arteries and arterioles in a state of partial contraction called sympathetic tone. Increased sympathetic stimulation increases vasoconstriction and SVR; decreased sympathetic stimulation allows vasodilatation, which decreases SVR.

Pathophysiology

When one or more cardiovascular components do not function properly, the body's hemodynamic properties are altered. Consequently, tissue perfusion may be inadequate to sustain normal cellular metabolism. The result is the clinical syndrome known as shock. The manifestations of shock result from the body's attempts to maintain vital organs (heart and brain) and to preserve life following a drop in cellular perfusion. However, if the injury or condition triggering shock is severe enough or of long enough duration, cellular hypoxia and cellular death occur.

Shock is triggered by a sustained drop in mean arterial pressure. This drop can occur after a decrease in cardiac output, a decrease in the circulating blood volume, or an increase in the size of the vascular bed due to peripheral vasodilatation. If intervention is timely and effective, the physiologic events that characterize shock may be stopped; if not, shock may lead to death.

Stage I: Early, Reversible, and Compensatory Shock

The initial stage of shock begins when baroreceptors in the aortic arch and the carotid sinus detect a sustained drop in MAP of less than 10 mmHg from normal levels. The circulating blood volume may decrease (usually to less then 500 mL), but not enough to cause serious effects.

The body reacts to the decrease in arterial pressure. The cerebral integration center initiates the body's response systems, causing the sympathetic nervous system to increase the heart rate and the force of cardiac contraction, thus increasing cardiac output. Sympathetic stimulation also causes peripheral vasoconstriction, resulting in increased systemic vascular resistance and a rise in arterial pressure. The net result is that the perfusion of cells, tissues, and organs is maintained. Symptoms are almost imperceptible during the early stage of shock. The pulse rate may be slightly elevated. If the injury is minor or of short duration, arterial pressure is usually maintained, and no further symptoms occur.

Compensatory shock begins after the MAP falls 10 to 15 mmHg below normal levels. The circulating blood volume is reduced by 25% to 35% (1000 mL or more), but compensatory mechanisms are able to maintain blood pressure and tissue perfusion to vital organs, thereby preventing cell damage.

■ Stimulation of the sympathetic nervous system results in the release of epinephrine from the adrenal medulla and the release of norepinephrine from the adrenal medulla and the sympathetic fibers. Both hormones rapidly stimulate the alpha- and beta-adrenergic fibers. Stimulated alpha-adrenergic fibers cause vasoconstriction in the blood vessels supplying the skin and most of the abdominal viscera. Perfusion of these areas decreases. Stimulated beta-adrenergic fibers cause vasodilatation in vessels supplying the heart and skeletal muscles (beta one response), and increase the heart rate and force of cardiac contraction (beta two response). Further, blood vessels in the respiratory system dilate, and the respiratory rate increases (beta two response). Thus, stimulation of the sympathetic nervous system results in increased cardiac output and oxygenation of these tissues.

■ The renin-angiotensin response occurs as the blood flow to the kidneys decreases. Renin released from the kidneys acts on angiotensinogen to form angiotensin I. This is converted by angiotensin converting enzyme in the lungs to angiotensin II, which causes vasoconstriction and stimulates the adrenal cortex to release aldosterone. Aldosterone causes the kidneys to reabsorb water and sodium and to lose potassium. The absorption of water maintains circulating blood volume while increased vasoconstriction increases SVR, maintaining central vascular volume and raising blood pressure.

■ The hypothalamus releases adrenocorticotropic hormone (ACTH), causing the adrenal glands to secrete aldosterone. Aldosterone promotes the reabsorption of water and sodium by the kidneys, preserving blood volume and pressure.

■ The posterior pituitary gland releases antidiuretic hormone (ADH), which increases renal reabsorption of water to increase intravascular volume. The combined effects of hormones released by the hypothalamus and posterior pituitary glands work to conserve central vascular volume.

■ As MAP falls in the compensatory stage of shock, decreased capillary hydrostatic pressure causes a fluid shift from the interstitial space into the capillaries. The net gain of fluid raises the blood volume.

Working together, these compensatory mechanisms can maintain MAP for only a short period of time. During this period, the perfusion and oxygenation of the heart and brain are adequate. If effective treatment is provided, the process is arrested, and no permanent damage occurs. However, unless the underlying cause of shock is reversed, these compensatory mechanisms soon become harmful, and shock perpetuates shock.

Stage II: Intermediate or Progressive Shock
The progressive stage of shock occurs after a sustained decrease in MAP of 20 mmHg or more below normal levels and a fluid loss of 35% to 50% (1800 to 2500 mL of fluid). Although the compensatory mechanisms in the previous state remain activated, they are no longer able to maintain MAP at a level sufficient to ensure perfusion of vital organs.

The vasoconstriction response that first helped sustain MAP eventually limits blood flow to the point that cells become oxygen deficient. To remain alive, the affected cells switch from aerobic to anaerobic metabolism. The lactic acid formed as a by-product of anaerobic metabolism contributes to an acidotic state at the cellular level. As a result, adenosine triphosphate (ATP), the source of cellular energy, is produced inefficiently. Lacking energy, the sodium-potassium pump fails. Potassium moves out of the cell, while sodium and water move inward. As this process continues, the cell swells, cell membrane integrity is lost, and cell organelles are damaged. Lysosomes within the cell spill out their digestive enzymes, which disintegrate any remaining organelles. Some enzymes spread to adjacent cells, where they erode and rupture cell membranes.

The acid by-products of anaerobic metabolism dilate the precapillary arterioles and constrict the postcapillary venules. This causes increased hydrostatic pressure within the capillary, and fluid shifts back into the interstitial space. The capillaries also become increasingly permeable, allowing serum proteins to shift from the vascular space into the interstitium. The buildup of plasma proteins increases the osmotic pressure in the interstitium, further accelerating the fluid shift out of the capillaries.

Throughout this period, the heart rate and vasoconstriction increase; however, perfusion of the skin, skeletal muscles, kidneys, and gastrointestinal organs is greatly diminished. Cells in the heart and brain become hypoxic while other body cells and tissues become ischemic and anoxic. A generalized state of acidosis and hyperkalemia ensues (∞ see Chapter 10). Unless this stage of shock is treated rapidly, the patient's chances of survival are poor.

Stage III: Refractory or Irreversible Shock
If shock progresses to the irreversible stage, tissue anoxia becomes so generalized and cellular death so widespread that no treatment can reverse the damage. Even if MAP is temporarily restored, too much cellular damage has occurred to maintain life. Death of cells is followed by death of tissues, which results in death of organs. Death of vital organs contributes to subsequent death of the body.

Effects of Shock on Body Systems
Whatever its causes, shock produces predictable effects on the body's organ systems. (See the Multisystem Effects of Shock feature on page 255.)

CARDIOVASCULAR SYSTEM The perfusion and oxygenation of the heart are adequate in the early stages of shock. As shock progresses, myocardial cells become hypoxic, and myocardial

MULTISYSTEM EFFECTS OF
Shock

Respiratory
- ↑ respiratory rate
- Respiratory acidosis

Potential Complication
- ARDS

Urinary
- ↓ renal perfusion
- ↓GFR

Late
- Oliguria

Potential Complications
- Acute tubular necrosis
- Kidney failure

Hepatic
Early
- ↑ glucose production

Progressive
- ↓glucose production= hypoglycemia
- ↓lactic acid conversion= metabolic acidosis

Potential Complication
- Destroyed Kupffer cells= systemic bacterial infections

Gastrointestinal
Early
- ↓GI motility

Late
- Paralytic ileus
- Ulceration of GI mucosa

Potential Complication
- Bowel necrosis

Neurologic
- ↓cognition
- ↓sympathetic activity
- ↓consciousness

Early
- Restlessness, apathy

Progressive
- Lethargy

Late
- Coma

Cardiovascular
Early
- No change

Progressive
- Slightly ↑BP
- Slowly ↑HR
- Sinus tachycardia
- Thready pulse

Late
- MAP <60 mmHg
- Steadily ↓BP
- Steadily ↓CO
- Imperceptible pulses

Integumentary
- Pallor (skin, lips, oral mucosa, nail beds, conjunctiva)
- Cool, moist skin

Late
- Edema

Metabolic Processes
- ↓temperature
- Thirst
- Acidosis (metabolic and respiratory)

muscle function diminishes. Initially, the blood pressure may be normal or even slightly elevated (as a result of compensatory mechanisms) and the heart rate only slightly increased. Sympathetic stimulation increases the heart rate (a sinus tachycardia of 120 beats per minute is common) in an effort to increase cardiac output. As a result of vasoconstriction and decreased blood volume, the palpated pulse is rapid, weak, and thready; as shock progresses, peripheral pulses are usually nonpalpable.

Tachycardia reduces the time available for left ventricular filling and coronary artery perfusion, further reducing cardiac output. With progressive shock, altered acid–base balance, hypoxia, and hyperkalemia damage the heart's electrical systems and contractility. Consequently, cardiac dysrhythmias may develop. Decreased blood volume with decreased venous return also decreases cardiac output, and blood pressure falls.

The blood pressure changes produced by shock are characterized by a progressive decrease in both systolic and diastolic pressures and a narrowing pulse pressure. Auscultation of blood pressure is often difficult or impossible and is an inaccurate reflection of blood pressure status. For this reason, hemodynamic monitoring is usually instituted to follow the patient's cardiovascular status accurately.

RESPIRATORY SYSTEM   During shock, impaired oxygen delivery to cells may occur due to a drop in circulating blood volume or, in the case of blood loss, by an insufficient number of red blood cells that carry oxygen. Although the respiratory rate increases because of compensatory mechanisms that promote oxygenation, the number of alveoli that are perfused decreases, and gas exchange is impaired. As a result, oxygen levels in the blood decrease, and carbon dioxide levels increase. As perfusion of the lungs diminishes, carbon dioxide is retained, and respiratory acidosis occurs.

A complication of decreased perfusion of the lungs is acute respiratory distress syndrome (ARDS), or "shock lung." ARDS is discussed in detail in ∞ Chapter 37. The exact mechanism that produces ARDS is unknown, but some contributing factors have been identified. This potentially lethal form of respiratory failure may result from any condition that causes hypoperfusion of the lungs, but it is more common in shock caused by hemorrhage, severe allergic responses, trauma, and infection.

GASTROINTESTINAL AND HEPATIC SYSTEMS   The gastrointestinal organs normally receive 25% of the cardiac output through the splanchnic circulation. Shock constricts the splanchnic arterioles and redirects arterial blood flow to the heart and brain. Consequently, gastrointestinal organs become ischemic and may be irreversibly damaged.

Gastric mucosa tends to ulcerate when it becomes ischemic. Lesions of the gastric and duodenal mucosa (called *stress ulcers*) can develop within hours of severe trauma, sepsis, or burns (Huether & McCance, 2008). Gastrointestinal ulcers may hemorrhage within 2 to 10 days following the original cause of shock. In addition, the permeability of damaged mucosa increases, allowing bacterial translocation to occur. During this process, enteric bacteria or their toxins enter the abdominal cavity, progress to the circulation, and can eventually result in sepsis.

Gastric and intestinal motility is impaired during shock, and paralytic ileus may result. If the episode of shock is prolonged, necrosis of the bowel may occur. In many cases, alterations in the structure and function of the gastrointestinal tract impair absorption of nutrients, such as protein and glucose.

Shock also alters the metabolic functions of the liver. Initially, *gluconeogenesis* (the process of forming glucose from noncarbohydrate sources) and *glycogenolysis* (the breakdown of glycogen into glucose) increase. This process allows blood glucose levels to increase as the body attempts to respond to the stressor; however, as shock progresses, liver functions are impaired, and hypoglycemia develops. Metabolism of fats and protein is impaired, and the liver can no longer effectively remove lactic acid, contributing to the development of metabolic acidosis.

The destruction of the liver's reticuloendothelial Kupffer cells (phagocytes that destroy bacteria) causes a further problem. Bacteria may proliferate within the circulatory system, causing overwhelming bacterial infection and toxicity.

NEUROLOGIC SYSTEM   The primary effects of shock on the neurologic system involve changes in mental status and orientation. Cerebral hypoxia produces altered levels of consciousness, beginning with apathy and lethargy and progressing to coma. A common early symptom of cerebral hypoxia is restlessness. Continued ischemia of brain cells eventually causes swelling, resulting in cerebral edema, neurotransmitter failure, and irreversible brain cell damage.

As cerebral ischemia worsens, the sympathetic activity and vasomotor centers are depressed. This leads to a loss of sympathetic tone, causing systemic vasodilatation and pooling of blood in the periphery. As a result, venous return and cardiac output further decrease.

PRACTICE ALERT

An early sign of shock is a change in the level of consciousness. Late signs of shock are mental status changes, hypotension, and marked tachycardia.

RENAL SYSTEM   Blood that normally perfuses the kidneys is shunted to the heart and brain during the progressive stage of shock, resulting in renal hypoperfusion. The drop in renal perfusion is reflected in a corresponding decrease in the glomerular filtration rate. Urine output is reduced, and the urine that is produced is highly concentrated. Oliguria of less than 20 mL per hour indicates progressive shock.

Healthy kidneys can tolerate a drop in perfusion for only about 20 minutes; thereafter, acute tubular necrosis develops (Huether & McCance, 2008). As tubular necrosis occurs, epithelial cells slough off and block the tubules, disrupting nephron function. The accumulating loss of functional nephrons eventually causes renal failure. Without normal renal function, metabolic waste products are retained in the plasma.

If treatment restores renal perfusion, the kidneys can regenerate the lost epithelial cells in the tubules, and renal function usually returns to normal. However, in the older or chronically ill patient or in the patient with sustained shock, loss of renal function may become permanent.

EFFECTS ON SKIN, TEMPERATURE, AND THIRST In most types of shock, blood vessels supplying the skin are vasoconstricted, and the sweat glands are activated. As a result, changes in skin color occur. The skin of Caucasian patients becomes pale. In people with darker skin (such as those of African, Hispanic, or Mediterranean descent), shock-related skin color changes may be assessed as paleness of the lips, oral mucous membranes, nail beds, and conjunctiva. The skin is usually cool and moist and, in the later stages of shock, often edematous.

The body temperature decreases as shock progresses, the result of a decrease in overall body metabolism. Some people in shock become thirsty, probably a response to decreased blood volume and increased serum osmolality (Huether & McCance, 2008).

Types of Shock

Shock is identified according to its underlying cause. All types of shock progress through the same stages and exert similar effects on body systems. Any differences are noted in the following discussion.

Hypovolemic Shock

Hypovolemic shock is caused by a decrease in intravascular volume of 15% or more (Huether & McCance, 2008). In hypovolemic shock, the venous blood returning to the heart decreases, and ventricular filling drops. As a result, stroke volume, cardiac output, and blood pressure decrease. Hypovolemic shock is the most common type of shock, and it often occurs simultaneously with other types.

The decrease in circulating blood volume that triggers hypovolemic shock may result from the following:

- Loss of blood volume from hemorrhage (from surgery, trauma, gastrointestinal bleeding, blood coagulation disorders, ruptured esophageal varices)
- Loss of intravascular fluid from the skin due to injuries such as burns (∞ see Chapter 17)
- Loss of intravascular volume from severe dehydration
- Loss of body fluid from the gastrointestinal system due to persistent and severe vomiting or diarrhea, or continuous nasogastric suctioning
- Renal losses of fluid due to the use of diuretics or to endocrine disorders such as diabetes insipidus
- Conditions causing fluid shifts from the intravascular compartment to the interstitial space
- Third spacing due to such disorders as liver diseases with ascites, pleural effusion, or intestinal obstruction

Hypovolemic shock affects all body systems. Its effects vary depending on the patient's age, general state of health, extent of injury or severity of illness, length of time before treatment is provided, and the rate of volume loss.

The manifestations of hypovolemic shock result directly from the decrease in circulating blood volume and the initiation of compensatory mechanisms (Figure 11–8 ■). The loss of circulating blood volume reduces cardiac output by decreasing venous return to the heart. As a result, blood pressure drops. The carotid and cardiac baroreceptors sense the decrease in blood pressure and communicate it to the vasomotor centers in the brainstem. The vasomotor centers then induce the sympathetic

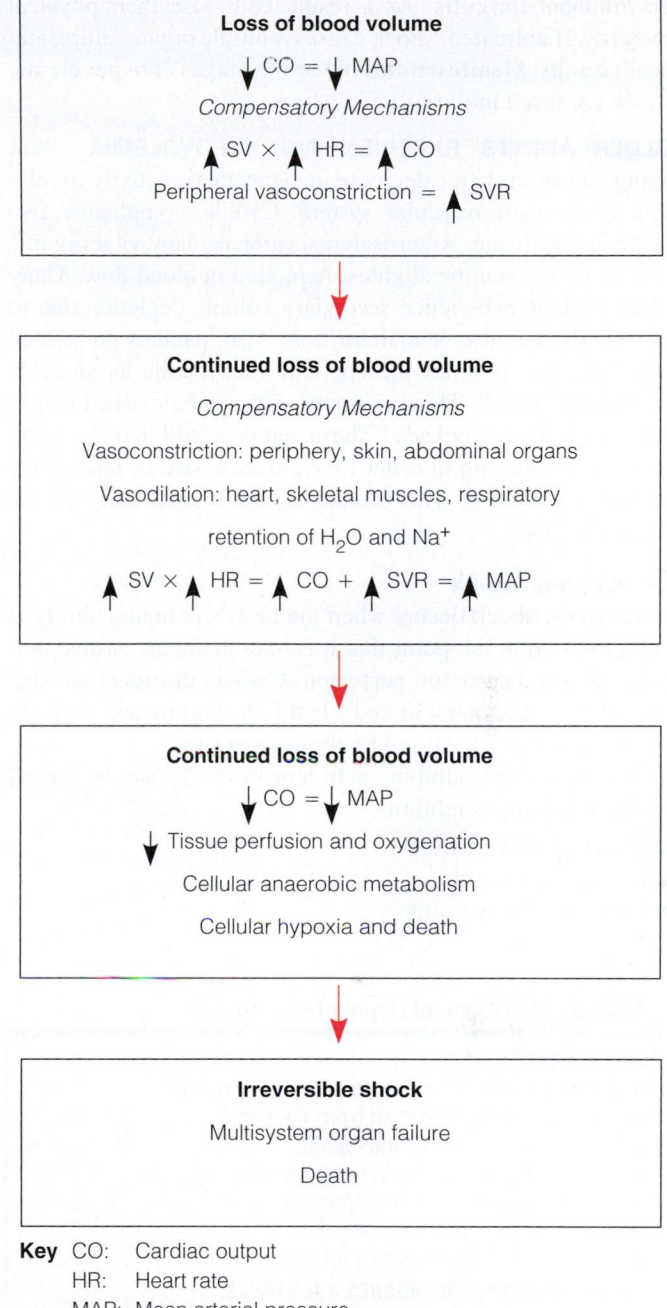

Key
CO:	Cardiac output
HR:	Heart rate
MAP:	Mean arterial pressure
SV:	Stroke volume
SVR:	Systemic vascular resistance

Figure 11–8 ■ The stages of hypovolemic shock.

compensatory responses. If the fluid loss is less than 500 mL, activation of the sympathetic response is generally adequate to restore cardiac output and blood pressure to near normal, although the heart rate may remain elevated.

With a sustained loss of blood volume (1000 mL or more), the shock stage progresses. Heart rate and vasoconstriction increase, and blood flow to the skin, skeletal muscles, kidneys, and abdominal organs decreases. Several renal mechanisms and a decline in capillary pressure help conserve blood volume. Eventually, the amount of blood flowing to cells is too low to oxygenate them and sustain production of cellular energy. Anaerobic metabolism begins, producing an acidotic environment for cells. As a result, cells lose their physical integrity. If untreated, shock causes multiple organ failure, and death results. Manifestations of various stages of hypovolemic shock are listed in the following box.

OLDER ADULTS EXPERIENCING HYPOVOLEMIA With aging comes a relative decrease in sympathetic activity in relation to the cardiovascular system. Cardiac compliance also decreases with age. Atherosclerosis affects many vital organs' sensitivity to even the slightest reduction in blood flow. Many older patients experience secondary volume depletion due to chronic diuretic use or malnutrition. Also, patients prescribed beta blockers may not present with tachycardia as an early indicator of shock. This important sign can be masked due to beta adrenergic blockade. These patients will require early invasive monitoring in order to avoid excessive or inadequate volume restoration. This should be considered early in the treatment phase.

Cardiogenic Shock

Cardiogenic shock occurs when the heart's pumping ability is compromised to the point that it cannot maintain cardiac output and adequate tissue perfusion. Cardiac disorders are discussed in ∞ Chapters 30 and 31; this section focuses only on the effects of shock caused by these disorders.

The loss of the pumping action of the heart may be caused by the following conditions:

- Myocardial infarction
- Cardiac tamponade
- Restrictive pericarditis

- Cardiac arrest
- Dysrhythmias, such as fibrillation or ventricular tachycardia
- Pathologic changes in the valves
- Cardiomyopathies from hypertension, alcohol, bacterial or viral infections, or ischemia
- Complications of cardiac surgery
- Electrolyte imbalances (especially changes in normal potassium and calcium levels)
- Drugs affecting cardiac muscle contractility
- Head injuries causing damage to the cardioregulatory center

Myocardial infarction is the most common cause of cardiogenic shock. Patients admitted to the hospital for treatment of myocardial infarction or cardiac surgery are at risk for cardiogenic shock. The severity and progression of shock are related to the amount of myocardial damage.

Whatever the cardiogenic cause, the decrease in cardiac output causes a decrease in MAP. Heart rate may increase in response to compensatory mechanisms. However, tachycardia increases myocardial oxygen consumption and decreases coronary perfusion. The myocardium becomes progressively depleted of oxygen, causing further myocardial ischemia and necrosis. The typical sequence of shock is essentially unchanged in cardiogenic shock.

Cyanosis, however, is more common in cardiogenic shock because stagnating blood increases extraction of oxygen from the hemoglobin at the capillary beds. As a result, the skin, lips, and nail beds may appear cyanotic. As cardiac failure (and cardiogenic shock) progresses, left ventricular end-diastolic pressure increases. The increase is transmitted to the pulmonary capillary bed, and pulmonary edema may occur. Retention of blood in the right side of the heart increases right atrial pressure, which leads to jugular venous distention as a result of backflow through the vena cava. Manifestations of cardiogenic shock are listed in the following box.

Obstructive Shock

Obstructive shock is caused by an obstruction in the heart or great vessels that either impedes venous return or prevents effective cardiac pumping action. The causes of obstructive shock are impaired diastolic filling (e.g., pericardial tamponade or pneumothorax), increased right ventricular afterload (e.g., pulmonary emboli), and increased left ventricular afterload (e.g., aortic stenosis, abdominal distention). The manifestations are the result of decreased cardiac output and blood pressure, with reduced tissue perfusion and cellular metabolism.

MANIFESTATIONS of Hypovolemic Shock

INITIAL STAGE
- Blood pressure: normal to slightly decreased
- Pulse: slightly increased from baseline
- Respirations: normal (baseline)
- Skin: cool, pale (in periphery), moist
- Mental status: alert and oriented
- Urine output: slight decrease
- Other: thirst, decreased capillary refill time

COMPENSATORY AND PROGRESSIVE STAGES
- Blood pressure: hypotension
- Pulse: rapid, thready
- Respirations: increased
- Skin: cool, pale (includes trunk); poor turgor with fluid loss, edematous with fluid shift
- Mental status: restless, anxious, confused, agitated
- Urine output: oliguria (less than 30 mL/hour)
- Other: marked thirst, acidosis, hyperkalemia, decreased capillary refill time, decreased or absent peripheral pulses

IRREVERSIBLE STAGE
- Blood pressure: severe hypotension (often, systolic pressure is below 80 mmHg)
- Pulse: very rapid, weak
- Respirations: rapid, shallow; crackles and wheezes
- Skin: cool, pale, mottled with cyanosis
- Mental status: disoriented, lethargic, comatose
- Urine output: anuria
- Other: loss of reflexes, decreased or absent peripheral pulses

MANIFESTATIONS of Cardiogenic Shock

- Blood pressure: hypotension, possible narrowing pulse pressures
- Pulse: rapid, thready; distention of veins of hands and neck
- Respirations: increased, labored; crackles and wheezes; pulmonary edema
- Skin: pale, cyanotic, cold, moist
- Mental status: restless, anxious, lethargic progressing to comatose
- Urine output: oliguria to anuria
- Other: dependent edema; elevated CVP; elevated pulmonary capillary wedge pressure; arrhythmias

Distributive Shock

Distributive shock (also called vasogenic shock) includes several types of shock that result from widespread vasodilatation and decreased peripheral resistance. As the blood volume does not change, relative hypovolemia results. Examples of distributive shock include septic, neurogenic, and anaphylactic shock. Treatment is based on the underlying pathogenesis.

Septic Shock

Septic shock, the leading cause of death for patients in intensive care units, is one part of a progressive syndrome called systemic inflammatory response syndrome (SIRS). This condition is most often the result of gram-negative bacterial infections (i.e., *Pseudomonas*, *E. coli*, *Klebsiella*), but may also follow gram-positive infections from *Staphylococcus* and *Streptococcus* bacteria. Gram-negative sepsis has greatly increased in the past 10 years, with a 60% mortality rate despite treatment. The pathophysiology of septic shock is complex and not completely understood.

Patients at risk for developing infections leading to septic shock include those who are hospitalized, have debilitating chronic illnesses, or have poor nutritional status. The risk is heightened after invasive procedures or surgery. Other patients at risk of septic shock include older adults and those who are immunocompromised. Portals of entry for infection that may lead to septic shock are as follows:

- Urinary system: catheterizations, suprapubic tubes, cystoscopy
- Respiratory system: suctioning, aspiration, tracheostomy, endotracheal tubes, respiratory therapy, mechanical ventilators
- Gastrointestinal system: peptic ulcers, ruptured appendix, peritonitis
- Integumentary system: surgical wounds, intravenous catheters, intra-arterial catheters, invasive monitoring, decubitus ulcers, burns, trauma
- Female reproductive system: elective surgical abortion, ascending infections from transmission of bacteria during the intrapartal and postpartal periods, tampon use, sexually transmitted diseases

Septic shock begins with *septicemia* (the presence of pathogens and their toxins in the blood). As pathogens are destroyed, their ruptured cell membranes allow endotoxins to leak into the plasma. The endotoxins disrupt the vascular system, coagulation mechanism, and immune system and trigger an immune and inflammatory response (∞ see Chapter 13 for more information). For this reason, the initial effects of septic shock differ from those of hypovolemic and cardiogenic shock; cardiac output is high and systemic vascular resistance is low.

Endotoxins directly damage the endothelial lining of small blood vessels first; the small blood vessels of the kidneys and lungs are most susceptible. Cellular damage stimulates the release of vasoactive proteins and activates coagulation factor XII. The vasoactive proteins stimulate peripheral vasodilatation and increase capillary permeability; the activation of coagulation factors results in the production of multiple intravascular blood clots.

As a result of the increased capillary permeability and vasodilatation, fluid shifts from the intravascular space to the interstitial space. Hypovolemia results as fluid volume is lost from the circulating blood. Hypovolemia and intravascular coagulation alter oxygenation and cellular metabolism, leading to anaerobic metabolism, lactic acidosis, and cellular death.

Septic shock has an early phase and a late phase. In early septic shock (sometimes called the *warm* phase), vasodilatation results in weakness and warm, flushed skin, and the septicemia often causes high fever and chills. In late septic shock (sometimes called the *cold* phase), hypovolemia and activity of the compensatory mechanisms result in typical shock manifestations, including cold, moist skin; oliguria; and changes in mental status. Death may result from respiratory failure, cardiac failure, or renal failure. Manifestations of septic shock are listed in the following box.

Toxic shock syndrome is an especially virulent form of septic shock, occurring most frequently in menstruating women who use tampons. It is thought that bacterial toxins diffuse from the site of infection in the vagina into the circulation. The toxins then trigger a widespread inflammatory response and septic shock. The manifestations of toxic shock syndrome include extreme hypotension, hyperpyrexia, headache, myalgia, confusion, skin rash, vomiting, and diarrhea (Huether & McCance, 2008).

Disseminated intravascular coagulation (DIC), a generalized response to injury, is a potential risk in septic shock. This condition is characterized by simultaneous bleeding and clotting throughout the vasculature. Sepsis injures blood cells, causing platelet aggregation and decreased blood flow. As a result, blood clots form throughout the microcirculation. The clotting slows circulation further while stimulating excess fibrinolysis. As the body's stores of clotting factors are depleted, generalized bleeding begins. DIC is further discussed in ∞ Chapter 33.

Neurogenic Shock

Neurogenic shock is the result of an imbalance between parasympathetic and sympathetic stimulation of vascular smooth muscle. If parasympathetic overstimulation or sympathetic understimulation persists, sustained vasodilatation occurs, and blood pools in the venous and capillary beds.

MANIFESTATIONS of Septic Shock

EARLY (WARM) SEPTIC SHOCK
- Blood pressure: normal to hypotension
- Pulse: increased, thready
- Respirations: rapid and deep
- Skin: warm, flushed
- Mental status: alert, oriented, anxious
- Urine output: normal
- Other: increased body temperature; chills; weakness; nausea, vomiting, diarrhea; decreased CVP

LATE (COLD) SEPTIC SHOCK
- Blood pressure: hypotension
- Pulse: tachycardia, arrhythmias
- Respirations: rapid, shallow, dyspneic
- Skin: cool, pale, edematous
- Mental status: lethargic to comatose
- Urine output: oliguria to anuria
- Other: normal to decreased body temperature; decreased CVP

Neurogenic shock causes dramatic reduction in systemic vascular resistance as the size of the vascular compartment increases. As systemic vascular resistance decreases, pressure in the blood vessels becomes too low to drive nutrients across capillary membranes, and cellular metabolism is impaired.

The following conditions can cause neurogenic shock by increasing parasympathetic stimulation or inhibiting sympathetic stimulation of the smooth muscle of blood vessels:

- Head injury
- Trauma to the spinal cord (spinal shock, a form of neurogenic shock, is described in ∞ Chapter 43)
- Insulin reactions (which cause hypoglycemia, decreasing glucose to the medulla)
- Central nervous system depressant drugs (such as sedatives, barbiturates, or narcotics)
- Anesthesia (spinal and general)
- Severe pain
- Prolonged exposure to heat

Bradycardia occurs early, but tachycardia begins as compensatory mechanisms are initiated. Central venous pressure drops as veins dilate, venous return to the heart decreases, stroke volume decreases, and MAP falls. In early stages, the extremities are warm and pink (from the pooling of blood), but as shock progresses, the skin becomes pale and cool. Manifestations of neurogenic shock are listed in the following box.

Anaphylactic Shock

Anaphylactic shock is the result of a widespread humorally mediated hypersensitivity reaction (called *anaphylaxis*). The pathophysiology in this type of shock includes vasodilatation, pooling of blood in the periphery, and hypovolemia with altered cellular metabolism. These physiologic alterations occur when a sensitized person has contact with an *allergen* (a foreign substance to which an individual is hypersensitive). Many different allergens can cause anaphylactic shock, including medications, blood administration, latex, foods, snake venom, and insect stings.

Anaphylactic shock does not occur with the first exposure to an allergen. With the first exposure to a foreign substance (the *antigen*), the body produces specific immunoglobulin E (IgE) antibodies against this antigen. The person is thus sensitized to that specific antigen. With subsequent exposure, the antigen reacts with the already formed IgE antibodies, disrupting cellular integrity. In addition, large amounts of histamine and other vasoactive amines are released and distributed through the circulatory system. These substances cause increased capillary permeability and massive vasodilatation, resulting in profound hypotension and eventual vascular collapse.

MANIFESTATIONS of Neurogenic Shock

- Blood pressure: hypotension
- Pulse: slow and bounding
- Respirations: vary
- Skin: warm, dry
- Mental status: anxious, restless, lethargic progressing to comatose
- Urine output: oliguria to anuria
- Other: lowered body temperature

MANIFESTATIONS of Anaphylactic Shock

- Blood pressure: hypotension
- Pulse: increased, dysrhythmias
- Respirations: dyspnea, stridor, wheezes, laryngospasm, bronchospasm, pulmonary edema
- Skin: warm, edematous (lips, eyelids, tongue, hands, feet, genitals)
- Mental status: restless, anxious, lethargic to comatose
- Urine output: oliguria to anuria
- Other: paresthesias; urticaria; pruritus; abdominal cramps, vomiting, diarrhea

---

Histamine also causes constriction of smooth muscles in the bladder, uterus, intestines, and bronchioles. Respiratory distress, bronchospasm, laryngospasm, and severe abdominal cramping result. Serotonin (a neurotransmitter with vasoconstrictive properties) is released, further affecting respiratory status by increasing capillary permeability in the lungs. As a result, plasma leaks into the alveoli, gas exchange is impaired, and pulmonary edema may occur.

Anaphylactic shock begins and progresses rapidly. Manifestations may begin within 20 minutes of contact with an antigen. Unless appropriate intervention is provided, death can occur within a matter of minutes. Because anaphylaxis is rapid and potentially lethal, people with known allergies should carry some form of warning (such as a MedicAlert bracelet) informing others of their susceptibility. Some patients carry an *Epi-pen* (epinephrine) to halt anaphylaxis. Healthcare providers should be extremely careful to assess and document allergies or previous drug reactions. Manifestations of anaphylactic shock are listed in the following box. Similar, but not related, are anaphylactoid reactions that are not humorally mediated and do not require prior exposure to a trigger. These can have similar symptoms and are treated in a similar manner.

Interdisciplinary Care

Medical care for the patient in shock focuses on treating the underlying cause, increasing arterial oxygenation, and improving tissue perfusion. Depending on the cause and type of shock, interventions include emergency care measures, oxygen therapy, fluid replacement, and medications. Emergency care is often the first course of collaborative action taken to arrest shock, as discussed earlier in this chapter. A *central venous catheter* may be used to aid in the differential diagnosis of shock and to provide information about the preload of the heart. A pulmonary artery catheter may be inserted to monitor cardiac dynamics, fluid balance, and the effects of vasoactive medications.

Diagnosis

The following diagnostic tests can help identify the type of shock and assess the patient's physical status. Measurements include the following:

- *Blood hemoglobin* and *hematocrit*, to detect the concentration that usually occurs in hypovolemic shock. These changes reflect the underlying etiology. In hypovolemic shock resulting from hemorrhage, the hemoglobin and hematocrit concentrations are lower than normal; in hypovolemic shock resulting from intravascular fluid loss, by contrast, the hemoglobin and hematocrit concentrations are higher than normal.

- *Arterial blood gases (ABGs)*, to determine oxygen and carbon dioxide levels and pH. The effects of shock and of the body's compensatory mechanisms cause a decrease in pH (indicating acidosis), a decrease in the partial pressure of oxygen (PaO_2) and in total oxygen saturation, and an increase in the partial pressure of carbon dioxide ($PaCO_2$).
- *Serum electrolytes*, to monitor the severity and progression of shock. As shock progresses, glucose levels decrease, sodium levels decrease, and potassium levels increase.
- *Blood urea nitrogen (BUN), serum creatinine levels, urine specific gravity*, and *osmolality*, to check renal function. As perfusion of the kidneys is decreased and renal function is reduced, the BUN and creatinine levels increase as does urine specific gravity and osmolality.
- *Blood cultures*, to identify the causative organism in septic shock.
- *White blood cell count* and *differential*, in the patient with septic or anaphylactic shock. The total WBC count is increased in septic shock. Elevated neutrophils indicate acute infection, increased monocytes indicate a bacterial infection, and increased eosinophils indicate an allergic response.
- *Serum cardiac enzymes*, which are elevated in cardiogenic shock: creatine kinase (CK), myoglobin, and c-reactive protein. Troponin can be elevated if the cause of cardiogenic shock is acute MI.

Other diagnostic tests may be ordered to determine the extent of injury or damage or to locate the site of internal hemorrhage. These tests might include x-ray studies, computerized tomography (CT) scans, magnetic resonance imaging (MRI), endoscopic examinations, and echocardiograms. Newer diagnostic methods for hypoperfusion include gastric tonometry and sublingual PCO_2. Gastric tonometry measures the partial pressure of carbon dioxide in the gastric lumen. The measurement of sublingual carbon dioxide correlates well with decreased MAP (Sole, Lamborn, & Hartshorn, 2001).

Medications

When fluid replacement alone is not sufficient to reverse shock, vasoactive drugs (drugs causing vasoconstriction or vasodilatation) and inotropic drugs (drugs improving cardiac contractility) may be administered. When used to treat shock, these drugs increase venous return through vasoconstriction of peripheral vessels; they also improve the pumping ability of the heart by facilitating myocardial contractility and by dilating coronary arteries to increase perfusion of the myocardium.

Drugs used to treat shock are discussed in the Medication Administration box on page 262. Other drugs that may be administered to the patient in shock include the following:

- Diuretics to increase urine output after fluid replacement has been initiated
- Sodium bicarbonate to treat acidosis
- Calcium to replace calcium lost as a result of blood transfusions
- Antiarrhythmic agents to stabilize heart rhythm
- Broad spectrum antibiotics to suppress organisms responsible for septic shock

- Epinephrine, antihistamines, and inhaled beta-2 agonists to treat anaphylactic shock
- Morphine to dilate veins and decrease anxiety

Oxygen Therapy

Establishing and maintaining a patent airway and ensuring adequate oxygenation are critical interventions in reversing shock. All patients in shock (even those with adequate respirations) should receive oxygen therapy (usually by mask or nasal cannula) to maintain the PaO_2 at greater than 80 mmHg during the first 4 to 6 hours of care. If the patient's unassisted respiration cannot maintain PaO_2 at this level, ventilatory assistance may be necessary. Care of the patient requiring ventilatory assistance is discussed in ∞ Chapter 37.

Fluid Resuscitation

The most effective treatment for the patient in hypovolemic shock is the administration of intravenous fluids or blood. Fluids also treat septic and, more judiciously, neurogenic shock. However, the patient with cardiogenic shock may require either fluid replacement or restriction, depending on pulmonary artery pressure.

Various fluids may be administered alone or in combination as part of fluid replacement therapy in treating shock. Fluid replacements are administered in massive amounts through two large-bore peripheral lines or through a central line. Current fluid resuscitation protocols include rapid crystalloid infusion followed by blood transfusion. Fluid replacements, such as crystalloid and colloid solutions, increase circulating blood volume and tissue perfusion. Whole blood or blood products increase the oxygen-carrying capacity of the blood and thus increase oxygenation of cells. However, these resuscitation fluids are not thought to minimize inflammation. Studies are underway to evaluate alternative resuscitation fluids such as a alternative colloid (hydroxyethyl starch [Hextend Biotime, Inc./Berkley, CA]), alternative crystalloid (Ringer's ethyl pyruvate), and hypertonic saline with dextran and polymerized hemoglobin.

EVIDENCE FOR NURSING CARE — The Patient with Cardiogenic Shock

Selected current resources that nurses may find helpful when planning evidence-based nursing care follow.

- Acute Coronary Syndromes. A National Clinical Guideline. (2008). *National Guideline Clearinghouse.* Retrieved November 3, 2009, from http://www.guideline.gov/summary/summary.aspx?doc_id=10585&nbr=005527&string=cardiogenic+AND+shock
- Cooper, B. E. (2008). Review and update on inotropes and vasopressors. *AACN Advanced Critical Care, 19*(1), 5–15.
- Ellender, T. J., & Skinner, J. C. (2008). The use of vasopressors and inotropes in the emergency medical treatment of shock. *Emergency Medicine Clinics of North America, 26*(3), 759–786.
- Gorman, D., Calhoun, K., Carassco, M., Niclaus, D., Neron, M., McNally, L., & Thompson, P. (2008). Take a rapid treatment approach to cardiogenic shock. *Nursing2008, 3*(4), 18–27.
- Spaniol, J. R., Knight, A. R., Zebley, J. L. Anderson, D., & Pierce, J. D. (2007). Fluid resuscitation therapy for hemorrhagic shock. *Journal of Trauma Nursing, 14*(3), 152–160.

MEDICATION ADMINISTRATION   The Patient in Shock

ADRENERGICS (SYMPATHOMIMETICS)

Vasoconstrictors

    Epinephrine (Adrenalin)

    Norepinephrine (Levophed)

    Metaraminol (Aramine)

    Vasopressin (Pitressin)

Inotropes

    Dopamine (Inotropin)

    Dobutamine (Dobutrex)

    Isoproterenol (Isuprel)

Adrenergic drugs (also called sympathomimetics) mimic the fight-or-flight response of the sympathetic nervous system, selectively stimulating alpha-adrenergic and beta-adrenergic receptors. Many of these drugs have both vasopressor (vaso-constricting) effects and positive inotropic effects. Stimulation of alpha-adrenergic receptors results in vasoconstriction and increased systemic blood pressure. Stimulation of beta-adrenergic receptors increases the force and rate of myocardial contraction.

The physiologic effect of these drugs includes improved perfusion and oxygenation of the heart, with increased stroke volume and heart rate, and increased cardiac output. Increased cardiac output in turn increases tissue perfusion and oxygenation. The major disadvantage is that increases in stroke volume and heart rate also increase the oxygen requirements of the myocardium. These drugs may be used in the early stages of shock, especially in types of shock characterized by vasodilation.

Nursing Responsibilities

- Carefully monitor responses in the older adult, who may be especially sensitive to sympathomimetics and require lower doses.
- When administering these drugs by the subcutaneous route, carefully aspirate the injection site to avoid injecting the drug directly into a blood vessel.
- Use the intravenous route only with continuous infusion pumps. Carefully adjust the dose to accommodate the patient's cardiovascular status (as ordered by the physician or by written protocol).
- Document lung sounds, vital signs, and hemodynamic parameters before starting the medication, and then according to institutional policy (usually every 5 to 15 minutes).
- Record and monitor urine output. Report output of less than 30 mL per hour.
- Be aware that the sympathomimetics are incompatible with sodium bicarbonate or alkaline solutions.
- When administering drugs that cause vasoconstriction, such as norepinephrine (Levophed) and metaraminol (Aramine), monitor the intravenous insertion site for

infiltration. If infiltration does occur, stop the infusion and notify the physician immediately. (Infiltration may cause ischemia and necrosis of tissue.)

Patient Teaching

- Because these drugs mimic a physiologic reaction to stress, they may cause feelings of anxiety.
- Close monitoring to adjust the dose will be carried out by qualified nurses using written protocols.
- Report heart palpitations or chest pain immediately.

Vasodilators

    Amnirone (Inocor)

    Nitroglycerin (Tridil)

    Nitroprusside (Nipride)

Drugs that cause vasodilation act directly on smooth muscle, affecting both arterioles and veins. Peripheral resistance, cardiac output, and pulmonary wedge pressure are all reduced as a result of the vasodilation. These effects decrease the oxygen need of the heart and decrease pulmonary congestion. Vasodilators are used primarily in the treatment of cardiogenic shock and may be combined with a sympathomimetic (e.g., dopamine).

Nursing Responsibilities

- Mix with D_5W or 0.9% saline.
- IV nitroglycerin must be mixed in glass bottles and infused through special, non-PVC tubing. Up to 40% to 80% of nitroglycerin can be absorbed by PVC bags or tubing.
- Infuse with an infusion pump, and use within 4 hours of reconstitution.
- Do not add other medications to the solution.
- Use cautiously in patients with increased intracranial pressure.
- Assess mental status, blood pressure, and pulse prior to initiating medication. Thereafter, assess blood pressure and pulse according to institutional policy (usually every 5 minutes initially, then every 15 minutes until stable, and then every hour).
- Monitor for confusion, dizziness, tachycardia, arrhythmias, hypotension, and adventitious breath sounds. Report these immediately if they occur, and slow infusion to a keep-open rate.
- Monitor patients receiving nitroprusside for signs of thiocyanate poisoning (nausea, disorientation, muscle spasms, decreased or absent reflexes) if infusion lasts longer than 72 hours.
- Keep patient in bed with side rails up.

Health Education for the Patient and Family

- It is important to stay in bed and change positions slowly to avoid dizziness.
- The blood pressure and pulse are taken frequently to adjust the dose of medication.
- Headache is a common side effect.

CRYSTALLOID SOLUTIONS Crystalloid solutions contain dextrose or electrolytes dissolved in water; they are hypertonic, isotonic, or hypotonic. Hypertonic solutions include 3% saline. Isotonic solutions include normal saline (0.9%), lactated Ringer's solution, and Ringer's solution. Hypotonic solutions include one-half normal saline (0.45%) and 5% dextrose in water (D5W).

Hypertonic crystalloid solutions pull fluid into the vascular space to promote excretion. Isotonic and hypotonic crystalloid solutions increase fluid volume in both the intravascular and the interstitial space. Of the total amount infused, only about 25% remains in the intravascular system; the remaining 75% moves into the interstitial space. Consequently, fluid volume is only minimally expanded and the potential for peripheral edema is increased when crystalloid solutions are used. However, Ringer's lactate (an electrolyte solution) and 0.9% saline are the fluids of choice in treating hypovolemic shock, especially in the emergency phase of care while blood is being typed and crossmatched. Large amounts of these solutions may be infused rapidly, increasing blood volume and tissue perfusion.

COLLOID SOLUTIONS   Colloid solutions contain substances (colloids) that should not diffuse through capillary walls. Hence, colloids tend to remain in the vascular system and increase the osmotic pressure of the serum, causing fluid to move into the vascular compartment from the interstitial space. As a result, plasma volume expands. Colloid solutions used to treat shock include 5% albumin, 25% albumin, hetastarch, plasma protein fraction, and dextran.

Colloid products reduce platelet adhesiveness and have been associated with reductions in blood coagulation. Consequently, the patient's prothrombin time (PT), INR, platelet count, and activated partial thromboplastin time (PTT) should be monitored when these solutions are administered. Normal values are as follows:

PT	10–15 seconds
INR	1–1.2 seconds
Platelets	150,000–400,000
APTT	< 35 seconds

See the following Medication Administration box for further information about colloid solutions and associated nursing responsibilities and patient teaching.

BLOOD AND BLOOD PRODUCTS   If hypovolemic shock is due to hemorrhage, the infusion of blood and blood products may be indicated. The goal of blood administration is to keep the hematocrit at 30% to 35% and the hemoglobin level between 12.5 and 14.5 g/100 mL. Available blood and blood products include fresh whole blood, stored whole blood, packed red blood cells, platelet concentrate, fresh-frozen plasma, and cryoprecipitate. Often, packed red blood cells are given to provide hemoglobin concentration and are supplemented with crystalloids to maintain an adequate circulatory volume (see the discussion of blood administration earlier in the chapter).

Nursing Care

Nursing assessments and interventions to prevent shock are an essential part of the nursing care of every patient. The primary nursing interventions to prevent shock are assessment and monitoring.

Health Promotion and Assessment

Nursing assessments are critical in preventing shock. Identifying patients at risk and making focused assessments are essential. Although shock may occur at any age, physiologic changes with aging make the older adult a high-risk population (see the following box).

■ *Hypovolemic shock:* Patients who have undergone surgery, have sustained multiple traumatic injuries, or have been seriously burned are most likely to develop hypovolemic shock. Monitoring fluid status is essential in preventing shock and includes daily assessments of weight, fluid intake by all routes, measurable fluid loss (e.g., urine, vomitus, wound drainage, gastric drainage, and chest tube drainage), and fluid loss that must be estimated, such as profuse perspiration and wound drainage. Assessments for the critically ill patient

---

MEDICATION ADMINISTRATION   **Colloid Solutions (Plasma Expanders)**

Albumin 5% (Albuminar-5, Buminate 5%)

Albumin 25% (Albuminar-25, Buminate 25%)

Dextran 40 (Gentran 40)

Dextran 70 (Gentran 70, Macrodex)

Dextran 75 (Gentran 75)

Hetastarch (Hespan [HES])

Plasma protein fraction (Plasmanate, Plasma-Plex, Plasmatein, Protenate)

These solutions are blood volume expanders and are used to treat hypovolemic shock due to surgery, hemorrhage, burns, or other trauma. Albumin and plasma protein fraction are prepared from healthy blood donors. Dextran and hetastarch are synthetically prepared large molecules. The solutions promote circulatory volume and tissue perfusion by rapidly expanding plasma volume. Dextran solutions are infrequently used.

Nursing Responsibilities
■ Before infusion begins, establish baseline of vital signs, lung sounds, heart sounds, and (if possible) CVP and pulmonary artery wedge pressure.
■ Start administration of ordered intravenous fluids, using a large-gauge (18-gauge or larger) infusion needle.
■ Obtain and record vital signs as required by institutional policy (usually every 15 to 60 minutes) and patient status.
■ Obtain and record intake and output every 1 to 2 hours.

■ Monitor for manifestations of congestive heart failure or pulmonary edema (dyspnea, cyanosis, cough, crackles, wheezes). If these manifestations appear, stop the fluids and notify the physician immediately.
■ Monitor for bleeding from new sites; an increase in blood pressure may cause bleeding in severed vessels that did not bleed with decreased blood pressure.
■ Monitor for manifestations of dehydration (dry lips; scant, dark-colored urine; loss of skin turgor). Increased intravenous fluids are usually ordered if the patient becomes dehydrated.
■ Monitor for manifestations of circulatory overload (jugular vein distention, increase in CVP, increase in pulmonary capillary wedge pressure). If these manifestations occur, slow rate of infusion and notify physician.
■ Monitor prothrombin time, partial thromboplastin time, and platelet counts.
■ If administering dextran or plasma protein fraction, have epinephrine and antihistamines readily available for any manifestations of a hypersensitivity reaction (fever, chills, rash, headache, wheezing, flushing).
■ Maintain patient on bed rest with side rails elevated.

Health Education for the Patient and Family
■ The solutions are given to replace lost serum protein, which helps maintain the volume of blood.
■ The vital signs are taken frequently to ensure the safety of the patient.

are ongoing and include fluid balance, hemodynamic values, and vital signs.

- *Cardiogenic shock:* Patients with left anterior wall myocardial infarctions are at risk for developing cardiogenic shock. Nursing care to prevent the development of cardiogenic shock focuses on maintaining or improving myocardial oxygen supply by providing immediate pain relief, maintaining rest, and administering supplemental oxygen.
- *Neurogenic shock:* The risk of neurogenic shock is increased in patients who have spinal cord injuries and those who have received spinal anesthesia. Preventive nursing care includes maintaining immobility of patients with spinal cord trauma and elevating the head of the bed 15 to 20 degrees following spinal anesthesia. Elevations of more than 20 degrees, however, can potentiate headaches following spinal anesthesia and should be avoided.
- *Anaphylactic shock:* Prevent anaphylactic shock by collecting information about allergies and drug reactions during the health history. Note these allergies clearly on all documents and place a special armband on the patient. Careful and frequent assessments during blood administration may prevent serious reactions to blood or blood products.
- *Septic shock:* Patients who are hospitalized, are debilitated, are chronically ill, or have undergone invasive procedures or tube insertions are at high risk for septic shock. Nursing care to prevent septic shock includes careful and consistent hand hygiene, the use of aseptic techniques for procedures (e.g., catheterizations, suctioning, changing dressings, starting and maintaining intravenous fluids or medications), and monitoring for local and systemic manifestations (e.g., white blood cell and differential counts) of infection.

Nursing Diagnoses and Interventions

Nursing care for the patient in shock focuses on assessing and monitoring overall tissue perfusion and on meeting psychosocial needs of the patient and the family. This section discusses nursing diagnoses that are appropriate for the patient with hypovolemic shock. See the accompanying Case Study & Nursing Care Plan on page 265.

EVIDENCE FOR NURSING CARE | **The Patient with Pneumothorax**

Selected resources that nurses may find helpful when planning evidence-based nursing care follow.

- Farrington, M., Lang, S., Cullen, L., & Stewart, S. (2009). Nasogastric tube placement verification in pediatric and neonatal patients. *Pediatric Nursing, 35*(1), 17–24.
- Global strategy for the diagnosis, management, and prevention of chronic obstructive pulmonary disease. (2008). National Guideline Clearinghouse. Retrieved from http://www.goldcopd.com
- Robinson, P. D, Cooper, P., & Ranganathan, S. C. (2009). Evidence-based management of paediatric primary spontaneous pneumothorax. *Paediatric Respiratory Reviews, 10*(3), 110–117.

Decreased Cardiac Output

Decreased cardiac output is the primary problem for the patient in shock. Although much of the care related to this diagnosis is collaborative, many independent nursing interventions are critical to the care of the patient in shock.

- *Assess and monitor cardiovascular function via the following:*
  - Blood pressure
  - Heart rate and rhythm
  - Pulse oximetry
  - Peripheral pulses
  - Hemodynamic monitoring of arterial pressures, pulmonary artery pressures, and central venous pressures (CVPs). *A baseline assessment is necessary to establish the stage of shock. If palpable peripheral pulses and audible (to auscultation) blood pressure are lost, inserting central arterial, venous, and pulmonary artery catheters is essential to establish progression of shock accurately and to evaluate the patient's response to therapy.*
- Measure and record intake and output (total output and urinary output) hourly. *A decrease in circulating blood volume with hypotension and the effect of the compensatory mechanisms associated with shock can cause renal failure. Urinary output of less than 30 mL per hour in an acutely ill adult indicates reduced renal blood flow.*
- Monitor bowel sounds, abdominal distention, and abdominal pain. *Decreased splanchnic blood flow reduces bowel motility and peristalsis; paralytic ileus may result.*
- Monitor for sudden sharp chest pain, dyspnea, cyanosis, anxiety, and restlessness. *Hemoconcentration and increased platelet aggregation may result in pulmonary emboli.*
  - Maintain bed rest and provide (to the extent possible) a calm, quiet environment. Place in a supine position with the legs elevated to about 20 degrees, trunk flat, and head and shoulders elevated higher than the chest (semi-fowler's can also be used with mechanically-ventilated patients) (Figure 11–9 ■). *Limiting activity and ensuring rest decreases the workload of the heart. The supine position with legs elevated increases venous return; however, this position should not be used for patients in cardiogenic shock. The Trendelenburg position is no longer recommended, because it causes the abdominal organs to press against the diaphragm (limiting respirations), decreases filling of the coronary arteries, and initiates aortic and carotid sinus reflexes.*

Figure 11–9 ■ The patient in shock should be positioned with the lower extremities elevated approximately 20 degrees (knees straight), trunk horizontal, and the head elevated about 10 degrees.

CASE STUDY & NURSING CARE PLAN   A Patient with Septic Shock

Huang Mei Lan is a 43-year-old unmarried female who lives alone in a major West Coast city. Ms. Huang came to America 15 years ago from China and now speaks English well. Her family still lives in China. She worked in a neighborhood sewing shop until 3 years ago, when she was diagnosed with breast cancer. Her treatment included mastectomy of the affected breast and follow-up chemotherapy.

Last month, Ms. Huang experienced a recurrence of cancer in the lymph glands of the affected side. Surgery to remove the glands was performed and chemotherapy started. Ms. Huang has a central line, a urinary catheter, and a surgical incision. She is underweight, weak, and depressed. Although she has multiple physical problems, she never complains or asks for any kind of medication.

ASSESSMENT

Ms. Huang's primary nurse, Robert O'Brien, enters her room early in the morning to make an initial assessment. He finds Ms. Huang huddled in the middle of the bed, shivering violently. Her vital signs are T 104° F, P 110, R 30, and BP 106/66. Her skin is hot, dry, and flushed with poor turgor. She is alert and oriented, but is restless and appears anxious. Ms. Huang states she is nauseated and suddenly begins vomiting and is incontinent of liquid stool. Laboratory data indicate leukocytosis, respiratory alkalosis, and reduced platelet count. Blood cultures, as well as cultures of Ms. Huang's sputum, urine, and wound drainage, are conducted. She is diagnosed as having septic shock.

Hetastarch is ordered per intravenous line, and intravenous broad-spectrum antibiotics are begun until the organism and its portal of entry can be determined. Despite treatment, Ms. Huang's condition worsens. Her blood pressure continues to drop, her skin becomes cool and cyanotic, and she begins to have periods of disorientation. She is transferred to the critical care unit. As she is being prepared for the transfer, she begins to cry and asks, "Am I going to die?"

DIAGNOSES

- *Ineffective Breathing Pattern* related to rapid respirations and progression of septic shock
- *Ineffective Tissue Perfusion* related to progression of septic shock with decreased cardiac output, hypotension, and massive vasodilatation
- *Deficient Fluid Volume* related to vomiting, diarrhea, high fever, and shift of intravascular volume to interstitial spaces

- *Anxiety* related to feelings that illness is worsening and is potentially life threatening, and the transfer to the critical care unit

EXPECTED OUTCOMES

- Regain and maintain blood gas parameters within normal limits.
- Maintain adequate circulating blood volume.
- Regain and maintain stable hemodynamic levels.
- Verbalize increased ability to cope with stressors.

PLANNING AND IMPLEMENTATION

- Monitor results of arterial blood gases, blood counts, clotting times, and platelet counts.
- Monitor respiratory status, including respiratory rate, rhythm, and breath sounds.
- Monitor neurologic status, including mental status and level of consciousness.
- Monitor cardiovascular status, including arterial blood pressure; rate, rhythm, and quality of pulses; central venous pressure; pulmonary artery pressure; and cardiac output.
- Monitor body temperature every 2 hours.
- Monitor urinary output hourly, reporting any output of less than 30 mL per hour.
- Monitor color and character of skin.
- Explain procedures and provide comfort measures (oral care, skin care, turning, positioning).

EVALUATION

Despite intensive nursing and medical care, Ms. Huang's condition remains critical. The interventions are continued.

CRITICAL THINKING IN THE NURSING PROCESS

1. Vasopressors may be used in the treatment of septic shock. Explain the rationale for their use.
2. While monitoring Ms. Huang's arterial blood gases, the nurse notes that her PaO_2 is < 60 mmHg and her $PaCO_2$ is > 50. What do these findings indicate, and why have they occurred?
3. Ms. Huang has been given large amounts of colloids intravenously. Hemodynamic monitoring indicates a higher than normal CVP and pulmonary artery pressure. What do these findings indicate? What physical assessments would you make to confirm the changes?

See Evaluating Your Response in Appendix C.

NURSING CARE OF THE OLDER ADULT   Variations in Assessment Findings—Shock

- Cardiac changes may include a thickened left ventricular wall, decreased elasticity of the myocardium, and more rigid valves. These changes result in a decreased stroke volume and cardiac output, thus decreasing responses to shock in general and increasing the risk of cardiogenic shock.
- Decreased arterial wall elasticity and vasomotor tone reduce the older adult's ability to respond to a decrease in oxygenation.

- Decreased elasticity and turgor of the skin make assessments of skin turgor more difficult.
- Previous medication and blood administration increase the risk of anaphylactic shock.
- Decreased immune system response increases the risk of septic shock.

Altered Tissue Perfusion

As shock progresses, diminished tissue perfusion causes ischemia and hypoxia of major organ systems. As shock worsens, blood flow and oxygenation of the lungs, heart, and brain are also impaired. Hypoxia and ischemia result from decreased tissue perfusion in the kidneys, brain, heart, lungs, gastrointestinal tract, and the periphery.

■ Monitor skin color, temperature, turgor, and moisture. *Decreased tissue perfusion is evidenced when the skin becomes pale, cool, and moist; as hemoglobin concentrations decrease, cyanosis occurs.*

■ Monitor cardiopulmonary function by assessing/monitoring the following:
  ■ Blood pressure (by auscultation or by hemodynamic monitoring)
  ■ Rate and depth of respirations
  ■ Lung sounds
  ■ Pulse oximetry and arterial blood gases
  ■ Peripheral pulses (brachial, radial, dorsalis pedis, and posterior tibial); include presence, equality, rate, rhythm, and quality (If unable to palpate pulses, use a device such as a Doppler ultrasound flowmeter to assess peripheral arterial blood flow.)
  ■ Jugular vein distention
  ■ CVP measurements

  Baseline vital signs are necessary to determine trends in subsequent findings. As shock progresses, the blood pressure decreases, and the pulse becomes rapid, weak, and thready. As perfusion of the lungs decreases, crackles, wheezes, and dyspnea are commonly assessed. Capillary refill is prolonged, and peripheral pulses are weak or nonpalpable. Neck veins that cannot be seen when the patient is in the supine position indicate decreased intravascular volume. CVP is an accurate means of determining fluid status in the patient in shock; the findings will be low (5–15 cmH$_2$O or 2–6 mmHG is normal) in hypovolemic shock because of the decreased blood volume. (∞ See Chapter 10 for a discussion of CVP.)

■ Monitor body temperature. *An elevated body temperature increases metabolic demands, depleting reserves of bodily energy. It also increases myocardial oxygen demand and may place the patient with previous cardiac problems at even greater risk for hypoperfusion.*

■ Monitor urinary output per Foley catheter hourly, using a urimeter. *Urine output is a reliable indicator of renal perfusion.*

■ Assess mental status and level of consciousness. *The appropriateness of the patient's behavior and responses reflects the adequacy of cerebral circulation. Restlessness and anxiety are common early in shock; in later stages, the patient may become lethargic and progress to a comatose state. Altered levels of consciousness are the result of both cerebral hypoxia and the effects of acidosis on brain cells.*

Anxiety

Many patients in hypovolemic shock have experienced some form of major trauma and may have multiple life-threatening injuries that result in emergency care and the potential for emergency surgery. Throughout this sequence of crisis events, treatment is invasive, and contact with family is minimal. Patient and family responses to these situations of uncertainty, instability, and change include anxiety, fear, and powerlessness. These responses are affected by age, developmental level, cultural and ethnic group, experience with illness and the healthcare system, and support systems.

■ Assess the cause(s) of the anxiety, and manipulate the environment to provide periods of rest. *Reducing stimuli that cause anxiety is calming and facilitates rest, which is necessary in the patient at risk for bleeding.*

■ Administer prescribed pain medications on a regular basis and implement any applicable nonpharmacologic comfort measures. *Pain precipitates and/or aggravates anxiety.*

■ Provide interventions to increase comfort and reduce restlessness:
  ■ Maintain a clean environment.
  ■ Provide skin and oral care.
  ■ Monitor the effectiveness of ventilation or oxygen therapy.
  ■ Eliminate all nonessential activities.
  ■ Remain with the patient during procedures.
  ■ Speak slowly and calmly, using short sentences.
  ■ Use touch to provide support.

  Unfamiliar sounds, sights, and odors can increase anxiety. Damp skin or a dry mouth increases discomfort. Inadequate gas exchange with a decrease in oxygen or an increase in carbon dioxide in the blood may cause the patient to experience a "feeling of doom." Activity increases the body's need for oxygen. Listening and touch provide support in an environment in which the patient often feels alone and abandoned. Severe anxiety interferes with the ability to understand others and to respond appropriately.

■ Provide support for the patient and family:
  ■ Provide time, space, and privacy for family members.
  ■ Allow family members access to the patient when feasible.
  ■ Encourage the expression of feelings and concerns. Provide anticipatory guidance to prepare for recovery or death and to support realistic hope.

NANDA, NIC, AND NOC LINKAGES
The Patient in Shock

NANDA

Risk for Ineffective Cerebral Tissue Perfusion

⬇

NIC

Cerebral Perfusion Promotion
Central Perfusion Monitoring
Fluid/Electrolyte Management
Hypovolemia Management
Shock Management

⬇

NOC

Tissue Perfusion: Cerebral, Ineffective
Circulation Status
Vital Signs
Neurological Status

Adapted from Bulechek, G., Butcher, H., & Dochterman, J. M. (Eds). (2008). *Nursing interventions classification (NIC)* (5th ed.). St. Louis: Mosby Elsevier; Moorhead, S., Johnson, M., Maas, M., & Swanson, E. (Eds). (2008). *Nursing outcomes classification (NOC)* (4th ed.). St. Louis: Mosby Elsevier; and Nanda International. (2009). *Nursing diagnoses: Definitions and classification 2009–2011.* Oxford, UK: Wiley-Blackwell.

- Acknowledge the beliefs, values, and expectations of the patient and family.

    Allowing the family access to the patient reduces anxiety and gives both the patient and the family some feeling of control. If prognosis is poor, access and involvement allow the family to begin the grieving process. If recovery is expected, contact provides the patient and family with a feeling of hope. Supporting the patient and family facilitates concrete problem solving, promotes acceptance of the illness and its implications, and helps them begin to establish ways of managing the illness experience.

- Provide information about the current setting to both the patient and family; give the family information about available resources (such as pastoral care, social services, temporary housing, meals). *Knowing what to expect and how to control the environment to meet basic needs reduces anxiety.*

Using NANDA, NIC, and NOC

Linkages between a selected NANDA nursing diagnosis, NIC, and NOC for the patient in shock are shown in the chart on the previous page.

Community-Based Care

Home care for the patient who has experienced shock is highly individualized, depending on the cause and the illness or injury that caused shock. Therefore, topics for consideration are not included in this section.

CHAPTER HIGHLIGHTS

- Trauma is defined as injury to human tissues and organs resulting from the transfer of energy from the environment. Energy sources can be mechanical, gravitational, thermal, electrical, physical, or chemical.
- Trauma types included minor trauma, which causes minimal damage to underlying tissues, or major/multiple trauma, which involves at minimum a serious single system injury or multiple trauma. Trauma can also be categorized as blunt and penetrating trauma. Blunt trauma is caused by forces like deceleration, acceleration, shearing, compression, or crushing. Penetrating trauma is the entrance into the body of a foreign object.
- Maintenance of the airway and cervical spine are the highest priority in the trauma patient, with airway assessment superseding all other interventions.
- The primary assessment conducted by the nurse identifies all life-threatening injuries and performance of appropriate interventions. The secondary assessment is when the nurse identifies all injuries in order to prioritize care.
- Shock is a clinical syndrome characterized by a systemic imbalance between oxygen supply and demand. This imbalance results in a state of inadequate blood flow to body organs and tissues, causing life-threatening cellular dysfunction.
- The symptoms of shock arise from the body's attempts to maintain vital organs (heart and brain) and to preserve life following a drop in oxygen delivery to the cells.
- An important early sign of shock is a change in the level of consciousness with restlessness a common symptom of cerebral hypoxia.
- Shock is defined in 3 stages: compensatory (stage 1), an early and reversible stage; progressive (stage 2), occurring after a fluid loss of 35% to 50% (1800 to 2500 mL of fluid), where the affected cells switch from aerobic to anaerobic metabolism in order to stay alive; and the final stage, refractory/irreversible (stage 3), where tissue anoxia and death becomes widespread.
- Hypovolemic shock is the most common type of shock and is caused by a decrease in circulating blood volume by 15% or greater.
- Cardiogenic shock is caused when the pumping ability of the heart is compromised to the point where adequate cardiac output cannot be maintained.
- Obstructive shock is caused by an obstruction in the heart or great vessels that either impedes venous return or prevents effective cardiac pumping action. Causes can include cardiac tamponade, pneumothorax, pulmonary embolism and aortic stenosis.
- Distributive shock includes several types of shock that result from widespread vasodilatation and decreased peripheral resistance. As the blood volume does not change, relative hypovolemia results, leading to altered cellular metabolism. Examples of distributive shock include septic, neurogenic, and anaphylactic shock.
- Septic shock is part of a progressive syndrome called systemic inflammatory response syndrome (SIRS), a condition most commonly caused by gram-negative infections.
- Anaphylactic shock is caused by a fulminating hypersensitivity reaction to a foreign substance.

TEST YOURSELF NCLEX-RN® REVIEW

1. What is the most common mechanical source of injury in adults of all ages?
    1. firearms
    2. accidental fire
    3. swimming pools
    4. motor vehicles

2. Severe facial injuries, such as those resulting from going through a windshield, increase the risk for all of the following. For which complication would you assess first?
    1. airway obstruction
    2. hemorrhage
    3. shallow respirations
    4. fractures

3. Which hospital intervention would be the priority?
   1. Verify cause of injury.
   2. Assess airway patency.
   3. Evaluate peripheral capillary refill.
   4. Check for hemorrhage.
4. You are monitoring blood administration to a trauma victim in shock. Which of the following assessment findings indicate a dangerous transfusion reaction?
   1. multiple urticaric, pruritic skin lesions
   2. an increase in body temperature by 3°
   3. decreasing dyspnea
   4. increasing blood pressure
5. Which of the following types of shock causes widespread vasodilatation and decreased peripheral resistance?
   1. cardiogenic shock
   2. septic shock
   3. hypovolemic shock
   4. obstructive shock
6. What is the best method to manage uncontrolled bleeding?
   1. Use direct pressure.
   2. Clamp a visible vessel.
   3. Apply a tourniquet.
   4. Elevate the injured part.

7. Trauma is defined as which of the following?
   1. an injury to human tissues from the transfer of energy
   2. the result of random chance vs. intention
   3. an accidental injury
   4. an intentional injury
8. Which of the following is a risk from a blood transfusion?
   1. pregnancy
   2. tuberculosis
   3. transfusion reaction
   4. weight gain
9. Distributive shock is caused from which of the following?
   1. blood loss
   2. widespread vasodilatation
   3. ineffective cardiac pumping action
   4. hypersensitivity reaction
10. Shock is defined as which of the following?
    1. systemic imbalance between oxygen supply and demand
    2. sufficient cardiac output
    3. controlled hemorrhage
    4. abnormal blood pressure

See Test Yourself answers in Appendix C.

Pearson Nursing Student Resources

Find additional review materials at
www.nursing.pearsonhighered.com
Prepare for success with additional NCLEX®-style practice questions, interactive assignments and activities, Web links, animations and videos, and more!

BIBLIOGRAPHY

American College of Emergency Physicians. (2009). Domestic Family Violence. Retrieved from http://www.acep.org/practres.aspx?id=29184

American Red Cross. (2003). Cryoprecipitate Transfusion Guidelines. Retrieved from http://www.newenglandblood.org/professional/cryoguide.htm

American Red Cross. (2003). Plasma Transfusion Guidelines. Retrieved from http://www.newenglandblood.org/professional/plasmaguide.htm

American Red Cross. (2003). Platelet Transfusion Guidelines. Retrieved from http://www.newenglandblood.org/professional/plateletguide.htm

American Red Cross. (2003). Red Cell Transfusion Guidelines. Retrieved from http://www.newenglandblood.org/professional/redcellguide.htm

American Red Cross. (2009). Blood types. Retrieved from http://www.givelife2.org/aboutblood/bloodtypes.aspAustralian Red Cross

Bickley, L. S. (2008). *Bates' guide to physical examination and history taking* (7th ed.). Philadelphia: Lippincott Williams & Wilkins.

Carcillo, J., Han, K., Lin, J., & Orr, R. (2007). Goal directed management of pediatric shock in the emergency department. *Clinical Pediatric Emergency Medicine* 8(3), 165–175.

Catenacci, M. H., & King, K. (2008). Severe sepsis and septic shock: Improving outcomes in the emergency department. *Emergency Medicine Clinics of North America, 26*(3), 603–623.

Cocci, M. N., Kimlin, E., Walsh, M., Donnino, M. W. (2007). Identification and resuscitation of the trauma patient in shock. *Emergency Medicine Clinics of North America,* 25(3), 623–642.

Deglin, J. H., & Vallerand, A. H. (2009). *Davis' drug guide* (10th Ed.). Philadelphia: F.A. Davis.

Department of Veterans' Affairs. (2009). Common reactions after trauma. Retrieved from http://ncptsd.va.gov/ncmain/ncdocs/fact_shts/fs_commonreactions.html

Dine, C. J., & Abella, B. S. (2009). Therapeutic hypothermia for neuroprotection. *Emergency Medicine Clinics of North America, 27*(1), 137–149.

Domino, F.J., Baldor, R. A., Golding, J., Grimes, J., & Taylor, J. S. (2010). *The 5-minute clinical consult* (18th ed.). Philadelphia: Lippincott, Williams & Wilkins.

Emergency Nurses Association. (2003). Core curriculum for pediatric emergency nursing. Chicago: Author.

Emergency Nurses Association. (2008). Emergency Nursing Core Curriculum (6th ed.). Philadelphia: Saunders.

Erickson, T. B., Thompson, T. M., Lu, J. J. (2007). The approach to the patient with the unknown overdose. *Emergency Medicine Clinics of North America, 25*(2), 249–281.

Fishman, A. P., Elias, J. A., Fishman, J. A., Grippi, M. A., Senior, S. M., & Pack, A. J. (2008). *Fishman's pulmonary diseases and disorders* (4th ed.). New York: McGraw-Hill Co.

Hildebrand, F., Pape, H. C., van Griensven, M., et al. (2005). Genetic predisposition for a compromised immune system after multiple trauma. *Shock, 24*(6), 518–522.

Huether, S. E., & McCance, K. L. (2008). *Understanding Pathophysiology* (4th ed.). St. Louis: Mosby Elsevier.

McGill, J. (2007). Airway management in trauma: An update. *Emergency Medicine Clinics of North America, 25*(3), 603–622.

Men Stopping Violence. (2009). The art of change. Retrieved from http://www.menstoppingviolence.org/index.php

NANDA International. (2009). *Nursing diagnoses: Definitions and classification 2009–2011* Oxford, UK: Wiley-Blackwell.

National Center of Health Statistics [NCHS]. (2009). *Health, United States, 2008* with chartbook. Hyattsville, MD: Author.

National Center for Patient Safety. (2004). Falls Toolkit. Retrieved from http://www.patientsafety.gov/SafetyTopics/fallstoolkit/index.html

National Highway Traffic Safety Administration. (2009). Child passenger safety studies and reports. Retrieved from http://www.nhtsa.dot.gov/portal/site/nhtsa/menuitem.9f8c7d6359e0e9bbbf30811060008a0c

National Institute of Mental Health. (2009). Men and depression. Retrieved from http://www.nimh.nih.gov/health/publications/men-and-depression/index.shtml

National Library of Medicine. (2009). Domestic Violence. Retrieved from http://www.nlm.nih.gov/medlineplus/domesticviolence.html

National Library of Medicine. (2009). Suicide. Retrieved from http://www.nlm.nih.gov/medlineplus/suicide.html

Papadakis, M. A., & McPhee, S. J. (2007). *Current consult medicine 2007.* New York: McGraw-Hill.

Perrin, K. O. (2009). *Understanding the essentials of critical care nursing.* Upper Saddle River, NJ: Pearson Prentice-Hall.

Sheehy S. A. B. (1984). Primary trauma survey and immediate intervention with the use of the mnemonic ABC4. *Journal of Emergency Nursing, 10*(4), 220–221.

Transfusion.com (2009). Transfusion update 2009: Cryoprecipitate. Retrieved from http://www.transfusion.com.au/Cryoprecipitate.aspx

Trzeciak, S., Dellinger, P., Abate, N. L., et al. (2007). Translating research to clinical practice: A 1-year experience with implementing early goal-directed therapy for septic shock in the emergency department. *Chest, 129*(2), 225–232.

Van Leeuwen, A. M., Kranpitz, T. R., & Smith, L. S. (2006). *Davis' laboratory and diagnostic tests* (2nd ed.). Philadelphia: F.A. Davis.

Nursing Care of Patients with Infections

LEARNING OUTCOMES

1. Explain the components and functions of the immune system and the immune response.
2. Compare antibody-mediated and cell-mediated immune responses.
3. Describe the pathophysiology of wound healing, inflammation, and infection.
4. Identify factors responsible for nosocomial infections.
5. Discuss the purposes, nursing implications, and health education for medications and treatments used to treat inflammations and infections.
6. Explain the nursing care necessary to prevent and/or monitor the status of infections.

CLINICAL COMPETENCIES

1. Apply standard precautions, particularly hand hygiene, to prevent the spread of infection within the patient, to other patients in the facility, and to members of the interdisciplinary team and visitors.
2. Use the nursing process as a framework to provide safe, effective individualized care for patients with inflammation and infection.
3. Collaborate with the interdisciplinary care team to integrate care of patients with infection.
4. Promote therapeutic levels and complete dosage of anti-inflammatory and anti-infective medication through prompt administration and patient and family teaching.
5. Assess for hypersensitivities to anti-infectives prior to administering and during administration.
6. Participate in quality improvement processes to reduce the rates and risk of infection for a patient group or population.

KEY TERMS

acquired immunity, *281*
active immunity, *281*
adaptive immune response, *270*
anergy, *283*
antibodies, *273*
antibody-mediated (humoral) immune response, *273*
antigens, *273*
B lymphocytes (B cells), *272*

cell-mediated (cellular) immune response, *273*
cytokines, *281*
endotoxins, *292*
exotoxins, *292*
immunity, *281*
immunocompetent, *278*
immunoglobulin (Ig), *278*
infection, *292*
innate adaptive immunity, *269*

lymphocyte, *272*
macrophages, *272*
natural killer cells (NK cells, null cells), *272*
nosocomial infections, *294*
passive immunity, *281*
pathogens, *291*
phagocytosis, *276*
T lymphocytes (T cells), *272*
vaccines, *283*

The human body is continually threatened by foreign substances, infectious agents, and abnormal cells. The immune system is the body's major defense mechanism against infectious organisms and abnormal or damaged cells. Recent years have seen the emergence of resistant microorganisms such as methicillin-resistant *Staphylococcus aureus* (MRSA) and altered strains of familiar diseases, such as multiple-drug-resistant tuberculosis. Other diseases have also emerged, including Lyme disease, *Clostridium difficile*, and human immunodeficiency virus (HIV).

A thorough knowledge of the immune system increases understanding of the local and systemic inflammatory response, resistance to infectious disease, and the importance of immunization. This foundation can help the nurse teach patients and families to follow recommended treatment regimens, to promote and maintain health, and to prevent disease. In addition, the nurse can prescribe appropriate rehabilitative measures, such as increased rest and attention to optimal nutrition.

Overview of the Immune System

The immune system is a complex and intricate network of specialized cells, tissues, and organs. Cells of the immune system seek out and destroy damaged cells and foreign tissue, yet recognize and preserve host cells (Porth, 2007). The immune system defends and protects the body from infection by bacteria, viruses, fungi, and parasites; removes and destroys damaged or dead cells; and identifies and destroys malignant cells, thereby preventing their further development into tumors.

The immune system is activated by minor injuries, such as small lacerations or bruises, or by major injuries, such as burns, surgeries, and systemic diseases (e.g., pneumonia). The response of the immune system may be innate or adaptive. Innate immunity provides a nonspecific, generic response to harmful events; adaptive immunity provides a specific response to unique organisms and includes memory as well as active and limited responses. **Innate adaptive immunity** responses prevent or limit the entry of invaders into the body, thereby limiting the extent of tissue damage and reducing the workload of the adaptive immune system. Inflammation is an innate, nonspecific response activated by both minor and major injuries. When the inflammatory process is unable to destroy invading organisms or toxins, a more specific response, called the **adaptive immune response**, is activated.

Immune System Components

The immune system consists of molecules, cells, and organs that produce the immune response (Table 12–1). These components may be involved in the innate inflammatory response, the adaptive immune response, or both.

Leukocytes

Leukocytes (white blood cells, WBCs) are the primary cells involved in both innate and adaptive immune system responses. Like all blood cells, leukocytes derive from stem cells, the hemocytoblasts, in the bone marrow (Figure 12–1 ■). Unlike red blood cells (RBCs), which are confined to the circulation, leukocytes use the circulation to transport themselves to the site of an inflammatory or immune response. As the mobile units of the immune system, leukocytes detect, attack, and destroy anything that is recognized as "foreign." They are able to move through tissue spaces, locating damaged tissue and infection by responding to chemicals released by other leukocytes and damaged tissue.

The normal number of circulating leukocytes is 4,500 to 10,000 cells per cubic millimeter (mm^3) of blood. Many more leukocytes are "marginated." Margination refers to adhesion of leukocytes to vascular epithelial cells along the vessel walls, in other tissue spaces, or in the lymph system. Marginated leukocytes migrate into injured areas or areas where pathogens infiltrate as part of the innate immune response. In the presence of an attack such as an infection, additional WBCs are released from the bone marrow, leading to *leukocytosis*, a WBC count of greater than 10,000/mm^3. As WBCs move out of the bone marrow into the blood, the bone marrow increases its production of additional leukocytes. A decrease in the number of circulating leukocytes, known as *leukopenia*, occurs when bone marrow activity is suppressed or when leukocyte destruction increases.

Leukocytes are divided into three major groups: granulocytes, monocytes, and lymphocytes. The granulocytes and monocytes derive from the myeloid stem cells of the bone marrow and are instrumental in the inflammatory response. Lymphocytes derive from the lymphoid stem cells of the bone marrow and are the primary cells involved in the specific immune response. In laboratory tests, the WBC count indicates the total number of circulating leukocytes. The WBC differential identifies the portion of the total represented by each type of leukocyte.

GRANULOCYTES Granulocytes constitute 60% to 80% of the total number of normal blood leukocytes. Their cytoplasm has a granular appearance, and their nuclei are distinctively multilobular (see Figure 12–1). Granulocytes have a short life span, measured in hours to days, compared to the life span of monocytes, which is measured in months to years. Granulocytes play a key role in protecting the body from harmful microorganisms

TABLE 12–1 Cells and Tissues of the Immune System

COMPONENT	LOCATION	FUNCTION
Leukocytes		
Granulocytes		
Neutrophils	Circulation	Phagocytosis and chemotaxis
Eosinophils	Circulation, respiratory tract, and gastrointestinal tract	Phagocytosis Protection against parasites Involved in allergic response
Basophils	Circulation	Release of chemotactic substances
Monocytes and macrophages	Circulation (monocytes) and body tissue, such as skin (histiocytes), liver (Kupffer cells), alveoli, spleen, tonsils, lymph nodes, bone, bone marrow, brain	Trapping and phagocytizing of foreign substances and cellular debris Secretion of interleukin-1 to stimulate lymphocyte growth
Lymphocytes	Circulation, lymph system, tissues	Activation of T and B cells
T cells (mature in thymus gland)		Control of viral infections and destruction of cancer cells Involved in hypersensitivity reactions and graft tissue rejection
B cells (mature in bone marrow)	Circulation, spleen	Production of antibodies (immunoglobulins) to specific antigens
NK (natural killer) cells	Circulation	Cytotoxic; killing of tumor cells, fungi, viral-infected cells, and foreign tissue
Lymphoid Tissues		
Primary or central lymphoid structures	Bone marrow and thymus gland	Production of immune cells; sites for cell maturation
Secondary or peripheral lymphoid structures	Lymph nodes, spleen, tonsils, intestinal lymphoid tissue, lymphoid tissue in other organs	Sites for activation of immune cells by antigens

Figure 12–1 ■ The development and differentiation of leukocytes from hemocytoblasts.

during acute inflammation and infection. There are three types of granulocytes: neutrophils, eosinophils, and basophils.

Neutrophils, also called polymorphonuclear leukocytes (PMNs or polys), are the most plentiful of the granulocytes, constituting 55% to 70% of the total number of circulating leukocytes. Neutrophils are *phagocytic* cells, responsible for engulfing and destroying foreign agents, particularly bacteria and small particles. Neutrophils are the first phagocytic cells to arrive at the site of invasion, drawn by chemicals released by damaged tissue and invading organisms.

Neutrophils are produced in the bone marrow and released into the circulation when they mature. Segmented neutrophils (or segs) are mature forms, and usually account for about 55% of total leukocytes. *Bands* are immature neutrophils and usually comprise 5% of leukocytes. As neutrophils mature, their nucleus changes from round to kidney-bean-shaped (banded) and then the nucleus separates into small, attached segments, thus the designations "banded" versus "segmented" neutrophils. It takes about 10 days for a neutrophil to mature and be released into the circulation. Once released, neutrophils have a circulating half-life of 6 to 10 hours. They cannot replicate and must be replaced constantly to maintain adequate numbers in the circulation. They do not return to the bone marrow.

Eosinophils account for 1% to 4% of the total number of circulating leukocytes. They mature in the bone marrow in 3 to 6 days before being released into the circulation. Eosinophils have a circulating half-life of 30 minutes and a tissue half-life of 12 days. They too are phagocytic cells, but are less efficient at this process than neutrophils. Eosinophils are found in large numbers in the respiratory and gastrointestinal tracts, where they are thought to be responsible for protecting the body from parasitic worms, including tapeworms, flukes, pinworms, and hookworms. Eosinophils surround the parasite and release toxic enzymes from their cytoplasmic granules. The parasite, although too large to be phagocytized, is destroyed. Eosinophils are also involved in a hypersensitivity response, inactivating some of the inflammatory chemicals released during the inflammatory response.

Basophils constitute about 0.5% to 1% of the circulating leukocytes. These cells are not phagocytic. Granules within basophils contain proteins and chemicals such as heparin, histamine, bradykinin, serotonin, and a slow-reacting substance of anaphylaxis (leukotrienes). These substances are released into the bloodstream during an acute hypersensitivity reaction or stress response.

MONOCYTES, MACROPHAGES, AND DENDRITIC CELLS
Monocytes, macrophages, and dendritic cells are the mediators of immunity. They recognize foreign matter (from molecules to cells) and initiate immune responses. *Monocytes* are the largest

of the leukocytes and constitute 2% to 3% of circulating leukocytes. After their release from the bone marrow, monocytes circulate in the serum for 1 to 2 days. They then migrate to various tissues throughout the body, attaching themselves to the tissues, where they remain for months or even years until they are activated. Monocytes mature into **macrophages** after settling into the tissues. Once they have migrated and matured, macrophages are differentiated by the tissues in which they reside. *Histiocytes* are tissue macrophages in loose connective tissue, *Kupffer cells* are found in the liver, *alveolar macrophages* in the lungs, and *microglia* in the brain. Tissue macrophages are also found in the spleen, tonsils, lymph nodes, and bone marrow. Osteoclasts are bone resorbing phagocytes of the monocyte/macrophage lineage (Porth & Matfin, 2009). These cells release a chemical that causes calcium removal from osteocytes (mature bone cells) and digestion of the collagen fibers that make up bone matrix. Dendritic cells are star-shaped cells that originate in both the myeloid and the lymphoid cell lines. Langerhans cells are specialized dendritic cells in the skin. Monocytes, macrophages, and dendritic cells are antigen-presenting cells (APCs), which activate immune responses in both B and T lymphocytes.

Monocytes, macrophages, and dendritic cells are actively phagocytic, with the capacity to phagocytize large foreign particles and cell debris. Once they are in the tissue, macrophages can multiply to encapsulate and trap foreign matter that cannot be phagocytized. Dendritic cells have long processes that can capture antigens and migrate to lymphoid tissue. They serve as sentinels for antigens in most organs including the heart, lungs, liver, kidney, and gastrointestinal tract. Like neutrophils, macrophages are drawn to an inflamed area by chemicals released from damaged tissue, a process known as chemotaxis. Monocytes and macrophages activate the immune response against chronic infections such as tuberculosis, viral infections, and certain intracellular parasitic infections; dendritic cells activate T cells against cancer, assist B lymphocytes to produce antibodies, and downregulate the immune system (DeMeyer & Buchsel, 2005).

LYMPHOCYTES The **lymphocytes** account for 20% to 40% of circulating leukocytes. Lymphocytes are the principal effector and regulator cells of specific immune responses to protect the body from microorganisms, foreign tissue, and cell mutations or alterations. Through a process known as immune surveillance, lymphocytes monitor the body for cancerous cells and eliminate or destroy them.

Like other leukocytes, lymphocytes derive from the stem cells in the bone marrow (Figure 12–2 ■). Lymphocytes have "homing" patterns: They constantly circulate, then return to concentrate in lymphoid tissues (the lymph nodes, spleen, thymus, tonsils, Peyer's patches in the submucosa of the distal ileum, and the appendix).

The three types of lymphocytes are **T lymphocytes (T cells)**, **B lymphocytes (B cells)**, and **natural killer cells (NK cells** or **null cells)**. None of these cells acts independently. Their functions are closely interrelated. T cells mature in the thymus gland, whereas B cells complete their maturation in the bone marrow. T cells and B cells are integral to the specific immune response and are

Figure 12–2 ■ The development and differentiation of lymphocytes from the lymphoid stem cell (lymphoblasts).

discussed further in that section of this chapter. On contact with an antigen, B lymphocytes are activated and mature into either plasma cells, which secrete antibodies, or memory cells. On contact with APCs, T lymphocytes mature into active T_{helper} cells, cytotoxic T cells, or memory T cells. Memory cells stay inactive, sometimes for years, but activate immediately with subsequent exposure to the same antigen. They then proliferate rapidly, producing an intense immune response. Memory cells are responsible for providing acquired immunity.

NK cells are large, granular cells found in the spleen, lymph nodes, bone marrow, and blood. They constitute 15% of circulating lymphocytes. NK cells are part of the innate immune system, provide immune surveillance and resistance to infection, and they play an important role in the destruction of early malignant cells. Like B cells and T cells, NK cells are cytotoxic, but unlike T cells do not require connection with an APC to become activated and kill cancer cells, virus-infected cells, and cells infected with microbes (Porth & Matfin, 2009). Fortunately, NK cells are inhibited when contact is made with normal host cells.

ANTIGENS Substances the immune system recognizes as foreign or "nonself" are called **antigens**; they provoke a specific immune response when introduced into the body. Typically, antigens are large protein molecules, although polysaccharides, polypeptides, and nucleic acids may also be antigenic. Many antigens are proteins found on the cell membrane or cell wall of microorganisms or tissues such as transplanted tissue or organs, incompatible blood cells, vaccines, pollen, egg white, and insect or snake venom.

Complete antigens, known as immunogens, have two characteristics: (1) *immunogenicity* is the ability to stimulate a specific immune response and (2) *specific reactivity* is the stimulation of specific immune system components. When an antigen is encountered in the body, generation of an effective immune response involves two major groups of cells: lymphocytes and antigen-presenting cells. Dendritic cells are APCs; two specific types of dendritic cells develop from pluripotent stem cells in the bone marrow. DC1s arise from monocytes, myeloid-type immune cells, and DC2s derive from lymphocyte precursors (DeMeyer & Buchsel, 2005). DC1s activate T cells against cancer cells. DC2s assist B lymphocytes to produce antibodies and to downregulate the immune system (Kimball, 2005). Downregulation of the immune response is very important to avoid autoimmune diseases.

Antigen-presenting cells are recognized by a specific receptor on a lymphocyte, and an immune response is generated by the lymphocytes. Two separate but overlapping immune responses may occur, depending on the antigen itself and the type of immune cell activated by contact with the antigen. The B cell or humoral branch of the immune system mainly eliminates extracellular antigens such as bacteria, bacterial toxins, and free viruses through the production of **antibodies**, molecules that bind with the antigen and inactivate it. There are five classes of antibodies: IgG, IgA, IgM, IgD, and IgE. These proteins make up the **antibody-mediated (humoral) immune response**. Intracellular pathogens, such as viral-infected cells, cancer cells, and foreign tissue, activate T lymphocytes, which are the primary agents of the **cell-mediated (cellular) immune response**.

In this immune response, the lymphocytes themselves, in the form of helper T cells, cytotoxic T cells, and NK cells, inactivate the antigen, either directly or indirectly.

Lymphoid System

The *lymphoid system* consists of the lymph nodes, spleen, thymus, tonsils, lymphoid tissue scattered in connective tissues and mucosa, and the bone marrow. The thymus and bone marrow, in which T cells and B cells mature, are considered central lymphoid organs. The spleen, lymph nodes, tonsils, and other peripheral lymphoid tissue are peripheral lymphoid organs (Figure 12–3 ■). This system exists to recover proteins such as albumin for the vascular system and to protect the bloodstream from invading organisms. Cells of the immune system such as neutrophils, macrophages, and dendritic cells carry antigens from interstitial space to lymph nodes for immune surveillance in the lymphatic circulation. Unlike the vascular tree, which has tight epithelial junctions, lymphatic epithelium is replete with open junctions that promote lymphocyte access and effectively protect the bloodstream from antigen entry.

Lymph nodes, the most numerous elements of the lymphoid system, are small, round or bean-shaped encapsulated bodies that vary in size from 1 mm to 2 cm. Distributed throughout the body, lymph nodes generally occur in groups at the junction of the lymphatic vessels. They can be found in the neck, axillae, abdomen, and groin.

Lymph nodes filter foreign products or antigens from the lymph and house and support proliferation of lymphocytes and macrophages. Lymph, a clear, protein-containing fluid transported within lymph vessels, enters the node through afferent

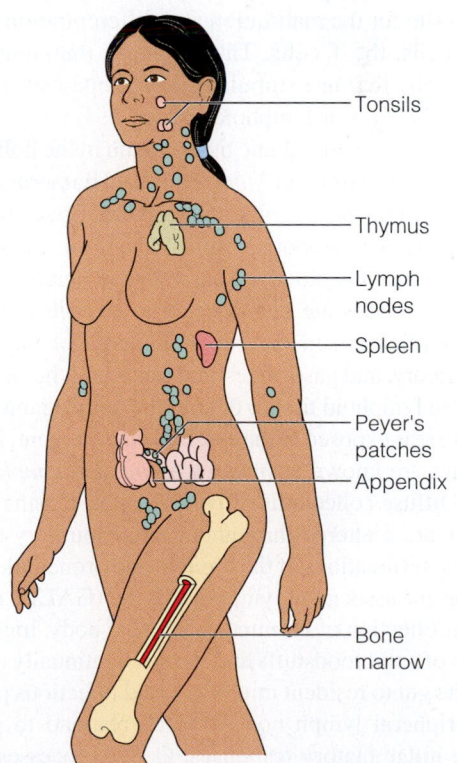

Figure 12–3 ■ The lymphoid system: the central organs of the thymus and bone marrow, and the peripheral organs, including the spleen, tonsils, lymph nodes, and Peyer's patches.

lymphatic vessels. Inside the node, the lymph flows through sinuses in the cortex of the lymph node where T and B lymphocytes and macrophages are abundant, then through sinuses of the medulla of the lymph node, which contains macrophages and plasma cells. The presence of a foreign antigen stimulates lymphocytes and macrophages to proliferate in the lymph nodes. Macrophages destroy the antigen by phagocytosis. Immune cells and lymph then leave the lymph node through efferent vessels. An abundant blood supply to the node also facilitates lymphocyte movement.

The *spleen* is the largest lymphoid organ in the body and the only lymphoid organ that can filter blood. The spleen is located in the upper left quadrant of the abdomen. The spleen has two kinds of tissue, white pulp and red pulp. White pulp is lymphoid tissue that serves as a site for lymphocyte proliferation and immune surveillance. B cells predominate in the white pulp. Blood filtration occurs in the red pulp. In blood-filled venous sinuses, phagocytic cells dispose of damaged or aged RBCs and platelets. Other debris and foreign matter, such as bacteria, viruses, and toxins, are also removed from the blood. The spleen also stores blood and the breakdown products of RBCs for future use. The spleen is not essential for life. If it is removed because of disease or trauma, the liver and the bone marrow assume its functions.

The *thymus gland* is located in the superior anterior mediastinal cavity beneath the sternum. It reaches its maximum size at puberty, then begins to atrophy slowly. By adulthood it is difficult to differentiate from surrounding adipose tissue even though it remains active. In the older adult, the vast majority of thymus tissue has been replaced by adipose and fibrous connective tissue. During fetal life and childhood, the thymus serves as a site for the maturation and differentiation of thymic lymphoid cells, the T cells. Thymosin, an immunoregulatory hormone of the thymus, stimulates lymphopoiesis, the formation of lymphocytes or lymphoid tissue.

Bone marrow is soft organic tissue found in the hollow cavity of the long bones, particularly the femur and humerus, as well as the flat bones of the pelvis, ribs, and sternum. Bone marrow produces and stores hematopoietic stem cells, from which all cellular components of the blood are derived (see Figure 12–1).

Lymphoid tissues are also located at key sites of potential invasion by microorganisms: the submucosa of the genitourinary, respiratory, and gastrointestinal tracts and the skin. Plasma cells in these lymphoid tissues defend the body against bacterial invasion at areas exposed to the external environment. In general, these tissues are known as *mucosa-associated lymphoid tissue* (MALT). Diffuse collections of lymphocytes, plasma cells, and phagocytes are scattered throughout the respiratory tract, concentrating at bifurcations of the bronchi and bronchioles. Peyer's patches, or gut-associated lymphoid tissue (GALT), comprises the largest collection of immune cells in the body. Ingestion and absorption of solid foodstuffs and liquids continually expose the lining of the gut to resident microflora and infectious pathogens. Unlike peripheral lymph nodes, which respond to pathogens with acute inflammatory responses, GALT processes common intestinal antigens without producing acute inflammation. Collections of immune cells make up the GALT. Intraepithelial lymphocytes fill the spaces between mucosal epithelial cells.

Beneath the basement membrane of gut epithelium lie abundant T cells and mature plasma cells, which are sources of IgA. Peyer's patches hold dense collections of lymphocytes in lymphoid nodules. As naïve B and T cells migrate through Peyer's patches, they are sensitized to specific antigens. In mesenteric lymph nodes these sensitized cells proliferate and circulate throughout the vascular tree where they produce secretory IgA. Secretory IgA coats mucosal cells and prevents attachment of intraluminal bacteria in the intestine, upper respiratory tract, the bronchi, mammary ducts, and salivary glands. Thus the GALT collection of immune cells effectively protects mucosa throughout the body that is exposed to resident and foreign pathogens.

Tonsils and adenoids protect the body from inhaled or ingested foreign agents. Skin-associated lymphoid tissue contains lymphocytes and dendritic cells such as Langerhans cells in the epidermis, which transport antigens to regional lymph nodes for destruction and development of specific immunity to the antigen.

Innate Immune Response

Innate immunity is the first line of defense. It is nonspecific and includes skin and mucosal barriers, vascular and cellular responses, and phagocytosis. Cells of the innate system include neutrophils, macrophages, and NK cells. NK cells indiscriminately kill pathogens but recognize self cells and leave them unharmed. Complement proteins and cytokines also function in the innate immune response.

Barrier protection is the body's defense against infection. Intact skin prevents invasion by external organisms. When the skin is damaged or lost (e.g., as a result of injury, surgery, or burns), infection is much more likely. The membranes lining inner surfaces of the body are protected by a barrier of mucus, which traps microorganisms and other foreign substances. These can then be removed by other protective mechanisms, such as ciliary movement or the washing action of tears or urine. In addition, many body fluids contain bactericidal substances that provide barrier protection. These include acid in gastric fluid, zinc in prostatic fluid, and lysozyme in tears, nasal secretions, saliva, and sweat (Porth & Matfin, 2009).

When these defenses are breached, the resulting tissue damage or foreign material entering the body induces inflammation. *Inflammation* is a response to injury that brings fluid, dissolved substances, and blood cells into the interstitial tissues where the invasion or damage has occurred. The response is called nonspecific because the same events occur regardless of cause of the inflammatory process. Through the inflammatory reaction, the invader is neutralized and eliminated, destroyed tissue removed, and the process of healing and repair initiated.

The inflammatory response has two stages: (1) a vascular response characterized by vasodilation and increased permeability of blood vessels, and (2) a cellular response. Phagocytosis sets the stage for healing (tissue repair).

Vascular Response

After tissue cells are damaged, local blood vessels briefly constrict. Vasodilation of the capillary arterioles and venules follows almost immediately as inflammatory mediators such as histamine and kinins are released from damaged tissue (Box 12–1).

BOX 12–1 Inflammatory Mediators

Many of the manifestations of inflammation are produced by *inflammatory mediators*, which are chemicals released as a result of immunologic processes or tissue injury or damage. These inflammatory mediators are broadly classified as follows:

- Vasoactive substances (e.g., histamine, prostaglandins, leukotrienes, and platelet-activating factor) produce smooth muscle constriction, postcapillary vasodilation, and increased capillary permeability.
- Chemotactic factors (e.g., complement fragments and chemokines) attract leukocytes to the damaged tissue.
- Plasma enzymes (proteases) activate the clotting cascade, plasminogen system, and complement system.
- Miscellaneous cell products (e.g., oxygen metabolites and lysosomal enzymes) damage surrounding tissue.

Increased blood flow causes vasocongestion at the injury site with resultant redness and heat. The congestion also increases local hydrostatic pressure. This, along with increased vessel permeability that results from chemical mediators, moves fluid out of the capillaries and into the interstitial spaces of the tissue. The escaping fluid, called fluid exudate, contains large amounts of protein. This protein increases osmotic pressure in the interstitial spaces, which draws water and causes local edema. Fluid exudate provides protection to the injured tissue by bringing certain nutrients needed for tissue healing, diluting bacterial toxins, and transporting cells needed for phagocytosis. Mild tissue damage such as a blister produces a *serous* exudate of primarily plasma fluid and a few proteins. With moderate to severe tissue damage, fluid exudate is *sanguineous* or *hemorrhagic*, containing large amounts of RBCs. A mixture of RBCs and serum is referred to as *serosanguineous* exudate. *Fibrinous* exudate forms a thick, sticky meshwork of fibrinogen, in effect "walling off" inflamed tissues and preventing the spread of infection (Porth, 2007). In more severe or acute inflammation, the fluid contains fibrin, RBCs, and dead and live bacteria. This type of exudate, called *purulent* exudate, has an odor and color characteristic of the bacteria present.

Many of the outward manifestations of inflammation result from vasoactive substances such as *histamine*, *serotonin*, and *leukotrienes* (formerly known as slow-reacting substance of anaphylaxis, or SRS-A). Stored in mast cells, basophils, and platelets, histamine is released when an injury occurs or with stimulation by the immune system. An important component of the early inflammatory response, histamine causes vasodilation and vascular permeability in the affected area. Histamine is also

a key factor in many hypersensitivity reactions. Serotonin is released from platelets and produces effects similar to those of histamine. The leukotrienes play a significant vasoactive role in the later stages of the inflammatory response.

Prostaglandins are chemotactic substances that draw leukocytes to the inflamed tissue. In addition, they play a vasoactive role and are pain and fever inducers. Aspirin and other non-steroidal anti-inflammatory drugs (NSAIDs) as well as the glucocorticoids inhibit prostaglandin synthesis, thereby reducing fever, pain, and inflammation.

Plasma factors such as Hageman factor activate the clotting cascade, plasminogen system (involved in the lysis of clots), and complement system. With activation of the clotting cascade, bacteria and other foreign substances are trapped in the area of tissue damage. Fibrin, which has vasoactive by-products, is also released. (∞ See Chapter 29 for a full description of the clotting process.) The complement system serves a chemotactic role and facilitates the phagocytic process.

Major chemical mediators of inflammation are summarized in Table 12–2.

The vascular response localizes invading bacteria and keeps them from spreading. Increased capillary permeability enhances the release of clotting factors such as fibrinogen, which converts to fibrin threads, entrapping the bacteria and walling them off from contact with the rest of the body.

Cellular Response

The cellular stage of the inflammatory process begins within less than an hour after the injury. This stage is marked by the margination and emigration of leukocytes into the damaged tissue, chemotaxis, and phagocytosis (Porth & Matfin, 2009).

As serous fluid escapes the capillaries, the viscosity of blood in the area increases and its flow becomes more sluggish. Leukocytes marginate, moving to the edges of the blood vessels, and begin to adhere to the capillary endothelium. This process is known as *pavementing*. After margination and pavementing, leukocytes emigrate from the blood vessel into the tissue spaces (Figure 12–4 ■). Within hours, millions of leukocytes emigrate into the area of inflammation.

Once leukocytes have emigrated, they are drawn to the damaged or inflamed tissues by chemotactic signals. Infectious agents, damaged tissues, and activated plasma substances such as complement fractions provide chemotaxic signals that attract an army of neutrophils, monocytes, and macrophages to the injury site.

TABLE 12–2 Major Chemical Mediators of Inflammation

FACTOR	SOURCE	EFFECT
Histamine	Mast cells, basophils, and platelets	Vasodilation and increased capillary permeability, producing tissue redness, warmth, and edema
Kinins (bradykinin and others)	Plasma protein factors	Histamine-like effects; chemotaxis and pain inducers
Prostaglandins	Metabolism of arachidonic acid from cell membranes	Histamine-like effects; chemotaxis, pain, and fever inducers
Leukotrienes	Arachidonic acid metabolism	Smooth muscle constriction (especially bronchoconstriction), increased vascular permeability, chemotaxis

A Leukocytes in circulation

B Margination and pavementing

C Emigration

Figure 12–4 ■ The process of leukocyte emigration at the site of inflammation. *A,* Normal blood flow with free movement of formed elements. *B,* As blood flow slows, leukocytes move toward the periphery of stream and begin to cling to capillary endothelium, a process known as margination and pavementing. *C,* Leukocytes emigrate from the vessel into inflamed tissues.

The number of neutrophils around the site increases to about 15,000 to 25,000/mm³, and they begin their role in phagocytosis within a few hours. Monocytes become transient macrophages to augment the activity of the fixed macrophages and dendritic cells; together they engulf dead cells, damaged tissue, nonfunctioning neutrophils, and invading bacteria.

Phagocytosis

Phagocytosis is a process by which a foreign agent or target cell is engulfed, destroyed, and digested. Neutrophils, macrophages, and dendritic cells, known as *phagocytes,* are the primary cells involved in phagocytosis. Once attracted to the inflammatory site, phagocytes select and engulf foreign material.

The following factors or processes help phagocytes differentiate foreign tissue from normal cells:

- *Smooth surface.* Normal tissue has a smooth surface that is resistant to phagocytosis, whereas the rough surface of a foreign agent or target cell promotes phagocytosis.

- *Surface charge.* Healthy body cells present an electronegative surface charge that repels phagocytes. Cellular debris and foreign agents, by contrast, have an electropositive charge that attracts them.

- *Opsonization.* This immune system process coats the surface of bacteria or target cells with a substance (an opsonin) as in the complement system (Box 12–2). Opsonization enables the phagocyte to bind tightly with the foreign tissue, facilitating phagocytosis (Figure 12–5A ■).

Phagocytes engulf the foreign agent or target cell by projecting pseudopodia ("false feet") in all directions around it (Figure 12–5B). This produces a chamber called a *phagosome* containing the antigen, which is ingested into the cytoplasm (Figure 12–5C). Once the phagosome has been engulfed, lysosomes fuse with the phagosome, killing any live organism and releasing digestive enzymes, which destroy the antigen (Figure 12–5D).

Phagocytes—in particular, neutrophils and macrophages—contain bactericidal agents that kill most of the bacteria they ingest before the bacteria can multiply and destroy the phagocyte itself. The phagocyte kills bacteria in a number of ways; for example, it alters the intracellular pH and produces bactericidal agents. Oxidizing agents, such as superoxide, hydrogen peroxide, and hydroxyl ions, are bactericidal. Two lysosomal substances that kill bacteria are lysozyme and phagocytin.

Some antigens, such as the tubercle bacterium, have coats or secrete substances that are resistant to lysosomal and bactericidal agents. To destroy such antigens, lysosomes release digestive enzymes into the phagosome. The lysosomes of neutrophils and macrophages contain an abundance of proteolytic

Figure 12–5 ■ The process of phagocytosis. *A,* Opsonization coats the surface of the bacterium with IgG (an antibody) and complement. *B,* The bacterium is bound to and engulfed by the phagocyte. *C,* The phagosome is ingested into the cytoplasm of the phagocyte. *D,* Lysosomes fuse with the phagosome, releasing digestive enzymes and destroying the antigen.

BOX 12–2 The Complement System

The *complement system* consists of approximately 20 complex plasma proteins that are activated by a tissue injury or antigen–antibody reaction. The complement system is involved in both innate and adaptive immune responses. Its activation results in the production of effector molecules that are involved in the processes of inflammation, phagocytosis, and cell lysis or destruction (Porth & Matfin, 2009). Specifically, complement activation leads to the following:

■ *Mediation of the inflammatory response.* When the complement system is activated, chemical mediators such as histamine are released from mast cells and basophils, leading to smooth muscle contraction, increased vascular permeability and edema, and the attraction of leukocytes.

■ *Opsonization (or coating) of microbes and antigen–antibody complexes to facilitate phagocytosis.*

■ *Alteration of the cell membrane or viral capsule.* When the cell surface is altered, a pore or channel is created for complement fluids and ions to enter the phagocytic cell and cause cell lysis and death. Bacteria and viruses are destroyed; certain normal cells, such as RBCs, platelets, and lymphocytes, that are damaged or old may also be destroyed through this process.

The complement system has three "arms," or pathways, of protein and enzyme reactions. The *classic pathway* is activated by antibody-containing immunoglobulins and other substances such as DNA and C-reactive protein. The *alternate* and *lectin pathways* do not use antibodies; are activated by tissue injury, polysaccharides, or enzymes; and are part of the innate immune system (Porth, 2007). When either pathway is activated, the result is mediation of the inflammatory process, attraction of phagocytes, facilitation of phagocytosis, and lysis of microbes.

(protein-destroying) enzymes that digest bacteria and other foreign protein components. The macrophage's lysosomes also contain lipases (fat-splitting enzymes) capable of digesting the thick lipid membranes of such bacteria as *Mycobacterium tuberculosis* and *Mycobacterium leprae*.

Once neutrophils have ingested toxic substances to their capacity, they in turn are killed. Neutrophils have the capacity to phagocytize 5 to 20 bacteria before they become inactive. Macrophages then digest the dead neutrophils. Monocytes or macrophages are capable of phagocytizing up to 100 bacteria. Because of their size, they can ingest larger particles than neutrophils can ingest, such as whole RBCs, necrotic tissue, cell fragments, malarial parasites, and dead neutrophils. Dendritic cells are also phagocytic and secrete Il-12, which is an important cytokine in the maturation of T_{helper} cells (Kimball, 2005). Macrophages have the ability to extrude (release) the toxic substances and lysosomal enzymes within their phagosomes. As a result, they can continue to function for months and even years.

Healing

During the initial inflammatory process, particulate matter, bacteria, damaged cells, and inflammatory exudate are removed by phagocytosis. This process, called *debridement*, prepares the wound for healing. Adequate nutrition is essential for inflammation and healing to proceed. Protein, glucose, and oxygen are needed by leukocytes for chemotaxis, phagocytosis, and intercellular killings. Persons with diabetes are at risk

for poor healing of wounds. Probable causes for this risk may be small vessel disease, which impairs microcirculation, and increased affinity for oxygen common to glycosylated hemoglobin. Oxygen circulation is impaired as well as release of oxygen to the cells.

The second phase of the healing process, known as *reconstruction*, may overlap the inflammatory phase. The ideal result of the healing process is *resolution*, the restoration of the original structure and function of the damaged tissue. Simple resolution occurs when there is no destruction of the normal tissue and the body is able to neutralize and remove the offending agent through the inflammatory process.

Resolution may also occur when the damaged tissue is capable of regeneration. The ability to regenerate, or replace lost *parenchyma* (functional tissue) with new, functional cells varies by tissue and cell type.

■ *Labile cells* continue to regenerate throughout life. These cells are found in tissues where there is a daily turnover of cells—namely, bone marrow and the epithelial cells of the skin, mucous membranes, cervix, gastrointestinal tract, and genitourinary tract.

■ *Stable cells* normally stop replicating when growth ceases, but are capable of regeneration when stimulated by an injury. Osteocytes (which are found in bone) and parenchymal cells of the kidneys, liver, and pancreas are stable cells.

■ *Permanent* or *fixed cells* are unable to regenerate. When these cells are destroyed, they are replaced by fibrous scar tissue. Nerve cells, skeletal muscle cells, and cardiac muscle cells are fixed cells (Porth & Matfin, 2009).

Researchers are searching for signaling molecules that will stimulate repair of permanent cells, allowing regeneration. Paralysis from spinal cord injury is often the stimulus for this research focus. When regeneration and complete resolution are not possible, healing occurs by replacement of the destroyed tissue with collagen scar tissue. This process is known as *repair*. Although tissue that has undergone repair lacks the physiologic function of the destroyed tissue, the scar fills the lesion and provides tensile tissue strength. The healing process is discussed further in ∞ Chapter 4.

Adaptive Immune Response

The introduction of antigens into the body causes a second, more specific reaction than the innate, nonspecific immune response. On the first exposure to an antigen, a change occurs in the host, resulting in a specific and rapid response following subsequent exposures. This specific response is known as the *adaptive immune response*.

The adaptive immune response to an antigen has the following distinctive properties:

■ The adaptive immune response typically is directed against materials recognized as foreign (i.e., from outside the body) and is not usually directed against the self (i.e., cells or structures produced by the body). This property is known as *self-recognition*.

■ The immune response is *specific*. It is initiated by and directed against particular antigens (such as a specific virus, bacterium, or transplanted tissue).

- Unlike a localized inflammatory response, the immune response is systemic. Immunity is generalized; it is not restricted to the initial site of infection or entry of foreign tissue.
- The immune response has memory. Repeated exposures to an antigen produce a more rapid response.

A patient whose immune system is able to identify antigens and effectively destroy or remove them is said to be **immunocompetent**. Health problems may occur when the immune response is altered (∞ see Chapter 13 for further discussion).

Antibody-Mediated Immune Response

The antibody-mediated (humoral) immune response is produced by B lymphocytes (B cells). B cells are constantly replaced through cell division and proliferation in the bone marrow. It is believed that B cells mature in the bone marrow and then migrate to the spleen to await activation. They normally constitute 10% to 15% of circulating lymphocytes.

B cells are activated by contact with an antigen and by T cells (discussed in the next section). Each B cell has receptor sites for a specific antigen or antigens. When the antigen is encountered, the activated B cell proliferates and differentiates into antibody-producing plasma cells and memory cells (Figure 12–6 ■). Plasma cells are short lived, lasting only about 1 day. While alive, however, they can produce thousands of antibody molecules per second. Memory cells retain antibody-producing information, allowing a rapid response if the antigen is again encountered.

An antibody is an **immunoglobulin (Ig)** molecule with the ability to bind to and inactivate a specific antigen. Immunoglobulins comprise the gamma globulin portion of the blood proteins. The immune system produces numerous antibodies, each active against a specific antigen. As mentioned earlier, antibodies fall into five classes of immunoglobulins: IgG, IgA, IgM, IgD, and IgE. Each has a slightly different structure and function. Their roles are summarized in Table 12–3.

Antibodies are Y-shaped molecules with two light and two heavy polypeptide chains (Figure 12–7 ■). The top portion of the Y, called the *Fab* or *antigen-binding fragment*, is chemically variable and specific to the antigen. The lower portion, the

Figure 12–6 ■ Antibody-mediated (humoral) immunity. On initial exposure to the antigen, B cells with appropriate receptor sites are activated to become plasma cells and produce antibodies or memory cells. This is known as the primary response. With subsequent exposures, memory cells respond rapidly with antibody production. This is known as the secondary response.

TABLE 12–3 Immunoglobulin Characteristics and Functions

CLASS	PERCENTAGE OF TOTAL	CHARACTERISTICS AND FUNCTION
IgG	75%	Most abundant Ig; also known as gamma globulin; found in blood, lymph, and intestines.
		Active against bacteria, bacterial toxins, and viruses.
		Activates complement and binds to macrophages.
		The only Ig to cross the placenta, providing immune protection to neonate.
IgA	10% to 15%	Found in saliva; tears; and bronchial, gastrointestinal, prostatic, and vaginal secretions, as well as blood and lymph.
		Provides local protection on exposed mucous membrane surfaces and potent antiviral activity by preventing binding of the virus to epithelial cells.
		Levels decrease during stress.
IgM	5% to 10%	Found in blood and lymph.
		First antibody produced with primary immune response.
		High concentrations early in infection, decreases within about a week.
		Mediates cytotoxic response and activates complement.
IgD	<1%	Found in blood, lymph, and surfaces of B cells.
		Exact function unknown; may be receptor-binding antigens to B-cell surface.
IgE	<0.1%	Found on mast cells and basophils.
		Involved in release of chemical mediators responsible for immediate hypersensitivity (allergic and anaphylactic) response and parasitic infections.

F_c, or *crystallized fragment*, is constant for its class of immunoglobulin and directs the biologic activity of the immunoglobulin (the manner in which it functions). For example, the lower portion of immunoglobulin molecules produced against hepatitis A and hepatitis B are the same (IgG), but the upper portion is different and specific to the virus.

The antibodies produced by B cells (see Figure 12–6) link with the antigen (Figure 12–8 ■) and inactivate it through one of the following processes:

- Promoting phagocytosis of the antigen by neutrophils
- Precipitation: combining with soluble antigens to form an insoluble complex or precipitate
- Neutralization: combining with a toxin to neutralize its effects; the antigen–antibody complex is then destroyed by the process of phagocytosis

- Lysis of the antigen cell membrane caused by combination with antibodies and complement proteins
- Agglutination (clumping) of antigens to form a noninvasive aggregate
- Opsonization: coating of the antigen with antibodies and complement, making them more susceptible to phagocytosis

The complete antibody-mediated response occurs in two phases. With initial exposure to an antigen, the primary response develops. B cells are activated to proliferate and begin producing antibodies. There is a latency period of 3 to 6 days before antibodies become detectable in the blood. Levels then continue to rise, peaking at 10 to 14 days after the initial exposure. With many illnesses (e.g., chickenpox), this peak correlates with recovery.

Figure 12–7 ■ An antibody molecule. The Fab section is unique, providing an antigen-specific binding site. The F_c section is common to each class of immunoglobulin (IgG, IgA, IgM, IgD, IgE).

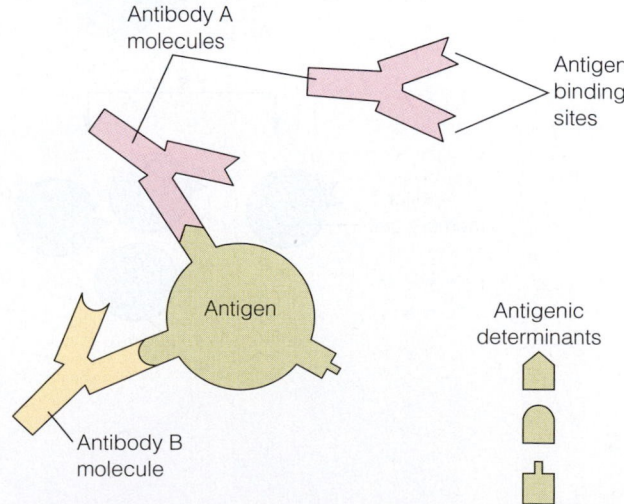

Figure 12–8 ■ Antigen–antibody binding. The unique Fab site on the antibody binds with specific receptor sites on the antigen. As shown, more than one kind of antibody may be produced to an antigen.

Subsequent exposure to the same antigen elicits a secondary response. Memory cells (see Figure 12–6) formed during the primary response stimulate the production of plasma cells, and an almost immediate rise in antibody levels occurs (Figure 12–9 ■). This rapid secondary response is the basis of acquired immunity and is instrumental in preventing disease. It is also the mechanism through which vaccines provide protection from disease.

Cell-Mediated Immune Response

Many antigens cannot stimulate the antibody-mediated response or are "hidden" from it because they live inside the body's cells (viruses and mycobacteria are examples of such antigens). The immune response providing protection against these antigens is the cell-mediated immune response, also called *cellular immunity*. T lymphocytes (T cells) initiate this type of immune response.

Approximately 70% to 80% of circulating lymphocytes are T cells. T cells migrate to the thymus during fetal and early life, establishing the lifetime pool of cells. T cells have a life span measured in years, maintaining their numbers through proliferation, primarily in the lymph nodes. T cells are much more complex than B cells. There are two major classes of T cells, *effector cells* and *regulator cells*. The main effector T cell is the *cytotoxic cell*, also called the *killer T cell*. Regulator T cells are further classified into two groups: *helper T cells* and *suppressor T cells*. T cells are antigen specific; that is, each subset is activated by a particular antigen. The antigens that activate T cells must be presented on another cell surface, such as pieces of virus presented on the surface of an

Figure 12–9 ■ Antibody production in the primary and secondary responses of the antibody-mediated immune response. Note the more rapid and effective production following subsequent exposure.

infected cell, or the histocompatibility locus antigen on a cell of transplanted tissue. When activated, T cells divide and proliferate, forming antigen-specific *clones* (Figure 12–10 ■). A clone is an exact copy of another cell.

Cytotoxic T cells bind with cell surface antigens on virus-infected or foreign cells. Killer T cells destroy the identified cell by combining with it and then either destroying its cell membrane or releasing cytotoxic substances into the cell. They are vital in the control of viral and bacterial infections.

Regulator T cells play a key role in controlling the immune response. The majority of regulator T cells are helper T cells. They stimulate the proliferation of other T cells, amplify the cytotoxic activity of killer T cells, and activate B cells to proliferate

Figure 12–10 ■ Cellular immune response. *A,* An infected cell, abnormal cell, or phagocyte presents antigen on its surface that binds with a receptor site on a killer T cell or a helper T cell. The killer T cell is activated to proliferate into memory cells or mature cytotoxic cells. *B,* The helper T cell is activated to augment the cytotoxic response and stimulate the antibody-mediated immune response.

and differentiate. They interact directly with B cells to promote their multiplication and conversion into plasma cells capable of producing antibodies. The other regulatory T-cell group, suppressor T cells, provides negative feedback, making the immune response a self-limiting process. Suppressor T cells release lymphokines, which inhibit the activity of other T cells and B cells.

On activation, both effector and regulator T cells synthesize and release lymphokines, a type of soluble protein. Lymphokines are a subgroup of nonspecific defense mechanisms known as **cytokines** (Box 12–3). Lymphokines secreted by cytotoxic and helper T cells are important in amplifying the immune response and the inflammatory response. They stimulate the following:

- B cells to become plasma cells and produce antibodies
- Macrophages to become activated macrophages (the most aggressive phagocyte)
- Proliferation of killer T cells

Although T cells can be activated only by specific antigens, much of the resulting effect is nonspecific—in other words, an enhanced inflammatory response. Like the antibody-mediated response, the cell-mediated response has memory. Subsequent exposures to an antigen result in a more rapid and effective inflammatory response and more effective phagocytosis by macrophages. This memory provides the basis for skin testing. A patient previously exposed to tuberculosis, for example, develops a more pronounced inflammatory response when minute amounts are injected under the skin.

BOX 12–3 Cytokines

Cytokines are hormone-like polypeptides produced primarily by cells of the immune system. Cytokines are also produced in small quantities in many different tissues throughout the body. Cytokines act as messengers of the immune system, facilitating communication between the cells to adjust or vary the inflammatory reaction or to initiate immune cell proliferation and differentiation. Cytokines are an essential component of an adequate immune response. The major cytokines and their functions are summarized in Table 12–4.

The inflammatory cytokines contribute to sickness behaviors. Patients respond to increases in these chemicals with increased sleep, seeking warmth, and reduced energy output to obtain and consume food or perform grooming activities. These are considered adaptive responses to illness; interventions to reduce or eliminate the production of certain cytokines are common. Aspirin or NSAIDs to reduce pain and fever are commonly used. Because some cytokines cross the blood–brain barrier, their increase may explain depression and anxiety experienced during illness. Prevention or limitation of these effects by prophylactic antidepressant medication may improve quality of life for patients receiving biologic therapy (cytokines such as Interleukin-2) as part of their treatment for rheumatoid arthritis, Crohn's disease, or cancer (Myers, 2008).

Interferons are a class of cytokine with broad antiviral and anticancer effects. A number of different forms of interferon exist, broadly grouped as alpha, beta, and gamma interferons. Interferon is synthesized by cells infected with a virus and secreted into extracellular fluid. It then binds to specific receptors on uninfected neighboring cells, protecting them from infection. The spread of the virus is thus inhibited, and recovery from infection enhanced. It appears that interferons also moderate the activity of NK cells and may be involved in preventing the spread of abnormal malignant cells.

The Patient with Natural or Acquired Immunity

Immunity refers to the protection of the body from disease. Immunity to disease may be either natural or acquired, active or passive.

Immunity develops from the activation of the body's immune response. Depending on the antigen, antibody-mediated or cell-mediated responses are activated. The immune response typically involves components of both. In the *immunocompetent* (having an immune system capable of responding to pathogens and tissue damage) patient, these responses inactivate and remove the antigen, allowing recovery to occur or preventing the development of disease. Patients with suppressed or impaired immune function are more susceptible to disease and require protection from exposure to environmental elements. Isolation techniques are employed to prevent the spread of disease and to protect immune-suppressed patients.

Pathophysiology

The processes of antibody-mediated and cell-mediated immunity result in the development of **acquired immunity** or **active immunity**. Active immunity occurs when the body produces antibodies or develops immune lymphocytes against specific antigens. Memory cells, which can produce an immediate immune response on re-exposure to the antigen, provide long-term immunity.

Active immunity can be naturally acquired, resulting from contact with the disease-producing antigen and subsequent development of the disease. Naturally acquired immunity is common for diseases such as chickenpox and hepatitis A, making the risk of developing the disease a second time very low.

For many diseases, the potential consequences of a single disease episode on the individual and society make prevention desirable, especially for highly contagious diseases capable of causing epidemics. In these instances, immunization or vaccination is used to provide artificially acquired immunity. The purpose of vaccination is to establish adequate levels of antibody and/or memory cells to provide effective immunity. Vaccination introduces the disease-producing antigen into the body in a manner that will stimulate the immune system to form antibodies and memory cells but will not produce disease. Vaccines may be made of killed organisms or of live organisms that have been *attenuated* or modified to reduce their disease-producing capability. Typhoid is an example of a killed organism vaccine; measles-mumps-rubella (MMR) vaccine, by contrast, is made from attenuated organisms. Many newer vaccines use subunits of the antigen; these are portions of the organism that have antigenic properties but are unable to produce disease.

Passive immunity provides temporary protection against disease-producing antigens. Passive immunity is provided by antibodies produced by other people or animals. These acquired antibodies are used up; they either combine with the antigen or are naturally degraded by the body, and their protection is gradually lost. Naturally acquired passive immunity is provided by the transfer of maternal antibodies via the placenta and breast milk to the infant. Rabies human immune

TABLE 12–4 Major Cytokines and Their Functions

CYTOKINE	WHERE PRODUCED	PRIMARY FUNCTIONS
Interleukin-1 (IL-1)	Monocytes, macrophages, and dendritic cells	Activates T and B cells
		Induces fever and tissue catabolism
		Enhances NK activity
		Attracts neutrophils, macrophages, and lymphocytes
		Stimulates bone marrow and endothelial cell growth, collagen, and collagenases
Interleukin-2 (IL-2)	Helper T cells	Stimulates T and B cell proliferation; aids in discriminating between self and nonself
		Activates killer T and NK cells
Interleukin-3 (IL-3)	T cells	Stimulates growth and differentiation of bone marrow stem cells
Interleukin-4 (IL-4)		Stimulates proliferation of T cells
		Increases IgE secretion by B cells
Interleukin-5 (IL-5)	T cells and activated mast cells	Promotes differentiation of B cells and eosinophils
		Stimulates production of IgA
Interleukin-6	T cells and macrophages	Pro-inflammatory and anti-inflammatory cytokine
		Induces fever
Interleukin-8	Macrophages	Mediator of the innate immune response
		Induces fever
		Angiogenic (stimulates vessel formation)
Gamma interferon	T and NK cells	Stimulates phagocytosis by neutrophils and macrocytes
		Activates NK cells
		Augments B cell proliferation, enhancing both cellular and humoral immune responses
Alpha and beta interferons	Virus-infected cells; macrophages	Activate macrophages and endothelial cells; β interferon induces fever
		Augment NK cell activity
		Act at gene level to protect neighboring cells from invasion by intracellular parasites, such as viruses, rickettsia, malaria
Macrophage inflammatory proteins (MIP-1-4CC)	Macrophages, dendritic cells, and lymphocytes	Chemokines (CC), which are small cytokines
		Promote inflammatory response, chemotaxis, and homeostasis (control migration of cells in maintenance and development)
Tumor necrosis factor (TNF)	Activated macrophages, T cells, and NK cells	Major chemical mediator of inflammatory response
		Stimulates T-cell activation, antibody production, and accumulation of leukocytes at inflammatory site
		Directly cytotoxic to some tumor cells
		Induces fever

globulin and hepatitis B immune globulin (HBIG) are examples of immunizations used to provide artificially acquired passive immunity. The types of active and passive immunity are summarized in Table 12–5.

Interdisciplinary Care

Collaborative care focuses primarily on assessing the patient's immune status and ensuring acquired immunity to prevent disease.

Diagnosis

A number of diagnostic tests can be performed to assess the patient's immune status.

- *Serum protein* measures the total protein in the blood, including albumin and globulins. Normal total protein levels for the adult are 6 to 8 g/dL; albumin is approximately 60% (3.2 to 4.5 g/dL) of the total serum protein, and globulins are normally 2.3 to 3.4 g/dL. Total protein levels, albumin,

and globulin are decreased in malnutrition and liver disease. Decreased globulin levels are noted with immunologic deficiencies.

- *Protein electrophoresis* analyzes protein content especially for albumin and gamma globulin and is used to assess immune function. Gamma globulins subjected to further electrophoresis separate into immunoglobulins: IgA, IgD, IgE, IgG, and IgM (see Table 12–2). Analysis of specific levels of each provides clues about the immune status of the patient. IgG levels are increased during acute infection. Decreased levels of IgG, IgA, and IgM are found in malignancies.

- *Antibody testing* is ordered to determine if a patient has developed antibodies in response to an infection or immunization. Antibodies for hepatitis, HIV, rubella, toxoplasmosis, and *Treponema pallidum* (the organism causing syphilis) can be identified. An elevated titer for hepatitis and rubella indicates immunity. For the other disorders and hepatitis, it may also be used to determine if the patient has the disease.

TABLE 12–5 Types of Acquired Immunity

TYPE OF IMMUNITY		HOW DEVELOPED	EXAMPLES
Active Immunity	Natural	Acquired by infection with an antigen, resulting in the production of antibodies	Chickenpox, hepatitis A
	Artificial	Acquired by immunization with an antigen, such as attenuated live virus vaccine	MMR, polio, DPT, hepatitis B vaccines
Passive Immunity	Natural	Acquired by transfer of maternal antibodies to the fetus or neonate via the placenta or breast milk	Neonate initially protected against MMR if mother immune
	Artificial	Acquired by administration of antibodies or antitoxins in immune globulin	Gamma globulin injection following hepatitis A exposure

■ *Skin testing* can assess cell-mediated immunity. A known antigen such as streptokinase, tuberculin purified protein derivative (PPD), or candida is injected intradermally. The site is then observed for induration and erythema, which typically peaks at 24 to 48 hours. An induration of at least 10 mm in diameter is a positive reaction indicating previous exposure and sensitization to the antigen. (∞ See Chapter 13 for further information on skin testing for hypersensitivity reactions.) No reaction, or **anergy**, indicates depressed cell-mediated immunity.

Immunizations

Vaccines are suspensions of whole or fractionated bacteria or viruses that have been treated to make them nonpathogenic. Vaccines are given to induce an immune response and subsequent immunity. Although vaccine development has been a major factor in improving public health, no vaccine is completely effective or entirely safe. Table 12–6 outlines the vaccines recommended for the adult patient to maintain optimal health and immune status (CDC, 2009).

Adults born before 1957 are generally considered to be immune to measles, mumps, and rubella by prior infection. For persons born after 1957 whose immunologic status is unclear or who are at significant risk of exposure to these diseases (e.g., persons entering healthcare careers), reimmunization is recommended by the CDC (Centers for Disease Control and Prevention). Adults who only received one dose of varicella (chickenpox) vaccine should receive a second dose. Adults aged 60 and older should receive zoster vaccine regardless of history of chickenpox or herpes zoster (shingles).

Tetanus and diphtheria (Td) toxoids are combined in a single immunization. The vaccine stimulates active immunity by inducing the production of antibodies and antitoxins. After an initial series of three immunizations, a booster injection is recommended every 10 years to maintain protection. Older patients, particularly those who never entered the workforce (e.g., older female adults), may have never received the initial series of Td vaccine. A resurgence of active cases of pertussis among adults and children has led the CDC to recommend that all adults receive one dose of tetanus/diphtheria/pertussis (Tdap) vaccine.

Hepatitis B (HB) vaccine is given as a series of three immunizations to promote active immunity to hepatitis B. It is mandated by the Occupational Health and Safety Administration (OSHA) for healthcare workers. High-risk populations include intravenous drug users, sexual partners of infected individuals, patients on hemodialysis, prison guards, and athletic coaches.

Influenza vaccine is recommended for persons at high risk for serious sequelae of influenza, including older adults, persons with lung disease or other chronic illness, and immunosuppressed individuals. The antigenic strain included in the influenza vaccine varies each year according to the predicted predominant strains affecting the population. Yearly reimmunization is therefore required. Pneumococcal vaccine is generally recommended for the same populations as influenza vaccine. A single dose of this vaccine confers lifetime immunity, although repeating immunization every 6 years may be considered for high-risk patients (including smokers and those with asthma). Pneumococcal vaccine for all senior citizens is a U.S. public health and Medicare goal. The purpose of immunization is to prevent respiratory infections and hospitalizations.

Human papillomavirus (HPV) vaccine has been shown to significantly reduce the risk for cervical cancer. HPV is recommended for all previously unvaccinated women through age 26 years.

In addition to routine immunizations, people traveling outside the United States and Canada should receive vaccines against diseases that are endemic in certain regions of the world.

Other immunologic substances may be administered as indicated. Immune globulins provide passive immunity as protection against a known or potential exposure to an antigen. Standard immune globulin is given to household contacts of patients with hepatitis A and persons traveling to areas in which it is endemic. HBIG contains higher titers of antibody to hepatitis B virus and is used for persons exposed by blood or sexual contact. Following confirmed or suspected contact with a pathogen, selected vaccines may be administered to stimulate an immediate immune response.

For most vaccines, a sensitivity test should be performed prior to administration to detect sensitivity to substances such as horse serum or eggs. The substance is injected intradermally; if after 20 minutes there is no evidence of a reaction, the selected vaccine can be administered.

Moderate to severe local reactions may occur following administration of an immunization. Common reactions include redness, swelling, tenderness, and muscle ache. Administering the vaccine in the dominant arm of the patient helps minimize local reactions because use and movement of the arm facilitates absorption of the solution. Applying heat to the site is also beneficial. Occasionally local ulcerations occur; when they do, warm, wet pack, or sterile wet-to-dry dressings may be prescribed.

TABLE 12–6 Recommended Immunizations for Adults

VACCINE	TYPE	DOSE	INDICATIONS	PRECAUTIONS AND NURSING IMPLICATIONS
Human papilloma virus (HPV)	Not a live virus	0.5 mL IM	Prior to exposure to HPV through sexual activity.	3 doses for females ≤ 26 years; IM in deltoid.
Measles-mumps-rubella (MMR)	Live virus	0.5 mL SC	All adults born after 1956, particularly those who are at risk for infection, such as college students and military recruits. Measles and mumps vaccination particularly recommended for males without history of previous infection; rubella vaccination recommended for all seronegative females.	As a live virus vaccine, should not be administered to pregnant women or immunocompromised patients. Do not administer to patients with a history of anaphylactic reaction to egg protein or neomycin. Give SC in fatty tissue over triceps.
Tetanus and diphtheria toxoids (Td); pertussis (Tdap)	Inactivated toxins	0.5 mL IM	Initial series of three injections (two doses, 4 to 6 weeks apart; third dose 6 to 12 months after dose 2) if never immunized; booster every 10 years; following a major or contaminated wound if more than 5 years since last booster. Replace one booster with Tdap.	Do not give in first trimester of pregnancy or to patients with a history of anaphylactic reaction to horse serum; administer deep IM in deltoid of dominant arm.
Hepatitis A		1 mL IM	Persons with liver disease or who receive clotting factors; travel to areas with high endemicity; illicit drug use or men who have sex with men.	Give IM in deltoid.
Hepatitis B (HB)	Inactive viral antigen	1.0 mL IM	Series of three doses: initial and at 1 and 6 months. Recommended for anyone at risk for exposure and for postexposure prophylaxis.	Use with caution in pregnant or lactating females, older patients, and patients with active infection; have epinephrine 1:1000 available on unit in case of anaphylaxis and laryngospasm.
Influenza	Inactivated virus or viral components	0.5 mL IM	Yearly for all patients over age 65 and those at risk for complications, including debilitated patients and patients with chronic disease.	Do not administer to acutely ill patients or patients with history of anaphylactic reaction to egg protein.
Pneumococcal	Bacterial polysaccharides	0.5 mL IM or SC	One dose for patients over age 65 and those at risk for pneumococcal pneumonia, including patients with chronic lung disease or other chronic diseases.	Do not administer to pregnant women.
Herpes zoster (shingles)		0.65 mL SC	Adults ≥ 60 years including those who report having had shingles.	Give in fatty tissue over triceps. Do not administer during pregnancy, immunocompromised, or HIV-infected persons.
Meningococcal vaccine (Menactra©)		0.5 mL IM	College students living in dormitories and military recruits.	Give in deltoid muscle; persons previously diagnosed with Guillain-Barré syndrome should not receive this vaccine.

⚕ Nursing Care

Maintaining a population that is fully immunized against common, potentially epidemic, and devastating diseases is a major public health task for nursing. Nurses not only recommend and administer vaccines to individual patients and their families, but also plan and implement preventive care for whole communities.

Although this process may appear to be straightforward, multiple issues affect society's ability to immunize the entire population. For some people, for example, religious beliefs may preclude the use of immunizations to prevent disease.

Also, people who are not citizens and the medically indigent population have difficulty accessing immunization services. Lack of immunization not only puts the individual at increased risk for infectious disease, but also increases the cost of medical services and the possibility of exposing immunocompromised people to disease.

Clinically important medical events including fever, injection-site hypersensitivity, unspecified rash, and injection-site edema that occur after vaccination should be reported to the Vaccine Adverse Event Reporting System (VAERS) by calling 1-800-822-7967 or by using the VAERS website. This report needs to be made even if the reporting person is not certain the event was caused by the vaccine. Approximately 14% of all reports describe serious adverse events, including life-threatening illness, hospitalization or prolongation of hospitalization, permanent disability, or death (Stokowski, 2008).

Health Promotion

In the public health setting, the nurse looks at the immunization needs and illness risk for an entire community. Communities include not only cities and localities but also groups of people, such as college populations and employees in a workplace. Public education needs may be met through presentations to groups of people, feature articles in newspapers and other local publications, advertising, radio presentations and public service announcements, and one-to-one discussion and teaching.

Assessment

Collect the following data through the health history and physical examination. Further focused assessments are described with nursing interventions in the next section.

- *Health history:* Age, medication use (corticosteroids and antibiotics) and blood transfusion, nutrition, known allergies, pregnancy status, infection, immunizations, autoimmune

disorders, chronic diseases such as asthma, diabetes mellitus, cancer, smoking history.
- *Physical assessment:* Skin lesions or rashes, breath sounds, respiratory rate.

Nursing Diagnoses and Interventions

Nursing care focuses on preventing injury from the immunization and educating the patient. See the accompanying Case Study & Nursing Care Plan.

Health-Seeking Behaviors: Immunization

For individual patients and their families, nurses promote immunocompetence by assessing immune status, recommending appropriate immunizations, and administering vaccines as ordered or indicated. Once a person reaches adulthood, routine immunizations often become a neglected part of health care.

- Determine knowledge level, understanding, attitudes, and religious beliefs about immunization. *This provides a basis for further education and determines if religious beliefs may contraindicate immunization.*
- Discuss the value and reasons for recommended immunizations. *Understanding promotes adherence.*

CASE STUDY & NURSING CARE PLAN   A Patient with Acquired Immunity

Terry Adams is a 48-year-old executive who is planning a trip to central Africa. In preparation, he contacts his local healthcare provider to obtain the necessary immunizations. Jane Wong, the registered nurse in the clinic, obtains a nursing history of Mr. Adams.

ASSESSMENT

Mr. Adams's history reveals that he has always been very healthy and active, apart from a mild case of asthma. As an adult, he has had little problem with his asthma "except for those rare occasions on which I am dumb enough to smoke more than one cigarette!" He is divorced and is not currently in a continuing relationship. He has two grown daughters with whom his relationship is good. Since contracting hepatitis A several years ago, he drinks alcohol only rarely, and never more than one or two drinks at any one time. He confesses to little organized exercise but plays golf two or three times a week and states that he is such a hyperactive workaholic that he rarely sits for any length of time. Mr. Adams has not seen a physician since recovering from the hepatitis and is unsure when he last received any immunizations. He does not know if he had all recommended childhood immunizations, but says his mother was "pretty conscientious" about health checkups. His physical examination reveals an alert and healthy individual with no abnormalities noted. His vital signs are as follows: T 97.4°F, P 64, R 14, and BP 142/82.

The physician orders the following immunizations for Mr. Adams:
- Measles-mumps-rubella (MMR)
- Combined tetanus and diphtheria toxoids with pertussis (Tdap)
- Yellow fever vaccine
- Typhoid vaccine
- Meningococcal meningitis vaccine

DIAGNOSES

- *Health-Seeking Behaviors:* Immunization related to impending international travel
- *Ineffective Health Maintenance* related to apparent lapse in immunization status
- *Risk for Injury* related to adverse response to immunization

EXPECTED OUTCOMES

- Obtain necessary immunizations.
- Verbalize a schedule for maintaining up-to-date immunization status.
- Experience no significant adverse effects from immunization.

PLANNING AND IMPLEMENTATION

- Administer MMR, Tdap, and meningococcal meningitis vaccines prior to discharge from clinic.
- Observe closely for 30 minutes following immunization for potential adverse responses.
- Schedule return visit in 1 week for typhoid vaccine.
- Provide referral to a registered vaccination center for yellow fever vaccine and documentation of vaccination.
- Provide instructions for comfort measures to relieve local and systemic adverse effects of vaccines. Provide written instructions on manifestations that should be reported to the physician.
- Document immunizations on a permanent record at the clinic and for the patient.

EVALUATION

Mr. Adams completes his prescribed immunizations without major adverse effects, although he does complain of fever, malaise, and general achiness for several days following the typhoid vaccination. His trip to Africa is successful, and he returns to the United States without contracting any infectious diseases.

CRITICAL THINKING IN THE NURSING PROCESS

1. Explain why it is important for adults to continue receiving immunizations throughout their life span.
2. If a patient says to you, "I don't believe in immunizations. I hear they are dangerous," how would you respond?
3. What manifestations would cause a patient to contact the primary caregiver after receiving an immunization? What is the rationale for the need to do this?

See Evaluating Your Response in Appendix C.

- Reinforce positive health-seeking behaviors. *This will help promote future health maintenance activities.*
- Using recommended immunization schedules, develop a plan to attain optimal immunization status. *Adherence with recommended schedules for immunization is important in preventing disease and disability.*
- Do not administer influenza vaccine if the patient is allergic to eggs, or tetanus antitoxin if sensitive to horse serum. *Vaccines prepared from chicken or duck embryos are contraindicated in patients who are allergic to eggs. Tetanus antitoxin is prepared from horse serum. Both will cause a severe allergic reaction.*
- Withhold administration of active immunologic products in the presence of an upper respiratory infection or other infection. *Active immunizations can cause a greater inflammatory reaction in the presence of infections.*
- Do not administer oral polio vaccine, MMR, or any live virus vaccine to immunosuppressed patients or to patients who are in close household contact with an immunosuppressed person. *Live virus vaccines can cause disease in the immunosuppressed patient. The virus may be transmitted from close household contacts during the initial postvaccination period.*
- Do not administer vaccines such as MMR, pneumococcal, or varicella to women who are pregnant. *Although the risk to the developing fetus is greatest during the first trimester, these vaccines are avoided throughout pregnancy.*
- Do not administer live attenuated virus vaccines and passive immunizations such as gamma globulin simultaneously. *Passive antibodies interfere with the response of the live attenuated virus.*
- Prior to administering prescribed vaccine, check the expiration date and manufacturer's instructions. *Outdated vaccines cannot provide adequate immunization protection. Certain injection sites have better absorption than others.*
- Keep epinephrine 1:1000 readily available for subcutaneous injection when administering immunizations. *Epinephrine causes vasoconstriction and reduces laryngospasm; in acute anaphylaxis, it can be lifesaving.*

> **SAFETY ALERT**
> Observe the patient for 20 to 30 minutes following vaccine administration to monitor for possible adverse reactions.

Helpful resources include state and county health departments, the CDC, and the National Institute of Allergy and Infectious Diseases.

Normal Immune Responses

The Patient with Tissue Inflammation

Inflammation is a nonspecific response to injury that serves to destroy, dilute, or contain the injurious agent or damaged tissue. Inflammation may be either acute or chronic. Acute inflammation is a short-term reaction of the body to all types of tissue damage. It is immediate and aimed at protecting the body and preventing further invasion or injury. Acute inflammation usually lasts less than 1 to 2 weeks. Once the injurious agent is removed, the inflammation subsides. Healing with tissue repair or scar formation occurs, and the body functions in normal or near-normal capacity.

Chronic inflammation is slower in onset and may not have an acute phase. Its clinical manifestations occur over months or years. It involves cell proliferation and is debilitating, with long-term adverse effects. There is increased cellular exudate, necrosis, fibrosis, and sometimes tissue scarring, resulting in severe tissue damage.

Pathophysiology and Manifestations

The tissue damage that evokes an inflammatory response may be caused by specific or nonspecific agents. These agents may be *exogenous*, from outside the body, or *endogenous*, from within the body. Causes of inflammation include the following:

- Mechanical injuries, such as cuts or surgical incisions
- Physical damage, such as burns
- Chemical injury from toxins or poisons
- Microorganisms, such as bacteria, viruses, or fungi
- Extremes of heat or cold
- Immunologic responses, such as hypersensitivity reactions
- Ischemic damage or trauma, such as a stroke or myocardial infarction

Acute Inflammation

Regardless of the cause, location, or extent of the injury, the acute inflammatory response follows the previously outlined sequence of vascular response, cellular and phagocytic response, and healing.

Many of the manifestations of inflammation are produced by inflammatory mediators such as histamine and prostaglandins released when tissue is damaged (see Box 12–1). The primary manifestations of inflammation include the following:

- Erythema (redness)
- Local heat caused by the increased blood flow to the injured area (hyperemia)
- Swelling due to accumulated fluid at the site
- Pain from tissue swelling and chemical irritation of nerve endings
- Loss of function caused by the swelling and pain

The degree of functional loss depends on the location and extent of the injury. With increased tissue damage, more fluid exudate is formed, resulting in increased swelling, pain, and functional impairment. Pain may be immediate or delayed. Prostaglandins intensify and prolong the pain. Kinins cause irritation to the nerve endings and contribute to the pain sensation.

Dead neutrophils, necrotic tissue, and (if the tissue is infected) digested bacteria accumulate as a result of inflammation and phagocytosis, forming *pus*. Pus usually forms and remains until after the infection subsides. Pus may push itself to the surface of the body or become internalized. In the latter case, pus is gradually autolyzed (self-digested) by enzymes over a period of days. The end product is then absorbed by the body. On occasion, pus may remain after the infection is resolved. Pockets of pus, called abscesses, may need to be artificially drained with a procedure called *incision and drainage (I&D)*.

Ectopic calcifications are another possible result of residual collections of pus.

Systemic responses to inflammation include an increase in the size of lymph nodes due to the proliferation of macrophages within the nodes in response to microorganisms in the lymph. Enlarged lymph nodes are usually noted in the groin, axillae, and neck. Fever, often precipitated by inflammatory mediators or bacterial toxins, inhibits the growth of many microorganisms and increases tissue repair functions. Loss of appetite and fatigue may occur in the effort to conserve energy during the inflammatory process. Leukocytosis occurs with increased WBC production to support inflammation and phagocytosis.

Chronic Inflammation

Whereas acute inflammation is a self-limiting process lasting less than 2 weeks, chronic inflammation tends to be self-perpetuating, lasting weeks to months or years. Chronic inflammation may develop when the acute inflammatory process has been ineffective in removing the offending agent. For example, mycobacteria have cell walls with high lipid and wax content, making them resistant to phagocytosis. Chronic inflammation and granuloma formation is common with *Mycobacterium tuberculosis* infection. Persistent irritation by chemicals, particulate matter, or physical irritants such as talc, asbestos, or silica may also result in chronic inflammation.

The chronic inflammatory process is characterized by a dense infiltration of the site by lymphocytes and macrophages. The macrophages mass or coalesce to form a multinucleated giant cell surrounded by lymphocytes, in a lesion called a *granuloma*. The granuloma is effective in walling off the offending agent, isolating it from the rest of the body; however, the infectious agent or offending irritant may not be destroyed and can survive within the granuloma for a long period of time. The granuloma formed in tuberculosis is called a tubercle. *M. tuberculosis* can survive for many years within the tubercle, emerging when the patient's immune system is no longer able to contain it. Rheumatoid arthritis is another condition marked by chronic inflammation. Inflammation in the joint capsule makes movement of the joint painful. The capsule is enlarged by inflammatory exudates, which cause stretching of the capsule.

Complications

Inflammation and wound healing are highly metabolic processes that may be affected by a number of factors. Without adequate nutrition, blood supply, and oxygenation, tissues cannot effectively complete the process. Impaired inflammatory and immune processes can interfere with phagocytosis and preparation of the wound for healing. Infection prolongs the inflammatory process and delays healing.

Chronic diseases may also impair healing. Diabetes mellitus is a prominent example. With high blood glucose levels associated with poorly controlled diabetes, chemotaxic and phagocytic function are decreased. Collagen formation and tensile strength of the wound are also impaired. Small blood vessel disease is common in people with diabetes, a factor that further impairs the healing process.

Drug therapy, particularly corticosteroid medications, may suppress the immune and inflammatory responses, delaying healing (Porth & Matfin, 2009). Other external factors, such as exposure to ionizing radiation and wound cleansing agents, can also affect healing. Table 12–7 summarizes major factors that affect the inflammatory process and wound healing.

Interdisciplinary Care

Management of the patient with inflamed tissue focuses on promoting healing. Care is generally supportive, allowing the patient's own physiologic processes to remove foreign matter and damaged cells. Wound care may be minimal, involving only simple cleaning, or extensive, involving irrigations and debridement. The patient is encouraged to rest, to increase fluid intake, and to eat a well-balanced, nutritious diet. Antibiotics may be prescribed to help eliminate infectious causes of inflammation.

Diagnosis

The following diagnostic tests may be ordered to identify the source and extent of inflammation. An important part of the assessment of the patient with an inflammation is monitoring the results of these tests.

TABLE 12–7 Factors That May Impair Healing

FACTOR	EFFECT
Malnutrition	
Protein deficit	Prolongs inflammation and impairs healing process
Carbohydrate and kilocalorie deficit	Impairs metabolic processes and promotes catabolism; proteins are used for energy rather than for healing
Fat deficit	Impairs cell membrane synthesis in tissue repair
Vitamin deficits	
Vitamin A	Limits epithelialization and capillary formation
B-Complex	Inhibits enzymatic reactions that contribute to wound healing
Vitamin C	Impairs collagen synthesis
Tissue hypoxia	Associated with an increased risk of infection and impaired healing, because oxygen is required to support cell function and collagen synthesis
Impaired blood supply	Inadequate delivery of oxygen and nutrients to healing tissues and removal of waste products
Impaired inflammatory and immune processes	Decreased phagocytosis and wound debridement; increased risk of infection; delayed healing

TABLE 12–8 The White Blood Cell Count and Differential

CELL TYPE AND NORMAL VALUE	INCREASED	DECREASED
Total WBCs: 4,000 to 10,000 per mm³	*Leukocytosis:* Infection or inflammation, leukemia, trauma or stress, tissue necrosis	*Leukopenia:* Bone marrow depression, overwhelming infection, viral infections, immunosuppression, autoimmune disease, dietary deficiency
Neutrophils (segs, PMNs, or polys): 55% to 70%	*Neutrophilia:* Acute infection or stress response, myelocytic leukemia, inflammatory or metabolic disorders	*Neutropenia:* Bone marrow depression, overwhelming bacterial infection, viral infection, Addison's disease
Eosinophils (eos): 1% to 4%	*Eosinophilia:* Parasitic infections, hypersensitivity reactions, autoimmune disorders	*Eosinopenia:* Cushing's syndrome, autoimmune disorders, stress, certain drugs
Basophils (basos): 0.5% to 1%	*Basophilia:* Hypersensitivity responses, chronic myelogenous leukemia, chickenpox or smallpox, splenectomy, hypothyroidism	*Basopenia:* Acute stress or hypersensitivity reactions, hyperthyroidism
Monocytes (monos): 2% to 8%	*Monocytosis:* Chronic inflammatory disorders, tuberculosis, viral infections, leukemia, Hodgkin's lymphoma, multiple myeloma	*Monocytopenia:* Bone marrow depression, corticosteroid therapy
Lymphocytes (lymphs): 20% to 40%	*Lymphocytosis:* Chronic bacterial infection, viral infections, lymphocytic leukemia	*Lymphocytopenia:* Bone marrow depression, immunodeficiency, leukemia, Cushing's syndrome, Hodgkin's lymphoma, renal failure

- *WBC with differential* provides information about the type and extent of inflammatory response. The differential count (the percentage of the total WBC made up by each type of leukocyte) provides further clues about inflammatory processes (Table 12–8).
- *Erythrocyte sedimentation rate (ESR or sed rate)* is a nonspecific test to detect inflammation. The rate at which RBCs fall to the bottom of a vertical tube is an indicator of inflammation. An increased ESR may indicate acute or chronic inflammation.
- *C-reactive protein (CRP) test* is used to detect CRP. This abnormal glycoprotein is produced by the liver and is excreted into the bloodstream during the acute phase of an inflammatory process. The expected result of this test is negative for CRP. A positive result indicates an acute or chronic inflammatory process. It may also indicate the patient's response to therapy, because it decreases when inflammation subsides.

In addition, cultures of the blood and other body fluids may be ordered to determine if infection is the cause of inflammation.

Medications

Medications may be prescribed for the patient with an inflammatory response to help alleviate distressing manifestations or destroy infectious agents.

Acetaminophen (Tylenol) may be administered to reduce the fever and pain associated with inflammation. Acetaminophen has no anti-inflammatory effect; it will not reduce the inflammatory process but will relieve associated manifestations. Acetaminophen decreases fever by acting directly on the hypothalamus heat-regulating center. It also works on the central nervous system to relieve pain sensations.

Antibiotics may be used either prophylactically to prevent infection from interfering with the healing process of damaged tissue, or therapeutically to treat the infection. If infection is present, the organism and its response or sensitivity to various antibiotics are used to guide therapy. Antibiotic therapy is discussed in the section of this chapter on infectious diseases.

Although inflammation is a beneficial process to prepare acutely injured tissue for healing, it can have damaging effects as well. When these effects are a concern or the manifestations of inflammation are deleterious to the patient, anti-inflammatory medications may be prescribed. Anti-inflammatory medications fall into three broad groups: salicylates, such as aspirin; other nonsteroidal anti-inflammatory drugs (NSAIDs); and corticosteroids.

Aspirin (acetylsalicylic acid, or ASA) is an NSAID that has antipyretic, analgesic, and antiplatelet effects. Its beneficial effects are largely dose related. Low doses (as little as 81 mg/day) inhibit platelet aggregation and normal blood clotting. Higher doses (650 to 1000 mg four to five times per day) are required to accomplish its anti-inflammatory effects. However, 650 mg of aspirin is an effective analgesic and antipyretic dosage. To relieve pain, aspirin acts primarily on peripheral sensory nerves by inhibiting the synthesis of prostaglandins and kinins, which are chemical stimuli of sensory nerves. As an antipyretic, aspirin acts both centrally and peripherally. It inhibits the formation of pyrogenic substances that raise the hypothalamic thermostat. It also dilates peripheral blood vessels and promotes diaphoresis, increasing the dissipation of heat (Wilson et al., 2009).

In therapeutic doses, aspirin mediates the inflammatory process by inhibiting the synthesis of prostaglandins and acting on the mobility and activation of leukocytes. Inflammation is reduced, along with the swelling, redness, and impaired function that accompanies it.

The other NSAIDs have activity similar to that of aspirin. They inhibit prostaglandin synthesis, reducing the inflammatory and pain response. Each NSAID has a slightly different mode of action for prostaglandin inhibition. Patients may have varying degrees of relief with different NSAIDs; sometimes, several different agents must be tried before the most effective is identified. Side effects also differ to a certain extent; however, all have a potential cross-sensitivity with aspirin, all irritate the gastrointestinal tract, and all cause some degree of sodium and water retention. They also are more costly than aspirin, but they have a longer duration of action; therefore, fewer daily doses are required to achieve the desired effect. Indomethacin and phenylbutazone are the most toxic of the NSAIDs. Their use is limited to short-term therapy. (∞ See Chapter 9 for further information on NSAIDs.)

For acute hypersensitivity reactions, such as reactions to poison ivy, or for inflammation that cannot be managed by aspirin or NSAID therapy, corticosteroid therapy may be prescribed. The glucocorticoids are hormones produced by the adrenal cortex that have widespread effects on body metabolism and the immune response. Glucocorticoids inhibit inflammation and may be life-saving in acute fulminating or chronic progressive inflammation. They do not cure disease; they are palliative to manage the inflammatory process. When glucocorticoids are prescribed to manage inflammation, the smallest possible effective dose is used. Whenever possible, a local-acting preparation such as a topical agent or intra-articular injection is prescribed to minimize its systemic effects. The incidence of potentially harmful side effects increases with higher doses and prolonged therapy. Wound healing is impaired, and the metabolism of fats, proteins, and carbohydrates is altered. Blood glucose control is impaired. Fat distribution changes, producing a cushingoid appearance with a moon face, increased truncal fat, and "buffalo hump." Fluid retention and hypertension are potential problems, as are osteoporosis, gastrointestinal bleeding, and emotional disturbances.

Nutrition

Healing depends on cell replication, protein synthesis, and the function of specific organs—the liver, heart, and lungs in particular. Weight loss and protein depletion are risk factors for poor healing and wound complications. Even a few days of severely impaired nutritional intake can noticeably affect healing. The patient with an inflammatory process or healing wound requires a well-balanced diet of sufficient kilocalories to meet the metabolic needs of the body (see Table 12–8). Inflammation often produces catabolism, a state in which body tissues are broken down. Healing, by contrast, is a process of anabolism or building up. Without sufficient kilocalories and nutrients, catabolism may predominate, impairing healing.

Carbohydrates are important to meet energy demands, as well as to support leukocyte function. However, hyperglycemia experienced in diabetes may impair healing. In diabetes, the glucose molecules bind the oxygen more tightly to the hemoglobin molecule and prevent adequate release of oxygen to the tissues for healing. Furthermore, neutrophils have diminished chemotactic and phagocytic functioning in hyperglycemia (Porth & Matfin, 2009). Adequate protein is necessary for tissue healing and the production of antibodies and WBCs. Lack of adequate protein increases the risk of infection. Complete protein sources, those that provide the essential amino acids, are preferred. Dietary fats are used in the synthesis of cell membranes.

Vitamins A, B-complex, C, and K are also important to the healing process. Vitamin A is necessary for capillary formation and epithelialization. B-complex vitamins promote wound healing, and vitamin C is necessary for collagen synthesis. Vitamin K provides a vital component for the synthesis of clotting factors in the liver.

Although it has been established that minerals contribute to the inflammatory and healing processes, less is known about required amounts. Zinc appears to be important for tissue growth, skin integrity, cell-mediated immunity, and other general immune mechanisms (Arnold & Barbul, 2006). However, the use of zinc supplements in smokers is cautioned against and sources in whole foods are recommended over supplements.

Oxygen is an important element in healing. Arterial and venous disorders impair oxygen availability to peripheral tissues and healing. White blood cells and fibroblasts for healing are impaired in ischemic conditions. In trauma, loss of blood flow to tissue causes ischemia and if prolonged, infection and cell death. Hyperbaric chambers increase oxygen above normal atmospheric pressure and promote healing. While 100% oxygen at atmospheric pressure saturates red blood cell hemoglobin, only hyperbaric pressures increase plasma transport of oxygen, making more available to tissues for immune function and healing.

Nursing Care

Acute inflammation may be self-limiting or extensive and require hospitalization. Nursing care includes teaching patients with acute and chronic inflammatory conditions self-management at home.

Health Promotion

Health promotion activities to prevent inflammation focus on reducing the risk for accidents and exposure to harmful agents that can result in subsequent injury. It is important to educate the public about potential hazards in both the work and home environments. In addition, safety education guidelines such as not drinking and driving, wearing a protective helmet when riding a bicycle, and using a safety belt in the car are important areas for discussion. Because most injuries occur at home, it is also important to discuss ways to make the home safer.

Assessment

The following data are collected through the health history and physical examination. Further focused assessments are described with nursing interventions in the next section.

- *Health history:* Risk factors, nutrition, medication use (anti-inflammatory and corticosteroids), location, duration, and type (redness, heat, pain, swelling, and impaired function) of manifestations
- *Physical assessment:* Movement of injured area, pain, circulation, wounds, lymph nodes.

Nursing Diagnoses and Interventions

The nursing care needs of the patient with an inflammation are related to the manifestations and altered tissue integrity. Priority nursing diagnoses include *Acute Pain*, *Impaired Tissue Integrity*, and *Risk for Infection*.

Acute Pain

Along with redness, warmth, swelling, and impaired function, pain is one of the primary manifestations of inflammation. Depending on the cause, affected area, and degree of inflammation, pain may be acute and immobilizing or chronic and demoralizing. It is important to remember that pain is a subjective experience and that patient responses to pain vary. (∞ Refer to Chapter 9 for more information about pain and pain management.)

- Assess pain using a scale of 0 to 10, with 0 being no pain and 10 being the worst pain; note the character, location, and duration of the pain. *Because pain is subjective, the patient provides the most accurate information regarding his or her pain experience.*
- Use physical and nonverbal cues to further assess the level of pain. *This intervention is especially important if the patient is nonverbal or tends to underreport pain.*
- Administer anti-inflammatory medications as prescribed. *These medications help reduce the pain resulting from acute inflammation.*
- Administer analgesic medications as prescribed. *Although most analgesics do little to reduce inflammation, they provide additional pain relief by reducing the perception of pain. Chest infections such as pneumonia may compromise breathing. In addition to administering oxygen at appropriate levels, relieving pain with opioid or NSAID analgesics helps increase the depth and slow the rate of respirations.*

PRACTICE ALERT

Because opioids can depress respirations, it is important to monitor oxygen saturation and encourage the patient to take deep breaths to keep oxygen saturation adequate.

- Provide comfort measures, such as back rubs, position changes, or relaxation techniques. *These measures reduce muscle tension, relieve areas of pressure, and provide distraction.*
- Encourage activities such as reading, watching television, and taking part in social interactions. *Such activities provide distraction from the pain experience.*
- Encourage rest. *Strenuous activity or exercising an inflamed body part may increase discomfort and tissue damage.*
- Provide cold or heat as pain-relief measures, as ordered. *For an acute injury, cold reduces swelling and relieves pain; after the initial stage, heat increases blood flow to the affected tissue and relieves pain and swelling by promoting absorption of edema. Do not apply either heat or cold for more than 20 minutes at a time and ensure there is a covering between the patient and the application*

SAFETY ALERT

Use heat or cold application cautiously in older patients who have fragile skin and are at risk for tissue injury.

- Elevate the inflamed area if possible. *Elevation promotes venous return and reduces swelling.*
- Teach about the appropriate use and expected effects of anti-inflammatory medications. *If the patient's pain continues after the initial doses of anti-inflammatory medication, he or she may become discouraged and stop taking the medication before it becomes fully effective.*

Impaired Tissue Integrity

The inflammatory response can either precipitate or result from impairment of the integrity of skin or other tissues. Whatever the cause of the tissue damage, it is vital that the nurse consider this alteration in delivering care.

- Assess general health and nutritional status. *Poor general health or chronic diseases such as diabetes mellitus or renal failure interfere with the healing processes and increase the risk of infection.*
- Assess circulation to the affected area. *Adequate tissue perfusion and oxygenation are necessary for healing.*
- Monitor the skin and surrounding tissue for increased manifestations of inflammation. *Inflammation can spread to adjacent tissues leading to conditions such as cellulitis.*
- Provide protection and support for inflamed tissue. *This reduces discomfort and decreases the risk of further tissue damage.*
- Clean inflamed tissue gently; if possible, use water, normal saline, or nontoxic wound cleansers such as Comfeel (Coloplast Corporation) only. *Soap and harsh cleansers such as povidone-iodine (Betadine) and hydrogen peroxide can cause further drying and tissue damage. Granulation tissue in a healing wound is fragile and easily damaged. (∞ See Chapters 4 and 16 for further discussion of wound care.)*
- Keep the inflamed area dry, and expose it to air as much as possible. *This promotes healing and helps prevent infection.*
- Balance rest with activity. *Rest decreases metabolic demands and allows for cell regeneration, while mobility helps to promote oxygenation and perfusion of the tissues.*
- Provide supplemental oxygen as ordered. *Supplemental oxygen improves tissue oxygenation and reduces hypoxia.*
- Provide a well-balanced diet with adequate kilocalories to meet the body's metabolic and healing needs. If the patient is allowed nothing by mouth (NPO), suggest parenteral or enteral nutrition. For the patient who is unable to consume an adequate diet, consult with a dietitian for between-meal supplements and/or multivitamin supplements. *Careful attention to diet and nutrient intake is important to provide the nutrients necessary for immune function and healing and to prevent catabolism.*

Risk for Infection

The inflammatory response often indicates that body defense mechanisms have been set in motion to protect against invading microorganisms. Wounds, whether traumatic or surgical in nature, are typically contaminated, as attested to by subsequent wound infections. The patient with a healing wound is at particular risk for infection.

- Assess the wound for specific manifestations of infection, including purulent drainage, foul odor, and delayed healing. *The normal inflammatory response can indicate infection and, on occasion, mask its presence.*
- Evaluate complete blood counts for adequate WBC response. *Leukocytosis may indicate infection or healthy response to injury and protection from infection. Immune-impaired patients may not respond with increased WBCs; manifestations of inflammation may be diminished in those individuals.*
- Monitor vital signs and pain level at least every 4 hours. *In response to the inflammatory process the temperature rises,*

usually in the range of 99°F (37.2°C) to 100.9°F (38.2°C). A temperature of 101.0°F (38.3°C) or above indicates infection. Fever is usually accompanied by increased heart and respiratory rates.

- Apply dry or moist heat to the affected area for no longer than 20 minutes several times a day. *Heat increases the circulation of blood to and from the inflamed tissue. Time is limited to prevent burns.*
- Provide and encourage fluid intake of 2500 mL/day. Older patients may limit fluid intake when mobility is impaired by illness or injury; high fluid intake increases the need for urination and patients may want to limit bathroom trips. *Teach the purpose and importance of hydration to promote blood flow and nutrient supply to the tissues and also dilution and removal of waste products and heat from the body.*
- Ensure adequate nutrition. *Adequate nutrition enhances the function and production of T cells and B cells, which are important in the immune response.*
- Use good hand hygiene techniques consistently. *Hand hygiene removes transient microorganisms and is the best mechanism to prevent the spread of infection to a susceptible person.*
- Use sterile technique when providing wound care. *Using sterile gloves and aseptic technique helps prevent further contamination of the wound and the spread of infection to other patients.*

Community-Based Care

Patient and family teaching enhances understanding of the inflammatory process, its cause, and its management. Teaching is also important to prevent further compromise that could result in infection.

Instructions, verbal and written, should include the following:

- Increase fluid intake to 2500 mL (approximately 2.5 quarts) per day, including that found in solid foods.
- Eat a well-balanced diet high in vitamins and minerals and with adequate protein and kilocalories for healing.
- Use good hand hygiene, particularly when caring for wounds or inflamed tissue and after using the bathroom.
- Elevate the inflamed area to reduce swelling and pain.
- Apply heat or cold for no longer than 20 minutes at a time to reduce the risk of tissue damage from burns or frostbite.
- Take all medications as prescribed, notifying the physician if adverse effects or hypersensitivity responses are noted. (See Moving Evidence into Action.)
- Rest acutely inflamed tissue; do not engage in strenuous activity until the inflammation has subsided.

The Patient with an Infection

Microorganisms—including bacteria, viruses, fungi, and parasites—often invade the human body and proliferate if undetected and controlled or eliminated by inflammatory and immune responses. In most cases, contact between humans and microorganisms is incidental and may even be beneficial to both organisms. Resident bacteria of the skin, mucous membranes, and gastrointestinal tract are an important part of the body's defense system. However, many microorganisms are virulent; that is, they have the ability to cause disease. **Pathogens** are virulent organisms rarely found in the absence of disease. Some microorganisms, known as opportunistic pathogens, rarely, if ever, cause harm to persons with intact immune systems, but are capable of producing infectious disease in the immunocompromised host (Porth & Matfin, 2009).

MOVING EVIDENCE INTO ACTION — Teaching to Take Antibiotics Appropriately

Nurses discharging patients from outpatient and acute care settings frequently teach patients to take a complete prescribed dose of oral antibiotics to manage acute infectious illness. Ingesting less than complete doses exposes patients to the risk of resistant infections and less than therapeutic outcomes. There are many potential restraining forces to the completion of antibiotic dosing: cost of purchase; difficulty swallowing the pills; multiple, frequent doses; and the potential for adverse, unpleasant side effects.

Because adherence is so important and nurses are patient educators, Aronson (2005) studied the experience of 11 patients who had just completed a short-term antibiotic regimen to treat a variety of acute infectious with various antibiotic regimens. The 11 subjects represent diverse gender and cultural backgrounds. The patients' descriptions, views, and experiences are the unique aspect of this research on adherence to antibiotic self-administration. The central theme that emerged was successful antibiotic self-administration. The patients integrated the dosing into their daily schedules and adapted to any unplanned circumstances. The primary categories involved in self-administration were (1) medication-taking behaviors, (2) factors influencing adherence, and (3) attitudes and beliefs about the medication and the value of completing the prescribed dose.

IMPLICATIONS FOR NURSING
Nurses teach patients about short-term antibiotic self-administration in outpatient and inpatient settings. The findings from this study can be used to guide educational interventions. Based on the findings in this study, encourage patient involvement in the decision to take short-term antibiotic medications to strengthen the relationship with the prescriber. Ask patients to identify the method they will use to remind themselves of each dose; inquire about their knowledge of and plans to manage side effects from the medication.

CRITICAL THINKING IN PATIENT CARE
1. Identify methods that patients can use to remind themselves of dosing schedules.
2. An 86-year-old woman is being discharged to her home following a respiratory infection. Identify the information she will need about short-term antibiotic medication when she is discharged.
3. Make a list of barriers to taking complete doses of antibiotics. What do you think is the single most important (to the patient) reason?
4. Discuss the interrelationship between malnutrition and immune system function (see the previous discussion of immune system function).

Source: Aronson, B. (2005). Medication management behaviors of adherent short-term antibiotic users. *Clinical Excellence for Nurse Practitioners, 9*(1), 23–30.

To a certain extent, modern medicine has contributed to the development of infectious diseases caused by antibiotic-resistant strains of microorganisms. Tuberculosis is on the rise in many countries, partially because organisms have become resistant to standard therapies. Patients receive immunosuppressive therapy following organ or tissue transplant or in the treatment of neoplasms, making them more susceptible to infection. Metal and plastic prosthetic devices are implanted, providing potential sites for colonization by disease-producing organisms. It has also become apparent that many diseases long considered unrelated to microorganisms may actually be infectious; for example, colonization of the gastric mucosa with *Helicobacter pylori* is the predominant cause of peptic ulcer disease, and oncogenic viruses have the ability to transform normal cells into malignant cells.

Pathophysiology

Infection occurs when an organism is able to colonize and multiply within a host. The host can be any organism capable of supporting the nutritional and physical growth requirements of the microorganism—for example, humans. When the host experiences injury, pathologic changes, inflammation, or organ dysfunction in response to an infection or from intoxication by cellular poisons produced by a pathogen, the host is said to have an infectious disease.

For a microorganism to cause infection, it must have disease-causing potential (virulence), be transmitted from its reservoir, and gain entry into a susceptible host. This is known as the chain of infection (Figure 12–11 ■).

PATHOGENS Pathogens capable of infecting and causing disease in a susceptible host include bacteria, viruses, mycoplasma, rickettsia, chlamydia, fungi, and parasites such as

protozoa, helminths (worms), and arthropods (Box 12–4). Each organism causes a different specific reaction in the host.

A number of different mechanisms have evolved in pathogens to facilitate their transmission and increase their ability to invade the host and cause disease. Factors influencing the transmission of an organism include its resistance to drying and to variations in environmental temperature. For example, spore-forming organisms are extremely resistant to drying.

Many microorganisms are capable of producing toxins or enzymes to facilitate their invasion of the host, increase their resistance to host defenses, and increase their ability to cause disease. Adhesion factors produced by or incorporated into the cell wall or membrane of the pathogen improve its ability to attach to and colonize the host. Pathogens may also produce enzymes to enhance their spread to local tissues, chemicals to block specific immune processes or deplete neutrophils and macrophages, or extracellular capsules to discourage phagocytosis.

Pathogens are often capable of producing toxins that alter or destroy the normal function of host cells and promote colonization, proliferation, and invasion by the pathogen. Toxins often increase the disease-producing capability of the pathogen and, in some cases, are totally responsible for it; for example, cholera, tetanus, and botulism result from bacterial toxins, not from the direct effects of the infection. **Exotoxins** are soluble proteins secreted into surrounding tissue by the microorganism. Exotoxins are highly poisonous, causing cell death or dysfunction. **Endotoxins** are found in the cell wall of gram-negative bacteria and are released only when the cell is disrupted. Endotoxins have less specific effects than exotoxins, but they act as activators of many human regulatory systems, producing fever; inflammation; and potentially clotting, bleeding, or hypotension when released in large quantities.

RESERVOIR AND TRANSMISSION The reservoir or source, where the pathogen lives and multiplies, may be either endogenous or exogenous. Organisms that reside on skin or mucosal surfaces of the host are endogenous. Exogenous sources can include other humans, animals, soil, water, intravenous fluid, or equipment. Infectious diseases are usually transmitted from human sources, that is, persons who have clinical disease or carriers with subclinical infection. Carriers harbor the pathogen without showing evidence of clinical disease. Pathogens exit human hosts via respiratory secretions, body fluids from the gastrointestinal and genitourinary tracts, skin or mucous membrane lesions, the placenta, and blood.

Organisms may be transmitted from the source to the susceptible host by direct or indirect contact, droplet or airborne transmission, or a vector. Direct contact includes person-to-person spread or contact with infected body fluids, as well as transmission from contaminated food or water. Indirect contact occurs when the infectious agent is contracted by use of inanimate objects, such as dirty eating utensils. Sneezing, talking, and coughing allow transmission by droplet contact when the host is within 2 to 3 feet of the source. Smaller respiratory particles that stay suspended in air and are carried via air currents allow airborne transmission. Vectors are insects and animals such as flies, mosquitoes, or rodents that act as intermediate hosts between the source and host. Microorganisms usually

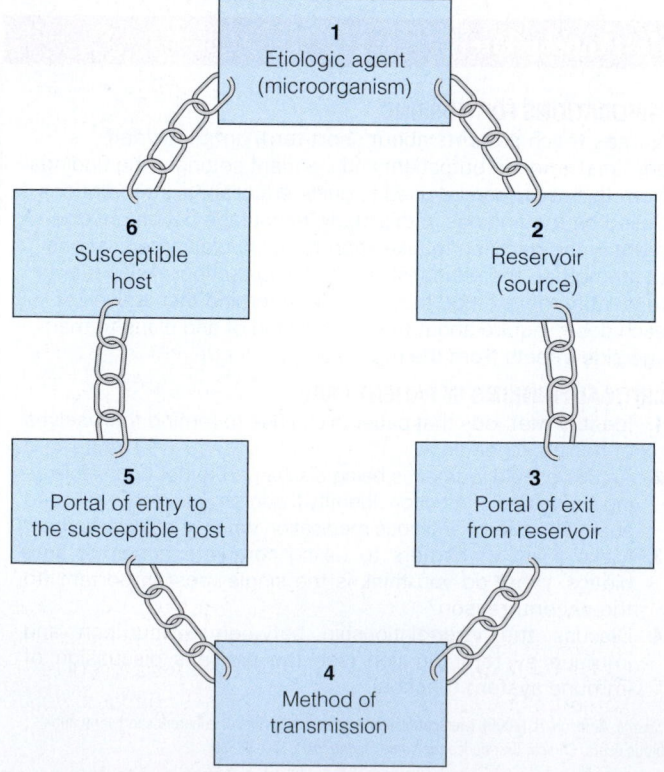

Figure 12–11 ■ The chain of infection.

BOX 12–4 Pathogenic Organisms

Bacteria
Bacteria are single-celled organisms capable of autonomous reproduction. Relatively small and simple organisms, they contain a single chromosome. A flexible cell membrane and rigid cell wall surrounds their cytoplasm, giving them a distinctive shape; some also have an extracellular capsule for additional protection. Bacteria have different characteristics and growth requirements: *aerobes* require oxygen for survival, whereas *anaerobes* cannot survive in the presence of oxygen; *gram-positive* bacteria stain purple when subjected to crystal violet stain, whereas *gram-negative* bacteria do not stain with crystal violet but turn red when subjected to safranin stain; the colonies formed by replicating bacteria differ from one another.

Prions
Prions are not independent organisms but small molecules that can modify host proteins. They primarily affect the neurologic system, causing neurologic degeneration in diseases such as mad cow disease (bovine spongiform encephalopathy) in animals and Creutzfeldt-Jacob in humans. These are slowly progressive, non-inflammatory conditions leading to dementia, lack of coordination, and death. Prion entry into the neurologic cells makes them resistant to the host immune system and anti-bacterial and anti-viral medications. They enter the host by injection, transplantation of contaminated tissue or medical devices, and possibly food (Porth & Matfin, 2009). They are very resistant to disinfection, requiring special procedures for sterilizing instruments, especially those used in CNS surgeries (Prusiner & Miller, 2007).

Viruses
Viruses are obligate intracellular parasites that are incapable of reproducing outside of a living cell. Viruses consist of a protein coat around a core of either DNA or RNA. Some viruses are shed continuously from infected cell surfaces; others, after inserting their genetic material into that of the infected cell, remain latent until they are stimulated to replicate. Viruses may or may not cause lysis and death of the host cell during replication. Oncogenic viruses are able to transform normal cells into malignant cells.

Mycoplasma
Although similar to bacteria, mycoplasma are smaller and have no cell wall, making them resistant to antibiotics that inhibit cell wall synthesis (e.g., penicillins).

Rickettsia and Chlamydia
As obligate intracellular parasites with a rigid cell wall, rickettsia and *Chlamydia* have some features of both bacteria and viruses. Rather than depending on the host cell for reproduction, they use vitamins, nutrients, or products of metabolism (e.g., ATP) from the host. *Chlamydia* are transmitted by direct contact, whereas many rickettsiae infect the cells of arthropods (e.g., fleas, ticks, and lice) and are transmitted from these vectors to humans.

Fungi
Fungi are prevalent throughout the world, but few are capable of causing disease in humans. Most fungal infections are self-limited, affecting the skin and subcutaneous tissue. Some fungi, such as *Pneumocystis jiroveci*, can cause life-threatening opportunistic infections in the immunocompromised host.

Parasites
The term *parasite* is typically applied to members of the animal kingdom that infect and cause disease in other animals. Protozoa, helminths, and arthropods are considered parasites. Protozoa are single-celled organisms transmitted via direct or indirect contact or an arthropod vector. Helminths are wormlike parasites: roundworms, tapeworms, and flukes are examples. They gain entry into humans primarily through ingestion of fertilized eggs or penetration of larvae through the skin or mucous membranes. Arthropod parasites, such as scabies (mites), lice, and fleas, typically infest external body surfaces, causing localized tissue damage and inflammation. Transmission is by direct contact with the arthropod or its eggs.

first colonize the portal of entry: nonintact skin; wounds; mucous membranes; and the respiratory, gastrointestinal, or genitourinary tracts.

HOST FACTORS   The susceptible host is the final link in the chain of infection. Exposure to pathogens does not automatically cause infection or infectious disease. The outcome of contact with a pathogenic microorganism is determined by the balance of microbial virulence and host resistance. Factors that can enable the host to resist infection include the following:

- Physical barriers, such as intact skin and mucous membranes
- The hostile environment created by acid stomach secretions, urine, and vaginal secretions
- Antimicrobial factors in saliva, tears, and prostatic fluid
- Respiratory defenses, including humidification, filtration, the mucociliary escalator, cough reflex, and alveolar macrophages
- Innate and adaptive immune responses to pathogenic invasion

Stages of the Infectious Process
When infectious disease develops in the host, it typically follows a predictable course with stages based on the progression and intensity of manifestations.

The initial stage is the incubation period, during which the pathogen begins active replication but does not yet cause manifestations. Depending on the organism and host factors, the incubation period may last from hours, as with salmonella, to years, as with HIV infection.

The prodromal stage follows, during which manifestations first begin to appear. At this stage, manifestations are often nonspecific and include general malaise, fever, myalgias, headache, and fatigue.

Maximal impact of the infectious process is felt during the acute phase as the pathogen proliferates and disseminates rapidly. Toxic by-products of microorganism metabolism and cell lysis, along with the immune response, produce tissue damage and inflammation during this stage (Porth & Matfin, 2009). Manifestations are more pronounced and specific to the infecting organism and site during the acute stage. Fever and chills may be significant during this phase. However, alcoholic patients and the very old may respond to severe infection by becoming hypothermic. The patient is often tachycardic and tachypneic because of increased metabolic demands. Localized manifestations include redness, heat, swelling, pain, and impaired function. When the infectious disease affects an internal organ, manifestations are related to inflammatory changes in that organ and surrounding tissue. The patient may experience tenderness to palpation over the site or show manifestations of impaired function, such as the hematuria and proteinuria characteristic of renal infections.

If the infectious process is prolonged, manifestations of the continuing immune response may become apparent. Catabolic and anorexic effects of the infection can lead to loss of body fat and muscle wasting. Immune complexes may be deposited at sites other than the primary infection, resulting in an inflammatory process. Glomerulonephritis (e.g., following strep throat) and vasculitis are possible results. Another possible consequence of prolonged infection and immune response is the triggering of an autoimmune disease process (discussed in ∞ Chapter 13), such as rheumatic cardiomyopathy or celiac disease. Type 1 diabetes mellitus is thought to be the result of such a response (Porth, 2007).

As the infection is contained and the pathogen eliminated, the convalescent stage of the disease occurs. During this stage, affected tissues are repaired and manifestations resolve. Resolution of the infection is total elimination of the pathogen from the body without residual manifestations. If a balance between organism and host factors occurs with neither predominating, chronic disease may develop or the organism may be driven into a protected site, such as an abscess. A carrier state develops when host defenses eliminate the infectious disease but the organism continues to multiply on mucosal sites.

Complications

Multiple and varied complications are associated with infectious diseases. They are typically specific to the infecting organism and the body system affected.

Acute invasion of the blood by certain microorganisms or their toxins can result in septicemia and septic shock. Whereas bacteremia, the presence of bacteria in the blood, may not have serious effects, septicemia refers to systemic disease associated with their presence or toxins. Septic shock indicates a state of hypotension and impaired organ perfusion resulting from sepsis. Unless treated aggressively, septic shock leads to diffuse cell and tissue injury, and potentially to organ failure. ∞ See Chapter 11 for an in-depth discussion of septic shock, other shock syndromes, and their management.

Nosocomial Infections

Nosocomial infections are acquired in a healthcare setting, such as a hospital or nursing home. Also called healthcare-associated infections (HAIs), nosocomial infections account for an estimated 1.7 million infections, 99,000 deaths, and $4.5 billion in excess healthcare costs annually. HAIs add hospital days, reduce admissions by occupying available beds, and add to the cost of health care (CDC, 2010; Klevens et al., 2007; Stone et al., 2005).

FAST FACTS

- Nosocomial infections typically manifest after 48 hours of hospitalization.
- Urinary tract infection is the most common type of HAI, followed by surgical site infection and pneumonia (CDC, 2009).
- *Clostridium difficile*–associated diarrhea is a frequently acquired nosocomial infection. It is an antibiotic-associated diarrhea and the risk of acquiring it increases with length of hospital stay, especially in an intensive care unit (ICU).

Patients entering hospitals are often the least able to mount immune defenses to infection. Immunologic responses may be compromised and normal defenses impaired in patients with, for example, cancer or chronic diseases, pressure ulcers, or organ transplants (McPhee, Papadakis, & Tierney, 2008). Nosocomial infections also occur when antibiotic therapy has altered natural defenses and impaired resistance to harmful microorganisms. Endogenous organisms outside their normal habitats (such as in *Escherichia coli* in the urinary tract) become a threat to the patient. Other pharmacologic and therapeutic procedures such as chemotherapy, the use of corticosteroids, or radiation therapy also contribute to nosocomial infections. Gram-negative enteric bacteria and gram-positive *Staphylococcus aureus* are the most common bacteria responsible.

Invasive procedures and altered immune defenses are the main factors contributing to infection. Urinary catheterization is the number one cause; cardiac catheterization, peripheral and central intravenous lines, respiratory care procedures, and surgical procedures are also closely linked to nosocomial infection. Consequently, the urinary tract, surgical wounds, respiratory tract, and invasive catheter sites on the skin are most often affected by hospital-acquired infection.

Surgical site infections rank second in frequency of healthcare associated infections (CDC, 2010). Superficial or deep wounds may be contaminated by endogenous or exogenous sources. Infections in body cavities or associated with prosthetics are difficult to diagnose; interventional radiology to obtain specimens of possible infected sites may be necessary (Weinstein, 2007).

Hospital-acquired pneumonia is the third most common nosocomial infection, accounting for 15% to 20% of these serious infections. Usually associated with ICU stays and mechanical ventilation, Sopina and Sobria (2005) found hospital-acquired pneumonia in non-ICU patients with severe underlying disease and a hospital stay greater than 5 days. Organisms causing the infection are often resistant to many drugs, not responding to antibiotics usually effective in treating infections acquired outside the hospital. There are more deaths associated with HA pneumonia than any other site of infection (Weinstein, 2007).

SAFETY ALERT

Since October 2002, alcohol-based hand rub has been recommended by the CDC as the preferred method for hand hygiene (CDC, 2002a). Antiseptic soaps and detergents are the next most effective agents and nonantiseptic soaps are the least effective. A soap and water wash is recommended for visibly soiled hands. Wearing gloves does not eliminate the need for hand hygiene.

Prevention is the most important control measure for nosocomial infections. The pathogens causing these infections are transmitted primarily by contact with hospital personnel and contaminated inanimate objects (Posani, 2004). *Effective hand hygiene is the single most important measure in infection control (Haas & Larsen, 2008)*. Although infections may also be transmitted by the airborne route, contaminated equipment, or from the environment, these are less significant causes. Invasive procedures and equipment should be used only when absolutely necessary; for example, it is not appropriate to insert an indwelling catheter when the only indication is incontinence. Peripheral intravenous equipment and sites must be kept

1. Central venous catheter infections have decreased by using chlorhexidine antiseptic for disinfection and maximal barrier precautions during insertion.
2. Ventilator-associated pneumonia is decreased by weaning patients off ventilators as soon as possible, limiting sedation of the patient, positioning patients to prevent gastric reflux and for maximal ventilation, and proper hand hygiene and sterile technique for all ventilator-associated care.
3. Surgical site infections are reduced by administering a prophylactic antibiotic 1 hour before the incision and discontinuing it within 24 hours after surgery, limiting hair removal (no shaving), controlling perioperative glucose levels (especially in cardiac surgeries), and ensuring normothermia for the patient during the perioperative period (especially in colorectal surgeries) (Weinstein, 2007).

clean and changed regularly: intravenous bags and bottles every 24 hours, tubing every 24 to 96 hours, and sites every 72 to 96 hours according to agency policy.

Antibiotic-Resistant Microorganisms

Antibiotic-resistant microorganisms are increasing at an alarming rate primarily due to prolonged or inappropriate use of antibiotic therapy. Although antibiotic therapy is expected to eradicate all targeted microorganisms, sometimes a few bacteria survive, leading to bacteria that reproduce with antibiotic resistance already encoded into their genetic makeup (Vrtis, 2008). Other bacteria produce enzymes that inactivate drugs, change drug binding sites, or alter their cell membrane to prevent drug absorption. It is important for infectious agents to be identified and treated with effective antibiotics; culture and sensitivity analysis guides prescription of effective antimicrobials. These reports need to be reviewed carefully and appropriate action taken if drug-resistant pathogens are found (Vrtis, 2008).

Standard precautions, most importantly hand hygiene and use of carefully selected antibiotics, are critical actions for stopping the spread of these diseases. Equipment such as stethoscopes, blood pressure cuffs, and thermometers should be restricted to use by each patient identified with one of these diseases. Personal protective gear used and disposed of appropriately are important safeguards.

Interdisciplinary Care

The goals of care for the patient with an infection are to identify the organ system affected by the infection; to identify the causative agent; and to achieve a cure by the least toxic, least expensive, and most effective means. Fortunately, most infectious diseases are self-limiting and will resolve with little or no medical care. However, medical treatment can be lifesaving in an overwhelming infection or immunocompromised host.

The body part or organ system affected by the infection is often obvious from the patient's history and presenting manifestations. Identifying the system allows the range of possible infecting organisms to be narrowed to those known to affect that system. Once the infecting agent has been identified, either positively or by probability, therapy can be specifically tailored to the patient's needs. Viral infections often resolve without treatment other than supportive care, such as providing rest and fluids. Skin infections may respond to a topical agent, avoiding the potential adverse effects of one administered systemically.

Diagnosis

To assess the patient's response to infection, identify the infecting organism, and monitor the progress of therapy, the following diagnostic tests may be ordered:

- *WBC count* provides clues about the infecting organism and the body's immune response to it.
- *WBC differential* is also ordered (see Table 12–8). Neutrophilia, increased numbers of circulating neutrophils (or PMNs), is a common response with infection or inflammation as the bone marrow responds to an increased need for phagocytes. Along with neutrophilia, a shift to the left is common in acute infection. This means that there are more immature neutrophils in circulation than normal, indicating an appropriate bone marrow response.

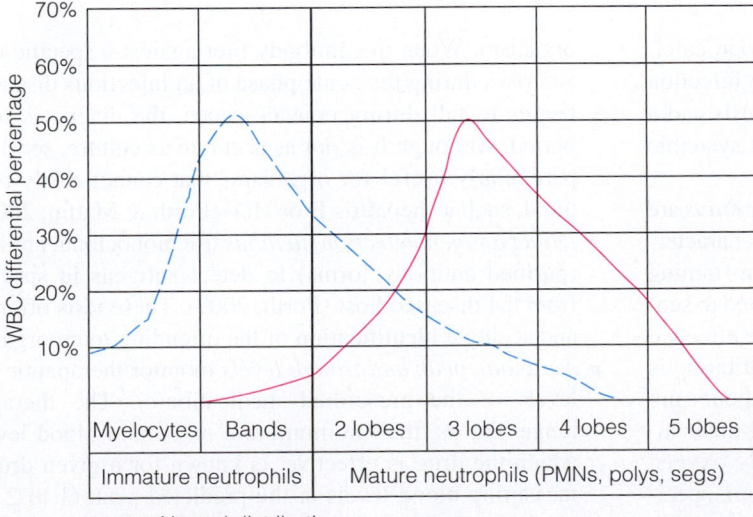

Type of WBC	Normal differential	Shift to left
Myelocytes	0%	Present
Band neutrophils (bands)	3% to 5%	Increased
Segmented neutrophils (segs, polys, PMNs)	50% to 65%	May be stable, increased, or decreased

Figure 12–12 ■ Neutrophils by stage of maturity and normal distribution in the blood.

NURSING CARE OF THE OLDER ADULT   **Infections in Older Adults**

Because immune function declines with aging, older adults are more susceptible to infections. Infections are among the top 10 causes for hospitalization and 1 of the 5 leading causes of death among people over 65 years of age. Additionally, the following changes that occur with aging place the older adult at greater risk of acquiring an infection than younger people.

- *Cardiovascular changes:*   decreased cardiac output, loss of capillaries, and decreased tissue perfusion delaying inflammatory response and healing.
- *Respiratory system changes:*   decreased mucociliary escalator, decreased elastic recoil, and a diminished cough reflex leading to decreased clearance of respiratory secretions. As a result of physiologic changes, the older adult with pneumonia may not present with cough or sputum production. The leading causes of pneumonia in older adults include *S. pneumoniae*, *Haemophilus influenzae*, *Klebsiella pneumoniae*, *S. aureus*, and pneumococci. Influenza A and B are prevalent in the aged; however, strain A accounts for greater illness severity and death (Eliopoulos, 2009). Older adults are at greater risk for developing pneumonia as a complication of influenza. Both pneumonia and influenza cause high mortality rates in the older person.
- *Genitourinary changes:*   loss of muscle tone, reduced bladder contractility, altered bladder reflexes, and prostatic hypertrophy in men leading to reduced bladder capacity and incomplete emptying. Urinary tract infection (UTI) is the most common infection and the leading cause of bacteremia and sepsis in older adults. Factors that contribute to UTI include poor hygiene, incomplete bladder emptying, inadequate fluid intake, and long-term indwelling catheters. In addition, chronic conditions and medications may contribute to retention, which can result in UTI.
- *Gastrointestinal system changes:*   impaired swallow reflex, decreased gastric acidity, and delayed gastric emptying, thus increasing the risk of aspiration with subsequent pneumonia.
- *Skin and subcutaneous tissue changes:*   thinning of skin, decreased cushioning, and decreased sensation leading to increased risk of injury and ulceration, especially in patients with limited mobility or with urinary or bowel incontinence.
- *Immune changes:*   decreased phagocytosis, reduced inflammatory response, and slowed or impaired healing processes. Immunoglobulin levels remain relatively stable, but primary and secondary antibody responses decline with aging. The thymus gland atrophies and some T-cell populations decrease or decline in function as the person ages. T-cell activation and the ability of T cells to proliferate following activation also decline with advancing age (Porth & Matfin, 2009). With these changes, cell-mediated immune function declines. The patient has reduced resistance to antigens such as *M. tuberculosis*, influenza and varicella-zoster viruses, malignant cells, and tissue grafts.

Other factors, such as a lower activity level, poor nutrition and an increased risk for dehydration, a higher prevalence of chronic diseases such as diabetes, use of multiple medications, and altered mentation contribute to the older adult's risk for infection.

Nosocomial infections are more common in older adults. The nurse must steadfastly adhere to principles of infection control. Nursing interventions should focus on prevention strategies such as (1) avoiding prolonged bed rest unless the medical condition contraindicates mobilization, (2) encouraging patients to take deep breaths, (3) providing adequate fluids, (4) providing regular toileting schedules with good hygiene, and (5) avoiding use of invasive devices such as indwelling catheters unless medically necessary.

The older adult may not exhibit the classic manifestations of inflammation and infection. The manifestations of inflammation—redness, heat, and swelling—tend to be diminished or absent in older adults. The classic manifestations of infection—fever and chills—may be absent altogether because of age-related changes in the immune system, loss of central temperature control mechanisms, decreased muscle mass, and loss of shivering ability. Rather than an elevated temperature to signal an infection, confusion and subtle changes in behavior such as restlessness may be observed. The older adult may have only subtle manifestations of sepsis, including changes in mental status, disorientation, and tachypnea.

In addition to monitoring for changes in the patient's mental status or behavior, the nurse should collect data on the amount of fluids consumed, urinary output, activity levels, complaints of fatigue, and respiratory status. Older adults are at increased risk for dehydration due to such factors as diminished thirst sensation and impaired water conservation by the kidneys. Carefully evaluate intake and output to determine if input is adequate (Spigt et al., 2006). A thorough assessment is necessary to facilitate an early diagnosis and prompt treatment that will improve outcomes for the older adult.

- *Procalcitonin (CTpr)* is a precursor of the hormone calcitonin. Procalcitonin increases dramatically during infection and sepsis and is accepted as both a marker of sepsis and a harmful mediator in lower respiratory tract and systemic infections.
- *Cultures of the wound, blood, or other infected body fluids* are used to identify probable microorganisms by their characteristics, such as shape, growth patterns, and Gram-staining qualities. After the organism is cultured, it is subjected to sensitivity testing using various antibiotics known to be effective against its particular strain to determine which antibiotic is likely to be most effective. Generally 24 to 48 hours are required to grow the organism, potentially delaying the institution of therapy. Because antibiotics (and possibly oxygen therapy) can alter the ability to culture an organism, specimens should be obtained before instituting therapy.
- *Serologic testing* provides an indirect means of identifying infecting agents by detecting antibodies to the suspected organism. When the antibody titer against a specific organism rises during the acute phase of an infectious disease and begins to fall during convalescence, the diagnosis is supported. Although it is not as accurate as culture, serology is particularly useful for organisms that cannot easily be cultured, such as hepatitis B or HIV (Porth & Matfin, 2009).
- *Direct antigen detection methods* use monoclonal antibodies (purified antibody forms) to detect antigens in specimens from the diseased host (Porth, 2007). These tests offer rapid and accurate identification of the offending microorganism.
- *Antibiotic peak and trough levels* monitor therapeutic blood levels of the prescribed medication(s). The therapeutic range, that is, the minimum and maximum blood levels at which the drug is effective, is known for a given drug. By measuring blood levels at the predicted peak (1 to 2 hours after oral administration, 1 hour after intramuscular administration, and 30 minutes after intravenous administration) and trough (lowest level, usually a few minutes before the next

scheduled dose), healthcare personnel can determine that the patient is maintaining a level within the therapeutic range at all times, ensuring maximal effect from the drug. It is also possible to determine whether the drug is reaching a toxic or harmful level during therapy, increasing the likelihood of adverse effects.

- *Radiologic examination of the chest, abdomen, or urinary system* may be ordered to detect organ abnormalities indicating an inflammatory response or tissue damage.
- *Lumbar puncture* is performed to obtain cerebrospinal fluid (CSF) for examination and culture if a central nervous system (CNS) infection, such as meningitis or encephalitis, is suspected.
- *Ultrasonic examination* is a noninvasive diagnostic test such as an echocardiogram or renal ultrasonography to identify an infectious site or evaluate the effects of infection on organ function.

Medications

After the infecting organism and affected body system have been identified, specific therapy to cure the infectious disease can be instituted. Antimicrobial preparations are broadly classified as bacteriostatic or bactericidal. *Bacteriostatic agents* inhibit the growth of the microorganism, leaving its destruction to the host's immune system. These agents are generally not indicated for the immunocompromised host. Tetracyclines, erythromycin, and chloramphenicol are bacteriostatic preparations. *Bactericidal agents* are capable of killing the organism without immune system intervention. These include the penicillins, cephalosporins, and aminoglycoside antibiotics.

The activity of antimicrobial agents on bacteria, fungi, and viruses falls under five basic mechanisms:

- Impairing cell wall synthesis, leading to lysis and cell destruction
- Inhibiting protein synthesis, causing impaired microbial function
- Altering cell membrane permeability, causing intracellular contents to leak
- Inhibiting the synthesis of nucleic acids
- Inhibiting cell metabolism and growth

Many microorganisms have the ability to develop resistance to an anti-infective agent; that is, the pathogen continues to live and grow in the presence of the anti-infective. Resistance develops as a result of a chance mutation by the pathogen, allowing a subpopulation of cells to survive. The chance of an organism's becoming resistant to an agent is partially related to the dose delivered. Resistance is less likely to occur when a lethal dose is administered; therefore, it is vital that patients understand the need to take all doses of the prescribed drug as ordered.

ANTIBIOTICS Medications used to treat bacterial infections are generally known as antibiotics. Most antibiotics are biologic substances, that is, substances produced by other microorganisms. Antibiotics fall into classes of drugs with related chemical structure and activity. Some are effective against only gram-positive bacteria, and others are effective against only gram-negative organisms. Broad-spectrum antibiotics have activity against a wide variety of bacteria, including both gram-positive

and gram-negative forms. No antibiotic is totally safe. Hypersensitivity responses occur; always check for allergies before administering the first dose. Some drugs are toxic to organ systems, exhibiting hepatotoxicity, nephrotoxicity, ototoxicity, or bone marrow suppression. The antibiotics presented in the following Medication Administration box are organized according to their antibacterial action.

ANTIVIRALS Most antibiotics have little effect on viruses because the virus has no cell wall and no cytoplasm, produces no enzymes, and sequesters itself in a host cell to reproduce. Antiviral agents must be very selective in differentiating normal cellular activity from viral activity. In addition, the immune function of the host is a vital component in fighting viral infections; antiviral therapy may be relatively ineffective in the severely immunocompromised host. Making a timely diagnosis to allow institution of antiviral therapy can be an additional problem because viruses are less easily identified using laboratory techniques. Antiviral agents in common use are summarized in the Medication Administration box on page 298. Antiretroviral agents used in the management of HIV and AIDS are presented in ∞ Chapter 13.

ANTIFUNGALS Antifungal agents are available in both topical and systemic forms. They act by interfering with the cytoplasmic membrane of the fungus. Topical agents include preparations for cutaneous use to treat candidiasis, tineas, and ringworm. Vaginal preparations to treat vulvovaginal candidiasis are also available, as are several nonprescription topical and vaginal antifungal agents.

Amphotericin B (Fungizone) is a systemic antifungal agent for parenteral administration. It is used to treat severe, life-threatening fungal infections including histoplasmosis, blastomycosis, and candidiasis. Another systemic antifungal in current use is flucytosine (Ancobon). Unlike amphotericin B, flucytosine can be administered orally. It is used to treat severe candidiasis infections such as candida septicemia, endocarditis, pulmonary or urinary tract infections, and *Cryptococcus* meningitis.

Fluconazole (Diflucan) has the broadest use as an antifungal agent. It can be administered either orally or parenterally and is used to treat candidiasis infections as well as *Cryptococcus* meningitis. It is generally better tolerated than other systemic antifungal medications.

ANTIPARASITICS Drugs used to treat parasitic infections are as varied as the organisms that cause them. Generally, agents classified as antiparasitic are both expensive and likely to be toxic. Quinine was one of the first antiparasitic drugs developed in the treatment of malaria. Quinine is highly toxic, but newer forms such as chloroquine (Aralen, Chlorcon) and hydroxychloroquine (Plaquenil) are widely used as antimalarial drugs. Metronidazole (e.g., Flagyl) is used to treat infections of protozoan parasites (see the preceding Medication Administration box).

Isolation Techniques

Controlling the spread of infectious diseases in the hospital or long-term care setting is particularly important to preventing nosocomial infection. Hand hygiene remains the single most important factor in preventing the transmission of infections. Not all infectious diseases spread readily, necessitating special techniques or procedures. However, diseases such as chickenpox

MEDICATION ADMINISTRATION Antibiotic Therapy

I. Cell Wall Synthesis Inhibitors

PENICILLINS

Penicillin G	Dicloxacillin (Dynapen)
Penicillin V	Methicillin (Staphcillin)
Amoxicillin (Amoxil)	Mezlocillin (Mezlin)
Nafcillin (Unipen)	Oxacillin (Prostaphlin)
Ampicillin (Polycillin)	Piperacillin (Pipracil)
Carbenicillin (Geopen, Geocillin)	Ticarcillin (Ticar)

Combination Agents

ampicillin and sulbactam (Unasyn)

ticarcillin and clavulanate (Timentin)

piperacillin and tazobactam (Zosyn)

amoxicillin and clavulanate (Augmentin)

Penicillins are bactericidal and interfere with cell wall synthesis and the enzymes involved in cell division and synthesis. They are more effective on gram-positive than gram-negative organisms. Penicillins are considered to be safe, effective, and of low toxicity. Resistance is now more common among *Streptococci* and *Staphylococci*. Penicillins and related antibiotics such as the cephalosporins (see below) contain a molecular structure known as a beta-lactam ring. Some bacteria produce enzymes (beta-lactamases or penicillinases) that cleave this ring, making the antibiotics ineffective. To combat this resistance, beta-lactamase or penicillinase inhibitors such as sulbactam and clavulanate are combined with some antibiotics to create an antibiotic effective against drug-resistant bacterial strains.

Nursing Responsibilities

- Monitor for hypersensitivity responses such as local erythema and itching at the site of injection, skin rashes, urticaria (hives), itching, fever, chills, and anaphylaxis.
- Observe patients receiving parenteral penicillin for at least 30 minutes.
- Discontinue the drug immediately if any hypersensitivity response occurs. Be prepared to administer antihistamines or corticosteroids for a mild reaction. Anaphylaxis is treated with epinephrine subcutaneously or intravenously and airway support.
- Do not administer penicillin to anyone with a history of a severe allergic reaction to any form of the drug; a cross-reactivity may occur in patients allergic to cephalosporin or carbapenem antibiotics.
- Assess for superinfection (vaginitis, stomatitis, or diarrhea) due to elimination of resident bacteria.

Health Education for the Patient and Family

- Notify the physician if you see white patches on the oral mucosa or if vaginitis develops. An antifungal drug may be prescribed and the antibiotic continued.
- Consuming yogurt or buttermilk may prevent superinfection. Do not take these products within 1 hour of taking the drug.

CEPHALOSPORINS

1st Generation	2nd Generation
Cephalexin (Keflex)	Cefotetan (Cefotan)
Cefazolin (Ancef)	Cefaclor (Ceclor)
Cefadroxil (Duricef)	Cefoxitin (Mefoxin)
Cefradine (Velocef)	Cefprozil (Cefzil)
	Cefuroxime (Ceftin)
	Cefixime (Cefixime)
	Cefotaxime (Claforan)

3rd Generation	4th Generation
Cefoperazone (Cefobid)	Cefepime (Maxipime)
Ceftazidime (Fortaz)	
Ceftriaxone (Rocephin)	

Cephalosporins are structurally similar to the penicillins and also inhibit cell wall synthesis. They are divided into four groups, or generations. First-generation cephalosporins act primarily against gram-positive organisms. Second- and third-generation drugs are more effective against gram-negative organisms than against gram-positive ones. Fourth-generation cephalosporins act effectively against both gram-positive and gram-negative organisms.

Nursing Responsibilities

- Monitor for previous hypersensitivity response to cephalosporins or penicillins.
- Assess intravenous site for phlebitis; intramuscular injection may cause local pain.
- Monitor laboratory results for adverse response, such as leukopenia and thrombocytopenia, nephrotoxicity (elevated BUN and serum creatinine), or hepatotoxicity (elevated bilirubin, LDH, ALT, AST, and alkaline phosphatase).
- Assess for manifestations of superinfections.

Health Education for the Patient and Family

- Take the medication on an empty stomach, 1 hour before or 2 hours after meals.
- Avoid alcohol while using cefmetazole, cefoperazone, or cefotetan because alcohol intolerance can develop with these antibiotics. These same drugs intensify bleeding tendencies.
- Space doses of the medication relatively evenly throughout the day and evening hours.
- Increase consumption of buttermilk or yogurt to prevent intestinal superinfection.

CARBAPENEMS

Imipenem (Primaxin)

Meropenem (Merrem)

Ertapenem (Invanz)

This newer class of antibiotics includes only three drugs and all must be given parenterally. Imipenem has the broadest antimicrobial spectrum of any drug. This makes it especially useful against mixed organism infections. These antibiotics cross the meninges and achieve therapeutic doses in CSF; they are effective against methicillin-resistant staphylococcus aureus (MRSA). These antibiotics cause bacterial cell wall lysis and subsequent death of the bacteria. Side effects include nausea and vomiting, diarrhea, hypersensitivity reactions, occasional superinfections with bacteria or fungi, and, rarely, seizures.

Nursing Responsibilities

- Ertapenem should not be mixed with dextrose or other drugs containing dextrose. IV infusions should be given over at least 30 minutes.
- Check for history of hypersensitivity to cephalosporins and penicillins and monitor for manifestations of reactions.
- Assess for manifestations of superinfection.
- Monitor laboratory indicators of renal function.

Health Education for the Patient and Family

- Report any manifestations of allergy such as skin rash, itching, or hives.

VANCOMYCIN

This antibiotic inhibits cell wall synthesis and is used for serious infections. It is only effective against gram-positive bacteria, especially *S. aureus* and *Staphylococcus epidermidis*,

MEDICATION ADMINISTRATION   Antibiotic Therapy (continued)

including the strains resistant to methicillin. *C. difficile* is also susceptible to this antibiotic, but infection with *C. difficile* is often treated first with metronidazole to delay emergence of resistance to vancomycin.

Nursing Responsibilities
■ Infuse slowly over 60 minutes or more to avoid "red man" syndrome. The syndrome is characterized by erythematous rash, flushing, tachycardia, and hypotension. Patients may become dizzy and agitated. The occurrence is usually associated with a first dose of vancomycin and is seen within 4 to 6 minutes of the start of a dose or after completion.
■ Ototoxicity is a serious adverse effect because hearing loss may be irreversible. Notify the physician immediately if the patient reports a sensation of fullness in the ears, as this indicates ototoxicity.

II. Bacterial Protein Synthesis Inhibitors

TETRACYCLINES

Tetracycline HCl (Sumycin)   Minocycline HCl (Minocin)
Doxycycline (Vibramycin)   Oxytetracycline (Terramycin)

Tetracyclines are active against many gram-positive and gram-negative bacteria, such as *Mycoplasma*, *Rickettsia*, and *Chlamydia*. They are bacteriostatic, interfering with microbial protein synthesis. Tetracycline binds readily with metal and solid elements in the bowel, limiting its absorption when administered with food; the other preparations are highly soluble in lipids and can be administered with food.

Nursing Responsibilities
■ Schedule doses 1 hour before or 2 hours after meals. Do not give with milk or milk products or antacids.
■ Monitor for manifestations of superinfection.
■ If the patient is taking an anticoagulant, monitor prothrombin time and for manifestations of bleeding.

Health Education for the Patient and Family
■ Avoid excessive sun exposure to reduce the risk of photosensitivity reactions.
■ Tetracyclines can stain the enamel of developing teeth when taken during pregnancy; although deciduous (baby) teeth are affected, permanent teeth are not.

MACROLIDES

Erythromycin (E-Mycin, Erythrocin)   Clarithromycin
Azithromycin (Zithromax)   Dirithromycin (Dynabac)
    Troleandomycin (Tao)

Macrolides are bacteriostatic and act effectively against gram-positive and gram-negative organisms. Erythromycin is used to treat *Streptococcal pharyngitis* in patients who are allergic to penicillin, and is the drug of choice for treating pertussis. Clarithromycin and azithromycin produce less nausea than erythromycin, increasing patient adherence.

Nursing Responsibilities
■ Administer erythromycin on an empty stomach or immediately before meals.
■ Give the drug with a full glass of water. Do not administer with acidic fruit juice.
■ Intravenous doses are very irritating to veins; give slowly (20 to 60 minutes per gram).

Health Education for the Patient and Family
■ Gastric distress is a common side effect with erythromycin.

AMINOGLYCOSIDES

Amikacin (Amikin)   Gentamicin (Garamycin)
Kanamycin (Kantrex)   Neomycin (Mycifradin)
Streptomycin   Tobramycin (Nebcin)

Aminoglycosides are bactericidal, interfering with protein synthesis in the pathogen. They are especially effective against gram-negative organisms. To provide a broader spectrum of activity, they are often combined with other antibiotics, especially penicillins. Aminoglycosides can be administered in multiple or single daily doses. They are ototoxic and nephrotoxic; the risk is highest for older adults, patients with preexisting renal disease, and persons receiving other ototoxic or nephrotoxic drugs.

Nursing Responsibilities
■ Assess renal function before and during aminoglycoside therapy. Monitor intake and output, daily weight, BUN, and serum creatinine.
■ Assess for adverse effects on hearing such as loss of perception of high tones, tinnitus, and vertigo.
■ Notify the physician if the patient is receiving other nephrotoxic or ototoxic drugs such as furosemide (Lasix) and ethacrynic acid (Edecrin).
■ Administer intravenous preparations separately from other drugs; flush tubing before and after administration.

Health Education for the Patient and Family
■ Monitor for a sudden weight gain that may indicate adverse effects on the kidney and report it to the physician.

OXAZOLIDINONES
Linezolid (Zyvox) is the first antibiotic in a class of antibiotics called oxazolidinones. This antibiotic inhibits protein synthesis and is effective against organisms that are resistant to both vancomycin and methicillin. Because of its usefulness against those organisms, its use should be reserved for infections caused by vancomycin-resistant enterococci (VRE) and MRSA.

Nursing Responsibilities
■ Monitor for side effects including nausea, diarrhea, hypertension, and headache.
■ Monitor platelets if patient is at risk for bleeding; this drug may cause thrombocytopenia.

Health Education for the Patient and Family
■ It can be taken with or without food.
■ Avoid taking ephedrine, pseudoephedrine, methylphenidate, or cocaine with this drug as high blood pressure may develop.

III. Bacterial Nucleic Acid Inhibitors

FLUOROQUINOLONES
Ciprofloxacin (Cipro)   Gatifloxacin (Tequin) (ophthalmic)
Levofloxacin (Levaquin)

Fluoroquinolones are bactericidal and especially active against gram-negative and some gram-positive organisms. They are used to manage infections of the respiratory, gastrointestinal, and genitourinary tracts. Cipro is approved to treat inhalation anthrax; infected individuals are not contagious (Lane & Fauci, 2008).

Nursing Responsibilities
■ Increase fluid intake to 2000 to 3000 mL/day unless contraindicated to prevent crystalluria.
■ Monitor laboratory results for hepatotoxicity (elevated ALT, AST).

Health Education for the Patient and Family
■ Drink six to eight glasses of water per day.
■ Avoid exposure to sunlight while taking these drugs.

SULFONAMIDES AND TRIMETHOPRIM
Sulfamethizole (Thiosulfil Forte)
Sulfamethoxazole (Gantanol; in combination with trimethoprim, TMP-SMZ, Bactrim, Septra)
Sulfisoxazole (Gantrisin)
Sulfadiazine (Coptin)

(continued)

MEDICATION ADMINISTRATION   Antibiotic Therapy (continued)

Sulfonamides are bacteriostatic. Trimethoprim is an antibiotic effective against most gram-positive and many gram-negative organisms. It is often combined with sulfamethoxazole to manage urinary tract infections, *P. jiroveci* pneumonia, and otitis media. Skin rashes and pruritus are the most common hypersensitivity reactions. Severe reactions include exfoliative dermatitis and Stevens-Johnson syndrome.

Nursing Responsibilities
- Assess for history of hypersensitivity to sulfonamides and related medications, such as thiazide diuretics and sulfonylurea preparations.
- Monitor intake and output. Maintain a fluid intake of at least 1500 mL/day to prevent crystalluria.
- Assess for evidence of bleeding, easy bruising, or systemic infection, and monitor blood count for possible bone marrow depression.

Health Education for the Patient and Family
- Take medication on an empty stomach with a full glass of water. Maintain a fluid intake of at least 2 quarts per day.
- Protect the skin from excessive sun exposure with clothing and sunscreens to reduce the risk of photosensitivity.

METRONIDAZOLE (FLAGYL)
Metronidazole is effective against anaerobic gram-negative bacteria and protozoan infections caused by amebiasis, giardiasis, and trichomoniasis. It is commonly used to prevent and treat infections following intestinal surgery, and is the drug of first choice with *C. difficile*.

Nursing Responsibilities
- Monitor for CNS effects of dizziness, headache, ataxia, confusion, depression, and peripheral neuropathy.
- Administer with food to minimize gastric distress and metallic taste. Infuse intravenous metronidazole over 60 minutes.
- Discontinue the medication and notify the physician if neurologic reactions occur.
- Increase fluid intake to 2500 mL/day to minimize the risk of nephrotoxicity.

Health Education for the Patient and Family
- This medication may turn urine reddish brown; this is expected and not harmful.
- Stop taking the drug and notify the physician if hypersensitivity reaction or adverse effects occur, such as changes in mentation or coordination, painful or frequent urination, painful or difficult intercourse, impotence.
- Do not drink alcohol while taking this medication; an Antabuse-type reaction (flushing, sweating, headache, vomiting, and abdominal cramps) may occur.
- Maintain a fluid intake of 2.5 to 3 quarts per day.
- When the drug is prescribed for *Trichomonas* infections, treatment of both partners is necessary. Use condoms to prevent cross-contamination during intercourse.

(varicella) are highly contagious and are spread by the airborne route, requiring special precautions to protect other hospitalized patients. Two additional airborne threats are SARS and avian flu. These are addressed in ∞ Chapter 36.

In determining the need for isolation precautions, healthcare personnel consider the usual reservoir or source of the microorganism, the mode of transmission, and susceptibility of hospital staff and other patients. For example, patients with *P. jiroveci* pneumonia do not require isolation, because immunocompetent persons are not susceptible to this infection.

The CDC has published guidelines for isolation precautions to be used in healthcare facilities (CDC, 2007). These guidelines include both *standard precautions* and *category-specific isolation precautions*.

Standard Precautions
Standard Precautions, published by the Hospital Infection Control Practices Advisory Committee of the Centers for Disease Control in 1996, provides guidelines for the handling of blood and other body fluids. These guidelines are used with all patients, regardless of whether they have a known infectious disease. The guidelines were developed in light of the realization that many patients with an infectious disease such as HIV or hepatitis B have no apparent manifestations, but can transmit the disease to others. Standard precautions are used by all healthcare workers who have direct contact with patients or with their body fluids or have indirect contact, such as by emptying trash, changing linens, or cleaning the room.

MEDICATION ADMINISTRATION   Antiviral Agents

AMANTADINE (SYMMETREL)
Amantadine is used to prevent and treat influenza A. It has been shown to be 55% to 80% or more effective in preventing the disease. When administered within 24 to 72 hours after the onset of manifestations, it reduces common manifestations of influenza. It is generally well tolerated; minimal CNS side effects, such as dizziness, anxiety, insomnia, and difficulty concentrating, may occur.

ACYCLOVIR (ZOVIRAX) AND GANCICLOVIR (CYTOVENE)
Acyclovir and ganciclovir are related compounds used primarily in the treatment of herpes viruses. Acyclovir is prescribed mainly in the treatment of genital herpes simplex infections. Although it does not kill the virus, acyclovir is effective in reducing the severity, duration, and frequency of recurrence of manifestations. Ganciclovir is indicated primarily in the treatment of cytomegalovirus infection. Although acyclovir is generally well tolerated with little toxicity, ganciclovir may profoundly suppress bone marrow function, and its use is therefore limited.

VIDARABINE (VIRA-A)
Vidarabine inhibits viral DNA synthesis and is effective against many herpesvirus infections. Its primary use is in treatment of herpes simplex encephalitis.

INTERFERONS
Interferons are naturally produced cytokines whose use as antiviral agents is being explored. When administered intranasally, interferons have been shown to be effective in preventing rhinovirus upper respiratory infections. Other uses being explored include treatment of human papillomavirus (genital warts) and preventing or reducing Kaposi's sarcoma in patients with AIDS. They are also used in combination biotherapy regimens for malignant melanoma.

Standard precautions apply to the following:

- Blood
- All body fluids, secretions, and excretions, regardless of whether they contain visible blood
- Nonintact skin
- Mucous membranes

Barrier protection is used to prevent exposing skin and mucous membrane surfaces to blood and body fluids. Barrier protection involves using gloves for touching or handling body fluids, and adding other protection such as gowns, masks, and goggles if splashing or spraying is likely. Needles and other sharp objects are not recapped or bent, but disposed of in puncture-proof containers to prevent inadvertent percutaneous (needle-stick) exposure. Standard precautions are presented in ∞ Appendix A.

Transmission-Based Precautions

In addition to hand hygiene and standard precautions, the nature and spread of some infectious diseases require that special techniques be used to protect uninfected patients and workers. The CDC identifies three types of transmission-based precautions: airborne, droplet, and contact precautions. Transmission-based precautions may be combined for diseases that have multiple routes of transmission. Indications for the use of transmission-based isolation precautions and the specific measures to be taken are outlined in Table 12–9.

∞ Nursing Care

Nursing management related to infectious disease focuses on prevention and health promotion and maintenance. Prevention is facilitated by assessing the patient's risk for infection based on underlying conditions, immune response, and prophylactic measures such as immunizations.

Health Promotion

Preventing infection requires education of not only healthcare personnel but also the general public. Part of an education program includes understanding the importance of immunizations, the guidelines for using antibiotics to prevent drug-resistant microorganisms, and the ways to prevent the spread of infection. Check immunization records for all family members and encourage them to keep immunizations up to date. Increase public awareness regarding appropriate antibiotic use. Guidelines for preventing the spread of infection to others include the following:

- Avoid crowds and contact with susceptible persons, especially those who are immunosuppressed (e.g., persons who have HIV infection, who are undergoing therapy for cancer, or who have had an organ transplant).
- Use disposable tissues to contain respiratory secretions when coughing or sneezing. Cough into the elbow or upper arm instead of the hand if disposable tissues are not available.
- Use appropriate food-handling precautions for diseases spread via the fecal–oral route, such as hepatitis A.
- Avoid contact with or sharing of body fluids. For example, do not share needles or razors; use a condom during sexual activity, or abstain; have each person clean his or her own blood spills or wounds if possible.

Assessment

The following data are collected through the health history and physical examination. Further focused assessments are described with nursing interventions in the next section.

- *Health history:* Current manifestations, age, medication use (antipyretics and anti-infectives), nutrition, exposure to infectious persons, immunizations, invasive procedures and therapies, chronic diseases such as diabetes mellitus, cancer.
- *Physical assessment:* Vital signs, body system(s) where infection is suspected, lymph node enlargement, and tenderness.

TABLE 12–9 Transmission-Based Precautions

CATEGORY	INFECTIOUS DISEASES	PURPOSE	PRECAUTIONS
Airborne precautions	Pulmonary tuberculosis, chickenpox (with contact precautions), measles, respiratory infections (pneumonia)	Reduce risk of airborne transmission of infectious agents. Airborne transmission occurs by dissemination of either airborne droplet nuclei or dust particles containing the infectious agent.	Private room with hand washing and toilet facilities, and special ventilation that does not allow air to circulate to general hospital ventilation; mask or special filter respirator for everyone entering room
Droplet precautions	Meningitis, pertussis	Reduce risk of droplet transmission of infectious agents. Droplet transmission involves contact of conjunctivae of the eyes or mucous membranes of the nose or mouth with large-particle droplets generated during coughing, sneezing, talking, or procedures such as suctioning.	Private room with hand washing and toilet facilities; mask, eye protection, and/or face shields worn by everyone entering room
Contact precautions	Acute diarrhea, chickenpox (with airborne precautions), respiratory syncytial virus (RSV); skin, wound, or urinary tract infection with multidrug-resistant organisms; *S. aureus* infections	Reduce risk of transmission by direct or indirect contact. Direct contact transmission involves skin-to-skin contact and physical transfer of organisms. It may occur between patients or during direct care activities such as bathing or turning patients. Indirect contact involves contact with a contaminated object.	Private room with hand washing and toilet facilities; gowns and protective apparel to provide barrier protection; disposable supplies or decontamination of all articles leaving room

Nursing Diagnoses and Interventions

Patients with an infection may be managed in the hospital or at home, depending on the severity of the infection. During the acute phase, nursing care includes administering prescribed antibiotics, implementing and maintaining aseptic technique and infection control measures, and encouraging a balance of rest and activity, good nutritional intake, and other general health measures to support immunologic function and healing. The key nursing diagnoses are *Risk for Infection*, *Anxiety*, and *Hyperthermia*.

Risk for Infection

The spread of infection is a risk in any facility that houses many people. It is a particular risk in hospitals, where many patients have at least some degree of immunosuppression and many drug-resistant strains of pathogens are prevalent. It is vital that nurses use good hand hygiene techniques at all times, employ standard precautions with all patients, and use category-specific isolation techniques as indicated to prevent infectious spread to other patients, themselves, and their families.

- Admit patients with known or suspected infections to a private room. *This is important to minimize the risk to other patients.*
- Perform hand hygiene using hand sanitizer on entering and leaving the patient's room. If visibly soiled, wash hands using a 10- to 15-second vigorous scrub with soap or antibacterial scrub solution. *A 10- to 15-second scrub removes transient microorganisms from the skin and helps prevent transmission of infection to or from the patient.*
- Use standard precautions and personal protective devices to reduce the risk of transmission. *Gloves, gowns, and masks are to be worn whenever there is a risk of skin or mucous membrane contamination by direct contact with infectious material, airborne spread of organisms, or droplet nuclei.*
- Explain the reasons for and importance of isolation procedures during hospitalization. *Patients with isolation precautions may feel neglected, dirty, or shunned. Explanation of reasons and procedures can enhance the patient's and family's understanding and acceptance.*
- Place a mask on the patient and/or cover all infectious lesions or wounds completely when transporting the patient to other parts of the facility for diagnostic or treatment procedures. *These measures help minimize air contamination and the risk to visitors and personnel.*
- Collect a culture and sensitivity (C&S) specimen as ordered or indicated by purulent drainage, pyuria, or other manifestations of infection. *C&S is performed to determine the presence and type of infectious organisms as well as antibiotics most likely to be effective in eradicating it.*

> **PRACTICE ALERT**
> Collect the specimen for C&S before the first dose of antibiotics is administered to ensure adequate organisms for culture.

- Administer prescribed anti-infective agents. *Anti-infectives are used to destroy the invading microorganism.*
- Inform all personnel having contact with the patient of the diagnosis. *This is particularly important for a patient with a disease requiring category-specific isolation so that personnel can take appropriate precautions.*
- Ensure that visitors don appropriate protective wear before they enter the patient's room. *Protective wear reduces their risk of infection.*
- Use appropriate measures for disposing of contaminated tissues, dressings, or other material and for removing soiled linens and equipment from the patient's room. *Check hospital policy or published guidelines for category-specific isolation.*
- Teach the importance of complying with prescribed treatment for the entire course of the regimen. *Because anti-infective agents kill only a portion of the pathogen population with each dose, completion of the entire course of therapy is necessary to reduce the risk of relapse and of creating drug-resistant organisms.*

Anxiety

The patient with an infectious disease may experience anxiety related to his or her manifestations, treatment measures, the prognosis, and expected outcome of the disease. The diagnosis of an infection can be traumatic, causing feelings of uneasiness, isolation, guilt (e.g., in regard to sexually transmitted infections), apprehension, or depression.

- Assess level of anxiety. *The level of anxiety influences the patient's response to and interpretation of the situation and degree of threat it poses.*
- Discuss the infection, treatments, prognosis, and outcomes. *Discussions help to allay fears and misconceptions.*
- Support and enhance the patient's coping strategies. *A person uses intrapersonal and interpersonal mechanisms to reduce or relieve anxiety.*
- Include significant others in the plan of care. *Inclusion of the patient and family members provides assurance and confidence, and promotes understanding of the unknown.*
- Explain isolation procedures, and answer any concerns. *Isolation may be necessary to prevent the spread of infection but can cause great anxiety for the patient and family members.*
- Provide referrals as needed for continuing care, for example, to home health agencies or for dressing changes or periodic assessment. *Referrals are often necessary to provide ongoing interventions and maintain continuity of care.*

Hyperthermia

Hyperthermia is an expected consequence of the infectious disease process. Fever may produce mild, short-term effects or, when prolonged, may cause serious life-threatening effects.

- Monitor temperature especially during episodes of chills; note heart rate and rhythm. *Chills indicate a rising temperature. Hyperthermia can cause dysrhythmias.*
- Administer prescribed antipyretic as indicated for elevated temperature. *Although antipyretics lower the temperature and enhance comfort for the patient, this benefit must be weighed against the possible beneficial effect of an elevated temperature in the immune response. Fever increases the motility and activity of WBCs, stimulates the production of interferon, and activates T cells. In addition, temperatures above the normal range inhibit the growth of many microorganisms (Porth & Matfin, 2009).*

- Promote body cooling through lowering the room temperature. *Rapid cooling stimulates the hypothalamus to increase the body's temperature; this increases both shivering and metabolic rate.*

> **PRACTICE ALERT**
> Use ice packs, cool/tepid baths, or a hypothermia blanket with caution to prevent unnecessary shivering.

- Monitor fluid loss; encourage increased fluid and electrolyte intake either orally or intravenously. *Hyperthermia causes fluid loss from evaporation and may result in dehydration and electrolyte imbalance.*
- If diaphoretic, bathe and provide dry clothing and bedding. *These measures increase patient comfort and decrease further water evaporation.*
- Promote rest periods. *Rest increases the energy reserve that is depleted by an increased metabolic, heart, and respiratory rate.*

Using NANDA, NIC, and NOC

Linkages between a selected NANDA nursing diagnosis, NIC, and NOC for the patient with an infection are shown in the chart that follows.

Community-Based Care

Patient and family teaching is directed toward helping the patient recover from the infection or disease, preventing its spread to others, and preventing life-threatening complications. Instructions should include the following points:

- Use good hand hygiene techniques, particularly after touching infected wounds or lesions, coughing, sneezing, blowing the nose, or using the bathroom. Wash hands thoroughly before eating or performing any procedures such as dressing changes. Wash hands with soap and water before and after preparing food or eating and before and after using the toilet or handling diapers. Do not share eating utensils.
- Take all prescribed antibiotics as ordered even after manifestations have subsided. Take the prescription at intervals around the clock as directed.
- Never allow anyone else to use your medications and never use anyone else's prescription even if they appear to be the same.

> **NANDA, NIC, AND NOC LINKAGES**
> **The Patient with an Infection**
>
> **NANDA** — Delayed Surgical Recovery
>
> **NIC** — Infection Control / Medication Administration / Vital Signs Monitoring / Wound Care
>
> **NOC** — Infection Severity / Wound Healing: Primary Intention / Post Procedure Recovery Status
>
> Data from NANDA International. (2009). *Nursing diagnoses: Definitions & classification 2009–2011.* Oxford, UK: Wiley-Blackwell; Bulechek, G. M., Butcher, H. K., & Dochterman, J. M. (Eds.). (2008). *Nursing interventions classification (NIC)* (5th ed.). St. Louis, MO: Mosby; and Moorhead, S., Johnson, M., Maas, M., & Swanson, E. (Eds.). (2008). *Nursing outcomes classification (NOC)* (4th ed.). St. Louis, MO: Elsevier Mosby.

- Notify your healthcare provider if
  - symptoms do not improve within 24 to 48 hours after antibiotic therapy is instituted, or they worsen.
  - manifestations of antibiotic allergy (itching, rash, difficulty breathing or swallowing, swelling of the face or tongue) occur. Discontinue medication and contact prescriber.
  - adverse responses, such as gastrointestinal distress or diarrhea interfere with completion of the prescription.
  - manifestations of infection recur after completing prescribed antibiotic.
- Report redness, swelling, or drainage around wounds or persistent high fever.
- Increase fluid intake to at least 2500 mL (2.5 quarts) per day.
- Report any manifestations of opportunistic infections: loose, watery, and foul-smelling diarrhea; vaginal discharge or itching; fuzzy growth or white plaques in mouth or on tongue; blood in urine; chills; fever; or unusual cough.
- In addition, suggest the following resources: County or public health department, Centers for Disease Control and Prevention.

CHAPTER HIGHLIGHTS

- The human body has a remarkable capacity to survive in an environment of deadly microorganisms and pathogens that can weaken and kill the body. Both natural barriers and the immune system prevent the invasion and replication of pathogens. The lymphatic system provides conduits for pathogens, isolating them from the bloodstream where they would grow rapidly.
- The adaptability and specificity of immune responses is possible because immune cells are genetically encoded to capture pathogens, move them to lymph nodes, and develop specific immune reactions. However, if the immune system's self-recognition fails, highly damaging autoimmune diseases can develop.
- A revolutionary increase in knowledge and understanding of the immune system has enabled progress in clinical medicine. Through scientific research concerning T and B lymphocytes, cytokines, antibodies, and other elements of the immune system, treatments are evolving for cancer, AIDS, organ transplantation, autoimmune diseases, infectious disease, and vaccines.
- Inflammation is a protective mechanism designed to prevent pathogens from entering the bloodstream and populating

functional tissues such as heart, liver, and kidney. Pain acts as a signal that tissue has been damaged and stimulates protective responses such as cleansing wounds and limiting function while healing progresses. Restoration occurs as the inflammatory process isolates the injury and repairs damaged tissue.

■ Localized infections may damage tissue and create pain, but systemic infections are life-threatening if they progress to septic shock. Unfortunately, hospitals are hazardous environments populated with collections of pathogens. Hospital-borne infections are often introduced into the body by medical procedures.

■ Hygiene, protection from harm, and nutrition support the immune defenses. Antimicrobial medications limit the spread of pathogens, but can lose their effectiveness when microbes mutate and develop resistance.

TEST YOURSELF NCLEX-RN® REVIEW

1. When a patient receives gamma globulin following exposure to hepatitis A, the nurse expects the patient to develop which of the following?
   1. natural passive immunity
   2. natural active immunity
   3. acquired passive immunity
   4. acquired active immunity

2. What would be the priority nursing intervention in the treatment of a patient with an infection?
   1. Administer prescribed anti-infective.
   2. Assess for history of hypersensitivities and allergies.
   3. Obtain specimen for culture and sensitivity.
   4. Monitor for reaction to anti-infective.

3. When administering medications, the nurse would know that which one of the following medications inhibits prostaglandin synthesis?
   1. acetaminophen (Tylenol)
   2. prednisone
   3. penicillin
   4. aspirin

4. The patient with an acute infection shows a shift to the left on the WBC differential count. The nurse recognizes a shift to the left because of which laboratory finding?
   1. increased band neutrophils
   2. increased eosinophils
   3. decreased leukocytes
   4. decreased monocytes

5. A patient is admitted with methicillin-resistant *Staphylococcus aureus* in a draining sacral wound. The patient should be placed in which type of isolation precautions?
   1. droplet precautions
   2. contact precautions
   3. airborne precautions
   4. protective precautions

6. The T cells of the immune system adapt to kill which type of organism?
   1. intracellular organisms
   2. interstitial microbes
   3. extracellular viruses
   4. protozoans

7. How would the nurse describe thrombocytosis?
   1. increased platelets
   2. decreased clotting time
   3. decreased platelets
   4. average number of platelets

8. A nurse makes the nursing diagnosis *Risk for Infection*. What group is he or she considering when making this diagnosis?
   1. the infected patient only
   2. healthcare workers in the facility
   3. patients hospitalized at the same time
   4. the infected patient, healthcare workers, and other patients

9. What does the nurse primarily monitor when administering antibiotics?
   1. compliance
   2. therapeutic levels
   3. oxygen desaturation
   4. hypersensitivities and teaching

10. All nurses are expected to follow standard precautions for all hospitalized patients. What do these include?
    1. hand hygiene, use of masks, and recapping needles
    2. use of masks and gowns, and spraying of disinfectant regularly
    3. use of gloves, gowns, and goggles with contaminated body fluids
    4. use of alcohol-based hand rub for visibly dirty or blood-contaminated hands

See Test Yourself answers in Appendix C.

Pearson Nursing Student Resources

Find additional review materials at
www.nursing.pearsonhighered.com

Prepare for success with additional NCLEX®-style practice questions, interactive assignments and activities, Web links, animations and videos, and more!

BIBLIOGRAPHY

Arnold, M., & Barbul, A. (2006). Nutrition and wound healing. *Plastic and Reconstructive Surgery, 117*(7 Suppl), 42S–58S.

Aronson, B. (2005). Medication management behaviors of adherent short-term antibiotic users. *Clinical Excellence for Nurse Practitioners, 9*(1), 23–30.

Bulechek, G. M., Butcher, H. K., & Dochterman, J. M. (Eds.). (2008). *Nursing interventions classification (NIC)* (5th ed.). St. Louis: Mosby Elsevier.

Centers for Disease Control and Prevention. (2002a). Guidelines for hand hygiene in health-care settings. *MMWR Recommendations and Reports, 51*(RR 16), 1–44.

Centers for Disease Control and Prevention. (2002b). *Guidelines for the prevention of intravascular catheter-related infections.* Retrieved from http://www.cdc.gov/mmwr/preview/mmwrhtml/mm5132a9.htm

Centers for Disease Control and Prevention. (2010). *Estimates of healthcare associated infections.* Retrieved from http://www.cdc.gov/ncidod/dhqp/hai.html

Centers for Disease Control and Prevention. (2007b). *Guideline for isolation precautions: Preventing transmission of infectious agents in healthcare settings.* Retrieved from http://www.cdc.gov/ncidod/dhqp/gl_isolation.html

Centers for Disease Control and Prevention. (2009). Recommended adult immunization schedule—United States, 2009. *MMWR, 57*(53).

Christ-Crain, M., Jaccard-Stolz, D., Bingisser, R., et al. (2004). Effect of procalcitonin-guided treatment on antibiotic use and outcome in lower respiratory tract infections: Cluster-randomised, single-blinded intervention trial. *Lancet, 363*(9409), 600–607.

Eliopoulos, C. (2009). *Gerontological nursing* (7th ed.). Philadelphia: Lippincott Williams & Wilkins.

Fauci, A., Braunwald, E., Kasper, D. L., et al. (Eds.). (2008). *Harrison's principles of internal medicine* (17th ed.). New York: McGraw-Hill.

George, E. L. (2005). Does a high WBC count signal infection? *Nursing2005, 35*(1), 20–21.

Haas, J. P., & Larson, E. L. (2008). Compliance with hand hygiene. *American Journal of Nursing 108*(8), 40–45.

Kee, J. (2009). *Prentice Hall handbook of laboratory and diagnostic tests with nursing implication.* Upper Saddle River, NJ: Pearson Prentice Hall.

Kjonegaard, R., & Myers III, F. E. (2005). Arresting drug-resistant organisms. *Nursing 2005, 35*(6), 48–50.

Lacy, C. F., Armstrong, L. L., Goldman, M. P., & Lance, L. L. (2008). *Drug information handbook: A comprehensive resource for all clinicians and healthcare professionals.* Hudson, Ohio: Lexi-Comp Inc.

Lane, H. C., & Fauci, A. S. (2008). Microbial terrorism. In Fauci, A., Braunwald, E., Kasper, D. L., Hauser, S. L., Longo, D. L., Jameson, J. L., & Loscalzo, J. (Eds.), *Harrison's Principles of Internal Medicine* (17th ed.). New York: McGraw-Hill.

McPhee, S., Papadakis, M., & Tierney, L., (Eds.). (2008). *Current medical diagnosis & treatment* (47th ed.). Stamford, CT: Appleton & Lange.

Moorhead, S., Johnson, M., Maas, M., & Swanson, E. (Eds.). (2008). *Nursing outcomes classification (NOC)* (4th ed.). St. Louis, MO: Mosby Elsevier.

NANDA International. (2009). *Nursing diagnoses: Definitions and classification 2009–2011.* Oxford, UK: Wiley-Blackwell.

Porth, C. (2007). *Essentials of pathophysiology: Concepts of altered health states* (2nd ed.). Philadelphia: Lippincott Williams & Wilkins.

Porth, C., & Matfin, G. (2009). *Pathophysiology: Concepts of altered health states* (8th ed.). Philadelphia: Lippincott Williams & Wilkins.

Posani, T. (2004). *Clostridium difficile*: Causes and interventions. *Critical Care Nursing Clinics of North America, 16*(4), 547–551.

Prusiner, S. B., & Miller, B. (2007). Prion diseases. In Fauci et al., (Eds.), *Harrison's Principles of Internal Medicine* (17th ed.) (2646–2651). New York: McGraw-Hill.

Rakel, R. E., & Bope, E. T. (2008). *Conn's current therapy.* Philadelphia: Sanders Elsevier.

Shorr, A. F. (2005). Preventing pneumonia. The role for pneumococcal and influenza vaccines. *Clinics in Chest Medicine, 26*(1), 123–134.

Skidmore-Roth, L. (2009). *Mosby's nursing drug reference.* St. Louis: Mosby Elsevier.

Spigt, M. G., Knottnerus, J. A., Westerterp, K. R., Rikkert, M., & van Schayck, C. P. (2006). The effects of 6 months of increased water intake on blood sodium, glomerular filtration rate, blood pressure, and quality of life in elderly (Aged 55–75) men. *Journal of the American Geriatric Society 54*, 438–443.

Stokowski, L. A. (2008). Promoting vaccine safety: Answers to common questions. Medscape Nurses; Nursing Perspectives. Retrieved from http://www.medscape.com/viewarticle/568534

Stone, P. W., Hedblom, E. C., Murphy, D. M., & Miller, S. B. (2005). The economic impact of infection control: Making the business case for increased infection control resources. *American Journal of Infection Control, 33*(9), 542–547.

Vrtis, M. C. (2008). Is your patient taking the right antimicrobial? *American Journal of Nursing, 108*(6), 49–55.

Weinstein, R. A. (2007). Healthcare associated infections. In Fauci et al., *Harrison's principles of internal medicine* (17th ed.) (835–841). New York: McGraw-Hill.

White, K. A. (2008). The growing threat of cephalosporin resistance. *American Nurse Today, 3*(4), 9–12.

Wilson, B., Shannon, M., & Shields, K. (2009). *Prentice Hall nurse's drug guide.* Upper Saddle River, NJ: Pearson Prentice Hall.

CHAPTER 13

Nursing Care of Patients with Altered Immunity

LEARNING OUTCOMES

1. Review the normal anatomy and physiology of the immune system.
2. Compare and contrast the four types of hypersensitivity reactions.
3. Explain the pathophysiology of autoimmune disorders and tissue transplant rejection.
4. Discuss the characteristics of immunodeficiencies.
5. Identify laboratory and diagnostic tests used to diagnose and monitor immune response.
6. Describe interdisciplinary therapies and medications used to treat patients with altered immunity.
7. Correlate the pathophysiologic alterations with the manifestations of HIV/AIDS infection.

CLINICAL COMPETENCIES

1. Assess functional health status of patients with altered immunity and monitor, document, and report abnormal manifestations.
2. Assess for hypersensitivities and anticipate interdisciplinary interventions if manifestations develop.
3. Provide patient teaching about hypersensitivities, avoidance of sensitizing agents, and prophylactic treatment.
4. Use appropriate interventions to protect patients who are immune suppressed.
5. Recognize the burden and benefit of highly active anti-retroviral drug therapy (HAART) for the patient with HIV infection.
6. Use the nursing process as a framework to provide safe and individualized care to patients with altered immune responses.
7. Revise plan of care as needed to provide safe and knowledgeable interventions to promote or restore functional health status to patients with altered immunity.

KEY TERMS

acquired immunodeficiency syndrome (AIDS), 324
allergy, 308
allograft, 317
anaphylaxis, 308

antigenic substances, 306
autograft, 317
autoimmune disorder, 315
histocompatibility, 317
human immunodeficiency virus (HIV), 324

hypersensitivity, 308
immunosuppression, 317
Kaposi's sarcoma (KS), 328
seroconversion, 325

Considering the complexity of the immune system, it is not surprising that abnormal or harmful responses occur. Altered immune system responses include those characterized by hyperresponsiveness of the immune system and those characterized by an impaired immune response. Allergies, autoimmune disorders, and reactions to organ or tissue transplants are all examples of hyperresponsive immune function. AIDS and other immunodeficiency disorders result from impairment of the immune system.

New diseases affecting the immune system have emerged in recent years. These diseases include human immunodeficiency virus (HIV) infection and altered strains of familiar diseases such as multiple-drug-resistant tuberculosis. At the same time, understanding of the components of the immune system and specific immune responses is increasing. Alterations of the immune system affect the functional health status of affected individuals in all areas; knowledge of the prevention and care of patients with disorders of the immune system is increasingly important in today's healthcare system.

Overview of the Immune System

The immune system protects the body from invasion by foreign antigens, identifies and destroys potentially harmful cells, and removes cellular debris. These functions are accomplished by the lymphoid organs and specifically designed lymphocytes through the processes of antibody-mediated immune response and cell-mediated immune response.

The effectiveness of the immune system depends on its ability to differentiate normal host tissue from abnormal or foreign tissue. Body cells, tissues, and fluids have unique antigenic properties recognized by the immune system as "self." **Antigenic substances** stimulate an immune system response, but when identified as "self" the competent immune system does not react. External agents, such as microorganisms, cells and tissues from other humans or animals, and some inorganic substances, have antigenic properties recognized by the immune system as "nonself."

Each body cell displays specific cell surface characteristics, or markers, that are unique to each person. These are known as *human leukocyte antigens (HLAs).* A person's HLA characteristics are coded within a large cluster of genes known as the major histocompatibility complex (MHC) located on chromosome 6. Chromosomes are paired, with each person inheriting one member of the pair from each parent. A chromosome pair contains multiple genes, each carrying instructions for production of one polypeptide chain. The number of genes in the MHC results in a multitude of HLA combinations. As a result, the possibility of two people having the same HLA type is extremely remote. Identical twins may be the exception, and some siblings have very similar HLA patterns. In tissue grafting and organ transplants, matching the HLA type as closely as possible tends to decrease rejection.

Immunocompetent people have an immune system that identifies antigens and effectively destroys or removes them. When the immune system functions improperly, the result may be an overreaction or a deficiency, resulting in health problems. Overreaction of the immune system leads to hypersensitivity disorders, such as allergies. When the immune system loses the ability to recognize self, autoimmune disorders may ensue (these disorders are discussed in later chapters of this book). Immunodeficiency diseases or malignancies can develop when the immune system is incompetent or unable to respond effectively, as is the case with acquired immunodeficiency disorder. These alterations in immunity are discussed later in this chapter.

As described in Chapter 12, the *antibody-mediated immune response* is accomplished by B lymphocytes (B cells) that are further divided into memory cells and plasma cells. They are activated by contact with an antigen and by T cells. B cells produce antibodies, also known as immunoglobulins (see Table 12–3), and serve to inactivate an invading antigen. One immunoglobulin in particular, IgM, forms natural antibodies, such as those for ABO blood group antigens, and is an important component of the immune system complexes seen in autoimmune disorders. Memory cells "remember" an antigen, and, when exposed to it a second time, immediately initiate the immune response. This action provides the foundation of acquired immunity.

The T cell component of the immune system identifies cells containing antigens and signals B cells and other components of the immune system to attack infected cells. T lymphocytes do not secrete antibodies. T lymphocytes are subdivided into effector cells and regulator cells. The cytotoxic cell or killer T cell is the primary effector cell. Regulator T cells are divided into two subsets known as helper T cells and suppressor T cells. In addition to destroying viruses within cells marked as "non self," cytotoxic T lymphocytes also attack malignant cells and are responsible for the rejection of transplanted organs and grafted tissues.

Immune function is also affected with aging, as described in the following Nursing Care of the Older Adult box.

Assessing Altered Immune System Function

Unlike body systems that are composed of closely related organs, the immune system is diverse and scattered. Optimal immune function depends on intact skin and mucous membrane barriers, adequate blood cell production and differentiation, a functional system of lymphatics and the spleen, and the ability to differentiate foreign tissue and pathogens from normal body tissue and flora. Because of this diversity of organs and function, assessment of the immune system is often integrated throughout the history and physical examination.

Health History

Before conducting the health history, review the biographic data, including age, gender, race, and ethnic background. Many autoimmune disorders are more prevalent in women than in men. Family history is also important because there is a genetic component in the etiology of many disorders affecting the immune system.

NURSING CARE OF THE OLDER ADULT — Changes in Immune Function in the Older Adult

Immune function declines with aging. External factors, such as nutritional status and the effects of chemical exposure, ultraviolet radiation, and environmental pollution, affect the older adult's immune status. Internal factors affect it as well, including genetics, the function of the neurologic and endocrine systems, chronic and prior illnesses, and individual anatomic and physiologic variations. These influences make it difficult to determine the effect of aging on the immune system. In some older individuals, the immune system is as effective as that of younger persons.

Immunosenescence refers to the decline in immune system effectiveness brought about by aging (Hakim & Gress, 2007). Changes associated with this decline include involution of the thymus with less competent T cell maturation, diminished antibody production and adhesion, and decreased tolerance of self antigens. Increased morbidity and mortality associated with infection and increases in cancer and autoimmune disorders result from these changes. Recent studies show improved immune function when elderly subjects receive a nutritional supplement formulated to stimulate the immune systems (Langkamp-Henken et al., 2006).

Many interview questions related to the immune system and disorders that affect it are of a sensitive nature. Be sure to provide privacy prior to the interview. If family members are present, request that they leave. Ask the least sensitive questions before moving into those that are more sensitive, such as those related to the use of illicit drugs or sexual activity. Cultural sensitivity is necessary for effective communication.

Physical Assessment

The techniques of inspection and palpation are used to assess a patient's immune system.

- Assess the general appearance; evident fatigue or weakness may indicate acute or chronic illness or immunodeficiency. Note whether the stated and apparent age coincide. Assess height, weight, and body type for apparent weight loss or wasting. Observe ease of movement and note any evident stiffness or difficulty moving. Check vital signs. An elevated temperature may indicate an infection or inflammatory response.
- Inspect the mucous membranes of the nose and mouth for color and condition. Pale, boggy (edematous) nasal mucosa is often associated with chronic allergies. Note petechiae, white patches, or lacy white plaques in the oral mucosa; they may indicate hemolysis or immunodeficiency.
- Assess skin color, temperature, and moisture. Pale or jaundiced skin may indicate a hemolytic reaction. Pallor may also indicate bone marrow suppression with accompanying immunodeficiency. Inspect the skin for evidence of rashes or lesions, such as petechiae; numerous bruises; purple or blue patches or lesions indicative of Kaposi's sarcoma; and wounds that are infected, inflamed, or unhealed. Note the location and distribution of any rashes or lesions.
- Inspect and palpate the cervical, axillae, and groin lymph nodes for evidence of lymphadenopathy (swelling) or tenderness.
- Inspect and palpate the joints for redness, swelling, tenderness, or deformity, which may indicate an autoimmune disorder such as rheumatoid arthritis or systemic lupus erythematosus. Assess joint range of motion, including the spine.

The Patient with a Hypersensitivity Reaction

Hypersensitivity is an altered immune response to an antigen that results in harm to the patient. When the antigen is environmental or exogenous, it is called an **allergy**, and the antigen is referred to as an *allergen*. The tissue response to a hypersensitivity reaction may be bothersome, causing a runny nose or itchy eyes, or it may be life threatening, leading to blood cell hemolysis or laryngospasm, an involuntary tightening of the muscles of larynx that causes difficulty inhaling.

Hypersensitivity reactions are primarily classified by the type of immune response that occurs on contact with the allergen. They may also be classified as immediate or delayed hypersensitivity responses. Anaphylaxis and transfusion reactions are examples of immediate hypersensitivity reactions; contact dermatitis is a typical delayed response. Allergies are sometimes referred to by the affected organ system (e.g., allergic rhinitis) or the allergen involved, as in hay fever. More than one type of reaction may occur simultaneously (King et al., 2005).

Pathophysiology

In a hypersensitivity reaction, an antigen–antibody or antigen–lymphocyte interaction causes a response that is damaging to body tissues. Antigen–antibody responses characterize types I, II, and III, also known as immediate hypersensitivity responses. Type IV hypersensitivity is an antigen–lymphocyte reaction, resulting in a delayed hypersensitivity response.

Type I IgE-Mediated Hypersensitivity

Common hypersensitivity reactions, such as allergic asthma, allergic rhinitis (hay fever), allergic conjunctivitis, hives (urticaria), and anaphylactic shock, are typical of type I or IgE-mediated hypersensitivity. This type of hypersensitivity response is triggered when an allergen interacts with IgE bound to mast cells and basophils. The antigen–antibody complex prompts release of histamine and other chemical mediators, complement, acetylcholine, kinins, and chemotactic factors (Figure 13–1 ■).

When a potent allergen such as bee or wasp venom or a drug is injected, resulting in widespread antibody–antigen reaction and response to these chemical mediators, a systemic response such as anaphylaxis, urticaria, or angioedema (localized, rapid swelling beneath the skin) results.

Anaphylaxis is an acute systemic type I response that occurs in highly sensitive persons following injection of a specific antigen. Substances known to trigger anaphylaxis are summarized in Box 13–1. Anaphylaxis rarely follows oral ingestion although this is possible. Food allergies are the cause of approximately 150 deaths per year in the United States (CDC, 2007).

The reaction begins within minutes of exposure to the allergen and may be almost instantaneous. The release of histamine and other mediators causes vasodilation and increased capillary permeability, smooth muscle contraction, and bronchial constriction. These chemical mediators cause the typical manifestations of anaphylaxis. Initially, a sense of foreboding or uneasiness, light-headedness, and itching palms and scalp may be noted. Hives may develop, along with angioedema of the eyelids, lips, tongue, hands, feet, and genitals. Swelling can also affect the uvula and larynx, impairing breathing. This is further complicated by bronchial constriction, manifested by air hunger, stridor and wheezing, and a barking cough. These respiratory effects can be lethal if the reaction is severe and intervention is not provided

---

BOX 13–1　Substances Known to Trigger Anaphylaxis in Sensitized Persons

- **Hormones:**　insulin, vasopressin, parathormone
- **Enzymes:**　trypsin, chymotrypsin, penicillinase
- **Pollens:**　ragweed, grass, trees
- **Foods:**　eggs, seafood, nuts, grains, beans, cottonseed oil, chocolate
- **Vitamins:**　thiamine, folic acid
- **Insect Venom:**　yellow jacket, hornet, paper wasp, honey bee
- **Occupational Agents:**　rubber, latex, industrial chemicals
- **Antibiotics:**　penicillins, cephalosporins, amphotericin B, nitrofurantoin
- **Local Anesthetics:**　procaine, lidocaine

Hypersensitivity Video

Sensitization stage

Antigen (allergen) invades body.

Plasma cells produce large amounts of class IgE antibodies against allergen.

IgE antibodies attach to mast cells in body tissues.

Subsequent (secondary) responses

More of same allergen invades body.

Allergen combines with IgE attached to mast cells, which triggers release of histamine (and other chemicals) from mast cell granules.

Histamine causes blood vessels to dilate and become leaky, which promotes edema; stimulates release of large amounts of mucus; and causes smooth muscles to contract (if respiratory system is site of allergen entry, asthma may ensue).

Mast cell with fixed IgE antibodies

IgE

Granules containing histamine

Antigen

Mast cell granules release contents after antigen binds with IgE anitbodies

Histamine and other chemical mediators

Outpouring of fluid from capillaries

Release of mucus

Constriction of small respiratory passages (bronchioles)

Figure 13–1 ■ Type I IgE-mediated hypersensitivity response.

immediately. Vasodilation and fluid loss from the vascular system can lead to impaired tissue perfusion and hypotension, a condition known as *anaphylactic shock* (∞ see Chapter 11).

Fortunately, localized responses are more common manifestations of type I hypersensitivity. Atopic reactions, which have a genetic predisposition, are localized, rather than systemic, IgE-mediated responses to an allergen. They are the result of contact of the allergen with cell-bound IgE in the bronchial tree, nasal mucosa, and conjunctival tissues. Chemical mediators are released locally, producing symptoms such as asthma, allergic rhinitis (hay fever), conjunctivitis, or atopic dermatitis. Allergens commonly associated with atopic reactions of this type include pollens, fungal spores, house dust

mites, animal dander, and feathers (Porth & Matfin, 2009). When an allergic response to food occurs in the digestive system, nausea, vomiting, diarrhea, and cramping may develop. If the gastrointestinal mucosa is altered by a local allergic response, then the allergen may be absorbed, leading to a systemic reaction. Urticaria (hives) is the most common systemic response to food allergies.

Type II Cytotoxic Hypersensitivity

A hemolytic transfusion reaction to blood of an incompatible type is characteristic of a type II or cytotoxic hypersensitivity reaction. IgG or IgM type antibodies are formed to a cell-bound antigen such as the ABO or Rh antigen. When these antibodies bind with the antigen, the complement cascade is activated, resulting in destruction of the target cell (Figure 13–2 ■).

Type II reactions may be stimulated by an exogenous antigen, such as foreign tissue or cells, or a drug reaction in which the drug forms an antigenic complex on the surface of a blood cell, stimulating the production of antibodies. The affected cell is then destroyed in the resulting antigen–antibody reaction; for example, hemolytic anemia is sometimes associated with the administration of drugs such as penicillins, cephalosporins, and streptomycin. Withdrawal of the drug stops the reaction and cell destruction (Porth, 2007).

Endogenous antigens can also stimulate a type II reaction, resulting in an autoimmune disorder such as Goodpasture's syndrome (pulmonary hemorrhage and glomerulonephritis), in which antigens are formed to specific tissues in the lungs and kidneys. Hashimoto's thyroiditis and autoimmune hemolytic anemia are additional examples of autoimmune type II reactions.

Type III Immune Complex–Mediated Hypersensitivity

Type III hypersensitivity reactions result from the formation of IgG or IgM antibody–antigen immune complexes in the circulation. When these complexes are deposited in vessel walls and extravascular tissues, complement is activated and chemical mediators of inflammation such as histamine are released. Chemotactic factors attract neutrophils to the site of inflammation. When neutrophils attempt to phagocytize the immune complexes, lysosomal enzymes are released, increasing tissue damage (Figure 13–3 ■).

Either systemic or local responses may be seen with type III reactions. For example, serum sickness is a systemic response, named because it was first identified after administration of foreign serum (e.g., horse antitetanus toxin). Although foreign serums are no longer administered, serum sickness still occurs in response to some drugs, such as penicillin and sulfonamides. Immune complexes are deposited in walls of small blood vessels, the kidneys, and joints. Manifestations of serum sickness include fever, urticaria or rash, arthralgias, myalgias, and lymphadenopathy.

Localized responses may occur at a number of different sites. As immune complexes accumulate in the glomerular basement membrane of the kidneys—for example, following a streptococcal infection or with systemic lupus erythematosus—glomerulonephritis develops. When an antigen such as dust from moldy hay is inhaled by agricultural workers, an acute alveolar inflammatory response can occur.

Type IV Delayed Hypersensitivity

Type IV reactions differ from other hypersensitivity responses in two ways. First, these reactions are cell mediated rather than antibody mediated, involving T cells of the immune system. Second, type IV reactions are delayed rather than immediate, developing 24 to 48 hours after exposure to the antigen. Type IV hypersensitivity responses result from an exaggerated interaction between an antigen and normal cell-mediated mechanisms. This exaggerated interaction results in the release of soluble inflammatory and immune

Figure 13–2 ■ Type II cytotoxic hypersensitivity response.

Antigens invade body and
bind to antibodies in
circulation. Antigen–antibody
complexes are formed.

Antigen

Antibody

Antigen–antibody
complex

Antigen–antibody complexes
are deposited in the basement
membrane of vessel walls and
other body tissues, activating
complement.

Basement
membrane

Complement activation leads
to release of inflammatory
chemical mediators. Infiltration
of polymorphonuclear
leukocytes (PMNs) is followed
by release of lysozymes.
Tissue damage may
be extensive.

Polymorphonuclear
leukocyte

Lysosome

Chemical
mediators

Release of lysosomal
granules

Figure 13–3 ■ Type III immune complex–mediated hypersensitivity response.

mediators (from the lysozymes within the macrophages) and recruitment of killer T cells, causing local tissue destruction (Figure 13–4 ■).

Contact dermatitis is a classic example of a type IV reaction. Intense redness, itching, blister formation, and thickening affect the skin in the area exposed to the antigen. Many antigens can provoke this response; poison ivy is a prime perpetrator. In the healthcare setting, an allergic response to latex can also produce contact dermatitis. An estimated 8% to 13% of healthcare workers are allergic to latex and sensitivity remains beyond 5 years, making continued avoidance very important (Smith et al., 2007). Other examples of cell-mediated responses include a positive tuberculin test and graft rejection episodes.

Latex Allergy

Although protective against infection, the repetitive use of latex gloves creates a persistent exposure to latex for healthcare workers. When gloves are powdered with cornstarch to facilitate donning and removing gloves, the cornstarch particles aerosolize when the gloves are removed. The cornstarch includes latex particles. This creates a respiratory exposure as well as dermal exposure to latex. In addition, chemicals used in the manufacture of latex products may be irritating. Products such as balloons, condoms, and rubber bands are commonly made of latex.

Sensitivity to latex develops without the user being aware until a rash appears on the hands. Type IV hypersensitivity (contact dermatitis) can progress to type I systemic allergic reactions without previous symptoms signaling an escalation. It is important to protect the patient and the healthcare worker who is allergic to latex. Prevention is aided by employers who select products free of latex. Nonlatex gloves are recommended for use where there is no contact with infectious materials or blood. Workers should be screened periodically to detect symptoms of allergy and educated about latex sources. Hand hygiene after using latex products limits exposure (NIOSH, 2008).

Antigen-presenting cell encounters cytotoxic T cell.

Antigen-presenting cell

T cell

Interaction causes release of lympho-kines, which attract macrophages.

Lymphokines

Lysozymes

Macrophage

Macrophages release lysozymes, resulting in local tissue damage.

Figure 13–4 ■ Type IV delayed hypersensitivity response.

Interdisciplinary Care

The focus of care for patients with allergic responses is to minimize exposure to the allergen, prevent the hypersensitivity response, and provide prompt, effective interventions for allergic responses. Identifying allergens for the individual to reduce the likelihood of exposure is a key aspect of management. A complete history of the patient's allergies is obtained, including medications, foods, animals, plants, and other materials. The type of hypersensitivity response is documented, as is its onset, manifestations, and usual treatment.

When a documented or suspected hypersensitivity reaction occurs, the allergen (e.g., intravenous medication or transfusion) is withdrawn immediately. With a type I hypersensitivity response, managing the patient's airway takes highest priority, followed by maintaining cardiac output. Type II hypersensitivity responses may necessitate aggressive management of bleeding or renal failure. A type III (immune complex) reaction is treated by removing the offending antigen and interrupting the inflammatory response.

With a hypersensitivity response, supportive care is important to relieve discomfort. This often involves the administration of selected antihistamine or anti-inflammatory medications.

Other therapies may be prescribed in selected instances, such as plasmapheresis, a procedure that involves continually withdrawing and reinfusing blood from the patient while removing the allergic components from the plasma portion.

Diagnosis

To identify possible allergens or hypersensitivity reactions, the following laboratory tests may be ordered:

■ *White blood cell (WBC) count with differential* can detect high levels of circulating eosinophils. Increased numbers of eosinophils are often present in patients with type I hypersensitivities.

■ *Radioallergosorbent test (RAST)* is a blood test that measures the amount of IgE directed toward specific allergens. Test results are compared with control values and used to identify hypersensitivities. RAST may also be used instead of skin testing if a severe allergic response is suspected (American Association of Clinical Chemistry, 2006).

■ *Blood type and crossmatch* are ordered prior to any anticipated transfusions. This diagnostic test is described in ∞ Chapter 11. Other blood tests associated with blood transfusions are a *Coombs' Direct* (to detect antibodies on red blood cells [RBCs]) and a *Coombs' Indirect* (to check recipient's and donor's blood for antibodies before a blood transfusion).

- *Immune complex assays* may be performed to detect the presence of circulating immune complexes in suspected type III hypersensitivity responses. The normal result is a test negative for circulating immune complexes. A negative test does not, however, rule out an immune complex hypersensitivity response.
- *Complement assay* is also useful in detecting immune complex disorders. In these disorders, complement is, in effect, used up by the development of antigen–antibody complexes. Decreased levels are seen on examination. Both total complement level and amounts of individual components of the complement cascade can be determined.

Skin Tests for Allergies

Skin tests are also used to determine causes of hypersensitivity reactions. These tests are used to identify specific allergens to which a person may be sensitive. Allergens for testing are selected according to the patient's history. Test solutions made from extracts of inhaled, ingested, or injected materials, such as pollens, mites, venoms, or some drugs, are used for the prick test and intradermal testing. Epicutaneous testing (prick testing) is generally done first to avoid a systemic reaction; it is followed by intradermal testing of allergens with a negative response to prick testing. Substances that cause a reaction to the prick test should not be tested intradermally.

- *Prick (epicutaneous or puncture) test:* A drop of diluted allergenic extract is placed on the skin, and the skin is then pricked or punctured through the drop. With a positive test, a localized pruritic (itchy) wheal and erythema occur. The response is maximal at 15 to 20 minutes.
- *Intradermal:* A small amount of allergen extract at a 1:500 or 1:1000 dilution is injected intradermally in the forearm or intrascapular area. If several allergens are being tested, injections are spaced 0.25 to 0.5 apart. As control measures, plain diluent (negative control) and histamine (positive control) are injected. If there is no response to a particular allergen at 15 to 20 minutes, the test is negative. The appearance of a wheal and erythema, with a wheal diameter at least 5 mm greater than that produced by the control, indicates a positive response (Figure 13–5 ■).
- *Patch:* A 1-inch patch impregnated with the allergen (e.g., perfume, cosmetics, detergents, or clothing fibers) is applied to the skin for 48 hours. Absence of a response indicates a negative test result. Positive responses are graded from mild (erythema in the exposed area) to severe (erythema, papules, vesicles, or ulceration).

Food Allergy Testing

Food allergy testing is performed when a food allergy is suspected but the source or implicated food item has not been clearly identified. Food allergy symptoms are typically demonstrated within hours of eating. The patient is asked to keep a diary of foods consumed and allergic responses for a week. An elimination diet, excluding most common food allergens and all suspected foods) is then prescribed for one week. If symptoms do not improve, a different variation of the elimination

Figure 13–5 ■ Skin testing on the forearm showing induration and erythema typical of a positive response to an antigen.

Source: Southern Illinois University/Photo Researchers, Inc.

diet is prescribed. If symptoms are relieved, foods are reintroduced to the diet one at a time until symptoms recur, indicating allergy to that food.

Medications

When it is impossible to avoid the offending allergen and allergic manifestations are severe or disrupt the patient's activities of daily living (ADLs), medications may be prescribed. *Immunotherapy*, also called hyposensitization or desensitization, consists of injecting an extract of the allergen(s) in gradually increasing doses. Immunotherapy is used primarily for allergic rhinitis or asthma related to inhaled allergens. It has also been shown to be effective in preventing anaphylactic responses to insect venom. With weekly or biweekly subcutaneous injections of the allergen, the patient develops IgG antibodies to the allergen that appear to block effectively the allergic IgE-mediated response. Once a therapy plateau is reached, injections may be discontinued or continued indefinitely either monthly or bimonthly.

Antihistamines are the major class of drugs used in treating the symptoms of hypersensitivity responses, type I in particular. They are also useful to some extent in relieving manifestations (such as urticaria) of some type II and type III reactions. Antihistamines block H_1-histamine receptors, acting as a competitive antagonist to histamine, but they do not affect the production or release of histamine. The prototype antihistamine is diphenhydramine (Benadryl). It and other antihistamines alleviate the systemic effects of histamine such as urticaria and angioedema (localized tissue swelling). They are also useful in relieving allergic rhinitis, drying respiratory secretions through an anticholinergic effect. The preferred route of administration is oral, although diphenhydramine and others can be given parenterally, particularly when immediate action is needed, as in anaphylaxis. Side effects include drowsiness and dry mouth. Antihistamines are not effective in relieving asthmatic responses to allergens and may actually worsen symptoms by their drying effect on respiratory secretions. Antihistamines are often combined with a sympathomimetic agent such as pseudoephedrine to improve their decongestant activity and counteract their sedative effect. Antihistamines and decongestants are discussed further in ∞ Chapter 35.

Hypersensitivity Video

Glucocorticoids (corticosteroids) are used in both systemic and topical forms for many types of hypersensitivity responses. Their anti-inflammatory effects, rather than their immunosuppressive effects, are of most benefit. A short course of corticosteroid therapy is often used for severe asthma, allergic contact dermatitis, and some immune-complex disorders; alternate-day dosing is preferred in long-term use (McPhee & Papadakis, 2009). Corticosteroids in topical forms or delivered by inhaler may be used for longer periods of time with few side effects; however, systemic absorption can occur.

Other Therapies

Other treatments used for hypersensitivity responses are generally dictated by the severity of the response and the organ system affected. Airway management takes highest priority for the patient with an acute anaphylactic reaction. Insertion of an endotracheal tube or emergency tracheostomy may be required to maintain airway patency with severe laryngospasm. Because anaphylaxis places the person at risk for vasomotor collapse and significant hypotension, it is necessary to insert an intravenous line and initiate fluid resuscitation with an isotonic solution such as Ringer's lactate.

Plasmapheresis, removal of harmful components in the plasma (also known as *plasma exchange therapy*), may be used to treat immune complex responses such as glomerulonephritis and Goodpasture's syndrome. Plasma and the glomerular-damaging antibody–antigen complexes are removed by passing the patient's blood through a blood cell separator. The RBCs are then returned to the patient along with an equal amount of albumin or human plasma. This procedure is usually done in a series rather than as a one-time treatment. It is not without risk, and informed consent is required. Potential complications of plasmapheresis include those associated with intravenous catheters, shifts in fluid balance, and alteration of blood clotting.

Treatment of Anaphylaxis

The immediate treatment for anaphylaxis is parenteral epinephrine, an adrenergic agonist (sympathomimetic) drug that has both vasoconstricting and bronchodilating effects. These qualities, combined with its rapid action, make epinephrine ideal for treating an anaphylactic reaction. For mild reactions with wheezing, pruritus, urticaria, and angioedema, a subcutaneous injection of 0.3 to 0.5 mL of 1:1000 epinephrine is generally sufficient. For patients with an injected toxin such as a bee sting, an additional amount equivalent to one-half the above may be injected directly into the site of the sting and a tourniquet applied above it to prevent further systemic absorption. Intravenous epinephrine using a 1:100,000 concentration may be used in the patient with a more severe anaphylactic reaction.

✍ Nursing Care

Nursing care related to hypersensitivity reactions is primarily directed toward prevention, early identification, and providing prompt, effective treatment.

Health Promotion

Health promotion activities include helping patients identify possible allergens that prompt a hypersensitivity response and discussing strategies to avoid these allergens. Anyone with severe food allergies may need referral to a dietitian to discuss necessary dietary changes and ways to continue meeting nutrient needs. It is important that persons with hypersensitivities inform healthcare personnel of all allergens. People who experience anaphylactic reactions should wear a Medic-Alert bracelet or tag at all times to identify the substance(s) that provokes this response. Patients who have experienced an anaphylactic reaction to insect venom or other potentially unavoidable allergens should carry a kit (commonly called a bee sting kit) for immediate treatment of future exposures. This kit typically includes a prefilled syringe of epinephrine and an epinephrine nebulizer, allowing prompt self-treatment.

Assessment

Collect the following data through the health history and physical examination. Further focused assessments are described with nursing interventions in the next section.

- *Health history:* risk factors, hypersensitivities (medications, household dust, bee stings, etc.), reaction (rash, hives, difficulty breathing), type of treatment for hypersensitivity reactions; allergy skin testing; asthma, hay fever, or dermatitis.
- *Physical assessment:* mucous membranes of nose and mouth, skin for lesions or rashes, eyes (tearing and redness), respiratory rate, and adventitious breath sounds.

Nursing Diagnoses and Interventions

Priority nursing diagnoses will vary according to the type of hypersensitivity reaction experienced by the patient. Because nurses are most likely to become involved with a patient experiencing a type I or type II response, this section focuses on diagnoses for these patients. Airway, breathing, and circulation (the ABCs) are of greatest importance for the patient with an anaphylactic reaction.

Ineffective Airway Clearance

In anaphylactic reactions, the airway may be obstructed due to facial angioedema, bronchospasm, or laryngeal edema. Establishing and maintaining a patent airway is of highest priority.

- Administer oxygen per nasal cannula at a rate of 2 to 4 L/min. Apply oxygen emergently and obtain a physician order for oxygen administration. *Providing external oxygen increases the alveolar oxygen and its availability to cells of the body.*
- Assess respiratory rate and pattern, level of consciousness and anxiety, nasal flaring, use of accessory muscles of respiration, chest wall movement, audible stridor; palpate for respiratory excursion; auscultate lung sounds and any adventitious sounds, such as wheezes. *Extreme anxiety or agitation, nasal flaring, stridor, and diminished lung sounds indicate air hunger and possible airway obstruction, necessitating immediate intervention.*
- Position in Fowler's to high Fowler's *to promote optimal lung expansion and ease of breathing.*
- Insert a nasopharyngeal or oropharyngeal airway, and arrange for immediate intubation as indicated. *Ensuring an adequate airway is vital to preserve life.*
- Administer subcutaneous epinephrine 1:1000, 0.3 to 0.5 mL, as prescribed. This may be repeated in 20 to 30 minutes if necessary. Administer parenteral diphenhydramine (deep intramuscular or intravenous) as prescribed. *Epinephrine is a*

potent vasoconstrictor and bronchodilator, counteracting the effects of histamine. Diphenhydramine is an antihistamine that blocks histamine receptors and their effect. These medications can be effective in rapidly reversing manifestations of anaphylaxis.

- Provide calm reassurance. *Hypoxemia and air hunger are terrifying for the patient. Anxiety can impair the patient's ability to cooperate with treatment and can increase the respiratory rate, making breathing less effective.*

Decreased Cardiac Output

Peripheral vasodilation and increased capillary permeability from the release of histamine can significantly impair cardiac output. When it falls to the degree that tissue perfusion becomes impaired and hypoxia results, a state of anaphylactic shock exists.

- Monitor vital signs frequently, noting fall in blood pressure, decreasing pulse pressure, tachycardia, and tachypnea. *These vital sign changes may indicate shock.*
- Assess skin color, temperature, capillary refill, edema, and other indicators of peripheral perfusion. *As cardiac output falls, peripheral vessels constrict and tissue perfusion is impaired.*
- Monitor level of consciousness. *A change in level of consciousness (lethargy, apprehension, or agitation) is often the first indicator of decreased cardiac output.*
- Insert one or more large-bore (18-gauge or larger) intravenous catheters as prescribed. *It is important to insert intravenous catheters as soon as possible to provide sites for rapid fluid replacement.*
- Administer warmed intravenous solutions of lactated Ringer's or normal saline, as prescribed. *These isotonic solutions help maintain intravascular volume. Warmed solutions are used to prevent hypothermia from the rapid administration of large amounts of fluid at room temperature (about 70°F, or 21.1°C).*
- Insert an indwelling catheter, and monitor urinary output frequently. *As the cardiac output drops, the glomerular filtration rate (GFR) falls. With an output of less than 30 mL/h, the patient is at risk for acute renal failure from ischemia.*

> **PRACTICE ALERT**
> Aggressive fluid therapy may lead to hypervolemia, resulting in pulmonary edema; assess for shortness of breath and crackles in the lungs.

Community-Based Care

Most hypersensitivity responses are appropriately treated by the patient or family members with self-care measures. Teaching is a vital component of care. If the patient is at risk for anaphylaxis, involving the family in teaching is essential because the response may occur with such rapidity that the patient will be unable to provide self-care. Include the following points in teaching the patient and family about managing hypersensitivities:

- When and how to use an anaphylaxis kit containing epinephrine and antihistamines in injectable, inhaler, and oral forms
- When to seek medical attention
- Use and adverse reactions of antihistamines and decongestants
- Advantages of autologous blood transfusion if future surgery is scheduled

- Skin care to prevent and care for contact dermatitis, as discussed in ∞ Chapter 16
- Helpful resources:
  - ALERT, Inc., Allergy to Latex Education and Resource Team (Toll free 1-888-97-ALERT)
  - Food Allergy and Anaphylaxis Network

The Patient with an Autoimmune Disorder

Maintaining optimal health and preventing disease depend not only on the immune system's ability to recognize and destroy foreign tissues and other antigens, but also on the immune system's ability to recognize self. When self-recognition is impaired and immune defenses are directed against normal host tissue, the result is an **autoimmune disorder**.

Autoimmune disorders can affect any tissue in the body. Some are tissue or organ specific, affecting a particular tissue or a particular organ. Hashimoto's thyroiditis is an example of an organ-specific autoimmune disorder. Circulating antibodies are formed to certain thyroid components, resulting ultimately in destruction of the gland. In other disorders, autoantibodies are formed that are not tissue specific, but tend to accumulate and cause an inflammatory response in certain tissue, for example, the renal glomeruli or the hepatic small bile ductules. Autoimmune disorders may also be systemic, with neither antibodies nor the resulting inflammatory lesions confined to any one organ. Rheumatologic disorders, such as rheumatoid arthritis and systemic lupus erythematosus (SLE), are characteristic of systemic autoimmune disorders.

Pathophysiology

The mechanism that causes the immune system to recognize host tissue as a foreign antigen is not clear. The following factors are under study as possible contributors to the development of autoimmune disorders:

- The release of previously "hidden" antigens into the circulation, such as DNA or other components of the cell nucleus, which elicits an immune response
- Chemical, physical, or biologic changes in host tissue that cause self-antigens to stimulate the production of autoantibodies
- The introduction of an antigen, such as a bacteria or virus, whose antigenic properties closely resemble those of host tissue, resulting in the production of antibodies that target not only the foreign antigen but also normal tissue. This is termed molecular mimicry. Heart damage in rheumatic fever and acute glomerulonephritis following beta-hemolytic streptococcal infections are examples of the development of antibodies against normal tissue (Porth & Matfin, 2009).
- A defect in normal cellular immune function that allows B cells to produce autoantibodies unchecked
- Initiation of the autoimmune response by very slow-growing mycobacteria

Although the exact mechanism producing autoimmunity is unclear, several characteristics of autoimmune diseases are known. It is apparent that genetics plays a role because a higher incidence is seen in family members of people with autoimmune disorders. More than one genetic change is likely occurring to cause development of these disorders. Autoimmune disorders are far more prevalent in females than in males. There is evidence that estrogen stimulates the immune response while androgens suppress the immune response (Porth, 2007).

The disorders tend to overlap, so that the patient with one autoimmune disorder may develop another or some manifestations of another. The onset of an autoimmune disorder is frequently associated with a physical or psychologic stressor. Autoimmune disorders are frequently characterized by periods of exacerbation and remission.

Specific autoimmune disorders are discussed in the sections of this textbook related to the affected organ systems or functional disruption.

Interdisciplinary Care

For the most part, the diagnosis of an autoimmune disorder is based on the patient's manifestations. Although the manifestations of these disorders can often be managed, a cure typically is not possible unless the affected target tissue is removed (e.g., colectomy for the patient with ulcerative colitis).

Diagnosis

Serologic assays are used to identify and measure antibodies directed toward host tissue antigens or normal cellular components. Many detectable autoantibodies are not specific to a single autoimmune disorder and are used to establish the autoimmune process rather than the specific disorder. Although healthy people often have low levels of autoantibodies, levels are much higher in patients affected by an autoimmune disorder. The following serologic assays may be ordered:

- *Antinuclear antibody (ANA)* detects antibodies produced to DNA and other nuclear material. These antibodies can cause tissue damage characteristic of autoimmune disorders such as SLE. The patient's serum is combined with nuclear material and tagged antihuman antibody to detect ANA-antihuman antibody complexes. A negative, or normal, result is a titer < 1:20. When complexes are detected at higher titer levels (> 1:20), the test is positive for ANA.
- *Lupus erythematosus (LE) cell test* is used to detect SLE and monitor its treatment. Neutrophils that contain large masses of phagocytized DNA from the nuclei of PMNs are called LE cells. Like the ANA, the LE cell test is nonspecific for SLE. A positive result may also be seen in rheumatoid arthritis (RA) or with medications such as isoniazid, clofibrate, penicillin, phenytoin, procainamide, streptomycin, tetracycline, trazodone, oral contraceptives, or sulfonamide drugs.
- *Rheumatoid factor (RF)* is an immunoglobulin present in the serum of approximately 80% of patients with rheumatoid arthritis. A person with RA may not have detectable RF (Porth & Matfin, 2009). Low titer levels (< 1:20) may normally be present in the older adult. An RF titer 1:80 or higher indicates RA. A titer between 1:20 and 1:80 could indicate SLE, scleroderma, or liver cirrhosis. Results are also reported as IU/ml; above 20 IU/ml is indicative of RA or Sjogren's syndrome, a disease in which autoantibodies attack the moisture-producing glands to cause dry eyes and dry mouth (Delaleu et al., 2009).

- *Complement assay* may also be useful in identifying autoimmune disorders. In these disorders, complement may be consumed in the development of antigen–antibody complexes. Decreased levels are seen on examination. Both total complement level and amounts of individual components of the complement cascade can be determined.
- *Anti CCP antibody test* is a blood test for RA. It measures anti-cyclic citrullinated peptide antibody in blood; the results are specific for RA. These antibodies replace normal protein in the joints of patients with RA.

Medications

Various approaches are used in the treatment of autoimmune disorders.

- Anti-inflammatory medications such as aspirin, nonsteroidal anti-inflammatory drugs (NSAIDs), and corticosteroids may be prescribed to reduce the inflammatory response and minimize tissue damage. When these agents are not effective or well tolerated by the patient, disease-modifying antirheumatic drugs or slow-acting anti-inflammatory medications may be prescribed.
- Cytotoxic drugs (described in the next section) may be used in combination with plasmapheresis in treating many autoimmune disorders.
- Disease-modifying antirheumatic drugs (DMARDs) reduce manifestations, reduce or prevent joint damage, and preserve the structure and function of the joints in patients with RA. The most common DMARDs in current use are methotrexate (Rheumatrex), sulfasalazine (Azulfidine), hydroxychloroquine (Plaquenil), leflunomide (Arava), and cyclosporine (Sandimmune, Neoral).
- Another class of antirheumatic drugs, referred to as *biologicals* or *biological response modifiers*, consists of laboratory-produced proteins that decrease the inflammatory process. These antibodies bind tumor necrosis factor alpha (TNF-α) and interleukin-1, both inflammatory elements. These medications include infliximab (Remicade) or adalimumab (Humira), etanercept (Enbrel), anakinra (Kineret), Rituxan, and abatacept (Orencia).
- Slow-acting anti-inflammatory drugs, including gold salts, hydroxychloroquine (Plaquenil), and penicillamine, may be used when other therapies are ineffective or not tolerated by the patient. These drugs, however, are relatively toxic and less frequently used.

Nursing Care

Nursing interventions for the patient with an autoimmune disorder are individualized and tailored to needs dictated by manifestations of the disorder. Nurses often will be involved with the patient in an outpatient setting, evaluating the patient's response to therapy and self-care management.

Consider the following nursing diagnoses in planning care for the patient with an autoimmune disorder:

- *Activity Intolerance* related to inflammatory effects of autoimmune disorder
- *Ineffective Coping* related to chronic disease process
- *Interrupted Family Processes* related to lack of understanding about autoimmune disorder and its effects
- *Ineffective Protection* related to disordered immune function

Community-Based Care

Because many autoimmune disorders are chronic, teaching the patient and family about the disorder and its management is a key nursing intervention. The patient may be taking drugs with multiple side effects or long-term effects, necessitating effective teaching. Patients with autoimmune disorders often do not appear to be ill, making it difficult for friends and families to understand their care needs. The chronicity of these disorders also puts the patient at high risk for unproven remedies and quackery. Provide psychologic support, listening, and teaching. In addition, suggest resources such as local support groups and the American Autoimmune Related Diseases Association.

The Patient with a Tissue Transplant

Since the first kidney transplant was performed from one identical twin to the other in 1954, organ and tissue transplantation have become increasingly popular and viable treatment options. The transplantation of avascular tissues, such as skin, cornea, bone, and heart valves, is considered routine, with little need for tissue matching and **immunosuppression** (the use of drugs to make the immune response less effective). Transplants of organs (e.g., the kidney, heart, heart and lung, liver, and bone marrow) are increasingly common. Commonly performed organ transplants are outlined in Table 13–1; success rates refer to survival of the transplant recipient.

Transplant success is closely tied to obtaining an organ with tissue antigens as close to those of the recipient as possible. Every body cell has cell surface antigens known as human leukocyte antigens (HLA) that are unique to the individual. Even though identical twins may have the same HLA type, a few of their antigens may be dissimilar enough to cause a transplant between them to be rejected. Matching the HLA type of the donor and recipient as closely as possible decreases the potential for rejection of the transplanted organ or tissue but does not eliminate it. Combining multiple organs for transplant such as liver-kidney, heart-liver, or heart-lung seems to be protective from rejection. The multiplicity of antigens seems to increase tolerance or may produce an "immune paralysis" (Rana et al., 2008).

Pathophysiology

An **autograft**, a transplant of the patient's own tissue, is the most successful type of tissue transplant. Skin grafts are the most common examples of autografts. Increasingly, autologous bone marrow transplants and blood transfusions are being used to reduce immunologic responses. When the donor and recipient are identical twins, the term *isograft* is used. Because of the high likelihood of an HLA match, the success of these grafts is good and rejection episodes are mild.

Few people, however, have an identical twin to provide tissue for donation, and when the need is for an organ such as the heart, liver, or lungs, a living-donor transplantation is not possible. Most often, organ and tissue transplants are **allografts**, which are grafts between members of the same species that have different genotypes and HLA. Allografts may come from living donors; examples are bone marrow, blood, and a kidney. Most often, organs for transplantation are obtained from a cadaver. Donors are typically people who meet the criteria for brain death; are less than 65 years old; and are free of systemic disease, malignancy, or infection, including HIV, hepatitis B, or hepatitis C. The organ is removed immediately before or after cardiac arrest and preserved until it is transplanted into the waiting recipient. Finally, *xenograft* is a transplant from an animal species to a human. These transplants are the least successful but may be used in selected instances, such as the use of pig skin as a temporary covering for a massive burn.

Tissue typing is used to determine **histocompatibility**, the ability of cells and tissues to survive transplantation without immunologic interference by the recipient. Tissue typing is performed in an attempt to match the donor and recipient as closely as possible for HLA type and blood type and to identify preformed antibodies to the donor's HLA.

Both antibody-mediated and cell-mediated immune responses are involved in the complex process of host-versus-graft transplant rejection. Host macrophages process donor antigen, presenting it to T and B lymphocytes. Activated lymphocytes (B and T cells) produce both antibody- and cell-mediated effects. Killer T cells bind with cells of the transplanted organ, resulting in cell lysis. Helper T cells stimulate the multiplication and differentiation of B cells, and

TABLE 13–1 Organ Transplant Indications and Success Rate

ORGAN	GRAFT TYPE	INDICATIONS FOR TRANSPLANT	SUCCESS RATE
Kidney	Allograft; may be isograft	End-stage renal disease	88.1% at 5 years
Heart	Allograft	End-stage cardiac disease refractory to medical management	74.4% at 5 years
Lung	Allograft	Pulmonary hypertension, cystic fibrosis, pulmonary fibrosis, chronic obstructive pulmonary disease	52.6 % at 5 years
Liver	Allograft	Severe liver dysfunction due to chronic active hepatitis, primary biliary cirrhosis, sclerosing cholangitis	73.6 % 5-year survival
Bone marrow	Autograft or allograft	Leukemia, aplastic anemia, congenital immunologic defects	30%–70% cure
Skin	Autograft, allograft, or xenograft	Severe burns, plastic surgery	> 95% at 5 years
Cornea	Allograft	Corneal ulceration and opacification	> 95% at 5 years
Pancreas	Allograft	Pancreatic insufficiency, diabetes	88.1% at 5 years
Islet cells	Allograft (multiple donor)	Type 1 diabetes mellitus	100% > 2 years

Source: US Transplant.org; Scientific registry of transplant recipients, http://www.ustransplant.org/

antibodies are produced to graft endothelium. Complement activation or antibody-dependent cell-mediated cytotoxicity leads to transplant cell destruction. Rejection typically begins after the first 24 hours of the transplant, although it may present immediately. Rejection episodes are characterized as hyperacute, acute, or chronic, as summarized in Table 13–2.

Hyperacute tissue rejection occurs immediately to 2 to 3 days after the transplant of new tissue. Hyperacute rejection is due to preformed antibodies and sensitized T cells to antigens in the donor organ. It is most likely to occur in patients who have had a previous organ or tissue transplant, such as a blood transfusion, and may be evident even before the transplant procedure is completed. The grafted organ initially appears pink and healthy, but soon becomes soft and cyanotic as blood flow is impaired. Organ function deteriorates rapidly, and manifestations of organ failure develop.

Acute tissue rejection is the most common and treatable type of rejection episode. It occurs between 4 days and 3 months after the transplant. Acute rejection is mediated primarily by the cellular immune response, resulting in transplant cell destruction. The patient experiencing acute rejection demonstrates manifestations of the inflammatory process, with fever, redness, swelling, and tenderness over the graft site. Signs of impaired function of the transplanted organ may be noted (e.g., elevated blood urea nitrogen [BUN] and creatinine, liver enzyme and bilirubin elevations, or elevated cardiac enzymes and signs of cardiac failure).

Chronic tissue rejection occurs from 4 months to years after transplant of new tissue. Chronic rejection is most likely the result of antibody-mediated immune responses. Antibodies and complement are deposited in transplant vessel walls, causing narrowing and decreased function of the organ due to ischemia. The gradual deterioration of transplanted organ function is seen with chronic tissue rejection.

Graft-versus-host disease (GVHD) is a frequent and potentially fatal complication of bone marrow transplant, some liver transplants, or transfusions with nonirradiated blood to immunocompromised patients (Porth & Matfin, 2009). When there is no close match between donor and recipient HLA, immunocompetent cells in the grafted tissue recognize host tissue as foreign and mount a cell-mediated immune response. If the host is immunocompromised, as is often the case when a bone marrow transplant is performed, host cells are unable to destroy the graft and instead become the targets of destruction.

Three important strategies for preventing or decreasing the severity of GVHD include (1) deleting donor T cells in the tissue or organ prior to infusion into the patient (however, this may increase the risk of graft failure and infection); (2) using umbilical cord stem cells in adult patients; and (3), closer HLA matching between donor and recipient. Acute GVHD occurs within the first 100 days following a transplant and primarily affects the skin, liver, and gastrointestinal tract. The patient develops a maculopapular pruritic rash beginning on the palms of the hands and soles of the feet. The rash may spread to involve the entire body and lead to desquamation. Gastrointestinal manifestations include abdominal pain, nausea, and bloody diarrhea. GVHD that lasts longer than 100 days is said to be chronic. If it is limited to the skin and liver, the prognosis is good. If multiple organs are involved, the prognosis is poor (Porth & Matfin, 2009).

Interdisciplinary Care

Pretransplant care and post-transplant care are directed toward reducing the risk that transplanted tissue will be rejected or result in GVHD. Diagnostic studies are directed first at identifying the potential recipient's blood type and histocompatibility. Potential donors are identified through diagnostic studies, and the recipient's immune response to the transplant is monitored. Immunosuppressive therapy with medications is a vital part of post-transplant care. The development of effective immunosuppressive drugs as well as improved methods of tissue typing are responsible for the success of organ transplants using allografts.

Diagnosis

Laboratories specializing in transplant are equipped to make the following diagnostic tests prior to organ or tissue transplantation:

- *Blood type* of both the donor and recipient are determined and they must match.
- *DNA sequencing* is made on blood cells to determine histocompatibility. Sequencing can be completed quickly. Quick response is important to minimize cold ischemia in cadaverous organs. Diagnostic testing of recipients can be made less urgently.
- *Crossmatching* of the patient's serum against the donor's lymphocytes is performed to identify any preformed antibodies against antigens on donor tissues. If present, these antibodies would likely result in an immediate or hyperacute graft rejection with probable loss of the transplant.

TABLE 13–2 Transplant Rejection Episodes

TYPE	CAUSE	PRESENTATION	TREATMENT
Hyperacute	Preexisting antibodies to donor ABO or HLA antigens	Occurs within minutes to hours or days of the transplant. Rapid deterioration of organ function	The transplant usually cannot be saved; prevent with crossmatch, and use antimetabolites or anti-inflammatory drugs before surgery.
Acute	Primarily a cell-mediated immune response to HLA antigens; antibody-mediated response may also contribute	Occurs within days to months after the transplant. Signs of inflammation and impaired organ function	Increase immunosuppression using steroids, cyclosporine, monoclonal antibodies, or anti-lymphocyte globulins.
Chronic	Probably antibody-mediated response; may also involve inflammatory damage to vessel endothelium	Occurs 4 months to years after the transplant. Gradual deterioration of organ function	None; loss of graft will occur, requiring retransplant.

- *HLA histocompatibility testing* identifies donors with an HLA type close to that of the recipient. It is used primarily to identify living donors for bone marrow and kidney transplant. Because of GVHD, histocompatibility tests to identify an identical or very close HLA match are particularly important in bone marrow transplant. HLA tests are performed using lymphocytes from a blood sample. The sample should not be obtained within 72 hours of a blood transfusion, because this will interfere with results.
- *Mixed lymphocyte culture (MLC) assay tests* also are used to determine histocompatibility between the donor and the allograft recipient. This test identifies whether lymphocytes of the recipient will react against the potential donor's leukocyte antigens (HLA). When a pretransplant test reveals a high potential for reaction, potent immunosuppression may prevent rejection. If the intended recipient is severely immunocompromised, the results may be falsely negative. Patients treated with chemotherapy within 2 weeks of specimen collection are potentially immunocompromised.
- *Ultrasonography* or *magnetic resonance imaging (MRI)* of the transplanted organ may be performed to evaluate its size, perfusion, and function.
- *Tissue biopsies* of the transplanted organ are performed routinely to assess for evidence of tissue rejection.

Medications

Prior to transplantation, several antibiotic and antiviral drugs may be prescribed, including the following:

- Trimethoprim-sulfamethoxazole (Septra, Bactrim) to decrease the incidence of gram-negative bacterial infections
- Acyclovir (Zovirax) to prevent the development of herpes simplex virus pneumonia in bone marrow transplant recipients
- Ganciclovir (Cytovene) to prevent the development of cytomegalovirus (CMV) pneumonia with bone marrow transplant recipients

The mainstays of drug therapy for patients following a tissue or organ transplant are immunosuppressive agents. See Figure 13–6 ■. Varying regimens of these drugs are used, depending on the transplanted tissue and the medical center; however, a combination of corticosteroids and cyclosporine is common for maintenance therapy. Antilymphocyte therapy and the use of monoclonal antibodies are increasingly common in the immediate post-transplant period and for treating steroid-resistant rejection episodes.

Corticosteroids, primarily prednisone (Deltasone, others) and methylprednisolone (Solu-Medrol, others) are important agents. The exact anti-inflammatory and immunosuppressive activity of corticosteroids is unknown but they are known to suppress production of interleukin-1 and -2, decrease monocyte migration, and suppress proliferative and cytotoxic T-cell activity. Although they are very effective, large doses of corticosteroids used post-transplant are associated with significant adverse effects. Wound healing is impaired, and the metabolism of fats, proteins, and carbohydrates is altered. Blood glucose increases with steroid use, impairing glucose control. Fat distribution changes, producing a cushingoid appearance with a moon face, increased truncal fat, and "buffalo hump." Fluid retention and hypertension are potential problems, as are osteoporosis, gastrointestinal bleeding, and emotional disturbances.

Cyclosporine inhibits T-cell function and the normal cell-mediated immune response. The incidence of cyclosporine toxicity and side effects is related to blood levels, so blood levels are monitored closely. Cyclosporine is both nephrotoxic and hepatotoxic, especially at high doses. Observable toxic effects include hypertension and central nervous system (CNS) symptoms such as flushing or tingling of the extremities, confusion, visual disturbances, and seizures or coma.

Azathioprine (Imuran) inhibits both cell-mediated and antibody-mediated immunity, although its activity is more specific for T cells than B cells. Because it is rapidly metabolized by the liver, azathioprine can be given to patients with impaired renal function but may not be effective in patients with impaired hepatic function. Bone marrow suppression is the most common adverse effect of this drug, necessitating frequent evaluation of the complete blood count (CBC). Hepatotoxicity, pancreatitis, and increased risk of neoplasm are also associated with azathioprine administration. Nursing responsibilities related to azathioprine are listed in the Medication Administration box on the following pages. Patients who cannot tolerate azathioprine may receive a newer immunosuppressant, mycophenolate mofetil (CellCept). Primarily, it is prescribed following renal and cardiac transplants.

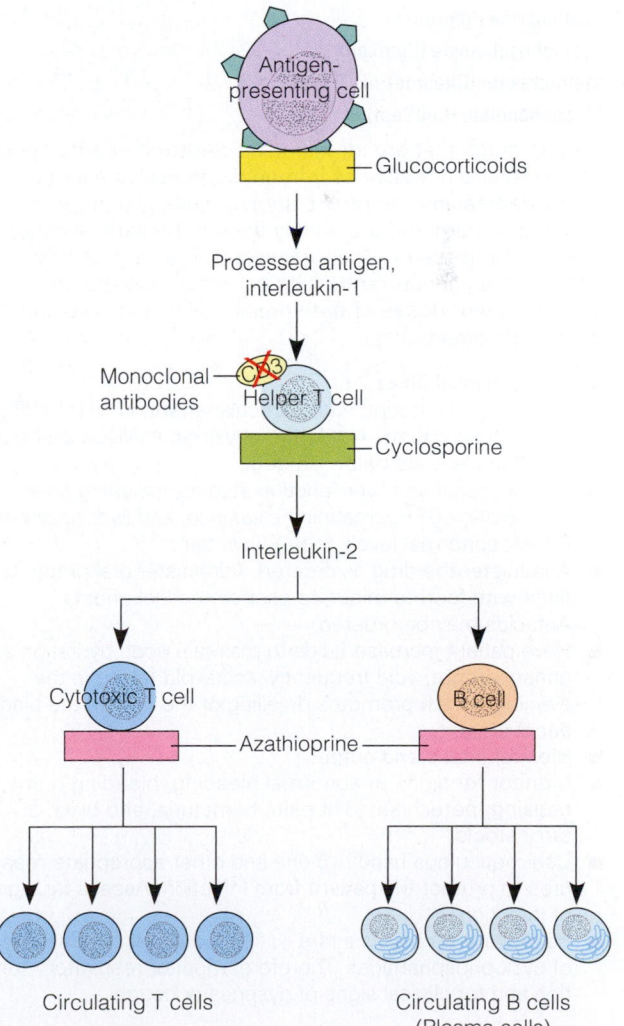

Figure 13–6 ■ Sites of action of immunosuppressive agents.

MEDICATION ADMINISTRATION   Immunosuppressive Agents

T-CELL SUPPRESSORS

Cyclosporine (Sandimmune)

Tacrolimus (Prograf)

Sirolimus (Rapamune)

These drugs inhibit T-cell development and activation. They are given concurrently with a glucocorticoid and in combination with other immunosuppressants and inhibit immune system activity and organ rejection.

Nursing Responsibilities

- Monitor BUN and creatinine for evidence of nephrotoxicity.
- Teach the signs and symptoms of infection unique to immune-suppressed individuals. A temperature of 100.6°F is significant evidence of infection. A sore throat may be a manifestation. Other signs and symptoms of inflammation and infection may be absent.
- Teach patients good hygiene to avoid infection with special emphasis on hand hygiene and avoiding infected individuals.
- Monitor blood pressure and availability and use of antihypertensive medications.
- Teach to avoid grapefruit juice, which can raise cyclosporine levels by 50% to 200% and increase the risk of toxicity. Sirolimus should not be taken with grapefruit juice. Sirolimus increases cholesterol and triglycerides. Lipid-lowering drugs may be necessary to prevent hyperlipidemias.

CYTOTOXIC AGENTS

Azathioprine (Imuran)

Cyclophosphamide (Cytoxan)

Methotrexate (Rheumatrex, Trexall)

Mycophenolate (CellCept)

Certain drugs that are identified as cytotoxic or antineoplastic agents are effective as immunosuppressive agents. They act by decreasing the proliferation of cells within the immune system and are widely used to prevent rejection following a tissue or organ transplant. They are usually administered concurrently with corticosteroid therapy, allowing lower doses of both preparations and resulting in fewer side effects.

Nursing Responsibilities

- Monitor blood count, with particular attention to the WBC and platelet counts. Notify the physician if WBCs fall below 4,000 or platelets below 75,000.
- Monitor renal and liver function studies, including creatinine, BUN, eGFR, creatinine clearance, and liver enzymes. Report abnormal levels to the physician.
- Administer the drug as ordered. Administer oral preparations with food to minimize gastrointestinal effects. Antacids may be ordered.
- Have patient increase fluids to maintain good hydration and urinary output, void frequently, and avoid taking in the evening, which promotes dwelling of the drug in the bladder overnight.
- Monitor intake and output.
- Monitor for signs of abnormal bleeding, bleeding gums, bruising, petechiae, joint pain, hematuria, and black or tarry stools.
- Use meticulous hand hygiene and other appropriate measures to protect the patient from infection. Assess for signs of infection.
- Pulmonary fibrosis is a rare (< 1%) potential adverse effect of cyclophosphamides. Therefore, monitor respiratory function and for clinical signs of dyspnea or cough.

Health Education for the Patient and Family

- Avoid large crowds and situations where exposure to infection is probable.
- Report signs of infection, such as chills, fever, sore throat, fatigue, or malaise, to the physician.
- Use contraceptive measures to prevent pregnancy while on immunosuppressive therapy; these drugs are teratogenic.
- Avoid the use of aspirin or ibuprofen while taking these drugs. Report any signs of bleeding to the physician. Check labels: Many over-the-counter products contain aspirin.
- With cyclophosphamide, amenorrhea may occur. The menses may resume after the drug is discontinued.
- If taking cyclophosphamide, report difficulty breathing or cough to the physician.

MONOCLONAL ANTIBODIES

Muromonab-CD3 (Orthoclone OKT3)

Basiliximab (Simulect)

Daclizumab (Zenapax)

Alemtuzumab (Campath)

Monoclonal antibodies are formed by immunizing a mouse with an antigen to produce a specific antibody. Lymphocytes producing the antibody are cloned, and the antibody is harvested. When injected into humans, the antibody binds with a surface antigen on T cells, removing them from circulation and inactivating those bound to allograft cells. Due to the high incidence of adverse effects, the first doses of the monoclonal antibody are administered by a physician and the patient closely observed for 2 hours following each dose. Alemtuzumab is used in bone marrow transplants, renal transplant, and in clinical trials for multiple sclerosis. This drug increases the risk of opportunistic infections such as cytomegalovirus.

Nursing Responsibilities

- Be sure a chest x-ray has been performed within 24 hours preceding initiation of monoclonal antibody therapy and that no pulmonary or cardiovascular congestion is present. The risk of anaphylaxis is greater in the patient with fluid overload.
- Premedicate as ordered with hydrocortisone, acetaminophen, and diphenhydramine to reduce potential adverse effects.
- Position a crash cart or code cart with emergency medications in the patient's room or in close proximity to it.
- After each of the first two doses, monitor vital signs every 15 minutes for 2 hours, then every 30 minutes for 2 hours.
- Observe closely for potential adverse effects, including chills and fever; tachycardia; headache and tremor; hypertension or hypotension; nausea, vomiting, and diarrhea; chest pain, dyspnea, and wheezing.
- OKT3 can also cause anaphylaxis; observe for evidence of urticaria, angioedema, laryngeal edema, wheezing, or other signs of anaphylactic reaction.
- Alemtuzumab infusion is potentially associated with chills, fever, rash, and hypotension. Adverse cardiac events and autoimmune reactions have been reported.
- Monitor CBC for evidence of leukopenia or pancytopenia.
- Assess for infection.

Health Education for the Patient and Family

- Teach about the drug and its purpose.
- Discuss potential adverse and side effects, and emphasize the need to report symptoms promptly.
- Inform the patient that adverse effects are most likely to occur following the first two doses, necessitating close observation at that time. Reassure the patient that this is standard protocol for this medication.

MEDICATION ADMINISTRATION Immunosuppressive Agents (continued)

ANTILYMPHOCYTE GLOBULINS

Antithymocyte globulin or ATG (ATGAM)

Antilymphocyte globulin or ALG

These globulins containing antilymphocyte antibodies are produced by immunizing horses (the main source), rabbits, or sheep with human lymphocytes to stimulate production of antibodies (see the following figure). Serum from the animal is then recovered, and the active IgG fraction is isolated, purified, and administered parenterally to the patient. It binds with peripheral lymphocytes and mononuclear cells, removing them from circulation.

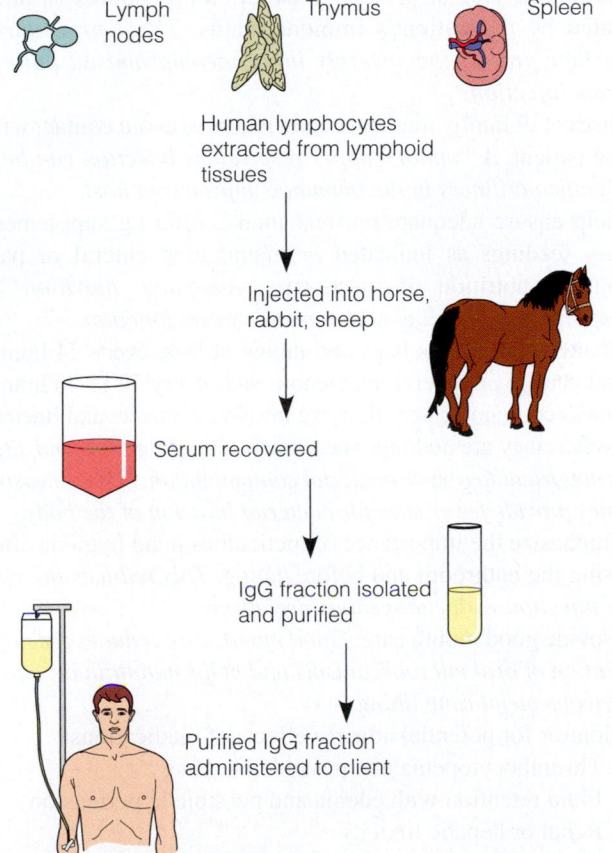

A horse is inoculated with washed human lymphocytes, stimulating the production of immunoglobulin with polyclonal antilymphocyte antibodies. These are then extracted from horse serum, purified, and administered intravenously to the patient.

ATG or ALG is used both to induce immunosuppression immediately following a transplant and to treat steroid-resistant rejection episodes. As with monoclonal antibody, multiple side effects are associated with ATG or ALG.

Nursing Responsibilities

- Perform a skin test for sensitivity to horse serum prior to initial dose. Report any positive reaction to the physician and hold administration until desensitization therapy has been completed.
- Premedicate as ordered with acetaminophen and diphenhydramine prior to each dose. Steroids may also be administered before the initial dose. Have epinephrine and hydrocortisone injections available at the bedside in case of anaphylactic reaction.
- Administer by intravenous infusion into a central line over 4 to 6 hours.
- Monitor vital signs hourly while medication is infusing.
- Assess for adverse effects, including chills and fever, erythema, and pruritus. Notify the physician; these may be treated symptomatically.
- Monitor CBC daily, notify the physician if WBC falls to less than 3000/mm^3 or platelet count to less than 100,000/mm^3. The medication may be stopped or reduced.
- Assess renal function studies to monitor for serum sickness. Report complaints of joint pain.
- Monitor for signs of infection, and report any signs promptly.

CORTICOSTEROIDS

Prednisone

Methylprednisolone (Medrol, Solu-Medrol)

Corticosteroids are immunosuppressants but also have dangerous side effects when high doses are used for a prolonged time. The mechanism of action is not fully identified but cytokine production is reduced, disabling an immune response. Adverse reactions include hypertension, hyperglycemia, and opportunistic infection. Too little corticosteroid can result in graft rejection. A few months after transplantation, patients can be weaned off corticosteroids without increasing the frequency of rejection episodes.

Health Education for the Patient and Family

- Explain the need for special precautions and close monitoring while this drug is being administered.
- Instruct the patient to report any adverse effects, including malaise or joint pain, promptly.
- Ask the patient to report any evidence of easy bruising, bleeding gums, or black stools.
- Teach family members about the importance of not exposing the patient to persons with infectious diseases.

Muromonab-CD3, also known as OKT3 or Orthoclone, is the first monoclonal antibody produced for therapeutic use in humans. As a monoclonal antibody, OKT3 is specific to T cells, blocking their generation and function. It binds with a surface antigen on T cells, inactivating and removing them from circulation. It also blocks killer T cells attached to the graft. Because of significant side effects, the use of OKT3 is limited primarily to treatment of steroid-resistant rejection. Two newer monoclonal antibodies, basiliximab (Simulect)

and daclizumab (Zenapax), are a combination of mouse and human antibodies and cause fewer side effects.

Polyclonal antilymphocyte antibodies are also used as adjunctive immunosuppressant therapy. These are administered as antilymphocyte globulin (ALG) or antithymocyte globulin (ATG). These globulins contain antibodies against both T and B cells, as well as other mononuclear leukocytes. When administered, they deplete circulating lymphocytes, platelets, and granulocytes.

✍ Nursing Care

The patient who has an organ or tissue transplant has both immediate and long-term nursing care needs. Both the patient and the family must be considered in providing nursing care.

Health Promotion

Part of the health promotion activities focus on preventing the need for a tissue transplant. It is important to increase public awareness regarding unhealthy lifestyle behaviors, such as excessive alcohol consumption and illegal drug use, and their relationship to organ failure. Patients with chronic diseases such as diabetes mellitus and hypertension must understand that inadequate management of these disorders could lead to end-stage renal disease. Other risk factors may simply relate to a person's heredity; understanding how heredity could affect future health might influence the patient's lifestyle choices.

Assessment

Assessment data collected following a tissue transplant focus on identifying potential rejection episodes. Further focused assessments are described with nursing interventions in the next section.

Nursing Diagnoses and Interventions

Because of the continuing risk of transplant rejection and the need for immunosuppression, *Ineffective Protection* and *Risk for Impaired Tissue Integrity* are priority nursing diagnoses. The patient's underlying disease process, the transplant, and the continuing need for immunosuppressive drug therapy also have emotional and psychologic consequences. Other nursing diagnoses, such as *Powerlessness* or *Ineffective Coping*, also may be appropriate.

Ineffective Protection

Ineffective protection is a problem for the transplant patient at all stages. Before the transplant occurs, failure of the affected organ may put the patient at risk for infection and other multisystemic problems. Incisions and invasive perioperative procedures impair skin and mucous membrane protection from infectious organisms and other antigens. Immunosuppressive drugs given postoperatively to prevent graft rejection disarm the immune response to a certain extent, increasing the risk of infections and neoplastic growths.

> **SAFETY ALERT**
> Use strict aseptic technique in changing dressings and caring for invasive catheters such as intravenous lines and indwelling urinary catheters to protect against external and resident host microorganisms.

- Wash hands and use hand sanitizer on entering room and before providing direct care. *Hand hygiene removes transient organisms from the skin, reducing the risk of transmission to the patient.*
- Assess frequently for manifestations of infection. Monitor vital signs, including temperature, every 4 hours. Assess for evidence of inflammation, abnormal wound drainage, changes in urine or other body secretions, complaints of pain, or behavior changes that may indicate infection. Culture abnormal wound drainage. *The patient on immunosuppressive therapy is more susceptible to infection, and usual manifestations may not be evident. Both the body temperature and inflammatory response can be suppressed by therapy. Prompt identification and intervention for infection is important in the immunosuppressed patient.*
- Monitor laboratory values, including CBC and tests of organ function; report changes to the physician. *An elevation in the WBC count with increased numbers of immature cells (bands) or a decline in function of the transplanted organ (e.g., a rising BUN and creatinine in the renal transplant patient) may be early indications of infection or transplant failure.*
- Initiate reverse or protective isolation procedures as indicated by the patient's immune status. *These procedures further protect the severely immunocompromised patient from infection.*
- Instruct ill family members and visitors to avoid contact with the patient. *A "minor" upper respiratory infection can be a significant illness in the immunocompromised host.*
- Help ensure adequate nutrient intake, offering supplementary feedings as indicated or maintaining enteral or parenteral nutrition if necessary. *Adequate nutrition is important for healing and immune system function.*
- Change intravenous bags and tubing at least every 24 hours, and change peripheral intravenous sites every 72 to 96 hours, unless contraindicated. Remove invasive catheters and lines as soon as they are no longer necessary. *Changing lines and sites is important to reduce bacterial contamination. Fewer invasive lines provide fewer sites for bacterial invasion of the body.*
- Emphasize the importance of meticulous hand hygiene after using the bathroom and before eating. *This reduces the risk of infection with endogenous organisms.*
- Provide good mouth care. *Good mouth care reduces the population of oral microorganisms and helps maintain an intact mucous membrane lining.*
- Monitor for potential adverse effects of medications:
  - Thrombocytopenia and possible bleeding
  - Fluid retention with edema and possible hypertension
  - Renal or hepatic toxicity
  - Cardiac effects, particularly in the presence of fluid retention and hypervolemia.
  Medications used to maintain immunosuppression and preserve the allograft have many potential adverse effects that can alter normal protective and homeostatic mechanisms.

Risk for Impaired Tissue Integrity: Allograft

The risk for transplant rejection is highest in the initial postoperative period, but it is never completely eliminated for the patient who has had an allograft. The patient who has had a bone marrow transplant has the additional risk of developing GVHD, which can affect the integrity of skin, mucous membranes, and other organs.

- Administer immunosuppressive therapy as prescribed. *Suppression of the immune response is necessary to reduce the risk of graft destruction by normal immune responses and to preserve the graft's function.*
- Assess for evidence of graft rejection, including tenderness, erythema, and swelling over the site; sudden weight gain,

edema, and hypertension; chills and fever; malaise; and an increased WBC count and sedimentation rate. Report any changes immediately. *Early identification of rejection allows adjustment of medication regimens and, possibly, preservation of the graft.*

- Monitor results of laboratory studies for function of the transplanted organ. *With a functional graft, results (e.g., renal or liver function studies) will improve; a functional decline may be an early indicator of rejection.*
- Assess for and report signs of GVHD immediately, including maculopapular rash, erythema of the skin and possible desquamation, hair loss, abdominal cramping and diarrhea, or jaundice with elevated bilirubin and liver enzymes (AST, ALT). *GVHD is a potentially lethal complication in the immunosuppressed patient and necessitates immediate intervention.*
- Stress the importance of maintaining immunosuppressive therapy and reporting signs of graft rejection promptly to the physician. *Continued immunosuppression and prompt treatment of rejection are vital to preserving graft function.*

Anxiety

The patient who undergoes an organ or tissue transplantation often faces the unwelcome choices of death from organ failure or receiving an organ that his or her body will likely attempt to reject. In most cases, the patient understands that to receive this transplant, someone else must die and be willing to give up an organ. When the transplant comes from a living donor (bone marrow or kidney), the patient may worry not only about him- or herself, but also about the condition of the donor. Fear of rejection and guilt may be even greater in this instance.

- Assess level of anxiety by noting such cues as expressions of apprehension, fear, or inadequacy; facial expression, tension, or shakiness; difficulty focusing; helplessness; poor eye contact; and restlessness. *Patients may have difficulty identifying or verbalizing feelings of fear and anxiety. Nonverbal cues are often useful in recognizing states of anxiety.*
- Provide opportunities to express feelings. Use opening statements such as "Facing an organ transplant must be very stressful," or "What concerns you most about this transplant?" Listen attentively. *Encouragement and active listening allow the patient to express feelings of anxiety or fear.*
- Arrange tasks to allow as much time with the patient as possible. When leaving, tell the patient when you will return. *Time spent with the patient facilitates the development of trust.*
- Provide clear, concise directions. *Highly anxious patients have difficulty focusing and retaining information.*
- Encourage involvement in care but do not request unnecessary decisions. *The patient needs to feel a sense of control but*

may become irritated if asked to make decisions unrelated to the situation.

- Encourage family members to remain with the patient as much as possible. *This can help reduce the patient's anxiety.*
- Encourage the use of coping behaviors that have been effective for the patient in the past. *Coping mechanisms and behaviors help lower anxiety to a more acceptable level.*
- Reduce or eliminate environmental stressors to the extent possible. *This gives the patient a better sense of control.*
- Assist with stress reduction and relaxation techniques, such as guided imagery, meditation, and muscle relaxation. *These techniques help the patient gain control over physical responses to anxiety.*
- Refer to a counselor, mental health specialist, or spiritual advisor as appropriate. *Counseling can help the patient identify and deal with his or her concerns and fears.*

Community-Based Care

Teaching the patient and family about an organ or tissue transplant begins before the transplant and continues throughout hospitalization and follow-up treatment. Transplant coordinators are nurses specializing in the transplant process and are excellent resources for patients, families, and nursing staff.

Initial teaching focuses on the options, risks, and potential benefits of the transplant itself. Include the procedure by which the organ is selected and obtained, as well as the procedure by which it is transplanted into the patient. If a living related donor is an option, discuss the risks and benefits for both the patient and the donor. Outline the post-transplant treatment regimen, including any lifestyle changes that may be necessary. Waiting for a cadaver organ is a tedious process; the patient must be ready to present for transplant when an organ is available. The transplant process is complex, expensive, and anxiety-provoking.

Following the transplant, provide verbal and written instructions, including the following:

- Manifestations of transplant rejection and the importance of notifying the physician
- Immunosuppressive drug regimen and side effects
- Wound care
- Avoiding exposure to infectious diseases, particularly respiratory infections, and wearing a mask when going outside
- Meticulous personal hygiene, hand hygiene technique, and frequent mouth care
- Wearing a Medic-Alert bracelet or tag
- Follow-up visits to the physician or clinic
- Helpful resources:
  - American Council on Transplantation
  - Local and state support groups related to specific organ transplant, such as the National Kidney Foundation

Impaired Immune Responses

Disorders of impaired immune system responses may be either congenital or acquired. Often the function of either T or B cells is impaired, reducing the body's ability to defend against foreign antigens or abnormal host tissue.

No matter what the cause, patients with immunodeficiency disorders demonstrate an unusual susceptibility to infection.

When the antibody-mediated response is primarily affected, the patient is at particular risk for severe and chronic bacterial infections. These patients do not develop long-lasting immunity to such diseases as chickenpox and are prone to recurrence of the diseases. Patients with a defect of cell-mediated immunity tend to develop disseminated viral infections such as herpes simplex and cytomegalovirus (CMV). Candidiasis (yeast) and other fungal infections are also common. Because T cells are involved with activating antibody-mediated immune responses as well, overwhelming bacterial infections may occur. Immunodeficiency in its most severe form occurs when both antibody-mediated and cell-mediated responses are impaired. Patients with combined immunodeficiency are susceptible to all varieties of infectious organisms, including those not normally considered to be pathogens.

Most immunodeficiency diseases are genetically determined and rare. They affect children more than adults. The noted exception is AIDS, an infectious disease caused by a virus.

The Patient with HIV Infection

In 1981, five cases of *Pneumocystis jiroveci* pneumonia (then known as *P. carinii* pneumonia or PJP) and 26 cases of a rare cancer, Kaposi's sarcoma, were diagnosed in young, previously healthy homosexual males in Los Angeles and New York City. The term **acquired immunodeficiency syndrome (AIDS)** was used to describe the immune system deficits associated with these opportunistic disorders. Prior to this time, both PJP and Kaposi's had been seen only in elderly, debilitated, or severely immunodeficient people. Other groups at risk for AIDS were soon identified: injection drug users, persons with hemophilia, recipients of blood transfusions, and immigrants from Haiti. Research to identify the cause of this apparently new disease progressed feverishly, and in 1983, a common antibody was identified in patients with AIDS. The **human immunodeficiency virus (HIV)** was isolated in 1984. It then became apparent that AIDS was the final, fatal stage of HIV infection. HIV is a retrovirus transmitted by direct contact with infected blood and body fluids. Significant concentrations of the virus are present in blood, semen, vaginal and cervical secretions, and cerebrospinal fluid (CSF) of infected individuals. It is also found in breast milk and saliva.

It began, like so many epidemics, with a few isolated cases, and has become a worldwide plague. (See the accompanying Focus on Cultural Diversity box.) Progression of HIV disease to AIDS has slowed because of the effectiveness of highly active antiretroviral therapy (HAART). Survival with AIDS has improved from 2.03 years with prophylactic treatment for opportunistic infections to more than 13 years with antiretroviral agents (Walensky, 2006).

Although the incidence of HIV has leveled and mortality due to AIDS has declined, the epidemic is far from over. In the United States it continues to disproportionately affect African Americans, men who have sex with men (MSM), people who engage in high-risk heterosexual behavior (sex with individuals known to be infected with HIV or at high risk for having HIV), and injection drug users. Two separate elements are reported in the surveillance data: HIV infection rate and AIDS occurrence. HIV infection is dependent on exposure to the virus; conversion to AIDS is related to access and use of HAART. HIV new cases are highest among MSM and high-risk heterosexuals; AIDS occurrence continues among MSM, high-risk heterosexuals, and African Americans (CDC, 2008).

Incidence and Prevalence

Through 2006, the CDC (2008) estimated that 1,106,400 persons in the United States were living with HIV/AIDS, with 21% undiagnosed and unaware of their HIV infection. There were 56,300 new cases of AIDS in 2006 in the United States. Deaths among people with AIDS had decreased from 50,610 in 1995 to 14,627 in 2006, more than likely the result of improved treatments rather than a decline in spread of the disease. A continued decline in deaths is dependent on access to quality care and treatment and continued development of treatments for those already heavily treated (McPhee & Papadakis, 2009).

The risk factors for HIV infection are behavioral. Among adults in the United States, 60% of reported cases are MSM, including homosexuals, bisexuals, and such groups as prison populations. Unprotected anal intercourse is the major route of transmission in this group. Injection drug use is the second leading risk factor, accounting for approximately 25% of cases, with sharing of needles and other drug paraphernalia the primary route of transmission. Heterosexual intercourse with an infected drug user and exchanging sex for drugs are major risk factors for women. Hemophiliacs who require large amounts of intravenous clotting factors and people infected through blood transfusion account for a small number of cases, approximately 2% (CDC, 2008).

Among risk groups, the most rapid increases are noted in young gay and bisexual men, women, and inner-city injection drug users, especially African Americans and Hispanics. In the United States, the rate of male adult/adolescent HIV/AIDS cases (per 100,000 population) reported was 83.7 among African Americans, 29.3 among Hispanics, 14.6 among Native Americans/Alaska Natives, 19.6 among Caucasians, and 10.3 among Asian and Pacific Islanders. The rapid increase of AIDS cases among women is of special concern: the reported rate of new cases among women in the United States per 100,000 population was 55.7 among African Americans, 14.4 among

---

FOCUS ON CULTURAL DIVERSITY
HIV/AIDS

- There are an estimated 33 million people infected with AIDS worldwide, with virtually every country in the world reporting cases (United Nations AIDS/WHO, 2007). The highest incidence is found in sub-Saharan Africa, South and Southeast Asia, the United States, western Europe, South America, and Canada.
- Approximately 67% of all people infected with HIV or who have AIDS live in sub-Saharan Africa, and another 15% live in South and Southeast Asia, largely in Thailand and India.
- The most common mode of transmission is heterosexual intercourse. The cofactors that increase the risk of HIV transmission include the presence of ulcerative or inflammatory sexually transmitted diseases, trauma, menses, and lack of male circumcision (McPhee & Papadakis, 2009; UNAIDS Report, 2007).

Hispanics, and 3.8 among Caucasians. The majority of women are infected through heterosexual contact (75%) with the remaining 25% through injection drug use (CDC, 2008).

In addition, AIDS in adults over age 50 accounts for approximately 29% of persons living with HIV/AIDS in the United States (CDC, 2008). Survival of persons infected earlier in their life accounts for a significant portion of these adults. Declining immune system function in older adults significantly increases their risk for contracting HIV/AIDS, along with the belief that they cannot be affected by it. Just as younger persons with HIV/AIDS contract the diseases primarily through sexual intercourse, so does the aging population. Because older adults are beyond childbearing years, they often fail to use condoms when engaging in sexual activity. Manifestations may be overlooked by healthcare professionals, leading to a delayed diagnosis and increased severity of the disease.

Less than 0.04% of people voluntarily donating blood (a process that generally excludes people with high-risk behavior) are found to be HIV positive. HIV is not transmitted by casual contact, nor is there any evidence of its transmission by vectors such as mosquitoes. Blood donation also poses no risk of contracting HIV to the donor, because only new sterile equipment is used. A small but real occupational risk exists for healthcare workers. Percutaneous exposure to infected blood or body fluids through a needle-stick injury or nonintact skin is the primary route of transmission. Documented evidence indicates that parenteral exposure poses a 1:300 risk of becoming HIV positive (McPhee & Papadakis, 2009). Mucosal exposures, such as splashing in the eyes or mouth, pose a much smaller risk.

Pathophysiology and Manifestations

HIV is a retrovirus, meaning it carries its genetic information in RNA. On entry into the body, the virus infects cells that have the CD4 antigen (T lymphocytes). Once inside the cell, the virus sheds its protein coat and uses an enzyme called *reverse transcriptase* to convert the RNA to DNA (Figure 13–7 ■). This viral DNA is then integrated into host cell DNA and duplicated during normal processes of cell division. Within the cell, the virus may remain latent or become activated to produce new RNA and to form *virions*. The virus then buds from the cell surface, disrupting its cell membrane and leading to destruction of the host cell.

Although the virus may remain inactive in infected cells for years, antibodies are produced to its proteins, a process known as **seroconversion**. These antibodies are usually detectable 6 weeks to 6 months after the initial infection. Helper T or CD4 cells are the primary cells infected by HIV, but it also infects macrophages, dendrites, and certain cells of the CNS. Helper T cells play a vital role in normal immune system function, recognizing foreign antigens and infected cells and activating antibody-producing B cells. They also direct cell-mediated immune activity and influence the phagocytic activity of monocytes and macrophages. The loss

---

PATHOPHYSIOLOGY LINKAGE HIV Infection/AIDS

MANIFESTATIONS	RELATED PATHOPHYSIOLOGY
Acute Retroviral Syndrome (ARS) or Primary HIV infection: fever, sore throat, arthralgias and myalgias, headache, rash, nausea, vomiting, and abdominal cramping. Difficult to diagnose; similar to infectious mononucleosis.	This is the first phase in the natural history of HIV/AIDS beginning about 14 days after infection. T_{helper} (CD4) cells are infected with a high load of rapidly replicating HIV RNA during ARS. Persistent generalized lymphadenopathy develops and the lining of the intestine is also damaged very quickly. Antibodies cannot be detected for 6 weeks to 6 months but the infected patient is highly contagious.
Asymptomatic infection (latency): From 3 years to more than 15 years, depending on availability and adherence to treatment with antiretroviral medications. No vaccine or cure is currently available.	A strong cell-mediated and humoral anti-HIV immune defense decreases viral load in the blood. However the virus harbors in lymphoid and neurologic tissues. The level of viral load achieved in this period is predictive of onset of full blown AIDS.

AIDS: HIV-associated neoplasms and opportunistic infections General malaise, fatigue, low grade fever, night sweats, involuntary weight loss, skin dryness, or rashes.
AIDS Dementia Complex
Opportunistic Infectious Diseases
   Pneumocystis jiroveci pneumonia
   Mycobacterium tuberculosis
   Mycobacterium avium complex
   Candidiasis
   Cryptosporidiosis
   Cryptococcosis
   Toxoplasmosis
   Herpes simplex or herpes zoster
   Cytomegalovirus
Secondary Cancers
   Kaposi's sarcoma
   Hodgkin's & non-Hodgkin's lymphoma
   Cervical dysplasia and cervical cancer
Other Conditions
   Pelvic inflammatory disease
   Human papillomavirus
	As the T4 cells fall below 200 per mm^3, virus titers rise rapidly and immune activity drops precipitously. It is the loss of immune competence that enables normally benign opportunistic parasites such as viruses, fungi or protozoa to cause infections. Malignancies develop as immune surveillance fails.

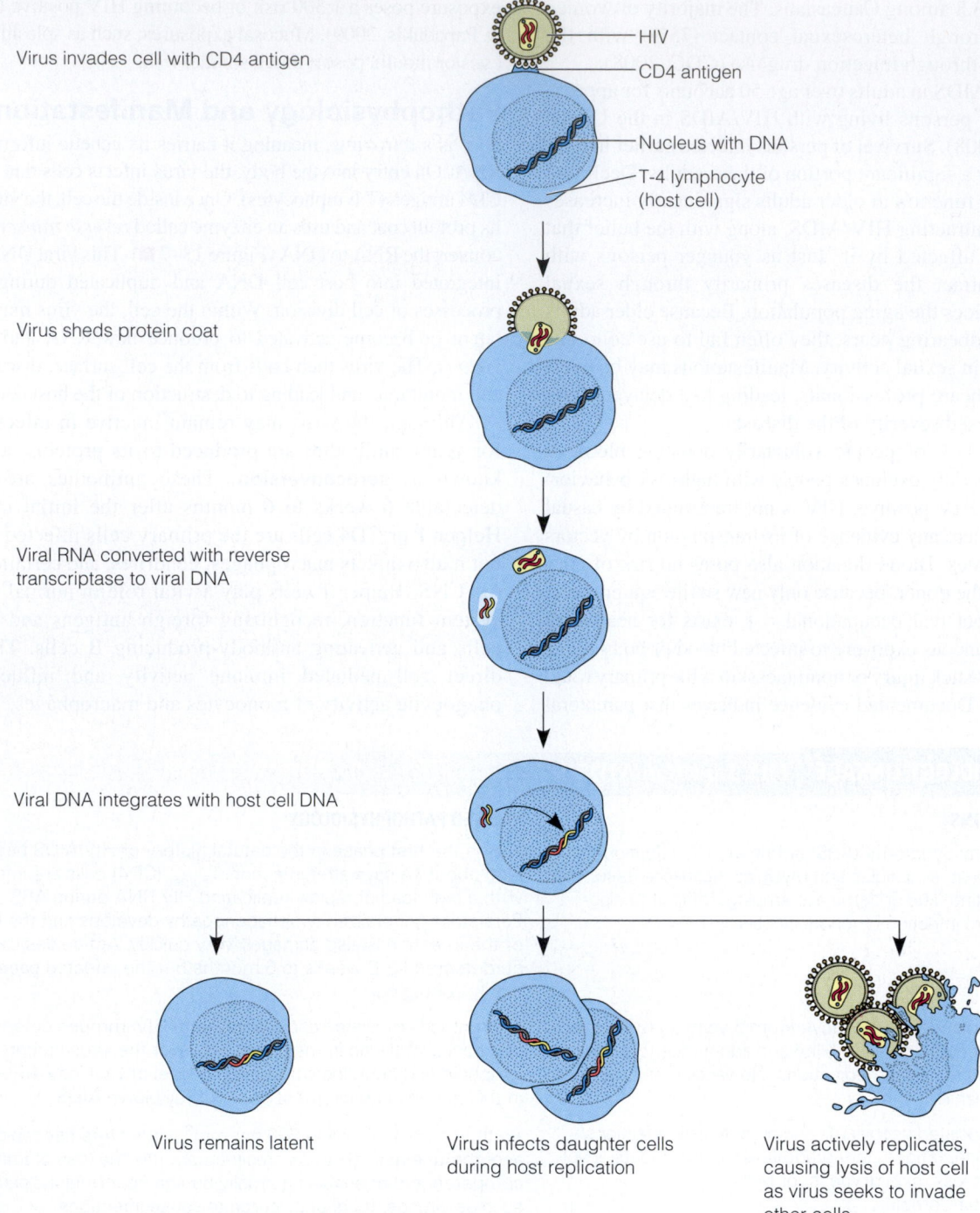

Virus invades cell with CD4 antigen

— HIV
— CD4 antigen

— Nucleus with DNA

— T-4 lymphocyte
   (host cell)

Virus sheds protein coat

Viral RNA converted with reverse
transcriptase to viral DNA

Viral DNA integrates with host cell DNA

Virus remains latent

Virus infects daughter cells
during host replication

Virus actively replicates,
causing lysis of host cell
as virus seeks to invade
other cells

Figure 13–7 ■ How HIV infects and destroys CD4 cells.

of these helper T cells leads to the immunodeficiencies seen with HIV infection. Figure 13–8 ■ illustrates the typical course of HIV infection.

The manifestations of HIV infection range from no symptoms to severe immunodeficiency with multiple opportunistic infections and cancers (see the Pathophysiology Linkage box on page 325). Most patients develop an acute mononucleosis-type illness within days to weeks after contracting the virus. Typical manifestations include fever, sore throat, arthralgias and myalgias, headache, rash, and lymphadenopathy. Pathologic changes are also noted in the CNS of many infected individuals although the mechanism of neurologic dysfunction is unclear. The patient

may also experience nausea, vomiting, and abdominal cramping. The patient often attributes this initial manifestation of HIV infection to a common viral illness such as influenza, upper respiratory infection, or stomach virus.

Following this acute illness, patients who are treated enter a long-lasting asymptomatic period. Although the virus is present and can be transmitted to others, the infected host has few or no symptoms. Most HIV-infected persons are in this stage of the disease. The length of the asymptomatic period varies widely, but its mean length is estimated to be 8 to 10 years.

Some patients with few other symptoms develop persistent generalized lymphadenopathy. This is defined as enlargement

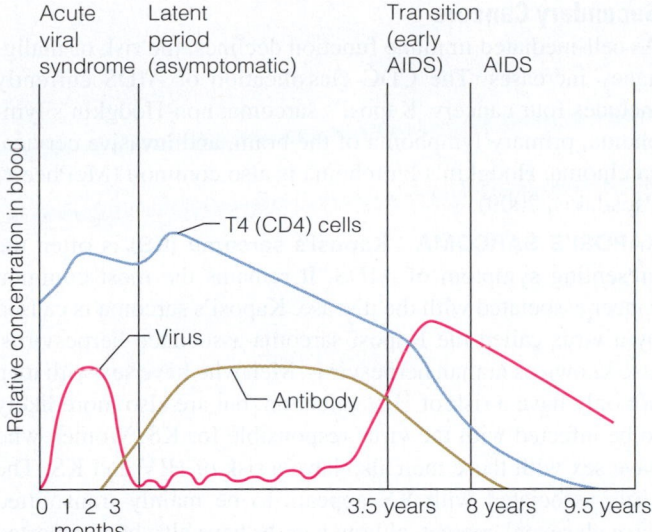

Acute viral syndrome | Latent period (asymptomatic) | Transition (early AIDS) | AIDS

Relative concentration in blood

T4 (CD4) cells

Virus

Antibody

0 1 2 3 months   3.5 years   8 years   9.5 years

Figure 13–8 ■ The progression of HIV infection. Acute illness develops shortly after the virus is contracted, corresponding with a rapid rise in viral levels. Antibodies are formed and remain present throughout the course of infection. Late in the disease, viral activation results in a marked increase in virus while CD4 (T4) cells diminish as they are destroyed with viral replication. Antibody levels gradually decrease as immune function is impaired.

of two or more lymph nodes outside the inguinal chain with no other illness or condition to account for the lymphadenopathy.

The move from asymptomatic disease or persistent lymphadenopathy to AIDS is often not clearly defined. The patient may complain of general malaise, fever, fatigue, night sweats, and involuntary weight loss (Figure 13–9 ■). Persistent skin dryness and rash may be a problem. Diarrhea is common, as are oral lesions such as hairy leukoplakia, candidiasis, and gingival inflammation and ulceration. The development of advanced HIV varies according to the viral load, rate of disease progression, and the development of resistance to antiretroviral therapy. Estimated survival time for newly-diagnosed patients who are treated with HAART is 20.4 years (Knoll, Lassmann, & Temesgen, 2007). This has increased from about 13 months at the start of the AIDS epidemic. With the development of significant constitutional disease, neurologic manifestations, or opportunistic infections or cancers, the patient has manifestations that are characteristic of

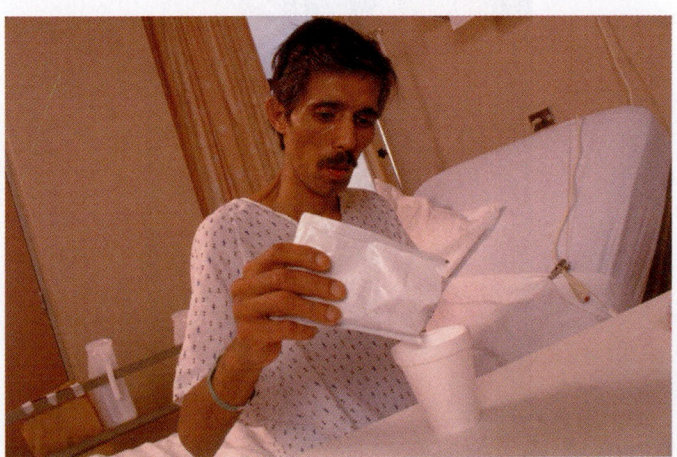

Figure 13–9 ■ Wasting syndrome in a patient with AIDS.

AIDS and a very poor prognosis. When manifestations develop, the outcome varies. With highly active antiretroviral therapy (HAART), many patients are living longer after being diagnosed with AIDS. Today *Pneumocystis carinii* or *jiroveci* pneumonia is most commonly diagnosed in those who are undiagnosed or have a late diagnosis of HIV infection or who fail to take prophylactic antibiotics when their CD4 count is < 200. HAART is credited with decreasing the incidence of opportunistic infections and improving survival (McPhee and Papadakis, 2009).

AIDS Dementia Complex and Neurologic Effects

Neurologic manifestations of HIV include dementia, delirium, and seizures. They result from both the direct effects of the virus on the nervous system and opportunistic infections.

AIDS dementia complex is the most common cause of mental status changes for patients with HIV infection. This dementia results from a direct effect of the virus on the brain and affects cognitive and motor function. Fluctuating memory loss, confusion, difficulty concentrating, lethargy, and diminished motor speed are typical manifestations of AIDS dementia complex. Patients become apathetic, losing interest in work and social and recreational activities. As the complex progresses, the patient develops severe dementia with motor disturbances such as ataxia, tremor, spasticity, incontinence, and paraplegia (Fauci et al., 2008; Porth, 2007).

Infections and lesions common with AIDS may also affect the CNS. Toxoplasmosis and non-Hodgkin's lymphoma are space-occupying lesions that may cause headache, altered mental status, and neurologic deficits. Cryptococcal meningitis and CMV infection also are common in people with AIDS. CNS complications have declined with the use of HAART therapy (McPhee & Papadakis, 2009) Peripheral nervous system manifestations are also common in HIV-infected patients. Sensory neuropathies with manifestations of numbness, tingling, and pain in the lower extremities affect about 30% of patients with AIDS. Weakness and paralysis progress and death occurs within 2 to 4 months (Porth, 2007).

Opportunistic Infections

Opportunistic infections are the most common manifestation of AIDS, often occurring simultaneously. The risk of opportunistic infections is predictable by the T4 or CD4 cell count. The normal CD4 cell count is greater than 1000/mm^3. When the CD4 count falls to less than 500/mm^3, manifestations of immunodeficiency are seen. With a count of less than 200/mm^3, opportunistic infections and cancers are likely.

PNEUMOCYSTIS JIROVECI PNEUMONIA *Pneumocystis jiroveci* (or *Pneumocystis carinii*) pneumonia is the most common opportunistic infection affecting patients with AIDS. When the CD4 count level cannot be maintained above 200 cells/mcl, PJP is likely to develop (McPhee & Papadakis, 2009). It tends to be recurrent, and is a major cause of death in patients with AIDS. PJP is caused by a common environmental fungus that is not pathogenic in patients with intact immune systems. Community-acquired bacterial or viral pneumonia rather than PJP is the most common cause of pulmonary disease in HIV infected persons treated with HAART (McPhee & Papadakis, 2009). Unlike many pneumonias, the manifestations of PJP are nonspecific and may progress insidiously.

Patients often present with fever, cough, dyspnea, tachypnea, and tachycardia. Complaints of mild chest pain and sputum may also be present. Breath sounds may initially be normal. With severe disease, the patient may present with cyanosis and significant respiratory distress.

TUBERCULOSIS (TB) An estimated 4% of patients with AIDS develop TB, contributing significantly to the rise in incidence of this disease in the United States (McPhee & Papadakis, 2009). In some patients, active TB results from reactivation of a prior infection. In other patients, it is a new, primary disease facilitated by impaired immune function. TB is the leading cause of death among HIV infected people (American Lung Association [ALA], 2007). Rapid progression, diffuse pulmonary infiltrates, and disseminated disease occur more commonly in patients with AIDS. Multiple-drug-resistant strains of tuberculosis present a significant problem.

Patients with pulmonary TB present with a cough productive of purulent sputum, fever, fatigue, weight loss, and lymphadenopathy. Disseminated disease affects the bone marrow, bone, joints, liver, spleen, CSF, skin, kidneys, gastrointestinal tract, lymph nodes, brain, and other sites.

OTHER INFECTIONS Herpes virus infections are common in patients with AIDS and may be severe. CMV can affect the retina, the gastrointestinal tract, or lungs. Disseminated herpes simplex or herpes zoster may occur, although severe mucocutaneous manifestations are more common.

Even for patients receiving HAART therapy, sinusitis is common and often frustrating. It manifests as headache, fever, and sinus congestion and discharge. Treatment includes antibiotics and guaifenesin to reduce sinus congestion.

Parasitic infections with *Toxoplasma gondii* and *Cryptococcus neoformans* commonly affect the CNS. Toxoplasmosis occurs as encephalitis or an intracerebral mass lesion. Changes in mental status, focal neurologic signs, and seizures may result. *Cryptococcus* infection may present as either meningitis or disseminated disease, primarily affecting the lungs. *Cryptosporidium*, a protozoon affecting the gastrointestinal tract, is an important cause of prolonged diarrhea in AIDS patients. Bacterial salmonella infections are also a relatively common cause of diarrhea.

Candida albicans infection is a common opportunistic infection in patients with AIDS. It is usually manifested as oral thrush or esophagitis. Oral thrush presents as white, friable plaques on the buccal mucosa or tongue and, in the HIV-infected patient, is often an early indication of progression to AIDS. Patients with esophagitis have difficulty swallowing and substernal pain or burning that increases with swallowing. Vaginal candidiasis is more common and more severe in women with HIV and is treated with topical or systemic medication.

Mycobacterium avium complex (MAC) is a major cause of "wasting syndrome" in persons with AIDS, typically occurring late in the course of the disease when CD4 cell counts are less than 50/mm^3. MAC is caused by organisms commonly found in food, water, and soil. Women with AIDS have a high incidence of pelvic inflammatory disease (PID). Although the pathogens appear to be the same as those in PID affecting non-HIV-infected women, the disease is more severe. Inpatient treatment with intravenous antibiotics is often necessary.

Secondary Cancers

As cell-mediated immune function declines, the risk of malignancy increases. The CDC classification of AIDS currently includes four cancers: Kaposi's sarcoma, non-Hodgkin's lymphoma, primary lymphoma of the brain, and invasive cervical carcinoma. Hodgkin's lymphoma is also common (McPhee & Papadakis, 2009).

KAPOSI'S SARCOMA Kaposi's sarcoma (KS) is often the presenting symptom of AIDS. It remains the most common cancer associated with the disease. Kaposi's sarcoma is caused by a virus called the Kaposi sarcoma-associated herpesvirus, also known as human herpesvirus. Men who have sex with men not only have a risk of HIV infection, but are also more likely to be infected with the virus responsible for KS. Women who have sex with these men also have a risk of HIV and KS. The virus associated with KS appears to be mainly transmitted through sexual contact, although cases have also been reported in injection drug users. People whose immune system is suppressed because they have received an organ transplant and are taking immunosuppressive medications are also at risk of developing KS (American Cancer Society, 2005).

A tumor of the endothelial cells lining small blood vessels, KS presents as vascular macules, papules, or violet lesions affecting the skin and viscera (Figure 13–10 ■). In people with dark skin, Kaposi's lesions appear more brown toned. In addition to the palate and toe webs, the face is a common site for skin lesions, especially the tip of the nose and pinnae of the ears. Common sites for visceral disease include the gastrointestinal tract, lungs, and lymphatic system.

The lesions of KS are usually painless initially, but may become painful as the disease progresses. Internally, the tumors may obstruct organ function or cause bleeding. When the lungs are involved, gas exchange may be severely impaired, resulting in pulmonary hemorrhage. This disease may progress slowly or rapidly. Rapidly progressing KS is treated with chemotherapy; milder forms may improve with the initiation of HAART therapy (McPhee & Papadakis, 2009).

LYMPHOMAS Lymphomas are malignancies of the lymphoid tissue, including lymphocytes, lymph nodes, and the lymphoid organs such as the spleen and bone marrow. In AIDS,

Figure 13–10 ■ Kaposi's sarcoma lesions.

Source: Zeva Oelbaum/Peter Arnold, Inc.

70% of lymphomas are outside the lymphatic system. Hodgkin's disease also occurs five times more frequently in patients with HIV infection than in those without (McPhee & Papadakis, 2009). The CNS is the usual site for these lymphomas, although they may be found in the bone marrow, gastrointestinal tract, liver, skin, and mucous membranes. They are aggressive tumors, growing and spreading rapidly. Headache and changes in mental status are common early symptoms of lymphomas affecting the CNS.

CERVICAL CANCER Cervical cancer develops frequently in women with HIV infection and tends to be aggressive. Women with concurrent HIV infection and cervical cancer usually die of the cervical cancer, not AIDS. Because of this, it is recommended that women with HIV infection have Papanicolaou (Pap) smears every 6 months and aggressive treatment of cervical dysplasia with colposcopic examination and cone biopsy.

CARDIOVASCULAR AND METABOLIC COMPLICATIONS
With the advances in HAART, AIDS has become a chronic disease and patients face increased risk for developing cardiovascular disease and metabolic diseases including diabetes. Dyslipidemia (high cholesterol, high triglycerides, low high-density lipoproteins, high levels of low-density lipoproteins) leads to atherosclerosis; these abnormalities develop secondary to some HAART medications, as well as in the absence of HAART. The protease inhibitor drugs make statin (medications used to lower hypercholesterolemia) therapy difficult because they impair metabolism of statins, leading to muscle toxicity.

AIDS NEPHROPATHY Nephropathy is a kidney disorder. HIV-associated nephropathy (HIVAN) manifests as excessive protein in the urine, excessive nitrogen in the blood (azotemia), normal-to-large kidneys on ultrasound images, normal blood pressure, and glomerular lesions revealed by renal biopsy. Before HAART, nephropathy rapidly progressed to renal failure and end-stage renal disease (ESRD), leading to the need for dialysis. HAART taken regularly from the time of diagnosis has decreased the incidence of nephropathy. Nucleoside reverse transcriptase inhibitors (NRTIs) and nonnucleoside reverse transcriptase inhibitors (NNRTIs) may require dose adjustments but are beneficial, even with renal insufficiency. Protease inhibitors may precipitate kidney stones, a painful but nonmetabolic disorder (Salifu, Pani, & Misra, 2007).

Interdisciplinary Care

Although multiple research studies to identify a cure for HIV infection and AIDS are under way, no cure is currently available. This fact, plus the apparent universally fatal nature of the disease, make prevention a vital strategy in HIV care. Search for a vaccine has not been successful to date. HIV infection is different from other viral diseases such as mumps and polio; there is a brief period after entry when viral infected cells are susceptible to the immune system. Following that brief period, latency develops, making an immune response ineffective. The goals of care for the patient with HIV disease are as follows:

- Early identification of the infection
- Promoting health-maintenance activities to prolong the asymptomatic period as long as possible

- Preventing opportunistic infections
- Treating disease complications, such as cancers
- Providing emotional and psychosocial support

Diagnosis

Diagnostic testing is used to screen and identify the infection, as well as to monitor the patient's disease and immune status. False-positive HIV test results are more likely in settings where the prevalence of HIV in the tested population is lower than in settings where the tested population prevalence is higher. When a preliminary, positive rapid test is explained to patients, phrases like "a good chance of being infected" or "very likely infected" can be used to indicate the likelihood of HIV infection, and qualified based on the HIV prevalence in the setting and the patient's individual risk. See Box 13–2 for CDC recommendations for HIV testing.

- *HIV rapid antibody test.* The rapid tests consist of test strips with embedded HIV antigen. If there are antibodies to HIV in the patient's blood, the strip turns a color indicating the test is positive. The results are interpreted visually. Confirmation of positive results is required with the Western blot antibody test. There are six FDA approved rapid tests (see Table 13–3). These tests are widely used because results can be given immediately and three of these can be performed by personnel without formal laboratory training (point-of-care testing). Immediate notification is critical because many patients tested for HIV do not return to learn the results; many cannot be located to receive the test results and be educated about safe behaviors whether they are positive or negative for HIV. Although confirmation of results is dependent on testing with a second source, enzyme-linked immunosorbent assay (ELISA) or Western blot test, learning results immediately gives the patient more information to make wise choices about his or her behaviors and self-care.

BOX 13–2 CDC Recommendations for HIV Testing of Adults and Adolescents

1. All persons aged 13–64, regardless of risk, should receive routine, voluntary screening for HIV in all health-care settings in which the prevalence of undiagnosed HIV infection is at least 0.1%.
2. All patients beginning treatment for TB should be screened for HIV.
3. All patients seeking treatment for sexually transmitted infections should be screened for HIV each time they seek such treatment.
4. Healthcare providers should encourage patients and their prospective sex partners to be tested before initiating a new sexual relationship.
5. Repeat HIV screening should be performed for patients with known risk at least annually. Persons likely to be at high risk include injection-drug users and their sex partners, persons who exchange sex for money or drugs, sex partners of HIV-infected persons, and men who have sex with men (MSM) or heterosexual persons who themselves or whose sex partners have had more than one sex partner since their most recent HIV test.

Source: Centers for Disease Control and Prevention. (2006). *Revised Recommendations for HIV Testing of Adults, Adolescents, and Pregnant Women in Health-care Settings.* Retrieved from http://www.cdc.gov/mmwr/preview/mmwrhtml/rr5514al.htm

TABLE 13–3 Rapid HIV Tests

TEST	SPECIMEN
OraQuick Advance Rapid HIV 1/2 Antibody Test	Whole blood (venipuncture or fingerstick), oral fluid or plasma
RevealG3 Rapid HIV-1 Antibody Test	Plasma or serum
Uni-Gold Recombigen HIV Test	Whole blood (venipuncture or fingerstick), plasma or serum
Multispot HIV-1/HIV-2 Rapid Test	Serum or plasma
Clearview HIV 1/2 STAT-PAK	Whole blood (venipuncture and fingerstick), serum or plasma
Clearview Complete HIV 1/2	Whole blood (venipuncture and fingerstick), serum or plasma

- *Enzyme-linked immunosorbent assay (ELISA)* is the most widely used screening test for HIV infection. ELISA tests for HIV antibodies; it does not detect the virus. Therefore, a patient may have a negative ELISA test early in the course of infection, before detectable antibodies have developed. The test has a 99.5% or higher sensitivity when performed at least 13 weeks after infection. This means that more than 99.5% of tests performed on blood containing HIV antibodies will show a positive result. False positives can occur; therefore, an initial positive result is always tested repeatedly and confirmed using a different method of antibody detection, usually the Western blot.
- *Western blot antibody testing* is more reliable but more time consuming and more expensive than ELISA. When combined with ELISA, however, a specificity of greater than 99.9% is achieved. Specificity is a measure of the probability that a negative test result indicates that no antibodies are present. In this test, the patient's serum is mixed with HIV proteins to detect reaction. If antibodies to HIV are present, a detectable antigen–antibody response will occur.
- *HIV viral load tests* measure the amount of actively replicating HIV. Levels correlate with disease progression and response to antiretroviral medications. Levels greater than 5,000 to 10,000 copies/mL indicate the need for treatment.
- *CBC* is performed to detect anemia, leukopenia, and thrombocytopenia, which are often present in HIV infection. Lymphopenia (or low levels of lymphocytes) is especially common in this disease.
- Absolute *CD4 lymphocyte count* is the most widely used test to monitor the progress of the disease and guide therapy. The CD4 cell count correlates very closely with the immunodeficiency disorders seen in AIDS. AIDS is now defined not only by the presence of opportunistic infections and other diseases indicative of immunodeficiency, but also by HIV-seropositive status and a CD4 count of less than $200/mm^3$ or a percentage of CD4 lymphocytes of less than 14%. CD4 counts are recommended every 3 to 6 months for all people with HIV disease.

- *Blood culture for HIV* provides the most specific diagnosis but is an expensive and cumbersome test that is not widely available in the United States.

Other diagnostic tests are used primarily to detect secondary cancers and opportunistic infections in the patient with HIV. Tests ordered are both general and specific to the patient's manifestations and may include the following:

- *Tuberculin skin testing* to detect possible tuberculosis infection
- *MRI* of the brain to identify lymphomas
- *Specific cultures and serology examinations for opportunistic infections* such as PJP, toxoplasmosis, and others
- *Pap smears* every 6 months for early detection of cervical cancer in women with cervical dysplasia (McPhee & Papadakis, 2009).

Medications

Pharmacologic management of the patient with HIV disease has four primary goals: (1) to suppress the infection itself, decreasing symptoms and prolonging life, (2) to provide prophylaxis of opportunistic infections, (3) to stimulate hematopoietic response, and (4) to treat opportunistic infections and malignancies. Today the drugs have been combined and dosing schedules simplified, which helps patients adhere to medication administration schedules.

The Panel on Antiretroviral Guidelines for Adults and Adolescents (2008) and the International AIDS Society—US Panel (2008) recommend initiation of treatment when the CD4 count falls to 350 mm^3. Effectiveness of treatment is monitored by viral load and CD4 cell counts; positive results are indicated by a reduction in viral load along with preserving the CD4 count above 350 mm^3. Starting treatment before immune failure, when the CD4 count is above 500 or 1000, may protect the immune system. Patients with a viral load higher than 100,000 copies, a rapidly declining CD4 cell count (> 100/μL per year), hepatitis B or C, cardiovascular disease risk, or HIV-associated nephropathy, and women who are pregnant, are treated regardless of their CD4 level or viral load. Monitoring these individuals may reveal higher levels of CD4 or lower viral load.

Six classes of drugs used in antiretroviral treatment include nucleoside reverse transcriptase inhibitors (NRTIs), nonnucleoside reverse transcriptase inhibitors (NNRTIs), protease inhibitors (PIs), and three types of entry inhibitors. HAART is a combination of three or more antiretroviral drugs. Combination therapies increase the likelihood of decreasing viral load and adherence to administration schedules has been eased by making various combinations available in one pill. Patients beginning the HAART protocol must understand the benefits, risks, costs, and effects on daily life. HAART does not eradicate HIV infection.

HAART medications are expensive; the newer triple combinations such as Trizivir (one pill twice a day) and Atripla (one pill once a day) cost between $1270 and $1600 for a 30-day supply. This cost does not include medications to prevent or treat opportunistic infections or cancer (McPhee & Papadakis, 2009). If medications are scheduled for specific times throughout the day, leading a normal life becomes a challenge. In addition, all HAART medications cause major adverse reactions leading to less than perfect adherence, as with most chronic diseases; in this case, however, the outcome could be fatal.

Each patient must be able to adhere to the treatment regimen. It may be preferable to delay initiating therapy until the patient is able to agree to adhere so irregular dosing does not lead to viral resistance. Some providers gauge patient ability to follow the HAART regimen by the patient's success with prophylaxis for an opportunistic infection. Discontinuation or interruption of HAART is considered dangerous; because of the burden of adverse reactions, patients may desire brief "holidays" from taking the medications. Periods without the drugs may result in acceleration of viral growth, immune failure, and clinical progression of the disease.

Another approach to adherence is the use of electronic monitoring devices (EMD) (Bova et al., 2005). By placing a microprocessor in a medication cap, records are created of the time, date, and frequency of bottle opening. Although this method does not guarantee that the medication will be taken even if the cap is removed, the record created is a source for follow-up and discussion between the provider and the patient. Whether the patient is asked to keep a diary of taking the medication, uses an EMD to keep a record, or relies on pill count, adherence to medication regimen is critically important.

Ingersoll and Heckman (2005) found the most effective provider–patient relationship for fostering adherence is a balance of appropriate challenge and support. Providers who were never confrontational seem to be perceived by patients as giving permission to be less adherent. Although depression, substance use, and financial considerations undoubtedly influence adherence to HAART therapy, and need to be addressed, provider–patient relationships seem to have the most influence on adherence behavior.

NUCLEOSIDE REVERSE TRANSCRIPTASE INHIBITORS The NRTIs (also called nucleoside analogs) inhibit the action of viral reverse transcriptase, a retroviral enzyme that catalyzes the substrates for conversion and copying of viral RNA to DNA sequences. This enzyme is necessary for viral integration into cellular DNA and replication. The nucleoside analogs act as a chemical decoy for building blocks of the formation of the DNA copy, preventing the RNA from being copied into DNA. Each drug substitutes for a particular nucleoside base at different points on the chain. See the accompanying Medication Administration box for this group of drugs.

Zidovudine (Retrovir, AZT), an antiretroviral agent approved for use with HIV infection, is generally reserved for second- or third-line regimens because it causes anemia and neutropenia. Zidovudine is often given in combination with lamivudine (Combivir) and the combination reduces the frequency of dosing. Zidovudine may also be used prophylactically following a documented parenteral exposure to HIV.

Abacavir causes hypersensitivities in genetically predisposed individuals. Before prescribing this medication, HLA B*5701 testing should be done; if the test is positive, the patient will have a hypersensitivity reaction and should not take the medication.

PROTEASE INHIBITORS Protease is a viral enzyme necessary for the formation of specific viral protein needed for viral assembly and maturation. PIs bond chemically with protease to block the function of the enzyme and result in the production of immature, noninfectious viral particles. When combined with other antiviral drugs, these chemicals increase the chance of eliminating the virus by interfering with different stages of its life cycle. However, viral resistance occurs rather quickly. PIs inhibit and induce metabolism of other drugs, so their use with other medications and the dose of those medications must be carefully planned. Some drugs will circulate longer because their metabolism is inhibited; others will be speedily metabolized and eliminated.

Protease inhibitors and nucleoside analogs are associated with serious metabolic derangements. These include elevated cholesterol and triglycerides, insulin resistance and diabetes mellitus, and changes in body fat composition, which are particularly distressing to the patients. These body fat changes are primarily abdominal obesity and skeletal wasting. This set of symptoms is referred to as lipodystrophy (McPhee & Papadakis, 2009). Elevated cholesterol should be treated with pravastatin or atorvastatin. Lovastatin and simvastatin react with PIs, so they need to be avoided. Reduction of dietary sources of cholesterol should be made. Unlike most PIs, atazanavir (Reyataz) has a beneficial effect on lipids, is effective in reducing viral load, and is usually well-tolerated by patients (Kirtin, 2008).

NONNUCLEOSIDE REVERSE TRANSCRIPTASE INHIBITORS Etravirine (Intelence), delavirdine (Rescriptor), efavirenz (Sustiva), and nevirapine (Viramune) are NNRTIs that may be used in combination with nucleoside analogs and protease inhibitors. However, one limitation to NNRTIs is the high incidence of cross-resistance to NRTIs. Some studies have shown that nevirapine and efavirenz may significantly reduce serum levels of the protease inhibitors. Only one NNRTI should be used at the same time. Nevirapine has a reported risk for liver toxicity and severe rash; it should not be used as a first line treatment for women whose CD4 count is > 250 cells/mcl (McPhee & Papadakis, 2009).

ENTRY INHIBITORS These newer antiviral drugs act by binding to the virus or the host cells and preventing viral entry into the host cells. Enfuvirtide (Fuzeon) blocks the HIV virus from entering human cells. This is the first of the entry inhibitors; unfortunately it can only be administered by injection twice a day and it is very expensive. Patients who develop resistance to HAART regimens are candidates for this regimen. Side effects include injection site pain, itching, and hardening of the tissue; allergic reactions; peripheral neuropathy; insomnia; depression; dyspnea; anorexia; and arthralgia (AIDSinfo, 2008).

Maraviroc (Selzentry) is the first antiretroviral drug that targets the host cells rather than targeting the virus directly. CCR5 antagonists block certain HIV viruses from entry to host immune cells. Certain forms of HIV viruses (R5 tropic viruses) require a CCR5 receptor as a "co-receptor" to gain entry to the cell; with this entry inhibitor, the R5 tropic virus cannot interact with the receptor and therefore is blocked from entering human cells. Before prescribing, a blood test is made to identify the type of viruses the patient carries; if the R5 form of the virus is found, the patient may be a candidate for taking this drug. This entry inhibitor is approved for use in treatment-experienced patients only. Preexisting cardiac and liver conditions are associated with adverse reactions (AIDS InfoNet, 2008).

NUCLEOSIDE REVERSE TRANSCRIPTASE INHIBITORS (NRTIs)

Zidovudine (AZT, Retrovir)

emtricitasbine (emtriva)

lamivudine (epivir)

zalcitabine (Hivid)

didanosine (Videx)

tenofovir disoproxil fumarate (Viread)

stavudine (Zerit)

abacavir sulfate (Ziagen)

COMBINATIONS OF NRTIs

lamivudine and zidovudine (combivir)

abacavir and lamivudine (Epzicom)

abacvir, zidovudine, and lamivudine (Trizivir)

Tenofovir disoproxil fumarate and emtricitabine (Truvada)

Nursing Responsibilities

- Assess for possible contraindications to therapy including allergic response, previous episodes of pancreatitis, and impaired renal or liver function.
- Abacavir sulfate causes allergic reactions in some patients. Prior to administering, HLA B*5701 testing should be made and if the test is positive, the patient should not take abacavir. Monitor for an allergic response: sudden fever, skin rash, severe tiredness or achiness, diarrhea, nausea, vomiting, stomach pain, sore throat, shortness of breath, cough, or general ill feeling. Stop the medication and inform the physician immediately.
- Administer with caution to patients taking vincristine (cancer drug), rifampin (Tb), pentamidine (*pneumocystis jiroveci*), ethambutol (Tb), or metronidazole (bacterial and protozoal infections). Concurrent use may increase the risk of acute and fatal pancreatitis.
- Assess for adverse effects. Nausea and headache are common. They may be self-limiting, decreasing with time, or significant and continuing, necessitating a change of therapy. Peripheral neuropathies may develop; these manifest as a sharp burning pain sensation in the hands and/or legs. Anemia and neutropenia are treated with erythropoietin (epoetin alpha) and G-CSF (filgrastim).
- Assess CBC with differential and serum chemistries for evidence of liver or pancreas changes. Lactic acidosis, an indication of liver disease may develop; monitor lactate levels and pH. Notify the physician of significant changes.
- Didanosine interferes with the absorption of ketoconazole and dapsone (given for opportunistic infection prophylaxis or treatment). Doses of these drugs should be scheduled at least 2 hours apart from didanosine doses. Do not use alcohol while taking didanosine; alcohol may increase the risk of pancreatitis.

Health Education for the Patient and Family

- Antiretroviral medications will not cure HIV infection but rather slow its progress and reduce significant symptoms.
- Follow individual drug guidelines for administration with or without food, swallowing whole, and dissolving a powder or chewing a tablet.
- You are still infective and can pass the infection to others. Use safer sex practices and other measures to prevent transmission to partners. Do not donate blood or breastfeed.
- Notify the physician if signs of an infection or adverse response develop: sore throat, swollen lymph glands, fever; unusual fatigue or weakness; easy bruising, bleeding gums, or an injury that will not heal; persistent or intractable nausea; muscle pain or wasting.

- Continue all scheduled follow-up visits and laboratory studies to monitor for drug toxicity.
- Check with the physician before taking any prescription or over-the-counter drug.

PROTEASE INHIBITORS (PIs)

Amprenavir (Agenerase)

Tipranavir (Aptivus)

Indinavir (Crixivan)

Saquinavir mesylate (Invirase)

Fosamprenavir calcium (Lexiva)

Ritonavir (Norvir)

Darunavir (Prezista)

Atazanavir sulfate (Reyataz)

Nelfinavir mesylate (Viracept)

Lopinavir/ritonavir (Kaletra)

Nursing Responsibilities

- Assess for evidence of cardiovascular or liver disease and diabetes mellitus. Most PIs are associated with lipodystrophy (enlarged abdomen, loss of tissue from the face, arms and legs) and diabetes mellitus (elevated blood glucose).
- The protease inhibitors are known to precipitate kidney stones. Monitor creatinine clearance and patient reports of colicky flank pain.
- Ritonavir is combined with other PIs—an approach called "PI boosting." The benefit of taking Ritonavir in combination with other PIs is the added strength and effectiveness of some drugs and decreased food interactions. However, Ritonavir interacts with many drugs, both prescription and over the counter.
- Administer by mouth. Follow individual drug guidelines for administration with or without food, swallowing whole, and dissolving a powder or chewing a tablet.
- Assess for adverse effects. Nausea and intestinal distress are common. Headache and peripheral neuropathies also are common. Skin reactions may be severe in about 1% of patients. Side effects may be self-limiting, decreasing with time, or significant and necessitating a change of therapy.

NONNUCLEOSIDE REVERSE TRANSCRIPTASE INHIBITORS (NNRTIs)

Etravirine (Intelence)

Delavirdine (Rescriptor)

Efavirenz (Sustiva)

Nevirapine (Viramune)

Nursing Responsibilities

- Assess for history of liver disease before administering these drugs.
- Administer by mouth. Follow individual drug guidelines for administering with or without food, swallowing whole, dissolving a powder or chewing a tablet.
- Assess for evidence of severe skin rash accompanied by blisters, fever, joint or muscle pain, redness and swelling of the eyes, sores in the mouth, and swelling; serious kidney problems; anemia; and liver and muscle problems. Individuals should tell a doctor if they have any of these side effects.
- Efavirenz side effects may include abnormal thinking, confusion, depression, hallucinations, memory loss, paranoid thinking, and thoughts of suicide.

MULTICLASS COMBINATION AGENTS

ATRIPLA: Efavirenz (NNRTI), emtricitabine (NRTI), and tenofovir disoproxil fumarate (NRTI)

TRIZIVIR: Abacavir (NRTI), lamivudine (NRTI), and zidovudine (NRTI)

Nursing Responsibilities
- Trizivir contains abacavir sulfate, which causes allergic reactions in some patients. Prior to administering, HLA B*5701 testing should be made and if the test is positive, the patient should not take abacavir. Monitor for an allergic response: sudden fever, skin rash, severe tiredness or achiness, diarrhea, nausea, vomiting, stomach pain, sore throat, shortness of breath, cough, or general ill feeling. Stop the medication and inform the physician immediately.
- NRTIs can cause a sometimes fatal lactic acidosis and liver disease as well as blood problems or muscle weakness. A doctor should be notified if an individual taking this medication experiences digestive system problems, joint or muscle pain and weakness, pain or tingling of hands or feet, headache, dizziness, and unusual tiredness.
- Administer by mouth.
- Assess for evidence of severe skin rash accompanied by blisters, fever, joint or muscle pain, redness and swelling of the eyes, sores in the mouth, and swelling; serious kidney problems; anemia; and liver and muscle problems.

ENTRY INHIBITORS
Enfuvirtide (Fuzeon)
Maraviroc (Selzentry)

Nursing Responsibilities
- Enfuvirtide is injected; Maraviroc is administered orally.
- Both Enfuvirtide and Maraviroc must be given in combination with other antiviral drugs.
- Enfuvirtide is supplied as a powder and must be dissolved in water for injection. Roll but do not shake the mixture because excessive foam may form. Inject when completely dissolved or refrigerate up to 24 hours. Do not inject solution until it warms to room temperature. Rotate sites.
- Side effects may include cough, fever, upper respiratory tract infections, abdominal pain, dizziness, and rash. These may indicate allergy. Musculoskeletal aches, stiffness, or weakness may indicate bone necrosis caused by the drugs. Instruct patient to report these to the doctor immediately.
- Monitor liver function (cirrhosis and hepatitis decrease liver function) tests including bilirubin, amylase, lipase, AST, and ALT.
- Monitor kidney function (serum creatinine and BUN).

INTEGRASE INHIBITORS
Raltegravir (Isentress)

Nursing Responsibilities
- Administer orally with or without food.
- Assess for side effects: headache, dizziness, diarrhea, and nausea.

HIV Integrase Strand Transfer Inhibitor

Raltegravir (Isentress) targets integrase, an HIV enzyme that integrates the viral genetic material into human DNA. Raltegravir is also called a "strand transfer inhibitor," referring to the process of DNA strand transfer from the virus to the host. It is taken orally twice daily and side effects include nausea, diarrhea, and headache. It is approved only for individuals who have developed resistance to HAART combinations. Like other types of HAART, raltegravir is not considered effective if used alone (AIDS InfoNet, 2008).

Other agents may also be administered in combination with antiretroviral therapy. Interferons, which are naturally occurring lymphokines, have been used alone and in combination. Alpha-interferon may be used to treat KS and in combination with zidovudine to slow disease progression. Gamma-interferon is also used. As more drugs become available, the burden to choose the best regimen increases for the healthcare provider. Referral to a physician who specializes in care of patients with HIV/AIDS is recommended. The most important limiting factor when choosing a regimen is patient adherence. Second to that is selecting an effective combination of drugs without overlapping toxicities or toxicities so debilitating that adherence will be further impaired.

Some patients undergoing HAART are developing body composition changes and metabolic abnormalities associated with the therapy, especially the PIs. Increased fat deposition in the midsection, breasts, and neck with atrophy in the face, buttocks, and extremities describes the body composition changes; metabolic abnormalities include increased low-density lipoprotein cholesterol and triglycerides and insulin resistance. The combination of changes is consistent with metabolic syndrome, which increases the risk of cardiovascular disease and diabetes. These conditions are commonly treated with medications. A number of pharmacologic agents are used to prevent and treat opportunistic infections and malignancies in the patient with HIV.

Many patients at some point require an implanted venous access device, such as a Groshong catheter, to facilitate blood sampling, intravenous medication administration, transfusions, and parenteral nutrition. See Chapter 14 for nursing care of the patient with an intravenous access device implant.

It is recommended that all HIV-infected patients receive pneumococcal, influenza, hepatitis B, and *Haemophilus influenzae b* vaccines. Persons with a positive PPD and negative chest x-ray are given prophylactic isoniazid. When the patient's CD4 cell count falls to less than 200, prophylactic treatment for PJP is begun, usually with trimethoprim-sulfamethoxazole. Patients with a CD4 count of less than 100 are started on prophylactic treatment for MAC.

Nursing Care

The patient with HIV and AIDS has many nursing care needs, including both physical and psychosocial support (see the Moving Evidence into Action box on page 334). Because there is as yet no cure for HIV disease, many of these needs fall within the realm of nursing to promote knowledge and understanding, self-care, comfort, and quality of life. As with many diseases that have an ultimately fatal outcome, the course of HIV infection may well be affected by the patient's social support systems, control, perceived self-efficacy in management, and coping mechanisms.

As the epidemic continues, nurses are providing care for increasing numbers of patients with HIV infection at various stages of disease including the undiagnosed. These patients are not only in special care settings, but also on general units, maternal–child units, hospice, and home settings. As patients with HIV disease live longer, nurses will increasingly encounter patients in whom HIV disease is a secondary diagnosis with another primary diagnosis, for example, seizures, heart disease, diabetes mellitus, or an operative procedure.

Prevention

To stop the spread of HIV it is important to identify those who are infected but undiagnosed (approximately 25% of HIV positive patients) and offer them treatment. In many states, requirements for documented informed consent and formalized counseling seem to discourage patient participation. The CDC has proposed "opt-out" testing for HIV. The test is made after informing the patient that (1) the test will be performed and (2) the patient may elect to decline or defer testing. Consent is inferred unless the patient declines testing. In opt-out testing, consent for screening is part of the general consent for care, without formalized pretest and posttest counseling performed by supplemental staff. Using existing nursing staff to obtain consent, provide pre-and post-test information, and perform point-of-care HIV testing has been tried and found effective in emergency room settings. HIV testing can be offered 24 hours a day, 7 days per week without hiring additional personnel. However, some states require documented informed consent that includes formalized pre- and posttest counseling by staff dedicated to this role (Kirton & Stevens, 2008).

To date, no safe immunization to protect against HIV infection has been developed. Education, counseling, and behavior modification are the primary tools for AIDS prevention. The benefit of education and behavior modification is evident in the homosexual male population. The incidence of new HIV infections in this population has declined dramatically in high-prevalence cities. Nurses play a vital role in providing education about this epidemic and infection prevention for individuals and communities.

All sexually active individuals need to know how HIV is spread. Following are the only *totally* safe sex practices:

- No sex
- Long-term mutually monogamous sexual relations between two uninfected people
- Mutual masturbation without direct contact

Patients who do engage in sexual activity need to know and practice safer sex. (∞ See Chapter 50 for safer sex guidelines.) Reducing the number of sexual partners—for example, by entering into and remaining in a long-term mutually monogamous relationship with an uninfected partner—reduces the risk. Patients should not engage in unprotected sex, especially if the HIV status of the partner is unknown. Latex condoms have been shown to reduce the risk of transmitting HIV. Their effectiveness is improved when nonoxynol-9, a spermicide, is used for lubrication; however, it may cause genital ulcers, which can facilitate HIV transmission. To be effective, condoms must be used with every sexual encounter involving vaginal, oral, or anal intercourse. They also need to be applied and removed properly. A female condom is also available for use.

Healthcare workers exposed to HIV infection or adults who experience a high-risk exposure to HIV may choose post-exposure prophylaxis. Risk of exposure for healthcare workers may be through needle sticks or cuts with a sharp object; mucous membrane or nonintact skin contact with semen, vaginal secretions, fluids contaminated with visible blood, and possibly CSF, synovial fluid, and pleural, peritoneal, pericardial, or amniotic fluids. CDC guidelines recommend treatment with HAART, which includes two NRTIs for lower risk exposures

MOVING EVIDENCE INTO ACTION Improving Dietary Habits in Disadvantaged Women with HIV/AIDS: The SMART/EST Women's Project

Women diagnosed with HIV/AIDS in the United States face many stresses. In a study (Segal-Isaacson, Tobin, Weiss et al., 2006), funded by the National Institutes of Mental Health, disadvantaged women with HIV/AIDS living in New York/New Jersey or Miami, Florida, were randomized to four treatment groups for assistance in learning effective coping strategies in phase I and to receive brief nutrition education in phase II. This study was the second SMART/EST (Stress Management and Relaxation Training/Expressive-Supportive Therapy) trial. Researchers learned in the first trial that the strategies they taught decreased depression and anxiety, and improved HIV-related self-care. These results were positively related to increased CD4 levels and decreased viral loads. A SMART/EST II trial was conducted to see if participation in training to improve stress management and expressive therapy would improve the subjects' ability to apply insights and information from health education counseling.

Nutritional practices were evaluated by self reports of intake by food groups (not by calories or nutrients) with a Rapid Eating and Activity Assessment for Patients—Short Version (REAP-S) questionnaire designed for a low literacy level. Significant changes were reported throughout the measurement points.

Improvement in lowering high fat intake and high sugar intake was made; no increase in fruit, vegetable, whole grains, or calcium-source intake was found. Those in groups did not report more change than those trained individually, suggesting that social support did not have a large effect

IMPLICATIONS FOR NURSING

Although wasting is a serious problem for many patients with HIV/AIDS, overweight and obesity are common and may impair quality of life for those living with HIV/AIDS. The researchers in this study observed that when empowered for greater self care, the participants improved their disease conditions. Perhaps the most encouraging aspect of these findings is the effect of brief nutritional information encounters. Nurses can affirm with each interaction that diet and exercise are beneficial and seek to learn the concerns and barriers patients face when attempting to meet their needs. A second and perhaps more urgent implication is the importance of healthy coping and self-care. When patients are discouraged, depressed, and denying the importance of self-care, nurses should help them obtain counseling services to address their needs. Advocating for mental health care is an important nursing intervention.

and the addition of a third drug for higher risk exposure. A 4-week course of treatment is recommended and should be started within 72 hours, preferably within 2 to 3 hours of exposure (Bartlett & Weber, 2005).

The most difficult group of high-risk people to reach and educate has been injection drug users. People in this group should never share needles, syringes, or other drug paraphernalia. Many cities have initiated needle-exchange programs, providing a sterile needle and syringe in exchange for a used one. A fresh solution of household bleach and water in a 1:10 ratio is effective to clean paraphernalia when sterile supplies are not available. It is important to also teach people in this population about safer sex practices, because most heterosexual HIV transmission occurs between injection drug users and their partners.

Screening of voluntary blood donors and donated blood supplies has reduced the risk of transmission by transfusion to 1 in 100,000. Because current blood-screening methods use antibody testing, receiving donated blood continues to carry a small risk. Patients in the *window period* between contraction of the virus and the development of detectable antibodies are able to transmit the virus to others, even though they do not yet test positive for HIV. This window period usually lasts from 6 weeks to 6 months; rarely, it lasts up to 1 year. When possible, encourage patients to use autologous transfusion, donating their own blood prior to an anticipated surgery.

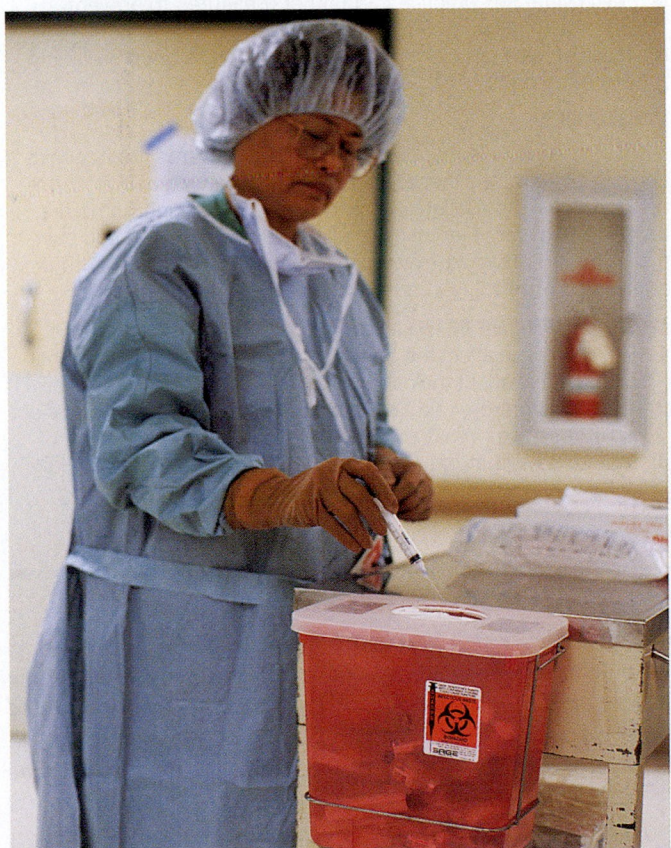

Figure 13–11 ■ This nurse is disposing of a needle and syringe in a special container, a necessary practice to avoid the transmission of HIV through needle sticks with contaminated needles.

Encourage HIV-positive patients to abstain from donating blood, organs, or sperm. They should understand tactics to avoid exchange of body fluids by not sharing needles or other drug paraphernalia, not sharing razors, and not obtaining a tattoo. Stress the importance of informing all medical personnel providing direct care (especially anyone performing a dental, surgical, or obstetric procedure) about the diagnosis.

Healthcare workers can prevent most exposures to HIV by using standard precautions (∞ refer to Appendix A and see Figure 13–11 ■). Testing to determine HIV status remains voluntary and relies on the use of antibody-screening methods. It is therefore impossible to identify every patient who is HIV positive. With standard precautions, all patients are treated alike, eliminating the need to know the patient's HIV status. All high-risk body fluids are treated as if they are infectious, and barrier precautions are used to prevent skin, mucous membrane, or percutaneous exposure to them. Counseling and testing are provided to healthcare workers with a documented needle-stick exposure. Some clinicians and facilities recommend prophylactic AZT therapy after needle-stick or splash exposure; however, it must be initiated immediately, and its effectiveness has yet to be established.

Assessment

Collect the following data through health history and physical examination. Further focused assessments are described with nursing interventions next.

- *Health history:* Risk factors (transfusion, unprotected sex, needle exposure), infections (sexually transmitted infections, hepatitis, tuberculosis), medications, recreational drug use, foreign travel, pets.
- *Physical assessment:* Height, weight, nutrition, skin and mucous membranes, vision, lymph nodes, breath sounds, abdominal tenderness, motor strength, coordination, cranial nerves, gait, deep tendon reflexes, genitourinary examination, mental status.

Nursing Diagnoses and Interventions

Nursing care needs for the patient with HIV infection change over the course of the disease. Preventive healthcare measures, health maintenance activities, education, and support of coping mechanisms are important in the early stages of the disease. Counseling the patient with a new diagnosis of HIV infection is vital. HIV infection and AIDS continue to carry a social stigma that may interfere with the patient's usual support systems and coping mechanisms. As the disease progresses and the patient experiences more physical symptoms, direct care needs become more important while the need for psychosocial support continues. Acute exacerbation of opportunistic infections may necessitate hospitalization, but typically the patient is managed at home. See the accompanying Nursing Case Study & Care Plan on page 336.

Ineffective Coping

On receiving the test results indicating HIV seropositive status, the person with HIV infection is faced with multiple issues rarely affecting other patients. HIV is a disease for which there is no known cure and which is, at this time, thought to be almost universally fatal. Social support systems, family relationships, and the ability to obtain and retain useful work and

CASE STUDY & NURSING CARE PLAN   A Patient with HIV Infection

Sara Lu is a 26-year-old elementary school teacher who lives with her parents and two younger sisters. Ms. Lu is very close to her parents and sisters; they share everything with each other. During the required physical for admission to graduate school, Ms. Lu tells her physician that lately she has felt fatigued. She also states that she has had a persistent sore throat, intermittent bouts of diarrhea, and mild shortness of breath for about a month. She takes no routine medications other than a daily multivitamin and an occasional acetaminophen tablet for a headache. She is active in a drama club in her community, and she jogs 3 miles three to four times a week. She is engaged to be married; her wedding date is 6 months away. Her fiancé is the only person with whom she has had sexual relations. Her sexual activity has been unprotected. Ms. Lu has a history of open heart surgery 7 years ago to correct a congenital valve defect. She has been physically healthy since that time, until about a month or two ago. The physician orders a mononucleosis test, ELISA, Western blot analysis, CD4 T-cell count, a p24 antigen test, and an erythrocyte sedimentation rate (ESR). She has been asked to return in 1 week for follow-up.

ASSESSMENT

On Ms. Lu's follow-up visit, Carole Kee, RN, obtains her nursing history. Ms. Lu continues to have flulike symptoms but has improved somewhat. She states that she just has not been as active as usual and is worried about her health. Her appetite has decreased because of soreness in her mouth, and she has noted some whitish patches on her tongue and cheeks.

A chest x-ray film reveals no abnormality. The results of her laboratory tests are as follows:

- ELISA: positive for antibodies against HIV
- Western blot analysis: positive for antibodies against HIV
- p24 antigen test: positive for circulating HIV antigens
- ESR: increased to 25 mm/h (normal for women is 15 to 20 mm/h; normal for men is 10 to 15 mm/h)
- CD4 T-cell count: 599/mm^3 (normal range is 600 to 1200 mm^3)

Ms. Lu's physical examination reveals that she has enlarged lymph nodes in her neck and white patches on her oral mucosa. Her skin is warm to the touch. Her vital signs are as follows: T 99.9°F (37.7°C), P 84, R 20, and BP 120/78.

Ms. Lu is told of the results of her laboratory tests and the medical diagnosis of HIV infection. Ms. Lu is obviously distressed and wants to know how this happened, its meaning, whether she has infected her loved ones, and whether she will get better.

DIAGNOSES

- *Imbalanced Nutrition: Less than Body Requirements* related to soreness in mouth
- *Risk for Deficient Fluid Volume* related to decreased fluid intake and diarrhea
- *Risk for Infection* related to altered immune protection
- *Anxiety* related to diagnosis and fear

- *Readiness for Enhanced Knowledge* about the HIV disease process and self-care

EXPECTED OUTCOMES

- Maintain adequate nutrition for optimal body and cellular function.
- Consume at least 2500 mL of fluid per day.
- Remain free of infections and their complications.
- Verbalize anxiety and use appropriate coping mechanisms.
- Verbalize and demonstrate knowledge of HIV disease.
- Verbalize measures to prevent HIV transmission to others, including safer sex practices.

PLANNING AND IMPLEMENTATION

- Monitor daily weight and intake and output.
- Monitor dietary habits and serum albumin levels.
- Teach Ms. Lu the importance of consuming a nutritionally balanced diet and maintaining adequate fluid intake.
- Provide dietary consultation referral.
- Encourage oral care before and after meals.
- Assess bowel sounds and monitor elimination pattern.
- Monitor for signs of dehydration, such as poor skin turgor, oliguria, and orthostatic hypotension.
- Increase fluid to 2500 mL daily.
- Use strict aseptic technique for all invasive procedures.
- Teach Ms. Lu to avoid exposure to infection and people with known illnesses.
- Monitor response to prescribed medications.
- Encourage regular physical exercise.
- Provide opportunities for Ms. Lu to verbalize her feelings.
- Avoid false reassurances.
- Provide appropriate and adequate information about HIV/AIDS.
- Teach safer sex practices and other measures to prevent HIV transmission.
- Teach anxiety-controlling techniques, such as deep breathing and meditation.

EVALUATION

Ms. Lu is eager to learn about her illness and wants her family to come with her for further explanation. She states that she is sure her fiancé will be available as well. Ms. Lu is taking home antifungal medication, diet plans, and a schedule for increased exercise. She will return in 1 week for counseling and in 1 month for a follow-up physical.

CRITICAL THINKING IN THE NURSING PROCESS

1. How does age affect the body's response to fighting HIV? What other factors affect the risk of HIV infection and its progression?
2. Are the laboratory results for Ms. Lu a true indication that she is HIV positive? What additional tests might be ordered?
3. Ms. Lu says that her fiancé would like to have a child. How will you counsel her regarding pregnancy and childbearing?

See Evaluating Your Response in Appendix C.

---

health insurance may be disrupted by the disease. The patient may experience guilt about his or her lifestyle and how the disease was contracted. As the disease progresses, social isolation, fatigue, body image changes, medication side effects, and multiple other issues affect the patient's ability to cope.

- Assess social support network and usual methods of coping. *This will help both the nurse and the patient identify people and mechanisms that can help the patient cope more effectively with the disease.*

- If possible, assign a primary nurse, whether the setting is home health, hospice, or acute care. *This helps promote the development of a therapeutic and trusting relationship and provides for continuity of care.*
- Plan for consistent, uninterrupted time with the patient. *Time and a consistent presence encourage the patient to express feelings and work through issues related to HIV infection.*
- Interact at every opportunity outside of providing specific nursing care treatments. *This purposeful interaction communicates caring and acceptance without fear of HIV disease.*

- Support the patient's social network. *Nontraditional families may offer more support than the traditional family. This in turn may necessitate a liberal interpretation of the term family if unit policy is immediate family only.*
- Promote interaction between the patient, significant others, and family. *Hospitalization and manifestations of HIV disease may bring about isolation from others and decrease the patient's ability to cope.*
- Encourage involvement in making care decisions. *This gives the patient a greater sense of self-worth and control over the situation, increasing coping abilities.*
- Set and maintain limits on manipulative and other destructive behaviors. *The patient who is unable to limit inappropriate behaviors needs the external control established by setting limits.*
- Assist to accept responsibility for actions without blaming others. *Effective coping cannot occur without accepting responsibility for one's actions.*
- Support positive coping behaviors, decisions, actions, and achievements. *As self-esteem is enhanced, coping improves* (Côté & Pepler, 2005).

Risk for Situational Low Self-Esteem

- Assess negative self-evaluation and statements of self-worth. *Statements of self-worth indicate level of self-esteem.*
- Reinforce personal strengths that are identified. *Focusing on personal strengths enables movement away from negative thoughts.*
- Assist in setting realistic goals. *Establishing and meeting realistic short-term goals is helpful in increasing self-confidence and decreasing negative self-talk.*
- Encourage active participation in plan of care. *Active participation reinforces sense of control and independence, increasing self-esteem.*
- Refer to clergy, social worker, clinical specialist, and/or counselor as appropriate. *Persons with expertise in counseling may be necessary to enable coping with current situation.*

Impaired Skin Integrity

Dryness, malnutrition, immobility from fatigue, and skin lesions on pressure sites contribute to impaired integrity of the skin for the patient with HIV disease. Maintaining skin integrity is important because of the progressive and debilitating nature of the disease. It is also a consideration both as the first line of defense against infection in an immunosuppressed patient and as a site for secondary manifestations such as KS and herpes.

- Assess the skin frequently for lesions and areas of breakdown. *Early identification of impaired skin integrity allows prompt intervention.*
- Monitor lesions for signs of infection or impaired healing. *Infection or poor tissue perfusion not only impairs healing but may lead to further skin breakdown.*
- Turn at least every 2 hours if unable to turn self, more frequently if necessary. *Turning decreases unrelieved pressure on bony prominences and improves circulation to the tissues.*
- Keep skin clean and dry using mild, nondrying soaps or oils for cleansing. *Night sweats and diarrhea, if present, can cause breakdown and damage to the skin. Frequent cleansing with nondrying products discourages bacterial growth, thus reducing the risk of infection.*

PRACTICE ALERT
Applying protective creams to reddened areas in the rectal area protects skin from the caustic effects of diarrhea.

- Massage around but not over affected pressure sites to increase circulation to the surrounding tissue. *Massaging over the affected area can cause skin breakdown.*
- If blisters are noted, leave intact, and dress with a hydrocolloid (e.g., DuoDERM) dressing. *Blisters provide natural sterile coverings for damaged tissue, improving healing and preventing bacterial invasion.*
- Caution against scratching. If confused, trim fingernails and use mitts or soft restraints to prevent scratching. Check for circulation of hands and fingers frequently if mitts or restraints are used. *Scratching and skin damage allow bacteria to be introduced into lesions, increasing the risk of infection. Tight or restrictive restraints or mitts may compromise circulation.*
- Avoid the use of heat or occlusive dressings. *Heat can further dry and damage the skin; occlusive dressings may impair circulation and lead to ulceration.*
- Prevent skin shearing by using a turnsheet and adequate personnel when repositioning. *Shearing causes tissue trauma that can lead to decubitus ulcers.*
- Encourage ambulation if possible; if the patient is confined to bed, encourage active or passive range-of-motion exercises. *Activity increases circulation, decreases pressure and skin breakdown, and helps maintain muscle tone.*
- Monitor nutritional intake and albumin levels. *Maintenance of optimal nutrition decreases the risk of tissue breakdown and improves resistance to infection.*

Imbalanced Nutrition: Less than Body Requirements

Many factors associated with HIV disease, including manifestations of the disease itself, put the patient at risk for altered nutrition and weight loss. Nausea and anorexia may be manifestations of the disease or the result of antiretroviral therapy. Chronic diarrhea is a common manifestation of HIV disease. Wasting syndrome is also common. It is manifested by involuntary weight loss of greater than 10% to 15% of baseline weight, severe diarrhea, fever, and chronic fatigue and weakness. The exact cause of wasting syndrome is unclear, but the diarrhea and fatigue contribute, as does the increased metabolic rate associated with fever. Oral and esophageal candidiasis and KS of the gastrointestinal tract may cause painful swallowing, making eating difficult and thereby contributing to anorexia. Poor nutritional status in the patient with HIV can ultimately result in altered comfort, a change in body image, muscle wasting, increased risk of infection, and higher mortality and morbidity.

- Assess nutritional status, including weight; body mass; caloric intake; and laboratory studies, such as total protein and albumin levels, hemoglobin, and hematocrit. *These factors provide a baseline to determine the effectiveness of interventions.*
- Identify possible causes of altered nutrition. *Identification of causes provides direction for planned interventions.*

- Administer prescribed medications for candidiasis and other manifestations as prescribed. *Eliminating this opportunistic infection improves comfort and facilitates food intake. Topical viscous anesthetic can help reduce pain and improve oral intake.*
- Administer antidiarrheal medications after stools and antiemetics prior to meals. Provide antipyretics as needed to control fever. *Reducing diarrhea will improve nutrient absorption; preprandial medication with an antiemetic reduces nausea and improves food intake. Reduction of fever lowers the body's metabolic demands.*

> **PRACTICE ALERT**
> High-fiber foods can increase intestinal motility and the incidence of diarrhea.

- Provide a diet high in protein and kilocalories. *A high-protein, high-kilocalorie diet provides the necessary nutrients to meet metabolic and tissue healing needs.*
- Offer soft foods and serve small portions. *Soft foods are easily digested. Small portions are more appealing to the anorectic or nauseated patient.*
- Involve in meal planning and encourage significant others to bring favorite foods from home. *The patient is more likely to consume adequate amounts of preferred foods. Allowing food choices enhances the patient's sense of control.*
- Assist with eating as needed. *Fatigue and weakness can prevent the patient from eating an adequate amount of food.*
- Provide supplementary vitamins and enteral feedings, such as Ensure. *This improves nutritional status and caloric intake.*
- Provide or assist with frequent oral hygiene. *Oral hygiene improves comfort and appetite, and reduces the risk of mucosal lesions.*
- Administer appetite stimulants, such as megestrol (Megace) and dronabinol (Marinol) as ordered. *Both drugs may increase appetite and promote weight gain.*

Ineffective Sexuality Pattern

The diagnosis of HIV infection can significantly alter the patient's expressions of sexuality. Guilt over the diagnosis may interfere with libido. The patient may be angry with a significant other or partner if that person was the probable source of infection. The patient may fear spreading the disease to others via sexual relations. As the disease progresses, its manifestations can affect body image and self-esteem, impairing sexuality. Other symptoms, such as nausea, fatigue, and weakness, may also interfere with libido and sexual satisfaction. If nurses are not comfortable discussing sexuality, referral to an appropriate counselor is appropriate.

- Examine own feelings about sexuality, role in dealing with a patient's sexuality, the patient's lifestyle, and sexual preferences. *To deal effectively with the patient's concerns, it is vital that the nurse be comfortable with his or her own feelings of sexuality and be able to accept the patient's lifestyle. Referring the patient to another nurse or counselor may be necessary.*
- Establish a trusting, therapeutic relationship through the use of time, active listening, caring, and self-disclosure. Maintain a nonthreatening, nonjudgmental attitude toward the patient.

Sexuality is a private issue that will be uncomfortable or impossible for the nurse and patient to discuss without a mutually trusting relationship.

- Provide factual information about HIV infection and its effects. *This helps the patient separate fears and myths from reality.*
- Discuss safer sex practices, including hugging, cuddling, nonsexual contact, the use of latex condoms and spermicidal lubricant, and mutual masturbation. *Alternative forms of sexual activity and expressing affection can allow the patient and significant other to remain close throughout the course of the disease.*
- Encourage discussion of fears and concerns with significant other. *Open communication helps him or her to deal with issues related to sexuality.*
- For the patient without a significant other, stress the need to continue to meet people and develop social relationships while practicing safer sex. *The risk of isolation is high in the patient with HIV infection, and relationships with others help the patient to cope with the disease.*
- Refer the patient and significant other to local support groups for people and partners of people with HIV. *Support groups provide a social and support network of people facing the same issues.*

Using NANDA, NIC, and NOC

Linkages between a selected NANDA nursing diagnosis, NIC, and NOC for the patient with an HIV infection are shown in the chart that follows.

Community-Based Care

Teaching needs for both the patient and significant other are extensive. The primary need is information about the disease, its spread, and its expected course. The patient and family need current factual information to plan realistically and to combat myths, misperceptions, and prejudices. At the same time, it is important to include information about current research and progress in treating the disease to maintain a sense of hopefulness.

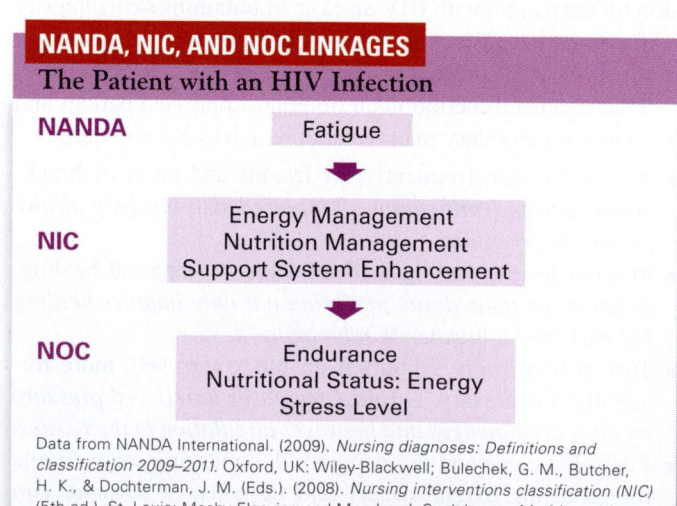

NANDA, NIC, AND NOC LINKAGES
The Patient with an HIV Infection

NANDA	Fatigue
NIC	Energy Management Nutrition Management Support System Enhancement
NOC	Endurance Nutritional Status: Energy Stress Level

Data from NANDA International. (2009). *Nursing diagnoses: Definitions and classification 2009–2011.* Oxford, UK: Wiley-Blackwell; Bulechek, G. M., Butcher, H. K., & Dochterman, J. M. (Eds.). (2008). *Nursing interventions classification (NIC)* (5th ed.). St. Louis: Mosby Elsevier; and Moorhead, S., Johnson, M., Maas, M., et al. (Eds.). (2008). *Nursing outcomes classification (NOC)* (4th ed.). St. Louis, MO: Mosby Elsevier.

The following topics should be discussed with the patient and family to prepare for home care:

- Guidelines for safer sex practices
- Nutrition, rest and exercise, stress reduction, lifestyle changes, and maintaining a positive outlook
- Infection prevention and transmission including hand hygiene and wearing gloves when handling patient's secretions or excretions
- Importance of regular medical follow-up and monitoring of immune status
- Signs and symptoms of opportunistic infections and malignancies, as well as other symptoms that should be reported
- Medications and adverse effects

- Use and care of implanted venous access devices, total parenteral nutrition, intravenous pumps and continuous medication delivery systems, and intravenous or aerosolized medications
- Cessation of smoking, alcohol, and recreational or illicit drug use
- Home health services
- Hospice and respite care services
- Community resources, such as support groups, social agencies, and counselors
- Helpful resources:
  - CDC National AIDS Hotline
  - Gay Men's Health Crisis Network
  - National Association of People with AIDS
  - National Organization on HIV over Fifty

CHAPTER HIGHLIGHTS

- The immune system is a complex combination of cellular and humoral components that protect against disease. Immunity develops when the body recognizes foreign proteins as "nonself" and develops nonspecific inflammatory responses and specific cellular responses to each foreign antigen.
- Patients suffer when the immune system is excessively or inadequately responsive, or when recognition of self fails and reactions escalate against self. The latter occurs in autoimmune diseases.
- With aging, there is a general decline in the sensitivity and regulation of the immune system, which may result in autoimmune disease.
- Hypersensitivities are excessive responses to antigens that result in harm to the patient. These range from benign to severely life threatening. Damage to host tissue is caused by chemicals of the immune response, destruction of cells, or creation of large antigen–antibody complexes that accumulate in the kidney glomerular capillaries.
- Allergic reactions are treated pharmacologically to prevent or moderate allergic responses. Another method of dampening allergic responses is by desensitization, a weekly process of introducing increasing amounts of known allergens subdermally.
- Patients must be taught that the safest practice is to avoid contact with all known allergens.
- Latex allergy is a problem for healthcare professionals. Repeated exposure to latex-containing equipment and gloves results in delayed hypersensitivity.

- Any type of allergic reaction has the potential to escalate to anaphylaxis. Respiratory arrest and cardiac failure are risks with full blown allergic reactions. Nurses must recognize early signs and symptoms and immediately signal for emergency care.
- Intentional immunosuppression is an essential step in preventing transplant rejection. The patient receiving a transplanted organ will be treated with immune-suppressing drugs to prevent initial rejection, to maintain the transplant, and to halt any rejection process that may develop. Patients will take the immune-suppressing, antirejection drugs for their lifetime. The drugs prevent cytokine production that upregulates an immune reaction and targets the transplanted organ. Most immunosuppressing drugs are nephrotoxic; immunosuppression places patients at greater risk for infection and cancers.
- HIV/AIDS continues to spread and many patients are unaware they have the virus. AIDS is a profoundly immune-suppressed condition that results from viral destruction of cellular components of host immunity.
- A major change in the AIDS epidemic is the disease profile, which has benefited from HAART. HAART is a combination of drugs that limits viral replication and host susceptibility to opportunistic infections and cancer. Patients are living much longer with the disease without progression to AIDS. The number of pills needed has decreased significantly by pharmaceutical combinations, but side effects of the combination of drugs that make up HAART are appearing as patients live longer.

TEST YOURSELF NCLEX-RN® REVIEW

1. Which one of the following conditions is caused by a type I IgE-mediated hypersensitivity reaction?
   1. autoimmune hemolytic anemia
   2. systemic lupus erythematosus
   3. graft rejection
   4. anaphylaxis
2. A patient received a liver transplant 1 day ago. If the patient were to develop an acute transplant rejection episode, when should the nurse expect to see the manifestations?
   1. approximately 4 days to 3 months later
   2. approximately 2 days later
   3. within the first 24 hours
   4. within the first 8 hours

3. The nurse notes a cough, shortness of breath, and tachypnea in a patient with AIDS. Which opportunistic infection is probably causing these manifestations?
   1. *Toxoplasma gondii*
   2. cytomegalovirus
   3. *Pneumocystis jiroveci*
   4. *Cryptococcus neoformans*
4. Which of the following explanations should the nurse give to a patient who has tested positive for HIV?
   1. "You have been diagnosed with AIDS."
   2. "At this point, AIDS is not active in your blood."
   3. "This means that you will not develop AIDS in the future."
   4. "Antibodies to the AIDS virus are present in the blood."

5. A patient is taking zidovudine (Retrovir). What would the nurse monitor to identify adverse reactions?
   1. cardiotoxicity
   2. leukopenia
   3. nephrotoxicity
   4. polycythemia

6. The order of administering antigens in allergy testing is based on prevention of anaphylaxis. Which method would a nurse expect to be used first?
   1. inhalation
   2. prick test
   3. intradermal injection
   4. subcutaneous injection

7. A hypersensitivity response is suspected when blood products are infusing. What priority intervention would the nurse perform?
   1. Discard the product immediately.
   2. Replace all tubing and attach a new line with NS.
   3. Backflush the line and run the NS attached at the Y tubing.
   4. Remove the intravenous catheter and establish access distal to the site.

8. Protease inhibitors and nucleoside analogs share correlations to metabolic abnormalities including which of the following?
   1. lactose intolerance
   2. diabetes mellitus
   3. Hashimoto's thyroiditis
   4. systemic lupus erythematosus

9. The priority when initiating or changing HIV drug therapy regimens is which of the following?
   1. cost of therapy
   2. access to dental care
   3. toxicities associated with each drug
   4. patient willingness to adhere to the drug regimen

10. Patients receiving kidney transplants will receive immunosuppressant therapy. What agent is used to induce immunosuppression immediately following a transplant?
    1. azathioprine
    2. corticosteroids
    3. muromonab-CD3
    4. antithymocyte globulin

See Test Yourself answers in Appendix C.

Pearson Nursing Student Resources

Find additional review materials at
www.nursing.pearsonhighered.com
Prepare for success with additional NCLEX®-style practice questions, interactive assignments and activities, Web links, animations and videos, and more!

BIBLIOGRAPHY

AIDS InfoNet. (2008). *Tropism tests.* Retrieved from http://www.aidsinfonet.org/fact_sheets/view/129

AIDSinfo. (2008). *AIDSinfo Drug Database.* US Department of Health and Human Services. Retrieved from http://www.aidsinfo.nih.gov/DrugsNew/Default.aspx?MenuItem=Drugs&Search=On

American Association for Clinical Chemistry. (2006). Lab Tests Online. Retrieved from http://www.labtestsonline.org/understanding/analytes/allergy/test.html

Bova, C. A., Fennie, K. P., Knafl, G. J., Dieckhaus, K. D., Wtrous, E., & Williams, A. B. (2005). Use of electronic monitoring devices to measure antiretroviral adherence: Practical considerations. *AIDS and Behavior, 9*(1), 103–110.

Branson, B. M. (2008). *Expanded HIV Testing—Implementing the CDC Recommendations: Guidance for Nurses.* Retrieved from http://www.medscape.com/viewarticle/572177

Bulechek, G. M., Butcher, H. K., & Dochterman, J. M. (Eds.). (2008). *Nursing interventions classification (NIC)* (5th ed.). St. Louis: Mosby Elsevier.

Centers for Disease Control and Prevention. (2006). Revised recommendations for HIV testing of adults, adolescents, and pregnant women in health-care settings. Retrieved from http://www.cdc.gov/mmwR/preview/mmwrhtml/rr5514a1.htm

Centers for Disease Control and Prevention. (2007). National Center for Chronic Disease Prevention and Health Promotion: Food Allergies. Retrieved from http://www.cdc.gov/HealthyYouth/foodallergies/

Centers for Disease Control and Prevention. (2008). HIV/AIDS. Retrieved from http://www.cdc.gov/hiv/topics/surveillance/.htm

Côté J. K., & Pepler, C. (2005). Cognitive coping intervention for acutely ill HIV-positive men. *Journal of Clinical Nursing, 14*(3), 321–326.

Department of Health and Human Services. (2008). *Panel on antiretroviral guidelines for adults and adolescents. Guidelines for the use of antiretroviral agents in HIV-1 infected adults and adolescents.* Retrieved from http://www.aidsinfo.nih.gov/ContentFiles/AdultandAdolescentGL.pdf

Fauci, A., Braunwald, E., Kasper, D., Hauser, S., Longo, D., Jameson, J., et al. (2008). *Harrison's principles of internal medicine* (17th ed.). New York, NY: McGraw Hill.

Hakin, F. T., & Gress, R. E. (2007). Immunosenescence: deficits in adaptive immunity in the elderly. *Tissue Antigens, 70*(3), 179–189.

Hammer, S. M., Eron, J. J., Reiss, P., Schooley, R. T., Thompson, M. A., Walmsley, S., Cahn, P., Fischl, M. A., Gatell, J. M., Hirsch, M. S., Jacobsen, D. M., Montaner, J. S., Richman, D. D., Yeni, P. G., & Volberding, P. A. (2008). Antiretroviral treatment of adult HIV infection; 2008 recommendations of the International AIDS Society—USA Panel. *Journal of the American Medical Association, 300*(5), 555–570.

Ingersoll, K. S., & Heckman, C. J. (2005). Patient-clinician relationships and treatment system effects on HIV medication adherence. *AIDS and Behavior, 9*(1), 89–101.

Kee, J. L. (2009). Prentice Hall handbook of laboratory and diagnostic tests with nursing implications. Upper Saddle River, NJ: Pearson Prentice Hall.

King, H. C., Mabry, R. L., Mabry, C. S., Gordon, B. R., & Marple, B. F. (2005). *Allergy in ENT practice: The basic guide* (2nd ed.). New York: Thieme Medical Publisher.

Kirton, C.A. (2008). Managing long-term complications of HIV. *Nursing, 38*(8), 44–50.

Kirton, C. A., & Stevens, L. C. (2008). *Implementing a rapid HIV testing program in the acute care setting: Nurses take the lead.* Retrieved from http://www.medscape.com/viewarticle/572180

Knoll, B., Lassmann, B., & Temesgen, Z. (2007). Current status of HIV infection: A review for non-HIV-treating physicians. *International Journal of Dermatology, 46*(12), 1219–1228.

Langkamp-Henken, B., Wood, S. M., Herlinger-Garcia, K. A., Thomas, D. J., Stechmiller, J. K., Bender, B. S., Gardner, E. M., DeMichele, S. J., Schaller, J. P., & Murasko, D. M. (2006). Nutritional formula improved immune profiles of seniors living in nursing homes. *Journal of the American Geriatric Society, 54*(12), 1861–1870.

McPhee, S. J., & Papadakis, M. (Eds.). (2009). *Current medical diagnosis & treatment* (48th ed.). New York: Lange-McGraw-Hill.

Moorhead, S., Johnson, M., Maas, M., & Swanson, E. (Eds.). (2008). *Nursing outcomes classification (NOC)* (4th ed.). St. Louis, MO: Mosby Elsevier.

NANDA International. (2009). *Nursing diagnoses: Definitions and classification 2009–2011.* Oxford, UK: Wiley-Blackwell.

Porth, C. M. (2007). *Essentials of pathophysiology: Concepts of altered health states* (2nd ed.). Philadelphia: Lippincott Williams & Wilkins.

Porth, C. M., & Matfin, G. (2009). *Pathophysiology: Concepts of altered health states.* (8th ed.). Philadelphia: Lippincott Williams & Wilkins.

Rana, A., Robles, S., Russo, M. J., Halazun, K. J., Woodland, D. C., Witkowski, P., Ratner, L. E., & Hardy, M. A. (2008). The combined organ effect: Protection against rejection? *Annals of Surgery, 248*(5), 871–879.

Robinson, F. P. (2005). Body composition changes in patients with HIV. *American Journal of Nursing, 105*(13), 69–72.

Salifu, M.O., Pani, S., & Misra, N. (2007). *HIV Nephropathy.* Retrieved from http://www.emedicine.com/med/TOPIC3203.HTM

Segal-Issacson, C., Tobin, J., Weiss, S., Brondolo, E., Vaughn, A., Wang, C., Camille, J., Gousse, Y., Ishii, M., Jones, D., LaPerriere, A., Lydston, D., Schneiderman, N., & Ironson, G. (2006). Improving dietary habits in disadvantaged women with HIV/AIDS: The SMART/EST women's project. *AIDS Behavior, 10*(5), 659–670.

Smith, A. M., Amin, H. S., Biagini, R. E., Hamilton, R. G., Arif, S. A., Yeang, H. Y., & Bernstein, D. I. (2007). Percutaneous reactivity to natural rubber latex proteins persists in health-care workers following avoidance of natural rubber latex. *Clinical & Experimental Allergy, 37*(9), 1349–1356.

Walensky, R. P., Paltiel, A. D., Losina, E., Mercincavage, L. M., Schackman, B. R., Sax, P. E., Weinstein, M. C., & Freedberg, K. A. (2006). The survival benefits of AIDS Treatment in the United States. *Journal of Infectious disease, 194*(1), 11–19.

WebMd. (2009). Allergy testing. Retrieved from http://www.webmd.com/allergies/allergy-tests

Wilkinson, J. M. (2008). *Nursing diagnosis handbook.* (9th ed.). Upper Saddle River, NJ: Pearson Prentice Hall.

Wilson, B., Shannon, M., & Shields, K. (2009). *Prentice Hall nurse's drug guide 2009.* Upper Saddle River, NJ: Pearson Prentice Hall.

Nursing Care of Patients with Cancer

LEARNING OUTCOMES

1. Define cancer and differentiate benign from malignant neoplasm.
2. Describe the theories of carcinogenesis.
3. Explain known carcinogens and identify risk factors for cancer.
4. Compare the mechanisms and characteristics of normal cells with those of malignant cells.
5. Describe physical and psychological effects of cancer.
6. Describe and compare laboratory and diagnostic tests for cancer.
7. Discuss the role of chemotherapy in cancer treatment and classify chemotherapeutic agents.
8. Compare and contrast the role of surgery, radiation therapy, and biotherapy in the treatment of cancer.
9. Explain causes and discuss the nursing interventions for common oncologic emergencies.
10. Design an appropriate care plan for patients with cancer and their families regarding cancer diagnosis, treatment, and coping strategies.

CLINICAL COMPETENCIES

1. Assess functional health status of patients with cancer, and monitor, document, and report abnormal manifestations.
2. Incorporate evidence-based research into the plan of nursing care for patients with cancer.
3. Prioritize nursing diagnosis based on assessment data and implement appropriate nursing interventions for patients with cancer during cancer diagnosis, treatment, and rehabilitation.
4. Safely administer medications for pain, nausea and vomiting, mucositis, or anemia.
5. Use the nursing process as a framework for planning and providing individualized care and integrating interdisciplinary care for patients with cancer to meet their healthcare needs.
6. Include cultural variation and diverse values in designing and implementing individualized plans of care for patients with cancer.
7. Design and provide individualized patient and family teaching to restore, promote, and maintain patients' functional status.
8. Revise plan of care as needed to provide effective interventions for patients with cancer and their families.

KEY TERMS

anaplasia, *346*
biotherapy, *365*
brachytherapy, *365*
cachexia, *351*
cancer, *341*
carcinogenesis, *346*
carcinogens, *346*
cell cycle, *346*

chemotherapy, *360*
differentiation, *346*
dysplasia, *346*
hospice, *380*
hyperplasia, *346*
metaplasia, *346*
metastasis, *348*
neoplasm, *348*

oncogene, *346*
oncologic emergencies, *376*
oncology, *342*
proto-oncogenes, *346*
radiation therapy, *364*
tumor marker, *355*
xerostomia, *375*

Cancer is a group of complex diseases characterized by uncontrolled growth and spread of abnormal cells (American Cancer Society [ACS], 2010a). Cancer can manifest in different ways depending on which body system is affected and the type of tumor cells involved. Cancer can affect people of any age, gender, ethnicity, or geographic region. Although the incidence and mortality rates of cancer have continued to decline since 1990, it remains one of the most feared diseases (ACS, 2010a). The fear engendered by even the suggestion of a cancer diagnosis often evokes feelings of hopelessness and helplessness (Fu, Xu, Liu, & Haber, 2008).

This chapter focuses on the general pathogenesis, pathophysiology, and etiology of cancer; identifies current diagnostic and treatment modalities; and discusses nursing care appropriate for patients with cancer. Discussions of cancers that affect specific body systems can be found in corresponding disorders chapters in the text.

Cancer occurs when normal cells mutate into abnormal cells with uncontrolled growth and spread in the body. Cancer can affect any body tissue. Nursing care of the patient with cancer is holistic and comprehensive, focusing on cancer as not one single disease, but as a constellation of many diseases. The nurse recognizes that cancer is a disruptive and life-threatening process affecting not only the person who is diagnosed with cancer, but also his or her significant others and family members. Nursing interventions are based on the understanding that cancer is a chronic disease with acute episodes, and that the patient is often treated with a combination of treatment modalities and in outpatient settings. Equally important, the nurse recognizes that caring for the patient with cancer involves prevention, early detection, risk reduction, treatment, patient education and counseling, long-term follow-up and rehabilitation, and comprehensive symptom management and palliation (Oncology Nursing Society [ONS], 2009).

Oncology is the study of cancer. The term is derived from the Greek word *oncoma* ("bulk"). Oncologists specialize in caring for patients with cancer; they may be medical doctors, surgeons, radiologists, immunologists, or researchers. The oncology nurse is an important and significant member of the oncology team. Oncology nurses are nurses who have received specialized training in cancer care and treatment. They have special skills in assisting the patient and family with physical and psychosocial issues associated with cancer, treatment, and palliation (ONS, 2009). Collaboration among healthcare professionals (e.g., surgeons, oncologists, nurses, social workers) ensures the most effective care and treatment for the patient with cancer.

Incidence and Mortality

In the United States, cancer is the second most common cause of death and about 1,529,560 new cancer cases are expected to be diagnosed in 2010 (ACS, 2010a). One in every four deaths in the United States is caused by cancer and more than 1500 people die of cancer each day (ACS, 2010a). Mortality rates for different cancers vary. Lung cancer remains the leading cause of all cancer deaths in both men and women, accounting for approximately 28% of all cancer deaths (ACS, 2010a).

Due to advances in cancer prevention, early detection, and treatment, the 5-year survival rate for individuals with cancers continues to improve in the United States. However, minority ethnic groups such as African American and Asian American populations have a disproportionate burden of cancer. African Americans have the highest mortality rate for all cancers and major cancers among all ethnic groups (ACS, 2010). For example, although breast cancer occurs more commonly in Caucasian women than in African American women, the survival rate is 90% for Caucasian women compared to only 77% for African Americans; breast cancer death rates are 32% higher in African American women than in White women (ACS, 2010). Similar disparities are seen in survival rates for colorectal, prostate, and endometrial cancers in these ethnic groups. Research has shown

that lack of health insurance, lower incomes, unequal access to health care, knowledge deficit, and cultural beliefs and attitudes are influential factors contributing to cancer disparity among African Americans (Ward et al., 2008). The Black–White disparity in overall cancer death rates have decreased from the early 1990s through 2004, especially in men. This reduction in disparity may be due to more rapid decreases in mortality from tobacco-related cancers in Black men than White men (DeLancey, Thun, Jemal, & Ward, 2008).

For information about diversity, cancer risk, and incidence see the accompanying Focus on Cultural Diversity box.

FAST FACTS

Cancer in the United States

- Breast cancer is the most frequently diagnosed cancer in women, with an estimated incidence of 207,090 new cases in 2010.
- Prostate cancer is the most frequently occurring cancer in men, with an estimated incidence of 217,730 new cases during 2010. The incidence rates of prostate cancer are significantly higher in African American men than in White men.
- Melanoma occurs mainly among Whites; the incidence rates are more than 10 times higher than African Americans.
- The incidence of bladder cancer is about four times higher in men than in women, and almost two times higher in Whites than in African Americans.

Source: American Cancer Society. (2010a). *Cancer facts and figures—2010*. Atlanta: Author.

Risk Factors

Risk factors are factors that make an individual or a population vulnerable to a specific disease or other unhealthy outcome. Risk factors can be divided into those that are controllable and those that are not controllable. Knowledge and assessment of risk factors are especially important in counseling patients and families about measures to prevent cancer. Figure 14–1 ■ summarizes the interaction of factors that promote cancer.

Heredity

It is estimated that 5% of all cancers have a strong hereditary component (ACS, 2010a). The familial pattern of some breast and colon cancers has been well documented. Lung, ovarian, and prostate cancers have also shown some familial relationships.

FOCUS ON CULTURAL DIVERSITY
Risk and Incidence of Cancer

- Hispanics have higher rates of cancers associated with infection, such as uterine, cervix, liver, and stomach.
- The incidence of liver cancer is almost twice as high in Hispanics compared to non-Hispanic Whites.
- African Americans are more likely to develop cancer than any other ethnic or racial group in the United States.
- African Americans have the highest death rate and shortest survival of any racial and ethnic group in the United States for most cancers.
- African Americans have the highest incidence and mortality for colorectal and lung cancers.
- Breast cancer occurrence is about 10% lower in African American women than in White women, but the mortality rate is approximately 37% higher.
- African American men are at least 59% more likely to develop prostate cancer than men of any other ethnic or racial group.
- Cancer incidence and mortality are lower in Native American men and women than in any other ethnic or racial group.

Sources: American Cancer Society. (2010a). *Cancer facts and figures—2009*. Atlanta: Author. American Cancer Society. (20010b). *Cancer facts and figures for African Americans—2009–2010*. Atlanta: Author. American Cancer Society. (2010c). *Cancer facts and figures for Hispanics/Latinos—2009–2010*. Atlanta: Author.

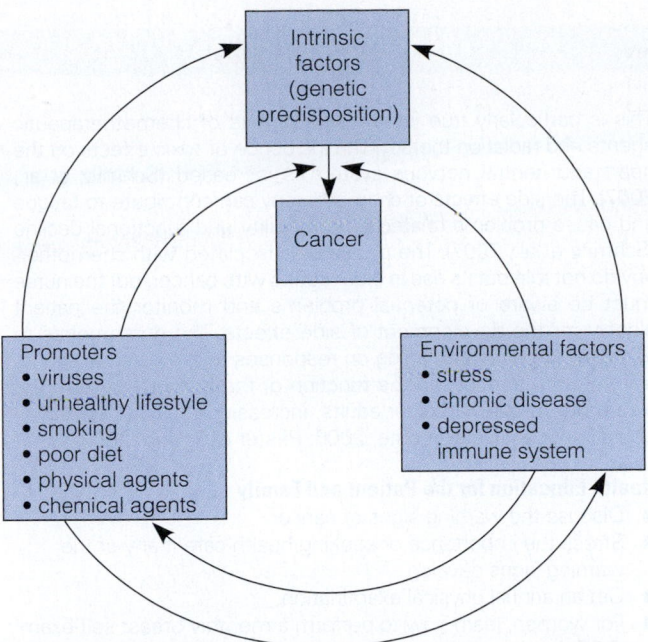

Figure 14–1 ■ Interaction of factors that promote cancer. Most people have immune systems that are competent enough to resist the establishment of cancer from an initiated cell. Cancer takes hold when a number of promotional factors occur together and over enough time to weaken immune resistance. Like factors are grouped together for ease of presentation but may occur in any combination.

The Human Genome Project has identified 50,000 genetic mutations linked to cancer through examination of 4,800 genes and 250,000 tumors (Forbes et al., 2008). For most cancers, research has yet to distinguish true genetic transfer from environmental causes. Although further research is needed to identify cancers that are due to the inheritance of defective genes, familial predisposition to malignancies should be counted among risk factors so that people at risk can reduce behaviors that promote cancer. For example, a patient with a family history of lung cancer should be counseled to avoid smoking, to avoid areas where smoking is allowed, and to avoid working in an occupation that may expose the patient to inhaled carcinogens.

Age

Cancer is a disease associated with aging; about 78% of cancer diagnoses occur after age 55 (ACS, 2010a). A number of factors are associated with this increased risk in older adults. One possible factor is that at least five cycles of genetic mutations seem necessary to cause permanent damage to the afflicted cells. In addition, long-term exposure to high doses of promotional agents is usually necessary to allow the cancer to take hold. In addition, poor overall immune response accompanies aging as a result of a progressive and overall diminution of immune functions that affect all cells and organs of the innate and adaptive immune system (Pfister & Savino, 2008). Another problem is that free radicals (molecules resulting from the body's metabolic and oxidative processes) tend to accumulate in the cells over time. Thus, with aging, the immune cells show an increase in oxidant and inflammatory compounds and a decrease in antioxidant defenses, causing cellular damage and mutation (De la Fuente, 2008).

Hormonal changes that occur with aging can be associated with cancer. Postmenopausal women receiving exogenous estrogen have an increased risk for breast and uterine cancers. Older men are at risk for prostate cancer, possibly due to breakdown of testosterone into carcinogenic forms. See the Nursing Care of the Older Adult box on page 344 for a discussion about older adults and cancer.

Stress resulting from severe and/or cumulative losses also is implicated in promoting cancer (Bauer, 2008). These losses, which are common to older adults, include the death of a spouse or friends, loss of position and status in society, and a decline in physical abilities. These repeated stressors are related to changes in the immune system that may lead to the development of cancer.

Gender

Gender is a risk factor for certain types of cancer. Breast cancer is the most frequently diagnosed cancer in women; prostate cancer in men. The incidence of bladder cancer is about four times higher in men than in women (ACS, 2010a). Thyroid cancer occurs more commonly among females, whereas bladder cancer is seen more often among males (ACS, 2010a). ∞ See Chapters 48 and 49 for more information on gender-specific cancers.

Poverty

The poor are at higher risk for cancer than the population in general. Lack of health insurance and inadequate access to health care, especially preventive screening and counseling, may be major factors (ACS, 2010a). Although other factors that may be involved, such as diet and stress, usually come under the category of controllable risks, these risks are frequently uncontrollable in this population.

Stress

Continuous unmanaged stress that keeps hormones such as epinephrine and cortisol at high levels can result in systematic "fatigue" and impaired immunologic surveillance. When the body attempts to adapt to physiologic and psychologic stressors, it goes through a series of stages called the general adaptation syndrome (Bauer, 2008). First, the "alarm reaction" occurs, in which adrenal hormones increase, allowing the body to cope with the stressor. Eventually, the body reaches the "stage of resistance," in which the stress hormones are significantly reduced, indicating that adaptation has occurred. If the physiologic adaptation is supported by appropriate coping strategies, the stressor is considered managed and body systems return to prealarm functioning. However, if adaptation continues and the stress hormones remain elevated, the "stage of exhaustion" sets in. This stage will maintain life, but at great expense to body systems, resulting in general wear-and-tear and depression of the immune system (Armaiz-Pena, Lutgendorf, Cole, & Sood, 2009).

Diet

Dietary factors appear to be one of the most important factors for cancer risk. A diet that is high in red meat and saturated fat appears to increase risk. Vegetables, fruits, fiber, folate, and calcium may be protective (ACS, 2010a). Some foods are considered genotoxic, such as the nitrosamines and nitrous indoles (a crystalline alkaloid compound) found in preserved meats and pickled, salted foods. Other foods, such as high-fat, low-fiber

Nurses need to be aware of how cancer and cancer treatments affect older adults. Cancer is the second leading cause of death in people over age 65 (ACS, 2010a). The incidence of cancer increases with advancing age, probably as a result of the accumulated exposure to carcinogens and to age-related declines in the action of the immune system (De la Fuente, 2008; Pfister & Savino, 2008). The most commonly seen cancers in older women are colorectal, breast, lung, pancreatic, and ovarian. In older men, lung, colorectal, prostate, pancreatic, and gastric cancers occur most frequently.

The importance of screening and early detection of cancer does not diminish with age. Unfortunately, older adults may be less likely to undergo cancer screening or seek treatment for cancer due to fear, depression, cognitive impairments, poor access to health care, or financial constraints (Sheinfeld et al., 2008). Some older adults (and healthcare providers) mistake cancer symptoms for normal age-related changes. Believing that little can be done, they do not seek health care for their symptoms. Fear of the cancer diagnosis also keeps older adults from seeking appropriate health care. When they do seek treatment, chronic conditions frequently seen in older adults may make the diagnosis of cancer more difficult by masking or confounding the usual symptoms associated with cancer.

Older adults are at greater risk for side effects associated with cancer treatment because of age-related physiologic changes and chronic conditions associated with aging (Schmitz et al., 2007).

This is particularly true for the side effects of chemotherapeutic agents and radiation therapy. The incidence of toxic effects on the heart and central nervous system is increased (Schmitz et al., 2007). The side effects of chemotherapy can contribute to fatigue and cause problems related to immobility and functional decline (Schmitz et al., 2007). The problems associated with chemotherapy do not rule out its use in older adults with cancer, but the nurse must be aware of potential problems and monitor the patient closely for the development of side effects. The nurse needs to consider the effects of aging on responses to the disease and its treatment. Alterations in the function of the immune system are also more frequent in older adults, increasing their risk for developing infection (De la Fuente, 2008; Pfister & Savino, 2008).

Health Education for the Patient and Family
- Discuss the warning signs of cancer.
- Stress the importance of seeking health care if any of the warning signs develop.
- Get an annual physical examination.
- For women, learn how to perform a monthly breast self-exam (BSE) and emphasize the importance of continuing BSE and regular mammography after menopause.
- Teach men the early signs of prostate cancer, and encourage them to have an annual digital rectal exam.

foods—the mainstay of many American diets—promote colon, breast, and sex hormone–dependent tumors. When fish and meat are excessively fried or broiled, potent carcinogenic compounds can form that may cause tumors in the mammary glands, colon, liver, pancreas, and bladder. Also, repeatedly using fat to fry foods at high temperatures produces high levels of polycyclic hydrocarbons, which increase cancer risk considerably. Other food-related substances believed to increase cancer risk include sodium saccharine, red food dyes, and both regular and decaffeinated coffee.

Occupation

Occupational risk might be considered to be either controllable or uncontrollable. For many people, both education and ability limit their choice of occupation; during times of high unemployment, moreover, changing one's occupation because it poses risk factors may not be a viable option. Federal standards are designed to protect workers from hazardous substances, but many believe that these standards are not strict enough and that inspections are not frequent enough to prevent violations.

Specific risks vary according to the occupation. For example, outdoor workers such as farmers and construction workers are exposed to solar radiation, healthcare workers such as x-ray technicians and biomedical researchers are exposed to ionizing radiation and carcinogenic substances, and exposure to asbestos is a problem for people who work in old buildings with asbestos insulation in the walls. Table 14–1 correlates known carcinogens and occupations.

Infection

A number of viruses have been linked to some cancers (Maeda et al., 2008). Avoiding those specific infections will decrease risk. Although some infections may be unavoidable (Epstein-Barr,

for example), others, such as genital herpes and human papillomavirus–induced genital warts, can often be avoided by following safer sex practices (e.g., the use of condoms) or obtaining a human papillomavirus (HPV) vaccine.

Tobacco Use

Smoking-related diseases remain the world's most preventable cause of death (ACS, 2010a). Lung cancer is considered highly preventable because of its relationship to smoking. The genotoxic carcinogenic substances in tobacco are considered weak; therefore, stopping smoking can reverse the damage it causes. However, many other substances in tobacco are highly promotional, so that the larger the dose and longer the use, the higher the risk for developing cancer. Research has shown a significantly lower lung cancer death risk for former smokers compared to current smokers.

Tobacco is also related to other forms of cancer. Smokers face an increased risk for oropharyngeal, esophageal, laryngeal, gastric, pancreatic, and bladder cancers (ACS, 2010a). Pipe and cigar smokers are especially susceptible to oropharyngeal and laryngeal cancers. Oral and esophageal cancers are more common among those who chew tobacco or use snuff. Smokers who have a genetic decrease in alpha-$_1$-antitrypsin (an enzyme that protects lung tissue) that results in emphysema face an even higher cancer risk than smokers without this defect.

Additional research has documented the deleterious effects of secondhand tobacco smoke (Van Hemelrijck et al., 2006). Tobacco-specific nitrosamines were recovered in the urine of children living with smokers. It is now accepted that nonsmokers exposed to tobacco smoke over long periods of time, whether in the workplace or the home, have an increased risk for lung or bladder cancers.

TABLE 14–1 Chemical Carcinogens and Relationship to Occupation

CHEMICAL AGENT	ACTION	OCCUPATION AFFECTED
Polycyclic hydrocarbons (smoke, soot, tobacco, smoked foods)	Genotoxic	Miners, coal/gas workers, chimney sweeps, migrant workers, workers in offices where smoking is allowed in closed areas
Benzopyrene		
Arsenic	Genotoxic	Pesticide manufacturers, mining
Vinyl chloride polymers	Promotional	Plastics workers
		Artists
Methylaminobenzine	Genotoxic	Fabric workers
		Rubber and glue workers
Asbestos	Promotional	Construction workers, workers in old, run-down buildings with asbestos insulation, insulation makers
Wood and leather dust	Promotional	Woodworkers, carpenters, leather toolers
Chemotherapy drugs	Genotoxic	Drug manufacturers, pharmacists, nurses

Alcohol Use

Alcohol promotes cancer by enhancing the contact between carcinogens such as those in tobacco and the stem cells that line the oral cavity, larynx, and esophagus. People who both smoke and drink a considerable amount of alcohol daily have an increased risk for oral, esophageal, and laryngeal cancers.

Recreational Drug Use

Recreational drug use often promotes an unhealthy lifestyle that increases general cancer risk; for example, drug users often do not maintain adequate nutrition. Furthermore, recreational drugs are implicated as promoters because of their suppressive effect on the immune system. Although it has not been directly implicated in cancer development, marijuana has been demonstrated to cause chromosomal damage that may over time also result in cancer-causing DNA damage and genetic mutations. Marijuana smoke is also more injurious to lung tissue than tobacco smoke.

Obesity

Overweight and obesity contribute to 14% to 20% of all cancer-related mortality in the United States (ACS, 2010a). Excessive body fat has been linked to an increased risk of hormone-dependent cancers. Because sex hormones are synthesized from fat, obese people often have excessive amounts of the hormones that feed hormone-dependent malignancies of the breast, bowel, ovary, endometrium, and prostate. Overweight and obesity are clearly associated with increased risk for developing many cancers, including cancers of the breast (in postmenopausal women), colon, endometrium, kidney, and adenocarcinoma of the esophagus (ACS, 2010a).

Sun Exposure

As the protective ozone layer thins, more of the sun's damaging ultraviolet radiation reaches the earth. As a consequence, the rate of skin cancers has increased. Sun-related skin cancers are now considered to be a problem for all people, regardless of skin color, but people of northern European extraction with very fair skin, blue or green eyes, and light-colored hair are most vulnerable. Elderly people with decreased pigment are also more at risk, even those with darker skin.

Pathophysiology

Cancer is a complex disease with hundreds of agents that can contribute to its pathogenesis. Advances in research have greatly increased the understanding of how cancer develops. It is now known that the development of cancer is a process in which normal cells are changed and acquire malignant properties. Before a discussion of the various theories of the causes of cancer, it is useful to review how normal cells divide and adapt to changing conditions.

Normal Cell Growth

Mature normal cells are uniform in size and have nuclei that are characteristic of the tissue to which the cells belong. Within the nucleus of normal cells, chromosomes containing deoxyribonucleic acid (DNA) molecules carry the genetic information that controls the synthesis of polypeptides (proteins). Genes are subunits of chromosomes and consist of portions of DNA that specify the production of particular sets of proteins. Thus, genes control the development of specific traits. The genetic code in the DNA of every gene is translated into protein structures that determine the type, maturity, and function of a cell. Any change or disruption in a gene can result in an inaccurate "blueprint" that can produce an aberrant cell, which may then become cancerous. Box 14–1 lists some of the functions of DNA.

The Cell Cycle

Two coordinated events are responsible for cellular reproduction. Reproduction occurs as the result of replication of cellular DNA and mitosis, when the cell divides into two daughter cells with identical DNA.

BOX 14–1 Functions of DNA

- Orders production of enzymes
- Instructs cells to produce specific chemicals
- Instructs cells to develop specific structures
- Determines individual traits and characteristics
- Controls other DNA by telling a cell to "switch on"

The **cell cycle** consists of four phases. In the gap 1 or G_1 phase, the cell enlarges and synthesizes proteins to prepare for DNA replication. During this phase the cell prepares to replicate and enter into the synthesis phase. During the synthesis (S) phase, DNA is replicated and the chromosomes in the cell are duplicated. During the gap 2 or G_2 phase, the cell prepares itself for mitosis. Finally, with all preparation complete, the cell begins mitosis in the M phase. This phase culminates in the division of the parent cell into two exact copies called daughter cells, each having identical genetic material. The cells then immediately enter G_1 where they begin the cell cycle again, or divert into a resting phase called G_0. The cell cycle is controlled by cyclins, which combine with and activate enzymes called cyclin-dependent kinases. Some cyclins cause a "braking" action and prevent the cycle from proceeding. Checkpoints in the cell cycle ensure that it proceeds in the correct order.

A malfunction of any of these regulators of cell growth and division can result in the rapid proliferation of immature cells. In some cases, these cells are considered cancerous (malignant). Knowledge of cell cycle events is used in the development of chemotherapeutic drugs, which are designed to disrupt the cancer cells during different stages of their cell cycle. These drugs and their use are discussed later in the chapter.

Differentiation

Differentiation is a normal process occurring over many cell cycles that allows cells to specialize in certain tasks. For example, some epithelial cells lining the lungs develop into tall columnar cells with cilia. These columnar cells sweep potentially dangerous debris out of the lungs. When adverse conditions occur in body tissues during differentiation, protective adaptations can produce alterations in cells. Some of these alterations are helpful, but in other cases the cells mutate beyond usefulness and become liabilities. Following are potentially unproductive cellular alterations that occur during cell differentiation:

- **Hyperplasia** is an increase in the number or density of normal cells. Hyperplasia occurs in response to stress, increased metabolic demands, or elevated levels of hormones. Examples include the hyperplasia of myocardial cells in response to a prolonged increase in the body's demand for oxygen, and hyperplasia of uterine cells in response to rising levels of estrogen during pregnancy. Hyperplastic cells are under normal DNA control.
- **Metaplasia** is a change in the normal pattern of differentiation such that dividing cells differentiate into cell types not normally found in that location in the body. The metaplastic cell is normal for its particular type, but it is not in its normal location. Some metaplastic cells are less functional than the cells they replace. Metaplasia is a protective response to adverse conditions. Metaplastic cells are under normal DNA control and are reversible when the stressor or other disruptive condition ceases.
- **Dysplasia** represents a loss of DNA control over differentiation occurring in response to adverse conditions. Dysplastic cells show abnormal variation in size, shape, and appearance and a disturbance in their usual arrangement. Examples of dysplasia include changes in the cervix in response to continued

irritation, such as from HPV, or leukoplakia on oral mucous membranes in response to chronic irritation from smoking.
- **Anaplasia** is the regression of a cell to an immature or undifferentiated cell type. Anaplastic cell division is no longer under DNA control. Anaplasia usually occurs when a damaging or transforming event takes place inside the dividing, still undifferentiated cell, leading to loss of useful function. Anaplasia may occur in response to overwhelmingly destructive conditions inside the cell or in surrounding tissue.

Although hyperplasia, metaplasia, and dysplasia often reverse after the irritating factor is eliminated, they can lead to malignancy under certain conditions. This is especially true of dysplasia, which represents a loss of DNA control. Anaplasia is not reversible, but the degree of anaplasia determines the potential risk for cancer.

Theories of Carcinogenesis

Factors that cause cancer are both external (chemicals, radiation, and viruses) and internal (hormones, immune conditions, and inherited mutations). Causal factors may act together or in sequence to initiate or promote **carcinogenesis**, a process by which normal cells are transformed into cancer cells. Often, more than 10 years pass between exposures or mutations and detectable cancer.

Cellular Mutation

The theory of cellular mutation suggests that certain agents cause mutations in cellular DNA and transform cells into cancer cells. Such agents are called **carcinogens**. It is believed that the carcinogenic process has three stages: initiation, promotion, and progression. The initiation stage involves permanent damage in the cellular DNA as a result of exposure to a carcinogen (e.g., radiation, chemicals) that was not repaired or had a defective repair. Promotion may last for years and includes conditions, such as smoking or alcohol use, that act repeatedly on the already affected cells. In the progression stage further inherited changes acquired during the cell replication develop into a cancer.

Oncogenes

Proto-oncogenes are normal genes that promote cell growth and repair. **Oncogenes** are abnormal genes that promote cell proliferation and are capable of triggering cancerous characteristics. Oncogenes can be classified according to their overall function. Several oncogenes and their relationship to human cancers have been identified. For example, BRCA-1 and BRCA-2 are oncogenes associated with breast cancer (Eccles, 2008).

A decrease in the body's immune surveillance may allow the expression of oncogenes; this can occur during times of stress or in response to certain carcinogens. For example, patients with AIDS, who have a decreased number of T-helper lymphocytes, have a much higher than normal incidence of certain cancers, including non-Hodgkin's lymphoma and Kaposi's sarcoma (Nowicki et al., 2008).

Tumor Suppressor Genes

Tumor suppressor genes normally block cell growth by suppressing oncogenes. They can become inactive by deletion or mutation. Inherited cancers have been associated with tumor suppressor genes. An example is p53, a suppressor gene that has been associated with sarcoma and cancer of the breast and brain.

Central to these theories are two important concepts about the etiology of cancer. First, damaged DNA, whether inherited or from external sources, sets up the necessary initial step for cancer to occur. Second, impairment of the human immune system, from whatever cause, lessens its ability to destroy abnormal cells.

Known Carcinogens

A number of agents are known to cause cancer, or at least are strongly linked to certain kinds of cancers. These known carcinogens include viruses, drugs, hormones, and chemical and physical agents. The National Toxicology Program (NTP) and the International Agency for Research on Cancer (IARC) play an important role in the identification and evaluation of carcinogens. See their respective websites for a list of substances known or reasonably anticipated to be human carcinogens.

Carcinogens can be categorized in two groups: Genotoxic carcinogens directly alter DNA and cause mutations, and promoter substances cause other adverse biologic effects, such as cytotoxicity, hormonal imbalances, altered immunity, or chronic tissue damage. Promoter substances do not cause cancer in the absence of previous cell damage (initiation) and often require high-level and long-term contact with the altered cells (NTP, 2005) (see Table 14–1). Although everyone comes in contact with a vast number of substances considered carcinogenic, not everyone develops cancer. Other factors, such as genetic predisposition, impairment of the immune response, and repeated exposure to the carcinogen, are necessary for a cancer to develop.

Viruses

Several viruses have been associated with the development of cancer. They damage cells and induce hyperplastic cell growth. Viral infection may play a role in cell mutation that can progress to malignant cells. Most people are able to suppress this progression. Box 14–2 identifies these viruses and the cancers with which they are associated. In addition, viruses play a

significant role in weakening immunologic defenses against neoplasms. For example, human immunodeficiency virus (HIV), which infects T-helper lymphocytes and monocytes, impairs the person's protection against certain cancers such as lymphoma and Kaposi's sarcoma (Nowicki et al., 2008).

Other viruses have also been associated with human malignancies. Hepatitis B virus integrates its DNA with liver cell DNA and is believed to cause primary hepatocellular carcinoma. Papillomaviruses cause plantar, common, and flat warts, which are benign and usually regress spontaneously; however, they also cause genital warts and laryngeal papillomas, which are associated with malignant melanoma and cervical, penile, and laryngeal cancers. Vaccines to prevent virus-induced cancers are being investigated in various cancers, such as melanoma, lung cancer, and osteosarcoma (Bodles-Brakhop & Draghia-Akli, 2008; di Pietro et al., 2008; Ullenhag et al., 2008). More research is needed to investigate the effectiveness of immunotherapy, such as vaccines.

Drugs and Hormones

Certain drugs can be either genotoxic or promotional. For example, chemotherapeutic drugs used to disrupt the cell cycle of malignant cells can be genotoxic for normal cells. They can also be promotional: By drastically reducing the number of leukocytes, they impair immune function. Examples of these chemotherapeutic drugs include busulfan, chlorambucil, and cyclophosphamide. Some recreational drugs also are implicated as carcinogens. These include the genotoxic betel nut chewed by many Pacific Islanders and the immunosuppressant promoters heroin and cocaine.

Hormones are also potential genotoxic carcinogens or promoters. Gonadotropic hormones often mediate cancers of the reproductive organs. Estrogen, both natural and synthetic, and diethylstilbestrol (DES) have been linked to cervical, endometrial, and breast cancers. Estrogen-containing contraceptive pills have been implicated in breast cancer, but they also have been shown to decrease the risk of ovarian cancer. Investigators have not reached a final conclusion about the cancer risk posed by contraceptives. Newer research suggests that alterations in the molecular structure of testosterone in older men may promote the development of prostate cancer. Also, glucocorticosteroids (cortisone) and anabolic steroids may act as promoters by altering the immune response or endocrine balance.

Chemical Agents

Many chemicals are both genotoxic and promotional. Because many of these substances are encountered in the workplace, they constitute occupational hazards. Examples of industrial and environmental carcinogens include polycyclic hydrocarbons, found in soot; benzopyrene, found in cigarette smoke; and arsenic, found in pesticides. These chemicals have some genotoxic action; some alter DNA replication. Other industrial and environmental chemicals are considered promotional agents, including wood and leather dust, polymer esters (used in plastics and paints), carbon tetrachloride, asbestos, and phenol (NTP, 2005). Polycyclic aromatic hydrocarbons, nitrosamines, phenols, and other chemicals in tobacco act as either carcinogens or promoters of cancer (see Table 14–1).

BOX 14–2 Cancers Associated with Different Viruses

Herpes Simplex Virus Types I and II (HSV-1 and HSV-2)
- Carcinoma of the lip
- Cervical carcinoma
- Kaposi's sarcoma

Human Cytomegalovirus (HCMV)
- Kaposi's sarcoma
- Prostate cancer

Epstein-Barr Virus (EBV)
- Burkitt's lymphoma

Human Herpesvirus-6 (HHV-6)
- Lymphoma

Hepatitis B Virus (HBV)
- Primary hepatocellular cancer

Papillomavirus
- Malignant melanoma
- Cervical, penile, and laryngeal cancers

Human T-Lymphotropic Viruses (HTLV)
- Adult T-cell leukemia and lymphoma
- T-cell variant of hairy-cell leukemia
- Kaposi's sarcoma

Natural substances in the body may also be carcinogenic or promotional. For example, end products of metabolism that are produced in excess amounts or are ineffectively eliminated, such as bile acids from a high-fat diet, may promote cancer.

Some foods contain carcinogens added during preparation or preservation. Examples include the sugar substitute sodium saccharine and nitrosamines and nitrous indoles, which are found in pickled, salted foods. In some cases, food contaminants produce carcinogenic chemicals. The *Aspergillus* fungi produce aflatoxin, a highly potent carcinogen. These organisms grow on improperly stored vegetable products, such as grains and peanuts.

Physical Agents

It has been well documented that excessive exposure to radiation causes increased rates of cancer by damaging the DNA in cells, by activating other oncogenetic factors, or by suppressing antitumor activity (protein inhibitors). Both solar radiation from ultraviolet rays and ionizing radiation from industrial or medical sources are carcinogenic. This fact has implications for workers exposed to these agents and for the population in general. Radon, a naturally formed radioactive gas found in the basements of many homes, is also a known carcinogen. People who have lived in areas where nuclear weapons have been tested or whose groundwater has been polluted by nuclear wastes are at risk for developing cancers. The effects of high-dose radiation exposure and subsequent cancer development have been demonstrated in the survivors of the atomic bombs at Nagasaki and Hiroshima and in workers exposed to radiation during the cleanup of nuclear disasters such as Chernobyl.

Types of Neoplasms

A **neoplasm** is a mass of new tissue (a collection of cells) that grows independently of its surrounding structures and has no physiologic purpose. The term *neoplasm* is often used interchangeably with *tumor*, from the Latin word meaning "swelling." Neoplasms are said to be autonomous because they grow at a rate uncoordinated with body needs, they share some of the properties of the parent cells but with altered size and shape, and they do not benefit the host and in some cases are harmful.

Neoplasms are not completely autonomous because they require a blood supply with nutrients and oxygen to sustain their growth. Neoplasms typically are classified as benign or malignant on the basis of their potential to damage the body and on their growth characteristics.

Benign Neoplasms

Benign neoplasms are localized growths. They form a solid mass, have well-defined borders, and frequently are encapsulated. Benign neoplasms tend to respond to the body's homeostatic controls. Thus, they often stop growing when they reach the boundaries of another tissue (a process called *contact inhibition*). They grow slowly and often remain stable in size. Because they are usually encapsulated, benign neoplasms often are easily removed and tend not to recur.

Although typically harmless, benign neoplasms nevertheless can be destructive if they crowd surrounding tissue and obstruct the function of organs. For example, a benign meningioma of the brain or spinal cord can cause increased intracranial pressure (IICP), which progressively impairs the person's

cerebral function. Unless the meningioma can be successfully removed, the steadily rising IICP will eventually lead to coma and death.

Malignant Neoplasms

In contrast to benign neoplasms, malignant neoplasms grow aggressively and do not respond to the body's homeostatic controls. Malignant neoplasms are not cohesive, and present with an irregular shape. Instead of slowly crowding other tissues aside, malignant neoplasms cut through surrounding tissues, causing bleeding, inflammation, and necrosis (tissue death) as they grow. This invasive quality of malignant neoplasms is reflected in the word origin of *cancer*, from the Greek *karkinos*, meaning "crab."

Malignant cells from the primary tumor may travel through the blood or lymph to invade other tissues and organs of the body and form a secondary tumor called a **metastasis**. This term also refers to the process by which such spreading of malignant neoplasms—perhaps their most destructive trait—occurs. Malignant neoplasms can recur after surgical removal of the primary and secondary tumors and after other treatments. Table 14–2 compares benign and malignant neoplasms.

Malignant neoplasms vary in their degree of differentiation from the parent tissue. Highly differentiated cancer cells try to mimic the specialized function of the parent tissue, but undifferentiated cancers, consisting of immature cells, have almost no resemblance to the parent tissue and so perform no useful function. Undifferentiated cancers rob the body of its energy and nutrition as they grow. Undifferentiated anaplastic cells have little structural or functional relationship to the parent cells and are the basis of many malignant neoplasms. The degree of differentiation of anaplastic cells is a consideration in the classification and staging of neoplasms, discussed later in this chapter.

Characteristics of Malignant Cells

Malignant neoplasms may be identified by the following predictable cellular characteristics:

- *Loss of regulation of the rate of mitosis.* This leads to rapid cell division and growth of the neoplasm.
- *Loss of specialization and differentiation.* Malignant cells do not perform typical cellular functions. Many produce hormones

TABLE 14–2 Comparison of Benign and Malignant Neoplasms	
BENIGN	**MALIGNANT**
Local	Invasive
Cohesive	Noncohesive
Well-defined borders	Does not stop at tissue border
Pushes other tissues out of the way	Invades and destroys surrounding tissues
Slow growth	Rapid growth
Encapsulated	Metastasizes to distant sites
Easily removed	Not always easy to remove
Does not recur	Can recur

and enzymes similar to those of the parent tissue, but usually in excessive amounts, possibly revealing their presence.

- *Loss of contact inhibition.* Malignant cells do not respect other cellular boundaries. They easily invade and destroy other tissues.
- *Progressive acquisition of a cancerous phenotype.* Cellular mutation seems to be a sequential process involving successive generations of cells, each generation becoming more deviant than the previous one. Additionally, malignant cells seem to be "immortal"; that is, they do not stop growing and die, as do normal cells, which have a genetically determined life span.
- *Irreversibility.* The transformation into a malignant cell is irreversible. Rarely does a malignant neoplasm revert to a benign state.
- *Altered cell structure.* Cytologic examination of malignant cells reveals distinct differences in the cell nucleus and cytoplasm as well as an overall cell shape that differs from that of normal cells of the particular tissue type.
- *Simplified metabolic activities.* The work of malignant cells is simpler than that of normal cells; they show an increased synthesis of substances needed for cell division, and they have no need to create proteins for the specialized functions of the tissues they invade.
- *Transplantability.* Malignant cells often break away from the primary tissue site and travel to other locations in the body, where they establish new growths.
- *Ability to promote their own survival.* Malignant cells may create ectopic sites to produce the hormones they need for their growth. By their very presence and their ability to initiate vascular permeability, malignant cells promote the development of nonneoplastic stroma, a connective tissue framework consisting of collagen and other components, which then supports the neoplasm. They may also create their own blood supply. Through a process called angiogenesis, tumor cells secrete a polypeptide angiogenic growth factor that stimulates blood vessels from surrounding normal tissue to grow into the tumor. Finally, malignant cells divert nutrition from the host to meet their own needs, by diffusion when the tumor is less than 1 mm and thereafter by means of the newly formed blood vessels. If unchecked, malignant cells eventually destroy their host.

The characteristics of malignant cells are summarized in Box 14–3.

BOX 14–3 Characteristics of Malignant Cells

- Loss of regulation of mitotic rate
- Loss of cell specialization
- Loss of contact inhibition
- Progressive acquisition of the cancerous phenotype and immortality
- Irreversibility of cancerous phenotype to greater aggressiveness
- Altered cell structure: differences in cell nucleus and cytoplasm
- Simplified metabolic activity
- Transplantability (metastasis)
- Ability to promote own survival

Tumor Invasion and Metastasis

Metastasis or the ability of cancer cells to invade adjacent tissues and travel to distant organs is considered their most ominous characteristic. This quality makes treatment a considerable challenge.

Invasion

Aggressive tumors possess several qualities that facilitate invasion (Figure 14–2 ■):

- *Ability to cause pressure atrophy.* The pressure of a growing tumor can cause atrophy and necrosis of adjacent tissues. The malignancy then moves into the vacated space.
- *Ability to disrupt the basement membrane of normal cells.* Many cancer cells can bind to elements of the basement membrane and secrete enzymes that degrade that physical barrier, thus facilitating their movement into normal tissues, lymph, and blood circulation.
- *Motility.* Because malignant cells are less tightly bound to each other than normal cells (reduced adhesiveness), they easily separate from the neoplasm and move into surrounding body fluids and tissues.
- *Response to chemical signals from adjacent tissues.* Chemotaxis (the movement of cells in response to a chemical stimulus) calls the tumor cells into the normal tissues, possibly as a result of the degrading of the basement membranes of the normal cells. This breakdown of normal cellular membranes releases the chemical stimulus physiologically designed to draw normal phagocytic cells to clean up the debris. (∞ See Chapter 12 on the inflammatory response for more information on chemotaxis.) Malignant cells are also known to respond chemotactically to the end product of cellular metabolism. Some cancer cells even produce a substance called autocrine motility factor, which calls other malignant cells to a normal tissue. The first invading cells produce this substance, which then actively draws other malignant cells from the primary tumor into the invaded normal tissue.

Metastasis

The factors that favor invasion also contribute to the process of metastasis. Metastasis can occur by means of one or more mechanisms including embolism in the blood or lymph, or spread by way of body cavities.

A blood- or lymph-borne metastasis allows a new tumor to be established in a distant organ. Figure 14–3 ■ shows metastasis through the bloodstream. A tumor's ability to metastasize in this manner requires the following steps:

1. Intravasation of malignant cells through blood or lymphatic vessel walls and into the circulation.
2. Survival of the malignant cells in the blood. (To survive, the cells must escape the notice of the body's immune surveillance; only about 1 in 1000 cells does so.)
3. Extravasation from the circulation and implantation in a new tissue.

The tumor cells tend to clump together, forming an embolus, and continue growing until their size prevents further travel in the vessel or lymph channel. The growing neoplastic mass then uses its invasive abilities (secreting enzymes and motility factor) to move into the nearest organ.

Figure 14–2 ■ How cancer cells invade normal tissue.

3 Motile cancer cells detach from primary tumor.

Primary tumor

Adjacent tissue layers

4 Motile cells attracted by chemotactic "signals" produced by activity within normal cells burrow through tissue membranes and begin to multiply.

1 Pressure necrosis of adjacent tissue layers. Cancer cells occupy vacated space.

2 Cancer cells release enzymes that lyse cell membranes of normal tissue.

About 60% of metastatic lesions tend to occur in a pattern that reflects blood or lymph circulation. However, it has been demonstrated that some malignant cells defy a bloodborne pattern and actually target specific organs to which they prefer to metastasize. For example, lung cancer frequently metastasizes to the adrenal glands, and breast cancer frequently metastasizes to bone. Malignant cells that gain access to

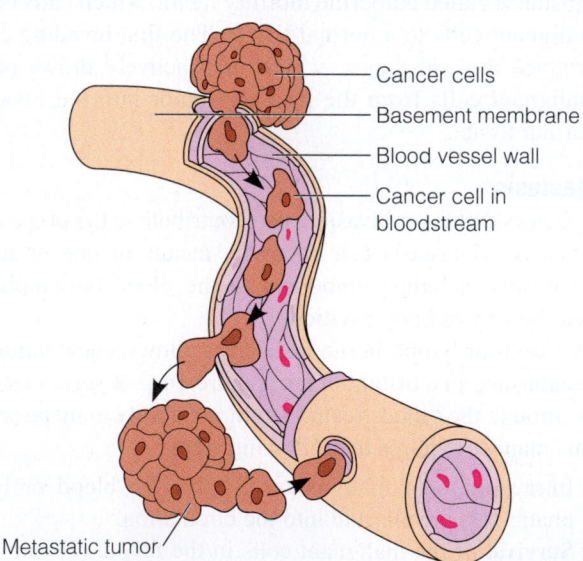

Cancer cells

Basement membrane

Blood vessel wall

Cancer cell in bloodstream

Metastatic tumor

Figure 14–3 ■ Metastasis through the bloodstream. Cancer cells secrete enzymes and a motility factor that disrupt the basement membrane in the blood vessel. In this way, the cancer cells gain access to the circulation. Once in the blood, only about 1 cell in 1000 escapes immune detection, but that can be enough. Undetected cells move out of the blood, again secreting enzymes and cutting through the vessel wall into new tissue. The tissue selected for establishing a new tumor may be downstream from the original tumor, or a chemical attraction may cause the malignant cells to target a specific site. Once in the new site, the malignant cells multiply and establish a metastatic tumor.

lymph channels may travel to a preferred organ and then move into it the same way they move through blood vessels. Alternatively, the malignant cells may become trapped in the lymph node and continue to grow. Eventually, the malignant cells replace the node's tissues. At this point, emboli from the cancerous node disseminate to other nodes, creating a cascade reaction. The malignant cascade causes widespread transfer of the tumor to uncharacteristic sites.

A malignant tumor may break through the walls of the organ in which it is primarily housed, shedding cells into the nearby body cavity. The cells then are free to establish new tumors in a distant area of that cavity. For example, malignant cells from a colon cancer may be seeded into the peritoneal cavity, establishing a new tumor in the mesenteric epithelium.

Metastatic lesions are differentiated from primary neoplasms by cell morphology: Metastatic cells do not resemble the tissue in which they reside. The most common sites of metastasis are the lymph nodes, liver, lungs, bones, and brain. Table 14–3 lists different cancers and common sites of metastasis.

For metastasis to occur, the cancerous cells must avoid detection by the immune system. Thus, impairment of the immune system is a major factor in the establishment of

TABLE 14–3 Various Cancers and Sites of Metastases

PRIMARY TUMOR	COMMON METASTATIC SITES
Bronchogenic (lung)	Spinal cord, brain, liver, bone
Breast	Regional lymph nodes, vertebrae, brain, liver, lung, bone
Colon	Liver, lung, brain, ovary, bone
Prostate	Bladder, bone (especially vertebrae), liver
Malignant melanoma	Lung, liver, spleen, regional lymph nodes, brain

BOX 14–4 Factors That May Weaken or Alter the Immune Response

- Accumulated stress
- Depression
- Increased age
- Pregnancy
- Chronic disease
- Chemotherapy treatment for the primary cancer

metastatic lesions. Cells may escape detection in several different ways:

- Aggressive cancer cells may compile a large mass (greater than 1 cm) so rapidly that the immune system is unable to overcome the tumor before it takes hold in a new tissue.
- For tumor cells to be recognized as foreign by the immune system, they must display on their surface a special antigen called tumor-associated antigen (TAA). TAA marks tumor cells for destruction by the lymphocytes. Some oncogenic viruses depress the expression of TAA on infected cells. Also, some tumors in advanced stages of growth no longer display TAA. Thus, such tumor cells escape detection as they travel through the blood or lymph.
- If the person's immune response is weakened or altered, then a metastatic tumor may take hold with little opposition. Factors that may weaken or alter the immune response are listed in Box 14–4.

An estimated 50% to 60% of all cancers have already metastasized by the time the primary tumor is identified. This may account for the current 50% death rate and certainly supports the need for patient education to facilitate early diagnosis. The time it takes for metastasis to occur is extremely variable and often difficult to predict. Some cancers, such as basal cell carcinomas, do not metastasize. The aggressiveness and location of the tumor, and the state of the person's immune system, determine whether and how rapidly metastasis takes place.

Physiologic and Psychologic Effects of Cancer

Much of the nursing care for patients with cancer is related to the effects of cancer disease and the side effects of cancer treatment. Although pathophysiologic effects of the cancer vary with the type and location of the cancer, the following effects usually are observed.

Disruption of Function

Physiologic functioning can be upset by obstruction or pressure. For example, a large tumor in the bowel can stop intestinal motility, resulting in a bowel obstruction. Prostatic tumors can obstruct the bladder neck or urethra, resulting in urine retention. Intracranial pressure can be dangerously increased by a glioma. Obstruction or pressure can cause anoxia and necrosis of surrounding tissues, which in turn cause a loss of function of the involved organ or tissue. For example, a kidney tumor may progress to renal failure. Pressure against the superior vena cava from an adjacent lung tumor or tumor-infiltrated lymph nodes can interrupt the blood flow to the heart.

In the liver, either a primary hepatocellular cancer or metastatic lesion can have several significant effects. In liver parenchymal tissue, it impairs the multiple life-sustaining functions of the liver, such as carbohydrate metabolism, synthesis of plasma proteins, detoxification, and immunologic functions. These functional impairments result in severe nutritional, hormonal, hematologic, and immunologic problems. (∞ See Chapter 25 for a more complete discussion of liver functions and effects of disruption.) Because more than 1 L of blood per minute passes through the liver via the portal vein, obstruction to this flow by a tumor can cause portal hypertension. This results in backup of fluid and increased pressure in the splanchnic circulation. The end result is ascites (third-spaced fluid in the peritoneal cavity) and varices (friable, overdistended blood vessels) of the esophageal, gastric, mesenteric, and hemorrhoidal vessels.

Hematologic Alterations

Hematologic alterations can impair the normal function of blood cells. For example, in leukemia, a malignant proliferative disease of the hematopoietic (blood cell–producing) system, the immature leukocytes cannot perform the normal protective phagocytic functions and immunity is compromised. The excessive numbers of immature leukocytes in the bone marrow diminish erythrocyte and thrombocyte (platelet) production, resulting in secondary anemia, neutropenia, and thrombocytopenia. In addition, gastrointestinal tumors disrupt the absorption of vitamin B_{12} and iron; growing tumors accumulate and store purines, depriving the bone marrow of substances needed for erythropoiesis (red blood cell production); and renal cell carcinoma produces its own erythropoietin hormone, resulting in production of an excessively large number of red blood cells and viscous blood, which impairs circulation, plugs small capillaries, and promotes thrombus formation (polycythemia).

Infection

If the tumor invades and connects two incompatible organs, such as the bowel and bladder, creating a fistula, infection becomes a serious problem. As they destroy viable tissue and thus their source of nutrition, tumors may become necrotic and septicemia may result. Some tumors are less efficient in creating capillaries; as a consequence, the center of the tumor may become necrotic and infected. When a tumor grows near the surface of the body, it may erode through to the surface, breaking down the natural defenses of intact skin and mucous membranes and providing a site for the entry of microorganisms. Any malignant involvement of the organs or tissues of immunity—such as the liver, bone marrow, Peyer's patches in the small intestine, spleen, or lymph nodes—can seriously impair the immune response, allowing infections to develop in vulnerable tissues.

Hemorrhage

Tumor erosion through blood vessels can cause extensive bleeding, giving rise to severe anemia. Hemorrhage can be serious enough to cause life-threatening hypovolemic shock.

Anorexia-Cachexia Syndrome

A characteristic feature of cancer is the wasted appearance of its victims, called **cachexia**. In many cases, unexplained rapid weight loss is the first manifestation that brings the patient to a healthcare provider. This can be due to a variety of problems associated with cancer, such as pain, infection, depression, or the side effects of chemotherapy and radiation. Usually the emaciation, malnutrition, and loss of energy are attributed to the anorexia-cachexia syndrome.

This syndrome is specific to cancer because of the effect of cancer cells on the host's metabolism. The neoplastic cells divert nutrition to their own use while causing changes that reduce the patient's appetite. Early in the disease, altered glucose metabolism leads to an increase in serum glucose levels, which creates negative feedback resulting in *anorexia* (loss of appetite). In addition, the tumor secretes substances that decrease appetite by altering taste and smell and producing early satiety. Pain, infection, and depression also contribute to anorexia. Some types of cancers cause specific food aversions, such as to red meat, coffee, or chocolate.

Avaricious cancer cells support their growth through widespread catabolism of the body's tissue and muscle proteins. This catabolism, coupled with inadequate nutrient intake, results in the typical cachexia. Normally, a starvation state reduces the body's basal metabolic rate. However, in many people with cancer, the metabolic rate is increased, probably because of the hyperactive metabolic and reproductive activities of the malignant cells. One theory suggests that cytokinins the body produces in response to the tumor are responsible for both early satiety and cachexia. One specific cytokine, called tumor necrosis factor alpha or cachectin, is believed to enhance the increased metabolic consumption of nutrients. Cancers of the gastrointestinal system further promote anorexia-cachexia by decreasing absorption and use of nutrients; the side effects of some treatment modalities enhance this effect. Figure 14–4 ■ shows the characteristic appearance of a cachectic person.

Paraneoplastic Syndromes

Paraneoplastic syndromes are indirect effects of cancer. They may be early warning signs of cancer or indicate complications or return of a malignancy. The most frequently occurring

paraneoplastic syndromes are endocrine, occurring when cancers set up ectopic sites of hormone production, and neurologic, occurring when cancer damages the nervous system (Toothaker & Rubin, 2009). Table 14–4 lists laboratory indicators of ectopic functioning. These ectopic sites produce excessive amounts of the hormone, which harm the host. Consider the following examples:

- Breast, ovarian, and renal cancers may set up ectopic parathyroid hormone sites, causing severe hypercalcemia.
- Oat cell and other lung cancers may produce ectopic secretions of insulin (causing hypoglycemia), parathyroid hormone (PTH), antidiuretic hormone (ADH, which causes excessive fluid retention, hypertension, and peripheral edema), and adrenocorticotropic hormone (ACTH). ∞ See Chapter 19 for the description of the multiple problems caused by excessive secretions of cortisone.

Other paraneoplastic syndromes include hematologic abnormalities such as anemia, thrombocytopenia, and coagulation abnormalities; nephrotic syndrome; cutaneous syndromes; and neurologic syndromes, such as distant tumors that produce IICP (Toothaker & Rubin, 2009).

Pain

Pain is a major healthcare problem for patients with cancer. Despite extensive progress in the scientific understanding of pain, more than 60% patients with cancer experience moderate to severe pain at some time during their illness (Deandrea, Montanari, Moja, Apolone, 2008; Paim et al., 2008). Despite recommendations of the World Health Organization (WHO) and even if effective treatments are available for 70% to 90% of cases, under-treatment is well documented and can involve up to 40% of patients (Deandrea et al., 2008). Under-treatment is usually attributed to an inappropriate use of opioids and barriers related to healthcare provider, patient, family, institution, and society (Eaton & Frieze, 2008). Communication and knowledge deficit are the major barriers to effective pain management. Because pain management for people with cancer has a reputation for being under-treated and ineffective, the anticipation of pain may engender fear in even the most stoic people.

Figure 14–4 ■ Cachectic person. Cancer robs its host of nutrients and increases body catabolism of fat and muscle to meet its metabolic needs.

Source: Simon Fraser/SPL/Photo Researchers, Inc.

TABLE 14–4 Laboratory Indicators of Ectopic Functioning

HORMONE	SPECIFIC LABORATORY TEST
Antidiuretic hormone (ADH)	Serum and urine osmolality
Adrenocorticotropic hormone (ACTH)	Plasma ACTH
	ACTH suppression test
	ACTH stimulation test
	Urine catecholamines
Calcitonin	Serum calcitonin
Insulin	Serum glucose Glucose tolerance test
Parathyroid hormone (PTH)	Serum PTH
	Serum calcium
Thyroxine	Serum thyroid-stimulating hormone (TSH), T_3, T_4

Types of Cancer Pain

Cancer pain can be divided into two main categories, acute and chronic, with subgroupings. These classifications serve to indicate appropriate therapeutic approaches. Acute pain has a well-defined pattern of onset, exhibits common signs and symptoms, and is often identified with hyperactivity of the autonomic system. Chronic pain, which lasts more than 6 months, frequently lacks the objective manifestations of acute pain, primarily because the autonomic nervous system adapts to this chronic stress. Chronic pain often results in personality changes, alterations in functional abilities, and lifestyle disruptions that can seriously affect compliance with treatment and the quality of life.

Most cancer patients who cite acute pain as the primary symptom that led to the diagnosis tend to associate pain with the introduction to their disease. If these patients experience pain during the illness or after treatment, they often perceive the pain as introducing another cancer, a recurrence of the original cancer, or a component of cancer treatments (Rosedale & Fu, 2010).

Chronic pain may be related to treatment or may indicate progression of the disease. Identifying the pain as treatment-related rather than tumor related is extremely important because it has a definite effect on the patient's psychological outlook. For the patient whose pain is due to the advancement of the disease, psychologic factors play an even more important role. Hopelessness and fear of impending death intensify physiologic pain and contribute to overall suffering (which goes well beyond just physical pain).

Three other categories used to classify patients with cancer pain include patients with preexisting pain, those with a history of drug abuse, and dying patients with cancer-related pain. The first two groups may have altered perceptions of pain and may not have the anticipated response to pain medication. For the dying patient, pain is strongly associated with both the patient's and family's confrontation of issues of hopelessness and death. Confronting these issues can intensify the perception of pain.

Causes of Cancer Pain

Direct tumor involvement is the primary cause of the pain experienced by people with cancer. This includes metastatic bone disease, nerve compression, and involvement of visceral organs. The pain from tumor involvement is believed to be mechanical, resulting from stretching of tissues and compression. Chemicals from ischemia or tumor metabolites and toxins that activate and sensitize nociceptors and mechanoreceptors are also responsible for tumor pain. ∞ See Chapter 9 for a more complete discussion of the mechanics of pain.

Side effects or toxic effects of cancer therapies (e.g., surgery, radiation, and chemotherapy) may also cause cancer pain. These are usually the result of traumatized tissue; one example of this is the oropharyngeal ulcerations that occur with some types of chemotherapy. However, these therapies may also be used to manage pain, such as radiation to decrease pain associated with bone metastasis.

Physical Stress

When the immune system discovers a neoplasm, it tries to destroy it using the resources of the body. The body mounts an all-out assault on the foreign invader, calling on many resources, including chemical mediators, hormones and enzymes, blood cells, antibodies, proteins, and inflammatory and immune responses. These protective responses mobilize fluid, electrolytes, and nutritional systems. This massive effort requires tremendous energy. If the neoplasm is small enough (i.e., microscopic), the immune system can destroy it, and a tumor will never manifest. A neoplasm of 1 cm is large enough to overwhelm most immune systems; however, the body will continue to try to fight it until it reaches the stage of exhaustion and is no longer capable (Selye, 1984). Thus, many patients with cancer present with fatigue, weight loss, anemia, dehydration, and altered blood chemistries (e.g., decreases in electrolytes).

Psychologic Stress

People confronted with the diagnosis of cancer exhibit a variety of psychologic and emotional responses. Some people see cancer as a death sentence and experience overwhelming grief, often giving up. Others may feel guilt, considering the cancer a punishment for past behaviors, such as smoking, unhealthy eating habits, or for delaying diagnosis or treatment. They may experience anger, especially if the person believes that he or she had been practicing a healthful lifestyle; beneath that anger may reside feelings of powerlessness. Fear is common: fear of the outcome of the illness, fear of the effects of treatment, fear of pain, fear of death. Some people feel isolated because of the stigma of cancer and old beliefs of contagion. Body image concerns and sexual dysfunction may be present but often are unexpressed, especially if the cancer is of the breast or sexual organs, or causes visible body changes.

Interdisciplinary Care

Interdisciplinary care for the patient with cancer begins with a variety of specialized laboratory and diagnostic tests.

Diagnosis

Several procedures are used to diagnose cancer. X-ray imaging, computed tomography (CT), ultrasonography, and magnetic resonance imaging (MRI) can locate abnormal tissues or tumors. However, only microscopic histologic examination of the tissue reveals the type of cell and its structural difference from the parent tissue. Tissue samples are acquired through biopsy, shedded cells (e.g., Papanicolaou smear), or collections of secretions (e.g., sputum). Lymph nodes are also biopsied to determine whether metastasis has begun. Simple screening procedures can be used to identify substances secreted by the tumor, such as the prostatic-specific antigen (PSA) blood test used to identify early prostatic cancers. Increases in enzymes or hormones released by normal tissues when they are damaged can also contribute to the diagnosis. Increased alkaline phosphatase noted in bone metastases and osteosarcoma is one example of an enzyme increase associated with cancer. Tumor markers are used for early diagnosis, for tracking responses to therapy, and for devising immunologic treatments.

CLASSIFICATION To help standardize diagnosis and treatment protocols, an elaborate identification system has been developed. This consists of naming the tumor (classification) and describing its aggressiveness (grading) and spread within or beyond the tissue of origin (staging).

Tumors are classified and named by the tissue or cell of origin. Tumor nomenclature often incorporates the Latin stem identifying the tissue from which the tumor arises. For example, a carcinoma arises from epithelial tissue; adjectives are added to further specify the location. A glandular malignancy arising from epithelial tissue is classified as an adenocarcinoma. A tumor arising from supportive tissues is called a sarcoma; the specific type of tissue is added as a prefix. For example, a cancer of fibrous connective tissue is called fibrosarcoma, and a smooth muscle cancer is a leiomyosarcoma. A tumor from seminal or germ tissue is called a seminoma. Table 14–5 compares the nomenclature of benign and malignant neoplasms.

Other names for tumors incorporate the name of the discoverer of that particular cancer, such as Burkitt's lymphoma or Hodgkin's disease. Hematopoietic malignancies (also known as "liquid tumors") are usually named by the type of immature blood cell that predominates. An example is myelocytic leukemia, named for the immature form of the granulocyte that is predominant in this malignancy.

GRADING AND STAGING   Grading evaluates the amount of differentiation (level of functional maturity) of the cell and estimates the rate of growth based on the mitotic rate. Cells that are the most differentiated—that is, most like the parent tissue and therefore the least malignant—are classified as grade 1 and are associated with a better prognosis. Grade 4 is reserved for the least differentiated and most aggressively malignant cells. Because of the differences inherent in tumor appearance and biologic behavior, grading criteria may vary with different locations and types of tumors.

Staging is used to classify solid tumors and refers to the relative size of the tumor and extent of the disease. The TNM classification system is an internationally recognized staging system: The T stands for the relative tumor size, depth of invasion, and surface spread; N indicates the presence and extent of lymph node involvement; and M denotes the presence or absence of distant metastases. Table 14–6 shows the basic outline of the TNM system; however, other systems are also used to differentiate types and locations of tumors (e.g., melanomas, cervical cancer, Hodgkin's disease).

CYTOLOGIC EXAMINATION   For the malignant tissues to be identified by name, grade, and stage, they must first be subjected to histologic and cytologic examination by light or electron microscope. Specimens are collected by three basic methods:

1. *Exfoliation from an epithelial surface.*   Examples include scraping cells from the cervix (Pap smear) or bronchial washings.
2. *Aspiration of fluid from body cavities or blood.*   Examples include white blood cells for evaluation of hematopoietic cancers, pleural fluid, and cerebrospinal fluid.
3. *Needle aspiration of solid tumors.*   This could include the breast, lung, or prostate.

TABLE 14–5 Nomenclature for Benign and Malignant Neoplasms

	TISSUE OF ORIGIN	BENIGN	MALIGNANT
Ectoderm/Endoderm	Epithelium	Papilloma	Carcinoma
	Gland	Adenoma	Adenocarcinoma
	Liver cells	Hepatocellular adenoma	Hepatocellular carcinoma
	Neuroglia	Glioma	Glioma
	Melanocytes	Melanoma	Malignant melanoma
	Basal cells		Basal cell carcinoma
	Germ cells	Tetroma	Seminoma
Mesoderm	Connective tissue		
	Adipose tissue	Lipoma	Liposarcoma
	Fibrous tissue	Fibroma	Fibrosarcoma
	Bone tissue	Osteoma	Osteosarcoma
	Cartilage	Chondroma	Chondrosarcoma
	Muscle		
	Smooth muscle	Leiomyoma	Leiomyosarcoma
	Striated muscle	Rhabdomyoma	Rhabdomyosarcoma
	Neural tissue		
	Nerve cells	Ganglioneuroma	Neuroblastoma
	Endothelial tissues		
	Blood vessels	Hemangioma	Angiosarcoma
			Kaposi's sarcoma
	Meninges	Meningioma	Malignant meningioma
Hematopoietic Tissues	Granulocytes	Granulocytosis	Leukemia
	Plasma cells		Multiple myeloma
	Lymphocytes		Lymphomas

TABLE 14–6 TNM Staging Classification System

	STAGE	MANIFESTATIONS
Tumor	T_0	No evidence of primary tumor
	T_{IS}	Tumor *in situ*
	T_1, T_2, T_3, T_4	Ascending degrees of tumor size and involvement
Nodes	N_0	No abnormal regional nodes
	N_{1a}, N_{2a}	Regional nodes—no metastasis
	N_{1b}, N_{2b}, N_{3b}	Regional lymph nodes—metastasis suspected
	N_x	Regional nodes cannot be assessed clinically
Metastasis	M_0	No evidence of distant metastasis
	M_1, M_2, M_3	Ascending degrees of metastatic involvement of the host, including distant nodes

Cytologic examination is also carried out on specimens from biopsied tissues or tumors and on collected body secretions, such as sputum or urine.

After collection, specimens are spread on a glass slide, fixed, and stained if necessary. The morphologic features of the cells are examined, with special attention to the nucleus and cytoplasm. Other special pathologic procedures can be carried out on the specimen, but they must be ordered ahead of time if special preparations of the specimen are necessary. Several special diagnostic cytologic procedures, such as cytogenetics, are proving useful in diagnosing and monitoring patient response to treatment.

TUMOR MARKERS A **tumor marker** is a protein molecule detectable in serum or other body fluids. This marker is used as a biochemical indicator of the presence of a malignancy. Small amounts of tumor marker proteins are found in normal body tissues or benign tumors and are not specific for malignancy.

However, high levels are suspicious and mandate follow-up diagnostic studies. Tumor marker tests are most useful for monitoring the patient's response to therapy and for detecting residual disease. However, one marker, PSA, is a detector of prostate cancer.

Tumor markers fall into two general categories: those derived from the tumor itself and those associated with host (immune) response to the tumor. Examples of tumor markers include the following:

- *Antigens.*   These are present in fetal tissue but normally are suppressed after birth. Thus, their presence in large amounts may reflect an anaplastic process in tumor cells. Alpha-fetoprotein (AFP) and carcinoembryonic antigen (CEA) are oncofetal antigens.
- *Hormones.*   Hormones are present in considerable amounts in human blood and tissues, but very high levels not related to other conditions may signify the presence of a hormone-secreting malignancy. Some common hormones seen as tumor markers include human chorionic gonadotropin (HCG), antidiuretic hormone (ADH), parathyroid hormone (PTH), calcitonin, and catecholamines.
- *Proteins.*   These narrow down the type of tissue that may be malignant, although they can also be increased in hyperplastic disorders. Examples of tissue-specific proteins include serum immunoglobulin and beta-2 microglobulin.
- *Enzymes.*   Rapid, excessive growth of a tissue may cause some of the enzymes and isoenzymes normally present in that particular tissue to spill into the bloodstream. Elevated levels can point to either hyperplasia of the tissue or cancer. Prostatic acid phosphatase (PAP) and neuron-specific enolase (NSE) are examples. Table 14–7 compares selected tumor-derived markers with their presence in neoplasms and other conditions.

ONCOLOGIC IMAGING Because physical assessment usually cannot detect cancer until the tumor has reached a size that poses a major risk for metastasis, radiologic examination is extremely important in early diagnosis. This diagnostic process

TABLE 14–7 Tumor-Derived Markers Associated with Specific Neoplasms

	TUMOR MARKER	ASSOCIATED NEOPLASM
Oncofetal Antigens	Carcinoembryonic antigen (CEA)	Adenocarcinomas of colon, lung, breast, ovary, stomach, pancreas
	Alpha-fetoprotein (AFP)	Hepatocellular carcinoma, gonadal germ cell tumors (seminoma)
Hormones	Human chorionic gonadotropin (HCG)	Gonadal germ cell tumors
	Calcitonin	Medullary cancer of thyroid
	Catecholamines/metabolites	Pheochromocytoma
Isoenzymes	Prostatic acid phosphatase (PAP)	Adenocarcinoma of prostate
	Neuron-specific enolase (NSE)	Small-cell lung carcinoma, neuroblastoma
Specific Proteins	Prostate-specific antigen (PSA)	Adenocarcinoma of prostate
	Immunoglobin	Multiple myeloma
	CA 125	Epithelial ovarian cancer
	CA 19-9	Adenocarcinoma of pancreas, colon
	CA 15-3	Breast cancer

Source: Adapted from Pfeifer, J. D., & Wick, M. R. (1995). The pathologic evaluation of neoplastic disease. In A. I. Holleb, D. J. Fink, & G. P. Murphy (Eds.), *American Cancer Society textbook of clinical oncology* (pp. 75–95). Atlanta: American Cancer Society.

may involve routine x-ray imaging (usually for screening only), CT, MRI, ultrasonography, nuclear imaging, angiography, and positron emission tomography. These diagnostic tests, including preparation and nursing implications, are discussed in the assessment chapters as well as with specific body system cancers throughout the book.

X-Ray Imaging Standard x-ray imaging is the method of choice for screening such body areas as the breast (mammography), lung, and bone to identify changes in tissue density that may indicate malignancies. X-ray imaging is still the method of choice for lung cancer, but does not usually reveal tumors until late in their development when they have reached about 1 cm in size.

Computed Tomography (CT) CT allows the visualization of cross sections of the anatomy. Because CT scans reveal subtle differences in tissue densities, they provide much greater accuracy in tumor diagnosis. This procedure is useful in screening for renal cell and most gastrointestinal tumors. CT scans are especially useful for evaluating possible lymph node involvement.

Magnetic Resonance Imaging (MRI) During an MRI, the patient is placed within a strong magnetic field, pulsed radio waves are directed at him or her, and transmitted signals based on tissue characteristics are analyzed by a computer. Related diagnostic imaging procedures—positron emission tomography (PET) and single photon emission computed tomography (SPECT)—create visible images by measuring electrical impulses from different body structures. MRI is the diagnostic tool of choice for both screening and follow-up of cranial and head and neck tumors.

Ultrasonography Ultrasonography measures sound waves as they bounce off various body structures, revealing abnormalities that indicate tumors. For example, transrectal ultrasonography has provided excellent imaging of early prostate cancers and is used to guide needle biopsy. Ultrasound imaging is more useful for detecting masses in the denser breast tissue of young women.

Nuclear Imaging Nuclear imaging involves the use of a special scanner in conjunction with the ingestion or injection of specific radioactive isotopes. This is an invasive but usually safe diagnostic method for identifying tumors in various body tissues. The procedure is often used to check for possible bone or other organ metastases.

Angiography Angiography is performed when the precise location of the tumor cannot be identified or there is a need to visualize the tumor's extent prior to surgery. The procedure involves injecting a radiopaque dye into a major blood vessel proximal to the organ or tissue to be examined. The movement of the dye through the vasculature of the organ or tissue is traced by means of fluoroscopy or serial x-ray films. Blockage to the flow of the dye indicates the tumor's location. Dye may be used to identify blood vessels supplying a tumor, allowing the surgeon to know where to safely ligate vessels.

DIRECT VISUALIZATION Direct visualization procedures are invasive but do not require the use of radiography. Examples include sigmoidoscopy (viewing the sigmoid colon with a fiber-optic flexible sigmoidoscope), cystoscopy (viewing the urethra and bladder), endoscopy (viewing the upper gastrointestinal tract), and bronchoscopy (inspecting the tracheobronchial tree). These methods allow the visual identification of the organs within the limits of the scope and usually permit biopsy of suspicious lesions or masses. Flexible fiber-optic scopes may be more useful because they allow deeper penetration than do traditional scopes. These procedures all require some patient preparation, cause moderate to considerable discomfort, and may require sedation or anesthesia, as in the case of bronchoscopy. Some procedures, such as sigmoidoscopy and cystoscopy, may be performed in the physician's office and therefore cost less, making them more accessible screening procedures.

When the tumor is exposed, a sample of tissue (biopsy) is sent to the pathology laboratory for a "frozen-section" histologic examination. This can be done rapidly while the patient remains on the operating table under anesthesia. If the initial report is negative, the benign mass is usually removed to prevent further symptoms. If the report is positive for cancer, the tumor and often adjacent lymph nodes are dissected, along with any other suspicious tissue. The tumor, nodes, and any other specimens are sent to the pathology laboratory for more in-depth analysis. The patient then receives the usual postoperative care.

LABORATORY TESTS Most laboratory tests of blood, urine, and other body fluids are used to rule out nutritional disorders and other noncancerous conditions that may be causing the patient's symptoms. In conjunction with other diagnostic studies, some laboratory tests can be quite useful either in screening for other pathologic conditions or for validating the cancer diagnosis. Table 14–8 identifies some useful laboratory tests, their normal values, and their possible indications.

PSYCHOLOGIC SUPPORT DURING DIAGNOSIS Preparing for and awaiting the results of diagnostic tests can create extreme anxiety. Many patients compare the experience to that of a prisoner awaiting trial and sentencing: After they know what the "sentence" is, then they can prepare for the future. In addition to coping with the possibility of a life-threatening disease, or at least a life-altering one, patients often also face the prospect of uncomfortable, even painful, diagnostic procedures. They have important decisions to make that depend on the outcome of those tests. Many unspoken questions may exist, including the following:

- Do I have cancer?
- If so, what kind, and how serious?
- Has it spread?
- Will I survive?
- What kind of treatment is needed?
- How will this affect my lifestyle?
- How will this affect family members and friends?

Denial or intellectualization can help some patients coping with cancer, but others display signs of anxiety and stress as they attempt to cope. The nurse can provide valuable support during this very difficult stage by helping patients become actively involved in managing their life and disease. Talk with patients as soon as they enter the healthcare system, asking what they know already about what is going to happen and soliciting questions from them. Taking this approach and encouraging patients to share what knowledge and experience

TABLE 14–8 Laboratory Tests Used for Cancer Diagnosis*

TEST	REFERENCE VALUE	ABNORMALITY INDICATED
Acid phosphatase (ACP)	0.0 to 0.8 unit/L	Elevated in prostate, breast, and bone cancer and in multiple myeloma
Adrenocorticotropic hormone (ACTH)	8 to 80 pg/mL	Decreased in adrenal cancer Elevated in pituitary cancer or with tumor that secretes ACTH (bronchiogenic cancer)
Alanine aminotransferase (ALT)	5 to 35 unit/mL (Frankel)	Moderate elevation in liver cancer
Albumin	3.5 to 5.0 g/dL	Decreased in malnutrition, metastatic liver cancer
Alkaline phosphatase (ALP)	20 to 90 unit/L	Elevated in cancer of liver, bone, breast, and prostate; in leukemia; and in multiple myeloma
Alpha-fetoprotein (AFP)	Male and nonpregnant female: < 15 ng/mL	Elevated in germ cell tumors (e.g., seminoma), testicular cancer
Aspartate aminotransferase (AST)	5 to 40 unit/mL (Frankel)	Elevated in liver cancer
Bilirubin	Total: 0.1 to1.2 mg/dL Direct: 0.0 to 0.3 mg/dL	Elevated in liver and gallbladder cancer
Bleeding time	Ivy method: 3 to 7 minutes	Prolonged in leukemia and metastatic liver cancer
Blood urea nitrogen (BUN)	5 to 25 mg/dL	Decreased in malnutrition; increased in renal cancer
Calcitonin	Male: < 40 pg/mL Female: < 20 pg/mL	Elevated to > 500 pg/mL in thyroid medullary cancer, breast cancer, and lung cancer
Calcium (Ca)	4.5 to 5.5 mEq/L 9.0 to 11.0 mg/dL	Elevated in bone cancer and ectopic parathyroid hormone production (paraplastic syndrome)
Carcinoembryonic antigen (CEA)	2.5 ng/mL in nonsmokers 5 ng/mL in smokers; > 12 ng/mL neoplasms	Elevated with GI cancers, lung, breast, bladder, kidney, cervical, leukemias Used to evaluate effectiveness of cancer treatment
Chloride (Cl)	95 to 105 mEq/L	Decreased in vomiting, diarrhea, syndrome of inappropriate antidiuretic hormone (SIADH)
C-reactive protein	> 1:2 titer is positive	Elevated in metastatic cancer and Burkitt's lymphoma
Creatinine	0.5 to 1.5 mg/dL	Decreased in malnutrition; elevated in most cancers
Dexamethasone suppression test	> 50% reduction in plasma cortisol	Nonsuppression in adrenal cancer and ACTH-producing tumors, severe stress
Estradiol-serum	Female: 20 to 300 pg/mL Menopausal female: < 20 pg/mL Male: 15 to 50 pg/mL	Elevated in estrogen-producing tumors and testicular tumors
Fibrinogen	200 to 400 mg/dL	Decreased in leukemia and as a side effect of chemotherapy
Gamma glutamyltransferase (GGT)	Male: 10 to 80 international unit/L Female: 5 to 25 international unit/L	Elevated in cancer of liver, pancreas, prostate, breast, kidney, lung, and brain
Fasting blood sugar	70 to 110 mg/dL	Decreased in malnutrition, cancer of stomach, liver, and lung
Haptoglobin	20 to 240 mg/dL	Elevated in Hodgkin's disease and cancer of lung, large intestine, stomach, breast, and liver
Hematocrit (Hct)	Male: 40% to 54% Female: 36% to 46%	Decreased in anemia, leukemia, Hodgkin's disease, lymphosarcoma, multiple myeloma, and malnutrition and as a side effect of chemotherapy
Hemoglobin (Hgb)	Male: 13.5 to 18 g/dL Female: 12 to 16 g/dL 1:3 ratio of Hgb:Hct	Decreased in anemia, many cancers, Hodgkin's disease, leukemia, and malnutrition and as a side effect of chemotherapy
Human chorionic gonadotropin (HCG)	Nonpregnant female <0.01 international unit/L	Elevated in choriocarcinoma
Insulin	5 to 25 microunit/mL	Elevated in insulinoma (islet cell tumor) and insulin-secreting cancers (e.g., lung cancer)
Lactic dehydrogenase (LDH)	100 to 190 international unit/L	Elevated in liver, brain, kidney, muscle cancers, acute leukemia, anemia
Occult blood	Negative	Positive in gastric and colon cancers

(continued)

TABLE 14–8 Laboratory Tests Used for Cancer Diagnosis* (continued)

TEST	REFERENCE VALUE	ABNORMALITY INDICATED
Serum osmolality	280 to 300 mOsm/kg H_2O	Decreased in SIADH
Urine osmolality	50 to 1200 mOsm/kg H_2O	Increased in SIADH
Parathyroid hormone (PTH)	400 to 900 pg/mL	Increased in PTH-secreting tumors
Platelet (thrombocyte) count	150,000/mm^3 to 400,000/mm^3	Decreased in bone, gastric, and brain cancer, in leukemia, and as a side effect of chemotherapy
Potassium (K)	3.5 to 5.0 mEq/L	Decreased in vomiting and diarrhea and in malnutrition
Prostatic-specific antigen (PSA)	0 to 4 ng/mL	Elevated from 10 to 120+ in prostate cancer
Total protein	6.0 to 8.0 g/dL	Decreased in malnutrition, gastrointestinal cancer, Hodgkin's disease; elevated in vomiting, diarrhea, multiple myeloma
Red blood cells (RBCs)	Male: 4.6 to 6.0 million/mm^3 Female: 4.0 to 5.0 million/mm^3	Decreased in anemia, leukemia, infection, multiple myeloma
Sodium (Na)	135 to 145 mEq/L	Decreased in SIADH, vomiting; elevated in dehydration
Uric acid	Male: 3.5 to 8.0 mg/dL Female: 2.8 to 6.8 mg/dL	Increased in leukemia, metastatic cancer, multiple myeloma, Burkitt's lymphoma, after vigorous chemotherapy
White blood cells (WBC)		
Total leukocytes	4500/mm^3 to 10,000/mm^3	Elevated in acute infection, leukemias, tissue necrosis; decreased as a side effect of chemotherapy
Neutrophils	50% to 70%	Elevated in bacterial infection and Hodgkin's disease; decreased in leukemia and malnutrition and as a side effect of chemotherapy
Eosinophils	1% to 3%	Elevated in cancer of bone, ovary, testes, and brain
Basophils	0.4% to 1.0%	Elevated in leukemia and healing stage of infection
Monocytes	4% to 6%	Elevated in infection, monocytic leukemia and cancer; decreased in lymphocytic leukemia and as a side effect of chemotherapy
Lymphocytes	25% to 35%	Elevated in lymphocytic leukemia, Hodgkin's disease, multiple myeloma, viral infections, and chronic infections; decreased in malnutrition, cancer, and other leukemias and as a side effect of chemotherapy

*All values refer to serum values unless otherwise indicated. Values are approximate; check the reference standards specified by your own agency's laboratory.

they have allows them to maintain control. From there, the nurse can provide the information needed.

As patients begin to feel more comfortable with the nurse, they may express concerns, fears, and other emotions. The nurse should actively listen and be supportive, but avoid giving advice and false reassurance, providing appropriate information when needed. For patients who are not ready to discuss concerns or for those who appear angry, being nonjudgmental and providing nonverbal support may facilitate more open communication. An atmosphere of calmness, warmth, caring, and respect can ease the tension and often unspoken terror of this initial period.

Support of and communication with the patient's significant others is extremely important. Often they try to be strong for the patient but have many fears and emotional concerns that they do not feel comfortable expressing. The nurse needs to be available to the family while the patient is undergoing diagnostic procedures. Allowing them to talk without the need to edit for the patient's benefit can help them manage their own difficulties in coping with their loved one's potential cancer diagnosis.

Cancer Treatment

The goals of cancer treatment are aimed at cure, control, or palliation of symptoms. These goals may overlap. Cancer may be treated through surgery, chemotherapy, radiation therapy, biotherapy, photodynamic therapy, bone marrow and stem cell transplants, hormonal therapy, and complementary therapies. Once cancer is diagnosed, the initial focus is on surgical and medical treatment. The goals of treatment are the following:

- Eliminating the tumor or malignant cells
- Preventing metastasis
- Reducing cellular growth and the tumor burden
- Promoting functional abilities and providing pain relief to those whose disease has not responded to treatment

SURGERY   Surgery remains an important approach in cancer care. Surgical resection is used for diagnosis and staging of more than 90% of all cancers and for primary treatment of more than 60% of cancers. The goals of surgery have also expanded to include prophylaxis, diagnosis, treatment, reconstruction, and palliation.

Prophylactic surgery aims to remove tissues or organs that are likely to develop cancer. Advances in identification of genetic markers make prophylactic surgery an option for individuals with a strong family history and genetic predisposition for the development of cancer. For example, a woman with a strong history of breast cancer, positive findings of BRCA-1 or BRCA-2, and abnormal finding on mammography may consider prophylactic mastectomy as one of the selective options. Other examples of prophylactic operations include colectomy and oophorectomy. With limited research on the long-term physiologic and psychological effects on individuals undergoing prophylactic surgery for cancer, it is vitally important for nurses and other healthcare professionals to discuss thoroughly with the patient and family potential risks and postoperative outcomes of the prophylactic surgery prior to the surgery. Nurses should respect the patient's decision whether or not to pursue the prophylactic surgery. For those patients who choose prophylactic surgery as a preventive measure for cancer, comprehensive preoperative teaching and counseling should be provided and long-term postoperative follow-up should be ensured to monitor the patient's physiologic and psychological adjustment to the surgery.

Diagnostic surgery aims to ensure histological diagnosis and staging of cancer through biopsy, endoscopy, laparoscopy, and open surgical exploration. Table 14–9 provides information about common surgical diagnostic procedures.

As a primary treatment for cancer, the goal of surgery is to remove the entire tumor and involved surrounding tissue and lymph nodes as much as possible and feasible. This sometimes necessitates mutilation of the body and the creation of new structures to assume function of the lost structures. For example, removal of the distal sigmoid colon and rectum requires a new means of bowel elimination, so the remaining healthy segment of the bowel is brought out through a created opening (stoma) in the abdominal wall, resulting in a permanent colostomy (∞ see Chapter 24). In like manner, when the bladder is removed, the ureters are transplanted into a created pouch just under the abdominal wall. This serves as a continent ileostomy, a substitute reservoir for urine (∞ see Chapter 27). Surgery can destroy sensitive nerve plexuses, resulting in alteration or loss of normal functioning; for example, prostate surgery may result in incontinence and impotence. Surgical removal of involved regional lymph nodes can lead to long-term lymphedema (swelling in the affected area) that greatly impacts cancer survivors' quality of life, for instance, lymphedema following surgery for breast cancer and melanoma (Norman et al., 2009).

Not all surgery results in such radical changes in functioning. The following surgeries can eliminate cancer successfully with less distressing results:

- Removing a nonessential portion of the organ or tissue containing the tumor, such as *in situ* small-bowel tumors
- Removing an organ whose function can be replaced chemically, such as the thyroid
- Resecting one of a pair of organs when the unaffected organ can take over the function of the missing one, such as a lung

Although the removal of any major body part has physiologic and psychological consequences, the alternative—terminal disease—is usually less desirable.

If the tumor is in a nonresectable location or deeply invaded with metastases, surgery may be done to achieve palliation to allow the involved organs to function as long as possible, to relieve pain, to provide comfort, or to bypass an obstruction. Surgery may also be done to reduce the bulk of the tumor in advanced disease, both at primary and metastatic sites. Decreasing the tumor size enhances the ability to control the remaining disease through other modalities. Surgery is often used in conjunction with other treatments to effect a cure. In cases when extensive removal of tissue is contraindicated (e.g., in surgical removal of a brain tumor), radiation may be used prior to surgery in an attempt to shrink the tumor before it is removed.

Surgical intervention may be used for reconstruction and rehabilitation to achieve more desirable functional and cosmetic effect after curative or radical surgery. One example is the construction of transabdominal myocutaneous (TRAM) flaps in conjunction with or following modified radical mastectomy (∞ see Chapter 49). For surgical interventions for cancers affecting specific body systems, refer to later chapters.

Surgical oncologists are working with researchers to identify premalignant disease earlier in high-risk populations and to conduct studies on ways to reverse oncogenic cell activity. Surgeons work with molecular biologists using sophisticated techniques to develop monoclonal antibodies. Laser technology is being explored for use in different types of cancer surgery because it minimizes blood loss, reduces deformity, increases the accuracy of tissue resection, and enhances healing. Lasers are currently being used to treat radical prostatectomy in order to preserve urinary continence and sexual functioning.

Another collaborative strategy is intraoperative radiation therapy, in which radiosensitive, nondiseased organs that may be damaged by radiation therapy are moved away from the radiation field and shielded. Radiation is administered while the patient is on the operating table. This technique allows

TABLE 14–9 Surgical Diagnostic Procedures

PROCEDURE	EXPLANATION
Fine-needle biopsy	Use of a very thin needle to aspirate a small amount of tissue from the tumors
Needle core biopsy	Use of a slightly larger needle than that used for a fine-needle biopsy to extract a small amount of tissue from tumors that cannot be aspirated by fine-needle aspiration
Incisional biopsy	Removal of part of a larger tumor by cutting through the skin
Excisional biopsy	Removal of an entire tumor through operation
Endoscopy	Use of a small viewing lens or video camera through natural body openings to view tumors such as cancer of the esophagus, stomach, or colon
Laparoscopy	Use of a small viewing lens or video camera through a small incision in the abdominal wall

more penetrating radiation to be directed to the malignant tumor with less trauma to normal, vulnerable tissues or organs.

Nursing responsibilities focus on preparing the patient physically and psychologically for surgery, as well as teaching routine postoperative care in which the patient is expected to participate (∞ see Chapter 4). Before surgery, the nurse should give the patient the opportunity to ask questions and to discuss concerns and fears. In some cases, the patient may want to discuss alternative treatment options. In the latter case, the nurse should contact the oncologist and the surgeon and set up a conference for the patient before surgery.

CHEMOTHERAPY   **Chemotherapy** involves the use of cytotoxic medications to cure liquid and solid cancers, such as leukemias, lymphomas, and breast and prostate cancer; to decrease tumor size, adjunctive to surgery or radiation therapy; or to prevent or treat suspected metastases. Chemotherapy may also be used in conjunction with biotherapy. All chemotherapy has side effects or toxic effects. The type and severity depend on the drugs used.

Chemotherapy disrupts the cell cycle in various phases by interrupting cell metabolism and replication. It also works by interfering with the ability of the malignant cell to synthesize vital enzymes and chemicals. Phase-specific drugs work during only some phases of the cell cycle; non-phase-specific drugs work through the entire cell cycle. Figure 14–5 ■ lists some of the drugs useful in each phase of the cell cycle.

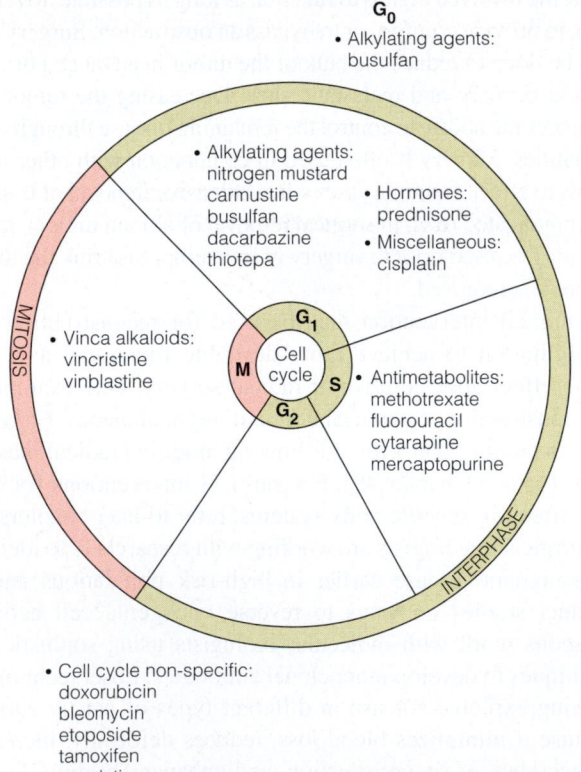

Figure 14–5 ■ Chemotherapeutic drugs useful in each phase of the cell cycle. Based on their chemical makeup and biologic activity, different drugs used for cancer treatment act in specific phases and subphases of the cell cycle. Some drugs, called non-phase-specific drugs, are generalized and act throughout the cycle. Chemotherapy often involves combinations of drugs designed to attack the cancer cells at many different times in the cycle to enhance effectiveness.

Most chemotherapy involves combinations of drugs administered over varying periods of time according to different protocols. One protocol for adult acute lymphocytic leukemia (ALL) uses the acronym DVPA: daunorubicin given on days 1 through 3; vincristine given on days 1, 8, 15, and 22; prednisone given on days 1 through 28, and asparaginase given on days 17 through 28. The treatment regimen is administered in cycles with rest periods, especially if toxic effects such as liver dysfunction or severe neutropenia (abnormally low amounts of neutrophils, a type of white blood cell) occur. The treatment is continued until the remission of the cancer is achieved. If the cancer progresses the particular protocol is abandoned and a new protocol may be tried.

Several courses of chemotherapy are necessary based on the hypothesis of cell-killing. A 1-cm tumor contains about 10^9 (10 billion) total cells, most of which are viable. During each cell cycle, the chemotherapy kills a fixed percentage of cells, always leaving some behind. With each reduction, the tumor burden of cells decreases until the number of viable, clonogenic cells (i.e., those that are able to clone daughter cells) becomes small enough to allow the body's immune system to finish the job. For this reason, oncologists usually give the maximum amount of chemotherapy tolerated by the patient. High-dose chemotherapy remains controversial.

CLASSES OF CHEMOTHERAPY DRUGS   Chemotherapeutic agents can be classified either by the effects of the agent on the cell or by the pharmacologic properties of the agent. According to the effects of the agent on the cell, chemotherapeutic agents can be divided into cell cycle–specific and cell cycle–nonspecific agents. Cell cycle–specific agents are effective at a specific phase (for example, S and M phases) in the cell cycle to prevent cell replication by damaging cellular DNA and blocking production of protein necessary for DNA and RNA synthesis. Cell cycle–nonspecific agents are effective throughout all the phases of the cell cycle, including the resting phase. Both cell cycle–specific and cell cycle–nonspecific agents are effective in rapidly dividing cells to prohibit the growth of fast-growing tumors.

The most common way of classifying chemotherapeutic agents is based on pharmacologic properties of the agent. The classifications include alkylating agents, antimetabolites, antitumor antibiotics, mitotic inhibitors, hormones and hormone antagonists, and miscellaneous agents.

Alkylating Agents   Alkylating agents are not phase specific and basically act on preformed nucleic acids by creating defects in tumor DNA. They cause crosslinking of DNA strands, which can permanently interfere with replication and transcription.

Alkylating agents work with both proliferating and nonproliferating cells (those in G_0 phase). Their toxicity relates to their ability to kill slowly cycling stem cells and manifests in delayed, prolonged, or permanent bone marrow failure. Toxicity can cause a mutagenic effect on bone marrow stem cells, culminating in a treatment-resistant form of acute myelogenous leukemia. Because of the alkylating agents' effect on stem cells, they also cause irreversible infertility. Other common adverse effects include nephrotoxicity (kidney damage) and hemorrhagic cystitis (bladder damage).

The several subclasses of alkylating agents include nitrogen mustard (mechlorethamine), nitrosoureas (carmustine), alkyl sulfonates (busulfan), triazines (dacarbazine), ethyleneamines (thiotepa), and cisplatin. Cisplatin is an alkylating agent containing platinum and chlorine atoms. It is most active in the G_1 subphase, but it is also not phase specific. Cisplatin binds to DNA and acts much like alkylating agents by forming intrastrand DNA crosslinks (gluing strands of DNA together so that they cannot separate). Its major toxic effect is reversible renal tubular necrosis. Cisplatin may be used alone or in combination with other chemotherapeutic drugs for testicular and ovarian cancers.

Antimetabolites The different types of antimetabolites include folic acid analogues (methotrexate), pyrimidine analogues (5-fluorouracil), cytosine arabinoside (ARA-C), and purine analogues (6-mercaptopurine). Antimetabolites, are phase specific, working best in the S phase and having little effect in G_0. They interfere with nucleic acid synthesis by either displacing normal metabolites at the regulatory site of a key enzyme or by substituting for a metabolite that is incorporated into DNA or RNA molecules. Toxic effects usually do not occur until very high levels of the drug are administered. Toxicity is more likely when the drugs accumulate in third-spaced fluid, such as pleural fluid (a characteristic that also makes them useful in treating malignant pleural effusions). Because the drug diffuses slowly from the third-spaced fluid, exposure of the tissue to the drug is prolonged. Most toxic effects relate to rapidly proliferating cells, such as cells in the gastrointestinal tract, hair, and skin and WBCs. Manifestations include nausea and vomiting, stomatitis, diarrhea, alopecia, and leukopenia. Some of the drugs can also cause liver and lung toxicity.

Antitumor Antibiotics Antitumor antibiotics are derived from natural sources that are generally too toxic to be used as antibacterial agents. They are not phase specific and act in several ways: They disrupt DNA replication and RNA transcription; create free radicals, which generate breaks in DNA and other forms of damage; and interfere with DNA repair. In addition, these drugs bind to cells and kill them, probably by damaging the cell membrane. Their main toxic effect is damage to the cardiac muscle. This limits the amount and duration of treatment. Examples of these antibiotics include actinomycin D, doxorubicin, bleomycin, mitomycin-C, and mithramycin.

Mitotic Inhibitors Mitotic inhibitors are drugs that act to prevent cell division during the M phase. Mitotic inhibitors include the plant alkaloids and taxoids. Plant alkaloids consist of medications extracted from plant sources: Vinca alkaloids (e.g., vincristine and vinblastine) and etoposide (also called VP-16). The Vinca alkaloids are phase specific, acting during mitosis. They bind to a specific protein in tumor cells that promotes chromosome migration during mitosis and serves as a conduit for neurotransmitter transport along axons. The toxicity of these drugs is characterized by depression of deep tendon reflexes, paresthesias (pain and altered sensation), motor weakness, cranial nerve disruptions, and paralytic ileus. Etoposide acts in all phases of the cell cycle, causing breaks in DNA and metaphase arrest. Although etoposide may cause bone marrow suppression and nausea and vomiting, the most common toxic effect is hypotension resulting from too rapid intravenous administration. The taxoids act during the G_2 phase to inhibit cell division. Paclitaxel is used for the treatment of Kaposi's sarcoma and metastatic breast and ovarian

cancer. Taxotere is used for breast cancer. Toxicities associated with these drugs include alopecia, bone marrow depression, and severe hypersensitivity reactions (e.g., hypotension, dyspnea, and urticaria).

Hormones and Hormone Antagonists The main hormones used in cancer therapy are the corticosteroids (e.g., prednisone), which are phase specific (G_1). These act by binding to specific intracellular receptors, repressing transcription of mRNA, and thereby altering cellular function and growth. Corticosteroids have multiple side effects such as impaired healing, hyperglycemia, hypertension, osteoporosis, and hirsutism.

Hormone antagonists work with hormone-binding tumors, usually those of the breast, prostate, and endometrium. They block the hormone's receptor site on the tumor and prevent it from receiving normal hormonal growth stimulation. These drugs do not cure, but cause regression of the tumor in about 40% of breast and endometrial tumors and 80% of prostate tumors. Tamoxifen competes with estradiol receptors in breast tumors. Raloxifene blocks estrogen in the breast. Diethylstilbestrol competes with hormone receptors in endometrial and prostate tumors. Aromatase inhibitors (Arimidex, Femara, and Aromasin) reduce the amount of estrogen produced in post-menopausal women. Antiandrogen (flutamide) and luteinizing hormone–releasing hormone block testosterone synthesis in prostate cancers. The main side effects of these drugs are alterations of the secondary sexual characteristics.

Miscellaneous Agents Several miscellaneous agents act at different phases in the cell cycle. L-Asparaginase and hydroxyurea are examples of miscellaneous agents.

EFFECTS OF CHEMOTHERAPEUTIC DRUGS The side effects and toxic effects of chemotherapy vary with the drug used and the length of treatment. Because most of these drugs act on fast-growing cells, the side effects are manifestations of damage to normal rapidly dividing somatic cells. The side effects of hormones express the action of the hormone used or suppression of the normal hormone, such as the masculinizing effects of male hormones administered for ovarian cancers.

Tissues usually affected by cytotoxic drugs include the following:

- Mucous membranes of the mouth, tongue, esophagus, stomach, intestine, and rectum. This may result in anorexia, loss of taste, aversion to food, erythema and painful ulcerations in any portion of the gastrointestinal tract, nausea, vomiting, and diarrhea.
- Hair cells, resulting in alopecia.
- Bone marrow depression affecting most blood cells (e.g., granulocytes, lymphocytes, thrombocytes, and erythrocytes). This results in an impaired ability to respond to infection, a diminished ability to clot blood, and severe anemia.
- Organs, such as heart, lungs, bladder, kidneys. This kind of damage is related to specific agents, such as cardiac toxicity with doxorubicin or pneumonitis with bleomycin.
- Reproductive organs, resulting in impaired reproductive ability or altered fetal development.

Table 14–10 gives the classifications of chemotherapeutic drugs, common examples, target malignancies, adverse effects

TABLE 14–10 Classifications of Chemotherapeutic Drugs

DRUG CLASSIFICATION	COMMON DRUGS	TARGET MALIGNANCIES	ADVERSE EFFECTS OR SIDE EFFECTS	NURSING IMPLICATIONS
Alkylating agents	Mechlorethamine (Mustargen)	Hodgkin's disease Lymphosarcoma Lung cancer Chronic leukemia	Nausea and vomiting Leukopenia Thrombocytopenia Hyperuricemia	Maintain good hydration. Alkalinize urine. Administer antiemetics prior to chemotherapy. Monitor WBC, uric acid. Assess for infection.
	Busulfan (Myleran)	Chronic myelogenous leukemia	Leukopenia Thrombocytopenia Renal failure Pulmonary fibrosis	Monitor WBCs, BUN. Maintain adequate fluid intake. Assess for infection. Assess lungs for fibrotic (coarse, loud) rales.
	Cyclophosphamide (Cytoxan)	Lymphomas Multiple myeloma Leukemias Adenocarcinoma of lung and breast	Hemorrhagic cystitis Renal failure Alopecia Stomatitis Liver dysfunction	Encourage daily fluid intake of 2 to 3 L during treatment. Monitor WBCs, BUN, liver enzymes. Teach ways to manage hair loss.
Antimetabolites	Methotrexate	Acute lymphoblastic leukemia Osteosarcoma Gestational trophoblastic carcinoma	Oral and gastrointestinal ulcerations Anorexia and nausea Leukopenia Thrombocytopenia Pancytopenia	Monitor CBC, WBC differential, BUN, uric acid, creatinine. Assess oral mucous membranes; treat ulcers prn. Assess for infection, bleeding.
	5-Fluorouracil (5-FU)	Colon carcinoma Rectal carcinoma Breast carcinoma Gastric carcinoma Pancreatic cancer	Stomatitis Alopecia Nausea and vomiting Gastritis Enteritis Diarrhea Anemia Leukopenia Thrombocytopenia	Monitor CBC with differential, BUN, uric acid. Administer antiemetics prn. Assess for bleeding; check stool occult blood. Evaluate hydration and nutrition status. Teach oral care for stomatitis. Assess for infection. Teach care for hair loss.
Antitumor antibiotics	Doxorubicin (Adriamycin)	Acute lymphoblastic leukemia (ALL) Acute myeloblastic leukemia Neuroblastoma Wilms' tumor Breast, ovarian, thyroid, lung cancer	Stomatitis Alopecia Nausea and vomiting Gastritis Enteritis Diarrhea Anemia Leukopenia Thrombocytopenia Cardiac toxicity	Monitor ECG; assess for arrhythmias, gallops, and congestive heart failure (CHF). Monitor CBC with differential, BUN, uric acid. Administer antiemetics prn. Assess for bleeding; check stool for occult blood. Evaluate hydration and nutrition status. Teach oral care for stomatitis. Assess for infection. Teach care for hair loss.
	Bleomycin (Blenoxane)	Squamous cell carcinoma Lymphosarcoma Reticulum cell sarcoma Testicular carcinoma Hodgkin's disease	Mucocutaneous ulcerations Alopecia Nausea and vomiting Chills and fever Pneumonitis and pulmonary fibrosis	Check for fever 3 to 6 hours after administration. Have chest x-ray films taken every 2 to 3 weeks. Assess respiratory status, and check for coarse rales. Evaluate hydration and nutrition status. Teach oral care for stomatitis. Assess for infection. Teach care for hair loss.
Plant alkaloids	Vincristine (Oncovin)	Combination therapy for acute leukemia, Hodgkin's and non-Hodgkin's lymphomas, rhabdomyosarcoma, neuroblastoma, Wilms' tumor	Areflexia Muscle weakness Peripheral neuritis Constipation Paralytic ileus Mild bone marrow Depression	Assess neuromuscular function. Monitor CBC with differential. Evaluate gastrointestinal function. Manage constipation.

TABLE 14–10 Classifications of Chemotherapeutic Drugs (continued)

DRUG CLASSIFICATION	COMMON DRUGS	TARGET MALIGNANCIES	ADVERSE EFFECTS OR SIDE EFFECTS	NURSING IMPLICATIONS
Plant alkaloids (*continued*)	Vinblastine (Velban)	Combination therapy for Hodgkin's disease, lymphocytic and histo-cytic lymphoma Kaposi's sarcoma, advanced testicular carcinoma, unresponsive breast cancer	Areflexia Alopecia Nausea and vomiting Bone marrow depression	Assess neuromuscular function. Monitor CBC with differential. Administer antiemetics prn. Teach ways to manage hair loss.
	Etoposide, also called VP-16 (VePesid)	Nonresponsive testicular tumors Small-cell lung cancer	Alopecia Hypotension with rapid infusion	Hydrate adequately before administration. Administer for 60 minutes. Monitor vital signs every 15 minutes during administration and every 2 to 4 hours thereafter. Teach ways to manage hair loss.
	Prednisone	Combination therapy for many tumors Leukemia Lymphoma	Fluid retention Hypertension Steroid diabetes Emotional lability Silent bleeding ulcers Increased risk for infection	Monitor vital signs. Administer diuretics prn. Check blood glucose regularly. Evaluate mental status. Administer oral medications with food. Administer hydrogen ion antagonist drugs (antacids) as ordered. Monitor WBC with differential. Check for signs of systemic infection.
	Diethylstilbestrol (DES)	Advanced breast and prostrate cancers	Fluid retention Feminization Uterine bleeding	Monitor vital signs. Administer diuretics prn as ordered. Explain reason for feminization to men, bleeding to women. Monitor for excessive bleeding.
	Tamoxifen (Nolvadex)	Breast cancer	Hot flashes Nausea and vomiting	Teach ways to manage hot flashes. Explain reason for hot flashes. Administer antiemetics as ordered.
Miscellaneous drugs	Cisplatin (CDDP) (Platinol)	Combination and single therapy for metastatic testicular and ovarian cancers, advanced bladder cancer, head and neck tumors, non-small-cell lung carcinoma, osteogenic sarcoma, neuroblastoma	Bone marrow depression: leukopenia and thrombocytopenia Renal tubular damage Deafness	Monitor WBC with differential and platelets, BUN, creatinine, uric acid. Watch for bleeding. Monitor for signs of infection. Evaluate hearing; check for tinnitus. Ensure that patient is well hydrated before drug is administered. Encourage 2 to 3 L of fluid intake daily.

and side effects, and nursing implications. Consult current pharmacology textbooks for additional drugs and for new combination therapies as they are developed.

PREPARATION AND ADMINISTRATION Many states and individual hospitals require that personnel be trained and certified to administer chemotherapy. Pharmacists in large hospitals and independent home care agencies usually prepare chemotherapeutic drugs for parenteral administration under specific safety guidelines established by the federal government or the Oncology Nursing Society. In some agencies, nurses both prepare and administer these drugs. Because of the potential carcinogenic effects, it is usually recommended that the healthcare professional wear gloves, a mask, and gown while preparing and

administering the drug and disposing of equipment. The nurse must use care when handling excretory products of patients undergoing chemotherapy and teach patients to dispose of their own body fluids safely. Oral medications pose a lesser risk of exposure, but a risk nonetheless, primarily through excretion in the urine.

Chemotherapeutic drugs can be administered orally, such as cyclophosphamide (Cytoxan) and chlorambucil (Leukeran). Other drugs, such as hormones or hormone-blocking agents, may also be given intramuscularly. However, many drugs require intravenous infusion or direct injection into intraperitoneal or intrapleural body cavities. Intravenous preparations can be given through large peripheral veins, but the risk of extravasation or irritation to the vein may preclude this method for long-term therapy. Many patients now receive vascular access devices (VADs), especially if their treatment requires several cycles over weeks or months. VADs are also useful for adjunctive parenteral nutrition in the patient who needs continuous intravenous infusions to manage pain or frequent blood drawing to monitor blood counts. Different types of VADs are available:

- Catheters that are inserted nonsurgically by threading them through a large peripheral vein into the vena cava. Called peripherally inserted central catheters (PICCs), they have multiple lumens that facilitate blood drawing. Placement is usually monitored by fluoroscopy.
- Catheters tunneled under the skin on the chest into a major vein, such as the subclavian vein. Hickman or Groshong catheters may be used.
- Surgically implanted ports are placed under the skin with a connected catheter inserted into a major vein. These are accessed by means of a special needle with a 90-degree angle inserted through the skin directly into the rubber dome of the port, which has a hard plastic back to prevent tissue damage.

Figure 14–6 ■ shows examples of different catheters and vascular access ports.

Risk of infection, catheter obstruction, and extravasation are the main problems associated with VADs. Nurses must teach patients and family members to observe for redness, swelling, pain, or exudate at the insertion site, which may indicate infection; to observe for swelling of the neck or skin near the VAD for extravasation and infiltration; and to flush catheters and provide site care (cleaning and dressing changes) on a regular basis. During each encounter with the patient, the nurse always inspects the site; observes for infection, infiltration, and catheter occlusion; and provides site care when necessary.

MANAGEMENT OF PATIENTS RECEIVING CHEMOTHERAPY
Nurses also help identify and manage toxic effects or side effects of the drugs and provide psychosocial support. Careful assessment and monitoring of the patient's manifestations, including appropriate laboratory tests, alert the nurse to the onset of toxicity. Nausea and vomiting, diarrhea, inflammation and ulceration of oral mucous membranes, hair loss, skin changes, anorexia, and fatigue require specific medical and nursing actions (discussed later in this chapter under the appropriate nursing diagnoses). Indicators of organ toxicities, such as nephrotoxicity, neurotoxicity, or cardiac toxicity, must be reported immediately to the physician. Another aspect of managing patients undergoing chemotherapy is to teach them how to care for access sites and to dispose of used equipment and excretions safely. Nurses teach patients to increase fluid intake to flush out the drugs; to get extra rest, which can both assist therapy and help the patient avoid other illnesses; to identify major complications of their particular drug protocol; to know when to call the physician or emergency medical services; and, if their WBC count is low, to limit their exposure to other people, especially children or those with infections.

During chemotherapy, a number of psychologic issues that can cause moderate to severe emotional distress may arise. The need to plan activities around chemotherapy treatments and their side effects can impair the patient's ability to work, manage a household or care for family members, function sexually, or participate in social and recreational activities. Weight loss and alopecia may prompt feelings of powerlessness and depression. The nurse can assist by carefully evaluating manifestations, providing specific interventions, and allowing patients opportunities to express their fears, concerns, and feelings. Patients should be encouraged to participate in their care and maintain control over their life as much as possible. Specific interventions will be discussed later in the chapter under the appropriate nursing diagnoses. Table 14–10 includes nursing implications for specific adverse effects of common chemotherapy drugs.

RADIATION THERAPY Still the treatment of choice for some tumors or by some oncologists, radiation may be used to kill the tumor, to reduce its size, to decrease pain, or to relieve obstruction. Lymph nodes and adjacent tissues are irradiated when beginning metastasis is suspected. **Radiation therapy**

Figure 14–6 ■ Vascular access devices. *A,* Single- and double-lumen catheters. *B,* Triple-lumen and Groshong catheters.

Source: Photos *A, B:* Courtesy of Bard Access Systems, Salt Lake City, UT.

consists of delivering ionizing radiations of gamma and x-rays in one of two ways:

- *External Radiation.* Also called *teletherapy*, involves delivery of radiation from a source at some distance from the patient. A relatively uniform dosage is delivered to the tumor.
- *Internal Radiation.* Also called **brachytherapy** in which radiation is given inside the body by implanting small amounts of radioactive material directly into a tumor or body cavity while avoiding scattering radiation to the surrounding tissues or organs. This technique allows delivery of high doses of radiation to the tumor while sparing adjacent tissue. Brachytherapy is referred to as internal, interstitial, or intracavitary radiation. The innovation of brachytherapy uses a MammoSite catheter to provide a 5-day accelerated partial breast irradiation and holds promise of reducing the risk of radiation-induced complications.

Lethal injury to DNA is believed to be the primary mechanism by which radiation kills cells, especially cells in faster growing tumors and tissues. As a result, when given over time, radiation can destroy not only rapidly multiplying cancer cells but also rapidly dividing normal cells, such as those of the skin and mucous membranes. A malignant tumor is considered cured when there are no surviving tumor stem cells. The goal of radiation therapy is to achieve maximum tumor control with a minimum of damage to normal tissue.

Implanted or ingested radiation can be dangerous for those living with, taking care of, or treating the patient. Caregivers must use protection by, for example, shielding themselves from the source of radiation, limiting the time of exposure to the patient, increasing the distance from the patient, and using specific safety procedures for handling secretions. Box 14–5 identifies safety principles to be followed by those caring for patients undergoing internal radiation.

BOX 14–5 Safety Principles for Radiation

These recommendations apply to caregivers working with patients receiving internal radiation (brachytherapy).
- Maintain the greatest possible distance from the source of radiation.
- Spend the minimum amount of time close to the radiation source.
- Shield yourself from the radiation with lead gloves and aprons when possible.
- If pregnant, avoid contact with radiation sources.
- If you work routinely near radiation, wear a monitoring device to measure whole-body exposure.
- Avoid direct exposure with radioisotope containers; for example, do not touch the container.
- Keep patients with implanted radioisotopes in a private room with private bath and as far away from other hospitalized persons as possible.
- Dispose of body fluids of patients with unsealed implanted radioisotopes with special care and in specially marked containers.
- Handle bed linen and clothing with care and according to agency protocol.
- Use long-handled forceps to place any dislodged implants into a lead container.
- Consult with the radiation therapy department for any questions or problems in caring for patients with radioactive implants.

Tumors have differing sensitivities to radiation. Tumors that have the greatest number of rapidly proliferating cancer cells usually exhibit the best early response to radiation. The decision to use radiation rather than other modalities is based on balancing the probability of controlling the tumor against the probability of causing complications, such as tissue damage. The decision is usually made by risk–benefit analysis. Planning for radiation therapy includes assessing the disease site, tumor size, and histologic findings. Treatment schedules vary based on these factors. The patient receiving external radiation may experience skin changes such as blanching, erythema, desquamation, sloughing, or hemorrhage. Ulcerations of mucous membranes may cause severe pain; in addition, oral secretions can decrease, making the patient more vulnerable to infection and dental caries. Gastrointestinal effects include nausea and vomiting, diarrhea, or bleeding. Lungs may develop interstitial exudate, a condition called radiation pneumonia. Occasionally, external radiation therapy may cause fistulas or necrosis of adjacent tissues. Implanted radioactive materials can lead to similar problems; moreover, the excretory products of these patients are usually considered dangerous and need special disposal. See the Nursing Care box on page 366 for nursing implications for patients receiving radiation therapy.

BIOTHERAPY **Biotherapy** modifies the biologic processes that result in malignant cells, primarily through enhancing the person's own immune responses. The development of this therapy was based on the immune surveillance hypothesis. Although it has been established that a competent immune system is the body's most important defense against any disease, the role that various immune cells play in combating different types of malignancies continues to be investigated. Currently, biotherapy is used for both hematologic malignancies, such as lymphoma and hairy-cell leukemia, and solid tumors, such as renal cancer, lung cancer, and melanoma (Trinh, 2008; Wu et al., 2008).

Tumor immunology has the following applications: detection screening in high-risk groups, differential diagnosis and classification of tumor cells, monitoring the course of the disease with early detection of recurrence, and active therapies to halt or limit the disease. The theory underlying tumor immunology is that most tumor cells have a structural appearance recognizable by the immune cells. Tumor-associated antigens exist on tumor cells but not on normal cells. TAAs elicit an immune response that, in a person with a competent immune system, destroys or inhibits tumor growth. Thus, TAAs can be isolated from serum and used for both diagnosis and various treatment modalities. The PSA is one such TAA currently in successful diagnostic use.

Tumor cells are often in a stage of arrested development (i.e., in the differentiation stage) for the cell type they represent; thus, they express antigens characteristic of that particular stage of development. The immaturity of the cells provides the physician with information about the relative aggressiveness of the cancer.

Another aspect of immunotherapy is the development of monoclonal antibodies that enhance the immune system's ability to fight the cancer. Monoclonal antibodies are developed by inoculating an animal with the tumor antigen and recovering the specific antibodies produced. The antibodies are then given to the person with that cancer to assist in the destruction of the tumor.

Monoclonal antibodies are also re-created, or cloned, in the genetic laboratory by recombining DNA to produce the specific antibody. Techniques involving recombinant DNA have been used to combine these antibodies with toxins and drugs that are then delivered selectively to the tumor sites. For example, approximately one fourth of all women diagnosed with early breast cancer present with tumors that are associated with Her-2/neu receptor overexpression. Overexpression of Her-2/neu results in a high risk of metastasis and poor prognosis, which represents a target for a selective monoclonal antibody therapy with trastuzumab (Herceptin) (Singer, Kostler, & Hudelist, 2008). Trastuzumab (Herceptin) a monoclonal antibody that inhibits Her-2 by binding to extracellular portion of the receptor to inhibit initial signal transduction, thus inhibit growth, proliferation, and angiogenesis. The combination of trastuzumab with chemotherapy has led to a considerable reduction of recurrences and to a significant reduction in breast cancer mortality (Singer et al., 2008).

A number of cytokines (normal growth-regulating molecules) with antitumor activity have been synthesized. Alpha interferon (IFN-α), bacillus Calmette-Guérin (BCG, which has been used for many years as an inoculation against tuberculosis), and interleukin-2 (IL-2) have shown some therapeutic benefit in eliciting increased immune responses. Combination strategies have also helped stimulate the function of macrophages. The use of hematopoietic growth factors (HGF) has been one of the most successful in biotherapy. HGF, such as granulocyte colony-stimulating factor and erythropoietin, offsets the suppression of granulocytes and erythrocytes that results from chemotherapy (Andres et al., 2008).

A promising discovery has been the natural killer (NK) cells. These cells are like large granular lymphocytes, but have a cell surface phenotype different from that of T lymphocytes or macrophages. They have demonstrated a spontaneous cytotoxic effect on some types of cancer cells. They provide a strong resistance to metastasis and secrete cytokines. Combining biotherapy (such as IL-2, IL-12) with chemotherapy show increased tumor destructive activity and treatment responses (Trinh, 2008; Wu, Jiang, Shi, & Xu, 2008).

NURSING CARE OF THE PATIENT   Receiving Radiation Therapy

NURSING RESPONSIBILITIES FOR EITHER EXTERNAL OR INTERNAL RADIATION THERAPY

- Assess and manage any complications, usually in collaboration with the radiation oncologist.
- Assist in documenting the results of the therapy; for example, patients receiving radiation for metastases to the spine will show improved neurologic functioning as tumor size diminishes.
- Provide emotional support, relief of physical and psychologic discomfort, and opportunities to talk about fears and concerns. For some patients, radiation therapy is a last chance for cure or even for relief of physical discomfort.

EXTERNAL RADIATION

Prior to the start of treatments, the treatment area will be specifically located by the radiation oncologist and marked with colored semipermanent ink or tattoos. Treatment is usually given 5 days per week for 15 to 30 minutes per day over 2 to 7 weeks.

Nursing Responsibilities

- Monitor for adverse effects: skin changes, such as blanching, erythema, desquamation, sloughing, or hemorrhage; ulcerations of mucous membranes; nausea and vomiting, diarrhea, or gastrointestinal bleeding.
- Assess lungs for rales, which may indicate interstitial exudate. Observe for any dyspnea or changes in respiratory pattern.
- Identify and record any medications that the patient will be taking during the radiation treatment.
- Monitor white blood cell counts and platelet counts for significant decreases.

Health Education for the Patient and Family

- Wash the skin that is marked as the radiation site only with plain water, no soap; do not apply deodorant, lotions, medications, perfume, or talcum powder to the site during the treatment period. Take care not to wash off the treatment marks.
- Do not rub, scratch, or scrub treated skin areas. If necessary, use only an electric razor to shave the treated area.
- Apply neither heat nor cold (e.g., heating pad or ice pack) to the treatment site.
- Inspect the skin for damage or serious changes, and report these to the radiologist or physician.

- Wear loose, soft clothing over the treated area.
- Protect skin from sun exposure during treatment and for at least 1 year after radiation therapy is discontinued. Cover skin with protective clothing during treatment; once radiation is discontinued, use sun-blocking agents with a sun protection factor (SPF) of at least 15.
- External radiation poses no risk to other people for radiation exposure, even with intimate physical contact.
- Be sure to get plenty of rest and eat a balanced diet.

INTERNAL RADIATION

The radiation source, called an implant, is placed into the affected tissue or body cavity and is sealed in tubes, containers, wires, seeds, capsules, or needles. An implant may be temporary or permanent. Internal radiation may also be ingested or injected as a solution into the bloodstream or a body cavity or be introduced into the tumor through a catheter. The radioactive substance may transmit rays outside the body or be excreted in body fluids.

Nursing Responsibilities

- Place the patient in a private room.
- Limit visits to 10 to 30 minutes, and have visitors sit at least 6 feet from the patient.
- Monitor for side effects such as burning sensations, excessive perspiration, chills and fever, nausea and vomiting, or diarrhea.
- Assess for fistulas or necrosis of adjacent tissues.

Health Education for the Patient and Family

- While a temporary implant is in place, stay in bed and rest quietly to avoid dislodging the implant.
- For outpatient treatments, avoid close contact with others until treatment has been discontinued.
- If the radiologist indicates the need for such measures, dispose of excretory materials in special containers or in a toilet not used by others.
- Carry out daily activities as able; get extra rest if feeling fatigued.
- Eat a balanced diet; frequent, small meals often are better tolerated.
- Contact the nurse or physician for any concerns or questions after discharge.

A combination of cytokines, particularly IFN-α and IL-2, with chemotherapy has been used to treat renal cell cancer, metastatic melanoma, and lung patients with promising results. Such a combination is referred to as either biochemotherapy or chemoimmunotherapy (Trinh, 2008; Wu et al., 2008). The rationale for biochemotherapy is based on the independent antitumor activity of both IFN-α and IL-2 against melanoma and their lack of cross-resistance with cytotoxic chemotherapy. Although the precise mechanism of antitumor effect of biochemotherapy regimens is less understood, two hypotheses have been proposed: (1) Chemotherapy enhances the antitumor effect of biologic agents and; (2) the biologic agents enhance the antitumor cytotoxic effect of chemotherapy.

As promising as these biotherapies or biochemotherapies are, they are accompanied by serious side effects and toxicities (Trinh, 2008; Wu et al., 2008). IL-2 can cause acute alterations in renal, cardiac, liver, gastrointestinal, and mental functioning. IFN-α causes mental slowing, confusion, and lethargy and, when used in combination with 5-fluorouracil or IL-2, severe flulike symptoms—chills and fever of 103°F to 106°F (39.4°C to 41.1°C), nausea, vomiting, diarrhea, anorexia, severe fatigue, and stomatitis—may result. The toxic effects are probably exaggerations of the normal systemic effects that these substances cause when fighting infection. For example, IL-2 is known to raise body temperature substantially in an attempt to create a hostile environment for foreign invaders.

The following Nursing Care box discusses nursing implications for patients receiving immunotherapy. For nursing care of specific problems, refer to the appropriate nursing diagnoses later in this chapter.

PHOTODYNAMIC THERAPY (PDT)
Photodynamic therapy is a method of treating certain kinds of superficial tumors. It is known by several different names: phototherapy, photoradiation, and photochemotherapy. Patients who have tumors growing on the surface of the bladder, peritoneal cavity, chest wall, pleura, bronchus, or head and neck are candidates for this treatment. The patient is given an intravenous dose of a photosensitizing compound, Photofrin, which is selectively retained in higher concentrations in malignant tissue. This drug is activated by a laser treatment that is started 3 days after the drug injection and administered for 3 days. The drug interacts with oxygen molecules in the tissue to produce a cytotoxic oxygen molecule called singlet oxygen.

At the time of the first intravenous injection, patients are observed for adverse hypersensitivity reactions, such as nausea, chills, and hives. Systemic or long-term toxicities are rare. The main side effects are local skin reactions and temporary photosensitivity, transiently elevated liver enzymes, and inflammatory responses of the tissues being treated, such as peritoneal or pleural tissues.

The major nursing responsibilities associated with photodynamic therapy are to address the patient and family's anxiety and to educate them in managing side effects. The drug remains in the subcutaneous tissues for 4 to 6 weeks after injection. Any direct or indirect exposure to the sun activates the drug, resulting in a chemical sunburn. Patients are taught to protect themselves from sunlight (even on cloudy days) by covering themselves from head to toe in opaque clothing, including a wide-brimmed

NURSING CARE OF THE PATIENT
Receiving Immunotherapy

Immunotherapy can consist of various substances used alone, such as IL-2, IL-12, or combination biotherapy, such as IFN-a with 5-fluorouracil. The nurse's role is to enhance the patient's quality of life.

Nursing Responsibilities
- Monitor for side effects: IFN-α may cause mental slowing, confusion, fatigue, and lethargy; combination therapy of 5-fluorouracil or IL-2 and IFN-α may cause severe flulike symptoms, with chills and fever of 103°F to 106°F (39.4°C to 41.1°C), nausea, vomiting, diarrhea, anorexia, severe fatigue, and stomatitis; erythropoietin may cause acute hypertension.
- Monitor enzymes and other appropriate biochemical indicators for acute alterations in renal, cardiac, liver, or gastrointestinal functioning, which can be side effects of IL-2.
- Evaluate response to therapy by conducting a thorough evaluation of patients' symptoms.
- Assess patients' coping behaviors and teach new strategies as needed.
- Manage fatigue and depression.
- Encourage self-care and participation in decision making.
- Provide close supervision for patients with altered mental functioning, either by caretakers or frequent nursing visits to the patient's home.
- If patient is unable to manage alone, teach medication administration and care of equipment to caregivers.

Health Education for the Patient and Family
- Minimize symptoms by managing fever and flulike symptoms: increase fluid intake, take analgesic and antipyretic medications, and maintain bed rest until symptoms abate.
- Seek help for serious problems not managed by usual means, such as dehydration from diarrhea.
- Use correct techniques for providing subcutaneous injections.
- Identify how to work and care for ambulatory pumps when medication is administered through an intercatheter or vascular access device.

hat, gloves, shoes and stockings, and sunglasses with 100% ultraviolet block. Long-term care of treated skin includes moisturizing lotions and protection from trauma or irritation.

BONE MARROW AND PERIPHERAL BLOOD STEM CELL TRANSPLANTATIONS
Bone marrow transplantation (BMT) is an accepted treatment to stimulate a nonfunctioning marrow or to replace marrow. BMT is given as an intravenous infusion of bone marrow cells from donor to patient. Most commonly used in leukemias, this therapy is being expanded to include treatment of other cancers including melanoma and testicular cancer. Chapter 33 provides an in-depth discussion of this procedure. Peripheral blood stem cell transplantation (PBSCT) is the process of removing circulating stem cells from the peripheral blood through apheresis and returning these cells to the patient after dose-intensive chemotherapy. PBSCT has fewer side effects, shorter hospitalization, and decreased cost compared to BMT.

COMPLEMENTARY THERAPIES
Although advances in cancer treatment have increased 5-year survival rates, the uncertainty of cure of cancer and cancer reoccurrence compels some

patients to look for complementary therapies. Complementary therapies refer to therapies that patients choose as a complement to medical treatment. Common complementary therapies for cancer can be categorized into botanical agents, nutritional supplements, dietary regimens, mind–body modalities, energy healing, spiritual approaches, and miscellaneous therapies. Box 14–6 provides information about complementary therapies.

To provide sensitive nursing care, nurses should be knowledgeable about common complementary therapies. It is important for nurses to provide truthful, nonjudgmental responses to the questions or inquiries about complementary therapies from patients with cancer. Nurses should encourage patients to report the use of any complementary therapies to their oncologist to prevent potential interactions of the those therapies with their medical treatment.

Pain Management

Pain management is an important component of oncology care and is considered a crucial part of the collaborative treatment plan. It is estimated that more than 60% of patients with early-stage cancer and up to 95% of patients with advanced cancer experience pain that requires analgesia (Eaton & Frieze, 2008). There are three main categories of pain syndromes in patients with cancer, and the category influences the type of treatment:

- *Pain associated with direct tumor involvement.* The most common causes are metastases to bone, nerve compression or infiltration, and involvement of hollow visceral organs.
- *Pain associated with treatment.* This may include postsurgical incisional or wound pain; peripheral neuropathy, ulceration of mucous membranes, and pain from herpes zoster outbreaks

secondary to chemotherapy; and pain in nerve plexuses, muscles, and peripheral nerves from radiation therapy.
- *Pain from a cause not related to either the cancer or therapy,* such as diabetic neuropathy.

The goal of pain therapy is to provide relief that allows patients to function as they wish and, in the case of terminally ill patients, to die relatively free of pain. With the emphasis on putting evidence into nursing practice, the Oncology Nursing Society (ONS, 2007) conducted a systematic review on cancer pain and concluded combinations of nonopioids, opioids, and coanalgesics are effective management of acute and persistent nociceptive and neuropathic pain that occurs as a result of cancer or cancer treatment. Other therapies include injection of anesthetic drugs into spinal cord or specific nerve plexuses, surgical severing of nerves, radiation to reduce tumor size and pressure, and behavioral approaches. Pharmacologic pain management follows these steps:

1. Conduct careful initial and ongoing assessment of the pain.
2. Evaluate the patient's functional goals.
3. Establish a plan with combinations of nonnarcotic drugs (such as aspirin or ibuprofen) with adjuvants (such as corticosteroids or antidepressants).
4. Evaluate the degree of pain relief.
5. Progress to stronger drugs as needed, from mild narcotics such as oxycodone (Percodan) or propoxyphene (Darvon) to strong narcotics such as morphine or hydromorphone (Dilaudid), and monitor side effects.
6. Continue to try combinations and escalate dosages until maximal pain relief balanced with patient's need to function is achieved.

BOX 14–6 Common Complementary Therapies for Cancer

Type	Description
Botanical agents	Herbs are believed to be the most "natural" and "safe" plants ingested with the hope for a cure of cancer. Commonly used botanical agents include echinacea, Essiac, ginseng, green tea, pau d'arco, and Hoxsey. The safety for many of these botanical agents has not been proven, especially as a complement to medical treatment.
Nutritional supplements	Chemical compounds include vitamins, minerals, enzymes, amino acids, and essential fatty acids, or proteins (such as shark cartilage). They are believed to have the ability to promote health and to help cure cancer. The safety of certain compounds such as vitamins has been established; however, in megadoses, many of the compounds can be toxic and have potential interactions with some therapeutic agents used for cancer such as chemotherapy.
Dietary regimens	The ingestion of only natural substances is believed to have the effect of purifying the body and slowing down the growth of cancer. Popular regimens include the grape diet, the carrot juice diet, and garlic, onions, and liver intake. The effectiveness of these dietary regimens remains to be established.
Mind–body modalities	The harmony of mind and body are believed to facilitate physiologic and psychological healing. Such modalities include relaxation, meditation, or imagery. Recent research has shown that these modalities helped individuals with cancer adjust to the experience of cancer.
Energy healing	The human body is believed to be an energy field and cancer might be the result of a disturbed energy field. Energy therapies, such as therapeutic touch and healing touch, can affect the energy field of the human body and promote physiologic healing. Therapeutic touch uses the hands on or near the body with the intent to promote healing. Healing touch uses energy healing techniques to heal by restoring the harmony and balance of the body. Clinical practice and research on energy healing have shown positive findings of energy healing in a variety of patients.
Spiritual approaches	Faith in God or a higher power of the universe is believed to help cancer healing. Spiritual approaches include faith healing, prayer to God, prayer groups, and chain prayer. Research has shown that faith in God or a higher power helped individuals with cancer to adjust to the experience of cancer.
Miscellaneous therapies	Aromatherapy has been used for patients with cancer to relieve nausea, vomiting, or retching and to decrease anxiety. However, aromatherapy might not be appropriate for patients who are highly sensitive to strong fragrance. Music, art, and humor therapies have been used to help patients with cancer to reduce anxiety, to express feeling of loss, and to promote optimism.

Medication usually is administered by the oral route as long as this route continues to be effective. Medication is given on a regular time schedule (e.g., every 4 hours) with additional medication prescribed to cover breakthrough pain. When the oral route alone becomes inadequate, the primary narcotic can be administered intramuscularly, subcutaneously, or rectally on an intermittent schedule; continuously by transdermal patches; or intravenously by a continuous drip, usually controlled by an infusion pump. Some newer pumps are portable, deliver medication continuously, and allow patients to control their breakthrough pain with a limited number of boluses. When narcotic doses are increased gradually, there is no limit to the amount the patient can receive, as long as adverse reactions can be managed. Patients have received up to 4800 mg daily (200 mg per hour) of morphine sulfate with up to six 200- to 400-mg breakthrough doses daily without major ill effects and with good pain control. The body develops tolerance to the sedative after a short period, and most patients are able to tolerate the level of medication needed to control the pain. Other side effects, such as constipation, nausea and vomiting, and itching, can be managed through the usual means and are discussed under the appropriate nursing diagnoses. If the patient has persistent untoward side effects that do not respond to treatment, or if the patient does not get adequate relief from the narcotic, different narcotics and combinations are tried. Morphine sulfate and transdermal fentanyl are the most commonly used drugs for relief of cancer pain (ONS, 2007). Patients receiving high-dose narcotics should not have the medication abruptly stopped, because withdrawal symptoms will occur. If the drug needs to be stopped, it must be tapered gradually. For more information on pain management, and on alternative therapies in particular, ∞ see Chapter 9.

✍ Nursing Care

Nurses face a major challenge in educating patients about preventive measures and lifestyle changes to reduce the risk of cancer. At the same time, patients with cancer must be reassured that they are not responsible for having acquired cancer.

Once a cancer diagnosis is established, nurses help patients recover and support them during the rehabilitation phase. In cases of terminal cancer, nurses provide comfort and facilitate positive growth for the patient and significant others.

Health Promotion

Early detection and treatment are considered the most important factors influencing the prognosis of those who have cancer. However, many people do not seek early diagnosis and treatment because of denial, fear and anxiety, stigma, or the absence of specific early signs such as pain or weight loss (which usually are late signs). For this reason, screening procedures such as mammograms, PSA, occult blood stool tests, and sigmoidoscopy may be lifesaving.

The ACS promotes early cancer detection through promotion of cancer awareness and guidelines for screening procedures. Although no longer in use by the ACS, the CAUTION model (Box 14–7) is helpful in promoting awareness of common symptoms that may indicate cancer. This model encourages people to seek medical attention when they discover signs and symptoms characteristic of cancer. For people without

---

BOX 14–7 Seven Warning Signs of Cancer

American Cancer Society CAUTION Model
Change in bowel or bladder habits
A sore that does not heal
Unusual bleeding or discharge
Thickening or lump in breast or elsewhere
Indigestion or difficulty swallowing
Obvious change in wart or mole
Nagging cough or hoarseness
If you have a warning signal, see your doctor!

Source: American Cancer Society.

---

symptoms, the ACS recommends incorporating a cancer checkup into periodic health examinations. This general cancer checkup includes health counseling, teaching self-examination techniques when appropriate, and, depending on age and gender, examination for cancers of the thyroid, oral cavity, skin, lymph nodes, testes, and ovaries (ACS, 2009a).

If a person is at special risk due to heredity, environment, occupation, or lifestyle, special tests or more frequent examinations may be necessary. A routine cancer checkup should include counseling to improve health behaviors and physical examination with related tests of the breast, uterus, cervix, colon, rectum, testes, prostate, skin, thyroid, and lymph nodes. Box 14–8 lists the tests recommended for a cancer checkup. Nurses have a special role in public education and should encourage everyone they come in contact with to schedule cancer checkups. Nurses must be familiar with the ACS guidelines so that they can advise patients, their families, and significant others.

Assessment

The assessment chapters in this text contain questions based on functional health patterns that include questions about manifestations and risk factors for cancer. Examples of appropriate questions to elicit information during a health history assessment follow:

Interview Questions

The following are appropriate questions to ask the patient during the initial interview and at subsequent assessments:

- "What brought you in to see the doctor?" Asking this question allows patients to tell their story in their own way, which may elicit more information than asking specific questions. The answer should elicit not only data about the signs and symptoms but also fears or concerns. If the cancer was discovered during a routine physical examination or checkup, the patient may have some difficulty accepting the disease, especially if there were no symptoms. For patients who offer insufficient information in response to this open-ended question, more specific questions may be necessary, such as "Did you have pain or any specific physical problems that caused you to seek health care?"
- "Do you have any other medical conditions or problems that are troubling you at this time?" It may be necessary to ask about specific diseases to help the patient focus. For example, "Do you have high blood pressure?" or "Are you having any problems with your lungs?" Information gained from these questions can help you anticipate problems and formulate potential nursing diagnoses related to other diseases that may interact with the cancer.

BOX 14–8   American Cancer Society Guidelines for Cancer Screening

Breast Cancer
- Yearly mammograms are recommended starting at age 40.
- A clinical breast exam should be part of a periodic health exam, about every 3 years for women in their 20s and 30s, and every year for women 40 and older.
- Women should know how their breasts normally feel and report any breast changes promptly to their healthcare providers. Breast self-exam is an option for women starting in their 20s.
- Screening MRI is recommended for women with an approximately 20% to 25% or greater lifetime risk of breast cancer, including women with a strong family history of breast or ovarian cancer and women who were treated for Hodgkin's disease.

Cervix/Uterus
- Screening should begin approximately three years after a woman begins having vaginal intercourse, but no later than 21 years of age.
- Screening should be done every year with regular Pap tests or every two years using liquid-based tests.
- At or after age 30, women who have had three normal test results in a row may get screened every 2 to 3 years. Doctors may suggest a woman get screened more frequently if she has certain risk factors, such as HIV infection or a weakened immune system.
- Women 70 and older who have had three or more consecutive Pap tests in the last 10 years may choose to stop cervical cancer screening.

- Screening after a total hysterectomy (with removal of the cervix) is not necessary unless the surgery was done as a treatment for cervical cancer.

Colon and Rectum
Beginning at age 50, men and women should follow one of the following examination schedules:
- A guaiac-based fecal occult blood test (FOBT) or a fecal immunochemical test (FIT) every year
- A flexible sigmoidoscopy (FSIG) every 5 years
- A colonoscopy every 10 years
- A double-contrast barium enema every 5 years
- A CT colonography every 5 years
- People who are at moderate or high risk for colorectal cancer should talk with their doctor about a more-frequent testing schedule for a stool DNA test (interval uncertain).

Prostate
- The prostate-specific antigen (PSA) test and the digital rectal examination (DRE) should be offered annually, beginning at age 50, to men who have a life expectancy of at least 10 years.
- Men at high risk (African American men and men with a strong family history of one or more first-degree relatives diagnosed with prostate cancer at an early age) should begin testing at age 45.
- For men at average risk and high risk, information should be provided about what is known and what is uncertain about the benefits and limitations of early detection and treatment of prostate cancer so that they can make an informed decision about testing.

Source: American Cancer Society, 2010a.

- "What kinds of physical problems are you having at this time? Do you have pain? Are you nauseated? Have you lost a great deal of weight? Are you so tired you have difficulty carrying on your daily activities? Are you feeling blue or discouraged because of your illness?" For each positive response, ask follow-up questions to narrow down or define the exact nature of the problem. This data helps identify what nursing diagnoses should be included in the care plan.
- "What options has your physician suggested for treating your cancer?" The answer will indicate patients' knowledge about their treatment and, possibly, their communication with the physician. Often, under the stress of a cancer diagnosis, patients do not hear or understand what the doctor is saying and are afraid to ask questions. Lack of knowledge indicates a need to collaborate with the physician to explain the information to the patient so that the patient can absorb and understand it. If the patient has a good understanding of the treatment plan, discussing how he or she feels about it can be useful in exposing fears, concerns, and emotional responses.
- "What do you expect to happen as a result of this treatment?" The answer may reveal unrealistic expectations or lack of understanding of consequences of the treatment.
- "What effects are the disease and/or treatment having on your ability to carry on with your usual daily activities?" Additional questions may be needed to pinpoint the types of limitations. The response to this question should provide information on the patient's functional status such as those shown in Box 14–9. This information can also be used to identify the need to collaborate with professionals from other disciplines. For example, if the patient is the sole financial support of the family and is unable to work, a social worker may be able to help with resources; if the patient is extremely weak, referral to a physical therapist may help with energy conservation strategies and strengthening exercises.
- "Who is available to help you at home and run errands for you? Who can provide transportation for you to get to your appointments or treatments? Who can you rely on to be a good listener when you're sad or to be a comfortable companion? Is there someone you would like to make healthcare decisions for you if there is a time when you are unable to make them for yourself?" It often seems that the person with cancer is the one who takes care of everyone else; asking for help may be difficult for this person. This information can identify how much support and help the patient has access to. The last question introduces the concept of advanced directives and durable power of attorney regarding health care (∞ see Chapter 5).
- "How do you manage your stress or your feelings of discomfort? What helps you feel better? Do you think these measures work well for you?" The responses to these questions provide information about the patient's coping strategies and may identify maladaptive strategies such as alcohol or drug use. Lack of appropriate coping methods can interfere with the patient's response to treatment and decrease overall quality of life.

Other assessment questions may be useful at different stages of the patient's illness. For example, if the patient is not expected to survive the cancer, it is important to ask whether the patient has made decisions about last wishes (e.g., for a funeral and burial), whether these have been discussed with significant others, and whether the patient has made out a will.

BOX 14–9 Two Scales of Functional Status for Cancer Patients

I. Karnofsky Scale: Criteria of Performance Status (PS)

100 Normal; no complaints; no evidence of disease.
90 Able to carry on normal activity; minor signs or symptoms of disease.
80 Able to carry on normal activity with effort; some signs or symptoms of disease.
70 Cares for self; unable to carry on normal activity or to do active work.
60 Requires occasional assistance but is able to care for most of own needs.
50 Requires considerable assistance and frequent medical care.
40 Disabled; requires special care and assistance.
30 Severely disabled; hospitalization indicated, although death not imminent.
20 Very sick; hospitalization necessary; active supportive treatment necessary.
10 Moribund; fatal processes progressing rapidly.
0 Dead.

II. Eastern Cooperative Oncology Group Scale (ECOG)

0 Fully active, able to carry on all predisease activities without restriction. (Karnofsky 90 to 100)
1 Restricted in physically strenuous activity, but ambulatory and able to carry out work of a light or sedentary nature, for example, light housework or office work. (Karnofsky 70 to 80)
2 Ambulatory and capable of all self-care, but unable to carry out work activities. Up and about more than 50% of waking hours. (Karnofsky 50 to 60)
3 Capable of only limited self-care, confined to bed or chair 50% or more of waking hours. (Karnofsky 30 to 40)
4 Completely disabled, cannot carry out any self-care, totally confined to bed or chair. (Karnofsky 10 to 20)

"Two Scales of Functional Status for Cancer Patients" from "Nitrogen Mustards in the Palliative Treatment of Carcinoma" by D. A. Karnofsky, L. Craver, & J. Burchenal, 1948. *Cancer*, 1(4), pp. 634-656. © American Cancer Society, reprinted by permission of Wiley-CISS, Inc., a subsidiary of John Wiley & Sons.

Physical Assessment

As soon as the patient is admitted to the healthcare service or agency, conduct a complete physical assessment to establish a baseline for subsequent evaluation of later changes. It is especially important to document the nutritional status of the patient using anthropomorphic measurements (i.e., frame size, height, weight, body fat, muscle mass, body mass index, and body composition), and to evaluate laboratory results and note any specific signs and symptoms. Table 14–11 compares the manifestations of good nutrition with those of malnutrition.

It is also important to assess the patient's hydration status, especially if the patient is not taking oral food and fluids well or is having bouts of vomiting. Box 14–10 lists specific assessments for hydration status. Other recommended assessments are discussed under the specific nursing diagnoses that follow. They can also be found in other chapters that address specific body systems affected by the cancer.

BOX 14–10 Factors to Consider in Assessing Hydration Status

- Intake and output
- Rapid weight changes
- Skin turgor and moisture
- Venous filling
- Vital sign changes
- Tongue furrows and moisture
- Eyeball softness
- Lung sounds
- Laboratory values

Nursing Diagnoses and Interventions

Nursing goals focus on supporting the whole person and providing interventions for specific problems such as pain, poor nutrition, dehydration, fatigue, adverse emotional responses, altered individual and family coping, and the side effects of medical

TABLE 14–11 Signs of Nutritional Status

SYSTEM	GOOD NUTRITION	POOR NUTRITION
General	Alert, energetic, good endurance, psychologically stable	Withdrawn, apathetic, easily fatigued, irritable
	Weight within range for height, age, body size	Over- or underweight
Integumentary	Skin glowing, good turgor, smooth, free of lesions	Skin dull, pasty, scaly-dry, bruises, multiple lesions
	Hair shiny, lustrous, minimal loss	Hair brittle, dull, falls out easily
Head, eyes, ears, nose, and throat	Eyes bright, clear, no fatigue circles	Eyes dull, conjunctiva pale, discoloration under eyes
	Oral mucous membranes pink-red and moist	Oral mucous membranes pale
	Gums pink, firm	Gums red, spongy, and bleed easily
	Tongue pink, moderately smooth, no swelling	Tongue bright to dark red, swollen
Abdomen	Abdomen flat, firm	Abdomen flaccid or distended (ascites)
Musculoskeletal	Firm, well-developed muscles	Flaccid muscles, wasted appearance
	Good posture	Stooped posture
	No skeletal changes	Skeletal malformations
Neurologic	Good attention span, good concentration, astute thought processes	Inattentive, easily distracted, impaired thought processes
	Good reflexes	Paresthesias, reflexes diminished or hyperactive

treatment. Nursing care also focuses on improving quality of life by promoting rehabilitation for survivors of cancer and helping those who succumb to the disease maintain their dignity in the dying process. Because cancer affects the whole family, nursing care includes everyone involved with the patient from the onset of diagnosis through the entire disease and treatment process and the ultimate outcome. Many diagnoses are pertinent to patients with cancer; this section addresses only the most common diagnoses. See the Case Study & Nursing Care Plan on page 378.

Anxiety

Early in the disease process (i.e., during diagnosis and treatment), threats to or changes in health status, physical comfort, role functioning, or even socioeconomic status can cause anxiety. Later, anxiety may result from the anticipation of pain, disfigurement, or the threat of death. In particular, patients whose coping skills have been poor in the past (e.g., in managing anger) may find themselves at a loss to manage this current crisis. The patient may manifest overt signs of anxiety: trembling, restlessness, irritability, hyperactivity, stimulation of the sympathetic nervous system (increased blood pressure, pulse, respiration, excessive perspiration, pallor), withdrawal, worried facial expressions, and poor eye contact. The patient may report insomnia and feelings of tension and apprehension, or express concerns regarding perceived changes brought about by the disease and fear of future events.

- Carefully assess the patient's level of anxiety (moderate anxiety, severe anxiety, or panic) and the reality of the threats represented in the patient's current situation. *The level of anxiety and the reality of the perceived threat influence the type of intervention that is appropriate for the patient. A patient in panic may need medical intervention with appropriate medications, whereas those with moderate or severe anxiety are often managed by the nurse through counseling and teaching new coping skills.*
- Establish a therapeutic relationship by conveying warmth and empathy and listening in a nonjudgmental manner. *A patient who feels safe in the relationship with the nurse more easily expresses feelings and thoughts. The patient will be able to trust the nurse and perhaps be willing to try new behaviors as suggested. The amount of time this relationship may take to develop depends on the patient's current emotional and mental state and the stage of the disease process.*
- Encourage the patient to acknowledge and express feelings, no matter how inappropriate they may seem to the patient. *Just by expressing their feelings, patients often can significantly diminish anxiety. Expressing feelings also allows the patient to direct energy toward healing and thus has a positive therapeutic effect. Moreover, by acknowledging feelings, especially those the patient considers unacceptable, the patient can lay the groundwork for new coping behaviors.*
- Review the coping strategies the patient has used in the past and build on past successful behaviors, introducing new strategies as appropriate. Explain why inappropriate strategies, such as repressing anger or turning to alcohol, are not helpful. *The patient will be more willing to make changes that build on what has already worked in the past. The patient will also be more willing to reject inappropriate strategies if he or she is given a persuasive reason why they have not had the desired effect in managing previous crises.*

- Identify resources in the community (such as crisis hotlines and support groups) that can help the patient manage anxiety-producing situations. *The patient may not have support systems available, or the patient's significant others may be having their own difficulties in dealing with the cancer diagnosis. Programs such as "I Can Cope," sponsored by the ACS in most communities, provide education, counseling, and support in a group setting with other cancer patients.*
- Provide specific information for the patient about the disease, its treatment, and what may be expected, especially for those patients with obvious misinformation. *Knowing what is to come gives the patient a sense of control and enables the patient to make decisions. Also, knowing that every effort will be made to keep the patient as free of pain as possible can do a great deal to relieve anxiety.*
- Provide a safe, calm, and quiet environment for the patient in panic. Remain with the patient and administer anti-anxiety medications as ordered. *Staying with the patient and displaying calmness and confidence can protect the patient from injury and prevent further panic. If the panic does not subside with the nurse's presence and support, referral to the physician for medication management may be necessary.*
- Use crisis intervention theory to promote growth in the patient and significant others, regardless of the outcome of the disease. *During a major crisis, people can, with assistance, transform the experience from one that causes defeat and despair to one that enhances personal and spiritual growth. If you are not skilled in this area, a referral to an appropriate mental health professional may be helpful to the patient and family.*

Disturbed Body Image

Cancer and cancer treatments frequently result in major physiologic and psychological body image changes. Loss of a body part (e.g., amputation, prostatectomy, or mastectomy), skin changes and hair loss from chemotherapy or radiation therapy, disfigurement of body part (e.g., lymphedema in the affected upper and lower extremities), or creation of unnatural openings on the body for elimination (e.g., colostomy or ileostomy) may have a major effect on the person's self-image. The gaunt, wasted appearance of the cachectic patient or draining, malodorous lesions that result when cancer breaks through the skin are other significant etiologies of body image disturbance. This may give rise to fear of rejection, which plays a major role in sexual dysfunction. In addition to all of the other afflictions the cancer brings about, the patient may undergo major changes in appearance and function. The patient may exhibit a visible physical alteration of some portion of the body, verbalize negative feelings about the body and/or fear of rejection by others, refuse to look at the affected site, and depersonalize the body change or lost part (e.g., by calling the colostomy "that thing").

- Discuss the meaning of the loss or change with the patient. *Doing so helps the nurse discover the best approach for this particular patient and involves the patient more actively in interventions. A small, seemingly trivial loss may have a big impact, especially when viewed in light of the other changes that are occurring in the patient's life. Likewise, a major loss may not be as important as the nurse might imagine. To ensure more appropriate and individualized care, evaluate each situation in terms of the reactions of the specific patient.*

■ Observe and evaluate interaction with significant others. People who are important to the patient may unintentionally reinforce negative feelings about body image; on the other hand, the patient may perceive rejection where none exists.

■ Allow denial, but do not participate in it; for example, if a patient does not want to look at the wound, the nurse may say, "I am going to change the dressing to your breast incision now." *During the initial stage of shock at the loss of a body part, denial is a protective mechanism and should not be challenged, nor should it be promoted. A matter-of-fact approach and an empathetic attitude will go far to facilitate the eventual acceptance of the change.*

■ Assist the patient and significant others to cope with the changes in appearance:
a. Provide a supportive environment.
b. Encourage the patient and significant others to express feelings about the situation.
c. Give matter-of-fact responses to questions and concerns.
d. Identify new coping strategies to resolve feelings.
e. Enlist family and friends in reaffirming the patient's worth. *A supportive, safe environment in which feelings are respected and new coping strategies can be tried promotes acceptance, as does reaffirming that the patient's worth is not diminished by any physical changes.*

■ Teach the patient or significant others to participate in the care of the afflicted body area. Provide support and validation of their efforts. *Active involvement in providing care, such as changing a dressing or emptying a colostomy bag, empowers the patient and/or significant others. This intimate involvement also desensitizes feelings about disfigurement and promotes acceptance. Involving significant others reduces the risk of their rejecting the patient and can promote closeness. Positive reinforcement from the nurse encourages them to continue these behaviors.*

■ Teach strategies for minimizing physical changes, such as providing skin care during radiation therapy and dressing to enhance appearance and minimize change in the body part. *Early intervention can limit the negative side effects of treatment and actually promote recovery. Involving the patient provides an additional way for the patient to be in control of a difficult situation.*

■ Teach ways to reduce the alopecia that results from chemotherapy and to enhance appearance until the hair grows back:
a. Discuss the pattern and timing of hair loss. *This allows the patient to cope with changes and incorporate them into daily activities.*
b. Encourage wearing cheerful, brightly colored head coverings; assist in color coordinating them with usual clothing. *Attractive head coverings protect the bald head while allowing the patient to feel stylish and well dressed.*
c. Refer to a good wig shop before hair loss is experienced. *Hair color and texture can be matched to minimize obvious changes in appearance.*
d. Refer to support programs such as "Look Good...Feel Better," which is sponsored by the ACS and the Cosmetic, Toilet, and Fragrance Association Foundation. *A support group can diminish feelings of isolation and provide practical tips for managing problems. For a list of community resources available to patients with cancer, refer to a local phone book.*
e. Reassure that hair will grow back after chemotherapy is discontinued, but also inform that the color and texture of the new hair may be different. Hair loss has been identified as the most distressing symptom by many patients. *Interventions to reduce that loss can have a significant impact on body image concerns. Moreover, knowing what to expect may decrease anxiety and distress.*

Anticipatory Grieving

Anticipatory grieving is a response to loss that has not yet occurred. Overall, only 50% of people with cancer fully recover, and certain types of cancer have a much higher death rate; thus, the patient with cancer is often confronted with facing death and making preparations for it. This can be a healthy response that allows the patient and family to work through the dying process and achieve growth in the final stage of life. Perceived changes in body image and lifestyle also can prompt anticipatory grieving. The patient or significant others may show sorrow, anger, depression, or withdrawal, expressing distress at the potential loss or verbalizing concern about unfinished life business. (∞ See Chapter 5 for more on nursing care of the patient who is grieving or dying.)

■ Use the therapeutic communication skills of active listening, silence, and nonverbal support to provide an open environment for the patient and significant others to discuss their feelings realistically and to express anger or other negative feelings appropriately. *This helps the patient and family to get in touch with feelings and confront the possibility of the loss or death.*

■ Answer questions about illness and prognosis honestly, but always encourage hope. *This allows for realistic appraisal of the situation and planning, and it also helps combat feelings of hopelessness and depression.*

■ Encourage the dying patient to make funeral and burial plans ahead of time and to be sure the will is in order. Make sure the necessary phone numbers can be easily located. *This gives a sense of control and relieves family members of these concerns at a time when the patient is most in need of their support and when they themselves are extremely stressed.*

■ Encourage the patient to continue taking part in activities he or she enjoys, including maintaining employment as long as possible. *This gives a sense of continuity of life even in the face of severe losses.*

Risk for Infection

Malnutrition, impaired skin and mucous membrane integrity, tumor necrosis, and suppression of the WBCs from chemotherapy or radiation may contribute to the risk for infection. Anorexia, as well as the disease itself, deprives the body of nutrients needed for healing, while impaired integrity of skin and mucous membranes (a result of chemotherapy and/or radiation therapy) compromise the first lines of defense against microbial invasion. Cells in the center of large or not very vascular tumors may die from malnutrition, eventually eroding through tissues to increase the risk of sepsis. Bone marrow depression due to the effects of certain types of cancers and chemotherapy undermine the body's ability to respond to infection. The patient may exhibit the classic signs of infection: lassitude, fever, anorexia, pain in the affected area, and physical evidence of infection, such as a purulent, draining lesion or wound. If the bone marrow is compromised, the usual signs and symptoms of infection may be absent or reduced.

- Monitor vital signs. *Fever and sympathetic nervous system responses, such as increased pulse and respiration, are usual early signs of infection. However, severely immunosuppressed patients may be unable to mount a fever; therefore, the absence of fever cannot rule out infection.*
- Monitor WBC counts frequently, especially if the patient is receiving chemotherapy known to cause bone marrow suppression. *This allows the nurse to notify the physician at the first sign of diminishing WBC counts so that corrective action can be taken.*
- Teach the patient to avoid crowds, small children, and people with infections when WBC count is at nadir (lowest point during chemotherapy) and to practice scrupulous personal hygiene. *During periods of leukopenia, the patient may lose immunity to his or her own natural flora. Careful attention to hygiene reduces the risk of infection. Crowds, which promote contact with a greater variety of infectious agents, and friends with minor infections can be very dangerous for the immunosuppressed. Small children should be avoided because they often have microbes to which most people are usually immune but which the patient may not be able to resist.*
- Protect skin and mucous membranes from injury. Teach appropriate skin care measures, such as good hygiene, use of a moisturizing lotion to prevent dryness and cracking, frequent changes of position for the bed-bound, and immediate attention to skin breaks or lesions. *Ensuring intact skin strengthens the first line of defense against infection.*
- Encourage the patient to consume a diet high in protein, minerals, and vitamins, especially vitamin C. *Improving nutrition decreases the risk of infection. Vitamin C has been shown to help prevent certain types of infection, such as colds.*

Risk for Injury

In addition to infection, cancer can pose a risk for injury from, for example, obstruction by a large tumor or one located in a limited body space (e.g., in the brain, bowel, or bronchial airways). If the cancer is one that creates ectopic sites of hormones, elevated levels of hormones that are not under the control of the pituitary gland can injure the patient in a variety of ways. Signs of obstruction depend on the organ involved: Bowel obstruction presents with pain, distention, and cessation of bowel activities; obstruction in the brain gives signs of increased intracranial pressure or personality/behavioral change; bronchial obstruction manifests as respiratory distress, cyanosis, and altered arterial blood gases. Ectopic production of parathyroid hormone manifests as high serum calcium levels as well as signs of hypercalcemia; ectopic production of antidiuretic hormone causes fluid retention and manifests as hypertension and peripheral and pulmonary edema.

- Assess frequently for signs and symptoms indicating problems with organ obstruction. *Early detection of major problems allows the nurse to seek medical help before the problem evolves into a physiologic crisis.*
- Teach to differentiate minor problems from those of a serious nature. Encourage the patient to consult with the nurse

or physician if in doubt or to call 911 if the patient becomes very ill. Box 14–11 provides guidelines to help patients identify serious problems. *Having guidelines for when to call the doctor provides an anxiety-reducing safety net for the patient and family and promotes early detection of complications.*

- Monitor laboratory values that may indicate the presence of ectopic functioning and report abnormal findings to physicians immediately. (See Table 14–4 for laboratory indicators of ectopic functions.) *Early detection promotes early medical intervention and prevents serious consequences from the ectopic secretion.* Refer to Chapters 10, 19, and 20 for specific signs and symptoms of electrolyte imbalances and endocrine disorders.

Imbalanced Nutrition: Less than Body Requirements

The anorexia-cachexia syndrome (described earlier in this chapter) is a common cause of malnutrition in cancer patients. Metabolism increases in response to increased cancer cell production while the cancer's parasitic activity reduces the nutrients available to the body. Loss of appetite, food aversion, nausea and vomiting, and painful oral lesions from chemotherapy or radiation may contribute to impaired nutrition. Tumors of the gastrointestinal tract that affect absorption also contribute to the problem. Manifestations include wasted appearance, considerable weight loss over a relatively short period of time, anthropometric measurements below 85% of standard for fat and muscle tissue, decreases in serum proteins, and negative responses to antigen testing.

- Assess current eating patterns, including usual likes and dislikes, and identify factors that impair food intake. *This allows for a more individualized plan based on needs and preferences.*
- Evaluate degree of malnutrition:
  a. Check laboratory values for total serum protein, serum albumin and globins, total lymphocyte count, serum

BOX 14–11 When to Call for Help

Instruct the patient or family member to call the nurse or physician if any of the following manifestations are experienced:
- Oral temperature greater than 101.5°F (38.6°C)
- Severe headache; significant increase in pain at usual site, especially if the pain is not relieved by the medication regimen; or severe pain at a new site
- Difficulty breathing
- New bleeding from any site, such as rectal or vaginal bleeding
- Confusion, irritability, or restlessness
- Withdrawal, greatly decreased activity level, or frequent crying
- Verbalizations of deep sadness or a desire to end life
- Changes in body functioning, such as the inability to void or severe diarrhea or constipation
- Changes in eating patterns, such as refusal to eat, extreme hunger, or a significant increase in nausea and vomiting
- Appearance of edema in the extremities or significant increase in edema already present

Instruct the patient or family member to call 911 if the patient
- is having much difficulty breathing or if the lips or face have a bluish tinge.
- becomes unconscious or has a convulsion.
- exhibits unmanageable behavior, such as being physically abusive, hurting self, or engaging in uncontrollable activity.

transferrin, hemoglobin, and hematocrit. *These values represent the laboratory values that are most likely to decrease with malnutrition.*

b. Calculate nitrogen balance and creatinine-height index. Calculate skeletal muscle mass, and compare findings to normal ranges. *Urinary creatinine is an index of lean body mass and decreases in malnutrition. Lean muscle mass is catabolized for energy in patients with cancer.*

c. Take anthropometric measurements and compare them to standards: height, weight, elbow breadth, arm circumference, triceps skinfold thickness, and arm muscle mass. *This estimates the degree of wasting; findings below 85% of standard are considered malnutrition.*

■ Teach the principles of maintaining good nutrition by using the Food Guide Pyramid and adapting the diet to medical restrictions and current preferences. *This tailors the food plan to the patient's needs and thereby promotes compliance.*

■ Manage problems that interfere with eating:

a. Encourage eating whatever is appealing and consider adding nutritional supplements such as Ensure Plus or Isocal to diet. *It is better to eat something even if it is not nutritionally balanced.*

b. Eat small, frequent meals. *These are more easily digested and absorbed and usually better tolerated by the patient with anorexia.*

c. Encourage to try icy cold foods (such as ice cream) or those that are more highly seasoned if food has no taste. *Chemotherapy and radiation therapy may harm taste buds and prevent distinguishing the taste of foods. Strong seasonings and coldness make food more enjoyable to the patient with diminished taste. However, spicy foods are not recommended for patients with stomatitis.*

d. Encourage cold and bland semisoft and liquid foods with painful oropharyngeal ulcers; use a nonalcohol anesthetic mouthwash prior to eating. *These foods are less irritating to sensitive mucous membranes; deadening the pain can make chewing and swallowing easier.*

e. Manage nausea and vomiting by administering antiemetic drugs (around-the-clock medication may be an effective preventive measure). Encourage patient to eat small, frequent, low-fat meals with dry foods such as crackers and toast, to avoid liquids with meals, and to sit upright for an hour after meals. Remove emesis basins, and encourage oral hygiene before eating. *Dry, low-fat foods are more readily tolerated when nauseated. Removing vomiting cues, such as odor and supplies associated with vomiting, can reduce nausea.*

■ Teach to supplement meals with nutritional supplements such as Ensure Plus or Isocal and to take multivitamin and mineral tablets with meals. Suggest increasing calories by adding ice cream or frozen yogurt to the liquid supplement or commercial protein-carbohydrate powders to milk or fruit juice. *Because the food intake is usually less than that needed to maintain or gain weight, these supplements can add calories in a manner often tolerated.*

■ Teach to keep a food diary to document daily intake. *If the patient can see how little is being consumed, he or she may eat more. A food diary also helps the nurse keep a calorie count and alert the physician if more drastic nutritional*

measures, such as a feeding tube or parenteral nutrition, need to be instituted.

■ Teach to administer parenteral nutrition via a central line or other VAD. Teach safety measures and care of the VAD, and explain how the pump delivering the solution works. Provide an emergency phone number for help with administration problems. (∞ See Chapter 22 for safety guidelines for administering parenteral nutrition.) *The patient with chronic or terminal cancer requiring parenteral nutrition is usually managed at home, so information on how to manage the entire process may be needed.*

Impaired Tissue Integrity

The most common impairment of tissue integrity occurs in the oral-pharyngeal-esophageal mucous membranes. It is secondary to the effects of some chemotherapeutic drugs and radiation treatment to the head and neck. The oral-pharyngeal-esophageal tissues are lined with cells with a high mitotic turnover rate and are therefore vulnerable to many chemotherapeutic drugs. Leukemias, bone marrow transplants, and herpes viral infections are other etiologic factors in the disruption of oral-pharyngeal-esophageal tissue. Manifestations of this problem may include the following:

■ Small ulcers occur on the tongue and mucous membranes in the mouth and throat.

■ Herpes simplex type 1 lesions or vesicles evolve into ulcerations.

■ Fungal infections, such as thrush (due to *Candida* infections), are manifested by a white, yellow, or tan coating with dry, red, fissured tissue underneath.

■ Red, swollen, friable gums bleed with minimal or no trauma.

■ **Xerostomia** is excessive dryness of the mucous membranes (due to chemotherapy or radiation).

Manage such problems with the following interventions:

■ Carefully assess and evaluate the type of tissue impairment present. Identify possible sources, such as chemotherapy or radiation therapy to head and neck. *This allows the nurse to implement corrective measures appropriate to the type of problem.*

■ Implement and teach measures for preventing oropharyngeal infection:

a. Observe for systemic signs of infection. Be suspicious of any fever that has no apparent cause. *This facilitates early identification of an infection before it spreads.*

b. Encourage cleaning teeth gently and using a nonalcohol mouthwash several times a day. This can be done after waking up in the morning, after any oral intake, and before bedtime. Soak dentures nightly in hydrogen peroxide and floss gently with waxed floss after meals and bedtime; this measure may be contraindicated for people with leukemia or thrombocytopenia. *Disrupted mucous membranes allow the normal oral bacterial flora into the systemic circulation, which can result in sepsis in the immunocompromised person. Reducing the oral flora by frequent hygiene decreases the risk of infection.*

c. Culture any oral lesions, and report the problem to the physician. Herpes lesions may not follow a typical pattern in immunosuppressed patients. *Identifying the cause of the infection, whether viral, fungal, or bacterial, allows the physician to prescribe the appropriate treatment.*

- Implement and teach measures for reducing trauma to delicate tissues:
  a. Counteract dry mouth (xerostomia) with lubricating and moisturizing agents, such as Gatorade, sugarless gum, and Blistex. *This protects mucous membranes from infection and trauma.*
  b. Avoid putting sharp instruments in the mouth. Use smooth plastic spoons and forks for eating, especially with a bleeding disorder. Dental work should be done by dental oncologists.
  c. Brush teeth with a very soft toothbrush and obtain a new toothbrush monthly. If gums are friable and bleeding, clean teeth with a soft cloth or toothpaste over finger. Chlorhexidine mouthwash (Peridex) may be used. *This protects gums from trauma and decreases risk of hemorrhage.*
- Administer specific medications as ordered to control infection and/or pain:
  a. Acyclovir is often used to treat viral infections.
  b. Systemic antibiotics are used to treat bacterial infections.
  c. Nystatin or clotrimazole solution for "swish and swallow" or lozenges that dissolve slowly in the mouth are used for fungal infections.
  d. Use viscous Xylocaine or various combination mouthwashes before meals and as needed. These agents reduce pain and inflammation. See Box 14–12 for the ingredients of combination mouthwashes. *Knowing the contents of each mouthwash can prevent hypersensitivity reactions (e.g., to lidocaine) and assist in patient teaching.*

Nursing Interventions for Oncologic Emergencies

In caring for patients with cancer, nurses may encounter a number of emergency situations in which their role may be pivotal to the patient's survival. Most of these emergencies require astute observations, accurate judgments, and rapid action once the problem has been identified. A brief description of the more common **oncologic emergencies** with nursing interventions follows. In all cases, immediate notification of the physician or emergency team is the first step.

BOX 14–12 Combination Mouthwashes for Oropharyngeal Pain Control

Kaiser Mouthwash
- Nystatin
- Hydrocortisone
- Tetracycline

Stanford Mouthwash
- Nystatin
- Tetracycline
- Lidocaine
- Hydrocortisone

Xyloxylin Suspension
- Benylin syrup
- Lidocaine
- Maalox suspension

Stomafate Suspension
- Sucralfate
- Sterile water
- Benylin syrup
- Maalox suspension

Pericardial Effusions and Neoplastic Cardiac Tamponade

Malignant pericardial effusion is an accumulation of excess fluid in the pericardial sac that compresses the heart, restricts heart movement, and results in a cardiac tamponade. The signs of cardiac tamponade are caused by compression of the heart, which leads to decreased cardiac output and impaired cardiac function. Signs include hypotension, tachycardia, tachypnea, dyspnea, cyanosis, increased central venous pressure, anxiety, restlessness, and impaired consciousness.

Interventions include the following:

- Start oxygen and alert respiratory therapy for other respiratory support as needed.
- Insert an intravenous catheter if one is not already in place.
- Monitor vital signs and initiate hemodynamic monitoring.
- Prepare vasopressor drugs.
- Bring emergency cart to bedside.
- Set up for and assist physician with a pericardial tap (pericardiocentesis).
- Reassure the patient.

Superior Vena Cava Syndrome

The superior vena cava can be compressed by mediastinal tumors or adjacent thoracic tumors. The most common cause is small-cell or squamous-cell lung cancers. Occasionally the problem is caused by thrombus around a central venous catheter that then plugs up the vena cava, resulting in obstruction and backup of the blood flowing into the superior vena cava.

Obstruction of the venous system causes increased venous pressure, venous stasis, and engorgement of veins that are drained by the superior vena cava. Signs and symptoms may develop slowly; facial, periorbital, and arm edema are early signs. As the problem progresses, respiratory distress, dyspnea, cyanosis, tachypnea, and altered consciousness and neurologic deficits may occur. Figure 14–7 ■ illustrates the superior venal cava syndrome.

Emergency measures include the following:

- Provide respiratory support with oxygen, and prepare for tracheostomy.
- Monitor vital signs.
- Administer corticosteroids (e.g., dexamethasone) to reduce edema.
- If the disorder is due to a clot, administer antifibrinolytic or anticoagulant drugs.
- Provide a safe environment, including seizure precautions.

After the emergency is managed, the patient often receives radiation or chemotherapy to reduce the tumor size.

Sepsis and Septic Shock

Tumor necrosis, immune deficiency, antineoplastic therapy, malnutrition, and comorbid conditions can lead to the development of sepsis. Bacteria gain entrance to the blood, grow rapidly, and produce septicemia. Because malignant tumors are more likely to use anaerobic metabolic pathways, the bacteria of tumor sepsis are usually gram negative and damage the body through a combination of bacterial endotoxins and an uncontrolled immune reaction. Gram-negative sepsis progresses to systemic shock and eventually results in multisystem failure. Signs and symptoms appear in two phases. The first phase is characterized by vasodilation with vascular dehydration, high fever, peripheral edema,

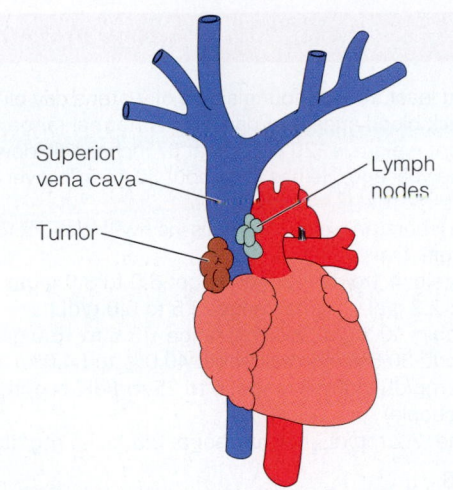

Figure 14–7 ■ The superior vena cava syndrome. The enlargement of a tumor adjacent to the superior vena cava (usually in the lung or mediastinum) compresses that major blood vessel, which leads into the right atrium of the heart. As a result, blood backs up into the venous system behind the obstruction, diminishing blood flow into the heart.

hypotension, tachycardia, tachypnea, hot flushed skin with creeping mottling beginning in the lower extremities, and anxiety or restlessness. Without treatment, the shock progresses to the second phase, which shows the more classic signs of shock: hypotension, rapid thready pulse, respiratory distress, cyanosis, subnormal temperature, cold clammy skin, decreased urinary output, and altered mentation. Identifying the problem while the patient is still in the hyperdynamic state is crucial to the patient's survival. ∞ See Chapter 11 for further discussion of septic shock.

Spinal Cord Compression

Spinal cord compression is most commonly associated with pressure from expanding tumors of the breast, lung, or prostate; lymphoma; or metastatic disease. Spinal cord compression constitutes an emergency because of the potential for irreversible paraplegia. Back pain is the initial symptom in almost all cases of spinal cord compression. This may progress to leg pain, numbness, paresthesias, and coldness. Later, bowel and bladder dysfunction occur and, finally, neurologic dysfunction progressing from weakness to paralysis. Treatment often consists of radiation or surgical decompression, but early detection is essential. ∞ See Chapter 43 for further discussion of spinal cord compression.

Obstructive Uropathy

Patients with intra-abdominal, retroperitoneal, or pelvic malignancies, such as prostate, cervical, or bladder cancers, may experience obstruction of the bladder neck or the ureters. Bladder neck obstruction usually manifests as urinary retention, flank pain, hematuria, or persistent urinary tract infections, but ureteral obstruction is not often evident until the patient is in renal failure. ∞ See Chapter 28 for further discussion of obstructive uropathy.

Hypercalcemia

Hypercalcemia in patients with cancer results from the excessive ectopic production of parathyroid hormone and is most commonly associated with cancers of the breast, lung, esophagus, thyroid, head, and neck and with multiple myeloma. Bone metastases may also cause hypercalcemia. When the rate of calcium mobilization

from the bone exceeds the renal threshold for excretion, serum calcium levels can become dangerously elevated. Patients with hypercalcemia often present with nonspecific symptoms of fatigue, anorexia, nausea, polyuria, and constipation. Neurologic symptoms include muscle weakness, lethargy, apathy, and diminished reflexes. Without treatment, hypercalcemia progresses to alterations in mental status, psychotic behavior, cardiac arrhythmias, seizures, coma, and death (∞ see Chapter 10).

Hyperuricemia

Hyperuricemia usually is a complication of rapid necrosis of tumor cells after vigorous chemotherapy for lymphomas and leukemias. Hyperuricemia may be related to increased uric acid production or to the tumor lysis syndrome associated with Burkitt's lymphoma. Uric acid crystals are deposited in the urinary tract, causing renal failure and uremia. Patients with hyperuricemia manifest with nausea, vomiting, lethargy, and oliguria.

Tumor Lysis Syndrome

Tumor lysis syndrome (TLS) is a life-threatening emergency for patients with cancer. TLS is characterized by a combination of two or more metabolic abnormalities, including hyperuricemia, hyperphosphatemia, hyperkalemia, and/or hypocalcemia (Cairo & Bishop, 2004). The syndrome develops because of massive and rapid destruction or death of cancer cells caused by cytotoxic treatment such as chemotherapy, radiation, biologic therapy, hormonal therapy, and surgery. It can occur spontaneously with sudden death of tumor cells. A high incidence of TLS occurs in patients with bulky, highly proliferating, and chemosensitive tumors such as high-grade lymphomas (Burkitt's lymphoma) and acute leukemia (ALL). Although the incidence of TLS in solid tumors is rare, cases of TLS following chemotherapy have been reported in patients with small-cell lung cancer, breast cancer, neuroblastoma, melanoma, and ovarian cancer.

The major cause of TLS is chemotherapy to tumors with a high proliferative rate, a relatively large tumor burden, and high sensitivity to cytotoxic agents, which leads to massive and rapid cell death. Usually, within a week of initiating chemotherapy, the body no longer can excrete the large amount of metabolic by-products from the cell death, resulting in the release of intracellular contents and metabolic by-products (such as potassium, phosphorus, and nucleic acid) into the bloodstream (Cairo & Bishop, 2004). As a result, a combination of metabolic derangements occurs, including hyperkalemia, hyperuricemia, and hyperphosphatemia with secondary hypocalcemia (Cairo & Bishop, 2004). These metabolic abnormalities put patients at risk for cardiac malfunction and renal failure.

Manifestations of TLS include nausea, vomiting, lethargy, edema, fluid overload, congestive heart failure, cardiac dysrhythmias, seizures, muscle cramps, tetany, syncope, and possible sudden death (Cairo & Bishop, 2004). Diagnosis of TLS mainly depends on laboratory tests and clinical signs and symptoms. Prevention is crucial in management of TLS. Patients at risk for TLS include those with bulky chemosensitive cancer such as high-grade lymphomas and acute leukemia, elevated serum uric acid, potassium, phosphorus, and renal deficiency. Preventive and management measures include identifying patients at risk, administration of allopurinol to inhibit the conversion of nucleic acid to uric acid, hydration and

CASE STUDY & NURSING CARE PLAN   A Patient with Cancer

James Casey, aged 72, is of northern European heritage. He has been receiving medical care for chronic obstructive pulmonary disease, chronic bronchitis, status postmyocardial infarction, and type I diabetes mellitus for over 15 years. He reports that he lost his wife from lung cancer 5 years ago and still "misses her terribly." He describes his bad habits as smoking two packs of cigarettes a day for 52 years (104 packs/year), one to two six-packs of beer a week, one "bourbon and water" a night, and "a lot of sugar-free junk food, like french fries." He assures the nurse that he quit smoking 2 years ago, when he could no longer walk a block without considerable shortness of breath, and just quit drinking alcohol a few weeks ago at his physician's insistence. About a year ago, he had a basal-cell carcinoma removed from his right ear. Six months ago, cancerous tumors were discovered in his bladder, and he underwent two 6-week chemotherapy courses of bladder instillations of BCG. His latest report indicates that the tumors have grown back and no further chemotherapy would be useful. The urologist had considered surgery but believed that Mr. Casey's other medical problems would compromise his chances of survival. Mr. Casey decides to let the disease run its course and to be managed at home through hospice care. Because he lives alone in a modest home, he asks his daughter, Mary, and her family to move in with him to provide care and support during his final months. The daughter accepts, saying she is glad to be able to spend this time with her father; she has been informed of the physical and emotional stress this will entail.

ASSESSMENT

Glynis Jackson, RN, the hospice nurse assigned as case manager for Mr. Casey, completes a health history and physical examination during her first two visits in his home, 1 day apart. She gathers this information over 2 days to conserve his strength and allow more time for Mr. Casey and his daughter to talk about their concerns.

During the physical assessment, Ms. Jackson notes that Mr. Casey is pale with pink mucous membranes, thin with a wasted appearance and a strained, worried facial expression. He complains of severe back pain no longer adequately relieved by Percodan and Vicodin alternating every 2 to 4 hours. His blood pressure is 90/50, right arm in the reclining position with no significant orthostatic change; his apical pulse is 102, regular and strong; respiratory rate 24 and unlabored; breath sounds are clear but diminished in the bases; oral temperature is 96.8°F.

A tunneled Groshong catheter as a VAD is present in the right anterior chest. There is no drainage, redness, or swelling at the site. The catheter was placed last week when the patient was being evaluated at the anesthesiologist's office for pain management, but no medication is running via the VAD. Mary reports that his urinary output is adequate. Approximately 200 mL of yellow, cloudy, nonmalodorous urine is present in the urinal at the bedside from his last voiding.

Mr. Casey states that he spends most of his time either in bed or sitting up in a chair in his room. He reports that he has no energy any more and is unable to walk to the bathroom unassisted, dress himself, or take care of his own personal hygiene. Ms. Jackson rates Mr. Casey's functional level at ECOG level 4: capable of only limited self-care, confined to bed or chair 50% or more of waking hours (Karnofsky 10 to 20). He tells the nurse that his daughter "is working day and night to help me and is looking awfully tired."

Mary reports that Mr. Casey is eating very poorly: He usually eats a small bowl of oatmeal with milk for breakfast and vegetable soup and crackers for lunch, but he tells her that he is too tired for dinner and wants only fruit juice. Mr. Casey tells the nurse that he has no appetite and eats just to please Mary. He

does drink at least three to four glasses of water a day plus juice. His fingerstick blood sugars remain within normal range.

His current weight is 120 pounds at 67 inches tall, down from 180 pounds a year ago. He has lost about 30 pounds over the last 2 months.

Available laboratory values from his visit with the doctor show the following:

Total protein: 4.1 g/dL (normal range: 6.0 to 8.0 g/dL)
Albumin: 2.2 g/dL (normal range: 3.5 to 5.0 g/dL)
Hemoglobin: 10.2 g/dL (normal range: 13.5 to 18.0 g/dL)
Hematocrit: 30.5% (normal range: 40.0% to 54.0%)
BUN: 30 mg/dL (normal range: 5 to 25 mg/dL, slightly higher in older people)
Creatinine: 2.2 mg/dL (normal range: 0.5 to 1.5 mg/dL)

DIAGNOSES

- *Imbalanced Nutrition: Less than Body Requirements* related to anorexia and fatigue
- *Risk for Caregiver Role Strain* related to severity of her father's illness and lack of help from other family members
- *Chronic Pain* related to progression of disease process
- *Impaired Physical Mobility* related to pain, fatigue, and beginning neuromuscular impairment
- *Risk for Impaired Skin Integrity* related to impaired physical mobility and malnourished state

EXPECTED OUTCOMES

- Increase oral intake and show improvement in serum protein values.
- Experience minimal pain for the rest of his life.
- Able to continue his current activity level.
- Maintain intact skin.
- Continue receiving support and care from his daughter.

PLANNING AND IMPLEMENTATION

- Ask about favorite foods, and ask Mary to offer a small portion of one of these foods each day.
- Encourage drinking up to four cans of liquid nutritional supplement with fiber a day, sipping them throughout the day.
- Talk with the physician about prescribing a medication to help stimulate the appetite.
- Refer to home health agency to have a home health aide come to the home, give him a shower or bed bath daily, and assist his daughter with some of the household chores.
- Talk with Mary about having her adult son and daughter relieve her of the housework and stay with Mr. Casey so that she can get out of the house occasionally. Offer to talk with them if she is uncomfortable doing so.
- Request a volunteer to spend up to 4 hours a day, twice a week with Mr. Casey so that Mary can attend to outside activities and chores.
- Talk with the anesthesiologist, and work out a pain control program, using the VAD and a CADD-PCA infusion pump with a continuous morphine infusion.
- Call the infusion therapist to set up the equipment and supplies (including the medication) for the morphine infusion.
- Teach how to use the pump and about the side effects of the morphine infusion, including those that require a call to the nurse for assistance. Teach which untoward effects should be reported.
- Request a physical therapy consultation to evaluate current level of functioning and determine how to maintain current level.
- Instruct Mary to allow ample rest periods for Mr. Casey between activities.
- Order a hospital bed with electronic controls to be delivered to the house.

CASE STUDY & NURSING CARE PLAN   A Patient with Cancer (continued)

- Order a special foam pad for bed and chair and a bedside commode from the medical supply house.
- Instruct Mary and the home health aide to inspect skin daily, give good skin care with emollient lotion after bathing, and report any beginning lesions immediately to the nurse.

EVALUATION

James Casey did increase his oral intake a little, sometimes eating the special treats his daughter prepared and drinking one or two cans of liquid nutritional supplement a day. However, his weight did not increase; it stayed at about 120 pounds until his death 2 weeks later. His daughter was very grateful for the extra help from the home health aide and the volunteer, though she could not bring herself to ask her son and daughter for help and did not want the nurse to do so. She did become more rested and reported that "Dad and I had some wonderful 3:00 AM talks when he couldn't sleep."

Mr. Casey was started on 20 mg of morphine per hour with boluses of 10 mg 4 times a day for breakthrough pain. This medication relieved his pain quite well; after 2 days he was alert enough most of the time to carry on a normal conversation and still walk to the bathroom with help up until 2 days before he died.

The hospital bed simplified Mr. Casey's care and made it much easier for him to rest comfortably and change position. His skin remained intact and in good condition.

Mary reported that Mr. Casey died peacefully in his sleep, about 2 weeks after care was started. She said spending the last weeks of his life together was a healing experience for both of them.

CRITICAL THINKING IN THE NURSING PROCESS

1. What other tests could be done to evaluate Mr. Casey's nutritional status?
2. Mr. Casey had severe back pain. What were the possible pathophysiologic reasons for his pain?
3. One of the specified interventions was to consult the physician regarding medication to increase Mr. Casey's appetite. What medications might fulfill that function? What side effects might they have that would contraindicate these medications for him?
4. If Mr. Casey had developed signs and symptoms of sepsis, what manifestations would you expect to see? As the nurse making the home visits, what would be your nursing actions, and in what order of priority?

See Evaluating Your Response in Appendix C.

---

diuretic therapy to promote urinary excretion of uric acid and phosphate, urine alkalinization to promote the urinary excretion of uric acid, administration of oral phosphate binder such as aluminum hydroxide to promote the excretion of phosphate through the bowel, administration of sodium polystyrene sulfonate (Kayexalate) to promote the excretion of potassium through the bowel, and initiation of hemodialysis to patients unresponsive to standard approaches to hyperkalemia, hyperuricemia, or hyperphosphatemia (Cairo & Bishop, 2004).

Using NANDA, NIC, and NOC

Linkages between a selected NANDA nursing diagnosis, NIC, and NOC for the patient with cancer are shown in the chart that follows.

NANDA, NIC, AND NOC LINKAGES
The Patient with Cancer

NANDA	Chronic Pain
NIC	Pain Management Medication Management
NOC	Pain Control Comfort Level Pain: Disruptive Effects Pain Occurrence Pain Severity Pain Distress Pain Experience

Adapted from Bulechek, G., Butcher, H., & Dochterman, J. M. (Eds.). (2008). *Nursing interventions classification (NIC)* (5th ed.). St. Louis: Mosby Elsevier; and Moorhead, S., Johnson, M., Maas, M., & Swanson, E. (Eds.). (2008). *Nursing outcomes classification (NOC)* (4th ed.). St. Louis: Mosby Elsevier. A full listing of interventions and outcomes may be found in these books.

Health Education for the Patient
Prevention

The ACS makes specific recommendations for cancer prevention in addition to the screening measures discussed earlier in this chapter (see Box 14–13). Encourage people to report to the public health department any known leaking of chemicals or radioactive materials into the water or air and any noted increase in the incidence of cancer, especially of one specific type, in their communities.

Rehabilitation and Survival

Rehabilitation from cancer not only involves regaining strength, recovering from surgery or chemotherapy, and learning to live with an altered body part or appliance, but also entails recovering from associated psychological and emotional turmoil.

Rehabilitation centers provide physical therapy, occupational therapy, speech therapy, job retraining, and an opportunity to recuperate before resuming full responsibilities. In addition, many patients go home to convalesce and receive in-home support in the form of nursing supervision, direct care, and teaching. Hygiene and home maintenance can be provided

BOX 14–13 American Cancer Society Dietary Guidelines to Prevent Cancer

- Avoid obesity.
- Cut down on total fat intake.
- Include a variety of vegetables and fruits in the daily diet.
- Eat more high-fiber foods, such as whole-grain cereals, vegetables, and fruits.
- Limit consumption of alcoholic beverages, if you drink at all.
- Limit consumption of salt-cured, smoked, and nitrate-cured foods.

Source: From the American Cancer Society, 2010a.

by a certified home health aide. Physical and occupational therapists provide muscle strengthening and mobility training (especially with prostheses), and home safety teaching.

Psychological rehabilitation of cancer survivors addresses quality-of-life issues. Three "seasons of cancer survival" have been described (Mullan, 1985). The first starts with diagnosis but is dominated by treatment. The second stage is one of extended survival, which occurs when treatment ends and the watchful waiting period begins. This period is characterized by fear of recurrence. Permanent survival is said to begin when the survival period has gone on long enough that the risk of recurrence is small. In this period, the patient has to deal with secondary problems related to health and social issues resulting from the cancer experience. Employment may be a problem, health insurance may be canceled, and life insurance may be difficult to get. Relationships may have suffered from the strain of the illness on significant others and the essential self-focusing required for recovery. Both the patient and significant others may have undergone a personal and spiritual growth that ushers in a new and enriching period of their lives.

New self-help groups are emerging in many communities to support others through their "seasons of survival." Many cancer survivors speak to groups about assisting other cancer survivors. Patients and families need to be informed about the resources available through community agencies as well as the survivor support groups.

Community-Based Care

Before the patient is discharged, teach both the patient and significant others or caregivers to manage the patient at home. Discuss problems that may result from the type of cancer and the treatment received, and provide information on how to manage these problems and when to call the physician.

- Teach wound care to the patient with an open wound or draining lesion, and provide a referral to a home health nurse to monitor progress.
- Explain special diets clearly, or refer the patient to a dietitian before discharge.
- Carefully review the physician's instructions with the patient and family, making sure they understand medications to be taken, any other treatments, and when to see the doctor for follow-up care.
- Provide or order equipment and supplies needed for home care, especially any specialized bed or equipment to aid mobility and ensure safety in the home.
- For the patient who will need complex care, such as parenteral nutrition, provide a referral to a home health nurse before discharge.

Because the hospital stay is often short, the patient and family will benefit from follow-up phone calls at home for several days. People do not learn well under the stress of going home; give the patient and family a number to call if they have concerns or questions.

Hospice Care

More and more patients with terminal cancer disease are electing to die at home. This decision has been made easier by the increased availability of **hospice** programs. When a patient and family or significant others elect hospice care, they are usually precluding additional hospitalizations other than those required to manage reversible problems.

Many hospice services are connected with an inpatient respite care unit, where the patient can receive 24-hour care for up to several weeks. This source provides the necessary care to the patient if a family member becomes ill or needs to be relieved temporarily of the tremendous burden of caring for a dying loved one. ∞ Chapter 5 provides more information on hospice care.

CHAPTER HIGHLIGHTS

- One in every four deaths in the United States is caused by cancer and more than 1500 people die of cancer each day. Cancer can affect people of any age, gender, ethnicity, or geographic region.
- Cancer is the second leading cause of death in people over age 65. The incidence of cancer increases with advancing age. The most commonly seen cancers in older women are colorectal, breast, lung, pancreatic, and ovarian. In older men, lung, colorectal, prostate, pancreatic, and gastric cancers occur most frequently.
- Oncogenes are genes that promote cell proliferation and are capable of triggering cancerous characteristics. Several oncogenes, such as BRCA-1 and BRCA-2, are associated with breast cancer.
- Tumor suppressor genes, which normally suppress oncogenes, can become inactive by deletion or mutation. Inherited cancers have been associated with tumor suppressor genes, such as p53, a suppressor gene that has been associated with sarcoma and cancer of the breast and brain.

- The diagnosis and treatment of cancer is a pivotal, life-changing event that prompts individuals to make immediate and ongoing adjustment to this life-threatening illness.
- Effective physical and psychosocial adjustment to cancer diagnosis and treatment has been shown to lead to successful completion of treatment, enhancement of cancer patients' ability to cope with disease, improvement of patients' quality of life, and ultimately, improvement of survival.
- The goals of cancer treatment are aimed at cure and control of cancer as well as management of cancer-related and treatment-related symptoms.
- Chemotherapy uses cytotoxic medications to cure or control cancer by interrupting cell metabolism and replication and by interfering with the ability of the malignant cell to synthesize vital enzymes and chemicals.

- Pain management is an important component of care for cancer patients. It is estimated that 20% to 50% of patients with early-stage cancer and up to 95% of patients with advanced cancer experience pain.
- Complementary therapies are therapies that patients choose as a complement to medical treatment. Common complementary therapies for cancer include botanical agents, nutritional supplements, dietary regimens, mind-body modalities, spiritual approaches, and miscellaneous therapies.

- Tumor lysis syndrome (TLS), a combination of two or more metabolic abnormalities, is a life-threatening emergency for patients with cancer. Patients at risk for TLS include those with bulky chemosensitive cancer such as high-degrade lymphomas and acute leukemia; elevated serum uric acid, potassium, and phosphorus; and renal deficiency.

TEST YOURSELF NCLEX-RN® REVIEW

1. A patient has a history of colon cancer. Cells from the colon tumor have traveled to his liver. What is this process called?
   1. carcinogenesis
   2. dysplasia
   3. metastasis
   4. mutation
2. A patient diagnosed with lung cancer reports he is having difficulty sleeping and often feels tense. What would be the most appropriate initial nursing intervention?
   1. Encourage the patient to express his feelings about the cancer diagnosis.
   2. Document the patient's report of difficulty sleeping and tenseness in the chart.
   3. Obtain an order for medication for sleep from the physician.
   4. Offer an anti-anxiety drug such as Ativan (lorazepam).
3. A patient is receiving external radiation for treatment of lung cancer. What would the nurse teach the patient about care of the skin in the marked area?
   1. Apply antibacterial ointment daily.
   2. Avoid contact with others.
   3. Avoid rubbing or scratching treated skin areas.
   4. Cleanse the skin with plain water.
4. A patient states she is having nausea and vomiting following her daily chemotherapy treatment. What would be the *most* appropriate nursing intervention?
   1. Keep the patient NPO until her daily chemotherapy is completed.
   2. Provide antiemetic medication 30 to 40 minutes prior to each treatment.
   3. Provide clear liquids until the chemotherapy is completed.
   4. Schedule chemotherapy administration for bedtime.
5. A patient experiences bone marrow depression as a result of chemotherapy. Which of the following assessments would the nurse expect to find?
   1. alopecia
   2. nausea and vomiting
   3. platelet count 50,000
   4. temperature 102°F

6. A 46-year-old businessman with a diagnosis of metastatic lung cancer is going to have chemotherapy tomorrow. To help him better understand the role of chemotherapeutic agents in treating cancer, the nurse has completed teaching him about chemotherapy. The nurse determines that the teaching is effective when the patient states which of the following?
   1. "Chemotherapy uses drugs that promote the normal growth of cells while killing the cancer cells."
   2. "Chemotherapy only uses a single drug to treat cancer because drug resistance is rare."
   3. "Chemotherapy includes drugs that not only attack cancer cells but also normal rapidly dividing cells."
   4. "Chemotherapy is a preferred therapy because it has fewer adverse effects than radiation therapy."
7. During training for new radiation nurses, the nurses learn about the delivery of high-energy radiation (e.g., electrons, x-rays, photons) to kill cancer cells by using a machine to focus a beam of radiation on the body. What is this called?
   1. external radiation therapy
   2. internal-beam radiation therapy
   3. brachytherapy
   4. biochemotherapy
8. A nurse is taking care of a patient who just received the first cycle of chemotherapy for acute leukemia 2 days ago. The patient's laboratory tests of uric acid, potassium, phosphorus, and calcium are closely monitored, based on the knowledge that the patient is at risk for what complication?
   1. spinal cord compression
   2. tumor lysis syndrome
   3. septic shock
   4. superior vena cava syndrome
9. In what phase of the cell cycle does DNA replicate to form two sets of chromosomes?
   1. G_1
   2. G_2
   3. S
   4. M
10. What is a characteristic of oncogenes?
    1. They promote cell growth when activated.
    2. They block cell growth.
    3. They stimulate a complex signaling process.
    4. They are strictly regulated.

See Test Yourself answers in Appendix C.

BIBLIOGRAPHY

American Cancer Society. (2010a). *Cancer facts and figures—2009.* Atlanta: Author.

American Cancer Society. (2009). *Cancer facts and figures for African Americans—2009–2010.* Atlanta: Author.

American Cancer Society. (2010b). *Cancer facts and figures for Hispanics/Latinos—2009–2010.* Atlanta: Author.

Andres, E., Federici, L., Weitten, T., Vogel, T., Alt, M. (2008). Recognition and management of drug-induced blood cytopenias: The example of drug-induced acute neutropenia and agranulocytosis. *Expert Opinion on Drug Safety, 7*(4), 481–489.

Armaiz-Pena, G. N., Lutgendorf, S. K., Cole, S. W., Sood, A. K. (2009). Neuroendocrine modulation of cancer progression. *Brain, Behavior, & Immunity, 23*(1), 10–15.

Bauer, M. E. (2008). Chronic stress and immunosenescence: A review. *Neuroimmunomodulation, 15*(4-6), 241–250.

Bodles-Brakhop, A. M., & Draghia-Akli, R. (2008). DNA vaccination and gene therapy: Optimization and delivery for cancer therapy. *Expert Review of Vaccines, 7*(7), 1085–1101.

Cairo, M. S., & Bishop, M. (2004). Tumour lysis syndrome: New therapeutic strategies and classification. *British Journal of Haematology, 127*(1), 3–11.

Deandrea, S., Montanari, M., Moja, L., Apolone, G. (2008). Prevalence of undertreatment in cancer pain. A review of published literature. *Annals of Oncology, 19*(12), 1985–1991.

De la Fuente, M. (2008). Role of neuroimmunomodulation in aging. *Neuroimmunomodulation, 15*(4-6), 213–223.

DeLancey, J. O., Thun, M. J., Jemal, A., & Ward, E. M. (2008). Recent trends in Black-White disparities in cancer mortality. *Cancer Epidemiology, Biomarkers & Prevention, 17*(11), 2908–2912.

di Pietro, A., Tosti, G., Ferrucci, P. F., Testori, A. (2008). Oncophage: Step to the future for vaccine therapy in melanoma. *Expert Opinion on Biological Therapy, 8*(12), 1973–1984.

Dragun, A. E., Harper, J. L., Jenrette, J. M., Sinha, D., & Cole, D. J. (2007). Predictors of cosmetic outcome following MammoSite breast brachytherapy: A single-institution experience of 100 patients with two years of follow-up. *International Journal of Radiation Oncology, Biology, Physics, 68*(2), 354–358.

Eaton, K. D., & Frieze, D. A. (2008). Cancer pain: Perspectives of a medical oncologist. *Current Pain & Headache Reports, 12*(4), 270–276.

Eccles, D. M. (2008). Identification of personal risk of breast cancer: Genetics. *Breast Cancer Research, 10,*(Suppl 4), S12.

Farquhar, C., Marjoribanks, J., Basser, R., Hetrick, S., & Lethaby, A. (2006). High dose chemotherapy and autologous bone marrow or stem cell transplantation versus conventional chemotherapy for women with metastatic breast cancer. *Cochrane Breast Cancer Group Cochrane Database of Systematic Reviews (3).*

Forbes, S. A. Bhamra, G., Bamford, S., Dawson, E., Kok, C., Clements, J., Menzies, A., Teague, J. W., Futreal, P. A., & Stratton, M. R. (2008). The Catalogue of Somatic Mutations in Cancer (COSMIC). *Current Protocols in Human Genetics* (Chapter 10: Unit 10.11).

Fu, M. R., Xu, B., Liu, Y., Haber, J. (2008). "Making the best of it": Chinese women's experiences of adjusting to breast cancer diagnosis and treatment. *Journal of Advanced Nursing, 63*(2), 155–165.

Karnofsky, D., Abelmann, W., Craver, L., & Burchenal, J. (1948). The use of nitrogen mustard in the palliative treatment of carcinoma. *Cancer, 1,* 634–656.

Kwitniewski, M., Juzeniene, A., Glosnicka, R., Moan, J. (2008). Immunotherapy: A way to improve the therapeutic outcome of photodynamic therapy? *Photochemical & Photobiological Sciences, 7*(9), 1011–1017.

Maeda, N., Fan, H., Yoshikai, Y. (2008). Oncogenesis by retroviruses: Old and new paradigms. *Reviews in Medical Virology, 18*(6), 387–405.

Misset, J., & Levi, F. (1995). Chronomodulated chemotherapy combining 5-fluorouracil, folinic acid, and oxaliplatin in advanced colorectal cancer: An overview of seven years of experience (Meeting abstract). *Cancer Investigation, 13*(Suppl 1), 49–50.

Mullan, F. (1985). Seasons of survival: Reflections of a physician with cancer. *New England Journal of Medicine, 313,* 270–273.

National Toxicology Program (NTP). (2005). *11th Report on Carcinogens.* Research Triangle Park. Retrieved from http://ntp.niehs.nih.gov/ntp/roc/toc11.html

Nowicki, M. J., Vigen, C., Mack, W. J., Seaberg, E., Landay, A., Anastos, K., Young, M., Minkoff, H., Greenblatt, R., Levine, A. M. (2008). Association of cells with natural killer (NK) and NKT immunophenotype with incident cancers in HIV-infected women. *AIDS Research & Human Retroviruses, 24*(2), 163–168.

Oncology Nursing Society. (2007).Pain: What are the pharmacologic interventions for nociceptive and neuropathic cancer pain in adults? Putting Evidence Into Practice (PEP Card). Retrieved March 23, 2009, from http://www.ons.org/outcomes/volume3/pain/pdf/ShortCard_pain.pdf

Oncology Nursing Society. (2009). Oncology Nursing Society position paper on quality cancer care. Retrieved March 10, 2009, from http://www.ons.org/publications/positions/QualityCancerCare.shtml

Paim, C. R., de Paula Lima, E. D., Fu, M. R., de Paula Lima, A., Cassali, G. D. (2008). Postlymphadenectomy complications and quality of life among breast cancer patients in Brazil. *Cancer Nursing, 31*(4), 302–309; quiz 310-1.

Pfister, G., & Savino, W. (2008). Can the immune system still be efficient in the elderly? An immunological and immunoendocrine therapeutic perspective. *Neuroimmunomodulation, 15*(4-6), 351–364.

Rosedale, M., & Fu, M. R. (2010). Confronting the unexpected: Temporal, situational, and attributive dimensions of breast cancer survivors' experiences of distressing symptoms. *Oncology Nursing Forum, 37*(1), E28–E33.

Schmitz, K. H., Cappola, A. R., Stricker, C. T., Sweeney, C., & Norman, S. A. (2007). The intersection of cancer and aging: Establishing the need for breast cancer rehabilitation. *Cancer Epidemiology, Biomarkers & Prevention, 16*(5), 866–872.

Selye, H. (1984). *The stress of life* (rev. 2nd ed.). New York: McGraw-Hill.

Sheinfeld, Gorin.S., Gauthier, J., Hay, J., Miles, A., & Wardle, J. (2008). Cancer screening and aging: Research barriers and opportunities. *Cancer, 113*(12 Suppl), 3493–3504.

Singer, C. F., Kostler, W. J., Hudelist, G. (2008). Predicting the efficacy of trastuzumab-based therapy in breast cancer: Current standards and future strategies. *Biochimica et Biophysica Acta, 1786*(2), 105–113.

Toothaker, T. B., & Rubin, M. (2009). Paraneoplastic neurological syndromes: A review *Neurologist, 15*(1), 21–33.

Trinh, V. A. (2008). Current management of metastatic melanoma. *American Journal of Health-System Pharmacy, 65*(24 Suppl 9), S3–8.

Ullenhag, G. J., Spendlove, I., Watson, N. F, Kallmeyer, C., Pritchard-Jones, K., Durrant, L. G. (2008). T-cell responses in osteosarcoma patients vaccinated with an anti-idiotypic antibody, 105AD7, mimicking CD55. *Clinical Immunology, 128*(2), 148–154.

Van Hemelrijck, M. J., Michaud, D. S., Connolly, G. N., Kabir, Z. (2009). Secondhand smoking, 4-aminobiphenyl, and bladder cancer: Two meta-analyses. *Cancer Epidemiology Biomarkers Prevention, 18*(4), 1312–1320.

Van Leeuwen, M. S. (2006). *Davis' comprehensive handbook to laboratory and diagnostic tests with nursing implications* (2nd ed.). St. Louis: C.V. Mosby.

Ward, E., Halpern, M., Schrag, N., Cokkinides, V., DeSantis, C., Bandi, P., Siegel, R., Stewart, A., & Jemal, A. (2008). Association of insurance with cancer care utilization and outcomes. *CA: A Cancer Journal for Clinicians, 58*(1), 9–31.

Wu, C., Jiang, J., Shi, L., Xu, N. (2008). Prospective study of chemotherapy in combination with cytokine-induced killer cells in patients suffering from advanced non-small-cell lung cancer. *Anticancer Research. 28*(6B), 3997–4002.

Building Clinical Competence
Pathophysiology and Patterns of Health

Functional Health Pattern: Health Perception-Health Management

Think about patients with altered health perception or health management for whom you have cared in your clinical experiences.

■ What were their major medical diagnoses? Had they been injured in an accident? Had they or will they be experiencing a loss of body function, loss of an important object, or loss of a family member? Had they had surgery? Did they have a genetic disorder?

■ What manifestations did each of these patients have? Were these manifestations similar or different?

■ How did the patients' healthcare behaviors interfere with their health status? Did the patient have a genetic disorder? Was there a family history of genetic disorders? Did the patient have genetic studies done? Did the patient complain of pain? If so, what type of pain? In what region of the body was the pain? Did the pain radiate? What was the quality and quantity of pain? What was the severity of the pain? What did the patient do to relieve pain? Did the patient have a significant body fluid loss? If so, what was the loss: vomiting, diarrhea, or hemorrhage? Did the patient have excess body fluid such as edema? Did the patient complain of cardiac dysrhythmias? Did the patient complain of muscle weakness or muscle spasms? Did the patient complain of numbness or tingling around the mouth or of the fingers and toes? Did the patient exhibit changes in respiratory patterns? Did the patient exhibit personality changes or confusion? Did the patient have any seizure activity? Did the patient have any traumatic injuries: multiple trauma injuries, abuse? Did the patient have a blood transfusion? Was the patient treated for shock? Was the patient treated for an infection? Did the patient have a problem with wound healing? Was the patient up-to-date with immunizations? Did the patient have allergies? Did the patient have any autoimmune disorders? Had the patient had an organ or tissue transplant? Had the patient been tested for HIV? Did the patient have HIV or AIDS?

The Health Perception-Health Management Functional Health Pattern includes healthcare behaviors such as health promotion and illness prevention activities, medical treatments, and follow-up care. Early intervention and health-promotion-focused care can result in a longer life and a better quality of life. Health perception and health maintenance are affected by perceived health status in two primary ways:

■ Factors that change or disrupt genes are genetic alterations (e.g., Down's syndrome, Turner syndrome, chronic myelogenous leukemia, Alzheimer's disease), autosomal dominant inheritance patterns (e.g., breast and ovarian cancer, neurofibromatosis, Huntington disease), autosomal recessive inheritance patterns (e.g., cystic fibrosis, sickle cell anemia), X-linked recessive inheritance (e.g., hemophilia), and monogenic inheritance (e.g., Prader-Willi syndrome).

■ Factors that change or disrupt cells are altered immune response (e.g., hypersensitivity, rheumatoid arthritis, systemic lupus erythematosus, HIV/AIDS), inflammation (e.g., osteoarthritis, *mycobacterium tuberculosis*, infection (e.g., influenza, meningitis), cancer (e.g., leukemia, lymphoma, sarcoma), trauma (e.g., rape, burns, fractures, gunshot wound), shock (e.g., hypovolemic, septic, anaphylactic), fluid volume (e.g., dehydration, edema), electrolyte imbalance (e.g., hyponatremia, hyperkalemia, hypocalcemia), and acid–base imbalance (e.g., respiratory acidosis, metabolic alkalosis).

The human body is continually threatened by foreign substances, infectious agents, and abnormal cells, resulting in alterations that cause abnormalities or disease processes. A patient's perceived pattern of health and well-being affects how health is managed, leading to manifestations such as the following:

■ Rapid weight loss (*neoplastic cells divert nutrition for own use causes increase in serum glucose and increased metabolic rate resulting in reduced appetite*)

■ Tachycardia (*shock or trauma causes vasoconstriction and decreased blood volume resulting in rapid, weak, and thready pulse to increase cardiac output*)

■ Tachypnea (*decreased perfusion of alveoli causes impaired gas exchange resulting in increased carbon dioxide and respiratory acidosis*)

Priority nursing diagnoses within the health perception and health management functional health pattern that may be appropriate for patients include the following:

■ *Risk for Infection* as evidenced by traumatized tissue, malnutrition, stasis of body tissue, leucopenia, and decreased hemoglobin

■ *Acute pain* as evidenced by guarding, facial grimacing, crying, diaphoresis, restlessness, and pupillary dilation

■ *Disturbed Body Image* as evidenced by verbalization of feelings, fear of rejection, preoccupation with loss, feelings of helplessness, and hiding body part

■ *Risk for Violence* as evidenced by verbal threats, physical injury to others, refusal to take medications, impulsivity, and clenching fists and jaw

Two nursing diagnoses from other functional health patterns often are of high priority for the patient with deficits in health perception or health maintenance:

■ *Impaired Tissue Integrity* (Nutritional-Metabolic Functional Health Pattern)

■ *Risk for Post-trauma Syndrome* (Cognitive-Perceptual Functional Health Pattern)

Question

1. Besides administration of medication, what did you do to help your patients manage their health related to pain, fever, inflammation, tachycardia, and tachypnea?

CLINICAL SCENARIO

Directions: *Read the following clinical scenarios and answer the questions that follow. To complete this exercise successfully, you will utilize not only knowledge of the content in this unit but also principles related to priority setting and maintaining patient safety.*

You have been assigned to work with the following four patients for the 0700 shift on a medical-surgical unit. Significant data obtained during report is as follows:

- Allen Barber is a 55-year-old patient with diabetes mellitus who is 4 days postoperative abdominal surgery with an inflammation of the incision site. Temperature is 101°F, pulse 94, respirations 24, blood pressure 138/82. The abdominal incision appears red with warmth and edema around the incision. The patient states his pain level is 8 on a pain scale of 0 to 10. Labs and wound cultures have been ordered.

- Tamra Sanders is a 22-year-old patient with Down syndrome. She is admitted in sickle cell crisis with a temperature of 102°F, pulse 90, respirations 30 and shallow, and blood pressure of 110/84. She is complaining of severe chest pain with shortness of breath. She states her pain scale level is 10 of 10. She has an order to begin morphine PCA.

- Mia Windham is a 26-year-old who was admitted yesterday with a maculopapular rash on her hands and feet that is spreading to her arms and legs. This morning she is complaining of abdominal pain, nausea, and bloody diarrhea. The patient has a history of having a bone marrow transplant 3 months ago as treatment for leukemia.

- Harry Anderson is a 40-year-old in late stages of AIDS. He is confused, incontinent, and is very spastic. He is on seizure precautions. He needs to be turned every 2 hours to prevent pressure sores. He is currently yelling that he needs help.

Questions

Priority Setting

1. In what order would you visit these patients after report?
   - A. _____
   - B. _____
   - C. _____
   - D. _____

Health Promotion

1. Harry Anderson, with HIV, has experienced weight loss. The dietician teaches him meal planning in which type of diet?
   - A. high protein, high fiber
   - B. high protein, high kilocalorie
   - C. low fiber, low protein
   - D. high carbohydrate, high vitamins

2. Before Allen Barber is discharged, what will the nurse encourage him to do at home to promote healing of his incision?

Nursing Process

1. Besides obtaining vital signs, what diagnosis-specific assessment data should be collected for each patient?
   - A. _____
   - B. _____
   - C. _____
   - D. _____

2. Identify one priority nursing diagnosis for each patient presented earlier. What is the rationale for your choices?

	Nursing Diagnosis	Rationale
Allen Barber		
Tamra Sanders		
Mia Windham		
Harry Anderson		

3. In what position should the nurse place Tamra Sanders to ease her breathing?

4. The nurse performs wound cleansing with which procedure?
   - A. Cleanse the wound with soap and water.
   - B. Use normal saline to cleanse the wound.
   - C. Cleanse the wound with povidone-iodine.
   - D. Hydrogen peroxide (1/2 strength) is used to cleanse the wound.

5. Due to diarrhea, Mia Windham's arterial blood gas results are pH – 7.30, pCO_2 – 35mmHg, pO_2 – 90mmHg, HCO_3^- 19mEq/L. Which does the nurse interpret these results as being?
   - A. metabolic acidosis
   - B. metabolic alkalosis
   - C. respiratory acidosis
   - D. respiratory alkalosis

6. Which laboratory studies would you expect to be drawn on a patient who is 4 days postoperative with an inflammation of the incision site?
   - A. white blood cell count/differential, erythrocyte sedimentation rate, C-reactive protein
   - B. troponins, metabolic panel for electrolytes, cultures of wound site
   - C. blood cultures, hematocrit and hemoglobin, blood glucose level
   - D. complete blood cell count, alkaline phosphatase, urine creatinine, and blood urea nitrogen

Communication

1. What information will you report to Mia Windham's doctor regarding her symptoms this morning?

2. The family of the patient with sickle cell anemia asks the nurse how sickle cell anemia is transmitted from one family member to another. Which statement by the nurse is the correct response?
   - A. "The mother carries the gene for sickle cell anemia and passes it to the children."
   - B. "The father carries the gene for sickle cell anemia and passes it to the children."
   - C. "Both parents carry the gene for sickle cell anemia and have a 25% chance of children getting the disease process."
   - D. "One parent has the disease and one parent carries the affected gene and they have a 50% chance of passing it to the children."

3. What communication techniques will you use when talking with Tamra Sanders because of her diagnosis of Down syndrome?

Delegation

1. What nursing interventions for each patient can be delegated to a CNA?
   A. _____
   B. _____
   C. _____
   D. _____

Related Questions

1. In which position does the nurse place the patient with hypovolemic shock?
   A. Semi-Fowler's position with legs straight
   B. Trendelenburg position with legs elevated 10 degrees
   C. left lateral position with legs bent toward chest
   D. supine position with legs elevated 20 degrees

2. Prior to administering cytotoxic agents, such as cyclophosphamide (Cytoxan), the nurse needs to notify the physician of which lab results?
   A. hemoglobin of 10.8g/dL, hematocrit of 35%
   B. potassium of 3.4mEq/L, sodium of 130mEq/L
   C. creatinine of 2mg/dL, blood urea nitrogen of 30mg/dL
   D. white blood cell count 3900mm^3, platelets of 74,000mm^3

3. The patient is admitted to the emergency department for a severe anaphylactic reaction to aspirin. Which medication is ordered to be administered?
   A. 0.5 mL of 1:1000 epinephrine subcutaneously
   B. 0.3 mL of 1:10,000 epinephrine subcutaneously
   C. Intravenous infusion of 1:10,000 epinephrine
   D. Intravenous infusion of 1:100,000 epinephrine

4. When administering a blood transfusion, what manifestations indicate a hemolytic reaction to the blood being administered?

5. The nurse teaches patients and families to decrease risk factors of cancer by following which cancer prevention recommendations? **Select all that apply.**
   A. Avoid tobacco and excessive alcohol use.
   B. Eat a diet low in fat and high in carbohydrates.
   C. Increase intake of vitamins A, D, E, and K.
   D. Limit exposure to sun from 11:00 AM to 3:00 PM.
   E. Increase vegetables and fruits in the diet.
   F. Eat meats grilled over charcoal fire instead of fried.

CASE STUDY: Herman Blount

Herman Blount is a 60-year-old African American construction worker who is seen in the physician's office with complaints of dull chest pain, shortness of breath, swelling of his hands and feet, weight loss, fatigue, and weakness. Upon physical assessment, vital signs are temperature 99.8°F, pulse 84, respirations 24, blood pressure 168/92. His height is 5' 11" and weight is 175 pounds. Mr. Blount states this is a loss of 35 pounds over the past 3 months. Wheezing is heard when breath sounds are auscultated. Coughing is noted with deep breathing. Remainder of the physical assessment is unremarkable. He has a medical history of high blood pressure for which he takes diltiazem and ramipril. He has a history of smoking 1 to 2 packs of cigarettes per day since he was 15 years old. He states he has been exposed to asbestos in his employment. Mr. Blount's nutrition assessment indicates that his diet consists of fried meats (especially chicken), green vegetables cooked in fatback, eggs, and bacon for breakfast, and at break time he eats doughnuts or cookies. His fluid intake consists of coffee for breakfast and break time, soda at lunch, and 3 to 4 beers at night.

Blood is drawn for a complete blood count, electrolytes, blood glucose, calcitonin, CEA, haptoglobulin, GGT, and creatinine. A sputum specimen is sent to the laboratory. A chest x-ray and CT scan are done. Based on the results of the chest x-ray, bronchoscopy and needle aspiration biopsies are performed to confirm the diagnosis of lung cancer. The pathophysiology of lung cancer is formation of tumors that begin as mucosal lesions that grow to form masses that obstruct the bronchi and invade adjacent lung tissue. The lung tumor can hemorrhage, causing hemoptysis. The cancer cells can spread via the lymph system to lymph nodes and other organs. Manifestations of lung cancer are chronic cough, hemoptysis, wheezing, shortness of breath, dull and aching chest pain, hoarseness, dysphagia, weight loss, anorexia, fatigue, weakness, bone pain, and clubbing of the fingers and toes. Complications of lung cancer are metastasis to other organs, superior vena cava syndrome, anemia, Cushing's syndrome, syndrome of inappropriate antidiuretic syndrome (SIADH), thrombophlebitis, osteoathropathy, peripheral neuropathy, and cerebellar degeneration.

As Mr. Blount is faced with decisions regarding treatment of his newly diagnosed lung cancer, the nursing diagnosis *Readiness for Enhanced Management of Therapeutic Regimen* is of highest priority at this time.

- Bronchial epithelial cell damage → cell mutation → progressive cell abnormalities → malignant cell forms clones which reproduce to form a tumor → tumor produces substances to support its growth → bronchial obstruction, replacement of normal lung tissue by tumor → cough and increasing dyspnea;

Mr. B.
60 y.o. male
Lung cancer

affects

leads to

assess

- C/o dull chest pain, SOB, peripheral edema, weight loss, fatigue and weakness.
- T 99.8° F, P 84, R 24, BP 168/92
- Ht 5' 11", wt 175 lb
- Wheezing and cough present
- Meds: diltiazem and ramipril for HTN
- 45-60 pack/year smoking history, consumes 3-4 beers/day, high fat diet
- Hx of occupational asbestos exposure

generates

- Ineffective Breathing Pattern as evidence by tachypnea
- Ineffective Airway Clearance as evidence by wheezing and cough
- Imbalanced Nutrition: Less than Body Requirements as evidenced by recent significant weight loss
- Ineffective Health Maintenance as evidenced by BP, smoking, alcohol and fat intake
- Readiness for Enhanced Coping related to new cancer diagnosis

generate nursing diagnosis

Readiness for Enhanced Management of Therapeutic Regimen

prioritized to

expected outcomes

- Actively participates in healthcare decisions, verbalizes understanding of planned treatment regimen
- Uses measures to reduce adverse effects of radiation and chemotherapy
- Joins smoking cessation program, enlisting family support for efforts to stop smoking.
- Takes antihypertensive medications as ordered, regularly monitors BP
- Discusses potential treatment outcomes and effects with family
- Meets, together with wife, with dietitian for menu planning to reduce fat and saturated fat intake

evaluate

- Joins smoking cessation program with wife; asks family and friends to avoid smoking in their presence
- Skin and mucous membranes remain intact during radiation therapy
- Weight remains stable, BP 152/84, R 20, P 80
- Stops drinking, stating "It doesn't even taste good without a cigarette."
- Increased intake of fresh fruit, vegetables, and whole grains

Independent Interventions
- Assess knowledge and understanding of disease, contributory factors, and treatment plan.
- Provide information and reinforce teaching as needed to promote understanding.
- Involve family in teaching and discussions.
- Teach measures to reduce/ manage adverse treatment effects
- Provide information about and referral to available smoking cessation programs.
- Assist client to plan for the future by providing information about usual course of illness and treatment.
- Facilitate communication among healthcare providers, client, and family.
- Teach coping/stress management techniques.
- Offer information about available community resources.

Activity:

1. After reviewing the concept map, go to the Pearson Nursing Student Resources for this book at www.nursing.pearson-highered.com to write a concept map based on the nursing diagnosis *Ineffective Breathing Pattern*.

   See answers and hints in Appendix C.

Nutritional and Metabolic Pattern

PART II

Functional Health Patterns with Related Nursing Diagnoses

HEALTH PERCEPTION HEALTH MANAGEMENT
- Perceived health status
- Perceived health management
- Health care behaviors: health promotion and illness prevention activities, medical treatments, follow-up care

VALUE-BELIEF
- Values, goals, or beliefs (including spirituality) that guide choices or decisions
- Perceived conflicts in values, beliefs, or expectations that are health related

COPING-STRESS-TOLERANCE
- Capacity to resist challenges to self-integrity
- Methods of handling stress
- Support systems
- Perceived ability to control and manage situations

NUTRITIONAL-METABOLIC
- Daily consumption of food and fluids
- Favorite foods
- Use of dietary supplements
- Skin lesions and ability to heal
- Condition of the integument
- Weight, height, temperature

PART II
Nutritional–Metabolic, Elimination (bowel) Patterns: Examples of related NANDA Nursing Diagnoses
- Anxiety
- Bowel Incontinence
- Constipation
- Diarrhea
- Disturbed Body Image
- Dysfunctional Gastrointestinal Motility
- Deficient Fluid Volume
- Hypothermia
- Hyperthermia
- Impaired Dentition
- Impaired Oral Mucous Membranes
- Impaired Skin Integrity
- Impaired Swallowing
- Ineffective Thermoregulation
- Impaired Tissue Integrity
- Risk for Electrolyte Imbalance
- Risk for Trauma
- Risk for Unstable Blood Glucose

SEXUALITY-REPRODUCTIVE
- Satisfaction with sexuality or sexual relationships
- Reproductive pattern
- Female menstrual and perimeno-pausal history

ELIMINATION
- Patterns of bowel and urinary excretion
- Perceived regularity or irregularity of elimination
- Use of laxatives or routines
- Changes in time, modes, quality or quantity of excretions
- Use of devices for control

ROLE-RELATIONSHIP
- Perception of major roles, relationships, and responsibilities in current life situation
- Satisfaction with or disturbances in roles and relationships

ACTIVITY-EXERCISE
- Patterns of personally relevant exercise, activity, leisure, and recreation
- ADLs which require energy expenditure
- Factors that interfere with the desired pattern (e.g., illness or injury)

SELF-PERCEPTION– SELF-CONCEPT
- Attitudes about self
- Perceived abilities, worth, self-image, emotions
- Body posture and movement, eye contact, voice and speech patterns

SLEEP-REST
- Patterns of sleep and rest/relaxation in a 24-hr period
- Perceptions of quality and quantity of sleep and rest
- Use of sleep aids and routines

COGNITIVE-PERCEPTUAL
- Adequacy of vision, hearing, taste, touch, smell
- Pain perception and management
- Language, judgment, memory, decisions

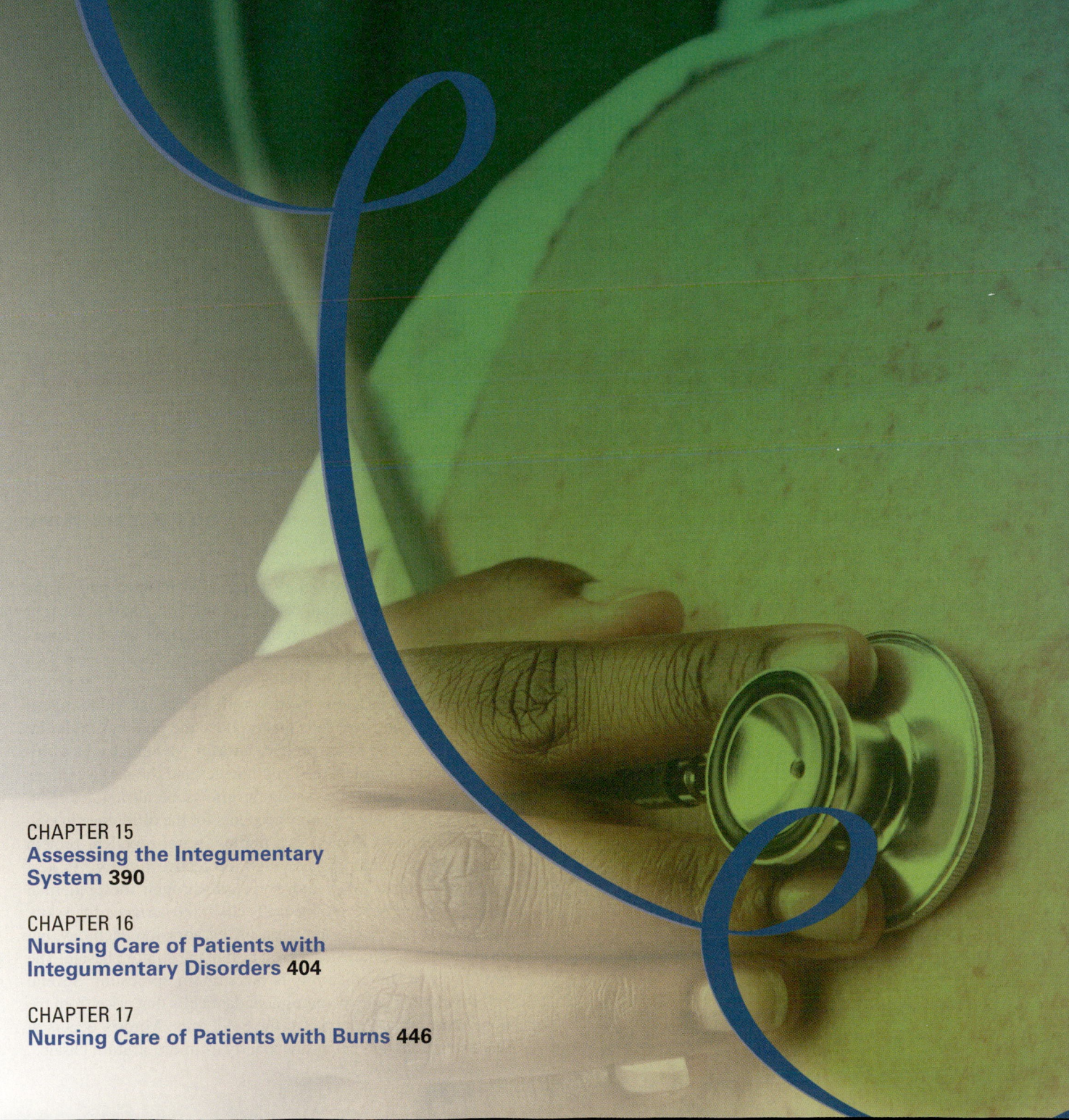

Responses to Altered Integumentary Structure and Function

LEARNING OUTCOMES

1. Describe the anatomy, physiology, and functions of the skin, hair, and nails.
2. Discuss factors that influence skin color.
3. Identify specific topics for a health history interview of the patient with problems involving the skin, hair, or nails.
4. Explain techniques for assessing the skin, hair, and nails.

5. Give examples of genetic disorders of the integumentary system.
6. Describe normal variations in assessment findings for the older adult.
7. Identify abnormal findings that may indicate impairment of the integumentary system.

CLINICAL COMPETENCIES

1. Conduct and document a health history for patients who have or are at risk for alterations in the skin, hair, or nails.
2. Conduct and document a physical assessment of the integumentary system.

3. Monitor the results of diagnostic tests and report abnormal findings.

EQUIPMENT NEEDED

- Disposable gloves
- Ruler
- Flashlight

KEY TERMS

alopecia, *399*	hirsutism, *399*	sebum, *392*
cyanosis, *392*	jaundice, *392*	urticaria, *398*
ecchymosis, *398*	keratin, *390*	vitiligo, *398*
edema, *398*	melanin, *390*	
erythema, *392*	pallor, *392*	

The skin, the hair, and the nails make up the integumentary system. The skin, the largest organ of the body, provides an external covering for the body, separating and protecting the body's organs and tissues from the external environment. Functions of the skin, hair, and nails are summarized in Table 15–1.

Anatomy, Physiology, and Functions of the Integumentary System

The Skin

The skin has a total surface area of 15 to 20 square feet and weighs about 9 pounds. It has been estimated that each square inch of skin contains 15 feet of blood vessels, 4 yards of nerves, 650 sweat glands, 100 oil glands, 1500 sensory receptors, and more than 3 million cells that are constantly dying and being replaced. The skin is composed of two regions: the epidermis and the dermis (Figure 15–1 ■). Alterations in the skin increase the risk for many physical and psychologic disorders, including fluid and electrolyte balance, temperature regulation, infection, wound healing, and self-concept.

The Epidermis

The epidermis, which is the surface or outermost part of the skin, consists of epithelial cells. The epidermis has either four or five layers, depending on its location; there are five layers over the palms of the hands and the soles of the feet, and four layers over the rest of the body.

The stratum basale is the deepest layer of the epidermis. It contains melanocytes, cells that produce the pigment **melanin**, and keratinocytes, which produce **keratin**. Melanin forms a protective shield to protect the keratinocytes and the nerve endings in the dermis from the damaging effects of ultraviolet light. Melanocyte activity probably accounts for the difference in skin color in humans. Keratin is a fibrous, water-repellent protein that gives the epidermis its tough, protective quality. As keratinocytes mature, they move upward through the epidermal layers, eventually becoming dead cells at the surface of the skin. Millions of these cells are worn off by abrasion each day, but millions are simultaneously produced in the stratum basale. The next layer of the epidermis is the stratum spinosum. Several cells thick, this layer contains abundant cells that arise from the bone marrow and migrate to the epidermis. Mitosis occurs at this layer, although not as abundantly as in the stratum basale.

TABLE 15–1 Functions of the Skin and Its Appendages

STRUCTURE	FUNCTIONS
Epidermis	Protects tissues from physical, chemical, and biologic damage.
	Prevents water loss and serves as a water-repellent layer.
	Stores melanin, which protects tissues from harmful effects of the ultraviolet radiation in sunlight.
	Converts cholesterol molecules to vitamin D when exposed to sunlight.
	Contains phagocytes, which prevent bacteria from penetrating the skin.
Dermis	Regulates body temperature by dilating and constricting capillaries.
	Transmits messages via nerve endings to the central nervous system.
Sebaceous (oil) glands	Secrete sebum, which lubricates skin and hair and plays a role in killing bacteria.
Eccrine sweat glands	Regulate body heat by excretion of perspiration.
Apocrine sweat glands	Remnants of sexual scent gland.
Hair	Cushions the scalp. Eyelashes and cilia protect the body from foreign particles. Provides insulation in cold weather.
Nails	Protect the fingers and toes, aid in grasping, and allow for various other activities, such as scratching the skin, picking up small items, peeling an orange, and so on.

The stratum granulosum is only two to three cells thick. The cells of the stratum granulosum contain a glycolipid that slows water loss across the epidermis. Keratinization, a thickening of the cells' plasma membranes, begins in the stratum granulosum. The stratum lucidum is present only in areas of thick skin. It is made up of flattened, dead keratinocytes. The outermost layer of the epidermis, the stratum corneum, is also the thickest, making up about 75% of the epidermis's total thickness. It consists of about 20 to 30 sheets of dead cells filled with keratin fragments arranged in "shingles" that flake off as dry skin.

The Dermis

The dermis is the second, deeper layer of skin. Made of a flexible connective tissue, this layer is richly supplied with blood cells, nerve fibers, and lymphatic vessels. Most of the

Figure 15–1 ■ Anatomy of the skin.

hair follicles, sebaceous glands, and sweat glands are located in the dermis. The dermis consists of a papillary and a reticular layer. The papillary layer contains capillaries and receptors for pain and touch. The deeper, reticular layer contains blood vessels, sweat and sebaceous glands, deep pressure receptors, and dense bundles of collagen fibers. The regions between these bundles form lines of cleavage in the skin. Surgical incisions parallel to these lines of cleavage heal more easily and with less scarring than incisions or traumatic wounds across cleavage lines.

Superficial Fascia

A layer of subcutaneous tissue called the superficial fascia lies under the dermis. It consists primarily of adipose (fat) tissue and helps the skin adhere to underlying structures.

Glands of the Skin

The skin contains sebaceous (oil) glands, sudoriferous (sweat) glands, and ceruminous glands. Each of these glands has a different function. Sebaceous glands are found all over the body except on the palms and soles. These glands secrete an oily substance called **sebum**, which usually is ducted into a hair follicle. Sebum softens and lubricates the skin and hair and also decreases water loss from the skin in low humidity. Sebum also protects the body from infection by killing bacteria. The secretion of sebum is stimulated by hormones, especially androgens. If a sebaceous gland becomes blocked, a pimple or whitehead appears on the surface of the skin; as the material oxidizes and dries, it forms a blackhead.

There are two types of sweat glands: eccrine and apocrine. Eccrine sweat glands are more numerous on the forehead, palms, and soles. The gland itself is located in the dermis; the duct to the skin rises through the epidermis to open in a pore at the surface. Sweat, the secretion of the eccrine glands, is composed mostly of water but also contains sodium, antibodies, small amounts of metabolic wastes, lactic acid, and vitamin C. The production of sweat is regulated by the sympathetic nervous system and serves to maintain normal body temperature. Sweating also occurs in response to emotions.

Most apocrine sweat glands are located in the axillary, anal, and genital areas. The secretions from apocrine glands are similar to those of sweat glands, but they also contain fatty acids and proteins. Apocrine glands are a remnant of sexual scent glands. Ceruminous glands, located in the skin of the external ear, are modified apocrine sweat glands. They secrete yellow-brown, waxy cerumen that provides a sticky trap for foreign materials.

Skin Color

Skin color varies among individuals and among people of different races, ranging from a pinkish white to various shades of brown and black. Areas of the skin that are normally exposed to the sun and environment, such as the face and hands, may have a slightly different color from areas that are usually covered with clothing. Special care must be taken when assessing changes in skin color in people with dark skin, such as Blacks, Hispanics, Native Americans, Asians, people of Mediterranean descent, and Whites who are deeply suntanned.

The color of the skin is the result of varying levels of pigmentation. Melanin, a yellow-to-brown pigment, is darker and is produced in greater amounts in persons with dark skin color than in those with light skin color. Exposure to the sun causes a buildup of melanin and a darkening or tanning of the skin in people with light skin. Carotene, a yellow-to-orange pigment, is found most in areas of the body where the stratum corneum is thickest, such as the palms of the hands. Carotene is more abundant in the skins of persons of Asian ancestry and, together with melanin, accounts for their golden skin tone. The epidermis in White skin has very little melanin and is almost transparent. Thus, the color of the hemoglobin found in red blood cells (RBCs) circulating through the dermis shows through, lending a pinkish skin tone.

Skin color is influenced by emotions and illnesses. **Erythema**, a reddening of the skin, may occur with embarrassment (blushing), fever, hypertension, or inflammation. It may also result from a drug reaction, sunburn, acne rosacea, or other factors. A bluish discoloration of the skin and mucous membranes, called **cyanosis**, results from poor oxygenation of hemoglobin. **Pallor**, or paleness of skin, may occur with shock, fear, or anger or in anemia and hypoxia. **Jaundice** is a yellow-to-orange color visible in the skin and mucous membranes; it is most often the result of a hepatic disorder. Table 15–2 further defines these terms and compares and contrasts skin color changes in people with light and dark skin.

The Hair

Hair is distributed all over the body, except the lips, nipples, parts of the external genitals, the palms of the hands, and the soles of the feet. Hair is produced by a hair bulb, and its root is enclosed in a hair follicle (Figure 15–2 ■). The exposed part,

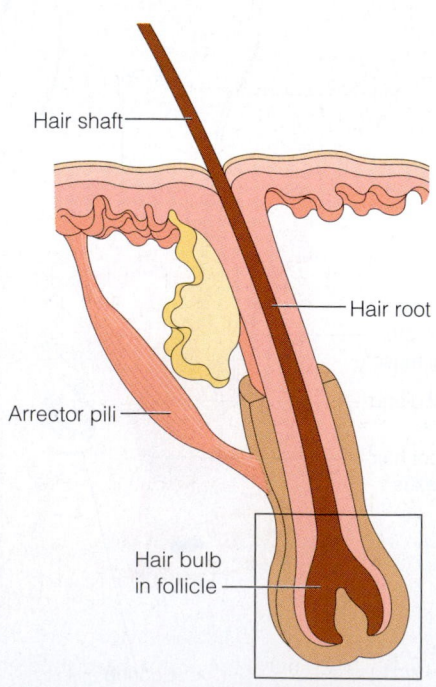

Figure 15–2 ■ Anatomy of a hair follicle.

Hair shaft

Hair root

Arrector pili

Hair bulb in follicle

TABLE 15–2 Skin Color Assessment Variations in People with Light and Dark Skin

PALLOR: *A decrease or absence in skin color as the result of a decrease in tissue perfusion; a decrease in shape, size, or amount of RBCs; or absence of melanin (local or generalized).*

DISORDER AND CAUSE	CHANGE IN LIGHT SKIN	CHANGE IN DARK SKIN
Anemia (decreased or abnormal size and shape of RBCs)	Generalized paleness	Brown skin is dull and has a yellow cast; black skin is dull and has an ashen gray cast.
Hemorrhage (decreased amount of circulating RBCs)	Generalized paleness	Brown skin is dull and has a yellow cast; black skin is dull and has an ashen gray cast
Shock (decreased amount of circulating RBCs or decreased perfusion)	Generalized paleness	Brown skin is dull and has a yellow cast; black skin is dull and has an ashen gray cast
Arterial insufficiency (trauma, acute arterial occlusion, or arteriosclerosis)	Local paleness	Dull, ashen gray
Vitiligo (patchy loss of melanocytes)	Patches of white spots, most often found over skin of the face, hands, or groin	Patches of white spots, most often found over skin of the face, hands, or groin
Albinism (total absence of melanin)	White/pink	Tan, cream, or white

CYANOSIS: *A bluish discoloration of the skin and mucous membranes resulting from a local or generalized excess of deoxygenated hemoglobin or a structural defect in the hemoglobin molecule.*

DISORDER AND CAUSE	CHANGE IN LIGHT SKIN	CHANGE IN DARK SKIN
Acute and chronic disorders of the structure and function of the heart and lungs (arterial insufficiency; exposure to cold, hypothermia)	Dusky blue (may be generalized or local, depending on cause)	Skin may appear darker, but will be dull; cyanosis is more readily assessed in the nail beds, oral mucous membranes, and conjunctivae

ERYTHEMA: *Redness of the skin or mucous membranes that is the result of dilatation and congestion of superficial capillaries.*

DISORDER AND CAUSE	CHANGE IN LIGHT SKIN	CHANGE IN DARK SKIN
Hyperemia (inflammation, increased body temperature, hot environmental temperature, embarrassment, alcohol ingestion)	Red or bright pink	Difficult to assess, skin may have dark red cast
Carbon monoxide poisoning (carbon monoxide displaces oxygen on the hemoglobin molecule, causing hypoxia, carboxyhemoglobinemia)	Cherry red in face and upper torso	Cherry red lips, oral mucous membranes, and nail beds
Venous stasis (inability of veins to return blood to heart; may result from edema, varicose veins, or pressure)	Dusky red	Difficult to assess

JAUNDICE: *Yellowish discoloration of the skin, mucous membranes, and sclerae of the eyes, caused by increased amounts of bilirubin or other pigments in the blood.*

DISORDER AND CAUSE	CHANGE IN LIGHT SKIN	CHANGE IN DARK SKIN
Increased serum bilirubin to >2–3 mg/ 100 mL (liver disease, pancreatic disease, gallbladder disease, hemolysis, such as following blood transfusion, severe burns or infections)	Yellowing of skin follows yellowing of sclerae and mucous membranes; may also be assessed in the fingernails and palms of the hands	Yellowing is best assessed at the junction of the hard palate and the soft palate or on the palms of the hands. Sclerae may be yellow near the limbus (do not confuse with normal yellow eye pigmentation)
Uremia (retained urochrome pigments in the blood)	Orange-green or gray cast to skin	Difficult to assess; may appear as yellowish green color in the scleral of the eye

called the shaft, consists mainly of dead cells. Hair follicles extend into the dermis and in some places, such as the scalp, below the dermis. Many factors, including nutrition and hormones, influence hair growth. Hair in various parts of the body has protective functions: The eyebrows and eyelashes protect the eyes, hair in the nose helps keep foreign materials out of the upper respiratory tract, and hair on the head protects the scalp from heat loss and sunlight.

The Nails

A nail is a modified scalelike epidermal structure. Like hair, nails consist mainly of dead cells. The body of the nail rests on the nail bed (Figure 15–3 ■). The proximal visible end of the nail has a white crescent, called a lunula. The sides of the nail are overlapped by skin, called nail folds. The proximal nail fold is thickened and is called the eponychium or cuticle. Nails form a protective coating over the dorsum of each digit on the fingers and toes.

Figure 15–3 ■ Anatomy of a nail.

Assessing the Integumentary System

The structures of the integumentary system are assessed by findings from diagnostic tests, a health assessment interview to collect subjective data, and a physical assessment to collect objective data. See the box that follows the physical assessment information for a sample documentation of an assessment of the integument.

Diagnosis

The results of diagnostic tests of the structure and function of the integumentary system are used to support the diagnosis of a specific injury or disease, to provide information to identify or modify the appropriate medication or treatments used to treat the disease, and to help nurses monitor the patients' responses to nursing care interventions. Some diagnostic tests are conducted to identify bacterial carriers. For example, if patients have repeated bacterial skin infections, or if a healthcare unit or agency experiences numerous bacterial infections of patients, nasal cultures may be performed to determine if the patients or the healthcare workers are carriers of the bacteria.

Regardless of the type of diagnostic test, the nurse is responsible for explaining the procedure and any special preparation needed, for assessing for medication use that may affect the outcome of the tests, for supporting the patient during the examination as necessary, for documenting the procedures as appropriate, and for monitoring the results of the tests.

Diagnostic tests to assess the integumentary system are described in the box on page 395. More information is included in the discussion of specific health problems or injuries in ∞ Chapters 16 and 17.

Genetic Considerations

When conducting a health assessment interview and physical assessment, it is important for the nurse to consider genetic influences on the health of the adult. During the health assessment interview, ask about integumentary disorders or abnormalities in immediate family members and also inquire about their gender. During the physical assessment, assess for any manifestations that indicate a genetic disorder (see the box Genetic Considerations: Examples of Integumentary Disorders). If data are found that indicate genetic risk factors or alterations, ask about genetic testing and refer for appropriate genetic counseling and evaluation. ∞ Chapter 8 provides further information about genetic implications in medical-surgical nursing.

Health Assessment Interview

A health assessment interview to determine problems with the integumentary system may be conducted as part of a health screening or total health assessment, or it may focus on a chief complaint (such as itching or a rash). If the patient has a skin problem, analyze its onset, characteristics and course, severity, precipitating and relieving factors, and note the timing and circumstances of any associated symptoms. For example, ask the patient the following:

- What type of itching have you experienced?
- When did you first notice a change in this mole?
- Did you change to any different kinds of shampoo or other hair products just before you started to lose your hair?

GENETIC CONSIDERATIONS
Examples of Integumentary Disorders

- Oculocutaneous albinism, an autosomal recessive inheritance disorder, causes hypopigmentation (albinism or absence of color) of the skin, hair, and eyes as a result of an inability to synthesize melanin.
- Keloids, which are elevated scars, have a familial tendency and are more commonly found in Blacks.
- Vitiligo, the sudden appearance of white patches on the skin, has a familial tendency.
- Male pattern baldness (the most common cause of baldness in men) is genetically predetermined.
- Hirsutism (excessive hair in women) may be genetically predetermined.
- Blacks may have very dry scalps and dry, fragile hair of genetic origin.
- A family history of skin cancer is a risk factor for skin cancer

DIAGNOSTIC TESTS of the Integumentary System

NAME OF TEST	PURPOSE & DESCRIPTION	RELATED NURSING INTERVENTIONS
Biopsy	A punch biopsy is done to differentiate benign lesions from skin cancers. An instrument is used to remove a small section of dermis and subcutaneous fat. Depending on size, the incision may be sutured with a single suture. An incisional biopsy is done to differentiate benign lesions from skin cancers. An incision is made and the skin lesion or tumor is removed for analysis. The incision is closed with sutures.	Apply dressing and provide information about self-care and when to return for suture removal.
Culture	A culture of scrapings from a lesion, from drainage, or of exudate is done to identify fungal, bacterial, or viral skin infections.	Obtain the culture with a sterile Culturette swab and culture tubes. Maintain strict asepsis while obtaining the culture.
Immunofluorescent Slides	Immunofluorescent studies of samples from skin and/or serum may be done to identify IgG antibodies (present in pemphigus vulgaris) and to identify varicella in skin cells (for herpes zoster). Skin or blood samples are placed on a slide and examined microscopically.	No special preparation is necessary.
Oil Slides	Oil slides are used to determine the type of skin infestation present. Scrapings of the lesion are placed on a slide with mineral oil and examined microscopically.	No special preparation is necessary.
Patch Test, Scratch Tests	These tests are used to determine a specific allergen. In a patch test, a small amount of the suspected material is placed on the skin under an occlusive bandage. In a scratch test, a needle is used to "scratch" small amounts of potentially allergic materials on the skin surface.	Explain to the patient the need to return in 48 hours to have the patched area or scratched areas evaluated.
Potassium Hydroxide (KOH)	A specimen from hair or nails is examined for a fungal infection. The specimen is obtained by placing material from a scraping on a slide, adding a potassium hydroxide solution, and examining it microscopically.	No special preparation is necessary.
Tzanck Test	This test is used to diagnose herpes infections, but it does not differentiate herpes simplex from herpes zoster. Fluid and cells from the vesicles are obtained, put on a slide, stained, and examined microscopically.	
Wood's Lamp	This test uses an ultraviolet light that causes certain organisms to fluoresce (such as *Pseudomonas* organisms and fungi). The skin is examined under a special lamp.	

Ask about any change in health, rashes, itching, color changes, dryness or oiliness, growth of or changes in warts or moles, and the presence of lesions. Precipitating causes, such as medications, the use of new soaps, skin care agents, cosmetics, pets, travel, stress, or dietary changes must also be explored. In assessing hair problems, ask about any thinning or baldness, excessive hair loss, change in distribution of hair, use of hair care products, diet, and dieting. When assessing nail problems, ask about nail splitting or breakage, discoloration, infection, diet, and exposure to chemicals.

The patient's medical history is important. Questions focus on previous problems, allergies, and lesions. Skin problems may be manifestations of other disorders, such as cardiovascular disease, endocrine disorders, hepatic disease, and hematologic disorders. Occupational and social history may provide cues to skin problems; ask the patient about

travel, exposure to toxic substances at work, use of alcohol, and responses to stress.

Assess the presence of risk factors for skin cancer carefully. These include male gender; age over 50; family history of skin cancer; extended exposure to sunlight; tendency to sunburn; history of sunburn or other skin trauma; light-colored hair or eyes; residence in high altitudes or near the equator; and exposure to radiation, x-rays, coal, tar, or petroleum products. (Risks for skin cancer are further discussed in ∞ Chapter 16.) Include specific questions to identify risk factors for malignant melanoma. These include a large number of moles, the presence of atypical moles, a family history of melanoma, prior melanoma, repeated severe sunburns, ease of freckling and sunburning, or inability to tan.

Interview questions categorized by functional health patterns follow. Responses should be documented in the patient's medical record.

FUNCTIONAL HEALTH PATTERN INTERVIEW Integumentary System

Functional Health Pattern	Interview Questions and Leading Statements
Health Perception-Health Management	■ Describe any health problems, injuries, or surgeries you have had. How were these treated? ■ Describe medications, herbs, and vitamins you currently are taking. ■ Describe your current problem. How long has it lasted? What have you done to treat it? ■ Do you have allergies to foods, plants, pets? Explain how the allergy affects you. ■ Describe what you do each day to care for your skin, hair, and nails.
Nutritional-Metabolic	■ Describe what you eat and how much and type of fluids you drink in a 24-hour period. ■ Do you have a history of food allergies? If so, describe what you are allergic to and how you respond. ■ Have you recently eaten any new foods? ■ Do you take any nutritional supplements, herbs, or vitamins? If so, what are they? ■ How well do your cuts and scratches heal?
Elimination	■ Is your skin and scalp dry or oily? ■ Have you noticed swelling around your eyes or ankles? ■ Do you perspire a lot?
Activity-Exercise	■ Describe your physical activities in a typical day. ■ Do you bruise easily? ■ Do you use a sunscreen when you are outside? If so, what SPF? ■ Do you visit tanning salons?
Sleep-Rest	■ How many hours do you sleep each night? ■ Do you have trouble sleeping because of itching or sweating?
Cognitive-Perceptual	■ Do you have any of the following: pain, discomfort, itching, tingling, burning, tenderness, or numbness? If so, where?
Self-Perception-Self-Concept	■ How does this condition make you feel about yourself?
Role-Relationships	■ How does this condition affect your relationships with others? ■ Is there anything in your work environment that may have caused this condition?
Sexuality-Reproductive	■ Has this condition interfered with your usual sexual activities?
Coping-Stress-Tolerance	■ Have you experienced any type of stress that may have worsened this condition? ■ Has this condition created stress for you? ■ Describe what you do when you feel stressed.
Value-Belief	■ Tell me how specific relationships or activities help you cope with this condition. ■ Describe specific cultural beliefs or practices that affect how you care for and feel about this condition. ■ Is there anything interfering with your spiritual beliefs, needs, or practices as a result of this condition? What can I or another caregiver do to help you with your spiritual needs? ■ Are there any specific treatments that you would not use to treat this condition?

Physical Assessment

Physical assessment of the skin, hair, and nails may be performed either as part of a total assessment or may be a focused assessment of the integument for patients with known or suspected problems. Physical assessment of the skin, hair, and nails is conducted by inspection and palpation. Assess the skin for color, presence of lesions (observable changes from normal skin structure), temperature, texture, moisture, turgor, and presence of edema. Characteristics of lesions to note include location and distribution, color, pattern, edges, size (measure with a ruler in centimeters), elevation, and type of exudate (if present). Common skin lesions of older adults are outlined in Box 15–1; see the box Nursing Care of the Older Adult for age-related integument changes. Examine the hair for color, texture, quality, and scalp lesions. Determine the shape, color, contour, and condition of the nails. Terminology of skin lesions with examples are outlined in Table 15–3.

The examination should be conducted in a warm, private room. The patient removes all clothing and puts on a gown or drape. The areas to be examined should be fully exposed, but protect the patient's modesty by keeping other areas covered. The patient may be standing, sitting, or lying down at various times of the examination. Don disposable gloves when

BOX 15–1 Common Skin Lesions of Older Adults

■ *Skin tags:* soft brown or flesh-colored benign papules
■ *Keratoses:* horny growth of keratinocytes, may be seborrheic (benign) or actinic (premalignant)
■ *Lentigines ("liver spots"):* brown or black benign macule with a defined border
■ *Angiomas (hemangioma):* benign vascular tumors with dilated blood vessels, found in the middle to upper dermis
■ *Telangiectases:* single dilated blood vessels, capillaries, or terminal arteries
■ *Venous lakes:* small, dark blue, slightly raised benign papules
■ *Photoaging:* wrinkling, mottling, pigmented areas, loss of elasticity, benign or malignant lesions

palpating open lesions, skin surfaces suspicious of infections or infestations, or discharge from lesions of the skin and mucous membranes. A ruler is used to measure the size of lesions. A flashlight is used to better visualize lesions.

SAMPLE DOCUMENTATION

Assessment of the Integumentary System

A 50-year-old man with no history of skin lesions, hair loss, or disorders of the nails. Took antibiotic for respiratory infection approximately 10 days ago and reports having a fine, raised, red rash on trunk and arms that itched. Nurse practitioner prescribed antihistamine and rash cleared in 3 days. Skin light brown, warm, dry, and elastic. Patches of vitiligo present over dorsum of hands. No lesions or edema noted. Healed scar on lower left abdomen (appendectomy as a young adult). Hair dark brown with gray at the temples, clean. Nails are smooth, hard, and immobile.

TABLE 15–3 Terminology of Skin Lesions with Associated Disorders

LESION	EXAMPLES OF DISORDERS
Pigmented	Freckle, seborrheic keratosis, nevus, melanoma
Scaly	Psoriasis, dermatitis, xerosis, tinea, actinic keratoses
Pustular	Acne vulgaris, folliculitis, candidiasis
Vesicular	Herpes simplex, herpes zoster, scabies
Nodular	Warts, basal cell carcinoma, acne
Weepy, crusted	Acute contact allergic dermatitis, impetigo
Figurate (shaped) erythema	Urticaria, cellulites
Bullous	Pemphigus, toxic epidermal necrolysis
Pruritic	Xerosis, scabies, pediculosis
Ulcerated	Pressure ulcer, skin cancer, herpes simplex

NURSING CARE OF THE OLDER ADULT — Age-Related Skin Changes

AGE-RELATED CHANGE	SIGNIFICANCE
Epidermis: ↓ thickness and miotic activity	■ Skin is more fragile and at greater risk for tears or injury ■ Delayed wound healing ■ Hyperkeratoses and skin cancers in sun-exposed areas are more evident
Epidermis: ↑ permeability, ↓ Langerhans cells	■ Increased risk of reactions to irritants ■ Decreased inflammatory response
Epidermis: ↓ number of active melanocytes	■ Increased susceptibility to sun exposure
Epidermis: hyperplasia of melanocytes, especially in sun-exposed areas	■ Small areas of hyperpigmentation ("liver spots") and hypopigmentation ("age spots"), especially on the hands
Epidermis: ↓ vitamin D production	■ Increased risk of osteomalacia, osteoporosis
Epidermis: dermal–epidermal junction flattens	■ Increased risk of skin tears, purpura, and pressure ulcers
Dermis: ↓ perfusion	■ More susceptible to dry skin ■ Decreased sensation (pain, touch, temperature, and peripheral vibration) ■ Increased risk of injury
Dermis: ↓ vasomotor response	■ Greater risk of hyperthermia and hypothermia
Dermis: elastic fibers degenerate	■ Decreased tone and elasticity, with wrinkle formation
Dermis: proliferation of capillaries	■ Cherry hemangiomas are common
Subcutaneous skin layer: thins	■ Greater risk of hypothermia ■ Increased risk of pressure ulcers
Subcutaneous skin layer: adipose tissue is redistributed	■ Cellulite forms ■ Bags over and under the eyes ■ Double chin forms ■ Abdominal fat increases ■ Breasts sag ■ Skin returns to normal more slowly when pinched (also called tenting)
Glands: ↓ eccrine and apocrine activity	■ Dry skin is common ■ Absent perspiration

TABLE 15–4 Integumentary Assessments

TECHNIQUE/NORMAL FINDINGS	ABNORMAL FINDINGS
Inspect skin color and note any odors coming from the skin. *Skin color should be even, appropriate to the age and race of the patient, without foul odors.*	■ A strong odor of perspiration may indicate poor hygiene and a need for patient teaching. A foul odor may indicate a disorder of the sweat glands. ■ Pallor and/or cyanosis are seen with exposure to cold and with decreased perfusion and oxygenation. In cyanotic dark-skinned patients, skin loses glow and appears dull. Cyanosis may be more visible in the mucous membranes and nail beds of these patients. ■ In dark-skinned patients, jaundice may be most apparent in the sclerae of the eyes. ■ Redness, swelling, and pain are seen with various rashes, inflammations, infections, and burns. First-degree burns cause areas of painful erythema and swelling. Red, painful blisters appear in second-degree burns, whereas white or blackened areas are common in third-degree burns. ■ **Vitiligo**, an abnormal loss of melanin in patches, typically occurs over the face, hands, or groin. Vitiligo is thought to be an autoimmune disorder.
Inspect the skin for lesions and alterations, including calluses, scars, tattoos, and piercings. Include inspection of skin creases and folds. *Skin should be intact without lesions.*	Primary, secondary, and vascular lesions are described and shown in Tables 15–5 through 15–7. ■ Pearly edged nodules with a central ulcer are seen in basal cell carcinoma. ■ Scaly, red, fast-growing papules are seen in squamous cell carcinoma. ■ Dark, asymmetric, multicolored patches (sometimes moles) with irregular edges appear in malignant melanoma. ■ Circular lesions are usually present in ringworm and in tinea versicolor. ■ Grouped vesicles may be seen in contact dermatitis. ■ Linear lesions appear in poison ivy and herpes zoster. ■ **Urticaria** (hives) appears as patches of pale, itchy wheals in an erythematous area. ■ In psoriasis, scaly red patches appear on the scalp, knees, back, and genitals. ■ In herpes zoster, vesicles appear along sensory nerve paths, turn into pustules, and then crust over. ■ Bruises (**ecchymosis**) are raised bluish or yellowish vascular lesions. Multiple bruises in various stages of healing suggest trauma or abuse.
Palpate skin temperature. *Skin should be warm.*	■ Skin is warm and red in inflammation and is generally warm with elevated body temperature. ■ Decreased blood flow decreases the skin temperature; this may be generalized, as in shock, or localized, as in arteriosclerosis.
Palpate skin texture. *Skin should be smooth.*	■ Changes in the texture of the skin may indicate irritation or trauma. ■ The skin is soft and smooth in hyperthyroidism and coarse in hypothyroidism.
Palpate skin moisture. *Skin should be dry.*	■ Excessively dry skin often is present in the elderly and patients with hypothyroidism. ■ Oily skin is common in adolescents and young adults. Oily skin may be a normal finding, or it may accompany a skin disorder such as acne vulgaris. ■ Excessive perspiration may be associated with shock, fever, increased activity, or anxiety.
Palpate skin turgor. *Skin fold should return rapidly to normal position.*	■ Pinch the patient's skin gently over the back of the hand or collarbone. Tenting, in which the skin remains pinched for a few moments before resuming its normal position, is common in older patients who are thin (Figure 15–4 ■). ■ Skin turgor is decreased in dehydration. It is increased in edema and scleroderma.

Figure 15–4 ■ Tenting in an older patient.

Assess for edema. *No edema should be present.*	■ Assess **edema** (accumulation of fluid in the body's tissues) by depressing the patient's skin (Figure 15–5 ■). Record findings as follows: 1+ Slight pitting, no obvious distortion 2+ Deeper pit, no obvious distortion 3+ Pit is obvious; extremities are swollen 4+ Pit remains with obvious distortion ■ Edema is common in cardiovascular disorders, renal failure, trauma, and cirrhosis of the liver. It also may be a side effect of certain drugs.

TABLE 15–4 Integumentary Assessments (continued)

TECHNIQUE/NORMAL FINDINGS	ABNORMAL FINDINGS

Slight pitting, no obvious distortion.	2mm ... 1+
Deeper pit, no obvious distortion.	4mm ... 2+
Pit is obvious; extremities are swollen.	6mm ... 3+
Pit remains with obvious distortion.	8mm ... 4+

A   B

Figure 15–5 ■ *A*, Degrees of pitting in edema. *B*, 4+ pitting.

Source: Dr. P. Marazzi/Science Photo Library/Photo Researchers, Inc.

Inspect distribution and quality of hair. *Hair should be evenly distributed for patient's gender.*	■ A deviation in the normal hair distribution in the male or female genital area may indicate an endocrine disorder. **Hirsutism** (increased growth of coarse hair, usually on the face and trunk) is seen in Cushing's syndrome, acromegaly, and ovarian dysfunction. **Alopecia** (hair loss) may be related to changes in hormones, chemical or drug treatment, or radiation. In adult males whose hair loss follows the normal male pattern, the cause is usually genetic.
Palpate hair texture. *Hair should be of even texture.*	■ Some systemic diseases change the texture of the hair. For instance, hypothyroidism causes the hair to coarsen, whereas hyperthyroidism causes the hair to become fine.
Inspect the scalp for lesions. *There should be no lesions on the scalp.*	■ Mild dandruff is normal, but excessive, greasy flakes indicate seborrhea. ■ Hair loss, pustules, and scales appear on the scalp in tinea capitis (scalp ringworm). ■ Red, swollen pustules appear around infected hair follicles and are called folliculitis. ■ Head lice may be seen as oval nits (eggs) adhering to the base of the hair shaft. Head lice are usually accompanied by itching.
Inspect nail curvature. *Nails should not be excessively curved.*	■ Clubbing (Figure 15–6 ■), in which the angle of the nail base is greater than 180 degrees, is seen in respiratory disorders, cardiovascular disorders, cirrhosis of the liver, colitis, and thyroid disease. The nail becomes thick, hard, shiny, and curved at the free end.

Flattened angle (180°)

Early clubbing

About 160°

Normal

A   B

Figure 15–6 ■ *A*, Assessing clubbing of the nails. *B*, Hand with nail clubbing.

Source: ISM/Phototake NYC.

Inspect the surface of the nails.	■ The nail folds become inflamed and swollen and the nail loosens in paronychia, an infection of the nails.

(continued)

TABLE 15–4 Integumentary Assessments (continued)

TECHNIQUE/NORMAL FINDINGS	ABNORMAL FINDINGS
Nail surfaces should be smooth and nail folds firm, without redness.	■ Inflammation and transverse rippling of the nail are associated with chronic paronychia and/or eczema. ■ The nail plate may separate from the nail bed in trauma, psoriasis, and *Pseudomonas* and *Candida* infections. This separation is called oncholysis. ■ Nail grooves may be caused by inflammation, by planus, or by nail biting. ■ Nail pitting may be seen with psoriasis. ■ A transverse groove (Beau's line) may be seen in trachoma and/or acute diseases. ■ Thin spoon-shaped nails (Figure 15–7 ■) may be seen in anemia. **Figure 15–7** ■ Spoon-shaped nails.
Inspect nail color. Nail color should be even. Pigmented bands are normally found in more than 90% of African Americans.	■ The sudden appearance of a pigmented band may indicate melanoma in people with light skin. ■ Yellowish nails are seen in psoriasis and fungal infections. ■ Dark nails occur with trauma, *Candida* infections, and hyperbilirubinemia. ■ Blackish-green nails are apparent in injury and in *Pseudomonas* infection. ■ Red splinter longitudinal hemorrhages may be seen in injury and/or psoriasis.
Inspect nail thickness. Nails should not be excessively thick.	■ Trauma to the nails usually causes thickening. Other causes of thick nails include psoriasis, fungal infections, and decreased peripheral vascular blood supply. ■ Thinning of the nails is seen in nutritional deficiencies.

TABLE 15–5 Primary Skin Lesions

Macule, Patch 	Flat, nonpalpable change in skin color. Macules are smaller than 1 cm, with a circumscribed border, and patches are larger than 1 cm and may have an irregular border. **Examples** Macules: freckles, measles, and petechiae. Patches: Mongolian spots, port-wine stains, vitiligo, and chloasma.	Vesicle, Bulla 	Elevated, fluid-filled, round or oval shaped, palpable mass with thin, translucent walls and circumscribed borders. Vesicles are smaller than 0.5 cm; bullae are larger than 0.5 cm. **Examples** Vesicles: herpes simplex/zoster, early chickenpox, poison ivy, and small burn blisters. Bullae: contact dermatitis, friction blisters, and large burn blisters.
Papule, Plaque 	Elevated, solid, palpable mass with circumscribed border. Papules are smaller than 0.5 cm; plaques are groups of papules that form lesions larger than 0.5 cm. **Examples** Papules: elevated moles, warts, and lichen planus. Plaques: psoriasis, actinic keratosis, and also lichen planus.	Wheal 	Elevated, often reddish area with irregular border caused by diffuse fluid in tissues rather than free fluid in a cavity, as in vesicles. Size varies. **Examples** Insect bites and hives (extensive wheals).
Nodule, Tumor 	Elevated, solid, hard or soft palpable mass extending deeper into the dermis than a papule. Nodules have circumscribed borders and are 0.5 to 2 cm; tumors may have irregular borders and are larger than 2 cm. **Examples** Nodules: small lipoma, squamous cell carcinoma, fibroma, and intradermal nevi. Tumors: large lipoma, carcinoma, and hemangioma.	Pustule 	Elevated, pus-filled vesicle or bulla with circumscribed border. Size varies. **Examples** Acne, impetigo, and carbuncles (large boils).
		Cyst 	Elevated, encapsulated, fluid-filled or semisolid mass originating in the subcutaneous tissue or dermis, usually 1 cm or larger. **Examples** Varieties include sebaceous cysts and epidermoid cysts.

TABLE 15–6 Secondary Skin Lesions

Atrophy

A translucent, dry, paper-like, sometimes wrinkled skin surface resulting from thinning or wasting of the skin due to loss of collagen and elastin.

Examples Striae, aged skin.

Ulcer

Deep, irregularly shaped area of skin loss extending into the dermis or subcutaneous tissue. May bleed. May leave scar.

Examples Decubitus ulcers (pressure sores), stasis ulcers, chancres.

Erosion

Wearing away of the superficial epidermis causing a moist, shallow depression. Because erosions do not extend into the dermis, they heal without scarring.

Examples Scratch marks, ruptured vesicles.

Fissure

Linear crack with sharp edges, extending into the dermis.

Examples Cracks at the corners of the mouth or in the hands, athlete's foot.

Lichenification

Rough, thickened, hardened area of epidermis resulting from chronic irritation such as scratching or rubbing.

Example Chronic dermatitis.

Scar

Flat, irregular area of connective tissue left after a lesion or wound has healed. New scars may be red or purple; older scars may be silvery or white.

Examples Healed surgical wound or injury, healed acne.

Scales

Shedding flakes of greasy, keratinized skin tissue. Color may be white, gray, or silver. Texture may vary from fine to thick.

Examples Dry skin, dandruff, psoriasis, and eczema.

Keloid

Elevated, irregular, darkened area of excess scar tissue caused by excessive collagen formation during healing. Extends beyond the site of the original injury. Higher incidence in people of African descent.

Examples Keloid from ear piercing or surgery.

Crust

Dry blood, serum, or pus left on the skin surface when vesicles or pustules burst. Can be red-brown, orange, or yellow. Large crusts that adhere to the skin surface are called scabs.

Examples Eczema, impetigo, herpes, or scabs following abrasion.

TABLE 15–7 Vascular Skin Lesions

Spider Angioma

Source: Custom Medical Stock Photo, Inc.

A flat, bright red dot with tiny radiating blood vessels ranging in size from a pinpoint to 2 cm. It blanches with pressure.

Cause A type of telangiectasis (vascular dilatation) caused by elevated estrogen levels, pregnancy, estrogen therapy, vitamin B deficiency, or liver disease, or may not be pathologic.

Localization/Distribution Most commonly appear on the upper half of the body.

Venous Star

Source: Photo Researchers, Inc.

A flat blue lesion with radiating, cascading, or linear veins extending from the center. It ranges in size from 3 to 25 cm.

Cause A type of telangiectasis (vascular dilatation) caused by increased intravenous pressure in superficial veins.

Localization/Distribution Most commonly appear on the anterior chest and the lower legs near varicose veins.

Petechiae

Source: Custom Medical Stock Photo, Inc.

Flat red or purple rounded "freckles" approximately 1 to 3 mm in diameter. Difficult to detect in dark skin. Do not blanch.

Cause Minute hemorrhages resulting from fragile capillaries, petechiae are caused by septicemias, liver disease, or vitamin C or K deficiency. They may also be caused by anticoagulant therapy.

Localization/Distribution Most commonly appear on the dependent surfaces of the body (e.g., back, buttocks). In the patient with dark skin, look for them in the oral mucosa and conjunctivae.

Purpura

Source: Custom Medical Stock Photo, Inc.

Flat, reddish blue, irregularly shaped extensive patches of varying size.

Cause Bleeding disorders, scurvy, and capillary fragility in the older adult (senile purpura).

Localization/Distribution May appear anywhere on the body, but are most noticeable on the legs, arms, and backs of hands.

Ecchymosis

Source: Photo Researchers, Inc.

A flat, irregularly shaped lesion of varying size with no pulsation. Does not blanch with pressure. In light skin, it begins as bluish purple mark that changes to greenish yellow. In brown skin, it varies from blue to deep purple. In black skin, it appears as a darkened area.

Cause Release of blood from superficial vessels into surrounding tissue due to trauma, hemophilia, liver disease, or deficiency of vitamin C or K.

Localization/Distribution Occurs anywhere on the body at the site of trauma or pressure.

TEST YOURSELF NCLEX-RN® REVIEW

1. Following a burn involving several layers of skin, the healed burn area does not grow hair or sweat. Which layer of the skin was a part of the burn?
   1. epidermis
   2. dermis
   3. stratum basale
   4. stratum spinosum
2. What pigment is responsible for skin tanning?
   1. carotene
   2. red blood cells
   3. melanin
   4. sebum
3. Which of the four assessment techniques are used during assessment of the integumentary system? **Select all that apply.**
   1. inspection
   2. palpation
   3. percussion
   4. auscultation
4. A nurse takes a patient's body temperature orally and finds it is elevated by 3 degrees. What other assessment would also be commonly found?
   1. erythema
   2. jaundice
   3. pallor
   4. cyanosis
5. A nurse is assessing a patient who is complaining of severe itching. What would be an appropriate interview question?
   1. "Tell me how this itch feels."
   2. "Why do you keep scratching it?"
   3. "Have you used a new soap?"
   4. "Describe your daily fluid intake."
6. A nurse is assessing the skin of an older adult patient for dehydration. What finding would indicate this condition?
   1. decreased turgor
   2. increased moisture
   3. presence of lesions
   4. pallor or cyanosis
7. A nurse is assessing for edema. What part of the body would he or she palpate?
   1. scalp
   2. fingers
   3. clavicle
   4. ankle/foot
8. A nurse documents that a patient with chronic dermatitis has rough, thickened areas of skin. What term would he or she use?
   1. ulcers
   2. papules
   3. atrophy
   4. lichenification
9. While making a home visit to an older woman, a nurse notices multiple angiomas on her arms and body. What might these indicate?
   1. high intake of vitamin A
   2. poor hygiene
   3. caregiver strain
   4. aging skin
10. While assessing the hair of a family, a nurse notices small white eggs on the hair shaft. What type of infestation is being assessed?
    1. bacterial
    2. viral
    3. head lice
    4. head lichens

See Test Yourself answers in Appendix C.

Pearson Nursing Student Resources

Find additional review materials at
www.nursing.pearsonhighered.com

Prepare for success with additional NCLEX®-style practice questions, interactive assignments and activities, Web links, animations and videos, and more!

BIBLIOGRAPHY

Armstrong, J., & Mitchell, E. (2008). Comprehensive nursing assessment in the care of older people. *Nursing Older People, (20)*1, 36–40.

Bickley, L., & Szilagyi, P. (2007). *Bates' guide to physical examination and history taking* (9th ed.). Philadelphia: Lippincott.

Fletcher, K. (2005). Skin: Geriatric self-learning module. *MEDSURG Nursing, 14*(2), 138–142.

Kee, J. (2009). *Prentice Hall handbook of laboratory & diagnostic tests with nursing implications.* (6th ed.). Upper Saddle River, NJ: Pearson Prentice Hall.

Khachemoune, A., & Ehrsam, E. (2005). Assessing malignant melanoma: A case study. *Dermatology Nursing, 17*(3), 188–190.

Kulkowski, K., & Ratliff, C. (2004). Wounds & skin care: Managing venous and neuropathic ulcers. *Nursing, 34*(8), 68.

Mirmirani, P. (2007). How to approach hair loss in women. *Dermatology Nursing, 19*(6), 531–535.

National Institute of Health. (2008). *Genes and Disease: Skin and Connective Tissue.* Available at http://www .ncbi.nlm.nih.gov/books/bookres.fegi/gnd/pdf.html

Nicol, N. (2005) Anatomy and physiology of the skin. *Dermatology Nursing, 17*(1), 62.

Osman, B., & Kernodle, M. (2007). A new look at pressure ulcers: Ultrasound technology can help detect skin integrity issues that are not apparent in a visual skin assessment. *Provider, 33*(4), 35–37.

Porth, C. (2007). Essentials of *Pathophysiology: Concepts of altered health states* (2nd ed.). Philadelphia: Lippincott.

Pullen, R. (2007). Assessing skin lesions. *Nursing, 37*(8), 44–45.

Rushing, J. (2008). Assessing a patient for lice infestation. *Nursing, 38*(7), 20.

Scanlon, E., & Stubbs, N. (2004). Pressure ulcer risk assessment in patients with darkly pigmented skin. *Professional Nurse, 19*(6), 339–341.

Scott, T. (2008). How do I differentiate normal aging of the skin from pathologic conditions? *Medscape Nurses.* Available at http://www.medscape.com/viewarticle/575293

Smith, M., & Nedorost, S. (2008). Hand dermatitis: Nursing support in the plan of care. *Dermatology Nursing, 20*(2), 121–125.

Snow, M. (2008). Fighting fungal infections: Stopping tinea in its tracks. *Nursing, 38*(7), 62–63.

Weber, J., & Kelley, J. (2006). *Health assessment in nursing* (3rd ed.). Philadelphia: Lippincott Williams &Wilkins.

Yoder, L. (2005). Be sun safe! Understand skin cancer prevention and detection. *MEDSURG Nursing, 14*(4), 254–256.

16 Nursing Care of Patients with Integumentary Disorders

LEARNING OUTCOMES

1. Describe the manifestations, self-care, and nursing care of common skin problems and lesions.
2. Compare and contrast the etiology, pathophysiology, interdisciplinary care and nursing care of patients with infections and infestations, inflammatory disorders, and malignancies of the skin.
3. Explain the risk factors for, pathophysiology of, and nursing interventions to prevent and care for pressure ulcers.

4. Discuss surgical options for excision of neoplasms, reconstruction of facial or body structures, and cosmetic procedures.
5. Explain the pathophysiology of selected disorders of the hair and nails.
6. Discuss the effects and nursing implications of medications and treatments used to treat disorders of the integument.

CLINICAL COMPETENCIES

1. Assess functional health status of patients with integumentary disorders, and monitor, document, and report abnormal manifestations.
2. Use research to plan and implement evidence-based nursing care for patients with pressure ulcers.
3. Use assessed data, patient values, evidence, and clinical expertise to determine priority nursing diagnoses and select and implement individualized nursing interventions for patients with integumentary disorders.
4. Administer topical, oral, and injectable medications used to treat integumentary disorders knowledgeably and safely.

5. Effectively communicate with and function within the interdisciplinary team to plan and provide care for patients with integumentary disorders.
6. Provide teaching appropriate for prevention and self-care of manifestations and disorders of the integumentary system.
7. Adapt individual and cultural variations, as well as expressed needs and preferences, into the plan of care for patients with integumentary disorders.
8. Revise the plan of care as needed to provide effective interventions to promote, maintain, or restore functional health status to patients with disorders of the integument.

KEY TERMS

acne, 421
actinic keratosis, 424
angioma, 407
basal cell cancer, 425
carbuncle, 411
cellulitis, 411
comedones, 421
cyst, 405
dermatitis, 419
dermatophytoses, 413
folliculitis, 410

frostbite, 439
furuncle, 411
herpes simplex, 416
herpes zoster, 416
keloids, 406
keratosis, 407
lichen planus, 423
malignant melanoma, 428
nevi, 407
paronychia, 443

pemphigus vulgaris, 422
pressure ulcer, 434
pruritus, 405
psoriasis, 407
scabies, 415
skin graft, 440
squamous cell cancer, 426
toxic epidermal necrolysis (TENS), 423
warts, 415
xerosis, 405

The skin and its accessory structures (the integumentary system) enclose and cover the body, providing protection by serving as a barrier between the internal and external environments. The skin contains receptors for touch and sensation, helps regulate body temperature, and maintains fluid and electrolyte balance. The skin also provides cues to racial and ethnic background, and plays a major role in determining self-concept, roles, and relationships.

Disorders of the integument range from dry skin to life-threatening cancer. Many disorders are treated in an outpatient setting or by self-care. This chapter discusses disorders of the skin, hair, and nails; ∞ Chapter 17 discusses the patient with burns. Primary and secondary skin lesions are described and illustrated in ∞ Chapter 15, Tables 15–5 and 15–6. These terms are used throughout this and the next chapter.

Common Skin Problems and Lesions

The disorders discussed in this section are those experienced by a large number of people. Although they are considered minor health problems in terms of health care, they may cause major

problems for the person experiencing a high level of discomfort and/or chronicity.

The Patient with Pruritus

Pruritus is a subjective itching sensation producing an urge to scratch. Pruritus may occur in a small, circumscribed area, or it may involve a widespread area; it may or may not be associated with a rash. The itch sensation begins in nerve endings in the skin, is carried to the dorsal horn of the spinal cord, and is then transmitted to the somatosensory cortex in the central nervous system (CNS). Itching may also be perceived by the brain but does not exist on the skin. Scratching is a neurologic reflex that can be controlled in varying degrees by the individual (Porth & Matfin, 2009).

Almost anything in the internal or external environment can cause pruritus. Insects, animals, plants, fabrics, metals, medications, allergies, and emotional distress are among the most common causes. Pruritus also may occur as a secondary manifestation of systemic disorders, such as certain types of cancer, diabetes mellitus, liver disease, and renal failure. Although the exact physiology is unknown, it is known that heat and prostaglandins trigger pruritus and that it is increased by histamine and morphine.

The pathophysiologic response of pruritus to stimulation or irritation follows a similar pathway, regardless of cause. The irritating agent stimulates receptors in the junction between the epidermis and dermis, and may also trigger the release of histamine and other chemical mediators that either further stimulate or mediate the itch response. The response of the person experiencing the itch is to scratch or rub the affected area. This may irritate the skin and cause further inflammation, which in turn sets off a cycle of increasingly intense itching and scratching, called the *itch-scratch-itch cycle*.

Secondary effects of scratching include skin excoriation, erythema (redness), wheals, changes in pigmentation, and infections. Persistent pruritus may interrupt sleep patterns because the itching sensation is often more intense at night. Long-term pruritus may be debilitating and increases the risk of infection as excoriation occurs.

Management of pruritus focuses on identifying and eliminating the cause and providing medications to relieve the itch. Antihistamines may relieve pruritus in some patients. Tranquilizers provide sedation, which may in turn relieve the emotional stress associated with pruritus; however, eliminating the stressors produces a more successful result. Topical or systemic antibiotics are used to treat the infection resulting from the scratching and excoriation. Topical medications that contain corticosteroids are often used to relieve the pruritus and inflammation. Topical medications may also be administered through therapeutic baths or soaks with agents that relieve pruritus, such as cornstarch and baking soda or coal tar concentrates. Creams containing a topical anesthetic or antibiotic may also be used. Therapeutic baths are discussed in the Medication Administration on page 406. Table 16–1 lists examples of topical agents used to treat skin disorders.

The Patient with Dry Skin (Xerosis)

Dry skin, also called **xerosis**, is most often a problem in the older adult from a decrease in the activity of sebaceous and sweat glands, reducing the skin's lubrication and moisture retention. However, dry skin may occur at any age from exposure to environmental heat and low humidity, sunlight, excessive bathing, and a decreased intake of liquids.

Two types of severe dry skin are xeroderma and ichthyosis. Xeroderma is a chronic skin condition characterized by dry, rough skin. Ichthyosis is an inherited dermatological condition in which the skin is dry, fissured, and hyperkeratotic; the surface of the skin has the appearance of fish scales.

The primary manifestation of dry skin is pruritus. Other manifestations include visible flaking of surface skin and an observable pattern of fine lines over the area. If the skin has been excessively dry and pruritic for a long period, the patient may have secondary skin lesions and lichenification (thickening).

Nursing care focuses on teaching the patient and family how to reduce the dry skin and relieve the pruritus, as outlined in Box 16–1.

The Patient with Benign Skin Lesions

The skin is subject to many different types and kinds of benign skin lesions, including cysts, keloids, nevi, angiomas, skin tags, and keratoses. Although these benign lesions are often considered more of a nuisance than an illness, they do require monitoring for an increase in size that interferes with the skin's appearance or function. Most benign skin lesions do not require treatment, although excision or laser surgery may be desired or necessary. Cysts may enlarge, skin tags may become irritated and bleed, nevi may change in appearance, or any of the lesions may cause discomfort with appearance.

Cysts

Cysts of the skin are benign closed sacs in or under the skin surface that are lined with epithelium and contain fluid or a semisolid material. Epidermal inclusion cysts and pilar cysts are the most common types.

TABLE 16–1 Medications Used to Treat Skin Disorders

TYPE	USE	EXAMPLES
Creams	Moisturize the skin	Aquacare, Curel, Nutraderm
Ointments	Lubricate the skin and retard water loss	Aquaphor, Vaseline
Lotions	Moisturize and lubricate the skin	Alpha-Keri, Dermassage, Lubriderm
Anesthetics	Relieve itching	Xylocaine
Antibiotics	Treat infection	Bacitracin, Polysporin, Gentamicin, Silvadene
Corticosteroids	Suppress inflammation and relieve itching	Dexamethasone, Clocortolone, Desonide

Epidermal inclusion cysts may occur anywhere on the body but are most often found on the head and trunk. Although they are painless, they may grow so large that they become irritated by contact with clothing (e.g., if located on the back of the neck) or cause obstruction (e.g., if located on the nose). The cysts contain a semisolid material mainly of keratin. Pilar cysts are found on the scalp and originate from sebaceous glands. They are also painless. Both types of cysts rarely require treatment unless they become large and bothersome.

Keloids

Keloids are elevated, irregularly shaped, progressively enlarging scars. They arise from excessive amounts of collagen in the stratum corneum during scar formation in connective tissue repair. These lesions are more common in young adults and appear within 1 year of the initial trauma.

This abnormal response most often occurs in people of African and Asian descent who sustain burns of the skin, but even seemingly minor trauma can result in keloid formation. There is a familial tendency to develop keloids. Other risk factors for keloid formation include excessive tension on a wound and poor alignment of skin edges following accidental or intentional skin trauma. Certain skin surfaces are also more likely to develop keloids: the chin, ears, shoulders, back, and lower legs.

The excessive scar formation is associated with increased metabolic activity of fibroplasts and increased type III collagen. The swollen appearance of the keloids is the result of an excess of extracellular material. The keloids first appear as red, firm, rubbery plaques that persist for several months after the initial trauma (Figure 16–1 ■). Uncontrolled overgrowth over time causes the keloids to extend beyond the original scar. Eventually, the keloid becomes smooth and hyperpigmented.

BOX 16–1 Teaching to Reduce Dry Skin and Relieve Pruritus

- Wash clothing in a mild detergent and rinse twice; do not use fabric softeners.
- Avoid using perfumes and lotions containing alcohol.
- Apply skin lubricants after a bath to help retain moisture.
- Soaps and hot water are drying. Clean the skin with tepid water and either a mild soap or cleansing creams. If soap is used, rinse it off carefully.
- It is not necessary to take a bath every day.
- If bath oils are used, add them to the bath water at the end of the bath (the moist skin is more likely to retain the oil). Use care not to slip in the tub.
- Use a humidifier to humidify the air.
- Apply creams and lotions when the skin is slightly damp after bathing.
- Increase fluid intake.
- Keep nails trimmed short, wear loose clothing, and keep the environment cool.
- A brief application of pressure or cold may relieve pruritus.
- Cotton gloves may be worn at night if scratching during sleep causes skin excoriation.
- Distraction or relaxation techniques may prove helpful.

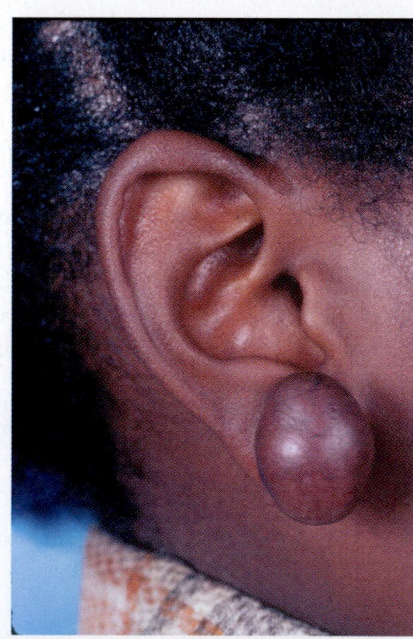

Figure 16–1 ■ Keloids form as a result of deposits of excessive amounts of collagen during scar formation.

Nevi

Nevi, more commonly called *moles*, are flat or raised macules or papules with rounded, well-defined borders (Figure 16–2 ■). Nevi arise from melanocytes during early childhood, with the cells initially accumulating at the junction of the dermis and epidermis. Over time, the cluster of cells moves into the dermis, and the lesion becomes visible. Nevi can occur on any skin surface of the body and may arise as single lesions or in groups. Almost all adults have nevi.

Nevocellular nevi are tan to deep brown, small in size, and grow in groups. Dysplastic nevi are larger than other nevi and may be flat, slightly raised, or appear as lesions with a darker, raised center and irregular border. Dysplastic nevi can transform into malignant lesions (see the later discussion about melanoma). It is important to monitor nevi for changes in size, thickness, color, bleeding, or itching. If any of these changes occur, the person should seek immediate professional assessment.

Angiomas

Angiomas, also called *hemangiomas*, are benign vascular tumors. They appear in the adult in different forms:

■ Nevus flammeus (port-wine stain) is a congenital vascular lesion that involves the capillaries. The lesions tend to occur on the upper body or face as macular patches that range from light red to dark purple. These lesions are present at birth and grow proportionately with the child into adulthood.
■ Cherry angiomas are small, rounded papules that may occur at any age, but they most commonly arise in the 40s and gradually increase in number. The lesions range in color from bright red to purple. These lesions are often found on the trunk.
■ Spider angiomas are dilated superficial arteries. They are common in pregnant women and in patients with hepatic disease. Spider angiomas occur most often on the face, neck, and upper chest. The lesions are usually small, bright red papules with radiating lines.
■ Telangiectases are single dilated capillaries or terminal arteries that appear most often on the cheeks and nose. These lesions are more common in older adults and result from photoaged (aging, sun-damaged) skin. The lesions look like broken veins.

■ Venous lakes are small, flat, blue blood vessels. They are seen on the exposed skin of the older adult: the ears, lips, and backs of the hands.

Skin Tags

Skin tags are soft papules on a pedicle. They can be as small as a pinhead or as large as a pea and are most often found on the front or side of the neck and in the axillae, as well as in areas where clothing (such as underwear) rubs the skin. These lesions have normal skin color and texture.

Keratoses

A **keratosis** is any skin condition in which there is a benign overgrowth and thickening of the cornified epithelium. These lesions most often appear in adults after age 50. *Seborrheic keratoses* appear as superficial flat, smooth, or warty-surfaced growths, 5 to 20 mm in diameter, most often on the face and trunk. The lesions may be tan, waxy yellow, dark brown, or flesh-colored, and they often appear greasy. They are most often seen in the older adult and do not appear to be related to damage from sun exposure.

The Patient with Psoriasis

Psoriasis is a chronic immune skin disorder characterized by raised, reddened, round circumscribed plaques covered by silvery white scales (Figure 16–3 ■). There are several different forms, but the most common is plaque psoriasis (psoriasis vulgaris), occurring in about 80% of cases (American Academy of Dermatology, 2009). As with any chronic illness, the skin manifestations may occur and disappear throughout life, with no discernible pattern to the recurrence.

As many as 7.5 million people in the United States have psoriasis; about 20% have moderate to severe forms (National Psoriasis Foundation, 2009).The incidence of psoriasis is lower in warm, sunny climates. The average age of onset is in the 30s, but it may occur at any age. Psoriasis occurs more often in Caucasians, and men and women are affected equally. Sunlight, stress, seasonal changes, hormone fluctuations, steroid withdrawal, and certain drugs (such as beta blockers, lithium, and chloroquine [an antimalarial]) appear to act as triggers to

Figure 16–2 ■ Nevi (moles) arise from melanocytes and are common in all adults.

Figure 16–3 ■ The characteristic lesions of psoriasis are raised, red, round plaques covered with thick, silvery scales.

development of the disorder. About one-third of patients have a family history of psoriasis. Trauma to the skin from such events as surgery, sunburn, or excoriation is also a common precipitating factor; lesions that result from trauma are called Koebner's reaction (Porth & Matfin, 2009).

Pathophysiology

Normally, the keratinocyte (an epidermal cell making up 95% of the epidermis) migrates from the basal cell to the stratum corneum (the outer skin layer) in about 14 days and is sloughed off 14 days later. Psoriatic skin cells, by contrast, have a shorter cycle of growth, completing the journey to the stratum corneum in only 4 to 7 days, a condition called hyperkeratosis. These immature cells produce an abnormal keratin that forms thick, flaky scales at the surface of the skin. The increased cell metabolism stimulates increased vascularity, which contributes to the erythema of the lesions.

Although the exact cause is unknown, there is increasing evidence that a T-lymphocyte-mediated reaction results in the production of chemical messengers that stimulate the growth of keratinocytes and dermal blood vessels. The accompanying inflammation further contributes to plaque formation. The lesions can be found anywhere on the skin but most commonly involve the skin over the elbows, knees, and scalp. Lesions involving the hand and foot are especially problematic for the patient. Initially, the lesions are papules that form into well-defined erythematous plaques with thick, silvery scales. The plaques in darker-skinned persons may appear purple.

Manifestations

The characteristic lesions in plaque psoriasis are well-demarcated regions of erythematous plaques that shed thick, silver-gray flakes. Pruritus is common over the psoriatic lesions. If the lesions are located in an intertriginous zone, such as between the toes, under the breasts, or in the perianal region, the psoriatic scales may soften, allowing painful fissures to form. When psoriasis affects the nails, pitting and a yellow or brown discoloration results. The nail may separate from the nail bed, thicken, and crumble. The involved nails, which are more often fingernails than toenails, are at high risk for infection. Psoriatic arthritis is a specific form of arthritis involving not only skin lesions but also inflammation of joints.

Interdisciplinary Care

Treatment is based on the type of psoriasis, the extent and location of the lesions, the age of the patient, and the degree of disfigurement or disability.

Diagnosis

Skin biopsy may be done if the patient presents with atypical manifestations, or to differentiate psoriasis from other inflammatory or infectious skin disorders. In addition, an ultrasound may reveal typical psoriatic changes in the stratus corneum and inflammation of the dermis.

Medications

A variety of medications and treatments may be prescribed, including topical medications and photochemotherapy. Although there is no cure, treatment decreases the severity and pain of the lesions. Corticosteroids, tar preparations, anthralin, calcipotriene (a vitamin D derivative) and tazarotene (a synthetic retinoid) are typically used. Ustekinumab, an injectable monoclonal antibody that decreases the immune response, is in advanced clinical trials for severe psoriasis.

Topical corticosteroids decrease inflammation, suppress mitotic activity of psoriatic cells, and delay the movement of keratinocytes to the surface of the skin (thus giving them time to mature and decreasing hyperkeratinosis). The most effective topical corticosteroids are potent preparations that are well absorbed through the skin and are used under an occlusive dressing. Corticosteroids may also be taken systemically or injected directly into the lesions. However, corticosteroids rarely cause a lasting remission and may cause the psoriasis to become unstable (McPhee, Papadakis, & Tierney, 2008). They are therefore used for repeated short periods of treatment and combined with other measures, such as tar preparations, occlusion, or a topical retinoid.

Tar preparations (such as Estar, Psorigel, and Fototar) suppress mitotic activity and are also anti-inflammatory. Their exact mechanism of action is unknown, but they are effective in removing scales and increasing remission time. Preparations made of coal tar are messy, cause staining, and have an unpleasant odor, but they are an effective form of treatment. Salex shampoo is prescribed for patients with scalp psoriasis to remove plaques and scales. Psorent is a non-prescription cream that is made from coal tar but does not stain or have an odor.

Calcipotriene (Dovonex) has been effective and safe in both the short-term and long-term treatment of psoriasis. It inhibits cell proliferation in the epidermis and facilitates cell differentiation. Although more irritating than calcipotriene, tazarotene gel (Avage, Tarorac) is a topical retinoid that may also be used to treat mild to moderate psoriasis.

Treatments

Psoriasis that is generalized (i.e., involves more than 30% of the body surface) is difficult to treat with topical medications. Treatments for generalized psoriasis include ultraviolet light therapy and photochemotherapy.

PHOTOTHERAPY Ultraviolet-B (UVB) light or narrow band UVB are treatments for generalized psoriasis. UVB light decreases the growth rate of epidermal cells, thereby decreasing hyperkeratosis. Mercury vapor lights or fluorescent UV tubes provide the UVB light; the latter are often arranged in a cabinet so the patient can stand and expose psoriatic lesions more easily. These units may be purchased or constructed to be used in the patient's home. Ultraviolet-A (PUVA) combines the oral or topical administration of psoralen (to make the skin more sensitive to light) with UVA, which penetrates deeper into the skin than UVB. PUVA requires fewer treatments for remission of lesions, but has more side effects and long-term use increases the risk of skin cancers.

The light therapy is administered in gradually increasing exposure times, until the patient experiences a mild erythema, like a mild sunburn. Treatments are given three times a week as an outpatient and are measured in seconds of exposure. The eyes are shielded during the treatment. The erythema response occurs in about 8 hours. Careful assessment is necessary to prevent more severe burning, which could exacerbate the psoriasis. In patients with extensive psoriasis, UVB treatments may be combined with tar preparations, which increase the photosensitivity of the skin.

PHOTOCHEMOTHERAPY   In photochemotherapy, a light-activated form of the drug methoxsalen is used. This drug is an antimetabolite that inhibits DNA synthesis and thereby prevents cell mitosis, decreasing hyperkeratosis. Exposure to ultraviolet-A (UVA) rays activates methoxsalen; it is administered orally, and the patient is exposed to UVA 2 hours later. Treatments are administered 2 to 3 times a week, for 10 to 20 total treatments. Treatment causes tanning, and direct sunlight must be avoided for 8 to 12 hours thereafter. Photochemotherapy has had a high success rate in achieving remission of psoriasis, but it can accelerate aging of exposed skin, induce cataract development, alter immune function, and increase the risk of melanoma.

Nursing Care

The patient with psoriasis requires nursing care to meet physical and psychologic responses to the illness. The nurse provides teaching for self-care and emotional support through nonjudgmental acceptance.

Nursing Diagnoses and Interventions

The nursing interventions discussed in this section focus on common problems of risk for impaired skin integrity and disturbed body image.

Impaired Skin Integrity

Psoriatic lesions range from several scales to large, open areas. Typical psoriatic skin lesions increase the risk of infection, which can compromise healing. In addition, certain treatments (e.g., the use of UVA or retinoids) may cause erythema or peeling of the skin, further altering skin integrity.

- Teach methods to reduce injury to the skin when taking therapeutic baths or treatments: Use warm, not hot, water; gently rub lesions with a soft washcloth, using a circular motion; dry the skin with a soft towel, using a blotting or patting motion; and keep the skin lubricated at all times. *Hot water and dry skin increase pruritus, further stimulating the itch-scratch-itch cycle. Dry skin also worsens psoriasis. Washing or drying the skin with rough linens or pressure may excoriate the skin over the psoriatic lesions.*
- Teach how to apply topical medications (see Box 16–2). *Applying a thin layer of medication more frequently is often more effective than applying a single thick layer of medication. The medications used to treat psoriasis may irritate the eyes and mucous membranes; when applied in skinfolds, they may also cause maceration (skin breakdown due to prolonged exposure to moisture).*
- Teach manifestations of infection and how to contact the healthcare provider if these occur: elevated temperature, increased swelling, redness, pain, increase in drainage, and any change in the color of the drainage. *The patient with skin lesions is at high risk for infection, as the skin is the body's first line of defense.*

BOX 16–2 General Guidelines for Applying Topical Medications

- Each time a medication is applied, the skin surface must be clean and dry. Remove the medication from the previous application. Remove creams by washing the skin with tap water; remove ointments by washing the skin first with mineral oil and then with a mild soap and water.
- To apply gels, creams, and pastes: Squeeze about 1/2 to 1 inch of the gel or cream into the palm of the hand. Rub the hands together until they are covered. Apply gels and creams to the affected areas with long strokes until the skin is thinly covered. Differences from these general guidelines follow:
  a. Corticosteroids are usually applied two to three times a day in small amounts and rubbed directly onto the lesions. Apply the medication after a bath and cover with an occlusive dressing.
  b. Apply medications containing tar in the direction of hair growth. Do not apply these medications to the face, to the genitals, or in skin folds. If the tar is water based or oil based, it will stain clothing.
  c. Wear gloves when applying anthralin stains.
- To apply lotions: Shake the bottle of lotion well. Pour a small amount into the palm of the hand, and pat the medication onto the skin. If the lotion is thin, apply it with a gauze pad.
- To apply sprays: Hold the container about 6 inches from the skin and apply the medication in a short spray.
- To apply medicated shampoo: Rinse out medication from the previous application. Apply the shampoo, massage into the hair and over the scalp carefully, and allow it to remain for the prescribed time. Rinse.
- To apply pastes: Use enough paste on an applicator (such as a wooden tongue depressor) to cover the lesion thinly.

- Teach manifestations of the complications of treatment: excoriation, increased erythema, increased peeling, and blister formation. *The topical medications or treatments may damage cells through chemical burns or excessive exposure to ultraviolet light. Times and methods of treatment need to be adjusted if these manifestations occur.*

Disturbed Body Image

The chronic skin lesions of psoriasis may cause patients to isolate themselves from social contacts, withdraw from normal roles and responsibilities, and feel helpless or powerless.

- Establish a trusting relationship by expressing acceptance of the patient, both verbally and nonverbally. For example, touch the patient during social communications, demonstrating that the lesions are not contagious or offensive. *One's body image is affected not only by self-perception but also by the responses of others. Nonjudgmental acceptance helps the patient adapt to the change in body image. By touching the patient during interactions, the nurse demonstrates acceptance.*
- Encourage expression of self-perception and the asking of questions about the disease and treatment in view of the chronic nature of psoriasis. *The patient adapts to a changed body image through a process of recognition, acceptance, and resolution. Each person responds individually to disfigurement and loss.*

- Promote social interaction through family involvement in care and referral to support groups of people with psoriasis or other chronic skin conditions. *Acceptance by others is critical to acceptance of self. Psoriasis treatment is lifelong, time consuming, and often unappealing. By becoming involved in care, the family communicates acceptance. Sharing experiences with others who have the same health problem is a source of strength in adjusting to a visible, chronic illness.*

Community-Based Care

Patient and family teaching focuses on treatments and skin care needs. The following topics should be addressed:

- The chronic nature of the disease, factors that may precipitate an exacerbation, and methods to reduce stress.

- Interventions for pruritus and dry skin, and specific care for psoriasis:
  - Expose the skin to sunlight, but avoid sunburn.
  - Avoid trauma to the skin (e.g., do not scrub off scales, and use only an electric razor).
  - Avoid exposure to contagious illnesses such as influenza and colds.
  - Discuss current medications with the healthcare provider. Certain drugs (such as indomethacin [Indocin], lithium, and beta-adrenergic blocking agents) are known to precipitate exacerbations of psoriasis.
- Suggest the National Psoriasis Foundation, the National Institutes of Health, or the American Academy of Dermatology as resources.

Infections and Infestations of the Skin

The skin's resistance to infections and infestations is provided by protective mechanisms, including skin flora, sebum, and the immune response. Although the skin is normally resistant to infections and infestations, these disorders may occur as a result of a break in the skin surface, a virulent agent, and/or decreased resistance due to a compromised immune system. This section discusses skin disorders resulting from bacterial infections, fungal infections, parasitic infestations, and viral infections.

The Patient with a Bacterial Infection of the Skin

A number of bacteria normally inhabit the skin and do not cause an infection. However, when a break in the skin allows invasion by pathogenic bacteria, an infection, called a *pyoderma*, may occur. The most common bacterial infections are caused by gram-positive *Staphylococcus aureus* and beta-hemolytic streptococci. Bacterial infections of the skin may be primary or secondary. Primary infections are caused by a single pathogen and arise from normal skin; secondary infections develop in traumatized or diseased skin.

Most bacterial infections are treated by a primary care provider, and the patient remains at home for care. If the infection becomes more serious, inpatient care may be required. In addition, nosocomial infections of wounds or open lesions in hospitalized patients are often the result of bacterial infections, especially by methicillin-resistant *Staphylococcus aureus (MRSA)*.

Pathophysiology

Bacterial infections of the skin arise from the hair follicle, where bacteria can accumulate and grow and cause a localized infection. However, the bacteria also can enter the body through open wounds, invade deeper tissues, and cause a systemic infection, a potentially life-threatening disorder. Various types of bacterial infections involve the skin, including folliculitis, furuncles and carbuncles, cellulitis, and *staphylococcus aureus*.

Folliculitis

Folliculitis is a bacterial infection of the hair follicle, most commonly caused by *Staphylococcus aureus*. The infection begins at the follicle opening and extends down into the follicle. The bacteria release enzymes and chemical agents that cause an inflammation. The lesions appear as pustules surrounded by an area of erythema on the surface of the skin (Figure 16–4 ■). The lesions are accompanied by discomfort ranging from slight burning to intense itching. A major complication is abscess formation. Folliculitis is found most often on the scalp and extremities. It is also often seen on the face of bearded men (called sycosis barbae), on the legs of women who shave, and on the eyelids (called a stye). Although folliculitis may appear without any apparent cause, contributing factors include poor hygiene, poor nutrition, prolonged skin

Figure 16–4 ■ The lesions of folliculitis are pustules surrounded by areas of erythema.

moisture, tight heavy fabrics on the upper legs, and trauma to the skin.

Furuncles and Carbuncles

Furuncles, often called boils, are inflammations of the hair follicle. They often begin as folliculitis, but the infection spreads down the hair shaft, through the wall of the follicle, and into the dermis. The causative organism is commonly *Staphylococcus aureus*. A furuncle is initially a deep, firm, red, painful nodule from 1 to 5 cm in diameter (Figure 16–5 ■). After a few days, the nodule changes into a large, painful cystic nodule. The cysts may drain substantial amounts of purulent drainage. One or more furuncles may occur on any part of the body that has hair. Contributing factors include poor hygiene, trauma to the skin, areas of excessive moisture (including perspiration), and systemic diseases such as diabetes mellitus and hematologic malignancies.

A **carbuncle** is a group of infected hair follicles. The lesion begins as a firm mass located in the subcutaneous tissue and the lower dermis. This mass becomes swollen and painful and has multiple openings to the skin surface. Carbuncles are most frequently found on the back of the neck, the upper back, and the lateral thighs. In addition to the local manifestations, the patient may experience chills, fever, and malaise. The contributing factors for carbuncles are the same as for furuncles. Both infections are more common in hot, humid climates.

Cellulitis

Cellulitis is a localized infection of the dermis and subcutaneous tissue. Cellulitis can occur following a wound or skin ulcer or as an extension of furuncles or carbuncles. The infection spreads as a result of a substance produced by the causative organism, called spreading factor (hyaluronidase). This factor breaks down the fibrin network and other barriers that normally localize the infection. The area of cellulitis is red, swollen, and painful (Figure 16–6 ■). In some cases, vesicles may form over the area of cellulitis. The patient may also experience fever, chills, malaise, headache, and swollen lymph glands.

Methicillin-resistant *Staphylococcus aureus* (MRSA) Infection

Methicillin-resistant *Staphylococcus aureus* (MRSA) infection is caused by the *S. aureus* bacteria, an organism resistant to the broad-spectrum antibiotics (such as methicillin, oxacillin, amoxicillin, and penicillin) usually used to treat it. This potentially fatal disease is divided into 2 types: Healthcare-associated infections (acquired in hospitals and other healthcare settings) (HA-MRSA) and community associated infections (acquired in the community in otherwise healthy people) (CA-MRSA). MRSA in hospitalized patients may lead to infections of wounds, skin around invasive tubes or catheters, the blood, the lungs, or the urinary system. MRSA in patients in the community is often manifested as skin infections and a potentially life-threatening pneumonia.

S. aureus are normally found on the skin and in the nose of about one-third of the population. If present, but not causing illness, the person is said to be colonized and capable of spreading the bacteria to other people. The bacteria are spread by direct contact with the bacteria or with contaminated equipment. The Association for Professionals in Infection Control (2007) reported that an estimated 1.2 million hospitalized patients acquired HA-MRSA and more than 425 were colonized (increasing the risk of infecting self or others). The incidence of CA-MRSA is about 5 per 100,000 people, but those numbers are increasing. The rates of both types are highest in healthcare workers, in males, in those over age 65, in Blacks, and in those with HIV and AIDS. The risk for CA-MRSA is increased in those who participate in contact sports, and in people sharing personal items and/or living in crowded or unsanitary conditions.

Figure 16–5 ■ A furuncle (boil) is a deep, firm, red, painful nodule.

Figure 16–6 ■ Cellulitis is a bacterial infection localized in the dermis and subcutaneous tissue. The involved area is red, swollen, and painful.

The infection usually begins as a small, raised, red nodule on the skin that resembles a pimple or spider bite. The nodule rapidly increases in size, becomes dark red, is painful, contains pus, and may become a deep abscess. Cellulitis involving the area containing the initial infection (such as an extremity) is common. Actions to prevent MRSA are outlined in Box 16–3.

Interdisciplinary Care

The diagnosis of a bacterial infection of the skin is made by assessing the appearance of the lesion and by identifying the causative organism. Antibiotics effective against the organism are used in treatment.

Diagnosis

Drainage from a lesion or a blood culture may be ordered to identify the causative organism and target the most effective antibiotic. People who experience repeated bacterial skin infections, or who provide care for others who exhibit infections, may have a culture taken from the external nares to determine whether they are carriers of bacteria (e.g., MRSA) and are reinfecting themselves or others.

Medications

The primary treatment for bacterial infections of the skin is an antibiotic specific to the organism. The antibiotic is usually taken orally, and may also be applied topically. Multiple furuncles and carbuncles may be treated with cloxacillin (a penicillinase-resistant penicillin); the cephalosporins also are often effective. MRSA infections may be treated with antimicrobial therapy, including trimethoprim-sulfamethoxazole (Bactrim), minocycline (Minocin), doxycycline (Vibramycin), or clindamycin (Cleocin). There are no recommended guidelines for treating colonization. For repeated infections in a household, treatment may include mupirocin ointment (Bactroban Nasal) and an antiseptic body wash (Leung-Chen, 2008).

BOX 16–3 Preventing MRSA in the Hospital and in the Community

In the Hospital:
- Wash your hands frequently.
- Ask all hospital staff to wash their hands or use an alcohol-based hand sanitizer every time before touching you or objects in your environment.
- Ensure all invasive tubes or needles are inserted under sterile conditions.

In the Community:
- Wash your hands often and for as long as it takes to hum the "Happy Birthday" song. Use a hand sanitizer with at least 60% alcohol for times when you can't wash your hands.
- Do not share personal items such as razors, towels, or athletic equipment.
- For athletes: Shower after practice or games with soap and water. Sit out practice or games if you have an infection of the skin. Wash towels and athletic clothing after every use with hot water and bleach.
- Keep cuts and scrapes covered with a dry sterile dressing until they are healed.
- Go to the doctor if you have a skin infection that is painful and getting worse. Ask about being tested for MRSA.
- Use antibiotics appropriately. Take the full prescribed dose. Do not share.

Nursing Care

Nursing care focuses on preventing the spread of infection and restoring normal skin integrity. Many patients provide self-care at home, but need education about preventing CA-MRSA.

Nursing Diagnosis and Interventions

Risk for Infection

- Practice good hand washing (hand hygiene) and teach its importance. *Careful hand hygiene is one of the most effective methods to reduce the spread of infection both in and out of the hospital setting. Healthcare providers must wash their hands with soap and water before and after patient care and between each patient contact. All patients, family members, and visitors (both in the home and hospital setting) should be taught the importance of hand hygiene, but it is even more important for the patient with a bacterial infection.*
- Assess for and teach how to identify an increase in infection, which may be manifested systemically by fever, tachycardia, chills, and malaise. Local manifestations of the spread of the infection include an increase in erythema, the size of the lesion, and drainage. *This assessment is especially important for older, debilitated, or immunosuppressed patients, and for those who have large or dirty wounds.*

SAFETY ALERT If a patient with a bacterial skin infection is hospitalized, place him or her on isolation precautions to limit the spread of the organisms to other patients.

- Cover draining lesions with a sterile dressing, and handle soiled dressings or linens according to standard precautions. When changing dressings, always wear disposable rubber gloves and masks. *These actions are necessary to prevent the spread of infection to other areas of the patient's body, to other patients, to visitors, and to the nurse providing care.*

Community-Based Care

The increasing numbers of people with community-associated MRSA have resulted in state laws about reporting of or screening for MRSA. Many state public health departments have guidelines available about the manifestations, prevention, and treatment of CA-MRSA, and the Centers for Disease Control and Prevention (CDC) has treatment guidelines. Teaching for any bacterial infection focuses on facilitating tissue healing and eliminating the infection. Address the following topics:

- The importance of maintaining good nutrition
- The importance of maintaining cleanliness through careful hand hygiene and proper handling and disposal of dressings
- Preventing the spread of infection by not sharing linens and towels and washing clothing and linens in hot water
- The importance of not squeezing or trying to open a pimple or boil
- The importance of taking the full course of prescribed antibiotics

EVIDENCE FOR NURSING CARE | The Patient with Bacterial Infection of the Skin

Selected resources that nurses may find helpful when planning evidence-based nursing care follow.

- Casey, M. L., & Chasens, E. R. (2009). Community-associated methicillin-resistant staphylococcus aureus: Implications for emergency department nursing. *Journal of Emergency Nursing, 35*(3), 224–229.
- Haas, J. P., & Larson, E. L. (2008). Compliance with hand hygiene. *The American Journal of Nursing, 108*(8), 40–44.
- Hodgkinson, B., Agnew, J., Godfrey, C., Goldie, B., Kenner, C., González, R. L., Ramirez, B. A., Maria, E. G., McInerney, P., & Robertson-Malt, S. (2007). Topical skin care in aged care facilities. *Best Practice, The Joanna Briggs Institute, 11*(3), 1–4. Retrieved from, http://www.joannabriggs.edu.au/pdf/BPISEng_11_3.pdf
- Johnson, D., Lineweaver, L., & Maze, L. M. (2009). Patients' bath basins as potential sources of infection: A multicenter sampling study. *American Journal of Critical Care, 18*(1), 31–38.

Figure 16–7 ■ Tinea pedis (athlete's foot) is a fungal infection that often occurs between the toes.

The Patient with a Fungal Infection

Fungi are free-living, plantlike organisms that live in the soil, on animals, and on humans. The fungi that cause superficial skin infections are called dermatophytes. In humans, the dermatophytes live on keratin in the stratum corneum, hair, and nails. Fungal disorders are also called *mycoses*.

Pathophysiology

Fungal infections include dermatophytoses (tinea or ringworm) and candidiasis (yeast) infections. The candidiasis infections may affect various parts of the body, but are more commonly seen in women as vaginal infections, discussed and illustrated in ∞ Chapter 50.

Dermatophytoses (Tinea)

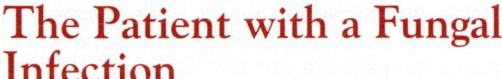

Superficial fungal infections of the skin are called **dermatophytoses** or, more commonly, ringworm. Fungal infections occur when a susceptible host comes in contact with the organism. The organism may be transmitted by direct contact with animals or other infected persons or by inanimate objects such as combs, pillowcases, towels, and hats. The most important factor in the development of the infection is moisture; the onset and spread of the fungal infection is greatest in areas where moisture content is high, such as within skinfolds, between the toes, and in the mouth. Other factors that increase the risk of a fungal infection include the use of broad-spectrum antibiotics that kill off normal flora and allow the fungi to grow, diabetes mellitus, immunodeficiencies, nutritional deficiencies, pregnancy, increasing age, and iron deficiency. The dermatophyte infections are named by the body part affected, for example:

- Tinea pedis is a fungal infection of the soles of the feet, the space between the toes, and/or the toenail (Figure 16–7 ■).

More often called athlete's foot, this is the most common tinea infection. The lesions vary from mild scaliness to painful fissures with drainage, and they are usually accompanied by pruritus and a foul odor. The infection is often chronic, absent in winter but reappearing in hot weather when perspiring feet are encased in shoes.

- Tinea corporis is a fungal infection of the body. It can be caused by several different fungi, and the lesions vary according to the causative organism. The most common lesions are large circular patches with raised red borders of vesicles, papules, or pustules. Pruritus and erythema are also present.
- Tinea cruris is a fungal infection of the groin that may extend to the inner thighs and buttocks. Often called "jock itch," it is often associated with tinea pedis and is more common in people who are physically active, are obese, and/or wear tight underclothing.

Interdisciplinary Care

Fungal infections are primarily diagnosed in outpatient settings and treated at home, but may also occur in hospitalized patients. The treatment is the same, regardless of the setting.

Diagnosis

Diagnostic tests are conducted to determine the causative fungi and may include cultures, microscopic examination using KOH and examination of the skin with ultraviolet light (Wood's lamp), described in ∞ Chapter 15.

Medications

Fungal infections of the skin are treated by topical or systemic antifungal medications. The over-the-counter (OTC) medications (such as miconazole, clotrimazole, butenafine, and terbinafine) are often less expensive and are effective (McPhee, Papadakis, & Tierney, 2008). Nursing implications for the antifungal medications are described in the Medication Administration Box on page 414.

EXAMPLES:
Butenafine (Mentax)
Clotrimazole (Mycelex)
Nystatin (Mycostatin, Nilstat)
Econazole (Spectazole)
Oxiconazole (Oxistat)
Miconazole (Monistat)
Undecylenic acid (Desenex)
Ketoconazole (Nizoral)
Fluconazole (Diflucan)
Amphotericin B (Fungizone)
Griseofulvin (Fulvicin)

Antifungal medications are prepared in a variety of forms, depending on the specific drug: powders, creams, shampoos, suspensions, troches, vaginal suppositories, and oral tablets. Some drugs interfere with the permeability of the fungal cell membrane, others interfere with DNA synthesis. Most of these medications are fungistatic but in large doses they may be fungicidal.

Nursing Responsibilities
- When taking the health history, ask about known hypersensitivity reactions to these agents; document carefully.
- Assess for side effects: skin rash, local irritation, gastrointestinal symptoms (if given PO), and mental status.
- Administer ketoconazole with food to minimize gastrointestinal irritation.

- Shake suspensions well before administration, and ask the patient to swish them around the mouth before swallowing.
- Tell the patient to allow oral tablets to dissolve in the mouth.

Health Education for the Patient and Family
- Therapy usually continues over a long period of time, but regular use of medications for the recommended period is necessary. Do not miss doses, and complete the full treatment.
- For griseofulvin: Take with meals or foods high in fat (such as ice cream) to avoid stomach upset and help with absorption. Avoid alcohol (which may cause rapid pulse and flushing) and exposure to sunlight (this drug causes increased sensitivity).
- For nystatin: Dissolve lozenges completely in the mouth. Hold suspensions in the mouth and swish throughout the mouth as long as possible before swallowing. Insert intravaginal medication high in the vagina. Continue with intravaginal applications throughout the menses.
- For antifungal shampoo: Use two times a week for 4 weeks, allowing at least 3 days between each shampoo. Wet hair, apply shampoo to produce lather, leave in place for 1 minute, and then rinse. Apply shampoo a second time, lather, leave in place for 3 minutes, and then rinse thoroughly.
- For topical application: Rub well into the affected areas, but do not get the medication in your eyes.
- For vaginal candidiasis infections: During therapy, refrain from sexual intercourse or advise partner to use a condom.
- Your sexual partner will need to be treated at the same time so that you do not pass the infection back and forth to each other.

Nursing Care

Many people treat themselves with OTC antifungal medications. It is recommended, however, that the person be professionally diagnosed the first time the infection occurs. If symptoms reappear, self-treatment is usually satisfactory. The interventions discussed for nursing care of the patient with a bacterial infection are also appropriate for the patient with a fungal infection. Teaching topics specific to fungal infections are as follows:

- Fungal diseases are contagious. Do not share linens or personal items with others.
- Use a clean towel and washcloth each day.
- Carefully dry all skinfolds, including those under the breasts, under the arms, and between the toes.
- Wear clean cotton underclothing each day.
- Fungi grow in moist environments, such as on sweaty feet. To prevent further infections, do not wear the same pair of shoes every day, wear socks that permit moisture to wick away from the skin surface, do not wear rubber- or plastic-soled shoes, and use talcum powder or an OTC antifungal powder twice a day.

The Patient with a Parasitic Infestation

Infestations of the skin by parasites are more common in developing countries but may occur in any geographic area of the world. They affect people of all social classes but are associated with crowded or unsanitary living conditions.

Pathophysiology

Two of the more common parasitic infestations of the skin are caused by lice and mites. These parasites do not normally live on the skin, but infest the skin through contact with an infested person or contact with clothing, linens, or objects infested with the parasites.

Pediculosis

Pediculosis is an infestation with lice, parasites that live on the blood of an animal or human host. The louse is a 2- to 4-mm oval organism with a stylet that pierces the skin; an anticoagulant in its saliva prevents host blood from clotting while it eats. The female louse lays its eggs (small pearl-gray or brown eggs, called nits) on hair shafts. The louse within the egg hatches, reaches the adult reproductive stage, and dies in 30 to 50 days (Porth & Matfin, 2009).

Two common types of human pediculosis follow:

- Pediculosis corporis is an infestation with body lice. This infestation is more common in people who do not have access to facilities for bathing or washing clothes, such as the homeless. The lice live in clothing fibers and are transmitted primarily by contact with infested clothing and bed linens. The skin lesions occur at the site of a louse bite; macules appear initially, followed by wheals and papules. Pruritus is common, and scratching often results in linear excoriations. The lesions are most often seen on the shoulders, trunk, and buttocks.
- Pediculosis pubis is an infestation with pubic lice (often called "crabs"). This infestation is spread through sexual activity with someone already infested or by contact with

infested clothing or linens. The lice are found in the pubic region and occasionally spread to the axillae or men's beards. The lice cause skin irritation and intense itching.

Scabies
Scabies is a parasitic infestation caused by a mite (Sarcoptes scabiei). The pregnant female mite burrows into the skin and lays two to three eggs each day for about a month. The eggs hatch in 3 to 5 days, and the larvae migrate to the surface of the skin but burrow into the skin for food or protection. The larvae develop, and the cycle repeats. Scabies infestation affects people of all socioeconomic classes. The infestation is found in webs between the fingers, the inner surfaces of the wrist and elbow, the axillae, the female nipple, the penis, the belt line, and the gluteal crease. The lesions are a small red-brown burrow, about 2 mm in length, sometimes covered with vesicles, which appears as a rash. Pruritus in response to the mite or its feces is common, especially at night, and excoriations may develop. The excoriations predispose the person to secondary bacterial infections. The incidence of scabies in residents of nursing homes and extended care facilities has increased.

Interdisciplinary Care
Parasitic infestations are diagnosed by identifying the organism and are treated with medications that kill the lice or mites.

Diagnosis
When a patient has manifestations of pediculosis, the hair shaft and the clothing are examined to identify the lice or the nits. Microscopic examination of the parasite provides a positive diagnosis. Scabies is diagnosed by skin scrapings and microscopic examination for the mites or their feces.

Medications
Lice are eradicated with agents that kill the parasite. Infestations of the body and pubic area are treated with topical medications that contain gamma benzene hexachloride, malathion (Prioderm lotion), or permethrin (NIX).

Infestations of the hair are treated with shampoos containing lindane, such as Kwell. A fine-toothed comb can be used to comb the dead nits off the hair shaft. Scabies may be eradicated by a single treatment of lindane lotion or Kwell applied to the entire skin surface for 12 hours. The associated itching is treated with systemic or topical medications, including corticosteroids. Secondary bacterial infections are treated with the appropriate antibiotic.

∾ Nursing Care
Nursing care for patients with a parasite infestation most often focuses on teaching to prevent infestation or to eradicate an existing infestation. For a hospitalized patient with pediculosis, isolation procedures are instituted until the patient no longer has the infestation.

Patient and family teaching is necessary to facilitate treatment at home, to prevent the spread of the infestation, and to dispel the myth that lice infest only people in dirty living conditions or with poor hygiene. Specific information includes the following:

- Wash clothing and linens in soap and hot water, or have them dry cleaned.
- Ironing the clothes kills any lice eggs.
- All family members and sexual partners must also be treated.
- Lice and mites may infest anyone.

The Patient with a Viral Infection
Viruses are pathogens that consist of an RNA or DNA core surrounded by a protein coat. They depend on live cells for reproduction and so are classified as intracellular pathogens. The viruses that cause skin lesions invade the keratinocyte, reproduce, and either increase cellular growth or cause cellular death.

An increase in the incidence of viral skin disorders has been attributed to a variety of causes. Some commonly used drugs, such as birth control medications and corticosteroids, are known to have immunosuppressive properties that allow the viruses to multiply. Other drugs, such as antibiotics, kill off normal skin bacteria that would otherwise serve as defense against viral infections.

Pathophysiology
Viral infections cause many different kinds of skin disorders, including warts, herpes simplex infections, and herpes zoster infections.

Warts
Warts, or verrucae, are lesions of the skin caused by the human papillomavirus (HPV). Warts may be nongenital or genital. Nongenital warts are benign lesions; genital warts may be precancerous. Warts are transmitted through skin contact. Wart lesions may be flat, fusiform (tapered at both ends), or round, but most are round and raised and have a rough, gray surface. There are many different types of warts; location and appearance of the warts depend on the causative virus. (Genital warts are discussed in ∾ Chapter 50.) Commonly occuring warts are as follows:

- A common wart (verruca vulgaris) may appear anywhere on the skin and mucous membranes of the body; they most commonly appear on the fingers. Common warts grow above the skin surface and may be dome-shaped with ragged borders (Figure 16–8 ■).
- Plantar warts occur at pressure points on the soles of the feet. The pressure of shoes and walking prevents these warts from growing outward, so they tend to extend deeper beneath the skin surface than do common warts. Plantar warts are often painful.
- A flat wart (verruca plana) is a small, flat lesion, usually seen on the forehead or dorsum of the hand.

Depending on their size, location, and any associated discomfort, warts may be treated with medications, cryotherapy, or electrodesiccation and curettage. A common method of wart removal is acid therapy, using a colloidal solution of 16% salicylic acid and 16% lactic acid. The solution is applied to the wart every 12 to 24 hours; the wart disappears in 2 to 3 weeks.

Figure 16–8 ■ The common wart, caused by a virus, appears as a raised, dome-shaped lesion.

Other methods of eradicating warts are cryosurgery, freezing with liquid nitrogen, and electrodesiccation of the wart with an electric current followed by excision of the dead tissue. Warts may also resolve spontaneously when immunity to the virus develops. This response may take up to 5 years.

Herpes Simplex

Herpes simplex (also called a fever blister or cold sore) virus infections of the skin and mucous membranes are caused by two types of herpesvirus: HSV I and HSV II. Most infections above the waist are caused by HSV I, with herpes simplex lesions most often found on the lips, face, and mouth. (Genital herpes infections, caused by HSV II) are discussed in ∞ Chapter 50.) The virus may be transmitted by physical contact, oral sex, or kissing.

The infection begins with a burning or tingling sensation, followed by the development of erythema, vesicle formation, and pain (Figure 16–9 ■). The vesicles progress through pustules, ulcers, and crusting until healing occurs in 10 to 14 days.

The initial infection is often severe and accompanied by systemic manifestations, such as fever and sore throat; recurrences are more localized and less severe. The virus lives in

nerve ganglia and may cause recurrent lesions in response to sunlight, menstruation, injury, or stress. Oral acyclovir may be used prophylactically to prevent reoccurrences and to treat recurrent outbreaks.

Herpes Zoster

Herpes zoster, also called *shingles*, is a viral infection of a dermatome section of the skin caused by varicella zoster (the herpesvirus that also causes chickenpox). The infection is believed to result from reactivation of a varicella virus remaining in the sensory dorsal ganglia after a childhood infection of chickenpox. When reactivated, the virus travels from the ganglia to the corresponding skin dermatome area.

Herpes zoster affects more than 1 million people in the United States each year, with more than half of the cases being in adults over the age of 60 (Porth & Matfin, 2009). Patients with Hodgkin's disease, certain types of leukemia, and lymphomas are more susceptible to an outbreak of the disease. Herpes zoster occurs more often in immunocompromised people, such as those with HIV infections, those receiving radiation therapy or chemotherapy, and those who have had major organ transplants. The appearance of the lesions in people with HIV infections may be one of the first manifestations of immune compromise. The herpes eruption lasts for about 2 to 3 weeks and usually does not recur.

Herpes zoster lesions are vesicles with an erythematous base. The vesicles appear on the skin area supplied by the neurons of a single or associated group of dorsal root ganglia (although they may occur beyond this area in immunosuppressed people). The lesions usually appear unilaterally on the face, trunk, and thorax (Figure 16–10 ■). New lesions continue to erupt for 3 to 5 days, then crust and dry. Recovery occurs in 2 to 3 weeks. The patient often experiences severe pain for up to 48 hours before and during eruption of the lesions. The pain may continue for weeks to months after the lesions have disappeared. The older adult is especially sensitive to the pain and often experiences more severe outbreaks of herpes zoster lesions.

Eruption of vesicles over a single dermatome usually only occurs one time. Generalized herpes zoster may indicate an

Figure 16–9 ■ Herpes simplex is a viral infection of the skin and mucous membranes.

Figure 16–10 ■ Herpes zoster is a viral infection of a dermatome section of the skin. The typical lesions are painful vesicles lying along the path of the nerve.

associated immunocompromised disease, such as Hodgkin's disease or HIV infection. Patients infected with HIV are 20 times more likely to develop herpes zoster (McPhee, Papadakis, & Tierney, 2008).

Complications of herpes zoster include postherpetic neuralgia (a sharp, spasmodic pain along the course of one or more nerves) and visual loss. The neuralgia, described as burning or stabbing, results from inflammation of the root ganglia. Permanent loss of vision may follow occurrence of lesions that arise from the ophthalmic division of the trigeminal nerve. The disease may disseminate in immunocompromised patients, causing lesions beyond the dermatome, visceral lesions, and encephalitis. This serious complication may cause death.

Interdisciplinary Care

The treatment for viral skin infections focuses on stopping viral replication and treating patient responses, such as itching and pain.

Diagnosis

Although diagnosis is usually based on manifestations and appearance of the lesions, laboratory tests may be necessary to differentiate herpes zoster from contact dermatitis and herpes simplex. The laboratory tests include a Tzanck smear, which identifies the herpes virus but does not distinguish herpes zoster from herpes simplex. Cultures of fluid from the vesicles and antibody tests are used to make the differential diagnosis of herpesvirus types. HIV testing should be considered if patients are under age 55 with a history of HIV risk factors. ∞ See Chapter 15 for more information about these tests.

Medications

Antiviral drugs are used to treat herpes zoster infections. Acyclovir (Zovirax) interferes with viral synthesis and replication. Although it does not cure herpes infections, it does decrease the severity of the illness and also decreases pain. It may be administered topically, orally, or parenterally. It is more effective if administration begins within the first 1 to 2 days after the first vesicles appear. Other antiviral medications include famciclovir (Famvir), and valacyclovir (Valtrex). Nerve blocks may be needed to treat initial pain. Narcotic and nonnarcotic analgesics are prescribed for pain management, and antihistamines may be administered for relief of pruritus. Patients with eye involvement are treated with topical steroid ophthalmic ointments and mydriatics.

Zostavax (a weakened form of varicella-zoster virus) is a vaccine used for adults age 60 years or older to prevent herpes zoster. It works by increasing the immune system response; if the patient experiences an outbreak of blisters despite being vaccinated, the nerve pain that follows may be prevented. The vaccine should not be taken by people who are allergic to any of the ingredients, gelatin, or neomycin; have a weaker immune system (such as those with AIDs or leukemia); or take steroids. Side effects include injection site manifestations (such as redness, itching, pain, bruising), headache, fever, hives at the injection site, joint or muscle pain, a rash, and swollen glands.

✆ Nursing Care

Patients with herpes zoster require nursing care for infection, pruritus, and pain. They also require teaching about preventing the spread of the virus to others. See page 418 for a case study and nursing care plan for the patient with herpes zoster.

Nursing Diagnoses and Interventions

This section focuses on the nursing diagnoses of acute pain and risk for infection.

Acute Pain

The patient with herpes zoster often experiences severe pain over the entire dermatome supplied by the affected nerve root. The pain is described as burning, tearing, or stabbing. The patient may avoid movement and does not want clothing or bed linens to touch the affected area.

- Monitor the location, duration, and intensity of the pain. *Each person experiences and expresses pain in his or her own manner. Pain tolerance is also individual. Accurate assessment of the patient's perception and tolerance of pain is essential in facilitating pain management.*
- Explain the rationale for taking prescribed medications on a regular schedule. *Delaying or withholding medications may allow the pain to reach an intensity at which the medication is less effective in promoting relief.*
- Teach measures to relieve pruritus: Take prescribed antipruritic medications, apply calamine lotion or wet compresses if prescribed, keep the room temperature cool, and use a bed cradle to keep sheets off affected areas of the body (see Box 16–10). *Pruritus is a common problem for patients with herpes zoster; scratching may excoriate the skin and increase the risk for secondary infections. Pruritus may intensify the experience of pain.*
- Encourage the use of distraction (such as music) or a specific relaxation technique (such as progressive muscle relaxation or deep breathing). *Noninvasive methods to relieve pain not only help the patient manage the pain experience but also increase the effectiveness of pain medications.*

Risk for Infection

Patients with herpes zoster have impaired skin integrity and pruritus with scratching and possible excoriation. These factors contribute to a high risk for secondary bacterial infection. In addition, the patient is contagious to others who did not have chickenpox as children.

- If hospitalized, monitor white blood cell count and assess for lymph gland enlargement.
  Secondary bacterial infections may occur in any patient with impaired skin integrity; if the patient is immunocompromised, the risk is even greater. Fever, changes in lesions or drainage, an increased white blood cell count, and lymph gland enlargement are manifestations of an infection.
- Teach interventions to decrease the itch-scratch-itch cycle, thereby decreasing the possibility of excoriation (see discussion about nursing care of patients with pruritus and psoriasis earlier in this chapter). *Excoriation from scratching provides an avenue for bacterial invasion.*

CASE STUDY & NURSING CARE PLAN A Patient with Herpes Zoster

Jesus Rivera is a 34-year-old migrant farm worker who currently lives in temporary housing in a rural area of the southwestern United States. His family includes his wife, Marta, who is 3 months pregnant, and two children, ages 3 and 5. He takes his wife to a medical clinic staffed by volunteer nurses, physicians, and students from a nearby university for a prenatal checkup. The clinic is open only on Saturday and provides care on a sliding fee scale or for free if the family is unable to pay. While Mrs. Rivera is being examined, Mr. Rivera asks the nurse to have someone look at some very painful blisters on his chest that developed about a week ago. He is afraid that exposure to pesticides has caused the sores.

ASSESSMENT

Mr. Rivera speaks Spanish and is able to communicate only slightly in English. The initial assessment of Mr. Rivera is performed by Anita Mendez, a student nurse fluent in Spanish. Mr. Rivera's history reveals problems with lower back pain but no significant past medical illnesses. He is not aware of any allergies and cannot remember having had chickenpox as a child. Two years ago, both children were sick and had blisters on their bodies, and a friend told them it was chickenpox. Mrs. Rivera thinks she had chickenpox as a child.

Because Mr. Rivera has not had any medical care for several years, baseline laboratory tests are ordered to screen for any other illnesses. The complete blood count (CBC), blood chemistry, and urinalysis are all within normal limits.

Mr. Rivera says that he did not feel well for several days before the blisters appeared, having experienced chills and general achiness. He had not taken his temperature because the family does not own a thermometer. Current vital signs are as follows: T 99°F (37.2°C), P 74, R 22, and BP 148/88.

Physical examination of the trunk reveals a bandlike pattern of lesions across the left thorax. Some of the lesions are vesicles filled with serous fluid; others are darker in color and are oozing a light yellow drainage. The skin around the lesions is red and inflamed. Mr. Rivera complains of a severe, burning pain with itching across his chest. He is diagnosed with herpes zoster.

DIAGNOSES

- *Risk for Infection* related to open oozing areas on the left thorax
- *Acute Pain* related to the presence of lesions and pruritus
- *Deficient Knowledge* of the cause of the skin disorder and recommended treatment
- *Anxiety* related to need to work in areas of pesticide application
- *Ineffective Health Maintenance* related to limited access to health care due to transitory work conditions and cultural and language barriers

EXPECTED OUTCOMES

- Skin lesions will heal without evidence of a secondary infection.
- Limit exposure (as much as possible) to his wife and children and to persons with debilitating illnesses to prevent the spread of the virus.
- Obtain relief of pain and pruritus with the proper use of medications.

- Verbalize an understanding of the disease process and participate in the treatment plan.
- Obtain follow-up care.
- Make an appointment for a referral for information about occupational hazards.

PLANNING AND IMPLEMENTATION

- Provide verbal and written instructions (in Spanish) for self-care:
  - Wear a clean cotton undershirt each day.
  - Trim the fingernails short, and keep the hands clean.
  - Wash the hands each time the infected area is touched.
  - Wash any soiled clothes or linens in hot water and soap.
  - Do not allow other family members to use your towels.
  - Take medications as prescribed for itching and pain.
  - Take the medicine for your sores every 4 hours, even during nighttime hours, for 7 days.
  - As much as possible, do not touch your wife and children until the sores are covered with scabs. Do not have sex with your wife while you have these sores.
- Teach how to take care of skin lesions:
  - Wear disposable gloves every time you do this treatment.
  - Wash the sores and the skin around them very gently with a soft washcloth and a mild soap.
  - Using your fingers, carefully rub the cream on the sores. Do this once every morning after breakfast and once every evening after supper.
  - Wash your hands carefully before and after each treatment.
- Make a follow-up appointment for the next week.
- Provide Mr. Rivera with the name and phone number of the Occupational Safety and Health Administration (OSHA) and recommend he call for an appointment to discuss his concerns about pesticides.

EVALUATION

Mrs. Rivera explains how she has taken care of her husband, and Mr. Rivera is careful to describe how he has followed the nurse's instructions. The skin lesions are dry and crusty, with no new blister formation. Mr. Rivera says he has not called OSHA and is not sure that he will, but he thanks Miss Mendez for the phone number. The nurses make an appointment in 1 month for a prenatal checkup for Mrs. Rivera and for follow-up of Mr. Rivera's herpes zoster. Mr. Rivera promises to return if they are still living close enough to keep the appointment.

CRITICAL THINKING IN THE NURSING PROCESS

1. Identify barriers to care present in this case study. How may nursing interventions promote healthcare delivery to disadvantaged populations?
2. Although most cases of herpes zoster are self-limiting, what further assessments and interventions might have been indicated had the lesions shown little improvement over time and/or the pain remained severe?
3. If Mr. Rivera is advised not to work until his lesions heal, the family may face economic and sociocultural hardships. Develop a plan of care for Mr. Rivera for the nursing diagnosis *Ineffective Role Performance*.

See Evaluating Your Response in Appendix C.

- Institute infection control procedures for patients who are hospitalized:
  - Maintain strict isolation for immunocompromised patients.
  - Wear gloves and gown if contact with lesions is likely.

- Instruct pregnant women to avoid exposure until lesions have crusted over.

Isolation procedures are instituted for the immunocompromised patient to prevent patient infection. Wear gloves and gown to prevent spreading the infection to self or others. Pregnant women must avoid exposure to people with herpes zoster because the herpes virus can cross the placental barrier.

Using NANDA, NIC, and NOC

Linkages between a selected NANDA nursing diagnosis, NIC, and NOC for the patient with herpes zoster are shown in the chart that follows.

Community-Based Care

Because most patients with viral infections provide self-care at home, the nurse focuses on teaching the patient and family how to provide the necessary care. With herpes zoster increasing in incidence in patients who are older or have a serious chronic illness, it may also be necessary to make a referral to a community health provider for continued support. Provide the following information and instructions:

- A vaccine is available to help prevent herpes zoster.
- The disease is usually self-limiting and heals completely. Second occurrences of herpes zoster are rare.
- Do not have social contact with children or pregnant women until crusts have formed over the blistered areas with herpes zoster, as the disease is contagious to people who have not had chickenpox.
- Use pain medications regularly.
- Follow suggestions to help reduce itching, scratching, and pain: Use medications as prescribed, wear lightweight cotton

clothing, keep room temperatures cool, wear cotton gloves at night if scratching is a problem, and practice relaxation and distraction activities.

- Report any increase in pain, fever, chills, drainage that smells bad and has pus, or a spread in the blisters to your healthcare provider.

NANDA, NIC, AND NOC LINKAGES
Herpes Zoster

NANDA — Acute Pain

↓

NIC — Pain Management
Analgesic Administration
Medication Management

↓

NOC — Comfort Status: Physical
Pain Control
Pain Level

Adapted from data from Bulechek, G., Butcher, H., & Dochterman, J. M. (Eds). (2008). *Nursing interventions classification (NIC)* (5th ed.) (pp. 128–129, 491, 532–533). St. Louis: Mosby Elsevier; Nanda International. (2009). *Nursing diagnoses: Definitions and classification 2009–2010*. Oxford, UK: Wiley-Blackwell; Moorhead, S., Johnson, M., Maas, M., & Swanson, E. (Eds). (2008). *Nursing outcomes classification (NOC)*. (4th ed.) (pp. 282, 536, 539–540). St. Louis: Mosby Elsevier.

Inflammatory Disorders of the Skin

The inflammatory skin disorders discussed in this section include dermatitis, acne, pemphigus, lichen planus, and toxic epidermal necrolysis.

The Patient with Dermatitis

Dermatitis is an inflammation of the skin characterized by erythema and pain or pruritus. Dermatitis may be acute or chronic.

Pathophysiology

Various exogenous and endogenous agents can cause an inflammatory response of the skin. Different types of skin eruptions occur, often specific to the causative allergen, infection, or disease. The initial skin responses to these agents or illnesses include erythema, formation of vesicles and scales, and pruritus (Figure 16–11 ■). Subsequently, irritation from scratching promotes edema, a serous discharge, and crusting. Long-term irritation in chronic dermatitis causes the skin to become thickened and leathery and darker in color.

Contact Dermatitis

Contact dermatitis is a type of dermatitis caused by a hypersensitivity response or chemical irritation. The major sources known to cause contact dermatitis are dyes, perfumes, poison plants (ivy, oak, sumac), chemicals, and metals (Box 16–4). A contact dermatitis common in the healthcare field is latex dermatitis.

FAST FACTS
Latex Allergy
- It is estimated that 5% to 10% of healthcare providers are allergic to latex (WebMD, 2009).
- The most common type of allergic response to latex gloves is Type IV, T-cell mediated contact dermatitis.
- Type I, IgE-mediated hypersensitivity, manifested by urticaria, rhinoconjunctivitis, asthma, or anaphylaxis, is far more serious than the T-cell mediated type.

Figure 16–11 ■ Dermatitis, may be a response to allergens, infections, or chemicals. This patient has contact dermatitis resulting from the metal salts in a ring.

Source: Biophoto Associates/Photo Researchers, Inc.

BOX 16–4   Common Causes of Contact Dermatitis

- Alkalis: soaps, detergents, household ammonia, lye, cleaners
- Cosmetics: perfumes, dyes, oils
- Hydrocarbons: crude petroleum, lubricating oil, mineral oil, paraffin, asphalt, tar
- Fabrics: wool, polyester, dyes, sizing
- Metal salts: calcium chloride, zinc chloride, copper, mercury, nickel, silver
- Plants: ragweed, poison oak, poison sumac, poison ivy, pine

Allergic contact dermatitis is a cell-mediated or delayed hypersensitivity to a wide variety of allergens. Sensitizing antigens include microorganisms, plants, chemicals, drugs, metals, or foreign proteins. On initial contact with the skin, the allergen binds to a carrier protein, forming a sensitizing antigen. The antigen is processed and carried to the T cells, which in turn become sensitized to the antigen. The first exposure is the sensitizing contact and the person does not experience manifestations, which occur with subsequent exposures. The manifestations include erythema, swelling, and pruritic vesicles in the area of allergen contact. For example, a person hypersensitive to metal may have lesions under a ring or watch.

Irritant contact dermatitis is an inflammation of the skin from irritants; it is not a hypersensitivity response. Common sources of irritant contact dermatitis include chemicals (such as acids), soaps, and detergents. The skin lesions are similar to those seen in allergic contact dermatitis.

Atopic Dermatitis

Atopic dermatitis is an inflammatory skin disorder that is also called eczema. The exact cause is unknown, but related factors include depressed cell-mediated immunity, elevated IgE levels, and increased histamine sensitivity. Patients with atopic dermatitis have a family history of hypersensitivity reactions, such as dry skin, eczema, asthma, and allergic rhinitis. Although up to one-third of patients with atopic dermatitis also have food allergies, a positive correlation has not been found.

The dermatitis results from a Type-1 hypersensitive reaction (∞ See Chapter 13). The immune response interacts with the allergen to create a chronic inflammatory condition. In the adult form of atopic dermatitis, characteristic lesions include chronic lichenification, erythema, and scaling, the result of pruritus and scratching. The lesions are usually found on the hands, feet, or flexor surfaces of the arms and legs. Scratching and excoriation increase the risk of secondary infections, as well as invasion of the skin by viruses such as herpes simplex. Serum studies may find elevated eosinophil and IgE levels.

Seborrheic Dermatitis

Seborrheic dermatitis is a chronic inflammatory disorder of the skin that involves the scalp, eyebrows, eyelids, ear canals, nasolabial folds, axillae, and trunk. The cause is unknown. Patients taking methyldopa (Aldomet) for hypertension occasionally develop this disorder, which is also a component of Parkinson's disease. Seborrheic dermatitis is also frequently seen in patients with AIDS.

The lesions are yellow or white plaques with scales and crusts. The scales are often yellow or orange and have a greasy appearance. Mild pruritus is also present. Diffuse dandruff with erythema of the scalp often accompanies the skin lesions.

Exfoliative Dermatitis

Exfoliative dermatitis is an inflammatory skin disorder characterized by excessive peeling or shedding of skin. The cause is unknown in about half of all cases, but a preexisting skin disorder (such as psoriasis, atopic dermatitis, contact dermatitis, or seborrheic dermatitis) is found in up to 63% of the cases (McPhee, Papadakis, & Tierney, 2008). Reactions to medications, such as sulfonamides, account for 20% to 40% of cases. Certain cancers (such as lymphoma) may also cause exfoliative dermatitis.

Both systemic and localized manifestations may appear. Systemic manifestations include weakness, malaise, fever, chills, and weight loss. Scaling, erythema, and pruritus may be localized or involve the entire body. In addition to peeling of skin, the patient may lose his or her hair and nails. Generalized exfoliative dermatitis may cause debility and dehydration. The impairment of skin integrity increases the risk for local and systemic infections.

Interdisciplinary Care

The patient with dermatitis is treated primarily with topical medications and therapeutic baths. If the dermatitis is due to hypersensitivity to an allergen, the patient avoids exposure to environmental irritants and suspected foods. The patient also discontinues as many medications as possible to determine whether the dermatitis is the result of a drug allergy.

Diagnosis

The diagnosis is often based on the manifestations of the disorder and on a history of exposure to a known allergen. Scratch tests and intradermal tests are used to identify a specific allergen.

Medications

The medications used depend on the cause of the dermatitis and the severity of the manifestations. Minor cases are treated with antipruritic medications, whereas more severe cases are treated with oral antihistamines, oral and/or topical corticosteroids, and wet dressings for weeping lesions. Topical immunosuppressive modulators (tacrolimus and pimecrolimus) are effective, but the FDA has published an alert about a possible link with skin cancer and lymphoma. Topical anti-infectives may be prescribed if necessary.

✎ Nursing Care

Nursing care of the patient with dermatitis focuses primarily on providing information for self-care at home. The patient is responsible for managing skin problems and requires education and support. Address the following topics:

- Medications and treatments do not cure the disease; they only relieve the symptoms.
- Dry skin increases pruritus, which stimulates scratching. Scratching may in turn cause excoriation, and excoriation increases the risk of infection.
- It may be necessary to change the diet or environment to avoid contact with allergens.
- When using steroid preparations, apply only a thin layer to slightly damp skin (e.g., after taking a bath).
- If occlusive dressings are necessary, a plastic suit may be used.
- When using oral corticosteroids, never abruptly stop taking the medication. Follow instructions to taper the dosage gradually.

- Advise to discuss use of topical steroids on the face for more than 2 weeks with healthcare provider to avoid adverse reactions, including steroid rosacea and steroid addiction syndrome (Smith, Nedorost, & Tackett, 2007).
- Antihistamines cause drowsiness. When using these medications, avoid alcohol and use caution when driving or working around machinery.

The Patient with Acne

Acne is a disorder of the pilosebaceous (hair and sebaceous gland) structure, which opens to the skin surface through a pore. Sebaceous glands are present over the entire skin surface except the soles of the feet and the palms of the hands, but the largest glands are on the face, scalp, and scrotum. The sebaceous glands, which empty directly into the hair follicle, produce sebum, a lipid substance. Sebum production is a response to direct hormonal stimulation by testicular androgens in men and adrenal and ovarian androgens in women.

Pathophysiology

Acne may be noninflammatory or inflammatory. Noninflammatory acne lesions are primarily **comedones**, more commonly called pimples, whiteheads, and blackheads. Whiteheads are pale, slightly elevated papules categorized as closed comedones. Blackheads are plugs of material that accumulate in the sebaceous glands. They are categorized as open comedones. The color is the result of the movement of melanin into the plug from surrounding epidermal cells. Inflammatory acne lesions include comedones, erythematous pustules, and cysts (Figure 16–12 ■). Inflammation close to the skin surface results in pustules; deeper inflammation results in cysts. The inflammation is believed to result from irritation from fatty acid constituents of the sebum and from substances produced by *Propionibacterium acnes* bacteria, both of which escape into the dermis when the follicular wall of closed comedones ruptures.

Several forms of acne occur at different periods of the life span. The most common are acne vulgaris, acne rosacea, and acne conglobata.

Figure 16–12 ■ Acne vulgaris lesions include comedones, erythematous pustules, and cysts.

Acne Vulgaris

Acne vulgaris is the form of acne common in adolescents and young to middle adults. The actual cause of acne vulgaris is unknown. Possible causes include androgenic influence on the sebaceous glands, increased sebum production, and proliferation of the organism *Propionibacterium acnes*. Many factors once thought to cause acne vulgaris, including high-fat diets, chocolate, infections, and cosmetics, have been disproved.

> **FAST FACTS**
> **Acne Vulgaris**
> - Acne vulgaris is the most common of all skin conditions.
> - Twelve percent of women and 3% of men over the age of 25 have acne vulgaris, and the rate does not begin to decrease until after age 44 (McPhee, Papadakis, & Tierney, 2008).
> - Scarring may be a sequelae of the disease, or may result from picking and manipulating the comedones by the patient.

Mild cases may involve only a few scattered comedones, but severe cases are manifested by multiple lesions of all types. Most acne vulgaris lesions form on the face and neck, but they also occur on the back, chest, and shoulders. Women in their 30s and 40s, often with no prior acne, may develop papular lesions on the chin and around the mouth. The lesions are usually mildly painful and may itch. The complications of acne vulgaris, especially in severe cases, are formation of cysts, pigment changes in persons with dark skin, severe scarring, and lowered self-concept from the skin eruptions.

Acne Rosacea

Acne rosacea is a chronic type of facial acne that occurs more often in middle and older adults. The cause is unknown. The lesions of acne rosacea begin with erythema over the cheeks and nose. Other skin lesions may or may not appear. Over years of time, the skin color changes to dark red, and the pores over the area become enlarged. The soft tissue of the nose may exhibit rhinophyma, an irregular bullous thickening.

Acne Conglobata

Acne conglobata is also a chronic type of acne of unknown cause that begins in middle adulthood. This type causes serious skin lesions: Comedones, papules, pustules, nodules, cysts, and scars occur primarily on the back, buttocks, and chest but may occur on other body surfaces. The comedones have multiple openings and a discharge that ranges from serous to purulent with a foul odor.

Interdisciplinary Care

The management of acne is similar, regardless of type. Because acne vulgaris is most common, the discussions of interdisciplinary and nursing care focus on that type. Treatment is based on the type and severity of the lesions.

Diagnosis

The disease is diagnosed by the typical location and appearance of lesions. If the patient has pustules, a culture of the drainage is performed to differentiate viral or bacterial dermatitis from acne.

TRETINOIN (AVITA, RENOVA, RETIN-A)

- Use the cream in a test area twice at night to test for sensitivity; if no reaction occurs, increase applications gradually to the prescribed frequency.
- A pea-sized amount of the cream is enough to cover the entire face.
- Apply the cream to clean, dry skin.
- Do not apply the cream to the eyes, mouth, angles of the nose, or mucous membranes.
- Wash your face no more than two to three times a day, using a mild soap. Do not use skin preparations (such as

aftershave lotion or perfumes) that contain alcohol, menthol, spice, or lime; they may irritate your skin.
- The medication may cause a temporary stinging or warm sensation but should not cause pain.
- The skin where you apply the cream will be mildly red and may peel; if you experience a more severe reaction, consult your healthcare provider.
- The medication may cause increased sensitivity to sunlight, use sunscreens and wear protective clothing when outdoors.
- Your acne may become worse during the first 2 weeks of treatment; this is an expected response.

Medications

The treatment of acne is tailored to the individual and is based on the severity of the lesions. For acne with comedones, tretinoin (retinoic acid, Retin-A) or benzoyl peroxide preparations are prescribed. Azelaic acid (Azelex) may also be used. The administration of these vitamin A analogues is discussed in the Medication Administration feature shown above. Benzoyl peroxide preparations are found in OTC medications such as Fostex, Acne-Dome, Desquam-X, Benzagel, Clear By Design, and Xerac BP. These products are keratolytic and loosen the comedones. Epiduo (a prescription gel) combines adapalene and benzoyl peroxide to treat acne vulgaris.

Mild forms of papular inflammatory acne are treated with topical clindamycin (Cleocin T), a bacteriostatic agent that decreases the amount of fatty acids on the skin surface. This medication may be combined with tretinoin therapy.

Moderate forms of papular inflammatory acne are treated with oral or topical antibiotics, such as tetracycline, erythromycin, and minocycline. These antibiotics are administered for 3 to 4 months; if the patient's skin is clear, the dose is lowered gradually to a maintenance dose that will maintain clear skin.

Treatments

Acne scars may alter the individual's self-concept. The scars may be removed by dermabrasion and laser treatment. (Dermabrasion is discussed in greater detail later in this chapter.)

✍ Nursing Care

Nursing care is individualized and is conducted primarily through teaching in clinics or healthcare provider offices. Regardless of the patient's age or gender, it is important to remember that almost all patients with acne are embarrassed by and self-conscious of their appearance. Prior to teaching, establish rapport with the patient and clarify beliefs; for example, the patient may believe the lesions result from poor hygiene, masturbation, use of cosmetics, eating the wrong types of foods, or lack of sexual activity. It is critical to teach the patient about the causes of and factors involved in acne prior to teaching self-care.

The teaching plan for the patient with acne includes general guidelines for skin care and health as well as specific guidelines for care of the acne lesions. The following topics should be addressed:

- Wash the skin with a mild soap and water at least twice a day to remove accumulated oils.

- Shampoo the hair often enough to prevent oiliness.
- Eat a regular, well-balanced diet. Foods do not cause or increase acne.
- Expose the skin to sunlight, but avoid sunburn.
- Get regular exercise and sleep.
- Try to avoid putting your hands on your face.
- Do not squeeze a pimple. Squeezing forces the material of the pimple deeper into the skin and may cause the pimple to become larger and infected.
- The treatment for acne lasts months, in some cases for the rest of one's life. It is very important to take the medications each day for the prescribed length of time.

The Patient with Pemphigus Vulgaris

Pemphigus vulgaris is a chronic disorder of the skin and oral mucous membranes characterized by blister formation. The disease is caused by autoantibodies that cause acantholysis (the separation of epidermal cells from one another). The disorder is associated with IgG antibodies and HLA-A10 antigen. Septicemia from an infection of *Staphylococcus aureus* is the most common cause of death. The disease occurs in middle and older adults of all races and ethnic backgrounds. The disorder has been associated with other autoimmune disorders and with the administration of certain drugs, such as penicillamine and captopril.

The blisters that form in pemphigus vulgaris usually appear first in the mouth and on the scalp and then spread in crops or waves to involve large areas of the body, including the face, back, chest, umbilicus, and groin. The blisters form in the epidermis and cause the epidermal cells to separate above the basal layer. These blisters rupture, leaving denuded skin, crusting, and oozing of fluid with a musty odor. The lesions are painful. Pressure on a blister causes it to spread to adjacent skin (Nikolsky's sign). The loss of fluid from the blisters may result in fluid and electrolyte imbalances. Secondary bacterial infections are a serious risk.

Interdisciplinary Care

The goals of treatment are to control the severity of the disease, to prevent infection and loss of fluids, and to promote healing. Patients who experience severe attacks or secondary infections are usually hospitalized. Although the disease cannot be cured, the manifestations can be controlled.

Diagnosis

Pemphigus vulgaris is diagnosed by manifestations and diagnostic tests, including immunofluorescence microscopy, which is done to identify the presence of IgG antibodies in the epidermis and serum, and skin biopsy (∞ see Chapter 15) to determine the presence of acantholysis.

Medications

Early lesions are treated with highly potent topical corticosteroids. As the disease becomes more severe, systemic corticosteroids or immunosuppressive agents (such as azathioprine or methotrexate) are prescribed. Secondary infections are treated with topical and/or systemic antibiotics.

Treatments

Plasmapheresis is occasionally used to treat pemphigus. In this procedure, the plasma is selectively removed from whole blood and reinfused into the patient. This decreases the serum level of antibodies for a period of time. Plasmapheresis with related nursing care is discussed in ∞ Chapter 44.

∞ Nursing Care

The hospitalized patient with pemphigus requires careful assessment of skin lesions and monitoring for manifestations of infection. Provide skin care through bathing and applying dressings to denuded areas, using aseptic technique to prevent infection. The patient may be placed on reverse isolation as a protective measure. Monitor the patient's hydration status to prevent fluid volume deficit and incorporate pain medications and noninvasive pain management techniques in the plan of care. Oral lesions often make eating difficult; the patient requires meticulous oral hygiene and nonirritating foods. The patient often is depressed and fearful; establishing a therapeutic relationship is essential, and referrals for counseling may be necessary.

Teaching the patient and family how to provide care at home also involves skin care, oral care, diet, pain management, prevention of infection and how to take prescribed medications. A referral to a home health agency or local health department may be necessary.

The Patient with Lichen Planus

Lichen planus is an inflammatory disorder of the mucous membranes and skin. It has no known cause but has been associated with exposure to drugs or to film processing chemicals. The disease affects adults of all ages.

The lesions first appear as violet papules, 2 to 10 mm in size, commonly occurring on the wrists, ankles, lower legs, and genitals. The lesions itch intensely. Over time, persistent lesions thicken and become dark red, forming hypertrophic lichen planus. Lesions on the oral mucous membranes appear as white, lacey rings; lesions may also appear on the mucous membranes of the vaginal area and the penis. The nails become thin and may shed.

Lichen planus lesions are self-limiting but last for an average of 12 to 18 months. The disorder is diagnosed by manifestations. Corticosteroids are used to control the inflammation, and antihistamines are used to control the pruritus.

The Patient with Toxic Epidermal Necrolysis

Toxic epidermal necrolysis (TEN) is a rare, life-threatening disease in which the epidermis peels off the dermis in sheets, leaving large areas of denuded skin. Conjunctivitis and mucositis of the mouth, upper airway, esophagus, and sometimes the genitourinary tract are often associated with TEN. The patient usually requires critical care, often in a burn center. The incidence of TEN has not been documented, but it is seen more often in men and in people of African descent. The mortality rate is decreasing because of current methods of care. The cause of death is almost always sepsis.

Although some cases have no known cause, most cases result from a drug reaction, and others are associated with a serious concomitant illness, such as cancer or AIDS. Drugs that have been associated with TEN are the sulfonamides, barbiturates, NSAIDs, phenytoin, allopurinol, and penicillin.

The pathophysiologic process in TEN is not completely understood, but the triggering mechanism is believed to be a hypersensitivity or immune response. TEN begins with a painful, localized erythema of the face and extremities, accompanied by fever, chills, muscle aches, and generalized malaise. A macular rash develops, followed by the formation of large, flaccid blisters over the body surface during the next 24 to 96 hours. The skin begins to slough, leaving the dermal surface exposed. Even in areas without blistering, the skin may peel off in layers. The skin sloughing continues over several days and can expose 95% or more of the dermal surface. Other manifestations include conjunctivitis, pharyngitis, stomatitis, and enlargement of lymph glands. Urethral slough is common, causing such painful voiding that the patient voluntarily retains urine. The patient is often disoriented, may be nearly comatose, and is seriously ill.

The loss of skin leads to fluid and electrolyte imbalances and secondary infections, as well as systemic effects on all other body systems. These complications may cause death. However, if the complications can be prevented, healing by epidermal regeneration occurs in about a month. The long-term complications of TEN include blindness, lacrimal duct occlusion, scarring and contractures, loss of nails, esophageal strictures, and glomerulonephritis.

The patient is hospitalized and requires rapid diagnosis and treatment. Any medication in use by the patient is stopped immediately. Interdisciplinary care involves fluid replacement, correction of electrolyte imbalances, prevention or management of infection, and pain control. The interdisciplinary and nursing care are essentially the same as for the patient with burns, discussed in ∞ Chapter 17.

Malignant Skin Disorders

The skin, despite its ability to protect the internal body from external damage, is a fragile organ and is subject to damage from ultraviolet radiation and chemicals. Over time, this damage results in alterations in cellular structure and function, and malignancies of the skin occur. Many of these lesions are found on skin surfaces that have undergone long-term exposure to the sun or the environment. Malignant skin tumors are the most common of all cancers.

The Patient with Actinic Keratosis

Actinic keratosis, also called senile or solar keratosis, is an epidermal skin lesion directly related to chronic sun exposure and photodamage. The prevalence is highest in people with light-colored skin; these lesions are rare in people with dark skin. About 20% of actinic keratoses convert to squamous cell carcinoma (Porth & Matfin, 2009). However, there is some thought that the lesions are all premalignant.

The lesions are erythematous rough macules a few millimeters in diameter. They are often shiny but may be scaly; if the scales are removed, the underlying skin bleeds. They occur in multiple patches, primarily on the face, dorsa of the hands, the forearms, and sometimes on the upper trunk (Figure 16–13 ■). Enlargement or ulceration of the lesions suggests transformation to malignancy. The lesions are usually treated by cryosurgery (freezing) or with 5-fluorouracil cream, which erodes the lesions.

The Patient with Nonmelanoma Skin Cancer

The nonmelanoma skin cancers are basal cell cancer and squamous cell cancer. Other types of nonmelanoma skin cancers, accounting for less than 1% of cases (ACS, 2008) are Merkel

Figure 16–13 ■ The effects of long-term sun exposure are illustrated in this epidermal skin lesion, called actinic keratosis.

cell carcinoma; Kaposi sarcoma; and lymphomas, sarcomas, and adnexal tumors of the skin. These uncommon tumors are not included in this discussion, but information can be found on the American Cancer Society website or the National Cancer Institute website.

Incidence

Nonmelanoma skin cancer is the most common malignant neoplasm found in fair-skinned Americans. The ACS (2008) estimates that more than 1 million new cases of nonmelanoma skin cancer are diagnosed in the United States each year. Of that number, about 80% are basal cell cancers and 20% are squamous cell cancers. Deaths from nonmelanoma skin cancer have dropped by 30% in the past 30 years. Men develop nonmelanoma skin cancer more often than do women, probably because of occupational exposures. Although nonmelanoma skin cancer may occur at any age, the incidence increases with each decade of life. Adults between the ages of 30 and 60 have the majority of these cancers.

Risk Factors

There are multiple etiologic factors involved in the development of nonmelanoma skin cancer, including environmental factors and host factors.

Environmental Factors

Ultraviolet radiation (UVR) from the sun is believed to be the cause of most nonmelanoma skin cancers. Sunlight contains both short-length rays (UVB) and long-length rays (UVA). UVB rays are absorbed by the top layer of skin and cause sunburn. UVA rays penetrate deeper into the skin layers, causing tissue damage. Both types of rays cause DNA alterations and suppress T-cell and B-cell immunity, allowing cancer cells to grow. Researchers have also discovered that many skin cancers contain changes in tumor suppressor genes (these genes normally help keep cells from growing out of control). The damaged gene found in basal cell cancer is p53, a gene that normally causes damaged cells to die. The damaged gene found in squamous cell cancer is the "patched" (PTCH) gene, which normally helps keep cell growth in check (ACS, 2008).

The amount of UVR reaching the earth is increasing, most likely from depletion of the ozone layer surrounding the planet. The U.S. Environmental Protection Agency predicts that for every 1% decrease in the ozone layer, a corresponding 1% to 3% increase in nonmelanoma skin cancer per year will occur.

Geographic, environmental, and lifestyle factors affect the amount of exposure to the sun and the risk for nonmelanoma skin cancer. People who live in latitudes close to the equator and those who live at higher altitudes receive greater UVR exposure. The amount of clothing worn, the time of day, and amount of time in the sun also determine the amount of exposure. Exposure to UVR in tanning booths is also implicated in the development of nonmelanoma skin cancer.

Certain chemicals have long been associated with nonmelanoma skin cancer. Polycyclic aromatic hydrocarbons, found in mixtures of coal, tar, asphalt, soot, and mineral oils, have been linked with skin cancers. Psoralens, used in conjunction with UVA for treatment of psoriasis and cutaneous T-cell lymphoma, increase the risk of squamous cell cancer. Other factors associated with nonmelanoma skin cancer are the use of ionizing radiation, viruses, and physical trauma. X-ray therapy for tinea capitis and the use of radium to treat other malignancies are risk factors. Human papillomavirus is implicated in the development of squamous cell cancer, as is damage to the skin from burns. Organ transplant recipients who undergo immunosuppression to prevent rejection are also at risk for the development of squamous cell cancer.

Host Factors

Skin pigmentation is an important factor in the development of nonmelanoma skin cancer. The amount of melanin pigment produced by the melanocytes determines a person's skin color. The more melanin, the more the skin is protected from the damage produced by ultraviolet rays. Thus, Asian and people of African and Mediterranean descent have a much lower incidence of nonmelanoma skin cancer than do people who have fair complexions and tend to freckle or sunburn easily, such as people of Irish, Scandinavian, or English ancestry.

Although most people have numerous pigmented lesions on their body, almost all of these are normal. However, a major risk factor in the development of nonmelanoma skin cancer is a change in an existing lesion or the presence of a premalignant lesion, such as actinic keratosis.

Pathophysiology

Basal cell cancer and squamous cell cancer arise from epithelial tissue but have different pathophysiology, classifications, and manifestations. These cancers are classified as keratinocyte cancers; when viewed under a microscope they share some features with keratinocytes, the most abundant skin cell type.

Basal Cell Cancer

Basal cell cancer is an epithelial tumor believed to originate either from the basal layer of the epidermis or from cells in the surrounding dermal structures. These tumors are characterized by an impaired ability of the basal cells of the epidermis to mature into keratinocytes, with mitotic division beyond the basal layer. This results in a bulky tumor that grows by direct extension and if untreated, destroys surrounding tissue, including healthy skin, nerves, blood vessels, lymphatic tissue, cartilage, and bone. Basal cell cancer is the most common but least aggressive type of skin cancer, rarely metastasizing. Although once seen only in middle to older adults, it is now being seen in younger people, probably due to increased sun exposure.

Basal cell cancers tend to recur. Tumors greater than 2 cm in diameter have a high recurrence rate. Predisposing factors for metastasis are the size of the tumor and the patient's resistance to treatment with surgery or chemotherapy. Even though they rarely metastasize, untreated basal cell cancers invade surrounding tissue and may destroy body parts, such as the nose or eyelid. Basal cell cancer is classified as nodular, superficial, pigmented, morpheaform, or keratotic.

Nodular basal cell cancer, the most common type of basal cell cancer, most often appears on the face, neck, and head. The tumor is made up of masses of cells that resemble epidermal basal cells and grow in a bulky, nodular form from lack of keratinization. In early stages, the tumor is a papule that looks like a smooth pimple. It is often pruritic and continues to grow at a steady rate, doubling in size every 6 to 12 months. As the tumor grows, the epidermis thins, but it remains intact. The skin over the tumor is shiny, and either pearly white, pink, or flesh colored. Telangiectasis may be visible over the area of the tumor. As the tumor continues to increase in size, the center or periphery may ulcerate, and the tumor develops well-circumscribed borders. It bleeds easily from mild injury.

Superficial basal cell cancer, found most often on the trunk and extremities, is the second most common type of basal cell cancer. This tumor is a proliferating tissue that attaches to the undersurface of the epithelium. The tumor is a flat papule or plaque, often erythematous, with well-defined borders. The tumor may ulcerate and be covered with crusts or shallow erosions (Figure 16–14 ■).

Pigmented basal cell cancer, found on the head, neck, and face, is less common. This tumor concentrates melanin pigment in the center of the basal cancer cells, giving it a dark brown, blue, or black appearance. The border of the tumor is shiny and well defined.

Morpheaform basal cell cancer, the rarest form of basal cell cancer, usually develops on the head and neck. The tumor forms fingerlike projections that extend in any direction along dermal tissue planes. The tumor resembles a flat ivory or flesh-colored scar. This form is more likely to extend into and destroy adjacent tissue, especially muscle, nerve, and bone. It is often more difficult to diagnose because of its appearance.

Keratotic basal cell cancer (basosquamous) is found on the preauricular and postauricular groove. It contains both basal cells and squamoid-appearing cells that keratinize. Its appearance is much like that of nodular basal cell cancer. This type of basal cell cancer tends to recur locally and also is the type most likely to metastasize.

Figure 16–14 ■ A superficial basal cell cancer is characterized by erythema, ulcerations, and well-defined borders.

Squamous Cell Cancer

Squamous cell cancer is a malignant tumor of the squamous epithelium of the skin or mucous membranes. It occurs most often on areas of skin exposed to ultraviolet rays and weather, such as the forehead, helix of the ear, top of the nose, lower lip, and back of the hands. Squamous cell cancer may also arise on skin that has been burned or has chronic inflammation. This is a much more aggressive cancer than basal cell cancer, with a faster growth rate and a much greater potential for metastasis if untreated. The tumors arise when the keratinizing cells of the squamous epithelium proliferate, producing a growth that eventually fills the epidermis and invades the dermal tissue planes. Keratinization of some cells is present, and the formation of keratin "pearls" is common. The keratin formation diminishes as the tumor grows. As the tumor grows, the tumor cells increase in number and rate of mitosis, forming odd shapes. An early form of squamous cell cancer is called Bowen's disease or cancer *in situ*.

Squamous cell cancer begins as a small, firm red nodule. The tumor may be crusted with keratin products. As it grows, it may ulcerate, bleed, and become painful. As the tumor extends into the surrounding tissue and becomes a nodule, the area around the nodule becomes indurated (hardened) (Figure 16–15 ■).

Recurrent squamous cell cancer can be invasive, increasing the risk of metastasis. Invasive squamous cell cancer may arise from preexisting skin lesions, such as scars and actinic keratosis, and extend into the dermis (called intraepidermal squamous cell cancer). This form appears as a slightly raised erythematous plaque with well-defined borders. Metastasis occurs most often via the lymphatics. The degree of risk for metastasis depends on the size and depth of penetration of the tumor.

Interdisciplinary Care

Treatment of nonmelanoma skin cancer focuses on removal of all malignant tissue using such methods as surgery, curettage and electrodesiccation, cryotherapy, or radiotherapy. These modalities offer a greater than 90% cure rate. After the malignant tissue is removed, the patient should have regular examinations for recurrence.

Figure 16–15 ■ As a squamous cell cancer grows, it tends to invade surrounding tissue. It also ulcerates, may bleed, and is painful.

Diagnosis

Nonmelanoma cancer is diagnosed by microscopic examination of tissue biopsied from the tumor. The biopsy is usually done as an office procedure under local anesthesia. The types of biopsy used are shave, punch, incisional, and excisional. Information about skin biopsy is provided in ∞ Chapter 15.

Treatments

Depending on the stage, type, size, and location of a non-melanoma cancer, it may be treated with surgical excision, Mohs' surgery, curettage and electrodessication, radiation, or other forms of local therapy.

SURGICAL EXCISION   Both basal cell and squamous cell cancers are excised surgically. The surgery may be minor or major, depending on the size and location of the tumor. Surgery for small tumors is most often performed in the outpatient surgery department or in the surgeon's office. Surgical excision allows rapid healing and yields good cosmetic results.

The goal of surgical excision is to remove the tumor completely, so some surrounding tissue is excised along with the tumor. If the tumor is on the face, the incision is made along normal wrinkle or anatomic lines so that the scars will be less obvious. The incision is closed in layers to leave the smallest possible scar. A pressure dressing is usually applied over the incision to provide support. If a large tumor is removed, a skin graft or skin flap may be performed to cover the excised area. If grafting is necessary, the patient is hospitalized.

MOHS' SURGERY   In Mohs' surgery, thin layers of the tumor are horizontally shaved off. A frozen section of the tissue is stained at each level to determine tumor margins. This method is the most accurate in assessing the extent of nonmelanoma skin cancer and the method that conserves the most normal tissue. It is often used in areas such as the nose, the nasolabial fold, the medial canthus, and the ear.

CURETTAGE AND ELECTRODESICCATION   Curettage and electrodesiccation are used to treat basal cell cancers that are less than 2 cm in diameter, are superficial, or recur because of poor margin control. It may also be used for primary squamous cell cancers that are less than 1 cm in diameter and have distinct borders. This type of treatment is most successful for tumors on anatomic sites over a fixed underlying surface, such as the ear, chest, and temple.

Abnormal tissue is scraped away (curettaged) within 1 to 2 mm of the margin and then a low-voltage electrode is used to abrade the tumor base (electrodesiccation). Curettage and electrodesiccation is not used for lesions where the dermis is thin (such as the eyelid) or where the tumor extends into the subcutaneous tissue.Curettage and electrodesiccation provide good cosmetic results and preserve normal tissue. However, healing time is longer, and it is difficult to ensure that all tumor margins have been removed.

Instead of a low-voltage electrode, some physicians use a carbon dioxide laser to vaporize the tumor. When used in conjunction with curettage, this treatment is effective on superficial basal cell cancers. Carbon dioxide vaporization results in minimal thermal injury to adjacent cells, less pain, and quicker healing.

RADIATION THERAPY Radiation is most often used for lesions that are inoperable because of their location (such as tumors on the corner of the nose, the eyelid, the canthus, and the lip) or size (between 1 cm and 8 cm). It is also used for patients who are older and of poor surgical risk. Radiation is painless and can be used to treat areas surrounding the tumor if necessary. However, the treatment is given over 3 to 4 weeks in a clinical facility, does not allow control of tumor margins, and may itself cause skin cancer.

OTHER FORMS OF LOCAL THERAPY Other forms of local therapy include the following:

- Cryosurgery, which involves applying liquid nitrogen to the tumor to freeze and kill abnormal cells.
- Photodynamic therapy (PDT) involves administering a topical or injectable chemical that collects in the tumor cells and makes them more sensitive to light. A light source is then focused on the tumor and the cells die.
- Topical chemotherapy means that an anti-cancer drug (usually 5-fluorouracil [5-FU]) is applied as a cream directly on the skin to kill the tumor cells.
- Immune response modifiers cause an immune response to the cancer, causing it to get smaller and die. The drugs used are imiquimod (Aldara) (a topical cream) and interferon (injected directly into the tumor).
- Laser surgery uses laser light to vaporize cancer cells.

Nursing Care

The increasing number of people with skin cancer means that nurses must be involved in prevention and early detection. Nurses have the opportunity to teach preventive behaviors in all settings, including the hospital, home, community, school, and clinic.

Nursing care for the patient with nonmelanoma skin cancer depends on the treatment used. Surgical excision is the most common form of treatment; nursing care depends on the extent of the procedure. However, regardless of the type of treatment, the patient will have impaired skin integrity, an increased risk for infection, and anxiety about the future following a diagnosis of cancer. Interventions with rationales for the patient with any type of skin cancer are discussed in the following section on melanoma.

Health Promotion

It is well known that cumulative sun exposure positively correlates with nonmelanoma skin cancers. Many skin cancers can be prevented by limiting exposure to risk factors. Primary prevention behaviors recommended by the ACS and the Skin Cancer Foundation are outlined in Box 16–5. In addition to these preventive behaviors, the ACS recommends "Slip! Slop! Slap! Wrap!" method: **slip** on a shirt, **slop** on 15 SPF (or higher) sunscreen, **slap** on a hat, and **wrap** on sunglasses before exposure to the sun. Information about sunscreen is listed in Box 16–6.

Nurses also provide patient and family education for early detection of nonmelanoma skin cancer. Numerous brochures describing the types of skin cancers, photographs of lesions, and prevention behaviors are available from the ACS, health education and support agencies, and pharmaceutical companies that manufacture sunscreen. Most of this literature is free.

BOX 16–5 Health Promotion: Preventing Skin Cancer

- Minimize sun exposure between the hours of 10 AM and 3 PM, when ultraviolet rays are the strongest.
- Cover up with a wide-brimmed hat, sunglasses, long-sleeved shirt, and long pants made of tightly woven materials when in the sun.
- Apply a waterproof or water-resistant sunscreen with an SPF of 15 or more at least 30 minutes before every exposure to the sun. If swimming or sweating heavily, reapply every hour. Apply sunscreen not only on sunny days but also on cloudy days (when ultraviolet rays can penetrate 70% to 80% of the cloud cover.
- Use sunscreen and protective clothing when you are on or near sand, snow, concrete, or water (which can reflect more than 50% of the ultraviolet rays onto your skin).
- Avoid tanning booths; UVR emitted by tanning booths damages the deep skin layers.

The patient or family at risk for or diagnosed with a skin cancer must be taught how to conduct a self-examination of the skin, described in Box 16–7, as well as the importance of conducting the examination on the same day of each month. Family members can help with areas that are hard to examine, such as the ears, scalp, and back.

BOX 16–6 Sunscreen Information

Types of Sunscreen

Chemical
Chemical sunscreens absorb ultraviolet light and act as a radiation filter. Examples follow:
- p-Aminobenzoic acid (PABA)
- Benzophenones
- Anthranilates
- Salicylates

Physical
Physical sunscreens reflect and scatter ultraviolet light. Examples follow:
- Zinc oxide
- Titanium dioxide
- Magnesium silicate
- Ferric chloride
- Kaolin
- Ichthyol

Adverse Reactions Associated with Sunscreens
Adverse reactions associated with sunscreens include contact and photocontact dermatitis. People with previous hypersensitivity reactions to benzocaine, procaine, sulfonamides, or para-phenylenediamine may develop hypersensitivity responses to PABA. People who are also taking systemic thiazide diuretics or sulfonamides may develop eczematous dermatitis.

Sunscreen Ratings
In the United States, the Food and Drug Administration rates commercial sunscreens according to their sun protection factor, or SPF. The SPF value is the ratio of the time required to produce minimal skin redness through a sunscreen product with the time required to produce the same degree of redness without the sunscreen. A person who can tolerate 1/2 hour of sun without a sunscreen should be able to tolerate 3 hours of sun when a sunscreen of SPF 6 is applied to the skin. SPF values of sunscreens range from 2 to 100. An SPF of 15 or greater is recommended.

BOX 16–7   Health Promotion: Skin Self-Examination

1. Choose the same day each month (such as the first day) to do the examination.
2. The best time to do the examination is after you take a bath or shower. Examine yourself in a well-lighted room in front of a full-length mirror. Have a hand mirror, a chair, and a hair dryer available. If you have difficulty seeing your back and scalp (or any other parts of your body), ask someone to help you.
3. Follow the same pattern with each examination:

Examine head and face, using one or both mirrors. Use blow dryer to inspect scalp.

Check hands, including nails. In full-length mirror, examine elbows, arms, underarms.

Focus on neck, chest, torso. Women: Check under breasts.

With back to the mirror, use hand mirror to inspect back of neck and back including buttocks.

Sitting down, check legs and feet, including soles, heels, and nails. Use hand mirror to examine genitals.

Community-Based Care

Teach the patient and family specific measures for self-care following surgery, including information about

- how and when to change dressings.
- the use of aseptic technique and careful hand hygiene when caring for the wound.
- symptoms to report (such as bleeding, fever, or signs of wound infection), and how to protect the operative site against trauma and irritations.

*(sidebar, vertical text)* Malignant Melanoma Video

The Patient with Melanoma

Melanoma (malignant melanoma) arises from melanocytes. This serious skin cancer is increasing in incidence each year. Melanoma accounts for less than 5% of skin cancers, but it causes a large majority of skin cancer deaths (ACS, 2008).

Incidence

This disease is over 10 times more common in fair-skinned people than in dark-skinned people. It is slightly more common in men than in women. Melanoma occurs more often in people who live in sunny climates, burn easily, and patronize tanning parlors. However, it may arise from already present lesions or from skin normally covered with clothing. Melanoma occurs in a wide age range, from adolescents to older adults, with the greatest rates in those over the age of 80.

Risk Factors

Although the exact cause of melanoma is unknown, it is known that certain risk factors are associated with the disease. The risk factors for melanoma are listed in Box 16–8.

Pathophysiology

Melanomas arise from melanocytes, cells located at or near the basal layer (the deepest epidermal layer). These cells produce melanin, the dark skin pigment. Melanin is made in granules and transferred to keratinocytes, where it accumulates on the superficial side of each keratinocyte and forms a shield of pigment over the nucleus as protection against ultraviolet rays. Melanomas can develop wherever there is pigment, but about one-third of them originate in existing nevi (moles).

Almost all melanomas are more than 6 mm in diameter, are asymmetric, and initially develop within the epidermis over a long period. While they are still confined to the epidermis, the lesions (called melanoma *in situ*) are flat and relatively benign. However, when they penetrate the dermis, they mingle with blood and lymph vessels and are capable of metastasizing. At this latter stage, the tumors develop a raised or nodular appearance and often have smaller nodules, called satellite lesions, around the periphery.

The prognosis for survival for people diagnosed with melanoma is determined by several variables, including location, tumor thickness, ulceration, metastasis, site, age, and gender.

BOX 16–8   Risk Factors for Melanoma Skin Cancer

- A high number of moles, or large moles
- Fair skin, freckling, blond hair, or blue eyes
- Close relative with the disease
- Men with gene changes from a family history of breast or ovarian cancer
- Treatment with medications that suppress the immune system
- Too much exposure to UV radiation from sunlight, tanning lamps, or tanning booths
- Over age 50
- Xeroderma pigmentosus, a rare inherited disease in which people are less able to repair damage caused by sunlight
- Past history of melanoma

Younger patients and women have a somewhat better chance of survival. Patients with tumors on the scalp and neck have a lower survival rate.

Precursor Lesions

The three specific precursor lesions for the development of melanoma are congenital nevi, dysplastic nevi, and lentigo maligna. A precursor lesion is also called a premalignant lesion, a name that indicates that the lesion's risk of becoming malignant is greater than normal.

CONGENITAL NEVI Congenital nevi are present at birth. Some lesions are small; others are large enough to cover an entire body area. Their color can range from brown to black. They are often slightly raised, with an irregular surface and a fairly regular border.

DYSPLASTIC NEVI Dysplastic nevi are also called atypical moles. Although dysplastic nevi are not present at birth, they appear as normal nevi during childhood and become dysplastic (having abnormal development) after puberty. A patient with classic dysplastic nevi has more than 100 nevi, at least one of which is larger than 8 mm in diameter, and at least one of which has the characteristics of melanoma (asymmetry, irregular border, color variegation, and a diameter greater than 6 mm). A familial tendency to dysplastic nevi increases the risk for the development of melanoma. Having many moles, whether normal or atypical, is a risk factor for melanoma.

Dysplastic nevi most often appear on the face, trunk, and arms but also are seen on the scalp, female breast, groin, and buttocks. The pigmentation of the nevi is irregular, with mixtures of tan, brown, black, red, and pink. An area of lighter pigmentation is surrounded by a papular area of deeper pigmentation (described as a "fried egg appearance"). The borders of the nevi are irregular.

LENTIGO MALIGNA Lentigo maligna, also called Hutchinson's freckle, is a tan or black patch on the skin that looks like a freckle. It grows slowly, becoming mottled, dark, thick, and nodular. It is usually seen on one side of the face of an older adult who has had a large amount of sun exposure.

Classification

Melanomas are classified into different types. The major types are superficial spreading melanoma, lentigo maligna melanoma, nodular melanoma, and acral lentiginous melanoma. Each of these tumors is characterized by a radial and/or vertical growth phase. During the initial radial phase, which may last from 1 to 25 years (depending on the type), the melanoma grows parallel to the skin surface. During this phase, the tumor rarely metastasizes and is often curable by surgical excision. However, during the vertical growth phase, atypical melanocytes rapidly penetrate into the dermis and subcutaneous tissue, greatly increasing the risk for metastasis and death.

SUPERFICIAL SPREADING MELANOMA Superficial spreading melanoma is the most common type, comprising 70% to 80% of all melanomas (Porth & Matfin, 2009). The lesions are usually flat and scaly or crusty and are about 2 cm in diameter. They often arise from a preexisting nevus. This type of melanoma is found on the trunk and back of men and on the legs of women. Superficial spreading melanomas occur more often in women than in men. The median age of occurrence is the 50s.

The radial growth phase lasts from 1 to 5 or more years. When the lesion enters the vertical growth phase, it grows rapidly, and its color changes from a mixture of tan, brown, and black to a characteristic red, white, and blue. The lesion also develops irregular borders and often has raised nodules and ulcerations (Figure 16–16 ■).

LENTIGO MALIGNA MELANOMA Lentigo maligna melanoma often arises from the precursor lesion, lentigo maligna. The lesions are large and tan with different shades of brown. This type of melanoma makes up 5% to 10% of malignant melanomas and is the least serious form (Porth & Matfin, 2009). It occurs on skin that has had long-term sun exposure, such as the face, neck, and sometimes the dorsal surface of the hands and lower extremities. Lentigo maligna melanoma affects women more than men. It is typically diagnosed in people in their 60s and 70s.

Lentigo maligna melanoma is characterized by a proliferation of atypical melanocytes parallel to the basal layer of the epidermis. The radial growth phase may last from 10 to 25 years, with the lesion growing to as large as 10 cm. The lesion becomes malignant as soon as the melanocytes invade the dermis. In the vertical growth phase, raised nodules may appear on the surface of the lesion. The lesion tends to acquire a freckled or mottled appearance.

NODULAR MELANOMA Nodular melanoma lesions are raised, dome-shaped, blue-black or red nodules on areas of the head, neck, and trunk that may or may not have been exposed to the sun. The lesions may look like a blood blister, or they may ulcerate and bleed. The lesions arise from unaffected skin rather than from a preexisting lesion. This type makes up 10% to 15% of malignant melanomas and is often diagnosed in people in their 50s (Porth & Matfin, 2009).

Nodular melanoma has only a vertical growth phase, but it grows aggressively during that phase. However, the absence of a radial growth phase makes this type more difficult to diagnose before it metastasizes.

ACRAL LENTIGINOUS MELANOMA Acral lentiginous melanoma, also called mucocutaneous melanoma, is less common in people with fair skin and more common in people with

Figure 16–16 ■ Malignant melanoma is a serious skin cancer that arises from melanocytes.

dark skin. The lesions progress from tan, brown, or black flat lesions to elevated nodules and are about 3 cm in diameter. The radial phase lasts from 2 to 5 years, and the lesions are found on the palms of the hands, soles of the feet, the mucous membranes, and the nailbeds. Acral lentiginous melanoma affects both men and women equally and is most often diagnosed in people in their 50s and 60s.

Interdisciplinary Care

The management of the patient with melanoma begins with identification, diagnosis, and tumor staging. If treatable, the tumor is removed through surgical excision. Melanoma is also treated with chemotherapy, immunotherapy, and radiation therapy. Other therapies used with success include biological therapies with interleukin-2 and interferon and therapeutic vaccines containing melanoma antigens.

Identification

Melanoma is most often found on the trunk of men and on the lower extremities of women. Nevertheless, it is important for the patient to have a complete physical examination and total skin assessment. In addition to a visual examination of all skin surfaces, palpation of regional lymph nodes, the liver, and the spleen is essential to assess for metastasis when a melanoma is suspected or found.

A change in the color or size of a nevus is reported in 70% of people diagnosed with a melanoma. The ABCDE rule is used to assess suspicious lesions.

> **FAST FACTS**
>
> **The ABCDE Rule + The Ugly Duckling Sign**
> Using the ABCDE rule to assess for melanoma:
> A = asymmetry (one half of the nevus does not match the other half)
> B = border irregularity (edges are ragged, blurred, or notched)
> C = color variation or dark black color
> D = diameter greater than 6 mm (size of a pencil eraser)
> E = evolving or changing
>
> The Ugly Duckling Sign = a mole that looks or feels different that other moles, or changes differently over time than other moles

Diagnosis

In addition to biopsy of any suspicious lesion, diagnostic tests are conducted to determine whether the tumor has metastasized. Because malignant melanoma may metastasize to any organ or tissue of the body, a variety of tests may be conducted, including microscopic examination, biopsy, and tests for metastasis (liver function tests and CT scan of the liver, a complete blood count, serum blood chemistry profile, chest x-ray, bone scan, and CT scan or MRI of the brain).

Microstaging

The term microstaging describes the assessment of the level of invasion of a malignant melanoma and the maximum tumor thickness. In one method, the Clark system of microstaging, the vertical growth of the lesion is measured from the epidermis to the subcutaneous tissue to determine the level of invasion (Figure 16–17 ■).

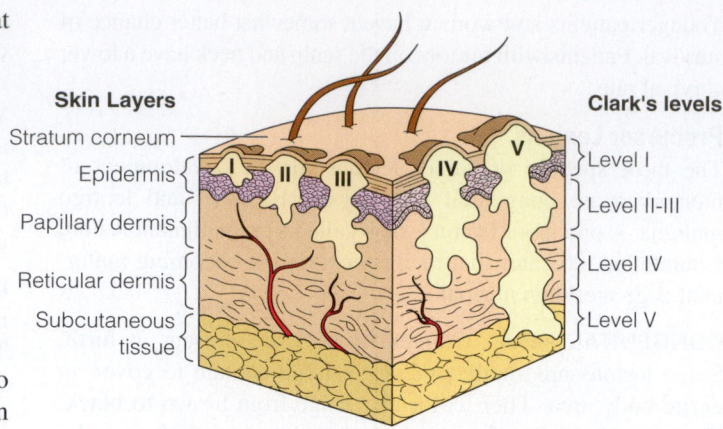

Figure 16–17 ■ Clark's levels for staging measure the invasion of a melanoma from the epidermis to the subcutaneous tissue.

Treatments

Surgical excision is the preferred treatment for malignant melanoma. Other methods of treatment include chemotherapy, immunotherapy, and radiation therapy.

SURGERY   If a biopsy identifies the lesion as a melanoma, a wide excision is performed that includes the full thickness of the skin and subcutaneous tissue. Regional lymph nodes are the most common sites for metastasis of melanoma. Standard surgical treatment for clinically suspicious lymph node involvement includes excision of the primary lesions as well as surgical dissection of the involved lymph nodes. Surgery also is indicated for palliative management of isolated metastasis. Removal of metastatic tumors in the brain, liver, lung, gastrointestinal tract, or subcutaneous tissue may relieve symptoms and prolong life. (See the Case Study & Nursing Care Plan that follows.)

IMMUNOTHERAPY   Immunotherapy is a relatively new treatment modality for melanoma. The role of the immunologic response initially was recognized because of the numerous spontaneous remissions seen in patients with melanoma—a higher occurrence than with any other adult tumor. In addition, researchers have recently identified tumor-specific antigen-antibodies in patients with melanoma.

Agents such as interferons, interleukins, monoclonal antibodies, bacille Calmette-Guérin (BCG), levamisole, transfer factors, and tumor vaccines have shown activity in melanoma, with varying response rates. The effectiveness of these agents, used either alone, in combination with chemotherapy, or in combination with each other, is under investigation. The use of immunotherapy in the treatment of melanoma is still new and requires further investigation.

RADIATION THERAPY   Melanoma responds to higher dose radiation, especially if the tumor is small. Response rates to radiation therapy depend on the site of the tumor, the thickness of the tumor, the type of melanoma, and the patient's general health, but may range from 0% to 71%. Radiation frequently is used for palliation of symptoms resulting from metastasis to the brain, bone, lymph nodes, gastrointestinal tract, skin, or subcutaneous tissue. Liver and lung metastases are not treated with radiation therapy because a loss of organ function may result.

BIOLOGICAL THERAPY Biological therapy is used to boost or restore the ability of the immune system to fight the cancer. Agents used include the monoclonal antibodies, growth factors, and vaccines. These agents may also have a direct antitumor effect.

NEW METHODS OF TREATMENT Melanoma skin cancer research is ongoing and directed toward more specific methods of diagnosis and treatment. Examples are as follows:

- *Gene therapy:* Clinical trials are in progress to test the effectiveness of adding certain genes to the malignant cells.
- *Melanoma DNA research*: Genes such as CDKN2A (also known as $_p16$) have been found to be mutated in some families with a high rate of melanoma.
- *Staging*: Very sensitive new tests can better detect the spread of melanoma to lymph nodes and can possibly better identify people who could be helped by a treatment such as immunotherapy after surgery.

∾ Nursing Care

Nurses have the opportunity to assess the skin of patients requiring care for many different health problems and may be the first healthcare provider to identify suspicious lesions. Wide excision and the high risk of metastasis from melanoma usually requires inpatient surgical treatment, with the nurse providing care and teaching. See the Evidence for Nursing Care box for selected resources related to the patient with malignant melanoma.

Health Promotion

The most important aspect of preventing melanoma is a health history and skin assessment. The ACS recommends that people between the ages of 20 and 40 see a skin specialist every 3 years and those over 40 have annual skin checkups. People with actinic keratoses should also have their skin checked regularly for any signs of change. Patients at risk (those with precancerous lesions and with personal risk factors), as well as those over the age of 40, should conduct a monthly skin self-examination (described in Box 16–7). When self-assessing for melanoma, the patient looks for a change in the following:

- Color, especially any lesion that becomes darker or variegated in shades of tan, brown, black, red, white, or blue
- Size, especially any lesion that becomes larger or spreads out

EVIDENCE FOR NURSING CARE — **The Patient with Malignant Melanoma**

Selected resources that nurses may find helpful when planning evidence-based nursing care follow.

- Rubin, K. (2009). Management of metastatic melanoma: Nursing challenges today and tomorrow. *Clinical Journal of Oncology Nursing, 13*(1), 81–89.
- Torrens, R., & Swan, B. A. (2009). Promoting prevention and early recognition of malignant melanoma. *Dermatology Nursing, 21*(3), 115–22. Retrieved from http://www.dermatologynursing.net/ceonline/2011/article21115122.pdf
- Zimmerman, L., & Britton, K. (2009). Prevention through vigilance: Malignant melanoma management. *Nursing Management, 40*(6), 26–29. Retrieved from http://www.nursingcenter.com/prodev/ce_article.asp?tid=865443

- Shape, especially any lesion that protrudes more from the skin or begins to have an irregular outline
- Appearance of a lesion, especially bleeding, drainage, oozing, ulceration, crusting, scaliness, or development of a mushrooming outward growth
- Consistency, especially any lesion that becomes softer or is more easily irritated
- Skin around a lesion, such as redness, swelling, or leaking of color from a lesion into the surrounding skin
- Sensation, such as itching or pain

Assessment

Skin assessment is discussed in ∾ Chapter 15. Specific health history questions and assessments for skin cancer are outlined in Box 16–9.

Nursing Diagnoses and Interventions

Although many different nursing diagnoses may be appropriate for the patient with a melanoma, common responses are impaired skin integrity, hopelessness, and anxiety. These diagnoses are also appropriate for use with patients with nonmelanoma skin cancer.

Impaired Skin Integrity

Melanomas not only destroy skin layers but also invade body structures. Certain types of melanomas may ulcerate prior to diagnosis, and treatment typically involves some type of surgical biopsy and excision. Any open lesion or incision increases the risk for secondary infection.

- Monitor for manifestations of infection: fever, tachycardia, malaise, incisional erythema, swelling, pain, or drainage that increases or becomes purulent. *Intact skin is the first line of defense against infection; impaired skin integrity increases the risk for infection. If infection is present, the patient may have both systemic and local manifestations.*
- Keep the incision line clean and dry by changing dressings as necessary. *Moisture increases the risk of infection.*
- Follow principles of medical and surgical asepsis when caring for patient's incision. Teach family members and visitors the importance of careful hand hygiene. Maintain standard precautions if drainage is present. *Careful hand hygiene is essential in preventing the spread of infection. Aseptic techniques are necessary when caring for any surgical incision to prevent infection.*
- Encourage and maintain adequate caloric and protein intake in the diet. Suggest a consultation with the dietitian if the patient does not want to eat. *Adequate calories and protein are necessary for proper healing. The patient with cancer has increased metabolic needs; if these needs are not met, nutritional problems that impair healing may result.*

Hopelessness

Hopelessness is an emotional state in which a person feels that there is no possibility that life will improve. Patients who experience hopelessness are often withdrawn, passive, and apathetic.

The diagnosis of melanoma threatens the quality and quantity of life as the patient faces the possibility or reality of metastasis; the possibility that the cancer may recur and cause death; and alterations in self-concept, roles, and relationships. Inspiring hope in patients during this health crisis is a legitimate nursing action.

BOX 16–9 Nursing Assessment for Skin Cancer

Interview Questions
- Have any members of your family ever been treated for skin cancer?
- Have you had a skin cancer removed from any part of your body?
- Have you noticed any change in the size, shape, or color of a mole, wart, birthmark, or scar?
- Do you have any moles, warts, birthmarks, or scars that itch, are painful, have crusting, or bleed?
- In what parts of the country or world have you lived?
- Have you ever been badly sunburned?
- Do you visit tanning salons?
- Are you exposed to any hazardous chemicals in your job?
- Have you been taught how to examine your skin? If so, how do you do this examination? How often?

Physical Assessment
1. Ask the patient to remove all clothing and put on an examination gown. Ensure good light; natural, bright light is best for inspection of lesions. The patient may sit, stand, or lie down.
2. Inspect and palpate the skin. Stretching the skin tightly during assessment facilitates assessment of nodular and scaly lesions and lesions in the dermis. Assess for the following:
   a. Obvious lesions
   b. Visible swellings
   c. Alterations in normal contour and borders of nevi
   d. Enlarged lymph glands
   e. Skin or mucosal discolorations
   f. Areas of ulceration, scaling, crusting, or erosion.
3. The order of assessment follows:
   a. Head and neck: entire scalp, eyelids, external ear, auditory canals, external surface of the nose, internal surface of the nose, the oral cavity, facial skin, the facial glands (parotid, submaxillary, sublingual)
   b. Thyroid and neck, including lymph glands
   c. Chest and abdomen, with special attention under pendulous breasts, in skin folds, and in areas covered with hair
   d. Back and buttocks, with special attention to the area between the buttocks
   e. Extremities, with special attention to the axillae, nail beds, webs between the fingers and toes, and soles of the feet
   f. External genitals, with special attention to skin folds, mucous membranes, and areas covered with hair
4. Measure and record a description of all skin lesions on an anatomic chart. Take photographs (if possible) of any suspicious lesion, and include them in the patient's record for future reference.

- Provide an environment that encourages the patient to identify and express feelings, concerns, and goals:
  - Use active listening, ask open-ended questions, and reflect on the patient's statements.
  - Acknowledge and respect feelings of apathy and/or anger as expressions of distress.
  - Convey an empathetic understanding of the fears and concerns.
  - Provide opportunities to express positive emotions: hope, faith, a sense of purpose, and the will to live.
  - Explore the patient's perceptions, and modify or clarify them if necessary by providing information and correcting misconceptions.
  - Encourage the patient to identify support systems and sources of strength and coping in the past.
  Verbalizing feelings, concerns, and goals allows others to validate or correct them, promotes a therapeutic nurse–patient relationship, and fosters feelings of self-worth. Expressing positive emotions and calling on support systems and sources of strength that were effective in coping with past crises help the person resolve the crisis and develop hope.
- Encourage active participation in self-care as well as in mutual decision making and goal setting. *Meeting self-care needs and making decisions about care increase personal confidence in one's capacity for coping.*
- Encourage a focus not only on the present but also on the future: Review past occasions for hope, discuss the patient's personal meaning of hope, establish and evaluate short-term goals with the patient and family, and encourage them to express hope for the future. *The nurse mobilizes the patient's resources to strengthen motivation, hope, and the will to live.*

Anxiety

The intensity of anxiety, aroused by a perceived threat, depends on the severity of the present situation and the patient's ability to handle the threat. Anxiety is one of the most common psychosocial responses in patients with cancer. Anxiety increases at the time of diagnosis and remains a constant emotion throughout the course of treatment, regardless of treatment type or setting. Interventions center on helping the patient recognize the manifestations of anxiety, determining whether the patient wishes to do anything about the anxiety, and facilitating coping strategies.

- Provide reassurance and comfort:
  - Set aside time to sit quietly with the patient.
  - Speak slowly and calmly.
  - Convey empathetic understanding by touch and supporting present coping mechanisms, such as crying and talking.
  - Do not make demands or expect the patient to make decisions.

Coping behaviors differ from situation to situation and from person to person. Anxiety at moderate to severe levels narrows perceptions and the ability to function.

- Decrease sensory stimuli by using short, simple sentences; focusing on the here and now; and providing concise information. *Higher levels of anxiety result in a focus on the present, inability to concentrate, and difficulty in understanding verbal communications.*
- Provide interventions that decrease anxiety levels and increase coping:
  - Provide accurate information about the illness, treatment, and expected length of recovery.
  - Encourage discussion of expected physical changes and ways to minimize disfigurement through cosmetics and clothing.

Geoff Sanders, aged 69, is retired from the postal service. He has always been an avid participant in outdoor sports: When he was younger he played baseball and tennis, and for the last 10 years he has played golf at least twice a week. He now lives in Connecticut, but as a younger man he lived in Florida for almost 15 years. Mr. Sanders has a variety of warts and moles and rarely pays attention to them. However, after taking a shower one day he noticed that a mole on his left lower leg looked bigger and darker. Mr. Sanders had just seen a public service announcement on television about the dangers of changes in moles, and he immediately called his primary care physician for an appointment at the dermatology clinic.

ASSESSMENT

On arriving at the clinic, Mr. Sanders is interviewed and examined by Tom Hall, a clinical nurse specialist. Following the assessment, Mr. Hall documents the following information.

Mr. Sanders has a family history of skin cancer; his father had several squamous cell cancers removed from his face. He has numerous nevi on his body; the one causing concern is located on the medial anterior left leg, 2 inches below the patella. Mr. Sanders states that the mole has been present for years but that he noticed just yesterday that it has become larger and darker. On further questioning, he states that the mole itches sometimes but has never hurt or bled. Mr. Sanders lived in Florida for 15 years and now experiences a sunburn early each summer before he tans. The sunburn involves the lower legs because Mr. Sanders wears shorts during his twice-weekly golf game.

A complete skin assessment reveals various freckles, warts, and nevi. With the exception of the nevus that prompted Mr. Sanders to come to the clinic, all lesions appear normal. The nevus in question is raised, 3 cm in diameter, with irregular borders and a nodular surface. It is variegated in color, with various shades of brown. The skin surrounding the nevus is slightly erythematous. Inguinal lymph nodes are not enlarged or painful. Mr. Hall takes a photograph of the lesion with Mr. Sanders's permission.

Following the assessment, Mr. Sanders discusses the lesion with a surgeon, who recommends excision. They discuss the possibility of skin cancer and the importance of early detection and treatment. Mr. Sanders is scheduled for a biopsy of the nevus under a local anesthetic the following morning. Following the biopsy, histologic examination reveals lentigo maligna melanoma. Staging of the tumor reveals that it is a melanoma *in situ*, with no metastasis to regional lymph nodes. Mr. Sanders undergoes a wide excision of the lesion the following afternoon.

DIAGNOSES

- *Impaired Skin Integrity* related to excision of melanoma from the left lower leg
- *Risk for Infection* related to surgical wound on left lower leg
- *Acute Pain* related to wide excision of melanoma on left lower leg
- *Anxiety* related to diagnosis of skin cancer

EXPECTED OUTCOMES

- Demonstrate complete healing of the incision without manifestations of infection.
- Verbalize relief of pain by the time the incision is healed.
- Verbalize fears and concerns about the diagnosis.

PLANNING AND IMPLEMENTATION

- Make the first dressing change, but ensure that Mr. Sanders can safely change the dressing himself prior to discharge the day after surgery.
- On discharge, provide adequate dressings and tape for the first home dressing change; include in discharge instructions necessary information about where to buy supplies and how many dressing supplies will be needed.
- Review and provide written instruction for prescribed systemic antibiotic and pain medication.
- Provide written instructions for dressing change, manifestations of infection, and phone number of clinic; stress importance of calling if any abnormal symptoms occur.
- Teach how to protect the incision from bumps and to protect the site from irritants.
- Discuss diagnosis, positive outlook for treatment of melanoma *in situ*, and the patient's concerns.
- Stress importance of lifelong regular healthcare evaluations to identify any recurrence or metastasis.

EVALUATION

Mr. Sanders returned to the dermatology clinic 1 week after his surgical incision. His incision is well approximated and shows no signs of infection. He is taking his antibiotic 4 times a day as prescribed and reports that his need for pain medications is decreasing. During his clinic visit the following week, Mr. Hall removes the sutures and assesses the wound as healed. Mr. Sanders completed his antibiotics and no longer requires pain medications. He says he is still "scared to death" about having cancer, but he has decided to join a local cancer support group. He also says he had gotten a list of skin safety rules from the American Cancer Society and will be sure to cover up and use sunscreens when he plays golf. Mr. Sanders makes an appointment for follow-up care in 3 months.

CRITICAL THINKING IN THE NURSING PROCESS

1. Consider reasons why people who notice a change in a skin lesion put off seeking health care. What can nurses do to effect change?
2. Design a teaching plan for young adults for preventing skin cancers.
3. What would you say to Mr. Sanders if he called the clinic and said that the antibiotics were making him sick and he didn't think he needed them anyway?
4. Design a nursing care plan for Mr. Sanders for the diagnosis *Powerlessness*.

See Evaluating Your Response in Appendix C.

- Include family members in teaching sessions.
- Encourage participation in care.

Although the prognosis and treatment of melanoma depend on various factors, the prognosis of complete cure is decreased with metastasis. Surgical incisions include excision with wide margins, which may cause disfigurement.

Active participation in care give the patient some control over the future and is often an effective means of coping with anxiety.

Using NANDA, NIC, and NOC

Linkages between a selected NANDA nursing diagnosis, NIC, and NOC for the patient with malignant melanoma are shown in the chart that follows.

Community-Based Care

Teaching the patient and family experiencing the diagnosis and treatment of melanoma focuses on self-care and ongoing self-monitoring. Education for the patient and family is specific to the type of treatment. In addition to wound care, patients who have had a lymph node dissection need instructions in how to protect the extremity from bleeding, trauma, and infection. Address the following topics:

- Schedule regular medical checkups every 3 months for the first 2 years, every 6 months for the next 5 years, and yearly thereafter.
- Proper self-care combined with regular medical care can help the patient lead a fairly normal life.
- If assistance for home care is necessary, provide referrals to a community health agency or a home care agency. In addition, refer the patient to a local cancer support group if desired. Other resources are the ACS, the Skin Cancer Foundation, and the National Cancer Institute.

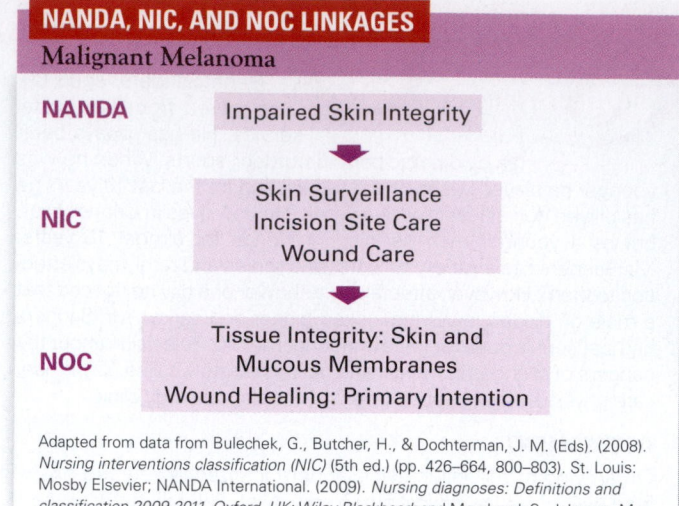

NANDA, NIC, AND NOC LINKAGES
Malignant Melanoma

NANDA — Impaired Skin Integrity

NIC — Skin Surveillance / Incision Site Care / Wound Care

NOC — Tissue Integrity: Skin and Mucous Membranes / Wound Healing: Primary Intention

Adapted from data from Bulechek, G., Butcher, H., & Dochterman, J. M. (Eds). (2008). *Nursing interventions classification (NIC)* (5th ed.) (pp. 426–664, 800–803). St. Louis: Mosby Elsevier; NANDA International. (2009). *Nursing diagnoses: Definitions and classification 2009-2011.* Oxford, UK: Wiley-Blackhead; and Moorhead; S., Johnson, M., Maas, M., & Swanson, E. (Eds). (2008). *Nursing outcomes classification (NOC)* (4th ed.) (pp. 699–700, 730–731). St. Louis: Mosby Elsevier.

Skin Trauma

Trauma to the skin can be unintentional or intentional (as in the case of surgery). Chemicals, radiation, pressure, or thermal changes cause skin trauma. This section discusses pressure ulcers and frostbite, as well as intentional trauma from cutaneous and plastic surgery or treatment. Thermal injury, or burns, is discussed in ∞ Chapter 17.

The Patient with a Pressure Ulcer

Pressure ulcers are ischemic lesions of the skin and underlying tissues caused by unrelieved pressure that impairs the flow of blood and lymph. The ischemia causes tissue necrosis and eventual ulceration. These ulcers, also called bed sores or decubitus ulcers, tend to develop over a bony prominence (such as the heels, greater trochanter, sacrum, and ischia), but they may appear on the skin of any part of the body subjected to external pressure, friction, or shearing forces.

Incidence

The increasing incidence of pressure ulcers in all healthcare settings, but especially in hospitals and long-term care facilities, has resulted in infection, loss of function, and pain for patients. These complications, in turn, have caused increased length of stay and costs. As a result, the Centers for Medicare and Medicaid will no longer make additional reimbursement payments to hospitals to cover the cost of pressure ulcers developed during a hospital stay.

FAST FACTS
Pressure Ulcers
- The incidence of pressure ulcers in hospitals is approximately 8%; the incidence in long-term care ranges from 2.4% to 23%.
- An estimated 60,000 patients die each year from pressure ulcer complications.
- The cost of treating these chronic wounds is about $11 billion a year.

(Ayello & Lyder, 2007; Porth & Matfin, 2009).

The prevention and treatment of pressure ulcers is a public health issue. The national health policy statement *Healthy People 2010* set a target of a 50% decrease in the prevalence of pressure ulcers in long-term care residents. The National Institute for Healthcare Improvement (NHI) has made preventing pressure ulcers one of 12 interventions to save lives. The NHI recommendations are described in the nursing care section that follows. Pressure ulcers are preventable, with nursing care being a major part of prevention.

Pathophysiology

Pressure ulcers develop from external pressure that compresses blood vessels or from friction and shearing forces that tear and injure vessels. Both types of pressure cause traumatic injury and initiate the process of pressure ulcer development.

External pressure that is greater than capillary pressure and arteriolar pressure interrupts blood flow in capillary beds. When pressure is applied to skin over a bony prominence for 2 hours, tissue ischemia and hypoxia from external pressure cause irreversible tissue damage. For example, when the body is in the supine position, the body's weight applies pressure to the sacrum. The same amount of pressure causes more damage when it is applied to a small area than when it is distributed over a large surface.

Shearing forces result when one tissue layer slides over another. The stretching and bending of blood vessels cause injury and thrombosis. Patients in hospital beds are subject to shearing forces when the head of the bed is elevated and the torso slides down toward the foot of the bed. Pulling the patient up in bed also subjects the patient to shearing forces. (For this reason, always lift patients up in bed). In both cases, friction and moisture cause the skin and superficial fascia to remain fixed to the bed sheet, while the deep fascia and bony skeleton slides in the direction of body movement.

When a person lies or sits in one position for an extended length of time without moving, pressure on the tissue between a bony prominence and the external surface of the body distorts capillaries and interferes with normal blood flow. If the pressure is relieved, blood flow to the area increases, and a brief period of reactive hyperemia occurs without permanent damage. However, if the pressure continues, platelets aggregate in the endothelial cells surrounding the capillaries and form microthrombi. These microthrombi impede blood flow, resulting in ischemia and hypoxia of tissues. Eventually, the cells and tissues of the immediate area of pressure and of the surrounding area die and become necrotic.

Alterations in the involved tissue depend on the depth of the injury. Injury to superficial layers of skin results in blister formation, whereas injury to deeper structures causes the pressure ulcer area to appear dark reddish-blue. As the tissues die, the ulcer becomes an open wound that may be deep enough to expose the muscles and bone. The necrotic tissue elicits an inflammatory response, and the patient experiences increases in temperature, pain, and white blood cell count. Secondary bacterial invasion is common. Enzymes from bacteria and macrophages dissolve necrotic tissue, resulting in a foul-smelling drainage.

Pressure ulcers are staged to classify the degree of tissue damage. The updated stages from the National Pressure Ulcer Advisory Panel (2007) are listed in Box 16–10.

BOX 16–10 **NPUAP's Updated Pressure Ulcer Staging**

STAGE I		A sign of risk. Intact skin with nonblanchable redness of a localized area, usually over a bony prominence. The area may be painful, firm, soft, warmer or cooler than adjacent tissue. May be difficult to detect in people with dark skin.
STAGE II		Partial thickness loss of dermis presenting as a shallow open ulcer with a red or pink wound bed. May also present as an intact or open blister. The ulcer may shiny or dry, without bruising or slough (loss of tissue).
STAGE III		Full-thickness tissue loss. Subcutaneous fat may be visible but bone, tendon, or muscle are *not* exposed. Slough may be present but does not obscure the depth of tissue loss. *May* include undermining and tunneling.
STAGE IV		Full-thickness skin loss with exposed bone, tendon or muscle. Slough or eschar (dead tissue such as a scab) may be present on some parts of the wound bed. Often includes undermining and tunneling.

Source: Text is from *Pressure Ulcers in Adults: Prediction and Prevention* by the Agency for Health Care Policy and Research, 1992 Rockville, MD: US Department of Health and Human Services. Photos courtesy of Karen Lou Kennedy, RN, FPN, www.kennedyterminalulcer.com.

Older adults are at a greater risk for developing pressure ulcers because of age-related changes in the integumentary system. Cell renewal slows, resulting in skin that has decreased elasticity. The margin between the epidermis and the dermis separates more easily, making the skin more prone to tearing. In addition, thinning subcutaneous tissue provides less cushioning over bony prominences. Water content decreases, and the skin becomes drier. These changes increase the older adult's susceptibility to skin trauma and prolong wound healing.

Chronic conditions associated with immobility and self-care deficit place older adults at risk of developing pressure ulcers. For example, bowel or bladder incontinence can produce regions of wet skin that are prone to infections and breakdown. Furthermore, sensory-perceptual alterations and impaired cognitive functioning may reduce the frequency with which the older adult shifts position when sitting or lying in bed. Finally, undernutrition, which is often seen in older adults, heightens the risk for developing pressure ulcers.

To prevent pressure ulcers, the skin of older adults should be kept clean, dry, and well hydrated. Moisturizers are recommended to keep the skin free of excessive dryness. Older adults should be taught to avoid bumping into furniture and to wear long skirts or pants to help protect the lower extremities from trauma.

When hospitalized, older adults should have a validated risk assessment for pressure ulcers completed on admission and as often as the tool suggests. A daily systematic skin inspection with particular attention to bony prominences should be completed.

Once pressure ulcers develop in older adults, the treatment is the same as for younger patients. However, additional steps may need to be taken. Because local perfusion to tissues is compromised, steps should be taken to prevent under- or overhydration. It is essential that optimal nutritional status be maintained. Also, keep in mind that it may take a longer time for the pressure ulcer to heal.

Risk Factors

Although a pressure ulcer may develop in an adult of any age who has an impairment in mobility, those most at risk are older adults with limited mobility and fractured hips, people with quadriplegia, and patients in the critical care setting (Porth & Matfin, 2009). Other patients prone to develop pressure ulcers are those with fractures of large bones (e.g., hip or femur) or who have undergone orthopedic surgery or sustained spinal cord injury. In addition to deficits in mobility and activity, incontinence and nutritional deficit also increase the risk of pressure ulcer development. Patients with chronic illnesses, such as renal failure and anemia, and those with edema or infection are also at increased risk. See nursing care of the older adult above for information about preventing pressure ulcer development in older adults.

Interdisciplinary Care

For the patient at risk for pressure ulcers, the goal is prevention. Existing ulcers require interdisciplinary treatment to promote healing and restore skin integrity.

Diagnosis

Diagnostic tests are conducted to determine the presence of a secondary infection and to differentiate the cause of the ulcer. If the ulcer is deep or appears infected, drainage or biopsied tissue is cultured to determine the causative organism.

Medications

Topical and systemic antibiotics specific to the infectious organism eradicate any infection present. Additionally, a variety of products promote healing. Examples are listed in Table 16–2.

TABLE 16–2 Products Used to Treat Pressure Ulcers

PRODUCT	PURPOSE
Hydrocolloid Dressings (such as DuoDerm)	May be used for stages I, II, III, and IV with minimal exudate. Forms a gel when coming into contact with wound exudate. Forms an occlusive barrier over the ulcer while maintaining a moist environment and preventing infection. Helps prevent friction and shear.
Alginate Dressings (such as SilvaSorb and Sorbsan)	May be used for stages II, III, and IV with moderate to heavy drainage, and in infected and non-infected wounds. Forms a gel when coming into contact with wound exudate. Should not be applied to dry or minimally draining wounds, as dehydration and delay in healing may result.
Hydrofibers (such as Aquacel)	May be used for stage II, III, and IV with moderate to heavy exudate. Can be used with actual or risk for infection. Combines the absorption of the hydrofiber with 1.2% silver as an antimicrobial agent.
Hydrogel Dressings (such as Intrasite gel)	May be used for stages II, III, IV. Rehydrate the wound bed and decrease pain. Promotes autolytic debridement.
Transparent Adhesive Dressings (such as OpSite and Tegrderm)	May be used in shallow I, II, and III ulcers. Provide a moist wound setting, prevent infection, and promote re-epithelialization. Minimize friction and shear.
Wet-to-Dry Dressings	Provide mechanical debridement.
Vacuum-assisted closure (VAC) sponges	Stimulate wound contracture while removing the exudate and wound edema.

Surgical Treatment

Surgical debridement may be necessary if the pressure ulcer is deep, if subcutaneous tissues are involved, or if an eschar has formed over the ulcer, preventing healing by granulation. Large wounds may require skin grafting for complete closure.

Nursing Care

The patient with one or more pressure ulcers not only has impaired skin integrity but also is at increased risk for infection, pain, and decreased mobility. Pressure ulcers prolong treatment for other health problems, increase healthcare costs, and diminish the patient's quality of life. See the nursing research box below for information on evidence-based interventions.

Nursing Diagnoses and Interventions

The following interventions and rationales are adapted from the clinical guidelines developed by the Agency for Health Care Policy and Research (1992, 1994) in identifying adults at risk and treating those with stage I pressure ulcers.

Risk for Impaired Skin Integrity

- Identify at-risk individuals needing prevention and the specific factors placing them at risk.
- Assess bed- and chair-bound patients, as well as those who are unable to reposition themselves, for additional risk factors: immobility, incontinence, nutritional factors (such as inadequate dietary intake and impaired nutritional status), and altered level of consciousness.
- Assess patients on admission to acute care and rehabilitation hospitals, nursing homes, home care programs, and other healthcare facilities.

- Use a systematic risk assessment by using a validated risk assessment tool (such as the Braden scale). See the information about predicting risk and using the Braden scale at the Nursing Center website (Stotts & Gunning berg, 2007).
- Document all assessments of risk. *Individuals at risk for pressure ulcers must be identified so that risk factors can be reduced through intervention. The primary risk factors for pressure ulcers are immobility and limited activity; therefore, assess patients who cannot reposition themselves or whose activity is limited to bed or chair. Validated tools ensure systematic evaluation of individual risk factors. The patient requires periodic reassessment for pressure ulcers. Accurate and complete documentation of all risk assessments ensures continuity of care and may be used as a foundation for the skin care plan.*
- Conduct a systematic skin inspection at least once a day, paying particular attention to the bony prominences. Systematic, comprehensive, and routine skin care may decrease pressure ulcer incidence Inspect the following to assess a pressure ulcer:
  - Location of any lesion or ulcer
  - Estimation of the stage
  - Dimensions of the ulcer: length, width, depth
  - Presence of any abnormal pathways in the wound:
  - Sinus tract: a cavity or channel underneath the wound
- Tunneling: a passageway or opening that may be visible at skin level, but with most of the tunnel under the surface of the skin
- Undermining: areas of tissue destruction underneath intact skin along wound margins
- Visible necrotic tissue (Slough is necrotic tissue that is in the process of separating from viable tissue.)
- Presence of an exudate

MOVING EVIDENCE INTO ACTION **Preventing Pressure Ulcers in Acute Care and Home Care Settings**

Despite advances in health care to extend life and improve functional status, older adults with chronic illnesses are at increased risk of developing pressure ulcers. The older adult, with age-related compromised cellular activity is especially vulnerable to impaired healing of injured tissue such as pressure ulcers. This article (Frantz, 2004) describes an evidence-based protocol designed to enhance the healing of pressure ulcers in older patients by using evidence-based interventions. The following interventions are recommended:

- Assess all individuals admitted to a healthcare facility with a pressure ulcer for the risk of developing additional pressure ulcers by using a standardized risk assessment scale.
- Perform a complete history and physical examination, combined with a detailed assessment of the ulcer characteristics (location, stage, type of tissue, presence of tunneling or tracts, exudate, odor, and condition of skin around the ulcer).
- Remove necrotic tissue and debris from the ulcer to decrease the growth of bacteria and remove foreign materials, such as exudates and metabolic wastes.
- Provide a moist wound environment to promote reepithelialization and healing.
- Control bacterial levels in the wound by using cleansing and debridment, as well as systemic and topical antibiotics.
- Supply essential substrates for tissue repair, including protein, calories, vitamins, and minerals. Maintain a positive nitrogen balance.
- Manage tissue loads by positioning to avoid external force on the ulcer.

IMPLICATIONS FOR NURSING

The design and implementation of a pressure ulcer prevention and treatment plan is essential for any person at risk, including older adults, those with debilitating or multiple illnesses, and those with health problems limiting mobility. To effectively implement a plan, it is important to prepare providers to use a standard protocol through educational programs, and to monitor indicators of improvement or deterioration in the ulcer and presence or absence of new ulcers. These outcomes should be assessed and recorded on a weekly basis.

CRITICAL THINKING IN PATIENT CARE

1. Describe the differences and similarities in a pressure ulcer prevention plan of care you would develop for two patients: a 76-year-old man in a nursing home who has had a stroke that paralyzed his left side, and a 36-year-old man with a spinal cord injury from a motorcycle accident who cannot walk and lives at home.
2. Consider the activities to treat pressure ulcers, and answer the following:
   a. What level of healthcare provider would you delegate to care for the patient?
   b. How much time in an 8-hour period would be needed for nursing care?
3. What would you teach family caregivers about providing care at home?

- Presence or absence of granulation tissue
  Skin inspection provides data the nurse uses in designing interventions to reduce risk and in evaluating outcomes of those interventions.
- Clean the skin at the time of soiling and at routine intervals, as frequently as the patient's need or preference dictates. Avoid hot water, use a mild cleansing agent, and clean the skin gently, applying as little force and friction as possible. *Metabolic wastes and environmental contaminants accumulate on the skin; these potentially irritating substances should be removed frequently. Feces and urine cause chemical irritation and should be removed as soon as possible. Hot water may cause skin injury. Mild cleansing agents are less likely to remove the skin's natural barrier.*
- Minimize environmental factors leading to skin drying, such as low humidity and exposure to cold. Treat dry skin with moisturizers. *Well-hydrated skin resists mechanical trauma. Hydration decreases as the ambient air temperature decreases, especially when the air humidity is low. Poorly hydrated skin is less pliable, and severe dryness is associated with fissuring and cracking of the stratum corneum. Moisturizers reduce dry skin.*
- Avoid massage over bony prominences. *Although massage has been practiced for years, evidence now suggests that massage over bony prominences may lead to deep tissue trauma in patients at risk for or with beginning skin manifestations of a pressure ulcer.*
- Minimize skin exposure to moisture due to incontinence, perspiration, or wound drainage. When these sources of moisture cannot be controlled, use underpads or briefs made of materials that absorb moisture and present a quick-drying surface to the skin. Change underpads and briefs frequently. Do not place plastic directly against the skin. *Moisture from incontinence, perspiration, or wound drainage may contain factors that irritate the skin; moisture alone can increase the susceptibility of the skin to injury.*
- To minimize skin injury due to friction and shearing forces, use proper positioning, transferring, and turning techniques. Lubricants (such as cornstarch or creams), protective films (such as transparent dressings and skin sealants), protective dressings (such as hydrocolloids), and protective padding may also reduce friction injuries. *Shear injury occurs when skin remains stationary and the underlying tissue shifts. This shift diminishes the blood supply to the skin and results in ischemia and tissue damage. Proper positioning, however, can eliminate most shear injuries. Friction injuries to the skin occur when it moves across a coarse surface, such as bed linens. Most friction injuries can be avoided by using appropriate techniques to move patients so that their skin is never dragged across the linens. Any agent that eliminates contact or decreases the friction between the skin and the linens reduces the potential for injury.*
- Assess factors involved in inadequate dietary intake of protein or kilocalories. Offer nutritional supplements, and support the patient during mealtimes. If dietary intake remains inadequate, consult with a dietitian about other dietary interventions. *The role nutrition plays in the development of (and to a lesser degree, the healing of) pressure ulcers is not understood, but poor dietary intake of*

kilocalories, protein, and iron has been associated with the development of pressure ulcers.
- Maintain the patient's current level of activity, mobility, and range of motion. *Frequent turning, repositioning, and movement are essential in reducing the risk of pressure ulcers.*
- For the patient on bed rest or who is immobile, provide interventions against the adverse effects of external mechanical forces of pressure, friction, and shear:
  - Reposition all at-risk patients at least every 2 hours, using a written schedule for systematic turning and repositioning.
  - For patients on bed rest, use positioning devices, such as pillows or foam wedges, to protect bony prominences.
- For completely immobile patients, use devices to totally relieve pressure on the heels (the most common method is to raise the heels off the bed). Do not use donut-type devices.
- Avoid placing patients in the side-lying position directly on the trochanter.
- Maintain the head of the bed at the lowest degree of elevation consistent with the patient's medical condition and other restrictions. Limit the amount of time the head of the bed is elevated.
- Use assistive devices, such as a trapeze or bed linen, to move patients in bed who cannot assist during transfers and position changes.
- Place any at-risk patient on a pressure-reducing device, such as foam, static air, alternating air, gel, or water mattress. *Data indicate that the more spontaneous movements that bedridden, older adult patients make, the lower the incidence of pressure ulcers and that fewer pressure ulcers develop in at-risk patients who are turned every 2 to 3 hours. Proper positioning can reduce pressure on bony prominences. It is difficult to redistribute pressure under heels; suspending the heels is the best method. Donut cushions are more likely to cause than to prevent pressure ulcers. Shearing forces are exerted on the body when the head of the bed is elevated. Lifting (rather than dragging) is less likely to cause injury from friction. Pressure-reducing devices and beds can decrease the incidence of pressure ulcers.*
- For chair-bound patients, use pressure-reducing devices. Consider postural alignment, distribution of weight, balance and stability, and pressure relief when positioning these patients. Avoid uninterrupted sitting in a chair or wheelchair. Reposition the patient every hour. Teach patients who can do so to shift their weight every 15 minutes. Use a written plan for positioning, movement, and the use of positioning devices. Do not use donut devices. *Prolonged, uninterrupted mechanical pressure results in tissue breakdown. The patient's weight should be shifted at least every hour.*

Community-Based Care

Patient and family teaching for care of a pressure ulcer also focuses on prevention and includes much of the same information presented in the preceding section. Because many patients with pressure ulcers are older or have other serious illnesses, a caregiver may require teaching on such topics as the following:

- Definition and description of pressure ulcers
- Common locations of pressure ulcers
- Risk factors for the development of pressure ulcers

- Skin care
- Ways to avoid injury
- Diet

Depending on the stage of the pressure ulcer, the nurse teaches the patient or caregiver how to care for ulcers that are already present: how to change wet-to-dry dressings, apply skin barriers, and avoid injury and infection. Referrals to a home health agency or community health department can help the family through the lengthy healing process.

The Patient with Frostbite

Frostbite is an injury of the skin from freezing. If the exposure to freezing temperatures is limited, only the skin and subcutaneous tissues become involved. However, as exposure increases, deeper structures freeze. The skin freezes when the temperature drops to 14°F to 24.8°F (210°C to 24°C). Frostbite is most common on exposed or peripheral areas of the body, such as the nose, ears, feet, and hands.

As human tissues freeze, ice crystals form and increase intracellular sodium content. Small blood vessels initially vasoconstrict but then vasodilate and become more permeable, causing cellular and tissue swelling. With continued exposure, vasoconstriction and increased viscosity of the blood cause infarction and necrosis of the affected tissue.

Superficial frostbite causes numbness, itching, and prickling. The skin appears cyanotic, reddened, or white. Deeper frostbite causes stiffness and paresthesias. As the skin and tissues thaw, the skin becomes white or yellow and loses its elasticity. The patient experiences burning pain. Edema, blisters, necrosis, and gangrene may appear.

Rapid thawing may significantly decrease tissue necrosis. General guidelines for rewarming areas of frostbite follow:

- If you are outdoors, treat superficial frostbite by applying firm pressure with a warm hand or by placing frostbitten hands in the axillae. If the feet are frostbitten, remove wet footwear, dry the feet, and put on dry footwear. Do not rub the areas with snow.
- In the hospital, rapidly rewarm affected areas in circulating warm water, 104°F to 105°F (40°C to 40.5°C) for 20 to 30 minutes. Do not rub or massage the areas.

Following rewarming, the patient is kept on bed rest with the affected parts elevated. Pain medications and anti-inflammatory agents are administered. Blisters are debrided. Whirlpool therapy may be used to clean the skin and debride necrotic tissue. Recovery from frostbite is usually complete if the involved area has not become necrotic. Necrotic tissue may require amputation.

The Patient Undergoing Cutaneous and Plastic Surgery

Although many skin disorders are so small and benign that no treatment is necessary, others require some type of surgery of the skin to remove the lesion. Other surgeries and treatments for skin lesions and deformities are used to restore function and change appearance. This section discusses both cutaneous and plastic surgery, as well as other types of treatment modalities used in the care of the patient with a skin disorder.

Cutaneous Surgery and Procedures

The basic types of cutaneous surgery described here are excision, electrosurgery, cryosurgery, curettage, and laser surgery. Two nonsurgical procedures, chemical destruction and sclerotherapy, are also discussed. Most of these procedures are performed in the office or outpatient clinic.

Fusiform Excision

Fusiform excision is the removal of a full thickness of the epidermis and dermis, usually with a thin layer of subcutaneous tissue. It is used to remove tissue for biopsies and for complete removal of benign and malignant lesions of the skin. Excision of small, superficial lesions is performed under a local anesthetic, and care is taken to place the incision in a way that will provide good cosmetic results.

Electrosurgery

Electrosurgery involves the destruction or removal of tissue with high-frequency alternating current. A variety of surgical procedures may be performed, including *electrodesiccation* (which produces superficial skin destruction), *electrocoagulation* (which produces deeper tissue destruction), and *electrosection* (which can cut through skin and tissue). Electrodesiccation is used to remove benign surface lesions, such as skin tags, keratoses, warts, and angiomas. It is also used to produce hemostasis for capillary bleeding. Electrocoagulation is used to remove telangiectases, warts, and superficial nonmelanoma skin cancers. Electrosection is used to make incisions, excise tissue, and perform biopsies.

Cryosurgery

Cryosurgery is the destruction of tissue by cold or freezing with agents such as fluorocarbon sprays, carbon dioxide snow, nitrous oxide, and liquid nitrogen. Cryosurgery is used to treat many skin lesions. The freezing agents are applied topically to the lesion. The effects depend on the degree of freeze. Light freezing causes damage to the epidermis with blistering or crusting that heals without scarring. Deeper freezes, used to treat malignant cells, cause edema, necrosis, and tissue slough. The effects of cryosurgery may not be obvious until 24 hours following the treatment. Postoperatively, infection is prevented by applying a topical antibiotic and keeping the treated areas clean. Healing occurs in 2 to 3 weeks.

Curettage

Curettage is the removal of lesions with a curette (a semisharp cutting instrument). It is used to remove benign and malignant superficial epidermal lesions. Benign lesions removed include keratoses, nevi, and angiomas. Nonmelanoma skin lesions are removed by curettage if they are small, well-defined, primary tumors. Curettage is also used to remove specimens of tissue for biopsy.

Following curettage, the wound may be treated with electrodesiccation to destroy any remaining malignant cells and to provide hemostasis. These wounds are not closed; rather, they are left open to heal by second intention. Topical antibiotic ointments and dressings may be used in the postoperative period.

Laser Surgery

Laser surgery is used to treat a variety of skin disorders. A laser is an intense light that produces a thermal injury on contact with tissue. The injury causes coagulation, vaporization, excision, and ablation (removal of a growth). Argon, pulsed dye, carbon dioxide, and Nd:YAG lasers are used in cutaneous and plastic surgery. A local anesthetic may be used, although pulsed dye laser causes minimal pain and rarely requires anesthesia.

Chemical Destruction

Chemical destruction is the application of a specific chemical to produce destruction of skin lesions. Chemical destruction is used to treat both benign and premalignant lesions. The chemical is applied to the lesion or is used to cause peeling. After application, the treated area forms a thin crust that sloughs off in about a week.

Sclerotherapy

Sclerotherapy is the removal of benign skin lesions with a sclerosing agent that causes inflammation with fibrosis of tissue. Agents that cause therapeutic sclerosis include aethoxysklerol (Sclerodex) and hypertonic sodium chloride. This type of treatment is used for telangiectases and superficial spider veins of the lower extremities. The solution is injected into the affected veins, causing a reaction that closes the lumen of the vein.

Plastic Surgery

Plastic surgery is the alteration, replacement, or restoration of visible portions of the body, performed to correct a structural or cosmetic defect. The word *plastic* comes from the Greek word *plastikos*, which means "able to be molded."

Many skin disorders discussed in this chapter cause changes in appearance. For example, acne may leave deep pitting scars, nevi and keloids are often disfiguring, and skin cancers may require wide excision and skin grafting. These scars, lesions, and wounds often cause embarrassment and alterations in body image. In addition, the removal of lesions may leave unsightly scars or areas of obviously missing tissue.

Cosmetic surgery involves procedures to enhance the attractiveness of normal features. There were almost 12 million surgical and nonsurgical cosmetic procedures performed in 2007 (American Society for Aesthetic Plastic Surgery, 2009). The most frequently performed procedures were Botox injections, liposuction, breast augmentation, and laser hair removal. Reconstructive surgery uses similar techniques; however, its purpose is to improve the function or appearance of parts of the body damaged by trauma, disease, or birth defects.

Many of the plastic surgeries permanently alter body image. To provide the patient with a preview of what surgery will accomplish, some surgeons integrate computer imaging into preoperative teaching. The computer projects a photograph of the targeted area onto a monitor and uses graphics to demonstrate how the size and or shape of the body part or area will change as a result of the surgery.

Skin Grafts and Flaps

Skin grafts and flaps are used to restore function while also maintaining an acceptable appearance. Both of these procedures involve the movement of skin from one part of the body to another part.

A **skin graft** is a surgical method of detaching skin from a donor site and placing it in a recipient site, where it develops a new blood supply from the base of the wound. Skin grafting is an effective way to cover wounds that have a good blood supply, that are not infected, and in which bleeding can be controlled.

Skin grafts may be either split thickness or full thickness. A split-thickness graft contains epidermis and only a portion of dermis of the donor site. A common donor site for a skin graft is the anterior thigh. Skin is removed in sheets from the donor site with a dermatome. A full-thickness graft contains both epidermis and dermis. These layers contain the greatest number of skin elements (sweat glands, sebaceous glands, or hair follicles) and are best able to withstand trauma. Areas of thin skin are the best donor sites for full-thickness skin grafts. The donor site must be surgically closed and will scar.

A skin flap is a piece of tissue whose free end is moved from a donor site to a recipient site while maintaining a continuous blood supply through its connection at the base or pedicle. Flaps carry their own blood supply and are therefore used to cover recipient sites that have a poor blood supply or have sustained a major tissue loss. They are often used for reconstruction or closure of large wounds. Microsurgical techniques, with anastomosis of small blood vessels and nerves, allow reconstruction with free flaps (in which the flap is completely removed from its donor site and moved to the recipient site).

Chemical Peeling

Chemical peeling is the application of a chemical to produce a controlled and predictable injury that alters the anatomy of the epidermis and superficial dermis. The result is skin that appears firmer, smoother, and less wrinkled. This form of cosmetic surgery is more useful in people who have fair, thin skin with fine wrinkling.Chemical agents used for peeling include phenol, trichloroacetic acid (TCA), and alpha-hydroxy acids (AHA).

Liposuction

Liposuction is a method of changing the contours of the body by aspirating fat from the subcutaneous layer of tissue. This treatment is used to remove excess fat from the buttocks, flanks, abdomen, thighs, upper arms, knees, ankles, and chin. It is not a cure for obesity and should not be used as a substitute for weight loss. The procedure is usually done for younger patients because their skin is more elastic. Liposuction may be performed on either an outpatient or inpatient basis.

To aspirate the fat, a small incision is made close to the area, and a suction cannula or curette is inserted and attached to a suction apparatus. The high vacuum pressure caused by the suction machine causes fat cells to emulsify, and they are aspirated out of the body. Following removal of the fat, a pressure dressing is applied to help the skin conform to the new tissue size.

Dermabrasion

Dermabrasion is a method of removing facial scars, severe acne, and pigment from unwanted tattoos. The area is sprayed with a chemical to cause light freezing and is then abraded with sandpaper or a revolving wire brush to remove the epidermis and a portion of the dermis.

Facial Cosmetic Surgery

Many different reconstructive surgeries may be performed to correct deformities or improve cosmetic appearance. Those discussed here are rhinoplasty, blepharoplasty, and rhytidectomy (face-lift).

■ A rhinoplasty is conducted to improve the appearance of the external nose. The nasal skeleton is reshaped, and the overlying skin and subcutaneous tissue are allowed to redrape over the new framework. A submucous resection of the nasal septum is often done at the same time; this surgery resects a segment of the septal cartilage to improve the nasal airway and also to alter the appearance of the nose. This surgery is done through incisions within the nose, so no visible scars remain after healing.

■ A blepharoplasty is a cosmetic surgery in which loose skin and protruding periorbital fat is removed from the upper and lower eyelids. With aging, the eyelid skin sags, allowing the periorbital fat to bulge; the skin of the upper eyelid can be so lax that it partially obstructs vision. The procedure is performed under local anesthesia, and excess skin and fat are excised. The incision is made in the normal eyelid lines so that scars are not visible after healing.

■ A rhytidectomy, or face-lift, is a cosmetic surgery done to improve appearance by removing excess skin (and sometimes fat) from the face and neck. As one ages, the skin of the face and neck tends to become loose and wrinkled. The procedure is usually performed with local anesthesia. To perform the surgery, bilateral incisions are made from the scalp at the temple, in front of the ear in the natural skin line, around the ear lobe, and to the occipital scalp. The skin is then elevated, fat is removed or suctioned, and excess skin is excised. The incision lines are sutured, and a pressure dressing is applied.

✺ Nursing Care

Nursing care for the patient having cutaneous or plastic surgery is highly individualized. It depends on the type of surgery or procedure performed, the type of deficit treated, the reason for the surgery or procedure, the expected results of the treatment, and the response of the patient to the lesion or surgery. Although some surgeries, such as skin grafts and flaps, require in-hospital care, many of the surgeries are carried out in the primary care setting, and the patient provides self-care at home following or between treatments.

Nursing Diagnoses and Interventions

A variety of nursing diagnoses may be appropriate for the patient having cutaneous or plastic surgery or procedures; the most common are Impaired Skin Integrity, Acute Pain, and Disturbed Body Image.

Impaired Skin Integrity

The patient having surgery of the skin has impaired skin integrity. Skin grafts and flaps are performed to repair large wounds, and it is necessary to inflict further wounds to collect the graft or flap from a donor site. Excisions and various cosmetic surgeries cause wounds. Skin is traumatized by freezing, chemicals, abrasion, sclerosing agents, electrical currents, and lasers. Although all of these treatment modalities are conducted to remove lesions, improve function, or improve appearance, they first impair the integrity of the skin. These impairments increase the risk for infection, which would further impair the skin integrity and may negate the benefits of surgery.

Nurses provide preoperative care and teaching, intraoperative assistance, and postoperative care and teaching; in each case, care and teaching are specific to the type of surgical treatment and the individual patient. In all cases, the nurse provides appropriate preoperative interventions to prepare the patient physically and emotionally for surgery and the postoperative period. The following interventions are appropriate for the patient having inpatient skin grafts or flaps.

■ Monitor incisions and graft, and flap donor and recipient sites, for manifestations of infection and necrosis:
  ■ Take and record vital signs every 4 hours.
  ■ Monitor all wounds for changes in color, consistency, amount, and odor of drainage every 4 to 8 hours.
  ■ Monitor wounds for increased swelling, redness, and pain every 4 to 8 hours.
  ■ Monitor and document assessment of graft every 4 hours.
  ■ Monitor and document temperature, turgor, color, dermal bleeding, and capillary refill of flaps every 4 hours.
  When bacterial infection is present, the inflammatory phase of wound healing is prolonged, retarding healing. Increased body temperature and tachycardia are manifestations of infection. The drainage in wounds that become infected is often increased in amount, purulent, thicker, and has a musty or foul odor. Tissue response to infection includes edema, increased erythema, and pain. Grafts and flaps that do not have adequate blood supply will appear black instead of the normal pink-red color.

■ Provide care for the donor site:
  ■ Position the patient to minimize pressure on the donor site.
  ■ Use a bed cradle to keep linens off the area.
  ■ If the donor site is left open and a heat lamp is to be applied to the area, place the lamp no closer than 2 feet from the wound.
  ■ Avoid moving the body part containing the donor site, if possible.
  ■ If the donor site is on the posterior portion of the body, place the patient on a special bed (such as a low-pressure or fluidized bed) to decrease pressure and allow air circulation around the donor site.
  Minimizing trauma from pressure and movement facilitates healing of the donor site. Leaving the site open to the air and providing heat increase healing. Special beds minimize ischemia and allow donor sites on the posterior side of the body to dry.

■ Encourage a diet high in protein, ascorbic acid, vitamins, and minerals. *An adequate protein intake is necessary to supply amino acids for tissue repair. Vitamin C is necessary for collagen formation and wound strength. Vitamins and minerals contribute to the healing process.*

■ Change dressings as prescribed, or if the frequency is not indicated, as necessary. Determine which dressings are not to be removed during the healing process and which are to be changed, and whether the wound is to be kept dry or moist.

  Use aseptic technique and follow standard precautions when changing dressings. Remove old dressings carefully and gently.

  Donor sites may be covered with an adherent gauze dressing that is allowed to dry and remains adherent through the healing process. Aseptic techniques prevent secondary bacterial infections. Standard precautions protect the nurse from HIV infection. Unless care is taken, the removal of adherent old dressings may damage the wound by traumatizing granulation tissue or wound edges. The use of semipermeable transparent dressings provides an environment that optimizes wound healing by promoting collagen synthesis and the formation of granulation tissue; it also increases cell migration and epithelial resurfacing and prevents the formation of scabs, crusts, and eschar.

Acute Pain

The patient having a graft or flap has two wounds; in fact, the donor site may be more painful than the recipient site. Cutaneous surgeries, dermabrasions, and chemical treatments result in blistering, swelling, and loss of epidermal tissue. The patient having facial reconstructive surgery has edema, with resultant pain.

- Administer pain medications on a regular basis, following guidelines for controlling pain in patients having operative procedures (∞ see Chapter 9). *Established, severe pain is difficult to control and has negative physical and psychological consequences.*
- Use alternative pain relief measures as appropriate and prescribed, such as ice bags or cold compresses. *Cold reduces swelling, acts as a local anesthetic, and decreases pain.*
- Teach noninvasive methods of pain relief, such as deep breathing, relaxation, and guided imagery. *Noninvasive methods of pain relief increase the effectiveness of pain medications and also allow the patient some control and self-management of pain.*

Disturbed Body Image

Cosmetic surgery is performed for a variety of reasons in adult patients of all ages. Changes in appearance, especially in a society that values youth and beauty, affect one's self-perception. Lesions or scars, especially of the face, may decrease self-esteem and cause a person to avoid social interactions and relationships. With aging, the skin becomes looser and wrinkles appear; this can be a source of anxiety and despair, especially to the woman who has always prided herself on her youthful appearance. Most patients cite one reason for having plastic surgery: to "feel better about myself."

- Provide preoperative teaching: Explain that bruising and swelling will be present and that it will be several weeks before these responses to surgery disappear. Explain that it may take a year for healing to complete and the final results to appear. *Expectations differ; many people expect immediate results. Knowledge of postoperative responses is necessary for the patient to adapt to change. The patient may need to make arrangements to take time off from work during the initial healing stage.*
- Provide time for the patient to verbalize feelings and concerns. Be empathetic, and listen nonjudgmentally. *Such nurse–patient interaction facilitates acceptance of changes in body image.*
- Refer to a consultant who can provide information on the use of cosmetics and apparel to enhance personal appearance. *Knowledgeable use of cosmetics and clothing can make scars much less noticeable. If the patient feels better about appearance, body image is improved.*

Community-Based Care

The nurse teaches the patient and family to provide self-care at home after cutaneous and plastic surgery and procedures. The nurse asks about the patient's expectations and stresses that final results will not be seen for several months, providing written instructions about wound care and manifestations of infection.

Hair and Nail Disorders

Disorders of the hair and nails are not serious threats to health, but they may cause embarrassment and a negative body image. Changes in hair growth and pattern as in nail growth and character occur as secondary responses to other illnesses or treatments and are also a part of the aging process.

The Patient with a Disorder of the Hair

Racial characteristics and gender influence the amount and type of hair one has. Caucasians typically have more facial and body hair than do Asians. People of Mongolian or Native American descent usually have straight hair, those of African descent have wavy to curly hair, and whites have straight to curly hair. In addition, male hair growth characteristics (such as facial hair and hair on the lower extremities) are normal in certain women of some races and families.

Pathophysiology

Hair color, growth, and pattern vary from person to person, and they are determined largely by genetic inheritance Changes such as hair loss in men or excess facial hair in women may seem minor, but they may create psychosocial problems for the person experiencing the changes.

Hirsutism

Hirsutism (hypertrichosis), is the appearance of excessive hair in women. Hirsutism most often occurs in a male distribution (that is, on the upper lip, chin, abdomen, and chest) in women. The excess hair is primarily the result of an increase in androgen levels (especially testosterone) that may be due to familial predisposition (considered normal); polycystic ovary syndrome; ovarian, adrenal, or pituitary tumors; Cushing's syndrome (an adrenal disorder); some central system disorders; and medications, such as minoxidil, cyclosporine, phenytoin, certain progestins, and anabolic steroids.

The manifestations of hirsutism include increased male pattern hair growth, acne, and menstrual irregularities. If the androgen excess is great, defeminization (a decrease in breast size and loss of normal adipose tissue) and virilization (frontal balding, increased muscle mass, deepening of the voice, and enlargement of the clitoris) may occur.

Alopecia

Alopecia is loss of hair, or baldness. Alopecia may result from scarring, various systemic diseases, or genetic predisposition. Scarring from trauma, radiation, and severe bacterial, fungal, or viral infections causes permanent and irreversible hair loss over the scarred area. Systemic diseases that may cause alopecia include systemic lupus erythematosus, thyroid disorders, and pituitary insufficiency. The hair loss from these disorders may be reversible. Hair loss from androgenic causes may also occur in the postmenopausal woman. Alopecia may be drug induced and is a side effect of a variety of medications (Box 16–11).

Examples of types of alopecia follow:

- Male pattern baldness is the most common cause of alopecia in men and is genetically predetermined. The hair loss begins at the temples, with recession of the hairline and baldness of the crown.
- Female pattern alopecia begins in women in their 20s and 30s, with progressive thinning and loss of hair over the central part of the scalp. Unlike men, women do not lose hair from the frontal hairline. Many of these women have elevated adrenal androgens.
- Alopecia areata is characterized by round or oval bald patches on the scalp as well as on other hairy parts of the body. The cause is unknown. This type of alopecia is usually self-limiting and reverses without treatment, although it often recurs.

Interdisciplinary Care

The patient with hirsutism is examined for hormone levels and indications of other systemic illnesses. Hirsutism is treated by addressing the underlying systemic disorder and stopping medications that may be causing the problem. Alopecia is diagnosed by assessing the appearance of the hair and hair loss and by assessing the patient for other systemic diseases and the use of medications that may cause hair loss. Various treatments are used to restore hair.

Diagnosis

Diagnostic tests that may be ordered for the woman with hirsutism include serum testosterone levels and an adrenal CT scan. Testosterone levels are measured and levels greater than 200 ng/dL indicate the need for further tests, such as a pelvic examination and tests of ovarian function. Adrenal tumors, a possible cause of hirsutism, are identified with an adrenal CT scan.

Medications

Hirsutism is treated with medications specific to the underlying cause. Oral contraceptives containing estrogen decrease ovarian androgen production and decrease free testosterone levels. Dexamethasone (Decadron) may be prescribed for people with high cortisol levels. Ketoconazole (Nizoral) inhibits androgen production. Antiandrogenic medications cause congenital abnormalities in male infants and are therefore given only to nonpregnant women, who are cautioned to avoid pregnancy while taking the medications.

BOX 16–11   Medications Causing Alopecia

■ Thallium	■ Allopurinol
■ Retinoids	■ Propranolol
■ Anticoagulants	■ Indomethacin
■ Antimitotic agents	■ Amphetamines
■ Antithyroid drugs	■ Salicylates
■ Oral contraceptives	■ Levopdopa
■ Trimethadone	■ Gentamicin
■ Excessive use of vitamin A	■ Chemotherapy

Male pattern baldness has been successfully treated with topical minoxidil (Loniten) or Rogaine Extra Strength, a commercial product that contains minoxidil. These drugs, which are vasodilators, stimulate vertex hair growth, probably by stimulating the epithelium of the hair follicle. About 40% of patients treated two times a day for a year will have moderate to dense regrowth of hair at the temples (McPhee, Papadakis & Tierney, 2008).

Surgery

Hair transplant techniques are used to restore hair or reduce the size of areas of alopecia. Transplanting hairs as small hair plugs or single hairs taken from the back or sides of the scalp is an effective means of replacing hair to areas of alopecia. This procedure is done in an outpatient office or clinic. Other types of surgical procedures include scalp reduction and flaps.

℘ Nursing Care

The patient with either hirsutism or alopecia is often self-conscious about appearance and tries a variety of OTC treatments before seeking medical care. Nursing care for the patient with hair disorders focuses on teaching the patient self-care and providing support during long-term care. Women with hirsutism are taught to use various means of removing unwanted hair, such as shaving, applying depilatories, waxing, or undergoing electrolysis. Women with mild hirsutism may bleach facial hair to make it less obvious. Patients with alopecia may wear hair pieces or wigs.

The Patient with a Disorder of the Nails

Nail disorders may be congenital or genetic, or they may be due to systemic diseases, trauma, allergies, or irritants. Nails may be discolored, multicolored, malformed, infected, or separated from underlying tissue.

Pathophysiology

The nail disorders discussed here are separation of the nail, infection, and ingrown toenails.

- Onycholysis is the separation of the distal nail plate from the nail bed. It occurs most often in the fingernails. This disorder may result from many different factors, including excessive or prolonged exposure to water, soaps, detergent, alkalies, and industrial keratolytic agents; Candida infections; nail hardeners; and thyroid disorders. Prolonged application of false fingernails may also cause this disorder.
- A **paronychia** is an infection of the cuticle of the fingernails or toenails. The disorder often follows a minor trauma and secondary infection with staphylococci, streptococci, or Candida. The acute form begins with a painful inflammation that may progress to an abscess. The chronic form is seen most often in people who have frequent exposure to water. In the chronic form, the skin around the nail is painful, edematous, and infected. The nail plate may become ridged and discolored.
- An onychomycosis is a fungal or dermatophyte infection of the nail plate. The nail plate elevates and becomes yellow or white. Psoriasis infections of the nail plate cause the nails to pit.

- An ingrown toenail (unguis incarnatus) results when the edge of the nail plate grows into the soft tissue of the toe. Pain and infection may occur. The infection, if untreated, may spread to the bone. This disorder is especially dangerous for the person with diabetes mellitus or peripheral vascular disease.

Interdisciplinary Care

The treatment of disorders of the nail vary from pharmacologic treatment to surgical removal. Infections of the nails are treated with antifungal or antibiotic medications. If the causative agent is a fungus or chronic dermatologic disorder, treatment is difficult and may not be effective. Persistently painful and/or infected nails are in some cases surgically removed.

✑ Nursing Care

Nursing care of the patient with a disorder of the nail focuses on teaching self-care. Patients with nail disorders that are caused by frequent exposure to water are taught to protect the hands or feet by wearing rubber gloves or boots and to keep the nails as clean and dry as possible. Patients with ingrown toenails are cautioned not to cut into the lateral nail bed, but rather to soak the nail twice a day and insert a piece of cotton or gauze under the softened nail until the nail has grown out enough to trim.

CHAPTER HIGHLIGHTS

- Pruritus (itching) accompanies dry skin (xerosis) and many skin disorders and may result in excoriation and infection as a result of scratching.
- Cysts, keloids, nevi, angiomas, skin tags, and keratoses are benign skin lesions. However, nevi should be monitored for changes indicating transformation into a malignant lesion.
- Psoriasis is a chronic immune skin disorder arising from keratinocytes. A variety of medications and treatments are used, with ultraviolet light therapy being most effective for generalized lesions.
- Skin disorders may be caused by a variety of bacteria, fungi, parasites, and viruses. The disorders are treated with organism-specific antibiotics, fungicides, anti-viral agents, or agents that kill the parasites. Herpes zoster, believed to follow a childhood infection with chickenpox, causes acute pain.
- Inflammatory disorders of the skin range from mild dermatitis to potentially lethal toxic epidermal necrolysis. Acne, a disorder of the hair and sebaceous glands opening to the skin surface, is characterized by comedones, pustules, and cysts.

- Malignant skin disorders include actinic keratosis, nonmelanoma skin cancer (basal cell cancer and squamous cell cancer), and malignant melanoma skin cancer. Skin cancer is the most common malignancy found in fair-skinned Americans. Prevention by avoiding sunburn, using sunscreen, and maintaining monthly skin self-examination is critical in preventing loss of tissue or metastasis and death.
- Skin trauma may be intentional (as in the case of cutaneous and plastic surgery) or unintentional (as from trauma, frostbite, and pressure). Older adults with limited mobility, as well as patients who are unable to move or who are in critical care units, are at greater risk for pressure ulcers. Prevention of pressure ulcers is the goal of both interdisciplinary and nursing care.
- Disorders of the hair include alopecia (loss of hair) and hirsutism (excess hair in women). Nails may be discolored, multicolored, malformed, infected, or separated from underlying tissue.

TEST YOURSELF NCLEX-RN® REVIEW

1. An elderly patient has severe xerosis. What topic should the nurse include in a teaching plan for this patient?
   1. Take a hot bath every day.
   2. Use fabric softeners when laundering clothing.
   3. Apply skin lotions after a bath.
   4. Maintain a warm environment.
2. A nurse assesses the following common skin lesions. Which lesion has the potential of becoming malignant?
   1. nevi
   2. angiomas
   3. skin tags
   4. keloids
3. A nurse has been asked to teach a woman with generalized psoriasis about ultraviolet light therapy (UVB). What should be included in the teaching?
   1. "The exact effect of UVB is unknown, but it decreases severe itching."
   2. "When combined with hot baths, UVB is very effective."
   3. "Treatments with UVB have to be given in the hospital to be safe."
   4. "UVB slows the growth of epidermal cells and decreases keratosis."

4. Which of the following skin lesions, if assessed, is a risk for skin cancer?
   1. lice infestation
   2. actinic keratosis
   3. pressure ulcer
   4. folliculitis
5. What question should the nurse include in a health history of a patient with a linear pattern of painful vesicles over the left thorax?
   1. "Do you remember being sunburned as a child?"
   2. "Are you a regular patron of tanning booths?"
   3. "Have you ever been diagnosed with acne?"
   4. "Did you have chickenpox when you were young?"
6. Which of the following statements would be appropriate for a nurse to make to a patient about a lice infestation?
   1. "Only dirty people have lice."
   2. "Anyone can have lice."
   3. "Lice do not like to live on humans."
   4. "Lice are a form of fungus."

7. Which assessments by the nurse would indicate a greater risk to develop a nonmelanoma skin cancer?
1. blond hair, freckles, fair skin
2. alopecia, thin hair, itching
3. dark hair, dark skin, dry skin
4. tanned skin, dark hair, edema

8. Of the following, which assessment is most significant to the development of a melanoma?
1. a change in the color or size of a nevus
2. sexual contact with a person who has a herpes virus infection
3. inadequate knowledge about infection prevention
4. a dietary intake of high-calorie foods

9. What is the rationale for a nurse lifting, rather than pulling, a patient up in bed?
1. Lifting a patient allows a brief period of increased capillary circulation.
2. Lifting a patient prevents tissue injury from shearing forces.
3. Pulling a patient up in bed decreases tissue ischemia and hypoxia.
4. Pulling a patient up in bed promotes capillary blood flow.

10. A nurse is caring for a young adult with acne scars. The patient asks about treatment to reduce the scarring. Which of the following might the nurse discuss?
1. liposuction
2. skin flap
3. dermabrasion
4. blepharoplasty

See Test Yourself answers in Appendix C.

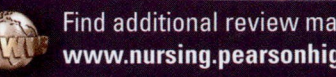

Pearson Nursing Student Resources
Find additional review materials at
www.nursing.pearsonhighered.com
Prepare for success with additional NCLEX®-style practice questions, interactive assignments and activities, Web links, animations and videos, and more!

BIBLIOGRAPHY

Agency for Health Care Policy and Research. (1992). *Pressure ulcers in adults: Prediction and prevention.* Rockville, MD: USDHHS.

Agency for Health Care Policy and Research. (1994). *Treatment of pressure ulcers.* Rockville, MD: USDHHS.

Allergies: Latex allergy. (2009). *WebMD.* Available at http://www.webmd.com/allergies/guide/latex-allergies

American Cancer Society. (2006). UV radiation & cancer. Retrieved from http://www.cancer.org

American Cancer Society. (2007). Skin cancer. Retrieved from http://www.cancer.org

American Cancer Society. (2008a). Melanoma skin cancer. Retrieved from http://www.cancer.org

American Cancer Society. (2008b). What are the key statistics about melanoma? Retrieved from http://www.cancer.org

American Cancer Society. (2008c). Skin cancer: Basal and squamous cell. Retrieved from http://www.cancer.org

American Society for Aesthetic Plastic Surgery. (2009). Cosmetic procedures in 2007. Retrieved from http://www.surgery.org/public/consumer/trends/cosmetic_procedures_in_2007

Ayello, E. A. (2007). Try this: Best practices in nursing care to older adults. Predicting pressure ulcer risk. *The Hartford Institute for Geriatric Nursing*, Issue 5, College of Nursing, New York University. Retrieved from http://www.hartfordign.org

Barklay, L. (2008). Management of atypical moles reviewed. *Medscape.* Retrieved from http://www.medscape.com/viewarticle/580864

Barclay, L. (2009). Use of topical corticosteroids for dermatologic conditions reviewed. *American Family Physician, 79*, 135–140.

Baron, E., Kirkland, E., & Domingo, D. (2008). Advances in photoprotection. *Dermatology Nursing, 20*(4), 265–273.

Barthel, D., & Crutchfield, C. (2004). Herpes zoster. *Dermatology Nursing, 16*(4), 362.

Black, J., Baharestani, M., Cuddigan, J., Dorner, B., Edsberg, L., Langemo, D., Posthauer, M., Ratliff, C., & Taler, G. (2007). National Pressure Ulcer Advisory Panel's updated pressure ulcer staging system. *Dermatology Nursing, 19*(4), 343–349.

Bolton, L. (2007). Evidence corner: Pressure ulcer risk scales. *Wounds, 19*(6), A15–A23.

Braden, B., & Bergstrom, N. (1988). *Braden scale for predicting pressure sore risk®.* Retrieved from http://www.bradenscale.com

Brown, J., Wimpenny, P., & Maughan, H. (2004). Skin problems in people with obesity. *Nursing Standard, 18*(35), 38–42.

Bulechek, G., Butcher, H., & Dochterman, J. (Eds.) (2008). *Nursing interventions classification (NIC)* (5th ed.). St. Louis: Mosby Elsevier.

Centers for Disease Control and Prevention. (2008a). *Community-associated methicillin resistant Staphylococcus aureus (CA-MRSA).* Retrieved from http://www.cdd.gov/ncidod/dhqp/ar_mrsa_ca.html

Centers for Disease Control and Prevention. (2008b). *Healthcare-associated methicillin resistant Staphylococcus aureus (HA-MRSA).* Retrieved from http://www.cdd.gov/ncidod/dhqp/ar_MRSA.html

Daus, L. (2008). Give them a hand: Patients with hand and foot psoriasis require special attention. *Dermatology Nursing, 20*(4), 291–193.

Gorgos, D. (2004). Top 3 causes of hair disorders identified. *Dermatology Nursing, 16*(4), 367–368.

Gould, D., Gldstone, L., Kelly, D., & Gammon, J. (2004). Examining the validity of pressure ulcer risk scales: A replication study. *International Journal of Nursing Studies, 41*(3), 3331–3339.

Hanson, D., Thompson, P., Langemo, D., Hunter, S., Tinkler, J., & Anderson, J. (2008). What you should know about psoriasis. *Nursing, 20*(6), 58–59.

Hess, C. (2009). Take steps to prevent pressure ulcers. *Nursing, 39*(1), 61.

Khachemoune, A., & Ehrsam, E. (2005). Assessing malignant melanoma: A case study. *Dermatology Nursing, 17*(3), 188–190.

Kucera, K. (2004). Managing common skin problems in the elderly. *Clincial Advisor, 7*(6), 23–24, 27–30.

McPhee, S., Papadakis, M., & Tierney, L. (Eds.). (2008). *Current medical diagnosis & treatment* (47th ed.). Stamford, CT: McGraw Hill Lange.

Moorhead, S., Johnson, M., Maas, M., & Swanson, E. (Eds.) (2008). *Nursing outcomes classification (NOC)* (4th ed.). St. Louis: Mosby Elsevier.

National Pressure Ulcer Advisory Panel. (2007). Pressure ulcer stages updated by NPUAP. Retrieved from http://www.npuap.org/pr2.htm

Nanda International. (2009). *Nursing diagnoses: Definitions & classification 2009–2011.* Oxford, UK: Wiley-Blackwell.

Porth, C. (2007). *Essentials of pathophysiology: Concepts of altered health states* (2nd ed.). Philadelphia: Lippincott Williams & Wilkins.

Porth, C., & Marfin, G. (2009). *Pathophysiology: Concepts of altered health states.* (8th ed.). Philadelphia: Lippincott Williams & Wilkins.

PsoriasisNet. (2008). *What is psoriasis?* Retrieved from http://www.skincarephysicians.com/psoriasisnet/whatis.html

Skin biopsy. (2008). *Harvard Health Publications,* Harvard Medical School. Retrieved from http://www.health.harvard.edu/diagnostic-tests/skin-biopsy.htm

Skin Cancer Foundation. (2008a). *Skin cancer facts.* Retrieved from http://www.skincancer.org/Skin-Cancer-Facts/

Skin Cancer Foundation. (2008b). *Melanoma.* Retrieved from http://www.skincancer.org/Melanoma/

Smith, M. (2008). Healthier aging. Taking a closer look for skin cancer. *Nursing, 37*(10), 58–60.

Smith, M., Nedorost, S., & Tackett, B. (2007). Facing up to withdrawal from topical steroids. *Nursing, 37*(9), 60–61.

Snow, M. (2008). Necrotizing fasciitis: Threatening life and limb. *Nursing, 38*(11), 23.

Stotts, N., & Gunningberg, L. (2007). Predicting pressure ulcer risk. *American Journal of Nursing, 107*(11), 40–48.

Tosanger, M., & Crutchfield, C. (2004a). Tinea corporis. *Dermatology Nursing, 16*(5), 453.

Tonanger, M., & Crutchfield, C. (2004b). Atrophic lichen planus. *Dermatology Nursing, 16*(1), 73–74.

Van Rijswijk, L., & Lyder, C. (2008). Pressure ulcers: Were they there on admission? *American Journal of Nursing, 108*(11), 27–28.

Wilson, B., Shannon, M., & Shields, K. (2010). *Prentice Hall's nurse's drug guide.* Upper Saddle River, NJ: Pearson Prentice Hall.

Wurster, J. (2007). What role can nurse leaders play in reducing the incidence of pressure sores? *Nursing Economics, 25*(5), 267–269.

Yamarmoto, L., & Marten, M. (2007). Listen up, MRSA. The bug stops here. *Nursing, 37*(12), 50–55.

Yarbo, C., Frogge, M., Goodman, M., & Groenwald, S. (Eds.) (2005). *Cancer nursing: Principles and practice.* (6th ed.). Sudbury, MA: Jones & Bartlett.

Zulkowski, K., & Gray-Leach, K. (2009). Staging pressure ulcers: What's the buzz in wound care? *American Journal of Nursing, 109*(1), 27–30.

17 Nursing Care of Patients with Burns

LEARNING OUTCOMES

1. Discuss the types and causative agents of burns.
2. Explain burn classification by depth and extent of injury.
3. Compare and contrast the pathophysiology and interdisciplinary care of a minor burn and a major burn.
4. Discuss the systemic pathophysiologic effects of a major burn and the stages of burn wound healing.
5. Explain the interdisciplinary care and nursing implications necessary during the emergent/resuscitative stage, the acute stage, and the rehabilitative stage of a major burn.

CLINICAL COMPETENCIES

1. Assess functional health status of patients with burns, and monitor, document, and report abnormal manifestations.
2. Use evidence-based research to plan and implement nursing care for patients with burns.
3. Determine priority nursing diagnoses, based on assessed data, to select and implement individualized nursing interventions for patient with burns.
4. Administer medications knowledgeably and safely to patients with burns.
5. Integrate interdisciplinary care into care of patients with burns.
6. Provide teaching appropriate for prevention of burns.
7. Revise plan of care as needed to provide effective interventions to promote, maintain, or restore functional health status to patients with burns.

KEY TERMS

allograft, *463*
autografting, *462*
burn, *446*
burn shock, *454*
compartment syndrome, *455*
contractures, *464*
Curling's ulcers, *455*
debridement, *463*

eschar, *454*
escharotomy, *460*
fascial excision, *460*
fasciectomy, *460*
fluid resuscitation, *458*
full-thickness burn, *449*
heterograft, *463*

homograft, *463*
hypertrophic scar, *452*
keloid, *452*
partial-thickness burn, *448*
superficial burn, *448*
surgical debridement, *460*
xenograft, *463*

A **burn** is an injury resulting from exposure to heat, chemicals, radiation, or electric current. A transfer of energy from a source of heat to the human body initiates a sequence of physiologic events that in the most severe cases leads to irreversible tissue destruction. Burns range in severity from a minor loss of small segments of the outermost layer of the skin to a complex injury involving all body systems. Treatments vary from simple application of a topical antiseptic agent in an outpatient clinic to an invasive, multisystem, interdisciplinary team approach in the aseptic environment of a burn center.

It is estimated that 500,000 million burn injuries that require medical intervention occur each year in the United States, and of those, about 40,000 require hospitalization with approximately 4000 of the burn injuries resulting in death (American Burn Association [ABA], 2007). The home is the most common site for fire-related burns (43%). Home fires cause 92.5% of all fire-related deaths. Most residential fires are caused by unattended cooking, resulting from combustible grease, cabinets, wall coverings, curtains, and paper or plastic bags. Smoking materials, including cigarettes, cigars, and pipes, are the leading cause of home fire deaths. Trash, mattresses, and upholstered furniture are frequently ignited materials in the home.

FAST FACTS
Causes of Home Fires
1. Cooking fires
2. Smoking
3. Heating equipment

Factors associated with deaths from burns are age (especially children under 5 and adults 65 and older), careless smoking, alcohol or drug intoxication, and physical and mental disabilities. A common source of burns in young children and older adults is from tap water scalds, while older children receive most burns from flame injuries. Older adults are more susceptible to deep burns from scalds because of their thinner skin. Fire injuries and deaths, occurring among college-age students, usually are due to alcohol use that impairs judgment and hampers escape (NFPA, 2004). Occupations involving work with chemicals, gasoline, or electricity pose another risk factor. Abuse is suspected when scald burns show a clear line of demarcation, indicating deliberate immersion. The presence of small, circular burns may be from cigarette burns inflicted by an abuser.

Older adults are more vulnerable to fire and burn injury because of decreased visual acuity, depth perception, sense of smell, and hearing, in addition to impaired mobility. All of these factors increase the risk for accidentally starting a fire and diminish the ability to survive it.

> **FAST FACTS**
> **Fire Deaths in Older Adults**
> - More than 1200 deaths in adults 65 and older occur each year.
> - Leading causes of fire-related deaths are smoking, heating, and cooking.
> - One-fifth of the deaths occur in bedridden or physically challenged older adults.

Infants and older adults have a greater risk of mortality. Morbidity increases in patients with pre-existing cardiac, pulmonary, or renal disorders, and diabetes mellitus. Patients who are alcoholics have lower survival rates of a major burn injury due to the development of more complications. Men account for 70% of burn patients versus 30% for women (ABA, 2007).

Types of Burn Injury

The four types of burn injury are thermal, chemical, electrical, and radiation. Although all four types can lead to generalized tissue damage and multisystem involvement, the causative agents and priority treatment measures are unique to each (Table 17–1).

Thermal Burns

Thermal burns result from exposure to dry heat (flames) or moist heat (steam and hot liquids). They are the most common burn injuries and occur most often in children and older adults. Direct exposure to the source of heat causes cellular destruction that can result in charring of vascular, bony, muscle, and nervous tissue.

Chemical Burns

Chemical burns are caused by direct skin contact with acids, alkaline agents, or organic compounds. More than 25,000 products found in the home or workplace can cause chemical burns. The chemical destroys tissue protein, leading to necrosis. Burns caused by alkalis (such as lye) are more difficult to neutralize than are burns caused by acids. They also tend to have deeper penetration with a correspondingly more severe burn than from acid. Organic compound burns, such as by petroleum distillates, cause cutaneous damage through fat solvent action and may also cause renal and liver failure if absorbed.

Chemical agents are further classified according to the manner by which they structurally alter proteins. Oxidizing agents, such as household bleach, alter protein configuration through the chemical process of reduction. Corrosives, such as lye, cause extensive protein denaturation. Protoplasmic poisons, such as organic compounds, form salts with proteins, inhibiting calcium and other ions needed for cell viability. The severity of the chemical burn is related to the type of agent, the concentration of the agent, the mechanism of action, the duration of contact, and the amount of body surface area exposed. Box 17–1 lists household cleaning agents that may cause burns.

Electrical Burns

The severity of electrical burns depends on the type and duration of current, and amount of voltage. It is particularly difficult to assess the extent of the electrical burn injury, because the destructive processes initiated by the electrical insult are concealed and may persist for weeks beyond the time of the incident. It is challenging to assess the depth and extent of the burn, as electricity follows the path of least resistance, which in the human body tends to lie along muscles, bone, blood vessels, and nerves. Entry and exit wounds tend to be small, masking widespread tissue damage underneath the wound. Tissue necrosis results from impaired blood flow, secondary to blood coagulation at the site of the electrical injury. Because electrical burn wounds of the extremities often cause severe tissue necrosis, they frequently develop gangrene that necessitates amputation (Bishop, 2004).

Alternating current (AC), as is found in conventional households, produces repeated electrical surges that lead to tetanic muscle contractions. Such sustained muscle contractions inhibit respiratory efforts for the duration of contact and result in respiratory arrest. The contractions also cause the person to clamp down on the power source (such as an electrical cord)

TABLE 17–1 Types, Causative Agents, and Priority Treatment Measures for Burns

TYPE	CAUSATIVE AGENT	PRIORITY TREATMENT
Thermal	Open flame	Extinguish flame (stop, drop, and roll).
	Steam	
	Hot liquids (water, grease, tar, metal)	Flush with cool water.
		Consult fire department.
Chemical	Acids	Neutralize or dilute chemical.
	Strong alkalis	Remove clothing.
	Organic compounds	Consult poison control center.
Electrical	Direct current	Disconnect source of current.
	Alternating current	Initiate CPR if necessary.
	Lightning	Move to area of safety.
		Consult electrical experts.
Radiation	Solar (ultraviolet)	Shield the skin appropriately.
	X-rays	Limit time of exposure.
	Radioactive agents	Move the patient away from the radiation source.
		Consult a radiation expert.

BOX 17–1 Household Cleaning Agents That May Cause Burns

- Drain cleaners
- Lye
- Industrial-strength ammonia
- Household ammonia
- Oven cleaners
- Toilet bowl cleaners
- Dishwasher detergents
- Bleach

Figure

CASE STUDY & NURSING CARE PLAN   A Patient with a Major Burn

Craig Howard, a 39-year-old truck driver, is admitted to the hospital following an accident in which the cab of his truck caught on fire. He was freed from the truck by a passing motorist, who stayed with him until the rescue team arrived and transported him to a local emergency department (ED). Mr. Howard's wife, Mary, and twin daughters, Jessica and Jane, aged 10, have been notified.

ASSESSMENT

On his admission to the ED, Mr. Howard is diagnosed with deep partial-thickness and full-thickness burns of the anterior chest, arms, and hands. A quick assessment based on the rule of nines estimates the extent of his burn injury at 36% of TBSA. His vital signs are as follows: T 96.2°F (35.6°C), P 140, R 40, and BP 98/60. In the field, the paramedics had inserted a large-bore central line into Mr. Howard's right subclavian vein and started the rapid infusion of lactated Ringer's solution. Mr. Howard is receiving 40% humidified oxygen via face mask. Initial ABGs are pH 7.49, PO_2 60 mmHg, PCO_2 32 mmHg, and bicarbonate 22 mEq/L. Lung sounds indicate inspiratory and expiratory wheezing, and a persistent cough reveals sooty sputum production. A Foley catheter is inserted and initially drains a moderate amount of dark, concentrated urine. A nasogastric tube is connected to low-intermittent suction. Mr. Howard is alert and oriented and complains of severe pain associated with the burn injuries. The burn unit is notified, and Mr. Howard is transferred there.

DIAGNOSIS

- *Risk for Ineffective Airway Clearance*, related to increasing lung congestion secondary to smoke inhalation
- *Deficient Fluid Volume*, related to abnormal fluid loss secondary to burn injury
- *Risk for Ineffective Tissue Perfusion (Peripheral)*, related to peripheral constriction secondary to circumferential burn wounds of the arms

EXPECTED OUTCOMES

- Demonstrate a patent airway, as evidenced by clear breath sounds; absence of cyanosis; and vital signs, chest x-ray findings, and ABGs within normal limits.
- Demonstrate adequate fluid volume and electrolyte balance, as evidenced by urine output, vital signs, mental status, and laboratory findings within normal limits.
- Demonstrate adequate tissue perfusion, as evidenced by palpable pulses, warm extremities, normal capillary refill, and absence of paresthesia.

PLANNING AND IMPLEMENTATION

- Prepare for prophylactic nasotracheal intubation to maintain airway patency.
- Initiate fluid resuscitation therapy using the Parkland formula to calculate intravenous fluid rate for the first 24 hours postburn.
- Assist the physician to perform escharotomies of both upper extremities.

EVALUATION

The nurse anesthetist inserted a nasotracheal tube and connected Mr. Howard to a T-piece delivering 40% oxygen. Vigorous respiratory toileting has significantly improved his ABGs. Bronchodilators have been parenterally administered and mucolytic agents added to his respiratory treatments. His tracheal secretions have begun to show evidence of clearing. Hourly urine outputs indicate adequate fluid resuscitation. Urine output has been maintained at 50 mL/h, and color and concentration have improved. CVP readings have been maintained at 6 cm H_2O, and blood pressure has increased to 100/64. The pulse rate has decreased to 100.

To improve tissue perfusion of both arms, the physician has performed bilateral escharotomies and the wounds are dressed, using sterile procedure. The extremities have demonstrated improved circulation.

CRITICAL THINKING IN THE NURSING PROCESS

1. Explain the rationale for the immediate insertion of a Foley catheter and nasogastric tube.
2. An escharotomy was performed on both arms. Why was this procedure necessary in Mr. Howard's case?
3. What is the rationale supporting the intravenous administration of narcotics to control Mr. Howard's pain?
4. Explain the sequence of events that led to a fluid and electrolyte shift during the first 24 to 48 hours after Mr. Howard sustained his injury.

See Evaluating Your Response in Appendix C.

NANDA, NIC, AND NOC LINKAGES
The Patient with a Major Burn

NANDA	Impaired Skin Integrity
↓	
NIC	Skin Surveillance Wound Care: Burns Infection Protection
↓	
NOC	Tissue Integrity: Skin & Mucous Membranes Wound Healing; Primary Intention

Adapted from Bulechek, G., Butcher, H., & Dochterman, J. M. (Eds.). (2008). *Nursing interventions classification (NIC)* (5th ed.). St. Louis: Mosby Elsevier; Moorhead, S., Johnson, M., Maas, M., & Swanson, E. (Eds.). (2008). *Nursing outcomes classification (NOC)* (4th ed.). St. Louis: Mosby Elsevier; and Nanda International. (2009). *Nursing diagnoses: Definitions and classification 2009–2011*. Oxford, UK: Wiley-Blackwell.

care. From admission to discharge, the nurse teaches the patient and family to assess all findings, implement therapies, and evaluate progress. The following topics should be addressed in preparing the patient and family for home care.

- The long-term goals of rehabilitation care: to prevent soft tissue deformity, protect skin grafts, maintain physiologic function, manage scars, and return the patient to an optimal level of independence
- Avoiding exposure to people with colds or infections and following aseptic technique meticulously when caring for the wound
- The need for progressive physical activity
- How to apply splints, pressure support garments, and other assistive devices
- Dietary requirements with required kcal
- Alternative pain control therapies, such as guided imagery, relaxation techniques, and diversional activities

- Care of the graft and donor sites
- Referral for occupational therapy, social service, clergy, and/or psychiatric services as appropriate

- Helpful resources:
  - American Burn Association
  - International Society for Burn Injuries
  - American Academy of Facial Plastic and Reconstructive Surgery

CHAPTER HIGHLIGHTS

- Four types of burn injuries are thermal, chemical, electrical, or radiation. The depth of the burn injury determines whether it is classified as a superficial, partial-thickness, or full-thickness burn.
- The "rule of nines" is used to estimate the extent of a burn by assigning percentages to different parts of the body.
- Major burns involve multiorgan pathophysiological alterations. Most critical is the fluid shift from the intracellular and intravascular compartments into the interstitium, resulting in a type of hypovolemic shock called burn shock. Other pathologic processes include an impaired immune system, disturbed functions of the skin, inhalation injury, gastrointestinal ulcerations and ileus, renal failure, and hypermetabolism.
- Interdisciplinary care focuses on manging the patient during the emergent/resuscitative, acute, and rehabilitative stages. To counter the effects of burn shock, fluid resuscitation using

guidelines such as the Parkland formula are initiated to replace fluid and electrolyte losses.
- Additional management for the patient with major burns includes preventing atelectasis, maintaining respiratory function, controlling pain, preventing infection and Curling's ulcer, promoting nutrition, and providing wound care.
- Extensive echar of an extremity or the torso, called circumferential wounds, can potentially occlude arterial flow or decrease respiratory function. An excharotomy is used to release tension, preventing additional complications.
- Surgical management of burn wounds include debridement and skin grafting. Biologic and biosynthetic dressings provide temporary covering and prepare the wound for permanent autografts.
- Continual psychological support of the patient and family is essential throughout convalescence and rehabilitation.

TEST YOURSELF NCLEX-RN® REVIEW

1. During the emergent phase of burn management, what diagnostic test result should the nurse expect to find?
   1. increased hematocrit
   2. serum albumin
   3. decreased serum potassium
   4. decreased blood urea nitrogen (BUN)
2. A patient is admitted with severe burns to the face and chest. The injured skin is dry and leathery, with no pain sensations present. The nurse recognizes that this burn is classified as which of the following?
   1. superficial
   2. superficial partial thickness
   3. deep partial thickness
   4. full thickness
3. Which of the following patients is at greatest risk for developing burn shock?
   1. 21-year-old with 90% superficial burn from a tanning bed
   2. 30-year-old with 10% TBSA from a gasoline explosion
   3. 39-year-old with radiation burns following treatment for cancer
   4. 48-year-old with > 50% TBSA from a high-voltage electrical accident
4. A patient with a major burn is receiving silver sulfadiazine (Silvadene) to the burns. What nursing action should be implemented when using this medication?
   1. premedicate for pain prior to application
   2. monitor WBC count daily
   3. observe for signs of dehydration
   4. monitor serum electrolyte levels daily

5. A patient with full-thickness burns over 50% of the body arrives in the ED. The patient weighs 70 kg. Using the Parkland formula, calculate the amount of fluid replacement that the nurse should deliver in the first 8 hours.
   1. 3500 mL
   2. 7000 mL
   3. 10,500 mL
   4. 14,000 mL
6. For a patient with a major burn, which of the following evaluation criteria indicate that fluid resuscitation is effective during the first 24 hours of care?
   1. urine output of 30 to 50 ml per hour
   2. central venous pressure of 18
   3. heart rate of 130 BPM
   4. blood pressure 96/70
7. A patient has deep partial-thickness burns to the entire left arm and left side of the back. What finding should be reported to the physician immediately?
   1. fluid-filled vesicles on the left arm
   2. pain in the left arm
   3. blanching when pressure applied to the left hand
   4. decreased left radial pulse
8. A patient received deep partial thickness burns to the anterior trunk, perineum, and left arm anterior and posterior. Using the "rule of nines," what is the percent of TBSA that was burned?
   1. 18%
   2. 28%
   3. 36%
   4. 40%

9. Which of the following topics should be included in a presentation on burn prevention at a senior citizen center? **Select all that apply.**
   1. Wear close-fitting clothing when cooking.
   2. Use a solar-powered nightlight.
   3. Set the water heater no higher than 120°F.
   4. Check smoke detectors annually.
   5. Install antiscald devices in bathroom plumbing.
   6. Have a neighbor routinely check for the odor of gas.

10. A patient has possible carbon monoxide poisoning secondary to smoke inhalation. What manifestation should the nurse expect to find in a patient with a 15% carbon monoxide level?
    1. dark red skin color
    2. drowsiness
    3. dizziness
    4. hypotension

Pearson Nursing Student Resources

Find additional review materials at
www.nursing.pearsonhighered.com

Prepare for success with additional NCLEX®-style practice questions, interactive assignments and activities, Web links, animations and videos, and more!

BIBLIOGRAPHY

American Burn Association. (2003). Senior safety. Retrieved from http://ameriburn.org

American Burn Association. (2007). Burn incidence and treatment in the US: 2007 fact sheet. Retrieved January 2, 2009, from, http://www.americanburn.org/resources_factsheet.php?

Bishop, J. F. (2004). Burn wound assessment and surgical management. Critical Care Nursing Clinics of North America, 16, 145–177.

Bulechek, G., Butcher, H., & Dochterman, J. M. (Eds.). (2008). Nursing interventions classification (NIC) (5th ed.). St. Louis: Mosby Elsevier.

Carrougher, G. J., Ptacek, J. T., Sharer, S. R., et al. (2003). Comparison of patient satisfaction and self-reports of pain in adult burn-injured patients. Journal of Burn Care and Rehabilitation, 24(1), 1–8.

Deglin, J. H., & Vallerand, A. H. (2009). Davis' drug guide (10th ed.). Philadelphia: F.A. Davis.

DeJong, A. E. E., Middlekoop, E., Faber, A. W., & Von Loey, N. E. E. (2007). Non-pharmacological nursing interventions for procedural pain relief in adults with burns: a systematic literature review. Burns, 33, 811–827.

Domino, F. J., Baldor, R. A., Golding, J., Grimes, J., & Taylor, J. S. (2010). The 5-minute clinical consult (18th ed.). Philadelphia: Lippincott, Williams & Wilkins.

Honari, S. (2004). Topical therapies and antimicrobials in the management of burn wounds. Critical Care Nursing Clinics of North America, 16, 1–11.

Huether, S. E., & McCance, K. L. (2008). Understanding Pathophysiology (4th ed.). St. Louis: Mosby Elsevier.

Joint Commission. (2009). 2006 patient safety goals. Retrieved from http://www.jointcommission.org/patientsafety/nationalpatientsafetygoals/

Montgomery, R. K. (2004). Pain management in burn injury. Critical Care Nursing Clinics of North America, 16, 39–49.

Moorhead, S., Johnson, M., Maas, M., & Swanson, E. (Eds.). (2008). Nursing outcomes classification (NOC) (4th ed.). St. Louis: Mosby Elsevier.

NANDA International. (2009). Nursing diagnoses: Definitions and classification 2009–2011. Oxford, UK: Wiley-Blackwell.

National Fire Protection Association. (2004). Leaving home: College fire safety and burn prevention campaign. Quincy, MA: NFPA.

National Fire Protection Association. (2005). Smoking material-related fires. Retrieved from http://www.nfpa.org/itemDetail.asp?categoryID=294&itemID19303&URL=Research%20&%20Reports/Fact%20sheets/Home%20safety/Smoking%20material-related%20fires

Osborn, K. (2003). Nursing burn injuries. Nursing Management, 34(5), 49–56.

Papadakis, M. A., & McPhee, S. J. (2007). Current consult medicine 2007. New York: McGraw-Hill.

Perrin, K. O. (2009). Understanding the essentials of critical care nursing. Upper Saddle River, NJ: Pearson Prentice-Hall.

Pham, T. N., Cancio, L. C., & Giban, N. S. (2008). American Burn Association practice guidelines burn shock resuscitation. Journal of Burn Care and Research 29(1), 257–266.

Supple, K. G. (2004). Physiologic response to burn injury. Critical Care Nursing Clinics of North America, 16, 119–126.

Van Leeuwen, A. M., & Poelhuis-Leth, D. J. (2009). Davis' laboratory and diagnostic tests (3rd ed.). Philadelphia: F.A. Davis.

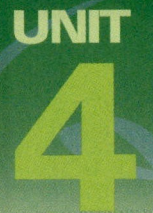

UNIT 4

Building Clinical Competence
Responses to Altered Integumentary Structure and Function

Functional Health Pattern: Nutritional-Metabolic

Think about patients with altered nutrition for whom you have cared in your clinical experiences.

- What were their major medical diagnoses (e.g., psoriasis, cysts, folliculitis, cellulitis, candidiasis, pediculosis, herpes zoster, seborrheic dermatitis, acne vulgaris, nonmelanoma skin cancer, malignant melanoma, basal cell carcinoma, pressure ulcers, hirsutism, alopecia, paronychia, or burn trauma)?

- What kinds of manifestations did each of these patients have? Were these manifestations similar or different?

- How did the patients' healthcare behaviors interfere with their integumentary system? What was their daily intake of foods and fluids? Were they gaining or losing weight? What medications or dietary supplements were they taking? What was the condition of their skin, hair, and nails? Did they complain of dry skin, itching, rashes, bruising easily, or hair loss? Had they noted any changes in moles or warts? Did they have any pressure areas on the sacrum, hips, or ankles? Did they have any previous skin disorders, and how were they treated? Did they use preventative measures to protect against temperature extremes?

The Nutritional-Metabolic Functional Health Pattern includes food and fluid consumption as needed to maintain the nutrition and metabolic needs that supply nutrients to the integumentary system. Breakdown of skin and its accessory structures leads to decreased protection between internal and external environments. Integumentary disorders are affected by nutritional and metabolic status in two primary ways:

- Lack of proper nutrients lowers the body's resistance to disorders and can result in integumentary disorders such as infection (e.g., viral, bacterial) or skin breakdown (e.g., pressure ulcers).

- Exposure to extremes of cold or heat can result in trauma to the skin and accessory structures (e.g., frostbite, burn trauma).

- Use of certain medications to treat disorders can result in hair distribution changes (e.g., hirsutism, alopecia).

Nutrients are used by the body to promote maintenance and repair. Improper intake of nutrients affects the integumentary system's ability to maintain protection, regulate body temperature, and maintain fluid and electrolyte balance. Exposure to environmental extremes breaks down the protective mechanism of the skin and interferes with sensory function. Due to these factors, the patient can develop skin, hair, and nail disorders, leading to manifestations such as the following:

- **Skin ulcerations** (*external pressure impairs the flow of blood and lymph or friction and shearing from sliding tears and injures vessels, causing tissue ischemia and hypoxia to occur, and resulting in tissue death and necrosis*)

- **Infection** (*microorganisms invade tissue and replicate, causing toxic by-products of microorganism metabolism, cell lysis, and immune response to occur, and resulting in inflammation and tissue damage*)

- **Alopecia** (*scarring from trauma, infection, radiation, medications affects rapidly growing cells in hair follicles; affected hair follicle cells slow down hair production, resulting in loss of hair*)

Priority nursing diagnoses within the Nutritional-Metabolic Health Pattern that may be appropriate for patients with integumentary disorders include the following:

- *Impaired Skin Integrity* as evidenced by disruption of skin surface, edema, delayed wound healing, itching, rashes

- *Risk for Infection* as evidenced by breakdown of skin, erythema of skin, warmth, edema, pain, red streaks from injury, fever, chills

- *Deficient Fluid Volume* as evidenced by draining wounds, limited intake of fluids, dry skin, increased skin turgor

- *Disturbed Body Image* as evidenced by altered body appearance, feelings of hopelessness, powerlessness

Two nursing diagnoses from other functional health patterns often are of high priority for the patient with integumentary disorders:

- *Acute Pain* (Cognitive-Perceptual Functional Health Pattern)

- *Ineffective Protection* (Activity-Exercise Functional Health Pattern)

Question

1. When the patient does not have adequate intake of food and fluids, what specifically can the nurse do to encourage nutrition?

CLINICAL SCENARIO

Directions: *Read the following clinical scenarios and answer the questions that follow. To complete this exercise successfully, you will utilize not only knowledge of the content in this unit, but also principles related to priority setting and maintaining patient safety.*

You have been assigned to work with the following four patients for the 0700 shift on a medical-surgical unit. Significant data obtained during report is as follows:

- Mr. Johnson is a 46-year-old who is hospitalized for surgery to release contractures at his elbows that resulted from a flash burn from a grill fire 3 years ago. He is scheduled for surgery at 0800 and needs vital signs, preoperative medication and the preoperative checklist completed.
- Mrs. Carter is a 35-year-old who was hospitalized 2 days ago with cellulitis in the right calf. Vital signs are temperature 100.4°F, pulse 80, respirations 20, and blood pressure 116/76. She is complaining of a headache and pain in the right calf. She was last medicated for pain at 0300.
- Mr. Jenkins is an 86-year-old with herpes zoster. He was admitted 4 days ago with lesions on his left neck and trunk areas. Vital signs are temperature 99°F, pulse 88, respirations 26, and blood pressure 158/90. He is complaining of burning pain across his back and is concerned more lesions are forming.
- Rami Ugandi is a 34-year-old African male who has a history of AIDS. He was transferred from the burn ICU to the medical-surgical unit at 0600 after being treated for toxic epidermal necrolysis for the past month. He will be discharged to his home with limited activity.

Questions

Priority Setting

1. In what order would you visit these patients after report? What is the rationale for your choice?
   - A. _____
   - B. _____
   - C. _____
   - D. _____

Health Promotion

1. A diet high in protein and iron may help to prevent pressure ulcers on the patient who is on prolonged bed rest. Which foods should you encourage Mr. Ugandi to eat to help prevent pressure ulcers?
   - A. eggs and chicken
   - B. broccoli and oranges
   - C. oatmeal and bananas
   - D. whole-grain bread and kidney beans

2. Mr. Jenkins is being discharged to home. About which of the following related to herpes zoster does the nurse need to teach Mr. Jenkins upon discharge?
   - A. "Continue taking the antiviral medication to cure the herpes zoster."
   - B. "You can attend church functions as herpes zoster is not contagious."
   - C. "Use narcotic pain medications only for severe pain so you do not become addicted to the medication."
   - D. "Wear cotton clothing and keep room temperatures cool to decrease the pain and itching from the herpes zoster lesions."

Nursing Process

1. What top priority nursing diagnoses would you choose for each of the patients presented earlier? What is the rationale for your choices?

	Nursing Diagnosis	Rationale
Mr. Johnson		
Mrs. Carter		
Mr. Jenkins		
Mr. Ugandi		

2. Mr. Johnson received partial-thickness and full-thickness flash burns on both anterior and posterior arms and his anterior trunk from a grill fire. Using the "rule of nines," what is the percentage of total body surface (TBSA) burned? _____%

3. Mrs. Carter was admitted with cellulitis in the right calf. Which clinical manifestations did the nurse assess for on admission?
   - A. redness, edema, and pain in the right calf
   - B. purulent drainage, pale skin, and pain in right calf
   - C. rash, redness, and swelling in right calf
   - D. itching, rash, and pain in right calf

4. The nurse applies mafenide acetate (Sulfamylon) to Mr. Ugandi's open skin wounds caused by toxic epidermal necrolysis. Which hypersensitivity reactions would require the nurse to discontinue the drug?
   - A. tachycardia and tachypnea
   - B. nausea and vomiting
   - C. facial edema and pruritis
   - D. diarrhea and *candidiasis*

Communication

1. Mr. Jenkins states, "I am tired of having these sores all over. Once they heal they won't ever come back will they? I think I would rather die than go through this again." How will you answer this question?

Delegation

1. What data collection and interventions can be delegated to a CNA for each patient?
   - A. _____
   - B. _____
   - C. _____
   - D. _____

Content-Specific Questions

1. Which serum laboratory values are decreased with inadequate nutritional intake, such as in a patient with severe burns? **Select all that apply.**
   - A. protein
   - B. potassium
   - C. iron
   - D. complete blood cell count
   - E. glucose
   - F. calcium

2. When a patient is admitted to the burn unit for treatment of severe burns, it is most important for the nurse to monitor the patient for which of the following?

   A. acute pain

   B. nausea and vomiting

   C. hypothermia

   D. fluid and electrolyte imbalance

3. Which of these patients is most at risk for skin breakdown leading to pressure ulcers?

   A. a 70-year-old who had a stroke with left-sided paralysis

   B. a quadriplegic admitted to the hospital with pneumonia

   C. a 56-year-old patient on dialysis three times a week

   D. an 84-year-old patient in traction for a hip fracture

4. Health promotion teaching for a patient at risk for skin cancer includes which interventions? **Select all that apply.**

   A. Wear long-sleeved shirts and a wide-brimmed hat in the sun.

   B. Apply sunscreen once a day.

   C. Avoid tanning booths or prolonged exposure to the sun.

   D. Minimize exposure to the sun between 1:00 PM and 4:00 PM.

   E. Apply sunscreen before and after swimming.

5. Morphine sulfate is a drug of choice for pain. Which clinical manifestation requires immediate nursing intervention?

   A. vomiting once after medication administered

   B. respiratory rate below 8 breaths per minute

   C. blood pressure of 110/70 after a baseline blood pressure of 120/80

   D. peripheral pulse of 68 after a baseline pulse of 78

CASE STUDY: Stephanie Chelen

Stephanie Chelen is a 23-year-old who is admitted to the medical-surgical unit after being exposed to the sun for a prolonged period of time. Due to the extent of the burns, she is admitted for observation and treatment. Upon admission, Ms. Chelen stated she fell asleep lying on her stomach while sunbathing at the beach. Her vital signs are temperature 100.6°F, pulse 94, respirations, 26, and blood pressure 116/76. Her height is 5'2" and weight is 125 lbs. Assessment shows that her back is red and slightly edematous with an area ~ 6 by 3 cm between the scapula that is beginning to develop blisters. The backs of her arms and legs and the soles of her feet are red and slightly edematous. She is complaining of pain on her back, arms, legs, and feet. She stated that she feels chilled, is nauseated, and has a headache. Labs are drawn for a complete blood count and electrolytes for baseline assessment. IV therapy is instituted to maintain hydration. The burn areas are washed with soap and water and an antibiotic ointment is applied. A mild analgesic is administered as ordered. The patient is covered to prevent further chilling and to prevent burned areas from exposure to air.

She is diagnosed with first degree and second degree burns. Using the "rule of nines," the partial thickness burned area on her back is classified as approximately 5% total body surface area. The superficial burns over the rest of the reddened areas are not classified. Superficial burns involve the epidermis layer of the skin. Superficial partial thickness burns involve the entire dermis and the papillae of the dermis. The pathophysiology of superficial and superficial partial thickness is the result of exposure to the sun for a prolonged time. An inflammatory response occurs caused by tissue injury. Platelets aggregate at the burn injury site, fibrin is deposited, and thrombus is formed. The thrombus along with vasoconstriction walls off the burn injury site. Then vasodilation occurs and with increased capillary permeability leads to redness and edema. Injury to the dermis from the superficial partial thickness burned area develops a moist, glistening appearance as blisters form. The burned area will blanch on pressure. There is pain in response to touch and temperature changes. The burned area should heal within 14 to 21 days with minimal or no scarring, but may have pigment changes. Manifestations of superficial and superficial partial thickness burns are skin redness, blister formation, local pain, headache, chills, nausea, and vomiting. Complications of superficial and superficial partial thickness burns are infection, hypothermia, dehydration, and fluid and electrolyte imbalances.

Due to the severity of tissue injury from the burns, the nursing diagnosis of *Impaired Skin Integrity* is appropriate for guiding nursing care.

- Inflammatory response to injury to dermis and epidermis
- Platelet aggregation and deposits of fibrin lead to hemostasis
- Fibroblasts are deposited and granulation tissue forms

affects

Ms. C.
23 y.o. female
Superficial and partial thickness burns

leads to

assess

- Partial thickness burns on back=5% TBS with redness and blistering
- Superficial burns with redness and blisters on posterior of arms, legs, and soles of feet
- Pain in burn areas

generates

- Acute Pain related to superficial and partial thickness burns
- Risk for Infection related to partial thickness burns
- Nausea related to effects of burns

generate nursing diagnosis

prioritized to

Impaired Skin Integrity

expected outcomes

- Burns heal within one month without manifestations of infection
- Provides wound care, including cleansing and application of topical medications
- Pain decreases to a 0 on a scale of 0 (least) to 10 (most) pain
- Verbalizes principles of safe sun exposure and risks of sunburn

evaluate

- Both superficial and partial thickness burns healed without infection
- Pain decreased within one week
- Verbalized understanding of safe sun exposure and risks of sunburn

Interdisciplinary Interventions
- Insert intravenous line and initiate fluids as prescribed.
- Wash burn area and apply prescribed topical medications.
- Administer prescribed analgesic for pain.

Independent Interventions
- Explain reason for intravenous fluids, cleansing burn area, and applying topical medications.
- Teach and request demonstration of wound care and application of topical medications (instruct patient's housemate as burns are on her back).
- Teach effects, side effects, and times for taking analgesic for pain.
- Teach manifestations of infection and need to notify healthcare provider if they occur.
- Instruct in methods of safe sun exposure and risks of sunburn.

Activity:

1. After reviewing the concept map above, is there anything you would change to make it more understandable? Would the care be different if patient was male, weighed 270 pounds, and was burned by an electric wire touching his back?

2. Go to the Pearson Nursing Student Resources for this book at www.nursing.pearsonhighered.com to write a concept map for this male patient.

See answers and hints in Appendix C.

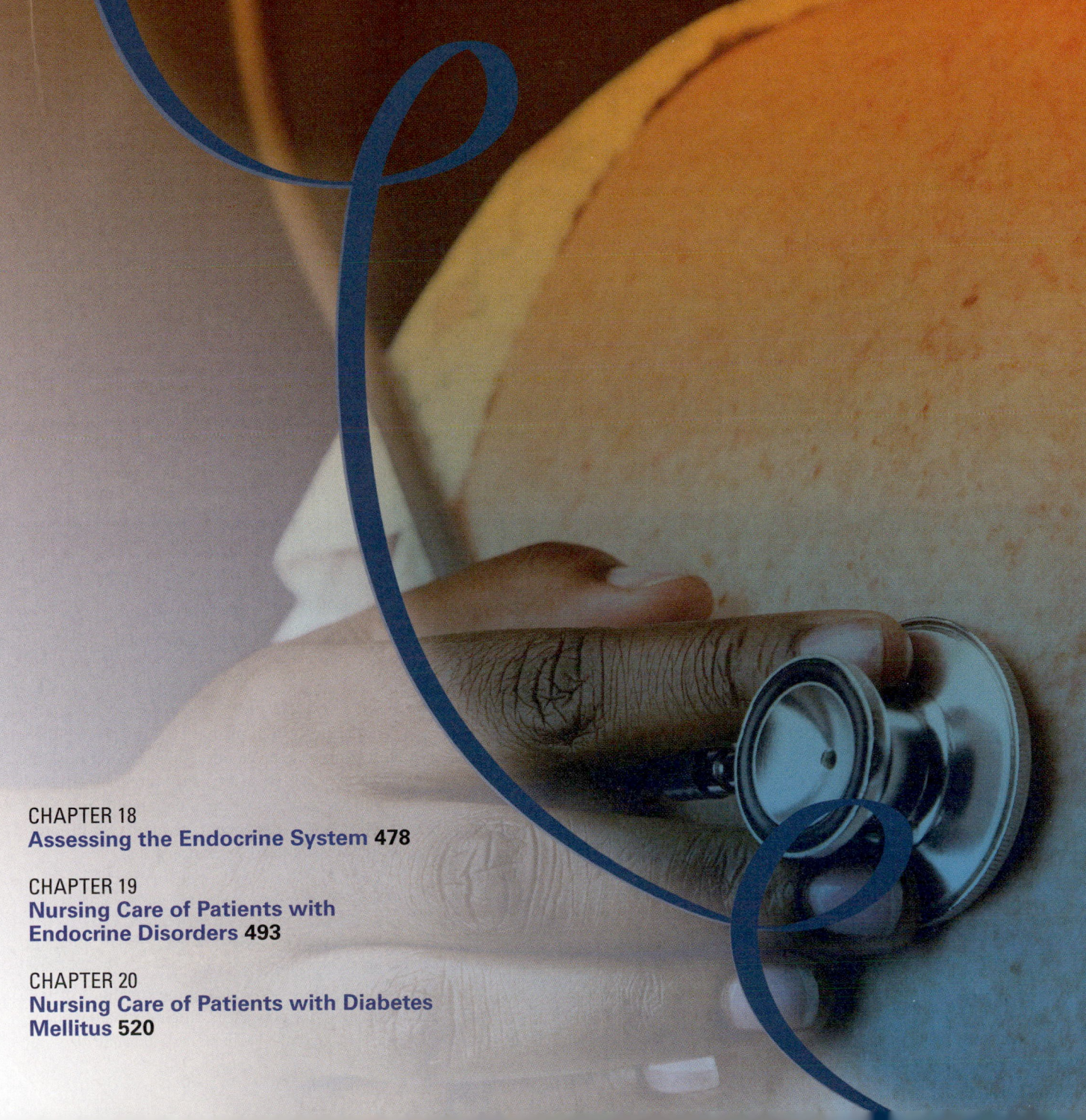

Responses to Altered Endocrine Function

UNIT 5

CHAPTER 18

Assessing the **Endocrine System**

LEARNING OUTCOMES

1. Describe the anatomy and physiology of the endocrine glands.
2. Summarize the functions of the hormones secreted by the endocrine glands.
3. Describe specific topics to consider during a health history interview of the patient with health problems involving endocrine function.
4. Explain techniques for assessing the thyroid gland and the effects of altered function of thyroid hormones.
5. Describe normal variations in endocrine assessment findings for the older adult.
6. Give examples of genetic disorders of the endocrine glands.
7. Identify abnormal findings that may indicate malfunction of the glands of the endocrine system.

CLINICAL COMPETENCIES

1. Conduct and document a health history for patients who have or are at risk for alterations in the structure or function of the endocrine glands.
2. Monitor the results of diagnostic tests and report abnormal findings.
3. Conduct and document a physical assessment of the structure of the thyroid gland and the effects of altered endocrine function on other body structures and functions.

EQUIPMENT NEEDED

- Reflex hammer
- Safety pin, cotton ball, containers with hot and cold water, tuning fork
- Blood pressure cuff
- Stethoscope

KEY TERMS

acromegaly, *490*	dwarfism, *491*	tetany, *491*
carpal spasm, *491*	exophthalmos, *490*	Trousseau's sign, *491*
Chvostek's sign, *491*	goiter, *490*	

The endocrine system is essential to the regulation of the body's internal environment. Through hormones secreted by its glands, the endocrine system regulates such varied functions as growth, reproduction, metabolism, fluid and electrolyte balance, and gender differentiation. It also has a role in adapting to constant alterations in the internal and external environment.

Disorders of the endocrine system primarily result from either too much or too little hormone production. These alterations in hormone levels affect a wide variety of human functions, including activity and exercise, nutrition and metabolism, elimination, self-perception and self-concept, sexuality and reproduction, coping with stress, and role-relationships.

Anatomy, Physiology, and Functions of the Endocrine System

The endocrine system is comprised of the pituitary gland, thyroid gland, parathyroid glands, adrenal glands, pancreas, and gonads (reproductive glands). The locations of these glands are illustrated in Figure 18–1 ■. Table 18–1 summarizes the functions of the endocrine glands and their hormones. Specific information about the ovaries and testes is found in ∞ Chapters 47 through 49.

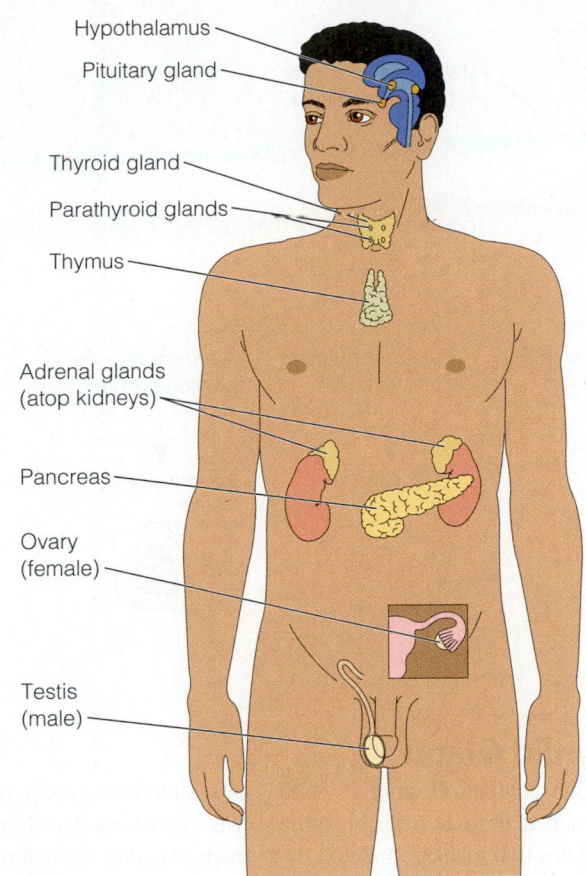

Hypothalamus
Pituitary gland
Thyroid gland
Parathyroid glands
Thymus
Adrenal glands (atop kidneys)
Pancreas
Ovary (female)
Testis (male)

Figure 18–1 ■ Location of the major endocrine glands.

Pituitary Gland

The pituitary gland (hypophysis) is located in the skull beneath the hypothalamus of the brain (Figure 18–2 ■). It often is called the "master gland" because its hormones regulate many body functions. The pituitary gland has two parts: the anterior pituitary (or adenohypophysis) and the

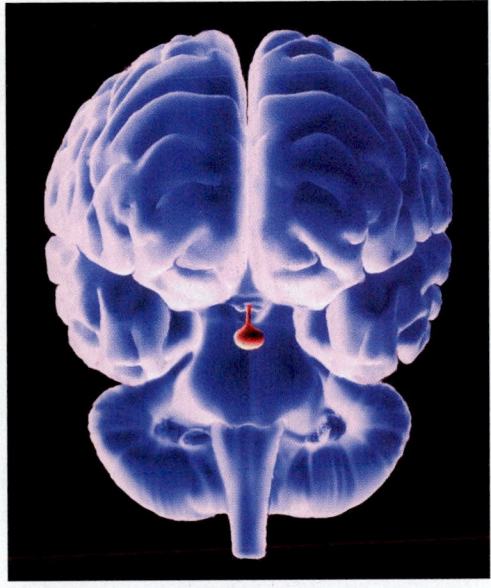

Figure 18–2 ■ Location of the pituitary gland.
Source: ISM/Phototake NYC.

TABLE 18–1 Organs, Hormones, Functions, and Feedback Mechanisms of the Endocrine System

ENDOCRINE GLAND	HORMONE SECRETED	TARGET ORGAN AND FEEDBACK MECHANISM
Thyroid gland	Thyroid hormone (TH): thyroxine (T_4) is the major hormone secreted by the thyroid gland. It is converted to triiodothyronine (T_3) at the target tissues.	Maintains metabolic rate and growth and development of all tissues. T_3 and T_4 are secreted in response to TSH.
	Calcitonin	Maintains serum calcium levels by decreasing bone resorption and decreasing resorption of calcium in the kidneys whenever levels of plasma calcium are elevated.
Parathyroid gland	Parathyroid hormone (PTH)	Maintains serum calcium levels by stimulating bone resorption and formation and by stimulating kidney resorption of calcium in response to falling levels of plasma calcium.
Adrenal cortex	Mineralocorticoids (e.g., aldosterone)	Promotes kidney tubule reabsorption of sodium and water and excretion of potassium in response to elevated levels of potassium and low levels of sodium, thereby increasing blood pressure and blood volume.
	Glucocorticoids (e.g., cortisol)	Helps regulate metabolism of carbohydrates, fats, and proteins. Activates anti-inflammatory responses to stressors. Low cortisol levels stimulate hypothalamic secretion of corticotropin-releasing hormone (CRH), which stimulates the anterior pituitary gland to release ACTH, which in turn stimulates the adrenal cortex to secrete cortisol.
	Gonadocorticoids (androgens and small amounts of estrogen and progesterone)	The quantity of sex hormones produced here is small, and the mechanism is not well understood.
Adrenal medulla	Catecholamines (epinephrine and norepinephrine)	Stimulates the heart, constricts blood vessels, inhibits visceral muscles, dilates bronchioles, increases respiration and metabolism, promotes hyperglycemia. Secreted in response to physical or psychologic stress.
Anterior pituitary (adenohypophysis)	Growth hormone (GH)	Promotes growth of body tissues by enhancing protein synthesis and promoting use of fat for energy and thus conserving glucose. Release is stimulated by growth hormone releasing hormone (GHRH) in response to low GH levels, hypoglycemia, increased amino acids, low fatty acids, and stress.

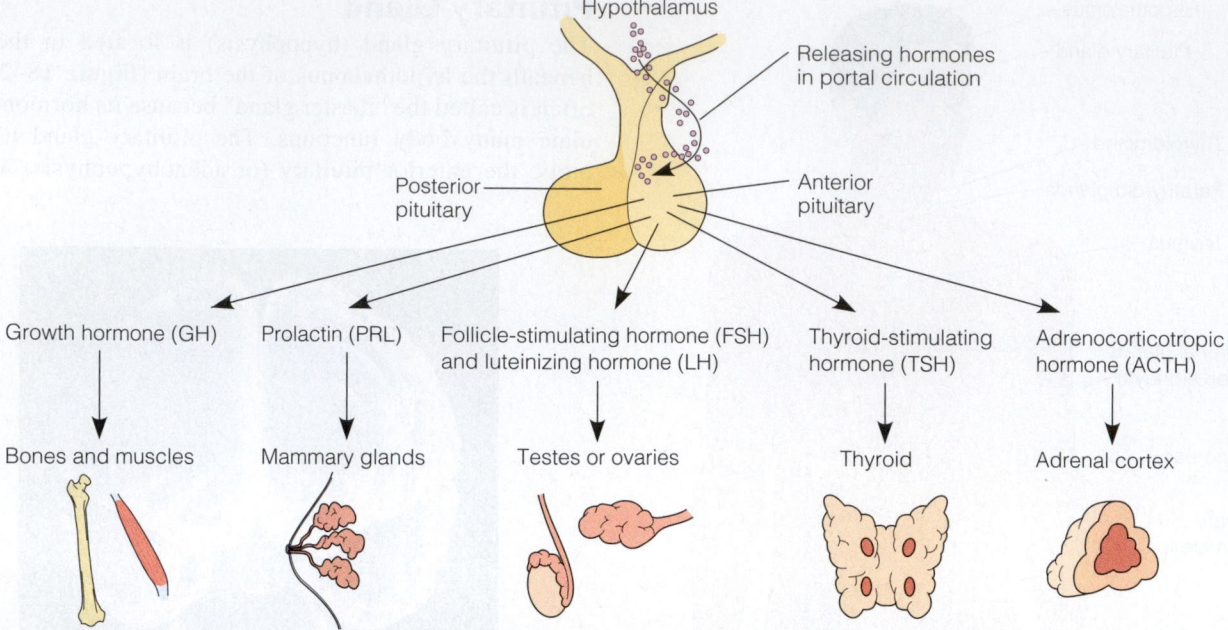

Figure 18–3 ■ Actions of the major hormones of the anterior pituitary.

posterior pituitary (or neurohypophysis). The anterior pituitary is glandular tissue; the posterior pituitary is an extension of the hypothalamus.

Anterior Pituitary

The anterior pituitary has several types of endocrine cells and secretes at least six major hormones (Figure 18–3 ■).

■ Somatotropic cells secrete growth hormone (GH) (also called somatotropin). GH stimulates growth of the body by signaling cells to increase protein production and by stimulating the epiphyseal plates of the long bones.

■ Lactotropic cells secrete prolactin (PRL). Prolactin stimulates the production of breast milk.

■ Thyrotropic cells secrete thyroid-stimulating hormone (TSH). TSH stimulates the synthesis and release of thyroid hormones from the thyroid gland.

■ Corticotropic cells secrete adrenocorticotropic hormone (ACTH). ACTH stimulates release of hormones, especially glucocorticoids, from the adrenal cortex.

■ Gonadotropic cells secrete the gonadotropin hormones, follicle-stimulating hormone (FSH), and luteinizing hormone (LH). These hormones stimulate the ovaries and testes (the gonads).

Posterior Pituitary

The posterior pituitary is made of nervous tissue. Its primary function is to store and release antidiuretic hormone (ADH) and oxytocin, produced in the hypothalamus:

■ ADH, also called vasopressin, decreases urine production by causing the renal tubules to reabsorb water from the urine and return it to the circulating blood.

■ Oxytocin induces contraction of the smooth muscles in the reproductive organs. In women, oxytocin stimulates the myometrium of the uterus to contract during labor. It also induces milk ejection from the breasts.

Thyroid Gland

The thyroid gland (Figure 18–4 ■) is anterior to the upper part of the trachea and just inferior to the larynx. This butterfly-shaped gland has two lobes connected by a structure called the isthmus.

The glandular tissue consists of follicles filled with a jelly-like colloid substance named thyroglobulin, a glycoprotein-iodine complex. Cells within the follicles secrete thyroid hormone (TH), a general name for two similar hormones: thyroxine (T_4) and triiodothyronine (T_3). The primary role of thyroid hormones in adults is to increase metabolism. TH secretion is initiated by

Figure 18–4 ■ The thyroid gland.

Source: Dorling Kindersley Media Library.

the release of TSH by the pituitary gland and is dependent on an adequate supply of iodine.

The thyroid gland also secretes calcitonin, a hormone that decreases excessive levels of calcium in the blood by slowing the calcium-releasing activity of bone cells, serves as a marker for sepsis, and is believed to be a mediator of inflammatory responses.

Parathyroid Glands

The parathyroid glands (usually four to six in number) are embedded on the posterior surface of the lobes of the thyroid gland. They secrete parathyroid hormone (PTH), or parathormone. When calcium levels in the plasma fall, PTH secretion increases. PTH also controls phosphate metabolism. It acts by increasing renal excretion of phosphate in the urine, by decreasing the excretion of calcium, and by increasing bone reabsorption to cause the release of calcium from bones. Normal levels of vitamin D are necessary for PTH to exert these effects on bone and kidneys.

Adrenal Glands

The two adrenal glands are pyramid-shaped organs that sit on top of the kidneys (Figure 18–5 ■). Each gland consists of two parts, an inner medulla and an outer cortex.

The adrenal medulla produces two hormones (also called catecholamines): epinephrine (adrenalin) and norepinephrine (noradrenalin). These hormones are similar to substances also released by the sympathetic nervous system and thus are not essential to life. Epinephrine increases blood glucose levels and stimulates the release of ACTH from the pituitary; ACTH in turn stimulates the adrenal cortex to release glucocorticoids. Epinephrine also increases the rate and force of cardiac contractions; constricts blood vessels in the skin, mucous membranes, and kidneys; and dilates blood vessels in the skeletal muscles, coronary arteries, and pulmonary arteries. Norepinephrine increases heart rate, increases the force of cardiac contractions, and vasoconstricts blood vessels throughout the body.

The adrenal cortex secretes several hormones, all corticosteroids. They are classified into two groups: mineralocorticoids and glucocorticoids. These hormones are essential to life.

The release of the mineralocorticoids is controlled primarily by renin (an enzyme). When a decrease in blood pressure or sodium is detected, specialized kidney cells release renin to act on angiotensinogen, manufactured by the liver. Angiotensinogen is modified by renin and other enzymes to become angiotensin, which stimulates the release of aldosterone from the adrenal cortex. Aldosterone prompts the distal tubules of the kidneys to release increased amounts of

water and sodium back into the circulating blood to increase circulating blood volume and pressure. This system (the renin–angiotensin–aldosterone system) is illustrated in ∞ Chapter 10 with the discussion of body fluid regulation.

The glucocorticoids include cortisol and cortisone. These hormones affect carbohydrate metabolism by regulating glucose use in body tissues, mobilizing fatty acids from fatty tissue, and shifting the source of energy for muscle cells from glucose to fatty acids. Glucocorticoids are released in times of stress. An excess of glucocorticoids in the body depresses the inflammatory response and inhibits the effectiveness of the immune system.

Pancreas

The pancreas, located behind the stomach between the spleen and the duodenum, is both an endocrine gland (producing hormones) and an exocrine gland (producing digestive enzymes). The digestive enzymes produced by the pancreas are discussed in ∞ Chapter 21. The content in this chapter discusses the endocrine pancreatic hormones.

The endocrine cells of the pancreas produce hormones that regulate carbohydrate metabolism. They are clustered in structures called pancreatic islets (or islets of Langerhans) scattered throughout the pancreas. Pancreatic islets have at least four different cell types:

- Alpha cells produce glucagon, which decreases glucose oxidation and promotes an increase in the blood glucose level by signaling the liver to release glucose from glycogen stores.
- Beta cells produce insulin, which facilitates the uptake and use of glucose by muscle, liver, and fat cells and prevents an excessive breakdown of glycogen in the liver and muscle. In this way, insulin decreases blood glucose levels. Insulin also facilitates lipid formation, inhibits the breakdown and mobilization of stored fat, and helps amino acids move into cells to promote protein synthesis. In general, the actions of glucagon and insulin oppose one another, helping to maintain a stable blood glucose level.
- Delta cells secrete somatostatin, which inhibits the secretion of glucagon and insulin by the alpha and beta cells.
- F cells secrete pancreatic polypeptide, which is believed to inhibit the exocrine activity of the pancreas.

Gonads

The gonads are the testes in men and the ovaries in women. These organs are the primary source of steroid sex hormones in the body. The hormones of the gonads are important in regulating body growth and promoting the onset of puberty. The structure and functions of the gonads are discussed in ∞ Chapter 47.

An Overview of Hormones

Hormones are chemical messengers secreted by the endocrine organs and transported throughout the body, where they exert their action on specific cells called target cells. Hormones do not cause reactions directly but rather regulate tissue responses. They may produce either generalized effects or local effects.

Hormones are transported from endocrine gland cells to target cells in the body in one of four ways:

- Endocrine glands release most hormones, including TH and insulin, into the bloodstream. Some hormones require a protein carrier.

Figure 18–5 ■ Location of the adrenal glands.

Source: Dorling Kindersley Media Library.

- Neurons release some hormones, such as epinephrine, into the bloodstream. This is called the neuroendocrine route.
- The hypothalamus releases its hormones directly to target cells in the posterior pituitary by nerve cell extension.
- With the paracrine method, released messengers diffuse through the interstitial fluid. This method of transport involves a number of hormonal peptides that are released throughout various organs and cells and act locally. An example is endorphins, which act to relieve pain.

Hormones that are released into the bloodstream circulate as either free, unbound molecules or as hormones attached to transport carriers. Peptide and protein hormones (such as insulin) circulate unbound, while steroid and thyroid hormones are carried by specific transport carriers synthesized by the liver. Hormone receptors are complex molecular structures, located on or inside target cells. They act by binding to specific receptor sites located on the surfaces of the target cells. These receptors recognize a specific hormone and translate the message into a cellular response. The receptor sites are structured so that they respond only to a specific hormone; for example, receptors in the thyroid gland are responsive to TSH but not to LH. Drugs that compete with a hormone for binding with transport carrier molecules increase hormone action by increasing the availability of the free, unbound hormone.

Hormone levels are controlled by the pituitary gland and by feedback mechanisms. Although most feedback mechanisms are negative, a few are positive. Negative feedback is controlled much as the thermostat in a house regulates temperature. Sensors in the endocrine system detect changes in hormone levels and adjust hormone secretion to maintain normal levels. When the sensors detect a decrease in hormone levels, they begin actions to cause an increase in hormone levels; when hormone levels rise above normal, the sensors cause a decrease in hormone production and release. For example, when the hypothalamus or

Figure 18–6 ■ Negative feedback.

anterior pituitary gland senses increased blood levels of TH, it releases hormones, causing a reduction in the secretion of TSH, which in turn prompts a decrease in the output of TH by the thyroid gland. See Figure 18–6 ■.

In positive feedback mechanisms, increasing levels of one hormone cause another gland to release a hormone. For example, the increased production of estradiol (a female ovarian hormone) during the follicular stage of the menstrual cycle in turn stimulates increased FSH production by the anterior pituitary gland. Estradiol levels continue to increase until the ovarian follicle disappears, eliminating the source of the stimulation for FSH, which then decreases.

Stimuli for hormone release may also be classified as hormonal, humoral, or neural (Figure 18–7 ■). In hormonal release,

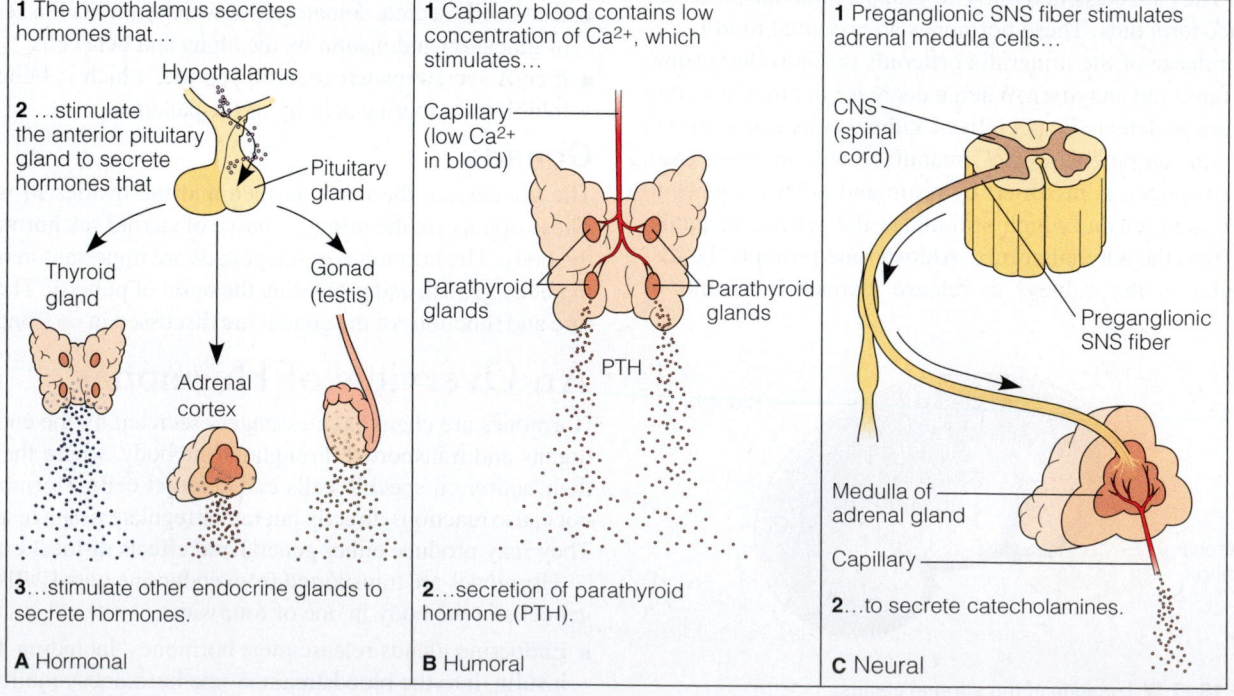

Figure 18–7 ■ Examples of three mechanisms of hormone release: *A*, hormonal; *B*, humoral; or *C*, neural.

hypothalamic hormones stimulate the anterior pituitary to release hormones. Fluctuations in the serum level of these hormones in turn prompt other endocrine glands to release hormones. In humoral release, fluctuations in the serum levels of certain ions and nutrients stimulate specific endocrine glands to release hormones to bring these levels back to normal. In neural release, nerve fibers stimulate the release of hormones.

Assessing Endocrine Function

The function of the endocrine glands is assessed by findings from diagnostic tests, a health assessment interview to collect subjective data, and a physical assessment to collect objective data. Hormones affect all body tissues and organs, and manifestations of dysfunction are often nonspecific, making assessment of endocrine function sometimes more difficult than assessment of other body systems.

Diagnostic Tests

The results of diagnostic tests of the endocrine system are used to support the diagnosis of a specific disease, to provide information to identify or modify the appropriate medication or therapy used to treat the disease, and to help nurses monitor the patient's responses to treatment and nursing care interventions. Diagnostic tests to assess the structure and function of the glands of the endocrine system are described in the following table. More information is included in the discussion of specific disorders in ∞ Chapters 19 and 20.

Regardless of the type of diagnostic test, the nurse is responsible for explaining the procedure and any special preparation needed, for assessing for medication use that may affect the outcome of the tests, for ensuring the consent form is signed (if necessary), for supporting the patient during the examination as necessary, for documenting the procedures as appropriate, and for monitoring the results of the tests. The nurse is also responsible for post-procedure care and patient teaching for self-care at home.

DIAGNOSTIC TESTS of the Endocrine System

PITUITARY TESTS

NAME OF TEST	PURPOSE & DESCRIPTION	RELATED NURSING INTERVENTIONS
Growth Hormone (GH), Human Growth Hormone (hGH)	In this blood serum test, GH levels (affected by food, stress, and activity) are measured to identify GH deficiency (dwarfism) or GH excess (gigantism, acromegaly). Normal value: Men: < 5 ng/mL Women: < 10 ng/mL	Tell patient not to eat or drink 8 to 10 hours prior to having blood drawn. Have patient rest for 30 to 60 minutes before blood is drawn.
Magnetic Resonance Imaging (MRI)	This radiographic study is done to identify tumors of the hypothalamus or pituitary gland.	Tell patient of need to lie still during the examination. Assess for any metallic implants (such as pacemakers, clips on brain aneurysms, body piercings, tattoos, shrapnel). If present, notify imaging physician. Remove transdermal medication patches (both OTC and prescribed) unless otherwise ordered (FDA, 2009). Replace the patch following the procedure. Ask the patient to tell the staff about the patch when making the appointment and when completing the admission information. Ask if patient is pregnant; if so the test is not performed. Ask about claustrophobia; if a problem, request patient to ask for a relaxing medication to take prior to the MRI.
Somatomedin C (Insulin-Like Growth Factor or IGF-1)	The results of this serum test are used to evaluate secretion of growth factor and to identify GH deficiency or excess (as discussed earlier). Normal value: 125–250 ng/mL	None; overnight fasting is preferred but not necessary.
Water Deprivation Test	This combination of blood and urine tests is used to identify causes of polyuria (increased urine output), including central diabetes insipidus, neurogenic diabetes insipidus, syndrome of inappropriate antidiuretic hormone (SIADH), and psychogenic polydipsia (drinking excessive amounts of fluids). ADH or vasopressin is given IM or subcutaneously. In patients without pathology, there is no change in urine and plasma osmolality. Urine osmolality increases in central diabetes insipidus and decreases in nephrogenic diabetes insipidus.	Tell patient not to smoke, eat, or drink after midnight, and that the test will take up to 8 hours. Every hour for ordered length of test assess weight, take postural BP (lying and standing measures separated by 2 minutes), assess urine for volume and specific gravity, and send samples of urine to the lab for osmolality. Blood samples for osmolality are taken when urine samples are collected and when patient demonstrates orthostatic hypotension. Coordinate specimen collection with the laboratory.

(continued)

DIAGNOSTIC TESTS of the Endocrine System (continued)

THYROID TESTS

NAME OF TEST	PURPOSE & DESCRIPTION	RELATED NURSING INTERVENTIONS
Magnetic Resonance Imaging (MRI)— thyroid	This radiographic study is done to identify tumors of the thyroid gland.	See information for MRI of the pituitary.
Radioactive Iodine Uptake (RIA)	This test provides a direct measure of thyroid activity and is useful in evaluating the activity of solitary thyroid nodules. Based on the rationale that the thyroid gland takes up iodine in any form, radioactive iodine is given orally or IV, and the thyroid gland uptake is measured with a scanner at several hourly intervals and at 24 hours. Normal value for uptake: 2–4 hours: 3%–19% 24 hours: 11%–30%	The patient should not eat or drink for 6 to 8 hours before the test, but can have food 1 hour after the oral dose is given. Tell patients not to take supplemental iodine several weeks before the test and thyroid medications should be discontinued.
Thyroid Antibodies (TA)	A blood test used to identify thyroid immune disease (Graves' disease, chronic thyroiditis, Hashimoto's thyroiditis). Normal values: Antithyroglobulin: negative to titer < 1:20 Antimicrosomal: negative to titer < 1:100	Assess for family history of thyroid disease and ask about recent viral infection (which could trigger autoimmune disease).
Thyroid Scan	This radiologic study evaluates thyroid nodules. Radioactive isotopes are given orally and a scanner is passed over the thyroid to make a graphic record of the radiation emitted. A normal thyroid scan has a homogeneous pattern of radiation with symmetric lobes. Benign lesions appear as warm spots (take up more radiation); malignant tumors appear as cold spots (less radiation taken up).	No special preparation is needed.
Thyroid-Stimulating Hormone (TSH)	In this blood test, levels of T_4 are measured to identify the circulating TSH, with levels above or below normal indicating thyroid disease. It is also used to compare TSH results with T_4 results to differentiate between pituitary and thyroid dysfunction. A decreased T_4 level and a normal or increased TSH level can indicate a thyroid disorder. A decreased T_4 level and a decreased TSH level can indicate a pituitary disorder. Normal value: < 3ng/ml	Tell patients to avoid shellfish for several days prior to the test. Assess medications: TSH value may be increased by aspirin, steroids, dopamine, and heparin; and decreased by lithium and potassium iodide.
Thyroid Suppression Test	Triiodothyronine (T_3) is taken for 7 to 10 days, and a reduction of its uptake to less than half of the initial uptake after that time is considered normal. The test is used to diagnose hyperthyroidism and hypothyroidism.	Explain the importance of taking the triiodothyronine for the length of time prescribed.
Thyrotropin-Releasing Hormone (TRH) Stimulation Test	A baseline TSH is measured; followed by an injection of TRH to stimulate the pituitary to release TSH. A second blood sample is drawn 20 to 30 minutes later and the TSH level is again measured. Levels higher or lower than normal are indicative of thyroid disease.	No special preparation is needed.
Thyroxine (T_4)	The results of this serum test are used to determine thyroid function and aid in the diagnosis of hyperthyroidism and hypothyroidism. Normal value: free T_4 1.0–2.3 ng/dL	Assess medications: Value may be decreased by cortisone, chlorpromazine (Thorazine), phenytoin (Dilantin), heparin, lithium, sulfonamides, reserpine (Serpasil), testosterone, propranolol (Inderal), tolbutamide (Orinase), and salicylates in high doses. Values may be increased by oral contraceptives, estrogen, clofibrate, and perphenazine (Trilafon).
Triiodothyronine (T_3)	The results of this blood serum test are used to diagnose hyperthyroidism and to compare T_3 with T_4 for diagnosis of thyroid disorder. Normal value: 80–200 ng/dL	Assess medications: Value can be decreased by propylthiouracil, methimazole (Tapazole), lithium, phenytoin (Dilantin), propranolol (Inderal), reserpine (Serpasil), large doses of aspirin, steroids, and sulfonamides. Value can be increased by estrogen, progestins, oral contraceptives, T_3, and methadone.

DIAGNOSTIC TESTS of the Endocrine System (continued)

NAME OF TEST	PURPOSE & DESCRIPTION	RELATED NURSING INTERVENTIONS
Triiodothyronine Resin Uptake (T_3RU)	This test is an indirect measure of free thyroxine (T_4). The patient's blood is mixed with radioactive T_3 and synthetic resin, and the radioactive T_3 will bind with available thyroid-binding globulin sites. The unbound radioactive T_3 is added to resin for T_3 uptake. In hyperthyroidism there are few binding sites left, more T_3 is taken up by the resin, and a high T_3 resin uptake results. The opposite occurs in hypothyroidism. Normal value: 25%–35% uptake	No special preparation is needed.

PARATHYROID TESTS

NAME OF TEST	PURPOSE & DESCRIPTION	RELATED NURSING INTERVENTIONS
Calcium (Ca)	This blood serum test is used to check for serum calcium excess or deficit in parathyroid and bone disorders, and to monitor calcium levels. Normal value: 9.0–11.0 mg/dL, 4.5–5.5 mEq/L, or 2.3–2.8 mmol/L (SI units)	Assess for manifestations of tetany, including positive Chvostek's and Trousseau's signs, if hypocalcemia is present (∞ see Chapter 10).
Magnetic Resonance Imaging (MRI)—parathyroid glands	This radiographic study is done to identify tumors of the parathyroid glands. See information for MRI of the pituitary for related nursing interventions.	
Parathyroid Hormone (PTH)	This blood test is used to identify hypoparathyroidism or hyperparathyroidism, and is also used to monitor response to PTH therapy. Normal value: Intact PTH: 11–54 pg/mL C-terminal PTH: 50–330 pg/mL N-terminal PTH: 8–24 pg/mL	Tell patients not to eat or drink for 8 hours before the test.

ADRENAL TESTS

NAME OF TEST	PURPOSE & DESCRIPTION	RELATED NURSING INTERVENTIONS
ACTH Stimulation	This test is conducted to check for pituitary hypofunction. The drug metyrapone (Metopirone) is given to block the production of cortisol, thus causing an increased ACTH secretion. If the ACTH level does not increase, the problem is pituitary insufficiency.	Assess medications as for ACTH test.
ACTH Suppression	This test is used to check for the origin of an endocrine disorder. The drug dexamethasone (Decadron) is given to suppress ACTH production. If an extremely high dose is needed, the cause is of pituitary origin; if the plasma cortisol continues to be high with ACTH suppression, the cause could be adrenal cortex hyperfunction (Cushing's syndrome). Normally, the plasma cortisol level should double in 1 hour.	Tell patients to avoid tea, caffeinated coffee, and chocolates; no other food or fluid restriction is needed. Assess medications: False positives may be caused by phenytoin, barbiturates, meprobamate, and carbamazepine. If dexamethasone causes gastric irritation, milk or antacids may be required.
Aldosterone	This blood test is done to identify a deficit or an excess of aldosterone, and to compare blood and urine levels with other lab data to evaluate overhydration with increased sodium and adrenal malfunction. Normal value: < 16 mcg/dL (fasting) A 24-hour urine test is considered a more reliable measure of aldosterone than a random aldosterone test. Normal value: 6–25 mcg/24 hours	Assess diet and lab results: Levels are increased by hyponatremia, hyperkalemia, and a low-salt diet. Assess medications: Values are increased by diuretics, hydralazine (Apresoline), diazoxide (Hyperstat), nitroprusside, and oral contraceptives. If a urine test is ordered, assess diet and lab results as for blood test. Assess medications: Urine aldosterone levels are increased by diuretics, lithium, and oral contraceptives. Refrigerate specimen during collection.

(continued)

DIAGNOSTIC TESTS of the Endocrine System (continued)

NAME OF TEST	PURPOSE & DESCRIPTION	RELATED NURSING INTERVENTIONS
Adrenocorticotropic Hormone (ACTH)	This blood serum test is used to determine if a decreased plasma level of cortisol is due to adrenal cortex hypofunction or pituitary hypofunction. Normal value: 7–10 AM: 8–80 pg/mL 4 PM: 5–30 pg/mL 10–12 PM: < 10 pg/mL	Tell the patient that food and fluids may be restricted, and to eat a low-carbohydrate diet for 24 hours prior to the test. Assess medications: ACTH values may be increased by metyrapone, vasopressin, and insulin, and decreased by steroids, estrogen amphetamines, and alcohol.
Computerized Tomography (CT) of the abdomen	This radiologic study is used to assess the adrenal gland for tumors (including size and metastasis).	Determine if contrast medium will be used; if so, assess patient for allergy to iodine (shellfish).
Cortisol	This blood serum test is used to measure the amount of total cortisol in the serum and to evaluate adrenal cortex function. Values are decreased in Addison's disease and hypothyroidism, and increased in Cushing's syndrome and hyperthyroidism. Normal value: 8–10 AM: 138–635 nmol 4–6 PM: 83–359 nmol A 24-hour urine test may be conducted to measure free (unbound) cortisol Normal value: < 100 mcg/24 hours	Tell patient not to eat or drink and to rest for 2 hours before the test. Evaluate medications: Cortisol is decreased by androgens, phenytoin (Dilantin), and increased by oral contraceptives, estrogen, spironolactone (Aldactone), and triparanol. Teach patient how to save urine for 24-hour period, to eat a low-sodium diet before the test, and to avoid stressful situations and physical activity for at least 24 hours prior to the test. Assess medications; values may be increased by reserpine (Serpasil), diuretics, phenothiazines, and amphetamines.
Late Night Cortisol Test	This test is used to differentiate the cause of adrenal disorders. A saliva specimen is collected at 11 PM and then dexamethasone 1 mg is administered orally. A serum cortisol is collected at 8 AM the next morning. The dexamethasone suppresses ACTH. If an extremely high dose of dexamethasone is required to suppress ACTH, the primary disorder is adrenal cortex hyperplasia (Cushing's disease). If ACTH is not suppressed with the synthetic cortisol, an adrenal tumor is suspected.	
17-Ketosteroids	This 24-hour urine test is done to measure metabolites in urine and evaluate adrenal cortex function. Normal value: Men: 5–25 mg in 24 hours Women: 5–15 mg in 24 hours	Instruct patient how to save urine (urine must contain a preservative and be refrigerated). Assess medications: Levels are affected by a variety of drugs (check information in agency protocol for test); if possible, these should be discontinued for 48 hours before the test. Women cannot have the test while menstruating because blood can cause a false-positive finding.
Magnetic Resonance Imaging (MRI)—adrenal glands	This radiographic study is done to identify tumors of the adrenal glands.	See information for MRI of the pituitary.
MIBG Scan	This nuclear medicine scan is used to detect the presence and location of adrenal pheochromocytomas. A special radioactive dye is given and concentrates on the tumor in the adrenal gland; the tumor can then be seen on x-ray.	Explain that the test takes about an hour a day for 3 or 4 days.

PANCREATIC ENDOCRINE TESTS

NAME OF TEST	PURPOSE & DESCRIPTION	RELATED NURSING INTERVENTIONS
Computed Tomography (CT) of the abdomen	This radiographic test is done to identify pancreatic tumors or cysts.	If contrast medium is used, assess for allergy to iodine (shellfish).

DIAGNOSTIC TESTS of the Endocrine System (continued)

NAME OF TEST	PURPOSE & DESCRIPTION	RELATED NURSING INTERVENTIONS
Fasting Blood Sugar (FBS)	This test of serum or plasma is used to identify or confirm a diagnosis of diabetes mellitus. It is also used to monitor treatment of diabetes mellitus. A finding of greater than 125 mg/dL, if confirmed with a repeated test on a different day, indicates diabetes mellitus. Normal value: Serum/plasma: 70–110 mg/dL (value varies in individual laboratories)	Tell the patient not to eat or drink for 12 hours before the test. Do not administer insulin until blood specimen is taken. Assess medications: FBS may be increased by cortisone, diuretics, ACTH, levodopa, epinephrine, anesthetics, and phenytoin (Dilantin).
Oral Glucose Tolerance Test (OGTT)	This blood and urine test is used to diagnose diabetes mellitus if prior fasting blood sugar (FBS) findings are increased or inconsistent.	**Nursing Implications for Oral** **Glucose Tolerance Test** The tests will not be done if patient's FBS is consistently high (> 200 mg/dL). The patient drinks a solution of 75 to 100 grams of glucose and samples of blood and urine are taken immediately and at 30, 60, and 120 minutes (or it may extend from 3 to 6 hours). Values for 2-hour plasma at 139 or below are considered normal; values at 200 or greater, if confirmed with a second test on a different day, are diagnostic of diabetes mellitus. Tell the patient not to eat or drink (except water) for 12 hours before the test. Assess medications: Drugs that may increase OGTT levels are steroids, oral contraceptives, estrogens, thiazide diuretics, and salicylates. Explain to the patient that he or she may feel weak and may perspire during the test and that these symptoms should be reported to the nurse. Although they usually are transitory, they may be manifestations of hyperinsulinism.
Glycosylated Hemoglobin (Hb A$_1$C)	This serum test is used to measure the effectiveness of treatment of diabetes mellitus. The results represent an average blood glucose level during a 1- to 4-month period; an elevated level indicates uncontrolled diabetes mellitus and increased risk for complications. Normal value: In most labs, the normal range is 4% to 5.9%. In poorly controlled diabetes, its 8.0% or above, and in well controlled patients it is less than 7.0%.	Monitor findings: Decreased levels can be caused by anemia, long-term blood loss, and chronic renal failure. Increased levels may result from hyperglycemia, alcohol ingestion, pregnancy, hemodialysis, and prolonged cortisone intake.
Magnetic Resonance Imaging (MRI)— pancreas	This radiographic study is done to identify tumors of the pancreas.	See information for MRI of the pituitary.

Genetic Considerations

When conducting a health assessment interview and physical assessment, it is important for the nurse to consider genetic influences on the health of the adult. During the health assessment interview, ask about endocrine disorders in immediate family members, including the family members' age of onset and gender. Ask the patient about a family history of such diseases as diabetes mellitus, diabetes insipidus, thyroid disorders, growth problems, hypertension, and obesity. Ask women about problems with pregnancy, menstruation, and/or menopause.

During the physical assessment, assess for any manifestations that might indicate a genetic disorder (see the following box). If data are found to indicate genetic risk factors or alterations, ask about genetic testing and refer for appropriate genetic counseling and evaluation. ∞ Chapter 8 provides further information about genetics in medical-surgical nursing.

Health Assessment Interview

A health assessment interview to determine problems with the endocrine system may be part of a health screening or total health assessment, or it may focus on a chief complaint (such as increased urination or changes in energy levels). If the patient has a problem with endocrine function, the nurse analyzes its onset, characteristics and course, severity, precipitating and relieving factors, and any associated symptoms, noting the timing and circumstances. For example, the nurse may ask the patient the following:

- "Describe the swelling you noticed in the front of your neck. When did it begin? Have you noticed any changes in your energy level? If so, describe them."
- "When did you first notice that your hands and feet were getting larger?"
- "Have you noticed that your appetite has increased even though you have lost weight?"

GENETIC CONSIDERATIONS
Examples of Endocrine System Disorders

- Type 1 and type 2 diabetes mellitus are classified as multifactorial inheritance disorders because both genetic and environmental factors are necessary for onset of the disorder.
- Pendred syndrome is an inherited disorder in which people have deafness and a thyroid goiter.
- Hashimoto's disease (chronic thyroiditis) is believed to have a genetic component.
- Multiple endocrine neoplasia is a group of rare diseases caused by genetic defects leading to hyperplasia and hyperfunction of two or more components of the endocrine system (especially the parathyroid, pancreas, and pituitary glands).
- Fragile X syndrome is a genetic condition that causes developmental problems including learning disabilities and mental retardation. Males are usually more severely affected than females.

The health history includes information about the patient's medical history, family history, and social and personal history. Ask the patient about any changes in normal growth and development as well as in height and weight. Changes in the size of extremities can often be detected by asking whether the patient has had to have rings enlarged or to buy increasingly larger gloves and shoes. Enlargement of the neck may be identified by asking whether the patient has difficulty finding shirts or blouses with a collar that fits. Also explore changes such as difficulty swallowing; increased or decreased thirst, appetite, and/or urination; visual changes; sleep disturbances; altered patterns of hair distribution (such as increased facial hair in women); changes in menstruation; changes in memory or ability to concentrate; and changes in hair and skin texture. Ask the patient about any injury or surgery of the head, as well as previous hospitalizations,

chemotherapy, radiation (especially to the neck), and the use of medications (especially hormones or steroids).

The nurse also asks about the patient's occupational and social history. Include questions about the patient's satisfaction with occupation, personal relationships, and lifestyle. Other areas of assessment include the patient's usual means of coping; use of alcohol, smoking, or drugs; diet (including weight gain or loss); exercise patterns; and sleep patterns. Although the patient may not recognize changes in behavior, family members may be able to provide important information.

Interview questions categorized by functional health patterns are listed on page 489.

Physical Assessment

Physical assessment of the endocrine system may be performed as part of a total health assessment or it may be a focused assessment of patients with known or suspected problems with endocrine function. Sample documentation of an assessment of the thyroid gland is included in the following box.

The only endocrine organ that can be palpated is the thyroid gland; however, other assessments that provide information about endocrine pathophysiology include inspection of the skin, hair, nails, facial appearance, reflexes, and musculoskeletal system. Measuring and monitoring trends in height and weight and vital signs also provide clues to altered endocrine system function.

The patient may sit during the examination. A reflex hammer is used to test deep tendon reflexes. Prior to the examination, the nurse collects the necessary equipment and explains the techniques to the patient to decrease anxiety. Additional techniques for assessing hypocalcemic tetany, a complication of endocrine disorders or surgery, are included here in the examination sequence. Normal age-related changes in assessment findings are described in Table 18–2.

Thyroid Disorders Video

NURSING CARE OF THE OLDER ADULT — Age-Related Endocrine Changes

AGE-RELATED CHANGE	SIGNIFICANCE
Pituitary: production of ACTH, TSH, FSH	Decreased secretion of glucocorticoids, 17-ketosteroids, progesterone, androgen, and estrogen (and thus lower levels on diagnostic tests)
Thyroid: in fibrosis and nodularity, in gland activity	Lower basal metabolic rate • Increased incidence of hypothyroidism • Palpable nodules on palpation
Adrenal medulla: secretion and level of norepinephrine, beta-adrenergic response to norepinephrine	Decreased response to beta-adrenergic and receptor blockers (medications) • May contribute to increased incidence of hypertension
Pancreas: calcification of blood vessels and distention and dilation of pancreatic ducts	Decreased production of lipase with reduced fat absorption and digestion, leading to intolerance of fatty foods and indigestion • Decreased absorption of fat-soluble vitamins
Pancreas: delayed and decreased insulin release; believed accompanied by decreased sensitivity to circulating insulin	Decreased ability to metabolize glucose with higher and more prolonged blood glucose levels may contribute to increased incidence of type 2 diabetes mellitus with aging (however, higher than normal blood glucose levels are not unusual in nondiabetic older adults)

FUNCTIONAL HEALTH PATTERN INTERVIEW Endocrine System

Functional Health Pattern	Interview Questions and Leading Statements
Health Perception-Health Management	■ Describe your overall state of health, rating it on a scale of 1 to 10 with 10 being the best health you have had. ■ Describe any problems you have had with an endocrine gland (pituitary, thyroid, parathyroid, adrenal, pancreas, ovaries, testes). ■ If you had a problem with any of these glands, how was it treated (medications, surgery, diet, hormone replacement)? ■ Do you smoke, drink alcohol, and/or use recreational drugs? If so, how much and what kind? ■ Have you ever been tested for high or low blood sugar?
Nutritional-Metabolic	■ Describe what you eat and how much (and type of) fluid you drink in a 24-hour period. ■ Do you take any nutritional supplements, herbs, or vitamins? ■ Have you noticed any change in your hunger or thirst? ■ Has your weight changed? If so, how many pounds and over what time period? ■ Have you noticed any change in your energy level? If so, explain. ■ Have you noticed any change in your ability to tolerate heat or cold? If so, describe the change. ■ Have you noticed any difficulty swallowing? Explain. ■ Have you noticed any changes in the texture of your skin? If so, what were they?
Elimination	■ Have you noticed any change in the color, odor, amount, or frequency of urination? If so, describe it. ■ Have you ever had kidney stones? If so, how were they treated? ■ Has there been a change in your bowel elimination (such as diarrhea or constipation)? If so, explain the change.
Activity-Exercise	■ Describe your physical activities in a usual day. ■ Has your energy level increased or decreased? Explain. ■ Do some activities make you very tired? Explain how you feel.
Sleep-Rest	■ How many hours of sleep do you get each night? ■ Do you feel nervous and unable to rest? Explain. ■ Have you ever sweated at night? Describe if so.
Cognitive-Perceptual	■ Have you noticed any problem with your memory? What was it? ■ Do you feel restless, anxious, or confused? Explain. ■ Have you noticed any change in your voice? Explain. ■ Have you noticed any change in the color or condition of your skin and hair (color, dryness, oiliness, bruises)? Describe if so. ■ Have you had any headaches, memory loss, changes in sensation, depression? Describe if so. ■ Have you noticed any change in your vision? Describe if so. ■ Have you had any heart palpitations? When did they occur? ■ Have you had any abdominal pain? What is it like and where is it located? ■ Have you had any pain or stiffness in your muscles and joints?
Self-Perception-Self-Concept	■ How does this condition make you feel about yourself? ■ How do you feel about taking medications?
Role-Relationships	■ How does this condition make you feel about yourself? How does this condition affect your relationships with others? ■ Does anyone in your family have an endocrine disorder? If so, when did it begin and how does it affect them? What family member is affected and at what age did it begin?
Coping-Stress-Tolerance	■ Does stress seem to make your condition worse? Explain. ■ Has this condition created stress for you? ■ Describe what you do when you feel stressed.
Value-Belief	■ Tell me how specific relationships or activities help you cope with this condition. ■ Describe specific cultural beliefs or practices that affect how you care for and feel about this condition. ■ Is there anything interfering with your spiritual beliefs, needs, or practices during your illness? What can I or another caregiver do to help you with your spiritual needs? ■ Are there any specific treatments that you would not use to treat this condition?

Endocrine Assessments

TABLE 18–2 Endocrine Assessments

TECHNIQUE/NORMAL FINDINGS	ABNORMAL FINDINGS
Skin Assessments	
Inspect skin color. *Skin color should be even and appropriate to age and race of the patient.*	■ Hyperpigmentation may be seen in patients with Addison's disease or Cushing's syndrome. ■ Hypopigmentation may be seen in diabetes mellitus, hyperthyroidism, or hypothyroidism. ■ A yellowish cast to the skin might indicate hypothyroidism. ■ Purple striae over the abdomen and bruising may be present in the patient with Cushing's syndrome.
Palpate the skin, assessing texture, moisture, and the presence of lesions. *Skin color should be appropriate to the patient's race, smooth, warm, dry, and intact without lesions.*	■ Rough, dry skin is often seen in patients with hypothyroidism, whereas smooth and flushed skin can be a sign of hyperthyroidism. ■ Lesions (such as ulcerations) on the lower extremities might indicate diabetes mellitus.
Nails and Hair Assessment	
Assess texture, distribution, and condition of nails and hair. *Hair should be of normal texture, appropriately distributed for gender; nail surfaces should have even color with smooth surfaces.*	■ Increased pigmentation of the nails is often seen in patients with Addison's disease. ■ Dry, thick, brittle nails and hair may be apparent in hypothyroidism; thin, brittle nails and thin, soft hair may be apparent in hyperthyroidism. ■ Hirsutism (excessive facial, chest, or abdominal hair) may be seen in Cushing's syndrome.
Facial Assessments	
Inspect the symmetry and form of the face. *Face should be bilaterally symmetrical.*	■ Variations of form and structure may indicate growth abnormalities such as **acromegaly** (continued growth of bone from growth hormone hypersecretion).
Inspect position of eyes. *Eyes should be equal in position on both sides of the face. Eyelids should close over eyes.*	■ **Exophthalmos** (protruding eyes) may be seen in hyperthyroidism.
Thyroid Gland Assessment	
Palpate the thyroid gland for size and consistency.	■ The thyroid may be enlarged in patients with Graves' disease or a **goiter** (enlarged thyroid gland).
Stand behind the patient and place your fingers on either side of the trachea below the thyroid cartilage (Figure 18–8 ■). Ask the patient to tilt his or her head to the right. Now ask the patient to swallow. As the patient swallows, displace the left lobe while palpating the right lobe. Repeat to palpate the left lobe. *Thyroid gland is not usually palpable. If it is, lobes should feel smooth, rubbery, and free of nodules.*	■ Multiple nodules may be seen in metabolic disorders, whereas the presence of only one nodule may indicate a cyst or a benign or malignant tumor. ■ A single enlarged nodule suggests malignancy. **Figure 18–8** ■ Palpating the thyroid gland from behind the patient.
Motor Function Assessment	
Assess the deep tendon reflexes. Deep tendon reflexes are assessed with the reflex hammer, and include the biceps reflex, brachioradialis reflex, triceps reflex, patellar reflex, and Achilles reflex. *Normal values range from 1+ (present, but decreased) to 2+ (normal) to 3+ (increased).* ∞ See Chapter 43 for guidelines and illustrations of deep tendon reflex assessment.	■ Increased reflexes may be seen in hyperthyroidism; decreased reflexes may be seen in hypothyroidism.

TABLE 18–2 Endocrine Assessments (continued)

TECHNIQUE/NORMAL FINDINGS	ABNORMAL FINDINGS
Sensory Function Assessment Test the patient's sensitivity to pain, temperature, vibration, light touch, and stereognosis (the ability to identify an object by touch). Compare symmetric areas on both sides of the body, and compare the distal to the proximal regions of the extremities. Ask the patient to close his or her eyes. *Sensory function should be bilaterally intact.* ■ To test pain, use the blunt and sharp ends of a new safety pin. Discard the pin after use. ■ To test temperature, use cups or other containers of cold and hot water. ■ To test vibration, use a tuning fork over one of the patient's finger or toe joints. ■ To test light touch, use a cotton wisp. ■ To test stereognosis, place in the patient's hand a simple, familiar object, such as a rubber band, cotton ball, or button. Ask the patient to identify the object.	■ Peripheral neuropathy and paresthesias (altered sensations) may occur in diabetes, hypothyroidism, or acromegaly.
Musculoskeletal Assessment Inspect the size and proportions of the patient's body structure. *Size and proportion of body structures should be bilaterally equal.*	■ Extremely short stature may indicate **dwarfism** (a condition characterized by short stature); insufficient pituitary growth hormone is one cause. ■ Extremely large bones may indicate acromegaly, caused by excessive growth hormone.
Assessing for Hypocalcemic Tetany Assess for **Trousseau's sign** (a test for hypocalcemia) with resulting **tetany** (tonic muscle spasms) by inflating a blood pressure cuff above the antecubital space to a point greater than systolic blood pressure for 2 to 5 minutes. Trousseau's sign is discussed in relation to hypocalcemia in ∞ Chapter 10. *A normal finding is no carpal spasm in response to compression of the arm by the blood pressure cuff.*	■ Decreased calcium levels cause the patient's hand and fingers to contract (**carpal spasm**).
Assess for **Chvostek's sign** (a test for hypocalcemia) by tapping your finger in front of the patient's ear at the angle of the jaw. A positive Chvostek's sign causes facial grimacing due to repeated contractions of the facial muscle. Chvostek's sign is discussed and illustrated in relation to hypocalcemia in ∞ Chapter 10. *A normal finding is no facial grimacing in response to tapping the patient's face in front of the ear.*	■ Decreased calcium levels cause the patient's lateral facial muscles to contract.

SAMPLE DOCUMENTATION
Assessment of the Thyroid Gland

A 37-year-old female presents at a community clinic for complaints of "always feeling so hot," "always hungry but losing weight," and "can't sleep at night—too jittery." Weight 110 lb (loss of 12 pounds in last 3 months). BP 90/78 (averages 84/72), P 96. Skin very warm and moist. Anterior neck has diffuse enlargement. Thyroid gland enlarged bilaterally on palpation. Referral made to endocrine clinic for further evaluation.

TEST YOURSELF NCLEX-RN® REVIEW

1. What assessment would the nurse expect if the pituitary produces an increased amount of ADH?
   1. increased output of urine
   2. decreased output of urine
   3. increased facial hair growth in women
   4. decreased production of testosterone

2. What assessment might a nurse make to identify low calcium levels?
   1. Save urine to measure 7-ketosteroids.
   2. Palpate turgor of skin.
   3. Conduct a Trousseau's sign test.
   4. Observe color of skin.

3. Excessive amounts of glucocorticoids, produced by the adrenal cortex, result in what pathophysiologic health problem?
   1. inhibited immune response
   2. increased response to glucagon
   3. delayed onset of puberty
   4. decreased metabolic rate

4. A nurse is conducting a health history focused on the endocrine system. Which of the following questions should be included?
   1. "When did you first notice the pain in your abdomen?"
   2. "Do your children have problems with urination?"
   3. "Have you noticed a change in your thirst?"
   4. "How did you get this scar on your leg?"

5. What assessments are made when the nurse palpates the thyroid gland?
   1. edema and movement
   2. size and consistency
   3. character and texture
   4. pain and pulse rate

6. Decreased calcium levels can be assessed with Chvostek's sign. What does the nurse do to conduct this assessment?
   1. inflates a blood pressure cuff above the antecubital space
   2. taps the finger in front of the patient's ear
   3. depresses the skin over the shin
   4. pinches a fold of skin over the sternum

7. Which of the following tests is the most accurate indicator of thyroid function?
   1. GH
   2. FBS
   3. aldosterone
   4. TSH

8. A nurse is conducting an assessment of the endocrine system in an older adult woman. What assessment is the result of aging?
   1. pituitary enlarged and firm
   2. normal heart tones
   3. thyroid nodules present
   4. decreased facial hair

9. A nurse is caring for a patient with newly diagnosed hypothyroidism. What skin assessment might be expected?
   1. increased hair growth
   2. rough, dry skin
   3. smooth, flushed skin
   4. cold and clammy skin

10. What endocrine disorder might the nurse assess by testing deep tendon reflexes?
    1. Cushing's syndrome
    2. acromegaly
    3. tetany
    4. hyperthyroidism

See Test Yourself answers in Appendix C.

Pearson Nursing Student Resources

Find additional review materials at
www.nursing.pearsonhighered.com

Prepare for success with additional NCLEX®-style practice questions, interactive assignments and activities, Web links, animations and videos, and more!

BIBLIOGRAPHY

Armstrong, J., & Mitchell, E. (2008). Comprehensive nursing assessment in the care of older people. *Nursing Older People, (20)*1, 36–40.

Bald, H. (2006). The process of conducting a physical assessment: A nursing perspective. *British Journal of Nursing, 15*(13), 710–714.

Bickley, L., & Szilagyi, P. (2007). *Bates' guide to physical examination and history taking* (9th ed.). Philadelphia: Lippincott.

Costello, T., & Coyne, I. (2008). Nurses' knowledge of mouth care practices. *British Journal of Nursing, 17*(4), 264–268.

Daddario, D. (2007). A review of the use of the health belief model for weight management. *MEDSURG Nursing, 16*(6), 363–366.

D'Amico, D., & Barbarito, C. (2007). *Health & physical assessment in nursing.* Upper Saddle River, NJ: Pearson Prentice Hall.

Dufour, D. (2007). Laboratory tests of thyroid function: Uses and limitations. *Endocrinology and Metabolism Clinics of North America, 36*(3), 579–594.

Eliopoulos, C. (2005). *Gerontological nursing* (6th ed.). Philadelphia: Lippincott.

Fletcher, J. (2006). Full nursing assessment of patients at risk of diabetic foot ulcers. *British Journal of Nursing, 15*(15). Tissue Viability Supplement: S18, S20–S21.

Galland, L. (2008). Mystery illness: When fatigue just won't go away. *Bottom Line/Health, 22*(4), 15.

Harrison, S., Cochrane, L., Abboud, R., & Leese, G. (2007). Do patients with diabetes wear shoes of the correct size? *International Journal of Clinical Practice, 61*(11), 1900–1904.

Karnath, B. M., & Hussain, N. (2006). Signs and symptoms of thyroid dysfunction. *Hospital Physician, 42*(10), 43–48.

Kee, J. (2009). *Prentice Hall handbook of laboratory & diagnostic tests with nursing implications* (6th ed.). Upper Saddle River, NJ: Pearson Prentice Hall.

Levin, N., & Greer, K. (2004). Cutaneous manifestations of endocrine disorders. *Dermatology Nursing, 13*(3), 185–186, 189–196, 201–202.

Lie, D. (2008). MRI may be more accurate than fine-needle biopsy in detection of thyroid cancer. Retrieved from http//www.medscape.com/viewarticle/566491

Lloyd, H., & Craig, S. (2007). A guide to taking a patient's history. *Nursing Standard, 22*(13), 42–48.

McClane, K. (2006). Screening instruments for use in a complete geriatric assessment. *Clinical Nurse Specialist, 20*(4), 201–207.

National Institute of Health. (2008). *Genes and disease: Nutritional and metabolic diseases; glands and hormones.* Retrieved from http://www.ncbi.nlm.nih.gov/books/bookres.fegi/gnd/pdf.html

Porth, C. M. (2007). *Essentials of pathophysiology: Concepts of altered health states* (2nd ed.). Philadelphia: Lippincott.

Porth, C. M., & Matfin, G. (2009). *Concepts of altered health states* (8th ed.). Philadelphia: Lippincott Williams & Wilkins.

Pullen, R. L. (2008). Preparing a patient for magnetic resonance imaging. *Nursing, 38,*10, 22.

U. S. Food and Drug Administration [FDA]. (2009). *FDA warns about risk of wearing medicated patches during MRIs.* Retrieved from http://www.fda.gov/bbs/topics/news/2009/new01967.html

Weber, J., & Kelley, J. (2009). *Health assessment in nursing* (4th ed.). Philadelphia: Lippincott Williams & Wilkins.

LEARNING OUTCOMES

1. Apply knowledge of normal anatomy, physiology, and assessments of the thyroid, parathyroid, adrenal, and pituitary glands when providing nursing care for patients with endocrine disorders.
2. Compare and contrast the manifestations of disorders that result from hyperfunction and hypofunction of the thyroid, parathyroid, adrenal, and pituitary glands.
3. Explain the nursing implications for medications prescribed to treat disorders of the thyroid and adrenal glands.
4. Provide appropriate nursing care for the patient before and after a subtotal thyroidectomy and an adrenalectomy.
5. Use the nursing process as a framework for providing individualized care to patients with disorders of the thyroid, parathyroid, adrenal, and pituitary glands.

CLINICAL COMPETENCIES

1. Assess functional health status of patients with endocrine disorders and monitor, document, and report abnormal manifestations.
2. Use assessed data, patient values, clinical expertise, and evidence to determine priority nursing diagnoses and select and implement nursing interventions.
3. Effectively communicate with and function within the interdisciplinary team to plan and provide patient care.
4. Administer medications knowledgeably and safely.
5. Plan and provide patient and family teaching to promote, restore, and maintain functional health status.
6. Monitor for respiratory problems and tetany in patients having a thyroidectomy.
7. Adapt individual and cultural values and variations as well as expressed needs and preferences into the plan of care.
8. Evaluate responses to care and use data to revise plan as needed.

KEY TERMS

acromegaly, 516
Addisonian crisis, 512
diabetes insipidus, 517
euthyroid, 496
exophthalmos, 494
gigantism, 516
goiter, 494

hyperparathyroidism, 505
hypoparathyroidism, 506
myxedema, 500
myxedema coma, 502
proptosis, 494
syndrome of inappropriate ADH
   secretion (SIADH), 516

tetany, 506
thyroid storm or crisis, 496
thyroidectomy, 497
thyroiditis, 496
thyrotoxicosis, 494

The thyroid, parathyroid, adrenal, and pituitary glands are part of the endocrine system. Disorders of the structure and function of these glands alter normal hormone levels and the way body tissues use those hormones. When hormone production increases or decreases, people experience alterations in health.

Patients with disorders of the glands discussed in this chapter require nursing care for multiple functional problems. They often face exhausting diagnostic tests, changes in physical appearance and emotional responses, and permanent alterations in lifestyle. Nursing care is directed toward meeting physiologic needs, providing education, and ensuring psychologic support for the patient and family. A holistic approach to the complex needs of patients with these endocrine disorders is an essential component of nursing care.

Disorders of the Thyroid Gland

Altered thyroid hormone (TH) production or use affects all major organ systems. In the adult, TH changes primarily affect metabolism, cardiovascular function, gastrointestinal function, and neuromuscular function. Thyroid disorders—both hyperthyroidism and hypothyroidism—are among the most common endocrine disorders.

The Patient with Hyperthyroidism

Hyperthyroidism (also called **thyrotoxicosis**) is a disorder caused by excessive delivery of TH to the tissues. Because the primary effect of TH is to increase metabolism and protein synthesis, hyperthyroidism affects all major organ systems of the body. The increase in metabolic rate and the alterations in cardiac output, peripheral blood flow, oxygen consumption, and body temperature are similar to those found in increased sympathetic nervous system activity (Porth & Matfin, 2009).

Pathophysiology and Manifestations

The effects of hyperthyroidism are the result of increased circulating levels of TH. This hormonal excess increases the metabolic rate and heightens the sympathetic nervous system's physiologic response to stimulation. The sensitizing effect of abnormally elevated TH levels increases the cardiac rate and stroke volume. As a result, cardiac output and peripheral blood flow increase. Elevated TH levels also increase carbohydrate, protein, and lipid metabolism. Lipids are depleted, and glucose tolerance decreases. Protein degradation increases, resulting in a negative nitrogen balance. Over time, the hypermetabolic effects of excess TH result in caloric and nutritional deficiencies.

Hyperthyroidism results from many different factors, including autoimmune stimulation (as in Graves' disease), excess secretion of thyroid-stimulating hormone (TSH) by the pituitary gland, thyroiditis, neoplasms (such as toxic multinodular goiter), side effect of certain drugs, and an excessive intake of thyroid medications. The most common etiologies of hyperthyroidism are Graves' disease and toxic multinodular goiter.

The patient with hyperthyroidism typically has an increased appetite and may gain weight, although weight loss is more typical, and may have hypermotile bowels and diarrhea. Additional manifestations related to hypermetabolism include emotional liability, heat intolerance, insomnia, palpitations, and increased sweating. The skin is smooth and warm, hair may become fine, and hair loss in the scalp, eyebrow, axilla, or pubic region is common.

Graves' Disease

Graves' disease, the most common cause of hyperthyroidism, is an autoimmune disorder, sometimes associated with the presence of other autoimmune disorders such as myasthenia gravis, diabetes mellitus, celiac, and pernicious anemia (McPhee & Papadakis, 2009). The serum of patients with Graves' disease has an antibody that binds to TSH receptors in the thyroid follicles and causes the thyroid cells to hyperfunction. When this antibody binds to the TSH receptors, it stimulates hormone synthesis and secretion, enlarging the gland. The cause is unknown, but there is a hereditary link. Graves' disease is seen eight times more often in women than in men and occurs most frequently between the ages of 20 and 40 (McPhee & Papadakis, 2009).

Patients with Graves' disease have an enlarged thyroid gland (**goiter**) and manifestations of hyperthyroidism. The goiter can result from excess TSH stimulation (when the amount of circulating TH is deficient), abnormal growth-stimulating immunoglobulins, or substances that inhibit TH synthesis. A goiter may be present in hyperthyroidism or hypothyroidism.

The eye pathophysiology of Graves' disease is manifested as proptosis and visual dysfunction. **Proptosis** (forward displacement) of the eye occurs in about one-third of cases (Porth, 2007). The forward protrusion of the eyeballs (**exophthalmos**) results from an accumulation of inflammation by-products in the retro-orbital tissues. The sclera may be visible above the iris, the upper lids may be retracted, and the person has a characteristic unblinking stare (Figure 19–1 ■). Exophthalmos is usually bilateral, but it may involve only one eye. The patient may experience blurred vision, diplopia, eye pain, lacrimation, and photophobia. The inability to close the eyelids completely over the protruding eyeballs increases the risk of corneal dryness, irritation, infection, and ulceration. Infiltration of the muscles that move the eye and of the optic nerve lead to paralysis and vision loss. The treatment of Graves' disease may stabilize the manifestations but generally does not reverse these changes in the eyes.

Other manifestations include fatigue, difficulty sleeping, hand tremors, and changes in menstruation ranging from decreased flow to amenorrhea. Older patients may present with atrial fibrillation, angina, or congestive heart failure.

Figure 19–1 ■ Exophthalmos in a patient with Graves' disease. The disease causes edema of fat deposits behind the eyes and inflammation of the extraocular muscles. The accumulating pressure forces the eyes outward from their orbits.

Source: University of Illinois, Custom Medical Stock Photo, Inc.

MULTISYSTEM EFFECTS OF
Hyperthyroidism

Endocrine
• Goiter

Respiratory
• Dyspnea

Gastrointestinal
• Nausea
• Vomiting
• Diarrhea
• Abdominal pain

Musculoskeletal
• Muscle wasting
• Weakness
• Fatigue

Neurologic
• Hand and eye tremors
• Nervousness
• Insomnia
• Emotional lability
• ↑ reflexes

Sensory
• Blurred vision
• Photophobia
• Lacrimation
• Exophthalmos (Graves' disease)

Cardiovascular
• Hypertension
• Tachycardia
• Dysrhythmias
• Palpitations

Reproductive
• Amenorrhea (female)
• ↓ fertility (female)
• ↓ libido (male)
• Impotence (male)

Integumentary
• Fine, thin hair
• Flushed, moist skin

Metabolic Processes
• Hyperthermia
• Diaphoresis
• Hunger
• Weight loss
• Fluid volume deficit

Toxic Multinodular Goiter

Toxic multinodular goiter (Figure 19–2 ■) is a thyroid tumor characterized by small, discrete, independently functioning nodules in the thyroid gland tissue that secrete excessive amounts of TH. It is not known how these nodules grow or become independent, but a genetic mutation of follicle cells is suspected. Elevated TH levels result in manifestations of hyperthyroidism; however, they are slower to develop and there is no pathophysiology involving the eyes or skin (Davis, Orlander, & Kermani, 2008). The patient with this type of hyperthyroidism is usually a woman in her 60s or 70s who has had a goiter for a number of years.

Thyroiditis

Thyroiditis (inflammation of the thyroid gland) is most often the result of a viral infection of the thyroid gland. The manifestations of thyroiditis are those of acute inflammation and the effects of increased TH. Thyroiditis is an acute disorder that may become chronic, resulting in a hypothyroid state as repeated infections destroy gland tissue. See the discussion of Hashimoto's thyroiditis later in this chapter.

Thyroid Crisis

Thyroid crisis (also called **thyroid storm**) is an extreme state of hyperthyroidism that is rare today because of improved diagnosis and treatment methods (Porth & Matfin, 2009). When it does occur, those affected are usually people with untreated hyperthyroidism (most often Graves' disease) and people with hyperthyroidism who have experienced a stressor, such as an infection, trauma, untreated diabetic ketoacidosis, or manipulation of the thyroid gland during surgery. Thyroid crisis is a life-threatening condition.

Figure 19–2 ■ Toxic multinodular goiter. The formation and growth of numerous nodules in the thyroid gland cause the characteristic massive enlargement of the neck.

The rapid increase in metabolic rate that results from the excessive TH causes the manifestations of thyroid crisis. The manifestations include hyperthermia, with body temperatures ranging from 102°F to 106°F (39°C to 41°C), tachycardia, systolic hypertension, dyspnea, and GI manifestations (abdominal pain, vomiting, diarrhea). Agitation, restlessness, and tremors are common, progressing to confusion, psychosis, delirium, and seizures. Unrecognized and untreated, the mortality rate is high. Rapid treatment of thyroid storm is essential to preserve life. Treatment includes cooling without aspirin (which increases free TH) or inducing shivering; replacing fluids, glucose, and electrolytes; relieving respiratory distress by administering oxygen; stabilizing cardiovascular function; and reducing TH synthesis and secretion.

> **MEMORY CUE**
> Excessive hormone amplifies manifestations of normal levels of the hormone.

Interdisciplinary Care

Treatment of hyperthyroidism focuses on reducing the production of TH by the thyroid gland, thus establishing a **euthyroid** (normal thyroid) state, and preventing or treating complications. Depending on the patient's age and physical status, either medications, radioactive iodine therapy, or surgery may be used.

Diagnosis

Hyperthyroidism is diagnosed according to the manifestations of the specific disorders causing excessive TH, and by the diagnostic test results described in ∞ Chapter 18. Elevated levels of TH (both T_3 and T_4) and increased radioactive iodine (RAI) uptake are diagnostic criteria of hyperthyroidism. In addition, a TSH (thyroid stimulating hormone) level may be measured and compared with thyroxine (T_4) to differentiate pituitary dysfunction from thyroid dysfunction. Other diagnostic tests include RAI, thyroid antibodies (TA), TSH, Triiodothyronine (T_3), T_4, and triiodothyronine resin uptake (T_3RU). Laboratory findings in hyperthyroidism are outlined in Table 19–1. A thyroid scan may be used to evaluate thyroid nodules and an MRI of the thyroid is used to identify thyroid tumors.

Medications

Hyperthyroidism is treated by administering antithyroid medications that reduce TH production. Because these drugs do not affect the release or activity of hormone that is already formed, therapeutic effects may not be seen for several weeks. To rapidly decrease the cardiovascular manifestations associated with hyperthyroidism, propanolol (Inderal) (a beta-blocker) or esmolol (a rapid-acting parenteral beta-blocker) is part of initial treatment. (∞ See Chapter 31 for information on beta-blockers.) Some commonly prescribed drugs, their actions, and nursing implications are shown in the Medication Administration box on page 497.

Radioactive Iodine Therapy

Because the thyroid gland takes up iodine in any form, radioactive iodine (^{131}I) concentrates in the thyroid gland and damages or destroys thyroid cells so that they produce less TH. Radioactive iodine is given orally. Results typically

TABLE 19–1 Laboratory Findings in Thyroid Disorders

TEST	NORMAL VALUES	HYPERTHYROIDISM	HYPOTHYROIDISM
Serum TA	Negative to 1:20	Increased	Normal
Serum TSH (sensitive assay)	2 to 10 mU/ml	Decreased in primary hyperthyroidism	Increased in primary hypothyroidism
Serum T_4	5 to 12 mcg/dL	Increased	Decreased
Serum T_3	80 to 200 ng/dL	Increased	Decreased
T_3 uptake (T_3RU)	25 to 35 relative percentage	Increased	Decreased
Thyroid suppression		Increased RAI uptake and T_4 levels	No change

occur in 6 to 8 weeks. In most instances, the patient is not hospitalized during treatment and does not require radiation precautions. This type of therapy is contraindicated in pregnant women because radioactive iodine crosses the placenta and can have negative effects on the developing fetal thyroid gland. Because the amount of gland destroyed is not readily controllable, the patient may develop hypothyroidism and require lifelong TH replacement. Adverse reactions include thyroiditis and cardiac instability due to liberation of stored thyroid hormone in the gland (Holcomb, 2006).

Surgery

Some hyperthyroid patients have such enlarged thyroid glands that pressure on the esophagus or trachea causes breathing or swallowing problems. In these cases, removal of all or part of the gland (**thyroidectomy**) is indicated. A subtotal thyroidectomy is usually performed. This procedure leaves enough of the gland in place to produce an adequate amount of TH. A total thyroidectomy is performed to treat cancer of the thyroid; the patient then requires lifelong hormone replacement (McPhee & Papadakis, 2009).

Before surgery, the patient should be in as nearly a euthyroid state as possible. The patient may be given antithyroid drugs to reduce hormone levels and iodine preparations to decrease the vascularity and size of the gland (which also reduces the risk of hemorrhage during and after surgery). Nursing care of the patient having a subtotal thyroidectomy is discussed in the box on page 499.

♋ Nursing Care

Health Promotion

Although hyperthyroidism is not preventable, it is important to teach patients the importance of regular healthcare provider visits and medication intake.

MEDICATION ADMINISTRATION Hyperthyroidism

IODINE SOURCES

Strong Iodine Solution (Lugol's Solution)

Potassium iodide (SSKI, Thyro-Block, Pima)

Large doses of iodine for a short term inhibit TH synthesis and release. Iodine also makes the hyperplastic thyroid less vascular prior to surgery and hastens the ability of other antithyroid drugs to reduce natural hormone output. It is also used in thyroid storm.

Nursing Responsibilities

■ Assess for hypersensitivity to iodine before giving medication; for example, ask patient about allergies to shellfish.

■ Dilute liquid iodine sources in water or orange juice to disguise bitter taste.

■ Monitor for increased bleeding tendencies if the patient is also taking anticoagulants; iodine increases their effect.

Health Education for the Patient and Family

■ The maximum effect of iodine in large doses usually occurs in 10 to 15 days.

■ Long-term iodine therapy is not effective in controlling hyperthyroidism.

ANTITHYROID DRUGS

Methimazole (Tapazole)

Carbimazole (converted to methimazole when absorbed)

Propylthiouracil (PTU, Propyl-Thyracil)

Antithyroid drugs inhibit TH production. They do not affect already formed hormones; thus, several weeks may elapse before the patient experiences therapeutic effects. Methimazole crosses the placenta and cannot be taken during pregnancy (Cooper, 2005).

Nursing Responsibilities

■ Monitor for side effects: agranulocytosis (reduction in neutrophils, eosinophils, or basophils), hypothyroidism, pruritus rash, elevated temperature, (for iodides) periorbital edema, anorexia, loss of taste, hair loss, changes in menstruation.

■ Administer drugs at the same time each day with meals to maintain stable blood levels.

■ Monitor for manifestations of hypothyroidism: fatigue, weight gain.

Health Education for the Patient and Family

■ Watch for unusual bleeding, redness, swelling, nausea, loss of taste, or epigastric pain. Report any such manifestations to the physician.

■ Propylthiouracil is associated with weight changes; check weight daily when starting this medication to determine effect. Report significant changes to physician.

■ If you are also taking warfarin, report any signs of bleeding.

■ If you are taking lithium, be aware of manifestations of hypothyroidism.

■ It may take up to 12 weeks before you experience the full effects of the drugs. Take the medication regularly and exactly as prescribed. Do not discontinue abruptly.

Assessment

The following data are collected through the health history and physical examination. Further focused assessments are described with nursing interventions.

- *Health history:* Other diseases, family history of thyroid disease, when manifestations began, severity of manifestations, intake of thyroid medications, menstrual history, changes in weight, bowel elimination.
- *Physical assessment:* Muscle strength, tremors, vital signs, cardiovascular and peripheral vascular systems, integument, size of thyroid, presence of bruit over thyroid, eyes and vision.

Nursing Diagnoses and Interventions

In planning and implementing nursing care for the patient with hyperthyroidism, the nurse considers the patient's responses to the systemic effects of the disorder. Although each patient may have different needs, nursing diagnoses discussed in this section focus on the most common health problems: cardiovascular problems, visual deficits, altered nutrition, and disturbed body image. See the accompanying Case Study & Nursing Care Plan on page 500.

Risk for Decreased Cardiac Output

The patient with hyperthyroidism is at risk for alterations in cardiac output. Excess TH directly affects the heart, resulting in increased rate and stroke volume. Increases in the metabolic demands and oxygen requirements of peripheral tissues increase the demands on the heart, and systolic hypertension, angina, dysrhythmias, or cardiac failure may occur. The patient often has palpitations and shortness of breath and is easily fatigued. The risk of complications is greater in patients with preexisting cardiovascular disorders.

- Monitor blood pressure, pulse rate and rhythm, respiratory rate, and breath sounds. Assess for peripheral edema, jugular vein distention, and increased activity intolerance. *Increased TH increases cardiac rate, stroke volume, and tissue demand for oxygen, causing stress on the heart. This may result in hypertension, arrhythmias, tachycardia, and congestive heart failure.*
- Suggest keeping the environment as cool and free of distraction as possible. Decrease stress by explaining interventions

EVIDENCE FOR NURSING CARE

The Patient with Thyroid Disorders (Hypo, Hyper, or Both)

Selected resources that nurses may find helpful when planning evidence-based nursing care follow.

- Kulie, T., Groff, A., Redmer, J. Hounshell, J., & Schrager, S. (2009). Vitamin D: An evidence-based review. *The Journal of the American Board of Family Medicine, 22*(6), 698–706.
- Surks, M. I., Ortiz, E., Daniels, G. H., Sawin, C. T., Col, N. F., Cobin, R. H., et al. (2004). Subclinical thyroid disease: Scientific review and guidelines for diagnosis and management. *National Clearinghouse Guideline.* Retrieved from http://www.guideline.gov/summary/summary.aspx?doc_id=5916&nbr=003902&string=hyperthyroid

and teaching relaxation procedures. *A physically comfortable and psychologically calm environment can reduce stimuli and stressors. Stress increases circulating catecholamines, which further increase cardiac workload.*

- Encourage a balance of activity with rest periods. *Rest periods decrease energy expenditure and tissue requirements for oxygen, decreasing demands cardiac workload.*

Disturbed Sensory Perception: Visual

Visual changes that occur in patients with hyperthyroidism include difficulty focusing, diplopia (double vision), or visual loss. If the patient is unable to close the eyelids because of exophthalmos, the risk of corneal dryness with resultant infection or injury increases. Visual deficits may also result from pressure on the optic nerve from retro-orbital edema. Although treatment of hyperthyroidism may stop the progression of eye changes, not all manifestations are reversible.

- Monitor visual acuity, photophobia (excessive sensitivity to light), integrity of the cornea, and lid closure. *The cornea is at risk for dryness, injury, conjunctivitis, and corneal infections. Injury and infection of the cornea can result in further loss of visual acuity.*
- Teach measures for protecting the eye from injury and maintaining visual acuity:
  - Use tinted glasses or shields as protection.
  - Use artificial tears to moisten the eyes.
  - Use cool, moist compresses to relieve irritation.
  - Promptly report any pain or changes in vision.

PRACTICE ALERT
Teach the patient to cover the eyes at night if they do not close, and to sleep with the head of the bed elevated 45 degrees (to decrease periorbital fluid accumulation).

The measures outlined decrease the risk of injury, provide comfort, decrease periorbital edema that can further compromise vision, and ensure immediate care for problems, thereby minimizing the risk of further visual loss.

Imbalanced Nutrition: Less than Body Requirements

The hypermetabolic state that occurs in hyperthyroidism causes gastrointestinal hypermotility, with nausea, vomiting, diarrhea, and abdominal pain. Although the patient may have an increased appetite and eat more than usual, weight loss continues.

- Ask the patient to weigh daily (at the same time each day), and keep a record of results. *The inability to meet metabolic demands results in loss of body weight.*
- In collaboration with a dietitian, teach the patient the need for a diet high in carbohydrates and protein and including between-meal snacks. Six small meals a day may be more desirable than three large meals. Caloric intake may need to be increased to 4000 kcal/day if weight loss exceeds 10% to 17% for height and frame. *Increased nutrients as part of a well-balanced diet are necessary to meet metabolic demands. Patients are often better able to increase food*

NURSING CARE OF THE PATIENT
Having a Subtotal Thyroidectomy

PREOPERATIVE CARE

- Administer ordered antithyroid medications and iodine preparations, and monitor their effects. *Antithyroid drugs are given before surgery to promote a euthyroid state. Iodine preparations are given to the patient before surgery to decrease vascularity of the gland, thereby decreasing the risk of hemorrhage.*
- Teach the patient to support the neck by placing both hands behind the neck when sitting up in bed, while moving about, and while coughing. *Placing the hands behind the neck eases tension on the suture line in the front of the neck.*
- Answer questions, and allow time for the patient to verbalize concerns. *Because the incision is made at the base of the throat, patients (especially women) are often concerned about their appearance after surgery. Explain that the scar will eventually be only a thin line and that jewelry or scarves may be used to cover the scar.*
- Teach the patient to expect hoarseness due to generalized swelling at the suture line. *This is expected to diminish with healing and is not caused by laryngeal nerve damage.*

POSTOPERATIVE CARE

- Provide comfort measures: Administer analgesic pain medications as ordered, and monitor their effectiveness; place the patient in a semi-Fowler's position after recovery from anesthesia; support head and neck with pillows. *Analgesic medications reduce the perception of pain and reduce physical stress during the postoperative period. Positioning the patient in a semi-Fowler's position and supporting the head and neck decrease strain on the suture line.*
- Perform focused assessments to monitor for complications:
  a. **Hemorrhage.** Assess dressing (if present) and the area behind and under the patient's neck and shoulders for drainage. Monitor blood pressure and pulse for manifestations of hypovolemic shock. Assess tightness of dressing (if present). *The vascularity of the gland increases the risk of hemorrhage. The location of the incision and the position of the patient may cause the drainage to run back and under the patient. The danger of hemorrhage is greatest in the first 12 to 24 hours after surgery.*
  b. **Respiratory distress.** Assess respiratory rate, rhythm, depth, and effort. Maintain humidification as ordered. Assist the patient with coughing and deep breathing. Have suction equipment, oxygen, and a tracheostomy set available for immediate use. *Respiratory distress may result from hemorrhage and edema, which may compress the trachea; from tetany and laryngeal spasms resulting from decreased hormones due to removal or damage to the parathyroid glands; and from damage to the laryngeal nerve, causing spasms of the vocal cords. Stridor is heard in acute obstructions. This is a high-pitched, squeaky sound and is a sign of airway obstruction. Equipment must be immediately available if the patient experiences respiratory distress that requires interventions and treatment.*
  c. **Laryngeal nerve damage.** Assess for the ability to speak aloud, noting quality and tone of voice. *The location of the laryngeal nerve increases the risk of damage during thyroid surgery. Although hoarseness may be due to edema or the endotracheal tube used during surgery and will subside, permanent hoarseness or loss of vocal volume is a potential danger.*
  d. **Tetany.** Assess for manifestations of latent tetany due to calcium deficiency, including tingling of toes, fingers, and lips; muscular twitches; positive Chvostek's and Trousseau's signs; and decreased serum calcium levels. Serum calcium levels will be monitored in the postoperative period. Keep calcium gluconate or calcium chloride available for immediate IV use, if necessary. *The parathyroid glands are located in and near the thyroid gland; surgery of the thyroid gland may injure or remove parathyroid glands, resulting in hypocalcemia and tetany. Tetany may occur in 1 to 7 days after thyroidectomy.*

---

intake by eating frequent, small meals. *A 1 lb weight gain requires approximately 3500 extra kilocalories.*

- Monitor nutritional status through results of laboratory data. Serum albumin, transferrin, and total lymphocyte counts are commonly lower than normal in nutritional deficits. *A negative nitrogen balance signifies a catabolic state in which protein is lost and metabolic demands are not being met.*

Disturbed Body Image and Anxiety

Physical changes common in hyperthyroidism include exophthalmos, goiter, tremors, hair loss, increased perspiration, loss of strength, fatigue, weight loss, and changes in reproductive and sexual function (amenorrhea in women and impotence in men). In addition, the patient often has mood changes and insomnia and is constantly nervous and anxious. There may even be periods of psychosis. These changes are frightening not only for the patient but also for family members.

- Establish a trusting relationship; encourage the patient to verbalize feelings about self and to ask questions about the illness and treatment. Provide reliable information and clarify misconceptions. *Establishing trust facilitates open sharing of feelings and perceptions.*

Community-Based Care

Patients with hyperthyroidism primarily provide self-care at home. Teaching is individualized to meet the patient's needs. Address the following topics:

- The patient taking oral medications must understand the need for lifelong treatment.
- The patient who has a thyroidectomy requires information about postoperative wound care.
- The patient having radioactive iodine therapy needs to know the manifestations of hypothyroidism.
- Depending on the age of the patient and the support systems available, referral to community healthcare agencies may be necessary.
- In addition, suggest the following resources, which are accessible via the Internet: the American Thyroid Association, the Thyroid Foundation of Canada, and the Endocrine Society.

Mrs. Juanita Manuel is a 33-year-old mother of four small children. She is a second-year student at the local community college, within one semester of completing the requirements for an associate's degree in child care. For the past 3 months, Mrs. Manuel has been constantly hungry and has eaten more than usual, but she has still lost 15 lb (6.8 kg). She has repeated bouts of diarrhea and often feels nauseated. Her hands shake, she can feel her heart beating rapidly, and she finds herself laughing or crying for no apparent reason.

Mrs. Manuel makes an appointment with her family physician. The nurse at the office completes a health history and physical assessment. When asked how she has been feeling, Mrs. Manuel replies, "Well, I don't know what's wrong with me—but I keep losing weight and I cry at the drop of a hat. I am also just so hot all the time, and I've never had that problem before. I hope I find out what's wrong and it's nothing serious."

ASSESSMENT

The health history indicates that although her appetite has increased, Mrs. Manuel has lost 15 lb (6.8 kg). She states that she has had diarrhea, nausea, palpitations, heat intolerance, and mood changes. Physical assessment findings include the following: T 101°F (38.3°C), P 110, R 24, and BP 162/86. Her skin is moist and warm, her hair thin and fine. She has visible tremors in her hands. Her eyeballs protrude, and she is unable to close her eyelids completely. Her thyroid is enlarged and palpable. Diagnostic tests reveal the following abnormal results: T_3, 350 g/dL (normal range: 80 to 200 ng/dL), T_4, 15.1 mg/dL (normal range: 5 to 12 mg/dL). A thyroid scan demonstrates an enlarged thyroid with increased iodine uptake. After the medical diagnosis of Graves' disease is made, Mrs. Manuel is started on the antithyroid medication propylthiouracil, 150 mg orally every 8 hours.

DIAGNOSES

- *Risk for Imbalanced Nutrition: Less than Body Requirements* related to weight loss of 15 lb (6.8 kg), with present weight 10% less than normal for height
- *Diarrhea* related to increased peristalsis as evidenced by 8 to 10 liquid stools per day
- *Risk for Disturbed Sensory Perception: Visual* related to an inability to close the eyelids completely
- *Anxiety* related to a lack of knowledge about disease process

EXPECTED OUTCOMES

- Gain at least 1 lb (0.45 kg) every 2 weeks.
- Regain normal bowel elimination patterns.
- Maintain normal vision (with no evidence of corneal damage) and verbalize measures to protect her eyes.
- Verbalize medical treatment and self-care needs.
- Verbalize a decrease in anxiety.

PLANNING AND IMPLEMENTATION

- Request that she keep a record of daily weight.
- Discuss adopting a high-kilocalorie diet. Identify food likes and dislikes, as well as foods that increase diarrhea, before instituting a plan to increase food intake.
- Request that she keep a stool chart, noting the time, type, and precipitating factors for diarrhea stools. Teach comfort measures for irritated anal area (clean washcloth and soap, nonirritating ointment).
- Teach how to apply eyedrops (artificial tears).
- Explain the need to elevate the head of the bed to 45 degrees at night, and tape eye shields over eyes before sleep.
- Teach about Graves' disease, the medication's effects and side effects, and the need for continued medical care.

EVALUATION

By her next office visit, Mrs. Manuel has gained 1 lb (0.45 kg) and has discussed her dietary needs with the nurse and her husband. She is having diarrhea less often. She has safely applied the eyedrops and states that she uses the eye shields and elevates the head of her bed at night. The office nurse reviewed the written and verbal information about Graves' disease and the medication prescribed. Mrs. Manuel verbalizes her understanding, stating, "I'll always take my medicine—I never want to feel like that again!" She says that she feels much less anxious now that she understands what has happened.

CRITICAL THINKING IN THE NURSING PROCESS

1. What is the pathophysiologic basis for Mrs. Manuel's abnormal vital signs?
2. What is the rationale for having the patient with exophthalmos elevate the head of the bed at night?
3. Outline a teaching plan that could be given to patients for home care following a subtotal thyroidectomy.

See Evaluating Your Response in Appendix C.

The Patient with Hypothyroidism

Hypothyroidism is a disorder that results when the thyroid gland produces an insufficient amount of TH. Because a decrease in TH levels decreases metabolic rate and heat production, hypothyroidism affects all body systems. Hypothyroidism is common in women between ages 30 and 60, with the incidence increasing after age 50. However, the disorder can occur at any stage of life. Careful evaluation of manifestations is important in the older adult because manifestations of hypothyroidism are often thought to be the result of aging instead of a pathologic process. The chronic, untreated hypothyroid state in adults is termed **myxedema**. The term reflects the characteristic accumulation of nonpitting edema in the connective tissues throughout the body. The edema is the result of water retention in mucoprotein (hydrophilic proteoglycans) deposits in the interstitial spaces. The face of a patient with myxedema appears puffy, the tongue is enlarged, and the voice is hoarse and husky (Porth & Matfin, 2009).

Pathophysiology and Manifestations

Hypothyroidism may be either primary or secondary. Primary hypothyroidism (which is more common) may be caused by congenital defects in the gland, loss of thyroid tissue following treatment for hyperthyroidism with surgery or radiation, antithyroid medications, thyroiditis, or endemic iodine deficiency. The cardiac drug amiodarone (Cordarone), which contains iodine, is increasingly being implicated in causing thyroid problems, especially hypothyroidism (Porth, 2007). Anabolic steroids, androgens, lithium, phenytoin, propanolol, interferon alpha, and interleukin-2 decrease T_4. The antithyroid drugs propylthiouracil and methimazole decrease T_4 measurement. Secondary hypothyroidism may result from pituitary TSH deficiency or peripheral resistance to thyroid hormones. (McPhee & Papadakis, 2009). Hypothyroidism has a slow onset, with manifestations occurring over months or even years. With treatment, the mental and physical manifestations rapidly reverse in patients of all ages.

MULTISYSTEM EFFECTS OF
Hypothyroidism

Endocrine
• Goiter

Respiratory
• Pleural effusion

Gastrointestinal
• Constipation

Musculoskeletal
• Muscle stiffness
• Weakness
• Fatigue

Neurologic
• Hand and foot paresthesias
• Lethargy
• Somnolence
• Confusion
• ↓ reflexes
• Slow speech
• Memory impairment

Sensory
• Periorbital edema

Cardiovascular
• Hypotension
• Bradycardia
• Dysrhythmias
• Enlarged heart
• Anemia

Reproductive
• Menorrhagia (female)
• Infertility (female)
• ↓ libido (male)

Integumentary
• Hair loss
• Brittle nails
• Coarse, dry skin
• Nonpitting edema

Metabolic Processes
• Hypothermia
• Anorexia
• Weight gain
• Systemic edema

When TH production decreases, the thyroid gland enlarges in a compensatory attempt to produce more hormone. The goiter that results is usually a simple or nontoxic form. People living in certain areas of the world where the soil is deficient in iodine, the substance necessary for TH synthesis and secretion, are more prone to become hypothyroid and develop simple goiter. (Iodine deficiency is discussed later.)

Patients with hypothyroidism characteristically have a goiter, fluid retention and edema, decreased appetite, weight gain, constipation, dry skin, dyspnea, pallor, hoarseness, and muscle stiffness. Many patients have a decreased sense of taste and smell, menstrual disorders, anemias, and cardiac enlargement. The pulse is typically slow. Deficient amounts of TH cause abnormalities in lipid metabolism, with elevated serum cholesterol and triglyceride levels. As a result, the patient is at increased risk for atherosclerosis and cardiac disorders. Decreased renal blood flow and glomerular filtration rate reduce the kidney's ability to excrete water, which may cause hyponatremia. Sleep apnea is more common in patients with hypothyroidism. Factors that result in decreased TH (in addition to those described) include iodine deficiency and Hashimoto's thyroiditis.

Iodine Deficiency

Iodine is necessary for TH synthesis and secretion. Iodine deficiency may result from certain goitrogenic drugs (which block TH synthesis); lithium carbonate, used to treat bipolar mental disorders; and antithyroid drugs. Goitrogenic compounds in foods such as turnips, rutabagas, and soybeans may also block TH synthesis if consumed in sufficient quantities. In areas of the world where the soil is deficient in iodine, dietary intake of iodine may be inadequate. The use of iodized salt has reduced this risk in the United States.

Hashimoto's Thyroiditis

Hashimoto's thyroiditis is the most common cause of goiter and primary hypothyroidism. In this autoimmune disorder, antibodies develop that destroy thyroid tissue. Functional thyroid tissue is replaced with fibrous tissue, and TH levels decrease. In addition, decreasing levels of TH in the early stages of the disease prompt the gland to enlarge to compensate, causing a goiter. However, as the disease progresses, the thyroid gland becomes smaller. This disorder is more common in women and has a familial link.

Myxedema Coma

Myxedema coma is a life-threatening complication of long-standing, untreated hypothyroidism. It is characterized by severe metabolic disorders (hyponatremia, hypoglycemia, lactic acidosis), hypothermia, cardiovascular collapse, impaired cognition, and coma. These patients are super sensitive to opioids and may die from normal doses. Myxedema coma may be precipitated by trauma, infection, failure to take thyroid replacement medications, the use of central nervous system depressants, and exposure to cold temperatures (Porth, 2007). The treatment of myxedema coma addresses the precipitating factors and manifestations and involves maintaining a patent airway; maintaining fluid, electrolyte, and acid–base balance; maintaining cardiovascular status; increasing body temperature; and increasing TH levels. If untreated, the mortality rate is high (Shah & Lettieri, 2007).

Interdisciplinary Care

The treatment of the patient with hypothyroidism focuses on diagnosis, prevention or treatment of complications, and replacement of the deficient TH. With early and continued treatment, both appearance and mental function return to normal.

Diagnosis

Hypothyroidism is diagnosed by the clinical manifestations and by a decrease in TH, especially T_4. TSH concentration often is increased because the negative hormonal feedback from TH is lost. The same laboratory and diagnostic tests used to diagnose hyperthyroidism are also used to diagnose hypothyroidism, with opposite results in most cases (refer to Table 19–1). ∞ See Chapter 18 for information on specific thyroid tests. Other laboratory tests associated with the diagnosis of hypothyroidism include elevated serum LDL cholesterol, triglycerides, and lipoproteins. Anemia, hypoglycemia, and hyponatremia are also common.

Medications

Hypothyroidism is treated with medications that replace TH. Levothyroxine (thyroxine, T_4) is the treatment of choice (Fitzgerald, 2007). Medications commonly used to treat hypothyroidism and their nursing implications are shown in the Medication Administration box on page 503. In the older adult, an age-related decrease in serum albumin and renal excretion can increase the amount of available drug and cause an exaggerated pharmacologic effect. Therefore, the older patient may require less thyroid medication than a younger patient.

Surgery

If the hypothyroid patient has a goiter large enough to cause respiratory difficulties or dysphagia, a subtotal thyroidectomy may be performed (see page 499).

∞ Nursing Care

Health Promotion

One of the most critical factors in preventing hypothyroidism is education of the public about the necessity of an adequate dietary intake of iodine. The use of iodized salt meets the requirements for hormone production. It is important to teach patients the importance of regular healthcare provider visits and medication intake.

Assessment

Collect the following data through the health history and physical examination (∞ see Chapter 18). Further focused assessments are described with nursing interventions that follow. When assessing the older patient, be aware of normal changes with aging, described in ∞ Chapter 18.

- *Health history:* Pituitary diseases (discussed later), history of hyperthyroidism and treatment with medications or radioactive iodine, thyroid surgery, treatment of head or neck cancer with radiation, diet, use of iodized salt, bowel elimination, depression, muscle or joint aching, cold intolerance, respiratory difficulties, heavy menstrual periods.
- *Physical assessment:* Muscle strength, deep tendon reflexes, vital signs, cardiovascular and peripheral vascular systems, integument, thyroid gland, weight.

THYROID PREPARATIONS

Levothyroxine sodium (T_4) (Levoxyl, Levothroid, Synthroid)

Liothyronine sodium (T_3) (Cytomel)

Liotrix (T_3–T_4) (Euthyroid, Thyrolar)

Thyroid preparations increase blood levels of TH, thus raising the patient's metabolic rate. As a result, cardiac output, oxygen consumption, and body temperature increase. Levothyroxine speeds the elimination of vitamin K–dependent clotting factors enhancing the effects of warfarin (Coumadin). Patients are at increased risk of bleeding if warfarin dosages are not appropriately reduced. The dosage depends on the drug chosen and the patient's degree of thyroid dysfunction, sensitivity to TH, age, body size, and health. The older adult may require lower doses.

Nursing Responsibilities

- Give 1 hour before meals or 2 hours after meals for best absorption.
- Thyroid preparations potentiate the effect of anticoagulant drugs. If the patient is also receiving an anticoagulant, monitor for bruising, bleeding gums, and blood in the urine.
- Thyroid medications potentiate the effect of digitalis. If the patient is also receiving a digitalis preparation, monitor for signs of digitalis toxicity.
- Monitor for manifestations of coronary insufficiency: chest pain, dyspnea, tachycardia.

- If the patient has insulin-dependent diabetes, monitor the effects of insulin. The effect of the insulin may change as thyroid function increases.
- During dose adjustment, take pulse before administering drug. Report pulse > 100.

Health Education for the Patient and Family

- Do not substitute brands of drugs or use generic equivalents without the physician's approval.
- The medications must be taken for the rest of one's life.
- Report manifestations of excess thyroid hormone to the physician: excess weight loss, palpitations, leg cramps, nervousness, or insomnia.
- If you have diabetes and use insulin, monitor blood glucose levels closely; the thyroid medications may alter the amount of insulin required.
- Thyroid preparations increase the risk of iodine toxicity. Do not use iodized salt or over-the-counter drugs containing iodine.
- If you are also taking an anticoagulant, report any signs of bleeding.
- Report any changes in menstrual periods.
- Take the thyroid preparation in the morning 30 minutes before eating to decrease the possibility of insomnia; take other medications such as calcium carbonate, iron, or antacids at least 4 hours before or after taking thyroid drugs; these medications may prevent absorption.
- Closely monitor blood pressure and pulse (older patients).
- Avoid excessive intake of foods that are known to inhibit TH utilization such as walnuts and high-fiber foods.

Nursing Diagnoses and Interventions

In planning and implementing care for patients with hypothyroidism, the nurse takes into account that the disorder affects all organ systems. Although many nursing diagnoses might be valid, this section focuses on patient problems with cardiovascular function, elimination, and skin integrity. See the accompanying Case Study & Nursing Care Plan on page 504.

Decreased Cardiac Output

A TH deficit causes a reduction in heart rate and stroke volume, resulting in decreased cardiac output. There may also be an accumulation of fluid in the pericardial sac (from the edema characteristic of hypothyroidism), and coronary artery disease may be present, further compromising cardiac function.

- Monitor blood pressure, rate and rhythm of apical and peripheral pulses, respiratory rate, and breath sounds. *Hypotension indicates decreasing peripheral blood flow. Fluid in the pericardial sac restricts cardiac function. Monopolysaccharide deposits in the respiratory system decrease vital capacity and hypoventilation.*
- Suggest the patient avoid chilling; increase room temperature, use additional bed covers, and avoid drafts. *Chilling increases metabolic rate and puts increased stress on the heart.*
- Explain the need to alternate activity with rest periods. Ask the patient to report any breathing difficulties, chest pain, heart palpitations, or dizziness. *Activity increases demands on the heart and should be balanced with rest. Manifestations of cardiac stress include dyspnea, chest pain, palpitations, and dizziness.*

Constipation

The hypothyroid patient is likely to have a reduced appetite and decreased food intake, a diminished activity level because of muscle aches and weakness, and reduced peristalsis to the point that fecal impactions may occur.

- Encourage a fluid intake of up to 2000 mL per day. Discuss preferred liquids and the best times of day to drink fluids. If kilocalorie intake is restricted, ensure that liquids have no or low kilocalories. *Sufficient fluid intake is necessary to promote proper stool consistency.*
- Discuss ways to maintain a high-fiber diet. *Diets high in fiber and fluid produce soft stools. Fiber that is not digested absorbs water, which adds bulk to the stool and assists in the movement of fecal material through the intestines. High fiber foods include beans, fruits, breads, cereals, popcorn, and rice. Consult nutritional labels for fiber content. Instruct not to eat high fiber foods within 4 hours of taking a thyroid hormone medication. These foods decrease absorption of thyroid hormone medications.*
- Encourage activity as tolerated. *Activity influences bowel elimination by improving muscle tone and stimulating peristalsis.*

Risk for Impaired Skin Integrity

The patient with hypothyroidism is at risk for impaired skin integrity related to the accumulation of fluid in the interstitial spaces and to dry, rough skin. Decreased peripheral circulation, decreased activity levels, and slow wound healing further increase the risk. These interventions are outlined here for the older patient who is hospitalized for surgery or severe hypothyroidism.

- Monitor skin surfaces for redness or lesions, especially if the patient's activity is greatly reduced. Use a pressure ulcer risk assessment scale to identify patients at risk. *Hypothyroidism causes dry, rough, edematous skin conditions that increase the risk of skin breakdown.*
- Provide or teach the immobile patient measures to promote optimal circulation:
  - Use a turning schedule if the patient is on bed rest, or teach the patient to change position every 2 hours.
  - Limit the time for sitting in one position; shift weight or lift the body using arm rests every 20 to 30 minutes.
  - Use pillows, pads, or sheepskin or foam cushions for bed and/or chair.
  - Teach and implement a schedule of range-of-motion exercises.
    Prolonged pressure, especially in patients with edema and circulatory impairment, can occlude capillaries and cause hypoxic tissue damage.
- Provide or teach the patient measures to maintain skin integrity:
  - Take baths only as necessary; use warm (not hot) water.
  - Use gentle motions when washing and drying skin.
  - Use alcohol-free skin oils and lotions.

Dry skin and edema increase the risk of skin breakdown. Hot water, rough massage, and alcohol-based preparations may increase skin dryness, further impairing the body's ability to maintain skin integrity.

Community-Based Care

Patients with hypothyroidism require lifelong care, primarily at home. Address the following topics:

- The need to take medications for the rest of one's life
- The need for periodic dosage reassessments
- If the patient is older or does not have a support system, helpful community resources
- Additional resources are the same as for the patient with hyperthyroidism.

The Patient with Cancer of the Thyroid

Thyroid cancer has an estimated incidence of slightly more than 37,200 new cases and accounted for more than 1,600 cancer deaths in 2009 (National Cancer Institute, 2009). The most consistent risk factor is exposure to ionizing radiation to the head and neck during childhood. For example, many adults in

CASE STUDY & NURSING CARE PLAN   A Patient with Hypothyroidism

Jane Lee is a 60-year-old retired nurse living with her husband and daughter on a farm that has been in the family for four generations. Mrs. Lee has gained 10 lb (4.5 kg) in the past few months, even though she is rarely hungry and eats much less than normal. She is always tired and weak—so tired that she has not even been able to help with the chores on the farm or do housework. She is concerned about her appearance and the way she sounds when she talks. Her face is puffy, and her tongue always feels thick. Mr. Lee convinces his wife to make an appointment at a health center in a nearby town.

ASSESSMENT

Brian Henning, RN, completes the health assessment for Mrs. Lee at the health center. He finds that she now weighs 150 lb (68 kg), an increase of 10 lb (4.5 kg) over her weight at her last visit 6 months earlier. Mrs. Lee states that she always feels cold, tired, and weak. She also states that she is constipated, has difficulty remembering things, and looks different. Physical assessment findings include a palpable and bilaterally enlarged thyroid; dry, yellowish skin; nonpitting edema of the face and lower legs; and slow, slurred speech. Diagnostic tests revealed the following abnormal findings: T_3, 56 ng/dL (normal range: 80 to 200 ng/dL); T_4, 3.1 (normal range: 5 to 12 mg/dL); TSH increased. The medical diagnosis of hypothyroidism is made, and Mrs. Lee is started on levothyroxine 0.05 mg daily.

DIAGNOSES

- *Constipation* related to decreased peristalsis, as evidenced by hard, formed stools every 4 days
- *Impaired Verbal Communication* related to changes in speech patterns and enlarged tongue
- *Situational Low Self-Esteem* related to changes in physical appearance and activity intolerance

EXPECTED OUTCOMES

- Regain normal bowel elimination patterns, having a soft, formed stool at least every other day.
- Experience improvement in verbal communication.
- Regain positive self-esteem as medication reduces physical changes and fatigue.

PLANNING AND IMPLEMENTATION

- Teach to increase fluids, bulk, and fiber in the diet to help regain a normal bowel elimination pattern of a soft, formed stool every other day.
- Take medication as prescribed and do not expect immediate reversal of manifestations affecting speech.
- Plan activities around rest periods. Encourage husband and daughter to help with housecleaning and cooking.

EVALUATION

On return to the health center 2 months later, Mrs. Lee reports that she is no longer constipated but that she is continuing to drink six glasses of water and eating oatmeal every day. She no longer feels cold, is regaining her normal energy, and even feels well enough to plant her garden. Her speech is clear and easy to understand. As she leaves the examining room, Mrs. Lee says, "It's hard to believe that I have changed so much—now I look and feel like the 'old' me!"

CRITICAL THINKING IN THE NURSING PROCESS

1. What physical changes that normally occur with aging are similar to the manifestations of hypothyroidism?
2. Describe the factors that put Mrs. Lee's safety at risk. What alterations in her home environment would you suggest to promote safety until the prescribed medication takes effect?
3. The patient taking oral thyroid medications may develop hyperthyroidism. List the manifestations you would include in a teaching plan to signal this condition.

See Evaluating Your Response in Appendix C.

their 60s, 70s, and 80s received x-ray treatments for colds, tonsillitis, acne, and sinus infections during childhood.

Of the several types of thyroid cancer, the most common types are listed here:

- Papillary thyroid carcinoma is the most common thyroid malignancy. It is usually detected as a single nodule, but may arise from a multinodular goiter. It is most often diagnosed in women between ages 30 and 50 (National Cancer Institute, 2009). Risks for the development of this form are exposure to external x-ray treatments to the head or neck as a child, childhood exposure to radioactive isotopes of iodine in nuclear fallout, and a family history. Papillary thyroid carcinoma is the least aggressive type, but does metastasize to local and regional lymph nodes and lungs.

- Follicular thyroid cancer is the second most common thyroid malignancy. It is diagnosed at a slightly older age (40 to 60) than papillary and more commonly in women. This form is more aggressive than papillary, with potential for vascular invasion and spread to lung and bone. Exposure to radiation is not considered a risk factor for this type of thyroid cancer.

- Medullary thyroid cancer arises from the cells of the thyroid that produce the hormone calcitonin; these cells do not uptake iodine and, therefore, are not susceptible to treatment with radioactive iodine. Persons with a family history of thyroid cancer have a change in a gene named RET and this can be passed from parent to child.

EVIDENCE FOR NURSING CARE The Patient with Thyroid Cancer

Selected resources that nurses may find helpful when planning evidence-based nursing care follow.

- Cooper, D. S., Doherty, G. M., Haugen, B. R., Kloos, R. T., Lee, S. L., Mandel, S J., et al. (2009). Revised American Thyroid Association management guidelines for patients with thyroid nodules and differentiated thyroid cancer. *Thyroid, 19*(11). DOI: 10.1089/thy.2009.0110. Retrieved from http://www.thyroid.org/professionals/publications/documents/ATA_Guidelines_DTC_2009.pdf

Thyroid cancer is manifested by a palpable, firm nontender nodule in the thyroid. If undetected, the tumor may grow and impinge on the esophagus or trachea, causing difficulty in swallowing or breathing. Most people with thyroid cancer do not have elevated thyroid hormone levels. The diagnosis is made by measuring thyroid hormones, performing thyroid scans, and by fine-needle biopsy of the nodule. The usual treatment is subtotal or total thyroidectomy. TSH suppression therapy with levothyroxine may be conducted prior to surgery. Radioactive iodine therapy (^{131}I) and chemotherapy are additional therapeutic options. While standard chemotherapy is not used often, new biologic chemotherapies offer promise of remission or cure for the more aggressive or refractory types of thyroid cancer (Pfister & Fagin, 2008). Nursing care for the patient with cancer is discussed in ∞ Chapter 14.

Disorders of the Parathyroid Glands

Disorders of the parathyroid glands, hyperparathyroidism and hypoparathyroidism, are not as common as those of the thyroid gland. Hypercalcemia and hypocalcemia (the primary results of alterations in parathyroid function) are discussed in ∞ Chapter 10.

The Patient with Hyperparathyroidism

Hyperparathyroidism results from an increase in the secretion of parathyroid hormone (PTH), which regulates normal serum levels of calcium. The increase in PTH affects the kidneys and bones, resulting in increased resorption of calcium and excretion of phosphate by the kidneys (increasing the risk of hypercalcemia and hypophosphatemia), increased bicarbonate excretion and decreased acid excretion by the kidneys (increasing the risk of metabolic acidosis and hypokalemia), increased release of calcium and phosphorus by bones with resultant bone decalcification, and deposits of calcium in soft tissues and the formation of renal calculi.

Pathophysiology and Manifestations

Hyperparathyroidism occurs more often in older adults and is three times more common in women. The disorder itself is not common. Primary hyperparathyroidism occurs when there is hyperplasia or an adenoma in one of the parathyroid glands. Secondary hyperparathyroidism is a compensatory response to chronic hypocalcemia. The tertiary form is most often seen in patients with chronic renal failure.

Many patients with hyperparathyroidism are asymptomatic. When manifestations occur, they are related to hypercalcemia and various musculoskeletal, renal, and gastrointestinal manifestations. Bone reabsorption results in pathologic fractures, while elevated calcium levels alter neural and muscular activity, leading to muscle weakness and atrophy. Proximal renal tubule function is altered, and metabolic acidosis, renal calculi formation, and polyuria occur.

Manifestations of the effect of hypercalcemia on the gastrointestinal tract include abdominal pain, constipation, anorexia, and peptic ulcer formation. Hypercalcemia also affects the cardiovascular system, causing dysrhythmias, hypertension, and increased sensitivity to cardiotonic glycosides (e.g., digitalis preparations).

Interdisciplinary Care

Hyperparathyroidism is diagnosed by excluding all other possible causes of hypercalcemia, by at least a 6-month history of manifestations, and by laboratory analysis of levels of serum calcium and PTH levels (McPhee & Papadakis, 2009).

Treatment of hyperparathyroidism focuses on decreasing the elevated serum calcium levels. Patients with mild hypercalcemia are urged to drink fluids and keep active. They should avoid immobilization, thiazide diuretics, large doses of vitamins A and D, antacids containing calcium, and calcium supplements. Severe hypercalcemia requires hospitalization and intensive treatment with intravenous saline. Medications to inhibit bone resorption and reduce hypercalcemia, such as pamidronate (Aredia), alendronate (Fosamax), and zoledronate (Zometa), are used for short-term treatment, improve bone density, and may relieve bone pain (Fitzgerald, 2007). Calcitonin, a hormone produced by the thyroid gland, decreases plasma levels of calcium by inhibiting bone resorption and increasing calcium excretion by the kidney (Lehne, 2004). A form of calcitonin from salmon is available as a nasal spray or IM/SQ injection. A medication for patients with hyperparathyroidism secondary to renal failure or parathyroid cancer is a calcimimetic. This drug increases the sensitivity of the calcium-sensing receptors of the parathyroid gland to serum calcium. The effect is decreased secretion of PTH and reduced serum calcium and phosphorus.

Surgical removal of the parathyroid glands affected by hyperplasia or adenoma treats primary hyperparathyroidism. The preoperative and postoperative nursing care of the patient having surgery of the parathyroids is essentially the same as that for the patient having a thyroidectomy (see page 499). Manipulation of the thyroid while removing the parathyroids may result in TH release, causing increased cardiac rate and stroke volume.

∞ Nursing Care

Nursing care of the patient with hypercalcemia is discussed in ∞ Chapter 10.

The Patient with Hypoparathyroidism

Hypoparathyroidism results from abnormally low PTH levels. The most common cause is damage to or inadvertent removal of all of the parathyroid glands during thyroidectomy. The lack of circulating PTH causes hypocalcemia and an elevated blood phosphate level.

Pathophysiology and Manifestations

Reduced levels of PTH result in impaired renal tubular regulation of calcium and phosphate. In addition, decreased activation of vitamin D results in decreased absorption of calcium by the intestines. The low calcium levels cause changes in neuromuscular activity, affecting peripheral motor and sensory nerves. Hypocalcemia lowers the threshold for nerve and muscle excitability; a slight stimulus anywhere along a nerve or muscle fiber initiates an impulse.

The neuromuscular manifestations that result include numbness and tingling around the mouth and in the fingertips, muscle spasms of the hands and feet, convulsions, and laryngeal spasms. **Tetany**, a continuous spasm of muscles, is the primary symptom of hypocalcemia. In severe cases of tetany, death may occur. Assessments for tetany include Chvostek's sign and Trousseau's sign (∞ see Chapter 18). The manifestations of hypoparathyroidism are summarized in the box on page 507.

Interdisciplinary Care

Hypoparathyroidism is diagnosed by low serum calcium levels and high phosphorous levels in the absence of renal failure, an absorption disorder, or a nutritional disorder.

Treatment of hypoparathyroidism focuses on increasing calcium levels. Intravenous calcium gluconate is given immediately to reduce tetany. Long-term therapy includes supplemental calcium, increased dietary calcium, and vitamin D therapy.

∞ Nursing Care

Nursing care for the patient with hypocalcemia is discussed in ∞ Chapter 10.

Disorders of the Adrenal Glands

Disorders of the adrenal cortex or adrenal medulla result in changes in the production of adrenocorticotropic hormone (ACTH). Hormones of the adrenal cortex are essential to life. They maintain homeostasis in response to stressors. Disorders of the adrenal cortex result in complex physical, psychologic, and

MOVING EVIDENCE INTO ACTION — **Serum Parathyroid Hormone Levels Predict Falls in Older Adults with Diabetes Mellitus**

In a retrospective analysis of data, Houston et al. (2008) found a positive correlation between higher levels of PTH and fall incidents in 492 independent-living older persons with an average age of 73.6 years who had diabetes mellitus (DM). The purpose of the study was to determine associations between body composition, weight-related health conditions, and reports of initial incidents causing functional limitations in older adults. Baseline assessments of physical performance and parathyroid hormone were among the data collected. Houston et al. found a positive correlation between increased parathyroid hormone level and the number of falls the subjects reported during the study period. They found no correlation between the physical performance scores of the subjects and the number of falls they reported. Neither gender nor race significantly affected the number of falls reported. However, participants with the highest PTH levels were more likely to be Black, to be sedentary, and have a higher body mass index (BMI).

IMPLICATIONS FOR NURSING

Falls are disconcerting to older adults even when no serious injury occurs. Nurses seek to prevent falls and would benefit from more precisely identifying those at risk for falling as well as decreasing fall potential. If correcting PTH to normal levels could prevent falls, treatment would be reasonable. The precise connection between serum PTH and falls is unknown; more studies are needed to reveal this important detail.

CRITICAL THINKING IN PATIENT CARE

1. What normal changes with aging combined with an increased parathyroid hormone level would increase the risk for falls?
2. What correlation might be considered between obesity, increased PTH levels, and falls?
3. What type of teaching is necessary to prevent falls in the home? How would this differ in the hospital or long-term care facility?

MANIFESTATIONS of Hypoparathyroidism

MUSCULOSKELETAL SYSTEM
- Muscle spasms
- Facial grimacing
- Carpopedal spasms
- Tetany or convulsions

INTEGUMENTARY SYSTEM
- Brittle nails
- Hair loss
- Dry, scaly skin

GASTROINTESTINAL SYSTEM
- Abdominal cramps
- Malabsorption

CARDIOVASCULAR SYSTEM
- Dysrhythmias

CENTRAL NERVOUS SYSTEM
- Paresthesias (lips, hands, feet)
- Mood disorders (irritability, depression, anxiety)
- Hyperactive reflexes
- Psychosis
- Increased intracranial pressure

metabolic alterations that are potentially life threatening. Hormones of the adrenal medulla are not essential to life, because the sympathetic nervous system produces similar body responses. The disorders that occur are hyperfunction and hypofunction of the adrenal cortex and hyperfunction of the adrenal medulla.

The Patient with Hypercortisolism (Cushing's Syndrome)

Cushing's syndrome is a chronic disorder in which hyperfunction of the adrenal cortex produces excessive amounts of circulating cortisol or ACTH. Cushing's syndrome is more common in women, with the average age of onset between 30 and 50 years (Figure 19–3 ■). However, the disorder may occur at any age, especially as the result of pharmacologic therapy. People who take steroids for long periods of time (e.g., for the treatment of arthritis, after an organ transplant, or as an adjunct to chemotherapy) are at increased risk for developing the disorder.

Pathophysiology

Cushing's syndrome may be the result of various causes. By far the most common cause is iatrogenic; only 2.6 new cases of Cushing's disease per million population are diagnosed yearly (McPhee & Papadakis, 2009). The most common etiologies of the disorder are as follows:

- Iatrogenic Cushing's syndrome, resulting from long-term therapy with potent pharmacologic glucocorticoid preparations.
- The pituitary form, with ACTH hypersecretion by a benign tumor of the pituitary (called *Cushing's disease*). This is most commonly caused by a small pituitary adenoma, with persistent but disorderly and random overproduction of ACTH. Forty-three percent of Cushing's disease is due to hypersecretion of ACTH by the pituitary.
- The ectopic form, caused by ACTH-secreting tumors (such as small-cell lung cancer). In this form, the ACTH is also random and episodic, but greater than in Cushing's disease.
- The adrenal form, resulting from excessive cortisol secretion by a benign or malignant adrenal tumor. The excess secretion suppresses pituitary ACTH production, resulting in atrophy of the uninvolved adrenal cortex.

Manifestations

The manifestations of Cushing's syndrome result from the ACTH or cortisol excess, and manifest as exaggerated cortisol actions. Obesity and a redistribution of body fat result in fat deposits in the

A   B

Figure 19–3 ■ A woman before and after developing Cushing's syndrome. In the photo at the right, notice the swollen facial features.

Courtesy of Dr. Charles Wilson, University of California, San Francisco.

PATHOPHYSIOLOGY LINKAGE   Cushing's Syndrome

MANIFESTATIONS	PATHOPHYSIOLOGY
Fat deposits in the abdominal region (central obesity), fat pads under the clavicles, a "buffalo hump" over the upper back, and a round "moon" face	Excess glucocorticoids affect normal carbohydrate metabolism, resulting in a redistribution of body fat and a breakdown of fats to fatty acids.
Muscle weakness and wasting, especially in the extremities	Excess cortisol results in changes in protein metabolism and protein catabolism from mobilization of amino acids for gluconeogenesis.
Thinning of skin, abdominal striae (purple "stretch marks"), easy bruising, poor wound healing, and frequent skin infections	Inhibition of fibroplasts by excess glucocorticoids with loss of collagen and connective tissue. Excess glucocorticoids depress the inflammatory response and inhibit immune system effectiveness.
Osteoporosis, compression fractures of the vertebrae, rib fractures	Excessive mineralocorticoids result in changes in absorption of calcium.
Hypokalemia	Loss of potassium.
Hypertension and hypernatremia	Excess aldosterone alters the absorption of sodium by the distal tubules of the kidneys (via the renin–angiotensin–aldosterone system) and sodium is retained. As potassium is lost, sodium is retained.
Hyperglycemia, polyuria, polydipsia	Altered glucose metabolism.
Increased risk of gastric ulcers	Increased gastric acid secretion.
Hirsutism (excessive hair growth; especially on the face in women), acne, menstrual irregularities	Increased androgen levels.
Emotional instability	Decreased response to stress.

abdominal region (central obesity), fat pads under the clavicle, a "buffalo hump" over the upper back, and a round "moon" face. Changes in protein metabolism cause muscle weakness and wasting, especially in the extremities. Glucocorticoid excess inhibits fibroblasts, resulting in loss of collagen and connective tissue. Thinning of skin, abdominal striae (reddish purple "stretch marks"), easy bruising, poor wound healing, and frequent skin infections result. Glucose metabolism is altered in the majority of patients, and diabetes mellitus may occur. Electrolyte imbalances also occur with the increased hormone levels. Changes in calcium absorption result in osteoporosis, compression fractures of the vertebrae, fractures of the ribs, and renal calculi. Hypokalemia and hypertension occur as potassium is lost and sodium is retained. Inhibited immune responses increase the risk of infection, and increased gastric acid secretion increases the risk of peptic ulcers. Emotional changes range from depression to psychosis. In women, increasing androgen levels cause hirsutism (excessive facial hair in particular), acne, and menstrual irregularities. The manifestations with related pathophysiology of Cushing's syndrome are outlined in the accompanying box.

The complications of untreated Cushing's syndrome include electrolyte imbalances (hyperglycemia, hypernatremia, and hypokalemia), hypertension, and emotional disturbances. Increased susceptibility to infections is also a factor. Compression fractures from osteoporosis and aseptic necrosis of the femoral head may result in serious disability. If the patient undergoes a bilateral adrenalectomy as a treatment for Cushing's syndrome, an acute deficit of cortisol (Addisonian crisis) may result.

Interdisciplinary Care

The treatment of Cushing's syndrome includes medications, radiation therapy, or surgery, depending on the etiologic origin of the disorder.

Diagnostic Tests

Cushing's syndrome is diagnosed through a variety of diagnostic tests. In addition to the laboratory tests described in ∞ Chapter 18 and in Table 19–2, a late night salivary cortisol test may be performed. A saliva specimen is collected at 11 PM; following the collection, dexamethasone 1 mg is given orally. A serum cortisol is collected at 8 AM the following morning. The dexamethasone *suppresses ACTH*. If an extremely high dose of cortisol is necessary to suppress ACTH, the primary disorder is adrenal cortex hyperplasia. If ACTH is not suppressed with the synthetic cortisol, an adrenal tumor is suspected. If the dexamethasone test is positive, a test for urinary free cortisol is made. This measures the amount of cortisol in the urine over 24 hours. Other diagnostic studies, including a CT scan or MRI of the abdomen, may be conducted to assess the adrenal gland for tumors.

Medications

Cushing's syndrome that results from a pituitary tumor is treated by medications as an adjunct to surgery or radiation. Medications are also used for patients with inoperable pituitary or adrenal malignancies. Although the drugs control manifestations, they do not effect a cure. Examples of some commonly prescribed drugs follow:

- Mitotane directly suppresses activity of the adrenal cortex and decreases peripheral metabolism of corticosteroids. It is used to treat metastatic adrenal cancer.
- Aminoglutethimide or ketoconazole (or both) inhibit cortisol synthesis by the adrenal cortex and may be administered to patients with ectopic ACTH-secreting tumors that cannot be surgically removed.
- Somatostatin analog (octreotide) suppresses ACTH secretion in some patients.

TABLE 19–2 Laboratory Findings in Adrenal Disorders

	TEST	NORMAL VALUES	HYPERFUNCTION (CUSHING'S SYNDROME)	HYPOFUNCTION (ADDISON'S DISEASE)
Serum	Cortisol	8 AM to 10 AM:	Increased	Decreased
		138 to 635 mmol		
		4 PM to 6 PM:		
		83 to 359 mmol		
	Blood urea nitrogen (BUN)	5 to 25 mg/dL	Normal	Increased
	Sodium	135 to 145 mEq/L	Increased	Decreased
	Potassium	3.5 to 5.0 mEq/L	Increased	Decreased
	Glucose (serum)	70 to 100 mg/dL	Increased	Decreased
Urine	Urinary free cortisol (UFS)	10 to 50 mcg/24 h	Increased	Low/absent
	17-KS	Male: 5 to 25 mg/24 h	Increased	Decreased
		Female: 5 to 15 mg/24 hr		
		Age > 65: 4 to 8 mg/24 hr		

Surgery

When Cushing's syndrome is caused by an adrenal cortex tumor, an adrenalectomy may be performed to remove the tumor. Only one adrenal gland is usually involved; however, if an ACTH-producing ectopic tumor is involved, a bilateral adrenalectomy is performed. Lifelong hormone replacement is necessary if both adrenal glands are removed. Nursing care of the patient having an adrenalectomy is discussed later.

Surgical removal of the pituitary gland (hypophysectomy) is indicated when Cushing's syndrome is the result of a pituitary disorder. The gland is removed either by a transsphenoidal route or by a craniotomy. Nursing care for the patient having cranial surgery is discussed in ∞ Chapter 42.

∞ Nursing Care

Health Promotion

Stress the risk of developing Cushing's syndrome for patients taking long-term steroids. The risk of abruptly discontinuing the medications is an essential component of teaching. For a review of glucocorticoid administration ∞ see Chapter 13.

Assessment

Collect the following data through the health history and physical examination (∞ see Chapter 18). Further focused assessments are described with nursing interventions later.

- *Health history:* History of pituitary, adrenal, pancreatic, or pulmonary tumor; frequent infections; gastrointestinal bleeding; stress fractures; pain; changes in weight distribution; change in height; fatigue; weakness; change in appearance; bruising; skin infections; menstrual history; sexual function.
- *Physical assessment:* Vital signs, behavior, appearance, fat distribution, face, skin, hair quantity and distribution, muscle size and strength, gait.

Nursing Diagnoses and Interventions

The nurse caring for the patient with Cushing's syndrome must take a holistic approach to plan and implement interventions for a wide variety of responses, including problems related to

fluid and electrolyte balance, injury, infection, and body image. For additional information about patients with alterations in fluid and electrolyte balance, ∞ see Chapter 10. Also, see the Case Study & Nursing Care Plan on page 511.

NURSING CARE OF THE PATIENT
Having an Adrenalectomy

PREOPERATIVE CARE

- Request a dietary consultation with the patient to discuss a diet high in vitamins and proteins. If hypokalemia exists, include foods high in potassium. *Glucocorticoid excess increases catabolism. Vitamins and proteins are necessary for tissue repair and wound healing following surgery.*
- Use medical and surgical asepsis when providing care and treatments. *Cortisol excess increases the risk of infection.*
- Monitor the results of laboratory tests of electrolytes and glucose levels. *Electrolyte and glucose imbalances are corrected before the patient has surgery.*
- Teach the patient to turn, cough, and perform deep-breathing exercises. *Although they are important for all surgical patients, these activities are even more important for the patient who is at risk for infection. Having the patient practice and demonstrate the activities increases postoperative compliance.*

POSTOPERATIVE CARE

- Take and record vital signs, measure intake and output, and monitor electrolytes on a frequent schedule, especially during the first 48 hours after surgery. *Removal of an adrenal gland, especially a bilateral adrenalectomy, results in adrenal insufficiency. Addisonian crisis and hypovolemic shock may occur. Cortisol is often given on the day of surgery and in the postoperative period to replace inadequate hormone levels. Intravenous fluids are also administered.*
- Assess body temperature, white blood cell (WBC) levels, and wound drainage. Change dressings using sterile technique. *Impaired wound healing increases the risk of infection in patients with adrenal disorders. Use aseptic technique to decrease this risk.*

Fluid Volume Excess

The excess cortisol secretion associated with Cushing's syndrome results in sodium and water reabsorption, causing fluid volume excess (Porth & Matfin, 2009). The patient will have weight gain, edema, and hypertension.

- Ask the patient to weigh at the same time each day, and maintain a record of results. *Body weight is an accurate indicator of fluid status. One liter of fluid retention corresponds to about 2 lb (0.9 kg) of body weight.*
- Monitor blood pressure, rate and rhythm of pulse, respiratory rate, and breath sounds. Assess for peripheral edema and jugular vein distention. *Extracellular fluid volume excess resulting from sodium and water retention is manifested by hypertension and a bounding, rapid pulse. There may also be crackles and wheezes, dependent edema, and venous distention.*
- Teach the patient and family the reasons for restricting fluid and the importance of limiting fluids if ordered. *Restricting fluid can help decrease the risk of fluid volume excess. Involving the patient and family in the plan of care and teaching the rationale for interventions helps achieve goals.*

Risk for Injury

The patient with Cushing's syndrome is at risk for injury from several causes. Excess cortisol causes increased absorption of calcium and demineralization of bones, resulting in risk of pathologic fractures. Muscle weakness and fatigue are common, increasing the potential for accidental falls. Teach the patient the following:

- Keep unnecessary clutter and equipment out of the way and off the floor.
- Ensure adequate lighting, especially at night.
- Use assistive devices for ambulation or to ask for help if needed.
- Be sure corrective lenses are available and clean.
- Use nonskid slippers or shoes.
- Watch for signs of fatigue (increased pulse and respirations); plan rest periods.
  A well-lighted environment free of clutter decreases the risk of falls and injury. Sensory and motor deficits increase the risk of falls; corrective lenses, assistive devices, and nonslip footwear can decrease this risk. Rest relieves fatigue. To reduce energy expenditure, include alternating periods of rest and activity in daily schedules.

Risk for Infection

Elevated cortisol levels impair the immune response and put the patient with Cushing's syndrome at increased risk for infection. Increased cortisol also affects protein synthesis, causing delayed wound healing, and inhibits collagen formation, which results in epidermal atrophy, further inhibiting resistance to infection. In addition, impaired blood flow to edematous tissue results in altered cellular nutrition, which increases the potential for infection. The following interventions are outlined for the patient with Cushing's syndrome who is hospitalized:

- Place in a private room, and limit visitors. *The patient must avoid exposure to environmental infection.*
- Monitor vital signs and verbalizations of subjective manifestations (e.g., the patient's response to "How do you feel?") every 4 hours. *Increased body temperature and pulse are systemic indicators of infection; however, because Cushing's syndrome impairs the normal inflammatory response, the usual indicators of inflammation may not be present.*
- Use principles of medical and sterile asepsis when caring for the patient, conducting procedures, or providing wound care. *Impaired skin and tissues make aseptic techniques even more necessary to decrease the risk of infection. Intact skin is the first line of defense against infection; if invasive procedures are performed or a wound is present, this defense is lost.*
- If wounds are present, assess the color, odor, and consistency of wound drainage, and look for increased pain in and around the wound. *Cortisol excess delays wound healing and closure.*
- Teach the importance of increasing intake of protein and vitamins C and A. *Protein, vitamin C, and vitamin A are necessary to collagen formation; collagen helps support and repair body tissues.*

> **PRACTICE ALERT**
> A generalized feeling of malaise may be the primary manifestation of infection, especially in the older adult.

Disturbed Body Image

The patient with Cushing's syndrome has obvious physical changes in appearance. The abnormal fat distribution, moon face, buffalo hump, striae, acne, and facial hair (in women) all contribute to disruptions in the way patients with this disorder perceive themselves.

- Encourage patients to express feelings and to ask questions about the disorder and its treatment. *The loss of one's normal body image may prompt feelings of hopelessness, powerlessness, anger, and depression. Understanding the disease and adapting to changes from that disease are the first steps in regaining control of one's own body.*
- Discuss strengths and previous coping strategies. Enlist the support of family or significant others in reaffirming the patient's worth. *Disturbances in body image are often accompanied by low self-esteem. Self-esteem derives from one's perception of competence and from appraisals of others.*
- Discuss signs of progress in controlling manifestations; for example, decreased facial edema or increased activity tolerance. *Many physical changes from cortisol excess disappear with treatment. Clearly communicate this fact, because the patient may believe changes are permanent.*

Using NANDA, NIC, and NOC

Linkages between a selected NANDA nursing diagnosis, NIC, and NOC for the patient with Cushing's syndrome are shown in the chart that follows.

Community-Based Care

The patient with Cushing's syndrome requires education about self-care at home specific to the type of treatment given. Address the following topics:

- Safety measures to prevent falls if fatigue, weakness, and osteoporosis are present.
- Taking medications as prescribed, with information about side effects. Patients often require medications for the rest of their lives, and dosage changes are highly likely.

- Having regular health assessments.
- Wearing a medical ID indicating the patient has Cushing's syndrome.
- Helping the older patient with referrals to social services or community health services because of the complexity of the treatment and care required.
- Providing helpful resources: The American Association of Clinical Endocrinologists, the Endocrine Society.

The Patient with Chronic Adrenocortical Insufficiency (Addison's Disease)

Addison's disease is a disorder resulting from destruction or dysfunction of the adrenal cortex. The result is chronic deficiency of cortisol, aldosterone, and adrenal androgens, accompanied by skin pigmentation. It can occur at any age, although it is more common in adults under the age of 60. Like

---

CASE STUDY & NURSING CARE PLAN   A Patient with Cushing's Syndrome

Sara Domico is a 30-year-old lawyer living in a major metropolitan area. She has never been married, and she shares her life with her cat, Beau, and her parents, who live nearby. Her physician recently diagnosed Ms. Domico as having Cushing's syndrome and admits her to the hospital for surgery for an adrenal cortex tumor (adrenalectomy). She has been having increased muscle weakness, so much so that she has difficulty climbing the one flight of stairs to her apartment. She has also had difficulty sleeping, irregular menstrual periods, and hypertension. Ms. Domico is especially concerned about her protruding abdomen, round face, development of facial hair, and the numerous bruises that have appeared on her skin.

ASSESSMENT
When Ms. Domico arrives at the hospital the morning of surgery, she is admitted by her case manager, Ann Sprengel, RN, CNS. Ms. Sprengel completes a physical assessment that includes abnormal findings of thin lower extremities, an enlarged abdomen, purple striae over the abdomen and buttocks, a round face, and obvious facial hair. Her blood pressure is 160/96. Ms. Domico tells Ms. Sprengel that she is always tired and that sometimes it "just wears me out to walk from the bedroom to the kitchen." Diagnostic tests conducted prior to admission reveal the following abnormal findings (all except cortisol levels are corrected before surgery):
   Glucose: 186 mg/dL (normal range: 70 to 110 mg/dL)
   Sodium: 152 mEq/L (normal range: 135 to 145 mEq/L)
   Potassium: 3.2 mEq/L (normal range: 3.5 to 5.0 mEq/L)
   Calcium: 4.3 mEq/L (normal range: 4.5 to 5.5 mEq/L)
   UFS > 100ug/24 hours (normal range 0–50 ug/24 hours)

DIAGNOSES
- *Fluid Volume Excess* related to sodium retention causing edema and hypertension
- *Risk for Injury* related to generalized fatigue and weakness
- *Risk for Infection* related to impaired immune response and edema
- *Disturbed Body Image* related to physical changes secondary to Cushing's syndrome

EXPECTED OUTCOMES
- Regain a normal body fluid balance.

- Remain free of injury.
- Remain free of infection.
- Verbalize understanding of the physical effects of the disease process and realistic expectations of desired changes in appearance.

PLANNING AND IMPLEMENTATION
- Weigh each morning, using the same scale.
- Maintain an accurate record of intake and output.
- Ensure adequate lighting in the room, and wear glasses and shoes when getting out of bed.
- Develop a written schedule of rest and activity periods.
- If agreeable, provide a private room, and restrict visitors to parents at this time.
- Use strict medical and surgical asepsis when providing care.
- Provide time for discussion of the disease and treatment; encourage verbalization of feelings and identify successful coping mechanisms used in the past.
- Encourage turning, coughing, and deep breathing and/or incentive spirometry every 2 to 4 hours.

EVALUATION
Ms. Domico states that she is "ready to have surgery and start feeling better." She has not fallen or injured herself, and she has remained free of infection. Although edema is still present, she has lost 8 lb (3.6 kg), and her blood pressure is decreased. Ms. Domico has openly discussed her concerns about the way she looks and feels; she understands that manifestations will improve following surgery. She has strong religious beliefs and family support, both of which provide strength and help her cope with the effects of the disorder and the need for any further treatment.

CRITICAL THINKING IN THE NURSING PROCESS
1. When Ms. Domico was admitted to the hospital, several of her test results were abnormal. Describe the pathophysiologic reason for those results.
2. List the assessments that nurses can make to determine body fluid balance.
3. Develop a plan of care for this patient for the nursing diagnosis *Fatigue*.

See Evaluating Your Response in Appendix C.

many endocrine disorders, Addison's disease is more common in women.

Pathophysiology

There are many possible causes of Addison's disease. The etiologies include the following:

- Autoimmune destruction of the adrenals. This is the most common cause. It may occur alone, or as part of a polyglandular autoimmune syndrome (PGA). Type 2 PGA is seen in adults, often associated with autoimmune thyroid disease (usually hypothyroidism), type 1 diabetes, primary ovarian or testicular failure, and pernicious anemia.
- Patients who are taking anticoagulants, have major trauma, sepsis, or are having open heart surgery may have bilateral adrenal hemorrhage.
- Adrenoleukodystrophy, an X-linked disorder characterized by an accumulation of very long chain fatty acids in the adrenal cortex, testes, brain, and spinal cord.
- ACTH deficit, resulting from pituitary tumors, pituitary surgery or irradiation, and the use of exogenous steroids.
- Abrupt withdrawal from long-term, high-dose steroid therapy, and tuberculosis or acquired immune deficiency syndrome (AIDS); the pathogens responsible for either disease can infiltrate and destroy adrenal tissue.

Adrenocortical destruction initially causes a decrease in adrenal glucocorticoid reserve. Basal glucocorticoid secretion is normal, but does not increase in response to stress and surgery. Trauma or infection can precipitate an adrenal crisis. As the destruction of the adrenal cortex continues, even basal secretion of glucocorticoids and mineralocorticoids is deficient. Decreasing plasma cortisol reduces the feedback inhibition of pituitary ACTH and plasma ACTH rises.

Secondary adrenocortical insufficiency occurs when either large doses or prolonged therapy with glucocorticoids are given for their anti-inflammatory and immunosuppressive effects to treat diseases such as arthritis and asthma. If the steroid medications are suddenly discontinued, the hypothalamus and pituitary cannot respond normally to the reduced level of circulating glucocorticoids.

Manifestations

The onset of Addison's disease is slow in most cases; the patient experiences manifestations after about 90% of the function of the gland is lost. The primary manifestations are the result of elevated ACTH levels and decreased aldosterone and cortisol (see the accompanying box). Aldosterone deficiency affects the ability of the distal tubules of the nephron to conserve sodium. Sodium is lost, potassium is retained, extracellular fluid is depleted, and the blood volume is decreased. Postural hypotension and syncope are common, and hypovolemic shock may occur. Hyponatremia causes dizziness, confusion, and neuromuscular irritability. Hyperkalemia causes cardiac dysrhthmias.

Cortisol insufficiency also causes decreased hepatic glyconeogenesis with hypoglycemia. The patient tolerates stress poorly and experiences lethargy, weakness, anorexia, nausea, vomiting, and diarrhea. The increased ACTH levels stimulate hyperpigmentation in more than 90% of patients with

---

MANIFESTATIONS of Addison's Disease

INTEGUMENTARY SYSTEM
- Delayed wound healing
- Hyperpigmentation

CARDIOVASCULAR SYSTEM
- Postural hypotension
- Arrhythmias
- Tachycardia

CENTRAL NERVOUS SYSTEM
- Lethargy
- Tremors
- Emotional lability
- Confusion

MUSCULOSKELETAL SYSTEM
- Weakness
- Muscle wasting
- Joint pain
- Muscle pain

GASTROINTESTINAL SYSTEM
- Anorexia
- Nausea and vomiting
- Diarrhea

REPRODUCTIVE SYSTEM
- Menstrual changes

METABOLIC EFFECTS
- Hyperkalemia
- Hyponatremia
- Hypoglycemia

Addison's disease (Porth & Matfin, 2009). In Caucasian patients, the skin looks deeply suntanned or bronzed in both exposed and unexposed areas.

Addisonian Crisis

Addisonian crisis is a life-threatening response to acute adrenal insufficiency. Triggers include surgery, acute systemic illness, trauma, or abrupt withdrawal of long-term corticosteroid therapy. The disorder is chronic after the acute episode resolves.

This response can occur in any person with Addison's disease; however, it is most commonly precipitated by major stressors, especially if the disease is poorly controlled. Addisonian crisis may also occur in patients who are abruptly withdrawn from glucocorticoid medications or who have hemorrhage into the adrenal glands from either septicemia or anticoagulant therapy.

The patient with Addisonian crisis may have any of the manifestations of Addison's disease, but the primary manifestations develop rapidly and are a high fever; weakness; severe, penetrating pain in the abdomen, lower back, and legs; severe vomiting; diarrhea; hypotension; and circulatory collapse, shock, and coma.

Treatment of the crisis is rapid intravenous replacement of fluids and glucocorticoids. Fluid balance is usually restored in 4 to 6 hours.

Interdisciplinary Care

The patient with Addison's disease requires early diagnosis and treatment. Medical treatment includes cortisol replacement therapy.

Diagnostic Tests

Addison's disease is diagnosed through findings of decreased levels of cortisol, aldosterone, and urinary 17-KS. Dehydration may result in increased hematocrit and blood urea nitrogen (BUN). Blood glucose levels are decreased, and potassium is increased. A list of laboratory findings in Addison's disease is shown in Table 19–2. The following diagnostic tests are used:

- *Serum cortisol levels,* which are decreased in adrenal insufficiency

- *Blood glucose levels,* which are decreased in adrenal insufficiency
- *Serum sodium levels,* which are decreased in adrenal insufficiency
- *Serum potassium levels,* which are increased in adrenal insufficiency
- *BUN levels,* which are increased in adrenal insufficiency
- *Urinary 17-hydroxycorticoids* and *17-KS levels,* which are decreased in adrenal insufficiency
- *Plasma ACTH levels,* which are increased in primary adrenal insufficiency (adrenal gland does not produce cortisol) but decreased in secondary adrenal insufficiency (ACTH is not adequately produced by the pituitary.)
- *ACTH stimulation test* is the most specific diagnostic test for Addison's disease. (Cortisol levels rise with pituitary deficiency but do not rise in primary adrenal insufficiency.)
- *CT scans* of the head, which identify any intracranial lesion impinging on the pituitary gland

Medications

The primary medical treatment of Addison's disease is replacement of corticosteroids and mineralocorticoids, accompanied by increased sodium in the diet. Hydrocortisone (Cortef) is given orally to replace cortisol; fludrocortisone (Florinef) is given orally to replace mineralocorticoids. Nursing implications in cortisol replacement are given in the following box.

ᘒ Nursing Care

Health Promotion

Health promotion interventions for the patient with or at risk for Addison's disease focus on careful assessments during anticoagulant therapy, open heart surgery, and trauma treatment. If the disease is present, teaching to prevent or treat an Addisonian crisis is essential.

Assessment

Collect the following data through the health history and physical examination (∞ see Chapter 18). Further focused assessments are described with nursing interventions in the following text.

- *Health history:* Weight loss, changes in skin color, nausea and vomiting, anorexia, diarrhea, abdominal pain, weakness, amenorrhea, changes in sexual desire, confusion, intolerance of stress.
- *Physical assessment:* Height and weight, vital signs, skin, hair quality and distribution, muscle size and strength.

MEDICATION ADMINISTRATION   **Addison's Disease**

CORTISOL REPLACEMENTS

Cortisone (Cortone, Cortogen)

Hydrocortisone (Cortisol, Hydrocortone, Cortef)

Fludrocortisone acetate (Florinef, F-Cortef)

Dexamethasone (Decadron, Hexadrol, Dexasone)

Prednisone (Meticorten, Deltasone, Orasone)

Prednisolone (Meticortelone)

Methylprednisolone (Medrol, Solu-Medrol)

Adrenocorticosteroids are used for replacement therapy in acute and chronic adrenal insufficiency. These drugs have anti-inflammatory and immunosuppressant effects. They also facilitate coping with stress.

   Because corticosteroids are immunosuppressants, their use is contraindicated when an infection is suspected because they mask the signs of infection. Immunizations with live vaccines should not be attempted. Corticosteroids are contraindicated in many other disorders, including peptic ulcer, Cushing's syndrome, cardiac disease, hyperthyroidism, hypothyroidism, and tuberculosis. Concurrent use with NSAIDs is contraindicated because of the effect on the gastrointestinal tract.

   When these drugs are administered in small doses for replacement therapy, side effects are uncommon. Large doses or prolonged therapy may cause a Cushing's-like syndrome, with atrophy of the adrenal cortex. Older patients, especially postmenopausal women, are more prone to develop hypertension and osteoporosis when undergoing glucocorticoid therapy. These drugs are used with caution in children and the older adult and are not usually administered to pregnant women.

Nursing Responsibilities
- Establish baseline data, including mental status, neurologic function, vital signs, and weight.

- Identify medications that might interact with corticosteroids: antidiabetic agents, cardiac glycosides, oral contraceptives, anticoagulants, NSAIDs.
- Document and report increased blood pressure, edema or weight gain, bleeding or bruising, weakness, or manifestations of Cushing's syndrome.
- Administer oral forms of the drug with food to minimize its ulcerogenic effect.
- Monitor electrolyte levels for increased sodium and decreased potassium.
- Monitor capillary blood glucose for hyperglycemia in the diabetic patient.

Health Education for the Patient and Family
- Take medications with food or milk, and report any gastric distress or dark stools.
- Most people need to take the medications for the rest of their lives.
- Consume a diet that is low in potassium, and higher in sodium and protein.
- Weigh yourself each day at the same time, and report any consistent weight gain, which indicates fluid retention.
- Use safety measures in the home to prevent falls and injuries.
- Corticosteroids may impair the effectiveness of oral contraceptives.
- Take the medication regularly and continuously. *Abruptly discontinuing the medication is dangerous.*
- Obtain a Medic-Alert bracelet.
- Monitor for increased stressors (infection, dental work, personal crisis) and increase the dose as indicated by the physician.
- Anticoagulant drugs or insulin may decrease the effectiveness of corticosteroids.
- Report the following to the physician: dizziness on sitting or standing, nausea and vomiting, pain, thirst, feelings of anxiety, malaise, infections.

Nursing Diagnoses and Interventions

The patient with Addison's disease requires nursing care for a wide variety of responses to the decrease in cortisol levels. Nursing diagnoses discussed in this section are directed toward problems with fluid and electrolyte balance and compliance with lifelong self-care. See the accompanying Case Study & Nursing Care Plan on page 515.

Deficient Fluid Volume

Fluid volume deficit in the patient with Addison's disease results from loss of water and sodium, as well as from vomiting and diarrhea. Extracellular fluid volume deficit, decreased cardiac output, hypotension, and hypovolemic shock may occur, especially in crisis situations. Interventions for this diagnosis are outlined for the patient who is hospitalized.

- Monitor intake and output, and assess for signs of dehydration: dry mucous membranes; thirst; poor skin turgor; sunken eyeballs; scanty, dark urine; increased urine specific gravity; weight loss; and increased hemoconcentration (increased hematocrit and BUN). *Glucocorticoid and mineralocorticoid depletion causes fluid volume deficit. Fluid volume deficit may reach crisis levels if undetected, causing altered tissue perfusion and hypovolemic shock.*

- Monitor cardiovascular status: Take and record vital signs, assess character of pulses, monitor potassium levels and ECGs. *Fluid volume deficit may lead to hypotension and a rapid, weak, or thready pulse. As aldosterone levels fall, renal excretion of potassium decreases, increasing blood levels of potassium.*

- Weigh the patient daily at the same time and in the same clothing. *Dehydration is manifested by weight loss.*

- Encourage an oral fluid intake of 3000 mL per day and an increased salt intake. *Cortisol deficiency increases fluid loss, leading to extracellular fluid volume depletion. Oral fluid replacement is necessary to balance this loss. An increase in dietary sodium can decrease the hyponatremia characteristic of adrenal insufficiency.*

- Teach to sit and stand slowly, and provide assistance as necessary. *Extracellular fluid volume deficit causes orthostatic hypotension, dizziness, and possible loss of consciousness. These manifestations increase the risk of injury from falls.*

PRACTICE ALERT
Hyperkalemia causes changes in cardiac muscle function, which are reflected in ECG changes. (ECGs are discussed in ∞ Chapter 30.)

Risk for Ineffective Therapeutic Regimen Management

Patients with Addison's disease must learn to provide lifelong self-care that involves varied components: medications, diet, and recognizing and responding to responses to stress. Changes in lifestyle are difficult to maintain permanently.

- Teach the effects of illness and treatment. Discuss patient and family concerns. *Lack of knowledge about the illness, as well as the possibility of complications from disregarding or altering the treatment, can negatively affect compliance.*

- Include the following in the teaching plan:
  - Self-administration of steroids
  - The importance of carrying at all times an emergency kit containing parenteral cortisone and a syringe/needle
  - Wearing a Medic-Alert bracelet that says "Adrenal insufficiency—takes hydrocortisone"
  - Increasing oral fluid intake and maintaining a diet high in sodium and low in potassium
  - The necessity of altering the medication dose when experiencing emotional or physical stressors
  - The importance of continuing health care
    One of the most important components of caring for the patient with Addison's disease is teaching both the patient and family to provide care. The length of treatment and the side effects of medications can discourage adherence to the regimen.

Community-Based Care

The patient with Addison's disease provides self-care at home. One of the most important components of caring for the patient with Addison's disease is teaching both the patient and family to provide care. Family stability, an awareness of the serious nature of the disease, and the effectiveness of treatment all promote adherence. The length of treatment and the side effects of medications, however, can discourage adherence. In addition to the information in the teaching topics included with nursing diagnoses and interventions, include the following topics:

- Referral to social worker, if appropriate
- Referral to community agencies for continued education and support
- Helpful resources: National Institute of Diabetes and Digestive and Kidney Diseases (Addison's disease), Endocrine Society, American Association of Clinical Endocrinologists

The Patient with Pheochromocytoma

Pheochromocytomas are tumors of chromaffin tissues in the adrenal medulla. These tumors, which are usually benign, produce catecholamines (epinephrine or norepinephrine) that stimulate the sympathetic nervous system. Although many organs are affected, the most dangerous effects are peripheral vasoconstriction and increased cardiac rate and contractility with resultant paroxysmal hypertension. Systolic blood pressure may rise to 200 to 300 mmHg, the diastolic to 150 to 175 mmHg. Attacks are often precipitated by physical, emotional, or environmental stimuli. This condition is life threatening.

A pheochromocytoma is diagnosed by increased catecholamine levels in the blood or urine, by x-ray studies, and by surgical exploration. Vanillylmandelic acid is the end product of metabolism of all catecholamine substances and is collected in a 24-hour urine sample. Removal of the tumor(s) by adrenalectomy is the treatment of choice.

CASE STUDY & NURSING CARE PLAN Addison's Disease

A 51-year-old unemployed salesman, Don Sardoff, is brought to the emergency room by his wife, Ellen, at 8 AM. Mrs. Sardoff tells the emergency room nurse that her husband has not been feeling well for the last week, but that when he got up this morning, he was so weak he couldn't dress himself and didn't know where he was. Mrs. Sardoff tells the nurse that her husband has been taking a cortisone drug for treatment of his rheumatoid arthritis for the past 2 years, but notes, "We didn't have the money to buy it this month."

ASSESSMENT

On admission to the emergency room, Mr. Sardoff is dehydrated, with dry oral mucous membranes and tongue, poor skin turgor, and sunken eyeballs. His blood pressure is 94/44, and his pulse is rapid and thready. He is weak, dizzy, and disoriented about time and place. Diagnostic tests reveal the following abnormal findings at 8:30 AM:

- EKG: widening QRS complex and increased PR interval
- Sodium: 129 mEq/L (normal range: 135 to 145 mEq/L)
- Glucose: 54 mg/dL (normal range: 70 to 110 mg/dL)
- Potassium: 5.3 mEq/L (normal range: 3.5 to 5 mEq/L)
- Cortisol: 2 mg/dL (normal for AM: 5 to 23 mg/dL)

The medical orders for Mr. Sardoff include intravenous administration of 5% dextrose in normal saline (D_5NS) at 250 mL/h and hydrocortisone (Solu-Cortef) 200 mg. After the fluids and medication are initiated, Mr. Sardoff is moved to an in-hospital medical bed.

DIAGNOSES

- *Deficient Fluid Volume* related to hypovolemia secondary to adrenal insufficiency
- *Ineffective Tissue Perfusion: Peripheral* related to fluid volume deficit
- *Anxiety* related to lack of knowledge about the effects and treatment of adrenal insufficiency

EXPECTED OUTCOMES

- Regain normal fluid balance.

- Regain normal peripheral perfusion with blood pressure within normal range.
- Verbalize knowledge of the causes and effects of adrenal insufficiency.

PLANNING AND IMPLEMENTATION

- Monitor intake and output closely.
- Take and record weight at the same time daily.
- Monitor blood pressure, pulses, and skin turgor every 2 hours until stable, then four times a day.
- Monitor electrolytes, and report abnormal results.
- Discuss a diet that is high in sodium, low in potassium, and has an increased fluid intake (3000 mL per day). Discuss the types of fluids desired and the best times for intake of increased fluids.
- Assist during activity to prevent falls.
- Provide verbal and written instructions, and encourage verbal feedback about the causes and effects of the disease, the effects of medications, the effects of not taking long-term cortisone drugs, the diet, and self-care at home.

EVALUATION

Following treatment for acute adrenal insufficiency, Mr. Sardoff is no longer dehydrated, and his blood pressure has returned to his normal reading of 132/88. He is alert and oriented, and anxious to learn to care for himself at home. After dietary instructions and teaching for self-care that included his wife, Mr. Sardoff verbalizes an understanding of his illness and the need to take his medication carefully and accurately. A referral is made to a social worker for assistance with costs of medications.

CRITICAL THINKING IN THE NURSING PROCESS

1. Adrenal insufficiency is often diagnosed only when the patient becomes seriously ill in response to a stressor. Explain why this statement is or is not true.
2. Describe the physical assessments that are found in the severely dehydrated patient.
3. Outline a teaching plan for Mr. Sardoff with foods for a high-sodium, low-potassium diet.

See Evaluating Your Response in Appendix C.

Disorders of the Pituitary Gland

The pituitary gland produces hormones that affect multiple body systems through regulation of endocrine function. Target tissues include the thyroid, adrenal cortex, ovary, uterus, mammary glands, testes, and kidneys. Disorders result from an excess or deficiency of one or more of the pituitary hormones due to a pathologic condition within the gland itself or to hypothalamic dysfunction.

Although disorders of the pituitary cause diverse and serious problems, they are not as common as disorders of other endocrine glands. Hyperpituitarism and hypopituitarism are discussed in this section.

The Patient with Disorders of the Anterior Pituitary Gland

Hyperfunction of the anterior pituitary gland, characterized by excess production and secretion of one or more trophic hormones, is usually the result of a pituitary tumor or pituitary

hyperplasia. The most common cause of hyperpituitarism is a benign adenoma. The manifestations result from pressure on the optic nerve causing visual changes or an excess of growth hormone (GH), prolactin (PRL), ACTH, or TSH.

Hypofunction of the anterior pituitary gland results in a deficiency of one or more of the gland's hormones. Conditions causing hypopituitarism include pituitary tumors; surgical removal of the pituitary gland; radiation; and pituitary infarction, infection, or trauma.

Pathophysiology and Manifestations

Growth hormone (somatotropin) is produced by cells in the anterior pituitary throughout life. GH stimulates the production of IGF-1 (an insulin-like growth factor) by the liver. GH is necessary for growth and also contributes to metabolic regulation. GH stimulates all aspects of cartilage growth, and one of its major effects is to stimulate the growth of the epiphyseal cartilage plates of long bones. In addition, other body tissues respond to the metabolic effect of GH and IGF-1 with increases in bone width and the growth of visceral and endocrine organs, skeletal and cardiac muscle, skin, and connective tissue. Gigantism and acromegaly (discussed next) result from over-stimulation. Growth retardation and short stature result from deficient production of GH.

Hypersecretion of PRL affects reproductive and sexual function. Women may have irregular or absent menses, difficulty becoming pregnant, and decreased libido. Men may be impotent and have decreased libido. PRL deficiency in post-partal women causes a failure to lactate.

An excess secretion of ACTH overstimulates the adrenal cortex, which in turn increases secretion of adrenal hormones. The result is Cushing's syndrome. Deficiencies of TSH are uncommon, but cause hypothyroidism.

Gigantism

Gigantism occurs when GH hypersecretion begins before puberty and the closure of the epiphyseal plates. The person becomes abnormally tall, often exceeding 7 ft (213 cm) in height, but body proportions are relatively normal. Most often the result of a tumor, the condition is rare today as a result of improved diagnosis and treatment.

Acromegaly

Acromegaly, which literally means "enlarged extremities," occurs when sustained GH and IGF-1hypersecretion begins during adulthood, most commonly because of pituitary tumors. IGF-1 causes most of the clinical manifestations of acromegaly (Porth, 2007). As a result of constant stimulation, the small bones of the hands and feet, the membranous bones of the skull, connective tissue, and soft tissues continue to grow. The forehead enlarges, the maxilla lengthens, the tongue enlarges, and the voice deepens. Overgrowth of bone and soft tissue in the hands and feet causes patients to buy increasingly larger rings, gloves, and shoes. This condition is different from Marfan's syndrome, a genetic disorder that results in elongated bones, optic changes, and severe cardiovascular effects. (∞ See Chapter 31 for nursing care of patients with cardiovascular disorders.)

Other manifestations include peripheral nerve damage from entrapment of nerves, headache, hypertension, congestive heart failure, skin thickening and copious sweating, seizures, and visual disturbances. Changes in appearance are subtle and diagnosis is usually made 10 years or more after onset of GH hypersecretion. Impaired glucose tolerance and diabetes may also develop. Arthralgias in the large joints develop secondary to the bone and connective tissue growth; manifestations may be relieved by treatment that halts excessive GH and IGF-1 production.

Interdisciplinary Care

Acromegaly is treated by surgical removal or irradiation of the pituitary tumor. A transsphenoidal or transfrontal surgical procedure is most commonly used. Somatostatin receptor binding drugs (SRBDs) suppress the anterior pituitary gland and decrease GH levels. These are administered by injection, and gastrointestinal side effects are common for the first couple of weeks. Gallstones may occur within a year of beginning treatment. Growth hormone receptor antagonists lower IGF-1 production and are used if manifestations persist with SRBDs. Radiation therapy is used when GH-producing tumors persist despite surgery or become resistant to medical therapies (Ben-Shlomo & Melmed, 2008).

∾ Nursing Care

Patients with anterior pituitary disorders require interventions to help in coping with physical and emotional changes, as well as to prevent complications involving other organs and functions of the endocrine system. Nursing care for the patient having cranial surgery is discussed in ∞ Chapter 42.

The Patient with Disorders of the Posterior Pituitary Gland

Disorders of the posterior pituitary are related primarily to excessive or deficient antidiuretic hormone (ADH) secretion. The disorders discussed here are the syndrome of inappropriate ADH secretion and diabetes insipidus.

Pathophysiology and Manifestations

Antidiuretic hormone is secreted in response to low circulatory volume, which is monitored by osmoreceptors in the hypothalamus. When a condition of hyperosmolality occurs, ADH secretion increases, and renal water is reabsorbed. Hypoosmolality causes the suppression of ADH, and renal water excretion increases. ADH, also known as vasopressin, causes the kidney to reabsorb water from the collecting ducts to increase circulatory volume.

Syndrome of Inappropriate ADH Secretion

The **syndrome of inappropriate ADH secretion (SIADH)** is characterized by high levels of ADH in the absence of serum hypo-osmolality. This disorder is most often caused by the ectopic production of ADH by malignant tumors (e.g., oat cell carcinoma of the lung, pancreatic carcinoma, leukemia, and Hodgkin's disease). A transient form may follow a head injury, pituitary surgery, or the use of medications such as barbiturates, anesthetics, or diuretics.

Manifestations of SIADH occur as a result of water retention, hyponatremia, and serum hypo-osmolality. Blood volume expands, but the plasma is diluted. Aldosterone is suppressed; as a result, renal excretion of sodium increases. Water moves from the hypotonic plasma and the interstitial spaces into the cells. Urinary output decreases and the urine becomes very concentrated.

Manifestations of SIADH (∞ see Chapter 10) are usually nonspecific but are related to hyponatremia and water intoxication. Despite fluid retention, the patient may experience thirst. Brain cells may swell, causing neurologic manifestations including headache, changes in mental status or personality, lethargy, and irritability. Weight gain results from the retention of fluid. Usually no edema is present, because water is distributed between the intracellular and extracellular spaces.

Treatment addresses the low serum sodium and intracellular swelling. Besides keeping the patient safe, nursing care involves teaching the patient about restricting fluids to 1 L/day. Fluid restriction continues until the source of ADH is successfully identified and if malignancy is the cause, destroyed. Furosemide and an intravenous infusion of half normal saline decrease circulatory volume and prevent sodium excretion (McAdams-Jones, 2008).

Demeclocycline (Declomycin) is a tetracycline antibiotic with the unique property of creating excessive urine flow. It is used as a treatment for SIADH when patients cannot adequately restrict water intake. Vasopressin antagonists may be given for SIADH. These drugs are especially beneficial for SIADH in persons with heart failure (McPhee & Papadakis, 2009). Sodium levels should be monitored and corrections of hyponatremia must be done cautiously to prevent cerebral osmotic demyelination.

Diabetes Insipidus

Diabetes insipidus is the result of ADH insufficiency. The two types are as follows:

- *Neurogenic diabetes insipidus* can either result from a disruption of the hypothalamus and pituitary gland (as from trauma, irradiation, or cranial surgery) or be idiopathic.
- *Nephrogenic diabetes insipidus* is a disorder in which the renal tubules are not sensitive to ADH. This may be familial in origin or the result of renal failure.

Diabetes insipidus may result from brain tumors or infections, pituitary surgery, cerebral vascular accidents, and renal and organ failure. It is also a complication of closed-head trauma with increased intracranial pressure.

A deficit of ADH causes excretion of large amounts of dilute urine (*polyuria*), in some instances as much as 12 L/day. The patient has extreme thirst and drinks large volumes of water (*polydipsia*). If unable to replace the water loss, the patient becomes dehydrated and hypernatremic. Even though

TABLE 19–3 Comparison of Posterior Pituitary Gland Disorders	
SIADH	**DIABETES INSIPIDUS**
Excessive ADH	Deficient ADH
Fluid volume excess	Fluid volume deficit
Restrict fluid intake	Encourage fluid intake
Demeclocycline (Declomycin) (oral agent) causes excessive urination	Desmopressin (DDAVP) (nasal spray) causes increased water reabsorption

hyperosmolality is present, the urine is dilute and has a low specific gravity.

If this disorder is caused by cerebral injury, manifestations commonly appear 3 to 6 days after the initial injury and last for 7 to 10 days. If the increased intracranial pressure is relieved, manifestations of diabetes insipidus usually disappear. However, diabetes insipidus may also be a chronic illness requiring lifelong treatment and care. See Table 19–3 for a comparison of posterior pituitary gland disorders.

Interdisciplinary Care

SIADH is treated by correcting underlying causes, treating the hyponatremia with intravenous hypertonic saline, and restricting oral fluids to less than 800 mL/day.

Diabetes insipidus is treated by correcting underlying causes, if possible. Other medical interventions include administering intravenous hypotonic fluids, increasing oral fluids, and replacing ADH hormone. Desmopressin acetate, administered intranasally, orally, or parenterally, is the treatment of choice.

✆ Nursing Care

Nursing care for the patient with SIADH and diabetes insipidus focuses on patient problems with fluid and electrolyte balance, as discussed in ∞ Chapter 10.

CHAPTER HIGHLIGHTS

- Hormones regulate growth, development, and metabolism. Homeostasis is dependent on a balanced level of each type of hormone. Not only do hormones affect organ function, but they also interact, and when excesses or deficits occur, manifestations of other endocrine disorders may occur.
- The pituitary gland, in conjunction with the hypothalamus, is the master gland of the body. Fifteen hormones and regulatory factors are synthesized in the anterior pituitary and hypothalamus; many are trophic hormones that stimulate the release of other hormones.

- Thyroid disorders are the most common endocrine disorders. Occurring mainly among women, these diseases change body image and impose upsets to energy levels, creating fatigue and exhaustion.
- Diagnostic tests and therapies are available to identify and treat thyroid disorders. Surgery, radiation therapy, and medications support good quality of life, but the medications must be used throughout the lifetime.
- The parathyroid glands synthesize parathormone, which maintains serum calcium. Thyroid tissues surrounding the parathyroids

synthesize a hormone, calcitonin, which decreases serum calcium to normal levels. These glands provide the proper level of serum calcium, which is vital for cardiac function, bone stability, nerve conduction, and muscle contraction.

- The adrenal glands regulate energy and fluid balance through corticosteroids and mineralocorticoids. Cushing's and Addison's

disease are polar opposites. Treatment eliminates the manifestations of one and creates the manifestations of the other. Patients with. these diseases require patient education until they fully grasp the significance of the condition and the importance of adhering to the treatment plan.

TEST YOURSELF NCLEX-RN® REVIEW

1. Graves' disease, the most common cause of hyperthyroidism, is categorized as what type of disorder?
   1. autoimmune
   2. infectious
   3. allergic
   4. genetic

2. What principle supports the treatment of hyperthyroidism with radioactive iodine?
   1. Radioactive iodine reduces the vascularity of the thyroid gland.
   2. Doses of radioactive iodine are too small to be hazardous to other body parts.
   3. The thyroid gland takes up iodine in any form.
   4. Irradiation of the thyroid gland decreases the risk of hypothyroidism.

3. You assess a patient with newly diagnosed hypothyroidism as having an enlarged thyroid gland (goiter). What physiologic process causes this enlargement?
   1. an excess of TH stimulates thyroid follicles
   2. an increased dietary iodine intake
   3. a compensatory effort to produce more TH
   4. tissue hypertrophy in response to increased TH

4. Mrs. Jonah has taken cortisone for her rheumatoid arthritis for several years. What endocrine disorder is she most at risk for developing?
   1. hyperthyroidism
   2. hypothyroidism
   3. acromegaly
   4. Cushing's syndrome

5. Which statement illustrates that the patient with Addison's disease understands your teaching?
   1. "I will be sure to stop taking my medications when I have an infection."
   2. "I have purchased an emergency kit and keep it with me all the time."
   3. "I know I should never alter my dose of medications."
   4. "I wonder why I look suntanned all the time."

6. Manifestations of hyponatremia found in SIADH include which of the following?
   1. weight loss
   2. irritability
   3. hyperkalemia
   4. constipation

7. A home health nurse is caring for a patient with hyperparathyroidism and osteoporosis. Which nursing diagnosis has priority with this patient?
   1. *Risk for Fear*
   2. *Risk for Injury*
   3. *Risk for Isolation*
   4. *Risk for Chronic Low Self-Esteem*

8. A nurse is monitoring a patient for signs of hypercalcemia. Which of the following is a sign of hypercalcemia?
   1. oliguria
   2. positive Chvostek's sign
   3. diminished bowel sounds
   4. hyperactive deep tendon reflexes

9. A patient with increased ACTH levels and Addison's disease is likely to manifest which of the following?
   1. tremor
   2. hair loss
   3. gingival hyperplasia
   4. dermal hyperpigmentation

10. Patients treated with glucocorticoids may be at risk for Addisonian crisis due to which of the following?
    1. rapid withdrawal of glucocorticoids
    2. excessive ACTH
    3. sodium retention
    4. hypokalemia

See Test Yourself answers in Appendix C.

Pearson Nursing Student Resources

Find additional review materials at
www.nursing.pearsonhighered.com

Prepare for success with additional NCLEX®-style practice questions, interactive assignments and activities, Web links, animations and videos, and more!

BIBLIOGRAPHY

American Cancer Society. (2007). Making treatment decisions: DHEA. Retrieved from http://www.cancer.org/docroot/ETO/content/ETO_5_3X_Dhea.asp?sitearea=ETO

American Thyroid Association. (2008). Thyroid function tests. Retrieved from http://www.thyroid.org/patients/patient_brochures/function_tests.html

Ben-Shlomo, A., & Melmed, S. (2008). Acromegaly. *Endocrinology and Metabolism Clinics, 37*(1), 101–122.

Bulechek, G. M., Butcher, H. K., & Dochterman, J. M. (Eds.). (2008). *Nursing interventions classification (NIC)* (5th ed.). St. Louis: Mosby Elsevier.

Davis, A. B., Orlander, P. R., & Kermani, A. (2008). Goiter, toxic nodular. eMedicine, WebMD. Retrieved from http://www.emedicine.com/MED/topic920.htm

Elamin, M. B., Murad, M. H., Mullan, R., Erickson, D., Harris, K., et al. (2008). Accuracy of diagnostic tests for Cushing's syndrome: A systematic review and meta-analyses. *The Journal of Clinical Endocrinology and Metabolism, 93*(5), 1553–1562.

Fatourechi, V. (2005). Pretibial myxedema: Pathophysiology and treatment options. *American Journal of Clinical Dermatology, 6*(5), 295–309.

Holcomb, S. S. (2006). Hospital nursing: Do the clues add up to Addison's disease? *Nursing, 36*(3), 64hn1–64hn4.

Houston, D. K., Schwartz, A. V., Cauley, J. A., Tylavsky, F. A., Simonsick, et al. (2008). Serum parathyroid hormone levels predict falls in older adults with diabetes mellitus. *Journal of the American Geriatric Society, 56*(11), 2027–2032.

Kee, J. L. (2010). *Handbook of laboratory and diagnostic tests with nursing implications.* Upper Saddle River, NJ: Pearson Prentice Hall.

McAdams-Jones, D. (2008). Rapid response: Reversing SIADH. *American Nurse Today, 3*(9), 40.

McPhee, S. J. Papadakis, M. A. (Eds.). (2009). *Current medical diagnosis & treatment* (48th ed.). New York: Lange Medical Books/McGraw-Hill.

Moorhead, S., Johnson, M., Maas, M., & Swanson, E. (Eds.). (2008). *Nursing outcomes classification (NOC)* (4th ed.). St. Louis, MO: Mosby Elsevier.

NANDA International. (2009). *Nursing diagnoses: Definitions and classification 2009–2011.* Oxford, UK: Wiley-Blackwell.

National Cancer Institute. (2009). Thyroid cancer. Retrieved from http://www.cancer.gov/cancertopics/types/thyroid

Nieman L. K., Biller, B. M., Findling, J. W., Newell-Price, J., Savage, M. O. et al. (2008). The diagnosis of Cushing's syndrome: An endocrine society clinical practice guideline. *The Journal of Clinical Endocrinology & Metabolism, 93*(5), 1526–1540.

Pfister, D. G., & Fagin, J. A. (2000). Refractory thyroid cancer: a paradigm shift in treatment is not far off. *Journal of Clinical Oncology, 26*(29), 4701–4704.

Porth, C. (2007). *Essentials of pathophysiology: Concepts of altered health states* (2nd ed.). Philadelphia: Lippincott, Williams and Wilkins.

Porth, C., & Matfin, G. (2009). *Pathophysiology: Concepts of altered health states* (8th ed.). Philadelphia: Lippincott Williams and Wilkins.

Shah, A. A., & Lettieri, C. J. (2007). Endocrine emergencies. Medscape Nurses. Retrieved from http://www.medscape.com/viewarticle/567307

Torres, P. U. (2006). Cinacalcet HCl: A novel treatment for secondary hyperparathyroidism caused by chronic kidney disease. *Journal of Renal Nutrition, 16*(3), 253–258.

Wilson, B., Shannon, M., & Shields, K. (2010). *Pearson's nurse's drug guide 2010.* Upper Saddle River, NJ: Pearson Prentice Hall.

20 Nursing Care of Patients with Diabetes Mellitus

LEARNING OUTCOMES

1. Describe the prevalence and incidence of diabetes mellitus (DM).
2. Explain the pathophysiology, risk factors, manifestations, and complications of type 1 and type 2 DM.
3. Provide rationale for diagnostic tests used for screening, diagnosis, and monitoring of DM.
4. Discuss the nursing implications for insulin and oral hypoglycemic agents used to treat patients with DM.
5. Discuss best practices of self-care management of DM related to diet planning, sick day management, and exercise.
6. Compare and contrast the manifestations of hypoglycemia, diabetic ketoacidosis (DKA), and hyperosmolar hyperglycemic state (HHS).

CLINICAL COMPETENCIES

1. Assess blood glucose levels and patterns of hyper- and hypoglycemia in patients with DM.
2. Use assessed data, patient values, clinical expertise, and evidence to determine priority nursing diagnoses and select and implement individualized nursing interventions.
3. Administer oral and injectable medications used to treat DM knowledgeably and safely.
4. Assess patients' ability to read markings on syringes and to identify correct insulin doses.
5. Provide individualized care to patients with hypoglycemia, diabetic ketoacidosis, and hyperosmolar hyperglycemic state.
6. Effectively communicate with and function within the interdisciplinary team to plan and provide patient care.
7. Provide appropriate teaching to facilitate self blood glucose monitoring, administration of oral and injectable hypoglycemic medications, diabetic diet, appropriate exercise, and effective foot care.
8. Adapt individual and cultural values and variations as well as expressed needs and preferences into the plan of care for patients with DM.
9. Revise plan of care as needed to provide effective interventions to promote, maintain, or restore normal glucose levels.

KEY TERMS

diabetes mellitus (DM), *520*
diabetic ketoacidosis (DKA), *541*
gastroparesis, *545*
gluconeogenesis, *521*
glucosuria, *523*

glycogenolysis, *521*
hyperglycemia, *522*
hyperosmolar hyperglycemic state (HHS), *542*
hypoglycemia, *543*

ketosis, *522*
polydipsia, *524*
polyphagia, *524*
polyuria, *523*

Diabetes Mellitus

Diabetes mellitus (DM) is a common chronic disease of adults requiring continuing medical supervision and patient self-care education. However, depending on the type of DM and the age of the patient, both patient needs and nursing care may vary greatly. Consider the following examples:

- Cheryl Draheim is a 45-year-old schoolteacher. She developed DM at age 34 after an automobile crash caused severe pancreatic injuries. Cheryl has always been very careful about taking her insulin, following her diet, and exercising regularly. However, she is beginning to notice that her vision is getting worse and that she is having increasing pain in her legs, especially after standing for long periods of time. Cheryl says that sometimes she believes the disease controls her more than she controls it.
- Tom Chang is 53 years old. Early in his 40s, Tom was diagnosed with type 2 DM. Although Tom was taught about the

disease and the importance of taking his oral medications, following his diet plan, and getting exercise, he rarely did more than take the medication. Five years ago, he was hospitalized for hyperglycemia and started taking insulin. Last year Tom had a stroke, leaving him unable to walk. Now, he has been admitted to the hospital for treatment of gangrene of the large toe on his left foot.
- Grace Staples is an independent 82-year-old woman who lives alone and happily takes care of her two cats. She is slightly overweight. Last year, during Grace's annual eye examination, eye changes typical for DM were found. She was referred to her family doctor, who diagnosed type 2 DM and started her on oral medications. Grace sticks to her diet, walks a mile every day, and plans to live to be 100.

As illustrated in these examples, DM is not a single disorder but a group of chronic disorders of the endocrine pancreas, all categorized under a broad diagnostic label. The condition is characterized by inappropriate hyperglycemia caused by a relative or absolute deficiency of insulin or by cellular resistance to the action of insulin. Of the several classifications of DM, this chapter will focus on type 1 and type 2. Type 1 DM is the result of pancreatic islet cell destruction and a total deficit of circulating insulin; type 2 DM results from insulin resistance with a defect in compensatory insulin secretion.

DM has been recognized as a disease for centuries, but it was not until 1921 that techniques were developed for extracting insulin from pancreatic tissue and for measuring blood glucose. At the same time, researchers discovered that insulin, when injected, produces a dramatic drop in blood glucose. This meant that DM was no longer a terminal illness, because hyperglycemia could now be controlled. Since that time, oral hypoglycemic drugs, human insulin products, insulin pumps, home blood glucose monitoring, and transplantation of the pancreas or of pancreatic islet or beta cells have advanced the treatment and care of people with DM.

Patients with DM face lifelong changes in lifestyle and health status. Nursing care is provided in many settings for the diagnosis and care of the disease and treatment of complications. A major role of the nurse is that of educator in both hospital and community settings.

Incidence and Prevalence

Approximately 1.6 million new cases of DM are diagnosed each year in the United States. This chronic illness affects an estimated 23.6 million people, of that number, 17.9 million have been diagnosed and an estimated 5.7 million are undiagnosed (National Institutes of Health [NIH], 2008). There is an increased prevalence of DM (especially type 2 DM) among older adults and in minority populations. See the following Focus on Cultural Diversity box.

DM is the sixth leading cause of death by disease in the United States, primarily because of the widespread cardiovascular effects that result in atherosclerosis, coronary artery disease, and stroke (CDC, 2009). People with DM are two to four times more likely to have heart disease, and two to four times more likely to have a stroke than people who do not have the disease. DM is the leading cause of end-stage renal disease (kidney failure), and the major cause of newly diagnosed blindness in people ages 20 to 74. DM also is the most frequent cause of nontraumatic amputations, with an estimated 71,000 amputations each year in people with DM (NIH, 2008).

Americans with DM use a disproportionate share of the nation's healthcare services. They visit outpatient services and physicians' offices more often than people who do not have the disease, and they require more frequent hospitalizations with longer days of in-hospital treatment. The cost of illness and resulting loss of productivity for people with DM exceeds $174 billion per year, according to an estimate by the American Diabetes Association (NIH, 2008).

Overview of Endocrine Pancreatic Hormones and Glucose Homeostasis

The hormones produced by several different cells of the endocrine pancreas, along with hormones produced by the small intestine, are responsible for glucose homeostasis in the body.

HORMONES The endocrine pancreas produces hormones necessary for the metabolism and cellular utilization of carbohydrates, proteins, and fats. The cells that produce these hormones are clustered in groups of cells called the islets of Langerhans. These islets have three different types of cells:

- Alpha cells produce the hormone *glucagon*, which stimulates the breakdown of glycogen in the liver, the formation of carbohydrates in the liver, and the breakdown of lipids in both the liver and adipose tissue. The primary function of glucagon is to decrease glucose oxidation and to increase blood glucose levels. Through **glycogenolysis** (the breakdown of liver glycogen) and **gluconeogenesis** (the formation of glucose from fats and proteins), glucagon prevents blood glucose from decreasing below a certain level when the body is fasting or in between meals. The action of glucagon is initiated in most people when blood glucose falls below about 70 mg/dL.
- Beta cells secrete the hormone *insulin*, which facilitates the movement of glucose across cell membranes into cells, decreasing blood glucose levels. Insulin prevents the excessive breakdown of glycogen in the liver and in muscle, facilitates lipid formation while inhibiting the breakdown of stored fats, and helps move amino acids into cells for protein synthesis. After secretion by the beta cells, insulin enters the portal circulation, travels directly to the liver, and is then released into the general circulation. Circulating insulin is rapidly bound to receptor sites on peripheral tissues (especially muscle and fat cells) or is destroyed by the liver or kidneys. Insulin release is regulated by blood glucose; it increases when blood glucose levels increase, and it decreases when blood glucose levels decrease. When a person eats food, insulin levels begin to rise in minutes, peak in 3 to 5 minutes, and return to baseline in 2 to 3 hours (Porth & Matfin, 2009). Amylin is a glucose-regulating hormone

also secreted by the beta cells with insulin that affects postprandial (postmeal) glucose levels. It impairs glucagon secretion and slows the rate at which glucose travels to the small intestine for absorption.

■ Delta cells produce *somatostatin*, which acts within the islets of Langerhan to inhibit the production of both glucagon and insulin. It also slows gastrointestinal motility, allowing more time for food to be absorbed.

In addition, the small intestine produces hormones that lower blood glucose following the intake of a meal. Glucagon-like peptide-1 (GLP-1) and glucose-dependent insulinotropic polypeptide (GIP) are secreted from the small intestine to increase insulin release after a meal has been ingested. This hormone-stimulated insulin increase following ingestion of food is called an incretin effect. An injectable form of these hormones, exenatide (Byetta), is an incretin mimetic used in the treatment of type II DM.

BLOOD GLUCOSE HOMEOSTASIS   All body tissues and organs require a constant supply of glucose; however, not all tissues require insulin for glucose uptake. The brain, liver, intestines, and renal tubules do not require insulin to transfer glucose into their cells. Skeletal muscle, cardiac muscle, and adipose tissue do require insulin for glucose movement into the cells.

Normal blood glucose is maintained in healthy people primarily through the actions of insulin and glucagon. Increased blood glucose levels, amino acids, and fatty acids stimulate pancreatic beta cells to produce insulin. As cells of cardiac muscle, skeletal muscle, and adipose tissue take up glucose, plasma levels of nutrients decrease, suppressing the stimulus to produce insulin. If blood glucose falls, glucagon is released to raise hepatic glucose output, raising glucose levels. Epinephrine,

growth hormone, thyroxine, and glucocorticoids (often referred to as glucose counterregulatory hormones) also stimulate an increase in glucose in times of hypoglycemia, stress, growth, or increased metabolic demand. The regulation of blood glucose levels by insulin and glucagon is illustrated in Figure 20–1 ■.

Pathophysiology of DM

DM is a group of metabolic diseases characterized by hyperglycemia resulting from defects in the secretion of insulin, the action of insulin, or both. There are four major types of DM. Type 1 DM (5% to 10% of diagnosed cases), type 2 DM (90% to 95% of diagnosed cases), gestational DM (2% to 5% of all pregnancies), and other specific types of DM (1% to 2% of diagnosed cases). The classification and characteristics of the four types are described in Table 20–1.

Type 1 Diabetes

Type 1 DM most often occurs in childhood and adolescence, but it may occur at any age, even in the 80s and 90s. This disorder is characterized by **hyperglycemia** (elevated blood glucose levels), a breakdown of body fats and proteins, and the development of **ketosis** (an accumulation of ketone bodies produced during the oxidation of fatty acids). Type 1 DM is the result of the destruction of the beta cells of the islets of Langerhans in the pancreas. When beta cells are destroyed, insulin is no longer produced. Although type 1 DM may be classified as either an autoimmune or idiopathic disorder, 90% of the cases are immune mediated. The disorder begins with insulitis, a chronic inflammatory process that occurs in response to the autoimmune destruction of islet cells. This process slowly destroys production of insulin, with the onset of hyperglycemia occurring when 80% to 90% of beta cell

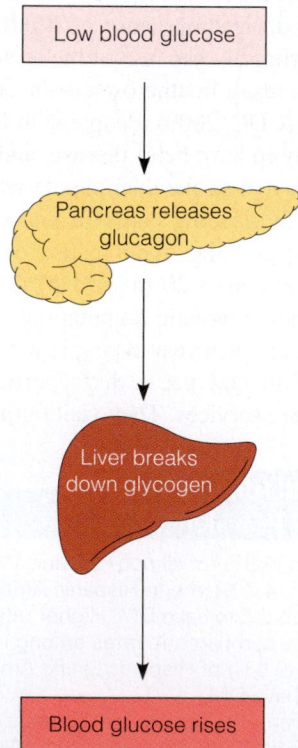

Figure 20–1 ■ Regulation (homeostasis) of blood glucose levels by insulin and glucagon. *A*, High blood glucose is lowered by insulin release. *B*, Low blood glucose is raised by glucagon release.

TABLE 20–1 Classification and Characteristics of Diabetes Mellitus

	CLASSIFICATION	CHARACTERISTICS
I. Type 1 DM	A. Immune-mediated	Beta cells are destroyed, usually leading to absolute insulin deficiency. Markers to the immune destruction of the beta cells include islet cell autoantibodies (ICAs) and insulin autoantibodies (IAAs). The rate of beta cell destruction is variable, usually more rapid in infants and children and slower in adults. Destruction of the beta cells has genetic predispositions and is also related to environmental factors as yet undefined.
	B. Idiopathic	Has no known etiologic causes. Most patients are of African or Asian descent. Is strongly inherited. Need for insulin may be intermittent.
II. Type 2 DM		May range from predominantly insulin resistance with relative insulin deficiency to a predominantly secretory defect with insulin resistance. There is no immune destruction of beta cells. Initially, and in some cases for the entire life, insulin is not necessary. Most people with this form are obese, or have an increased amount of abdominal fat. Risks for development include increasing age, obesity, and a sedentary lifestyle. Occurs more frequently in women who have had gestational DM, and in people with lipid disorders or hypertension. There is a strong genetic predisposition.
III. Other specific types	A. Genetic defects of beta cell	Hyperglycemia occurs at an early age (usually before age 25). This type is referred to as maturity-onset DM of the young (MODY).
	B. Genetic defects in insulin action	Are genetically determined. Dysfunctions may range from hyperinsulinemia to severe DM.
	C. Diseases of the exocrine pancreas	Acquired processes causing DM include pancreatitis, trauma, infection, pancreatectomy, and pancreatic cancer. Severe forms of cystic fibrosis and hemochromatosis may also damage beta cells and impair insulin secretion.
	D. Endocrine disorders	Excess amount of hormones (e.g., growth hormone, cortisol, glucagon, and epinephrine) impair insulin secretion, resulting in DM in people with Cushing's syndrome, acromegaly, and pheochromocytoma.
	E. Drug or chemical induced	Many drugs impair insulin secretion, precipitating DM in people with predisposing insulin resistance. Examples are nicotinic acid, glucocorticoids, thyroid hormone, thiazides, and phenytoin.
	F. Infections	Certain viruses may cause beta cell destruction, including congenital measles, cytomegalovirus, adenovirus, and mumps.
IV. Gestational diabetes mellitus (GDM)		Any degree of glucose intolerance with onset or first recognition during pregnancy.

function is lost. This process usually occurs over a long preclinical period. It is believed that both alpha-cell and beta-cell functions are abnormal, with a lack of insulin and a relative excess of glucagon resulting in hyperglycemia.

RISK FACTORS   Genetic predisposition plays a role in the development of type 1 DM. Although the risk in the general population ranges from 1 in 400 to 1 in 1000, the child of a person with DM has a 1 in 20 to 1 in 50 risk. Genetic markers that determine immune responses have been found in most people diagnosed with type 1 DM. Although the presence of these markers does not guarantee that the person will develop type 1 DM, they do indicate increased susceptibility (Porth & Matfin, 2009).

Environmental factors are believed to trigger the development of type 1A DM. The trigger can be a viral infection (mumps, rubella, or coxsackievirus B4) or a chemical toxin, such as those found in smoked and cured meats. As a result of exposure to the virus or chemical, an abnormal autoimmune response occurs in which antibodies respond to normal islet beta cells as though they were foreign substances, destroying them. The manifestations of type 1 DM appear when approximately 90% of the beta cells are destroyed. However, manifestations may appear at any time during the loss of beta cells if an acute illness or stress increases the demand for insulin beyond the reserves of the damaged cells. The actual cause and exact sequence are not completely understood, but research continues to identify the genetic markers of this disorder and to investigate ways of altering the immune response to prevent or cure type 1 DM.

Type IB DM, a rare form, is strongly inherited and affects people of African and Asian descent. It is not an autoimmune disorder; beta cell destruction varies and periods of ketoacidosis develop.

MANIFESTATIONS   The manifestations of type 1 DM are the result of a lack of insulin to transport glucose across the cell membrane into the cells (Figure 20–2 ■). Glucose molecules accumulate in the circulating blood, resulting in hyperglycemia. Hyperglycemia causes serum hyperosmolality, drawing water from the intracellular spaces into the general circulation. The increased blood volume increases renal blood flow, and the hyperglycemia acts as an osmotic diuretic. The resulting osmotic diuresis increases urine output. This condition is called **polyuria**. When the blood glucose level exceeds the renal threshold for glucose—usually about 180 mg/dL—glucose is excreted in the urine, a condition called **glucosuria**. The decrease in intracellular volume and the increased urinary

Insulin deficit

+

Associated risk factors

↓

↑ Glucose production and ↓ Glucose utilization

↓

Hyperglycemia

↓

Osmotic diuresis

↓

Extracellular dehydration

Renal insufficiency   Hypovolemia

↓   ↓

Severe hyperosmolarity   Shock

↓   ↓

Fluid shifts   Tissue hypoxia

↓   ↓

Intracellular dehydration   Lactic acidosis

COMA

Figure 20–2 ■ Pathophysiologic results of type 1 DM.

output cause dehydration. The mouth becomes dry and thirst sensors are activated, causing the person to drink increased amounts of fluid (**polydipsia**).

Because glucose cannot enter the cell without insulin, energy production decreases. This decrease in energy stimulates hunger, and the person eats more food (**polyphagia**). Despite increased food intake, the person loses weight as the body loses water and breaks down proteins and fats in an attempt to restore energy sources. Malaise and fatigue accompany the decrease in energy. Blurred vision is also common, resulting from osmotic affects that cause swelling of the lenses of the eyes.

Thus, the classic manifestations are polyuria, polydipsia, and polyphagia, accompanied by weight loss, malaise, and fatigue. Depending on the degree of insulin lack, the manifestations vary from slight to severe. People with type 1 DM require an exogenous (external) source of insulin to maintain life.

Type 2 DM

Type 2 DM is a condition of fasting hyperglycemia that occurs despite the availability of endogenous insulin. Type 2 DM can occur at any age but it is usually seen in middle age and older people. It is the most common form of DM. Heredity plays a role in its transmission. The level of insulin produced varies in type 2 DM, and despite its availability, its function is impaired by insulin resistance in peripheral tissues.

The liver produces more glucose than normal, dietary carbohydrates are not metabolized well, and eventually the pancreas secretes less than adequate amounts of insulin (Porth, 2007). Whatever the cause, there is sufficient insulin production to prevent the breakdown of fats with resultant ketosis; thus, type 2 DM is characterized as a nonketotic form of DM. However, the amount of insulin available is not sufficient to lower blood glucose levels through the uptake of glucose by muscle and fat cells.

A major factor in the development of type 2 DM is cellular resistance to the effect of insulin. This resistance is increased by obesity, inactivity, illnesses, medications, and increasing age. In obesity, insulin has a decreased ability to influence glucose absorption and metabolism by the liver, skeletal muscles, and adipose tissue. Hyperglycemia increases gradually and may exist over a long time before DM is diagnosed, thus approximately half the newly diagnosed type 2 diabetics already have complications (Capriotti, 2005). Treatment usually begins with prescriptions for weight loss and increased activity. If these changes can be sustained, no further treatment will be necessary for many individuals. Hypoglycemic medications are begun when lifestyle changes are insufficient. Often, a combination of insulin and hypoglycemic medication is used to achieve the best glycemic control in the patient with type 2 DM.

RISK FACTORS The major risk factors for type 2 DM are the following:

- History of DM in parents or siblings. Although there is no identified HLA linkage, the children of a person with type 2 DM have a two to fourfold increased risk of developing type 2 DM and a 30% risk of developing a glucose intolerance (the inability to metabolize carbohydrate normally).
- Obesity, defined as being at least 20% over desired body weight or having a body mass index (BMI) of at least 27 kg/m^2. Obesity, especially visceral obesity (abdominal fat), is associated with increased insulin resistance.
- Physical inactivity.
- Race/ethnicity (see the box on page 521).
- In women, a history of gestational DM, polycystic ovary syndrome, or delivering a baby weighing more than 9 lb.
- Hypertension ($\geq$ 130/85 in adults), HDL cholesterol of $\geq$ 35 mg/dL, and/or a triglyceride level of $\geq$ 250 mg/dL.
- Metabolic syndrome, a cluster of manifestations associated with type 2 DM. Hypertension, visceral obesity, low levels of high-density lipoproteins, high levels of triglycerides, elevated C-reactive protein, and a fasting blood glucose greater than 110 mg/dL increases the risk of DM, coronary heart disease, and stroke (Porth & Matfin, 2009).

MANIFESTATIONS The person with type 2 DM experiences a slow onset of manifestations and is often unaware of the disease until seeking health care for some other problem. The hyperglycemia in type 2 DM is usually not as severe as in type 1 DM, but similar manifestations occur, especially polyuria and polydipsia. Polyphagia is not often seen, and weight loss is uncommon. Other manifestations are also the result of hyperglycemia: blurred vision, fatigue, paresthesias, and skin infections.

Type 2 DM Video

MULTISYSTEM EFFECTS OF
Diabetes Mellitus

Early Manifestations
- Type 1 DM
  - Polyuria
  - Polydipsia
  - Polyphagia
  - Weight loss
  - Glycosuria
  - Fatigue
- Type 2 DM
  - Polyuria
  - Polydipsia
  - Blurred vision

Progressive Complications
- Hyperglycemia
  - Diabetic ketoacidosis
  - Hyperglycemic hyperosmolar nonketotic coma
- Hypoglycemia

Late Complications
Neurologic
- Somatic neuropathies
  - Paresthesias
  - Pain
  - Loss of cutaneous sensation
  - Loss of fine motor control
- Visceral neuropathies
  - Sweating dysfunction
  - Pupillary constriction
  - Fixed heart rate
  - Constipation
  - Diarrhea
  - Incomplete bladder emptying
  - Sexual dysfunction

Sensory
- Diabetic retinopathy
- Cataracts
- Glaucoma

Cardiovascular
- Orthostatic hypotension
- Accelerated atherosclerosis
- Cerebrovascular disease (stroke)
- Coronary artery disease (MI)
- Peripheral vascular disease
- Blood viscosity and platelet disorders

Renal
- Hypertension
- Albuminuria
- Edema
- Chronic renal failure

Musculoskeletal
- Joint contractures

Integumentary
- Foot ulcers
- Gangrene of the feet
- Atrophic changes

Immune System
- Impaired healing
- Chronic skin infections
- Periodontal disease
- Urinary tract infections
- Lung infections
- Vaginitis

DM in the Older Adult

Although the older adult may have either type 1 or type 2 DM, most often he or she has type 2. The National Institute of Diabetes and Digestive and Kidney Diseases estimates that nearly 23.1% of the U.S. population over 60 have DM (NIH, 2008). It is predicted that the number of older adults with DM will continue to increase because the incidence of the disease increases with age and because the number of people over 65 is increasing.

The normal physiologic changes of aging may mask manifestations of the onset of DM. Manifestations of DM in older adults may not include the classic symptoms of polyuria and thirst. Conditions such as orthostatic hypotension, periodontal disease, infections, stroke, slow gastric emptying (gastroparesis), impotence, neuropathy, confusion, and glaucoma should be considered potential indicators of DM (Eliopoulos, 2005), and may also increase the potential for complications from the disease or its treatment. Common problems in the older adult that make the diagnosis and management of DM more difficult are described in the following Nursing Care of the Older Adult box. The older adult with DM also has a longer recovery period after surgery or serious illness, often requiring insulin to maintain blood glucose levels. The benefits and risks of treatment to maintain glycemic control as well as blood pressure and lipid management must be carefully balanced.

Interdisciplinary Care

The results of a 10-year DM Control and Complications Trial (DCCT), sponsored by the National Institutes of Health (NIH), have significant implications for the management of type 1 DM. People in the study who kept their blood glucose levels close to normal by frequent monitoring, several daily insulin injections, and lifestyle changes that included exercise and a healthier diet reduced by 60% their risk for the development and progression of complications involving the eyes, the kidneys, and the nervous system. Treatment of the patient with DM focuses on maintaining blood glucose at levels as nearly normal as possible through medications, dietary management, and exercise.

Type 2 DM benefits from similar levels of control. Studies of patients with DM who have gastrointestinal surgery for morbid obesity show complete remission of type 2 DM in over 3⁄4 of the cases. Laparoscopic adjustable gastric banding (LAGB) and Roux-en-Y gastric bypass (RYGB) result in remarkable reductions in blood glucose levels and HgbA1C. RYGB, which alters gastrointestinal anatomy, improves insulin sensitivity and is associated with total remission of DM in a significant percentage of patients (Cummings & Flum, 2008; ADA, 2009).

Diagnosis

Diagnostic tests are conducted for screening purposes to diagnose DM, and ongoing laboratory tests are conducted to evaluate the effectiveness of diabetic management. Definitions of

NURSING CARE OF THE OLDER ADULT   Diabetes Mellitus

HEALTH PROBLEM/COMPLICATION	IMPLICATIONS FOR NURSING CARE
Urinary incontinence	Polyuria, a classic manifestation of DM, often is ignored. This problem also often leads to social isolation.
Decreased thirst	Polydipsia, a classic manifestation of DM, often is ignored. This further increases the risk of dehydration and electrolyte imbalances.
Decreased hunger and weight loss	Polyphagia, a classic manifestation of DM, often is ignored. The aging process, medications, depression, or lack of socialization may decrease hunger. Weight loss may be gradual and go unnoticed.
Fatigue and depression	Fatigue and depression are common symptoms of DM but may be blamed on increased age.
Hypoglycemia	The older adult may have either very mild manifestations or none at all, or there may be an inability to sense or respond to hypoglycemia. As a result, hypoglycemia is often ignored until it causes serious effects.
Peripheral neuropathy	Manifestations may be thought to be due to arthritis, and over-the-counter drugs often are used to self-medicate. The risk of falls increases, as does the risk of gangrene and amputation.
Peripheral vascular disease	May go undetected if the person does not get enough exercise to cause claudication. May also impair abilities to climb stairs and walk.
Diabetic retinopathy	May be undetected if the person has cataracts. Diabetic patients also have an increased incidence of cataracts and glaucoma. Deficits in vision threaten independence, mobility, and social interactions. Yellowing of the lens with age makes it difficult to read colored test strips; numeric meters are preferable. Filling insulin syringes may be impossible for the patient with macular degeneration or other causes of visual loss.
Hypertension	Treatment with diuretics may further impair glucose tolerance and result in electrolyte imbalances.
Persistent pain	Older adults may believe the pain from arthritis to be more important than the DM management. Also, depression from chronic pain as well as inactivity and loss of appetite may interfere with DM self-care.
Parkinson's disease	The tremors and rigidity of this disease make self-care involving fine and gross motor skills difficult or impossible.
Polypharmacy	Older adults commonly take more than one type of medication and are at increased risk for problems relating to drug interactions.
Cognitive impairment	Delirium or dementia can prevent the patient from communicating or performing self care.

normal blood glucose levels vary in clinical practice, depending on the laboratory that performs the assay.

DIAGNOSTIC SCREENING Three diagnostic tests may be used to diagnose DM, and each must be confirmed, on a subsequent day, with one of the three tests. The diagnostic criteria recommended by the American Diabetes Association (ADA) (2009) are the following:

1. Manifestations of hyperglycemia (polyuria, polydipsia, and unexplained weight loss) and a casual plasma glucose (PG) concentration > 200 mg/dL (11.1 mmol/L). Causal is defined as any time of day without regard to time since last meal.
2. Fasting plasma glucose (FPG) > 126 mg/dL (7.0 mmol/L). Fasting is defined as no caloric intake for 8 hours.
3. Two-hour PG > 200 mg/dL (11.1 mmol/L) during an oral glucose tolerance test (OGTT). The test should be performed with a glucose load containing the equivalent of 75 anhydrous glucose dissolved in water. See Procedure 20–1 on the following page.

When using these criteria, the following levels are used for the FPG:

- Normal fasting glucose = 100 mg/dL (6.1 mmol/L)
- Impaired fasting glucose (IFG) = > 100 (6.1 mmol/L) and < 126 mg/dL (7.0 mmol/L)
- Diagnosis of DM = > 126 mg/dL (7.0 mmol/L)

When using these criteria, the following levels are used for the OGTT:

- Normal glucose tolerance = 2-hr PG: < 140 mg/dL (7.8 mmol/L)
- Impaired glucose tolerance (IGT) = 2-hr PG: ≥ 140 (7.8 mmol/L) and < 200 mg/dL (11.1 mmol/L)
- Diagnosis of DM = 2-hr PG: ≥ 200 mg/dL (11.1 mmol/L)

In addition, the ADA (2010) recommends measuring levels of glycosylated hemoglobin (A1C), with a level of 6.5% enough to make a diagnosis of diabetes. Levels of 5.7% to 6.49% indicate a high risk for developing both diabetes and cardiovascular disease, and are a marker for prediabetes.

Prediabetes Prediabetes is a term used to describe people who are at increased risk of developing DM. Prediabetes is characterized by increased levels of A1C, increased fasting blood glucose (IFG), and impaired (IGT) plasma glucose. The results of these tests may not be high enough to be classified as DM. These test results indicate there is a risk for progression to DM, but it is not inevitable. Studies suggest that weight loss and increased physical activity may prevent or delay DM and may return blood glucose levels to normal. People with prediabetes are already at increased risk for other adverse health outcomes such as heart disease and stroke (ADA, 2009).

DIAGNOSTIC TESTS TO MONITOR DM MANAGEMENT Diagnostic tests used to diagnose and monitor DM include a fasting blood glucose (FBG), an oral glucose tolerance test, and a glycosylated hemoglobin (A1C). Normal values for these tests as well as nursing implications are described in ∞ Chapter 18.

Other tests that may be used are urine tests for glucose, ketones, and albumin. Although not as accurate as blood tests, urine analysis for increased glucose and ketones indicate hyperglycemia. Urine tests for albumin are used to detect the early inset of kidney damage. Serum cholesterol and tyiglyceride levels, if elevated, indicate an increased risk of cardiovascular impairments.

Monitoring Blood Glucose

People with DM must monitor their condition daily by testing glucose levels. Two types of tests are available. The first type, long used prior to the development of devices to directly measure blood glucose, is urine testing for glucose and ketones. Urine testing is less commonly used today. The second type, direct measurement of blood glucose, is widely used in all types of healthcare settings and in the home.

URINE TESTING FOR KETONES AND GLUCOSE Urine testing for glucose and ketones was at one time the only available method for evaluating the management of DM. An inexpensive, noninvasive, and painless test, it has unpredictable results and cannot be used to detect or measure hypoglycemia. In the healthy state, glucose is not present in the urine because insulin maintains serum glucose below the renal threshold of 180mg/dl. The accuracy of this measurement is not reliable in DM because the renal threshold may rise with aging or secondary to DM. Urine testing is recommended to monitor hyperglycemia and ketoacidosis in people with type 1 DM who have unexplained hyperglycemia during illness or pregnancy. Ketones may be detected through urine testing and reflect the presence of DKA. People who choose not to self-monitor blood glucose by other methods may use urine testing. (See Procedure 20–1.)

SELF-MONITORING OF BLOOD GLUCOSE Self-monitoring of blood glucose (SMBG) allows the person with DM to monitor and achieve metabolic control and decrease the danger of hypoglycemia. The ADA recommends that all patients with DM be taught some method of monitoring glycemic control. The timing of SMBG is highly individualized, depending on the person's diagnosis, general disease control, and physical state. SMBG is recommended three or more times a day for patients with type 1 DM using multiple insulin injections or insulin pump therapy. Monitoring by patients with type 2 DM who are not using insulin should be sufficient to help them reach glucose goals. Postprandial blood glucose is often the most useful information for evaluating level of glycemic control in the type 2 DM patient (ADA, 2009). If patients only check their fasting glucose, they would be unaware of the postprandial results.

When adding or modifying therapy, patients with both types of DM should test more often than usual. SMBG is also useful when the person is ill or pregnant, or has manifestations of hypoglycemia or hyperglycemia. Both hypoglycemia and hyperglycemia may contribute to complications and decrease quality of life. With the information assessed with SMBG, patients can alter their diet, their physical activity, and even their medication to reduce the postprandial increases, reduce their risk for complications, and feel better because they are no longer experiencing wide swings in glucose levels (Pearson, 2009).

The ADA annually publishes a comprehensive list of currently available blood glucose monitoring machines and strips with approximate prices in *Diabetes Forecast*. Most medical insurance policies cover the cost of these machines and the test strips. Many companies provide a machine free of cost. Testing

PROCEDURE 20–1 Testing Urine for Ketones and Glucose

TO TEST THE URINE FOR KETONES

1. Ask the patient to void, discard the urine, and drink a full glass of water.
2. Thirty minutes later, collect a urine sample.
3. For acid test tablets: Place the tablet on a white paper towel, place one drop of urine on the tablet, and wait

30 seconds. If the tablet turns any shade from lavender to deep purple, the test is positive for ketones.

4. For Ketostix: Dip the reagent stick into the urine sample. Wait 15 seconds, and compare the color of the pad at the end of the stick to an accompanying color chart. Purple is indicative of ketones.

TO TEST THE URINE FOR GLUCOSE

1. Follow the same procedure to collect a urine sample.
2. Dip the reagent stick into the urine sample, and wait the time indicated. Compare the color of the pad on the end of

the reagent stick with an accompanying color chart. The glucose is expressed as a percentage (for example, 0.5%, 1%, 2%). Remember that normally no glucose is found in the urine, so the presence of glucose is an abnormal manifestation indicating hyperglycemia.

---

supplies are specific to each machine and this obligates the recipient to purchase supplies for that machine.

A new technology for continuous blood glucose monitoring (CGM) is available. The CGM has a sensor that is inserted under the skin. This sensor continuously sends data useful as a warning for high or low glucose levels. Finger-stick measurements are required before making therapy adjustments (McPhee & Papadakis, 2009). The CGM may be used for diagnostic evaluation; patients wear the pump for 3 days under the supervision of physicians and nurses. The data reveal patterns of glycemic control useful for treatment.

Following is the equipment needed for SMBG:

- Some type of lancet device to perform a finger-stick for obtaining a drop of blood (such as an Autolet, Penlet, or Soft Touch).
- Chemically impregnated test strips that change color when they come into contact with glucose or that can be read by machine (e.g., Glucostix and Chemstrip bG). The strip may also be read by comparing its color with a color chart on the side of the container or on an insert packed with the strips (Figure 20–3 ■).
- A blood glucose monitor (e.g., the Glucometer, the AccuChek, or the One Touch) if the most accurate measurement is desired

Figure 20–3 ■ Determination of blood glucose levels by visual reading. The color of the strip is compared with the color chart on the side of the container.

or recommended. The manufacturer's instructions must be followed carefully. If the timing of the blood on the strip is not exact, the test will not be accurate. In addition, the machine must be cleaned according to the manufacturer's directions to ensure accuracy. Monitors that use no-wipe technology improve the accuracy of glucose measurement. Other monitors are computerized and/or include a memory of previous glucose readings to show a pattern of control.

FACTORS THAT AFFECT GLUCOSE METER PERFORMANCE

According to the U.S. Food and Drug Administration (FDA), several factors affect the accuracy of blood glucose test results. The quality of the meter and test strips, and training to use the meter contribute to the degree of accuracy. Other factors can create falsely positive or negative readings.

Hematocrit   Patients with higher hematocrit values will usually test falsely low in blood glucose and patients with lower hematocrit will test falsely higher. Anemia and sickle cell anemia are two conditions that can affect hematocrit values.

Other Substances   Overdoses of many medications will cause inaccurate results. Meters and supplies vary in sensitivity to medications. Uric acid (a natural substance in the body that can be more concentrated in some people with DM), glutathione (an anti-oxidant also called GSH), and ascorbic acid (vitamin C) are known to interfere.

Using Correct Supplies and Sample Volume   The test strips must be compatible with the glucose meter, are not outdated, or have been exposed to air and humidity, which can alter strip sensitivity. Insufficient amounts of blood on the testing strip causes inaccurate results. Although a meter may indicate a sufficient amount of blood on the test strip, it is best to observe that the recepticle is full of capillary blood. Yared, Aljaberi, Renouf, and Yale (2005) found that meters read significantly smaller than reference volumes and gave results varying 40% to 68% from the reference volume results. The erroneous results underestimated the true glucose value.

Medications

The pharmacologic treatment for DM depends on the type of DM. People with type 1 must have insulin; those with type 2 are usually able to control glucose levels with an oral hypoglycemic medication, but they may require insulin if control is inadequate or if they are subjected to a stressor, such as surgery.

INSULIN   The person with type 1 DM requires a lifelong exogenous source of the insulin hormone to maintain life. Insulin is not a cure for DM; rather, it is a means of controlling hyperglycemia. Insulin is also necessary in other situations, such as the following:

- People who are unable to control glucose levels with oral antidiabetic drugs and/or diet
- People who are experiencing physical stress (such as an infection or surgery) or who are taking corticosteroids
- Women with gestational DM who are unable to control glucose with diet
- People with DKA or HHS
- People who are receiving high-calorie tube feedings or parenteral nutrition

Sources of Insulin   Preparations of insulin are derived from animal (pork pancreas) or synthesized in the laboratory from either an alteration of pork insulin or recombinant DNA technology, using strains of *E. coli* to form biosynthetic human insulin. Insulin analogs have been developed by modifying the amino acid sequence of the insulin molecule. Although different types are prescribed on an individualized basis, it is standard practice to prescribe human insulin.

Insulin Preparations   Insulins are available in rapid-acting, short-acting, intermediate-acting, and long-acting preparations. The trade names and times of onset, peak, and duration of action are listed in Table 20–2.

Insulin lispro (Humalog) is a human insulin analog that is derived from genetically altered *E. coli* that includes the gene for insulin lispro. It is classified as rapid-acting or ultra-short-acting insulin. Compared to regular insulin, lispro has a more rapid onset (< 15 minutes), an earlier peak of glucose lowering (30 to 60 minutes), and a shorter duration of activity (3 to 4 hours). This means that lispro should be administered within 15 minutes before a meal (rather than 30 to 60 minutes before as recommended for regular insulin). Patients with type 1 DM usually also require concurrent use of a longer-acting insulin product. Lispro is much less likely than regular insulin to cause tissue changes

and may lower the risk of nocturnal hypoglycemia in patients with type 1 DM.

Regular insulin is unmodified crystalline insulin, classified as a short-acting insulin. Regular insulin is clear in appearance and is the only insulin preparation that can be given by the IV route; the other types are suspensions and could be harmful if given by this route. Regular insulin is also used to treat DKA, to initiate treatment for newly diagnosed type 1 DM, and in combination with intermediate-acting insulins to provide better glucose control.

The onset, peak and duration of action of insulin can be changed by adding acetate buffers and protamine. Zinc and protamine are added to NPH insulin to prolong their action, and they are classified as intermediate- or long-acting insulins. These preparations appear cloudy when properly mixed prior to injection. Protamine and zinc are foreign substances and may cause hypersensitivity reactions. Insulin detemir, the newest long acting insulin (17–24 hours), is a clear insulin and must not be mixed with other insulins and cannot be used in insulin pumps. Doses may be administered once or twice daily. Insulin glargine (Lantus) is a 24-hour long-acting DNA human insulin analog that is given subcutaneously once or twice a day, usually at bedtime, to treat patients with both type 1 and type 2 DM. It has a relatively constant effect (meaning it does not have a peak time of effect). It is not recommended for use in pregnancy. Glargine should not be mixed with other insulins; the pH is incompatible (McPhee & Papadakis, 2009). Glargine cannot be used in insulin pumps.

> **SAFETY ALERT**
> Insulin glargine and insulin detemir are clear, unlike other intermediate or long-acting insulins. Do not mistake these for regular insulin. Do not mix with *any* other insulins. Do not inject IV, only subcutaneously.

Concentrations of Insulin   Insulin is dispensed as 100 U/mL (U-100) and 500 U/mL (U-500) in the United States. U-100 is the standard insulin concentration used; there are 100 units of insulin in 1 mL. U-500 insulin is only used in rare cases of insulin resistance when patients require very large doses.

TABLE 20–2 Insulin Preparations

PREPARATION	NAME	ONSET (h)	PEAK (h)	DURATION (h)
Rapid acting	Lispro	0.25	1–1.5	3–4
	Aspart (NovoLog)	0.25	40–50 minutes	3–5
	Glulisine (Apidra)	0.25	1–1.5	3–5
Short acting	Regular (Novolin-R, Humulin-R)	0.5–1.0	2–3	4–6
Intermediate acting	NPH (Humulin (N) NPH	2	6–8	12–16
	detemir (Levemir)	(onset and peak not defined)		17–24
Long acting	glargine (Lantus)	(onset and peak not defined)		24
Combinations	Humulin 50/50	0.5	3	22–24
	Humulin 70/30	0.5	4–8	24
	Novolin 70/30	0.5	4–8	24

U-500 and the insulin analog lispro are the only insulins that require a prescription.

Insulin Administration Nursing implications for administering insulin are outlined in the following Medication Administration box and further discussion follows in the chapter. The considerations for administering insulin include routes of administration, syringe and needle selection, preparing the injection, sites of injection, mixing insulins, and insulin regimens.

Routes of Administration All insulins are given parenterally, although current research is investigating the development of a nasal spray and an oral preparation of insulin. Only regular insulin is given by both subcutaneous and IV routes; all others are given only subcutaneously. If the IV route is not available, regular insulin may also be administered IM in an emergency situation.

CONTINUOUS SUBCUTANEOUS INSULIN INFUSION
Regular or rapid-acting insulins are used in continuous subcutaneous insulin infusion (CSII) devices, often called insulin pumps (e.g., MiniMed and Disetronic pumps). CSII devices have a small pump that holds a syringe of insulin, connected to a subcutaneous needle by tubing. The pump is about the size of a pager and can be worn on a belt or tucked into a pocket. The needle is placed in the skin, usually in the abdomen, and is changed every 3 days. This device delivers a constant amount of programmed insulin throughout each 24-hour period. It also can be used to deliver a bolus of insulin manually (e.g., before meals).

MEDICATION ADMINISTRATION   **Insulin**

Nursing Responsibilities
- Discard vials of insulin that have been open for several weeks or whose expiration date has passed.
- Refrigerate extra insulin vials not currently in use, but do not freeze them.
- Store insulin in a cool place, and avoid exposure to temperature extremes or sunlight.
- Store compatible mixtures of insulin for no longer than 1 month at room temperature or 3 months at 36°F to 46°F (2°C to 8°C).
- Discard any vials with discoloration, clumping, granules, or solid deposits on the sides.
- If breakfast is delayed, also delay the administration of rapid-acting insulin.
- Monitor and maintain a record of blood glucose readings 30 minutes before each meal and bedtime (or as prescribed).
- Monitor food intake, and notify the physician if food is not being consumed.
- Monitor electrolytes (especially potassium) and creatinine.
- Observe injection sites for manifestations of hypersensitivity, lipodystrophy, and lipoatrophy.
- If manifestations of hypoglycemia occur, confirm by testing blood glucose level, and administer an oral source of a fast-acting carbohydrate, such as juice, milk, or crackers. Hypoglycemic manifestations are described later under complications, but commonly include feelings of shakiness, hunger, and/or nervousness accompanied by sweating, tachycardia, or palpitations.
- If manifestations of hyperglycemia occur, confirm by testing blood glucose level, and notify the physician.

Health Education for the Patient and Family
- The manifestations of DM.
- Self-administration of insulin, with a return demonstration.
  a. Wash hands carefully.
  b. Have a vial of insulin, the insulin syringe with needle, and alcohol pads ready to use.
  c. Remove the cover from the needle.
  d. Fill the syringe with an amount of air equal to the number of units of insulin, and insert the needle into the vial.
  e. Push air into the vial, invert the vial, and withdraw the prescribed units of insulin.
  f. Replace the cover over the needle.
  g. Wipe the selected site with alcohol. The injection is less likely to be painful if the alcohol is allowed to dry.
  h. Pinch up a fold of skin, and insert the needle into the tissue at the recommended angle.
  i. Insert the insulin.
  j. Withdraw the needle; if desired, apply firm pressure to the site for a few seconds.
  k. Recap the needle. Many people with DM reuse disposable syringes with attached needles without adverse effects. The primary reason for discarding after several uses is that the needle becomes dull and makes the injection painful.
  l. Insulin pens may be more convenient to us. The dose is selected with a dial on the pen. Needles should be changed with each use and insulins, except commercially-mixed such as 70/30, cannot be mixed in a pen.
- Follow instructions for mixing insulins (refer to the box on page 542).
- Always keep an extra vial or cartridge of insulin available; refrigerate insulins not in use. Discard insulin pens kept at room temperature for current use at 28 days. Discard vials of insulin kept at room temperature for 30 days. Stored, refrigerated vials and cartridges should be discarded if their expiration date is exceeded.
- Always have a vial of regular insulin available for emergencies.
- Be aware of the signs of hypersensitivity responses, hypoglycemia, and hyperglycemia.
- Keep candy or a sugar source available at all times to treat hypoglycemia, if it occurs. Eat within 15 minutes of injecting rapid-acting insulins.
- Vision may be blurred during the first 6 to 8 weeks of insulin therapy; this is the result of fluid changes in the eye and should clear up in 8 weeks.
- Avoid alcoholic beverages, which may cause hypoglycemia.
- Follow these guidelines for sick days:
  a. Never omit insulin.
  b. Always monitor blood glucose and/or urine ketones at least every 2 to 4 hours.
  c. Always drink plenty of fluids, try to drink at least one glass of water or other calorie-free, caffeine-free liquid each hour.
  d. Get as much rest as possible.
  e. Contact the physician if there is persistent fever, vomiting, shortness of breath, severe pain in the abdomen, dehydration, loss of vision, chest pain, persistent diarrhea, blood glucose levels above 250, or ketones in the urine.
- Establish a plan for rotating injection sites, and observe closely for changes in tissues such as hardness, dimpling, or sunken areas.

CORRECTIONAL DOSES OF INSULIN Maintaining normal blood glucose prior to and during hospitalization decreases the risk of postoperative infections and shortens hospital stays. Healing is impaired when hemoglobin is glycosylated as glycosylated Hgb has an increased affinity for oxygen, putting tissues at risk for ischemia and decreases the effectiveness of white blood cells (increasing the risk of infection).

Treatment of hospitalized type 1 and type 2 patients requires a medication regimen that is responsive to glycemic changes secondary to the admitting condition and its treatment, including surgery (Braithwaite et al., 2007). People with type 2 DM may not be able to manage with oral medications during hospitalization because of the risk of hypoglycemia from not eating and the slow response of these medications to correct hyperglycemia. Researchers found significantly less mortality and significantly reduced acquired kidney injury when normal blood glucoses (80–110 mg/dl) were maintained by intensive insulin therapy (intravenous regular insulin) in surgical ICU patients; in critically ill surgical patients, blood glucoses should be kept close to 110 mg/dl and not exceed 140 mg/dl (ADA, 2009). It is recommended that critically ill patients maintain blood glucose levels equal to or < 140 mg/dl (ADA, 2009).

When hospitalized patients who are eating or have some source of oral intake experience periods of hyperglycemia outside the ICU, it is preferable to provide subcutaneous basal-prandial-correction therapy (Umpierrez et al., 2007).

The basal dose is a once or twice daily subcutaneous insulin such as insulin glargine (once daily) or NPH (twice daily). The prandial or mealtime dose is a portion of 1/2 the total daily dose of insulin. Correctional doses are combined with prandial doses, based on carbohydrate intake and are given postprandially. This method is employed to keep serum glucose below 180 mg/dl (ADA, 2009; Braithwaite et al., 2007). If the patient is requiring correction doses, the prandial dose needs to be increased until correction doses are eliminated. See Box 20–1 for methods to calculate basal, prandial, and correction doses for hospitalized patients on scheduled subcutaneous insulin doses and patients with insulin pumps.

Programming the amount of insulin to be delivered with a pump is determined by frequent blood glucose monitoring. Several different pumps are available, and each has rechargeable batteries, a syringe, a programmable computer, and a motor and drive mechanism. The rapid-acting insulin analog lispro is an appropriate insulin for insulin pumps, and short-acting regular insulin may also be used. Lispro is not approved for use in pregnancy.

Many people with DM believe the pump allows more normal regulation of blood glucose and provides greater lifestyle flexibility. Pumps are as safe as multiple-injection therapy when recommended procedures are followed. A potential complication is an undetected interruption in insulin delivery, which may result in a rapid onset of DKA. The needle site

---

BOX 20–1 Insulin Total Daily Dose (ITDD)

1. The total amount of insulin that the patient administered daily by injection (rapid- or short-acting with intermediate- or long-acting); for example, 48 units (30 units NPH and 18 units regular insulin).
   OR
2. 0.5–1 units/kg (normal kidney/liver function already on insulin) 48 units for 96-kg patient
   OR
3. 0.3–0.5 units/kg (reduced kidney/liver function or initial insulin therapy)
   Test blood glucose with test strip AC and HS.

Basal Dose: 40%–50% of the ITDD
1. Insulin pump. Multiply the ITDD by 50% (48.0 × 0.5 = 24 units). The basal insulin pump dose for this patient is 24 units. Divide the basal insulin pump dose by 24 to get the hourly basal pump dose and rate (24/24 = 1.0 unit/hour). Use rapid-acting or regular insulin.
2. Subcutaneous Insulin. Multiply the ITDD by 50% (48.0 × 0.5 = 24 units). This will be administered as one insulin glargine SQ injection daily or NPH injections of 12 units each twice daily. These basal doses are made with long-acting or intermediate-acting insulins.

Mealtime Bolus Dose
1. Insulin pump: To calculate bolus doses, take the remaining 50% of insulin and divide it by four doses according to the patient's meal plan for the day. For example, the remaining 50% could be divided thus: 20% at breakfast = 10 units; 10% at lunch = 5 units; 15% at dinner = 8 units, and 5% with a bedtime snack = 2 units.
   To calculate the units for each of these four daily bolus doses, multiply the percent of each meal bolus times the

total daily insulin pump dose. For example, for 48 units for a total daily dose:
   Breakfast dose is 20% (or 0.2) × 48 units = 10 units
   Lunch dose is 10% (or 0.1) × 48 units = 5 units
   Dinner dose is 15% (or 0.15) × 48 units = 8 units
   Bedtime snack dose is 5% (or 0.05) × 48 = 2 units
   (Nursing, 2005)
   Correction doses may be needed if the patient is hyperglycemic.
2. Subcutaneous insulin mealtime dose: Divide half of the ITDD into three mealtime doses.
   Breakfast = 8 units; Lunch = 8 units; Supper = 8 units. No bedtime dose is given.
   Rapid-acting insulin (regular or aspart) is given in conjunction with the meal.

Mealtime Correction Dose
This is different from sliding scale dosing because it is given before hyperglycemia develops and with a scheduled insulin dose. It is given with rapid-acting insulin combined with the mealtime dose.
1. Test blood glucose prior to each meal.
   If blood glucose mg/dl is < 80 or symptomatic for hypoglycemia follow hypoglycemia protocol.

81–100	no correction dose needed
101–150	add 1 unit or 2 units if mealtime dose is > 20 units
151–200	add 2 units or 3 units if mealtime dose is > 20 units
201–250	add 3 units or 4 units if mealtime dose is > 20 units
251–300	add 4 units or 5 units if mealtime dose is > 20 units
> 300	add 5 units or 10 units if mealtime dose is > 20 units

Note: When correction doses are needed, the scheduled doses of rapid-acting insulin need to be re-ordered at higher doses.

must be kept clean and changed on a regular basis (usually every 2 to 3 days) to prevent inflammation and infection. Although the patient who chooses an insulin pump has more to learn, many are very satisfied with having more normal glucose control.

SYRINGE AND NEEDLE SELECTION

Insulin is administered by sterile, single-use needles and either disposable insulin syringes or a multiple dose insulin pen (Figure 20–4 ■), calibrated in units per milliliter. This means that in U-100 insulin, there are 100 U of insulin in 1 mL. Syringes for administering U-100 insulin can be purchased in either 0.3 mL (30 U), 0.5 mL (50 U), or 1.0 mL (100 U) size. The advantage of the 0.3 mL and 0.5 mL sizes is that the distance between unit markings is greater, making it easier to measure the dose accurately.

Most insulin syringes are manufactured with the needle permanently attached in a 25- to 27-gauge, 0.5-inch size. If this type of syringe is not available, an insulin syringe and a 25-gauge, 0.5-inch, or 0.75-inch needle should be used. Some hospitals and many patients are using insulin pens instead of insulin syringes to administer insulin. The pens, either reusable or disposable, contain prefilled cartridges of insulin; the desired dose is adjusted on the pen's dial prior to injection. A disposal needle is replaced for each injection and handling the needles creates a risk of needle sticks. Insulin types cannot be mixed in a pen; separate injections must be made if more than one type of insulin is needed (BDdiabetes.com).

Insulin pens are convenient to use, eliminating the need to carry an insulin vial and fill a syringe. The insulin in the cartridges is more stable than insulin packaged in vials. Cartridges in use should be stored at room temperature and must be discarded at 28 days. Cartridges not in current use may be stored in the refrigerator.

Other special injection products are available for people with physical handicaps. These products include automatic injectors and jet spray injectors. Prefilled syringes or pens are useful for people who are visually impaired or traveling. Prefilled syringes are stable for up to 30 days if stored in the refrigerator.

PREPARING THE INJECTION

The vial of insulin in use may be kept at room temperature for up to 4 weeks. Stored vials should be kept in the refrigerator and brought to room temperature prior to administration.

Regular insulin does not require mixing. If the solution is cloudy or discolored, the vial should be discarded. The other types of insulin must be mixed to disperse the particles evenly throughout the solution. Mix the vial by gently rolling it between the hands; vigorous shaking causes bubble formation, which makes the dose inaccurate. It is critical that no air bubbles remain in the prepared dose, because even a small bubble can displace several units of insulin.

SITES OF INJECTION

Although in theory any area of the body with subcutaneous tissue may be used for injections of insulin, certain sites are recommended (Figure 20–5 ■). The rate of absorption and peak of action of insulin differs according to the site. The site that allows the most rapid absorption is the abdomen, followed by the deltoid muscle, then the thigh, and then the hip. Because of the rapid absorption, the abdomen is the recommended site. See Box 20–2 for techniques to minimize painful injections.

When administering insulin, gently pinch a fold of skin and inject the needle at a 90-degree angle. If the person is very thin, a 45-degree angle may be required to avoid injecting into muscle. Aspiration to check for blood is not necessary. Do not massage the site after administering the injection, because this may interfere with absorption; rotation within sites is recommended. The distance between injections should be about 1 inch (avoiding the area within a 2-inch radius around the umbilicus). Insulin should not be injected into an area to be exercised (such as the thigh before a vigorous walk) or to which heat will be applied; exercise or heat may increase the rate of absorption and cause a more rapid onset and peak of action.

Figure 20–4 ■ Insulin pen with adjustable dose.

Source: Courtesy of Novo Nordisk Inc.

Figure 20–5 ■ Sites of insulin injection. The abdomen is the preferred site.

Lipodystrophy Lipodystrophy (hypertrophy of subcutaneous tissue) or lipoatrophy (atrophy of subcutaneous tissue) may result if the same injection sites are used repeatedly. The tissues become hardened and have an orange-peel appearance. The use of refrigerated insulin may trigger the development of tissue atrophy or hypertrophy. These problems rarely occur with the use of human insulins. Lipodystrophy and lipoatrophy alter insulin absorption, delaying its onset or retaining the insulin in the tissue for a period of time instead of allowing it to be absorbed into the body. Lipodystrophy usually resolves if the area is unused for a minimum of 6 months.

MIXING INSULINS When a person with DM requires more than one type of insulin, mixing is recommended to avoid administering two injections per dose. Two different concentrations are administered, because a single dose of intermediate-acting or long-acting insulin rarely provides adequate control of blood glucose levels. The procedure for mixing insulins is described in Box 20–3. Following are some general guidelines:

- Commercially mixed insulins are recommended if the insulin ratio is appropriate for the requirements of the patient.
- Regular insulin may be mixed with all types of insulin except glargine and detemir; it may be injected immediately after mixing or stored for future use.
- NPH insulin and PZI insulin may be mixed only with regular insulin.
- Always withdraw regular insulin first to avoid contaminating the regular insulin with intermediate-acting insulin.

INSULIN REGIMENS Individualizing the appropriate insulin dosage is achieved through a balance among insulin, diet, and exercise. For most people with DM, the timing of insulin action requires two or more injections each day, often a mixture of rapid-acting and intermediate-acting insulins. Timing of the injections depends on blood glucose levels, food consumption, exercise, and types of insulin used. The objective is to avoid daytime and nighttime hypoglycemia while achieving adequate blood glucose control. Typical insulin regimens are outlined in Table 20–3.

HYPERSENSITIVITY RESPONSES When injected, insulin may cause local and systemic hypersensitivity responses. Manifestations of local reactions are a hardening and reddening of the area that develops over several hours. Local reactions result from a contaminant in the insulin and are more likely to occur when less purified insulin products are used.

Systemic reactions occur rapidly and are characterized by widespread red, intensely pruritic welts. Respiratory difficulty may occur. Systemic responses are due to an allergy to the insulin

BOX 20–3 Mixing Insulins: 10 Units of Regular and 20 Units of NPH

1. Wash hands.
2. Inspect regular insulin for clarity.
3. Gently rotate NPH insulin to mix well.
4. Wipe off the top of both vials with an alcohol pad.
5. Draw 20 U of air into the syringe, and inject air into the NPH vial (Figure *A*). Withdraw needle.
6. Draw 10 U of air into the syringe, and inject air into the regular vial (Figure *B*).
7. Invert the vial, and withdraw 10 U of regular insulin (Figure *C*). Withdraw the needle.
8. Insert the needle into the NPH vial, and carefully withdraw 20 U of NPH insulin (Figure *D*).
9. Don disposable gloves.
10. Administer the insulin.
11. Discard gloves, wash hands, and properly dispose of the syringe.
12. Document insulin administration.

20 Units

A Injecting air into the NPH vial.

10 Units

B Injecting air into the regular insulin vial.

C Withdrawing regular insulin.

10 Units regular insulin

D Withdrawing NPH insulin.

20 Units NPH insulin
10 Units regular insulin
30 Units total dosage

TABLE 20–3 Insulin Regimens

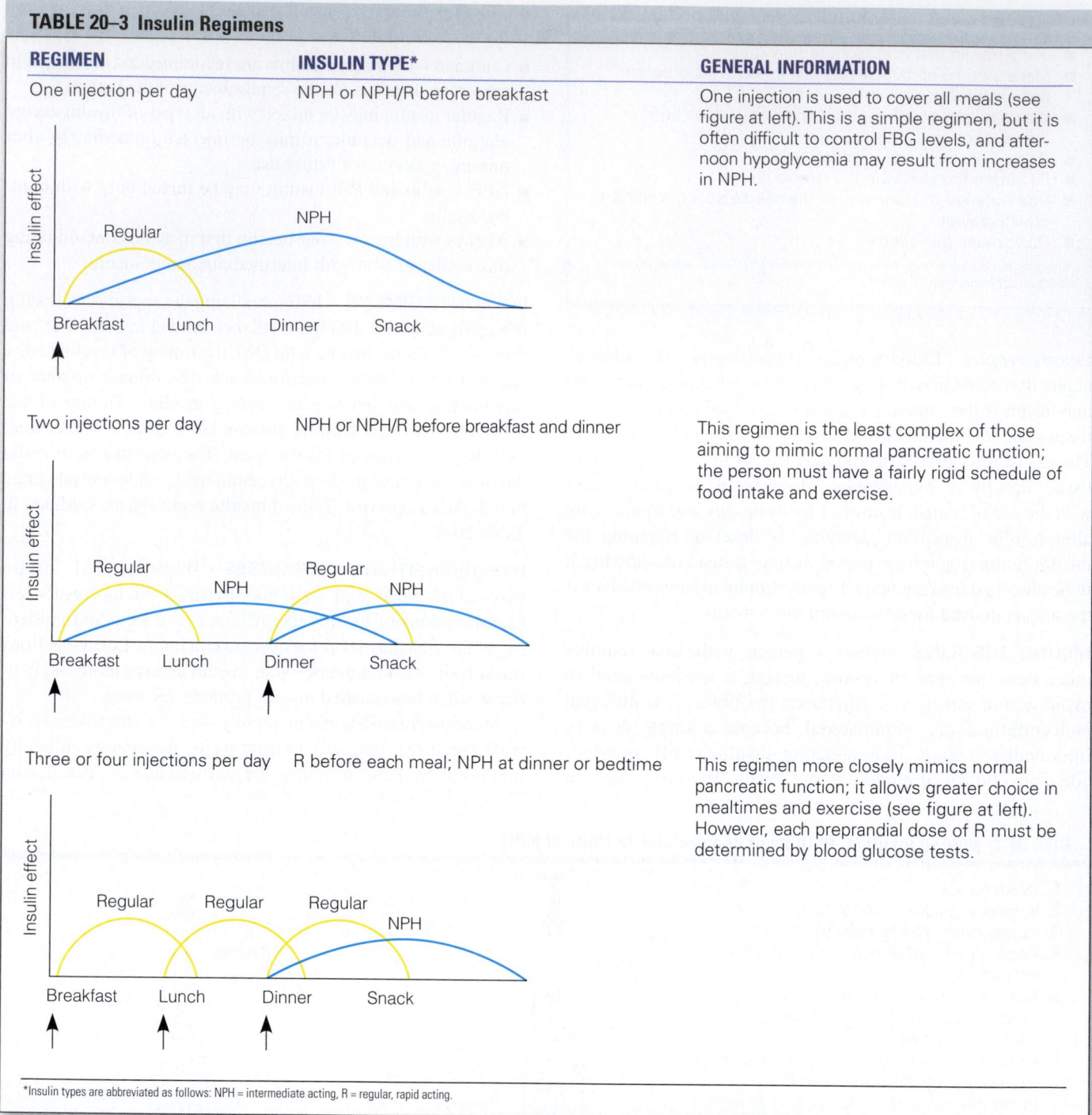

REGIMEN	INSULIN TYPE*	GENERAL INFORMATION
One injection per day	NPH or NPH/R before breakfast	One injection is used to cover all meals (see figure at left). This is a simple regimen, but it is often difficult to control FBG levels, and after-noon hypoglycemia may result from increases in NPH.
Two injections per day	NPH or NPH/R before breakfast and dinner	This regimen is the least complex of those aiming to mimic normal pancreatic function; the person must have a fairly rigid schedule of food intake and exercise.
Three or four injections per day	R before each meal; NPH at dinner or bedtime	This regimen more closely mimics normal pancreatic function; it allows greater choice in mealtimes and exercise (see figure at left). However, each prandial dose of R must be determined by blood glucose tests.

*Insulin types are abbreviated as follows: NPH = intermediate acting, R = regular, rapid acting.

itself. The patient can be desensitized by administering small doses of human insulin, followed by progressively larger doses.

Hypoglycemic Agents

Hypoglycemic agents are used to treat people with type 2 DM. Nursing implications for this category of drugs are discussed in the Medication Administration box on page 535. These medications lower blood sugar by stimulating or increasing insulin secretion, preventing breakdown of glycogen to glucose by the liver, and increasing peripheral uptake of glucose by making cells less resistant to insulin. Peripheral uptake refers to uptake by muscles and fat in the arms and legs rather than in the trunk. Some hypoglycemics keep blood sugar low by blocking absorption of carbohydrates in the intestines. A hypoglycemic agent that is only available as an injectable is exenatide (Byetta). It has several modes of action: (1) signals the pancreas to make insulin when nutrients are ingested and stop insulin release as blood sugar normalizes, (2) stops liver conversion of glycogen to glucose, and (3) decreases absorption of sugar from the intestines.

ASPIRIN THERAPY   Cardiovascular disease is the most common cause of morbidity and mortality in people with DM (ADA, 2009). It is recommended that a once daily dose of 81 to 325 mg of enteric-coated aspirin be considered as primary prevention for patients at risk for heart disease: most men over the age of 50 and most women over the age of 60 with at least one additional risk factor (family history of cardiovascular disease, smoking, hypertension, dyslipidemia, or albuminuria) (ADA, 2010). Aspirin therapy is contraindicated for patients with aspirin allergy, bleeding tendency, anticoagulant therapy, recent gastrointestinal bleeding, or active liver disease.

Nutrition

The management of DM requires a careful balance between the intake of nutrients, the expenditure of energy, and the dose and timing of insulin or oral antidiabetic agents. Although everyone has the same need for basic nutrition, the person with DM must eat a more structured diet to prevent hyperglycemia. The goals for dietary management for adults with DM, based on guidelines established by the ADA, are as follows:

- Achieve and maintain as near normal blood glucose levels as safely possible by balancing food intake with insulin or oral glucose.
- Achieve and maintain optimal serum lipid levels to reduce the risk of vascular disease.
- Achieve and maintain blood pressure levels in the normal range.

MEDICATION ADMINISTRATION Non-Insulin Hypoglycemic Agents

SULFONYLUREAS

Glimepiride (Amaryl)

Glipizide (Glucotrol, Glucotrol XL)

Glyburide (Diabeta, Micronase)

Tolazamide (Tolinase)

Tolbutamide (Orinase)

These drugs are used primarily to treat mild, nonketotic type 2 DM in people who are not obese. Glyburide, glipizide, and glimepiride are 100 to 200 times more potent than tolbutamide. These patients cannot control the manifestations by diet alone, but they do not require insulin. The drugs act by stimulating the pancreatic cells to secrete more insulin and by increasing the sensitivity of peripheral tissues to insulin. Dose adjustments must be made gradually and therefore these drugs are not useful for meeting acute changes that occur in illness or surgery. The most common side effect is hypoglycemia and this is exacerbated by NPO status. They are also associated with weight gain. These drugs are usually suspended during hospitalization (ADA, 2009).

MEGLITINIDES

Repaglinide (Prandin)

This drug lowers blood glucose levels by stimulating release of insulin from the pancreatic islet cells.

BIGUANIDES

Metformin (Glucophage)

Metformin reduces both the FBG and the degree of postprandial hyperglycemia in patients with type 2 DM. It primarily decreases the overproduction of glucose by the liver, and may also make insulin more effective in peripheral tissues. If renal insufficiency develops, metformin must be discontinued. It is used as an adjunct to diet, especially in patients who are obese or not responding to the sulfonylureas. Because of an increased risk of metformin-induced lactic acidosis, metformin is usually suspended during hospitalization. It should be discontinued temporarily before and for 48 hours after using intra-arterial iodinated contrast media for diagnostic imaging and anesthesia due to a small but significant risk of renal failure. In the Diabetes Prevention Program, some people treated with metformin reduced their risk of developing DM. An ADA panel recommends Metformin for prevention only for very-high-risk individuals (those with combined IGT and IFG, BMI > 35, and under 60 years of age with at least one other risk factor for DM). Lifestyle changes including diet and regular moderate exercise are part of preventing or delaying the onset of DM (ADA, 2009).

ALPHA-GLUCOSIDE INHIBITORS

Acarbose (Precose)

Miglitol (Glyset)

These drugs work locally in the small intestine to slow carbohydrate digestion and delay glucose absorption. As a result, postprandial glucose and glycosylated hemoglobin are better controlled, reducing the risk of long-term complications. They do not cause hypoglycemia but diminishing gastrointestinal side effects such as flatulence, diarrhea, and abdominal discomfort may occur.

D-PHENYLALANINE (AMINO ACID) DERIVATIVE

Nateglinide (Starlix)

Repaglinide (Prandin)

This is a new class of oral medications for treatment of type 2 DM. They stimulate rapid and short insulin secretion from the pancreatic beta cells to decrease spikes in glucose following meals and also reduce the overall blood glucose level. They should be taken shortly before meals; without a meal, hypoglycemia is a risk. Side effects may occur and diminish with nateglinide; these include nausea, vomiting, diarrhea, joint pain, and flu-like symptoms. Repaglinide is associated with temporary weight gain, diarrhea, and joint pain.

INCRETIN MIMETICS

Exenatide (Byetta) Injectable only

This medication signals the pancreas to make the right amount of insulin after meals to help lower blood sugar closer to normal levels. It limits liver conversion of glycogen to glucose, and slows the rate at which sugar enters the bloodstream, avoiding high blood sugar spikes.

DPP-4 INHIBITORS

Sitagliptin (Januvia)

Saxagliptin (Onglyza)

The enzyme DPP-4 degrades incretin hormones. Incretin is described in the discussion of exenatide and promotes insulin secretion. These drugs inhibit the DPP-IV enzyme, causing more stable glucose levels by decreasing liver release of glucose and increasing insulin secretion. Side effects may include headache, nasopharyngitis, and urinary tract infections; there may also be allergic-like reactions such as rash and hives. They are taken once daily in combination with diet and exercise.

SYNTHETIC AMYLIN HORMONE

Pramlintide (Symlin)

This medication is a synthetic form of Amylin, a hormone co-secreted with insulin from the B cells in the pancreas. It complements the role of insulin in limiting glucose levels by delaying gastric emptying and suppressing glucagon secretion after food intake. Patients with type 1 DM almost totally lack this hormone. It is used with insulin as a subcutaneous injection at mealtime for type 1 and type 2 DM and increases the risk of severe hypoglycemia.

Nursing Responsibilities

- Assess patients taking oral hypoglycemic agents closely for the first 7 days to determine therapeutic response.

(continued)

MEDICATION ADMINISTRATION Non-Insulin Hypoglycemic Agents (continued)

- Administer the drug with food.
- Teach the patient the importance of maintaining a prescribed diet and exercise program.
- Monitor for hypoglycemia if the patient is also taking nonsteroidal anti-inflammatory agents (NSAIDs), sulfonamide antibiotics, ranitidine, cimetidine, or beta blockers; these drugs intensify the action of sulfonylureas.
- Monitor for hyperglycemia if the patient is also taking calcium channel blockers, oral contraceptives, glucocorticoids, phenothiazines, or thiazide diuretics; these drugs decrease the hypoglycemic responses to sulfonylureas.
- Do not administer these drugs to pregnant or lactating women.
- Assess for side effects: nausea, heartburn, diarrhea, dizziness, fever, headache, jaundice, skin rash, urticaria, photophobia, thrombocytopenia, leukopenia, or anemia.
- If the patient is to have a thyroid test, determine whether the drug has been taken; sulfonylureas interfere with the uptake of radioactive iodine.
- Monitor for hypoglycemia with concurrent administration of an oral antidiabetic agent and insulin.

- Temporarily hold metformin for 2 days prior to injection of any radiocontrast agent to avoid potential lactic acidosis if renal failure occurs.

Health Education for the Patient and Family
- Maintain prescribed diet and exercise regimen.
- You may need insulin if you have surgery, trauma, fever, or infection.
- Follow instructions to monitor blood glucose.
- Report illness or side effects to the healthcare provider.
- Undergo periodic laboratory evaluations as prescribed by your healthcare provider.
- Avoid alcohol intake, which may cause a reaction involving flushing, palpitations, and nausea.
- The medication interferes with the effectiveness of oral contraceptives; other birth control measures may be required.
- Mild manifestations of hyperglycemia may appear if a different agent is begun.
- Take medications as prescribed; for example, once a day at the same time each day. If you are taking acarbose, take the pill with the first bite of food at breakfast, lunch, and dinner.

- Prevent or at least slow the rate of development of chronic complications of DM by modifying nutrient intake and lifestyle.
- Prevent and treat the acute complications of insulin-treated DM, short-term illnesses, and exercise-related problems.
- Address individual nutrition needs, taking into account personal and cultural preferences and willingness to change.
- Maintain the pleasure of eating by only limiting food choices when indicated by scientific evidence (ADA, 2008).

CARBOHYDRATES The ADA recommends that carbohydrates should be individualized to the patient's needs, with recommended allowances of 45% to 65% of the daily diet. Carbohydrates contain 4 kcal per gram and intake should not be restricted to less than 130 g/day (ADA, 2008). This group of nutrients consists of plant foods (grains, fruits, vegetables), milk, and some dairy products. Carbohydrates can be divided into simple sugars and complex carbohydrates. Glycemic index is the rate a food raises blood glucose, and thus insulin. Proponents of low carbohydrate diets use the glycemic index as the scientific foundation for decreasing intake of foods with a high glycemic index. However, many factors effect the digestion of carbohydrates; to date research does not support using glycemic index as a basis for therapy.

The use of sucrose as part of the total carbohydrate content in the diet does not impair blood glucose control in people with DM. Sucrose and sucrose-containing foods must be substituted for other carbohydrates gram for gram. Dietary fructose (from fruits and vegetables or from fructose-sweetened foods) produces a smaller rise in plasma glucose than sucrose and most starches, so it may offer an advantage as a sweetening agent. However, large amounts of fructose have potentially adverse effects on serum cholesterol and LDL cholesterol, so amounts used should be controlled.

PROTEIN The recommended daily protein intake is 15% to 20% of total daily kcal intake. Protein has 4 kcal per gram. Sources of protein should be low in fat, low in saturated fat, and low in cholesterol. Although this amount of protein is much less than that which most people normally consume, it is recommended to help prevent or delay renal complications. To help the patient accept the decrease in the amount of protein, the nurse may suggest a less severe restriction at diagnosis with a gradual decrease to take place over a period of years.

FATS Dietary fats should be low in saturated fat, trans fatty acids, and cholesterol. Saturated and trans fatty acids are the principal dietary determinants of plasma LDL cholesterol. Saturated fats should be no higher than 10% of the total kcal allowed per day, intake of trans fatty acids should be minimal, and dietary cholesterol intake less than 300 mg per day. Fat has 9 kcal per gram. Sources of the different types of fat include the following:

- *Saturated fat.* Animal meats (butter fats, lard, bacon), cocoa butter, coconut oil, palm oil, and hydrogenated oils.
- *Polyunsaturated fat.* Oils of corn, safflower, sunflower, soybean, sesame seed, and cottonseed.
- *Trans fatty acids.* Partially hydrogenated vegetable oils such as shortenings and in animal fats. Trans fats lower HDL cholesterol and increase LDL cholesterol leading to coronary heart disease.
- *Monosaturated fat.* Peanut oil, olive oil, and canola oil.

Limiting fat and cholesterol intake may help prevent or delay the onset of atherosclerosis, a common complication of DM.

FIBER Dietary fiber may be helpful in treating or preventing constipation and other gastrointestinal disorders, including colon cancer. It also helps provide a feeling of fullness, and large amounts of soluble fiber may be beneficial to serum lipids. Soluble fiber is found in dried beans, oats, barley, and in some vegetables and fruits (e.g., peas, corn, zucchini, cauliflower, broccoli, prunes, pears, apples, bananas, oranges). Insoluble fiber, which is found in wheat, corn, and in some vegetables and fruits (e.g., carrots, brussels sprouts, eggplant, green beans, pears, apples, strawberries), does facilitate intestinal motility and give a feeling of fullness.

The ideal level of fiber has not been determined, but an intake of 14 g/1000 kcal per day is recommended (ADA, 2008). An increase in fiber may cause nausea, diarrhea or constipation, and increased flatulence, especially if the person does not also increase fluid intake. Fiber should be increased gradually.

SODIUM Although the body requires sodium, most people consume much more than is needed each day, especially in processed foods. The recommended daily intake is 1000 mg of sodium per 1000 kcal, not to exceed 3000 mg per day, with lower levels (1500 mg) for people with hypertension. The primary concern with sodium is its association with hypertension, a common health problem in people with DM. It is suggested that table salt (which is 40% sodium) and processed foods high in sodium be avoided in the DM meal plan.

SWEETENERS The diet plan for people with DM restricts the amount of refined sugars. As a result, many people use noncaloric sweeteners and foods or drinks made with noncaloric sweeteners. The Food and Drug Administration (FDA) has approved commercially produced nonnutritive sweeteners. Although questions have been raised about the safety of these substances in laboratory animal studies, they are considered safe for use by humans. Included in this category of sweeteners are saccharin (Sweet & Low), aspartame or neotame (NutraSweet, Equal), sucralose (Splenda), and acesulfame potassium (Sunnette). The nonnutritive sweeteners have negligible amounts of or no kilocalories, do not produce dental caries, and produce very little or no changes in blood glucose levels.

People with DM also use nutritive sweeteners, including fructose, sorbitol, and xylitol. The kcal content of these substances is similar to that of table sugar (sucrose), but they cause less elevation in blood glucose. They are often included in foods labeled as "sugar free." Sorbitol may cause flatulence and diarrhea.

Researchers are continuing to study the safety and effectiveness of the sweeteners. In addition, the FDA recommends that the food industry label products with the amount of each ingredient in milligrams per serving and the number of servings per container. When teaching patients about diet, the nurse should include information about the kilocalorie content of sweeteners and the meaning of such words as sugar free and dietetic on labels.

ALCOHOL Although drinking alcoholic beverages is not encouraged, neither is it totally prohibited for the patient with DM. Alcohol consumption may potentiate the hypoglycemic effects of insulin and oral agents. The ADA recommends that men with DM consume no more than two drinks and women with DM no more than one drink per day.

In the following list are guidelines for people who include alcohol in their diet plan.

- The signs of intoxication and hypoglycemia are similar; thus, the person with type 1 DM is at increased risk for an insulin reaction.
- Two oral hypoglycemic agents (chlorpropamide and tolbutamide) may interact with the alcohol, causing headache, flushing, and nausea.
- Liqueurs, sweet wines, wine coolers, and sweet mixes contain large amounts of carbohydrate.
- Light beer is the recommended alcoholic drink.
- Alcohol should be consumed with meals and added to the daily food intake. In most instances, the alcohol is substituted for fat in calculating the diet; a drink with 1.5 oz of alcohol is the equivalent of two fat exchanges (90 kcal). (Food exchanges are discussed next.)

MEAL PLANNING Several different systems for meal planning are available to the person with DM. These systems include a consistent-carbohydrate DM meal plan, exchange lists, point systems, food groups, carbohydrate counting, and calorie counting. No matter what system is used, however, it must take into account the person's individualized eating habits, diet history, food values, and special needs. Altering foods and meal patterns are often one of the most difficult parts of DM management; careful consideration of individualized preferences enhances compliance with the diet. Although the ADA recommends that a registered dietitian provide the nutrition prescription, nurses must know what is prescribed and be able to reinforce teaching and answer questions.

The Consistent-Carbohydrate DM Meal Plan The consistent-carbohydrate DM meal plan, which is replacing the traditional exchange list plan, focuses on carbohydrate content. The patient eats a similar amount of carbohydrates at each meal or snack each day, based on an individual diet prescription and the food guide pyramid. Carbohydrates in a meal have the most effect on postprandial (after meals) blood glucose levels. They also determine, to a greater extent than do proteins and fats, insulin requirements before meals. Patients should be taught to count carbohydrates so they can administer 1 unit of regular insulin or insulin lispro for each 10 or 15 g of carbohydrate eaten at a meal. This method provides a better connection between food, medications, and exercise.

The Exchange Lists The exchange list diet is based on the person's ideal (or reasonable) weight, activity level, age, and occupation. These factors determine the total kilocalories that the person may consume each day. After the calories have been determined, the proportions of carbohydrates, proteins, and fats are calculated, using guidelines established by the American Diabetes Association and the American Dietetic Association.

The distribution of foods throughout the day is based on exchange lists. The name and quantity of food that make up one exchange (or serving) are listed; standard household measurements are used. One food portion on the list can be substituted (exchanged) for another with very little difference in calories or amount of carbohydrates, proteins, and fats. The meal plan prescribes how many exchanges are allowed for each food group per meal and snacks.

Diet Plan for Type 1 DM   Diet and insulin prescription must be integrated for optimal energy metabolism and the prevention of hyperglycemia or hypoglycemia. The goals of the diet plan are to achieve optimal glucose and lipid levels, improve overall health, and maintain reasonable body weight. To meet these goals, the following strategies must be implemented:

- Glucose regulation requires correlating eating patterns with insulin onset and peak of action.
- Meals, snacks, and insulin regimens should be based on the person's lifestyle.
- Meal planning depends on the specific insulin regimen prescribed.
- Snacks are an important consideration in relation to the amount and timing of exercise.
- The diet plan must consider the availability of foods, based on occupational, financial, religious, and ethnic constraints.
- SMBG levels help the patient make adjustments for planned and unplanned changes in routines.

Diet Plan for Type 2 DM   The goals of the diet plan are to improve blood glucose levels, improve overall health, prevent or delay complications, and attain or maintain reasonable body weight. Because the majority of these patients are overweight, weight loss is important and facilitates achieving the other goals.

There are no specific guidelines for the type 2 diet, but in addition to decreasing kilocalories, it is recommended that the patient consume three meals of equal size, evenly spaced approximately 4 to 5 hours apart, with one or two snacks. The person with type 2 DM should also decrease fat intake. If the exchange list is difficult to use, calorie counting or designing the diet by grams of fat may be more useful.

SICK-DAY MANAGEMENT   When the person with DM is sick or has surgery, blood glucose levels increase, even though food intake decreases. The person often mistakenly alters or omits the insulin dose, causing further problems. The guidelines for dietary management during illness focus on preventing dehydration and providing nutrition for promoting recovery. In general, sick-day management includes the following:

- Monitoring blood glucose at least four times a day throughout an illness
- Testing urine for ketones if blood glucose is greater than 240 mg/dL
- Continuing to take the usual insulin dose or oral hypoglycemic agent
- Sipping 8 to 12 oz of fluid each hour
- Substituting easily digested liquids or soft foods if solid foods are not tolerated (The substituted liquids and foods should be carbohydrate equivalents, for example, 1/2 cup sweetened gelatin, 1/2 cup fruit juice, one Popsicle, 1/4 cup sherbet, and 1/2 cup regular soft drink.)
- Calling the healthcare provider if the patient is unable to eat for more than 24 hours or if vomiting and diarrhea last for more than 6 hours

DIET PLAN FOR THE OLDER ADULT   The majority of older adults with diabetes have type 2 DM and should follow the general guidelines for that diet plan. However, special considerations for the older adult are important if the diet plan is to be followed, including dietary likes and dislikes, changes in taste perception, dental health, available income, and who prepares the food. Other factors to consider in planning the diet for the older adult include the age-related decline in kcal requirements, decline in physical activity due to age and/or chronic illnesses, and the onset or progression of other chronic illnesses. The older adult who is overweight should reduce kcal intake to ensure weight loss, but at the same time, careful monitoring for malnutrition is necessary. It is possible for the older adult to revert to normal glucose tolerance if ideal body weight is regained.

Exercise

The third component of DM management is a regular exercise program consisting of at least 150 minutes per week (ADA, 2009). The benefits of exercise are the same for everyone, with or without DM: improved physical fitness, improved emotional state, weight control, and improved work capacity. In people with DM, exercise increases the uptake of glucose by muscle cells, potentially reducing the need for insulin. Exercise also decreases cholesterol and triglycerides, reducing the risk of cardiovascular disorders. People with DM should consult their primary healthcare provider before beginning or changing an exercise program. The ability to maintain an exercise program is affected by many different factors, including fatigue and glucose levels. It is as important to assess the person's usual lifestyle before establishing an exercise program as it is before planning a diet. Factors to consider include the patient's usual exercise habits, living environment, and community programs. The exercise that the person enjoys most is probably the one that he or she will continue throughout life. Use proper footwear, inspect the feet daily and after exercise, avoid exercise in extreme heat or cold, and avoid exercise during periods of poor glucose control.

TYPE 1 DM   In the person with type 1 DM, glycemic responses to exercise vary according to the type, intensity, and duration of the exercise. Other factors that influence responses include the timing of exercise in relation to meals and insulin injections, and the time of day of the activity. Unless these factors are integrated into the exercise program, the person with type 1 DM has an increased risk of hypoglycemia and hyperglycemia. Following are general guidelines for an exercise program.

- People who have frequent hyperglycemia or hypoglycemia should avoid prolonged exercise until glucose control improves.
- The risk of exercise-induced hypoglycemia is lowest before breakfast, when free-insulin levels tend to be lower than they are before meals later in the day or at bedtime.
- Exercise should be moderate and regular; brief, intense exercise tends to cause mild hyperglycemia, and prolonged exercise can lead to hypoglycemia.
- Exercising at a peak insulin action time may lead to hypoglycemia.
- SMBG is essential both before and after exercise.
- Food intake may need to be increased to compensate for the activity.
- Fluid intake, especially water, is essential.

Young adults may continue participating in sports with some modifications in diet and insulin dosage. Athletes should begin training slowly, extend activity over a prolonged period, take a carbohydrate source (such as a drink consisting of 5% to 10% carbohydrate) after about 1 hour of exercise, and monitor blood glucose levels for possible adjustments. In addition, a snack should be available after the activity is completed. It may be necessary to omit the usual regular insulin dose prior to an athletic event; even if the athlete is hyperglycemic at the beginning of the event, blood glucose levels will fall to normal after the first 60 to 90 minutes of exercise.

TYPE 2 DM   An exercise program for the person with type 2 DM is especially important. The benefits of regular exercise include weight loss in those who are overweight, improved glycemic control, increased well-being, socialization with others, and a reduction of cardiovascular risk factors. A combination of diet, exercise, and weight loss often decreases the need for oral hypoglycemic agents. This decrease is due to an increased sensitivity to insulin, increased kcal expenditure, and increased self-esteem. Regular exercise may prevent type 2 DM in high-risk individuals (ADA, 2009).

Following are general guidelines for an exercise program:

- Before beginning the program, have a medical screening for previously undiagnosed hypertension, neuropathy, retinopathy, and nephropathy.
- Begin the program with mild exercises, and gradually increase intensity and duration.
- Exercise at least 150 minutes a week in regular, shorter time sessions.
- Include resistance exercise (muscle-strengthening) and low-impact aerobic exercises in the program.

Treatments

SURGERY   Surgical management of DM includes surgically revising the GI tract as well as replacing or transplanting the pancreas, pancreatic cells, or beta cells. Although it is still in the investigative stage, many researchers believe that transplantation of the tail of the pancreas is the most promising technique for achieving long-term disease control. Islet cell transplantation has had moderate success, and research is continuing. A diabetic patient can receive a portion of a pancreas from a living relative, often as part of a kidney transplant. The transplanted pancreas may protect the new kidney from damage. Transplants of more than one organ survive better than solo transplants (ADA, 2008). Other research is being conducted in the use of an internally implanted artificial pancreas, or closed-loop artificial beta cell.

Surgery is a stressor that often alters self-management and glycemic control in people with DM. In response to stress, levels of catecholamines, cortisol, glucagon, and growth hormones increase, as does insulin resistance. Hyperglycemia occurs, and protein stores are decreased. In addition, diet and activity patterns change, and medication types and dosages vary. As a result, surgical patients who have DM are at increased risk for postoperative infection, delayed wound healing, fluid and electrolyte imbalances, hyper- and hypoglycemia, and DKA (Loh-Trivedi & Rothenberg, 2008).

Preoperatively, all patients should be in the best possible metabolic state. Screening for complications and regular blood glucose monitoring are part of preoperative preparation. Oral hypoglycemic agents may be withheld for 1 or 2 days before

surgery, and regular insulin is often administered to the patient with type 2 DM, and those with hyperglycemia but not diagnosed with DM, during the perioperative period. All patients with hyperglycemia whether diagnosed with DM or not follow a carefully prescribed insulin regimen individualized to specific needs.

The insulin regimen in the perioperative period is individualized. When the patient is NPO, short-acting insulin should not be given without intravenous glucose. Patients with type 1 DM and type 2 DM, and patients with hyperglycemia who are critically ill in the perioperative period should receive IV glucose and insulin infusion in an intensive care unit. The target blood glucose level during surgery is between 110 and 140 mg/dL. This avoids hypoglycemia, which is difficult to detect under anesthesia, and prevents glycosuria, dehydration, and impaired wound healing. IV infusion of glucose, insulin, and added potassium is appropriate for all hyperglycemic patients undergoing surgery (ADA, 2009).

The surgical procedure should be scheduled for as early as possible in the morning to minimize the length of fasting. If there is no food intake after surgery, intravenous dextrose should be administered, accompanied by subcutaneous regular insulin every 6 hours for the noncritically ill surgical patient. The dose can be adjusted to blood glucose levels. Although kcal intake is decreased postoperatively, stress can increase insulin requirements. Glucose control is also affected postoperatively by nausea and vomiting, anorexia, and gastrointestinal suction.

During the postoperative period, the patient with type 2 DM may continue to require insulin or may resume oral medications, depending on glucose control. The patient with type 1 DM may require reduced insulin as healing progresses and stress diminishes. Regular blood glucose monitoring is essential, as are assessments for hypoglycemia.

Complications of Diabetes Mellitus

The person with DM, regardless of type, is at increased risk for complications involving many different body systems. Alterations in blood glucose levels, alterations in the cardiovascular system, neuropathies, an increased susceptibility to infection, and periodontal disease are common. In addition, the interaction of several complications can cause problems of the feet. The Multisystem Effects of Diabetes Mellitus illustration on page 525 shows the progression from cardinal signs to acute and late complications for the patient with DM. A discussion of each of these complications follows; related interdisciplinary care and nursing care are discussed later in the chapter.

Acute Complications: Alterations in Blood Glucose Levels

The following discussion provides additional information about hyperglycemia and hypoglycemia. Table 20–4 compares DKA, HHS, and hypoglycemia.

HYPERGLYCEMIA   The major problems resulting from hyperglycemia in the person with DM are DKA and HHS. Two other problems are the dawn phenomenon and the Somogyi phenomenon.

TABLE 20–4 DKA, HHS, and Hypoglycemia Compared

		DKA	HHS	HYPOGLYCEMIA
DM Type		Primary Type 1	Type 2	Both
Onset		Slow	Slow	Rapid
Cause		↓ Insulin	↓ Insulin	↑ Insulin
		Infection	Older age	Omitted meal/snack
				Error in insulin dose
Risk Factors		Surgery	Surgery	Surgery
		Trauma	Trauma	Trauma
		Illness	Illness	Illness
		Omitted insulin	Dehydration	Exercise
		Stress	Medications	Medications
			Dialysis	Lipodystrophy
			Hyperalimentation	Renal failure
				Alcohol intake
Assessments	Skin	Flushed; dry; warm	Flushed; dry; warm	Pallor; moist; cool
	Perspiration	None	None	Profuse
	Thirst	Increased	Increased	Normal
	Breath	Fruity	Normal	Normal
	Vital signs	BP ↓	BP ↓	BP ↓
		P ↑	P ↑	P ↑
		R Kussmaul's	R normal	R normal
	Mental status	Confused	Lethargic	Anxious; restless
	Thirst	Increased	Increased	Normal
	Fluid intake	Increased	Increased	Normal
	Gastrointestinal effects	Nausea/vomiting; abdominal pain	Nausea/vomiting; abdominal pain	Hunger
	Fluid loss	Moderate	Profound:	Normal
	Level of consciousness	Decreasing	Decreasing	Decreasing
	Energy level	Weak	Weak	Fatigue
	Other	Weight loss	Weight loss	Headache
		Blurred vision	Malaise	Altered vision
			Extreme thirst	Mood changes
			Seizures	Seizures
Laboratory Findings	Blood glucose	> 300 mg/dL	> 600 mg/dL	< 50 mg/dL
	Plasma ketones	Increased	Normal	Normal
	Urine glucose	Increased	Increased	Normal
	Urine ketones	Increased	Normal	Normal
	Serum potassium	Abnormal	Abnormal	Normal
	Serum sodium	Abnormal	Abnormal	Normal
	Serum chloride	Abnormal	Abnormal	Normal
	Plasma pH	< 7.3	Normal	Normal
	Osmolality	> 340 mOsm/L	> 340 mOsm/L	Normal
Treatment		Insulin	Insulin	Glucagon
		Intravenous fluids	Intravenous fluids	Rapid-acting carbohydrate
		Electrolytes	Electrolytes	Intravenous solution of 50% glucose

The dawn phenomenon is a rise in blood glucose between 4 AM and 8 AM that is not a response to hypoglycemia. This condition occurs in people with both type 1 and type 2 DM. The exact cause is unknown but is believed to be related to nocturnal increases in growth hormone, which decreases peripheral uptake of glucose. The Somogyi phenomenon is a combination of hypoglycemia during the night with a rebound morning rise in blood glucose to hyperglycemic levels. The hyperglycemia stimulates the counterregulatory hormones, which stimulate gluconeogenesis and glycogenolysis and also inhibit peripheral glucose use. This may cause insulin resistance for 12 to 48 hours.

Diabetic Ketoacidosis As the pathophysiology of untreated type 1 DM continues, the insulin deficit causes fat stores to break down to provide energy, resulting in continued hyperglycemia and mobilization of fatty acids with a subsequent ketosis (see Figure 20–2). **Diabetic ketoacidosis (DKA)** develops when there is an absolute deficiency of insulin and an increase in the insulin counterregulatory hormones (cortisol). Glucose production by the liver increases, peripheral glucose use decreases, fat mobilization increases, and ketogenesis (ketone formation) is stimulated. Increased glucagon levels activate the gluconeogenic and ketogenic pathways in the liver.

In the presence of insulin deficiency, hepatic overproduction of beta-hydroxybutyrate and acetoacetic acids (ketone bodies) causes increased ketone concentrations and an increased release of free fatty acids. As a result of a loss of bicarbonate (which occurs when the ketone is formed), bicarbonate buffering does not occur, and a metabolic acidosis occurs, called DKA. Depression of the central nervous system (CNS) from the accumulation of ketones and the resulting acidosis may cause coma and death if left untreated (Porth & Matfin, 2009). The impact of DKA is illustrated in Figure 20–6 ■.

DKA also may occur in a person with diagnosed DM when energy requirements increase during physical or emotional stress. Stress states initiate the release of gluconeogenic hormones, resulting in the formation of carbohydrates from protein or fat. The person who is sick, has an infection (the most frequent cause of DKA), or who decreases or omits insulin doses is at a greatly increased risk for developing DKA.

DKA involves four metabolic problems:

- Hyperosmolarity from hyperglycemia and dehydration
- Metabolic acidosis from an accumulation of ketoacids
- Extracellular volume depletion from osmotic diuresis
- Electrolyte imbalances (such as loss of potassium and sodium) from osmotic diuresis

A Decreased uptake of glucose results in breakdown of protein to amino acids for use as energy source (gluconeogenesis).

B Increased breakdown of fats (lypolysis) results in glycerol for use as energy (gluconeogenesis).

Glucose

Osmotic diuresis

Loss of water and electrolytes

Dehydration

Circulatory failure

Metabolic acidosis from increased ketoacids

CNS depression and coma

Figure 20–6 ■ DKA Impact.

MANIFESTATIONS of Diabetic Ketoacidosis (DKA)

DEHYDRATION (FROM HYPERGLYCEMIA)
- Thirst
- Warm, dry skin with poor turgor
- Soft eyeballs
- Dry mucous membranes
- Weakness
- Malaise
- Rapid, weak pulse
- Hypotension

METABOLIC ACIDOSIS (FROM KETOSIS)
- Nausea and vomiting
- Ketone (fruity, alcohol-like) breath odor
- Lethargy
- Coma

OTHER MANIFESTATIONS
- Abdominal pain (cause unknown)
- Kussmaul's respirations (increased rate and depth of respirations, with a longer expiration; a compensatory response to prevent a further decrease in pH)

Manifestations of DKA result from severe dehydration and acidosis. These manifestations are summarized in the box above. Laboratory findings include the following:

- Blood glucose levels higher than 250 mg/dL
- Plasma pH less than 7.3
- Plasma bicarbonate less than 15 mEq/L
- Presence of serum ketones
- Presence of urine ketones and glucose
- Abnormal levels of serum sodium, potassium, and chloride

TREATMENT OF DKA DKA requires immediate medical attention. Admission to the hospital is appropriate when the person has a blood glucose of greater than 250 mg/dL, a decreasing pH, and ketones in the urine. If the patient is alert and conscious, fluids may be replaced orally. In the first 12 hours of treatment, adults usually require 8–10 L of fluid to replace losses from polyuria and vomiting. The initial fluid replacement may be accomplished by administering 0.9% saline solution at a rate of 500 to 1000 mL/h. After 2 to 3 hours (or when blood pressure is returning to normal), the administration of 0.45% saline at 200 to 500 mL/h may continue for several more hours. When the blood glucose levels reach 250 mg/dL, dextrose is added to prevent rapid decreases in glucose; there is a risk of fatal cerebral edema if fluids are given too rapidly or excessively.

Regular insulin is used in the management of DKA and may be given by various routes, depending on the severity of the condition. Mild ketosis may be treated with subcutaneous insulin, whereas severe ketosis requires intravenous insulin infusion. Nursing responsibilities for the patient receiving intravenous insulin are described in the following Medication Administration box.

When renal function and blood pressure are restored, potassium and sodium can be corrected. The electrolyte imbalance of primary concern is depletion of body stores of potassium. Initially, serum potassium levels may be normal, but they decrease during treatment. Insulin causes potassium to be shifted into the cells, increasing hypokalemia. In DKA (and from rehydration), the body loses potassium from increased urinary output, acidosis, catabolic state, and vomiting or diarrhea. Potassium replacement is begun early in the course of treatment, usually by adding potassium to the rehydration fluids. Replacement is essential for preventing cardiac dysrhythmias secondary to hypokalemia. Cardiac rhythms and potassium levels must be monitored every 2 to 4 hours.

Hyperosmolar Hyperglycemic State (HHS) The metabolic problem called **hyperosmolar hyperglycemic state (HHS)** occurs in people who have type 2 DM. HHS is characterized by a plasma osmolarity of 340 mOsm/L or greater (the normal range is 280 to 300 mOsm/L), greatly elevated blood glucose levels (over 600 mg/dL and often 1000 to 2000 mg/dL), and altered levels of consciousness. HHS is a serious, life-threatening medical emergency and has a higher mortality rate than DKA. Mortality is high not only because the metabolic changes are serious but also because people with DM are usually older and have other medical problems that either cause or are caused by HHS. The precipitating factors associated with HHS include infection, therapeutic agents that cause hyperglycemia, therapeutic procedures, acute illness, and chronic illness (Box 20–4). The most common precipitating factor is infection. The manifestations of this disorder may be slow to appear, with onset ranging from 24 hours to 2 weeks. The manifestations are initiated by hyperglycemia, which causes increased urine output. With increased output, plasma volume decreases and glomerular filtration rate (GFR) drops. As a result, glucose is retained and water is lost. Glucose and sodium accumulate in the blood and increase serum osmolarity.

MEDICATION ADMINISTRATION Intravenous Insulin

General Guidelines
- Regular insulin may be given undiluted directly into the vein or through a Y-tube or three-way stopcock.
- Insulin is usually diluted in 0.9% saline or 0.45% saline solution for infusion.
- Because glass or plastic infusion containers and plastic tubing may reduce insulin potency by at least 20% and possibly by up to 80% before the insulin reaches the venous system, tubing should be flushed to the intravenous catheter connection with the insulin solution prior to starting an infusion.

Nursing Responsibilities
- Monitor blood glucose levels hourly.
- Infuse the insulin solution separately from the hydration solution.
- Flush the intravenous tubing with 50 mL of insulin mixed with normal saline solution to saturate binding sites on the tubing before administering the insulin to the patient; this step increases the amount of insulin delivered over the first few hours.
- Do not discontinue the intravenous infusion until subcutaneous administration of insulin is resumed.
- Monitor for manifestations of hypoglycemia.
- Ensure that glucagons and D50 is readily available as an antidote for insulin overdose.

BOX 20–4 Factors Associated with Hyperosmolar Hyperglycemic State (HHS)

Therapeutic Agents
- Glucocorticoids
- Diuretics
- Beta-adrenergic blocking agents
- Immunosuppressants
- Chlorpromazine
- Diazoxide

Therapeutic Procedures
- Peritoneal dialysis
- Hemodialysis
- Hyperosmolar alimentation (oral or parenteral)
- Surgery

Acute Illness
- Infection
- Gangrene
- Urinary infection
- Burns
- Gastrointestinal bleeding
- Myocardial infarction
- Pancreatitis
- Stroke

Chronic Illness
- Renal disease
- Cardiac disease
- Hypertension
- Previous stroke
- Alcoholism

Serum hyperosmolarity results in severe dehydration, reducing intracellular water in all tissues, including the brain. The person has dry skin and mucous membranes, extreme thirst, and altered levels of consciousness (progressing from lethargy to coma). Neurologic deficits may include hyperthermia, motor and sensory impairment, positive Babinski's sign, and seizures. Metabolic acidosis is not part of the pathology; despite elevated blood glucose, sufficient insulin is present to prevent metabolism of fats with the resulting fatty acids and ketones of DKA. Treatment is directed toward correcting fluid and electrolyte imbalances, lowering blood glucose levels with insulin, and treating underlying conditions.

TREATMENT OF HHS HHS is a serious, life-threatening metabolic condition. The patient admitted to the intensive care unit for treatment typically manifests blood glucose levels over 700 mg/dL, increased serum osmolarity, and altered levels of consciousness or seizures. Treatment is similar to that of DKA: correcting fluid and electrolyte imbalances and providing insulin to lower hyperglycemia. In general, treatment modalities include the following:

- Establishing and maintaining adequate ventilation
- Correcting shock with adequate intravenous fluids
- Instituting nasogastric suction if comatose to prevent aspiration
- Maintaining fluid volume with intravenous isotonic or colloid solutions
- Administering potassium intravenously to replace losses
- Administering insulin to reduce blood glucose, usually discontinuing administration when blood glucose levels reach 250 mg/dL (Because ketosis is not present, there is no need to continue insulin, as with DKA.)

Hypoglycemia

Hypoglycemia (low blood glucose levels) is common in people with type 1 DM and occasionally occurs in people with type 2 DM who are treated with certain oral hypoglycemic agents. This condition is often called insulin shock, insulin reaction, or "the lows" in patients with type 1 DM. Hypoglycemia results primarily from a mismatch between insulin intake (e.g., an error in insulin dose), physical activity, and lack of carbohydrate availability (e.g., omitting a meal). The intake of alcohol and drugs such as chloramphenicol (Chloromycetin), Coumadin, monoamine oxidase (MAO) inhibitors, probenecid (Benemid), salicylates, and sulfonamides can also cause hypoglycemia.

The manifestations of hypoglycemia (see the following box) result from a compensatory autonomic nervous system (ANS) response and from impaired cerebral function due to a decrease in glucose available for use by the brain. The manifestations vary, particularly in older adults. The onset is sudden, and blood glucose is usually less than 45 to 60 mg/dL. Severe hypoglycemia may cause death.

People who have type 1 DM for 4 or 5 years fail to secrete glucagon in response to a decrease in blood glucose. They then depend on epinephrine to serve as a counterregulatory response to hypoglycemia. However, this compensatory response can become absent or blunted. The person then develops a syndrome called hypoglycemia unawareness. The person does not experience manifestations of hypoglycemia, even though it is present. Because treatment is not initiated in the absence of manifestations, the person is likely to have episodes of severe hypoglycemia.

TREATMENT OF HYPOGLYCEMIA
Mild Hypoglycemia When mild hypoglycemia occurs, immediate treatment is necessary. People experiencing hypoglycemia should take about 15 g of a rapid-acting sugar. This amount of sugar is found, for example, in three glucose tablets, 1/2 cup (4 ounces) of fruit juice or regular soda, 8 oz of skim milk, five Life Savers candies, three large marshmallows, or 3 tsp of sugar or honey. Sugar should not be added to fruit juice. Adding sugar to the fruit sugar already in the juice could cause a rapid rise in blood glucose, with persistent hyperglycemia.

MANIFESTATIONS of Hypoglycemia

MANIFESTATIONS CAUSED BY RESPONSES OF THE AUTONOMIC NERVOUS SYSTEM
- Hunger
- Nausea
- Anxiety
- Pale, cool skin
- Sweating
- Shakiness
- Irritability
- Rapid pulse
- Hypotension

MANIFESTATIONS CAUSED BY IMPAIRED CEREBRAL FUNCTION
- Strange or unusual feelings
- Headache
- Difficulty in thinking
- Inability to concentrate
- Change in emotional behavior
- Slurred speech
- Blurred vision
- Decreasing levels of consciousness
- Seizures
- Coma

If the manifestations continue, the 15/15 rule should be followed: Wait 15 minutes, monitor blood glucose, and, if it is low, eat another 15 g of carbohydrate. This procedure can be repeated until blood glucose levels return to normal (McPhee & Papadakis, 2009). BG should be tested 1 hour after the BG has reached $\geq$ 70 mg/dl because BG levels will start to fall again after 1 hour (Anthony, 2007). People with DM should have some source of carbohydrate readily available at all times so that hypoglycemic manifestations can be quickly reversed. If hypoglycemia occurs more than two or three times a week, the DM management plan should be adjusted.

Severe Hypoglycemia People with DM who have severe hypoglycemia are often hospitalized. The criteria for hospitalization are one or more of the following:

- Blood glucose is less than 50 mg/dL, and the prompt treatment of hypoglycemia has not resulted in recovery of sensorium.
- The patient has coma, seizures, or altered behavior.
- The hypoglycemia has been treated, but a responsible adult cannot be with the patient for the following 12 hours.
- The hypoglycemia was caused by a sulfonylurea drug.

If the patient is conscious and alert, 10 to 15 g of an oral carbohydrate may be given. If the patient has altered levels of consciousness, parenteral glucose or glucagon is administered. Glucose is administered intravenously as a 50 ml of 50% (D50) solution, usually at a rate of 10 mL over 1 minute by intravenous push (McPhee & Papadakis, 2009). This is the most rapid method of increasing blood glucose levels.

Glucagon is an antihypoglycemic agent that raises blood glucose by promoting the conversion of hepatic glycogen to glucose. It is used in severe insulin-induced hypoglycemia and may be given in the recommended dose of 1 mg by the subcutaneous, intramuscular, or intravenous route. Glucagon has a short period of action; an oral (if the patient is conscious) or intravenous carbohydrate should be administered following the glucagon to prevent a recurrence of hypoglycemia. If the patient has been unconscious, glucagon may cause vomiting when consciousness returns.

Chronic Complications

Alterations in the Cardiovascular System

The macrocirculation (large blood vessels) in people with DM undergoes changes due to atherosclerosis; abnormalities in platelets, red blood cells and clotting factors; and changes in arterial walls. It has been established that atherosclerosis has an increased incidence and earlier age of onset in people with DM (although the reason is unknown). Other risk factors that contribute to the development of macrovascular disease of DM are hypertension, hyperlipidemia, cigarette smoking, and obesity. Alterations in the vascular system increase the risk of the long-term complications of coronary artery disease, cerebral vascular disease, and peripheral vascular disease.

Alterations in the microcirculation in the person with DM involve structural defects in the basement membrane of smaller blood vessels and capillaries. (The basement membrane is the structure that supports and serves as the boundary around the space occupied by epithelial cells.) These defects cause the capillary basement membrane to thicken, eventually resulting

in decreased tissue perfusion. The effects of alterations in the microcirculation affect all body tissues but are seen primarily in the eyes and the kidneys.

CORONARY ARTERY DISEASE Coronary artery disease is a major risk factor in the development of myocardial infarction in people with DM, especially in the middle to older adult with type 2 DM. Coronary artery disease is the most common cause of death in people with type 2 DM (McPhee & Papadakis, 2009). People with DM who have myocardial infarction are more prone to develop congestive heart failure as a complication of the infarction and are also less likely to survive in the period immediately following the infarction. (Myocardial infarction is discussed in ∞ Chapter 30.)

HYPERTENSION Hypertension is a common complication of DM. It affects 75% of all people with DM, and is a major risk factor for cardiovascular disease and microvascular complications such as retinopathy and nephropathy. Hypertension may be reduced by weight loss, exercise, and decreasing sodium intake and alcohol consumption. If these methods are not effective, treatment with antihypertensive medications is necessary.

STROKE (CEREBROVASCULAR ACCIDENT) People with DM, especially older adults with type 2 DM, are two to four times more likely to have a stroke (CDC, 2007). Although the exact relationship between DM and cerebral vascular disease is unknown, hypertension (a risk factor for stroke) is a common health problem in those who have DM. In addition, atherosclerosis of the cerebral vessels develops at an earlier age and is more extensive in people with DM (Porth & Matfin, 2009).

The manifestations of impaired cerebral circulation (∞ see Chapter 42) are often similar to those of hypoglycemia or HHS: blurred vision, slurred speech, weakness, and dizziness. People with these manifestations have potentially life-threatening health problems and require medical attention.

Peripheral Vascular Disease

Peripheral vascular disease of the lower extremities accompanies both types of DM, but the incidence is greater in people with type 2 DM. Atherosclerosis of vessels in the legs of people with DM begins at an earlier age, advances more rapidly, and is equally common in both men and women. Impaired peripheral vascular circulation leads to peripheral vascular insufficiency with intermittent claudication (pain) in the lower legs and ulcerations of the feet. Occlusion and thrombosis of large vessels and small arteries and arterioles, as well as alterations in neurologic function and infection, result in gangrene (necrosis, or the death of tissue). Gangrene from DM is the most common cause of nontraumatic amputations of the lower leg. In people with DM, dry gangrene is most common, manifested by cold, dry, shriveled, and black tissues of the toes and feet. The gangrene usually begins in the toes and moves proximally into the foot.

DIABETIC RETINOPATHY Diabetic retinopathy is the name for the changes in the retina that occur in the person with DM. The retinal capillary structure undergoes alterations in blood flow, leading to retinal ischemia and a breakdown in the blood-retinal barrier. Diabetic retinopathy is the leading cause of blindness in people between ages 20 and 74 (CDC, 2007).

After 20 years of DM, almost all patients with type 1 DM and more than 60% of patients with type 2 DM will have some degree of retinopathy, in most cases without vision loss (Porth& Matfin, 2009). If exudate, edema, hemorrhage, or ischemia occurs near the fovea, the person experiences visual impairment at any stage. In addition, the person with DM is at increased risk for developing cataracts (opacity of the lens) as a result of increased glucose levels within the lens itself. Screening for retinopathy is important, as laser photocoagulation surgery has proven beneficial in preventing loss of vision.

DIABETIC NEPHROPATHY Diabetic nephropathy is a disease of the kidneys characterized by the presence of albumin in the urine, hypertension, edema, and progressive renal insufficiency. This disorder accounts for 44% of new cases of end stage renal disease; 40% of patients requiring dialysis or transplantation in the United States have DM (Porth & Matfin, 2009). Nephropathy occurs in 30%–40% of people with type 1 DM and 15%–20% of those with type 2 (McPhee & Papadakis, 2009).

Despite research, the exact pathologic origin of diabetic nephropathy is unknown, but it is known that thickening of the basement membrane of the glomeruli eventually impairs renal function. It is suggested that an increased intracellular concentration of glucose supports the formation of abnormal glycoproteins in the basement membrane and mesangium. The accumulation of these large proteins stimulates glomerulosclerosis (fibrosis of the glomerular tissue). Glomerulosclerosis thickens the basement membrane and simultaneously makes it functionally leaky, allowing large molecules such as protein to be lost in the urine. Kimmelstiel-Wilson syndrome is a type of glomerulosclerosis found only in people with DM. In advanced nephropathy, tubular atrophy occurs, and end-stage renal disease results. (Renal failure is discussed in ∞ Chapter 28.)

The first indication of nephropathy is microalbuminuria, an abnormal level of albumin in the urine. Without specific interventions, people with type 1 DM with sustained microalbuminuria will develop nephropathy, accompanied by hypertension, over a period of 10 to 15 years. People with type 2 DM often have microalbuminuria and nephropathy shortly after diagnosis, because the DM has often been present but undiagnosed for many years. Because the hypertension accelerates the progress of diabetic nephropathy, aggressive antihypertensive management should be instituted. Management includes control of hypertension with ACE inhibitors such as captopril (Capoten), weight loss, reduced salt intake, and exercise.

Alterations in the Peripheral and Autonomic Nervous Systems

Peripheral and visceral neuropathies are disorders of the peripheral nerves and the autonomic nervous system. In people with DM, these disorders are often called diabetic neuropathies The etiology of diabetic neuropathies involves (1) a thickening of the walls of the blood vessels that supply nerves, causing a decrease in nutrients; (2) demyelinization of the Schwann cells that surround and insulate nerves, slowing nerve conduction; and (3) the formation and accumulation of sorbitol within the Schwann cells, impairing nerve conduction. The manifestations depend on the locations of the lesions.

The peripheral neuropathies (also called *somatic neuropathies*) include polyneuropathies and mononeuropathies. *Polyneuropathies*, the most common type of neuropathy associated with DM, are bilateral sensory disorders. The manifestations appear first in the toes and feet and progress upward. The fingers and hands may also be involved, but usually only in later stages of DM. The manifestations of polyneuropathy depend on the nerve fibers involved. The lack of sensation prevents awareness of injury and for this reason, people with diabetes must be taught to visually inspect their feet and legs daily, looking for evidence of injury.

The person with polyneuropathy commonly has distal paresthesias (a change in sensation, such as numbness or tingling); pain described as aching, burning, or shooting; and feelings of cold feet. Other manifestations may include impaired sensations of pain, light touch, two-point discrimination, and vibration. There is no specific treatment for polyneuropathy.

Mononeuropathies are isolated peripheral neuropathies that affect a single nerve. Depending on the nerve involved, manifestations may include the following:

- Palsy of the third cranial (oculomotor) nerve, with headache, eye pain, and an inability to move the eye up, down, or medially
- Radiculopathy, with pain over a dermatome and loss of cutaneous sensation, most often located in the chest
- Diabetic femoral neuropathy, with motor and sensory deficits (pain, weakness, areflexia) in the anterior thigh and medial calf
- Entrapment or compression of the medial nerve at the wrist, resulting in carpal tunnel syndrome with pain and weakness of the hand; the ulnar nerve at the elbow, with weakness and loss of sensation over the palmar surface of the fourth and fifth fingers; and the peroneal nerve at the head of the fibula, with foot drop.

VISCERAL NEUROPATHIES The visceral neuropathies (also called autonomic neuropathies) cause various manifestations, depending on the area of the ANS involved. These neuropathies may include the following:

- Sweating dysfunction, with an absence of sweating (anhidrosis) on the hands and feet and increased sweating on the face or trunk
- Abnormal pupillary function, most commonly seen as constricted pupils that dilate slowly in the dark
- Cardiovascular dysfunction, resulting in such abnormalities as a fixed cardiac rate that does not change with exercise, postural hypotension, and a failure to increase cardiac output or vascular tone with exercise
- Gastrointestinal dysfunction, with changes in upper GI motility (**gastroparesis**) resulting in dysphagia, anorexia, heartburn, nausea, and vomiting and altered blood glucose control. Constipation is one of the most common GI manifestations associated with DM, possibly a result of hypomotility of the bowel. Diabetic diarrhea is not as common, but it does occur and is often associated with fecal incontinence during sleep due to a defect in internal sphincter function.

■ Genitourinary dysfunction, resulting in changes in bladder function and sexual function. Bladder function changes include an inability to empty the bladder completely, loss of sensation of bladder fullness, and an increased risk of urinary tract infections. Sexual dysfunctions in men include ejaculatory changes and impotence. Sexual dysfunctions in women include changes in arousal patterns, vaginal lubrication, and orgasm. Alterations in sexual function in people with DM are the result of both neurologic and vascular changes.

MOOD ALTERATIONS Persons with DM, both type 1 and type 2, endure the chronic strains of living with complex self-care and are at increased risk for depression and DM-specific emotional distress. Major depression and depressive symptoms affect 20% of people with DM making it twice as prevalent among people with DM as among the general population (Weinger, 2007). Depression affects the ability to self manage DM; depressed patients tend to forget to take their medications or run out of medications because they forget to refill their prescriptions in a timely manner. Treating depression has been associated with better control of serum glucose so screening for depression is an important part of assessing the individual's ability to manage the disease. Tests to identify the scope of depression are available (ADA, 2009; Weinger, 2007).

Interventions to help patients with depression include antidepressant medications and psychotherapy focused on restoring logical thinking and problem solving skills. But treating the depression alone does not improve self-management. Stress management programs and self-management of DM education are positively correlated with improved self care (Weinger, 2007). Nurses can assist depressed patients by correcting misconceptions about depression, identifying individual strengths in managing DM, acknowledging negative feelings that may be expressed, suggesting problem-solving behaviors to better manage the disease, and referring to appropriate resources.

INCREASED SUSCEPTIBILITY TO INFECTION The person with DM has an increased risk of developing infections. The exact relationship between infection and DM is not clear, but many dysfunctions that result from diabetic complications predispose the person to develop an infection. Vascular and neurologic impairments, hyperglycemia, and altered neutrophil function are believed to be responsible (Porth & Matfin, 2009).

The person with DM may have sensory deficits resulting in inattention to trauma, and vascular deficits that decrease circulation to the injured area; as a result, the normal inflammatory response is diminished and healing is slowed. Nephrosclerosis and inadequate bladder emptying with retention of urine predispose the person with DM to pyelonephritis and urinary tract infections. Bacterial and fungal infections of the skin, nails, and mucous membranes are common. Tuberculosis is more prevalent in people with DM than in the general population. Surgical patients with a blood glucose value greater than 220 mg /dL have higher infection rates (ADA, 2009).

PERIODONTAL DISEASE Although periodontal disease does not occur more often in people with DM, it does progress more rapidly, especially if the DM is poorly controlled. It is believed to be caused by microangiopathy, with changes in vascularization of the gums. As a result, gingivitis (inflammation of the gums) and periodontitis (inflammation of the bone underlying the gums) occur.

Complications Involving the Feet

The high incidence of both amputations and problems with the feet in people with DM is the result of angiopathy, neuropathy, and infection. People with DM are at high risk for amputation of a lower extremity, with increased risk in those who have had DM for more than 10 years, are male, have poor glucose control, or have cardiovascular, retinal, or renal complications.

Vascular changes in the lower extremities of the person with DM result in arteriosclerosis. DM-induced arteriosclerosis tends to occur at an earlier age, occurs equally in men and women, is usually bilateral, and progresses more rapidly. The blood vessels most often affected are located below the knee. Blockages form in the large, medium, and small arteries of the lower legs and feet. Multiple occlusions with decreased blood flow result in the manifestations of peripheral vascular disease (see the box on page 547). Peripheral vascular disease is discussed in ∞ Chapter 32.

Diabetic neuropathy of the foot produces multiple problems. Because the sense of touch and perception of pain is absent, the person with DM may have some type of foot trauma without being aware of it. The person thus is at increased risk for trauma to tissues of the feet, leading to ulcer development. Infections commonly occur in traumatized or ulcerated tissue (see Figure 20–7 ■).

Despite the many potential sources of foot trauma in the person with DM, the most common are cracks and fissures caused by dry skin or infections such as athlete's foot, blisters caused by improperly fitting shoes, pressure from stockings or shoes, ingrown toenails, and direct trauma (cuts, bruises, or burns). It is important to remember that the person with diabetic neuropathy who has lost the perception of pain may not be aware that these injuries have occurred. In addition, when a part of the

Figure 20–7 ■ Ulceration following trauma in the foot of the person with diabetes.

Source: Harry Przekop, Medichrome/The Stock Shop, Inc.

MANIFESTATIONS of Peripheral Vascular Disease

- Loss of hair on lower leg, feet, and toes
- Atrophic skin changes: shininess and thinning
- Cold feet
- Feet and ankles darker than leg
- Dependent rubor, blanching on elevation
- Thick toenails
- Diminished or absent pulses
- Nocturnal pain
- Pain at rest, relieved by standing or walking
- Intermittent claudication
- Patchy areas of gangrene on feet and toes

body loses sensation, the person tends to dissociate from or ignore the part, so that an injury may go unattended for days or weeks. The injury may even be forgotten entirely.

Foot lesions usually begin as a superficial skin ulcer. In time, the ulcer extends deeper into muscles and bone, leading to abscess or osteomyelitis. Gangrene can develop on one or more toes; if untreated, the whole foot eventually becomes

gangrenous. (Care of the feet, an essential part of patient and family education, is discussed later in the chapter.)

Nursing Care

DM is a chronic condition and the plan of care is dedicated to preventing complications and maintaining or improving quality of life. The responses of the person with DM to the illness are often complex and individual, involving multiple body systems. Assessments, planning, and implementation differ for the person with newly diagnosed DM, the person with long-term DM, and the person with acute complications of DM. The plan of care and content of teaching also differ according to the type of DM, the person's age and culture, and the person's intellectual, psychological, and social resources. Nurses who are DM specialists and generalists are relied upon to teach patients to successfully manage living with DM. In order to teach and support patients in their efforts to manage DM, all nurses need to understand DM, learn effective behavioral change strategies, and know appropriate interventions (Seley & Weinger, 2007). The following box describes a nursing study of hypoglycemia in hospitalized adults.

MOVING EVIDENCE INTO ACTION — Hypoglycemia in Hospitalized Adults

Until recently most hospitalized patients with type 2 DM or hyperglycemia were treated with supplemental insulin prescribed by a sliding-scale protocol when they experienced hyperglycemia. These patients are at risk for hypoglycemic events, usually because of inadequate carbohydrate (CHO) intake relative to insulin administration or oral hypoglycemic medications. Newer strategies for tighter control of blood glucose in hospitalized patients increase the incidence of hypoglycemic events. Nurses are the professionals who usually detect the onset of hypoglycemia, either by its manifestations or through routine blood glucose monitoring.

In a study at two midwestern hospitals, Anthony (2007) discovered that nurses failed to provide fully appropriate responses to all of the 410 incidents of hypoglycemia that occurred in 105 patients at each hospital. The acceptable, accurate response to a hypoglycemic event (blood glucose ≤ 70mg/dl) defined at both institutions by their hospital-approved practice guidelines involves five elements: (1) administration of 15 g of CHO, (2) blood glucose (BG) retest performed in 15 minutes, (3) BG performed 1 hour after hypoglycemia resolved, (4) physician notified, and (5) hypoglycemic event documented in the patient record. Step 1 is repeated until the BG is ≥ 70 mg/dl.

There were failures to adhere to each of these five guidelines. First, the correct dose of CHO was only given to 17% of the patients in hospital A and 3% in hospital B. Follow-up BG tests confirming that hypoglycemia had been successfully treated was only recorded in 9% of cases at hospital A and 6% at hospital B. In both institutions, some patients were discharged following a hypoglycemic event without a follow-up BG test. The recommended BG test 1 hour after evidence of normal BG was documented in 25% of events at hospital A and in 16% of events at hospital B. None of the recorded tests was drawn within the 50- to 70-minute window defined for the 1 hour post test. At hospital A, 54% of the events were documented in the patients' medical records; at hospital B, documentation was made in 71% of the events. Physician notification was only documented in 15% of events at hospital A and 28% of events at hospital B.

IMPLICATIONS FOR NURSING
Multiple and complex issues characterize the clinical care of patients with hypoglycemia. Because of the nearly epidemic rise in type 2 DM, and the prevalence of tighter blood glucose control among hospitalized patients, caring correctly for patients with hypoglycemia is very important. This includes preventing hypoglycemia as well as responding to it. Giving the incorrect dose of CHO is attributable to lack of knowledge. Verification that BG has returned to a normal level may be based on the patient's self report that he or she is "fine now." In the hurried practice of staff nursing, accepting a self report as evidence of normal BG is understandable but not acceptable. Someone may feel fine with a blood glucose that is climbing to 200 mg/dl or dropping below 70. Monitoring BG is a professional nursing responsibility, although performing the test can be delegated to trained assistants. Today's DM climate is crowded with new and improved ideas and thousands of newly diagnosed patients who need to adapt to increased levels of self-care and who require expert healthcare guidance. Each nurse must be knowledgeable and willing to teach, mentor, support and refer patients to appropriate professionals in the DM team.

CRITICAL THINKING IN PATIENT CARE
1. You are caring for two patients with DM who are receiving home care for complications of long-term DM. One patient follows the medical regimen faithfully, the other adapts it to his own schedule and needs. What differences can you identify in your own reaction to these two different patients? How would these reactions affect your relationship with the patients?
2. Imagine you have just been diagnosed with type 1 DM. Make a list of the questions you would have and the areas that would cause you the most difficulty in complying with your medical care.
3. How would you respond if your patient tells you, "Sometimes I eat whatever I want to for several days." What do you think this behavior indicates?

EVIDENCE FOR NURSING CARE — The Patient with Type 1 DM

Selected resources that nurses may find helpful when planning evidence-based nursing care follow.

■ Holzinger, U., Feldbacher, M., Bachlechner, A., Kitzberger, R., Fuhrmann, V., & Madl, C. (2008). Improvement of glucose control in the intensive care unit: An interdisciplinary collaboration study. *American Journal of Critical Care, 17*(2), 150–156. Retrieved from http://ajcc.aacnjournals.org/misc/journalclub.shtml

Health Promotion

Health promotion activities primarily focus on preventing the onset and complications of DM. The prevention of type 2 disease has been shown in randomized controlled trials to be achievable in a significant number of persons at risk. A combination of lifestyle changes (weight loss and increased physical activity) and medications (especially metformin) prevents or delays the onset of type 2 DM (ADA, 2009). Prevention of progression to DM is dependent on at-risk persons accepting responsibility to learn and sustain lifestyle changes through self management education, counseling and coaching. Blood glucose screening at 3-year intervals beginning at age 45 is recommended for those not in the high-risk group.

Assessment

The following data are collected through the health history and physical examination (∞ see Chapter 18). Further focused assessments are described next with nursing interventions. When assessing the older patient, be aware of normal aging changes in all body systems that may alter interpretation of findings.

■ *Health history:* Family history of DM; history of hypertension or other cardiovascular problems; history of any change in vision (e.g. blurring) or speech, dizziness, numbness or tingling in hands or feet; pain when walking; frequent voiding; change in weight, appetite, infections, and healing; problems with gastrointestinal function or urination; or altered sexual function.

■ *Physical assessment:* Height/weight ratio, vital signs, visual acuity, cranial nerves, sensory ability (touch, hot/cold, vibration) of extremities, peripheral pulses, skin and mucous membranes (hair loss, appearance, lesions, rash, itching, vaginal discharge).

Nursing Diagnoses and Interventions

Although many different nursing diagnoses are appropriate for the person with DM, those discussed in this section address problems with skin integrity, infection, injury, sexuality, coping, and health maintenance. The goals of care are to maintain function, prevent complications, and teach self-management. See the accompanying Case Study & Nursing Care Plan for more information.

Risk for Impaired Skin Integrity

The person with DM is at increased risk for altered skin integrity as a result of decreased or absent sensation from neuropathies, decreased tissue perfusion from cardiovascular complications, and infection. In addition, poor vision increases the risk of trauma, and an open lesion is more prone to infection

EVIDENCE FOR NURSING CARE — The Patient with Type 2 DM

Selected resources that nurses may find helpful when planning evidence-based nursing care follow.

■ Gazmararian, J., Zimmer, D., & Barnes, C. (2009). Perception of barriers to self-care management among diabetic patients. *The Diabetes Educator, 35*(5), 778–788.

and delayed healing. Impaired skin and tissue integrity, with resultant gangrene, is especially common in the feet and lower extremities. Conduct baseline and ongoing assessments of the feet, including the following:

■ Musculoskeletal assessment that includes foot and ankle joint range of motion, bone abnormalities (bunions, hammertoes, overlapping digits), gait patterns, use of assistive devices for walking, and abnormal wear patterns on shoes.

■ Neurologic assessment that includes sensations of touch and position, pain, and temperature.

■ Vascular examination that includes assessment of lower-extremity pulses, capillary refill, color and temperature of skin, lesions, and edema.

■ Hydration status, including dryness or excessive perspiration.

■ Lesions, fissures between toes, corns, calluses, plantar warts, ingrown or overgrown toenails, redness over pressure points, blisters, cellulitis, or gangrene.

People with DM are at significant risk for lower-extremity gangrene. Peripheral neuropathies may result in alterations in the perception of pain, loss of deep tendon reflexes, loss of cutaneous pressure and position sensation, foot drop, changes in the shape of the foot, and changes in bones and joints. Peripheral vascular disease may cause intermittent claudication, absent pulses, delayed venous filling on elevation, dependent rubor, and gangrene. Injuries, lesions, and changes in skin hydration potentiate infections, delayed healing, and tissue loss in the person with DM.

■ Teach foot hygiene. Wash the feet daily with lukewarm water and mild hand soap; pat dry, and dry well between the toes. Always test the water temperature in the shower or bath before stepping in. Apply a very thin coat of lubricating cream if dryness is present (but not between the toes). *Proper hygiene decreases the chance of infection. Temperature receptors may be impaired, so the water should always be tested before use.*

■ Discuss the importance of not smoking if patient smokes. *Nicotine in tobacco causes vasoconstriction, further decreasing the blood supply to the feet.*

■ Discuss the importance of maintaining blood glucose levels through prescribed diet, medication, and exercise. *Hyperglycemia promotes the growth of microorganisms.*

■ Conduct foot care teaching sessions as often as necessary (see the previous box). If the person has visual deficits, is obese, or cannot reach the feet, teach the caregiver how to inspect and care for the feet. Feet should be inspected daily. *Foot care is a priority in DM management to prevent serious problems. Many people with DM are unaware of lesions or injury until infection and compromised circulation are far advanced. The hows and whys of each component must*

MEETING INDIVIDUALIZED NEEDS Foot Care Teaching Session

BUYING AND WEARING SHOES AND STOCKINGS

- Shoes that allow 1/2 to 3/4 inch of toe room are best; there should be room for toes to spread out and wiggle. The lining and inside stitching should be smooth, and the insole soft. The sole should be flexible and cushion the foot. The heel should fit snugly, and the arch support should give good support.
- Do not wear open-toed shoes, sandals, high heels, or thongs; they increase the risk of trauma.
- Buy shoes late in the afternoon, when feet are at their largest; always buy shoes that feel comfortable and do not need to be "broken in."
- Shoes made of natural fibers (leather, canvas) allow perspiration to escape.
- Check the shoes before each wearing for foreign objects, wrinkled insoles, and cracks that might cause lesions.
- Stockings made of wool or cotton allow perspiration to dry.
- Do not wear garters, knee stockings, or panty hose; they may interfere with circulation.
- Wear insulated boots in the winter.

INSPECTING THE FEET

- Check the feet daily for red areas, cuts, blisters, corns, calluses, or cracks in the skin. Check between the toes for cracks or reddened areas.
- Check the skin of the feet for dry or damp areas.
- Use a mirror to check each sole and the back of each heel.
- If you are unable to inspect the feet daily, be sure that someone else does so.

CARE OF TOENAILS

- Cut the toenails after washing, when they are softer and easier to trim.
- Cut the nails straight across with a clipper, and smooth edges and corners with an emery board.
- Do not use razor blades to trim the toenails.
- If you are unable to see well or to reach the feet easily, have someone else trim the nails. If the nails are very thick or ingrown, if the toes overlap, or if circulation is poor, get professional care from a podiatrist.

GENERAL INFORMATION

- Never go barefoot. Wear slippers when leaving the bed during the night.
- Do not use commercial corn medicines or pads, chemicals (such as boric acid, iodine, or hydrogen peroxide), or over-the-counter cortisone medications on the feet.
- Do not put heating pads, hot water bottles, or ice packs on the feet. If the feet become cold at night, wear socks or use extra blankets.
- Do not allow the feet to become sunburned.
- Do not put tape on the feet.
- Do not sit with the legs crossed at the knees or ankles.

---

be included in teaching. A variety of methods may be used, including demonstration, return demonstration, audiovisual aids, and written lists. If the person is wearing shoes and socks, ask him or her to remove them to practice foot care effectively.

PRACTICE ALERT
Suggest the use of a hand mirror to check the bottom of the feet and the back of the heels.

Risk for Infection

The person with DM is at increased risk for infection. The risk of infection is believed to be due to vascular insufficiency that limits the inflammatory response, neurologic abnormalities that limit the awareness of trauma, and a predisposition to bacterial and fungal infections.

- Use and teach meticulous hand hygiene. *Hand hygiene is the single most effective method for preventing the spread of infection.*
- Monitor for manifestations of infection: increased temperature, pain, malaise, swelling, redness, discharge, cough. *Early diagnosis and treatment of infections can control their severity and decrease complications.*
- Discuss the importance of skin care. Keep the skin clean and dry, using lukewarm water and mild soap. *People with DM are more prone to develop furuncles and carbuncles; the infection often increases the need for insulin. Clean, intact skin and mucous membranes are the first line of defense against infection.*

- Teach dental health measures:
  - Obtain a dental examination every 4 to 6 months.
  - Maintain careful oral hygiene, which includes brushing the teeth with a soft toothbrush and fluoridated toothpaste at least twice a day and flossing as recommended.
  - Be aware of the manifestations requiring dental care: bad breath; unpleasant taste in the mouth; bleeding, red, or sore gums; and tooth pain.
  - If dental surgery is necessary, monitor for need to make adjustments in insulin. *All people with DM need to be taught proper oral hygiene, the risk of periodontal disease, and the importance of obtaining dental care for manifestations of oral or dental problems.*
- Teach women with DM about the manifestations and preventive measures for vaginitis caused by *Candida albicans*. The manifestations are an odorless, white or yellow cheeselike discharge and itching. *DM is a predisposing factor for* Candida albicans *vaginitis, the most common form of vaginitis. Poor personal hygiene and wearing clothing that keeps the vaginal area warm and moist increase the risk of vaginitis. The infection may spread to the urinary tract, resulting in urinary tract infections; preventing and treating vaginitis decrease this risk.*

PRACTICE ALERT
Teach women with DM to take preventive measures by maintaining good personal hygiene, wiping front to back after voiding, wearing cotton underwear, avoiding tight jeans and nylon pantyhose, and avoiding douching.

Risk for Injury

The person with DM is at risk for injury from multiple factors. Neuropathies may alter sensation, gait, and muscle control. Cataracts or retinopathy may cause visual deficits. Hyperglycemia often causes osmotic changes in the lenses of the eye, resulting in blurred vision. In addition, changes in blood glucose alter levels of consciousness and may cause seizures. The impaired mobility, sensory deficits, and neurologic effects of complications of DM increase the risk of accidents, burns, falls, and trauma.

- Assess for the presence of contributing or causative factors that increase the risk of injury: blurred vision, cataracts, decreased adaptation to dark, decreased tactile sensitivity, hypoglycemia, hyperglycemia, hypovolemia, joint immobility, unstable gait. *A knowledge base is necessary to develop an individualized plan of care. The risk of injury increases with the number of factors identified.*
- Reduce environmental hazards in the healthcare facility, and teach the patient about safety in the home and in the community.

IN THE HEALTHCARE FACILITY

- Orient the patient to new surroundings on admission.
- Keep the bed at the lowest level.
- Keep the floors free of objects.
- Use a night light.
- Check the temperature of the bath or shower water before the patient uses it.
- Instruct the patient to wear shoes or slippers when out of bed.
- Monitor blood glucose levels regularly.
- Monitor for side effects of prescribed medications, such as dizziness or drowsiness.

IN THE HOME AND COMMUNITY

- Use a night light, preferably one with a soft, nonglare bulb.
- Turn the head away when switching on a bright light.
- Avoid directly looking into headlights when driving at night.
- Test the temperature of the bath or shower water before use.
- Conduct a daily foot inspection.
- Wear shoes and slippers with nonskid soles.
- Do not use throw rugs.
- Install hand grips in the tub and shower and next to the toilet.
- Wear a seat belt when driving or riding in a car.
  Strange environments and the presence of hazardous environmental factors increase the risk of falls or other accidents. Glare is often responsible for falls in people with visual deficits. The nurse can reduce factors that increase the risk of injury by implementing care and teaching safe practices during the activities of daily life.
- Monitor for and teach the patient and family to recognize and seek care for the manifestations of DKA in the patient with type 1 DM: hyperglycemia, thirst, headaches, nausea and vomiting, increased urine output, ketonuria, dehydration, and decreasing level of consciousness. *Blood glucose levels increase if the insulin need is unmet or insufficiently met; the cellular use of fats for fuel results in ketosis. Osmotic diuresis increases urinary output, resulting in thirst and dehydration.*
- Monitor for and teach the patient and family to recognize and seek care for the manifestations of HHS in the patient with type 2 DM: extreme hyperglycemia, increased urinary output, thirst, dehydration, hypotension, seizures, and decreasing level of consciousness. *HHS is a life-threatening condition requiring recognition and treatment.*
- Monitor for and teach the patient and family to recognize and treat the manifestations of hypoglycemia: low blood glucose, anxiety, headache, uncoordinated movements, sweating, rapid pulse, drowsiness, and visual changes. Teach patient and family to carry some form of rapid-acting sugar source at all times. *Severe hypoglycemia causes a decrease in the level of consciousness. The decrease in blood glucose most often results from too much insulin, too little food, or too much exercise.*
- Recommend that the patient wear a MedicAlert bracelet or necklace identifying self as a person with DM. *In case of sudden, severe illness or accident, a MedicAlert bracelet can allow immediate medical attention for DM to be instituted.*

Sexual Dysfunction

Sexuality is a complex and inseparable part of every person. It involves not only physical sexual activities but also a person's self-perception as male or female, roles and relationships, and attractiveness and desirability. Changes in sexual function and in sexuality have been identified in both men and women with DM.

Alterations in erectile ability occur in approximately 50% of all men with DM. The incidence of impotence increases with the duration of the DM and is often associated with peripheral neuropathy. Libido is usually unaffected, even when impotence is present. Women with DM also have alterations in sexual function, although the reason is less clear. The problems reported by women involve decreased desire and decreased vaginal lubrication. Women with DM are also at increased risk for vaginitis and may avoid sexual intercourse in order to avoid pain.

- Include a sexual history as a part of the initial and ongoing assessment of the patient with DM. A specific history form may be used that addresses sexual development, personal and family values, current sexual practices and concerns, and changes desired. Ask a nonthreatening, open-ended question to elicit information, such as, "Tell me about your experience with sexual function since you have been diagnosed with DM." *Obtaining accurate information to assess the sexual health of a patient is necessary before counseling can begin or referrals can be made. Patients may not discuss problems with sexual function unless the nurse initiates the conversation.*
- Provide information about the actual and potential physical effects of DM on sexual function. Include the effect of poor control of blood glucose on sexual function as part of any teaching plan. *Patients benefit from basic information about male and female anatomy and the sexual response cycle, and how DM can affect this part of the body. Changes in blood glucose levels not only may cause changes in desire and physical response but also may alter sexual responses as a result of depression, anxiety, and fatigue.*
- Provide counseling or make referrals as appropriate. The nurse is responsible for knowing about sexuality and sexual health throughout the life span and provides information based on knowledge of the effects of illness and treatment on sexual function. For example, men who are impotent may regain the ability to have sexual intercourse through penile implants, suction apparatus, the use of drugs that facilitate gaining and maintaining an erection, such as sildenafil citrate

(Viagra), or injections of medications (such as yohimbine, an alpha-2 adrenergic blocker) that increase vascular blood flow into the corpus of the penis. Women with decreased vaginal lubrication can decrease painful intercourse by using vaginal lubricants (such as K-Y Jelly) or estrogen creams.

The nurse may make specific suggestions to facilitate positive sexual functioning, referring the patient to the appropriate healthcare provider as necessary for intensive therapy.

Ineffective Coping

Coping is the process of responding to internal or environmental stressors or potential stressors. When coping responses are ineffective, the stressors exceed the individual's available resources for responding. The person diagnosed with DM is faced with lifelong changes in many parts of his or her life. Diet, exercise habits, and medications must be integrated into the person's lifestyle and be carefully controlled. Daily injections may be a reality. Fear of potential complications and of negative effects on the future is common.

If the person is unable to cope successfully with these changes, emotional stress can interfere with glycemic control. In addition, unsuccessful coping often results in noncompliance with prescribed treatment modalities, further impairing glycemic control and increasing the potential for acute and chronic complications.

- Assess the patient's psychosocial resources, including emotional resources, support resources, lifestyle, and communication skills. *Chronic illness affects all dimensions of a person's life, as well as the lives of family members and significant others. A comprehensive assessment of strengths and weaknesses is the first step in developing an individualized plan of care to facilitate coping.*

- Explore with the patient and family the effects (actual and perceived) of the diagnosis and treatment of DM on finances, occupation, energy levels, and relationships. *Common frustrations associated with DM are the disease itself, the treatment modalities, and the healthcare system. Effective coping involves maintaining a healthy self-concept and satisfying relationships, emotional balance, and handling emotional stress.*

- Teach constructive problem-solving techniques. *Problem-focused behaviors include setting attainable and realistic goals, learning about all aspects of the problem, learning new procedures or skills that increase self-esteem, and reaching out to others for support.*

- Provide information about support groups and resources, such as suppliers of products, journals, books, and cookbooks for people with DM. *Sharing with others who have similar problems provides opportunities for mutual support and problem solving. Using available resources improves the ability to cope.*

Using NANDA, NIC, and NOC

Linkages between a selected NANDA nursing diagnosis, NIC, and NOC for the patient with DM are shown in the chart that follows.

Community-Based Care

Teaching the patient and family to self-manage DM is a healthcare team responsibility. Nurses are very important resources and must be knowledgeable and up-to-date on their understanding of

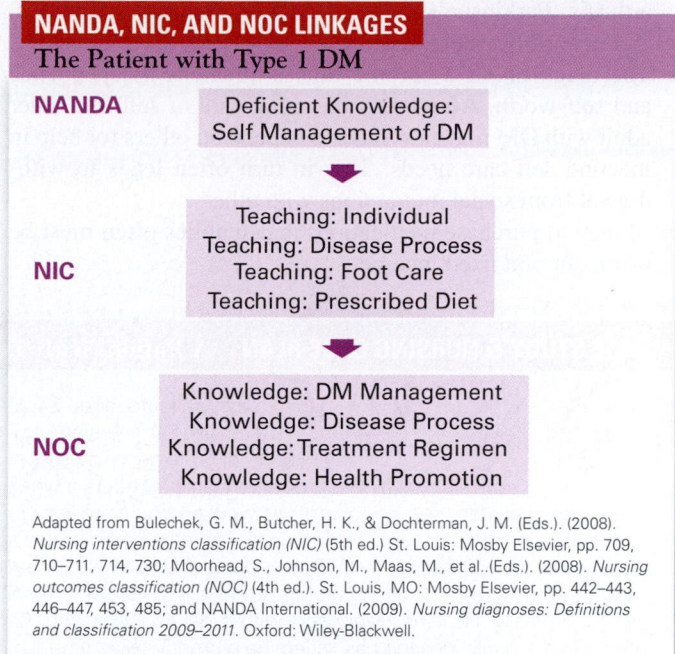

NANDA, NIC, AND NOC LINKAGES
The Patient with Type 1 DM

NANDA → Deficient Knowledge: Self Management of DM

NIC → Teaching: Individual
Teaching: Disease Process
Teaching: Foot Care
Teaching: Prescribed Diet

NOC → Knowledge: DM Management
Knowledge: Disease Process
Knowledge: Treatment Regimen
Knowledge: Health Promotion

Adapted from Bulechek, G. M., Butcher, H. K., & Dochterman, J. M. (Eds.). (2008). *Nursing interventions classification (NIC)* (5th ed.) St. Louis: Mosby Elsevier, pp. 709, 710–711, 714, 730; Moorhead, S., Johnson, M., Maas, M., et al..(Eds.). (2008). *Nursing outcomes classification (NOC)* (4th ed.). St. Louis, MO: Mosby Elsevier, pp. 442–443, 446–447, 453, 485; and NANDA International. (2009). *Nursing diagnoses: Definitions and classification 2009–2011.* Oxford: Wiley-Blackwell.

DM care. Even if a formal teaching plan is developed and implemented by diabetes nurse educators, all nurses must be able to reinforce knowledge and answer questions. Teaching is necessary for both the person who is newly diagnosed and for the person who has had DM for years. In fact, the latter may need almost as much teaching as the newly diagnosed person. Products for DM care, especially insulins, have changed dramatically and knowledge about risk reduction to prevent complications has increased.

The American Diabetes Association recommends that teaching be carried out on three levels. The first level focuses on survival skills, with the person learning basic knowledge and skills to be able to provide DM management for the first week or two while adjusting to the idea of having the disease. The second level focuses on home management, emphasizing self-reliance and independence in the daily management of DM. The third level aims at improving lifestyle and educating patients to individualize self-management of the illness.

Teaching may have to be adapted to the special needs of the older adult. Because 40% of all people with DM are over the age of 65, considering the special needs of this population is essential. Uncontrolled DM in the older adult increases the potential for functional loss, social disengagement, and increased morbidity and mortality. Education for self-care allows the older adult to be more actively involved in his or her DM management and decreases the potential for acute and long-term complications from the disease. Considerations for teaching the older adult with DM include the following:

- Changes in diet may be difficult to implement for many reasons. Balanced meals at regular intervals may not have been part of the patient's lifestyle. Purchasing, storing, and preparing foods may be a problem. Dentures may not fit well. Changes in taste sensation often cause the patient to increase the use of salt and sugar.

- Exercise of any type may not have been part of the activities of daily living. Exercise must be individualized for any physical limitations imposed by other chronic illnesses, such as arthritis, Parkinson's disease, chronic respiratory diseases, and/or cardiovascular diseases.

- The diagnosis of a chronic illness threatens independence and self-worth. After years of taking care of self, the older adult with DM may now have to depend on others for help in meeting self-care needs. This in turn often leads to withdrawal from social interactions with others.
- Money to purchase medications and supplies often must be taken out of a fixed income.

- Visual deficits make insulin administration difficult or impossible. Visual deficits also interfere with blood glucose monitoring, food preparation, exercises, and foot care.

It is important that the nurse and patient mutually establish goals based on the assessment data. Inquiries about patient and family priorities can be made effectively with the simple question, "What concerns you most about having diabetes?" The topics of concern range from medications to economics. Addressing topics of greatest concern first increases

---

CASE STUDY & NURSING CARE PLAN   A Patient with Type 1 DM

Jim Meligrito, aged 24, is a third-year nursing student at a large midwestern university. Mr. Meligrito also works 20 hours a week as a campus student security guard. His working hours are 8 PM to midnight, five nights a week. He lives with his father, who is also a student. Neither of the two men likes to cook, and they usually eat "whatever is handy." Mr. Meligrito has smoked 8 to 10 cigarettes a day for 5 years. He was diagnosed with type 1 DM at age 12. Although his insulin dosage has varied, he currently takes a total of 32 units of insulin each day, 10 U of NPH and 6 U of regular insulin each morning and evening. He monitors his blood glucose about three times a week. He feels that he is too busy for a regular exercise program and that he gets enough exercise in clinicals and in weekend sports activities. He has not seen a healthcare provider for over a year.

One day during a 6-hour clinical laboratory in pediatrics, Mr. Meligrito notices that he is urinating frequently, is thirsty, and has blurred vision. He also is very tired but blames all his manifestations on drinking a couple of beers and having had only 4 hours of sleep the night before while studying for an examination, and the stress he has been under lately from school and work. When he remembers that he had forgotten to take his insulin that morning, he realizes he must have hyperglycemia but decides that he will be all right until he gets home in the afternoon. Around noon, he begins having abdominal pain, feels weak, has a rapid pulse, and vomits. When he reports his physical manifestations to his clinical instructor, she sends him immediately to the hospital emergency department, accompanied by another student.

ASSESSMENT

As soon as Mr. Meligrito arrives at the emergency department, his blood glucose level is measured at 300 mg/dL. Urine samples and additional blood samples are sent to the laboratory for analysis. Blood glucose is 330 mg/dL, HgbA1c is 9.5%, urine shows the presence of ketones, electrolytes are normal, and pH is 7.1. His vital signs are as follows: T 99°F (37.2°C), P 140, R 28, and BP 102/52. An intravenous infusion of 1000 mL normal (0.9%) saline with 40 mEq of KCl is started at a rate of 400 mL/h. Intravenous regular insulin at 5 U/h (diluted in 0.9% saline) is begun. Hourly blood glucose monitoring is initiated. Mr. Meligrito is nauseated and lethargic but remains oriented. Three hours later, he has a blood glucose level of 160, and his pulse and blood pressure are normal. He is dismissed from the emergency department after making an appointment for the next morning with the hospital's DM nurse educator. When he meets with the DM educator, he says that he no longer feels in control of the DM or his future goal to become a nurse anesthetist.

DIAGNOSIS

- *Powerlessness* related to a perceived lack of control of DM due to present demands on time
- *Deficient Knowledge*: Self-management of DM
- *Risk for Ineffective Role Performance* related to uncertainty about capacity to achieve desired role as registered nurse

EXPECTED OUTCOMES

- Identify those aspects of DM that can be controlled and participate in making decisions about self-managing care.
- Demonstrate an understanding of DM self-management through planned medication, diet, exercise, and blood glucose self-monitoring activities.
- Explore and clarify Mr. Meligrito's perceptions of his role as a student nurse, verbalizing his ability to meet his expectations.

PLANNING AND IMPLEMENTATION

- Mutually establish specific and individualized short-term and long-term goals for self-management of blood glucose.
- Provide opportunities to express feelings about himself and his illness.
- Explore perceptions of his own ability to control his illness and his future, and clarify these perceptions by providing information about resources and support groups.
- Facilitate decision-making abilities in self-managing his prescribed treatment regimen.
- Provide positive reinforcement for increasing involvement in self-care activities.
- Provide relevant learning activities about insulin administration, dietary management, exercise, self-monitoring of blood glucose, and healthy lifestyle.

EVALUATION

After taking an active part in the weekly educational meetings for 2 months, Mr. Meligrito has greatly enhanced his understanding of and compliance with self-management of his DM. He states that he finally understands how insulin, food, and exercise affect his body, having previously thought they were "just things I should do when I wanted to." He decides to perform self-management activities one week at a time, rather than think too far into (and thereby feel overwhelmed by) the future. Both son and father have developed a workable meal schedule and weekly grocery list, and they have begun eating breakfast and dinner together. Mr. Meligrito and a friend have arranged to walk 2 to 3 miles three times a week on a community hiking trail. To gain a sense of control over his illness, he has also worked out a schedule that allows time for school, health care, and himself.

CRITICAL THINKING IN THE NURSING PROCESS

1. What is the pathophysiologic basis for the changes in temperature, pulse, respirations, and blood pressure that occurred on Mr. Meligrito's admission to the hospital emergency department?
2. How can smoking and poor self-management of DM increase the risk of long-term complications?
3. Is powerlessness a common response to a chronic illness? Why or why not?
4. Consider that you are teaching Mr. Meligrito and another patient, Mr. McDaniel (aged 75, newly diagnosed with type 2 DM). What components of your teaching plan would be the same and what components would be different?

See Evaluating Your Response in Appendix C.

the patient's and family's confidence that the information provided will be useful. It is equally important that family members understand that the responsibility for daily management lies with the patient and that the primary role of the family is supportive. The patient is the person with the disease, and it is the patient who each day must take medications or inject insulin, test blood or urine, calculate and balance foods, exercise, adjust medications, inspect the body for injury, and determine whether and when medical assistance is needed. However, family members require the same knowledge so that they can provide emotional support as well as physical care if necessary.

The following should be included in teaching the patient and family about care at home:

- Information about normal metabolism, DM, and how DM changes metabolism
- Diet plan: how diet helps keep blood glucose in normal range; number of kcal required and why; amount of carbohydrates, meats, and fats allowed and why; and how to calculate the diet, integrating personal food preferences

- Exercise: how it helps lower blood glucose, the importance of a regular program, types of exercise, integrating personal exercise preferences, how to handle increased activity
- Self-monitoring of blood glucose: how to perform the tests accurately, how to care for equipment, what to do for high or low blood glucose
- Medications:
  - Insulin: type, dosage, mixing instructions (if necessary), times of onset and peak actions, how to get and care for equipment, how to give injections, where to give injections
  - Oral agents: type, dosage, side effects, interaction with other drugs
- Manifestations of acute complications of hypoglycemia and hyperglycemia; what to do when they occur
- Hygiene: skin care, dental care, foot care
- Sick days: what to do about food, fluids, and medications
- Helpful resources: The American Diabetes Association, the American Dietetic Association, National Diabetes Information Clearinghouse, Indian Health Service, and the National Council of La Raza.

CHAPTER HIGHLIGHTS

- Approximately 1.3 million new cases of DM are diagnosed each year in the United States. DM is the sixth leading cause of death by disease in the United States, primarily due to widespread cardiovascular effects.
- The incidence of type 2 diabetes mellitus (DM) is increasing in epidemic proportions in all racial and ethnic groups in the United States.
- Type 2 DM has a hereditary link and is characterized by obesity and sedentary lifestyles. Unlike Type 1 DM, in which the onset is often sudden, the development of type 2 manifestations that bring patients to their healthcare providers for evaluation is slow; it is estimated that 50% of newly diagnosed

type 2 DM have already developed complications secondary to hyperglycemia.
- Tighter, more intensive glycemic control is increasingly the focus of care for hospitalized patients with hyperglycemia.
- New products for patients with DM include insulins, noninsulin hypoglycemics, and blood glucose monitoring devices. Nurses must be familiar with these products and help patients become proficient in their use.
- Motivation for self-care by the patient with DM continues to be a challenge because treatment commonly includes life style changes. Through education and support, patients can achieve control of DM and avoid complications.

TEST YOURSELF NCLEX-RN® REVIEW

1. Increased susceptibility to the development of type 1 DM is indicated by which of the following?
   1. genetic markers that determine immune response
   2. persistent obesity throughout the adolescent years
   3. delivery of a baby that weighs less than 6 lb
   4. excessive amounts of plasma glucagon
2. Diabetic ketoacidosis is the result of which pathologic process?
   1. An excess amount of insulin drives all glucose into the cells.
   2. A decreased amount of glucagon causes low protein levels.
   3. A deficit of insulin causes fat stores to be used as an energy source.
   4. An increase occurs in the breakdown of glucose molecules with hypoglycemia.

3. Which of the following patients would be most at risk for the development of type 2 DM?
   1. young adult who is a professional basketball player
   2. middle-aged man who maintains normal weight
   3. middle-aged woman who is the sole caretaker of her parents
   4. woman over age 70 who is overweight and sedentary
4. A nurse notes that a patient has a nursing diagnosis of *Peripheral Neurovascular Dysfunction* involving both feet. Which of the following assessments would support this diagnosis?
   1. normal sensation to touch
   2. loss of normal reflexes
   3. states "I can't feel my feet anymore."
   4. states "I have been having chest pain."

5. Which of the following statements would indicate that a patient understands teaching about foot care at home?
    1. "I will walk barefooted as long as I am in the house."
    2. "I always buy my shoes as soon as the stores open."
    3. "I will check my feet for cuts and bruises every night."
    4. "If I get a blister, I just put alcohol on it and bandage it."

6. Lantus and detemir insulin, long-acting insulins, have a unique insulin characteristic that increases the risk for administration error. The nurse understands that which of the following applies to this long-acting insulin?
    1. It is combined with glucose to raise energy levels.
    2. It is subject to being inactivated by light and must be kept cold.
    3. It is a clear solution like regular insulin, unlike other intermediate and long-acting insulins.
    4. It is activated by vigorous agitation.

7. The nurse is preparing an insulin infusion for a patient in diabetic ketoacidosis (DKA). She is careful to select which type of insulin that can be administered intravenously?
    1. glargine
    2. NPH
    3. regular
    4. Humalog

8. Glycosylated hemoglobin (A1C) is useful for evaluating the degree of blood glucose control the patient with DM has been maintaining for the previous 2 to 3 months. The ADA recommends a diagnosis of DM at what A1C level?
    1. > 15%
    2. > 9%
    3. > 6.5%
    4. > 2.25%

9. When the insulin-dependent patient is NPO on the day of surgery, which of the following should be done with short-acting regular insulin?
    1. It should be given intravenously.
    2. It should be chilled to slow absorption.
    3. It should be given with intravenous glucose.
    4. It should be combined with long-acting insulin.

10. Subcutaneous injections of insulin can be made in several locations in the body. The nurse teaches the patient that the most rapid absorption occurs in which of the following?
    1. hip
    2. thigh
    3. deltoid
    4. abdomen

See Test Yourself answers in Appendix C.

Pearson Nursing Student Resources

Find additional review materials at
www.nursing.pearsonhighered.com

Prepare for success with additional NCLEX®-style practice questions, interactive assignments and activities, Web links, animations and videos, and more!

BIBLIOGRAPHY

American Diabetes Association (ADA). (2008a). Pancreas transplantation. Retrieved from http://www.diabetes.org/

American Diabetes Association (ADA). (2008b). Nutrition recommendations for DM. *Diabetes Care, 31*(Supplement 1), S61–S78.

American Diabetes Association (ADA). (2009). Standards of medical care in diabetes—2009. *Diabetes Care, 32*(Supplement 1), S13–S41.

American Diabetes Association (ADA). (2010). Standards of medical care in diabetes—2010. *Diabetes Care, 33*(Supplement 1), S11–S61.

Anthony, M. (2007). Treatment of hypoglycemia in hospitalized adults. *The Diabetes Educator, 33*(4), 709–715.

BD Diabetes. (2009). *Insulin pens.* Retrieved from http://www.bddiabetes.com/US/main.aspx?cat=1&id=254

Boulton, A. J., & Malik, R. A. (2010). Neuropathy of impaired glucose tolerance and its measurement. *Diabetes Care, 33*(1), 207–209.

Braithwaite, S. S., Robertson, B., Mehrotra, H. P., McElveen, L. M., & Thompson, C. L. (2007). Managing hyperglycemia in hospitalized patients. *Clinical Cornerstone 8*(2), 55–57.

Bulechek, G. M., Butcher, H. K., & Dochterman, J. M. (Eds.). (2008). *Nursing interventions classification (NIC)* (5th ed.). St. Louis: Mosby Elsevier.

Centers for Disease Control and Prevention (CDC). (2007). *National diabetes fact sheet 2007.* Retrieved from http://www.cdc.gov/diabetes/pubs/pdf/ndfs_2007.pdf

Centers for Disease Control and Prevention (CDC). (2008). State-specific incidence of diabetes among adults—participating states, 1995–1997 and 2005–2007. *Morbidity and Mortality Weekly Reports,* October 31, 2008/57(43), 1169–1173.

Cummings, D. E., & Flum, D. R. (2008). Gastrointestinal surgery as a treatment for diabetes. *Journal of the American Medical Association (JAMA), 299*(3), 341–343.

Dixon, J. B., O'Brien, P. E., Playfair, L. J., Chapman, L., Schachter, L. M., et al. (2008). Adjustable gastric banding and conventional therapy for type 2 diabetes: A randomized controlled trial. *Journal of the American Medical Association, 299*(3), 316–323.

Green, D. E. (2007). New therapies for diabetes. *Clinical Cornerstone, 8*(2), 58–63.

Haas, L. (2007). Functional decline in older adults with diabetes. *American Journal of Nursing, 107*(6S), 50–54.

Jain, V., Sharma, D., Prabhakar, H., & Dash, H. H. (2008). Metformin-associated lactic acidosis following contrast media-induced nephrotoxicity. *European Journal of Anaesthesiology, 25*(2), 166–167.

Kitabchi, A. E., Umpierrez, G. E., Murphy, M. B., Barrett, E. J., Kreisberg, R. A., et al (2004). American Diabetes Association Position Statement: Hyperglycemic crises in diabetes. *Diabetes Care, 27*(S1), S94–S102.

Loh-Trivedi, M., & Rothenberg, D. M. (2008). Perioperative management of the diabetic patient. Retrieved from http://emedicine.medscape.com/article/284451-overview

McPhee, S., & Papadakis, M. (Eds.). (2009). *Current medical diagnosis & treatment* (48th ed.). New York: McGraw Hill Medical.

Medtronic MiniMed, Inc. (2006). *MiniMed Paradigm® REAL-Time Insulin Pump and Continuous Glucose Monitoring System.* Retrieved from http://www.minimed.com/products/insulinpumps/realtime/index.html

Miller, D. K. (2009). Are you ready to care for a patient with an insulin pump? *Nursing, 10*(39), 57–60.

Moorhead, S., Johnson, M., Maas, M., & Swanson, E. (Eds.). (2008). *Nursing outcomes classification (NOC)* (4th ed.). St. Louis: Mosby Elsevier.

NANDA International. (2009). *Nursing diagnoses: Definitions and classification 2009–2011.* Oxford: Wiley-Blackwell.

National Eye Institute. (2006). Diabetic retinopathy. Retrieved from http://www.neil.nih.gov

National Institutes of Health (NIH). (2008). *Diabetes statistics in the United States.* Retrieved from http://diabetes.niddk.nih.gov/dm/pubs/statistics/

Pearson, T. L. (2009). Motivating patients to monitor their blood glucose. Retrieved from http://www.medscape.com/viewarticle/588565?src=mp&spon=24&uac=116901HG

Peeples, M, & Seley, J. J. (2007). Diabetes care: The need for change. *American Journal of Nursing, 107*(6S), S13–S15, S17–S19.

Porth, C. (2007). *Essentials of Pathophysiology: Concepts of altered health states* (2nd ed.). Philadelphia: Lippincott Williams & Wilkins.

Porth, C., & Matfin, G. (2009). *Pathophysiology: Concepts of altered health states* (8th ed). Philadelphia: Lippincott Williams & Wilkins.

Seley, J. J., & Weinger, K. (2007). Executive summary: The state of the science on nursing best practices for diabetes self-management. *American Journal of Nursing, 107*(6S), 6–11.

Umpierrez, G. E., Smiley, D., Zisman, A., Prieto, L. M., et al. (2007). Randomized study of basal-bolus insulin therapy in the inpatient management of patients with type 2 diabetes. *Diabetes Care, 30,* 2181–2186.

Van Praet, J. T. & De Vriese, A. S. (2007). Prevention of contrast-induced nephropathy: A critical review. *Current Opinion in Nephrology & Hypertension, 16*(4), 336–347.

WebMD, Diabetes Health Center. (2009). *New type 2 diabetes drug Onglyza approved.* Retrieved from http://diabetes.webmd.com/news/20090731/new-type-2-diabetes-drug-onglyza-approved

Weinger, K. (2007). Psychosocial issues and self-care. *American Journal of Nursing, 107*(6S), 34–38.

Wiener, R. S., Wiener, D. C., & Larson, R. J. (2008). Benefits and risks of tight glucose control in critically ill adults: A meta-analysis. *JAMA, 300*(8), 933–944.

Yared, Z., Aljaberi, K., Renouf, N., & Yale, J. (2005). The effect of blood sample volume on 11 glucose monitoring systems. *Diabetes Care, 28,* 1836–1837.

Functional Health Pattern: Nutritional-Metabolic

Think about patients with altered endocrine function for whom you have cared in your clinical experiences.

- What were their major medical diagnoses (e.g., Graves' disease, myxedema coma, cancer of the thyroid, hyperparathyroidism, hypoparathyroidism, Cushing's syndrome, Addison's disease, pheochromocytoma, gigantism, syndrome of inappropriate antidiuretic hormone secretion, diabetes insipidus, and diabetes mellitus)?

- What kinds of manifestations did each of these patients have? Were these manifestations similar or different?

- How did the patients' healthcare behaviors interfere with their nutritional and metabolic status? Were they on a prescribed diet? What was their daily intake of foods and fluids? Did they have an increased appetite with loss of weight? Did they notice their hands and feet getting larger? Did they have difficulty swallowing or notice swelling in the front of their neck? Did they note an increase or decrease in urination? Did they note a change in energy levels? Had they noticed any visual changes? Did they complain of sleep disturbances? Had they had any changes in hair distribution, such as facial hair or changes in skin texture? Had there been a change in memory or the ability to concentrate? Did the patients use hormones or steroids? Was there a family history of diabetes mellitus, diabetes insipidus, thyroid problems, hypertension, or obesity?

The Nutritional-Metabolic Functional Health Pattern includes metabolism, which is the biochemical processes that take place in the body due to hormones produced and released by the endocrine glands. These processes relate to the distribution of nutrients after digestion of carbohydrates, proteins, and fats. The endocrine system regulates growth, reproduction, metabolism, fluid and electrolyte balance, and gender differentiation. Endocrine disorders affect the metabolic status in two primary ways:

- Lack of hormones can result in endocrine disorders of the thyroid gland (e.g., hypothyroidism), disorders of the parathyroid gland (e.g., hypoparathyroidism), disorders of the adrenal gland (e.g., chronic adrenocortical insufficiency), disorders of the pituitary gland (e.g., hypopituitarism, diabetes insipidus), or disorders of the pancreas (e.g., hypoglycemia).

- Excess hormones can result in endocrine disorders of the thyroid gland (e.g., hyperthyroidism), disorders of the parathyroid gland (e.g., hyperparathyroidism), disorders of the adrenal

gland (e.g., hypercortisolism), disorders of the pituitary gland (e.g., hyperpituitarism, SIADH) or disorders of the pancreas (e.g., hyperglycemia).

Hormones are chemical substances, secreted by the endocrine glands, that initiate or regulate functioning of a target organ by binding to a receptor site located on the surface of the target organ. They are regulated by a negative or positive feedback system in which decreased or increased hormone levels signal the release of hormones to maintain homeostasis of the body's internal environment. Imbalance of hormones can result in endocrine disorders, leading to manifestations such as the following:

- **Weight loss** (*increased thyroid hormones cause an increase in metabolism of carbohydrates, proteins, and lipids resulting in caloric and nutritional deficiencies*)

- **Blurred vision** (*lack of insulin production by the pancreas causes osmotic effects to the eye tissue resulting in swelling of the lenses of the eyes*)

- **Increased urination** (*deficit of antidiuretic hormones causes excretion of large amounts of urine resulting in dehydration and hypernatremia*)

Priority nursing diagnoses within the Nutritional-Metabolic Functional Health Pattern that may be appropriate for patients with endocrine disorders include the following:

- *Imbalanced Nutrition: Less than Body Requirements* as evidenced by increased food intake with weight loss or loss of appetite

- *Deficient Fluid Volume* as evidenced by dry mucous membranes, increased skin turgor, thirst, and decreased urine output

- *Hyperthermia* as evidenced by body temperatures ranging from 102°F (39°C) to 106°F (41°C)

- *Impaired Skin Integrity* as evidenced by dry, rough, reddened, and edematous skin

Two nursing diagnoses from other functional health patterns often are of high priority for the patient with endocrine disorders:

- *Disturbed Body Image* (Self-Perception-Self-Concept Functional Health Pattern)

- *Ineffective Therapeutic Regimen Management* (Health Perception, Health Management, Functional Health Pattern)

Question

1. What did you do to help your patient manage his or her nutritional needs?

CLINICAL SCENARIO

Directions: *Read the following clinical scenarios and answer the questions that follow. To complete this exercise successfully, you will utilize not only knowledge of the content in this unit, but also principles related to priority setting and maintaining patient safety.*

You have been assigned to work with the following four patients for the 0700 shift on a medical-surgical unit. Significant data obtained during report is as follows:

- Mr. Blew is a 54-year-old who is admitted with complaints of polydipsia, polyuria, and polyphagia. There is a fruity odor to his breath and he seems confused at times. Vital signs on admission are temperature 99°F, pulse 90, respirations 30 and deep, and blood pressure 110/68. His blood glucose is 650 on admission at 0630.
- Mrs. Rant is a 65-year-old who is admitted with severe back pain in the flank area on the right side, nausea, and vomiting. She is being evaluated for treatment due to renal calculi. She

has a history of hyperparathyroidism. Vital signs are temperature 97.6°F with clammy skin, pulse 100, respirations 24, and blood pressure of 168/94. She is requesting pain medication for the back pain.

- Mrs. Fox is an 86-year-old who was transferred from the medical ICU yesterday. She was admitted after being found in a comatose state by her daughter. On admission her blood sugar was 45, serum sodium was 128, temperature was 96.6°F, and she had a heart rate of 50. Vital signs this AM are temperature 98.4°F, pulse 78, respirations 18, and blood pressure 140/86. She is due for electrolytes to be drawn at 0730.
- Mr. Rite is a 56-year-old who was admitted 4 days ago after falling from a ladder and hitting his head. He is complaining of a headache and thirst even after drinking 2000 ml of fluids during the night. Vital signs are temperature 100°F, pulse 98, respirations 14, and blood pressure 114/84.

Questions

Priority Setting

1. In what order would you visit these patients after report?
   A. _____
   B. _____
   C. _____
   D. _____

Health Promotion

1. Mr. Blew is diagnosed with diabetes mellitus. Besides diet and medication administration, what other teaching is necessary in order for him to maintain a high level of health?

2. The nurse explains to Mrs. Rant the dietary treatment for hyperparathyroidism. Which is the appropriate dietary teaching for this patient?
   A. Increase fluids in the diet and avoid taking vitamin D supplements.
   B. Increase potassium in the diet and avoid taking vitamin C supplements.
   C. Decrease sodium in the diet and take vitamin B6 supplements.
   D. Decrease phosphorus in the diet and take vitamin A supplements.

Nursing Process

1. What top priority nursing diagnoses would you choose for each of the patients presented earlier? Explain the rationale for your choices.

	Nursing Diagnosis	Rationale
Mr. Blew		
Mrs. Rant		
Mrs. Fox		
Mr. Rite		

2. If Mr. Blew's blood glucose drops to 50, which manifestations might he exhibit?
   A. Bradycardia, nausea, and vomiting
   B. Tachycardia, hypotension, and shakiness
   C. Thirst, diarrhea, and fatigue
   D. Hypertension, edema, and dyspnea

3. Due to the manifestations of headache and excessive thirst that Mr. Rite is exhibiting 4 days after his fall, the nurse should monitor for symptoms of which complication?
   A. Migraine headache
   B. Hypertensive crisis
   C. Increased intracranial pressure
   D. Infection

4. A prescription for levothyroxine sodium (Synthroid) is given to Mrs. Fox after being diagnosed with hypothyroidism. The patient voices understanding of how to take the medication when she states which of the following?
   A. "I must take the medication with meals."
   B. "I must take my pulse before taking the medication and report to the doctor a pulse > 100."
   C. "I will only need to take this medication until my thyroid blood levels are back to normal."
   D. "I can eat any food I choose as foods do not interfere with the medications."

5. Which laboratory studies would be conducted for Mr. Blew to monitor his diabetes management? **Select all that apply.**
   A. Fasting blood glucose
   B. Glycosylated hemoglobin (c)
   C. Urinalysis
   D. Complete blood cell count
   E. Serum electrolytes
   F. Serum cholesterol and triglyceride levels

Communication

1. Mr. Blew understands diabetic teaching implemented by the nurse when he states which of the following?
   A. "I will check my blood glucose before every meal."
   B. "If I follow my prescribed diet, I will not have to check my blood sugar."
   C. "If my blood glucose drops below 60, I can drink juice or milk to raise it."
   D. "If my blood sugar is over 200, I can eat graham crackers to lower it."

2. Mrs. Fox's daughter asks if her mother will be able to go home alone or if she will need to be sent to a nursing home to live. How will you answer?

Delegation

1. For each patient, what assessment data and nursing interventions can be delegated to a certified nursing assistant (CNA)?

Related Questions

1. The nurse assessing a patient with hyperthyroidism may find which manifestations?
   A. diaphoresis, diarrhea, alopecia, weight loss
   B. dry skin, constipation, hirsutism, obesity
   C. hypertension, abdominal pain, constipation, anorexia
   D. dry skin, numbness around mouth and fingertips, tetany

2. In postoperative thyroidectomy nursing care, it is most important for the nurse to monitor the patient for which of these complications?
   A. bleeding
   B. laryngeal nerve damage
   C. tetany
   D. respiratory distress

3. Metabolic syndrome is a cluster of manifestations associated with type 2 diabetes mellitus. Which manifestations are indicative of metabolic syndrome?
   A. hypertension, abdominal obesity, blood glucose > 110 mg/dL
   B. tachycardia, weight gain, blood glucose < 110 mg/dL
   C. hypotension, weight loss, blood glucose >150 mg/dL
   D. bradycardia, stomach obesity, blood glucose < 100 mg/dL

4. Which of the following laboratory value results may be seen in a patient with untreated Cushing's syndrome?
   A. serum sodium level of 150 mEq/L, serum potassium level of 2.8 mEq/L
   B. blood glucose of 68mg/dL, blood urea nitrogen level of 28 mg/dL
   C. serum calcium level of 9.0 mg/dL, serum sodium level of 130 mEq/L
   D. blood glucose of 350mg/dL, serum potassium level of 5.2 mEq/L

CASE STUDY: Louis Gregg

Louis Gregg is a 65-year-old African American male who was admitted with complaints of increased urination, increased thirst, fatigue, blurred vision, and numbness in his feet. He states that he retired 9 months ago after 45 years as a construction worker. He now leads a sedentary lifestyle and doesn't have as much energy as he used to have. He has gained 50 pounds since retirement. Upon assessment, Mr. Gregg weighs 255 pounds and is 5'11" tall. Vital signs are T 98.8°F, P 88, R 20, and BP 150/90. Decreased pulses are noted in dorsal pedis and posterior tibial pulses. Both feet are pale pink in color and cool to touch. Assessment findings are documented in the patient's record and reported to the physician. The following laboratory studies are ordered to determine the diagnosis of type 2 diabetes mellitus: plasma glucose concentration, fasting blood glucose, and oral glucose tolerance test.

Type 2 DM is a disease of fasting hyperglycemia, with some but not enough insulin production by the endocrine pancreas. With increased age, obesity, and a sedentary lifestyle, cells become resistant to insulin. Glucose uptake by muscle and fat cells is not sufficient to lower blood glucose, while insulin has a decreased ability to influence glucose metabolism by the liver, skeletal muscles, and adipose tissue. The manifestations of type 2 DM include polyuria, polydipsia, blurred vision, fatigue, paresthesias, and skin infections. In times of physical stress, the patient may develop HHS. Complications include myocardial infarction, hypertension, stroke, peripheral vascular disease, renal disease, and blindness.

Based on Mr. Gregg's manifestations and weight gain, a nursing diagnosis of *Imbalanced Nutrition: More than Body Requirements* is appropriate for guiding nursing care for this patient.

- Beta cells decrease insulin production; cells become less sensitive to insulin
- Glucose accumulates in blood; chronic hyperglycemia affects function of cells and tissues

Mr. G.
65 y.o. male
Type 2 diabetes mellitus

affects

leads to

assess

- Ineffective Tissue Perfusion related to effects of chronic hyperglycemia
- Deficient Knowledge: Cause and effects of Type 2 DM
- Deficient Knowledge: Self-care of Type 2 DM

- Ht: 5', 11", Wt: 255
- Retired, sedentary lifestyle
- States he has gained 50 pounds in 9 months
- Lab findings of hyperglycemia

generates

assess

generates

generate nursing diagnosis

prioritized to

Imbalanced Nutrition: More than Body Requirements

expected outcomes

- Loses 2 pounds per week for the next month
- Takes part in exercise program at local fitness center
- Walks each day for a minimum of 30 minutes
- Discusses diet requirements with dietitian
- Verbalizes importance of a balance of diet, exercise, and medications for type 2 diabetes mellitus

evaluate

- Verbalized cause and effects of DM
- Enrolled in both fitness class and support group
- Has lost 15 pounds in 8 weeks
- Walks briskly for 45 minutes each day

Interdisciplinary Interventions
- Make referral to dietitian to discuss appropriate diet.

Independent Interventions
- Discuss understanding of balance of diet, exercise, and medications in controlling illness.
- Suggest enrollment in senior wellness activities at community recreation center.
- Encourage to weigh self at least every 2 days and maintain record of weights.
- Teach pathophysiology, manifestations, and complications of type 2 diabetes mellitus.
- Teach effects and guidelines for taking oral hypoglycemic medications.

Activity:

1. After reviewing the concept map, is there anything you would change to make it more understandable?

2. Go to the Pearson Nursing Student Resources for this book at www.nursing.pearsonhighered.com to write a concept map using the nursing diagnosis *Risk for Peripheral Neurovascular Dysfunction*.

See answers and hints in Appendix C.

Responses to Altered Gastrointestinal Function

UNIT 6

CHAPTER 21

Assessing the **Gastrointestinal** System

LEARNING OUTCOMES

1. Describe the anatomy, physiology, and functions of the gastrointestinal (GI) system and the accessory digestive organs.
2. Identify specific topics to consider during a health history interview of the patient with GI disorders.
3. Explain techniques used for assessing nutritional status and GI function.
4. Give examples of genetic disorders of the GI system.
5. Describe normal variations in GI assessment findings for the older adult.
6. Identify abnormal findings that may indicate alterations in GI function.

CLINICAL COMPETENCIES

1. Conduct and document a health history for patients who have or are at risk for alterations in GI function.
2. Conduct and document a physical assessment of nutritional status and the GI system.
3. Monitor the results of diagnostic tests and report abnormal findings.

EQUIPMENT NEEDED

- Stethoscope
- Balance scale with height measuring attachment
- Tape measure
- Skin fold calipers
- Water-soluble lubricant
- Occult blood test, such as Occultest or Hemocult II
- Disposable gloves

KEY TERMS

bile, *567*
borborygmus, *581*
bruit, *581*
cheilosis, *579*
flatus, *569*

gingivitis, *579*
glossitis, *579*
hernia, *584*
leukoplakia, *579*
melena, *585*

nutrition, *560*
ostomy, *569*
steatorrhea, *585*
striae, *580*
Valsalva's maneuver, *567*

The GI system consists of the mouth, pharynx, esophagus, stomach, small intestine, and large intestine. The accessory digestive organs include the liver, gallbladder, and pancreas (Figure 21–1 ■). **Nutrition** is the process by which the body, via the GI system and the accessory digestive organs, ingests, absorbs, transports, uses, and eliminates nutrients in food.

Nutrients

Nutrients are substances found in food and are used by the body to promote growth, maintenance, and repair. The categories of nutrients are carbohydrates, proteins, fats, vitamins, minerals, and water.

Carbohydrates

The primary sources of carbohydrates (sugars and starches) are plant foods. Monosaccharides and disaccharides come from milk, sugar cane, sugar beets, honey, and fruits. Polysaccharide starch is found in grains, legumes, and root vegetables. Following ingestion, digestion, and metabolism, carbohydrates are converted primarily to glucose, the molecule body cells use to make adenosine triphosphate (ATP). Excess glucose in the healthy person is converted to glycogen or fat. Glycogen is stored in the liver and muscles; fat is stored as adipose tissue. Carbohydrate use by the body is shown in Figure 21–2A ■.

Excess intake of carbohydrates over time can result in obesity, dental caries, and elevated plasma triglycerides. In comparison, long standing carbohydrate deficiencies lead to tissue wasting from protein breakdown and metabolic acidosis from an excess of ketones as a by-product of fat breakdown.

Proteins

Proteins are classified as either complete or incomplete. Complete proteins are found in animal products such as eggs, milk, milk products, and meat. They contain the greatest amount

Figure 21–1 ■ Organs of the gastrointestinal system and accessory digestive organs.

of amino acids and meet the body's requirements for tissue growth and maintenance. Incomplete proteins are found in legumes, nuts, grains, cereals, and vegetables. These sources are low in or lack one or more of the amino acids essential for building complete proteins.

The body uses proteins to build many different structures, including skin keratin, the collagen and elastin in connective tissues, and muscles. They also are used to make enzymes, hemoglobin, plasma proteins, and some hormones. Protein use by the body is shown in Figure 21–2*B*.

Healthy people with adequate caloric intake have an equal rate of protein synthesis and protein breakdown and loss, reflected as nitrogen balance. If the breakdown and loss of proteins exceed intake, a negative nitrogen balance results. This may be due to starvation, altered physical states (e.g., from injury or illness), and altered emotional states (such as depression or anxiety). A positive nitrogen balance, which results when protein intake exceeds breakdown, is normal during growth, tissue repair, and pregnancy. Anabolic steroids affect the rate of protein use; for example, the adrenal corticosteroids are released in times of stress to increase protein breakdown and conversion of amino acids to glucose. Excessive intake of

proteins may lead to obesity, whereas deficits cause weight loss and tissue wasting, edema, and anemia.

Fats (Lipids)

Fats (lipids) include phospholipids, steroids (such as cholesterol), and neutral fats, more commonly known as triglycerides. Neutral fats are the most abundant fats in the diet. They may be either saturated or unsaturated. Saturated fats are found in animal products (milk and meats) and in some plant products (such as coconut). Unsaturated fats are found in seeds, nuts, and most vegetable oils. Sources of cholesterol include meats, milk products, and egg yolks. Fat use by the body is shown in Figure 21–2*C*.

When a person consumes more fats than the body requires, the excess is stored as adipose tissue, increasing the risk of obesity and other chronic illnesses, including cardiovascular disease. A deficit of fats may cause excessive weight loss and skin lesions.

Fats are a necessary part of the structure and function of the body. For example,

- Phospholipids are a part of all cell membranes.
- Triglycerides are the major energy source for hepatocytes and skeletal muscle cells.

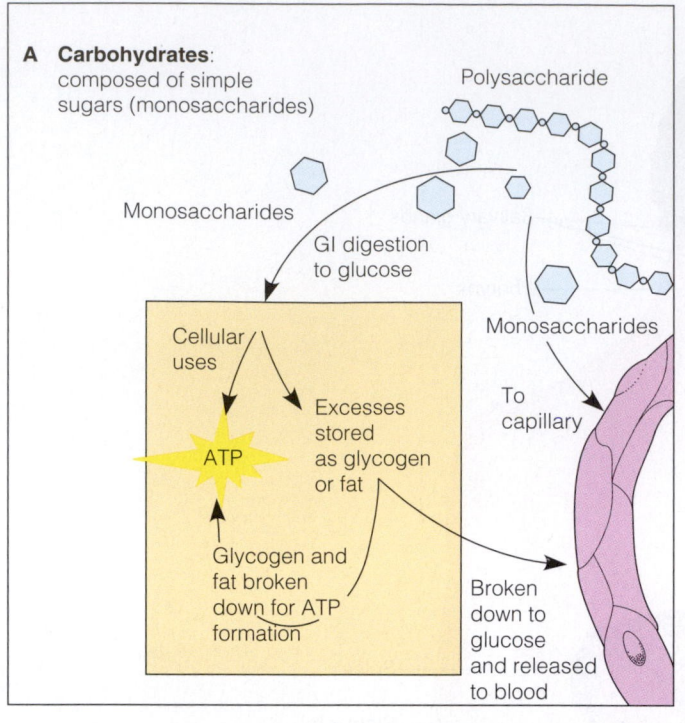

A Carbohydrates: composed of simple sugars (monosaccharides)

Polysaccharide

Monosaccharides

GI digestion to glucose

Cellular uses

ATP

Excesses stored as glycogen or fat

Glycogen and fat broken down for ATP formation

Monosaccharides

To capillary

Broken down to glucose and released to blood

B Proteins: polymers of amino acids

Protein

GI digestion to amino acids

Normally infrequent

Cellular uses

Structural proteins build and repair body tissues (e.g., connective tissue fibers, muscle proteins)

Functional proteins (e.g., enzymes, antibodies, hemoglobin)

ATP

ATP formation if inadequate glucose and fats or if some essential amino acids are lacking

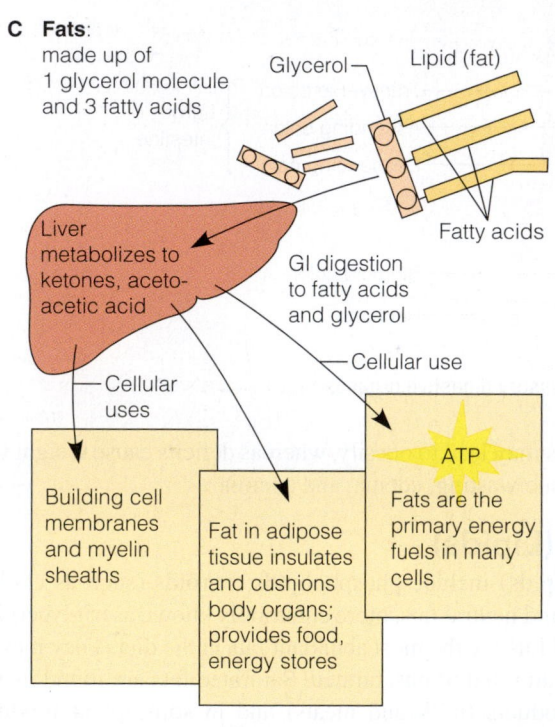

C Fats: made up of 1 glycerol molecule and 3 fatty acids

Glycerol — Lipid (fat)

Fatty acids

Liver metabolizes to ketones, aceto-acetic acid

GI digestion to fatty acids and glycerol

Cellular use

Cellular uses

Building cell membranes and myelin sheaths

Fat in adipose tissue insulates and cushions body organs; provides food, energy stores

ATP

Fats are the primary energy fuels in many cells

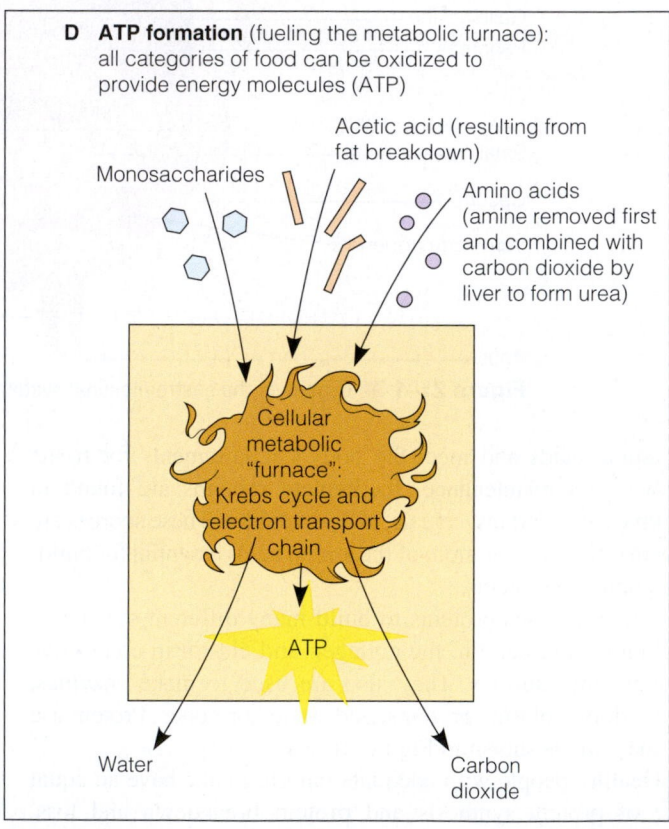

D ATP formation (fueling the metabolic furnace): all categories of food can be oxidized to provide energy molecules (ATP)

Monosaccharides

Acetic acid (resulting from fat breakdown)

Amino acids (amine removed first and combined with carbon dioxide by liver to form urea)

Cellular metabolic "furnace": Krebs cycle and electron transport chain

ATP

Water

Carbon dioxide

Figure 21–2 ■ A schematic overview of nutrient use by body cells, including *A,* carbohydrates; *B,* proteins; *C,* fats; and *D,* ATP formation.

- Dietary fats facilitate absorption of fat-soluble vitamins.
- Linoleic acid, an essential fatty acid, helps form prostaglandins, regulatory molecules that assist in smooth muscle contraction, maintenance of blood pressure, and control of inflammatory responses.
- Cholesterol is the essential component of bile salts, steroid hormones, and vitamin D.

- Adipose tissue serves as a protection around body organs, as a layer of insulation under the skin, and as a concentrated source of fuel for cellular energy.

Vitamins

Vitamins are organic compounds that facilitate the body's use of carbohydrates, proteins, and fats. All of the vitamins except vitamins D and K must be ingested in foods or taken as supplements.

TABLE 21–1 Recommended Daily Intake of Fat-Soluble Vitamins

NAME	SOURCE	FUNCTION	MINIMUM RECOMMENDED DAILY INTAKE (M = MEN, W = WOMEN)
Vitamin A (retinol)	■ Fish liver oils ■ Egg yolk ■ Liver ■ Fortified milk ■ Margarine	Necessary for vision, integrity of skin and mucous membranes, cell membrane function, and reproductive function	M = 900 mcg W = 700 mcg
Vitamin D	■ The action of sunshine on cholesterol in the skin	Necessary for blood calcium homeostasis (in turn necessary for blood clotting), bone formation, and neuromuscular function	M and W, 50 and under = 5 mcg M and W, 51 to 70 years of age = 10 mcg M and W, 70+ years of age = 15 mcg
Vitamin E	■ Vegetable oils ■ Margarine ■ Whole grains ■ Dark green leafy vegetables	As an antioxidant, helps prevent the oxidation of vitamins A and C in the intestines and decreases the oxidation of unsaturated fatty acids to facilitate cell membrane integrity	M and W = 15 mg
Vitamin K	■ Synthesized by coliform bacteria in the large intestine ■ Green, leafy vegetables ■ Cabbage ■ Cauliflower ■ Pork	Essential for the formation of clotting proteins in the liver	M = 120 mcg W = 90 mcg

Vitamin D is made by ultraviolet irradiation of cholesterol molecules in the skin, and vitamin K is synthesized by bacteria in the intestine.

Vitamins are categorized as either fat soluble or water soluble. The fat-soluble vitamins (A, D, E, and K) bind to ingested fats and are absorbed as the fats are absorbed. Water-soluble vitamins (the B complex and C) are absorbed with water in the GI system (however, vitamin B_{12} must become attached to intrinsic factor to be absorbed). Fat-soluble vitamins are stored in the body, and excesses may cause toxicity; water-soluble vitamins in excess of body requirements are excreted in the urine.

The recommended amounts of vitamins are labeled by the National Academy of Sciences as dietary reference intakes (DRIs) per day. The source, function, and minimum daily recommended intake levels are provided for each vitamin in Table 21–1 and Table 21–2. The recommended DRIs serve as a reference point and should be individualized to each person's lifestyle, medical status, and current knowledge of research about vitamins. It should also be noted that DRIs differ by recommending source.

Minerals

Minerals work with other nutrients to maintain the structure and function of the body. An adequate supply of calcium, phosphorus, potassium, sulfur, sodium, chloride, and magnesium—as well as other trace elements such as iron, iodine, copper, and zinc—is necessary to health. Most minerals in the body are found in body fluids or are bound to organic compounds. The best sources of minerals are vegetables, legumes, milk, and some meats. Dietary sources for the major minerals are discussed in ∞ Chapter 10. The recommended daily intake for minerals is outlined in Table 21–3.

Anatomy, Physiology, and Functions of the GI System

The GI system is a continuous hollow tube, extending from the mouth to the anus. Once foods are placed in the mouth, they are subjected to a variety of processes that move them and break them down into end products that can be absorbed from the lumen of the small intestine into the blood or lymph. These digestive processes are ingestion of food; movement of food and wastes; secretion of mucus, water, and enzymes; mechanical and chemical digestion of food; and absorption of digested food.

The Mouth

The mouth, also called the oral or buccal cavity, is lined with mucous membranes and is enclosed by the lips, cheeks, palate, and tongue (Figure 21–3 ■).

The lips and cheeks are skeletal muscle covered externally by skin. Their function is to keep food in the mouth during chewing. The palate consists of the hard palate and the soft palate. The hard palate covers bone in the roof of the mouth and provides a hard surface against which the tongue forces food. The soft palate, extending from the hard palate and ending at the back of the mouth as a fold called the uvula, is primarily muscle. When food is swallowed, the soft palate rises as a reflex to close off the oropharynx.

The tongue, composed of skeletal muscle and connective tissue, contains mucous and serous glands, taste buds, and papillae. The tongue mixes food with saliva during chewing, forms the food into a bolus (a mass) and initiates swallowing. Some papillae provide surface roughness to facilitate licking and moving food; other papillae house the taste buds.

TABLE 21–2 Recommended Daily Intake of Water-Soluble Vitamins

NAME	SOURCE	FUNCTION	MINIMUM RECOMMENDED DAILY INTAKE (M = MEN, W = WOMEN)
Vitamin B$_1$ (thiamin)	■ Lean meats ■ Liver ■ Eggs ■ Green leafy vegetables ■ Legumes ■ Whole grains	An essential coenzyme for carbohydrate metabolism and use; also for healthy function of nerves, muscles, and the heart	M = 1.5 mg W = 1.1 mg
Vitamin B$_2$ (riboflavin)	■ Liver ■ Egg white ■ Whole grains ■ Meat ■ Poultry ■ Fish ■ Milk	Involved in the catabolism and use of carbohydrates, fats, and proteins; the use of other B vitamins; and is important for the production of adrenal hormones	M = 1.8 mg W = 1.4 mg
Vitamin B$_6$ (pyridoxine)	■ Meat ■ Poultry ■ Fish ■ Potatoes ■ Tomatoes ■ Sweet potatoes ■ Spinach	Necessary for amino acid metabolism, formation of antibodies, and formation of hemoglobin	M = 2.0 mg W = 1.5 mg
Vitamin B$_{12}$ (cyanocobalamin)	■ Liver ■ Meat ■ Poultry ■ Dairy foods (except butter) ■ Eggs	Essential for the production of nucleic acids and red blood cells in the bone marrow; also plays an important role in the use of folic acid and carbohydrates, and in healthy function of the nervous system	M and W = .2.0 mcg
Vitamin C (ascorbic acid)	■ Citrus fruits ■ Potatoes ■ Tomatoes ■ Green leafy vegetables	Acts as an antioxidant and vasoconstrictor; also serves in the formation of connective tissue, conversion for cholesterol to bile salts, iron absorption and use, and conversion of folic acid to an active form	M and W = 60 mg
Vitamin B$_3$ niacin (nicotinamide)	■ Meat ■ Poultry ■ Fish ■ Liver ■ Peanuts ■ Green leafy vegetables	Plays an important role in the metabolism of carbohydrates and fats; inhibits cholesterol synthesis; important for integumentary, nervous, and digestive system health; assists in the manufacture of reproductive hormones	M = 20 mg W = 14 mg
Biotin	■ Liver ■ Eggs ■ Nuts ■ Legumes	Essential for the catabolism of fatty acids and carbohydrates, and helps dispose of the waste products of protein catabolism	M and W = 30 mcg
Pantothenic acid	■ Meats ■ Whole grains ■ Egg yolk ■ Liver ■ Yeast ■ Legumes	Assists in the synthesis of steroids and of the heme in hemoglobin; is essential for the metabolism of carbohydrates and fats, and for the manufacture of reproductive hormones	M and W = 5 mg
Folic acid (folate)	■ Liver ■ Dark green vegetables ■ Lean beef ■ Eggs ■ Veal ■ Whole grains ■ Synthesized by bacteria in the intestine	The basis of a coenzyme necessary to the manufacture of nucleic acids and so is essential for the formation of red blood cells, growth and development, and nervous system health	M = 200 mcg W = 180 mcg

Figure 21–3 ■ Structures of the mouth, the pharynx, and the esophagus.

Saliva moistens food so it can be made into a bolus, dissolves food chemicals so they can be tasted, and provides enzymes (such as amylase) that begin the chemical breakdown of starches. Saliva is produced by salivary glands (parotid, submaxillarly, and sublingual), most of which lie superior or inferior to the mouth and drain into it. Adults have 32 permanent teeth. The teeth chew (masticate) and grind food to break it down into smaller parts, mixed with saliva.

The Pharynx

The pharynx consists of the oropharynx and the laryngopharynx (see Figure 21–3). Both structures provide passageways for food, fluids, and air. The pharynx is made of skeletal muscles

and is lined with mucous membranes. The skeletal muscles move food to the esophagus via the pharynx through peristalsis (alternating waves of contraction and relaxation of involuntary muscle). The mucosa of the pharynx contains mucous-producing glands that provide fluid to facilitate the passage of the bolus of food as it is swallowed.

The Esophagus

The esophagus, a muscular tube about 10 inches (25 cm) long, serves as a passageway for food from the pharynx to the stomach (see Figures 21–1 and 21–3). The epiglottis, a flap of cartilage over the top of the larynx, keeps food out of the larynx during swallowing. The esophagus descends through the thorax and diaphragm, entering the stomach at the cardiac orifice. The gastroesophageal sphincter surrounds this opening. This sphincter, along with the diaphragm, keeps the orifice closed when food is not being swallowed.

The Stomach

The stomach, located high on the left side of the abdominal cavity, is connected to the esophagus at the upper end and to the small intestine at the lower end (Figure 21–4 ■). Normally about 10 inches (25 cm) long, the stomach is a distensible organ that can expand to hold up to 4 L of food and fluid. The stomach may be divided into the cardiac region, fundus, body, and pylorus (see Figure 21–4). The pyloric sphincter controls emptying of the stomach into the duodenal portion of the small intestine. The stomach is a storage reservoir for food, continues the mechanical breakdown of food, begins the process of protein digestion, and mixes the food with gastric juices into a thick fluid called chyme.

The stomach is lined with columnar epithelial, mucous-producing cells. Millions of openings in the lining lead to gastric glands that can produce 4 to 5 L of gastric juice each day. The gastric glands contain a variety of secretory cells that produce substances to protect the stomach from being digested

TABLE 21–3 Recommended Daily Intake of Minerals

NAME	MINIMUM RECOMMENDED DAILY INTAKE (M = MEN, W = WOMEN)
Calcium	M and W = 1000 mg, W > menopause = 1200 mg
Phosphorus	M and W = 1000 mg
Iron	M = 8 mg/d, W = 18 mg
Zinc	M = 11 mg/d, W = 8 mg
Manganese	M = 2.3 mg/d, W = 1.8 mg
Molybdenum	M and W = 45 mcg
Chromium	M = 35 mcg/d, W = 25 mcg
Iodine	M and W = 150 mcg
Selenium	M and W = 70 mcg
Magnesium	M and W = 400 mg
Copper	M and W = 900 mcg
Chloride	M and W = 3400 mg
Sodium	M and W = 1100 to 3000 mg, depending on health status and recommending body

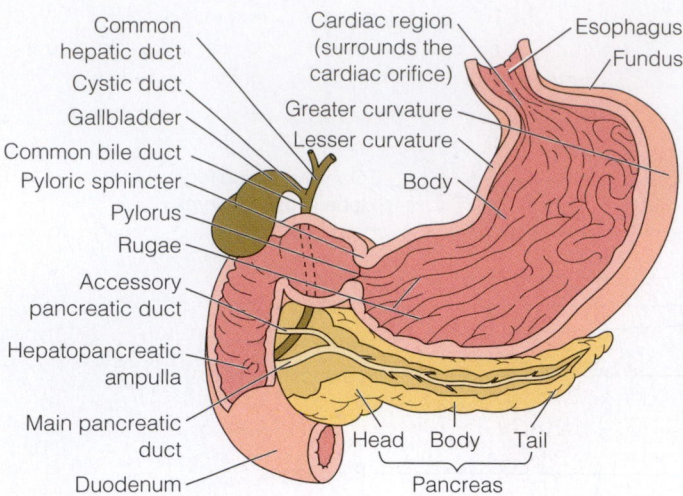

Figure 21–4 ■ The internal anatomic structures of the stomach, including the pancreatic, cystic, and hepatic ducts; the pancreas; and the gallbladder.

by gastric juice, secrete hydrochloric acid and intrinsic factor, and help regulate gastric motility.

The secretion of gastric juice is under both neural and endocrine control. Stimulation of the parasympathetic vagus nerve increases secretory activity; in contrast, stimulation of sympathetic nerves decreases secretions. Mechanical digestion is accomplished by peristaltic movements that churn and mix the food with the gastric juices to form chyme. After a person eats a well-balanced meal, the stomach empties completely in approximately 4 to 6 hours. Gastric emptying depends on the volume, chemical composition, and osmotic pressure of the gastric contents. The stomach empties large volumes of liquid content more rapidly, while gastric emptying is slowed by solids and fats.

The Small Intestine

The small intestine begins at the pyloric sphincter and ends at the ileocecal junction at the entrance of the large intestine (see Figure 21–1). The small intestine is about 20 ft (6 m) long but only about 1 inch (2.5 cm) in diameter. This long tube hangs in coils in the abdominal cavity, suspended by the mesentery and surrounded by the large intestine. The small intestine has three regions: the duodenum, the jejunum, and the ileum. The duodenum begins at the pyloric sphincter and extends around the head of the pancreas for about 10 inches (25 cm). Both pancreatic enzymes and bile from the liver enter the small intestine at the duodenum. The jejunum, the middle region of the small intestine, extends for about 8 ft (2.4 m). The ileum, the terminal end of the small intestine, is approximately 12 ft (3.6 m) long and meets the large intestine at the ileocecal valve.

Food is chemically digested and most of it absorbed as it moves through the small intestine. Circular folds containing, villi (finger-like projections of the mucosa cells), and microvilli (tiny projections of the mucosa cells) increase the surface area of the small intestine to enhance absorption of food. Although up to 10 L of food, liquids, and secretions enter the GI system each day, less than 1 L reaches the large intestine.

Enzymes in the small intestine break down carbohydrates, proteins, lipids, and nucleic acids. Pancreatic amylase acts on starches, converting them to maltose, dextrins, and oligosaccharides; the intestinal enzymes dextrinase, glucoamylase, maltase, sucrase, and lactase further break down these products into monosaccharides. Pancreatic enzymes (trypsin and chymotrypsin) and intestinal enzymes continue to break down proteins into peptides. Pancreatic lipases digest lipids in the small intestine. Triglycerides enter as fat globules and are coated by bile salts and emulsified. Nucleic acids are hydrolyzed by pancreatic enzymes and then broken apart by intestinal enzymes. Both pancreatic enzymes and bile are excreted into the duodenum in response to the secretion of secretin and cholecystokinin, hormones produced by the intestinal mucosa cells when chyme enters the small intestine.

Nutrients are absorbed through the mucosa of the intestinal villi into the blood or lymph by active transport, facilitated transport, and passive diffusion. Almost all food products and water, as well as vitamins and most electrolytes, are absorbed in the small intestine, leaving only indigestible fibers, some water, and bacteria to enter the large intestine.

The Large Intestine

The large intestine (colon) begins at the ileocecal valve and terminates at the anus (Figure 21–5 ■). It is about 5 feet (1.5 m) long. The large intestine includes the cecum, the appendix, the colon, the rectum, and the anal canal. The colon is divided into ascending, transverse, and descending segments. The rectum is a mucosa-lined tube approximately 12 cm in length (Figure 21–6 ■). The rectum ends at the anal canal, which terminates at the anus, a hairless, dark-skinned area. The anorectal junction separates the rectum from the anal canal and may be the site of internal hemorrhoids (clusters of dilated veins in swollen anal tissue).

The major function of the large intestine is to eliminate indigestible food residue from the body. The large intestine absorbs water, salts, and vitamins formed by the food residue and bacteria. The semiliquid chyme that passes through the ileocecal valve is formed into feces as it moves through the large intestine by peristalsis. Goblet cells lining the large intestine secrete mucous to facilitate the lubrication and passage of feces.

The defecation reflex is initiated when feces enter the rectum and stretch the rectal wall. This spinal cord reflex causes the walls of the sigmoid colon to contract and the anal sphincters to relax. This reflex can be suppressed by voluntary control of the external sphincter. Closing the glottis and contracting the diaphragm and abdominal muscles to increase intra-abdominal

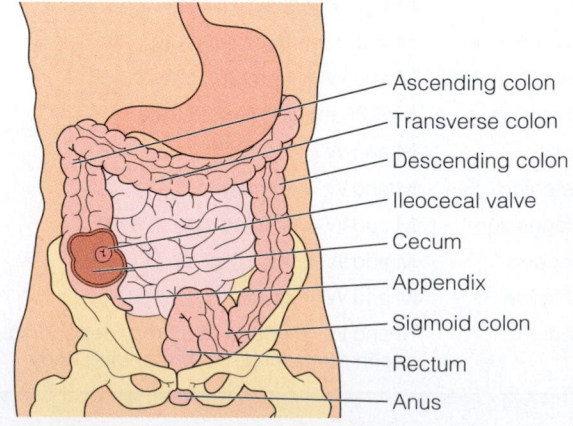

Figure 21–5 ■ Anatomy of the large intestine.

Ascending colon
Transverse colon
Descending colon
Ileocecal valve
Cecum
Appendix
Sigmoid colon
Rectum
Anus

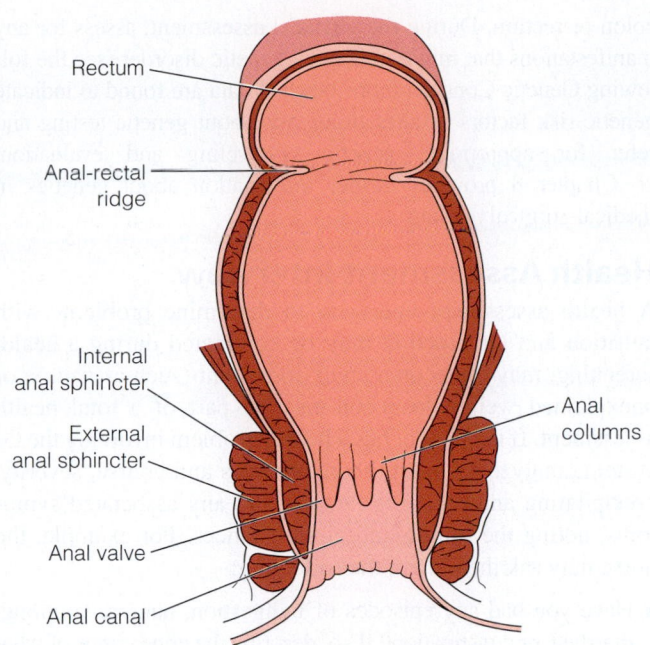

Rectum

Anal-rectal ridge

Internal anal sphincter

External anal sphincter

Anal valve

Anal canal

Anal columns

Figure 21–6 ■ Structure of the rectum and anus.

pressure (**Valsalva's maneuver**) facilitates expulsion of feces. Prolonged suppression of defecation can result in a weakened reflex that may in turn lead to constipation (infrequent and often uncomfortable passage of hard, dry stool). Frequent bouts of constipation may lead to external hemorrhoids.

The Accessory Digestive Organs

The liver, gallbladder, and exocrine pancreas are accessory digestive organs. The liver produces bile, necessary for fat digestion and absorption, and stores it in the gallbladder. The liver also receives nutrients absorbed by the small intestine and metabolizes or synthesizes these nutrients so they are in a form that can be used by the cells of the body. The exocrine pancreas produces enzymes necessary for digestion of fats, proteins, and carbohydrates.

The Liver and Gallbladder

The liver weighs about 3 lb (1.4 kg) in the average-sized adult. It is located in the right side of the abdomen, inferior to the diaphragm and anterior to the stomach (see Figure 21–1). A mesenteric ligament separates the right and left lobes and suspends the liver from the diaphragm and anterior abdominal wall. The liver is encased in a fibroelastic capsule, called the Glisson capsule. This capsule contains blood vessels, lymphatics, and nerves.

Liver tissue consists of units called lobules, which are composed of plates of hepatocytes (liver cells). A branch of the hepatic artery, a branch of the hepatic portal vein, and a bile duct communicate with each lobule. Sinusoids, blood-filled spaces within the lobules, are lined with Kupffer cells. These phagocytic cells remove debris from the blood.

Bile production is the liver's primary digestive function. **Bile** is a greenish, watery solution containing bile salts, cholesterol, bilirubin, electrolytes, water, and phospholipids. These substances are necessary to emulsify and promote the absorption of fats. Liver cells make from 700 to 1200 mL of bile daily. When bile is not needed for digestion, the sphincter of Oddi (located at the point at which bile enters the duodenum) is

closed, and the bile backs up the cystic duct into the gallbladder for storage. Bile is concentrated and stored in the gallbladder, a small sac cupped in the inferior surface of the liver. When food containing fats enters the duodenum, hormones stimulate the gallbladder to secrete bile into the cystic duct. The cystic duct joins the hepatic duct to form the common bile duct, from which bile enters into the duodenum (see Figure 21–4).

The major digestive and metabolic functions of the liver are outlined in Box 21–1. These functions require a large amount of blood, with the liver receiving blood from both venous and arterial blood vessels. The hepatic artery, branching from the abdominal aorta, provides oxygenated blood at the rate of 400 to 500 mL/min. The hepatic portal vein delivers about 1000 to 1200 mL/min of deoxygenated blood to the liver from the inferior and superior mesenteric veins and the splenic vein.

The Exocrine Pancreas

The pancreas, a gland located between the stomach and small intestine, is the primary enzyme-producing organ of the digestive system. It is a triangular gland extending across the abdomen, with its tail next to the spleen and its head next to the duodenum (see Figure 21–4). The body and tail of the pancreas are retroperitoneal, lying behind the greater curvature of the stomach. The pancreas is actually two organs in one, having both exocrine and endocrine structures and functions. The exocrine portion of the pancreas, through secretory units called acini, secretes alkaline pancreatic juice containing many different enzymes. The acini, clusters of secretory cells surrounding ducts, drain into the pancreatic duct. The pancreatic duct joins with the common bile duct just before it enters the duodenum (so that pancreatic juice and bile from the liver enter the small intestine together). The endocrine functions of the pancreas are discussed in ∞ Chapter 18.

The pancreas produces from 1 to 1.5 L of pancreatic juice daily. Pancreatic juice is clear and has high bicarbonate content. This alkaline fluid neutralizes the acidic chyme as it enters the duodenum, optimizing the pH for intestinal and pancreatic

---

BOX 21–1 Major Metabolic and Digestive Functions of the Liver

- Secretes bile
- Stores fat-soluble vitamins (A, D, E, and K)
- Metabolizes bilirubin
- Stores blood and releases blood into the general circulation during hemorrhage
- Synthesizes plasma proteins to maintain plasma oncotic pressure
- Synthesizes prothrombin, fibrinogen, and factors I, II, VII, IX, and X, which are necessary for blood clotting
- Synthesizes fats from carbohydrates and proteins to be either used for energy or stored as adipose tissue
- Synthesizes phospholipids and cholesterol necessary for the production of bile salts, steroid hormones, and plasma membranes
- Converts amino acids to carbohydrates through deamination
- Releases glucose during times of hypoglycemia
- Takes up glucose during times of hyperglycemia and stores it as glycogen or converts it to fat
- Alters chemicals, foreign molecules, and hormones to make them less toxic
- Stores iron as ferritin, which is released as needed for the production of red blood cells

enzyme activity. The secretion of pancreatic juice is controlled by the vagus nerve and the intestinal hormones secretin and cholecystokinin. Pancreatic juice contains enzymes that aid in the digestion of all categories of foods: lipase promotes fat breakdown and absorption; amylase completes starch digestion; and trypsin, chymotrypsin, and carboxypeptidase are responsible for half of all protein digestion. Nucleases break down nucleic acids.

Metabolism

After carbohydrates, fats, and proteins are ingested, digested, absorbed, and transported across cell membranes, they must be metabolized to produce and provide energy to maintain life. Metabolism is the process of biochemical reactions occurring in the body's cells. Metabolic processes are either catabolic or anabolic. Catabolism involves the breakdown of complex structures into simpler forms, for example, the breakdown of carbohydrates to produce ATP, an energy molecule that fuels cellular activity. In the process of anabolism, simpler molecules combine to build more complex structures; for example, amino acids bond to form proteins.

The biochemical reactions of metabolism produce water, carbon dioxide, and ATP (see Figure 21–2D on page 562). The energy value of foods is measured in kilocalories (kcal). A kilocalorie is defined as the amount of heat energy needed to raise the temperature of 1 kilogram (kg) of water 1 degree centigrade.

Assessing Gastrointestinal Function

The GI system is assessed by findings from diagnostic tests, a health assessment interview to collect subjective data, and a physical assessment to collect objective data.

Diagnostic Tests

The results of diagnostic tests of nutritional status and GI function are used to support the diagnosis of a specific disease, to provide information to identify or modify the appropriate medication or therapy used to treat the disease, and to help nurses monitor the patient's responses to treatment and nursing care interventions. Diagnostic tests to assess nutritional status and function of the GI system and the accessory organs are described on pages 571–574. More information, including specific laboratory tests, is included in the discussion of disorders in ∞ Chapters 22, 23, 24, and 25.

Regardless of the type of diagnostic test, the nurse is responsible for explaining the procedure and any special preparation needed, ensuring the consent form is signed (if necessary), supporting the patient during the examination as necessary, documenting the procedure as appropriate, and monitoring the results of the test. The nurse is also responsible for post-procedure care and patient teaching for self-care at home.

Genetic Considerations

When conducting a health assessment interview and physical assessment, it is important for the nurse to consider genetic influences on the health of the adult. During the health assessment interview, ask about family members with known abnormalities of copper accumulation in the body, hypercholesteremia, abnormal cholesterol or fat metabolism, obesity, or cancer of the pancreas,

colon or rectum. During the physical assessment, assess for any manifestations that might indicate a genetic disorder (see the following Genetic Considerations box). If data are found to indicate genetic risk factors or alterations, ask about genetic testing and refer for appropriate genetic counseling and evaluation. ∞ Chapter 8 provides further information about genetics in medical-surgical nursing.

Health Assessment Interview

A health assessment interview to determine problems with nutrition and GI function may be conducted during a health screening, may focus on a chief complaint (such as nausea or unexplained weight loss), or may be part of a total health assessment. If the patient has a health problem involving the GI system, analyze its onset, characteristics and course, severity, precipitating and relieving factors, and any associated symptoms, noting the timing and circumstances. For example, the nurse may ask the patient the following:

- Have you had any episodes of indigestion, nausea, vomiting, diarrhea, or constipation? If so, describe the appearance of what was vomited or the stools and anything that makes these problems better or worse. How long have you had these problems?
- What is your usual dietary intake pattern during a 24-hour period?
- Have you ever had bleeding from your rectum? If so, describe the amount and color of the blood (for example, was it bright red or dark red?).

When collecting information about the patient's current health status, ask about any changes in weight, appetite, and the ability to taste, chew, or swallow. What is the patient's perception of the role of nutrition in maintaining health? Who buys and prepares the food? What medications (prescribed, over-the-counter, or vitamins) is the patient currently taking? Does the patient take any vitamins, herbal supplements, or other "health food" items? Does the patient consume alcohol (how much and type)? If the patient has experienced nausea or vomiting, ask whether the vomitus contains bright red blood, dark (old) blood, bile, or fecal material. If the patient is very thin or verbalizes concerns about body size incongruent with the ratio of height to weight, ask whether the patient induces vomiting or uses laxatives to control weight. Ask whether the patient has braces, bridges, or dentures, and what self-care measures are used for such appliances, as well as oral hygiene practices and frequency of dental visits. Ask about any medical conditions that may influence the patient's bowel elimination pattern, such as a stroke or spinal cord impairment, inflammatory GI diseases, endocrine disorders, and allergies. Note any recent travel to other countries. Assess the patient's lifestyle for any patterns of psychologic stress and/or depression, which may alter bowel elimination. Depression may be associated with constipation, whereas diarrhea (frequent passage of loose, watery stools) may occur in situations of high stress and anxiety. Explore the patient's activities of daily living (ADLs), including exercise, sleep–rest patterns, and dietary and fluid intake. Ask the patient to describe the frequency and character of the stools. Ask about any history of diarrhea, constipation, or bleeding from the rectum, and collect information about the use of medications, laxatives, suppositories, or enemas. Anticholinergic drugs, antihistamines, tranquilizers, or narcotics may cause constipation.

Determine whether the patient has had any lower abdominal pain or rectal pain. Crampy, colicky pains occur with diarrhea and/or constipation. A sudden onset of lower abdominal cramping occurs in obstruction of the colon. Left lower abdominal pain is associated with diverticulitis. Rectal pain may occur with stool retention and/or hemorrhoids. ∞ See Chapter 9 for further information about pain assessment.

If the patient has an **ostomy** (surgical opening into the bowel), ask about skin care problems, consistency of stool, foods that cause problems with diarrhea or **flatus** (intestinal gas), the number of times that the patient empties the appliance bag each day, and irrigation habits. It is also important to explore the patient's feelings about the appliance.

Explore any family history of colon cancer, colitis, gallbladder disease, or malabsorption syndromes, such as lactose intolerance and celiac sprue. Assess the patient's risk factors for cancer, including age greater than 50; family member with colon cancer; history of endometrial, ovarian, or breast cancer; and previous diagnoses of colon inflammation, polyps, or cancer.

Ask the patient to describe any heartburn, indigestion, abdominal discomfort, or pain. Explore the location of the pain, the type of pain, the time it occurs, foods that aggravate or relieve it, and how it is relieved. Abdominal pain is often referred to other sites (∞ see Chapter 9). For example, a patient with a liver disorder may

GENETIC CONSIDERATIONS
Examples of Gastrointestinal Disorders

- An autosomal recessive disorder, Wilson's disease is an abnormality of copper transport, resulting in copper accumulation and toxicity to the liver and grain. Neurologic disease results in adults.
- Lynch syndrome (hereditary nonpolyposis colorectal cancer) is a type of inherited cancer of the GI system, especially the colon and rectum. Colon polyps occur at an earlier age and are more likely to become malignant.
- Tangier disease is a disease of cholesterol transport, leading to characteristic orange tonsils, very low levels of high-density lipoprotein, and an enlarged liver and spleen.
- Hypercholesterolemia has a familial tendency.
- About 90% of human pancreatic cancers show a chromosome defect.
- Obesity is believed to result from a variety of factors, including genetics.
- Familial adenomatous polyposis (FAP) and hereditary nonpolyposis colorectal cancer (HNPCC) are inherited disorders in which there is progressive development of colorectal adenomas. Unless treated, colorectal cancer inevitably occurs by the fourth or fifth decade of life.
- In about 20% of cases, Crohn's disease (an inflammatory bowel disease) appears to be familial in origin.
- Colon cancer is one of the most common inherited cancer syndromes.
- Celiac disease (CD) is a genetic, inheritable disease responsible for the malabsorption of nutrients resulting in malnutrition. If people with CD eat certain types of proteins (glutens, found in wheat, barley, rye, and oats) an autoimmune response causes damage to the small intestine, so that nutrients are not absorbed.
- Gaucher disease, more common in descendants of Jewish people from eastern Europe, results in lack of an enzyme to break down fats. Fats accumulate in the liver, spleen, and bone marrow, causing pain, fatigue, jaundice, bone damage, anemia, and even death.

experience pain over the right shoulder (Kehr's sign). Epigastric (middle upper abdominal) pain is experienced in cases of acute gastritis, obstruction of the small intestine, and acute pancreatitis. Pain in the right upper quadrant is associated with cholecystitis. Pain in the left upper quadrant may be related to a gastric ulcer.

The health history should include questions about any prior surgeries or trauma of the GI system. Explore the past history of any medical condition that may affect the patient's ingestion, digestion, and/or metabolism (for example, Crohn's disease, diabetes mellitus, irritable bowel syndrome, peptic ulcers, or pancreatitis). Other areas significant to assessment are food allergies (especially to milk, which is evidenced as lactose intolerance with abdominal cramping, excessive flatus, and loose stools) and a family history that may provide clues to increased risk for health problems.

In addition to other factors assessed in the health history, culture and ethnicity are important components of nutritional status and GI health. Nutritional diversity is common among cultural and ethnic groups and questions should be included to identify specific customs, food likes and dislikes, and how foods are prepared and served. For example, in some ethnic groups, dietary substances are used to protect health, such as eating raw garlic or onions (Spector, 2009). In other cultures, dietary balance is believed to be necessary to keep the body in balance or harmony. It is necessary that nurses know about specific culturally related nutritional values and practices, and ask questions to identify health-related concerns specific to individualized dietary intake.

Interview questions categorized by functional health patterns are listed in the box on page 575.

Physical Assessment
Physical assessment of the GI system may be performed as part of a total health assessment, as a focused assessment of patients with known or suspected health problems, in combination with assessment of the urinary and reproductive systems (problems that may cause manifestations similar to those of the GI system), or alone for patients with known or suspected health problems. The techniques of inspection, auscultation, percussion, and palpation are used. Palpation is the last method used in assessing the abdomen. Figure 21–11 ■ illustrates the four quadrants of the abdomen with the organs contained in each quadrant.

PRACTICE ALERT
When assessing the abdomen, use palpation last, because pressure on the abdominal wall and contents may interfere with bowel sounds and cause pain, ending the examination.

Collect objective data by obtaining anthropometric measurements (height, weight, triceps skin folds, and midarm circumference) and by examining the mouth and abdomen. Prior to the examination, collect all necessary equipment and explain techniques to the patient to decrease anxiety. Ask the patient to void.

The patient may be seated during assessment of the mouth, but is supine during the abdominal assessment. Have the patient turn to the left lateral (Sims') position for the rectal examination. The older patient or the patient with limited mobility may need assistance in assuming this position. The patient should be standing to assess for an inguinal hernia.

FUNCTIONAL HEALTH PATTERN INTERVIEW   Nutritional Status and Gastrointestinal System

Functional Health Pattern	Interview Questions and Leading Statements
Health Perception-Health Management	■ Have you had any illness or surgery that affects your nutrition, digestion, or bowel elimination? If so, how were these treated? ■ Describe your current problem; how long has it lasted; what have you done to treat it? ■ (Depending on age): Have you had your colon screened for cancer (such as a colonoscopy)? When was it last done? ■ What medications do you take? Do you take antacids? Do you take laxatives or use enemas? If so, what do you use them for and how often do you take them? ■ Do you have allergies to foods? What are they and how do you react? ■ Do you have tooth or gum pain that interferes with your ability to eat? When was your last dental examination? Describe what you do each day to take care of your teeth. ■ Do you use any treatment for hemorrhoids? Describe.
Nutritional-Metabolic	■ Describe what you eat and how much (and type) of fluids you drink in a 24-hour period. ■ Describe herbs, vitamins, and dietary supplements you currently are taking. ■ Have you noticed any change in your appetite? Explain. ■ What is your current weight? What do you feel your ideal weight would be? Have you had a recent gain or loss? Explain. ■ If patient has an ostomy: Do certain foods cause gas or diarrhea? Descibe. Describe your skin around the stoma. ■ Do you have any of the following: indigestion, belching, nausea, vomiting, difficulty swallowing? If so, what causes this and how do you treat it? ■ Do you drink alcohol? If so, what type? Describe your average number of drinks each day. ■ Questions specific to the patient's culture and ethnic group would be included in this functional health pattern area, such as what types of food are preferred or not eaten, what types of foods are never eaten together, and what types of foods are eaten to remain healthy.
Elimination	■ How often do you have a bowel movement? Are your bowel movements affected by what you eat? Explain. ■ Have you noticed any change in the color of your bowel movements? Explain. Have you noticed bright red blood in your bowel movement? ■ Have you ever used laxatives or made yourself vomit to control your weight? Explain.
Activity-Exercise	■ Describe your activities on a typical day. ■ What type of exercise do you get and how often? ■ Do you smoke? If so, what and how many cigarettes per day?
Sleep-Rest	■ Do you wake up hungry during the night? ■ Does abdominal pain, cramping, nausea, or diarrhea ever interfere with your sleep? Explain.
Cognitive-Perceptual	■ Describe the amount and type of foods you should eat each day. ■ Rate your ability to taste and smell foods on a scale of 1 to 10 (with 10 being excellent). ■ Describe any pain you have had in your mouth, stomach, abdomen, or rectum. What type of pain was it (dull, crampy, achy, burning)? What seems to cause it? What do you do to relieve it?
Self-Perception-Self-Concept	■ Are you satisfied with your appearance in terms of weight? If no, why? ■ Have you been successful in the past in gaining or losing weight? ■ How does this condition make you feel about yourself?
Role-Relationships	■ How does this condition affect your relationships with others? ■ Do you eat with others regularly? If so, who?
Sexuality-Reproductive	■ Has this condition interfered with your usual sexual activities?
Coping-Stress-Tolerance	■ Have you experienced any type of stress that may have worsened this condition? ■ Has having this condition created stress for you? ■ Describe what you do when you feel stressed.
Value-Belief	■ Tell me how specific relationships or activities help you cope with this problem. ■ Describe specific cultural beliefs or practices that affect how you care for and feel about this condition. ■ Is there anything interfering with your spiritual beliefs, needs, or practices during your illness? What can I or another caregiver do to help you with your spiritual needs? ■ Are there any specific treatments that you would not use to treat this condition?

DIAGNOSTIC TESTS of the Gastrointestinal System

THE ESOPHAGUS AND STOMACH

NAME OF TEST	PURPOSE & DESCRIPTION	RELATED NURSING INTERVENTION
Barium Swallow or Upper GI Series	These tests are conducted to diagnose esophageal varices, inflammation, ulcerations, hiatal hernia, foreign bodies, polyps, diverticula, and tumors of the esophagus, stomach, and duodenal bulb. The patient drinks 16 to 20 ounces of a chalky liquid (barium sulfate or meglumine diatrizoate [Gastrografin]) before the exam. These radiologic studies are done by observing the movement of a contrast medium with a fluoroscope (Figure 21–7 ■).	Instruct the patient not to eat or drink fluids or smoke for 8 to 12 hours before the test. Tell the patient not to take narcotics or anticholinergic medications for 24 hours pretest and not to take any medications for 8 hours pretest. Following the test, ensure the patient eliminates the barium by taking laxatives and forcing fluids as appropriate.

Figure 21–7 ■ A barium x-ray of a healthy stomach.
Source: Biophoto Associates/Photo Researchers, Inc.

Esophageal Acidity, Esophageal Manometry, Acid Perfusion (Bernstein Test)	Esophageal acidity is measured to diagnose problems of the lower esophageal sphincter and chronic reflux esophagitis. A catheter with a pH electrode is inserted into the esophagus through the mouth. The measurement may be one time, or over a 24-hour period. Esophageal manometry is done to measure esophageal sphincter pressure and peristaltic contractions for diagnosis of esophageal motility problems, such as achalasia. A manometric catheter with a pressure transducer is inserted into the esophagus through the mouth and esophageal pressure is measured before and after swallowing. Acid perfusion (Bernstein test) tests are done to distinguish between gastric acid reflux and cardiac involvement. A catheter is inserted through the nose into the esophagus. A saline solution, followed by an HCL solution, is dripped into the catheter and the patient is asked to indicate when pain occurs. Normal esophageal pH is 5 to 6.	Advise the patient to be NPO and to avoid alcohol intake for 8 to 12 hours prior to the exam. Assess medications: Results of the tests may be affected by antacids, anticholinergics, and cimetidine-like drugs, which increase the pH, reducing acidity and causing false test results.

(continued)

DIAGNOSTIC TESTS of the Gastrointestinal System (continued)

NAME OF TEST	PURPOSE & DESCRIPTION	RELATED NURSING INTERVENTION
Gastric Analysis Normal values: Fasting: 1.0–5.0 mEq/L/per hour Stimulation: 10–25 mEq/L/per hour	This test is used to evaluate gastric secretions for an increase or decrease of free hydrochloric acid by inserting a nasogastric tube into the stomach and aspirating stomach fluids. A stimulation gastric analysis may follow, with a gastric stimulant (such as Histalog or pentagastrin) administered and several gastric samples aspirated.	Instruct the patient to not smoke, eat, or drink fluids for 8 to 12 hours prior to the test. Assess medications and fluid intake: Anticholinergics, cholinergics, adrenergic blockers, antacids, steroids, alcohol, and coffee can alter results. Remove loose dentures. Insert nasogastric tube. Aspirate gastric contents at 15- to 20-minute intervals as ordered.
Gastric Emptying Studies	To evaluate the ability of the stomach to empty liquids or solids. In this nuclear imaging study, the patient is asked to eat a cooked egg containing Tc-^{99m} (solids) or to drink orange juice with Tc^{99m} (liquids). Sequential images are recorded with a gamma camera every 2 minutes for up to an hour.	Explain to the patient that the substances contain only very small amounts of radioactivity and are not hazardous.
Magnetic Resonance Imaging (MRI)—Stomach	An MRI of the stomach may be conducted to identify the source of gastric bleeding.	Inform the patient of the need to lie still during the examination. Assess for any metallic implants (such as pacemakers, clips on brain aneurysms, body piercing, tattoos, shrapnel). If present, notify imaging physician. Remove transdermal medication patches (both OTC and prescribed) unless otherwise ordered (FDA, 2009). Replace the patch following the procedure. Tell the patient to inform the staff about the patch when making the appointment and when completing the admission information. Ask if the patient is pregnant; if so the test is not performed. Ask about claustrophobia; if a problem, request that the patient ask for a relaxing medication to take prior to the MRI.
Upper GI Endoscopy (Esophagogastroduodenoscopy [EGD]), Gastroscopy	These tests directly visualize the mucous membrane lining of the esophagus, stomach, and duodenum. A flexible fiber-optic endoscope is used to visualize inflammations, ulcerations, tumors, or varices, and video imaging may illustrate gastric motility. They may also be combined with an ultrasound examination by attaching an ultrasound transducer to the endoscope.	Schedule this test at least 2 days after a barium swallow or upper GI series. Remove dentures and eyeglasses. Inform the patient not to eat food or drink fluids for 6 to 8 hours before the procedure. Tell the patient that the procedure takes about 20 to 30 minutes and that a local anesthetic will be administered to the throat to help prevent discomfort. After the procedure the patient is allowed to eat and drink as soon as he or she can swallow safely. Mild bloating, belching, or flatulence may occur after the procedure. Tell the patient to contact the physician postexamination for difficulty swallowing; epigastric, substernal, or shoulder pain; fever; vomiting blood; or having black tarry stools.

THE INTESTINES

NAME OF TEST	PURPOSE & DESCRIPTION	RELATED NURSING INTERVENTION
Abdominal Ultrasound	This test is used to identify abdominal masses, ascites, and disorders of the appendix. A lubricant gel is applied to the skin and a transducer is placed over the area of interest. High-frequency sound waves pass through the body structures and are recorded as they are reflected.	Tell the patient not to eat, drink, smoke, or chew gum for 6 hours prior to the examination and to eat a fat-free meal the evening before the test. Ensure that the patient has not had any other tests that might interfere with results, such as an upper GI series.
Barium Enema (Ba Enema)	A barium enema is conducted to identify structural abnormalities of the rectum and colon. This fluoroscopic radiologic examination of the colon is done by administering a contrast medium rectally. Double-contrast or air-contrast studies are the examination of choice, with air being infused after the barium is evacuated.	Inform the patient to follow a clear liquid diet for 24 hours and then to not eat or drink fluid for 8 hours before the procedure. Instruct in the administration of the prescribed laxatives, enemas, or suppositories the evening before the procedure. Following the procedure, the patient should increase fluid intake and take a laxative, if prescribed. Stools may be white until all the barium is expelled.

DIAGNOSTIC TESTS of the Gastrointestinal System (continued)

NAME OF TEST	PURPOSE & DESCRIPTION	RELATED NURSING INTERVENTION
Colonoscopy	A visual examination of the entire colon to the ileocecal valve is conducted to identify tumors, polyps, and inflammatory bowel disease and to dilate strictures. A flexible endoscope is inserted anally and advanced through the colon. Polyps are removed during the procedure to prevent future malignancies.	Tell the patient to follow the examining physician's order for preparation (this varies by physician or clinic), which may include a liquid diet the day prior to the examination, remaining NPO for 8 hours before the procedure, and a bowel preparation by, for example, citrate of magnesia, laxatives, or polyethylene glycol. (Be aware that the FDA has issued a "black box" warning for oral phosphate solutions sometimes used as bowel preparation; these drugs may damage kidney function, especially in older adults, or those who are dehydrated, have kidney disease or colitis, or are taking medications that affect kidney function [Khurana et al., 2008]). Explain that sedation is usually given during the procedure and that polyps (if present) will be removed. Instruct the patient to refrain from eating prepared foods that contain olestra (a synthetic fat additive used in products such as potato chips); the chemical may cover tissue lesions and also cause adhesive plaques to form on the colonoscopy instruments. Inform the patient that after the procedure increased flatus is common, and to report to the healthcare provider any abdominal pain, chills, fever, rectal bleeding, or mucopurulent discharge. If polyps were removed, the patient should avoid high-fiber foods for 1 to 2 days and do no heavy lifting for 7 days.
Guaiac Fecal Occult Blood Test (G-FOBT)	In this test, feces are tested for occult (hidden) blood. This is often done as a screening test for colon cancer. A stool specimen may be sent to the laboratory, or the test may be done with a commercial kit such as Hemoccult II or Occultest.	When testing for occult blood with a commercial kit, place a smear of stool on the designated area and drop the reagent on the area. A blue color that develops in response to the reagent indicates the presence of blood. If the test is done at home, tell the patient to avoid (if recommended by the healthcare provider) taking aspirin, NSAIDs, anticoagulants, red meats, fish, broccoli and other high fiber vegetables, mushrooms, vitamin C supplements, and iron supplements for 3 days prior to the stool collection.
Immunochemical Fecal Occult Blood Test (I-FOBT)	An I-FOBT is a test used to test for blood in the stool, and is considered to be more effective in detecting colon cancer than is the guaiac fecal occult blood test. A brush is used to collect water drops around the surface of a stool while it is still in the toilet bowl. The sample is then sent to the laboratory for analysis.	No special preparation is necessary. The specimen is collected and sent to the laboratory.
Magnetic Resonance Imaging (MRI)—Abdominal	An abdominal MRI may be done to identify sources of GI bleeding and to stage colon cancer.	See previous information about MRI of the stomach.
Sigmoidoscopy	A sigmoidoscopy is a visual examination of the anus, rectum, and sigmoid colon to identify tumors, polyps, infections, inflammations, hemorrhoids, and fissures. The test is done by using a flexible sigmoidoscope. Specimens are obtained and polyps removed during the procedure.	Instruct the patient to eat a clear liquid or light diet the evening before the procedure and to take prescribed laxatives. An enema or rectal suppository may be required the morning of the procedure. Explain to the patient that after the procedure large amounts of flatus may be expelled if air was instilled into the bowel, and to report any abdominal pain, fever, or rectal bleeding to the healthcare provider. If a polyp is removed, the patient should avoid heavy lifting for 7 days, and avoid high-fiber foods for 1 to 2 days.
Small-Bowel Series	This radiologic examination is done to diagnose abnormalities of the small intestine. The patient drinks a contrast medium and films are taken every 20 minutes until the medium reaches the terminal ileum. It may also be done in conjunction with an upper GI series or barium swallow.	Inform the patient that a low-residue diet should be eaten as prescribed (usually up to 48 hours pre-procedure), and not to eat for 8 hours or drink fluids for 4 hours before the test. Tell the patient about the procedure: it takes several hours to complete, and barium may be given orally, into the bowel via an endoscope, or through a weighted tube. Following the procedure the patient should increase oral fluid intake and take a prescribed laxative to facilitate evacuation of the barium. The stools will be white for up to 72 hours after the examination; normal color will return when all the barium is evacuated.

(continued)

DIAGNOSTIC TESTS of the Gastrointestinal System (continued)

NAME OF TEST	PURPOSE & DESCRIPTION	RELATED NURSING INTERVENTION
Stool Specimen, Stool Culture	A sample of stool is collected for gross and microscopic examination, as well as for form, consistency, and color. Gross examination includes volume and water content, and the presence of any blood, pus, mucus, or excess fat. Microscopic examination identifies the presence of WBCs, unabsorbed fat, and parasites. When an enteric pathogen is suspected, a stool culture is done.	Ask the patient to provide a fresh stool sample. A sterile container should be used to collect a stool sample for a culture. Ask women of childbearing age if they are having their menstrual period; if so, note this on the laboratory request.
Stool DNA test (sDNA)	This test involves examining a stool specimen for DNA changes. Premalignant polyps and malignant lesions of the bowel shed cells that have been identified as DNA markers for bowel and rectal cancer. The patient uses a kit containing an ice pack (that must be frozen for several hours before use), collects one bowel movement in a special container, then mails or brings the container with the ice pack in a provided box to the laboratory.	No special preparation is needed. Explain the procedure to the patient.
Virtual Colonoscopy (VC)	A VC is used to diagnose polyps, diverticulosis, and cancer. X-rays and computers are used to produce two- and three-dimensional images of the colon on a screen. If abnormalities are found, a conventional colonoscopy may be needed (such as to remove polyps or do a biopsy).	Explain to the patient that laxatives or other oral agents are taken the day before the procedure and a rectal suppository used the morning of the procedure. Inform the patient that a tube is inserted into the rectum, air is instilled to inflate the colon, and scans are taken.

THE GALLBLADDER AND PANCREAS

NAME OF TEST	PURPOSE & DESCRIPTION	RELATED NURSING INTERVENTION
Abdominal Ultrasound, Hepatobiliary Ultrasound, Gallbladder Ultrasound	Abdominal ultrasound is used to detect abdominal tumors, cysts, and ascites. Hepatobiliary ultrasound is used to visualize the biliary ducts, and to detect subphrenic abscesses, cysts, tumors, and cirrhosis of the liver. Gallbladder ultrasound is used to detect gallstones. These noninvasive procedures record ultrasound waves as they are reflected off body structures. A conductive gel is applied to the skin and a transducer placed on the area of interest.	Instruct the patient to remain NPO for 8 to 12 hours prior to the test.
Cholangiography ■ Percutaneous Transhepatic Cholangiogram (PTC) ■ Surgical Cholangiogram	A PTC is done to evaluate filling of the hepatic and biliary ducts. Using local anesthesia, the liver and bile duct is entered with a long needle (using fluoroscopy), bile is withdrawn, and a contrast medium is injected into the bile duct. During a surgical cholangiogram with general anesthesia, contrast medium is injected into the common bile duct to evaluate filling of the duct.	Assess for allergy to iodine, seafood, or x-ray dye (many contain iodine). Assess medications: Oral hypoglycemic agents are contraindicated for use with iodinated contrast. Monitor for bile leakage or hemorrhage following the tests.
Cholecystography (Oral) (GB Series)	The test is used to detect gallbladder stones, inflammation or tumors, and obstruction of the cystic duct. Radiopaque tablets (for example, iopanoic acid [Telepaque], sodium ipodate [Oragrafin], iodoalphionic acid [Priodax], or iodipamide meglumine [Cholografin]) are given the evening before the test; x-rays are taken the following morning. A high-fat meal may be given after the fasting x-rays are completed and further x-rays taken to determine how rapidly the GB expels the dye.	*If the patient is also having GI x-rays with barium, the GB tests should be done first, because barium would interfere with the test.* Instruct the patient to eat a fat-free diet 24 hours prior to test. No food or fluids except sips of water should be taken 12 hours before the test. Radiopaque tablets are to be taken 2 hours after the evening meal. Assess for allergy to iodine, seafood, or x-ray dye (many contain iodine). Assess medications: Oral hypoglycemic agents are contraindicated for use with iodinated contrast.

DIAGNOSTIC TESTS of the Gastrointestinal System (continued)

NAME OF TEST	PURPOSE & DESCRIPTION	RELATED NURSING INTERVENTION
Computed Tomography (CT)	This is a noninvasive procedure using radio-frequency waves and a magnetic field is used to evaluate disorders of the GB, pancreas, and liver.	No special preparation is needed.
Endoscopic Retrograde Cholangiopancreatography (ERCP)	An ERCP is done to directly visualize GI structures, and to retrieve gallstones from the distal common bile duct, dilate structures, and biopsy tumors. A fiber-optic endoscope is inserted through the mouth, the esophagus, stomach, and descending duodenum, and the common bile ducts and pancreatic ducts. Contrast medium is injected into the ducts and structures are visualized.	Tell the patient not to drink fluids or eat for 8 hours before the test. Assess patient for allergy to iodine, seafood, or x-ray dye (many contain iodine). Assess medications: Oral hypoglycemic agents are contraindicated for use with iodinated contrast. Assess gag reflex prior to giving food or fluids. If atropine was given, assess for manifestations of urinary retention. Tell the patient that a sore throat may be present for a few days after the test; suggest warm saline gargles to ease discomfort.
Magnetic Resonance Cholangiopancreatography (MRCP)	This noninvasive MRI study is done to evaluate the biliary and pancreatic ducts.	See previous information for MRI of the stomach.
Serum Amylase Normal value: 0–130 Unit/L	This blood test is used to measure the secretion of amylase by the pancreas. It is used to diagnose acute pancreatitis, when amylase level peaks in 24 hours and then drops to normal in 48 to 72 hours.	No special preparation is needed.
Serum Lipase Normal value: 0–160 Unit/L	This blood test is used to measure the secretion of lipase by the pancreas.	No special preparation is needed.

THE LIVER

NAME OF TEST	PURPOSE & DESCRIPTION	RELATED NURSING INTERVENTION
Liver Biopsy	A liver biopsy is performed to rule out metastatic cancer or to detect a cyst or cirrhosis of the liver. The procedure is considered minor surgery, and is done at a hospital. Using ultrasound, a biopsy needle is inserted into the liver and guided to the pathologic site. See Figure 21–8 ■.	Inform the patient to tell the doctor about any anticoagulants taken, and to withhold aspirin and ibuprofen for a week before the procedure. Food and fluids are withheld for 4 to 6 hours before the procedure, assess and record baseline vital signs, and review prothrombin time and platelet count. Administer vitamin K as prescribed. Ask the patient to void immediately before the procedure. After the needle is removed, pressure is applied; place the patient on the right side for 1 to 2 hours to maintain pressure on the insertion site. Explain to the patient that pain may be experienced in the right shoulder as the local anesthetic loses effect, that the dressing will be assessed frequently, that food and fluids are withheld for 2 hours after the biopsy, and that coughing, lifting, or straining should be avoided for 1 to 2 weeks. The patient will not be allowed to drive home, and must go directly to bed for 8 to 10 hours (or as prescribed by the physician).

Figure 21–8 ■ Liver biopsy. *A,* The patient exhales completely, and then holds his or her breath. This brings the liver and diaphragm to their highest position. *B,* The biopsy needle is inserted into the liver. *C,* Approximately 1 mL of saline is injected to clear the needle of blood and tissue. *D,* The needle is advanced, and a tissue sample is aspirated. Pressure is applied to the site immediately after the needle is withdrawn. The specimen is sent to the laboratory for analysis.

Note: A wide variety of blood tests are used to diagnose and monitor liver disease. These are discussed in appropriate interdisciplinary care sections in ∞ Chapter 25.

Explain what will happen during the examination, and encourage the patient to take deep, regular breaths to increase relaxation. Explain that during the rectal examination, it may feel as though the patient is about to have a bowel movement and sometimes flatus (gas) is passed. Assure the patient that this is normal. Ensure that the examination area is private and the patient is draped properly to prevent unnecessary exposure.

Physical assessment of the integumentary system, nervous system, musculoskeletal system, cardiovascular system, and respiratory system may reflect the patient's nutritional status. Table 21–4 summarizes abnormal nutritional assessment findings related to these body systems. Normal age-related findings for the older adult are summarized in the Nursing Care of the Older Adult box.

TABLE 21–4 Assessment Findings Due to Malnutrition

BODY SYSTEM	ASSESSMENT FINDINGS
Nails	Soft and spoon shaped in iron deficiency. Splinter hemorrhages in vitamin C deficiency.
Hair	Dry, dull, and scarce in zinc, protein, and linoleic acid deficiencies.
Skin	Flaky and dry in vitamin A, vitamin B, and/or linoleic acid deficiency. Cracks and/or hyperpigmentation in niacin deficiency. Bruising in vitamin C or vitamin K deficiency.
Eyes	Eyes become dry and soft with decrease in vitamin A. Conjunctiva is pale with a decrease in iron, and red with a decrease in riboflavin.
Nervous system	Reflexes are decreased and patient may have peripheral neuropathies with thiamine deficiency. Patient may be irritable and/or disoriented with thiamine deficiency.
Musculoskeletal system	Muscle wasting is seen with deficits in protein, carbohydrate, and fat metabolism. Calf pain occurs with thiamine deficiency; joint pain may occur with vitamin C deficiency.
Cardiovascular system	Heart size and rate may increase with thiamine deficiency. Diastolic blood pressure may be increased with a high intake of fat. Lowered cardiac output and decreased blood pressure may occur with caloric deficiencies over a long time period.
GI system	Cheilosis (sores at corner of mouth) seen in vitamin B-complex deficiencies, especially riboflavin. Stomatitis and spongy, bleeding gums may also be seen in malnutrition.

NURSING CARE OF THE OLDER ADULT   Age-Related Gastrointestinal Changes

AGE-RELATED CHANGE

Teeth: ▲ number of root cavities and cavities around existing dental work; tooth enamel harder and more brittle; dentin is more fibrous; tooth cusps flatten; root pulp shrinks; ▲ loss of bone supporting teeth

Gums: Gingiva retracts

Taste: Less acute as tongue atrophies, especially for sweet sensations

Saliva: ▼ amount is produced (1/3 of that produced in younger years)

Esophageal motility: ▼ intensity of propulsive waves and slower emptying time, weaker gag reflex

Stomach: Mucosa atrophies, ▼ production of hydrochloric acid and pepsin leading to higher pH in stomach

Liver: Less efficient handling of cholesterol

Small intestine: ▼ number of absorbing cells on intestinal wall, slowed fat absorption, faulty absorption of vitamin B$_{12}$, vitamin D, calcium, and iron

Large intestine: ▼ mucous secretion and elasticity of the wall of the rectum, loss of tone in internal sphincter with decreased awareness of need to defecate

SIGNIFICANCE

Increase in periodontal disease and tooth loss
Increase in fractures of teeth
Increased incidence of dentures

Increase in periodontal disease

Excessive seasoning of foods

Decreased ability to break down starches
Swallowing may take longer

Discomfort when swallowing food
Increased risk of aspiration

Increase in incidence of gastric irritation

Increased incidence of gallstones

- Decreased ability to absorb vitamins A, D, E, and K
- Increased risk of osteoporosis and fractures (▼ calcium and vitamin D)
- Increased risk of iron-deficiency anemia (weakness, lassitude, pallor) (▼ iron)
- Increased risk of pernicious anemia (weakness, dyspnea, glossitis, numbness, dementia, depression) (▼ vitamin B$_{12}$)

- Increased tendency for constipation

Gastrointestinal Assessments

Technique/Normal Findings	Abnormal Findings

Anthropometric Assessment

Weigh the patient and measure the patient's height. Compare the patient's actual weight to ideal body weight (IBW) (Table 21–5). *Weight should be appropriate to height as indicated on a standardized table.*

- A weight 10% to 20% less than ideal body weight indicates malnutrition.
- A weight 10% above ideal body weight is considered overweight.
- A weight 20% above ideal body weight is considered obese.

TABLE 21–5 Example of a Height and Weight Table

	HEIGHT		WEIGHT		
	FEET	**INCHES**	**SMALL FRAME**	**MEDIUM FRAME**	**LARGE FRAME**
Men (ages 25–29)	5	2	128–134	131–134	138–150
	5	3	130–136	133–143	140–153
	5	4	132–138	135–145	142–156
	5	5	134–140	137–148	144–160
	5	6	136–142	139–151	146–164
	5	7	138–145	142–154	149–168
	5	8	140–148	145–157	152–172
	5	9	142–151	148–160	155–176
	5	10	144–154	151–163	158–180
	5	11	146–157	154–166	161–184
	6	0	149–160	157–170	164–188
	6	1	152–164	160–174	168–192
	6	2	155–168	164–178	172–197
	6	3	158–172	167–182	176–202
	6	4	162–176	171–187	181–207
Women (ages 25–29)	4	10	102–111	109–121	118–131
	4	11	103–113	111–123	120–134
	5	0	104–115	113–126	122–137
	5	1	106–118	115–129	125–140
	5	2	108–121	118–132	128–143
	5	3	111–124	121–135	131–147
	5	4	114–127	124–138	134–151
	5	5	117–130	127–141	137–155
	5	6	120–133	130–144	140–159
	5	7	123–136	133–147	143–163
	5	8	126–139	136–150	146–167
	5	9	129–142	139–153	149–170
	5	10	132–145	142–156	152–173
	5	11	135–148	145–159	155–176
	6	0	138–151	148–162	158–179

Technique/Normal Findings	Abnormal Findings
Calculate the patient's percentage of ideal body weight (%IBW). To calculate IBW, (1) determine the height and weight of the patient, (2) multiply the height times 2, (3) divide the body weight by the answer obtained in step 2, and (4) multiply the answer from step 3 by 703. The result is the patient's IBW. *Ideal body weight should be within normal range (19–25).*	A healthy IBW is from 19 to 25. Underweight is considered anything below 18, 25 to 29 is considered overweight, and anything over 30 is considered obese. *Note:* This is one of several ways used to calculate IBW.

Measure body mass index (BMI). Determine BMI by using one of the following formulas. *BMI should be between 20 and 25.*

- A BMI of 25 to 29.9 kg/m² indicates overweight.
- A BMI of 30 kg/m² indicates obesity.

$$\frac{\text{Weight in kilograms}}{\text{Height in meters}^2} = BMI$$

$$\frac{\text{Weight in pounds} \times 705}{\text{Height in inches}^2} = BMI$$

Measure triceps skinfold thickness (TSF). Find the midpoint between the patient's olecranon and acromion processes. Grasp the skin and fat, and pull it away from the muscle. Apply skinfold calipers for 3 seconds, and record the reading (Figure 21–9 ■). Repeat three times, and average the three readings. Compare the patient's reading to the standard values shown in Table 21–6. *TSF should be within normal range as compared to standard values.*

- Triceps readings are 10% or more below standards in malnutrition and 10% or more above standards in obesity or overnutrition.

Figure 21–9 ■ Measuring the triceps skinfold thickness with calipers.

TABLE 21–6 Values for Anthropometric Measurements

MEASUREMENT	STANDARD VALUE	
	MALE	FEMALE
Triceps skinfold thickness	12.5 mm	16.5 mm
Midarm circumference	29.3 cm	28.5 cm
Midarm muscle circumference	25.3 cm	23.2 cm

Measure midarm circumference (MAC). Find the midpoint between the patient's olecranon and acromion processes. Wind tape measure around arm (Figure 21–10 ■). Compare the patient's reading to the standard values shown in Table 21–6. *MAC should be within normal range as compared to standard values.*

- MAC decreases with malnutrition and increases with obesity.

Figure 21–10 ■ Measuring MAC with a tape measure.

Technique/Normal Findings	Abnormal Findings

Calculate midarm muscle circumference (MAMC). Use the patient's triceps skinfold measurement and midarm circumference readings to calculate the patient's MAMC.

Compare the result to the standard values shown in Table 21–6. *MAMC should be within normal range as compared to standard values.*

- In mild malnutrition, the MAMC is 90% of the standard; in moderate malnutrition, 60% to 90%. In severe malnutrition (muscle wasting), the MAMC is less than 60% of the standard.

$$MAMC = MAC - (0.314 \times TSF)$$

Determine waist-to-hip ratio. With the patient standing, measure the waist, and then measure the hips midway between the iliac crest and the greater trochanter. Use the following formula to calculate the waist-to-hip ratio. *Normal findings: females, waist ratio less than or equal to 0.80; males, waist ratio less than or equal to 1.0.*

- Females with a ratio greater than 0.80 and males with a ratio greater than 1.0 have a three to five times greater risk for having a heart attack or stroke (Weber & Kelley, 2009).

$$\frac{\text{Waist circumference}}{\text{Hip circumference}} = \text{waist-to-hip ratio}$$

SAMPLE DOCUMENTATION

Assessment of Nutritional Status

Twenty-two-year-old female visiting health clinic for regular check-up. Height 5 feet, 5 inches (165 cm); Weight 128 pounds (58 kg). BMI: 24. MAC: 28 cm. Waist-to-hip ratio: 0.6. Skin is warm, moist, and smooth without lesions other than well-healed scar on RLQ of abdomen from appendectomy, age 15. Oral mucosa and tongue pink and moist. No breath odor. All teeth present with evidence of dental care. Abdomen slightly concave when lying on back, bowel sounds present in all four quadrants, liver nonpalpable, tympany over lower abdomen on percussion.

Oral Assessment

Inspect and palpate the lips. *Lips should be of normal color for race without lesions.*

- **Cheilosis** (painful lesions at corners of mouth) is seen with riboflavin and/or niacin deficiency.
- Cold sores or clear vesicles with a red base are seen in herpes simplex 1.

Inspect and palpate the tongue. *Tongue should be pink, smooth, and have good turgor.*

- Atrophic smooth **glossitis** is characterized by a bright red tongue. It is seen in B_{12}, folic acid, and iron deficiencies.
- Vertical fissures are seen in dehydration.
- A black, hairy tongue may be seen following antibiotic therapy.

Inspect and palpate the buccal mucosa. *Mucosa should be moist, without lesions and of appropriate color.*

- **Leukoplakia** (small white patches) may be a sign of a premalignant condition.
- A reddened, dry, swollen mucosa may be seen in stomatitis.
- Candidiases (white cheesy patches that bleed when scraped) may be seen in immune-suppressed patients receiving antibiotics or chemotherapy and in terminally ill patients.

Inspect and palpate the teeth. *Teeth should be in a state of good hygiene without caries.*

- Cavities and excessive plaque are seen with poor nutrition and/or poor oral hygiene.

Inspect and palpate the gums. *Gums should be of even color without swelling.*

- Swollen, red gums that bleed easily (**gingivitis**) are seen in periodontal disease, vitamin C deficiencies, or with hormonal changes.

Inspect the throat and tonsils. *Tonsils (if present) should be of appropriate color and size.*

- In acute infections, tonsils are red and swollen and may have white spots.

Note the patient's breath. *Breath should not have unusual or foul odors.*

- Sweet, fruity breath is noted in diabetic ketoacidosis.
- Acetone breath may be a sign of uremia.
- Foul breath may result from liver disease, respiratory infections, and poor oral hygiene.

Abdominal Assessment

Right Upper Quadrant
Liver and gallbladder
Pylorus
Duodenum
Head of pancreas
Right adrenal gland
Portion of right kidney
Hepatic flexure of colon
Portions of ascending and
   transverse colon

Left Upper Quadrant
Left lobe of liver
Spleen
Stomach
Body of pancreas
Left adrenal gland
Portion of left kidney
Splenic flexure of colon
Portions of transverse and
   descending colon

Right Lower Quadrant
Lower pole of right kidney
Cecum and appendix
Portion of ascending colon
Bladder (if distended)
Right ovary and salpinx
Right spermatic cord
Right ureter

Left Lower Quadrant
Lower pole of left kidney
Sigmoid colon
Portion of descending colon
Bladder (if distended)
Left ovary and salpinx
Uterus (if enlarged)
Left spermatic cord
Left ureter

Midline
Aorta
Bladder
Uterus

○ = Umbilicus

Figure 21–11 ■ The four quadrants of the abdomen.

BOX 21–2 Guidelines for Assessing the Abdomen

Ask the patient to empty the bladder before beginning the examination. Assist the patient to the dorsal recumbent (supine) position, with a small pillow under the head, a pillow under the knees (if desired), and the arms at the sides of the body. Warm the stethoscope before applying it to the patient's skin. Ask the patient to point to areas that are painful, and explain that those areas will be examined last. Expose the abdomen from below the breasts to the pubic symphysis, and drape the patient's thoracic and genital areas. When you document your findings, specify the location by abdominal quadrant.

General guidelines for abdominal assessment are as follows:

1. Inspect the abdomen under a good light source that is shining across the abdomen. Sit at the right side of the patient, and note symmetry, distention, masses, visible peristalsis, and respiratory movements. If masses are detected, ask the patient to take a deep breath, which decreases the size of the abdominal cavity and makes any abnormality more visible.
2. Auscultate each quadrant of the abdomen, using the diaphragm of the stethoscope. Listen for bowel sounds, arterial bruits, venous hums, and friction rubs.

3. Percuss several areas within each quadrant of the abdomen, using a systematic path. (For example, always begin in the lower left quadrant, then proceed to the lower right quadrant, upper right quadrant, and upper left quadrant, respectively). The predominant percussion tones for the entire abdomen are tympany and dullness. Tympany is present over gas-filled intestines. Dullness is present over the liver, the spleen, an enlarged kidney, or a full stomach. Percuss for fluid, gaseous distention, and masses.
4. Palpate each quadrant of the abdomen for shape, position, mobility, size, consistency, and tenderness of the major abdominal organs. Begin this part of the assessment with light palpation, and increase the depth of palpation to elicit tenderness or better identify organ size and shape. Deep palpation should be conducted only by nurses with considerable experience. Remember to palpate areas of indicated tenderness last and to use gentle pressure. Palpation may be difficult or impossible if the patient exhibits muscle guarding from pain or is ticklish. The gallbladder and the spleen are normally not palpable.

Technique/Normal Findings	Abnormal Findings
Inspect abdominal contour, skin integrity, venous pattern, and aortic pulsation. *Abdomen should be slightly concave or rounded with intact skin. There should not be distended veins or obvious aortic pulsations.*	■ Generalized abdominal distention may be seen in gas retention or obesity. ■ Lower abdominal distention is seen in bladder distention, pregnancy, or ovarian mass. ■ General distention and an everted umbilicus are seen with ascites and/or tumors. ■ A scaphoid (sunken) abdomen is seen in malnutrition or when fat is replaced with muscle. ■ **Striae** (whitish-silver stretch marks) are seen in obesity and during or after pregnancy. ■ Spider angiomas may be seen in liver disease. ■ Dilated veins are prominent in cirrhosis of the liver, ascites, portal hypertension, or venocaval obstruction. ■ Pulsation is increased in aortic aneurysm.

Technique/Normal Findings	Abnormal Findings

Auscultate all four quadrants of the abdomen with the diaphragm of the stethoscope (Figure 21–12 ■). Begin in the lower right quadrant, where bowel sounds are almost always present. If bowel sounds are not heard, ask a colleage to check your findings. *Normal bowel sounds (gurgling or clicking) occur every 5 to 15 seconds. Listen for at least 5 minutes in each of the four quadrants to confirm the absence of bowel sounds.*

- **Borborygmus** (hyperactive high-pitched, tinkling, rushing, or growling bowel sounds) is heard in diarrhea or at the onset of bowel obstruction.
- Bowel sounds may be absent later in bowel obstruction, with an inflamed peritoneum, and/or following surgery of the abdomen

Figure 21–12 ■ Auscultating the abdomen with the diaphragm of the stethoscope.

Auscultate the abdomen for vascular sounds with the bell of the stethoscope (Figure 21–13 ■). *No sounds (bruits, venous hum, or friction rub) other than bowel sounds should be auscultated.*

- **Bruits** (blowing sound due to restriction of blood flow through vessels) may be heard over constricted arteries. A bruit over the liver may be heard in hepatic carcinoma.
- A venous hum (continuous medium-pitched sound) may be heard over a cirrhotic liver.
- Friction rubs (rough grating sounds) may be heard over an inflamed liver or spleen.

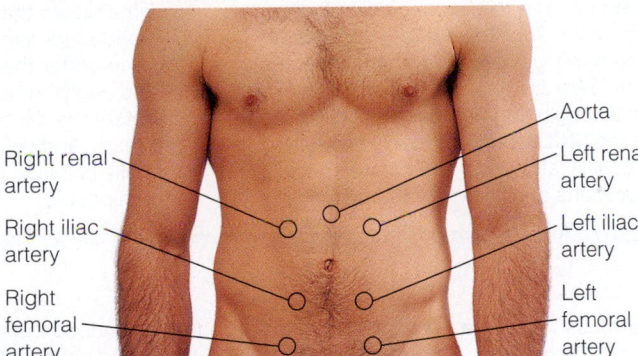

Figure 21–13 ■ Location of placement of the stethoscope for auscultation of arteries of the abdomen.

Percuss the abdomen in all four quadrants (Figure 21–14 ■). *Normally, tympany is heard over the stomach and gas-filled bowels.*

- Dullness is heard when the bowel is displaced with fluid or tumors or filled with a fecal mass.

Figure 21–14 ■ Location of sites for systematic percussion of all four quadrants.

Technique/Normal Findings	Abnormal Findings

Percuss the liver (see Box 21–3 for guidelines for liver percussion and palpation; see Figure 21–15 ■ for landmarks). *The lower border of liver dullness is located at the costal margin to 1 to 2 cm below.*

- In cirrhosis and/or hepatitis, the liver is greater than 6 to 10 cm in the MCL and greater than 4 to 8 cm in the midsternal line (MSL).

Figure 21–15 ■ Anatomic location of the liver, with the mid-clavicular line (MCL) and midsternal line (MSL) superimposed. The normal liver span is 6 to 12 cm.

BOX 21–3 Guidelines for Percussing and Palpating the Liver

The size of the liver may be determined by percussion and palpation, as follows:

1. Percuss, in the midclavicular line (MCL), beginning below the umbilicus (see Figure 21–15). Begin to percuss over a region of tympany, and move upward. The first dull percussion tone occurs at the lower border of the liver. Determine the upper liver border by beginning percussion over an area of lung resonance (in the MCL) and percussing downward to the first dull tone, usually at the 5th to 7th interspace. Mark each of these locations and measure the distance

from one mark to the other to determine liver size. The normal liver size is 6 to 12 cm in the MCL; however, men have larger livers than women.

2. Conduct bimanual palpation of the liver by placing your left hand under the patient at the level of the 11th to 12th ribs and applying upward pressure. Place your right hand below the costal margin, ask the patient to take a deep breath, and palpate for the liver border. The liver is not normally palpable in a healthy adult, although it may be in very thin people.

Percuss the spleen for dullness posterior to the midaxillary line at the level of the 6th to 11th rib (Figure 21–16 ■). *The spleen is percussed as an oval area of dullness approximately 7 cm wide near the left 10th rib and slightly posterior to the midaxillary line.*

- A large area of dullness that extends to the left anterior axillary line on inspiration is associated with an enlarged spleen and may be related to trauma, infection, or mononucleosis.

Figure 21–16 ■ Percussing the spleen.

Technique/Normal Findings	Abnormal Findings

Percuss for shifting dullness (Figure 21–17 ■). *If ascites is not present, the borders between tympany and dullness remain relatively constant despite position changes.*

- In a patient with ascites, the level of dullness increases when the patient turns to the side.

Figure 21–17 ■ Percussing for shifting dullness in ascites. *A,* Common percussion tones when the patient is lying supine; *B,* changes in percussion tones (shifting dullness) when the patient turns to the side.

Palpate the abdomen in all four quadrants (Figure 21–18 ■). If the patient tightens the abdominal muscles (called "guarding") flexing the knees may relax the muscles. *There should be no abdominal masses or pain on palpation.*

- In cases of peritoneal inflammation, palpation causes abdominal pain and involuntary muscle spasms.
- Abnormal masses include aortic aneurysms, neoplastic tumors of the colon or uterus, and a distended bladder or distended bowel due to obstruction.
- A rigid, boardlike abdomen may be palpated when the patient has a perforated duodenal ulcer.

Figure 21–18 ■ Light to moderate palpation of the abdomen. *A,* In light palpation, the examiner, keeping the fingers approximated, gently depresses the abdominal wall about 1 cm to assess for large masses, slight tenderness, and muscle guarding. *B,* The examiner performs moderate palpation by using the palm or the side of the hand to depress the abdominal wall to a slightly greater depth than in light palpation. This technique is useful for assessing abdominal organs that move with respiration (such as the liver and the spleen).

Use a circular motion to move the abdominal wall over underlying structures, Feel for masses and note any tenderness or pain the patient may have during this part of the exam. Palpate lightly at first (0.5 to 5 inch), then deeply (1.5 to 2 inches) with caution. If a mass is palpated, ask the patient to raise head and shoulders. A mass in the abdomen may become more prominent with this maneuver, as will a ventral abdominal wall hernia. If the mass is no longer palpable, it is deeper in the abdomen. *There should be no palpable masses or pain.*

Technique/Normal Findings   **Abnormal Findings**

Palpate for rebound tenderness. Press the fingers into the abdomen slowly and release the pressure quickly. *Releasing pressure should not cause or increase pain.*

- In peritoneal inflammation, pain occurs when the fingers are withdrawn.
- Right upper quadrant pain occurs with acute cholecystitis.
- Upper middle abdominal pain occurs with acute pancreatitis.
- Right lower quadrant pain occurs with acute appendicitis.
- Left lower quadrant pain is seen in acute diverticulitis.

Palpate the liver. Box 21–3 provides guidelines for liver assessment (also see Figure 21–19 ■). Note whether the patient guards the abdomen or reports any sharp pain, especially on inspiration. *The abdomen should be nontender, and the liver is usually nonpalpable.*

- An enlarged liver with a smooth, tender edge may indicate hepatitis or venous congestion.
- An enlarged, nontender liver may be felt in a malignant condition.
- The patient with inflammation of the gallbladder feels sharp pain on inspiration and stops inspiring. This is called Murphy's sign.

Figure 21–19 ■ Palpating the liver with the bimanual method.

Inguinal Area Assessment

Inspect the inguinal area for bulges after asking the patient to bear down. *The inguinal area is normally free of bulges.*

- Bulges that appear in the inguinal area when the patient bears down may indicate a **hernia** (a defect in the abdominal wall that allows abdominal contents to protrude outward).

Palpate the inguinal area with the gloved hand. Ask the patient to shift weight to the left to palpate the right inguinal area and vice versa. Place your right index finger upward into the inguinal area and ask the patient to bear down or cough. *Bulging or masses are normally not palpable.*

- A bulge or mass may indicate a hernia.

Perianal Assessment

Inspect the perianal area. Wearing gloves, spread the patient's buttocks apart. Observe the area, and ask patient to bear down as if trying to have a bowel movement. *The perianal area should be intact, without obvious lesions.*

- Swollen, painful, longitudinal breaks in the anal area may appear in patients with anal fissures. (These are caused by the passing of large, hard stools or by diarrhea.)
- Dilated anal veins appear with hemorrhoids.
- A red mass may appear with prolapsed internal hemorrhoids.
- Doughnut-shaped red tissue at the anal area may appear with a prolapsed rectum.

Palpate the anus and rectum.

Technique/Normal Findings	Abnormal Findings

Lubricate the gloved index finger and ask the patient to bear down. Touch the tip of your finger to the patient's anal opening. Flex the index finger, and slowly insert it into the anus, pointing the finger toward the umbilicus (Figure 21–20 ■). Rotate the finger in both directions to palpate any lesions or masses. *There should be no masses in the anus or rectum.*

- Movable, soft masses may be polyps.
- Hard, firm, irregular embedded masses may indicate carcinoma.

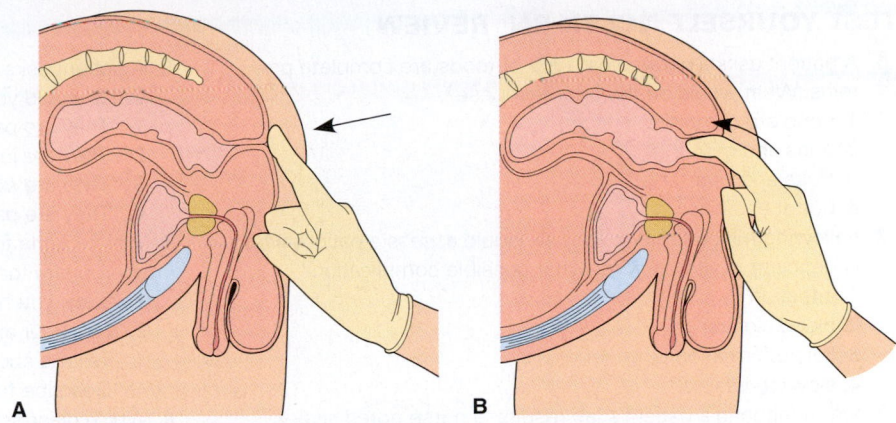

Figure 21–20 ■ Digital examination of the *A,* anus, and *B,* rectum.

Fecal Assessment

Inspect the patient's feces. After palpating the rectum, withdraw your finger gently. Inspect any feces on the glove. Note color and/or presence of blood. Also use gloved fingers to note consistency. *Stool should be soft with no blood present.*

- See Box 21–4 for information about stool characteristics.

Test the feces for occult blood. Use a testing kit such as Occultest or Hemoccult II. *There should be no occult blood in the feces.*

- A positive occult blood test requires further testing for colon cancer or GI bleeding due to peptic ulcers, ulcerative colitis, or diverticulosis.

Note the odor of the feces. *No distinctly foul odors should be present.*

- Distinctly foul odors may be noted with stools containing blood or extra fat or in cases of colon cancer.

SAMPLE DOCUMENTATION

Abdominal Assessment

Seventy-two-year-old female, currently a resident in an extended care facility, states she has not had a bowel movement for a week, and normally has one every other day. She also says she has lost her appetite and "just feels terrible." Abdominal assessment reveals a firm, slightly distended abdomen. Bowel sounds are active with gurgles in all four quadrants. Slight dullness to percussion in LLQ (sigmoid colon). States she has some generalized abdominal discomfort with moderate palpation. Hard stool present in rectum. Stool negative for occult blood.

BOX 21–4 Assessing Stool Characteristics

Inspect feces for color, odor, and consistency after the rectal exam or after defecation. Both hands are gloved.

Color

- Blood *on* the stool results from bleeding from the sigmoid colon, anus, or rectum. Blood *within* the stool indicates bleeding from the colon due to ulcerative colitis, diverticulosis, or tumors. Black, tarry stools, called **melena**, occur with upper GI bleeding. Oral iron may turn stools black and mask melena.
- Grayish or whitish stools can result from biliary obstruction due to lack of bile in stool.
- Greasy, frothy, yellow stools, called **steatorrhea**, may appear with fat malabsorption.

Odor

- Distinct, foul odors may be noted with stools containing blood or extra fat or in cases of colon cancer.

Consistency

- Hard stools or long, flat stools may result from a spastic colon or bowel obstruction due to a tumor or hemorrhoids. Hard stools may also result from ingestion of oral iron.
- Mucousy, slimy feces may indicate inflammation and occur in irritable bowel syndrome.
- Watery, diarrhea stools appear with malabsorption problems, irritable bowel syndrome, emotional or psychologic stress, ingestion of spoiled foods, or lactose intolerance.

TEST YOURSELF NCLEX-RN® REVIEW

1. A patient asks a nurse what type of foods are complete proteins. What would be the best response?
   1. none are complete
   2. eggs and milk
   3. fruits and vegetables
   4. butter and oils

2. Following minor surgery, a nurse would assess a patient who is deficient in vitamin K for what possible complication?
   1. infection
   2. blood clotting
   3. keloid formation
   4. slow peristalsis

3. On monitoring a patient's lab results, a nurse noted a very high serum amylase level. What disease does this indicate?
   1. cheilosis
   2. gastric reflux
   3. gallstones
   4. acute pancreatitis

4. While assessing an older woman, the nurse noticed her teeth have obvious caries and she has difficulty swallowing. She says, "My mouth is so dry." What health problem might result from these findings?
   1. nutritional deficit
   2. acute pain
   3. altered elimination
   4. risk for infection

5. What percussion sound would the nurse expect to hear when assessing the abdomen of a patient with ascites?
   1. flatness
   2. resonance
   3. alternating amplitude
   4. shifting dullness

6. A patient asks you to tell her what internal hemorrhoids are. What would you say?
   1. "They are part of the arteries of the body."
   2. "They are just bits of tissue that occur for no reason."
   3. "They are swollen veins in the anal canal."
   4. "They are part of the lymphatic system."

7. Which of the following questions or statements would be appropriate for the patient with an ostomy?
   1. "Have you had any bleeding from your hemorrhoids?"
   2. "Has your appetite changed lately?"
   3. "Tell me about your family."
   4. "Describe the consistency of your stools."

8. Which diagnostic test would be most appropriate to detect intestinal parasites?
   1. colonoscopy
   2. CT of the abdomen
   3. barium enema
   4. stool specimen

9. Why is removal of polyps during a colonoscopy important?
   1. to identify genetic disorders
   2. to prevent the development of cancer
   3. to facilitate further examination of the bowel
   4. to decrease future problems with constipation

10. A nurse is conducting a health history and states, "Tell me about any colon cancer in your family." Is this an appropriate question?
    1. No, colon cancer is rarely found in family members.
    2. No, this question should only be asked by physicians.
    3. Yes, but it should wait for further diagnostic testing.
    4. Yes, colon cancer is a common inherited disorder.

See Test Yourself answers in Appendix C.

Pearson Nursing Student Resources

Find additional review materials at
www.nursing.pearsonhighered.com

Prepare for success with additional NCLEX®-style practice questions, interactive assignments and activities, Web links, animations and videos, and more!

BIBLIOGRAPHY

Amella, E. (2007). Assessing nutrition in older adults. *Best Practices in Nursing Care to Older Adults.* The Hartford Institute for Geriatric Nursing. Retrieved from www.hartfordign.org

American Cancer Society. (2009). *American Cancer Society guidelines for the early detection of cancer (colon and rectal cancer).* Retrieved from http://cancer.org/docroot/ped/content/ped_2_3x_acs_cancer_detection_guidelines_3

American Society for Gastrointestinal Endoscopy. (2008). *Colonoscopy.* Manchester, MA: American Society for Gastrointestinal Endoscopy.

Armstrong, J., & Mitchell, E. (2008). Comprehensive nursing assessment in the care of older people. *Nursing Older People, (20)*1, 36–40.

Ayden, N., & Karaoz, S. (2008). Nutritional assessment of patients before gastrointestinal surgery and nurses' approach to this issue. *Journal of Clinical Nursing, 17*(5), 608–617.

Bazensky, I., Shoobridge-Moran, C., & Yoder, L. (2007). Colorectal cancer: An overview of the epidemiology, risk factors, symptoms, and screening guidelines. *MEDSURG Nursing, 16*(1), 46–52.

Berman, H., Brooks, L., & Silver, S. (2007). A rational approach to constipation. *Geriatrics & Aging, 10*(10), 654–660.

Camillo, P. (2007). Should a rectal exam be a routine part of a pelvic examination? *Medscape Nurses.* Retrieved from http://www.medscape.com/viewarticle?562990

Costello, T., & Coyne, I. (2008). Nurses' knowledge of mouth care practices. *British Journal of Nursing, 17*(4), 264–268.

Daly, J., Merchant, M., & Barcey, T. L. (2009). Colorectal cancer screening. *American Journal of Nursing, 10*(109), 60–62.

D'Amico, D., & Barbarito, C. (2007). *Health & physical assessment in nursing.* Upper Saddle River, NJ: Pearson Prentice Hall.

Eliopoulos, C. (2005). *Gerontological nursing* (6th ed). Philadelphia: Lippincott Williams & Wilkins.

Foster, D., Parr, J., & Wright, L. (2005). Tackling malnutrition. *Nursing Management, 12*(5), 28–30.

Grams, L., & Spremulli, M. (2008). Assessing a patient for dysphagia. *Nursing, 38*(8), 15.

Greenwald, B. (2006). A pilot study evaluating two alternate methods of stool collection for the fecal occult blood test. *MEDSURG Nursing, 15*(2), 89–94.

Holcomb, S. S. (2008). Acute abdomen: What a pain! *Nursing, 38*(9), 34–40.

Kee, J. (2009). *Prentice Hall handbook of laboratory & diagnostic tests with nursing implications* (6th ed.). Upper Saddle River, NJ: Pearson Prentice Hall.

Khurana, A., McLean, L., Atkinson, S., & Foulks, C. (2008). The effects of oral sodium phosphate drug products on renal function in adults undergoing bowel endoscopy. *Archives of Internal Medicine, 168*(6), 593–597.

Lee, D. (2008). Colon cancer: The genetic factor. *MedicineNet.com.* Retrieved from http://www.medicinenet.com/script/main/art.asp?articlekey=46105&pf=3&page=1

Lou, M., Dai, Y., Huang, G., & Yu, P. (2007). Nutritional status and health outcomes for older people with dementia living in institutions. *Journal of Advanced Nursing, 60*(5), 470–477.

McCarron, K. (2007). Jaundice: More than meets the eye. *Nursing Made Incredibly Easy! 5*(3), 25–27.

MedicineNet.com. (2008). Colon cancer: The genetic factor. Retrieved from http://www.medicinenet.com

Molle, E. (2005). Healthier aging: Caring for older adults. Getting down to the lower GI tract. *Nursing, 35*(11), 20–21.

National Digestive Diseases Information Clearinghouse. (2004). Liver biopsy. NIH Publication No. 05-4731.

National Institute of Health. (2008). *Genes and disease; Nutritional and metabolic diseases; The digestive system.* Retrieved from http://www.ncbi.nlm.nih.gov/books/bookres.fegi/gnd/pdf.html

Nelson, R., & Vega, C. (2007). Virtual colonscopy may be used first in screening for colorectal cancer. *Medscape Medical News.* Retrieved from http://www.medscape.com/viewarticle/564041

Porth, C. M., & Matfin, (2009). *Concepts of altered health states* (8th ed.). Philadelphia: Lippincott Williams & Wilkins.

Pullen, R. L. (2008). Preparing a patient for magnetic resonance imaging. *Nursing, 38*(10), 22.

Schoch, L., & Whiteman, K. (2007). Monitoring liver function. *Nursing, 37*(11), 22–23.

Spector, R. E. (2009). *Cultural diversity in health and illness* (7th ed). Upper Saddle River, NJ: Pearson Prentice Hall.

U.S. Department of Health. (2005). *Dietary guidelines for Americans 2005. Key recommendations for the general population.* Retrieved from http://www.health.gov/dietaryguidelines/dga2005/recommendations.htm

U. S. Food and Drug Administration [FDA]. (2009). *FDA warns about risk of wearing medicated patches during MRIs.* Retrieved from http://www.fda.gov/bbs/topics/news/2009/new01967.htm

Weber, J., & Kelley, J. (2009). *Health assessment in nursing* (4th ed.). Philadelphia: Lippincott Williams & Wilkins.

Nursing Care of Patients with Nutritional Disorders

LEARNING OUTCOMES

1. Compare and contrast the pathophysiology and manifestations of nutritional disorders.
2. Identify causes and predict effects of nutritional disorders on patient health status.
3. Explain interdisciplinary care for patients with nutritional disorders.
4. Develop strategies to promote nutrition for patient populations.

CLINICAL COMPETENCIES

1. Assess the functional health status of patients with nutritional disorders.
2. Monitor nutritional status and responses to care; document and report abnormal or unexpected responses.
3. Use assessed data to determine priority nursing diagnoses and implement evidence-based nursing interventions.
4. Administer medications and enteral and parenteral nutrition knowledgeably and safely.
5. Integrate interdisciplinary care in the plan of care.
6. Adapt cultural values and variations into the plan of care for patients with nutritional disorders.
7. Plan and provide patient-centered teaching to restore, promote, and maintain functional health status.
8. Evaluate responses to care and use data to revise plan of care as needed.

 KEY TERMS

anorexia nervosa, *607*
bariatrics, *588*
basal metabolic rate (BMR), *590*
binge-eating disorder, *607*
body mass index (BMI), *588*
bulimia nervosa, *607*

catabolism, *599*
enteral nutrition, *600*
lower body obesity, *590*
malnutrition, *598*
nutrients, *589*
obesity, *588*

parenteral nutrition (PN), *604*
protein-calorie malnutrition (PCM), *599*
starvation, *599*
triglycerides, *590*
upper body obesity, *590*
very low calorie diet (VLCD), *593*

Obesity and malnutrition, the major nutritional disorders in the world today, affect many systems and organs. They often cause serious health problems, such as hypertension, heart disease, fluid and electrolyte imbalances, disability, and death.

Patients with nutritional disorders require complex, skilled nursing care. Developmental, sociocultural, psychologic, and physiologic factors may play a role in these disorders: A holistic approach to nursing care is vital. Before proceeding with the discussion of obesity and malnutrition, review the sections on metabolism and nutrients in ∞ Chapter 21.

The Patient with Obesity

Obesity, an excess of adipose tissue, is one of the most prevalent, preventable health problems in the United States. Obesity has serious physiologic and psychologic consequences, and is associated with increased morbidity and mortality. It contributes to poor health-related quality of life to a greater extent than smoking, excess alcohol use, or poverty. The obesity epidemic has prompted rapid growth in **bariatrics**, the healthcare science that focuses on patients who are extremely obese.

Health-related problems associated with obesity are listed in Table 22–1.

While obesity is often defined by weight, it is more accurately defined by the **body mass index (BMI)**, an indirect measure of the amount of body fat, or adipose tissue. Adipose tissue is created when energy consumption exceeds energy expenditure. A BMI of 25 to 29.9 kg/m^2 is classified as *overweight*; obesity is a BMI of 30 kg/m^2 or greater (Centers for Disease Control and Prevention [CDC], 2009). The terms *overweight* and *obese* are not mutually exclusive; a patient who is obese also is overweight.

FAST FACTS
Prevalence of overweight and obesity in the United States:
- Women
  - Black: 78.2%
  - Hispanic: 76.1%
  - White: 61.2%
- Men
  - Black: 68.5%
  - Hispanic: 79.3%
  - White: 72.6%

TABLE 22–1 Health-Related Problems Associated with Obesity

BODY SYSTEM	OBESITY-RELATED PROBLEMS
Cardiovascular	Atherosclerosis, hypercholesterolemia
	Coronary heart disease
	Heart failure
	Hypertension
	Stroke
	Varicosities
	Venous thrombosis
Respiratory	Asthma
	Sleep apnea
Gastrointestinal	Gallbladder disease
	Hiatal hernia
	Colon cancer
Genitourinary	Prostate cancer
	Stress incontinence
Musculoskeletal	Low back pain
	Muscle strains and sprains
	Osteoarthritis
Endocrine and Reproductive	Diabetes mellitus, type 2
	Breast and endometrial cancers
	Polycystic ovarian syndrome
	Complications of pregnancy
Other	Depression
	Postoperative complications

Incidence and Prevalence

More than 30% of the adult population in the United States is obese; nearly two-thirds of all adults in the United States are overweight. The prevalence of obesity is higher in women and in economically disadvantaged people of all races. While the prevalence of overweight has been increasing since 1960, the prevalence of obesity is increasing to a greater extent, particularly during the past 10 to 15 years (Weight-control Information Network [WIN], 2010). Of particular concern is the increasing incidence of obesity in children and young adults. The prevalence of overweight and obesity varies among ethnic and cultural groups. Adults of Asian heritage generally have a lower incidence of overweight and obesity. See the Focus on Cultural Diversity box that follows.

Risk Factors

Many factors contribute to obesity, including genetic, physiologic, psychologic, environmental, and sociocultural factors. Heredity may contribute up to 40% of the risk for obesity (NHLBI, 1998). The inheritance of obesity does not usually follow a clear Mendelian pattern. There is, however, a strong correlation between the weight of adopted children and their biologic parents, and identical twins tend to have similar BMIs, whether raised together or apart. While several genes that contribute to appetite and fat deposition have been identified, obesity as a purely genetic condition is rare (Fauci et al., 2008).

Physical inactivity is probably the most important factor contributing to obesity. Inactive people may consume fewer calories than active people and continue to gain weight due to lack of energy expenditure. Cultural and environmental factors such as reliance on the automobile for transportation and increased time spent using the computer contribute to decreased energy expenditure among adults in the United States. Increased time spent watching television is seen as a major contributing factor to the increased incidence of obesity among children and adolescents (Fauci et al., 2008).

Environmental influences, such as an abundant and readily accessible food supply, fast-food restaurants, advertising, and vending machines, contribute to increased food intake. Sociocultural influences that contribute to obesity include increased consumption of restaurant meals, overeating at family meals, rewarding behavior with food, religious and family gatherings that promote food intake, and sedentary lifestyles. Socioeconomic status also tends to correlate with the risk for overweight and obesity: In the United States, women with low incomes are more likely to be obese than those of higher socioeconomic status (NHLBI, 2010). The association between socioeconomic status and obesity is less clear in men.

Psychologic factors, such as low self-esteem, also play a role in obesity. Low self-esteem may precipitate unhealthy eating behaviors, and the resulting weight gain in turn may diminish self-image even further. A person may overeat as a result of anxiety, depression, guilt, or boredom, or as a means of getting attention. Some experts characterize overeating as a food addiction and as a coping mechanism for stressful life events.

Overview of Normal Physiology

All body activities require energy, including activities of daily living, as well as those necessary to maintain cell and tissue function. **Nutrients** in food (or enteral or parenteral feedings) provide this energy and are the building blocks for growth and tissue repair. The body stores excess nutrients and energy (measured as kilocalories) to meet the body's needs when required nutrients are unavailable. This ability to store and release energy is important to maintaining body function. A significant portion of daily energy expenditure is fixed: More

FOCUS ON CULTURAL DIVERSITY
Obesity

While the prevalence of overweight and obesity has increased among nearly all populations in the United States, Black women have the highest prevalence (Flegal, Carroll, Ogden, et al., 2010). Cultural factors play a role; historically, large Black women were viewed as wealthy, valued, and able to carry a pregnancy to term (Johnson & Broadnax, 2003). Differences in perception of body image and weight-related concerns also play a role. In general, Black girls and women report less social pressure to be slim, less dissatisfaction with weight and body image, and fewer incidents of discrimination related to weight (Thomas, Moseley, Stallings, Nichols-English, & Wagner, 2008). A sedentary lifestyle also contributes to the rate of obesity. Among African Americans, women of all ages report less regular exercise participation than White women, and men aged 45 and older report less regular exercise than White women (American Obesity Association, 2002).

than 70% of the energy expended each day goes to maintaining the **basal metabolic rate (BMR)**, essentially the "cost" (in kilocalories) of being alive. Physical activity accounts for only 5% to 10% of the energy spent daily (Fauci et al., 2008).

Energy is primarily stored as fat in adipose tissue. Although mature fat cells (adipocytes) do not multiply, the immature cells in adipose tissue can multiply, particularly when exposed to estrogen during puberty, in late adolescence, during breastfeeding, and in middle-aged adults who are overweight. Fat cells store excess energy as **triglycerides**, formed from dietary fats and carbohydrates. The body breaks down the triglycerides in fat cells when needed to provide energy (Porth & Matfin, 2009).

Pathophysiology

Obesity occurs when excess calories are stored as fat. It can result from excess energy intake, decreased energy expenditure, or a combination of both. The etiology of obesity is not as simple as excess kilocalorie intake in relation to energy expenditure.

Energy intake and energy expenditure are regulated by a complex interaction of endocrine and neural signals. In the absence of external influences, these regulatory mechanisms increase appetite and reduce energy expenditure when weight loss occurs, and suppress appetite and increase energy expenditure after overfeeding. In a society where food is abundant and physical activity is limited, the latter is less effective.

Appetite, which affects food intake, is regulated by the central nervous system and by emotional factors. The hunger center in the hypothalamus stimulates appetite in response to stimuli such as hypoglycemia and peptides produced in the gut. As nutrient levels rise, the satiety center (also in the hypothalamus) sends the message to stop eating. Gastrointestinal filling and hormonal factors also signal *satiety* (a sensation of fullness). Appetite may have little relationship to hunger or physical signals, however, people may eat to relieve depression or anxiety.

Several hormones are involved in regulating obesity, including thyroid hormone, insulin, and leptin (a peptide produced by fatty tissue that suppresses appetite and increases energy expenditure). Some studies suggest that leptin resistance is a cause of obesity. Insulin is associated with body fat distribution. The two major types of body fat distribution are upper body and lower body obesity.

Upper body obesity (also called *central obesity*) is identified by a waist-to-hip ratio of greater than 1 in men or 0.8 in women. (∞ See Chapter 21 for a method to calculate the waist-to-hip ratio.) People with upper body obesity tend to have more intra-abdominal fat and higher levels of circulating free fatty acids (Porth & Matfin, 2009). As a result, upper body obesity is associated with a greater risk of complications such as hypertension, abnormal blood lipid levels, heart disease, stroke, and elevated insulin levels. Men tend to have more intra-abdominal fat than women, although women develop a central fat distribution pattern after menopause.

Lower body obesity (also known as *peripheral obesity*), in which the waist-to-hip ratio is less than 0.8, is more commonly seen in women. The risk for hyperinsulinemia, abnormal lipids, and heart disease is lower in people with lower body obesity

than in those with upper body obesity. Lower body obesity may be more difficult to treat, however.

Complications of Obesity

Obesity is a major health risk factor, increasing the risk of mortality from all causes over that of normal-weight people. As obesity increases, so does the risk of dying.

CARDIOVASCULAR DISEASE Obesity is a significant risk factor for cardiovascular disease, including hypertension, coronary heart disease (CHD), and heart failure. The prevalence of hypertension in obese men and women is approximately twice that in people with a BMI of less than 25 (NHLBI, 1998). Several factors contribute to hypertension in obese individuals, including sodium retention with associated increased vascular resistance, blood volume, and cardiac output. The increases in blood pressure seen with obesity increase the risk for CHD and stroke.

Patients who are obese, particularly those who have abdominal obesity, often have a lipid profile that promotes atherosclerosis. Levels of low-density lipoprotein (LDL) and very low density lipoprotein (VLDL) cholesterol and triglycerides are increased, and levels of high density lipoprotein (HDL or desirable) cholesterol are reduced. Furthermore, adipose tissue secretes cytokines that stimulate the liver to produce C-reactive protein (CRP), now recognized as a risk factor for CHD.

These factors account for the fact that many obese individuals have *metabolic syndrome*, a constellation of cardiovascular risk factors, including increased waist circumference, hypertension, elevated blood triglycerides and fasting blood glucose, and low HDL cholesterol. The metabolic syndrome is an identified risk factor for atherosclerosis and CHD.

Obesity increases the risk for heart failure. Left ventricular muscle mass increases, and the ventricle dilates in obese individuals, possibly related to increased blood volume and cardiac output.

RESPIRATORY DISORDERS Overweight and obesity increase the risk for developing asthma in both adults and children. The relationship between obesity and asthma is not clear, but may be related to genetic factors and the connection between obesity and inflammation. Obesity is the major risk factor for obstructive sleep apnea, intermittent airflow obstruction due to upper airway collapse during sleep. Not only is obesity a risk factor for sleep apnea, the reverse also may be true: sleep apnea may predispose patients for weight gain (NHLBI, 2004).

DIABETES MELLITUS Obesity increases the risk of insulin resistance and type 2 diabetes. While not all obese people develop diabetes, up to 80% of people with type 2 diabetes are obese. Both weight gain in adulthood and abdominal (central) obesity are positively correlated with the risk for developing type 2 diabetes (Fauci et al., 2008).

OTHER DISORDERS Obesity affects reproductive function in both men and women. Androgen (male sex hormone) levels are reduced in obese men; menstrual irregularities and polycystic ovarian syndrome (PCOS) are more common in obese women. PCOS is an additional risk factor for hyperinsulinemia and insulin resistance. Increased weight increases the risk for developing gallstones in both men and women. The risk for developing several types of cancer, including colon, breast, and endometrial, increases in obesity. Increased weight places abnormal stress on joints, increasing the prevalence of joint pain and osteoarthritis, particularly in weight-bearing joints (especially the knee joints). Other health-related problems associated with obesity are listed in Table 22–1.

Interdisciplinary Care

Obesity treatment is far more complex than just reducing food consumption. Most experts recommend an individualized program of exercise, diet, and behavior modification designed to meet the patient's specific needs.

Diagnosis

Although body weight may be used to identify obesity, measures of body fat are more accurate. Males at ideal body weight have 10% to 20% body fat, whereas females at ideal body weight have 20% to 30% body fat.

- *Body mass index* is used to identify excess adipose tissue. BMI is calculated by dividing the weight (in kilograms) by the height in meters squared (m^2). See Box 22–1. BMI calculations may not as accurately reflect the extent of adipose tissue in people who are highly muscular (e.g., body builders) or in those who have lost muscle mass (e.g., older adults).
- *Anthropometry* includes measurements of height, weight, bone size, and skinfold to estimate subcutaneous fat. ∞ See Chapter 21 for more information about anthropometric measurements.
- *Underwater weighing (hydrodensitometry)* is considered the most accurate way to determine body fat. This technique involves submerging the whole body and then measuring the amount of displaced water.
- *Bioelectrical impedance* uses a low-energy electrical impulse to determine the percentage of body fat by measuring the electrical resistance of the body.
- *Waist circumference* is measured to determine body fat distribution. Men with a waist measurement of 40 inches (102 cm) or greater and women with a waist measurement of 35 inches (88 cm) or greater have a higher risk for complications of obesity.

Other diagnostic tests may be done to help identify a physiologic cause of obesity, as well as complications of obesity.

- A *thyroid profile* is done to rule out thyroid disease (∞ see Chapter 18).
- *Serum glucose* is measured to identify coexisting diabetes mellitus.

BOX 22–1 Calculating Body Mass Index (BMI)

BMI = weight (kg)/height^2 (m^2)
Normal = BMI 18.5–24.9 kg/m^2
Overweight = BMI 25–29.9 kg/m^2
Obese = BMI > 30 kg/m^2
Extreme obesity = BMI > 40 kg/m^2

- *Serum cholesterol* is measured to assess for elevated levels.
- A *lipid profile* is ordered; high-density lipoprotein (HDL) levels may be reduced in obese patients, whereas low-density lipoprotein (LDL) levels are elevated.
- An *electrocardiogram (ECG)* is performed to detect effects of obesity on the heart, such as rate or rhythm disruptions, myocardial infarction, or heart enlargement.

Medications

Drug therapy may be used when the patient is at increased medical risk as a result of obesity; it is not recommended for "cosmetic" weight loss. When used in combination with diet and exercise, drugs can help promote weight loss. Prescription weight loss drugs are approved for use only in patients with a BMI of 30 and above, and those with a BMI of 27 or higher and an obesity-related condition such as hypertension, type 2 diabetes, or an abnormal lipid profile. Weight-loss drugs generally fall into one of two classes: appetite suppressants and lipase inhibitors.

Sibutramine (Meridia) is an appetite suppressant that acts on the CNS. Sibutramine may increase the metabolic rate, promoting weight loss, and it has an antidepressant effect. Sibutramine increases the pulse rate and blood pressure, potentially limiting its use in patients with hypertension, CHD, or heart failure. Other drugs used as appetite suppressants include amphetamines and nonamphetamines, and antidepressants such a bupropion (Wellbutrin, Zyban) and fluoxetine (Prozac). None of these drugs are approved for long-term use as appetite suppressants. Amphetamines carry a high abuse potential and are not approved for treating obesity. Nonamphetamines such as diethylpropion (Tenuate) and phentermine (Adipex-P) may be used, but also increase pulse rate and blood pressure.

Orlistat (Xenical) is a lipase inhibitor, reducing fat absorption from the GI tract, leading to weight loss. It reduces blood glucose and total and LDL cholesterol levels, and lowers blood pressure. The adverse effects of orlistat relate to its inhibition of fat absorption: oily stools, flatulence, and fecal urgency. These effects tend to diminish when dietary fat intake is limited. See the Medication Administration box on page 593 for the nursing implications of these drugs.

Rimonabant (Acomplia) is a new drug currently under review by the FDA for use in weight loss, smoking cessation, and to lower cholesterol. The drug works in the brain to suppress appetite and the craving for nicotine, and in the periphery to decrease insulin resistance and improve the lipid profile (Lehne, 2007).

Treatments

Successful treatment of obesity (sustained achievement of normal body weight without adverse consequences) is rarely achieved. Treatment focuses on reducing the health risks associated with obesity by changing both eating and exercise habits. A pound of body fat is equivalent to 3500 kcal. To lose 1 pound a person must reduce daily caloric intake by 500 kcal for 7 days or increase activity enough to burn the equivalent kilocalories. A weight loss goal of 1 to 2 pounds per week and a 10% reduction in body weight in 6 months of therapy is recommended (NHLBI, 2000). A combination of physical activity, dietary therapy, behavior modification, pharmacology, and, in some cases, surgery is required to achieve and maintain weight loss (Table 22–2).

MEDICATION ADMINISTRATION **Drugs to Treat Obesity**

APPETITE SUPPRESSANTS
Phentermine (Adipex-P, Fastin, Ionamin, Obestin-30, Oby-Trim, others)
Sibutramine (Meridia)

Phentermine acts directly on the appetite-control center in the CNS to suppress the appetite and reduce hunger. Sibutramine reduces hunger and increases sensations of satiety by inhibiting the uptake of serotonin, norepinephrine, and dopamine. These drugs may be used to treat obesity in patients with a BMI of > 30 kg/m^2 and obese patients who have risk factors such as diabetes or hypertension.

Nursing Responsibilities
- Assess for contraindications, such as pregnancy or lactation, use of other appetite suppressants, impaired liver or kidney function, history of CHD, or alcohol abuse.
- Regularly monitor blood pressure and heart rate during treatment. Increases may indicate need to reduce dose or discontinue treatment.

Health Education for the Patient and Family
- Take as directed; do not exceed recommended dose. Do not take if you may be pregnant or are nursing.
- Take your last dose no later than 4 PM to avoid insomnia.
- You may experience difficulty sleeping, nervousness, or palpitations while taking this drug.

- Increase your fluid intake to reduce possible side effects of dry mouth and constipation.
- This drug does not replace diet and exercise for weight loss; continue to follow your prescribed regimen.

LIPASE INHIBITOR
Orlistat (Alli, Xenical)

Orlistat inhibits lipases necessary for the breakdown and absorption of fat, thus decreasing the absorption of dietary fat. Its action is primarily local, within the GI tract, with few systemic effects.

Nursing Responsibilities
- Administer with meals or up to 1 hour following a meal.
- Provide a fat-soluble vitamin supplement (A, D, E, and K) daily. Separate administration time from orlistat by at least 2 hours.

Health Education for the Patient and Family
- Take as directed; do not increase dose. You may skip a dose if you do not consume a meal.
- Use in conjunction with a low-calorie, low-fat diet.
- Common gastrointestinal side effects include oily or fatty stools, flatulence, oily discharge, or frequent stools with difficulty controlling defecation. These side effects may diminish with time or increase if a meal high in fat is consumed.
- Notify your healthcare provider if you become pregnant while taking this medication.

EXERCISE Exercise is a critical element in weight loss and maintenance. Physical activity increases energy consumption and promotes weight loss while preserving lean body mass. Physical activity improves physical fitness, decreases appetite, promotes self-esteem, and increases the basal metabolic rate. The Centers for Disease Control and Prevention (CDC) recommend that all adults engage in both aerobic and muscle-strengthening activities each week. Table 22–3 outlines CDC activity recommendations and gives example activities to achieve goals. Activities should be spread throughout the week, and may be spread over the course of the day; however, it is important to expend moderate or vigorous effort for at least 10 minutes at a time when exercising (CDC, 2008).

Because fitness levels differ, patients may be taught to use their target heart rate or perceived exertion to "measure" the vigor of activities. The *target heart rate* is calculated based on maximum heart rate; in turn, maximum heart rate is estimated

using the formula 220 minus age in years. For example, while the maximum heart rate for a 35-year-old is 185 beats per minute (bpm), it would be 155 bpm for someone who is 65 years old. While the target heart rate for the 35-year-old engaging in vigorous intensity activity would be 130 to 157 bpm, it would be 108 to 132 bpm for the older adult. Perceived exertion is a subjective rating of activity intensity, using self evaluation of factors such as heart and respiratory rate, sweating, and muscle fatigue (CDC, 2008).

NUTRITION The diet is planned to create a daily 500- to 1000-kcal deficit. Ideally, the diet should be low in kilocalories and fat and contain adequate nutrients, minerals, and fiber. The patient should eat regular meals with small servings. A gradual, slow weight loss of no more than 1 to 2 pounds per week is recommended. This means a diet of 1000 to 1200 kcal/day for most women, and 1200 to 1600 kcal/day for most men. Fewer

TABLE 22–2 Treatment Recommendations for Overweight and Obesity

TREATMENT	BMI				
	25–26.9	27–29.9	30–34.9	35–39.9	≥40
Diet, exercise, and behavior modification	With two or more comorbidities[1]	With two or more comorbidities[1]	Yes	Yes	Yes
Pharmacotherapy[2]		With two or more comorbidities[1]	Yes	Yes	Yes
Surgery				With two or more comorbidities[1]	

[1]For example, hypertension, hyperlipidemia, diabetes, and other obesity-related complications.

[2]Considered when 6 months of combined therapy has not produced a loss of 1 pound per week.

Source: Adapted from National Institutes of Health; National Heart, Lung, and Blood Institute; North American Association for the Study of Obesity. (2000). *The practical guide: Identification, evaluation, and treatment of overweight and obesity in adults.* Bethesda, MD: NIH.

TABLE 22–3 CDC Physical Activity Recommendations for Adults

ACTIVITY	RECOMMENDATION	EXAMPLES
Aerobic activity:	Engage in moderate- or vigorous-intensity activity for at least the recommended amount of time weekly, or in an equivalent combination of moderate- and vigorous-intensity activity.	
■ Moderate-intensity aerobic activity (target heart rate of 50% to 70% of maximum heart rate)	2 hours and 30 minutes (150 minutes) every week	■ Walking fast ■ Water aerobics ■ Bicycle riding on level ground ■ Doubles tennis ■ Ballroom dancing ■ Pushing a lawn mower ■ General gardening
■ Vigorous-intensity aerobic activity (target heart rate of 70% to 85% of maximum heart rate)	1 hour and 15 minutes (75 minutes) every week	■ Race walking, jogging, running ■ Swimming laps ■ Singles tennis ■ Aerobic dancing ■ Bicycling 10 mph or faster ■ Heavy gardening (continuous hoeing or digging) ■ Hiking uphill
Muscle-strengthening activities	2 or more days per week: at least one set of 8 to 12 repetitions for all major muscle groups	■ Lifting weights ■ Using resistance bands ■ Exercises that use body weight for resistance (push-ups, sit-ups) ■ Heavy gardening ■ Yoga

Source: Centers for Disease Control and Prevention (CDC). (2008). *Physical activity for everyone.* Atlanta, GA: Author.

than 1200 kcal each day may lead to loss of lean tissue and nutritional deficiencies. The recommended diet generally is low in fat and high in dietary fiber (Table 22–4). Recent research shows equivalent weight loss among different diets (e.g., low-fat, low-carbohydrate, or high-protein diets); adherence to the diet and participation in group sessions were shown to be the significant factors (Sacks et al., 2009). Excessive calorie restrictions can lead to failure to follow the prescribed diet, feelings of guilt, and

overeating. "Yo-yo" dieting (repeated cycles of weight loss and gain) may lead to a metabolic deficiency that makes subsequent weight loss efforts increasingly difficult.

Very low calorie diets (VLCDs) are generally reserved for patients who have a BMI greater than 30 (WIN, 2008). This type of program offers a protein-sparing modified fast (800 kcal/day or less) under close medical supervision. VLCDs typically use commercially prepared formulas (liquid shakes or bars) to replace all food intake for several weeks or months, resulting in rapid weight loss while maintaining lean body mass. Exercise, nutrition, and behavior modification counseling should accompany the diet. Benefits include decreased blood pressure, blood glucose, and cholesterol and triglyceride levels, along with improved exercise tolerance. VLCDs may not be appropriate for use in people over age 50 due to normal loss of lean body mass and adverse effects such as fatigue, constipation, nausea, diarrhea, and gallstone formation. In the long term, weight gain is common, and VLCDs may be no more effective for weight loss than a diet that includes 800 to 1000 daily kcal (WIN, 2008).

BEHAVIOR MODIFICATION Behavior modification is a critical component of successful weight management. See the research box on p. 592. Strategies such as keeping food records, eliminating cues that precipitate eating, and changing the act of eating are often helpful.

Recording food intake, amount, location of eating, and situations that induce eating often help the patient gain self-control. Researchers have found that most overweight people are stimulated to eat by external cues, such as the proximity to food and the time of day. In contrast, hunger and satiety are the cues that regulate eating in adults of normal weight. Strategies to control food cues include keeping food out of view, eliminating snack

TABLE 22–4 Recommended Nutrient Intake for Weight Loss

NUTRIENT	RECOMMENDED INTAKE
Calories	1000 to 1600 per day or approximately 500 to 1000 less than usual daily intake
Total fat	30% or less of total calories
Saturated fats	10% or less of total calories
Cholesterol	< 300 mg/day
Protein (from plant and lean animal sources)	Approximately 15% of total calories
Carbohydrate (complex carbohydrates from vegetables, fruits, and whole grains)	55% or more of total calories
Fiber (e.g., oat bran, legumes, barley, most fruits and vegetables)	20 to 30 g/day
Sodium chloride	< 2.4 g sodium or 6 g sodium chloride/day
Calcium	1000 to 1500 mg/day

Source: Adapted from National Institutes of Health; National Heart, Lung, and Blood Institute; North American Association for the Study of Obesity. (2000). *The practical guide: Identification, evaluation, and treatment of overweight and obesity in adults.* Bethesda, MD: NIH.

MOVING EVIDENCE INTO ACTION   The Overweight Patient

What are the most effective strategies to promote weight loss? The type and number of strategies are as diverse as the population, with avid proponents of each. Recent research by Sacks et al. (2008) of the Harvard School of Public Health showed virtually no difference in the amount of weight loss, satiety, hunger, or satisfaction with the diet for groups following diets that emphasized specific nutrients (fat, protein, or carbohydrate). All participants lost weight and their cardiovascular risk factors improved. The strongest predictor of weight loss was attendance at group sessions. A study by Turner, Thomas, Wagner, & Moseley (2008) produced further evidence to support the importance of behavior change to effective weight loss. In their study, patients were allowed to choose their preferred diet from among a low-calorie, low-fat, or low-carbohydrate plan. All patients participated in weekly groups presenting behavior change strategies; fitness activities and a group session with an aerobics instructor were available as part of the program. No significant difference in weight loss was found among the different diet plans. Participating in exercise, on the other hand, made a significant difference. Average weight loss ranged from 2.1 lbs for participants who did not attend the exercise program at all to 9.4 lbs for those who attended three sessions.

IMPLICATIONS FOR NURSING

Achieving and maintaining significant weight loss is a struggle for most overweight and obese patients. Patients frequently seek advice from nurses and other healthcare practitioners about the "best" diet and the "best" way to meet their weight-loss goals. Current evidence points to the importance of using a multidisciplinary approach to behavior change and weight loss: reduced calorie intake, regular exercise, and support groups or programs to help identify and maintain changes in eating behaviors.

CRITICAL THINKING IN PATIENT CARE

1. Although research shows that reducing total calorie intake is more important than emphasizing or limiting intake of fats, carbohydrate, or protein, many people "swear by" a specific diet plan. What factors do you think contribute to the belief that one specific diet is more effective than another?
2. Exercise is consistently shown to be a significant factor in achieving and maintaining weight loss. How does exercise contribute to weight loss?
3. Develop a teaching plan to help a 72-year-old woman with osteoarthritis of her knees achieve CDC recommendations for aerobic and muscle-strengthening activities (see Table 22–4).

foods, and eating only in designated areas. See Box 22–2 for a list of behavior modification strategies.

Other strategies focus on helping patients examine factors such as lifestyle, personality, and environment that affect eating behaviors. The goal is to empower the overweight individual to choose activities that are not related to food.

Social support and group programs such as Weight Watchers, Overeaters Anonymous, and Take Off Pounds Sensibly (TOPS) promote weight loss success through peer support. Most organized programs require participants to pay a fee, which may improve compliance.

SURGERY   Surgical treatment of obesity (*bariatric surgery*) generally is limited to extremely obese patients (BMI of over 40 kg/m^2) or those who have serious obesity-related problems such as type 2 diabetes, coronary heart disease, or severe sleep apnea (WIN, 2008). In addition, patients must be able to tolerate surgery and be free of addiction to alcohol or other drugs. The benefits of surgery include major weight loss and improved blood pressure, plus a reduced risk of diabetes, sleep apnea, angina, heart failure, blood lipid levels, and venous disease. Bariatric surgery, however, is not without risk, and the decision to undergo surgery is a significant one.

The most common bariatric surgical procedures are adjustable gastric banding, gastric bypass, gastric sleeve, and biliopancreatic bypass with duodenal switch. These procedures restrict stomach capacity, limiting food intake, and, in most cases, bypass a portion of the small intestine to restrict absorption of calories and nutrients. In many cases, they can be performed laparoscopically.

In the Roux-en-Y gastric bypass (RGB, Figure 22–1A ■), a small stomach pouch is created to restrict food intake. A Y-shaped section of the jejunum is then attached to the pouch to allow food to bypass the lower stomach and duodenum. As

BOX 22–2   Behavioral Change Strategies for the Obese Patient

Controlling the Environment
- Purchase low-calorie foods.
- Shop from a prepared list and on a full stomach.
- Keep all foods in the kitchen.
- Store all foods in the refrigerator or in the cabinets in opaque containers.
- Prepare exact portions of food to eliminate leftovers.
- Eat all foods in the same place, avoid eating in the kitchen.
- Avoid eating when watching television or reading.
- Reduce frequency of eating out at restaurants, parties, and picnics.

Controlling Physiologic Responses to Food
- Eat slowly by taking small bites, allowing 20 minutes for a meal.
- Eat a salad or drink a hot beverage before a meal.
- Chew each bite thoroughly and slowly.
- Put eating utensils or food down between bites.
- Concentrate on the eating process, savor the food.
- Stop eating with the first feelings of fullness.

Controlling Psychologic Responses to Food
- Appreciate the aesthetic experience of eating.
- Use attractive dinnerware, and prepare a formal setting for eating.
- Use small plates and cups to make servings of food look larger.
- Concentrate on conversations and socialization during the meal.
- Use nonfood rewards for meeting a goal.
- Acknowledge small successes and improvements in all behavior.
- Substitute other activities for eating (e.g., reading, exercise, hobbies).

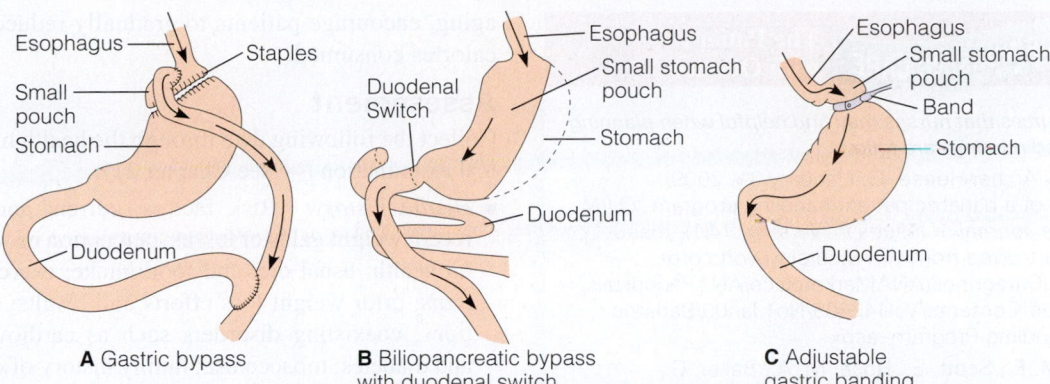

Figure 22–1 ■ Surgical procedures to treat obesity. *A*, Roux-en-Y gastric bypass surgery; *B*, Biliopancreatic diversion; *C*, Adjustable gastric banding.

a result, calorie and nutrient absorption is limited. The biliopancreatic diversion (BPD, Figure 22–1*B*) is a more complex procedure and carries a higher risk of nutritional deficiencies. This surgery may be performed in two stages, with the majority of the stomach removed and a gastric sleeve created during the first stage. In BPD, the duodenum and jejunum are bypassed by connecting the ileum directly to the stomach pouch or just distal to the pyloric valve.

These surgeries that restrict nutrient intake and absorption produce rapid weight loss that is maintained over time. Many patients maintain a significant weight loss for 10 years or more, with improvement in obesity-associated health problems such as type 2 diabetes, hypertension, and sleep apnea. Because these procedures allow food to bypass the duodenum and jejunum, nutrient deficiencies are common, particularly of iron, calcium, vitamin B$_{12}$, and, possibly, the fat-soluble vitamins.

Restrictive procedures, such as adjustable gastric banding (AGB, Figure 22–1*C*), are safer but generally less effective in the long term. In AGB, a hollow band of silicone rubber is placed around the upper (proximal) portion of the stomach. The band is inflated with saline solution to create a small stomach pouch with a narrow passage through to the rest of the stomach. The amount of band inflation can be adjusted using a port implanted under the skin. Few nutritional deficiencies are associated with restrictive bariatric procedures. Vomiting is a common postoperative risk with restrictive procedures. The band may slip or break, necessitating a return to surgery. While patients typically lose about 50% of their excess body weight within the first year after these procedures, fewer maintain that weight loss over a 10-year period than those undergoing gastric bypass.

Although the risk for postoperative complications is high, the mortality rate for bariatric procedures is low (less than 1% for restrictive surgeries and up to 5% for combination procedures). Possible postoperative complications include anastomosis leak with peritonitis, abdominal wall hernia, gallstones, wound infections, deep venous thrombosis, nutritional deficiencies, and gastrointestinal symptoms. Dumping syndrome, which can be precipitated by a meal high in simple carbohydrates, may develop following gastric bypass surgeries. In dumping syndrome, stomach contents move rapidly through the small intestine, drawing fluid into the intestine by osmosis. The patient experiences nausea, bloating, abdominal pain, weakness, sweating, and possibly syncope. ∞ See Chapter 23 for more information about dumping syndrome.

Nursing care for the patient who has undergone bariatric surgery is substantially the same as for a patient who has undergone a gastric resection. ∞ See Chapter 23 for more information about gastric resection and associated nursing care. Bariatric patients have additional nursing care needs related to their obesity. See the box on page 596.

Maintaining Weight Loss

Losing weight and maintaining that loss are two separate but related issues. Most experts agree that the majority of dieters regain lost weight within a 2-year period. The potential risks associated with regaining weight make maintenance a critical issue. Patients are encouraged to continue exercise, self-monitoring, and treatment support. Long-term weight loss and maintenance mean a lifelong commitment to significant lifestyle changes, including food and eating habits, activity and exercise routines, and behavior modification. Failure to maintain weight loss can lead to feelings of inadequacy, powerlessness, and hopelessness.

✍ Nursing Care

Health Promotion

Maintaining a healthy weight throughout the life span begins in childhood. Obese children and teenagers become obese adults. Promote healthy eating, including a diet rich in whole grains, fruits, and vegetables and low in fat. The USDA Food Guide Pyramid (∞ Chapter 2) and the Healthy Eating Pyramid provide visual guidance for appropriate food choices to maintain a healthy, well-balanced diet. Encourage all children and adults to maintain an active lifestyle, engaging in at least 30 minutes of aerobic activity daily. Encourage parents to limit time children spend watching television, using the computer, and playing video games. Discuss the effects of smoking and excess alcohol use on nutrition and activity. To reduce weight gain commonly associated with

EVIDENCE FOR NURSING CARE — The Patient with Obesity

Selected resources that nurses may find helpful when planning evidence-based nursing care follow.

- Muir, M. & Archer-Heese, G. (January 31, 2009). Essentials of a bariatric patient handling program. *OJIN: The Online Journal of Issues in Nursing, 14*(1), manuscript 5. Retrieved from www.nursingworld.org/MainMenuCategories/ANAMarketplace/ANAPeriodicals/OJIN/TableofContents/Vol142009/No1Jan09/Bariatric-Patient-Handling-Program-.aspx
- Pokorny, M. E., Scott, E., Rose, M. A., Baker, G., Swanson, M., Waters, W., et al. (2009). Challenges in caring for morbidly obese patients. *Home Healthcare Nurse: The Journal for the Home Care and Hospice Professional, 27*(1), 43–52.

aging, encourage patients to gradually reduce the amount of calories consumed.

Assessment

Collect the following data through the health history and physical examination (∞ see Chapter 21):

- *Health history:* Risk factors; current and usual weight; recent weight gains or losses; perception of weight and effect on health; usual diet and food intake; exercise/activity patterns; prior weight loss efforts and results; current medications; coexisting disorders such as cardiovascular disease and diabetes; tobacco use; family history of overweight, diabetes, and weight-related morbidity.
- *Physical examination:* Vital signs; weight (use a scale of adequate capacity) and height; skinfold measurements; waist-to-hip ratio; BMI; inspect skin under the breasts and abdominal folds.

NURSING CARE
The Bariatric Patient Undergoing Surgery

Severely obese patients undergoing bariatric or general surgery have unique nursing care needs to ensure personal and caregiver safety.

- Obtain a thorough preoperative health history and physical assessment (including skin assessment). Note any limitations of mobility or assistive devices used. *Bariatric patients often have multiple chronic health problems that may affect postoperative assessment and recovery. Skin folds are at high risk for fungal infections that may compromise immune protection. Knowing about and providing assistive devices to accommodate mobility limitations will help promote early postoperative mobilization and reduce the risk for complications.*
- Obtain equipment of appropriate size and weight capacity, including bed, mechanical lifts, expanded-capacity wheelchair, walker, commode, bedside chair (without arms), sphygmomanometer, and scale. Clearly label any equipment provided by the patient. *Appropriately sized equipment is vital to promote the patient's comfort and safety. Equipment made to meet the needs of patients who are within normal weight and BMI measurements may fail or the patient may not be able to sit or recline without the risk of falling.*
- Provide friction-reducing devises such as sliders, foam, or pressure-reducing mattresses. *Following surgery, mobility may be limited. Special equipment facilitates skin care while helping maintain patient and caregiver safety.*
- Ensure training and availability of nursing staff in adequate numbers to ensure patient and caregiver safety during position changes, transfers, and caregiving activities such as hygiene. *Even with use of appropriate lifts, sliders, and other devices, as many as six to eight caregivers may be necessary to safely move and transfer the bariatric patient.*
- Elevate the head of the bed. Apply continuous positive airway pressure (CPAP) device as ordered. *Thoracic and abdominal fat may restrict lung capacity, particularly when the patient is supine. Elevating the head of the bed reduces the pressure of abdominal fat on the diaphragm. Patients who are obese are at risk for obstructive sleep apnea due to upper airway collapse; CPAP helps maintain upper airway patency.*
- Frequently monitor level of consciousness and respiratory status (rate, breath sounds, oxygen saturation). *The postsurgical bariatric patient may sequester anesthetic agents in fatty tissue, increasing the risk for respiratory depression after surgery.*
- Initiate cardiac monitoring and compare heart rhythm to preoperative ECG. Promptly report changes in rate or rhythm, such as frequent PVCs (∞ see Chapter 30). *The obese patient is at significant risk for coronary heart disease; surgery and anesthesia place an additional risk for cardiovascular complications. Development of dysrhythmias not seen preoperatively may indicate myocardial ischemia, hypoxia, or electrolyte imbalance.*
- Assess peripheral pulses, skin color, and temperature of extremities. Apply elastic compression stockings or sequential compression device of appropriate size for the patient. Teach and remind to perform foot and leg exercises. *The obese patient is at significant risk for developing deep venous thrombosis due to alterations in clotting and immobility. Furthermore, multiple risk factors for atherosclerosis increase the likelihood of peripheral vascular disease and impaired circulation.*
- Assess pain level and analgesic effectiveness frequently. *Maintaining adequate pain relief is important to promote lung expansion and prevent respiratory complications in the bariatric patient.*
- Regularly monitor blood glucose levels, administering insulin as ordered. *Surgery is a physiologic stressor that causes increased cortisol levels that, in turn, can increase blood glucose levels.*
- Provide meticulous wound care, using strict aseptic technique and frequently assessing for signs of infection. *Excess adipose tissue impairs healing and immune function. Wound infection further delays healing and can be difficult to eradicate.*

Nursing Diagnoses and Interventions

Nursing care for overweight and obese patients is community based and holistic, focusing on both physiologic and psychologic responses to weight and appearance. See the following Case Study & Nursing Care Plan for the patient with obesity.

Imbalanced Nutrition: More than Body Requirements

Although many factors contribute to obesity, it always involves an imbalance of kcal consumption to energy expenditure.

- Encourage the patient to identify the factors that contribute to excess food intake. *Identification of cues to eating helps the patient eliminate or reduce these cues.*
- Establish realistic weight loss goals and exercise/activity objectives. *Small, reasonable goals, such as loss of 1 to 2 pounds per week, increase the likelihood of success.*
- Assess the patient's knowledge and discuss diet plan options. Provide necessary teaching about diet. *Current research (Sacks et al., 2009) shows no significant difference in the efficacy of selected diet plans. Offering a selection of appropriate diet plans empowers the patient to choose a plan that best matches food preferences and lifestyle.*
- Discuss behavior modification strategies, such as self-monitoring and environmental management. *Behavior modification, diet, and exercise are critical to promoting successful, long-term weight loss.*
- Monitor weight loss, blood pressure, and laboratory data, including blood glucose and lipid levels. *Continuing assessment not only is important to evaluate the safety of weight loss strategies, but also to reinforce positive benefits of weight loss.*

Activity Intolerance

Obese patients may experience excess fatigue, tachycardia, and shortness of breath with activity due to the physiologic effects of excess weight as well as a sedentary lifestyle. A medical evaluation may be needed before beginning an exercise program.

- Assess current activity level and tolerance of that activity. Assess vital signs. *This provides baseline information to plan an activity program and assess response to that activity.*
- After medical clearance, plan with the patient a program of regular, gradually increasing exercise. If desired, plan several 10 to 15 minute exercise periods over the course of the day. Develop plans for gradually increasing the duration and intensity of exercise. Consider a consultation with an exercise physiologist. *An individualized exercise program promotes activities within the patient's physical capabilities.*

Ineffective Therapeutic Regimen Management

Most overweight or obese patients experience some difficulty integrating all the components of a weight loss program into a daily routine. To be successful, the overweight patient must modify dietary intake in a world of daily temptations. There may be many obstacles to exercise, including a busy schedule, activity intolerance, impaired physical mobility, lack of equipment, and the embarrassment of being fat.

- Discuss ability and willingness to incorporate changes into daily patterns of diet, exercise, and lifestyle. *This provides data from which to set realistic goals with the patient.*
- Help the patient identify behavior modification strategies and support systems for weight loss and maintenance. *Weight loss and maintenance are most successful if the patient establishes lifestyle patterns that promote interest and motivation and thus exercise and diet management. Family and social support is critical to successful adherence to the therapeutic regime (Turner, Thomas, Wagner, & Moseley, 2008).*
- Have the patient establish strategies for dealing with "stress" eating or interruptions in the therapeutic regime. *A sense of failure associated with overeating or lack of exercise can lead to further overeating. Identifying positive strategies to deal with these situations promotes self-acceptance and limits self-punishment through overeating.*

Chronic Low Self-Esteem

Most overweight and obese individuals verbalize the experience of "fat prejudice," ridicule, embarrassment, and health problems attributed to being "fat." These experiences, coupled with problems such as finding attractive clothing or a chair large enough to sit on can affect self-esteem. Many patients report that "fat" jokes or comments contribute to a sense of negative self-worth.

- Encourage the patient to verbalize the experience of being overweight, and validate the patient's experience. *This provides baseline data to use in developing individualized interventions to address self-esteem issues.*
- Set small goals with the patient and offer positive feedback and encouragement. *Small goals provide more opportunities for success. Positive feedback and encouragement provide a comfortable environment in which to develop self-esteem.*
- Refer for counseling as appropriate. *Many patients benefit from counseling for issues related to self-esteem.*

Using NANDA, NIC, and NOC

Linkages between a selected NANDA nursing diagnosis, NIC, and NOC for the patient for obese patients are shown in the chart that follows.

Community-Based Care

Weight reduction usually occurs in community-based settings. Weight loss and maintenance require a long-term commitment by the patient, family, and support systems. Address the following topics with the patient and family:

- Lifestyle changes are more effective than diets. Fad diets promote rapid weight loss but often are not nutritionally sound or may be difficult to maintain for a lifetime.

NANDA, NIC, AND NOC LINKAGES
The Patient with Obesity

NANDA

Imbalanced Nutrition:
More than Body Requirements

NIC

Nutrition Management
Weight Reduction Assistance
Behavior Modification
Body Image Enhancement
Self-Esteem Enhancement

NOC

Nutrition Status
Nutritional Status: Nutrient Intake
Weight Loss Behavior
Body Image
Self-Esteem

Data from NANDA International. (2009). *Nursing diagnoses: Definitions & classification 2009–2011.* Oxford, UK: Wiley-Blackwell; Bulechek, G., Butcher, H., & Dochterman, J. (Eds.). (2008). *Nursing interventions classification (NIC)* (5th ed.). St. Louis, MO: Mosby; and Moorhead, S., Johnson, M., Maas, M., & Swanson, E. (Eds.). (2008). *Nursing outcomes classification (NOC)* (4th ed.). St. Louis, MO: Mosby.

- All household members should consume a diet that is nutritionally sound, low in fat, and high in fiber.
- Establish realistic weight loss goals and a system of nonfood rewards for achieving each goal.
- Identify an "exercise buddy" or support system to promote continued physical activity.
- Expect occasional failures. Resume prescribed diet and exercise routine as soon as possible; the goal is long-term weight management.
- Community resources such as Weight Watchers, TOPS, or health-care-based programs provide information, strategies, and support for successful weight management.

The Patient with Malnutrition

Malnutrition results from inadequate intake of nutrients. There may be a lack of major nutrients (calories, carbohydrates, proteins, and fats) or micronutrients such as vitamins and minerals. Malnutrition may be caused by inadequate nutrient intake; impaired absorption and use of nutrients; loss of nutrients due to diarrhea, hemorrhage, or renal failure; or increased metabolic needs (e.g., infection or physiologic stressors).

CASE STUDY & NURSING CARE PLAN   A Patient with Obesity

Sam Elliott, aged 57, has gained 30 pounds since his retirement 2 years ago.

The most active thing he does each day is "puttering around" and "walking to the end of the driveway to get the mail." His diet includes juice, oatmeal, muffin, and coffee with cream for breakfast; donuts and coffee with friends mid-morning; a bologna-and-cheese sandwich with chips and a root beer for lunch; and cheese, crackers, and wine before a dinner of meat, potatoes, vegetables, and dessert. He tells the nurse, "I have never had to diet. I just don't know how to get this weight off."

ASSESSMENT

Mr. Elliott is 5' 8" (173 cm) tall and weighs 201 lb (91.2 kg). His BMI is 30.1 kg/m². His cholesterol is 240 mg/dL (normal 150 to 200 mg/dL) with an HDL of 37 mg/dL (normal male value > 45 mg/dL) and an LDL of 180 mg/dL (normal < 130 mg/dL). His BP is 138/90. His fasting blood glucose is normal at 103 mg/dL. His ECG shows normal sinus rhythm. He reports fatigue and shortness of breath with activity. His healthcare provider has advised a weight loss of 30 pounds and a regular exercise program.

DIAGNOSES

- *Imbalanced Nutrition: More than Body Requirements* related to food intake in excess of energy expenditure
- *Risk for Ineffective Therapeutic Regimen Management* related to knowledge deficit
- *Activity Intolerance* related to sedentary lifestyle

EXPECTED OUTCOMES

- Lose 1 pound each week.
- Walk 30 minutes 5 days each week.
- Verbalize an understanding of the relationship between weight loss, weight control, and exercise.
- Identify behavior modification strategies to avoid overeating.
- Identify support systems for behavior modification.

PLANNING AND IMPLEMENTATION

- Assess weight and blood pressure once or twice each week.
- Discuss current eating habits and strategies to reduce fat and calorie intake.
- Discuss cues that promote eating. Identify strategies to eliminate or reduce eating cues.
- Teach to keep a food diary to examine and change eating habits.
- Discuss the role of regular exercise in weight loss and weight control. Instruct to maintain an exercise record to track the intensity and duration of activity.
- Discuss lifestyle and behavior modification strategies to promote successful weight loss and control.

EVALUATION

Two weeks after changing his diet and beginning to exercise, Mr. Elliott has lost 2 pounds. He has maintained a food diary. He has identified boredom as a cue to eating. In light of that fact, he has started volunteering at the local hospital, where he is working with children. He is walking for 30 minutes 5 days a week. He plans to increase his activity periods to 45 minutes. He verbalizes commitment to a lifelong plan of exercising and eating a low-fat diet. His BP has ranged from 132/76 to 136/84. He plans to have the employee health nurse at the hospital check his weight and BP each week and to join Weight Watchers for ongoing support.

CRITICAL THINKING IN THE NURSING PROCESS

1. What are some possible pathophysiologic bases for Mr. Elliott's abnormal cholesterol, HDL, and LDL levels?
2. Develop a teaching plan for a group of overweight men and women.
3. Identify potential barriers to losing weight and strategies to reduce or eliminate these barriers.

See Evaluating Your Response in Appendix C.

Incidence and Prevalence

Malnutrition is a widespread cause of disease and mortality throughout the world. It is endemic in regions affected by famine. Groups at risk for malnutrition in the United States include the young, poor, elderly, homeless, low-income women, and ethnic minorities. Even when food is plentiful, patients may be undernourished because of poor food choices.

It is estimated that one-third to one-half of all hospitalized patients are malnourished (Fauci et al., 2008). Malnutrition may be present on admission or develop as a result of surgery or serious illness. Malnutrition increases both mortality and the incidence of complications in both medical and surgical patients. The incidence of malnutrition is even higher in long-term care residents, where up to 85% of residents may be malnourished (DiMaria-Ghalili & Amella, 2005).

Risk Factors

Risk factors for malnutrition include the following:

- Age—older adults are at greater risk for malnutrition due to a variety of factors (See the accompanying Meeting Individualized Needs box.)
- Poverty, homelessness, inadequate food storage and preparation facilities
- Functional health problems that limit mobility or vision
- History of weight loss of more than 20% of usual weight
- Oral or gastrointestinal problems that affect food intake, digestion, and absorption
- Inability to eat for 5 or more days
- Chronic pain or chronic diseases such as pulmonary, cardiovascular, renal, or endocrine disorders, or cancer
- Dementia, mental health disorders, eating disorders
- Medications or treatments that affect appetite
- Alcohol or drug addition
- Acute problems such as infection, surgery, or trauma

Pathophysiology

Carbohydrates and fats in the diet are the body's primary energy source. Approximately 15% to 25% of the body is fat, the body's energy reservoir. The remainder (muscles, bones, other body tissues and organs) is lean body mass, metabolically active tissue. Proteins in the diet primarily are used to maintain this tissue. Glycogen and proteins in this lean body mass also act as energy stores.

When dietary intake of nutrients does not meet the body's energy needs, the body uses glycogen, body proteins, and lipids (fats) to support metabolism. In **starvation** (inadequate dietary intake), glycogen initially is used to provide energy. After the first 24 hours of starvation, gluconeogenesis (formation of glucose from proteins) is the major source of energy. As starvation continues, the body breaks down fats into free fatty acids and ketones, which provide energy for the brain. The size of all body compartments is reduced as body fats and muscle proteins are used to meet energy needs. As lean body mass is reduced, metabolically active tissue is lost, and energy expenditure decreases.

The stress of acute illness, surgery, or trauma produces a different response. The acute stress response produces a state of hypermetabolism and **catabolism** (cell and tissue breakdown). This hypermetabolic state increases energy expenditure and nutrient needs, resulting in **protein-calorie malnutrition (PCM)**. In PCM, both protein and calories are deficient. Lean body mass is broken down to meet these needs. If untreated, up to half of the body's protein stores can be used within 3 weeks. Visceral protein stores also are converted to energy, with loss of protein from organs such as the liver, gastrointestinal tract, kidneys, and heart. Loss of protein from the liver affects its ability to produce plasma proteins. Immune cells decrease, and wound healing is impaired. Atrophy of gastrointestinal mucosa leads to malabsorption, further compounding the protein deficit. Myocardial contractility and cardiac output decline, and respiratory function is compromised (Porth & Matfin, 2009).

Chronic protein deficiency with adequate calories to meet energy needs is called *kwashiorkor*. When both proteins and calories are insufficient to meet the body's needs, PCM is known as *marasmus*.

Manifestations

The manifestations of malnutrition may vary among patients. Weight loss is the most apparent manifestation: The malnourished patient may have a body weight of less than 90% of ideal. Body mass also is reduced (see Box 22–1), as is skinfold thickness. Other manifestations include a wasted appearance, dry

Nutrition for the Older Adult

Older adults are at greater risk for malnutrition. Age-related changes that contribute to this problem include changes in taste and smell, poor oral health, loss of teeth or ill-fitting dentures, medication-related anorexia, and functional limitations that impair the ability to shop and cook. Older adults living on fixed incomes may not be able to afford well-balanced meals. Depression, social isolation, and loneliness often contribute to loss of appetite. Eating is a social event, and older adults who eat alone may not eat as well as those who share meals with companions.

Conduct a thorough assessment to determine nutritional status. Assess psychologic factors that influence eating habits, such as loneliness, isolation, and depression. Note the patient's general appearance and obtain a diet history, including information about foods and nutrients the patient consumes, and recent weight loss or gain. Review laboratory values, including complete blood count, total protein, prealbumin, and albumin levels.

TEACHING FOR HOME CARE

To maintain nutritional status, advise the older patient to do the following:

- Eat a well-balanced diet with fresh fruits and vegetables.
- Shop wisely to get the most value for the money.
- Avoid processed foods and foods high in fat.
- Drink adequate fluids.
- Exercise regularly.
- Contact local agencies for the availability of congregate meals (e.g., at local senior centers) or home-delivered meals (e.g., Meals on Wheels).

and brittle hair, and pale mucous membranes. Peripheral or abdominal edema may be present. Older adults may show general symptoms of frailty, including weakness, slow walking speed, low physical activity level, unintentional weight loss, and exhaustion. Manifestations of specific nutrient deficiencies may be present (see the accompanying box). See page 601 for the Multisystem Effects of Malnutrition.

Subcutaneous fat and muscle proteins are broken down in PCM, impairing mobility and increasing the risk for skin and tissue breakdown (pressure ulcers). Protein synthesis is inhibited and wound healing delayed. Serum albumin levels fall, leading to abdominal edema, diarrhea, and impaired nutrient absorption. Immune function is impaired, increasing the risk of infection. Cardiac output falls, and the risk for postural hypotension increases.

Interdisciplinary Care

The goal of treatment for the malnourished patient is to restore ideal body weight while replacing and restoring depleted nutrients and minerals. The patient's age, severity of malnutrition, and coexisting health problems help determine interventions. Treatment may include oral supplementation, tube feedings, or parenteral nutrition.

Diagnosis

A nutrition screening tool such as the one in Box 22–3 can help identify patients at risk for malnutrition. As with obesity, the standard measurements to assess for malnutrition include height, weight, calculation of BMI, and skinfold measurements. A BMI of less than 18 to 20 kg/m^2 may indicate malnutrition. The following laboratory studies also may be ordered:

- *Serum albumin* is reduced in PCM, and may be below 3.0 g/dL.
- *Prealbumin* (also known as *transthyretin*) is a transport protein and precursor to albumin. It has a short (2-day) half-life, and is sensitive to acute changes in nutritional status. A prealbumin level of less than 10 mg/dl indicates severe nutritional deficiency; a level lower than 5 mg/dl is seen in severe protein depletion (Kee, 2009).
- The *total lymphocyte count* is reduced in PCM.
- *Serum electrolytes* are measured. Potassium levels are low in severe malnutrition.

The following specialized procedures to evaluate the extent of malnutrition may be ordered:

- *Bioelectric impedance analysis* measures body fat and total body water.
- *Total daily energy expenditure* (which includes resting energy expenditure, energy needed for digestion, plus physical activity needs) may be measured to help determine the patient's calorie intake needs.

Medications

Malnourished patients generally require supplemental vitamins and minerals to restore these essential micronutrients. A multivitamin and mineral supplement may be given, or therapy may be tailored to correct specific deficiencies. See the Medication Administration box on page 602 for nursing implications of vitamin and mineral supplements.

MANIFESTATIONS of Specific Nutrient Deficiencies

DEFICIENCY	ASSESSMENT DATA
Calorie	Weight loss
	Weakness, listlessness
	Loss of subcutaneous fat
	Muscle wasting
Protein	Thin or sparse hair
	Flaking skin
	Hepatomegaly
Vitamin A	Night blindness
	Altered taste and smell
	Dry, scaling, rough skin
Thiamine	Confusion, apathy
	Cardiomegaly, dyspnea
	Muscle cramping and wasting
	Paresthesias, neuropathy
	Ataxia
Riboflavin	Cheilosis, stomatitis
	Neuropathy, glossitis
Vitamin C	Swollen, bleeding gums
	Delayed wound healing
	Weakness, depression
	Easy bruising
Iron	Smooth tongue
	Listlessness, fatigue
	Dyspnea

Nutrition

Fluids and nutrients are carefully reintroduced in severely malnourished patients. Refeeding can precipitate fluid and electrolyte imbalances, heart failure, malabsorption, and diarrhea.

First, fluid and electrolyte imbalances are corrected, with particular attention paid to restoring normal potassium, magnesium, and calcium levels, as well as acid–base balance. Once fluid and electrolyte imbalances are corrected, protein and calories are gradually reintroduced into the diet. Initial feedings are limited amounts (100 mL) of liquid formula to prevent diarrhea. Vitamin and mineral supplements at about twice the Dietary Reference Intake (DRI) are provided along with refeeding. Fat and lactose are reintroduced into the diet last. Lactose intolerance may develop in severely malnourished patients; yogurt may be tolerated better than a milk-based formula.

Food intake is gradually increased until the patient is able to consume about 5000 kcal per day, and is gaining 3 to 5 pounds (1.5 to 2.0 kg) weekly. Commercially available nutritional supplements (such as Ensure or Sustacal) may supplement protein and calorie intake.

ENTERAL NUTRITION **Enteral nutrition**, or tube feeding, may be used to meet calorie and protein requirements in patients unable to consume adequate food. Indications for tube feedings include difficulty swallowing, unresponsiveness, oral or neck surgery or trauma, anorexia, or serious illness. Tube feedings

MULTISYSTEM EFFECTS OF
Malnutrition

Neurologic
- ↓Cognition
- ↓Consciousness (drowsiness, lethargy)
- Tremors
- Paresthesias
- Impaired coordination

Endocrine
- ↓Thyroid hormones
- ↓Testosterone (male)
- ↓Estrogen (female)

Integumentary
- Hair: brittle, dull, dry, loss of color
- Nails: fragile, brittle, spoon-shaped
- Petechiae
- Poor wound healing

Respiratory
- ↓Respiratory rate
- ↓Vital capacity

Hepatic
- Hepatomegaly
- ↓Bile synthesis

Cardiovascular
- Dysrythmias and conduction disturbances
- ↓ HR
- ↓ BP
- Enlarged heart

Potential Complication
- Heart failure

Gastrointestinal
Oral/esophageal:
- Cheilosis
- Glossitis
- Gingivitis
Stomach/intestines:
- Ascites
- Constipation
- Intestinal atrophy
- Steatorrhea
- ↓Gastric and pancreatic secretions

Potential Complication
- Malabsorption syndrome

Reproductive
- Amenorrhea

Musculoskeletal
- Muscle wasting
- Tenderness
- Impaired strength

Metabolic Processes
- ↓Weight
- ↓Core body temperature
- Edema

Immune System
- ↓Cell-mediated and humoral immunity
- ↑Susceptibility to infections

BOX 22–3 Mini-Nutritional Assessment MNA®

A. Has food intake declined over the past three months due to loss of appetite, digestive problems, chewing or swallowing difficulties?
  0 = severe loss of appetite
  1 = moderate loss of appetite
  2 = no loss of appetite
B. Weight loss during last three months
  0 = weight loss greater than 3 kg (6.6 lbs)
  1 = does not know
  2 = weight loss between 1 and 3 kg (2.2 and 6.6 lbs)
  3 = no weight loss
C. Mobility
  0 = bed or chair bound
  1 = able to get out of bed/chair but does not go out
  2 = goes out

D. Has suffered psychological stress or acute disease in the past three months
  0 = yes
  2 = no
E. Neuropsychological problems
  0 = severe dementia or depression
  1 = mild dementia
  2 = no psychological problems
F. Body Mass Index (BMI)
  0 = BMI less than 19
  1 = BMI 19 to less than 21
  2 = BMI 21 to less than 23
  3 = BMI 23 or greater
Screening score (subtotal maximum of 14 points)
12 points or greater: Normal—no need for further assessment
11 points or below: Possible malnutrition – continue assessment

Used with permission by Société des Produits Nestlé S.A., Vevey Switzerland, 2007.

MEDICATION ADMINISTRATION **Vitamin and Mineral Supplements**

FAT-SOLUBLE VITAMINS

Vitamin A

Vitamin D

Vitamin E

Vitamin K

The fat-soluble vitamins are absorbed in the gastrointestinal tract. Vitamins A and D are stored in the liver.

All fat-soluble vitamins may become toxic if taken in excess amounts.

Nursing Responsibilities

- Monitor for manifestations of vitamin excess as well as for adverse effects from vitamin administration.
- Monitor carefully for hypersensitivity reactions during the parenteral administration. Have emergency equipment available.
- Administer vitamin A with food.
- Do not administer vitamin K intravenously.

Health Education for the Patient and Family

- Teach the importance of eating a well-balanced diet. If indicated, provide lists of foods high in specific vitamins.
- Caution that excessive intake of these vitamins may lead to toxicity.

WATER-SOLUBLE VITAMINS

Vitamin C (ascorbic acid)

Vitamin B complex:

  Thiamine (B_1)

  Riboflavin (B_2)

  Niacin (nicotinic acid)

  Pyridoxine hydrochloride (B_6)

  Pantothenic acid

  Biotin

These vitamins are used to prevent or treat deficiency problems. If the diet is deficient in one vitamin, it is usually deficient in other vitamins as well; therefore, multivitamin preparations are often administered. Most of these vitamins are well absorbed from the gastrointestinal tract.

Nursing Responsibilities

- Monitor for responses to replacement therapy.
- Monitor for hypersensitivity reactions from parenteral administration. Have emergency equipment available.

Health Education for the Patient and Family

- Do not exceed the recommended daily intake for the specific vitamin.

MINERALS

Sodium	Copper
Manganese	Potassium
Fluoride	Chromium
Magnesium	Iodine
Selenium	Calcium
Zinc	

Minerals are inorganic chemicals that are vital to a variety of physiologic functions. Also called trace elements, these minerals are part of a balanced diet. Recommended daily intakes have not been established for all mineral substances. The dosage of prescribed minerals depends on the specific deficiency, route of administration, and the patient's general health.

Nursing Responsibilities

- Monitor for manifestations of mineral imbalance.
- Prior to administration, dilute oral mineral preparations.
- Prior to the administration of iodine, assess for history of hypersensitivity to iodine or seafood; if hypersensitive, notify the physician.

Health Education for the Patient and Family

- Encourage the patient to avoid exceeding the known recommended daily intake of the mineral.
- Instruct the patient to take minerals other than fluoride and zinc with or after meals.

Figure 22–2 ■ A nasoduodenal tube and a jejunostomy tube.

Courtesy of Michal Heron/Pearson Education/PH College

BOX 22–4 **Measures to Verify Feeding Tube Placement**

After inserting the feeding tube and verifying appropriate placement through pH of the aspirate and an x-ray, mark the feeding tube position with indelible marker. Prior to each feeding (or every 8 to 12 hours if continuous feedings are being administered), assess the abdomen and tube placement. Use the following steps to assess tube placement:

■ Assess the abdomen for distention, bowel sounds, and tenderness using the sequence of inspection, auscultation, percussion, and palpation.

■ Assess tube condition and placement by verifying that the indelible mark remains at the same position. Ask the patient to open the mouth, and inspect the position of the tube in the oropharynx. Do not administer a feeding if the patient is having difficulty speaking or is coughing.

■ Using a 60 mL syringe, inject 30 mL of air into the feeding tube, then aspirate a small amount of gut contents and check the pH of the aspirate.

Reassess tube placement if the patient vomits or retches, requires oropharyngeal suctioning, complains of discomfort or reflux into the mouth, or develops signs of respiratory distress.

may provide part or all of a patient's nutritional needs. Enteral feedings provide nutrients directly to the gut and other digestive organs, support immune function, promote blood flow to the gut, and support other functions of the GI tract such as the release of hormones and epidermal growth factor (Fauci et al., 2008).

Tube feedings are usually administered through a soft, small-caliber nasogastric or nasoduodenal tube with a weighted tip (Figure 22–2 ■). They also can be administered through a gastrostomy or jejunostomy tube. Small-bore feeding tubes are easily displaced; appropriate tube placement should be periodically checked by aspirating the tube and checking the pH of aspirated contents. A pH of < 4 indicates placement in the stomach; pH > 6 indicates the tube is in the jejunum. See Box 22–4.

Most tube feeding formulas provide 1 kcal/mL with approximately 14% of the calories from protein, 60% from carbohydrates, and 25% to 30% from fat. Administering 1500 mL per day provides the recommended daily intake of all vitamins and minerals. Formulas that provide more calories per milliliter, more grams of protein, added fiber, or lower fat also are available (Table 22–5). Commercial products provide instructions for initiating therapy. Enteral feedings may initially be started with smaller volumes to prevent diarrhea, with the volume gradually increased to provide the required calories for maintenance and healing. Formulas may be administered as a bolus feeding or as a continuous-drip feeding regulated by a feeding pump (Figure 22–3 ■).

Aspiration and diarrhea are the most common complications of enteral feedings. Continuous infusion of the formula reduces the risk of aspiration. The risk also is reduced by placing the feeding tube in the jejunum rather than the stomach. To avoid aspiration, the nurse elevates the head of the bed at least 30 degrees during feeding and for at least 1 hour after feeding. Dual-lumen tubes that allow gastric suction with simultaneous instillation of an enteral feeding into the jejunum also reduce the risk for aspiration. Formulas that contain fiber can reduce the incidence of diarrhea. Fluid and

TABLE 22–5 Selected Enteral Feeding Formulas

FORMULA TYPE	CONTAINS	EXAMPLES
Complete—suitable for most patients requiring enteral feedings	■ 1 kcal/mL ■ Protein: ~ 14% total kcal ■ Fat: ~ 30% total kcal ■ Carbohydrate: ~ 60% total kcal ■ Recommended daily intake of all minerals and vitamins in 1500 mL/day	Compleat, Ensure, Isocal, Nutren, Isolan, Sustacal, Resource
High-calorie complete—appropriate for patients on fluid restriction	As above; provides 1.5 to 2 kcal/mL	Ensure Plus, Sustacal HC, Comply, Nutren 1.5, Resource Plus, Isocal HCN, Magnacal, TwoCal HN
Complete lactose-free, high-residue—used to prevent/treat diarrhea, constipation	As above; provides fiber	Jevity, Profiber, Nutren 1.0 with fiber, Fiberlan, Sustacal with fiber, Ultracal, Ensure with fiber, Fibersource, Accupep HPF, Reabfin, others
Disease-specific formulas:		
Renal failure	Contain essential amino acids	Amin-Aid, Travasorb Renal, Aminess
Respiratory failure	Fat: > 50% total kcal	Pulmocare, NutriVent
Liver failure with hepatic encephalopathy	High amounts of branched-chain amino acids	Hepatic-Acid II, Travasorb Hepatic

Figure 22–3 ■ The nurse secures the feeding tube of a patient receiving a continuous enteral feeding.

Courtesy of Michal Heron/Pearson Education/PH College

electrolyte status is monitored carefully, and additional water is administered as needed.

PARENTERAL NUTRITION **Parenteral nutrition (PN)** is the intravenous administration of amino acids, often with added carbohydrates, fats, electrolytes, vitamins, and minerals. These hypertonic solutions usually are administered through a central vein, such as the subclavian vein (Figure 22–4 ■), particularly when therapy may be prolonged. A peripherally inserted central catheter (PICC) line may be used for short-term PN.

Fat emulsion

Parenteral nutrition solution

Subclavian vein

Clavicle

Superior vena cava

Pump

Filter

Right atrium

Y site for piggyback

Subcutaneous tunnel

Figure 22–4 ■ Parenteral nutrition infusing through a catheter in the right subclavian vein.

PN is initiated when a patient's nutritional requirements cannot be met through diet or enteral feedings. Increasingly, PN may be used concurrently with enteral nutrition. Patients who have undergone major surgery or trauma or are seriously undernourished are often candidates for PN. PN is used for both short- and long-term management of nutritional deficiencies.

To begin therapy, a peripheral or central venous catheter is inserted under aseptic conditions. The location of the catheter tip is confirmed by x-ray. Parenteral nutrition solutions are mixed in the pharmacy and commonly contain 3% to 11.4% amino acids (a mixture of essential and nonessential amino acids), 10% or more dextrose, and added electrolytes, minerals, and vitamins. Fat emulsions (lipids) may be added to the solution, although they often are administered separately. The sterility of the solution is maintained, and no medication is added to the solution after it is mixed or to the lumen through which the PN is being administered. When given separately, fat emulsions may be administered either through a peripheral vein or via the same intravenous catheter as PN. PN solutions are always administered with an infusion pump to ensure the correct rate of infusion.

Complications The patient receiving parenteral nutrition is at risk for infectious, metabolic, and mechanical complications. Disruption of the skin barrier and administration of a solution high in glucose presents a risk for infection in patients receiving PN. Infection may be local, limited to the insertion site or the catheter itself, or may be systemic. Meticulous sterile technique when inserting the catheter, preparing and administering PN solutions, and during site and catheter care reduces the risk for infection. Using a catheter impregnated with antiseptics and an in-line filter also reduce the risk for infection. The insertion site and the patient's temperature are monitored for evidence of infection. Cultures of the solution, catheter, and blood may be obtained if infection is suspected.

Glucose intolerance may develop, particularly early in the course of PN. The concentration of glucose in PN solutions may be gradually increased to reduce this risk. Blood and urine glucose levels are measured every 6 hours until insulin production adjusts to the increased glucose load. Patients with impaired kidney function or liver disease may develop excessively high blood urea nitrogen (BUN) levels or metabolic acidosis. Hyperlipidemia is a common complication of fat infusions; these solutions are given intermittently to allow fats to clear from the blood between infusions. Fluid overload or dehydration may develop, particularly in older adults. PN formulas can cause electrolyte shifts, with resulting imbalances.

Pneumothorax, brachial plexus injury, and improper position are possible mechanical complications of central venous catheter insertion. Once in place, a thrombus (clot) or fibrin sheath may form within or around the catheter. The catheter also can be mechanically occluded, or may dislodge, leak, or break and become an embolus.

∞ Nursing Care

Health Promotion

Aggressive nursing assessment and interventions can help prevent malnutrition associated with hospitalization or long-term care. In hospitalized patients, carefully monitor food intake. When the patient is placed on NPO status for surgery or tests, ask the care provider to restore diet orders as soon as possible. If allowed, encourage family members to provide favorite foods to promote intake. In long-term care settings, promote socialization during meals. Assess food likes and dislikes for patients, and provide foods they are likely to eat.

Assessment

Collect nutritional assessment data on admission and periodically (once or twice a week) during long-term institutionalization.

■ *Health history:* Usual daily dietary pattern (type and amount of foods consumed); usual weight and recent changes; appetite and food tolerance; specific food likes and dislikes; difficulty swallowing; problems such as anorexia, nausea, diarrhea, or constipation; history of surgery and/or chronic diseases (e.g., chronic lung disease) and medications.

■ *Physical examination:* Height, weight, skinfold thickness, BMI; vital signs; general appearance, muscle wasting, mobility; skin and mucous membranes; bowel sounds; laboratory studies.

Use of a nutritional assessment tool can help identify patients (older adults in particular) at risk for malnutrition (see Box 22–3).

Nursing Diagnoses and Interventions

The complex effects of malnutrition on multiple body systems place the patient at high risk for a number of other problems. This section addresses problems with nutrition, infections, fluid

---

EVIDENCE FOR NURSING CARE | **The Patient with Malnutrition**

Selected resources that nurses may find helpful when planning evidence-based nursing care follow.

■ Capra, S., Collins, C., Lamb, M., Vanderkroft, D., & Chan, S. W-C. (2007). Effectiveness of interventions for undernourished older inpatients in the hospital setting. *Best Practice, The Joanna Briggs Institute, 11*(2), 1–4. Retrieved from http://www.joannabriggs.edu.au/pdf/BPISEng_11_2.pdf

■ Johnson, A. D. (2009). Assessing gastric residual volumes. *Critical Care Nurse, 29*(5), 72–73.

■ DiMaria-Ghalili, R. (2008). *Nutrition in the elderly: Nutrition standard of practice protocol: Nutrition in aging.* New York, NY: Hartford Institute for Geriatric Nursing, New York University College of Nursing. Retrieved from www.consultgerirn.org/topics/nutrition_in_the_elderly/want_to_know_more

■ Winkelman, C., & Best, K. (2009). Formula for success: Deliver enterable nutrition using best practices. *American Nurse Today, 4*(3), 18–23.

---

volume, and skin integrity. See page 607 for a Case Study & Nursing Care Plan for the patient with malnutrition.

Imbalanced Nutrition: Less than Body Requirements

The nurse plays a critical role in the ongoing assessment of the malnourished patient, while collaborating with the multidisciplinary team to provide nutritional therapies.

■ If the patient is able to eat, provide an environment and nursing measures that encourage eating, for example, adequate staff to assist with meals, sitting at the bedside or in a common area, and providing favorite foods. *Measures to promote a more "normal" and social dining experience support the patient's intake (DiMaria-Ghalili, 2008).*

■ Eliminate foul odors, provide oral hygiene before and after meals, make meals appetizing, and offer frequent, small meals including preferred foods. Consult with the nutrition support team to provide adequate protein, calories, minerals, and vitamins. *Oral hygiene and a pleasant environment make food more appetizing. Small, frequent meals are generally more appealing and less overwhelming to a patient with anorexia. Many patients require complicated nutritional therapy such as enteral or parenteral therapy to meet nutritional needs.*

■ Provide a rest period before and after meals. *Eating requires energy, and the malnourished patient may have decreased physical strength and energy.*

■ Assess knowledge and provide appropriate teaching. *Lack of knowledge often contributes to undernutrition. Education empowers the patient to make healthy choices.*

Risk for Infection

Malnourished patients have a much higher risk for infection than well-nourished people. Malnutrition affects many components of the immune system, including the skin, mucous membranes, and lymph tissue and cells.

■ Monitor temperature and assess for manifestations of infection every 4 hours. *Although the baseline temperature may be subnormal in malnourished patients, any elevation from baseline may indicate infection. Manifestations of infection may include chills, malaise, erythema, and leukocytosis. Early detection of infection may prevent complications.*

■ Maintain medical asepsis when providing care and surgical asepsis when carrying out procedures. *Hand hygiene is the best strategy to prevent the spread of pathogens. Sterile technique is required for procedures such as inserting central lines and changing dressings.*

■ Teach the signs and symptoms of infection, hand hygiene, and factors that increase the risk for infection. *Knowledge empowers the patient to participate in self-care, thus reducing exposure to infectious pathogens.*

Risk for Deficient Fluid Volume

The patient with malnutrition may also have a fluid volume deficit. Difficulty swallowing food and fluids or administration of hyperosmolar nutritional solutions may lead to dehydration or electrolyte disturbances.

■ Monitor oral mucous membranes, urine specific gravity, level of consciousness, and laboratory findings every 4 to 8 hours. *Dry mucous membranes, increased urine specific gravity, decreased level of consciousness, and electrolyte imbalances may indicate dehydration.*

- Weigh daily and monitor intake and output. *Daily weights and intake and output measurements help monitor fluid balance.*
- If allowed, offer fluids frequently in small amounts, considering the patient's preferences. *Frequent, small amounts of fluids are better tolerated and promote adequate intake.*

Risk for Impaired Skin Integrity

Skin integrity depends on adequate nutrition. Loss of subcutaneous tissue and muscle increase the risk of pressure ulcers. In addition, healing is impaired in malnourished patients.

- Assess skin every 4 hours. *Baseline and ongoing assessments allow prompt identification of early manifestations of skin breakdown.*
- Turn and reposition at least every 2 hours. Encourage passive and active range-of-motion exercises. *These measures reduce pressure and promote oxygenation of cells.*
- Keep skin dry and clean, and minimize shearing forces. Keep linens smooth, clean, and dry. Provide therapeutic beds, mattresses, or pads. *These nursing measures promote comfort and reduce the risk of skin breakdown.*

Using NANDA, NIC, and NOC

Linkages between a selected NANDA nursing diagnosis, NIC, and NOC for the patient with malnutrition are shown in the chart that follows.

Community-Based Care

Community-dwelling older adults, homeless people, and other disadvantaged populations are at particular risk for being malnourished. See the accompanying nursing research box.

Patients with malnutrition may be cared for at home or in the hospital with diet, enteral, or parenteral therapy. Each year, it is

---

NANDA, NIC, AND NOC LINKAGES
The Patient with Malnutrition

NANDA
> Imbalanced Nutrition: Less than Body Requirements

NIC
> Weight Gain Assistance
> Fluid/Electrolyte Management
> Nutrition Therapy
> Infection Protection

NOC
> Nutritional Status
> Nutritional Status: Nutrient Intake
> Electrolyte & Acid/Base Balance
> Immune Status

Data from NANDA International. (2009). *Nursing diagnoses: Definitions & classification 2009–2011.* Oxford, UK: Wiley-Blackwell; Bulechek, G., Butcher, H., & Dochterman J. (Eds.). (2008). *Nursing interventions classification (NIC)* (5th ed.). St. Louis, MO: Mosby; and Moorhead, S., Johnson, M., Maas, M., & Swanson, E. (Eds.). (2008). *Nursing outcomes classification (NOC)* (4th ed.). St. Louis, MO: Mosby.

---

more common to see patients managing tube feeding or PN at home. Teaching for the patient and family includes the following topics:

- Diet recommendations and use of nutritional supplements
- Where to obtain recommended foods and nutritional supplements
- If continuing enteral or parenteral nutrition, (1) how to prepare and/or handle solutions, (2) how to add them to either the feeding tube or central line, (3) how to manage infusion pumps, (4) how to care for the feeding tube or central catheter, (5) how to recognize and manage problems and complications, and (6) how and when to notify the healthcare provider of problems

---

MOVING EVIDENCE INTO ACTION | **Patients with Malnutrition**

The percentage of older adults who have risk factors for malnutrition is higher than in young and middle adults. These risk factors include functional limitations, chronic disease, and psychosocial factors. A study of community-dwelling low- and underweight older adults by Martin, Kayser-Jones, Stotts, Porter, & Froelicher (2007) found three variables in particular to have a clear association with being severely underweight: an illness or condition that affected food intake, a 10-lb or greater unintentional weight loss within the past 6 months, and an inability to travel outside the home without assistance.

IMPLICATIONS FOR NURSING

This study provides information that can be especially useful for nurses in community-based care settings. Using a brief nutritional screening tool (see Box 22–3) and weighing the patient on a regular basis can alert the nurse to the need for referral or additional support to prevent malnutrition. A patient whose food intake has been affected by chronic disease

should be referred to a dietician for assistance with meal planning. Measures such as encouraging use of nutritional supplements (e.g., Ensure) can help stop or even reverse unintentional weight loss.

CRITICAL THINKING IN PATIENT CARE

1. What essential information should you collect from patients in an ambulatory care setting (e.g., physician's office or clinic) to screen for those who are at risk for becoming malnourished?
2. This study found that participants who needed assistance traveling outside the home were at significant risk for being underweight. Identify nursing interventions and community resources to reduce this risk for an older adult in your community.
3. Develop a teaching plan to prepare caregivers in a residential care facility to use the Mini Nutritional Assessment Screening tool outlined in Box 22–3 for screening residents.

CASE STUDY & NURSING CARE PLAN   A Patient with Malnutrition

Rose Morris is an 88-year-old widow who lives alone. She typically rises early and has a cup of tea before spending her morning puttering in her garden. She consumes her main meal of the day at lunch, which usually includes rice and some vegetables. For dinner, she generally eats a bowl of rice with "whatever seems to be in the refrigerator." She admits to little interest in cooking or eating since her husband died 10 years ago and her group of friends has been "dying off too."

ASSESSMENT

Mrs. Morris weighs 95 lb (43.1 kg) and is 5'3" (160 cm) tall, for a BMI of 16.8. She reports weighing 118 lb (53.5 kg) 5 years ago. Her triceps skinfold thickness measurement is 11 mm (normal values for a female: > 13 mm). Her skin is pale, and she appears thin and wasted. Her temperature is 97°F (36.°C). Diagnostic test results include serum albumin 2.9 g/dL (normal 3.4 to 4.8 g/dL) and serum cholesterol 130 mg/dL (normal 150 to 200 mg/dL). A diagnosis of protein-calorie malnutrition is made, and a 1500-calorie per day diet is recommended.

DIAGNOSES

- *Imbalanced Nutrition: Less than Body Requirements* related to lack of knowledge and inadequate food intake
- *Risk for Infection* related to protein-calorie malnutrition
- *Impaired Social Interaction* related to widowhood and reduced social support group

EXPECTED OUTCOMES

- Gain at least 1 pound per week.
- Verbalize understanding of nutritional requirements and identify strategies to incorporate requirements into daily diet after discharge.

- Remain infection free, evidenced by normal vital signs.
- Identify strategies to increase social interaction, such as participating in senior citizens' lunches at local senior center.

PLANNING AND IMPLEMENTATION

- Weigh weekly at a consistent time of day.
- Refer to dietitian for evaluation of nutritional needs.
- Teach about nutritional requirements, and plan an eating program that includes high-calorie, high-protein foods and supplements and reflects her food preferences. Encourage small, frequent meals.
- Encourage to keep a food intake diary.
- Teach strategies to reduce risks for infection.
- Provide information about communal meals available to seniors in the community, and help Mrs. Morris develop a plan to participate.

EVALUATION

One month later, Mrs. Morris has gained 3 pounds and reports feeling "more energetic." A friend is helping her shop to ensure that she purchases foods to maintain her protein, calorie, and nutrient intake. She has begun attending senior lunches twice a week, and is enjoying "being around people again." Although she still doesn't enjoy cooking like she used to, she is using prepared foods and supplements to maintain her nutrient intake.

CRITICAL THINKING IN THE NURSING PROCESS

1. What is the physiologic basis for Mrs. Morris's low albumin and cholesterol levels?
2. Mrs. Morris asks, "Can I get better by just taking more vitamins?" How will you respond?
3. Design a teaching plan for a Hispanic patient with protein-calorie malnutrition.

See Evaluating Your Response in Appendix C.

The Patient with an Eating Disorder

Eating disorders are characterized by severely disturbed eating behavior and weight management. Eating disorders are more common in affluent societies where food is plentiful. Women are much more commonly affected than men. **Anorexia nervosa** is characterized by a refusal to maintain a minimally normal body weight, a distorted body image, and an intense fear of gaining weight or of loss of control over food intake. Anorexia nervosa affects about 1% of women in the United States at some time in their lives (Fauci et al., 2008). **Bulimia nervosa**, which affects 1% to 3% of women in the United States, is characterized by recurring episodes of binge eating followed by purge behaviors such as self-induced vomiting, use of laxatives or diuretics, fasting, or excessive exercise. A third eating disorder, **binge-eating disorder**, is believed to affect many more people than either anorexia or bulimia. Binge-eating disorder is characterized by recurrent episodes of binge eating—eating an excessive amount of food during a defined period of time and a sense of loss of control over eating during binge episodes (National Institute of Mental Health [NIMH], 2007).

Anorexia Nervosa

Anorexia nervosa typically begins during mid to late adolescence. Patients with anorexia nervosa have a distorted body image and irrational fear of gaining weight. Refusal to maintain body weight at or above a minimally normal level for height and body type is a common manifestation of anorexia nervosa. Patients maintain weight loss by restricted calorie intake, often accompanied by excessive exercise. Some may exhibit binge–purge behavior.

Although its cause is unknown, psychologic, biologic, genetic, and cultural risk factors have been identified for anorexia nervosa. A history of sexual or physical abuse and family history of mood disorders are nonspecific risk factors. Abnormal levels of neurotransmitters and other hormones may play a role. Genetic factors are suggested by a higher incidence within families and in the monozygotic twin of an affected individual. Women who develop anorexia nervosa tend to be obsessive and perfectionistic, and often feel inadequate or unable to maintain control in their lives. Family, social, or occupational (e.g., a career in modeling or ballet) pressures to maintain low body weight also contribute.

The manifestations and complications of anorexia nervosa are listed in the box on page 608. Patients who engage in binge–purge behavior have a higher risk for complications.

Eating Disorder Video

MANIFESTATIONS AND COMPLICATIONS of Eating Disorders

DISORDER	MANIFESTATIONS	COMPLICATIONS
Anorexia Nervosa	■ Weight < 85% of normal, muscle wasting ■ Fear of weight gain, refusal to eat ■ Disturbed body image, excessive exercise ■ Amenorrhea ■ Skin and hair changes ■ Hypotension, bradycardia ■ Hypothermia, cold intolerance ■ Constipation ■ Insomnia	■ Electrolyte and acid–base disturbances ■ Reduced cardiac output, dysrhythmias ■ Elevated BUN, serum creatinine levels ■ Anemia ■ Hypoglycemia, elevated serum uric acid levels ■ Osteoporosis ■ Enlarged salivary glands ■ Delayed gastric emptying ■ Abnormal liver function
Bulimia Nervosa	■ Weight often normal; may be slightly overweight ■ Binge–purge behavior ■ Oligomenorrhea or amenorrhea ■ Lacerations of palate; callous on fingers or dorsum of hand	■ Enlarged salivary glands ■ Stomatitis, loss of dental enamel ■ Fluid, electrolyte, and acid–base imbalances ■ Dysrhythmias ■ Esophageal tears, stomach rupture
Binge-Eating Disorder	■ Usually overweight or obese ■ Recurrent episodes of binge eating (2 or more days a week for 6 months) ■ Episodes characterized by the following: 　■ Eating more rapidly than usual 　■ Eating until uncomfortably full 　■ Eating large amounts of food when not physically hungry 　■ Eating alone due to embarrassment over quantity 　■ Disgust, depression, or guilt following a binge episode 　■ Marked distress about binging behavior	■ Type 2 diabetes ■ Hypertension, hyperlipidemia ■ Coronary heart disease, heart failure ■ Gallbladder disease ■ Depression, social isolation

Bulimia Nervosa

Bulimia nervosa develops in late adolescence or early adulthood. Unlike patients with anorexia nervosa, the weight of patients with bulimia is within or above the normal range. Like anorexia nervosa, however, the cause likely is multifactorial, including cultural, psychosocial, and biologic factors. The patient with bulimia often restricts caloric intake, leading to increased hunger and overeating. Foods consumed during a binge often are high calorie, high fat, and sweet. After binge eating, the patient induces vomiting (usually by stimulating the gag reflex), or may take excessive quantities of laxatives or diuretics. Fluid and electrolyte balance may be severely disrupted by loss of fluid and gastrointestinal secretions. The complications of bulimia nervosa (see the preceding box) primarily result from the purging behavior.

Binge-Eating Disorder

Binge-eating disorder (BED) shares many of the characteristics of bulimia; however, patients with BED do not purge. BED commonly affects obese middle-aged adults. It affects Blacks and Whites equally. The cause of BED is unknown, although genetics may play a role in its development. Psychosocial factors contribute; people with BED often are depressed, anxious, or have a personality disorder. People with BED consume an excessive amount of food during binging episodes, eating even when not hungry and continuing to eat until uncomfortably full. Binging often occurs when the person is alone. After overeating, the patient may feel disgusted or guilty about the amount of food consumed, and depressed about the inability to control eating.

Interdisciplinary Care

Eating disorders, anorexia nervosa in particular, are difficult to effectively treat. Because of the intense fear of weight gain and the distorted body image of patients with anorexia, they strongly resist increasing food intake. While community-based care is appropriate for most patients with an eating disorder, complications of the disorder or resistance to treatment may necessitate hospitalization for some patients. In all cases, a comprehensive treatment plan for eating disorders includes medical care and monitoring, psychosocial interventions, and nutrition counseling.

Diagnosis

There is no specific diagnostic test for anorexia, bulimia, or binge-eating disorder. Laboratory studies in patients with anorexia or bulimia may show anemia and leukopenia on CBC, abnormal serum electrolyte levels, and elevated BUN and serum creatinine. In patients with BED, the blood glucose and lipid levels may be elevated. The BMI usually is above the normal range, and may identify the patient as obese.

A mental health evaluation is indicated for patients with eating disorders to identify contributing factors and help direct treatment.

Treatment

Patients with anorexia nervosa may require hospitalization, particularly if their weight is less than 75% of normal. Refeeding is gradually introduced to avoid complications such as heart failure. Multivitamins are given along with calcium and vitamin D supplements to minimize bone loss. Meals must be supervised and a firm but empathetic attitude conveyed about the importance of adequate food intake. Intravenous feeding may be required in some cases. Psychologic treatment focuses on providing emotional support during weight gain and helping patients base their self-esteem on factors other than weight (e.g., personal relationships, satisfaction with achieving occupational goals) (Fauci et al., 2008). Cognitive-behavioral therapy or psychotherapy may be used; families often are included in the treatment program. A tricyclic antidepressant, selective serotonin reuptake inhibitor (SSRI) such as fluoxetine (Prozac) or sertraline (Zoloft), or lithium carbonate may be prescribed to facilitate weight maintenance and reduce anxiety.

The goal of bulimia treatment is to reduce or eliminate binge eating and purging behavior. A combination of nutritional counseling and therapy, psychosocial interventions, and medications may be used. Nutritional counseling is directed at establishing a regular meal pattern and encouraging an appropriate amount of regular exercise. An antidepressant drug such as fluoxetine (Prozac) may benefit the patient with bulimia nervosa and help prevent relapse. Cognitive-behavioral therapy also is used to treat bulimia, focusing on excessive concerns about weight, persistent dieting, and binge–purge behaviors.

Treatment for patients with binge-eating disorder focuses on establishing healthy eating patterns, psychosocial therapy (including cognitive-behavioral therapy and group counseling) to address underlying issues, and management of obesity and its complications. Patients with BED also may benefit from an SSRI or other antidepressant drug.

✌ Nursing Care

Nurses can be instrumental in identifying patients with eating disorders and referring them for treatment. It is particularly important to identify these disorders early to prevent adverse effects on growth and increase the success of treatment.

The nurse is an integral part of the eating disorders treatment team. *Imbalanced Nutrition: Less than Body Requirements* is a primary nursing diagnosis for patients with anorexia or bulimia, and *Imbalanced Nutrition: More than Body Requirements* is a priority nursing diagnosis for patients with binge-eating disorder. The following nursing diagnoses also should be considered:

- *Ineffective Therapeutic Regimen Management*
- *Chronic Low Self-Esteem*
- *Disturbed Body Image*
- *Dysfunctional Family Processes*
- *Powerlessness*

When planning and implementing care, consider the following nursing activities.

- Regularly monitor weight, using standard conditions. *Weight gain or loss provides information about the effectiveness of care, as well as the patient's risk for complications.*
- Monitor food intake during meals, recording percentage of meal and snack consumed. Maintain close observation for at least 1 hour following meals; do not allow patient alone in bathroom. *Observing the patient during and after meals helps prevent disposal of food and purging behavior after eating. Recording actual food intake allows accurate calculation of calorie intake.*
- Serve balanced meals, including all nutrient groups. Increase serving size gradually. *The patient may find "normal" food servings overwhelming, reducing the desire to eat. Calorie intake is initially limited to prevent complications associated with refeeding, then gradually increased.*
- Serve frequent, small feedings of cold or room temperature foods. *Cool foods reduce sensations of early satiety, promoting greater food intake at a meal or snack.*
- Administer a multivitamin and mineral supplement to replace losses.

Patients with eating disorders require extended treatment of the disorder. Involvement of the family and social support persons is vital to success. Encourage family members to participate in teaching and nutritional counseling sessions. Discuss the value of family therapy to address issues that have contributed to the disorder. Emphasize the need to provide consistent messages of support for healthy eating habits. Discuss using rewards for food and calorie intake rather than weight gain. Provide referrals to a dietitian, nutritional support team, counseling, and support groups for people with eating disorders.

CHAPTER HIGHLIGHTS

- Nutritional disorders are common, affecting people worldwide, and contributing significantly to mortality and morbidity. While malnutrition is a serious problem in underdeveloped nations, obesity and its consequences are more prevalent in the United States and other industrialized societies.
- Obesity, defined as excess adipose tissue and a BMI greater than 30 kg/m^2, is linked with many disorders, including type 2 diabetes, coronary heart disease, gallbladder disease, and osteoarthritis.
- Exercise and reduced kilocalorie intake are the mainstays of obesity treatment. Drugs that suppress the appetite or interfere with fat absorption in the gut may be used to facilitate weight loss in patients with multiple risk factors for obesity complications or people who have had difficulty achieving weight loss through diet and exercise.

- Bariatric surgery is a treatment option for morbidly obese patients. The primary types of bariatric surgery used in the United States are restrictive procedures that limit stomach capacity and food consumption, and combination restrictive/malabsorptive procedures that limit both capacity and nutrient absorption.
- Nursing care for obese patients focuses on health promotion, education, and support of the prescribed treatment plan.
- In the United States, protein-calorie malnutrition is a common problem among hospitalized patients. Malnutrition increases the risk for complications and impairs healing. Early identification and prevention are the primary focuses of treatment; nurses can be instrumental in identifying at-risk patients (e.g., the elderly, patients living alone, people on extended NPO status).

- Refeeding of malnourished patients is a gradual process. Enteral feedings (oral or by feeding tube) are preferred whenever possible. Parenteral nutrition may be required when enteral feeding is not possible or not tolerated by the patient.
- Eating disorders, including anorexia nervosa, bulimia nervosa, and binge-eating disorder, can be difficult to effectively treat and maintain in remission. While patients with anorexia typically are underweight and malnourished, resisting efforts to achieve a normal weight, patients with bulimia are more likely to be of normal weight and those with binge-eating disorder are more likely to be overweight or obese.
- Treatment for eating disorders is multifaceted, including physical care to restore electrolyte balance and treat complications, nutritional counseling and therapy, psychosocial therapy, family support, and possibly medications.

TEST YOURSELF NCLEX-RN® REVIEW

1. Of the following noted in a patient's history, which does the nurse identify as the greatest risk factor for obesity?
    1. adopted at 2 months of age
    2. usual diet includes "fast-food" lunches twice a week
    3. does not engage in regular activity
    4. allergic to chocolate and strawberries
2. A patient on a reduced-calorie diet asks the nurse what she can do to lose weight faster, because most weeks she loses no more than 0.5 lb. "At this rate, it will take me years to get to my goal!" The most appropriate response by the nurse would be which of the following?
    1. "Let's reevaluate your long-term goal. Perhaps it was set too low for you."
    2. "A pound of body fat equals 3500 calories. Let's reevaluate your diet and exercise plan for calorie intake and expenditure."
    3. "Perhaps we should look into a diet supplement since you are unable to stick with your prescribed diet plan."
    4. "You sound frustrated. Would you like to take some time off from your diet and exercise plan?"
3. An expected finding in a patient admitted with a diagnosis of protein-calorie malnutrition would be which of the following?
    1. recent 5-lb weight loss
    2. increased skinfold thickness measurements
    3. hyperactive bowel sounds
    4. anxiety and agitation
4. Before administering an intermittent enteral feeding, the nurse confirms placement of the small-bore feeding tube in the stomach by doing which of the following?
    1. instilling water and listening for the gastric gurgle
    2. withdrawing the tube slightly, then reinserting it
    3. aspirating gastric contents and checking for a pH of < 4
    4. obtaining a flat-plate x-ray of the stomach
5. The nurse identifies which of the following as a realistic goal for a patient with anorexia nervosa?
    1. Will consume 100% of a 2500-calorie diet.
    2. Will gain 2 pounds per week.
    3. Will rest alone in room following meals.
    4. Will participate in family counseling.

6. The nurse identifies which nursing diagnosis as high priority for a patient with a BMI of 30.4 kg/m^2 and a waist–hip ratio of 1.1?
    1. *Health-Seeking Behaviors: Weight Loss*
    2. *Risk for Impaired Tissue Perfusion: Cardiovascular*
    3. *Ineffective Coping*
    4. *Deficient Knowledge: Diet*
7. The nurse teaching a patient about sibutramine (Meridia) includes which of the following instructions? **Select all that apply.**
    1. You may skip a dose of the drug if you skip a meal.
    2. Do not consume alcohol while taking this drug.
    3. Do not drive while taking this drug because the drug may increase sleepiness.
    4. Increase your intake of water and other fluids while taking this drug.
    5. Continue to follow your prescribed diet while taking this drug.
8. The nurse caring for a home-bound older adult who is losing an unplanned 1 to 2 pounds monthly plans for which of the following? **Select all that apply.**
    1. Meals on Wheels deliveries
    2. Ensure nutritional supplements
    3. placement in a residential care facility
    4. transportation to congregate senior meals
    5. follow-up by primary care physician
    6. referral for diagnostic studies
9. Which of the following is a high-priority nursing intervention to prevent malnutrition in the surgical patient?
    1. aggressive pain management
    2. daily weights
    3. maintaining intravenous flow
    4. requesting early restoration of oral intake
10. Three days after gastric bypass surgery, the patient complains of increasing abdominal pain. Bowel sounds are absent; the abdomen is firm and very tender. The nurse should do which of the following?
    1. Report findings to the surgeon.
    2. Ambulate the patient to promote peristalsis.
    3. Chart assessment data and continue to monitor.
    4. Evaluate the effectiveness of analgesia.

See Test Yourself answers in Appendix C.

Pearson Nursing Student Resources

Find additional review materials at
www.nursing.pearsonhighered.com

Prepare for success with additional NCLEX®-style practice questions, interactive assignments and activities, Web links, animations and videos, and more!

BIBLIOGRAPHY

Amella, E. (2007). Assessing nutrition in older adults. *Try this: Best practices in nursing care to older adults, 9*(2007). The Hartford Institute for Geriatric Nursing, New York University, College of Nursing. Retrieved from www.ConsultGeriRN.org

American Psychiatric Association. (2006). Practice guideline for the treatment of patients with eating disorders. (3rd ed.) Washington, DC: American Psychiatric Association (APA);

Arzouman, J., Lacovara, J., Blackett, A., McDonald, P., Traver, G., & Bartholomeaux, F. (2006). Developing a comprehensive bariatric protocol: A template for improving patient care. *MEDSURG Nursing, 15*(1), 21–26.

Baugh, N., Zuelzer, H., Meador, J., & Blankenship, J. (2007). Wounds in surgical patients who are obese. *American Journal of Nursing, 107*(6), 40–50.

Brown, A., & Siahpush, M. (2007). Risk factors for overweight and obesity: Results from the 2001 National Health Survey. *Public Health, 121,* 603–613.

Budd, G. (2007). Disordered eating: Young women's search for control and connection. *Journal of Child and Adolescent Psychiatric Nursing, 20*(2), 96–106.

Centers for Disease Control and Prevention [CDC]. (2008). *2008 Physical activity guidelines for Americans.* Atlanta, GA: Author. Retrieved from www.cdc.gov./physicalactivity

CDC. (2009a). Obesity. Halting the epidemic by making health easier. National Center for Chronic Disease Prevention and Health Promotion. Retrieved from www.cdc.gov/nccdphp

CDC. (2009b). Obesity. Introduction. Retrieved from www.cdc.gov

CDC. (2009c). Preventing obesity and chronic diseases through good nutrition and physical activity. Retrieved from www.cdc.gov

Clinical update. Effectiveness of interventions for under nourished older inpatients in the hospital setting. (2007). *Australian Nursing Journal, 15*(5), 28–31.

Differences in prevalence of obesity among Black, White, and Hispanic adults – United States, 2006–2008. (2009, July 17). *MMWR: Mortality and Morbidity Weekly Report, 58*(27). Retrieved from www.cdc.gov/mmwr

DiMaria-Ghalili, R. (2008). Nutrition in the elderly. Nursing standard of practice protocol: Nutrition in aging. Hartford Institute for Geriatric Nursing, New York University College of Nursing. Retrieved from consultgerirn.org/topics/nutrition_in_the_elderly

DiMaria-Ghalili, R., & Guenter, P. (2008). The mini nutritional assessment. *American Journal of Nursing, 108*(2), 50–59.

Dorner, B. (2007). The obesity challenge. Retrieved from www.nursinghomesmagazine.com

Fauci, A. S., Braunwald, E., Kasper, D. L., Hauser, S. L., Longo, D. L., Jameson, J. L., et al. (Eds.). (2008). *Harrison's principles of internal medicine* (17th ed.). New York: McGraw-Hill.

Flegal, K., Carroll, M., Ogden, C., & Curtin, L. (2010, January 20). Prevalence and trends in obesity among US adults, 1999–2008. *JAMA, 303*(3), 235–241.

Flood, M., & Newman, A. (2007). Obesity in older adults: Synthesis of findings and recommendations for clinical practice. *Journal of Gerontological Nursing, December 2007,* 19–35.

Grindel, M., & Grindel, C. (2006). Nursing care of the person having bariatric surgery. *MEDSURG Nursing, 15*(3), 129–145.

Harrington, L. (2006). Postoperative care of patients undergoing bariatric surgery. *MEDSURG Nursing, 15*(6), 357–363.

Jarosz, P., & Bellar, A. (2008). Age-appropriate obesity treatment. *The Nurse Practitioner, 33*(5), 24–31.

Kumanyika, S., Obarzanek, E., Stettler, N., Bell, R., Field, A., Fortmann, S., et al. (2008). Population-based prevention of obesity: The need for comprehensive promotion of healthful eating, physical activity, and energy balance: A scientific statement from American Heart Association Council on Epidemiology and Prevneiton, Interdisciplinary Committee for Prevention. *Circulation, 118,* 428–464. Retrieved from www.circ.ahajournals.org

Lehne, R. (2007). *Pharmacology for nursing care* (6th ed.). St. Louis, MO: Saunders.

Martin, C., Kayser-Jones, J., Stotts, N., Porter, C., & Froelicher, E. (2007). Risk for low weight in community-dwelling, older adults. *Clinical Nurse Specialist, 21*(4), 203–211.

McPhee, S. J., Papadakis, M. A., & Tierney, L. M. (2008). *Current medical diagnosis & treatment* (47th ed.). New York: Lange Medical Books/McGraw-Hill.

McWilliams, B. (2008). Assessing the benefits of a malnutrition screening tool. *Nursing Times: NT, 104*(24), 30–32.

Menifield, C., Doty, N., & Fletcher, A. (2008). Obesity in America. *The ABNF Journal, Summer 2008,* 83–88.

Metheny, N. A., Dahms, T. E., Stewart, B. J., Stone, K. S., Frank, P. A., & Clouse, R. E. (2005). Verification of inefficacy of the glucose method in detecting aspiration associated with tube feedings. *MEDSURG Nursing, 14*(2), 112–121.

Muir, M., Heese, G., McLean, D., Bodnar, S., & Rock, B. (2007). Handling of the bariatric patient in critical care: A case study of lessons learned. *Critical Care Nursing Clinics of North America, 19*(2), 223–240.

National Center for Health Statistics [NCHS]. (2008). NCHS Data on eating behaviors. Retrieved from www.cdc.gov/nchs

National Heart, Lung, and Blood Institute [NHLBI]. (1998). *Clinical guidelines on the identification, evaluation, and treatment of overweight and obesity in adults: The evidence report* (National Institutes of Health: Publication No. 98-4083). Retrieved from http://www.nhlbi.nih.gov

NHLBI. (2009). *Overweight and obesity.* Retrieved from www.nhlbi.nih.gov/health/dci/Diseases/obe/obe_all.html

NHLBI. (2000). *The practical guide. Identification, evaluation, and treatment of overweight and obesity in adults* (NIH Publication No. 00-4084). Retrieved from www.nhlbi.nih.gov

NHLBI. (2004). *Think tank on enhancing obesity research at the National Heart, Lung, and Blood Institute.* (NIH Publication No. 04-5249). Retrieved from www.nhlbi.nih.gov

National Institute of Diabetes and Digestive and Kidney Diseases [NIDDK]. (2008). Longitudinal assessment of bariatric surgery (LABS). (NIH Publication No. 04-5573). Retrieved from www.win.niddk.nih.gov

National Institute of Mental Health [NIMH]. (2007). Eating disorders. (NIH Publication No. 07-4901). Retrieved from www.nimh.nih.gov

Noble, K. (2008). The obesity epidemic: The impact of obesity on the perianesthesia patient. *Journal of PeriAnesthesia Nursing, 23*(6), 418–425.

North American Nursing Diagnosis Association. (2009). *Nursing diagnoses: Definitions & classification 2009–2011.* Oxford, UK: Wiley-Blackwell.

The Obesity Society. (2009a). Obesity, bias, and stigmatization. Retrieved from www.obesity.org

The Obesity Society. (2009b). Obesity statistics. Retrieved from www.obesity.org

Obden, C., Carroll, M., McDowell, M., & Flegal, K. (2007). Obesity among adults in the United States—No statistically significant changes since 2003–2004. NCHS Data Brief No 1. Hayattsville, MD: National Center for Health Statistics.

Pettit, E. (2009). Treating morbid obesity. *RN, 72*(2), 30–34.

Porth, C. M., & Matfin, G. (2009). *Pathophysiology: Concepts of altered health states* (7th ed.). Philadelphia: Lippincott.

Price, D. (2008). Protein-energy malnutrition among the elderly: Implications for nursing care. *Holistic Nursing Practice, 22*(6), 355–360.

Sacks, F., Bray, G., Carey, V., Smith, S., Ryan, D., Anton, S., et al. (2009). Comparison of weight-loss diets with different compositions of fat, protein, and carbohydrates. *New England Journal of Medicine, 360*(9), 859–873.

Thomas, A., Moseley, G., Stallings, R., Nichols-English, G., & Wagner, P. (2008). Perceptions of obesity: Black and White differences. *Journal of Cultural Diversity, 15*(4), 174–180.

Tozzo, M. (2007). Battling obesity: Small steps, big rewards. *Nursing2007, 37*(3), 68–69.

Turner, S., Thomas, A., Wagner, P., & Moseley, G. (2008). A collaborative approach to wellness: Diet, exercise, and education to impact behavior change. *Journal of the American Academy of Nurse Practitioners, 20*(2008), 339–344.

Weight-control Information Network [WIN]. (2007a). *Medical care for obese patients.* (NIH Publication No. 03-4159). Bethesda, MD: National Institutes of Health.

WIN. (2007b). *Prescription medications for the treatment of obesity.* (NIH Publication No. 07-4191). Bethesda, MD: National Institutes of Health.

WIN. (2010). Overweight and obesity statistics. Bethesda, MD: National Institutes of Health. Retrieved from www.win.niddk.nih.gov

WIN. (2008a). *Bariatric surgery for severe obesity.* (NIH Publication No. 08-4006). Bethesda, MD: National Institutes of Health.

WIN. (2008b). *Very low-calorie diets.* (NIH Publication No. 03-3894). Bethesda, MD: National Institutes of Health.

Wilkinson, J., & Ahern, N. (2009). *Nursing diagnosis handbook* (9th ed.). Upper Saddle River, NJ: Pearson Prentice Hall.

Nursing Care of Patients with Upper Gastrointestinal Disorders

LEARNING OUTCOMES

1. Describe the pathophysiology of common disorders of the mouth, esophagus, and stomach.
2. Relate manifestations and diagnostic test results to the pathophysiologic processes involved in upper gastrointestinal disorders.
3. Explain interdisciplinary care for patients with upper gastrointestinal disorders.
4. Describe the role of the nurse in interdisciplinary care of patients with upper gastrointestinal disorders.

CLINICAL COMPETENCIES

1. Assess the functional health status of patients with upper gastrointestinal disorders.
2. Monitor, document, and, as needed, report manifestations of upper gastrointestinal disorders and their complications.
3. Plan patient-centered nursing care using an evidence base, research, and, as appropriate, decision-support technology.
4. Determine priority nursing diagnoses and interventions based on assessed data.
5. Administer medications and prescribed care knowledgeably and safely.
6. Coordinate and integrate interdisciplinary care into plan of care.
7. Construct and revise individualized plans of care considering the culture and values of the patient.
8. Plan and provide patient and family teaching to promote, maintain, and restore functional health.

KEY TERMS

achalasia, 627
anorexia, 642
Curling's ulcers, 642
Cushing's ulcers, 642
dumping syndrome, 645
dysphagia, 627
erosive (stress-induced) gastritis, 642
gastric mucosal barrier, 630

gastritis, 641
gastroesophageal reflux, 622
hematemesis, 630
hematochezia, 630
melena, 630
nausea, 612
occult bleeding, 630
partial gastrectomy, 645

peptic ulcer disease (PUD), 633
peptic ulcers, 633
steatorrhea, 635
stomatitis, 616
total gastrectomy, 645
ulcer, 634
vomiting, 612
Zollinger-Ellison syndrome, 635

The upper gastrointestinal tract includes the mouth, esophagus, stomach, and proximal small intestine. Food and fluids, ingested through the mouth, move through the esophagus to the stomach. The stomach and upper intestinal tract (duodenum and jejunum) are responsible for the majority of food digestion. When an acute or chronic condition or disease process interferes with the function of this portion of the gastrointestinal (GI) tract, nutritional status can be affected and the patient may experience symptoms that interfere with functional status and lifestyle.

Nurses provide acute care for the hospitalized patient, coordinate care in ambulatory and long-term care settings, and teach the skills and knowledge needed to manage these conditions at home.

The Patient with Nausea and Vomiting

Nausea and vomiting are common gastrointestinal symptoms. **Nausea** is a vague but unpleasant sensation of sickness or queasiness. It may or may not be accompanied by (and possibly relieved by) vomiting. **Vomiting** is the forceful expulsion of the contents of the upper GI tract resulting from contraction of muscles in the gut and abdominal wall. Nausea and vomiting without abdominal pain are commonly associated with food poisoning, infectious gastroenteritis (discussed in Chapter 24), gallbladder disease, or ingestion of toxins (such as drugs or alcohol). When associated with severe abdominal pain, they may indicate a serious disorder such as peritonitis, acute gastrointestinal obstruction, or pancreatitis.

Pathophysiology

Nausea, an unpleasant subjective sensation, occurs when the vomiting center in the medulla of the brain is stimulated. Distention of the duodenum is a common stimulus for nausea. The vomiting center can be stimulated by input from several different sources:

- The GI tract, produced by distention, irritation, or infection
- The vestibular system of the ear
- Higher central nervous system centers in response to certain sights, smells, or emotional experiences

- Chemoreceptors outside the blood–brain barrier that are stimulated by drugs, chemotherapeutic agents, toxins, systemic disorders, and pregnancy
- Disorders such as acute myocardial infarction and heart failure commonly produce nausea and vomiting, possibly due to direct stimulation of the vomiting center by hypoxia
- Increased intracranial pressure (e.g., due to intracranial bleeding or a tumor) produces vomiting that may or may not be accompanied by nausea

Anorexia, loss of appetite, commonly precedes nausea, just as nausea frequently precedes vomiting. Vomiting, a response that requires coordinated movements of the thorax and abdominal wall, the gut, the pharynx, and muscles of the mouth and face, is coordinated by the brainstem. *Emesis* (or *vomitus*) is produced when inspiratory muscles of the thorax (including the diaphragm) and abdomen contract, increasing intrathoracic and intra-abdominal pressures. The gastroesophageal sphincter relaxes, and the larynx moves upward to facilitate oral expulsion of gastric contents.

In addition to the subjective sensation of queasiness, nausea frequently is accompanied by autonomic nervous system manifestations such as pallor, sweating, tachycardia, and increased salivation. Vomiting, which stimulates the vagus nerve and parasympathetic nervous system, may be accompanied by dizziness, light-headedness, hypotension, and bradycardia.

Potential complications of vomiting include dehydration, hypokalemia, metabolic alkalosis (from loss of hydrochloric acid from the stomach), aspiration with resulting pneumonia, and rupture or tears of the esophagus.

Interdisciplinary Care

In most cases, nausea and vomiting are self-limited and require no treatment. If vomiting is severe or accompanied by other symptoms, acute care may be required to determine the underlying problem and prevent or treat complications.

Diagnostic tests may include serum electrolytes; pregnancy testing if indicated; liver, pancreatic, and renal function studies; and imaging studies (flat plate of the abdomen, abdominal CT scan) to detect gastrointestinal obstruction. An upper endoscopy may be performed (∞ see Chapter 21 for nursing care of the patient undergoing upper endoscopy). CT scan or MRI of the head may be ordered if an intracranial problem is suspected as the cause. Specialized testing such as gastrointestinal motility studies may be indicated when other diagnostic studies are negative for an anatomic cause of nausea and vomiting.

Food is initially withheld, although clear liquids in small quantities are encouraged to prevent dehydration. Dry foods such as soda crackers may reduce nausea and promote comfort.

Medications

Unless vomiting is associated with pregnancy, antiemetic medications may be prescribed to prevent or control nausea and vomiting. These drugs fall into a number of different classes, and often are more effective when given in combination.

- Serotonin receptor antagonists are the most effective drugs available for patients experiencing nausea and vomiting due to chemotherapy. They are effective when given only once or

twice a day, an additional advantage. Ondansetron (Zofran) is a prototype drug in this class.
- Dopamine antagonists include the phenothiazines (e.g., prochlorperazine [Compazine] and thiethylperazine [Torcan]), butyrophenones (haloperidol [Haldol] and droperidol [Inapsine]), and other drugs such as metoclopramide (Reglan). These drugs, while effective, can produce extrapyramidal symptoms, sedation, and hypotension.
- Antihistamines such as meclizine (Antivert), hydroxyzine (Vistaril, Atarax), and dimenhydrinate (Dramamine) are primarily used to treat nausea and vomiting arising from vestibular center stimuli (e.g., motion sickness).
- Two drugs classed as cannabinoids, related to marijuana, are approved to treat nausea and vomiting associated with chemotherapy. These drugs, dronabinol (Marinol) and nabilone (Cesamet), may produce unpleasant psychiatric effects such as dissociation and dysphoria, and are contraindicated for patients with psychiatric disorders. Tachycardia and hypotension are additional possible side effects.
- While corticosteroids are not approved as a class for treating nausea and vomiting, methylprednisolone (Solu-Medrol) and dexamethasone (Decadron) may be used in combination to treat vomiting associated with cancer treatment.
- Lorazepam (Ativan) is a benzodiazepine drug approved for use as an antiemetic. It produces a degree of sedation, but can suppress anticipatory vomiting (e.g., before chemotherapy). It also helps control extrapyramidal symptoms associated with the phenothiazine antiemetics.
- A new class of antiemetics, neurokinin receptor antagonists, primarily are used to prevent nausea and vomiting associated with chemotherapy. Aprepitant (Emend) is a prototype of this class.

Nursing responsibilities and patient education for antiemetic drugs are outlined in the accompanying Medication Administration box.

Complementary and Alternative Medicine

Mind–body interventions such as biofeedback, guided imagery, music therapy, and hypnosis may be effective for some patients with nausea. Biofeedback uses machinery to translate physiologic processes into audible or visible signals to teach the patient to exert conscious control over those processes. In guided imagery, the patient uses imagination to invoke specific images to modify physiologic responses. Music therapy employs creating or listening to music to affect physiologic and psychologic responses. In hypnosis, an altered mind state is induced to make the patient receptive to suggestions. A study by Suzanne Dibble and colleagues (2007) suggests that acupressure may help relieve chemotherapy-induced nausea and vomiting when combined with standard therapies. See the accompanying box.

Ginger, an aromatic root frequently used in cooking, may also be helpful in relieving nausea and vomiting, particularly when due to motion sickness (Fontaine, 2005; Spencer & Jacobs, 2003). In limited clinical trials, it has been shown to be safe for reducing nausea associated with pregnancy. It may help relieve nausea associated with cancer chemotherapy. Ginger can inhibit platelet aggregation, and may increase the risk of bleeding in patients taking antiplatelet or anticoagulant drugs (Lehne, 2007).

Chemotherapy-Induced Nausea and Vomiting

Patients undergoing chemotherapy regimens for cancer treatment often experience treatment-related nausea and vomiting. While newer antiemetic drugs are increasingly effective in preventing and treating chemotherapy-induced nausea and vomiting (CINV), many patients still experience both acute and delayed CINV. A study by Suzanne Dibble and colleagues (2007) looked at the effectiveness of acupressure in relieving CINV in women undergoing treatment for breast cancer.

Acupressure is a noninvasive Chinese medicine technique used to restore energy (*Qi*) balance in the body. It is believed that acupressure on P6, a specific point on the wrist, restores energy balance, relieving nausea. Acupressure may be applied using the thumbs, fingers, hands, or passive devices such as wrist bands.

All women in the study received standard CINV therapy. The study group was taught to apply acupressure to P6; a placebo group applied acupressure to a point on the side of the hand (S13), and the control group received standard therapy without acupressure. Although no significant differences were found in the acute nausea experiences among the groups, acupressure on the P6 point was found to be useful in

reducing delayed nausea and vomiting and hastening recovery after chemotherapy.

IMPLICATIONS FOR NURSING

Several studies have found acupressure to be an effective adjunct for relieving CINV. Nurses working in oncology units or with patients undergoing chemotherapy can teach patients how to use this noninvasive technique to promote comfort. Furthermore, patients may be less reluctant to start and continue chemotherapy if they perceive the ability to help control at least some of its unpleasant adverse effects.

CRITICAL THINKING IN PATIENT CARE

1. What are the mechanisms by which chemotherapy produces nausea and vomiting? Why are some regimens associated with more CINV than others?
2. Why is *preventing* CINV from the onset of chemotherapy so important?
3. Do you think acupressure is likely to be effective in a patient who doesn't "believe in all that alternative medicine stuff?" Why or why not?
4. Develop a teaching plan for a patient who will be starting chemotherapy using a drug known to produce nausea and vomiting in most patients who receive it.

⁀ Nursing Care

Assessment of the patient is vital to help determine the cause of nausea and vomiting, and to rule out underlying systemic disease or acute conditions that require immediate care (e.g., bowel obstruction). When the cause is known or no other acute symptoms are present, nursing interventions can promote comfort and prevent complications.

Nausea

The nursing diagnosis of nausea is defined as a subjective, unpleasant, wavelike sensation in the throat, epigastric region, or abdomen that may lead to vomiting (Wilkinson & Ahern, 2009).

- Monitor subjective complaints of nausea. *Nausea is a subjective sensation best described by the patient.*
- Monitor vital signs, skin turgor and condition, and weight. Maintain accurate intake and output records. Monitor amount, color, and specific gravity of urine. *Nausea can cause aversion to food and fluids, leading to dehydration even when it is not accompanied by vomiting.*
- Administer antiemetic medication as ordered, prior to meals and before treatments or procedures known to stimulate nausea. *Preventing nausea is particularly important for patients receiving chemotherapy, to avoid the association between the treatment and nausea.*
- Instruct to deep breathe to voluntarily suppress the vomiting reflex. *Controlling vomiting helps prevent dehydration and other complications associated with prolonged or severe vomiting.*
- Instruct to consume small quantities of clear fluids and dry foods at separate times. *Separating the intake of dry foods and fluids helps reduce the nausea stimulus.*

Community-Based Care

Instruct the patient to restrict intake to small quantities of clear liquids (tea, apple juice, broth, Jell-O) and dry foods such as soda crackers to help reduce nausea and prevent vomiting. Teach to avoid food-preparation odors if they produce nausea. Advise to restrict fluid intake for 1 hour before and after meals. Stress the need to maintain fluid intake to prevent dehydration and the importance of seeking additional medical help if unable to take in fluids or keep food down. Provide information about electrolyte replacement solutions such as sports drinks and commercially available electrolyte replacement solutions.

EVIDENCE FOR NURSING CARE **The Patient with Nausea and Vomiting**

Selected resources that nurses may find helpful when planning evidence-based nursing care follow.

- Association of Comprehensive Cancer Centres (ACCC). (2006, Jan 12). *Editorial Board Palliative Care: Practice Guidelines. Nausea and vomiting.* Utrecht, The Netherlands. Retrieved from http://www.guideline.gov/summary/summary.aspx?doc_id=11793&nbr=006067&string=
- Abraham, J. (2008 December). Acupressure and acupuncture in preventing and managing postoperative nausea and vomiting in adults. *Journal of Perioperative Practice, 18*(12), 543–551.
- Dibble, S., Lucy, J., Cooper, B., Israel, J., Cohen, M., Nussey, B., et al. (2007). Acupressure for chemotherapy-induced nausea and vomiting: A randomized clinical trial. *Oncology Nursing Forum, 34*(4), 813–820.

SEROTONIN RECEPTOR ANTAGONISTS

Dolasetron (Anzemet)

Granisetron (Kytril)

Ondansetron (Zofran)

Palonosetron (Aloxi)

The serotonin receptor antagonists suppress nausea and vomiting by blocking the effect of serotonin on vagal afferent nerves that stimulate the vomiting center. Their primary uses are to prevent vomiting associated with chemotherapy, radiation therapy, and surgery.

Nursing Responsibilities

- Administer 30 to 60 minutes prior to chemotherapy or surgery as directed.
- May be given orally or intravenously (push or infusion; follow directions specific to the drug used).
- Monitor liver function and clotting studies; report abnormal levels to the physician.

Health Education for the Patient and Family

- Take this drug exactly as directed.
- This drug may be taken without regard to food intake.
- Headache is a common side effect of these drugs, use acetaminophen or another mild analgesic as directed by your physician.

DOPAMINE ANTAGONISTS

Chlorpromazine (Thorazine)

Perphenazine (Trilafon)

Prochlorperazine (Compazine)

Promethazine (Phenergan)

Thiethylperazine (Torcan)

Haloperidol (Haldol)

Droperidol (Inapsine)

Metoclopramide (Reglan)

These drugs act by blocking dopamine receptors in the chemoreceptor trigger zone (CTZ). Their primary uses are to suppress nausea and vomiting associated with surgery, cancer chemotherapy, and toxins. The major adverse effects associated with these drugs are sedation, hypotension, and extrapyramidal reactions. Older adults are more sensitive to the effects of these drugs; a lower dose often is indicated.

Nursing Responsibilities

- Administer orally or parenterally as ordered before surgery or before meals and procedures known to produce nausea and vomiting.
- These drugs may interact with a number of other medications, often increasing their sedative and hypotensive effects.
- Administer with caution to older adults, closely monitoring for adverse effects such as confusion, agitation, changes in vital signs.
- Monitor for evidence of extrapyramidal symptoms, including tremor, restlessness, hyperactivity, anxiety, impaired coordination; notify physician if symptoms develop.

Health Education for the Patient and Family

- Use the drug as ordered; do not increase your dose without consulting your primary care provider.
- These drugs may cause drowsiness. Avoid using other central nervous system (CNS) depressants such as alcohol while taking these drugs.
- Change positions from lying to sitting and sitting to standing slowly because these drugs can cause light-headedness or dizziness.

- Promptly report changes in coordination, tremors, difficulty speaking or swallowing, or weakness to your physician.

SUBSTANCE P/NEUROKININ RECEPTOR ANTAGONIST

Aprepitant (Emend)

Aprepitant is a new drug that can prevent both acute and delayed chemotherapy-induced nausea and vomiting when given in combination with other antiemetic drugs. It is well-absorbed when given orally, and has a prolonged duration of action.

Nursing Responsibilities

- Administer daily for 3 days, giving the first dose 1 hour before chemotherapy.
- Can be given with food or on an empty stomach.
- Monitor for toxic and desired effects of other drugs, including chemotherapy drugs, corticosteroids, and warfarin (Coumadin), as aprepitant can affect their metabolism and blood levels.

Health Education for the Patient and Family

- Use barrier contraception while taking this drug as oral contraceptives will be less effective.
- Promptly contact your physician if you develop skin rash, difficulty breathing, changes in heart beat or blood pressure, dizziness or confusion, leg or abdominal pain, or rectal bleeding.
- Contact your physician before taking any new prescription, over-the-counter, or herbal preparations.

ANTIHISTAMINES

Buclizine (Bucladin-S)

Cyclizine (Marezine)

Dimenhydrinate (Dramamine)

Diphenhydramine (Benadryl)

Hydroxyzine (Vistaril, Atarax)

Meclizine (Antivert)

Antihistamines are primarily used to treat nausea and vomiting associated with motion sickness. They act by blocking histamine and acetylcholine (muscarinic) receptors in the neural pathway from the inner ear to the vomiting center in the brainstem.

Nursing Responsibilities

- Do not administer these drugs to patients for whom anticholinergic drugs are contraindicated: people with narrow-angle glaucoma, urinary retention, bowel obstruction.
- May be administered orally, parenterally, or rectally, depending on the preparation and the patient's ability to tolerate oral preparations.
- Use with caution in patients who are taking other CNS depressants or antihistamine preparations, tricyclic antidepressants, or monoamine oxidase inhibitors.

Health Education for the Patient and Family

- These drugs frequently cause drowsiness. Use caution when operating machinery or performing tasks requiring mental alertness.
- Avoid using alcohol or other substances that cause drowsiness or sedation while taking these drugs.
- The medication may cause dry mouth. Sips of water, ice chips, hard candies, and sugarless gum can be used for comfort.
- Use sunscreen and protective clothing to protect from sunburn while using these drugs.

(continued)

CANNABINOIDS

Dronabinol (Marinol)

Nabilone (Cesamet)

Drugs in this class, which contain the same active ingredient as marijuana, are reserved for use to relieve nausea and vomiting associated with cancer chemotherapy in patients who have not responded to treatment with other antiemetics. Their action is thought to result from inhibition of the vomiting center in the medulla.

Nursing Responsibilities

- Use with caution in older adults and people with a history of cardiovascular disease or substance abuse. These drugs are contraindicated for patients with a history of psychiatric disorders.

- Monitor for adverse effects such as dizziness, tachycardia, hypotension, impaired thinking and judgment, incoordination, irritability, depersonalization, distorted vision, and hallucinations.

Health Education for the Patient and Family

- Take the drug 1 to 3 hours before chemotherapy.
- Change positions slowly after taking this drug to prevent dizziness.
- You may experience distorted thinking, visual disturbances, confusion, and other mental symptoms while taking this drug.
- Keep this and all drugs out of the reach of children. Do not share this drug with anyone else.

Disorders of the Mouth

Inflammations, infections, and neoplastic lesions of the mouth affect food ingestion and nutrition. Oral lesions may have a variety of causes, including infection, trauma, irritants such as alcohol, and hypersensitivity. Appropriate treatment of the disorder, any underlying factors, and associated symptoms is essential.

The Patient with Stomatitis

Stomatitis, inflammation and ulcers of the oral mucosa, is a common disorder of the mouth. Viral infection is the most common cause. Other causes include bacterial or fungal infections, mechanical trauma (e.g., cheek biting), irritants (e.g., tobacco or ill-fitting dentures), nutritional deficiencies, and chemotherapeutic agents. Stomatitis often affects people who are immunocompromised (e.g., patients with HIV disease or who have cancer, and frail older adults). Box 23–1 lists common risk factors for stomatitis.

FAST FACTS

- Herpes simplex ("cold sore") is the most frequent viral cause of stomatitis; others include primary varicella zoster (chickenpox), Epstein-Barr virus, influenza, cytomegalovirus, and HIV.
- Overgrowth of *Candida albicans* is the most frequent fungal cause of stomatitis, usually following antibiotic or corticosteroid therapy.
- About 40% of people undergoing chemotherapy to treat cancer experience *oral mucositis*, a type of stomatitis; 75% of those undergoing chemotherapy in preparation for bone marrow or stem cell transplant develop oral mucositis.
- Most patients undergoing radiation therapy of the head and neck develop oral mucositis.

Pathophysiology and Manifestations

The oral mucosa, which lines the oral cavity, is a relatively thin, fragile layer of stratified squamous epithelial cells that constantly is being replaced. The blood supply to the oral mucosa is rich. As epithelial cells slough, stem cells in the submucosa develop into epithelial cells to replace those that are lost.

Frequent exposure to the environment, a rich blood supply, and the oral mucosa's delicate nature increase the risk of infection or inflammation, reaction to toxins, and trauma. Stomatitis results from persistent damage to oral mucosal cells. Damage is initially superficial, progressing to ulceration and involvement of the entire epithelium. Finally, healing begins within 2 to 4 weeks.

Oral mucositis progresses through identifiable stages. Radiotherapy and chemotherapy damage the DNA of epithelial cells, resulting in necrosis and death of some cells. This stimulates the release of inflammatory mediators that further damage tissues, causing additional epithelial cells to die. As a result, the oral mucosa thins. Tumor necrosis factor alpha (TNF-α) is released, which activates additional inflammatory cytokines. Tissues below the mucosa are damaged as well. In the ulcerative stage of oral mucositis, irregular ulcers that extend from the epithelium into the submucosa develop. As nerve endings are exposed, this stage is accompanied by significant pain. During the final healing stage, cells in the epithelium proliferate, and the normal thickness of the oral mucosa is restored.

The clinical manifestations of stomatitis vary according to its cause. Table 23–1 outlines common causes of stomatitis with their manifestations and treatment. Chemotherapy or chemical irritation may result in initial generalized redness and swelling, followed by development of deep, irregular ulcerations. Ulcers may be covered with pseudomembranes. Oral pain associated with stomatitis can interfere with the ability to eat, drink, and swallow normally.

Potential complications of stomatitis include malnutrition, fluid and electrolyte imbalance, sepsis, and bacterial endocarditis.

BOX 23–1 Risk Factors for Stomatitis

- Age > 65 years
- Impaired immune status (HIV disease, cancer, diabetes)
- Chronic renal failure or heart failure
- Chemotherapy, radiation therapy, stem cell transplant
- Oxygen therapy, mouth breathing
- Medications (antibiotics, phenytoin, anticholinergics, corticosteroids)
- Poor oral hygiene, ill-fitting dentures
- Tobacco or alcohol use

TABLE 23–1 Manifestations and Treatment of Common Stomatitis Conditions

TYPE	CAUSE	MANIFESTATIONS	TREATMENT
Cold sore, fever blister	Herpes simplex virus	■ Initial burning at site ■ Clustered vesicular lesions on lip or oral mucosa	■ Self-limiting ■ Acyclovir, famciclovir, valacyclovir to shorten course
Aphthous ulcer (canker sore, ulcerative stomatitis)	Unknown; may be type of herpes virus	■ Well-circumscribed, shallow erosions with white or yellow center encircled by red ring ■ Less than 1 cm in diameter ■ Painful	■ Topical steroid ointment ■ Amlexanox oral paste (Aphthasol) ■ Oral prednisone
Candidiasis (thrush)	*Candida albicans*	■ Creamy white, curdlike patches ■ Red, erythematous mucosa	■ Fluconazole (Diflucan) ■ Ketoconazole (Nizoral) ■ Clotrimazole troches ■ Nystatin vaginal troches (dissolved orally) or mouth rinse
Necrotizing ulcerative gingivitis (trench mouth, Vincent's infection)	Infection with spirochetes and bacilli or systemic infection	■ Acute gingival inflammation and necrosis ■ Bleeding, halitosis ■ Fever ■ Cervical lymphadenopathy	■ Correct any underlying disorders ■ Warm, half-strength peroxide mouthwashes ■ Oral penicillin
Oral mucositis	Damage to epithelial cells and stem cells in the submucosa caused by chemotherapy or radiation therapy	■ Erythema and inflammation of oral mucosa ■ Painful, irregularly shaped ulcerations, initially superficial, progressing to deep ulcers that may be confluent (overlapping with one another) ■ Pseudomembranes covering ulcers ■ Tissue necrosis with spontaneous bleeding, potential sepsis	■ Regular oral hygiene with brushing and flossing ■ Saline or sodium bicarbonate solution mouth rinses after and between meals ■ Gelclair mouth rinse before meals for analgesia ■ Palifermin, an epithelial cell growth factor ■ Low-level laser therapy

Interdisciplinary Care

Stomatitis is diagnosed by direct physical examination and, if indicated, cultures, smears, and evaluation for systemic illness. Treatment addresses both the underlying cause and any coexisting illnesses. An undiagnosed oral lesion present for more than 1 week and that does not respond to therapy must be evaluated for malignancy.

Direct smears and cultures of lesions may be obtained to identify causative organisms. If systemic illness is suspected, a variety of diagnostic tests may be ordered to identify the underlying cause.

General treatment measures include providing meticulous oral hygiene, with brushing using a soft brush and flossing (as tolerated). A solution of saline, sodium bicarbonate, or a combination of saline/bicarbonate promotes comfort and healing when used after and between meals.

Medications

Using a topical anesthetic, such as a mouthwash of 2% viscous lidocaine diluted with water, diphenhydramine (Benadryl) solution, or benzocaine spray or gel can promote comfort and the ability to consume oral food and fluids.

> **SAFETY ALERT**
> Instruct patients to expectorate lidocaine solution, not swallow it, to avoid impairment of swallowing.

Amlexanox (Aphthasol, OraDisc A) or Orabase, a protective paste, may be applied to oral ulcers to promote comfort.

Amlexanox speeds healing of aphthous ulcers as well. Triamcinolone acetonide may be mixed in Orabase to reduce inflammation and promote healing. Other coating agents include Amphojel or Kaopectate. Sodium bicarbonate mouthwashes may provide relief and promote cleansing, whereas alcohol-based mouthwashes may cause pain and burning and should be avoided. Agents that form a film over exposed nerve endings and deep ulcerations (e.g., Zilactin, Gelclair) may be used in patients with oral mucositis.

Fungal infections often are treated with a nystatin oral suspension; patients are instructed to "swish and swallow" the solution. Clotrimazole lozenges also treat oral fungal infections. If the infection does not resolve, oral antifungal medications such as fluconazole or ketoconazole may be used. Antifungals are usually continued for at least 3 days after symptoms disappear.

Herpetic lesions may be treated with topical or oral acyclovir (Zovirax), famciclovir (Famvir), or valacyclovir (Valtrex). Acyclovir ointment provides comfort and lubrication while limiting the spread of the virus. Oral preparations reduce the severity of symptoms and the duration of the lesions.

Bacterial infections are treated with antibiotics based on cultures and smears. Oral penicillin is the treatment of choice if the patient is not allergic and the cultured bacteria are sensitive. Nursing implications for selected drugs used to treat stomatitis are outlined on page 618.

An epithelial cell growth-stimulating factor, palifermin (Kepivance), reduces the incidence and duration of oral mucositis in patients undergoing high-dose chemotherapy in preparation for bone marrow or stem cell transplant.

∞ Nursing Care

Health Promotion

Nurses can help prevent stomatitis by identifying patients at risk and suggesting measures to reduce the likelihood that stomatitis will develop. Teach and encourage all patients to regularly perform mouth care, including teeth brushing and flossing. Provide frequent mouth care with nondrying agents for patients who are unable to provide self-care. Encourage patients with ill-fitting dentures or other dental prostheses (such as partial plates) to see a qualified dentist or denturist. Suggest patients taking an extended course of antibiotic therapy or who have impaired immune function consume 8 oz of yogurt containing live bacterial cultures or 8 oz of buttermilk daily unless contraindicated. Discuss dietary modifications, such as limiting consumption of highly spiced or acidic foods and avoiding very hot beverages. Patients undergoing chemotherapy or radiation therapy should avoid use of alcohol and tobacco because these substances further damage oral mucosa, increasing the risk for oral mucositis.

Assessment

Oral assessment is important not only for patients who have been diagnosed with stomatitis, but also for those with risk factors, manifestations, or evidence of possible complications (e.g., recent weight loss).

- *Health history:* Complaints of mouth pain, altered taste, lack of appetite, malaise; presence of dentures, regularity of dental care; current health status including chronic diseases; current medications; use of alcohol or tobacco.

- *Physical examination:* Inspect lips, gums, teeth, interior cheeks, tongue and base of tongue, soft and hard palate; tonsils, and oral pharynx. Observe and assess general health status including temperature, weight.

- *Diagnostic tests:* WBC, sedimentation rate, serum albumin.

Nursing Diagnoses and Interventions

Nursing care for the patient with stomatitis or oral mucositis focuses not only on the oral inflammation, but also on any underlying systemic diseases and the effects of the condition on the patient's comfort and nutrition.

Impaired Oral Mucous Membrane

Stomatitis and oral mucositis disrupt the integrity of the oral mucous membrane. Regardless of cause, the pain and symptoms must be relieved to promote comfort as well as food and fluid intake.

- Assess and document oral mucous membranes and the character of any lesions every 4 to 8 hours. *Baseline and ongoing assessment data provide the basis for evaluation.*

- Assist with thorough mouth care after meals, at bedtime, and every 2 to 4 hours while awake. If unable to tolerate a toothbrush, offer sponge or gauze toothettes. Avoid using alcohol-based mouthwashes or lemon-glycerin swabs. Provide saline or sodium bicarbonate rinse or a combined saline/sodium bicarbonate rinse after every meal and between meals. *Mouth care promotes hygiene, comfort, and healing. Alcohol-based mouthwashes and lemon-glycerin swabs may dry and irritate mucous membranes, causing pain and further tissue*

MEDICATION ADMINISTRATION   **Drugs Used to Treat Stomatitis**

TOPICAL ORAL ANESTHETICS

Orajel

Viscous lidocaine

Anbesol

Triamcinolone acetonide

These drugs reduce the pain associated with mucous membrane lesions or stomatitis. They provide temporary relief of pain. Any oral lesion that persists longer than 1 week should be evaluated by an oral surgeon.

Nursing Responsibilities
- Instruct the patient to seek medical attention for any oral lesion that does not heal within 1 week.
- Monitor for local hypersensitivity reactions, and discontinue use if they occur.

Health Education for the Patient and Family
- Apply every 1 to 2 hours as needed.
- Perform oral hygiene after meals and at bedtime.

TOPICAL ANTIFUNGAL AGENTS

Clotrimazole

Nystatin

These products help in the topical treatment of candidiasis. Their effects are primarily local rather than systemic.

Nursing Responsibilities
- Instruct the patient to dissolve lozenges in the mouth.

- Instruct the patient to rinse mouth with oral suspension for at least 2 minutes and expectorate or swallow as directed.
- These drugs are contraindicated in pregnancy.

Health Education for the Patient and Family
- Take medication as prescribed.
- Do not eat or drink 30 minutes after medication.
- Contact physician if symptoms worsen.
- Perform good oral hygiene after meals and at bedtime; remove dentures at bedtime.

ANTIVIRAL AGENTS

Acyclovir (Zovirax)

Famciclovir (Famvir)

Valacyclovir (Valtrex)

Acyclovir, famciclovir, and valacyclovir are useful in the treatment of oral herpes simplex virus. They help reduce the severity and frequency of infections. These antiviral agents interfere with the DNA synthesis of herpes simplex virus.

Nursing Responsibilities
- Start therapy as soon as herpetic lesions are noted.
- Administer with food or on an empty stomach.

Health Education for the Patient and Family
- The virus remains latent and can recur during stressful events, fever, trauma, sunlight exposure, and treatment with immunosuppressive drugs.
- Take the medication as ordered, and contact the physician if symptoms worsen.

damage, whereas saline or bicarbonate rinses promote comfort and healing (Cawley & Benson, 2005).

- Assess knowledge and teach about condition, mouth care, and treatments. Instruct to avoid alcohol, tobacco, and spicy or irritating foods. *Knowledge promotes patient participation in the plan of care and compliance. Alcohol, tobacco, and hot, spicy, or rough foods may injure the inflamed mucous membranes.*

Imbalanced Nutrition: Less than Body Requirements

Oral lesions and pain may limit oral intake, which may in turn lead to nutritional deficits. Anorexia and general malaise may also contribute to decreased intake.

- Assess food intake as well as the patient's ability to chew and swallow. Weigh daily. Provide appropriate assistive devices such as straws or feeding syringes. *Adequate nutrition is essential for healing. Daily weights allow monitoring of the adequacy of food intake. Assistive devices may allow food intake while avoiding irritation of ulcerations or lesions.*
- Encourage a high-calorie, high-protein diet considerate of food preferences. Offer soft, lukewarm, or cool foods or liquids such as eggnogs, milk shakes, nutritional supplements, popsicles, and puddings frequently in small amounts. Obtain nutritional consultation. *Oral intake may be limited, and enriched foods and liquids enhance nutrition. A nutritional consultation can help ensure an adequate diet and assist in meeting nutritional needs.*
- Provide analgesics for pain relief as needed. *Significant pain associated with stomatitis or oral mucositis can interfere with effective mouth care and food and fluid intake. Pain management is a vital part of nursing care.*

Using NANDA, NIC, and NOC

Linkages between a selected NANDA nursing diagnosis, NIC, and NOC for the patient with stomatitis are shown in the chart that follows.

NANDA, NIC, AND NOC LINKAGES
The Patient with Stomatitis

NANDA Impaired Oral Mucous Membrane

NIC Oral Health Restoration
Nutrition Management
Fluid Monitoring

NOC Oral Hygiene
Self-Care: Oral Hygiene
Tissue Integrity: Skin & Mucous Membranes
Nutritional Status: Food and Fluid Intake

Data from NANDA International. (2009). *Nursing diagnoses: Definitions & classification 2009–2011.* Oxford, UK: Wiley-Blackwell; Bulechek, G., Butcher, H., & Dochterman, J. (Eds.). (2008). *Nursing interventions classification (NIC)* (5th ed.). St. Louis, MO: Mosby; and Moorhead, S., Johnson, M., Maas, M., & Swanson, E. (Eds.). (2008). *Nursing outcomes classification (NOC)* (4th ed.). St. Louis, MO: Mosby.

Community-Based Care

Patients with mild stomatitis generally provide self-care. While patients with cancer-treatment-related oral mucositis may require more aggressive therapy, the patient and caregivers often are able to manage the regimen in home- or community-based settings. Include the following topics in teaching for home care:

- Managing any underlying health conditions and ongoing treatments such as chemotherapy
- The recommended diet and oral hygiene regime, including foods and substances (e.g., alcohol, tobacco products) to avoid
- Nutritional supplements to help meet nutritional requirements
- Prescribed medication, its route, side effects, frequency of administration, and signs and symptoms to report
- The importance of completing the full course of antibiotic, antiviral, or antifungal treatment
- Manifestations to report and the importance of follow-up care

The Patient with Oral Cancer

Oral cancer, malignancy of the oral mucosa, may develop on the lips, tongue, floor of the mouth, or other oral tissues. It is uncommon, accounting for only 3% of all new cancers diagnosed in men and 2% in women during 2008. It has, however, a high rate of morbidity and mortality. It is seen more often in people over age 40. Although a lesion can develop in any area of the mouth, the most common sites are the lower lip, tongue, and floor of the mouth. The stage of an oral cancer determines the prognosis, treatment, and degree of disability. The primary risk factors for oral cancer are smoking, drinking alcohol, and chewing tobacco. Marijuana use, occupational exposures to chemicals, and viruses such as human papilloma virus (HPV) also may contribute to the risk for oral cancer.

Pathophysiology and Manifestations

More than 90% of oral and oropharyngeal tumors are a squamous cell carcinoma. Most early cancers present as inflamed areas with irregular, ill-defined borders. These lesions typically are not painful. More advanced cancers appear as deep ulcers that are fixed to deeper tissues. Early lesions involve the mucosa or submucosa, whereas more advanced tumors may invade and destroy underlying tissues, including muscles and bones of the face. Tumors frequently metastasize to regional lymph nodes. Other cancerous lesions, including lymphoma, malignant melanoma, and Kaposi's sarcoma, may

MANIFESTATIONS of Oral Cancer

- White patches (leukoplakia)
- Red patches (erythroplakia)
- Ulcers
- Masses
- Pigmented areas (brownish or black)
- Fissures
- Asymmetry of the head, face, jaws, or neck

Figure 23–1 ■ Oral cancer.

Source: Biophoto Associates/Photo Researchers, Inc.

BOX 23–2 Oral Cancer Staging

Stage 0	Carcinoma *in situ*
Stage I	Tumor ≤ 2 cm; no regional node involvement
Stage II	Tumor > 2 cm to ≤ 4 cm; no regional node involvement
Stage III	Tumor ≤ 2 cm to > 4 cm; one involved lymph node
Stage IVA & B	Tumor may invade adjacent structures; one or more nodes involved
Stage IVC	Distant metastasis present

develop in the mouth, although less frequently than squamous cell carcinoma.

The earliest symptom of oral cancer is a painless oral ulceration or lesion (Figure 23–1 ■). Later symptoms vary and may include difficulty speaking, swallowing, or chewing; swollen lymph nodes; and blood-tinged sputum. See the accompanying box for other manifestations of oral cancer. Any oral lesion that does not heal or respond to treatment within 1 to 2 weeks should be evaluated for malignancy.

Interdisciplinary Care

The first component of treatment is eliminating any causative factors such as chewing tobacco, smoking, or drinking alcohol. Tumor staging then determines therapy. The TNM (tumor, nodes, metastasis) classification is used to stage oral cancer. See Box 23–2. A biopsy of the oral lesion allows direct visualization of cells to determine the presence or absence of cancerous cells. Staging may require additional diagnostic studies such as computed tomography (CT) scans or magnetic resonance imaging (MRI).

Early cancers (stages I and II) are highly curable using surgery or radiation therapy. The treatment choice is based on the expected functional and cosmetic results of treatment. More advanced tumors (stages III and IV) generally require a treatment combination of surgery, radiation, and possibly chemotherapy. ∞ See Chapter 14 for more information about radiation and chemotherapy to treat cancer.

Following biopsy and staging of the tumor, surgery is often indicated, although an advanced or extensive tumor may be considered unresectable. If the tumor involves surrounding tissues, the cosmetic effects of surgery are important considerations. The goal of surgery is removal of the lesion and potentially cancerous surrounding tissue or lymph nodes. Advanced carcinomas may require extensive excision or a *radical neck dissection*, a potentially disfiguring procedure in which the lymph nodes and muscles of the neck are removed. A tracheostomy is performed at the time of surgery. The tracheostomy may be temporary, but often is permanent. ∞ See Chapter 35 for more information about caring for a patient following radical neck dissection and a tracheostomy.

✍ Nursing Care

Health Promotion

Reducing or eliminating tobacco use (smoking and smokeless tobacco) and excess alcohol consumption can significantly reduce the incidence of oral cancer. Teach children and adolescents about the dangers of using tobacco and alcohol. Emphasize the relationship between smokeless tobacco and oral cancer. Discuss strategies to deal with peer pressure to use tobacco and alcohol.

To promote early identification of and intervention for oral cancer, teach patients about the risk factors for and manifestations of the disease. This is a particularly important nursing strategy in older men who have the highest incidence, and in populations in whom the disease often is advanced when detected (people of lower socioeconomic status, people who rarely see a dentist, and African American men).

Assessment

Early precancerous oral lesions are very treatable. Unfortunately, these lesions usually are painless, so diagnosis and treatment often is delayed. Assess the oral cavity of all patients, particularly those with risk factors for oral cancer.

- *Health history:* Complaints of oral lesions that fail to heal; use (current or past) of tobacco products or excess alcohol.
- *Physical examination:* Inspect and palpate lips and oral mucosa (including tongue and floor of mouth under the tongue) for tumors or lesions. Lesions may appear as velvety red or white patches that do not scrape off, or as ulcers or areas of necrosis.

Nursing Diagnoses and Interventions

The mouth allows food ingestion, and the lips are integral to verbal and nonverbal expression. The head, mouth, and lips are important to self-perception and body image. Nursing diagnoses discussed in this section consider such problems as airway clearance, nutrition, communication, and body image. See the accompanying Case Study & Nursing Care Plan.

Risk for Ineffective Airway Clearance

The location and the extent of an oral cancer and its excision may compromise the airway. Swelling of adjacent tissues, increased oral secretions, or difficulty swallowing may contribute to respiratory distress. If extensive surgery is performed, a tracheostomy usually is performed to maintain airway patency.

Juan Chavez, a married 44-year-old farmer, has two adult children. He and his wife raise and sell fruits and vegetables. Two months ago, Mr. Chavez developed a sore on his tongue that would not heal. Mr. Chavez tells his admission nurse, Sara Bucklin, "The doctor says he will have to remove part of my tongue," and anxiously asks, "Will I ever look the same? How will I be able to talk?"

ASSESSMENT

Mr. Chavez's admission history reveals that he has been healthy, but has smoked two packs of cigarettes a day for more than 20 years, and usually drinks two to four beers per day. He admits to being anxious and tearful of surgery and its outcomes. He says he quit smoking and drinking 2 weeks ago. The biopsy report is positive for squamous cell carcinoma of the tongue. Mr. Chavez has no enlarged cervical nodes and says he has no bloody sputum or saliva, difficulty swallowing, chewing, or talking. His weight is in the normal range for his height. A wide excision of the oral lesion is planned.

DIAGNOSES

- *Risk for Ineffective Airway Clearance* related to oral surgery
- *Risk for Imbalanced Nutrition: Less than Body Requirements* related to oral surgery
- *Impaired Verbal Communication* related to excision of a portion of the tongue
- *Disturbed Body Image* related to surgical excision of the tongue

EXPECTED OUTCOMES

- Maintain a patent airway and remain free of respiratory distress.
- Maintain a stable weight and level of hydration.
- Effectively communicate with staff and family using a magic slate and flash cards.
- Communicate an increased ability to accept changes in body image.

PLANNING AND IMPLEMENTATION

- Assess airway patency and respiratory status every hour until stable.

- Maintain semi-Fowler's position, supporting arms. Encourage to turn, cough, and deep breathe every 2 to 4 hours.
- Teach the importance of activity, turning, coughing, and deep breathing.
- Monitor daily weights.
- Consult with dietitian to assess calorie needs and plan appropriate enteral feeding. Assess response to enteral feedings.
- Demonstrate and allow to practice using magic slate and flash cards prior to surgery.
- Allow adequate time for communication efforts.
- Keep emergency call system in reach at all times and answer light promptly. Alert all staff of inability to respond verbally.
- Encourage expression of feelings regarding perceived and actual changes.
- Provide emotional support and encourage self-care and participation in decision making.

EVALUATION

At the time of discharge, Mr. Chavez has maintained his weight and has started on oral liquids, including supplements and enriched liquids. His airway has remained clear, and he is effectively coughing and deep breathing. He has used the magic slate to communicate throughout his hospital stay. He is regaining use of his tongue, and can speak a few words. Although initially distressed, he is communicating an increased ability to cope with loss of part of his tongue. He and his wife say they understand his discharge instructions, including diet, activity, follow-up care, and signs and symptoms to report.

CRITICAL THINKING IN THE NURSING PROCESS

1. What measures can you, as a nurse, implement to reduce the incidence of oral cancer?
2. Plan a health education program for young athletes who chew tobacco.
3. Mr. Chavez's wife calls you 2 weeks after discharge. She tells you that he refuses to try to talk and is relying on his magic slate to communicate. How will you respond?

See Evaluating Your Response in Appendix C.

PRACTICE ALERT

In the initial postoperative period, assess airway patency and respiratory status at least hourly. A patent airway is vital to maintain respirations and oxygenation of tissues. Frequent assessment allows early identification of possible airway compromise.

- Unless contraindicated, place in Fowler's position, supporting arms. Assist the patient to turn, cough, and deep breathe at least every 2 to 4 hours. *Fowler's position promotes lung expansion. Turning, coughing, and deep breathing help maintain a patent airway by preventing pooling of secretions.*
- Maintain adequate hydration (2000 to 3000 mL per day unless contraindicated) and humidity of inspired air. *Adequate hydration helps thin and loosen secretions.*

Imbalanced Nutrition: Less than Body Requirements

Surgery affects oral food and fluid intake. Enteral feedings or parenteral nutrition may be required. A gastrostomy tube usually is inserted during surgery to maintain nutrition. If an oral diet is permitted, anorexia or pain may affect intake.

- Weigh daily. Assess oral intake for adequacy of protein, calories, and nutrients. *Daily weights and nutritional assessments provide information about the adequacy of diet.*
- Offer soft, bland foods with supplements as indicated. Provide small, frequent feedings, making mealtimes pleasant. *Soft, bland foods may be better tolerated following oral surgery. Large meals may be overwhelming; small, frequent meals promote food and nutrient intake.*
- Provide enteral feedings per gastrostomy tube as ordered. Elevate the head of the bed 30 to 40 degrees. *Enteral feedings maintain nutritional status in the patient who is unable to consume foods orally. Elevating the head of the bed reduces the risk of regurgitation and aspiration of gastric contents.*
- Assess for gastric residual volume per facility protocol for the type of feeding (intermittent or continuous). Notify the physician of volumes greater than 200 mL or 50% of previous feeding if feeding is intermittent. *Excess residual volume may increase the risk for aspiration.*
- Consider a nutritional consultation to assess diet and plan appropriate supplements. *A registered dietitian can calculate energy requirements and develop an individualized diet plan to meet nutritional requirements.*

Impaired Verbal Communication

Oral surgery can interfere with communication. Effective communication is vital to postoperative recovery and prevention of complications.

- Before surgery, establish and practice a communication plan such as using a magic slate or flash cards. *Practicing communication techniques reduces fear and anxiety while promoting communication.*
- Provide ample time for communication efforts and do not answer for the patient. Be alert for nonverbal communications. Use yes/no questions and simple phrases. *Providing adequate time allows the patient opportunity to express ideas and thoughts. Nonverbal communication provides cues regarding comfort or other needs. Simple yes/no questions are easily answered nonverbally.*
- If indicated, refer to or consult with a speech therapist. *A speech therapist can help promote or restore effective communication.*

PRACTICE ALERT

Provide an emergency call system and respond promptly. Make all staff aware that the patient cannot respond over an intercom system by posting an alert on the intercom. Nonverbal patients rely on an emergency call system to summon help. Answering promptly reduces fear and anxiety and maintains safety.

Disturbed Body Image

Radical surgery of the head or neck seriously affects body image. An altered speech pattern and any disfigurement affect the ability to feel attractive or effective in work or social roles.

Patients may defer lifesaving surgery to postpone disfiguring interventions or therapies.

- Assess coping style, self-perception, and responses to altered appearance or function. *This information can be used to identify appropriate interventions and care.*
- Encourage verbalization of feelings regarding perceived and actual changes. *Nonjudgmental acceptance of feelings and fears helps establish trust.*
- Provide emotional support, encourage self-care, and provide decision-making opportunities. *Self-care promotes self-acceptance and independence. Giving choices empowers the patient to participate in care.*

Community-Based Care

Discharge planning for the patient with oral cancer depends on the type of treatment planned and surgery performed. Depending on the patient's age, condition, and availability of support systems, referral to a rehabilitation center and community healthcare agencies may be an essential component of care. Visits from home care nurses can assist in meeting healthcare needs.

Discuss the following topics with the patient and family members or care providers:

- Diagnosis and prescribed care
- Monitoring for new lesions or recurrences
- Diet, nutrition, and activity
- Pain management
- Airway management, care of incision, and signs and symptoms to report

Disorders of the Esophagus

The esophagus plays an essential role in the ingestion of food and liquids. Disorders of the esophagus can be inflammatory, mechanical, or cancerous. Because of its location and neighboring organs, the symptoms of esophageal disorders may mimic those of a variety of other illnesses.

The Patient with Gastroesophageal Reflux Disease

Gastroesophageal reflux is the backward flowing of gastric contents into the esophagus. When this occurs, the patient experiences heartburn. Many people with gastroesophageal reflux have few symptoms, while others develop inflammatory esophagitis as a result of exposure to gastric juices. *Gastroesophageal reflux disease (GERD)* is a common gastrointestinal disorder.

FAST FACTS

- GERD affects 15% to 20% of adults.
- Up to 7% of people experience daily symptoms such as heartburn, regurgitation, and indigestion, and as many as 15% to 20% have symptoms weekly (Fauci et al., 2008; McPhee et al., 2008).

Pathophysiology

Normally, the lower esophageal sphincter remains closed except during swallowing. Reflux (backflow) of gastric contents into the esophagus is prevented by pressure differences between the stomach and the lower esophagus. The diaphragm, the lower esophageal sphincter, and the location of the gastroesophageal junction below the diaphragm help maintain this pressure difference (Figure 23–2 ■).

Gastroesophageal reflux may result from transient relaxation of the lower esophageal sphincter, an incompetent lower esophageal sphincter, and/or increased pressure within the stomach. Factors contributing to gastroesophageal reflux include increased gastric volume (e.g., after meals), positioning that allows gastric contents to remain close to the gastroesophageal junction (e.g., bending over, lying down), and increased gastric pressure (e.g., obesity or wearing tight clothing). A hiatal hernia may contribute to GERD.

Gastric juices contain acid, pepsin, and bile, which are corrosive substances. Esophageal peristalsis and bicarbonate in salivary secretions normally clear and neutralize gastric juices in the esophagus. During sleep and in patients with impaired esophageal peristalsis or decreased salivation, the esophageal mucosa is damaged by gastric juices, causing an inflammatory response (Figure 23–3 ■). With prolonged exposure, reflux esophagitis develops. In nonerosive reflux disease, the mucosa remains normal or mildly inflamed. Erosive esophagitis, however,

Figure 23–2 ■ The esophagus. The inset shows a closer view of the lower esophageal sphincter.

is characterized by red, friable (easily torn) mucosa and superficial ulcers. If untreated, scarring occurs, and esophageal stricture may develop.

Manifestations

GERD causes heartburn, usually after meals, with bending over, or when reclining. Regurgitation of sour material into the mouth, or difficulty and pain with swallowing may develop. Other manifestations may include atypical chest pain, sore throat, and hoarseness. See the following table illustrating links between the pathophysiology of GERD and its symptoms. Aspiration of gastric contents can cause hoarseness or respiratory symptoms.

Complications include esophageal strictures and Barrett's esophagus. Strictures, caused by scar tissue, edema, and spasm, can lead to dysphagia. Barrett's esophagus is characterized by changes in the cells lining the esophagus and an increased risk of developing esophageal cancer (Porth & Matfin, 2009).

Interdisciplinary Care

Often the diagnosis of GERD is made by the history of symptoms and predisposing factors. Interdisciplinary care focuses on lifestyle changes, diet modification, and for more severe cases, drug therapy. Surgery is reserved for patients who develop serious complications.

Diagnosis

Diagnostic tests that may be ordered for patients with manifestations of GERD include the following:

- *Barium swallow* to evaluate the esophagus, stomach, and upper small intestine.
- *Upper endoscopy* to permit direct visualization of the esophagus. Tissue may be obtained for biopsy to establish the diagnosis and rule out malignancy. ∞ See Chapter 21 for nursing care of the patient undergoing an upper endoscopy.

- In the *Bernstein test*, saline and dilute acid solutions are instilled into the esophagus. In patients with GERD, the acid solution produces symptoms of heartburn, whereas the saline solution does not; neither solution produces symptoms in patients who do not have GERD.
- *24-hour ambulatory pH monitoring* may be performed to establish the diagnosis of GERD. For this test, a small tube with a pH electrode is inserted through the nose into the esophagus. The electrode is attached to a small box worn on the belt that records the data. The data are later analyzed by computer.

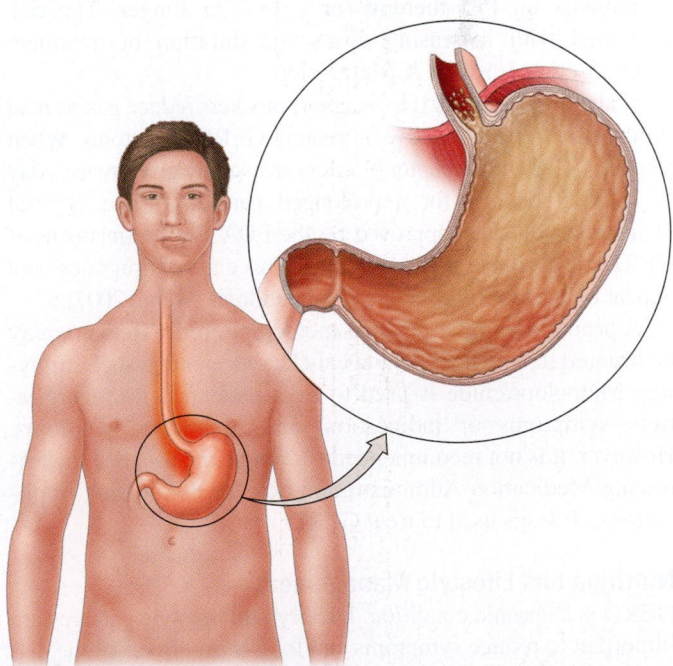

Figure 23–3 ■ In gastroesophageal reflux disease, reflux of corrosive gastric secretions into the lower esophagus causes inflammation of esophageal mucosa.

MANIFESTATIONS AND PATHOPHYSIOLOGY of GERD

MANIFESTATION	PATHOPHYSIOLOGY
Heartburn Chest pain Regurgitation Belching	Reflux of gastric juices through the lower esophageal (cardiac) sphincter into the lower esophagus exposes esophageal mucosa to corrosive pepsin, acid, and bile. Gastric juices normally are cleared by esophageal peristalsis or neutralized by saliva; when these mechanisms are impaired, esophageal mucosa becomes inflamed, and eventually may ulcerate. Further exposure of the inflamed and ulcerated mucosa to corrosive gastric juices leads to heartburn or angina-like or atypical chest pain.
Dysphagia	Untreated esophagitis leads to inflammatory cell infiltrates, fibrosis, and scaring of esophageal tissue, constricting its lumen and causing difficult, painful swallowing.
Pain after eating	Increased gastric volume increases pressure within the stomach relative to the ability of the lower esophageal sphincter to prevent reflux into the esophagus. Reflux irritates already inflamed tissue, causing pain.
Chronic cough Hoarseness Laryngitis, pharyngitis	Reflux of gastric contents into the pharynx and mouth allows aspiration of gastric contents into the tracheobronchial tree. This usually occurs during sleep, when a recumbent position increases gastroesophageal reflux, and relaxation of tissues and muscles in the oropharynx increases the risk of aspiration.

- *Esophageal manometry* measures pressures of the esophageal sphincters and esophageal peristalsis.

Medications

Antacids, such as Mylanta or Maalox, relieve mild or moderate symptoms by neutralizing stomach acid. Gaviscon, which forms a floating barrier between the gastric contents and the esophageal mucosa when the patient is upright, may be used.

Proton-pump inhibitors (PPIs) such as omeprazole (Prilosec) and lansoprazole (Prevacid) reduce gastric secretions. PPIs promote healing of erosive esophagitis and relieve symptoms. An 8-week course of treatment is initially prescribed, although some patients may require 3 to 6 months of therapy. Relapse is common after PPI therapy is discontinued. Although these drugs have minimal side effects, they may interfere with absorption of calcium and vitamin B_{12}. A study by Yang and associates showed an increased risk of hip fracture in patients on PPI therapy for a year or longer. The risk increased with increasing doses and duration of treatment (Yang, Lewis, Epstein, & Metz, 2006).

Histamine$_2$-receptor (H$_2$-receptor) blockers reduce gastric acid production and are effective in treating GERD symptoms. When treating GERD, H$_2$-receptor blockers are usually given twice a day or more frequently for a prolonged period of time. Several H$_2$-receptor blockers approved by the FDA for the treatment of GERD are available over the counter. This class of drugs does not appear to increase hip-fracture risk (Gendreau-Webb, 2007).

A promotility agent, such as metoclopramide (Reglan), may be ordered to enhance esophageal clearance and gastric emptying. Metoclopramide is used to treat patients with regurgitation, symptoms of indigestion, and nighttime symptoms. However, it is not recommended for long-time use. See the following Medication Administration box for the nursing implications of drugs used to treat GERD.

Nutrition and Lifestyle Management

GERD is a chronic condition. Dietary and lifestyle changes are important to reduce symptoms and long-term effects of the disorder. Acidic foods such as tomato products, citrus fruits, spicy foods, and coffee are eliminated from the diet. Fatty foods, chocolate, peppermint, and alcohol relax the lower esophageal

sphincter or delay gastric emptying, so they should be avoided. The patient is advised to maintain ideal body weight, eat smaller meals, refrain from eating for 3 hours before bedtime, and stay upright for 2 hours after meals. Elevating the head of the bed on 6- to 8-inch blocks often is beneficial. Stopping smoking is a necessary lifestyle change. Avoiding tight clothing and avoiding bending may help to relieve symptoms.

Surgery

Surgery may be used for patients who do not respond to pharmacologic and lifestyle management. Antireflux surgeries increase pressure in the lower esophagus, inhibiting gastric content reflux. Laparoscopic fundoplication, a procedure in which the gastric fundus is wrapped around the distal esophagus, is the treatment of choice for GERD. An open surgical procedure known as Nissen fundoplication also may be done (Figure 23–4 ■). Other laparoscopic procedures to tighten the lower esophageal sphincter may include use of an endoscopic suturing system or burning spots on the muscle surrounding the sphincter to create scar tissue. Surgery or ablation therapy also is recommended to reduce the risk of esophageal cancer in patients with persistent cell changes in the distal esophagus.

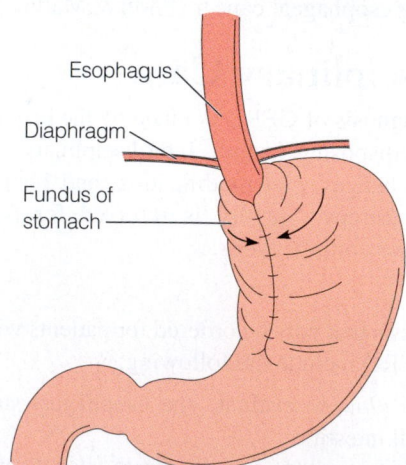

Figure 23–4 ■ Nissen fundoplication. The fundus of the stomach is wrapped around the lower esophagus and the edges are sutured together.

PROTON-PUMP INHIBITORS

Esomeprazole (Nexium)

Lansoprazole (Prevacid)

Omeprazole (Prilosec)

Pantoprazole (Protonix)

Rabeprazole (AcipHex)

Proton-pump inhibitors are the drugs of choice for severe GERD. PPIs inhibit the hydrogen-potassium-ATP pump, reducing gastric acid secretion. If the patient's symptoms do not improve with treatment, the dose may be increased.

Nursing Responsibilities

- Administer 30 minutes before breakfast (and at bedtime if ordered twice a day).
- Do not crush tablets.
- Monitor liver function tests for possible abnormal values, including increased AST, ALT, alkaline phosphatase, and bilirubin levels.

Health Education for the Patient and Family

- Take the drug as ordered for the full course of therapy, even if symptoms are relieved.
- Do not crush, break, or chew tablets.
- Increase your calcium intake or take a calcium supplement while using this drug as it can interfere with calcium absorption.
- Avoid cigarette smoking, alcohol, aspirin, and NSAIDs while taking this drug because these substances may interfere with healing.
- Report black tarry stools, diarrhea, or abdominal pain to your primary care provider.

H₂-RECEPTOR BLOCKERS

Cimetidine (Tagamet)   Ranitidine (Zantac)

Famotidine (Pepcid)   Nizatidine (Axid)

H_2-receptor blockers reduce acidity of gastric juices by blocking the ability of histamine to stimulate acid secretion by the gastric parietal cells. As a result, both the volume and concentration of hydrochloric acid in gastric juice are reduced. H_2-receptor blockers are given orally or intravenously. Both prescription and over-the-counter preparations are available.

Nursing Responsibilities

- To ensure absorption, do not give an antacid within 1 hour before or after giving an H_2-receptor blocker.
- When administered intravenously, do not mix with other drugs. Administer in 20 to 100 mL of solution over 15 to 30 minutes. Rapid intravenous injection as a bolus may cause dysrhythmias and hypotension.
- Monitor for interaction with such drugs as oral anticoagulants, beta-blockers, benzodiazepines, tricyclic antidepressants, and others. H_2-receptor blockers may inhibit the metabolism of other drugs, increasing the risk of toxicity.

Health Education for the Patient and Family

- Take the drug as directed, even if pain and gastric discomfort are relieved early in the course of therapy.
- Take at bedtime if once-a-day dosing is ordered. If spaced through the day, take before meals. Avoid taking antacids for 1 hour before and 1 hour after taking this drug.
- To promote healing, avoid cigarette smoking (which increases gastric acid secretion) and gastric mucosal irritants such as alcohol, aspirin, and NSAIDs.

- Long-term use of these drugs can lead to gynecomastia (breast enlargement) and impotence in men and breast tenderness in women. Discontinuing the drug will reverse these effects.
- Report possible adverse effects such as diarrhea, confusion, rash, fatigue, malaise, or bruising to your care provider.

ANTIULCER AGENT

Sucralfate (Carafate)

Sucralfate reacts with gastric acid to form a thick paste that adheres to damaged gastric mucosal tissue. It protects gastric mucosa and promotes healing through this local action.

Nursing Responsibilities

- Administer on an empty stomach, 1 hour before meals and at bedtime.
- Do not crush tablets.
- Separate administration time from antacids by at least 30 minutes.

Health Education for the Patient and Family

- Take as directed, even after symptoms have been relieved.
- Do not crush or chew tablets; shake suspension well.
- Increase your intake of fluids and dietary fiber to prevent constipation.

ANTACIDS

Maalox	Gaviscon	Gelusil	Tums
Mylanta	Aludrox	Riopan	Amphojel

Antacids buffer or neutralize gastric acid, usually acting locally. Antacids are used in GERD, gastritis, and peptic ulcer disease to relieve pain and prevent further damage to esophageal and gastric mucosa.

Nursing Responsibilities

- Antacids interfere with the absorption of many drugs given orally; separate administration times by at least 2 hours.
- Monitor for constipation or diarrhea resulting from antacid therapy. Notify the physician should either develop; a different antacid may be ordered.
- Although most antacids have little systemic effect, electrolyte imbalances can develop. Monitor serum electrolytes, particularly sodium, calcium, and magnesium levels.

Health Education for the Patient and Family

- Take your antacid frequently as prescribed, 1 to 3 hours after meals and at bedtime. To be effective, the antacid must be in your stomach.
- Avoid taking an antacid for approximately 2 hours before and 1 hour after taking another medication.
- Shake suspensions well prior to administration.
- Chew tablets thoroughly, and follow with 4 to 6 ounces of water.
- Report worsening symptoms, diarrhea, or constipation to your primary care provider.
- Continue taking the antacid for the duration prescribed. Although pain and discomfort often are relieved soon after treatment begins, healing takes 6 to 8 weeks.

PROMOTILITY AGENT

Metoclopramide (Reglan)

By acting on the central nervous system, metoclopramide stimulates upper gastrointestinal motility and gastric emptying. As a result, nausea, vomiting, and symptoms of GERD are reduced.

(continued)

MEDICATION ADMINISTRATION   Drugs Used to Treat GERD, Gastritis, and Peptic Ulcer Disease (continued)

Nursing Implications

- Do not administer this drug to patients with possible gastrointestinal obstruction or bleeding, or a history of seizure disorders, pheochromocytoma, or Parkinson's disease.
- Monitor for extrapyramidal side effects (e.g., difficulty speaking or swallowing, loss of balance, gait disruptions, twitching or twisting movements, weakness of arms or legs) or manifestations of tardive dyskinesia (uncontrolled rhythmic facial movement, lip-smacking, tongue rolling). Report immediately.
- Give oral doses 30 minutes before meals and at bedtime.
- May be given by direct intravenous push over 1 to 2 minutes, or diluted by slow infusion over 15 to 30 minutes.

Health Education for the Patient and Family

- Take this drug as directed. If you miss a dose, take as soon as you remember unless it is close to the time for the next dose.
- Do not drive or engage in other activities that require alertness if this drug makes you drowsy.
- Avoid using alcohol or other CNS depressants while you are taking this drug.
- Immediately contact your healthcare provider if you develop involuntary movements of your eyes, face, or limbs.

Nursing Care

Assessment

Assessment data related to GERD include the following:

- *Health history:* Manifestations such as frequent heartburn or atypical chest pain; intolerance of foods that are acidic, spicy, or fatty; regurgitation of acidic gastric juice; increased symptoms when bending over, lying down, or wearing tight clothing; difficulty swallowing; possible hoarseness.
- *Physical assessment:* Epigastric tenderness.

Nursing Diagnoses and Interventions

Relieving the discomfort associated with GERD is the priority of nursing care. Teaching focuses on preventing symptoms and long-term consequences of the disorder.

Acute Pain

The epigastric pain associated with GERD can be severe, interfering with rest and causing anxiety.

- Provide small, frequent meals. Restrict intake of fat, acidic foods, coffee, and alcohol. *Limiting the size of meals reduces pressure in the stomach, reducing esophageal reflux. Fatty, acidic foods, coffee, and alcohol increase gastric acidity and interfere with gastric emptying, increasing the incidence of gastroesophageal reflux.*

- Instruct to stop smoking. Refer to a smoking cessation clinic or program as needed. *Cigarette smoking increases gastric acidity and interferes with healing of damaged mucosa.*
- Administer antacids, H_2-receptor blockers, and PPIs as ordered. Instruct patient to continue therapy as prescribed, even after symptoms have been relieved. *These drugs neutralize or reduce gastric acid secretion, relieving symptoms and promoting healing.*
- Discuss the long-term nature of GERD and its management. *Lifestyle changes need to be continued after healing and symptom relief to manage the long-term effects of GERD.*

Using NANDA, NIC, and NOC

Linkages between a selected NANDA nursing diagnosis, NIC, and NOC for the patient with GERD are shown in the chart that follows.

Community-Based Care

GERD is a lifelong condition best managed by the patient. Teach the patient and family about continuing management strategies, including dietary changes, remaining upright after meals, and avoiding eating for at least 3 hours before bedtime. Suggest elevating the head of the bed on 6- to 8-inch wooden blocks placed under the legs. Discuss the need for continued gastric acid reduction using antacids, H_2-receptor blockers, or

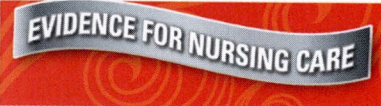

EVIDENCE FOR NURSING CARE   The Patient with Gastrointestinal Reflux Disease

Selected resources that nurses may find helpful when planning evidence-based nursing care follow.

- Kahrilas, P., Shaheen, N., Vaezi, M., Hiltz, S., Black, E., Modlin, I., et al. (2008, October). American Gastroenterological Association Medical Position Statement on the management of gastroesophageal reflux disease. *Gastroenterology, 135*(4), 1383–1391. Retrieved from www.guideline.gov/summary/summary .aspx?doc_id=13315&nbr=006759&string=heartburn
- Scottish Intercollegiate Guidelines Network (SIGN). (2003; reaffirmed 2007). *Dyspepsia. A national clinical guideline.* Edinburgh, Scotland: Scottish Intercollegiate Guidelines Network. Retrieved from www.guideline.gov/summary/ summary.aspx?doc_id=3723&nbr=002949&string= dyspepsia

NANDA, NIC, AND NOC LINKAGES
The Patient with GERD

NANDA — Chronic Pain

NIC — Behavior Modification / Nutrition Monitoring / Teaching: Individual

NOC — Pain: Disruptive Effects / Symptom Control / Knowledge: Treatment Regimen

Data from NANDA International. (2009). *Nursing diagnoses: Definitions & classification 2009–2001.* Oxford, UK: Wiley-Blackwell; Bulechek, G., Butcher, H., & Dochterman, J. (Eds.). (2008). *Nursing interventions classification (NIC)* (5th ed.). St. Louis, MO: Mosby; and Moorhead, S., Johnson, M., Mass, M., & Swanson, E. (Eds.). (2004). *Nursing outcomes classification (NOC)* (4th ed.). St. Louis, MO: Mosby.

PPIs. All are effective to reduce the acidity of gastric juices. Antacids, the most cost-effective measure, require frequent doses to neutralize gastric acid. H$_2$-receptor blockers, also available over the counter, are a cost-effective management strategy that require only twice-a-day dosing.

The Patient with Hiatal Hernia

A *hiatal hernia* occurs when part of the stomach protrudes through the esophageal hiatus of the diaphragm into the thoracic cavity. Although hiatal hernia is thought to be a common problem, most affected individuals are asymptomatic. The incidence of hiatal hernia increases with age.

In a *sliding hiatal hernia*, the gastroesophageal junction and the fundus of the stomach slide upward through the esophageal hiatus (Figure 23–5 ■). Several factors may contribute to a sliding hiatal hernia, including weakened anchors of the gastroesophageal junction to the diaphragm, shortening of the esophagus, or increased intra-abdominal pressure. Small sliding hiatal hernias produce few symptoms.

In a *paraesophageal hiatal hernia*, the junction between the esophagus and stomach remains in its normal position below the diaphragm while a part of the stomach herniates through the esophageal hiatus. A paraesophageal hernia can become incarcerated (constricted) and strangulate, impairing blood flow to the herniated tissue. Patients with paraesophageal hernia may develop gastritis, or chronic or acute gastrointestinal bleeding. The manifestations of hiatal hernias are listed in the following box.

A barium swallow or an upper endoscopy may be done to diagnose hiatal hernia. Many patients with hiatal hernia require no treatment. If symptoms are present, treatment

measures such as those for patients with GERD may be ordered. If medical management is ineffective or the hernia becomes incarcerated, surgery may be required. The most common surgical procedure is the Nissen fundoplication (see Figure 23–4). This surgery, which may be done laparoscopically, prevents the gastroesophageal junction from slipping into the thoracic cavity.

Nursing care for the patient with a hiatal hernia is similar to that for the patient with GERD. If surgery is performed, nursing care is similar to that for patients undergoing gastric or thoracic surgery (∞ see Chapter 4).

The Patient with Impaired Esophageal Motility

Disorders of esophageal motility can cause **dysphagia** (difficult or painful swallowing) or chest pain. It is estimated that nearly 75% of patients hospitalized with stroke experience dysphagia. Other neurologic disorders such as Parkinson's disease, amyotrophic lateral sclerosis, and Alzheimer's disease also can cause dysphagia.

Primary disorders of swallowing are less common. **Achalasia**, a disorder of unknown etiology, is characterized by impaired peristalsis of the smooth muscle of the esophagus and impaired relaxation of the lower esophageal sphincter (LES). The patient experiences gradually increasing dysphagia with both solid foods and liquids. Fullness in the chest during meals, chest pain, and nighttime cough are additional manifestations. Other patients may experience *diffuse esophageal spasm* that causes nonperistaltic contraction of esophageal smooth muscle. This disorder causes chest pain and/or dysphagia. The chest pain can be severe, and usually occurs at rest.

Treatment of achalasia may include endoscopically guided injection of botulinum toxin into the lower esophageal sphincter or balloon dilation of the LES. Botulinum toxin injection lowers LES pressure, but may need to be repeated every 6 to 9 months. Balloon dilation tears muscle fibers in the LES, reducing its pressure (Figure 23–6 ■). A laparoscopic myotomy (incision into the circular muscle layer of the LES) also reduces pressure and relieves symptoms.

The Patient with Esophageal Cancer

Cancer of the esophagus is a relatively uncommon malignancy in the United States. It does, however, have a high mortality rate, primarily because symptoms often are not recognized until late in the course of the disease.

MANIFESTATIONS of Hiatal Hernia
- Reflux, heartburn
- Feeling of fullness
- Substernal chest pain
- Dysphagia
- Occult bleeding
- Belching, indigestion

Figure 23–5 ■ Hiatal hernia. The gastroesophageal junction and fundus of the stomach slide upward through the diaphragm, allowing gastric juices to reflux into the lower esophagus.

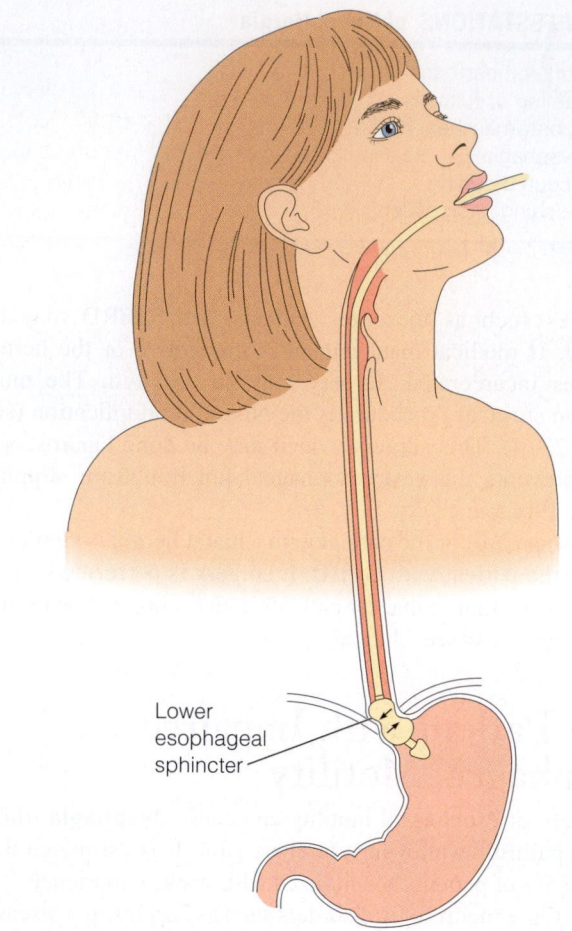

Lower
esophageal
sphincter

Figure 23–6 ■ Balloon dilation of the lower esophageal sphincter.

> **FAST FACTS**
> - Esophageal cancer is the seventh leading cause of death in men.
> - It accounted for an estimated 11,490 deaths in 2009 (American Cancer Society, 2008).
> - Esophageal cancer usually occurs after age 50; it is more common in men than in women and in Blacks than in Whites.
> - Most esophageal tumors develop in the lower third of the esophagus.

Pathophysiology

There are two types of esophageal tumors, adenocarcinoma and squamous cell carcinoma. Over the past two decades, the incidence of squamous cell tumors of the esophagus has been decreasing, whereas the incidence of adenocarcinoma has increased dramatically, particularly among white males (Fauci et al., 2008). Cigarette smoking and chronic alcohol use are strong risk factors for squamous cell esophageal tumors, and also appear to contribute to the risk of developing adenocarcinoma. Box 23–3 lists major identified risk factors for esophageal cancer.

Only about 10% of esophageal tumors develop in the upper portion of the esophagus; about 35% develop in the midportion. The lower third of the esophagus is the most common site, accounting for about 55% of tumors. Adenocarcinomas tend to develop in dysplastic (abnormal) columnar epithelium in the

> **BOX 23–3 Risk Factors for Esophageal Cancer**
> - Excess alcohol consumption
> - Cigarette smoking
> - Ingested carcinogens such as nitrates and industrial chemicals
> - Smoked opiates
> - Physical mucosal damage (e.g., hot tea, lye ingestion, radiation damage, chronic achalasia)
> - Congenital disorders
> - Chronic gastric reflux

distal esophagus. It is commonly associated with Barrett's esophagus, a possible complication of chronic GERD and achalasia.

The disease usually spreads to adjacent and supraclavicular lymph nodes, the liver, lungs, and the pleura.

Manifestations

The most common symptoms of esophageal carcinoma are progressive dysphagia and recent weight loss. Other manifestations are listed in the box that follows. The cancer often is advanced and incurable by the time the disease is diagnosed because symptoms such as difficulty swallowing don't develop until more than 60% of the circumference of the esophagus is affected by tumor (Fauci et al., 2008).

Tracheoesophageal fistulas may develop as the disease progresses, leading to aspiration and pneumonia. Paraneoplastic symptoms such as hypercalcemia may accompany advanced esophageal cancer.

Interdisciplinary Care

Controlling dysphagia and maintaining nutritional status are essential goals of therapy for patients with esophageal cancer, regardless of the stage of the disease. Treatment may involve surgery, radiation therapy, and/or chemotherapy.

Diagnosis

Diagnostic and staging procedures for esophageal cancer may include esophagography, bronchoscopy, and scans to detect metastasis. The following diagnostic tests may be performed (∞ see Chapter 21):

- *Barium swallow* to identify irregular mucosal patterns or narrowing of the lumen, which suggests esophageal cancer.
- *Esophagoscopy* to allow direct visualization of the tumor and obtain tissue for biopsy.
- *Chest x-ray*, *CT scans*, or *MRI* to identify possible tumor metastases to other organs or tissues.
- *Complete blood count (CBC)* may indicate anemia due to chronic blood loss. *Serum albumin levels* may be low due to malnutrition, and *liver function tests (ALT, alkaline phosphatase, AST, and bilirubin)* are elevated if liver metastases are present.

MANIFESTATIONS of Esophageal Cancer

■ Dysphagia	■ Regurgitation
■ Anemia	■ Anorexia
■ Weight loss	■ Chest pain
■ GERD-like symptoms	■ Persistent cough

Treatments

The treatment of esophageal cancer is challenging; fewer than 5% of patients survive 5 years after it is diagnosed (Fauci et al., 2008). A combination of chemotherapy and radiation, followed by surgery to resect the tumor appears to be more effective than any single form of therapy.

Surgery involves resection of the affected portion of the esophagus (*esophagectomy*) and possible anastomosis of the stomach to the remaining esophagus. Mediastinal lymph nodes may be resected at the time of surgery. Esophagectomy is not without risk; potential surgical complications include anastomosis leak, respiratory complications such as pneumonia or acute respiratory distress syndrome, gastric necrosis or bleeding, cardiac dysrhythmias, and infection and sepsis. Intensive nursing care is required postoperatively to prevent and rapidly identify and treat complications that do develop.

The effectiveness of primary radiation therapy is similar to that with radical surgery. Complications associated with radiation therapy to the esophagus include perforation, hemorrhage, and strictures. When used, combination chemotherapy regimens are more effective in reducing tumor mass than single-drug regimens. When the tumor has spread locally or to distant sites, palliative therapy relieves dysphagia and pain (McPhee et al., 2008). Palliative therapy may include local treatments such as endoscopic dilation, wire stents or laser therapy to keep the esophagus patent, and placement of a gastrostomy or jejunostomy for enteral feeding and fluids.

✎ Nursing Care

Health Promotion

Health promotion measures to reduce the risk for and incidence of esophageal cancer include educating people (especially young people) about the dangers of cigarette smoking and excess alcohol use. Refer to smoking cessation and alcohol treatment programs as indicated. Educate patients with GERD about the relationship between chronic damage to the esophagus due to reflux and esophageal cancer, and stress the importance of effective disease management.

Assessment

Early diagnosis and treatment of esophageal cancer can make a difference in the patient's prognosis. Collect the following assessment data related to esophageal cancer:

- *Health history:* Current symptoms such as chest pain, dysphagia, odynophagia (pain with swallowing), coughing or hoarseness; duration of symptoms; recent weight loss; smoking history; current and past patterns of alcohol consumption.
- *Physical examination:* Weight; general health status; skin color; supraclavicular and cervical lymph nodes for lymphadenopathy.

Nursing Diagnoses and Interventions

Disruption of the integrity and function of the esophagus and the discomfort associated with swallowing in patients with esophageal cancer affect the patient's ability to maintain adequate nutritional status, and, potentially, a patent airway.

Imbalanced Nutrition: Less than Body Requirements

The patient diagnosed with esophageal cancer may already suffer from some degree of malnutrition because of difficulty and pain with swallowing. Enteral nutrition via nasogastric feeding tube or gastrostomy tube or parenteral nutrition maintain nutritional status after surgery or if the tumor is inoperable and obstruction occurs. ∞ See Chapter 22 for nursing interventions related to enteral and parenteral feedings.

Risk for Ineffective Airway Clearance

After surgery for esophageal cancer, the patient is at high risk for aspiration and difficulty maintaining a patent airway due to disruption of the esophagus and incision into the thoracic cavity.

- Assess mental and respiratory status (including rate, depth, breath sounds, and oxygen saturation levels) at least every hour during the initial postoperative period. *Altered mental status increases the risk for aspiration. An increased respiratory rate, dyspnea, diminished breath sounds, or decreased oxygen saturation levels may indicate impaired airway clearance or possible aspiration pneumonia.*
- Provide aggressive pulmonary hygiene measures, including endotracheal suctioning and chest physiotherapy as indicated or ordered. Following extubation, encourage frequent coughing, deep breathing, and use of the incentive spirometer. *Respiratory complications are a frequent complication of esophagectomy. Aggressive nursing care helps mobilize secretions and prevent atelectasis and possible pneumonia.*
- If present, monitor chest tube function and drainage. Promptly report drainage that is bright red and excessive in amount (> 70 mL/h) or purulent. Maintain patency of chest tubes per unit protocol or physician's order. *If a thoracic incision has been used, chest tubes are placed to promote lung reinflation. Proper chest tube function is necessary to prevent pneumothorax and impaired lung inflation.*
- Monitor cardiopulmonary status and hemodynamic pressures. Administer intravenous fluids and fluid boluses as ordered. *Fluid volume imbalances that compromise cardiopulmonary status may develop following esophagectomy. Maintaining adequate fluid intake and preventing fluid overload are important postoperatively. The patient also is at risk for acute respiratory distress syndrome, a critical complication that can further compromise ventilation, gas exchange, and circulation.*
- Do not move or manipulate the nasogastric tube. Maintain low gastric suction as ordered. *Manipulating or moving the nasogastric tube may disrupt suture lines, resulting in a leak into the mediastinum.*
- Verify enteral tube feeding placement by checking the pH of gastric aspirate (∞ see Chapter 22). Stop enteral feedings if feelings of fullness or nausea occur. Suction gastrointestinal contents as needed, positioning the patient on the side. *Overdistention of the stomach or delayed gastric emptying may result in regurgitation of stomach contents. Nausea or a feeling of fullness may indicate stomach overdistention. Suctioning and positioning limit the risk of aspiration.*

Anticipatory Grieving

Upon a diagnosis of cancer, the patient and family may experience a grief reaction. The pessimistic prognosis associated with esophageal cancer and the disruptions in relationships may result in an intense sense of loss. ∞ Chapter 5 discusses care of patient experiencing grief and loss.

Community-Based Care

Most care for patients with esophageal cancer is provided in community-based and home settings. Include the following topics in patient and family teaching for home care:

- Planned treatment options including the risks, benefits, and potential adverse effects of each

- Wound and follow-up care following surgery
- Prevention and manifestations of complications such as wound or chest infection, anastomosis leak, deep venous thrombosis
- How to prepare, implement, and care for tube feedings or home parenteral nutrition

Based on the patient's needs and prognosis, referral to a home health agency and/or hospice may be appropriate.

Disorders of the Stomach and Duodenum

The stomach and upper small intestine (duodenum and jejunum) are responsible for the majority of food digestion. The major disorders that affect digestion are nausea and vomiting, gastritis, peptic ulcer disease, and cancer of the stomach. Nursing roles in managing these disorders include both acute care for the hospitalized patient and teaching to give the patient the skills and knowledge to manage these conditions at home.

Overview of Normal Physiology

Normally, the stomach is protected from the digestive substances it secretes—namely, hydrochloric acid and pepsin—by the **gastric mucosal barrier**. The gastric mucosal barrier includes the following:

- An impermeable hydrophobic lipid layer that covers gastric epithelial cells. This lipid layer prevents diffusion of water-soluble molecules, but substances such as aspirin and alcohol can diffuse through it.
- Bicarbonate ions secreted in response to hydrochloric acid secretion by the parietal cells of the stomach. When bicarbonate (HCO_3^-) secretion is equal to hydrogen ion (H^+) secretion, the gastric mucosa remains intact. Prostaglandins, chemical messengers involved in the inflammatory response, support bicarbonate production and blood flow to the gastric mucosa.
- Mucous gel that protects the surface of the stomach lining from the damaging effects of pepsin and traps bicarbonate to neutralize hydrochloric acid. This gel also acts as a lubricant, preventing mechanical damage to the stomach lining from its contents.

When an acute or chronic irritant disrupts the mucosal barrier, or when disease alters the processes that maintain the barrier, the gastric mucosa becomes irritated and inflamed. Lipid-soluble substances such as aspirin and alcohol penetrate the gastric mucosal barrier, leading to irritation and possible inflammation. Bile acids also break down the lipids in the mucosal barrier, increasing the potential for irritation (Porth & Matfin, 2009). In addition, aspirin and other nonsteroidal anti-inflammatory drugs (NSAIDs) inhibit prostaglandins. Aspirin and NSAIDs alter the nature of gastric mucus, affecting its protective function.

The Patient with Gastrointestinal Bleeding

Because of its constant exposure to the environment, the gastrointestinal tract can be subjected to trauma, exposure to toxins, infection with pathogens such as *Helicobacter pylori*,

inflammatory processes, and insults such as ischemia due to systemic diseases. While the mucosal lining of the GI tract is remarkably able to withstand these insults and heal rapidly, its rich supply of blood can result in significant bleeding when a vessel is eroded or abnormally distended (*varices*). Gastrointestinal hemorrhage is a relatively common admitting diagnosis and complication of critical illnesses. It is a medical emergency requiring aggressive medical and nursing care.

Although bleeding and hemorrhage can occur anywhere in the GI tract, the upper portion of the tract is more commonly affected. The three primary disorders leading to upper (UGI) hemorrhage are erosive gastritis, peptic ulcer disease, and esophageal varices. Erosive gastritis and peptic ulcer disease are discussed in the following sections of this chapter; esophageal varices, usually seen as a complication of cirrhosis of the liver, are discussed in ∞ Chapter 25.

FAST FACTS
- About 50% of UGI bleeds are due to peptic ulcer disease.
- Erosive gastritis is the second leading cause of UGI hemorrhage, responsible for about 20% of bleeds.
- The third leading cause, esophageal varices, has the highest mortality rate, between 40% and 70%.

Pathophysiology

Blood in the GI tract has several effects. It is irritating to the stomach, and typically leads to nausea and vomiting (**hematemesis**, vomiting blood). If the blood has been present in the stomach for a period of time and is partially digested, it may have a "coffee-grounds" appearance, rather than presenting as bright red blood. The accumulation of blood in the GI tract stimulates peristasis, leading to hyperactive bowel sounds and diarrhea. Stools may be black and tarry (**melena**) or frankly bloody (**hematochezia**); stool containing partially digested blood has a characteristic odor. With significant upper GI bleeding, digestion of blood proteins increases blood urea nitrogen (BUN) levels.

Physiologic responses to an upper GI bleed depend on the rapidity and magnitude of the blood loss. GI bleeding resulting from erosion of a small vessel typically is slow, and may not be identified until the patient presents with manifestations of blood loss anemia due to depletion of iron stores. (∞ See Chapter 33 for further discussion of blood loss anemia.) Although no visible blood may be present in the stool, **occult** (or hidden) **bleeding** may be detected by chemical means.

GI hemorrhage, with loss of a significant amount of blood within a few hours, rapidly depletes blood volume, producing manifestations of decreased cardiac output: tachycardia, hypotension, pallor, and decreased urine output. Peripheral blood vessels constrict to maintain perfusion of vital organs. Unless the blood volume is restored, hypovolemic shock progresses, leading to acidosis, renal failure, bowel infarction, acute coronary syndrome, coma, and death. ∞ See Chapter 11 for more information about shock and its management.

Interdisciplinary Care

The acuity of the bleed and the patient's condition dictate the timing and extent of diagnostic testing and interventions. A patient with a massive GI hemorrhage is admitted to the critical care unit and aggressively treated to stem bleeding, restore blood volume, and stabilize the cardiovascular system. Identifying the cause of the bleeding is postponed in many cases until the patient's condition has been stabilized.

When the bleeding is slow or chronic, diagnostic testing and treatment may be managed in a community-based setting.

Diagnosis

Diagnostic testing focuses on determining the extent and effects of the bleed, as well as its cause.

- A *complete blood count with hemoglobin and hematocrit* are obtained. In an acute bleed, the CBC, hemoglobin, and hematocrit may not initially indicate the extent of blood loss because plasma is lost along with blood cells.
- *Blood type and crossmatch* are performed to prepare for transfusion as necessary.
- *Serum electrolytes, osmolality,* and *BUN* are obtained to determine the effects of the blood loss and protein digestion on blood chemistries.
- *Liver function studies* and a *coagulation profile* may be obtained to help determine the cause of the bleeding.
- An *upper endoscopy* is performed as soon as possible to identify and, if possible, treat the source of bleeding. ∞ See Chapter 21 for nursing care of the patient undergoing upper endoscopy.

Treatments

In acute GI hemorrhage, initial treatment focuses on stemming the bleeding and restoring cardiovascular stability. Intravenous fluids such as normal saline or a balanced electrolyte solution are administered through a large-bore intravenous catheter. Fresh whole blood, which contains clotting factors, is administered to restore blood volume and components in an acute hemorrhage. In less acute situations, packed red cells may be administered to restore the oxygen-carrying capacity of the blood.

Hemostasis is achieved using upper endoscopy whenever possible. A sclerosing agent may be injected into the bleeding vessel, or the vessel may be sealed using a heated probe, electrocautery, or laser. Rarely, emergency surgery is required to stop hemorrhage.

GASTRIC LAVAGE Gastric lavage, washing out of stomach contents, may be done in patients with upper GI hemorrhage to remove blood from the GI tract, prevent vomiting, and prepare for upper endoscopy. See Procedure 23–1 for nursing responsibilities related to gastric lavage.

♻ Nursing Care

Health Promotion

Preventing gastrointestinal bleeding is the most important step in reducing the mortality and morbidity associated with an acute GI hemorrhage. Identifying patients at risk and instituting regular gastric pH monitoring and maintenance of drug therapy to reduce gastric acidity are important preventive measures. All critically ill patients should be considered to be at risk for stress-related erosive gastritis.

Assessment

Assessment of the patient experiencing an acute GI hemorrhage is very focused on the immediate crisis. The ability to obtain subjective information may be limited; however, it is important to identify possible contributing factors such as use of aspirin, other platelet inhibitors, or anticoagulant medications and the presence of any acute or chronic conditions that may contribute to bleeding (e.g., hypertension, a clotting disorder, peptic ulcer disease, chronic hepatitis, or cirrhosis of the liver). If possible, identify all current medications and their purpose, as well as any allergies to medications or other substances.

Physical examination focuses on the effect of the bleeding on cardiovascular status. Obtain vital signs and orthostatic vital signs (an early sign of hypovolemia). Place the acutely ill patient on a cardiac monitor and obtain a rhythm strip. Obtain oxygen saturation level. Assess peripheral pulse strength, as well as color, temperature, and capillary refill of extremities. Evaluate mental status, including level of consciousness and orientation. An indwelling catheter may be inserted to evaluate urine output.

Nursing Diagnoses and Interventions

Nursing care priorities for the patient with an acute GI bleed focus on restoring and maintaining an effective cardiac output and tissue perfusion, and on stopping the hemorrhage and preventing further bleeding.

Risk for Shock

Significant amounts of blood may be lost in a very short time with an acute GI hemorrhage. Because some of the blood enters the bowel, it may be difficult to accurately estimate the amount of blood lost by measuring emesis, gastric suction return, and blood expelled as feces. As blood volume drops, venous return decreases. The heart rate increases to maintain the cardiac output, and peripheral blood vessels constrict to improve venous return and cardiac output.

- Frequently assess and document vital signs, including blood pressure, pulse rate and cardiac rhythm, respiratory rate, and oxygen saturation levels. Obtain hemodynamic pressure measurements as ordered, reporting trends and changes. *The vital signs, oxygen saturation levels, and hemodynamic pressure values provide indicators of the effectiveness of peripheral tissue perfusion, oxygenation, and fluid replacement.*
- Monitor for and report changes in skin color, temperature, and moisture, or slow capillary refill. *Peripheral vasoconstriction and activation of the sympathetic nervous system typically cause pale, cool, and moist or diaphoretic skin. Development of cyanosis or mottling indicates a further decrease in tissue perfusion and oxygenation.*

PROCEDURE 23–1 Gastric Lavage

When it is important to remove or dilute gastric contents rapidly, gastric lavage (irrigation or washing out of the stomach) may be indicated. In acute poisoning or ingestion of a caustic substance, a large-bore 30- to 36-Fr. nasogastric tube is inserted, and lavage performed. An 18-Fr. nasogastric tube may be used when the procedure is performed to remove blood from the upper GI tract. Because the GI tract is not sterile, clean technique is appropriate for use, although the solution used will generally be sterile.

■ Obtain baseline assessment, including vital signs, abdominal inspection, girth, and bowel sounds. *It is important to have assessment data documented prior to instituting the procedure for comparison.*

■ Explain the procedure, answering questions and clarifying perceptions. Instruct to report any pain, difficulty breathing, or other problems during the procedure. *A patient who is able to understand and cooperate with the procedure will tolerate lavage better. The patient may be aware of symptoms of complications such as perforation or tube displacement before they are evident to the nurse.*

■ Place in semi-Fowler's or Fowler's position. If unable to tolerate elevation of the head of the bed because of hypotension, place in left side-lying position. *Elevating of the head of the bed or sidelying position will minimize the risk of aspiration.*

■ Insert a nasogastric tube if one is not already in place. Verify tube placement by aspirating gastric contents and test pH of aspirate. *Proper placement is vital to prevent aspiration or overdistention of the small bowel with irrigating solution.*

■ Irrigate the stomach, using either a closed or an open system technique.

CLOSED-SYSTEM IRRIGATION

■ Wearing clean gloves, connect bag or bottle of normal saline irrigating solution to nasogastric tube using a Y connector. Attach drainage or suction tube to other arm of connector (Figure 23–7 ■). Empty the stomach, clamp drain tube or turn off suction, and allow 50 to 200 mL of solution to run into stomach by gravity. Stop solution and allow to drain or

suction out. Repeat until ordered amount has been used or desired results are obtained, for example, no further clots and solution returns clear or light pink. Measure the amount of drainage, subtracting the amount of irrigant instilled, to obtain gastric output. *The closed system minimizes the risk of contact with body fluids for the nurse. Measuring gastric output is important in monitoring fluid balance.*

INTERMITTENT OPEN SYSTEM

■ Wearing clean gloves and other personal protective equipment as necessary (gown and face protection), empty the stomach using suction or a 50-mL catheter-tip syringe. Measure and discard the aspirate. Using the syringe, draw up approximately 50 mL of irrigation solution, and instill it using gentle pressure. Aspirate the nasogastric tube, and discard the solution into a measuring container. Continue this procedure until the desired amount of irrigant has been instilled or desired results have been obtained. *Manual irrigation with a catheter-tip syringe may be more effective than gravity flow in removing clots from the stomach and nasogastric tube.*

■ Continue to monitor vital signs (including temperature), tolerance of the procedure, and other assessment data. *The patient may be unstable and require continuous reevaluation. Gastric lavage may cause hypothermia; therefore, monitor temperature and indications of hypothermia, such as lethargy and changes in cardiac rate and rhythm.*

■ If the aspirate has not cleared to light pink or pink tinged after 20 to 30 minutes of lavage or if the patient is unable to tolerate the procedure, notify the physician. *Medical or surgical intervention may be necessary to stop hemorrhage in some instances.*

■ On completion of lavage, provide mouth and nares care. Continue to monitor vital signs, abdominal status, and other assessment data.

■ Document the procedure, including the amount and type of irrigant used, gastric output character and amount, and the patient's condition and tolerance of the procedure.

Figure 23–7 ■ The patient with a closed-system gastric lavage.

- Insert an indwelling urinary catheter and measure urine output hourly. Report an output of less than 30 mL for two consecutive hours. *A fall in urine output may indicate further reduction in cardiac output. As cardiac output falls, the kidneys become ischemic and acute renal failure may develop.*
- Unless contraindicated, insert a nasogastric tube and connect to low suction. Measure gastric output hourly unless otherwise directed. *Measuring gastric output provides information about the amount of blood and fluid lost. This information helps determine fluid and blood replacement needs.*
- Maintain two peripheral intravenous lines with large-bore catheters or a central venous catheter for fluid and blood administration as ordered. Frequently monitor vital signs, respiratory status, and hemodynamic pressure measurements, reporting changes in status. *Rapid administration of isotonic intravenous fluids, blood, and blood products can lead to fluid overload and potential heart failure.*
- Replace gastric drainage with balanced electrolyte intravenous solutions as ordered. *GI losses are replaced in addition to fluids given to meet daily requirements to prevent fluid volume deficiency.*

Risk for Bleeding

- Maintain gastric suction and drainage and patency of nasogastric tube. *Blood is irritating to the GI tract, precipitating vomiting and stimulating peristalsis, leading to diarrhea. In addition, digested blood can increase BUN levels, potentially leading to confusion and altered mental status.*
- Irrigate the nasogastric tube with room temperature saline or tap water as ordered. Calculate intake and output, subtracting the amount of irrigant from gastric output. *Irrigation of the nasogastric tube helps remove irritating blood from the gut and produces a degree of vasoconstriction in stomach mucosa, slowing bleeding.*
- Prepare for upper endoscopy or surgery as planned. *Endoscopy or emergency surgery may be performed to repair the bleeding site or sclerose bleeding vessels.*
- Following an acute bleed and in patients at risk for GI bleeding, monitor gastric pH as ordered and check vomitus and feces for the presence of occult blood. Maintain infusions of drugs to reduce gastric acidity as ordered. *The patient remains at risk for GI bleeding. Monitoring for occult blood helps identify slow bleeding or recurrent hemorrhage. Reducing the acidity of gastric secretions reduces irritation of the gastric mucosa, reducing the risk of bleeding.*

Community-Based Care

Following an acute GI hemorrhage, continuing care focuses on resolving the underlying disease process if possible and preventing future episodes of GI bleeding. If a bleeding gastric ulcer was identified, testing for *H. pylori* infection will be done, and a treatment regimen prescribed to eradicate the infection (see the section on peptic ulcer disease later that follows). The patient who experienced an episode of erosive stress gastritis will often be discharged with instructions to continue taking a gastric acid–reducing medication and avoid known gastric irritants such as aspirin and alcohol. The patient with esophageal varices due to cirrhosis or chronic hepatitis needs additional instructions (∞ see Chapter 25).

Patients with minor or slow GI bleeding often are managed in the community. Provide teaching about the cause of the bleeding and measures to prevent future episodes. Provide verbal and written instructions for prescribed medications such as acid reducers and oral iron supplements. Discuss appropriate nutrition; while a special diet to "soothe the stomach" rarely is indicated, foods rich in iron may be recommended to treat the resulting anemia.

Discuss indicators of GI bleeding to be reported to the physician. If the source of bleeding has not been identified, provide instructions about prescribed follow-up diagnostic testing.

The Patient with Peptic Ulcer Disease

Peptic ulcer disease (PUD), a break in the mucous lining of the gastrointestinal tract where it comes in contact with gastric juice, is a chronic health problem. PUD affects approximately 10% of the population or 4 million people in the United States every year, primarily those between ages 25 and 64 years. Furthermore, its complications account for an estimated 15,000 deaths annually (Fauci et al., 2008; Ramakrishnan & Salinas, 2007).

Peptic ulcers occur in any area of the gastrointestinal tract exposed to acid-pepsin secretions, including the esophagus, stomach, or duodenum. *Duodenal ulcers* are the most common. They usually develop between the ages of 30 and 55, and are more common in men than women. *Gastric ulcers* more often affect older patients, between the ages of 55 and 70. Ulcers are more common in people who smoke and who are chronic users of NSAIDs. Alcohol and dietary intake do not seem to cause PUD, and the role of stress is uncertain. Although the incidence of PUD has dramatically decreased, the incidence of gastric ulcers is increasing, believed due to the widespread use of NSAIDs (McPhee et al., 2008).

Risk Factors

Chronic *H. pylori* infection and use of aspirin and NSAIDs are the major risk factors for PUD. Contributing risk factors are listed in Box 23–4. Overall, an estimated 10% to 15% of patients infected with *H. pylori* develop PUD. Of the NSAIDs, aspirin is the most ulcerogenic. A strong familial pattern suggests a genetic factor in the development of PUD. Cigarette smoking is a significant risk factor, doubling the risk of PUD. Cigarette smoking inhibits the secretion of bicarbonate by the pancreas and possibly causes more rapid transit of gastric acid into the duodenum.

Pathophysiology

The innermost layer of the stomach wall, the gastric mucosa, consists of columnar epithelial cells, supported by a middle layer of blood vessels and glands, and a thin outer layer of smooth muscle. The mucosal barrier of the stomach, a thin coating of mucous gel and bicarbonate, protects the gastric mucosa. The mucosal barrier is maintained by bicarbonate secreted by the epithelial cells, by mucous gel production stimulated by

- *H. pylori* infection
  - Older age
  - Low socioeconomic status
  - Birth in a developing country
  - Crowded, unsanitary living conditions
  - Unclean food or water
- Use of aspirin
- History of ulcer
- Concurrent use of drugs such as glucocorticoids or NSAIDs
- Cigarette smoking
- Family history of PUD

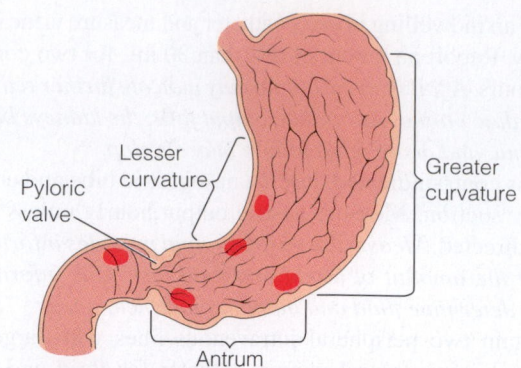

Figure 23–8 ■ Common sites affected by peptic ulcer disease.

prostaglandins, and by an adequate blood supply to the mucosa (see the overview of normal physiology on page 630).

An **ulcer**, or break in the gastrointestinal mucosa, develops when the mucosal barrier is unable to protect the mucosa from damage by hydrochloric acid and pepsin, the gastric digestive juices. See the accompanying Pathophysiology Illustrated: Peptic Ulcer Disease feature on pages 636–637.

H. pylori infection, found in about 50% of people who have PUD, is unique in colonizing the stomach. It is spread person to person (oral–oral or fecal–oral), and contributes to ulcer formation in several ways. The bacteria produce enzymes that reduce the efficacy of mucous gel in protecting the gastric mucosa. In addition, the host's inflammatory response to *H. pylori* contributes to gastric epithelial cell damage without producing immunity to the infection. Although the gastric mucosa is the usual site for *H. pylori* infection, this infection also contributes to duodenal ulcers. This is possibly related to increased gastric acid production associated with *H. pylori* infection.

NSAIDs contribute to PUD through both systemic and topical mechanisms. Prostaglandins are necessary for maintaining the gastric mucosal barrier. NSAIDs interrupt prostaglandin synthesis by disrupting the action of the enzyme cyclooxygenase (COX). The two forms of this enzyme are COX-1 and COX-2. The COX-1 enzyme is necessary to maintain the integrity of the gastric mucosa, but the anti-inflammatory effects of NSAIDs are due to their ability to inhibit the COX-2 enzyme. The COX-2–selective NSAIDs may be less damaging to the gastric mucosa because they have less effect on the COX-1 enzyme. In addition to their systemic effect, aspirin and many NSAIDs cross the lipid membranes of gastric epithelial cells, damaging the cells themselves.

The ulcers of PUD may affect the esophagus, stomach, or duodenum. They may be superficial or deep, affecting all layers of the mucosa (see Pathophysiology Illustrated: Peptic Ulcer Disease). Duodenal ulcers, the most common, usually develop in the proximal portion of the duodenum, close to the pylorus (Figure 23–8 ■). They are sharply demarcated and usually less than 1 cm in diameter (Figure 23–9 ■). Gastric ulcers often are found on the lesser curvature and the area immediately proximal to the pylorus. Gastric ulcers are associated with an increased incidence of gastric cancer.

Peptic ulcer disease may be chronic, with spontaneous remissions and exacerbations. Exacerbations of the disease may be associated with trauma, infection, or other physical or psychologic stressors.

Manifestations

Pain is the classic symptom of peptic ulcer disease. The pain is typically described as gnawing, burning, aching, or hunger-like and is experienced in the epigastric region, sometimes radiating to the back. The pain occurs when the stomach is empty (2 to 3 hours after meals and in the middle of the night) and is relieved by eating with a classic "pain–food–relief" pattern. The patient may complain of heartburn or regurgitation and may vomit.

The presentation of peptic ulcer disease in the older adult is often less clear, with vague and poorly localized discomfort, perhaps chest pain or dysphagia, weight loss, or anemia. In the older adult, a complication of PUD such as upper GI hemorrhage or perforation of the stomach or duodenum may be the presenting symptom.

Complications

The complications associated with peptic ulcers include hemorrhage, obstruction, and perforation. See the following box for the manifestations of these complications.

Among people with PUD, 10% to 20% experience hemorrhage as a result of ulceration and erosion into the blood vessels of the gastric mucosa. Bleeding is the most frequent complication in older adults. It is the presenting symptom in up to 20% of people with PUD (Fauci et al., 2008). When small blood vessels erode, blood loss may be slow and insidious, with occult blood in the stool the only initial sign. If

Figure 23–9 ■ A superficial peptic ulcer.
Source: SPL/Photo Researchers, Inc.

bleeding continues, the patient becomes anemic and experiences symptoms of weakness, fatigue, dizziness, and orthostatic hypotension. Erosion into a larger vessel can lead to sudden and severe bleeding with hematemesis, melena, or hematochezia (blood in the stool), and signs of hypovolemic shock.

Gastric outlet obstruction may result from edema surrounding the ulcer, smooth muscle spasm, or scar tissue. Generally, obstruction is a gradual rather than an acute process. Symptoms include a feeling of epigastric fullness, accentuated ulcer symptoms, and nausea. If the obstruction becomes complete, vomiting occurs. Hydrochloric acid, sodium, and potassium are lost in vomitus, potentially leading to fluid and electrolyte imbalance and metabolic alkalosis.

The most lethal complication of PUD is *perforation* of the ulcer through the mucosal wall. When perforation occurs, gastric or duodenal contents enter the peritoneum, causing an inflammatory process and peritonitis. Chemical peritonitis from the hydrochloric acid, pepsin, bile, and pancreatic fluid is immediate; bacterial peritonitis follows within 6 to 12 hours from gastric contaminants entering the normally sterile peritoneal cavity. When an ulcer perforates, the patient has immediate, severe upper abdominal pain, radiating throughout the abdomen and possibly to the shoulder. The abdomen becomes rigid and boardlike, with absent bowel sounds. Signs of shock may be present, including diaphoresis, tachycardia, and rapid, shallow respirations. Classic symptoms of perforation may not be present in an older adult. The older adult may instead present with mental confusion and other nonspecific symptoms. This atypical presentation can lead to delays in diagnosis and treatment, increasing the associated mortality rate.

Zollinger-Ellison Syndrome

Zollinger-Ellison syndrome is peptic ulcer disease caused by a gastrinoma, or gastrin-secreting tumor of the pancreas, stomach, or intestines. More than 60% of gastrinomas are malignant tumors. Gastrin is a hormone that stimulates the secretion of pepsin and hydrochloric acid. The increased gastrin levels

MANIFESTATIONS of PUD Complications

HEMORRHAGE
- Occult or obvious blood in the stool
- Hematemesis
- Fatigue
- Weakness, dizziness
- Orthostatic hypotension
- Hypovolemic shock

OBSTRUCTION
- Sensations of epigastric fullness
- Nausea and vomiting
- Electrolyte imbalances
- Metabolic alkalosis

PERFORATION
- Severe upper abdominal pain, radiating to the shoulder
- Rigid, boardlike abdomen
- Absence of bowel sounds
- Diaphoresis
- Tachycardia
- Rapid, shallow respirations
- Fever

associated with these tumors result in hypersecretion of gastric acid, which in turn causes mucosal ulceration.

The peptic ulcers of Zollinger-Ellison syndrome may affect any portion of the stomach or duodenum, as well as the esophagus or jejunum. Characteristic ulcer-like pain is common. The high levels of hydrochloric acid entering the duodenum may cause diarrhea and **steatorrhea** (excess fat in the feces) from impaired fat digestion and absorption. Complications of bleeding and perforation are often seen with Zollinger-Ellison syndrome. Fluid and electrolyte imbalances may result from persistent diarrhea with resultant losses of potassium and sodium in particular.

Interdisciplinary Care

Treatment for PUD focuses on eradicating *H. pylori* infection and treating or preventing ulcers related to use of NSAIDs.

Diagnosis

- *Upper GI series* using barium as a contrast medium can detect 80% to 90% of peptic ulcers. It commonly is the diagnostic procedure chosen first; it is less costly and less invasive than endoscopy. Small or very superficial ulcers may be missed, however.
- *Endoscopy* allows visualization of the esophageal, gastric, and duodenal mucosa and direct inspection of ulcers. Tissue also can be obtained for biopsy. Nursing care of the patient undergoing endoscopy is outlined in ∞ Chapter 21.
- Biopsy specimens obtained during an endoscopy can be tested for the presence of *H. pylori* using a *biopsy urease test*, which is more than 90% accurate in diagnosing the infection. It is, however, invasive and costly.
- Noninvasive methods of detecting *H. pylori* infection include fecal *H. pylori* antigen tests (to detect antigens to *H. pylori* in the feces), and the *urea breath test*. In this test, radiolabeled urea is given orally. The urease produced by *H. pylori* bacteria converts the urea to ammonia and radiolabeled carbon dioxide, which can then be measured as the patient exhales. These tests also can be used to evaluate the effectiveness of treatment to eradicate *H. pylori*. Treatment with PPIs interferes with urea breath test and fecal antigen test results, so these drugs should be discontinued for 7 or more days prior to testing (McPhee et al., 2008).
- If Zollinger-Ellison syndrome is suspected, *gastric analysis* may be performed to evaluate gastric acid secretion. Stomach contents are aspirated through a nasogastric tube and analyzed. In Zollinger-Ellison syndrome, gastric acid levels are very high.

Medications

The medications used to treat PUD include agents to eradicate *H. pylori*, drugs to decrease gastric acid content, and agents that protect the mucosa. Nursing responsibilities related to selected drugs to treat GERD, gastritis, and PUD are found in the Medication Administration box on pages 625–626.

Eradication of *H. pylori* generally requires 14 days of therapy using a combination of two antibiotics with a proton-pump inhibitor or a bismuth compound (e.g., a PPI, clarithromycin, and amoxicillin, or a PPI, bismuth subsalicylate, tetracycline, and metronidazole). With complete eradication of *H. pylori*, reinfection rates are less than 0.5% per year.

PATHOPHYSIOLOGY ILLUSTRATED
Peptic Ulcer Disease

Normal gastric mucosa

In the stomach and duodenum, the mucosal barrier protects the gastric mucosa (including the epithelial, vascular, and smooth muscle layers) from damage. Specialized mucous cells throughout the gastric mucosa produce a mucus (a mixture of water, lipids, and glycoproteins) that serves as a barrier to the diffusion of ions (such as hydrogen ion) and molecules (such as pepsin). A thin layer of bicarbonate, secreted by surface epithelial cells, forms between the mucus and cell membranes. Blood flow to the gastric mucosa is vital to maintain this barrier. Prostaglandins and nitric oxide stimulate mucus and bicarbonate production, helping maintain it as well. The mucosal barrier constantly bathes surfaces of the gastric epithelial lining.

pH 2

Mucosal barrier

pH 7

Gastric mucosa

Mucus gel layer

Bicarbonate layer

Epithelial layer

Growth factors (e.g. nitric oxide)

Prostaglandins

Subepithelial layer

Muscularis mucosae

Submucosa (vascular) layer

Oblique muscle layer

Circular muscle layer

Longitudinal muscle layer

Serosa (visceral peritoneum)

Aspirin
Alcohol
Bile acids

H. pylori

Thinning and disruption of mucosal barrier

Decreased prostaglandins due to
• Aspirin
• NSAIDs

Ischemia due to
• Hemorrhage
• Hypotension
• Shock

Disruption of mucosal barrier

The mucosal barrier can be disrupted by a number of factors. Ischemia of the gastric mucosa (e.g., due to hemorrhage, hypotension, or shock) impairs mucous production, increasing the risk of damage to the mucosa. Aspirin disrupts the mucosal barrier, and, along with other nonsteroidal anti-inflammatory drugs, inhibits prostaglandins which are necessary to maintain mucous production. Alcohol and bile acids also damage the mucous barrier. *Helicobacter pylori*, a common pathogen to infect the gastric mucosa, disrupts the mucosal barrier.

Vasoconstriction

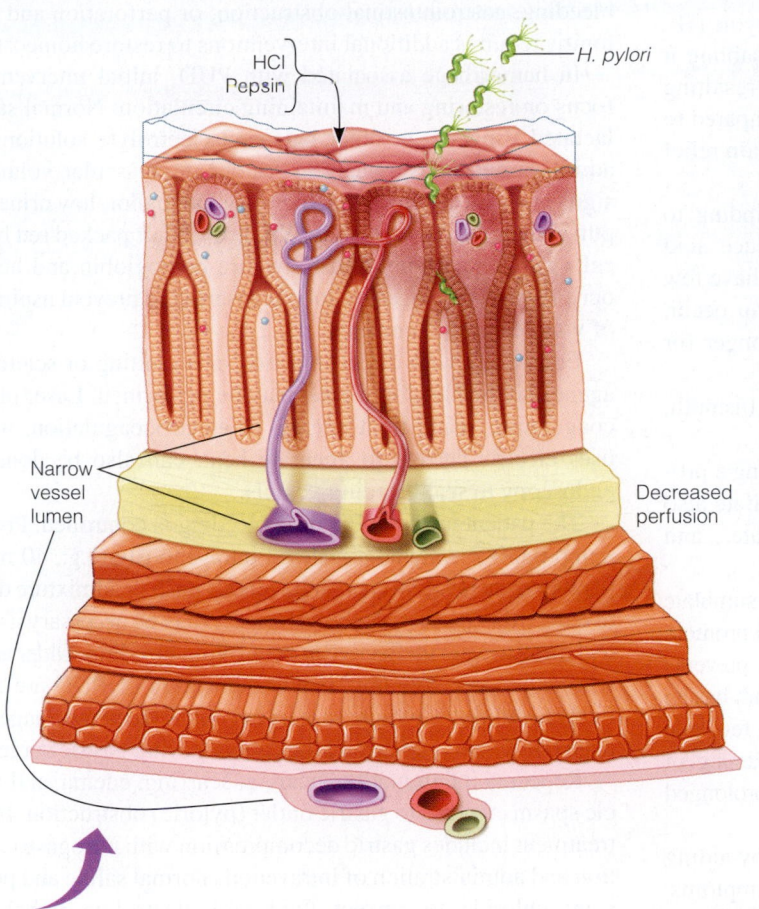

HCl
Pepsin

H. pylori

Narrow
vessel
lumen

Decreased
perfusion

Inflammatory process

When the mucosal barrier is damaged, gastric acid and digestive juices disrupt the epithelial cell membranes, allowing acid to diffuse into cell walls. An acute inflammatory process results. Gastric epithelial cells migrate to the damaged area, a process known as restitution. Adequate blood flow and an alkaline environment are necessary for this repair process. Prostaglandins play an important role in epithelial repair. In the presence of *H. pylori* infection, excess acid production, inadequate blood flow, inhibition of prostaglandins, and other factors that are less clear, the inflammatory process further damages gastric and duodenal epithelial cells, leading to ulceration of the mucosa.

Erosion and ulcer formation

Superficial ulcers (erosions) erode the mucosa, but do not penetrate the muscularis mucosae. True ulcers extend through the muscularis mucosae and into deeper layers of the gastrointestinal wall, damaging blood vessels and potentially penetrating the entire wall. Hemorrhage and peritonitis are potential acute complications of peptic ulcers.

Acute ulcer   Erosion   Chronic ulcer

Mucosal
barrier

Gastric
mucosa

Muscularis
mucosae

Scarring

Serosa

In patients who have NSAID-induced ulcers, the NSAID in use should be discontinued if at all possible. If this is not possible, twice-daily PPIs enable ulcer healing.

Medications that decrease gastric acid content include PPIs and the H_2-receptor antagonists.

- Proton-pump inhibitors bind the acid-secreting enzyme (H^+, K^+ ATPase) that functions as the proton pump, disabling it for up to 24 hours. These drugs are very effective, resulting in more than 90% ulcer healing after 4 weeks. Compared to the H_2-receptor blockers, the PPIs provide faster pain relief and more rapid ulcer healing.
- Histamine$_2$-receptor blockers inhibit histamine binding to the receptors on the gastric parietal cells to reduce acid secretion. These drugs are very well tolerated and have few serious side effects; however, drug interactions can occur. These drugs must be continued for 8 weeks or longer for ulcer healing.

Agents that protect the mucosa include sucralfate, bismuth, antacids, and prostaglandin analogs.

- Sucralfate binds to proteins in the ulcer base, forming a protective barrier against acid, bile, and pepsin. Sucralfate also stimulates the secretion of mucus, bicarbonate, and prostaglandin.
- Bismuth compounds (e.g., Pepto-Bismol, CBS, BBS) stimulate mucosal bicarbonate and prostaglandin production to promote ulcer healing, and likely provide a coating action that prevents further damage by HCl and pepsin. In addition, bismuth has an antibacterial action against *H. pylori*. There are very few side effects, other than constipation and a harmless darkening of stools and the tongue. When used in high doses for a prolonged period, bismuth compounds may be neurotoxic.
- Antacids stimulate gastric mucosal defenses, thereby aiding in ulcer healing. They provide rapid relief of ulcer symptoms, and are often used as needed to supplement other antiulcer medications. Antacids are inexpensive, but patients often have difficulty with a regular regimen because the drugs must be taken frequently and may cause either constipation (from the aluminum-type antacids) or diarrhea (from the magnesium-based antacids). Antacids also interfere with the absorption of iron, digoxin, some antibiotics, and other drugs.
- Prostaglandin analogs (misoprostol) promote ulcer healing by stimulating mucus and bicarbonate secretions and by inhibiting acid secretion. Although not as effective as the other drugs discussed, misoprostol is used to prevent NSAID-induced ulcers.

Treatments

NUTRITION In addition to pharmacologic treatment, patients are encouraged to maintain good nutrition, consuming balanced meals at regular intervals. It is important to teach patients that bland or restrictive diets are unnecessary. Mild alcohol intake is not harmful. Smoking should be discouraged, because it slows the rate of healing and increases the frequency of relapses.

SURGERY The identification of *H. pylori* as a cause of PUD and the availability of drugs to treat the infection and heal peptic ulcers has all but eliminated surgery as a primary treatment option for peptic ulcer disease. Surgery may be required to treat a complication of PUD, such as hemorrhage, perforation, or gastric outlet obstruction. See the section on gastric cancer for more information about gastric surgery and related nursing care.

Treatment of Complications

The patient hospitalized with a complication of PUD such as bleeding, gastrointestinal obstruction, or perforation and peritonitis requires additional interventions to restore homeostasis.

In hemorrhage associated with PUD, initial interventions focus on restoring and maintaining circulation. Normal saline, lactated Ringer's, or other balanced electrolyte solutions are administered intravenously to restore intravascular volume if signs of shock (tachycardia, hypotension, pallor, low urine output, and anxiety) are present. Whole blood or packed red blood cells may be administered to restore hemoglobin and hematocrit levels. A nasogastric tube is inserted to prevent aspiration of vomited gastric contents.

Endoscopy with direct injection of a clotting or sclerosing agent into the bleeding vessel may be performed. Laser photocoagulation, using light energy, or electrocoagulation, which uses electric current to generate heat, can also be done via endoscopy to seal bleeding vessels.

The patient is kept NPO until bleeding is controlled. Proton-pump inhibitors are administered intravenously (e.g., 40 mg of pantoprazole [Protonix] per intravenous push or admixture daily) to reduce the risk of rebleeding. Surgery may be necessary if medical measures are ineffective in controlling bleeding. Older adults who experience bleeding as a complication of PUD are more likely to rebleed or require surgery to control the hemorrhage. See page 646 for nursing care of the patient having gastric surgery.

Repeated inflammation, healing, scarring, edema, and muscle spasm can lead to gastric outlet (pyloric) obstruction. Initial treatment includes gastric decompression with nasogastric suction and administration of intravenous normal saline and potassium chloride to correct fluid and electrolyte imbalance. H_2-receptor blockers are given intravenously as well. Balloon dilation of the gastric outlet may be done via upper endoscopy. If these measures are unsuccessful in relieving obstruction, surgery may be required.

Gastric or duodenal perforation resulting in contamination of the peritoneum with gastrointestinal contents often requires immediate intervention to restore homeostasis and minimize peritonitis. Intravenous fluids maintain fluid and electrolyte balance. Nasogastric suction removes gastric contents and minimizes peritoneal contamination. Placing the patient in Fowler's or semi-Fowler's position allows peritoneal contaminants to pool in the pelvis. Intravenous antibiotics aggressively treat bacterial infection from intestinal flora. Laparoscopic surgery or an open laparotomy may be performed to close the perforation.

✑ Nursing Care

Health Promotion

Although it is difficult to predict which patients will develop peptic ulcer disease, promote health by advising patients to avoid risk factors such as excessive aspirin or NSAID use and cigarette smoking. In addition, encourage patients to seek treatment for manifestations of GERD or chronic gastritis, both of which are associated with *H. pylori* infection.

Assessment

Collect the following subjective and objective data when assessing the patient with peptic ulcer disease:

- *Health history:* Complaints of epigastric or left upper quadrant pain, heartburn, or discomfort; its character, severity, timing and relationship to eating; measures used for relief; nausea or vomiting, presence of bright blood or "coffee-grounds" material in vomitus; current medications including use of aspirin or other NSAIDs; cigarette smoking and use of alcohol or other drugs.
- *Physical examination:* General appearance including height and weight relationship; vital signs including orthostatic measurements; abdominal examination including shape and contour, bowel sounds, and tenderness to palpation; presence of obvious or occult blood in vomitus and stool.

Nursing Diagnoses and Interventions

The priorities of nursing care for the patient with peptic ulcer disease are reducing discomfort, maintaining nutritional status, and preventing or rapidly identifying and intervening for potential complications. See the accompanying Case Study & Nursing Care Plan.

Acute Pain

The pain of peptic ulcer disease is often predictable and preventable. Pain is typically experienced 2 to 4 hours after eating, as high levels of gastric acid and pepsin irritate the exposed mucosa. Measures to neutralize the acid, minimize its production, or protect the mucosa often relieve this pain, minimizing the need for analgesics.

- Assess pain, including location, type, severity, frequency, and duration, and its relationship to food intake or other contributing factors.

> **PRACTICE ALERT**
> Avoid making assumptions about pain. Acute pain may indicate a complication, such as perforation (often heralded by sudden, severe epigastric pain and a rigid, boardlike abdomen) or it may be totally unrelated to PUD (e.g., angina, gallbladder disease, or pancreatitis).

- Administer PPIs, H$_2$-receptor antagonists, antacids, or mucosal protective agents as ordered. Monitor for effectiveness and side effects or adverse reactions. *The pain associated with PUD is generally caused by the effect of gastric juices on exposed mucosal tissue. These medications reduce pain and promote healing by reducing acid production, neutralizing acid, or providing a barrier for the damaged mucosa.*
- Teach relaxation, stress reduction, and lifestyle management techniques. Refer for stress management counseling or classes as indicated. *Although there is no clear relationship between stress and PUD, measures to relieve stress and promote physical and emotional rest help reduce the perception of pain and may reduce ulcer genesis.*

Disturbed Sleep Pattern

Nighttime ulcer pain, which typically occurs between 1:00 and 3:00 AM, may disrupt the sleep cycle and result in inadequate rest. Anticipation of pain may lead to insomnia or other sleep disruptions.

> **EVIDENCE FOR NURSING CARE** | The Patient with Peptic Ulcer Disease
>
> *Selected resources that nurses may find helpful when planning evidence-based nursing care follow.*
>
> - University of Michigan Health System. (2005). *Peptic ulcer disease.* Ann Arbor, MI: University of Michigan Health System. Retrieved from http://www.guideline.gov/summary/summary.aspx?doc_id=7406&nbr=004376&string=peptic+AND+ulcer+AND+disease
> - Stanley, A. J., Ashley, D., Dalton, H. R., Mowat, C., Gaya, D. R., Thompson, E., et al. (2009). Outpatient management of patients with low-risk upper-gastrointestinal haemorrhage: Multicentre validation and prospective evaluation. *Lancet, 373*(9657), 42–7. doi:10.1016/S0140-6736(08)61769-9
> - Yang, Y., Lewis, J., Epstein, S., & Metz, D. (2006, December 27). Long-term proton pump inhibitor therapy and risk of hip fracture. *JAMA: Journal of the American Medical Association, 296*(24), 2947–2953.

- Stress the importance of taking medications as prescribed. *The bedtime dose of PPI or H$_2$-receptor blocker minimizes hydrochloric acid production during the night, reducing nighttime pain.*
- Instruct to limit food intake after the evening meal, eliminating any bedtime snack. *Eating before bed can stimulate the production of gastric acid and pepsin, increasing the likelihood of nighttime pain.*
- Encourage use of relaxation techniques and comfort measures such as soft music as needed to promote sleep. *Once the pain associated with PUD has been controlled, these measures help reduce anxiety and reestablish a normal sleep pattern.*

Imbalanced Nutrition: Less than Body Requirements

In an attempt to avoid discomfort, the patient with peptic ulcer disease may gradually reduce food intake, sometimes jeopardizing nutritional status. Anorexia and early satiety are additional problems associated with PUD.

- Assess current diet, including pattern of food intake, eating schedule, and foods that precipitate pain or are being avoided in anticipation of pain. *The patient may not realize the extent of self-imposed dietary limitations, especially if symptoms have persisted for an extended time. Assessment increases awareness and also helps identify the adequacy of nutrient intake.*
- Refer to a dietitian for meal planning to minimize PUD symptoms and meet nutritional needs. Consider normal eating patterns and preferences in meal planning. *Although no specific diet is recommended for PUD, patients should avoid foods that increase pain. Six small meals per day often help increase food tolerance and decrease postprandial discomfort.*
- Monitor for complaints of anorexia, fullness, nausea, and vomiting. Adjust dietary intake or medication schedule as indicated. *PUD and resultant scarring can lead to impaired gastric emptying, necessitating a treatment change.*

■ Monitor laboratory values for indications of anemia or other nutritional deficits. Monitor for therapeutic and side effects of treatment measures such as oral iron replacement. Instruct the patient taking oral iron replacement to avoid using an antacid within 1 to 2 hours of taking the iron preparation. *Anemia can result from poor nutrient absorption or chronic blood loss in patients with PUD. Oral iron supplements may cause GI distress, nausea, and vomiting; if these side effects are intolerable, notify the physician for a possible change of therapy. Antacids bind with oral iron preparations, blocking absorption.*

Risk for Bleeding

Erosion of a blood vessel with resultant hemorrhage is a significant risk for the patient with peptic ulcer disease. Acute bleeding can lead to hypovolemia and fluid volume deficit, which can lead to a decrease in cardiac output and impaired tissue perfusion.

■ Monitor stools and gastric drainage for overt and occult blood. Assess gastric drainage (vomitus or from a nasogastric tube) to estimate the amount and rapidity of hemorrhage. *Drainage is bright red with possible clots in acute hemorrhage; dark red or the color of coffee grounds when blood has been in the stomach for a period of time. Hematochezia (stool containing red blood and clots) is present in acute hemorrhage; melena (black, tarry stool) is an indicator of less acute bleeding. When small vessels are disrupted, bleeding may be slow and not overtly evident. With chronic or slow gastrointestinal bleeding, the risk of a fluid volume deficit is minimal; anemia and activity intolerance are more likely.*

■ Maintain intravenous therapy with fluid volume and electrolyte replacement solutions; administer whole blood or packed cells as ordered. *Both fluids and electrolytes are lost through vomiting, nasogastric drainage, and diarrhea in an episode of acute bleeding. To prevent shock, it is essential to maintain a blood volume and cardiac output sufficient to perfuse body tissues. Whole blood and packed cells replace both blood volume and red blood cells, providing additional oxygen-carrying capacity to meet cell needs.*

■ Insert a nasogastric tube and maintain its position and patency. Initially, measure and record gastric output every hour, then every 4 to 8 hours. *Nasogastric suction removes blood from the gastrointestinal tract, preventing vomiting and possible aspiration. Gastric output is replaced milliliter for milliliter with a balanced electrolyte solution to maintain homeostasis.*

■ Monitor hemoglobin and hematocrit, serum electrolytes, BUN, and creatinine values. Report abnormal findings. *Hemoglobin and hematocrit are lower than normal with acute or chronic GI bleeding. In acute hemorrhage, initial results may be within normal range because both cells and plasma are lost. Loss of fluids and electrolytes with gastric drainage and diarrhea will alter normal levels. Digestion and absorption of blood in the GI tract may result in elevated BUN and creatinine levels.*

■ Assess abdomen, including bowel sounds, distention, girth, and tenderness every 4 hours and record findings. *Borborygmi or hyperactive bowel sounds with abdominal tenderness are common with acute GI bleeding. Increased distention, increasing abdominal girth, absent bowel sounds, or extreme tenderness with a rigid, boardlike abdomen may indicate perforation.*

■ Maintain bed rest with the head of the bed elevated. Ensure safety. *Loss of blood volume may cause orthostatic hypotension with resultant syncope or dizziness upon standing.*

Using NANDA, NIC, and NOC

Linkages between a selected NANDA nursing diagnosis, NIC, and NOC for the patient with peptic ulcer disease are shown in the chart that follows.

Community-Based Care

Peptic ulcer disease is managed in home and community-based settings; only its complications typically require treatment in an acute care setting. Provide the following information when preparing the patient for home care:

■ Prescribed medication regimen, including desired and potential adverse effects

■ Importance of continuing therapy even when symptoms are relieved

■ Relationship between peptic ulcers and factors such as NSAID use and smoking. If indicated, refer to a smoking cessation clinic or program.

NANDA, NIC, AND NOC LINKAGES
The Patient with Peptic Ulcer Disease

NANDA
Ineffective Health Maintenance

NIC
Bleeding Reduction: Gastrointestinal
Medication Management
Fluid/Electrolyte Management
Teaching: Disease Process

NOC
Nutritional Status: Food and Fluid Intake
Hydration
Knowledge: Treatment Regimen
Treatment Behavior: Illness or Injury

Data from NANDA International. (2009). *Nursing diagnoses: Definitions & classification 2009–2011.* Oxford, UK: Wiley-Blackwell; Bulechek, G. M., Butcher, H., & Dochterman, J. (Eds.). (2008). *Nursing interventions classification (NIC)* (5th ed.). St. Louis, MO: Mosby; and Moorhead, S., Johnson, M., Mass, M., & Swanson, E. (Eds.). (2008). *Nursing outcomes classification (NOC)* (4th ed.). St. Louis, MO: Mosby.

CASE STUDY & NURSING CARE PLAN   A Patient with Peptic Ulcer Disease

Sean O'Donnell is a 47-year-old police officer who lives and works in a metropolitan area. Mr. O'Donnell has had "heartburn" and abdominal discomfort for years, but thought it went along with his job. Last year, after becoming weak, light-headed, and short of breath, he was found to be anemic and was diagnosed as having a duodenal ulcer. He took omeprazole (Prilosec) and ferrous sulfate for 3 months before stopping both, saying he had "never felt better in his life." Mr. O'Donnell has now been admitted to the hospital with active upper GI bleeding.

ASSESSMENT

Rachel Clark is Mr. O'Donnell's admitting nurse and case manager. On initial assessment, Mr. O'Donnell is alert and oriented, though very apprehensive about his condition. Skin pale and cool; BP 136/78, P 98; abdomen distended and tender with hyperactive bowel sounds; 200 mL bright red blood obtained on nasogastric tube insertion. Hemoglobin 8.2 g/dL and hematocrit 23% on admission. Mr. O'Donnell is taken to the endoscopy lab where his bleeding is controlled using laser photocoagulation. On his return to the nursing unit, he receives two units of packed RBCs and intravenous fluids to restore blood volume. A 5-day course of high-dose oral omeprazole (40 mg bid) is ordered to prevent rebleeding, and Mr. O'Donnell is allowed to begin a clear liquid diet 24 hours after his endoscopy. Tissue biopsy obtained during endoscopy confirms the presence of *H. pylori* infection.

DIAGNOSES

- *Deficient Fluid Volume* related to acutely bleeding duodenal ulcer
- *Risk for Injury* related to acute blood loss
- *Fear* related to threat to well-being
- *Ineffective Self Health Management* related to lack of knowledge regarding PUD and its treatment

EXPECTED OUTCOMES

- Maintains normal blood pressure, pulse, and urine output (> 30 mL/h)
- Remains free of injury
- Seeks information to reduce fear
- Identifies and uses coping strategies to manage fear
- Describes prescribed therapeutic regimen
- Verbalizes ability to manage prescribed regimen

PLANNING AND IMPLEMENTATION

- Place call light within reach and encourage to ask for help when getting up or ambulating. Remind to rise slowly from lying to sitting and sitting to standing.
- Discuss situation and provide information about all procedures and treatments.
- Reassure about the effectiveness of treatment in reducing the risk for further bleeding.
- Discuss current and planned treatment measures; stress the importance of completing the prescribed treatment to reduce the risk of further ulcer development.
- Encourage to avoid using aspirin or NSAIDs in the future; suggest alternative medications such as acetaminophen.
- Discuss stress reduction techniques and refer for stress reduction counseling or workshops as indicated.

EVALUATION

Mr. O'Donnell is discharged 48 hours after admission. He has had no further evidence of bleeding, and has resumed a regular diet. His hemoglobin and hematocrit remain low, and he has a prescription for ferrous sulfate. He will complete the prescribed high-dose omeprazole regimen at home, then begin treatment with omeprazole, amoxicillin, and clarithromycin (Biaxin) to eradicate the *H. pylori* infection detected during endoscopy. After 2 weeks of this regimen, he will continue taking omeprazole at bedtime for 4 to 8 weeks. He verbalizes a good understanding of his treatment and the importance of completing the entire regimen. Mr. O'Donnell expresses concern about his ability to "keep his cool on the inside" when under stress. Ms. Clark, his case manager, gives him the names of several resources to help with stress management in case he wants help.

CRITICAL THINKING IN THE NURSING PROCESS

1. How does *H. pylori* infection contribute to the development of peptic ulcers?
2. Describe the physiologic responses to fear and anxiety. Why is it important to alleviate fear and its physical consequences in patients with PUD?
3. What suggestions can you make to help Mr. O'Donnell manage his complex treatment regimen during the next 3 months?
4. Develop a teaching plan that includes stress reduction techniques Mr. O'Donnell can use while performing his duties as a police officer.

See Evaluating Your Response in Appendix C.

- Importance of avoiding aspirin and other NSAIDs; stress the necessity of reading the labels of over-the-counter medications for possible aspirin content
- Manifestations of complications that should be reported to the care provider, including increased abdominal pain or distention, vomiting, black or tarry stools, light-headedness, or fainting
- Stress and lifestyle management techniques that may help prevent exacerbation. Refer to resources for stress management, such as classes, counseling, and formal or informal groups.

The Patient with Gastritis

Gastritis, inflammation of the stomach lining, results from irritation of the gastric mucosa. Gastritis is common, and may be caused by a variety of factors. The most common form of gastritis, *acute gastritis*, is generally a benign, self-limiting disorder associated with the ingestion of gastric irritants such as aspirin, alcohol, caffeine, or foods contaminated with certain bacteria. Manifestations of acute gastritis may range from asymptomatic to mild heartburn to severe gastric distress, vomiting, and bleeding with hematemesis (vomiting blood).

Chronic gastritis is a separate group of disorders characterized by progressive and irreversible changes in the gastric mucosa (Porth & Matfin, 2009). Chronic gastritis is more common in the elderly, chronic alcoholics, and cigarette smokers. When symptoms of chronic gastritis occur, they are often vague, ranging from a feeling of heaviness in the epigastric region after meals to gnawing, burning, ulcer-like epigastric pain unrelieved by antacids.

Pathophysiology

Acute Gastritis

Acute gastritis is characterized by disruption of the mucosal barrier by a local irritant. This disruption allows hydrochloric acid and pepsin to come into contact with the gastric tissue, resulting in irritation, inflammation, and superficial erosions. The gastric mucosa rapidly regenerates, generally making acute gastritis a self-limiting disorder, with resolution and healing occurring within several days.

The ingestion of aspirin or other NSAIDs, corticosteroids, alcohol, and caffeine is commonly associated with the development of acute gastritis. Accidental or purposeful ingestion of a corrosive alkali (such as ammonia, lye, Lysol, and other cleaning agents) or acid leads to severe inflammation and possible necrosis of the stomach. Gastric perforation, hemorrhage, and peritonitis are possible results. Iatrogenic causes of acute gastritis include radiation therapy and administration of certain chemotherapeutic agents.

Erosive Gastritis

A severe form of acute gastritis, **erosive (stress-induced) gastritis**, occurs as a complication of other life-threatening conditions such as shock, severe trauma, major surgery, sepsis, burns, or head injury. When these erosions follow a major burn, they are called **Curling's ulcers**, after Thomas Curling, a British physician, who first described them in 1842. When stress ulcers occur following head injury or CNS surgery, they are referred to as **Cushing's ulcers**, after Harvey Cushing, a U.S. surgeon.

The primary mechanisms leading to erosive gastritis appear to be ischemia of the gastric mucosa resulting from sympathetic vasoconstriction, and tissue injury due to gastric acid. As a result, multiple superficial erosions of the gastric mucosa develop. Maintaining the gastric pH at greater than 3.5 and inhibiting gastric acid secretion with medications help prevent erosive gastritis.

MANIFESTATIONS The patient with acute gastritis may have mild symptoms such as **anorexia** (loss of appetite), or mild epigastric discomfort relieved by belching or defecating. More severe manifestations include abdominal pain, nausea, and vomiting. Gastric bleeding may occur, with hematemesis or melena (black, tarry stool that contains blood). Erosive gastritis is not typically associated with pain. The initial symptom often is painless gastric bleeding occurring 2 or more days after the initial stressor. Bleeding typically is minimal, but can be massive. Corrosive gastritis can cause severe bleeding, signs of shock, and an *acute abdomen* (severely painful, rigid, boardlike abdomen) if perforation occurs. See the following Manifestations box.

MANIFESTATIONS of Acute and Chronic Gastritis

ACUTE GASTRITIS

Gastrointestinal
- Anorexia
- Nausea and vomiting
- Hematemesis
- Melena
- Abdominal pain

Systemic
- Possible shock

CHRONIC GASTRITIS

Gastrointestinal
- Vague discomfort after eating; may be asymptomatic

Systemic
- Anemia
- Fatigue

Chronic Gastritis

Unrelated to acute gastritis, chronic gastritis is a progressive disorder that begins with superficial inflammation and gradually leads to atrophy of gastric tissues. The initial stage is characterized by superficial changes in the gastric mucosa and a decrease in mucus. As the disease evolves, glands of the gastric mucosa are disrupted and destroyed. The inflammatory process involves deep portions of the mucosa, which thins and atrophies. There are several types of chronic gastritis; *H. pylori* gastritis and autoimmune gastritis are the most commonly seen.

H. pylori gastritis is the most common form of chronic gastritis. Its incidence increases with age, and is significantly higher in developing countries than in industrialized countries (Porth & Matfin, 2009). It is caused by chronic infection of the gastric mucosa by *H. pylori*, a gram-negative spiral bacterium. *H. pylori* infection causes inflammation of the gastric mucosa, with infiltration by neutrophils and lymphocytes. The outermost layer of gastric mucosa thins and atrophies, providing a less effective barrier against the autodigestive properties of hydrochloric acid and pepsin.

Infection with *H. pylori* also is associated with peptic ulcer disease and an increased risk of developing gastric cancer.

Autoimmune gastritis is a less common form of chronic gastritis, accounting for about 10% of patients with chronic gastritis (Porth & Matfin, 2009). In autoimmune gastritis, the body produces antibodies to parietal cells and intrinsic factor. These antibodies destroy gastric mucosal cells, resulting in tissue atrophy and the loss of hydrochloric acid and pepsin secretion. Production of intrinsic factor also is affected in most cases. Because intrinsic factor is required for the absorption of vitamin B_{12}, this immune response results in pernicious anemia. For further discussion of pernicious anemia, ∞ see Chapter 33.

MANIFESTATIONS Chronic gastritis is often asymptomatic until atrophy is sufficiently advanced to interfere with digestion and gastric emptying. The patient may complain of vague gastric distress, epigastric heaviness after meals, or ulcer-like symptoms. These symptoms typically are not relieved by antacids. In addition, the patient may experience fatigue and other symptoms of anemia. If intrinsic factor is lacking, paresthesias and other neurologic manifestations of vitamin B_{12} deficiency may be present. See the previous Manifestations box.

Interdisciplinary Care

Acute gastritis is usually diagnosed by the history and clinical presentation. In contrast, the vague symptoms of chronic gastritis may require more extensive diagnostic testing.

Patients with acute and chronic gastritis are generally managed in community settings. The patient requires acute care only when nausea and vomiting are severe enough to interfere with normal fluid and electrolyte balance and nutritional status. If hemorrhage results, surgical intervention may be required.

Diagnosis

Diagnostic tests that may be ordered for the patient with gastritis include the following:

- *Testing* for *H. pylori* infection, including urea breath tests, serologic testing, and fecal antigen testing.

- *Gastric analysis* to assess hydrochloric acid secretion. Secretion may be decreased in patients with chronic gastritis.
- *Hemoglobin, hematocrit,* and *red blood cell (RBC) indices* are evaluated for evidence of anemia. The patient with gastritis may develop pernicious anemia because of parietal cell destruction, or iron-deficiency anemia because of chronic blood loss.
- *Serum vitamin B$_{12}$ levels* are measured to evaluate for possible pernicious anemia. Normal values for vitamin B$_{12}$ are 200 to 1000 pg/mL, with lower levels seen in older adults.
- *Upper endoscopy* may be done to inspect the gastric mucosa for changes, identify areas of bleeding, and obtain tissue for biopsy. Bleeding sites may be treated with electro- or laser coagulation or injected with a sclerosing agent during the procedure.

∞ See Chapter 21 for patient preparation and teaching related to diagnostic tests for upper GI disorders.

Medications

Drugs such as a PPI, H$_2$-receptor blocker, or sucralfate may be ordered to prevent or treat acute stress gastritis. PPIs and H$_2$ receptor blockers reduce the amount or effects of hydrochloric acid on the gastric mucosa. Lansoprazole (Prevacid), esomeprazole (Nexium), and omeprazole (Prilosec) are examples of PPIs. H$_2$-receptor blockers include cimetidine (Tagamet), ranitidine (Zantac), famotidine (Pepcid), and nizatidine (Axid). These drugs also are available in nonprescription strength. Sucralfate (Carafate) works locally to prevent the damaging effects of acid and pepsin on gastric tissue. It does not neutralize or reduce acid secretion. Nursing implications for drugs commonly used in managing gastritis are included in the Medication Administration box on pages 625–626.

Chronic *H. pylori* infection may be treated using combination therapy that includes two antibiotics (such as metronidazole, amoxicillin, clarithromycin, or tetracycline), a bismuth compound, and possibly a PPI. In some cases, eradication of the infection is not warranted, and the patient is treated symptomatically.

Treatments

In acute gastritis, gastrointestinal tract rest is provided by 6 to 12 hours of NPO status, then slow reintroduction of clear liquids (broth, tea, gelatin, carbonated beverages), followed by ingestion of heavier liquids (cream soups, puddings, milk), and finally a gradual reintroduction of solid food.

If nausea and vomiting threaten fluid and electrolyte balance, intravenous fluids and electrolytes are ordered.

GASTRIC LAVAGE   Acute gastritis resulting from ingestion of a poisonous or corrosive substance (acid or strong alkali) is treated with immediate dilution and removal of the substance. Vomiting is not induced because it might further damage the esophagus and possibly the trachea; instead, gastric lavage, washing out of the stomach contents, is performed. See Procedure 23–1.

COMPLEMENTARY THERAPIES   Complementary therapies such as herbal remedies or aromatherapy may be appropriate to recommend for patients with gastritis. Refer the patient to a healthcare provider trained in natural and herbal remedies or to an aromatherapist for an individualized treatment plan. Recommendations may include the following:

- Chamomile tea or the essential oil used in aromatherapy
- Garlic; one clove chopped fine and taken daily at bedtime
- Ginger, powdered or in capsules or made into a tea taken before or after meals
- Mint oil aromatherapy via a diffuser, in a bath, or diluted with a carrier oil and used for a soothing massage

✍ Nursing Care

Health Promotion

Teach all patients and community members about measures to prevent acute gastritis. Food contaminated with bacteria is a significant cause of acute gastritis. Discuss food safety measures such as fully cooking meats and egg products, and promptly refrigerating foods after cooking to avoid bacterial growth. Stress that food contaminated with potential pathogens often looks, smells, and tastes good, making it difficult to identify. Teach patients to abstain from eating or drinking anything during an acute episode of vomiting, then reintroduce clear liquids gradually once vomiting has stopped (2 to 4 hours after the last episode of vomiting). Suggest using liquids such as Pedialyte or a sport drink to replace lost electrolytes and fluid. Instruct patients to avoid milk and milk products until they easily tolerate clear liquids and solid foods such as dry toast or saltine crackers.

Assessment

Assessment data to collect for patients with acute or chronic gastritis include the following:

- *Health history:* Current symptoms and their duration; relieving and aggravating factors; history of ingestion of toxins, contaminated food, alcohol, aspirin, or NSAIDs; other medications.
- *Physical examination:* Vital signs including orthostatic vitals if indicated; peripheral pulses; general appearance; abdominal assessment including appearance, bowel sounds, and tenderness.

Nursing Diagnoses and Interventions

In planning and implementing nursing care for the patient with acute or chronic gastritis, consider both the direct effects of the disorder on the gastrointestinal system and nutritional status as well as its effects on lifestyle and psychosocial integrity. This section focuses on problems related to nausea and anorexia associated with gastritis.

Nausea

Nausea, vomiting, and abdominal distress are the primary manifestations of acute gastritis. Patients with chronic gastritis often experience anorexia and nausea that can interfere with food intake and nutritional status.

- Monitor subjective complaints of nausea. *Nausea is a subjective sensation best described by the patient.*
- For the patient with acute gastritis, monitor vital signs, skin turgor and condition, and weight. Maintain accurate intake and output records. Monitor amount, color, and specific

gravity of urine. *Nausea and vomiting associated with acute gastritis can significantly affect food and fluid intake, leading to dehydration.*

- Administer antiemetic medication as ordered, prior to meals and before treatments or procedures known to stimulate nausea. *Preventing nausea is particularly important for patients receiving chemotherapy to avoid the association between the treatment and nausea.*
- Instruct to consume small quantities of clear fluids and dry foods at separate times. *Separating the intake of dry foods and fluids helps reduce the nausea stimulus.*

Imbalanced Nutrition: Less than Body Requirements
Manifestations of chronic gastritis may lead to reduced food intake and malnutrition. The patient often associates these unpleasant sensations with eating, and may gradually reduce food intake. Associated anorexia also contributes to poor food intake.

- Monitor and record food and fluid intake and any abnormal losses (such as vomiting). *Careful monitoring can help in developing a dietary plan to meet the caloric needs of the patient.*
- Monitor weight and laboratory studies such as serum albumin, hemoglobin, and RBC indices. *Weights and laboratory values provide data regarding nutritional status and the effectiveness of interventions.*
- Arrange for dietary consultation to determine caloric and nutrient needs and develop a dietary plan. Consider food preferences and tolerances in menu planning. *A diet high in protein, vitamins, and minerals may be prescribed to meet nutritional needs of the patient with chronic gastritis. In addition, specific food intolerances may need to be considered. Planning to include preferred foods in the diet helps ensure consumption of the prescribed diet.*
- Provide nutritional supplements between meals or frequent small feedings as needed. *Many patients with chronic gastritis tolerate small, frequent feedings better than three large meals per day.*
- Maintain tube feedings or parenteral nutrition as ordered. ∞ Refer to Chapter 22 for further information on enteral and parenteral feedings.

Community-Based Care
Because acute or chronic gastritis is usually managed in community-based settings, teaching is vital. For the patient with acute gastritis, teaching focuses on managing acute symptoms, reintroducing fluids and solid foods, identifying indicators of possible complications (e.g., continued vomiting, signs of fluid and electrolyte imbalance), and preventing future episodes.

Provide the following information for patients with chronic gastritis:

- Maintaining optimal nutrition
- Helpful dietary modifications
- Using prescribed medications
- Avoiding known gastric irritants, such as aspirin, alcohol, and cigarette smoking

Referral to smoking cessation classes or programs to treat alcohol abuse may be necessary.

The Patient with Cancer of the Stomach
Worldwide, cancer of the stomach is the most common cancer (after skin cancer), but it is less common in the United States.

> **FAST FACTS**
> - An estimated 21,130 new cases of stomach cancer are diagnosed annually in the United States (ACS, 2009).
> - Its incidence is highest in Hispanics, African Americans, and Asian Americans.
> - Men are affected nearly twice as often as women.

Older adults are more likely to develop gastric cancer: The mean age at time of diagnosis is 63. People in lower socioeconomic groups are more often affected by gastric cancer.

Risk Factors
H. pylori infection is a major risk factor for cancer of the distal portion of the stomach; 35% to 89% of cases can be attributed to this infection. Other risk factors are a genetic predisposition, chronic gastritis, pernicious anemia, gastric polyps, and carcinogenic factors in the diet (such as smoked foods and nitrates). Achlorhydria, a lack of hydrochloric acid in the stomach, is a known risk factor. The risk for gastric cancer also is increased in people who have had a partial gastric resection.

Pathophysiology
Adenocarcinoma, which involves the mucus-producing cells of the stomach, is the most common form of gastric cancer. These carcinomas may arise anywhere on the mucosal surface of the stomach but are most frequently found in the distal portion. More than half of all gastric cancers occur in the antrum or pyloric region (Porth & Matfin, 2009). Gastric cancer begins as a localized lesion (*in situ*), then progresses to involve the

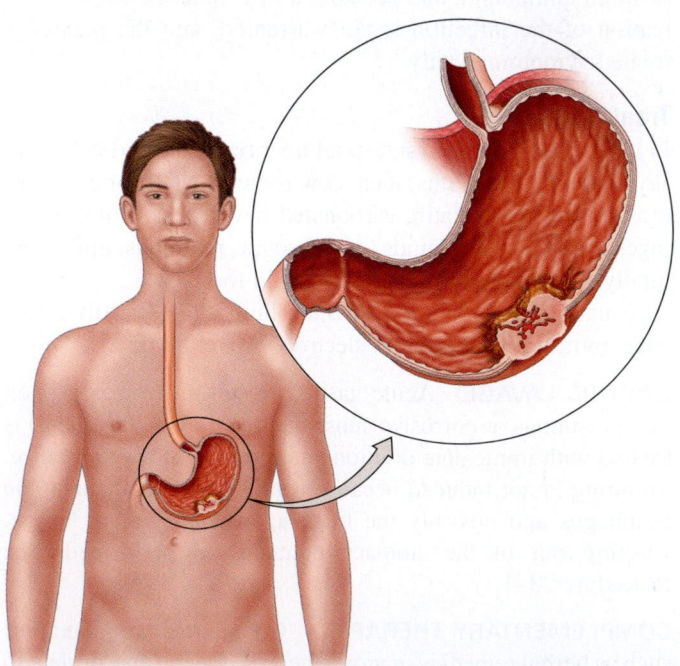

Figure 23–10 ■ Gastric cancer affecting the antrum of the stomach.
Source: Robert Margulies/Phototake NYC.

mucosa or submucosa (early gastric carcinoma). Lesions may spread by direct extension to tissues surrounding the stomach, the liver in particular. The lesion may ulcerate or appear as a polypoid (polyp-like) mass (Figure 23–10 ■). Lymph node involvement and metastasis occur early due to the rich blood and lymphatic supply to the stomach. Metastatic lesions are often found in the liver, lungs, ovaries, and peritoneum.

Manifestations

Gastric cancer has few manifestations. Unfortunately, the disease is often quite advanced and metastases are usually present at the time of diagnosis. Early symptoms are vague, including feelings of early satiety, anorexia, indigestion, and possibly vomiting. The patient may experience ulcer-like pain unrelieved by antacids, typically occurring after meals. As the disease progresses, weight loss occurs, and the patient may be *cachectic* (in very poor health and malnourished) at the time of diagnosis. An abdominal mass may be palpable, and occult blood may be present in the stool, indicating gastrointestinal bleeding.

Interdisciplinary Care

Diagnosis

Anemia detected by a CBC often is the first indication of gastric cancer. An upper GI x-ray with barium swallow is useful to identify lesions, and ultrasound or other radiologic techniques may identify a mass. Upper endoscopy with visualization and biopsy of the lesion provides the definitive diagnosis.

Surgery

When gastric cancer is identified prior to the development of metastasis, surgical removal of part or all of the stomach and regional lymph nodes is the treatment of choice. **Partial gastrectomy** involves removal of a portion of the stomach, usually the distal half to two-thirds. In partial gastrectomy, the surgeon constructs an anastomosis from the remainder of the stomach directly to the duodenum or to the proximal jejunum. The *gastroduodenostomy* (Billroth I) and the *gastrojejunostomy* (Billroth II) are commonly used partial gastrectomy procedures (Figures 23–11*A* and *B* ■).

A **total gastrectomy**, removal of the entire stomach, may be done for diffuse cancer that is spread throughout the gastric mucosa but limited to the stomach. In a total gastrectomy, the surgeon constructs an anastomosis from the esophagus to the duodenum or jejunum. Total gastrectomy with *esophagojejunostomy* is illustrated in Figure 23–11*C*.

Nursing care of the patient who has undergone gastric surgery is outlined in the following box.

COMPLICATIONS Several long-term complications may develop following gastrectomy procedures. **Dumping syndrome** is the most common problem. It may follow a partial gastrectomy with duodenal or jejunal anastomosis. When the pylorus has been resected or bypassed, a hypertonic, undigested food bolus may rapidly enter the duodenum or jejunum. Water is pulled into the lumen of the intestine by the hyperosmolar character of the chyme, resulting in decreased blood volume and intestinal dilation. Peristalsis is stimulated, and intestinal motility is increased.

Early symptoms of dumping syndrome occur within 5 to 30 minutes after eating. These symptoms result from intestinal dilation, peristaltic stimulation, and hypovolemia caused by undigested food in the proximal small intestine. Manifestations include nausea with possible vomiting, epigastric pain with cramping and *borborygmi* (loud, hyperactive bowel sounds), and diarrhea. Systemic symptoms from the hypovolemia and reflex sympathetic stimulation include tachycardia, orthostatic hypotension, dizziness, flushing, and diaphoresis.

The entry of hyperosmolar chyme into the jejunum also causes a rapid rise in the blood glucose. This stimulates the release of an excessive amount of insulin, leading to hypoglycemic symptoms 2 to 3 hours after the meal. The pathogenesis and clinical manifestations of dumping syndrome are represented in Figure 23–12 ■. Dumping syndrome is typically self-limiting, lasting 6 to 12 months after surgery; however, a small percentage of people continue to experience long-term symptoms.

Dumping syndrome is managed primarily by a dietary pattern that delays gastric emptying and allows smaller boluses of undigested food to enter the intestine. Meals should be small and more frequent. Liquids and solids are taken at separate times instead of together during a meal. The amount of proteins and fats in the diet is increased, because they exit the stomach more slowly than carbohydrates. Carbohydrates, especially simple sugars, are reduced. The patient is instructed to rest in a recumbent or semirecumbent

Figure 23–11 ■ Partial and total gastrectomy procedures. *A,* Partial gastrectomy with anastomosis to the duodenum. *B,* Partial gastrectomy with anastomosis to the jejunum. *C,* Total gastrectomy with anastomosis of the esophagus to the jejunum.

NURSING CARE OF THE PATIENT   Having Gastric Surgery

PREOPERATIVE NURSING CARE

- ∞ See Chapter 4 for routine preoperative care and teaching.
- Insert a nasogastric tube if ordered preoperatively. *Although it is often inserted in the surgical suite just prior to surgery, the nasogastric tube may be placed preoperatively to remove secretions and empty stomach contents.*

POSTOPERATIVE NURSING CARE

- Provide routine care for the surgical patient as outlined in ∞ Chapter 4.
- Assess position and patency of nasogastric tube, connecting it to low suction. Gently irrigate with sterile normal saline if tube becomes clogged. *The nasogastric tube will be placed in surgery to avoid disruption of the gastric suture lines and should be well secured. If repositioning or tube replacement is needed, notify the surgeon. Patency must be maintained to keep the stomach decompressed, reducing pressure on sutures.*
- Assess color, amount, and odor of gastric drainage, noting any changes in these parameters or the presence of clots or bright bleeding. *Initial drainage is bright red. It becomes dark, then clear or greenish-yellow over the first 2 to 3 days. A change in the color, amount, or odor may indicate a complication such as hemorrhage, intestinal obstruction, or infection.*
- Maintain intravenous fluids while nasogastric suction is in place. *The patient on nasogastric suction is not only unable to take oral food and fluids but also is losing electrolyte-rich fluid through the nasogastric tube. If replacement fluid and electrolytes are not maintained, the patient is at risk for dehydration; imbalances of sodium, potassium, and chloride; and metabolic alkalosis.*

- Provide antiulcer and antibiotic therapy as ordered. *These medications may be ordered for the postoperative patient, depending on the procedure performed. Antibiotic therapy is a common preventive measure for infection that may result from contamination of the abdominal cavity with gastric contents.*
- Monitor bowel sounds and abdominal distention. *Bowel sounds indicate resumption of peristalsis. Increasing distention may indicate third spacing, obstruction, or infection.*
- Resume oral food and fluids as ordered. Initial feedings are clear liquids, progressing to full liquids and then frequent small feedings of regular foods. Monitor bowel sounds and for abdominal distention frequently during this period. *Oral feedings are reintroduced slowly to minimize trauma to the suture lines by possible gastric distension.*
- Encourage ambulation. *Ambulation stimulates peristalsis.*
- Begin discharge planning and teaching. Consult with a dietitian for diet instructions and menu planning; reinforce teaching. Teach the patient about potential postoperative complications, such as abdominal abscess, dumping syndrome, postprandial hypoglycemia, or pernicious anemia. Also, teach the patient to recognize signs and symptoms and preventive measures. *The patient's gastric capacity is reduced after partial gastrectomy, necessitating a corresponding reduction in meal size. Changes in gastric emptying and reduction in gastric secretions may change the patient's tolerance for many foods, requiring slow reintroduction of these foods. Dumping syndrome, postprandial hypoglycemia, and pernicious anemia are possible long-term complications of partial gastrectomy. For most patients, dietary modifications can control both dumping syndrome and postprandial hypoglycemia.*

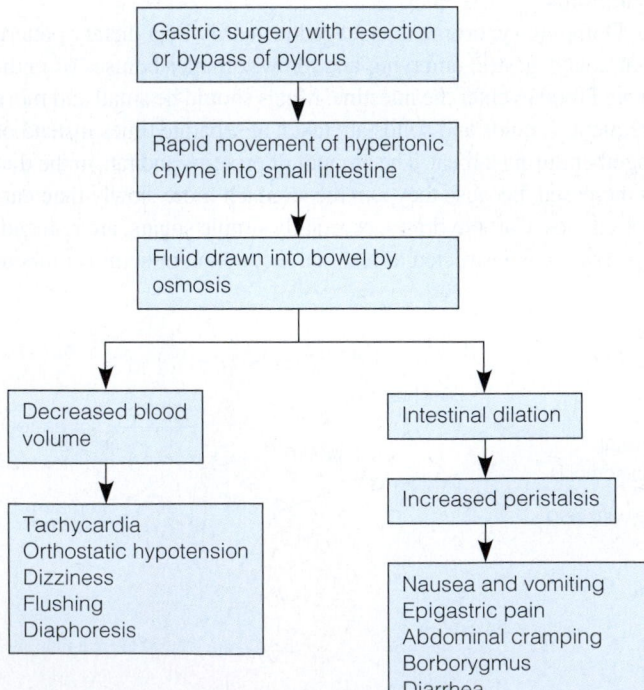

Figure 23–12 ■ The pathogenesis and manifestations of dumping syndrome.

position for 30 to 60 minutes after meals. Anticholinergics, sedatives, and antispasmodics may be prescribed.

Anemia may be a chronic problem after a major gastric resection. Iron is absorbed primarily in the duodenum and proximal jejunum; rapid gastric emptying or a gastrojejunostomy may interfere with adequate absorption.

The cells of the stomach produce intrinsic factor, required for the absorption of vitamin B_{12}. Vitamin B_{12} deficiency leads to pernicious anemia. Because of hepatic stores of vitamin B_{12}, symptoms of anemia may not be seen for 1 to 2 years after surgery. Vitamin B_{12} levels are routinely monitored following extensive gastric resections.

Other nutritional problems seen following surgery include folic acid deficiency and decreased absorption of calcium and vitamin D. Poor absorption of nutrients, combined with the inability to eat large meals, puts the patient at risk for weight loss in addition to the more specific nutrient deficiencies. Nearly 50% of patients who have gastric surgery experience significant weight loss, primarily because of insufficient calorie intake. Factors contributing to insufficient intake of calories include early satiety (feeling of fullness), decreased stomach size, and altered emptying patterns.

Other Therapies

Combination chemotherapy administered before surgery and in combination with radiation therapy after surgery has been found to reduce tumor recurrence and prolong survival (Fauci

NURSING CARE OF THE PATIENT   With a Gastrostomy or Jejunostomy Tube

Patients who have had extensive gastric surgery or who require long-term enteral feedings to maintain nutrition may have a gastrostomy or jejunostomy tube inserted.

PROCEDURE

Gastrostomy tubes are surgically placed in the stomach, with the stoma in the epigastric region of the abdomen (see Figure 23–13 ■). Jejunostomy tubes are placed in the proximal jejunum. Immediately following the procedure, the tube may be connected to low suction or plugged. If the patient has been receiving tube feedings, these may be reinitiated shortly after tube placement.

NURSING CARE

- Assess tube placement by aspirating stomach contents and checking the pH of aspirate to determine gastric or intestinal placement. A pH of 5 or less indicates gastric placement; the pH is generally 7 or higher with intestinal placement. *Recent studies show auscultation to be ineffective in determining feeding tube placement. Measuring the pH of aspirate from the tube is more reliable as a means of determining tube placement.*
- Inspect the skin surrounding the insertion site for healing, redness, swelling, and the presence of any drainage. If drainage is present, note the color, amount, consistency, and odor. *Changes in the insertion site, drainage, or lack of healing may indicate an infection.*
- Assess the abdomen for distention, bowel sounds, and tenderness *to evaluate functioning of the gastrointestinal tract.*
- Until the stoma is well healed, use sterile technique for dressing changes and site care. Clean technique is appropriate for use once healing is complete. *Sterile technique reduces the risk of wound contamination by pathogens that can lead to infection. Once healing has occurred, clean technique is*

acceptable because the gastrointestinal tract is not a sterile body cavity.

- Wearing clean gloves, remove old dressing. Cleanse the site with saline or soap and water, and rinse as appropriate. A well-healed stoma may be cleansed in the shower with the tube clamped or plugged. Pat dry with 4 × 4 gauze pads, and allow to air dry. Apply Stomahesive, karaya, or other protective agents around tube as needed to protect the skin. *Gastric acid and other wound drainage is irritating to the skin. Meticulous care is important to maintain the integrity of the skin surrounding the stoma.*
- Redress the wound using a stoma dressing or folded 4 × 4 gauze pads. *Do not cut gauze pads, because threads may enter the wound, causing irritation and increasing the risk of inflammation.*
- Irrigate the tube with 30 to 50 mL of water, and clean the tube inside and out as indicated or ordered. Soft gastric tubes may require cleaning of the inner lumen with a special brush to maintain patency. *Tube feeding formulas may coat the inside of the gastrostomy tube and eventually cause it to become occluded. Regular irrigation with water and brushing as indicated maintain tube patency.*
- Provide mouth care or remind the patient to do so. *When feedings are not being taken orally, the usual stimulus to do mouth care is lost. In addition, salivary fluids may not be as abundant, and oral mucous membranes may become dry and cracked.*
- If indicated, teach the patient and family how to care for the tube and feedings. Refer to a home health agency or visiting nurse for support and reinforcement of learning. *Gastrostomy tubes are often in place long term. When the patient and family are able to assume care, independence and self-image are enhanced.*

et al., 2008). For the patient with more advanced disease, treatment is palliative and may include surgery, radiation therapy, and chemotherapy. These patients may require a gastrostomy or jejunostomy feeding tube (Figure 23–13). See the box on for nursing care of the patient with a gastrostomy or jejunostomy tube.

Figure 23–13 ■ Gastrostomy. *A,* Gastrostomy tube placement. *B,* The tube is fixed against both the abdomen and stomach walls by cross bars.

Because gastric cancer is generally advanced by the time of diagnosis, the prognosis is poor. The 5-year survival rate of all patients treated for gastric carcinoma is 10%.

ᘒ Nursing Care

Health Promotion

Although the exact causes of gastric cancer are unknown, contributing factors such as *H. pylori* infection and consumption of foods preserved with nitrates have been identified. To reduce their risk of developing gastric cancer, encourage patients with known *H. pylori* infection to complete the prescribed course of treatment and verify that it has eradicated the infection. With all patients, discuss the relationship between gastric cancer and consumption of foods preserved with nitrates (such as bacon and other processed meats), and encourage limited consumption of these products.

Assessment

Assessment data related to gastric cancer include the following:

- *Health history:* Manifestations such as anorexia, early satiety, indigestion, or vomiting; epigastric pain after meals; recent unintentional weight loss.

CASE STUDY & NURSING CARE PLAN   A Patient with Gastric Cancer

George Harvey is a 61-year-old estate attorney who lives with his wife, Harriet. For the last 3 months, Mr. Harvey has had increasing anorexia and difficulty eating. He has lost 10 pounds. His physician has diagnosed gastric cancer, and Mr. Harvey is admitted for a partial gastrectomy and gastrojejunostomy. The oncologist has recommended postoperative chemotherapy and radiation. Mr. Harvey reports that the doctor told him "that will give me the best chance for cure."

ASSESSMENT

On admission before surgery, Mr. Harvey tells his nurse, Lauren Walsh, that he has eaten very little in the past few weeks. He asks, "What will happen to my wife if something happens to me? I'm afraid this cancer will get me." Mr. Harvey weighs 147 lb (67 kg) and is 72 inches (183 cm) tall. He is pale and thin; his vital signs are BP 148/86, P 92, R 18, and T 97.8°F PO. A firm mass is palpable in the left epigastric region. The rest of his physical assessment data are within normal limits. Mr. Harvey's hemoglobin is 12.8 g/dL, hematocrit is 39%, and serum albumin level is 3.2 g/dL, indicating that he is mildly malnourished. All other preoperative laboratory and diagnostic studies are within normal limits.

DIAGNOSES

- *Imbalanced Nutrition: Less than Body Requirements* related to anorexia and difficulty eating
- *Acute Pain* related to surgical incision and manipulation of abdominal organs
- *Risk for Ineffective Airway Clearance* related to upper abdominal surgery
- *Grieving* related to recent diagnosis of cancer

EXPECTED OUTCOMES

- Maintain present weight during hospitalization.
- Resume a high-calorie, high-protein diet by time of discharge.
- Verbalize effective pain management, maintaining a reported pain level of 3 or less on a scale of 1 to 10.
- Maintain a patent airway and clear breath sounds.
- Verbalize feelings regarding diagnosis and participate in decision making.

PLANNING AND IMPLEMENTATION

- Weigh daily.
- Maintain nasogastric tube placement, patency, and suction as ordered.

- Maintain intravenous fluids and parenteral nutrition as ordered until oral food intake is resumed.
- Arrange for diet teaching, including strategies to prevent dumping syndrome, before discharge.
- Maintain patient-controlled analgesia until able to take oral analgesics.
- Assess respiratory status including rate, depth, and breath sounds every hour initially, then every 4 hours.
- Assist to cough, deep breathe, and use inspirometer every 2 to 4 hours and as needed. Splint abdomen during coughing.
- Encourage verbalization of feelings about diagnosis and perceived losses.
- Encourage participation in decision making.

EVALUATION

Mr. Harvey's weight remained stable through his hospitalization. On discharge he is taking a high-protein, high-calorie diet in six small feedings per day. He and his wife have reviewed his diet with the dietitian and are planning on using some dietary supplements at home to meet protein needs. He verbalizes an understanding of measures to prevent dumping syndrome, including separating his intake of solid foods and liquids. Mr. Harvey is using oral analgesics in the morning and at bedtime to control his pain. He and his wife have begun to discuss the meaning of his diagnosis. Mrs. Harvey tells the discharge nurse, "We are going to go to a support group called 'Coping with Cancer' when George is stronger."

CRITICAL THINKING IN THE NURSING PROCESS

1. What is the rationale for maintaining nasogastric suction after gastrojejunostomy?
2. Develop a preoperative teaching plan for a patient undergoing a partial gastrectomy.
3. Mr. Harvey calls you just before the initial dose of chemotherapy and says, "Everyone tells me that chemotherapy will cause vomiting, and I don't think I can take being sick again." How would you respond?
4. Design interventions to ensure adequate nutrition for people with advanced gastric cancer.

See Evaluating Your Response in Appendix C.

- *Physical assessment:* General appearance, weight for height; abdominal distention or a palpable upper abdominal mass; occult blood in stool or vomitus.

Nursing Diagnoses and Interventions

Priorities of nursing care for the patient with gastric cancer focus on effects of the disease and its treatment on nutritional status, and on the effects of a potentially fatal disease on the patient and family. See the accompanying Case Study & Nursing Care Plan above.

Imbalanced Nutrition: Less than Body Requirements

The patient with gastric cancer may be malnourished because of anorexia, early satiety, and increased metabolic needs related to the tumor. Extensive gastric resection also makes it difficult

to consume an adequate diet. Malnourishment, in turn, impairs healing and the patient's ability to tolerate cancer treatment.

- Consult with dietitian for a complete nutrition assessment and diet planning. *The patient is at risk for protein-calorie malnutrition, which impairs the ability to heal and recover from extensive surgery.*
- Weigh daily. Monitor laboratory values such as hemoglobin, hematocrit, and serum albumin levels. *Daily weights are a valuable measurement of both fluid and nutritional status. Laboratory values provide further evidence of nutritional status.*
- Provide preferred foods; have family prepare meals when possible. Provide supplemental feedings between meals. *Small, frequent feedings and preferred foods encourage intake of nutrients.*

- Arrange for visitors to be present during meals. *Eating is a social function as well as a physiologic one. Companionship often improves food intake.*
- Administer pain and antiemetic medications as needed before meals. *Pain and nausea suppress the appetite; relief promotes food intake.*

Grieving

- Encourage family members to spend as much time as possible with the patient. *The family may feel helpless and ineffectual. Supporting family members' presence can encourage this vital interaction.*
- Do not negate denial if present. *Denial is a coping mechanism that protects the patient from hopelessness.*
- Allow patients to talk openly if desired about their condition and the prognosis. *Acceptance of the patients' fears helps reduce anxiety and promote coping behaviors.*

- Actively listen to the patient's and family's expressions of grieving. Avoid interrupting or offering meaningless words of consolation. *Being present and listening actively are often the most effective interventions for the grieving patient.*

Community-Based Care

Although the patient with gastric cancer may be hospitalized for surgery, most care is provided in the home and community-based settings such as hospice care. When preparing the patient and family for home care, discuss the following topics:

- Care of incision and feeding tube (if present) or central venous line
- Maintaining nutrition and preventing complications of surgery such as dumping syndrome
- Pain management
- Provide referrals to home care agencies, hospice, and cancer support groups as appropriate
- Provide information about services available through the local chapter of the American Cancer Society

CHAPTER HIGHLIGHTS

- Nausea and vomiting, common GI symptoms, may be indicative of disorders affecting many organ systems, including the GI tract, inner ear, CNS, or heart. Nausea and vomiting also are frequently related to medical interventions, such as drugs and cancer therapies. Complications such as dehydration, electrolyte imbalance, and aspiration of gastric contents are primary concerns in treating nausea and vomiting.
- Stomatitis and oral mucositis are common disorders of the mouth, potentially having a significant effect on comfort and nutrition. In most cases, management is symptomatic and supportive, directed toward promoting comfort and maintaining nutritional status.
- Tobacco and alcohol use contribute to a number of upper GI disorders, including GERD, oral and esophageal cancers, and peptic ulcer disease. Encourage all patients to stop smoking or using smokeless tobacco and to consume alcohol in moderate amounts if at all to reduce their risk or these disorders.
- Gastroesophageal reflux disease (GERD) is common. While it often is considered to be a benign condition, prolonged exposure of the lower esophagus to gastric juices can lead to esophagitis, hemorrhage, and scarring.
- Both esophageal and gastric cancer often are diagnosed late in the disease because their symptoms may be vague. Encourage patients with complaints of dysphagia, a sensation of gastric fullness, or heartburn to seek medical evaluation. Surgical resection

of the cancerous portion of the esophagus or stomach is the treatment of choice when the tumor is diagnosed early.
- Upper gastrointestinal bleeding can lead to significant blood loss and shock. Peptic ulcer disease accounts for the majority of UGI hemorrhage, although erosive gastritis and esophageal varices also are common causes. Nursing care focuses on monitoring and promoting cardiovascular stability and preventing further hemorrhage.
- Acute gastritis, often associated with aspirin or NSAID use, is generally benign and self-limited. Erosive gastritis, a complication of critical conditions such as shock, trauma, a major burn, or head injury, can lead to unexpected gastric hemorrhage. Prophylactic therapy with proton pump inhibitors or H_2-receptor blockers is important to prevent erosive gastritis in at risk patients. Chronic gastritis is an unrelated disorder usually associated with *H. pylori* infection.
- *H. pylori* infection also is a major risk factor for peptic ulcer disease and gastric cancer. Effectively treating the infection can reduce or eliminate the risk of future exacerbations of PUD.
- An acute change in the nature of abdominal pain in a patient with PUD, especially when accompanied by vomiting, guarding of the abdomen, or a change in bowel sounds, could indicate an obstruction or perforation and release of gastric contents into the peritoneal cavity.

TEST YOURSELF NCLEX-RN® REVIEW

1. The nurse assessing for oral cancer risk factors in a patient with a persistent sore on his tongue asks about which of the following?
   1. consumption of highly spiced foods
   2. thumb sucking or pacifier use as a child
   3. regular use of dental floss
   4. tobacco use in any form

2. The nurse teaching a patient with gastroesophageal reflux disease includes which of the following instructions? **Select all that apply.**
   1. This is a benign disease requiring no treatment.
   2. Elevate the head of the bed on 6- to 8-inch blocks.
   3. Stop taking the prescribed proton-pump inhibitor once symptoms are relieved.
   4. Peppermint and chocolate candies can help relieve symptoms.
   5. Avoid lying down for several hours after eating.

3. The nurse evaluates his teaching of a patient with acute stress gastritis as effective when the patient states that she will do which of the following?
   1. Avoid using aspirin or NSAIDs for routine pain relief.
   2. Consume only bland foods.
   3. Return for yearly upper endoscopy exams.
   4. Fully cook all meat, poultry, and egg products.

4. The nurse identifies which of the following nursing diagnoses as highest priority for the patient admitted with peptic ulcer disease and possible perforation?
   1. *Acute Pain*
   2. *Ineffective Health Maintenance*
   3. *Nausea*
   4. *Impaired Tissue Integrity: Gastrointestinal*

5. Following a partial gastrectomy for gastric cancer, a patient complains of nausea, abdominal pain and cramping, and diarrhea after eating. Recognizing manifestations of dumping syndrome, the nurse recommends which of the following?
   1. fasting for a period of 6 to 12 hours before meals
   2. decreasing the protein content of meals
   3. frequent small meals that contain solid foods or liquids, but not both
   4. a diet rich in carbohydrates to maintain blood glucose levels

6. The nurse caring for a patient with esophageal cancer affecting the middle portion of the esophagus would immediately report which of the following?
   1. crackles in the base of the right lung
   2. bright bleeding from the mouth
   3. weight loss
   4. difficulty swallowing solid foods

7. The physician has ordered omeprazole 20 mg twice daily, clarithromycin 500 mg twice daily, and amoxicillin 1 g daily for a patient with peptic ulcer disease. It is most important for the nurse to instruct the patient to do which of the following?
   1. Stop the drugs immediately and notify the physician if a rash, hives, or itching develop.
   2. Consume 8 oz of yogurt or buttermilk daily while taking these drugs.
   3. Take the drugs on an empty stomach, 1 hour before breakfast and at least 2 hours after dinner.
   4. Take the drugs with a full glass of water.

8. When planning care for a patient with stomatitis, the nurse identifies which of the following as a priority intervention?
   1. Assist to cleanse mouth with mouthwash following meals.
   2. Allow patient to select appealing foods from a menu.
   3. Provide viscous lidocaine to relieve mouth pain before meals.
   4. Refer the patient to a smoking cessation program.

9. The evening following a gastric resection, the nurse notes that there has been no drainage from the nasogastric tube for the past 3 hours. The nurse should do which of the following?
   1. Chart the finding.
   2. Reposition the nasogastric tube.
   3. Gently irrigate the tube with normal saline.
   4. Notify the surgeon.

10. A patient with a history of peptic ulcer disease suddenly begins to complain of severe abdominal pain. The nurse should do which of the following? **Select all that apply.**
    1. Administer the prescribed proton-pump inhibitor.
    2. Obtain an order for a narcotic analgesic.
    3. Withhold oral food and fluids.
    4. Place the patient in Fowler's position.
    5. Notify the physician.

See Test Yourself answers in Appendix C.

BIBLIOGRAPHY

Abraham, J. (2008 December). Acupressure and acupuncture in preventing and managing postoperative nausea and vomiting in adults. *Journal of Perioperative Practice, 18*(12), 543–551.

Adams, M. P., Holland, L. N., Jr., & Bostwick, P. M. (2008). *Pharmacology for nurses: A pathophysiologic approach* (2nd ed.). Upper Saddle River, NJ: Pearson Prentice Hall.

Agarwal, K., & Agarwal, S. (2008 February). *Helicobacter pylori* vaccine: From past to future. *Mayo Clinic Proceedings, 83*(2), 168–175.

American Cancer Society. (2009). *Cancer facts and figures 2009*. Atlanta: Author.

American College of Physicians (ACP). (2008 August). In the clinic. Gastroesophageal reflux disease. *Annals of Internal Medicine, 5 August 2008,* ITC2-1– ITC2-14.

American Medical Directors Association (AMDA) (2006). Gastrointestinal disorders. Columbia, MD: AMDA.

Barba, K., Fitzgerald, P., & Wood, S. (2007 July). Managing peptic ulcer disease. *Nursing2007.* Retrieved from www.nursing2007.com

Barclay, L., & Vega, C. (2007 April). Peppermint oil may relieve digestive symptoms, headaches. *Medscape Medical News, 2007.* Retrieved from www.medscape.com

Boparai, V., Rajagopalan, J., & Triadafilopoulos, G. (2008). Guide to the use of proton pump inhibitors in adult patients. *Drugs 2008, 68*(7), 925–947.

Bulechek, G. M., Butcher, H. K., & Dochterman, J. M. (Eds.). (2008). *Nursing interventions classification (NIC)* (5th ed.). St. Louis, MO: Mosby.

Cawley, M. M., & Benson, L. M. (2005). Current trends in managing oral mucositis. *Clinical Journal of Oncology Nursing, 9*(5), 584–594.

Copstead, L. C., & Banasik, J. L. (2010). *Pathophysiology* (4th ed.). St. Louis, MO: Elsevier/Saunders.

Dibble, S., Lucy, J., Cooper, B., Israel, J., Cohen, M., Nussey, B., et al. (2007). Acupressure for chemotherapy-induced nausea and vomiting: A randomized clinical trial. *Oncology Nursing Forum, 34*(4), 813–820.

Dodd, V., Watson, J., Choi, Y., Tomar, S., & Logan, H. (2008). Oral cancer in African Americans: Addressing health disparities. *American Journal of Health Behavior, 32*(6), 684–692.

Edmondson, D., & Schiech, L. (2008 April). Esophageal cancer: A tough pill to swallow. *Nursing2008, 38*(4), 44–48.

Edwards, S. J., & Metheny, N. A. (2000). Measurement of gastric residual volume: State of the science. *MEDSURG Nursing, 9*(3), 125–128.

Fauci, A. S., Braunwald, E., Kasper, D. L., Hauser, S. L., Longo, D. L., Jameson, J. L., et al. (2008). *Harrison's principles of internal medicine* (17th ed.). New York: McGraw-Hill.

Fontaine, K. L. (2005). *Healing practices: Alternative therapies for nursing* (2nd ed.). Upper Saddle River, NJ: Prentice Hall Health.

Gendreau-Webb, R. (2007 October). Bone up on proton pump inhibitors and fracture risk. *Nursing2007, 37*(10), 60–61.

Harris, D., Eilers, J., Harriman, A., Cashavelly, B., & Maxwell, C. (2008 February). Putting evidence into practice®: Evidence-based interventions for the management of oral mucositis. *Clinical Journal of Oncology Nursing, 12*(1), 141–152.

Kahrilas, P. (2008 October). Gastroesophageal reflux disease. *New England Journal of Medicine, 359*(16), 1700–1707.

Kee, J. L. (2009). *Handbook of Laboratory and diagnostic tests with nursing implications* (6th ed.). Upper Saddle River, NJ: Pearson Prentice Hall.

Khvorova, Y., & Neill, J. (2008 July). A review of the effect of peppermint oil in various gastrointestinal conditions. *J. GENCA, 18*(3), 6–15.

Knudtson, M., & Davis, Jr., R. H. (2005). Frequent heartburn: An evidence-based approach to cost-effective management. *American Journal for Nurse Practitioners, 9*(1), 137–144.

Lehne, R. A. (2007). *Pharmacology for nursing care* (6th ed.). St. Louis, MO: Elsevier.

Mackenzie, D. J., Popplewell, P. K., & Billingsley, K. G. (2004). Care of patients after esophagectomy. *Critical Care Nurse, 24*(1), 16, 18–31.

McCance, K. L., & Huether, S. E. (2006). *Pathophysiology* (5th ed.). St. Louis, MO: Mosby.

McGinley, S. R. (2003). The other tobacco threat. Smokeless does not mean harmless. *Advance for Nurse Practitioners, 11*(4), 29–30, 34, 90.

McPhee, S. J., Papadakis, M. A., & Tierney, L. M. (2008). *Current medical diagnosis & treatment* (47th ed.). New York: Lange Medical Books/McGraw-Hill.

Moorhead, S., Johnson, M., Maas, M., & Swanson, E. (Eds.). (2008). *Nursing outcomes classification (NOC)* (4th ed.). St. Louis, MO: Mosby.

National Cancer Institute. (2008). Lip and oral cavity cancer treatment (PDQ®). Health professional version. Retrieved from www.cancer.gov

National Cancer Institute. (2008). Oral cancer prevention (PDQ®). Health Professional version. Retrieved from www.cancer.gov

NANDA International. (2009). *Nursing diagnoses: Definitions & classification 2005–2006.* Philadelphia: Author.

Palmer, J. L., & Metheny, N. A. (2008 February). Preventing aspiration in older adults with dysphagia. *American Journal of Nursing, 108*(2), 40–48.

Porth, C. M., & Matfin, G. (2009). *Pathophysiology: Concepts of altered health states* (8th ed.). Philadelphia: Lippincott.

Ramakrishnan, K. (2007 October). Peptic ulcer disease. *American Family Physician, 76*(7), 1005–1012.

Rothrock, J. C. (2007). *Alexander's care of the patient in surgery* (13th ed.). St. Louis, MO: Mosby.

Schlansky, B., & Hwang, J. H. (2009). Prevention of nonsteroidal anti-inflammatory drug-induced gastropathy. *Journal of Gastroenterology, 44*(Suppl XIX), 44–52.

Spencer, J. W., & Jacobs, J. J. (2003). *Complementary and alternative medicine: An evidence-based approach* (2nd ed.). St. Louis, MO: Mosby.

Stovall, M. (2008 April). Diagnosing gastric carcinoma. *Clinical Journal of Oncology Nursing, 12*(2), 209–212.

Sugano, K. (2008 July). Gastric cancer: Pathogenesis, screening, and treatment. *Gastrointestinal Endoscopy Clinics of North America, 18*(3), 513–522.

Treister, N. S., & Woo, S. B. (2008). Chemotherapy-induced oral mucositis. Medscape. Retrieved from www.emdicine.medscape.com

University of Michigan Health System. (2005). Peptic ulcer disease. Ann Arbor, MI: Author. Retrieved from www.guidline.gov

Urden, L. D., Stacy, K. M., & Lough, M. E. (2006). *Thelan's critical care nursing* (5th ed). St. Louis, MO: Mosby.

Use evidence-based clinical guidelines to prevent and treat oral mucositis. *ONS News, 20*(2), 7.

Way, L. W., & Doherty, G. M. (2003). *Current surgical diagnosis & treatment* (11th ed.). New York: McGraw-Hill.

White, G., O-Rourke, F., Ong, B., Cordato, D., & Chan, D. (2008 May). Dysphagia: Causes, assessment, treatment, and management. *Geriatrics, 63*(5), 15–20.

Wilkinson, J. M., & Ahern, N. R. (2009). *Nursing diagnosis handbook* (9th ed.). Upper Saddle River, NJ: Prentice Hall Health.

Yang, Y., Lewis, J., Epstein, S., & Metz, D. (2006 December 27). Long-term proton pump inhibitor therapy and risk of hip fracture. *JAMA: Journal of the American Medical Association, 296*(24), 2947–2953.

Nursing Care of Patients with Bowel Disorders

LEARNING OUTCOMES

1. Compare and contrast the causes, pathophysiology, manifestations, interdisciplinary and nursing care of patients with disorders of bowel motility.
2. Explain the pathophysiology, manifestations, complications, interdisciplinary care, and nursing care of patients with acute or chronic inflammatory bowel disorders, neoplastic disorders, and structural and obstructive bowel disorders.
3. Discuss the purposes, nursing implications, and health education for the patient and family related to medications used to treat bowel disorders.
4. Explain the rationale for using selected diets, including those for diarrhea and constipation and low-residue, gluten-free, and high-fiber diets.
5. Describe selected surgical procedures of the bowel, including colectomy, colostomy, ileostomy, and perianal surgery.

CLINICAL COMPETENCIES

1. Assess the functional status of patients with bowel disorders, and recognize, document, and report unexpected or abnormal findings.
2. Use assessed data to determine priority nursing diagnoses, identify and implement patient-centered evidence-based nursing interventions, and revise the plan of care for patients with bowel disorders.
3. Integrate interdisciplinary care and administer medications knowledgeably and safely for patients with bowel disorders.
4. Provide skilled care to patients having bowel surgery, an ostomy, or perianal surgery.
5. Provide culturally appropriate teaching to promote nutrition, prevent acute and chronic bowel disorders, encourage screening, and facilitate community-based care related to bowel disorders.

KEY TERMS

borborygmi, 656
colectomy, 684
colostomy, 704
constipation, 657
diarrhea, 652

hematochezia, 690
ileostomy, 686
inflammatory bowel disease (IBD), 679
malabsorption, 695

paralytic ileus, 669
peritonitis, 667
steatorrhea, 655
stoma, 686

Disorders of intestinal absorption and bowel elimination can affect functional elimination status and other health patterns such as health perception-health management, nutritional-metabolic, activity-exercise, self-perception-self-concept, and sexuality-reproductive. Bowel function can be affected by inflammations, infections, tumors, obstructions, or changes in structure.

Patients with intestinal disorders often face extensive diagnostic testing, surgery, and permanent changes in physical appearance and lifestyle. Nursing care is directed toward meeting the patient's physiologic needs, providing emotional support, and educating the patient to adapt to changes in lifestyle.

Disorders of Intestinal Motility

Few body functions respond as readily to internal and external influences as the process of defecation. Factors affecting the gastrointestinal (GI) tract directly, such as food intake and bacterial population, affect the number and consistency of stools. Indirect factors, such as psychologic stress or voluntary postponement of defecation, also affect elimination.

In modern society, normal bowel elimination patterns vary widely. For some patients, two to three stools per day is the usual pattern. Others may normally have as few as three stools per week. It is important to evaluate each patient's bowel elimination against his or her own normal pattern.

The Patient with Diarrhea

Diarrhea is an increase in the frequency, volume, and fluid content of the stool. In diarrhea, the water content of feces is increased, usually due to either malabsorption or water secretion in the bowel. It is a manifestation rather than a primary disorder.

Diarrhea may be acute or chronic. Acute diarrhea, which lasts less than a week, is usually due to an infectious agent. Chronic diarrhea (diarrhea that persists longer than 3 to 4 weeks) may be caused by inflammatory bowel disorders, malabsorption, or endocrine disorders.

Pathophysiology

About 1500 mL of digested material enters the large intestine daily. Normally, most of the water and some of the solutes are reabsorbed in the bowel, leaving only about 200 mL of feces to be eliminated.

Large-volume diarrhea, characterized by both increased numbers and volume of stools, is caused by increased water content of the stool. This increased water content may result from either osmotic or secretory processes. Water may be pulled into the bowel lumen by osmosis when the feces contain osmotically active molecules. Some stool softeners and laxatives work on this principle. When the lactose in milk is not broken down and absorbed, the lactose molecules exert an osmotic pull, causing diarrhea. The diarrhea associated with cholera and *Escherichia coli* infection is caused by increased water secretion in the small and large intestines. Unabsorbed dietary fat, some cathartics and other drugs, and other factors can cause secretory diarrhea.

Small-volume diarrhea, characterized by frequent small stools, is usually caused by inflammation or disease of the colon. Diseases that affect the intestinal mucosa, such as inflammatory bowel disease, cause an exudative diarrhea. The mucosal inflammation causes plasma, serum proteins, blood, and mucus to accumulate in the bowel, increasing fecal bulk and fluidity. An increased rate of propulsion within the bowel can also decrease the amount of water normally absorbed from the chyme, leading to diarrhea. For this reason, laxatives that increase bowel motility and bowel resection or bypass can lead to diarrhea.

Antibiotic-associated diarrhea may occur as a result of disruption of normal intestinal flora by antibiotic therapy. Loss of normal flora can affect food digestion, leading to diarrhea, or can allow overgrowth of pathogens such as *Clostridium difficile* (see the section on gastroenteritis for more information about *C. difficile*). The accompanying nursing research box presents information about other possible causes of diarrhea in hospitalized patients.

Manifestations

The manifestations of diarrhea depend on its cause, duration, and severity, as well as the area of bowel affected and the patient's general health. Diarrhea can present as several large, watery stools daily, or very frequent small stools that contain blood, mucus, or exudate.

Complications

Diarrhea can have devastating effects. Water and electrolytes are lost in diarrheal stool. This can lead to dehydration, particularly in the very young, the older adult, or the debilitated patient unable to respond to thirst. With severe diarrhea, vascular collapse and hypovolemic shock may occur. Potassium and magnesium are lost, potentially leading to hypokalemia and hypomagnesemia. The loss of bicarbonate in the stool can lead to metabolic acidosis. ∞ See Chapter 10 for further discussion of the effects of these imbalances.

> **SAFETY ALERT**
> Monitor orthostatic vital signs, skin turgor, serum electrolytes and osmolality, and urinalysis to identify and respond to possible adverse effects of diarrhea.

Interdisciplinary Care

Management of diarrhea focuses on identifying and treating the underlying cause. In addition, the diarrhea itself may need to be treated to promote comfort and to prevent complications. The history (including the onset and associated circumstances of

---

MOVING EVIDENCE INTO ACTION | Diarrhea

Hospitalized patients often have a number of risk factors for diarrhea. *Clostridium difficile* is now recognized as the cause of a significant portion of treatment-related diarrhea; it does not, however, account for all cases. Previous studies have demonstrated a relationship between diarrhea and enteral tube feedings, medications containing sorbitol, lactose intolerance, and other factors. A prospective study by Thorson, Bliss, and Savik (2008) looked at the risk for developing diarrhea among patients receiving enteral tube feeding and a control group without enteral tube feeding. Findings of the study illustrate the contributory effects of severe illness and the combination of sorbitol-containing medications and enteral tube feeding.

IMPLICATIONS FOR NURSING

Severely ill patients often require enteral tube feedings for nutritional support. Healing and immune function require adequate nutrition; other studies point to the beneficial effects of enteral nutrition for the majority of patients. Discontinuing enteral feedings due to diarrhea is not a desirable option. In some cases, changing the enteral feeding formula or adding probiotic (cultures of beneficial yeasts or bacteria) supplements may help

normalize bowel function. Other options include antidiarrheal medications or soluble fiber supplements.

CRITICAL THINKING IN PATIENT CARE

1. Administering medications containing sorbitol, a sugar that is not absorbed by the gut, are associated with an increased risk of developing diarrhea among hospitalized patients. How does sorbitol increase the risk for diarrhea? What would you do if you realized that your seriously ill patient is receiving enteral tube feeding and medications containing sorbitol?

2. The position of the feeding tube tip in the gut also is identified as a risk factor for diarrhea associated with enteral tube feedings. Thinking about the functions of the stomach, pyloric valve, duodenum, and jejunum, which type of tube (gastric, duodenal, or jejunal) might carry the highest risk for diarrhea? The lowest? What other enteral tube feeding risk factors are considered in tube placement?

3. Your patient is being discharged home with a gastrostomy tube and directions for enteral feedings. What teaching will you provide to the patient and family regarding tube care, feeding administration, and bowel management?

the diarrhea) and physical examination often provide enough information to identify its cause.

Diagnosis

Diagnostic tests that may be ordered to help identify the cause of diarrhea include a stool specimen analysis and culture. A sigmoidoscopy may be conducted to directly visualize the bowel mucosa. (∞ See Chapter 21 for further information on diagnostic tests.) Tissue biopsy may be performed to identify chronic inflammatory processes, infection, and other causes of diarrhea. In addition, laboratory tests of serum electrolytes, serum osmolality, and arterial blood gases (ABGs) may be ordered to assess for adverse effects of diarrhea. Increased serum osmolality indicates water loss and dehydration.

Medications

Antidiarrheal medications are used sparingly or not at all until the cause of diarrhea has been identified. In diarrhea associated with botulism or bacillary dysentery, giving an antidiarrheal agent can worsen or prolong the disease by slowing elimination of the toxin from the bowel. Once the underlying cause for diarrhea has been established, specific medications may be ordered to treat the underlying cause. Antibiotics are used with caution because they alter the normal bacterial population of the bowel and may actually worsen diarrhea. A balanced electrolyte solution may be required to replace fluid losses. Intravenous or oral potassium preparations may be prescribed.

Opium and some of its derivatives, anticholinergics, absorbents, and demulcents are commonly used as antidiarrheal preparations. Specific preparations, their method of action, and the nursing implications for these medications are outlined in the Medication Administration box on page 655.

Nutrition

Fluid replacement is of primary importance in managing the patient with diarrhea. If the patient is able to tolerate oral fluids (i.e., if the patient is not experiencing nausea and vomiting), an oral glucose/balanced electrolyte solution provides the best fluid replacement. Commercial preparations such as Gatorade and other sports drinks are available, as are pediatric solutions (e.g., Pedialyte), which can be used for adults as well as children. A solution of 5 mL (1 teaspoon) each of table salt and baking soda and 4 teaspoons (20 mL) of granulated sugar added with desired flavoring (such as lemon extract or juice) to 1 quart (1 L) of water can be made at home to replace water and electrolytes.

Solid food is withheld in the first 24 hours of acute diarrhea to rest the bowel. After that time, frequent, small, soft feedings can be added. Milk and milk products are added last, because the lactose they contain frequently aggravates the diarrhea. Raw fruits and vegetables, fried foods, bran, whole-grain cereals, condiments, spices, coffee, and alcoholic beverages are avoided during the recovery period.

Patients with chronic diarrhea may benefit by eliminating specific foods from the diet. Foods and nonfood substances that may aggravate diarrhea are outlined in Table 24–1. The diet should be high in calories and nutritional value. Vitamin supplements may be necessary, particularly the fat-soluble vitamins (A, D, E, and K). Patients with severe chronic diarrhea may require parenteral nutrition (∞ see Chapter 21).

Complementary and Alternative Therapies

Herbal or homeopathic therapies may be used to help relieve diarrhea. Patients who are lactose intolerant (discussed later in the chapter) may use lactase enzyme tablets or drops when consuming milk products. Herbal treatments may include a strong tea of black pepper, chamomile, coriander, rosemary, sandalwood, or thyme. Ginger in the form of tea or capsules can be helpful in reducing intestinal inflammation and lessens the effects of food poisoning. Homeopathic practitioners may use podophyllum tablets to treat diarrhea. Probiotics, live microorganisms similar to those normally found in the gut, may be used to prevent or treat antibiotic-associated diarrhea (National Center for Complementary and Alternative Medicine [NCCAM], 2008; Rowland et al., 2008). Probiotics are available as dietary supplements and foods (e.g., yogurt, yogurt drinks). Refer the patient to a qualified practitioner for more information about using complementary and alternative therapies to treat diarrhea.

∞ Nursing Care

Diarrhea is a common problem that may complicate patient care.

Health Promotion

Teach all patients about the importance of hand hygiene as a measure to prevent the spread of infectious diseases, including those that cause diarrhea. Teach safe food handling techniques

---

TABLE 24–1 Foods That May Aggravate Chronic Diarrhea

FOODS	REASON
Milk, ice cream, yogurt, soft cheeses, cottage cheese	Contain lactose; not tolerated by patients with lactase deficiency who cannot digest lactose.
Apple juice, pear juice, grapes, honey, dates, nuts, figs, fruit-flavored soft drinks	Contain fructose; when consumed in large quantities, fructose may not be totally absorbed, causing an osmotic pull of fluid into the bowel.
Table sugar	Contains sucrose; not tolerated by patients with sucrase deficiency.
Apple juice, pear juice, sugarless gums, and mints	May contain sorbitol or mannitol, sugars that are not absorbed and can cause osmotic draw.
Antacids	Magnesium-containing antacids decrease bowel transit time and contain poorly absorbed salts that can exert an osmotic draw.
Coffee, tea, cola drinks, over-the-counter analgesics	Contain caffeine, which can decrease bowel transit time.

to prevent bacterial contamination, and discuss measures to ensure safe drinking water. For patients planning to travel outside the United States or to wilderness areas, teach measures to purify water for drinking and cooking.

Assessment

The nursing assessment can help identify the cause of the patient's diarrhea, as well as early signs of complications. Collect the following assessment data:

- *Health history:* Duration and extent of diarrhea; associated manifestations; dietary intake; recent travel out of the country or to wilderness areas; previous history of diarrhea; chronic diseases; prescription and nonprescription medications.
- *Physical examination:* Vital signs (including orthostatic blood pressure); peripheral pulses; skin temperature, moisture, turgor; color and moisture of mucous membranes;

abdominal contour and girth; bowel sounds; stool for obvious or occult blood, pus, mucus, or **steatorrhea** (bulky, foul-smelling stool).

Nursing Diagnoses and Interventions

Nursing care of the patient with diarrhea focuses on identifying the cause, relieving the manifestations, preventing complications, and preventing the potential spread of infection to others.

Diarrhea

Nursing interventions for diarrhea are provided to help the patient recover a normal elimination pattern without adverse consequences.

- Monitor and record the frequency and characteristics of bowel movements *to provide a measure of the effectiveness of treatment.*

MEDICATION ADMINISTRATION | Antidiarrheal Preparations

ABSORBENTS AND PROTECTANTS

Kaolin and pectin (Kaopectate, Donnagel-MB)

Polycarbophil (FigerNorm, Equalactin)

Absorbent preparations act locally in the intestines to bind substances that can cause diarrhea. Absorbents are safe and are generally available over the counter, although their efficacy has not been proved.

Nursing Responsibilities

- Assess for contraindications to antidiarrheal therapy, such as some infections or chronic inflammatory bowel disease, including ulcerative colitis.
- If fever is present, check with physician before giving the medication.
- Administer these medications at least 1 hour before or 2 hours after other oral medications; they may interfere with the absorption of other drugs.
- Observe the patient's response to the medication. Constipation is a potential problem.

Health Education for the Patient and Family

- Take the recommended dosage at the onset of diarrhea and after each loose stool.
- Do not take any of these preparations for more than 48 hours. If diarrhea persists, notify the physician.
- Do not give antidiarrheal medications to debilitated older patients without physician supervision.

ANTISECRETORY

Bismuth subsalicylate (Pepto-Bismol)

Bismuth subsalicylate, available without a prescription, has antisecretory, anti-inflammatory, and antibacterial effects. It is widely used to control traveler's diarrhea. Although it is generally safe at recommended doses, bismuth subsalicylate has potential toxic effects and interacts with drugs such as aspirin and oral anticoagulants.

Nursing Responsibilities

- Administer as ordered.
- Do not administer within 1 hour of other drugs, as it may interfere with their absorption.
- Monitor for increased anticoagulant effect when given with Coumadin or aspirin.

Health Education for the Patient and Family

- Chew bismuth subsalicylate tablets, rather than swallowing them whole, for maximal effectiveness.

- This drug may cause harmless darkening of your tongue and stools.
- If you are allergic to aspirin, use bismuth subsalicylate with caution. Do not use aspirin while you are taking this drug unless directed to do so by your physician. Contact your physician if diarrhea persists for more than 2 days.

OPIUM AND OPIUM DERIVATIVES

Camphorated tincture of opium (Paregoric)

Tincture of opium (laudanum, opium tincture)

Difenoxin (Motofen)

Diphenoxylate (Lomotil, Lotrol, others)

Loperamide hydrochloride (Imodium)

Opium and its derivatives act on the central nervous system (CNS) to decrease the motility of the ileum and colon, slowing transit time and promoting more water absorption. They also decrease the sensation of a full rectum and increase anal sphincter tone. Paregoric and tincture of opium have a greater potential for abuse and are prescription drugs subject to controls under the federal Controlled Substance Act of 1970. Difenoxin, diphenoxylate, and loperamide are derivatives of opium with few analgesic, euphoric, or abuse-promoting effects and are in more common use today.

Nursing Responsibilities

- Assess for contraindications to antidiarrheal or narcotic medications prior to giving these drugs.
- Administer paregoric undiluted with water.
- Do not administer difenoxin and diphenoxylate to patients receiving monoamine oxidase inhibitors (MAOIs); hypertensive crises may occur.
- Observe closely for increased effects of other CNS depressants, such as alcohol, narcotic analgesics, or barbiturate sedatives.
- Observe for abdominal distention; toxic megacolon may occur if these drugs are given to the patient with ulcerative colitis.

Health Education for the Patient and Family

- Take the medication as recommended at the onset of diarrhea and after each loose stool.
- These drugs may be habit forming; use for no more than 48 hours.
- Avoid using alcohol and over-the-counter cold preparations while taking these drugs.
- These preparations may cause drowsiness; avoid driving or operating machinery while taking them.

- Measure abdominal girth and auscultate bowel sounds every 8 hours as indicated. Loud, rushing bowel sounds (**borborygmi**) indicate increased peristalsis, and may be heard in patients with acute diarrhea. *Diminished or absent bowel sounds may indicate a complication of treatment, such as constipation or toxic megacolon.*
- Use standard precautions, including gloves and hand hygiene. *Standard precautions help prevent the spread of infection to others.*
- Provide ready access to bathroom, commode, or bedpan. *The patient may have little warning of the need to defecate. Easily accessed toileting facilities reduce the risk for soiling or injury.*
- Administer antidiarrheal medications as prescribed *to promote comfort and prevent excess fluid loss.*
- Limit food intake if the diarrhea is acute, reintroducing solid foods slowly, in small amounts, *to allow the bowel to rest and mucosa to heal in acute diarrhea states.*

Risk for Deficient Fluid Volume

The increased water content of diarrheal stool places the patient at risk for fluid deficit.

- Record intake and output; weigh daily; assess skin turgor, mucous membranes, and urine specific gravity every 8 hours. *These assessments are used to monitor fluid volume.*

> **PRACTICE ALERT**
> Assess skin turgor over the sternum in the older adult. Loss of subcutaneous fat associated with aging makes skin turgor assessment on the arms or hands less reliable.

- Monitor vital signs, including orthostatic blood pressures. *Orthostatic hypotension is identified by a drop in BP of more than 10 mmHg and pulse increase of 10 beats per minute (bpm) when changing from a lying to a sitting position or from a sitting to a standing position. It is an indicator of fluid volume deficit.*

> **SAFETY ALERT**
> Institute safety precautions such as providing assistance when ambulating the patient with orthostatic hypotension. The fall in blood pressure with position changes can cause light-headedness and syncope.

- Provide fluid and electrolyte replacement solutions as indicated. Ensure ready access to fluids; assist the debilitated patient with fluid intake. Notify the care provider if the patient is unable to tolerate oral fluids. *Oral fluids are encouraged as tolerated to prevent dehydration. Intravenous fluids are necessary if oral fluids are not tolerated. An intake of 3000 mL/day or more is often needed to replace fluid losses.*

Risk for Impaired Skin Integrity

Decreased extracellular fluid volume and the irritating effects of diarrheal stool increase the risk for skin breakdown.

- Assist with cleaning the perianal area as needed. Use warm water, a gentle cleanser, and soft cloths. *Cleansing removes*

irritating substances in the stool. Gentle cleansing helps maintain integrity of dehydrated skin.

- Apply protective ointment to the perianal area. *Moisture-barrier ointments or creams protect the skin from excoriation and help prevent tissue breakdown.*

Using NANDA, NIC, and NOC

Linkages between a selected NANDA nursing diagnosis, NIC, and NOC for the patient with diarrhea are shown in the chart that follows.

Community-Based Care

Acute and chronic diarrhea generally are managed by the patient in the home. Teach the patient and family members about the following subjects:

- Causes of diarrhea (as directed by the diagnosis)
- Importance of hand washing and other hygiene measures
- Importance of maintaining adequate fluid intake to replace lost water and electrolytes
- Use of a balanced electrolyte solution such as Gatorade or a similar product (purchased or home prepared) for fluid replacement
- Recommendations to limit food intake during acute diarrhea, and resume gradually with small feedings of foods that have a constipating effect: applesauce, bananas, crackers, rice, potatoes
- To avoid foods high in fiber, milk products, and caffeine
- Ways to maintain nutrition if chronic diarrhea is a problem: frequent small meals, nutritional supplements, vitamin supplements
- Precautions and limitations of antidiarrheal preparations
- Importance of seeking medical intervention if diarrhea continues or recurs

NANDA, NIC, AND NOC LINKAGES
The Patient with Altered Bowel Motility

NANDA — Diarrhea

NIC
Diarrhea Management
Electrolyte Monitoring
Fluid/Electrolyte Management
Medication Management
Perineal Care

NOC
Bowel Continence
Electrolyte & Acid–Base Balance
Fluid Balance
Medication Response
Symptom Severity

Data from NANDA International. (2009). *Nursing diagnoses: Definitions & classification 2009–2011.* Oxford, UK: Wiley-Blackwell; Bulechek, G., Butcher, H., & Dochterman, J. (Eds.). (2008). *Nursing interventions classification (NIC)* (5th ed.). St. Louis, MO: Mosby; and Moorhead, S., Johnson, M., Maas, M., & Swanson, E. (Eds.). (2008). *Nursing outcomes classification (NOC)* (4th ed.). St. Louis, MO: Mosby.

The Patient with Constipation

Constipation is defined as the infrequent (two or fewer bowel movements weekly) or difficult passage of stools. Constipation affects older adults more frequently than younger people. Recent studies indicate that approximately 20% to 35% of people over age 65 report recurrent constipation and laxative use. Although fecal transit in the large intestine slows with aging, the increased incidence of constipation is thought to relate more to impaired general health status, increased medication use, and decreased physical activity in the older adult.

Pathophysiology

Constipation may be a primary problem or a manifestation of another disease or condition. Acute constipation, a definite change in the bowel elimination pattern, often is caused by an organic process. A change in bowel patterns that persists or becomes more frequent or severe may be due to a tumor or other partial bowel obstruction. With chronic constipation, functional causes that impair storage, transport, and evacuation mechanisms impede the normal passage of stools. Common causes of constipation are listed in Table 24–2.

Psychogenic factors are the most frequent causes of chronic constipation. These factors include postponing defecation when the urge is felt, and the perception of satisfaction with defecation. Patients often use laxatives and enemas to stimulate a bowel movement when constipation is perceived. Overuse of these measures can lead to real intestinal problems that worsen the condition. For example, *cathartic colon* (impaired colonic motility and changes in bowel structure) mimics ulcerative colitis in that the normal pouchlike or saccular appearance of the colon is lost. *Melanosis coli* is a brownish-black discoloration of the colon mucosa. Both conditions may be caused by long-term laxative use.

TABLE 24–2 Selected Causes of Constipation

FACTOR	RELATED CAUSE
Activity	Lack of exercise: bed rest
Dietary	Highly refined, low-fiber foods; inadequate fluid intake
Drugs	Antacids containing aluminum or calcium salts; narcotic analgesics; anticholinergics; many antidepressants, tranquilizers, and sedatives; antihypertensives, such as ganglionic blockers, calcium-channel blockers, beta-adrenergic blockers, and diuretics; iron salts
Large bowel	Diverticular disease, inflammatory disease, tumor, obstruction; changes in rectal or anal structure or function
Psychogenic	Voluntary suppression of urge; perceived need to defecate on schedule; depression
Systemic	Advanced age; pregnancy; neurologic conditions (trauma, multiple sclerosis, tumors, cerebrovascular accident, parkinsonism); endocrine and metabolic disorders (hypothyroidism, hypercalcemia, uremia, porphyria)
Other	Chronic laxative or enema use

Manifestations and Complications

The manifestations of constipation include having bowel movements less often than the usual pattern, frequent flatus, abdominal discomfort, anorexia, straining to have a bowel movement, and the passage of hard, dry stools.

With significant constipation or long-term dependence on laxatives or enemas, fecal impaction may develop. Impaction may also occur following barium administration for radiologic exam. The impaction is felt as a rock-hard or putty-like mass of feces in the rectum. Abdominal cramping and a full sensation in the rectal area may be manifestations of impaction. Watery mucus or foul-smelling liquid stool may be passed around the impaction, causing the patient to complain of diarrhea.

Interdisciplinary Care

Initial evaluation of constipation is based on the history and physical examination. The abdomen may appear somewhat distended, and bowel sounds may be reduced. If an impaction is present, digital examination of the rectum reveals a palpable, hard or putty-like fecal mass.

Simple or chronic constipation is treated with education (a daily bowel movement is not necessary for health), and modification of diet and exercise routines. If the problem is acute or does not resolve, further diagnostic examination may be ordered.

Diagnosis

A barium enema may be ordered to identify bowel structure, tumors, or diverticula. If the problem is acute, a sigmoidoscopy or colonoscopy may be used for evaluation and biopsy. (∞ See Chapter 21 for nursing implications of these tests.)

Medications

Laxative and cathartic preparations are used to promote stool evacuation. Milder preparations are generally known as laxatives; cathartics have a stronger effect. Most laxatives are appropriate only for short-term use. Cathartics and enemas interfere with normal bowel reflexes and should not be used for simple constipation. Laxatives should not be given if a patient has an undiagnosed intestinal obstruction, abdominal pain, fecal impaction, rectal fissures, ulcerated hemorrhoids, Crohn's disease, ulcerative colitis, or chronic inflammatory bowel disease. When the bowel is obstructed, laxatives or cathartics may cause serious mechanical damage and perforate the bowel.

The only laxatives that are appropriate and safe for long-term use are bulking agents, such as psyllium seed, calcium polycarbophil, and methylcellulose. These agents act by increasing the bulk of the feces and drawing water into the bowel to soften it. Commonly prescribed laxatives and cathartics are discussed in the following Medication Administration box.

Nutrition

Foods that have a high fiber content are recommended. Vegetable fiber is largely indigestible and unabsorbable, so it increases stool bulk. Fiber also helps draw water into the fecal mass, softening the stool and making defecation easier. Raw fruits and vegetables are good sources of dietary fiber, as is cereal bran. Use 2 to 3 teaspoons of unprocessed bran with meals (sprinkled on fruit or cereal) or up to 1/4 cup daily to supply adequate fiber.

BULK-FORMING AGENTS

Calcium polycarbophil (Fibercon, others)

Methylcellulose (Citrucel)

Psyllium (Metamucil, others)

Bulk-forming agents contain vegetable fiber, which is not digested or absorbed in the gut. This natural fiber creates bulk and draws water into the intestine, softening the stool mass.

Nursing Responsibilities

■ Mix the agent with a full glass of cool liquid just prior to administering.

■ Do not administer to patients with possible stool impaction or bowel obstruction.

Health Education for the Patient and Family

■ Drink at least 6 to 8 full glasses of nonalcoholic fluid per day. Adequate hydration is necessary to produce the drug's laxative effect.

■ These agents may be mixed with water, milk, or fruit juice.

■ Take the drug in the morning or with meals. To reduce the risk of impaction, do not take at bedtime.

■ Because of the increased risk of impaction, check with the physician before increasing dietary fiber while you are taking these agents.

WETTING AGENTS

Docusate (Colace, Surfak, Doxidan, others)

Wetting agents reduce stool surface tension and form an emulsion of fat and water, softening the stool. They are used primarily to prevent straining and reduce the discomfort of expelling hard stools.

Nursing Responsibilities

■ Administer with ample fluids to promote softening effect.

■ Wetting agents may alter the absorption of other drugs. Do not administer within 1 hour of other oral medications.

■ Do not attempt to crush or open caplets; a liquid form is available for patients who cannot swallow pills or capsules.

Health Education for the Patient and Family

■ Do not use for more than 1 week unless specifically recommended by the physician.

■ Take the medication in the morning or evening, but avoid taking it with other medications.

■ Adequate fluid is necessary to obtain the beneficial effect of the drug. Drink 6 to 8 glasses of nonalcoholic fluid per day.

OSMOTIC AND SALINE LAXATIVES/CATHARTICS

Lactulose (Rhodialose)

Sorbitol

Magnesium hydroxide (Milk of Magnesia)

Polyethylene glycol (Klean-Prep)

Laxatives in this group contain poorly absorbed salts or carbohydrates that remain in the bowel, increasing osmotic pressure and drawing water into the intestine. Stool volume increases, consistency decreases, and peristalsis is stimulated. Many of these agents also have an irritant effect on the bowel, further stimulating peristalsis. They are used to stimulate rapid or complete bowel evacuation to relieve constipation and to prepare the bowel for diagnostic and surgical procedures. They should be limited to acute, short-term use; chronic use may suppress normal bowel reflexes.

Nursing Responsibilities

■ Assess for possible contraindications to osmotic or saline laxatives, including bowel ulceration or obstruction, dehydration, electrolyte imbalances, heart failure (which may be aggravated by the sodium content), or renal failure.

■ Administer with a full glass of liquid, preferably in the morning to avoid sleep disturbance.

■ Monitor fluid and electrolyte status: skin turgor, mucous membranes, intake and output; daily weight; and laboratory studies, such as hemoglobin and hematocrit levels, serum osmolality and electrolytes, and urine specific gravity.

Health Education for the Patient and Family

■ Do not use these agents on a routine basis to treat or prevent constipation.

■ Chill the solution to increase its palatability.

■ Expect some abdominal cramping.

■ Use only as directed. Increase fluid intake to at least 6 to 8 glasses of nonalcoholic fluid.

■ Notify the physician if adverse effects occur, including abdominal pain, bloody stool, excessive skin or mucous membrane dryness, rapid weight loss, dizziness, or other unusual symptoms.

■ These agents work in 3 to 6 hours; take them in the morning or early evening to avoid sleep disturbance.

IRRITANT OR STIMULANT LAXATIVES

Bisacodyl (Dulcolax, Bisco-Lax, Carter's Liver Pills, Codylax, others)

Phenolphthalein (Evac-U-Gen, Evac-U-Lax, Feen-A-Mint, Phenolax, others)

Senna (Senna laxative, Fletcher's Castoria)

Castor oil

Stimulant laxatives work by stimulating the motility and secretion of intestinal mucosa. Their use results in watery stool, often accompanied by abdominal cramping and pain. They are used to relieve constipation, although they should not be used as the initial treatment. Stimulant laxatives are also used for preparing the bowel for diagnostic testing.

Nursing Responsibilities

■ Assess for potential contraindications to these laxatives, including abdominal pain and cramping, nausea and vomiting, and anal or rectal fissures.

■ Administer on an empty stomach to minimize the effects of food on its dissolution and absorption.

■ Do not crush enteric-coated bisacodyl tablets or administer with alkaline products. This may hasten their dissolution in the stomach, leading to gastric distress.

Health Education for the Patient and Family

■ Discourage the use of this type of laxative, even in over-the-counter preparations, for the initial or continuing relief of constipation.

■ Do not use the laxative for more than 1 week; chronic use can be habit forming and may suppress normal bowel reflexes.

■ These laxatives are excreted in breast milk and should not be used by lactating women.

■ Phenolphthalein-containing products may discolor the urine pink or red. Report possible hypersensitivity manifestations, such as difficulty breathing, dizziness or light-headedness, or skin rashes, to the primary care provider, and stop taking the medication.

LUBRICANTS

Mineral oil

Mineral oil acts by forming an oily coat on the fecal mass, preventing the reabsorption of water, and resulting in softer stool. Problems associated with the use of mineral oil as a laxative include reduced absorption of the fat-soluble vitamins A, D, E, and K; possible damage to the liver and spleen due to systemic absorption; and potential pneumonitis from aspiration of oil droplets into the lungs.

Nursing Responsibilities
- Assess for possible contraindications to use of mineral oil, including advanced age, preexisting lung disease, and hemorrhoids or other rectal lesions.
- Do not give mineral oil concurrently with wetting agents or stool softeners, because these increase the potential for systemic absorption and increase the effects of the mineral oil.
- Administer mineral oil in the evening before bedtime to reduce the effect on the absorption of fat-soluble vitamins and minimize the risk of aspiration.

- Assess for manifestations of vitamin deficiency. Monitor the patient taking oral anticoagulants for evidence of increased bleeding, such as bleeding gums, easy bruising, or melena.

Health Education for the Patient and Family
- Long-term use of mineral oil is not recommended because of its risks and adverse effects.
- Do not use mineral oil if hemorrhoids or rectal lesions are present; leakage of the oil through the anal sphincter may cause itching and interfere with healing.
- Suck on a lemon or orange slice after taking oral mineral oil to reduce the oily aftertaste.

Fluids are also important to maintain bowel motility and soft stools. The patient should drink 6 to 8 glasses of fluid per day. It is important to advise the patient to increase fluid intake when dietary fiber is initially increased to decrease flatus and help maintain softer stools.

In older adults, constipation may be due to inadequate food intake. Carefully evaluate diet history and usual daily intake.

Enemas

Significant or chronic constipation or a fecal impaction may require the administration of an enema. As a general rule, enemas are used only in acute situations and only on a short-term basis. They may also be ordered to prepare the bowel for diagnostic testing or examination. The following types of enemas may be prescribed:

- A *saline enema* using 500 to 2000 mL of warmed physiologic saline solution is the least irritating to the bowel.
- *Tap-water enemas* use 500 to 1000 mL of water to soften feces and irritate the bowel mucosa, stimulating peristalsis and evacuation.
- *Soap-suds enemas* consist of a tap-water solution to which soap is added as a further irritant.
- *Phosphate enemas* (e.g., Fleet) use a hypertonic saline solution to draw fluid into the bowel and irritate the mucosa, leading to evacuation.
- *Oil retention enemas* instill mineral or vegetable oil into the bowel to soften the fecal mass. The instilled oil is retained overnight or for several hours before evacuation.

The repeated use of enemas can lead not only to impaired bowel function, but also to fluid and electrolyte imbalances. Tap-water and phosphate enemas are particularly likely to cause these problems. In acute conditions with risk of bowel obstruction, perforation, ulceration, or other problem, enemas should not be administered until their safe use can be established.

Complementary and Alternative Therapies

Herbal or homeopathic therapies may be used to help relieve constipation. Flaxseed oil lubricates the colon for easier passage of stool. Patients are instructed to take 1 to 2 tablespoons daily. Flax seeds are a lesser known but a highly concentrated source of fiber, and 1 to 2 tablespoons of ground flaxseeds can be sprinkled on cereals or salads daily, followed by 10 ounces of water.

Acupressure, massage, reflexology, aromatherapy, and stress management therapies can also be very beneficial in relieving constipation (Balch & Stengler, 2004). Other recommendations include exercise to stimulate intestinal contractions.

Nursing Care

Health Promotion

Education can prevent constipation. Teach patients the importance of maintaining a diet high in natural fiber. Foods such as fresh fruits, vegetables, whole-grain products, and bran provide natural fiber. Encourage reducing consumption of meats and refined foods, which are low in fiber and can be constipating. Emphasize the need to maintain a high fluid intake every day, particularly during hot weather and exercise. Discuss the relationship between exercise and bowel regularity. Encourage patients to engage in some form of exercise, such as walking daily.

Discuss normal bowel habits, and explain that a daily bowel movement is not the norm for all people. Encourage patients to respond to the urge to defecate when it occurs. Suggest setting aside a time, usually following a meal, for elimination.

Assessment

To assess the patient with real or perceived constipation, collect the following data:

- *Health history:* Usual and current pattern of defecation, including time of day, amount, and stool consistency; usual diet, fluid intake, and activity pattern; possible contributing factors such as opioid analgesics, activity limitations, painful hemorrhoids, perianal surgery; chronic diseases such as endocrine or neurologic disorders; prescribed and nonprescription medications.
- *Physical examination:* Abdominal girth and shape, bowel sounds, tenderness, and percussion tone; digital exam of the rectum if impaction is suspected.

For discussion of constipation in the older adult see Meeting Individualized Needs on page 660.

Nursing Diagnoses and Interventions

Nursing interventions for the patient with constipation focus chiefly on education.

MEETING INDIVIDUALIZED NEEDS — Constipation and the Older Adult

Constipation and perceived constipation are common problems in older adults. Although constipation is not a normal consequence of aging, factors such as slowed peristalsis, lowered activity levels, reduced food and fluid intake, and decreased sensory perception contribute to the higher incidence of constipation seen in the elderly. Chronic diseases such as diabetes, mobility problems, and medications also increase the risk of constipation in older adults.

Cultural influences and advertising lead many older adults to believe that a daily bowel movement is important for health. This belief contributes to an increased incidence of perceived constipation in the elderly. Because of this perception, the older adult may come to rely on laxatives, suppositories, or enemas to facilitate regular bowel movements. These external aids to defecation can further impair the ability to maintain "normal" bowel habits: a movement of soft stool every 2 to 3 days.

Constipation

Whether real or perceived, constipation is disruptive to the patient's activities of daily living (ADLs) and life satisfaction.

- Monitor pattern of defecation and stool consistency. *This information helps establish the patient's usual pattern of defecation and differentiate between actual and perceived constipation.*
- Provide additional fluids to maintain an intake of at least 2500 mL per day. *A generous fluid intake helps maintain soft stool consistency and promote intestinal motility.*
- Encourage drinking a glass of warm water before breakfast. Provide time and privacy following breakfast for bowel elimination. *This helps develop a pattern of natural elimination; the warm water provides mild stimulation of bowel peristalsis.*
- Consult with the dietitian to provide a diet high in natural fiber unless contraindicated. Provide foods such as natural bran, prunes, or prune juice. *Natural fiber adds bulk to the stool and has a mild stimulant effect.*
- Encourage activities such as ambulation or chair exercises (e.g., range of motion, stretching, wheelchair lifts) as tolerated. *Activity stimulates peristalsis and strengthens abdominal muscles, facilitating elimination.*
- If indicated, consult with primary care provider about the use of bulk laxatives, stool softeners, or other laxatives as needed. *Laxatives may be necessary to relieve acute constipation. Patients with long-term activity or diet restrictions or impaired abdominal muscle strength may need a bulk-forming laxative to maintain normal elimination patterns and prevent constipation.*

Community-Based Care

Include the following topics when teaching self-care measures to prevent and treat constipation:

- Increasing dietary fiber intake by including fresh fruits and vegetables, whole grains, high-fiber breakfast cereals, and unprocessed bran in the diet (Bran can be sprinkled on cereals, mixed into bread or muffin recipes, or mixed with fruit juice to increase its palatability.)
- Maintaining fluid intake of 6 to 8 glasses of water per day (unless contraindicated)
- Suggestions for remaining physically active to promote bowel function and maintain muscle tone
- Responding to the urge to defecate when perceived
- Appropriate use of laxatives:
  - Do not use laxatives, suppositories, or enemas on a regular basis.

- Bulk-forming agents provide insoluble fiber, and are safe for long-term use; it is important to drink at least 6 to 8 glasses of water daily when using these (or any) laxatives.
- Other laxatives such as milk of magnesia, docusate (Colace, DSS), bisacodyl (Dulcolax), cascara, or castor oil should be used only occasionally to relieve constipation.
- Reporting any change in bowel habits such as new or persistent constipation or diarrhea, abdominal pain, black or bloody stools, nausea or anorexia, weakness, or unexplained weight loss to the primary care provider

The Patient with Irritable Bowel Syndrome

Irritable bowel syndrome (IBS), also known as spastic bowel or mucous colitis, is a motility disorder of the lower GI tract. It is a chronic disorder with no identifiable organic cause. IBS is characterized by abdominal pain and bloating with constipation, diarrhea, or both.

Irritable bowel syndrome is common, affecting up to 20% of people in Western civilization. It usually affects young people, with about 50% of patients diagnosed before age 35. There is a higher prevalence of IBS in women than in men (American College of Physicians [ACP], 2007).

Pathophysiology

In IBS, it appears that CNS regulation of the motor and sensory functions of the bowel is altered. Patients with IBS often experience increased motor reactivity of the small bowel and colon in response to stimuli such as food intake, hormonal influences, and physiologic or psychologic stress. IBS is characterized by visceral hypersensitivity and hyperactivity of the GI tract. Hypersecretion of colonic mucus is a common feature of the syndrome.

IBS may develop as a sequela of gastroenteritis, particularly when the infection is caused by *Campylobacter*, *Salmonella*, or *Shigella*.

A lower visceral pain threshold is often found in patients with IBS. Patients may complain of pain, bloating, and distention when intestinal gas levels are normal. Serotonin, a neurotransmitter involved in regulating GI motility, and visceral perception may play a role in IBS. Higher than expected postprandial plasma serotonin levels are noted in some patients with IBS (Fauci et al., 2008).

Psychologic factors such as depression or anxiety have been linked to IBS; however, they have not been identified as causes of the disorder. Recent research does indicate a correlation between emotional, physical, and sexual abuse and IBS.

Manifestations

IBS is characterized by abdominal pain that often is relieved by defecation and a change in bowel habits (see the accompanying Manifestations box). The pain may be either colicky, occurring in spasms, or dull and continuous. Altered patterns of defecation may include the following:

- A change in frequency
- Abnormal stool form (hard or lumpy, loose or watery)
- Altered stool passage (straining, urgency, or a sensation of incomplete evacuation)
- Passage of mucus

The patient may also complain of abdominal bloating and excess gas. Other manifestations include nausea, vomiting, anorexia, fatigue, headache, depression, or anxiety. The abdomen is often tender to palpation, particularly over the sigmoid colon.

Interdisciplinary Care

Irritable bowel syndrome is diagnosed based on the presence of abdominal pain or discomfort at least 3 days per month in the past 3 months that has at least two of the following characteristics: (1) improved with defecation; (2) associated with a change in frequency of elimination; (3) associated with a change in stool form (Fauci et al., 2008). Management is directed toward relieving manifestations and reducing or eliminating precipitating factors. Many patients benefit from cognitive behavioral therapy or psychotherapy (Moynihan, Callahan, Kalsmith, & Moses, 2008).

Diagnosis

The primary purpose of diagnostic testing is to rule out other causes of abdominal pain and altered fecal elimination. The stools may be examined for occult blood, ova and parasites, and white blood cells (WBCs). A sigmoidoscopy, colonoscopy, and/or a small-bowel series (upper GI series with small-bowel follow-through) and barium enema may be performed to visually examine the bowel mucosa, measure intraluminal pressures, and biopsy suspicious lesions. Nursing care for these procedures is outlined in ∞ Chapter 21. Laboratory tests include a complete blood count (CBC) with differential and erythrocyte sedimentation rate to evaluate for anemia from bleeding or a possible tumor. Increased WBCs indicate a bacterial infection.

MANIFESTATIONS of Irritable Bowel Syndrome

- Abdominal pain
  - May be relieved by defecation
  - May be intermittent and colicky or dull and continuous
- Altered bowel elimination
  - Constipation
  - Diarrhea
  - Mucous stools
- Abdominal bloating and flatulence
- Abdominal tenderness, especially over sigmoid colon
- Possible nausea, vomiting

Medications

Although not curative, medications may be prescribed to manage the manifestations of IBS. Bulk-forming laxatives (such as bran, methylcellulose, or psyllium) may help reduce bowel spasm and normalize the number and form of bowel movements. An anticholinergic drug such as dicyclomine (Antispas, Bentyl) or hyoscyamine (Anaspaz) may be ordered to inhibit bowel motility by interfering with parasympathetic stimulation of the gastrointestinal tract. It relieves postprandial abdominal pain when given 30 to 60 minutes before meals. Because of side effects such as dry mouth, blurred vision, and urinary hesitancy, these drugs are used with caution in older adults. In patients with diarrhea, loperamide (Imodium) or diphenoxylate (Lomotil) may be used prophylactically to prevent diarrhea in selected situations.

Antidepressant drugs, including tricyclics and selective serotonin reuptake inhibitors (SSRIs), may help relieve abdominal pain associated with IBS. Although the anticholinergic side effects of the tricyclics (such as desipramine [Norpramin] and imipramine [Tofranil]) may help decrease diarrhea, they have more adverse effects than SSRIs such as sertraline (Zoloft) and fluoxetine (Prozac). Alosetron (Lotronex) is a serotonin receptor antagonist that reduces abdominal pain and diarrhea in patients with IBS. Its use is limited, however, by its association with ischemic colitis.

Nutrition

Many patients with IBS benefit from additional dietary fiber. Adding bran to meals provides added bulk and water content to the stool, reducing the incidence of both loose diarrheal stools and hard, constipated stools. Other dietary changes are specific to individual triggers for IBS manifestations. Some patients may benefit from limiting lactose, fructose, or sorbitol intake (see Table 24–1). When excess gas and flatulence are problems, reducing the intake of gas-forming foods, such as beans, cabbage, apple and grape juices, nuts, and raisins, may be helpful. Caffeinated drinks, such as coffee, tea, and soft drinks, act as gastrointestinal stimulants; limiting intake of these fluids may prove beneficial.

Complementary and Alternative Therapies

Herbal preparations may provide some benefit for patients with IBS. Herbs with an antispasmodic effect, such as anise, chamomile, peppermint, and sage, may be used to reduce the manifestations of IBS. Ginger root can be consumed as a tea or capsule to assist with reduction of gas, bloating, and diarrhea and to improve the functioning of the stomach. Probiotic therapies (such as yogurt with active bacterial cultures) have been shown to benefit patients with IBS, as has hypnosis (Moynihan et al., 2008).

Nursing Care

Patients with IBS rarely require acute care for it as a primary problem. However, nurses frequently interact with these patients in clinics and other community settings.

Assessment

Careful assessment is important to help identify the effects of IBS on the patient. Collect the following assessment data:

- *Health history:* Current manifestations, their onset and duration; current treatment measures; effect of manifestations on

MOVING EVIDENCE INTO ACTION | **Irritable Bowel Syndrome**

Irritable bowel syndrome is a functional disorder; while the patient's symptoms are real, physical findings often are absent or limited. Consensus groups of physicians practicing in western Europe developed and revised diagnostic criteria for IBS. These criteria include recurrent abdominal pain or discomfort that improves with defecation, a change in the frequency of defecation, and/or a change in the appearance of the stool. Barakzai, Gregory, and Fraser (2007) noted that the prevalence of IBS is lower in Mexican Americans, and wondered if this reflects a cultural bias in the criteria. Using a retrospective study of the medical records of 139 Mexican Americans diagnosed with IBS, they found significant variation in how these patients described their symptoms. While diarrhea, constipation, and abdominal pain frequently were reported, patients also presented with complaints such as dizziness, myalgias, headache, and more vague complaints such as cold bones and cold stomach. Symptoms related by more than half of the patients studied did not meet the current criteria for diagnosing IBS.

IMPLICATIONS FOR NURSING

Culture influences what people perceive, how they interpret it, and what they choose to report as symptoms. As nurses, it is important to remember that culture not only affects what the

patient reports, but also how we hear and interpret what is said. To develop an accurate diagnostic picture, it is important to obtain a complete history, maintain a nonjudgmental attitude about how symptoms are reported, and use a skilled interpreter.

CRITICAL THINKING IN PATIENT CARE

1. In this study, researchers found presenting complaints such as "nervousness" that initially may appear to be vague or unrelated to the ultimate diagnosis. What follow-up questions could you ask when the patient describes such symptoms as "nervousness," or "cold stomach"?
2. When you are talking with your non-native English-speaking patient, she describes a symptom in her native tongue. When you ask her to translate what she said to English, she tells you there is no corresponding English word for what she is describing. How will you proceed?
3. As you are talking with your patient with IBS symptoms, she says, "I might as well just go home and learn to live with this, because nobody seems to believe me, and all of the tests come back normal. I guess I'm just crazy." How will you respond?

lifestyle; careful exploration of history of emotional, physical, or sexual abuse. The accompanying nursing research box illustrates the importance of culture in how the patient may relate his or her symptoms.

- *Physical examination:* Apparent general state of health; abdominal shape and contour, bowel sounds, tenderness.

Nursing Diagnoses and Intervention

The primary nursing responsibility to patients with IBS is education; providing referrals and counseling are additional nursing responsibilities. See the previous sections on diarrhea and constipation for selected nursing interventions.

Community-Based Care

Include the following topics in teaching for the patient with IBS:

- The nature of the disorder and the reality of the patient's manifestations

EVIDENCE FOR NURSING CARE | **The Patient with Irritable Bowel Syndrome**

Selected resources that nurses may find helpful when planning evidence-based nursing care follow.

- National Collaborating Centre for Nursing and Supportive Care. (2008, February). *Irritable bowel syndrome in adults. Diagnosis and management of irritable bowel syndrome in primary care.* London, UK: National Institute for Health and Clinical Excellence (NICE). Retrieved from http://www.guideline.gov/summary/summary.aspx?doc_id=13703
- Dalrymple, J., & Bullock, I. (2008 March). Diagnosis and management of irritable bowel syndrome in adults in primary care: Summary of NICE guidance. *BMJ: British Medical Journal, 336*(7643), 556–558.

- Stress and anxiety reduction techniques, such as meditation, visualization, exercise, "time-out," and progressive relaxation
- Dietary influences that may contribute to IBS and suggested dietary changes, such as additional fiber and water intake
- The use and role of prescribed medications, their adverse effects, and when to contact the physician
- The importance of routine follow-up appointments and of notifying the primary care provider if manifestations change (such as blood in the stool, significant constipation or diarrhea, increasing abdominal pain, or weight loss)

If needed, refer the patient to a counselor or other mental health professional for assistance in dealing with psychologic factors.

The Patient with Fecal Incontinence

Fecal incontinence, the loss of voluntary control of defecation, occurs less frequently than urinary incontinence but is no less distressing to the patient. Multiple factors may contribute to fecal incontinence (Box 24–1). Bowel incontinence is usually considered a symptom, not a disease or disorder. Patients often do not reveal fecal incontinence in discussing health concerns. Little information is available about its incidence and prevalence. Because many of the etiologic factors are more prevalent in the older adult, older patients are more often affected.

Pathophysiology

To understand the pathophysiology of fecal incontinence, it is necessary to understand the normal mechanisms of defecation. The rectum is normally empty. When it is distended by feces entering from the sigmoid colon, the defecation reflex is stimulated. This reflex causes involuntary relaxation of the internal sphincter and stimulates the urge to defecate. When the external

BOX 24–1 Selected Causes of Fecal Incontinence

Neurologic Causes
- Spinal cord injury or disease
- Head injury, stroke, or brain tumor
- Degenerative neurologic disease, such as multiple sclerosis, amyotrophic lateral sclerosis (ALS), dementia
- Diabetic neuropathy

Local Trauma
- Obstetric tears
- Anorectal injury
- Anorectal surgery with sphincter damage

Inflammatory Processes
- Infection
- Radiation

Other Causes
- Diarrhea
- Stool impaction
- Pelvic floor relaxation or loss of sphincter tone
- Tumors

sphincter, which is under both somatic (voluntary) and autonomic (involuntary) control, relaxes, defecation occurs. Adults normally can override the defecation reflex by voluntary contraction of the external sphincter and pelvic floor muscles. The wall of the rectum gradually relaxes, and the urge to defecate subsides.

The most common causes of fecal incontinence are those that interfere with either sensory or motor control of the rectum and anal sphincters. If the external sphincter is paralyzed as a result of spinal cord injury or disease, defecation occurs automatically when the internal sphincter relaxes with the defecation reflex. If sphincter muscles have been damaged or excessive pelvic floor relaxation has occurred, it may not be possible to override the defecation reflex with voluntary control.

Age-related changes in anal sphincter tone and response to rectal distention increase the risk for fecal incontinence in older adults. Resting and maximal anal sphincter pressures are decreased, particularly in older women. In addition, less rectal distension is needed to produce sustained relaxation of the anal sphincter in older females.

Interdisciplinary Care

The diagnosis of fecal incontinence is based on the patient's history. Physical examination of the pelvic floor and anus is performed to evaluate muscle tone and rule out a fecal impaction. Impaired sphincter muscle may be palpable on digital exam. Anorectal manometry or a rectal motility test may be used to evaluate the functional ability of the sphincter muscles. In this test, a small, flexible balloon catheter is introduced into the rectum, and pressures are measured in the rectum and internal and external sphincters. Normally, rectal dilation causes the internal sphincter to relax and the external sphincter to contract. Sigmoidoscopy may be used to examine the rectum and anal canal.

Management of fecal incontinence is directed toward the identified cause. Medications to relieve diarrhea or constipation may be prescribed. A high-fiber diet, ample fluids, and regular exercise are helpful for many patients. Exercises to improve sphincter and pelvic floor muscle tone (Kegel exercises) may be of long-term benefit. ∞ See Chapter 27 for more information about Kegel exercises.

Patients may benefit from using loperamide before meals and prophylactically before running errands or leaving the house. Biofeedback therapy may be used for mentally alert patients with intact sphincter muscles but low muscle tone. With motivation and reinforcement, patients achieve improved sphincter control in response to a stimulus. The goal of biofeedback is to improve sensation, coordination, and strength of the sphincter muscle.

When damage to the sphincter or rectal prolapse (protrusion of rectal mucous membrane through the anus) is the cause of fecal incontinence, surgical repair is the treatment of choice. Surgery may be indicated when conservative measures have not been effective. Permanent colostomy, the creation of an opening from the large bowel on the abdominal wall, is a last choice option for some patients, but it can control fecal output when other measures fail.

✆ Nursing Care

Health Promotion

A bowel training program to establish a regular pattern of elimination often is effective in relieving fecal incontinence. Teach the patient to establish a regular time of day for elimination, usually 15 to 30 minutes after breakfast. A stimulant, such as a cup of coffee, a rectal suppository, or even a phosphate enema, may be given to prompt defecation. Patients with neurologic incontinence may learn to stimulate the anal canal digitally to initiate defecation.

Dietary changes may be useful in managing fecal incontinence. If incontinence occurs only with mild loose or liquid stools, increasing dietary fiber or using a bulking agent to increase stool bulk and solidity may be effective. The majority of the fiber should come from a fiber-rich diet because fiber supplements provide only a limited amount of additional fiber. When incontinence of solid stool occurs, a low-residue diet of foods that are easily digested and absorbed may be prescribed to reduce the frequency of defecation.

Assessment

- *Health history:* Extent, onset, and duration of incontinence; identified contributing factors; history of spinal cord or anorectal injury or surgery; chronic diseases such as diabetes, multiple sclerosis, or other neurologic disorders.
- *Physical examination:* Mental status; general health; examination of perianal tissues; digital rectal examination.

Nursing Diagnoses and Interventions

Bowel Incontinence

Nurses are often responsible for instituting bowel training programs and other measures to manage fecal incontinence.

- Teach caregivers to place the patient on a toilet or commode and provide for privacy at a certain time of day. *Placing the patient in a normal position to defecate at a consistent time of day stimulates the defecation reflex and helps reestablish a pattern of stool evacuation.*
- If necessary, insert a glycerin or bisacodyl (Dulcolax) suppository 15 to 20 minutes before positioning on the toilet or commode. *This helps to stimulate evacuation. Once a regular*

elimination pattern is established, it may be possible to discontinue suppository use.

- Maintain a caring, nonjudgmental manner in providing care. *This promotes a feeling of acceptance when the patient may feel unacceptable.*

> **PRACTICE ALERT**
> Provide room odor control with deodorizer tablets, sprays, or other devices. Controlling odor is important to preserve the patient's self-esteem.

Risk for Impaired Skin Integrity

Good skin care is vital for the patient with fecal incontinence. Stool contains enzymes and other irritating substances that promote skin breakdown when they are not promptly removed. This can lead to pressure ulcers, particularly when a neurologic disorder (such as spinal cord injury, dementia, or stroke) impairs mobility.

- Clean the skin thoroughly with mild soap and water after each bowel movement. *Toilet tissue may be more irritating to the skin and less effective in removing fecal material.*
- Apply a skin barrier cream or ointment after each bowel movement. *These help protect the skin from irritating substances in the feces.*
- If incontinence pads or briefs are used, check frequently for soiling and change when feces is noted. *Although these help protect bedding and clothing from soiling, they can contribute to skin breakdown if they are not checked and changed frequently.*

Community-Based Care

Managing fecal incontinence is a challenging problem for the patient and family caregivers. For the patient with intact cognition, it can be psychologically devastating. The patient may become socially isolated from fear of odor or soiling clothing. Self-esteem may suffer from a sense of lost control over body functions and the inability to provide self-care. It is important to stress that incontinence is never normal (i.e., aging alone is not a cause of incontinence) and often is treatable. Encourage the patient to seek medical evaluation of the problem.

Topics of patient and family education include the following:

- Recommended dietary measures such as consuming a high-fiber diet and ample fluids to maintain soft, formed stool, or a low-residue diet to reduce the number of stools.
- Suggestions for regular exercise to stimulate bowel peristalsis and regular evacuation.
- Use of bulk-forming laxatives, such as psyllium seed (Metamucil), to provide stool bulk and reduce the number of small, liquid stools.
- Prescribed medications (such as loperamide to reduce the number of stools), their appropriate use, and management of adverse effects (such as constipation).
- Bowel training program instructions, including techniques for digital anal stimulation, inserting suppositories, or administering enemas as recommended. For digital anal simulation, teach to insert a lubricated gloved finger through the anal sphincter into the rectum 1.5 to 2 inches while seated on the toilet or commode, then use a circular side-to-side movement to gently stretch the rectal wall until the internal sphincter relaxes.
- The importance of good skin care, particularly if neurologic impairment is present.
- The potential benefits and associated risks of biofeedback and surgical treatment, if recommended.
- Provide referrals for home care or community health services as indicated.

Acute Inflammatory and Infectious Bowel Disorders

The GI tract is particularly vulnerable to inflammation and infection because of its continual exposure to the external environment. Although most pathogens affecting the GI tract are ingested in food or water, infection also may be spread by direct contact, possibly by the respiratory route. Pathogens may also be transmitted sexually through anal intercourse.

Acute disease of the GI tract may be caused by the pathogen itself or by a bacterial or other toxin. Acute inflammatory disorders such as appendicitis and peritonitis result from contamination of damaged or normally sterile tissue by the patient's own endogenous or resident bacteria.

The Patient with Appendicitis

Appendicitis, inflammation of the vermiform appendix, is a common cause of acute abdominal pain. It is the most common reason for emergency abdominal surgery, affecting 10% of the population (McPhee et al., 2008). Appendicitis can occur at any age, but is more common in adolescents and young adults and slightly more common in males than females.

Pathophysiology

The appendix is a tubelike pouch attached to the cecum just below the ileocecal valve. It is usually located in the right iliac region, at an area designated as McBurney's point (Figure 24–1 ■). The function of the appendix is not fully understood, although it may serve as a type of reservoir for beneficial intestinal bacteria.

Obstruction of the proximal lumen of the appendix is apparent in most acutely inflamed appendices. The obstruction is often caused by a *fecalith*, or hard mass of feces. Other obstructive causes include a calculus or stone, a foreign body, inflammation, a tumor, parasites (e.g., pinworms), or edema of lymphoid tissue. Following obstruction, the appendix becomes distended with fluid secreted by its mucosa. Pressure within the lumen of the appendix increases, impairing its blood supply and leading to inflammation, edema, ulceration, and infection. Purulent exudate forms, further distending the appendix. Within 24 to 36 hours, tissue necrosis and gangrene result, leading to perforation if treatment is not initiated. Perforation results in bacterial peritonitis.

Appendicitis can be classified as simple, gangrenous, or perforated, depending on the stage of the process. In simple appendicitis, the appendix is inflamed but intact. When areas of tissue

Figure 24–1 ■ McBurney's point, located midway between the umbilicus and the anterior iliac crest in the right lower quadrant. It is the usual site for localized pain and rebound tenderness due to appendicitis.

necrosis and microscopic perforations are present in the appendix, the disorder is called gangrenous appendicitis. A perforated appendix shows evidence of gross perforation and contamination of the peritoneal cavity.

Manifestations

Continuous mild generalized or upper abdominal pain is the initial characteristic manifestation of acute appendicitis. Over the next 4 hours, the pain intensifies and localizes in the right lower quadrant of the abdomen. It is aggravated by moving, walking, or coughing. On palpation, localized and rebound tenderness are noted at McBurney's point. *Rebound tenderness* is demonstrated by relief of pain with direct palpation of McBurney's point followed by pain on release of pressure. Extension or internal rotation of the right hip increases the pain. In addition to pain, a low-grade temperature, anorexia, nausea, and vomiting are often present.

Pain and local tenderness may be less acute in older adults, delaying the diagnosis, and leading to a 15% mortality of perforated appendicitis in the older adult (McPhee et al., 2008). This can present a significant problem; the course of acute appendicitis in older adults is more virulent and complications develop sooner. Pregnant women may develop right lower quadrant, periumbilical, or right subcostal (under the rib cage) pain due to possible displacement of the appendix by the distended uterus.

Complications

Perforation, peritonitis, and abscess are possible complications of acute appendicitis. Perforation is manifested by increased pain and a high fever. It can lead to a small, localized abscess, local

peritonitis, or significant generalized peritonitis. (Peritonitis is discussed in the next section of this chapter.)

A less common disorder is chronic appendicitis, characterized by chronic abdominal pain and recurrent acute attacks at intervals of several months or more. Other conditions, such as inflammatory bowel disease and renal disorders, often cause manifestations attributed to chronic appendicitis.

Interdisciplinary Care

The acutely inflamed appendix can perforate within 24 hours, so rapid diagnosis and treatment are important. Because of this urgency and the low incidence of surgical complications, diagnostic testing and preoperative treatment may be limited. The patient is admitted to the hospital, and intravenous fluids and antibiotics are initiated. Oral food and fluids are withheld until a diagnosis is confirmed. Once the diagnosis is established, an appendectomy is performed.

Diagnosis

Diagnostic and laboratory tests are used to help confirm the diagnosis and rule out other possible causes for the manifestations. Abdominal ultrasound is the most effective test for diagnosing acute appendicitis. Ultrasound examination has reduced the incidence of exploratory surgery and is particularly useful with patients with atypical symptoms, such as older adults. Other diagnostic tests used to accurately diagnose appendicitis include abdominal x-rays, an intravenous pyelogram, a urinalysis, and a pelvic examination. In addition, a WBC count with differential is obtained. With appendicitis, the total white count is elevated (10,000 to 20,000/mm^3), with an increased number of immature WBC (bands).

Medications

Prior to surgery, intravenous fluids are given to restore or maintain vascular volume and prevent electrolyte imbalance. Antibiotic therapy with a third-generation cephalosporin effective against many gram-negative bacteria, such as cefoperazone (Cefobid), cefotaxime (Claforan), ceftazidime (Fortaz), or ceftriaxone (Rocephin), is initiated prior to surgery. The antibiotic is repeated during surgery and continued for at least 48 hours postoperatively. (The nursing implications for cephalosporin antibiotics are discussed in ∞ Chapter 12.) Pain medications are administered as prescribed.

Surgery

The treatment of choice for acute appendicitis is an *appendectomy*, surgical removal of the appendix. Either a laparoscopic approach (insertion of an endoscope to view abdominal contents) or laparotomy (surgical opening of the abdomen) may be used for appendectomy. Laparoscopic appendectomy requires a very small incision through which the laparoscope is inserted. This procedure has several advantages: (1) Direct visualization of the appendix allows definitive diagnosis without laparotomy; (2) postoperative hospitalization is short; (3) postoperative complications are infrequent; and (4) recovery and resumption of normal activities is rapid.

An open appendectomy is performed by laparotomy. A small transverse incision is made at McBurney's point (Figure 24–1); the appendix is isolated and ligated (tied off) to prevent contamination of the site with bowel contents, and then removed. Laparotomy generally is used when the appendix has ruptured. It allows removal of contaminants from the peritoneal cavity by irrigation with sterile normal saline. Occasionally the wound may be left unsutured for periodic irrigation. Recovery is generally uneventful. ∞ Refer to Chapter 4 for discussion of preoperative and postoperative nursing care.

ᏍᏛ Nursing Care

A Case Study & Nursing Care Plan for a patient with appendicitis is included on page 667.

Assessment

Because appendicitis can rapidly progress from inflammation to perforation, prompt assessment is vital. Obtain the following assessment data:

- *Health history:* Current manifestations, including onset, duration, progression, and aggravating or relieving factors; most recent food or fluid intake; known medication or other allergies; current medications; history of chronic diseases.
- *Physical examination:* Vital signs including temperature; apparent general health; abdominal shape and contour, bowel sounds, tenderness to light palpation.

Nursing Diagnoses and Interventions

Preoperative nursing care is directed toward preparing the patient physically and psychologically for emergency surgery. Limited time is available for preoperative teaching.

> **PRACTICE ALERT**
> Keep the patient with suspected appendicitis NPO, and do not administer laxatives or enemas, which may cause perforation of the appendix. No heat should be applied to the abdomen; this may increase circulation to the appendix and also cause perforation.

Risk for Infection

Preventing complications during the preoperative and postoperative periods is a primary nursing care goal. Perforation and peritonitis are the most likely preoperative complications; postoperative complications include wound infection, abscess, and possible peritonitis.

> **PRACTICE ALERT**
> Assess abdominal status frequently, including distention, bowel sounds, and tenderness. Increasing generalized pain, a rigid, boardlike abdomen, and abdominal distention may indicate developing peritonitis.

- Monitor vital signs, including temperature. *Tachycardia and rapid shallow respirations may indicate perforation of the appendix with resulting peritonitis. Fever may develop as well, and the blood pressure may fall if sepsis is present.*
- Maintain intravenous infusion until oral intake is adequate. *Intravenous fluids are given to maintain vascular volume and to provide a route for antibiotic administration.*

- Assess wound, abdominal girth, and postoperative pain. *Swelling of the wound, increased abdominal girth, or an increase in pain may indicate infection or peritonitis.*

Acute Pain

The patient with appendicitis experiences pain before and after surgery. Analgesia is limited until the diagnosis is established. Postoperative pain is controlled by narcotic or nonnarcotic analgesics.

- Assess pain, including its character, location, severity, and duration. Report any unexpected changes in the nature of pain. *Both preoperatively and postoperatively, the patient's pain provides important clues about the diagnosis and possible complications such as rupture of the appendix or peritonitis.*

> **PRACTICE ALERT**
> Sudden relief of preoperative pain may signal rupture of the distended and edematous appendix.

- Administer analgesics as ordered. *Preoperatively, pain medication can be given after a diagnosis is established. Postoperatively, provide analgesics to maintain comfort and enhance mobility.*
- Assess effectiveness of medication 30 minutes after administration. Report unrelieved pain. *Pain unrelieved by prescribed analgesic may indicate a complication or the need for further assessment. For example, continued abdominal discomfort and distention may indicate excess intestinal gas that may be better relieved by ambulation.*

Using NANDA, NIC, and NOC

Linkages between a selected NANDA nursing diagnosis, NIC, and NOC for the patient with appendicitis are shown in the chart that follows.

Community-Based Care

Preoperative teaching may be limited by pain and the urgent nature of surgery. Explain why food and fluids are not permitted during this time. If time allows, teach postoperative turning, coughing, deep breathing, and pain management.

> **NANDA, NIC, AND NOC LINKAGES**
> **The Patient with Appendicitis or Peritonitis**
>
> **NANDA** — Acute Pain
>
> ⬇
>
> **NIC** — Analgesic Administration / Pain Management / Vital Signs Monitoring
>
> ⬇
>
> **NOC** — Pain Control / Comfort Status: Physical / Vital Signs
>
> Data from NANDA International. (2009). *Nursing diagnoses: Definitions & classification 2009–2011.* Oxford, UK: Wiley-Blackwell; Bulechek, G., Butcher, H., & Dochterman, J. (Eds.). (2008). *Nursing interventions classification (NIC)* (5th ed.). St. Louis, MO: Mosby; and Moorhead, S., Johnson, M., Maas, M., & Swanson, E. (Eds.). (2008). *Nursing outcomes classification (NOC)* (4th ed.). St. Louis, MO: Mosby.

Jamie Lynn is a 19-year-old college student majoring in physical therapy. Ms. Lynn arrives at the emergency department at 1:00 AM complaining of general lower abdominal pain that had started the previous evening. By midnight, the pain was more localized over the right lower quadrant. She also reports nausea and vomiting.

ASSESSMENT

Sue Grady, RN, completes the admission assessment in the emergency department. Ms. Lynn is complaining of nausea and severe abdominal pain, stating, "Walking makes my stomach hurt worse." Physical assessment findings include T 100.2°F (37.8°C), P 84, R 16, and BP 110/70; skin warm to touch; abdomen flat and guarded, with marked tenderness in right lower quadrant. Ms. Lynn's CBC shows WBC 14,000/mm^3; neutrophils 81.1%; lymphocytes 12.5%. The diagnosis of acute appendicitis is made, and Ms. Lynn is transferred to surgery for a laparoscopic appendectomy.

DIAGNOSES

- *Impaired Skin Integrity* related to surgical incision
- *Acute Pain* related to surgical intervention
- *Anxiety* related to situational crisis

EXPECTED OUTCOMES

- Incision will heal without infection or complications
- Will verbalize adequate pain relief
- Will verbalize decreased anxiety
- Will return to preoperative activities

PLANNING AND IMPLEMENTATION

- Assess pain using a pain scale; provide analgesics as needed.
- Teach pain management following discharge.
- Teach abdominal splinting during coughing, turning, or ambulating as needed.
- Teach home care of incision.
- Discuss activity limitations as ordered.
- Instruct to report fever or warmth, redness, or drainage from the incision.

EVALUATION

On discharge the following evening, Ms. Lynn is fully ambulatory. Her appetite has returned, and she is tolerating food and fluids well. Her temperature is normal. The nurse provides Ms. Lynn with written and verbal information on postoperative care following an appendectomy.

CRITICAL THINKING IN THE NURSING PROCESS

1. What is the pathophysiologic basis for Ms. Lynn's elevated WBC?
2. How would Ms. Lynn's postoperative care and teaching differ if she had undergone a laparotomy instead of a laparoscopic appendectomy?
3. Outline a teaching plan to give to patients for home care following an appendectomy.
4. Develop a care plan for Ms. Lynn for the nursing diagnosis *Anxiety* related to a situational crisis.

See Evaluating Your Response in Appendix C.

With uncomplicated appendectomy, the patient often is discharged either the day of surgery or the day following surgery. Postoperative teaching includes the following:

- Wound or incision care, including hand hygiene and dressing change procedures as indicated
- Instructions to report fever, increased abdominal pain, swelling, redness, drainage, bleeding, or warmth of the operative site to the physician
- Activity limitations (e.g., lifting, driving), if any
- Returning to work if appropriate

The Patient with Peritonitis

Peritonitis, inflammation of the peritoneum, is a serious complication of many acute abdominal disorders. It is usually caused by enteric bacteria entering the peritoneal cavity through a perforated ulcer, ruptured appendix, perforated diverticulum (discussed later in this chapter), necrotic bowel, or during abdominal surgery. Pelvic inflammatory disease, gallbladder rupture, abdominal trauma, or peritoneal dialysis can also lead to peritonitis.

Pathophysiology

The peritoneum is a double-layered serous membrane lining the walls (parietal peritoneum) and organs (visceral peritoneum) of the abdominal cavity. There is a potential space between the parietal and visceral layers of the peritoneum that contains a small amount of serous fluid. This space, the peritoneal cavity, normally is sterile.

Peritonitis results from contamination of the normally sterile peritoneal cavity by infection or a chemical irritant. Chemical peritonitis often precedes bacterial peritonitis. Perforation of a peptic ulcer or rupture of the gallbladder releases gastric juices (hydrochloric acid and pepsin) or bile into the peritoneal cavity, causing an acute inflammatory response.

Bacterial peritonitis usually is caused by infection by *Escherichia coli*, *Klebsiella*, *Proteus*, or *Pseudomonas* bacteria, which normally inhabit the bowel. Inflammatory and immune defense mechanisms are activated when bacteria enter the peritoneal space. These defenses can effectively eliminate small numbers of bacteria, but may be overwhelmed by massive or continued contamination. When this occurs, mast cells release histamine and other vasoactive substances, causing local vasodilation and increased capillary permeability. Polymorphonuclear leukocytes (a type of WBC) infiltrate the peritoneum to phagocytize bacteria and foreign matter. Fibrinogen-rich plasma exudate promotes bacterial destruction and forms fibrin clots to seal off and segregate the bacteria. This process helps limit and localize the infection, allowing host defenses to eradicate it. Continued contamination, however, leads to generalized inflammation of the peritoneal cavity. The inflammatory process causes fluid to shift into the peritoneal space (third spacing). Circulating blood volume is depleted, leading to hypovolemia. *Septicemia*, a systemic disease caused by pathogens or their toxins in the blood, may follow.

Manifestations

Manifestations of peritonitis depend on the severity and extent of the infection, as well as the age and general health of the patient. Both local and systemic manifestations are present (see the accompanying box). The patient often presents with evidence of an *acute abdomen*, an abrupt onset of diffuse, severe abdominal pain. The pain may localize and intensify near the area of infection. Movement may intensify the pain. The entire abdomen is tender, with guarding or rigidity of abdominal muscles. The acute abdomen is often described as boardlike. Rebound tenderness may be present over the area of inflammation. Peritoneal inflammation inhibits peristalsis, resulting in a paralytic ileus. (Paralytic ileus is discussed in a later section of this chapter.) Bowel sounds are markedly diminished or absent, and progressive abdominal distention is noted. Pooling of GI secretions may cause nausea and vomiting. Systemic manifestations of peritonitis include fever, malaise, tachycardia and tachypnea, restlessness, and possible disorientation. The patient may be oliguric (having little urine output) and show signs of dehydration and shock.

The older, chronically debilitated, or immunosuppressed patient may present with few of the classic signs of peritonitis. Increased confusion and restlessness, decreased urinary output, and vague abdominal complaints may be the only manifestations present. These patients are at increased risk for delayed diagnosis, contributing to a higher mortality rate.

Complications

Complications of peritonitis may be life threatening. Abscess formation is common. The very defense mechanisms designed to isolate and localize the infection can protect it from immune responses and systemic antibiotics. Fibrous adhesions in the abdominal cavity are a late complication and may lead to subsequent obstruction.

Without prompt and effective treatment, septicemia and septic shock can develop. Fluid loss into the abdominal cavity may lead to hypovolemic shock. These potentially lethal complications require immediate, aggressive intervention to prevent multiple organ failure and death. Septicemia, shock, and its management are discussed in ∞ Chapter 11.

Interdisciplinary Care

Care of the patient with peritonitis focuses on establishing the diagnosis and identifying and treating its cause as well as the peritonitis. Preventing complications is an important aspect of care.

Diagnosis

Diagnostic tests are performed to establish the diagnosis of peritonitis, rule out other disorders, and help identify the cause. The tests that may be ordered include a WBC count (elevated to approximately 20,000/mm^3 in peritonitis), blood cultures, abdominal CT scan, liver and renal function studies, serum electrolytes, and a paracentesis (in peritonitis, peritoneal fluid will contain increased protein and WBCs). Increased numbers of immature blood cells are present as the bone marrow releases them in response to the infection.

Medications

Until the infecting organism has been identified, a broad-spectrum antibiotic effective against organisms commonly implicated in peritonitis is prescribed. A beta-lactam antibiotic such as imipenem (Primaxin) or meropenem (Merrem), which has a very broad spectrum of action, may be used. Once culture results have been obtained, antibiotic therapy is modified to the specific organism(s) responsible. Antibiotics that may be ordered include ampicillin (e.g., Omnipen, Polycillin), metronidazole (Flagyl), ciprofloxacin (Cipro), clindamycin (Cleocin), a cephalosporin such as ceftriaxone (Rocephin) or an aminoglycoside antibiotic such as gentamicin (Garamycin) or amikacin (Amikin). Nursing implications for antibiotic therapy are discussed in ∞ Chapter 12. Analgesics are prescribed to promote comfort.

Surgery

If the cause of peritonitis is a perforation, gangrenous bowel, or inflamed appendix, a laparotomy is done to close the perforation or remove the damaged and inflamed tissue. If an abscess is present, it also may be surgically drained or removed.

Peritoneal lavage, washing of the peritoneal cavity with copious amounts of warm isotonic fluid, may be done during surgery. This procedure dilutes residual bacteria and removes gross contaminants, blood, and fibrin clots. In rare instances, peritoneal lavage may be continued for several days following surgery. The solution is infused into the upper portion of the peritoneal cavity and removed via drains in the pelvic cul-de-sac. Careful attention to fluid and electrolyte status and strict aseptic technique are necessary.

Patients who have had laparotomy for peritonitis often return from surgery with either Penrose or closed drain systems such as a Jackson-Pratt drain. In some cases, the incision may be left unsutured. With severe and long-standing peritonitis, the abdomen may be closed temporarily with polypropylene mesh containing a nylon zipper or Velcro to allow repeated exploration of the abdomen and drainage of infectious sites.

Nutrition
Intravenous fluids and electrolyte replacements are administered to maintain vascular volume and fluid and electrolyte balance. Parenteral nutrition is given until adequate oral intake resumes.

Other Treatments
The patient is placed on bed rest in Fowler's position to help localize the infection and promote lung ventilation. Oxygen is often ordered to facilitate cellular metabolism and healing.

INTESTINAL DECOMPRESSION   The inflammatory process of peritonitis often draws large amounts of fluid into the abdominal cavity and the bowel. In addition, peristaltic activity of the bowel is slowed or halted by the inflammation, causing **paralytic ileus** (or *ileus*), impaired propulsion or forward movement of bowel contents. Intestinal decompression is used to relieve abdominal distention, facilitate closure, and minimize postoperative respiratory problems. A nasogastric or long intestinal tube is inserted and connected to continuous drainage (Figure 24–2 ■). If prolonged intestinal decompression is

Weighted
Balloon

Figure 24–2 ■ The weighted tip or inflated balloon at the end of an intestinal tube is drawn into the intestine by gravity and peristalsis.

anticipated, a jejunostomy may be performed for comfort. Suction is maintained until peristalsis resumes, bowel sounds are present, and the patient is passing flatus. Food and fluids are withheld until intestinal motility has returned and suction is discontinued.

Nursing Care
Peritonitis is a serious illness. Early recognition and treatment are important to minimize the risk of complications.

Assessment
- *Health history:* Pain, its onset, character, severity, location, aggravating and relieving factors; associated symptoms such as anorexia, nausea, vomiting; current and previous history of peptic ulcer disease, gallbladder disease, chronic diseases; current medications.
- *Physical examination:* Vital signs including temperature; level of consciousness; skin color, temperature, warmth, capillary refill and turgor; abdominal shape, contour, bowel sounds, tenderness, tympany, and guarding.

Nursing Diagnoses and Interventions
Patients with peritonitis require intensive nursing and medical care to prevent complications and recover fully. Nursing care priorities include interventions to manage pain, altered fluid balance, altered protection due to infection, and anxiety.

Acute Pain
Abdominal distention and acute inflammation contribute to the pain associated with peritonitis. Surgery further disrupts abdominal muscles and other tissues, causing pain. Effective pain management promotes immune function, healing, mobility, and recovery.

- Assess pain, including its location, severity (using a standard pain scale), and type. Monitor analgesic effectiveness. Report changes to the primary care provider.

> **PRACTICE ALERT**
> Unrelieved pain or a change in the location, severity, or type of pain may indicate spread of infection, abscess formation, or other complications of peritonitis.

- Place in Fowler's or semi-Fowler's position with the knees and feet elevated. *This position reduces stress on abdominal structures and facilitates respirations, promoting comfort.*
- Administer analgesics as ordered on a routine basis or using patient-controlled analgesia (PCA). *Routine analgesic administration maintains a therapeutic blood level and helps maintain comfort, facilitating healing and movement.*
- Teach and assist with adjunctive pain management techniques such as meditation, visualization, massage, and progressive relaxation. *Adjunctive measures augment analgesics and help promote a sense of control over pain.*

Deficient Fluid Volume

In peritonitis, significant amounts of fluid are drawn into the abdominal cavity and bowel, reducing vascular volume and cardiac output. This fluid also may be lost from the body by intestinal suction or through drains placed in the abdomen during surgery. An unsutured incision causes additional significant fluid loss.

- Maintain accurate intake and output records. Measure urine output every 1 to 2 hours; report output of less than 30 mL/h. Measure gastrointestinal output at least every 4 hours. *Intake and output records provide valuable information about fluid volume status.*

> **PRACTICE ALERT**
> Urine output of less than 30 mL/hr may indicate hypovolemia, decreased cardiac output, and impaired tissue perfusion.

- Monitor vital signs and hemodynamic parameters such as central venous pressure, cardiac output, and pulmonary artery pressures every hour or as indicated. *These measurements provide important information about fluid and vascular volumes as well as cardiovascular status.*
- Weigh daily. *Weight is an accurate indicator of fluid status. Rapid weight gains or losses reflect changes in fluid volume.*
- Assess skin turgor, color, temperature, and mucous membranes at least every 8 hours. *Warm, dry skin with poor turgor and dry, shiny mucous membranes indicate dehydration.*
- Measure or estimate fluid losses through abdominal drains and on dressings. *Significant amounts of exudative fluid may be lost.*
- Monitor laboratory values, including hemoglobin and hematocrit, urine specific gravity, serum osmolality and electrolytes, and ABGs. Report changes to the physician. *Laboratory results provide information about fluid and electrolyte status and acid–base balance.*
- Administer intravenous fluids and electrolytes as ordered. Gastrointestinal drainage may be replaced milliliter for milliliter with a balanced electrolyte solution. *Intravenous fluids are necessary to meet daily fluid intake needs, as well as replace continuing losses of water and electrolytes.*
- Provide good skin care and frequent oral hygiene. *Fluid deficit increases the risk of skin breakdown and ulceration of mucous membranes.*

Delayed Surgical Recovery

Repeated surgeries, an unsutured incision, and the presence of drains interrupt skin integrity and the body's first line of defense against microorganisms. In addition, immune defenses are stressed by the infection and potential malnutrition. As a result, the risk for impaired healing and further infection is increased.

- Monitor temperature, pulse rate, and for localized signs of infection such as redness and swelling around incisions and drain sites, increased or purulent drainage, and cloudy or malodorous urine. *Impaired defenses increase the risk for extension of the infection or unrelated infections.*

- Obtain cultures of purulent drainage from any site. *Early identification of any additional infection allows timely intervention.*
- Monitor WBC and differential, serum protein, and albumin. *An increased WBC with a higher percentage of immature cells present in the blood is an indicator of infection and normal immune response. Serum albumin and protein levels are indicators of nutritional status as well as immune function.*
- Practice meticulous hand hygiene and use standard precautions at all times. *Hand hygiene reduces transient bacteria on the skin and remains the most important method of controlling infection. Standard precautions reduce the risk of spreading infection to or from the patient.*
- Use strict aseptic technique for dressing changes, wound care, and irrigations. *Disruption of the protective barrier of the skin increases the risk of contamination and further infection.*
- Maintain fluid balance and nutritional status through enteral or parenteral feedings, as indicated. See the following research box for evidence-based recommendations for care of enterally fed patients. *Adequate nutrition and fluid balance are necessary for optimal immune system function.*

> **PRACTICE ALERT**
> An acute infection such as peritonitis causes a stress response with excess energy expenditure and loss of body proteins and cell mass. Glycogen stores are rapidly depleted, and body proteins are used to meet energy needs. Withholding food further complicates this process, leading to rapid development of protein-calorie malnutrition (PCM). PCM impairs the immune response and slows healing.

Anxiety

The severity and potential threat to life associated with peritonitis present a situational crisis for the patient and family. Anxiety is a common response.

- Assess the patient's and family's anxiety level and present coping skills. *Interventions need to be tailored to the needs and strengths of the patient and family.*
- Present a calm, reassuring manner. Encourage expression of concerns; listen carefully, and acknowledge their validity. *This helps establish trust.*
- Maintain consistent caregiver assignments. *Consistency of nursing care and care providers helps reduce anxiety. Complex wound care and irrigation procedures are best performed by people who are very familiar with prescribed techniques.*
- Explain all treatments, procedures, tests, and examinations. *An increased understanding of what is being done can reduce anxiety.*
- Reinforce and clarify information as needed. *This improves understanding and promotes acceptance.*
- Teach and assist with relaxation techniques such as meditation, visualization, and progressive relaxation. *These measures promote positive coping skills and reduce physical manifestations of anxiety.*

Enterally Fed, Critically Ill Patient

A vital component of the treatment and care of critically ill patients (such as those with peritonitis) is providing nutritional support, primarily through enteral feedings. Although this remains the method of choice for this population, and has many advantages, enteral feeding also comes with the risk of bronchopulmonary aspiration as a complication. Aspiration occurs in as many as 40% of patients and up to 50% to 75% of patients who have an endotracheal tube in place. Several methods are currently used to detect aspiration, but not as much information has been published about how to prevent aspiration in enterally fed patients. This study (Sanko, 2004) was conducted to review and synthesize current research in order to make recommendations to improve the quality and safety of administering enteral nutrition to critically ill patients. Recommended prevention techniques included the following:

- Preventing aspiration with feeding tube placement by verifying placement with an x-ray. After verifying the placement, the tube should be securely taped and the external tube length should be measured, noted, and marked on the tube as a reference point for further tube placement checks. If the position of the tube is questioned, the x-ray should be repeated.
- Maintaining the head of the bed at an angle of at least 30 degrees, with 45% being ideal, and stopping feedings 30 to 60 minutes before placing the patient in the supine position.
- Maintaining cuff pressure in patients with artificial airways at 20 to 30 cm H_2O.

Based on published findings, there is not sufficient evidence to support placement of feeding tubes beyond the pylorus or using small-bore tubes to prevent aspiration.

IMPLICATIONS FOR NURSING
Based on this review of the relevant research, it is obvious that more research is needed in this area of care. However, daily assessments of the patient and the feeding tube with multiple methods (including x-ray, external length marking, pH testing, aspirate characteristics, or trypsin/pepsin levels) should be conducted by caregivers who have the knowledge to accurately interpret the results.

CRITICAL THINKING IN PATIENT CARE
1. Aspiration is defined as the inhalation of oropharyngeal or gastric contents into the larynx and lower respiratory tract. The result is usually aspiration pneumonitis or aspiration pneumonia. What assessments would you conduct and monitor to identify these complications?
2. You are on a committee that is evaluating the practice of adding blue dye to feeding solutions in order to better detect aspiration. The literature does not support this method. How and what would you do to convince the committee that this practice should not be continued?
3. What principle supports elevating the head of the bed to prevent aspiration? (Consider gravity and the placement of internal organs with the patient in this position.)

Community-Based Care
Teaching for home care includes the following topics:

- Wound care procedures, including dressing changes or irrigations. Provide verbal and written instructions on how to change dressings or do irrigations as well as where to obtain supplies, and allow opportunities to practice and demonstrate the procedure prior to discharge.
- Prescribed medications, including name and purpose of the drug, potential adverse effects, and their management.
- Manifestations of further infection (redness, heat, swelling, purulent drainage, chills, and fever) and potential complications to be reported to the care provider.
- Prescribed activity restrictions.
- Instructions for a high-calorie, high-protein diet for healing and optimal immune function.

Provide a referral to home health services for assessment, wound care, and further teaching, as needed.

The Patient with Gastroenteritis

Gastroenteritis, or *enteritis*, is an inflammation of the stomach and small intestine. Enteritis may be caused by bacteria, viruses, parasites, or toxins. Upper GI manifestations such as anorexia, nausea, and vomiting are common. Diarrhea of varying intensity and abdominal discomfort are nearly universal features of gastroenteritis.

The infectious organism usually enters the body in contaminated water or food. For this reason, gastroenteritis often is called food poisoning. Viruses commonly cause acute diarrheal illness. Diarrhea due to rotaviruses or the Norwalk virus occurs year-round in both adults and children. These illnesses are generally mild and self-limited, but can have severe consequences in the very young, the very old, or in people with impaired immune function.

Pathophysiology
Bacterial or viral infection of the GI tract produces inflammation, tissue damage, and manifestations by two primary mechanisms:

- *The production of exotoxins.* A number of bacteria produce and excrete an exotoxin that enters the surrounding environment (intestinal lumen), causing damage and inflammation. Exotoxins in the GI tract are often referred to as *enterotoxins*. They impair intestinal absorption and can cause secretion of significant amounts of electrolytes and water into the bowel, resulting in diarrhea and fluid loss. Common bacterial enterotoxins include those produced by *Staphylococcus, Clostridium perfringens, Clostridium botulinum*, some strains of *Escherichia coli*, *Vibrio cholera*, and *C. difficile*.
- *Invasion and ulceration of the mucosa.* Other bacteria, including some *Shigella, Salmonella*, and *E. coli* species, damage tissue more directly. They invade the intestinal mucosa of the small bowel or colon, producing microscopic ulceration, bleeding, fluid exudate, and water and electrolyte secretion.

In some cases, the mechanism of injury is unclear. It may be a combination of direct and toxic damage. For example, the Norwalk virus damages the mucosa of the jejunum, with fluid and electrolyte secretion.

Manifestations

Although the manifestations of bacterial and viral enteritis vary according to the organism involved, several features are common (see the following Manifestations box). Anorexia, nausea, and vomiting are caused by distention of the upper GI tract by unabsorbed chyme and excess water. Bowel distention, along with irritation of the bowel mucosa and gas production due to fermentation of undigested food, lead to abdominal pain and cramping. Borborygmi, excessively loud and hyperactive bowel sounds, are another result. The abdomen is often distended and tender.

Diarrhea is usually predominant with enteritis. Fluid is secreted into the bowel lumen, and the unabsorbed chyme and electrolytes create an osmotic pull of fluid into the bowel. Motility is stimulated, and stools become watery and frequent. Loss of fluids and electrolytes through diarrhea can lead to the most serious manifestations of enteritis. Fluid volume can be rapidly depleted, leading to dehydration and hypovolemia. Orthostatic hypotension and fever may be noted initially. If fluid loss continues, hypovolemic shock may develop.

Complications

Electrolyte and acid–base imbalances may result from gastroenteritis. Extensive vomiting can lead to metabolic alkalosis due to the loss of hydrochloric acid from the stomach. When diarrhea predominates, metabolic acidosis is more likely. Potassium is lost in either case, leading to hypokalemia. Hyponatremia may develop if fluids are replaced with pure water. Headache, cardiac irregularities, changes in respiratory rate and pattern, malaise and weakness, muscle aching, and signs of neuromuscular irritability are the possible manifestations of these disturbances in homeostasis.

Specific Types of Gastrointestinal Infections

Several gastrointestinal infections produce specific effects that are discussed below and summarized in Table 24–3.

TRAVELER'S DIARRHEA   People traveling to another country frequently develop diarrhea within 2 to 10 days, particularly when there is a significant difference in climate, sanitation standards, or food and drink. Strains of enterotoxin-producing *E. coli*, *Shigella* species, *Salmonella*, and *Campylobacter* are the most frequent causes of traveler's diarrhea (Yates, 2005). Other bacteria and viruses also may cause traveler's diarrhea.

MANIFESTATIONS of Gastroenteritis

GASTROINTESTINAL EFFECTS
- Anorexia, nausea, and vomiting
- Abdominal pain and cramping
- Borborygmi
- Diarrhea

GENERAL EFFECTS
- Malaise, weakness, and muscle aches
- Headache
- Dry skin and mucous membranes
- Poor skin turgor
- Orthostatic hypotension, tachycardia
- Fever

Up to 10 or more loose stools per day and abdominal cramping are common manifestations. Nausea and vomiting are less frequent; fever is rare. Manifestations usually resolve within 2 to 5 days. Complications are rare.

ESCHERICHIA COLI HEMORRHAGIC COLITIS   Most pathologic forms of *E. coli* bacteria cause little more than common traveler's diarrhea. However, some strains, such as serotype 0157:H7, produce a potent enterotoxin in the large intestine after being ingested. This toxin damages bowel mucosa and the endothelial cells of blood vessels in the GI tract. If absorbed, the toxin can damage other blood vessels as well, such as those of the kidney.

Cattle provide the reservoir for *E. coli* 0157:H7. It is usually spread through undercooked beef (hamburger in particular) and unpasteurized milk or apple juice. It may also be spread by direct contact via the fecal–oral route. The onset of hemorrhagic colitis is abrupt, with severe abdominal cramping and watery diarrhea that becomes grossly bloody within 24 hours. Fever may be present.

Hemolytic uremic syndrome and thrombotic thrombocytopenic purpura are significant complications of *E. coli* hemorrhagic colitis, affecting about 5% of people with the disease. Older adults have the highest risk for developing complications.

STAPHYLOCOCCAL FOOD POISONING   Certain foods provide an excellent medium for staphylococcal growth when contaminated and left at room temperature. Examples include meats and fish, dairy products (e.g., custards), and bakery products (e.g., cream-filled pastries). The organism itself does not affect the bowel; the toxin it produces, however, impairs intestinal absorption and acts on receptors in the gut, stimulating the medullary center to produce vomiting.

The onset of staphylococcal food poisoning is abrupt, occurring within 2 to 8 hours after consuming the contaminated food. Nausea and vomiting are severe. Manifestations typically last 3 to 6 hours, and include abdominal cramping, diarrhea, headache, and fever. Complications such as fluid and electrolyte imbalances are rare, but may develop in older adults and people with underlying chronic disease processes.

CHOLERA   *Cholera* is an acute diarrheal illness caused by strains of *Vibrio cholerae*. It is endemic in parts of Asia, the Middle East, and Africa. Cholera is spread by the fecal–oral route through contaminated water or food. The organism produces an enterotoxin, enzymes, and other substances that affect the entire small intestine. Water and electrolytes are secreted into the bowel lumen in response to the toxin. The enzymes and other substances produced by the bacteria may affect mucous protection of bowel endothelium.

Cholera ranges in severity from very mild, with few or no manifestations, to acute and fulminant. Its onset is typically abrupt, with severe, frequent, watery diarrhea. Up to 1 L of stool may be passed in an hour, rapidly depleting fluid volume. Stool is often described as "rice water stool" and is characteristically gray and cloudy, with no fecal odor, blood, or pus. Vomiting may accompany the diarrhea. Other manifestations relate to the loss of fluid and electrolytes: thirst, oliguria, muscle cramps, weakness, and significant signs of dehydration.

TABLE 24–3 Selected Bacterial Infections of the Bowel

DISEASE AND ORGANISM	INCUBATION	PATHOGENESIS	MANIFESTATIONS	MANAGEMENT
Traveler's diarrhea: *Escherichia coli*	24 to 72 hours	Enterotoxin causes hyper-secretion of the small intestine.	Abrupt onset of diarrhea; vomiting rare	Prophylactic bismuth subsalicylate; antidiarrheal such as loperamide; 3-day course of norfloxacin, ciprofloxacin, or azithromycin
Hemorrhagic colitis: *E. coli* 0157:H7	1 to 3 days	Enterotoxin causes direct mucosal damage in large intestine; also toxic to vascular endothelial cells.	Severe abdominal cramping, watery diarrhea that becomes grossly bloody; fever; possible complications: hemolytic uremic syndrome and thrombotic thrombocytopenic purpura	Supportive care with fluid replacement and bland diet; may require dialysis or plasmapheresis for complications
Staphylococcal food poisoning	2 to 8 hours	Enterotoxin impairs intestinal absorption and affects vomiting centers in the brain.	Severe nausea and vomiting; abdominal cramping and diarrhea; headache and fever	Fluid and electrolyte replacement as needed
Cholera: *Vibrio cholerae*	1 to 3 days	Enterotoxin affects entire small intestine, causing secretion of water and electrolytes into bowel lumen.	Severe diarrhea with "rice water stool," gray, cloudy, odorless, with no blood or pus; vomiting; thirst, oliguria, muscle cramps, weakness; dehydration and vascular collapse	Oral or intravenous rehydration; possible antimicrobial therapy with tetracycline, doxycycline, or ciprofloxacin, others
Salmonellosis: *Salmonella*	8 to 48 hours	Superficial infection of the GI tract without invasion or production of toxins.	Diarrhea with abdominal cramping, nausea, and vomiting; low-grade fever, chills, weakness	Treatment of symptoms; a third-generation cephalosporin or a fluoroquinolone antibiotic for severe illness
Shigellosis (bacillary dysentery): *Shigella*	1 to 4 days	Local tissue invasion, primarily involving large intestine and distal ileum; endotoxin causes fluid and electrolyte secretion into bowel lumen.	Watery diarrhea with severe abdominal cramping and tenesmus; lethargy	Fluid and electrolyte replacement; correction of acidosis; antibiotic therapy with ciprofloxacin, ceftriaxone, others
Clostridium difficile colitis (*C. difficile*)	1 to 2 weeks	Antibiotic therapy interferes with normal protective bacteria in the colon; *C. difficile* colonizes and releases toxins that cause mucosal inflammation and damage	Diarrhea, abdominal cramps, malaise, fever, anorexia	Cessation of the causative antibiotic; antibiotic therapy with vancomycin or metronidazole (specific for *C. difficile*)

Metabolic acidosis and hypokalemia develop. If untreated, circulatory collapse and acute renal failure may occur.

Recovery from cholera usually occurs spontaneously within 3 to 6 days. With prompt and adequate fluid replacement, mortality is less than 1%.

CLOSTRIDIUM DIFFICILE COLITIS *Clostridium difficile colitis* (*C. difficile* colitis) is associated with antibiotic therapy. Treatment with antibiotics (especially broad-spectrum antibiotics) predisposes to interference with the normal protective bacteria of the colon, leading to colonization by *C. difficile* by the oral–fecal route. Subsequent release of toxins by the bacteria causes mucous damage and inflammation. This is primarily a problem in hospitalized patients, causing diarrhea and abdominal cramping. These manifestations commonly begin within 1 to 2 weeks of antibiotic treatment. It is also being seen in the community in healthy adults. The bacteria can be identified in the stool.

SALMONELLOSIS *Salmonellosis* is food poisoning caused by ingesting raw or improperly cooked foods contaminated with *Salmonella* bacteria. Meat, poultry, eggs, and dairy products commonly are implicated in salmonellosis; recent outbreaks

have been linked to products such as peanuts and alfalfa sprouts. These bacteria cause superficial infection of the GI tract, rarely invading further. They do not produce a toxin.

Manifestations develop 8 to 48 hours after ingesting the bacteria. Diarrhea may be violent with abdominal cramping, nausea, and vomiting. A low-grade fever, chills, and weakness may accompany GI manifestations. The disease usually is self-limited, resolving within 3 to 5 days, although bacteremia may develop.

SHIGELLOSIS (BACILLARY DYSENTERY) *Shigellosis* (or bacillary dysentery) occurs worldwide, and may be endemic or occur in epidemics. Humans are the reservoir for *Shigella* organisms, which are spread directly via the fecal–oral route or indirectly through contaminated food, fomites (inanimate objects), and vectors (such as fleas). The incubation period for shigellosis is 1 to 4 days.

Shigella organisms infect the distal ilium and lower intestine. They invade the tissue, causing inflammation, and they produce an enterotoxin. The result is watery diarrhea containing blood, mucus, and inflammatory exudate. The onset of diarrhea is abrupt, with severe abdominal cramping, and *tenesmus*, a sensation of urgent and continuing need to defecate. Lethargy is common; rarely, neurologic manifestations occur.

In adults, shigellosis is usually mild and self-limiting. Older adults and debilitated patients are at risk for volume depletion and electrolyte imbalances. Secondary infection is another potential complication, as is acute blood loss from mucosal ulcerations.

NOROVIRUS Norovirus-associated gastroenteritis is a highly contagious disease that often occurs in outbreaks within an institution or facility. It is characterized by acute vomiting, watery, nonbloody diarrhea, abdominal cramps, and nausea. Systemic manifestations such as myalgia, malaise, headache, and low-grade fever are common.

Noroviruses are transmitted primarily by the fecal–oral route, either through direct contact or via contaminated food or water. The average incubation period is 12 to 48 hours. The disease tends to be self-limiting, with dehydration its most common complication.

Interdisciplinary Care

The goals of care for gastroenteritis are to manage the manifestations, prevent complications, identify the cause of the infection, and prevent its spread. The history and manifestations provide valuable cues about the cause. Diagnostic testing is used to identify the pathogen and evaluate its effects. In most cases, treatment is supportive, directed toward relieving manifestations, restoring fluid and electrolyte balance, and maintaining function.

Diagnosis

If manifestations are severe or do not resolve within about 48 hours, laboratory testing is used to identify the causative organism and to assess fluid, electrolyte, and acid–base balance. A stool specimen for culture, ova and parasites, and

fecal leukocytes usually reveals the infective organism, but may require up to 6 weeks to identify some bacteria. In infections such as botulism, the toxin itself may be isolated in the stool. Contamination of the stool by urine or treatment with antibiotics, bismuth subsalicylate (Pepto-Bismol), or mineral oil may interfere with pathogen growth, altering stool culture results. Use a clean bedpan or collection device to obtain the stool specimen, and instruct the patient to avoid mixing the stool with urine or toilet tissue.

A sigmoidoscopy may be done to differentiate inflammatory bowel disease from infectious processes. It does not replace stool cultures, because the lesions associated with some infectious processes are indistinguishable from those of ulcerative colitis. (Nursing care of the patient having a sigmoidoscopy is discussed in ∞ Chapter 21.)

Serum osmolality and electrolytes and ABGs are done to assess and monitor fluid, electrolyte, and acid–base balance. Common imbalances associated with enteritis and diarrhea are outlined in Table 24–4.

Medications

Acute enteritis usually resolves spontaneously, and no drug treatment is required. If the patient is severely ill and manifestations are prolonged, medications may be prescribed.

Antibiotic therapy specific to the organism may be used to treat bacterial colitis, cholera, salmonellosis, or shigellosis. Ciprofloxacin (Cipro), clarithromycin (Biaxin), erythromycin, amoxicillin/clavulanate (Augmentin), or another antibiotic may be prescribed. Stool culture is obtained prior to starting antibiotics, but treatment may begin before culture results are available. A presumptive diagnosis based on history and presenting manifestations guides the choice of antibiotic.

An antidiarrheal drug may be prescribed to promote comfort and reduce fluid loss. Nursing measures related to antidiarrheal medications are outlined in the Medication Administration box on page 655.

TABLE 24–4 Laboratory Values Associated with Enteritis and Diarrhea

TEST	NORMAL VALUE	CHANGE WITH SIGNIFICANT DIARRHEA
Serum osmolality	280 to 300 mOsm/kg	Increased; levels above 320 mOsm/kg indicate significant dehydration.
Serum potassium	3.5 to 5.3 mEq/L	Decreased due to loss through stool and vomitus; levels below 2.5 mEq/L are critical.
Serum sodium	135 to 145 mEq/L	Decreased due to loss through stool and vomitus; may be significant when fluid losses are replaced with pure water; levels below 120 mEq/L may be critical.
Serum chloride	95 to 105 mEq/L	Increased when sodium loss is greater than chloride loss; decreased with severe diarrhea and with vomiting; possible critical values are below 80 mEq/L or above 115 mEq/L.
Blood gases		
■ pH	Arterial: 7.35 to 7.45	Decreased in metabolic acidosis, a possible result of severe diarrhea; increased in metabolic alkalosis, a possible result of severe vomiting and chloride loss; values below 7.25 or above 7.55 are critical.
■ PCO_2	Arterial: 35 to 45 mmHg	Typically decreased in metabolic acidosis as the body attempts to eliminate excess acid by "blowing off" CO_2; increased with metabolic alkalosis as the body retains CO_2 in an attempt to normalize pH.
■ Bicarbonate	24 to 28 mEq/L	Decreased in metabolic acidosis; increased in metabolic alkalosis.
Hematocrit	Males: 40% to 54%	Increased with dehydration and hypovolemia as a result of concentration of blood cells.
	Females: 36% to 46%	
Urine specific gravity	1.005 to 1.030	Increased with dehydration and hypovolemia as kidneys attempt to conserve fluid.

Nutrition and Fluids

Replacing lost fluids and electrolytes is vital when vomiting and/or diarrhea are severe or prolonged. In many cases of enteritis, fluid and electrolyte replacement are all that is required until the infection resolves.

Oral rehydration is preferred for replacing physiologic fluids. An oral glucose-electrolyte solution is often well tolerated in sips, even when vomiting is present. Commercial preparations such as Gatorade, All-Sport, and Pedialyte are available. A solution of 5 mL (1 teaspoon) table salt, 5 mL baking soda, 20 mL (4 teaspoons) granulated sugar, and flavoring (such as lemon extract or juice) to 1 L (1 quart) of water also is effective.

Intravenous rehydration may be necessary with severe diarrhea and fluid loss. In some cases, a combination of oral and intravenous fluids may be used to replace lost fluids and maintain vascular volume. Balanced electrolyte solutions, such as glucose in normal saline and Ringer's solution, are used. Lactated Ringer's solution or another alkalinizing solution may be ordered if metabolic acidosis is present.

Gastric Lavage

Gastric lavage and catharsis—in effect, "washing out" the stomach and intestines—may be performed to remove unabsorbed toxin from the GI tract if botulism is suspected. The patient with botulism is closely observed for signs of respiratory distress. Respiratory support with endotracheal intubation or tracheostomy and mechanical ventilation may be required (∞ see Chapter 37).

Plasmapheresis

Plasmapheresis (plasma exchange therapy) may be performed to remove circulating toxins for hemorrhagic colitis caused by *E. coli*. ∞ See Chapter 44 for the nursing care of a patient having this procedure. Potential complications include those associated with intravenous catheters, shifts in fluid balance, and altered blood clotting.

Dialysis

Acute tubular necrosis and renal failure associated with hemorrhagic colitis may necessitate dialysis to remove wastes and prevent severe fluid and electrolyte imbalances and metabolic acidosis. Although acute renal failure often resolves spontaneously and renal function resumes, dialysis can be lifesaving. Either hemodialysis or peritoneal dialysis may be used, generally as a temporary measure. Nursing care related to acute renal failure and dialysis is discussed in ∞ Chapter 28.

∞ Nursing Care

Although *C. difficile* colitis bacterial infections usually are hospital acquired, few patients with acute enteritis require hospitalization. Most are treated in community settings. Assessment, education, and support of self-care measures are major nursing responsibilities.

Health Promotion

Nurses play a significant role in preventing enteritis as educators, community health providers, and advocates for environmental safety.

Teach the importance of proper food handling and maintaining appropriate temperatures. Raw fruits and vegetables should be thoroughly washed before consuming. Adequate cooking of meat products is vital to prevent disorders such as staphylococcal food poisoning, *E. coli* hemorrhagic colitis, and salmonellosis. Emphasize the importance of not consuming raw meat products, and cooking hamburger, in particular, to the point that no redness is noted in the meat. The highly pathogenic *E. coli* serotype 0157:H7 is present in the gut of infected animals. Meats from the animal may be contaminated with bowel contents. The organism is readily destroyed by heat, so cuts of meat such as steaks or roasts are less likely to cause infection, since the organism is on the outside of the meat. However, the process of grinding hamburger allows *E. coli* to be mixed throughout the meat. Thorough cooking destroys the organism. This pathogen (and others) may be spread through unpasteurized milk. Discuss the dangers of consuming milk that has not been pasteurized and encourage patients to avoid it.

Dairy products, eggs, and egg products left at room temperature provide a good growth medium for bacteria. Discuss the importance of prompt refrigeration of meats and these products to minimize this risk. Many gastrointestinal infections are spread through contaminated water. Encourage travelers to consume only bottled water unless local water supplies are clearly safe. Water purification tablets are available for hikers and campers, and may be used when traveling abroad.

Assessment

- *Health history:* Onset, duration, and severity of manifestations; recent activities such as attending a picnic or potluck, international travel, or camping; other affected members of the household; measures taken to relieve manifestations or replace fluids.
- *Physical examination:* Vital signs including temperature and orthostatic blood pressure; skin color, temperature, moisture, and turgor; peripheral pulses and capillary refill; abdominal shape, contour, bowel sounds, tenderness.

Nursing Diagnoses and Interventions

Diarrhea and fluid volume deficit are priority nursing diagnoses. See the earlier section of this chapter on diarrhea for specific nursing interventions related to these diagnoses. Nausea and vomiting frequently accompany the diarrhea associate with gastroenteritis. Nursing care of the patient experiencing nausea and vomiting is detailed in ∞ Chapter 23.

Community-Based Care

Discuss the following topics with the patient for self-care:

- The importance of good hand hygiene, particularly before handling food and after each bowel movement
- The need to wash clothing and linens contaminated with feces separately in hot water and detergent

- Oral solutions to replace lost fluids and electrolytes
- Appropriate use of antidiarrheal medications if recommended
- Manifestations of complications to report to the healthcare provider

The Patient with a Protozoal Bowel Infection

Parasites live within, on, or at the expense of other organisms. Parasitic intestinal infections are common in developing countries. They include both protozoal and helminthic (parasitic worms) infections. Parasites that infect the bowel usually enter the GI tract through the mouth by the fecal–oral route; some are spread by direct contact or through sexual activity.

Of the protozoal bowel infections, only giardiasis is common in the United States. Amebiasis is found chiefly in the tropics and where sanitation is poor. Cryptosporidiosis, a form of coccidiosis, is an important worldwide cause of sporadic mild diarrhea, traveler's diarrhea, and severe diarrhea in people who are immunocompromised.

Pathophysiology and Manifestations

The most common protozoal infections of the bowel are discussed next and summarized in Table 24–5.

Giardiasis

Giardiasis is a protozoal infection of the upper small intestine caused by *Giardia lamblia*. It is the most common intestinal protozoal pathogen in the United States. Humans and other mammals are the reservoir for *Giardia*. It is spread by the fecal–oral route, usually in contaminated food or water. It is also spread by direct contact. When the cyst form of the organism is ingested, trophozoites emerge in the duodenum and jejunum, attaching themselves to the intestinal mucosa. This leads to superficial invasion, inflammation, and destruction of the mucosa of the small intestine.

Giardiasis may be asymptomatic, although manifestations may develop suddenly or insidiously. Diarrhea is common. It is usually mild, with one or more large, loose stools per day. Diarrhea may be severe, however, with frequent, copious, frothy, malodorous, and greasy stools. Other manifestations include weight loss and weakness; anorexia, nausea, and vomiting; epigastric pain, abdominal cramping and distention, flatulence, and belching. Malabsorption may develop.

Amebiasis

Amebiasis (amebic dysentery) is caused by the protozoon *Entamoeba histolytica*. Several strains of the protozoon have been identified. Humans are the host for this parasite. It usually is transmitted through food or water contaminated by feces and by person-to-person contact. The parasite enters the intestines, where it may live without causing disease, or it may invade the intestinal wall to cause ulceration and inflammation. The cecum, appendix, ascending colon, sigmoid colon, and rectum are most often affected. Ulcers may spread to cause hemorrhage, edema, and mucosal sloughing. The infection may spread via the blood to the liver, lungs, or brain.

Amebiasis is usually asymptomatic. Mild manifestations include abdominal cramps, flatulence, and intermittent diarrhea containing blood and mucus. Severe manifestations of amebic dysentery include frequent watery stools containing blood, mucus, and necrotic tissue; colic, tenesmus, and abdominal tenderness; nausea and vomiting; and fever. The liver may be enlarged and tender to palpation.

Complications are rare, but may include appendicitis, bowel perforation with peritonitis, and fulminating colitis.

TABLE 24–5 Common Protozoal Infections of the Bowel

DISEASE AND ORGANISM	INCUBATION	PATHOGENESIS	MANIFESTATIONS	MANAGEMENT
Giardiasis: *Giardia lamblia*	1 to 3 weeks or more	Trophozoite attaches to mucosa in duodenum and jejunum, causing superficial invasion, inflammation, and tissue destruction.	Diarrhea, mild or severe, daily or intermittent; anorexia, nausea, vomiting; epigastric pain, cramping, distention; flatulence and belching; may be asymptomatic	Metronidazole (Flagyl, others), tinidazole (Tindamax), nitazoxanide (Alinia)
Amebiasis: *Entamoeba histolytica*	2 to 4 weeks	Organisms may reside in large intestine without causing disease or can invade colon wall, causing ulceration; may be carried via blood to liver to produce abscess.	Usually asymptomatic; diarrhea may be mild, with few semiformed mucus-containing stools per day, or severe, with 10 to 20 blood-streaked liquid stools per day; abdominal cramps and flatulence; colic, tenesmus, vomiting, tenderness; fatigue, weight loss; prostration and toxicity	Metronidazole and paromomycin (Humatin) or iodoquinol (Diiodohydroxyquin, Yodoxin); metronidazole or tinidazole for hepatic abscess
Cryptosporidiosis: *Cryptosporidium*	2 to 10 days	Organisms attach to epithelial surface of small bowel (jejunum), causing villous atrophy and mild inflammatory changes; may secrete enterotoxin.	In immunocompetent patients: asymptomatic to profuse, watery diarrhea of sudden onset, abdominal cramping; malaise, fever; anorexia, nausea, vomiting. In immunodeficient patients: profuse watery diarrhea with loss of up to 15 to 20 L/day; severe malabsorption, electrolyte imbalance; weight loss; lymphadenopathy	Self-limiting in immunocompetent patients. For immunodeficient patients: spiramycin, zidovudine (AZT), paromomycin (Humatin), octreotide, eflornithine; fluid and electrolyte replacement; parenteral nutrition as needed

Cryptosporidiosis (Coccidiosis)

Cryptosporidiosis causes sporadic mild diarrhea and traveler's diarrhea in all age groups. In people with impaired immune function, such as those with human immunodeficiency virus (HIV) disease, it causes severe diarrhea, malabsorption, and significant weight loss.

This organism is transmitted by the fecal–oral route. Contaminated water is a frequent source of infection. The organism attaches to epithelium of the small bowel, causing surface damage and inflammation and characteristic watery diarrhea. The disease is self-limited in people with competent immune systems. Watery diarrhea may be accompanied by low-grade fever, nausea, vomiting, abdominal cramps, and general malaise.

Immunocompromised patients develop profuse watery diarrhea with significant fluid and electrolyte losses and severe malabsorption. The organism may be found in the respiratory tract, large intestines, and biliary tract of immunocompromised people. Lymphadenopathy (enlarged lymph nodes) may develop.

Interdisciplinary Care

Management of protozoal bowel infections includes identifying the causative organism and administering medications.

Diagnosis

Diagnostic testing includes a stool examination for ova and parasites, and possibly for their antigens. Many protozoa are shed intermittently rather than continuously; stools are collected sequentially (e.g., every other day for a total of three specimens). These organisms often are fragile, requiring a fresh stool specimen. Serology testing for an immune response to the suspected parasite also may be performed. A sigmoidoscopy may be done to examine the bowel mucosa and collect a stool specimen for examination (in this case, no bowel prep is done prior to the test). When giardiasis is suspected, duodenal aspirate may be stained and examined microscopically for the protozoa. Small bowel biopsy can identify giardiasis or *Cryptosporidium* infection.

MEDICATION ADMINISTRATION   **Antiprotozoal Agents**

LOCAL (GASTROINTESTINAL) AGENTS

Iodoquinol (Yodoxin, Amebaquin)

Paromomycin (Humatin)

These drugs exert a local amebicidal effect in the intestines and are poorly absorbed when administered orally. Local agents have the advantage of provoking fewer side effects than systemically active agents.

Nursing Responsibilities

- Assess for potential contraindications:
  a. Hypersensitivity to the drug or drug class
  b. Iodoquinol: malnutrition, thyroid disorders; hepatic or renal impairment, optic neuropathy, or hypersensitivity to iodine
  c. Paromomycin: ulcerative bowel lesions; hypersensitivity to aminoglycoside antibiotics, impaired renal function, intestinal obstruction
- Observe for adverse effects: anorexia, nausea, vomiting, abdominal cramping, diarrhea, and increased flatulence; report skin rash, visual disturbances, or changes in blood work to primary care provider.

Health Education for the Patient and Family

- Take as prescribed for the full course of therapy.
- Take with food to reduce gastrointestinal effects.
- Keep follow-up appointments as recommended to evaluate the effects of treatment.
- Report adverse effects to the physician:
  a. Any change in vision
  b. Numbness, tingling, or pain in extremities
  c. Chills, fever, skin rash or boils
  d. A change in urination or character of urine
  e. Diminished hearing or tinnitus
  f. Weight loss, diarrhea, fatty stools
  g. Candidiasis of the mouth or vagina
- Practice good hand hygiene, particularly after using the toilet, to prevent spreading the disease to others.

SYSTEMIC AGENTS

Metronidazole (Flagyl, Satric, Metzol, others)

Furazolidone (Furoxone), albendazole (Albenza)

Patients with symptomatic protozoal infections are generally treated with a systemic antiprotozoal agent. Metronidazole is the most widely used of these antiprotozoal agents and is the drug of choice for treating amebiasis.

Nursing Responsibilities

- Assess for possible contraindications to therapy:
  a. Hypersensitivity to the prescribed agent or related drugs
  b. Liver dysfunction or blood dyscrasias
  c. Concurrent use of alcohol or an MAOI
  d. Pregnancy
- Administer as ordered.
  a. Metronidazole may be given orally after meals or as a continuous or intermittent intravenous infusion.
  b. Administer furazolidone and albendazole orally with meals to minimize gastric distress.
- Observe for possible adverse effects; notify the physician if significant. Gastrointestinal effects are common.
  a. Peripheral neuropathy and CNS effects may occur with metronidazole.
  b. Blood dyscrasias may develop with furazolidone or albendazole; monitor CBC and report abnormal results.
  c. Furazolidone can cause hypoglycemia; carefully monitor blood glucose in diabetic patients.
  d. Report abnormal liver function test results.
- Monitor the character and number of stools; obtain specimens as ordered to evaluate the effectiveness of therapy.

Health Education for the Patient and Family

- Take the drug as prescribed for the full duration of the prescription.
- Taking oral preparations after meals helps minimize gastrointestinal side effects. Notify the physician if nausea and vomiting continue.
- Do not use alcohol while taking these drugs. An antabuse-type response with severe headache, flushing, and vomiting may occur.
- Report adverse effects to the physician, including dizziness and other nervous system changes, sore throats, fatigue, bruising, or infection.
- Candidiasis of the mouth or vagina may occur with metronidazole therapy. Report symptoms to the physician.
- A harmless change in urine color to deep yellow (quinacrine) or rust or brown (metronidazole or chloroquine) may occur while taking these drugs.
- If you are diabetic taking furazolidone, carefully monitor blood glucose levels because hypoglycemia may develop.
- Practice good hand hygiene, particularly after using the toilet, to prevent transmitting the protozoa to others.

Medications

Pharmacologic treatment includes both local and systemic antiparasitic drugs, such as iodoquinol (Amebaquin), paromomycin (Humatin), metronidazole (Flagyl), tinidazole (Tindamax), or nitazoxanide (Alinia). Treatment is usually provided on an outpatient basis. Severe amebic dysentery may require hospitalization for intravenous fluid and electrolyte replacements. Nursing care related to common antiprotozoal drugs is outlined in the Medication Administration box on page 677.

ᑭ Nursing Care

Nursing assessment, diagnoses, and interventions for the patient with a protozoal GI infection are similar to those indicated for patients with bacterial or viral infections. *Diarrhea* and *Risk for Deficient Fluid Volume* are priority nursing diagnoses. See previous sections of this chapter for specific nursing interventions related to these diagnoses.

Nurses need to teach the public how parasitic diseases are transmitted and how to avoid spreading the infection. Prevention of amebiasis and giardiasis involves the following:

- Provision of safe water supplies
- Appropriate disposal of human feces
- Safe food storage, handling, and preparation
- Adequate hand hygiene after defecating and before handling food

Instruct people living in high-risk areas (e.g., tropical climates, areas with untreated water supplies) to boil, filter, or treat water supplies with iodine to eliminate protozoal contamination. Instruct them to avoid foods that cannot be peeled or cooked. Teach the manifestations of protozoal infections and where to obtain treatment.

Emphasize the importance of keeping toilet areas clean and maintaining good personal hygiene. Advise the patient to avoid rectal contact during sexual activity. Other household members should have stool specimens examined for parasites. Contaminated recreational water (swimming pools, water slides) is increasingly recognized as a potential source of cryptosporidiosis; advise immunocompromised individuals to avoid this exposure.

The Patient with a Helminthic Disorder

Helminths are parasitic worms, capable of causing infectious diseases in humans. Helminths are subclassified as round worms (nematodes), flukes (trematodes), or tapeworms (cestodes).

Pathophysiology

Although all helminths can infect humans, the definitive host and intermediate hosts vary with each organism. In nearly all instances of helminthic disorders, the organism enters the body through the GI tract in contaminated and inadequately cooked foods. Some of these organisms remain in the intestinal tract; others migrate to infect the liver, lungs, or other structures. Table 24–6 summarizes the most common helminths and their effects.

Interdisciplinary Care

The management of helminthic disorders includes diagnostic testing and medications.

Diagnosis

The primary means of diagnosing helminthic disorders is examination of the stool for ova and parasites. Enterobiasis is diagnosed by the presence of the parasite's eggs on the perianal skin or on cellulose tape placed over the anus. A CBC may also be ordered. Anemia may be present, particularly with hookworm disease. *Eosinophilia* (an increased percentage of eosinophils in the blood) is common in helminthic disorders. With trichinosis, serum muscle enzymes such as the creatinine kinase (CK) and aspartate aminotransferase (AST) are typically elevated. Serologic testing for antibodies to the worm may also be performed. Blood, duodenal washings, and cerebrospinal fluid (CSF) may be examined for the presence of the trichinosis larvae. Inflamed muscle may be biopsied.

Medications

Helminthic infections often are treated with a single oral dose or 3-day course of pyrantel pamoate (Antiminth), albendazole (Albenza), or mebendazole (Vermox). Doses may need to be repeated every 2 weeks for patients with heavy infections. These drugs are generally safe, requiring few precautions. Giving the drug after meals minimizes GI side effects. Treatment is followed by a stool culture at 2 weeks to evaluate effectiveness. If necessary, an additional course of the drug is prescribed. Other members of the household are generally also treated.

Most patients with trichinosis recover spontaneously without long-term effects. The intestinal phase of the disease is treated with albendazole, taken twice daily for as long as 60 days, or a 13-day course of mebendazole. Hospitalization may be required during the muscle invasion phase of the disease if the infection is severe. Corticosteroids may be used to reduce the inflammation and manage the manifestations.

ᑭ Nursing Care

Because many patients with these disorders are asymptomatic, nurses need to be alert for histories that indicate risk and subtle manifestations of the disorder. Use standard precautions to minimize the risk of spreading these infections to other patients. Wear gloves and gowns as necessary to prevent fecal contamination of hands and clothing. On rare occasions, parasites may be present in the sputum or vomitus, so handle these secretions with care. Disinfect toilets, toilet seats, and commodes after use. Teach the patient the importance of hand hygiene after using the toilet and before handling food to prevent reinfection.

Discuss measures to prevent spread of the disease in the household. Emphasize the importance of hygiene measures including changing bedding, daily cleaning of toilets with disinfectant, and hand hygiene.

Many helminthic disorders are acquired by consuming food that has been fecally contaminated or contains larvae of the organism. Explain the importance of not fertilizing food or grain crops with fecal material, particularly human feces. Teach

TABLE 24–6 Selected Helminthic Diseases

	INFECTION	HOST	AREA	PATHOGENESIS	MANIFESTATIONS
Nematode infections	Ascariasis	Humans	Worldwide, cosmopolitan; warm, moist climates	Eggs are ingested in fecally contaminated food and drink; motile larvae migrate to lungs and back to small intestine, where they mature to produce more eggs.	Pulmonary: low-grade fever, cough, blood-tinged sputum, wheezing, dyspnea, substernal chest pain. GI: ulcer-like epigastric pain, vomiting, abdominal distention
	Enterobiasis (pinworm infection)	Humans	Worldwide, cosmopolitan	Infect cecum; eggs deposit on perianal skin, organisms may be transmitted to others or reinfect host by oral ingestion.	Nocturnal perianal and perineal pruritus; insomnia, irritability, restlessness
	Hookworm disease	Humans	Tropics and subtropics	Larvae enter through skin or by ingestion and migrate to lungs, up bronchial tree, and down esophagus to mature in upper small bowel, where they attach and suck blood.	Skin: pruritic dermatitis at site of entry Pulmonary: dry cough, wheezing, blood-tinged sputum GI: anorexia, diarrhea, abdominal pain Systemic: anemia, pallor, cardiac insufficiency
	Trichinosis	Pigs, dogs, cats, rats, many wild animals	Temperate areas where pork is consumed	Larvae are ingested in undercooked meat; adult female burrows into mucosa of small intestine to produce larvae that disseminate via blood and lymphatic system to body tissues and become encysted in striated muscle.	GI: diarrhea, abdominal cramps, malaise Muscle: fever; muscle pain, tenderness, edema, and spasm Systemic: periorbital and facial edema, sweating; photophobia and conjunctivitis; manifestations of inflammation in tissues invaded by larvae
Cestode infections	Fasciolopsiasis (intestinal fluke) Tapeworm	Humans; other mammals and fish	Worldwide	Organism is ingested by eating uncooked fish or meat containing embryo cysts, by fecal contamination, or by swallowing infected intermediate hosts, such as arthropods, fleas, or lice; head (scolex) of adult worm attaches in upper small intestine, and eggs form in individual segments.	Large tapeworms: often asymptomatic; infection may cause mild nausea, diarrhea, abdominal pain; anemia, thrombocytopenia, and mild leukopenia Small tapeworms: may be asymptomatic; diarrhea, abdominal pain, anorexia, vomiting, weight loss, and irritability

patients to cook all meats and fish adequately to destroy possible larvae. In general, pickled or salt-preserved meats and fish are no safer than raw. Smoking, another means of preserving fish and meat, may not achieve temperatures high enough to destroy the organisms. Vegetables grown in soil that may be contaminated with eggs or larvae should be peeled or cooked prior to eating.

Emphasize the importance of safe water supplies. Encourage people traveling to areas in which water supplies are questionable to drink only bottled water or carry purification tablets. Work with patients who have private water systems to protect water from fecal contamination by either humans or animals.

The patient with a helminthic disorder may feel dirty or be ashamed of the disease. Emphasize the prevalence of these disorders, and assure the patient that infection can occur despite good health practices when the eggs or larva of the organism are prevalent.

Chronic Inflammatory Bowel Disorders

The Patient with Inflammatory Bowel Disease

Chronic **inflammatory bowel disease (IBD)** includes two separate but closely related conditions: ulcerative colitis and Crohn's disease. These conditions have a number of similarities.

The etiology of both illnesses is unknown, although current evidence implicates both genetic and environmental factors. IBD occurs more frequently in the United States and northern European nations than it does in southern Europe and countries in the Southern Hemisphere. IBD affects certain ethnic groups more than others, as outlined in the following

Focus on Cultural Diversity box. As many as 1 million Americans have IBD, with that number divided about equally between ulcerative colitis and Crohn's disease (Crohn's & Colitis Foundation of America [CCFA], 2009). It tends to run in families, with 15% to 25% of patients having a close relative with one of the types of IBD (CCFA, 2009). Factors such as an abnormal immune response to microorganisms normally found in the gut are thought to play a role in the development of IBD. Factors such as smoking and oral contraceptive use also affect the risk for IBD.

The peak incidence of IBD is in adolescents and young adults between the ages of 15 and 30 years but it also affects older adults (Fauci et al., 2008). IBD is a chronic and recurrent disease process. Responses to physiologic or psychologic stresses do not cause IBD, but often play a role in exacerbations of the disease.

Despite the similarities, ulcerative colitis and Crohn's disease have distinct differences. Ulcerative colitis primarily affects the large bowel in a continuous pattern, progressing distally to proximally. In Crohn's disease, a patchy pattern of involvement is seen, affecting primarily the small intestine. Ulcerative colitis shows mainly mucosal involvement; in Crohn's disease, the submucosal layers of the bowel are affected. A comparison of ulcerative colitis and Crohn's disease is found in Table 24–7. The Multisystem Effects of Inflammatory Bowel Disease are illustrated on page 682.

Ulcerative Colitis

Ulcerative colitis is a chronic inflammatory bowel disorder that affects the mucosa and submucosa of the colon and rectum. Most people with ulcerative colitis have mild or moderate disease, with six or fewer stools per day. Its onset usually is insidious, with attacks that last 1 to 3 months occurring at intervals of months to years. Typically, only the distal colon is affected, with few systemic manifestations of the disease. Approximately 15% of people with ulcerative colitis develop *fulminant colitis*, with involvement of the entire colon, severe bloody diarrhea, acute abdominal pain, and fever. Patients with fulminant disease are at high risk for complications.

Pathophysiology

The inflammatory process of ulcerative colitis begins at the rectosigmoid area of the anal canal and progresses proximally. In most patients, the disease is confined to the rectum and sigmoid colon. It may progress to involve the entire colon, stopping at the ileocecal junction.

Ulcerative colitis begins with inflammation at the base of the crypts of Lieberkühn in the distal large intestine and rectum. Microscopic, pinpoint mucosal hemorrhages occur, and crypt

TABLE 24–7 Characteristics of Ulcerative Colitis and Crohn's Disease

	CHARACTERISTIC	ULCERATIVE COLITIS	CROHN'S DISEASE
Clinical	Gender	Equal	Equal
	Age at onset	15 to 30 years; secondary peak 60 to 80 years	15 to 30 years; secondary peak 60 to 80 years
	Course of disease	Typically chronic and intermittent	Slowly progressive, relapsing
	Diarrhea	5 to 30 stools per day with blood and mucus	Common, usually less severe than colitis, with no obvious blood or mucus in stool
	Abdominal pain	Cramping in left lower quadrant; relieved by defecation	Cramping or steady right lower quadrant or periumbilical pain; tenderness and mass noted in right lower quadrant
	Nutritional deficit	Common; involves anemia, hypoalbuminemia, and weight loss	Common and significant: involves anemia, weight loss, and multiple vitamin and mineral deficits
	Constitutional manifestations	Fever rare; may have associated arthritic, skin, or other organ involvement, such as erythema nodosum or uveitis	Fever, malaise, fatigue; may have some associated conditions plus urinary complications
Pathologic	Depth of involvement	Mucosa and submucosa	Transmural (entire bowel wall)
	Portion of bowel involved	Typically rectum and sigmoid colon; may extend to involve entire large bowel	Any portion of GI tract; terminal ileum and ascending colon involvement predominates
	Distribution	Continuous from rectum	Patchy; skip lesions
	Appearance of mucosa	Granular, dull, hyperemic, friable; disease uniform in affected bowel; pseudopolyps may be seen	Cobblestone appearance, with areas of normal tissue surrounded by ulceration and fissures
Complications	Acute	Toxic megacolon, perforation, massive hemorrhage	Obstruction, fistulization, abscess formation, malabsorption
	Long term	Colorectal cancer	Colon cancer

abscesses develop (Figure 24–3 ■). These abscesses penetrate the superficial submucosa and spread laterally, leading to necrosis and sloughing of bowel mucosa. Further tissue damage is caused by inflammatory exudates and the release of inflammatory mediators, such as prostaglandins and other cytokines (∞ see Chapter 12 for further discussion of the inflammatory process). The mucosa is red and edematous due to vascular congestion, friable (easily broken), and ulcerated. It bleeds easily, and hemorrhage is common. Edema creates a granular appearance. Pseudopolyps, tonguelike projections of bowel mucosa into the lumen, may develop as the epithelial lining of the bowel regenerates. Chronic inflammation leads to atrophy, narrowing, and shortening of the colon, with loss of its normal haustra.

Manifestations

Diarrhea is the predominant manifestation of ulcerative colitis. Stools contain both blood and mucus. Nocturnal diarrhea may occur. Mild ulcerative colitis is characterized by fewer than 4 stools per day, intermittent rectal bleeding and mucus, and few systemic manifestations. Severe ulcerative colitis can lead to more than 6 to 10 bloody stools per day, extensive colon involvement, anemia, hypovolemia, and malnutrition. Rectal inflammation causes fecal urgency and tenesmus. Left lower quadrant cramping relieved by defecation is common. Other manifestations include fatigue, anorexia, and weakness.

Patients with severe disease may also have systemic manifestations such as arthritis involving one or several joints, skin and mucous membrane lesions, or *uveitis* (inflammation of the uvea, the vascular layer of the eye, which may also involve the sclera and cornea). Some patients develop thromboemboli, with blood vessel obstruction due to clots carried from the site of their formation. The liver and biliary system may be affected by the disease, as may the kidneys, with an increased risk for gallstones, cirrhosis, kidney stones, and ureteral obstruction (Fauci et al., 2008).

Complications

Acute complications of ulcerative colitis include hemorrhage, toxic megacolon, and colon perforation. Massive hemorrhage may occur with severe attacks of the disease. *Toxic megacolon*, a condition characterized by acute motor paralysis and dilation of the colon to greater than 6 cm, may affect part or all of the colon. The transverse segment of the bowel is most often affected. Toxic megacolon may be triggered by the use of laxatives, narcotics, and electrolyte imbalances (Fauci et al., 2008). Manifestations of toxic megacolon include fever, tachycardia, hypotension, dehydration, abdominal tenderness and cramping, and a change in the number of stools per day. Perforation is rare, but the risk of this dangerous complication is increased with toxic megacolon. Perforation leads to peritonitis.

The risk for colorectal cancer is increased in patients with ulcerative colitis. Beginning 8 to 15 years after the diagnosis, annual or biennial colonoscopies with biopsy to detect masses or cell dysplasia are recommended for patients who have extensive ulcerative colitis (Fauci et al., 2008).

Crohn's Disease

Like ulcerative colitis, Crohn's disease, also known as regional enteritis, is a chronic, relapsing inflammatory disorder affecting the gastrointestinal tract. Crohn's disease can affect any portion of the GI tract from the mouth to the anus, but usually affects the terminal ileum and ascending colon. Only the small bowel is involved in nearly 40% of patients with Crohn's disease. The disease is limited to the colon bowel in 30% of those affected. Both the small and large intestine are involved in the remaining 30% of patients (Porth & Matfin, 2009).

Figure 24–3 ■ *A,* Photomicrograph of the mucosa of the large intestine showing the entrances to the crypts of Lieberkühn. The crypts are the focal points for *B,* ulcerative colitis and *C,* Crohn's disease.

Source: B, Dr. E. Walker/Photo Researchers, Inc.; *C,* Javier Domingo/Photo Researchers, Inc.

MULTISYSTEM EFFECTS OF
Irritable Bowel Disease

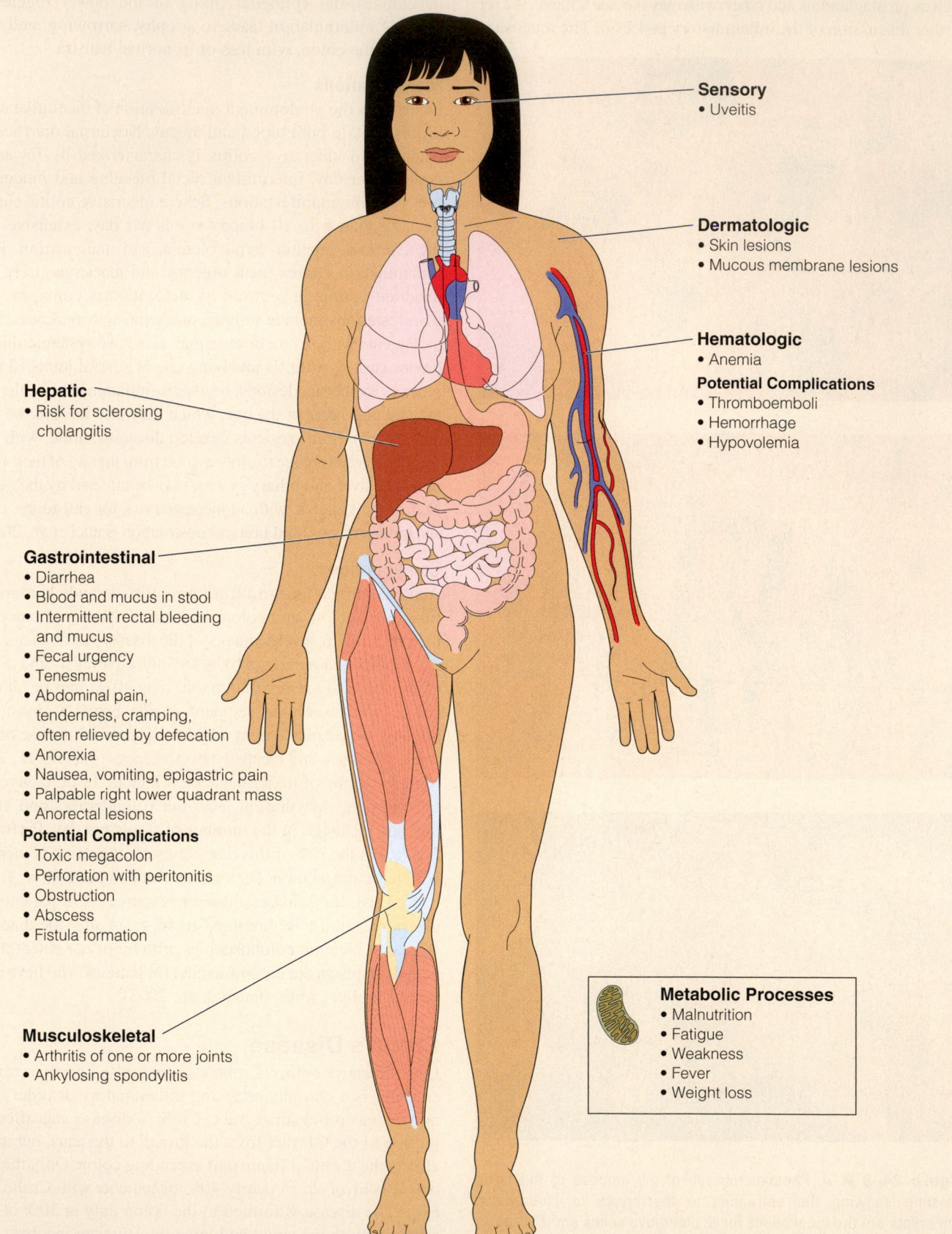

Sensory
- Uveitis

Dermatologic
- Skin lesions
- Mucous membrane lesions

Hematologic
- Anemia

Potential Complications
- Thromboemboli
- Hemorrhage
- Hypovolemia

Hepatic
- Risk for sclerosing cholangitis

Gastrointestinal
- Diarrhea
- Blood and mucus in stool
- Intermittent rectal bleeding and mucus
- Fecal urgency
- Tenesmus
- Abdominal pain, tenderness, cramping, often relieved by defecation
- Anorexia
- Nausea, vomiting, epigastric pain
- Palpable right lower quadrant mass
- Anorectal lesions

Potential Complications
- Toxic megacolon
- Perforation with peritonitis
- Obstruction
- Abscess
- Fistula formation

Musculoskeletal
- Arthritis of one or more joints
- Ankylosing spondylitis

Metabolic Processes
- Malnutrition
- Fatigue
- Weakness
- Fever
- Weight loss

Pathophysiology

Crohn's disease typically begins as a small inflammatory *aphthoid lesion* (shallow ulcers with a white base and elevated margin, similar to a canker sore) of the mucosa and submucosa of the bowel. These initial lesions may regress, or the inflammatory process can progress to involve all layers of the intestinal wall. Deeper ulcerations, granulomatous lesions, and fissures (knife-like clefts that extend deeply into the bowel wall) develop. The inflammatory process involves the entire bowel wall (transmural).

The lumen of the affected bowel assumes a "cobblestone appearance" as fissures and ulcers surround islands of intact mucosa over edematous submucosa. The inflammatory lesions of Crohn's disease are not continuous; rather, they often occur as "skip" lesions with intervening areas of normal-appearing bowel. Some evidence suggests that despite its normal appearance, the entire bowel is affected by this disorder.

As the disease progresses, fibrotic changes in the bowel wall cause it to thicken and lose flexibility, taking on an appearance that has been likened to a rubber hose. The inflammation, edema, and fibrosis can lead to local obstruction, abscess development, and the formation of fistulas between loops of bowel or bowel and other organs (Figure 24–4 ■). Fistulas between loops of bowel are known as enteroenteric fistulas; those that occur between bowel and bladder are known as enterovesical fistulas; and fistulas that occur between bowel and skin are known as enterocutaneous fistulas. Perineal fistulas are relatively common, originating in the ileum.

Depending on the severity and extent of the disease, malabsorption and malnutrition may develop as the ulcers prevent absorption of nutrients. When the jejunum and ileum are affected, the absorption of multiple nutrients may be impaired, including carbohydrates, proteins, fats, vitamins, and folate. Disease in the terminal ileum can lead to vitamin B_{12} malabsorption and bile salt reabsorption. The ulcerations can also lead to protein loss and chronic, slow blood loss with consequent anemia.

Manifestations

Because the GI system involvement in Crohn's disease can be so diverse, manifestations vary among patients. The majority of people with Crohn's disease experience persistent diarrhea. Stools are liquid or semiformed and typically do not contain blood, although blood may be passed if the colon is involved. Abdominal pain and tenderness are also common. The pain may be located in the right lower quadrant and relieved by defecation. A palpable right lower quadrant mass is often present. Systemic manifestations such as fever, fatigue, malaise, weight loss, and anemia are common. Anorectal lesions such as fissures, ulcers, fistulas, and abscesses also are common and may occur years before intestinal disease is apparent. If the stomach and duodenum are involved, nausea, vomiting, and epigastric pain may occur.

Complications

Certain complications of Crohn's disease (e.g., intestinal obstruction, abscess, and fistula) are so common that they are considered part of the disease process. For many patients, the disease initially presents with one of these complications. Intestinal obstruction is a common complication caused by repeated inflammation and scarring of the bowel that leads to fibrosis and stricture. Obstruction of the bowel lumen causes abdominal distention, cramping pain, and borborygmi. Nausea and vomiting may occur.

Fistulas may be asymptomatic, particularly if they occur between loops of small bowel. When fistulization causes an abscess, chills and fever, a tender abdominal mass, and leukocytosis develop. A fistula between the small bowel and colon may exacerbate diarrhea, weight loss, and malnutrition. When the bladder is involved, recurrent urinary tract infections occur.

Perforation of the bowel is uncommon, but can lead to generalized peritonitis. Massive hemorrhage also is an uncommon complication of Crohn's disease. Long-standing Crohn's disease increases the risk of cancer of the small intestine or colon by five to six times. This cancer risk, however, is significantly lower than the risk associated with ulcerative colitis.

Interdisciplinary Care

Interdisciplinary care for inflammatory bowel disease begins by establishing the diagnosis and the extent and severity of the disease. Treatment is supportive, including medications and dietary measures to decrease inflammation, promote intestinal rest and healing, and reduce intestinal motility. Many patients with IBD require surgery at some point to manage the disease or its complications.

Diagnosis

Diagnostic testing is used to establish the diagnosis of IBD, assess the extent of the disease, and evaluate the effects of the disorder. A sigmoidoscopy, colonoscopy, or a barium upper and lower x-ray series is performed to inspect the bowel mucosa for characteristic changes of IBD. (Nursing implications for these diagnostic tests are outlined in ∞ Chapter 21).

Laboratory tests to differentiate IBD and to identify effects and complications of the disease include a stool examination

Figure 24–4 ■ The progression of Crohn's disease.

for blood and mucus, and stool cultures to rule out infectious causes of bowel inflammation and diarrhea. CBC with hemoglobin and hematocrit shows anemia from chronic inflammation, blood loss, and malnutrition, and leukocytosis due to inflammation and possible abscess formation. The sedimentation rate and levels of C-reactive protein are typically elevated during periods of acute inflammation. Serum albumin may be decreased because of malabsorption, malnutrition, protein loss through intestinal lesions, and chronic inflammation. Folic acid and serum levels of most vitamins, including A, B complex, C, and the fat-soluble vitamins, often are decreased due to malabsorption. Additional tests for renal and hepatic function may be done if the patient has significant systemic manifestations of the disease.

Medications

The ultimate goal of care is to achieve and maintain remission of the disease and its symptoms. Drug therapy plays a key role in achieving this goal. Locally acting and systemic anti-inflammatory drugs are the primary medications used to manage mild to moderate IBD. Drugs to suppress the immune response may be used to treat patients with severe disease.

Sulfasalazine (Azulfidine) is a sulfonamide antibiotic and anti-inflammatory that is poorly absorbed from the gastrointestinal tract and acts topically on the colonic mucosa to inhibit the inflammatory process. The active anti-inflammatory ingredient in sulfasalazine, 5-aminosalicylic acid (5-ASA), also is available in preparations that do not contain sulfa, such as olsalazine and mesalamine. They have the advantage of causing fewer adverse effects than sulfasalazine. Azo compounds, such as balsalazide and olsalazine, are 5-ASA compounds that are released in the colon and are especially useful to treat ulcerative colitis. Mesalamine (Canasa, Rowasa) is an orally or rectally administered 5-ASA compound that provides topical anti-inflammatory action in the colon of patients with ulcerative colitis. Specific preparations, their method of action, and nursing implications for these medications are outlined in the Medication Administration box on page 685.

For acute exacerbations of IBD, corticosteroids are given to reduce inflammation and induce remission. For ulcerative colitis, the drug may be administered rectally for its local effect and to minimize systemic effects. Hydrocortisone can be administered rectally. Intravenous corticosteroids may be required to treat severe disease; oral preparations are used for less severe manifestations and long-term therapy. Corticosteroids are tapered off once remission has been achieved.

Mercaptopurine (6-MP, Purinethol) and other immunosuppressive agents such as azathioprine (Imuran), methotrexate, and cyclosporine (Sandimmune) can be used to treat patients who have not responded to other treatments or who require chronic steroid therapy. These drugs may allow withdrawal from corticosteroids, maintain remission, and facilitate healing. Long-term therapy may be required to produce a beneficial effect. For more information about immunosuppressive drugs, ∞ see Chapter 13.

Newer treatments for IBD employ other immune response modifiers, such as the monoclonal antibody infliximab (Remicade) to suppress tumor necrosis factor (TNF, an inflammatory mediator substance) in patients who have not responded to standard therapies. Although antibiotic therapy generally is not indicated in IBD, metronidazole (Flagyl) has active anti-inflammatory effects. It may be prescribed to help prevent remission after ileal resection in Crohn's disease. Ciprofloxacin (Cipro) is an alternative to metronidazole.

Antidiarrheal agents, such as loperamide and diphenoxylate, may be given to slow gastrointestinal motility and reduce diarrhea. These drugs are safe for patients with mild, chronic manifestations, but they are not given during acute attacks because they may precipitate toxic dilation of the colon.

Nutrition

Antigens in the diet may stimulate the immune response in the bowel, exacerbating IBD. As a result, dietary management for inflammatory bowel disease is individualized. Some patients benefit from eliminating all milk and milk products from the diet. Increased dietary fiber may help reduce diarrhea and relieve rectal manifestations, but is contraindicated for patients with intestinal strictures caused by repeated inflammation and scarring.

All food may be withheld to promote bowel rest during an acute exacerbation of Crohn's disease. Nutritional status is maintained using enteral or total parenteral nutrition (TPN). ∞ See Chapter 22 for more information about enteral feedings and TPN. TPN carries a higher risk of complications than does enteral nutrition. An elemental diet such as Ensure, which contains all essential nutrients in a residue-free formula, may be prescribed. Elemental diets provide essential nutrients to the small intestine to support cell growth, but are not always palatable.

Surgery

Surgical interventions for IBD differ, depending on the primary disease process and the portion of the bowel affected. Generally, surgery is performed only when necessitated by complications of the disease or failure of conservative treatment measures.

Bowel obstruction is the leading indication for surgery in Crohn's disease. Other complications that may require surgical intervention include perforation, internal or external fistula, abscess, and perianal complications. Resection of the affected portion of bowel with an end-to-end anastomosis to preserve as much bowel as possible is the usual treatment. The disease process tends to recur in other areas following removal of affected bowel segments. There is an increased risk of fistula formation following surgery. Bowel strictures may be treated with a strictureplasty. In this procedure, longitudinal incisions are made in the narrowed segment to relieve the stricture while preserving bowel.

COLECTOMY Patients with extensive chronic ulcerative colitis may require a total **colectomy** (surgical resection and removal of the colon) to treat the disease itself; for complications such as toxic megacolon, perforation, or hemorrhage; or as a prophylactic measure due to the high colon cancer risk associated with extensive ulcerative colitis.

The surgical procedure of choice for extensive ulcerative colitis is a *total colectomy with an ileal pouch-anal anastomosis (IPAA)*. In this procedure, the entire colon and rectum are

MEDICATION ADMINISTRATION Inflammatory Bowel Disease

SULFASALAZINE (AZULFIDINE)

Sulfasalazine is an anti-inflammatory drug used for its local effect on the intestinal mucosa in inflammatory bowel disease. The active part of the drug is 5-ASA, which inhibits prostaglandin production in the bowel. Prostaglandin is an important mediator of the inflammatory process; blocking its production reduces inflammation.

Nursing Responsibilities

- Assess for contraindications, including pregnancy or a history of hypersensitivity to sulfonamides or salicylates.
- Assess baseline values for renal function tests (serum creatinine, BUN, urinalysis), liver function tests, and CBC.
- Administer as ordered. Suppositories or retention enemas may be administered at bedtime. Administer oral forms with a full glass of water.
- Have resuscitation equipment available; anaphylactic responses may occur.
- Evaluate for therapeutic response, including reduced number of stools, reduced mucus and blood, and improved stool consistency.
- Monitor for possible adverse responses:
  - a. Headache, anorexia, nausea, or vomiting
  - b. Skin rash, dermatitis, urticaria, or pruritus
  - c. Evidence of blood dyscrasias, such as bleeding, easy bruising, fever
  - d. Leukopenia, thrombocytopenia, hemolytic anemia, or agranulocytosis
  - e. Changes in urinary output or renal function studies
  - f. Evidence of hepatitis or myocarditis

Health Education for the Patient and Family

- Take oral preparations after meals to decrease gastric distress.
- Drink at least 2 quarts of fluid per day to reduce the risk of kidney damage.
- Use sunscreen to prevent burns; this drug increases sensitivity to sun.
- Do not take aspirin, vitamin C, or any other over-the-counter medications containing aspirin or vitamin C without consulting your doctor.
- This medication may interfere with the effectiveness of oral contraceptives; use alternative methods of contraception.
- Notify your doctor if you develop headache, anorexia, nausea, vomiting, skin rash or hives, sore throat or mouth, bleeding gums, joint pain, easy bruising, or fever.

MESALAMINE (ASACOL ROWASA) AND OLSALAZINE (DIPENTUM)

Mesalamine and olsalazine contain the same active ingredient, 5-ASA, as sulfasalazine, but cause fewer adverse effects. Their mechanism of action is the same as that of sulfasalazine. These drugs are available as suppositories, suspension for enema, or oral tablets.

Nursing Responsibilities

- Assess for possible contraindications such as pregnancy, lactation, or hypersensitivity to these drugs or aspirin.
- Administer as ordered. If more than one dose per day is ordered, space doses evenly over the 24-hour period.
- Evaluate for desired effects (as for sulfasalazine) and potential adverse effects.
  - a. Nausea, diarrhea, abdominal cramps, or flatulence
  - b. CNS effects including headache, dizziness, insomnia, weakness, or fatigue
  - c. Rash or itching
  - d. Flulike symptoms, general malaise

Health Education for the Patient and Family

- Teach the recommended method of administration, including how to insert rectal suppositories or administer a retention enema.

- Shake suspension forms well prior to using.
- Diarrhea is the most common side effect of these drugs. Notify your doctor if adverse effects occur.

CORTICOSTEROIDS

Methylprednisolone (Medrol, Solu-Medrol)

Prednisolone (Delta-Cortel) Prednisone

Glucocorticoids are hormones produced by the adrenal cortex. These hormones are necessary for the stress response. Cortisol, the main glucocorticoid, has potent anti-inflammatory effects. Corticosteroids are used to treat acute episodes of IBD. Because of their multiple and significant side effects, they are not used to maintain remission.

Nursing Responsibilities

- Assess for conditions that may be adversely affected by corticosteroid drugs: peptic ulcer disease, glaucoma or cataracts, diabetes, or psychiatric disorders.
- Obtain baseline vital signs and weight; monitor both routinely during therapy. Hypertension and weight gain may result from salt and water retention.
- Monitor for edema.
- Administer as ordered. For daily or alternate-day dosing, administer in the morning, when physiologic glucocorticoid levels are highest, to reduce adrenal cortisone suppression.
- Administer oral preparations with food to decrease gastrointestinal side effects. Antacids or histamine H_2-receptor blocking agents, such as cimetidine (Tagamet), may be prescribed during corticosteroid therapy.
- Monitor for desired effects: reduced diarrhea, less blood and mucus in the stool, and less abdominal cramping.
- Monitor for adverse effects:
  - a. Increased susceptibility to infection and masking of early signs of infection
  - b. Hyperglycemia
  - c. Hypokalemia, as manifested by muscle weakness, nausea, vomiting, and cardiac rhythm disturbances
  - d. Edema, hypertension, and signs of heart failure
  - e. Peptic ulcer formation and possible gastrointestinal hemorrhage (abdominal pain, black or tarry stools, and signs of bleeding)
  - f. Changes in mental status, including depression, euphoria, aggression, and behavioral changes
  - g. With long-term use, cushingoid effects, such as abnormal fat deposits in the face (moon faces) and trunk (buffalo hump), muscle wasting and thin extremities, thinning of the skin, and osteoporosis

Health Education for the Patient and Family

- Take as prescribed; do not change the dose or time of day. Do not stop the medication abruptly. The dose will be tapered down gradually when the drug is discontinued.
- Notify the physician if adverse or cushingoid effects occur.
- Take with food or at mealtimes to decrease the gastrointestinal effects.
- Monitor weight. If a gain of more than 5 pounds is noted, notify the physician.
- Moderate salt intake and avoid foods and snacks high in sodium, such as processed meats and potato chips. Increase intake of foods high in potassium, such as fruits, vegetables, and lean meats.
- Carry a card or wear a bracelet or tag at all times identifying corticosteroid use.

Figure 24–5 ■ Ileal pouch-anal anastomosis (IPAA).

removed; a pouch is formed from the terminal ileum; and the pouch is brought into the pelvis and anastomosed to the anal canal (Figure 24–5 ■). A temporary or loop ileostomy (described in the next section) is generally performed at the same time and is maintained for 2 to 3 months to allow the anal anastomosis to heal. When the healing is complete, the ileostomy is closed, and the patient has six to eight daily bowel movements through the anus. Advanced age, obesity, or other factors may preclude an IPAA. For these patients, a permanent ileostomy or continent ileostomy may be created.

OSTOMY   An intestinal ostomy is a surgically created opening between the intestine and the abdominal wall that allows the passage of fecal material. The surface opening is called a **stoma** (Figure 24–6 ■). The precise name of the ostomy depends on the location of the stoma. An **ileostomy** is an ostomy made in the ileum of the small intestine. In an ileostomy, the colon, rectum, and anus are usually completely removed (*total proctocolectomy with permanent ileostomy*). The anal canal is closed, and the end of the terminal ileum is brought to the body surface through the right abdominal wall to form the stoma. A temporary or *loop ileostomy* may be formed to eliminate feces and allow tissue healing for 2 to 3 months following an IPAA. A loop of ileum is brought to the body surface to form a stoma and allow stool drainage into an external pouch. When the ileostomy is no longer necessary, a second surgery is performed to close the stoma and repair the bowel, restoring fecal elimination through the anus.

In a *continent ileostomy* (Figure 24–7 ■), an intra-abdominal reservoir is constructed and a nipple valve formed (the ileum folded back on itself) from the terminal ileum, before it is brought to the surface of the abdominal wall. Stool collects in the internal pouch; the nipple valve prevents it from leaking through the stoma. A catheter is inserted into the pouch to drain the stool.

Nursing care of the patient with an ileostomy is outlined in the following box. Procedure 24–1 on page 688 describes how to apply one- and two-piece drainable ostomy pouches.

Figure 24–6 ■ A healthy-appearing stoma.
Courtesy of Carol Williams, RN, BS, UC Davis Medical Center.

Complementary and Alternative Therapies

The chronic nature of IBD and adverse effects of many prescribed treatments lead up to 50% of patients with IBD to seek or use complementary and alternative therapies. The most common complementary therapies used by patients with IBD include herbal therapies, nutritional supplements, probiotics, and fish oil (Langmead & Rampton, 2006; Mayo Clinic, 2008). Herbal remedies such as aloe vera gel and curcumin appear to have a beneficial effect, as do Chinese traditional medicine including Jian Pi Ling tablets and Yukui tang tablets. Probiotics, bacteria similar to those normally found in the gut, appear to have a beneficial anti-inflammatory effect in the bowel (Connelly, 2008). Probiotics are available in foods such as yogurt, miso, and soy beverages, as well as in dietary supplements. Results have been mixed in studies of the beneficial effect of fish oil or Omega-3 fatty acid supplements for IBD. Peppermint tea is an excellent tonic for reducing nausea, relieving abdominal pain, and providing a calming effect. Chamomile tea helps to reduce intestinal inflammation (Balch & Stengler, 2004). Anecdotal evidence supports the use of homeopathy to promote comfort in patients with IBD. Acupuncture improves perceived well-being in patients with IBD, but does not appear to effect remission (Langmead & Rampton, 2006). Many complementary and alternative therapies for IBD may interact with prescribed medications; instruct the patient to discuss all potential therapies with the primary care provider. Acupressure, body massage, reflexology, aromatherapy, and stress reduction therapies can also aid in reducing manifestations of IBD.

Figure 24–7 ■ Continent (Kock's) ileostomy.

NURSING CARE OF THE PATIENT   Having an Ileostomy

PREOPERATIVE CARE

■ Provide routine preoperative care and teaching as outlined in ∞ Chapter 4.

■ Refer to an enterostomal therapist for marking and teaching about the stoma location, ostomy care, and options for ostomy appliances. *It is important to begin teaching prior to surgery to facilitate learning and acceptance of the ostomy postoperatively.*

■ Discuss the availability of a local United Ostomy Association chapter, and provide a referral as necessary or desired. *Local chapters often have members with ostomies who are willing to provide both preoperative and postoperative teaching, listening, and support.*

■ Provide preoperative bowel preparation as ordered. *Cathartics, enemas, and preoperative antibiotics are often ordered to reduce the risk of abdominal contamination and infection after surgery.*

POSTOPERATIVE CARE

■ Provide routine postoperative care and teaching as outlined in ∞ Chapter 4.

■ Apply an ostomy pouch over the stoma. (See Procedure 24–1.) *Stool from an ileostomy is expressed continuously or irregularly, and it is liquid in nature; continuous use of a pouch to collect the drainage is necessary.*

■ Assess frequently for bleeding, stoma viability, and function. In the early postoperative period, small amounts of blood in the pouch are expected. A healthy stoma appears pink or red and moist as a result of mucous production (Figure 24–6). It should protrude approximately 2 cm from the abdominal wall. *Frequent assessment is particularly important in the initial postoperative period to ensure stoma health and monitor for possible complications. A dusky, brown, black, or white stoma indicates circulatory compromise. Other possible stoma complications include retraction (indentation or loss of the external portion of the stoma) or prolapse (outward telescoping of the stoma, that is, an abnormally long stoma).*

■ As the stoma starts to function, empty the pouch, explaining the procedure to the patient. Initial drainage is dark green, viscid, and usually odorless. Drainage gradually thickens and becomes yellow-brown. Empty the pouch when it is one-third full. Measure drainage, and include it as output on intake and output records. Rinse the pouch and reapply the clamp. *Emptying the pouch when it is no more than one-third full helps prevent the skin seal from breaking as a result of the weight of the pouch. Because of the potential for excess fluid loss through ileostomy drainage, it is important to include it as fluid output.*

■ Assess the peristomal skin. Skin around the stoma should remain clean and pink and free of irritation, rashes, inflammation, or excoriation. *Skin complications may arise from appliance irritation or hypersensitivity, excoriation from a leaking appliance, or* Candida albicans, *a yeast infection.*

■ Protect peristomal skin from enzymes and bile salts in the ileostomy effluent. Using a skin barrier on the pouch is essential. Change the pouch if leakage occurs or if the patient complains of burning or itching skin. *Enzymes and bile salts normally reabsorbed in the large intestine are irritating to the skin. Excoriation of skin surrounding the stoma impairs the first line of defense against microorganisms and can interfere with the ability to achieve a tight skin seal and prevent pouch leakage.*

■ Report the following abnormal assessment findings to the physician:
  a. Allergic or contact dermatitis. *A rash may result from contact with fecal drainage or indicate sensitivity to pouch, paste, tape, or sealant.*
  b. Purulent ulcerated areas surrounding the stoma. *Disruption of the protective barrier of the skin allows bacterial entry.*
  c. A red, bumpy, itchy rash or white-coated area. *This is a manifestation of* Candida albicans, *a yeast infection.*
  d. Bulging around the stoma. *This finding may indicate herniation, caused by loops of intestine protruding through the abdominal wall.*

■ Apply protective ointments to the perirectal area of patients with newly functioning ileoanal reservoirs and anastomoses. *This helps protect the skin from the initial stools. As stools thicken and become fewer per day, the patient experiences less perirectal irritation.*

Health Education for the Patient and Family

■ While caring for the ostomy, explain procedures to the patient. *Teaching is immediate and ongoing to facilitate acceptance of the ostomy and self-care.*

■ Teach to manage the pouch clamp, and to empty, rinse, and perform pouch changes. *Self-care is vital to independence and self-esteem.*

■ Instruct how to use an electric razor to shave the peristomal hair if necessary. *An electric razor prevents accidental cutting of the stoma with a razor blade.*

■ Teach to check the stoma and peristomal skin with each pouch change. *Ongoing assessment is important for optimal health and function of the stoma and surrounding skin. Stripping of tape or excessively frequent pouch removal may cause mechanical trauma to peristomal skin. Chronic skin irritation by ileostomy effluent may lead to pseudoverracous lesions, or wartlike nodules.*

■ Instruct to report abnormal appearance of the stoma or surrounding skin to the physician:
  a. Narrowing of the stoma lumen. *This indicates stenosis and may interfere with fecal elimination.*
  b. Lacerations or cuts in the stoma. *The stoma contains no nerves, so trauma may occur without pain.*
  c. Separation of the stoma from the abdominal surface. *This potential complication may require surgical repair.*

■ Emphasize the importance of adequate fluid and salt intake; the risk for dehydration and hyponatremia is increased particularly during hot weather, when fluid is lost through perspiration as well as ileostomy drainage. Water intake should be sufficient to maintain pale urine and an output of at least 1 quart per day. When exercising in hot weather, the patient should consume extra water and salt. High-potassium foods, such as bananas and oranges, may be recommended. *Loss of the reabsorptive surface of the large bowel increases the amount of water and sodium loss in the stool. If the ileostomy is high (more proximal in the ileum), additional potassium losses may also occur.*

■ Discuss manifestations of fluid and electrolyte imbalances:
  a. Extreme thirst
  b. Dry skin and oral mucous membrane
  c. Decreased urine output
  d. Weakness, fatigue
  e. Muscle cramps
  f. Abdominal cramps, nausea, vomiting
  g. Shortness of breath
  h. Orthostatic hypotension (feeling faint when suddenly changing positions)

(continued)

NURSING CARE OF THE PATIENT Having an Ileostomy (continued)

- Discuss dietary concerns. A low-residue diet is recommended initially (see Table 24–8). Foods that may cause excessive odor or gas are typically avoided as well. *Because food blockage is a potential problem, high-fiber foods are limited, and foods that may cause blockage, such as popcorn, corn, nuts, cucumbers, celery, fresh tomatoes, figs, strawberries, blackberries, and caraway seeds, are avoided. Symptoms of food blockage include abdominal cramping, swelling of the stoma, and absence of ileostomy output for over 4 to 6 hours.*
- Teach self-care measures to relieve food blockage:
  a. Take a warm shower or tub bath. *This can help relax the abdominal muscles.*
  b. Assume a knee–chest position. *The knee–chest position reduces intra-abdominal pressure.*
  c. Drink warm fluids or grape juice if not vomiting. *This provides a mild cathartic effect.*

  d. Massage peristomal area. *Massage may stimulate peristalsis and fecal elimination.*
  e. Remove pouch if the stoma is swollen, and apply a pouch with a larger opening. *If the stoma swells, the pouch may create a mechanical obstruction to output.*
- Notify the physician or enterostomal therapy nurse of the following:
  a. The previous measures fail to relieve the obstruction.
  b. Signs of a partial obstruction persist, including high-volume odorous fluid output, abdominal cramps, nausea, and vomiting.
  c. There is no ileostomy output for 4 to 6 hours.
  d. Signs of fluid and electrolyte imbalance occur, such as weakness, dizziness, lightheadedness, or headache.
  Should self-care measures not succeed in breaking up a blockage, ileostomy lavage, as described in Procedure 24–2, may be required.

PROCEDURE 24–1 Changing a One- or Two-Piece Drainable Ostomy Pouch

GATHER SUPPLIES
- Disposable gloves
- One- or two-piece pouch
- Skin barrier paste
- Skin prep
- Clamp
- Pouch deodorant
- Measuring guide
- Adhesive remover
- Skin cleanser
- Washcloths
- Plastic bag

BEFORE THE PROCEDURE
Explain the procedure and provide for privacy.

Follow standard precautions. Don gloves.

PROCEDURE
1. Remove soiled pouch (and the flange if a two-piece pouch) by gently pulling on the pouch or flange and pushing on skin. Use adhesive remover to remove skin barrier paste.
2. Empty pouch, discarding it and the flange (if applicable) in a plastic bag. Save the tail closure clamp. The pouch from a two-piece system may be cleaned out and reused.
3. Cleanse skin and stoma with warm water and skin cleanser or mild soap. Rinse skin and stoma, and pat dry.
4. Note stoma color and peristomal skin condition.
5. If necessary, clip or shave peristomal hair.
6. Use measuring guide or previous pattern to check size of stoma.
   a. Presized pouch: check to verify that size is correct.
   b. Cut-to-fit pouch or flange: Trace the correct size of the stoma onto the back of the flange, and cut the opening to match the pattern. The opening should be no more than 1/8 inch larger than stoma.

7. Apply skin prep to skin covered by a wafer, pouch, or tape. Allow to dry.
8. Remove backings from pouch or flange.
9. Apply a bead of skin barrier paste around the stoma base or around the opening of the pouch or flange. Allow the paste to air-dry for 1 to 2 minutes.
10. Center the pouch or flange over the stoma, and press to adhere.
11. For a two-piece pouch, snap the pouch onto skin barrier flange.
12. Place deodorizing tablets or a few drops of liquid pouch deodorizer (in some cases, antiseptic mouthwash may be used) in the pouch. Apply the clamp.
13. "Picture frame" the pouch with tape to provide extra security.

TABLE 24–8 Low-Residue Diet

FOOD GROUP	ALLOWED	AVOID
Beverages	Coffee, teas, juices, carbonated beverages; milk limited to 2 cups per day	Alcohol, prune juice
Breads and cereals	Products made from refined flours (white bread, crackers) or finely milled grains (e.g., corn flakes, crisp rice cereal, puffed wheat)	Whole-grain breads, rolls, or cereal; breads or rolls with seeds, nuts, or bran
Desserts	Gelatins, tapioca, plain custards, or puddings; angel-food or sponge cake; ice cream or frozen desserts without fruit or nuts	Any desserts containing dried fruits, nuts, seeds, or coconut; rich pastries, pies
Fruits	Fruit juices and strained fruits; cooked or canned apples, apricots, cherries, peaches, pears; bananas	All other raw or cooked fruits
Meats and other protein sources	Roasted, baked, or broiled tender or ground beef, veal, pork, lamb, poultry, or fish; smooth peanut butter; cottage, cream, American, or mild cheddar cheeses in small amounts	Tough or spiced meats and those prepared by frying; highly flavored cheeses; nuts
Potatoes, rice, and pasta	Peeled potatoes; white rice; most pasta products	Potato skins, potato chips, or fried potatoes; brown rice; whole-grain pasta products
Sweets	Sugar, honey, jelly, hard candy and gumdrops, plain chocolates	Jam, marmalade; candy made with seeds, nuts, coconut
Vegetables	Vegetable juices and strained vegetables; cooked or canned vegetables	Raw or whole cooked vegetables
Other	Salt, ground seasonings; cream sauce and plain gravy	Chili sauce, horseradish; popcorn, seeds of any kind; whole spices, olives, vinegar

PROCEDURE 24–2 Ileostomy Lavage

GATHER SUPPLIES
- Disposable gloves
- Disposable irrigation sleeve
- 60 mL catheter-tipped syringe
- #14 Fr. catheter
- Water-soluble lubricant
- Normal saline for irrigation
- Bedpan
- Clean ostomy pouch

BEFORE THE PROCEDURE
Explain the procedure and provide for privacy.

Follow standard precautions. Don gloves.

PROCEDURE
1. Remove the pouch. Apply disposable irrigation sleeve.
2. Clamp the bottom of the sleeve, or place it into the bedpan.
3. Gently examine stoma digitally to break up any fecal mass proximal to stoma and determine direction of the bowel.

4. Lubricate catheter, and insert into stoma until blockage is reached. If the catheter does not reach the blockage after 8 to 10 cm, notify the physician. This may indicate a more proximal obstruction.
5. Instill 30 to 50 mL normal saline.
6. Remove catheter. Allow stoma to drain.
7. Repeat the procedure until the mass is removed.
8. When the blockage is removed, remove the irrigation sleeve.
9. Clean peristomal skin.
10. Apply pouch and clamp.

AFTER THE PROCEDURE
1. Document the procedure, amount of solution used, consistency of results, and the patient's tolerance of the procedure.
2. Discuss dietary intake to help determine cause of blockage.

Nursing Care

Health Promotion
Although IBD cannot, at this time, be predicted or prevented, effective management may help the patient avoid complications of the disease. Stress the importance of complying with the prescribed treatment regimen and promptly reporting manifestations of exacerbations to the physician.

Assessment
Assessment data related to IBD includes the following subjective and objective data:
- *Health history:* Current manifestations, including onset, duration, severity (number of stools per day, presence of blood or mucus in stool, abdominal pain or cramping, tenesmus); usual diet, ability to maintain weight and nutrition, food intolerances; associated manifestations such as

arthralgias, fatigue, malaise; current medications; previous treatment and diagnostic tests.

- *Physical examination:* General appearance; weight; vital signs including orthostatic vitals and temperature; abdominal assessment including shape, contour, bowel sounds, palpation for tenderness and masses, presence of stoma or scars.

Nursing Diagnoses and Interventions

When planning nursing care for the patient with IBD, it is vital to consider the chronic, recurrent nature of the disorder. Teaching is a major aspect of care. Diarrhea and disturbed body image are significant nursing care problems for the patient with IBD. With severe disease, impaired nutrition must be considered a priority problem as well. See the accompanying Case Study & Nursing Care Plan for a patient with ulcerative colitis.

Diarrhea

During an acute exacerbation of IBD, diarrhea can be frequent and painful. The frequency of defecation and associated abdominal pain and cramping may interfere with ADLs and increase the risk for fluid volume deficit and impaired skin integrity.

- Record the frequency, amount, and color of stools using a stool chart. Measure and record liquid stool as output. *The severity of diarrhea is an indicator of the severity of the disease and helps determine the need for fluid replacement.*

> **PRACTICE ALERT**
> Observe stools for obvious blood and test for occult blood as indicated. Report grossly bloody stools (**hematochezia**), which may indicate hemorrhage and necessitate emergency surgery.

- Monitor vital signs every 4 hours. *Tachycardia, tachypnea, and fever may be indicators of fluid volume deficit.*

EVIDENCE FOR NURSING CARE The Patient with Inflammatory Bowel Disease

Selected resources that nurses may find helpful when planning evidence-based nursing care follow.

- Belling, R., McLaren, S., & Woods, L. (2009). Specialist nursing interventions for inflammatory bowel disease. *Cochrane Database of Systemic Reviews*, 4. Art. No.: CD006597. DOI: 10.1002/14651858.CD006597.pub2. Retrieved from http://www.cochrane.org/reviews/en/ab006597.html
- Singh, S., Graff, L. A., & Bernstein, C. N. (2009). Do NSAIDs, antibiotics, infections, or stress trigger flares in IBD? *The American Journal of Gastroenterology, 104,* 1298–1313.
- Smith, G. D., Watson, R., Roger, D., McRorie, E., Hurst, N., Luman, W., & Palmer, K. R. (2002). Impact of a nurse-led counseling service on quality of life in patients with inflammatory bowel disease. *Journal of Advanced Nursing, 38*(2), 152–160. Retrieved from http://www.ncbi.nlm.nih.gov/pubmed

- Weigh daily and record. *Rapid weight loss (over days to a week) usually indicates fluid loss, whereas weight loss over weeks to months may indicate malnutrition.*
- Assess for other indications of fluid deficit: warm, dry skin, poor skin turgor, dry shiny mucous membranes, weakness, lethargy, complaints of thirst. *The extent of fluid loss may not be readily evident with diarrhea, particularly if the patient uses the bathroom without assistance. Systemic manifestations of fluid volume deficit may be the first indicators of the problem.*
- Maintain bowel rest by keeping NPO or limiting oral intake to elemental feedings as indicated. *Bowel rest during an acute exacerbation of IBD promotes healing and reduces diarrhea and other manifestations.*
- Administer prescribed anti-inflammatory and antidiarrheal medications as indicated. *Anti-inflammatory medications reduce the extent of bowel inflammation and diarrhea. Unless contraindicated, antidiarrheal medications help reduce fluid loss and increase comfort.*

> **PRACTICE ALERT**
> When giving antidiarrheal medications to a patient with ulcerative colitis, closely observe for manifestations of toxic megacolon: fever, tachycardia, hypotension, dehydration, abdominal pain and cramping, and an abrupt relief of diarrhea.

- Maintain fluid intake by mouth or intravenously as indicated. *The patient with IBD requires fluid to replace ongoing losses, as well as fluid to meet the usual daily needs of the body. If an elemental diet or total parenteral nutrition is prescribed, additional fluids may be required to meet fluid intake needs.*
- Provide good skin care. *Fluid deficit and tissue dehydration increase the risk for skin excoriations or breakdown.*
- Assess perianal area for irritation or denuded skin from the diarrhea. Use gentle cleansing agents, such as Peri-Wash or Tucks, diaper wipes, or cotton balls saturated with witch hazel. Apply a protective cream, such as zinc oxide–based preparations, to protect skin from the irritating effects of diarrheal stool. *Digestive enzymes in the stool are very corrosive, increasing the risk of skin breakdown where exposed to diarrheal stool.*

Disturbed Body Image

The patient with IBD may experience frustration at not being able to control, or even predict, fecal elimination, particularly when the disease is severe. Diarrhea can interfere with the ability to complete tasks, maintain employment or engage in social activities, and even meet basic needs such as eating, sleeping, and sexual activity. Body image can suffer as a result. Treatment of IBD, be it total colectomy with ileal pouch-anal anastomosis, ileostomy, or chronic corticosteroid therapy, can affect the view of self.

- Accept feelings and perception of self. *Negating or denying the reality of the patient's perception impairs trust.*
- Encourage discussion of physical changes and their consequences as they relate to self-concept. *This demonstrates acceptance and provides an opportunity to express the impact of the disease and its treatment on the patient's life.*

- Encourage discussion about concerns regarding the effect of the disease or treatment on close personal relationships. *This demonstrates understanding and provides an opportunity for the patient to express feelings about the impact of the disease on relationships and significant others.*
- Encourage the patient to make choices and decisions regarding care. *This increases the patient's sense of control over the disease and his or her future.*
- Discuss possible treatment options and their effects openly and honestly. *Open discussion allows more informed decisions.*
- Involve the patient in care, teaching and demonstrating as needed. *This encourages and facilitates independence and decision making.*
- Provide care in an accepting, nonjudgmental manner. *Acceptance of the patient despite potential embarrassment about odors or diarrhea enhances self-esteem.*
- Arrange for interaction with other patients or groups of people with IBD or ostomies. *The patient may feel that no one who has not experienced a similar problem can understand his or her feelings.*
- Teach coping strategies (odor control, dietary modifications, and so on), and support their use. *This facilitates healthy adaptation to the disease.*

Imbalanced Nutrition: Less than Body Requirements
Crohn's disease can significantly alter the bowel's ability to absorb nutrients. In both forms of IBD, blood and protein-rich fluid may be lost in diarrheal stools. With malabsorption and continuing nutrient losses, multiple nutrient deficits can develop, affecting growth and development, healing, muscle mass, bone density, and electrolyte balances.

- Monitor laboratory results, including hemoglobin and hematocrit, serum electrolytes, and total serum protein and albumin levels. *These studies provide an indicator of nutritional status.*
- Provide the prescribed diet: high-kilocalorie, high-protein, low-fat diet with restricted milk and milk products if lactose intolerance is present. *Calories and protein are important to replace lost nutrients. Fat restriction helps reduce diarrhea and nutrient loss, particularly when significant portions of the terminal ileum have been resected.*
- Provide parenteral nutrition as necessary if the patient is unable to absorb enteral nutrients. *Parenteral nutrition can help reverse nutritional deficits and promote weight gain and healing in the patient with acute manifestations.*
- Arrange for dietary consultation. Consider food preferences as allowed. *Providing preferred foods in the prescribed diet increases intake and supports nutritional status.*
- Provide or administer elemental enteral nutrition and supplements as ordered. *Elemental enteral nutritional supplements support healing while providing for bowel rest. They can replace losses and improve nutritional status more rapidly than diet alone.*
- Include family members, the primary food preparer in particular, in teaching and dietary discussions. *Families can reinforce teaching and help the patient maintain required restrictions or kilocalorie intake.*

Using NANDA, NIC, and NOC
Linkages between a selected NANDA nursing diagnosis, NIC, and NOC for the patient with IBD are shown in the chart that follows.

Community-Based Care
IBD is a chronic condition for which the patient provides daily self-management. For this reason, teaching is a vital component of care. Teach the patient and family about the following topics:

- The type of IBD affecting the patient, including the disease process, short- and long-term effects, the relationship of stress to disease exacerbations, and the manifestations of complications
- Prescribed medications, including drug names, desired effects, schedules for tapering the doses if ordered (as with corticosteroids), and possible side effects or adverse reactions and their management
- The recommended diet and the rationale for any specific restrictions
- Use of nutritional supplements such as Ensure to maintain weight and nutritional status
- Indicators of malabsorption and impaired nutrition; recommendations for self-care and when to seek medical intervention
- If discharged with a central catheter and home parenteral nutrition, written and verbal instructions on catheter care, troubleshooting, and parenteral nutrition administration (Have the patient and a family member demonstrate catheter care and parenteral nutrition maintenance.)
- The importance of maintaining a fluid intake of at least 2 to 3 quarts per day, increasing fluid intake during warm weather, exercise, or strenuous work, and when fever is present
- The increased risk for colorectal cancer and importance of regular bowel exams
- Risks and benefits of various treatment options

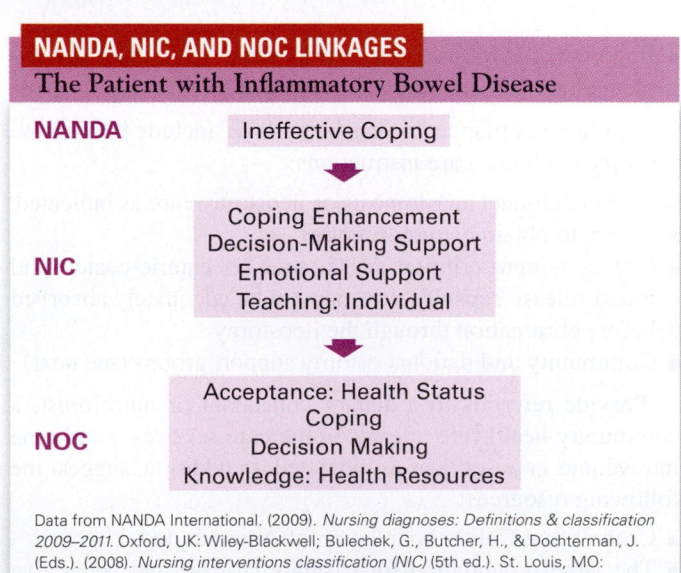

NANDA, NIC, AND NOC LINKAGES
The Patient with Inflammatory Bowel Disease

NANDA Ineffective Coping

NIC Coping Enhancement / Decision-Making Support / Emotional Support / Teaching: Individual

NOC Acceptance: Health Status / Coping / Decision Making / Knowledge: Health Resources

Data from NANDA International. (2009). *Nursing diagnoses: Definitions & classification 2009–2011.* Oxford, UK: Wiley-Blackwell; Bulechek, G., Butcher, H., & Dochterman, J. (Eds.). (2008). *Nursing interventions classification (NIC)* (5th ed.). St. Louis, MO: Mosby; and Moorhead, S., Johnson, M., Maas, M., & Swanson, E. (Eds.). (2008). *Nursing outcomes classification (NOC)* (4th ed.). St. Louis, MO: Mosby.

CASE STUDY & NURSING CARE PLAN   A Patient with Ulcerative Colitis

Cortez Lewis is a 42-year-old real estate agent and mother of three school-age children. She has had ulcerative colitis for 18 years and has been treated with prednisone and sulfasalazine. Over the past 4 months she has been having abdominal pain and cramping and frequent bloody diarrhea stools. During the same period, she has lost 20 lb (9 kg); and has had difficulty maintaining her career. She recently developed several lesions of the lower leg identified as erythema nodosum. A recent colonoscopy revealed extensive involvement of the entire colon. On admission, Mrs. Lewis states, "I'm tired of fighting this disease. I am a prisoner in my home because of the diarrhea." She is admitted for a total proctocolectomy and ileal pouch-anal anastomosis.

ASSESSMENT

Janet Wheeler, RN, completes the admission assessment. Mrs. Lewis now weighs 115 lb (52.2 kg). She complains of abdominal cramping, pain, and frequent bloody diarrhea stools. Several reddened lesions are noted on her lower legs. Physical assessment findings include T 98°F (36.6°C), P 72, R 20, and BP 104/72. Skin cool and pale. Abnormal laboratory findings include hemoglobin 7.3 g/dL (normal 11.7 to 15.7 g/dL); hematocrit 23.3% (normal 35% to 47%); WBC 15,580/mm^3 (normal 3500 to 11,000/mm^3); platelet count 995,000/mm^3 (normal 150,000 to 450,000/mm^3); serum protein 4.6 g/dL (normal 6 to 8 g/dL); serum albumin 2.4 g/dL (normal 3.5 to 5 g/dL). Preparation for surgery is begun.

DIAGNOSES

- *Imbalanced Nutrition: Less than Body Requirements* related to impaired absorption
- *Diarrhea* related to inflammation of bowel
- *Risk for Deficient Fluid Volume* related to abnormal fluid loss
- *Risk for Impaired Tissue Integrity* related to drainage from temporary ileostomy
- *Acute Pain* related to surgical intervention
- *Risk for Sexual Dysfunction* related to temporary ileostomy

EXPECTED OUTCOMES

- Resume prescribed diet within 5 days after surgery.
- Demonstrate normal fecal elimination through the temporary ileostomy.
- Maintain adequate fluid balance.

- Demonstrate appropriate ostomy care prior to discharge.
- Report a tolerable level of discomfort.
- Verbalize feelings about sexuality and acknowledge importance of discussing sexual issues with husband.

PLANNING AND IMPLEMENTATION

- Discuss dietary modifications related to nutritional status and presence of ileostomy. Provide referral to dietitian for diet planning and teaching.
- Teach importance of maintaining a high fluid intake and manifestations of dehydration.
- Teach to empty and change ostomy pouch of choice.
- Teach stoma and peristomal skin assessment with each pouch change.
- Teach food blockage management.
- Refer to local United Ostomy Association.
- Provide list of local medical suppliers for ostomy appliances.

EVALUATION

On discharge, Mrs. Lewis is caring for her ileostomy by demonstrating her ability to empty, rinse, and change the pouch. The enterostomal therapy (ET) nurse has provided written and verbal instructions on ileostomy care. Mrs. Lewis verbalizes her understanding of the recommended diet and the need to limit high-fiber food intake and avoid enteric-coated and timed-release medications. The ET nurse has discussed sexual aspects of having an ileostomy and has given Mrs. Lewis a booklet, "Sex and the Female Ostomate," available through the United Ostomy Association. Mrs. Lewis is looking forward to the planned surgery to close the temporary ileostomy.

CRITICAL THINKING IN THE NURSING PROCESS

1. Why is the patient with an ileostomy at risk for dehydration? How can Mrs. Lewis monitor her fluid status at home?
2. Why were Mrs. Lewis's hemoglobin and hematocrit low on admission? If her hemoglobin had been low but her hematocrit normal on admission, what might be the explanation?
3. Outline a teaching plan that could be given to patients for home care of an ileostomy.
4. Develop a care plan for Mrs. Lewis for the nursing diagnosis *Risk for Impaired Skin Integrity*.

See Evaluating Your Response in Appendix C.

- Importance of informing interdisciplinary care team of complementary and alternative therapy use

If surgery is planned or has been done, include the following topics in home care instructions:

- Ileal pouch-anal anastomosis or ileostomy care as indicated
- Where to obtain ostomy supplies
- Use of nonprescription drugs, such as enteric-coated and timed-release capsules that may not be adequately absorbed before elimination through the ileostomy
- Community and national ostomy support groups (see next)

Provide referrals to a dietary consultant or nutritionist, a community healthcare agency, home care services, and home intravenous care services as indicated. In addition, suggest the following resources:

- Crohn's and Colitis Foundation of America, Inc.
- The Israel Foundation for Crohn's Disease and Ulcerative Colitis
- United Ostomy Association, Inc.

The Patient with Diverticular Disease

Diverticula are small (0.5- to 1.0-cm) outpouchings of the colon that occur in rows (Figure 24–8 ■). Diverticula may occur anywhere in the intestinal tract, excluding the rectum. The vast majority, however, affect the large intestine, with 85% to 95% occurring in the sigmoid colon (Fauci et al., 2008; McPhee, 2008).

FAST FACTS

Diverticular Disease
- People in the United States, Australia, the United Kingdom, and France have high and increasing incidence rates of diverticular disease.
- The incidence of diverticula increases with age, with 5% to 10% of the population older than 45 years of age and almost 80% of those older than 85 years of age experiencing it.
- Most of the people diagnosed with diverticular disease remain asymptomatic.
- Men and women are equally affected.

Figure 24–8 ■ Diverticula of the colon.

Diverticulitis

Diverticulitis is inflammation in and around the diverticular sac. It typically affects only one diverticulum, usually in the sigmoid colon. Undigested food and bacteria collect in the diverticula, forming a hard mass that impairs the mucosal blood supply, allowing bacterial invasion. Mucosal ischemia leads to perforation. With microscopic perforation, inflammation is localized. Gross perforation of a diverticulum results in more extensive bacterial contamination and can lead to abscess formation or peritonitis.

MANIFESTATIONS Pain is a common manifestation of diverticulitis. It is usually left-sided and may be mild to severe and either steady or cramping. The patient may also experience either constipation or increased frequency of defecation. Depending on the location and severity of the inflammation, nausea, vomiting, and a low-grade fever may occur. On examination, the abdomen may be distended, with tenderness and a palpable mass in the left lower quadrant resulting from the inflammatory response.

The older adult may have less specific manifestations, complaining of vague abdominal pain. A palpable mass and signs of a large bowel obstruction may be present.

COMPLICATIONS Complications associated with diverticulitis (in addition to peritonitis and abscess formation) include bowel obstruction, fistula formation, and hemorrhage. Severe or repeated episodes of diverticulitis may lead to scarring and fibrosis of the bowel wall, further narrowing the bowel lumen. This increases the risk for obstruction of the large bowel. Acutely inflamed tissue may adhere to the small bowel, increasing the potential for small-bowel obstruction as well. Fistulas may form, usually between the sigmoid colon and the bladder. Urinary tract infection is the usual sign of a colovesical fistula. Fistulas may also perforate into the small intestine, ureter, vagina, perineum, or abdominal wall. Bleeding from perforation of a vessel wall can occur with diverticulitis. Although it may be significant, bleeding usually stops spontaneously.

Cultural factors, diet in particular, are thought to play an important role in the development of diverticula. A diet consisting of highly refined and fiber-deficient foods is believed to be the major factor contributing to the disease. Decreased activity levels and delaying defecation have been suggested as contributing factors. The increasing incidence of diverticula with aging suggests that dietary factors (lack of fiber), a decrease in physical activity, poor bowel habits (neglecting the urge to defecate), and the effects of aging contribute to development of the disease (Porth & Matfin, 2009).

Pathophysiology

Diverticula form when increased pressure within the bowel lumen causes bowel mucosa to herniate through defects in the colon wall. The circular and longitudinal muscles often thicken or hypertrophy in the area affected by diverticula. This narrows the bowel lumen, increasing intraluminal pressure. Deficient dietary fiber and a lack of fecal bulk contribute to muscle hypertrophy and narrowing of the bowel. Contraction of the muscles in response to normal stimuli such as meals may occlude the narrowed lumen, further increasing intraluminal pressure. The high pressure causes mucosa to herniate through the muscle wall, forming a diverticulum. Areas where nutrient blood vessels penetrate the circular muscle layer are the most common sites for diverticula formation.

Diverticulosis

Diverticulosis indicates the presence of diverticula. More than two-thirds of patients with diverticulosis are asymptomatic. When manifestations such as episodic pain (usually left-sided), constipation, and diarrhea occur, they often can be attributed to irritable bowel syndrome (IBS), which commonly accompanies diverticular disease. (IBS is discussed earlier in this chapter.) As the disease progresses, abdominal cramping, narrow stools (decrease in caliber), increased constipation, bleeding in the stools, weakness, and fatigue may develop.

Complications of diverticulosis include hemorrhage and diverticulitis. A diverticulum may bleed, whether it is inflamed or not, possibly due to erosion of an adjacent blood vessel by a fecalith (hard mass) in the diverticulum.

Interdisciplinary Care

Management of diverticular disease varies from no prescribed treatment to surgical resection of affected colon, depending on the severity of the disease and its complications.

Diagnosis

Diagnostic testing is used to identify diverticular disease when the disease is symptomatic or complications develop. In addition to illustrating diverticula, a barium enema and x-rays can reveal segmental spasm and muscular thickening with a narrowed bowel lumen. Flexible sigmoidoscopy or colonoscopy may be done to detect diverticulosis, assess for strictures or bleeding, and rule out tumor as the cause of the patient's manifestations. Abdominal x-ray films may show free abdominal air associated with diverticulitis and perforation. CT scan may be done with or without contrast media to assess inflammation and detect an abscess or fistula.

Flexible Sigmoidoscopy Video

Laboratory tests include hemoccult or guaiac testing of stool to identify the presence of occult blood, and a WBC count, which may show leukocytosis with a left shift (an increased number of immature WBCs) due to inflammation in diverticulitis.

Medications

Systemic broad-spectrum antibiotics effective against usual bowel flora are prescribed to treat acute diverticulitis. Oral antibiotics such as metronidazole (Flagyl) and ciprofloxacin (Cipro) or trimethoprim-sulfamethoxazole (Septra, Bactrim) may be prescribed if manifestations are mild. Rifixamin (Xifaxan) is a poorly absorbed antibiotic that may be used together with fiber to treat uncomplicated diverticular disease. Severe, acute attacks often necessitate hospitalization and treatment with intravenous fluids and antibiotics effective against anaerobic and gram-negative bacteria. Therapy may include a second-generation cephalosporin such as cefoxitin (Mefoxin), or another antibiotic such as piperacillin-tazobactam (Zosyn) or ticarcillin-clavulanate (Timentin). Antibiotics and their nursing implications are discussed in ∞ Chapter 12.

Although a stool softener such as docusate sodium (Colace) may be prescribed, it is important to note that laxatives (which can further increase intraluminal pressure in the colon) are avoided for the patient with diverticular disease.

Nutrition

Dietary modification is central to the management of diverticular disease. It appears that dietary changes can reduce the risk of complications of diverticulosis. A high-fiber diet is recommended; it increases stool bulk, decreases intraluminal pressures, and may reduce spasm (Table 24–9). Bran is a low-cost fiber supplement that can be added to cereal, soups, salads, or other foods. Commercial bulk-forming products, such as psyllium seed (Metamucil) or methylcellulose also may be recommended. These products are discussed in the Medication Administration box on pages 658–659. The patient often is advised to avoid foods with small seeds (such as popcorn, caraway seeds, figs, or berries), which could obstruct diverticula.

Bowel rest is prescribed during an acute episode of diverticulitis. The patient initially may be NPO with intravenous fluids and possibly parenteral nutrition. Feeding is resumed gradually. Initially, a clear liquid diet is prescribed with gradual advancement to a soft, low-roughage diet (i.e., a diet low in insoluble fiber) with daily added psyllium seed to soften stool and increase its bulk. Among the foods the patient should avoid are wheat and corn bran, vegetable and fruit skins, nuts, and dry beans. The high-fiber diet is resumed following full recovery.

Surgery

Patients with acute diverticulitis may require surgery, usually to treat generalized peritonitis or an abscess that fails to respond to medical treatment. Hemorrhage that recurs or cannot be controlled may also necessitate surgery. Elective surgery may be performed for recurrent episodes of diverticulitis or persistent diverticulitis with continuing pain, tenderness, and a palpable mass.

The affected bowel segment is resected, and if possible an anastomosis of the proximal and distal portions is performed. When an acute infection and diverticulitis are present, a two-stage Hartmann procedure is required. A temporary colostomy is created and anastomosis delayed until the inflammation has subsided. A second surgery is performed 2 to 3 months later to reconnect the bowel and close the temporary colostomy.

∂ Nursing Care

Health Promotion

Teaching patients about the benefits of a high-fiber diet is important primary prevention for diverticular disease. Nurses working with groups and individuals in the community should emphasize the importance of a high-fiber diet and its benefits in preventing diverticular disease and other disorders. In facilities such as residential settings, the nurse can work with dietary staff and care providers to increase the amount of fiber in residents' diets, unless this is contraindicated by a preexisting condition.

Assessment

Because most patients with diverticular disease have few or no manifestations, nursing assessment focuses on manifestations of complications.

- *Health history:* Abdominal pain or cramping, chronic constipation or irregular bowel habits; nausea and vomiting; history of diverticular disease or irritable bowel syndrome.
- *Physical examination:* Bowel sounds, presence of abdominal tenderness of masses and location; stool for occult blood.

Nursing Diagnoses and Interventions

Patients with acute diverticulitis are acutely ill and have multiple nursing care needs. The risk of perforation and resulting peritonitis or abscess formation is high. Priority nursing diagnoses include *Acute Pain* and *Anxiety* related to the possibility of a significant complication or possible surgery.

Potential Complication: Perforation

During an acute attack of diverticulitis, inflammation and mucosal ischemia place the patient at risk for perforation and peritonitis. In addition to maintaining bowel rest to reduce the risk of perforation, the nurse monitors for manifestations of perforation and possible sepsis.

- Monitor vital signs including temperature at least every 4 hours. *Tachycardia and tachypnea may be early indications of*

TABLE 24–9 Foods Recommended in a High-Fiber, High-Residue Diet	
FOOD GROUP	**RECOMMENDED FOODS**
Cereals and grains	Wheat or oat bran; cooked cereals, such as oatmeal; dry cereals, such as bran buds or flakes, corn flakes, shredded wheat; whole-grain breads or crackers; brown rice
Fruits	Unpeeled raw apples, peaches, and pears; oranges; blackberries, raspberries, strawberries (may be restricted for the patient with diverticulosis)
Vegetables	Dried beans (navy, kidney, pinto), lima beans; broccoli; peas; corn; squash; raw vegetables, such as carrots, celery, and tomatoes; potatoes (with skins)

increased inflammation and resulting fluid shift. Fever greater than 101°F (38.3°C) may indicate increased inflammation or spread of inflammation. Note, however, that little temperature elevation may occur in the older patient. A change in behavior or increasing lethargy may be subtle indications of infection in the older adult.

- Assess abdomen every 4 to 8 hours or more often as indicated, including measuring abdominal girth, auscultating bowel sounds, and palpating for tenderness. Promptly report significant changes to the physician. *Increasing abdominal distention, a decrease or change in the quality of bowel sounds, and/or increasing tenderness or guarding may indicate spread of the infectious process or peritonitis.*
- Assess for evidence of lower intestinal bleeding by visual examination and guaiac testing of stools for occult blood. *Perforation of a diverticulum may produce either intestinal or intra-abdominal bleeding and require immediate treatment such as surgery.*
- Maintain intravenous fluids, TPN, and accurate intake and output records. *During acute diverticulitis, oral intake is usually prohibited or restricted. Intravenous fluids are given to maintain fluid and electrolyte balance; TPN is used to maintain nutritional status, facilitating healing and recovery.*

Acute Pain

Pain is a common manifestation of acute diverticulitis. It results from inflammation of the bowel and edema of affected tissues. If surgery is required, postoperative pain is managed with narcotic analgesics.

- Ask the patient to rate pain using a 0 to 10 pain scale. Document the level of pain, and note any changes in location or character of pain. *The perception and response to pain is individual and is affected by past experiences, culture, ethnic background, and many other factors. A change in the character or intensity of the pain may indicate a complication such as perforation or abscess formation.*
- Administer prescribed analgesic or maintain PCA as ordered. Assess analgesic effectiveness. Avoid administering morphine. Provide adjunctive medications as ordered, and encourage use of adjunctive techniques, such as relaxation, positioning, and distraction. Notify the physician if pain management is inadequate. *If patient has not obtained adequate pain relief, further assessment and intervention are required.*
- Maintain bowel rest and total body rest (bed rest with limited activity). *Rest helps reduce inflammation and promote healing, increasing comfort.*
- Reintroduce oral foods and fluids slowly, providing a soft, low-fiber diet with bulk-forming agents. *This allows continued healing of the affected bowel while promoting soft, easily expelled stools.*

Anxiety

The patient with acute diverticulitis faces not only hospitalization, but also potential serious complications such as peritonitis and hemorrhage. Surgery and formation of a temporary colostomy may be necessary. Furthermore, episodes of acute diverticulitis are often recurrent, and the patient may fear future problems.

- Assess and document level of anxiety. *Severe anxiety or panic states can interfere with the ability to respond to instructions and assist with care. Low to moderate anxiety levels enhance learning and compliance with prescribed interventions.*
- Demonstrate empathy and awareness of the perceived threat to health. *It is important to recognize and respect the patient's feelings and perceptions as reality.*
- Attend to physical care needs. *This provides reassurance that these needs will be met and relieves concerns about them.*
- Spend as much time as possible with the patient. *Presence of a caring nurse helps relieve fears of abandonment or that help will not be available if needed. It also enhances trust and provides opportunity for expression of fears or concerns.*
- Assess level of understanding about disease and condition. *This allows misperceptions that may contribute to anxiety to be corrected.*
- Encourage supportive family and friends to remain with the patient as much as possible. *This provides a supportive environment for the patient and also distracts from physical concerns.*
- Assist the patient to identify and use appropriate coping mechanisms. *Coping mechanisms provide immediate relief of anxiety while the patient adapts to the situation.*
- Involve the patient and family (as appropriate) in care decisions. *This increases the patient's sense of control over the situation.*

Community-Based Care

The patient with diverticular disease is responsible for self-care. Discuss the following topics for home care:

- Prescribed high-fiber diet and the need to maintain the diet for life to reduce the incidence of complications, including ways to increase dietary fiber
- Complications of diverticular disease and its manifestations

Provide a referral to a dietitian for teaching as indicated. Prior to discharge of the patient with acute diverticulitis, discuss the following:

- Food and fluid limitations, including recommendations for a low-residue diet during the initial period of healing.
- Colostomy management (if a temporary colostomy has been created), including where to obtain supplies and dietary management.
- Planned procedure to reanastomose the colon and revise the colostomy. Refer to community healthcare agencies as indicated.

Malabsorption Syndromes

Malabsorption is a condition in which the intestinal mucosa ineffectively absorbs nutrients—including carbohydrates, proteins, fats, water, electrolytes, minerals, and vitamins—resulting in their excretion in the stool. Many bowel disorders can lead to malabsorption.

Diseases of the small intestine often cause malabsorption. Other medical and/or surgical conditions can result in malabsorption if they affect digestion or the intestinal mucosa. Primary diseases of the small-bowel mucosa, such as sprue, Crohn's disease, and acute infections, can lead to malabsorption.

TABLE 24–10 Selected Causes of Malabsorption

CAUSE	RELATED FACTORS OR CONDITIONS
Impaired absorption	Sprue
	Short bowel syndrome
	Acute enteritis and other bowel infections or infestations
	AIDS-related opportunistic infections and Kaposi's sarcoma
	Celiac disease
	Crohn's disease
	Intestinal ischemia or infarction
	Scleroderma
Impaired digestion	Lactose intolerance
	Gastrectomy
	Chronic pancreatitis, cancer of the pancreas
	Cystic fibrosis
	Biliary obstruction
	Cirrhosis, hepatitis, or liver failure
	Zollinger-Ellison syndrome

It can also result from *maldigestion*, inadequate preparation of chyme for absorption. For example, major gastric resections, pancreatic disorders with impaired pancreatic enzyme secretion, and biliary disorders that affect bile secretion can impair digestion and absorption of chyme. Selected causes of impaired absorption and digestion are listed in Table 24–10.

Regardless of the cause, malabsorption causes common manifestations resulting from impaired absorption of chyme and the nutrients it contains (see Pathophysiology Linkage). Predominant GI manifestations include anorexia; abdominal bloating; diarrhea with loose, bulky, foul-smelling stools; and steatorrhea (fatty stools). Weight loss, weakness, general malaise, muscle cramps, bone pain, abnormal bleeding, and anemia are common systemic manifestations of malabsorption. These manifestations result from malnutrition and fluid loss due to poor absorption.

Three common malabsorption disorders in adults are celiac disease, lactose intolerance, and short bowel syndrome.

The Patient with Celiac Disease

Celiac disease, also known as celiac sprue or nontropical sprue, is a chronic immune-mediated disorder of the small intestine in which the absorption of nutrients, particularly fats, is impaired. It is characterized by sensitivity to the gliadin fraction of gluten, a cereal protein. Gluten is found in wheat, rye, barley, and oats. It is also used as a filler in many prepared foods and in medications.

The cause of celiac disease is unknown; however, genetic and immune factors are known to play a role in its development. Caucasians of European descent are most commonly affected (McPhee et al., 2008). Having a first-degree relative with celiac disease significantly increases the risk. Nearly all people with celiac disease share the HAL-DQ2 allele, although only a small percentage of people with this allele actually have celiac disease (Fauci et al., 2008).

Manifestations of celiac disease often develop in childhood, but may develop at any age. The severity of the disease depends on the extent of mucosal involvement in the intestine and the duration of the disease.

Pathophysiology

Most absorption of nutrients occurs in the small intestine. The mucosa of the small intestine is arranged in microscopic folds, which in turn contain even smaller finger-like projections called villi. The cells of the villi are covered with microscopic hairs, microvilli, projecting from the cell membrane. The folds, villi, and microvilli of the intestinal mucosa provide a huge surface area for nutrient absorption. Cells of the intestines are specialized to absorb different nutrients. Readily digested nutrients are absorbed in the proximal intestine; others are absorbed more distally in the intestines. Nutrients are absorbed by the processes of simple diffusion (water and small lipids), facilitated diffusion (water-soluble vitamins), and active transport (glucose and amino acids). Once absorbed into the cells of the villi, nutrients enter the blood or lymph for systemic distribution.

PATHOPHYSIOLOGY LINKAGE   Local and Systemic Manifestations of Malabsorption

CATEGORY	MANIFESTATION	CAUSE
Local (GI)	Diarrhea	Disruption of bowel mucosa impairs absorption of fluid and electrolytes, leading to excess water in the stool
	Abdominal distention	Gas formation from fermentation of undigested carbohydrates
	Steatorrhea	Impaired fat absorption leading to excess fat in feces
Systemic	Weight loss	Carbohydrate, protein, and fat deficit
	Weakness and malaise	Kilocalorie deficit; impaired absorption of micronutrients (vitamins and minerals) leading to nutrient deficiencies, anemia; fluid and electrolyte losses
	Anemia	Vitamin B_{12}, folic acid, and iron deficits impair erythropoiesis
	Bone pain	Calcium and vitamin D deficits lead to bone demineralization
	Muscle cramps, paresthesias	Protein wasting, vitamin B_{12} and electrolyte deficits impair neuromuscular function
	Easy bruising and bleeding	Vitamin K deficit
	Glossitis, cheilosis	Iron, folic acid, and vitamin B_{12} deficits

In celiac disease, it the intestinal mucosa is damaged by an immunologic response. Gliadin acts as an antigen (a substance that induces the formation of antibodies that interact specifically with it), prompting an inappropriate T-cell mediated immune response. People with celiac disease have increased antibodies to other antigens as well. The immune response prompts an inflammatory response in the small bowel, resulting in loss of villi and microvilli. The villi shorten and atrophy, resulting in loss of intestinal folds and absorptive surface. Digestive enzyme production, including disaccharidase and particularly lactase, is reduced as well. The proximal small bowel is affected to the greatest extent, likely due to its greater exposure to dietary gluten.

Manifestations

Manifestations of celiac disease may develop at any age. Local manifestations include abdominal bloating and cramps, diarrhea, and steatorrhea. Systemic manifestations result from the effects of malabsorption and resulting deficiencies. Anemia is common. Patients with celiac disease are often small in stature, and may have delayed maturity. Other signs of nutrient deficiencies include tetany, vitamin deficiencies, muscle wasting, and rickets (impaired bone development). When gluten is removed from the diet, the manifestations resolve.

Gastrointestinal malignancies and intestinal lymphoma are potential complications of celiac disease. Other complications include intestinal ulceration and development of refractory disease, or disease that no longer responds to a gluten-free diet.

Interdisciplinary Care

With any malabsorptive disorder, the initial focus of management is to identify the cause. Once this has been determined, specific therapy can be prescribed.

Diagnosis

Laboratory and diagnostic testing are used to make the differential diagnosis for various causes of malabsorption syndromes and to determine the severity of nutrient deficiencies.

An enteroscopy permits direct examination of intestinal mucosa and collection of a tissue specimen for biopsy. Tissue biopsy is necessary to establish the diagnosis of celiac disease.

Upper GI series with small-bowel follow-through may be done to evaluate the structures of the upper GI tract. With celiac disease, the typical "feathery" pattern of barium in the small bowel is lost, and the barium may precipitate and clump. Nursing implications of diagnostic tests are included in ∞ Chapter 21.

Laboratory tests are used to identify pathophysiologic effects of the disease. Fecal fat is measured to document the presence of steatorrhea. The fat content of stool is increased in many malabsorptive disorders, including celiac disease. Serologic testing for IgA endomysial antibodies and IgG and IgA antigliadin antibodies is used to diagnose celiac disease and evaluate compliance with the prescribed gluten-free diet. Serum levels of protein, albumin, cholesterol, electrolytes, and iron may be ordered to evaluate for nutrient deficiencies. The hemoglobin, hematocrit, and RBC indices are used to evaluate anemia. Prothrombin time is increased in vitamin K deficiency.

Medications

Patients with severe nutritional deficits may require vitamin and mineral supplements, as well as iron and folic acid to correct anemia. Vitamin K may be administered parenterally if the prothrombin time is prolonged. In patients whose disease fails to respond to dietary management, corticosteroids may be ordered to suppress the inflammatory response.

Nutrition

The patient with celiac disease is placed on a gluten-free diet. This treatment is generally successful, as long as the patient avoids gluten totally. Gluten is so widely used in prepared foods that this may be no easy task. Consultation with a dietitian and detailed dietary instructions are necessary. Patients need to become aware of hidden sources of gluten and to analyze dietary labels. Common sources of gluten and foods to be avoided are indicated in Table 24–11.

The prescribed diet is high in calories and protein to correct nutrient deficits. Fat content is restricted to minimize steatorrhea. The diet usually is restricted in lactose as well to compensate for the loss of lactase-containing microvilli. Foods containing lactose may be reintroduced once remission has occurred. Patients with refractory disease may benefit from restriction of other dietary proteins such as soy (Fauci et al., 2008).

TABLE 24–11 Dietary Sources of Gluten

FOOD GROUP	CONTAINS GLUTEN	MAY CONTAIN GLUTEN
Cereals, grains, and grain products	Bread, crackers, cereal, and pasta containing wheat, rye, or barley grain or flour	Seasoned rice and potato mixes
Beverages	Malt, Postum, Ovaltine, beers, and ales	Commercial chocolate milk, cocoa, and other beverage mixes, such as instant tea mix, dietary supplements
Desserts	Cakes, cookies, and pastries made with wheat, rye, or barley flour	Commercial ice cream and sherbet
Meats and other protein sources		Meat loaf, cold cuts and prepared meats, breaded meats; cheese products; soy protein meat substitutes; commercial egg products
Fruits and vegetables		Commercial seasoned vegetable mixes or vegetables with sauce; canned baked beans; commercial pie fillings
Miscellaneous		Commercial salad dressings and mayonnaise; ketchup and prepared mustard; gravy, white sauce; nondairy creamer; syrups; commercial pickles

✌ Nursing Care

Nursing care for the patient with celiac disease focuses on the effects of the disorder on health and nutrition, as well as the patient's ability to manage the disease.

Assessment

- *Health history:* Onset, duration, and severity of manifestations; number and character of stools; previous teaching related to disorder; current treatment and diet.
- *Physical examination:* Vital signs; abdominal shape, contour, bowel sounds; manifestations of malnutrition (e.g., anemia, small stature, muscle wasting, signs of other nutrient deficiencies).

Nursing Diagnoses and Interventions

Diarrhea and malnutrition are significant problems for the patient with celiac disease and the priority foci for nursing intervention.

Diarrhea

Steatorrhea and diarrhea typically occur with celiac disease because fat, water, and other nutrients are poorly absorbed, remaining in the bowel to be eliminated in the stool. Diarrhea can interfere with lifestyle, ADLs, skin integrity, and fluid and electrolyte balance.

- Assess and document the frequency and nature of stools. *Bowel elimination reflects the severity of the disease and efficacy of treatment. With effective treatment, stools become less frequent and more normal in color and appearance.*
- Weigh daily, monitor intake and output, and assess skin turgor and mucous membranes for indications of fluid balance. *Diarrhea increases the risk for hypovolemia and dehydration resulting from excess fluid loss in the stool.*
- Assess and document perianal skin condition. *Frequent defecation can irritate skin and mucous membranes, increasing the risk of breakdown.*
- Encourage a liberal fluid intake. *Oral fluids help replace fluid lost through diarrheal stool.*

Imbalanced Nutrition: Less than Body Requirements

Celiac disease is a chronic condition. With continuing malabsorption, multiple nutrient deficits may occur, resulting in impaired growth and development, impaired healing, muscle wasting, bone disease, and electrolyte imbalances.

- Maintain accurate dietary intake records. *Assessment of dietary intake provides information about compliance with the prescribed diet as well as the adequacy of nutrient intake.*
- Monitor laboratory results, including hemoglobin and hematocrit, serum electrolytes, total serum protein, and albumin levels. *These studies provide information about nutritional status.*
- Arrange for dietary consultation. Provide for food preferences as allowed. *An individualized diet developed to address the patient's food preferences as well as nutrient needs will promote appetite and food intake.*
- Provide the prescribed high-kilocalorie, high-protein, low-fat, gluten-free diet for the patient with celiac sprue. Restrict lactose (dairy product) intake as indicated. *Calories and protein are important to replace lost nutrients. Fat restriction helps reduce diarrhea and nutrient loss. Lactose may be restricted during initial treatment, then slowly reintroduced into the diet as the gut heals and its normal structure is restored.*
- Provide parenteral nutrition as ordered if the patient is unable to absorb enteral nutrients. *Parenteral nutrition can help reverse nutritional deficits and promote weight gain when manifestations are acute.*
- Encourage nutritional supplements. *Nutritional supplements often are necessary to replace losses and restore nutrient levels to normal more rapidly than diet alone can achieve.*
- Include family members, the primary food preparer in particular, in teaching and dietary discussions. *Families can reinforce teaching and help the patient maintain required restrictions or kilocalorie intake.*

Community-Based Care

The patient with celiac disease has a chronic condition that requires continuing dietary management.

Provide a detailed list of foods that contain gluten and need to be eliminated from the diet, as well as foods that are allowed. Teach the patient and family how to identify gluten-containing commercial products by reading labels and lists of ingredients. Encourage the purchase and use of a gluten-free cookbook. Discuss potential long-term complications of the disorder and manifestations to be reported to the primary care provider.

If corticosteroids have been prescribed, stress the importance of taking the medication as ordered. Emphasize the need to avoid stopping the medication abruptly and to notify all caregivers that a corticosteroid is part of the patient's medication regimen. Instruct to frequently monitor weight. A weight gain of 5 lb (2.3 kg) or more in less than a week usually reflects fluid gain, a possible adverse effect of corticosteroids. Other potential effects include decreased resistance to infection, an impaired inflammatory response, and changes in the metabolism of carbohydrates, proteins, and fats.

The Patient with Lactase Deficiency

For carbohydrates to be absorbed from the small intestine, they first must be broken down into simple sugars, or monosaccharides. Lactose is the primary carbohydrate in milk and milk products. It is a disaccharide, requiring the enzyme lactase for digestion and absorption. Lactase deficiency can lead to *lactose intolerance* and manifestations of malabsorption. Lactase deficiency usually is genetic in origin, but also occurs secondarily to celiac disease, Crohn's disease, and other disorders affecting the mucosa of the small intestine. There is a racial/ethnic component to the disorder, as described in the following Focus on Cultural Diversity box.

Manifestations

Many people with lactase deficiency are asymptomatic. Small to moderate amounts of milk (one to two 8-ounce glasses) may be well tolerated. Manifestations of lactose intolerance include lower abdominal cramping, pain, and diarrhea following milk ingestion. Undigested lactose ferments in the intestine, forming gases that contribute to bloating and flatus. Lactic and fatty acids produced by this fermentation irritate the bowel, leading to increased motility and abdominal cramping. The undigested lactose draws water into the intestine, which contributes to increased motility and diarrhea. The diarrhea associated with lactose intolerance may be explosive.

Interdisciplinary Care

The diagnosis of lactase deficiency usually is based on a history of intolerance to milk and milk products, and a trial of a lactose-free diet. If manifestations resolve when lactose intake is eliminated, the diagnosis of lactase deficiency is confirmed.

Diagnosis

The lactose breath test is a noninvasive test that may be used to diagnose lactase deficiency. Expired hydrogen gas (H_2) is measured following oral administration of 50 g of lactose. If lactose is digested and absorbed normally, then little change occurs in the amount of exhaled H_2 from fasting to postlactose administration. With lactose intolerance, exhaled H_2 increases following lactose administration as the sugar ferments in the bowel.

For the lactose tolerance test, 100 g of lactose solution is orally administered, followed by measurement of blood glucose levels at intervals of 30, 60, and 120 minutes. If lactose is digested and absorbed normally, the blood glucose rises more than 20 mg/dL. The expected blood glucose elevation does not occur in lactase deficiency.

Nutrition

A lactose-free or reduced lactose diet relieves the manifestations of the disorder. Some patients require total elimination of milk and milk products from the diet. Many can tolerate limited amounts of lactose. Milk pretreated with lactase is readily available. Nonprescription lactase enzyme preparations are available to improve milk tolerance. Yogurt containing bacterial lactases may be well tolerated. Calcium supplements are often recommended, particularly for women on a reduced-lactose or lactose-free diet.

✍ Nursing Care

Nursing care for the patient with lactose intolerance focuses on providing education and support. Discuss sources of lactose: Milk, ice cream, and cottage cheese are high in lactose; aged cheese and yogurt contain much smaller amounts. Potential hidden sources of lactose include sherbets, desserts made from milk and milk chocolate, sauces and gravies, and cream soups. Suggest a trial of lactase-treated milk or lactase enzyme supplements. Emphasize the importance of obtaining nutrients

contained in dairy products from other sources. Proteins may be obtained from meats, eggs, legumes, and grains. Other sources of calcium include sardines, oysters, and salmon, as well as plant sources such as beans, cauliflower, rhubarb, and green leafy vegetables.

The Patient with Short Bowel Syndrome

The small bowel may be resected due to tumors, infarction of bowel mucosa, incarcerated hernias, Crohn's disease, trauma, and enteropathy resulting from radiation therapy. Resection of significant portions of the small intestine may result in a condition known as *short bowel syndrome*. The severity of the disorder depends on the total amount of bowel resected, as well as the portions of bowel removed. Removal of the proximal portions, including the duodenum, jejunum, and proximal ileum, and the distal portion of the ileum is associated with more severe malabsorption and manifestations than is resection of midportions of the ileum.

Resection of the small intestine affects the absorption of water, nutrients, vitamins, and minerals. Transit time of ingested foods and fluids is reduced, and digestive processes are impaired. The bowel undergoes an adaptive process in which the remaining villi enlarge and lengthen to increase absorptive surface following resection. For many patients, absorption and bowel function return to preoperative or near-normal levels. Others have continued significant impairment of digestion and absorption, leading to nutrient deficiencies, weight loss, and diarrhea. Short bowel syndrome is associated with an increased risk for kidney stones and gallstones.

Interdisciplinary Care

Management of short bowel syndrome focuses on alleviating manifestations. Patients often simply require frequent, small, high-kilocalorie, high-protein feedings.

Diagnosis

Laboratory and diagnostic studies are used to evaluate nutrient deficiencies. Total serum proteins and albumin are reduced, as are serum levels of folate, iron, vitamins, minerals, and electrolytes. Anemia and a prolonged prothrombin time (indicative of vitamin K deficiency) may develop.

Medications

Multivitamin and mineral supplementation is frequently necessary. Antidiarrheal medications are used to reduce bowel motility, allowing a greater amount of time for nutrient absorption. Some patients are affected by gastric hypersecretion following bowel resection. For these patients, a proton-pump inhibitor such as omeprazole (Prilosec) may be ordered. Patients with severe manifestations of short bowel syndrome may require parenteral nutrition.

✍ Nursing Care

Nursing care for the patient with short bowel syndrome focuses on the problems of potential fluid volume deficit, malnutrition, and diarrhea.

Fluid losses are generally greatest in the initial periods following surgery, warranting the closest attention at that time. Close monitoring of vital signs, intake and output, daily weights, skin turgor, and condition of mucous membranes is vital. It is important to remember that the risk also is high when other abnormal fluid losses occur through, for example, fever, draining wounds, or excess perspiration.

Document nutritional status, including weight, anthropometric measurements, laboratory values, and kilocalorie intake. Provide nutritional supplementation with enteral feedings as needed. Maintain central lines and PN, using aseptic technique.

For diarrhea, document the number and character of stools. Administer antidiarrheal medications as ordered. If the patient is lactose intolerant, limit intake of milk and milk products. Provide good skin care of the perianal region to prevent breakdown from frequent bowel movements. Refer to the discussion of nursing care for the patient with celiac disease for other measures for altered nutrition and diarrhea.

The patient and family affected by this condition require extensive education. Because there is no way to cure or replace the lost bowel at this time, the patient must manage the disorder on a day-to-day basis. Provide instructions about the recommended diet and medication regimen. Emphasize the importance of maintaining an adequate fluid intake, particularly in hot weather or during strenuous exercise. Teach the patient to monitor his or her weight frequently and report changes. Include teaching about possible manifestations of dehydration and nutrient deficiencies that should be reported to the physician. Referring the patient to a dietitian or counselor can help the person cope with what may be a lifelong problem.

Neoplastic Disorders

Cancer remains the second leading cause of death in the United States, preceded only by heart disease. Although cancer may affect any portion of the digestive tract, the large intestine and rectum are the most common sites. Malignant neoplasms of the lower bowel are the second leading cause of death from cancer (after lung cancer), making this a significant healthcare concern.

The Patient with Polyps

A *polyp* is a mass of tissue that arises from the bowel wall and protrudes into the lumen. Polyps may develop in any portion of the bowel, but they occur most often in the sigmoid colon and rectum. They vary considerably in size and may be single or multiple. It is estimated that approximately 30% of people over the age of 50 have polyps. Although most polyps are benign, some have the potential to become malignant. Familial adenomatous polyposis (FAP) is a syndrome with a dominant inheritance pattern that leads to the development of hundreds to thousands of adenomatous polyps. Some of these polyps will inevitably become malignant (Fauci et al., 2008).

Pathophysiology

Polyps are identified by their structure and tissue type. Most polyps are adenomas, benign epithelial tumors that are considered premalignant lesions. Greater than 95% of adenocarcinomas arise from adenomas; however, less than 1% of polyps ever become malignant (Fauci et al., 2008). Of polyps that are removed during colonoscopy, more than 70% are adenomatous (McPhee et al., 2008).

Adenomatous polyps represent disruption of the normal process of cell proliferation to replace epithelial cells lining the intestine. Cells are constantly being reproduced to replace those shed as feces move through the colon. Disruption of the normal process of cell division and maturation can lead to formation of a polyp composed of tightly packed epithelial cells. The cells may appear grossly normal or show signs of dysplasia. Polyps may develop as tubular, villous, or tubulovillous adenomas. Polyps may be named by the way they are attached to the bowel wall as either sessile (raised nodules) or pedunculated (attached by a stalk) (Figure 24–9 ■).

Tubular adenomas (also called pedunculated polyps) are more common than sessile polyps and account for about 65% of benign polyps of the large intestine (Porth & Matfin, 2009).

A

B

Figure 24–9 ■ *A,* Tubular (or pedumculated) and *B,* villous (or sessile) polyps.

A tubular adenoma is a globelike structure attached to the intestinal wall by a thin, stalk-like stem. The incidence of this type of polyp increases with age, although it occurs in all age groups and in both genders. Most are small, 1 cm or less in diameter, although they may be as large as 4 to 5 cm. The malignant potential of these polyps seems to be related to their size. Small adenomas less than 1 cm have a low risk of being malignant, and larger adenomas greater than 1 cm have a much higher risk of harboring malignancy or a high-grade dysplasia.

Villous adenomas (also called sessile polyps) have a broad base and an elevated, cauliflower-like surface (Figure 24–9B). They typically develop in the rectosigmoid colon. This type of polyp is often larger than tubular adenomas, usually more than 5 cm. Villous adenomas are not common, accounting for about 10% of colon polyps. They have a higher malignant potential than tubular adenomas. Some adenomatous polyps contain both tubular epithelium and villi and are known as *tubulovillous adenomas*.

Manifestations

Most polyps are asymptomatic, found coincidentally during routine examination or diagnostic testing. Intermittent painless rectal bleeding, bright or dark red, is the most common presenting complaint. A large polyp may cause abdominal cramping, pain, or manifestations of obstruction. Diarrhea and mucous discharge may be associated with a large villous adenoma.

Interdisciplinary Care

The diagnosis of intestinal polyps is generally based on diagnostic studies such as sigmoidoscopy or colonoscopy. A rectal polyp may be palpable on digital examination, but further studies are necessary to determine its size and type and the extent of colon involvement, and to assess for malignancy. Genetic testing and counseling is offered to patients with or a family history of FAP. First degree relatives of a patient with FAP undergo annual sigmoidoscopy beginning at age 10 years.

Once identified, polyps are removed because of the risk of malignancy. Pedunculated polyps and small villous lesions may be removed during colonoscopy using an electrocautery snare or hot biopsy forceps passed through the scope. This relatively safe procedure has less than a 2% risk of complications such as perforation or hemorrhage. Large villous adenomas are completely excised and examined histologically for evidence of malignancy. In some cases, the colon segment containing the polyp is resected. Patients with FAP usually undergo a total colectomy with ileorectal anastomosis before age 20 years to significantly reduce their risk for developing colon cancer.

Treatment following polypectomy depends on histologic examination of the excised tissue. Because polyps tend to recur, follow-up colonoscopy is recommended in 3 years and then every 5 years if no further polyps are detected. When the polyp is found to be malignant, follow-up care is determined by the tissue type and degree of invasion.

∾ Nursing Care

Health Promotion

The incidence of intestinal polyps increases with age. They affect men and women equally. It is believed that an adenomatous polyp requires more than 5 years of growth to become significant in size and malignant potential. Advise all patients to have a screening for colorectal cancer (with a colonoscopy being the "gold standard" for diagnosis) at age 50 and as recommended thereafter for early detection of polyps (American Cancer Society [ACS], 2008).

Assessment

Polyps are a "silent" disease, with few or no manifestations.

- *Health history:* Rectal bleeding; personal or family history of intestinal polyps or colorectal cancer.

Nursing Diagnoses and Interventions

Nursing care for the patient with polyps focuses on education and assisting the patient through diagnostic testing and polyp removal. Before and after colonoscopy and polypectomy, provide direct care and teaching about the procedure, expected sensations during the procedure, and anticipated postoperative care. Cathartics are prescribed prior to colonoscopy; cleansing enemas may be ordered. Observe for evidence of fluid and electrolyte imbalance during preoperative preparation. If enemas are ordered, use normal saline (not tap water) to reduce the risk of electrolyte imbalances. Following polypectomy, observe closely for possible complications such as hemorrhage.

Community-Based Care

Include the following topics when teaching for home care:

- The significance of polyps and their relationship to colorectal cancer
- The importance of keeping follow-up appointments and undergoing repeat colonoscopy as recommended: at 3 years following polypectomy, then every 5 to 10 years unless additional polyps are found
- Manifestations to report to the physician, such as diarrhea, pain, rectal bleeding, light-headedness, or other indications of possible blood loss

The Patient with Colorectal Cancer

Colorectal cancer (cancer of the colon or rectum) is the third most common cancer diagnosed in the United States. In the United States about 146,970 new cases of colorectal cancer were diagnosed in 2009, and it was expected to cause about 49,920 deaths during that year (ACS, 2009). Earlier diagnosis and improved treatment have improved the survival rate for colorectal cancer. Its incidence, which is nearly equal among men and women, has been declining in the United States for the past 15 years. The incidence of colorectal cancer varies among ethnic groups; see the following Focus on Cultural Diversity box. Colorectal cancer occurs most frequently after age 50. The incidence continues to rise with increasing age. With early diagnosis and treatment, the 5-year survival rate for colorectal cancer is 90%; however, only 39% of colorectal cancers are diagnosed at this early stage.

Although the specific cause of colorectal cancer is unknown, a number of risk factors have been identified (Box 24–2). Genetic factors are linked to the risk for colorectal cancer. Up to 25% of people who develop colorectal cancer have a family history of the disease (Fauci et al., 2008). Persons with familial adenomatous polyposis inevitably will develop colon cancer unless the colon is removed. Hereditary nonpolyposis colorectal cancer (also known as Lynch syndrome) is an autosomal dominant disorder that significantly increases the risk for developing colorectal and other cancers. Tumors associated with Lynch syndrome often affect the ascending colon, and tend to occur at an earlier age. Inflammatory bowel diseases increase the risk of colorectal cancer.

Diet plays a role in the development of colorectal cancer. The disease is prevalent in economically prosperous countries where people consume diets high in calories, meat proteins, and fats. This dietary pattern, common in the United States, is thought to increase the population of anaerobic bacteria in the gut. These anaerobes convert bile acids into carcinogens. Diets high in fruits and vegetables, folic acid, and calcium appear to reduce the risk of colorectal cancer. Cereal fiber, once thought to reduce colorectal cancer risk, does not now appear to play a role either way in its development. Other factors that may reduce the risk of colorectal cancer include regular exercise, taking a daily multivitamin, and the use of aspirin and other NSAIDs.

Pathophysiology

Nearly all colorectal cancers that begin as adenomatous polyps are adenocarcinomas. Most tumors develop in the rectum and sigmoid colon, although any portion of the colon may be affected (Figure 24–10 ■). The tumor typically grows undetected, producing few manifestations. By the time manifestations occur, the disease may have spread into deeper layers of the bowel tissue and adjacent organs. Colorectal cancer spreads by direct extension to involve the entire

BOX 24–2   Risk Factors for Colorectal Cancer

- Age over 50 years
- Polyps of the colon and/or rectum
- Family history of colorectal cancer
- Personal history of colorectal, ovarian, endometrial, or breast cancer
- Inflammatory bowel disease
- Exposure to radiation
- Diet: high animal fat and kilocalorie intake
- Obesity, smoking, and alcohol use

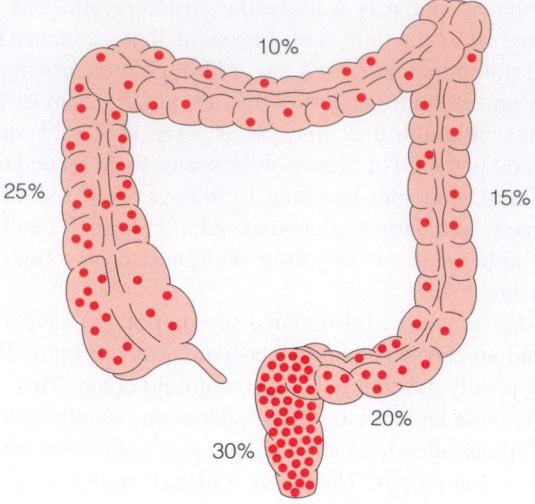

Figure 24–10 ■ The distribution and frequency of cancer of the colon and rectum.

bowel circumference, the submucosa, and outer bowel wall layers. Neighboring structures such as the liver, greater curvature of the stomach, duodenum, small intestine, pancreas, spleen, genitourinary tract, and abdominal wall also may be involved by direct extension. Metastasis to regional lymph nodes is the most common form of tumor spread. This is not always an orderly process; distal nodes may contain cancer cells while regional nodes remain normal. Cancerous cells from the primary tumor may spread by way of the lymphatic system or circulatory system to secondary sites such as the liver, lungs, brain, bones, and kidneys. "Seeding" of the tumor to other areas of the peritoneal cavity can occur when the tumor extends through the serosa or during surgical resection.

Manifestations

Bowel cancer often produces no manifestations until it is advanced. Because it grows slowly, 5 to 15 years of growth may occur before manifestations develop. The manifestations depend on its location, type and extent, and complications. Rectal bleeding is often the initial manifestation that prompts patients to seek medical care. Other common early manifestations include a change in bowel habits, either diarrhea or constipation. Pain, anorexia, and weight loss are characteristic in advanced disease. A palpable abdominal or rectal mass may be present. Occasionally the patient presents with anemia from occult bleeding.

Complications

The primary complications associated with colorectal cancer are (1) bowel obstruction due to narrowing of the bowel lumen by the lesion; (2) perforation of the bowel wall by the tumor, allowing contamination of the peritoneal cavity by bowel contents; and (3) direct extension of the tumor to involve adjacent organs.

Most recurrences of colorectal cancer after tumor removal occur within the first 4 years. The size of the primary tumor does not necessarily relate to long-term survival. The number of involved lymph nodes, penetration of the tumor through the bowel wall, and tumor adherence to adjacent organs are better predictors of the prognosis for the disease.

Interdisciplinary Care

The focus of interdisciplinary care for colorectal cancer is prevention, early detection, and intervention. Colorectal cancer is always treated by surgical resection, with chemotherapy and radiation therapy used as adjuncts.

Prevention

Measures to prevent colon cancer that are considered to be effective and safe include consuming a diet high in fruits and vegetables and low in saturated fat and red meat, regular exercise, maintaining a healthy weight, limiting alcohol consumption, and quitting smoking. Consuming fiber supplements, minerals such as calcium, vitamins, and nonsteroidal anti-inflammatory drugs may help prevent colorectal cancer, but their effect is not yet proven (ACS, 2009). Although considered safe, these measures are the subject of further research to demonstrate conclusive proof of effectiveness.

Screening

The ACS (2008) recommends one of the following testing schedules for the early detection of colorectal cancer, beginning at age 50. These options are acceptable choices for average-risk adults.

- Yearly fecal occult blood test (FOBT) or fecal immunochemical test (FIT) or stool DNA test (sDNA).
- Flexible sigmoidoscopy every 5 years, *or*
- double-contrast barium enema every 5 years, *or*
- CT colonography (virtual colonoscopy) every 5 years, *or*
- colonoscopy every 10 years.

Diagnosis

Diagnostic and laboratory tests are used for screening, diagnosis, and monitoring purposes. Diagnostic tests include a sigmoidoscopy or colonoscopy as the primary diagnostic test used to detect and visualize tumors. While flexible sigmoidoscopy can detect 50% to 65% of colorectal cancers, many clinicians recommend colonoscopy. Tissue for biopsy is obtained at the time of endoscopy to confirm cancerous tissue and evaluate cell differentiation (∞ see Chapter 14). Current staging methods primarily use the TNM system, as outlined in Table 24–12. Radiologic examinations may include a chest x-ray to detect tumor metastasis to the lung. Computed tomography (CT) scan, magnetic resonance imaging (MRI), or ultrasonic examination may be used to assess tumor depth and involvement of other organs by direct extension or metastasis.

Laboratory tests used are a fecal occult blood (by guaiac or hemoccult testing) to detect blood in the feces and a CBC to detect anemia resulting from chronic blood loss and tumor growth. Carcinoembryonic antigen (CEA) is a tumor marker that can be detected in the blood of patients with colorectal cancer. CEA levels are used to estimate prognosis, monitor treatment, and detect cancer recurrence.

Surgery

Surgical resection of the tumor, adjacent colon, and regional lymph nodes is the treatment of choice for colorectal cancer. Options for surgical treatment vary from destruction of the tumor by laser photocoagulation performed during endoscopy to abdominoperineal resection with permanent colostomy. When possible, the anal sphincter is preserved and colostomy avoided.

Laser photocoagulation uses a very small, intense beam of light to generate heat in tissues toward which it is directed. The heat generated by the laser beam can be used to destroy small tumors. It is also used for palliative surgery of advanced tumors to remove obstruction. Laser photocoagulation can be performed endoscopically and is useful for patients who cannot tolerate major surgery.

Other surgical treatment options for small, localized tumors include local excision and fulguration. These procedures also may be performed during endoscopy, eliminating the need for abdominal surgery. Local excision may be used to remove a disk of rectum containing a tumor in patients with a small,

TABLE 24–12 The TNM Classification for Colorectal Cancer

STAGE	PRIMARY TUMOR (T)	REGIONAL LYMPH NODES (N)	DISTANT METASTASIS (M)
	TX—Primary tumor cannot be assessed	NX—Regional lymph nodes cannot be assessed	MX—Presence of distant metastasis cannot be assessed
	T0—No evidence of primary tumor		
Stage 0	Tis—Carcinoma *in situ*	N0—No regional lymph node metastasis	M0—No distant metastasis
Stage I	T1—Tumor invades submucosa		
	T2—Tumor invades muscularis propria		
Stage II	T3—Tumor invades through muscularis propria into subserosa or into non peritonealized pericolic or perirectal tissues		
	T4—Tumor perforates visceral peritoneum or directly invades other organs or structures		
Stage III	Any T	N1—Metastasis in one to three pericolic or perirectal lymph nodes	
		N2—Metastasis in four or more pericolic or perirectal lymph nodes	
Stage IV	Any T	Any N	M1—Distant metastasis

well-differentiated, mobile polypoid lesion. *Fulguration* or electrocoagulation is used to reduce the size of some large tumors for patients who are poor surgical risks. This procedure requires general anesthesia and may need to be repeated at intervals.

Most patients with colorectal cancer undergo surgical resection of the colon with anastomosis of remaining bowel as a curative procedure. The distribution of regional lymph nodes determines the extent of resection because these may contain metastatic lesions. Most tumors of the ascending, transverse, descending, and sigmoid colon can be resected.

Tumors of the rectum usually are treated with an abdominoperineal resection in which the sigmoid colon, rectum, and anus are removed through both abdominal and perineal incisions. A permanent sigmoid colostomy is performed to provide for elimination of feces. Nursing care of the patient having bowel surgery is outlined in the accompanying box below.

COLOSTOMY Surgical resection of the bowel may be accompanied by a colostomy for diversion of fecal contents. A **colostomy** is an ostomy made in the colon. It may be created if the bowel is obstructed by the tumor, as a temporary measure to promote healing of anastomoses, or as a permanent means of

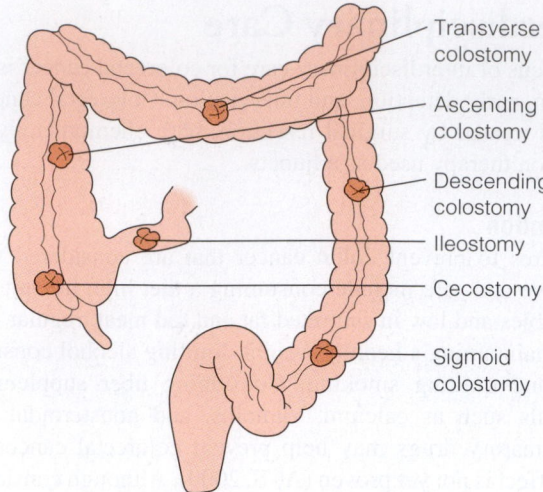

Figure 24–11 ■ Various ostomy levels and sites.

fecal evacuation when the distal colon and rectum are removed. Colostomies take the name of the portion of the colon from which they are formed: ascending colostomy, transverse colostomy, descending colostomy, and sigmoid colostomy (Figure 24–11 ■).

NURSING CARE OF THE PATIENT Having Bowel Surgery

PREOPERATIVE NURSING CARE
- Provide routine preoperative care for the surgical patient as outlined in ∞ Chapter 4.
- Arrange for consultation with ET specialist if appropriate. *The ET nurse is trained to identify and mark an appropriate stoma location, taking into consideration the level of ostomy, skinfolds, and the patient's clothing preferences. Initial ostomy care teaching also is provided by the ET nurse during the preoperative visit.*
- Insert a nasogastric tube if ordered. *Although it is often inserted in the surgical suite just prior to surgery, the nasogastric tube may be placed preoperatively to remove secretions and empty stomach contents.*
- Perform bowel preparation procedures as ordered. *Oral and parenteral antibiotics as well as cathartics and enemas may be prescribed preoperatively to clean the bowel and reduce the risk of peritoneal contamination by bowel contents during surgery.*

POSTOPERATIVE NURSING CARE
- Provide routine care for the surgical patient (∞ Chapter 4).
- Monitor bowel sounds and degree of abdominal distention. *Surgical manipulation of the bowel disrupts peristalsis, resulting in an initial ileus. Bowel sounds and the passage of flatus indicate a return of peristalsis.*
- Assess the position and patency of the nasogastric tube, connecting it to low suction. If the tube becomes clogged, gently irrigate with sterile normal saline. *A nasogastric or gastrostomy tube is used postoperatively to provide gastrointestinal decompression and facilitate healing of the anastomosis. Ensuring its patency is important for comfort and healing.*
- Assess color, amount, and odor of drainage from surgical drains and the colostomy (if present), noting any changes or the presence of clots or bright bleeding. *Initial drainage may be bright red and then become dark and finally clear or*

greenish yellow over the first 2 to 3 days. A change in the color, amount, or odor of the drainage may indicate a complication such as hemorrhage, intestinal obstruction, or infection.*
- Alert all personnel caring for the patient with an abdominoperineal resection to avoid rectal temperatures, suppositories, or other rectal procedures. *These procedures could disrupt the anal suture line, causing bleeding, infection, or impaired healing.*
- Maintain intravenous fluids while nasogastric suction is in place. *The patient on nasogastric suction is unable to take oral food and fluids and, moreover, is losing electrolyte-rich fluid through the nasogastric tube. If replacement fluid and electrolytes are not maintained, the patient is at risk for dehydration, sodium, potassium, and chloride imbalance, and metabolic alkalosis.*
- Provide antacids, histamine₂ receptor antagonists, and antibiotic therapy as ordered. *These medications may be ordered for the postoperative patient, depending on the procedure performed. Antibiotic therapy is a common measure to prevent infection resulting from contamination of the abdominal cavity with gastric contents.*
- Resume oral food and fluids as ordered. Initial feedings may be clear liquids, progressing to full liquids, and then frequent small feedings of regular foods. Monitor bowel sounds and monitor for abdominal distention frequently during this period. *Oral feedings are reintroduced slowly to minimize abdominal distention and trauma to the suture lines.*
- Begin discharge planning and teaching. Consult with a dietitian for instructions and menu planning; reinforce teaching. Teach about potential postoperative complications such as abdominal abscess, or bowel obstruction, their signs and symptoms, and preventive measures.

A *sigmoid colostomy* is the most common permanent colostomy performed, particularly for cancer of the rectum. It is usually created during an abdominoperineal resection. This procedure involves the removal of the sigmoid colon, rectum, and anus through abdominal and perineal incisions. The anal canal is closed, and a stoma formed from the proximal sigmoid colon. The stoma usually is located on the lower left quadrant of the abdomen.

When a *double-barrel colostomy* is performed, two separate stomas are created (Figure 24–12 ■). The distal colon is not removed, but bypassed. The proximal stoma, which is functional, diverts feces to the abdominal wall. The distal stoma, also called the mucous fistula, expels mucus from the distal colon. It may be pouched or dressed with a 4 × 4 gauge dressing. A double-barrel colostomy may be created for cases of trauma, tumor, or inflammation, and it may be temporary or permanent.

An emergency procedure used to relieve an intestinal obstruction or perforation is called a *transverse loop colostomy*. During this procedure, a loop of the transverse colon is brought out from the abdominal wall and suspended over a plastic rod or bridge, which prevents the loop from slipping back into the abdominal cavity. The loop stoma may be opened at the time of surgery or a few days later at the patient's bedside. The bridge may be removed in 1 to 2 weeks. Transverse loop colostomies are typically temporary.

In a *Hartmann procedure*, a common temporary colostomy procedure, the distal portion of the colon is left in place and is oversewn for closure. A temporary colostomy may be done to allow bowel rest or healing, such as following tumor resection or inflammation of the bowel. It also may be created following traumatic injury to the colon, such as a gunshot wound. Anastomosis of the severed portions of the colon is delayed because bacterial colonization of the colon would prevent proper healing of the anastomosis. About 3 to 6 months following a temporary colostomy, the colostomy is closed and the colon is reconnected. Patients with temporary colostomies require the same care as patients with permanent colostomies. See nursing care for a patient with a colostomy on page 706.

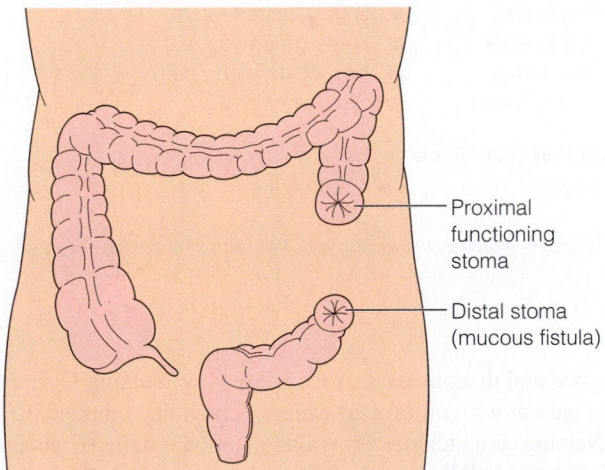

Figure 24–12 ■ A double-barrel colostomy. The proximal stoma is the functioning stoma; the distal stoma expels mucus from the distal colon.

— Proximal functioning stoma

— Distal stoma (mucous fistula)

Radiation Therapy

Although radiation therapy is not used as a primary treatment for colon cancer, it is used with surgical resection for treating rectal tumors. Small rectal cancers may be treated with intracavitary, external, or implantation radiation. Rectal cancer has a high rate of regional recurrence following complete surgical resection, particularly when the tumor has invaded tissues outside the bowel wall or regional lymph nodes. Pre- or postoperative radiation therapy reduces the recurrence of pelvic tumors, although the effect of radiation therapy on long-term survival is less clear. Radiation therapy is used preoperatively to shrink large rectal tumors enough to permit surgical removal of the tumor.

Chemotherapy

Chemotherapeutic agents, such as intravenous fluorouracil (5-FU) and folinic acid (leucovorin), are also used postoperatively as adjunctive therapy for colorectal cancer. When combined with radiation therapy, chemotherapy reduces the rate of tumor recurrence and prolongs survival for patients with stage II and stage III rectal tumors. The benefit for colon cancers is less clear, but chemotherapy may be used to reduce its spread to the liver and prevent recurrence. Irinotecan (CPT-11) or oxaliplatin may be used in chemotherapy regimens for colorectal cancer. Further discussion about chemotherapy and nursing implications is included in ∞ Chapter 14.

✐ Nursing Care

Health Promotion

Primary prevention of colorectal cancer is a significant nursing care issue. Teach patients the importance of maintaining an optimal weight and staying physically active. Discuss dietary recommendations provided by the ACS for the prevention of colorectal cancer. These recommendations include decreasing the amount of fat, refined sugar, and red meats in the diet while increasing intake of dietary fiber. Foods that contain high amounts of fiber include raw fruits and vegetables, legumes, and whole-grain products.

Stress the importance of regular health examinations, including digital rectal exams. Discuss recommendations for regular hemoccult testing of stool after age 40. Include the importance of seeking medical treatment if blood is noted in or on the stool. Teach patients the warning signs for cancer, including those specific to bowel cancer, such as a change in bowel habits.

Assessment

- *Health history:* Usual bowel patterns and any recent changes; weight loss, fatigue, decreased activity tolerance; presence of blood in the stool; pain with defecation, abdominal discomfort, perineal pain; usual diet; family history of colon cancer, other specific risk factors such as inflammatory bowel disease or colon polyps.
- *Physical examination:* General appearance; weight; abdominal shape, contour; bowel sounds, abdominal tenderness; stool hemoccult or guaiac.

NURSING CARE OF THE PATIENT with a Colostomy

- Assess the location of the stoma and the type of colostomy performed. *Stoma location is an indicator of the section of bowel in which it is located and a predictor of the type of fecal drainage to expect.*
- Assess stoma appearance and surrounding skin condition frequently (see the box on page 687). *Assessment of stoma and skin condition is particularly important in the early postoperative period, when complications are most likely to occur and are most treatable.*
- Position a collection bag or drainable pouch over the stoma. *Initial drainage may contain more mucus and serosanguineous fluid than fecal material. As the bowel starts to resume function, drainage becomes fecal in nature. The consistency of drainage depends on the stoma location in the bowel.*
- If ordered, irrigate the colostomy, instilling water into the colon similar to an enema procedure. *The water stimulates the colon to empty.*
- When a colostomy irrigation is ordered for a patient with a double-barrel or loop colostomy, irrigate the proximal stoma. Digital assessment of the bowel direction from the stoma can assist in determining which is the proximal stoma. *The distal bowel carries no fecal contents and does not need irrigation. It may be irrigated for cleansing just prior to reanastomosis.*
- Empty a drainable pouch or replace the colostomy bag as needed or when it is no more than one-third full. *If the pouch is allowed to overfill, its weight may impair the seal and cause leakage.*
- Provide stomal and skin care for the patient with a colostomy as for the patient with an ileostomy (see the box on page 687). *Good skin and stoma care is important to maintain skin integrity and function as the first line of defense against infection.*
- Use caulking agents, such as Stomahesive or karaya paste, and a skin barrier wafer as needed to maintain a secure ostomy pouch. This may be particularly important for the patient with a loop colostomy. *The main challenge for a patient with a transverse loop colostomy is to maintain a secure ostomy pouch over the plastic bridge.*
- A small needle hole high on the colostomy pouch will allow flatus to escape. This hole may be closed with a Band-Aid and opened only while the patient is in the bathroom for odor control. *Ostomy bags may "balloon" out, disrupting the skin seal, if excess gas collects.*

Health Education for the Patient and Family

- Prior to discharge, provide written, verbal, and psychomotor instruction on colostomy care, pouch management, skin care, and irrigation for the patient. *Whether the colostomy is temporary or permanent, the patient will be responsible for its management. Good understanding of procedures and*

care enhances the ability to provide self-care, as well as self-esteem and control.
- Allow ample time for the patient (and family, if necessary) to practice changing the pouch, either on the patient or a model. *Practice of psychomotor skills improves learning and confidence.*
- If an abdominoperineal resection has been performed, emphasize the importance of using no rectal suppositories, rectal temperatures, or enemas. Suggest that the patient carry medical identification or a Medic-Alert tag or bracelet. *These measures are important to prevent trauma to the tissues when the rectum has been removed.*
- The diet for a patient with a colostomy is individualized and may require no alteration from that consumed preoperatively. Dietary teaching should, however, include information on foods that cause stool odor and gas and foods that thicken and loosen stools. Foods that cause these effects on ostomy output are listed next.

Foods That Increase Stool Odor
- Asparagus
- Beans
- Cabbage
- Eggs
- Fish
- Garlic
- Onions
- Some spices

Foods That Increase Intestinal Gas
- Beer
- Broccoli
- Brussels sprouts
- Cabbage
- Carbonated drinks
- Cauliflower
- Corn
- Cucumbers
- Dairy products
- Dried beans
- Peas
- Radishes
- Spinach

Foods That Thicken Stools
- Applesauce
- Bananas
- Bread
- Cheese
- Yogurt
- Pasta
- Pretzels
- Rice
- Tapioca
- Creamy peanut butter

Foods That Loosen Stools
- Chocolate
- Dried beans
- Fried foods
- Greasy foods
- Highly spiced foods
- Leafy green vegetables
- Raw fruits and juices
- Raw vegetables

Foods That Color Stools
- Beets
- Red gelatin

Nursing Diagnoses and Interventions

In planning and implementing care, consider both physical care needs and emotional response to the diagnosis. Because colorectal cancer is often advanced at the time of diagnosis, the prognosis, even with treatment, may be poor. Denial and anger are common. Extensive abdominal surgery and potentially a colostomy may be necessary, and the effects of chemotherapy and radiation therapy can leave the patient

fatigued and discouraged. A Case Study & Nursing Care Plan for a patient with colorectal cancer is included on page 707.

Nursing care includes providing emotional support, teaching, and direct care before and after diagnostic procedures and surgery and during adjunctive treatments. Priority nursing diagnoses include *Acute Pain, Imbalanced Nutrition*, and *Anticipatory Grieving. Risk for Sexual Dysfunction* should be considered as a priority diagnosis if a colostomy has been created.

- Monitor for adequate pain relief. Use subjective and objective information, including the location, intensity, and character of the pain, as well as nonverbal signs, such as grimacing; muscle tension; apparent dozing; changes in pulse or blood pressure; or rapid, shallow respirations. *The patient may assume that pain is to be expected or tolerated or may fear becoming addicted to analgesic medications. Careful questioning and assessment can provide accurate information about pain status, allowing better control of discomfort.*
- Ask patient to rate pain using a 0 to 10 pain scale. Document the level of pain. *Pain is a subjective experience. Patients perceive and respond to pain differently. Religion and ethnic background may affect the response to pain.*
- Monitor analgesic effectiveness 30 minutes after administration. Monitor for pain relief and adverse effects. *The method*

EVIDENCE FOR NURSING CARE — The Patient with Colorectal Cancer

Selected resources that nurses may find helpful when planning evidence-based nursing care follow.

- Daly, J. M., Merchant, M. L., & Levy, B. T. (2009). Colorectal cancer screening. *The American Journal of Nursing, 109*(10), 60–62. doi:10.1097/01.NAJ.0000361496.60341.84
- National Cancer Institute. (2008). *Colon cancer treatment (PDQ®). Health professional version.* Retrieved from www.cancer.gov/cancertopics/pdq/treatment/colon/ healthprofessional/

of delivery, dosage, or medication itself may need to be adjusted to provide adequate pain relief.

- Assess the incision for inflammation or swelling; assess drainage catheters and tubes for patency. *Poorly controlled pain or pain that changes may be related to organ distention from an obstructed nasogastric tube, urinary catheter, or wound drain, or may indicate an infection.*

CASE STUDY & NURSING CARE PLAN   A Patient with Colorectal Cancer

William Cunningham is a 65-year-old retired railroad employee, husband, and father of three grown children. For the past 3 months, Mr. Cunningham has noticed small amounts of blood and occasional mucus in his stools. He has a sensation of pressure in the rectum, and notices that his stools are smaller in diameter, about the size of pencil. After palpating a mass on digital examination of the rectum, the physician orders a colonoscopy. A large sessile lesion is found in the rectum and biopsied. The pathology report shows the lesion to be adenocarcinoma. Mr. Cunningham is scheduled for an abdominoperineal resection and sigmoid colostomy.

ASSESSMENT

Madonna Hart, RN, completes the admission assessment. Mr. Cunningham states that his bowel habits have recently changed, but denies pain or other symptoms. Physical assessment findings include T 98.4°F (36.9°C), P 82, R 18, and BP 118/78. He is 70 inches (178 cm) tall and weighs 185 lb (84 kg). Laboratory findings are normal except for the previous pathology report of adenocarcinoma of rectal lesion.

Mr. Cunningham states, "I really don't want a colostomy, but if that is what it takes to get rid of this, I'm ready to get it over with."

DIAGNOSES

- *Acute Pain* related to surgical intervention
- *Risk for Impaired Skin Integrity (Peristomal)* related to fecal drainage and pouch adhesive
- *Risk for Constipation/Diarrhea* related to effects of surgery on bowel function
- *Disturbed Body Image* related to colostomy
- *Risk for Sexual Dysfunction* related to wide rectal incision, radiation therapy, and colostomy

EXPECTED OUTCOMES

- Report pain within an acceptable range that allows ease of movement and ambulation.

- Perform colostomy care using correct technique.
- Demonstrate willingness to discuss changes in sexual function.
- Wear clothing to enhance physical and emotional self-esteem.

PLANNING AND IMPLEMENTATION

- Provide analgesia as ordered, evaluating its effectiveness.
- Discuss foods that cause odor and gas.
- Teach colostomy care.
- Maintain consistent nursing personnel assignment to facilitate trust.
- Refer to the local United Ostomy Association.
- Provide a list of local medical supply companies for ostomy supplies.
- Provide for privacy when teaching and discussing concerns about ostomy.

EVALUATION

On discharge, Mr. Cunningham is able to empty and rinse out his colostomy pouch. He is changing the pouch and caring for surrounding skin appropriately. Ms. Hart has given him verbal and written instructions on colostomy care. He verbalizes understanding of phantom rectal pain, and the importance of avoiding rectal suppositories. He expresses an understanding of the need to avoid heavy lifting, and the importance of follow-up care. Ms. Hart has referred Mr. Cunningham to a home health agency in his community for further questions and follow-up care.

CRITICAL THINKING IN THE NURSING PROCESS

1. What is the cause of phantom rectal pain?
2. Why is it important to discuss dietary concerns with a patient with a colostomy, especially odor- and gas-forming foods?
3. Outline a plan to teach Mr. Cunningham how to irrigate a colostomy.
4. Develop a care plan for Mr. Cunningham for the nursing diagnosis *Disturbed Body Image*.

See Evaluating Your Response in Appendix C.

- Assess the abdomen for distention, tenderness, and bowel sounds. *Intra-abdominal bleeding, peritonitis, or paralytic ileus can cause pain that may be confused with incisional pain.*
- Administer analgesia prior to an activity or procedure. *Adequate pain relief reduces muscle tension, allowing for more comfortable participation in activities.*
- Assist with adjunctive comfort measures, such as positioning, diversional activities, management of environmental stimuli, guided imagery, and teaching relaxation techniques. *These measures enhance the effects of analgesia by reducing muscle tension.*
- Splint incision with a pillow, and teach the patient how to self-splint when coughing and deep breathing *to prevent respiratory complications related to fear of pain.*

Imbalanced Nutrition: Less than Body Requirements

Bowel preparation for diagnostic procedures, surgery, radiation therapy, and chemotherapy place the patient with colorectal cancer at risk for nutritional deficiencies. Fluid and electrolyte replacement is provided following surgery, along with possible PN (∞ see Chapter 22). Adequate kilocalorie and nutrient intake are necessary for healing after surgery. Additionally, if the tumor is advanced, metabolic needs may be increased and the appetite decreased.

- Assess nutritional status, using data such as height and weight, skinfold measurements, body mass index (BMI) calculation (∞ see Chapter 21), and laboratory data including serum albumin level. Refer to dietitian or nutritionist for dietary management. *The patient who is malnourished before beginning aggressive cancer treatment requires more vigorous nutrition management to promote healing.*
- Assess readiness for resumption of oral intake after surgery or procedures using data such as statements of hunger, presence of bowel sounds, passage of flatus, and minimal abdominal distention. *Manipulation of the bowel interrupts peristalsis of the GI tract. It is important to ensure that peristalsis has resumed prior to resumption of oral intake.*
- Monitor and document food and fluid intake. *Documentation helps identify the adequacy of kilocalories and other nutrient intake.*
- Weigh daily. *Weight fluctuation may indicate adequate or inadequate dietary intake.*
- Maintain PN and central intravenous lines as ordered. *Parenteral nutrition prevents tissue catabolism and promotes healing when food intake is disrupted for more than 2 to 3 days.*
- When oral intake resumes, help the patient develop a meal plan that incorporates food preferences and considers the patient's schedule and environment. *Consideration of likes, dislikes, and circumstances in meal planning promotes adequate intake.*

Grieving

When a bowel resection is performed for colorectal cancer, the patient needs to adjust to the loss of a major body part as well as to the diagnosis of cancer. Even when the prognosis for recovery is good, many people perceive cancer as fatal. Supporting the patient and family during the initial stages of grieving can improve physical recovery as well as psychologic coping and eventual adaptation.

- Work to develop a trusting relationship with the patient and family. *This increases the nurse's effectiveness in helping them work through the grieving process.*
- Listen actively, encouraging the patient and family to express their fears and concerns. Assist to identify strengths, past experiences, and support systems:
  - Demonstrate respect for cultural, spiritual, and religious values and beliefs; encourage use of these resources to cope with losses.
  - Encourage discussion of the potential impact of loss on individual family members, family structure, and family function. Assist family members to share concerns with one another.
  - Refer to cancer support groups, social services, or counseling as appropriate.

  These resources can be used throughout the grieving process.

Risk for Sexual Dysfunction

Colorectal cancer and ostomy surgery increase the risk for sexual dysfunction, defined as a change in sexual function so that it becomes unsatisfying, unrewarding, or inadequate (NANDA, 2009). Physical factors that can lead to sexual dysfunction include disruption of nerves and blood vessels that supply the genitals, radiation therapy, chemotherapy, and other medications prescribed after surgery.

Psychologically, an *ostomate* (patient with an ostomy) experiences an altered body image and may develop low self-esteem. The patient may feel undesirable and fear rejection. He or she may be concerned about odors or pouch leakage during sexual activity. This emotional stress can contribute to sexual dysfunction.

- Provide opportunities for the patient and family to express feelings about the cancer diagnosis, ostomy, and effects of other treatments. *Encouraging verbalization of feelings about the diagnosis, ostomy, and treatments provides an opportunity to validate that feelings of anger and depression are normal responses to the diagnosis and change in body function.*
- Provide consistent colostomy care. *An accepting attitude and consistent care that provides a secure appliance and controls odor and leakage instill a sense of confidence in the patient.*
- Encourage expression of sexual concerns. Provide privacy and caregivers who have established trust with the patient and family and are comfortable with discussions about sexual concerns. *Sexuality is a very private concern to most people. The patient and family are not likely to express their concerns openly unless trust has been established.*
- Reassure the patient and significant other that the effect of physical illness and prescribed interventions on sexuality usually is temporary. *The patient and partner may misinterpret an initial decrease in libido as evidence that sexual activity will not be possible or resume following recovery.*
- Refer the patient and partner to social services or a family counselor for further interventions. *Patients are often discharged from acute care settings well before concerns about sexual activity surface. Ongoing counseling provides a continuing resource.*

- Arrange for a visit from a member of the United Ostomy Association. *People who are living and coping with an ostomy can provide information and support, helping the new ostomate overcome feelings of isolation and rejection.*

Using NANDA, NIC, and NOC

Linkages between a selected NANDA nursing diagnosis, NIC, and NOC for the patient with colorectal cancer are shown in the chart that follows.

Community-Based Care

During the diagnostic and preoperative periods, provide instruction about the following topics:

- Tests to be performed and preparatory procedures, including dietary restrictions, laxatives, enemas, and food and fluid restrictions just prior to the procedure
- Recommended postprocedure care and potential adverse effects to report
- Preoperative care, such as intestinal preparation and food and fluid restrictions

If a colostomy is planned, refer to an enterostomal therapist for stoma placement and initial teaching.

Once treatment has been initiated, include the following topics (as appropriate) in teaching for home care:

- Pain management
- Skin care and management of potential adverse effects of radiation therapy and/or chemotherapy (∞ Refer to

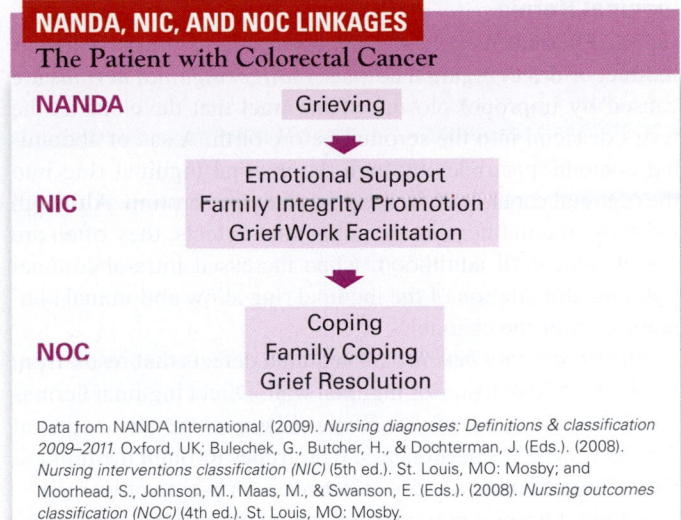

NANDA, NIC, AND NOC LINKAGES
The Patient with Colorectal Cancer

NANDA	Grieving
NIC	Emotional Support Family Integrity Promotion Grief Work Facilitation
NOC	Coping Family Coping Grief Resolution

Data from NANDA International. (2009). *Nursing diagnoses: Definitions & classification 2009–2011.* Oxford, UK; Bulechek, G., Butcher, H., & Dochterman, J. (Eds.). (2008). *Nursing interventions classification (NIC)* (5th ed.). St. Louis, MO: Mosby; and Moorhead, S., Johnson, M., Maas, M., & Swanson, E. (Eds.). (2008). *Nursing outcomes classification (NOC)* (4th ed.). St. Louis, MO: Mosby.

Chapter 14 for further discussion of teaching needs related to these therapies.)
- Incision and ostomy care
- Recommended diet
- Follow-up appointments and care

If the tumor is inoperable or a cure is not anticipated, provide information about pain and symptom management. Discuss the hospice philosophy and available services. Provide a referral to a local hospice or home health department.

Structural and Obstructive Bowel Disorders

Any portion of the intestines may be affected by a structural or obstructive disorder. Defects in the abdominal wall may allow intra-abdominal contents (such as loops of bowel) to protrude, indirectly affecting bowel function. Likewise, obstructions may result from disease of the bowel itself or from obstruction of the bowel lumen by an external force.

The Patient with a Hernia

A *hernia* is a defect in the abdominal wall that allows abdominal contents to protrude out of the abdominal cavity. Trauma, surgery, and increased intra-abdominal pressure caused by such conditions as pregnancy, obesity, weight lifting, or tumors are risk factors for hernia formation.

Pathophysiology

Hernias are classified by location (Figure 24–13 ■), and may be congenital or acquired. Most hernias occur in the groin (inguinal or femoral hernias). Inguinal hernias often are congenital, caused by improper closure of the tract that develops as the testes descend into the scrotum during fetal development. Groin hernias may be acquired, resulting from weakness of fascia in a region called Hesselbach's area or from dilation of the femoral ring (e.g., during pregnancy and childbirth). Ventral or incisional hernias of the abdominal wall generally are acquired, caused by weakening of normal abdominal wall musculature. Umbilical hernias also are congenital, and usually are

detected in infancy. Hiatal hernias develop in the diaphragm (∞ see Chapter 23).

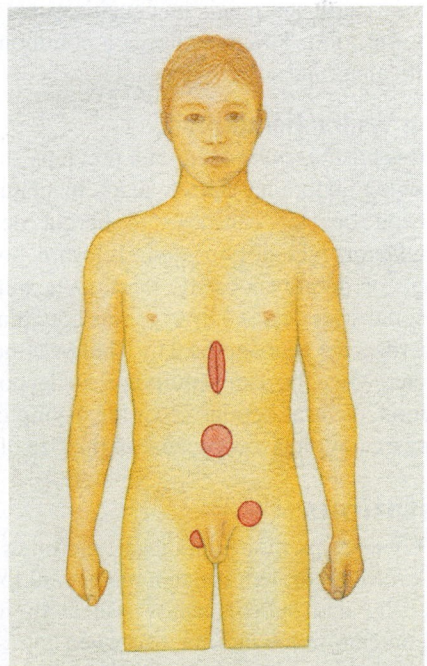

Figure 24–13 ■ An abdominal wall (ventral or incisional) hernia and an inguinal hernia.

Inguinal Hernia

Inguinal hernias usually affect males, and may be classified as indirect or direct inguinal hernias. *Indirect inguinal hernias* are caused by improper closure of the tract that develops as the testes descend into the scrotum before birth. A sac of abdominal contents protrudes through the internal inguinal ring into the inguinal canal. It often descends into the scrotum. Although indirect inguinal hernias are congenital defects, they often are not evident until adulthood, when increased intra-abdominal pressure and dilation of the inguinal ring allow abdominal contents to enter the channel.

Direct inguinal hernias are acquired defects that result from weakness of the posterior inguinal wall. Direct inguinal hernias usually affect older adults. *Femoral hernias* are also acquired defects in which a peritoneal sac protrudes through the femoral ring. These hernias usually affect obese or pregnant women.

Inguinal hernias may produce no symptoms and are discovered during routine physical examination. They may cause a lump, swelling, or bulge in the groin, particularly with lifting or straining. An inguinal hernia may cause sharp pain or a dull ache that radiates into the scrotum. A palpable mass may be present in the groin, although it may be felt only with increased intra-abdominal pressure (as occurs during coughing) and invagination of the scrotum toward the inguinal ring.

Umbilical Hernia

Pregnancy and obesity contribute to the development of umbilical hernias in adults. *Umbilical hernias* may be congenital and evident during infancy, or acquired as the tissue closing the umbilical ring weakens, allowing protrusion of abdominal contents. These hernias are more common in women. Other predisposing factors include multiple pregnancies with prolonged labor, ascites, and large intra-abdominal tumors.

Umbilical hernias tend to enlarge steadily and contain omentum, although they may also contain small or large bowel. The hernia may cause sharp pain on coughing or straining or a dull, aching sensation. Strangulation is a common complication of umbilical hernias.

Incisional or Ventral Hernia

Incisional or *ventral hernias* occur at a previous surgical incision or following abdominal muscle tears. Inadequate healing of the incision or tear can lead to hernia development. Contributing factors include poor wound closure, postoperative infection, age or debility, obesity, inadequate nutrition, and excess incisional stress caused by vigorous coughing.

Ventral hernias are characterized by a bulge at the incisional site, often noted when the patient pulls to a sitting position from a lying position. Ventral hernias often are asymptomatic, and the risk of incarceration is low because of the size of the defect.

Manifestations

Abdominal contents (peritoneum, bowel, and other abdominal organs) can protrude through the abdominal wall to form a sac covered by skin and subcutaneous tissues. In most cases, abdominal contents move into the sac when intra-abdominal pressure increases, then return to the abdominal cavity when pressure returns to normal or when manual pressure is placed on the bulging sac. This is known as a *reducible hernia*.

Complications

The risk for complications is low with a reducible hernia. If the contents of a hernia cannot be returned to the abdominal cavity, it is said to be *incarcerated*. Contents of an incarcerated hernia are trapped, usually by a narrow neck or opening to the hernia. Incarceration increases the risk of complications, including obstruction and strangulation. Obstruction occurs when the lumen of the bowel contained within the hernia becomes occluded, much like the crimping of a hose. A *strangulated hernia* develops when blood supply to bowel and other tissues in the hernia sac is compromised, leading to necrosis. The affected bowel can infarct, leading to perforation with contamination of the peritoneal cavity. Manifestations of a strangulated hernia include severe abdominal pain and distention, nausea, vomiting, tachycardia, and fever.

Interdisciplinary Care

The diagnosis of a hernia is made by a physical examination. The patient is examined in a supine or standing position. A bulge may be seen or felt when the patient coughs or bears down. No laboratory or diagnostic testing is usually required, unless bowel obstruction or strangulation is suspected.

Surgical repair, or *herniorrhaphy*, is the usual treatment of hernia. Surgery is generally well tolerated by people of all ages and carries a much lower risk than the complications of incarceration, obstruction, and strangulation. Emergency surgery is indicated for a hernia that is incarcerated, painful, or tender. In a herniorrhaphy, the abdominal wall defect is closed by suturing or with wire or mesh over the defect. If incarceration has occurred or strangulation is suspected, the abdomen is explored at the time of surgery and any infarcted bowel resected. Heavy lifting and heavy manual labor are restricted for approximately 3 weeks after surgery.

When surgery is contraindicated, the patient may be taught to reduce the hernia by lying down and gently pushing against the mass. A binder or truss may be worn to prevent or control the protrusion. An incarcerated hernia should not be reduced by the patient.

✤ Nursing Care

Assessment

- *Health history:* Manifestations of hernia, such as bulging in the groin or of the abdominal wall when coughing, straining, or moving from lying to standing; pain (abdominal, groin, or scrotal); history of hernia or abdominal surgery.
- *Physical examination:* Observe for bulging of the abdominal wall or around the umbilicus when raising head and shoulders from supine position; wearing gloves, palpate inguinal region for bulges when the patient coughs or bears down (Valsalva maneuver) while standing.

Nursing Diagnoses and Interventions

Herniorrhaphy is generally an uncomplicated procedure, usually performed as same-day surgery. Preoperative assessment and teaching and immediate postoperative care are the primary nursing care needs. Care is similar to that provided for a patient with an appendectomy.

Risk for Ineffective Gastrointestinal Perfusion

When providing care for a patient with a known hernia, the possibility of obstruction and strangulation must be considered throughout nursing assessments. Although nursing interventions may not be able to prevent these complications, rapid identification of the problem allows timely surgical treatment. Prompt treatment may prevent major complications related to infection and peritoneal contamination by bowel contents.

- Assess bowel sounds and abdominal distention at least every 8 hours. *A change in bowel sounds—either cessation of sounds or an onset of hyperactive, high-pitched sounds—may indicate obstruction. With obstruction, abdominal girth may increase.*

> **PRACTICE ALERT**
> Promptly report any acute increase in abdominal, groin, perineal, or scrotal pain. An abrupt increase in the intensity of pain may indicate bowel ischemia due to strangulation.

- Notify primary care provider if the hernia becomes painful or tender. *Pain and tenderness may indicate incarceration and increased risk for strangulation.*
- If signs of possible obstruction or strangulation occur, notify the physician. Place patient in supine position with the hips elevated and knees slightly bent. Withhold all food and fluids (NPO), and begin preparations for surgery. *This position helps relax abdominal muscles and may facilitate reduction of the hernia. Strangulation or obstruction require immediate surgical intervention.*

Community-Based Care

Include the following topics when teaching patients about hernias and home care:

- Rationale for examining the groin and abdomen for bulges
- The nature of hernias, risk factors, and manifestations
- Surgical intervention for hernias
- How to reduce a hernia if necessary
- The importance of seeking immediate medical intervention for signs of strangulation or obstruction
- The need to notify the physician if upper respiratory infection and cough develop preoperatively (forceful coughing is not recommended postoperatively)
- Postoperative pain management and activity restrictions

The Patient with Intestinal Obstruction

Intestinal obstruction is failure of intestinal contents to move through the bowel lumen. Intestinal obstructions may affect either the large or small bowel. The small intestine is more commonly affected; however, bowel obstructions may also occur in the large intestine. Obstruction is the most common reason for small-bowel surgery.

Pathophysiology

Intestinal obstructions may be either mechanical or functional in nature. *Mechanical* obstructions may be caused by (1) problems outside the intestine, such as bands of scar tissue (adhesions) or hernias; (2) problems within the intestine, such as tumors or inflammatory bowel disease; or (3) obstruction of the intestinal lumen. The obstruction may be partial or complete. In some mechanical obstructions, such as a strangulated hernia, blood supply to the affected portion of bowel also is impaired, resulting in necrosis of the affected segment. *Functional* obstruction occurs when peristalsis fails to propel intestinal contents although there is no mechanical obstruction. *Adynamic ileus* (also known as *paralytic ileus* or simply *ileus*) is the most common functional obstruction after abdominal surgery. Obstructions are further classified by the portion of intestine affected.

When the intestine is obstructed, gas and fluid accumulate proximal to and within the obstructed segment, distending the bowel. Swallowed air accounts for most of the gas. Ingested fluid, saliva, gastric juice, and pancreatic secretions contribute to accumulated fluid. Water and sodium are drawn into the bowel lumen, contributing to fluid accumulation, distention, and vascular fluid losses. Distention of the bowel lumen interferes with peristaltic movement, leading to atony and further distention. Significant distention of the bowel lumen compromises blood flow to mucosa, eventually leading to necrosis. Gangrenous bowel may perforate with resulting peritonitis. Rapid bacterial growth in the obstructed bowel can lead to sepsis and death.

Significant bowel distention, vomiting, and third spacing of fluids in the bowel and peritoneal cavity can lead to massive loss of fluids and electrolytes with resulting hypovolemia, hypokalemia, renal insufficiency, and shock.

Small-Bowel Obstruction

Adhesions, or bands of scar tissue, and hernias account for most mechanical small bowel obstructions. In adults, adhesions develop following abdominal surgery or inflammatory processes. Adhesions usually produce a *simple obstruction*, or single blockage in one portion of the intestine (Figure 24–14A ■). The obstruction produced by an incarcerated hernia is a *closed-loop obstruction*, with two different portions of the bowel lumen obstructed (Figure 24–14B).

Tumors, either intrinsic (of the bowel itself) or extrinsic (of another organ but affecting the bowel because of their size), can progressively occlude the bowel lumen and eventually obstruct it (Figure 24–14C). Other, less common causes of bowel obstruction include intussusception (rare in adults) (Figure 24–14D); volvulus, which is the rotation of loops of bowel about a fixed point (Figure 24–14E); foreign bodies; stricture; and inflammatory bowel disease.

Both volvulus and an incarcerated hernia can cause a *strangulated obstruction*. In a strangulated obstruction, not only is the lumen of the bowel obstructed, but the blood supply to the affected portion is also compromised.

In a functional obstruction or adynamic ileus, peristalsis stops due to either neurogenic or muscular impairment. The bowel lumen remains patent, but contents are not propelled forward.

Figure 24–14 ■ Selected causes of mechanical obstruction. *A*, adhesions; *B*, incarcerated hernia; *C*, tumor; *D*, intussusception; and *E*, volvulus.

Temporary ileus commonly follows gastrointestinal surgery. It may result from tissue anoxia or peritoneal irritation due to hemorrhage, peritonitis, or perforation of an organ. Other conditions that can precipitate paralytic ileus include renal colic, spinal cord injuries, uremia, and electrolyte imbalances, hypokalemia in particular. In addition, the effects of some narcotics, anticholinergic drugs, and antidiarrheal medications such as diphenoxylate can produce a functional obstruction.

MANIFESTATIONS   The manifestations of a small-bowel obstruction vary, depending on the type and level of obstruction and how rapidly it develops. Cramping or colicky abdominal pain that may be intermittent or increasing in intensity is

common. Vomiting is common, particularly in high or proximal obstructions, because distention of the lumen stimulates the vomiting center. In a high obstruction, vomitus contains bile and mucus. As bacterial fermentation occurs, vomitus often contains fecal matter, particularly with a low or distal obstruction. Flatus and feces already present in the lower bowel may be expelled early in the obstructive process, but this expulsion ceases as the obstruction continues.

Early in the course of a mechanical obstruction, borborygmi and high-pitched tinkling bowel sounds often are present. Borborygmi may coincide with waves of colicky abdominal pain as the intestine attempts to propel contents past the obstruction. Visible peristaltic waves may be noted in the distended loops of bowel in thin patients. In the later stages, the bowel becomes silent. With a paralytic ileus, bowel sounds are greatly diminished or absent throughout the process. Abdominal distention is minimal with proximal obstructions, but may be pronounced with distal obstruction and paralytic ileus. The abdomen may be tender to palpation as well.

In addition to abdominal and gastrointestinal manifestations, signs of fluid and electrolyte imbalance develop. Hypovolemia can develop rapidly as extracellular fluid is sequestered in the bowel and vomiting occurs. Although early vital signs may be normal, changes are noted as dehydration and hypovolemia develop. The patient becomes tachycardic and tachypneic, and blood pressure falls. Temperature may be elevated. Urine output drops, and signs of hypovolemic shock may be seen. The manifestations of mechanical small bowel obstruction are outlined with their accompanying pathophysiologic processes in the Pathophysiology Linkage box that follows.

COMPLICATIONS   Hypovolemia and hypovolemic shock with multiple organ dysfunction is a significant complication of bowel obstruction and can lead to death. Renal insufficiency from hypovolemia can lead to acute renal failure. Pulmonary

PATHOPHYSIOLOGY LINKAGE   Small Bowel Obstruction

MANIFESTATION	PATHOPHYSIOLOGY
Abdominal pain: intermittent midabdominal, colicky; intensity may initially decrease, then become severe and steady	Peristaltic waves attempt to propel bowel contents past the obstruction. As the bowel becomes increasingly distended, peristalsis is inhibited and pain may decrease in intensity. If unrelieved, distention of bowel lumen impairs mucosal blood supply, leading to ischemia and necrosis. Bowel infarction or perforation may occur, leading to chemical and bacterial peritonitis.
Bowel sounds: initially loud, possibly high-pitched; may correspond with waves of abdominal pain; later infrequent or absent	Initial distention of the bowel proximal to the obstruction stimulates peristalsis as the bowel attempts to propel contents past the obstruction. With further distention and resulting electrolyte imbalances, peristalsis is inhibited and bowel sounds become less frequent to inaudible.
Vomiting	Distention of the bowel stimulates the vomiting center of the brain, which, in turn, stimulates the vomiting reflex.
Abdominal distention	Fluid (saliva, gastric juice, bile, pancreatic secretions) and air are trapped in the bowel proximal to the obstruction.
Hypovolemia, electrolyte imbalance	Normal movement of water and sodium from the bowel lumen to the interstitial and intravascular spaces is initially inhibited. Fluids and electrolytes are lost through vomiting. With continued obstruction and bowel distention, sodium and water move from the vascular system into the bowel lumen, further distending it. Intestinal venous return is inhibited, leading to tissue edema and accumulation of fluid and electrolytes within the peritoneal cavity.

ventilation may be impaired because abdominal distention elevates the diaphragm and interferes with respiratory processes.

Strangulation associated with incarcerated hernia or volvulus impairs the blood supply to the bowel. Gangrene may rapidly result, causing bleeding into the bowel lumen and peritoneal cavity and eventual perforation. With perforation, bacteria and toxins from the strangulated intestine enter the peritoneum and, potentially, the circulation, resulting in peritonitis and possible septic shock. Strangulation greatly increases the risk of mortality.

Large-Bowel Obstruction

Obstruction of the large intestine occurs much less frequently than small-bowel obstruction. Although any portion of the colon may be affected, obstruction usually occurs in the sigmoid segment. Cancer of the bowel is the most common cause; other causes include volvulus, diverticular disease, inflammatory disorders, and fecal impaction.

MANIFESTATIONS Constipation and colicky abdominal pain are usual manifestations of large-bowel obstruction. The pain is often deep and cramping; severe, continuous pain may signal bowel ischemia and possible perforation. Vomiting is a late sign, if it occurs at all. The abdomen is distended, with high-pitched, tinkling bowel sounds with rushes and gurgles. On palpation, localized tenderness or a mass may be noted.

COMPLICATIONS If the ileocecal valve between the small and large intestines is competent, distention proximal to the obstruction is limited to the colon itself. This is known as a *closed-loop obstruction*. It can lead to massive colon dilation as the ileum continues to empty gas and fluid into the colon. Increasing pressure within the obstructed colon impairs circulation to the bowel wall. Gangrene, perforation and peritonitis are potential complications. Massive distention can impair function of the diaphragm, leading to atelectasis. Pressure on the inferior vena cava may impair venous return.

Interdisciplinary Care

The management of a bowel obstruction focuses on relieving the pressure and obstruction, and providing supportive care. The intestine is decompressed, and fluid and electrolyte balance is restored. Surgery may be necessary to relieve a mechanical obstruction or if strangulation is suspected.

Diagnosis

Radiologic studies (x-rays and CT scan) are used to confirm the diagnosis of bowel obstruction. Laboratory testing is used to evaluate for the presence of infection and fluid and electrolyte imbalances.

An abdominal x-ray often shows distended loops of intestine with fluid and gas in a small-bowel obstruction. Free air under the diaphragm indicates a perforation. X-ray or CT scan with contrast media may be required to confirm a mechanical obstruction and assess the completeness of the obstruction. Gastrografin is often used to provide contrast rather than barium when a bowel obstruction is suspected.

Laboratory tests used are WBC, serum amylase, serum osmolality, electrolytes, and arterial blood gases. These tests will show the following results with a bowel obstruction:

- *WBC* often shows mild leukocytosis due to an inflammatory response to changes within the obstructed bowel lumen. With strangulation, leukocytosis is marked.
- *Serum amylase levels* may be elevated, particularly when strangulation is present.
- *Serum osmolality* and *electrolyte levels* are affected by fluid and electrolyte losses from vomiting and fluid sequestering in the bowel lumen. With hypovolemia, the serum osmolality and urine specific gravity increase. Potassium and chloride are lost through vomiting, leading to hypokalemia and hypochloremia.
- ABGs may reveal metabolic alkalosis (pH > 7.45, bicarbonate > 24 mEq/L, PCO_2 > 45 mmHg) with small-bowel obstruction due to loss of hydrochloric acid from the stomach.

Gastrointestinal Decompression

Most partial small-bowel obstructions are successfully treated with gastrointestinal decompression using a nasogastric tube. Functional obstructions respond to treatment with bowel rest and intestinal decompression as well. Current evidence indicates that a standard nasogastric tube is as effective for gastrointestinal decompression as a longer intestinal tube. Collected fluid and gas are removed using low suction until peristalsis resumes or the obstruction is relieved.

Surgery

Surgical intervention is required for complete mechanical obstructions as well as for strangulated or incarcerated obstructions of the small intestine. Patients with incomplete mechanical obstruction may also require surgery if the obstruction persists.

Prior to surgery, a nasogastric tube is inserted to relieve vomiting and abdominal distention and to prevent aspiration of intestinal contents. Fluid and electrolyte balance must be restored before surgery. Isotonic intravenous fluids, such as normal (physiologic) saline, Ringer's solution, or other balanced electrolyte solutions, are used. Additional electrolytes may be added to the solution to correct low levels. It is particularly important to correct hypokalemia prior to surgery. Acid–base imbalances are also addressed, often using intravenous acidifiers or alkalinizing agents. If strangulation has occurred, the patient may require plasma or blood replacement. Intravenous broad-spectrum antibiotics are administered prophylactically (see the section on peritonitis).

Simple mechanical obstruction due to adhesions may be relieved using laparoscopic surgery to remove or lyse the scar tissue. A laparotomy may be performed to allow inspection of the small intestine and removal of infarcted or gangrenous tissue. Obstructing tumors are resected, and foreign bodies are removed. Any bowel that appears to be gangrenous is resected, usually followed by an end-to-end anastomosis of remaining intestine. If a large tumor mass or dense adhesions are found, the area of obstruction may be bypassed by anastomosis of proximal small bowel to small or large intestine distal to the obstruction. Nursing care of the patient having bowel surgery is included in the box on page 704.

Obstructions of the large intestine usually necessitate surgery. The primary goal is to relieve colonic distention and prevent perforation; the secondary goal is to remove the obstructing lesion. In some cases, colonoscopy may be used to relieve the distention. If the patient's condition prohibits major surgery or the obstructing tumor is advanced, laser photocoagulation may be used to enlarge the bowel lumen and a stent inserted to reduce the risk of reobstruction. Removal of the obstructing lesion is the preferred treatment. The proximal and distal bowel segments may be anastomosed, or a permanent colostomy or ileostomy may be required.

✍ Nursing Care

Health Promotion

Teach health promotion activities, such as increasing dietary fiber intake, maintaining a generous fluid intake, and exercising daily to help prevent constipation and possible large-bowel obstruction, particularly in the older adult. Stress the importance of complying with dietary restrictions (such as avoiding popcorn) for patients who experience repeated small-bowel obstructions.

Assessment

Nurses may be instrumental in the early identification of intestinal obstructions in older adults, the homebound patient, or the institutionalized patient. Early identification and intervention significantly reduce morbidity from bowel obstruction.

- *Health history:* Complaints of abdominal pain and bloating, constipation; previous history of bowel obstruction or risk factors such as hernia, inflammatory bowel disease, diverticulosis, or previous abdominal surgery; current medications.
- *Physical examination:* Vital signs including orthostatic blood pressure, temperature; skin color, temperature, texture, and turgor; color and moisture of mucous membranes; abdominal shape, contour, bowel sounds, presence of tenderness or masses on palpation.

Nursing Diagnoses and Interventions

In patients with a suspected or confirmed bowel obstruction, frequent assessment for complications such as fluid and electrolyte imbalance, acid–base imbalances, hypovolemic shock, perforation, and peritonitis is necessary.

Deficient Fluid Volume

Because of the large collection of fluid in the bowel proximal to an obstruction, the accompanying vomiting, and nasogastric suction, the patient with an intestinal obstruction often has a fluid volume deficit. If not corrected promptly, hypovolemic shock, acute renal failure, and multiple organ system dysfunction from poor tissue perfusion may result.

- Monitor vital signs, pulmonary artery pressures, cardiac output (CO), and central venous pressure (CVP) hourly. *A decrease in blood pressure, tachycardia, and tachypnea may indicate hypovolemia. Although invasive, hemodynamic parameters such as pulmonary artery pressures, CO, and CVP allow accurate assessment of fluid volume status.*

- Measure urinary output hourly and nasogastric drainage every 2 to 4 hours. *A urinary output of 30 mL per hour or more usually indicates an adequate glomerular filtration rate (GFR), another indicator of fluid volume. Nasogastric output provides a tool for evaluating fluid replacement needs.*

> **PRACTICE ALERT**
> Promptly report urine output of less than 30 mL per hour. This often indicates hypovolemia and an increased risk for shock and acute renal failure.

- Maintain intravenous fluids and blood volume expanders as ordered. The amount of fluid administered is calculated to meet ongoing fluid needs and replace previous and current losses. *Restoration and maintenance of blood volume are necessary to maintain cardiac output and tissue and organ perfusion.*
- Measure abdominal girth every 4 to 8 hours. Mark the level of measurement on the abdomen. *A reference mark allows consistent, accurate measurements. An increase in abdominal girth indicates increasing intestinal distention.*
- Notify the physician of changes in status. *Changes in vital signs, pain, and signs of increasing distention can indicate the need for immediate surgical intervention.*

Ineffective Gastrointestinal Perfusion

Perfusion of the intestinal wall and mucosa may be impaired by the obstructive process itself (e.g., strangulation or volvulus) or by significant intestinal distention. The goal is to maintain tissue perfusion and promote normal peristalsis and bowel elimination.

- Monitor vital signs hourly. Assess peripheral pulses, skin color, temperature, and capillary refill. *Cardiovascular assessment is vital to detect early signs of hypovolemic shock resulting from sequestering large volumes of fluid in the intestines. Hypovolemia and shock can convert mild bowel ischemia to infarction as the blood supply to the tissue falls.*
- Monitor urine output hourly. Report output of less than 30 mL per hour. *Urine output is a good indicator of the GFR and tissue perfusion. The urine output often falls before vital sign changes are apparent in hypovolemia.*
- Monitor temperature at least every 4 hours. *An elevated temperature may be an early indication of sepsis from bowel perforation as a result of gangrene.*
- Frequently assess pain. *A change in the character of pain or a rapid increase in its intensity may signal bowel infarction or perforation.*
- Maintain NPO status until peristalsis resumes. *Enteral food or fluids may increase distention and bowel ischemia. They also are restricted until the possibility of perforation is eliminated.*

Ineffective Breathing Pattern

Significant abdominal distention from a bowel obstruction can cause the diaphragm to flatten, impairing pulmonary ventilation. Following surgery, splinting of abdominal muscles to avoid pain can lead to shallow respirations. These factors, plus the risk of aspiration of gastrointestinal contents during vomiting, place the patient at high risk for respiratory complications, particularly with a small-bowel obstruction.

- Assess respiratory rate, pattern, and lung sounds at least every 2 to 4 hours. *Tachypnea, shortness of breath, or apparent dyspnea may be early signs of respiratory compromise. Diminished breath sounds, particularly in the bases of the lungs, or crackles indicate poor lung expansion and possible impaired ventilation.*
- Monitor ABG results for possible effects of altered respiratory status. *Tachypnea may lead to respiratory alkalosis as excess carbon dioxide is eliminated. Conversely, impaired chest expansion can lead to respiratory acidosis because of alveolar hypoventilation.*
- Elevate the head of the bed. *Elevating the head of the bed reduces the work of breathing and improves alveolar ventilation by reducing the pressure of abdominal distention on the diaphragm.*
- Provide a pillow or folded bath blanket to use in splinting the abdomen while coughing postoperatively. *Splinting abdominal muscles and incisions improves the ease and effectiveness of coughing postoperatively.*
- Maintain nasogastric or intestinal tube patency. *Maintaining gastrointestinal suction helps reduce abdominal distention and prevent aspiration associated with vomiting.*

- Encourage use of incentive spirometer or other assistive device hourly. *These devices encourage deep breathing, opening distal airways and preventing atelectasis.*
- Contact respiratory therapy as indicated. *The respiratory therapist may suggest or perform additional measures to maintain effective pulmonary ventilation.*
- Provide good oral care at least every 4 hours. *Dehydration and nasogastric suction dry the mucous membranes of the mouth and throat, increasing the risk of bacterial growth. Many respiratory infections result from aspirated organisms.*

Community-Based Care

Include the following topics when teaching the patient with intestinal obstruction in preparation for home care:

- Wound care
- Activity level, return to work, and any other recommended restrictions
- Recommended follow-up care
- Care of temporary colostomy (if appropriate) and planned reanastomosis
- For recurrent obstructions, their cause, early identification of manifestations, and possible preventive measures

Anorectal Disorders

Anorectal lesions include hemorrhoids, a normal condition common to all adults that may become enlarged and painful; anal fissure; anorectal abscess; anorectal fistulas; and pilonidal disease.

The Patient with Hemorrhoids

The anus and anal canal contain two superficial venous plexuses with the hemorrhoidal veins. When pressure on these veins is increased or venous return impeded, they can develop *varices*, or varicosities, becoming weak and distended. This condition is commonly known as *hemorrhoids*, or "piles." When asymptomatic, hemorrhoids are considered to be a normal condition found in all adults.

Pathophysiology and Manifestations

Hemorrhoids develop when venous return from the anal canal is impaired. Straining to defecate increases venous pressure and is the most common cause of distended hemorrhoids. Pregnancy increases intra-abdominal pressure, raising venous pressure, and is another cause of hemorrhoids. Other factors that may contribute to symptomatic hemorrhoids include prolonged sitting, obesity, chronic constipation, and a low-fiber diet.

Hemorrhoids are classed as either internal or external. *Internal* hemorrhoids affect the venous plexus above the mucocutaneous junction of the anus (Figure 24–15 ■). Internal hemorrhoids rarely cause pain, usually presenting with bleeding. Bleeding from internal hemorrhoids is bright red and unmixed with the stool. It can vary in quantity from streaks on toilet tissue to enough to color the water in the

toilet. Recurrent bleeding of internal hemorrhoids may be sufficient to cause anemia. Mucous discharge and a feeling of incomplete evacuation of stool also may be manifestations of internal hemorrhoids.

External hemorrhoids affect the inferior hemorrhoidal plexus below the mucocutaneous junction. Bleeding is rare with external hemorrhoids. Anal irritation, a feeling of pressure, and difficulty cleaning the anal region may be manifestations of external hemorrhoids.

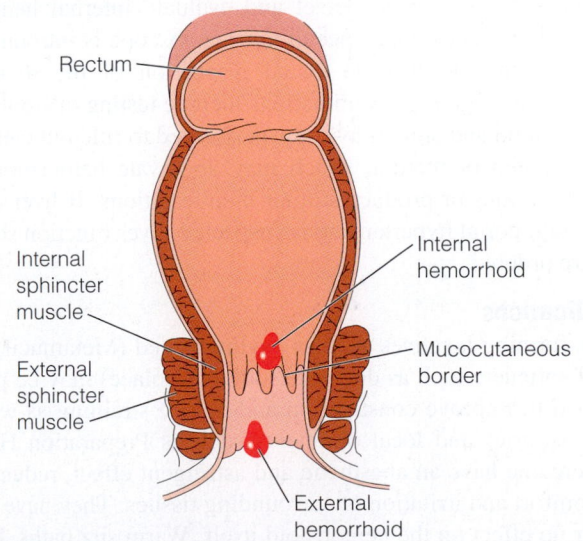

Figure 24–15 ■ The location of internal and external hemorrhoids.

As they enlarge, hemorrhoids may prolapse or protrude through the anus. Initially, prolapse occurs only with defecation and the hemorrhoids spontaneously regress back into the anal canal. Eventually, the patient may need to manually replace internal hemorrhoids after defecation, or they may become permanently prolapsed, in which case replacement is not possible. Manifestations of permanently prolapsed hemorrhoids include mucous discharge and clothing soilage.

Normal hemorrhoids are not painful. Prolapsed hemorrhoids may become strangulated as a result of congestion and edema, leading to thrombosis. Hemorrhoidal thrombosis causes extreme pain and may lead to infarction of skin and mucosa overlying the hemorrhoid. Internal hemorrhoids associated with portal hypertension in liver disease may bleed profusely if ruptured. (∞ See Chapter 25 for further discussion of portal hypertension.)

A *thrombosed external hemorrhoid* is a thrombosis of the subcutaneous external hemorrhoidal veins of the anal canal, rather than a true hemorrhoid. It appears as a painful bluish hematoma beneath the skin and typically occurs following a sudden increase in venous pressure, for example, heavy lifting, coughing, or straining. Pain is significant at onset but gradually subsides. Spontaneous rupture with bleeding may occur. Thrombosed external hemorrhoids resolve without intervention.

Interdisciplinary Care

Because hemorrhoids are a normal condition, management is conservative unless complications such as permanent prolapse or thrombosis occur.

Diagnosis

Hemorrhoids are diagnosed by the patient's history and by examination of the anorectal area. External hemorrhoids can be seen on visual inspection, especially if thrombosed. The patient is asked to strain (Valsalva's maneuver) during the examination to detect prolapse. Internal hemorrhoids are usually not palpable or tender on digital examination of the rectum. Anoscopic examination is used to detect and evaluate internal hemorrhoids. For this exam, a speculum or endoscope is introduced into the anus to provide visual inspection of the tissues. Additional diagnostic examinations include testing of stool for occult blood and sigmoidoscopy, performed to rule out cancer of the colon or rectum, which may aggravate hemorrhoidal manifestations or produce similar manifestations. If liver disease with portal hypertension is suspected, liver function studies are ordered.

Medications

Bulk-forming laxatives such as psyllium seed (Metamucil) or stool softeners such as docusate sodium (Colace) may be prescribed to improve constipation and reduce straining as well. Suppositories and local ointments such as Preparation H or Nupercaine have an anesthetic and astringent effect, reducing discomfort and irritation of surrounding tissues. They have little or no effect on the hemorrhoid itself. Warm sitz baths, bed rest, and local astringent compresses may be recommended to reduce the swelling of edematous prolapsed hemorrhoids after digital reduction.

Nutrition

Hemorrhoids that are not permanently prolapsed or acutely thrombosed generally are treated conservatively. A high-fiber diet and increased water intake to increase stool bulk, improve its softness, and reduce straining is effective for most patients with internal or external hemorrhoids.

Sclerotherapy

Hemorrhoids that are permanently prolapsed, are thrombosed, or produce significant manifestations may be treated more aggressively. *Sclerotherapy* involves injecting a chemical irritant into tissues surrounding the hemorrhoid to induce inflammation and eventual fibrosis and scarring. It is used to treat recurrent bleeding and early prolapse of internal hemorrhoids. The treatment produces minimal pain. Enlarged or prolapsing hemorrhoids also may be treated with rubber band ligation. A rubber band is placed snugly around the hemorrhoidal plexus and surrounding mucosa, causing the tissue to necrose and slough within 7 to 10 days. Treatment is limited to one hemorrhoidal complex at a time, so repeat treatments may be necessary. Pain should be minimal if the band is placed appropriately; persistent pain following band ligation may signal an infection. Bleeding can occur as the hemorrhoid sloughs. Other procedures used to treat hemorrhoids include cryosurgery, in which hemorrhoids are necrosed by freezing with a cryoprobe; infrared photocoagulation; or electrocoagulation.

Hemorrhoidectomy

Patients with chronic manifestations, permanent prolapse, chronic bleeding and anemia, or painful thrombosed hemorrhoids may be treated surgically with a *hemorrhoidectomy*. In this procedure, hemorrhoids are surgically excised, leaving normal skin and surrounding tissues. This procedure may use conventional techniques or a laser to remove both internal and external hemorrhoids. Few complications are associated with hemorrhoidectomy.

∞ Nursing Care

Primary prevention of symptomatic hemorrhoids involves education of patients of all ages. Stress the importance of maintaining an adequate intake of dietary fiber, a liberal fluid intake, and regular exercise to maintain stool bulk, softness, and regularity. Discuss the need to respond to the urge to defecate rather than postponing defecation. Teach appropriate constipation management, including the use of bulk-forming laxatives.

Most patients with hemorrhoids are treated in community settings where the primary nursing focus is educational. Discuss the appropriate use of over-the-counter preparations and sitz baths for the relief of minor hemorrhoidal manifestations. If necessary, teach patients how to reduce prolapsed hemorrhoids digitally.

Teach manifestations of possible hemorrhoidal complications, such as chronic bleeding, prolapse, and thrombosis. Stress the need to seek medical evaluation if manifestations persist. Discuss the link between manifestations of hemorrhoids and colorectal cancer, and urge the patient to seek medical intervention for persistent, unresolved, or progressive manifestations.

When a hemorrhoidectomy is performed, the patient requires more direct nursing intervention. Postoperative care of

BOX 24–3 Perianal Postoperative Care

Assessment
- Monitor vital signs every 4 hours for 24 hours.
- Inspect rectal dressing every 2 to 3 hours for 24 hours.
- Monitor urinary output.

Pain Control
- Assist to position of comfort, usually side-lying.
- Provide analgesics as prescribed.
- Keep fresh ice packs over the rectal dressing as ordered.
- Assist with sitz bath three to four times per day.
- Provide a flotation pad for use when sitting.

Elimination
- Give stool softeners as prescribed.
- Give an analgesic before the first postoperative bowel movement if possible.
- When tolerated, encourage fluid intake of at least 2000 mL per day.

Patient and Family Teaching
- Take sitz bath after each bowel movement for 1 to 2 weeks after surgery.
- Drink at least 2 quarts of fluid per day.
- Eat adequate dietary fiber, and exercise moderately.
- Take stool softeners as prescribed.
- Report to the physician the following symptoms: rectal bleeding, continued pain on defecation, fever greater than 101°F (38.3°C), purulent rectal drainage.

the patient with perianal surgery is outlined in Box 24–3. Anal packing may be in place for the first 24 hours following the procedure. When removed, observe the patient closely for bleeding. Pain is a common postoperative problem. Although the operative procedure is minor, postoperative discomfort can be significant because the anal region is richly innervated and muscle spasms may occur. In addition to systemic analgesics, sitz baths usually are ordered. These not only help promote relaxation and reduce discomfort but also clean the anal area. Use of a rubber ring or donut device minimizes pressure on the surgical site while the patient sits in the bath.

The patient may remain hospitalized until after the first postoperative bowel movement. Stool softeners, adequate fluids, and analgesia before defecation can reduce anxiety and discomfort. Adequate cleaning following defecation, usually with a sitz bath, is vital.

Whether caring for a patient with hemorrhoids or a hemorrhoidectomy, consider the following nursing diagnoses:

- *Acute* or *Chronic Pain* related to inflamed anal tissues
- *Constipation* related to dietary habits and/or delay of defecation
- *Risk for Infection* related to disruption of anal tissue

The Patient with an Anorectal Lesion

Unlike the rectum, which is relatively insensitive to pain, the anal canal is richly supplied with sensory nerves and highly sensitive to painful stimuli. Lesions of the anorectal area may cause significant pain, particularly with defecation. Infection is a potential complication of anorectal lesions because of contamination by fecal bacteria. The superior boundary of the anal canal (the anorectal juncture or pectinate line) contains 8 to 12 anal crypts where anorectal abscesses or fistulas can form. Lesions of the anorectal area include fissures, abscesses, fistulas, and pilonidal disease.

Anal Fissure

Anal fissures or ulcers occur when the epithelium of the anal canal over the internal sphincter becomes denuded or abraded. Irritating diarrheal stools and tightening of the anal canal with increased sphincter tension are frequent causes of anal fissures. Other factors that may contribute to their development include childbirth trauma, habitual cathartic use, laceration by a foreign body, and anal intercourse. Chronic inflammation and infection of surrounding tissues accompanies an anal fissure.

Patients with anal fissures typically have periods of exacerbation and remission. Because they occur below the mucocutaneous line, anal fissures are painful. The pain occurs with defecation and may be described as tearing, burning, or cutting. Bright red bleeding is noted with a bowel movement. Bleeding is typically minor and noted on toilet tissue. Because of fear of defecation, the patient may develop constipation, which further disrupts normal bowel habits and aggravates manifestations.

The diagnosis of anal fissure is made on gentle digital examination of the anal canal and anoscopy using a small anoscope. Treatment is usually conservative, involving dietary changes to increase fiber intake and stool bulk, increased fluid intake, and use of bulk-forming laxatives. A topical agent such as hydrocortisone cream may be prescribed. Surgical intervention with an internal sphincterotomy, an incision into the internal sphincter to increase its diameter, is considered when the fissure does not heal with medical intervention.

Anorectal Abscess

Invasion of the pararectal spaces by pathogenic bacteria can lead to an *anorectal abscess*. Commonly caused by infection that extends from the anal crypt into a pararectal space, the abscess may appear small but often contains a large amount of pus. Multiple pathogens may be present, including *Escherichia coli*, *Proteus*, streptococci, and staphylococci. Other factors that may contribute to the development of an anorectal abscess include infection of a hair follicle, sebaceous gland, or sweat gland, and abrasions, fissures, or anal trauma. The incidence of anorectal abscess is higher in men.

Pain is the primary manifestation of an anorectal abscess. Sitting or walking may aggravate the pain, but it is unrelated to defecation. External swelling, redness, heat, and tenderness are apparent on examination. With a deeper abscess, swelling may not be visible, but the abscess is palpable on digital examination.

If the abscess either does not drain spontaneously or is not drained surgically, adjacent anatomic spaces will be affected. Systemic sepsis is also a potential complication.

Incision and drainage is the treatment of choice for an anorectal abscess because it rarely resolves with antibiotic therapy alone. This treatment often leads to a persistent fistula, which is surgically closed after the infection has cleared.

Anorectal Fistula

A fistula is a tunnel or tubelike tract with openings at each end. *Anorectal fistulas* have one opening in the anal canal with the other usually found in perianal skin. Most occur spontaneously or as a result of anorectal abscess drainage. Crohn's disease is a predisposing factor to fistula development.

The primary manifestation of an anorectal fistula is intermittent or constant drainage or discharge, which may be purulent. This may be accompanied by local itching, tenderness, and pain associated with defecation.

Digital and anoscopic examination with gentle probing of the fistula tract are used to establish the diagnosis. Although some fistulas may heal spontaneously, the treatment of choice is a fistulotomy. The primary opening of the fistula is removed, and the tract is opened to allow it to heal by secondary intention, from the inside outward. If the sphincter is involved, a two-stage operation may be done to preserve the muscle and prevent fecal incontinence.

Pilonidal Disease

The patient with *pilonidal disease* has an acute abscess or chronic draining sinus in the sacrococcygeal area. Underlying the abscess or sinus is a cyst with granulation tissue, fibrosis, and, often, hair tufts. This disease usually affects young hirsute (hairy) males and is probably due to hair entrapment in deep tissues of the sacrococcygeal area. Some researchers believe that it is a congenital disorder.

The lesion of pilonidal disease is generally asymptomatic unless it becomes acutely infected. Manifestations of acute inflammation accompany infection, including pain, tenderness, redness, heat, and swelling of the affected area. Purulent discharge may be noted from one or more sinuses or openings in the midline.

The preferred treatment option for pilonidal disease is incision and drainage. The sinus tract and underlying cyst are excised and closed by either primary- or secondary-intention healing. The patient may be instructed to remove hair from the area routinely by shaving or using a depilatory to prevent further hair entrapment and recurrence of the problem.

Nursing Care

Patients with anorectal disorders are often treated in the community, and the primary nursing responsibility is education. Teach the importance of maintaining a high-fiber diet and liberal fluid intake to increase stool bulk and softness and thereby decrease discomfort with defecation. Stress the importance of responding to the urge to defecate to prevent constipation.

Following surgical treatment of any of these disorders, teach the patient to keep the perianal region clean and dry. If a dressing is in place, instruct to avoid soiling it with urine or feces during elimination. Following removal of the dressing, teach to clean the area gently with soap and water following a bowel movement. Discuss the use of sitz baths for cleaning and comfort. Suggest taking an analgesic if necessary prior to defecation, but caution that some analgesics may promote constipation. Teach manifestations of infection or other possible complications to report to the physician. If an antibiotic has been prescribed, provide written and verbal instructions about its use, its desired and possible adverse effects, and their management.

CHAPTER HIGHLIGHTS

■ Disorders of intestinal motility include diarrhea, constipation, irritable bowel syndrome, and fecal incontinence. Diarrhea is a manifestation of many other bowel disorders, including lactose intolerance, infections, and inflammatory diseases of the bowel. Constipation may be a primary problem (especially for the older adult) or a manifestation of another disorder. Irritable bowel syndrome (IBS) is a functional disorder without any identifiable organic cause. Fecal incontinence is usually considered to be the manifestation of a disorder rather than a disorder itself.

■ Appendicitis is an acute inflammation of the vermiform appendix, manifested by abdominal pain that localizes in the right lower quadrant of the abdomen. On palpation, localized and rebound tenderness is present at McBurney's point. It is treated most often with an appendectomy.

■ Peritonitis (inflammation of the peritoneum from infection or chemical irritant) is a serious complication of a wide variety of acute abdominal disorders, including perforated ulcer, ruptured appendix, abdominal trauma or surgery, or necrotic bowel. Complications may be life threatening; without prompt and effective treatment, septicemia and septic shock may occur.

■ Gastroenteritis, which may result from bacterial or viral infections, parasites, or toxins, is often the result of consuming contaminated water or food. Manifestations include nausea and vomiting, diarrhea, and abdominal discomfort.

■ Nurses provide education to help prevent protozoal infections (such as giardiasis, amebiasis, and coccidiosis) and helminthic infestations (roundworms, flukes, or tapeworms). Both types of bowel disorders are treated with medications.

■ Chronic inflammatory bowel disease (IBD) includes two separate but closely related conditions: ulcerative colitis and Crohn's disease. Ulcerative colitis affects the mucosa and submucosa of the colon and rectum. Crohn's disease can affect any part of the GI tract, but usually involves the terminal ilium and ascending colon. Diarrhea is common to both disorders. A colectomy (removal of the large colon) may be performed to treat ulcerative colitis; an ileostomy (artificial opening from the abdomen to the ileum) may be performed to treat Crohn's disease.

■ Diverticula are saclike projections of mucosa through the muscular layer of the colon. When these sacs become inflamed, the condition is labeled diverticulitis. A diet high in fiber is recommended for self-care.

- Malabsorption syndromes, in which the intestinal mucosa ineffectively absorbs nutrients, may be caused by a wide variety of diseases. However, three common malabsorption disorders in adults are celiac disease, lactase deficiency with resulting lactose intolerance of milk and milk products, and short bowel syndrome (a condition that can develop following resection of the small bowel).
- Malignant tumors of the lower bowel are the second leading cause of death from cancer. The risk of colon cancer may be reduced through health-related screenings and a diet high in fruits, vegetables, folic acid, and calcium. Rectal bleeding is the most common initial manifestation but may not occur until the cancer is well advanced. Surgical treatment is through resection of the bowel, accompanied by a colostomy for diversion of fecal contents.

- A hernia is a defect in the abdominal wall that allows intra-abdominal contents to protrude out of the abdominal cavity. Hernias may follow trauma, surgery, and increased intra-abdominal pressure (as from pregnancy or obesity). Hernias may be congenital or acquired, and may be inguinal, umbilical, incisional, or ventral.
- Intestinal obstructions occur when intestinal contents cannot move through the lumen of the bowel. They may occur in either the large or small intestine, may be partial or complete, and are caused by many factors, ranging from surgical ileus following abdominal surgery to adhesions or tumors.
- Anorectal disorders include hemorrhoids, anorectal lesions (fissures, abscess, and fistula), and pilonidal disease. These disorders are painful and pose a risk for bleeding and infection.

TEST YOURSELF NCLEX-RN® REVIEW

1. A patient presents at the urgent care clinic with complaints of diarrhea for the past week. The nurse should first do which of the following?
   1. Advise the patient to abstain from all food intake until the diarrhea subsides.
   2. Ask the patient to describe the number and character of daily stools.
   3. Question the patient about possible exposure to an enterotoxin or protozoal infection.
   4. Recommend an over-the-counter antidiarrheal preparation such as Pepto-Bismol.
2. Which of the following is of highest priority when caring for a patient admitted with possible appendicitis?
   1. Perform preoperative skin preparation.
   2. Teach postoperative coughing, deep breathing, and exercise.
   3. Withhold all food and fluids.
   4. Insert saline lock for intravenous antibiotic therapy.
3. When teaching a patient with inflammatory bowel disease about prescribed sulfasalazine, the nurse instructs the patient to do which of the following?
   1. Use a sunscreen while taking the drug.
   2. Take the drug on an empty stomach.
   3. Limit fluid intake to 1500 mL per day or less.
   4. Take vitamin C while on the drug.
4. A patient reports frequent large, fatty, foul-smelling stools. The nurse inquires further about which of the following?
   1. possible exposure to enterotoxins in food or water
   2. a history of alternating diarrhea and constipation
   3. known family history of colorectal cancer
   4. the relationship of episodes to particular foods
5. A patient tells the nurse that both his father and grandfather died of colon cancer, and he is worried that he is going to die from "the same horrible disease." Which of the following does the nurse include in her recommendations?
   1. The genetic link is weak in colon cancer, so he should simply follow the usual recommendations for screening.
   2. He should plan for annual digital rectal exams and periodic colonoscopy for early identification of possible tumors.
   3. He should have annual CEA levels drawn to screen for early tumor development.
   4. Significantly increasing his intake of dietary fiber can reduce his risk of developing colon cancer within 5 years.

6. A patient has a nasogastric tube in place to maintain gastric decompression. Which nursing actions are important in monitoring responses to *Deficient Fluid Volume* when caring for this patient? **Select all that apply.**
   1. Low suction is used to decompress the stomach.
   2. Give the patient as much water as he or she wants to drink.
   3. Listen to bowel sounds prior to checking the placement of the NG tube.
   4. Document the amount and color of NG tube drainage every shift.
   5. Keep an accurate record of intake and output every 2 to 4 hours.
   6. Measure abdominal girth every 4 to 8 hours.
7. A patient has developed a paralytic ileus following a recent abdominal surgery. What is the most important nursing consideration when caring for this patient?
   1. Ensure that the patient is able to eat a clear liquid diet.
   2. Maintain the patient on strict bedrest.
   3. Monitor bowel sounds every hour.
   4. Ensure nasogastric tube is functioning.
8. Mrs. Jones has a history of diverticulosis and has been having abdominal pain recently. When educating Mrs. Jones about her diet prior to discharge from the hospital, what type of foods should be excluded from Mrs. Jones's diet?
   1. whole-wheat bread
   2. raspberries
   3. soup
   4. apples
9. Your 85-year-old patient Mr. Allen was admitted with a diagnosis of constipation. Which of the following is important in your discharge education for this patient? **Select all that apply.**
   1. Eat plenty of fresh fruits and vegetables daily.
   2. Take a bisacodyl (Dulcolax) daily.
   3. Drink six to eight glasses of nonalcoholic fluid daily.
   4. Take docusate (Colace) at nighttime only.
   5. Eat whole-wheat bread instead of white bread.
   6. Eat a bran cereal for breakfast.
10. Which of the following nursing interventions are of highest priority when caring for a patient with a small bowel obstruction?
    1. placing the patient in semi-Fowler's position
    2. maintaining nasogastric suction
    3. keeping strict intake and output records
    4. administering prescribed analgesics

See Test Yourself answers in Appendix C.

BIBLIOGRAPHY

American Cancer Society. (2006). *Cancer facts & figures for Hispanics/Latinos 2006–2008.* Atlanta, GA: Author.

American Cancer Society. (2007). *Cancer facts & figures for African Americans 2007–2008.* Atlanta, GA: Author.

American Cancer Society. (2009). *Cancer facts & figures 2009.* Atlanta, GA: Author.

American Cancer Society. (2008). *Colorectal cancer facts & figures 2008-1010.* Atlanta, GA: Author.

American College of Physicians. (2007). In the clinic. Irritable bowel syndrome. *Annals of Internal Medicine, 3 July 2007*, ITC7-1-ITC7-16.

Balch, J. F., & Stengler, M. (2004). *Prescription for natural cures: A self-care guide for treating health problems with natural remedies including diet and nutrition, nutritional supplements, bodywork, and more.* Hoboken, NJ: Wiley & Sons.

Banning, M. (2008). Ageing and the gut. *Nursing Older People, 20*(1), 17–21.

Barakzai, M., Gregory, J., & Fraser, D. (2007). The effect of culture on symptom reporting: Hispanics and irritable bowel syndrome. *Journal of the American Academy of Nurse Practitioners, 19*(2007), 261–267.

Bazensky, I., Shoobridge-Moran, C., & Yoder, L. (2007 February). Colorectal cancer: An overview of the epidemiology, risk factors, symptoms, and screening guidelines. *Medsurg Nursing, 16*(1), 46–51.

Bulechek, G., Butcher, H., & Dochterman, J. (Eds.). (2008). *Nursing interventions classification (NIC)* (5th ed.). St. Louis, MO: Mosby.

Calfee, D. (2008 September). *Clostridium difficile*: A reemerging pathogen. *Geriatrics, 63*(9), 10–14, 21.

Centers for Disease Control and Prevention. (2006). Noroviruses. Retrieved from http://www.cdc.gov/ncidod/dvrd/revb/gastro/norovirus-factsheet.htm

Centers for Disease Control and Prevention. (2009 May 7). Outbreak of *Salmonella* serotype Saintpaul infections associated with eating alfalfa sprouts – United States, 2009. *Morbidity and Mortality Weekly Report, 58*(Early Release May 7, 2009). Retrieved from www.cdc.gov/mmwr

Cokkinides, V., Bandi, P., Siegel, R., Ward E., & Thun, M. (2007). *Cancer prevention & early detection facts & figures 2008.* Atlanta, GA: American Cancer Society.

Connelly, P. (2008 June). *Lactobacillus plantarum*– A literature review of therapeutic benefits. *Journal of the Australian Traditional-Medicine Society, 14*(2), 79–82.

Crohn's & Colitis Foundation of America. (2008). *About ulcerative colitis & procitis.* Retrieved from www.ccfa.org/info/about/ucp

Crohn's & Colitis Foundation of America. (2009). *About Crohn's disease.* Retrieved from http://www.ccfa.org/info/about/crohns

Dalrymple, J., & Bullock, I. (2008 March). Diagnosis and management of irritable bowel syndrome in adults in primary care: Summary of NICE guidance. *BMJ: British Medical Journal, 336*(7643), 556–558.

Dupont, H. (2008). Systematic review: Prevention of travellers' diarrhorea. *Alimentary Pharmacology & Therapeutics, 27*, 741–751.

Fauci, A., Braunwald, E., Kasper, D., Hauser, S., Longo, D., Jameson, J., et al. (2008). *Harrison's principles of internal medicine* (17th ed.). New York, NY: McGraw Hill.

Freeman, L. (2007 May). Responding to small-bowel obstruction. *Nursing 2007, 37*(5), 56hn1–56hn2, 56hn4, 56hn6.

Ginsberg, D., Phillips, S., Wallace, J., & Josephson, K. (2007 June). Evaluating and managing constipation in the elderly. *Urologic Nursing, 27*(3), 191–200.

Guarino, A., Vecchio, A., & Canani, R. (2009 April). Probiotics as prevention and treatment for diarrhea. *Current Opinion in Gastroenterology, 25*(1). Retrieved from www.medscape.com

Heitkemper, M., & Wolff, J. (2007 April). Challenges in chronic constipation. *The Nurse Practitioner, 32*(4), 36–42.

Higgins, R. (2009 February). Abdominal assessment and diagnosis of appendicitis. *Emergency Nurse, 16*(9), 22–24.

Holman, C., Roberts, S., & Nicol, M. (2008 June). Preventing and treating constipation in later life. *Nursing Older People, 20*(5), 22–24.

Kee, J. (2009). *Handbook of laboratory and diagnostic tests with nursing implications* (6th ed.). Upper Saddle River, NJ: Prentice Hall.

Kyle, G. (2009 January). Common bowel problems in older adult care. *Nursing & Residential Care, 11*(1), 22–25.

Kyle, G. (2009 February). Common bowel problems: Constipation risk assessment. *Nursing & Residential Care, 11*(2), 76–79.

Langmead, L., & Rampton, D. (2006). Review article: Complementary and alternative therapies for inflammatory bowel disease. *Alimentary Pharmacology & Therapeutics, 23*, 341–349.

Lindberg, D. (2009 January/February). Hydrogen breath testing in adults. *Gastroenterology Nursing, 32*(1), 19–24.

Managing constipation in the elderly. (2007). *Geriatrics Supplement*, August 2007.

Martin, S. (2008). Against the grain: An overview of celiac disease. *Journal of the American Academy of Nurse Practitioners, 20*(2008), 243–250.

Mayo Clinic. (2008). *Ulcerative colitis.* Retrieved from www.mayoclinic.com/health/ulcerative-colitis/

McPhee, S. Papadakis, M., & Tierney, L., Jr. (2008). *Current medical diagnosis & treatment* (47th ed.). New York, NY: McGraw Hill.

Moorhead, S., Johnson, M., Maas, M., & Swanson, E. (Eds.). (2008). *Nursing outcomes classification (NOC)* (4th ed.). St. Louis, MO: Mosby.

Moynihan, N., Callahan, M., Kalsmith, B., & Moses, P. (2008 February). How do you spell relief for irritable bowel syndrome? C-A-R-E-F-U-L-L-Y. *The Journal of Family Practice, 57*(2), 100–108.

NANDA International. (2009). *Nursing diagnoses: Definitions & classification 2009–2011.* Oxford, UK: Wiley-Blackwell.

National Cancer Institute. (2008). *Colon cancer treatment (PDQ®). Health professional version.* Retrieved from www.cancer.gov/cancertopics/pdq/treatment/colon/healthprofessional/

National Center for Complementary and Alternative Medicine (NCCAM). (2008). *An introduction to probiotics.* Retrieved from http://nccam.nih.gov/health/probiotics

Pontieri-Lewis, V. (2006 August). Basics of ostomy care. *Medsurg Nursing, 15*(4), 199–202.

Porth, C. M., & Matfin, G. (2009). *Pathophysiology: Concepts of altered health states* (8th ed.). Philadelphia, PA: Lippincott.

Rowland, I., Melton, L., Gray, J., Bulpitt, C., Hickson, M., Smith, M., et al. (2008 February). Latest research and thinking into the power of probiotics. *Practice Nurse, 35*(Supplement), 1–4.

Sabol, V., & Carlson, K. (2007 January–March). Diarrhea: Applying research to bedside practice. *AACN Advanced Critical Care, 18*(1), 32–44.

Stahlfeld, K., Hower, J., Homitsky, S., & Madden, J. (2007 June). Is acute appendicitis a surgical emergency? *The American Surgeon, 73*, 626–630.

Thorson, M., Bliss, D., & Savik, K. (2008). Re-examination of risk factors for non-*Clostridium difficile*-associated diarrhea in hospitalized patients. *JAN: Original Research*, 354–364.

Westwood, N., & Travis, S. (2008). Review article: What do patients with inflammatory bowel disease want for their clinical management? *Alimentary Pharmacology & Therapeutics, 27*(Supplement 1), 1–8.

Wilkinson, J., & Ahern, N. (2009). *Prentice Hall nursing diagnosis handbook* (9th ed.). Upper Saddle River, NJ: Prentice Hall.

Willcox, A., & Hayward, M. (2008 July). A guide to travel health. *Emergency Nurse, 16*(4), 30–37.

Wilson, B., Shannon, M., Shields, K., & Stang, C. (2008). *Prentice Hall nurse's drug guide 2008.* Upper Saddle River, NJ: Prentice Hall.

Yantis, M., & Velander, R. (2009 March). Probiotics can thwart antibiotic-associated diarrhea. *Nursing 2009, 39*(3), 58–59.

Yarbo, C., Frogge, M., & Goodman, M. (2005). *Cancer nursing: Principles and practice* (6th ed.). Sudbury, MA: Jones & Bartlett.

Yates, J., (2005). Traveler's diarrhea. *American Family Physician, 71*(11), 2095–2100.

CHAPTER 25

Nursing Care of Patients with Gallbladder, Liver, and Pancreatic Disorders

LEARNING OUTCOMES

1. Describe the pathophysiology of commonly occurring disorders of the gallbladder, liver, and exocrine pancreas.
2. Use knowledge of normal anatomy and physiology to understand the manifestations and effects of biliary, hepatic, and pancreatic disorders.
3. Relate changes in normal assessment data to the pathophysiology and manifestations of gallbladder, liver, and exocrine pancreatic disorders.

CLINICAL COMPETENCIES

1. Assess functional health status of patients with gallbladder, liver, or pancreatic disease.
2. Monitor for, recognize, document, and report expected and unexpected manifestations in patients with gallbladder, liver, or pancreatic disease.
3. Provide appropriate, evidence-based teaching about diagnostic tests and test results for patients with gallbladder, liver, and pancreatic disorders.
4. Integrate appropriate dietary, pharmacologic, and other interdisciplinary measures into nursing care and teaching of the patient with a gallbladder, liver, or pancreatic disorder.
5. Provide safe, patient-centered nursing care for the patient who has surgery of the gallbladder, liver, or pancreas.
6. Integrate psychosocial, cultural, and spiritual considerations into the plan of care for a patient with a gallbladder, liver, or pancreatic disorder.
7. Use evidence-based practice, technology, and information management tools to develop, implement, evaluate, and, as needed, revise the plan of care for patients with disorders of the gallbladder, liver, or pancreas.
8. Provide appropriate patient and family teaching to promote, maintain, and restore functional health status for patients with gallbladder, liver, and pancreatic disorders.

KEY TERMS

ascites, 727
biliary colic, 722
cholecystitis, 722
cholelithiasis, 721
cirrhosis, 736

esophageal varices, 728
hepatitis, 729
jaundice, 728
pancreatitis, 751
paracentesis, 743

portal hypertension, 728
portal systemic encephalopathy, 728
steatorrhea, 753

Gallbladder, liver, and exocrine pancreatic disorders may occur as primary disorders, or develop secondarily to other disease processes. The functioning of one organ frequently affects that of another. Duct inflammation or obstruction, and changes in the multiple functions of these organs, can cause significant health effects.

Patients with a gallbladder, liver, or pancreatic disorder may experience pain, metabolic and nutritional disturbances, and altered body image. Nursing care addresses physiologic, emotional, and psychosocial needs of the patient and family.

Gallbladder Disorders

Altered bile flow through the hepatic, cystic, or common bile duct is a common problem and a frequent cause of hospitalization. It often leads to inflammation and other complications. Gallstones are the most common cause of obstructed flow. Tumors and abscesses also can obstruct bile flow.

The Patient with Gallstones

Cholelithiasis is the formation of stones (*calculi* or *gallstones*) within the gallbladder or biliary duct system. Cholelithiasis is a common problem in the United States, affecting more than 10%

of men and 20% of women by age 65 (McPhee et al., 2008). Box 25–1 lists risk factors for gallstones. The incidence of gallstones varies among people of different ethnic backgrounds; see the accompanying Focus on Cultural Diversity box.

Physiology Review

Normally, bile is formed by the liver and stored in the gallbladder. Bile contains bile salts, bilirubin, water, electrolytes, cholesterol, fatty acids, and lecithin. In the gallbladder, some of the water and electrolytes are absorbed, further concentrating

Figure 25–1 ■ Common locations of gallstones.

the bile. Food entering the intestine stimulates the gallbladder to contract and release bile through the common bile duct and sphincter of Oddi into the intestine. The bile salts in bile increase the solubility and absorption of dietary fats.

Pathophysiology and Manifestations

Cholelithiasis

Gallstones form when several factors interact: abnormal bile composition, biliary stasis, and inflammation of the gallbladder. Most gallstones (80%) consist primarily of cholesterol; the rest contain a mixture of bile components. Excess cholesterol in bile is associated with obesity, a high-calorie and high-cholesterol diet, and drugs that lower serum cholesterol levels. When bile is supersaturated with cholesterol, it can precipitate out to form stones. Biliary stasis, or slowed emptying of the gallbladder, contributes to cholelithiasis. Stones do not form when the gallbladder empties completely in response to hormonal stimulation. Slowed or incomplete emptying allows cholesterol to concentrate and increases the risk of stone formation. Finally, inflammation of the gallbladder allows excess water and bile salt reabsorption, increasing the risk for lithiasis.

> **PRACTICE ALERT**
> Certain very-low-calorie diets are associated with a high risk of cholelithiasis. Increased cholesterol concentration in the bile and decreased gallbladder contractions associated with fasting increase the risk of gallstone formation.

Most gallstones are formed in the gallbladder. They then may migrate into the ducts (Figure 25–1 ■), leading to *cholangitis* (duct inflammation). Although some people with cholelithiasis are asymptomatic, many develop manifestations.

> **FOCUS ON CULTURAL DIVERSITY**
> **Gallstones**
>
> Native Americans in both the Northern and Southern Hemispheres, and those of the Pima tribe in particular, have a higher incidence of gallstones than do Caucasians of American or European heritage. This is thought to result from genes that promote efficient calorie use and fat storage—a beneficial trait when the availability of adequate food varies over time. Gallstones composed of cholesterol are less common in African Americans, and Asians have a low incidence of the disease (McPhee et al., 2008).

Early manifestations of gallstones may be vague: epigastric fullness or mild gastric distress after eating a large or fatty meal. Stones that obstruct the cystic duct or common bile duct lead to distention and increased pressure behind the stone. This causes **biliary colic**, a severe, steady pain in the epigastric region or right upper quadrant of the abdomen. The pain may radiate to the back, right scapula, or shoulder. The pain often begins suddenly following a meal, and may last as long as 5 hours. It often is accompanied by nausea and vomiting.

Obstruction of the common bile duct may cause bile reflux into the liver, leading to jaundice, pain, and possible liver damage. If the common duct is obstructed, pancreatic enzymes will be unable to enter the small intestine, and pancreatitis (discussed later in this chapter) becomes a potential complication.

Cholecystitis

Cholecystitis is inflammation of the gallbladder. *Acute cholecystitis* usually follows obstruction of the cystic duct by a stone. The obstruction increases pressure within the gallbladder, leading to ischemia of the gallbladder wall and mucosa. Retained bile causes chemical irritation and bacterial inflammation often follows. The ischemia can lead to necrosis and perforation of the gallbladder wall.

Acute cholecystitis usually begins with an attack of biliary colic. The pain involves the entire right upper quadrant (RUQ), and may radiate to the back, right scapula, or shoulder. Movement or deep breathing may aggravate the pain. The pain usually lasts longer than biliary colic, continuing for 12 to 18 hours. Anorexia, nausea, and vomiting are common. Fever often is present, and may be accompanied by chills. The RUQ is tender to palpation.

Chronic cholecystitis may result from repeated bouts of acute cholecystitis or from persistent irritation of the gallbladder wall by stones. Bacteria may be present in the bile as well. Chronic cholecystitis often is asymptomatic.

Complications of cholecystitis include *empyema*, a collection of infected fluid within the gallbladder; gangrene and perforation with resulting peritonitis or abscess formation; formation of a fistula into an adjacent organ (such as the duodenum, colon, or stomach); or obstruction of the small intestine by a large gallstone (*gallstone ileus*). Table 25–1 compares the manifestations and complications of acute cholelithiasis with those of cholecystitis.

TABLE 25–1 Manifestations and Complications of Cholelithiasis and Cholecystitis

MANIFESTATIONS	CHOLELITHIASIS	CHOLECYSTITIS
Pain	■ Abrupt onset ■ Severe, steady ■ Localized to epigastrium and RUQ of abdomen ■ May radiate to back, right scapula, and shoulder ■ Lasts 30 minutes to 5 hours	■ Abrupt onset ■ Severe, steady ■ Generalized in RUQ of abdomen ■ May radiate to back, right scapula, and shoulder ■ Lasts 12 to 18 hours ■ Aggravated by movement, breathing
Associated symptoms	■ Nausea, vomiting	■ Anorexia, nausea, vomiting ■ RUQ tenderness and guarding ■ Chills and fever
Complications	■ Cholecystitis ■ Common bile duct obstruction with possible jaundice and liver damage ■ Common duct obstruction with pancreatitis	■ Gangrene and perforation with peritonitis ■ Chronic cholecystitis ■ Empyema ■ Fistula formation ■ Gallstone ileus

Interdisciplinary Care

Treatment of the patient with gallstones depends of the acuity of the condition and the patient's overall health status. When gallstones are present but asymptomatic and the patient has a low risk for complications, conservative treatment is indicated. However, when the patient experiences frequent symptoms, has acute cholecystitis, or has very large stones, the gallbladder and stones are usually surgically removed.

Diagnosis

Diagnostic tests are ordered to identify the presence and location of stones, identify possible complications, and help differentiate gallbladder disease from other disorders.

■ *Serum bilirubin* is measured. Elevated direct (conjugated) bilirubin may indicate obstructed bile flow in the biliary duct system (Box 25–2).

■ *Complete blood count (CBC)* may show an elevated WBC count in the presence of inflammation and infection.

■ *Serum amylase* and *lipase* are measured to identify possible pancreatitis related to common duct obstruction.

■ *Ultrasonography of the gallbladder* is a noninvasive exam that can accurately diagnose cholelithiasis with more than 95% accuracy. It also can be used to assess emptying of the gallbladder.

■ *Abdominal x-ray* (flat plate of the abdomen) may show gallstones that have a high calcium content.

■ *Gallbladder scans* (e.g., HIDA, DIDA, or DISIDA scans) use an intravenous radioactive solution that is rapidly extracted from the blood and excreted into the biliary tree to diagnose cystic duct obstruction and acute or chronic cholecystitis.

∞ See Chapter 21 for more information about and the nursing implications of these diagnostic tests.

Medications

Patients who refuse surgery or for whom surgery is inappropriate may be treated with a drug to dissolve the gallstones. Ursodiol (Actigall) and chenodiol (Chenix) reduce the cholesterol content of gallstones, leading to their gradual dissolution. These drugs act by reducing cholesterol production in the liver, thus reducing the cholesterol content of bile. Consequently,

these drugs are most effective in treating stones with high cholesterol content. They are less effective in treating radiopaque stones with high calcium salt content. Ursodiol is generally well-tolerated with few side effects, whereas chenodiol has a high incidence of diarrhea at therapeutic doses. It also is hepatotoxic, so periodic liver function studies are required during therapy.

The primary disadvantages of pharmacologic treatment for gallstones include its cost, long duration (2 years or more), and the high incidence of recurrent stone formation when treatment is discontinued. If infection is suspected, antibiotics may be ordered to cure the infection and reduce associated inflammation and edema. Patients with pruritus (itching) due to severe obstructive jaundice and an accumulation of bile salts on the skin may be given cholestyramine (Questran). This drug binds with bile salts to promote their excretion in the feces. A opioid analgesic such as morphine may be required for pain relief during an acute attack of cholecystitis.

BOX 25–2 Sorting Out Total, Direct, and Indirect Bilirubin Levels

When serum bilirubin levels are drawn, the results usually are reported as the total bilirubin, direct bilirubin, and indirect bilirubin levels. Most bilirubin is formed from hemoglobin, as aging or abnormal RBCs are removed from circulation and destroyed. It is then bound to protein and transported to the liver. This protein-bound bilirubin is called *indirect* or *unconjugated* bilirubin. Once in the liver, bilirubin is separated from the protein and converted to a soluble form, *direct* or *conjugated* bilirubin. Conjugated bilirubin is then excreted in the bile.

■ Total (serum) bilirubin includes both indirect and direct forms. In adults, the normal total bilirubin is 0.1 to 1.2 mg/dL. Total bilirubin levels increase when more is being produced (e.g., RBC hemolysis), or when its metabolism or excretion are impaired (e.g., liver disease or biliary obstruction).

■ Direct (conjugated) bilirubin levels, normally 0.1 to 0.3 mg/dL in adults, rise when its excretion is impaired by obstruction within the liver (e.g., in cirrhosis, hepatitis, exposure to hepatotoxins) or in the biliary system.

■ Indirect (unconjugated) bilirubin levels, normally < 1.0 mg/dL in adults, rise in RBC hemolysis (e.g., sickle cell disease or transfusion reaction).

Treatments

SURGERY   *Laparoscopic cholecystectomy* (removal of the gallbladder) is the treatment of choice for symptomatic cholelithiasis or cholecystitis. This minimally invasive procedure has a low risk of complications and generally requires a hospital stay of less than 24 hours. Not all patients are candidates for laparoscopic cholecystectomy, and there is a risk that a laparoscopic cholecystectomy may be converted to a *laparotomy* (surgical opening into the abdomen) during the procedure. See the accompanying box for nursing care for a patient having a laparoscopic cholecystectomy.

When stones are lodged within the ducts, a cholecystectomy with common bile duct exploration may be done. A T-tube (Figure 25–2 ■) is inserted to maintain patency of the duct and promote bile passage while the edema decreases. Excess bile is collected in a drainage bag secured below the surgical site. If it is suspected that a stone has been retained following surgery, a postoperative cholangiogram via the T-tube or direct visualization of the duct with an endoscope may be performed. See the box on page 725 for nursing care for a patient with a T-tube.

Some patients who are poor surgical risks and for whom laparoscopic cholecystectomy is inappropriate may have either a *cholecystostomy* to drain the gallbladder, or a *choledochostomy* to remove stones and position a T-tube in the common bile duct.

NUTRITION   Food intake may be eliminated during an acute attack of cholecystitis, and a nasogastric tube inserted to relieve nausea and vomiting. Dietary fat intake may be limited, especially if the patient is obese. If bile flow is obstructed, fat-soluble vitamins (A, D, E, and K) and bile salts may need to be administered.

OTHER THERAPIES   In some cases, shock wave lithotripsy may be used with drug therapy to dissolve large gallstones. In *extracorporeal shock wave lithotripsy*, ultrasound is used to align the stones with the source of shock waves and the computerized lithotripter. Positioning is of prime importance throughout the procedure, which usually takes an hour. Mild

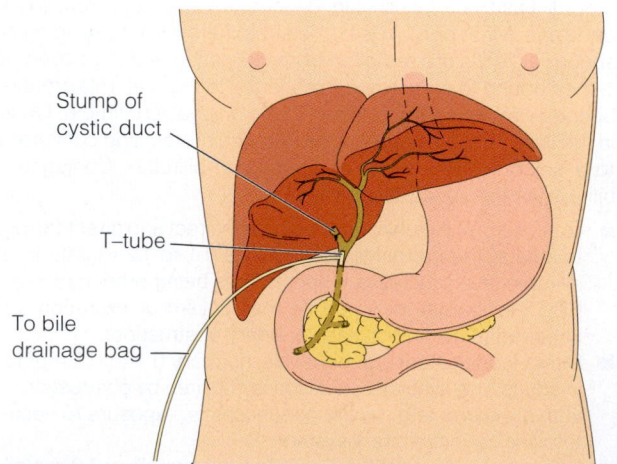

Figure 25–2 ■ T-tube placement in the common bile duct. Bile fluid flows with gravity into a drainage collection device below the level of the common bile duct.

Stump of cystic duct
T–tube
To bile drainage bag

NURSING CARE OF THE PATIENT
Having Laparoscopic Cholecystectomy

PREOPERATIVE CARE
- Provide routine preoperative care as ordered (∞ see Chapter 4).
- Assess for manifestations of cholecystitis and other complications of gallstones. *An acutely inflamed gallbladder and ductal system increases surgical complexity and may necessitate open cholecystectomy.*
- Reinforce teaching about the procedure and postoperative expectations, including pain management, deep breathing, and mobilization. *Preoperative teaching reduces anxiety and promotes rapid postoperative recovery.*

POSTOPERATIVE CARE
- Provide routine postoperative recovery care as outlined in ∞ Chapter 4.
- Treat postoperative pain and nausea and vomiting prophylactically and as needed to relieve symptoms. *Postoperative pain is common during the first 24 to 48 hours after surgery. Manipulation of the bowel and insufflation of the abdomen with gas commonly lead to postoperative nausea (Graham, 2008).*
- Assist to chair at bedside as allowed. *Early mobilization promotes lung ventilation and circulation, reducing the potential for postoperative complications.*
- Advance oral intake from ice chips to regular diet as tolerated. *Oral intake can be rapidly resumed due to minimal disruption of the gastrointestinal tract during surgery.*
- Provide and reinforce teaching: pain management, incision care, activity level, postoperative follow-up appointments. *With early discharge, the patient and family assume responsibility for the majority of postoperative care. A clear understanding of this care and expected needs reduces anxiety and the risk of postoperative complications.*
- Initiate follow-up contact 24 to 48 hours after discharge to evaluate adequacy of pain control, incision management, and discharge understanding. *Contact following discharge provides an opportunity to evaluate care and reinforce teaching.*

sedation may be given during the procedure. Nursing care after the procedure includes monitoring for biliary colic, which can result from the gallbladder contracting to remove stone fragments; nausea; and transient hematuria. *Percutaneous cholecystostomy*, ultrasound-guided drainage of the gallbladder, may be done in high-risk patients to postpone or even eliminate the need for surgery.

COMPLEMENTARY THERAPIES   The herb goldenseal has been used in treating cholecystitis. One of the active ingredients in goldenseal, berberine, stimulates secretion of bile and bilirubin. It also inhibits the growth of many common pathogens, including those known to infect the gallbladder. A study of the effectiveness of berberine in patients with cholecystitis demonstrated relief of all symptoms. Goldenseal can stimulate the uterus, so it is contraindicated for use during pregnancy and lactation. An herbal formula composed of peppermint and wormwood extracts is believed by some to promote emptying of the gallbladder and increase bile salts, thereby reducing the recurrence and growth of gallstones (Chi, 2008).

NURSING CARE OF THE PATIENT
with a T-Tube

- Ensure that the T-tube is properly connected to a sterile container; keep the tube below the level of the surgical wound. *This position promotes the flow of bile and prevents backflow or seepage of caustic bile onto the skin. The tube itself decreases biliary tree pressure.*
- Monitor drainage from the T-tube for color and consistency; record as output. Normally, the tube may drain up to 500 mL in the first 24 hours after surgery; drainage decreases to less than 200 mL in 2 to 3 days, and is minimal thereafter. Drainage may be blood tinged initially, changing to green-brown. Report excessive drainage immediately (after 48 hours, drainage greater than 500 mL is considered excessive). *Stones or edema and inflammation can obstruct ducts below the tube, requiring treatment.*
- Place in Fowler's position. *This promotes gravity drainage of bile.*
- Assess skin for bile leakage during dressing changes. *Bile irritates the skin; it may be necessary to apply skin protection with karaya or another barrier product.*
- Teach patient how to manage the tube when turning, ambulating, and performing activities of daily living. *Direct pulling or traction on the tube must be avoided.*
- If indicated, teach care of the T-tube, how to clamp it, and signs of infection. *Patients may be discharged home with the tube in place. Reporting early signs of infection facilitates prompt treatment.*

♨ Nursing Care

In addition to the nursing care discussed in this section, a Case Study & Nursing Care Plan for a patient with cholelithiasis is found on page 727.

Health Promotion

Although most risk factors for cholelithiasis cannot be controlled or modified, several can. Modifiable risk factors include obesity, hyperlipidemia, extremely low-calorie diets, and diets high in cholesterol. By contrast, physical activity, a high-fiber and low carbohydrate diet, and consumption of unsaturated fats all appear to have a protective effect, reducing the incidence of gallstones and cholecystitis. Discuss the dangers of "yo-yo" dieting, with cycles of weight loss followed by weight gain, and of extremely low-calorie diets. Encourage patients with high serum cholesterol levels to discuss using cholesterol-lowering drugs with their primary care provider.

Assessment

Assessment data related to cholelithiasis and cholecystitis include the following:

- *Health history:* Current manifestations, including RUQ pain, its character and relationship to meals, duration, and radiation, nausea and vomiting, or other symptoms; duration of symptoms; risk factors or previous history of symptoms; chronic diseases such as diabetes, cirrhosis, or inflammatory bowel disease; current diet; use of oral contraceptives or possibility of pregnancy.

- *Physical assessment:* Current weight; color of skin and sclera; abdominal assessment including light palpation for tenderness; color of urine and stool.
- *Diagnostic tests:* Monitor results of WBC, serum bilirubin, liver enzymes, and pancreatic enzymes (amylase and lipase).

Nursing Diagnoses and Interventions

Priority nursing diagnoses for the patient with cholelithiasis or cholecystitis often include pain related to biliary colic or surgery, imbalanced nutrition related to the effects of altered bile flow and to nausea and anorexia, and risk for infection related to potential rupture of an acutely inflamed gallbladder. Nursing interventions for the patient who has undergone a laparoscopic or open cholecystectomy are similar to those for other patients having abdominal surgery. (∞ See Chapter 4.)

Pain

The pain associated with cholelithiasis can be severe. Sometimes a combination of interventions is indicated.

- Discuss the relationship between fat intake and the pain. Teach ways to reduce fat intake (Box 25–3). *Fat entering the duodenum initiates gallbladder contractions, causing pain when gallstones are present in the ducts.*
- Withhold oral food and fluids during episodes of acute pain. Insert nasogastric tube and connect to low suction if ordered. *Emptying the stomach reduces the amount of chyme entering the duodenum and the stimulus for gallbladder contractions, thus reducing pain.*
- For severe pain, administer morphine, fentanyl, or other narcotic analgesia as ordered. *Recent research indicates that morphine is no more likely to cause spasms of the sphincter of Oddi than meperidine.*
- Place in Fowler's position. *Fowler's position decreases pressure on the inflamed gallbladder.*
- Monitor vital signs, including temperature, at least every 4 hours. *Bacterial infection often is present in acute cholecystitis, and may cause an elevated temperature and respiratory rate.*

Imbalanced Nutrition: Less than Body Requirements

The patient with severe gallbladder disease may develop nutritional imbalances related to anorexia, pain, and nausea following meals, and impaired bile flow that alters absorption of fat and fat-soluble vitamins (A, D, E, and K) from the gut.

EVIDENCE FOR NURSING CARE — The Patient with Gallstones

Selected resources that nurses may find helpful when planning evidence-based nursing care follow.

- Holcomb, S. S. (2008). Acute abdomen: What a pain! *Nursing2008, 38*(9), 34–40.
- Society of American Gastrointestinal and Endoscopic Surgeons (SAGES). (2007, November). *Diagnostic laparoscopy for acute abdominal pain. In: Diagnostic laparoscopy guidelines.* Los Angeles, CA: Society of American Gastrointestinal and Endoscopic Surgeons (SAGES).

BOX 25–3 Examples of High-Fat Foods

- Whole-milk products (e.g., cream, ice cream, cheese)
- Doughnuts, deep-fried
- Avocados
- Sausage, bacon, hot dogs
- Gravies with fat, cream
- Most nuts (e.g., pecans, cashews)
- Corn chips and potato chips
- Butter and cooking oils
- Fried foods (e.g., cheeseburgers, hamburgers, french fries)
- Peanut butter
- Chocolate candies

- Assess nutritional status, including diet history, height and weight, and skinfold measurements (∞ see Chapters 21 and 22). *Even though often obese, patients with gallbladder disease may have an imbalanced diet or may have specific vitamin deficiencies, particularly of the fat-soluble vitamins.*
- Evaluate laboratory results, including serum bilirubin, albumin, glucose, and cholesterol levels. Report abnormal results to the primary care provider. *Elevated serum bilirubin may indicate impaired bilirubin excretion due to obstructed bile flow. A low serum albumin may indicate poor nutritional status. Glucose intolerance and hypercholesterolemia are risk factors for cholelithiasis.*
- Refer to a dietitian or nutritionist for diet counseling to promote healthy weight loss and reduce pain episodes. *A low-carbohydrate, low-fat, higher protein diet reduces symptoms of cholecystitis. While fasting and very-low-calorie diets are contraindicated, a moderate reduction in calorie intake and increased activity levels promote weight loss.*
- Administer vitamin supplements as ordered. *Patients who do not absorb fat well due to obstructed bile flow may require supplements of the fat-soluble vitamins.*

Risk for Infection

An acutely inflamed gallbladder may become necrotic and rupture, releasing its contents into the abdominal cavity. While the resulting infection often remains localized, peritonitis can result from chemical irritation and bacterial contamination of the peritoneal cavity.

PRACTICE ALERT
Rupture of an acutely inflamed gallbladder may be heralded by abrupt but transient pain relief as contents are released from the distended gallbladder into the abdomen. Promptly report this change to the physician.

Following open cholecystectomy (*laparotomy*), the risk for pulmonary infection is significant due to the high abdominal incision.

- Monitor vital signs including temperature every 4 hours. Promptly report vital sign changes or temperature elevation. *Tachycardia, increased respiratory rate, or an elevated temperature may indicate an infectious process.*
- Assess abdomen every 4 hours and as indicated (e.g., when pain level changes abruptly). *Increasing abdominal* tenderness or a rigid, boardlike abdomen may indicate rupture of the gallbladder with peritonitis.
- Assist to cough and deep breathe or use incentive spirometer every 1 to 2 hours while awake. Splint abdominal incision with a blanket or pillow during coughing. *The high abdominal incision of an open cholecystectomy interferes with effective coughing and deep breathing, increasing the risk of atelectasis and respiratory infections such as pneumonia.*
- Place in Fowler's position and encourage ambulation as allowed. *Fowler's position and ambulating promote lung expansion and airway clearance, reducing the risk of respiratory infections.*
- Administer antibiotics as ordered. *Antibiotics may be given preoperatively to reduce the risk of infection from infected gallbladder contents, and may be continued postoperatively to prevent infection.*

Community-Based Care

Teaching varies, depending on the choice of treatment options for cholelithiasis and cholecystitis. If surgery is not an option, teach about medications that dissolve stones, their use and adverse effects (diarrhea is a common side effect), and maintaining a low-fat and low-carbohydrate diet if indicated. Include an explanation about the role of bile and the function of the gallbladder in terms that the patient and family can understand.

Provide appropriate preoperative teaching for the planned procedure. Discuss the possibility of open cholecystectomy even when a laparoscopic procedure is planned. Teach postoperative self-care measures to manage pain and prevent complications. If the patient will be discharged with a T-tube, provide instructions about its care (see the Nursing Care box on page 725). Discuss manifestations of complications to report to the physician. Stress the importance of follow-up appointments.

Following cholecystectomy, a low-fat diet may be initially recommended. Refer the patient and food preparer to a dietitian to review low-fat foods. (See Box 25–3 for examples of high-fat foods to avoid.) Higher fat foods may be gradually added to the diet as tolerated.

The Patient with Cancer of the Gallbladder

Gallbladder cancer is rare, primarily affecting people over age 65. Women are more likely to develop the disorder. Manifestations of gallbladder cancer include intense pain and a palpable mass in the RUQ of the abdomen. Jaundice and weight loss are common. Gallbladder cancers spread by direct extension to the liver, and metastasize via the blood and lymph system.

At the time of diagnosis, the cancer usually is too advanced to treat surgically. Ninety-five percent of patients with primary cancer of the gallbladder die within 1 year. Radical and extensive surgical interventions may be performed, but the prognosis is poor regardless of treatment. Nursing care is palliative, focusing on maintaining comfort and independence to the extent possible.

CASE STUDY & NURSING CARE PLAN   A Patient with Cholelithiasis

Joyce Red Wing is a 44-year-old married mother of three children. A member of the Chickasaw tribe, she is active in tribal activities and works part time as a cook at a community kitchen. Recently Mrs. Red Wing has noticed a dull pain in her upper abdomen that gets worse after eating fatty foods; nausea and sometimes vomiting accompany the pain. She had a similar pain after the birth of her last child. She is diagnosed with cholelithiasis, and is admitted for a laparoscopic cholecystectomy.

ASSESSMENT

David Corbin, RN, takes Mrs. Red Wing's admission history. It includes intolerance to fatty foods and intermittent "stabbing" abdominal pain that radiates to her back. Her usual diet includes tacos or fried bread and biscuits with gravy for breakfast. She reports "not wanting to eat much of anything lately." She states she has never had surgery before and hopes "everything goes well." Physical assessment includes T 100°F (37.7°C), P 88, R 20, and BP 130/84. She has had a recent 5 lb weight loss, currently weighing 130 lb (59 kg). She is 63 inches (160 cm) tall. Abdominal examination elicits tenderness in the right upper abdominal quadrant. She has no jaundice, chills, or evidence of complications.

DIAGNOSES

- *Imbalanced Nutrition: Less than Body Requirements* related to anorexia and recent weight loss
- *Acute Pain* related to inflamed gallbladder and surgical incisions
- *Risk for Infection* related to potential bacterial contamination of abdominal cavity
- *Anxiety* related to lack of information about perioperative experience

EXPECTED OUTCOMES

- Maintain present weight within 5 lb (2.3 kg) over the next 3 weeks.
- Resume regular diet, decreasing intake of foods high in fat.
- Verbalize adequate pain control after surgery and with activity resumption.
- Remain free of infection.
- Verbalize a decrease in anxiety before surgery.

PLANNING AND IMPLEMENTATION

- Teach about the gallbladder and the function of bile.
- Discuss pre- and postoperative care, including self-care following discharge.
- Promote mobility as soon as allowed after surgery.
- Teach home care of incisions and recognition of signs of infection.
- Review specific high-fat foods to avoid and ways to maintain her weight.
- Provide analgesia as needed postoperatively. Teach appropriate analgesic use after discharge.

EVALUATION

Mrs. Red Wing is discharged the morning after her surgery. She is afebrile, has no signs of infection, and is able to appropriately care for her incisions. She identifies signs of infection and talks about ways to reduce her fat intake while keeping her weight stable. She verbalizes understanding of initial activity restrictions and resumption of normal activities. Mrs. Red Wing states, "It wasn't as bad as I thought it would be at first." She has an appointment to see her surgeon in 1 week.

CRITICAL THINKING IN THE NURSING PROCESS

1. What is the rationale for a low-fat diet with cholelithiasis? Discuss nutritional practices as they relate to the medical problem and Mrs. Red Wing's culture.
2. How would your discharge teaching for Mrs. Red Wing differ if she had had an open cholecystectomy instead of a laparoscopic cholecystectomy?
3. Design a nursing care plan for Mrs. Red Wing for the nursing diagnosis *Fatigue*.

See Evaluating Your Response in Appendix C.

Liver Disorders

The liver is a complex organ with multiple metabolic and regulatory functions. Optimal liver function is essential to health. Because of the significant amount of blood in the liver at all times, it is exposed to the effects of pathogens, drugs, toxins, and possibly malignant cells. As a result, liver cells may become inflamed or damaged, or cancerous tumors may develop.

Physiology Review

The essential functions of the liver include the metabolism of proteins, carbohydrates, and fats. It also is responsible for the metabolism of steroid hormones and most drugs. It synthesizes essential blood proteins, including albumin and clotting factors in particular. The liver detoxifies alcohol and other toxic substances. Ammonia, a toxic by-product of protein metabolism, is converted to urea in the liver for elimination by the kidneys. The liver produces bile, an essential substance for absorbing fats and eliminating bilirubin from the body. Minerals and fat-soluble vitamins are stored in the liver, as is glycogen (stored carbohydrate for energy reserves). The Kupffer cells that line the sinusoids phagocytize foreign cells and damaged blood cells. ∞ See Chapter 21 for more information about the liver.

Common Manifestations of Liver Disorders

Although many different disorders can disrupt liver function, their manifestations relate to three primary effects: disrupted liver cell function, impaired bilirubin conversion and excretion leading to jaundice, and disrupted blood flow through the liver, with resulting portal hypertension.

Hepatocellular Failure

The liver is vital to digestion and metabolism of nutrients; the production of plasma proteins, including those involved in clotting; and the metabolism and excretion of compounds such as bilirubin, steroid hormones, and ammonia, as well as toxins (such as alcohol) and drugs. Impaired function of liver cells has multiple effects, including the following:

- Impaired protein metabolism with decreased production of albumin and clotting factors. Low albumin levels contribute to edema in peripheral tissues and **ascites**, accumulation of fluid in the abdomen (Figure 25–3 ■), as plasma oncotic pressure is reduced. Impaired clotting factor production increases the risk for bleeding.

Figure 25–3 ■ In ascites, serous fluid collects in the abdominal cavity, causing uniform distension.

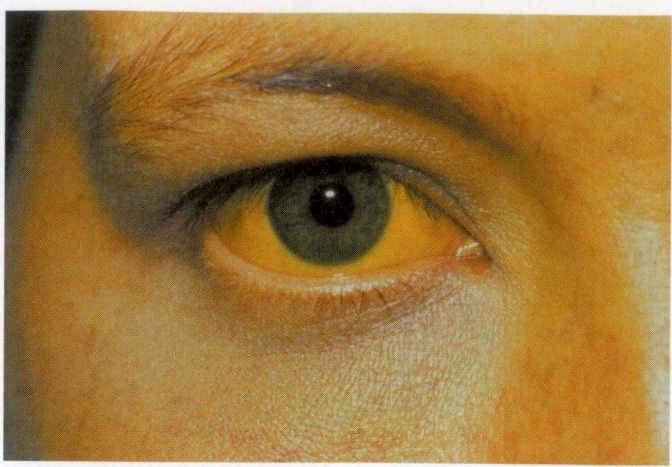

Figure 25–4 ■ Jaundice. Note the yellowing of the white (sclera) of the eye and of the surrounding facial skin.

- Disrupted glucose metabolism and storage with resulting alterations in blood glucose levels (either hyperglycemia or hypoglycemia).
- Reduced bile production that impairs the absorption of lipids and fat-soluble vitamins. Inadequate vitamin K, a fat-soluble vitamin, affects the production of clotting factors, leading to a bleeding tendency.
- Impaired metabolism of steroid hormones (including estrogen and testosterone) leads to feminization in men and irregular menses in women.

Jaundice

Disrupted metabolism and excretion of bilirubin allows it to accumulate in tissues, leading to **jaundice**, yellow staining of tissues (Figure 25–4 ■). Jaundice (also called *icterus*) often is first noticeable in the sclera of the eyes, then the skin.

When RBCs are destroyed (due to cell aging or disease), hemoglobin is released. The hemoglobin molecule breaks up into globin, a protein, and heme, the iron-containing portion of the molecule. In this process, biliverdin, later converted to fat-soluble bilirubin (*unconjugated bilirubin*), is released. The bilirubin binds with albumin to be transported to the liver. In the liver, it is converted to a water-soluble form (*conjugated bilirubin*) to be excreted in the bile. See Box 25–2 for more information about bilirubin metabolism.

Jaundice can result from disruptions at any point in the production and metabolism of bilirubin:

- *Hemolytic jaundice* develops when excess RBC destruction (hemolysis) releases more bilirubin into circulation than the liver is able to process. High blood levels of unconjugated bilirubin are seen.
- *Hepatic jaundice* occurs when impaired liver cell (*hepatocyte*) function disrupts the conversion and excretion of bilirubin. Blood levels of both conjugated and unconjugated bilirubin may be elevated. Stools may appear normal or clay colored, and urine is dark because the conjugated bilirubin is excreted by the kidneys.

- Obstruction of bile flow within the biliary system (the gallbladder and bile ducts) impairs bilirubin excretion, leading to *obstructive jaundice*. Levels of conjugated bilirubin are elevated. Stools are light or clay colored due to lack of bile pigment; and urine is dark because the kidneys excrete bilirubin.

Portal Hypertension

Impaired blood flow through the liver increases pressure in the portal venous system that drains the gastrointestinal tract, the spleen, and surface veins of the abdomen. **Portal hypertension**, increased pressure in the portal system, has several effects when it is prolonged:

- Dilation of veins in the gastrointestinal tract and the abdominal wall. This congestion tends to suppress the appetite and lead to formation of collateral vessels in the distal esophagus, stomach, and rectum. The dilated, congested vessels in the esophagus are known as **esophageal varices**; in the rectum, they lead to the development of hemorrhoids. In advanced liver failure, superficial varices may develop around the umbilicus, a feature known as *caput medusae*.
- Splenomegaly, or enlargement of the spleen.
- Ascites, accumulation of fluid in the peritoneal cavity. Increased hydrostatic pressure in abdominal vessels forces fluid out of the vessels and into the peritoneal cavity. Low serum albumin levels (*hypoalbuminemia*) contribute to fluid accumulation by reducing the osmotic draw of fluid back into vessels.
- **Portal systemic encephalopathy** (or *hepatic encephalopathy*), impaired consciousness and mental status due to the accumulation of toxic waste products in the blood (ammonia in particular) as blood bypasses the congested liver. It appears that factors other than elevated ammonia levels contribute, including toxic fatty acids, altered neurotransmitters, and an imbalance of plasma amino acid ratios. Cerebral edema develops late in the course of liver failure, resulting from both the accumulation of toxins and vascular mechanisms. As cerebral edema

progresses, intracranial pressure increases, cerebral perfusion decreases, and brain cells become hypoxic.

- *Hepatorenal syndrome* is acute renal failure due to disrupted blood flow to the kidneys. ∞ See Chapter 28 for more information about renal failure.

See the section of this chapter on cirrhosis for more information about the effects and complications associated with portal hypertension.

The Patient with Hepatitis

Hepatitis is inflammation of the liver. It is usually caused by a virus, although it may result from exposure to alcohol, drugs and toxins, or other pathogens. Hepatitis may be acute or chronic in nature. Cirrhosis, discussed in the next section, is a potential consequence of severe hepatocellular damage. Chronic hepatitis also increases the risk for developing liver cancer.

Pathophysiology and Manifestations

The inflammatory process of hepatitis, whether caused by a virus, toxin, or other mechanism, damages hepatic cells and disrupts liver function. Cell-mediated immune responses damage hepatocytes and Kupffer cells, leading to hyperplasia, necrosis, and cellular regeneration. The flow of bile through bile canaliculi and into the biliary system can be impaired by the inflammatory process, leading to jaundice. When the inflammatory process is mild (e.g., hepatitis A), the liver parenchyma is not significantly damaged. The inflammatory processes associated with hepatitis B and hepatitis C, however, can lead to severe liver damage. The metabolism of nutrients, drugs, alcohol, and toxins and the process of bile elimination are disrupted by the inflammation of hepatitis. ∞ See Chapter 21 for more information about the liver, and the preceding section for more information about the effects of disrupted liver function.

Viral Hepatitis

Viral hepatitis is nearly always caused by one of five viruses: hepatitis A virus (HAV), hepatitis B virus (HBV), hepatitis C virus (HCV), the hepatitis B-associated delta virus (HDV), and hepatitis E virus (HEV). With the exception of HBV, all of the hepatitis viruses are RNA viruses; HBV is a DNA virus. The viruses differ from one another in mode of transmission, incubation period, the severity and type of liver damage they cause, and their ability to become chronic or develop a carrier (asymptomatic) state. The illnesses they cause, however, are clinically very similar. Table 25–2 identifies unique features of the primary hepatitis viruses.

> **FAST FACTS**
> In the United States, hepatitis A, hepatitis B, and hepatitis C dominate.
> - Hepatitis A is less common than hepatitis B, with a reported 2,979 acute cases reported in 2007. The rate of hepatitis A infections per 100,000 population has fallen steadily since the introduction of hepatitis A vaccine, to the lowest ever reported rate of 1.0 in 2007.
> - There were 4,519 reported cases of hepatitis B in 2007. The rate of reported hepatitis B infections peaked at 11.5 per 100,000 population in 1985, since then falling to 1.5.
> - In 2007, 849 cases of hepatitis C were reported, for a national rate of 0.3 per 100,000 population.
> - The estimated number of actual new cases of viral hepatitis is significantly higher than the number of reported cases: An estimated 25,000 new cases of hepatitis A, 43,000 new cases of hepatitis B, and 17,000 new cases of hepatitis C are believed to have developed in 2007 (Centers for Disease Control and Prevention [CDC], 2009).

Hepatitis viruses replicate in the liver, indirectly damaging liver cells (hepatocytes). The viruses provoke an immune response that causes inflammation and necrosis of hepatocytes, leading to the clinical presentation of acute disease. Although the extent of damage and the immune response vary among the different hepatitis viruses, the disease itself usually follows a predictable pattern.

No manifestations are present during the incubation period after exposure to the virus. The *prodromal* or *preicteric* (before jaundice) *phase* may begin abruptly or insidiously, with general malaise, anorexia, fatigue, and muscle and body aches.

TABLE 25–2 Comparison of Types of Viral Hepatitis

VIRUS	HEPATITIS A (HAV)	HEPATITIS B (HBV)	HEPATITIS C (HCV)	HEPATITIS D (HDV)	HEPATITIS E (HEV)
Mode of transmission	Fecal–oral	Blood and body fluids; perinatal	Blood and body fluids	Blood and body fluids; perinatal	Fecal–oral
Incubation (in weeks)	2–6	6–24	5–12	3–13	3–6
Onset	Abrupt	Slow	Slow	Abrupt	Abrupt
Carrier state	No	Yes	Yes	Yes	Yes
Possible complications	Rare	Chronic hepatitis Cirrhosis Liver cancer	Chronic hepatitis Cirrhosis Liver cancer	Chronic hepatitis Cirrhosis Fulminant hepatitis	May be severe in pregnant women
Laboratory findings	Anti-HAV antibodies present	Positive HBsAg (HB surface antigen); anti-HBV antibodies present	Anti-HCV antibodies present	Positive HDVAg (delta antigen) early; anti-HDV antibodies later	Anti-HEV antibodies present

These manifestations often are mistaken for the flu. Nausea, vomiting, diarrhea, or constipation may develop, as well as mild RUQ abdominal pain. Chills and fever may be present.

The *icteric* (jaundiced) *phase* usually begins 5 to 10 days after the onset of symptoms. It is heralded by jaundice of the sclera, skin, and mucous membranes. Inflammation of the liver and bile ducts prevents bilirubin from being excreted into the small intestine. As a result, the serum bilirubin levels are elevated, causing yellowing of the skin and mucous membranes. Pruritus may develop due to deposition of bile salts on the skin. The stools are light brown or clay colored because bile pigment is not excreted through the normal fecal pathway. Instead, the pigment is excreted by the kidneys, causing the urine to turn brown. Whereas patients with acute hepatitis A or B are likely to develop jaundice, many people with hepatitis C do not develop jaundice. As a result, the infection may go undiagnosed for an extended period of time.

During the icteric phase, the initial prodromal manifestations usually diminish even though the serum bilirubin increases. The appetite increases, and the temperature returns to normal. When uncomplicated, spontaneous recovery usually begins within 2 weeks of the onset of jaundice.

The *convalescent phase* follows jaundice and lasts several weeks. During this time, manifestations gradually improve: Serum enzymes decrease, liver pain decreases, and gastrointestinal symptoms and weakness subside. See the accompanying box for the manifestations of each phase of hepatitis.

HEPATITIS A

Hepatitis A, or *infectious hepatitis,* is transmitted by the fecal–oral route via contaminated food, water, shellfish, and direct contact with an infected person. International travel is the primary risk factor for developing hepatitis A; others include close household or sexual contact with an infected partner (CDC, 2009). The virus is in the stool of infected persons up to 2 weeks before symptoms develop. Once jaundice develops, the amount of virus in the stool and the risk of spreading the disease decrease significantly. Although hepatitis A usually has an abrupt onset, it is typically a benign and self-limited disease with few long-term consequences. Symptoms last up to 2 months.

HEPATITIS B

Hepatitis B can cause acute hepatitis, chronic hepatitis, *fulminant* (rapidly progressive) hepatitis, or a carrier state. Less than 5% of adults infected with hepatitis B develop chronic hepatitis (National Institutes of Health [NIH], 2008). In a *carrier state*, the person harbors the active virus and is capable of spreading it to others, even though there are no discernible manifestations of the disease. It is more likely to develop when the virus is acquired at birth from an infected mother (Fauci et al., 2008). This virus is spread through contact with infected blood and body fluids. High-risk groups for hepatitis B include injection drug users, people with multiple sex partners, men who have sex with other men, and people frequently exposed to blood products (such as people on hemodialysis). Healthcare workers are at risk through exposure to blood and needle-stick injuries. Hepatitis B is a risk factor for primary liver cancer, particularly in people who are infected perinatally (Fauci et al., 2008).

In hepatitis B, liver cells are damaged by the immune response to this antigen. Damage may affect only portions or the majority

of the liver. The liver shows evidence of injury and scarring, regeneration, and proliferation of inflammatory cells. During the prodromal period, patients with HBV may experience such immune-mediated manifestations as urticaria and other rashes, arthralgias, serum sickness, or glomerulonephritis (Copstead & Banasik, 2010). The disease itself may be asymptomatic.

HEPATITIS C

Hepatitis C, formerly known as non-A, non-B hepatitis, is the primary worldwide cause of chronic hepatitis, cirrhosis, and liver cancer (Porth & Matfin, 2009). It is transmitted through infected blood and body fluids. Injection drug use is the primary risk factor for HCV infection, accounting for nearly half of all new infections (CDC, 2009). Acute hepatitis C usually is asymptomatic; if symptoms do develop, they often are mild and nonspecific. The disease often is recognized long after exposure occurred, when secondary effects of the disease (such as chronic hepatitis or cirrhosis) develop. Only about 15% of acute infections completely resolve; most progress to chronic active hepatitis (Copstead & Banasik, 2010).

> **SAFETY ALERT**
> Nurses frequently care for patients whose hepatitis antigen status is unknown or who have a secondary diagnosis of chronic hepatitis B or C. Exercise Standard Precautions including hand hygiene and personal protective equipment use with all patients to reduce the risk of exposure to these blood borne pathogens.

HEPATITIS DELTA

Hepatitis delta only causes infection in people who also are infected with hepatitis B. It can cause acute or chronic infection, and can increase the severity of HBV infection (Porth & Matfin, 2009). It is transmitted in the same manner as HBV; as the number of people with immunity to HBV has increased, the incidence of hepatitis delta has decreased (Fauci et al., 2008).

HEPATITIS E

Hepatitis E is rare in the United States. It is transmitted by fecal contamination of water supplies in developing areas such as southeast Asia, parts of Africa, and Central

MANIFESTATIONS of Acute Hepatitis

PREICTERIC PHASE
- "Flulike" symptoms: malaise, fatigue, fever
- Gastrointestinal: anorexia, nausea, vomiting, diarrhea, constipation
- Muscle aches, polyarthritis
- Mild right upper abdominal pain and tenderness

ICTERIC PHASE
- Jaundice
- Pruritus
- Clay-colored stools
- Brown urine
- Decrease in preicteric phase symptoms (e.g., appetite improves; no fever)

POSTICTERIC/CONVALESCENT PHASE
- Serum bilirubin and enzymes return to normal levels
- Energy level increases
- Pain subsides
- Gastrointestinal: minimal to absent

America. Person-to-person transmission is rare. It primarily affects young adults. It can cause fulminant, fatal hepatitis in pregnant women.

Chronic Hepatitis

Chronic hepatitis is chronic infection of the liver. Although it may cause few symptoms, it is the primary cause of liver damage leading to cirrhosis, liver cancer, and liver transplantation. Three of the known hepatitis viruses cause chronic hepatitis: HBV, HCV, and HDV. Patients with chronic hepatitis may have periods of active liver disease interspersed with periods of inactivity. Liver damage and fibrosis variably progress during periods of disease activity (NIH, 2008). Manifestations of chronic hepatitis include malaise, fatigue, and hepatomegaly. Occasional icteric (jaundiced) periods may occur. Liver enzymes, particularly serum aminotransferase levels, typically are elevated.

In chronic active hepatitis, inflammation extends to involve entire hepatic lobules. Chronic active hepatitis usually leads to cirrhosis and end-stage liver failure.

Fulminant Hepatitis

Fulminant hepatitis is a rapidly progressive disease, with liver failure developing within 2 to 3 weeks after the onset of symptoms. Although uncommon, it is usually related to HBV with concurrent HDV infection.

Toxic Hepatitis

Many substances, including alcohol, certain drugs, and other toxins, can directly damage liver cells. Alcoholic hepatitis can result from chronic alcohol abuse or from an acute toxic reaction to alcohol. Alcoholic hepatitis causes necrosis of hepatocytes and inflammation of the liver parenchyma (functional tissue). Unless alcohol intake is avoided, progression to cirrhosis is common.

Other potential hepatotoxins include acetaminophen, benzene, carbon tetrachloride, halothane, chloroform, and poisonous mushrooms. These substances directly damage liver cells, leading to necrosis. The degree of damage often depends on age and the extent of exposure (dose) to the hepatotoxin. Acetaminophen overdose is the leading cause of acute liver failure.

Autoimmune Hepatitis

Autoimmune hepatitis is a chronic disorder in which a cell-mediated immune response directed against liver cells causes persistent inflammation and necrosis with fibrosis and scarring. Circulating autoantibodies such as antinuclear antibody (ANA) usually are present. Many affected individuals have a personal or family history of other autoimmune disorders, such as rheumatoid arthritis or thyroiditis, suggesting a genetic link to the disorder. Chronic autoimmune hepatitis can ultimately lead to cirrhosis and liver failure.

Interdisciplinary Care

Management of hepatitis focuses on determining its cause, providing appropriate treatment and support, and teaching strategies to prevent further liver damage. Effective management begins with thorough assessment of diagnostic and laboratory data.

Diagnosis

Liver function tests, such as blood levels of bilirubin and enzymes commonly released when liver cells are damaged, are obtained. These include the following:

- *Alanine aminotransferase (ALT)* is an enzyme contained within each liver cell. When liver cells are damaged, ALT is released into the blood. Levels may exceed 1000 U/L or more in acute hepatitis.
- *Aspartate aminotransferase (AST)* is an enzyme found predominantly in heart and liver cells. AST levels rise when liver cells are damaged; with severe damage, blood levels may be 20 to 100 times normal values.
- *Alkaline phosphatase (ALP)* is an enzyme present in liver cells and bone. Serum ALP levels often are elevated in hepatitis, and may remain elevated after ALT and AST levels have returned to normal ranges.
- *Serum bilirubin* levels, including *conjugated* and *unconjugated*, are elevated in viral hepatitis due to impaired bilirubin metabolism and obstruction of the hepatobiliary ducts by inflammation and edema. The bilirubin level decreases as inflammation and edema subside.
- Laboratory tests for viral antigens and their specific antibodies may be done to identify the infecting virus and its state of activity. These tests are summarized in Table 25–2.
- A *liver biopsy* may be done to detect and evaluate chronic hepatitis. (Nursing implications for this test are outlined in ∞ Chapter 21.)

∞ See Chapter 21 for more information about diagnostic tests and their nursing implications.

Medications

PREVENTION Hepatitis A and hepatitis B are preventable diseases. Vaccines are available, as are preparations to prevent the disease following known or suspected exposure.

Vaccines Hepatitis A vaccine provides long-term protection against HAV infection. It is an inactivated whole-virus vaccine available in pediatric and adult formulations. Although more than 95% of adults achieve immunity after one dose of the vaccine, two doses are recommended for full protection. See Table 25–3.

Three doses of hepatitis B vaccine provide immunity to HBV infection in 90% of healthy adults. Because the hepatitis delta virus requires the presence of the hepatitis B virus, hepatitis B vaccine also protects against HDV. Hepatitis B vaccine is a recombinant vaccine. Vaccines produced by different manufacturers may be used interchangeably, although their dosages differ. Older adults are less likely to achieve immunity than younger adults. Patients on hemodialysis and people who are immunocompromised may need larger or more doses of the vaccine to achieve adequate protection. Serologic testing for immunity is recommended on completion of the series for people in these high-risk groups.

A combined hepatitis A and hepatitis B vaccine is available for use. It is recommended for the same high-risk populations as the single vaccines. Three doses are given: the initial dose, followed by doses no sooner than 4 weeks and 6 months later.

TABLE 25–3 CDC Recommendations for Hepatitis Prevention in Adults

DISEASE/STRATEGY	IMMUNIZATION	ADVERSE REACTIONS	POPULATION RECOMMENDATIONS
Hepatitis A			
Prevention	Hepatitis A vaccine (Havrix; VAQTA), 2 doses with at least 6 months between doses Injected IM into deltoid muscle Combined hepatitis A and hepatitis B vaccine (Twinrix), 3 doses (initial dose followed by doses 4 weeks and 6 months later) given IM into deltoid muscle	Pain at injection site	■ Everyone who desires protection from HAV infection ■ International travelers ■ Men who have sex with men ■ Illegal drug users ■ Persons with clotting-factor disorders, chronic liver disease ■ Persons with occupational risk
Postexposure prophylaxis	Standard immune globulin IM into large muscle mass within 2 weeks of exposure Hepatitis A vaccine may be used in healthy people 40 years old and younger	Rare; risk of anaphylaxis in people with IgA deficiency	■ Close contacts of people with known hepatitis A ■ People potentially exposed to hepatitis A at child care center or restaurant with infected food handler
Hepatitis B			
Prevention	Recombinant hepatitis B vaccine (Recombivax HB; Engerix-B), 3 doses (minimum of 16 weeks between dose #1 and #3) given IM into deltoid muscle Combined hepatitis A and hepatitis B vaccine (Twinrix), 3 doses (initial dose followed by doses 4 weeks and 6 months later) given IM into deltoid muscle	Pain at injection site; fatigue, headache	■ Infants and adolescents ■ Adults seeking protection from HBV infection ■ Persons with chronic liver disease ■ Men who have sex with men ■ Prostitutes; heterosexuals with multiple sexual partners ■ People with an STI ■ Injection drug users ■ Long-term male prisoners ■ People on hemodialysis ■ Healthcare workers
Postexposure prophylaxis	Hepatitis B immune globulin (HBIG) given IM into large muscle mass within 24 hours of exposure; concurrent initiation of hepatitis B vaccine series	Infrequent; muscle stiffness, pain	■ Infants born to women with HBV infection ■ Percutaneous or permucosal exposure to HBV when unvaccinated or antibody response is negative or unknown

Source: Centers for Disease Control and Prevention. (2009). *Epidemiology and prevention of vaccine-preventable diseases* (11th ed.). (Atkinson, J., Wolfe, S., Hamborsky, J., & McIntyre, L. Eds.). Washington, DC: Public Health Foundation.

Postexposure Prophylaxis Postexposure prophylaxis may be recommended for household or sexual contacts of people with HAV or HBV and other people who are known to have been exposed to these viruses. It is not necessary if the exposed person has been vaccinated and is known to be immune.

Hepatitis A prophylaxis is provided by a single dose of immune globulin (IG) given within 2 weeks after exposure. IG is recommended for all people with household or sexual contact with a person known to be infected with hepatitis A. See Table 25–3 for further recommendations.

Hepatitis B postexposure prophylaxis is indicated for people exposed to the hepatitis B virus. Hepatitis B immune globulin (HBIG) is given to provide for short-term immunity. HBV vaccine may be given concurrently. Candidates for postexposure prophylaxis include those with known or suspected percutaneous or permucosal contact with infected blood, sexual partners of patients with acute HBV or who are HBV carriers, and household contacts of patients with acute HBV infection (National Immunization Program, 2005).

DISEASE TREATMENT Nearly all people with acute viral hepatitis recover fully without pharmacologic treatment. Severe cases of acute hepatitis B may be treated with an antiretroviral drug such as lamivudine (Epiver, Heptovir), adefovir (Hepsera), entecavir (Baraclude), tenofovir (Viread) or telbivudine (Tyzeka). Treatment is not indicated for mild to moderate cases (Fauci et al., 2008). Acute hepatitis C generally is treated with interferon alpha, an antiviral agent, to reduce the risk of chronic hepatitis C. While single drug treatment with interferon α is common, a long-acting interferon (peginterferon or Pegasys) may be combined with the antiviral drug ribavirin (Rebetol, Virazole). Combination therapy with peginterferon and ribavirin is the treatment of choice for chronic hepatitis C. See the accompanying Medication Administration feature for nursing responsibilities related to interferons and antiviral drugs.

Interferon α interferes with viral replication, reducing the viral load. It is given by intramuscular or subcutaneous injection. Virtually all patients treated with interferon develop a

MEDICATION ADMINISTRATION Drugs to Treat Chronic Hepatitis

INTERFERON ALPHA

Conventional interferons

Interferon alfa-2a (Roferon-A)

Interferon alfa-2b (Intron A)

Interferon alfacon-1 (Infergen)

Long-acting interferons:

Peginterferon alfa-2a (Pegasys)

Peginterferon alfa-2b (PEG-Intron)

Human interferons have antiviral, immunosuppressive, and antineoplastic activity. Interferon alpha interferes with viral replication by blocking the virus from entering host cells, inhibiting syntheses of viral RNA and proteins, and viral release from host cells. Conventional interferons have a short half-life and must be administered several times weekly; long-acting preparations can be given once weekly. Long-acting preparations have a higher incidence of adverse effects, however.

Nursing Responsibilities
- Administer by subcutaneous injection. Do not use if solution is discolored or contains visible particulates.
- Monitor for manifestations of hypersensitivity (e.g., angioedema or bronchoconstriction); immediately notify physician and administer emergency treatment as needed to maintain cardiorespiratory status.
- Monitor CBC, platelet count, and renal and liver function studies. Frequently assess mental status. Withhold the drug and notify the physician of significant changes in lab values, manifestations of neuropsychiatric effects, severe abdominal pain, or changes in vision.

Patient Education
- This drug may cause flulike symptoms with fever, fatigue, body aches, headache, and chills. These symptoms tend to diminish over time with continued use of the drug. If approved by your physician, acetaminophen may be used to promote comfort.
- Notify your doctor immediately if you become severely depressed or develop thoughts of suicide, have severe chest pain or difficulty breathing, notice unusual bleeding or

bruising or have bloody diarrhea, notice a change in your vision, develop severe stomach or lower back pain, or notice a new or worsening skin condition.
- Keep all appointments for lab tests and follow-up visits to your doctor.
- Women: Use a reliable means of birth control and notify your physician immediately if you become pregnant.

ANTIRETROVIRAL DRUGS (NUCLEOSIDE/NUCLEOTIDE ANALOGS)

Lamivudine (Epiver-HBV)

Adefovir (Hepsera)

Entecavir (Baraclude)

Tenofovir (Viread)

Telbivudine (Tyzeka)

The nucleoside/nucleotide analog antiretroviral drugs were originally developed for treating HIV infection and now also are approved for HBV treatment, although the recommended doses differ for these two uses. These drugs inhibit synthesis of viral DNA. Therapy with antiretroviral drugs may be prolonged as relapse is common when the drug is stopped. Viral resistance to the drug also is a concern.

Nursing Responsibilities
- Administer PO as ordered.
- Monitor baseline and periodic renal and liver function tests, CBC with differential, blood chemistries, and serum electrolytes. Notify the physician of significant changes.
- Lactic acidosis is a risk with these drugs; monitor for manifestations such as hyperventilation, lethargy, and ABG values indicative of metabolic acidosis. Withhold the drug and notify the physician if manifestations of lactic acidosis develop.

Patient Teaching
- Take the drug as prescribed.
- Notify your doctor if you develop severe abdominal pain, nausea, vomiting or anorexia, or if you become jaundiced.
- Symptoms of recurrent hepatitis B may develop after you stop taking this drug; notify your physician if this occurs.

flulike syndrome with fever, fatigue, muscle aches, headache, and chills. Acetaminophen helps alleviate some of these adverse effects, which tend to decrease over time. Depression also is a common adverse effect of this drug. Instruct patients to contact their physician if suicidal thoughts or manifestations of depression develop. Ribavirin has two major adverse effects: hemolytic anemia and birth defects. Blood counts are obtained before and during treatment to detect early signs of hemolytic anemia. Because of the risk for birth defects, this drug is contraindicated for use during pregnancy, and two reliable methods of birth control must be used by women taking the drug and female sexual partners of men taking the drug.

In addition to interferon α or peginterferon, options for treating chronic hepatitis B include antiviral drugs such as lamivudine or adefovir. Using an antiviral drug in combination with an interferon reduces liver inflammation and fibrosis. Although side effects are minimal, patients may become resistant to the beneficial effects of these drugs. Entecavir is the most potent of the HBV antivirals and may be used as an alternate to lamivudine or adefovir. Treatment of acute hepatitis also includes as-needed bed rest, adequate nutrition as tolerated, and avoidance of strenuous activity, alcohol, and agents that

are toxic to the liver. In most cases, clinical recovery takes 3 to 16 weeks.

Complementary Therapies

Milk thistle, with its active ingredient silymarin, has been used by herbalists to treat liver disease for over 2000 years. Clinical studies have demonstrated that treatment with silymarin promotes quality of life and reduces symptoms in patients with hepatitis C. It also is beneficial for patients who have liver damage due to toxins, cirrhosis, and alcoholic liver disease. Silymarin is a powerful antioxidant that also promotes liver cell growth; it has not been shown, however, to decrease viral activity or reduce liver inflammation (National Center for Complementary and Alternative Medicine, 2008).

Herbalists also may use licorice root to treat hepatitis. It has both antiviral and anti-inflammatory effects. Long-term use of licorice root, however, can lead to hypertension and affect fluid and electrolyte balance.

Herbal preparations also may be used to relieve the adverse effects of interferon alpha. Ginger can help relieve nausea, and St. John's wort is used for the depression associated with interferon alpha.

ℰℴ Nursing Care

Health Promotion

Nurses play an instrumental role in preventing the spread of hepatitis. Stress the importance of hygiene measures such as hand hygiene after toileting and before all food handling. Discuss the dangers of injection drug use and, with drug users, of sharing needles or other equipment. Encourage all sexually active patients to use safer sexual practices such as abstinence, mutual monogamy, and barrier protection (such as male or female condoms).

Discuss recommendations for hepatitis A and hepatitis B vaccine with people in high or moderate risk groups for these infections. Ensure that nurses and other healthcare workers at risk for exposure to blood and body fluids are effectively vaccinated against hepatitis A and B. Encourage all people with known or probable exposure to HAV or HBV to obtain postexposure prophylaxis. See the accompanying nursing research feature for a study of healthcare workers' attitudes toward infected peers.

Assessment

Collect assessment data related to hepatitis, such as the following:

- *Health history:* Current manifestations, including anorexia, nausea, vomiting, abdominal discomfort, changes in bowel elimination or color of stools; muscle or joint pain; fatigue; changes in color of skin or sclera; duration of symptoms; known exposure to hepatitis; high-risk behaviors such as injection drug use or multiple sexual partners; previous history of liver disorders; current medications, prescription and over the counter.
- *Physical assessment:* Vital signs including temperature; color of sclera and mucous membranes; skin color and condition; abdominal contour and tenderness; color of stool and urine.
- *Diagnostic tests:* Serum bilirubin, liver function tests, serologic antibody–antigen levels.

Nursing Diagnoses and Interventions

Patients with acute or chronic hepatitis usually are treated in community settings; rarely is hospitalization required. Nursing care focuses on preventing spread of the infection to others and promoting the patient's comfort and ability to provide self-care.

Risk for Infection (Transmission)

An important goal when caring for patients with acute viral hepatitis is preventing spread of the infection.

- Use standard precautions. Practice meticulous hand hygiene. *The hepatitis viruses are spread by direct contact with feces or blood and body fluids. Standard precautions and good hand hygiene protect both healthcare workers and other patients from exposure to the virus.*
- For patients with HAV or HEV, use standard precautions and contact isolation if fecal incontinence is present. *The fecal–oral route is the primary mode of transmission of these viruses. Other hepatitis viruses are transmitted through blood and other body fluids.*
- Encourage prophylactic treatment of all members of household and intimate sexual contacts. *Prophylactic treatment of people in close contact with the patient decreases their risk of contacting the disease or, if already infected, the severity of the disease.*

> **SAFETY ALERT**
> If the patient diagnosed with hepatitis A is employed as a food handler or child care worker, contact the local health department to report possible exposure of patrons. Maintain confidentiality. Prophylactic treatment of people who have possibly been exposed to the virus can prevent a local epidemic of the disease.

MOVING EVIDENCE INTO ACTION **Applying Evidence to Practice**

Although the number of healthcare workers infected with blood borne pathogens such as HBV and HCV is small, those instances in which the infection has been transmitted to patients by the infected worker have received widespread publicity. Calls for testing of all healthcare workers or for restricting the practice of infected workers have been raised.

Kagan, Ovadia, and Kaneti (2008) studied nurses' and physicians' knowledge, attitudes, and opinions regarding disclosure and practice restrictions of healthcare workers infected with a blood borne pathogen. Although a correlation was found between knowledge about blood borne pathogens and attitudes toward infected healthcare workers, this study did not find a correlation between knowledge and opinions about disclosure of infection status or practice restrictions. There was, however, a correlation noted between attitudes toward infected workers and opinions regarding disclosure and oractuce restrictions.

IMPLICATIONS FOR NURSING

Of the major blood borne pathogens, HBV is associated with a significantly higher risk of transmission to and from healthcare workers than are HCV or HIV. Interestingly, participants in this study were more likely to have a positive attitude toward

healthcare workers infected with HBV and less likely to endorse self-disclosure and practice restrictions. Nurses need appropriate information and knowledge in order to accurately respond to patient's questions and concerns about blood borne pathogens.

CRITICAL THINKING IN PATIENT CARE

1. In this study, participants reported a more positive attitude toward healthcare workers infected with HBV than those infected with HCV or HIV. What factors do you think may have contributed toward this difference in attitudes?
2. Do you believe that nurses infected with a blood borne pathogen should disclose their status to patients for whom they provide care? Why or why not? Should a physician with HBV or HCV restrict his or her practice? If so, in what ways?
3. A coworker you know to be infected with HBV tells you that she is considering a position in a hemodialysis clinic. You know that patients undergoing hemodialysis fall within a high risk group for contracting hepatitis B. How will you respond to your coworker? What additional knowledge or information do you need to develop your response?

Source: Kagan, H., Ovadia, K., & Kaneti, T. (2008). Physicians' and nurses' vies on infected health care workers. *Nursing Ethics, 15*(5), 573–585.

EVIDENCE FOR NURSING CARE The Patient with Hepatitis

Selected resources that nurses may find helpful when planning evidence-based nursing care follow.

■ Davenport, A. & Myers, F. (2009). How to protect yourself after body fluid exposure. *Nursing2009, 39*(5), 22–28.
■ National Institutes of Health. (2008 October). NIH Consensus Development Conference statement on management of hepatitis B. *NIH Consensus and State-of-the-Science Statement, 25*(2), 1–29.

Fatigue

Fatigue and possible weakness are common in acute hepatitis. Although bed rest is rarely indicated, adequate rest periods and limitation of activities may be necessary. Many patients with acute hepatitis may be unable to resume normal activity levels for 4 or more weeks.

■ Encourage planned rest periods throughout the day. *Adequate rest is necessary for optimal immune function.*
■ Assist to identify essential activities and those that can be deferred or delegated to others. *Identifying essential and nonessential activities promotes the patient's sense of control.*
■ Suggest using level of fatigue to determine activity level, with gradual resumption of activities as fatigue and sense of well-being improves. *Fatigue associated with activity is an indicator of appropriate and inappropriate activity levels. As recovery progresses, increasing activity levels are tolerated with less fatigue.*

Imbalanced Nutrition: Less than Body Requirements

Adequate nutrition is important for immune function and healing in patients with acute or chronic hepatitis.

■ Help plan a diet of appealing foods that provides a high-kilocalorie intake of approximately 16 carbohydrate kilocalories per kilogram of ideal body weight. *Sufficient energy is required for healing; adequate carbohydrate intake can spare protein.*
■ Encourage planning food intake according to symptoms of the disease. Discuss eating smaller meals and using between-meal snacks to maintain nutrient and calorie intake. *Patients with acute hepatitis often are more anorexic and nauseated in the afternoon and evening; planning the majority of calorie intake in the morning helps maintain adequate intake. Limiting fat intake and the size of meals may reduce the incidence of nausea.*
■ Instruct to avoid alcohol intake and diet drinks. *Alcohol avoidance is vital to prevent further liver damage and promote healing. Diet drinks (e.g., diet sodas or juice drinks) provide few calories when an increased calorie intake is needed for healing.*
■ Encourage use of nutritional supplements such as Ensure or instant breakfast drinks to maintain calorie and nutrient intake. *Nutritional supplement drinks are an additional source of concentrated calories and nutrients.*

Disturbed Body Image

Jaundice and associated rashes and itching can affect the patient's body image. Nursing measures to prevent skin breakdown and address body image are discussed in the following section on cirrhosis.

Using NANDA, NIC, and NOC

Linkages between a selected NANDA nursing diagnosis, NIC, and NOC for the patient with viral hepatitis are shown in the chart that follows.

Community-Based Care

Provide discharge teaching to patients and their families for home care. Include the following topics:

■ Recommended prophylactic treatment
■ Infection control measures such as frequent hand hygiene; not sharing eating utensils; avoiding food handling or preparation activities by the patient with hepatitis A; abstaining from sexual relations during acute infection; and using barrier protection if a carrier or for chronic infection
■ Managing fatigue and limited activity
■ Managing pruritus and maintaining skin integrity: use warm, not hot water when bathing; use mild or no soap; limit duration of baths and showers; pat dry, do not rub, apply an alcohol-free lotion soon after bathing to retain skin moisture; wear loose cotton garments that allow moisture to evaporate from skin; reduce room temperature, especially at night, to prevent overheating; keep fingernails short, and wear cotton mittens or gloves as needed to prevent scratching during sleep
■ Promoting nutrient intake
■ Avoiding hepatic toxins such as alcohol, acetaminophen, and selected other drugs; encourage to alert all care providers to presence of infection
■ Recommended follow-up

If chronic hepatitis B or C is being treated with medications, teach how to administer the drug, its dosing schedule, precautions, and management of adverse effects. Stress the importance of keeping follow-up appointments, including recommended laboratory testing.

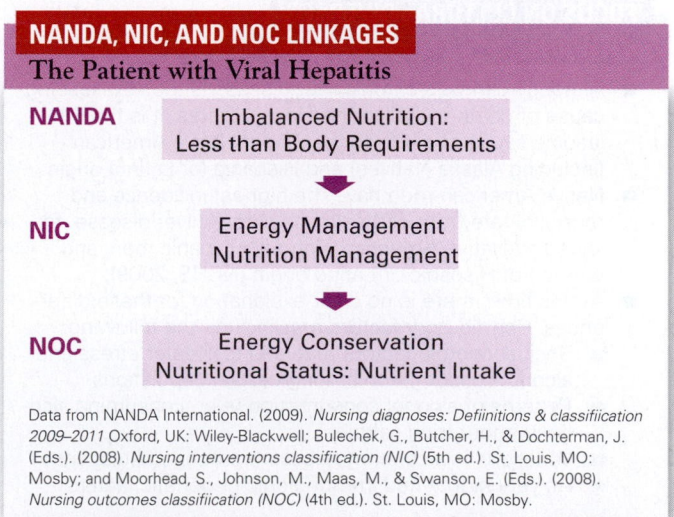

NANDA, NIC, AND NOC LINKAGES
The Patient with Viral Hepatitis

NANDA	Imbalanced Nutrition: Less than Body Requirements
NIC	Energy Management Nutrition Management
NOC	Energy Conservation Nutritional Status: Nutrient Intake

Data from NANDA International. (2009). *Nursing diagnoses: Defiinitions & classifiication 2009–2011* Oxford, UK: Wiley-Blackwell; Bulechek, G., Butcher, H., & Dochterman, J. (Eds.). (2008). *Nursing interventions classifiication (NIC)* (5th ed.). St. Louis, MO: Mosby; and Moorhead, S., Johnson, M., Maas, M., & Swanson, E. (Eds.). (2008). *Nursing outcomes classifiication (NOC)* (4th ed.). St. Louis, MO: Mosby.

The Patient with Cirrhosis

Cirrhosis is characterized by fibrosis of liver tissue leading to decreased mass, impaired liver function, and altered blood flow. Cirrhosis was previously thought to be an irreversible condition; now, however, it is recognized that fibrosis may be reversed when the underlying cause is eliminated (Fauci et al., 2008).

> ### FAST FACTS
> - Cirrhosis is the 12th leading cause of death in the United States overall.
> - In adults ages 25 to 64 years, however, cirrhosis/chronic liver disease is the 7th leading cause of death.
> - Overall, the death rate due to cirrhosis and chronic liver disease in men is more than twice that of women (National Center for Health Statistics [NCHS], 2009).

Alcoholic cirrhosis is the most common type of cirrhosis in the United States. Chronic hepatitis B or C also are leading causes of cirrhosis, particularly in people who consume alcohol excessively. Other causes include prolonged obstruction of the biliary (bile drainage) system; long-term, severe right heart failure, and uncommon liver disorders. The incidence and mortality attributable to cirrhosis and chronic liver disease vary significantly among populations. See the accompanying Focus on Cultural Diversity box.

Pathophysiology

In cirrhosis, functional liver tissue is gradually destroyed and replaced by fibrous scar tissue. As hepatocytes and liver lobules are destroyed, the metabolic functions of the liver are lost. Structurally abnormal nodules encircled by connective tissue develop. This fibrous connective tissue forms constrictive bands that disrupt blood and bile flow within liver lobules. Blood no longer flows freely through the liver to the inferior vena cava. This restricted blood flow leads to portal hypertension, increased pressure in the portal venous system.

Alcoholic Cirrhosis

Alcoholic or Laënnec's cirrhosis is the end result of alcoholic liver disease. Its development is directly related to alcohol consumption: total amount of alcohol consumed, number of years

> ### FOCUS ON CULTURAL DIVERSITY
> #### Cirrhosis
>
> - Although cirrhosis/chronic liver disease is the 12th leading cause of death overall in the United States, it is the 6th leading cause of death for people of Native American (including Alaska Natives) and Hispanic (or Latino) origin.
> - Native American men have the highest incidence and mortality rate from cirrhosis and chronic liver disease, followed by Native American women, Hispanic men, and women of Hispanic or Latino origin (NCHS, 2009).
> - At this time, there is no clear explanation for these differences. Contributory factors may include the following:
>   - Socioeconomic factors that lead to greater stress and alcohol consumption among certain populations
>   - Patterns of alcohol consumption (e.g., consuming alcohol without food calories)
>   - Variations in alcohol metabolism among populations
>   - As yet unidentified immunologic or genetic factors

of excessive alcohol consumption, and blood alcohol levels. Women develop cirrhosis at lower overall levels of alcohol use than men. This may relate to the effects of estrogen and less effective metabolism of alcohol in women, resulting in higher blood alcohol levels.

Alcohol causes metabolic changes in the liver: Triglyceride and fatty acid synthesis increases, and the formation and release of lipoproteins decrease, leading to fatty infiltration of hepatocytes (fatty liver). At this stage, abstinence from alcohol can allow the liver to heal. With continued alcohol abuse, the disease progresses. Inflammatory cells infiltrate the liver (alcoholic hepatitis), causing necrosis, fibrosis, and destruction of functional liver tissue. In the final stage of alcoholic cirrhosis, regenerative nodules form, and the liver shrinks and develops a nodular appearance. Malnutrition commonly accompanies alcoholic cirrhosis. See Pathophysiology Linkage: Cirrhosis, and Pathophysiology Illustrated: Cirrhosis and Portal Hypertension on the following pages.

Posthepatic Cirrhosis

Advanced progressive liver disease resulting from chronic hepatitis B or C, autoimmune hepatitis, or from nonalcoholic fatty liver disease is known as posthepatic or postnecrotic cirrhosis. Chronic viral hepatitis is the leading cause of posthepatic cirrhosis in the United States. About 25% of persons with chronic hepatitis B or C will eventually develop cirrhosis. The immune response is responsible for producing liver damage and fibrosis in chronic and autoimmune hepatitis. The liver is shrunken and nodular, with extensive liver cell loss and fibrosis. The obesity epidemic is seen as a major factor contributing to an increased incidence of cirrhosis due to nonalcoholic fatty liver disease.

Biliary Cirrhosis

When bile flow is obstructed within the liver or in the biliary system, retained bile damages and destroys liver cells close to the interlobular bile ducts. This leads to inflammation, fibrosis, and formation of regenerative nodules. Within the liver, bile ducts are narrowed or obstructed, leading to elevated bilirubin levels and progressive liver failure.

Manifestations and Complications

Early in the course of cirrhosis, few manifestations may be present. The liver usually is enlarged and may be tender. A dull, aching pain in the epigastric area or RUQ may be present. Other early signs include weight loss, weakness, and anorexia. Bowel function is disrupted with diarrhea or constipation.

As the disease progresses, manifestations related to liver cell failure and portal hypertension develop. Impaired metabolism causes such manifestations as bleeding, ascites, gynecomastia (breast enlargement) in men and infertility in women, jaundice, and neurologic changes. Portal hypertension accounts from such manifestations as ascites, peripheral edema, anemia, and low WBC and platelet counts. See Multisystem Effects of Cirrhosis on page 738.

Portal Hypertension

Increased pressure in the portal system causes blood to be rerouted to adjoining lower pressure vessels. This *shunting* of blood involves collateral vessels. Affected veins, which become

PATHOPHYSIOLOGY LINKAGE Cirrhosis

MANIFESTATIONS	UNDERLYING PATHOPHYSIOLOGY
Edema, ascites	■ Impaired hepatocyte function impairs plasma protein synthesis (hypoalbuminemia) ■ Disrupted hormone balance due to loss of metabolic and detoxification functions ■ Metabolism of aldosterone is impaired, leading to salt and water retention; disrupted renal blood flow contributes to fluid retention ■ Increased hydrostatic pressure in portal venous system
Bleeding, bruising	■ Decreased clotting factor synthesis related to impaired hepatocyte function ■ Increased platelet destruction by enlarged spleen ■ Impaired vitamin K absorption and storage
Esophageal varices, hemorrhoids	■ Increased pressure in portal venous system with development of weak, thin-walled vessels, particularly in the lower esophagus, rectum, and abdominal wall
Gastritis, anorexia, diarrhea	■ Engorged veins in gastrointestinal system disrupt normal appetite mechanisms ■ Alcohol ingestion ■ Impaired bile synthesis and fat absorption
Abdominal wall vein distention (caput medusae)	■ Portal hypertension
Jaundice	■ Impaired bilirubin metabolism due to disrupted hepatocyte function ■ Bile excretion is impaired by fibrosis and obstruction of biliary channels
Malnutrition, muscle wasting	■ Impaired nutrient metabolism ■ Impaired fat absorption ■ Impaired hormone metabolism
Anemia, leukopenia, increased risk for infection	■ Bleeding ■ Increased blood cell destruction by spleen
Asterixis, encephalopathy	■ Accumulated metabolic toxins ■ Impaired ammonia metabolism and excretion
Gynecomastia, infertility, impotence	■ Altered sex hormone metabolism

engorged and congested, are located in the esophagus, rectum, and abdomen. Portal hypertension increases the hydrostatic pressure in vessels of the portal system. Increased hydrostatic pressure in the capillaries pushes fluid out, contributing to ascites formation.

Splenomegaly

The spleen enlarges (splenomegaly) because portal hypertension causes blood to be shunted into the splenic vein. Splenomegaly increases the rate at which red and white blood cells and platelets are removed from circulation and destroyed. This increased blood cell destruction leads to anemia, leukopenia, and thrombocytopenia.

Ascites

Ascites is the accumulation of plasma-rich fluid in the abdominal cavity. Although portal hypertension is the primary cause of ascites, decreased serum proteins and increased aldosterone also contribute to the fluid accumulation. *Hypoalbuminemia*, low serum albumin, decreases the colloidal osmotic pressure of plasma. This pressure normally holds fluid in the intravascular compartment; when plasma colloidal osmotic pressure decreases, fluid escapes into extravascular compartments. *Hyperaldosteronism*, an increase in aldosterone levels, causes sodium and water retention, contributing to ascites and generalized edema.

Esophageal Varices

Esophageal varices are enlarged, thin-walled veins that form in the submucosa of the esophagus. These collateral vessels form when blood is shunted from the portal system due to portal hypertension. The thin-walled varices may rupture, causing massive hemorrhage; even eating high-roughage foods can precipitate bleeding. Thrombocytopenia, platelet deficiency, and impaired production of clotting factors by the liver contribute to the risk for hemorrhage.

Portal Systemic Encephalopathy

Portal systemic encephalopathy (*hepatic encephalopathy*) results from accumulation of neurotoxins in the blood and cerebral edema. Ammonia, a by-product of protein metabolism, contributes to hepatic encephalopathy. Ammonium ion is produced as proteins and amino acids are broken down by bacteria in the intestinal tract. Normally, the ammonia produced is then converted by the liver to urea before entering the general circulation. As functional liver tissue is destroyed, ammonia can no longer be converted to urea, and it accumulates in the blood. Other nervous system depressants, such as narcotics and tranquilizers, also can contribute to hepatic encephalopathy. Box 25–4 lists selected precipitating factors for hepatic encephalopathy. Accumulation of other metabolic toxins are thought to contribute as well.

PATHOPHYSIOLOGY ILLUSTRATED
Cirrhosis and Portal Hypertension

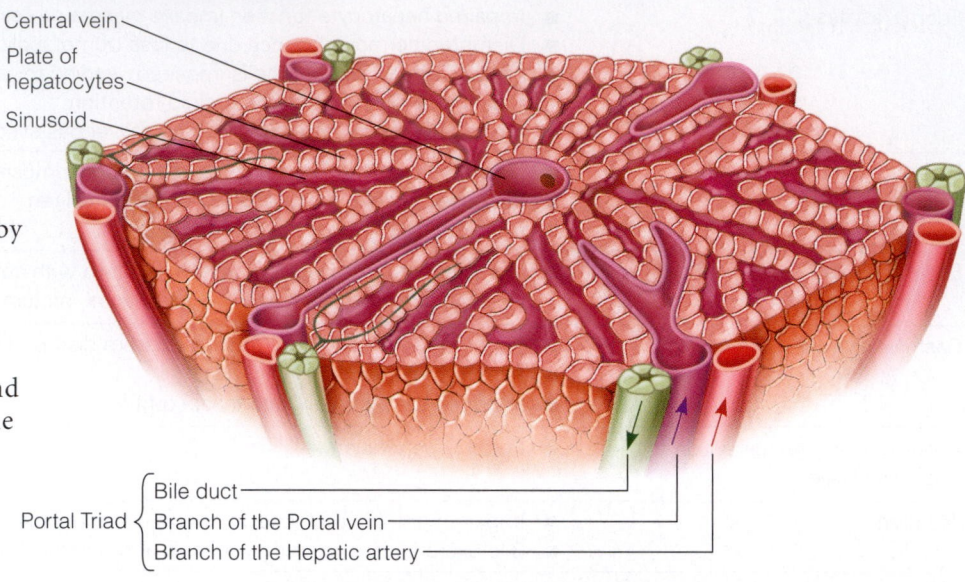

Central vein
Plate of hepatocytes
Sinusoid

Normal liver

The liver contains multiple lobules made up of plates of hepatocytes, the functional cells of the liver, surrounded by small capillaries called sinusoids. These sinusoids receive a mixture of venous and arterial blood from branches of the portal vein and hepatic artery. Blood from the sinusoids drains into the central vein of the lobule. Hepatocytes produce bile, which drains outward to bile ducts.

Portal Triad {
Bile duct
Branch of the Portal vein
Branch of the Hepatic artery

Fatty liver

Ingested alcohol is primarily metabolized in the liver. Acetaldehyde, formed when alcohol is metabolized, damages hepatocytes and impairs the oxidation of fatty acids. As a result, fat accumulates within hepatocytes and liver lobules. Other alcohol metabolism byproducts, including oxygen free radicals, promote inflammation and may stimulate autoantibody production.

◆ Auto-antibodies

▲ Free radicals

Alcoholic hepatitis

With continued alcohol intake, liver cells degenerate and spotty cellular necrosis occurs. Inflammatory cells such as polymorphonuclear leukocytes and lymphocytes infiltrate the lobule.

Alcoholic cirrhosis

Cellular necrosis and inflammation transform some liver cells into fibroblasts that produce and deposit collagen. Weblike bands of connective tissue develop around the portal triads and central vein, eventually connecting with one another. Small islands of liver cells continue to regenerate, forming nodules. Hepatocyte destruction outpaces regeneration. As a result of cell loss, fibrosis and scarring, the liver shrinks and becomes hard and nodular.

Nodule formation

Cellular necrosis

Fibrous bands of connective tissue

Portal hypertension

Bands of fibrotic scar tissue obstruct the sinusoids and blood flow from the portal vein to the hepatic vein. Pressure in the portal venous system, which drains the gastrointestinal tract, pancreas, and spleen, increases. This increased pressure opens collateral vessels in the esophagus, anterior abdominal wall, and rectum, allowing blood to bypass the obstructed portal vessels. Prolonged portal hypertension leads to the development of (1) varices (fragile, distended veins) in the lower esophagus, stomach, and rectum; (2) splenomegaly (an enlarged spleen); (3) ascites (accumulation of fluid in the abdomen); and (4) portal systemic encephalopathy (disrupted CNS function with altered consciousness).

Fibrous bands of connective tissue

Esophageal varices

Splenomegaly

Nodular cirrhosis

Ascites

Hemorrhoids

MULTISYSTEM EFFECTS OF
Cirrhosis

Neurologic
- Portal systemic encephalopathy
  (agitation → lethargy → stupor → coma)
- Paresthesias
- Sensory disturbances
- Asterixis ("liver flap")

Endocrine
- Gynecomastia in males

Potential Complication
- Diabetes mellitus

Respiratory
- Dyspnea

Cardiovascular
- Bounding pulse
- Pulmonary hypertension
- Portal hypertension
- Dysrhythmias

Hepatic
- Atrophic, nodular liver
- Splenomegaly

Potential Complication
- Liver cancer

Hematologic
- ↓clotting factors
- Thrombocytopenia
- Anemia

Potential Complication
- Disseminated intravascular
  coagulation

Gastrointestinal
Esophageal:
- Esophageal varices
Stomach/intestines:
- Abdominal pain
- Anorexia
- Ascites
- Nausea
- Clay-colored stools
- Peptic ulcers
- GI bleeding
- Hemorrhoids

Reproductive
- Oligomenorrhea (female)
- Testicular atrophy (male)

Integumentary
- Jaundice (skin, sclera of eyes)
- Erythema of palms
- Spider angioma
- Decreased body hair
- Pruritis
- Ecchymoses
- Caput medusae (dilated veins around
  the umbilicus)

Immune System
- Leukocytopenia
- ↑ susceptibility
  to infections

Metabolic Processes
- Fluid and electrolyte imbalances
  – Hypoalbuminemia
  – Hypokalemia
  – Hypocalcemia
- Malnutrition
- Muscle wasting

Asterixis (liver flap), a muscle tremor that interferes with the ability to maintain a fixed position of the extremities and causes involuntary jerking movements, is an early sign of portal systemic encephalopathy. Asterixis primarily affects the upper extremities, but also may affect the tongue and feet. Asterixis is elicited by instructing the patient to extend the arms and dorsiflex the wrists. If present, asterixis causes a downward flapping of the hands (Figure 25–5 ■). Changes in personality and mentation develop; agitation, restlessness, impaired judgment, and slurred speech also are early manifestations of hepatic encephalopathy. As it progresses, confusion, disorientation, and incoherence develop. Cerebral edema that leads to increased intracranial pressure and cerebral hypoxia is the leading cause of death in people with portal systemic encephalopathy and liver failure.

Hepatorenal Syndrome

Although the cause is unclear, renal failure with azotemia (excess nitrogenous waste products in the blood), sodium retention, oliguria, and hypotension may develop in patients with advanced cirrhosis and ascites. Hepatorenal syndrome appears to be the result of imbalanced blood flow, leading to constriction of vessels leading to and within the kidneys. The syndrome may be precipitated by gastrointestinal bleeding, aggressive diuretic therapy, or by an unknown cause.

Spontaneous Bacterial Peritonitis

Patients with cirrhosis and ascites may develop bacterial peritonitis, even in the absence of known contamination of the peritoneal cavity or other specific risk factors (e.g., paracentesis). The inflammatory response to peritonitis worsens ascites by increasing the permeability of capillaries in the mesentery. The manifestations of spontaneous bacterial peritonitis may be subtle, with increased abdominal discomfort or pain, fever, increasing ascites, worsening encephalopathy, and an overall decline in condition.

Interdisciplinary Care

Care for the patient with cirrhosis is holistic, addressing physiologic, psychosocial, and spiritual needs. The importance of including the family in the plan of care cannot be overemphasized, particularly if alcohol abuse is identified as the cause. Alcohol abstinence is critical: Fewer than 50% of patients who have experienced complications of cirrhosis and who continue to drink will survive for 5 years. The prognosis improves with abstinence, and liver transplant may be a treatment option in abstinent patients (Fauci et al., 2008).

Treatment of cirrhosis is supportive, directed at slowing the progression to liver failure and reducing complications. Treatment includes medications to help regulate protein metabolism, maintenance of fluid and electrolyte balance, and supportive therapies, including treatment of underlying problems, such as malnutrition, anemia, bleeding, encephalopathy, renal failure, and infections.

Diagnosis

Studies to confirm the diagnosis of cirrhosis and identify its cause and effects are performed. Diagnostic tests may include the following:

- *Liver function studies* include *ALT*, *AST*, and *ALP*. All may be elevated in cirrhosis, but usually not as severely as in acute hepatitis. Elevations in these enzymes may not correlate well with the extent of liver damage in cirrhosis.
- *CBC with platelets* is done. A low RBC count, hemoglobin, and hematocrit demonstrate anemia related to bone marrow suppression, increased RBC destruction, bleeding, and deficiencies of folic acid and vitamin B_{12}. Platelets are low, related to increased destruction by the spleen. Leukopenia (low WBC count) also relates to splenomegaly.
- *Coagulation studies* show a prolonged prothrombin time due to impaired production of coagulation proteins and lack of vitamin K.
- *Serum electrolytes* are measured. Hyponatremia is common, due to hemodilution. Hypokalemia, hypophosphatemia, and hypomagnesemia also are frequently seen, related to malnutrition and altered renal excretion of these electrolytes.
- *Bilirubin* levels are usually elevated in severe cirrhosis, including both direct (conjugated) and indirect (unconjugated) bilirubin.
- *Serum albumin* levels show hypoalbuminemia due to impaired liver production.
- *Serum ammonia* levels are elevated because the liver fails to effectively convert ammonia to urea for renal excretion.
- *Serum glucose* and *cholesterol* levels frequently are abnormal in patients with cirrhosis.

Figure 25–5 ■ Asterixis. Note the downward tremor of the hand on dorsiflexion of the wrist.

- *Abdominal ultrasound* is performed to evaluate liver size, detect ascites, and identify liver nodules. Ultrasound may be used in conjunction with *Doppler studies* to evaluate blood flow through the liver and spleen.
- *Esophagoscopy* (upper endoscopy) may be done to determine the presence of esophageal varices.
- *Liver biopsy* is not always necessary to diagnose cirrhosis, but may be done to distinguish cirrhosis from other forms of liver disease. See page 575 for nursing implications for a patient having a liver biopsy. Figure 21–8 shows the site and position for liver biopsy. Biopsy may be deferred if the bleeding time is prolonged (such as a prothrombin time [PT] greater than 3 seconds over the control).

∞ See Chapter 21 for more information about and the nursing implications of the aforementioned diagnostic tests.

Medications

Medications are used to treat the complications and effects of cirrhosis; they do not reverse or slow the process of cirrhosis itself. Known hepatotoxic drugs and alcohol are avoided, as are drugs metabolized by the liver (e.g., barbiturates, sedatives, hypnotics, and acetaminophen). Several groups of drugs are commonly prescribed. See the Medication Administration box for nursing responsibilities and patient teaching for commonly used drugs in patients with cirrhosis.

- Diuretics reduce fluid retention and ascites. Spironolactone (Aldactone) is frequently the drug of first choice because it addresses one of the causes of ascites—increased aldosterone levels. If additional diuresis is necessary, a loop diuretic such as furosemide (Lasix) may be added to the regimen.
- Medications to reduce the nitrogenous load and lower serum ammonia levels are added when manifestations of hepatic encephalopathy develop. Commonly administered medications are lactulose and antibiotics such as neomycin, metronidazole, or rifaximin. Lactulose reduces the number of ammonia-forming organisms in the bowel and increases the acidity of colon contents, converting ammonia into ammonium ion. Ammonium ion is not absorbable, and is excreted in the feces. Neomycin sulfate is a locally acting antibiotic that also reduces the number of ammonia-forming bacteria in the bowel. Because it is toxic to the kidneys and auditory system, it is alternated with metronidazole. Metronidazole is a systemic antibiotic effective against common Gram-negative bacteria that inhabit the bowel. Peripheral neuropathy is a

---

MEDICATION ADMINISTRATION **The Patient with Cirrhosis**

DIURETICS
Spironolactone (Aldactone)

Furosemide (Lasix)

Spironolactone is a potassium-sparing diuretic that competes with aldosterone. It reduces ascites by increasing renal excretion of fluid and decreasing aldosterone levels. Furosemide is a loop diuretic that promotes the excretion of potassium. Drugs may be given in combination if serum potassium level permits.

Nursing Responsibilities
- Monitor ECG, serum potassium, BUN, creatinine levels, and hydration status.
- Weigh daily.
- Carefully monitor intake and output.
- Monitor for signs of hyperkalemia if taking spironolactone alone: bradycardia; widening QRS, spiking T waves, or ST segment depression on ECG; diarrhea; and muscle twitching.
- Assess for hyponatremia: confusion, lethargy, apprehension.

Health Education for the Patient and Family
- Maintain diet and fluid restrictions as prescribed.
- Report increases in weight or edema.
- Immediately report signs of hyponatremia, hyperkalemia, or hypokalemia (∞ see Chapter 10).
- Expect increased urinary output; take medications in morning hours to avoid nocturia.

LAXATIVES
Lactulose (Cephulac, Chronulac)

Lactulose is a disaccharide laxative that is not absorbed by the gastrointestinal tract. It reduces the number of ammonia-producing bacteria and lowers the pH in the colon. The lower pH (increased acidity) converts ammonia to ammonium ion, a nonabsorbable form that is excreted in the feces. Lactulose also pulls water into the bowel lumen, increasing the number of daily stools.

Nursing Responsibilities
- Assess bowel sounds and abdominal girth.
- Maintain accurate stool chart.
- Adjust dose to achieve two to four soft stools per day.
- Monitor electrolytes and hydration.

Health Education for the Patient and Family
- Drink adequate fluids.
- Report diarrhea; if present, decrease dose. You should have an average of two to four stools per day.
- This drug may cause nausea. Continue taking the drug; taking it with crackers or a soft drink may reduce nausea.

ANTI-INFECTIVE AGENTS
Neomycin sulfate (Neo Tabs)

Metronidazole (Flagyl)

Rifaximin (Xifaxan)

These antibiotics act in the gut to reduce intestinal bacteria and decrease ammonia production in the bowel lumen. Neomycin may be administered as an oral or rectal preparation; metronidazole and rifaximin are administered orally.

Nursing Responsibilities
- Monitor hearing, renal, and neurologic functions. Neomycin is ototoxic, nephrotoxic, and neurotoxic. Metronidazole is neurotoxic.
- Prior to administration, check for previous hypersensitivity reaction.
- Monitor intake and output.
- Monitor BUN and creatinine levels.

Health Education for the Patient and Family
- Report dizziness, tinnitus (ringing in ears), hearing loss, headaches, tremors, vision changes or extremity numbness and tingling immediately.
- Keep follow-up appointments.
- Maintain fluids; avoid dehydration. (Teach signs of dehydration.)

potential toxic effect of metronidazole. Rifaximin, a poorly absorbed antibiotic, acts locally within the bowel and has few adverse or toxic effects.

- A beta-blocker such as nadolol (Corgard) or propranolol (Inderal) may be given to reduce portal hypertension and prevent bleeding of esophageal varices.
- Ferrous sulfate and folic acid are given as indicated to treat anemia. Vitamin K may be ordered to reduce the risk of bleeding. When bleeding is acute, packed RBCs, fresh frozen plasma, or platelets may be administered to restore blood components and promote hemostasis.
- Antacids are prescribed as indicated. A drug regimen to treat *H. pylori* infection may also be effective (∞ see Chapter 23).
- Oxazepam (Serax), a benzodiazepine antianxiety/sedative drug, is not metabolized by the liver, and may be used to treat acute agitation.

Nutrition and Fluid Management

Dietary support is an essential part of care for the patient with cirrhosis. Dietary needs change as hepatic function fluctuates.

- Sodium intake is restricted to under 2 g/day, and fluids are restricted as necessary to reduce ascites and generalized edema. Fluids are often limited to 1500 mL/day. Fluid needs are calculated based on response to diuretic therapy, urine output, and serum electrolyte values.
- Unless serum ammonia levels are high, a palatable diet with adequate calories and protein is recommended. Although dietary protein restriction has previously been recommended for patients with cirrhosis and hepatic encephalopathy, it is now recognized that the effects of protein-calorie malnutrition are more damaging than protein consumption (Fauci et al., 2008; Wolf, 2008). Vegetable proteins may be recommended along with restricted red meat consumption. Parenteral nutrition is used as needed to maintain nutritional status when food intake is limited.
- Vitamin and mineral supplements are ordered based on laboratory values. Deficiencies in the B-complex vitamins, particularly thiamin, folate, and B_{12}, and the fat-soluble vitamins A, D, and E are common. These vitamins may need to be administered in a water-soluble form. Patients with alcohol-induced cirrhosis are at high risk for magnesium deficiency, which needs to be replaced.

Complication Management

ASCITES   **Paracentesis**, aspiration of fluid from the peritoneal cavity, may be a diagnostic or a therapeutic procedure. It may be done therapeutically to relieve severe ascites that does not respond to diuretic therapy. The goal of paracentesis is to relieve respiratory distress caused by excess fluid in the abdomen. Ascites fluid may be withdrawn in moderate amounts of 500 mL to 1 L daily to reduce the risk of fluid and electrolyte imbalances. Large-volume paracentesis, withdrawal of 4 to 6 L of fluid at one time, may be used. Albumin is often administered intravenously during large-volume paracentesis to maintain intravascular volume as the pressure of the ascites fluid in the abdomen is relieved. Nursing care for the patient undergoing paracentesis are listed in the accompanying box. Figure 25–6 ■ shows insertion sites and patient positioning during paracentesis.

Figure 25–6 ■ Sites and position for paracentesis. *A,* Potential sites of needle or trocar insertion to avoid abdominal organ damage. *B,* The patient sits comfortably; in this position, the intestines float back and away from the insertion site.

ESOPHAGEAL VARICES   Primary care for esophageal varices involves screening with endoscopy. When varices are identified, beta blocker therapy may be initiated to lower portal venous pressure or endoscopic variceal ligation or sclerotherapy may be performed. In *variceal ligation* or *banding,* small rubber bands are placed on varices to occlude blood flow. *Endoscopic sclerosis* involves injecting a sclerosing agent directly into the varices to induce inflammation and clotting. ∞ See Chapter 21 for the nursing implications of endoscopy.

Bleeding esophageal varices are life threatening and require intensive care management. Restoration of hemodynamic stability is the first priority. A central line is inserted and central venous and pulmonary artery pressures are monitored (∞ see Chapter 31). Blood is given to restore blood volume, and fresh frozen plasma may be administered to restore clotting factors. Somatostatin or octreotide, drugs that constrict blood vessels in the gut, are given intravenously to reduce blood flow in the portal venous system.

When the blood pressure and cardiac output have stabilized, upper endoscopy is performed to evaluate and treat the varices. A large nasogastric tube is inserted prior to endoscopy, and gastric lavage (irrigation of the stomach with large quantities of normal saline) is performed to improve visualization. During endoscopy, the varices may be banded or sclerosed to reduce the risk of recurrent bleeding. *Balloon tamponade* of bleeding varices may be used if bleeding cannot be controlled through vasoconstriction or if endoscopy is unavailable or contraindicated by the patient's condition. A multiple-lumen nasogastric (NG) tube (such as a Sengstaken-Blakemore tube or a Minnesota tube) is inserted, and the gastric and esophageal balloons are inflated to apply direct pressure on the bleeding varices (Figure 25–7 ■). Tension is applied to the tube to further compress the varices. Balloon tamponade carries a number of risks, including aspiration,

NURSING CARE OF THE PATIENT Undergoing Paracentesis

PREPARATION

- Verify presence of an informed consent. *Paracentesis is an invasive procedure requiring informed consent.*
- Describe what to expect during paracentesis: Following cleansing and local anesthesia, a small incision may be made and a needle or trocar inserted to withdraw fluid. The trocar is connected to tubing and a collection bottle; specimens may be sent to laboratory. Blood pressure is monitored during the procedure. *A clear understanding of the procedure and its purpose reduces anxiety and facilitates cooperation during the procedure.*
- Weigh prior to paracentesis. Measure abdominal girth at the level of the umbilicus. *Weight is an accurate means of determining fluid balance, particularly in patients with edema. Abdominal girth provides an additional measure of the effectiveness of paracentesis.*
- Assess vital signs for baseline. *Fluid shifts during and after paracentesis can affect cardiovascular stability. Baseline vital signs provide a reference for subsequent measurements.*
- Have patient void immediately prior to the test. *The bladder must be empty prior to paracentesis to reduce the risk for bladder puncture.*

- Position seated, either on the side of the bed or in a chair, with feet supported. *The sitting position allows ascites fluid to collect in the lower abdomen, facilitating its removal.*

AFTER THE PROCEDURE

- A small dressing is placed over the puncture site after the needle is withdrawn. There may be some fluid leakage from the site. *Depending on the size of the trocar inserted and the amount of remaining ascites fluid, the insertion puncture may not immediately seal, allowing fluid to escape.*
- Monitor vital signs every 15 minutes for 1 hour, every 30 minutes for 1 hour, then every 4 hours. Measure abdominal girth and obtain weight. *Removal of large amounts of fluid from the abdominal cavity can cause significant fluid shifts with resulting vascular instability. Weight and abdominal girth measurements provide information about fluid balance.*
- Salt-poor albumin may be given after the procedure to replace lost protein. *Removing ascites fluid reduces pressure within the peritoneal cavity. In the patient with hypoalbuminemia and portal hypertension, a significant amount of vascular fluid can escape as a result, leading to hypovolemia. Albumin is given to increase plasma oncotic pressure, helping retain fluid within the vascular system.*

---

airway obstruction, and tissue ischemia and necrosis. An endotracheal tube is inserted prior to nasogastric intubation to support the airway and reduce the risk of aspiration. This short-term measure is used only until more definitive treatment can be done. Without definitive treatment, rebleeding is common when balloon tamponade is discontinued.

Figure 25–7 ■ Triple-lumen nasogastric tube (Sengstaken-Blakemore) used to control bleeding esophageal varices.

SAFETY ALERT
When caring for a patient with a multiple-lumen NG tube, always deflate the esophageal balloon before the gastric balloon. This practice prevents the balloon from becoming misplaced and occluding the airway. Always keep an appropriate syringe at the bedside to deflate the esophageal balloon should the patient develop respiratory distress.

PORTAL HYPERTENSION *Transjugular intrahepatic portosystemic shunt (TIPS)* may be used as an emergency measure to relieve portal hypertension and its complications of esophageal varices and ascites. A channel is created through the liver tissue using a needle inserted transcutaneously (Figure 25–8 ■). An expandable metal stent is inserted into this channel to allow blood to flow directly from the portal vein into the hepatic vein, bypassing the cirrhotic liver. The shunt relieves pressure in esophageal varices and allows better control of fluid retention with diuretic therapy. Stenosis and occlusion of the shunt are frequent complications. TIPS also increases the risk of developing hepatic encephalopathy (due to decreased perfusion of the liver and impaired ammonia metabolism) and may reduce long-term survival. It generally is used as a short-term measure until liver transplant is performed.

Surgery

Liver transplantation is indicated for some patients with irreversible, progressive cirrhosis. A decline in functional status, increasing bilirubin levels, falling albumin levels, and increasing problems with complications that respond poorly to treatment

Figure 25–8 ■ Transjugular intrahepatic portosystemic shunt (TIPS). *A,* Guided by angiography, a balloon catheter inserted via the jugular vein is advanced to the hepatic veins and through the substance of the liver to create a portacaval (portal vein-to-vena cava) channel. *B,* A metal stent is positioned into the channel, and expanded by inflating the balloon. *C,* The stent remains in place after the catheter is removed, creating a shunt for blood to flow directly from the portal vein into the hepatic vein.

are indications for liver transplantation. Malignancy, active alcohol or drug abuse, and poor surgical risk are contraindications for the surgery. See the box for nursing care of the patient undergoing a liver transplant.

Nursing Care

In addition to the nursing care discussed in this section, a Case Study & Nursing Care Plan for a patient with alcoholic cirrhosis is found on page 748.

Health Promotion

For most patients, high-risk behaviors are the risk factors for cirrhosis. With all patients (including children and young adults), stress the relationship between alcohol and drug abuse and liver disorders. While many patients tolerate alcohol use in moderation with no adverse effects on the liver, excess alcohol use is the leading cause of cirrhosis. Injection drug use also is a significant risk factor, increasing the risk for contracting blood-borne hepatitis (B, C, or D). These types of viral hepatitis can lead to chronic hepatitis and, ultimately, to cirrhosis. Provide information and referral as appropriate for hepatitis B immunization. Discuss abstinence or safer sex practices as another measure to prevent viral hepatitis and potential liver damage.

Assessment

Assessment data related to cirrhosis include the following:

- *Health history:* Current manifestations, including abdominal pain or discomfort, recent weight loss, weakness, and anorexia; altered bowel elimination; excess bleeding or bruising; abdominal distention; jaundice, pruritus; altered libido or impotence; duration of symptoms; history of liver or gallbladder disease; pattern and extent of alcohol or injection drug use; use of other prescription and nonprescription drugs.
- *Physical assessment:* Vital signs; mental status; color and condition of skin and mucous membranes; peripheral pulses and presence of peripheral edema; abdominal assessment including appearance, shape and contour, bowel sounds, abdominal girth, percussion for liver borders, and palpation for tenderness and liver size.

Nursing Diagnoses and Interventions

Nursing care of the patient with cirrhosis presents many challenges because liver function affects all body systems. The nurse is responsible for coordinating care among care providers. Many nursing diagnoses may apply. The diagnoses discussed in this section focus on problems with fluid and electrolyte balance, disturbed thought processes, risk for bleeding, skin integrity, and nutrition.

Excess Fluid Volume

Cirrhosis affects water and salt regulation due to portal hypertension, hypoalbuminemia, and hyperaldosteronism. Signs of fluid volume overload and portal hypertension may develop: ascites, peripheral edema, internal hemorrhoids and varices, and prominent abdominal wall veins. Careful monitoring is necessary, because treatment measures can lead to further fluid and electrolyte imbalances.

EVIDENCE FOR NURSING CARE **The Patient with Cirrhosis**

Selected resources that nurses may find helpful when planning evidence-based nursing care follow.

- Garcia-Tsao, G., & Bosch, J. (2010). Management of varices and variceal hemorrhage in cirrhosis. *New England Journal of Medicine, 362*(9), 823–832.
- Les, I., Doval, E., Flavià, M., Jacas, C., Cárdenas, G., Esteban, R., et al. (2010). Quality of life in cirrhosis is related to potentially treatable factors. *European Journal of Gastroenterology & Hepatology, 22*(2), 221–227.
- O'Shea, R., Dasarathy, S., McCullough, A., (2010, January). Alcoholic liver disease. *Hepatology, 51*(1), 307–28. Retrieved from http://www.guideline.gov/summary/summary.aspx?ss=15&doc_id=15477&nbr=007577&string=cirrhosis
- Runyon, B., & AASLD Practice Guidelines Committee. (2009, June). Management of adult patients with ascites due to cirrhosis: An update. *Hepatology, 49*(6), 2087-107. Retrieved from http://www.guideline.gov/summary/summary.aspx?ss=15&doc_id=14887&nbr=007373&string=cirrhosis

NURSING CARE OF THE PATIENT   Undergoing Liver Transplantation

PREOPERATIVE CARE

- Obtain a complete nursing history and physical examination. *A complete preoperative nursing assessment provides baseline data for comparison after surgery.*
- Provide routine preoperative care as ordered (∞ see Chapter 4). *Preoperative care is similar to that provided for other patients undergoing major surgery.*
- Discuss preoperative and postoperative expectations with the patient and family. Introduce to the intensive care unit, and discuss anticipated drainage tubes and supportive measures in the immediate postoperative period. Provide information about visiting policies and family accommodations (if available). *Preoperative teaching helps relieve anxiety in the patient and family members. Patients return from surgery to an intensive care or specialized care unit. Restrictions on the number of visitors and the time they may spend with the patient are common.*
- Once a donor liver is located, check for evidence of infection; if no infection is present, begin preoperative antibiotics as ordered. *An acute or chronic infection may contraindicate liver transplantation as drugs given postoperatively to suppress rejection of the transplanted organ also impair the ability to fight infection.*

POSTOPERATIVE CARE

- Provide routine postoperative care as outlined in ∞ Chapter 4.
- Maintain airway and ventilatory support until awake and alert. *Until the new liver clears the anesthesia, the patient requires measures to support respirations and ventilation.*
- Monitor temperature and implement rewarming measures (such as warming blankets, heating lamps, and head covers) as indicated. *The patient often is hypothermic after liver transplant, necessitating careful rewarming while maintaining hemodynamic stability.*
- Frequently monitor hemodynamic pressures, including arterial blood pressure, central venous pressure, and pulmonary artery pressures. *Postoperative fluid volume status may be difficult to determine without careful pressure measurements. The rate and type of fluids administered are determined by hemodynamic status.*

- Monitor urine output hourly; maintain careful intake and output records. Weigh daily. *Urine output and weight provide additional information about fluid volume status. In addition, renal function may be altered after liver transplant; acute renal failure is a significant risk.* ∞ *See Chapter 28 for more information about acute renal failure and its management.*
- Monitor for signs of active bleeding, including excess drainage, increasing abdominal girth, bloody nasogastric drainage, black tarry stools, tachypnea, tachycardia, diminished peripheral pulses, or pallor. Report immediately. *Altered coagulation in the early postoperative period increases the risk for bleeding. Blood products to replace volume and clotting factors may be necessary.*
- Monitor serum electrolytes and laboratory values related to blood coagulation, liver function, and renal function. Report abnormal results or significant changes immediately. *Electrolyte imbalances are common postoperatively. Altered liver or renal function tests may indicate rejection of the transplanted liver or acute renal failure. Other early signs of transplant rejection include fever, a drop in bile output, or a change in bile color and viscosity.*
- Monitor neurologic status. *With good function of the transplanted organ, mental status should clear within days of the transplant.*
- Provide discharge teaching:
  a. Teach how to reduce risk of infection, and signs of infection to report.
  b. Instruct how to recognize and report signs of organ rejection.
  c. Discuss all medications, including their purpose, schedule, adverse effects, and potential long-term effects. Stress the importance of complying with all prescribed medications and postoperative precautions for the remainder of the patient's life.
  d. Discuss possible changes in body image and psychologic responses to receiving a transplanted organ. Refer to a counselor or support group as indicated.
  e. Refer for home health services for continued assessment and teaching.
  f. Stress importance of continued follow-up with transplant team and primary care provider.

- Weigh daily. Assess for jugular vein distention, measure abdominal girth daily, and check for peripheral edema. Monitor intake and output. *Careful assessment is important to detect fluid shifts.*
- Assess urine specific gravity. *Specific gravity measures the concentration of urine, an indicator of hydration.*

> ### PRACTICE ALERT
> Monitor the patient with cirrhosis for signs of impaired renal function, such as oliguria, a fixed specific gravity of about 1.012, central edema (around the eyes and of the face), and increasing serum creatinine and BUN levels. Such signs may indicate hepatorenal syndrome or acute renal failure from another cause.

- Provide a low-sodium diet (500 to 2000 mg/day) and restrict fluids as ordered. *Excess sodium leads to water retention, and can increase fluid volume, ascites, and portal hypertension.*

Risk for Acute Confusion

Accumulated nitrogenous waste products and other metabolites affect mental status and thought processes. Effects of portal systemic encephalopathy can range from mild confusion to agitation to coma.

- Assess neurologic status, including level of consciousness and mental status. Observe for signs of early encephalopathy: changes in handwriting, speech, and asterixis. *Early identification of evidence of encephalopathy allows prompt intervention—subtle changes in neurologic functioning are important!*

> ### PRACTICE ALERT
> Closely monitor patients who have experienced gastrointestinal bleeding for signs of portal systemic encephalopathy. Blood in the intestinal tract is digested as a protein, increasing serum ammonia levels and the risk for portal systemic encephalopathy.

■ Avoid factors that may precipitate portal systemic encephalopathy. Avoid hepatotoxic medications and CNS depressant drugs. *Cautious use of medications and close monitoring can eliminate iatrogenic causes of encephalopathy.*

■ If possible, plan for consistent nursing care assignments. *Consistent care providers facilitate early identification of subtle neurologic changes indicative of portal systemic encephalopathy.*

■ Administer medications or enemas as ordered to reduce nitrogenous products. Monitor bowel function and provide measures to promote regular elimination and prevent constipation. *Oral or rectally administered (per enema) medications are ordered to reduce intestinal bacteria and the ammonia they produce. Regular bowel elimination promotes protein and ammonia elimination in the feces.*

■ Orient to surroundings, person, and place; provide simple explanations and reassurance. *Modification of verbal interactions to level of understanding and mental status may reduce anxiety and agitation.*

Risk for Bleeding
Impaired coagulation, esophageal varices, and possible acute gastritis place the patient with cirrhosis at significant risk for hemorrhage. Clotting is altered by vitamin K deficiency; impaired manufacture of coagulation Factors II, VII, IX, and X; and increased platelet destruction due to splenomegaly.

■ Monitor vital signs; report tachycardia or hypotension. *Increased pulse and decreasing blood pressure may indicate hypovolemia due to hemorrhage.*

■ Institute bleeding precautions (Box 25–6). *Preventive measures can decrease the risk for active bleeding.*

■ Monitor coagulation studies and platelet count. Report abnormal results. *Coagulation studies help determine the risk for bleeding and the need for treatment.*

■ Carefully monitor the patient who has had bleeding esophageal varices for evidence of rebleeding: hematemesis, hematochezia (bright blood in the stool) or tarry stools, signs of hypovolemia or shock. *Rebleeding is common following variceal hemorrhage, especially within the first week.*

PRACTICE ALERT
Carefully monitor the respiratory status of the patient with a Sengstaken-Blakemore or Minnesota tube. Displacement of the tube can obstruct the airway unless an endotracheal tube is in place. The esophageal balloon prevents the patient from swallowing oral secretions, increasing the risk for aspiration. Keep the head of the bed elevated to 45 degrees to reduce the risk of aspiration and promote gas exchange.

Impaired Skin Integrity
Severe jaundice with bile salt deposits on the skin may cause pruritus. Scratching related to the pruritus damages the skin and impairs its integrity. Malnutrition, particularly protein deficiency, and edema also increase the risk for tissue breakdown and impaired skin integrity.

BOX 25–5 Bleeding Precautions

■ Prevent constipation.
■ Avoid rectal temperatures or enemas.
■ Avoid injections; if needed, use small-gauge needle and apply gentle pressure.
■ Monitor platelet count, PT, and aPPT.
■ Assess for ecchymotic areas and areas of purpura.
■ Apply pressure to bleeding sites. After venipuncture, apply direct pressure for at least 5 minutes.
■ Use only a soft toothbrush.
■ Avoid blowing nose.
■ Assess oral cavity for bleeding gums.

■ Use warm water rather than hot water when bathing. *Hot water increases pruritus.*

■ Use measures to prevent dry skin: Apply an emollient or lubricant as needed to keep skin moist, avoid soap or preparations with alcohol, and do not rub the skin. *Dry skin contributes to pruritus.*

■ If indicated, apply mittens to the hands to prevent scratching. *Patients with encephalopathy may not understand the need to refrain from scratching.*

■ Institute measures to prevent skin and tissue breakdown: Turn at least every 2 hours, use an alternating pressure mattress, and frequently assess skin condition. *Frequent position changes relieve pressure and promote circulation and tissue oxygenation.*

■ Administer prescribed antihistamine (to relieve pruritus) cautiously. *Decreased liver function increases the risk for altered drug responses.*

Imbalanced Nutrition: Less than Body Requirements
The patient with cirrhosis is at risk for malnutrition for a number of reasons: possible chronic alcohol use, anorexia, impaired vitamin and mineral absorption, and impaired protein metabolism. In addition, salt restrictions may make the diet less palatable and appealing to the patient.

■ Weigh daily. Instruct to weigh at least weekly at home. *Weight is a good indicator of both nutritional status and fluid balance. Short-term weight fluctuations tend to reflect fluid balance, while longer term changes in weight are more reflective of nutritional status.*

■ Provide small meals with between-meal snacks. *A small meal is more appealing for an anorexic patient. Between-meal snacks help maintain adequate calorie and nutrient intake.*

■ Unless protein is restricted due to impending portal systemic encephalopathy, promote protein and nutrient intake by providing nutritional supplements such as Ensure or instant breakfasts. *The sodium and protein content of all meals and snacks must be calculated when maintaining restrictions of these nutrients.*

■ Arrange for consultation with a dietitian for diet planning while hospitalized and at home. *The dietitian can provide detailed instructions, sample menus, and suggestions for improving the palatability of the diet and promoting intake.*

CASE STUDY & NURSING CARE PLAN   A Patient with Alcoholic Cirrhosis

Richard Wright is a 48-year-old divorced father of two teenagers. Mr. Wright has been admitted to the community hospital with ascites and malnutrition. He has had three previous hospital stays for cirrhosis, the most recent being 6 months ago.

ASSESSMENT

Mr. Wright is lethargic but responds appropriately to verbal stimuli. He complains of "spitting up blood the past week or so" and says, "I'm just not hungry." He has lost 20 lb (9 kg) since his previous admission. He is jaundiced and has petechiae and ecchymoses on his arms and legs. Liz Mowdi, Mr. Wright's nurse, notes pitting pretibial edema. Abdominal assessment reveals a tight, protuberant abdomen with caput medusae. The liver margin is not palpable; the spleen is enlarged. Vital signs are T 100°F (37.7°C), P 110, R 25, and BP 110/70.

Abnormal laboratory results include WBC 3700/mm³ (normal 4300 to 10,800/mm³); RBC 4.0 million/mm³ (normal 4.6 to 5.9 million/mm³); platelets 75,000/mm³ (normal 150,000 to 350,000/mm³); serum ammonia 105 μm/dL (normal 35 to 65 μm/dL); total bilirubin 4.9 mcg/dL (normal 0.1 to 1.0 mcg/dL); and serum sodium 150 mEq/L (normal 135 to 145 mEq/L). Potassium, hemoglobin, hematocrit, total protein, and albumin levels are markedly decreased. Hepatic enzymes are elevated. Blood urea nitrogen and creatinine levels are marginally elevated. Oxygen saturation (O_2 sat) is 88% (normal range: 96% to 100%) per pulse oximetry.

Endoscopy shows bleeding from gastric ulcer, and the diagnosis of alcoholic cirrhosis with gastritis is made. Mr. Wright is started on Aldactone, 25 mg PO q8h; Riopan, 30 mL 2 h p.c. and hs; lactulose, 30 mL qh until onset of diarrhea, then 15 mL tid; and 800 mg sodium diet; fluid restriction of 1500 mL/day.

DIAGNOSES

- *Impaired Gas Exchange* related to pressure of ascites fluid on the diaphragm as manifested by tachypnea and decreased oxygen saturation
- *Excess Fluid Volume* related to electrolyte imbalance and hypoalbuminemia as manifested by ascites and peripheral edema
- *Imbalanced Nutrition: Less than Body Requirements* related to anorexia and possible alcohol abuse as manifested by weight loss and low serum protein levels
- *Risk for Acute Confusion* related to effects of high ammonia levels as manifested by lethargy
- *Risk for Bleeding* related to impaired platelet formation and portal hypertension

EXPECTED OUTCOMES

- Respiratory rate and O_2 sats will be within normal limits.
- Abdominal girth will decrease by 1 to 2 cm per day; peripheral edema will decrease.
- Will gain 1 lb (0.45 kg) per week without evidence of increased fluid retention. Serum albumin levels will return to normal range.
- Will be alert and oriented; serum ammonia levels are within normal range.
- Will demonstrate no further evidence of active bleeding.
- Will verbalize willingness to join a community support group.

PLANNING AND IMPLEMENTATION

- Weigh daily.
- Provide high-calorie, low-salt, low-protein diet with between-meal snacks.
- Maintain stool chart.
- Assign same nurses to care as much as possible to facilitate evaluation of mental status. Promptly report changes in status or laboratory values.
- Measure abdominal girth every 8 hours, marking level of measurement.
- Institute bleeding precautions.
- Elevate head of bed; assist to chair with legs elevated tid as tolerated.
- Include significant others in care and teaching; refer to community agencies for discharge follow-up.

EVALUATION

A week after admission, Mr. Wright's ascites has decreased and no further active bleeding is noted. His serum protein levels have increased, and his laboratory values are improving. No further bruising is noted during hospitalization. Although he shows a 5-lb weight loss as excess water is eliminated, he is consuming 100% of his diet. His serum ammonia levels have returned to normal. On discharge, O_2 sat is 96%; respirations are 18. Lactulose will be continued on discharge.

Ms. Mowdi provides both written and verbal information about the medication and cirrhosis, including measures to prevent complications. Mr. Wright and his children express interest in Alcoholics Anonymous and Al-Anon and are referred to those agencies. Prior to discharge, follow-up appointments are made with a psychiatric social worker and a primary caregiver.

CRITICAL THINKING IN THE NURSING PROCESS

1. Describe the relationship between portal hypertension, liver dysfunction, and ascites.
2. Outline a 1-day menu for a low-protein, low-sodium, high-calorie diet.
3. What is the pathophysiologic basis for portal systemic encephalopathy? What are the nursing responsibilities related to lactulose and neomycin?
4. Design a nursing care plan for Mr. Wright for the diagnosis *Ineffective Coping.*

See Evaluating Your Response in Appendix C.

Using NANDA, NIC, and NOC

Linkages between a selected NANDA nursing diagnosis, NIC, and NOC for the patient with cirrhosis are shown in the chart that follows.

Community-Based Care

Cirrhosis is a chronic, progressive disease. As such, the patient and family assume major roles in managing the disease and its manifestations and in preventing complications. Teaching topics for home care include the following:

- The absolute necessity of avoiding alcohol and other hepatotoxic drugs. Suggest inpatient or community-based alcohol treatment programs and Alcoholics Anonymous as indicated.
- Diet and fluid intake restrictions and recommendations. Include suggestions to promote nutritional intake and increase the flavor of food when sodium is restricted.
- Prescribed medications, their timing, intended and adverse effects, and manifestations to report to the primary care provider.
- Bleeding precautions (see Box 25–5).

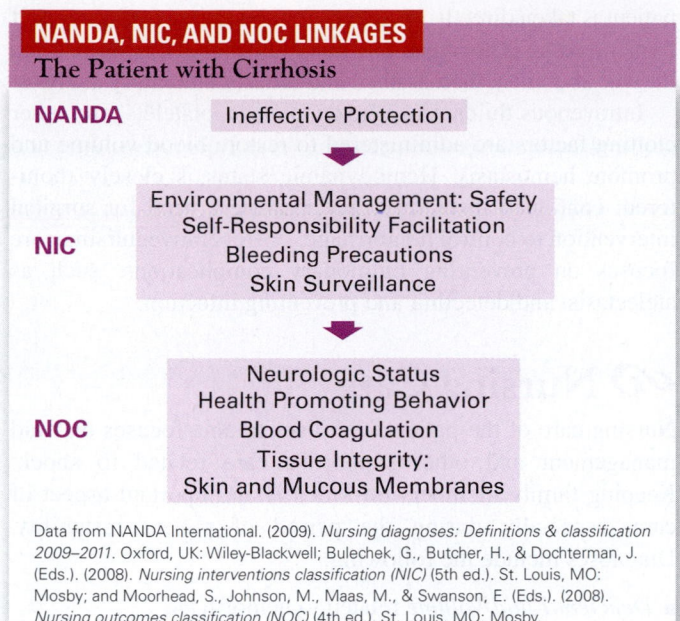

Data from NANDA International. (2009). *Nursing diagnoses: Definitions & classification 2009–2011*. Oxford, UK: Wiley-Blackwell; Bulechek, G., Butcher, H., & Dochterman, J. (Eds.). (2008). *Nursing interventions classification (NIC)* (5th ed.). St. Louis, MO: Mosby; and Moorhead, S., Johnson, M., Maas, M., & Swanson, E. (Eds.). (2008). *Nursing outcomes classification (NOC)* (4th ed.). St. Louis, MO: Mosby.

- Manifestations of potential complications to be reported to the primary care provider. Stress the importance of promptly reporting evidence of gastrointestinal bleeding for prompt intervention for potential hemorrhage.
- Skin care techniques to reduce pruritus and the risk of damage.
- Ways to manage fatigue and conserve energy.

Provide referrals for home health services, dietary consultation, social services, and counseling as needed by the patient and family. Suggest local support groups where available. If appropriate, suggest hospice services for the patient with end-stage liver disease.

The Patient with Cancer of the Liver

Primary liver cancer is uncommon in the United States, accounting for only 0.5% to 2% of all cancers (American Cancer Society [ACS], 2009). It is, however, a common malignancy worldwide. Hepatocellular carcinoma is common in parts of Asia and Africa, where the incidence is as high as 500 cases per 100,000 people. This higher incidence is linked to chronic hepatitis B or C infection. The incidence of primary liver cancer in men is nearly double that in women. The incidence of liver cancer is higher in Hispanics than it is in Black and non-Hispanic Whites; Blacks have a higher incidence than Whites (ACS, 2006; ACS 2007). The prognosis for primary liver cancer is poor, in part because the disease often is advanced at the time of diagnosis. Metastasis to the liver from primary tumors of the lung, breast, and gastrointestinal tract are relatively common.

Pathophysiology

About 80% to 90% of primary hepatic cancers arise from the liver's parenchymal cells (hepatocellular carcinoma); the remainder form in the bile ducts (cholangiocarcinoma). Regardless of the origin, the progress of the disease is similar.

BOX 25–6 Suspected Causes of Primary Liver Cancer

- Chronic hepatitis C infection
- Chronic hepatitis B infection
- Cirrhosis, regardless of type
- Aflatoxin (a toxin produced by *Aspergillus* molds) exposure
- Chronic ethanol consumption
- Nonalcoholic fatty liver (steatohepatitis or NASH)

Several etiologic factors have been identified (Box 25–6). Most primary liver cancer in the United States is related to alcoholic cirrhosis, HBV, or HCV.

The underlying pathophysiology of primary liver cancer is damage to hepatocellular DNA. This damage may be caused by integration of HBV or HCV into the DNA or by repeated cycles of cell necrosis and regeneration that facilitate DNA mutations. HBV and aflatoxins damage a specific tumor suppressor gene, p53. Tumors may be limited to one specific area, may occur as nodules throughout the liver, or may develop as surface infiltrates. The tumor interferes with normal hepatic function, leading to biliary obstruction and jaundice, portal hypertension, and metabolic disruptions (hypoalbuminemia, hypoglycemia, and bleeding disorders). It also may secrete bile products and produce hormones (paraneoplastic syndrome) that may lead to polycythemia, hypoglycemia, and hypercalcemia. Tumors usually grow rapidly and metastasize early.

Manifestations

Initial manifestations of liver cancer develop insidiously and often are masked by the presence of cirrhosis or chronic hepatitis. Weakness, anorexia, weight loss, fatigue, and malaise are common early manifestations. Abdominal pain and a palpable mass in the right upper quadrant are common presenting symptoms. See the following box for manifestations of primary liver cancer. Ascites and jaundice may be present at diagnosis. Signs of liver failure with portal hypertension, splenomegaly, and altered metabolism develop as the tumor progresses.

Interdisciplinary Care

Ultrasound of the liver is used as a screening tool for liver cancer. CT scan with contrast and MRI are used to determine tumor size and extent. A liver biopsy is done to confirm the diagnosis and identify the tumor type or origin. See the box on page 575 for the nursing implications of liver biopsy. Serum alpha-fetoprotein (AFP) levels, normally low in nonpregnant adults, rise in most patients with hepatocellular cancer.

MANIFESTATIONS of Primary Liver Cancer

- Malaise
- Anorexia
- Lethargy
- Weight loss
- Fever of unknown origin
- Jaundice
- Feeling of abdominal fullness
- Painful right upper quadrant mass
- Manifestations of liver failure

Small, localized tumors may be surgically resected, or destroyed using radiofrequency ablation or injection of an agent such as ethanol directly into the tumor. Most tumors, however, have spread extensively or have distant metastasis at the time of diagnosis, so this is frequently not an option. Additionally, patients with underlying liver disease such as cirrhosis may not tolerate loss of additional functional liver tissue. Liver transplantation may be done for stage I or II tumors (no apparent lymph node involvement or distant metastasis). Liver transplantation is limited as a treatment option by the availability of donor organs.

Radiation therapy may be used to shrink the tumor, decreasing pressure on surrounding organs and reducing pain. Chemotherapy may be used as primary treatment for advanced tumors. Direct continuous hepatic arterial infusion with an implanted pump has shown promise in prolonging survival rates. ∞ See Chapter 14 for nursing care for patients receiving radiation therapy or chemotherapy.

ᐳ Nursing Care

Encourage patients with risk factors for primary liver cancer to avoid alcohol and other substances that may further damage the liver. Urge them to discuss regular screening for liver tumors (such as serum AFP levels) with their primary care physician.

Both the patient and the family need extensive nursing support. Controlling pain is a priority. Because of the poor prognosis, early referral for hospice services may be appropriate.

Nursing diagnoses, interventions, and teaching for the patient with liver cancer are similar to those for patients with cirrhosis (see pages 745–749).

The Patient with Liver Trauma

Blunt or penetrating trauma to the abdomen can damage the liver. Liver trauma is frequently seen in combination with injuries to other abdominal organs. Motor vehicle crashes, stab or gunshot wounds, and iatrogenic sources such as liver biopsy are among the causes of these injuries.

Pathophysiology and Manifestations

Liver trauma generally causes bleeding due to the vascularity of the organ. Liver injury may cause a surface hematoma, hematoma within the liver parenchyma, laceration of liver tissue, or disruption of vessels leading to or from the liver. Severe bleeding can rapidly disrupt hemodynamic stability and lead to shock.

> **PRACTICE ALERT**
> Bleeding due to liver trauma may not be immediately apparent. Instruct the patient with apparent or potential liver trauma to immediately report light-headedness, rapid heart rate, shortness of breath, thirst, or increasing abdominal pain.

Interdisciplinary Care

Diagnostic peritoneal lavage is often used along with CT scan to diagnose liver trauma. The procedure is performed by making a small abdominal incision into the peritoneum (after the bladder has been emptied), and inserting a small catheter into the peritoneal cavity. If blood is immediately detected, the patient is taken directly to surgery for abdominal exploration. If frank bleeding is not apparent, a liter of isotonic fluid is instilled into the abdomen, then drained and sent for laboratory analysis.

Intravenous fluids, fresh frozen plasma, platelets, and other clotting factors are administered to restore blood volume and promote hemostasis. Hemodynamic status is closely monitored; continued instability may indicate a need for surgical intervention to control hemorrhage. Postoperative nursing care focuses on preventing pulmonary complications, such as atelectasis, and detecting and preventing infection.

ᐳ Nursing Care

Nursing care of the patient with liver trauma focuses on fluid management and other supportive care related to shock. Keeping family members informed is an important aspect of care, especially during the period of patient instability. Diagnoses include the following:

- *Deficient Fluid Volume* related to hemorrhage
- *Risk for Infection* related to wound or abdominal contamination
- *Risk for Bleeding* related to impaired coagulation

The Patient with Liver Abscess

Liver abscesses usually are bacterial or amoebic (protozoal) in origin. Bacterial abscesses may follow trauma or surgical procedures, including biopsy. Multiple or single abscesses occur most commonly in the right lobe. Amoebic abscesses most frequently occur following infestation of the liver by *Entamoeba histolytica*. Amoebic infestation is associated with poor hygiene, unsafe sexual practices, or travel in areas where drinking water is contaminated.

Pathophysiology and Manifestations

Following bacterial or amoebic invasion of the liver, healthy tissue is destroyed, leaving an area of necrosis, inflammatory exudate, and blood. This damaged region becomes walled off from the healthy liver tissue. Pyogenic (bacterial) liver abscess may be caused by cholangitis, or distant or intra-abdominal infections, such as peritonitis or diverticulitis. *Escherichia coli* is the most frequently identified causative organism. The onset of pyogenic abscess is usually sudden, causing acute symptoms such as fever, malaise, vomiting, hyperbilirubinemia, and pain in the right upper abdomen.

The infection pathway for amoebic hepatic abscesses usually is the portal venous circulation from the right colon. Generally, the onset of amoebic abscess is insidious.

Interdisciplinary Care

Hepatic abscess is diagnosed through biopsy, hepatic aspirate, blood and fecal cultures, and CT scan and ultrasound studies. Therapy is based on identifying the causative organism through laboratory cultures. Pyogenic abscesses are treated with antibiotics to which the causative organism is sensitive.

Pharmacologic agents used for amebic hepatic abscess are the same as those used for intestinal amebic infestation (∞ see Chapter 24); combination therapy is commonly used. Two commonly used drugs for treating amebic liver abscesses are metronidazole (Flagyl) and iodoquinol (Diquinol). Both medications can cause gastrointestinal symptoms. Bone marrow suppression is a risk with metronidazole.

If the abscess does not respond to antibiotic therapy, percutaneous aspiration or surgical drainage may be done. In these procedures, a *percutaneous closed-catheter drain* is placed in the abscess to promote drainage of purulent material.

♋ Nursing Care

A major aspect of nursing care is prevention; teaching patients to avoid contaminated water and foods is especially important. Nursing interventions include teaching hikers to treat water and food handlers to wash hands thoroughly.

Patients who have a liver abscess require supportive care to prevent dehydration from the accompanying fever, nausea, vomiting, and anorexia. Careful monitoring of fluid and electrolyte status is indicated, as are comfort measures for abdominal pain. Possible nursing diagnoses include the following:

- *Risk for Deficient Fluid Volume* related to effects of prolonged fever and vomiting
- *Readiness for Enhanced Knowledge* related to transmission of amebic abscess
- *Activity Intolerance* related to pain and weakness

Exocrine Pancreas Disorders

The pancreas is both an exocrine and an endocrine gland. It is made up of two basic cell types, each having different functions. The exocrine cells produce enzymes that empty through ducts into the small intestine, whereas the endocrine cells produce hormones that enter the bloodstream directly. Disorders of the exocrine pancreas affect the secretion and glandular control of digestive enzymes, whereas disorders of the endocrine pancreas affect the production of hormones necessary for normal carbohydrate, protein, and fat metabolism. Disorders of the exocrine pancreas are discussed in this section of the chapter; diabetes mellitus, a disorder of the endocrine pancreas, is discussed in ∞ Chapter 20.

The Patient with Pancreatitis

Pancreatitis, or inflammation of the pancreas, is characterized by the release of pancreatic enzymes into the tissue of the pancreas itself, leading to hemorrhage and necrosis. Pancreatitis may be either acute or chronic. About 5000 new cases of acute pancreatitis are diagnosed every year in the United States. It is a serious disease, with a mortality rate of approximately 10% (Fauci et al., 2008). Hospitalizations for acute pancreatitis have increased over the past 15 years. Additionally, the incidence of hospitalization for acute pancreatitis is higher in Blacks than it is in Whites (Fagenholz et al., 2007). Alcoholism and gallstones are the primary risk factors for acute pancreatitis, however, the etiology of about 30% of cases is unclear.

The incidence of chronic pancreatitis is less clear because many people with chronic pancreatitis do not have classic manifestations of the disease. Patients with chronic pancreatitis may have long-term effects of the disease, with chronic changes in enzyme and hormone production.

Physiology Review

Knowledge of the normal structure and functions of the exocrine pancreas is important to understand how inflammation affects it and the patient. The exocrine pancreas consists of lobules of acinar cells. The acinar cells secrete digestive enzymes and fluids (pancreatic juices) into ducts that empty into the main pancreatic duct (the duct of Wirsung). The pancreatic duct joins the common bile duct and empties into the

duodenum through the ampulla of Vater (in some people the main pancreatic duct empties directly into the duodenum). The epithelial lining of the pancreatic ducts secretes water and bicarbonate to modify the composition of the pancreatic secretions. Pancreatic enzymes are secreted primarily in an inactive form and are activated in the intestine, a modification that prevents digestion of pancreatic tissue by its own enzymes (Porth & Matfin, 2009). The pancreatic enzymes, with related functions, are as follows:

- Proteolytic enzymes, including trypsin, chymotrypsin, carboxypolypeptidase, ribonuclease, and deoxyribonuclease, which break down dietary proteins
- Pancreatic amylase, which breaks down starch
- Lipase, which breaks down fats into glycerol and fatty acids

Pathophysiology
Acute Pancreatitis

Acute pancreatitis is an inflammatory disorder that involves self-destruction of the pancreas by its own enzymes through autodigestion. The milder form of acute pancreatitis, *interstitial edematous pancreatitis*, leads to inflammation and edema of pancreatic tissue. It often is self-limiting. The more severe form, *necrotizing pancreatitis*, is characterized by inflammation, hemorrhage, and ultimately necrosis of pancreatic tissue.

Acute pancreatitis is more common in middle adults; its incidence is higher in men than in women. Gallstones are the leading cause of acute pancreatitis, with alcohol being the second leading cause (Fauci et al., 2008). Some patients recover completely, others experience recurring attacks, and still others develop chronic pancreatitis. The mortality and symptoms depend on the severity and type of pancreatitis, as well as the patient's age and general health. Organ failure (respiratory failure in particular) is the leading cause of death in acute pancreatitis (Fauci et al., 2008).

Although the exact cause of pancreatitis is not known, the following factors may activate pancreatic enzymes within the pancreas, leading to autodigestion, inflammation, edema, and/or necrosis.

- Gallstones may obstruct the pancreatic duct or cause bile reflux, activating pancreatic enzymes in the pancreatic duct system.

■ Alcohol causes duodenal edema, and may increase pressure and spasm in the sphincter of Oddi, obstructing pancreatic outflow. It also stimulates pancreatic enzyme production, thus raising pressure within the pancreas.

Other factors associated with acute pancreatitis include tissue ischemia or anoxia, trauma or surgery, pancreatic tumors, third-trimester pregnancy, infectious agents (viral, bacterial, or parasitic), elevated calcium levels, and hyperlipidemia. Some medications have been linked with this disorder, including thiazide diuretics, estrogen, steroids, salicylates, and NSAIDs.

Regardless of the precipitating factor, the pathophysiologic process begins with the release of activated pancreatic enzymes into pancreatic tissue. Activated proteolytic enzymes, trypsin in particular, digest pancreatic tissue and activate other enzymes such as phospholipase A, which digests cell membrane phospholipids, and elastase, which digests the elastic tissue of blood vessel walls. This leads to proteolysis, edema, vascular damage and hemorrhage, and necrosis of parenchymal cells. Cellular damage and necrosis release activated enzymes and vasoactive substances that produce vasodilation, increase vascular permeability, and cause edema. A large volume of fluid may shift from circulating blood into the retroperitoneal space, the peripancreatic spaces, and the abdominal cavity.

MANIFESTATIONS Acute pancreatitis develops suddenly, typically with an abrupt onset of continuous severe epigastric and abdominal pain. This pain commonly radiates to the back and is relieved somewhat by sitting up and leaning forward. The pain often is initiated by a fatty meal or excessive alcohol intake.

Other manifestations include nausea and vomiting; abdominal distention and rigidity; decreased bowel sounds; tachycardia; hypotension; elevated temperature; and cold, clammy skin. Within 24 hours, mild jaundice may appear. Retroperitoneal bleeding may occur 3 to 6 days after the onset of acute pancreatitis; signs of bleeding include bruising in the flanks (Turner's sign) or around the umbilicus (Cullen's sign). See the accompanying Manifestations box below.

COMPLICATIONS Systemic complications of acute pancreatitis include intravascular volume depletion with shock, acute tubular necrosis and renal failure (∞ see Chapter 28 for more information about acute renal failure), and acute respiratory distress syndrome (ARDS). Hypovolemic shock and acute renal failure usually develop within 24 hours after the onset of acute pancreatitis. Manifestations of ARDS may be seen 3 to 7 days after its onset, particularly in patients who have experienced severe volume depletion. ∞ See Chapter 38 for more information about ARDS.

Localized complications include pancreatic necrosis, abscess, pseudocysts, and pancreatic ascites. Pancreatic necrosis causes an inflammatory mass that may be infected. It may lead to shock and multiple organ failure. A pancreatic abscess may form late in the course of the disease (6 or more weeks after its onset), causing an epigastric mass and tenderness (McPhee et al., 2008). Pancreatic pseudocysts, encapsulated collections of fluid, may develop both within the pancreas itself and in the abdominal cavity (Figure 25–9 ■). They may impinge on other structures, or may rupture, causing generalized peritonitis. Rupture of a pseudocyst or of the pancreatic duct can lead to pancreatic ascites. Pancreatic ascites is recognized by gradually increasing abdominal girth and persistent elevation of the serum amylase level without abdominal pain.

Chronic Pancreatitis

Chronic pancreatitis is characterized by chronic inflammation, fibrosis, and gradual destruction of functional pancreatic tissue. In contrast to acute pancreatitis, which is reversible, chronic pancreatitis is an irreversible process that eventually leads to pancreatic insufficiency. Alcoholism is the primary risk factor for chronic pancreatitis in the United States. Malnutrition is a major worldwide risk factor. About 10% to 20% of chronic pancreatitis is idiopathic, with no identified cause. A genetic mutation on a gene associated with cystic fibrosis may play a role in these cases. Children or young adults with cystic fibrosis may develop chronic pancreatitis as well.

MANIFESTATIONS of Acute and Chronic Pancreatitis

ACUTE PANCREATITIS
- Abrupt onset of severe epigastric and left upper quadrant pain, may radiate to back
- Nausea, vomiting; fever
- Decreased bowel sounds; abdominal distention and rigidity
- Tachycardia, hypotension; cold, clammy skin
- Possible jaundice
- Positive Turner's sign (flank ecchymosis) or Cullen's sign (periumbilical ecchymosis)

CHRONIC PANCREATITIS
- Recurrent epigastric and LUQ pain, radiates to back
- Anorexia, nausea and vomiting, weight loss
- Flatulence, constipation
- Steatorrhea

Figure 25–9 ■ Acute pancreatitis. Gross clinical specimen of a pancreas affected by acute pancreatitis. Pseudocyst, a pus-filled bleb seen as the yellow area (lower left center), is a potential complication of acute pancreatitis.

In chronic pancreatitis related to alcoholism, pancreatic secretions have an increased concentration of insoluble proteins. These proteins calcify, forming plugs that block pancreatic ducts and the flow of pancreatic juices. This blockage leads to inflammation and fibrosis of pancreatic tissue. In other cases, a stricture or stone may block pancreatic outflow, causing chronic obstructive pancreatitis. In chronic pancreatitis, recurrent episodes of inflammation eventually lead to fibrotic changes in the parenchyma of the pancreas, with loss of exocrine function. This leads to malabsorption from pancreatic insufficiency. If endocrine function is disrupted as well, clinical diabetes mellitus may develop.

MANIFESTATIONS Chronic pancreatitis typically causes recurrent episodes of epigastric and left upper abdominal pain that radiates to the back. This pain may last for days to weeks. As the disease progresses, the interval between episodes of pain becomes shorter. Other manifestations include anorexia, nausea and vomiting, weight loss, flatulence, constipation, and **steatorrhea** (fatty, frothy, foul-smelling stools caused by a decrease in pancreatic enzyme secretion).

COMPLICATIONS Complications of chronic pancreatitis include malabsorption, malnutrition, and possible peptic ulcer disease. Pancreatic pseudocyst or abscess may form, or stricture of the common bile duct may develop. Diabetes mellitus may develop, and there is an increased risk for pancreatic cancer. Opioid addiction related to frequent, severe pain episodes is common.

Interdisciplinary Care

Acute pancreatitis often is a mild, self-limiting disease. Treatment focuses on reducing pancreatic secretions and providing supportive care. Treatment to eliminate the causative factor is begun after the acute inflammatory process resolves. Severe necrotizing pancreatitis may require intensive care management. Treatment for chronic pancreatitis often focuses on managing pain and treating malabsorption and malnutrition.

Diagnosis

The laboratory tests that may be ordered when pancreatitis is suspected are summarized in Table 25–4. Diagnostic studies include the following:

- *Ultrasonography* can identify gallstones, a pancreatic mass, or pseudocyst.
- *Endoscopic ultrasonography* can detect changes indicative of chronic pancreatitis in the pancreatic duct and parenchyma.
- *Contrast-enhanced CT scan* may be ordered to identify pancreatic enlargement, ductal calcifications, fluid collections in or around the pancreas, and perfusion deficits in areas of necrosis.
- *Magnetic resonance cholangiopancreatography (MRCP)* is a noninvasive test that allows visualization of the bile and pancreatic ducts.
- *Endoscopic retrograde cholangiopancreatography (ERCP)* may be performed to diagnose chronic pancreatitis and to differentiate inflammation and fibrosis from carcinoma.
- *Percutaneous fine-needle aspiration biopsy* may be performed to differentiate chronic pancreatitis from cancer of the pancreas; the cells that are aspirated are examined for malignancy.

More information about these tests and their nursing implications can be found in ∞ Chapter 21.

Medications

The treatment of acute pancreatitis is largely supportive. Opioid analgesics such as morphine sulfate or hydromorphone (Dilaudid) are used as needed to control pain. Prophylactic antibiotics are prescribed for patients with severe or necrotizing pancreatitis to prevent infection.

Patients with chronic pancreatitis may also require analgesics, but are closely monitored to prevent drug dependence. Pancreatic enzyme supplements are given to manage abdominal pain and reduce steatorrhea (see the Medication Administration box on page 754). Patients with chronic pancreatitis may need to remain on pancreatic enzyme supplements for life. H_2 blockers such as cimetidine (Tagamet) and ranitidine (Zantac), and proton-pump inhibitors such as omeprazole

TABLE 25–4 Laboratory Tests in Exocrine Pancreatic Disorders

TEST	NORMAL VALUE	SIGNIFICANCE
Serum amylase	30 to 170 units/L	Rises within 2 to 12 hours of onset of acute pancreatitis to two to three times normal. Returns to normal in 3 to 4 days.
Serum lipase	14 to 280 units/L	Levels rise in acute pancreatitis; remain elevated for 7 to 14 days.
Urine amylase	4 to 37 units/L/2h	Urine amylase levels rise in acute pancreatitis.
Serum glucose	70 to 110 mg/dL	May be transient elevation in acute pancreatitis.
Serum bilirubin	0.1 to 1.2 mg/dL	Compression of the common duct may increase bilirubin levels in acute pancreatitis.
Serum alkaline phosphatase (ALP)	42 to 136 units/L	Compression of the common duct may increase levels in acute pancreatitis.
Serum calcium	9 to 11 mg/dL or 4.5 to 5.5 mEq/L	Hypocalcemia develops in up to 25% of patients with acute pancreatitis.
White blood cells	4500/mm^3 to 10,000/mm^3	Leukocytosis indicates inflammation and is usually present in acute pancreatitis.

MEDICATION ADMINISTRATION The Patient with Chronic Pancreatitis

PANCREATIC ENZYME REPLACEMENT

Pancrelipase (Lipancreatin)

Pancrelipase enhances the digestion of starches and fats in the gastrointestinal tract by supplying an exogenous source of the enzymes protease, amylase, and lipase. The drug promotes nutrition and decreases the number of bowel movements.

Nursing Responsibilities
- Assess for allergy to pork protein.
- Monitor frequency and consistency of stools.
- Weigh every other day. Record weights.

- Give with meals; if not enteric coated, H_2 antagonists or antacids may be given concurrently to prevent destruction of the enzymes by hydrochloric acid.
- Monitor for side effects: rash, hives, respiratory difficulty, hematuria, hyperuricemia, or joint pain.

Health Education for the Patient and Family
- Take with meals or snacks.
- If medicine is enteric coated, do not crush, chew, or mix with alkaline foods (e.g., milk, ice cream).
- Be sure to follow prescribed diet.
- Continue taking this drug until or unless advised by physician that it is no longer necessary.

(Prilosec) may be given to neutralize or decrease gastric secretions. Octreotide (Sandostatin), a synthetic hormone, suppresses pancreatic enzyme secretion and may also be used to relieve pain in chronic pancreatitis.

Treatments

NUTRITION Oral food and fluids generally are withheld during acute episodes of pancreatitis to reduce pancreatic secretions and promote rest of the organ. A nasogastric tube may be inserted and connected to suction. Intravenous fluids are administered to maintain vascular volume, and total parenteral nutrition (TPN) is initiated. Oral food and fluids are begun once the serum amylase levels have returned to normal, bowel sounds are present, and pain disappears. A low-fat diet is ordered, and alcohol intake is strictly prohibited.

SURGERY If the pancreatitis is the result of a gallstone lodged in the sphincter of Oddi, an *endoscopic transduodenal sphincterotomy* may be performed to remove the stone. When cholelithiasis is identified as a causative factor, a cholecystectomy is performed once the acute pancreatitis has resolved. Surgical procedures to promote drainage of pancreatic enzymes into the duodenum or resection of all or part of the pancreas may be done to provide pain relief in patients with chronic pancreatitis. Large pancreatic pseudocysts may be drained endoscopically or surgically.

COMPLEMENTARY THERAPIES Several complementary therapies may be used in conjunction with traditional treatments for patients with acute or chronic pancreatitis. Fasting or use of low-salt, low-fat vegetarian diets may reduce episodes of recurrent pain. Qigong, a system of gentle exercise, meditation, and controlled breathing, is believed to balance the flow of qi (a vital life force) through the body. Qigong lowers the metabolic rate, and may reduce the stimulation of pancreatic enzyme secretion. Magnetic field therapy also may be employed for patients with pancreatitis. All complementary therapies should be prescribed by a trained and competent practitioner.

⌀ Nursing Care

In addition to the nursing care discussed in this section, a Case Study & Nursing Care Plan for a patient with acute pancreatitis is found on page 755.

Health Promotion

Teach patients who abuse alcohol about the risk for developing pancreatitis. Advise abstinence to reduce this risk, and refer to an alcohol treatment program or Alcoholics Anonymous.

Assessment

Assessment data related to acute or chronic pancreatitis include the following:

- *Health history:* Current manifestations; abdominal pain (location, nature, onset and duration, identified precipitating factors); anorexia, nausea, or vomiting; flatulence, diarrhea, constipation, or stool changes; recent weight loss; history of previous episodes or gallstones; alcohol use (extent and duration); current medications.
- *Physical assessment:* Vital signs including orthostatic vitals and peripheral pulses; temperature; skin temperature and color, presence of any flank or periumbilical ecchymoses; abdominal assessment including bowel sounds, presence of distention, tenderness, or guarding.

Nursing Diagnoses and Interventions

Nursing care for the patient with acute pancreatitis focuses on managing pain, nutrition, and maintaining fluid balance.

Acute Pain

Obstruction of pancreatic ducts and inflammation, edema, and swelling of the pancreas caused by pancreatic autodigestion cause severe epigastric, left upper abdominal, or midscapular back pain. The pain often is accompanied by nausea and vomiting, abdominal tenderness, and muscle guarding.

- Using a standard pain scale (∞ see Chapter 9), assess pain, including location, radiation, duration, and character. Note nonverbal cues of pain: restlessness or remaining rigidly still; tense facial features; clenched fists; rapid, shallow respirations; tachycardia; and diaphoresis. Administer analgesics on a regular schedule. *Pain assessment before and after analgesic administration measures its effectiveness. Administering analgesics on a regular schedule prevents pain from becoming established, severe, and difficult to control. Unrelieved pain has negative consequences; for example, pain, anxiety, and restlessness may increase pancreatic enzyme secretion.*

CASE STUDY & NURSING CARE PLAN   A Patient with Acute Pancreatitis

Rose Schliefer is a 59-year-old wife, mother of three, and grandmother of four. She has been hospitalized for the past 6 weeks for acute hemorrhagic pancreatitis and pseudocyst. The pancreatitis was caused by gallstones. Mrs. Schliefer spent 3 weeks in intensive care, and then underwent surgery to remove the gallstones and to insert drains into the pseudocyst. Prior to discharge, she had progressed to a soft, high-carbohydrate, low-fat diet; had all drains removed; and was able to walk in the hall. Mrs. Schliefer was referred to a community health agency in her home town for continued follow-up.

ASSESSMENT

Lee Quinn, the community health nurse, assesses Mrs. Schliefer at home after discharge. Mrs. Schliefer is thin and appears anxious and tired. She states that she lost 30 lb (13.6 kg) in the hospital and now weighs only 102 lb (46 kg). She is 66 inches (168 cm) tall. Her vital signs are within normal limits. Mrs. Schliefer has a well-healed upper abdominal scar and two small wounds (from drains) on each side of her abdomen. The wounds are closed but still have scabs. Her skin is cool and dry, and turgor is poor. She is alert and oriented and responds appropriately to questions. Blood glucose levels are normal. Mrs. Schliefer states that her main problems are lack of energy and lack of appetite for the low-fat diet that has been ordered. Mrs. Schliefer's husband and daughters express concern about their ability to provide care. Although they have been taught all about the disease and how to provide care, they still are not sure they know exactly what should be done now that Mrs. Schliefer is at home.

DIAGNOSES

- *Fatigue* related to decreased metabolic energy production
- *Imbalanced Nutrition: Less than Body Requirements* related to prolonged hospitalization, dietary restrictions, and impaired digestion
- *Bathing Self-Care Deficit* (Level II: requires help of another person, supervision, and teaching) related to decreased strength and endurance
- *Risk for Caregiver Role Strain* related to inexperience with caregiving tasks

EXPECTED OUTCOMES

- Set priorities for daily and weekly activities, and incorporate a rest period into daily activity.
- Gain 1 to 2 lbs per week.
- Bathe and maintain personal hygiene without assistance.
- Family members will verbalize comfort with providing necessary care.

PLANNING AND IMPLEMENTATION

- Explain causes of fatigue. Review effects of pancreatitis, surgery, and acute illness on energy levels.

- Develop activity goals, incorporating small, incremental steps toward achieving goals. Mrs. Schliefer indicates that she wants to cook a meal for the whole family. To reach this goal, she will do the following:
  a. Schedule the meal when her energy level is highest.
  b. List actions necessary to prepare the meal and delegate difficult tasks to family members.
  c. Ask daughters to reorganize the kitchen to avoid unnecessary steps.
  d. Plan the meal no sooner than the third week after being home.
- Instruct her to do the following:
  a. Rest in bed each day from 1:00 PM to 3:00 PM.
  b. Eat six small meals a day with family members or friends.
  c. Sit and rest quietly for 15 minutes before eating.
- Discuss dietary restrictions and how to adapt them to usual diet.
- Advise to use shower chair and develop self-care goals for bathing and hygiene in small steps. Add self-care tasks gradually as tolerated.
- Discuss division of responsibilities for physical care, home maintenance, and medical care with family members.
- Encourage family discussion of concerns about future; acknowledge family strengths.

EVALUATION

One month after discharge, Mrs. Schliefer and her family have established new routines based on her energy levels. Mrs. Schliefer now fixes lunch because she feels best during midday. She and her husband share this time together without interruption. Mrs. Schliefer still rests during the day but can now provide self-care. She has gained only 2 lb, but states that she is getting used to the new diet and that "things are even starting to taste good without butter." She also says that sitting quietly before meals is helpful and that she prefers eating six small meals a day. Mr. and Mrs. Schliefer and their daughters agree that their initial worries about Mrs. Schliefer's care have been resolved; now they all know what they must do, and the future looks much brighter.

CRITICAL THINKING IN THE NURSING PROCESS

1. Your patient with acute pancreatitis is also an alcoholic. Describe assessments that indicate the beginnings of withdrawal.
2. Discuss the pathophysiologic basis of hypovolemic shock in acute necrotic pancreatitis.
3. Outline a teaching plan that includes specific foods to omit and to include in a high-carbohydrate, low-protein, low-fat diet.
4. Develop a plan of care for the nursing diagnosis *Impaired Home Maintenance*.

See Evaluating Your Response in Appendix C.

PRACTICE ALERT

Regularly assess respiratory status (at least every 4 to 8 hours), including respiratory rate, depth, and pattern; breath sounds; oxygen saturation; and arterial blood gas results. Report tachypnea, adventitious or absent breath sounds, oxygen saturation levels below 92%, $PaO_2 < 70$ mmHg or $PaCO_2 > 45$ mmHg. Severe abdominal pain causes shallow respirations and hypoventilation, and suppresses cough effectiveness, which can lead to pooling of secretions, atelectasis, and pneumonia.

- Maintain NPO status and nasogastric tube patency as ordered. *Gastric secretions stimulate hormones that stimulate pancreatic secretion, aggravating pain. Eliminating oral intake and maintaining gastric suction reduce gastric secretions. Nasogastric suction also decreases nausea, vomiting, and intestinal distention.*
- Maintain bed rest in a calm, quiet environment. Encourage use of nonpharmacologic pain management techniques such as meditation and guided imagery. *Decreasing physical movement and mental stimulation decreases metabolic rate,*

gastrointestinal secretion, pancreatic secretions, and resulting pain. Adjunctive pain relief measures enhance the effectiveness of analgesics (∞ see Chapter 9).

■ Assist to a comfortable position, such as a side-lying position with knees flexed and head elevated 45 degrees. *Sitting up, leaning forward, or lying in a fetal position tends to decrease pain caused by stretching of the peritoneum by edema and swelling.*

■ Remind family and visitors to avoid bringing food into the patient's room. *The sight or smell of food may stimulate secretory activity of the pancreas through the cephalic phase of digestion.*

Imbalanced Nutrition: Less than Body Requirements

The effects of pancreatitis and its treatment may result in malnutrition. Inflammation increases metabolic demand and frequently causes nausea, vomiting, and diarrhea. At a time of increased metabolic demand, NPO status and gastric suction further decrease available nutrients. In the patient with chronic pancreatitis, loss of digestive enzymes affects the digestion and use of nutrients.

■ Monitor laboratory values: serum albumin, serum transferrin, hemoglobin, and hematocrit. *Serum albumin, serum transferrin (which transports iron in the blood), hemoglobin, and hematocrit levels are decreased in malnutrition. Decreased pancreatic enzymes affect protein catabolism and absorption; decreased transferrin affects iron absorption and transport, thereby decreasing hematocrit and hemoglobin levels.*

■ Weigh daily or every other day. *Short-term weight changes (over hours to days) accurately reflect fluid balance, whereas weight changes over days to weeks reflect nutritional status.*

■ Maintain stool chart; note frequency, color, odor, and consistency of stools. *Protein and fat metabolism are impaired in pancreatitis; undigested fats are excreted in the stool. Steatorrhea indicates impaired digestion and, possibly, an increase in the severity of pancreatitis.*

■ Monitor bowel sounds. *The return of bowel sounds indicates return of peristalsis; nasogastric suction usually is discontinued within 24 to 48 hours thereafter.*

■ Administer prescribed intravenous fluids and/or TPN. *Intravenous fluids are given to maintain hydration. TPN is used to provide fluids, electrolytes, and kilocalories when fasting is prolonged (more than 2 to 3 days).*

■ Provide oral and nasal care every 1 to 2 hours. *Fasting and nasogastric suction increase the risk for mucous membrane irritation and breakdown.*

■ When oral intake resumes, offer small, frequent feedings. Provide oral hygiene before and after meals. *Oral hygiene decreases oral microorganisms that can cause foul odor and taste, decreasing appetite. Small, frequent feedings reduce pancreatic enzyme secretion and are more easily digested and absorbed.*

Risk for Deficient Fluid Volume

Acute pancreatitis can lead to a fluid shift from the intravascular space into the abdominal cavity (third spacing). Third spacing of fluid may cause hypovolemic shock, affecting cardiovascular function, respiratory function, renal function, and mental status.

■ Assess cardiovascular status every 4 hours or as indicated, including vital signs, cardiac rhythm, hemodynamic parameters (central venous and pulmonary artery pressures); peripheral pulses and capillary refill; and skin color, temperature, moisture, and turgor. *These measurements are indicative of fluid volume status and are used to monitor response to treatment. Stable values are as follows: heart rate less than 100; blood pressure within 10 mmHg of baseline; central venous pressure 0 to 8 mmHg; pulmonary wedge pressure 8 to 12 mmHg; cardiac output approximately 5 L/min; and skin warm, dry, with good turgor and color. (∞ See Chapter 11 for a full discussion of hypovolemic shock.)*

■ Monitor renal function. Obtain hourly urine output; report if less than 30 mL per hour. Weigh daily. *Urine output of less than 30 mL per hour indicates decreased renal perfusion or acute renal failure, a major complication of acute pancreatitis. Weight changes are an effective indicator of fluid volume status.*

■ Monitor neurologic function, including mental status, level of consciousness, and behavior. *Hypotension and hypoxemia may decrease cerebral perfusion, causing changes in mental status, decreased level of consciousness, and changes in behavior. In addition, alcohol withdrawal is a risk in the patient with acute pancreatitis.*

Using NANDA, NIC, and NOC

Linkages between a selected NANDA nursing diagnosis, NIC, and NOC for the patient with pancreatitis are shown in the chart that follows.

Community-Based Care

The patient with pancreatitis is often acutely ill and, along with family members, needs information about both hospital procedures and self-care at home following discharge. During the acute stage, keep explanations brief and simple.

Prior to discharge, teach the patient and family about the disease and how to prevent further attacks of inflammation. Include the following topics as appropriate:

■ Alcohol can cause stones to form, blocking pancreatic ducts and the outflow of pancreatic juice. Continued alcohol intake is likely to cause further inflammation and destruction of the pancreas. Avoid alcohol entirely.

NANDA, NIC, AND NOC LINKAGES
The Patient with Pancreatitis

NANDA → Acute/Chronic Pain

NIC → Pain Management
Respiratory Monitoring

NOC → Pain Control
Respiratory Status: Ventilation

Data from NANDA International. (2009). *Nursing diagnoses: Definitions & classification 2009–201.* Oxford, UK: Wiley-Blackwell; Bulechek, G. M., Butcher, H., & Dochterman, J. (Eds.). (2008). *Nursing Interventions Classification (NIC)* (5th ed.). St. Louis, MO: Mosby; and Moorhead, S., Johnson, M., Maas, M., & Swanson, E. (Eds.). (2008). *Nursing Outcomes Classification (NOC)* (4th ed.). St. Louis, MO: Mosby.

- Smoking and stress stimulate the pancreas and should be avoided.
- If pancreatic function has been severely impaired, discuss appropriate use of pancreatic enzymes, including timing, dose, potential side effects, and monitoring of effectiveness.
- A low-fat diet is recommended. Provide a list of high-fat foods to avoid. Crash dieting and binge eating also should be avoided as they may sometimes precipitate attacks. Spicy foods, coffee, tea, or colas, and gas-forming foods stimulate gastric and pancreatic secretions and may precipitate pain. Avoid them if this occurs.
- Report symptoms of infection (fever of 102°F [38.8°C] or more, pain, rapid pulse, malaise) because a pancreatic abscess can develop after initial recovery.

Refer to a dietitian or nutritionist for diet teaching as needed. If appropriate, refer to community agencies, such as Alcoholics Anonymous, or to an alcohol treatment program. Provide referrals to community or home health agencies as needed for continued monitoring and teaching at home.

The Patient with Pancreatic Cancer

Cancer of the pancreas accounts for approximately 3% of all cancers. It is, however, one of the most lethal cancers: The 5-year survival rate is only about 5%. An estimated 42,470 new cases occurred in the United States in 2009, with approximately 35,240 deaths from cancer of the pancreas occurring the same year (American Cancer Society, 2009). The incidence of pancreatic cancer increases after age 50. The incidence is higher in Blacks than in Whites.

> **FAST FACTS**
> Identified risk factors for pancreatic cancer include:
> - Cigarette smoking—the incidence is twice as high in smokers as in nonsmokers
> - Chronic pancreatitis
> - Diabetes mellitus
> - Cirrhosis
> - Obesity, high-fat diet; possibly red meat consumption
> - Genetic predisposition

In contrast to acute and chronic pancreatitis, alcohol abuse and gallstones are not identified risk factors for pancreatic cancer.

Pathophysiology and Manifestations

Most cancers of the pancreas occur in the exocrine pancreas, are adenocarcinomas, and are fatal within 1 to 3 years after diagnosis.

Cancer of the pancreas often causes few symptoms until advanced. Early manifestations are nonspecific, including anorexia, nausea, weight loss, flatulence, and dull epigastric pain. The pain increases in severity as the tumor grows. Other manifestations depend on the location of the tumor. Cancer of the head of the pancreas, which is the most common site, often obstructs bile flow through the common bile duct and the ampulla of Vater, resulting in jaundice, clay-colored stools, dark urine, and pruritus. Cancer of the body of the pancreas presses on the celiac ganglion, causing pain that increases when the person eats or lies supine. Cancer of the tail of the pancreas often causes no symptoms until it has metastasized. Other late manifestations include a palpable abdominal mass and ascites. Because the manifestations are nonspecific, up to 85% of patients with cancer of the pancreas do not seek health care until the cancer becomes too far advanced for a cure.

Interdisciplinary Care

Early cancers of the head of the pancreas may be resectable. A pancreatoduodenectomy (commonly called Whipple's procedure) is performed to remove the head of the pancreas, the entire duodenum, the distal third of the stomach, a portion of the jejunum, and the lower half of the common bile duct. The common bile duct is then sutured to the end of the jejunum, and the remaining pancreas and stomach are sutured to the side of the jejunum (Figure 25–10 ■). Radiation and chemotherapy are often used in addition to surgery.

Postoperative nursing care of the patient undergoing Whipple's procedure is outlined on page 758. Immediate postoperative care is often provided in the intensive care unit.

The patient with pancreatic cancer has multiple problems requiring nursing care. ∞ Chapter 14 provides a discussion of care of the patient with cancer; the nursing diagnoses and interventions discussed for the patient with pancreatitis are also appropriate for the patient with pancreatic cancer.

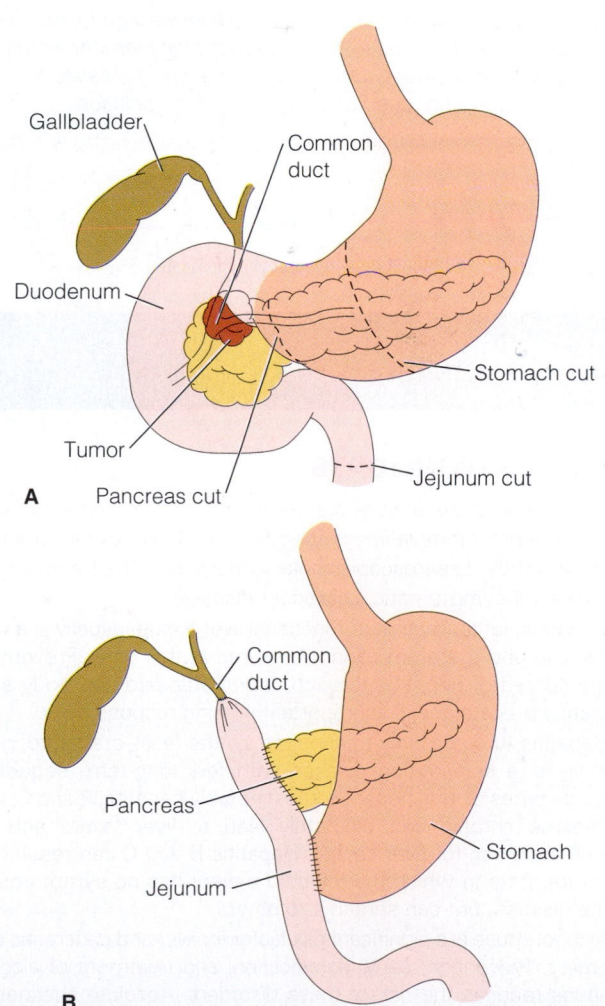

Figure 25–10 ■ Pancreatoduodenectomy (Whipple's procedure): *A*, areas of resection; *B*, appearance following resection.

NURSING CARE OF THE PATIENT   Undergoing Whipple's Procedure

PREOPERATIVE CARE

- Provide routine preoperative nursing care as outlined in ∞ Chapter 4.
- Clarify teaching and learning as needed. Provide psychologic support for patient and family. *The patient and family faced with a diagnosis of pancreatic cancer may require reinforcement of teaching as anxiety, fear, and possible denial can interfere with learning.*

POSTOPERATIVE CARE

- Provide postoperative care as outlined in ∞ Chapter 4.
- Maintain in semi-Fowler's position. *Semi-Fowler's position facilitates lung expansion and reduces stress on the anastomosis and suture line.*
- Maintain low gastrointestinal suction. If drainage is not adequate, obtain an order to irrigate, using minimal pressure. Do not reposition nasogastric tube. *Pressure within the operative area from retained secretions increases intraluminal pressure and places stress on the suture line. Forceful irrigations and repositioning of the nasogastric tube may disrupt the suture line.*
- Maintain pain control using analgesics as prescribed (PCA, infusion, or given on a regular basis). Assess effectiveness of pain management. *Doses higher than normal may be required if narcotic analgesics have been used prior to surgery to manage pain. Increased pain may indicate complications such as disruption of suture line, leakage from anastomosis, or peritonitis. Adequate pain management increases resistance to stress, facilitates healing, and increases the ability to cough, deep breathe, and change position.*

- Assist with coughing, deep breathing, and changing position every 1 to 2 hours. Splint incision during coughing and deep breathing. *The location of the incision makes coughing and deep breathing more painful. The prolonged surgical procedure, anesthesia, location of incision, and immobility increase the risk of retained secretions, atelectasis, and pneumonia. Changing position facilitates drainage of secretions; effective coughing and deep breathing remove secretions and open distal alveoli.*
- Monitor for complications:
  a. Take vital signs every 2 to 4 hours or as indicated; immediately report changes (such as elevated temperature; hypotension; weak, thready pulse; increased or difficult respirations).
  b. Assess skin color, temperature, moisture, and turgor.
  c. Measure urinary output, gastrointestinal output, and drainage from any other tubes; monitor amount and type of wound drainage.
  d. Assess level of consciousness.
  e. Assess abdomen, including contour, bowel sounds, tenderness. Report increasing abdominal pain or signs of acute abdomen (rigid, board-like abdomen).
  f. Monitor results of laboratory tests, especially arterial blood gases, hemoglobin, and hematocrit.

  The major complications following Whipple's procedure are hemorrhage, bile leak, hypovolemic shock, and hepatorenal failure. The assessments listed provide information about the patient's status and alert the nurse to abnormal findings that signal the onset of these complications.

CHAPTER HIGHLIGHTS

- Gallstones (cholelithiasis) are common and often unrecognized until the patient develops manifestations of biliary colic or acute cholecystitis. Laparoscopic cholecystectomy is the treatment of choice for symptomatic gallbladder disease.
- Hepatitis, inflammation of functional liver tissue, usually is a viral disease and therefore cannot be cured at this time. Preventing the spread of hepatitis through use of standard and body substance precautions is an important nursing responsibility.
- Hepatitis A, commonly transmitted via the fecal–oral route, generally is a self-limiting disease with few long-term sequelae. Some types of viral hepatitis, most notably hepatitis B and C, can become chronic and ultimately lead to liver failure and an increased risk for liver cancer. Hepatitis B and C can result in a carrier state in which the infected patient has no symptoms of the disease, but can spread it to others.
- Alcohol abuse is a significant risk factor for liver and pancreatic disorders. Prevention, early identification, and treatment of alcohol abuse reduces the risk of these disorders. Absolute abstinence from alcohol is an important part of the treatment plan for patients with liver and pancreatic disorders.

- Cirrhosis leads to portal hypertension and liver failure, which, in turn, account for most of the manifestations and complications of the disorder. Complications such as ascites, splenomegaly, esophageal varices, and portal systemic encephalopathy affect multiple body systems and significantly contribute to mortality and morbidity associated with cirrhosis.
- Bleeding from esophageal varices may be massive, resulting in a medical emergency and requiring prompt control to maintain cardiac output.
- Acute pancreatitis often develops as a complication of gallstones. Acute pancreatitis often resolves with no long term consequences. Chronic pancreatitis is more frequently related to alcohol abuse and can lead to continuing pain and digestive disruptions.
- All of the accessory organs of digestion (the gallbladder, liver, and pancreas) can be a primary site of malignancy. Cancer of the gallbladder is uncommon; hepatocellular and pancreatic cancer are more common and their incidence is increasing. These cancers often are advanced when diagnosed, reducing treatment options and the chance for cure.

TEST YOURSELF NCLEX-RN® REVIEW

1. When assessing the patient admitted for a laparoscopic cholecystectomy, the nurse would expect to find which of the following?
   1. a history of right upper quadrant pain
   2. obvious jaundice of the sclera and skin
   3. complaints of recurrent heartburn and acid reflux
   4. complaints of chills, fever, nausea, and vomiting

2. Which of the following does the nurse include in her teaching for a patient with acute cholecystitis? **Select all that apply.**
   1. Avoid consumption of foods high in fat such as gravies and peanut butter.
   2. Limit your intake to dry crackers and clear liquids during episodes of acute pain.
   3. A low-carbohydrate diet such as the Atkins diet is recommended for weight loss.
   4. Call your doctor if you develop severe abdominal pain and a temperature.
   5. Surgery for gallstones is optional; they pose little risk when fat intake is minimal.

3. During an outbreak of hepatitis A traced to a food handler at a local restaurant, the nurse teaches staff at the restaurant that the most cost-effective means of protecting customers from further outbreaks is to do which of the following?
   1. insist that all food handlers be immunized against hepatitis A
   2. test all new employees for hepatitis A antigen
   3. wash hands thoroughly before handling food and after using the bathroom
   4. use gloves for handling food if any cuts or scrapes are on hands

4. The nurse would evaluate teaching as effective when a patient with chronic hepatitis C states which of the following?
   1. "I will reduce my alcohol intake and use only acetaminophen for pain relief."
   2. "I understand that I must return to the doctor every year for a follow-up liver biopsy."
   3. "Even though no treatment is available for this disease, I plan to live a long life."
   4. "I will avoid donating blood and will use barrier protection during sex."

5. When evaluating for people possibly exposed to hepatitis A by a recently diagnosed patient, the nurse inquires about which of the following?
   1. sexual partners within the past 6 months
   2. close household contacts within the past 4 weeks
   3. food preparation activities since the development of jaundice
   4. immunization status of the patient

6. A patient hospitalized with cirrhosis, ascites, and mild hepatic encephalopathy suddenly vomits 200 mL of bright red blood. Which of the following should the nurse do first?
   1. Insert a nasogastric tube.
   2. Place in Fowler's position.
   3. Contact the physician.
   4. Check stool for occult blood.

7. The nurse caring for a patient scheduled for an abdominal paracentesis instructs the patient to do which of the following?
   1. avoid eating or drinking fluid for 6 hours prior to the procedure
   2. scrub the abdomen with antiseptic soap before the procedure
   3. empty the bladder before the procedure
   4. report excess flatus following the procedure to the physician

8. A patient hospitalized with severe ascites due to cirrhosis develops a fever and confusion. The nurse should do which of the following?
   1. auscultate bowel sounds and palpate for abdominal tenderness
   2. inquire about headache and check for nuchal rigidity
   3. observe for neck vein distention and auscultate lung sounds
   4. measure abdominal girth and percuss for shifting dullness

9. A 54-year-old woman admitted with acute pancreatitis says, "I don't understand how I got this disease. I thought alcoholics got pancreatitis—I never drink." Which of the following is the most appropriate response by the nurse?
   1. "Was there a time in your life that you did drink heavily?"
   2. "It also is prevalent in smokers; do you smoke cigarettes?"
   3. "Gallstones also are a risk factor. We'll evaluate for them."
   4. "Intravenous drug use is a risk factor. Do you use drugs by injection?"

10. The nurse caring for a patient returning to the unit following Whipple's procedure identifies which of the following as of highest priority in the plan of care?
    1. referral to a smoking cessation program
    2. frequent turning, coughing, and deep breathing exercises
    3. early mobilization including ambulation as tolerated
    4. maintaining patency of the nasogastric tube

See Test Yourself answers in Appendix C.

Pearson Nursing Student Resources

Find additional review materials at
www.nursing.pearsonhighered.com
Prepare for success with additional NCLEX®-style practice questions, interactive assignments and activities, Web links, animations and videos, and more!

BIBLIOGRAPHY

American Cancer Society. (2009). *Cancer facts and figures 2009*. Atlanta, GA: Author.

American Cancer Society. (2007). *Cancer facts & figures for African Americans 2007–2008*. Atlanta, GA: Author.

American Cancer Society. (2006). *Cancer facts & figures for Hispanics/Latinos 2006–2008*. Atlanta, GA: Author.

American College of Physicians. (2008). In the clinic. Hepatitis C. *Annals of Internal Medicine, 3 June 2008*, ITC1-ITC16.

Baltimore, J., & Davidson, J. (2007 March). Caring for a patient with acute cholecystitis. *Nursing2007, 37*(3), 64hn1-64hn2, 64hn4.

Belogia, E., Costa, J., Gareen I., Grem, J., Inadomi, J., Kern, E., et al. (2009). National Institutes of Health Consensus Development Conference Statement: Management of hepatitis B. *Annals of Internal Medicine 2009, 150*, 104–110.

Brenner, Z., & Krenzer, M. (2010, January). Understanding acute pancreatitis. *Nursing, 40*(1), 32-37.

Bulechek, G., Butcher, H., & Dochterman, J. (2008). *Nursing interventions classification (NIC)* (5th ed.). St. Louis, MO: Mosby.

Cainelli, F. (2008). Hepatitis C virus infection in the elderly: Epidemiology, natural history and management. *Drugs Aging 2008, 25*(1), 9–18.

Centers for Disease Control and Prevention. (2009). *Epidemiology and prevention of vaccine-preventable diseases* (11th ed.). (Atkinson, W., Wolfe, S., Hamborski, J., & McIntyre, L., Eds.). Washington, DC: Public Health Foundation.

Centers for Disease Control and Prevention. (2009 May 22). Surveillance for acute viral hepatitis – United States, 2007. *MMWR 2009, 58*(SS-3).

Chi, T. (2008 April). Efficacy of an herbal extract formula on gallbladder conditions. *Nutritional Perspectives: Journal of the Council on Nutrition of the American Chiropractic Association, 31*(2), 4–5, 7–9.

Chronic pancreatitis. (2007 December 1). *American Family Physician, 76*(11), 1679–1688.

Copstead, L. C., & Banasick, J. L. (2010). *Pathophysiology* (4th ed.). St. Louis, MO: Saunders.

Diestag, J. (2008 October 2). Hepatitis B virus infection. *New England Journal of Medicine, 359*(14), 1486–1500.

DiPiro, J., Talbert, R., Yee, G., Matzke, G., Wells, B., & Posey, L. (2008). *Pharmacotherapy: A pathophysiologic approach* (7th ed.). New York, NY: McGraw Hill.

Elwood, D. (2008 December). Cholecystitis. *Surgical Clinics of North America, 88*(6), 1241–1252.

Fagenholz, P., Castillo, C., Harris, N., Pelletier, A., & Camargo, C., Jr. (2007 July). Increasing United States hospital admissions for acute pancreatitis, 1988–2003. *Annals of Epidemiology, 17*(7), 491–197.

Fauci, A., Kasper, D., Braunwald, E., Hauser, S., Longo, D., Jameson, J., et al. (Eds.). (2008). *Harrison's principles of internal medicine* (17th ed.). New York, NY: McGraw-Hill.

Fontaine, K. L. (2005). *Complementary & alternative therapies for nursing* (2nd ed.). Upper Saddle River, NJ: Prentice Hall Health.

Goenka, N., Subramanian, S., Weston, P., & Vora, J. (2007 July–August). Nonalcoholic fatty liver disease: More than 'just a bit of fatty liver.' *Practical Diabetes International, 24*(6), 305–308.

Graham, L. (2009 October 22). Care of patients undergoing laparoscopic cholecystectomy. *Nursing Standard, 23*(7), 41–48.

Lambou-Gianoukos, S., & Heller, S. (2008 December). Lithogenesis and bile metabolism. *Surgical Clinics of North America, 88*(6), 1175–1194.

Lehne, R. (2007). *Pharmacology for nursing care* (6th ed.). St. Louis, MO: Saunders.

Maheshwari, A., Ray, S., & Thuluvath, P. (2008 July 26). Acute hepatitis C. *Lancet, 372*(9635), 321–332.

Marchiondo, K. (2010, January). Acute Pancreatitis. *MEDSURG Nursing, 19*(1), 54-55.

McCance, K. L., & Huether, S. E. (2006). *Pathophysiology: The biologic basis for disease in adults & children* (5th ed.). St. Louis, MO: Mosby.

McPhee, S., Papadakis, M., & Tierney, L. (2008). *Current medical diagnosis & treatment* (47th ed.). New York, NY: Lange Medical Books/McGraw-Hill.

Moorhead, S., Johnson, M., Maas, M., & Swanson, E. (2008). *Nursing outcomes classification (NOC)* (4th ed.). St. Louis, MO: Mosby.

Nair, R., Lawler, L., & Miller, M. (2007 December 1). Chronic pancreatitis. *American Family Physician, 76*(11), 1679–1688.

NANDA International. (2009). *Nursing diagnoses: Definitions & classification 2009–2011*. Oxford, UK: Wiley-Blackwell.

National Center for Complementary and Alternative Medicine, National Institutes of Health. (2008). *Get the facts. CAM and hepatitis C: A focus on herbal supplements*. (NCCAM Pub. No. D422). Retrieved from www.nccam.nih.gov

National Center for Complementary and Alternative Medicine, National Institutes of Health. (2008). *Herbs at a glance. Milk thistle*. Retrieved from www.nccam.nih.gov

National Center for Health Statistics. (2009 April). Deaths: Final data for 2006. *National Vital Statistics Reports, 57*(14).

National Center for Health Statistics. (2009). *Health, United States, 2008, with chartbook*. Hyattsville, MD: Author.

National Institute of Diabetes and Digestive and Kidney Diseases. (2007 Winter). NIDDK explores causes, treatment, and research challenges for acute liver failure. *Digestive Diseases News*, Winter 2007, 1–2, 6.

National Institutes of Health. (2008 October). NIH Consensus Development Conference statement on management of hepatitis B. *NIH Consensus and State-of-the-Science Statement, 25*(2), 1–29.

Poll, R. (2009). Improving awareness of the hepatitis C virus. *Practice Nursing, 20*(3), 131–132.

Porth, C., & Matfin, G. (2009). *Pathophysiology: Concepts of altered health states* (8th ed.). Philadelphia: Lippincott.

Riehl, M. (2007 April). Help your patient cope with pancreatic cancer. *Nursing2007, 37*(4). 54–57.

Ross, S. (2008 September). Milk thistle (silybum marianum): An ancient botanical medicine for modern times. *Holistic Nursing Practice, 22*(5), 299–300.

Rothrock, J. (2007). *Alexander's care of the patient in surgery* (13th ed.). St. Louis, MO: Mosby.

Rustgi, V. (2007). The epidemiology of hepatitis C infection in the United States. *Journal of Gastroenterology 2007, 42*, 513–521.

Sanders, G., & Kingsnorth, A. (2007 August 11). Gallstones. *BMJ: British Medical Journal, 335*(7614), 295–299. See, A., & Irvine, L. (2010). Modern management of acute biliary pancreatitis in pregnancy. *Journal of Obstetrics & Gynaecology, 30*(4), 410–411.

Sun, V., & Sarna, L. (2008 October). Symptom management in hepatocellular carcinoma. *Clinical Journal of Oncology Nursing, 12*(5), 759–766.

Ward, J. (1008 May). Editorial. Time for renewed commitment to viral hepatitis prevention. *American Journal of Public Health, 98*(5), 779–780.

Wilkinson, J., & Ahern, N. (2009). *Nursing diagnosis handbook* (9th ed.). Upper Saddle River, NJ: Prentice Hall Health.

Wolf, D. (2008 August). Encephalopathy, hepatic. *eMedicine Gastroenterology*, August 14, 2008. Retrieved from http://emedicine.medscape.com

Functional Health Pattern: Nutritional-Metabolic

Think about patients with altered gastrointestinal function for whom you have cared in your clinical experiences.

- What were their major medical diagnoses?
- What kinds of manifestations did each of these patients have? Were these signs and symptoms similar or very different?
- How did the patients' manifestations and eating behaviors affect their nutritional status? Were they on a prescribed diet? Did they use dietary supplements? Did they have difficulty chewing or swallowing? Were they gaining or losing weight?
- How did the patients' health status affect their elimination patterns? Had the bowel routine changed recently? If so, how? Did they use laxatives? If so, how often and what type? Did they use any medications that affect bowel movements? Had they had a colonoscopy or other diagnostic tests of the rectum or colon? Did they have an ostomy?

Responses to altered gastrointestinal function commonly affect the nutritional-metabolic and the elimination health patterns. The Nutritional-Metabolic Health Pattern describes the pattern of food and fluid consumption in relation to metabolic need. Nutritional and gastrointestinal disorders affect nutritional status in two primary ways:

- Lack of proper nutrients (e.g., poor eating habits, anorexia or nausea, impaired GI absorption) can lead to nutritional disorders such as malnutrition, reduced energy, and impaired tissue repair and healing.
- Excess intake of nutrients can result in nutritional disorders such as obesity, alcoholic cirrhosis, or cholelithiasis.

The Elimination Health Pattern describes patterns of excretory function, including bowel function and the patient's perception of what is "normal." Bowel elimination can be affected by food and fluid intake, GI disorders, medications, and indirect factors such as perception, psychologic status, and exercise patterns. Bowel disorders affect the elimination pattern in two primary ways:

- Interfering with formation of a formed fecal mass, leading to diarrhea.
- Interfering with bowel transit and defecation, resulting in constipation.

The purposes of the gastrointestinal system are to intake food, break the food into molecules of nutrients, absorb these nutrients into the blood, and finally to excrete solid waste. The nutrients promote growth, maintenance, and repair damaged tissue of the body. Categories of nutrients include proteins, carbohydrates, fats, vitamins, and minerals. Manifestations such as the following affect nutrient intake:

- Nausea (*unpleasant, wave-like sensations in the stomach; feelings of urge or need to vomit*)
- Heartburn (*backflow of gastric contents into esophagus causes high acidity of stomach contents in esophagus resulting in pain and irritation of mucosa lining the esophagus*)
- Pain (*swollen tissue, inflammatory changes cause tissue damage, which stimulates pain receptors that transmit pain impulses to the brain*)

Bowel elimination is the end process of digestion. Nutrients are absorbed during digestion and indigestible materials are eliminated from the body through the gastrointestinal tract. Bowel disorders interrupt normal patterns of elimination, leading to manifestations such as the following:

- Diarrhea (*mucosal inflammation causes plasma, serum protein, blood, and mucus to increase fluidity and bulk of stool, which results in increased rate of propulsion of loose, watery stool*)
- Constipation (*decreased motility, denial of urge to defecate, or decreased fluid intake causes hard, dry stool, which results in difficulty passing stool*)
- Flatus (*excessive amount of air or gas in the intestines causes distention of the intestines with mild to moderate pain, which results in passage of excessive air or gas*)

Priority nursing diagnoses within the Nutritional-Metabolic Health Pattern that may be appropriate for patients with gastrointestinal disorders follow:

- *Imbalanced Nutrition*: *Less than Body Requirements* as evidenced by decreased food intake, weight loss, dry and brittle hair, weakness
- *Deficient Fluid Volume* as evidenced by dry mucous membranes, poor skin turgor, thirst, increased body temperature
- *Impaired Skin Integrity* as evidenced by disruption of skin surface, pain, itching
- *Impaired Tissue Integrity* as evidenced by poor wound healing

Nursing diagnoses from other health patterns often are of high priority for patients with gastrointestinal disorders include the following:

- *Acute Pain* (Cognitive-Perceptual Health Pattern)
- *Nausea* (Cognitive-Perceptual Health Pattern)
- *Fatigue* (Activity-Exercise Health Pattern)

Priority nursing diagnoses within the Elimination Health Pattern that may be appropriate for patients with bowel disorders include the following:

- *Bowel Incontinence* as evidenced by urgency, inability to delay defecation, or fecal staining of clothing.
- *Diarrhea* as evidenced by frequent, large or watery stools, abdominal cramping, and hyperactive bowel sounds.
- *Constipation* as evidenced by difficulty defecating, hard and dry stool, distended abdomen, or excessive flatus.
- *Risk for Impaired Liver Function* as evidenced by excess alcohol intake, exposure to viral hepatitis, or presence of gallstones.

Nursing diagnoses from other functional health patterns may be of high priority for patients with bowel elimination disorders follow:

- *Acute Pain* (Cognitive-Perceptual Health Pattern)
- *Anxiety* (Self-Perception-Self-Concept Health Pattern)
- *Imbalanced Nutrition*: *Less than Body Requirements* (Nutritional-Metabolic Health Pattern)

CLINICAL SCENARIO

Directions: *Read the following clinical scenario and answer the questions that follow. To complete this exercise successfully you will not only use knowledge of the content in this unit, but also principles related to setting priorities and maintaining patient safety.*

You have been assigned to work with the following four patients for the 0700 shift on a medical-surgical unit. Significant data obtained during report is as follows:

- Thomas Jones, aged 56, was admitted with cirrhosis of the liver. He transferred to your unit yesterday after a 3-day stay in ICU for treatment of esophageal varices. Significant history includes daily alcohol consumption (6 to 12-pack of beer or a pint of liquor daily for several years) and history of smoking (2 packs per day for the past 30 years). Current vital signs are T100°F, P 96, R 28, BP 150/90. He complains of abdominal tenderness and dyspnea. Treatment for the bleeding problems has been successful but he appears anxious and irritable.

- Tonya Cooper, aged 21, was admitted yesterday with dehydration, weakness, and fainting. Upon assessment her weight is 90 lbs (40.9 kg) and height is 5'5". Her vital signs are T 97° F, P 70, R 26, BP 90/56 mm Hg with orthostatic BP of 70/48 mm Hg. She has a history of bouts of anorexia nervosa and laxative use for 3 years. She has an IV infusing with 0.9% NaCl with added KCL. She is to be monitored for food intake and watched for one hour after meals. She is ringing her call light to get up to the bathroom.

- Paul Bruner, age 86, was admitted the previous evening with sharp abdominal pain. During the admission assessment, a mass was palpated in his abdomen. His vital signs on admission were temperature 100.4°F, pulse 88, respirations 26, and blood pressure 150/86. He is scheduled for surgery at 10:30 and needs two enemas prior to surgery.

- Grace Freeman is a 36-year-old who had a temporary colostomy placed five days ago due to an abdominal injury from a motor vehicle accident. Vital signs at 0400 were temperature 98.6°F, pulse 78, respirations 14, and blood pressure 112/78. She put on her call light for assistance as her colostomy bag is full and she needs help emptying it.

Question

1. What life style changes did your patients need to make in order to improve their nutritional status? How did you help them identify these changes? How did your assist each patient to meet their elimination needs?

Questions

Priority Setting

1. In what order would you visit these patients after report? What is the rationale for your choice?
   A. _____
   B. _____
   C. _____
   D. _____

Health Promotion

1. Besides nutrition teaching, what other health promotion topics should be discussed with each patient?
   A. _____
   B. _____
   C. _____
   D. _____

2. Teaching appropriate constipation management includes which actions? **Select all that apply.**
   A. Decrease dietary fiber.
   B. Increase fluid intake.
   C. Increase exercise activity.
   D. Use bulk-forming laxatives.
   E. Use enemas daily.

3. When teaching the importance of early detection of malignant tumors, the nurse should include which of the following as the most common initial clinical manifestation of malignant tumors of the lower bowel?
   A. rectal bleeding
   B. diarrhea
   C. rectal pain
   D. constipation

Nursing Process

1. What priority nursing diagnoses would you choose for each of the patients presented previously? Explain the rationale for your choices.

	Nursing Diagnosis	Rationale
Thomas Jones		
Tonya Cooper		
Paul Bruner		
Grace Freeman		

2. When Mr. Jones was admitted to the emergency department, which laboratory studies would you expect to draw? **Select all that apply.**
   A. AST
   B. troponins
   C. ALK
   D. Complete blood cell count
   E. LDH
   F. ADH

3. To prepare Mr. Jones for an esophagoscopy, the nurse institutes which the following interventions?
   A. Explains that it is not a painful procedure but he will be medicated for pain
   B. Keeps the patient NPO for 12 hours prior to the procedure
   C. Inserts a large nasogastric tube and irrigates the stomach to improve visualization
   D. Positions the patient in a supine position with the head slightly hyperextended

4. Write a discharge teaching plan for Mrs. Freeman regarding how to take care of the colostomy at home.

Communication

1. In planning discharge for Ms. Cooper, the family and patient participate in teaching and diet counseling sessions. Which is the priority item for the family and Ms. Cooper to follow after discharge?
   A. Monitor weight regularly to determine further weight loss.
   B. Use rewards for food and caloric intake rather than for weight gain.
   C. Gradually increase the amount of food taken at meals.
   D. Attend support groups for people with eating disorders.

2. If Ms. Cooper says to you, "I don't know why everyone is so concerned about what I do with my life." How will you respond?

3. While giving Mr. Bruner an enema he states, "I'm not sure I need this surgery. If I have cancer I might as well die. It's my daughter who thinks I should do this." How should the nurse respond?

Delegation

1. For each patient, what assessment data and nursing interventions can be delegated to a nursing assistant?

2. What instruction will you give the nursing assistant assisting Ms. Cooper with her meals?

Content-Specific Questions

1. While performing a venipuncture on a patient with hepatitis B, a nurse receives a needle stick. What steps should be taken to provide safety for the nurse?

2. Patients with celiac disease are placed on a gluten-free diet. The patient understands dietary instructions when the patient chooses which meal?
   A. Corned beef sandwich on rye bread
   B. Tossed green salad with oatmeal raisin cookie
   C. Eggs and bacon with whole wheat toast
   D. Tomato soup with cornbread

3. Patients with severe diarrhea may develop metabolic acidosis. Which arterial blood gases indicate metabolic acidosis?
   A. pH 7.45, PCO2 40 mmHg, Bicarbonate 25 mEq/L
   B. pH 7.28, PCO2 30 mmHg, Bicarbonate 19 mEq/L
   C. pH 7.55, PCO2 50 mmHg, Bicarbonate 30 mEq/L
   D. pH 7.33, PCO2 36 mmHg, Bicarbonate 24 mEq/L

4. To prepare a patient for a colonoscopy, the nurse teaches the patient to implement which interventions?
   A. Maintain a liquid diet for 4 days prior to the procedure.
   B. Remain NPO for 4 hours prior to the procedure.
   C. Administer bowel preparation the evening before the procedure.
   D. Administer a cleansing enema the evening before the procedure.

5. When assessing a patient with large bowel obstruction, which clinical manifestations are noted on assessment?
   A. tachycardia and diarrhea
   B. colicky abdominal pain and constipation
   C. severe abdominal cramping and vomiting
   D. dull bowel sounds and nausea

CASE STUDY: Joseph Brown

Joseph Brown, aged 82, has a history of hypertension and angina pectoris for which he takes furosemide, atenolol, and Nitrostat. His son brings him to the hospital after finding him weak, confused, and in need of good hygiene. Mr. Brown feels that he cooked some outdated food that made him ill. He states he has had nausea, vomiting, and diarrhea for the past 2 days. He also states he has not been able to take his medications for the past 2 days and feels that his heart is beating too fast.

Admission assessment shows temperature 101.6°F, pulse 102, respirations 20, and blood pressure 130/70. His height is 5'10" and he weighs 150 lbs. He states that his usual weight is 165 lbs. His skin color is pale. His abdomen is distended, tender to palpation, and has hyperactive bowel sounds. He complains of nausea and a sore rectum from bouts of diarrhea. He appears tired and listless.

Mr. Brown is diagnosed with acute gastroenteritis. In acute gastroenteritis, bacterial or viral infection damages GI mucosa directly or produces exotoxins that inflame and damage the GI mucosa. Intestinal absorption is impaired and water and electrolytes are secreted into the bowel, leading to diarrhea and fluid loss. Manifestations of acute gastroenteritis are nausea, vomiting, anorexia, diarrhea, and abdominal pain. Complications include dehydration, fluid and electrolyte imbalances, acid–base imbalance, and possible hypovolemic shock. Due to Mr. Brown's nausea, diarrhea, and weight loss, the nursing diagnosis of *Imbalanced Nutrition: Less than Body Requirements* is a priority for nursing care.

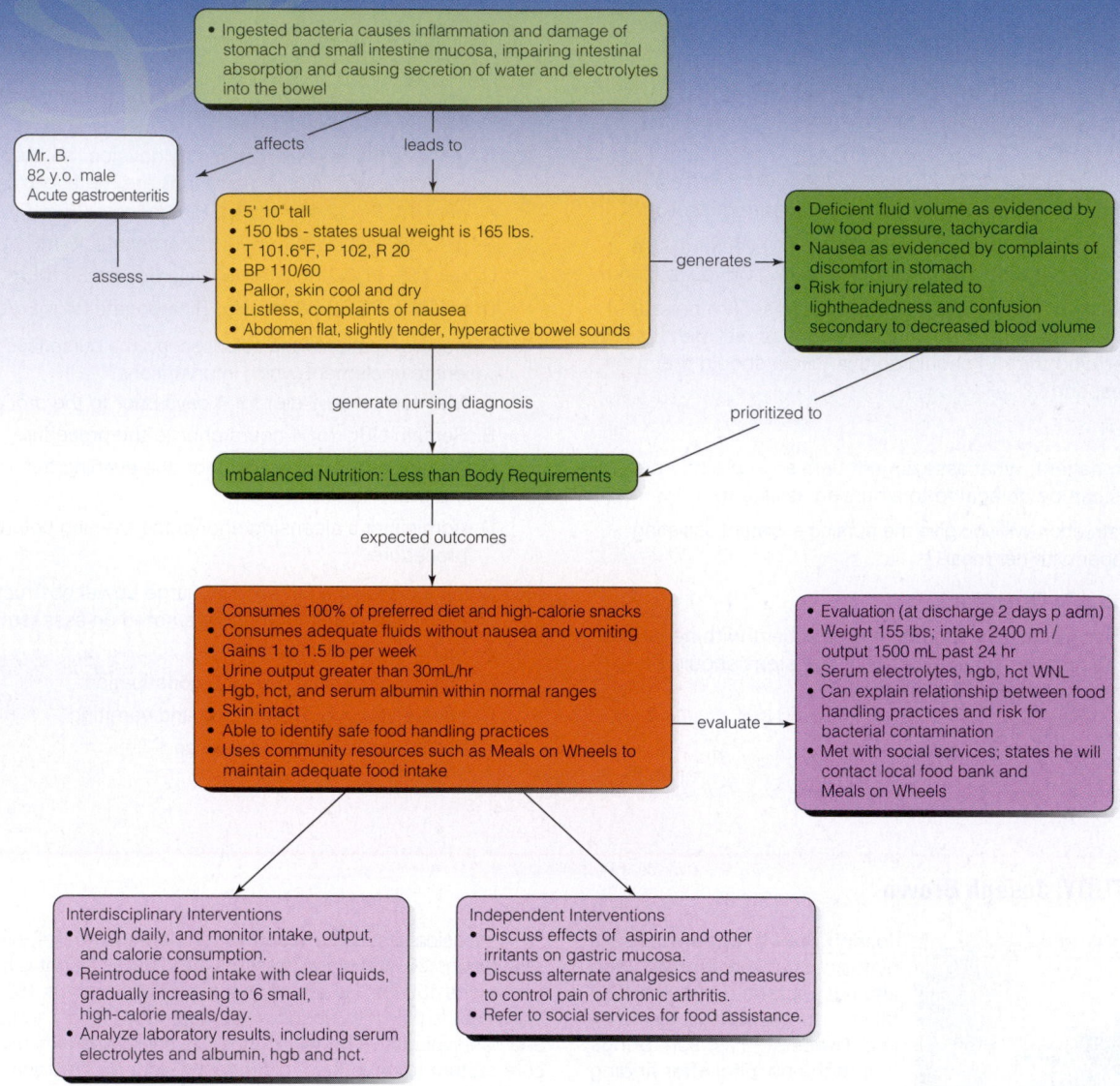

- Ingested bacteria causes inflammation and damage of stomach and small intestine mucosa, impairing intestinal absorption and causing secretion of water and electrolytes into the bowel

Mr. B.
82 y.o. male
Acute gastroenteritis

affects

leads to

assess

- 5' 10" tall
- 150 lbs - states usual weight is 165 lbs.
- T 101.6°F, P 102, R 20
- BP 110/60
- Pallor, skin cool and dry
- Listless, complaints of nausea
- Abdomen flat, slightly tender, hyperactive bowel sounds

generates

- Deficient fluid volume as evidenced by low food pressure, tachycardia
- Nausea as evidenced by complaints of discomfort in stomach
- Risk for injury related to lightheadedness and confusion secondary to decreased blood volume

generate nursing diagnosis

prioritized to

Imbalanced Nutrition: Less than Body Requirements

expected outcomes

- Consumes 100% of preferred diet and high-calorie snacks
- Consumes adequate fluids without nausea and vomiting
- Gains 1 to 1.5 lb per week
- Urine output greater than 30mL/hr
- Hgb, hct, and serum albumin within normal ranges
- Skin intact
- Able to identify safe food handling practices
- Uses community resources such as Meals on Wheels to maintain adequate food intake

evaluate

- Evaluation (at discharge 2 days p adm)
- Weight 155 lbs; intake 2400 ml / output 1500 mL past 24 hr
- Serum electrolytes, hgb, hct WNL
- Can explain relationship between food handling practices and risk for bacterial contamination
- Met with social services; states he will contact local food bank and Meals on Wheels

Interdisciplinary Interventions
- Weigh daily, and monitor intake, output, and calorie consumption.
- Reintroduce food intake with clear liquids, gradually increasing to 6 small, high-calorie meals/day.
- Analyze laboratory results, including serum electrolytes and albumin, hgb and hct.

Independent Interventions
- Discuss effects of aspirin and other irritants on gastric mucosa.
- Discuss alternate analgesics and measures to control pain of chronic arthritis.
- Refer to social services for food assistance.

Activity:

1. After reviewing the case study and concept map, do you agree that *Imbalanced Nutrition: Less than Body Requirements* is the highest priority nursing diagnosis for this patient? Why or why not?

2. Go to the Pearson Nursing Student Resources for this book at www.nursing.pearsonhighered.com to write a concept map using the nursing diagnosis *Deficient Fluid Volume*.

See answers and hints in Appendix C.

Elimination Pattern

PART
III

Functional Health Patterns with Related Nursing Diagnoses

HEALTH PERCEPTION HEALTH MANAGEMENT

- Perceived health status
- Perceived health management
- Health care behaviors: health promotion and illness prevention activities, medical treatments, follow-up care

VALUE-BELIEF

- Values, goals, or beliefs (including spirituality) that guide choices or decisions
- Perceived conflicts in values, beliefs, or expectations that are health related

COPING-STRESS-TOLERANCE

- Capacity to resist challenges to self-integrity
- Methods of handling stress
- Support systems
- Perceived ability to control and manage situations

NUTRITIONAL-METABOLIC

- Daily consumption of food and fluids
- Favorite foods
- Use of dietary supplements
- Skin lesions and ability to heal
- Condition of the integument
- Weight, height, temperature

PART III

Elimination (Urinary) Patterns: Examples of related NANDA Nursing Diagnoses

- Deficient Fluid Volume
- Excess Fluid Volume
- Functional Urinary Incontinence
- Impaired Urinary Elimination
- Overflow Urinary Incontinence
- Reflex urinary Incontinence
- Stress Urinary Incontinence
- Risk for Electrolyte Imbalance
- Risk for Imbalance Fluid Volume
- Risk for Ineffective Renal Perfusion
- Urinary Retention

SEXUALITY-REPRODUCTIVE

- Satisfaction with sexuality or sexual relationships
- Reproductive pattern
- Female menstrual and perimeno-pausal history

ELIMINATION

- Patterns of bowel and urinary excretion
- Perceived regularity or irregularity of elimination
- Use of laxatives or routines
- Changes in time, modes, quality or quantity of excretions
- Use of devices for control

ROLE-RELATIONSHIP

- Perception of major roles, relationships, and responsibilities in current life situation
- Satisfaction with or disturbances in roles and relationships

ACTIVITY-EXERCISE

- Patterns of personally relevant exercise, activity, leisure, and recreation
- ADLs which require energy expenditure
- Factors that interfere with the desired pattern (e.g., illness or injury)

SELF-PERCEPTION– SELF-CONCEPT

- Attitudes about self
- Perceived abilities, worth, self-image, emotions
- Body posture and movement, eye contact, voice and speech patterns

SLEEP-REST

- Patterns of sleep and rest/relaxation in a 24-hr period
- Perceptions of quality and quantity of sleep and rest
- Use of sleep aids and routines

COGNITIVE-PERCEPTUAL

- Adequacy of vision, hearing, taste, touch, smell
- Pain perception and management
- Language, judgment, memory, decisions

Responses to Altered Urinary Elimination

UNIT 7

LEARNING OUTCOMES

1. Describe the anatomy, physiology, and functions of the renal system.
2. Identify specific topics for consideration during a health history interview of the patient with health problems involving the renal system.
3. Describe techniques used to assess the integrity and function of the renal system.
4. Give examples of genetic disorders of the renal system.
5. Describe normal variations in assessment findings for the older adult.
6. Identify abnormal findings that may indicate alterations in urinary elimination.

CLINICAL COMPETENCIES

1. Conduct and document a health history for patients who have or are at risk for alterations in renal function.
2. Conduct and document a physical assessment of the renal system.
3. Monitor the results of diagnostic tests and report abnormal findings.

EQUIPMENT NEEDED

- Urine specimen cup
- Disposable gloves
- Stethoscope

KEY TERMS

dysuria, 777
hematuria, 771

micturition, 773
nocturia, 779

urea, 772

The functions of the renal system (also called the urinary system) are to regulate body fluids, to filter metabolic wastes from the bloodstream, to reabsorb needed substances and water into the bloodstream, and to eliminate metabolic wastes and water as urine. Disorders of the renal system affect the whole body, and may result in alterations in fluid and electrolyte balance, cardiovascular function, and nutritional status. In turn, healthy renal system function depends on the health of other body systems, especially the circulatory, endocrine, and nervous systems.

Anatomy, Physiology, and Functions of the Renal System

The organs of the renal system are the paired kidneys, the paired ureters, the urinary bladder, and the urethra (Figure 26–1 ■). Each structure is essential to the total functioning of the renal system.

The Kidneys

The two kidneys are located outside the peritoneal cavity and on either side of the vertebral column at the levels of T_{12} through L_3. These highly vascular, bean-shaped organs are approximately 4.5 inches (11.4 cm) long and 2.5 inches (6.4 cm) wide. The lateral surface of the kidney is convex; the medial surface is concave and forms a vertical cleft, the hilum. The ureter, renal artery, renal vein, lymphatic vessels, and nerves enter or exit the kidney at the level of the hilum.

Internally, each kidney has three distinct regions: the cortex, medulla, and pelvis. The outer region, or renal cortex, is light in color and has a granular appearance (Figure 26–2 ■). This region of the kidney contains the glomeruli, small clusters of

Figure 26–1 ■ The renal system. *A,* Anterior view of the renal system in a female. *B,* The kidneys are shown in relation to the vertebrae and ribs.

capillaries. The glomeruli bring blood to and carry waste products from the nephrons, the functional units of the kidney.

The renal medulla, just below the cortex, contains cone-shaped tissue masses called renal pyramids, formed almost entirely of bundles of collecting tubules. The collecting tubules that make up the pyramids channel urine into the innermost region, the renal pelvis. The renal pelvis is continuous with the ureter as it leaves the hilum. Branches of the pelvis, the calyces, extend toward the medulla and serve to collect urine and empty it into the pelvis. From the pelvis, urine is channeled through the ureter and into the bladder for storage. The walls of the calyces, the renal pelvis, and the ureter contain smooth muscle that moves urine along by peristalsis.

Formation of Urine

Each kidney contains approximately 1 million nephrons, which process the blood to make urine (Figure 26–3 ■). Each nephron contains a tuft of capillaries called the glomerulus, which is completely surrounded by the glomerular capsule (or Bowman's space). The complex structures of the kidneys process about 180 L (47 gal) of blood-derived fluid each day. Of this amount, only 1% is excreted as urine; the rest is returned to the circulation. (Normal and abnormal findings of urine on laboratory analysis are listed in Table 26–1.) Urine formation is accomplished entirely by the nephron through three processes: glomerular filtration, tubular reabsorption, and tubular secretion (Figure 26–4 ■).

GLOMERULAR FILTRATION   Glomerular filtration is a passive process in which hydrostatic pressure forces fluid and solutes through a membrane. The amount of fluid filtered from the blood into the capsule per minute is called the glomerular filtration rate (GFR). Three factors influence this rate: the total surface area available for filtration, the permeability of the filtration membrane, and the net filtration pressure.

Net filtration pressure is responsible for the formation of filtrate and is determined by two forces: hydrostatic pressure (push) and osmotic pressure (pull). The glomerular hydrostatic pressure pushes water and solutes across the membrane. This pressure is opposed by the osmotic pressure in the glomerulus (primarily the colloid osmotic pressure of plasma proteins in the glomerular blood) and the capsular hydrostatic pressure exerted by fluids within the glomerular capsule. The difference between these forces determines the net filtration pressure, which is directly proportional to the GFR.

Figure 26–2 ■ Internal anatomy of the kidney.

The normal GFR in both kidneys is 120 to 125 mL/min in adults. This rate is held constant under normal conditions by renal autoregulation. The myogenic mechanism, which responds to pressure changes in the renal blood vessels, controls the diameter of the afferent arterioles to achieve autoregulation. An increase in systemic blood pressure causes the renal vessels to constrict, whereas a decrease in blood pressure causes the afferent arterioles to dilate. These changes adjust the glomerular hydrostatic pressure and, indirectly, maintain the GFR.

Another control of the GFR is the result of the renin–angiotensin mechanism at work in the kidneys. The juxtaglomerular apparatus, located in the distal tubules, responds to slow filtrate flow by releasing chemicals that cause intense vasodilation of the afferent arterioles. Conversely, an increase in the flow of filtrate promotes vasoconstriction, decreasing the GFR. A sustained drop in systemic blood pressure triggers the juxtaglomerular cells to release renin. Renin acts on a plasma globulin, angiotensinogen, to release angiotensin I, which is in turn converted to angiotensin II. As a vasoconstrictor, angiotensin II activates vascular smooth muscle throughout the body, causing systemic blood pressure to rise.

Glomerular filtration is also controlled by the sympathetic nervous system (SNS). During periods of extreme stress or emergency, SNS system stimulation constricts the afferent arterioles and inhibits filtrate formation. The SNS also stimulates the juxtaglomerular cells to release renin, increasing systemic blood pressure.

TUBULAR REABSORPTION   Tubular reabsorption is a process that begins as the filtrate enters the proximal tubules. In healthy kidneys, almost all organic nutrients such as glucose

Figure 26–3 ■ The structure of a nephron, showing the glomerulus within the glomerular capsule.

Figure 26–4 ■ Schematic view of the three major mechanisms by which the kidneys adjust to the composition of plasma: *A,* glomerular filtration; *B,* tubular reabsorption; and *C,* tubular secretion.

TABLE 26–1 Normal Results and Abnormal Findings: Urinalysis

CHARACTERISTIC OR COMPONENT	NORMAL RESULTS	ABNORMAL FINDING WITH POSSIBLE CAUSE
Color	Light straw to amber yellow	■ Red, dark, smoky color may be the result of blood in the urine (**hematuria** or menstrual blood). ■ Cloudy urine occurs from infection (pyuria) ■ Colorless urine indicates very dilute urine, such as in overhydration, kidney disease, alcohol ingestion, or diabetes insipidus. ■ Very dark yellow urine indicates dehydration and/or fever. ■ Red or red brown urine may be caused by sulfisoxazole-phenazopyridine (Azo Gantrisin), phenytoin (Dilantin), cascara, chlorpromazine (Thorazine), docusate calcium, and phenolphthalein (Doxidan); and by carrots, rhubarb, and food coloring. ■ Orange urine is caused by fever, urobilin, phenazopyridine (Pyridium), amidopyrine, nitrofurantoin, sulfonamides, carrots, beets, and food coloring. ■ Blue or green urine is caused by *Pseudomonas*, amitriptyline (Elavil), methylene blue, methocarbamol (Robaxin), and yeast concentrate. ■ Brown or black urine is caused by Lysol poisoning, melanin, bilirubin, methemoglobin, porphyrin, cascara, and injectable iron.
Appearance	Clear	■ Hazy or cloudy urine indicates bacteria, pus, RBCs, WBCs, phosphates, prostatic fluid spermatozoa, or urates. ■ Milky urine is the result of fats or pyuria. ■ Yellow foam results from bilirubin, bile, or severe cirrhosis of the liver. ■ A dark yellow to brownish color is seen with deficient fluid volume.
Odor	Aromatic	■ Ammonia smell increases as urine stands outside the body. ■ Urinary tract infection (UTI) causes a foul or unpleasant odor, depending on the causative organism. ■ Asparagus causes a distinctive odor. ■ Mousy odors result from phenylketonuria. ■ Sweet or fruity odors occur in starvation and diabetic ketoacidosis.
pH	4.5–8.0	■ < 4.5: metabolic acidosis, respiratory acidosis, diet high in meat protein, ammonium chloride, and mandelic acid ■ > 8.0: bacteriuria, UTI, antibiotics (neomycin, kanamycin), sulfonamides, sodium bicarbonate, acetazolamide (Diamox), potassium citrate
Specific gravity	1.005–1.030	■ < 1.005: diabetes insipidus, overhydration, renal disease, severe potassium deficit ■ > 1.030: dehydration, fever, diabetes mellitus, vomiting, diarrhea, contrast media
Protein	2–8 mg/dL	■ > 8 mg/dL: proteinuria, exercise, fever, stress, acute infection, kidney disease, lupus erythematosus, leukemia, multiple myeloma, cardiac disease, toxemia of pregnancy, septicemia, lead, mercury, neomycin, barbiturates, sulfonamides
Glucose	Negative	■ > 15 mg/dL or + 4: diabetes mellitus, stroke, Cushing's syndrome, anesthesia, glucose infusions, severe stress, infections, ascorbic acid, aspirin, cephalosporins, and epinephrine
Ketones	Negative	■ + 1 to 3: ketoacidosis, starvation, high-protein diet
RBCs	Rare	■ > 2 per low-power field: kidney trauma, kidney diseases, renal calculi, cystitis, excess aspirin, anticoagulants, sulfonamides, menstrual contamination
WBCs	3–4	■ > 4 per low-power field: UTI, fever, strenuous exercise, kidney diseases
Casts	Occasional hyaline	■ Fever, kidney diseases, heart failure

and amino acids are reabsorbed. However, the tubules constantly regulate and adjust the rate and degree of water and ion reabsorption in response to hormonal signals. Reabsorption may be active or passive. Substances reclaimed through active tubular reabsorption are usually moving against electrical and/or chemical gradients. These substances, including glucose, amino acids, lactate, vitamins, and most ions, require an ATP-dependent carrier to be transported into the interstitial space. In passive tubular reabsorption, which includes diffusion and osmosis, substances move along their gradient without expenditure of energy.

TUBULAR SECRETION   The final process in urine formation is tubular secretion, which is essentially reabsorption in reverse. Substances such as hydrogen and potassium ions, creatinine, ammonia, and organic acids move from the blood of the peritubular capillaries into the tubules themselves as filtrate. Thus, urine consists of both filtered and secreted substances. Tubular secretion is important for disposing of substances not already in the filtrate, such as medications. This process eliminates undesirable substances that have been reabsorbed by passive processes and rids the body of excessive potassium ions. It is also a vital force in the regulation of blood pH.

Maintaining Normal Composition and Volume of Urine

Maintaining the normal composition and volume of urine involves a countercurrent exchange system. In this system, fluid flows in opposite directions through the parallel tubes of the loop of Henle and the vasa recta, tiny capillaries that run along the loop of Henle. Fluid is exchanged across these parallel membranes in response to a concentration gradient (Figure 26–5 ■). When the filtrate enters the proximal convoluted tubule, its osmolality (at 300 mOsm/kg) is essentially the same as that of the plasma and the interstitial fluid of the renal cortex.

Urine is composed, by volume, of about 95% water and 5% solutes. The largest component of urine by weight is **urea** (a nitrogenous waste product formed in the liver from the breakdown of amino acids). Other solutes normally excreted in the urine include sodium, potassium, phosphate, sulfate, creatinine, uric acid, calcium, magnesium, and bicarbonate.

Clearing Waste Products

The kidneys excrete water-soluble waste products and other chemicals or substances from the body. This process is called renal plasma clearance, which refers to the ability of the kidneys to clear (cleanse) a given amount of plasma of a particular substance in a given time (usually 1 minute). The kidneys clear 25 to 30 g of urea each day. They also clear creatinine (an end product of creatine phosphate, found in skeletal muscle), uric acid (a metabolite of nucleic acid metabolism), and ammonia as well as bacterial toxins and water-soluble drugs.

Renal Hormones

Hormones either activated or synthesized by the kidneys include the active form of vitamin D, erythropoietin, and natriuretic hormone.

Vitamin D is necessary for the absorption of calcium and phosphate by the small intestine. In an inactive form, vitamin D enters the body either by dietary intake or through the action of ultraviolet rays on cholesterol in the skin. Activation occurs in two steps, the first in the liver and the second in the kidneys. The renal step is stimulated by parathyroid hormone, which in turn responds to a decreased plasma calcium level. Erythropoietin stimulates the bone marrow to produce red blood cells in response to tissue hypoxia. The stimulus for the production of erythropoietin by the kidneys is decreased oxygen delivery to kidney cells. The right atria of the heart releases natriuretic hormone in response to increased volume and

Figure 26–5 ■ The countercurrent exchange system is responsible for establishing and maintaining an osmotic gradient necessary to the composition, volume, and pH of urine.

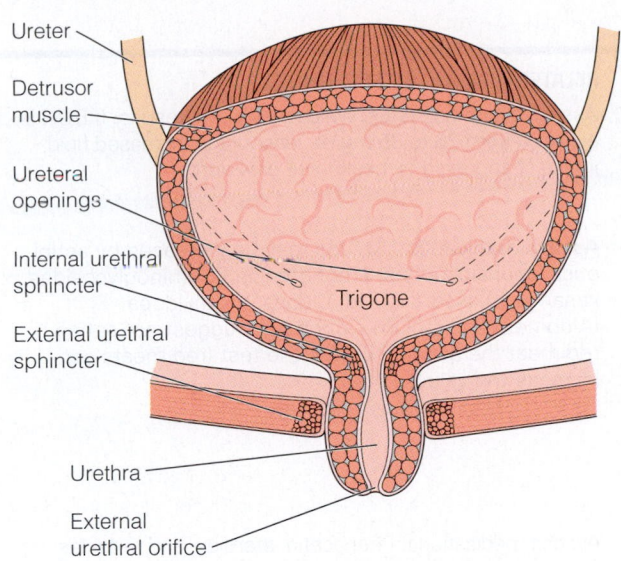

Ureter

Detrusor
muscle

Ureteral
openings

Internal urethral
sphincter

Trigone

External urethral
sphincter

Urethra

External
urethral orifice

Figure 26–6 ■ Internal view of the urinary bladder and trigone.

stretch, as occurs in increased extracellular volume. This hormone inhibits ADH secretion, so that the collecting tubules are less porous and a large amount of dilute urine is produced.

The Ureters, Urinary Bladder, and Urethra

The ureters are bilateral tubes approximately 10 to 12 inches (26 to 30 cm) long. They transport urine from the kidney to the bladder through peristaltic waves originating in the renal pelvis. The wall of the ureter has three layers: an inner epithelial mucosa, a middle layer of smooth muscle, and an outer layer of fibrous connective tissue. The urinary bladder is posterior to the symphysis pubis and serves as a storage site for urine. In males, the bladder lies immediately in front of the rectum; in females, the bladder lies in front of the vagina and the uterus. Openings for the ureters and the urethra are inside the bladder: The trigone is the smooth triangular portion of the base of the bladder outlined by the openings for the ureters and urinary bladder. (See Figure 26–6 ■.)

The size of the bladder varies with the amount of urine it contains. In healthy adults, the bladder holds about 300 to 500 mL of urine before internal pressure rises and signals the need to empty the bladder through **micturition** (also called urination or voiding). However, the bladder can hold more than twice that amount if necessary. The bladder has an internal urethral sphincter that relaxes in response to a full bladder and signals the need to urinate. A second external urethral sphincter is formed by skeletal muscle and is under voluntary control.

The urethra is a thin-walled muscular tube that channels urine to the outside of the body. It extends from the base of the bladder to the external urinary meatus. In females, the urethra is approximately 1.5 inches (3 to 5 cm) long, and the urinary meatus is anterior to the vaginal orifice. In males, the urethra is approximately 8 inches (20 cm) long and serves as a channel for semen as well as urine. The prostate gland encircles the urethra at the base of the bladder in males. The male urinary meatus is located at the end of the glans penis.

Assessing Renal System Function

Renal system function is assessed by findings from diagnostic tests, a health assessment interview to collect subjective data, and a physical assessment to collect objective data.

Diagnostic Tests

The results of diagnostic tests of renal system function are used to support the diagnosis of a specific disease, to provide information to identify or modify the appropriate medication or therapy used to treat the disease, and to help nurses monitor the patient's responses to treatment and nursing care interventions. Diagnostic tests to assess the structures and functions of the renal system are described in the box. More information is included in the discussion of specific disorders in ∞ Chapters 27 and 28.

Regardless of the type of diagnostic test, the nurse is responsible for explaining the procedure and any special preparation needed, assessing for medication use that may affect the outcome of the tests, ensuring the consent form is signed (if necessary), supporting the patient during the examination as necessary, documenting the procedures as appropriate, and monitoring the results of the tests. The nurse is also responsible for postprocedure care and patient teaching for self-care at home.

Genetic Considerations

When conducting a health assessment interview and physical assessment, it is important for the nurse to consider genetic influences on adult health. During the health assessment interview, ask about family members with health problems affecting kidney function, or of family members diagnosed with polycystic disease or diabetes mellitus. During the physical assessment, assess for any manifestations that might indicate a genetic disorder (see Genetic Considerations). If data are found to indicate genetic risk factors or alterations, ask about genetic testing and refer for appropriate genetic counseling and evaluation. ∞ Chapter 8 provides further information about genetics in medical-surgical nursing.

GENETIC CONSIDERATIONS
Examples of Renal System Disorders

- Adult polycystic kidney disease (APKD) is linked to a familial chromosome 16 disorder. The disease is characterized by large cysts in one or both kidneys and a gradual loss of kidney tissue with resultant chronic renal failure.
- Chronic renal failure may be a complication of type 1 and type 2 diabetes mellitus (DM), but is seen more often in patients with type 1 DM. Type 1 and type 2 DM are classified as multifactorial inheritance disorders because both genetic and environmental factors are necessary for onset of the disorder.
- Bladder cancer is the fourth most common type of cancer in men and the ninth most common cancer in women. Genetic factors related to chromosome 9 are interrelated with risk factors such as smoking and exposure to industrial chemicals to cause bladder cancer.

DIAGNOSTIC TESTS of the Renal System

NAME OF TEST	PURPOSE & DESCRIPTION	RELATED NURSING INTERVENTIONS
Blood urea nitrogen (BUN)	This blood test measures urea. Increased levels may result from dehydration, vomiting, diarrhea, digested blood, or prerenal/renal failure. **Normal values:** 5–25 mg/dL	Assess hydration status, which may affect results. If BUN is elevated from 26 to 35 mg/dL, encourage increased fluid intake (if approved by healthcare provider).
Creatinine (serum)	This blood test is used to diagnose kidney dysfunction. Creatinine is a by-product of the breakdown of muscle and is excreted by the kidneys. When 50% or more nephrons are destroyed, serum creatinine levels rise. Normal BUN/creatine ratio is 10:1. Values are not affected by hydration status. **Normal value:** Serum: 0.5–1.5 mg/dL. (Older adults and women may have decreased values due to decreased muscle mass.)	Assess medications; values may be increased by antibiotics (cephalosporins, amphotericin B, aminoglycosides, kanamycin) ascorbic acid, L-dopa, methyldopa (Aldomet), and lithium carbonate. Suggest not eating red meat the evening before the test (red meats can increase the value).
Creatinine clearance	A 24-hour urine test to identify renal dysfunction and to monitor renal function. **Normal value:** 85–135/min Women and older adults may have slightly lower values.	Assess medications: Phenacetin, steroids, and thiazides may decrease creatinine clearance; ascorbic acid, steroids, L-dopa, methyldopa (Aldomet), and cefoxitin may increase creatinine clearance. Levels of creatinine are elevated in hypothyroidism, hypertension, pregnancy, and exercise. Ask the patient to void and discard first voiding. Instruct patient, family, and staff (if hospitalized) to save all urine for a clearly designated 24-hour period, maintaining the specimen in the container on ice or in the refrigerator.
Cystatin C	This blood test may be used as an alternative to creatinine and creatinine clearance to screen for and monitor kidney dysfunction in people suspected of having kidney diseases. Cystatin C is a cysteine proteinase inhibitor that is filtered by the kidneys; increased concentrations in the blood indicate kidney dysfunction. Results of the test are not affected by muscle mass, gender, age or race.	No special preparation is required.
CT scan of kidneys	The CT scan allows evaluation of kidney size, tumors, abscesses, suprarenal masses, and obstructions. A contrast dye may be administered orally or injected IV, allowing increased visualization of the density of renal tissue and masses in comparison to an ultrasound.	Assess the patient for allergies to iodine, x-ray contrast dye, and seafood. Assess medications: Oral hypoglycemic agents are contraindicated for use with iodinated contrast. Ensure that serum creatinine and BUN levels are available. Tell the patient to remain NPO for 4 hours prior to the test, and that laxatives or enemas may be ordered to remove gas or fecal material from the bowel. Posttest, monitor for and tell the patient to report allergic reactions to the dye (rash, itching, headache, vomiting), and to increase fluid intake to help excrete the dye.
Cystometrogram (CMG) (voiding cystogram)	This test is conducted to evaluate bladder capacity and neuromuscular functions of the bladder, urethral pressures, and causes of bladder dysfunction. A measured quantity of fluid is instilled into the bladder, and the filling capacity and voiding pressures are measured. **Normal value:** Urine stream strong and uninterrupted, normal filling pattern and sensation of fullness; bladder capacity: 300–600 mL; urge to void: >150 mL; fullness felt: 300 mL.	Tell patient that the bladder will be filled and during filling he or she will be asked to describe the first urge to void, and the sensation of being unable to delay urination any longer.

DIAGNOSTIC TESTS of the Renal System (continued)

NAME OF TEST	PURPOSE & DESCRIPTION	RELATED NURSING INTERVENTIONS
Cystoscopy (cystogram), cystography	Direct visualization of the bladder wall and urethra is accomplished by using a cystoscope. During the procedure small renal calculi can be removed from the ureter, bladder, or urethra, and tissue biopsy can be done. It also permits determination of the cause of hematuria or UTI. A stent may be inserted during the procedure to facilitate urinary drainage past an obstruction. A retrograde pyelogram may be done during the cystoscopy. By instilling a contrast dye into the bladder (cystography), neurogenic bladder, fistulas, tumors, or ruptures can be identified. The test may be done with either local or general anesthesia.	Assess history of cystitis or prostatitis (these disorders could result in sepsis after the procedure), hypersensitivity to anesthetics, and urinary patterns (amount, color, odor). Take and record vital signs. Following the procedure, assess for complications (hemorrhage, bladder perforation, urinary retention) and report gross hematuria (blood in the urine). Apply heat to the lower abdomen or assist with sitz bath if ordered to relieve pain and muscle spasms. Tell the patient to avoid alcoholic drinks for 2 days, to increase fluid intake, and that a slight burning sensation with voiding may occur for a day or two. Instruct the patient to immediately notify the physician if the urine remains bloody for more than three voidings after the procedure, or if bright bleeding, low urine output, abdominal or flank pain, chills, or fever develops.
GFR, estimated GFR (eGFR)	A measured GFR is considered the most accurate means of detecting changes in kidney function. Because the GFR is a complicated measurement to obtain, an eGFR can be used. The eGFR is calculated based on the serum creatinine, age, gender, and (in some instances) racial origin. The National Kidney Foundation recommends that the eGFR be calculated automatically every time a creatinine test is done. **Normal Value:** 90–120 mL/min	No special preparation is necessary.
Intravenous pyelogram (IVP), retrograde pyelogram	An IVP is a radiologic examination done to visualize the entire renal tract to identify abnormal size, shape, and function of the kidneys or to detect renal calculi (stones), tumors, or cysts. A radiopaque substance is injected IV and a series of x-rays taken. A retrograde pyelogram is a radiologic examination done to evaluate the structures of the ureters and kidney pelvis. It may be performed alone or in conjunction with a cystoscopy.	Schedule IVP prior to any ordered barium test or gallbladder studies using contrast material. Ask about allergy to seafood, iodine, or radiologic contrast dye. Notify physician or radiologist if allergies are known. Assess medications: Oral hypoglycemic agents are contraindicated for use with iodinated contrast. Assess renal and fluid status, including serum osmolality, creatinine, and blood urea nitrogen (BUN) levels. Notify the physician of any abnormal values. Instruct the patient to complete ordered pretest bowel preparation, including prescribed laxative or cathartic the evening before the test, and an enema or suppository the morning of the test. Tell the patient not to eat food for 8 to 12 hours prior to the test; clear liquids are allowed. Take and record vital signs. Instruct the patient to contact the healthcare provider for any delayed reactions to the dye (breathing difficulty, rash, itching, rapid heart beat).
MRI of the kidneys	An MRI is used to visualize the kidneys by assessing computer-generated films of radiofrequency waves and changes in magnetic fields.	Inform patient of need to lie still during the examination. Assess for any metallic implants (such as pacemakers, clips on brain aneurysms, body piercings, tattoos, shrapnel). If present, notify imaging physician. Remove transdermal medication patches (both OTC and prescribed) unless otherwise ordered (FDA, 2009). Replace the patch following the procedure. Tell the patient to inform the staff about the patch when making the appointment and when completing the admission information. Ask if patient is pregnant; if so the test is not performed. Ask about claustrophobia; if this is a problem request the patient to ask for a relaxing medication to take prior to the MRI.
Portable ultrasonic bladder scan	This test is used to obtain information about residual urine. Warmed ultrasound gel is applied over the lower abdomen, and the ultrasound probe is placed just above the pubic bone. The scanner shows an outline of the bladder and displays the amount of urine in the bladder in milliliters. Obtain several readings and use the largest (the most accurate). Print the information, place it on the patient's chart, and document the residual urine amount.	No special preparation is needed, but the test is usually not used for pregnant women. Report a residual amount more than 100 mL.

(continued)

DIAGNOSTIC TESTS of the Renal System (continued)

NAME OF TEST	PURPOSE & DESCRIPTION	RELATED NURSING INTERVENTIONS
Renal arteriogram or angiogram	This radiologic test is done to visualize renal blood vessels to detect renal artery stenosis, renal thrombosis or embolism, tumors, cysts, or aneurysm; to determine the causative factor for hypertension; and to evaluate renal circulation. A contrast medium is injected into the femoral artery.	Assess for allergy to iodine, seafood, or other contrast dye from other x-ray procedures. Assess medications: Oral hypoglycemic agents are contraindicated for use with iodinated contrast; anticoagulants should be discontinued. Instruct the patient to take a laxative or cleansing enema the night before the test (if ordered) and to remain NPO for 8 to 12 hours prior to the test. Take and record vital signs. Ask the patient to void and remove dentures and jewelry before the test. After the test, monitor for bleeding from the femoral artery, restrict activity for a day, assess peripheral pulses, and monitor urine output. Instruct the patient to contact the healthcare provider for any delayed reactions to the dye (such as breathing difficulty, rash, itching, rapid heart beat, decreased urine output).
Renal biopsy	A renal biopsy is performed to determine the cause of renal disease, to rule out cancer metastasis to the kidney, or if rejection is occurring with a kidney transplant. It is performed by using a cystoscope, excising a wedge of kidney tissue, or through the skin with a biopsy needle (percutaneous route).	If a general anesthetic is used, ask the patient not to eat or drink fluids for 8 to 12 hours before the biopsy. Take and record vital signs. Note hemoglobin and hematocrit values and report abnormal findings. After the biopsy, if the percutaneous route was used, apply pressure to the site for about 20 minutes to prevent bleeding. Assess bowel sounds if surgical interventions were used. Tell the patient to increase oral fluid intake and to report decreased urination or burning on urination.
Renal scan	This test is done to evaluate kidney blood flow, location, size, and shape; and to assess kidney perfusion and urine production. Radioactive isotopes are injected IV and radiation detector probes are placed over the kidneys to monitor activity in the kidneys. Radioisotope distribution in the kidneys is scanned and graphed. Nonfunctioning tissue, such as in tumors and cysts, appears as cold spots.	Ask patient to drink several glasses of water prior to the test. Obtain weight and have patient void. After the procedure, increase fluid intake.
Renal ultrasound	This noninvasive test is conducted to detect renal or perirenal masses, identify obstructions, and diagnose renal cysts and solid masses. It is done by applying a conductive gel to the skin and placing a small external ultrasound probe on the patient's skin. Sound waves are recorded on a computer as they are reflected off tissues.	No special preparation is needed.
Residual urine (postvoiding residual urine)	A residual urine test is conducted to measure the amount of urine left in the bladder after voiding. **Normal value:** < 50 mL	Ask the patient to void in a collection device and measure the amount. Immediately after voiding, catheterize using sterile technique and a straight catheter. Drain bladder completely. Document time, amount voided, amount obtained on catheterization, color, clarity, odor, and any other significant data. Report amount of residual urine if it is more than 100 mL.
Urinalysis (UA)	An examination of the constituents of a sample of urine in order to establish a baseline, to provide data for diagnosis, or to monitor results of treatment. Normal findings and abnormal findings with causes are outlined in Table 26–1.	Provide a clean specimen cup for a sample of urine. An early morning specimen is preferred. Note on the laboratory slip if the patient is menstruating (some menstrual blood may be present in the urine sample if so). Assess medications, fluid status, and foods that might affect urinalysis results. Tell the patient to refrigerate the specimen until it can be taken for analysis.

DIAGNOSTIC TESTS of the Renal System (continued)

NAME OF TEST	PURPOSE & DESCRIPTION	RELATED NURSING INTERVENTIONS
Urine culture (midstream, clean-catch)	A culture of a urine sample is conducted to identify the causative organism of a UTI. Normal value: <10,000 organisms/mL (urine is sterile but urethra contains bacteria and a few WBCs) Values of >100,000 organisms/mL indicate UTI	Provide a sterile container for the urine sample. Ask women to separate labia with one hand and clean labia with other hand, using sterile cotton sponges saturated with a cleansing solution, and wiping three times front to back. Ask men to retract the foreskin and cleanse glans with three cotton sponges saturated with a cleansing solution, using a circular motion. After cleaning, tell patient to begin voiding and then collect specimen in the container (initial voiding will contain urethral contaminants). If patient is unable to void, it may be necessary to obtain a specimen by urinary catheterization. Ask the patient to wait to take antibiotics or sulfonamides until after the specimen is taken and to refrigerate the specimen until it can be taken for testing. If the patient is taking antibiotics, it should be listed on the laboratory slip.
Uroflowmetry	This test measures the volume of urine voided per second.	Ask the patient to increase fluid intake and refrain from voiding for several hours before the test to ensure a full bladder and a strong urge to void during testing. Tell the patient he or she will be asked to urinate into a funnel.

Health Assessment Interview

A health assessment interview to determine problems with renal structure and function may be conducted during a health screening, may focus on a chief complaint (such as burning on urination or difficulty starting the stream when urinating), or may be part of a total health assessment. As with alterations in bowel function, patients with problems with renal system function may be embarrassed to talk about renal elimination patterns. It is often helpful to discuss less personal information first.

Assess the patient's current urinary status. Focus questions on changes in patterns of urination, changes in the urine, and pain. Assess changes in patterns of urination by asking the patient the following questions: How many times a day do you urinate? Do you feel that you empty your bladder each time? How many times do you get up at night to urinate? Do you experience a very strong desire to urinate and feel that you just cannot wait? Have you noticed that you urinate small amounts of dark, strong-smelling urine?

Changes in the urine that should be explored include the presence of blood or a cloudy appearance of the urine. If the patient has noticed blood, explore the use of medications (such as anticoagulants or dye-containing drugs) or bleeding problems. Cloudy, foul-smelling urine often indicates infection (pyuria); ask the patient about temperature elevations, chills, and general malaise. Cloudy urine in men may result from retrograde ejaculation (when semen is discharged into the bladder instead of from the penis) during intercourse.

If the patient reports pain (**dysuria**), explore its location, duration, and intensity. Kidney pain is experienced in the back and the costovertebral angle (the angle between the lower ribs and adjacent vertebrae) and may spread toward the umbilicus. Renal colic (pain in response to renal calculi moving through the ureter) is severe, sharp, stabbing, and excruciating; often it is felt in the flank, bladder, urethra, testes, or ovaries. Bladder and urethral pain is usually dull and continuous but may be experienced as spasms. The patient with a distended bladder experiences constant pain increased by any pressure over the bladder.

Information about surgeries or other treatment of previous renal problems is essential to the health history, as is a family history of altered structure or function. A family history of renal problems may be the first clue to abnormalities in the patient's renal function. Explore information regarding family occurrence of end-stage renal disease, renal calculi, and frequent infections as well as related problems such as hypertension and diabetes mellitus.

Questions about lifestyle, diet, and work history should explore cigarette smoking and/or exposure to toxic industrial or environmental chemicals (to identify risks for cancer), usual fluid intake, type of fluid intake, and self-care measures to replace fluids lost during work or physical activity in hot temperatures.

Interview questions categorized by functional health patterns are listed in the box on page 778.

Physical Assessment

The structure and function of the renal system is assessed by examination of the skin, abdomen, kidneys, bladder, and urinary meatus. Guidelines for abdominal assessment are outlined in ∞ Chapter 21. Normal age-related findings for the older adult are summarized in the Nursing Care of the Older Adult box on page 779.

Physical assessment of the renal system may be performed as part of a total health assessment, as part of an abdominal assessment, or as part of the back examination (for the kidneys). The techniques of inspection, auscultation, palpation, and percussion are used.

PRACTICE ALERT
Auscultate immediately after inspection because percussion or palpation may increase bowel motility and interfere with sound transmission during auscultation.

Before beginning the assessment, ask the patient to provide a clean-catch urine specimen (if ordered) and give the patient a specimen cup. Assess the specimen for color, odor, and clarity before you send it to the laboratory.

FUNCTIONAL HEALTH PATTERN INTERVIEW Renal System

Functional Health Pattern	Interview Questions and Leading Statements
Health Perception-Health Management	■ Have you ever had a bladder or kidney disease, injury, or surgery? Describe. ■ If so, how was the problem treated? ■ Describe your usual intake of fluids for a 24-hour period. What type of fluids do you drink? ■ Have you ever smoked? If so, how many cigarettes per day? ■ Describe the problem you are having with your kidneys or bladder. ■ Are you taking medications for this or any other health problem? If so, what do you take and how often? ■ *For women:* Describe how you care for yourself when you urinate (for example, direction of wiping with tissue). ■ If you have a surgical diversion of urine, describe how you care for yourself (what skin and appliance care do you do, how often do you empty the bag?). ■ Do you wear or have you ever worn an external catheter, indwelling catheter, or incontinence briefs? Explain. ■ Have you ever done self-catheterization? If so, why and how often?
Nutritional-Metabolic	■ How much coffee, tea, or alcohol do you drink in a 24-hour period? ■ Have you ever limited your fluid intake? Explain. ■ Do you limit the amount of salt you eat? Explain. ■ Do you have swelling in your ankles? If so, what do you do?
Elimination	■ How many times a day do you urinate? Has there been a change in your usual pattern of urination? ■ Do you experience a sudden urge to urinate? ■ Has there been a change in your urine, such as a change in amount, color, or odor? Have you ever noticed blood in your urine or on the tissue after you wipe? ■ Is it difficult for you to begin or end your flow of urine? ■ Have you ever had problems controlling your urine when you laugh, sneeze, or cough? ■ Do you have any discharge from your urethra? Explain.
Activity-Exercise	■ Do your urinary problems interfere with your activities of daily living? Explain. ■ Describe your usual energy level. Has there been a change? Explain. ■ Have you ever been taught to do Kegel exercises to help you control your urination? If so, how often do you practice these?
Sleep-Rest	■ Does a problem with urination interfere with your ability to sleep and rest? Explain. ■ Has there been a change in the number of times you wake up at night to urinate? Explain.
Cognitive-Perceptual	■ Do you have any pain or burning when you urinate? ■ Have you experienced any tenderness or pain over the lower sides of your back or severe pain that spreads over your lower abdomen? If so, describe its location, intensity, aggravating factors, and duration.
Self-Perception-Self-Concept	■ How does having this condition make you feel about yourself?
Role-Relationships	■ How does having this condition affect your relationships with others?
Sexuality-Reproductive	■ Has this condition interfered with your usual sexual activity?
Coping-Stress-Tolerance	■ Has having this condition created stress for you? ■ Have you experienced any kind of stress that makes this condition worse? Explain. ■ Describe what you do when you feel stressed.
Value-Belief	■ Describe how specific relationships or activities help you cope with this problem. ■ Describe specific cultural beliefs or practices that affect how you care for and feel about this problem. ■ Is there anything interfering with your spiritual beliefs, needs or practices during your illness? What can I or another caregiver do to help you with your spiritual needs? ■ Are there any specific treatments that you would not use to treat this condition?

At the beginning of the assessment, the patient may be sitting or lying supine. Prior to the examination, collect all necessary equipment and explain the techniques to the patient to decrease anxiety. Because the examination involves exposure of the genital area, give the patient a gown and drape the patient appropriately to minimize exposure.

Guidelines for percussion and palpation of the kidneys are outlined in Box 26–1.

Age-Related Renal System Changes

AGE-RELATED CHANGE

Kidneys: ← size of renal cortex and number of nephrons, ← growth of renal tissue, → risk of atherosclerosis, all of which may result in atrophy of the kidneys.

Renal tubules: ← function, with less effective exchange of substances, water and sodium conservation and suppression of ADH secretion in presence of hypoosmolality.

Bladder:
- Muscles weaken and bladder capacity decreases.
- More difficult to empty bladder.
- Delayed micturition reflex.

SIGNIFICANCE

- Decreased renal blood flow.
- Decreased GFR by about 50% between ages 20 and 90.

- Risk of hyponatremia and **nocturia** (voiding more often at night).
- Effects of medications may be altered (with decreased filtration).
- Decreased reabsorption of glucose may result in 1+ proteinuria and glycosuria, which are not of major clinical significance.

- Urinary retention is more common.
- Urinary frequency, urgency, and nocturia are more common with aging.
- Larger amounts of residual urine present after voiding.
- Some stress incontinence may occur, especially in women who have had several children.
- Urinary incontinence is *not* a normal outcome of aging.

BOX 26–1 Guidelines for Physical Assessment of the Kidneys

Percussion of the Kidneys

Percussion of the kidneys helps assess pain or tenderness. Assist the patient to a sitting position, and stand behind the patient. For indirect percussion, place the palm of your nondominant hand over the costovertebral angle (see Figure A). Strike this area with the ulnar surface of your dominant hand, curled into a fist (see Figure B). For direct percussion, also strike the area over the costovertebral angle with the ulnar surface of your dominant hand, curled into a fist. Repeat the technique for the other kidney. You should do percussion of the kidneys with only enough force so the patient feels a gentle thud. Percussion is usually done at the end of the assessment.

Palpation of the Kidneys

Although the technique of palpation of the kidneys is outlined here, this technique is best performed by an advanced practitioner, because it involves deep palpation. In addition, the kidneys are difficult to palpate.

Assist the patient to the supine position and stand at the right side of the patient. To palpate the left kidney, reach across the patient and place your left hand under the patient's left flank with your palm upward. Elevate the left flank with your fingers, displacing the kidney upward. Ask the patient to take a deep breath and use the palmer surface of your right hand to palpate the kidney (Figure C). Repeat the technique for the right kidney.

12th rib

A
Costovertebral angle

C

Renal Assessments

Technique/Normal Findings	Abnormal Findings

Skin Assessment

Inspect the skin and mucous membranes, noting color, turgor, and excretions. *The color of skin and mucous membranes should be even and appropriate to the age and race of the patient; skin should be dry with no visible excretions.*

- Pallor of the skin and mucous membranes may indicate kidney disease with resultant anemia.
- Decreased turgor of the skin may indicate dehydration.
- Edema (generalized or in the lower extremities) may indicate fluid volume excess. (Changes in skin turgor may indicate renal insufficiency with either excess fluid loss or retention.)
- An accumulation of uric acid crystals, called uremic frost, may be seen on the skin of the patient with late-stage renal failure.

Abdominal Assessment

Inspect the abdomen, noting size, symmetry, masses or lumps, swelling, distention, glistening, or skin tightness.

The abdomen should be slightly concave, symmetric, and without distention or masses.

- Enlargements or asymmetry may indicate a hernia or superficial mass.
- If the urinary bladder is distended, it rises above the symphysis pubis as a rounded mass.
- Distention, glistening, or skin tightness may be associated with fluid retention.
- Ascites is an accumulation of fluid in the peritoneal cavity.

Urinary Meatus Assessment

This technique is not part of a routine assessment, but it is an important component in patients with health problems of the renal system.

For the male patient: With the patient in a sitting or standing position, compress the tip of the glans penis with the gloved hand to open the urinary meatus (Figure 26–7 ■).

For the female patient: With the patient in the dorsal lithotomy position, spread the labia with your gloved hand to expose the urinary meatus.

The urinary meatus should be midline and free of redness, lesions, or discharge.

- Increased redness, swelling, or discharge from the urinary meatus may indicate infection or sexually transmitted infection.
- Ulceration of the urinary meatus may indicate a sexually transmitted infection.
- Hypospadias is displacement of the urinary meatus to the ventral surface of the penis.
- Epispadias is displacement of the urinary meatus to the dorsal surface of the penis.

Figure 26–7 ■ Inspecting the urinary meatus of the male.

Kidney Assessment

See Box 26–1 for assessment guidelines for percussion and palpation of the kidneys.

Auscultate the renal arteries by placing the bell of the stethoscope lightly in the areas of the renal arteries, located in the left and right upper abdominal quadrants. *Bruits are not normally heard over the renal arteries.*

Percuss the kidneys for tenderness or pain. *No tenderness or pain should be elicited.*

- Systolic bruits ("whooshing" sounds) may indicate renal artery stenosis.

- Tenderness and pain on percussion of the costovertebral angle suggest glomerulonephritis or glomerulonephrosis.

Technique/Normal Findings	Abnormal Findings
Palpate the kidneys. The lower pole of the right kidney may be palpable with deep palpation; the remaining right kidney and the left kidney are normally not palpable. *If palpable, they should be nontender, bilaterally of appropriate size and density, and without palpable masses.*	■ A mass or lump may indicate a tumor or cyst. ■ Tenderness or pain on palpation may suggest an inflammatory process. ■ A soft kidney that feels spongy may indicate chronic renal disease. ■ Bilaterally enlarged kidneys may suggest polycystic kidney disease. ■ Unequal kidney size may indicate hydronephrosis.
Bladder Assessment Percuss the bladder for tone and position. *The bladder should be midline without dullness.*	■ A dull percussion tone over the bladder of a patient who has just urinated may indicate urinary retention. ■ A distended bladder may be palpated at any point from the symphysis pubis to the umbilicus and is felt as a firm, rounded organ. It indicates urinary retention.

SAMPLE DOCUMENTATION

Assessment of Renal System Function

Home visit made to 66-year-old woman with end-stage chronic kidney failure. Skin pale and oral mucous membranes dry. 4+ edema in ankles and feet. Eyelids swollen. Skin tight and shiny over abdomen and bilateral lower extremities. Abdomen distended and tender on light palpation; further palpation deferred. Urinary bladder not palpable. Urine output for past 24 hours is 15 mL.

TEST YOURSELF NCLEX-RN® REVIEW

1. A nurse is assessing the renal system of an older woman. Which statement by the woman would indicate a health problem?
   1. "I sometimes have to get up at night to urinate."
   2. "When I have to urinate, I really feel an urge to go."
   3. "My doctor told me I have a slight amount of protein in my urine."
   4. "I leak urine all the time."
2. A patient has been vomiting for 4 hours. What hormone is increased as a result?
   1. thyroxine
   2. renin
   3. aldosterone
   4. ADH
3. What diagnostic test can be used to determine GFR as well as glomerular damage?
   1. routine urinalysis
   2. renal scan
   3. creatinine clearance
   4. renal biopsy
4. What gland encircles the male urethra at the base of the bladder?
   1. spleen
   2. pancreas
   3. prostate
   4. adrenal
5. During a health history interview, a patient tells the nurse that she has to get up to void several times a night. This finding is documented as which of the following?
   1. polyuria
   2. nocturia
   3. dysuria
   4. hematuria
6. What question would the nurse ask a patient prior to an IVP?
   1. "Are you allergic to shellfish?"
   2. "Do you have burning on urination?"
   3. "Have you ever had kidney stones?"
   4. "Why are you having this test?"
7. Before beginning the physical assessment of the renal system, the nurse should ask the patient to do which of the following?
   1. empty the bladder
   2. take several deep breaths
   3. provide a urine specimen
   4. drink several glasses of water
8. Following surgery, a patient has not voided for 12 hours. What assessment should the nurse make?
   1. Palpate for bladder distention.
   2. Auscultate for bowel sounds.
   3. Inspect for edema of the urethra.
   4. Percuss for gastric tympany.

9. Which renal system disorder is believed to be the result of genetic and environmental factors?
1. hematuria
2. incontinence
3. kidney infection
4. bladder cancer

10. What assessment would the nurse use to assess hydration status of a patient?
1. auscultation of renal arteries
2. palpation for skin turgor
3. percussion for dullness over bladder
4. palpation of both kidneys

See Test Yourself answers in Appendix C.

Pearson Nursing Student Resources

Find additional review materials at
www.nursing.pearsonhighered.com
Prepare for success with additional NCLEX®-style practice questions, interactive assignments and activities, Web links, animations and videos, and more!

BIBLIOGRAPHY

Armstrong, J., & Mitchell, E. (2008). Comprehensive nursing assessment in the care of older people. *Nursing Older People, (20)*1, 36–40.

Bently, J. (2007). History taking in the Australian outback: Haematuria. *British Journal of Nursing, 16*(4), 231.

Bickley, L., & Szilagyi, P. (2005). *Bates' guide to physical examination and history taking* (9th ed.). Philadelphia: Lippincott.

Dowling-Castronovo, A. (2004). Try this: Best practices in nursing care to older adults from the Hartford Institute for Geriatric Nursing. Urinary incontinence assessment. *Dermatology Nursing, 16*(1), 97–98.

Eliopoulos, C. (2006). *Gerontological nursing* (6th ed.). Philadelphia: Lippincott Williams & Wilkins.

Flasar, C. (2008). What is urine specific gravity? *Nursing, 38*(7), 14.

Holcomb, S. S. (2008a). Acute abdomen: What a pain! *Nursing, 38*(9), 34–40.

Holcomb, S. S. (2008b). Third spacing: When body fluid shifts. *Nursing, 37*(8), 50–53.

Ind, D. (2006). Fluid assessment. *Renal Society of Australian Journal, 2*(3), 51–52.

Johnson, V. (2007). Voiding dysfunction. *Urologic Nursing, 27*(1), 84.

Kee, J. (2009). *Prentice Hall handbook of laboratory & diagnostic tests with nursing implications.* (6th ed.). Upper Saddle River, NJ: Pearson Prentice Hall.

Naish, W., & Haliam, M. (2007). Urinary tract infection: Diagnosis and management. *Nursing Standard, 21*(23), 50–59, 60.

National Institute of Health. (2008). *Genes and Disease: Glands and Hormones.* Available http://www.ncbi.nlm.nih.gov/books/bookres.fegi/gnd/pdf.html

Nursing guidelines for assessment and management of urinary retention in hospitalized older adults. (2007). *Australian Nursing Journal, 15*(2), 22–23.

Palmer, M. (2004). Physiologic and psychologic age-related changes that affect urologic patients. *Urologic Nursing, 24*(4), 247–252, 257.

Perform abdominal assessment, or risk missing life-threatening trauma injury: Don't allow "invisible" injuries to escape detection in your ED. (2004). *ED Nursing, 7*(7), 73–75.

Porth, C. (2007). Essentials of *pathophysiology: Concepts of altered health states* (2nd ed.). Philadelphia: Lippincott. Williams & Wilkins.

Weber, J., & Kelley, J. (2009). *Health assessment in nursing* (4th ed.). Philadelphia: Lippincott Williams & Wilkins.

Wilson, L. A. (2005). Urinalysis. *Nursing Standard, 19*(35), 51–54.

Nursing Care of Patients with Urinary Tract Disorders

LEARNING OUTCOMES

1. Identify populations at risk for common urinary tract disorders and behaviors that increase the risk.
2. Explain the pathophysiology of common urinary tract disorders.
3. Describe the manifestations of urinary tract disorders, relating manifestations to the pathophysiology of the disorder.
4. Discuss the nursing implications of medications and treatments prescribed for patients with urinary tract disorders.
5. Describe invasive and surgical procedures used in treating urinary tract disorders.

CLINICAL COMPETENCIES

1. Assess the functional health status of patients with urinary tract disorders, using data to determine priority nursing diagnoses and select individualized nursing interventions.
2. Identify, report, and document abnormal or unexpected assessments, monitoring patient status.
3. Use evidence-based research to plan and implement nursing care for patients with urinary tract disorders.
4. Integrate the interdisciplinary plan of care into care for patients with urinary tract disorders.
5. Knowledgeably and safely administer prescribed medications and treatments for patients with urinary tract disorders.
6. Provide effective nursing care for patients undergoing invasive procedures or surgery of the urinary tract.
7. Plan and provide appropriate teaching for prevention of and self-care of urinary tract disorders.
8. Evaluate patient responses, revising plan of care as needed to promote, maintain, or restore functional health of patients with urinary tract disorders.

KEY TERMS

cystectomy, 802
cystitis, 785
dysuria, 785
hematuria, 785
hydronephrosis, 794
lithiasis, 792

lithotripsy, 795
neurogenic bladder, 807
nocturia, 785
pyelonephritis, 785
renal colic, 794
ureteral stent, 787

ureteroplasty, 787
urgency, 785
urinary calculi, 792
urinary diversion, 802
urinary incontinence (UI), 809

The urinary system includes the kidneys, ureters, urinary bladder, and urethra. This organ system can be affected by a variety of disorders, including congenital malformations, infections, obstructions, trauma, tumors, and neurologic conditions. Any portion of the system—from the kidney through the urethra—can be affected with serious or even life-threatening consequences unless the problem is appropriately diagnosed and treated. Kidney disorders can affect urine production and waste elimination directly, and are discussed in the next chapter. Disorders of the urinary drainage system (the kidney pelvis, ureters, bladder, and urethra) may obstruct urine flow or spread to the kidneys, affecting urine production and elimination. The anatomy and physiology and nursing assessment related to the urinary tract is presented in ∞ Chapter 26.

When caring for patients with urinary tract disorders, it is important to consider the patient's modesty in voiding, possible difficulty in discussing the genitals, embarrassment about being exposed for examination and testing, and fear of changes in body image or function. These psychosocial issues may interfere with the patient's willingness to seek help, discuss treatment, and learn about preventive measures.

Nursing interventions for patients with urinary tract disorders are directed toward primary prevention, early detection, and management of the disorder through health teaching and nursing care.

The Patient with a Urinary Tract Infection

Bacterial infections of the urinary tract are a common reason for seeking health services, second only to upper respiratory infections. Community acquired urinary tract infections (UTIs) are common in young women, and unusual in men under the age of 50.

Risk Factors for UTI

Patients can be predisposed to UTI by a variety of factors (Box 27–1). Some risk factors cannot be changed (e.g., aging and the short urethra of the female). In women, sexual activity increases the risk for UTI, thought to result from bacteria introduced into the bladder via the urethra during sexual intercourse. Use of spermicidal compounds with a diaphragm, cervical cap, or condom alters the normal bacterial flora of the vagina and perineal tissues and further increases the risk for UTI. Some females lack a normally protective mucosal enzyme and have decreased levels of cervicovaginal antibodies to enterobacteria, further increasing their risk. Prostatic hypertrophy and bacterial prostatitis are risk factors among males. Circumcision appears to have a protective effect. Unprotected anal intercourse also is a risk factor. Congenital or acquired factors contributing to the risk of infection include urinary tract obstruction by tumors or calculi, structural abnormalities such as strictures, impaired bladder innervation, bowel incontinence, and chronic diseases such as diabetes mellitus. Pregnancy increases the risk of UTI and asymptomatic bacteriuria due to hormonal effects, physical compression by the expanding uterus, and pregnancy-related changes in the bladder mucosa (Rahn, 2008).

Instrumentation of the urinary tract (e.g., catheterization or cystoscopy) is a major risk factor for UTI. Even when performed under strict aseptic conditions, catheterization can result in bladder infection. The placement of the catheter prevents the flushing action of voiding, and bacteria may ascend to the bladder either through the catheter lumen or via exudate between the urethral mucosa and the catheter.

Older patients have an increased incidence of UTI. The greatest degree of increase is seen in men, as the ratio of female-to-male UTI in older adults changes from 50:1 to less than 5:1. An increased risk of urinary stasis, chronic disease states (such as diabetes mellitus), and an impaired immune response contribute to the higher incidence of UTI in the older adult. In men, the prostate typically enlarges with aging, potentially resulting in urinary retention as the urethra narrows. Prostatic secretions are lessened, diminishing their protective, antibacterial effect. In older women, loss of tissue elasticity and weakening of perineal muscles often contribute to the development of a cystocele or rectocele. Resulting changes in bladder and urethral position increase the risk of incomplete bladder emptying.

Physiology Review

The urinary tract is normally sterile above the urethra. Adequate urine volume, a free flow from the kidneys through the urinary meatus, and complete bladder emptying are the most important mechanisms maintaining sterility. Pathogens that enter and contaminate the distal urethra are washed out during voiding. Other defenses for maintaining sterile urine include its normal acidity and bacteriostatic properties of the bladder and urethral cells. The peristaltic activity of the ureters and a competent vesicoureteral junction help maintain sterility of the upper urinary tract. As the ureter enters the bladder, its distal portion tunnels between the mucosa and muscle layers of the bladder wall (Figure 27–1 ■). During voiding, increased *intravesicular* (within the bladder) pressure compresses the ureter, preventing *reflux*, or backflow of urine toward the kidneys. In males, a long urethra and the antibacterial effect of zinc in prostatic fluid also help prevent contamination of this normally sterile environment.

BOX 27–1 Risk Factors for UTI

Female
- Short, straight urethra
- Proximity of urinary meatus to vagina and anus
- Sexual intercourse
- Use of diaphragm and spermicidal compounds for birth control
- Pregnancy

Male
- Being uncircumcised
- Prostatic hypertrophy

Both
- Aging
- Urinary tract obstruction
- Neurogenic bladder dysfunction
- Vesicoureteral reflux
- Genetic factors
- Catheterization
- Anal intercourse

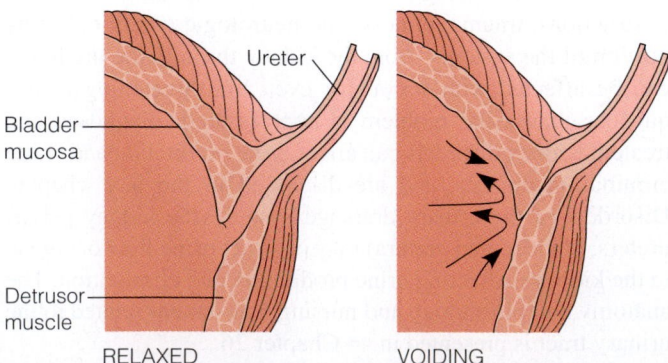

Figure 27–1 ■ A competent vesicoureteral junction. Note how increased intravesicular pressure during voiding occludes the distal portion of the ureter, preventing reflux.

Pathophysiology and Manifestations

Pathogens usually enter the urinary tract by ascending from the mucous membranes of the perineal area into the lower urinary tract. Bacteria that have colonized the urethra, vagina, or perineal tissues are the usual source of infection (Porth & Matfin, 2009). From the bladder, bacteria may continue to ascend the urinary tract, eventually infecting the *parenchyma* (functional tissue) of the kidneys. Hematogenous spread of infection to the urinary tract is rare. Infections introduced in this manner are usually associated with previous damage or scarring of the urinary tract. Bacteria introduced into the urinary tract may cause asymptomatic bacteriuria or an inflammatory response with manifestations of UTI. Asymptomatic bacteriuria is commonly found in pregnant women, the elderly, and patients with diabetes mellitus or who have an indwelling urinary catheter (Lin & Fajardo, 2008).

UTIs can be categorized in several ways. Anatomically, they may affect the lower or the upper urinary tract. Lower urinary tract infections include *urethritis*, inflammation of the urethra; *prostatitis*, inflammation of the prostate gland (discussed in ∞ Chapter 48); and **cystitis**, inflammation of the urinary bladder. The most common upper urinary tract infection is **pyelonephritis**, inflammation of the kidney and renal pelvis. The infection may involve superficial tissues such as the bladder mucosa, or may invade other tissues such as prostate or renal tissues. Epidemiologically, UTIs are identified as community acquired or catheter associated.

Cystitis

Cystitis, inflammation of the urinary bladder, is the most common UTI. The infection tends to remain superficial, involving the bladder mucosa. The mucosa becomes hyperemic (red) and may hemorrhage (Figure 27–2 ■), and the inflammatory response causes pus to form. This process causes the classic manifestations associated with cystitis. Typical presenting symptoms of cystitis include **dysuria** (painful or difficult urination), urinary frequency and **urgency** (a sudden, compelling need to urinate), and **nocturia** (voiding two or more times at night). In addition, the urine may have a foul odor and appear cloudy (*pyuria*) or bloody (**hematuria**) because of mucus, excess white cells in the urine, and bleeding of the inflamed bladder wall. Suprapubic pain and tenderness also may be present. See the following box for manifestations of cystitis.

Cystitis in adult females usually results from colonization of the bladder by bacteria normally found in the lower gastrointestinal tract. These bacteria gain entry by ascending the short, straight female urethra. In addition to the risk factors listed on page 784, personal hygiene practices and voluntary urinary retention can contribute to the risk for UTI in women.

Older patients may not experience the classic symptoms of cystitis. Instead, they often present with nonspecific manifestations such as nocturia, incontinence, confusion, behavior change, lethargy, anorexia, or "just not feeling right." Fever may be present; however, hypothermia also may develop in an older adult.

Although the bacteriostatic effect of prostatic fluid and a longer urethra provide an effective barrier to bladder infection for adult males, in elderly men an enlarged prostate can impede urine flow, leading to incomplete bladder emptying and urinary stasis. Bacteria are not completely flushed with voiding, allowing colonization of the bladder.

Cystitis is usually uncomplicated and readily responds to treatment. When left untreated, the infection can ascend to involve the kidneys. Severe or prolonged infection may lead to sloughing of bladder mucosa and ulcer formation. Chronic cystitis can lead to bladder stones (discussed later in this chapter).

Catheter-Associated UTI

At least 10% to 15% of hospitalized patients with indwelling urinary catheters develop bacteriuria. The longer the catheter remains in place, the greater the risk for infection. Bacteria, including *E. coli*, *Proteus*, *Pseudomonas*, and *Klebsiella*, reach the bladder by either migrating through the column of urine within the catheter or by moving up the mucous sheath of the urethra outside the catheter. Bacteria enter the catheter system at the connection between the catheter and drainage system or through the emptying tube of the drainage bag. Colonization of perineal skin by bowel flora is a common source of infection in catheterized women. Causative organisms associated with catheter-associated UTI are more likely to demonstrate antibiotic resistance than those found in community-acquired UTI (Fauci et al., 2008).

Catheter-associated UTIs often are asymptomatic. Gram-negative bacteremia is the most significant complication associated with these UTIs. Most catheter-associated UTIs resolve quickly when the catheter is removed and a short course of antibiotic is administered. Intermittent catheterization carries a lower risk of infection than does an indwelling catheter, and is preferred for patients who are unable to empty their bladder by voiding.

Figure 27–2 ■ Appearance of the bladder wall affected by cystitis.
Source: Craig Zuckerman/Phototake NYC.

MANIFESTATIONS of Cystitis

- Dysuria
- Pyuria
- Frequency
- Hematuria
- Urgency
- Suprapubic discomfort
- Nocturia

Pyelonephritis

Pyelonephritis is inflammation of the renal pelvis and parenchyma, the functional kidney tissue. *Acute pyelonephritis* is a bacterial infection of the kidney; *chronic pyelonephritis* is associated with nonbacterial infections and inflammatory processes that may be metabolic, chemical, or immunologic in origin.

ACUTE PYELONEPHRITIS   Acute pyelonephritis usually results from an infection that ascends to the kidney from the lower urinary tract. Asymptomatic bacteriuria or cystitis can lead to acute pyelonephritis. Risk factors include pregnancy (because of slowed ureteral peristalsis), urinary tract obstruction, and congenital malformation. Urinary tract trauma, scarring, calculi (stones), kidney disorders such as polycystic or hypertensive kidney disease, and chronic diseases such as diabetes may also contribute to pyelonephritis. *Vesicoureteral reflux*, a condition in which urine moves from the bladder back toward the kidney, is a common risk factor in children who develop pyelonephritis and is also seen in adults when bladder outflow is obstructed.

The infection spreads from the renal pelvis to the renal cortex. The pelvis, calyces, and medulla of the kidney are primarily affected, with white blood cell (WBC) infiltration and inflammation. The kidney becomes grossly edematous. Localized abscesses may develop on the cortical surface of the kidney. As with cystitis, *E. coli* is the organism responsible for 85% of the cases of acute pyelonephritis. Other organisms commonly found include *Proteus* and *Klebsiella*, bacteria that normally inhabit the intestinal tract.

The onset of acute pyelonephritis is typically rapid, with chills and fever, malaise, vomiting, flank pain, costovertebral tenderness, urinary frequency, and dysuria (see the following Manifestations box). Symptoms of cystitis also may be present. The older adult may present with a change in behavior, acute confusion, incontinence, or a general deterioration in condition.

CHRONIC PYELONEPHRITIS   Chronic pyelonephritis involves chronic inflammation and scarring of the tubules and interstitial tissues of the kidney. It is a common cause of chronic kidney disease. It may develop as a result of UTIs or other conditions that damage the kidneys, such as hypertension or vascular conditions, severe vesicoureteral reflux, or obstruction of the urinary tract.

The patient with chronic pyelonephritis may be asymptomatic or have mild manifestations such as urinary frequency, dysuria, and flank pain. Hypertension can develop as kidney tissue is destroyed.

MANIFESTATIONS of Acute Pyelonephritis

URINARY	SYSTEMIC
■ Urinary frequency	■ Vomiting
■ Dysuria	■ Diarrhea
■ Pyuria	■ Acute fever
■ Hematuria	■ Shaking chills
■ Flank pain	■ Malaise
■ Costovertebral tenderness	

Interdisciplinary Care

Treatment of UTI focuses on eliminating the causative organism, preventing relapse or reinfection, and identifying and correcting any contributing factors. Drug treatment with antibiotics and urinary anti-infectives is commonly used. In some cases, surgery may be indicated to correct contributing factors.

Diagnosis

Laboratory testing for UTI includes the following:

■ *Urinalysis* to assess for pyuria, bacteria, and blood cells in the urine. A bacteria count greater than 100,000 (10^5) per milliliter is indicative of infection. Rapid tests for bacteria in the urine include using a *nitrite dipstick* (which turns pink in the presence of bacteria) and the *leukocyte esterase test*, an indirect method of detecting bacteria by identifying lysed or intact WBCs in the urine.

Urine should be collected via suprapubic aspiration or by midstream clean-catch specimen; if necessary, straight catheterization or "mini-cath," with strict aseptic technique, may be used. Catheterization is avoided if possible to reduce the risk of further infection. ∞ See Chapter 26 for nursing care related to collecting a urinalysis specimen.

■ *Gram stain of the urine* may be done to identify the infecting organism by shape and characteristic (gram-positive or gram-negative).

■ *Urine culture and sensitivity* tests may be ordered to identify the infecting organism and the most effective antibiotic. Culture requires 24 to 72 hours, so treatment to eliminate the most common organisms often is initiated without culture.

> **SAFETY ALERT**
> Obtain urine specimens from a patient with an indwelling urinary catheter by briefly (15 minutes or less) clamping the proximal drainage tubing, then withdrawing urine directly from the port using sterile technique. Sterile technique is necessary to reduce the risk of catheter-associated UTI.

■ *WBC with differential* may be done to detect typical changes associated with infection, such as *leukocytosis* (elevated WBC) and increased numbers of neutrophils.

In men and in adult women with recurrent infections or persistent bacteriuria, additional diagnostic testing may be ordered to evaluate for structural abnormalities and other contributing factors:

■ *Intravenous pyelography (IVP)* is used to evaluate for structural or functional abnormalities, such as vesicoureteral reflux, of the kidneys, ureters, and bladder.

■ *Voiding cystourethrography* may be ordered to detect structural or functional abnormalities of the bladder and urethral strictures. This test has a lower risk of allergic response to the contrast dye than IVP.

■ *Cystoscopy* may be used to diagnose conditions such as prostatic hypertrophy, urethral strictures, bladder calculi, tumors, polyps or diverticula, and congenital abnormalities. A tissue biopsy may be obtained during the procedure, and other interventions performed (e.g., stone removal or stricture dilation).

- *Manual pelvic* or *prostate examinations* are done to assess for structural changes of the genitourinary tract, such as prostatic enlargement, cystocele, or rectocele.

Nursing implications for these diagnostic procedures are presented in ∞ Chapter 26.

Medications

Most acute uncomplicated infections of the lower urinary tract can be treated with a short course of antibiotic therapy. Upper urinary tract infections, in contrast, usually require longer treatment to eradicate the infecting organism and prevent recurrence.

Short-course therapy (a 3-day course of treatment) reduces treatment cost, increases compliance, and has a lower rate of side effects. Oral trimethoprim-sulfamethoxazole (TMP-SMX), SMX, TMP, or a quinolone antibiotic such as ciprofloxacin (Cipro), norfloxacin (Noroxin), or levofloxacin (Levaquin, Quixin) may be ordered.

Men and women with pyelonephritis, urinary tract abnormalities or stones, or a history of previous infections with antibiotic-resistant infections require a 7- to 10-day course of a fluoroquinolone antibiotic such as ciprofloxacin, levofloxacin, or an alternate antibiotic. The patient with severe illness may need hospitalization and intravenous antibiotic therapy. Imipenem-cilastatin (Primaxin), or an antibiotic combination such as IV ampicillin and gentamicin or ceftriaxone (Rocephin) may be prescribed for severe illness or sepsis associated with UTI. ∞ See Chapter 12 for the nursing implications for antibiotic therapy.

The outcome of treatment for UTI is determined by follow-up urinalysis and culture. *Cure*, as evidenced by no pathogens present in the urine, is the desired outcome. Treatment *failure* occurs when therapy fails to eradicate bacteria in the urine. *Recurrent infection* occurs when a persistent source of infection causes repeated infection after initial cure. *Reinfection* is the development of a new infection with a different pathogen following successful UTI treatment.

> ### PRACTICE ALERT
> Follow-up urine culture is scheduled 10 days to 2 weeks following completion of antibiotic therapy for UTI to ensure that bacteria have been eradicated from the urinary tract.

Patients who experience frequent symptomatic UTIs may be treated with prophylactic antibiotic therapy with a drug such as TMP-SMZ, TMP, or nitrofurantoin (Furadantin, Macrodantin, Macrobid). TMP and nitrofurantoin do not achieve effective plasma concentrations at recommended doses, but do reach effective concentrations in the urine. Nitrofurantoin also may be used to treat UTI in pregnant women. Nursing implications for these urinary anti-infectives and for phenazopyridine (Pyridium), a urinary analgesic, are outlined in the following Medication Administration box.

Antibiotics and urinary anti-infectives are not generally recommended to treat asymptomatic bacteriuria except in pregnant women. The preferred treatment for catheter-associated UTI is removal of the indwelling catheter followed by a 10- to 14-day course of antibiotic therapy to eliminate the infection.

Surgery

Surgery may be indicated for recurrent UTI if diagnostic testing indicates calculi, structural anomalies, or strictures that contribute to the risk of infection. Table 27–1 lists major causes of urinary tract obstruction that may contribute to UTI.

Stones, or *calculi*, in the renal pelvis or in the bladder are an irritant and provide a matrix for bacterial colonization. Treatment may include surgical removal of a large calculus from the renal pelvis or cystoscopic removal of bladder calculi. *Percutaneous ultrasonic pyelolithotomy* or *extracorporeal shock wave lithotripsy* (described in the next section of this chapter) may be used instead of surgery to crush and remove stones. (See the Diagnostic Tests box on pages 774–777 for nursing care related to cystoscopy.)

Ureteroplasty, surgical repair of a ureter, may be indicated for structural abnormality or stricture of a ureter. This may be combined with a ureteral reimplantation if vesicoureteral reflux is present. The patient returns from these surgeries with an indwelling urinary catheter (Foley or suprapubic) and a **ureteral stent** (a thin catheter inserted into the ureter to provide for urine flow and ureteral support), which remains in place for 3 to 5 days. Care of the patient with a ureteral stent is outlined in the box on page 789.

COMPLEMENTARY THERAPIES Complementary therapies such as aromatherapy or herbal preparations may be used in conjunction with antibiotics to treat UTI. Research supports the use of cranberry products to prevent UTI in women with recurrent symptomatic infections. Blueberry juice also is commonly used to prevent and treat UTI. Adding bergamot, sandalwood, lavender, or juniper oil to bath water helps relieve the discomfort of UTI. Herbal supplements such as saw palmetto have a urinary antiseptic effect, and may be beneficial in treating or preventing UTI. Consult a qualified herbologist for recommended doses and appropriate use.

TABLE 27–1 Major Causes of Urinary Tract Obstruction by Location

LOCATION	OBSTRUCTIVE PROCESS
Kidney pelvis	Calculi (stones)
	Polycystic kidney disease
	Infection and scarring
Ureters	Calculi
	Scarring and stricture
	Congenital defects or strictures
	External processes such as pregnancy, tumors, lymph node enlargement
Bladder	Neurogenic bladder
	Tumors
	Calculi and other foreign bodies
Urethra	Benign prostatic hypertrophy
	Tumors
	Scarring and stricture
	Trauma

URINARY ANTI-INFECTIVES

Nitrofurantoin (Furadantin, Macrodantin, Macrobid)

Trimethoprim (Proloprim, Trimpex)

Urinary anti-infectives are usually used prophylactically to prevent recurrence of UTI in patients with frequent symptomatic infections. Nitrofurantoin also may be used to treat UTI in pregnant women.

Nursing Responsibilities

- Ensure adequate fluid intake (1500 to 2000 mL/day) to maintain a urine output of at least 1500 mL of urine per 24 hours. Do not overhydrate.
- Administer with meals to minimize GI side effects, such as nausea, gastric upset, and abdominal cramping.
- Trimethoprim is contraindicated for use in patients with renal or hepatic impairment; nitrofurantoin is contraindicated for patients with impaired renal function. Report abnormal laboratory values such as elevated creatinine or BUN, bilirubin, alanine aminotransferase (ALT), aspartate aminotransferase (AST), and lactic dehydrogenase (LDH).
- Use with caution in older or chronically ill patients. Monitor closely for adverse effects.
- Do not administer trimethoprim to pregnant women because of possible adverse effects on the fetus.
- Monitor the patient taking nitrofurantoin for an acute or chronic pulmonary reaction with manifestations of dyspnea, cough, chills, fever, and chest pain. Discontinue the drug and notify the physician.
- Nitrofurantoin may cause peripheral neuropathy, especially in older patients and adult diabetics. Notify the physician if symptoms develop.
- Nitrofurantoin oral suspension may stain the teeth; have the patient rinse the mouth thoroughly after administering.
- Monitor for signs of phenytoin toxicity (sedation, ataxia, and increased blood levels) if trimethoprim is given concurrently. Phenytoin doses may need to be reduced.

Health Education for the Patient and Family

- These drugs are used along with hygiene practices to prevent recurrent UTI. Take as directed, even when no symptoms are present.
- Drink six to eight glasses of water or fluid per day while taking these drugs.
- Take the drug with meals or food to reduce gastric effects; however, avoid milk products because they may interfere with absorption.

- Trimethoprim should not be taken during pregnancy. Contact your physician before attempting to become pregnant.
- Contact your doctor if you develop any of the following: chest pain, difficulty breathing, cough, chills, and fever; numbness and tingling or weakness of the extremities; rash or pruritus (itching).
- If you are taking an oral suspension of nitrofurantoin, rinse your mouth thoroughly after each dose to avoid staining the teeth.
- Nitrofurantoin turns the urine brown. This is not harmful and subsides when the drug is discontinued.
- If you are taking trimethoprim along with phenytoin (Dilantin) or a related anticonvulsant, contact your doctor if you become sedated or begin to stagger.

URINARY ANALGESIC

Phenazopyridine (Pyridium)

Phenazopyridine is a urinary tract analgesic that may be used for symptomatic relief of the pain, burning, frequency, and urgency associated with UTI during the first 24 to 48 hours of therapy. Its use is somewhat controversial because it does not treat the infection and may delay effective treatment in the patient with recurrent UTI who saves a dose or two "for the next time."

Nursing Responsibilities

- Monitor renal function (urine output, weight, serum creatinine, and BUN) during treatment; report changes.
- Stop the drug and contact the physician if sclera or skin become yellow tinged. This may indicate reduced excretion and toxicity.

Health Education for the Patient and Family

- Take with meals to minimize gastric upset.
- Consume 2 to 3 quarts of fluid daily while taking this drug.
- If you are a diabetic, check your blood sugars regularly while taking this drug.
- This drug turns urine orange or red. Protect your clothing from staining.
- Contact lenses may become stained if worn while taking this drug.
- Promptly contact your doctor if symptoms of UTI recur; do not take phenazopyridine before you seek medical treatment.
- If you develop itching or notice a yellow tinge to your skin or eyes, stop taking the drug and notify the physician.

℘ Nursing Care

Health Promotion

Teach measures to prevent UTI to all patients, particularly to young, sexually active women. Encourage patients to maintain a generous fluid intake of 2.0 to 2.5 quarts per day, increasing intake during hot weather or strenuous activity. Discuss the need to avoid voluntary urinary retention, emptying the bladder every 3 to 4 hours. Instruct women to cleanse the perineal area from front to back after voiding and defecating. Teach to void before and after sexual intercourse to flush out bacteria introduced into the urethra and bladder. Teach measures to maintain the integrity of perineal tissues: Avoid bubble baths, feminine hygiene sprays, and vaginal douches; wear cotton briefs, avoid synthetic materials; if postmenopausal, use hormone replacement therapy or estrogen cream. Unless contraindicated, suggest measures to

maintain acid urine: Drink two glasses of low-sugar cranberry juice daily; take ascorbic acid (vitamin C), and avoid excess intake of milk and milk products, other fruit juices, and sodium bicarbonate (baking soda).

Assessment

Focused assessment data for the patient with a UTI includes the following:

- *Health history:* Current symptoms, including frequency, urgency, burning on urination, voidings per night; color, clarity, and odor of urine; other manifestations such as lower abdominal, back, or flank pain; nausea or vomiting; fever; duration of symptoms and any treatment attempted; history of previous UTIs and their frequency; possibility of pregnancy and type of birth control used; chronic diseases such as diabetes; current medications and any known allergies.

NURSING CARE OF THE PATIENT with a Ureteral Stent

Ureteral stents are used to maintain patency and promote healing of the ureters (see the following figure). A stent may be temporary, used during and after a surgical procedure, or it may be used for longer periods in patients with ureteral obstruction due to tumors, strictures, or other causes.

Stents may be positioned during surgery or cystoscopy. They are made of a nontoxic material such as silicone or polyurethane, with side drainage holes placed along the length of the stent. Stents are radiopaque for easy radiographic identification. One or both ends of the stent may be pigtail or J shaped to prevent migration.

- Label all drainage tubes including stents for easy identification. Attach each catheter and stent to a separate closed drainage system. *Careful labeling allows close monitoring of output from all sources and reservoirs. Separate drainage systems minimize the risk of infection.*
- If the stent has been brought to the surface, secure it and maintain its position. *The stent is usually placed in the renal pelvis. It is important to secure it well to prevent trauma to the kidney, inadvertent removal of the stent, and ureter obstruction.*
- Monitor urine output, including color, consistency, and odor. Monitor for signs of infection or bleeding: fever, tachycardia, pain, hematuria, and cloudy or malodorous urine. *The stent facilitates urine flow but may become obstructed because of bleeding, calculi, or sediment. Obstruction may result in hydronephrosis and kidney damage. The stent itself is a foreign body in the urinary tract and can increase the risk of UTI.*
- Maintain fluid intake, encouraging fluids that acidify urine, such as low-sugar apple, cranberry, and blueberry juice.

The stent can precipitate calculus formation as well as UTI. Increasing fluid intake and acidifying the urine help prevent these complications.

- For an indwelling stent, stress the need for regular follow-up to monitor for and prevent complications such as UTI and calculi. *The patient with an indwelling stent may tend to forget that the stent is in place and become lax in compliance with follow-up and preventive measures.*

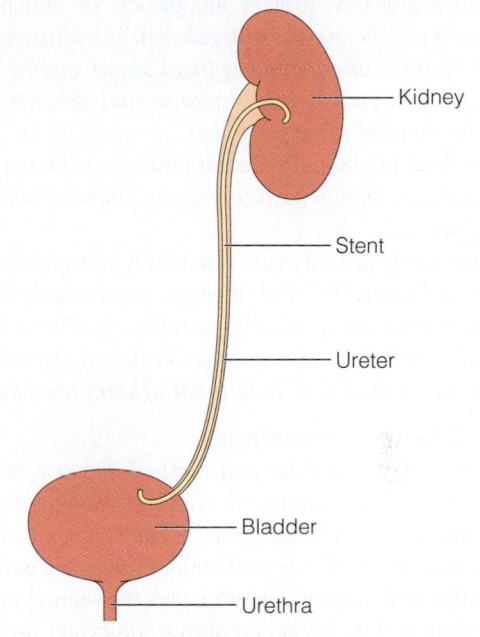

- *Physical examination:* General health; vital signs including temperature; abdominal shape, contour, tenderness to palpation (especially suprapubic); percuss for costovertebral tenderness (see Box 26–1).

∞ See Chapter 26 for complete nursing assessment of the urinary system.

Nursing Diagnoses and Interventions

The patient's general health, abilities for self-care, and risk factors that may contribute to UTI are considered when planning and implementing nursing care for the patient with a UTI. Priority nursing diagnoses focus on comfort, urinary elimination, and teaching/learning needs. A Case Study & Nursing Care Plan for the patient with cystitis can be found on page 792.

Acute Pain

Pain is a common manifestation of both lower and upper UTI. Urinary tract pain is caused primarily by distention and increased pressure within the tract. The severity of the pain is related to the rate at which inflammation and distention develop, not their degree.

In cystitis, inflammation causes a sensation of fullness; dull, constant suprapubic pain; and possibly low back pain. The inflamed bladder wall and urethra cause dysuria, pain, and burning on urination. Bladder spasms may develop, causing periodic severe, stabbing discomfort. Pain associated with pyelonephritis is often steady and dull, localized to the outer abdomen or flank region. Urologic disorders rarely cause central abdominal pain.

- Assess pain: timing, quality, intensity, location, duration, and aggravating and alleviating factors. *A change in the nature, location, or intensity of the pain could indicate an extension of the infection or a related but separate problem.*

EVIDENCE FOR NURSING CARE **The Patient with Urinary Tract Infection**

Selected resources that nurses may find helpful when planning evidence-based nursing care follow.

- American College of Obstetricians and Gynecologists (ACOG). (2008 March). *Treatment of urinary tract infections in nonpregnant women.* Washington, DC: Author.
- Gotelli, J., Merryman, P., Carr, C., McElveen, L., Epperson, C., & Bynum, D. (2008 December). A quality improvement project to reduce the complications associated with indwelling urinary catheters. *Urologic Nursing, 28*(6), 465–467, 473.
- Lin, K., & Fajardo, K. (2008 July 1). Clinical guidelines. Screening for asymptomatic bacteriuria in adults: Evidence for the U. S. Preventive Services Task Force reaffirmation recommendation statement. *Annals of Internal Medicine, 149*(1), W-20–W-24.
- Robinson, S., Allen, L., Barnes, M., Berry, T., Foster, T., Friedrich, L., et al. (2007 June). Development of an evidence-based protocol for reduction of indwelling urinary catheter usage. *MEDSURG Nursing, 16*(3), 157–161.

- Teach or provide comfort measures such as warm sitz baths, warm packs or heating pads, and balanced rest and activity. Systemic analgesics, urinary analgesics, or antispasmodic medication may be used as ordered. *Warmth relaxes muscles, relieves spasms, and increases local blood supply. Because pain can stimulate a stress response and delay healing, it should be relieved when possible.*
- Increase fluid intake unless contraindicated. *Increased fluid dilutes urine, reducing irritation of the inflamed bladder and urethral mucosa.*
- Instruct to notify primary care provider if pain and discomfort continue or intensify after therapy is initiated. *Pain and discomfort in voiding typically are relieved within 24 hours of the initiation of antibiotic therapy. Continued discomfort may indicate a complicated UTI or other urinary tract disorder.*

Impaired Urinary Elimination

Inflammation of the bladder and urethral mucosa affects the normal process and patterns of voiding, causing frequency, urgency, and burning on urination, as well as nocturia. Urine may be blood tinged, cloudy, and malodorous. The patient with short- or long-term urinary retention (see the section on urinary retention later in this chapter) requires additional measures to assess for and prevent UTI.

- Monitor (or instruct the patient to monitor) color, clarity, and odor of urine. *Urine should return to clear yellow within 48 hours, unless drug therapy causes a change in the color of urine. If clarity does not return, further investigation may be necessary.*

- Instruct to avoid caffeinated drinks, including coffee, tea, and cola; citrus juices; drinks containing artificial sweeteners; and alcoholic beverages. *Caffeine, citrus juices, and artificial sweeteners irritate bladder mucosa and the detrusor muscle, and can increase urgency and bladder spasms.*
- Use strict aseptic technique and a closed urinary drainage system when inserting a straight or indwelling urinary catheter. Insert indwelling catheters to the full recommended length (4 or more inches in women and to the bifurcation in men) before inflating the balloon. *Bacteria colonizing the perineal tissues or on the nurse's hands can be introduced into the bladder during catheterization. Aseptic technique reduces this risk. Inflation of the balloon while in the urethra damages urethral tissues and can cause significant discomfort for the patient.*

- When possible, use intermittent straight catheterization to relieve urinary retention. Remove indwelling urinary catheters as soon as possible. *Using intermittent straight catheterization allows the bladder to fill and completely empty in a more normal manner, maintaining physiologic function. The risk of infection associated with an indwelling catheter is about 3% to 5% per day of catheterization (Fauci et al., 2008). See the accompanying box for evidence-based practice for reducing the risk of catheter-associated UTI.*
- Maintain the closed urinary drainage system, and use aseptic technique when emptying the catheter drainage bag. Maintain gravity flow, preventing reflux of urine into the bladder from the drainage system. *Bacteria can enter the drainage system when its integrity is interrupted (e.g., disconnecting the catheter from the drainage system) or during emptying of the drainage bag. These bacteria can ascend the column of urine to the bladder, causing UTI.*
- Provide perineal care on a regular basis and following defecation. Use antiseptic preparations only as ordered. *Regular cleansing of perineal tissues reduces the risk of colonization by bowel or other bacteria. While antiseptic solutions may be ordered for catheter care, they can dry perineal tissues and reduce normal flora, increasing the risk of colonization by pathogens, and should not routinely be used.*

Readiness for Enhanced Self Health Maintenance

The patient with a urinary tract infection is at an increased risk for future UTI and needs to understand the disease process, risk factors, measures to prevent recurrent infection, diagnostic procedures, and home care. In addition, once the manifestations of UTI are relieved, motivation to continue the treatment plan declines. Failure to complete the full course of therapy and recommended follow-up can lead to continued bacteriuria and recurrent infections.

- Teach how to obtain a midstream clean-catch urine specimen. *Cleansing of the urinary meatus and perineal area reduces contamination of the specimen by external cells and bacteria. Ninety percent of urethral bacteria are cleared in the first 10 mL of voided urine; a midstream specimen is representative of urine in the bladder.*
- Assess knowledge about the disease process, risk factors, and preventive measures. *The patient may have little understanding of UTI, its causes, and contributing factors.*
- Discuss the prescribed treatment plan and the importance of taking all prescribed antibiotics.

MOVING EVIDENCE INTO ACTION — Reducing Catheter-Associated Complications

Insertion of an indwelling (retention) catheter is a commonly performed procedure in hospitals, with up to 25% of patients having an indwelling catheter at some time during hospitalization. Furthermore, catheters often remain in place when there is no clear indication for their continued use. Indwelling catheters are not only associated with an increased risk for UTI, but also often affect the patient's comfort and mobility as well. Nurses on an older adult acute care unit determined that approximately 24% of the patients were catheterized at any one time (Gotelli et al., 2008). Of these, more than half had no clear indication for catheterization. Using a nurse-driven protocol, the need for catheterization was assessed using specific criteria (e.g., aggressive diuretic or fluid therapy, accurate monitoring of intake and output, management of urinary incontinence with stage 3 pressure ulcers), and the catheter removed when criteria were no longer met. As a result, the prevalence of catheterization dropped from 24% at any given time to just over 16%.

IMPLICATIONS FOR NURSING

Although a physician's order is required for inserting an indwelling catheter, nurses often are in the best position to evaluate the need for continued catheterization as the patient progresses. This study demonstrated the effectiveness of (1) providing nurses with clear criteria for assessing the need for catheterization, and (2) empowering nurses to remove an indwelling catheter and implement a bladder retraining program when criteria are no longer met. These nursing actions can have a positive impact on patient outcomes, reducing the risk for catheter-associated infection and other complications.

CRITICAL THINKING IN PATIENT CARE

1. This summary notes several of the criteria used to determine the continued need for an indwelling urinary catheter. What other criteria would you consider in determining the appropriateness of continued catheterization? Provide justification for the criteria you identify.
2. An indwelling urinary catheter has been called a "one-point restraint." Identify why this is the case, and discuss potential noninfectious complications of urinary catheterization.
3. Patients who have had a urinary catheter in place for an extended period may require a bladder retraining program. Develop such a program for an older adult in an acute care or post-acute care setting.

Source: Gotelli, J., Merryman, P., Carr, C., McElveen, L., Epperson, C., & Bynum, D. (2008 December). A quality improvement project to reduce the complications associated with indwelling urinary catheters. *Urologic Nursing, 28* (6), 465–467, 473.

- Help the patient develop a plan for taking medications, such as taking them with meals (unless contraindicated) or setting out all doses for the day in the morning. *Missed doses of antibiotic can result in subtherapeutic blood levels and reduced effectiveness. Taking medication in association with a regular daily activity such as meals helps patients remember doses.*
- Instruct to keep appointments for follow-up and urine culture. *Follow-up urine culture, often scheduled 7 to 14 days after completion of antibiotic therapy, is vital to ensure complete eradication of bacteria and prevent relapse or recurrence.*
- Teach measures to prevent future UTI (see the preceding Health Promotion section). *Keeping urine dilute and acidic and voiding regularly flush bacteria out of the bladder and urethra. The proximity of the female urethral meatus to the vagina and anus increases the risk of bacterial contamination, especially during intercourse. Bubble baths, feminine hygiene sprays, synthetic fibers, and douches may dry and irritate perineal tissues, promoting bacterial growth.*

Using NANDA, NIC, and NOC

Linkages between a selected NANDA nursing diagnosis, NIC, and NOC for the patient with a urinary tract infection are shown in the chart that follows.

Community-Based Care

Because both upper and lower urinary tract infections are usually managed in the community, teaching is the most important nursing intervention. Provide instruction on the following topics:

- Risk factors for UTI and how to minimize or eliminate these factors through increased fluid intake, regular elimination, and personal hygiene measures
- Early manifestations of UTI and the importance of seeking medical intervention promptly
- Maintaining optimal immune system function by attending to physical and psychosocial stressors, such as lack of adequate rest, poor nutrition, and high levels of emotional stress
- The importance of completing the prescribed treatment and keeping follow-up appointments
- Minimizing the risk of UTI when an indwelling urinary catheter is necessary:
  - Use alternatives to an indwelling catheter when possible. For urinary incontinence, try scheduled toileting, incontinence pads or diapers, and external catheters if possible. For urinary retention, teach the patient or a family member to perform straight catheterization every 3 to 4 hours using clean technique.
  - Teach care measures such as perineal care, managing and emptying the collection chamber, maintaining a closed system, and bladder irrigation or flushing if ordered when an indwelling catheter is necessary.

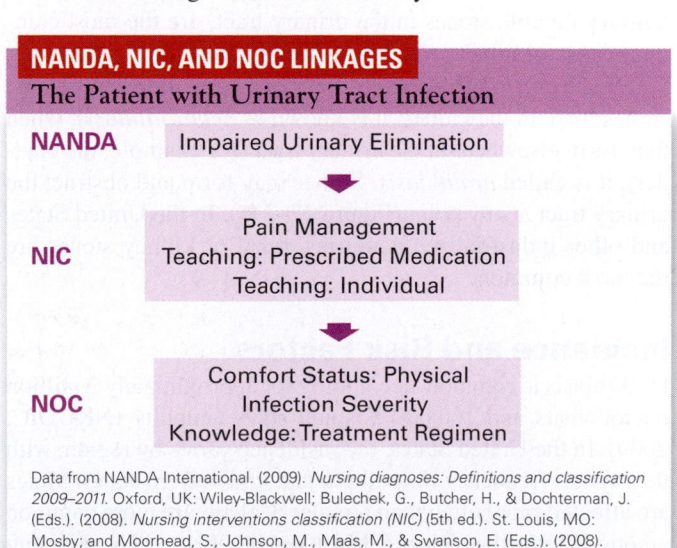

NANDA, NIC, AND NOC LINKAGES
The Patient with Urinary Tract Infection

NANDA — Impaired Urinary Elimination

NIC — Pain Management / Teaching: Prescribed Medication / Teaching: Individual

NOC — Comfort Status: Physical / Infection Severity / Knowledge: Treatment Regimen

Data from NANDA International. (2009). *Nursing diagnoses: Definitions and classification 2009–2011.* Oxford, UK: Wiley-Blackwell; Bulechek, G., Butcher, H., & Dochterman, J. (Eds.). (2008). *Nursing interventions classification (NIC)* (5th ed.). St. Louis, MO: Mosby; and Moorhead, S., Johnson, M., Maas, M., & Swanson, E. (Eds.). (2008). *Nursing outcomes classification (NOC)* (4th ed.). St. Louis, MO: Mosby.

CASE STUDY & NURSING CARE PLAN   A Patient with Cystitis

Miija Waisanen is a 25-year-old second-year nursing student. She was recently married, and she and her husband live in an apartment near the college she attends. Mrs. Waisanen has never been pregnant, and she is using a diaphragm for birth control. She presents at the local urgent care clinic complaining of low back pain, frequency, urgency, and burning on urination that began the day before.

ASSESSMENT

Patrice Ramiros, RN, admits Mrs. Waisanen to the clinic. Mrs. Waisanen denies having had similar symptoms in the past or ever having been diagnosed with a UTI. She describes her pain as a constant, dull ache that does not change with movement. She feels the need to urinate almost constantly, but experiences difficulty in starting her stream, and burning pain and cramping when voiding. She reports getting up four times the night before to urinate. She denies painful intercourse and states that her last menstrual period began only 2 weeks ago. Physical examination reveals: BP 112/68; P 90 and regular, afebrile. Suprapubic tenderness noted but no flank or costovertebral angle tenderness. Clean-catch urine specimen shows hematuria, multiple WBCs, and a bacteria count greater than 10^5 per milliliter.

The nurse practitioner prescribes trimethoprim-sulfamethoxazole (TMP-SMZ) 160 mg/800 mg PO bid for 3 days, and aspirin or acetaminophen 650 mg PO every 4 hours as needed for pain. Mrs. Waisanen is instructed to return to the clinic in 7 days for a follow-up urine culture, or sooner if her symptoms do not improve.

DIAGNOSES

- *Acute Pain* related to infection and inflammatory process in the urinary tract
- *Impaired Urinary Elimination* related to inflammation as evidenced by frequency, urgency, nocturia, and dysuria
- *Readiness for Enhanced Self Health Management* related to risk factors for and treatment of UTI

EXPECTED OUTCOMES

- Report relief of low back pain and burning on urination.
- Regain a normal voiding pattern without frequency, urgency, nocturia, and abnormal urine characteristics.

- Verbalize understanding of the disease process, related risk factors, follow-up instructions, and symptoms of recurrence indicating the need for medical attention.

PLANNING AND IMPLEMENTATION

- Teach comfort measures: warm sitz baths, a heating pad on low heat applied to her lower back or abdomen, rest, increased fluid intake, avoiding caffeinated beverages, and aspirin or acetaminophen as ordered.
- Advise to refrain from sexual intercourse until infection and inflammation have cleared to avoid further irritation of inflamed tissues.
- Discuss the possible relationship between using a diaphragm for birth control and UTI in women.
- Discuss dietary and hygiene practices to prevent UTI, symptoms indicating the need for further intervention, and the risks of undertreatment.

EVALUATION

Six months later, Mrs. Waisanen rotates through the urgent care clinic for her community-based nursing experience. Ms. Ramiros asks how she is doing. Mrs. Waisanen reports that her symptoms and urine cleared within about a day after starting the antibiotic and she has had no further problems. She has seen her women's healthcare nurse practitioner to change her birth control to oral contraceptives, increased her intake of fluid and vitamin C, and no longer puts off urinating until she "has time to go!"

CRITICAL THINKING IN THE NURSING PROCESS

1. What physiologic and psychosocial factors put Mrs. Waisanen at risk for developing a UTI?
2. Compare and contrast the benefits and drawbacks to short-course therapy versus conventional therapy for UTI.
3. Develop a care plan for Mrs. Waisanen for the nursing diagnosis *Ineffective Health Maintenance*.

See Evaluating Your Response in Appendix C.

The Patient with Urinary Calculi

Urinary calculi, stones in the urinary tract, are the most common cause of upper urinary tract obstruction (Porth & Matfin, 2009). The term **lithiasis** means "stone formation." When the stones form in the kidney, it is known as *nephrolithiasis*; when they form elsewhere in the urinary tract (for example, the bladder), it is called *urolithiasis*. Stones may form and obstruct the urinary tract at any point (Figure 27–3 ■). In the United States and other industrialized countries, renal or kidney stones are the most common.

Incidence and Risk Factors

Urolithiasis is common, accounting for approximately 2 million doctor visits and 166,000 hospital stays annually (NKUDIC, 2009). In the United States, the incidence varies by region, with the highest frequency in southern and midwestern states. Males are affected more often than females. Calculi are more common among Whites than Blacks. Most people affected are in young or middle adulthood.

Although the majority of stones are idiopathic (having no demonstrable cause), a number of risk factors have been identified. The greatest risk factor for stone formation is a prior personal or family history of urinary calculi. A genetic predisposition toward the accumulation of certain mineral substances in the urine or a congenital lack of protective factors may explain the familial link. Other identified risk factors include dehydration with resultant increased urine concentration, immobility, and excess dietary intake of calcium, oxalate, or proteins. Gout, hyperparathyroidism, and urinary stasis or repeated infections also contribute to calculus formation.

Physiology Review

Normally, a balance exists in the kidneys between the need to conserve water and to eliminate poorly soluble materials such as calcium salts. This balance is affected by factors such as diet, environmental temperature, and activity. Protective inorganic and organic substances in the urine, such as pyrophosphate, citrate, and glycoproteins, normally inhibit stone formation.

Stone
in calyx

Stone free
in pelvis

Staghorn

Hydroureter

Ureteral
stone

Bladder stones

Urethral stone

Figure 27–3 ■ Development and location of calculi within the urinary tract.

Source: Dr. E. Walker/Photo Researchers, Inc.

Pathophysiology

Three factors contribute to urolithiasis: supersaturation, nucleation, and lack of inhibitory substances in the urine.

When the concentration of an insoluble salt in the urine is very high, that is, when the urine is supersaturated, crystals may form. Usually, these crystals disperse and are eliminated because the bonds holding them together are weak. However, a nucleus of crystals may develop stable bonds to form a stone. More often, crystals form around an organic matrix or mucoprotein nucleus to become a stone. The stimulus required to initiate crystallization in supersaturated urine may be minimal. Ingesting a meal high in insoluble salt, or decreased fluid intake as occurs

during sleep, allows the concentration to increase to the point where precipitation occurs and stones are formed and grow. When fluid intake is adequate, no stone growth occurs. The acidity or alkalinity of the urine and the presence or absence of calculus-inhibiting compounds also affect lithiasis.

Most (70% to 80%) kidney stones are *calcium stones*, composed of calcium oxalate and/or calcium phosphate. These stones are generally associated with high concentrations of calcium in the blood or urine. *Uric acid stones* develop when the urine concentration of uric acid is high. They are more common in men, and may be associated with gout. Genetic factors contribute to the development of uric acid stones and calcium stones. *Struvite* (magnesium-ammonium phosphate) *stones* are associated with UTI caused by urease-producing bacteria such as *Proteus*. These stones can grow to become very large, filling the renal pelvis and calyces. They often are called *staghorn stones* because of their shape (see Figure 27–3 ■). *Cystine stones* are rare, and are associated with a genetic defect. The types of renal calculi, contributing factors, and recommended dietary modifications are listed in Table 27–2.

> **MEMORY CUE**
> - Most urinary stones form in the renal pelvis and are composed primarily of calcium salts.
> - Men are more frequently affected by urinary stones than women.
> - Loss of calcium from the bones (e.g., due to immobility) and dehydration are major risk factors for urinary stones.

TABLE 27–2 Risk Factors and Interventions for Renal Calculi

STONE TYPE AND INCIDENCE	RISK FACTORS	MANAGEMENT
Calcium phosphate and/or oxalate 70%–80%	Hypercalciuria and hypercalcemia: hyperparathyroidism, immobility, bone disease, vitamin D intoxication, multiple myeloma, renal tubular acidosis, prolonged steroid intake Alkaline urine Dehydration Inflammatory bowel disease	Pharmacology: Thiazide diuretics, phosphates Dietary: Limit foods high in sodium and protein, increase foods that acidify urine Other: Increase hydration, exercise
Struvite 15%–20%	UTIs, especially *Proteus* infections	Pharmacology: Antibiotic therapy for UTI Other: Surgical intervention or lithotripsy to remove stone
Uric acid 5%–10%	Gout, increased purine intake, acid urine	Pharmacology: Potassium citrate, allopurinol Dietary: Low purine diet Other: Increase hydration
Cystine (uncommon)	Genetic defect, acid urine	Pharmacology: Penicillamine, sodium bicarbonate Dietary: Sodium restriction Other: Increase hydration

Manifestations

The symptoms caused by urinary calculi vary with their size and location (see the following Manifestations box). Manifestations develop as a result of obstructed urine flow with resulting distention, and tissue trauma caused by passage of the rough-edged, crystalline stone.

Calculi affecting the kidney calyces and pelvis may cause few symptoms. If the stone has gradually or partially obstructed urinary flow, dull, aching flank pain may be present, but renal calculi often are silent, without symptoms. Bladder calculi may cause few symptoms other than dull suprapubic pain with exercise or after voiding.

Renal colic, acute, severe flank pain on the affected side, develops when a stone obstructs the ureter, causing ureteral spasm. The pain of renal colic may radiate to the suprapubic region, groin, and external genitals (the scrotum or labia). The severity of the pain often causes a sympathetic response with associated nausea, vomiting, pallor, and cool, clammy skin.

Manifestations of UTI, including chills and fever, frequency, urgency, and dysuria, may accompany urinary calculi at any level. Trauma to the urinary tract by the calculi may cause gross or microscopic hematuria. Gross hematuria is often the only sign of bladder stones.

Complications

Urinary stones may obstruct urine flow at any point of the urinary tract, leading to complications such as hydronephrosis and urinary stasis with subsequent infection.

Obstruction

Stones can obstruct the urinary tract at any point from the calyces of the kidney to the distal urethra, impeding the outflow of urine. If the obstruction develops slowly, there may be few or no symptoms, whereas sudden obstruction (e.g., blockage of a ureter by a passing stone) may cause severe manifestations. Urinary tract obstruction can ultimately lead to renal failure. The degree of obstruction, its location, and the duration of impaired urine flow determine the effect on renal function.

HYDRONEPHROSIS The kidneys continue to produce urine, causing increased pressure and distention of the urinary tract behind the obstruction. **Hydronephrosis**, distention of the renal pelvis and calyces, and *hydroureter*, distention of the ureter, are possible results. If the pressure is unrelieved, the collecting tubules, proximal tubules, and glomeruli of the kidney are damaged, causing a gradual loss of renal function.

Acute hydronephrosis typically causes colicky pain on the affected side. The pain may radiate into the groin. Chronic hydronephrosis develops slowly, and may have few manifestations other than dull, aching back or flank pain. When hydronephrosis is significant, a palpable mass may be felt in the flank region. Hematuria and signs of UTI such as pyuria, fever, and discomfort may occur. Gastrointestinal symptoms such as nausea, vomiting, and abdominal pain may accompany hydronephrosis (see the following Manifestations box).

INFECTION The urinary stasis associated with partial or complete obstruction increases the risk of urinary tract infection. Either upper or lower UTI may develop.

Interdisciplinary Care

Management of urinary calculi focuses on relieving acute symptoms, destroying or removing stones, and preventing further stone formation. Asymptomatic stones (those not causing pain, infection, or obstruction) are treated conservatively.

Diagnosis

Laboratory and diagnostic tests that may be ordered when urinary calculi are suspected include the following:

- *Urinalysis* to assess for hematuria and the presence of WBCs and crystal fragments. The urine pH is helpful in identifying the type of stone.
- *Chemical analysis* of any stones passed in the urine determines the type of stone and suggests measures to prevent further stone formation. Retrieving stones or teaching the patient to do so is a nursing responsibility. All urine is strained and may be saved. Any visible stones or sediment are sent for analysis.
- *Urine calcium*, *uric acid*, and *oxalate* levels measure the amount of these substances excreted over a 24-hour period, and may be assessed to help identify possible causes of lithiasis. Elevated calcium levels occur in hyperparathyroidism, Cushing's syndrome, and osteoporosis, all of which may contribute to lithiasis. Uric acid levels may be elevated in

---

MANIFESTATIONS of Urinary Calculi

KIDNEY STONES
- Often asymptomatic
- Dull, aching flank pain
- Microscopic hematuria
- Manifestations of UTI

URETERAL STONES
- Renal colic
  - Acute, severe flank pain on affected side
  - Often radiates to suprapubic region, groin, and external genitals
- Nausea, vomiting, pallor, and cool, clammy skin

BLADDER STONES
- May be asymptomatic
- Dull suprapubic pain, possibly associated with exercise or voiding
- Gross or microscopic hematuria
- Manifestations of UTI

MANIFESTATIONS of Acute and Chronic Hydronephrosis

ACUTE
- Acute, colicky pain; may radiate into groin
- Hematuria, pyuria
- Fever
- Nausea, vomiting, abdominal pain

CHRONIC
- Dull, aching flank pain
- Hematuria, pyuria
- Fever
- Palpable flank mass

patients with gout and those at risk for forming uric acid calculi. Urine oxalate excretion may help to differentiate calcium oxalate from calcium phosphate stones.

- *Serum calcium*, *phosphorus*, and *uric acid* levels may be obtained to help identify factors contributing to calculus formation.
- *KUB* (kidneys, ureters, and bladder) x-ray of the lower abdomen may show calculi as opacities in the kidneys, ureters, and bladder.
- *Renal ultrasonography* uses reflected sound waves to detect stones and evaluate the kidneys for possible hydronephrosis.
- *Spiral computed tomography (CT) scan* of the kidney, with or without contrast medium, shows calculi, ureteral obstruction, and other renal disorders.
- *Cystoscopy* is used to visualize and possibly remove calculi from the urinary bladder and distal ureters.

Nursing implications and care for patients undergoing these tests and procedures is outlined in ∞ Chapter 26.

Medications

An acute episode of renal colic is treated with analgesia, medications to promote stone passage, and hydration. A narcotic analgesic such as morphine sulfate is given, often intravenously, to relieve pain and reduce ureteral spasm. Indomethacin, a nonsteroidal anti-inflammatory drug (NSAID), given as a suppository, may reduce the amount of narcotic analgesia required for acute renal colic. An oral alpha-adrenergic blocker such as tamsulosin (Flomax) or a calcium-channel blocker such as nifedipine (Adalat CC, Procardia) is prescribed to relax ureteral muscle and promote passage of the stone (Stevermer & Ewigman, 2008). Oral or intravenous fluids reduce the risk of further stone formation and promote urine output.

After analysis of the calculus, various medications may be ordered to inhibit or prevent further lithiasis. A thiazide diuretic, frequently prescribed for calcium calculi, acts to reduce urinary calcium excretion and is very effective in preventing further stones. Potassium citrate alkalinizes urine (raises the pH) and is often prescribed to prevent stones that tend to form in acidic urine (uric acid, cystine, and some forms of calcium stones). See Table 27–2 for other preparations related to types of stones. Nursing responsibilities focus on teaching the patient about the prescribed medication, its importance in preventing further stone formation, and potential adverse effects.

Nutrition and Fluid Management

Diet modifications may be prescribed to change the character of the urine and prevent further lithiasis.

Increased fluid intake of 2.5 to 3.0 L per day is recommended, regardless of stone composition. A fluid intake to ensure the production of approximately 2.0 to 2.5 L of urine a day prevents the stone-forming salts from becoming concentrated enough to precipitate. Fluid intake should be spaced throughout the day and evening. Some authorities recommend that patients drink one to two glasses of water at night to prevent concentration of urine during sleep.

Recommended dietary changes may include reduced intake of the primary substance forming the calculi. For calcium stones, however, restricting dietary calcium may actually increase the risk of stone formation while promoting bone loss. A low-sodium restricted-protein diet has been shown to be more effective in preventing the recurrence of calcium stones. Dietary sodium also is restricted in patients who form cystine stones (Fauci et al., 2008).

The patient with uric acid stones requires a diet low in purines. Organ meats, sardines, and other high-purine foods are eliminated from the diet. Foods with moderate levels of purines, such as red and white meats and some seafood, may be limited.

In addition to limiting certain foods, the diet may be modified to maintain a urinary pH that does not promote lithiasis. Uric acid and cystine stones tend to form in acid urine. Foods that tend to alkalinize the urine may be recommended. Because alkaline urine promotes formation of calcium stones and urinary tract infections, the diet may be modified to lower the pH of the urine. Foods that affect urinary pH and foods high in various stone components are summarized in Table 27–3.

Treatment

Treatment of existing calculi depends on the location of the stone, the extent of obstruction, renal function, the presence or absence of UTI, and the patient's general state of health. In general, the stone is removed if it is causing severe obstruction, infection, unrelieved pain, or serious bleeding.

Lithotripsy, using sound or shock waves to crush a stone, is the preferred treatment for urinary calculi. Several techniques are available. *Extracorporeal shock wave lithotripsy (ESWL)* is a noninvasive technique for fragmenting kidney stones using shock waves generated outside the body. Acoustic shock waves are aimed under fluoroscopic guidance at the stone (Figure 27–4 ■). These shock waves travel through soft tissue without causing damage, but shatter the stone as its greater density stops their progress. Repeated shock waves pulverize the stone into fragments small enough to be eliminated in the urine. The procedure may require 30 minutes to 2 hours to complete. Intravenous sedation generally is adequate to maintain comfort during the procedure. See the box on page 796 for nursing care of the patient undergoing a lithotripsy procedure.

TABLE 27–3 Teaching Patients with Urolithiasis: Possible Food and Fluid Modifications

Foods high in oxalate	Asparagus, beer and colas, beets, cabbage, celery, chocolate and cocoa, fruits, green beans, nuts, tea, tomatoes
Purine-rich foods	Goose, organ meats, sardines and herring, venison; moderate in beef, chicken, crab, pork, salmon, veal
Acidifying foods	Cheese, cranberries, eggs, grapes, meat and poultry, plums and prunes, tomatoes, whole grains
Alkalinizing foods	Green vegetables, fruit (except as noted above), legumes, milk and milk products, rhubarb

Figure 27–4 ■ Extracorporeal shock-wave lithotripsy. Acoustic shock waves generated by the shock wave generator travel through soft tissue to shatter the urinary stone into fragments, which are then eliminated in the urine.

Source: Visuals Unlimited.

Figure 27–5 ■ Percutaneous ultrasonic lithotripsy. A nephroscope is inserted into the renal pelvis, and ultrasonic waves are used to fragment the stone. The fragments then are removed through the nephroscope.

Lithotripsy also may be performed using a percutaneous ultrasonic or laser technique. *Percutaneous nephrolithotomy* uses a nephroscope inserted into the kidney pelvis through a small flank incision (Figure 27–5 ■). The stone is fragmented using a small ultrasonic transducer or laser, and the fragments are removed through the nephroscope. In a *ureteroscopy* procedure, laser beams are used to disintegrate the stone, without damaging soft tissue. A ureteroscope (passed up the ureter from the bladder during cystoscopy) is used to guide the laser probe into direct contact with the stone.

A double J stent may be inserted into the affected ureter to maintain its patency following ESWL or other lithotripsy procedures. (See the box on page 789 for nursing care of the patient with a ureteral stent.)

On rare occasions, surgical intervention is necessary to remove a calculus in the renal pelvis or ureter. *Ureterolithotomy* is incision in the affected ureter to remove a calculus. *Pyelolithotomy* is incision into and removal of a stone from the kidney pelvis. A staghorn calculus that invades the calyces and renal parenchyma may require a *nephrolithotomy* for removal. ∞ See Chapter 4 for care of the surgical patient.

NURSING CARE OF THE PATIENT Having Lithotripsy

PREOPERATIVE CARE
- Assess knowledge and understanding of the procedure, providing information as needed. *Anxiety is reduced, and recovery is enhanced and hastened when the patient is fully prepared for surgery.*
- Follow directions from the radiology department, physician, or anesthetist for withholding food and fluids and for bowel preparation prior to surgery. *Conscious sedation, general anesthesia, or spinal anesthesia may be required, depending on the procedure. Fecal material in the bowel may impede fluoroscopic visualization of the kidney and stone.*

POSTOPERATIVE CARE
- In the initial period, monitor vital signs frequently. *The kidney is highly vascular; therefore, hemorrhage and resulting shock are potential complications of lithotripsy. Bleeding may be internal or retroperitoneal and difficult to detect.*
- Monitor amount, color, and clarity of urine output. *Urine is often bright red initially, but bleeding should diminish within 48 to 72 hours. Cloudy urine may indicate the presence of an infection.*

- Maintain placement and patency of urinary catheters. Anchor ureteral catheters or nephrostomy tubes securely. Irrigate gently if ordered. *A kinked or plugged catheter may result in hydroureter, hydronephrosis, and kidney damage. Decreased urinary output and flank pain are possible symptoms of obstructed urine flow. Excessive force in irrigation may cause trauma and bleeding.*
- Prepare for discharge by teaching care of the indwelling catheter, urine-collection device, and incision site (if present). Teach signs and symptoms to report: urine leakage from incision for more than 4 days, symptoms of infection, pain, bright hematuria. *Many patients are discharged with dressings and catheters in place. The patient and family need necessary information to provide self-care.*
- Teach measures to reduce the risk of further lithiasis. *Many patients have repeated episodes of lithiasis and renal colic. Prevention of stone formation is important to preserve renal function.*

Bladder stones may be removed using an instrument passed through a cystoscope to crush the stones. The remaining stone fragments are then irrigated out of the bladder using an acid solution to counteract the alkalinity that precipitated stone formation.

Nursing Care

Nursing care for the patient with urolithiasis is directed at providing for comfort during acute renal colic, assisting with diagnostic procedures, ensuring adequate urinary output, and teaching the patient information necessary to prevent future stone formation.

Health Promotion

Discuss the importance of maintaining an adequate fluid intake with all patients. Stress the need to increase fluid intake during warm weather and strenuous exercise or physical labor. Discuss the relationship between weight-bearing activity and retention of calcium in the bones. Encourage all patients to remain as physically active as possible to prevent bone resorption (loss) and possible hypercalciuria.

Instruct patients with known gout to maintain a generous fluid intake so as to produce at least 2 L of urine every day. Discuss the risk of lithiasis with patients who have frequent UTIs, and teach measures to reduce the incidence of UTI and the risk for lithiasis.

Assessment

Obtain subjective and objective assessment data specific to urolithiasis:

- *Health history:* Complaints of flank, back, or abdominal pain, radiation, characteristics and timing, aggravating or relieving factors; other symptoms such as nausea and vomiting; possible contributing factors such as dehydration; previous or family history of kidney stones; current or previous treatment measures.
- *Physical examination:* General appearance including position, vital signs; skin color, temperature, moisture, turgor; abdominal, flank, or costovertebral tenderness; amount, color, and characteristics of urine (presence of hematuria, bacteria, pyuria, pH).

Nursing Diagnoses and Interventions

See the Case Study & Nursing Care Plan on page 799 for additional nursing diagnoses and interventions.

Acute Pain

Pain is the primary outward manifestation of urolithiasis, particularly when a stone lodges within a ureter, causing acute obstruction and distention. Invasive and noninvasive procedures to remove or crush stones also may be painful. Patients undergoing surgery also experience incisional pain.

- Assess pain using a standard pain scale and its characteristics. Administer analgesia as ordered and monitor its effectiveness. *The intensity, type of pain, and its responsiveness to analgesia provide valuable clues as to its cause. Regular administration of prescribed analgesics controls pain more effectively than waiting until pain becomes intolerable. Administering an ordered NSAID on a routine schedule may significantly reduce the need for narcotic analgesia in patients with renal colic.*
- Unless contraindicated, encourage fluid intake and ambulation in the patient with renal colic. *Increased fluids and ambulation increase urinary output, facilitating movement of the calculus through the ureter and decreasing pain.*
- Use nonpharmacologic measures such as positioning, moist heat, relaxation techniques, guided imagery, and diversion as adjunctive therapy for pain relief. *Adjunctive pain relief measures can enhance the effectiveness of analgesics and other prescribed treatment.*
- If surgery has been performed, monitor urinary output, catheters, incision, and wound drainage. *Pain may be a symptom of proximal distention due to a blocked catheter. Infection or hematoma at the surgical site can significantly increase perceived pain.*

Impaired Urinary Elimination

Obstruction of the urinary tract is the primary problem associated with urolithiasis. Obstruction can ultimately lead to stasis, infection, or irreversible renal damage.

- Monitor amount and character of urine output. If catheterized, measure output hourly. Document any hematuria, dysuria, frequency, urgency, and pyuria. Strain all urine for stones, saving any recovered stones for laboratory analysis. *The amount of urine output helps determine possible urinary*

EVIDENCE FOR NURSING CARE — The Patient with Urinary Calculi

Selected resources that nurses may find helpful when planning evidence-based nursing care follow.
- Baumgarten, D. A., Francis, I. R., Bluth, E. I., Bush, Jr., W. H., Casalino, D. D., Curry, N. S., et al. (2007). ACR Appropriateness Criteria® acute onset flank pain, suspicion of stone disease. *National Guideline Clearinghouse.* Retrieved from http://www.guideline.gov/summary/summary.aspx?doc_id=11563&nbr=005991&string=urinary+AND+calculi
- Tiselius, H., Alken, P., Buck C, Gallucci, M., Knoll, T., Sarica, K., et al. (2008 March). *Guidelines on urolithiasis.* Arnhem, The Netherlands: European Association of Urology (EAU. Retrieved from http://www.guideline.gov/summary/summary.aspx?ss=15&doc_id=12528&nbr=006452&string=urolithiasis

tract obstruction and adequacy of hydration. Hematuria, gross or microscopic, is often associated with calculi and with procedures used to remove stones, such as cystoscopy or lithotripsy. A change in the amount of hematuria may indicate stone passage or a complication. Dysuria, frequency, urgency, and cloudy urine are symptoms of UTI, often associated with urolithiasis. Antibiotic therapy may be required. Analysis of stones recovered from the urine can direct measures to prevent further lithiasis.

PRACTICE ALERT
A stone that completely obstructs the ureter can lead to hydronephrosis and kidney damage on the affected side. Report symptoms of hydronephrosis such as dull flank pain or aching and changes in renal function studies (BUN and serum creatinine). Because the other kidney continues to function, urine output may not fall significantly with obstruction of one ureter. A drop in eGFR or rising BUN and serum creatinine levels may be early signs of renal failure.

■ Maintain patency and integrity of all catheter systems. Secure catheters well, label as indicated, and use sterile technique for all ordered irrigations or other procedures. *A kinked or plugged catheter, particularly a ureteral catheter or nephrostomy tube, may damage the urinary system. Labeling catheters can prevent mistakes, such as inappropriate irrigation or clamping. Any catheter increases the risk of infection; aseptic technique in all procedures reduces this risk.*

Readiness for Enhanced Knowledge
The patient with urolithiasis has multiple learning needs. These include information about the disease and its possible consequences, any diagnostic or therapeutic procedures performed, and strategies to prevent future lithiasis.

■ Assess understanding and previous learning. *Relating information to previously learned material enhances retention and understanding.*
■ Present all material in a manner appropriate to knowledge base, developmental and educational level, and current needs. *Learning is an active process that requires the patient's participation. Tailoring teaching to the individual increases involvement.*
■ Teach about all diagnostic and treatment procedures. *Knowing what to expect reduces anxiety, enhances compliance, and hastens recovery.*
■ If the patient will be managed in the community, teach to
  ■ collect and strain all urine, saving any stones.
  ■ report stone passage to the physician and bring the stone in for analysis.
  ■ report any changes in the amount or character of urine output to physician.
  When pain can be managed with oral analgesics, urinary stones are managed in the community. The patient needs to know how and why to collect the calculus and indicators of complications, such as reduced urine output and cloudy or bloody urine.

■ Teach measures to prevent further urolithiasis:
  ■ Increase fluid intake to 2500 to 3500 mL per day.
  ■ Follow recommended dietary guidelines.
  ■ Maintain activity level to prevent urinary stasis and bone resorption.
  ■ Take medications as prescribed.
The risk of recurrent lithiasis is approximately 50%; however, this risk can be reduced by measures to prevent conditions favoring stone formation.
■ Teach about the relationship between urinary calculi and UTI, emphasizing preventive measures and the importance of prompt treatment. *Urinary tract infection promotes urolithiasis and thus requires prompt treatment to reduce this risk.*

Using NANDA, NIC, and NOC
Linkages between a selected NANDA nursing diagnosis, NIC, and NOC for the patient with urinary calculi are shown in the chart that follows.

Community-Based Care
The patient with urinary calculi needs to know how to manage existing stones and what to do to reduce the risk of future stone formation. Discuss the following topics to prepare the patient and family for home care:

■ Importance of maintaining a fluid intake adequate to produce 2.0 to 2.5 quarts of urine per day
■ Prescribed medications, their management, and potential adverse effects
■ Dietary recommendations
■ Prevention, recognition, and management of UTI
■ Any further diagnostic or treatment measures planned

When the patient is to be discharged with dressings, a nephrostomy tube, or a catheter, teach the patient and family about the following:

■ How to change dressings, maintaining aseptic technique
■ Assessment of the wound and skin for healing and possible complications such as infection or skin breakdown

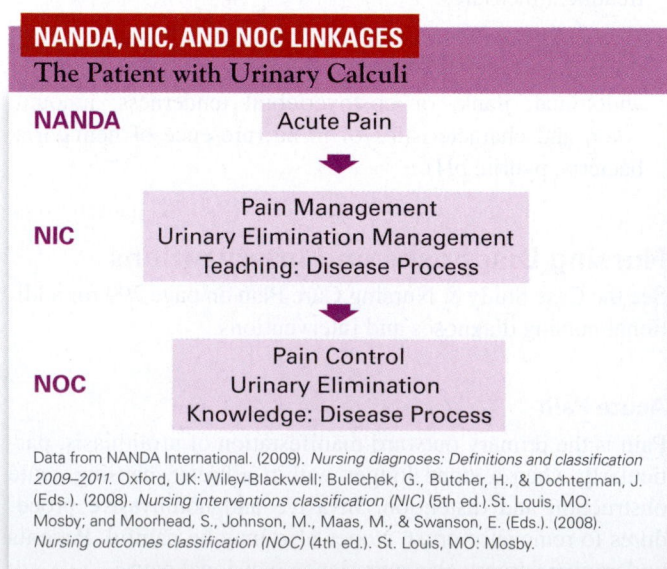

NANDA, NIC, AND NOC LINKAGES
The Patient with Urinary Calculi

NANDA → Acute Pain

NIC → Pain Management
Urinary Elimination Management
Teaching: Disease Process

NOC → Pain Control
Urinary Elimination
Knowledge: Disease Process

Data from NANDA International. (2009). *Nursing diagnoses: Definitions and classification 2009–2011.* Oxford, UK: Wiley-Blackwell; Bulechek, G., Butcher, H., & Dochterman, J. (Eds.). (2008). *Nursing interventions classification (NIC)* (5th ed.).St. Louis, MO: Mosby; and Moorhead, S., Johnson, M., Maas, M., & Swanson, E. (Eds.). (2008). *Nursing outcomes classification (NOC)* (4th ed.). St. Louis, MO: Mosby.

Figure 27–7 ■ Stages of bladde[r]... ness, beginning at the 3 o'clock pos[ition]... in a clockwise manner.

Tumors of the urinary tract typ[ically]... and may not be discovered unt[il]... flank pain or renal failure.

PRACTICE ALERT

Intermittent painless hematuria [is]... ing symptom of bladder cancer [...] less hematuria to contact their [...]

Interdisciplinary C[are]

Treatment of the patient with a t[umor depends]... on removing or destroying the can[cer]... invasion or metastasis, and mainta[ining]...

Diagnosis

When a urinary tract tumor is [suspected, diag]... nostic tests may be ordered:

- *Urinalysis* is done to evaluate [for hematuria. Micro]... scopic hematuria is often the [earliest sign of a tumor of]... the urinary tract.
- *Urine cytology*, microscopi[c examination of cells in the]... urine, is performed to iden[tify]...

TABLE 27–5 Surgical Proced[ures]

PROCEDURE	I[MPLICATIONS]
Transurethral resection of bladder tumor	D[...] b[...] b[...]
Partial cystectomy	R[...] s[...] t[...]
Complete or radical cystectomy	R[...] i[...]

Richard Leton, aged 44, owns a small business. He is admitted to the medical unit from the emergency department (ED) after awakening at 4:00 AM with severe right-sided pain. His CBC is normal, and urinalysis reveals microscopic hematuria, but no protein or bacteria. A renal ultrasound shows a 4- to 5-mm stone partially obstructing the right ureter.

Stephen Phillips, Mr. Leton's admitting nurse, notes that he is pale, diaphoretic, and very anxious. He complains of nausea and asks for an emesis basin. Mr. Leton received 4 mg of intravenous morphine sulphate and 20 mg nifedipine PO shortly after admission to the ED, approximately 2.5 hours ago. He denies pain at this time, but says, "I'm scared to death that it'll come back—I couldn't even move, it hurt so bad."

ASSESSMENT

Mr. Leton's history reveals no previous episodes of renal calculi. He felt well until the pain awakened him during the night. He admits that he has been working under a deadline to complete a construction project and that he probably has not been drinking enough fluids "considering how hot it's been." Physical assessment findings include T 100.4°F (38.0°C) PO, P 98, R 24, and BP 160/86. Color is pale to ashen, skin cool and moist. Abdomen firm with moderate tenderness in the right upper outer quadrant. The ED physician orders an IV of 5% dextrose in 1/2 normal saline at 200 mL/h until nausea relieved, then PO fluids of at least 3000 mL/24 h; nifedipine 20 mg PO every 8 hours; morphine sulfate (MS) 2 to 10 mg IV prn severe pain; indomethacin (Indocin) 50 mg per rectal suppository q8h; promethazine (Phenergan) 25 mg PO or per suppository q6h prn nausea; activity to tolerance; and strain all urine, sending recovered stones for analysis.

DIAGNOSES

- *Anxiety* related to anticipation of recurrent severe pain
- *Risk for Imbalanced Nutrition: Less than Body Requirements* related to nausea
- *Acute Pain* related to partial obstruction of right ureter by calculus
- *Impaired Urinary Elimination* related to partial obstruction of ureter by calculus
- *Readiness for Enhanced Knowledge* about disease process, contributing factors, and management

EXPECTED OUTCOMES

- Demonstrate reduced anxiety by relaxed facial expression, vital signs within his normal range, and ability to rest when not disturbed.
- Consume at least 50% of diet and 100% of ordered fluids without nausea or vomiting.
- Request analgesia as needed at onset of pain; report effective pain relief.
- Maintain urine output of 2500 mL/24 h with no signs of infection or obstruction (such as increased pain, dysuria, pyuria, or hematuria).
- Relate an understanding of the process of urolithiasis and contributing factors.
- Verbalize dietary and fluid intake, and other measures to reduce risk of future stone formation.

PLANNING AND IMPLEMENTATION

- Reassure that measures to prevent further episodes of renal colic are being implemented, and that medication is available to relieve pain promptly.
- Assess the effectiveness of analgesia and its adverse effects, especially nausea.
- Maintain IV as ordered until oral fluid intake exceeds 200 mL of fluid per hour while awake.
- Measure and strain all urine. Assess urine for color, clarity, and odor.
- Teach about urolithiasis and its risk factors, especially as they relate to Mr. Leton.
- Teach the importance of maintaining a high fluid intake, especially when working outdoors in hot weather, recommended dietary modifications and their rationale, ordered medications and their effects, how to identify and prevent UTI, and symptoms that should be reported to the physician.

EVALUATION

Mr. Leton passed the obstructing stone the evening after admission and is discharged the following day. On discharge, he denies pain or nausea, his urine is clear and pale yellow, and urinalysis is normal. Laboratory analysis shows that the calculus was calcium oxalate. Mr. Leton is able to state the importance of continuing a high fluid intake. He verbalizes that he will reduce his intake of sodium, modify his protein intake, and that he will increase his intake of foods to acidify his urine. He is able to list foods to include in his diet. He states, "You'd better believe I'll follow my diet, drink my water, and make sure I don't get an infection. I hope to never feel pain like that again!"

CRITICAL THINKING IN THE NURSING PROCESS

1. What factors contributed to the onset and timing of Mr. Leton's ureteral colic?
2. What is the rationale for administering indomethacin, an NSAID, to a patient with ureteral colic?
3. Why did Mr. Phillips include a nursing intervention to assess for a relationship between Mr. Leton's nausea, his pain, and the ordered analgesic agent?

See Evaluating Your Response in Appendix C.

- How to manage drainage systems and maintain their patency
- Emptying drainage bags and assessing urine output
- When to contact the physician and recommendations for follow-up care

The Patient with a Urinary Tract Tumor

A malignancy can develop in any part of the urinary tract; however, 90% develop in the bladder, about 8% develop in the renal pelvis, and only 2% develop in the ureter or urethra (Fauci et al., 2008). When diagnosed early, the 5-year survival rate for bladder cancer is 93% (American Cancer Society [ACS], 2009).

Incidence and Risk Factors

An estimated 70,980 new cases of bladder cancer were diagnosed in the United States in 2009, and 14,330 people died as a result of the disease. The incidence of bladder cancer is nearly four times higher in men than it is in women, and about twice as high in White men as it is in Black men (ACS, 2009). Most people who develop bladder cancer are over age 60.

Two major factors are implicated in the development of bladder cancer: the presence of carcinogens in the urine and chronic

inflammation or infection of bla
ing is the primary risk factor f
smokers is twice that of nonsm
cals and dyes used in the plastic
substances in the work environ
finishers, spray painters, and pe
els of arsenic in drinking water a
risk. Additional risk factors for b
in an urban area, chronic UTIs, a
Schistosoma haematobium, end
also increases the risk for blac
2009). The risk for bladder ca
increasing the intake of fluids an

FAST FACTS

The major risk factors for bladde
- Male gender, aged > 60, res
- Cigarette smoking
- Occupational exposure to dy
- Chronic UTI or bladder calcul

Pathophysiology

Most urinary tract malignancie
Transitional epithelium lines th
pelvis through the urethra. Carc
of certain chemicals and from ci
the urine and stored in the blad
influence on abnormal cell devel
noma of the urinary tract occur
tional epithelial cell tumors.

Urinary tract tumors begin as
that develop into either flat or pa
may be either superficial or invas
papillary lesions (*papillomas*), a
by a stalk to the bladder mucosa
are generally superficial, noninva
and frequently recur (Fauci et al.
to become invasive, and the prog

Carcinoma *in situ* (CIS), whic
poorly differentiated flat tumor
associated with a poorer progno
tially present as superficial le

TABLE 27–4 Bladder Tumor St

DEPTH OF INVOLVEMENT	STAGE
Superficial	Cis
	I
Invasive	II
	III
	IV

NURSING CARE OF THE PATIENT   Having a Cystectomy and Urinary Diversion

PREOPERATIVE CARE

- Provide routine preoperative care as outlined in ∞ Chapter 4.
- Assess knowledge of the proposed surgery and its long-term implications, clarifying misunderstandings and discussing concerns. *Patients having surgery for cancer of the urinary tract are trying to cope with the diagnosis of cancer and may not fully understand the surgery and its potential effects. Open discussion can facilitate postoperative recovery and adjustment.*
- Begin teaching about postoperative tubes and drains, self-care of stoma, and control of drainage and odor. *Postoperative physiologic and psychologic stressors may interfere with learning. A basic understanding of what to expect in the way of tubes, drains, and procedures reduces stress in the immediate postoperative period. Preoperative teaching can enhance recall and postoperative learning.*
- Assist in identifying stoma site, avoiding folds of skin, bones, scar tissue, and the waistline or belt area. Be sure to consider the patient's occupation and style of clothing. The site should be visible to the patient and accessible for manipulation. *Stoma placement is a vital component of adjustment and self-care. Care is taken to place the stoma away from areas of constant irritation by clothing or movement. It should be located so that the patient can cover and disguise the collecting device, maintain the seal to prevent leakage, and effectively cleanse and maintain the site.*
- Perform bowel-preparation activities as ordered. *Bowel preparation is done to prevent fecal contamination of the peritoneal cavity and to decompress the bowel during surgery.*

POSTOPERATIVE CARE

- Provide routine postoperative care (∞ see Chapter 4).
- Monitor intake and output carefully, assessing urine output every hour for the first 24 hours, then every 4 hours or as ordered. Call the physician if urine output is less than 30 mL per hour. *Tissue edema and bleeding may interfere with urinary output from stoma, catheters, or drains. Maintenance of urine outflow is vital to prevent hydronephrosis and possible renal damage. A urine output of at least 30 mL per hour is necessary for effective renal function.*
- Assess color and consistency of urine. Expect pink or bright red urine fading to pink and then clearing by the third postoperative day. Urine may be cloudy due to mucus production by bowel mucosa. *Bright red blood in the urine from a urinary diversion may indicate hemorrhage, necessitating further surgery. Excessive cloudiness or malodorous urine may indicate infection.*
- Assess size, color, and condition of the stoma and surrounding skin every 2 hours for the first 24 hours, then every 4 hours for 48 to 72 hours. Expect the stoma to appear bright red and slightly edematous initially. Slight bleeding during cleansing is normal. *Compromised circulation causes the stoma to appear pale, gray, or cyanotic or blanch when touched. Other complications, such as infection or impaired healing, may be evidenced by a change in the appearance of the stoma or incision.*
- Irrigate the ileal diversion catheter with 30 to 60 mL of normal saline every 4 hours or as ordered. *Mucus produced by the bowel wall may accumulate in the newly devised reservoir or obstruct catheters.*
- Monitor serum electrolyte values, acid–base balance, and renal function tests such as BUN and serum creatinine. *Reabsorption of electrolytes from reservoirs created by portions of bowel may result in electrolyte imbalance and metabolic acidosis. Optimal renal function is necessary to maintain a normal state of homeostasis.*
- Teach the patient and family about stoma and urinary diversion care, including odor management, skin care, increased fluid intake, pouch application and leakage prevention, self-catheterization for patients with continent reservoirs, and signs of infection and other complications. *The ability to provide self-care is a significant factor in the adjustment to a changed body image. Teaching family members facilitates acceptance and adjustment. The family also needs this knowledge in case illness or disability interferes with the self-care capacity.*

---

effect on skin. In addition, adhesives and sealants used to prevent pouch leakage may irritate the skin.

- Assess peristomal skin for redness, excoriation, or signs of breakdown. Assess for urine leakage from catheters, stents, or drains. Keep the skin clean and dry. Change wet dressings. *Intact skin is the first line of defense against infection. Impaired skin integrity may lead to local or systemic infection and impaired healing.*
- Ensure gravity drainage of urine collection device or empty bag every 2 hours. *Overfilling of the collection bag may damage the seal, allowing leakage and contact of urine with skin.*
- Change urine collection appliance as needed, removing any mucus from stoma. See Box 27–2 for care of a urinary drainage stoma. *Meticulous care and protection of skin surrounding stoma can maintain integrity and prevent breakdown.*

Disturbed Body Image

A radical cystectomy and urinary diversion affect the patient's body image. In most cases, an abdominal stoma is created, requiring either a drainage appliance or regular catheterization of the stoma to drain urine. Removal of the prostate and seminal vesicles or the uterus and ovaries leaves the patient sterile. If radiation or chemotherapy is planned as adjunctive therapy, the patient may experience hair loss, stomatitis, nausea and vomiting, or other disturbing side effects of therapy.

- Use therapeutic communication techniques, actively listening and responding to the patient's and family's concerns. *Patients must know their feelings and concerns are respected and valued. Denial, anger, guilt, bargaining, or depression are common during grieving and normal for a patient undergoing a significant change in body image.*
- Recognize and accept behaviors that indicate use of coping mechanisms, encouraging adaptive mechanisms. *The patient may initially use defensive coping mechanisms such as denial, minimization, and dissociation from the immediate situation to reduce anxiety and maintain psychologic integrity. Adaptive mechanisms include learning as much as possible about the surgery and its effects, practicing procedures, setting realistic goals, and rehearsing various alternative outcomes.*

CASE STUDY & NURSING CARE PLAN   A Patient with a Bladder Tumor

Ben Hussain is a 61-year-old automobile salesman. He is married and has five children, all of whom are grown and living away from home. One week ago, Mr. Hussain became alarmed when his urine became bright red. Even though he had no other symptoms, he called his physician. The physician ordered a urinalysis and urine cytology, revealing gross hematuria and poorly differentiated abnormal cells. Cystoscopy and tissue biopsy confirm a stage C tumor involving the bladder trigone. Mr. Hussain is admitted for a radical cystectomy and continent urinary diversion.

ASSESSMENT

Mr. Hussain's admission history, obtained by Tara Mills, RN, his primary nurse, indicates that he has lost 10 to 15 pounds during the last few months. He smoked two to three packs of cigarettes per day for 40 years, but cut back to a pack a day about a year ago. He says he could not quit smoking entirely. He drinks five to six cups of coffee daily and consumes a moderate amount of alcohol, averaging three to four drinks a day. Mr. Hussain says that he is "a little nervous about surgery and what they're going to find." Ms. Mills notes that he fidgets and talks rapidly throughout their interview. He also expresses concern about how he will handle the pain after surgery, because he had never been hospitalized before his cystoscopy. Physical assessment findings include T 98.2°F (36.7°C) PO, P 84, R 18, and BP 154/86. Examinations of the skin, neuromuscular, and cardiac systems are within normal limits. Scattered expiratory crackles are noted on auscultation of lung fields. Bowel sounds are very active; Mr. Hussain explains that he began taking his bowel-preparation laxative the day before admission. Slight tenderness is noted in the suprapubic region. Mr. Hussain's urine is clear and bright pink. CBC and chemistry screening results are within normal limits. Surgery is planned for 9:00 AM the following day.

DIAGNOSES

- *Anxiety* related to undetermined extent of disease and fear of pain
- *Readiness for Enhanced Knowledge* related to care and management of continent urinary diversion
- *Impaired Urinary Elimination* related to cystectomy and urinary diversion
- *Risk for Impaired Gas Exchange* related to smoking history and effects of anesthesia

EXPECTED OUTCOMES

- Verbalize decreased feelings of anxiety.
- Demonstrate appropriate postoperative pain relief through subjective reports of pain severity and objective findings.
- Be able to care for urinary diversion and surrounding skin prior to discharge.
- Demonstrate self-catheterization of stoma using appropriate technique prior to discharge.

- Maintain normal urine output with acceptable color and clarity and no signs of infection.
- Maintain adequate gas exchange as evidenced by good skin color, O_2 saturation greater than 95%, and clear lung sounds on auscultation.

PLANNING AND IMPLEMENTATION

- Spend as much time as possible with Mr. Hussain and his family preoperatively, answering questions fully and encouraging expression of fears.
- Provide written and verbal explanations when feasible.
- Administer analgesia on a regular basis for the first 48 to 72 hours. Monitor for objective signs of unrelieved pain.
- Explain all procedures related to stoma and diversion care as they are being performed.
- Encourage Mr. Hussain to look at stoma and touch it when ready.
- Teach stoma and skin care, as well as self-catheterization, emphasizing measures to prevent skin irritation and urinary tract infection.
- Monitor urine output, color, clarity, and consistency every hour for first 24 hours, then every 4 hours for 24 hours, then every 8 hours. Report output of less than 30 mL per hour, bright bleeding, excessively cloudy or malodorous urine.
- Assist with use of incentive spirometer every hour while awake. Ambulate as soon as possible. Assess lung sounds every 4 hours, reporting increased crackles or diminished breath sounds.
- Refer Mr. and Mrs. Hussain to local stoma group on discharge.

EVALUATION

On discharge, Mr. Hussain has performed self-catheterization and stoma and skin care several times. His wife also is able to catheterize the stoma and demonstrate skin care. His urine is pale yellow and slightly cloudy. Mr. Hussain is ambulating independently and using oxycodone (Percocet) twice a day for pain relief. His lungs are clear, and he is very proud of having "survived" 7 days without a cigarette. He says, "Now I'm going to shoot for 7 weeks, then 7 months, then 7 years without a smoke!" A home health referral is made to continue teaching Mr. Hussain to care for his diversion and appliance.

CRITICAL THINKING IN THE NURSING PROCESS

1. How does cigarette smoking contribute to the increased risk of urinary tract tumors?
2. Suppose Mr. Hussain had become confused, disoriented, and tremorous and had begun to experience visual hallucinations 2 to 3 days postoperatively. What would you suspect the cause to be? What would be the appropriate response?
3. Develop a care plan for Mr. Hussain for the nursing diagnosis *Risk for Sexual Dysfunction*.

See Evaluating Your Response in Appendix C.

- Encourage looking at, touching, and caring for the stoma and appliance as soon as possible. Allow the patient to proceed gradually, providing support and encouragement. *Accepting the stoma as part of the self is vital to adapting to the changed body image and is indicated by a willingness to provide self-care.*
- Discuss concerns about returning to usual activities, perceived relationship changes, and resumption of sexual relations. Provide referral to support group or provide for contact with someone who has successfully adjusted to a urinary

diversion. *Patients and families may be reluctant to discuss topics of concern. An atmosphere of openness and acceptance facilitates expression of concerns and anxieties related to the changed body image.*

Risk for Infection

Diagnostic instrumentation procedures, surgical manipulation, and disruption of normal urinary tract defense mechanisms increase the risk of ascending urinary tract infection. When an ileal conduit or artificial bladder is created using bowel tissue, the normal bacteriostatic activity of bladder mucosa is lost. In addition, the peristaltic action of the ureters may be disrupted, and the vesicoureteral junction no longer prevents urine reflux. Adjunctive chemotherapy or radiation treatments may impair normal immune function and further increase the risk of infection.

- Maintain separate closed drainage systems, keeping drainage bags lower than the kidney, and prevent loops or kinks in drainage tubing, which impede urine flow. *Although urine is sterile when it leaves the kidney, bacteria grow rapidly in urine. Prevention of urine reflux is essential to preventing UTI.*
- Monitor for signs of infection: elevated temperature, cloudy or foul-smelling urine, hematuria, general malaise, back or abdominal pain, and nausea and vomiting. *Infection undermines the healing process. Early detection and treatment help prevent long-term consequences such as chronic pyelonephritis.*

PRACTICE ALERT
Impaired immune function (due to aging or the effects of chemotherapy) and urine cloudiness (related to the effects of urine on ileal mucosa) can mask usual signs of UTI such as fever and altered urine clarity. Be alert for more generalized manifestations such as increased fatigue and malaise.

- Teach signs and symptoms of infection and self-care measures to prevent UTI. *The patient with a cystectomy and ileal diversion, urostomy, or continent reservoir is at risk of UTI for life because of impaired urinary defense mechanisms. Using clean or aseptic technique in providing care, increasing fluid intake, and using measures to acidify urine minimize this risk to a certain degree but do not eliminate it.*

Community-Based Care
The need for individual and family teaching for the patient who has had surgery to treat a urinary tract tumor is significant. For many patients, surgery means a lifelong change in urinary elimination. Even the patient who has undergone transurethral excision of bladder tumors requires follow-up cystoscopy on a regular basis and needs to be alert for signs of tumor recurrence.

The patient who has had a urinary diversion needs teaching about care of the stoma and surrounding skin, prevention of urine reflux and infection, signs and symptoms of UTI and renal calculi, and, in some cases, self-catheterization using clean technique.

The Patient with Urinary Retention

Urinary retention, incomplete emptying of the bladder, can lead to overdistention of the bladder, poor detrusor muscle contractility, and inability to urinate. If the problem persists, hydroureter and hydronephrosis can result.

Physiology Review
Normally, bladder emptying is controlled by the interaction of muscle tone and the autonomic nervous system. The sympathetic nervous system (SNS) relaxes the detrusor muscle, allowing the bladder to fill with urine. The internal sphincter, a

continuation of the detrusor muscle, remains closed during filling. Pressures within the bladder remain low during filling, in contrast to high sphincter and urethral pressures. Voluntary muscles of the external sphincter and pelvic floor help maintain these high pressures. When the bladder contains 150 to 300 mL of urine, signals from stretch receptors in the bladder wall are transmitted to the spinal cord and cerebral cortex. Reflexive bladder emptying can be consciously inhibited. During *micturition* (bladder emptying), parasympathetic stimulation causes the detrusor muscle of the bladder fundus to contract, opening the internal sphincter. The external sphincter then relaxes, allowing urine to flow out.

Pathophysiology
Either mechanical obstruction of the bladder outlet or a functional problem can cause urinary retention. *Benign prostatic hypertrophy (BPH)* is a common cause; difficulty initiating and maintaining urine flow is often the presenting complaint in men with BPH. Fecal impaction may be a contributing factor in urinary retention, particularly in older adults or immobile patients. Acute inflammation associated with infection or trauma of the bladder, urethra, or perineal tissues may also interfere with micturition. Scarring due to repeated UTI can lead to urethral stricture and a mechanical obstruction. Bladder calculi may also obstruct the urethral opening from the bladder.

Surgery, particularly abdominal or pelvic surgery, may disrupt detrusor muscle function, leading to urine retention. Drugs also may interfere with its function. Anticholinergic medications such as atropine, glycopyrrolate (Robinul), propantheline bromide (Pro-Banthine), scopolamine hydrochloride (Transderm-Scop), and others can lead to acute urinary retention and bladder distention. Many other drug groups have anticholinergic side effects and may cause urinary retention. Among these are antianxiety agents such as diazepam (Valium), antidepressant and tricyclic drugs such as imipramine (Tofranil), antiparkinsonian drugs, antipsychotic agents, and some sedative/hypnotic drugs. In addition, antihistamines common in over-the-counter cough, cold, allergy, and sleep-promoting drugs have anticholinergic effects and may interfere with bladder emptying. Diphenhydramine (Benadryl) is an example of a nonprescription antihistamine.

Voluntary urinary retention (particularly common among nurses!) may lead to overfilling of the bladder and a loss of detrusor muscle tone.

Manifestations
The patient with urinary retention is unable to empty the bladder completely. Overflow voiding or incontinence may occur, with 25 to 50 mL of urine eliminated at frequent intervals. Assessment reveals a firm, distended bladder that may be displaced to one side of midline. Percussion of the lower abdomen reveals a dull tone, reflective of fluid in the bladder.

Severe urinary retention with resulting bladder distention impairs the ability of the vesicoureteral junction to prevent backflow of urine into the ureters (see Figure 27–1 on page 784). Reflux of urine from the distended bladder distends the ureters (hydroureter) and kidneys (hydronephrosis).

Hydronephrosis impairs renal function, and acute renal failure can result. ∞ See Chapter 28 for more information about acute renal failure.

Interdisciplinary Care

Urinary retention is confirmed using a bladder scan or by inserting a urinary catheter (if possible) and measuring the urine output. Use of a bladder scan is preferred to reduce the risk of UTI.

An indwelling urinary catheter or intermittent straight catheterization can prevent urinary retention and overdistention of the bladder. Cholinergic medications such as bethanechol chloride (Urecholine), which promote detrusor muscle contraction and bladder emptying, may be used. A medication with no anticholinergic side effects may be substituted when urinary retention is related to drug therapy.

Mechanical obstructions are treated by removing or repairing the obstruction when possible. Resection of the prostate gland may be done for urinary retention related to BPH. Bladder calculi are removed, and measures to prevent their formation are instituted.

℘ Nursing Care

Health promotion measures to prevent urinary retention include monitoring urine output in at-risk patients and evaluating drug regimens for medications known to interfere with detrusor muscle function. Pay particular attention to elimination when these drugs are ordered for (or used by) a patient with BPH or other mechanical obstruction of urine flow.

Impaired Urinary Elimination

Nursing measures to promote urination include placing the patient in normal voiding position and providing for privacy. Additional measures include running water, placing the patient's hands in warm water, pouring warm water over the perineum, or taking a warm sitz bath.

In acute urinary retention, catheterization may be necessary to relieve bladder distention and prevent hydronephrosis. Use a relatively small catheter (16 Fr. for a man, 14 Fr. for a woman). A coudé-tipped catheter is passed more easily in the older man with an enlarged prostate. Using 2% lidocaine gel (10 mL injected into the male urethra or 6 mL injected into the female urethra) reduces discomfort during catheterization and the risk of catheter-associated infection and promotes pelvic muscle relaxation (Bardsley, 2005). Carefully observe the patient as the distended bladder drains.

> **PRACTICE ALERT**
> Some patients may experience a vasovagal response, becoming pale, sweaty, and hypotensive if the bladder is rapidly drained. Draining urine in 500-mL increments and clamping the catheter for 5 to 10 minutes between increments may prevent this response. Hematuria also may occur with rapid bladder decompression. Promptly notify the physician if hematuria develops.

Home care for the patient with urinary retention varies, depending on the cause. Some patients may be taught intermittent self-catheterization. Instruct all patients who have experienced urinary retention to avoid over-the-counter drugs that affect micturition, especially those with an anticholinergic effect (allergy and cold medications, many nonprescription sleep aids). Other home care measures include double-voiding (urinate, remain on the toilet for 2 to 5 minutes, then urinate again), scheduled voiding, or, when other measures fail, an indwelling catheter. When an indwelling catheter is necessary, teach the patient and family to use clean technique when changing from overnight bag to leg bag, and to promptly report signs of UTI to the primary care provider.

The Patient with Neurogenic Bladder

The neurologic connections influencing bladder filling, the perception of fullness and the need to void, and bladder emptying are complex. Disruption of the central or peripheral nervous systems may interfere with normal mechanisms, causing **neurogenic bladder**.

Pathophysiology

As noted in the physiology section on urinary retention, bladder filling and emptying are controlled by the central nervous system (CNS). This neurologic control can be disrupted at any level: the cerebral cortex (voluntary impulses), the micturition center of the midbrain, the spinal cord tracts, or the peripheral nerves of the bladder itself.

Spastic Bladder Dysfunction

A simple reflex arc exists between the bladder and the spinal cord at levels S_2 through S_4. The stimulus of more than 400 mL of urine in the bladder causes reflex contraction of the detrusor muscle and bladder emptying unless voluntary control (cerebral input) is used to suppress it. Disruption of CNS transmission above the sacral spinal cord segment typically leads to *spastic neurogenic bladder*. Both sensory and voluntary control of urination are interrupted partially or totally, while the sacral reflex arc remains intact. The stimuli generated by bladder filling cause frequent spontaneous detrusor muscle contraction and involuntary bladder emptying. Spinal cord injury above the sacral segment is the most common cause of a spastic bladder. Other causes include stroke, multiple sclerosis, and other CNS lesions.

Flaccid Bladder Dysfunction

Damage to the sacral spinal cord at the level of the reflex arc, the cauda equina, or the sacral nerve roots causes loss of detrusor muscle tone and a *flaccid neurogenic bladder*. The perception of bladder fullness is lost, and the bladder becomes overdistended, with weak and ineffective detrusor muscle contractions. Flaccid neurogenic bladder is seen with myelomeningocele and during the spinal shock phase of a spinal cord injury above the sacral region. During the spinal shock phase, all reflex activity below the level of spinal cord injury is suppressed.

Peripheral neuropathies may also cause bladder atony and overfilling. Either sensory or motor pathways (or both) may be disrupted, leading to incomplete bladder emptying and large residual volumes after voiding. Diabetes mellitus is the most common cause of peripheral bladder neuropathy. Other causes include multiple sclerosis, chronic alcoholism, and prolonged overdistention of the bladder.

Interdisciplinary Care

Management of neurogenic bladder focuses on maintaining continence and avoiding complications associated with over-filling or incomplete emptying of the bladder. Because self-care is the goal, teaching is a primary intervention for the healthcare team.

Diagnosis

The following diagnostic tests may be ordered for the patient with a neurogenic bladder:

- *Urine culture* to detect possible UTI related to impaired bladder function.
- *Urinalysis* and *eGFR, serum creatinine* and *BUN* to evaluate renal function. See Table 28–2 on page 826 for normal BUN and creatinine levels. Ascending infection or hydronephrosis

resulting from bladder overfilling and vesicoureteral reflux can damage the kidneys. Impaired renal function may lead to blood cells or protein in the urine, and elevated BUN and creatinine levels.

- *Postvoid bladder scan* to measure residual urine. Amounts greater than 50 mL may indicate ineffective detrusor muscle contractions, common in neurogenic bladder.
- *Cystometrography* to evaluate bladder filling and the detrusor muscle tone and function. See page 774 for nursing care of the patient undergoing cystometrography.

Medications

Medications may be prescribed to increase or decrease the contractility of the detrusor muscle, to increase or decrease the tone of the internal sphincter, or to relax the external urethral sphincter.

Bethanechol, a cholinergic drug, stimulates detrusor muscle contraction in flaccid neurogenic bladder. It is generally used to manage short-term urinary retention (e.g., following surgery or childbirth). It may be used in combination with bladder-training techniques to promote complete emptying of a neurogenic

---

MEDICATION ADMINISTRATION   **The Patient with Neurogenic Bladder**

ANTICHOLINERGIC DRUGS TO TREAT SPASTIC BLADDER

Darifenacin (Enablex)

Oxybutynin (Ditropan, Ditropan XL)

Solifenacin succinate (VESIcare)

Trospium (Sanctura)

Tolterodine (Detrol, Detrol LA)

Propantheline bromide (Pro-Banthine)

Flavoxate hydrochloride (Urispas)

Anticholinergic drugs inhibit the response to acetylcholine, relaxing the detrusor muscle and increasing internal sphincter tone. The combination of detrusor relaxation and internal sphincter contraction increases the bladder capacity of patients with spastic or hyperreflexive neurogenic bladder. Of these medications, darifenacin, solifenacin succinate, and tolterodine have the most specific effects on the detrusor muscle with fewer anticholinergic side effects.

Nursing Responsibilities

- Assess for contraindications, such as glaucoma, gastrointestinal or urinary tract obstruction, severe ulcerative colitis or toxic megacolon, unstable cardiovascular status, or myasthenia gravis.
- Observe for the desired effect of increased bladder capacity with decreased incontinence and spasm.
- Monitor for possible interaction with other drugs such as narcotic analgesics, antidysrhythmic medications, antihistamines, antidepressants, or psychoactive drugs.
- Monitor heart rate and blood pressure, especially when given to patients with known cardiovascular disease.
- Assess for adverse effects such as urinary hesitancy or retention, dysrhythmias, mental status changes, and gastrointestinal disturbances.

Health Education for the Patient and Family

- Take the drug as ordered. Some of these drugs (e.g., trospium) need to be taken on an empty stomach for optimal absorption, others may be taken irrespective of food intake.
- Promptly report eye pain, rapid heart beat, difficulty breathing, rash or hives, or changes in mental function to your primary care provider.

- These drugs may cause drowsiness or blurred vision. Use caution when driving, operating machinery, or performing other tasks requiring mental acuity.
- Hard candies help relieve dry mouth associated with these drugs.
- Do not use alcohol or nonprescription antihistamines while taking these drugs.

CHOLINERGIC DRUGS TO STIMULATE MICTURITION

Bethanechol chloride (Urecholine)

Bethanechol stimulates the parasympathetic nervous system, increasing detrusor muscle tone and producing a contraction strong enough to initiate micturition. It is used primarily to treat acute postoperative and postpartum urinary retention.

Nursing Responsibilities

- Assess for contraindications, including hypersensitivity, hyperthyroidism, peptic ulcer disease, asthma, significant bradycardia or hypotension, coronary heart disease, epilepsy, and parkinsonism.
- Do not give to patients who have had recent gastrointestinal or bladder surgery or those with possible gastrointestinal or urinary tract obstruction.
- Give oral forms on an empty stomach to reduce the risk of nausea and vomiting.
- Administer parenteral bethanechol subcutaneously. Keep atropine, the antidote for bethanechol overdose or toxicity, available.
- Observe for desired effect within 30 to 60 minutes after oral administration, 5 to 15 minutes after injection.
- Assess for adverse effects such as malaise, headache, abdominal cramping, nausea, hypotension with reflex tachycardia, wheezing, and dyspnea.

Health Education for the Patient and Family

- Take the medication 1 hour before or 2 hours after meals.
- Use caution when rising from a recumbent or sitting position; you may feel dizzy or light-headed.

bladder. Anticholinesterase drugs such as neostigmine (Prostigmin) and pyridostigmine (Mestinon) also may be used to increase detrusor muscle tone.

Anticholinergic drugs (parasympathetic blockers) relax the detrusor muscle and contract the internal sphincter, increasing bladder capacity in patients with spastic bladder dysfunction. Oxybutynin (Ditropan), tolterodine (Detrol), darifenacin (Enablex), solifenacin succinate (VESIcare), and trospium (Sanctura) inhibit the muscarinic effects of acetylcholine on smooth muscle, reducing detrusor muscle spasticity and promoting bladder filling. Other anticholinergic drugs also may be used, including propantheline (Pro-Banthine) or flavoxate (Urispas). Dry mouth, blurred vision, and constipation are potential adverse effects of anticholinergic medications. See the Medication Administration box for drugs used to modify detrusor muscle activity on the previous page.

Nutrition

Dietary measures to reduce the risk for UTI and urinary calculi may be suggested for the patient with neurogenic bladder. A moderate to high fluid intake and a diet that acidifies the urine are helpful. Cranberry juice is recommended to maintain urine acidity. See Table 27–3 for additional foods to include or avoid in the diet to help prevent UTI and urolithiasis. The timing of fluid intake may be regulated to promote continence.

Bladder Retraining

Patients with spastic neurogenic bladder may use measures to stimulate reflex voiding, allowing scheduled toileting. Techniques include using trigger points, for example, stroking or pinching the abdomen, inner thigh, or glans penis. Pulling pubic hairs, tapping the suprapubic region, or inserting a gloved finger into the rectum and gently stretching the anal sphincter can also stimulate urination.

The *Credé's method* (applying pressure to the suprapubic region with the fingers of one or both hands), manual pressure on the abdomen, and the Valsalva maneuver (bearing down while holding one's breath) promote bladder emptying for the patient with a spastic or flaccid bladder.

> **PRACTICE ALERT**
> Increasing lower abdominal and bladder pressure with the Credé's method can stimulate autonomic dysreflexia in some patients with spinal cord injuries. Autonomic dysreflexia is a medical emergency in which the blood pressure rises rapidly due to SNS stimulation.

See Chapter 44 for a discussion of autonomic dysreflexia.

The patient with a flaccid bladder may require catheterization to completely empty the bladder. An indwelling catheter may be used initially, but intermittent catheterization is preferred. Clean intermittent self-catheterization is performed every 3 to 4 hours to prevent overdistention of the bladder (see Procedure 43–1).

Surgery

Surgery may be required when urination cannot be effectively managed using more conservative measures. *Rhizotomy*, or destruction of the nerve supply to the detrusor muscle or the external sphincter, may be used for patients with hyperreflexia

or spasticity. Urinary diversion is another surgical technique used when conservative management fails. Implantation of an artificial sphincter may be useful for some patients with neurogenic bladder. See Table 27–6 for urinary diversion techniques and page 802 for nursing care of the patient undergoing a urinary diversion.

Nursing Care

Nursing care of the patient with a neurogenic bladder is directed toward promoting urinary drainage and continence, preventing complications, and teaching the patient and family self-care techniques.

Assessment

Nursing assessment for neurogenic bladder includes obtaining a complete nursing history, focusing on information related to CNS or spinal cord injury or disease, as well as disorders that affect the peripheral nervous system (e.g., diabetes). Ask about measures used to stimulate or control urination. Inspect and palpate the lower abdomen and suprapubic region for tenderness or bladder distention. Percuss the suprapubic region for a dull percussion tone indicative of a full bladder. Dullness up to the level of the umbilicus indicates at least 500 mL of urine in the bladder (Gray, 2000). Assess urine for color, clarity, and odor. Collect a specimen for analysis as indicated.

Nursing Diagnoses and Interventions

Although each patient has individual nursing care needs, examples of nursing diagnoses appropriate for the patient with a neurogenic bladder include the following:

- *Impaired Urinary Elimination* related to impaired bladder innervation
- *Toileting Self-Care Deficit* related to neurologic injury
- *Risk for Impaired Skin Integrity* related to urinary incontinence
- *Risk for Infection* related to impaired urination reflex

Community-Based Care

Include the following in teaching for the patient with neurogenic bladder and family members:

- Measures to stimulate reflex voiding and promote bladder emptying
- Use of prescribed medications, including desired and adverse effects, and interactions with other drugs
- Manifestations of UTI or urolithiasis, and measures to reduce the risk of these complications

The Patient with Urinary Incontinence

The most common manifestation of impaired bladder control is **urinary incontinence (UI)**, or involuntary urination. UI can have a significant impact on patients, leading to physical problems such as skin breakdown, infection, and rashes. Psychosocial consequences include embarrassment, isolation and withdrawal, feelings of worthlessness and helplessness, and depression.

NURSING CARE OF THE OLDER ADULT   **Minimizing the Risk for UTI and UI**

Older adults have a higher incidence of two common urinary tract disorders: UTI and UI.

URINARY TRACT INFECTION

Aging affects normal protective mechanisms to prevent UTI. The pH of urine increases with aging, allowing bacteria to grow and multiply more readily. Glucosuria, more common in older adults due to the higher incidence of diabetes, facilitates bacterial growth. Incomplete bladder emptying and urinary retention are more common due to problems such as prostatic hypertrophy in men, bladder prolapse in women, and neurogenic bladder in both sexes. Changes in vaginal pH in women and decreased prostatic secretions in men may also contribute to an increased incidence of UTI.

While many UTIs in older adults are asymptomatic and self-limited, infections can lead to bacteremia, sepsis, and shock. Manifestations of UTI in the elderly include dysuria, urgency, frequency, incontinence, occasional hematuria, and confusion. Symptoms such as fever, chills, and flank pain and tenderness may be absent. Dementia may make diagnosis more difficult.

URINARY INCONTINENCE

UI, the involuntary loss of urine, is a common problem in older adults. While incontinence should never be considered a *normal* consequence of aging, age-related changes contribute to its development. Bladder capacity tends to decline with age and involuntary bladder muscle contractions are more common. Fluid ingested during the day tends to be excreted later in the day and into the night. In women, decreased estrogen levels and pelvic muscle relaxation decrease bladder outlet and urethral resistance pressures. Decreased estrogen also causes atrophic vaginitis and urethritis, with manifestations of dysuria and urgency. In men, the prostate enlarges with aging. Other risk factors for UI in older adults include impaired mobility and chronic degenerative diseases, impaired cognition, medications, low fluid intake, diabetes, and stroke.

Assessing for Home Care

Assessment for urinary problems in the older adult focuses on risk factors, the extent and manifestations of the disorder, and contributing factors. Using clear language, ask about problems with urine loss, its frequency, and any contributing factors. Inquire about frequency, urgency, and burning on urination. Identify current medications and the time of day each is taken. Assess patterns of fluid intake and output. Assess the abdomen for evidence of bladder distention or tenderness. Perform a mental status examination if indicated.

Assess the home environment (whether in the community or a residential living facility) for possible barriers to urinary elimination:

- Inadequate lighting, particularly at night
- Narrow doorways that may interfere with access to the toilet
- Inadequate toilet facilities
- The need for mobility aids such as safety bars, a raised toilet seat, or a bedside commode

Teaching for Home Care

Discuss the following points to help prevent UTI and UI in the older adult:

- Maintain a generous fluid intake. Reduce or eliminate fluid intake after the evening meal to reduce nocturia.
- Wear comfortable clothing that is easy to remove for toileting.
- Maintain good hygiene, but do not bathe more often than necessary; frequent bathing and feminine hygiene sprays or douches may dry perineal tissues, increasing the risk of UTI or UI.
- Perform pelvic muscle exercises (Kegel exercises) several times a day to increase perineal muscle tone.
- Reduce consumption of caffeine-containing beverages (coffee, tea, colas), citrus juices, and artificially sweetened beverages containing NutraSweet.
- Use behavioral techniques such as scheduled toileting, habit training, and bladder training to reduce the frequency of incontinence. *Scheduled toileting* is toileting at regular intervals (e.g., every 2 to 4 hours). *Habit training* is toileting the patient on a schedule that corresponds with the normal pattern. *Bladder training* gradually increases the bladder capacity by increasing the intervals between voidings and resisting the urge to void.
- See your primary care provider regularly for a pelvic or prostate exam.
- For women, discuss possible benefits and risks of hormone replacement therapy, physical therapy, or surgery to treat incontinence.
- Report a change in urine color, odor, or clarity, or symptoms such as burning, frequency, or urgency to your primary care provider.

Resources for Home Care

- National Association for Continence website

Incidence and Prevalence

Up to 25 million people in the United States have some degree of urinary incontinence. The estimated cost of managing UI is $14.2 billion yearly (Bradway et al., 2008). UI is especially common among older patients (see the box above). UI often leads to institutionalization; in long-term care, foster care, and homebound populations, the incidence is more than 50% (National Association for Continence, 2009; NKUDIC, 2009). The actual prevalence of urinary incontinence is nearly impossible to determine. Embarrassment and the availability of products to protect clothing and prevent detection contribute to patients' not seeking evaluation of and treatment for incontinence.

FAST FACTS

- UI is especially common among older patients. Although the prevalence of urinary incontinence increases in older adults, it is *not* a normal consequence of aging and it *can* be treated.
- An estimated 38% or more of women aged 60 and older experience UI.
- Among men aged 60 and older, the prevalence is about 17%.
- Annual healthcare costs associated with UI exceed $463 million; when the amount spent on commercial products to manage UI is included, spending likely exceeds $14 billion annually.

Pathophysiology

Urinary continence requires input from the CNS, a bladder able to expand and contract and sphincters that can maintain a urethral pressure higher than that in the bladder. Intact cognition, mobility, motivation, and manual dexterity also are necessary to maintain continence. Mechanically, incontinence results when the pressure within the urinary bladder exceeds urethral resistance, allowing urine to escape. Any condition causing higher than normal bladder pressures or reduced urethral resistance can potentially result in incontinence. Relaxation of the pelvic musculature, disruption of cerebral and nervous system control, and disturbances of the bladder and its musculature are common contributing factors.

Incontinence may be an acute, self-limited disorder, or it may be chronic. The causes may be congenital or acquired, reversible or irreversible. Congenital disorders associated with incontinence include *epispadias* (absence of the upper wall of the urethra), and *meningomyelocele* (a neural tube defect in which a portion of the spinal cord and its surrounding meninges protrude through the vertebral column). CNS or spinal cord trauma, stroke, and chronic neurologic disorders such as multiple sclerosis and Parkinson's disease are examples of acquired, irreversible causes of incontinence. Reversible causes include acute confusion, medications such as diuretics or sedatives, prostatic enlargement, vaginal and urethral atrophy, UTI, and fecal impaction.

Incontinence is commonly categorized as stress incontinence, urge incontinence (also known as overactive bladder), overflow incontinence, and functional incontinence. Table 27–7 summarizes each type with its physiologic cause and associated factors. *Mixed incontinence*, with elements of both stress and urge incontinence, is common. *Total incontinence* is loss of all voluntary control over urination, with urine loss occurring without stimulus and in all positions.

Incontinence is associated with an increased risk for falls, fractures, pressure ulcers, urinary tract infection, and depression. It contributes to the stress of caregivers, and often is a factor in institutionalizing the patient.

Interdisciplinary Care

UI management is directed at identifying and correcting the cause if possible. If the underlying disorder cannot be corrected, techniques to manage urine output can often be taught.

Evaluation for incontinence begins with a complete history, including specific questions about lower urinary tract symptoms and the duration, frequency, volume, and associated circumstances of urine loss. A voiding diary (Figure 27–9 ■) is often used to collect detailed information. The history also includes information about chronic or acute illnesses, previous surgeries, and current medication use, both prescription and over the counter.

Physical assessment includes abdominal, rectal, and pelvic assessment as well as evaluation of mental and neurologic status, mobility, and dexterity. Findings often associated with incontinence in women include weak abdominal and pelvic muscle tone, cystocele or urethrocele, and atrophic vaginitis. In men, an enlarged prostate gland is the physical finding most commonly associated with incontinence.

See the Moving Evidence into Action feature on page 813 for evidence-based practice for diagnosing lower urinary tract symptoms in women.

TABLE 27–7 Types of Urinary Incontinence

	DESCRIPTION	PATHOPHYSIOLOGY	CONTRIBUTING FACTORS
Stress	Loss of urine associated with increased intra-abdominal pressure during sneezing, coughing, lifting. Quantity of urine lost is usually small.	Relaxation of pelvic musculature and weakness of urethra and surrounding muscles and tissues leads to decreased urethral resistance.	■ Multiple pregnancies ■ Decreased estrogen levels ■ Short urethra, change in angle between bladder and urethra ■ Abdominal wall weakness ■ Prostate surgery ■ Increased intra-abdominal pressure due to tumor, ascites, obesity
Urge	Involuntary loss of urine associated with a strong urge to void	Hypertonic or overactive detrusor muscle leads to increased pressure within bladder and inability to inhibit voiding.	■ Neurologic disorders such as stroke, Parkinson's disease, multiple sclerosis; peripheral nervous system disorders ■ Detrusor muscle overactivity associated with bladder outlet obstruction, aging, or disorders such as diabetes
Overflow	Inability to empty bladder, resulting in overdistention and frequent loss of small amounts of urine	Outlet obstruction or lack of normal detrusor activity leads to overfilling of bladder and increased pressure.	■ Spinal cord injuries below S_2 ■ Diabetic neuropathy ■ Prostatic hypertrophy ■ Fecal impaction ■ Drugs, especially those with anticholinergic effect
Functional	Incontinence resulting from physical, environmental, or psychosocial causes	Ability to respond to the need to urinate is impaired.	■ Confusion or dementia ■ Physical disability or impaired mobility ■ Therapy or sedation ■ Depression ■ Regression

Your Daily Voiding Diary

Date _____

This diary will help you and your healthcare team identify factors causing bladder control problems. Choose a 24-hour period when you can record your fluid intake (type and amount), urine output and episodes of urine leakage, any strong urge to void just prior to leaking, and your activity when leak episodes occur. The line below illustrates how to use your diary.

Time	Fluid Intake		Urine Output			Leaks			Urge		Activity
(clock)	Amount	Type	(restroom icon)			(face icon)			Yes	No	(bicycle icon)
7 am	2 cups	coffee	sm	(med)	lg	(sm)	med	lg	Yes		walking
			sm	med	lg	sm	med	lg			
			sm	med	lg	sm	med	lg			
			sm	med	lg	sm	med	lg			
			sm	med	lg	sm	med	lg			
			sm	med	lg	sm	med	lg			
			sm	med	lg	sm	med	lg			
			sm	med	lg	sm	med	lg			
			sm	med	lg	sm	med	lg			
			sm	med	lg	sm	med	lg			
			sm	med	lg	sm	med	lg			
			sm	med	lg	sm	med	lg			
			sm	med	lg	sm	med	lg			
			sm	med	lg	sm	med	lg			
			sm	med	lg	sm	med	lg			
			sm	med	lg	sm	med	lg			
			sm	med	lg	sm	med	lg			
			sm	med	lg	sm	med	lg			

I used____pads today.   I used____diapers today.

Questions to ask my health care team: _____

_____

_____

Figure 27–9 ■ A sample voiding diary.

Source: Adapted from *Your Daily Bladder Diary*, National Kidney and Urologic Diseases Information Center, National Institute of Diabetes and Digestive and Kidney Disease (NIDDK), National Institutes of Health.

Diagnosis

With an appropriate history and physical examination, diagnostic testing rarely is required. Certain tests may, however, be done to rule out UTI or to guide treatment.

- *Urinalysis* and *urine culture* using a clean-catch specimen are done to rule out infection and other acute causes of incontinence.
- *Postvoiding residual (PVR) volume* is measured to determine how completely the bladder empties with voiding. Less than 50 mL PVR is expected; when 100 mL or more is obtained, further testing is indicated.
- *Cystometrography* is used to assess neuromuscular function of the bladder by evaluating detrusor muscle function, pressure within the bladder, and the filling pattern of the bladder.
- *Uroflowmetry* is a noninvasive test used to evaluate voiding patterns.
- *Cystoscopy* or *ultrasonography* may be ordered to identify structural disorders contributing to incontinence, such as an enlarged prostate or a tumor.

Nursing implications for the specialized studies for urinary incontinence are outlined in ∞ Chapter 26.

Medications

Both stress and urge incontinence may improve with drug treatment.

Drugs that contract the smooth muscles of the bladder neck may reduce episodes of mild stress incontinence. Duloxetine (Cymbalta), a drug that inhibits the uptake of both norepinephrine and serotonin, is the drug of choice for treating stress UI that is not fully controlled with nonpharmacologic treatment (e.g., teaching, pelvic muscle exercise). In clinical trials, this drug reduced the frequency of UI and the number of voidings per day, particularly when combined with pelvic floor muscle training. Adverse effects such as nausea, headache, insomnia and constipation are common with duloxetine, limiting its usefulness for many patients (DiPiro et al., 2008).

When incontinence is associated with postmenopausal atrophic vaginitis, estrogen therapy may be effective. Both systemic estrogens and local creams are used.

Patients with urge incontinence may be treated with preparations that increase bladder capacity. Anticholinergic drugs inhibit muscarinic receptors of the parasympathetic nervous system, reducing detrusor muscle contractions. A number of drugs have been approved to treat urge UI, including oxybutynin (Ditropan

| **Lower Urinary Tract Symptoms in Women**

The underdiagnosis and inadequate treatment of UI is a commonly recognized problem; less well recognized is the extent to which women experience lower urinary tract symptoms (LUTS) with or without accompanying UI. LUTS include storage symptoms (e.g., frequency, urgency, and nocturia), voiding symptoms (slow stream, hesitancy, straining, and terminal dribble), and postmicturition symptoms (incomplete bladder emptying, postvoiding dribble). Various studies have indicated that up to 67% of women over age 18 years experience LUTS; the prevalence increases with aging. Many women are reluctant to seek treatment for LUTS; when they do, primary care providers often do not offer appropriate treatment information.

IMPLICATIONS FOR NURSING

Asking specific questions about LUTS can facilitate identification of symptoms affecting the patient's qualify of life. Accurate assessment and diagnosis is vital to planning and implementing appropriate care and achieving the desired outcomes of continence and quality of life. Successful treatment promotes self-esteem and provides positive reinforcement for continuing planned strategies.

CRITICAL THINKING IN PATIENT CARE

1. Identify at least five questions you should ask a patient to determine the presence of LUTS. How will you follow up to identify the potential effect of LUTS on the patient's quality of life (consider activities of daily living [ADLs], employment, social interactions, intimate relationships)?
2. Identify patient teaching for a woman who experiences frequency, urgency, nocturia and postvoid dribbling but who only occasionally loses urine.
3. What nursing care measures and patient teaching will you provide for the patient with stress incontinence that may not be appropriate or necessary for the patient with urge incontinence? For the patient with urge incontinence but not stress incontinence?
4. Develop a nursing care and teaching plan using the nursing diagnosis *Readiness for Enhanced Urinary Elimination*.

Source: Bradway, C., Coyne, K., Irwin, D., & Kopp, Z. (2008). Lower urinary tract symptoms in women–A common but neglected problem. *Journal of the American Academy of Nurse Practitioners, 20*(2008), 311–318.

and the extended release form, Ditropan XL), tolterodine (Detrol and its longer acting form, Detrol LA), trospium (Sanctura), darifenacin (Enablex), and solifenacin (VESIcare). These drugs can be taken once or twice a day, and have fewer side effects than less specific anticholinergic drugs. These drugs are contraindicated for the patient with acute glaucoma. Urinary retention is a potential side effect that must be considered when these drugs are used (see the Medication Administration box on page 808). Studies about the use and effectiveness of botulinum toxin A to control detrusor muscle overactivity are currently underway in the United States and Europe. Botulinum toxin A is injected directly into the muscle; its effects last for a period of 3 to 9 months, necessitating repeated injections (DiPiro et al., 2008).

Surgery

Surgery may be used to treat stress incontinence associated with cystocele or urethrocele and overflow incontinence associated with an enlarged prostate gland.

Suspension of the bladder neck, a technique that brings the angle between the bladder and urethra closer to normal, is effective in treating stress incontinence associated with urethrocele in 80% to 95% of patients. A laparoscopic, vaginal, or abdominal approach may be used to perform this surgery. Care of the patient with a bladder neck suspension is outlined in the accompanying box.

Prostatectomy, using either the transurethral or suprapubic approach, is indicated for the patient who is experiencing overflow incontinence as a result of an enlarged prostate gland and urethral obstruction. Care of the patient with a prostatectomy is outlined in ∞ Chapter 49.

Other surgical procedures of potential benefit in the treatment of incontinence include implantation of an artificial sphincter, formation of a urethral sling to elevate and compress the urethra, and augmentation of the bladder with bowel segments to increase bladder capacity.

NURSING CARE OF THE PATIENT
Having a Bladder Neck Suspension

PREOPERATIVE CARE

- Provide routine preoperative care and teaching as outlined in ∞ Chapter 4.
- Discuss the need to avoid straining and the Valsalva maneuver postoperatively. Suggest measures such as increasing fluid and fiber intake and using a stool softener to prevent postoperative constipation. *Straining and increased abdominal pressure during the Valsalva maneuver may place excessive stress on suture lines and interfere with healing.*

POSTOPERATIVE CARE

- Provide routine postoperative care as outlined in ∞ Chapter 4.
- Monitor urine output, including quantity, color, and clarity. Expect urine to be pink initially, gradually clearing. *Bright red urine, excessive vaginal drainage, or incisional bleeding may indicate hemorrhage. Instrumentation of the urinary tract increases the potential for UTI; cloudy urine may be an early sign.*
- Maintain stability and patency of suprapubic and/or urethral catheters. Secure catheters in position. *Maintaining bladder decompression eliminates pressure on suture lines. Preventing movement or pulling on catheters reduces the risk for resultant pressure on surgical incisions.*
- Carefully monitor urine output after catheter removal. *Difficulty voiding is common following catheter removal. Early intervention to prevent bladder distention is important to prevent pressure on suture lines.*
- If the urethral or suprapubic catheter will remain in place on discharge, teach proper care to the patient and family members as needed. *Appropriate self-care and early recognition of problems reduce the risk for significant complications.*

Complementary Therapies

Biofeedback and relaxation techniques may help reduce episodes of UI. Biofeedback uses electronic monitors to teach conscious control over physiologic responses of which the individual is not normally aware. Developing awareness of perceptible information allows the patient to gain voluntary control over urination. Biofeedback is widely used to manage urinary incontinence.

♪ Nursing Care

Health Promotion

Although UI rarely causes serious physical effects, it frequently has significant psychosocial effects, and can lead to lowered self-esteem, social isolation, and even institutionalization. Get the word out—inform all patients that UI is not a normal consequence of aging and that treatments are available. To reduce the incidence of UI, teach all women to perform pelvic floor muscle (Kegel) exercises (Box 27–3) to improve perineal muscle tone. Advise women to seek advice from their women's healthcare or primary care practitioner about using topical hormone therapy during menopause to maintain perineal tissue integrity. Advise older men to have routine prostate examinations to prevent urethral obstruction and overflow incontinence. Pelvic floor muscle exercises also may benefit men who experience UI following prostatectomy, but evidence supporting this is limited.

Assessment

Nursing assessment for the patient with UI includes both subjective and objective data:

- *Health history:* Voiding diary; frequency of incontinent episodes, amount of urine loss and activities associated with incontinence; methods used to deal with incontinence; use of Kegel exercises or medications; any chronic diseases, related surgeries, etc.; effects of incontinence on usual activities, including social activities.

BOX 27–3 Pelvic Floor Muscle (Kegel) Exercises

- Identify the pelvic muscles with these techniques:
  - Stop the flow of urine during voiding and hold for a few seconds.
  - Tighten the muscles at the vaginal entrance around a gloved finger or tampon.
  - Tighten the muscles around the anus as though resisting defecation.
- Perform exercises by tightening pelvic muscles, holding for 10 seconds, and relaxing for 10 to 15 seconds. Continue the sequence (tighten, hold, relax) for 10 repetitions.
- Keep abdominal muscles and breathing relaxed while performing exercises.
- Initially, exercises should be performed twice per day, working up to four times a day.
- Encourage exercising at a specific time each day or in conjunction with another daily activity (such as bathing or watching the news). Establish a routine because these exercises should be continued for life.
- Assistive devices, such as vaginal cones and biofeedback, may be useful for patients who have difficulty identifying appropriate muscle groups.

- *Physical examination:*   Physical and mental status, including any physical limitations or impaired cognition; inspect, palpate, and percuss abdomen for bladder distention; inspect perineal tissues for redness, irritation, or tissue breakdown; observe for bulging of bladder into vagina when bearing down; assess pelvic muscle tone as indicated.

Nursing Diagnoses and Interventions

In planning nursing care, consider the patient's mental status, mobility, and motivation. Behavioral techniques can be effective, but require long-term commitment and the physical and mental capability to use them.

Nursing care and modification of routines can restore continence fully or partially even in the institutionalized patient. Scheduled toileting, bladder training, and prompted voiding combined with positive reinforcement such as praise can reduce the need for diapers, incontinence pads, and indwelling catheters.

See the Case Study & Nursing Care Plan on page 816 for additional nursing diagnoses and interventions for the patient with urinary incontinence.

Readiness for Enhanced Urinary Elimination

Exercises to strengthen pelvic floor muscles, dietary modifications, and bladder training programs often are effective to restore and maintain continence.

- Instruct to keep a voiding diary, recording the time and amount of all fluid intake and urinary output, status at the time of voiding (dry or wet) and on arising from sleep, and activities. *Voiding diaries provide valuable information for identifying the type of incontinence and possible measures to reduce or eliminate incontinent episodes.*
- Teach pelvic floor muscle exercises (see Box 27–3). Instruct to consciously tighten pelvic muscles when the need to void is perceived and to relax the abdomen while walking to the bathroom. *Improved pelvic muscle strength helps retain urine and prevent stress incontinence by increasing urethral pressure. Exercises also decrease abnormal detrusor muscle contractions, decreasing pressure within the bladder.*

PRACTICE ALERT
Do not advise patients who have difficulty emptying the bladder completely to stop urine flow while voiding to identify pelvic floor muscles. Repeated interruption of micturition can interfere with complete bladder emptying and increase the risk for UTI.

EVIDENCE FOR NURSING CARE **The Patient with Urinary Incontinence**

Selected resources that nurses may find helpful when planning evidence-based nursing care follow.

- Dowling-Castronovo, A., & Bradway, C. (2008). Urinary Incontinence. *Nursing Standard of Practice Protocol: Urinary incontinence (UI) in older adults admitted to acute care.* Hartford Institute for Geriatric Nursing, New York University College of Nursing.

CHAPTER 27 / Nursing Care of Patients with Urinary Tract Disorders **815**

Using the patient's voiding diary, suggest dietary and fluid intake modifications to reduce stress and urge incontinence. Include limiting caffeine, alcohol, citrus juice, and artificial sweetener consumption; limiting fluid intake to no less than 1.5 to 2.0 L per day; and limiting evening fluid intake. *Caffeine, alcohol, and citrus juices are bladder irritants and tend to promote detrusor instability, increasing the risk of urge incontinence. Artificial sweeteners may also irritate the bladder. Fluid intake of 1.5 to 2.0 L per day is adequate to maintain health for most patients; excess fluid may increase stress incontinence if bathroom facilities are not readily available.*

PRACTICE ALERT
Limiting total fluid intake to less than 1.5 to 2.0 L per day is not recommended for patients with UI. Inadequate fluid increases urine concentration, leading to bladder wall irritation and possibly increasing problems of urge incontinence.

Toileting Self-Care Deficit

Functional incontinence may be the predominant problem in an institutionalized older adult. Limited mobility, impaired vision, dementia, lack of access to facilities and privacy, and tight staffing patterns increase the risk for incontinence in previously continent residents. The primary problem in functional incontinence is an outside factor that interferes with the ability to respond normally to the urge to void. An immobilized patient may wet the bed if a call light is not within reach; a patient with Alzheimer's disease may perceive the urge to void but be unable to interpret its meaning or respond by seeking a bathroom. For these patients, self-care deficit in toileting is a primary problem.

- Assess physical and mental abilities and limitations, usual voiding pattern, and ability to assist with toileting. *A thorough assessment allows planned interventions to address specific needs and promote independence.*
- Provide assistive devices as needed to facilitate independence, such as raised toilet seats, grab bars, a bedside commode, or night-lights. *Fostering independence in toileting bolsters self-concept and maintains a positive body image.*
- Plan a toileting schedule based on the patient's normal elimination patterns to achieve approximately 300 mL of urine output with each voiding. *Allowing the bladder to fill to a point at which the urge to void is experienced and then emptying it completely helps maintain normal bladder capacity and bacteriostatic functions.*
- Position for ease of voiding—sitting for females, standing for males—and provide privacy. *Normal positioning, usual toileting facilities, and privacy enhance the ability to void on schedule and empty the bladder completely.*
- Adjust fluid intake so that the majority of fluids are consumed during times of the day when the patient is most able to remain continent. Unless fluids are restricted, maintain a fluid intake of at least 1.5 to 2.0 L per day. *An adequate fluid intake is vital to promote hydration and urinary function. Overly concentrated urine can irritate the bladder, increasing incontinence.*
- Assist with clothing that is easily removed (e.g., elastic-waist pants or loose dresses). Velcro and zipper fasteners may be easier to use than snaps and buttons. *Clothing that is difficult*

to remove can increase the risk of incontinence in the patient with mobility problems or impaired dexterity.

Impaired Social Interaction

Urinary incontinence increases the risk for social isolation due to embarrassment, fear of not having ready access to a bathroom, body odor, or other factors. Social isolation, in turn, can increase problems of incontinence, because normal cues and relationships are lost, and the need to remain dry is less strongly felt.

- Assess reasons for and extent of social isolation. Verify the degree of social isolation with the patient or significant other. *Do not assume that social isolation is only related to urinary incontinence. Other problems frequently associated with aging (such as a hearing deficit) may be primary or contributing factors.*
- Refer patient for urologic examination and incontinence evaluation. *Patients who assume that urinary incontinence is a normal part of the aging process may not be aware of treatment options.*
- Explore alternative coping strategies with patient, significant other, staff, and other healthcare team members. *Protective pads or shields, good perineal hygiene, scheduled voiding, and clothing that does not interfere with toileting can enhance continence.*

Using NANDA, NIC, and NOC

Linkages between a selected NANDA nursing diagnosis, NIC, and NOC for the patient with urinary incontinence are shown in the chart that follows.

Community-Based Care

Because UI is a contributing factor in the institutionalization of many older people, patient and family teaching can have a significant impact on maintaining independence and residence in the community. Address possible causes of incontinence and appropriate treatment measures. Refer for urologic examination if not already completed. Discuss fluid intake management, perineal care, and products for clothing protection.

NANDA, NIC, AND NOC LINKAGES
The Patient with Urinary Incontinence

NANDA
Readiness for Enhanced Urinary Elimination

NIC
Urinary Elimination Management
Urinary Habit Training
Self-Efficacy Enhancement

NOC
Urinary Continence
Self-Care: Toileting
Social Involvement

Data from NANDA International. (2009). *Nursing diagnoses: Definitions & classification 2009–2011.* Oxford, UK: Wiley-Blackwell; Bulechek, G., Butcher, H., & Dochterman, J. (Eds.). (2008). *Nursing interventions classification (NIC)* (5th ed.). St. Louis, MO: Mosby; and Moorhead, S., Johnson, M., Maas, M., & Sullivan, E. (Eds.). (2008). *Nursing outcomes classification (NOC)* (4th ed.).St. Louis, MO: Mosby.

CASE STUDY & NURSING CARE PLAN   A Patient with Urinary Incontinence

Anna Giovanni, a 76-year-old retired teacher, has been widowed for 10 years and lives alone. Mrs. Giovanni's eldest daughter expresses concern that her mother seems increasingly reluctant to leave her apartment to visit friends and family. She reports a strong odor of urine throughout her mother's apartment and that her mother's bed is often wet. She expresses worry about needing to place her mother in a nursing home if she cannot continue to live independently.

ASSESSMENT

Jane Oberle, RN, a nurse practitioner, examines Mrs. Giovanni who admits that she has problems with urine leakage when laughing and coughing, and a strong urge to void on hearing the sound of running water. At night, her urge to void is so strong that she often cannot reach the bathroom in time. Mrs. Giovanni denies a history of UTIs, neurologic disorders, or difficulty with her bowels. She had a hysterectomy at age 52 and was on hormone replacement therapy for about 10 years afterward. She is taking digoxin 0.125 mg daily, furosemide 40 mg twice daily, and potassium chloride 20 mEq three times daily for mild heart failure.

Physical assessment reveals a moderate cystourethrocele and atrophy of vaginal and vulvar tissues. Moderate perineal dermatitis is noted. Pelvic floor strength is weak. Urinalysis is within normal limits, and postvoiding residual urine is 5 mL.

Analysis of Mrs. Giovanni's voiding diary shows moderate consumption of tea and juices throughout the day, with nine daytime voidings and four night voidings with an average volume of about 250 mL per void. She notices urine leakage most often in the late afternoon and at night. Ms. Oberle identifies a diagnosis of stress incontinence with an urgency component and decides to try a conservative approach before referring Mrs. Giovanni for further testing and possible cystourethrocele repair. She prescribes estrogen cream, tolterodine (Detrol), and a barrier cream to treat Mrs. Giovanni's vulvitis.

DIAGNOSES

- *Stress Urinary Incontinence* related to weak pelvic floor musculature and tissue atrophy
- *Urge Urinary Incontinence* related to excess intake of caffeine and citrus juices
- *Impaired Skin Integrity* related to constant contact of urine with perineal tissues
- *Ineffective Coping* related to inability to control urine leakage

EXPECTED OUTCOMES

- Remain dry between voidings and at night.
- Demonstrate improved perineal muscle strength.
- Regain and maintain perineal skin integrity.
- Return to her previous level of social activity.

PLANNING AND IMPLEMENTATION

- Teach how to identify pelvic floor muscles and how to perform Kegel exercises.
- Suggest drinking decaffeinated tea and noncitrus fruit juices (grape, apple, and cranberry).
- Encourage to minimize fluid intake after evening meal.
- Change afternoon dose of furosemide from 9:00 PM to 3:00 PM.
- Instruct to void by the clock, gradually increasing intervals from every 45 to 60 minutes to every 2 to 2.5 hours. Advise to maintain shorter voiding intervals for 2 to 3 hours after furosemide doses.
- Teach to cleanse perineal area, wiping front to back, after each voiding or incident of urine leakage.
- Introduce commercial products available for clothing and furniture protection, encouraging experimentation to identify the most helpful product(s).
- Provide a commode for bedside at night and adequate lighting to prevent injury.
- Schedule follow-up visits and evaluations to reinforce teaching.

EVALUATION

Three months after her initial visit, Mrs. Giovanni states that she is doing very well, experiencing only occasional leakage of small amounts of urine, primarily when sneezing, coughing, or laughing. She finds a minipad adequate for protection and is often able to remain dry all day. She has had no further problems with enuresis since changing her evening furosemide dose to late afternoon and limiting her fluids after dinner. She can make it to the bathroom and no longer needs the bedside commode. Her perineal tissue is intact, and she demonstrates improved muscle strength. Her daughter says her mother is beginning to resume her normal social activities, and that she is no longer worried about her mother's ability to care for herself independently.

CRITICAL THINKING IN THE NURSING PROCESS

1. What factors in Mrs. Giovanni's past medical history and current medication regimen contributed to her nighttime incontinence?
2. What is the rationale for including an intervention to teach Mrs. Giovanni about perineal cleansing as part of her care plan?
3. Develop a care plan for Mrs. Giovanni for the nursing diagnosis *Situational Low Self-Esteem* related to urinary incontinence.

See Evaluating Your Response in Appendix C.

CHAPTER HIGHLIGHTS

- Urinary tract infections are very common and are a leading complication among hospitalized patients. Short-course antibiotic therapy is appropriate for uncomplicated infections of the lower urinary tract that are not associated with the presence of an indwelling urinary catheter.
- Teach patients about perineal hygiene and the importance of maintaining adequate fluid intake as measures to help prevent UTI.
- Urinary stones (most commonly kidney stones in the United States) can obstruct the urinary tract at any level, and cause significant pain as they move from the kidney through the ureter.

Instruct patients who have had a kidney stone to maintain a generous fluid intake, particularly during exercise and warm weather, to reduce the risk of further stone formation.

■ The risk for bladder cancer is greater among men than women, and cigarette smoking is the most significant risk factor for bladder cancer. Most tumors can be resected transurethrally if diagnosed early, before spreading to deeper layers of the bladder wall, the lymph nodes, and adjacent tissue.

■ When resection of the urinary bladder is necessary, a urinary diversion is created to collect urine. A collection appliance must be worn constantly on an ileal conduit; when a continent urinary diversion is created, the pouch is emptied by intermittent catheterization of the stoma.

■ Urinary retention may occur as a result of some medications, neurologic damage or disease, or obstruction (e.g., an enlarged prostate gland). If the underlying condition cannot be treated, medications or intermittent catheterization are used to promote bladder emptying.

■ Older adults in particular are at risk for urinary incontinence, a treatable condition. A health history, voiding diary, and diagnostic testing are used to establish the type of urinary incontinence and direct treatments such as surgery, pelvic floor muscle exercises, medications, and scheduled toileting.

TEST YOURSELF NCLEX-RN® REVIEW

1. A 23-year-old woman presents to the urgency clinic with symptoms of a UTI. The nursing history reveals that the patient was treated 3 months previously for a UTI. What additional question should the nurse ask?
   1. "Did you complete your antibiotic prescription for your first UTI?"
   2. "What form of birth control are you using?"
   3. "Does your partner have similar symptoms?"
   4. "How much fluid do you drink each day?"

2. A 58-year-old woman presents at her primary care provider's office with symptoms of frequency, urgency, nocturia, dysuria, and cloudy, rust-colored urine for the third time in the past 2 years. The nurse should plan to include which of the following in her teaching for this patient? **Select all that apply.**
   1. return to the office in 10 days for follow-up culture
   2. preprocedure instruction for an IVP
   3. the potential benefits of estrogen vaginal cream
   4. recommendations for perineal cleansing
   5. recommendations for screening cystoscopy

3. Recognizing the risk for urolithiasis in the immobilized patient, the nurse appropriately plans to do which of the following?
   1. Administer a calcium supplement.
   2. Regularly monitor urine pH.
   3. Maintain an indwelling urinary catheter.
   4. Increase fluid intake to 3000 mL per day.

4. A patient admitted with possible kidney stones develops sudden complaints of acute crampy pain on the left side that radiates into the groin. He is nauseated, and vomits clear fluid. On voiding, his urine is pink. The most appropriate response by the nurse is which of the following?
   1. Obtain a bladder scan to assess for residual urine.
   2. Administer the prescribed narcotic analgesic.
   3. Notify the physician.
   4. Strain all urine.

5. The nurse teaching a group of community members about wellness and disease prevention includes which of the following as a measure to reduce the risk for bladder cancer?
   1. Do not start smoking; if you smoke, stop.
   2. Avoid using hair dyes and pesticides in the home.
   3. Limit your intake of coffee and other caffeinated beverages.
   4. Empty your bladder every 2 hours.

6. At a local health fair, a man remarks to the nurse that his urine occasionally appears pink. He wonders if this is anything to be concerned about. How should the nurse respond?
   1. Instruct the man to notify his physician if he develops pain or difficulty voiding.
   2. Advise the man to make an appointment to see his physician.
   3. Instruct the man to track the relationship between urine color and his activities.
   4. Tell the man to increase his fluid intake to 2 1/2 to 3 quarts per day.

7. The nurse evaluates her teaching as effective when the patient with a newly created continent ileal diversion is able to do which of the following?
   1. Demonstrate care for the collection device.
   2. State the importance of promptly reporting cloudy urine to the physician.
   3. Demonstrate self-catheterization of the stoma.
   4. Identify factors contributing to his risk for bladder cancer.

8. The nurse identifies which of the following as a high-priority goal for a patient with stress incontinence?
   1. can identify products for protecting clothing and furniture
   2. states chronic and benign nature of the disorder
   3. performs pelvic floor muscle exercises as taught at least twice a day
   4. limits intake of beverages containing artificial sweeteners

9. A patient tells the nurse that she has difficulty getting to the bathroom in time to prevent urine leaks once she feels the need to void. What teaching should the nurse provide?
   1. Limit intake of caffeine-containing beverages, particularly in the evening.
   2. Establish a voiding schedule, emptying her bladder at least every 2 hours.
   3. Discuss potential benefits of bladder suspension surgery with her physician.
   4. Wear clothing that is easily removed for toileting.

10. The nurse caring for a patient in the spinal shock phase following spinal cord injury appropriately plans to do which of the following?
    1. Insert a Foley catheter to accurately measure output.
    2. Stimulate voiding using Credé's method.
    3. Assess for urinary retention following each voiding.
    4. Catheterize with straight catheter every 3 to 4 hours.

See Test Yourself answers in Appendix C.

Pearson Nursing Student Resources

Find additional review materials at
www.nursing.pearsonhighered.com

Prepare for success with additional NCLEX®-style practice questions, interactive assignments and activities, Web links, animations and videos, and more!

BIBLIOGRAPHY

American Cancer Society. (2009). *Cancer facts and figures 2009*. Atlanta: Author.

American College of Obstetricians and Gynecologists (ACOG). (2008 March). Treatment of urinary tract infections in nonpregnant women. Washington, DC: Author.

Barclay, L. (2008 March 17). New guidelines for management of urinary tract infection in nonpregnant women. *Medscape Medical News*. Retrieved from www.medscape.com

Bardsley, A. (2005). Use of lubricant gels in urinary catheterization. *Nursing Standard, 20*(8), 41–46.

Bishop, T. (2008 June 6). Urinalysis (urine testing) can provide valuable information about a patient's condition, allowing the detection of systemic disease and infection. *Practice Nurse 2008, 35*(12), 18–20.

Bradway, C., Coyne, K., & Kopp, Z. (2008). Lower urinary tract symptoms in women–A common but neglected problem. *Journal of the American Academy of Nurse Practitioners, 20*(2008), 311–318.

Bulechek, G., Butche, H., & Dochterman, J. (Eds.). (2008). *Nursing interventions classification (NIC)* (5th ed.). St. Louis, MO: Mosby.

Copstead, L. & Banasik, J. (2010). *Pathophysiology* (4th ed.). St. Louis, MO: Elsevier/Saunders.

Davis, C. (2008 April). The cost of containment. *Nursing Older People, 20*(3), 24–26.

DiPiro, J., Talbert, R., Yee, G., Matzke, G., Wells, B., & Posey, L. M. (2008). *Pharmacotherapy: A pathophysiologic approach* (7th ed.). New York, NY: McGraw-Hill.

Dowling-Castronovo, A., & Bradway, C. (2008). Urinary Incontinence. Nursing Standard of Practice Protocol: Urinary incontinence (UI) in older adults admitted to acute care. Hartford Institute for Geriatric Nursing, New York University College of Nursing.

Dowling-Castronovo, A., & Specht, J. (2009 February). Assessment of transient urinary incontinence in older adults. *American Journal of Nursing, 109*(2), 62–71.

Fauci, A., Kasper, D., Braunwald, E., Hauser, S., Longo, D., Jameson, J., et al. (Eds.). (2008). *Harrison's principles of internal medicine* (17th ed.). New York, NY: McGraw-Hill.

Fontaine, K. L. (2005). *Complementary & alternative therapies for nursing practice* (2nd ed.). Upper Saddle River, NJ: Prentice Hall.

Gotelli, J., Merryman, P., Carr, C., McElveen, L., Epperson, C., & Bynum, D. (2008 December). A quality improvement project to reduce the complications associated with indwelling urinary catheters. *Urologic Nursing, 28*(6), 465–467, 473.

Katz, A. (2009 March). When worlds collide: Urinary incontinence and female sexuality. *American Journal of Nursing, 109*(3), 59–63.

Kee, J. (2009). *Handbook of laboratory and diagnostic tests with nursing implications* (6th ed.). Upper Saddle River, NJ: Pearson Prentice Hall.

Lajiness, M. (2008 October). Common antibiotics for the treatment of urinary tract infections. *Urologic Nursing, 28*(5), 387–389.

Lin, K., & Fajardo, K. (2008 July 1). Clinical guidelines. Screening for asymptomatic bacteriuria in adults: Evidence for the U. S. Preventive Services Task Force reaffirmation recommendation statement. *Annals of Internal Medicine, 149*(1), W-20–W-24.

McPhee, S., Papadakis, M., & Tierney, L., Jr. (Eds.). (2008). *Current medical diagnosis & treatment* (47th ed.). New York, NY: McGraw Hill.

Moorhead, S., Johnson, M., Maas, M., & Swanson, E. (Eds.). (2008). *Nursing outcomes classification (NOC)* (4th ed.). St. Louis, MO: Mosby.

NANDA International. (2009). *Nursing diagnoses definitions and classification 2009–2011*. Oxford, UK: Wiley-Blackwell.

National Kidney and Urologic Diseases Information Clearinghouse. (2009). *Kidney and urologic diseases statistics for the United States*. Retrieved from www.kidney.niddk.nih.gov

National Kidney Foundation. (2008). *The problem of kidney and urologic disease*. Retrieved from www.kidney.org

Nursing guidelines for assessment and management of urinary retention in hospitalized older adults. (2007 August). *Australian Nursing Journal, 15*(2), 22–23.

Paige, N., & Nagami, G. (2009 February). The top 10 things nephrologists wish every primary care physician knew. *Mayo Clinic Proceedings, 84*(2), 180–186.

Palmer, M. (2008). Urinary incontinence quality improvement in nursing homes: Where have we been? Where are we going? *Urologic Nursing, 28*(6), 439–444.

Palmer, M., & Newman, D. (2007 March). Bladder matters: Urinary incontinence and estrogen. *American Journal of Nursing, 107*(3), 35–36, 38.

Pickett, S. (2008 October 17). The basics. Urinary tract infection. *GP: General Practitioner, October 2007, 37,* 39.

Porth, C., & Matfin, G. (2009). *Pathophysiology: Concepts of altered health states* (8th ed.). Philadelphia: Lippincott.

Rahn, D. (2008 October). Urinary tract infections: Contemporary management. *Urologic Nursing, 28*(5), 333–341.

Research backs cranberries for preventing urinary tract infections in women. (2008 April). *Harvard Women's Health Watch*. Retrieved from www.health.harvard.edu

Richards, S. (2008 June 6). Urinary tract infection. *Practice Nurse, 35*(11), 16–18.

Robinson, S., Allen, L., Barnes, M., Berry, T., Foster, T., Friedrich, L., et al. (2007 June). Development of an evidence-based protocol for reduction of indwelling urinary catheter usage. *MEDSURG Nursing, 16*(3), 157–161.

Rosh, A. (2009 April 5). Suprapubic aspiration. Retrieved from www.emedicine.medscape.com

Rothrock, J. C. (2007). *Alexander's care of the patient in surgery* (13th ed.). St. Louis, MO: Mosby.

Spencer, J. W., & Jacobs, J. J. (2003). *Complementary and alternative medicine: An evidence-based approach* (2nd ed.). St. Louis, MO: Mosby.

Stevemer, J., & Ewigman, B. (2008 April). Drugs help pass more ureteral stones. *The Journal of Family Practice, 57*(4), 224–227.

Stokowski, L. (2009). Preventing catheter-associated urinary tract infections. *Medscape Nurses 2009*. Retrieved from www.medscape.com

Wilkinson, J., & Ahern, N. (2009). *Nursing diagnosis handbook* (9th ed.). Upper Saddle River, NJ: Prentice Hall.

Wilson, B., Shannon, M., Shields, K., & Stang, C. (2008). *Nurse's drug guide*. Upper Saddle River, NJ: Prentice Hall.

Nursing Care of Patients with
Kidney Disorders

LEARNING OUTCOMES

1. Describe the pathophysiology of common kidney disorders, relating pathophysiology to normal functions and manifestations of the disorder.
2. Discuss risk factors for kidney disorders and nursing measures to reduce these risks.
3. Explain diagnostic studies used to identify disorders of the kidneys and their effects.
4. Discuss the effects and nursing implications for medications and treatments used for patients with kidney disorders.
5. Compare and contrast renal replacement therapies, including dialysis and kidney transplant, to manage acute and chronic renal failure.

CLINICAL COMPETENCIES

1. Assess the functional health status of patients with kidney disorders.
2. Recognize, monitor, document, and report unexpected or abnormal manifestations in patients with kidney disorders.
3. Provide safe and effective nursing care for patients undergoing renal replacement therapies, surgery involving the kidneys, or renal transplant.
4. Using assessed data and current standards of practice, determine priority nursing diagnoses and interventions for patients with renal disorders.
5. Plan and implement evidence-based nursing care for patients with renal disorders using research and best practices.
6. Collaborate and coordinate with the patient and other members of the interdisciplinary team to prioritize and implement care.
7. Provide teaching appropriate to the patient and situation for patients with kidney disorders.
8. Evaluate patient responses to care, revising the plan of care as needed to promote, maintain, or restore functional health status for patients with renal disorders.

KEY TERMS

acute renal failure, *836*
acute tubular necrosis, *837*
azotemia, *822*
chronic kidney disease (CKD), *848*
dialysis, *840*
glomerular filtration rate, *820*

glomerulonephritis, *822*
hematuria, *821*
hemodialysis, *840*
nephrectomy, *832*
nephrotic syndrome, *824*
oliguria, *822*

peritoneal dialysis, *840*
proteinuria, *821*
renal failure, *835*
ultrafiltration, *840*
uremia, *849*

The internal environment of the body normally remains in a relatively constant or *homeostatic* state. The kidneys help maintain homeostasis by regulating the composition and volume of extracellular fluid. They excrete excess water and solutes and also can conserve water and solutes when deficits occur. In addition, the kidneys help regulate acid–base balance and they excrete metabolic wastes. Regulation of blood pressure is also a key function of the kidneys.

Both primary kidney disorders (such as glomerulonephritis) and systemic diseases (such as diabetes mellitus) can affect renal function. In the United States, more than 23 million people (about 13% of adults) have chronic kidney disease (National Kidney and Urologic Diseases Information Clearinghouse [NKUDIC], 2009). Every year, approximately 1 in every 1000 people in the United States develops end-stage renal disease (ESRD), the final phase of chronic renal disease in which little or no kidney function remains. Chronic renal disease accounted for more than 87,500 deaths in 2006, and is a major cause of lost work time and wages (NKUDIC, 2009). Ironically, the increased prevalence of chronic renal disease in recent years is partially related to the success of dialysis and transplantation.

doses and longer dosing intervals. Common medications affected by decreased GFR include the following:

- Cardiac drugs: digoxin, procainamide
- Antibiotics: aminoglycosides, tetracyclines, cephalosporins
- Histamine H_2 antagonists: cimetidine
- Antidiabetic agents: chlorpropamide.

When caring for older adults, it is especially important to monitor drugs that are toxic to the renal tubules. Radiologic dyes and aminoglycoside, tetracycline, and the cephalosporin antibiotics are part of this group.

Age-related changes in renal function and related nursing implications are summarized in Table 28–1.

Age-Related Changes in Kidney Function

Glomeruli in the renal cortex (∞ see Chapter 26 for a review of normal kidney structure and function) are lost with aging, reducing kidney mass. Because of the large functional reserve of the kidneys, however, renal function remains adequate unless additional stressors affect the renal system. The **glomerular filtration rate (GFR)**, the amount of filtrate made by the kidneys per minute, declines due to age-related factors affecting the renovascular system (such as arteriosclerosis, decreased renal vascularity, and decreased cardiac output). By age 80, the GFR may be less than half of what it was at age 30.

Age-related changes in renal function have significant implications. The kidneys are less able to concentrate urine and compensate for increased or decreased salt intake. When combined with diminished effectiveness of antidiuretic hormone (ADH) and a reduced thirst response, both common in aging, this decreased ability to concentrate urine increases the risk for dehydration. Potassium excretion may be decreased because of lower aldosterone levels. As a result, fluid and electrolyte imbalances are more common and potentially critical in the older patient.

Decreased GFR in the older adult also reduces the clearance of drugs excreted through the kidneys. This reduced clearance prolongs the half-life of drugs and may necessitate lower drug

The Patient with Polycystic Kidney Disease

Polycystic kidney disease, a hereditary disease characterized by formation of fluid-filled cysts and massive kidney enlargement, affects both children and adults. This disease has two forms: The autosomal dominant form primarily affects adults; the autosomal recessive form is present at birth (Porth & Matfin, 2009). Autosomal recessive polycystic kidney disease is rare. It usually is diagnosed prenatally or in infancy. Renal failure generally develops during childhood, necessitating kidney transplant or dialysis. Autosomal dominant polycystic kidney disease (ADPKD) is relatively common, affecting 1 in every 400 to 1000 people and accounting for approximately 4.5% of patients with ESRD in the United States (Fauci et al., 2008; NKUDIC, 2009). See the genetics box that follows. This section focuses on autosomal dominant polycystic kidney disease, the more common form of the disorder.

Pathophysiology

Renal cysts are fluid-filled sacs affecting the nephron, the functional unit of the kidneys. The cysts, which arise from tubular epithelial cells, may range in size from microscopic to several centimeters in diameter and affect the renal cortex and medulla of both kidneys. Cysts may detach from the tubule, continuing to enlarge by active fluid secretion. As the cysts enlarge and multiply, the kidneys also enlarge. Although only a small percentage of nephrons are involved, the cysts compress adjacent

TABLE 28–1 Nursing Implications of Age-Related Changes in Kidney Function

FUNCTIONAL CHANGE	EFFECT	IMPLICATIONS
Decreased GFR	Decreased clearance of drugs excreted primarily through the kidneys increases drug half-life and blood levels, and risk of drug toxicity	Monitor carefully for signs of toxicity, especially when administering digoxin, aminoglycoside antibiotics, tetracycline, vancomycin, chlorpropamide, procainamide, cimetidine, and cephalosporin antibiotics.
Decreased number of functional nephrons; lower levels of aldosterone; increased resistance to ADH	Decreased ability to conserve water and sodium; impaired potassium excretion; and decreased hydrogen ion excretion, resulting in reduced ability to compensate for acidosis	Monitor for dehydration and hyponatremia; maintain fluid intake of 1500 to 2500 mL/day unless contraindicated; monitor for hyperkalemia, especially if taking a potassium-sparing diuretic, heparin, angiotensin-converting enzyme (ACE) inhibitor, beta-blocker, or NSAID; increased risk for acidosis.
Reduced numbers of functional nephrons	Decreased renal reserve with increased risk of failure	Avoid giving nephrotoxic drugs if possible; monitor urine output and blood chemistries for early signs of renal failure.

renal parenchyma. Renal blood vessels and nephrons are compressed and obstructed, leading to tissue ischemia. This activates the renin-angiotensin system within the kidney. Functional tissue is destroyed, with compression, ischemia, and accumulation of inflammatory mediators likely playing a role (Figure 28–1 ■).

People affected by polycystic kidney disease often develop cysts elsewhere in the body, including the liver, spleen, pancreas, lungs, and reproductive organs. Up to 40% of people with ADPKD develop liver cysts, which may bleed or become infected. Diverticular disease of the colon is common, and may lead to perforation of the bowel (Fauci et al., 2008). About 25% of people with polycystic kidney disease have cardiac valve abnormalities, including mitral valve prolapse ("floppy" mitral valves) and aortic valve insufficiency. The risk of subarachnoid or cerebral hemorrhage from a ruptured cerebral aneurysm is significantly increased in patients with ADPKD.

Manifestations

Polycystic kidney disease is slowly progressive. Symptoms usually develop by age 40 to 50. Common manifestations include flank pain, microscopic or gross **hematuria** (blood in the urine), **proteinuria** (proteins in the urine), and *polyuria* and

Figure 28–1 ■ A polycystic kidney. The functional tissue of the kidneys is gradually destroyed and replaced with fluid-filled cysts.

Source: A. Glauberman/Photo Researchers, Inc.

nocturia, as the concentrating ability of the kidney is impaired. Urinary tract infection and renal calculi are common, as cysts interfere with normal urine drainage. Most patients develop hypertension from disruption of renal vessels. The kidneys become palpable, enlarged, and knobby. Symptoms of renal insufficiency and chronic renal failure typically develop by age 60 to 70. The progression to ESRD tends to occur more rapidly in Blacks and in men.

Interdisciplinary Care

Diagnostic tests used to determine the extent of polycystic kidney disease include the following:

- *Renal ultrasonography* is the diagnostic procedure of choice for polycystic kidney disease.
- *Computed tomography (CT) scan* of the kidney may be used to detect cystic disease at an earlier stage when there is a positive family history.
- *Genetic testing* for ADPKD type 1 and type 2 is available, and is particularly important when a family member is being considered as a potential kidney donor.

∞ See Chapter 26 for the nursing implications of these tests.

Management of adult polycystic kidney disease is largely supportive. Care is taken to avoid further renal damage by nephrotoxic substances, UTI, obstruction, or hypertension. A fluid intake of 2000 to 2500 mL per day is encouraged to help prevent UTI and lithiasis. Hypertension associated with polycystic disease is generally controlled using a multidrug regimen that includes an angiotensin-converting enzyme (ACE) inhibitor or angiotensin receptor blocker (ARB) (∞ see Chapter 32). Ultimately, dialysis or renal transplantation is required. Patients with polycystic kidney disease are typically good candidates for transplantation because of the absence of associated systemic disease, but may still experience effects of the extrarenal elements of the disease.

∞ Nursing Care

For those with adult polycystic kidney disease, an autosomal dominant disorder, discuss genetic counseling and screening of family members for evidence of the disease. Consider the following nursing diagnoses when planning care for the patient with polycystic kidney disease:

- *Excess Fluid Volume* related to impaired renal function
- *Grieving* related to potential loss of kidney function
- *Readiness for Enhanced Knowledge* regarding measures to help preserve kidney function
- *Risk for Ineffective Coping* related to potential genetic transmission of the disorder to offspring.

Teach the patient with polycystic kidney disease about the disease, its genetic nature, and usual course. Discuss measures to maintain optimal renal function. Instruct to maintain a fluid intake of at least 2500 mL per day. Include additional information about preventing UTI (such as hygiene measures) and early manifestations of UTI. Stress the importance of seeking treatment to prevent further kidney damage. Advise to avoid drugs that are potentially toxic to the kidneys and to check with the primary care provider before taking any new drug. Discuss the potential benefits of genetic counseling with the patient and family.

The Patient with a Glomerular Disorder

Disorders and diseases involving the glomerulus are the leading cause of chronic kidney disease in the United States. They are the underlying disease process for more than half of those people needing dialysis and result in a significant number of deaths per year (NKUDIC, 2009).

Glomerular disorders may be either primary, involving mainly the kidney, or secondary to a multisystem disease or hereditary condition. Primary glomerular disease is often immunologic or idiopathic in origin. Diabetes mellitus, undiagnosed or inadequately treated hypertension, systemic lupus erythematosus (SLE), and Goodpasture's syndrome are frequently implicated in secondary glomerular disorders.

> **FAST FACTS**
> - Glomerular disorders and diseases are the leading cause of chronic kidney disease in the United States.
> - Hematuria, proteinuria, and hypertension often are early manifestations of glomerular disorders.
> - Acute poststreptococcal glomerulonephritis (also called acute proliferative glomerulonephritis) is the most common primary glomerular disorder.
> - Diabetes mellitus, hypertension, and SLE are common causes of secondary glomerulonephritis.

Physiology Review

The glomerulus is a tuft of capillaries surrounded by a thin, double-walled capsule (Bowman's capsule) (see Figure 26–3). About 20% of the resting cardiac output flows through the glomeruli of the kidneys, forming approximately 180 L of plasma ultrafiltrate. More than 99% of this filtrate is reabsorbed in the renal tubules. The rate of glomerular filtration is controlled by opposing forces: The pressure and amount of blood flowing through the glomeruli promote filtration, and the pressure in Bowman's capsule and colloid osmotic (*oncotic*) pressure of the blood oppose it. The total surface area of glomerular capillaries also affects the GFR. The glomerular capillary membrane has three layers: the capillary endothelial layer, the basement membrane, and the capsule epithelial layer. Water and the smallest solutes (such as electrolytes) pass freely across this membrane, whereas larger molecules (such as plasma proteins) are retained in the blood.

Pathophysiology

Glomerular disease affects both the structure and function of the glomerulus, disrupting glomerular filtration. The capillary membrane becomes more permeable to plasma proteins and blood cells. This increased permeability in the glomerulus causes the manifestations common to glomerular disorders: hematuria, proteinuria, and edema. The GFR falls, leading to **azotemia** (increased blood levels of nitrogenous waste products) and hypertension. Glomerular involvement may be diffuse (involving all glomeruli) or focal (involving some glomeruli while others remain essentially normal).

Both hematuria and proteinuria are caused by glomerular capillary membrane damage, which allows blood cells and proteins to escape from the blood into the glomerular filtrate. Hematuria may be either gross or microscopic. Proteinuria is considered to be the most important indicator of glomerular injury, because it increases progressively with increased glomerular damage. Loss of plasma proteins leads to *hypoalbuminemia* (low serum albumin levels), which in turn reduces the plasma oncotic pressure (osmotic pressure created by plasma proteins), leading to edema.

As plasma proteins are lost, the forces opposing filtration diminish, and the amount of filtrate increases. The increased flow of filtrate stimulates the renin–angiotensin–aldosterone mechanism (∞ see Chapter 26), producing vasoconstriction and a resulting fall in GFR. Increased aldosterone production causes salt and water retention, which further contribute to edema. As the GFR falls, filtration and elimination of nitrogenous wastes, including urea, decrease, causing azotemia. **Oliguria**, urine output of less than 400 mL in 24 hours, may result from the decreased GFR. Hypertension results from fluid retention and disruption of the renin–angiotensin system, a key regulator of blood pressure.

The major primary glomerular disorders include acute glomerulonephritis, rapidly progressive glomerulonephritis, nephrotic syndrome, and chronic glomerulonephritis. Diabetic nephropathy and lupus nephritis are the most common secondary forms of glomerular disease.

Acute Postinfectious Glomerulonephritis

Glomerulonephritis is inflammation of the glomerular capillary membrane. Acute glomerulonephritis can result from systemic diseases or primary glomerular diseases, but acute postinfectious glomerulonephritis (also known as acute poststreptococcal glomerulonephritis) is the most common form. Infection of the pharynx or skin with group A beta-hemolytic streptococcus is the usual initiating event for this disorder. Staphylococcal or viral infections, such as hepatitis B, mumps, or varicella (chickenpox), can lead to a similar postinfectious acute glomerulonephritis. This primarily childhood disease also can affect adults.

In acute postinfectious glomerulonephritis, circulating antigen–antibody immune complexes formed during the primary infection become trapped in the glomerular membrane, leading to an inflammatory response. The complement system is activated, and vasoactive substances and inflammatory mediators are released. Endothelial cells proliferate, and the glomerular membrane swells and becomes permeable to plasma proteins and blood cells. Renal involvement is diffuse, spread throughout the kidneys. See Pathophysiology Illustrated: Acute Glomerulonephritis on page 823.

MANIFESTATIONS AND COMPLICATIONS Acute postinfectious glomerulonephritis is characterized by an abrupt onset of hematuria, proteinuria, salt and water retention, and evidence of azotemia occurring 10 to 14 days after the initial infection. The urine often appears brown or cola-colored. Salt and water retention increase extracellular fluid volume, leading to hypertension and edema. The edema is primarily noted in the face, particularly around the eyes (*periorbital* edema). Dependent

PATHOPHYSIOLOGY ILLUSTRATED
Acute Postinfectious Glomerulonephritis

Infection from group A beta-hemolytic Streptococcus causes an immune response that causes inflammation and damage to the glomeruli. Protein and red blood cells are allowed to pass through the glomeruli. Blood flow to the glomeruli is reduced due to obstruction with damaged cells and renal insufficiency results, leading to the retention of sodium, water, and waste.

Kidney
Glomerulus

INFECTION

IMMUNE RESPONSE
Antigen–antibody complexes are deposited into the glomerular capillary filtration membrane

Monocyte (leukocyte)
Membrane
IgG (ab-antigen)

Coagulation system may be activated, leading to a proliferation of cells in the glomerular membrane

Inflammation and attack on the glomerular membrane occurs by neutrophils and monocytes

Subepithelial deposits of gamma globulins (immune complex)

Neutrophil
Endothelial cell proliferation
Mesangial cell proliferation

Enzymes are released that damage glomerular cell walls

Increased membrane permeability permits the passage of protein and red blood cells into the urine

RBC
Protein
Leukocyte
RBCs and leukocytes leak into capsular space causing edema

Capillary lumen occluded with proliferating cells and leukocytes

Renal blood flow and glomerular filtration are decreased

Renal insufficiency; retention of sodium, water, and waste

edema, affecting the hands and upper extremities in particular, may also be noted. Other manifestations may include fatigue, anorexia, nausea and vomiting, and headache (see the Pathophysiology Linkages table on page 824).

The older adult may have less apparent symptoms. Nausea, malaise, arthralgias, and proteinuria are common manifestations; hypertension and edema are seen less often. Pulmonary infiltrates may occur early in the disorder, often due to worsening of a preexisting condition such as heart failure.

The prognosis for adults with acute glomerulonephritis is less favorable than it is for children. The symptoms may resolve spontaneously within 10 to 14 days. Full recovery is usual in children, whereas 60% or more affected adults recover completely. The remainder have persistent symptoms, and some have permanent kidney damage (Porth & Matfin, 2009).

Rapidly Progressive Glomerulonephritis

Rapidly progressive glomerulonephritis (RPGN), which also may be known as crescentic glomerulonephritis, is characterized by manifestations of severe glomerular injury without a specific, identifiable cause. This type of glomerulonephritis often progresses to renal failure within months. It may be idiopathic

MANIFESTATION	RELATED PATHOPHYSIOLOGY
Hematuria, cola-colored urine	Disruption of the glomerular capillary membrane allows red blood cells to escape from the vascular system into Bowman's capsule, ultimately being excreted in the urine
Proteinuria	Plasma proteins cross the damaged glomerular capillary membrane, becoming part of the filtrate and excreted urine
Salt and water retention	Loss of plasma proteins reduces plasma oncotic pressure, reducing this oppositional force to filtration. The amount of filtrate increases, stimulating the renin-angiotensin-aldosterone system and prompting salt and water retention.
Edema, periorbital and facial, dependent	Increased vascular volume due to salt and water retention coupled with decreased plasma oncotic pressure forces more fluid out of capillaries into interstitial tissues.
Hypertension	Activation of the renin-angiotensin-aldosterone system leads to vasoconstriction and increased peripheral vascular resistance, as well as increased vascular volume due to salt and water retention.
Azotemia	Vasoconstriction reduces renal blood flow, reducing filtration and excretion of metabolic waste products.
Fatigue, anorexia, nausea, and vomiting	Retained metabolic waste products and fluid and electrolyte and acid–base imbalances affect energy production and vomiting centers in the CNS.
Headache	Increased intravascular volume and fluid and electrolyte and acid–base imbalances lead to intracranial vasodilation.

(primary), or secondary to a systemic disorder such as SLE or Goodpasture's syndrome. It affects people of all ages.

In RPGN, glomerular cells proliferate and, together with macrophages, form crescent-shaped lesions that obliterate Bowman's space. Glomerular damage is diffuse, leading to a rapid, progressive decline in renal function. Irreversible renal failure often develops over weeks to months.

Patients with RPGN typically present with complaints of weakness, nausea, and vomiting. Some may relate a history of a flulike illness preceding the onset of the glomerulonephritis. Other symptoms include oliguria and abdominal or flank pain. Moderate hypertension may develop. On urinalysis, hematuria and massive proteinuria are noted.

GOODPASTURE'S SYNDROME *Goodpasture's syndrome* is a rare autoimmune disorder of unknown etiology. It is characterized by formation of antibodies to the glomerular basement membrane. These antibodies also may bind to alveolar basement membranes, damaging alveoli and causing pulmonary hemorrhage. Goodpasture's syndrome usually affects young men between ages 18 and 35, as well as men and women in their 60s or 70s.

Although the glomeruli may be nearly normal in appearance and function in Goodpasture's syndrome, extensive cell proliferation and crescent formation characteristic of rapidly progressive glomerulonephritis are more common. Renal manifestations include hematuria, proteinuria, and edema. Rapid progression to renal failure may occur. Alveolar membrane damage can lead to mild or life-threatening pulmonary hemorrhage. Cough, shortness of breath, and hemoptysis (bloody sputum) are early respiratory manifestations.

Nephrotic Syndrome

Nephrotic syndrome is a group of clinical findings as opposed to a specific disorder. It is characterized by massive proteinuria, hypoalbuminemia, hyperlipidemia, and edema. A number of

disorders can affect the glomerular capillary membrane, changing its porosity and allowing plasma proteins to escape into the urine.

Minimal change disease (MCD) is the most common cause of nephrotic syndrome in children but accounts for only 10% to 15% of adults with nephrotic syndrome. In MCD, the size and form of glomeruli appear normal by light microscopy. Relapse, common in children, occurs less frequently in adults. When it occurs, however, relapse can be resistant to effective treatment.

In White, non-Hispanic adults, *membranous glomerulonephropathy* is the most common cause of nephrotic syndrome. The glomerular basement membrane thickens, although no inflammation is present. This form of nephrotic syndrome develops secondarily to malignancy, infection, or an autoimmune disorder in up to 30% of cases. The cause often cannot be identified (idiopathic). *Focal sclerosis*, in which scarring (sclerosis) of glomeruli occurs, and *membranoproliferative glomerulonephritis*, caused by thickening and proliferation of glomerular basement membrane cells, are additional forms of nephrotic syndrome.

With plasma protein loss in the urine and resulting hypoalbuminemia, the oncotic pressure of the plasma falls. Fluid shifts from the vascular compartment to interstitial spaces, causing the edema characteristic of nephrotic syndrome. Salt and water retention, possibly due to activation of the renin–angiotensin system, contribute to the edema. Edema may be severe, affecting the face and periorbital area as well as dependent tissues (Figure 28–2 ■).

Loss of plasma proteins stimulates the liver to increase albumin production and lipoprotein synthesis. As a result, serum triglyceride and low-density lipoprotein (LDL) levels increase, as do urine lipids (*lipiduria*). Hyperlipidemia increases the risk for atherosclerosis in patients with nephrotic syndrome.

Thromboemboli (mobilized blood clots) are a relatively common complication of nephrotic syndrome. Loss of clotting and anticlotting factors along with plasma proteins are thought to disrupt the coagulation system, increasing the risk for renal venous thrombosis, deep venous thrombosis, and pulmonary

Figure 28–2 ■ Severe edema characteristic of nephrotic syndrome.

embolism. Renal venous thrombosis can cause flank or groin pain on one or both sides, gross hematuria, and a reduced GFR.

Nephrotic syndrome usually resolves without long-term effects in children. The prognosis for adults is less optimistic because the syndrome often occurs secondarily to another disorder. Many adults do not recover completely, experiencing persistent proteinuria and potentially, progressive renal impairment.

Chronic Glomerulonephritis

Chronic glomerulonephritis is typically the result of progressive glomerular disorders such as RPGN, lupus nephritis, or diabetic nephropathy. In many cases, however, no previous glomerular disease has been identified.

Slow, progressive destruction of the glomeruli and a gradual decline in renal function are characteristic of chronic glomerulonephritis. The kidneys decrease in size symmetrically, and their surfaces become granular or roughened. Eventually, entire nephrons are lost.

Symptoms develop insidiously, and the disease is often not recognized until signs of renal failure develop. Chronic glomerulonephritis may also be diagnosed when hypertension and impaired renal function are found coincidentally during a routine physical examination or treatment for an unrelated disorder. Viral or bacterial infectious diseases can exacerbate the disorder, prompting its diagnosis.

The course of chronic glomerulonephritis varies, with years to decades between the diagnosis and the development of end-stage renal failure.

Diabetic Nephropathy

Diabetic nephropathy, kidney disease common in the later stages of diabetes mellitus (DM), is the leading cause of chronic kidney disease in North America. About 40% of patients with diabetes develop nephropathy; because type 2 diabetes is more prevalent, it accounts for a higher portion of patients with chronic kidney disease. Diabetes-associated kidney lesions are more common in Blacks, Native Americans, and Pacific Islanders (Fauci et al., 2008).

Initial evidence of microproteinuria indicating renal damage is typically seen within 5 to 10 years after the onset of diabetes. Overt proteinuria and nephropathy generally develop within another 5 to 10 years of the onset of microproteinuria.

The characteristic lesion of diabetic nephropathy is glomerulosclerosis and thickening of the glomerular basement membrane. As the disease progresses, the glomerular capillary lumen narrows, reducing the surface area for glomerular filtration. Arteriosclerosis, a common feature of long-term diabetes and hypertension, contributes to the disease, as do nephritis and tubular lesions. Pyelonephritis, inflammation of the kidney, is also implicated in the development of diabetic nephropathy. A further discussion of diabetic nephropathy is found in ∞ Chapter 20.

Lupus Nephritis

Systemic lupus erythematosus (SLE) is an inflammatory autoimmune disorder affecting the connective tissue of the body. Most patients with SLE develop kidney abnormalities related to their disease; many develop manifestations of nephritis (Fauci et al., 2008). Circulating immune complexes deposited in the glomerulus as well as those that form within the glomerular capillary wall trigger an inflammatory response leading to glomerular injury in SLE. Manifestations of lupus nephritis range from microscopic hematuria to massive proteinuria. Its progression may be slow and chronic or *fulminant*, with a sudden onset and the rapid development of renal failure. End-stage kidney disease eventually develops in about 20% of patients with lupus nephritis. Improved management of the underlying disease, immunotherapy, dialysis, and renal transplantation have significantly improved the prognosis in recent years.

Interdisciplinary Care

Management of all types of glomerulonephritis, acute and chronic, primary and secondary, focuses on identifying the underlying disease process and preserving kidney function. In most glomerular disorders, there is no specific treatment to achieve a cure. Treatment goals are to maintain renal function, prevent complications, and support the healing process.

Diagnosis

Laboratory and diagnostic testing are valuable to identify the cause of glomerulonephritis and evaluate kidney function.

The following studies may be ordered to help identify the underlying cause or etiology:

- *Throat or skin cultures* detect infection by group A beta-hemolytic streptococci. Although poststreptococcal glomerulonephritis typically follows the acute infection by 1 to 2 weeks, treatment to eradicate any remaining organisms is initiated to minimize antibody production.
- *Antistreptolysin O (ASO) titer* and other tests detect streptococcal *exoenzymes* (bacterial enzymes that stimulate the immune response in acute poststreptococcal glomerulonephritis). Other titers such as antistreptokinase (ASK) or antideoxyribonuclease B (ADNAase B) may be obtained as well.
- *Erythrocyte sedimentation rate (ESR)* may be elevated in acute poststreptococcal glomerulonephritis and in lupus nephritis.
- *KUB* (kidney, ureter, bladder) *abdominal x-ray* may show enlarged kidneys in acute glomerulonephritis, whereas bilateral small kidneys are typical of late chronic glomerulonephritis.

- *Kidney scan* demonstrates delayed uptake and excretion of the radioactive material in glomerular diseases.
- *Biopsy* is the most reliable diagnostic procedure for glomerular disorders. Biopsy helps determine the type of glomerulonephritis, the prognosis, and appropriate treatment.

∞ See Chapter 26 for the nursing implications of diagnostic tests used to evaluate glomerular disorders.

The following studies are used to evaluate kidney function:

- *Blood urea nitrogen (BUN)* is measured. Urea is eliminated from the body by filtration in the glomerulus; minimal amounts are reabsorbed in the renal tubules. Glomerular diseases interfere with filtration and elimination of urea nitrogen, causing blood levels to rise. Normal BUN values are listed in Table 28–2. Levels up to 50 mg/dL or 17.7 mmol/L indicate mild azotemia, and levels higher than 100 mg/dL or 35.7 mmol/L indicate severe renal impairment.
- *Serum creatinine* is a good indicator of kidney function. Levels greater than 4 mg/dL indicate serious renal impairment.
- *Urine creatinine* levels decrease when renal function is impaired because it is not effectively eliminated from the body.
- *eGFR (estimated GFR)* is a calculated value used to evaluate renal function. Four variables are used to calculate the eGFR: serum creatinine, age in years, gender, and race (African American or other). Values of 60 mL/min/1.73 m^2 or higher are within the normal range for adults (20 years old and above), and may simply be reported as > 60 mL/min/1.73 m^2.
- *Creatinine clearance* may be used to evaluate the GFR. The *clearance*, or amount of blood cleared of creatinine in 1 minute, depends on the amount and pressure of blood being filtered and the filtering ability of the glomeruli. Disorders such as glomerulonephritis affect glomerular filtration, decreasing the creatinine clearance.
- *Serum electrolytes* are evaluated because impaired kidney function alters their excretion.
- *Urinalysis* often shows red blood cells (RBCs) and proteins in the urine of patients with a glomerular disorder. These substances, normally too large to enter glomerular filtrate, escape due to increased porosity of glomerular capillaries in glomerular disorders.

Medications

Although no drugs are available to cure glomerular disorders, medications are used to treat underlying disorders, reduce inflammation, and manage the symptoms.

Antibiotics are prescribed for the patient with poststreptococcal glomerulonephritis to eradicate any remaining bacteria, removing the stimulus for antibody production. Nephrotoxic antibiotics, such as the aminoglycoside antibiotics, streptomycin, and some cephalosporins, are avoided.

Aggressive immunosuppressive therapy is used to treat acute inflammatory processes such as rapidly progressive glomerulonephritis, Goodpasture's syndrome, and exacerbations of SLE. When begun early, immunosuppressive therapy significantly reduces the risk of end-stage renal disease and renal failure. Prednisone, a glucocorticoid, is prescribed in relatively large doses of 1 mg per kilogram of body weight per day (e.g., a 160-pound man would receive 70 to 75 mg per day). Other immunosuppressive agents such as cyclophosphamide (Cytoxan) or azathioprine (Imuran) are prescribed in conjunction with corticosteroids. Corticosteroid use in poststreptococcal glomerulonephritis may actually worsen the condition, so it is avoided.

TABLE 28–2 Changes in Laboratory Values Associated with Kidney Disease

TEST	NORMAL VALUE	VALUE IN RENAL DISEASE
Blood urea nitrogen (BUN)	5–25 mg/dL Slightly higher in older adults	25–50 mg/dL or higher
BUN/Creatinine ratio	10:1 (BUN:creatinine) to 20:1	Decreased ratio in acute tubular necrosis; increased in glomerular disease, azotemia
Creatinine, serum	0.5–1.5 mg/dL Slightly lower in females, older adults	Elevated; levels > 4 mg/dL indicate severe impairment of renal function
Creatinine clearance	85–135 mL/min Slightly lower in females Values decline in older adults	Reduced renal reserve: 32.5–85.0 mL/min Renal insufficiency: 6.5–32.5 mL/min Renal failure: < 6.5 mL/min
eGFR	≥ 60 mL/min/1.73 m^2	Decreased in renal impairment
Serum albumin	3.5–5 g/dL; lower in older adults	Decreased in nephrotic syndrome
Serum electrolytes	Potassium: 3.5–5.3 mEq/L Sodium: 135–145 mEq/L Calcium: 4.5–5.5 mEq/L or 9–11 mg/dL Phosphorus: 2.5–4.5 mg/dL	Increased in renal insufficiency Decreased in nephrotic syndrome Decreased in renal failure Increased in renal failure
Red blood cell count	Female: 4.0–5.0 million/mm^3 Male: 4.6–6.0 million/mm^3	Decreased in chronic kidney disease
Urine creatinine	1 – 2 g/24 hours	Decreased in disorders of impaired renal function
Urine protein	25–150 mg/24 hours	Increased in disorders of impaired renal function
Urine red blood cells	< 2/HPF; no RBC casts	Present in glomerular disorders

Oral glucocorticoids such as prednisone also are used in high doses to induce remission of nephrotic syndrome. When glucocorticoids alone are ineffective, other immunosuppressive agents such as cyclophosphamide or chlorambucil (Leukeran) may be used to induce or maintain remission. ∞ See Chapter 13 for more information about corticosteroids and other immunosuppressive drugs.

ACE inhibitors or angiotensin-receptor blockers (ARBs) may be ordered to reduce protein loss associated with nephrotic syndrome and slow the progression of renal failure. They have a protective effect on the kidney in patients with diabetic nephropathy.

Antihypertensives are prescribed to maintain the blood pressure within normal levels. Blood pressure management is important because systemic and renal hypertension are associated with a poorer prognosis in patients with glomerular disorders.

Treatments

Restricted activity may be recommended during the acute phase of poststreptococcal glomerulonephritis. When the edema of nephrotic syndrome is significant or the patient is hypertensive, sodium intake may be restricted to 1 to 2 g per day. Dietary protein may be restricted if azotemia is present. When proteins are restricted, those included in the diet should be complete or high-value proteins. Complete proteins supply the essential amino acids required for growth and tissue maintenance. Complete and incomplete proteins are compared in Table 28–3.

Plasma exchange therapy (also called *plasmapheresis*), a procedure to remove damaging antibodies from the plasma, is used in conjunction with immunosuppressive therapy to treat RPGN and Goodpasture's syndrome. Plasma and glomerular-damaging antibodies are removed using a blood cell separator. The RBCs are then returned to the patient along with albumin or human plasma to replace the plasma removed. This procedure is usually done in a series of treatments. It is not without risk, and informed consent is required. Potential complications of plasma exchange therapy include those associated with intravenous catheters, fluid volume shifts, and altered coagulation.

Renal failure resulting from a glomerular disorder may necessitate dialysis to restore fluid and electrolyte balance and remove waste products from the body. Dialysis procedures and related nursing care are explained in the acute renal failure section later in this chapter.

Nursing Care

Health Promotion

Discuss the importance of effectively treating streptococcal infections in all age groups to help reduce the risk for acute glomerulonephritis. Stress the importance of completing the full course of antibiotic therapy to eradicate the infecting bacteria. Teach patients with diabetes mellitus and SLE about potential renal effects of their disease. Discuss measures to reduce the risk of associated nephritis, such as effectively managing the disease, treating hypertension, and avoiding drugs and substances that are potentially toxic to the kidneys.

Assessment

∞ Review Chapter 26 for complete assessment of the renal and urinary systems. Focused assessment data related to glomerular disorders include the following:

- *Health history:* Complaints of facial or peripheral edema or weight gain, fatigue, nausea and vomiting, headache, general malaise, abdominal or flank pain; cough or shortness of breath; changes in amount, color, or character of urine (e.g., frothy urine); history of skin or pharyngeal streptococcal infection, diabetes, SLE, or kidney disease; current medications.
- *Physical examination:* General appearance; vital signs; weight; presence of periorbital, facial, or peripheral edema; inspect skin for lesions, infection; inspect throat, obtain culture as indicated; obtain urine specimen for color, character, odor.

Nursing Diagnoses and Interventions

Nursing care is supportive and educational. Monitoring renal function and fluid volume status are key components of care, as is protecting the patient from infection. Both manifestations of glomerular disorders and their treatment can interfere with a patient's ability to maintain usual roles and responsibilities. For additional potential nursing diagnoses and interventions, see the Case Study & Nursing Care Plan on page 829.

Excess Fluid Volume

Excess fluid volume and resulting edema are common manifestations of glomerular disorders. When proteins are lost in the urine, the oncotic pressure of plasma falls, and fluid shifts into the interstitial spaces. The body responds to this fluid shift by

TABLE 28–3 Complete and Incomplete Protein Sources

	COMPLETE PROTEINS	INCOMPLETE PROTEINS
Definition	Provide all essential amino acids needed for growth and tissue maintenance	Lack one or more essential amino acids or contain inadequate proportions
Examples	Milk, eggs, cheese, meats, poultry, fish, and soy	Vegetables, breads, cereals and grains, legumes, seeds, and nuts

EVIDENCE FOR NURSING CARE — The Patient with Glomerulonephritis

Selected resources that nurses may find helpful when planning evidence-based nursing care follow.

- Nguyen, T., & Toto, R. (2008). Slowing chronic kidney disease progression: results of prospective clinical trials in adults. *Pediatric Nephrology, 23*(9), 1409–1422.
- Singapore Ministry of Health. (2007 March). *Glomerulonephritis.* Singapore: Singapore Ministry of Health. Retrieved from http://www.guideline.gov/summary/summary.aspx?doc_id=10845&nbr=005660&string=glomerulonephritis

View from back

Incision

A   B   C

Figure 28–4 ■ Incisions used for kidney surgery: *A*, flank; *B*, lumbar; and *C*, thoracoabdominal.

■ Encourage frequent (every 1 to 2 hours) deep breathing, spirometer use, and coughing. Assist to splint the incision. *These measures promote alveolar ventilation, gas exchange, and airway clearance.*

Risk for Impaired Urinary Elimination

Surgery involving the urinary tract increases the risk for altered renal function and urine elimination. In addition, removal of one kidney dictates extra caution to maintain renal circulation, a sterile urinary tract, and free urine flow.

■ Monitor vital signs, CVP, and urine output every 1 to 2 hours initially, then every 4 hours. *Hypovolemia due to hemorrhage, diuresis, or fluid sequestering (third spacing) reduces blood flow to the kidney and increases the risk of renal ischemia with possible acute tubular necrosis and acute renal failure.*

■ Frequently assess the amount and nature of drainage on surgical dressings and from drainage tubes, stents, and catheters. Measure and record output from each drain or catheter separately. *Frequent and accurate assessment of drainage helps to identify excess bleeding, abnormal fluid loss, infection, or other potential surgical complications.*

> **PRACTICE ALERT**
> Prevent kinking, twisting, or tension on drains and tubes. Do not clamp. Irrigate carefully and only with a physician's order. Notify the physician immediately if any tube becomes dislodged. It is vital to maintain the patency of drains, particularly any affecting the remaining kidney, to prevent the excess pressure of hydronephrosis.

■ Maintain fluid intake with intravenous fluids until oral intake is resumed. Encourage an intake of 2000 to 2500 mL per day as soon as the patient tolerates oral liquids. *A liberal fluid intake prevents dehydration, helps to dilute any nephrotoxic substances, and promotes good urinary output.*

■ Use strict aseptic technique in caring for all urinary catheters, tubes, stents, drains, and incisions. *Asepsis is vital to prevent infection and possible compromise of the remaining kidney.*

■ Following catheter removal, assess frequently for urinary retention. Notify the physician if the patient is unable to void within 4 to 6 hours or if manifestations of retention (distended bladder, discomfort, urinary dribbling) develop. *Maintenance of urine output is vital to prevent stasis and possible complications such as infection and hydronephrosis.*

■ Monitor laboratory results, including urinalysis, BUN, serum creatinine, and serum electrolytes. Report abnormal findings to the physician. *Abnormal values may indicate early acute renal failure; prompt intervention is necessary to preserve renal function.*

Grieving

The patient having a radical nephrectomy for renal cancer not only loses a major organ but also has to adjust to the diagnosis of cancer. Although the prognosis for recovery may be good, many people perceive cancer as always fatal. Providing support for the patient and family during the initial stages of grieving can improve physical recovery, psychologic coping, and eventual adaptation.

■ Work to develop a trusting relationship with the patient and family. *Trust increases the nurse's effectiveness in helping them work through the process of grieving.*

■ Listen actively, encouraging the patient and family to express fears and concerns. *As they begin to express their concerns, patient and family can begin to deal more effectively with them.*

■ Assist the patient and family to identify strengths, past experiences, and support systems. *These resources can be employed in working through the grieving process.*

■ Demonstrate respect for cultural, spiritual, and religious values and beliefs; encourage use of these resources to cope with losses. *Value and belief systems can provide a structure and form for dealing with the grieving process.*

Having A Nephrectomy

PREOPERATIVE CARE

■ Provide routine preoperative care as outlined in ∞ Chapter 4.

■ Report abnormal laboratory values to the surgeon. *Bacteriuria, blood coagulation abnormalities, or other significant abnormal values may affect surgery and postoperative care.*

■ Discuss operative and postoperative expectations as indicated, including the location of the incision (Figure 28–4) and anticipated tubes, stents, and drains. *Preoperative teaching about postoperative expectations reduces anxiety for the patient and family during the early postoperative period.*

POSTOPERATIVE CARE

■ Provide routine postoperative care as described in ∞ Chapter 4.

■ Frequently assess urine color, amount, and character, noting any hematuria, pyuria, or sediment. Promptly report oliguria or anuria, as well as changes in urine color or clarity. *Preserving function of the remaining kidney is critical; frequent assessment allows early intervention for potential problems.*

■ Note the placement, status, and drainage from ureteral catheters, stents, nephrostomy tubes, or drains. Label each clearly. Maintain gravity drainage; irrigate only as ordered. *Maintaining drainage tube patency is vital to prevent potential hydronephrosis. Bright bleeding o+r unexpected drainage may indicate a surgical complication.*

■ Support the grieving process and adjustment to the loss of a kidney. *Loss of a major organ leads to a body image change and grief response. When renal cancer is the underlying diagnosis, the patient may also grieve the loss of health and potential loss of life.*

■ Provide the following home care instructions for the patient and family:

a. The importance of protecting the remaining kidney by preventing UTI, renal calculi, and trauma. ∞ See Chapter 27 for measures to prevent UTI and calculi. *Damage to the remaining kidney by UTI, renal calculi, or trauma can lead to renal failure.*

b. Maintain a fluid intake of 2000 to 2500 mL per day. *This important measure helps prevent dehydration and maintain good urine flow.*

c. Gradually increase exercise to tolerance, avoiding heavy lifting for a year after surgery. Participation in contact sports is not recommended to reduce the risk of injury to the remaining kidney. *Lifting is avoided to allow full tissue healing. Trauma to the remaining kidney could seriously jeopardize renal function.*

d. Care of the incision and any remaining drainage tubes, catheters, or stents. *This routine postoperative instruction is vital to prepare the patient for self-care and prevent complications.*

e. Report signs and symptoms to the physician, including manifestations of UTI (dysuria, frequency, urgency, nocturia, cloudy, malodorous urine) or systemic infection (fever, general malaise, fatigue), redness, swelling, pain, or drainage from the incision or any catheter or drain tube site. *Prompt treatment of postoperative infection is vital to allow continued healing and prevent compromise of the remaining kidney.*

■ Encourage discussion of the potential impact of loss on the patient and the family structure and function. Assist family members to share concerns with one another. *Sharing of fears and concerns among family members promotes involvement and support of the entire family unit so that the individual is not left to cope alone.*

■ Refer to cancer support groups, social services, or counseling as appropriate. *Support groups and counseling services provide additional resources for coping.*

Community-Based Care

If renal cancer was detected at an early stage and cure is anticipated, teaching for home care focuses on protecting the remaining kidney. Include the following measures to prevent infection, renal calculi, hydronephrosis, and trauma:

■ Maintain a fluid intake of 2000 to 2500 mL per day, increasing the amount during hot weather or strenuous exercise.

■ Urinate when the urge is perceived, and before and after sexual intercourse.

■ Properly clean the perineal area.

■ Watch for manifestations of UTI and understand the importance of early and appropriate evaluation and intervention.

■ If the patient is an older adult male, he should watch for manifestations of prostatic hypertrophy, a major cause of urinary tract obstruction. Stress the importance of routine screening examinations.

■ Avoid contact sports such as football or hockey; use measures to prevent motor vehicle accidents and falls, which could damage the kidney.

Renal Failure

Renal failure is a condition in which the kidneys are unable to remove accumulated metabolites from the blood, leading to altered fluid, electrolyte, and acid–base balance. The cause may be a primary kidney disorder, or renal failure may occur secondary to a systemic disease or other urologic defects. Renal failure may be either acute or chronic. Acute renal failure has an abrupt onset and with prompt intervention is often reversible. Chronic kidney disease (CKD) which may culminate in renal failure, develops slowly and insidiously, often producing few symptoms until the kidneys are severely damaged and unable to meet the excretory needs of the body. Acute renal failure and the final stages of chronic kidney disease are characterized by azotemia, increased levels of nitrogenous wastes in the blood.

Acute Renal Failure Video

Renal failure is common and costly. In 2006, more than 110,800 new patients began receiving treatment for end-stage renal disease (ESRD). Annually, more than 354,700 patients with ESRD undergo dialysis, about 18,000 have kidney transplants, and another 77,650 are awaiting kidney transplants. The annual cost of ESRD treatment (in 2006 dollars) is $33.6 billion. The cost is also measured in lives and lifestyle. The 5-year survival rate for patients undergoing dialysis is about 33% (NKUDIC, 2009). Although many patients report satisfaction with their quality of life, often patients on dialysis are unable to work, and the family structure may disintegrate under the strain of treatment.

The Patient with Acute Renal Failure

Acute renal failure (ARF) is a rapid decline in renal function (over hours to days) with azotemia and fluid and electrolyte imbalances. The most common causes of acute renal failure are ischemia and nephrotoxins. The kidney is particularly vulnerable to both because of the amount of blood that passes through it. A fall in blood pressure or volume can cause ischemia of kidney tissues. Nephrotoxins in the blood damage renal tissue directly.

Incidence and Risk Factors

Approximately 5% to 7% of all hospitalized patients develop ARF; the incidence jumps to as much as 30% in critical and special care units (Fauci et al., 2008). The mortality rate for ARF in seriously ill patients is up to 60%. This high death rate is probably more related to the populations affected by ARF—older patients and the critically ill—than to the disorder itself (Porth & Matfin, 2009).

Major trauma or surgery, infection, hemorrhage, severe heart failure, severe liver disease, and lower urinary tract obstruction are risk factors for ARF. Drugs and radiologic contrast media that are toxic to the kidney (*nephrotoxic*) also increase the risk for ARF. Older adults develop ARF more frequently due to their higher incidence of serious illness, hypotension, major surgeries, diagnostic procedures, and treatment with nephrotoxic drugs. The older adult also may have some degree of preexisting renal insufficiency associated with aging.

Physiology Review

The functional unit of the kidneys, the nephron (see Figure 26–3), produces urine through three processes: glomerular filtration, tubular reabsorption, and tubular secretion. In the

glomerulus, a filtrate of water and small solutes is formed. The solute concentration of this filtrate is equal to that of plasma, with the exception of large molecules such as plasma proteins and blood cells. The GFR, the amount of filtrate formed per minute, is affected by blood volume and pressure, the autonomic nervous system, and other factors. From the glomerulus, the filtrate flows into the *tubules*, where its composition is changed by the processes of *tubular reabsorption* and *tubular secretion*. Most water and many filtered solutes such as electrolytes and glucose are reabsorbed. Metabolic waste products such as urea, hydrogen ion, ammonia, and some creatinine are secreted into the tubule for elimination. By the time urine exits the collecting duct into the renal pelvis, 99% of the filtrate has been reabsorbed.

Pathophysiology

The causes and pathophysiology of acute renal failure are commonly categorized as prerenal, intrinsic, and postrenal ARF. Prerenal ARF is the most common, accounting for about 55% of the total. In *prerenal ARF*, hypoperfusion and ischemia lead to acute renal failure without directly affecting the integrity of kidney tissues. *Intrinsic* (or *intrarenal*) *ARF*, due to direct damage to functional kidney tissue, is responsible for another 40%. Urinary tract obstruction with resulting kidney damage is the precipitating factor for *postrenal ARF*, the least common form (~5%). Table 28–5 summarizes the causes of acute renal failure.

Prerenal ARF

Prerenal ARF results from conditions that affect renal blood flow and perfusion. Any disorder that significantly decreases vascular volume, cardiac output, or systemic vascular resistance can affect renal blood flow. The kidneys normally receive 20% to 25% of the cardiac output to maintain the GFR. A drop in renal blood flow to less than 20% of normal causes the GFR to fall. As the filtration of substances by the glomeruli is reduced, less reabsorption of substances in the tubule is required. As a result, kidney cells require less energy and oxygen, and their metabolism slows. Prerenal ARF is rapidly reversed when blood flow is restored, and the renal parenchyma remains undamaged. Continued ischemia can lead to tubular cell necrosis and significant nephron damage. Intrinsic ARF due to ischemic injury may result. See Pathophysiology Illustrated: Acute Renal Failure on page 838.

Postrenal ARF

Obstructive causes of acute renal failure are classified as postrenal. Any condition that prevents urine excretion can lead to postrenal ARF. Benign prostatic hypertrophy is the most

TABLE 28–5 Causes of Acute Renal Failure

	CAUSE	EXAMPLES
Prerenal	Hypovolemia	Hemorrhage, dehydration, excess fluid loss from GI tract, burns, wounds
	Low cardiac output	Heart failure, cardiogenic shock
	Altered vascular resistance	Sepsis, anaphylaxis, vasoactive drugs
Intrarenal	Glomerular/microvascular injury	Glomerulonephritis, DIC, vasculitis, hypertension, toxemia of pregnancy, hemolytic uremic syndrome
	Acute tubular necrosis	Ischemia due to conditions associated with prerenal failure; toxins such as drugs, heavy metals; hemolysis, rhabdomyolysis (muscle cell breakdown)
	Interstitial nephritis	Acute pyelonephritis, toxins, metabolic imbalances, idiopathic
Postrenal	Ureteral obstruction	Calculi, cancer, external compression
	Urethral obstruction	Prostatic enlargement, calculi, cancer, stricture, blood clot

common precipitating factor. Others include renal or urinary tract calculi and tumors. ∞ See Chapter 27 for further discussion of urinary tract obstruction.

Intrinsic (Intrarenal) ARF

Intrinsic or intrarenal failure is characterized by acute damage to the renal parenchyma and nephrons. Intrarenal causes include diseases of the kidney itself and acute tubular necrosis, the most common intrarenal cause of ARF.

In acute glomerulonephritis, glomerular inflammation can reduce renal blood flow and cause ARF. Vascular disorders affecting the kidney, such as vasculitis (inflammation of the blood vessels), malignant hypertension, and arterial or venous occlusion, can damage nephrons sufficiently to result in acute renal failure.

ACUTE TUBULAR NECROSIS Nephrons are especially susceptible to injury from ischemia or exposure to nephrotoxins. **Acute tubular necrosis (ATN)**, destruction of tubular epithelial cells, causes an abrupt and progressive decline of renal function. Prolonged ischemia is the primary cause of ATN. When ischemia and nephrotoxin exposure occur concurrently, the risk for ATN and tubular dysfunction is especially high. Risk factors for ischemic ATN include major surgery, severe hypovolemia, sepsis, trauma, and burns. The impact of ischemia resulting from vasodilation and fluid loss in sepsis, trauma, and burns often is compounded by toxins released by bacteria or from damaged tissue.

Ischemia lasting more than 2 hours causes severe and irreversible damage to kidney tubules with patchy cellular necrosis and sloughing. The GFR is significantly reduced as a result of (1) ischemia, (2) activation of the renin–angiotensin system, and (3) tubular obstruction by cellular debris, which raises the pressure in the glomerular capsule.

Common nephrotoxins associated with ATN include the aminoglycoside antibiotics and radiologic contrast media. Many other drugs (e.g., NSAIDs and some chemotherapy drugs), heavy metals such as mercury and gold, and some common chemicals such as ethylene glycol (antifreeze) are also potentially toxic to the renal tubule. The risk for ATN is higher when nephrotoxic drugs are given to older patients or patients with preexisting renal insufficiency, and when used in combination with other nephrotoxins. Dehydration increases the risk by increasing the toxin concentration in nephrons.

Nephrotoxins destroy tubular cells by both direct and indirect effects. As tubular cells are damaged and lost through necrosis and sloughing, the tubule becomes more permeable. This increased permeability results in filtrate reabsorption, further reducing the ability of the nephron to eliminate wastes.

Rhabdomyolysis caused by release of excess myoglobin from injured skeletal muscles can cause ATN. Myoglobin is a protein that acts as the oxygen reservoir for muscle fibers, much as hemoglobin does for the blood. Muscle trauma, strenuous exercise, hyperthermia or hypothermia, drug overdose, infection, and other factors can precipitate rhabdomyolysis. The myoglobin clogs renal tubules causing ischemic injury, and contains an iron pigment that directly damages the tubules. *Hemolysis*, red blood cell destruction, releases hemoglobin into the circulation with much the same effect as rhabdomyolysis.

Course and Manifestations

The course of acute renal failure due to ATN typically includes three phases: initiation, maintenance, and recovery.

Initiation Phase

The initiation phase may last hours to days. It begins with the initiating event (e.g., hemorrhage) and ends when tubular injury occurs. If ARF is recognized and the initiating event is effectively treated during this phase, the prognosis is good. The initiation phase of ARF has few symptoms; in fact, it is often identified only when manifestations of the maintenance phase develop.

Maintenance Phase

The maintenance phase of ARF is characterized by a significant fall in GFR and tubular necrosis. Oliguria may develop, although many patients continue to produce normal or near-normal amounts of urine (nonoliguric ARF). Even though urine may be produced, the kidney cannot efficiently eliminate metabolic wastes, water, electrolytes, and acids from the body during the maintenance phase of ARF. Azotemia, fluid retention, electrolyte imbalances, and metabolic acidosis develop. These abnormalities are more severe in the oliguric patient than in the nonoliguric one, leading to a poorer prognosis with oliguria.

BOX 28–1   How Deceased Donor Kidneys Are Allocated for Transplant

The scarcity of organs for transplant raises questions about how deceased donor kidneys are allocated—who receives a kidney and who does not. Past inequities in the allocation process (e.g., more men than women, more Caucasians than people of other ethnicities, more rich than poor, and more young than old) led to the development of the United Network for Organ Sharing (UNOS) in 1986. UNOS has policies for organ distribution, including kidneys, hearts, livers, and other transplanted organs.

UNOS maintains national, regional, and local lists of patients awaiting transplants. When an organ becomes available, donor information is entered into the UNOS computer. The computer then runs a match program, generating a list of patients ranked by criteria such as blood and tissue type, organ size, and medical urgency of the patient. Factors such as time on the waiting list and distance between the donor and the transplant center also are considered. A candidate with a perfect match (six HLAs in common) and compatible blood type gets priority for the kidney, regardless of region or geographic area. Otherwise, the list

of patients in the local area is checked first, then the regional list of patients awaiting transplant. If no match is found in the region, the organ becomes available to patients nationwide.

The UNOS allocation system, standardized fees, and Medicare coverage for transplantation have done much to ensure equitable access to available kidneys. Still, controversy exists. Patients with resources for travel may register in several different regions for an organ. Up to 10% of patients receiving a transplant in any center may be foreign nationals competing with U.S. citizens for scarce organ resources. A transplant center can accept or reject a candidate for transplant who has lost a kidney because of noncompliance.

As long as the demand for kidneys exceeds the supply of donor organs, it is likely that controversy will exist regarding their allocation. Nurses can help by identifying potential donors and contacting the transplant coordinator. In addition, nurses can inform the public about organ donation and the allocation system, and encourage donation.

recipient has a greater than 91.7% probability of survival after 2 years. At 5 years, the difference is even greater: 33.1% for dialysis compared with more than 80.2% for transplant (NKU-DIC, 2008). The transplant patient is no longer tethered to a dialysis catheter, machine, or center. Dietary and fluid restrictions are reduced, and the body image is more "whole."

Most transplanted kidneys are obtained from deceased donors; however, transplants from living donors are increasing. In 2009, of transplanted kidneys, 45% came from living donors, most of whom were related to the recipient (OPTN, 2009). With both deceased and living donor transplants, a close match between blood and tissue type is desired. Human leukocyte antigens (HLAs) are compared between the donor and recipient; six antigens in common is considered to be a "perfect" match. The success of well-matched living-donor transplants is better than for deceased donor organ transplants, with a 1-year graft survival of 95.1% compared to 89% for deceased donor transplants (OPTN, 2009). Close tissue matching probably accounts for the better outcome with living donors. People with normal kidneys who are in good physical health may donate a kidney. Predonation counseling is vital: Nephrectomy is major surgery and involves a risk that trauma or disease may damage the remaining kidney in the future. If the transplant fails, the psychologic impact on the donor can be significant. Nursing care of the patient having a nephrectomy is summarized in the box on page 835.

Ideally, deceased donor kidneys are obtained from people who meet the criteria for brain death, are less than 65 years old, and are free of systemic disease, malignancy, or infection, including HIV and hepatitis B or C. Expanded deceased donor criteria may allow donation of a kidney from a deceased donor who is older than 65 years or who has cardiovascular disease (hypertension or stroke) or an elevated serum creatinine (UNOS, 2008). Kidneys are removed after brain death has been determined, and are preserved by hypothermia or a technique called continuous hypothermic pulsatile perfusion. A kidney preserved by hypothermia is transplanted within 24 to 48 hours. Continuous pulsatile perfusion allows up to 3 days before transplantation. The system used to allocate deceased donor kidneys for transplantation is outlined in Box 28–1.

The donor kidney is placed in the lower abdominal cavity of the recipient, and the renal artery, vein, and ureter are anastomosed (Figure 28–10 ■). The renal artery of the donor kidney is connected to the hypogastric artery, and the renal vein to the iliac vein. The ureter is connected to one of the recipient's ureters or directly to the bladder, using a tunnel technique to prevent reflux. Nursing care for the patient having a kidney transplant is outlined in the box on page 855.

Unless the donor and recipient are identical twins, the grafted organ stimulates an immune response to reject the transplanted organ. Immunosuppressive drugs minimize this response. Azathioprine or mycophenolate mofetil are commonly used, often in combination with prednisone, a corticosteroid. Cyclosporine, a potent immunosuppressive, also may be used. These drugs suppress a portion of the immune system and

Transplanted kidney

Internal iliac artery and vein

External iliac artery and vein

Grafted ureter

Figure 28–10 ■ Placement of a transplanted kidney in the iliac fossa with anastomosis to the hypogastric artery, iliac vein, and bladder.

the inflammatory response, increasing the risk for infections and cancers with long-term therapy. The nursing implications of immunosuppressive therapy are outlined in ∞ Chapter 13.

Glucocorticoids such as prednisone and methylprednisolone are used for both maintenance of immunosuppression and to treat acute rejection episodes. Side effects of long-term corticosteroid use include impaired wound healing, emotional disturbances, osteoporosis, and cushingoid effects on glucose, protein, and fat metabolism.

Azathioprine inhibits both cellular and humoral immunity. Because this drug is rapidly metabolized by the liver, the dose may not need to be altered in the presence of renal failure. Bone marrow suppression, abnormalities of liver function, and alopecia are the primary significant adverse effects for azathioprine. The action of mycophenolate mofetil is similar to that of azathioprine. Its advantages are minimal bone marrow suppression and increased potency in preventing or reversing rejection of the transplanted organ (Fauci et al., 2008).

Cyclosporine primarily affects cellular immunity, the helper T cells in particular. Among its many adverse effects, which include hepatotoxicity and hirsutism, nephrotoxicity is a primary concern for the kidney transplant patient.

Even with immunosuppressive therapy, the transplanted kidney can be rejected at any time. Either acute or chronic rejection may develop. *Acute rejection* develops within months of the transplant. It is caused by a cellular immune response with T-lymphocyte proliferation (Porth & Matfin, 2009). Few manifestations may be apparent other than a rise in serum creatinine and possible oliguria. Methylprednisolone, a glucocorticoid, and OKT3 monoclonal antibody (∞ see Chapter 13) are used to manage acute rejection episodes. OKT3 can cause severe systemic reactions, including chills, fever, hypotension, headache, and possible pulmonary edema (Fauci et al., 2008). *Chronic rejection*, which may develop months to years following the transplant, is a major cause of graft loss. Both humoral and cellular immune responses are involved in chronic rejection. It does not respond to increased immunosuppression. The presenting manifestations of chronic rejection—progressive azotemia, proteinuria, and hypertension—are those of progressive renal failure.

Hypertension is a possible complication of kidney transplant, resulting from graft rejection, renal artery stenosis, or renal vasoconstriction. Patients may develop glomerular lesions and manifestations of nephrosis. Hypertension and altered blood lipids (increased LDLs and decreased HDLs) increase the risk of death from myocardial infarction and stroke following transplant (Fauci et al., 2008).

Long-term immunosuppression has adverse effects as well. Infection is a continuing threat. Bacterial and viral infections may develop, as well as fungal infections of the blood, lungs, and CNS. Tumors are also common, with carcinoma *in situ* of the cervix, lymphomas, and skin cancers most prevalent. The risk of congenital anomalies is increased in infants whose mothers have undergone immunosuppressive therapy. Corticosteroid use may lead to bone problems, gastrointestinal disorders such as peptic ulcer disease, and cataract formation.

✑ Nursing Care

Health Promotion

Measures to reduce the risk of CKD focus on preventing kidney disease and appropriately managing diabetes and hypertension. Promote early and effective treatment of all infections, particularly skin and pharyngeal infections caused by streptococcal bacteria. Discuss measures to reduce the risk for urinary tract infections, and stress the importance of prompt treatment to eradicate the infecting organism. Discuss the relationship between diabetes, hypertension, and kidney disease. Emphasize that maintaining blood glucose levels and the blood pressure within the recommended ranges reduces the risk of adverse effects on the kidneys. Ensure that all patients with less than optimal renal function are well-hydrated, particularly when a nephrotoxic drug is prescribed or anticipated. Finally, encourage the patient with ESRD to investigate options for early transplantation to avoid long-term dialysis.

Assessment

Both subjective and objective data are used to assess the patient with CKD:

- *Health history:* Complaints of anorexia, nausea, weight gain, or edema; current treatment (if any), including type and frequency of dialysis or previous kidney transplant; chronic diseases such as diabetes, heart failure, or kidney disease.
- *Physical examination:* Mental status; vital signs including temperature, heart and lung sounds, and peripheral pulses; urine output (if any); weight; skin color, moisture, condition; presence of edema (periorbital or dependent); bowel tones; presence and location of an AV fistula, shunt, graft, or peritoneal catheter.

See the box on page 859 for assessment of the older adult with ESRD.

EVIDENCE FOR NURSING CARE — The Patient with Chronic Renal Failure

Selected resources that nurses may find helpful when planning evidence-based nursing care follow.

- Lin, Y-F., Wu, V-C., Ko, W-J, Chen, Y-S., Chen, Y-M., Li, W-Y. et al. (2009). Residual urine output and postoperative mortality in maintenance hemodialysis patients. *American Journal of Critical Care*, 18(5), 446–55.
- Michigan Quality Improvement Consortium. (2008 November). *Diagnosis and management of adults with chronic kidney disease*. Southfield, MI: Michigan Quality Improvement Consortium. Retrieved from http://www.guideline.gov/summary/summary.aspx?ss=15&doc_id=13824&nbr=&string=
- National Collaborating Centre for Chronic Conditions. (2008 September). *Chronic kidney disease. Early identification and management of chronic kidney disease in adults in primary and secondary care*. London, UK: National Institute for Health and Clinical Excellence (NICE). Retrieved from http://www.guideline.gov/summary/summary.aspx?ss=15&doc_id=14330&nbr=&string=

Nursing Diagnoses and Interventions

Whether the patient with ESRD is facing long-term dialysis or renal transplantation, a number of nursing care needs can be identified. This section focuses on nursing care related to impaired renal function, nutritional deficits due to dietary restrictions and nausea, increased risk for infection, and changes in body image. Also see the Case Study & Nursing Care Plan on page 860 for additional potential nursing diagnoses and interventions for the patient with chronic kidney disease.

Risk for Ineffective Renal Perfusion

Capillaries are an integral part of the nephron. As nephrons are destroyed, kidney perfusion progressively declines. As renal perfusion and nephron function fall, the kidney is less able to maintain fluid and electrolyte balance and eliminate waste products from the body.

■ Monitor intake and output, vital signs including orthostatic blood pressures, and weight. *These provide important data to identify changes in fluid volume.*

PRACTICE ALERT
Weight changes are a more accurate indicator of fluid volume status in the oliguric or anuric patient than intake and output measurements.

■ Restrict fluids as ordered. *As renal function declines, the ability to eliminate excess fluid is impaired.*
■ Monitor respiratory status, including lung sounds, every 4 to 8 hours. *Fluid volume overload may lead to heart failure and possible pulmonary edema.*
■ Monitor BUN, serum creatinine, eGFR, pH, electrolytes, and CBC. Report significant changes. *As renal function declines, the GFR falls and progressive azotemia with increasing BUN and serum creatinine is seen. Metabolic acidosis develops as the kidney is unable to eliminate hydrogen ions and conserve bicarbonate. Hyponatremia, hyperkalemia, hyperphosphatemia, and hypocalcemia are associated with renal failure. The RBC count, hemoglobin, and hematocrit decline due to deficient erythropoietin to stimulate cell production in the bone marrow. An acute fall in hemoglobin and hematocrit may indicate GI bleeding, a risk in patients with ESRD.*
■ Report manifestations of electrolyte imbalances, such as cardiac dysrhythmias and other ECG changes, muscle tremors and possible tetany, and Kussmaul's respirations. *Manifestations of electrolyte imbalance may indicate the need for intervention.*
■ Administer medications to treat electrolyte imbalances as ordered. *Medications may be prescribed to help maintain electrolyte and acid–base balance and prevent adverse effects of imbalances.*

SAFETY ALERT
Monitor carefully for desired and adverse effects of all medications. Impaired renal function affects drug elimination and increases the risk for toxic effects.

■ Administer antihypertensive medications as ordered. *Hypertension management is an important factor in slowing the progression of CKD.*

■ Time activities and procedures to allow rest periods. *The anemia associated with CKD may cause significant fatigue and activity intolerance.*

Imbalanced Nutrition: Less than Body Requirements

Anorexia, nausea, and vomiting are common manifestations of CKD and uremia. The patient often has a metallic taste and bad breath, which also diminish appetite. A diet restricted in protein and sodium will compound these problems. Food intake may be insufficient to meet metabolic needs. Catabolism, the breakdown of body proteins to meet energy needs, exacerbates azotemia and uremia.

■ Monitor food and nutrient intake as well as episodes of vomiting. *Careful monitoring helps determine the adequacy of intake.*
■ Weigh daily before breakfast. *This provides the most accurate measurement. Remember that a gain of 2 pounds or more over a 24-hour period is more likely to reflect fluid retention than a gain in body mass.*
■ Administer antiemetic agents 30 to 60 minutes before eating. *Antiemetics reduce nausea and the risk of vomiting with food intake.*
■ Assist with mouth care prior to meals and at bedtime. *Mouth care improves taste, stimulates the appetite, and maintains the integrity of oral mucous membranes.*
■ Serve small meals and provide between-meal snacks. *Small meals are less likely to prompt nausea and help improve food intake.*
■ Arrange for a dietary consultation. Provide preferred foods to the extent possible, and involve the patient in planning daily menus. Encourage family members to bring food as dietary restrictions allow. *Providing preferred foods within restrictions promotes intake.*
■ Monitor nutritional status by tracking weight, laboratory values such as serum albumin and BUN, and anthropometric measurements (∞ see Chapters 21 and 22). *Indicators of impaired nutrition develop gradually and may be subtle. Careful assessment is important.*
■ Administer parenteral nutrition as prescribed. Routinely monitor blood glucose levels, and use strict aseptic technique when handling the solution and venous access site. *Parenteral nutrition may be necessary to prevent catabolism and increasing azotemia. Hyperglycemia and infection are risks associated with parenteral nutrition (∞ see Chapter 22). Immune system suppression associated with renal failure further increases the risk for infection.*

Risk for Infection

Chronic kidney disease affects the immune system and leukocyte function, increasing susceptibility to infection. Invasive devices required for hemodialysis or peritoneal dialysis add to this risk. The patient who has had a kidney transplant remains on immunosuppressive therapy for life, further depressing the immune system and increasing the risk for infection.

■ Use standard precautions and good hand hygiene technique at all times. *Hand hygiene is a primary means of preventing the transfer of organisms. Patients who are on hemodialysis or who have had multiple blood transfusions to treat anemia have an increased risk for hepatitis B, hepatitis C, and HIV infection.*

CASE STUDY & NURSING CARE PLAN   A Patient with End-Stage Renal Disease

Walter Cohen, 45 years old, is the print shop manager at a local community college. He has been a type 1 diabetic since the age of 20, and was diagnosed with diabetic nephropathy 10 years ago. Despite blood pressure control with antihypertensive medications and frequent blood glucose monitoring with insulin coverage, he developed overt proteinuria 5 years ago and has now progressed to end-stage renal disease. He enters the nephrology unit for temporary hemodialysis to relieve uremic symptoms. While there, a CAPD catheter will be inserted. Mr. Cohen's desire to continue working is the primary factor in his choice of CAPD over hemodialysis.

ASSESSMENT

Richard Gonzalez, Mr. Cohen's care manager, obtains a nursing assessment. Mr. Cohen states that his diabetes has always been difficult to control. He has had numerous hypoglycemic episodes and has been hospitalized "four or five times" for ketoacidosis. Recently he has developed symptoms of peripheral neuropathy and increasing retinopathy. He attributed his lack of appetite, nausea, vomiting, and fatigue over the past month to "a touch of the flu." His weight remained stable, so he did not worry about not eating much.

Physical assessment findings include T 97.8°F (36.5°C) PO, P 96, R 20, and BP 178/100. Skin cool and dry, with minor excoriations on forearms and lower legs. Breath odor fetid. Scattered fine rales noted in bilateral lung bases. Soft S_3 gallop noted at cardiac apex. Bilateral pitting edema of lower extremities to just below the knees; fingers and hands also edematous. Abdominal assessment essentially normal, with hypoactive bowel sounds. Urinalysis shows a specific gravity of 1.011, gross proteinuria, and multiple cell casts. CBC results: RBC 2.9 million/mm³; hemoglobin 9.4 g/dL; hematocrit 28%. Blood chemistry abnormalities include BUN 198 mg/dL; creatinine 18.5 mg/dL; sodium 125 mEq/L; potassium 5.7 mEq/L; calcium 7.1 mg/dL; phosphate 6.8 mg/dL. A temporary jugular venous catheter will be placed for hemodialysis the next day, followed by peritoneal catheter insertion later in the week.

DIAGNOSES

- *Excess Fluid Volume* related to failure of kidneys to eliminate excess body fluid
- *Imbalanced Nutrition: Less than Body Requirements* related to effects of uremia
- *Impaired Skin Integrity* of lower extremities related to dry skin and itching
- *Risk for Infection* related to invasive catheters and impaired immune function

EXPECTED OUTCOMES

- Adhere to the prescribed fluid restriction of 750 mL per day.
- Demonstrate reduced extracellular fluid volume by weight loss, decreased peripheral edema, clear lung sounds, and normal heart sounds.
- Consume and retain 100% of prescribed diet, including snacks.
- Demonstrate healing of lower extremity skin lesions.
- Remain free of infection.
- Demonstrate appropriate peritoneal catheter care and CAPD.

PLANNING AND IMPLEMENTATION

- Space fluids, allowing 400 mL from 0700 to 1500, 200 mL from 1500 to 2300, and 100 mL from 2300 to 0700.
- Provide mouth care at least every 4 hours and before every meal.
- Keep sugarless hard candy and ice chips at the bedside; include ice consumed as fluid intake.
- Weigh daily before breakfast; monitor vital signs, and heart and lung sounds, every 4 hours.
- Document intake and output every 4 hours.
- Arrange dietary consultation for menu planning.
- Administer prescribed antiemetic 1 hour before meals.
- Monitor food intake, noting percentage and types of food consumed.
- Clean lesions on lower extremities every 8 hours and assess healing.
- Teach CAPD procedure and peritoneal catheter care.
- Assist to identify strengths and needs in health regimen management.

EVALUATION

Mr. Cohen was hospitalized for 2 weeks, undergoing four hemodialysis sessions to reduce uremic symptoms. An arteriovenous fistula has been created in his left arm in case he should need hemodialysis in the future. He begins peritoneal dialysis the second week, and by discharge he is able to manage the catheter care and dialysis runs with the help of his wife. His heart and lung sounds are normal, and he has minimal peripheral edema on discharge. The excoriations on his legs have healed. His temperature is normal, and no evidence of infection is noted. Mr. Cohen remains anorectic and slightly nauseated, but is eating most of his prescribed diet and snacks. He has lost 10 pounds with excess fluid removal by dialysis, but his weight remains stable during the second week. Mr. Cohen and his wife have been introduced to another patient who has been on CAPD for several years and promises to help them with problem solving.

CRITICAL THINKING IN THE NURSING PROCESS

1. How does diabetes mellitus damage the kidneys and lead to CKD? Why is this more significant for a patient with type 1 diabetes than for someone with type 2 diabetes (∞ see Chapter 20)?
2. Why do high levels of urea in the blood often cause changes in cognition and mental status? What manifestations of encephalopathy would you expect to see?
3. How might Mr. Cohen's insulin dosage and diet need to be changed with the institution of peritoneal dialysis? Why?
4. Develop a care plan for the nursing diagnosis *Disturbed Body Image*.

See Evaluating Your Response in Appendix C.

SAFETY ALERT
Use strict aseptic technique when managing ports, catheters, and incisions, to reduce the risk of introducing infectious organisms when immune responses are impaired.

- Monitor temperature and vital signs at least every 4 hours. *A low-grade fever or increased pulse rate may indicate an infection in the immunosuppressed patient.*

- Monitor WBC count and differential. *Increased WBCs may indicate a bacterial infection; decreased WBCs may indicate a viral infection. A shift in the differential showing more immature WBCs (bands) in circulation is another indicator of infection.*
- Culture urine, peritoneal dialysis fluid, and other drainage as indicated. *Culture is done to verify the presence of pathogens.*

MOVING EVIDENCE INTO ACTION   Patients with Early Chronic Kidney Disease

In a study of patients with early CKD, nurse researchers in Canada looked at patients' perceptions of health, kidney disease, and the supports these patients needed to manage their disease (Costantini et al., 2008). The study included 14 patients between ages 19 and 69.

The researchers identified that these patients went through a process they termed "renegotiating life with chronic kidney disease." Soon after the initial diagnosis, patients engaged in a discovery process, searching for evidence of the disease (when the patient often was free of symptoms) and coming to realize the life-long nature of their disease. Discovery both required disease-specific information and prompted realization of the need for additional information on self-care and managing the disease. Researchers identified this as the process of learning to live with kidney disease and assuming increasing responsibility for managing the disease.

IMPLICATIONS FOR NURSING

Patients with any chronic disease, including CKD need information and support to become effective self-health managers. While the disease may have a common name, each individual has unique

needs—the information and support desired by a 19-year-old with CKD may be very different than that for a 69-year-old. Treating all patients with ESRD holistically, respecting their individual and unique characteristics and experience, is vital to promote acceptance and autonomy. Listen carefully, responding to each person's concerns. Discuss the effects of the disease and its treatment on the patient's life, marital and family relationships, and socialization. Suggest strategies to manage prescribed medications, diet and fluid restrictions, and day-to-day symptoms. Whenever appropriate, provide information about treatment options, allowing the patient to determine the preferred alternative.

CRITICAL THINKING IN PATIENT CARE

1. Identify assessment tools and data you could use to evaluate the knowledge and learning readiness of a patient with early CKD.
2. What interventions can you, as the nurse, implement to promote autonomy and acceptance in the patient with CKD? How might these interventions differ for young, middle, and older adults?
3. Develop a teaching plan for a 19-year-old single woman newly diagnosed with CKD and a teaching plan for a 69-year-old married man with newly identified CKD.

PRACTICE ALERT
Monitor clarity of dialysate return. Dialysate should return clear in the patient undergoing peritoneal dialysis. Cloudy dialysate may indicate peritonitis, the most common complication of peritoneal dialysis, and should be reported and cultured.

- Provide good respiratory hygiene including position changes, coughing, and deep breathing. *These measures improve clearance of respiratory secretions, reducing the risk for infection.*
- Restrict visits from obviously ill people. Teach the patient and family about the risk for infection and measures to reduce the spread of infection. *The patient's resistance to infection is impaired, necessitating extra caution in preventing unnecessary exposures.*

Disturbed Body Image

Chronic disease and impaired kidney function can affect the patient's body image. Hemodialysis requires an arteriovenous fistula or shunt; a permanent peritoneal catheter is required for peritoneal dialysis. While kidney transplant can restore an image of wholeness, a visible scar remains and the organ may be perceived as "foreign."

- Involve the patient in care, including meal planning, dialysis, and catheter, port, or incision care to the extent possible. *Involvement improves acceptance and stimulates discussion about the effect of the disease and treatment measures on the patient's life.*
- Encourage expression of feelings and concerns, accepting perceptions and feelings without criticism. *Self-expression enhances the patient's self-worth and acceptance.*
- Include the patient in decision making and encourage self-care. *Increased autonomy enhances the patient's sense of control, independence, and self-worth.*
- Support positive gains, but do not support denial. *The patient may have difficulty accepting the renal failure, but adaptation to the loss is important.*

- Help the patient develop and achieve realistic goals. *Realistic goals allow the patient to see progress.*
- Provide positive reinforcement and feedback. *These measures support growth and adaptation.*
- Reinforce effective coping strategies. *Reinforcement helps the patient develop positive versus negative strategies for coping.*
- Facilitate contact with a support group or other community members affected by renal failure. *The patient benefits by providing and receiving support in a group of people going through similar circumstances.*
- Refer for mental health counseling as indicated or desired. *Counseling can help the patient develop effective coping and adaptation strategies.*

Using NANDA, NIC, and NOC

Linkages between a selected NANDA nursing diagnosis, NIC, and NOC for the patient with chronic kidney disease are shown in the chart that follows.

Community-Based Care

Chronic renal failure and ESRD are long-term processes that require patient management. No matter what treatment option is chosen (hemodialysis, peritoneal dialysis, or renal transplantation), day-to-day management falls to the patient and family. See the accompanying Nursing Research box. Teaching for home care includes the following topics:

- Nature of chronic kidney disease and renal failure, including expected progression and effects
- Monitoring weight, vital signs, and temperature
- Prescribed medications, including purpose, intended effect, and potential adverse effects and their management
- Prescribed dietary and fluid restrictions (Involve the patient, a dietitian, and the family member usually responsible for cooking. Include strategies to manage nausea and relieve thirst within allowed fluid limits.)

- How to assess and protect a fistula or shunt for hemodialysis (or the extremity to be used if one is anticipated)
- Peritoneal catheter care and the procedure for peritoneal dialysis as indicated (Include a family member or significant other, in case the patient is unable to perform the procedure independently at some time.)
- Following kidney transplant, prescribed medications, adverse effects and their management, infection prevention, graft protection, and manifestations of organ rejection

Refer to a dietitian for diet planning and counseling. If home hemodialysis is planned, refer the designated dialysis helper for formal training. Both the National Kidney Foundation and the American Association of Kidney Patients may be able to provide support and educational materials for the patient with ESRD (see the box on page 859). Local and state chapters of these organizations can provide additional support.

NANDA, NIC, AND NOC LINKAGES
The Patient with Chronic Kidney Disease

NANDA — Ineffective Coping

NIC — Anticipatory Guidance
Coping Enhancement
Decision-Making Support

NOC — Coping
Decision Making
Psychosocial Adjustment: Life Change

Data from NANDA International. (2009). *Nursing diagnoses: Definitions and classification 2009–2011*. Oxford, UK: Wiley-Blackwell; Bulechek, G., Butcher, H., and Dochterman, J. (Eds.). (2008). *Nursing interventions classification (NIC)* (5th ed.). St. Louis, MO: Mosby; and Moorhead, S., Johnson, M., Maas, M., and Swanson, E. (Eds.). (2008). *Nursing outcomes classification (NOC)* (4th ed.). St. Louis, MO: Mosby.

CHAPTER HIGHLIGHTS

- Congenital and acquired disorders of the kidneys can profoundly affect urinary elimination and ultimately all body systems.
- Glomerulonephritis, inflammation of the glomerulus of the kidney, leads to loss of proteins and blood cells in the urine, a decrease in the glomerular filtration rate, and severe edema.
- The renal and cardiovascular systems are closely interrelated. Vascular disorders, such as hypertension, renal artery stenosis, or obstruction of the renal artery or vein, can have serious consequences in terms of renal function.
- Renal cell malignancies, while uncommon, often are not evident until the cancer is advanced and has metastasized to other sites.

- Acute renal failure is a frequent complication of critical illnesses, typically occurring in people with no prior history of kidney disorders. Ischemic and nephrotoxic damage to the kidney are the most common precipitating factors for ARF.
- Chronic kidney disease can be the result of numerous systemic and kidney disorders, such as diabetes mellitus, hypertension, systemic lupus erythematosus, and chronic glomerulonephritis.
- When the kidneys fail, renal replacement therapies are necessary to eliminate metabolic waste products and sustain life. Dialysis and kidney transplant are the primary renal replacement therapies used.

TEST YOURSELF NCLEX-RN® REVIEW

1. The physician orders digoxin 0.125 mg three times per week for an 82-year-old patient with heart failure. Which of the following is an appropriate response by the nurse?
   1. Question the order because older patients may require larger doses due to protein loss in the urine.
   2. Administer the drug as ordered, monitoring the patient for manifestations of toxicity.
   3. Assess the patient's eGFR before administering the drug at this dose.
   4. Use 0.25-mg digoxin tablets, cutting the tablet in half to save money for the patient.
2. A patient newly diagnosed with polycystic kidney disease asks if there is anything his children need to know about their risk for getting the disorder. How should the nurse respond?
   1. Because the condition was just diagnosed, there is no risk of passing the condition on to his children.
   2. When his children prepare to marry, they and their potential partners should undergo genetic testing to determine if their children will be at risk.
   3. The adult form of this disorder is transmitted as a dominant gene; each child has a 50% risk of having inherited the defective gene.
   4. His children would have developed symptoms of the disorder *in utero* or shortly after birth if they had inherited the defective gene.

3. In obtaining a nursing history from a 22-year-old patient admitted with a diagnosis of acute glomerulonephritis, the nurse specifically asks the patient about a recent history of which of the following?
   1. urinary tract infection
   2. strep throat
   3. x-ray using contrast media
   4. illicit drug use
4. The nurse evaluates his teaching for a patient with acute glomerulonephritis as effective when the patient does which of the following?
   1. chooses soy or animal proteins for allowed grams of protein in diet
   2. states the need to remain on bed rest until his urine returns to clear yellow
   3. demonstrates care for the vascular shunt or peritoneal catheter
   4. limits fluid intake to less than 1500 mL per day

5. Which of the following is an appropriate postoperative nursing intervention for the patient who has had a partial or total nephrectomy?
   1. connecting all catheters and drains to a single collection device
   2. routine irrigation of all catheters with sterile normal saline
   3. administering cough suppressant medication as needed
   4. labeling and securing all catheters, tubes, and drains

6. Important nursing interventions to prevent acute renal failure in the critically ill patient include which of the following?
   1. maintaining fluid volume and cardiac output
   2. avoiding all potentially nephrotoxic drugs
   3. administering antihypertensive drugs
   4. assessing for a history of diabetes or hypertension

7. The nurse evaluates her teaching as effective when the patient recovering from acute renal failure states that he will do which of the following?
   1. Limit his fluid intake to 1500 mL or less per day.
   2. Consume only vegetable proteins.
   3. Avoid taking drugs that may be nephrotoxic.
   4. Self-catheterize for residual urine at least once a week.

8. The nurse caring for a patient preparing to undergo hemodialysis includes which of the following in the plan of care? **Select all that apply.**
   1. Obtain weight and orthostatic vital signs.
   2. Assess blood pressure of extremity where fistula has been created.
   3. Monitor serum creatinine, BUN, and hematocrit levels.
   4. Determine urine specific gravity and pH.
   5. Restrict fluid and protein intake.

9. An appropriate goal of nursing care for a patient with end-stage renal disease is the patient will be able to do which of the following?
   1. Identify a live-in caregiver.
   2. State the advantages and disadvantages of types of renal replacement therapies.
   3. Demonstrate the ability to independently perform hemodialysis in the home.
   4. Relate the hospice philosophy and identify indicators of the need for hospice care.

10. Following a kidney transplant, the nurse notes that the patient's urine is cloudy. How should the nurse respond?
    1. Record the finding.
    2. Increase the intravenous flow rate.
    3. Irrigate the urinary catheter.
    4. Notify the physician.

Pearson Nursing Student Resources
Find additional review materials at
www.nursing.pearsonhighered.com
Prepare for success with additional NCLEX®-style practice questions, interactive assignments and activities, Web links, animations and videos, and more!

BIBLIOGRAPHY

American Cancer Society. (2009). *Cancer facts and figures 2009.* Atlanta, GA: Author.

Barone, C. P., Martin-Watson, A. L., & Barone, G. W. (2004). The postoperative care of the adult renal transplant recipient. *Medsurg Nursing, 13*(5), 286–302.

Brown, D., & Martindale, A. (2008). Urinary tract trauma – diagnosis and management. *Trauma, 10,* 5–11.

Bulechek, G., Butcher, H., & Dochterman, J. (Eds.). (2008). *Nursing interventions classification (NIC)* (5th ed.). St. Louis, MO: Mosby.

Cheung, C., Ponnusamy, A., & Anderton, J. (2008). Management of acute renal failure in the elderly patient: A clinician's guide. *Drugs & Aging, 25*(6), 455–476.

Copstead, L. C., & Banasik, J. L. (2010). *Pathophysiology* (4th ed.). St. Louis, MO: Elsevier/Saunders.

Costantini, L., Beanlands, H., McCay, E., Cattran, D., Hladunewich, M., & Francis, D. (2008, March–April). The self-management experience of people with mild to moderate chronic kidney disease. *Nephrology Nursing Journal, 35*(2), 147–155.

DiPiro, J., Talbert, R., Yee, G., Matzke, G., Wells, B., & Posey, L. (2008). *Pharmacotherapy: A pathophysiologic approach* (7th ed.). New York, NY: McGraw Hill.

Fauci, A., Kasper, D., Braunwald, E., Hauser, S., Longo, D., Jameson, J., et al. (Eds.). (2008). *Harrison's principles of internal medicine* (17th ed.). New York: McGraw-Hill.

Kendrick, M. (2008 September 24). What's the point of measuring eGFR? *Pulse, 24 September 2008.* Available at www.pulsetoday.co.uk.

Kinzner, C., & Hain, D. (2007 November–December). Understanding the eGFR. *Nephrology Nursing Journal, 34*(6), 655–657.

Kohtz, C., & Thompson, M. (2007 September). Preventing contrast medium-induced nephropathy. *American Journal of Nursing, 107*(9), 40–49.

Lu, D., McCarthy, A., Lanning, L., Delaney, C., & Porter, C. (2007 May–June). A descriptive study of individuals with membranoproliferative glomerulonephritis. *Nephrology Nursing Journal, 34*(3), 295–302.

Marshall, M., Golper, T., Shaver, M., Alam, M., & Chatoth, D. (2001). Sustained low-efficiency dialysis for critically ill patients requiring renal replacement therapy. *Kidney International, 60,* 777–785.

McCance, K. L., & Huether, S. E. (2010). *Pathophysiology: The biologic basis for disease in adults & children* (6th ed.). St. Louis, MO: Mosby.

McPhee, S., Papadakis, M., & Tierney, L., Jr. (Eds.). (2008). *Current medical diagnosis & treatment* (47th ed.). New York: McGraw-Hill.

Menezes, F., Wey, S., Peres, C., Medina-Pestana, J., & Camargo, L. (2008 August). Risk factors for surgical site infection in kidney transplant recipients. *Infection Control & Hospital Epidemiology, 29*(8), 771–773.

Moorhead, S., Johnson, M., Maas, M., & Swanson, E. (Eds.). (2008). *Nursing outcomes classification (NOC)* (4th ed.). St. Louis, MO: Mosby.

NANDA International. (2009). *Nursing diagnoses: Definitions and classification 2009–2011.* Oxford, UK: Wiley-Blackwell.

National Kidney Disease Education Program. (2008). Health professionals. Chronic kidney disease (CKD) information. Retrieved from www.nkdep.nih.gov.

National Kidney and Urologic Diseases Information Clearinghouse. (2009). *Kidney and urologic disease statistics for the United States* (NIH Publication No. 09-3895). Retrieved from http://www.niddk.nih.gov/kudiseases/kidney/pubs/kustats

National Kidney Foundation. (2002). K/DOQI Clinical practice guidelines for chronic kidney disease: Evaluation, classification and stratification. *American Journal of Kidney Disease, 39*(supplement 1), S1-S266. Retrieved from www.kdoqi.org

National Kidney Foundation. (2009). The problem of kidney and urologic disease. Retrieved from www.kidney.org

Olson, D. (2007 March). Arranging live organ donation over the internet. *American Journal of Nursing, 107*(3), 69–72.

Organ Procurement and Transplantation Network. (2009 August). Donors recovered in the U.S. by donor type. Retrieved from http://optn.transplant.hrsa.gov/

Organ Procurement and Transplantation Network. (2009 August). Kidney Kaplan-Meyer graft survival rates for transplants performed 1997–2004. Retrieved from http://optn.transplant.hrsa.gov/

Peiffer, K. (2007 March). Brain death and organ procurement. *American Journal of Nursing, 107*(3), 58–67.

Phillips, A. (2009 January–February). Autosomal dominant polycystic kidney disease: A case study. *Nephrology Nursing Journal, 36*(1), 41–47.

Porth, C., & Matfin, G. (2009). *Pathophysiology: Concepts of altered health states* (8th ed.). Philadelphia: Lippincott.

Racial differences in trends of end-stage renal disease by primary diagnosis – United States, 1994–2004. (2007 March 23). *MMWR: Morbidity & Mortality Weekly Report, 56*(11), 253–256.

Russell, S. (2008 February). Responding to 2 threats to the kidney. *Nursing, 38*(2), 36–40.

Spencer, J. W., & Jacobs, J. J. (2003). *Complementary and alternative medicine: An evidence-based approach* (2nd ed.). St. Louis, MO: Mosby.

Sque, M., Long, T., Payne, S., & Allardyce, D. (2007). Why relatives do not donate organs for transplants: 'Sacrifice' or 'gift of life'? *Journal of Advanced Nursing, 61*(2), 134–144.

United Network for Organ Sharing: Policies. (2008–2009). Retrieved from www.unos.org

U.S. Renal Data System. (2008). *USRDS 2008 Annual data report: Atlas of chronic kidney disease and end-stage renal disease in the United States.* Bethesda, MD: National Institutes of Health, National Institute of Diabetes and Digestive and Kidney Diseases.

Wilkinson, J., & Ahern, N. (2009). *Nursing diagnosis handbook* (9th ed.). Upper Saddle River, NJ: Prentice Hall.

Functional Health Pattern: Elimination

Think about patients with altered urinary elimination for whom you have cared.

- What were their major medical diagnoses? Was the urinary elimination problem their primary diagnosis or a secondary one? Was it present on admission of the patients to the healthcare system or did it develop during the course of care?
- What kinds of manifestations did each of these patients have? Were these manifestations similar or different?
- Which health care behaviors affected the patients' elimination status? What was their amount and type of fluid intake? Did they take any medications?
- The Elimination Health Pattern includes patterns of urinary elimination, including urine formation, flow, and micturition. It is affected by disorders of the kidneys, ureters, urinary bladder, and urethra. The urinary system regulates body fluids, filters metabolic wastes from the bloodstream, reabsorbs essential substances and water back into the bloodstream, and eliminates metabolic wastes and water as urine.
- Kidney disorders affect the production of urine, elimination of waste products from the body, and regulatory processes such as fluid and electrolyte and acid–base balance, blood pressure, and RBC formation. Disorders of the urinary tract (kidneys, ureters, urinary bladder, and urethra) can interfere with the flow and excretion of urine produced in the kidneys.

Alterations in the structure and function of the urinary system may cause either local or systemic manifestations such as the following:

- **Dysuria** (inflamed urinary tract tissue causes the release of inflammatory chemicals, which causes irritation of nociceptors and leads to pain)
- **Hematuria** (inflamed or damaged urinary tract tissue leads to increased capillary permeability, which causes RBCs to be released into the urine)
- **Proteinuria** (damage to glomerulus allows large protein molecules to enter filtrate; protein is detectable in the urine)
- **Hypertension** (impaired water and electrolyte excretion, disruption of the renin-angiotensin-aldosterone system cause hypervolemia and increased peripheral vascular resistance, which results in increased blood pressure)

Priority nursing diagnoses within the elimination functional health pattern that may be appropriate for patients with urinary disorders include the following:

- *Impaired Urinary Elimination*
- *Urinary Incontinence (Stress, Urge, Total)*
- *Urinary Retention*

Nursing diagnoses from other functional health patterns that often are of high priority for the patient with a urinary elimination disorder include the following:

- *Ineffective Health Maintenance* (Health Perception-Health Management Pattern)
- *Acute Pain* (Cognitive-Perceptual Pattern)
- *Excess Fluid Volume* (Nutritional-Metabolic Pattern)

Question

1. When the patient has difficulty starting the urinary stream, what can the nurse do to assist with voiding?

Questions

Refer to the Clinical Scenario on the next page to answer the following questions.

Priority Setting

1. In what order would you visit these patients after report?
   A. _____
   B. _____
   C. _____
   D. _____

Health Promotion

1. In order to prevent urinary tract infection, what should Agnes Smith be taught?
2. In order to prevent further kidney stones, what should Joseph Rouse be taught about his diet?
3. In order to prevent further kidney damage, what should Angela Baldwin be taught about her diet?

Nursing Process

1. What priority nursing diagnoses would you choose for each of the patients presented? What is the rationale for your choice?

	Nursing Diagnosis	Rationale
Phillip Jones		
Agnes Smith		
Joseph Rouse		
Angela Baldwin		

2. Philip Jones is complaining of inability to void. A bladder scan indicates that there is 800 mL of urine in the bladder. Which interventions does the nurse perform?
   A. Insert a urinary catheter and completely drain the bladder at once.
   B. Insert a urinary catheter and drain urine in 500 mL increments.
   C. Ambulate Mr. Jones to the bathroom to try to void and run water in the sink.
   D. Give Mr. Jones a glass of water to drink to encourage voiding.

CLINICAL SCENARIO

Directions: *Read the following clinical scenario and answer the questions that follow. To complete this exercise successfully you will not only use knowledge of the content in this unit, but also principles related to setting priorities and maintaining patient safety.*

You have been assigned to work with the following four patients for the 0700 shift on a renal medical-surgical unit. Significant data obtained during report is as follows:

■ Phillip Jones is a 45-year-old who was admitted two days ago after a fall from a deer hunting stand. He experienced a bruised right kidney and numerous ecchymotic areas to the right side from the fall. His vital signs are temperature 99°F, pulse 98, respirations 28, and blood pressure 110/68. He is complaining of abdominal pain and difficulty urinating.

■ Agnes Smith is an 84-year-old who was admitted 2 hours ago with complaints of urinary incontinence, anorexia, confusion and lethargy. Her vital signs on admission were temperature 97°F, pulse 88, respirations 20, and blood pressure 148/90. The physician ordered trimethoprim-sulfamethoxazole (Bactrim) to be started as soon as possible.

■ Joseph Rouse is a 45-year-old who is to undergo surgery for removal of uric acid stones after having a failed lithotripsy. His vital signs are temperature 99.6°F, pulse 94, respirations 24, blood pressure 112/68. His skin is pale, cool and clammy. He is complaining of nausea, severe left-sided flank pain with spasms, and lightheadedness.

■ Angela Baldwin is a 34-year-old who has a medical history of systemic lupus erythematosus. She was admitted with complaints of left flank pain and generalized edema. Urinalysis results indicate hematuria and proteinuria. Vital signs are temperature 100°F, pulse 88, respirations 26, and blood pressure 144/90. She is admitted for aggressive immunosuppressive therapy.

3. Which nursing actions are instituted for Philip Jones following kidney trauma?
   A. Monitor level of consciousness and urine output.
   B. Monitor vital signs for hypotension and bradycardia.
   C. Observe for hypertension and check urine for hematuria.
   D. Observe urine for oliguria and proteinuria.

4. After Joseph Rouse returned from surgery, the nurse needs to report which urinary output?
   A. 20 mL per hour
   B. 40 mL per hour
   C. 300 mL per 8 hours
   D. 400 mL per 8 hours

Communication

1. The physician ordered trimethoprim-sulfamethoxazole (Bactrim) for Agnes Smith's uncomplicated cystitis. Mrs. Smith understands the length of antibiotic therapy when she verbalizes which statement?
   A. "I should be able to return home after three days of antibiotics."
   B. "I can be discharged after five days of antibiotics."
   C. "I need to stay in the hospital for one week to finish the antibiotics."
   D. "I can stay in the hospital for five days of antibiotics and take five days of antibiotics at home."

2. If Angela Baldwin asks, "Are these urinary problems I am having an indication that the lupus is getting worse?" How will you respond?

Delegation

1. What data collection and interventions can be delegated to a nursing assistant for each patient?
   A. _____
   B. _____

C. _____
D. _____

Content-Specific Questions

1. The physician orders phenazopyridine (Pyridium) for relief of pain and burning with cystitis. What should the nurse teach the patient about the use of this medication?
   A. Take the medication with antacids to prevent stomach upset.
   B. Drink less fluid to allow the drug to concentrate in the bladder.
   C. The drug turns the urine and other body secretions orange or red.
   D. Stop taking the drug if nausea and diarrhea occur.

2. The patient diagnosed with uric acid stones is ordered to follow a diet low in purines. Which is the meal plan lowest in purines?
   A. liver with onions and potatoes
   B. chicken sandwich with French fries
   C. spaghetti with ground beef meat sauce
   D. macaroni and cheese with stewed tomatoes

3. When assessing a patient with glomerulonephritis, which manifestations are indicative of an early disease process?
   A. pyuria, leukocytosis, and hyperthermia
   B. hematuria, proteinuria, and hypertension
   C. dysuria, hyperglycemia, and hypertension
   D. oliguria, flank pain, and hypotension

4. Which are risk factors of urinary tract infections? **Select all that apply.**
   A. Circumcision in males
   B. decreased cervicovaginal antibodies
   C. sexual intercourse in women
   D. short urethra in men
   E. aging in men
   F. urinary catheterization

5. Which is the most accurate indicator of fluid volume status in the oliguric or aneuric patient?
   A. intake and output
   B. weight changes
   C. restrict fluids
   D. BUN and creatinine levels

6. The most reliable diagnostic procedure to determine glomerular disorders is which diagnostic test?
   A. kidney scan
   B. antistreptolysin O titer
   C. kidney biopsy
   D. blood urea nitrogen

CASE STUDY: Amos Jenkins

Amos Jenkins is a 45-year-old Black male who has been a truck driver for the past 20 years. He is admitted to the hospital with complaints of nausea for one week, weakness, fatigue, loss of appetite, and feeling very depressed. He has a past medical history of type 1 diabetes mellitus, hypertension, and diabetic neuropathy. Upon admission, his vital signs are temperature 98.7°F, pulse 96, respirations 20, and blood pressure 170/100. He has bilateral pitting edema to lower extremities. His fingers and hands are also edematous. He complains of dry and itching skin. His urine is collected for a urinalysis and blood work is drawn and sent to the laboratory. Results returned with a specific gravity of 1.011, gross hematuria, BUN 198 mg/dL, and creatinine 18.5 mg/dL.

Based on his past medical history and current findings, a medical diagnosis of chronic kidney disease is determined. In CKD, entire nephron units are gradually destroyed. In the early stages remaining functional nephrons hypertrophy. Glomerular capillary flow and pressure increase in the nephrons to compensate for lost renal mass. Increased demand on the remaining nephrons leads to glomerular sclerosis or scarring with eventual nephron destruction. As the disease progresses, renal insufficiency develops, with eventual renal failure. The manifestations of CKD are nausea, apathy, weakness, fatigue, proteinuria, hematuria, polyuria, nocturia, and pale and dry skin. As the disease progresses, manifestations uremia develop, including vomiting, increasing weakness, paresthesias, lethargy, confusion, headache, abdominal pain, urine-like breath odor, and uremic frost. Complications of chronic renal failure are fluid and electrolyte imbalance, acid–base imbalance, hypertension, hyperlipidemia, glucose intolerance, pulmonary edema, anemia, bleeding disorders, osteodystrophy, sexual impotence, psychotic symptoms, seizures, and coma.

Based on Mr. Jenkins's assessment and past medical history, the nursing diagnosis of *Impaired Urinary Elimination* is appropriate for planning nursing interventions.

- Glomerulosclerosis, thickening of glomerular asement membrane → glomerular capillary lumen narrows → reduced surface area for glomerular filtration and gradual loss of nephron units → eventual renal insufficiency and failure

Mr. A.J.
45 y.o. male
Chronic renal failure

affects

leads to

assess →

- C/o nausea, weakness, fatigue, anorexia
- States "feeling depressed"
- T 98.7°F, P 96, R 20, BP 170/110
- Bilateral pitting edema of hands, fingers, & lower extremities
- Skin dry, excoriated
- Scanty output of dark, frothy urine; sp grav 1.011, gross hematuria, 3+ protein
- BUN 198 mg/dL, serum creatinine 18.5 mg/dL

← generates →

- Excess Fluid Volume as evidenced by peripheral edema
- Nausea as evidenced by subjective complaints and anorexia
- Impaired Skin Integrity as evidenced by dry, excoriated skin
- Powerlessness as evidenced by complaints of feeling depressed

generate nursing diagnosis

prioritized to

Impaired Urinary Elimination

expected outcomes

- Adheres to prescribed fluid and dietary restrictions
- Demonstrates reduced extracellular fluid volume: weight loss, reduced edema, clear lung sounds
- Verbalizes understanding of renal replacement options and selects preferred option from those presented by nephrologist
- Demonstrates ability to effectively manage diabetes and maintain blood glucose within acceptable range

← evaluate →

- 5 days after admission:
- Weight down 6 lb
- BP 150/88, P 82, R 18
- Peripheral edema 1 + or less to ankles
- Has undergone 2 hemodialysis sessions; preparing for peritoneal catheter placement
- Met with dietitian and diabetic educator X 3

Interdisciplinary Interventions
- Space fluid intake, considering total allowed intake and client preferences.
- Request dietary consult to plan palatable menus within prescribed restrictions of proteins and simple carbohydrates.
- Weigh q12h under standard conditions.
- Administer diuretics and antihypertensives as ordered.

Independent Interventions
- Discuss renal replacement therapy options with client and family, assisting them to determine the most feasible.
- Refer to diabetic educator for teaching and management of treatment regimen.

Activity:

1. After reviewing the concept map, is there anything you would change to make it more understandable?

2. Go to the Pearson Nursing Student Resources for this book at www.nursing.pearsonhighered.com to write a concept map addressing the nursing diagnosis *Readiness for Enhanced Knowledge* related to planned peritoneal dialysis.

   See answers and hints in Appendix C.

Activity–Exercise Pattern

PART IV

Functional Health Patterns with Related Nursing Diagnoses

HEALTH PERCEPTION HEALTH MANAGEMENT

- Perceived health status
- Perceived health management
- Health care behaviors: health promotion and illness prevention activities, medical treatments, follow-up care

VALUE-BELIEF

- Values, goals, or beliefs (including spirituality) that guide choices or decisions
- Perceived conflicts in values, beliefs, or expectations that are health related

COPING-STRESS-TOLERANCE

- Capacity to resist challenges to self-integrity
- Methods of handling stress
- Support systems
- Perceived ability to control and manage situations

NUTRITIONAL-METABOLIC

- Daily consumption of food and fluids
- Favorite foods
- Use of dietary supplements
- Skin lesions and ability to heal
- Condition of the integument
- Weight, height, temperature

PART IV

Activity-Exercise Patterns: Examples of Related NANDA Nursing Diagnosis

- Activity Intolerance
- Acute Pain
- Delayed Surgical Recovery
- Decreased Cardiac Output
- Deficient Diversional Activity
- Dysfunctional Ventilatory Weaning Response
- Fatigue
- Impaired Bed Mobility
- Impaired Gas Exchange
- Impaired Home Maintenance
- Impaired Physical Mobility
- Impaired Spontaneous Ventilation
- Impaired Transfer Ability
- Impaired Walking
- Ineffective Breathing Pattern
- Ineffective Peripheral; Tissue Perfusion
- Risk for Decreased Cardiac Perfusion
- Risk for Shock
- Risk for Vascular Trauma
- Sedentary Life Style
- Self-Care Deficit

SEXUALITY-REPRODUCTIVE

- Satisfaction with sexuality or sexual relationships
- Reproductive pattern
- Female menstrual and perimeno-pausal history

ELIMINATION

- Patterns of bowel and urinary excretion
- Perceived regularity or irregularity of elimination
- Use of laxatives or routines
- Changes in time, modes, quality or quantity of excretions
- Use of devices for control

ROLE-RELATIONSHIP

- Perception of major roles, relationships, and responsibilities in current life situation
- Satisfaction with or disturbances in roles and relationships

ACTIVITY-EXERCISE

- Patterns of personally relevant exercise, activity, leisure, and recreation
- ADLs which require energy expenditure
- Factors that interfere with the desired pattern (e.g., illness or injury)

SELF-PERCEPTION– SELF-CONCEPT

- Attitudes about self
- Perceived abilities, worth, self-image, emotions
- Body posture and movement, eye contact, voice and speech patterns

SLEEP-REST

- Patterns of sleep and rest/relaxation in a 24-hr period
- Perceptions of quality and quantity of sleep and rest
- Use of sleep aids and routines

COGNITIVE-PERCEPTUAL

- Adequacy of vision, hearing, taste, touch, smell
- Pain perception and management
- Language, judgment, memory, decisions

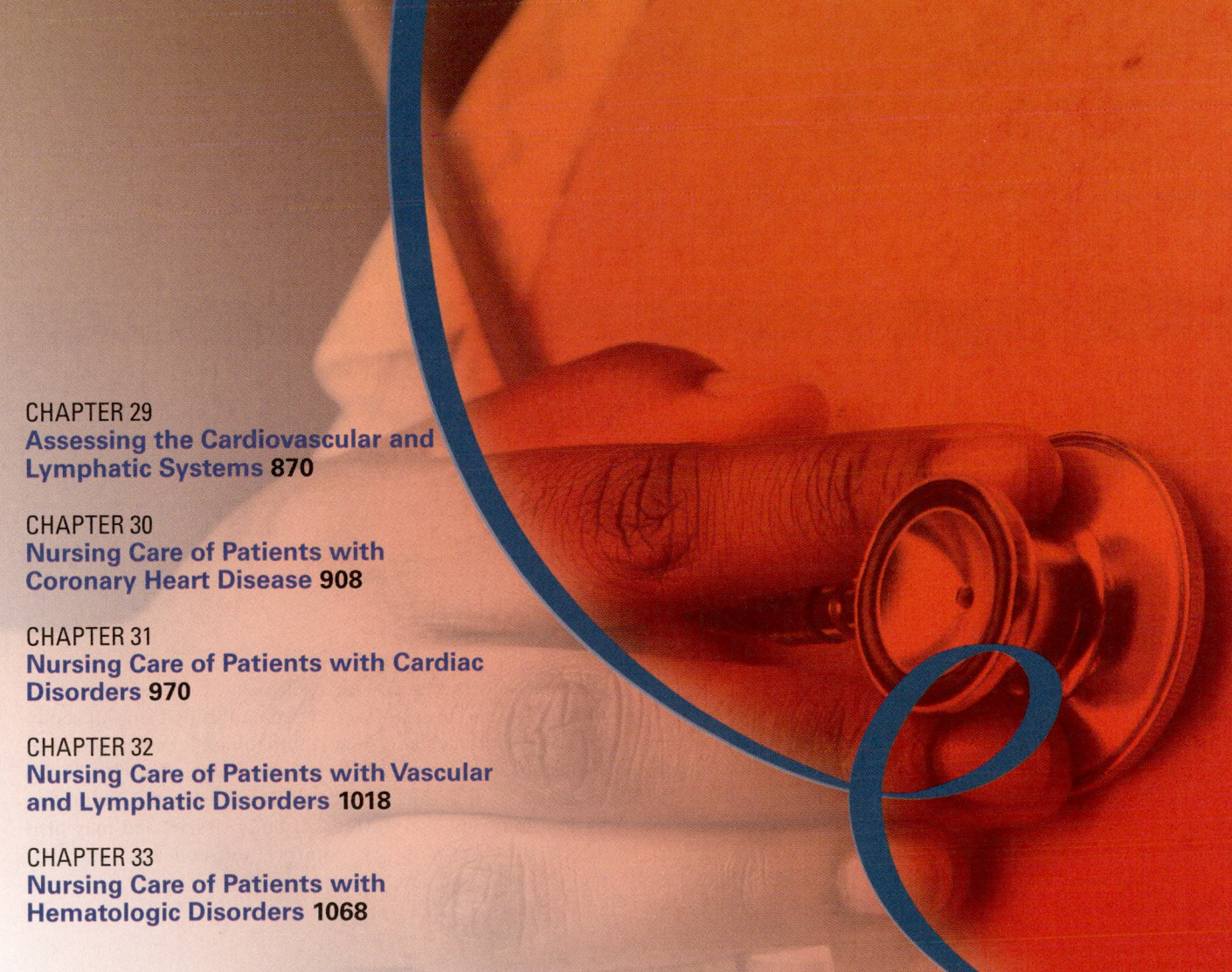

Responses to Altered Cardiovascular Function

UNIT 8

CHAPTER 29

Assessing the **Cardiovascular** and **Lymphatic Systems**

LEARNING OUTCOMES

1. Describe the anatomy, physiology, and functions of the cardiovascular and lymphatic systems.
2. Describe normal variations in cardiovascular assessment findings for the older adult.
3. Give examples of genetic disorders of the cardiovascular system.
4. Identify specific topics for consideration during a health history assessment interview of the patient with cardiovascular or lymphatic disorders.
5. Explain techniques used to assess cardiovascular and lymphatic structure and function.
6. Identify manifestations of impaired cardiovascular structure and functions.

CLINICAL COMPETENCIES

1. Assess an ECG strip and identify normal rhythm and cardiac events and abnormal cardiac rhythm.
2. Conduct and document a health history for patients having alterations in the structure and functions of the cardiovascular or lymphatic systems.
3. Conduct and document a physical assessment of cardiovascular and lymphatic status.
4. Monitor the results of diagnostic tests and report abnormal findings.

EQUIPMENT NEEDED

- Stethoscope with a diaphragm and a bell
- Blood pressure cuff
- Good light source
- Watch with a second hand
- Centimeter ruler
- Tape measure
- Doppler ultrasound device (if needed) and transducer gel

KEY TERMS

apical impulse, *894*
cardiac index (CI), *875*
cardiac output (CO), *874*
dysrhythmia, *897*
heave, *894*

hemostasis, *883*
ischemic, *874*
Korotkoff's sounds, *900*
lift, *894*
lymphadenopathy, *905*

lymphedema, *900*
orthostatic hypotension, *900*
retraction, *894*
thrill, *897*
thrust, *894*

The cardiovascular system is comprised of the heart (the system's pump), the peripheral vascular system (a network of arteries, veins, and capillaries) and the hematologic system (blood and blood components). The lymphatic system (the lymph, lymph nodes, and spleen) is a special vascular system that helps maintain sufficient blood volume in the cardiovascular system by picking up excess tissue fluid and returning it to the bloodstream.

The heart beats an average of 80 times per minute, or once every 0.86 second, every minute of a person's life. As the heart ejects blood with each beat, a closed system of blood vessels transports oxygenated blood to all body organs and tissues and then returns deoxygenated blood to the heart for reoxygenation in the lungs. Deficits in the structure or function of the cardiovascular and lymphatic system may adversely affect all body tissues and may also affect self-care, mobility, comfort, self-concept, sexuality, and role performance.

Anatomy, Physiology, and Functions of the Heart

The Heart

The heart is a hollow, cone-shaped organ approximately the size of an adult man's fist. Beating from 60 to 100 beats each minute for a lifetime, it moves more than 1800 gallons of blood each day (Porth, 2007). Located in the mediastinum of the thoracic cavity, between the vertebral column and the sternum, the heart is flanked laterally by the lungs. Two-thirds of the heart mass lies to the left of the sternum; the upper base lies beneath the second rib, and the pointed apex is approximate with the fifth intercostal space, midpoint to the clavicle (Figure 29–1 ■).

The heart is covered by the pericardium, a double layer of fibroserous membrane (Figure 29–2 ■). The pericardium encases the heart and anchors it to surrounding structures, forming the pericardial sac. The snug fit of the pericardium prevents the heart from overfilling with blood. The outermost layer is the parietal pericardium; the visceral pericardium (or epicardium) adheres to the heart surface. The small space between the visceral and parietal layers of the pericardium is called the pericardial cavity. A serous lubricating fluid produced in this space cushions the heart as it beats.

The heart wall consists of three layers of tissue: the epicardium, the myocardium, and the endocardium (see Figure 29–2). The epicardium covers the entire heart and great vessels, and then folds over to form the parietal layer that lines the pericardium and adheres to the heart surface. The myocardium, the middle layer of the heart wall, consists of specialized cardiac muscle cells (myofibrils) that provide

the bulk of contractile heart muscle. The endocardium is a thin three-layer membrane that lines the inside of the heart's chambers and great vessels.

Chambers and Valves of the Heart

The heart has two upper atria and two lower ventricles. They are separated longitudinally by the interventricular septum (Figure 29–3 ■). The right atrium receives deoxygenated blood from the veins of the body: The superior vena cava returns blood from the body area above the diaphragm, the inferior vena cava returns blood from the body below the diaphragm, and the coronary sinus drains blood from the heart. The left atrium receives freshly oxygenated blood from the lungs through the pulmonary veins. The right ventricle receives deoxygenated blood from the right atrium and pumps it through the pulmonary artery to the pulmonary capillary bed for oxygenation. The newly oxygenated blood then travels through the pulmonary veins to the left atrium. Blood enters the left atrium and crosses the mitral (bicuspid) valve into the left ventricle. Blood is then pumped out of the aorta to the arterial circulation.

Each of the heart's chambers is separated by a valve that allows unidirectional blood flow to the next chamber or great vessel (see Figure 29–3). The atria are separated from the ventricles by the two atrioventricular (AV) valves; the tricuspid valve is on the right side, and the bicuspid (or mitral) valve is on the left. The flaps of each of these valves are anchored to the papillary muscles of the ventricles by the chordae tendineae.

Figure 29–1 ■ Location of the heart in the mediastinum of the thorax. *A,* Relationship of the heart to the sternum, ribs, and diaphragm. *B,* Cross-sectional view showing relative position of the heart in the thorax. *C,* Relationship of the heart and great vessels to the lungs.

Systemic, Pulmonary, and Coronary Circulation

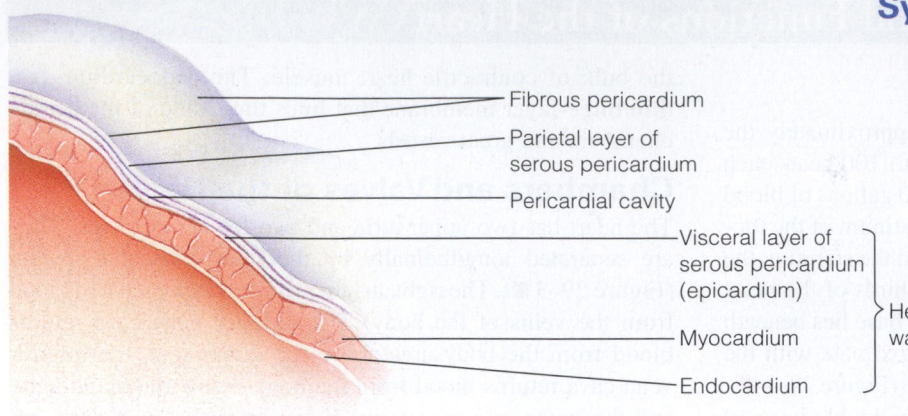

Figure 29-2 ■ Coverings and layers of the heart.

These structures control the movement of the AV valves to prevent backflow of blood. The ventricles are connected to their great vessels by the semilunar valves. On the right, the pulmonary (pulmonic) valve joins the right ventricle with the pulmonary artery. On the left, the aortic valve joins the left ventricle to the aorta. Closure of the AV valves at the onset of contraction (systole) produces the first heart sound, or S_1 (characterized by the syllable "lub"); closure of the semilunar valves at the onset of relaxation (diastole) produces the second heart sound, or S_2 (characterized by the syllable "dub").

Because each side of the heart both receives and ejects blood, the heart is often described as a double pump. Blood enters the right atrium and moves to the pulmonary bed at almost the exact same time that blood is entering the left atrium. The circulatory system has two parts: the systemic circulation (a high-pressure system), which supplies blood to all other body tissues, and the pulmonary circulation (a low pressure system). The systemic circulation consists of the left side of the heart, the aorta and its branches, the capillaries that supply the brain and peripheral tissues, the systemic venous system, and the vena cava. The pulmonary circulation consists of the right side of the heart, the pulmonary artery, the pulmonary capillaries, and the pulmonary vein. Pulmonary circulation begins with the right side of the heart. Deoxygenated blood from the venous system enters the right atrium through two large veins, the superior and inferior venae cavae, and is transported to the lungs via the pulmonary artery and its branches (Figure 29-4 ■). After oxygen and carbon dioxide are exchanged in the pulmonary capillaries, oxygen-rich blood returns to the left atrium through several pulmonary veins. Blood is then pumped out of the left ventricle through the aorta and its major branches to supply all body tissues by the systemic circulation.

Figure 29-3 ■ The internal anatomy of the heart, frontal section.

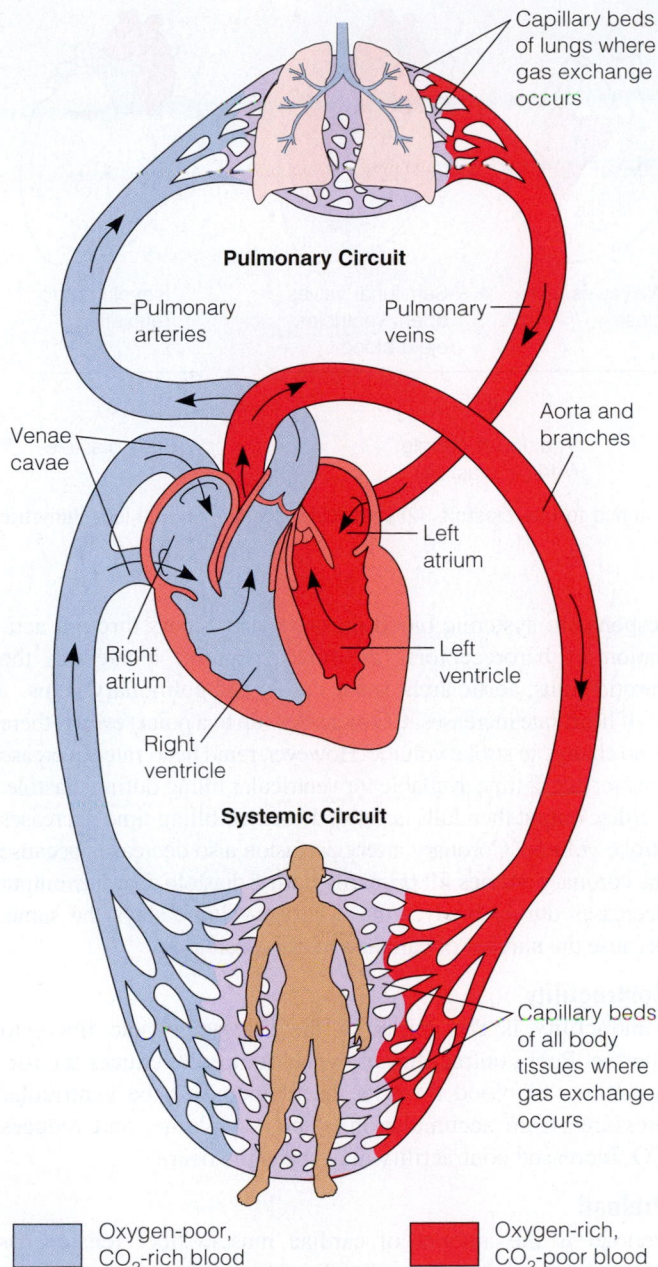

Figure 29–4 ■ Pulmonary and systemic circulation.

Oxygen-poor, CO₂-rich blood

Oxygen-rich, CO₂-poor blood

The heart muscle is supplied by its own network of vessels through the coronary circulation. The left and right coronary arteries originate at the base of the aorta and branch out to encircle the myocardium (Figure 29–5A ■), supplying it with blood, oxygen, and nutrients. The left main coronary artery divides to form the anterior descending and circumflex arteries. The anterior descending artery supplies the anterior interventricular septum and the left ventricle. The circumflex branch supplies the left lateral wall of the left ventricle. The right coronary artery supplies the right ventricle and forms the posterior descending artery. The posterior descending artery supplies the posterior portion of the heart. While ventricular contraction delivers blood through the pulmonary circulation and the systemic circulation, it is during ventricular relaxation that the coronary arteries fill with oxygenated blood. After the blood perfuses the heart muscle, the cardiac veins drain the blood into

the coronary sinus, which empties into the right atrium of the heart (Figure 29–5B). Blood flow through the coronary arteries is regulated by several factors. Aortic pressure is the primary factor. Other factors include the heart rate (most flow occurs during diastole, when the muscle is relaxed), metabolic activity of the heart, and blood vessel tone (constriction).

The Cardiac Cycle and Cardiac Output

The contraction and relaxation of the heart constitutes one heartbeat and is called the cardiac cycle (Figure 29–6 ■). Ventricular filling is followed by ventricular systole, a phase during which the ventricles contract and eject blood into the pulmonary and systemic circuits. Systole is followed by a relaxation phase known as diastole, during which the ventricles refill, the atria contract, and the myocardium is perfused. Normally, the complete cardiac cycle occurs about 70 to 80 times per minute, measured as the heart rate (HR).

Figure 29–5 ■ Coronary circulation. *A,* Coronary arteries; *B,* coronary veins.

Left atrium
Right atrium
Left ventricle
Right ventricle

Passive filling | Atrial contraction

AV valves close | Semilunar valves open; ventricles eject blood

Isovolumetric relaxation

1
Mid-to-late diastole
(Ventricular filling)

2
Ventricular systole
(Atria in diastole)

3
Early diastole

Figure 29–6 ■ The cardiac cycle has three events: (1) ventricular filling in mid-to-late diastole, (2) ventricular systole, and (3) isovolumetric relaxation in early diastole.

During diastole, the volume in the ventricles is increased to about 120 mL (the end-diastolic volume), and at the end of systole, about 50 mL of blood remains in the ventricles (the end-systolic volume). The difference between the end-diastolic volume and the end-systolic volume is called the stroke volume (SV). Stroke volume ranges from 60 to 100 mL/beat and averages about 70 mL/beat in an adult. The ejection fraction is the stroke volume divided by the end-diastolic volume and represents the fraction or percent of the diastolic volume that is ejected from the heart during systole (Porth & Matfin, 2009). For example, an end-diastolic volume of 120 mL divided by a stroke volume of 80 mL equals an ejection fraction of 66%. The normal ejection fraction ranges from 50% to 70%.

The **cardiac output (CO)** is the amount of blood pumped by the ventricles into the pulmonary and systemic circulations in 1 minute. Multiplying the HR by the SV determines the cardiac output: HR × SV = CO. The average adult CO ranges from 4 to 8 L/min. Cardiac output is an indicator of how well the heart is functioning as a pump. If the heart cannot pump effectively, CO and tissue perfusion are decreased. Body tissues that do not receive enough blood and oxygen (carried in the blood on hemoglobin) become **ischemic** (deprived of oxygen). If the tissues do not receive enough blood flow to maintain the functions of the cells, the cells die, resulting in necrosis (infarction).

Activity level, metabolic rate, physiologic and psychologic stress responses, age, and body size all influence CO. In addition, CO is determined by the interaction of four major factors: heart rate, preload, afterload, and contractility. Changes in each of these variables influence CO intrinsically, and each also can be manipulated to affect CO. The heart's ability to respond to the body's changing need for CO is called cardiac reserve.

Heart Rate

Heart rate is affected by both direct and indirect autonomic nervous system stimulation. Direct stimulation is accomplished through the innervation of the heart muscle by sympathetic and parasympathetic nerves. The sympathetic nervous system increases the heart rate, whereas the parasympathetic vagal tone slows the heart rate. Reflex regulation of the heart rate in response to systemic blood pressure also occurs through activation of baroreceptors (pressure receptors) located in the carotid sinus, aortic arch, venae cavae, and pulmonary veins.

If heart rate increases, CO increases (up to a point) even if there is no change in stroke volume. However, rapid heart rates decrease the amount of time available for ventricular filling during diastole. Cardiac output then falls because decreased filling time decreases stroke volume. Coronary artery perfusion also decreases because the coronary arteries fill primarily during diastole. Cardiac output decreases during bradycardia if stroke volume stays the same, because the number of cardiac cycles is decreased.

Contractility

Contractility is the ability of the cardiac muscle fibers to shorten. Poor contractility of the heart muscle reduces the forward flow of blood from the heart, increases the ventricular pressures from accumulation of blood volume, and reduces CO. Increased contractility may stress the heart.

Preload

Preload is the amount of cardiac muscle fiber tension, or stretch, that exists at the end of diastole, just before contraction of the ventricles. Preload is influenced by venous return and the compliance of the ventricles. It is related to the total volume of blood in the ventricles: The greater the volume, the greater the stretch of the cardiac muscle fibers, and the greater the force with which the fibers contract to accomplish emptying. This principle is called Starling's law of the heart. Disorders such as renal disease and congestive heart failure result in sodium and water retention and increased preload. Vasoconstriction also increases venous return and preload.

> **MEMORY CUE**
> This mechanism has a physiologic limit. Just as continuous overstretching of a rubber band causes the band to relax and lose its ability to recoil, overstretching of the cardiac muscle fibers eventually results in ineffective contraction.

Too little circulating blood volume results in a decreased venous return and therefore a decreased preload. A decreased preload reduces stroke volume and thus cardiac output. Decreased preload may result from hemorrhage or misdistribution of blood volume, as occurs in third spacing (∞ see Chapter 10).

Afterload

Afterload is the force the ventricles must overcome to eject their blood volume. It is the pressure in the arterial system ahead of the ventricles. The right ventricle must generate enough tension to open the pulmonary valve and eject its volume into the low-pressure pulmonary arteries. Right ventricle afterload is measured as pulmonary vascular resistance (PVR). The left ventricle, in contrast, ejects its load by overcoming the pressure behind the aortic valve. Afterload of the left ventricle is measured as systemic vascular resistance (SVR). Arterial pressures are much higher than pulmonary pressures; thus, the left ventricle has to work much harder than the right ventricle.

Alterations in vascular tone affect afterload and ventricular work. As the pulmonary or arterial blood pressure increases (e.g., through vasoconstriction), PVR and/or SVR increases, and the work of the ventricles increases. As workload increases, consumption of myocardial oxygen also increases. A compromised heart cannot effectively meet this increased oxygen demand, and a vicious cycle ensues. By contrast, a very low afterload decreases the forward flow of blood into the systemic circulation and the coronary arteries.

Clinical Indicators of Cardiac Output

For many critically ill patients, invasive hemodynamic monitoring catheters are used to measure CO in quantifiable numbers. However, advanced technology is not the only way to identify and assess compromised blood flow. Because CO perfuses the body's tissues, clinical indicators of low CO may be manifested by changes in organ function that result from compromised blood flow. For example, a decrease in blood flow to the brain presents as a change in level of consciousness. Other manifestations of decreased CO are discussed in ∞ Chapters 10 and 30.

Cardiac index (CI) is the CO adjusted for the patient's body size, also called the patient's body surface area (BSA). Because it takes into account the patient's BSA, the cardiac index provides more meaningful data about the heart's ability to perfuse the tissues and therefore is a more accurate indicator of the effectiveness of the circulation.

BSA is stated in square meters (m^2), and cardiac index is calculated as CO divided by BSA. Cardiac measurements are considered adequate when they fall within the range of 2.5 to 4.2 L/min/m^2. For example, two patients are determined to have a CO of 4 L/min. This parameter is within normal limits. However, one patient is 5 feet, 2 inches (157 cm) tall and weighs 120 lb (54.5 kg), with a BSA of 1.54 m^2. This patient's cardiac index is 4 ÷ 1.54, or 2.6 L/min/m^2. The second patient is 6 feet, 2 inches (188 cm) tall and weighs 280 lb (81.7 kg), with a BSA of 2.52 m^2. This patient's cardiac index is 4 ÷ 2.52, or 1.6 L/min/m^2. The cardiac index results show that the same CO of 4 L/min is adequate for the first patient but grossly inadequate for the second patient.

The Conduction System of the Heart

The cardiac cycle is perpetuated by a complex electrical circuit commonly known as the intrinsic conduction system of the heart. Cardiac muscle cells possess an inherent characteristic of self-excitation, which enables them to initiate and transmit impulses independent of a stimulus. However, specialized areas of myocardial cells typically exert a controlling influence in this electrical pathway.

One of these specialized areas is the sinoatrial (SA) node, located at the junction of the superior vena cava and right atrium (Figure 29–7 ■). The SA node acts as the normal "pacemaker" of the heart, usually generating an impulse 60 to 100 times per minute. This impulse travels across the atria via internodal pathways to the atrioventricular (AV) node, in the floor of the interatrial septum. The very small junctional fibers of the AV node slow the impulse, slightly delaying its transmission to the ventricles. It then passes through the bundle of His at the atrioventricular junction and continues down the interventricular septum through the right and left bundle branches and out to the Purkinje fibers in the ventricular muscle walls.

This path of electrical transmission produces a series of changes in ion concentration across the membrane of each cardiac muscle cell. The electrical stimulus increases the permeability of the cell membrane, creating an action potential (electrical potential). The result is an exchange of sodium, potassium, and calcium ions across the cell membrane, which changes the intracellular electrical charge to a positive state. This process of depolarization results in myocardial contraction. As the ion exchange reverses and the cell returns to its resting state of electronegativity, the cell is repolarized, and cardiac muscle relaxes. The cellular action potential serves as the basis for electrocardiography (ECG), a diagnostic test of cardiac function.

Sinoatrial node (pacemaker)

Internodal pathways

Atrioventricular node

Atrioventricular bundle (bundle of His)

Right bundle branch

Left bundle branch

Purkinje fibers

Figure 29–7 ■ The intrinsic conduction system of the heart.

The Peripheral Vascular System

The two components of the peripheral vascular system are the arterial network and the venous network. The arterial network begins with the major arteries that branch from the aorta. The major arteries of the systemic circulation are illustrated in Figure 29–8 ■. These major arteries branch into successively smaller arteries, which in turn subdivide into the smallest of the arterial vessels, called *arterioles*. The smallest arterioles feed into beds of hairlike capillaries in the body's organs and tissues.

In the capillary beds, oxygen and nutrients are exchanged for metabolic wastes, and deoxygenated blood moves back to the heart through venules, the smallest vessels of the venous network. Venules join the smallest of veins, which in turn join larger and larger veins. The blood transported by the veins empties into the superior and inferior venae cavae entering the right side of the heart. The major veins of the systemic circulation are shown in Figure 29–9 ■.

Structure of Blood Vessels

The structure of blood vessels reflects their different functions within the circulatory system (Figure 29–10 ■). Except for the tiniest vessels, blood vessel walls have three layers: the tunica intima, the tunica media, and the tunica adventitia. The tunica intima, the innermost layer, is made of endothelium that provides a slick surface to facilitate the flow of blood. In arteries, the middle layer, or tunica media, is made of smooth muscle and is thicker than the tunica media of veins. This makes arteries more elastic than veins and allows the arteries to alternately expand and recoil as the heart contracts and relaxes with each beat, producing a pressure wave that can be felt as a pulse over an artery. The smaller arterioles are less elastic than arteries but contain more smooth muscle, which promotes their constriction and dilation. In fact, arterioles exert the major control over arterial blood pressure. The tunica adventitia, or outermost layer, is made of connective tissue and serves to protect and anchor the vessel. Veins have a thicker tunica adventitia than do arteries.

Blood in the veins travels at a much lower pressure than does blood in the arteries. Veins have thinner walls, a larger lumen, and greater capacity, and many are supplied with valves that help blood flow against gravity back to the heart. The "milking" action of skeletal muscle contraction also supports venous return. When skeletal muscles contract against veins, the valves proximal to the contraction open, and blood is propelled toward the heart. The abdominal and thoracic pressure changes that occur with breathing also propel blood toward the heart.

The tiny capillaries, which connect the arterioles and venules, contain only one thin layer of tunica intima that is permeable to the gases and molecules exchanged between blood and tissue cells. Capillaries typically are found in interwoven networks. They filter and shunt blood from precapillary arterioles to postcapillary venules.

Arterial Circulation

The factors that affect arterial circulation are blood flow, peripheral vascular resistance, and blood pressure. Blood flow refers to the volume of blood transported in a vessel, in an organ, or throughout the entire circulation over a given period of time. It is commonly expressed as liters or milliliters per minute or cubic centimeters per second.

Peripheral vascular resistance (PVR) refers to the opposing forces or impedance to blood flow as the arterial channels become more and more distant from the heart. Peripheral vascular resistance is determined by three factors:

- *Blood viscosity:* The greater the viscosity, or thickness, of the blood, the greater its resistance to moving and flowing.
- *Length of the vessel:* The longer the vessel, the greater the resistance to blood flow.
- *Diameter of the vessel:* The smaller the diameter of a vessel, the greater the friction against the walls of the vessel and, thus, the greater the impedance to blood flow.

Blood pressure (BP) is the force exerted against the walls of the arteries by the blood as it is pumped from the heart. It is most accurately referred to as mean arterial pressure (MAP). The highest pressure exerted against the arterial walls at the peak of ventricular contraction (systole) is called the systolic BP. The lowest pressure exerted during ventricular relaxation (diastole) is the diastolic BP.

Mean arterial blood pressure is regulated mainly by CO and peripheral vascular resistance (PVR), as represented in this formula: MAP = CO × PVR. For clinical use, the MAP may be estimated by calculating the diastolic blood pressure plus one-third of the pulse pressure (the difference between the systolic and diastolic blood pressure).

Factors Influencing Arterial Blood Pressure

Blood flow, peripheral vascular resistance, and BP, which influence arterial circulation, are in turn influenced by various factors, as follows:

- The sympathetic and parasympathetic nervous systems are the primary mechanisms that regulate BP. Stimulation of the sympathetic nervous system exerts a major effect on peripheral resistance by causing vasoconstriction of the arterioles, thereby increasing BP. Parasympathetic stimulation causes vasodilation of the arterioles, lowering BP.
- Baroreceptors and chemoreceptors in the aortic arch, carotid sinus, and other large vessels are sensitive to pressure and chemical changes and cause reflex sympathetic stimulation, resulting in vasoconstriction, increased heart rate, and increased BP.
- The kidneys help maintain BP by excreting or conserving sodium and water. When BP decreases, the kidneys initiate the renin–angiotensin mechanism. This stimulates vasoconstriction, resulting in the release of the hormone aldosterone from the adrenal cortex, increasing sodium ion reabsorption and water retention. In addition, pituitary release of antidiuretic hormone (ADH) promotes renal reabsorption of water. The net result is an increase in blood volume and a consequent increase in CO and BP.
- Temperatures may affect peripheral resistance: Cold causes vasoconstriction, whereas warmth produces vasodilation.
- Many chemicals, hormones, and drugs influence BP by affecting CO and/or PVR. For example, epinephrine causes vasoconstriction and increased heart rate; prostaglandins dilate blood

Figure 29–8 ■ Major arteries of the systemic circulation.

Dural sinuses

External jugular vein
Vertebral vein
Internal jugular vein

Superior vena cava

Axillary vein

Great cardiac vein

Hepatic veins

Hepatic portal vein
Superior mesenteric vein

Inferior vena cava

Ulnar vein
Radial vein

Common iliac vein
External iliac vein
Internal iliac vein

Digital veins

Femoral vein

Great saphenous vein

Popliteal vein

Posterior tibial vein

Anterior tibial vein

Peroneal vein

Dorsal venous arch

Subclavian vein
Right and left
brachiocephalic veins
Cephalic vein
Brachial vein

Basilic vein
Splenic vein
Median cubital vein
Renal vein

Inferior mesenteric vein

Dorsal digital
veins

Figure 29–9 ■ Major veins of the systemic circulation.

Figure 29–10 ■ Structure of arteries, veins, and capillaries. Capillaries are composed of only a fine tunica intima. Notice that the tunica media is thicker in arteries than in veins.

vessel diameter (by relaxing vascular smooth muscle); endothelin, a chemical released by the inner lining of vessels, is a potent vasoconstrictor; nicotine causes vasoconstriction; and alcohol and histamine cause vasodilation.

■ Dietary factors such as intake of salt, saturated fats, and cholesterol elevate BP by affecting blood volume and vessel diameter.

■ Race, gender, age, weight, time of day, position, exercise, and emotional state may also affect BP. These factors influence the arterial pressure. Systemic venous pressure, though it is much lower, is also influenced by such factors as blood volume, venous tone, and right atrial pressure.

The Lymphatic System

The structures of the lymphatic system include the lymph, lymph nodes, the spleen, the thymus, the tonsils, and the Peyer's patches of the small intestine. Lymph nodes are small aggregates of specialized cells that assist the immune system by removing foreign material, infectious organisms, and tumor cells from lymph. Lymph nodes are distributed along the lymphatic vessels, forming clusters in certain body regions such as the neck, axilla, and groin (see Figure 29–11 ■).

The spleen, the largest lymphoid organ, is in the upper left quadrant of the abdomen under the thorax. The main function of the spleen is to filter the blood by breaking down old red blood cells and storing or releasing to the liver their by-products (such as iron). The spleen also synthesizes lymphocytes, stores platelets for blood clotting, and serves as a reservoir of blood. The thymus gland is in the lower throat and is most active in childhood, producing hormones (such as thymosin) that facilitate the immune action of lymphocytes. The tonsils of the pharynx and Peyer's patches of the small intestine are lymphoid organs that protect the upper respiratory and digestive tracts from foreign pathogens.

The lymphatic vessels, or lymphatics, form a network around the arterial and venous channels and interweave at the capillary beds. They collect and

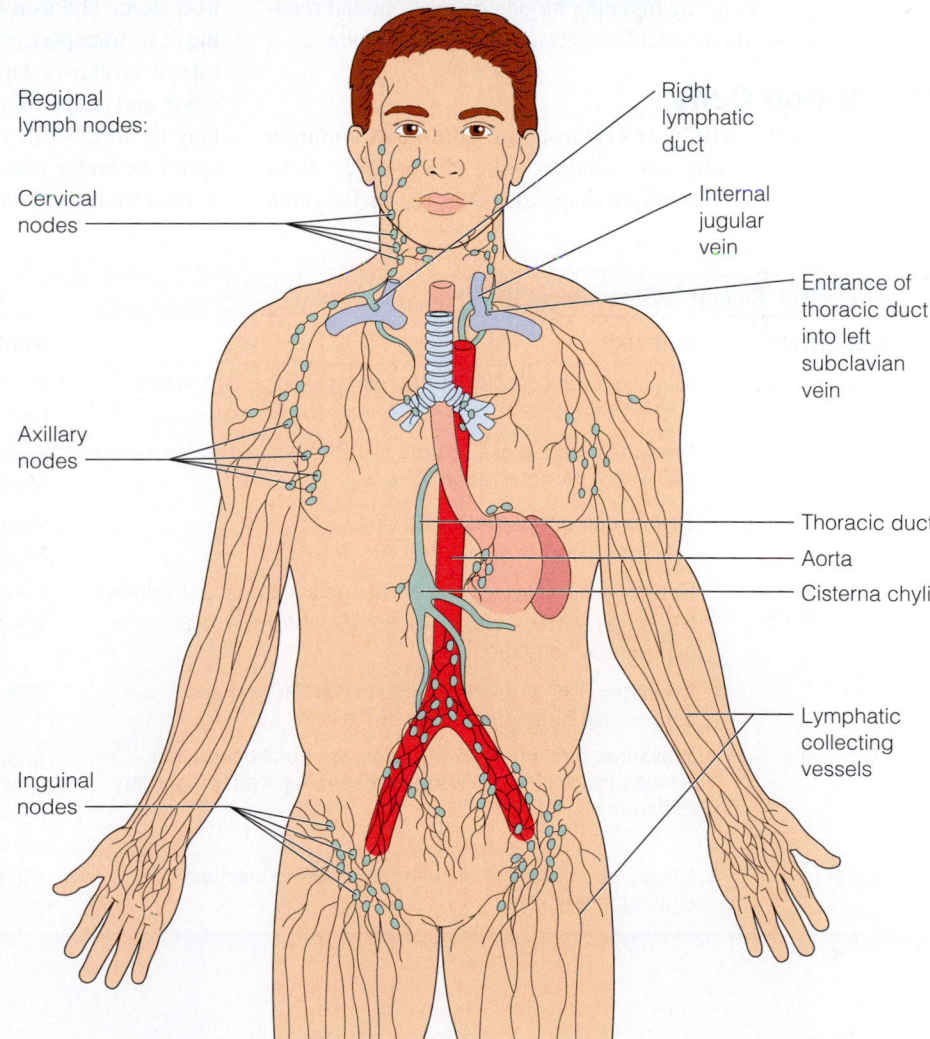

Figure 29–11 ■ The lymphatic system.

drain excess tissue fluid, called lymph, that "leaks" from the cardiovascular system and accumulates at the venous end of the capillary bed. The lymphatics return this fluid to the heart through a one-way system of lymphatic venules and veins that eventually drain into the right lymphatic duct and left thoracic duct, both of which empty into their respective subclavian veins. Lymphatics are a low-pressure system without a pump; their fluid transport depends on the rhythmic contraction of their smooth muscle and the muscular and respiratory movements that assist venous circulation.

The Hematologic System

Blood consists of plasma, solutes (e.g., proteins, electrolytes, and organic constituents), red blood cells, white blood cells, and platelets (which are fragments of cells). The hematopoietic (blood-forming) system includes the bone marrow (myeloid) tissues, where blood cells form, and the lymphoid tissues of the lymph nodes, where white blood cells mature and circulate. All blood cells originate from cells in the bone marrow called stem cells, or hemocytoblasts. The origin of the cellular components of blood is illustrated in Figure 29–12 ■. Normal laboratory values for blood components are found in Table 29–1.

Regulatory mechanisms cause stem cells to differentiate into families of parent cells, each of which gives rise to one of the formed elements of the blood (red blood cells, platelets, and white blood cells). The functions of blood include transporting oxygen, nutrients, hormones, and metabolic wastes; protecting against invasion of pathogens; maintaining blood coagulation; and regulating fluids, electrolytes, acids, bases, and body temperature.

Red Blood Cells

Red blood cells (RBC), or erythrocytes, (the most common type of blood cell) are shaped like biconcave disks (Figure 29–13 ■). This unique shape increases the surface area of the cell and allows the cell to pass through very small capillaries without disrupting the cell membrane. RBCs and the hemoglobin molecules they contain transport oxygen to body tissues. Hemoglobin also binds with some carbon dioxide, carrying it to the lungs for excretion. Abnormal numbers of RBCs, changes in their size and shape, or altered hemoglobin content or structure can adversely affect health. Anemia, the most common RBC disorder, is an abnormally low RBC count or reduced hemoglobin content. Polycythemia is an abnormally high RBC count.

Hemoglobin, synthesized within the RBC, is the oxygen-carrying protein. It consists of the heme molecule and globin, a protein molecule. Globin is made of four polypeptide chains—two alpha chains and two beta chains (Figure 29–14 ■). Each of the four polypeptide chains contains a heme unit containing an iron atom. The iron atom binds reversibly with oxygen, allowing it to transport oxygen as oxyhemoglobin to the cells. The rate of synthesis depends on the availability of iron. The size, color, and shape of stained RBCs also may be analyzed. RBCs may be normocytic (normal size), smaller than normal (microcytic), or larger than normal (macrocytic). Their color may be normal (normochromic) or diminished (hypochromic).

TABLE 29–1 Complete Blood Count (CBC)

COMPONENT	PURPOSE	NORMAL VALUES
Hemoglobin (Hb)	Measures the capacity of the hemoglobin to carry gases	Women: 12–16 g/dL Men: 13.5–18 g/dL
Hematocrit (Hct)	Measures packed cell volume of RBCs, expressed as a percent of the total blood volume	Women: 38%–47% Men: 40%–54%
Total RBC count	Counts number of circulating RBCs	Women: $4–5 \times 10^6/\mu L$ Men: $4.5–6 \times 10^6/\mu L$
Red cell indices: MCV 10^6MCH	Determines relative size of MCV (mean corpuscular volume)	82–98 fl
	Measures average weight of Hb/RBC (MCH = mean corpuscular hemoglobin)	27–29 pg
MCHC	Evaluates RBC saturation with Hb (MC HC = mean corpuscular hemoglobin concentration)	32%–36%
WBC count	Measures total number of leukocytes (total count) and whether each kind of WBC is present in proper proportion (differential)	Total WBC count: 4000–11,000/ μL ($4–11 \times 10^9$/L) WBC differential: Neutrophils: 50%–70% Eosinophils: 2%–4% Basophils: 0%–2% Lymphocytes: 20%–40% Monocytes: 4%–8%
Platelets	Measures number of platelets available to maintain clotting functions	150,000–400,000/μL ($150–400 \times 10^9$/L)

Figure 29–12 ■ Blood cell formation from stem cells. Regulatory factors control the differentiation of stem cells into blasts. Each of the five kinds of blasts is committed to producing one type of mature blood cell. Erythroblasts, for example, can differentiate only into RBCs; megakaryoblasts can differentiate only into platelets.

Top view

Side view

Figure 29–13 ■ Top and side view of a red blood cell (erythrocyte). Note the distinctive biconcave shape.

Red Blood Cell Production and Regulation

In adults, RBC production (erythropoiesis) (Figure 29–15 ■) begins in red bone marrow of the vertebrae, sternum, ribs, and pelvis, and is completed in the blood or spleen. Erythroblasts begin forming hemoglobin while they are in the bone marrow, a process that continues throughout the RBC life span. The cells enter the circulation as reticulocytes, which fully mature in about 48 hours. The complete sequence from stem cell to RBC takes 3 to 5 days.

The stimulus for increased RBC production is tissue hypoxia. The hormone erythropoietin is released by the kidneys in response to hypoxia. It stimulates the bone marrow to produce RBCs. However, the process of RBC production takes about 5 days to maximize. During periods of increased RBC

Figure 29–14 ■ The hemoglobin molecule includes globin (a protein) and heme, which contains iron. Globin is made of four subunits, two alpha and two beta polypeptide chains. A heme disk containing an iron atom (red dot) nests within the folds of each protein subunit. The iron atoms combine reversibly with oxygen, transporting it to the cells.

production, the percentage of reticulocytes (immature RBCs) in the blood exceeds that of mature cells.

Red Blood Cell Destruction

RBCs have a life span of about 120 days. Old or damaged RBCs are lysed (destroyed) by phagocytes in the spleen, liver, bone marrow, and lymph nodes. The process of RBC destruction is called hemolysis. Phagocytes save and reuse amino acids and iron from heme units in the lysed RBCs. Most of the heme unit is converted to bilirubin, an orange-yellow pigment that is removed from the blood by the liver and excreted in the bile. During disease processes causing increased hemolysis or impaired liver function, bilirubin accumulates in the serum, causing jaundice, a yellowish appearance of the skin and sclera.

White Blood Cells

White blood cells (WBCs, leukocytes) originate from hemopoietic stem cells in the bone marrow and differentiate into the various types of white blood cells. They are a part of the body's defense against microorganisms. Leukocytosis is a higher than normal WBC count; leukopenia is a WBC count that is lower than normal.

The two basic types of WBCs are granular leukocytes (or granulocytes) and nongranular leukocytes. Stimulated by granulocyte-macrophage colony-stimulating factor (GM-CSF) and granulocyte colony-stimulating factor (G-CSF), granulocytes mature fully in the bone marrow before being released into the bloodstream. The three types of granulocytes are as follows:

■ Neutrophils (also called polymorphonuclear [PMN] or segmented [segs] leukocytes) are active phagocytes, the first cells to arrive at a site of injury. Their numbers increase during inflammation. Immature forms of neutrophils (bands) are released during inflammation or infections, and are referred to as having a shift to the left (so named because immature cell frequencies appear on the left side of the graph) on a differential blood count. Neutrophils have a life span of only about 10 hours and are constantly being replaced.

■ Eosinophils are found in large numbers in the mucosa of the intestines and lungs. Their numbers increase during allergic reactions and parasitic infestations.

■ Basophils contain histamine, heparin, and other inflammatory mediators. Basophils increase in numbers during allergic and inflammatory reactions.

Nongranular WBCs (agranulocytes) include the monocytes and lymphocytes. They enter the blood stream before final maturation. These cells are an active part of the inflammatory and immune responses and are discussed in ∞ Chapters 12 and 13.

Platelets

Platelets (thrombocytes) produce ATP and release mediators required for clotting. Platelets are formed in the bone marrow as pinched-off portions of large megakaryocytes. Platelet production is controlled by thrombopoietin, a protein produced by the liver, kidney, smooth muscle, and bone

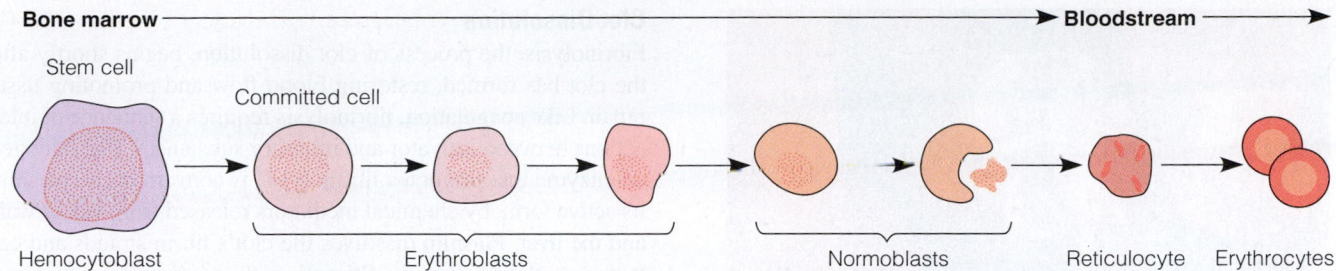

Bone marrow ————————————————————————————————— **Bloodstream** →

Stem cell

Committed cell

Hemocytoblast | Erythroblasts | Normoblasts | Reticulocyte | Erythrocytes

Figure 29–15 ■ Erythropoiesis. RBCs begin as erythroblasts within the bone marrow, maturing into normoblasts, which eventually eject their nucleus and organellas to become reticulocytes. Reticulocytes mature within the blood or spleen to become erythrocytes.

marrow. The number of circulating platelets controls thrombopoietin release. Platelets live up to 10 days in circulation. An excess of platelets is thrombocytosis. A deficit of platelets is thrombocytopenia.

Hemostasis

Platelet and coagulation disorders affect **hemostasis** (control of bleeding). Hemostasis is a series of complex interactions between platelets and clotting mechanisms that maintains a relatively steady state of blood volume, BP, and blood flow through injured vessels. The five stages of hemostasis are (1) vessel spasm, (2) formation of the platelet plug, (3) development of an insoluble fibrin clot, (4) clot retraction, and (5) clot dissolution.

Vessel Spasm

When a blood vessel is damaged, thromboxane A_2 (TXA_2) is released from platelets and cells, causing vessel spasm. This spasm constricts the damaged vessel for about 1 minute, reducing blood flow.

Formation of the Platelet Plug

Platelets attracted to the damaged vessel wall change from smooth disks to spiny spheres. Receptors on the activated platelets bind with von Willebrand's factor (a protein molecule) and exposed collagen fibers at the site of injury to form the platelet plug (Figure 29–16 ■). The platelets release adenosine diphosphate (ADP) and TXA_2 to activate nearby platelets, adhering them to the developing plug. Activation of the clotting pathway on the platelet surface converts fibrinogen to fibrin. Fibrin, in turn, forms a meshwork that binds the platelets and other blood cells to form a stable plug (Figure 29–17 ■).

Development of the Fibrin Clot

The process of coagulation creates a meshwork of fibrin strands that cements the blood components to form an insoluble clot. Coagulation requires many interactive reactions and two clotting pathways (Figure 29–18 ■). The slower intrinsic pathway is activated when blood contacts collagen in the injured vessel wall; the faster extrinsic pathway is activated when blood is exposed to tissues. The final outcome of both pathways is fibrin clot formation. Each procoagulation substance is activated in sequence; the activation of one coagulation factor activates another in turn. Table 29–2 lists

Injury to vessel lining exposes collagen fibers; platelets adhere

Platelet plug forms

Fibrin clot with trapped red blood cells

Collagen fibers

Platelets

Fibrin

Chemical release increases platelet adhesion

| Mediating factors from platelets and thromboplastin from damaged cells | + | Calcium and other clotting factors in blood plasma |

Coagulation

1 — Prothrombin activator

2 — Prothrombin → Thrombin

3 — Fibrinogen (soluble) → Fibrin (insoluble)

Figure 29–16 ■ Platelet plug formation and blood clotting. The flow diagram summarizes the events leading to fibrin clot formation. PF_3 (blue arrow) released from damaged tissue combines with other clotting factors to release prothrombin activator, the first step of coagulation. Second, prothrombin is converted into thrombin. Finally, thrombin transforms soluble fibrinogen into insoluble fibrin (red arrow) to form a clot.

Figure 29–17 ■ Scanning electron micrograph of a RBC trapped in a fibrin mesh. The spherical gray object at top is a platelet.
Source: Copyright © Boehniger Ingelheim; photo Lennart Nilsson, Albert Bonniers Förlog AB.

known factors, their origin, and their function or pathway. A deficiency of one or more factors or inappropriate inactivation of any factor alters normal coagulation.

Clot Retraction

After the clot is stabilized (within about 30 minutes), trapped platelets contract. Platelet contraction squeezes the fibrin strands, pulling the broken portions of the ruptured blood vessel closer together. Growth factors released by the platelets stimulate cell division and tissue repair of the damaged vessel.

Clot Dissolution

Fibrinolysis, the process of clot dissolution, begins shortly after the clot has formed, restoring blood flow and promoting tissue repair. Like coagulation, fibrinolysis requires a sequence of interactions between activator and inhibitor substances. Plasminogen, an enzyme that promotes fibrinolysis, is converted into plasmin, its active form, by chemical mediators released from vessel walls and the liver. Plasmin dissolves the clot's fibrin strands and certain coagulation factors. Stimuli such as exercise, fever, and vasoactive drugs promote plasminogen activator release. The liver and endothelium also produce fibrinolytic inhibitors.

Assessing Cardiovascular and Lymphatic Function

Cardiovascular function is assessed by findings from diagnostic tests, a health assessment interview to collect subjective data, and a physical assessment to collect objective data.

Diagnostic Tests

The results of diagnostic tests of cardiac function are used to support the diagnosis of a specific disease, to provide information to identify or modify the appropriate medications or therapy used to treat the disease, and to help nurses monitor the patient's responses to treatment and nursing care interventions. Diagnostic tests to assess the structures and functions of the heart are described on page 886. More information is included in the discussion of specific disorders in ∞ Chapters 30, 31, 32, and 33.

Regardless of the type of diagnostic test, the nurse is responsible for explaining the procedure and any special preparation needed, ensuring the consent form is signed (if necessary), supporting the patient during the examination as necessary, documenting the procedure as appropriate, and monitoring the results of the test. The nurse is also responsible for postprocedure care and patient teaching for self-care at home.

Genetic Considerations

When conducting a health assessment interview and physical assessment, it is important for the nurse to consider genetic influences on the health of the adult. Ask about family members

TABLE 29–2 Blood Coagulation Factors

FACTOR	NAME	FUNCTION OR PATHWAY
I	Fibrinogen	Converted to fibrin strands
II	Prothrombin	Converted to thrombin
III	Thromboplastin	Catalyzes conversion of thrombin
IV	Calcium ions	Needed for all steps of coagulation
V	Proaccelerin	Extrinsic/intrinsic pathways
VII	Serum prothrombin conversion accelerator	Extrinsic pathway
VIII	Antihemophilic factor	Intrinsic pathway
IX	Plasma prothrombin component	Intrinsic pathway
X	Stuart factor	Extrinsic/intrinsic pathways
XI	Plasma prothrombin antecedent	Intrinsic pathway
XII	Hageman factor	Intrinsic pathway
XIII	Fibrin stabilizing factor	Cross-links fibrin strands to form insoluble clot

Intrinsic Pathway (slow)

Blood is exposed to collagen in wall of damaged vessel

XII → Activated XII

XI → Activated XI

IX → Activated IX

Mediating factors from aggregated platelets

Ca²⁺

V

VIII Complex

Extrinsic Pathway (rapid)

Blood is exposed to extravascular tissue

Thromboplastin III released

Ca²⁺

VII

VII Complex

X → Activated X

Ca²⁺

V

Common Pathway

Prothrombin activator

Prothrombin II

Thrombin

Ca²⁺

Fibrinogen I

Fibrin

XIII

Activated XIII

Cross-linked fibrin clot

Figure 29–18 ■ Clot formation. Both the slower intrinsic pathway and the more rapid extrinsic pathway activate factor X. Factor X then combines with other factors to form prothrombin activator. Prothrombin activator transforms prothrombin into thrombin, which then transforms fibrinogen into long fibrin strands. Thrombin also activates Factor XIII, which draws the fibrin strands together into a dense meshwork. The complete process of clot formation occurs within 3 to 6 minutes after blood vessel damage.

with health problems affecting the cardiovascular system, such as high BP, high cholesterol levels, leukemia, or early onset CAD. Depending on the racial and ethnic background of the patient, ask about any family members with sickle cell anemia or thalassemia. During the physical assessment, assess for any manifestations that might indicate a genetic disorder (see the box on page 890). If data are found to indicate genetic risk factors or alterations, ask about genetic testing and refer for appropriate genetic counseling and evaluation. ∞ Chapter 8 provides further information about genetics in medical-surgical nursing.

The Health Assessment Interview

A health assessment interview to determine problems with cardiovascular or lymphatic structure and function may be conducted during a health screening, may focus on a chief complaint (such as chest pain or leg pain when walking), or

may be part of a total health assessment. If the patient has a problem with cardiovascular or lymphatic function, analyze its onset, characteristics, course, severity, precipitating and relieving factors, and any associated symptoms, noting the timing and circumstances. For example, ask the patient the following:

■ What is the location of the chest pain you experienced? Did it move up to your jaw or into your left arm?
■ Describe the type of activity that brings on your chest pain.
■ Does the leg pain occur only with activities such as walking, or during rest?
■ Have you felt light-headed during the times your heart is racing?

The interview begins by exploring the patient's chief complaint (e.g., chest pain, leg pain, or fatigue). Describe the patient's chest pain or leg pain in terms of location, quality or character, timing, setting or precipitating factors, severity,

DIAGNOSTIC TESTS of the Cardiovascular and Lymphatic System

THE HEART AND PERIPHERAL VASCULAR SYSTEM

NAME OF TEST	PURPOSE & DESCRIPTION	RELATED NURSING INTERVENTIONS
Blood pool imaging	This test is useful for evaluation of cardiac status following myocardial infarction and congestive heart failure and effectiveness of cardiac medications Following IV injection of technetium 99m pertechnetate, sequential evaluation of the heart can be performed for several hours. It can be done at the patient's bedside.	No special preparation is needed.
Cardiac catheterization (coronary angiography, coronary arteriography)	A cardiac catheterization may be performed to identify coronary artery disease (CAD) or cardiac valvular disease, to determine pulmonary artery or heart chamber pressures, to obtain a myocardial biopsy, to evaluate artificial valves, or to perform angioplasty or stent an area of CAD. The test is performed by inserting a long catheter into a vein or artery (depending on whether the right side or the left side of the heart is being examined) in the arm or leg. Using fluoroscopy, the catheter is then threaded to the heart chambers or coronary arteries or both. Contrast dye is injected and heart structures are visualized and heart activity is filmed. The test is done in the hospital for diagnosis and before heart surgery. *Right cardiac catheterization:* The catheter is inserted into the femoral vein or antecubital vein and then threaded through the inferior vena cava into the right atrium to the pulmonary artery. Pressures are measured at each site and blood samples can be obtained for the right side of the heart. The functions of the tricuspid and pulmonary valves can be observed. *Left cardiac catheterization:* The catheter is inserted into the brachial or femoral artery and advanced retrograde through the aorta to the coronary arteries and/or left ventricle. The patency of the coronary arteries and/or functions of the aortic and mitral valves and left ventricle can be observed.	Inform the patient that food and fluids should not be taken for 6 to 8 hours before the test. Assess for allergies to seafood, iodine, or iodine contrast dyes. If an allergic response to the dye is possible, antihistamines (such as Benadryl) or steroids may be administered the evening before and the morning of the test. Assess for use of aspirin or NSAIDs (risk of bleeding), Viagra (risk of heart problems), or history of kidney disease (dye used may be toxic to the kidneys). Take and record vital signs, including peripheral pulses. Explain that the patient is positioned on a padded table that tilts. A local anesthetic is used at the site of catheter insertion. ECG leads are applied and vital signs are monitored during the procedure. The patient lies supine and is asked to cough and deep breathe frequently. The procedure takes 1/2 to 3 hours. After the procedure, monitor vital signs every 15 minutes for the first hour and then every 30 minutes until stable. Assess cardiac rhythm and rate for alterations. Assess peripheral pulses distal to the insertion site. Assess for chest heaviness, dyspnea, and abdominal or groin pain. Monitor catheter insertion site for bleeding or hematoma. Administer pain medications as prescribed. Instruct patient to increase fluid intake and restrict activity as ordered.
Cardiolite scan	This test is used to evaluate blood flow in different parts of the heart. Cardiolite (technetium 99m sestamibi) is injected IV. In a dipyridamole cardiolite scan, dipyridamole (Persantine) is injected to increase blood flow to coronary arteries. These scans may be done in conjunction with a treadmill test.	See information in this table for treadmill test. Instruct the patient to avoid intake of caffeine for 12 hours before having a test with dipyridamole cardiolite.
Chest x-ray	An x-ray of the thorax can illustrate the contours, placement, and chambers of the heart. It may be done to identify heart displacement or hypertrophy, or fluid in the pericardial sac.	No special preparation is needed.
Computed tomography (CT) scan—thoracic	A thoracic CT scan may be conducted to quantify calcium deposits in coronary arteries.	Assess for allergy to iodine or seafood if contrast medium is to be administered. If allergy exists, follow orders for times and types of medications. For IV contrast studies, instruct patient not to eat or drink for 4 hours prior to the test. Assess medications: oral hypoglycemic agents are contraindicated for use with iodinated contrast. Request patient remove hairpins, earrings, and dentures.

DIAGNOSTIC TESTS of the Cardiovascular and Lymphatic System **(continued)**

NAME OF TEST	PURPOSE & DESCRIPTION	RELATED NURSING INTERVENTIONS
Echocardiogram ■ M-mode ■ Two-dimensional (2-D) ■ Cardiac Doppler ■ Color Doppler ■ Stress echocardiogram	Echocardiograms use a transducer to record waves that are bounced off the heart, and to record the direction and flow of blood through the heart in audio and graphic data. An *M(motion)-mode echocardiogram* records the motion, wall thickness, and chamber size of the heart. A *2-D echocardiogram* provides a cross-sectional view of the heart. *Color flow imaging* combines 2-D echocardiography and Doppler technology to evaluate the speed and direction of blood flow through the heart, which can identify pathology such as leaky valves. *Stress echocardiography* combines a treadmill test with ultrasound images to evaluate segmental function and wall motion. If the patient is not physically able to exercise, IV dobutamine may be administered and ultrasound images takes.	No special preparation is needed; see related nursing care for the patient having a treadmill test for a stress echocardiogram.
Electrocardiogram (ECG)	See Boxes 29–1 and 29–2.	No special preparation is needed.
Lipids	Blood lipids are cholesterol, triglycerides, and phospholipids. They circulate bound to proteins, and so are known as lipoproteins. Lipids are measured to evaluate risk for CAD and to monitor effectiveness of anticholesterol medications. **Normal values:** Cholesterol: 140–200 mg/dL Triglycerides: 40–190 mg/dL HDL: Men = 37–70 mg/dL Women = 40–88 mg/dL LDL: < 1 mg/dL (*Note:* Normal values may vary by laboratory.)	Recommend a low-fat meal the evening prior to the test, then no food for 8–12 hours. Instruct the patient to have no alcohol intake for 24 hours prior to the test. Assess medications. Blood lipids may be increased by thyroxine, estrogens, aspirin, antibiotics (tetracycline and neomycin), nicotinic acid, heparin, and colchicine.
Magnetic resonance imaging (MRI)	An MRI may be used to identify and locate areas of myocardial infarction, perfusion of the heart, and patency of coronary arteries after coronary grafts.	Assess for any metallic implants (such as clips on brain aneurysms, pacemaker, body piercing, tatoos, and shrapnel). If present, notify physician. Remove transdermal medication patches (both OTC and prescribed) unless otherwise ordered. (FDA, 2009). Replace the patch following the procedure. Tell the patient to inform the staff about the patch when making the appointment and when completing the admission information. Ask if patient is pregnant; if so the test is not performed. Ask about claustrophobia; if a problem exists, request patient ask the referring physician for a relaxing medication prior to the MRI. If the patient is very claustrophobic, obese, or confused, an open MRI may be used.
Nuclear dobutamine stress test	Dobutamine is an adrenergic drug that increases myocardial contractility, heart rate, and systolic BP, which increases coronary oxygen consumption and thus increases coronary blood flow.	Instruct the patient to not eat food or drink fluids other than water after midnight. Tell the patient to discontinue beta-blockers, calcium channel blockers, and ACE inhibitors for 36 hours prior to the test. If hospitalized, do not administer nitrates for 6 hours prior to the test.
Nuclear persantine [dipyridamole] stress test	This test is used when the patient is not physically able to walk on the treadmill. Persantine, given IV, dilates the coronary arteries and increases myocardial blood flow. Coronary arteries that are narrowed from CAD cannot dilate to increase myocardial perfusion.	Patient is NPO after midnight except for water. Food, fluids, and drugs that contain caffeine should be avoided for 24 hours prior to the test, as should decaffeinated fluids. Some drugs, such as theophylline preparations, are discontinued for 36 hours prior to the test.

(continued)

DIAGNOSTIC TESTS of the Cardiovascular and Lymphatic System (continued)

NAME OF TEST	PURPOSE & DESCRIPTION	RELATED NURSING INTERVENTIONS
Pericardiocentesis	This procedure is performed in the hospital to remove fluid from the pericardial sac for diagnostic or therapeutic purposes. It may also be done as an emergency procedure for the patient with cardiac tamponade (which may result in death). A large-gauge (16 to 18) needle is inserted to the left of the xiphoid process into the pericardial sac and excess fluid is withdrawn (see Figure 29–19 ■).	Take and record baseline vital signs. Assess for history of cardiac problems. Explain to patient the need to remain still during the procedure, that the procedure takes about 30 minutes, and that a local anesthetic will be used at the needle insertion site. Monitor the ECG during and after the procedure and report abnormal findings to the physician. Monitor vital signs after the procedure as ordered. Notify the physician of changes in cardiac rhythm, BP, heart rate, or level of consciousness. If the procedure is to treat an emergency, monitor central venous pressure (CVP) and BP closely. As the effusion is relieved, CVP will decrease and BP will increase.

Myocardium

Pericardial sac

16–18 gauge needle

Figure 29–19 ■ Pericardiocentesis.

NAME OF TEST	PURPOSE & DESCRIPTION	RELATED NURSING INTERVENTIONS
Positron emission tomography (PET)	Two scans are performed following injection of radionuclides, and the resulting images are compared for myocardial perfusion and myocardial metabolic function. A stress test (treadmill) may be a part of the test. If the myocardium is ischemic or damaged, the images will be different. Normally, the images will be the same.	Assess the patient's blood glucose: For accurate metabolic activity images, the blood glucose level must be between 60 and 140 mg/dL. If exercise is included in the test, instruct the patient to be NPO and avoid smoking and caffeine for 24 hours prior to the test.
Thallium/technetium stress test (myocardial imaging perfusion test, cardiac blood pool imaging)	*Thallium stress test:* Thallium-201, a radioisotope that accumulates in myocardial cells, is used during the stress test to evaluate myocardial perfusion. Second scans are done 2 to 3 hours later when the heart is at rest; this is to differentiate between an ischemic area and an infarcted or scarred area of myocardium. *Exercise technetium perfusion test:* Technetium 99m-laced compounds are administered and a scan is done to evaluate cardiac perfusion, wall motion, and ejection fraction. This is probably the most useful noninvasive test to diagnose and monitor CAD.	Assess medications; those that affect the BP or heart rate should be discontinued for 24 to 36 hours prior to the test (unless the test is being done to monitor the effectiveness of the medications). See treadmill test for other interventions.
Treadmill test (stress test)	Stress testing is based on the theory that coronary artery disease results in depression of the ST segment with exercise. Depression of the ST segment and depression or inversion of the T wave indicates myocardial ischemia. When the patient is walking on a treadmill machine, the work rate of the heart is changed every 3 minutes for 15 minutes by increasing the speed and degree of incline by 3% each time. Patients exercise until they are fatigued, develop symptoms, or reach their maximum predicted heart rate.	Ask the patient to wear comfortable shoes, and to avoid food, fluids, and smoking for 2 to 3 hours before the test. Assess for events that contraindicate the tests: recent myocardial infarction; severe, unstable angina; controlled dysrhythmias; congestive heart failure; or recent pulmonary embolism.

DIAGNOSTIC TESTS of the Cardiovascular and Lymphatic System (continued)

NAME OF TEST	PURPOSE & DESCRIPTION	RELATED NURSING INTERVENTIONS
Transesophageal echocardiography (TEE)	A TEE allows visualization of adjacent cardiac and extracardiac structures to identify or monitor mitral and aortic valve pathology, left atrium intracardiac thrombus, acute dissection of the aorta, endocarditis, perioperative left ventricular function, and intracardiac repairs during surgery. A transducer (probe) attached to an endoscope is inserted into the esophagus, and images are taken. Concurrent IV contrast medium, Doppler ultrasound, and color flow imaging may be used.	Instruct the patient to not eat or drink fluids for 4 hours before the test. Explain that a sedative will be given before the test. Take and record vital signs.

THE LYMPHATIC SYSTEM

NAME OF TEST	PURPOSE & DESCRIPTION	RELATED NURSING INTERVENTIONS
Abdominal or thoracic CT scan	A radiologic study used to assess the liver or spleen and enlarged lymph nodes in the mediastinum.	Tell the patient not to eat or drink for 4 hours before the test. Oral hypoglycemic agents should not be taken if iodionated contrast is used. Assess for allergy to iodine products and notify physician if so. Administer oral contrast as prescribed. Following the test, tell the patient to increase oral intake of fluids to help flush out the dye, and to report any allergic reactions to the dye (such as skin rash, headache, vomiting, or kidney dysfunction).
Lymph node biopsy	A lymph node biopsy is done to obtain tissue for histologic examination for diagnosis and treatment. It may be open (performed in the operating room) or closed (needle) by needle aspiration of tissue from a lymph node.	Use sterile technique when changing dressings.
Lymphangiography (lymphangiogram)	This is an x-ray examination of the lymphatic vessels and lymph nodes, used to assess metastasis of the lymph nodes, to identify malignant lymphoma, and to identify the cause of lymphedema. An iodine contrast substance is injected at various sites and fluoroscopy is used to visualize lymphatic filling.	Ask the patient about allergies to seafood, iodine, or contrast medium used in a previous x-ray test. Tell the patient that the blue contrast dye discolors the urine and possibly the skin for a few days. Take and record vital signs. Ask patient to void before the test. After the test, monitor for dyspnea, pain and hypotension; assess incision sites for manifestations of infection, and assess for leg edema. Elevate lower extremities as indicated.
Magnetic resonance imaging (MRI)—liver, spleen, lymph nodes	A radiologic study used to visualize the liver, spleen, and lymph nodes. It does not require injection of contrast medium.	Assess for any metallic implants (such as clips on brain aneurysms, pacemaker, body piercing, tattoos, and shrapnel). If present, notify physician. Remove transdermal medication patches (both OTC and prescribed) unless otherwise ordered (FDA, 2009). Replace the patch following the procedure. Tell the patient to inform the staff about the patch when making the appointment and when completing the admission information, Ask if patient is pregnant; if so the test is not performed. Ask about claustrophobia; if a problem exists, request patient ask the referring physician for a relaxing medication prior to the MRI. If the patient is very claustrophobic, obese, or confused, an open MRI may be used.

(continued)

GENETIC CONSIDERATIONS
Examples of Cardiovascular Disorders

- Familial hypercholesterolemia is a single gene disorder that results in atherosclerosis and CAD, which may occur at an earlier age than in the general population (i.e., before age 55 in men and age 65 in women). However, increased cholesterol levels may also be inherited and are a risk factor for CAD in both men and women.
- Marfan's syndrome is an autosomal-dominant inherited disorder that affects the skeleton, the eyes, and the cardiovascular system. The cardiovascular effects are a dilatation of the proximal aorta and aortic dissection associated with degeneration of the elastic fibers in the tunica media of the aorta. There may also be thoracic aortic aneurysms.
- Hypertrophic cardiomyopathy, a disease of sarcomere proteins, has a genetic transmission.
- Long QT syndrome (LQTS) is an inherited genetic disorder that results from structural abnormalities of the potassium channels in the heart, leading to dysrhythmias. This can result in unconsciousness, and may cause sudden cardiac death in teenagers and young adults when exposed to stressors ranging from exercise to loud sounds.
- Sickle cell anemia is the most common inherited blood disorder in the United States, affecting 1 in 500 people of African descent. It is characterized by episodes of pain, chronic hemolytic anemia, and severe infections.
- Gaucher disease, more common in descendants of Eastern European Jewish people, is an inherited illness caused by a gene mutation. The gene is responsible for an enzyme that breaks down a specific fat. When the fat is not broken down, it accumulates in the liver, spleen, and bone marrow, causing pain, fatigue, jaundice, bone damage, anemia, and even death.
- Hemophilia A is a hereditary blood disorder, primarily affecting males, characterized by a deficiency of the blood clotting factor named Factor VIII. Abnormal bleeding results.
- Chronic myeloid leukemia (CML), a cancer of blood cells, is characterized by replacement of bone marrow with malignant, leukemic cells. Leukemic cells also circulate in the blood, causing enlargement of the spleen, liver, and other organs. This leukemia is the result of chromosomal abnormality called the Philadelphia chromosome.
- Thalassemia, an inherited disease of faulty hemoglobin synthesis, is more often found in descendants of people living near the Mediterranean Sea, Africa, the Middle East, and Asia. It comprises a group of disorders that range from very mild blood abnormalities to severe or fatal anemia.

DIAGNOSTIC TESTS   of the Cardiovascular and Lymphatic System (continued)

THE HEMATOLOGIC SYSTEM

NAME OF TEST	PURPOSE & DESCRIPTION	RELATED NURSING INTERVENTIONS
Bone marrow examination	A bone marrow examination is conducted to evaluate blood-forming tissue; to diagnose multiple myeloma, leukemia, and some lymphomas; and to assess effectiveness of therapy for leukemia. Bone marrow specimens are obtained by either aspiration or biopsy. The preferred site for bone marrow aspiration is the posterior iliac crest; the sternum may also be used. The procedure is performed by inserting a needle into the bone and drawing out a sample of the blood in the marrow. A bone marrow biopsy is performed by making a small incision over the bone and screwing a core biopsy instrument into the bone to obtain a specimen. Bone marrow studies are used to diagnose leukemias, metastatic cancer, lymphoma, aplastic anemia, and Hodgkin's disease.	Explain that the procedure (either aspiration or biopsy) takes about 20 minutes, a sedative may be given prior to the procedure, and that it is important to remain very still during the procedure to prevent accidental injury. Tell the patient that although the area will be anesthetized with a local anesthetic, insertion of the needle will be painful for a short time. Taking deep breaths may make this part of the procedure less painful. The aspiration site may ache for 1 or 2 days. Take and record vital signs and ask the patient to void. If specimen is taken from the sternum or iliac crest place patient in the supine position; if the posterior iliac crest is used, place patient in the prone position. After the procedure apply pressure to the puncture site for 5 to 10 minutes. Apply a sterile dressing to the puncture site and monitor for bleeding for 24 hours.
Complete blood count (CBC)	This is a blood test that measures blood components. See Table 29–1.	None
Erythrocyte sedimentation rate (ESR)	This blood test is done as a measure of inflammation, and is increased in many illnesses, including cancer, heart disease, and kidney disease. **Normal values:** Women: 1–20 mm in 1 hour Men: 1–15 mm in 1 hour	None
Magnetic resonance angiography (MRA)	An MRA is used to visualize vascular occlusive disease and aneurysms of the abdominal aorta. The procedure is done by using a non-iodine-based contrast medium injected IV.	See MRI

BOX 29–1 Electrocardiogram

The electrocardiogram (ECG) is a graphic record of the heart's activity. Electrodes applied to the body surface are used to obtain a graphic representation of cardiac electrical activity. These electrodes detect the magnitude and direction of electrical currents produced in the heart. They attach to the electrocardiograph by an insulated wire called a lead. The electrocardiograph converts the electrical impulses it receives into a series of waveforms that represent cardiac depolarization and repolarization. Placement of electrodes on different parts of the body allows different views of this electrical activity, much like turning the head while holding a camera provides different views of the scenery. ECG waveforms and patterns are examined to detect dysrhythmias as well as myocardial damage, the effects of drugs, and electrolyte imbalances.

ECG waveforms reflect the direction of electrical flow in relation to a positive electrode. Current flowing toward the positive electrode produces an upward (positive) waveform; current flowing away from the positive electrode produces a downward (negative) waveform. Current flowing perpendicular to the positive pole produces a biphasic (both positive and negative) waveform. Absence of electrical activity is represented by a straight line called the isoelectric line.

ECG waveforms are recorded by a heated stylus on heat-sensitive paper. The paper is marked at standard intervals that represent time and voltage or amplitude (see Figure 1). Each small box is 1 mm². The recording speed of the standard ECG is 25 mm/second, so each small box represents 0.04 second. Five small boxes horizontally and vertically make one large box, equivalent to 0.20 second. Five large boxes represent 1 full second. Measured vertically, each small box represents 0.1 mV.

Both bipolar and unipolar leads are used in recording the ECG. A bipolar lead uses two electrodes of opposite polarity (negative and positive). In a *unipolar* lead, one positive electrode and a negative reference point at the center of the heart are used. The electrical potential between the two monitoring points is graphically recorded as the ECG waveform.

1 large box or 5 mm = 0.5 mV

1 large box or 5 mm = 0.20 Second

1 small box or 1 mm = 0.04 Second

1 mm = 0.1 mV

1) Time and voltage measurements on ECG paper at a recording speed of 25 mm/second.

The heart can be viewed from both the frontal plane and the horizontal plane (see Figure 2). Each plane provides a unique perspective of the heart muscle. The frontal plane is an imaginary cut through the body that views the heart from top to bottom (superior–inferior) and side to side (right–left). This perspective of the heart is analogous to a paper doll cutout. It provides information about the inferior and lateral walls of the heart. The horizontal plane is a cross-sectional view of the heart from front to back (anterior–posterior) and side to side (right–left). Information regarding the anterior, septal, and lateral walls of the heart, as well as the posterior wall, is obtained from this view.

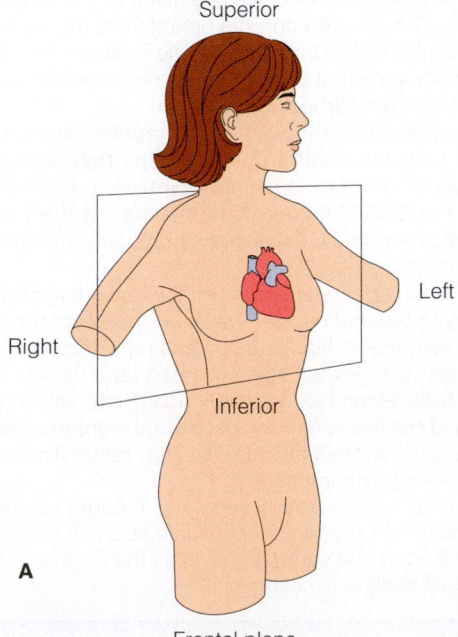

Superior

Right

Left

Inferior

A

Frontal plane

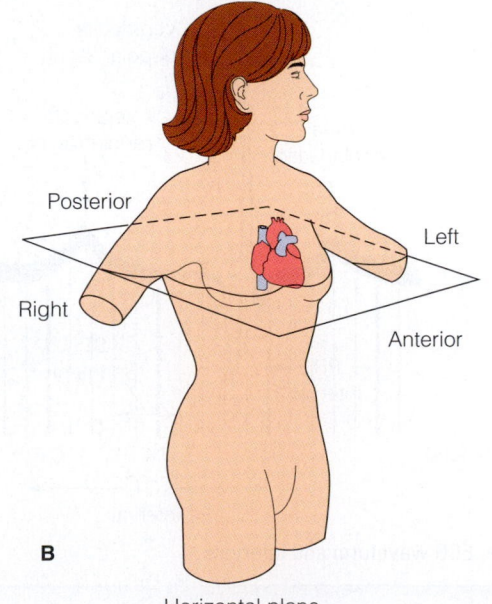

Posterior

Right

Left

Anterior

B

Horizontal plane

2) Planes of the heart. *A,* Frontal plane, *B,* horizontal plane.

(continued)

BOX 29–1 **Electrocardiogram** (continued)

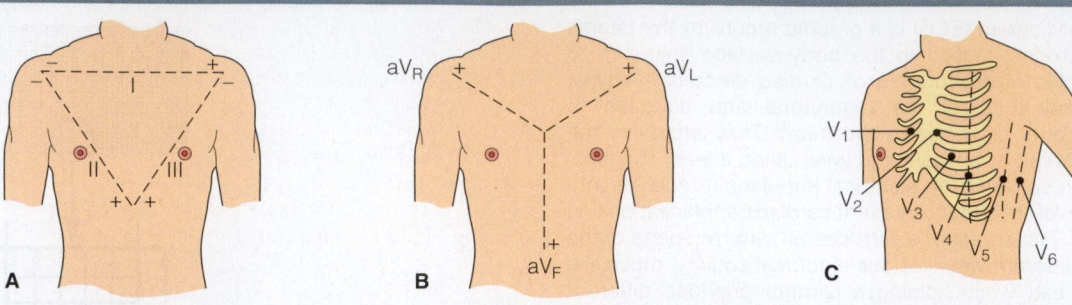

3) Leads of the 12-lead ECG. *A,* Bipolar limb leads I, II, III; *B,* Unipolar limb leads aV$_R$, aV$_L$, aV$_F$; *C,* Unipolar precordial leads V$_1$ to V$_6$.

A standard 12-lead ECG provides a simultaneous recording of six limb leads and six precordial leads (see Figure 3). The limb leads provide information about the heart in the frontal plane and include three bipolar leads (I, II, III) and three unipolar leads (aV$_R$, aV$_L$, and aV$_F$). The bipolar limb leads measure electrical activity between a negative lead on one extremity and a positive lead on another. The unipolar limb leads (called augmented leads) measure the electrical activity between a single positive electrode on a limb (right arm [R], left arm [L], or left leg [F for foot]), and the center of the heart.

The precordial leads, also known as chest leads or V leads, view the heart in the horizontal plane. They include six unipolar leads (V$_1$, V$_2$, V$_3$, V$_4$, V$_5$, and V$_6$), which measure electrical activity between the center of the heart and a positive electrode on the chest wall.

The cardiac cycle is depicted as a series of waveforms, the P, Q, R, S, and T waves (see Figure 4).

■ The *P wave* represents atrial depolarization and contraction. The impulse is from the sinus node. The P wave precedes the

QRS complex and is normally smooth, round, and upright. P waves may be absent when the SA node is not acting as the pacemaker. Atrial repolarization occurs during ventricular depolarization and usually is not seen on the ECG.

■ The *PR interval* represents the time required for the sinus impulse to travel to the AV node and into the Purkinje fibers. This interval is measured from beginning of P wave to beginning of QRS complex. If no Q wave is seen, the beginning of the R wave is used. The PR interval is normally 0.12 to 0.20 second (up to 0.24 second is considered normal in patients over age 65). PR intervals greater than 0.20 second indicate a delay in conduction from the SA node to the ventricles.

■ The *QRS complex* represents ventricular depolarization and contraction. The QRS complex includes three separate waves: The Q wave is the first negative deflection, the R wave is the positive or upright deflection, and the S wave is the first negative deflection after the R wave. Not all QRS complexes have all three waves; nonetheless, the complex is called a QRS complex. The normal duration of a QRS complex is from 0.06 to 0.10 second. QRS complexes greater than 0.10 second indicate delays in transmitting the impulse through the ventricular conduction system.

■ The *ST segment* signifies the beginning of ventricular repolarization. The ST segment, the period from the end of the QRS complex to the beginning of the T wave, should be isoelectric. An abnormal ST segment is displaced (elevated or depressed) from the isoelectric line.

■ The *T wave* represents ventricular repolarization. It normally has a smooth, rounded shape that is usually less than 10 mm tall. It usually points in the same direction as the QRS complex. Abnormalities of the T wave may indicate myocardial ischemia or injury, or electrolyte imbalances.

■ The *QT interval* is measured from the beginning of the QRS complex to the end of the T wave. It represents the total time of ventricular depolarization and repolarization. Its duration varies with gender, age, and heart rate; usually, it is 0.32 to 0.44 second long. Prolonged QT intervals indicate a prolonged relative refractory period and a greater risk of dysrhythmias. Shortened QT intervals may result from medications or electrolyte imbalances.

■ The *U wave* is not normally seen. It is thought to signify repolarization of the terminal Purkinje fibers. If present, the U wave follows the same direction as the T wave. It is most commonly seen in hypokalemia.

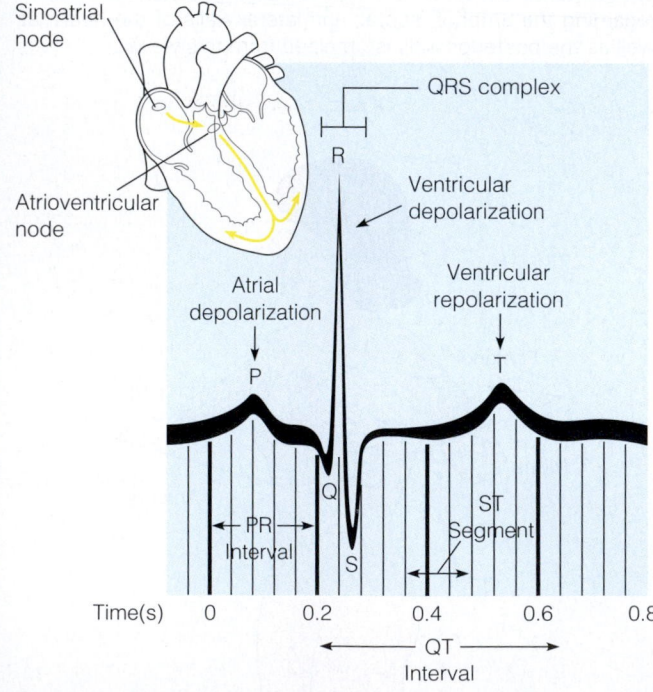

4) Normal ECG waveform and intervals.

BOX 29–2 Interpreting an ECG

Interpreting an ECG strip to determine the cardiac rhythm is a skill that takes practice to learn and master. Many methods are used to analyze ECGs. It is important to use a consistent method for ECG analysis. Identifying and interpreting complex dysrhythmias requires advanced skills and knowledge obtained through further education. One method follows:

- *Step 1: Determine rate.* Assess heart rate. Use P waves to determine the atrial rate and R waves for the ventricular rate. Several approaches can determine the heart rate.
- Count the number of complexes in a 6-second rhythm strip (the top margin of ECG paper is marked at 3-second intervals), and multiply by 10. This provides an estimate of the rate and is particularly valuable if rhythms are irregular.
- Count the number of large boxes between two consecutive complexes, and divide 0 (the number of large boxes in 1 minute) by this number. For example, there are 6 large boxes between two R waves; 0 divided by 6 equals a ventricular rate of 50 bpm. Memorize the following sequence for rapid rate determination: 0, 150, 100, 75, 60, 50, 43. One large box between complexes equals a rate of 0; two, a rate of 150; three, a rate of 100; and so on.
- Count the number of small boxes between two consecutive complexes, and divide 1500 (the number of small boxes in 1 minute) by this number. For example, there are 19 small boxes between two R waves; 1500 divided by 19 equals a ventricular rate of 79 bpm. This is the most precise measurement of heart rate.
- *Step 2: Determine regularity.* Regularity is the consistency with which the P waves or QRS complexes occur. In a regular rhythm, all waves occur at a consistent rate. Rhythm regularity is determined by measuring the interval between consecutive waves. Place one point of an ECG caliper (a measuring device) on the peak of the P wave (for atrial rhythm) or the R wave (for ventricular rhythm). Adjust the other point to the peak of the next wave, P to P or R to R. Keeping the calipers set at this distance, evaluate intervals between consecutive waves. The rhythm is *regular* if all caliper points fall on succeeding wave peaks. Alternately, use a strip of blank paper on top of the ECG strip, marking the peaks of two or three consecutive waves. Then move

the paper along the strip to consecutive waves. Wave peaks that vary by more than one to three small boxes (depending on the rate) are *irregular*. Irregular rhythms may be *irregularly irregular* (if the intervals have no pattern) or *regularly irregular* (if a consistent pattern to the irregularity can be identified).

- *Step 3: Assess P wave.* The presence or absence of P waves helps determine origin of the rhythm. All the P waves should be alike in size and shape (*morphology*). If P waves are not seen or they differ in shape, the rhythm may not originate in the sinus node.
- *Step 4: Assess P to QRS relationship.* Determine the relationship between P waves and QRS complexes. There should be one and only one P wave for every QRS complex, because the normal stimulus for ventricular contraction originates in the sinus node.
- *Step 5: Determine interval durations.* To evaluate impulse transmission through the cardiac conduction system, measure the PR interval, QRS duration, and QT interval. To measure, count the number of small boxes from the beginning of the interval to the end, and multiply by 0.04 second. Then determine whether the interval duration is within its normal limits. For example, the PR interval is 3.5 small boxes wide, or 0.14 second. This is within the normal limits of 0.12 to 0.20 second. This interval should be consistent, not varying from beat to beat. A PR interval greater than 0.20 second or one that varies from beat to beat is abnormal.

  The QRS complex duration is normally between 0.06 and 0.10 second. A QRS complex greater than 0.12 second indicates delayed ventricular conduction.

  The QT interval is normally 0.32 to 0.44 second. It varies inversely with the heart rate: The faster the heart rate, the shorter the QT interval. As a general rule, the QT interval should be no more than half the previous R–R interval. A prolonged QT interval indicates a prolonged relative refractory period of the heart.

- *Step 6: Identify abnormalities.* Note the presence and frequency of *ectopic* (extra) beats, deviation of the ST segment above or below the baseline, and abnormalities in waveform shape and duration.

---

aggravating and relieving factors, and associated symptoms (Table 29–3 ■).

Explore the patient's medical history for any cardiovascular disorders such as angina, heart attack, congestive heart failure (CHF), stroke, hypertension (HTN), peripheral vascular disease (PVD), or other chronic illnesses (such as diabetes or bleeding disorders). Ask the patient about previous heart surgery or illnesses, such as rheumatic fever, scarlet fever, or recurrent streptococcal throat infections, and radiation treatment for breast cancer. Review the patient's family history for CAD, HTN, stroke, hyperlipidemia, diabetes, congenital heart disease, or sudden death.

Ask the patient about past or present occurrence of cardiovascular symptoms, such as chest pain, shortness of breath, difficulty breathing, cough, palpitations, fatigue, light-headedness or dizziness, fainting, heart murmur, blood clots, leg cramps or swelling, changes in skin color or temperature, varicose veins, or edema. Because cardiovascular function affects all other body systems, a full history may need to explore other related systems, such as respiratory function. Ask about past or present bleeding (from the nose, gums or mouth, or rectum) as well as associated symptoms (such as pallor, dizziness, fatigue), lymph node changes (swelling, pain, heat), swelling of extremities, and recurrent infections.

Review the patient's personal habits and nutritional history, including body weight; eating patterns; dietary intake of fats, salt, fluids; dietary restrictions; hypersensitivities or intolerances to food or medication; and the use of caffeine and alcohol. If the patient uses tobacco products, ask about type (cigarettes, pipe, cigars, snuff), duration, amount, and efforts to quit. If the patient uses street drugs, ask about type, method of intake (e.g., inhaled or injected), duration of use, and efforts to quit. Include questions about the patient's activity level and tolerance, recreational activities, and relaxation habits. Assess the patient's sleep patterns for interruptions in sleep due to dyspnea, cough, discomfort, urination, or stress. Ask how many pillows the patient uses when sleeping.

It is important to consider socioeconomic factors that may precipitate or aggravate circulatory problems, such as inadequate clothing, shoes, or shelter; and occupational levels such as prolonged sitting or standing, exposure to radiation or extremes of temperature. Lifestyle, including intravenous drug use or sexual practices may be significant in determining the risk for diseases associated with bleeding and impaired lymphatic function.

Interview questions categorized by functional health patterns are listed in the table on page 895.

TABLE 29–3 Assessing Chest Pain

CHARACTERISTIC	EXAMPLES
Location	Substernal, precordial, jaw, back
	Localized or diffuse
	Radiation to neck, jaw, shoulder, arm
Character/quality	Pressure; tightness; crushing, burning, or aching quality; heaviness; dullness; "heartburn" or indigestion
Timing: onset, duration, and frequency	Onset: Sudden or gradual?
	Duration: How many minutes does the pain last?
	Frequency: Is the pain continuous or periodic?
Setting/precipitating factors	Awake, at rest, sleep interrupted?
	With activity? With eating, exertion, exercise, elimination, emotional upset?
Intensity/severity	Can range from 0 (no pain) to 10 (worst pain ever felt)
Aggravating factors	Activity, breathing, temperature
Relieving factors	Medication (nitroglycerin, antacid), rest; there may be no relieving factors
Associated symptoms	Fatigue, shortness of breath, palpitations, nausea and vomiting, sweating, anxiety, light-headedness or dizziness

Physical Assessment

Physical assessment of cardiovascular function may be performed either as part of a total assessment or alone for patients with suspected or known problems with heart, peripheral vascular, lymphatic, or hematologic function. The patient may sit or lie in the supine position. Before beginning the assessment, collect all required equipment and explain the techniques to the patient to decrease anxiety.

Assess the heart through inspection, palpation, and auscultation over the precordium (the area of the chest wall overlying the heart) (see Figure 29–20 ■). Movements over the precordium may be more easily seen with tangential lighting (in which the light is directed at a right angle to the area being observed, producing shadows). A quiet environment is essential to hear and assess heart sounds accurately. Assess the heart and thorax for the following:

- The **apical impulse** is a normal, visible pulsation (**thrust**) in the area of the midclavicular line in the left fifth intercostal space. It can be seen on inspection in about half of the adult population. (The apical impulse was previously called the point of maximal impulse [PMI] but this is no longer used because a maximal impulse may occur in other areas of the precordium as a result of abnormal conditions.)
- **Retraction** is a pulling in of the tissue of the precordium; a slight retraction just medial to the midclavicular line at the area of the apical impulse is normal and is more likely to be visible in thin patients.
- Pulsations (other than the normal apical pulsations), which may be called **heaves** or **lifts**, are considered abnormal. They may occur as the result of an enlarged ventricle.

The techniques used to assess the peripheral vascular and lymphatic systems include inspecting the skin for such changes as edema, ulcerations, or alterations in color and temperature; auscultating BP; and palpating the major pulse points of the body (Figure 29–21 ■) and lymph nodes. The patient may be

Figure 29–20 ■ Areas for inspection and palpation of the precordium, indicating the sequence for palpation.

Labels: RSB, 2nd ICS; LSB, 2nd ICS; LSB, 3rd ICS; LSB, 4th ICS; MCL, 5th ICS

Figure 29–21 ■ Body sites at which peripheral pulses are most easily palpated.

Labels: Temporal, Carotid, Apical, Brachial, Radial, Femoral, Popliteal, Posterior tibial, Dorsalis pedis

FUNCTIONAL HEALTH PATTERN INTERVIEW   The Cardiovascular and Lymphatic Systems

Functional Health Pattern	Interview Questions and Leading Statements
Health Perception-Health Management	■ Have you ever had any problems with your heart, blood vessels, lymph glands, or blood? If so, describe. What was used to treat these problems? ■ Have you been diagnosed with high blood pressure? If so, how is it treated? ■ Do you have a history of diabetes, rheumatic fever, scarlet fever, or strep throat infections? If so, describe them and their treatment. ■ Have you had your cholesterol checked recently? What is it? If you have high cholesterol, how is it treated? ■ Describe any problems you have with chest pain, fatigue, bleeding, bruising, swollen glands, or circulation. ■ Do you take any medications to make your heart function more effectively, such as aspirin, those to control your heart rate, anticoagulants, or diuretics? How often do you take them? ■ Do you have a pacemaker? At what age did you get it and for what problem? How do you check the batteries? ■ Do you smoke, chew tobacco, or use snuff? If so, how often and how much? ■ Do you drink alcohol? If so, what type, how much, and for how long? ■ Are you able to manage your activities of daily living and work independently? Explain.
Nutritional-Metabolic	■ Describe your food and liquid intake in a 24-hour period. How often do you eat fried foods, fast foods, or red meat? ■ How much salt do you use on food? ■ Do you eat high-fiber foods? If so, what are they and how often? ■ Have you had a recent weight gain or loss? Explain. ■ Have you noticed any change in color of your skin; for example, pale or dusky or flushed? If so, do you know what causes this? ■ Have you had any swelling in your feet or legs? Where and how much? What do you do to relieve it? ■ Have you noticed any loss of hair or sores on your legs? Are your toenails thick? Have you ever worn support stockings?
Elimination	■ Has a heart problem interfered with your usual bowel and bladder elimination? Explain.
Activity-Exercise	■ Describe your usual activity in a 24-hour period. Do you exercise regularly? If so, how often and how long? ■ Has there been any change in your ability, energy, or strength to perform your usual activities (such as bathing, cleaning house, yard work, shopping)? If so, explain. ■ Do you ever have to stop and rest while doing daily activities? Explain. Have you ever had leg pain when you walk? If so, how far can you walk before the pain begins? ■ Do you notice shortness of breath with certain activities? If so, what are they? How long does this last? What do you do to breathe better? ■ Describe any cough you have had. Was it dry or wet? Do you cough up mucus? If so, what color is it? How long have you had the cough? ■ Have you experienced any numbness or tingling, dizziness or light-headedness, or palpitations? Describe if so. ■ Have you ever used oxygen?
Sleep-Rest	■ How long do you sleep each night? Do you feel rested after you sleep? ■ Does your heart problem interfere with your ability to sleep and rest? Explain. ■ How many pillows do you use at night? ■ Where do you sleep at night (e.g., in a recliner to breathe more easily)? ■ Do you ever feel short of breath while you are resting or sleeping? Does this wake you up if so? Explain.
Cognitive-Perceptual	■ Describe any chest pain you have experienced. When did it occur? Where was it located? On a scale of 0 to 10, with 10 being the worst pain you have ever had, rate the pain and describe it (for example, burning, crushing, stabbing, squeezing, heavy, tight). ■ What were you doing when the pain began; for example, were you working or resting? Did it begin suddenly or gradually? How long did it last? ■ Did you have any other symptoms with the pain, such as nausea or vomiting, sweating, racing heart, pale skin, palpitations? ■ Do you have any of these sensations in your legs or feet: pain, cramps, burning, tingling, numbness? If so, when do they occur and what do you to relieve them?
Self-Perception-Self-Concept	■ How does having this condition make you feel about yourself?
Role-Relationships	■ How does this condition affect your relationships with others? ■ Has having this condition interfered with your ability to work? Explain.
Sexuality-Reproductive	■ Has this condition interfered with your usual sexual activity? ■ Have you ever had chest pain during sexual activity? What do you do for it? ■ Do you use a slower pace or different positions that are less stressful for you during sexual activities? Does this help?

(continued)

FUNCTIONAL HEALTH PATTERN INTERVIEW   The Cardiovascular and Lymphatic Systems (continued)

Functional Health Pattern	Interview Questions and Leading Statements
Coping-Stress-Tolerance	■ Has having this condition created stress for you? ■ Have you experienced any kind of stress that makes this condition worse? Explain. ■ Describe what you do when you feel stressed.
Value-Belief	■ Describe how specific relationships or activities help you cope with this problem. ■ Describe specific cultural beliefs or practices that affect how you care for and feel about this problem. ■ Is there anything interfering with your spiritual beliefs, needs, or practices during your illness? What can I or another caregiver do to help you with your spiritual needs? ■ Are there any specific treatments that you would not use to treat this problem?

NURSING CARE OF THE OLDER ADULT   Age-Related Cardiovascular Changes

AGE-RELATED CHANGE	SIGNIFICANCE
Myocardium: � efficiency and contractibility.	■ Decreased CO when under physiologic stress with resulting tachycardia that lasts longer. The person may require rest time between physical activities.

AGE-RELATED CHANGE

Myocardium: ➜ efficiency and contractibility.

Sinus node: ➜ in thickness of shell surrounding the node, and a ➜ in the number of pacemaker cells.

Left ventricle: Slight hypertrophy, prolonged isometric contraction phase and relaxation time; ➜ time for diastolic filling and systolic emptying cycle.

Valves and blood vessels: Aorta is elongated and dilated, valves are thicker and more rigid, and resistance to peripheral blood flow increases by 1% per year.

Bone marrow: ➜ ability of bone marrow to respond to need for increased RBCs, WBCs, and platelets.

Blood vessels:

Tunica intima: fibrosis, calcium and lipid accumulation, cellular proliferation.

Tunica media: thins, elastin fibers calcify; increase in calcium results in stiffening. Baroreceptor function is impaired and peripheral resistance increases.

Immune system

Impaired function of B and T lymphocytes.

➜ production of antibodies.

SIGNIFICANCE

■ Decreased CO when under physiologic stress with resulting tachycardia that lasts longer. The person may require rest time between physical activities.

■ Stroke volume may increase to compensate for tachycardia, leading to increased BP.

■ BP increases to compensate for increased peripheral resistance and decreased CO.

■ Anemia may result.

■ As a result of age-related changes, the systolic BP rises. Decreased arterial elasticity results in vascular changes in the heart, kidneys, and pituitary gland. Decreased baroreceptor function results in postural hypotension. Vessels in the head, neck, and extremities are more prominent.

■ Inefficient vasoconstriction, decreased CO, and reduced muscle mass and subcutaneous tissue lead to a reduced ability to respond to cold temperatures.

■ With a decrease in BP and changes in blood vessel walls, tissue perfusion may be inadequate, leading to edema, inflammation, pressure ulcers, and changes in effects of medications.

■ Increased risk for infection, with decreased manifestations of an actual infection.

■ Increased incidence of cancers.

assessed in the supine, sitting, and standing positions. Physical assessment of the lymphatic system, using inspection and palpation, is usually integrated into the assessment of other body systems. For example, the tonsils are inspected with the pharynx during the head and neck assessment; the regional lymph nodes are evaluated with corresponding body regions (e.g., occipital, auricular, and cervical nodes are evaluated with assessment of the head and neck, axillary nodes with assessment of the breast or thorax, epitrochlear node with assessment of the peripheral vascular exam of the arms, and inguinal nodes with assessment of the abdomen); and the spleen can be palpated during the abdominal assessment. Normal age-related findings for the older adult are summarized in the Nursing Care of the Older Adult box.

Cardiovascular Assessments

Technique/Normal Findings	Abnormal Findings

Apical Impulse Assessment

First using the palmar surface and then repeating with finger pads, palpate the precordium for symmetry of movement and the apical impulse for location, size, amplitude, and duration. The sequence for palpation is shown in Figure 29–20. To locate the apical impulse, ask the patient to assume a left lateral recumbent position. Simultaneous palpation of the carotid pulse may also be helpful. *The apical impulse is not palpable in all patients. The apical impulse may be palpated in the mitral area, and has only a brief small amplitude.*

- An enlarged or displaced heart is associated with an apical impulse lateral to the midclavicular line (MCL) or below the fifth left intercostal space (ICS).
- Increased size, amplitude, and duration of the apical impulse are associated with left ventricular volume overload (increased afterload) in conditions such as HTN and aortic stenosis, and with pressure overload (increased preload) in conditions such as aortic or mitral regurgitation.
- Increased amplitude alone may occur with hyperkinetic states, such as anxiety, hyperthyroidism, and anemia.
- Decreased amplitude is associated with a dilated heart in cardiomyopathy.
- Displacement alone may also occur with dextrocardia, diaphragmatic hernia, gastric distention, or chronic lung disease.
- A **thrill** (a palpable vibration over the precordium or an artery) may accompany severe valve stenosis.
- A marked increase in amplitude of the apical impulse at the right ventricular area occurs with right ventricular volume overload in atrial septal defect.
- An increase in amplitude and duration occurs with right ventricular pressure overload in pulmonic stenosis and pulmonary hypertension. A lift or heave may also be seen in these conditions (and in chronic lung disease).
- A palpable thrill in this area occurs with ventricular septal defect.

Palpate the subxiphoid area with the index and middle finger. *No pulsations or vibrations should be palpated.*

- Right ventricular enlargement may produce a downward pulsation against the fingertips.
- An accentuated pulsation at the pulmonary area may be present in hyperkinetic states.
- A prominent pulsation reflects increased flow or dilation of the pulmonary artery.
- A thrill may be associated with aortic or pulmonary stenosis, aortic stenosis, pulmonary HTN, or atrial septal defect.
- Increased pulsation at the aortic area may suggest aortic aneurysm.
- A palpable second heart sound (S_2) may be noted with systemic HTN.

Cardiac Rate and Rhythm Assessment

Auscultate heart rate (Figure 29–22 ■). *The heart rate should be 60 to 100 beats per minute with regular rhythm.*

- A heart rate exceeding 100 beats per minute (beats/min) is tachycardia. A heart rate less than 60 beats/min is bradycardia.

Figure 29–22 ■ Areas for auscultation of the heart.

Simultaneously palpate the radial pulse while listening to the apical pulse. *The radial and apical pulses should be equal.*

- If the radial pulse falls behind the apical rate, the patient has a pulse deficit, indicating weak, ineffective contractions of the left ventricle.

Auscultate heart rhythm. *The heart rhythm should be regular.*

- **Dysrhythmias** (abnormal heart rate or rhythm) may be regular or irregular in rhythm; their rates may be slow or fast. Irregular rhythms may occur in a pattern (e.g., an early beat every second beat, called bigeminy), sporadically, or with frequency and disorganization (e.g., atrial fibrillation). A pattern of gradual increase and decrease in heart rate that is within normal heart rate and that correlates with inspiration and expiration is called sinus arrhythmia.

Technique/Normal Findings	Abnormal Findings

Heart Sounds Assessment
See guidelines for cardiac auscultation in Box 29–3.

BOX 29–3 Guidelines for Cardiac Auscultation

1. Locate the major auscultatory areas on the precordium (see Figure 29–22).
2. Choose a sequence of listening. Either begin from the apex and move upward along the sternal border to the base, or begin at the base and move downward to the apex. One suggested sequence is shown in Figure 29–22.
3. Listen first with the patient in the sitting or supine position. Then ask the patient to lie on the left side, and focus on the apex. Lastly, ask the patient to sit up and lean forward. These position changes bring the heart closer to the chest wall and enhance auscultation. Carry out the following steps when the patient assumes each of these positions:
   a. First, auscultate each area with the diaphragm of the stethoscope to listen for high-pitched sounds: S_1, S_2, murmurs, pericardial friction rubs.
   b. Next, auscultate each area with the bell of the stethoscope to listen for lower pitched sounds: S_3, S_4, murmurs.
   c. Listen for the effect of respirations on each sound; while the patient is sitting up and leaning forward, ask him or her to exhale and hold the breath while you listen to heart sounds.

Identify S_1 (first heart sound) and note its intensity. At each auscultatory area, listen for several cardiac cycles. *S_1 is loudest at the apex of the heart.*

- An accentuated S_1 occurs with tachycardia, states in which CO is high (fever, anxiety, exercise, anemia, hyperthyroidism), complete heart block, and mitral stenosis.
- A diminished S_1 occurs with first-degree heart block, mitral regurgitation, CHF, CAD, and pulmonary or systemic HTN. The intensity is also decreased with obesity, emphysema, and pericardial effusion. Varying intensity of S_1 occurs with complete heart block and grossly irregular rhythms.

Listen for splitting of S_1. *Splitting of S_1 may occur during inspiration.*

- Abnormal splitting of S_1 may be heard with right bundle branch block and premature ventricular contractions.

Identify S_2 (second heart sound) and note its intensity. *S_2 immediately follows S_1 and is loudest at the base of the heart.*

- An accentuated S_2 may be heard with HTN, exercise, excitement, and conditions of pulmonary HTN such as CHF and cor pulmonale.
- A diminished S_2 occurs with aortic stenosis, a fall in systolic BP (shock), and increased anteroposterior chest diameter.

Listen for splitting of S_2. *No splitting of S_2 should be heard.*

- Wide splitting of S_2 is associated with delayed emptying of the right ventricle, resulting in delayed pulmonary valve closure (e.g., mitral regurgitation, pulmonary stenosis, and right bundle branch block).
- Fixed splitting occurs when right ventricular output is greater than left ventricular output and pulmonary valve closure is delayed (e.g., with atrial septal defect and right ventricular failure).
- Paradoxical splitting occurs when closure of the aortic valve is delayed (e.g., left bundle branch block).

Identify extra heart sounds in systole. *Extra heart sounds are not present in systole.*

- Ejection sounds (or clicks) result from the opening of deformed semilunar valves (e.g., aortic and pulmonary stenosis).
- A midsystolic click is heard with mitral valve prolapse (MVP).

Identify the presence of extra heart sounds in diastole. *Extra heart sounds are not present in diastole.*

- An opening snap results from the opening sound of a stenotic mitral valve.
- A pathologic S_3 (a third heart sound that immediately follows S_2, called a ventricular gallop) results from myocardial failure and ventricular volume overload (e.g., CHF, mitral or tricuspid regurgitation).
- An S_4 (a fourth heart sound that immediately precedes S_1, called an atrial gallop) results from increased resistance to ventricular filling after atrial contraction (e.g., HTN, CAD, aortic stenosis, and cardiomyopathy).
- A combined S_3 and S_4 is called a summation gallop and occurs with severe CHF.
- A pericardial friction rub results from inflammation of the pericardial sac, as with pericarditis.

Technique/Normal Findings	Abnormal Findings

Murmur Assessment

Identify any murmurs. Note location, timing, presence during systole or diastole, and intensity. Use the following scale to grade murmurs:

I = Barely heard

II = Quietly heard

III = Clearly heard

IV = Loud

V = Very loud

VI = Loudest; may be heard with stethoscope off the chest. A thrill may accompany murmurs of grade IV to grade VI.

Note pitch (low, medium, high), and quality (harsh, blowing, or musical). Note pattern/shape, crescendo, decrescendo, and radiation/transmission (to axilla, neck). *No murmurs should be heard.*

- Midsystolic murmurs are heard with semilunar valve disease (e.g., aortic and pulmonary stenosis) and with hypertrophic cardiomyopathy.
- Pansystolic (holosystolic) murmurs are heard with AV valve disease (e.g., mitral and tricuspid regurgitation, ventricular septal defect).
- A late systolic murmur is heard with MVP.
- Early diastolic murmurs occur with regurgitant flow across incompetent semilunar valves (e.g., aortic regurgitation).
- Middiastolic and presystolic murmurs, such as with mitral stenosis, occur with turbulent flow across the AV valves.
- Continuous murmurs throughout systole and all or part of diastole occur with patent ductus arteriosus.

Blood Pressure and Pulse Pressure Assessment

See Box 29–4 for blood pressure measurement guidelines.

BOX 29–4 Guidelines for Blood Pressure Assessment

Review of Korotkoff's Sounds

The first sound heard is the systolic pressure; at least two consecutive sounds should be clear. If the sound disappears and then is heard again 10 to 15 mm later, an auscultatory gap is present; this may be a normal variant, or it may be associated with hypertension. The first diastolic sound is heard as a muffling of the Korotkoff's sound and is considered the best approximation of the true diastolic pressure. The second diastolic sound is the level at which sounds are no longer heard.

The American Heart Association recommends documenting all three readings when measuring BP, for example, 120/72/64. If only two readings are documented, the systolic and the second diastolic pressure are taken, for example, 120/64.

Technique Reminders

- Choose a cuff of an appropriate size: The cuff should snugly cover two-thirds of the upper arm, and the bladder should completely encircle the arm. The bladder should be centered over the brachial artery, with the lower edge 2 to 3 cm above the antecubital space.
- The patient's arm should be slightly flexed and supported (on a table or by the examiner) at heart level.
- To determine how high to inflate the cuff, palpate the brachial pulse, and inflate the cuff to the point on the manometer at which the pulse is no longer felt; then, add 30 mmHg to this reading, and use the sum as the target for inflation. Wait 15 seconds before reinflating the cuff to auscultate the BP.
- To recheck a BP, wait at least 30 seconds before attempting another inflation.
- Always inflate the cuff completely, and then deflate it. Once deflation begins, allow it to continue; do not try to reinflate the cuff if the first systolic sound is not heard or if the cuff inadvertently deflates.
- The bell of the stethoscope more effectively transmits the low-pitched sounds of BP.

Sources of Error

- Falsely high readings can occur if the cuff is too small, too loose, or if the patient supports his or her own arm.
- Falsely low readings can occur if a standard cuff is used on a patient with thin arms.

- Inadequate inflation may result in underestimation of the systolic pressure or overestimation of the diastolic pressure if an auscultatory gap is present.
- Rapid deflation and repeated or slow inflations (causing venous congestion) can lead to underestimation of the systolic BP and overestimation of the diastolic BP.

Factors Altering Blood Pressure

- A change from the horizontal to upright position causes a slight decrease (5 to 10 mm) in systolic BP; the diastolic BP remains unchanged or rises slightly.
- BP taken in the arm is lower when the patient is standing.
- If the BP is taken with the patient in the lateral recumbent position, a lower BP reading may be obtained in both arms; this is especially apparent in the right arm with the patient in the left lateral position.
- Factors that increase BP include exercise, caffeine, cold environment, eating a large meal, painful stimuli, and emotions.
- Factors that lower BP include sleep (by 20 mmHg) and very fast, slow, or irregular heart rates.
- BP tends to be higher in taller or heavier patients.

Alternative Methods of Blood Pressure Measurement

- The palpatory method may be necessary if severe hypotension is present and the BP is inaudible. Palpate the brachial pulse, and inflate the cuff 30 mm above the point where the pulse disappears; deflate the cuff, and note the point on the manometer where the pulse becomes palpable again. Record this as the palpatory systolic BP.
- Leg BP measurement may be needed when there is injury of the arms or to rule out coarctation of the aorta or aortic insufficiency when arm diastolic BP is over 90 mmHg. Place the patient in the prone or supine position with the leg slightly flexed. Place a large leg cuff on the thigh with the bladder centered over the popliteal artery. Place the bell of the stethoscope over the popliteal space. Normal leg systolic BP is higher than arm BP; diastolic BP should be equal to or lower than arm BP. Abnormally low leg BP occurs with aortic insufficiency and coarctation of the aorta.

Technique/Normal Findings	Abnormal Findings
Auscultate BP in each arm with the patient seated. *The normal BP is considered to be < 120/< 80*	■ Consistent BP readings over 140/90 in adults under age 40 is considered hypertension. ■ BP under 90/60 is considered hypotension. ■ An auscultatory gap—a temporary disappearance of sound between the systolic and diastolic BP—may be a normal variation, or it may be associated with systolic HTN or a drop in diastolic BP due to aortic stenosis. ■ **Korotkoff's sounds** (see Box 29–4) may be heard down to zero with cardiac valve replacements, hyperkinetic states, thyrotoxicosis, and severe anemia, as well as after vigorous exercise. ■ The sounds of aortic regurgitation may obscure the diastolic BP. ■ A difference of over 10 mmHg between arms suggests arterial compression on the side of the lower reading, aortic dissection, or coarctation of the aorta.
Auscultate BP in each arm with the patient standing. If orthostatic changes occur, measure the BP with the patient supine, legs dangling, and again with the patient standing, 1 to 3 minutes apart. *A decrease of systolic BP is expected, but should be < 10 mmHg; diastolic BP should not drop on standing.* Observe the pulse pressure. The pulse pressure is the difference between the systolic and diastolic BP. For example, if the BP is 140/80, the pulse pressure is 60. *A normal pulse pressure is one-third the systolic measurement.*	■ A decrease in systolic BP of over 10 to 15 mmHg and a drop in diastolic BP on standing are called **orthostatic hypotension**. Causes include antihypertensive medications, volume depletion, PVD, prolonged bed rest, and aging. ■ A widened pulse pressure with an elevated systolic BP occurs with exercise, arteriosclerosis, severe anemia, thyrotoxicosis, and increased intracranial pressure. ■ A narrowed pulse pressure with a decreased systolic BP occurs with shock, cardiac failure, and pulmonary embolus. **PRACTICE ALERT** If unable to auscultate BP or palpate pulses, a Doppler ultrasound device may be used to evaluate blood flow. Apply a dime-sized amount of gel over the blood vessel to be assessed and lightly place the probe over the gel. Listen for a whooshing (artery) or rushing (vein) sound.
Skin Assessment	
Inspect the color of the skin. *The skin color should be appropriate to the patient's age and race.*	■ Pallor reflects constriction of peripheral blood flow (e.g., due to syncope or shock) or decreased circulating oxyhemoglobin (e.g., due to hemorrhage or anemia). ■ Central cyanosis of the lips, earlobes, oral mucosa, and tongue suggests chronic cardiopulmonary disease. (See Box 29–5 for abnormal findings associated with peripheral vascular and lymphatic assessment.)

BOX 29–5 Abnormal Findings Associated with Peripheral Vascular and Lymphatic Assessment

■ *Pallor* is an absence of color of the skin. The degree of pallor depends on the patient's normal skin color and health status. Dark skin may appear ashen or have a yellowish tinge.
■ *Cyanosis* is a bluish discoloration of the skin and mucous membranes in people with light skin. In people with dark skin, cyanosis may be difficult to observe. Inspect the nail beds and conjunctiva.
■ *Edema* is an abnormal accumulation of fluid in the interstitial spaces of body tissues. It is often most apparent in the lower extremities.
■ *Varicose veins* are tortuous and dilated veins that have incompetent valves. The saphenous veins of the legs are most commonly affected.
■ *Enlarged lymph nodes* result from infection or malignancy.

■ *Atrophic changes* are changes in size or activity of body tissues as the result of pathology or injury. Decreased blood flow and oxygenation of the lower extremities often cause atrophic changes of loss of hair, thickened toe nails, changes in pigmentation, and ulcerations.
■ *Gangrene* is the necrosis (or death) of tissue, most often the result of loss of blood supply and infection. Gangrene often begins in the most distal of the tissues of the extremities.
■ *Pressure ulcers*, also called decubitus ulcers or bed sores, are the result of ischemia and hypoxia of tissue following prolonged pressure. These ulcers often are located over bony prominences. If untreated, the tissue changes proceed from red skin to deep, crater-like ulcers.

Inspect the skin of the extremities and over the regional lymph nodes, noting any edema, erythema, red streaks, or skin lesions. *There should be no edema, redness, or lesions over the regional lymph nodes.*	■ Lymphangitis (inflammation of a lymphatic vessel) may produce a red streak with induration (hardness) following the course of the lymphatic collecting duct; infected skin lesions may be present, particularly between the digits. ■ **Lymphedema** (swelling due to lymphatic obstruction) occurs with congenital lymphatic anomaly (Milroy's disease) or with trauma to the regional lymphatic ducts from surgery or metastasis (e.g., arm lymphedema after radical mastectomy with axillary node removal). ■ Edema of lymphatic origin is usually not pitting, and the skin may be thickened; one example is the taut swelling of the face and body that occurs with myxedema, associated with hypothyroidism.

Technique/Normal Findings	**Abnormal Findings**

Artery and Vein Assessment

Palpate the temporal arteries. *There should be no redness, swelling, nodules, or variations in pulse amplitude.*

■ Redness, swelling, nodularity, and variations in pulse amplitude may occur with temporal arteritis.

Inspect and palpate the carotid arteries. Note symmetry, the pulse rate, rhythm, volume, and amplitude. *Note any variation with respiration. Describe all pulses as increased, normal, diminished, or absent. Scales ranging from 0 to 4+ are sometimes used as follows:*

0 = Absent
1+ = Diminished
2+ = Normal
3+ = Increased
4+ = Bounding

Pulse waveforms are shown in Box 29–6. *The carotid pulses should be bilaterally equal in rate, rhythm, volume, and amplitude.*

BOX 29–6   Types of Pulse Patterns

A Normal pulse

B Hypokinetic (weak) pulse

C Hyperkinetic (bounding) pulse

D Bigeminal pulse

E Pulsus alternans

F Waterhammer (collapsing) pulse

G Pulsus bisferiens

■ A unilateral pulsating bulge is seen with a tortuous or kinked carotid artery.

■ Alterations in pulse rate or rhythm are due to cardiac dysrhythmias.

■ An absent pulse indicates arterial occlusion.

■ A hypokinetic (weak) pulse is associated with decreased stroke volume (Box 29–6 *B*). This may be due to congestive heart failure (CHF), aortic stenosis, or hypovolemia; to increased peripheral resistance, which may result from cold temperatures; or to arterial narrowing, commonly found with atherosclerosis.

■ A hyperkinetic (bounding) pulse occurs with increased stroke volume and/or decreased peripheral resistance (Box 29–6 *C*). This may result from states in which CO is high or from aortic regurgitation. It also may occur with anemia, hyperthyroidism, bradycardia, or reduced compliance, as with atherosclerosis.

■ A bigeminal pulse is marked by decreased amplitude of every second beat (Box 29–6 *D*). This may be due to premature contractions (usually ventricular).

■ Pulsus alternans is a regular pulse with alternating strong and weak beats (Box 29–6 *E*). This may be due to left ventricular failure and severe HTN.

Auscultate the carotid arteries, using the bell of the stethoscope. *No bruits should be heard.*

■ A murmuring or blowing sound heard over stenosed peripheral vessels is known as a *bruit*. A bruit heard over the middle to upper carotid artery suggests atherosclerosis.

Inspect and palpate the internal and external jugular veins for venous pressure. *See Box 29–7 for guidelines for assessing jugular venous pressure (JVP).*

■ An increase in jugular venous pressure (JVP) over 3 cm and located above the sternal angle reflects increased right atrial pressure. This occurs with right ventricular failure or, less commonly, with constrictive pericarditis, tricuspid stenosis, and superior venae cavae obstruction.

Technique/Normal Findings	Abnormal Findings
If venous pressure is elevated, assess the hepatojugular reflex. (Compress the liver in the right upper abdominal quadrant with the palm of the hand for 30 to 60 seconds while observing the jugular veins.)	■ A decrease in venous pressure reflects reduced left ventricular output or blood volume. ■ Unilateral neck vein distention suggests local compression or anatomic anomaly. ■ A rise in the column of neck vein distention over 1 cm with liver compression indicates right heart failure.

Upper Extremity Assessment

Inspect and palpate the arms and hands, noting size and symmetry, skin color, and temperature. *Arms and hands should be symmetrical in size and shape, warm, and of appropriate skin color.*	■ Unilateral swelling with venous prominence occurs with venous obstruction. ■ Cyanosis of the nail beds reflects chronic cardiopulmonary disease. ■ Unilateral swelling with venous prominence occurs with venous obstruction. ■ Cold temperature of the hands and fingers occurs with vasoconstriction.
Palpate the nail beds for capillary refill. (Apply pressure to the patient's fingertips. Watch for blanching of the nail beds. Release the pressure. Note the time it takes for capillary refill, indicated by the return of pink color on release of the pressure.) *Capillary refill should be less than 2 seconds (i.e., immediate).*	■ Capillary refill that takes less than 3 seconds reflects circulatory compromise, such as hypovolemia or anemia.
Assess venous pattern and pressure. (Elevate one of the patient's arms over the head for a few seconds. Slowly lower the arm. Observe the filling of the patient's hand veins.) *Hand veins should fill equally and immediately.*	■ Distention of hand veins at elevations over 9 cm above heart level reflects an increase in systemic venous pressure.

BOX 29–7 **Assessing Jugular Venous Pressure**

When a patient with normal venous pressure lies in the supine position, full neck veins are normally visible, but as the head of the bed is elevated, the pulsations disappear. In the patient with greatly elevated venous pressure, visible pulsations of the jugular vein are present even in the upright position. To conduct the inspection, do the following:

1. Remove clothing from the patient's neck and chest. Elevate the head of the bed 30 to 45 degrees, and turn the patient's head to the opposite side. Shine a light tangentially across the neck to increase shadows. If the external jugular veins are distended, they will be visible vertically between the mandible and outer clavicle.
2. If jugular distention is present, assess the JVP by measuring from the highest point of visible distention to the sternal angle (the point at which the clavicles meet) on both sides of the neck (see the accompanying figure). Bilateral measurements above 3 cm are considered elevated and indicate increased venous pressure; distention on only one side may indicate obstruction.

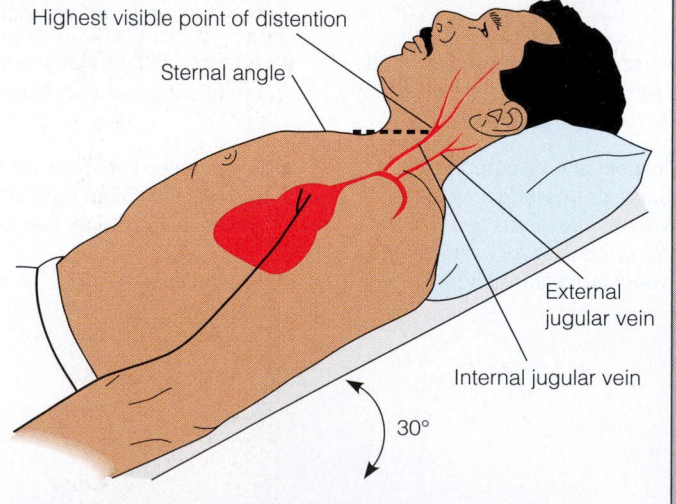

Highest visible point of distention

Sternal angle

External jugular vein

Internal jugular vein

30°

Assessment of the highest point of jugular vein distention

Technique/Normal Findings	Abnormal Findings
Palpate the radial and brachial pulses. Note rate, rhythm, volume amplitude, symmetry, variations with respiration. (See Box 29–6 for pulse patterns.) *Radial and brachial pulses should have equal and normal rate, be strong, and not vary with respirations.*	■ Alterations in pulse rate or rhythm are due to cardiac dysrhythmias (such as atrial fibrillation, atrial flutter, and premature ventricular contractions). A pulse rate over 100 bpm is tachycardia; a pulse rate below 60 bpm is bradycardia. ■ A pulse deficit (slower radial rate than apical rate) occurs with dysrhythmias and CHF. ■ Irregularities of rhythm produce early beats and pauses (skipped beats) in the pulse, which may be regular in pattern, sporadic, or grossly irregular. ■ Diminished or absent radial pulses may be due to thromboangiitis obliterans (Buerger's disease) or acute arterial occlusion. ■ A weak and thready pulse, often with tachycardia, reflects decreased CO. ■ A bounding pulse occurs with hyperkinetic states and atherosclerosis. ■ Unequal pulses between extremities suggest arterial narrowing or obstruction on one side. ■ In sinus dysrhythmia (a normal variant, especially in young adults), the pulse rate increases with inspiration and decreases with expiration.
If arterial insufficiency is suspected, palpate the ulnar pulse and perform the Allen test: ■ Have the patient make a tight fist. ■ Compress both the radial and ulnar arteries. ■ Have the patient open the hand to a slightly flexed position. ■ Observe for pallor and manifestations of pain. ■ Release the ulnar artery and observe for the return of pink color within 3 to 5 seconds. ■ Repeat the procedure on the radial artery. *Color should return within 3 to 5 seconds in both the ulnar and the radial arteries.*	■ The normal ulnar artery may or may not have a palpable pulse. ■ Persistent pallor with the Allen test suggests ulnar artery occlusion.
Lower Extremity Assessment	
Inspect and palpate each leg, noting size, shape, and symmetry; arterial pattern; skin color, temperature, and texture; hair pattern; pigmentation; rashes; ulcers, sensation; and capillary refill. *Legs should be symmetric in size and shape, arterial pattern, appropriate color, warm, without lesions. Capillary refill on toenails should be immediate.*	■ Chronic arterial insufficiency may be due to arteriosclerosis or autonomic dysfunction, or to acute occlusion resulting from thrombosis, embolus, or aneurysm. ■ Signs of arterial disruption include pallor, dependent rubor (dusky redness); cool to cold temperature; and atrophic changes, such as hair loss with shiny and smooth texture, thickened nails, sensory loss, slow capillary refill, and muscle atrophy. ■ Ulcers with symmetric margins, a deep base, black or necrotic tissue, and absence of bleeding may occur at pressure points on or between the toes, on the heel, on the lateral malleolar or tibial area, over the metatarsal heads, or along the side or sole of the foot. ■ Gangrene due to complete arterial occlusion presents as black, dry, hard skin; pregangrenous color changes include deep cyanosis and purple-black discoloration.
With the patient supine, assess the venous pattern of the legs. Repeat with the patient standing. *Venous pattern on both legs should be symmetric, and there should be no edema, cyanosis, or lesions.*	■ Signs of venous insufficiency include swelling, thickened skin, cyanosis, stasis dermatitis (brown pigmentation, erythema, and scaling), and superficial ankle ulcers located predominantly at the medial malleolus with uneven margins, ruddy granulation tissue, and bleeding. ■ Varicose veins appear as dilated, tortuous, and thickened veins, which are more prominent in a dependent position.
Palpate the femoral, popliteal, posterior tibial, and dorsalis pedis pulses for volume, amplitude, and symmetry (see Figure 29–21). *All lower extremity pulses should be strong and equal in amplitude.*	■ Diminished or absent leg pulses suggest partial or complete arterial occlusion of the proximal vessel and are often due to arteriosclerosis obliterans. ■ Increased and widened femoral and popliteal pulsations suggest aneurysm. ■ Absence of a posterior tibial pulse with signs and symptoms of arterial insufficiency is usually due to acute occlusion by thrombosis or embolus. ■ Diminished or absent pedal pulses are often due to popliteal occlusion associated with diabetes mellitus.

Technique/Normal Findings	Abnormal Findings
If pulses are diminished, observe for postural color changes. Elevate both legs 60 degrees, and observe the color of the soles of the feet. Have the patient sit and dangle the legs; note the return of color to the feet.	■ Extensive pallor on elevation is suggestive of arterial insufficiency. ■ Rubor (dusky redness) of the toes and feet along with delayed venous return (over 45 seconds) suggests arterial insufficiency.
If arterial insufficiency is suspected, auscultate the femoral arteries. *No bruits should be heard.*	■ Femoral bruits suggest arterial narrowing due to arteriosclerosis.
Inspect and gently palpate the calves. *There should be no redness or swelling, heat, or pain in the calves of the legs.*	■ Redness, warmth, swelling, tenderness, and cords along a superficial vein suggest thrombophlebitis or deep venous thrombosis.
Inspect and palpate for edema. Use your thumb to compress the dorsum of the patient's foot, around the ankles, and along the tibia (Figure 29–23A). A depression in the skin that does not immediately refill is called pitting edema. *Normally, there is no edema.*	Edema can be graded on a scale from 1+ to 4+ (Figure 29–23 ■): 1+ (–2 mm depression) No visible change in the leg; slight pitting 2+ (–4 mm depression) No marked change in the shape of the leg; pitting slightly deeper 3+ (–6 mm depression) Leg visibly swollen; pitting deep 4+ (–8 mm depression) Leg very swollen; pitting very deep ■ Edema may be caused by disease of the cardiovascular system such as CHF; by renal, hepatic, or lymphatic problems; or by infection. ■ Venous distention suggests venous insufficiency or incompetence.

2 mm
1+

4 mm
2+

6 mm
3+

8 mm
4+

A

B

Figure 29–23 ■ Evaluation of edema. *A,* Palpating for edema over the tibia. *B,* Four-point scale for grading edema.

Abdominal Assessment

Inspect and palpate the abdominal aorta. Note size, width, and any visible pulsations or bulging. *Abdominal aorta should be of appropriate size without visible pulsations or bulging.*	■ A pulsating mass in the upper abdomen suggests an aortic aneurysm, particularly in the older adult. ■ An aorta greater than 2.5 to 3 cm in width reflects pathologic dilation, most likely due to arteriosclerosis.

Technique/Normal Findings	Abnormal Findings

Auscultate the epigastrium and each abdominal quadrant, using the bell of the stethoscope (Figure 29–24 ■). *No bruits should be heard over the abdominal aorta.*

- Abdominal bruits reflect turbulent blood flow associated with partial arterial occlusion.
- A bruit heard over the aorta suggests an aneurysm.
- A bruit heard over the epigastrium and radiating laterally, especially with HTN, suggests renal artery stenosis.
- Bruits heard in the lower abdominal quadrants suggest partial occlusion of the iliac arteries.

Aorta

Renal artery

Iliac artery

Femoral artery

Figure 29–24 ■ Auscultation sites of the abdominal aorta and its branches.

Lymph Node Assessment

Palpate the regional lymph nodes of the head and neck, axillae, arms, and groin. Use firm, circular movements of the finger pads and note size, shape, symmetry, consistency, delineation, mobility, tenderness, sensation, and condition of overlying skin. *Nodes should not be enlarged or painful.*

- **Lymphadenopathy** refers to the enlargement of lymph nodes (over 1 cm) with or without tenderness. It may be caused by inflammation, infection, or malignancy of the nodes or the regions drained by the nodes.
- Lymph node enlargement with tenderness suggests inflammation (*lymphadenitis*). With bacterial infection, the nodes may be warm and matted with localized swelling.
- Malignant or metastatic nodes may be hard, indicating lymphoma; rubbery, indicating Hodgkin's disease; or fixed to adjacent structures. Usually they are not tender.
- Ear infections and scalp and facial lesions, such as acne, may cause enlargement of the preauricular and cervical nodes.
- Anterior cervical nodes are enlarged and infected with streptococcal pharyngitis and mononucleosis.
- Lymphadenitis of the cervical and submandibular nodes occurs with herpes simplex lesions.
- Enlargement of supraclavicular nodes, especially the left, is highly suggestive of metastatic disease from abdominal and thoracic cancer.
- Axillary lymphadenopathy is associated with breast cancer.
- Lesions of the genitals may produce enlargement of the inguinal nodes.
- Persistent generalized lymphadenopathy is associated with acquired immune deficiency syndrome (AIDS) and AIDS-related complex.

Spleen Assessment

Palpate for the spleen, in the upper left quadrant of the abdomen. *The spleen is normally not palpable.*

A palpable spleen in the left upper abdominal quadrant of an adult may indicate abnormal enlargement (splenomegaly) and may be associated with cancer, blood dyscrasias, and viral infection, such as mononucleosis.

Percuss for splenic dullness in the lowest left intercostal space (ICS) at the anterior axillary line or in the ninth to tenth ICS at the midaxillary line (Figure 29–25 ■). *Normally, tympany is heard.*

A dull percussion note in the lowest left ICS at the anterior axillary line or below the tenth rib at the midaxillary line suggests splenic enlargement.

Figure 29–25 ■ Percussing the spleen.

SAMPLE DOCUMENTATION
Assessment of Cardiac Function

56-year-old male admitted to cardiac critical care unit from ED to rule out myocardial infarction. States he has pain in the middle of his chest that is "like a heavy pressure"; 6 on a 10-point scale. Skin cool, slightly moist. BP 190/94 right arm and 186/92 left arm (both reclining). Apical pulse 92, regular and strong. No pulse deficit. Respirations 28. Apical impulse nonpalpable, no visible heaves or thrusts. S_1 and S_2 auscultated without murmurs or clicks. S_4 noted.

TEST YOURSELF NCLEX-RN® REVIEW

1. A patient who is hemorrhaging has decreased preload. What physiologic event will follow?
   1. increased afterload
   2. increased ejection fraction
   3. decreased CO
   4. decreased action potential
2. A nurse is assessing chest pain. What question will provide information about pain intensity?
   1. "Did the pain move into your left arm?"
   2. "Was your pain relieved by resting or worse when you were busy?"
   3. "On a scale of 0 (no pain) to 10 (worst pain), what number was your pain?"
   4. "Was the pain a pressure, a burning, or a tightness?"
3. A nurse is assessing the apical pulse. What anatomic location would be used?
   1. left midclavicular, fifth intercostal space
   2. left substernal, sixth intercostal space
   3. right midaxillary, second intercostal space
   4. right nipple line, any intercostal space
4. A patient's pulse rate is 50. The nurse would document this as which of the following?
   1. tachycardia
   2. bradycardia
   3. hypertension
   4. hypotension
5. A patient has a very low RBC count. What subjective manifestation would be elicited during a health history?
   1. sore throat
   2. chest pain
   3. fatigue
   4. nausea
6. A patient has a low platelet count. What would the nurse likely find on physical assessment?
   1. enlarged lymph nodes
   2. excessive bruising
   3. varicose veins
   4. changes in pulse pressure
7. An older adult is severely dehydrated and, as a result, has increased blood viscosity. How will this affect the peripheral vascular resistance (PVR)?
   1. increased PVR
   2. decreased PVR
   3. no change
   4. depends on gender
8. What method would be most appropriate to assess the carotid arteries?
   1. Inspect for absence of movement.
   2. Auscultate with the bell of the stethoscope.
   3. Palpate with firm pressure.
   4. Percuss lightly over each artery.
9. When auscultating the abdominal aorta, the nurse hears a murmuring or blowing sound. This sound should be documented as which of the following?
   1. hypokinetic pulse
   2. bigeminal pulse
   3. bruit
   4. dysrhythmia
10. The nurse is assessing a man who has severe leg pain. The leg is cool and cyanotic, and the femoral pulse can not be palpated. What would be the priority intervention based on these assessments?
    1. Document the findings.
    2. Ask the family about this problem.
    3. Teach the man relaxation techniques.
    4. Notify the physician immediately.

See Test Yourself answers in Appendix C.

Pearson Nursing Student Resources

Find additional review materials at
www.nursing.pearsonhighered.com

Prepare for success with additional NCLEX®-style practice questions, interactive assignments and activities, Web links, animations and videos, and more!

BIBLIOGRAPHY

Armstrong, J., & Mitchell, E. (2008). Comprehensive nursing assessment in the care of older people. *Nursing Older People, (20)*1, 36–40.

Assessment of the neck and lymph nodes in the elderly patient. (2007). *Medscape.* Retrieved from http://www.medscape.com/viewprogram/7808_pnt

Ballas, M., & Kraut, E. (2008). Bleeding and bruising: A diagnostic workup. *American Family Physician, 77*(8), 1117–1124.

Bickley, L., & Szilagyi, P. (2007). *Bates' guide to physical examination and history taking* (9th ed.). Philadelphia: Lippincott.

Closs, S., Nelson, E., & Briggs, M. (2008). Can venous and arterial leg ulcers be differentiated by the characteristics of the pain they produce? *Journal of Clinical Nursing, 17*(5), 637–645.

Coviello, J. (2004). Cardiac assessment 101: A new look at the guidelines for cardiac homecare patients. *Home Healthcare Nurse, 22*(2), 116–123.

Dulak, S. (2004). Hands-on help assessing heart sounds. *RN, 67*(8), 24ac1–4.

Eagle, M. (2006). Doppler ultrasound–basics revisited. *British Journal of Nursing, 15*(11), Tissue Viability Supplement, S24–30.

Edwards, W. L. (2007). What comprises a preventative cardiovascular assessment for an adult? *Medscape Nurses.* Retrieved from http://www.medscape.com/viewarticle?564859

Eliopoulos, E. (2005). *Gerontological nursing* (6th ed.). Philadelphia: Lippincott Williams & Wilkins.

Geiter, H. (2009). Complete blood count: Getting beyond the basics. What the shapes of RBCs can tell you. *American Nurse Today, 4*(1), 10–11.

Hackam, D. (2007). The ankle-brachial index independently predicted all–cause mortality in high-risk patients with peripheral vascular disease. *ACP Journal Club, 147*(3), 81.

Jevon, P., & Cunningham, A. (2007). Inspection and palpation of the precordium. *Nursing Times, 103*(26), 26–27.

Kee, J. (2009). *Prentice Hall handbook of laboratory & diagnostic tests with nursing implications* (6th ed.). Upper Saddle River, NJ: Prentice Hall.

Kwabe, H., & Saito, I. (2007). What measurement of home blood pressure should be used for clinical evaluation when multiple measurements are made? *Journal of Hypertension, 25*(7), 1369–1374.

Lindsey, J. (2005). Heart sounds: Do you hear what I see? *Journal of Emergency Medical Services,* (4), 104, 106.

MacDonald, S., Yates, J., Lance, R., Giganti, N., & Chepurko, D. (2005). Are you asking the right admission questions when assessing dyspnea? *Heart & Lung, 34*(4), 260–269.

McCarron, K. (2007). Clues in the blood: Know your CBCs. *Nursing Made Incredibly Easy! 5*(3), 13–15, 17.

National Institute of Health. (2008). *Genes and Disease: The Heart and Blood Vessels; Blood and Lymph Diseases.* Retrieved from http://www.ncbi.nlm.nih.gov/books/bookres.fegi/gnd/pdf.html

Ott, L. (2008). Assessing blood flow with CT angiography. *Nursing, 38*(1), 26.

Overbaugh, K. J. (2009). Acute coronary syndrome. *American Journal of Nursing, 109*(5), 42–52.

Porth, C. (2007). *Essentials of pathophysiology: Concepts of altered health states* (2nd ed.). Philadelphia: Lippincott Williams & Wilkins.

Porth, C., & Matfin, G. (2009). *Pathophysiology: Concepts of altered health states* (8th ed). Philadelphia: Lippincott Williams & Wilkins.

Rice, K. (2005). How to measure ankle/brachial index. *Nursing, 35*(1), 56–57.

Rushing, J. (2005). Clinical do's & dont's. Assessing for orthostatic hypotension. *Nursing, 35*(1), 30.

Scott, C. & Macinnes, J. (2006). Cardiac patient assessment: Putting the patient first. *British Journal of Nursing, 15*(9), 502–508.

Southeimer, D. (2006). Peripheral vascular disease: Diagnosis and treatment. *American Family Physician, 73*(11), 1971–1976, 1887–1890.

Weber, J., & Kelley, J. (2009). *Health assessment in nursing* (4th ed.). Philadelphia: Lippincott Williams & Wilkins.

Williams, M. (2007). Assessment of the neck and lymph nodes in the elderly patient. Medscape. Retrieved from http://www.medscape.com/viewprogram/7808_pnt

Worley, C. (2006). "It hurts when I walk": Venous stasis disease—etiology and assessment. *Dermatoloby Nursing, 18*(5), 480–481, 490.

CHAPTER 30

Nursing Care of Patient with Coronary Heart Disease

LEARNING OUTCOMES

1. Discuss the coronary circulation and electrical properties of the heart.
2. Compare and contrast the pathophysiology and manifestations of coronary heart disease and common cardiac dysrhythmias.
3. Describe interdisciplinary and nursing care for patients with coronary heart disease and or cardiac dysrhythmias.
4. Relate the outcomes of diagnostic tests and procedures to the pathophysiology of cardiac disorders and implications for patient responses to the disorder.
5. Discuss nursing implications for medications and treatments used to prevent and treat coronary heart disease and dysrhythmias.
6. Describe nursing care for the patient undergoing diagnostic testing, an interventional procedure, or surgery for coronary heart disease or a dysrhythmia.

CLINICAL COMPETENCIES

1. Assess functional health status of patients with coronary heart disease and/or a dysrhythmia, including the impact of the disorder on the patient's ability to perform activities of daily living and usual tasks.
2. Use knowledge of the normal anatomy and physiology of the heart in caring for patients with coronary heart disease.
3. Monitor patients with coronary heart disease or dysrhythmias for expected and unexpected manifestations, reporting and recording findings as indicated.
4. Use assessed data to select nursing diagnoses, determine priorities of care, and develop and implement individualized nursing interventions for patients with coronary heart disease and dysrhythmias.
5. Administer medications and treatments for patients with coronary heart disease and dysrhythmias safely and knowledgably.
6. Integrate interdisciplinary care into nursing care planning and implementation for patients with coronary heart disease and dysrhythmias.
7. Provide appropriate teaching for prevention, health promotion, and self-care related to coronary heart disease and dysrhythmias.
8. Evaluate the effectiveness of nursing interventions, revising or modifying the plan of care as needed to promote, maintain, or restore functional health for patients with coronary heart disease or dysrhythmias.

KEY TERMS

acute coronary syndrome (ACS), *925*
acute myocardial infarction (AMI), *934*
angina pectoris, *920*
atherosclerosis, *909*
atrial kick, *946*
cardiac arrest, *952*

cardiac rehabilitation, *940*
cardiovascular disease (CVD), *908*
collateral channels, *909*
coronary heart disease (CHD), *909*
dysrhythmia, *935*
ectopic beats, *946*

heart block, *946*
ischemia, *920*
pacemaker, *957*
paroxysmal, *950*
sudden cardiac death (SCD), *965*

Impaired blood flow to the myocardium, changes in the conduction of electrical impulses through the heart, and structural changes in the heart itself affect the heart's ability to fulfill its major purpose: to pump enough blood to meet the body's demand for oxygen and nutrients. Impaired cardiac function, no matter what the underlying cause, affects the patient's ability to participate in exercise and activities and to fulfill life roles. Disruptions in cardiac function affect other organ systems as well, potentially leading to organ system failure and death.

Cardiovascular disease (CVD) is a generic term for disorders of the heart and blood vessels. CVD is the leading cause of death and disability in the United States. About 80 million people (or 1 in 3) have some type of cardiovascular disease.

The direct and indirect CVD costs in 2008 were estimated to be $475.3 billion dollars (American Heart Association [AHA], 2009).

FAST FACTS

- Heart disease accounted for 864,500 U.S. deaths in 2005.
- CVD has accounted for more deaths than any other single cause yearly since 1900 (except 1918).
- In 2005, more women in the United States died of CVD than cancer, chronic lung diseases, Alzheimer's disease, accidents, and diabetes combined.
- If all major forms of CVD were eliminated, life expectancy would rise almost 7 years.

On an encouraging note, the incidence of new CVD cases per year is decreasing. Public education aimed at reducing fat intake, increasing exercise, and lowering cholesterol levels have made people more aware of risk factors associated with CVD. The mortality rate from heart disease peaked in 1963 and has shown a slow but steady decline since that time.

This chapter focuses on disorders of myocardial blood flow (coronary heart disease) and cardiac rhythm. Disorders of cardiac structure and function are discussed in ∞ Chapter 31. Review the normal anatomy and physiology and nursing assessment of the heart in ∞ Chapter 29 before proceeding with this chapter.

Disorders of Myocardial Perfusion

The Patient with Coronary Heart Disease

Coronary heart disease (CHD), or *coronary artery disease (CAD)*, affects 16.8 million people in the United States and causes more than 607,000 deaths annually (AHA, 2009). CHD is caused by impaired blood flow to the myocardium. Accumulation of atherosclerotic plaque in the coronary arteries is the usual cause. CHD may be asymptomatic, or may lead to angina pectoris, acute coronary syndrome, myocardial infarction (MI or heart attack), dysrhythmias, heart failure, and even sudden death.

Physiology Review

The two main coronary arteries, the left and the right, supply blood, oxygen, and nutrients to the myocardium. They originate in the root of the aorta, just outside the aortic valve. The *left main coronary artery* divides to form the anterior descending and circumflex arteries. The *anterior descending* artery supplies the anterior interventricular septum and the left ventricle, including the apex of the heart. The *circumflex* branch supplies the lateral wall of the left ventricle. The *right coronary artery* supplies the right ventricle and forms the posterior descending artery. The *posterior descending* artery supplies the posterior portion of the heart (see Figure 29–5).

Blood flow through the coronary arteries is primarily regulated by aortic pressure. Other factors include the heart rate (most flow occurs during diastole, when the muscle is relaxed), metabolic activity of the heart, blood vessel tone (constriction), and collateral circulation. Although there are no connections between the large coronary arteries, small arteries are joined by **collateral channels**. If large vessels are gradually occluded, these channels enlarge, providing alternative routes for blood flow (Heuther & McCance, 2008).

Pathophysiology

Coronary atherosclerosis is the most common cause of reduced coronary blood flow.

Atherosclerosis

Atherosclerosis is a progressive disease characterized by *atheroma* (plaque) formation, which affects the intimal and medial layers of large and midsize arteries. See Pathophysiology Illustrated.

Atherosclerosis is initiated by unknown precipitating factors that cause lipoproteins and fibrous tissue to accumulate in the arterial wall. Although the precise mechanisms are unknown, abnormal lipid metabolism and injury to or inflammation of endothelial cells lining the artery appear to be key to its development.

In the bloodstream, lipids are transported attached to proteins called apoproteins. High levels of certain *lipoproteins*, a type of apoprotein, increase the risk of atherosclerosis. *Low-density lipoproteins*, which are high in cholesterol, carry cholesterol to peripheral tissues where some of it is released to be taken up and incorporated into cells for use in producing energy. *Very-low-density lipoproteins*, large molecules primarily composed of triglycerides and cholesterol, carry triglycerides to muscle and fat cells. When the triglycerides are released into these tissues, the remainder of the molecule is a low-density lipoprotein. *High-density lipoproteins*, in contrast, attract cholesterol, returning it from peripheral tissues to the liver.

Hyperlipidemia itself may damage arterial endothelium. Other potential mechanisms of vessel injury include excessive pressures within the arterial system (hypertension), toxins found in cigarette smoke, infections, and inflammation (Huether & McCance, 2008). Endothelial damage promotes platelet adhesion and aggregation, and attracts leukocytes to the area.

At the site of injury, *atherogenic* (atherosclerosis-promoting) lipoproteins collect in the intimal lining of the artery, binding to the extracellular portion of the vessel endothelium. Macrophages migrate to the injured site as part of the inflammatory process. Contact with platelets, cholesterol, and other blood components stimulates abnormal proliferation of smooth muscle cells and connective tissue within the vessel wall. Although blood flow is not affected at this stage, this early lesion appears as a yellowish fatty streak on the inner lining of the artery. Fibrous plaque develops as smooth muscle cells enlarge, collagen fibers proliferate, and blood lipids accumulate. The lesion protrudes into the arterial lumen and is fixed to the inner wall of the intima. It may invade the muscular media layer of the vessel as well. The developing plaque not only gradually occludes the vessel lumen but also impairs the vessel's ability to dilate in response to increased oxygen demands. Fibrous plaque lesions often develop at arterial bifurcations or curves or in areas of narrowing. As the plaque expands, it can produce severe stenosis or total occlusion of the artery.

The final stage of the process is the development of *atheromas*, complex lesions consisting of lipids, fibrous tissue, collagen, calcium, cellular debris, and capillaries. These calcified lesions can ulcerate or rupture, stimulating thrombosis. The vessel lumen may be rapidly occluded by the thrombus, or it may embolize to occlude a distal vessel.

Plaque formation may be *eccentric*, located in a specific, asymmetric region of the vessel wall, or *concentric*, involving the entire vessel circumference. Manifestations of the process usually do not appear until about 75% of the arterial lumen has been occluded.

Atherosclerosis Animation

PATHOPHYSIOLOGY ILLUSTRATED
Coronary Heart Disease

Coronary heart disease usually is due to *atherosclerosis*, occlusion of the coronary arteries by fibrous, fatty plaque. Coronary heart disease is manifested by *angina pectoris, acute coronary syndrome,* and/or *myocardial infarction*. Risk factors for coronary heart disease include age (over 50 years), heredity, smoking, obesity, high serum cholesterol levels, hypertension, and diabetes mellitus. Other factors, such as diet and lack of exercise, also contribute to the risk of CHD.

Coronary artery

Adventitia

Media

Intima

Plaque

Atherosclerosis

In atherosclerosis, lipids accumulate in the intimal layer of arteries. Fibroblasts in the area respond by producing collagen, and smooth muscle cells proliferate, together forming a complex lesion called plaque. Plaque consists mostly of cholesterol, triglycerides, phospholipids, collagen, and smooth muscle cells.

Plaque reduces the size of the lumen of the affected artery, impairing blood flow. In addition, plaque may ulcerate, causing a thrombus to form that may completely occlude the vessel.

Endothelium

Collagen

Smooth muscle cell

Cholesterol crystal

Lipid

Plaque

Internal elastic lamina (damaged)

Fibrosis

Angina Pectoris

Angina is characterized by episodes of chest pain, usually precipitated by exercise and relieved by rest. When myocardial oxygen needs are greater than partially occluded vessels can supply, myocardial cells become ischemic and shift to anaerobic metabolism. Anaerobic metabolism produces lactic acid that stimulates nerve endings in the muscle, causing pain. The pain subsides when the oxygen supply again meets myocardial demand.

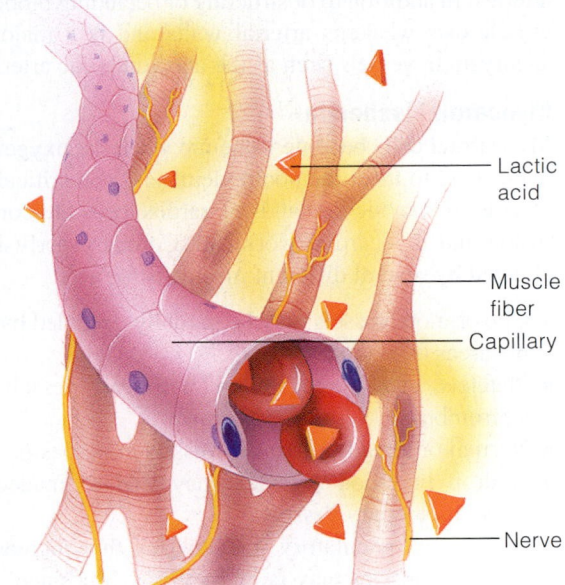

Lactic acid

Muscle fiber

Capillary

Nerve

Myocardial Infarction

Myocardial infarction occurs when complete obstruction of a coronary artery interrupts blood supply to an area of myocardium. Affected tissue becomes ischemic and eventually dies (infarcts) if the blood supply is not restored. The necrotic area is bordered by an area of injured or damaged tissue, which is in turn surrounded by an area of ischemic tissue.

As myocardial cells die, they lyse and release various cardiac isoenzymes into the circulation. Elevated serum levels of creatinine kinase (CK) and cardiac-specific troponins are specific indicators of myocardial infarction.

Infarcted myocardium

Ischemic myocardium

Injured (stunned) myocardium

Capillary

Muscle fiber

Potassium

Creatinine kinase isoenzyme (CK)

Lactic dehydrogenase isoenzyme (LDH)

Atherosclerosis tends to develop where arteries *bifurcate* or branch. Certain vessels have a higher likelihood of being affected, including the coronary arteries (the left anterior descending artery in particular), the renal arteries, the bifurcation of the carotid arteries, and branching sections of peripheral arteries. In addition to obstructing or occluding blood flow, atherosclerosis weakens arterial walls and is a major cause of aneurysm in vessels such as the aorta and iliac arteries.

Myocardial Ischemia

Myocardial cells become ischemic when the oxygen supply is inadequate to meet metabolic demands. The critical factors in meeting metabolic demands of cardiac cells are coronary perfusion and myocardial workload. Coronary perfusion can be affected by several different mechanisms:

- One or more vessels may be partially occluded by large, stable areas of plaque.
- Platelets can aggregate in narrowed vessels, forming a thrombus.
- Normal or already narrowed vessels may spasm.
- A drop in blood pressure may lead to inadequate flow through coronary vessels.
- Normal autoregulatory mechanisms that increase flow to working muscles may fail (Huether & McCance, 2008).

Workload is affected by the heart rate, myocardial contractility, preload (the amount of blood in the ventricles just prior to systole), and afterload (the peripheral pressure that must be overcome to move blood out of the heart into the circulation). The oxygen content of the blood and hematocrit are contributing factors to myocardial ischemia. Table 30–1 lists factors that may lead to myocardial ischemia.

Myocardial cells have a limited supply of adenosine triphosphate (ATP). When myocardial workload increases or the supply of blood and oxygen falls, cellular ATP stores are quickly depleted, affecting contractility. Cellular metabolism switches from an efficient aerobic process to anaerobic metabolism. Lactic acid accumulates, and cells are damaged. If blood flow is restored within 20 minutes, aerobic metabolism and contractility are restored, and cellular repair begins (McCance & Huether, 2006). Continued ischemia results in cell necrosis and death (infarction).

Coronary heart disease is generally divided into two categories, chronic ischemic heart disease and acute coronary syndromes. *Chronic ischemic heart disease* includes stable and vasospastic angina, and silent myocardial ischemia. In women, angina is the most common presenting symptom of CHD. *Acute coronary syndromes* range from unstable angina to myocardial infarction (Heuther & McCance, 2008). Acute coronary syndromes and myocardial infarction are the most common presenting symptoms of CHD in men. These disorders are discussed in the following sections of this chapter.

FOCUS ON CULTURAL DIVERSITY
Heart Disease

- Native Americans (American Indians and Alaska Natives) have the highest prevalence of coronary heart disease, followed by Whites, African Americans, Mexican Americans, native Hawaiians, and Asian Americans.
- People with less than a high school diploma have the highest rate of CHD; people with a bachelor's degree or higher have the lowest.
- Economic status is a factor; the rate of CHD in people with a family income less than $35,000 per year have a significantly higher rate than those with incomes greater than $75,000 per year.
- Regionally, the rate of CHD is highest in the South and lowest in the West.

Incidence and Prevalence

Many risk factors for CHD can be controlled through lifestyle modification. In fact, with increased public awareness of risk factors related to CHD, mortality rates are declining by about 3.3% per year. Nevertheless, CHD remains a major public health problem. Heart disease is the leading cause of death for all U.S. ethnic groups except Asian females (AHA, 2009). See the accompanying box. Nurses are in a prime position to encourage and support positive lifestyle changes by teaching and promoting healthy living practices. Individual choices can and do affect health.

The highest incidence of CHD is in the Western world, mainly in White males aged 45 and older. Both men and women are affected by coronary heart disease; in women, however, the onset is about 10 years later because of the heart-protective effects of estrogen. After menopause, women's risk is equal to that of men.

Risk Factors

The causes of atherosclerosis are not known, but certain risk factors have been linked with the development of atherosclerotic plaques. The Framingham Heart Study provided vital research into the relationship between risk factors and the development of heart disease (Box 30–1). Research into CHD is ongoing, looking at causative factors, manifestations, and protective measures for many populations.

Risk factors for CHD are frequently classified as *nonmodifiable*, or factors that cannot be changed, and *modifiable*, those factors that can be changed (Table 30–2).

TABLE 30–1 Factors Contributing to Myocardial Ischemia

CORONARY PERFUSION	MYOCARDIAL WORKLOAD	BLOOD OXYGEN CONTENT
■ Atherosclerosis	■ Rapid heart rate	■ Reduced atmospheric oxygen pressure
■ Thrombosis	■ Increased preload, afterload, or contractility	■ Impaired gas exchange
■ Vasospasm	■ Increased metabolic demands	■ Low red blood cells and hemoglobin content
■ Poor perfusion pressure	(e.g., hyperthyroidism)	

BOX 30–1 The Framingham Heart Study

The Framingham Heart Study (FHS) is an ongoing, significant clinical research study that has provided data about cardiovascular disease for over 50 years. The study was initiated in 1948 with an original study group of 5209 participants in the town of Framingham, Massachusetts. Every 2 years, this original group is evaluated for cardiovascular "events" via their medical history, physical findings, and diagnostic testing. Children of the original group have also been studied as part of the Framingham Offspring Study. It was in reports of the FHS that the term "risk factor" first appeared.

Implications for Nursing

The data collected from both the FHS and the Framingham Offspring Study provide a rich database from which to develop evidence-based approaches for patients with heart disease. A major application of these research findings to practice is in primary preventive education, for example, through community cardiovascular health programs. As noted in the text, although research shows that increased public awareness of cardiovascular risk factors has lowered morbidity and mortality from heart disease, heart disease remains the number-one killer in the United States. Education about the effects of lifestyle on the cardiovascular system must begin in the early school years and be reinforced throughout the formative years. When healthy choices become habit, cardiac disease will be reduced.

A second application of these findings is in collaborative treatment. Nurses should keep up to date on the latest strategies for medical treatment so that they can provide accurate rationales to patients and formulate effective nursing treatment plans that complement medical management strategies. The result is better communication, a sense of collegiality and teamwork, and positive patient outcomes.

Critical Thinking in Patient Care

1. What kinds of strategies can be used in elementary school settings to teach cardiovascular health in a fun, informative manner?
2. Which healthcare providers should be included in a multidisciplinary effort to encourage patients to modify their lifestyles?
3. What changes do you need to make in your lifestyle to role model heart healthy living?

Nonmodifiable Risk Factors

Age is a nonmodifiable risk factor. Over 50% of heart attack victims are 65 or older; 80% of deaths due to myocardial infarction occur in this age group. *Gender* and *genetic factors* also are nonmodifiable risk factors for CHD. Men are affected by CHD at an earlier age than women. A family history of CHD in a male first-degree relative younger than age 55 or a female first-degree relative younger than 65 years is identified as a risk factor for CHD (National Cholesterol Education Program [NCEP], 2002). Chromosome p921.3 has been associated with CHD. The region containing this chromosome also contains gene sequences for cyclin-dependent kinase inhibitors, which are implicated in the pathogenesis of atherosclerosis (Samani, Erdman, Hall, et al., 2007).

Modifiable Risk Factors

Modifiable risk factors include lifestyle factors and pathologic conditions that predispose the patient to developing CHD. Disease conditions that contribute to CHD include hypertension, diabetes mellitus, and hyperlipidemia. Although these conditions are not a matter of choice, they are modifiable risk factors that can often be controlled through medication, weight control, diet, and exercise.

Behavioral or lifestyle factors can be controlled or completely eliminated. Lifestyle changes require significant commitment by the patient; ongoing support from the healthcare team is vital for success.

HYPERTENSION *Hypertension* is consistent blood pressure readings greater than 140 mmHg systolic or 90 mmHg diastolic. Hypertension is common, affecting more than one-third of people over age 50 in the United States. Its prevalence is higher in African Americans than in Hispanics, and higher in Hispanics than in White Americans. Hypertension damages the endothelial cells of arteries, possibly by excess pressure and altered characteristics of blood flow. This damage can stimulate the development of atherosclerotic plaque.

TABLE 30–2 Risk Factors for Coronary Heart Disease

NONMODIFIABLE		MODIFIABLE	
	PATHOPHYSIOLOGIC		LIFESTYLE
Age	Hyperlipidemia		Cigarette smoking
Men ≥ 45 years	Elevated LDL cholesterol		Obesity
Women ≥ 55 years	Elevated triglycerides		Physical inactivity
	Low HDL cholesterol		Atherogenic diet
Gender	Hypertension		Women only: use of oral contraceptives, hormone replacement therapy
Heredity	Diabetes mellitus		
	Women only: premature menopause		
	Emerging risk factors:		
	Elevated homocysteine levels		
	Thrombogenic factors		
	Inflammatory factors		
	Impaired fasting glucose		

DIABETES *Diabetes mellitus* contributes to CHD in several ways. Diabetes is associated with higher blood lipid levels, a higher incidence of hypertension, and obesity—all risk factors in their own right. In addition, diabetes affects the endothelium of blood vessels, contributing to the process of atherosclerosis. Hyperglycemia and hyperinsulinemia, altered platelet function, elevated fibrinogen levels, and inflammation also are thought to play a role in the development of atherosclerosis in people with diabetes.

ABNORMAL BLOOD LIPIDS *Hyperlipidemia* is an abnormally high level of blood lipids and lipoproteins. Lipoproteins carry cholesterol in the blood. Low-density lipoproteins (LDLs) are the primary carriers of cholesterol. High levels of LDL promote atherosclerosis because LDL deposits cholesterol on artery walls. Table 30–3 lists desirable and high-risk levels for total and LDL cholesterol. In contrast, high-density lipoproteins help clear cholesterol from the arteries, transporting it to the liver for excretion. HDL levels above 35 mg/dL have a protective effect, reducing the risk of CHD; in contrast, HDL levels lower than 35 mg/dL are associated with an increased risk for CHD. Triglycerides, compounds of fatty acids bound to glycerol and used for fat storage by the body, are carried on very low-density lipoprotein (VLDL) molecules. Elevated triglycerides also contribute to the risk for CHD.

> **MEMORY CUE**
>
> LDLs = less desirable lipoproteins
> HDLs = highly desirable lipoproteins

CIGARETTE SMOKING *Cigarette smoking* is an independent risk factor for CHD, responsible for more deaths from CHD than from lung cancer or pulmonary disease (Woods, Froclicher, Motzer, & Bridges, 2009). The effects of smoking on the cardiovascular system are dose dependent (NCEP, 2002). The male cigarette smoker has two to three times the risk of developing heart disease than the nonsmoker; the female who smokes has up to four times the risk. For both men and women who stop smoking, the risk of mortality from CHD is reduced by half. Second-hand (or environmental) tobacco smoke also increases the risk of death from CHD by as much as 30% (Woods et al., 2009). Tobacco smoke promotes CHD in several ways. Carbon monoxide damages vascular endothelium, promoting cholesterol deposition. Nicotine stimulates catecholamine release, increasing blood pressure, heart rate, and myocardial oxygen use. Nicotine also constricts arteries, limiting tissue perfusion (blood flow and oxygen delivery). Furthermore, nicotine reduces HDL levels and increases platelet aggregation, increasing the risk of thrombus formation.

> **FAST FACTS**
>
> Cigarette smoking is the leading independent risk factor for coronary heart disease and a primary target of risk factor management.

OBESITY *Obesity* (excess adipose tissue), generally defined as a body mass index (BMI) of 30 kg/m^2 or greater, and fat distribution affect the risk for CHD. Obese people have higher rates of hypertension, diabetes, and hyperlipidemia. In the Framingham study, obese men over age 50 had twice the incidence of CHD and acute MI of those who were within 10% of their ideal weight. Central obesity, or intra-abdominal fat, is associated with an increased risk for CHD. The best indicator of central obesity is the waist circumference. A waist-to-hip ratio of greater than 0.8 (women) or 0.9 (men) increases the risk for CHD.

PHYSICAL INACTIVITY *Physical inactivity* is associated with higher risk of CHD. Research data indicate that people who maintain a regular program of physical activity are less prone to developing CHD than sedentary people. Cardiovascular benefits of exercise include increased availability of oxygen to the heart muscle, decreased oxygen demand and cardiac workload, and increased myocardial function and electrical stability. Other positive effects of regular physical activity include decreased blood pressure, blood lipids, insulin levels, platelet aggregation, and weight.

DIET *Diet* is a risk factor for CHD, independent of fat and cholesterol intake. Diets high in fruits, vegetables, whole grains, and unsaturated fatty acids appear to have a protective effect. The underlying factors are not clear, but probably relate to nutrients such as antioxidants, folic acid, other B vitamins, omega-3 fatty acids, and other unidentified micronutrients (American Heart Association Nutrition Committee, 2006).

EMERGING RISK FACTORS Recent research demonstrates a link between elevated serum *homocysteine levels* and CHD. Until menopause, women have lower homocysteine levels than men, which may partially explain their lower risk for CHD. Homocysteine levels are negatively correlated with serum folate and dietary folate intake; that is, increasing folate intake lowers homocysteine levels.

Based on evidence that aspirin and antiplatelet therapies reduce the risk for myocardial infarction, *clot-promoting factors*

TABLE 30–3 Classification of Serum Cholesterol and Triglyceride Values*

	TOTAL CHOLESTEROL (MG/DL)	LDL CHOLESTEROL (MG/DL)	TRIGLYCERIDE (MG/DL)
Optimal		Less than 100	
Desirable	Under 200	100–129	< 150
Borderline	200 to 239	130 to 159	150 to 199
High	240 or higher	160 to 189	200 to 499
Very High		> 190	≥ 500

*As defined by the National Blood, Lung, and Heart Institute's National Cholesterol Education Program.

BOX 30–2 Characteristics of the Metabolic Syndrome

- Abdominal obesity
- Abnormal blood lipids (low HDL, high triglycerides)
- Hypertension
- Elevated fasting blood glucose
- Clotting tendency
- Inflammatory factors

are identified as CHD risk factors. *Inflammation* also has recently been identified as a risk factor. Inflammatory processes may increase the development of atherosclerotic plaque, and are implicated in plaque rupture (NCEP, 2002). Inflammation also promotes clot formation at the site of ruptured plaque. Although identified as risk factors, it is not generally recommended that patients routinely be tested for these factors.

METABOLIC SYNDROME   The *metabolic syndrome*, a group of metabolic risk factors occurring in an individual, is a strong risk factor for CHD (Box 30–2). The metabolic syndrome has emerged as a risk factor for premature CHD that is equal to cigarette smoking. Three underlying causes of metabolic syndrome are identified: overweight/obesity, physical inactivity, and genetic factors. It is closely associated with *insulin resistance*, impaired tissue responses to insulin. Genetic factors play a role in insulin resistance, as do the acquired factors of abdominal obesity and physical inactivity (NCEP, 2002).

RISK FACTORS UNIQUE TO WOMEN   Risk factors unique to women include *premature menopause*, *oral contraceptive use*, and *hormone replacement therapy (HRT)*. At menopause, serum HDL levels drop and LDL levels rise, increasing the risk of CHD. Early menopause (natural or surgically induced) increases the risk of CHD and MI. Women who have bilateral oophorectomy before age 35 without hormone replacement are eight times more likely to have an MI than women experiencing natural menopause. Estrogen replacement therapy reduces the risk of CHD and MI in these women. Oral contraceptives, by contrast, increase the risk for MI, particularly in women who also smoke. This increased risk is due to the tendency of oral contraceptives to promote clotting, increase blood pressure, serum lipids, and glucose tolerance (Woods et al., 2009). The Women's Health Initiative randomized trial of HRT showed an increased risk for CHD in previously healthy women taking a commonly prescribed combination of estrogen and progestin (Writing Group, 2002). This well-controlled research study (see the following box) was terminated early when it showed a small but significant increase risk for CHD, stroke, pulmonary embolism, and invasive breast cancer in women taking HRT.

FAST FACTS

- Risk factors for coronary heart disease are those factors that promote atherosclerosis and plaque development.
- Angina pectoris, acute coronary syndromes, and myocardial infarction are the manifestations of myocardial ischemia and coronary heart disease due to atherosclerosis.
- Atherosclerosis also is the primary underlying cause of stroke and peripheral vascular disease; therefore, the risk factors for atherosclerosis also are the risk factors for coronary heart disease, including angina, acute coronary syndromes, and myocardial infarction.

Interdisciplinary Care

Care of patients with coronary heart disease focuses on aggressive risk factor management to slow the atherosclerotic process and maintain myocardial perfusion. Until manifestations of chronic or acute ischemia are experienced, the

---

MOVING EVIDENCE INTO ACTION   The Postmenopausal Woman

The Women's Health Initiative (WHI) is studying the risks and benefits of strategies to reduce the incidence of heart disease, breast and colorectal cancer, and fractures in postmenopausal women (Rossouw et al., 2007). A group of 161,809 postmenopausal women between age 50 and 79 were originally enrolled in WHI trials. Of these women, a subgroup of 16,608 women with intact uteri became part of a randomized trial to assess the risks and benefits of HRT, using the most frequently prescribed combined hormone (estrogen and progestin [Prempro]) replacement in the United States.

   After a mean of 5.2 years of follow-up, this study was stopped due to convincing evidence that the risk for invasive breast cancer exceeded the benefits of HRT. The study also demonstrated increased risks for coronary heart disease, stroke, deep vein thrombosis, and pulmonary embolism, although overall mortality was not affected. HRT reduced the risk for colorectal cancer and hip fracture in this study group. The risk for CHD appears to be independent of other CHD risk factors such as age, ethnicity, hypertension, diabetes, smoking, obesity, and other identified risk factors.

IMPLICATIONS FOR NURSING

Nurses often are in position of advising women about menopause, its manifestations, and hormone replacement therapy. While HRT does reduce unpleasant menopausal effects such as night sweats and hot flashes, and it reduces the risk of osteoporosis and subsequent fractures, it carries associated risks. Advise each patient about the risks and benefits of HRT, clearly presenting the evidence. Suggest alternative strategies to reduce menopausal symptoms, such as complementary medicines (∞ see Chapter 49). Encourage measures such as weight-bearing exercise, calcium supplements, and a diet high in fiber and antioxidants to reduce the risks for osteoporosis, fracture, and colorectal cancer. Ultimately, each patient will make her own decision about postmenopausal HRT.

CRITICAL THINKING IN PATIENT CARE

1. What factors might you suggest that a patient consider when deciding whether to use HRT for menopausal manifestations and risks?
2. In this study, the increased risk for CHD was not related to the duration of time taking HRT, whereas the increased risk for stroke and invasive breast cancer emerged more than 1 year after randomization (stroke in the second through fifth year of the study, breast cancer within several years following randomization). Will this data affect your advice to menopausal women inquiring about HRT? If so, how?

diagnosis often is presumptive, based on history and the presence of risk factors.

Diagnosis

Laboratory testing assesses for risk factors such as an abnormal blood lipid profile (elevated triglyceride and LDL levels and decreased HDL levels).

- *Total serum cholesterol* is elevated in hyperlipidemia. A *lipid profile* includes triglyceride, HDL, and LDL levels, and enables calculation of the ratio of HDL to total cholesterol. The ratio should be at least 1:5, with 1:3 being the ideal ratio. Elevated lipid levels are associated with an increased risk of atherosclerosis (see Table 30–3). In patients with a strong family history of premature CHD or familial hypercholesterolemia, *lipoprotein (a)* also may be measured. Elevated levels of Lp(a) may independently increase the risk of CHD. Other subsets of blood lipids may also be measured in selected patients. See the Diagnostic Tests table in ∞ Chapter 29 for nursing care related to lipid profile studies.

Diagnostic tests to identify subclinical (asymptomatic) CHD may be indicated when multiple risk factors are present.

- *C-reactive protein* is a serum protein associated with inflammatory processes. Recent evidence suggests that elevated blood levels of this protein may be predictive of CHD.
- The *ankle-brachial blood pressure index (ABI)* is an inexpensive, noninvasive test for peripheral vascular disease that may be predictive of CHD. The systolic blood pressure in the brachial, posterior tibial, and dorsalis pedis arteries is measured by Doppler. An ABI of < 0.9 in either leg indicates the presence of peripheral arterial disease and a significant risk for CHD.
- *Exercise ECG testing* assesses the cardiac response to increased workload induced by exercise. The test is considered "positive" for CHD if myocardial ischemia is detected on the ECG (depression of the ST segment by greater than 3 mm; see Figure 30–1 ■), the patient develops chest pain, or the test is stopped due to excess fatigue, dysrhythmias, or other symptoms before the predicted maximal heart rate is achieved.
- *Electron beam computed tomography (EBCT)* creates a three-dimensional image of the heart and coronary arteries that can reveal coronary artery calcification and other abnormalities. A coronary artery calcium score can be calculated from this test, providing additional important information in the diagnosis of CHD. This noninvasive test requires no special preparation, and can identify patients at risk for developing myocardial ischemia.
- *Myocardial perfusion imaging* (see the section on angina that follows) evaluates myocardial blood flow and perfusion, both at rest and during stress testing (exercise or mental stress). These diagnostic tests are further explained in ∞ Chapter 29 and the section on angina. Perfusion imaging studies are costly, and therefore not recommended for routine CHD risk assessment.

Risk Factor Management

Conservative management of CHD focuses on risk factor modification, including smoking, diet, exercise, and management of comorbidities.

SMOKING Smoking cessation reduces the risk for CHD within months after quitting and improves cardiovascular status. People who quit reduce their risk by 50%, regardless of how long they smoked before quitting. For women, the risk becomes equivalent to a nonsmoker within 3 to 5 years of smoking cessation (Woods et al., 2009). In addition, stopping smoking improves HDL levels, lowers LDL levels, and reduces blood viscosity. All smokers are advised to quit with health promotion activities focused on prevention.

DIET The National Cholesterol Education Program (2002) recommend reduced saturated fat and cholesterol intake with strategies to lower LDL levels (Table 30–4). Most fats are a mixture of saturated and unsaturated fatty acids. The highest proportions of saturated fat are found in whole-milk products, red meats, and coconut oil. Recommended proteins include nonfat dairy products, fish, and poultry. Solidified vegetable fats (e.g., margarine, shortening) contain *trans* fatty acids, which behave more like saturated fats. Soft margarines and vegetable oil spreads contain low levels of trans fatty acids, and should be used instead of butter, stick margarine, and shortening. Monounsaturated fats, found in olive, canola, and peanut oils, actually lower LDL and cholesterol levels. Certain cold-water fish, such as tuna, salmon, and mackerel, contain high levels of omega-3 (or n-3) fatty acids, which help raise HDL levels and decrease serum triglycerides, total serum cholesterol, and blood pressure.

In addition, increased intake of soluble fiber (found in oats, psyllium, pectin-rich fruit, and beans) and insoluble fiber (found in whole grains, vegetables, and fruit) is recommended. Folic acid and vitamins B_6 and B_{12} affect homocysteine metabolism, reducing serum levels. Leafy green vegetables (e.g., spinach and broccoli) and legumes (e.g., black-eyed peas, dried beans, and lentils) are rich sources of folate. Meat, fish, and poultry are rich in vitamins B_6 and B_{12}. Vitamin B_6 also is found in soy products; B_{12} is in fortified cereals. Increased intake of antioxidant nutrients (vitamin E, in particular) and foods rich in antioxidants (fruits

TABLE 30–4 Dietary Recommendations to Reduce Total Cholesterol, LDL Levels, and CHD Risk

NUTRIENT	RECOMMENDATION
Calories	Adjusted to attain/maintain desirable body weight
Total fat	25%–35% of total calories
■ Saturated fats	■ < 7% of total calories
■ Polyunsaturated fat	■ Up to 10% of total calories
■ Monounsaturated fat	■ Up to 20% of total calories
■ Cholesterol	■ < 200 mg/day
Carbohydrate (primarily complex carbohydrates, such as whole grains, fruits, and vegetables)	50%–60% of total calories
Dietary fiber	20–30 g/day
Protein	About 15% of total calories

Note: Compiled from Adult Treatment Panel III Final Report by the National Cholesterol Education Program, 2002.

and vegetables) appears to increase HDL levels and have a protective effect on CHD.

In middle-aged and older adults, moderate alcohol intake may reduce the risk for CHD (National Cholesterol Education Program, 2002). Consumption of no more than two drinks per day for men or one drink per day for women is recommended. A drink is 5 ounces of wine, 12 ounces of beer, or 1 1/2 ounces of whiskey. People who do not drink alcohol, however, should not be encouraged to start consuming it as a heart-protective measure.

People who are overweight or obese are encouraged to lose weight through a combination of reduced calorie intake (maintaining a nutritionally sound diet) and increased exercise. High-protein, high-fat weight loss programs are not recommended for weight reduction.

EXERCISE Regular physical exercise reduces the risk for CHD in several ways. It lowers VLDL, LDL, and triglyceride levels, and raises HDL levels. Regular exercise reduces blood pressure and insulin resistance. Unless contraindicated, all patients are encouraged to participate in at least 30 minutes of moderate intensity physical activity 5 to 6 days each week. To achieve weight loss and prevent weight gain, 60 to 90 minutes of moderate intensity exercise daily is recommended (US Department of Health & Human Services, 2005).

HYPERTENSION Although hypertension often cannot be prevented or cured, it can be controlled. Hypertension control (maintaining a blood pressure lower than 140/90 mmHg) is vital to reduce atherosclerosis-promoting effects and to reduce the workload of the heart. Management strategies include reducing sodium intake, increasing calcium intake, regular exercise, stress management, and medications. Hypertension management is discussed in ∞ Chapter 32.

DIABETES Diabetes increases the risk of CHD by accelerating the atherosclerotic process. Weight loss (if appropriate), reduced fat intake, and exercise are particularly important for the diabetic patient. Because hyperglycemia apparently contributes to atherosclerosis, consistent blood glucose management is vital. ∞ See Chapter 20 for detailed discussion about diabetes and blood glucose management.

Medications

Medication to lower total serum cholesterol and LDL levels and to raise HDL levels is an integral part of CHD management. Based on the patient's overall risk for CHD, drug therapy is used in conjunction with diet and other lifestyle changes.

Drugs used to treat hyperlipidemia act specifically by lowering LDL levels. The goal of treatment is to achieve an LDL level of < 130 mg/dL (NCEP, 2002). Medications to treat hyperlipidemia are not inexpensive; the cost–benefit ratio needs to be considered, as long-term treatment may be required. The four major classes of cholesterol-lowering drugs are statins, bile acid sequestrants, nicotinic acid, and fibrates. The nursing implications and patient teaching for these drug classes are outlined in the Medication Administration box on page 918.

The statins, including lovastatin (Mevacor), pravastatin (Pravachol), simvastatin (Zocor), and others, are first-line drugs for treating hyperlipidemia. They effectively lower LDL levels

and may increase in HDL levels. The statins can cause myopathy; all patients are instructed to report muscle pain and weakness or brown urine. Liver function tests are monitored during therapy, as these drugs may increase liver enzyme levels.

The other cholesterol-lowering drugs, such as the bile acid sequestrants, nicotinic acid, and fibrates, are primarily used when combination therapy is required to lower serum cholesterol levels. They also may be used for selected patients, such as younger adults, women who wish to become pregnant, or to specifically lower triglyceride levels.

Patients at high risk for MI are often started on prophylactic low-dose aspirin therapy. The dose ranges from 80 to 325 mg/day. In women, the benefit of low-dose aspirin in reducing the risk for CHD is not clear prior to age 65 (Mosca et al., 2007). Aspirin is contraindicated for patients who have a history of aspirin sensitivity, bleeding disorders, or active peptic ulcer disease. Angiotensin-converting enzyme (ACE) inhibitors or angiotensin receptor blockers also may be prescribed for high-risk patients, including diabetics with other CHD risk factors.

Complementary Therapies

Diet and exercise programs that emphasize physical conditioning and a low-fat diet rich in antioxidants have been shown to be effective in managing CHD (Box 30–3). Supplements of vitamins C, E, B$_6$, B$_{12}$, and folic acid may be beneficial. Other potentially helpful complementary therapies include red wine or grape juice, foods containing bioflavonoids, green tea, nuts, and herbals such as ginkgo biloba, garlic, and curcumin. Emphasize the need for patients to talk to their physician prior to taking any herbal preparations, as interactions with prescribed drugs are common. Behavioral therapies of benefit for patients with CHD include relaxation and stress management; guided imagery; treatment of depression; anger/hostility management; and meditation, tai chi, and yoga.

BOX 30–3 Complementary Therapies: Diet for CHD

Two diet programs have been shown to have a beneficial effect on CHD. The *Pritikin diet* is basically vegetarian, high in complex carbohydrates and fiber, low in cholesterol, and extremely low in fat (< 10% of daily calories). Egg whites and limited amounts of nonfat dairy or soy products are allowed. The Pritikin program requires 45 minutes of walking daily and recommends multivitamin supplements, including vitamins C and E and folate.

The *Ornish diet* also is vegetarian, although egg whites and a cup of nonfat milk or yogurt per day are allowed. No oil or fat is permitted, even for cooking. Two ounces of alcohol a day are permitted. The Ornish program also calls for stress reduction, emotional social support systems, daily stretching, and walking for 1 hour three times a week.

Hypertension is a major, modifiable risk factor for CHD. When used with other lifestyle changes The DASH (Dietary Approaches to Stop Hypertension) eating plan can help to prevent and control blood pressure. The diet is heavy on grains (six to eight servings daily), vegetables (four to five servings daily) and fruits (four to five servings daily) and limiting sodium (1500 to 2300 milligrams daily), fats, meats and sweets. Refer to the U.S. Department of Health and Human Services website for a complete brochure.

MEDICATION ADMINISTRATION Cholesterol-Lowering Drugs

STATINS

Atorvastatin (Lipitor)

Fluvastatin (Lescol)

Lovastatin (Mevacor)

Pravastatin (Pravachol)

Rosuvastatin (Crestor)

Simvastatin (Zocor)

Statins inhibit the enzyme HMG-CoA reductase in the liver, lowering LDL synthesis and serum levels. The statins are first-line treatment for elevated LDL, used in conjunction with diet and lifestyle changes. Although their side effects are minimal, they may cause increased serum liver enzyme levels and myopathy.

Nursing Responsibilities

- Monitor serum cholesterol and liver enzyme levels before and during therapy. Report elevated liver enzyme levels.
- Assess for muscle pain and tenderness. Monitor CPK level if present.
- If taking digoxin concurrently, monitor for and report digoxin toxicity.

Health Education for the Patient and Family

- Promptly report muscle pain, tenderness, or weakness; skin rash or hives, or changes in skin color; abdominal pain, nausea, or vomiting.
- Do not use these drugs if you are pregnant or plan to become pregnant.
- Inform your doctor if you are taking any other medications concurrently.

BILE ACID SEQUESTRANTS

Cholestyramine (Questran)

Colestipol (Colestid)

Colesevelam (Welchol)

Bile acid sequestrants lower LDL levels by binding bile acids in the intestine, reducing its reabsorption and cholesterol production in the liver. They are used in combination therapy regimens and for women who are considering pregnancy. Their primary disadvantages are inconvenience of administration due to bulk and gastrointestinal side effects such as constipation.

Nursing Responsibilities

- Mix cholestyramine and colestipol powders with 4 to 6 oz of water or juice; administer once or twice a day as ordered with meals.
- Store in a tightly closed container.

Health Education for the Patient and Family

- Promptly report constipation, severe gastric distress with nausea and vomiting, unexplained weight loss, black or bloody stools, or sudden back pain to your doctor.
- Drinking ample amounts of fluid while taking these drugs reduces problems of constipation and bloating.
- Do not omit doses as this may affect the absorption of other drugs you are taking.

CHOLESTEROL ABSORPTION INHIBITORS

Ezetimibe (Zetia)

Cholesterol absorption inhibitors block absorption in the small intestine. Contraindicated with acute liver disease or hepatic insufficiency.

Nursing Responsibilities

- Can initially increase liver enzymes when used with statins, resolves with continued use.
- Can be taken without regard to meals.

NICOTINIC ACID

Niacin (Nicobid, Nicolar, Niaspan, others)

Nicotinic acid in both prescription and nonprescription forms lowers total and LDL cholesterol and triglyceride levels. The crystalline form and Niaspan, a prescription extended-release tablet, also raise HDL levels. Because the doses required to achieve significant cholesterol-lowering effects are associated with multiple side effects, nicotinic acid generally is used in combination therapy, particularly with the statin drugs.

Nursing Responsibilities

- Give oral preparations with meals and accompanied by a cold beverage to minimize GI effects.
- Administer with caution to patients with active liver disease, peptic ulcer disease, gout, or type 2 diabetes.
- Monitor blood glucose, uric acid levels, and liver function tests during treatment.

Patient and Family Teaching

- Flushing of face, neck, and ears may occur within 2 hours following dose; these effects generally subside as treatment continues. Alcohol use during nicotinic acid therapy may worsen this effect.
- Report weakness or dizziness with changes in posture (lying to sitting; sitting to standing) to your doctor. Change positions slowly to reduce the risk of injury.

FIBRIC ACID DERIVATIVES

Gemfibrozil (Lopid)

Fenofibrate (Tricor, Lipofen)

Clofibrate (Atromid-S)

The fibrates are used to lower serum triglyceride levels; they have only a slight to modest effect on LDL. They affect lipid regulation by blocking triglyceride synthesis. They are used to treat very high triglyceride levels, and may be used in combination with statins.

Nursing Responsibilities

- Monitor serum LDL and VLDL levels, electrolytes, glucose, liver enzymes, renal function tests, and CBC during therapy. Report abnormal values.
- Up to 2 months of treatment may be required to achieve a therapeutic effect; rebound, with decreasing benefit, may occur in the second or third month of treatment.

Patient and Family Teaching

- Take with meals if the drug causes gastric distress.
- Promptly report flulike symptoms (fatigue, muscle aching, soreness, or weakness) to your doctor.
- Do not use this drug if you are pregnant or plan to become pregnant. Use reliable birth control measures while taking this drug.
- Contact your doctor before stopping this drug and before taking any over-the-counter preparations.

✍ Nursing Care

Nurses are instrumental in educating adults about their risk for coronary heart disease, promoting participation in screening programs to identify that risk, and teaching all patients measures to reduce their risk for CHD.

Health Promotion

Present information about healthy lifestyle habits to community and religious groups, school children (grades K through 12), and the media. Work with local governments and organizations to create venues and opportunities that promote a healthy life style. Walking and bicycle lanes are a safe alternative to driving that incorporates exercise into the daily routine. Lobby with smoking prevention/cessation groups against tobacco advertising aimed at youth. While promoting a healthy diet, work with school systems to remove high fructose drinks and fat laden snacks from school vending machines. Be a model of healthy life style habits, taking care of yourself, exercising and eating right. In promoting healthy lifestyle habits, nurses can positively affect the incidence, morbidity, and mortality from CHD.

Strongly encourage all patients to avoid smoking in the first place, and to stop all forms of tobacco use. Discuss the adverse effects of smoking and the benefits of quitting. Provide information about dietary recommendations to maintain a healthy weight and optimal cholesterol levels. Discuss the benefits and importance of regular exercise. Finally, encourage patients with cardiovascular risk factors to undergo regular screening for hypertension, diabetes, and abnormal blood lipids.

Assessment

Nursing assessment for CHD focuses on identifying risk factors.

- *Health history:* Current manifestations such as chest pain or heaviness, shortness of breath, weakness; current diet, exercise patterns, and medications; smoking history and pattern of alcohol intake; history of heart disease, hypertension, or diabetes; family history of CHD or other cardiac problems.
- *Physical examination:* Current weight and its appropriateness for height; body mass index; waist-to-hip ratio; blood pressure; strength and equality of peripheral pulses.

Nursing Diagnoses and Interventions

Imbalanced Nutrition: More than Body Requirements

This nursing diagnosis may be appropriate for patients who are obese, have a waist-to-hip ratio greater than 0.8 (female) or 0.9 (male), or whose diet history or serum cholesterol levels indicate a need to reduce fat and cholesterol intake. ∞ See Chapters 21 and 22 for more information about assessing obesity.

- Encourage assessment of food intake and eating patterns to help identify areas that can be improved. *Patients often are unaware of their fat and cholesterol intake, particularly when many meals are eaten away from home. Careful assessment increases awareness and allows the patient to make conscious changes.*
- Discuss AHA and therapeutic lifestyle change (TLC) dietary recommendations, emphasizing the role of diet in heart disease. Provide guidance regarding specific food choices with healthy alternatives. *Specific diet information and suggestions help the patient make better food choices.*
- Refer to clinical dietitian for diet planning and further teaching. Suggest cookbooks that offer low-fat recipes to encourage healthier eating, and provide AHA and American Cancer Society recipe pamphlets and information on low-fat eating. *These resources provide tools for the patient to use as eating patterns change.*
- Encourage gradual but progressive dietary changes. *Drastic changes in eating patterns may cause frustration and discourage the patient from maintaining a healthy diet over the long term.*
- Discourage use of high-fat, low-carbohydrate, or other fad diets for weight loss. *These diets may adversely affect serum cholesterol and triglyceride levels, and often are too drastic to maintain over the long term.*
- Encourage reasonable goals for weight loss (e.g., 1.0 to 1.5 lb per week and a 10% weight loss over 6 months). Provide information about weight loss programs and support groups such as Weight Watchers and Take Off Pounds Sensibly (TOPS). *Gradual but steady weight loss is more likely to be sustained. Recognized programs that emphasize healthy eating provide support and incentive for making lifetime dietary changes.*

Ineffective Health Maintenance

Patients with risk factors for CHD may be unable to identify or independently manage their risk factors.

- Discuss risk factors for CHD, stressing that changing or managing those factors that can be modified reduces the patient's overall risk for the disease. *Patients with significant nonmodifiable risk factors may be discouraged, reducing their ability to eliminate or control modifiable risk factors.*
- Discuss the immediate benefits of smoking cessation. Provide resource materials from the AHA, the American Lung Association, and the American Cancer Society. Refer

---

EVIDENCE FOR NURSING CARE — **The Patient with Atherosclerosis**

Selected resources that nurses may find helpful when planning evidence-based nursing care follow.

- Brackbill, M. L., Sytsma, C. S., & Sykes, K. (2009). Perioperative outcomes of coronary artery bypass grafting: Effects of metabolic syndrome and patient's sex. *American Journal of Critical Care, 18*(5), 468–473.
- Eastwood, J., Doering, L., Roper, J., & Hays, R. D. (2008). Uncertainty and health-related quality of life 1 year after coronary angiography. *American Journal of Critical Care.* Retrieved from http://ajcc.aacnjournals.org/misc/journalclub.shtml
- Palatnik, A. M. (2009). Too fast, too slow, too ugly: Dysrhythmias that every nurse should recognize. *Nursing2009, 39*(9), 38–45.
- Prevention of secondary disease: Lipid screening and cardiovascular risk. (2007). *New York State Department of Health—State/Local Government Agency [U.S.]. National Guideline Clearinghouse.* Retrieved from http://www.guideline.gov/summary/summary.aspx?doc_id=10963&nbr=005743&string=arteriosclerosis

to a structured smoking cessation program to increase the likelihood of success in quitting. *Long-time smokers may assume that the damage from smoking has already been done, and quitting would not be "worth the price."*

■ Help the patient identify specific sources of psychosocial and physical support for smoking cessation, dietary, and lifestyle changes. *Support persons, groups, and aids such as nicotine patches help the patient achieve success and provide encouragement during difficult times (such as withdrawal symptoms).*

■ Discuss the benefits of regular exercise for cardiovascular health and weight loss. Help identify favorite forms of exercise or physical activity. Encourage planning for 30 minutes of continuous aerobic activity (i.e., walking, running, bicycling, swimming) four to five times a week. Encourage identification of an "exercise buddy" to help maintain motivation. *Engaging in preferred activities with a partner maintains motivation and increases the likelihood of maintaining an exercise program. Encourage continuation of the plan, even when days are missed. Exercise is cumulative, so increasing the duration of exercise on subsequent days can "make up" for a lost day.*

■ Provide information and teaching about prescribed medications such as cholesterol-lowering drugs. Discuss the relationship between hypertension, diabetes, and CHD. *Teaching is important to promote understanding of and compliance with the prescribed drug regimen.*

Community-Based Care

Encourage participation in some form of cardiac rehabilitation program. Formal programs provide comprehensive assessment of, interventions for, and teaching of patients with cardiac disease. Monitored exercise and information about risk factors help patients identify ways to lower their risk for CHD.

Because patients themselves are primarily responsible for maintaining the lifestyle changes necessary to reduce the risk of CHD, provide teaching and support as outlined in the previous section. Assist the patient to make healthy choices and reinforce positive changes. Emphasize the importance of regular follow-up appointments to monitor progress.

The Patient with Angina Pectoris

Angina pectoris, or *angina*, is chest pain resulting from reduced coronary blood flow, which causes a temporary imbalance between myocardial blood supply and demand. The imbalance may be due to coronary heart disease, atherosclerosis, or vessel constriction that impairs myocardial blood supply. Hypermetabolic conditions such as exercise, thyrotoxicosis, stimulant abuse (e.g., cocaine), hyperthyroidism, and emotional stress can increase myocardial oxygen demand, precipitating angina. Anemia, heart failure, ventricular hypertrophy, or pulmonary diseases may affect blood and oxygen supplies as well, causing angina.

Pathophysiology

The imbalance between myocardial blood supply and demand causes temporary and reversible myocardial ischemia. **Ischemia**, deficient blood flow to tissue, may be caused by partial obstruction of a coronary artery, coronary artery spasm, or a thrombus.

Obstruction of a coronary artery deprives cells in the region of the heart normally supplied by that vessel of oxygen and nutrients needed for metabolic processes. Cellular processes are compromised as ATP stores are depleted. Reduced oxygen causes cells to switch from aerobic metabolism to anaerobic metabolism. Anaerobic metabolism causes lactic acid to build up in the cells. It also affects cell membrane permeability, releasing substances such as histamine, kinins, and specific enzymes that stimulate terminal nerve fibers in the cardiac muscle and send pain impulses to the central nervous system. The pain radiates to the upper body because the heart shares the same dermatome as this region. Return of adequate circulation provides the nutrients needed by cells, and clears the waste products. More than 30 minutes of ischemia irreversibly damages myocardial cells (necrosis).

Three types of angina have been identified:

■ *Stable angina* is the most common and predictable form of angina. It occurs with a predictable amount of activity or stress, and is a common manifestation of CHD. Stable angina usually occurs when the work of the heart is increased by physical exertion, exposure to cold, or by stress. Stable angina is relieved by rest and nitrates.

■ *Prinzmetal's (variant) angina* is atypical angina that occurs unpredictably (unrelated to activity), and often at night. It is caused by coronary artery spasm with or without an atherosclerotic lesion. The exact mechanism of coronary artery spasm is unknown. It may result from hyperactive sympathetic nervous system responses, altered calcium flow in smooth muscle, or reduced prostaglandins that promote vasodilation.

■ *Unstable angina* occurs with increasing frequency, severity, and duration. Pain is unpredictable and occurs with decreasing levels of activity or stress and may occur at rest. Patients with unstable angina are at risk for myocardial infarction. Unstable angina is discussed further in the section on acute coronary syndromes.

Silent myocardial ischemia, or asymptomatic ischemia, is thought to be common in people with CHD. Silent ischemia may occur with either activity or with mental stress. Mental stress increases the heart rate and blood pressure, increasing myocardial oxygen demand (McCance & Huether, 2006). Like symptomatic angina, silent myocardial ischemia is associated with an increased chance of myocardial infarction and death.

> **FAST FACTS**
> ■ Stable angina occurs with a predictable amount of activity or stress.
> ■ Unstable angina occurs with increasing frequency and severity; it may occur at times unrelated to activity or stress.
> ■ Prinzmetal's angina is the only type of angina not necessarily related to coronary heart disease and atherosclerosis, developing due to coronary artery spasm.

Course and Manifestations

The cardinal manifestation of angina is chest pain. The pain typically is precipitated by an identifiable event, such as physical activity, strong emotion, stress, eating a heavy meal, or

MANIFESTATIONS of Angina

- Chest pain: Substernal or precordial (across the chest wall); may radiate to neck, arms, shoulders, or jaw
- Quality: Tight, squeezing, constricting, or heavy sensation; may also be described as burning, aching, choking, dull, or constant
- Associated manifestations: Dyspnea, pallor, tachycardia, anxiety, and fear
- Atypical manifestations: Indigestion, nausea, vomiting, upper back pain
- Precipitating factors: Exercise or activity, strong emotion, stress, cold, heavy meal
- Relieving factors: Rest, position change, nitroglycerine

exposure to cold. The classic sequence of angina is activity–pain, rest–relief. The patient may describe the pain as a tight, squeezing, heavy pressure, or constricting sensation. It characteristically begins beneath the sternum and may radiate to the jaw, neck, shoulder or arm. Less characteristically, the pain may be felt in the jaw, epigastric region, or back. Anginal pain usually occurs in a *crescendo-decrescendo* pattern (increasing to a peak, then gradually decreasing) lasting typically 2 to 5 minutes. It is generally relieved by rest. Additional manifestations of angina include dyspnea, pallor, tachycardia, and great anxiety and fear.

Women frequently present with atypical symptoms of angina, including indigestion or nausea, vomiting, and upper back pain. The manifestations of angina are summarized in the following box.

The severity of angina can be graded by the degree to which it limits the patient's activities. Class I angina does not occur with ordinary physical activities. It is prompted by strenuous, rapid, or prolonged physical exertion. Class II angina may develop with rapid or prolonged walking or stair climbing, whereas Class III angina significantly limits ordinary physical activities. The patient with Class IV angina may have angina at rest, as well as with physical activity.

Interdisciplinary Care

The management of stable angina focuses on maintaining coronary blood flow and cardiac function. Stable angina often can be managed by medical therapy. Measures to restore coronary blood flow are discussed in the section on acute coronary syndrome. As for CHD, risk factor management is a vital component of care for the patient with angina (see the preceding section of this chapter).

Diagnosis

The diagnosis of angina is based on past medical history and family history, a comprehensive description of the chest pain, and physical assessment findings. Laboratory tests may confirm the presence of risk factors, such as an abnormal blood lipid profile and elevated blood glucose. Diagnostic tests provide information about overall cardiac function.

Common diagnostic tests to assess for coronary heart disease and angina include electrocardiography, stress testing, nuclear medicine studies, echocardiography (ultrasound), and coronary angiography.

ELECTROCARDIOGRAPHY A resting ECG may be normal, may show nonspecific changes in the ST segment and T wave, or may show evidence of previous myocardial infarction. Characteristic ECG changes are seen during anginal episodes. During periods of ischemia, the ST segment is depressed or downsloping, and the T wave may flatten or invert (Figure 30–1). These changes reverse when ischemia is relieved. For more details about the ECG, its waveforms, and its uses, ∞ see Chapter 29.

STRESS ELECTROCARDIOGRAPHY Stress electrocardiography (exercise stress test) uses ECGs to monitor the cardiac response to an increased workload during progressive exercise. See Diagnostic Tests in the previous chapter for more information about exercise stress tests.

RADIONUCLIDE TESTING Radionuclide testing is a safe, noninvasive technique to evaluate myocardial perfusion and left ventricular function. The amount of radioisotope injected is very small; no special radiation precautions are required during or after the scan. Thallium-201 or a technetium-based radiocompound is injected intravenously, and the heart is scanned with a radiation detector. Ischemic or infarcted cells of the myocardium do not take up the substance normally, appearing as a "cold spot" on the scan. If the ischemia is transient, these spots gradually fill in, indicating the reversibility of the process. With severe ischemia or a myocardial infarction, these areas remain devoid of radioactivity.

Figure 30–1 ■ ECG changes during an episode of angina. Note characteristic T-wave inversion and ST-segment depression of myocardial ischemia.

Left ventricular function can also be evaluated. Whereas the ejection fraction (portion of blood ejected from the left ventricle during systole), normally increases during exercise, it may actually decrease in coronary heart disease and stress-induced ischemia.

Radionuclide testing may be combined with pharmacologic stress testing for patients who are physically unable to exercise or to detect subclinical myocardial ischemia. A vasodilator is injected to induce the same ischemic changes that occur with exercise in the diseased heart. Coronary arteries unaffected by atherosclerosis dilate in response to the drugs, increasing blood flow to already well-perfused tissue. This reduces flow to ischemic muscle, called *myocardial steal syndrome*.

ECHOCARDIOGRAPHY *Echocardiography* is a noninvasive test that uses ultrasound to evaluate cardiac structure and function. It may be done at rest, during supine exercise, or immediately following upright exercise to evaluate movement of the myocardial wall and assess for possible ischemia or infarction.

Transesophageal echocardiography (TEE) uses ultrasound to identify abnormal blood flow patterns as well as cardiac structures. In TEE, the probe is on the tip of an endoscope inserted into the esophagus, positioning it close to the posterior heart (especially the left atrium and the aorta). It avoids interference by breasts, ribs, or lungs. ∞ See Diagnostic Tests in Chapter 29 for more information about these tests and the nursing implications.

CORONARY ANGIOGRAPHY *Coronary angiography* is the gold standard for evaluating the coronary arteries. Guided by fluoroscopy, a catheter introduced into the femoral or brachial artery is threaded into the coronary artery. Dye is injected into each coronary opening, allowing visualization of the main coronary branches and any abnormalities, such as stenosis or obstruction. Narrowing of the vessel lumen by more than 50% is considered significant; most lesions that cause symptoms involve more than 70% narrowing. Vessel obstructions are noted on a coronary artery "map" that provides a guide for tracking disease progression and for elective treatment with angioplasty or cardiac surgery. During angiogram, the drug ergonovine maleate may be injected to induce coronary artery spasm and diagnose Prinzmetal's angina. Nursing care of the patient undergoing a coronary angiogram is summarized in the box on page 923.

Medications

Drugs may be used for both acute and long-term relief of angina. The goal of drug treatment is to reduce oxygen demand and increase oxygen supply to the myocardium. Three main classes of drugs are used to treat angina: nitrates, beta blockers, and calcium channel blockers.

NITRATES Nitrates, including nitroglycerin and longer-acting nitrate preparations, are used to treat acute anginal attacks and prevent angina.

Sublingual nitroglycerin is the drug of choice to treat acute angina. It acts within 1 to 2 minutes, decreasing myocardial work and oxygen demand through venous and arterial dilation,

which in turn reduce preload and afterload. It may also improve myocardial oxygen supply by dilating collateral blood vessels and reducing stenosis. Rapid-acting nitroglycerin is also available as a buccal spray in a metered system. For some patients, this may be easier to handle than small nitroglycerin tablets.

> **PRACTICE ALERT**
> Sublingual nitroglycerin tablets and nitroglycerine spray are the only medications appropriate to treat an acute anginal attack.

Longer-acting nitroglycerin preparations (oral tablets, ointment, or transdermal patches) are used to prevent attacks of angina, not to treat an acute attack. The primary problem with longterm nitrate use is the development of *tolerance*, a decreasing effect from the same dose of medication. Tolerance can be limited by a dosing schedule that allows a nitrate-free period of at least 8 to 10 hours daily. This is usually scheduled at night, when angina is less likely to occur.

Headache is a common side effect of nitrates, and may limit their usefulness. Nausea, dizziness, and hypotension are also common effects of therapy.

BETA BLOCKERS Beta blockers, including propranolol, metoprolol, nadolol, and atenolol, are considered first-line drugs to treat stable angina. They block the cardiac-stimulating effects of norepinephrine and epinephrine, preventing anginal attacks by reducing heart rate, myocardial contractility, and blood pressure, thus reducing myocardial oxygen demand. Beta blockers may be used alone or with other medications to prevent angina.

Beta blockers are contraindicated for patients with asthma or severe COPD (∞ see Chapter 37) because they may cause severe bronchospasm. They are not used in patients with significant bradycardia, or AV conduction blocks, and are used cautiously in heart failure, Beta blockers are not used to treat Prinzmetal's angina because they may make it worse.

CALCIUM CHANNEL BLOCKERS Calcium channel blockers reduce myocardial oxygen demand and increase myocardial blood and oxygen supply. These drugs, which include verapamil, diltiazem, and nifedipine, lower blood pressure, reduce myocardial contractility, and, in some cases, lower the heart rate, decreasing myocardial oxygen demand. They are also potent coronary vasodilators, effectively increasing oxygen supply. Like beta blockers, calcium channel blockers act too slowly to effectively treat an acute attack of angina; they are used for long-term prophylaxis. Because they may actually increase ischemia and mortality in patients with heart failure or left ventricular dysfunction, these drugs are not usually prescribed in the initial treatment of angina. They are used cautiously in patients with dysrhythmias, heart failure, or hypotension.

The nursing implications of antianginal medications are summarized in the Medication Administration box on page 923.

ASPIRIN The patient with angina, particularly unstable angina, is at risk for myocardial infarction because of significant narrowing of the coronary arteries. Low-dose aspirin (80 to 325 mg/day) is often prescribed to reduce the risk of platelet aggregation and thrombus formation.

MEDICATION ADMINISTRATION   Antianginal Medications

ORGANIC NITRATES

Nitroglycerin (Nitropaste, Nitro-Dur, Nitro-Bid, Nitrol, Transderm-Nitro, Nitrogard, Nitrodisc, Tridil)

Isosorbide dinitrate (Isordil)

Isosorbide mononitrate (ISMO)

Amyl nitrite

Nitrates dilate both arterial and venous vessels, depending on the dose. Coronary artery vasodilation increases blood flow and myocardial oxygen supply. Venous dilation allows peripheral blood pooling, reducing venous return, preload, and cardiac work. Arterial dilation reduces vascular resistance and afterload, also reducing cardiac work. Sublingual nitroglycerin (NTG) tablets are used to treat and prevent acute anginal attacks (when taken prophylactically before activity). Nitrates are administered sublingually, by buccal spray, or intravenously for immediate effect, or orally or topically for sustained effect.

Nursing Responsibilities

- Dilute intravenous nitroglycerin before infusing; use only glass bottles for the mixture. Nitroglycerin adheres to PVC bags and tubing, affecting the amount of drug that is delivered. Use non-PVC infusion tubing.
- Wear gloves when applying nitroglycerin paste or ointment to prevent absorbing the drug through the skin. Measure dose carefully and spread evenly in a 2-by-3 inch area.
- Remove nitroglycerin patches or ointment at night to help prevent tolerance.

Health Education for the Patient and Family

- Use only the sublingual, buccal, and spray forms of nitrates to treat acute angina.
- If the first nitrate dose does not relieve angina within 5 minutes, take a second dose. After 5 more minutes, you may take a third dose if needed. If the pain is unrelieved or lasts for 20 minutes or longer, seek medical assistance immediately.
- Carry a supply of nitroglycerin tablets with you. Dissolve sublingual nitroglycerin tablets under the tongue or between the upper lip and gum. Do not eat, drink, or smoke until the tablet is completely dissolved.
- Keep sublingual tablets in their original amber glass bottle to protect them from heat, light, and moisture. Replace your supply every 6 months.
- You may experience a burning or tingling sensation under the tongue and develop a transient headache when you take the drug. These are expected; the headache will diminish over time.
- Use caution when standing from a sitting position; nitroglycerine may make you lightheaded.
- Rotate ointment or transdermal patch application sites. Apply to a hairless area; spread ointment evenly without rubbing or massaging. Remove the patch or residual ointment at bedtime daily. Apply a fresh dose in the morning.
- If you are using a long-acting nitrate, keep a supply of immediate-acting nitrates to treat acute angina.

BETA BLOCKERS

Atenolol (Tenormin)

Carvedilol (Coreg)

Metoprolol (Lopressor, Toprol)

Nadolol (Corgard)

Propranolol (Inderal)

Beta blockers decrease cardiac workload by blocking beta receptors on the heart muscle, decreasing heart rate, contractility, myocardial oxygen consumption, and blood pressure. Beta blockers also reduce *reflex tachycardia* (an increased heart rate in response to stimuli such as increased SNS activity or vasodilation), which may develop with other antianginal drugs. Beta blockers are frequently prescribed as antianginal and antihypertensive agents.

Nursing Responsibilities

- Document heart rate and blood pressure before administering the medication. Withhold drug if the heart rate is below 50 BPM or the blood pressure is below prescribed limits. Notify the physician.
- Assess for and report possible contraindications to therapy, including heart failure, bradycardia, AV block, asthma, or COPD.
- Concurrent use of beta blockers and calcium channel blockers increases the risk for heart failure; notify the physician if these drugs are prescribed together.
- Do not abruptly discontinue these drugs after long-term therapy, as this can increase heart rate, contractility, and blood pressure, and cause fatal dysrhythmia, myocardial infarction, or stroke.

Health Education for the Patient and Family

- Beta blockers help prevent angina but will not relieve an acute attack. Keep a supply of fast-acting nitrates on hand for acute anginal attacks.
- Do not suddenly stop taking this medication. Discuss discontinuing this medication with your doctor.
- Take your pulse daily. Do not take the drug, and contact your doctor if your heart rate is below 50 BPM. Check your blood pressure frequently.
- Report a slow or irregular pulse, swelling or weight gain, or difficulty breathing to your doctor.

CALCIUM CHANNEL BLOCKERS

Amlodipine (Norvasc)

Bepridil (Vascor)

Diltiazem (Cardizem)

Felodipine (Plendil)

Isradipine (DynaCirc)

Nicardipine (Cardene)

Nifedipine (Adalat, Procardia)

Nimodipine (Nimotop)

Verapamil (Isoptin, Calan)

Calcium channel blockers are used to control angina, hypertension, and dysrhythmias. By blocking the entry of calcium into cells, these drugs reduce contractility, slow the heart rate and conduction, and cause vasodilation. Calcium channel blockers increase myocardial oxygen supply by dilating the coronary arteries; they decrease the workload of the heart by lowering vascular resistance and oxygen demand. Calcium channel blockers are often prescribed for patients with coronary artery spasm (Prinzmetal's angina).

Nursing Responsibilities

- Do not mix verapamil in any solution containing sodium bicarbonate. Administer IV push verapamil over 2 to 3 minutes.

(continued)

- Document blood pressure and heart rate before administering the drug. Withhold the drug if the heart rate is below 50 BPM. Notify the physician.
- The nifedipine capsule may be punctured and administered by extracting the liquid with a syringe and squirting the dose under the patient's tongue (discard the needle first!).
- Use caution when giving a calcium channel blocker with other cardiac depressants, such as beta blockers. Concomitant administration with nitrates may cause excessive vasodilation.
- Manifestations of toxicity include nausea, generalized weakness, signs of decreased cardiac output, hypotension, bradycardia, and AV block. Report these findings immediately. Maintain intravenous access, and slowly administer intravenous calcium chloride. Do not infuse large volumes of fluid to treat hypotension as heart failure may result.

Health Education for the Patient and Family
- Take your pulse before taking the drug. Do not take the drug, and notify physician if your heart rate drops below 50 BPM.
- Keep a fresh supply of immediate-acting nitrate available to treat acute anginal attacks. Calcium channel blockers will not work fast enough to relieve an acute attack.

Nursing Care

The focus of nursing care for patients with angina is similar to the collaborative care focus: to reduce myocardial oxygen demand and improve the oxygen supply. Angina usually is treated in community settings; the primary nursing focus is education.

Health Promotion

In addition to health promotion measures, emphasize the importance of active CHD risk factor management to slow progression of the disease. Encourage patients to stop smoking. Discuss the use of cholesterol-lowering drug therapy with patients who have hypercholesterolemia. Encourage regular aerobic exercise and a diet based on AHA or National Cholesterol Education Program guidelines.

Assessment

Focused assessment data for the patient with angina includes the following:

- *Health history:* Chest pain, including type, intensity, duration, frequency, aggravating factors and relief measures; associated symptoms; history of other cardiovascular disorders, peripheral vascular disease, or stroke; current medications and treatment; usual diet, exercise, and alcohol intake patterns; smoking history; use of other recreational drugs.
- *Physical assessment:* Vital signs and heart sounds; strength and equality of peripheral pulses; skin color and temperature (central and peripheral); physical appearance during pain episode (e.g., shortness of breath, apparent anxiety, color, diaphoresis).

Nursing Diagnoses and Interventions

High-priority nursing diagnoses for patients with angina include ineffective cardiac tissue perfusion and management of the prescribed therapeutic regimen.

Ineffective Tissue Perfusion: Cardiac

Anginal pain results from impaired blood flow and oxygen supply to the myocardium. Nursing interventions can both prevent ischemia and shorten the duration of pain.

- Keep prescribed nitroglycerin tablets at the patient's side so one can be taken at the onset of pain. *Anginal pain indicates myocardial ischemia. Nitroglycerin reduces cardiac work and may improve myocardial blood flow, relieving ischemia and pain.*

- Start oxygen at 4 to 6 L/min per nasal cannula or as prescribed. *Supplemental oxygen reduces myocardial hypoxia.*
- Space activities to allow rest between them. *Activity increases cardiac work and may precipitate angina. Spacing of activities allows the heart to recover.*
- Teach about prescribed medications to maintain myocardial perfusion and reduce cardiac work. Emphasize that long-acting nitrates, beta blockers, and calcium channel blockers are used to *prevent* anginal attacks, not to *treat* an acute attack. *It is important for the patient to understand the purpose and use of prescribed drugs to maintain optimal myocardial perfusion.*
- Instruct to take sublingual nitroglycerin before engaging in activities that precipitate angina (e.g., climbing stairs, sexual intercourse). *This prophylactic dose of nitroglycerin helps maintain cardiac perfusion when increased work is anticipated, preventing ischemia and chest pain.*
- Encourage to implement and maintain a progressive exercise program under the supervision of the primary care provider or a cardiac rehabilitation professional. *Exercise slows the atherosclerotic process and helps develop collateral circulation to the heart muscle.*
- Refer to a smoking cessation program as indicated. *Nicotine causes vasoconstriction and increases the heart rate, decreasing myocardial perfusion and increasing cardiac workload.*

Risk for Ineffective Therapeutic Regimen Management

Denial may be strong in the patient with angina pectoris. Because many people think of the heart as the locus of life itself, problems such as angina remind people of their mortality, an uncomfortable fact. Denial may lead to "forgetting" to take prescribed medications or to attempting activities that will precipitate angina. Some patients, by contrast, may become "cardiac cripples," afraid to engage in activities because of anticipated chest pain. Their inactivity may actually hasten the atherosclerotic process and inhibit collateral circulation development, worsening angina.

- Assess knowledge and understanding of angina. *Assessment allows tailoring of teaching and interventions to the needs of the patient.*
- Teach about angina and atherosclerosis as needed, building on current knowledge base. *This can help the patient understand*

that angina is a manageable disease and that pain can usually be controlled and the disease progress slowed.

- Provide written and verbal instructions about prescribed medications and their use. *Written instructions reinforce teaching and are available to the patient for future reference.*
- Stress the importance of taking chest pains seriously while maintaining a positive attitude. *Although it is vital to recognize the significance of chest pain and deal with it appropriately, it is also important to maintain a positive outlook.*
- Refer to a cardiac rehabilitation program or other organized activities and support groups for patients with coronary artery disease. *Programs such as these help the patient develop risk factor management strategies, maintain a program of supervised activity, and gain coping skills.*

Community-Based Care

Many patients with stable angina manage their pain effectively, continuing to live active and productive lives. To promote effective management of this disorder, include the following topics in teaching for home care.

- Coronary heart disease and the processes that cause chest pain, including the relationship between the pain and reduced blood flow to the heart muscle.
- Use and effects (desired and adverse) of prescribed medications; importance of not discontinuing medications abruptly.
- Nitroglycerine use for acute angina: Always carry several tablets (not the entire supply); prophylactic use before activities that often cause chest pain; take tablet at first indication of pain rather than waiting to see if the pain develops; seek immediate medical assistance if three nitroglycerin tablets over 15 to 20 minutes do not relieve the pain. Instruct patient to not continue the series of nitroglycerin if dizziness or light-headedness develops but to seek immediate medical assistance.
- The importance of calling 911 or going to the emergency department immediately for unrelieved chest pain.
- Appropriate storage of nitroglycerin: This unstable compound needs to be stored in a cool, dry, dark place; no more than a 6-month supply should be kept on hand.

For the patient who has undergone cardiac surgery, also include the following:

- Respiratory care, activity, and pain management
- The importance of actively participating in rehabilitation
- Manifestations of infection or other potential complications and their management

The Patient with Acute Coronary Syndrome

Acute coronary syndrome (ACS) is a condition of unstable cardiac ischemia. ACS includes unstable angina and acute myocardial ischemia with or without significant injury of myocardial tissue. Although the term ACS may, in some cases, be applied to acute myocardial infarction (myocardial tissue death), myocardial infarction is discussed separately in the next section of this chapter. An estimated 1.5 million Americans are admitted to the hospital annually with ACS (AHA, 2009).

FAST FACTS

- Acute coronary syndrome (severe cardiac ischemia), a common cause of hospital admission, includes unstable angina and acute myocardial infarction.
- Unstable angina is characterized by injury to myocardial cells; with prompt restoration of blood flow, muscle tissue recovers.
- Myocardial infarction is characterized by necrosis and death of myocardial cells; scar tissue forms and functional muscle is lost.
- ACS is the most common identified cause of sudden cardiac death (AHA, 2009).

Pathophysiology

ACS is a dynamic state in which coronary blood flow is acutely reduced, but not fully occluded. Myocardial cells are injured by the acute ischemia that results. Most people affected by ACS have significant stenosis of one or more coronary arteries.

ACS is precipitated by one or more of the following processes: (1) rupture or erosion of atherosclerotic plaque with formation of a blood clot that does not fully occlude the vessel; (2) coronary artery spasm (e.g. Prinzmetal's angina); (3) progressive vessel obstruction by atherosclerotic plaque or restenosis following a percutaneous revascularization (PCR) procedure; (4) inflammation of a coronary artery; or (5) increased myocardial oxygen demand and/or decreased supply (e.g. acute blood loss or anemia). Of these, ruptured or eroded plaque is the predominant pathophysiology underlying ACS (AHA, 2005). Plaque rupture often is triggered by hemodynamic factors such as increased heart rate, blood flow, and blood pressure in response to a surge of sympathetic nervous system activity. Increased SNS activity also is thought to contribute to the higher incidence of plaque rupture within the first hour of arising from bed in the morning (Heuther & McCance, 2008).

When atherosclerotic plaque ruptures or erodes, the exposed lipid core of the plaque stimulates platelet aggregation and the extrinsic clotting pathway. Thrombin is generated and fibrin is deposited, forming a clot that severely impairs or obstructs blood flow to tissue distal to the area of plaque rupture. As a result, these cells become ischemic.

Injured myocardial cells contract less effectively, potentially reducing cardiac output if a large area of myocardium is affected. Lactic acid released from ischemic cells stimulates pain receptors, causing chest pain. Ischemia and injury affect electrical impulse conduction, producing inversion of the T wave and possibly elevation of the ST segment on the ECG.

Manifestations

The cardinal manifestation of ACS is chest pain, usually substernal or epigastric. The pain often radiates to the neck, left shoulder, and/or left arm. The pain may occur at rest and typically lasts longer than 10 to 20 minutes. In ACS, the chest pain is more severe and prolonged than that previously experienced by the patient. It may be a new onset of pain, or may represent a pattern of increasing frequency and severity of anginal pain. Dyspnea, diaphoresis, pallor, and cool skin may be present.

TABLE 30–5 Comparing Stable Angina, Acute Coronary Syndrome, and Acute Myocardial Infarction

	STABLE ANGINA	ACUTE CORONARY SYNDROME	ACUTE MYOCARDIAL INFARCTION
Pathophysiology	Myocardial ischemia occurs with increased workload (e.g., during exercise) due to stable atherosclerotic plaque narrowing coronary arteries.	Coronary artery spasm or partial occlusion by unstable plaque and thrombus formation with increasing myocardial ischemia.	Obstruction of a coronary artery by a thrombus blocks blood supply to a portion of myocardium, resulting in necrosis.
Chest pain	Stable and predictable, occurring with exertion or emotion Crescendo-decrescendo pattern May radiate to neck, shoulder, arms Usually lasts 5 to 10 minutes, relieved by rest	Occurs at rest; increasing frequency and severity Lasts 10 minutes or longer Radiates to neck, left shoulder, and arm Lasts longer than 10 minutes	Begins abruptly, unrelated to rest or exercise Severe, "crushing" Unrelieved by rest or nitroglycerine Radiates to arms, neck, jaw
Other Manifestations	Indigestion, nausea Possible shortness of breath Anxiety	Epigastric pain Dyspnea Tachycardia, hypotension Cool, pale skin	Epigastric pain, nausea Dyspnea Pallor, diaphoresis Tachycardia or bradycardia, hyper- or hypotension
Diagnosis	ECG: T-wave inversion during anginal episodes Cardiac markers: within normal range	ECG: ST-segment depression, T-wave inversion Cardiac markers: within normal range or transient elevation	ECG: ST-segment elevation, possible Q wave Cardiac markers: elevated

Tachycardia and hypotension may occur. The patient may be nauseated or feel light-headed. Table 30–5 compares the features of stable angina, ACS, and acute myocardial infarction.

Interdisciplinary Care

The patient with ACS generally presents at the emergency department or physician's office with complaints of severe chest pain. The pain may be unrelieved by nitroglycerine or may be more severe and of longer duration than previous anginal episodes. The ECG is used in conjunction with blood levels of cardiac markers to differentiate between unstable angina and acute myocardial infarction. Patients with unstable angina generally are admitted to the acute care unit on bed rest with cardiac monitoring for 12 to 24 hours. Coronary revascularization procedures may be performed within 48 hours if significant CHD is identified.

Diagnosis

The ECG and serum cardiac markers are the primary tests used to establish the diagnosis of ACS. Serum cardiac markers, proteins released from injured and necrotic heart muscle, can be measured (see the following section on acute myocardial infarction and Table 30–6 for more information about serum cardiac markers).

- Cardiac muscle troponins, *cardiac-specific troponin T (cT_nT)* and *cardiac-specific troponin I (cT_nI)*, are sensitive indicators of myocardial damage. Troponins may be elevated in ACS or may be within normal limits if chest pain is due to unstable angina.
- Creatine kinase (CK) and CK-MB (specific to myocardial muscle) levels are likely to be within normal limits or demonstrate transient elevation, returning to normal levels within 12 to 24 hours.

The ECG, particularly when done during the acute episode of chest pain, is a valuable diagnostic tool for ACS. ST-segment changes (elevation or depression) during chest pain that resolve when the pain abates usually indicate acute myocardial ischemia and severe underlying CHD.

Medications

Medications include drugs to reduce myocardial ischemia and those to reduce the risk for blood clotting. Fibrinolytic drugs (that is, drugs that break down the fibrin in blood clots) may be given prior to or on admission to the emergency department. These drugs restore blood flow to ischemic cardiac muscle and can prevent permanent damage. See the section on myocardial infarction and Nursing Care of the Patient Receiving Fibrinolytic Therapy for more information about fibrinolytic drugs and their nursing implications.

Nitrates and beta blockers are used to restore blood flow to the ischemic myocardium and reduce the workload of the heart. Nitroglycerin is given by sublingual tablet or buccal spray. If chest pain is unrelieved after three doses 5 minutes apart, an intravenous nitroglycerin infusion is initiated. The infusion may be continued until the chest pain is relieved or for 12 to 24 hours. Topical or oral nitrates are then initiated. Beta-adrenergic blockers are initially given intravenously, followed by oral beta-blockers. See the Medication Administration box on page 923 for the nursing implications of these drugs.

Aspirin, other antiplatelet drugs, and heparin are given to inhibit blood clotting and reduce the risk of thrombus formation. Aspirin and clopidogrel (Plavix) are given to patients with ACS who do not have an excessive bleeding risk. Aspirin and clopidogrel suppress platelet aggregation, interrupting the process of forming a stable blood clot. Both increase the risk of serious hemorrhage; for most patients, however, the benefit

MEDICATION ADMINISTRATION Antiplatelet Drugs

ORAL ANTIPLATELET DRUGS

Aspirin

Clopidogrel (Plavix)

Dipyridamole (Persantine)

Ticlopidine (Ticlid)

Antiplatelet drugs suppress platelet aggregation in arteries, preventing the development of an arterial thrombus. Aspirin, clopidogrel, and dipyridamole block different platelet activation pathways to inhibit platelet aggregation and clot formation. Ticlopidine alters the function of platelet membranes. The dose of aspirin given to achieve antiplatelet effects is low, typically 80 to 325 mg/day.

Nursing Responsibilities

- Inquire about a history of intracranial hemorrhage, upper gastrointestinal bleeding, peptic ulcer disease, or known bleeding tendency.
- Observe for and report increased bruising, petechiae, purpura, and apparent or occult bleeding (e.g. melana, hematemesis).
- Only dipyridamole can be used concurrently with warfarin (Coumadin).

Health Education for the Patient and Family

- Take as directed. Take aspirin with food or milk; clopidogrel may be taken at any time of day.
- Do not use nonsteroidal anti-inflammatory drugs (NSAIDs) or other over-the-counter drugs that may contain aspirin or an NSAID unless prescribed by your physician.
- Check with your physician before taking any herbal remedies such as evening primrose oil, feverfew, garlic, ginkgo biloba, or grapeseed extract while taking these medications.
- Report unusual bruising or excessive bleeding.
- Inform all care providers (including dental professionals) of use of these drugs.

INTRAVENOUS ANTIPLATELET DRUGS

Abciximab (ReoPro)

Eptifibatide (Integrilin)

Tirofiban (Aggrastat)

The intravenously administered antiplatelet drugs, abciximab, epi-dibatide, and tirofiban, block the final common pathway of platelet activation, and thus are more effective. However, the risk of bleeding is greater than with the orally administered antiplatelet drugs.

Nursing Responsibilities

- Determine history of bleeding disorders, intracranial hemorrhage, recent trauma, or surgery.
- Inquire about recent use of oral antiplatelet or anticoagulant drugs.
- Monitor CBC including hemoglobin, hematocrit, and platelet count; clotting studies, including PT, INR, PTT; vital signs; and ECG during therapy.
- Maintain a separate intravenous line for blood draws and administration of other drugs during infusion.
- Closely observe for and immediately report anaphylaxis or bleeding uncontrolled by pressure. Keep resuscitation equipment readily available.
- Maintain bed rest during infusion.

Health Education for the Patient and Family

- This drug is given to reduce the risk of clotting and myocardial infarction. It helps maintain blood flow through the affected vessel following angioplasty and stent placement.
- Immediately report any chest tightness, difficulty breathing, shortness of breath, or itching that develops during the infusion.
- Your risk of bleeding should return to normal within about 2 days following the infusion.
- Immediately report any unusual bruising or bleeding to your doctor.

---

outweighs the risk. Intravenous antiplatelet drugs such as abciximab (ReoPro), eptifibatide (Integrilin), or tirofiban (Aggrastat) may be used when an invasive coronary revascularization procedure is anticipated in the immediate or near future. Nursing implications for the antiplatelet drugs are outlined in the accompanying box on page 927.

Revascularization Procedures

Several procedures may be used to restore blood flow and oxygen to ischemic tissue. Nonsurgical techniques include transluminal coronary angioplasty, laser angioplasty, coronary atherectomy, and intracoronary stents. Coronary artery bypass grafting (CABG) is a surgical procedure that may be used.

PERCUTANEOUS CORONARY REVASCULARIZATION

Percutaneous coronary revascularization (PCR) procedures are used to restore blood flow to the ischemic myocardium in patients with CHD. Approximately 600,000 PCR procedures are done annually in the United States. PCR is used to treat patients with the following:

- Moderately severe, chronic stable angina unrelieved by medical therapy

- Unstable angina
- Acute myocardial infarction
- Significant stenosis of the left anterior descending coronary artery
- Stenosis of a coronary artery bypass graft (Masoudi et al., 2008)

PCR procedures are similar to the procedure used for coronary angiography. A catheter introduced into the arterial circulation is guided into the opening of the narrowed coronary artery. A flexible guide wire is inserted through the catheter lumen into the affected vessel. The guide wire is then used to thread an angioplasty balloon, arterial stent, or other therapeutic device into the narrowed segment of the artery. The procedure is performed in the cardiac catheterization laboratory using local anesthesia. The hospital stay is short (1 to 2 days), minimizing costs.

In a *percutaneous transluminal coronary angioplasty (PTCA)*, a balloon-tipped catheter is threaded over the guide wire, with the balloon positioned across the area of narrowing (Figure 30–2 ■). The balloon is inflated in a step-by-step fashion for about 30 seconds to 2 minutes to compress the plaque against the arterial wall, with a goal of reducing the vessel

Artery cross-section

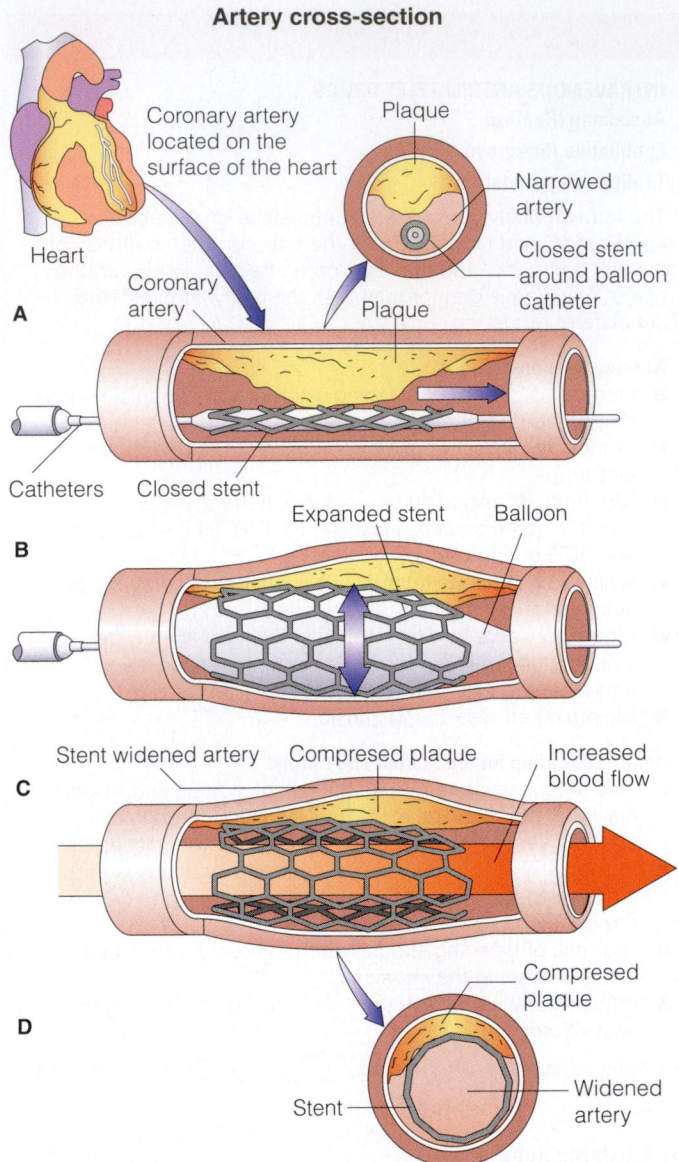

Figure 30–2 ■ Percutaneous coronary revascularization. *A,* The balloon catheter with the stent is threaded into the affected coronary artery. *B, C,* The stent is positioned across the blockage and expanded. *D,* The balloon is deflated and removed, leaving the stent in place.

obstruction to less than 50% of the arterial lumen. PTCA typically is accompanied by placement of a stent. *Intracoronary stents* are metallic scaffolds used to maintain an open arterial lumen. Stents reduce the rate of restenosis following angioplasty by about one-third, and are now used in the majority of all PCR procedures (Masoudi et al., 2008). The stent is placed over a balloon catheter, guided into position, and expanded as the balloon is inflated. It then remains in the artery as a prop after the balloon is removed. Endothelial cells will completely line the inner wall of the stent to produce a smooth inner lining. Antiplatelet medications (aspirin and ticlopidine) are given following stent insertion to reduce the risk of thrombus formation at the site.

In contrast to stent procedures that enlarge the artery by displacing plaque, *atherectomy* procedures remove plaque from

the identified lesion. The directional atherectomy catheter shaves the plaque off vessel walls using a rotary cutting head, retaining the fragments in its housing and removing them from the vessel. Rotational atherectomy catheters pulverize plaque into particles small enough to pass through the coronary microcirculation. Laser atherectomy devices use laser energy to remove plaque.

Complications following PCR procedures include hematoma at the catheter insertion site, pseudoaneurysm, embolism, hypersensitivity to contrast dye, dysrhythmias, bleeding, vessel perforation, and restenosis, or reocclusion of the treated vessel.

Nursing care of the patient undergoing PCR is outlined in the box on page 929.

CORONARY ARTERY BYPASS GRAFTING Surgery for coronary heart disease involves using a section of a vein or an artery to create a connection (or bypass) between the aorta and the coronary artery beyond the obstruction (Figure 30–3 ■). This then allows blood to perfuse the ischemic portion of the heart. The internal mammary artery in the chest and the saphenous vein from the leg are the vessels most commonly used for coronary artery bypass grafting (CABG).

Bypass grafts are safe and effective. Angina is totally relieved or significantly reduced in 90% of patients who undergo complete revascularization. While anginal pain may recur within 3 years, it rarely is as severe as before surgery. CABG has a positive effect on mortality in many cases. It is recommended for patients who have multiple vessel disease and impaired left ventricular function or diabetes, and for patients who have significant obstruction of the left main coronary artery (Perrin, 2009).

A median sternotomy commonly is used to access the heart. The heart is usually stopped during surgery. The *cardiopulmonary bypass (CPB) pump* is used to maintain perfusion to the rest of the organs during open-heart surgery.

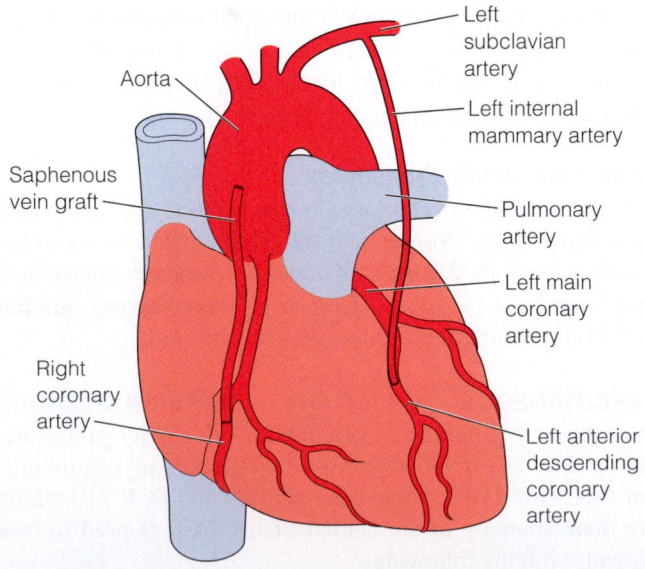

Figure 30–3 ■ Coronary artery bypass grafting using the internal mammary artery and a saphenous vein graft.

NURSING CARE OF THE PATIENT Having PCR

BEFORE THE PROCEDURE

- Assess knowledge of the procedure and expectations of treatment. *This allows information to be tailored to the patient's needs and provides an opportunity to clarify misconceptions.*
- Describe the cardiac catheterization laboratory and the planned PCR procedure, including the following:
  - Preoperative preparation (∞ see Chapter 4)
  - Planned anesthesia or sedation to be used
  - Drugs that may be given during the procedure, such as anticoagulants to reduce the risk of thrombus formation, and intravenous nitroglycerine and a calcium channel blocker to dilate coronary arteries and prevent anginal pain
- Discuss possible sensations during the procedure, including flushing or warmth and a metallic taste in the mouth as the contrast dye is injected, and a feeling of pressure or chest pain during balloon inflation. *Advanced preparation for expected sensations reduces anxiety and improves outcomes.*
- Perform a comprehensive assessment, including hydration status (skin and mucous membrane moisture, turgor) and peripheral circulation (color, warmth, sensation, pulses, and capillary refill).

AFTER THE PROCEDURE

- Complete a head-to-toe assessment. Note any complaints of chest pain, or evidence of decreased cardiac output or myocardial infarction. *Assessment provides a baseline for subsequent assessments and allows early identification of possible complications.*
- Monitor vital signs and cardiac rhythm continuously. Treat dysrhythmias as ordered. Obtain a 12-lead ECG if signs of ischemia develop, and notify physician. *Vital signs reflect cardiac output. Dysrhythmias may develop with reperfusion of the ischemic myocardium. ECG changes may indicate infarction or restenosis of the affected vessel.*
- Maintain intravenous nitroglycerin infusion. Administer anticoagulant and antiplatelet medications, nitrates, and calcium channel blockers as ordered. *These drugs decrease*

oxygen demand and increase oxygen supply by dilating the coronary arteries and systemic vasculature. They also reduce the risk of thrombus formation.
- Monitor for and treat or report chest pain as indicated. *Chest pain may indicate ischemia and possible myocardial infarction.*
- Maintain bed rest as ordered with the head of the bed at 30 degrees or less. Prevent flexion of the leg on the affected side. Following sheath removal, follow protocol for pressure dressing or device or sandbag placement. *A large puncture wound occurs at the insertion site. Immobilization allows the wound to seal; a pressure dressing helps prevent bleeding.*
- Monitor distal pulses, color, movement, sensation, and temperature of the affected leg, and insertion site every 15 minutes for the first hour, every 30 minutes for the next hour, every hour for the next 8 hours, and then every 4 hours. *A clot may form at the site, reducing perfusion of the affected leg. The site and dressing are monitored for excessive bleeding hematoma formation or pseudoaneurysm. Pseudoaneurysm occurs as a result of inadequate hemostasis after catheter removal.*
- Monitor intake and output, serum electrolytes, blood urea nitrogen (BUN), creatinine, complete blood count (CBC), partial thromboplastin time (PTT), and cardiac enzymes. Report abnormal results to the physician. *Contrast dye causes osmotic diuresis and may cause renal damage or a hypersensitivity reaction. Electrolyte imbalances increase the risk of dysrhythmias. Cardiac enzymes are monitored for indications of possible myocardial damage during the procedure. The PTT monitors the effectiveness of heparin therapy.*
- Monitor for bradycardia, lightheadedness, hypotension, diaphoresis, and loss of consciousness during sheath removal. Keep atropine at bedside during sheath removal. *Bradycardia and signs of decreased cardiac output may occur during sheath removal because of a vasovagal reaction. Atropine decreases vagal tone and increases heart rate.*

Venous blood is removed from the body through a cannula placed in the right atrium or the superior and inferior venae cavae. Blood then circulates through the CPB pump, where it is oxygenated, its temperature is regulated, and it is filtered. Oxygenated blood is returned to the body through a cannula in the ascending aorta (Figure 30–4 ■). Cardiopulmonary bypass enables surgeons to operate on a quiet heart and a relatively bloodless field. Hypothermia can be maintained to reduce the metabolic rate and decrease oxygen demand during surgery.

Newer techniques have been developed that allow surgeons to perform CABG without cardioplegia (stopping the heart) and CPB. Off-pump coronary artery bypass (OPCAB) allows use of a smaller incision for access. Although cardiopulmonary bypass is employed for the majority of coronary artery bypass procedures, OPCAB is a promising alternative. Controlled studies demonstrate lower mortality and morbidity rates and

faster recovery for patients undergoing OPCAB as compared to CABG with cardiopulmonary bypass (Eagle et al., 2004).

When the saphenous vein is used, it is excised from its normal attachments in the leg, flushed with a cold heparinized saline solution, and then reversed so that its valves do not interfere with blood flow. When appropriate, a laparoscopic approach may be used to remove the vein. The vein is *anastomosed* (grafted) to the aorta and the coronary artery, distal to the occlusion (see Figure 30–3). This provides a bridge or conduit for blood flow past the obstruction. If the internal mammary artery (IMA) is used, its distal end is excised and anastomosed to the coronary artery distal to the obstruction. The IMA often is used to revascularize the left coronary artery because of the greater oxygen demand of the left ventricle.

Once grafting is completed, cardiopulmonary bypass is discontinued and the patient is rewarmed. Rewarming stimulates the heart to resume beating. Temporary pacing wires are

Figure 30–4 ■ A diagrammatic representation of cardiopulmonary bypass. A cannula in the superior and inferior venae cavae removes venous blood, which is then pumped through an oxygenator and heat exchanger. After filtering, oxygenated blood is returned to the ascending aorta.

sutured in place and passed through the chest wall in case temporary pacing is necessary. Chest tubes are placed in the pleural space and mediastinum to drain blood and reestablish negative pressure in the thoracic cavity. The sternum is closed using heavy wires and bone wax, the skin is closed with sutures or staples, and sterile dressings are applied over sternal and leg incisions.

Pre- and postoperative nursing care and teaching for the patient having a coronary artery bypass graft or other open-heart surgery are outlined on pages 931–933.

MINIMALLY INVASIVE CORONARY ARTERY SURGERY
Minimally invasive coronary artery surgery is a potential future alternative to CABG. Two approaches may be used: *Port-access coronary artery bypass* uses several small holes, or "ports" in the chest wall to access vessels for connection to the CPB pump and the surgical site; alternatively, the femoral artery and femoral vein may be used for CPB (Eagle et al., 2004). CPB is avoided altogether using the *minimally invasive coronary artery bypass (MIDCAB)* approach. With MIDCAB, a small surgical incision and several chest wall ports are used to graft a chest wall artery to the affected coronary vessel while the heart continues to beat.

TRANSMYOCARDIAL LASER REVASCULARIZATION
A new development in myocardial revascularization techniques is called *transmyocardial laser revascularization (TMLR)*. In this procedure, a laser is used to drill tiny holes into the myocardial muscle itself to provide collateral blood flow to ischemic

muscle. Patients whose coronary artery obstructions are too diffuse to bypass are candidates for this new surgical treatment.

✏ Nursing Care

Health promotion, assessment, nursing diagnoses, and interventions for the patient with ACS are similar to those identified for patients with angina and with acute myocardial infarction. See the preceding and subsequent sections of this chapter for specific nursing care activities, as well as the Case Study & Nursing Care Plan that follows.

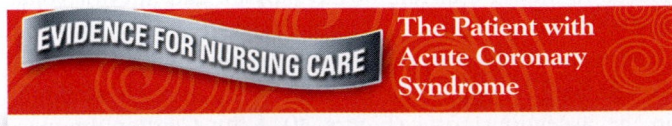

EVIDENCE FOR NURSING CARE — **The Patient with Acute Coronary Syndrome**

Selected resources that nurses may find helpful when planning evidence-based nursing care follow.

- Acute Coronary Syndromes. *AACN Practice Alert.* Retrieved from http://www.aacn.org/WD/Practice/Content/practicealerts.pcms?menu=Practice
- Cheek, D. J., Hawkins, J. S., & Sherrod, M. M. (2009). Unlocking the secrets of common cardiac conditions. *Nursing2009, 39*(1), 52–56.
- DeVon, H. A., Ryan, C. J., Ochs, A. L., & Shapiro, M. (2008). Symptoms across the continuum of acute coronary syndromes: Differences between women and men. *American Journal of Critical Care, 17*(10), 14–24.

NURSING CARE OF THE PATIENT Having a Coronary Artery Bypass Graft

PREOPERATIVE CARE

■ Provide routine preoperative care and teaching as outlined in ∞ Chapter 4.

■ Verify presence of laboratory and diagnostic test results in the chart, including CBC, coagulation profile, urinalysis, chest x-ray, and coronary angiogram. *These baseline data are important for comparison of postoperative results and values.*

■ Type and crossmatch four or more units of blood as ordered. *Blood is made available for use during and after surgery as needed.*

■ Provide specific patient and family teaching related to procedure and postoperative care. Include the following topics:
  ■ Cardiac recovery unit; sensory stimuli, personnel; noise and alarms; visiting policies
  ■ Tubes, drains, and general appearance
  ■ Monitoring equipment, including cardiac and hemodynamic monitoring systems
  ■ Respiratory support: ventilator, endotracheal tube, suctioning; communication while intubated
  ■ Incisions and dressings
  ■ Pain management

Preoperative teaching reduces anxiety and prepares the patient and family for the postoperative environment and expected sensations.

POSTOPERATIVE CARE

■ Provide routine postoperative care as outlined in ∞ Chapter 4. In addition to the care needs of all patients having major surgery, the cardiac surgery patient has specific care needs related to open-heart and thoracic surgery. These are outlined under the nursing diagnoses identified next.

Decreased Cardiac Output

Cardiac output may be compromised postoperatively due to bleeding and fluid loss; depression of myocardial function by drugs, hypothermia, and surgical manipulation; dysrhythmias; increased vascular resistance; and a potential complication, *cardiac tamponade,* compression of the heart due to collected blood or fluid in the pericardium.

■ Monitor vital signs, oxygen saturation, and hemodynamic parameters every 15 minutes. Note trends and report significant changes to the physician. *Initial hypothermia and bradycardia are expected; the heart rate should return to the normal range with rewarming. The blood pressure may fall during rewarming as vasodilation occurs. Hypotension and tachycardia, however, may indicate low cardiac output. Pulmonary artery pressure (PAP), pulmonary artery wedge pressure (PAWP), cardiac output, and oxygen saturation are monitored to evaluate fluid volume, cardiac function, and gas exchange. Hemodynamic monitoring is further discussed in ∞ Chapter 31.*

■ Auscultate heart and breath sounds on admission and at least every 4 hours. *A ventricular gallop, or S3, is an early sign of heart failure; an S4 may indicate decreased ventricular compliance. Muffled heart sounds may be an early indication of cardiac tamponade. Adventitious breath sounds (wheezes, crackles, or rales) may be a manifestation of heart failure or respiratory compromise.*

■ Assess skin color and temperature, peripheral pulses, and level of consciousness with vital signs. *Pale, mottled, or cyanotic coloring, cool and clammy skin, and diminished pulse amplitude are indicators of decreased cardiac output.*

■ Continuously monitor and document cardiac rhythm. *Dysrhythmias are common, and may interfere with cardiac filling and contractility, decreasing the cardiac output.*

■ Measure intake and output hourly. Report urine output less than 30 mL/h for 2 consecutive hours. *Intake and output measurements help evaluate fluid volume status. A fall in urine output may be an early indicator of decreased cardiac output.*

■ Record chest tube output hourly. *Chest tube drainage greater than 70 mL/h or that is warm, red, and free flowing indicates hemorrhage and may necessitate a return to surgery. A sudden drop in chest tube output may indicate impending cardiac tamponade.*

■ Monitor hemoglobin, hematocrit, and serum electrolytes. *A drop in hemoglobin and hematocrit may indicate hemorrhage that is not otherwise obvious. Electrolyte imbalances, potassium, calcium, and magnesium in particular, affect cardiac rhythm and contractility.*

■ Administer intravenous fluids, fluid boluses, and blood transfusions as ordered. *Fluid and blood replacement helps ensure adequate blood volume and oxygen-carrying capacity.*

■ Administer medications as ordered. *Medications ordered in the early postoperative period to maintain the cardiac output include inotropic drugs (e.g., dopamine, dobutamine) to increase the force of myocardial contractions; vasodilators (e.g., nitroprusside or nitroglycerin) to decrease vascular resistance and after-load; and antidysrhythmics to correct dysrhythmias that affect cardiac output.*

■ Keep a temporary pacemaker at the bedside; initiate pacing as indicated. *Temporary pacing may be needed to maintain the cardiac output with bradydysrhythmias, such as high-level AV blocks.*

PRACTICE ALERT

Assess for signs of cardiac tamponade: increased heart rate, decreased BP, decreased urine output, increased central venous pressure, a sudden decrease in chest tube output, muffled/distant heart sounds, and diminished peripheral pulses. Notify physician immediately. Cardiac tamponade is a life-threatening complication that may develop postoperatively. Cardiac tamponade interferes with ventricular filling and contraction, decreasing cardiac output. Untreated, cardiac tamponade leads to cardiogenic shock and possible cardiac arrest.

Hypothermia

Hypothermia is maintained during cardiac surgery to reduce the metabolic rate and protect vital organs from ischemic damage. Although rewarming is instituted on completion of the surgery, the patient often remains hypothermic on admission to cardiac recovery. Gradual rewarming is necessary to prevent peripheral vasodilation and hypotension.

■ Monitor core body temperature (e.g., tympanic membrane, pulmonary artery, bladder) for the first 8 hours following surgery. *Oral and rectal temperature measurements are not reliable indicators of core body temperature during this period.*

■ Institute rewarming measures (e.g., warmed intravenous solutions or blood transfusion, warm blankets, warm inspired gases, radiant heat lamps) as needed to maintain a temperature above 96.8°F (36°C). Administer thorazine, morphine, or diltiazem as ordered to relieve shivering. *Low body temperature may cause shivering, increasing oxygen demand and consumption. Hypothermia also increases the risk for hypoxia, metabolic acidosis, vasoconstriction and increased cardiac work, altered clotting, and dysrhythmias.*

(continued)

NURSING CARE OF THE PATIENT Having a Coronary Artery Bypass Graft (continued)

Acute Pain

Following a CABG, pain is experienced due to both the thoracic incision and removal of the saphenous vein from the leg. Dissection of the internal mammary artery (usually the left IMA) from the chest wall also causes chest pain on the affected side. Chest tube sites are also uncomfortable. The leg from which the saphenous vein graft was obtained may be more painful than the chest incision.

- Frequently assess for pain, including its location and character. Document its intensity using a standard pain scale. Assess for verbal and nonverbal indicators of pain. Validate pain cues with the patient. *Pain is subjective, and differs among individuals. Incisional pain is expected; however, anginal pain also may develop. It is important to differentiate the type of pain.*

> **PRACTICE ALERT**
> Promptly report anginal or cardiac pain. Cardiac pain may indicate a perioperative or postoperative myocardial infarction.

- Administer analgesics on a scheduled basis, by PCA, or by continuous infusion for the first 24 to 48 hours. *Research demonstrates that adequate pain management in the immediate postoperative period reduces complications from sympathetic stimulation and allows faster recovery. Pain causes muscle tension and vasoconstriction, impairing circulation and tissue perfusion, slowing wound healing, and increasing cardiac work.*
- Premedicate 30 minutes before activities or planned procedures. *Premedication and the subsequent reduction of pain improves patient participation and cooperation with care.*

Ineffective Airway Clearance/Impaired Gas Exchange

Atelectasis due to impaired ventilation and airway clearance is a common pulmonary complication of cardiac surgery. Gas exchange may also be affected by blood loss and decreased oxygen-carrying capacity following surgery. Phrenic nerve paralysis is a potential complication of cardiac surgery that may also contribute to impaired ventilation and gas exchange.

- Evaluate respiratory rate, depth, effort, symmetry of chest expansion, and breath sounds frequently. *Pain, anxiety, excess fluid volume, surgical injury, narcotics and anesthesia, and altered homeostasis can affect respiratory rate, depth, and effort postoperatively. Decreased chest expansion or asymmetrical movement may indicate impaired ventilation of one lung, and needs further evaluation.*
- Note endotracheal tube (ETT) placement on chest x-ray. Mark tube position and secure in place. Insert an oral airway if an oral ETT is used. *The chest x-ray documents correct ETT placement above the bifurcation to the right and left mainstem bronchus. Marking its appropriate placement allows evaluation of potential tube movement. Secure the tube firmly in place to prevent slippage or inadvertent removal. An oral airway helps prevent obstruction of an oral ETT by biting.*
- Maintain ventilator settings as ordered. Monitor arterial blood gases (ABGs) as ordered. *Mechanical ventilation promotes optimal lung expansion and oxygenation postoperatively. ABGs are used to evaluate oxygenation and acid–base balance.*
- Suction as needed. *Suctioning is performed only as indicated to clear airway secretions.*
- Prepare for ventilator weaning and extubation, as appropriate. *The patient is removed from the ventilator and extubated as soon as possible to reduce complications associated with mechanical ventilation and intubation.*
- After extubation, teach use of the incentive spirometer, and encourage use every 2 hours. Encourage deep breathing; advise against vigorous coughing. Teach use of a "cough pillow" to splint chest incision and decrease pain. Frequently turn and encourage movement. Dangle on postoperative day 1. *Deep breathing, controlled coughing, and position changes improve ventilation and airway clearance and help prevent complications. Vigorous coughing may excessively increase intrathoracic pressure and cause sternal instability.*

Risk for Infection

Following an open chest procedure, a sternal infection may develop that can progress to involve the mediastinum. Incisions for removal of the saphenous vein also may become infected. Patients with IMA grafts, who are diabetic, are older, or malnourished are at high risk: Harvesting of IMA disrupts blood supply to the sternum, and these patients have impaired immune responses and healing.

- Assess sternal incision and leg wounds every shift. Document redness, warmth, swelling, and/or drainage from the site. Note wound approximation. *These assessments provide indicators of inflammation and healing.*
- Maintain a sterile dressing for the first 48 hours, and then leave the incision open to air. Use Steri-Strips as needed to maintain approximation of the wound edges. *The sterile dressing prevents early contamination of the wound, whereas exposing the incision after 48 hours promotes healing.*
- Report signs of wound infection: a swollen, reddened area that is hot and painful to the touch, drainage from the wound, impaired healing, or healed areas that reopen. *Evidence of infection or impaired healing requires further evaluation and treatment.*
- Culture wound drainage as indicated. *Identifying the infective organism facilitates appropriate antibiotic therapy.*
- Collaborate with the dietitian to promote nutrition and fluid intake. *Good nutritional status is vital to healing and immune function.*

Disturbed Thought Processes

Many factors affect neuropsychologic function after CABG, including the length of cardiopulmonary bypass, age, presurgery organic brain dysfunction, severity of illness, and decreased cardiac output. Sensory overload and deprivation, sleep disruption, and numerous drugs also affect thinking and mental clarity.

- Frequently reorient during initial recovery period. State that surgery is over and that the patient is in the recovery area. *Frequent reorientation provides emotional support and reality checks.*
- Explain all procedures before performing them. Speak in a clear, calm voice. Encourage questions, and give honest answers. *These measures provide information, decrease anxiety, and establish trust.*
- Secure all intravenous lines and invasive catheters/tubes (e.g., ETT, Foley catheter, nasogastric tube). *Disoriented patients may tug or pull at invasive equipment, disrupting them and increasing the risk of injury.*
- Note verbal responses to questions. Correct misconceptions immediately (e.g., "Mr. Snow, look at all the special equipment in this room. Does this room look like your bedroom at home?"). *Helping the patient recognize differences in the hospital environment offers a basis for continual reality checks.*

NURSING CARE OF THE PATIENT Having a Coronary Artery Bypass Graft (continued)

- Maintain a calendar and clock within the patient's view. *This provides current information regarding day, date, and time.*
- Involve family members in providing reorientation. Place familiar objects and photographs within view. Encourage family presence. *The family provides reassurance and contact with the familiar, assisting with orientation.*
- Promote patient participation in care and decision making as appropriate. *This allows the patient to maintain a degree of power and control and enables the patient to take an active role in recovery.*

- Report signs of hallucinations, delusions, depression, or agitation. *These may indicate progressive deterioration of mental status.*
- Administer sedatives cautiously. *Mild sedation may help prevent injury. Some sedatives may, however, have adverse effects, increasing confusion and disorientation.*
- Reevaluate neurologic status every shift. *These data allow evaluation of the effect of interventions.*

CASE STUDY & NURSING CARE PLAN A Patient with Coronary Artery Bypass Surgery

Six weeks ago, John Clements, aged 50, was discharged from the hospital after emergency triple bypass surgery. Despite having emergency surgery, his postoperative recovery was uneventful, and he was discharged 6 days after admission. He returns to the clinic for a postoperative stress test and to discuss his cardiac rehabilitation program. Anne Wagner, RN, CNS, a cardiac clinical nurse specialist and the program coordinator, meets Mr. Clements to obtain specific information regarding his medical status.

ASSESSMENT

Mr. Clements's medical history reveals significant CHD, an anterior wall myocardial infarction that led to his emergency triple bypass, and hyperlipidemia. Current medications include Cardizem, Isordil, Ecotrin, and Transderm-Nitro 5. The ECG reveals sinus rhythm with some ST-segment and T-wave flattening. Resting heart rate 68, and blood pressure 136/84.

Mr. Clements has a strong family history of CHD. He does not smoke and uses alcohol occasionally in social situations. He enjoys "good Southern-style cooking" and watching television. Mr. Clements states his only regular exercise used to be an evening of dancing with his wife and friends about once a month, "But I get short of breath walking around the block now, so I guess I can't go dancing anymore!"

Mr. Clements owns his own contracting business and states that he typically works about 50 to 60 hours per week. He tells Ms. Wagner, "I don't know what this program is supposed to do for me. I have got to get back to work! You just can't sit around in my business—you have to make sure that the work is getting done on time, and you have to check on supplies and equipment and the like. But I feel like a weakling—I need to get my energy back!"

DIAGNOSES

- *Activity Intolerance* related to general weakness and fatigue
- *Ineffective Role Performance* related to health crisis

EXPECTED OUTCOMES

- Verbalize an understanding of the definition and components of his structured cardiac rehabilitation program.
- Verbalize a desire to make lifestyle changes.
- Identify resources available in the community to assist with lifestyle changes.
- Participate in his activity program without suffering any complications.
- Verbalize an increase in energy after 6 weeks on the program.
- Accept the reality of the temporary change in his usual work responsibilities.

PLANNING AND IMPLEMENTATION

- Define the purpose and components of a cardiac rehabilitation program.
- Enroll in "heart health" classes, including cardiac anatomy, physiology, and coronary heart disease; exercise and activity prescriptions; lifestyle modifications, including diet counseling and stress management; emotional reactions to CAD; sexual activity; use of cardiac medications; and self-responsibility for health.
- Plan an exercise program based on stress test results, physical examination, and interview.
- Encourage to schedule rest periods before and after activity/exercise.
- Review signs and symptoms of overexertion.
- Provide information about community resources for emotional and educational support.
- Assist to identify strategies for dealing with concerns about his business role.

EVALUATION

Mr. Clements decides to "give the rehab program a try." Ms. Wagner and an exercise physiologist work with him to plan an individualized exercise/activity program. A registered dietitian provides dietary counseling. Ms. Wagner emphasizes stress management strategies. Mr. Clements is able to list manifestations of overexertion and states that he realizes the need for gradual activity progression.

After 6 weeks, Mr. Clements has reported a significant increase in energy and strength. "I am feeling much stronger, and have been sleeping better. Mary and I are taking evening walks around the neighborhood. My chest soreness is also gone." He has completed the 12-week cardiac rehabilitation program, and another stress test indicates that his cardiac function is adequate. Mr. Clements has joined the local Mended Hearts support group and states that he is now incorporating "heart-healthy" considerations into his daily routines.

CRITICAL THINKING IN THE NURSING PROCESS

1. Develop a personalized risk factor reduction plan for Mr. Clements.
2. How might denial affect Mr. Clements's ability to (a) accept the need for cardiac rehabilitation, (b) comply with the proposed lifestyle changes, and (c) make permanent adjustments to his daily life?
3. How does spousal support influence a patient's compliance with a structured cardiac rehabilitation program?
4. Mr. Clements tells you that since the surgery, his wife has been afraid that sexual activity will induce another heart attack. How would you respond to these concerns?

See Evaluating Your Response in Appendix C.

The Patient with Acute Myocardial Infarction

Acute MI Animation

An **acute myocardial infarction (AMI)**, necrosis (death) of myocardial cells, is a life-threatening event. If circulation to the affected myocardium is not promptly restored, loss of functional myocardium affects the heart's ability to maintain an effective cardiac output. This may ultimately lead to cardiogenic shock and death.

Heart disease remains the leading cause of death in the United States. Of the major heart diseases, myocardial infarction (MI) or *heart attack*, and other forms of ischemic heart disease cause the majority of deaths. Annually, approximately 785,000 people in the United States experience their first MI; another 470,000 suffer an MI subsequent to the initial one. It is estimated that 195,000 silent attacks occur each year (AHA, 2009).

The majority of deaths from MI occur during the initial period after symptoms begin: approximately 60% within the first hour, and 40% prior to hospitalization. Heightening public awareness of the manifestations of MI, the importance of seeking immediate medical assistance, and training in cardiopulmonary resuscitation (CPR) techniques are vital to decrease deaths due to MI.

Myocardial infarction rarely occurs without preexisting coronary heart disease. While no specific cause has been identified, the risk factors for MI are those for coronary heart disease: age, gender, heredity, race, smoking, obesity, hyperlipidemia, hypertension, diabetes, sedentary lifestyle, diet, and others. See the previous section of this chapter on coronary heart disease for further discussion of these risk factors.

Pathophysiology

Atherosclerotic plaque may form stable or unstable lesions. *Stable* lesions progress by gradually occluding the vessel lumen, whereas *unstable* (or *complicated*) lesions are prone to rupture and thrombus formation. Stable lesions often cause angina (discussed in the previous sections); unstable lesions often lead to acute coronary syndromes or acute ischemic heart diseases. Acute coronary syndromes include unstable angina, myocardial infarction, and sudden cardiac death (Anderson et al., 2007).

Myocardial infarction occurs when blood flow to a portion of cardiac muscle is completely blocked, resulting in prolonged tissue ischemia and irreversible cell damage. Coronary occlusion is usually caused by ulceration or rupture of a complicated atherosclerotic lesion. When an atherosclerotic lesion ruptures or ulcerates, substances are released that stimulate platelet aggregation, thrombin generation, and local vasomotor tone. As a result, the vessel constricts, and a thrombus (clot) forms, occluding the vessel and interrupting blood flow to the myocardium distal to the obstruction.

Cellular injury occurs when the cells are denied adequate oxygen and nutrients. With prolonged ischemia lasting more than 20 to 45 minutes, irreversible hypoxemia causes cellular death and tissue necrosis. Oxygen, glycogen, and ATP stores of ischemic cells are rapidly depleted. Cellular metabolism shifts to an anaerobic process, producing hydrogen ions and lactic acid. Cellular acidosis increases cells' vulnerability to further damage with release of intracellular enzymes through the damaged cell membranes.

Cellular acidosis, electrolyte imbalances, and hormones released in response to cellular ischemia affect impulse conduction and myocardial contractility. Myocardial contractility decreases, increasing the risk for dysrhythmias, subsequently reducing stroke volume, cardiac output, blood pressure, and tissue perfusion.

Within 20 minutes of injury the subendocardium, being most susceptible to changes in coronary blood flow, suffers the initial damage. If blood flow is restored at this point, the infarction is limited to subendocardial tissue (a *subendocardial* or *non-Q-wave infarction*). The damage progresses to the epicardium within 1 to 6 hours. When all layers of the myocardium are affected, it is known as a *transmural infarction*. A significant Q wave develops with a transmural infarction, so this also may be called a *Q-wave MI*. Complications such as heart failure are more frequently associated with Q-wave MIs; however, patients with non-Q-wave MIs frequently experience recurrent ischemia or subsequent MI within weeks or months of the event (Woods et al., 2009).

The necrotic, infarcted tissue is surrounded by regions of injured and ischemic tissues. Tissue in the ischemic area is potentially viable; restoration of blood flow minimizes the amount of tissue lost. The surrounding tissue also undergoes metabolic changes. It may be *stunned*, its contractility impaired for hours to days following reperfusion, or *hibernating*, a process that protects myocytes until perfusion is restored.

MEETING INDIVIDUALIZED NEEDS   Recognizing a Myocardial Infarction in Women and Older Adults

Women and older adults often present with atypical manifestations of MI. However, heart disease is the number one cause of death in both groups, making early recognition and aggressive treatment vital.

Women are more likely than men to have a "silent" or unrecognized heart attack, or to present in cardiac arrest or with cardiogenic shock. Women often experience epigastric pain and nausea, causing them to blame their discomfort on heartburn. Shortness of breath is common, as is fatigue and weakness of the shoulders and upper arms.

Older people often seek treatment for vague complaints of difficulty breathing, confusion, fainting, dizziness, abdominal pain, or cough. They often attribute their symptoms to a stroke. The prevalence of silent ischemia is greater in older adults.

Stress the importance of seeking medical help promptly for atypical manifestations of MI. Prompt diagnosis and intervention reduces the mortality and morbidity of MI in women and older adults, just as it does in men. Despite this fact, both women and older adults are more likely to delay seeking treatment and are less likely to be accurately diagnosed and aggressively treated for CHD. Younger women are a particularly important group to reach; their mortality rate when MI occurs is twice that of men (Jensen & Moser, 2009).

Myocardial remodeling may occur, with cellular hypertrophy and loss of contractility in regions distant from the infarction. Rapid restoration of blood flow limits these changes (McCance & Huether, 2006).

When a larger artery is compromised, *collateral vessels* connecting smaller arteries in the coronary system dilate to maintain blood flow to the cardiac muscle. The degree of collateral circulation helps determine the extent of myocardial damage from ischemia. Acute occlusion of a coronary artery without any collateral flow results in massive tissue damage and possible death. Progressive narrowing of the larger coronary arteries allows collateral vessels to develop and enlarge, meeting the demand for blood flow. Good collateral circulation can limit the size of an MI.

MI usually affects the left ventricle because it is the major "workhorse" of the heart; its muscle mass is greater, as are its oxygen demands.

MIs are described by the damaged area of the heart. The coronary artery that is occluded determines the area of damage. Occlusion of the left anterior descending (LAD) artery affects blood flow to the anterior wall of the left ventricle (an *anterior MI*) and part of the interventricular septum. Occlusion of the left circumflex artery (LCA) causes a *lateral MI. Right ventricular, inferior*, and *posterior infarcts* involve occlusions of the right coronary artery (RCA) and posterior descending artery (PDA). Occlusion of the left main coronary artery is the most devastating, causing ischemia of the entire left ventricle, and a grave prognosis. Identifying the infarct site helps predict possible complications and determine appropriate therapy.

Cocaine-Induced MI

AMI may develop due to cocaine intoxication. Cocaine increases sympathetic nervous system activity by both increasing the release of catecholamines from central and peripheral stores and interfering with the reuptake of catecholamines. This increased catecholamine concentration stimulates the heart rate and increases its contractility, increases the automaticity of cardiac tissues and the risk of dysrhythmias, and causes vasoconstriction and hypertension. The patient with cocaine-induced MI may present with an altered level of consciousness, confusion and restlessness, seizure activity, tachycardia, hypotension, increased respiratory rate, and respiratory crackles.

Manifestations

Pain is a classic manifestation of MI. Chest pain due to MI is more severe than anginal pain. However, it is not the intensity of the chest pain that distinguishes MI from angina or acute coronary syndrome, but its duration and its continuous nature. The onset of pain is sudden and usually is not associated with activity. In fact, most MIs occur in the early morning. Patients with a history of angina may have more frequent anginal attacks in the days or weeks prior to an MI (unstable angina or ACS). Chest pain may be described as crushing and severe; as a pressure, heavy, or squeezing sensation; or as chest tightness or burning. The pain often begins in the center of the chest (*substernal*), and may radiate to the shoulders, neck, jaw, or arms. It lasts more than 15 to 20 minutes and is not relieved by rest or nitroglycerin.

Women and older adults often experience atypical chest pain, presenting with complaints of indigestion, heartburn, nausea, and

---

MANIFESTATIONS of Acute Myocardial Infarction

- Chest pain: substernal or precordial (across the entire chest wall); may radiate to neck, jaw, shoulder(s), or left arm
- Tachycardia, tachypnea
- Dyspnea, shortness of breath
- Nausea and vomiting
- Anxiety, sense of impending doom
- Diaphoresis
- Cool, mottled skin; diminished peripheral pulses
- Hypotension or hypertension
- Palpitations, dysrhythmias
- Signs of left heart failure
- Decreased level of consciousness

---

vomiting (see the accompanying box). Up to 25% of patients with acute MI deny chest discomfort (Woods et al., 2009).

Compensatory mechanisms cause many of the other symptoms of MI. Sympathetic nervous system stimulation causes anxiety, tachycardia, and vasoconstriction producing a cool, clammy, mottled skin. Pain and blood chemistry changes stimulate the respiratory center, causing tachypnea. The patient often has a sense of impending doom and death. Tissue necrosis causes an inflammatory reaction that increases the white blood cell (WBC) count and elevates the temperature. Serum cardiac enzyme levels rise as enzymes are released from necrotic cardiac cells.

Other manifestations may vary, depending on the location and amount of infarcted tissue. Hypertension, hypotension, or signs of heart failure may develop. Vagal stimulation may cause nausea and vomiting, bradycardia, and hypotension. Hiccupping may develop due to diaphragmatic irritation. If a large vessel is occluded, the first sign of MI may be sudden death. Typical manifestations of MI are listed in the box on page 935.

Complications

The risk of complications associated with MI is related to its size and location.

Dysrhythmias

Dysrhythmias, disturbances or irregularities of heart rhythm, are the most frequent complication of MI. Dysrhythmias are discussed in detail in the next section of this chapter.

Infarcted tissue is *arrhythmogenic*; that is, it alters the generation and conduction of electrical impulses in the heart, increasing the risk of dysrhythmias. Premature ventricular contractions (PVCs) are common following an MI, developing in more than 90% of patients with an AMI. While not dangerous in themselves, they may be predictive of more dangerous dysrhythmias such as ventricular tachycardia or ventricular fibrillation (Woods et al., 2009). Ventricular fibrillation (VF) is a frequent cause of sudden cardiac death. The risk of ventricular fibrillation is greatest in the first hour after MI, declining with time. Infarction around a conduction pathway will affect electrical conduction. Atrioventricular (AV) block may occur following anterior wall infarction. First-degree and Mobitz I (Wenckebach) blocks are most common, although complete heart block can occur. Bradydysrhythmias (abnormal slow rhythms) may develop when the inferior wall of the ventricle is affected.

NURSING CARE OF THE PATIENT | Having A Permanent Pacemaker Implant

PREOPERATIVE CARE

- Provide routine preoperative care and teaching as outlined in ∞ Chapter 4.
- Assess knowledge and understanding of the procedure, clarifying and expanding on existing knowledge as needed. *Clarifying knowledge, providing information, and conveying emotional support reduces anxiety and fear and allows the patient to develop a realistic outlook regarding pacer therapy.*
- Place ECG monitor electrodes away from potential incision sites. *This helps preserve skin integrity.*
- Teach range-of-motion (ROM) exercises for the affected side. *ROM exercises of the affected arm and shoulder prevent stiffness and impaired function following pacemaker insertion.*

POSTOPERATIVE CARE

- Provide postoperative monitoring, analgesia, and care as outlined in ∞ Chapter 4.
- Obtain a chest x-ray as ordered. *A postoperative chest x-ray is used to identify lead location and detect possible complications, such as pneumothorax or pleural effusion.*
- Position for comfort. Minimize movement of the affected arm and shoulder during the initial postoperative period. *Restricting movement minimizes discomfort on the operative side and allows the leads to become anchored, reducing the risk of dislodging.*
- Assist with gentle ROM exercises at least three times daily, beginning 24 hours after pacemaker implantation. *ROM exercises help restore normal shoulder movement and prevent contractures on the affected side.*
- Monitor pacemaker function with cardiac monitoring or intermittent ECGs. Report pacemaker problems to the physician:
  - Failure to pace. *This may indicate battery depletion, damage or dislodgement of pacer wires, or inappropriate sensing.*
  - Failure to capture (the pacemaker stimulus is not followed by ventricular depolarization). *The electrical output of the pacemaker may not be adequate, or the lead may be dislodged.*
  - Improper sensing (the pacemaker is firing or not firing, regardless of the intrinsic rate). *This increases the risk for decreased cardiac output and dysrhythmias.*
  - Runaway pacemaker (a pacemaker firing at a rapid rate). *This may by due to generator malfunction or problems with sensing.*
  - Hiccups. *A lead positioned near the diaphragm can stimulate it, causing hiccups. Hiccups may occur in extremely thin patients or may indicate a medical emergency with perforation of the right ventricle by the pacing electrode tip.*
- Assess for dysrhythmias and treat as indicated. *Until the catheter is "seated" or adheres to the myocardium, its movement may cause myocardial irritability and dysrhythmias. Fibrotic tissue develops within 2 to 3 days.*

- Document the date of pacemaker insertion, the model and type, and settings. *This information is important for future reference.*
- Immediately report signs of potential complications, including myocardial perforation, cardiac tamponade, pneumothorax, hemothorax, emboli, skin breakdown, bleeding, infection, endocarditis, or poor wound healing (∞ see Chapter 31 for more information about cardiac tamponade and endocarditis, and ∞ Chapter 36 for pneumothorax and hemothorax). *Early identification of complications allows for aggressive intervention.*
- Provide a pacemaker identification card including the manufacturer's name, model number, mode of operation, rate parameters, and expected battery life. *This card provides a reference for the patient and future healthcare providers.*

HOME CARE

Provide appropriate teaching for the patient and family about the following:

- Placement of the pacemaker generator and leads in relation to the heart.
- How the pacemaker works and the rate at which it is set.
- Battery replacement. Most pacemaker batteries last 6 to 12 years. Replacement requires outpatient surgery to open the subcutaneous pocket and replace the battery.
- Notify healthcare provider of weakness, dizziness, or light-headedness.
- How to take and record the pulse rate. Instruct to assess pulse daily before arising and notify the physician if 5 or more BPM slower than the preset pacemaker rate.
- Incision care and signs of infection. Bruising may be present following surgery.
- Signs of pacemaker malfunction to report, including dizziness, fainting, fatigue, weakness, chest pain, or palpitations.
- Activity restrictions as ordered. This usually is limited to contact sports (which may damage the generator) and avoiding heavy lifting for 2 months after surgery.
- Resume sexual activity as recommended by the physician. Avoid positions that cause pressure on the site.
- Avoid tight-fitting clothing over the pacemaker site to reduce irritation and avoid skin breakdown.
- Carry the pacemaker identification card at all times, and wear a MedicAlert bracelet or tag.
- Notify all care providers of the pacemaker.
- Do not hold or use certain electrical devices over the pacemaker site, including household appliances or tools, garage door openers, antitheft devices, or burglar alarms. A pacemaker will set off airport security detectors; notify security officials of its presence.
- Maintain follow-up care with the physician as recommended.

∞ Nursing Care

Caring for the patient with cardiac dysrhythmias requires the ability to recognize, identify, and promptly treat the dysrhythmia. The urgency of intervention is determined by the effects of the dysrhythmia on the patient. Nursing care focuses on maintaining cardiac output, monitoring the response to therapy, and teaching. See the Case Study & Nursing Care Plan for a patient with a dysrhythmia.

Health Promotion

Health promotion measures to prevent CHD also reduce the risk for dysrhythmias. In most cases, dysrhythmias develop as a result of ischemic or structural changes in the heart, rather than in isolation. Advise patients who are at risk or who complain of occasional palpitations or "flutters" in their chest to reduce their intake of caffeine and other sympathetic nervous system stimulants, such as excess chocolate.

Assessment

Assessment is vital before treating any suspected dysrhythmia. What appears to be ventricular tachycardia on the monitor may be the patient scratching or brushing his or her teeth. Apparent asystole on the monitor may be due to a loose electrode patch. Similarly, a heart rate of 52 BPM may not affect the overall cardiac output in some patients. ∞ Review Chapter 29 for complete assessment of the patient with a cardiac problem.

- *Health history:* Complaints of palpitations (ask for further definition of palpitations), "fluttering" sensations, or a sensation of the heart racing; episodes of dizziness, lightheadedness, or syncope (fainting); timing (duration, time of day); correlation with food or beverage intake, activity; presence of chest pain, shortness of breath, or other associated symptoms; history of heart or endocrine disease (such as hyperthyroidism); current medications.
- *Physical examination:* Level of consciousness (LOC); vital signs, including apical pulse for a full minute; regularity and amplitude of peripheral pulses; color; presence of dyspnea, adventitious lung sounds; ECG rhythm analysis; oxygen saturation levels.

Nursing Diagnoses and Interventions

The effect of the dysrhythmia on cardiac output is the priority of nursing care. Other potential nursing diagnoses related to dysrhythmias may include *Ineffective Tissue Perfusion*, *Activity Intolerance*, and *Fear* or *Anxiety*.

Decreased Cardiac Output

Dysrhythmias can affect cardiac output. Bradycardias decrease cardiac output if the stroke volume does not increase to compensate for the slow heart rate. Tachycardia reduces diastolic filling time, affecting stroke volume and coronary artery perfusion. Loss of the atrial kick in junctional rhythms, atrial fibrillation, and AV blocks also decreases ventricular filling and cardiac output. In ventricular fibrillation, loss of ventricular contractions causes cardiac arrest and no cardiac output.

> **PRACTICE ALERT**
> Before treating any dysrhythmia, assess the patient, not just the monitor! Loose electrode pads, disconnected leads or cables, and muscle movement can simulate critical dysrhythmias. The patient's condition is the best indicator of the need for treatment.

- Assess for decreased cardiac output: decreased LOC; tachycardia; tachypnea; hypotension; low oxygen saturation; diaphoresis; low urine output; cool, clammy, mottled skin; pallor or cyanosis; and diminished peripheral pulses. *Initial signs of decreased cardiac output may be subtle, such as decreased LOC. Early recognition of the dysrhythmia's effect on cardiac output facilitates appropriate treatment and may prevent further adverse effects.*
- Monitor ECG; post ECG strip every shift and when rhythm changes occur. *Documenting cardiac rhythm provides a record of disease progression and treatment effectiveness.*

> **PRACTICE ALERT**
> Assess vital signs, ECG, and oxygen saturation every 5 to 15 minutes during acute dysrhythmic episodes and during antidysrhythmic drug infusions. These data provide a record of cardiac output during the dysrhythmia. Antidysrhythmic drugs can adversely affect heart rate, rhythm, and blood pressure, further decreasing cardiac output.

- Assess for underlying causes of dysrhythmias, such as hypovolemia, hypoxia, anemia, electrolyte imbalance, vagal stimulation, or medications. *Sinus tachycardia often develops in response to tissue hypoxia. Vagal stimulation (such as the Valsalva maneuver) can precipitate bradycardia.*
- Assess serum electrolytes (especially potassium, calcium, and magnesium) and digitalis and antidysrhythmic drug levels as indicated. Report abnormal values. *Electrolyte imbalances affect cardiac depolarization and repolarization and may cause dysrhythmias. Toxic levels of digitalis and antidysrhythmic drugs can precipitate further dysrhythmias. Impaired renal or hepatic function increases the risk for toxicity, as does aging.*
- Be prepared to administer antidysrhythmic medications as indicated. Implement Advanced Cardiac Life Support (ACLS) protocols as needed. *Emergency drugs should be readily available, especially on units with high-risk patients. See Table 30–7 and the Medication Administration box on page 956 for drugs used to treat common dysrhythmias that may affect cardiac output.*
- If appropriate, instruct to perform the Valsalva maneuver (bear down as if straining or coughing) for supraventricular tachycardia or ventricular tachycardia without angina. *Vagal maneuvers stimulate the parasympathetic system and may terminate some dysrhythmias. The Valsalva maneuver is contraindicated if chest pain occurs with the dysrhythmia.*
- Prepare to assist with cardioversion. Prepare the patient per orders or hospital protocol (see Procedure 30–2). Explain the procedure to reduce anxiety. Have emergency equipment readily available. *Elective or emergency cardioversion is a treatment of choice for certain dysrhythmias.*

> **PRACTICE ALERT**
> On recognizing ventricular fibrillation and cardiac arrest, begin emergency procedures. Call for help. Obtain defibrillator and immediately defibrillate. If the defibrillator will be brought by another healthcare provider, begin CPR. Initiate ACLS protocols and assist with resuscitation measures as directed. Cardiac output ceases with ventricular fibrillation. Immediate or early defibrillation has been shown to have the greatest impact on survival following cardiac arrest.

- After cardiac arrest, transfer to critical care. Perform and document head-to-toe assessment; obtain laboratory tests, 12-lead ECG, and chest x-ray as ordered; monitor and maintain oxygenation and intravenous infusions; and monitor vital signs and cardiac rhythm. *The period following resuscitation is critical, necessitating careful monitoring. Postarrest assessment allows comparison of the patient's condition with prearrest status and may identify CPR-related injuries. Correcting electrolyte disturbances, hypoxia, and acid–base imbalances is*

CASE STUDY & NURSING CARE PLAN   A Patient with Supraventricular Tachycardia

Elisa Vasquez, 53 years old, is admitted to the cardiac unit with complaints of palpitations, lightheadedness, and shortness of breath. Her history reveals rheumatic fever at age 12 with subsequent rheumatic heart disease and mitral stenosis. An intravenous line is in place and she is receiving oxygen. Marcia Lewin, RN, is assigned to Ms. Vasquez.

ASSESSMENT

Ms. Lewin's assessment reveals that Ms. Vasquez is moderately anxious. Her ECG shows supraventricular tachycardia (SVT) with a rate of 154. Vital signs: T 98.8° F (37.1°C), R 26, BP 95/60. Peripheral pulses weak but equal, mucous membranes pale pink, skin cool and dry. Fine crackles noted in both lung bases. A loud S_3 gallop and a diastolic murmur are noted. Ms. Vasquez is still complaining of palpitations and tells Ms. Lewin, "I feel so nervous and weak and dizzy." Ms. Vasquez's cardiologist orders 2.5 mg of verapamil to be given slowly via intravenous push and tells Ms. Lewin to prepare to assist with synchronized cardioversion if drug therapy does not control the ventricular rate.

DIAGNOSIS

- *Decreased Cardiac Output* related to inadequate ventricular filling associated with rapid tachycardia
- *Ineffective Tissue Perfusion: Cerebral/Cardiopulmonary/Peripheral* related to decreased cardiac output
- *Anxiety* related to unknown outcome of altered health state

EXPECTED OUTCOMES

- Maintain adequate cardiac output and tissue perfusion.
- Demonstrate a ventricular rate within normal limits and stable vital signs.
- Verbalize reduced anxiety.
- Verbalize an understanding of the rationale for the treatment measures to control the heart rate.

PLANNING AND IMPLEMENTATION

- Provide oxygen per nasal cannula at 4 L/min.
- Continuously monitor ECG for rate, rhythm, and conduction. Assess vital signs and associated symptoms with changes in ECG. Report findings to physician.
- Explain the importance of rapidly reducing the heart rate. Explain the cardioversion procedure and encourage questions.

- Encourage verbalization of fears and concerns. Answer questions honestly, correcting misconceptions about the disease process, treatment, or prognosis.
- Administer intravenous diazepam as ordered before cardioversion.
- Document pretreatment vital signs, level of consciousness, and peripheral pulses.
- Place emergency cart with drugs and airway management supplies in patient unit.
- Assist with cardioversion as indicated.
- Assess LOC, level of sedation, cardiovascular and respiratory status, and skin condition following cardioversion.
- Document procedure and postcardioversion rhythm, and response to intervention.

EVALUATION

Intravenous verapamil lowers Ms. Vasquez's heart rate to 138 for a short time, after which it increases to 164 with BP of 82/64. Her cardiologist, Dr. Mullins, performs carotid sinus massage. The ventricular rate slows to 126 for 2 minutes, revealing atrial flutter waves, and then returns to a rate of 150. Dr. Mullins explains the treatment options, including synchronized cardioversion. Ms. Vasquez agrees to the procedure.

Ms. Vasquez is lightly sedated and synchronized cardioversion is performed. One countershock converts Ms. Vasquez to regular sinus rhythm at 96 BPM with BP 112/60.

Ms. Vasquez is sleepy from the sedation but recovers without incident. She states that she feels "much better," and her vital signs return to her normal levels. She remains in NSR with a rate of 86 to 92 for the remainder of her hospital stay. Dr. Mullins places Ms. Vasquez on furosemide to treat manifestations of mild heart failure.

CRITICAL THINKING IN THE NURSING PROCESS

1. What is the scientific basis for using carotid massage to treat supraventricular tachycardias? Was this an appropriate maneuver in the case of Ms. Vasquez?
2. What other treatment options might the physician have used to treat Ms. Vasquez's supraventricular tachycardia if she had been asymptomatic with stable vital signs?
3. Develop a teaching plan for Ms. Vasquez related to her prescription for furosemide.

See Evaluating Your Response in Appendix C.

important to prevent further dysrhythmias and potential adverse effects on cardiac output. Intravenous access is crucial to maintain drug infusions. Hemodynamic monitoring may be instituted. The 12-lead ECG documents myocardial status, and the chest x-ray provides information about pulmonary status and possible thoracic injury due to CPR.

- Notify the family of significant changes in the patient's condition or cardiac arrest, providing up-to-date information. Prepare family members prior to visits by explaining interventions (such as invasive tubes, a ventilator, or additional equipment) implemented since the last visit. *Concern for the family and significant others is part of holistic nursing. Researchers studying the needs of families have found that one of the most important needs was information about their loved one's condition. Patients and families need and appreciate honest communication and compassionate care. Preparing the family for critical changes in the patient's condition and plan of care helps them to cope with a situational crisis.*

Community-Based Care

Dysrhythmias have a significant physical and psychologic impact on the patient and all family members. Many of these patients and their families are under a great deal of stress from frequent hospitalizations, experimentation with therapies, frustration, and the fear of sudden cardiac death. A major teaching effort focuses on coping strategies and lifestyle changes, as well as specific management of prescribed therapies. Include the following topics as appropriate when teaching the patient and family for home care:

- Function, maintenance, precautions, and signs of malfunction or complications of any implanted device such as a pacemaker or ICD
- Monitoring pulse rate and rhythm
- Activity or dietary restrictions, and any potential effects of the dysrhythmia or its treatment on lifestyle
- Medication management to reduce the risk of dysrhythmias, including the desired and potential adverse effects of antidysrhythmic drugs

- Specific instructions related to planned diagnostic tests or procedures
- The importance of follow-up visits with the cardiologist
- The importance of and where to obtain CPR training for the patient and family members

In addition, discuss fears related to treatment or implanted devices, such as that of shocking a significant other during close contact or sexual activity. Explain that if a shock occurs, the partner may feel a slight buzz or tingling but should not be harmed. Refer to and encourage the patient and family to attend a peer support group for the specific condition.

The Patient with Sudden Cardiac Death

Sudden cardiac death (SCD) is defined as unexpected death occurring within 1 hour of the onset of cardiovascular symptoms. It usually is caused by ventricular fibrillation and cardiac arrest. *Cardiac arrest* is the sudden collapse, loss of consciousness, and cessation of effective circulation that precedes biologic death. Worldwide, less than 6% of out-of-hospital cardiac arrest victims survive. In communities of North America that have organized lay rescuer and automated AED programs, the survival rate is significantly better, ranging from 49% to 74% when a witnessed arrest due to ventricular fibrillation occurs (AHA, 2005).

Almost 50% of all deaths due to CHD are attributed to SCD. CHD causes up to 80% of all sudden cardiac deaths in the United States. Other cardiac pathologies such as cardiomyopathy and valvular disorders also may lead to SCD. Noncardiac causes of sudden death include electrocution, pulmonary embolism, and rapid blood loss from a ruptured aortic aneurysm.

Ventricular fibrillation is the most common dysrhythmia associated with SCD, accounting for 65% to 80% of cardiac arrests. Sustained severe bradydysrhythmias, *asystole* or cardiac standstill, and pulseless electrical activity (organized cardiac electrical activity without a mechanical response) are responsible for most remaining SCDs (EHRA et al., 2006). Selected cardiac and noncardiac causes of sudden cardiac death are listed in Box 30–6.

Risk factors for SCD are those associated with CHD (see the first section of this chapter). Advancing age and male gender are powerful risk factors. After age 65, the gap between male and female incidence of SCD narrows (EHRA et al., 2006). Patients with dysrhythmias such as recurrent VT may have a higher risk of SCD. Women with AMI, however, are more likely to present with cardiac arrest and cardiogenic shock than with ventricular tachycardia (Jensen & Moser, 2008).

Pathophysiology

Evidence of CHD with significant atherosclerosis and narrowing of two or more major coronary arteries is found in 75% of SCD victims. Although most have had prior MI, only 20% to 30% have recent AMI. An acute change in cardiovascular status precedes cardiac arrest by up to 1 hour; however, often the onset is instantaneous or abrupt. Tachycardia develops, and the

---

BOX 30–6 **Selected Causes of Sudden Cardiac Death**

Cardiac Causes
- Coronary heart disease
- Reperfusion following ischemia
- Myocardial hypertrophy
- Cardiomyopathy
- Inflammatory myocardial disorders
- Valve disorders
- Primary electrical disorders
- Dissecting or ruptured aortic or ventricular aneurysm
- Cardiac drug toxicity

Noncardiac Causes
- Pulmonary embolism
- Cerebral hemorrhage
- Autonomic dysfunction
- Choking
- Electrical shock
- Electrolyte and acid–base imbalances

---

number of PVCs increase. This is followed by a run of VT that deteriorates into VF (Perrin, 2009).

Abnormalities of myocardial structure or function also contribute. Structural abnormalities include infarction, hypertrophy, myopathy, and electrical anomalies. Functional deviations are caused by such factors as ischemia followed by reperfusion, altered homeostasis, autonomic nervous system and hormone interactions, and toxic effects. The interactions of the two cause myocardial instability and may precipitate fatal dysrhythmias.

Manifestations

SCD may be preceded by typical manifestations of ACS or MI, including severe chest pain, dyspnea or orthopnea, and palpitations or light-headedness. The event itself is abrupt, with complete loss of consciousness and death within minutes. If VT precedes cardiac arrest, consciousness and mentation may be impaired prior to collapse and loss of consciousness.

Interdisciplinary Care

The goal of care is to restore cardiac output and tissue perfusion. Treatment measures are initiated as soon as clinical cardiac arrest is verified by the absence of respirations and carotid or femoral pulses. Basic and advanced cardiac life support measures must be instituted within 2 to 4 minutes of cardiac arrest to prevent permanent neurologic damage and ischemic injury to other organs.

Basic Life Support

Basic life support (BLS) begins with identification of the cardiac arrest and initiation of an emergency response.

Providers trained in use of the *automated external defibrillator (AED)* should immediately defibrillate the patient in VF. Self-adhesive conductive pads attached to connecting cables are positioned on the chest (Figure 30–13 ■). The AED analyzes the rhythm and advises the provider to charge the device if VF is detected. After warning all personnel to stand clear, the shock button is depressed to deliver a shock. Following the shock, CPR is immediately initiated. After approximately 2 minutes or five cycles of CPR, the rhythm is evaluated and circulation checked. The sequence of analysis, shock, and CPR is continued and ACLS protocols are initiated (AHA, 2005).

Figure 30–13 ■ Schematic of an automated external defibrillator (AED) attached to a patient.

Cardiopulmonary resuscitation (CPR) is a mechanical attempt to maintain tissue perfusion and oxygenation using oral resuscitation and external cardiac compressions. All healthcare providers need to be proficient in CPR. The technique should be performed according to AHA guidelines and hospital protocol (see Box 30–7). Research demonstrates clear benefit from sustained, effective chest compressions, yet compressions often are interrupted for ventilation, assessment of pulses, and other measures. Many patients are excessively ventilated and under-perfused during CPR (Sanders & Ewy, 2005).

CPR carries a high risk for both cardiac and noncardiac trauma. CPR-related complications include injuries to the skin, thorax, upper airway, abdomen, lungs, heart, and great vessels. These complications can be minimized by adhering to accepted CPR techniques.

Advanced Life Support

Advanced life support (ALS), provided by specially trained healthcare personnel, includes advanced airway support (insertion of a laryngeal mask airway [LMA], esophageal-tracheal Combitube, or endotracheal intubation) to maintain the airway and oxygenation, use of intravenous drugs following specific protocols, and additional interventions such as repeated defibrillation procedures and cardiac pacing. Epinephrine, vasopressin, sodium bicarbonate, and antidysrhythmic drugs such as amiodarone, bretylium, lidocaine, procainamide, magnesium sulfate, and atropine are used to attempt to restore and maintain an effective cardiac rhythm.

Postresuscitation Care

Patients who experience SCD associated with ventricular fibrillation and acute MI have the best prognosis (EHRA et al., 2006). The patient is transferred to a coronary care unit and MI treatment measures are instituted. Antidysrhythmic drugs may be continued for 24 to 48 hours to reduce the risk of subsequent episodes of VF.

Because the risk for recurrent SCD is significant in survivors, extensive diagnostic testing and interventions such as angioplasty or surgical revascularization of the myocardium, ablation, or an implantable cardioverter-defibrillator may be indicated.

✍ Nursing Care

Nursing care of the patient experiencing SCD requires prompt recognition of the event and immediate initiation of BLS and ALS protocols. As noted before, fast and effective cardiac compressions and early defibrillation of unstable VT and VF are the most important keys to survival of cardiac arrest victims. Important concepts of emergency cardiac care follow.

- Treat the patient, not the monitor. Recognize signs and symptoms of cardiac compromise early.
- Activate the emergency medical services system (i.e., call a code or call 911).
- Begin and continue basic cardiac life support principles throughout the resuscitation effort.
- Continually assess the effectiveness of emergency interventions.
- Defibrillate pulseless VT or VF as soon as possible.
- Initiate ALS protocols early.

The family is not forgotten during resuscitation. If the family is present, they are usually offered a private consultation room in which to await the outcome. If the family is not present, they are notified that their family member is not doing well and asked to come to the hospital as soon as possible. The situation is presented in a careful manner to prevent the family from racing to the hospital, precipitating an automobile crash. Pastoral care or the family's choice of spiritual support is offered to help during this difficult time. Attendance of family members during resuscitation efforts is controversial, and depends on institutional protocols and family desires.

After successful resuscitation, the nurse provides care specific to the patient's underlying disease processes and needs. Intravenous infusions such as lidocaine, bretylium, or dopamine may be ordered to prevent further dysrhythmias and maintain hemodynamic stability.

If the patient does not survive the arrest, the nurse provides postmortem care and emotional and spiritual support to the family.

BOX 30–7 Cardiopulmonary Resuscitation

1. Assess for responsiveness; shake the patient and shout.
2. Call for help. Dial 911 (if outside the healthcare facility) or initiate the institutional code or cardiac arrest procedure.
3. Open the airway using the head-tilt/chin-lift maneuvers. Simultaneously press down on the forehead with one hand while lifting the chin upward with the other (part *A* of the accompanying figure).
4. Check for breathing; look and listen. Inspect the chest for rise and fall with respirations; listen and feel for air movement through the nose or mouth. This step should take no more than 10 seconds.
5. If not breathing, begin rescue breathing using a pocket mask, mouth shield, or bag-valve mask (see part *B* of the figure). Administer two breaths (1 second per breath), observing for rise of the chest with each breath.
6. Check the carotid or femoral artery for a pulse (≤ 10 sec).
7. If a pulse is present, continue rescue breathing, administering 8 to 10 breaths per minute, until help arrives or spontaneous respirations resume. Recheck the carotid pulse every 2 minutes.
8. If no pulse is present, analyze rhythm and defibrillate or, if unwitnessed arrest or AED unavailable, initiate external cardiac compressions. Place on a firm surface. Position the heel of one hand in the center of the chest between the nipples (child and adult), with the other hand on top and the fingers either interlocked or extended.
9. Initiate hard and fast cardiac compressions, pressing straight down to depress the sternum 1.5 to 2 inches, keeping the elbows locked and positioning the shoulders directly over the hands (part *C* of the figure). Release pressure completely between compressions but do not lift the hands from the chest.
10. Compress the chest at a rate of approximately 100 times per minute. With one- or two-rescuer CPR, provide two breaths after each 30 compressions. Assess the pulse after five complete cycles of 30 compressions and two breaths; continue CPR until help arrives.

A, Head-tilt/Chin-lift maneuver and using a bag-valve mask.
B, Placement of hands on the sternum between nipples.
C, Arm, hand, and shoulder position for cardiac massage.

Nursing diagnoses to consider for the patient experiencing SCD include the following:

- *Ineffective Tissue Perfusion: Cerebral* related to ineffective cardiac output
- *Impaired Spontaneous Ventilation* related to cardiac arrest
- *Spiritual Distress* related to unexplained sudden cardiac death
- *Disturbed Thought Processes* related to compromised cerebral circulation
- *Fear* related to risk for future episodes of sudden cardiac death

The risk for a future episode of SCD requires careful and effective teaching for home care prior to discharge. Discuss the following topics with the patient and family:

- Risk factor reduction for CHD
- Planned diagnostic studies to identify the cause of SCD, and possible interventions

- The risks and benefits of an ICD if appropriate
- The importance of carrying a card at all times listing all current medications and the healthcare provider
- Early manifestations or warning signs of cardiac arrest
- The importance of CPR training and maintaining proficiency in performing CPR (Provide referral to local CPR training providers or scheduled classes through the American Heart Association or American Red Cross.)

Nurses can impact death rates from cardiac arrest through community teaching as well. Survival rates from SCD improve in communities in which a significant portion of the population is trained in CPR and early response by EMS agencies is stressed. Work with community groups and individuals can help create a population of people able to perform effective CPR.

CHAPTER HIGHLIGHTS

- Atherosclerosis is the primary underlying process in coronary heart disease, impaired perfusion of myocardial tissue.
- The risk factors for coronary heart disease are those for atherosclerosis: age, gender, and genetic factors; hypertension, diabetes, abnormal blood lipids; cigarette smoking, obesity, physical inactivity, and diet; and emerging risk factors such as the metabolic syndrome and homocysteine levels.
- Smoking cessation, exercise, diet modification, weight loss, medications to achieve desired blood lipid values, and effective hypertension and diabetes management are the primary treatment measures for coronary heart disease.
- Atherosclerosis of coronary vessels impairs the supply of blood, oxygen, and nutrients to the myocardium. Myocardial ischemia results in the manifestations of coronary heart disease, angina pectoris, acute coronary syndrome, and myocardial infarction.
- Stable angina develops with a predictable amount of activity or stress, and typically follows an activity–pain, rest–relief pattern. Stable angina often can be managed effectively by medications and risk factor modification. The nursing focus is on education.
- Acute coronary syndrome or unstable angina is characterized by increasingly severe chest pain that occurs unpredictably. Acute coronary syndrome often requires aggressive interventions such as percutaneous coronary revascularization or coronary artery bypass surgery.
- Myocardial infarction, necrosis of myocardial tissue, results from complete blockage of a coronary artery, usually due to atherosclerotic plaque rupture and thrombus formation. Prompt restoration of blood flow through a revascularization procedure or administration of a fibrinolytic drug to dissolve the blood clot is necessary to preserve functional muscle tissue.

- The nursing focus for patients with acute coronary syndrome and myocardial infarction is on reducing myocardial work through measures such as pain relief and activity limitation, promoting blood flow and oxygenation through medication and oxygen administration and positioning, and early recognition and treatment of complications.
- Cardiac dysrhythmias may arise anywhere in conductive tissue of the myocardium. Dysrhythmias may be either benign or fatal, depending on their effect on cardiac output.
- Tachycardias increase the workload of the heart and may interfere with cardiac output if ventricular filling is impaired by the rapid rate.
- Bradycardias can affect cardiac output when the rate is too slow to meet the metabolic needs of the body.
- Atrial fibrillation is a common dysrhythmia that can lead to formation of blood clots within the heart and subsequent stroke if these clots lodge in cerebral blood vessels.
- Frequent ventricular dysrhythmias may indicate an increased risk for ventricular fibrillation and cardiac arrest.
- AV conduction blocks interfere with conduction of the sinus or atrial impulse through the AV node and to the ventricles.
- Although many antidysrhythmic medications are available, all increase the risk of dysrhythmia development, so they are used sparingly.
- The nurse's role in caring for patients with cardiac dysrhythmias focuses on prompt identification of the rhythm disruption, assessment of its effect on the patient, administration of medications and other treatment measures, and institution of life support procedures as indicated.

TEST YOURSELF NCLEX-RN® REVIEW

1. The nurse evaluates her teaching as effective when a patient identifies which of the following modifiable risk factors for coronary heart disease (CHD) as contributing to the greatest extent?
   1. obesity
   2. diet
   3. smoking
   4. stress
2. When teaching a patient about lovastatin (Mevacor), the nurse instructs the patient to do which of the following?
   1. Promptly report muscle pain or tenderness to the physician.
   2. Consume a diet that includes no more than 20% of calories from saturated fat.
   3. Abstain from alcohol use while taking this drug.
   4. Take the drug with meals to minimize gastric distress.
3. When assessing a patient with stable angina, the nurse would expect to find which of the following?
   1. persistent ECG changes
   2. correlation between activity level and pain
   3. increasing nocturnal pain
   4. evidence of impaired cardiac output such as weak peripheral pulses

4. The nurse caring for a patient with acute coronary syndrome identifies which of the following nursing diagnoses as of highest priority?
   1. *Anxiety* related to unknown outcome of disorder
   2. *Ineffective Health Maintenance* related to lack of knowledge about coronary heart disease
   3. *Decreased Cardiac Output* related to myocardial ischemia
   4. *Ineffective Tissue Perfusion: Cardiopulmonary* related to underlying coronary heart disease
5. The nurse caring for a patient returning from a coronary angioplasty with stent placement plans which of the following interventions?
   1. securing chest tubes to bedding
   2. maintaining leg extension on the affected side
   3. discontinuing intravenous lines when taking oral fluids
   4. treating chest pain with intravenous morphine as needed
6. In planning care for the patient with acute myocardial infarction (AMI), the nurse identifies the highest priority goal of care as which of the following?
   1. stable ECG rhythm
   2. ability to verbalize causes and effects of CHD
   3. compliance with prescribed bed rest
   4. relief of pain

7. Which of the following nursing diagnoses is of highest priority for the patient undergoing fibrinolytic therapy?
1. *Ineffective Protection*
2. *Ineffective Health Maintenance*
3. *Risk for Powerlessness*
4. *Anxiety*

8. In reviewing laboratory results for a patient admitted with acute chest pain, the nurse is most concerned about which of the following?
1. hematocrit 35%
2. AST 65 U/L
3. CK 320 U/L
4. APTT 35 seconds

9. The nurse recognizes second-degree AV block, type II (Mobitz II), and intervenes appropriately when he does which of the following?
1. records the finding in the chart
2. prepares for temporary pacemaker insertion
3. administers a class IB antidysrhythmic drug
4. places the patient in Fowler's position

10. On identifying sinus bradycardia at a rate of 45 BPM, the nurse should do which of the following?
1. Assess mental status and blood pressure.
2. Assess peripheral pulses on all four extremities.
3. Determine if an apical-radial pulse deficit is present.
4. Prepare to administer intravenous atropine.

See Test Yourself answers in Appendix C.

Pearson Nursing Student Resources

Find additional review materials at
www.nursing.pearsonhighered.com

Prepare for success with additional NCLEX®-style practice questions, interactive assignments and activities, Web links, animations and videos, and more!

BIBLIOGRAPHY

American College of Cardiology/American Heart Association Task Force and the European Society of Cardiology. (2006). Guidelines for the management of patients with atrial fibrillation. *Journal of the American College of Cardiology, 48*(4), 854–906.

American Heart Association. (2005). Acute Coronary Syndromes. In: 2005 International Consensus Conference on cardiopulmonary resuscitation and emergency cardiovascular care Science with treatment recommendations. *Circulation, 112*(22 Suppl), III55–III72.

American Heart Association. (2009). Heart disease and stroke statistics—2009 update. *Circulation, 119,* e21–e181.

American Heart Association Nutrition Committee. (2006). Diet and lifestyle recommendations revision 2006: A scientific statement from the American Heart Association Nutrition Committee. *Circulation, 114*(1), 82–96.

Anderson, J. L., Adams, C. D., Antman, E. M., Bridges, C. R., Califf, R. M., Casey, D. E., et al. (2007). ACC/AHA 2007 guidelines for the management of patients with unstable angina/non-ST-elevation myocardial infarction: A report of the American College of Cardiology. *Journal of the American College of Cardiology, 50*(7), e1–e157.

Bonow, R. O., Carabello, B. A., Chatterjee, K., de Leon, A. C., Faxon, D. P., Freed, M. D., et al. (2006). ACC/AHA 2006 guideline for the management of patients with valvular heart disease. *Journal of the American College of Cardiology, 48*(3), e1–e148.

Bulechek, G., Butcher, H., & Dochterman, J. M. (Eds.). (2008). *Nursing interventions classification (NIC)* (5th ed.). St. Louis: Mosby Elsevier.

Chan, D. S., Chan, J. P., & Chang, A.M. (2005). Acute coronary syndromes: Cardiac rehabilitation programmes and quality of life. *Journal of Advanced Nursing, 49*(6), 591–599.

Deglin, J. H., & Vallerand, A. H. (2009). *Davis's drug guide*. Philadelphia: F.A. Davis.

Domino, F. J., Baldor, R. A., Golding, J., Grimes, J., & Taylor, J. S. (2010). *The 5-minute clinical consult* (18th ed.). Philadelphia: Lippincott, Williams & Wilkins.

Eagle, K. A., Guyton, R. A., Davidoff, R., Edwards, F. H., Ewy, G. A., Gardner, T. J., et al. (2004). ACC/AHA 2004 guideline update for coronary artery bypass graft surgery: A report of the American College of Cardiology/American Heart Association Task Force on Practice Guidelines. Retrieved from www.acc.org/clinical/guidelines/cabg/cabg.pdf

Epstein, A. E., DiMarco, J. P., Ellenbogen, K. A., Estes, N. A., Freedman, R. A. Gettes, L. S., et al. (2008). ACC/AHA/HRS 2008 guidelines for device-based therapy of cardiac rhythm abnormalities: A report so the American College of Cardiology/American Heart Association Task Force. *Journal of the American College of Cardiology, 51*(21), e1–e62.

European Heart Rhythm Association, Heart Rhythm Society, Zipes, D. P., et al. (2006). ACC/AHA/ESC 2006 Guidelines for the management of patients with ventricular arrhythmias and the prevention of sudden cardiac death: A report of the American College of Cardiology/American Heart Association Task Force and the European Society of Cardiology. *American Journal of the College of Cardiology, 48*(5), e247–e346.

Foley, S. (2005). Update on risk factors for atherosclerosis: The role of inflammation and apolipoprotein E. *Medsurg Nursing, 14*(1), 43–50.

Hardin-Fanning, F. (2008). The effects of a Mediterranean-style dietary pattern on cardiovascular risk. *Nursing Clinics of North America, 43*(1), 105–115.

Jensen, L. A., & Moser, D. A. (2008). Gender differences in knowledge, attitudes, and beliefs about heart disease. *Nursing Clinics of North America, 43*(1), 77–104.

Greenland, P., Bonow, R. O., Brundage, B. H., Budoff, J., Eisenberg, M. J., Grundy, S. M., et al. (2007). ACCF/AHA 2007 clinical expert consensus document on coronary artery calcium scoring by computed tomography in global cardiovascular risk assessment and in evaluation of patients with chest pain. *Journal of the American College of Cardiology, 49*(3), 378–402.

Grines, C. L., Bonow, R. O., Casey D. E., Gardner, T. J., Lockhart, P. B., Moliterno, D. J., et al. (2007). Prevention of premature discontinuation of dual antiplatelet therapy in patients with coronary artery stents. *Circulation, 115*(6), 813–818.

Hart, P. L. (2005). Women's perceptions of coronary heart disease: An integrative review. *Journal of Cardiovascular Nursing, 20*(3), 170–176.

Householder-Hughes, S. (2006). Non-ST segment elevation acute coronary syndromes: Management strategies for optimal outcomes. *Critical Care Nurse Supplement*, 8–36.

Huether, S. E., & McCance, K. L. (2008). *Understanding Pathophysiology* (4th ed.). St. Louis: Mosby Elsevier.

King, S. B., Smith, S. C., Hirshfeld, J.W., Jacobs, A. K., Morrison, D. A., Williams, D. O., et al. (2008). 2007 focused update of the ACC/AHA/SCAI 2005 guideline update for percutaneous coronary intervention: A report of the American College of Cardiology/American Heart Association Task Force on practice guidelines. *Journal of the American College of Cardiology, 51*(2), 172–209.

Kligfield, P., Gettes, L. S., Bailey, J. J., Childers, R., Deal, B. J., Hancock, E. W., et al. (2007). Recommendations for the standardization and interpretation of the electrocardiogram: part I: The electrocardiogram and its technology. *Circulation, 115*(10), 1306–1324.

Leon, A. S., Franklin, B. A., Costa, F., et al. (2005). Cardiac rehabilitation and secondary prevention of coronary heart disease: An American Heart Association scientific statement from the council on clinical cardiology. *Circulation, 111,* 369–376.

Masoudi, F. A., Bonow, R. O., Brindis, R. G., Cannon, C. P., DeBuhr, J., Fitzgerald, S. (2008). ACC/AHA 2008 statement on performance measurement and reperfusion therapy: A report of the ACC/AHA Task Force on performance measures. *Journal of the American College of Cardiology, 52,* 2100–2122.

Moorhead, S., Johnson, M., Maas, M., & Swanson, E. (Eds). (2008). *Nursing outcomes classification (NOC)* (4th ed.). St. Louis: Mosby Elsevier.

Mosca, L., Banka, C. L., Benjamin, E. J., Berra, K., Bushnell, C., Dolor, R. J., et al. (2007). Evidence-based guidelines for cardiovascular disease prevention in women: 2007 update. *Circulation, 115*(11), 1481–1501.

National Cholesterol Education Program. (2002). *Third report of the National Cholesterol Education Program (NCEP) Expert Panel on detection, evaluation, and treatment of high blood cholesterol in adults (Adult Treatment Panel III). Final report.* Bethesda, MD: National Heart, Lung, and Blood Institute, National Institutes of Health.

National High Blood Pressure Education Program. (2004). *The seventh report of the Joint National Committee on Prevention, Detection, Evaluation, and Treatment of High Blood Pressure.* Bethesda, MD: National Heart, Lung, and Blood Institute, National Institutes of Health.

NANDA International. (2009). *Nursing diagnoses: Definitions and classification 2009–2011.* Oxford, UK: Wiley-Blackwell.

Papadakis, M. A., & McPhee, S. J. (2007). *Current Consult Medicine 2007.* New York: McGraw-Hill.

Perrin, K. O. (2009). *Understanding the essentials of critical care nursing.* Upper Saddle River, NJ: Pearson Prentice Hall.

Rossouw, J. E., Prentice, R. L., Manson, J. E., Wu, L. L., Barad, D., Barnabei, V. M., et al. (2007). Postmenopausal hormone therapy and risk of cardiovascular disease by age and years since menopause. *JAMA, 297,* 1465–1477.

Samani, N. J., Erdmann, J., Hall, A. S., et al. (2007). Genomewide association analysis of coronary artery disease. *New England Journal of Medicine, 35* (5), 443–453.

Sanders, A. B., & Ewy, G. A. (2005). Cardiopulmonary resuscitation in the real world: When will the guidelines get the message? *JAMA, 293*(3), 363–365.

Smith S. C., et al. (2006). AHA/ACC guidelines for secondary prevention for patients with coronary and other atherosclerotic vascular disease: 2006 update: Endorsed by the National Heart, Lung and Blood Institute. *Circulation, 113*(19), 2363–2372.

U.S. Department of Health & Human Services. (2005). *Dietary guidelines for Americans 2005.* U.S. Department of Agriculture. Retrieved from www.healthierus.gov/dietaryguidelines

Witherell, C. L. (1994). Cardiac rhythm control devices. *Critical Care Nursing Clinics of North America, 6*(1), 92–105.

Woods, S. L., Froelicher, E. S., Motzer, S. A., & Bridges, E. J. (2009). *Cardiac nursing* (6th ed.). Philadelphia: Lippincott.

31 Nursing Care of Patients with Cardiac Disorders

LEARNING OUTCOMES

1. Compare and contrast the etiology, pathophysiology, and manifestations of common cardiac disorders, including heart failure, structural disorders, and inflammatory disorders.
2. Explain risk factors and preventive measures for cardiac disorders such as heart failure, inflammatory disorders, and valve disorders.

3. Discuss indications for and management of patients with hemodynamic monitoring.
4. Discuss the effects and nursing implications for medications commonly prescribed for patients with cardiac disorders.
5. Describe nursing care for the patient undergoing cardiac surgery or cardiac transplant.

CLINICAL COMPETENCIES

1. Apply knowledge of normal cardiac anatomy and physiology and assessment techniques in caring for patients with cardiac disorders.
2. Assess functional health status of patients with cardiac disorders, documenting and reporting deviations for expected findings.
3. Based on patient assessment and knowledge of the disorder, determine priority nursing diagnoses.
4. Plan, prioritize, and provide evidence-based, individualized care for patients with cardiac disorders.

5. Safely and knowledgeably administer prescribed medications and treatments to patients with cardiac disorders.
6. Actively participate in planning and coordinating interdisciplinary care for patients with cardiac disorders.
7. Provide appropriate teaching and community-based care for patients with cardiac disorders and their families.
8. Evaluate the effectiveness of nursing care, revising the plan of care as needed to promote, maintain, or restore functional health status of patients with cardiac disorders.

KEY TERMS

aortic valve, *1001*
cardiac tamponade, *998*
cardiomyopathy, *1012*
endocarditis, *992*
heart failure, *971*
hemodynamics, *977*
mean arterial pressure (MAP), *978*

mitral valve, *1001*
murmur, *1002*
myocarditis, *996*
orthopnea, *974*
paroxysmal nocturnal dyspnea (PND), *975*
pericarditis, *997*
pulmonary edema, *988*

pulmonic valve, *1001*
regurgitation, *990*
rheumatic fever, *990*
rheumatic heart disease (RHD), *990*
stenosis, *990*
tricuspid valve, *1001*
valvular heart disease, *1001*

Cardiac disorders affect the structure and/or function of the heart. These disorders interfere with the heart's primary purpose: to pump enough blood to meet the body's demand for oxygen and nutrients. Disruptions in cardiac function affect the functioning of other organs and tissues, potentially leading to organ system failure and death. Emergence of symptoms (fatigue, dyspnea, chest pain) is common with the progression of cardiac disorders. The New York Heart Association (NYHA) classification is commonly used to describe the severity of exertional symptoms observed. (See Table 31–1.)

Heart failure is the most common cardiac disorder. Other cardiac disorders discussed in this chapter include structural cardiac disorders, such as valve disorders and cardiomyopathy, and inflammatory cardiac disorders, such as endocarditis and

pericarditis. Before continuing with this chapter, please review the heart's anatomy and physiology, nursing assessment, and diagnostic tests in ∞ Chapter 29.

TABLE 31–1 New York Heart Association Classification

CLASS	SEVERITY OF SYMPTOMS
I	No limitation in physical activity/asymptomatic
II	Symptoms with strenuous activity
III	Symptoms with mild activity
IV	Symptoms at rest

Heart Failure

Heart failure is a complex syndrome resulting from cardiac disorders that impair the ventricles' ability to fill with and effectively pump blood (Hunt et al., 2005). In heart failure, the heart is unable to pump enough blood to meet the metabolic demands of the body. It is the end result of many conditions. Frequently, it is a long-term effect of coronary heart disease and myocardial infarction when left ventricular damage is extensive enough to impair cardiac output (∞ see Chapter 29). Other diseases of the heart also may cause heart failure, including structural and inflammatory disorders. In normal hearts, failure can result from excessive demands placed on the heart. Heart failure may be acute or chronic.

The Patient with Heart Failure

As mentioned, heart failure develops when the heart cannot effectively fill or contract with adequate strength to function as a pump to meet the needs of the body. As a result, cardiac output falls, leading to decreased tissue perfusion. The body initially adjusts to reduced cardiac output by activating inherent compensatory mechanisms to restore tissue perfusion. These normal mechanisms may result in vascular congestion—hence, the commonly used term *congestive heart failure (CHF)*. As these mechanisms are exhausted, heart failure ensues, with increased morbidity and mortality.

Heart failure is a disorder of cardiac function. It frequently is due to *impaired myocardial contraction*, which may result from coronary heart disease and myocardial ischemia or infarct or from a primary cardiac muscle disorder such as cardiomyopathy or myocarditis. Structural cardiac disorders, such as valve disorders or congenital heart defects, and hypertension also can lead to heart failure when the heart muscle is damaged by the long-standing *excessive workload* associated with these conditions. Other patients without a primary abnormality of myocardial function may present with manifestations of heart failure due to *acute excess demands* placed on the myocardium, such as volume overload, hyperthyroidism, and massive pulmonary embolus (see Table 31–2). Hypertension and coronary heart disease are the leading causes of heart failure in the United States. The high prevalence of hypertension in African Americans contributes significantly to their risk for and incidence of heart failure.

Incidence, Prevalence, and Risk Factors

More than 5.7 million people in the United States are currently living with heart failure; approximately 550,000 new cases of heart failure are diagnosed annually (American Heart Association [AHA], 2009). Its incidence and prevalence increase with age: Less than 5% of people between ages 55 and 64 have heart failure, whereas 6% to 10% of people older than 65 are affected (see the box on the following page). At 40, the lifetime risk of developing heart failure is one in five (AHA, 2009). The estimated direct and indirect costs of heart failure in the U.S. in 2006 was 29.6 billion dollars. The prevalence and mortality rate for heart failure is higher in African Americans than in Whites. See the accompanying box.

Ischemic heart disease (coronary heart disease) is the leading risk factor for heart failure. Up to 75% of persons with heart failure have a history of hypertension.

The prognosis for a patient with heart failure depends on its underlying cause and how effectively precipitating factors can be treated. Most patients with heart failure die within 8 years of the diagnosis. The risk for sudden cardiac death is dramatically increased, occurring at a rate six to nine times that of the general population. In 2005, one in eight death certificates in the U.S. mentioned heart failure as the primary or a contributing cause of death (AHA, 2009).

Physiology Review

The mechanical pumping action of cardiac muscle propels the blood it receives to the pulmonary and systemic vascular systems for reoxygenation and delivery to the tissues. *Cardiac output (CO)* is the amount of blood pumped from the ventricles in 1 minute. Cardiac output is used to assess cardiac performance, especially left ventricular function. Effective cardiac output depends on adequate functional muscle mass and the ability of the ventricles to work together. Cardiac output normally is regulated by the oxygen needs of the body: As oxygen use increases, cardiac output increases to maintain cellular function. *Cardiac reserve* is the ability of the heart to increase CO to meet metabolic demand. Ventricular damage reduces the cardiac reserve.

Cardiac output is a product of heart rate and stroke volume. *Heart rate* affects cardiac output by controlling the number of ventricular contractions per minute. It is influenced by the autonomic nervous system, catecholamines, and thyroid hormones. Activation of a stress response (e.g., hypovolemia or fear) stimulates the sympathetic nervous system, increasing the heart rate and its contractility. Elevated heart rates increase cardiac output. Very rapid heart rates, however, shorten ventricular filling time (diastole), reducing stroke volume and cardiac output. On the other hand, a slow heart rate reduces cardiac output simply because of fewer cardiac cycles.

Stroke volume, the volume of blood ejected with each heartbeat, is determined by preload, afterload, and myocardial contractility. *Preload* is the volume of blood in the ventricles at

TABLE 31–2 Selected Causes of Heart Failure

IMPAIRED MYOCARDIAL FUNCTION	INCREASED CARDIAC WORKLOAD	ACUTE NONCARDIAC CONDITIONS
■ Coronary heart disease	■ Hypertension	■ Volume overload
■ Cardiomyopathies	■ Valve disorders	■ Hyperthyroidism
■ Rheumatic fever	■ Anemias	■ Fever, infection
■ Infective endocarditis	■ Congenital heart defects	■ Massive pulmonary embolus

- Up to 5.7 million Americans have heart failure; of these, about 800,000 (15%) are African Americans.
- In African Americans:
  - Manifestations of heart failure develop at an earlier age.
  - The disease progresses more rapidly.
  - More hospital visits are attributed to heart failure.
  - The mortality rate is higher than in White men and women.

BOX 31–1 Explaining Physiologic Terms Using Practical Examples

The concepts of preload, the Frank-Starling mechanism, compliance, and afterload can be difficult to understand and to explain to patients. Use common analogies to make these concepts easier to understand:

- *Preload:* Think about a new rubber band. As you stretch the rubber band further, it snaps back into shape with greater force.
- *Frank-Starling mechanism:* When you repeatedly stretch that rubber band beyond a certain limit, it loses some elasticity and fails to return to its original shape and size.
- *Compliance:* Use a new rubber balloon to illustrate this concept. A new balloon is not very compliant—it takes a lot of work (force) to inflate it. As the balloon is repeatedly stretched, it becomes more compliant, expanding easily with less force.
- *Afterload:* When a hose is crimped or plugged, more force is required to eject a stream of water out its end.

end-diastole (just prior to contraction). The blood in the ventricles exerts pressure on the ventricle walls, stretching muscle fibers. The greater the blood volume, the greater force with which the ventricle contracts to expel the blood. End diastolic volume (EDV) depends on the amount of blood returning to the ventricles (*venous return*), and the distensibility or stiffness of the ventricles (*compliance*). (See Box 31–1.)

Afterload is the force needed to eject blood into the circulation. This force must be great enough to overcome arterial pressures within the pulmonary and systemic vascular systems. The right ventricle must generate enough force to open the pulmonary valve and eject its blood into the pulmonary artery. The left ventricle ejects its blood into the systemic circulation by overcoming the arterial resistance behind the aortic valve. Increased systemic vascular resistance (e.g., hypertension) increases afterload, impairing stroke volume and increasing myocardial work.

Contractility is the natural ability of cardiac muscle fibers to shorten during systole. Contractility is necessary to overcome arterial pressures and eject blood during systole. Impaired contractility affects cardiac output by reducing stroke volume. The *ejection fraction (EF)* is the percentage of blood in the ventricle that is ejected during systole. A normal ejection fraction is approximately 60%.

Pathophysiology

When the heart begins to fail, mechanisms are activated to compensate for the impaired function and maintain the cardiac output. The primary compensatory mechanisms are (1) the Frank-Starling mechanism; (2) neuroendocrine responses including activation of the sympathetic nervous system and the RAAS; and (3) myocardial hypertrophy. These mechanisms and their effects are summarized in Table 31–3.

Decreased cardiac output initially stimulates aortic baroreceptors, which in turn stimulate the sympathetic nervous system (SNS). SNS stimulation produces both cardiac and vascular responses through the release of norepinephrine. Norepinephrine increases heart rate and contractility by stimulating cardiac beta receptors. Cardiac output improves as both heart rate and stroke volume increase. Norepinephrine also causes arterial and venous vasoconstriction, increasing venous

Heart failure is common in older adults, affecting nearly 10% of people over the age of 75 years.

Aging affects cardiac function. Diastolic filling is impaired by decreased ventricular compliance. With aging, the heart is less responsive to sympathetic nervous system stimulation. As a result, maximal heart rate, cardiac reserve, and exercise tolerance are reduced. Concurrent health problems such as arthritis that affect stamina or mobility often contribute to a more sedentary lifestyle, further decreasing the heart's ability to respond to increased stress.

Assessing for Home Care

The older adult with heart failure may not be dyspneic, instead presenting with weakness and fatigue, somnolence, confusion, disorientation, or worsening dementia. Dependent edema and respiratory crackles may or may not indicate heart failure in older adults.

Assess the diet of the older adult. Decreased taste may lead to increased use of salt to bring out food flavors. Limited mobility or visual acuity may cause the older adult to rely on prepared foods that are high in sodium such as canned soups and frozen meals. Discuss normal daily activities and assess

sleep and rest patterns. It is also important to assess the environment for the following:

- Safe roads or neighborhoods for walking
- Access to pharmacy, medical care, and assistive services such as a cardiac rehabilitation program or structured exercise programs designed for older adults

Patient and Family Teaching

Teaching for the older adult with heart failure focuses on maintaining function and promptly identifying and treating episodes of heart failure. Teach patients how to adapt to changes in cardiovascular function associated with aging, such as the following:

- Allowing longer warm-up and cool-down periods during exercise
- Engaging in regular exercise such as walking 5 or more times a week
- Resting with feet elevated (e.g., in a recliner) when fatigued
- Maintaining adequate fluid intake
- Preventing infection through pneumococcal and influenza immunizations

TABLE 31–3 Compensatory Mechanisms Activated in Heart Failure

MECHANISM	PHYSIOLOGY	EFFECT ON BODY SYSTEMS	COMPLICATIONS
Frank-Starling mechanism	The greater the stretch of cardiac muscle fibers, the greater the force of contraction.	■ Increased contractile force leading to increased CO	■ Increased myocardial oxygen demand ■ Limited by overstretching
Neuroendocrine response	Decreased CO stimulates the sympathetic nervous system and catecholamine release.	■ Increased HR, BP, and contractility ■ Increased vascular resistance ■ Increased venous return	■ Tachycardia with decreased filling time and decreased CO ■ Increased vascular resistance ■ Increased myocardial work and oxygen demand
	Decreased CO and decreased renal perfusion stimulate renin/angiotensin system.	■ Vasoconstriction and increased BP	■ Increased myocardial work ■ Renal vasoconstriction and decreased renal perfusion
	Angiotensin stimulates aldosterone release from adrenal cortex.	■ Salt and water retention by the kidneys ■ Increased vascular volume	■ Increased preload and afterload ■ Pulmonary congestion
	ADH is released from posterior pituitary. Atrial natriuretic factor is released.	■ Water excretion inhibited ■ Increased sodium excretion ■ Diuresis	■ Fluid retention and increased preload and afterload
	Blood flow is redistributed to vital organs (heart and brain).	■ Decreased perfusion of other organ systems ■ Decreased perfusion of skin and muscles	■ Renal failure ■ Anaerobic metabolism and lactic acidosis
Ventricular hypertrophy	Increased cardiac workload causes myocardial muscle to hypertrophy and ventricles to dilate.	■ Increased contractile force to maintain CO	■ Increased myocardial oxygen demand ■ Cellular enlargement

return to the heart. Increased venous return increases ventricular filling and myocardial stretch, increasing the force of contraction (the Frank-Starling mechanism). Overstretching the muscle fibers past their physiologic limit results in an ineffective contraction.

Blood flow is redistributed to the brain and the heart to maintain perfusion of these vital organs. Decreased renal perfusion causes renin to be released from the kidneys. Activation of the renin-angiotensin-aldosterone system produces additional vasoconstriction and stimulates the adrenal cortex to produce aldosterone (RAAS) and the posterior pituitary to release antidiuretic hormone (ADH). Aldosterone stimulates sodium reabsorption in renal tubules, promoting water retention. ADH acts on the distal tubule to inhibit water excretion and causes vasoconstriction. The effect of these hormones is significant vasoconstriction and salt and water retention, with a resulting increase in vascular volume. Increased ventricular filling increases the force of contraction, improving cardiac output. The increased vascular volume and venous return also increase atrial pressures, stimulating the release of an additional hormone, *atrial natriuretic factor (ANF)* or *atriopeptin*. Atrial natriuretic factor balances the effects of the other hormones to a certain extent, promoting sodium and water excretion and inhibiting the release of norepinephrine, renin, and ADH. This hormone is thought to be a natural preventive that delays severe cardiac decompensation.

Ventricular remodeling occurs as the heart chambers and myocardium adapt to fluid volume and pressure increases. The chambers dilate to accommodate excess fluid resulting from increased vascular volume and incomplete emptying. Initially, this additional stretch causes more effective contractions. *Ventricular hypertrophy* occurs as existing cardiac muscle cells enlarge, increasing their contractile elements (actin and myosin) and force of contraction.

Although these responses may help in the short-term regulation of cardiac output, it is now recognized that they hasten the deterioration of cardiac function. The onset of heart failure is heralded by *decompensation*, the loss of effective compensation. Heart failure progresses due to the very mechanisms that initially maintained circulatory stability.

The rapid heart rate shortens diastolic filling time, compromises coronary artery perfusion, and increases myocardial oxygen demand. Resulting ischemia further impairs cardiac output. Beta-receptors in the heart become less sensitive to continued SNS stimulation, decreasing heart rate and contractility. As the beta-receptors become less sensitive, norepinephrine stores in the cardiac muscle become depleted. In contrast, alpha-receptors on peripheral blood vessels become increasingly sensitive to persistent stimulation, promoting vasoconstriction and increasing afterload and cardiac work.

Initially, ventricular hypertrophy and dilation increase cardiac output, but chronic distention causes the ventricular wall eventually to thin and degenerate. The purpose of hypertrophy is thus defeated. In addition, chronic overloading of the dilated ventricle eventually stretches the fibers beyond the optimal point for effective contraction. The ventricles continue to dilate to accommodate the excess fluid, but the heart loses the ability to contract forcefully. The heart muscle may eventually become so large that the coronary blood supply is inadequate, causing ischemia.

Chronic distention exhausts atrial stores of ANF. The effects of norepinephrine, renin, and ADH prevail, and the renin-angiotensin pathway is continually stimulated. This mechanism ultimately raises the hemodynamic stress on the heart by increasing both preload and afterload. As heart function deteriorates, less blood is delivered to the tissues and to the heart itself. Ischemia and necrosis of the myocardium further weaken the already failing heart, and the cycle repeats.

In normal hearts, the cardiac reserve allows the heart to adjust its output to meet metabolic needs of the body, increasing the cardiac output by up to 5 times the basal level during exercise. Patients with heart failure have minimal to no cardiac reserve. At rest, they may be unaffected; however, any stressor (e.g., exercise, illness) taxes their ability to meet the demand for oxygen and nutrients. Manifestations of activity intolerance when the person is at rest indicate a critical level of cardiac decompensation.

Classifications and Manifestations of Heart Failure

Heart failure is commonly classified in several different ways, depending on the underlying pathology. Classifications include systolic versus diastolic failure, left-sided versus right-sided failure, high-output versus low-output failure, and acute versus chronic failure.

FAST FACTS

Terms used to describe or classify heart failure are as follows:
- Systolic or diastolic failure
- Left ventricular (or sided) or right ventricular (or sided) failure
- Low-output or high-output failure
- Acute or chronic failure
- Forward or backward effects

Systolic versus Diastolic Failure

Systolic failure occurs when the ventricle fails to contract adequately to eject a sufficient blood volume into the arterial system. Systolic function is affected by loss of myocardial cells due to ischemia and infarction, cardiomyopathy, or inflammation. The manifestations of systolic failure are those of decreased cardiac output: weakness, fatigue, and decreased exercise tolerance.

Diastolic failure results when the heart cannot completely relax in diastole, disrupting normal filling. Passive diastolic filling decreases, increasing the importance of atrial contraction to preload. Diastolic dysfunction results from decreased ventricular compliance due to hypertrophic and cellular changes and impaired relaxation of the heart muscle. Its manifestations result from increased pressure and congestion behind the ventricle: shortness of breath, tachypnea, and respiratory crackles if the left ventricle is affected; distended neck veins, liver enlargement, anorexia, and nausea if the right ventricle is affected. Many patients have components of both systolic and diastolic failure.

Left-Sided versus Right-Sided Failure

Depending on the pathophysiology involved, either the left or the right ventricle may be primarily affected. In chronic heart failure, however, both ventricles typically are impaired to some degree. Coronary heart disease and hypertension are common causes of *left-sided heart failure*, whereas *right-sided heart failure* often is caused by conditions that restrict blood flow to the lungs, such as acute or chronic pulmonary disease. Left-sided heart failure also can lead to right-sided failure as pressures in the pulmonary vascular system increase with congestion behind the failing left ventricle.

As left ventricular function fails, cardiac output falls. Pressures in the left ventricle and atrium increase as the amount of blood remaining in the ventricle after systole increases. These increased pressures impair filling, causing congestion and increased pressures in the pulmonary vascular system. Increased pressures in this normally low-pressure system increase fluid movement from the blood vessels into interstitial tissues and the alveoli (Figure 31–1 ■).

The manifestations of left-sided heart failure result from pulmonary congestion (*backward effects*) and decreased cardiac output (*forward effects*). Fatigue and activity intolerance are common early manifestations. Dizziness and syncope also may result from decreased cardiac output. Pulmonary congestion causes dyspnea, shortness of breath, and a cough. The patient may develop **orthopnea** (difficulty breathing while lying

Pulmonary circulation

Pulmonary artery

Pulmonary vein congestion

Diminished cardiac output

Heart

Portal circulation

Systemic circulation

Figure 31–1 ■ The hemodynamic effects of left-sided heart failure.

down), prompting use of two or three pillows or a recliner for sleeping. Cyanosis from impaired gas exchange may be noted. On auscultation of the lungs, inspiratory crackles (rales) and wheezes may be heard in lung bases. An S_3 gallop may be present, reflecting the heart's attempts to fill an already distended ventricle.

In right-sided heart failure, increased pressures in the pulmonary vasculature or right ventricular muscle damage impair the right ventricle's ability to pump blood into the pulmonary circulation. The right ventricle and atrium become distended, and blood accumulates in the systemic venous system. Increased venous pressures cause abdominal organs to become congested and peripheral tissue edema to develop (Figure 31–2 ■).

Dependent tissues tend to be affected because of the effects of gravity; edema develops in the feet and legs, or if the patient is bedridden, in the sacrum. Congestion of gastrointestinal tract vessels causes anorexia and nausea. Right upper quadrant pain may result from liver engorgement. Neck veins distend and become visible even when the patient is upright due to increased venous pressure.

Low-Output versus High-Output Failure

Patients with heart failure due to coronary heart disease, hypertension, cardiomyopathy, and other primary cardiac disorders develop *low-output failure* and manifestations such as those

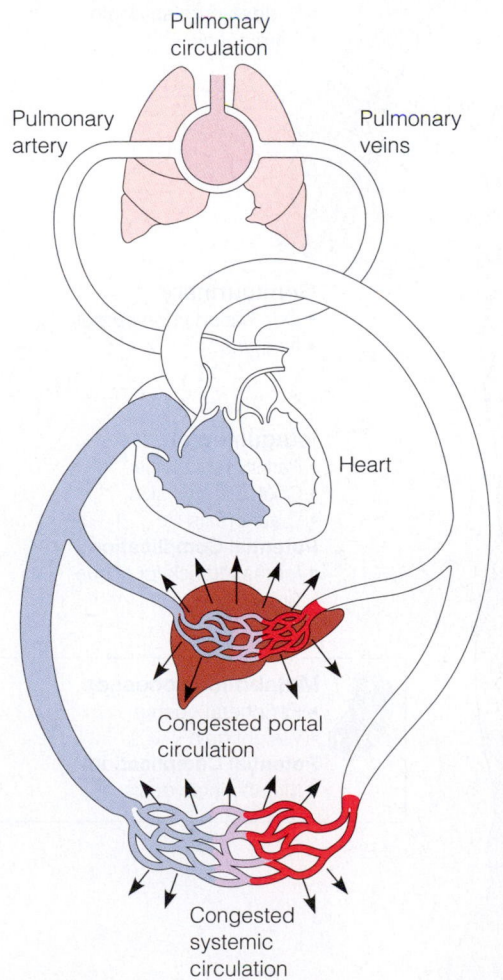

Figure 31–2 ■ The hemodynamic effects of right-sided heart failure.

Labels in figure: Pulmonary circulation; Pulmonary artery; Pulmonary veins; Heart; Congested portal circulation; Congested systemic circulation

previously described. Patients in hypermetabolic states (e.g., hyperthyroidism, infection, anemia, or pregnancy) require increased cardiac output to maintain blood flow and oxygen to the tissues. If the increased blood flow cannot meet the oxygen demands of the tissues, compensatory mechanisms are activated to further increase cardiac output, which in turn further increases oxygen demand. Thus, even though cardiac output is high, the heart is unable to meet increased oxygen demands. This condition is known as *high-output failure.*

Acute versus Chronic Failure

Acute failure is the abrupt onset of a myocardial injury (such as a massive MI) resulting in suddenly decreased cardiac function and signs of decreased cardiac output. *Chronic failure* is a progressive deterioration of the heart muscle due to cardiomyopathies, valvular disease, or CHD.

Other Manifestations

In addition to the previous manifestations for the various classifications of heart failure, other signs and symptoms commonly are seen.

A fall in cardiac output activates mechanisms that cause increased salt and water retention. This causes weight gain and further increases pressures in the capillaries, resulting in edema. *Nocturia*, voiding more than one time at night, develops as edema fluid from dependent tissues is reabsorbed when the patient is supine. **Paroxysmal nocturnal dyspnea (PND)**, a frightening condition in which the patient awakens at night acutely short of breath, also may develop. Paroxysmal nocturnal dyspnea occurs when edema fluid that has accumulated during the day is reabsorbed into the circulation at night, causing fluid overload and pulmonary congestion. Severe heart failure may cause dyspnea at rest as well as with activity, signifying little or no cardiac reserve. Both an S_3 and an S_4 gallop may be heard on auscultation.

See page 976 for the Multisystem Effects of Heart Failure.

Complications

The compensatory mechanisms initiated in heart failure can lead to complications in other body systems. Congestive hepatomegaly and splenomegaly caused by engorgement of the portal venous system results in increased abdominal pressure, ascites, and gastrointestinal problems. With prolonged right-sided heart failure, liver function may be impaired. Myocardial distention can precipitate dysrhythmias, further impairing cardiac output. Pleural effusions and other pulmonary problems may develop. Major complications of severe heart failure are cardiogenic shock (∞ described in Chapter 11) and acute pulmonary edema, a medical emergency described in the next section of this chapter.

Interdisciplinary Care

The main goals for care of heart failure are to slow its progression, reduce cardiac workload, improve cardiac function, and control fluid retention. Treatment strategies are based on the evolution and progression of heart failure (Table 31–4).

MULTISYSTEM EFFECTS OF
Heart Failure

Respiratory
- Dyspnea on exertion
- Shortness of breath
- Tachypnea
- Orthopnea
- Dry cough
- Crackles (rales) in lung bases

Potential Complications
- Pulmonary edema
- Pneumonia
- Cardiac asthma
- Pleural effusion
- Cheyne-Stokes respirations
- Respiratory acidosis

Gastrointestinal
- Anorexia, nausea
- Abdominal distention
- Liver enlargement
- Right upper quadrant pain

Potential Complications
- Malnutrition
- Ascites
- Liver dysfunction

Musculoskeletal
- Fatigue
- Weakness

Neurologic
- Confusion
- Impaired memory
- Anxiety, restlessness
- Insomnia

Cardiovascular
- Activity intolerance
- Tachycardia
- Palpitations
- S_3, S_4 heart sounds
- Elevated central venous pressure
- Neck vein distention
- Hepatojugular reflux
- Splenomegaly

Potential Complications
- Angina
- Dysrhythmias
- Sudden cardiac death
- Cardiogenic shock

Genitourinary
- Decreased urine output
- Nocturia

Integumentary
- Pallor or cyanosis
- Cool, clammy skin
- Diaphoresis

Potential Complications
- Increased risk for tissue breakdown

Metabolic Processes
- Peripheral edema
- Weight gain

Potential Complication
- Metabolic acidosis

TABLE 31–4 Stages of Heart Failure

STAGE	DESCRIPTION	RECOMMENDED TREATMENT MEASURES
A	Patients at high risk for developing heart failure, but without structural heart disease or symptoms of heart failure (patients with hypertension, CHD, diabetes, obesity, metabolic syndrome, or who have a family history of cardiomyopathy, or who are taking cardiotoxic drugs)	Treat underlying risk factors (e.g., hypertension) including lipid disorders ACE inhibitor or angiotensin-receptor blocker (ARB) therapy as appropriate Exercise Salt restriction Smoking cessation Discourage alcohol, illicit drug use Control blood glucose in patients with metabolic syndrome
B	Patients with structural heart disease but no manifestations of heart failure (patients with previous MI, asymptomatic valve disease, or left ventricular dysfunction)	As for stage A ACE inhibitor or ARB therapy as appropriate Beta-blocker therapy if indicated
C	Patients with structural heart disease and current or prior symptoms of heart failure (shortness of breath, fatigue, decreased exercise tolerance)	As for stages A and B Drug therapy with a diuretic, ACE inhibitor, and/or beta blocker Additional drugs as indicated, such as an aldosterone antagonist, ARB, digitalis, hydralazine, nitrates Ventricular pacing or an implantable defibrillator (ICD) as indicated
D	Refractory heart failure (patients with manifestations of heart failure at rest despite aggressive treatment)	As for stages A, B, and C as appropriate Hospice care Hemodynamic monitoring Continual infusion of positive inotropic agents Valve replacement, cardiac transplant as indicated Permanent mechanical support; experimental surgery or drug therapy

Note: Adapted from Hunt, S. A., Abraham, W. T., Chin, M. H., Feldman, A. M., Francis, G. S., Ganiats, T. G., Jessup, M., Konstam, M. A., Mancini, D. M., Michl, K., Silver, M. A., Stevenson, L. W., and Yancy, C. W. (2005). ACC/AHA 2005 guideline update for the diagnosis and management of chronic heart failure in the adult: Executive summary: A report of the American College of Cardiology/American Heart Association task force on practice guidelines (writing committee to update the 2001 guidelines for the evaluation and management of heart failure). American College of Cardiology website. Retrieved from http://content.onlinejacc.org/cgi/reprint/46/6/e1.pdf

Diagnosis

Diagnosis of heart failure is based on the history, physical examination, and diagnostic findings.

- *Atrial natriuretic factor (ANF)*, also called *atrial natriuretic hormone (ANH)*, and *B-type natriuretic peptide (BNP)* are hormones released by the heart muscle in response to changes in blood volume. Blood levels of these hormones increase in heart failure, however, it is important to remember that BNP levels may be elevated in women and in people over age 60 who do not have heart failure. Therefore, an elevated BNP cannot be used alone to diagnosis heart failure (Hunt et al., 2005).
- *Serum electrolytes* are measured to evaluate fluid and electrolyte status. Serum osmolality may be low due to fluid retention. Sodium, potassium, and chloride levels provide a baseline for evaluating the effects of treatment; serum calcium and magnesium are measured as well.
- *Urinalysis, blood urea nitrogen (BUN)*, and *serum creatinine* are obtained to evaluate renal function.
- *Liver function tests*, including ALT, AST, LDH, serum bilirubin, and total protein and albumin levels, are obtained to evaluate possible effects of heart failure on liver function.
- Thyroid function tests, including TSH and TH levels, are obtained because both hyperthyroidism and hypothyroidism can be either a primary or a contributing cause of heart failure (Hunt et al., 2005).
- In acute heart failure, *arterial blood gases (ABGs)* are drawn to evaluate gas exchange in the lungs and tissues.

- *Chest x-ray* may show pulmonary vascular congestion and cardiomegaly in heart failure.
- *Electrocardiography* is used to identify ECG changes associated with ventricular enlargement and to detect dysrhythmias, myocardial ischemia, or infarction.
- *Echocardiography with Doppler flow studies* are performed to evaluate left ventricular function. Either *transthoracic echocardiography* or *transesophageal echocardiography* may be used.
- *Radionuclide imaging* is used to evaluate ventricular function and size. ∞ See Chapter 29 for more information and the nursing implications of these tests.

Hemodynamic Monitoring

Hemodynamics is the study of forces involved in blood circulation. Hemodynamic monitoring is used to assess cardiovascular function in the critically ill or unstable patient. The main goals of invasive hemodynamic monitoring are to evaluate cardiac and circulatory function and the response to interventions.

Hemodynamic parameters include heart rate, arterial blood pressure, central venous or right atrial pressure, pulmonary pressures, and cardiac output. *Direct* hemodynamic parameters are obtained straight from the monitoring device (e.g., heart rate, arterial and venous pressures). *Indirect* or *derived* measurements are calculated using the direct data (e.g., the cardiac index, mean arterial blood pressure [MAP], and stroke volume). Invasive hemodynamic monitoring is routinely used in critical care units.

Hemodynamic monitoring systems measure the pressure within a vessel and convert this signal into an electrical waveform that is amplified and displayed. The electrical signal may be graphically recorded on graph paper and displayed digitally on the monitor. System components include an invasive catheter threaded into an artery or vein connected to a transducer by stiff, high-pressure tubing. The pressure transducer translates pressures into an electrical signal that is relayed to the monitor. Additional components of the system include stopcocks and a continuous flush system with normal saline or heparinized saline and an infusion pressure bag to prevent clots from forming in the catheter. Figure 31–3 ■ illustrates a pressure transducer and typical hemodynamic monitoring system.

Hemodynamic pressure monitoring may be used to measure peripheral arterial pressures, or central pressures, such as central venous pressure (CVP) or right atrial pressure (RAP) and pulmonary artery pressure (PAP). Although the information obtained from invasive monitoring is valuable, the procedure is not without risk. Nursing care of the patient undergoing hemodynamic monitoring is outlined on page 979. Box 31–2 lists potential complications of central pressure monitoring. Pressure monitoring systems require calibration, leveling and zeroing of the transducer to the level of the patient's left atrium. This is called the phlebostatic axis.

INTRA-ARTERIAL PRESSURE MONITORING
Intra-arterial pressure monitoring is commonly used in intensive and coronary care units. An indwelling arterial line, commonly called an *art line* or an *A line*, allows direct and continuous monitoring of systolic, diastolic, and mean arterial blood pressure and provides easy access for arterial blood sampling. Arterial lines are used to assess blood volume, monitor the effects of vasoactive drugs, and to obtain frequent arterial blood gas determinations. Because the invasive catheter is inserted directly into the artery, it offers immediate access for blood gas measurements and blood testing.

BOX 31–2 Potential Complications of Central Catheters

- Bleeding
- Hematoma
- Pneumothorax
- Hemothorax
- Arterial puncture
- Dysrhythmias

- Venospasm
- Infection
- Air embolism
- Thromboembolism
- Brachial nerve injury
- Thoracic duct injury

The arterial blood pressure reflects the cardiac output and the resistance to blood flow created by the elastic arterial walls (*systemic vascular resistance, SVR*). Cardiac output is determined by the blood volume and the ability of the ventricles to fill and effectively pump that blood. Systemic vascular resistance is primarily determined by vessel diameter and distensibility (compliance). Factors such as sympathetic nervous system input, circulating hormones (e.g., epinephrine, norepinephrine, atrial natriuretic factor, and vasopressin), and the RAAS affect SVR.

The systolic blood pressure, normally about 120 mmHg in healthy adults, reflects the pressure generated during ventricular systole. During diastole, elastic arterial walls keep a minimum pressure within the vessel (diastolic blood pressure) to maintain blood flow through the capillary beds. The average diastolic pressure in a healthy adult is 80 mmHg. The **mean arterial pressure (MAP)** is the average pressure in the arterial circulation throughout the cardiac cycle. It reflects the driving pressure, or perfusion pressure, an indicator of tissue perfusion. The formula MAP = CO × SVR often is used to show the relationships between factors determining the blood pressure. Mean arterial pressure can be calculated by adding one-third of the pulse pressure to the diastolic pressure (MAP = DBP+PP/3). For example, a blood pressure of 120/80 results in a mean arterial pressure of 93. Mean arterial pressures of 70 to 90 mmHg are desirable. Perfusion to vital organs is severely jeopardized at MAPs of 50 or less; MAPs greater than 105 mmHg may indicate hypertension or vasoconstriction.

VENOUS PRESSURE MONITORING
Central venous pressure (CVP) and *right atrial pressure (RAP)* are measures of blood volume and venous return. They also reflect right heart filling pressures. Pressures are elevated in right-sided heart failure. CVP and RAP are primarily used to monitor fluid volume status. To measure venous and atrial pressures, a catheter is inserted in the internal jugular or subclavian vein. The distal tip of the catheter is positioned in the superior vena cava just above or just inside the right atrium. CVP may be measured in either centimeters of water (cm H_2O) or in millimeters of mercury (mmHg). A water manometer is a clear tube with calibrated markings that is attached between a central catheter and the intravenous fluid bag. Pressure in the venous system causes fluid in the manometer to rise or fall. The CVP is recorded by noting the fluid level in

Pressure bag around bag of flush solution

Manometer for bag

Intravenous solution tubing

Hand bulb for pressurizing bag

Pressure monitor

Two-way stopcock

Pressure transducer

Flush device

Nondistensible tubing

Three-way stopcock for blood samples

Catheter

Figure 31–3 ■ A hemodynamic monitoring setup.

NURSING CARE OF THE PATIENT   Undergoing Hemodynamic Monitoring

- Calibrate and level the system at least once a shift using the right atrium as a constant reference level. Relevel the transducer after a change in position. Mark the right atrial position (at the fourth intercostal space, midaxillary line) on the chest wall, and use this as a reference point for all readings. *Calibration and leveling ensure that accurate pressures are recorded. Marking the right atrial level provides a consistent reference point for all caregivers.*
- Measure all pressures between breaths. *This ensures that intrathoracic pressure does not influence pressure readings.*
- Maintain 300 mmHg of pressure on the flush solution at all times. *This ensures a continuous flow of flush solution through the pressure tubing and catheter to prevent clot formation and catheter occlusion.*
- Monitor pressure trends rather than individual readings. *Individual readings may not reflect the patient's true status. Trends in pressure readings along with clinical observations provide a better overall picture of the patient's status.*
- Obtain a chest x-ray before infusing intravenous fluid into any newly placed central line. *Chest x-ray verifies the location of the catheter and helps prevent pulmonary complications of incorrect catheter placement such as pneumothorax.*
- Set alarm limits for monitored hemodynamic variables. Turn alarms on. *Alarms warn of hemodynamic instability. Always investigate alarms. They may be temporarily silenced to change tubing or draw blood but should never be turned off.*
- Use aseptic technique during catheter insertion and site care. *Aseptic technique is important to prevent infection.*

- Assess and document appearance of the insertion site at least every shift; observe for signs of infiltration, infection, or phlebitis. *Frequent assessment allows early detection and prompt treatment of complications.*
- Change intravenous solutions every 24 hours, site dressing every 48 hours, and tubing to the insertion site every 72 hours. Label solution, tubing, and dressing with date and time of change. *These measures help prevent infection.*
- Thoroughly flush stopcock ports after drawing blood samples from the pressure line. *Flushing prevents colonization of bacteria and occlusion of the catheter.*
- Assess pulse and perfusion distal to the monitoring site. *Frequent assessment is vital to ensure perfusion of the distal extremity.*
- When discontinuing the pressure line, apply manual pressure to the insertion site as soon as the catheter tip is out. Hold pressure for 5 to 15 minutes or until the bleeding stops. *This is particularly important for arterial lines to prevent bleeding and hematoma formation.*
- Secure all connections and stopcocks. *This is done to prevent disconnection of the invasive line and potential hemorrhage.*
- Ensure that electrical equipment is grounded, intact, and operating as expected. *This helps prevent electrical injury.*
- Loosely restrain the affected extremity if the patient pulls on the catheter or connections. *Restraints may be necessary to prevent injury from accidental or intentional disconnection or discontinuation of invasive lines (i.e., if the patient has dementia or is agitated).*
- Keep tubing free of kinks and tension. This prevents the catheter from becoming clotted or inadvertently dislodged.

---

the manometer. If the central line is connected to a pressure transducer, venous pressure is displayed digitally in millimeters of mercury.

The normal range for CVP is 2 to 8 cm H_2O or 2 to 6 mmHg, but CVP varies in individual patients. Hypovolemia and shock decrease the CVP; fluid overload, vasoconstriction, and cardiac tamponade increase CVP.

PULMONARY ARTERY PRESSURE MONITORING The pulmonary artery (PA) catheter is a flow-directed, balloon-tipped catheter first used in the early 1970s. The PA catheter is often called a *Swan-Ganz catheter*, after the physicians who developed it. The PA catheter is used to evaluate left ventricular and overall cardiac function. The PA catheter is inserted into a central vein, usually the internal jugular or subclavian vein, and threaded into the right atrium. A small balloon at the tip of the catheter allows the catheter to be drawn into the right ventricle and from there into the pulmonary artery (Figure 31–4 ■). The inflated balloon carries the catheter forward until the balloon wedges in a small branch of pulmonary vasculature. Once in place, the balloon is deflated, and multiple lumens of the catheter allow measurement of pressures in the right atrium, pulmonary artery, and left ventricle. The normal PA pressure is around 25/10 mmHg; normal mean pulmonary artery pressure is about 15 mmHg (Figure 31–5A ■). Pulmonary artery pressure is increased in left-sided heart failure.

Inflation of the balloon effectively blocks pressure from behind the balloon and allows measurement of pressures generated by the left ventricle. This is known as pulmonary artery wedge pressure (PAWP or PWP) and is used to assess left ventricular function. The normal pulmonary artery wedge pressure is 8 to 12 mmHg (Figure 31–5B). PAWP is increased in left ventricular failure and pericardial tamponade, and decreased in hypovolemia.

Cardiac output also can be measured with the PA catheter using a technique called thermodilution. Cardiac output and the

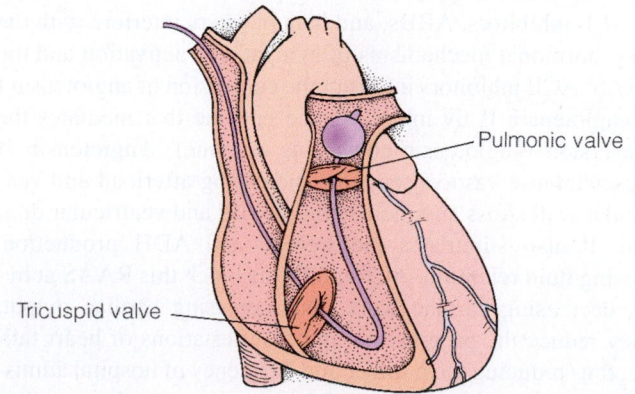

Figure 31–4 ■ Inflation of the balloon on the flow-directed catheter allows it to be carried through the pulmonic valve into the pulmonary artery.

Pulmonary Artery Pressure (PAP)

A

Pulmonary Capillary Wedge Pressure (PCWP)

B

Figure 31–5 ■ Typical waveforms seen when measuring *A*, pulmonary artery pressure, and *B*, pulmonary wedge pressure.

cardiac index are used to assess the heart's ability to meet the body's oxygen demands. Because body size affects overall cardiac output, the cardiac index is a more precise measure of heart function. The *cardiac index* is a calculation of cardiac output per square meter of body surface area. The normal cardiac index is 2.8 to 4.2 L/min/m².

Medications

Patients with heart failure often receive multiple medications to reduce cardiac work and improve cardiac function. The main drug classes used to treat heart failure are the angiotensin-converting enzyme (ACE) inhibitors, angiotensin II receptor blockers (ARBs), beta blockers, diuretics, inotropic medications (including digitalis, sympathomimetic agents, and phosphodiesterase inhibitors), direct vasodilators, and antidysrhythmic drugs. Nursing implications for ACE inhibitors and ARBs, diuretics, and inotropic medications are found in the Medication Administration box on page 981.

ACE inhibitors, ARBs, and beta blockers interfere with the neurohormonal mechanisms of sympathetic activation and the RAAS. ACE inhibitors interrupt the conversion of angiotensin I to angiotensin II by inhibiting the enzyme that mediates the conversion (angiotensin-converting enzyme). Angiotensin II causes intense vasoconstriction, increasing afterload and ventricular wall stress and increasing preload and ventricular dilation. It also stimulates aldosterone and ADH production, causing fluid retention. ACE inhibitors block this RAAS activity, decreasing cardiac work and increasing cardiac output. They reduce the progression and manifestations of heart failure, thus reducing the number and frequency of hospital admissions, decreasing mortality rates, and preventing cardiac complications (Deglin & Vallerand, 2009). However, ACE inhibitors should be used with caution in African Americans due to increased risk for developing angioedema.

In contrast to ACE inhibitors, ARBs do not block the production of angiotensin II; instead, they block its action. The pharmacologic effect is similar, and they also are used in heart failure to slow its progression, reduce manifestations, and prevent cardiac complications.

Beta blockers improve cardiac function in heart failure by inhibiting SNS activity. This prevents the long-term deleterious effects of sympathetic stimulation. Because beta blockers reduce the force of myocardial contraction and may actually worsen symptoms, they are used in low doses. Beta blockers are indicated for all classes of heart failure patients. The combination of ACE inhibitors and beta blockers improves patient outcomes. Beta blockers are discussed on pages 922 and 923 of ∞ Chapter 30.

Patients with symptomatic heart failure often are treated with diuretics as well. Diuretics relieve symptoms related to fluid retention. They may, however, cause significant electrolyte imbalances and rapid fluid loss. Patients with severe heart failure are often treated with a loop, or high-ceiling, diuretic such as furosemide (Lasix), bumetanide (Bumex), torsemide (Demadex), or ethacrynic acid (Edecrin). These drugs have a rapid onset of action, inhibiting chloride reabsorption in the ascending loop of Henle, prompting sodium and water excretion. Their major drawback is their efficacy in promoting diuresis; loss of vascular volume can stimulate the SNS. Thiazide diuretics may be used for patients with less severe manifestations of heart failure. These agents promote fluid excretion by blocking sodium reabsorption in the terminal loop of Henle and the distal tubule.

Vasodilators relax smooth muscle in blood vessels, causing dilation. Arterial dilation reduces peripheral vascular resistance and afterload, reducing myocardial work. Venous dilation reduces venous return and preload. Pulmonary vascular relaxation reduces pulmonary capillary pressure, allowing reabsorption of fluid from interstitial tissues and the alveoli. Vasodilators include nitrates, hydralazine, and prazosin, an alpha-adrenergic blocker. ∞ See Chapter 32 for more information about vasodilators.

Nitrates produce both arterial and venous vasodilation. They may be given by nasal spray or the sublingual, oral, or intravenous route. Sodium nitroprusside is a potent vasodilator that may be used to treat acute heart failure. It can cause excessive hypotension, so is often given along with dopamine or dobutamine to maintain the blood pressure. Isosorbide or nitroglycerin ointment may be used in long-term management of heart failure. (∞ See Chapter 30 page 922.)

In 2005, the FDA approved a new drug for treatment of heart failure in African Americans. This drug, known as BiDil is a combination of two vasodilators, hydralazine and isosorbide, in fixed doses. In a study of African Americans with severe heart failure, BiDil improved symptoms and significantly reduced the number of hospitalizations and deaths attributed to heart failure. The accompanying cultural diversity box discusses the nursing implications for BiDil.

Digitalis glycosides are used judiciously in symptomatic heart failure. Digitalis has a *positive inotropic effect* on the heart, increasing the strength of myocardial contraction by increasing the intracellular calcium concentrations. Digitalis also decreases SA node automaticity and slows conduction through the AV node, increasing ventricular filling time.

MEDICATION ADMINISTRATION Heart Failure

ANGIOTENSIN-CONVERTING ENZYME (ACE) INHIBITORS

Enalapril (Vasotec)

Captopril (Capoten)

Moexipril (Univasc)

Quinapril (Accupril)

Trandolapril (Mavik)

Lisinopril (Prinivil, Zestril)

Fosinopril (Monopril)

Perindopril (Aceon)

Ramipril (Altace)

ANGIOTENSIN II RECEPTOR BLOCKERS (ARBS)

Candesartan (Atacand)

Losartan (Cozaar)

Telmisartan (Micardis)

Irbesartan (Avapro)

Nesiritide (Natrecor)

Valsartan (Diovan)

ACE inhibitors and ARBs prevent acute coronary events and reduce mortality in heart failure. ACE inhibitors interfere with production of angiotensin II, resulting in vasodilation, reduced blood volume, and prevention of its effects in the heart and blood vessels. In heart failure, ACE inhibitors reduce afterload and improve cardiac output and renal blood flow. They also reduce pulmonary congestion and peripheral edema. ACE inhibitors suppress myocyte growth and reduce ventricular remodeling in heart failure. While the pharmacologic effect of ARBs is similar, they block the action of angiotensin II at the receptor rather than interfering with its production.

Nursing Responsibilities

- Do not give these drugs to women in the second and third trimesters of pregnancy.
- Carefully monitor patients who are volume depleted or who have impaired renal function.
- Use an infusion pump when administering ACE inhibitors intravenously.
- Monitor blood pressure closely for 2 hours following first dose and as indicated thereafter.
- Monitor serum potassium levels; ACE inhibitors can cause hyperkalemia (this is less of a concern with ARBs).
- Monitor white blood cell (WBC) count for potential neutropenia. Report to the physician.

Health Education for the Patient and Family

- Take the drug at the same time every day to ensure a stable blood level.
- Monitor your blood pressure and weight weekly. Report significant changes to your doctor.
- Avoid making sudden position changes; for example, rise from bed slowly. Lie down if you become dizzy or lightheaded, particularly after the first dose.
- Report any signs of easy bruising and bleeding, sore throat or fever, edema, or skin rash. Immediately report swelling of the face, lips, or eyelids, and itching or breathing problems.
- A persistent, dry cough may develop if you are taking an ACE inhibitor. Contact your doctor if this becomes a problem.
- Take captopril or moexipril 1 hour before meals.

DIURETICS

Chlorothiazide (Diuril)

Furosemide (Lasix)

Ethacrynic acid (Edecrin)

Bumetanide (Bumex)

Toresemide (Demedex)

Hydrochlorothiazide (HydroDIURIL)

Spironolactone (Aldactone)

Triamterene (Dyrenium)

Amiloride (Midamor)

Acetazolamide (Diamox)

Metolazone (Zaroxolyn)

Diuretics act on different portions of the kidney tubule to inhibit the reabsorption of sodium and water and promote their excretion. With the exception of the potassium-sparing diuretics—spironolactone, triamterene, and amiloride—diuretics also promote potassium excretion, increasing the risk of hypokalemia. Spironolactone, an aldosterone receptor blocker, reduces symptoms and slows progression of heart failure. Aldosterone receptors in the heart and blood vessels promote myocardial remodeling and fibrosis, activate the sympathetic nervous system, and promote vascular fibrosis (which decreases compliance) and baroreceptor dysfunction.

Nursing Responsibilities

- Obtain baseline weight and vital signs.
- Monitor blood pressure, intake and output, weight, skin turgor, and edema as indicators of fluid volume status.
- Assess for volume depletion, particularly with loop diuretics (furosemide, ethacrynic acid, and bumetanide): dizziness, orthostatic hypotension, tachycardia, and muscle cramping.
- Report abnormal serum electrolyte levels to the physician. Replace electrolytes as indicated.
- Do not administer potassium replacements to patients receiving a potassium-sparing diuretic.
- Evaluate renal function by assessing urine output, BUN, and serum creatinine.
- Administer intravenous furosemide slowly, no faster than 20 mg/minute. Evaluate for signs of ototoxicity. Do not administer this drug or ethacrynic acid concurrently with aminoglycoside antibiotics (e.g., gentamicin), which are also ototoxic.

Health Education for the Patient and Family

- Drink at least six to eight glasses of water per day.
- Take your diuretic at times that will be the least disruptive to your lifestyle, usually in the morning and early afternoon if a second dose is ordered. Take with meals to decrease gastric upset.
- Monitor your blood pressure, pulse, and weight weekly. Report significant weight changes to your doctor.
- Report any of the following to your doctor: severe abdominal pain, jaundice, dark urine, abnormal bleeding or bruising, flulike symptoms, signs of hypokalemia, hyponatremia, and dehydration (thirst, salt craving, dizziness, weakness, rapid pulse). ∞ See Chapter 10 for manifestations of electrolyte imbalances.
- Avoid sudden position changes. You may experience dizziness, lightheadedness, or feelings of faintness.
- Unless you are taking a potassium-sparing diuretic, integrate foods rich in potassium into your diet (∞ see Chapter 10). Limit sodium use.

POSITIVE INOTROPIC AGENTS

Digitalis Glycosides

Digoxin (Lanoxin)

Digitalis improves myocardial contractility by interfering with ATPase in the myocardial cell membrane and increasing the amount of calcium available for contraction. The increased force of contraction causes the heart to empty more completely,

(continued)

increasing stroke volume and cardiac output. Improved cardiac output improves renal perfusion, decreasing renin secretion. This decreases preload and afterload, reducing cardiac work. Digitalis also has electrophysiologic effects, slowing conduction through the AV node. This decreases the heart rate and reduces oxygen consumption.

Nursing Responsibilities
- Assess apical pulse before administering. Withhold digitalis and notify the physician if heart rate is below 60 BPM and/or manifestations of decreased cardiac output are noted. Record apical rate on medication record.
- Evaluate ECG for scooped (spoon-shaped) ST segment, AV block, bradycardia, and other dysrhythmias (especially PVCs and atrial tachycardias).
- Report manifestations of digitalis toxicity: anorexia, nausea, vomiting, abdominal pain, weakness, vision changes (diplopia, blurred vision, yellow-green or white halos seen around objects), and new-onset dysrhythmias.
- Assess potassium, magnesium, calcium, and serum digoxin levels before giving digitalis. Hypokalemia can precipitate toxicity even when the serum digitalis level is in the "normal" range.
- Monitor patients with renal insufficiency or renal failure and older adults carefully for digitalis toxicity.
- Prepare to administer digoxin immune fab (Digibind) for digoxin toxicity.

Health Education for the Patient and Family
- Take your pulse daily before taking your digoxin. Do not take the digoxin if your pulse is below 60 or if you are weak, fatigued, lightheaded, dizzy, short of breath, or having chest pain. Notify your physician immediately.
- Contact your doctor if you develop manifestations of digitalis toxicity: palpitations, weakness, loss of appetite, nausea, vomiting, abdominal pain, blurred or colored vision, or double vision.
- Avoid using antacids and laxatives; they decrease digoxin absorption.
- Notify your physician immediately if you develop manifestations of potassium deficiency: weakness, lethargy, thirst, depression, muscle cramps, or vomiting.

- Incorporate foods high in potassium into your diet: fresh orange or tomato juice, bananas, raisins, dates, figs, prunes, apricots, spinach, cauliflower, and potatoes.

Sympathomimetic Agents
Dopamine (Inotropin)
Dobutamine (Dobutrex)

Sympathomimetic agents stimulate the heart, improving the force of contraction. Dobutamine is preferred in managing heart failure because it does not increase the heart rate as much as dopamine, and it has a mild vasodilatory effect. These drugs are given by intravenous infusion and may be titrated to obtain their optimal effects.

Phosphodiesterase Inhibitors
Inamrinone (Inocor)
Milrinone (Primacor)

Phosphodiesterase inhibitors are used in treating acute heart failure to increase myocardial contractility and cause vasodilation. The net effects are an increase in cardiac output and a decrease in afterload.

Nursing Responsibilities
- Use an infusion pump to administer these agents. Monitor hemodynamic parameters carefully.
- Avoid discontinuing these drugs abruptly.
- Change solutions and tubing every 24 hours.
- Inamrinone is given as an intravenous bolus over 2 to 3 minutes, followed by an infusion of 5 to 10 mg/kg/min.
- Inamrinone may be infused full strength or diluted in normal saline or half-strength saline. Do not mix this drug with dextrose solutions. After dilution, amnirone can be piggybacked into a line containing a dextrose solution.
- Monitor liver function and platelet counts; inamrinone may cause hepatotoxicity and thrombocytopenia.

Health Education for the Patient and Family
- Notify the nursing staff if you experience abdominal pain or notice a skin rash or bruising.

Digitalis has a narrow therapeutic index; in other words, therapeutic levels are very close to toxic levels. Early manifestations of digitalis toxicity include anorexia, nausea and vomiting, headache, altered vision, and confusion. A number of cardiac dysrhythmias are also associated with digitalis toxicity, including sinus arrest, supraventricular and ventricular tachycardias, and high levels of AV block. Low serum potassium levels increase the risk of digitalis toxicity, as do low magnesium and high calcium levels. Older adults are at particular risk for digitalis toxicity. In 2005, the AHA Heart Failure guidelines noted that the risk of toxicity outweighs the benefits of this class of drug (AHA, 2005). Digitalis levels may be affected by a number of other drugs; check for potential interactions.

Dysrhythmias are common in patients with heart failure. Although PVCs may be frequent, they are often not associated with an increased risk of ventricular tachycardia and fibrillation. Because many antidysrhythmic medications depress left ventricular function, PVCs are frequently left untreated in heart failure. Amiodarone is the drug of choice to treat nonsustained

ventricular tachycardia, which is associated with a poor prognosis. (See Chapter 30 page 956.)

Nutrition and Activity

A sodium-restricted diet is recommended to minimize sodium and water retention. Intake is generally limited to 1.5 to 2 g of sodium per day, a moderate restriction. Box 10–2 includes patient teaching regarding a sodium-restricted diet.

Exercise intolerance, decreased ability to participate in activities using large skeletal muscles due to fatigue or dyspnea, is a common early manifestation of heart failure. Activity may be restricted to bed rest during acute episodes of heart failure to reduce cardiac workload and allow the heart to recompensate. Prolonged bed rest and continued activity limitations, however, are not recommended. A moderate, progressive activity program is prescribed to improve myocardial function. Exercise should be performed 3 to 5 days per week, and each session should include a 10 to 15 minute warm-up period, 20 to 30 minutes of exercise at the recommended intensity, and a cool-down period. Walking is encouraged on nontraining days (Lichtenstein et al., 2006).

FOCUS ON CULTURAL DIVERSITY
BiDil for Treating Heart Failure in African Americans

BiDil, a fixed-dose combination of two vasodilators (hydralazine and isosorbide), is indicated as an adjunctive treatment in African Americans with heart failure. It has been shown to reduce symptoms, decrease the number of hospitalizations, and prolong life in Blacks. The recommended dose is one to two tablets three times per day, although the dose may be as low as ½ tablet three times a day if side effects are intolerable.

Nursing Implications
- Assess vital signs and fluid volume status before administering this drug, as hypotension (orthostatic hypotension in particular) is a common effect.
- Notify the physician if manifestations of systemic lupus erythematosus, glomerulonephritis, or peripheral neuropathy develop.
- Use caution when administering concurrently with MAO inhibitors
- Closely monitor for hypotension when administered concurrently with any potent parenteral antihypertensive agent.

Patient and Family Teaching
- Take this drug as prescribed.
- Headache is a common adverse effect of this drug, particularly when first starting therapy. Headaches tend to subside with continued treatment.
- Notify your doctor if headaches continue after the first few weeks of therapy, or if you develop chest pain or palpitations while taking this drug.
- This drug can cause a drop in blood pressure, particularly when changing positions from lying to sitting or sitting to standing. Change positions slowly and use caution to prevent falls.
- Do not use drugs such as sildenafil (Viagra, Revatio), vardenafil (Levitra), or tadalafil (Cialis) while taking this medication as the combination may cause an extreme drop in blood pressure leading to fainting, chest pain, or a heart attack.

Other Treatments

In end-stage heart failure, devices to provide circulatory assistance or surgery may be required. Surgery may be used to treat the underlying cause of failure (e.g., replacement of diseased valves) or to improve quality of life. Valve replacement is discussed later in this chapter. Heart transplant is currently the only clearly effective surgical treatment for end-stage heart failure; its use is limited by the availability of donor hearts.

CIRCULATORY ASSISTANCE Devices such as the intra-aortic balloon pump or a left-ventricular assist device may be used when the patient is expected to recover or as a bridge to transplant. (∞ See Chapter 30.) Newer devices that will allow longer term support outside the hospital are in the developmental stages. These devices will serve either as a bridge to transplant or allow the myocardium to heal over an extended period of time.

CARDIAC TRANSPLANTATION Heart transplant is the treatment of choice for end-stage heart disease. Survival rates are good: 83% at 1 year and 76% at 3 years. More than 90% of patients return to normal, unrestricted functional abilities

following transplant (Papadakis & McPhee, 2007). The most frequently used transplant procedure leaves posterior walls of the atria, the superior and inferior vena cavae, and pulmonary veins of the recipient intact (Figure 31–6A ■). The atrial walls of the donor heart are then anastomosed to the recipient's atria (Figure 31–6B). The donor pulmonary artery and aorta are anastomosed to the recipient vessels (Figure 31–6C). Care is taken to avoid damaging the sinus node of the donor heart and to ensure integrity of the suture line to prevent postoperative bleeding. Donor organs are obtained from persons with no evidence of cardiac trauma.

Nursing care of the heart transplant patient is similar to care of any cardiac surgery patient (∞ see Chapter 30 page 931). Bleeding is a major concern in the early postoperative period. Chest tube drainage is frequently monitored (initially every 15 minutes), as are the cardiac output, pulmonary artery pressures, and CVP. Cardiac tamponade (compression of the heart) can develop, presenting as either a sudden event or a gradual process. Chest tubes are gently milked (not stripped) as needed to maintain patency. Atrial dysrhythmias are relatively common following cardiac transplant. Temporary pacing wires are placed

Figure 31–6 ■ Cardiac transplantation. *A,* The heart is removed, leaving the posterior walls of the atria intact. The donor heart is anastomosed to the atria, *B,* and the great vessels, *C.*

during surgery as the conduction system may be disrupted by surgical manipulation or postoperative swelling. Hypothermia is induced during surgery; postoperatively, the patient is gradually rewarmed over a 1 to 2 hour period. Prevention of rapid rewarming and shivering are important to maintain hemo-dynamic stability and reduce oxygen consumption. Cardiac function is impaired in up to 50% of transplanted hearts during the early postoperative period. Inotropic agents such as low-dose dopamine, dobutamine, or milrinone may be required to support cardiac function and circulation (Wade et al., 2004).

Infection and rejection are major postoperative concerns; these are the chief causes of mortality in transplant patients. Rejection may develop immediately after transplant (a rare occurrence), within weeks to months, or years after the transplant. Acute rejection usually presents within weeks of the transplant, developing when the transplanted organ is recognized by the immune system as foreign. Lymphocytes infiltrate the organ, and myocardial cell necrosis can be detected on biopsy. Acute rejection often can be treated using immunosuppressive drugs (Wade et al., 2004). These drugs also are given to prevent rejection of the transplanted organ, even when the tissue match is good (∞ see Chapter 12). Although immunosuppressive medications help prevent organ rejection, they impair the patient's defenses against infection. Early postoperative infections commonly are bacterial or fungal (*candida*). Multiple invasive lines, prolonged ventilator support, and immunosuppressive therapy contribute to the transplant recipient's risk for infection. Aggressive nursing care directed at prevention of infection is vital: limiting visitors with communicable diseases, pulmonary hygiene measures, early ambulation, and strict aseptic technique (Wade et al., 2004).

The donor heart is denervated during the transplant procedure. Lack of innervation by the autonomic nervous system affects the heart rate (usually between 90 and 110 bpm in transplanted hearts), its response to position changes, stress, exercise, and certain drugs.

OTHER PROCEDURES Other surgical procedures such as cardiomyoplasty and ventricular reduction surgery do not improve the prognosis or quality of life in patients with end-stage heart failure. *Cardiomyoplasty* involves wrapping the latissimus dorsi muscle around the heart to support the failing myocardium. The muscle is stimulated in synchrony with the heart, providing a more forceful contraction and increasing cardiac output. In ventricular reduction surgery (or *partial ventriculectomy*), a portion of the anteriolateral left ventricular wall is resected to improve cardiac function (Papadakis & McPhee, 2007).

Complementary Therapies
Strong evidence supports the use of several complementary therapies for heart failure. Hawthorn, a shrubby tree, contains natural cardiotonic ingredients in its blossoms, leaves, and fruit. It increases the force of myocardial contraction, dilates blood vessels, and has a natural ACE inhibitor. Hawthorn should never be used without consulting an experienced herb practitioner and advising the physician (Fontaine, 2005). Nutritional supplements of coenzyme Q10, magnesium, and thiamine may be used in conjunction with other treatments. Coenzyme Q10 improves mitochondria function and energy production.

End-of-Life Care
Unless a cardiac transplant is performed, chronic heart failure is ultimately a terminal disease. The patient and family need honest discussions about the anticipated course of the disease and treatment options. It is important to discuss advance directives such as the living will and medical power of attorney, differentiating potential acute events from which recovery would be anticipated (e.g., reversible exacerbation of heart failure, sudden cardiac arrest) from prolonged life support without reasonable expectation of functional recovery. Hospice services are available for patients with heart failure, and should be offered when appropriate. Severe dyspnea is common in the final stages of the disease. It may be managed with narcotic analgesics or with frequent intravenous diuretics and continuous infusion of a positive inotropic agent (Hunt et al., 2005).

∞ Nursing Care

Health Promotion
Health promotion activities to reduce the risk for and incidence of heart failure are directed at the risk factors. Teach patients about coronary heart disease, the primary underlying cause of heart failure. Discuss CHD risk factors, and ways to reduce those risk factors (∞ see Chapter 30).

Hypertension also is a major cause of heart failure. Routinely screen patients for elevated blood pressure, and refer patients to a primary care provider as indicated. Discuss the importance of effectively managing hypertension to reduce the future risk for heart failure. Likewise, stress the relationship between effective diabetes management and reduced risk of heart failure.

Assessment
Obtain both subjective and objective data when assessing the patient with heart failure.

- *Health history:* Complaints of increasing shortness of breath, dyspnea with exertion, decreasing activity tolerance, or paroxysmal nocturnal dyspnea; number of pillows used for sleeping; recent weight gain; presence of a cough; chest or abdominal pain; anorexia or nausea; history of cardiac disease, previous episodes of heart failure; other risk factors such as hypertension or diabetes; current medications; usual diet and activity and recent changes. Determine patient's NYHA class.

EVIDENCE FOR NURSING CARE **The Patient with Heart Failure**

Selected resources that nurses may find helpful when planning evidence-based nursing care follow.

- Moss, A. J., Hall, W. J., Cannom, D. S., Klein, H., Brown, M. W., Daubert, J. P., et al. (2009). Cardiac-resynchronization therapy for the prevention of heart-failure events. *The New England Journal of Medicine, 361*(14), 1329–1338. Retrieved from http://content.nejm.org/cgi/reprint/361/14/1329.pdf
- Whitten, S. E. (2008). Systolic heart failure in a patient with hypertrophic obstructive cardiomyopathy: A potentially life-threatening complication. *Critical Care Nurse, 28*(5), 44–52.

■ *Physical examination:* General appearance; ease of breathing, conversing, changing positions; apparent anxiety; vital signs including apical pulse; color of skin and mucous membranes; neck vein distension, peripheral pulses, capillary refill, presence and degree of edema; heart and breath sounds; abdominal contour, bowel sounds, tenderness; right upper abdominal tenderness, liver enlargement.

Nursing Diagnoses and Interventions

Heart failure impacts quality of life, interfering with such daily activities as self-care and role performance. Reducing the oxygen demand of the heart is a major nursing care goal for the patient in acute heart failure. This includes providing rest and carrying out prescribed treatment measures to reduce cardiac work, improve contractility, and manage symptoms. See also the accompanying Case Study & Nursing Care Plan for additional nursing diagnoses and interventions for the patient with heart failure.

Decreased Cardiac Output

As the heart fails as a pump, stroke volume and tissue perfusion decrease.

■ Monitor vital signs and oxygen saturation as indicated. *Decreased cardiac output stimulates the SNS to increase the heart rate in an attempt to restore CO. Tachycardia at rest is common. Diastolic blood pressure may initially be elevated because of vasoconstriction; in late stages, compensatory mechanisms fail, and BP falls. Oxygen saturation levels provide a measure of gas exchange and tissue perfusion.*

■ Auscultate heart and breath sounds regularly. *S_1 and S_2 may be diminished if cardiac function is poor. A ventricular gallop (S_3) is an early sign of heart failure; atrial gallop (S_4) may also be present. Crackles are often heard in the lung bases; increasing crackles, dyspnea, and shortness of breath indicate worsening failure.*

> **PRACTICE ALERT**
> Report manifestations of decreased cardiac output and tissue perfusion: changes in mentation; decreased urine output; cool, clammy skin; diminished pulses; pallor or cyanosis; or dysrhythmias. These are manifestations of decreased tissue perfusion to organ systems.

■ Administer supplemental oxygen as needed. *This improves oxygenation of the blood, decreasing the effects of hypoxia and ischemia.*

■ Administer prescribed medications as ordered. *Drugs are used to decrease the cardiac workload and increase the effectiveness of contractions.*

■ Encourage rest, explaining the rationale. Elevate the head of the bed to reduce the work of breathing. Provide a bedside commode, and assist with ADLs. Instruct to avoid the Valsalva maneuver. *These measures reduce cardiac workload.*

> **PRACTICE ALERT**
> Promote psychologic rest and decrease anxiety. Maintain a quiet environment; encourage expression of fears and feelings. Explain care measures and their purpose. Psychologic rest decreases oxygen consumption and improves cardiac function.

Excess Fluid Volume

As cardiac output falls, compensatory mechanisms cause salt and water retention, increasing blood volume. This increased fluid volume places additional stress on the already failing ventricles, making them work harder to move the fluid load.

■ Assess respiratory status and auscultate lung sounds at least every 4 hours. Notify the physician of significant changes in condition. *Declining respiratory status indicates worsening left heart failure.*

> **PRACTICE ALERT**
> Immediately notify the physician if the patient develops air hunger, an overwhelming sense of impending doom or panic, tachypnea, severe orthopnea, or a cough productive of large amounts of pink, frothy sputum. Acute pulmonary edema, a medical emergency, can develop rapidly, necessitating immediate intervention to preserve life.

■ Monitor intake and output. Notify the physician if urine output is less than 30 mL/h. Weigh daily. *Careful monitoring of fluid volume is important during treatment of heart failure. Diuretics may reduce circulating volume, producing hypovolemia despite persistent peripheral edema. A fall in urine output may indicate significantly reduced cardiac output and renal ischemia. Weight is an objective measure of fluid status: 1 L of fluid is equal to 2.2 lb of weight.*

■ Record abdominal girth every shift. Note complaints of a loss of appetite, abdominal discomfort, or nausea. *Venous congestion can lead to ascites and may affect gastrointestinal function and nutritional status.*

■ Monitor and record hemodynamic measurements. Report significant changes and negative trends. *Hemodynamic measurements provide a means of monitoring condition and response to treatment.*

■ Restrict fluids as ordered. Allow choices of fluid type and timing of intake, scheduling most fluid intake during morning and afternoon hours. Offer ice chips and frequent mouth care; provide hard candies if allowed. *Providing choices increases the patient's sense of control. Ice chips, hard candies, and mouth care relieve dry mouth and thirst and promote comfort.*

Activity Intolerance

Patients with heart failure have little or no cardiac reserve to meet increased oxygen demands. As the disease progresses and cardiac function is further compromised, activity intolerance increases. The low cardiac output and inability to participate in activities may hinder self-care.

> **PRACTICE ALERT**
> Monitor vital signs and cardiac rhythm during and after activities. Tachycardia, dysrhythmias, increasing dyspnea, changes in blood pressure, diaphoresis, pallor, complaints of chest pain, excessive fatigue, or palpitations indicate activity intolerance. Instruct to rest if manifestations are noted. The failing heart is unable to increase cardiac output to meet increased oxygen demands associated with activity. Assessing response to activities helps evaluate cardiac function. Decreasing activity tolerance may signal deterioration of cardiac function, not overexertion.

- Organize nursing care to allow rest periods. *Grouping activities together allows adequate time to "recharge."*
- Assist with ADLs as needed. Encourage independence within prescribed limits. *Assisting with ADLs helps ensure that care needs are met while reducing cardiac workload. Involving the patient promotes a sense of control and reduces helplessness.*
- Plan and implement progressive activities. Use passive and active ROM exercises as appropriate. Consult with physical therapist on activity plan. *Progressive activity slowly increases exercise capacity by strengthening and improving cardiac function without strain. Activity also helps prevent skeletal muscle atrophy. ROM exercises prevent complications of immobility in severely compromised patients.*
- Provide written and verbal information about activity after discharge. *Written information provides a reference for important information. Verbal information allows clarification and validation of the material.*

Deficient Knowledge: Low-Sodium Diet

Diet is an important part of long-term management of heart failure to manage fluid retention.

- Discuss the rationale for sodium restrictions. *Understanding fosters compliance with the prescribed diet.*
- Consult with dietitian to plan and teach a low-sodium and, if necessary for weight control, low-kcal diet. Provide a list of high-sodium, high-fat, high-cholesterol foods to avoid. Provide American Heart Association materials. *Dietary planning and teaching increases the patient's sense of control and participation in disease management. Food lists are useful memory aids.*

> **PRACTICE ALERT**
> Teach how to read food labels for nutritional information. Many processed foods contain hidden sodium, which can be identified by careful label reading.

- Assist the patient to construct a 2-day meal plan choosing foods low in sodium. *This allows learning assessment, clarification of misunderstandings, and reinforcement of teaching.*

> **NANDA, NIC, AND NOC LINKAGES**
> The Patient with Heart Failure
>
> **NANDA**   Activity Intolerance
>
> **NIC**   Cardiac care: Rehabilitative
> Energy Management
> Self-Care Assistance
> Teaching: Prescribed Activity/Exercise
>
> **NOC**   Activity Tolerance
> Endurance
> Energy Conservation
> Self-Care: Activities of Daily Living (ADLs)
> Knowledge: Treatment Regimen
>
> Adapted from Bulechek, G., Butcher, H., & Dochterman, J. M. (Eds). (2008). *Nursing interventions classification (NIC)* (5th ed.). St. Louis: Mosby Elsevier; Moorhead, S., Johnson, M., Maas, M., & Swanson, E. (Eds). (2008). *Nursing outcomes classification (NOC)* (4th ed.). St. Louis: Mosby Elsevier; and NANDA International. (2009). *Nursing diagnoses: Definitions and classification 2009–2011*. Oxford, UK: Wiley-Blackwell.

- Encourage small, frequent meals rather than three heavy meals per day. *Small, frequent meals provide continuing energy resources and decrease the work required to digest a large meal.*

Using NANDA, NIC, and NOC

Linkages between a selected NANDA nursing diagnosis, NIC, and NOC for the patient with heart failure are shown in the chart that follows.

Community-Based Care

Heart failure is a chronic condition requiring active participation by the patient and family for effective management. In teaching for home care, include the following topics:

- The disease process and its effects on the patient's life
- Warning signals of cardiac decompensation that require treatment

BOX 31–3 Home Activity Guidelines for the Patient with Heart Failure

- Perform as many activities as independently as you can.
- Space your meals and activities.
  a. Eat six small meals a day.
  b. Allow time during the day for periods of rest and relaxation.
- Perform all activities at a comfortable pace.
  a. If you get tired during any activity, stop what you are doing and rest for 15 minutes.
  b. Resume activity only if you feel up to it.
- Stop any activity that causes chest pain, shortness of breath, dizziness, faintness, excessive weakness, or sweating. Rest. Notify your physician if your activity tolerance changes and if symptoms continue after rest.
- Avoid straining. Do not lift heavy objects. Eat a high-fiber diet and drink plenty of water to prevent constipation. Use laxatives or stool softeners, as approved by your physician, to avoid constipation and straining during bowel movements.
- Begin a graded exercise program. Walking is good exercise that does not require any special equipment (except a good pair of

walking shoes). Plan to walk twice a day at a comfortable, slow pace for the first couple of weeks at home, and then gradually increase the distance and pace. A suggested schedule is provided next—but progress at your own speed. Take your time. Aim for walking at least 3 times per week (every other day).

Week 1	200 to 400 ft (1/4 mile)	Twice a day, slow leisurely pace
Week 2	1/4 mile	15 min, minimum of 3 times per week
Weeks 2 to 3	1/2 mile	30 min, minimum of 3 times per week
Weeks 3 to 4	1 mile	30 min, minimum of 3 times per week
Weeks 4 to 5	1 1/2 mile	30 min, minimum of 3 times per week
Weeks 5 to 6	2 miles	40 min, minimum of 3 times per week

CASE STUDY & NURSING CARE PLAN   A Patient with Heart Failure

One year ago, Arthur Jackson, 67 years old, had a large anterior wall MI and underwent subsequent coronary artery bypass surgery. On discharge, he was started on a regimen of enalapril (Vasotec), digoxin, furosemide (Lasix), coumadin, and a potassium chloride supplement. He is now in the cardiac unit complaining of severe shortness of breath, hemoptysis, and poor appetite for 1 week. He is diagnosed with acute heart failure.

ASSESSMENT

Mr. Jackson refuses to settle in bed, preferring to sit in the bedside recliner in high Fowler's position. He states, "Lately, this is the only way I can breathe." Mr. Jackson states that he has not been able to work in his garden without getting short of breath. He complains of his shoes and belt being too tight.

When Ms. Takashi, RN (Mr. Jackson's nurse), obtains his nursing history, Mr. Jackson insists that he takes his medications regularly. He states that he normally works in his garden for light exercise. In his diet history, Mr. Jackson admits fondness for bacon and Chinese food and sheepishly admits to snacking between meals "even though I need to lose weight."

Mr. Jackson's vital signs are BP 95/72 mmHg, HR 124 and irregular, R 28 and labored, and T 97.5°F (36.5°C). The cardiac monitor shows atrial fibrillation. An S_3 is noted on auscultation; the cardiac impulse is left of the midclavicular line. He has crackles and diminished breath sounds in the bases of both lungs. Significant jugular venous distention, 3+ pitting edema of feet and ankles, and abdominal distention are noted. Liver size is within normal limits by percussion. Skin cool and diaphoretic. Chest x-ray shows cardiomegaly and pulmonary infiltrates.

DIAGNOSES

- *Excess Fluid Volume* related to impaired cardiac pump and salt and water retention
- *Activity Intolerance* related to impaired cardiac output
- *Impaired Health Maintenance* related to lack of knowledge about diet restrictions

EXPECTED OUTCOMES

- Demonstrate loss of excess fluid by weight loss and decreases in edema, jugular venous distention, and abdominal distention.
- Demonstrate improved activity tolerance.
- Verbalize understanding of diet restrictions.

PLANNING AND IMPLEMENTATION

- Take hourly vital signs and hemodynamic pressure measurements.
- Administer and monitor effects of prescribed diuretics and vasodilators.
- Weigh daily; strict intake and output.

- Enforce fluid restriction of 1500 mL/24 hours: 600 mL day shift, 600 mL evening shift, 300 mL at night.
- Auscultate heart and breath sounds every 4 hours and as indicated.
- Administer oxygen per nasal cannula at 2 L/min. Monitor oxygen saturation continuously. Notify physician if less than 94%.
- Place in high Fowler's or position of comfort.
- Notify physician of significant changes in laboratory values.
- Teach about all medications and how to take and record pulse. Provide information about anticoagulant therapy and signs of bleeding.
- Design an activity plan with Mr. Jackson that incorporates preferred activities and scheduled rest periods.
- Instruct about sodium-restricted diet. Allow meal choices within allowed limits.
- Consult dietitian for planning and teaching Mr. and Mrs. Jackson about low-sodium diet.

EVALUATION

Mr. Jackson is discharged after 3 days in the cardiac unit. He has lost 8 pounds during his stay and states it is much easier to breathe and his shoes fit better. He is able to sleep in semi-Fowler's position with only one pillow. His peripheral edema has resolved. Mr. and Mrs. Jackson met with the dietitian, who helped them develop a realistic eating plan to limit sodium, sugar, and fats. The dietitian also provided a list of high-sodium foods to avoid. Mr. Jackson is relieved to know that he can still enjoy Chinese food prepared without monosodium glutamate (MSG) or added salt. Ms. Takashi and the physical therapist designed a progressive activity plan with Mr. Jackson that he will continue at home. He remains in atrial fibrillation, a chronic condition. His knowledge of digoxin and coumadin has been assessed and reinforced. Ms. Takashi confirms that he is able to accurately check his pulse and can list signs of digoxin toxicity and excessive bleeding.

CRITICAL THINKING IN THE NURSING PROCESS

1. Mr. Jackson's medication regimen remains the same after discharge. What specific teaching does he need related to potential interactions of these drugs?
2. Mr. Jackson tells you, "Talk to my wife about my medications—she's Tarzan and I'm Jane now." How would you respond?
3. Design an exercise plan for Mr. Jackson to prevent deconditioning and conserve energy.
4. Mr. Jackson tells you, "Sometimes I forget whether I have taken my aspirin, so I'll take another just to be sure. After all, they are only baby aspirin. One or two extra a day shouldn't hurt, right?" What is your response?
5. Mr. Jackson is admitted to the neuro unit 6 months later with a cerebral vascular accident (CVA). What is the probable cause of his stroke?

See Evaluating Your Response in Appendix C.

- Desired and adverse effects of prescribed drugs; monitoring for effects; importance of compliance with drug regimen to prevent acute and long-term complications of heart failure
- Prescribed diet and sodium restriction; practical suggestions for reducing salt intake; recommend American Heart Association materials and recipes
- Exercise recommendations to strengthen the heart muscle and improve aerobic capacity (Box 31–3)

- The importance of keeping scheduled follow-up appointments to monitor disease progression and effects of therapy

Provide referrals for home health care and household assistance (shopping, transportation, personal needs, and housekeeping) as indicated. Referrals to community agencies, such as local cardiac rehabilitation programs, heart support groups, or the AHA, can provide with additional materials and psychosocial support.

The Patient with Pulmonary Edema

Pulmonary edema is an abnormal accumulation of fluid in the interstitial tissue and alveoli of the lung. Both cardiac and non-cardiac disorders can cause pulmonary edema. Cardiac causes include acute myocardial infarction, acute heart failure, and valvular disease. *Cardiogenic pulmonary edema*, the focus of this section, is a sign of severe cardiac decompensation. Noncardiac causes of pulmonary edema include primary pulmonary disorders, such as acute respiratory distress syndrome (ARDS), trauma, sepsis, drug overdose, or neurologic sequelae. Pulmonary edema due to ARDS is discussed in ∞ Chapter 37.

MANIFESTATIONS of Pulmonary Edema

RESPIRATORY
- Tachypnea
- Labored respirations
- Dyspnea
- Orthopnea
- Paroxysmal nocturnal dyspnea
- Cough productive of frothy, pink sputum
- Crackles, wheezes

CARDIOVASCULAR
- Tachycardia
- Hypotension
- Cyanosis
- Cool, clammy skin
- Hypoxemia
- Ventricular gallop

NEUROLOGIC
- Restlessness
- Anxiety
- Feeling of impending doom

FAST FACTS
- Cardiogenic pulmonary edema is a severe form of heart failure. Risk factors are those associated with heart failure, and treatment focuses on maintaining oxygenation and improving cardiac function.
- Noncardiogenic pulmonary edema is a primary or secondary lung disorder. It usually occurs secondarily to a critical event such as major trauma, shock, or DIC. Treatment focuses on maintaining oxygenation and the primary, underlying disorder.

Pulmonary edema is a medical emergency: The patient is literally drowning in the fluid in the alveolar and interstitial pulmonary spaces. Its onset may be acute or gradual, progressing to severe respiratory distress. Immediate treatment is necessary.

Pathophysiology

In cardiogenic pulmonary edema, the contractility of the left ventricle is severely impaired. The ejection fraction falls as the ventricle is unable to eject the blood that enters it, causing a sharp rise in end-diastolic volume and pressure. Pulmonary hydrostatic pressures rise, ultimately exceeding the osmotic pressure of the blood. As a result, fluid leaking from the pulmonary capillaries congests interstitial tissues, decreasing lung compliance, and interfering with gas exchange. As capillary and interstitial pressures increase further, the tight junctions of the alveolar walls are disrupted, and the fluid enters the alveoli, along with large red blood cells and protein molecules. Ventilation and gas exchange are severely disrupted, and hypoxia worsens.

Manifestations

The patient with acute pulmonary edema presents with classic manifestations (see the accompanying box). Dyspnea, shortness of breath, and labored respirations are acute and severe, accompanied by orthopnea, the inability to breathe when lying down. Cyanosis is present, and the skin is cool, clammy, and diaphoretic. A productive cough with pink, frothy sputum develops due to fluid, RBCs, and plasma proteins in the alveoli and airways. Crackles are heard throughout the lung fields on auscultation. As the condition worsens, lung sounds become harsher. The patient often is restless and highly anxious, although severe hypoxia may cause confusion or lethargy.

As noted earlier, pulmonary edema is a medical emergency. Without rapid and effective intervention, severe tissue hypoxia and acidosis will lead to organ system failure and death.

Interdisciplinary Care

Immediate treatment for acute pulmonary edema focuses on restoring effective gas exchange and reducing fluid and pressure in the pulmonary vascular system. The patient is placed in an upright sitting position with the legs dangling to reduce venous return by trapping some excess fluid in the lower extremities. This position also facilitates breathing.

Diagnostic testing is limited to assessment of the acute situation. *Arterial blood gases (ABGs)* are drawn to assess gas exchange and acid–base balance. Oxygen tension (PaO_2) is usually low. Initially, carbon dioxide levels ($PaCO_2$) may also be reduced because of rapid respirations. As the condition progresses, the $PaCO_2$ rises and respiratory acidosis develops (∞ see Chapter 10). *Oxygen saturation* levels also are continuously monitored. The *chest x-ray* shows pulmonary vascular congestion and alveolar edema. Provided the patient's condition allows, *hemodynamic monitoring* is instituted. In cardiogenic pulmonary edema, the pulmonary artery wedge pressure (PAWP) is elevated, usually over 25 mmHg. Cardiac output may be decreased.

Morphine is administered intravenously to relieve anxiety and improve the efficacy of breathing. It also is a vasodilator that reduces venous return and lowers left atrial pressure. Although morphine is very effective for patients with cardiogenic pulmonary edema, naloxone, its antidote, is kept readily available in case respiratory depression occurs.

Oxygen is administered using a positive pressure system that can achieve a 100% oxygen concentration. A continuous positive airway pressure (CPAP) mask system may be used, or the patient may be intubated and mechanical ventilation employed (∞ see Chapter 37). Positive pressure increases alveolar pressures and gas exchange while decreasing fluid diffusion into the alveoli.

Potent loop diuretics such as furosemide, ethacrynic acid, or bumetanide are administered intravenously to promote rapid diuresis. Furosemide is also a venous dilator, reducing venous return to the heart. Vasodilators such as intravenous nitroprusside are given to improve cardiac output by reducing afterload. Dopamine or dobutamine and possibly digoxin are administered to improve the myocardial contractility and cardiac output. Intravenous aminophylline may be used cautiously to reduce bronchospasm and decrease wheezing.

When the patient's condition has stabilized, further diagnostic tests may be done to determine the underlying cause of pulmonary edema, and specific treatment measures directed at the cause instituted.

∞ Nursing Care

Nursing care of the patient with acute pulmonary edema focuses on relieving the pulmonary effects of the disorder. Interventions are directed toward improving oxygenation, reducing fluid volume, and providing emotional support.

The nurse often is instrumental in recognizing early manifestations of pulmonary edema and initiating treatment. As with many critical conditions, emergent care is directed toward the ABCs: airway, breathing, and circulation.

Nursing Diagnoses and Interventions

Promoting effective gas exchange and restoring an effective cardiac output are the priorities for nursing and interdisciplinary care of the patient with cardiogenic pulmonary edema. The experience of acute dyspnea and shortness of breath is terrifying for the patient; the nurse is instrumental in providing emotional support and reassurance.

Impaired Gas Exchange

Accumulated fluid in the alveoli and airways interfere with ventilation of the lungs. As a result, alveolar oxygen levels fall and carbon dioxide levels may rise. Reduced alveolar oxygen decreases diffusion of the gas into pulmonary capillaries. In addition, pulmonary edema increases the distance over which gases must diffuse to cross the alveolar-capillary membrane, further reducing oxygen levels in the blood and oxygen delivery to the tissues.

■ Ensure airway patency. *A patent airway is absolutely vital for pulmonary function, including ventilation and gas exchange.*

> **PRACTICE ALERT**
> Assess the effectiveness of respiratory efforts and airway clearance. Pulmonary edema increases the work of breathing. This increased effort can lead to fatigue and decreased respiratory effort.

■ Assess respiratory status frequently, including rate, effort, use of accessory muscles, sputum characteristics, lung sounds, and skin color. *The status of a patient in acute pulmonary edema can change rapidly for the better or worse.*
■ Place in high-Fowler's position with the legs dangling. *The upright position facilitates breathing and decreases venous return.*
■ Administer oxygen as ordered by mask, CPAP mask, or ventilator. *Supplemental oxygen promotes gas exchange; positive pressure increases the pressure within the alveoli, airways, and thoracic cavity, decreasing venous return, pulmonary capillary pressure, and fluid leak into the alveoli.*
■ Encourage patient to cough up secretions; provide nasotracheal suctioning if necessary. *Coughing moves secretions from smaller airways into larger airways where they can be suctioned out if necessary.*

> **PRACTICE ALERT**
> Have emergency equipment readily available in case of respiratory arrest. Be prepared to assist with intubation and initiation of mechanical ventilation. Fatigue, impaired gas exchange, and respiratory acidosis can lead to respiratory and cardiac arrest.

Decreased Cardiac Output

Cardiogenic pulmonary edema usually is caused by either an acute decrease in myocardial contractility or increased workload that exceeds the ability of the left ventricle. The significant decrease in cardiac output increases pressure within the pulmonary vascular system and triggers compensatory mechanisms that increase the heart rate and blood volume. These compensatory mechanisms further increase the workload of the failing heart.

■ Monitor vital signs, hemodynamic status, and rhythm continuously. *Acute pulmonary edema is a critical condition, and cardiovascular status can change rapidly.*
■ Assess heart sounds for possible S_3, S_4, or murmurs. *These abnormal heart sounds may be due to excess work or may indicate the cause of the acute pulmonary edema.*
■ Initiate an intravenous line for medication administration. Administer morphine, diuretics, vasodilators, bronchodilators, and positive inotropic medications (e.g., digoxin) as ordered. *These drugs reduce cardiac work and improve contractility.*

> **PRACTICE ALERT**
> Insert an indwelling catheter; record output hourly. Urine output of less than 30 mL/hr indicates impaired renal perfusion due to severely impaired cardiac output and a risk for renal failure or other complications.

■ Keep accurate intake and output records. Restrict fluids as ordered. *Fluids may be restricted to reduce vascular volume and cardiac work.*

Fear

Acute pulmonary edema is a very frightening experience for everyone (including the nurse).

■ Provide emotional support for the patient and family members. *Fear and anxiety stimulate the sympathetic nervous system, which can lead to ineffective respiratory patterns and interfere with cooperation with care measures.*
■ Explain all procedures and the reasons to the patient and family members. Keep information brief and to the point. Use short sentences and a reassuring tone. *Anxiety and fear interfere with the ability to assimilate information; brief, factual information and reassurance reduce anxiety and fear.*
■ Maintain close contact with the patient and family, providing reassurance that recovery from acute pulmonary edema is often as dramatic as its onset.
■ Answer questions, and provide accurate information in a caring manner. *Knowledge reduces anxiety and psychologic stress associated with this critical condition.*

Community-Based Care

During the acute period, teaching is limited to immediate care measures. Once the acute episode of pulmonary edema has resolved, teach the patient and family about its underlying cause and prevention of future episodes. If pulmonary edema follows an acute MI, include information related to CHD and the AMI, as well as information related to heart failure. Review the teaching and home care for patients with these disorders for further information.

Inflammatory Heart Disorders

Any layer of cardiac tissue—the endocardium, myocardium, or pericardium—can become inflamed, thus damaging the heart valves, heart muscle, or pericardial lining. Manifestations of inflammatory heart disorders range from very mild to life threatening. This section discusses the causes and management of rheumatic heart disease, endocarditis, myocarditis, and pericarditis.

The Patient with Rheumatic Fever and Rheumatic Heart Disease

Rheumatic fever is a systemic inflammatory disease caused by an abnormal immune response to pharyngeal infection by group A beta-hemolytic streptococci. Rheumatic fever usually is a self-limiting disorder, although it may become recurrent or chronic. Although the heart commonly is involved in the acute inflammatory process, only about 10% of people with rheumatic fever develop rheumatic heart disease (Huether & McCance, 2008). Rheumatic heart disease frequently damages the heart valves and is a major cause of mitral and aortic valve disorders discussed in the next section of this chapter.

Incidence, Prevalence, and Risk Factors

In the United States and other industrialized nations, rheumatic fever and its sequelae are rare. The peak incidence of rheumatic fever is between ages 5 and 15; although it is rare after age 40, it may affect people of any age. About 3% of people with untreated group A streptococcal pharyngitis develop rheumatic fever (Papadakis & McPhee, 2007). Rheumatic fever and rheumatic heart disease remain significant public health problems in many developing countries. Highly virulent strains of group A streptococci have caused scattered outbreaks in the United States in recent years (Huether & McCance, 2008).

Risk factors for streptococcal infections of the pharynx include environmental and economic factors such as crowded living conditions, malnutrition, immunodeficiency, and poor access to health care. Evidence also suggests an unknown genetic factor in susceptibility to rheumatic fever.

FAST FACTS

- The peak incidence of rheumatic fever is in children ages 5 to 15.
- Young adults (in late adolescence and the early twenties) are the primary adult population affected by rheumatic fever.
- People past age 40 rarely develop the disease, unless it is a case of recurrent rheumatic fever.
- Although crowded living conditions and lower socioeconomic status are risk factors, a relatively recent outbreak in the United States occurred in people with ready access to health care.

Pathophysiology

The pathophysiology of rheumatic fever is not yet totally understood. It is thought to result from an abnormal immune response to M proteins on group A β-hemolytic streptococcal bacteria. These antigens can bind to cells in the heart, muscles, and brain. They also bind with receptors in synovial joints, provoking an autoimmune response (Huether & McCance, 2008). The resulting immune response to the bacteria also leads to inflammation in tissues containing these M proteins. Inflammatory lesions develop in connective tissues on the heart, joints, and skin. The antibodies may remain in the serum for up to 6 months following the initiating event. ∞ See Chapters 11 and 12 for more information about the immune system and inflammatory response.

Carditis, inflammation of the heart, develops in about 50% of people with rheumatic fever. The inflammatory process usually involves all three layers of the heart—the pericardium, myocardium, and endocardium. *Aschoff bodies*, localized areas of tissue necrosis surrounded by immune cells, develop in cardiac tissues. Pericardial and myocardial inflammation tends to be mild and self-limiting. Endocardial inflammation, however, causes swelling and erythema of valve structures and small vegetative lesions on valve leaflets. As the inflammatory process resolves, fibrous scarring occurs, causing deformity.

Rheumatic heart disease (RHD) is a slowly progressive valvular deformity that may follow acute or repeated attacks of rheumatic fever. Valve leaflets become rigid and deformed; commissures (openings) fuse, and the chordae tendineae fibrose and shorten. This results in stenosis or regurgitation of the valve. In **stenosis**, a narrowed fused valve obstructs forward blood flow. **Regurgitation** occurs when the valve fails to close properly (an *incompetent* valve), allowing blood to flow back through it. Valves on the left side of the heart are usually affected; the mitral valve is most frequently involved.

Manifestations

Manifestations of rheumatic fever typically follow the initial streptococcal infection by about 2 to 3 weeks. Fever and migratory joint pain are often initial manifestations. The knees, ankles, hips, and elbows are common sites of swelling and inflammation. *Erythema marginatum* is a temporary nonpruritic skin rash characterized by red lesions with clear borders and blanched centers usually found on the trunk and proximal extremities. Neurologic symptoms of rheumatic fever, although

---

MANIFESTATIONS of Rheumatic Fever

CARDIAC
- Chest pain
- Friction rub
- Heart murmur

MUSCULOSKELETAL
- *Migratory polyarthritis:* redness, heat, swelling, pain, and tenderness of more than one joint
- Usually affects large joints of extremities

SKIN
- *Erythema marginatum:* transitory pink, nonpruritic, macular lesions on trunk or inner aspect of upper arms or thighs
- *Subcutaneous nodules* over extensors of wrist, elbow, ankle, and knee joints

NEUROLOGIC
- *Sydenham's chorea:* irritability; behavior changes; sudden, jerky, involuntary movements

rare in adults, may range from irritability and an inability to concentrate to clumsiness and involuntary muscle spasms.

Manifestations of carditis include chest pain, tachycardia, a pericardial friction rub, or evidence of heart failure. On auscultation, an S_3, S_4, or a heart murmur may be heard. Cardiomegaly or pericardial effusion may develop. Other manifestations of rheumatic fever are listed in the accompanying box.

Interdisciplinary Care

Management of the patient with rheumatic heart disease focuses on eradicating the streptococcal infection and managing the manifestations of the disease. Carditis and resulting heart failure are treated with measures to reduce the inflammatory process and manage the heart failure. Activities are limited, but bed rest is not generally ordered.

Diagnosis

In addition to the history and physical examination, a number of laboratory and diagnostic tests may be ordered for the patient with suspected rheumatic fever. Table 31–5 identifies tests and values indicative of carditis associated with rheumatic fever.

- *Complete blood count (CBC)* and *erythrocyte sedimentation rate (ESR)* are indicators of the inflammatory process. The white blood cell count is elevated, and the number of red blood cells may be low due to the inflammatory inhibition of erythropoiesis. The ESR, a general indicator of inflammation, is elevated.
- *C-reactive protein (CRP)* is positive in an active inflammatory process.
- *Antistreptolysin (ASO) titer* is a test for streptococcal antibodies. It rises within 2 months of the onset and is positive in most patients with rheumatic fever.
- Throat culture is positive for group A β-hemolytic streptococcus in only 25% to 40% of patients with acute rheumatic fever (Papadakis & McPhee, 2007).

Medications

As soon as rheumatic fever is diagnosed, antibiotics are started to eliminate the streptococcal infection. Penicillin is the antibiotic of choice to treat group A streptococci. Antibiotics are prescribed for at least 10 days. Erythromycin or clindamycin is used if the patient is allergic to penicillin. Prophylactic antibiotic therapy is

continued for 5 to 10 years to prevent recurrences. Recurrences after 5 years or age 25 are rare (Papadakis & McPhee, 2007). Penicillin G, 1.2 million units injected intramuscularly every 3 to 4 weeks, is the prophylaxis of choice. Oral penicillin, amoxicillin, sulfadiazine, or erythromycin may also be used.

Joint pain and fever are treated with salicylates (e.g., aspirin), ibuprofen, or another nonsteroidal anti-inflammatory drug (NSAID); corticosteroids may be used for severe pain due to inflammation or carditis. ∞ See Chapter 9 for information about the use of these anti-inflammatory medications.

❧ Nursing Care

Health Promotion

Rheumatic fever is preventable. Prompt identification and treatment of streptococcal throat infections helps decrease spread of the pathogen and the risk for rheumatic fever. Characteristics of streptococcal sore throat include a red, fiery-looking throat, pain with swallowing, enlarged and tender cervical lymph nodes, fever range of 101° to 104°F (38.3° to 40.0°C), and headache. Emphasize the importance of finishing the complete course of medication to eradicate the pathogen.

Assessment

Assess patients at risk for rheumatic fever (prolonged, untreated or recurrent pharyngitis) for possible manifestations.

- *Health history:* Complaints of recent sore throat with fever, difficulty swallowing, and general malaise; treatment measures; previous history of strep throat or rheumatic fever; history of heart murmur or other cardiac problems; current medications.
- *Physical examination:* Vital signs including temperature; skin color, presence of rash on trunk or proximal extremities; mental status; evidence of inflamed joints; heart and lung sounds.

Nursing Diagnoses and Interventions

The nursing care focus for the patient with RHD is on providing supportive care and preventing complications. Teaching to prevent recurrence of rheumatic fever is extremely important. *Pain* and *Activity Intolerance* are priority nursing diagnoses for the patient with rheumatic fever and RHD.

TABLE 31–5 Diagnostic Tests for Rheumatic Heart Disease

TEST	VALUES CHARACTERISTIC OF RHEUMATIC HEART DISEASE
White blood cell count (WBC)	Greater than 10,000/mm^3
Red blood cell count (RBC)	Less than 4 million/mm^3
Erythrocyte sedimentation rate (ESR)	More than 20 mm/h
C-reactive protein	Positive
Antistreptolysin (ASO) titer	Above 250 IU/mL
Throat culture	Usually positive for group A beta-hemolytic streptococci
Cardiac enzymes	Elevated in severe carditis
ECG changes	Prolonged PR interval
Chest x-ray	May show cardiac enlargement
Echocardiogram	May show valvular damage, enlarged chambers, decreased ventricular function, or pericardial effusion

Acute Pain

Joint and chest pain due to acute inflammation is common in rheumatic fever. Pain and inflammation may interfere with rest and healing.

- Administer anti-inflammatory drugs as ordered. Promptly report manifestations of aspirin toxicity, including tinnitus, vomiting, and gastrointestinal bleeding. Give aspirin and other NSAIDs with food, milk, or antacids to minimize gastric irritation. *Joint pain and fever may be treated with anti-inflammatory agents such as aspirin and NSAIDs. When used for its anti-inflammatory effect, aspirin doses may be high, and it is given around the clock (e.g., every 4 hours). Steroids may be prescribed for severe carditis.*
- Provide warm, moist compresses for local pain relief of acutely inflamed joints. *Moist heat helps relieve pain associated with inflamed joints by reducing inflammation.*
- Auscultate heart sounds as indicated (every shift or each home visit). Notify the physician if a pericardial friction rub or a new murmur develops. *A friction rub is produced as inflamed pericardial surfaces rub against each other. This also stimulates pain receptors, and may increase discomfort.*

Activity Intolerance

The patient with acute carditis or RHD may develop heart failure if the heart is unable to supply enough oxygen to meet the body's demand. Manifestations of fatigue, weakness, and dyspnea on exertion may result.

- Explain the importance of activity limitations and reinforce teaching as needed. *Activities are limited during the acute phase of carditis to reduce the workload of the heart. Understanding the rationale improves cooperation with the limitations.*
- Encourage social and diversional activities such as visits with friends and family, reading, playing cards or board games, watching television, and listening to music or audio books. *Diversional activities provide a focus for the patient whose physical activities must be limited.*
- Encourage gradual increases in activity, monitoring for evidence of intolerance or heart failure. Consult a cardiac rehabilitation specialist to help design an activity progression schedule. *Gradual activity progression is encouraged as the patient's condition improves. Activity tolerance is monitored and activities modified as needed.*

Community-Based Care

Most patients with rheumatic fever and carditis do not require hospitalization. Teaching for home care focuses on both acute care and preventing recurrences and further tissue damage. Include the following topics:

- The importance of completing the full course of antibiotic therapy and continuing antibiotic prophylaxis as prescribed for the patient with chronic RHD include the importance of antibiotic prophylaxis for invasive procedures (e.g., dental care, endoscopy, or surgery) to prevent bacterial endocarditis. Pamphlets on endocarditis prevention are helpful reminders, and are available from the American Heart Association.
- Preventive dental care and good oral hygiene to maintain oral health and prevent gingival infections, which can lead to recurrence of the disease.

- Early recognition of streptococcal sore throat and appropriate treatment for both the patient and family members.
- Early manifestations of heart failure to report to the physician.
- Prescribed medications, including their dosage, route, intended and potential adverse effects, and manifestations to report to the physician.
- Dietary sodium restriction if ordered or recommended. A high-carbohydrate, high-protein diet may be recommended to facilitate healing and combat fatigue.

Refer for home health services or household assistance as indicated.

The Patient with Infective Endocarditis

Endocarditis, inflammation of the endocardium, can involve any portion of the endothelial lining of the heart. The valves usually are affected. Endocarditis is usually infectious in nature, characterized by colonization or invasion of the endocardium and heart valves by a pathogen.

> **FAST FACTS**
> - Subacute bacterial endocarditis develops more slowly and usually occurs in people with previous heart valve damage.
> - Acute bacterial endocarditis has an abrupt onset and typically affects people with no previous history of heart problems.

Incidence and Risk Factors

Endocarditis is relatively uncommon, with an incidence of 1.5 to 6.2 cases per 100,000 people in developed countries (Papadakis & McPhee, 2007). The greatest risk factor for endocarditis is previous heart damage. Lesions develop on deformed valves, on valve prostheses, or in areas of tissue damage due to congenital deformities or ischemic disease. The left side of the heart, the mitral valve in particular, is usually affected. Intravenous drug use also is a significant risk factor. The right side of the heart usually is affected in these patients. Other risk factors include invasive catheters (e.g., a central venous catheter, hemodynamic monitoring, or an indwelling urinary catheter), dental procedures or poor dental health, and recent heart surgery.

Prosthetic valve endocarditis (PVE) may occur in patients with a mechanical or tissue valve replacement. This infection may develop in the early postoperative period (within 2 months after surgery) or late. Prosthetic valve endocarditis accounts for 10% to 20% of endocarditis cases. It usually affects males over the age of 60, and is more frequently associated with aortic valve prostheses than with mitral valve replacements. Early PVE is usually due to prosthetic valve contamination during surgery or perioperative bacteremia. Its course often is rapid, and mortality is high. Late-onset PVE more closely resembles subacute endocarditis.

Pathophysiology

Entry of pathogens into the bloodstream is required for infective endocarditis to develop. Bacteria may enter through oral lesions, during dental work or invasive procedures, such as intravenous catheter insertion, surgery, or urinary catheterization; during intravenous drug use; or as a result of infectious processes such as urinary tract or upper respiratory infection.

The initial lesion is a sterile platelet-fibrin vegetation formed on damaged endothelium (Figure 31–7 ■). In acute infective endocarditis, these lesions develop on healthy valve structures, although the mechanism is unknown. In subacute endocarditis, they usually develop on already damaged valves or in endocardial tissue that has been damaged by abnormal pressures or blood flow within the heart.

Organisms that have invaded the blood colonize these vegetations. The vegetation enlarges as more platelets and fibrin are attracted to the site and cover the infecting organism. This covering "protects" the bacteria from quick removal by immune defenses such as phagocytosis by neutrophils, antibodies, and complement. Vegetations may be singular or multiple. They expand while loosely attached to edges of the valve. Friable vegetations can break or shear off, embolizing and traveling through the bloodstream to other organ systems. When they lodge in small vessels, they may cause hemorrhages, infarcts, or abscesses. Ultimately, the vegetations scar and deform the valves and cause turbulence of blood flowing through the heart. Heart valve function is affected, either obstructing forward blood flow, or closing incompletely.

Endocarditis is classified by its acuity and disease course (Table 31–6). *Acute infective endocarditis* has an abrupt onset and is a rapidly progressive, severe disease. Although almost any organism can cause infective endocarditis, virulent organisms such as *Staphylococcus aureus* cause a more abrupt onset and destructive course. *S. aureus* is commonly the infective organism in acute endocarditis. In contrast, *subacute infective endocarditis* has a more gradual onset, with predominant systemic manifestations. It is more likely to occur in patients with preexisting heart disease. *Streptococcus viridans*, enterococci, other gram-negative and gram-positive bacilli, yeasts, and fungi tend to cause the subacute forms of endocarditis (Huether & McCance, 2008).

Manifestations

The manifestations of infective endocarditis often are nonspecific (see the accompanying box). A temperature above 101.5°F (39.4°C) and flulike symptoms develop, accompanied by cough, shortness of breath, and joint pain. The presentation of acute staphylococcal endocarditis is more severe, with a sudden onset, chills, and a high fever. Heart murmurs are heard in 90%

Figure 31–7 ■ A vegetative lesion of bacterial endocarditis.
Source: M. English/Custom Medical Stock Photo, Inc.

of persons with infective endocarditis. An existing murmur may worsen, or a new murmur may develop.

Splenomegaly is common in chronic disease. Peripheral manifestations of infective endocarditis result from microemboli or circulating immune complexes. These manifestations include the following:

- *Petechiae*—small, purplish-red hemorrhagic spots on the trunk, conjunctiva, and mucous membranes
- *Splinter hemorrhage*—hemorrhagic streaks under the fingernails or toenails
- *Osler's nodes*—small, reddened, painful raised growths on finger and toe pads
- *Janeway lesions*—small, nontender, purplish-red macular lesions on the palms of the hands and soles of the feet
- *Roth's spots*—small, whitish spots (cotton-wool spots) seen on the retina

Complications

Embolization of vegetative fragments may affect any organ system, particularly the lungs, brain, kidneys, and the skin and mucous membranes, with resulting organ infarction. Other common complications of infective endocarditis include heart failure, abscess, and aneurysms due to infiltration of the arterial wall by organisms. Without treatment, endocarditis is almost universally fatal; fortunately, antibiotic therapy is usually effective to treat this disease.

TABLE 31–6 Classifications of Infective Endocarditis

	ACUTE INFECTIVE ENDOCARDITIS	SUBACUTE INFECTIVE ENDOCARDITIS
Onset	Sudden	Gradual
Usual organism	*Staphylococcus aureus*	*Streptococcus viridans*, enterococci, gram-negative and gram-positive bacilli, fungi, yeasts
Risk factors	Usually occurs in previously normal heart; intravenous drug use, infected intravenous sites	Usually occurs in damaged or deformed hearts; dental work, invasive procedures, and infections
Pathologic process	Rapid valve destruction	Valve destruction leading to regurgitation; embolization of friable vegetations
Presentation	Abrupt onset with spiking fever and chills; manifestations of heart failure	Gradual onset of febrile illness with cough, dyspnea, arthralgias, abdominal pain

MANIFESTATIONS of Infective Endocarditis

- Chills and fever
- General malaise, fatigue
- Arthralgias
- Cough, dyspnea
- Heart murmur
- Anorexia, abdominal pain
- Petechiae, splinter hemorrhages
- Splenomegaly

Interdisciplinary Care

Eradicating the infecting organism and minimizing valve damage and other adverse consequences of infective endocarditis are the priorities of care.

Diagnosis

There are no definitive tests for infective endocarditis, but diagnostic tests help establish the diagnosis.

- *Blood cultures* usually are positive for bacteria or other pathogens. Blood cultures are considered positive when a typical infecting organism is identified from two or more separate blood cultures (drawn from different sites and/or at different times, e.g., 12-hour intervals).
- *Echocardiography* (either transthoracic or transesophageal) to visualize vegetations can be diagnostic for infective endocarditis when combined with positive blood cultures. ∞ See Chapter 29 for more information about echocardiography.
- *Serologic immune testing* for circulating antigens to assess for typical infective organisms may be done.

Other diagnostic tests may include the CBC, ESR, serum creatinine, chest x-ray, and an electrocardiogram.

Medications

Preventing endocarditis in patients at high risk is important. Antibiotics are commonly prescribed for patients with preexisting valve damage or heart disease prior to high risk procedures. In 2007, the AHA significantly altered the recommendations for endocarditis prophylaxis, reducing the groups of patients who require antibiotics prior to procedures (Wilson et al., 2007). (See Table 31–7.)

Antibiotic therapy effectively treats infective endocarditis in most cases. The goal of therapy is to eradicate the infecting organism from the blood and vegetative lesions in the heart. The fibrin covering that protects colonies of organisms from immune defenses also protects them from antibiotic therapy. Therefore, an extended course of multiple intravenous antibiotics is required.

Following blood cultures, antibiotic therapy is initiated with drugs known to be effective against the most common infecting organisms: staphylococci, streptococci, and enterococci. The initial regimen may include nafcillin or oxacillin, penicillin or ampicillin, and gentamicin. Once the organism has been identified, therapy is tailored to that organism. Staphylococcal and enterococcal infections are treated with a combination of penicillin and gentamicin. If the patient is allergic to penicillin, ceftriaxone, cefazolin, or vancomycin may be used. Staphyloccoal infections are treated with nafcillin or oxacillin and gentamicin; cefazolin or vancomycin may be used if penicillin allergy is present. Intravenous drug therapy is continued for 2 to 8 weeks, depending on the infecting organism, the drugs used, and the results of repeat blood cultures. ∞ See Chapter 12 for the nursing implications for antibiotic therapy.

The patient with prosthetic valve endocarditis requires extended treatment, usually 6 to 8 weeks. Combination therapy using vancomycin, rifampin, and gentamicin is used to treat these resistant infections.

Surgery

Some patients with infective endocarditis require the following from surgery:

- Replace severely damaged valves.
- Remove large vegetations at risk for embolization.
- Remove a valve that is a continuing source of infection that does not respond to antibiotic therapy.

The most common indication for surgery is valvular regurgitation that causes heart failure and does not respond to medical therapy. When the infection has not responded to antibiotic therapy within 7 to 10 days, the infected valve may be replaced to facilitate eradication of the organism. Patients with fungal endocarditis usually require surgical intervention. More information on valve replacement surgery is provided in the section on valve disorders.

TABLE 31–7 Updated Recommendations for Antibiotic Prophylaxis for Infective Endocarditis

INDICATIONS FOR PROPHYLAXIS	SELECTED PROCEDURES FOR WHICH PROPHYLAXIS IS RECOMMENDED	SUGGESTED ANTIBIOTICS
Prosthetic valves	Dental procedures in which bleeding is likely, including cleaning	Amoxicillin
Previous episode(s) of infective endocarditis		Erythromycin
Congenital heart disease	Most surgeries	Ampicillin
Unrepaired, cyanotic	Bronchoscopy (only with incision of the respiratory tract mucosa)	Clindamycin
Completely repaired up to 6 months post-repair		Vancomycin (recommended for MRSA)
Repaired with residual defects	Cystoscopy	(*Note:* Choice of antibiotic depends on procedure)
Cardiac transplant	Urinary catheterization when infection is present	
	Incision and drainage of infected tissue	
	Vaginal delivery if infection is present	

Nursing Care

Health Promotion

Prevention of endocarditis is vital in susceptible people. Education is a key part of prevention. Use every opportunity to educate individuals and the public about the risks of intravenous drug use, including endocarditis. Discuss preventive measures with all patients with specific risk factors, such as a history of valve replacement, congenital heart defects, or cardiac transplantation (Wilson et al., 2007).

Assessment

Assessment related to ineffective endocarditis includes identifying risk factors and manifestations of the disease.

- *Health history:* Complaints of persistent flulike symptoms, fatigue, shortness of breath, and activity intolerance; history of recent dental work or other invasive procedures; known heart murmur, valve or other heart disorder; recent intravenous drug use.
- *Physical examination:* Vital signs including temperature; apical pulse and heart sounds; rate and ease of respirations, lung sounds; skin color, temperature, and presence of petechiae or splinter hemorrhages.

Nursing Diagnoses and Interventions

Nursing care focuses on managing the manifestations of endocarditis, administering antibiotics, and teaching the patient and family members about the disorder. In addition to the diagnoses identified next, nursing diagnoses and interventions for heart failure also may be appropriate for patients with infective endocarditis.

Risk for Imbalanced Body Temperature

Fever is common in patients with infective endocarditis. It may be acutely elevated and accompanied by chills, particularly with acute infective endocarditis. The inflammatory process initiates a cycle of events that affects the regulation of temperature and causes discomfort.

- Record temperature every 2 to 4 hours. Report temperature above 101.5°F (39.4°C). Assess for complaints of discomfort. *Fever is usually low grade (below 101.5°F [39.4°C]) in infective endocarditis; higher temperatures may cause discomfort. The temperature usually returns to normal within 1 week after initiation of antibiotic therapy. Continued fever may indicate a need to modify the treatment regimen.*
- Obtain blood cultures as ordered, before initial antibiotic dose. *Initial blood cultures are obtained before antibiotic therapy is started to obtain adequate organisms to culture and identify. Follow-up cultures are used to assess the effectiveness of therapy.*
- Provide anti-inflammatory or antipyretic agents as prescribed. *Fever may be treated with anti-inflammatory or antipyretic agents such as aspirin, ibuprofen, or acetaminophen.*
- Administer antibiotics as ordered; obtain peak and trough drug levels as indicated. *Intravenous antibiotics are given to eradicate the pathogen. Peak and trough levels are used to evaluate the dose effectiveness in maintaining a therapeutic blood level.*

Risk for Ineffective Tissue Perfusion

Embolization of vegetative lesions can threaten tissue and organ perfusion. Vegetations from the left heart may lodge in arterioles or capillaries of the brain, kidneys, or peripheral tissues, causing infarction or abscess. A large embolism can cause manifestations of stroke or transient ischemic attack, renal failure, or tissue ischemia. Emboli from the right side of the heart become entrapped in pulmonary vasculature, causing manifestations of pulmonary embolism.

- Assess for, document, and report manifestations of decreased organ system perfusion:
  a. Neurologic: changes in level of consciousness, numbness or tingling in extremities, hemiplegia, visual disturbances, or manifestations of stroke
  b. Renal: decreased urine output, hematuria, elevated BUN or creatinine
  c. Pulmonary: dyspnea, hemoptysis, shortness of breath, diminished breath sounds, restlessness, sudden chest or shoulder pain
  d. Cardiovascular: chest pain radiating to jaw or arms, tachycardia, anxiety, tachypnea, hypotension
  All major organs and tissues, and the microcirculation may be affected by emboli when vegetations break off due to turbulent blood flow. Emboli may cause manifestations of organ dysfunction. The most devastating effects of emboli are in the brain and the myocardium, with resulting infarctions. Intravenous drug users have a high risk of pulmonary emboli as a result of right-sided endocardial fragments.
- Assess and document skin color and temperature, quality of peripheral pulses, and capillary refill. *Peripheral emboli affect tissue perfusion, with a risk for tissue necrosis and possible extremity loss.*

Ineffective Health Maintenance

The patient with endocarditis often is treated in the community. Teaching about disease management and prevention of possible recurrences of endocarditis is vital.

- Demonstrate intravenous catheter site care and intermittent antibiotic administration if the patient and family will manage therapy. Have the patient and/or significant other redemonstrate appropriate techniques. *Intermittent antibiotic infusions may be managed by the patient or family members, or the patient may go to an outpatient facility to receive the infusions. Appropriate site care is necessary to reduce the risk of trauma and infection.*
- Explain the actions, doses, administration, and desired and adverse effects of prescribed drugs. Identify manifestations to be reported to the physician. Provide practical information about measures to reduce the risk of superinfection (e.g., consuming 8 oz of yogurt or buttermilk containing live bacterial cultures daily). *Careful compliance with prescribed drug therapy is vital to eradicate the infecting organism. Antibiotic therapy can, however, cause superinfections such as candidiasis due to elimination of normal body flora.*
- Teach about the function of heart valves and the effects of endocarditis on heart function. Include a simple definition of endocarditis, and explain the risk for its recurrence.

Information helps the patient and family understand endocarditis, its treatment, and its effects. Understanding increases compliance.

- Describe the manifestations of heart failure to be reported to the physician. *Evidence of heart failure may necessitate modification of the treatment regimen or replacement of infected valves.*

> ### PRACTICE ALERT
> Stress the importance of notifying all care providers of valve disease, heart murmur, or valve replacement before undergoing invasive procedures. Invasive procedures provide a portal of entry for bacteria. A history of valve disease increases the risk for the development or recurrence of endocarditis.

- Encourage good dental hygiene and mouth care and regular dental checkups. Teach how to prevent bleeding from the gums and avoid developing mouth ulcers (e.g., gentle tooth brushing, ensuring that dentures fit properly, and avoiding toothpicks, dental floss, and high-flow water devices). *The oropharynx harbors streptococci, which are common causes of endocarditis. Bleeding gums offer an opportunity for bacteria to enter the bloodstream.*
- Encourage the patient to avoid people with upper respiratory infections. *Streptococci are normal pathogens in the upper respiratory tract; exposure to people with upper respiratory infections may increase the risk of infection.*
- If anticoagulant therapy is ordered, explain its actions, administration, and major side effects. Identify manifestations of bleeding to be promptly reported to the physician. *Patients with valve disease or a prosthetic valve following infective endocarditis may require continued anticoagulant therapy to prevent thrombi and emboli. Knowledge is vital for appropriate management of anticoagulant therapy and prevention of complications.*

Community-Based Care

When preparing the patient with infective endocarditis for home care, provide teaching as outlined for the nursing diagnosis, *Ineffective Health Maintenance.* In addition, discuss the following topics:

- Although serious and frightening, infective endocarditis can usually be treated effectively with intravenous antibiotics.
- The importance of promptly reporting any unusual manifestation, such as a change in vision, sudden pain, or weakness, so that interventions to control complications can be promptly implemented.
- The rationale for all treatments and procedures.
- Preventing recurrences of infective endocarditis.
- The importance of maintaining contact with the physician for follow-up care and monitoring for long-term effects such as progressive valve damage and dysfunction.
- If appropriate, explain the risks associated with intravenous drug use.

Provide educational materials on infective endocarditis from the American Heart Association. Refer as appropriate to home health or home intravenous therapy services. Refer the patient and family members or significant others as appropriate to a drug or substance abuse treatment program or facility. Provide follow-up care to ensure compliance with the referral and treatment plan.

The Patient with Myocarditis

Myocarditis is inflammation of the heart muscle. It usually results from an infectious process, but also may occur as an immunologic response, or due to the effects of radiation, toxins, or drugs. In the United States, myocarditis is usually viral, caused by coxsackievirus B. Approximately 10% of people with HIV disease develop myocarditis due to infiltration of the myocardium by the virus. Bacterial myocarditis, much less common, may be associated with endocarditis caused by *Staphylococcus aureus*, or with diphtheria. Parasitic infections caused by *Trypanosoma cruzi* (Chagas' disease) are common in Central and South America (Kasper et al., 2005).

Incidence and Risk Factors

Myocarditis may occur at any age, and it is more common in men than women. Factors that alter immune response (e.g., malnutrition, alcohol use, immunosuppressive drugs, exposure to radiation, stress, and advanced age) increase the risk for myocarditis. It also is a common complication of rheumatic fever and pericarditis.

Pathophysiology

In myocarditis, myocardial cells are damaged by an inflammatory process that causes local or diffuse swelling and damage. Infectious agents infiltrate interstitial tissues, forming abscesses. Autoimmune injury may occur when the immune system destroys not only the invading pathogen but also myocardial cells. The extent of damage to cardiac muscle ultimately determines the long-term outcome of the disease. Viral myocarditis usually is self-limited; it may progress, however, to become chronic, leading to dilated cardiomyopathy (see the section of this chapter that follows). Severe myocarditis may lead to heart failure.

Manifestations

The manifestations of myocarditis depend on the degree of myocardial damage. The patient may be asymptomatic. Nonspecific manifestations of inflammation such as fever, fatigue, general malaise, dyspnea, palpitations, arthralgias, and sore throat may be present. A nonspecific febrile illness or upper respiratory infection often precedes the onset of myocarditis symptoms. Abnormal heart sounds such as muffled S_1, an S_3, murmur, and pericardial friction rub may be heard. In some cases, manifestations of myocardial infarction, including chest pain, may occur.

Interdisciplinary Care

Myocarditis treatment focuses on resolving the inflammatory process to prevent further damage to the myocardium.

Diagnostic studies may be ordered to help diagnose myocarditis.

- *Electrocardiography* may show transient ST segment and T wave changes, as well as dysrhythmias and possible heart block.
- *Cardiac markers*, such as the creatinine kinase, troponin T, and troponin I, may be elevated, indicating myocardial cell damage.
- *Endomyocardial biopsy* to examine myocardial cells is necessary to establish a definitive diagnosis; patchy cell necrosis and the inflammatory process can be identified.

If appropriate, antimicrobial therapy is used to eradicate the infecting organism. Antiviral therapy with interferon-α may be instituted. Immunosuppressive therapy with corticosteroids or other immunosuppressive agents (∞ see Chapter 13) may be used to minimize the inflammatory response. Heart failure is treated as needed, using ACE inhibitors and drugs. Patients with myocarditis often are particularly sensitive to the effects of digitalis, so it is used with caution. Other medications used in treating myocarditis include antidysrhythmic agents as to control dysrhythmias and anticoagulants to prevent emboli.

Bed rest and activity restrictions are ordered during the acute inflammatory process to reduce myocardial work and prevent myocardial damage. Activities may be limited for as long as 6 months to a year (Huether & McCance, 2008).

🙷 Nursing Care

Nursing care is directed at decreasing myocardial work and maintaining cardiac output. Both physical and emotional rest are indicated, because anxiety increases myocardial oxygen demand. Hemodynamic parameters and the ECG are monitored closely, especially during the acute phase of the illness. Activity tolerance, urine output, and heart and breath sounds are frequently assessed for manifestations of heart failure. Consider the following nursing diagnoses for the patient with myocarditis.

- *Activity Intolerance* related to impaired cardiac muscle function
- *Decreased Cardiac Output* related to myocardial inflammation
- *Fatigue* related to inflammation and impaired cardiac output
- *Anxiety* related to possible long-term effects of the disorder
- *Excess Fluid Volume* related to compensatory mechanisms for decreased cardiac output

Community-Based Care

Include the following topics when preparing the patient with myocarditis for home care.

- Activity restrictions and other prescribed measures to reduce cardiac workload
- Early manifestations of heart failure to report to the physician
- The importance of following the prescribed treatment regimen
- Any recommended dietary modifications (such as a low-sodium diet for heart failure)
- Prescribed medications, their purpose, doses, and possible adverse effects

- The importance of adhering to the treatment plan and recommended follow-up appointments to reduce the risk of long-term consequences such as cardiomyopathy

The Patient with Pericarditis

The pericardium is the outermost layer of the heart. It is a two-layered membranous sac with a thin layer of serous fluid (normally no more than 30 to 50 mL) separating the layers. It protects and cushions the heart and the great vessels, provides a barrier to infectious processes in adjacent structures, prevents displacement of the myocardium and blood vessels, and prevents sudden distention of the heart.

Pericarditis is the inflammation of the pericardium. Pericarditis may be a primary disorder or develop secondarily to another cardiac or systemic disorder. Some possible causes of pericarditis are listed in Box 31–4. Acute pericarditis is usually viral and affects men (usually under the age of 50) more frequently than women (Papadakis & McPhee, 2007). Pericarditis affects 40% to 50% of patients with end-stage renal disease and uremia. Postmyocardial infarction pericarditis and postcardiotomy (following open-heart surgery) pericarditis also are common.

Pathophysiology

Pericardial tissue damage triggers an inflammatory response. Inflammatory mediators released from the injured tissue cause vasodilation, hyperemia, and edema. Capillary permeability increases, allowing plasma proteins, including fibrinogen, to escape into the pericardial space. White blood cells amass at the site of injury to destroy the causative agent. Exudate is formed, usually fibrinous or serofibrinous (a mixture of serous fluid and fibrinous exudate). In some cases, the exudate may contain red blood cells or, if infectious, purulent material. The inflammatory process may resolve without long-term effects, or scar tissue and adhesions may form between the pericardial layers.

Fibrosis and scarring of the pericardium may restrict cardiac function. Pericardial effusions may develop as serous or purulent exudate (depending on the causative agent) collects in the pericardial sac. Pericardial effusion may be recurrent. Chronic inflammation causes the pericardium to become rigid.

BOX 31–4 Selected Causes of Pericarditis

Infectious
- Viruses
- Bacteria
- Tuberculosis
- Syphilis
- Parasites

Noninfectious
- Myocardial and pericardial injury
- Rheumatic fever
- Uremia
- Neoplasms
- Radiation
- Trauma or surgery
- Myxedema
- Autoimmune disorders
- Connective tissue diseases
- Prescription and nonprescription drugs
- Postcardiac injury

Manifestations

Classic manifestations of acute pericarditis include chest pain, a pericardial friction rub, and fever. Chest pain, the most common symptom, has an abrupt onset. It is caused by inflammation of nerve fibers in the lower parietal pericardium and pleura covering the diaphragm. The pain is usually sharp, may be steady or intermittent, and may radiate to the back or neck. The pain can mimic myocardial ischemia; careful assessment is important to rule out myocardial infarction. Pericardial pain is aggravated by respiratory movements (i.e., deep inspiration and/or coughing), changes in body position, or swallowing. Sitting upright and leaning forward reduces the discomfort by moving the heart away from the diaphragmatic side of the lung pleura.

Although not always present, a *pericardial friction rub* is the characteristic sign of pericarditis. A pericardial friction rub is a leathery, grating sound produced by the inflamed pericardial layers rubbing against the chest wall or pleura. It is heard most clearly at the left lower sternal border with the patient sitting up or leaning forward. The rub is usually heard on expiration and may be constant or intermittent.

A low-grade fever (below 100°F [38.4°C]) often develops due to the inflammatory process. Dyspnea and tachycardia are common.

Complications

Pericardial effusion, cardiac tamponade, and constrictive pericarditis are possible complications of acute pericarditis.

Pericardial Effusion

A *pericardial effusion* is an abnormal collection of fluid between the pericardial layers that threatens normal cardiac function. The fluid may consist of pus, blood, serum, lymph, or a combination. The manifestations of a pericardial effusion depend on the rate at which the fluid collects. Although the pericardium normally contains about 30 to 50 mL of fluid, the sac can stretch to accommodate a gradual accumulation of fluid. Over time, the pericardial sac can accommodate up to 2 L of fluid without immediate adverse effects. Conversely, a rapid buildup of pericardial fluid (as little as 100 mL) does not allow the sac to stretch and can compress the heart, interfering with myocardial function. This compression of the heart is known as **cardiac tamponade**. Slowly developing pericardial effusion is often painless and has few manifestations. Heart sounds may be distant or muffled. The patient may have a cough or mild dyspnea.

Cardiac Tamponade

Cardiac tamponade is a medical emergency that must be aggressively treated to preserve life. Cardiac tamponade may result from pericardial effusion, trauma, cardiac rupture, or hemorrhage. Rapid collection of fluid in the pericardial sac interferes with ventricular filling and pumping, critically reducing cardiac output.

Classic manifestations of cardiac tamponade result from rising intracardiac pressures, decreased diastolic filling, and decreased cardiac output. A hallmark of cardiac tamponade is a paradoxical pulse, or *pulsus paradoxus*. A paradoxical pulse markedly decreases in amplitude during inspiration. Intrathoracic pressure normally drops during inspiration, enhancing venous

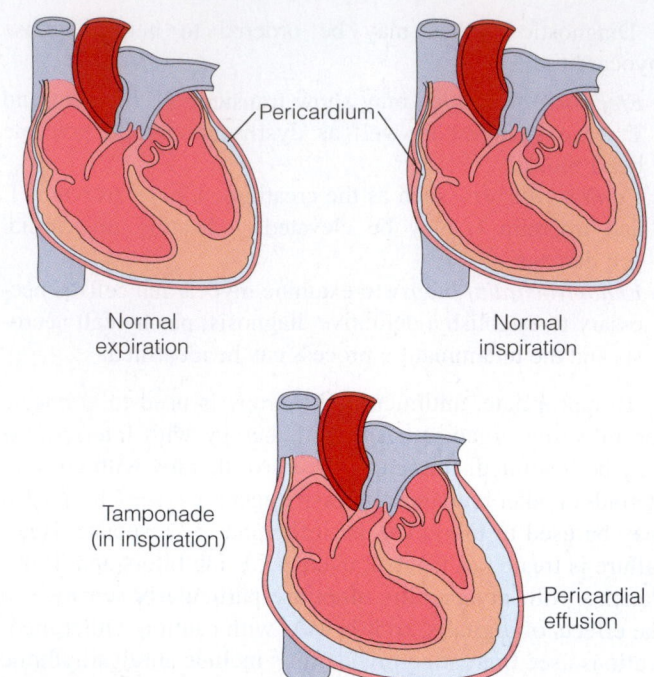

Figure 31–8 ■ Cardiac tamponade. Note increased volume in the right ventricle during inspiration in both the normal heart and the heart affected by a pericardial effusion. In tamponade, fluid in the pericardial sac and the distended right ventricle restrict filling of the left ventricle and consequently, cardiac output.

return to the right heart. This draws more blood into the right side of the heart than the left, causing the interventricular septum to bulge slightly into the left ventricle. When ventricular filling is impaired by excess fluid in the pericardial sac, this bulging of the interventricular septum decreases cardiac output during inspiration (Figure 31–8 ■). On palpation of the carotid or femoral artery, the pulse is diminished or absent during inspiration. A drop in systolic blood pressure of more than 10 mmHg during inspiration also indicates pulsus paradoxus.

Other manifestations of cardiac tamponade include muffled heart sounds, dyspnea and tachypnea, tachycardia, a narrowed pulse pressure, and distended neck veins (see the accompanying box).

Chronic Constrictive Pericarditis

Chronic pericardial inflammation can lead to scar tissue formation between the pericardial layers. This scar tissue eventually contracts, restricting diastolic filling and elevating venous

---

MANIFESTATIONS of Cardiac Tamponade

- Paradoxical pulse
- Narrowed pulse pressure, hypotension
- Tachycardia
- Weak peripheral pulses
- Distant, muffled heart sounds
- Jugular venous distention
- High central venous pressure
- Decreased level of consciousness
- Low urine output
- Cool, mottled skin

pressure. Constrictive pericarditis may follow viral infection, radiation therapy, or heart surgery. Its manifestations include progressive dyspnea, fatigue, and weakness. Ascites is common; peripheral edema may develop. Neck veins are distended, and may be particularly noticeable during inspiration (*Kussmaul's sign*). This occurs because the right atrium is unable to dilate to accommodate increased venous return during inspiration. See Figure 31–9 ■.

Interdisciplinary Care

Care for the patient with pericarditis focuses on identifying its cause if possible, reducing inflammation, relieving symptoms, and preventing complications. The patient is closely monitored for early manifestations of cardiac tamponade so that it can be treated promptly.

Diagnosis

There are no specific laboratory tests to diagnose pericarditis, but tests are often performed to differentiate pericarditis from myocardial infarction.

- *CBC* shows elevated WBCs and an ESR greater than 20 mm/h indicating acute inflammation.
- *Cardiac enzymes* may be slightly elevated because the inflammatory process extends to involve the epicardial surface of the heart. Cardiac enzymes are typically much lower in pericarditis than in myocardial infarction.
- *Electrocardiography* shows typical changes associated with pericarditis, such as diffuse ST segment elevation in all leads. This resolves more quickly than changes of acute MI and is not associated with the QRS complex and T wave changes typically seen in MI. With a large pericardial effusion, the QRS amplitude may be decreased. Atrial dysrhythmias may occur in acute pericarditis.

Figure 31–9 ■ Constrictive pericarditis.

- *Echocardiography* is used to assess heart motion, for pericardial effusion, and the extent of restriction.
- *Hemodynamic monitoring* may be used in acute pericarditis or pericardial effusion to assess pressures and cardiac output. Elevated pulmonary artery pressures and venous pressures occur with impaired filling due to pericardial effusion or constrictive pericarditis.
- *Chest x-ray* may show cardiac enlargement if a pericardial effusion is present.
- *Computed tomography (CT scan)* or *magnetic resonance imaging (MRI)* may be used to identify pericardial effusion or constrictive pericarditis.

Medications

Drug treatment for pericarditis addresses its manifestations. Aspirin and acetaminophen may be used to reduce fever. Nonsteroidal anti-inflammatory drugs (NSAIDs) are used to reduce inflammation and promote comfort. In severe cases or with recurrent pericarditis, corticosteroids may be given to suppress the inflammatory response.

Pericardiocentesis

Pericardiocentesis may be done to remove fluid from the pericardial sac for diagnostic or therapeutic purposes (see Figure 29–19). The physician inserts a large (16 to 18 gauge) needle into the pericardial sac and withdraws excess fluid. The needle is attached to an ECG monitoring lead to help determine if the needle is touching the epicardial surface, which helps prevent piercing the myocardium. Pericardiocentesis may be an emergency procedure for the patient with cardiac tamponade. Nursing implications for pericardiocentesis are outlined in the box on page 888 of ∞ Chapter 29.

Surgery

For recurrent pericarditis or recurrent pericardial effusion, a rectangular piece of the pericardium, or "window," may be excised to allow collected fluid to drain into the pleural space. Constrictive pericarditis may necessitate a partial or total *pericardiectomy,* removal of part or all of the pericardium, to relieve the ventricular compression and allow adequate filling.

∽ Nursing Care

Health Promotion

While it may not yet be possible to identify many patients at risk for acute pericarditis or to prevent it, early identification and treatment of the disorder can reduce the risk of complications. Promptly report a pericardial friction rub or other manifestations of pericarditis in patients with recent AMI, cardiac surgery, or systemic diseases associated with a risk for pericarditis.

Assessment

Assessment data to collect from the patient with suspected pericarditis includes the following:

- *Health history:* Complaints of acute substernal or precordial chest pain, effect of movement and breathing on discomfort, pain radiation, associated symptoms; recent AMI, heart surgery, or other cardiac disorder; current medications; chronic conditions such as renal failure or a connective tissue or autoimmune disorder.

■ *Physical examination:* Vital signs including temperature, variation in systolic BP with respirations; strength of peripheral pulses, variations with respiratory movement; apical pulse, clarity, changes with respiratory movement, presence of a friction rub; neck vein distension; level of consciousness, skin color, and other indicators of cardiac output.

Nursing Diagnoses and Interventions

Nursing care for the patient with pericarditis may occur in the acute or community setting. Closely observe for early manifestations of increasing effusion or cardiac tamponade. Priority nursing diagnoses relate to comfort, the risk for tamponade, and effects of the acute inflammatory process.

Acute Pain

Inflamed pericardial layers rubbing against each other and the lung pleura stimulate phrenic nerve pain fibers in the lower portion of the parietal pericardium. Pain is usually acute and may be severe until inflammation resolves.

■ Assess chest pain using a standard pain scale and noting the quality and radiation of the pain. Note nonverbal cues of pain (grimacing, guarding behaviors), and validate with the patient. *Careful assessment helps identify the cause of pain. The pain of pericarditis may radiate to the neck or back and is aggravated by movement, coughing, or deep breathing. A pain scale allows evaluation of the effectiveness of interventions.*

■ Auscultate heart sounds every 4 hours. *Presence of a pericardial friction rub often correlates with the location and severity of the pain.*

■ Administer NSAIDs on a regular basis as prescribed with food. Document effectiveness. *NSAIDs reduce fever, inflammation, and pericardial pain. They are most effective when administered around the clock on a consistent basis. Administering the medications with food helps decrease gastric distress.*

■ Maintain a quiet, calm environment, and position of comfort. Offer back rubs, heat/cold therapy, diversional activity, and emotional support. *Supportive interventions enhance the effects of the medication, may decrease pain perception, and convey a sense of caring.*

Ineffective Breathing Pattern

Respiratory movement intensifies pericardial pain. In an effort to decrease pain, the patient often breathes shallowly, increasing the risk for pulmonary complications.

> **PRACTICE ALERT**
> Document respiratory rate, effort, and breath sounds every 2 to 4 hours. Report adventitious or diminished breath sounds. Shallow, guarded respirations may lead to increased respiratory rate and effort. Poor ventilation of peripheral alveoli may lead to congestion or atelectasis.

■ Encourage deep breathing and use of the incentive spirometer. Provide pain medication before respiratory therapy, as needed. *Deep breathing and an incentive spirometer promote alveolar ventilation and prevent atelectasis. Analgesia prior*

to respiratory treatments improves their effectiveness by decreasing guarding.

■ Administer oxygen as needed. *Supplementary oxygen promotes optimal gas exchange and tissue oxygenation.*

■ Place in Fowler's or high Fowler's position. Assist to a position of comfort. *Appropriate positioning reduces the work of breathing and decreases chest pain due to pericarditis.*

Risk for Decreased Cardiac Output

The acute inflammatory process of pericarditis can lead to significant pericardial effusion and cardiac tamponade. This potentially fatal complication can also occur with chronic pericardial effusion if the amount of fluid exceeds the ability of the pericardial sac to expand. Constrictive pericarditis increases the risk for decreased cardiac output because of restricted cardiac filling.

■ Document vital signs hourly during the acute inflammatory processes. *Frequent assessment allows early recognition of manifestations of decreased cardiac output, such as tachycardia, hypotension, or changes in pulse pressure.*

> **PRACTICE ALERT**
> Assess heart sounds and peripheral pulses, and observe for neck vein distention and paradoxical pulse hourly. Promptly report distant, muffled heart sounds, new murmurs or extra heart sounds, decreasing quality of peripheral pulses, and distended neck veins. Acute pericardial effusion interferes with normal cardiac filling and pumping, causing venous congestion and decreased cardiac output. As the amount of fluid increases in the pericardial sac, heart sounds are obscured. A drop in systolic blood pressure of more than 10 mmHg on inspiration signifies an abnormal response to changes in intrathoracic pressure.

■ Report significant changes or trends in hemodynamic parameters and dysrhythmias. *Compression of the heart interferes with venous return, increasing CVP and right atrial pressures; dysrhythmias may also occur.*

■ Promptly report other signs of decreased cardiac output: decreased level of consciousness; decreased urine output; cold, clammy, mottled skin; delayed capillary refill; and weak peripheral pulses. *These signs of decreased organ and tissue perfusion indicate a significant drop in cardiac output.*

■ Maintain at least one patent intravenous access site. *The patient in cardiac tamponade may require rapid intravenous fluid infusion to restore blood volume and administration of emergency drugs to support the circulation.*

■ Prepare for emergency pericardiocentesis and/or surgery as necessary. Provide appropriate explanations and reassurance. Observe for adverse responses during pericardiocentesis. *Excess pericardial fluid must be rapidly evacuated to prevent further compromise of cardiac output and death. Emotional support and explanations reduce the patient's and family's anxiety and promote a caring atmosphere.*

Activity Intolerance

In chronic constrictive pericarditis, pericardial adhesions and scarring restrict pericardial compliance, restricting heart filling and movement. Restricted filling and ineffective cardiac contraction decrease the cardiac output. The heart cannot compensate for increased metabolic demands by increasing cardiac output, and cardiac reserve falls significantly.

■ Document vital signs, cardiac rhythm, skin color, and temperature before and after activity. Note any subjective complaints of fatigue, shortness of breath, chest pain, palpitations, or other symptoms with activity. *These parameters help determine the response to increased cardiac work. Increased heart rate and respiratory rate and effort, decreased blood pressure, and dysrhythmias are indicators of activity intolerance. Pallor or cyanosis and cool, clammy, mottled skin are signs of decreased tissue perfusion. Complaints of weakness, shortness of breath, fatigue, dizziness, or palpitations are further evidence of activity intolerance.*

■ Work with the patient and physical therapist to develop a realistic, progressive activity plan. Monitor response. Encourage independence, but provide assistance as needed. *Patient involvement in planning increases the likelihood of success, as well as the patient's self-esteem and sense of control. Promoting self-care provides additional control and independence and enhances self-image. Activity that significantly increases the heart rate (more than 20 BPM over resting) should be stopped and reassessed for intensity.*

■ Plan interventions and care activities to allow uninterrupted rest and sleep. *This supports healing and restoration of physical and emotional health.*

Community-Based Care

Include the following topics when teaching the patient and family in preparation for home care.

■ The importance of continuing anti-inflammatory medications as ordered. Advise to take NSAIDs with food, milk, or antacids to minimize gastric distress, and to notify the physician if unable to tolerate the drug. Instruct to avoid aspirin or preparations containing aspirin while taking NSAIDs because it may interfere with activity.

■ Prescribed medications, including dose, desired and possible adverse effects, and interactions with other drugs or food.

■ Monitoring weight twice weekly because NSAIDs may cause fluid retention.

■ Maintaining fluid intake of at least 2500 mL per day to minimize the risk of renal toxicity due to NSAID use.

■ Measures to maintain activity restriction if ordered. Activity will be gradually increased once the inflammatory process has resolved.

■ Manifestations of recurrent pericarditis, and the importance of reporting these manifestations promptly to the physician.

Disorders of Cardiac Structure

The Patient with Valvular Heart Disease

Proper heart valve function ensures one-way blood flow through the heart and vascular system. **Valvular heart disease** interferes with blood flow to and from the heart. Acquired valvular disorders can result from acute conditions, such as infective endocarditis, or from chronic conditions, such as rheumatic heart disease. Rheumatic heart disease is the most common cause of valvular disease (Huether & McCance, 2008; Bonow et al., 2006). Acute myocardial infarction also can damage heart valves, causing tearing, ischemia, or damage to the papillary muscles that affects valve leaflet function. Congenital heart defects may affect the heart valves, often with no manifestations until adulthood. Aging affects heart structure and function, and also increases the risk for valvular disease.

Physiology Review

The heart valves direct blood flow within and out of the heart. The valves are fibroelastic tissue supported by a ring of fibrous tissue (the annulus) that provides support.

The atrioventricular (AV) valves, the **mitral** (or *bicuspid*) **valve** on the left and the **tricuspid valve** on the right, separate the atria from the ventricles. These valves normally are fully open during diastole, allowing blood to flow freely from the atria into the ventricles. Rising pressure within the ventricles at the onset of systole (contraction) closes the AV valves, creating the S_1 heart sound ("lub"). The leaflets of the AV valves are connected to ventricular papillary muscles by fibrous *chordae*

tendineae. The chordae tendineae prevent the valve leaflets from bulging back into the atria during systole.

The semilunar valves, the **aortic** and **pulmonic valves**, separate the ventricles from the great vessels. They open during systole, allowing blood to flow out of the heart with ventricular contraction. As the ventricle relaxes and intraventricular pressure falls at the beginning of diastole, the higher pressure within the great vessels (the aorta and pulmonary artery) closes these valves, creating the S_2 heart sound ("dup").

Pathophysiology

Valvular heart disease occurs as two major types of disorders: stenosis and regurgitation. Stenosis occurs when valve leaflets fuse together and cannot fully open or close. The valve opening narrows and becomes rigid (Figure 31–10A ■). Scarring of the valves from endocarditis or infarction, and calcium deposits can lead to stenosis. Stenotic valves impede the forward flow of blood, decreasing cardiac output because of impaired ventricular filling or ejection and stroke volume. Because stenotic valves also do not close completely, some backflow of blood occurs when the valve should be fully closed.

Regurgitant valves (also called *insufficient* or *incompetent* valves) do not close completely (Figure 31–10B). This allows regurgitation, or backflow of blood, through the valve into the area it just left. Regurgitation can result from deformity or erosion of valve cusps caused by the vegetative lesions of bacterial endocarditis, by scarring or tearing from myocardial infarction, or by cardiac dilation. As the heart enlarges, the

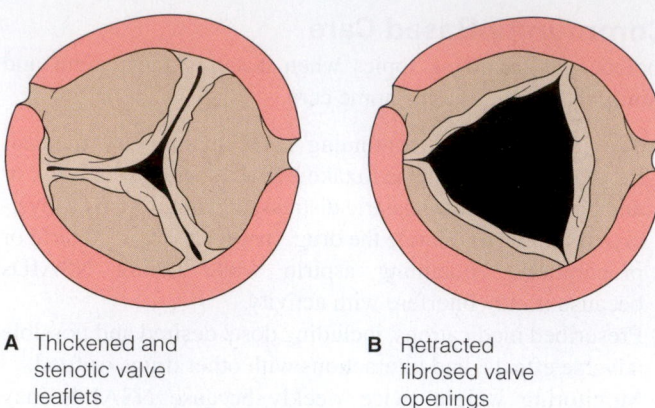

A Thickened and stenotic valve leaflets

B Retracted fibrosed valve openings

Figure 31–10 ■ Valvular heart disorders. *A,* Stenosis of a heart valve. *B,* An incompetent or regurgitant heart valve.

valve *annulus* (supporting ring of the valve) is stretched, and the valve edges no longer meet to allow complete closure.

Valvular disease causes hemodynamic changes both in front of and behind the affected valve. Blood volume and pressures are reduced in front of the valve, because flow is obstructed through a stenotic valve and backflow occurs through a regurgitant valve. By contrast, volumes and pressures characteristically increase behind the diseased valve. These hemodynamic changes may lead to pulmonary complications or heart failure. Higher pressures and compensatory changes to maintain cardiac output lead to remodeling and hypertrophy of the heart muscle.

Stenosis increases the work of the chamber behind the affected valve as the heart attempts to move blood through the narrowed opening. Excess blood volume behind regurgitant valves causes dilation of the chamber. In mitral stenosis, for

example, the left atrium hypertrophies to generate enough pressure to open and deliver its blood through the narrowed mitral valve. Not all of the blood is delivered before the valve closes, leaving blood to accumulate in the left atrium. This chamber dilates to accommodate the excess volume.

Eventually, cardiac output falls as compensatory mechanisms become less effective. The normal balance of oxygen supply and demand is upset, and the heart begins to fail. Increased muscle mass and size increase myocardial oxygen consumption. The size and workload of the heart exceed its blood supply, causing ischemia and chest pain. Eventually, necrosis occurs and functional muscle is lost. Contractile force, stroke volume, and cardiac output decrease. High pressures on the left side of the heart are reflected backward into the pulmonary system, causing pulmonary edema, pulmonary hypertension, and, eventually, right ventricular failure.

Valvular disorders interfere with the smooth flow of blood through the heart. The flow becomes turbulent, causing a **murmur**, a characteristic manifestation of valvular disease. Table 31–8 describes the murmurs associated with various types of valvular disorders.

Blood forced through the narrowed opening of a stenotic valve or regurgitated from a higher pressure chamber through an incompetent valve creates a jet stream effect (much like water spurting out of a partially occluded hose opening). The physical force of this jet stream damages the endocardium of the receiving chamber, increasing the risk for infective endocarditis.

The higher pressures on the left side of the heart subject its valves (the mitral and aortic valves) to more stress and damage than those on the right side of the heart (the tricuspid and pulmonic). Pulmonic valve disease is the least common of the valvular disorders.

TABLE 31–8 Heart Murmur Timing and Characteristics

MURMUR	CARDIAC CYCLE TIMING	AUSCULTATION SITE	CONFIGURATION OF SOUND	CONTINUITY
Mitral stenosis	Diastole	Apical	S_2 ——— S_1	Rumble that increases in sound toward the end, continuous
Mitral regurgitation	Systole	Apex	S_1 ——— S_2	Holosystolic (occurs throughout systole), continuous
Aortic stenosis	Midsystolic	Right sternal border (RSB) 2nd intercostal space (ICS)	S_1 ——— S_2	Crescendo-decrescendo, continuous
Aortic regurgitation	Diastole (early)	3rd ICS, LSB	S_2 ——— S_1	Decrescendo, continuous
Tricuspid stenosis	Diastole	Lower LSB	S_2 ——— S_1	Rumble that increases in sound toward the end, continuous
Tricuspid regurgitation	Systole	4th ICS, LSB	S_1 ——— S_2	Holosystolic, continuous

Mitral Stenosis

Mitral stenosis narrows the mitral valve, obstructing blood flow from the left atrium into the left ventricle during diastole. It is usually caused by rheumatic heart disease or bacterial endocarditis; it rarely results from congenital defects. It affects females more frequently (66%) than males (Bonow et al., 2006; Papadakis & McPhee, 2007). Mitral stenosis is chronic and progressive.

In mitral valve stenosis, fibrous tissue replaces normal valve tissue, causing valve leaflets to stiffen and fuse. Resulting changes in blood flow through the valve lead to calcification of the valve leaflets. As calcium is deposited in and on the valve, the leaflets become more rigid and narrow the opening further. As the valve leaflets become less mobile, the chordae tendineae fuse, thicken, and shorten. Thromboemboli may form on the calcified leaflets.

The narrowed mitral opening impairs blood flow into the left ventricle, reducing end-diastolic volume and pressure, and decreasing stroke volume. The narrowed opening also forces the left atrium to generate higher pressure to deliver blood to the left ventricle. This leads to left atrial hypertrophy. The left atrium also dilates as obstructed blood flow increases its volume. As the resistance to blood flow increases, high atrial pressures are reflected back into the pulmonary vessels, increasing pulmonary pressures (Figure 31–11 ■). Pulmonary hypertension increases the workload of the right ventricle, causing it to dilate and hypertrophy. Eventually, heart failure occurs.

MANIFESTATIONS Mitral stenosis may be asymptomatic or cause severe impairment. Its manifestations depend on cardiac output and pulmonary vascular pressures. Dyspnea on exertion (DOE) is typically the earliest manifestation. Others include cough, hemoptysis, frequent pulmonary infections such as bronchitis and pneumonia, paroxysmal nocturnal dyspnea, orthopnea, weakness, fatigue, and palpitations. As the stenosis worsens, manifestations of right heart failure, including jugular venous distension, hepatomegaly, ascites, and peripheral edema develop. Crackles may be heard in the lung bases. In severe mitral stenosis, cyanosis of the face and extremities may be noted. Chest pain is rare but may occur.

On auscultation, a loud S_1, a split S_2, and a mitral opening snap may be heard. The opening snap reflects high left atrial pressure. The murmur of mitral stenosis occurs during diastole, and is typically low-pitched, rumbling, crescendo-decrescendo. It is heard best with the bell of the stethoscope in the apical region. It may be accompanied by a palpable thrill (vibration).

COMPLICATIONS Atrial dysrhythmias, particularly atrial fibrillation, are common due to chronic atrial distention. Thrombi may form and subsequently embolize to the brain, coronary arteries, kidneys, spleen, and extremities—potentially devastating complications.

Women with mitral stenosis may be asymptomatic until pregnancy. As the heart tries to compensate for increased circulating volume (30% more in pregnancy) by increasing cardiac output, left atrial pressures rise, tachycardia reduces ventricular filling and stroke volume, and pulmonary pressures increase. Sudden pulmonary edema and heart failure may threaten the lives of the mother and fetus.

→ Blood flow
→ Reduced blood flow
⇉ Backward pressure against flow

Figure 31–11 ■ Mitral stenosis. Narrowing of the mitral valve orifice (1) reduces blood volume to left ventricle (2), which reduces cardiac output (3). Rising pressure in the left atrium (4) causes left atrial hypertrophy and pulmonary congestion. Increased pressure in pulmonary vessels (5), causes hypertrophy of the right ventricle and right atrium.

Mitral Regurgitation

Mitral regurgitation or *insufficiency* allows blood to flow back into the left atrium during systole because the valve does not close fully. Rheumatic heart disease is a common cause of mitral regurgitation. Men develop mitral regurgitation more frequently than women. Degenerative calcification of the mitral annulus may cause mitral regurgitation in older women. Processes that dilate the mitral annulus or affect the supporting structures, papillary muscles, or the chordae tendineae may cause mitral regurgitation (e.g., left ventricular hypertrophy and MI). Congenital defects also may cause mitral regurgitation.

In mitral regurgitation, blood flows into both the systemic circulation and back into the left atrium through the deformed valve during systole. This increases left atrial volume (Figure 31–12 ■). The left atrium dilates to accommodate its extra volume, pulling the posterior valve leaflet further away from the valve opening and worsening the defect. The left ventricle dilates to accommodate its increased preload and low cardiac output, further aggravating the problem.

MANIFESTATIONS Mitral regurgitation may be asymptomatic or cause symptoms such as fatigue, weakness, exertional dyspnea, and orthopnea. In severe or acute regurgitation,

Blood flow
Reduced blood flow
Backward pressure against flow

Figure 31–12 ■ Mitral regurgitation. The mitral valve closes incompletely (1), allowing blood to regurgitate during systole from the left ventricle to the left atrium (2). Cardiac output falls; to compensate, the left ventricle hypertrophies (3). Rising left atrial pressure (4) causes left atrial hypertrophy and pulmonary congestion. Elevated pulmonary artery pressure (5) causes slight enlargement of the right ventricle.

manifestations of left-sided heart failure develop, including pulmonary congestion and edema. High pulmonary pressures may lead to manifestations of right-sided heart failure.

The murmur of mitral regurgitation is usually loud, high pitched, rumbling, and holosystolic (occurring throughout systole). It is often accompanied by a palpable thrill and is heard most clearly at the cardiac apex. It may be characterized as a cooing or gull-like sound or have a musical quality (Bonow et al., 2006; Papadakis & McPhee, 2007).

Mitral Valve Prolapse

Mitral valve prolapse (MVP) is a type of mitral insufficiency that occurs when one or both mitral valve cusps billow into the atrium during ventricular systole. MVP is more common in young women between ages 14 and 30; its incidence declines with age. Its cause often is unclear. It also can result from acute or chronic rheumatic damage, ischemic heart disease, or other cardiac disorders. It commonly affects people with inherited connective tissue disorders such as Marfan syndrome (see the Genetic Considerations box). Mitral valve prolapse usually is benign, but about 0.01% to 0.02% of people with MVP have thickened mitral leaflets and a significant risk of morbidity and sudden death.

GENETIC CONSIDERATIONS
Patients with Marfan Syndrome

Marfan syndrome is a genetic (autosomal dominant) connective tissue disorder that affects the skeleton, eyes, and cardiovascular system. Skeletal characteristics include a long, thin body, with long extremities and long, tapering fingers, sometimes called *arachnodactyly* (spider fingers). Joints are hyperextensible, and skeletal deformities such as kyphosis, scoliosis, pigeon chest, or pectus excavatum are common. The potentially life-threatening cardiovascular effects of Marfan syndrome include mitral valve prolapse, progressive dilation of the aortic valve ring, and weakness of arterial walls. People with Marfan syndrome frequently die young, between 30 and 40 years, often due to dissection and rupture of the aorta (Huether & McCance, 2008).

Excess collagen tissue in the valve leaflets and elongated chordae tendineae impair closure of the mitral valve, allowing the leaflets to billow into the left atrium during systole. Some ventricular blood volume regurgitates into the left atrium (Figure 31–13 ■).

MANIFESTATIONS AND COMPLICATIONS Mitral valve prolapse usually is asymptomatic. A midsystolic ejection click or murmur may be audible. A high-pitched late systolic murmur, sometimes described as a "whoop" or "honk," due to the

Blood flow
Reduced blood flow

Figure 31–13 ■ Mitral valve prolapse. Excess tissue in the valve leaflets (1) and elongated cordae tendineae (2) impair mitral valve closure during systole. Some ventricular blood regurgitates into the left atrium (3).

regurgitation of blood through the valve, may develop in MVP. Atypical chest pain is the most common symptom of MVP. It may be left sided or substernal, and is frequently related to fatigue, not exertion. Tachydysrhythmias may develop with MVP, causing palpitations, lightheadedness, and syncope. Increased sympathetic nervous system tone may cause a sense of anxiety (Bonow et al., 2006).

Mitral valve prolapse increases the risk for bacterial endocarditis. Progressive worsening of regurgitation can lead to heart failure. Thrombi may form on prolapsed valve leaflets; embolization may cause transient ischemic attacks (TIAs).

Aortic Stenosis

Aortic stenosis obstructs blood flow from the left ventricle into the aorta during systole. Aortic stenosis is more common in males (80%) than females (Kasper et al., 2005). Aortic stenosis may be idiopathic, or due to a congenital defect, rheumatic damage, or degenerative changes. When rheumatic heart disease is the cause, mitral valve deformity is also often present. Rheumatic heart disease destroys aortic valve leaflets, with fibrosis and calcification causing rigidity and scarring. In the older adult, calcific aortic stenosis may result from degenerative changes associated with aging. Constant "wear and tear" on this valve can lead to fibrosis and calcification. Idiopathic calcific stenosis generally is mild and does not impair cardiac output.

As aortic stenosis progresses, the valve annulus decreases in size, increasing the work of the left ventricle to eject its volume through the narrowed opening into the aorta. To compensate, the ventricle hypertrophies to maintain an adequate stroke volume and cardiac output (Figure 31–14 ■). Left ventricular compliance also decreases. The additional workload increases myocardial oxygen consumption, which can precipitate myocardial ischemia. Coronary blood flow may also decrease in aortic stenosis. As left ventricular end-diastolic pressure increases because of reduced stroke volume, left atrial pressures increase. These pressures also affect the pulmonary vascular system; pulmonary vascular congestion and pulmonary edema may result.

COURSE AND MANIFESTATIONS Aortic stenosis may be asymptomatic for many years. As the disease progresses and compensation fails, usually between age 50 and 70, obstructed cardiac output causes manifestations of left ventricular failure. Dyspnea on exertion, angina pectoris, and exertional syncope are classic manifestations of aortic stenosis. Pulse pressure, an indicator of stroke volume, narrows to 30 mmHg or less. Hemodynamic monitors show increased left atrial pressure and pulmonary artery wedge pressure, as well as decreased stroke volume and cardiac output.

Aortic stenosis produces a harsh systolic murmur best heard in the second intercostal space to the right of the sternum. This crescendo-decrescendo murmur is produced by turbulence of blood entering the aorta through the stenotic valve. A palpable thrill is often felt. The murmur may radiate to the carotid arteries. Ventricular hypertrophy displaces the cardiac impulse to the left of the midclavicular line. As aortic stenosis progresses, S_3 and S_4 heart sounds may be heard, indicating heart failure and reduced left ventricular compliance.

	Blood flow
	Reduced blood flow
	Backward pressure against flow

Figure 31–14 ■ Aortic stenosis. The narrowed aortic valve orifice (1) decreases the left ventricular ejection fraction during systole (2) and cardiac output (3). The left ventricle hypertrophies (4). Incomplete emptying of the left atrium (5) causes backward pressure through pulmonary veins and pulmonary hypertension. Elevated pulmonary artery pressure (6) causes right ventricular strain.

As cardiac output falls, tissue perfusion decreases. Late in the disease, pulmonary hypertension and right ventricular failure develop. Untreated, symptomatic aortic stenosis has a poor prognosis; 10% to 20% of these patients experience sudden cardiac death (Bonow et al., 2006; Papadakis & McPhee, 2007).

Aortic Regurgitation

Aortic regurgitation, also called *aortic insufficiency*, allows blood to flow back into the left ventricle from the aorta during diastole. It is more common in males (75%) in its "pure" form; in females, it is commonly associated with coexisting mitral valve disease. Most aortic regurgitation (67%) results from rheumatic heart disease (Bonow et al., 2006; Papadakis & McPhee, 2007). Other causes include congenital disorders, infective endocarditis, blunt chest trauma, aortic aneurysm, syphilis, Marfan syndrome, and chronic hypertension.

In aortic regurgitation, thickened and contracted valve cusps, scarring, fibrosis, and calcification impede complete valve closure. Chronic hypertension and aortic aneurysm may dilate and stretch the aortic valve opening, increasing the degree of regurgitation.

In aortic regurgitation, volume overload affects the left ventricle as blood from the aorta adds to blood received from the atrium during diastole. This increases diastolic left ventricular pressure. Increased preload causes more forceful contractions and a high stroke volume (Figure 31–15 ■). With time, muscle cells hypertrophy to compensate for increased cardiac work and afterload; eventually this hypertrophy compromises cardiac output and increases regurgitation.

High left-ventricular pressures increase left atrial workload and pressure. This pressure is transmitted to the pulmonary vessels causing pulmonary congestion. The workload of the right ventricle increases as a result, and right-sided heart failure may develop. Acute aortic regurgitation from traumatic injury or infective endocarditis causes a rapid decline in hemodynamic status from acute heart failure and pulmonary edema, because compensatory mechanisms do not have time to develop.

MANIFESTATIONS Aortic regurgitation may be asymptomatic for many years, even when severe. The increased stroke volume may cause complaints of persistent palpitations, especially when recumbent. A throbbing pulse may be visible in arteries of the neck; the force of contraction may cause a characteristic head bob (Musset's sign) and shake the whole body. Other symptoms include dizziness, and exercise intolerance.

Fatigue, exertional dyspnea, orthopnea, and paroxysmal nocturnal dyspnea are common in aortic regurgitation. Anginal pain may result from excessive cardiac work and decreased coronary perfusion. Unlike CAD, angina often occurs at night and may not respond to conventional therapy.

The murmur of aortic regurgitation is heard during diastole as blood flows back into the left ventricle from the aorta. It is a "blowing," high-pitched sound heard most clearly at the third left intercostal space. A palpable thrill and ventricular heave may be noted. An S_3 and S_4 may be heard as the heart fails and ventricular compliance diminishes. The apical impulse is displaced to the left.

High systolic and low diastolic pressures cause a widened pulse pressure. The arterial pressure waveform has a rapid upstroke and quickly collapsing downstroke, known as a *water-hammer pulse*. It is caused by the force of rapid and early delivery of the stroke volume into the aorta.

Tricuspid Valve Disorders

Tricuspid stenosis obstructs blood flow from the right atrium to the right ventricle. It usually results from rheumatic heart disease; mitral stenosis often occurs concurrently with tricuspid stenosis.

Fibrosed, retracted tricuspid valve cusps and fused leaflets narrow the valve orifice and prevent complete closure. Right ventricular filling is impaired during diastole, and during systole, some blood regurgitates back into the right atrium. Pressure in the right atrium increases, and it enlarges in response to the increased pressure and workload. This increased right atrial pressure is reflected backward into the systemic circulation. Right ventricular stroke volume decreases, reducing the volume delivered to the pulmonary system and left heart. Stroke volume, cardiac output, and tissue perfusion fall.

Manifestations of tricuspid stenosis relate to systemic congestion and right-sided heart failure. They include increased central venous pressure, jugular venous distention, ascites, hepatomegaly, and peripheral edema. Low cardiac output causes fatigue and weakness. The low-pitched, rumbling diastolic murmur of tricuspid stenosis is most clearly heard in the fourth intercostal space at the left sternal border or over the xiphoid process.

Tricuspid regurgitation usually occurs secondarily to right ventricular dilation. Stretching distorts the valve and its supporting structures, preventing complete valve closure. Left ventricular failure is the usual cause of right ventricular overload; pulmonary hypertension is another cause. The valve may also be damaged by rheumatic heart disease, infective endocarditis, inferior MI, trauma, or other conditions.

Tricuspid regurgitation allows blood to flow back into the right atrium during systole, increasing right atrial pressures. Increased right atrial pressure causes manifestations of right-sided heart failure, including systemic venous congestion and low cardiac output. Atrial fibrillation due to atrial distention is common. The retrograde flow of blood over the deformed tricuspid valve causes a high-pitched, blowing systolic murmur heard over the tricuspid or xiphoid area.

Pulmonic Valve Disorders

Pulmonic stenosis obstructs blood flow from the right ventricle into the pulmonary system. It usually is a congenital disorder, although rheumatic heart disease or cancer also may

■ Blood flow
■ Reduced blood flow
■ Backward pressure against flow

Figure 31–15 ■ Aortic regurgitation. The cusps of the aortic valve widen and fail to close during diastole (1). Blood regurgitates from the aorta into the left ventricle (2) increasing left ventricular volume and decreasing cardiac output (3). The left ventricle dilates and hypertrophies (4) in response to the increase in blood volume and workload.

cause pulmonic stenosis. The right ventricle hypertrophies to generate the pressure needed to pump blood into the pulmonary system. The right atrium also hypertrophies to overcome the high pressures generated in the right ventricle. Right-sided heart failure occurs when the ventricle can no longer generate adequate pressure to force blood past the narrowed valve opening.

Pulmonic stenosis typically is asymptomatic unless severe. Dyspnea on exertion and fatigue are early signs. As the condition progresses, right-sided heart failure develops, with peripheral edema, ascites, hepatomegaly, and increased venous pressures. Turbulent blood flow caused by the narrowed valve generates a harsh, systolic crescendo-decrescendo murmur heard in the pulmonic area, the second left intercostal space.

Pulmonic regurgitation is more common than pulmonary stenosis. It is a complication of pulmonary hypertension, which stretches and dilates the pulmonary orifice, causing incomplete valve closure. Infective endocarditis, pulmonary artery aneurysm, and syphilis also may cause pulmonic regurgitation.

Incomplete valve closure allows blood to flow back into the right ventricle during diastole, decreasing blood flow to the pulmonary circuit. The extra blood increases right ventricular end-diastolic volume. When the ventricle can no longer compensate for the increased volume, right-sided heart failure develops. The murmur of pulmonic regurgitation is a high-pitched, decrescendo, blowing sound heard along the left sternal border during diastole.

Interdisciplinary Care

A heart murmur identified during routine physical examination often is the initial indication of valvular disease. If no symptoms are present, close observation for disease progression and prophylactic therapy to prevent infection of the diseased heart may be the only treatment.

Manifestations of heart failure are treated with diet and medications (see the preceding section on heart failure). When medical management is no longer effective, surgery is considered.

Diagnosis

The following diagnostic tests help to identify and diagnose valvular disease. ∞ See Chapter 30 for more information about these tests and related nursing care.

- *Echocardiography* is used routinely to diagnose valvular disease. Thickened valve leaflets, vegetations or growths on valve leaflets, myocardial function, and chamber size can be determined, and pressure gradients across valves and pulmonary artery pressures can be estimated. Either transthoracic or transesophageal echocardiography may be used.
- *Chest x-ray* can identify cardiac hypertrophy, chamber and great vessel enlargement, and dilation of the pulmonary vasculature. Calcification of the valve leaflets and annular openings may also be visible.
- *Electrocardiography* can demonstrate atrial and ventricular hypertrophy, conduction defects, and dysrhythmias associated with valvular disease.
- *Cardiac catheterization* may be used to assess contractility and to determine the pressure gradients across the heart

valves, in the heart chambers, and in the pulmonary system. It is used prevalvular surgery to assess CAD risk.
- *Exercise testing* should be used only with asymptomatic patients to assess for exercise-induced symptoms and abnormal blood pressure response. It is contraindicated for symptomatic aortic stenosis patients.

Medications

Heart failure resulting from valvular disease is treated with diuretics, ACE inhibitors, vasodilators, and possibly digitalis glycosides. Digitalis increases the force of myocardial contraction to maintain cardiac output. Diuretics, ACE inhibitors, and vasodilators reduce preload and afterload. (See the Medication Administration box on pages 981–982.)

In patients with valvular disorders, atrial distention often causes atrial fibrillation. Digitalis or small doses of beta blockers are given to slow the ventricular response (∞ see Chapter 32 for more information about atrial fibrillation and its treatment). Anticoagulant therapy is added to prevent clot and embolus formation, a common complication of atrial fibrillation as blood pools in the noncontracting atria. Anticoagulant therapy also is required following insertion of a mechanical heart valve. ∞ See Chapter 33 for more information about anticoagulant therapy.

Valvular damage increases the risk for infective endocarditis as altered blood flow allows bacterial colonization. Antibiotics are prescribed prophylactically prior to any dental work, invasive procedures, or surgery to minimize the risk of bacteremia (bacteria in the blood) and subsequent endocarditis.

Percutaneous Balloon Valvotomy

Percutaneous balloon valvotomy is an invasive procedure performed in the cardiac catheterization laboratory. A balloon catheter similar to that used in coronary angioplasty procedures is inserted into the femoral vein or artery. Guided by fluoroscopy, the catheter is advanced into the heart and positioned with the balloon straddling the stenotic valve. The balloon is then inflated for approximately 90 seconds to divide the fused leaflets and enlarge the valve orifice (Figure 31–16 ■). Balloon valvotomy is the treatment of choice for symptomatic mitral valve stenosis. It is used to treat children and young adults with aortic stenosis, and may be indicated for older adults who are poor surgical risks, and as a "bridge to surgery" when heart function is severely compromised (Bonow et al., 2006; Papadakis & McPhee, 2007). Nursing care of the patient with a balloon valvotomy is similar to that of the patient following coronary revascularization (∞ see Chapter 30 page 926).

Surgery

Surgery to repair or replace the diseased valve may be done to restore valve function, alleviate symptoms, and prevent complications and death. Ideally, diseased valves are repaired or replaced before cardiopulmonary function is severely compromised. The diseased valve is repaired when possible, because the risk for surgical mortality and complications is lower than with valve replacement.

RECONSTRUCTIVE SURGERY *Valvuloplasty* is a general term for reconstruction or repair of a heart valve. Methods include "patching" the perforated portion of the leaflet, resecting excess tissue, debriding vegetations or calcification, and other techniques.

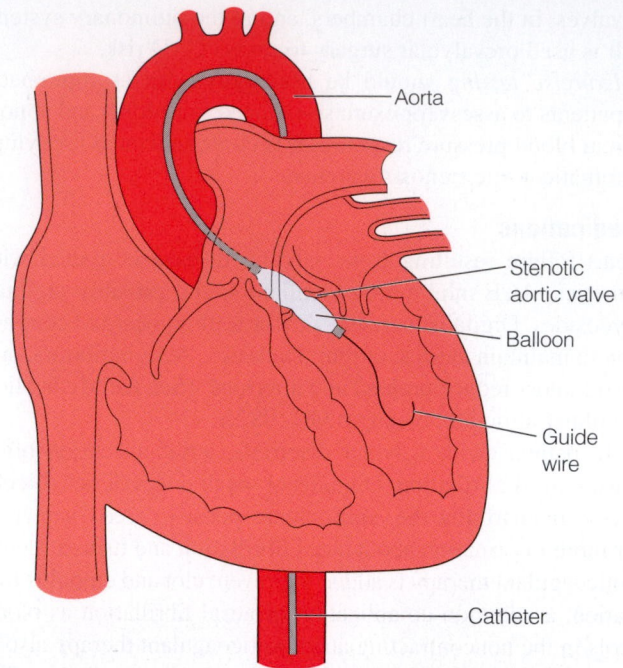

Figure 31–16 ■ Balloon valvotomy. The balloon catheter is guided into position straddling the stenosed valve. The balloon is then inflated to increase the size of the valve opening.

Valvuloplasty may be used for stenotic or regurgitant mitral and tricuspid valves, mitral valve prolapse, and aortic stenosis. Common valvuloplasty procedures include the following:

■ *Open commissurotomy*, surgical division of fused valve leaflets, is done to open stenotic valves. Fused commissures (junctions between valve leaflets or cusps) are incised, and calcium deposits are debrided as needed.

■ *Annuloplasty* repairs a narrowed or an enlarged or dilated valve annulus, the supporting ring of the valve. A prosthetic ring may be used to resize the opening, or stitches and purse-string sutures may be used to reduce and gather excess tissue. Annuloplasty may be used for either stenotic or regurgitant valves.

VALVE REPLACEMENT   Valve replacement is indicated when manifestations of valve dysfunction develop, preferably before left heart function is seriously impaired. In general, three factors determine the outcome of valve replacement surgery: (1) heart

function at the time of surgery, (2) intraoperative and postoperative care, and (3) characteristics and durability of the replacement valve.

Many different prosthetic heart valves are available, including mechanical and biologic tissue valves. Selection depends on the valve hemodynamics, resistance to clot formation, ease of insertion, anatomic suitability, and patient acceptance. The patient's age, underlying condition, and contraindications to anticoagulation (such as a desire to become pregnant) also are considered in selecting the appropriate prosthesis. Table 31–9 lists the advantages and disadvantages of biologic and mechanical valves.

Biologic tissue valves may be *heterografts*, excised from a pig (Figure 31–17*A* ■) or made of calf pericardium, or *homografts* from a human (obtained from a cadaver or during heart transplant). Biologic valves allow more normal blood flow and have a low risk of thrombus formation. As a result, long-term anticoagulation rarely is necessary. They are less durable, however, than mechanical valves. Up to 50% of biologic valves must be replaced by 15 years.

Mechanical prosthetic valves have the major advantage of long-term durability. These valves are frequently used when life expectancy exceeds 10 years. Their major disadvantage is the need for lifetime anticoagulation to prevent the development of clots on the valve.

Most mechanical valves are either a tilting disk or a ball and cage design. The tilting-disc valve designs are frequently used because they have a lower profile than the caged-ball types, allowing blood to flow through the valve with less obstruction (Figures 31–17*B*). The St. Jude bileaflet design has good hemodynamics and low risk for clot formation. Both biologic and mechanical valves increase the risk of endocarditis, although its incidence is fairly low.

Nursing Care

Health Promotion

Preventing rheumatic heart disease is a key element in preventing heart valve disorders. Rheumatic heart disease is a consequence of rheumatic fever (see the previous section of this chapter), an immune process that may be a sequela to β-hemolytic streptococcal infection of the pharynx (strep throat). Early treatment of strep throat prevents rheumatic fever. Teach individual patients, families, and communities about the importance of

TABLE 31–9 Advantages and Disadvantages of Prosthetic Heart Valves

CATEGORY	TYPES	ADVANTAGES	DISADVANTAGES
Mechanical valves	Ball-and-cage	Long-term durability	Lifetime anticoagulation
	Tilting disc	Good hemodynamics	Audible click
			Risk of thromboembolism
			Infections are harder to treat
Biologic tissue valves	Porcine heterograft	Low incidence of thromboembolism	Prone to deterioration
	Bovine heterograft	No long-term anticoagulation	Frequent replacement is required
	Human aortic homograft	Good hemodynamics	
		Quiet	
		Infections are easier to treat	

A   **B**

Figure 31–17 ■ Prosthetic heart valves. *A,* Carpentier-Edwards porcine xenograft. *B,* St. Jude Medical valve.

Courtesy of Baxter (A); and St. Jude Medical (B).

timely and effective treatment of strep throat. Emphasize the importance of completing the full prescription of antibiotics to prevent development of resistant bacteria. Prophylactic antibiotic therapy before invasive procedures to prevent infectious endocarditis is an important health promotion measure for patients with preexisting heart disease.

Assessment

Assessment data related to valvular heart disease includes the following:

- *Health history:* Complaints of decreasing exercise tolerance, dyspnea on exertion, palpitations; history of frequent respiratory infections; previous history of rheumatic heart disease, endocarditis, or a heart murmur.
- *Physical examination:* Vital signs; skin color and temperature, evidence of clubbing or peripheral edema; neck vein distention; breath sounds; heart sounds and presence of S_3, S_4, or murmur; timing, grade, and characteristics of any murmur; palpate for cardiac heave and thrills; abdominal contour, liver and spleen size.

Nursing Diagnoses and Interventions

Nursing priorities include maintaining cardiac output, managing manifestations of the disorder, teaching about the disease process and its management, and preventing complications. Nursing care of the patient undergoing valve surgery is similar to that of the patient having other types of open-heart surgery (∞ see Chapter 30 page 931), with increased attention to anticoagulation and preventing endocarditis.

Decreased Cardiac Output

Nearly all valve disorders affect ventricular filling and/or emptying, reducing cardiac output. Stenosis of the AV valves impairs ventricular filling and increases atrial pressures. Regurgitation of these valves reduces cardiac output as a portion of the blood in the ventricle regurgitates into the atria during systole. Stenosis of the semilunar valves obstructs ventricular outflow to the great vessels; regurgitation allows blood to flow

back into the ventricles, creating higher filling pressures. When compensatory measures fail, heart failure develops.

- Monitor vital signs and hemodynamic parameters, reporting changes from the baseline. *A fall in systolic blood pressure and tachycardia may indicate decreased cardiac output. Increasing pulmonary artery and pulmonary wedge pressures may also indicate decreased cardiac output, causing increased congestion and pressure in the pulmonary vascular system.*

> **PRACTICE ALERT**
> Promptly report changes in level of consciousness; distended neck veins; dyspnea or respiratory crackles; urine output less than 30 mL/h; cool, clammy, or cyanotic skin; diminished peripheral pulses; or slow capillary refill. These findings indicate decreased cardiac output and impaired tissue and organ perfusion.

- Monitor intake and output; weigh daily. Report weight gain of 3 to 5 lb within 24 hours. *Fluid retention is a compensatory mechanism that occurs when cardiac output decreases; 2.2 lb (1 kg) of weight equals 1 L of fluid.*
- Restrict fluids as ordered. *Fluid intake may be restricted to reduce cardiac workload and pressures within the heart and pulmonary circuit.*

EVIDENCE FOR NURSING CARE — **The Patient with Valvular Heart Disease**

Selected resources that nurses may find helpful when planning evidence-based nursing care follow.

- Hill, K. M. (2009). Mitral valve repair: A new choice. *American Nurse Today; 2009, 4*(5), 8–10.
- McRae, M. E., Rodger, M., & Bailey, B. B. (2009). Transcatheter and transapical aortic valve replacement. *Critical Care Nurse, 29*(1), 22–36.

- Monitor oxygen saturation continuously and arterial blood gases as ordered. Report oxygen saturation less than 95% (or as specified) and abnormal ABG results. *Oxygen saturation levels and ABGs allow assessment of oxygenation.*
- Elevate the head of the bed. Administer supplemental oxygen as ordered. *These measures improve alveolar ventilation and oxygenation.*
- Provide for physical, emotional, and mental rest. *Physical and psychologic rest decreases the cardiac workload.*
- Administer prescribed medications as ordered to reduce cardiac workload. *Diuretics, ACE inhibitors, and direct vasodilators may be prescribed to reduce fluid volume and afterload, reducing cardiac work.*

Activity Intolerance

Altered blood flow through the heart impairs delivery of oxygen and nutrients to the tissues. As the heart muscle fails and is unable to compensate for altered blood flow, tissue perfusion is further compromised. Dyspnea on exertion is often an early symptom of valvular disease.

- Monitor vital signs before and during activities. *A change in heart rate of more than 20 BPM, a change of 20 mmHg or more in systolic BP, and complaints of dyspnea, shortness of breath, excessive fatigue, chest pain, diaphoresis, dizziness, or syncope may indicate activity intolerance.*
- Encourage self-care and gradually increasing activities as allowed and tolerated. Provide for rest periods, uninterrupted sleep, and adequate nutritional intake. *Gradual progression of activities avoids excessive cardiac stress. Encouraging self-care increases the patient's self-esteem and sense of power. Adequate rest and nutrition facilitate healing, decrease fatigue, and increase energy reserves.*
- Provide assistance as needed. Suggest use of a shower chair, sitting while brushing hair or teeth, and other energy-saving measures. *Reducing energy expenditure helps maintain a balance of oxygen supply and demand.*
- Consult with cardiac rehabilitation specialist or physical therapist for in-bed exercises and an activity plan. *In-bed exercises may help improve strength.*
- Discuss ways to conserve energy at home. *Information provides practical ways to deal with activity limitations and empowers the patient to manage these limitations.*

Risk for Infection

Damaged and deformed valve leaflets and turbulent blood flow through the heart significantly increase the risk of infective endocarditis. Invasive diagnostic and monitoring lines (e.g., cardiac catheterization, hemodynamic monitoring) and disrupted skin with surgery also increase the risk of infection.

- Use aseptic technique for all invasive procedures. *Invasive procedures breach the body's protective mechanisms, potentially allowing bacteria to enter. Aseptic technique reduces this risk.*

PRACTICE ALERT
Record temperature every 4 hours; notify physician if temperature exceeds 100.5°F (38.5°C). Fever may be an early indication of infection.

- Assess wounds and catheter sites for redness, swelling, warmth, pain, or evidence of drainage. *These signs of inflammation may signal infection.*
- Administer antibiotics as ordered. Ensure completion of the full course. *Antibiotics are used to prevent and treat infection. Completion of the full course of therapy prevents drug-resistant organisms from multiplying.*
- Monitor WBC and differential. Notify physician of leukocytosis or leukopenia. *A high WBC and increased percentage of immature WBCs (bands) may indicate bacterial infection; a low WBC count may indicate an impaired immune response and increased susceptibility to infection.*

Ineffective Protection

Anticoagulant therapy commonly is prescribed for patients with chronic atrial fibrillation, a history of emboli, and following valve replacement surgery. Although chronic anticoagulant therapy decreases the risk of clots and emboli, it increases the risk for bleeding and hemorrhage.

PRACTICE ALERT
Monitor the International Normalized Ratio (INR) or prothrombin time (PT or protime). Report an INR > 3.5 or a PT > 2.5 times the normal to the physician. An excessively high INR or PT indicate excessive anticoagulation and an increased risk for bleeding.

- Test stools and vomitus for occult blood. *Bleeding due to excessive anticoagulation may not be apparent.*
- Instruct to avoid using aspirin or other nonsteroidal anti-inflammatory drugs (NSAIDs). Encourage reading ingredient labels on over-the-counter drugs; many contain aspirin. *Aspirin and other NSAIDs interfere with clotting and may potentiate the effects of the anticoagulant therapy.*
- Advise using a soft-bristled toothbrush, electric razor, and gentle touch when cleaning fragile skin. *These measures decrease the risk of skin or gum trauma and bleeding.*

PRACTICE ALERT
Monitor hemoglobin, hematocrit, and platelet count as ordered. Notify the physician of decreasing hemoglobin and hematocrit levels or if the platelet count falls below 50,000/mm³. Low hemoglobin and hematocrit indicate blood loss. Platelet counts below 50,000/mm³ significantly increase the risk of bleeding.

Community-Based Care

For most patients, valvular disease is a chronic condition. The patient has primary responsibility for managing effects of the disorder. To prepare the patient and family for home care, discuss the following topics.

- Management of symptoms, including any necessary activity restrictions or lifestyle changes
- The importance of adequate rest to prevent fatigue
- Diet restrictions to reduce fluid retention and symptoms of heart failure

CASE STUDY & NURSING CARE PLAN A Patient with Mitral Valve Prolapse

Julie Snow, a 22-year-old college student, sees a nurse practitioner at the college health clinic for a physical examination after experiencing palpitations, fatigue, and a headache during midterm examinations. Ms. Snow tells Lakisha Johnson, FNP, "I'm scared that something is wrong with me."

Over the last few months, Ms. Snow has had occasional palpitations that she describes as "feeling like my heart is doing flip-flops." Rarely, these palpitations have been accompanied by a sharp, stabbing pain in her chest that lasts only a few seconds. She initially attributed her symptoms to stress, but she is increasingly concerned because the "attacks" are becoming more frequent. Ms. Snow states that she has "always been healthy," does not smoke, uses alcohol socially, and exercises, albeit intermittently. Ms. Snow admits that she has been drinking a lot of coffee and cola and eating a lot of "junk food" lately.

ASSESSMENT

Ms. Johnson's assessment of Ms. Snow documents the following: height 66 in. (168 cm), weight 140 lb (63.6 kg), T 99.3, BP 118/64, P 82, and R 18. Slightly anxious but in no acute distress. Systolic click and soft crescendo murmur grade II/VI noted on auscultation. Apical impulse at 5th ICS left MCL. Lungs clear to auscultation. Review of remaining systems reveals no apparent abnormalities. An ECG shows sinus rhythm with occasional PACs. Based on the admission history, manifestations, and physical assessment, Ms. Johnson suspects mitral valve prolapse (MVP).

DIAGNOSES

- *Anxiety* related to fear of heart disease and implications for lifestyle
- *Powerlessness* related to unpredictability of symptoms
- *Risk of Infection (endocarditis)* related to altered valve function

EXPECTED OUTCOMES

- Verbalize an understanding of MVP and its management.
- Discuss ways to decrease or relieve MVP symptoms.
- Acknowledge the risk for endocarditis and identify precautions to prevent it.

PLANNING AND IMPLEMENTATION

- Consult with and refer to the cardiologist for continued monitoring and follow-up.
- Teach about MVP, including heart valve anatomy, physiology, and function, common manifestations of MVP, and treatment rationale.
- Discuss symptoms of progressive mitral regurgitation, and the need to report these to the cardiologist.
- Discuss recommended follow-up care and its rationale.

- Allow to verbalize feelings and share concerns about MVP. Encourage to attend an MVP support group meeting.
- Discuss the prognosis for MVP, emphasizing that most patients live normal lives using diet and lifestyle management.
- Instruct to keep a weekly record of symptoms and their frequency for 1 month.
- Discuss lifestyle changes to manage symptoms: aerobic exercise with warm-up and cool down periods; maintaining adequate fluid intake, especially during hot weather or exercise; relaxation techniques (e.g., meditation, deep-breathing exercises, music therapy, yoga, guided imagery, heat therapy, or progressive muscle relaxation) to perform daily; avoiding caffeine and crash diets; forming healthy eating habits.
- Teach about infective endocarditis risk and prevention with prophylactic antibiotics. Encourage notifying dentist and other healthcare providers of MVP before dental or any invasive procedure.

EVALUATION

After several educational sessions at the college health clinic, Ms. Snow verbalizes an understanding of MVP by explaining heart valve function, listing common manifestations of MVP, and describing indications of deteriorating heart function. She states she will report these manifestations to her cardiologist if they occur. She is given a booklet on MVP for additional reading. She verbalizes understanding of the risk of endocarditis, and states that she will notify her doctors of her MVP and the need for antibiotics before invasive procedures. Ms. Snow is attending a monthly MVP support group (led by a cardiology clinical nurse specialist) on campus and states, "I am so glad to know I'm not alone! It really helps to know that others are living well with MVP." Her weekly symptom log shows her symptoms are associated with late-night studying and drinking large amounts of coffee and cola. Ms. Snow has moderated her caffeine intake and increased her fluids, relieving her symptoms. In addition, Ms. Snow is taking a relaxation music therapy class. Ms. Snow states that she realizes that she has "the ability to control my life through the choices I make."

CRITICAL THINKING IN THE NURSING PROCESS

1. Develop an action plan for Ms. Snow that outlines specific activities she can use to manage symptoms of MVP.
2. Why are patients with symptomatic MVP encouraged to include regular exercise in their health habits?
3. How does the support of family, friends, and other people with MVP assist MVP patients in managing their condition?
4. What manifestations would indicate a progressive worsening of Ms. Snow's mitral regurgitation?

See Evaluating Your Response in Appendix C.

- Information about prescribed medications, including purpose, desired and possible adverse effects, scheduling, and possible interactions with other drugs
- The importance of keeping follow-up appointments to monitor the disease and its treatment
- Notifying all healthcare providers about valve disease or surgery to facilitate prescription of prophylactic antibiotics before invasive procedures or dental work
- Manifestations to immediately report to the healthcare provider: increasing severity of symptoms, especially of worsening heart failure or pulmonary edema; signs of transient ischemic attacks or other embolic events; evidence of bleeding, such as joint pain, easy bruising, black and tarry stools, bleeding gums, or blood in the urine or sputum

Provide referrals to community resources such as home maintenance services, home health services, and structured cardiac rehabilitation programs. Refer the patient and family (especially the primary food preparer) to a dietitian or nutritionist for teaching and assistance with menu planning. See the accompanying Case Study & Nursing Care Plan for additional nursing care and teaching for a patient with mitral valve prolapse.

The Patient with Cardiomyopathy

Cardiomyopathies are disorders that affect the heart muscle itself. They are a diverse group of disorders that affect both systolic and diastolic functions. Cardiomyopathies may be either primary or secondary in origin. Primary cardiomyopathies are idiopathic; their cause is unknown. Secondary cardiomyopathies occur as a result of other processes, such as ischemia, infectious disease, exposure to toxins, connective tissue disorders, metabolic disorders, or nutritional deficiencies. In many cases, the cause of cardiomyopathy is unknown. Close to 27,000 deaths annually are directly attributed to cardiomyopathy. Mortality associated with cardiomyopathy is higher in older adults, men, and African Americans (AHA, 2009).

Pathophysiology

The cardiomyopathies are categorized by their pathophysiology and presentation into three groups: dilated, hypertrophic, and restrictive. Table 31–10 compares the causes, pathophysiology, manifestations, and management of the cardiomyopathies.

Dilated Cardiomyopathy

Dilated cardiomyopathy is the most common type of cardiomyopathy, accounting for 87% of cases (AHA, 2004). Dilated cardiomyopathy also is a common cause of heart failure, accounting for about one in three cases. It is primarily a disease of middle age males; African American males have a higher risk than Whites (Papadakis & McPhee, 2007).

The cause of dilated cardiomyopathy is unknown, although it appears to frequently result from toxins, metabolic conditions, or infection. Reversible dilated cardiomyopathy may develop due to alcohol and cocaine abuse, chemotherapeutic drugs, pregnancy, and systemic hypertension. Up to 20% of cases of dilated cardiomyopathy may be genetic in origin, most commonly transmitted in an autosomal dominant pattern, although autosomal recessive, X-linked, and mitochondrial patterns of inheritance also are seen (Huether & McCance, 2008).

In dilated cardiomyopathy, heart chambers dilate and ventricular contraction is impaired. Both end-diastolic and end-systolic volumes increase, and the left ventricular ejection fraction is substantially reduced, decreasing cardiac output.

TABLE 31–10 Classifications of Cardiomyopathy

	DILATED	HYPERTROPHIC	RESTRICTIVE
Causes	Usually idiopathic; may be secondary to chronic alcoholism or myocarditis	Hereditary; may be secondary to chronic hypertension	Usually secondary to amyloidosis, radiation, or myocardial fibrosis
Pathophysiology	Scarring and atrophy of myocardial cells Thickening of ventricular wall Dilation of heart chambers Impaired ventricular pumping Increased end-diastolic and end-systolic volumes Mural thrombi common	Hypertrophy of ventricular muscle mass Small left ventricular volume Septal hypertrophy may obstruct left ventricular outflow Left atrial dilation	Excess rigidity of ventricular walls restricts filling Myocardial contractility remains relatively normal
Manifestations	Heart failure Cardiomegaly Dysrhythmias S_3 and S_4 gallop; murmur of mitral regurgitation	Dyspnea, anginal pain, syncope Left ventricular hypertrophy Dysrhythmias Loud S_4 Sudden death	Dyspnea, fatigue Right-sided heart failure Mild to moderate cardiomegaly S_3 and S_4 Mitral regurgitation murmur
Management	Management of heart failure Implantable cardioverter-defibrillator (ICD) as needed Cardiac transplantation	Beta-blockers Calcium channel blockers Antidysrhythmic agents ICD, dual-chamber pacing Surgical excision of part of the ventricular septum	Management of heart failure Exercise restriction

Left ventricular dilation is prominent; left ventricular hypertrophy is usually minimal. The right ventricle also may be enlarged. Extensive interstitial fibrosis (scarring) is evident; necrotic myocardial cells also may be seen (Papadakis & McPhee, 2007).

MANIFESTATIONS AND COURSE Manifestations of dilated cardiomyopathy develop gradually. Heart failure often presents years after the onset of dilation and pump failure. Both right- and left-sided failure occur, with dyspnea on exertion, orthopnea, paroxysmal nocturnal dyspnea, weakness, fatigue, peripheral edema, and ascites. Both S_3 and S_4 heart sounds are commonly heard, as well as an AV regurgitation murmur. Dysrhythmias are common, including supraventricular tachycardias, atrial fibrillation, and complex ventricular tachycardias. Untreated dysrhythmias can lead to sudden death (Huether & McCance, 2008). Mural thrombi (blood clots in the heart wall) may form in the left ventricular apex and embolize to other parts of the body.

The prognosis of dilated cardiomyopathy is grim; most patients get progressively worse and 50% die within 5 years after the diagnosis; 75% die within 10 years (AHA, 2009).

Hypertrophic Cardiomyopathy

Hypertrophic cardiomyopathy is characterized by decreased compliance of the left ventricle and hypertrophy of the ventricular muscle mass. This impairs ventricular filling, leading to small end-diastolic volumes, and low cardiac output. About half of all patients with hypertrophic cardiomyopathy have a family history of the disease. It is genetically transmitted in an autosomal dominant pattern (Papadakis & McPhee, 2007).

The pattern of left ventricular hypertrophy is unique in that the muscle may not hypertrophy "equally." In a majority of patients, the interventricular septal mass, especially the upper portion, increases to a greater extent than the free wall of the ventricle. The enlarged upper septum narrows the passageway of blood into the aorta, impairing ventricular outflow. For this reason, this disorder is also known as *idiopathic hypertrophic subaortic stenosis (IHSS)* or *hypertrophic obstructive cardiomyopathy (HOCM)*.

MANIFESTATIONS AND COURSE Hypertrophic cardiomyopathy may be asymptomatic for many years. Symptoms typically occur when increased oxygen demand causes increased ventricular contractility. They may develop suddenly during or after physical activity; in children and young adults, sudden cardiac death may be the first sign of the disorder. Hypertrophic cardiomyopathy is the probable or definite cause of death in 36% of young athletes who die suddenly (AHA, 2009). It is hypothesized that sudden cardiac death is due to ventricular dysrhythmias or hemodynamic factors. Predictors of sudden cardiac death in this population include age of less than 30 years, a family history of sudden death, syncopal episodes, severe ventricular hypertrophy, and ventricular tachycardia seen on ambulatory ECG monitoring (Papadakis & McPhee, 2007). For a brief synopsis of a nursing research study regarding family presence during CPR and invasive procedures, see the box on that follows.

The usual manifestations of hypertrophic cardiomyopathy are dyspnea, angina, and syncope. Angina may result from ischemia due to overgrowth of the ventricular muscle, coronary artery abnormalities, or decreased coronary artery perfusion. Syncope may occur when the outflow tract obstruction severely decreases cardiac output and blood flow to the brain. Ventricular dysrhythmias are common; atrial fibrillation also may develop. Other manifestations of hypertrophic cardiomyopathy include fatigue, dizziness, and palpitations. A harsh, crescendo-decrescendo systolic murmur of variable intensity heard best at the lower left sternal border and apex is characteristic in hypertrophic cardiomyopathy. An S_4 may also be noted on auscultation.

MOVING EVIDENCE INTO ACTION | **Sudden Cardiac Death**

When cardiac arrest occurs or invasive procedures are performed, family members typically are asked to leave the patient's care unit. The traditional rationale for this practice is fear of disrupted clinical interventions, trauma of the witnesses, and risk for increased hospital liability. However, in 1995, the Emergency Nurses Association (ENA) adopted a position supporting family presence during invasive procedures, including resuscitation efforts (CPR), as a means of maintaining family integrity and dignity. This study evaluated the responses of families, nurses, and physicians to family presence during invasive procedures and CPR.

Results of the study showed that families saw their presence as a positive experience and their right. They viewed themselves as active care partners, and being present met their needs for information and providing comfort and connection with the patient. Nurses overwhelmingly supported family presence; attending physicians also demonstrated a positive response. Physician residents were the least supportive of family presence.

IMPLICATIONS FOR NURSING
Family members often are asked to leave the patient's side during invasive procedures and CPR with the intention of protecting them from the trauma of witnessing painful or distressing events.

This study clearly showed being present as a positive experience, even when the ultimate outcome was the patient's death.

Offering the opportunity to be present and providing information, psychologic and emotional support to an appropriate family member during invasive procedures and CPR supports the family unit and the patient during times of crisis. Screening is important: People who are combative, emotionally unstable, or have altered mental status (e.g., dementia, alcohol intoxication) probably are not appropriate. It also is important to allow families to decline the invitation without guilt.

CRITICAL THINKING IN PATIENT CARE
1. Identify procedures and situations in which family members are often asked to leave the patient's side. When would it be appropriate to allow at least one significant other to remain with the patient?
2. How would you present the option and prepare a family member for being present during a traumatic event such as CPR following the sudden death of a young adult with undiagnosed hypertrophic cardiomyopathy?
3. You support family presence during traumatic events and procedures, but your charge nurse does not. What steps might you use to effect a change in policy on your unit?

Restrictive Cardiomyopathy

The least common form of cardiomyopathy, *restrictive cardiomyopathy* is characterized by rigid ventricular walls that impair diastolic filling. Causes of restrictive cardiomyopathy include myocardial fibrosis and infiltrative processes, such as amyloidosis. Fibrosis of the myocardium and endocardium causes excessive stiffness and rigidity of the ventricles. Decreased ventricular compliance impairs filling, with decreased ventricular size, elevated end-diastolic pressures, and decreased cardiac output. Contractility is unaffected, and the ejection fraction is normal.

MANIFESTATIONS AND COURSE The manifestations of restrictive cardiomyopathy are those of heart failure and decreased tissue perfusion. Dyspnea on exertion and exercise intolerance are common. Jugular venous pressure is elevated, and S_3 and S_4 are common. The prognosis for restrictive cardiomyopathy is poor. Most patients die within 3 years, and the systemic nature of the underlying disease process precludes effective treatment.

Interdisciplinary Care

With the exception of treating an underlying cause, little can be done to treat either dilated or restrictive cardiomyopathies. For these disorders, treatment focuses on managing heart failure and treating dysrhythmias. Refer to the section of this chapter on heart failure and ∞ Chapter 30 for specific treatment strategies. Treatment of hypertrophic cardiomyopathy focuses on reducing contractility and preventing sudden cardiac death. Strenuous physical exertion is restricted, as it may precipitate dysrhythmias or sudden cardiac death. Dietary and sodium restrictions may help diminish the manifestations.

Diagnosis

Diagnosis begins with a history and physical assessment to rule out known causes of heart failure. Other tests may include the following:

- *Echocardiography* is done to assess chamber size and thickness, ventricular wall motion, valvular function, and systolic and diastolic function of the heart.
- *Electrocardiography* and *ambulatory ECG monitoring* demonstrate cardiac enlargement and detect dysrhythmias.
- *Chest x-ray* shows cardiomegaly, enlargement of the heart, and any pulmonary congestion or edema.
- *Hemodynamic studies* are used to assess cardiac output and pressures in the cardiac chambers and pulmonary vascular system.
- *Radionuclear scans* help identify changes in ventricular volume and mass, as well as perfusion deficits.
- *Cardiac catheterization* and *coronary angiography* may be done to evaluate coronary perfusion, the cardiac chambers, valves, and great vessels for function and structure, pressure relationships, and cardiac output.
- *Myocardial biopsy* uses the transvenous route to obtain myocardial tissue for biopsy. The cells are examined for infiltration, fibrosis, or inflammation.

Medications

The drug regimen used to treat heart failure also is used for dilated or restrictive cardiomyopathy. This includes ACE inhibitors, vasodilators, and digitalis (see the previous section of this chapter). Beta blockers also may be used with caution in patients with dilated cardiomyopathy. Anticoagulants are given to reduce the risk of thrombus formation and embolization. Antidysrhythmic drugs are avoided if possible due to their tendency to precipitate further dysrhythmias (Deglin & Vallerand, 2009).

Beta blockers are the drugs of choice to reduce anginal symptoms and syncopal episodes associated with hypertrophic cardiomyopathy. The negative inotropic effects of beta blockers and calcium channel blockers decrease the myocardial contractility, decreasing obstruction of the outflow tract. Beta blockers also decrease heart rate and increase ventricular compliance, increasing diastolic filling time and cardiac output. Vasodilators, digitalis, nitrates, and diuretics are contraindicated. Amiodarone may be used to treat ventricular dysrhythmias (Deglin & Vallerand, 2009).

Surgery

Without definitive treatment, patients with cardiomyopathy develop end-stage heart failure. Cardiac transplant is the definitive treatment for dilated cardiomyopathy. Ventricular assist devices may be used to support cardiac output until a donor heart is available. Transplantation is not a viable option for restrictive cardiomyopathy because transplantation does not eliminate the underlying process causing infiltration or fibrosis, and eventually the transplanted organ is affected as well. See the section on heart failure for more information about cardiac transplantation.

In severely symptomatic patients with obstructive hypertrophic cardiomyopathy, excess muscle may be surgically resected from the aortic valve outflow tract. The septum is incised, and tissue is removed. This procedure provides lasting improvement in about 75% of patients (Papadakis & McPhee, 2007).

An implantable cardioverter-defibrillator (ICD) often is inserted to treat potentially lethal dysrhythmias, reducing the need for antidysrhythmic medications. A dual-chamber pacemaker also may be used for to treat hypertrophic cardiomyopathy.

∽ Nursing Care

Nursing assessment and care for patients with dilated and restrictive cardiomyopathy is similar to that for patients with heart failure. Teaching about the disease process and its management is vital. Some degree of activity restriction often is necessary; assist to conserve energy while encouraging self-care. Support coping skills and adaptation to required lifestyle changes. Provide information and support for decision making about cardiac transplantation if that is an option. Discuss the toxic and vasodilator effects of alcohol, and encourage abstinence. See the nursing care section for heart failure for nursing diagnoses and suggested interventions.

The patient with hypertrophic cardiomyopathy requires care similar to that provided for myocardial ischemia; nitrates and other vasodilators, however, are avoided. If surgery is performed, nursing care is similar to that for any patient undergoing open-heart surgery or cardiac transplant. Discuss the genetic transmission of hypertrophic cardiomyopathy, and suggest screening of close relatives (parents and siblings).

Provide pre- and postoperative care and teaching as appropriate for patients undergoing invasive procedures or surgery for cardiomyopathy.

Nursing diagnoses that may be appropriate for patients with cardiomyopathy include the following:

- *Decreased Cardiac Output* related to impaired left ventricular filling, contractility, or outflow obstruction
- *Fatigue* related to decreased cardiac output
- *Ineffective Breathing Pattern* related to heart failure
- *Fear* related to risk for sudden cardiac death
- *Ineffective Role Performance* related to decreasing cardiac function and activity restrictions
- *Anticipatory Grieving* related to poor prognosis

Community-Based Care

Cardiomyopathies are chronic, progressive disorders generally managed in home and community care settings unless surgery or transplant are planned or end-stage heart failure develops.

When teaching the patient and family for home care, include the following topics.

- Activity restrictions and dietary changes to reduce manifestations and prevent complications
- Prescribed drug regimen, its rationale, intended and possible adverse effects
- The disease process, its expected ultimate outcome, and treatment options
- Cardiac transplantation, including the procedure, the need for lifetime immunosuppression to prevent transplant rejection, and the risks of postoperative infection and long-term immunosuppression
- Symptoms to report to the physician or for which immediate care is needed.
- Cardiopulmonary resuscitation procedures and available training sites

Refer the patient and family for home and social services and counseling as indicated. Provide community resources such as support groups or the AHA.

CHAPTER HIGHLIGHTS

- Heart failure is the most common cardiac disorder, a condition in which the heart is unable to pump effectively to meet the body's needs for blood and oxygen to the tissues.
- Heart failure is due to *impaired myocardial contraction* and is most commonly caused by coronary heart disease and myocardial ischemia or infarct.
- Heart failure can also occur due to long standing *excessive workload* of the heart muscle such as in hypertension or valvular disorders.
- When the heart starts to fail, compensatory mechanisms are activated to help maintain tissue perfusion. While these mechanisms, including increased contractile force, vasoconstriction, sodium and water retention, and remodeling of the heart, effectively maintain cardiac output in the short term, in the long term they hasten deterioration of heart function.
- Goals of heart failure management are to reduce the workload and improve its function. Medical management includes medication use including ACE inhibitors, beta blockers, diuretics and vasodilators to reduce the cardiac workload.
- In 2005, the AHA updated the heart failure guidelines with digitalis no longer recommended due to the risk for digitalis toxicity outweighing the benefit due to the narrow therapeutic window.
- Nursing care of the patient with heart failure is primarily supportive and educative, providing the patient and family with the necessary knowledge and resources to manage this chronic condition.
- Cardiogenic pulmonary edema, a manifestation of severe cardiac decompensation, is a medical emergency, requiring immediate

and effective treatment to preserve life. The nurse's role in managing pulmonary edema focuses on supporting respiratory and cardiac function through careful assessment and early intervention, administering prescribed medications, and providing reassurance to the patient and family.

- Inflammatory and infectious processes, such as rheumatic fever, endocarditis, myocarditis, and pericarditis, can affect any layer of the heart. While some, such as myocarditis and pericarditis, typically are mild and self-limiting, others can have long-term effects on cardiac structure and function.
- Processes such as rheumatic heart disease, endocarditis, and congenital conditions can affect the structure and function of the heart valves, resulting in either stenosis (narrowing) of the valve and restricted flow through it, or regurgitation, backflow of blood through a valve that does not fully close. The mitral and aortic valves are commonly affected due to the higher pressures and increased workload of the left side of the heart.
- Valve disorders may be mild, producing a heart murmur but no functional impairment for the patient, or severe, causing symptoms of heart failure even at rest. Repair or replacement of the valve may ultimately be required.
- Cardiomyopathies affect the heart muscle and its ability to stretch during filling and contact effectively. Dilated cardiomyopathy, the most common type, is progressive, ultimately necessitating heart transplant. Hypertrophic cardiomyopathy affects both ventricular filling and outflow through the aortic valve. Surgical resection of excess tissue may relieve its manifestations.

TEST YOURSELF NCLEX-RN® REVIEW

1. In reviewing the physician's admitting notes for a patient with heart failure, the nurse notes that the patient has an ejection fraction of 25%. The nurse recognizes this as meaning which of the following?
   1. Ventricular function is severely impaired.
   2. The amount of blood being ejected from the ventricles is within normal limits.
   3. Twenty-five percent of the blood entering the ventricle remains in the ventricle after systole.
   4. Cardiac output is greater than normal, overtaxing the heart.

2. In assessing a patient admitted 24 hours previously with heart failure, the nurse notes that the patient has lost 2.5 lb (1 kg) of weight, his heart rate is 88 (HR was 105 on admission), and he now has crackles in the bases of his lung fields only. The nurse correctly interprets this data as indicating which of the following?
   1. The patient's condition is unchanged from admission.
   2. More aggressive treatment is needed.
   3. The treatment regimen is achieving the desired effect.
   4. No further treatment is required at this time as the failure has resolved.

3. The nurse assessing a patient admitted with left ventricular failure would recognize which of the following findings as consistent with the diagnosis? **Select all that apply.**
   1. 5 cm jugular vein distention at 30°
   2. complaints of shortness of breath with minimal exertion
   3. substernal chest pain during exercise
   4. bilateral inspiratory crackles to midscapulae
   5. fatigue

4. The nurse caring for a patient undergoing pulmonary artery pressure monitoring provides appropriate care when he or she does which of the following?
   1. secures the intravenous line to the bed linens
   2. maintains flush solution flow by gravity
   3. reports waveform dampening during wedge pressure measurements
   4. calibrates and levels the system every shift

5. Morphine 2 to 5 mg IV as needed for pain and dyspnea is ordered for a patient in acute pulmonary edema. The nurse appropriately does which of the following?
   1. questions this order because no time intervals have been specified
   2. administers the drug as ordered, monitoring respiratory status
   3. withholds the drug until the patient's respiratory status improves
   4. administers the drug only when the patient complains of chest pain

6. The nurse notes a grating heart sound when auscultating the apical pulse of a patient with pericarditis. The most appropriate response is to do which of the following?
   1. Note the finding in the patient's medical record.
   2. Obtain an electrocardiogram.
   3. Immediately notify the physician.
   4. Initiate resuscitation measures.

7. An appropriate goal of nursing care for the patient with acute infective endocarditis would be which of the following?
   1. "Will resume usual activities within 1 week of treatment."
   2. "Will relate the benign and self-limiting nature of the disease."
   3. "Will consider cardiac transplantation as a viable treatment option."
   4. "Will state the importance of continuing intravenous antibiotic therapy as ordered."

8. An expected assessment finding in a patient with mitral stenosis being admitted for a valve replacement would be which of the following?
   1. muffled heart sounds
   2. S_3 and S_4 heart sounds
   3. diastolic murmur heard at the apex
   4. cardiac heave

9. A patient facing heart valve replacement asks the nurse which type of valve is the best, biologic or mechanical. An appropriate response would be which of the following?
   1. The need to take drugs to prevent rejection of biologic tissue is a major consideration.
   2. Clotting is a risk with mechanical valves, necessitating anticoagulant drug therapy after insertion.
   3. Biologic valves tend to be more durable than mechanical valves.
   4. Endocarditis is a risk following valve replacement; it is more easily treated with mechanical valves.

10. The parents of a young athlete who collapsed and died due to hypertrophic cardiomyopathy ask the nurse how it is possible that their son had no symptoms of this disorder before experiencing sudden cardiac death. The nurse responds with which of the following?
    1. "Exercise causes the heart to contract more forcefully, and can lead to changes in the heart's rhythm or the outflow of blood from the heart in people with hypertrophic cardiomyopathy."
    2. "It is likely that your son had symptoms of the disorder before he died, but he may not have thought them important enough to tell someone about."
    3. "In this type of cardiomyopathy, the ventricle does not fill normally. During exercise, the heart may not be able to meet the body's needs for blood and oxygen."
    4. "Cardiomyopathy results in destruction and scarring of cardiac muscle cells. As a result, the ventricle may rupture during strenuous exercise, leading to sudden death."

See Test Yourself answers in Appendix C.

Pearson Nursing Student Resources
Find additional review materials at
www.nursing.pearsonhighered.com
Prepare for success with additional NCLEX®-style practice questions, interactive assignments and activities, Web links, animations and videos, and more!

BIBLIOGRAPHY

American Heart Association. (2009). Heart disease and stroke statistics – 2009 update. *Circulation 119*, e21–e181.

Bonow, R. O., Carabello, B. A., Chatterjee, K., de Leon, A. C., Faxon, D. P., Freed, M. D., et al. (2006). ACC/AHA 2006 guideline for the management of patients with valvular heart disease. *Journal of the American College of Cardiology, 48*(3), e1–e148.

Bulechek, G., Butcher, H., & Dochterman, J. M. (Eds.). (2008). *Nursing interventions classification (NIC)* (5th ed.). St. Louis: Mosby Elsevier.

Brown, H. (2005). Action stat. Cardiac tamponade. *Nursing, 35*(3), 88.

Carter, T., & Brooks, C. A. (2005). Pericarditis: Inflammation or infarction? *Journal of Cardiovascular Nursing, 20*(4), 239–244.

D'Amico, C. L. (2005). Cardiac transplantation: Patient selection in the current era. *Journal of Cardiovascular Nursing 20*(5 Suppl), S4–S13.

Dearani, J. A., Connolly, H. M., Martinez, R., Fontanet, H. & Webb, G. D. (2007). Caring for adults with congenital cardiac disease: Successes and challenges for 2007 and beyond. *Cardiology in the Young 17*(Suppl 2), 87–96.

Deglin, J. H., & Vallerand, A. H. (2009). *Davis' Drug Guide* (10th ed.). Philadelphia: F.A. Davis.

Domino, F. J., Baldor, R. A., Golding, J., Grimes, J., & Taylor, J. S. (2010). *The 5-minute clinical consult* (18th ed.). Philadelphia: Lippincott, Williams & Wilkins.

Dunbar, S. B., Clark, P. C., Deaton, C., Smith, A. L., De, A. K., & O'Brien, M. C. (2005). Family education and support interventions in heart failure: A pilot study. *Nursing Research, 54*(3), 158–166.

Fontaine, K. L. (2005). *Healing practices: Alternative therapies for nursing* (2nd ed.). Upper Saddle River, NJ: Prentice Hall Health.

Gardetto, N. J. & Carroll, K. C. (2007). Management strategies to meet the core heart failure measures for acute decompensated heart failure: A nursing perspective. *Critical Care Nursing Quarterly 30*(4), 307–320.

Hayes, D. D. (2007). New guidelines for preventing endocarditis. *Nursing 37*(8), 22–23.

Hill, K. M. (2007). Surgical repair of cardiac valves. *Critical Care Nursing Clinics of North America 19*(4), 353–360.

Huether, S. E. & McCance, K. L. (2008). *Understanding Pathophysiology* (4th ed.). St. Louis: Mosby Elsevier.

Hunt, S. A., Abraham, W. T., Chin, M. H., Feldman, A. M., Francis, G. S., Ganiats, T. G., et al. (2005). ACC/AHA 2005 guideline update for the diagnosis and management of chronic heart failure in the adult: A report of the American College of Cardiology / American Heart Association Task Force on Practice Guidelines (Writing Committee to Update the 2001 Guidelines for the Evaluation and Management of Heart Failure). American College of Cardiology website. Retrieved from http://content.onlinejacc.org/cgi/reprint/46/6/e1.pdf

Hodges, P. (2009). Heart failure: Epidemiologic update. *Critical Care Nursing Quarterly 32*(1), 24–32.

Konick-McMahan, J., Bixby, B., & McKenna, C. (2003). Heart failure in older adults. Providing nursing care to improve outcomes. *Journal of Gerontology Nursing, 29*(12), 35–41.

Lichtenstein, A. H., Appel, L. J., Brands, M., Carnethon, M., Daniels, S., France, H. A., et al. (2006). Diet and lifestyle recommendations revision 2006: A scientific statement from the American Heart Association Nutrition Committee. *Circulation 114*(1), 82–96.

McCalmont, V. & Ohler, L. (2008). Cardiac transplantation: Candidate identification, evaluation, and management. *Critical Care Nursing Quarterly 31*(3), 216–219.

Moorhead, S., Johnson, M., Maas, M., & Swanson, E. (Eds.). (2008). *Nursing outcomes classification (NOC)* (4th ed.). St. Louis: Mosby Elsevier.

NANDA International. (2009). *Nursing diagnoses: Definitions and classification 2009–2011.* Oxford, UK: Wiley-Blackwell.

National Heart, Lung, and Blood Institute. National Institutes of Health. (2007). *Morbidity & mortality: 2007 chart book of cardiovascular, lung, and blood diseases.* Bethesda, MD: Author.

Papadakis, M. A. & McPhee, S. J. (2007). *Current consult medicine 2007.* New York: McGraw-Hill.

Payne-Emerson, H. & Lennie, T. A. (2008). Nutritional considerations in heart failure. *Nursing Clinics of North America, 43*(1), 117–132.

Perrin, K. O. (2009). *Understanding the Essentials of Critical Care Nursing.* Upper Saddle River, NJ: Pearson Prentice-Hall.

Quinn, B. (2007). Pharmacological treatment of heart failure. *Critical Care Nursing Quarterly 30*(4), 299–306.

Reimer-Kent, J. (2007). Infective endocarditis: A review and update of a clinical enigma. *Canadian Journal of Cardiovascular Nursing 17*(3), 5–12.

Rock-Prior, P. (2004). Variables predictive of poor postdischarge outcomes for hospitalized elders in heart failure. *Western Journal of Nursing Research, 26*(5), 533–546.

Sauls, J. L., & Rone, T. (2005). Emerging trends in the management of heart failure: Beta blocker therapy. *Nursing Clinics of North America, 40*(1), 135–148.

Scott, L. D., Setter-Kline, K., & Britton, A. S. (2004). The effects of nursing interventions to enhance mental health and quality of life among individuals with heart failure. *Applied Nursing Research, 17*(4), 248–256.

Simmonds-Holcomb, S. (2006). Recognizing and managing different types of carditis. *Nursing, 36*(Suppl Cardiac), 4–9.

Sims, J. M. & Miracle, V. A. (2007). An overview of mitral valve prolapse. *Dimensions of Critical Care Nursing 26*(4), 145–149.

Spencer, J. W., & Jacobs, J. J. (2003). *Complementary and alternative medicine: An evidence-based approach* (2nd ed.). St. Louis: Mosby.

Stahovich, M., Chillcott, S., Dembitsky, W. P. (2007). The next treatment option: Using ventricular assist devices for heart failure. *Critical Care Nursing Quarterly, 30*(4), 337–346.

Wadas, T. M. (2005). The implantable hemodynamic monitoring system. *Critical care Nurse, 25*(5), 14–16, 18–20, 22–24, 26.

Wade, C. R., Reith, K. K., Sikora, J. H., & Augustine, S. M. (2004). Postoperative nursing care of the cardiac transplant recipient. *Critical Care Nursing Quarterly, 27*(1), 17–28.

Warnes, C. A., Williams, R. G., Bashore, T. M., Child, J. S., Connolly, H. M., Dearani, J. A., et al. (2008). ACC/AHA 2008 guidelines for the management of adults with congenital heart disease: A report of the American College of Cardiology/American Heart Association Task Force on Practice Guidelines. *Journal of the American College of Cardiology 52* (23), e1-e121.

Way, L. W., & Doherty, G. M. (2003). *Current surgical diagnosis & treatment* (11th ed.). New York: Lange Medical/McGraw-Hill.

Wheeler, E. C., Klemm, P., Hardic, T., Plowfield, L., Birney, M., Polek, C., & Lynch, K. G. (2004). Racial disparities in hospitalized elderly patients with chronic heart failure. *Journal of Transcultural Nursing, 15*(4), 291–297.

White, R. M. (2005). The role of brain natriuretic peptide in systolic heart failure. *Dimensions of Critical Care Nursing, 24*(4), 171–174.

Wilson, W., Taubert, K. A., Gewitz, M. Lockhart, P. B., Baddour, L. M., Levison, M. et al. (2007). Prevention of infective endocarditis: Guidelines from the American Heart Association. *Circulation, 116*(15), 1736–1754.

Winters, M. & Obriot, P. (2007). Mitral valve repair. *AORN Journal 85*(1), 152–166.

Woods, S. L., Froelicher, E. S., Motzer, S. A., & Bridges, E. (2004). *Cardiac nursing* (5th ed.). Philadelphia: Lippincott.

Wu, J-R., Moser, D. K., Lennie, T. A. & Burkhart, P. V. (2008). Medication adherence in patients who have heart failure: A review of the literature. *Nursing Clinics of North America 43*(1), 133–153.

32 Nursing Care of Patients with Vascular and Lymphatic Disorders

LEARNING OUTCOMES

1. Compare and contrast the manifestations and effects of disorders affecting large and small vessels, arteries, and veins.
2. Explain risk factors for and measures to prevent peripheral vascular disorders and their complications.
3. Explain the nursing implications for medications and other interdisciplinary treatments used for patients with peripheral vascular disorders.
4. Describe preoperative and postoperative nursing care of patients having vascular surgery.
5. Relate the manifestations and diagnostic test results to the etiology, and pathophysiology of common peripheral vascular and lymphatic disorders.

CLINICAL COMPETENCIES

1. Assess patients with peripheral vascular disorders, using data to select and prioritize appropriate nursing diagnoses and identify desired outcomes of care.
2. Identify the effects of peripheral vascular disorders on the functional health status of assigned patients.
3. Use research and an evidence base to plan and provide individualized care for patients with peripheral vascular disorders.
4. Collaborate with the interdisciplinary care team in planning and providing care for patients with peripheral vascular disorders.
5. Safely and knowledgably administer medications and prescribed treatments for patients with peripheral vascular disorders.
6. Provide patient and family teaching to promote, maintain, and restore health in patients with common peripheral vascular disorders.

KEY TERMS

aneurysm, *1034*
atherosclerosis, *1040*
blood pressure, *1018*
chronic venous insufficiency, *1057*
deep venous thrombosis (DVT), *1050*
diastolic blood pressure, *1019*
dissection, *1036*
embolism, *1047*
hypertension, *1019*

intermittent claudication, *1036*
lymphedema, *1062*
mean arterial pressure (MAP), *1019*
peripheral vascular disease (PVD), *1040*
primary hypertension, *1019*
pulse pressure, *1019*
Raynaud's disease/phenomenon, *1046*
secondary hypertension, *1032*

systolic blood pressure, *1019*
thromboangiitis obliterans, *1045*
thromboembolus, *1047*
thrombus, *1047*
varicose veins, *1059*
vasoconstriction, *1040*
vasodilation, *1040*
venous thrombosis, *1050*

The major processes that interfere with peripheral blood flow and that of lymphatic fluid include constriction, obstruction, inflammation, and vasospasm. These conditions lead to disorders of blood pressure regulation, peripheral artery function, aortic structure, venous circulation, and lymphatic circulation.

A holistic approach is important when caring for patients with disorders of the peripheral vascular and lymphatic systems. The focus of care is on teaching long-term care measures, pain relief, improving peripheral blood and lymphatic circulation, preventing tissue damage, and promoting healing. The prescribed treatment may have emotional, social, and economic effects on the patient and family.

Disorders of Blood Pressure Regulation

Blood flows through the circulatory system from areas of higher pressure to areas of lower pressure. The amount of pressure in any portion of the vascular system is affected by a number of factors, including blood volume, vascular resistance, and cardiac output. The **blood pressure** is the tension or pressure exerted by blood against arterial walls. A certain amount of pressure within the system is necessary to maintain open vessels, capillary perfusion, and oxygenation of all body tissues. Excess pressure, however, has harmful effects, increasing the workload of the heart, altering the structure of the vessels, and affecting sensitive body tissues such as the kidneys, eyes, and central nervous system.

This section focuses on **hypertension**, or excess pressure in the arterial portion of systemic circulation. Excessively low blood pressure, *hypotension*, is discussed in the shock section of ∞ Chapter 11. Altered pulmonary vascular pressures are discussed in ∞ Chapter 37.

Physiology Review

Blood flow through the circulatory system requires *sufficient blood volume* to fill the blood vessels and *pressure differences* within the system that allow blood to move forward. The arterial, or supply side, of the circulation has relatively high pressures created by the thick elastic walls of the arteries and arterioles. The venous, or return side of the system, on the other hand, is a low pressure system of thin-walled, distensible veins. Blood flows through the capillaries linking these two systems from the higher pressure arterial side to the lower pressure venous side.

The arterial blood pressure is created by the ejection of blood from the heart during systole (*cardiac output* or *CO*) and the tension, or resistance to blood flow, created by the elastic arterial walls (*systemic vascular resistance* or *SVR*). The blood pressure rises as the heart contracts during systole, ejecting its blood. This pressure wave, or the **systolic blood pressure**, is felt as the peripheral pulse and heard as the Korotkoff's sounds during blood pressure measurement. In healthy adults the average systolic pressure is less than 120 mmHg. During diastole, or cardiac relaxation and filling, elastic arterial walls maintain a minimum pressure, the **diastolic blood pressure**, to maintain blood flow through the capillary beds. The average diastolic pressure in a healthy adult is less than 80 mmHg. The difference between the systolic and diastolic pressure, normally about 40 mmHg, is known as the **pulse pressure**. The **mean arterial pressure (MAP)** is the average pressure in the arterial circulation throughout the cardiac cycle. It can be calculated using the formula [systolic BP + 2 (diastolic BP)] / 3.

> **FAST FACTS**
> - Cardiac output and systemic (or peripheral) vascular resistance are the primary factors that determine blood pressure.
> - A decrease in cardiac output (e.g., due to hemorrhage) or decreased peripheral vascular resistance (e.g., systemic vasodilation) cause the blood pressure to fall.

Increased cardiac output (e.g., during exercise) or increased peripheral vascular resistance (e.g., vasoconstriction due to drug administration) cause the blood pressure to rise. Cardiac output is determined by the blood volume and the ability of the ventricles to fill and effectively pump that blood. A number of factors contribute to systemic vascular resistance, including vessel length, blood viscosity, and vessel diameter and distensibility (compliance). While vessel length and blood viscosity remain relatively constant, vessel diameter and compliance are subject to normal regulatory activities and disease.

The arterioles normally determine the SVR as their diameter changes in response to a variety of stimuli:

- *Sympathetic nervous system (SNS)* stimulation. Baroreceptors in the aortic arch and carotid sinus signal the SNS via the cardiovascular control center in the medulla when the MAP changes. A drop in MAP stimulates the SNS, increasing the heart rate, cardiac output, and constricting arterioles (except in skeletal muscle). As a result, BP rises. A rise in MAP has the opposite effect, decreasing the heart rate and cardiac output, and causing arteriolar vasodilation.
- *Circulating epinephrine and norepinephrine* from the adrenal cortex (e.g., the fight-or-flight response) have the same effect as SNS stimulation.
- *Renin-angiotensin-aldosterone system* responds to renal perfusion. A drop in renal perfusion stimulates renin release. Renin converts angiotensinogen to angiotensin I, which is subsequently converted to angiotensin II in the lungs by angiotensin-converting enzyme (ACE). Angiotensin II is a potent vasoconstrictor. It also promotes sodium and water retention both directly and by stimulating the adrenal medulla to release aldosterone. Both SVR and CO increase, raising BP.
- *Atrial natriuretic peptide* is released from atrial cells in response to stretching by excess blood volume. It promotes vasodilation and sodium and water excretion, lowering BP.
- *Adrenomedullin* is a peptide synthesized and released by endothelial and smooth muscle cells in blood vessels. It is a potent vasodilator.
- *Vasopressin* or *antidiuretic hormone* (from the posterior pituitary gland) promotes water retention and vasoconstriction, raising BP.
- *Local factors* such as inflammatory mediators and various metabolites can promote vasodilation, affecting BP.

In addition to the preceding stimuli, the primary factor affecting vessel compliance is the extent of arteriosclerosis (hardening of the arteries) and atherosclerosis (plaque accumulation). Figure 32–1 ■ summarizes the interrelationships of major factors regulating blood pressure.

> **FAST FACTS**
> - Sympathetic nervous system stimulation, epinephrine and norepinephrine, and the hormones angiotensin II and vasopressin (antidiuretic hormone or ADH) are *vasoconstrictors*, increasing the blood pressure.
> - Parasympathetic nervous system stimulation and the hormones atrial natriuretic peptide and adrenomedullin are *vasodilators*, decreasing the blood pressure
> - The hormones aldosterone and ADH promote sodium and water retention, increasing the blood pressure.

The Patient with Primary Hypertension

Primary hypertension, also known as *essential hypertension*, is a persistently elevated systemic blood pressure. One in three or 73.6 million people in the United States have hypertension (American Heart Association [AHA], 2009). More than 90% of these have primary hypertension, which has no identified cause.

Hypertension is defined as systolic blood pressure of 140 mmHg or higher, or diastolic pressure of 90 mmHg or higher, based on the average of three or more readings taken on separate occasions (NHLBI, 2004). Exceptions include patients

Figure 32–1 ■ Factors affecting blood pressure.

being treated for hypertension and an initial reading of a systolic pressure of 210 mmHg or higher and/or a diastolic blood pressure of 120 mmHg or higher. Table 32–1 identifies classifications of blood pressure for adults aged 18 and older as defined by the Joint National Committee.

Hypertension is an important public health issue: While it rarely causes symptoms or noticeably limits the patient's functional health, hypertension is a major risk factor for coronary heart disease, heart failure, stroke, and renal failure. Hypertension and its consequences are not unique to the United States. The World Health Organization identifies blood pressure above optimal levels (a systolic BP > 115 mmHg) as responsible for 62% of cerebrovascular disease and 49% of ischemic heart disease worldwide (NHLBI, 2004).

While the identification and treatment of hypertension in the United States has improved significantly in the past 25 years,

approximately 30% of hypertensive adults remain unaware of their condition. Although 59% of hypertensive adults are being treated for the disorder, effective blood pressure control is achieved in only about 34% (NHLBI, 2004).

Pathophysiology

Primary hypertension is thought to develop from complex interactions among factors that regulate cardiac output and systemic vascular resistance. These interactions may include the following:

- Excess sympathetic nervous system with overstimulation of α- and β-adrenergic receptors, resulting in vasoconstriction and increased cardiac output.
- Altered function of the renin-angiotensin-aldosterone system and its responsiveness to factors such as sodium intake and overall fluid volume. The renin-angiotensin-aldosterone system affects vasomotor tone and salt and water excretion. Chronically high levels of angiotensin II lead to arteriolar remodeling, which permanently increases SVR. In approximately 20% of people with primary hypertension, renin levels are lower than normal. Increased sodium intake increases the blood pressure in these patients. Low plasma renin levels are more commonly seen in African Americans than in Whites. Another 15% of patients with hypertension have higher than normal plasma renin levels. For these patients, salt intake has less of an effect on blood pressure (Huether & McCance, 2008). Most people with hypertension have normal levels of renin activity.
- Other chemical mediators of vasomotor tone and blood volume such as atrial natriuretic peptide (factor) also play a role by affecting vasomotor tone and sodium and water excretion. Vascular endothelium itself produces hormones (*endothelins*)

TABLE 32–1 Classification of Blood Pressure for Adults*

CATEGORY	SYSTOLIC (mmHG)		DIASTOLIC (mmHG)
Normal	< 120	and	< 80
Prehypertension	120–139	or	80–89
Hypertension‡			
Stage 1	140–159	or	90–99
Stage 2	≥ 160	or	≥ 100

*When systolic and diastolic blood pressures fall into different categories, the higher category is used to classify blood pressure status.

‡Based on the average of two or more readings taken at each of two or more visits after an initial screening.

Note: Adapted from NHLBI. (2004). *The Seventh Report of the Joint Cardional Committee on Prevention, Detection, Education, and Treatment of High Blood Pressure,* NIH Publication No. 04-5250. Bethesda, MD: National Institutes of Health. Retrieved from http://www.nhlbi.nih.gov/guidelines/hypertension

that also affect vasomotor tone. Endothelin-1 is a potent vasoconstrictor (Huether & McCance, 2008).

■ The interaction between insulin resistance, hyperinsulinemia and endothelial function may be a primary cause of hypertension. Excess insulin has several effects that potentially contribute to hypertension: (1) sodium retention by the kidneys, (2) increased sympathetic nervous system activity, (3) hypertrophy of vascular smooth muscle, and (4) changes in ion transport across cell membranes (Huether & McCance, 2008).

The result is sustained increases in blood volume and peripheral resistance. The cardiovascular system adapts to increased blood volume by increasing cardiac output. Autoregulatory mechanisms in the systemic arteries react to the increased volume, causing vasoconstriction. The increased systemic vascular resistance causes hypertension.

It appears unlikely that one single cause and pathologic process will be found to account for essential hypertension. Increasingly, evidence points to hypertension as a diverse group of pathophysiologic mechanisms resulting in the common manifestation of elevated blood pressure.

Manifestations

The early stages of primary hypertension typically are asymptomatic, marked only by elevated blood pressure. Blood pressure elevations are initially transient but eventually become permanent. When symptoms do appear, they are usually vague. Headache, usually in the back of the head and neck, may be present on awakening, subsiding during the day. Other symptoms result from target organ damage, and may include nocturia, confusion, nausea and vomiting, and visual disturbances. Examination of the retina of the eye may reveal narrowed arterioles, hemorrhages, exudates, and *papilledema* (swelling of the optic nerve).

Complications

Sustained hypertension affects the cardiovascular, neurologic, and renal systems. The rate of atherosclerosis accelerates, increasing the risk for coronary heart disease and stroke. The workload of the left ventricle increases, leading to ventricular hypertrophy, which then increases the risk for coronary heart disease, dysrhythmias, and heart failure. The diastolic blood pressure is a significant cardiovascular risk factor until age 50; the systolic pressure then becomes the more important factor contributing to cardiovascular risk (NHLBI, 2004). Most deaths due to hypertension result from coronary heart disease and acute myocardial infarction or heart failure.

Accelerated atherosclerosis associated with hypertension increases the risk for cerebral infarction (stroke). Increased pressure in the cerebral vessels can lead to development of microaneurysms and an increased risk for cerebral hemorrhage. *Hypertensive encephalopathy*, a syndrome characterized by extremely high blood pressure; altered level of consciousness, increased intracranial pressure, papilledema, and seizures may develop. Its etiology is unclear.

Hypertension also can lead to nephrosclerosis and renal insufficiency. Proteinuria and microscopic hematuria develop, as well as signs of chronic renal failure. African Americans experience hypertensive kidney disease more frequently than Whites.

Incidence and Risk Factors

Hypertension primarily affects middle-aged and older adults: More than 50% of people age 60 to 74 and about 75% of those 75 and older are hypertensive (AHA, 2009). An age-related increase in the systolic blood pressure is the primary factor leading to the high incidence of hypertension in older adults. Unlike the diastolic blood pressure, which tends to rise until approximately age 50, then level off, the systolic blood pressure continues to rise with aging (NHLBI, 2004).

The prevalence of hypertension is significantly higher in Blacks than in Whites and Hispanics. Nearly 40% of Black adults are hypertensive, whereas less than 30% of adult White and Hispanic people are affected. In Whites and Hispanics, more males than females are hypertensive; in Blacks, more women than men are affected (NHLBI, 2004b).

FAST FACTS
■ Almost 1/3 of the adult population in the United States has hypertension.
■ The prevalence of hypertension is highest in African American females and lowest in people of Asian ancestry.
■ The prevalence of hypertension is higher among people who live in the southeastern United States.
■ Up until age 45, more men than women are affected by hypertension; after that it affects more women than men.
■ Hypertension increases the risk of stroke to about four times that of people with normal blood pressure, and the risk for heart failure by two to three times that of people with normal blood pressure (AHA, 2009).

A number of risk factors have been identified for primary hypertension (Box 32–1). Genetics play a role, as do environmental factors.

■ *Family history.* Studies show a genetic link in up to 40% of people with primary hypertension (Huether & McCance, 2008). Genes involved in the renin-angiotensin-aldosterone system and others that affect vascular tone, salt and water transportation in the kidney, obesity, and insulin resistance are likely involved in the development of hypertension, although no consistent genetic linkages have been found.

■ *Age.* The incidence of hypertension rises with increasing age. Aging affects baroreceptors involved in blood pressure regulation as well as arterial compliance. As the arteries become less compliant, pressure within the vessels increases. This is often most apparent as a gradual increase in the systolic pressure with aging. See the Nursing Care of the Older Adult box on page 1022.

BOX 32–1 Factors Contributing to Hypertension

Modifiable Factors
■ High sodium intake
■ Low potassium, calcium, and magnesium intake
■ Obesity
■ Excess alcohol consumption
■ Insulin resistance

Nonmodifiable Factors
■ Genetic factors
■ Family history
■ Age
■ Race

- *Race.* Primary hypertension is more common and more severe in Blacks than in people of other ethnic backgrounds (see the accompanying diversity box). It also tends to develop at an earlier age, and is associated with more cardiovascular and renal damage. More African Americans with hypertension have low renin levels and altered renal excretion of sodium at normal blood pressure levels. This genetic tendency to conserve salt may have developed as an adaptation to working in a warm environment, when salt and water conservation are beneficial (Huether & McCance, 2008).
- *Mineral intake.* High sodium intake often is associated with fluid retention. Hypertension related to sodium intake involves a number of different physiologic mechanisms, including the renin-angiotensin-aldosterone system, nitric oxide, catecholamines, endothelin, and atrial natriuretic peptide. Low potassium, calcium, and magnesium intakes also contribute to hypertension by unknown mechanisms. The ratio of sodium to potassium intake appears to play a role, possibly through the effects of increased potassium intake on sodium excretion. Potassium also promotes vasodilation by reducing responses to catacholamines and angiotensin II. Calcium also has a vasodilator effect. While magnesium has been shown to reduce the blood pressure, the mechanism of action is unclear (Huether & McCance, 2008).
- *Obesity.* Central obesity (fat cell deposits in the abdomen), determined by an increased waist-to-hip ratio, has a stronger correlation with hypertension than body mass index or skinfold thickness. Although a clear correlation exists between obesity and hypertension, the relationship may be one common cause: Genetic factors appear to play a role in the common triad of obesity, hypertension, and insulin resistance.
- *Insulin resistance.* Insulin resistance with resulting hyperinsulinemia is linked with hypertension by its effects on the sympathetic nervous system, vascular smooth muscle, renal regulation of sodium and water, and changes ion transport across cell membranes. Insulin resistance may be a genetic or an acquired trait. While it is more commonly seen in obese individuals, insulin resistance also has been found in people of normal weight.
- *Excess alcohol consumption.* Regular consumption of three or more drinks a day increases the risk of hypertension.

FOCUS ON CULTURAL DIVERSITY
Hypertension in African Americans

- The prevalence of hypertension among Blacks living in the United States is among the highest in the world: In Black adults, 41.8% of males and 45.4% of females are hypertensive.
- African Americans with the highest risk for hypertension tend to be the following:
  - Middle aged or older
  - Less educated
  - Overweight or obese
  - Physically inactive
  - Affected by diabetes (AHA, 2005)

Decreasing or discontinuing alcohol consumption reduces the blood pressure, particularly systolic readings. Lifestyle factors associated with excessive alcohol intake (obesity and lack of exercise) may contribute to hypertension as well.

- *Stress.* Physical and emotional stress cause transient elevations of blood pressure, but the role of stress in primary hypertension is less clear. Blood pressure normally fluctuates throughout the day, increasing with activity, discomfort, or emotional responses such as anger. Frequent or continued stress may cause vascular smooth muscle hypertrophy or affect central integrative pathways of the brain.

Interdisciplinary Care

Hypertension management focuses on reducing the blood pressure to less than 140 mmHg systolic and 90 mmHg diastolic. The ultimate goal of hypertension management is to reduce cardiovascular and renal morbidity and mortality. The risk of cardiovascular complications (coronary heart disease, heart failure, stroke) decreases when the average blood pressure is less than 140/90; when the patient also has diabetes or renal disease, the treatment goal is a blood pressure less than 130/80. It now is recognized that most people with hypertension will require a combination of two or more drugs along with lifestyle changes to achieve recommended blood pressure levels (NHLBI, 2004). While there is no cure for hypertension, it can be controlled. Figure 32–2 ■ shows the recommended algorithm for hypertension management.

NURSING CARE OF THE OLDER ADULT   Hypertension

Controlling high blood pressure is as important in the older adult as in younger adults. In the United States, the lifetime risk of hypertension is about 90% in men and women who live to age 80 to 85 (AHA 2009). Systolic hypertension is common, as is an elevated pulse pressure (systolic BP minus diastolic BP), indicating decreased compliance of large arteries. Despite this fact, less than two-thirds of people over age 80 who have high blood pressure are being treated and only 38% of men and 23% of women undergoing treatment had blood pressures that met established targets (NHLBI, 2005).

The Framingham Heart Study shows that cardiovascular deaths are two to five times more common in older adults with isolated systolic hypertension than in people with normal blood pressures. Stroke also is more common in older adults with systolic hypertension. These findings appear to relate to changes in blood vessels associated with aging: decreased compliance and decreased baroreceptor sensitivity. Decreased compliance impairs the ability of the vessels to expand and contract with varying amounts of blood, increasing peripheral vascular resistance and decreasing renal blood flow.

To obtain accurate blood pressure readings for older patients, slightly different procedures may be required. Palpation of the artery during cuff inflation is recommended to prevent inaccurate systolic readings due to an auscultatory gap, present in many older adults. The reflexes that maintain blood pressure during position changes diminish with aging. Allow the older patient to sit upright or stand for two to five minutes before evaluating the blood pressure for true orthostatic readings.

Figure 32–2 ■ Algorithm for treating hypertension.

Note: Adapted from National Heart, Lung, and Blood Institute. (2004). *The Seventh Report of the Joint National Committee on Prevention, Detection, Evaluation, and Treatment of High Blood Pressure.* Bethesda, MD: National Institutes of Health.

Diagnosis

The patient with hypertension is evaluated for the presence of identifiable causes of hypertension, cardiovascular risk factors, and the presence or absence of target organ damage (heart, brain, kidneys, peripheral vascular systems, and retina of the eye). Before treatment is started, the following diagnostic tests are performed:

- Electrocardiogram (ECG)
- Urinalysis
- Blood glucose
- Hematocrit
- Serum potassium, creatinine, and calcium
- Cholesterol and lipoprotein profile, including HDL, LDL, and triglycerides

Additional tests that may be done include urinary albumin excretion, evaluation of the glomerular filtration rate (such as

the creatinine clearance), and tests for emerging cardiovascular risk factors such as C-reactive protein and homocystine levels.

Lifestyle Modifications

Lifestyle modifications are recommended for all patients whose blood pressure falls within the prehypertension range (120–139/80–89) and everyone with intermittent or sustained hypertension. These modifications include weight loss, dietary changes, restricted alcohol use and cigarette smoking, increased physical activity, and stress reduction (Box 32–2).

DIET Dietary approaches to managing hypertension focus on reducing sodium intake, maintaining adequate potassium and calcium intakes, and reducing total and saturated fat intake. A mild to moderate sodium restriction (no added salt) lowers blood pressure and potentiates the effect of antihypertensive drugs for most hypertensive patients. The DASH (Dietary

- Maintain normal body weight; lose weight if overweight.
- Make dietary modifications:
  - Eat a diet rich in fruits, vegetables, and low-fat dairy products.
  - Reduce sodium intake.
  - Reduce intake of cholesterol, total and saturated fat.
- Limit alcohol intake to no more than 1 oz of ethanol (1/2 oz for women and lighter weight people) per day.
- Engage in aerobic exercise for 30 minutes most days of the week (5 to 6).
- Stop smoking.
- Use stress management techniques such as relaxation therapy.

Approaches to Stop Hypertension) diet has proven beneficial effects in lowering blood pressure. This diet (Box 32–3) focuses on whole foods rather than individual nutrients. It is rich in fruits and vegetables (up to 10 servings per day), and low in total and saturated fats (NHLBI, 2003).

Weight loss is recommended for patients who are obese. Loss of as little as 10 pounds (4.5 kg) reduces blood pressure in many people (NHLBI, 2004). A balanced diet such as the DASH diet is recommended for weight loss.

PHYSICAL ACTIVITY   Regular exercise (such as walking, cycling, jogging, or swimming) reduces blood pressure and contributes to weight loss, stress reduction, and feelings of overall well-being. Previously sedentary patients are encouraged to engage in aerobic exercise for 30 to 45 minutes per day most days of the week (5 to 6 days). Isometric exercise (such as weight training) may not be appropriate, as it can raise the systolic blood pressure.

ALCOHOL AND TOBACCO USE   The recommended alcohol intake for patients with hypertension is no more than one ounce of ethanol or two drinks per day. A drink is 12 oz of beer, 5 oz of wine, or 1.5 oz of 80-proof whiskey. Women and lighter-weight people should reduce this limit by half. Although alcohol withdrawal may increase blood pressure, this is usually temporary and diminishes as abstinence or restricted intake continues.

Although nicotine is a vasoconstrictor, substantial data linking smoking to hypertension are lacking. A definitive link exists between smoking and heart disease, however. Patients who smoke are strongly urged to quit. Smoking also reduces the effect of some antihypertensive medications such as propranolol (Inderal). Smoking cessation aids such as nicotine patches and gum contain lower amounts of nicotine and usually do not raise blood pressure.

- Grains—seven to eight servings per day
- Vegetables—four to five servings per day
- Fruits—four to five servings per day
- Nonfat/low-fat dairy products—two to three servings per day
- Meats, poultry, and fish—two or less 3 oz servings per day
- Nuts, seeds, and dry beans—four to five servings per week
- Fats and oils—two to three servings per day
- Sweets—five servings per week (should be low in fat)

STRESS REDUCTION   Stress stimulates the sympathetic nervous system, increasing vasoconstriction, systemic vascular resistance, cardiac output, and the blood pressure. Regular, moderate exercise is the treatment of choice for reducing stress in hypertensive patients. Relaxation techniques such as biofeedback, therapeutic touch, yoga, and meditation to relax both mind and body may also lower blood pressure, although their effect has not been proven in hypertension management.

Medications

Current pharmacologic treatment of hypertension involves using one or more of the following drug classes: diuretics, beta-adrenergic blockers, centrally acting sympatholytics, vasodilators, angiotensin-converting enzyme (ACE) inhibitors, angiotensin II receptor blockers (ARBs), and calcium channel blockers. For most patients, two or more antihypertensive drugs selected from different drug classes are necessary to achieve effective control. These drug classes have different sites of action (Figure 32–3 ■). Nursing implications for administration of antihypertensive drugs (other than diuretics) are outlined in the Medication Administration feature on pages 1025–1026.

DRUG CLASSES   Diuretics are the preferred treatment for systolic hypertension in older adults. Diuretics are relatively safe and well-tolerated drugs; in addition, most are relatively inexpensive. Thiazide diuretics, such as hydrochlorothiazide (HydroDIURIL), are widely used. In major clinical studies, treatment with a single diuretic controlled blood pressure in about 50% of the patients and reduced hypertension-linked morbidity and mortality related to coronary heart disease. Diuretics control hypertension primarily by preventing tubular reabsorption of sodium, thus promoting sodium and water excretion and reducing blood volume. Thiazide diuretics also reduce systemic vascular resistance through an unknown mechanism. Diuretics are particularly effective in Blacks and in patients who are obese, older, or who have increased plasma volume or low renin activity. The adverse effects of diuretics generally are dose related. In addition to hypokalemia, diuretics may affect serum levels of glucose, triglycerides, uric acid, low-density lipoproteins, and insulin. More information about diuretics can be found in ∞ Chapters 10 and 28.

Patients with heart failure, coronary heart disease, or diabetes may initially be treated with a beta blocker. These drugs lower blood pressure, apparently by reducing peripheral vascular resistance. They may also reduce the amount of renin released by the kidneys by blocking beta$_1$ receptors in the kidney. Beta blockers reduce the risk of complications such as heart failure and stroke. They are, however, relatively contraindicated for patients with asthma or chronic obstructive pulmonary disease, as they promote bronchial constriction.

ACE inhibitors and ARBs also are commonly used in initial treatment of hypertension, particularly for patients who are diabetic or who have heart failure, a history of MI, or chronic kidney disease. ACE inhibitors block formation of angiotensin II by inhibiting the action of angiotensin-converting enzyme. Angiotensin II is a potent vasoconstrictor that also stimulates aldosterone release from the adrenal gland; blocking its action prevents vasoconstriction and sodium and water retention resulting from aldosterone release. ARBs have a very similar effect,

MEDICATION ADMINISTRATION Antihypertensive Drugs

ALPHA-ADRENERGIC BLOCKERS

Doxazosin (Cardura)

Prazosin (Minipress)

Terazosin (Hytrin)

Alpha-adrenergic blocking agents block alpha receptors in vascular smooth muscle, decreasing vasomotor tone and vasoconstriction. They also reduce serum levels of low-density (LDL) and very low-density lipoproteins (VLDL). However, vasodilation may cause orthostatic hypotension and reflex stimulation of the heart, resulting in tachycardia and palpitations. A beta blocker may be ordered to minimize this effect.

Nursing Responsibilities

- Give the first dose at bedtime to minimize risk of fainting (called "first-dose syncope"). If the first dose is given in the daytime (or if the dose is increased), instruct to remain in bed for 3 to 4 hours.
- Assess blood pressure and apical pulse before each dose and as indicated thereafter.

Health Education for the Patient and Family

- There is a risk of fainting after taking the first dose of this drug. Take the drug at bedtime to reduce this risk, and do not drive or engage in other hazardous activities for 12 to 24 hours after the first dose.
- This drug may cause dizziness or lightheadedness. Change positions slowly, and sit down if you become dizzy or lightheaded.
- Notify your primary care provider if you develop nasal congestion or impotence while taking this drug.
- Notify your primary care provider before discontinuing this medication.

ANGIOTENSIN-CONVERTING ENZYME (ACE) INHIBITORS

Benazepril (Lotensin)	Moexipril (Univasc)
Captopril (Capoten)	Perindopril (Aceon)
Enalapril (Vasotec)	Quinapril (Accupril)
Fosinopril (Monopril)	Ramipril (Altace)
Lisinopril (Prinivil, Zestril)	Trandolapril (Mavik)

Angiotensin II Receptor Blockers (ARBs)

Candesartan (Atacand)	Olmesartan (Benicar)
Eprosartan (Teveten)	Telmisartan (Micardis)
Irbersartan (Avapro)	Valsartan (Diovan)
Losartan (Cozaar)	

The ACE inhibitors lower blood pressure by preventing conversion of angiotensin I to angiotensin II. This in turn prevents vasoconstriction and sodium and water retention. Angiotensin II receptor blockers (ARBs) have the same effect, but they act by blocking the effect of angiotensin II on receptors. Both ACE inhibitors and ARBs are less effective in Black patients and are contraindicated in pregnancy (Deglin & Vallerand, 2009). Their primary adverse effects are persistent cough, first-dose hypotension, and hyperkalemia.

Nursing Responsibilities

- Assess blood pressure and WBC before giving the first dose. Monitor blood pressure for 2 hours after the first dose and regularly thereafter.
- Administer PO 1 hour before meals; tablets may be crushed.

- Report changes in WBC or differential, hyperkalemia, or changes in BUN or serum creatinine to the primary care provider.
- Do not administer to patients with renal artery stenosis or who are pregnant.
- Immediately report and treat manifestations of angioedema (giant wheals and edema of the tongue, glottis, and pharynx). Initiate resuscitation measures as needed. Discontinue drug immediately and do not use in the future.

Health Education for the Patient and Family

- Report peripheral edema, signs of infection, or difficulty breathing to your primary care provider.
- Change position (lying to sitting and sitting to standing) slowly to prevent dizziness; sit down if dizziness or light-headedness develops.
- Do not take a potassium supplement or use a potassium-based salt substitute while taking this drug unless prescribed by your healthcare provider.
- Notify your healthcare provider if you become pregnant while taking this drug. Although it is safe early in pregnancy, taking the drug during the second and third trimesters may harm the fetus.

BETA-ADRENERGIC BLOCKING AGENTS

Acebutolol (Sectral)	Nadolol (Corgard)
Atenolol (Tenormin)	Nebivolol (Bystolic)
Betaxolol (Kerlone)	Penbutolol (Levatol)
Bisoprolol (Zebeta)	Pindolol (Visken)
Carteolol (Cartrol)	Propranolol (Inderal)
Esmolol (Brevibloc)	Sotalol (Betapace)
Metoprolol tartrate (Lopressor)	Timolol (Blocadren)

Combined with an alpha-blocker:

Carvedilol (Coreg)   Labetalol (Normodyne)

Beta-adrenergic blockers are commonly used to control hypertension. Beta blockers reduce blood pressure by preventing beta-receptor stimulation in the heart, thereby decreasing heart rate and cardiac output. Beta blockers also interfere with renin release by the kidneys, decreasing the effects of angiotensin and aldosterone. Potential adverse effects of beta blockers include bronchospasm, fatigue, sleep disturbances, nightmares, bradycardia, heart block, worsening of heart failure, gastrointestinal disturbances, impotence, and increased triglyceride levels.

Nursing Responsibilities

- Before giving initial dose, assess for contraindications to beta blockers such as asthma, chronic lung disease, bradycardia, or heart block.
- Assess blood pressure and apical pulse before giving dosage; notify primary care provider if vital signs are outside established parameters.
- Report adverse effects such as bradycardia, decreased cardiac output (fatigue, dyspnea with exertion, hypotension, decreased level of consciousness), heart failure, heart block, bronchoconstriction (wheezing, dyspnea), or altered blood glucose levels (in diabetic patients).
- Carefully monitor responses of the older patient.

Health Education for the Patient and Family

- Monitor blood pressure and pulse daily as instructed.
- Change position (lying to sitting and sitting to standing) slowly to prevent dizziness and possible falls.

(continued)

- Report effects such as fatigue, lethargy, and impotence to your primary care provider.
- Notify your healthcare provider if you become short of breath or develop a cough or swelling of your extremities.
- If you have diabetes, check blood glucose levels more frequently as hypoglycemia may develop with few symptoms.
- Talk to your primary care provider before taking any over-the-counter medications.
- Carry an adequate supply of the drug when traveling. Do not stop taking this drug without notifying your primary care provider.

CALCIUM CHANNEL BLOCKERS

Amlodipine (Norvasc)	Nicardipine (Cardene)
Clevidipine (Cleviprex)	Nifedipine (Procardia)
Diltiazem (Cardizem)	Nisoldipine (Sular)
Felodipine (Plendil)	Verapamil (Isoptin)
Isradipine (DynaCirc)	

Calcium channel blockers inhibit the flow of calcium ions across the cell membrane of vascular tissue and cardiac cells. In doing so, they relax arterial smooth muscle, lowering peripheral resistance through vasodilation. Calcium channel blockers can cause reflex tachycardia, and some (e.g., verapamil and diltiazem) may impair cardiac function, worsening heart failure.

Nursing Responsibilities
- Assess blood pressure, apical pulse, and liver and renal function tests prior to giving these drugs.
- Calcium channel blockers may be given orally or intravenously.
- Do not administer verapamil or diltiazem to patients with severe hypotension, sinus, or atrioventricular blocks. Administer with caution to patients also taking digoxin or a beta blocker.
- Periodically monitor blood pressure and apical pulse during therapy. Promptly report signs of bradycardia, AV block, or heart failure to the healthcare provider.

Health Education for the Patient and Family
- Take blood pressure and pulse daily as taught. Notify your healthcare provider if your pulse is less than 60 BPM or your blood pressure is not within the specified range.
- This drug may cause constipation. Drink six to eight glasses of water each day, and increase fiber in diet.
- Report shortness of breath, weight gain, or swelling in feet or ankles to your primary care provider.

CENTRALLY ACTING SYMPATHOLYTICS

Clonidine (Catapres)	Methyldopa (Aldomet)
Guanfacine (Tenex)	Reserpine (generic)

The centrally acting sympatholytics stimulate the α_2 receptors in the CNS to suppress sympathetic outflow to the heart and blood vessels. A fall in cardiac output and vasodilation result, reducing blood pressure. Dry mouth and sedation are common adverse effects. Severe reflex hypertension may occur if abruptly discontinued. Clonidine is contraindicated during pregnancy; methyldopa is contraindicated for patients with active liver disease.

Nursing Responsibilities
- Assess for contraindications to therapy. Obtain baseline blood pressure, CBC, Coomb's test, and liver function studies.
- Administer oral doses at bedtime to minimize effects of sedation.
- Methyldopa may be given intravenously for hypertensive emergencies.
- Apply transdermal clonidine patch to dry, hairless area of intact skin on the chest or upper arm. Assess for rash, which indicates allergy, at area of application.
- Promptly report changes in laboratory values to the healthcare provider. Discontinue methyldopa if manifestations of liver dysfunction develop.

Health Education for the Patient and Family
- Relieve dry mouth by sipping water or chewing sugarless gum.
- Take with meals if gastric upset or nausea develop.
- Change position (lying to sitting and sitting to standing) slowly to prevent dizziness and possible falls.
- Do not suddenly discontinue medication or skip doses; this could cause serious hypertension.
- Report mental depression or decreased mental acuity to your healthcare provider.
- Side effects (such as dry mouth, nausea, and dizziness) tend to diminish over time.
- Do not drive a car if the medications cause drowsiness.

VASODILATORS

Hydralazine (Apresoline)

Minoxidil (Loniten)

Vasodilators reduce blood pressure by relaxing vascular smooth muscle (especially in the arterioles), and decreasing peripheral vascular resistance. These drugs are often prescribed in combination with a diuretic or beta blocker, because they can cause reflex tachycardia and fluid retention. Because these drugs can have significant toxic effects, they are not routinely used to manage chronic hypertension.

Nursing Responsibilities
- Hydralazine may be given orally or intravenously; minoxidil is given orally.
- Assess blood pressure and pulse before giving the drug and monitor during therapy as indicated. Report tachycardia or hypotension to the healthcare provider.
- Report peripheral edema and manifestations of volume overload and heart failure.
- Immediately report muffled heart sounds or paradoxical pulse as pericardial effusion and possible cardiac tamponade may develop during minoxidil therapy.
- Discontinue hydralazine and report manifestations of a SLE-like syndrome: muscle or joint pain, fever, or symptoms of nephritis or pericarditis.

Health Education for the Patient and Family
- Change position (lying to sitting and sitting to standing) slowly to prevent dizziness and possible falls.
- Report muscle, joint aches, and fever to your healthcare provider.
- Headache, palpitations, and rapid pulse may develop but should abate in about 10 days.
- Do not discontinue the medication without talking to your healthcare provider.
- Minoxidil may cause excessive hair growth. Contact your healthcare provider if this becomes troublesome.

Figure 32–3 ■ Sites of antihypertensive drug action.

although their action is to block angiotensin II receptors, thus preventing its vasoconstrictive and volume expansion effects.

Several drug classes work through their ability to promote vasodilation and reduce peripheral vascular resistance. Alpha blockers such as prazosin and terazosin block stimulation of alpha-1 receptors on arterioles and veins, preventing vasoconstriction. Because of their ability to dilate both arterioles and veins, alpha blockers can cause significant orthostatic hypotension, particularly following the initial dose. Calcium channel blockers promote dilation of arterioles, the primary regulators of peripheral vascular resistance. These drugs can cause reflex tachycardia. Some calcium channel blockers, verapamil and diltiazem in particular, also suppress heart function, reducing stroke volume and cardiac output. Reflex tachycardia is minimal with these calcium channel blockers. Direct-acting vasodilators such as hydralazine and minoxidil also directly affect the arterioles, reducing peripheral vascular resistance. These drugs have little effect on veins, so the risk of orthostatic hypotension is minimal. They are, however, associated with reflex tachycardia and fluid retention, so rarely are administered as in single-drug treatment regimens.

Other factors considered in selecting drugs for treating hypertension include demographic characteristics of the patient, concurrent conditions, quality of life, cost, and possible interactions among prescribed drugs. In general, diuretics and calcium channel blockers are more effective for treating hypertension in Blacks than beta blockers or ACE inhibitors. Beta blockers are preferred to treat hypertension with concurrent coronary heart disease and angina, but are contraindicated for patients who have asthma or depression. Beta blockers also reduce exercise tolerance and may adversely affect lifestyle for some patients.

DRUG REGIMENS Treatment usually is initiated using a single antihypertensive drug at a low dose. Unless otherwise indicated, a diuretic is recommended as the initial drug of choice. The dose is slowly increased until optimal blood pressure control is achieved. If the drug does not effectively lower the blood pressure or has troubling side effects, a different drug from another class of antihypertensive medications is substituted. If, on the other hand, the drug is tolerated well but has not lowered blood pressure to the desired level, a second drug from another class may be added to the treatment regimen.

Treatment of patients with stage 2 hypertension generally is more aggressive to minimize the risk of MI, heart failure, or stroke. When the average blood pressure is greater than 200/120, immediate therapy, and possible hospitalization, is vital.

After a year of effective hypertension control, an effort may be made to reduce the dosage and number of drugs. This is known as step-down therapy. It is more successful in patients who have made lifestyle modifications. Careful blood pressure monitoring is necessary during and after step-down therapy, as the blood pressure often rises again to hypertensive levels.

Complementary Therapies

Behavioral and mind-body therapies may be helpful for some patients in lowering blood pressure (see the Moving Evidence into Action box). The blood pressure increases in response to physiologic and psychologic stress and anxiety. Mind-body therapies such as yoga and t'ai chi, meditation, and guided imagery are designed to modify both physiologic and cognitive aspects of the stress response. In a study of older African American men and women with moderate hypertension, transcendental mediation was shown to reduce the blood pressure.

MOVING EVIDENCE INTO ACTION   **The Patient with Primary Hypertension**

Standard therapies for hypertension include lifestyle changes and medications. Patients often are advised to reduce stress levels in their lives, but rarely are provided with the tools to do so. This study (Yucha, Tsai, Calderon, & Tian, 2005) sought to identify those patients that were most likely to benefit (reduced blood pressure in both clinic and ambulatory settings) from biofeedback-assisted relaxation training. Participants, all of whom had stage 1 or 2 hypertension, received 8 weeks of relaxation training with biofeedback provided by measurements of finger temperature, muscle tension, and respiratory sinus arrhythmia. The biggest benefit (greatest reduction in BP) occurred in participants who were not taking antihypertensive medication, had lower starting finger temperatures, had less daytime blood pressure variation, and who had a more external health locus of control.

IMPLICATIONS FOR NURSING

Predicting which patients would benefit from biofeedback-assisted relaxation training to lower blood pressure could potentially reduce the risk that these patients will go on to develop stage 1 or 2 hypertension. While biofeedback-assisted relaxation training is expensive and may not be covered by insurance, its benefits in reducing the overall costs of treating hypertension and its potential consequences are significant.

Nurses are in a position to identify patients with prehypertension through blood pressure screening. It is very appropriate to suggest mind-body therapies such as relaxation training with biofeedback to these patients, most of whom do not require medication.

CRITICAL THINKING IN PATIENT CARE

1. This study found that patients who were not taking antihypertensive medications were more likely to benefit from training in biofeedback-assisted relaxation. Think about the different ways in which antihypertensive medications work. Why do you think more benefit was seen in those patients who were not taking drugs?
2. Another finding of the study showed more benefit in patients with a more external health locus of control. Compare characteristics of patients with an internal health locus of control and those with an external health locus. What differences in these patients might account for this finding?
3. While you are discussing life-style modifications and the use of mind-body therapies with a patient with prehypertension, he tells you that he thinks all this is nonsense. How would you respond?

Adapted from Yucha, C. B., Tsai, P. S., Calderon, K. S., & Tian, L. (2005). Biofeedback-assisted relaxation training for essential hypertension: Who is most likely to benefit? *Journal of Cardiovascular Nursing, 20*(3), 198–205.

Eastern exercises such as yoga and t'ai chi, which often combine imagery, meditation, and physical exercise, have been shown to reduce sympathetic nervous system activity, blood pressure, and heart and respiratory rates (Spencer & Jacobs, 2003). A nursing research study of hypertensive patients in Thailand demonstrated the effectiveness of yoga to reduce blood pressure, heart rate, and body mass index (McCaffrey, Ruknui, Hatthakit, & Kasetsomboon, 2005).

ॐ Nursing Care

Health Promotion

Health promotion teaching and activities focus on the modifiable risk factors for hypertension. Advise all patients (as well as children and adolescents) to stop or never start smoking. Discuss the risks of obesity, excess alcohol intake, and a sedentary lifestyle with patients. Encourage all patients to eat a diet rich in fruits and vegetables and low in total and saturated fat.

Discuss the potential benefits of following the DASH diet or a similar eating plan. Advise all patients to remain active and engage in aerobic exercise 5 or more days a week. Discuss the stress-reducing benefits of exercise.

Offer blood pressure screening, and refer patients for follow-up as indicated (Table 32–2).

Assessment

Focused assessment of the patient with hypertension includes the following:

- *Health history:* Complaints of morning headache, cervical pain; cardiovascular or central nervous system manifestations; history of hypertension, renal disease, diabetes; family history of high blood pressure, heart failure, or kidney disease; current medications.

- *Physical examination:* Vital signs including blood pressure in both arms, apical and peripheral pulses; ophthalmologic exam of retinal fundus as appropriate.

TABLE 32–2 Recommended Blood Pressure Follow-Up

CATEGORY	BLOOD PRESSURE (mmHG)	RECOMMENDED FOLLOW-UP
Normal	< 120/80	Recheck in 2 years
Prehypertension	120–139/80–89	Recheck in 1 year
Stage 1 hypertension	140–159/90–99	Confirm within 2 months
Stage 2 hypertension	≥ 160/≥ 100	Evaluate or refer to care provider within 1 month; for higher pressures (e.g., ≥ 180/≥ 110), evaluate or refer to care provider immediately or within 1 week as indicated

Note: NHLBI. (2004). Adapted from *The Seventh Report of the Joint National Committee on Prevention, Detection, Education, and Treatment of High Blood Pressure,* NIH Publication No. 04-5250, Bethesda, MD: National Institutes of Health. Retrieved from http://www.nhlbi.nih.gov/guidelines/hypertension

■ *Laboratory data:* Serum electrolytes, glucose, and creatinine; cholesterol and lipoprotein profile; urinalysis.

Nursing Diagnoses and Interventions

All patients with primary hypertension and their families need significant teaching to manage this chronic condition. Health maintenance is a high-priority problem. Depending on the stage of hypertension and concurrent illnesses, other appropriate nursing diagnoses may include imbalanced nutrition, fluid volume excess, and risk for noncompliance.

Ineffective Health Maintenance

Unhealthy lifestyle and behaviors can contribute to health problems such as hypertension. When hypertension has been identified, knowledge of the disease and its management is vital for the patient. Willingness to take responsibility for hypertension management is central to effective blood pressure control. Adopting healthy lifestyle changes enhances drug therapy; in some cases, the need for medications may be eliminated or reduced. Because hypertension is often an asymptomatic disease and many antihypertensive drugs have unpleasant side effects, it is vital that the patient understand the chronic progressive nature of the disease and its long-term consequences.

■ Assist with identifying current behaviors that contribute to hypertension. *The patient must first identify contributory behaviors before he or she can change them. Using knowledge of hypertension risk factors, the nurse can help identify behaviors and factors contributing to hypertension that can be changed. Including the family in this process is important to reduce potential sabotage of the patient's efforts to adopt healthier behaviors.*

■ Assist in developing a realistic health maintenance plan. *Preparing a health maintenance plan for the patient does little to encourage personal responsibility for health. However, nurses can guide patients in developing realistic goals and expectations for the treatment plan and modifying risk factors such as smoking, exercise, diet, and stress.*

■ Help the patient and family identify strengths and weaknesses in maintaining health. *Discussing areas of the health maintenance plan that are working well and those that present difficulties can help to identify necessary changes in the plan and additional strategies for implementing it.*

Risk for Noncompliance

Noncompliance, or failure to follow the identified treatment plan, is a continuing risk for any patient with a chronic disease. Recommended lifestyle changes such as diet, exercise,

restricted alcohol intake, stress reduction, and smoking cessation often are difficult to maintain on a continuing basis. In addition, prescribed medications may have undesirable effects whereas hypertension itself often has no symptoms or noticeable effects.

■ Inquire about reasons for noncompliance with the recommended treatment plan. Listen openly and without judging. *Nonthreatening discussion of factors contributing to noncompliance validates the patient's self-esteem and partnership in the treatment plan.*

> **PRACTICE ALERT**
> Assess factors contributing to noncompliance, such as adverse drug effects. Suggest measures to manage adverse effects or, if indicated, contact the primary care provider about possible alternative drugs. Some adverse effects of antihypertensive drugs, such as gastric upset, lightheadedness, or nocturia may be easily managed by changing the timing of the drug dose. Others, such as fatigue, decreased exercise tolerance, or impotence may interfere with lifestyle and life roles to the extent that the patient finds them intolerable.

■ Evaluate knowledge of hypertension, its long-term effects, and treatment. Provide additional information and reinforce teaching as needed. *Knowledge increases the sense of control, which also increases the likelihood of compliance with treatment.*

■ Assist to develop realistic short-term goals for lifestyle changes. *Attempting to lose weight, exercise daily, stop smoking, and dramatically change the diet all at the same time may be overwhelming, leading to a sense of failure. Smaller, gradual changes are more easily incorporated into lifestyle and daily activities, improving compliance.*

■ Work with the patient to develop mutual outcomes for the treatment plan. Discuss measures to improve compliance. The patient has absolute control over compliance with the treatment plan. *Demonstrating respect and involving the patient in decision making and planning can improve compliance.*

■ Help the patient identify cues and develop reminders (e.g., written notes, a medication box filled weekly) to assist with maintaining a schedule for exercise and medications. *Cues and other devices provide helpful reminders of activities and schedules until they are incorporated into habits.*

■ Reassure the patient that relapse into old habits and behaviors is common. Encourage avoiding feelings of guilt associated with relapse, and use the circumstance to renew efforts to comply with treatment. *Guilt and feelings of failure can lead to further noncompliance unless the event is used to identify reasons for noncompliance and ways to prevent it from recurring in the future.*

Imbalanced Nutrition: More than Body Requirements

The relationship between obesity, excess alcohol intake, and hypertension is well-documented. Hypertension is particularly associated with central obesity, identified by waist circumference greater than hip circumference. While weight loss is difficult and takes commitment to changing eating and exercise habits, it is possible for most patients to achieve.

EVIDENCE FOR NURSING CARE / **The Patient with Hypertension**

Selected resources that nurses may find helpful when planning evidence-based nursing care follow.

■ Dumont, C. & Hardware, J. (2009). Teaching patients to tame their hypertension. *American Nurse Today, 4*(7), 20–24.

■ Held, M. L., & Sturtz, M. (2009). Managing acute decompensated heart failure. *American Nurse Today, 4*(2), 18–22.

■ Horne, E. M., & Gordon, P. M. (2009). Taking aim at hypertensive crises. *Nursing2009, 39*(3), 48–53.

- Assess usual daily food intake, and discuss possible contributing factors to excess weight, such as sedentary lifestyle, or using food as a reward or stress reliever. Inquire about diversional activities, exercise patterns, and previous weight reduction efforts (e.g., participation in weight reduction programs or using fad or crash diets). *Assessment data provides clues about contributing factors to obesity, the patient's knowledge base about the relationship between eating and exercise habits and weight, and safe weight loss strategies. This provides direction for further teaching and for developing a realistic weight reduction plan.*

- Mutually determine with the patient a realistic target weight (e.g., loss of 10% of current body weight over a 6-month period). Regularly monitor weight. Encourage a system of nonfood rewards for achieving small, incremental goals. *Setting weight loss goals helps formalize the process and provides motivation for continued progress. Developing realistic goals may be difficult; unrealistic goals, however, set the patient up for failure. Continuous incremental weight loss provides reassurance that it can be achieved and promotes permanent weight reduction.*

- Refer to a dietitian for information about low-fat, low-calorie foods and eating plans. Focus on changing eating habits as opposed to "following a diet." *Focusing on changing eating habits promotes the sense that low-fat, low-calorie eating patterns should become a part of lifestyle rather than a short-term measure to be endured until the weight loss goal is achieved.*

- Recommend participating in an approved weight loss program such as Weight Watchers, Overeaters Anonymous, or Take off Pounds Sensibly (TOPS). *Organized weight loss programs provide structure for a balanced weight reduction program, as well as mutual support from others trying to lose weight.*

Excess Fluid Volume

Excess fluid volume often contributes to hypertension by increasing the cardiac output. A number of factors associated with hypertension can cause excess fluid volume, including sodium retention and disruption of the renin-angiotensin-aldosterone system. In addition, some antihypertensive drugs, such as calcium channel blockers and vasodilators, can contribute to excess fluid in the interstitial spaces and peripheral edema.

PRACTICE ALERT
Monitor blood pressure and other vital signs as indicated: every 1 to 2 hours or more frequently during acute hypertensive states; or once a week or more frequently during initial treatment outside of the hospital setting. Vital signs are an indicator of fluid balance and the effectiveness of treatment. An elevated blood pressure, pulse, and respiratory rate may indicate fluid retention, whereas orthostatic hypotension and tachycardia may indicate fluid volume deficit.

- Monitor intake and output, and weigh daily (if in an acute or long-term care facility) or weekly (in the community). *Rapid weight changes (over days) more accurately reflect fluid balance than intake and output records. One liter of fluid weighs 1 kg (2.2 lb). Weight changes and intake and output records help monitor the effects of therapy.*

- Monitor for peripheral edema (sacral edema in the bedridden patient). *Drugs such as vasodilators can cause fluid accumulation in interstitial tissues, leading to peripheral or dependent edema. Adding a diuretic to the treatment plan may be necessary.*

- Refer to a dietitian for teaching about a restricted sodium diet. Discuss the relationship between sodium intake and fluid retention. Provide opportunities to choose low-sodium foods from simulated menus. Support efforts, and reassure that lifestyle changes such as consuming less sodium take time. *Knowledge provides the power to take control of sodium intake. Patience and perseverance are needed to succeed; positive reinforcement of efforts to change long-standing dietary patterns is important.*

- Monitor laboratory values, such as blood urea nitrogen (BUN), urine specific gravity, creatinine, electrolytes, and hematocrit and hemoglobin. Hypertension can alter renal perfusion and function, leading to fluid retention and altered laboratory values. *Changes in BUN and creatinine indicate impaired renal function, whereas changes in hematocrit and hemoglobin often reflect changes in fluid volume.*

- Discuss the importance of adhering to treatment plans such as dietary restrictions and medication schedules. *Understanding the rationale for treatment measures promotes the patient's sense of control and encourages compliance with the treatment regimen.*

Using NANDA, NIC, and NOC

Linkages between a selected NANDA nursing diagnosis, NIC, and NOC for the patient with hypertension are shown in the chart that follows.

Community-Based Care

Effective control of hypertension requires the patient to not only participate in the plan of care, but also to take an active role in managing the disease. Treatment is managed in community

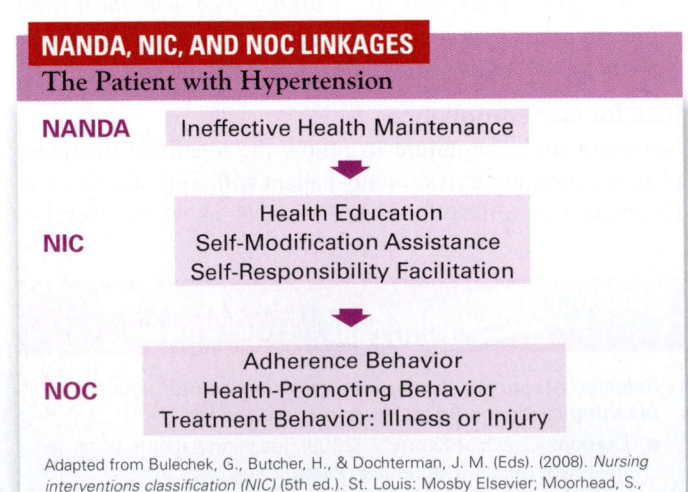

NANDA, NIC, AND NOC LINKAGES
The Patient with Hypertension

NANDA — Ineffective Health Maintenance

NIC — Health Education / Self-Modification Assistance / Self-Responsibility Facilitation

NOC — Adherence Behavior / Health-Promoting Behavior / Treatment Behavior: Illness or Injury

Adapted from Bulechek, G., Butcher, H., & Dochterman, J. M. (Eds). (2008). *Nursing interventions classification (NIC)* (5th ed.). St. Louis: Mosby Elsevier; Moorhead, S., Johnson, M., Maas, M., & Swanson, E. (Eds). (2008). *Nursing outcomes classification (NOC)* (4th ed.). St. Louis: Mosby Elsevier; Nanda International. (2009). *Nursing diagnoses: Definitions and classification 2009–2011*. Oxford, UK: Wiley-Blackwell; and Dochterman, J., & Bulechek, G. (2004). *Nursing interventions classification (NIC)* (4th ed.). St. Louis: Mosby.

CASE STUDY & NURSING CARE PLAN   A Patient with Hypertension

Margaret Spezia is a married, 49-year-old Italian American with eight children whose ages range from 3 to 18 years. For the past 2 months, Mrs. Spezia has had frequent morning headaches, and occasional dizziness and blurred vision. At her annual physical examination 1 month ago, her blood pressure was 168/104 and 156/94. She was instructed to reduce her fat and cholesterol intake, to avoid using salt at the table, and to start walking for 30 to 45 minutes daily. Mrs. Spezia returns to the clinic for a follow-up.

ASSESSMENT

While escorting Mrs. Spezia to the exam room and obtaining her weight, blood pressure, and history, Lisa Christos, RN, notices that Mrs. Spezia seems restless and upset. Ms. Christos says, "You look upset about something. Is everything OK?" Mrs. Spezia responds, "Well, my head is throbbing, and I'm sort of dizzy. I think I'm just overdoing it and not getting enough rest. You know, raising eight children is a lot of work and expense. I just started working part time so we wouldn't get behind in our bills. I thought the extra money might relieve some of my stress, but I'm not so sure that's really happening. I'm not getting any better and I'm worried that I'll lose my job or become disabled and that my husband won't be able to manage the children by himself. I really need to go home, but first, I want to get rid of this awful headache. Would you please get me a couple of aspirin or something?"

Mrs. Spezia's history shows a steady weight gain over the past 18 years. She has no known family history of hypertension. Physical findings include height 63 inches (160 cm), weight 225 lb (102 kg), T 99°F (37.2°C), P 100 regular, R 16, BP 180/115 (lying), 170/110 (sitting), 165/105 (standing), average 10-point difference in readings between right and left arm (lower on left). Skin cool and dry, capillary refill 4 seconds right hand, 3 seconds left hand. Mrs. Spezia's total serum cholesterol is 245 mg/dL (normal < 200 mg/dL). All other blood and urine studies are within normal limits. Based on analysis of the data, Mrs. Spezia is started on enalapril 5 mg and hydrochlorothiazide 12.5 mg in a combination drug (Vaseretic), and placed on a low-fat, low-cholesterol, no-added-salt diet.

DIAGNOSES

- *Fatigue* related to effects of hypertension and stresses of daily life
- *Imbalanced Nutrition: More than Body Requirements* related to excessive food intake
- *Ineffective Health Maintenance* related to inability to modify lifestyle
- *Deficient Knowledge* related to effects of prescribed treatment

EXPECTED OUTCOMES

- Reduce blood pressure readings to less than 150 systolic and 90 diastolic by return visit next week.

- Incorporate low-sodium and low-fat foods from a list provided into her diet.
- Develop a plan for regular exercise.
- Verbalize understanding of the effects of prescribed drug, dietary restrictions, exercise, and follow-up visits to help control hypertension.

PLANNING AND IMPLEMENTATION

- Teach to take own blood pressure daily and record it, bringing the record to scheduled clinic visits.
- Teach name, dose, action, and side effects of her antihypertensive medication.
- Instruct to walk for 15 minutes each day this week, and to investigate swimming classes at the local pool.
- Discuss strategies for achieving a realistic weight loss goal.
- Refer a dietary consultation for further teaching about fat and sodium restrictions.
- Discuss stress-reducing techniques, helping identify possible choices.

EVALUATION

Mrs. Spezia returns to the clinic 1 week later. Her average blood pressure is now 148/88 mmHg. She has lost 1.5 lb, and states that her oldest daughter has suggested that they join a weight reduction program together. Mrs. Spezia is walking for an average of 20 minutes at a local mall each day. She verbalizes an understanding of her medication, and is taking it in the morning and before dinner each day. She met with the dietitian and discussed ways to reduce the sodium and fat in her diet. The dietitian provided a list of low-fat, low-sodium foods and recommended cookbooks to help Mrs. Spezia modify her cooking. Mrs. Spezia tells Ms. Christos, "I just can't believe how much better I feel already. My headaches are gone, I've actually lost some weight, and I feel motivated to keep going. If I had only known how much better I could feel! I don't expect I'll ever go back to my old habits again; it's just not worth it!"

CRITICAL THINKING IN THE NURSING PROCESS

1. Identify the factors that contributed to Mrs. Spezia's hypertension. Which were modifiable and which were not?
2. What is the rationale for reducing sodium and fat in Mrs. Spezia's diet?
3. Suppose your hypertensive patient is homeless and has no source of income. How could you help ensure your patient would follow the treatment plan? What would you do if the patient did not follow it?
4. Discuss the role of stress in hypertension. What factors in Mrs. Spezia's life contribute to her stress level?
5. Develop a plan of care for the diagnosis, *Situational Low Self-Esteem* related to obesity.

See Evaluating Your Response in Appendix C.

---

settings, with regular visits to a clinic or office to monitor blood pressure and effects of treatment measures. Include the following topics when teaching the patient and family about hypertension:

- Specific lifestyle changes recommended for the patient and suggestions for implementing them. For example, consider the following:
  - Increase activity gradually. Develop a realistic exercise program that is enjoyable and fits into lifestyle. Identify an exercise buddy for additional motivation. Activity and exercise, through a gradual conditioning of muscles and

blood vessels, lower blood pressure by reducing peripheral vascular resistance. As the heart becomes conditioned and pumps more efficiently, kidney perfusion improves and intravascular volume falls, further reducing blood pressure. Exercise also reduces stress and contributes to weight loss and maintenance. Aerobic exercise, such as walking, jogging, swimming, and cycling are appropriate; isometric activities (such as weight lifting) should be avoided without healthcare provider approval.

- Adopt healthy eating patterns, following a low-fat, low-cholesterol, moderate sodium diet that also is rich in fruits and vegetables and includes at least two servings of low-fat milk or milk products daily. Do not give up if you slip into old eating habits on occasion; use such occasions to identify ways to avoid future lapses.

- Stop smoking. Participating in organized smoking cessation programs or using aids such as nicotine patches can help.
- Use alcohol in moderation if at all, consuming no more than 1.5 oz of hard liquor, 5 to 10 oz of wine, or 12 to 20 oz of beer per day.
- Use stress-reducing techniques such as meditation, relaxation, deep breathing, and exercise to manage stress. Anger and hostility intensify vasoconstriction; channeling these emotions into more positive responses such as using a change process to modify factors that provoke these emotions can reduce their harmful effects on blood pressure.
- Prescribed medications, their intended effect, dose and timing, interactions, and possible adverse effects. Discuss effects that should be reported to the healthcare provider, and those that can be managed by the patient or that will diminish over time.
- The importance of monitoring blood pressure and regular visits to the primary care provider or hypertension clinic to monitor treatment. During follow-up visits, assess the blood pressure and specific laboratory work (such as serum creatinine, BUN, and/or serum electrolytes) to evaluate the disease and the effects of antihypertensive medications.

Refer the patient to community blood pressure clinics, and to home health services as needed for regular follow-up and reinforcement of teaching. Refer to a dietitian or to an organized weight loss program as indicated for further teaching and weight loss support. The accompanying Case Study & Nursing Care Plan provides additional information about community-based care for the patient with high blood pressure.

The Patient with Secondary Hypertension

Secondary hypertension is elevated blood pressure resulting from an identifiable underlying process. It accounts for only 5% to 10% of identified cases of hypertension. Kidney disease is the most common identifiable cause of high blood pressure in both adults and children (Huether & McCance, 2008). Other common identifiable causes of hypertension in adults include renovascular disease (reduced blood flow to the kidneys), disorders of the adrenal cortex, pheochromocytoma, coarctation of the aorta, and sleep apnea. The pathophysiology of selected causes of high blood pressure are summarized as follows:

- *Kidney disease.* Any disease that affects renal blood flow (e.g., renal artery stenosis) or renal function (e.g., glomerulonephritis, renal failure) can lead to hypertension. Disruption of the blood supply stimulates the renin-angiotensin-aldosterone system, with resulting vasoconstriction and sodium and water retention. Altered kidney function affects the elimination of water and electrolytes, leading to hypertension.
- *Coarctation of the aorta.* Coarctation of the aorta is narrowing of the aorta, usually just distal to the subclavian arteries.

Reduced renal and peripheral blood flow stimulates the renin-angiotensin-aldosterone system and local vasoconstrictive responses, raising the blood pressure. A marked difference between pressures in the upper and lower extremities is common, with weak pulses and poor capillary refill in the lower extremities.

- *Endocrine disorders.* Adrenal gland disorders such as Cushing's syndrome and primary aldosteronism can cause hypertension. A rare tumor of the adrenal medulla, *pheochromocytoma*, causes persistent or intermittent hypertension. Other endocrine disorders such as hyperthyroidism and pituitary disorders also can lead to hypertension.
- *Neurologic disorders.* Increased intracranial pressure causes an elevated blood pressure as the body attempts to maintain cerebral blood flow. Disorders that interfere with autonomic nervous system regulation (such as high spinal cord injury) may allow the sympathetic nervous system to predominate, increasing systemic vascular resistance and blood pressure.
- *Drug use.* Estrogen and oral contraceptive use may lead to hypertension, possibly by prompting sodium and water retention and affecting the renin-angiotensin-aldosterone system. Stimulant drugs, such as cocaine and methamphetamines, increase systemic vascular resistance and cardiac output, resulting in hypertension.
- *Pregnancy.* About 10% of all pregnant women are hypertensive. Hypertension may predate pregnancy or occur as a direct response to the pregnancy. The mechanism of pregnancy-induced hypertension (PIH) is unclear. It is a significant cause of maternal and fetal morbidity and mortality and requires careful perinatal management.

The pattern of secondary hypertension varies, depending on its cause. Pheochromocytoma may cause attacks of hypertension that last for minutes to hours, accompanied by anxiety, palpitations, diaphoresis, pallor, and nausea and vomiting. Primary aldosteronism may cause hypertension, weakness, paresthesias, polyuria, and nocturia (∞ see Chapter 19). Symptoms of kidney disease accompany hypertension when a renal disorder is the cause.

The following diagnostic tests may be ordered to differentiate primary from secondary hypertension.

- *Renal function studies* and *urinalysis* identify renal causes of hypertension. Elevated serum creatinine and BUN, reduced creatinine clearance, and hematuria, proteinuria, and casts often indicate kidney disease.
- *Serum potassium* is decreased in hyperaldosteronism.
- *Blood chemistries*, including serum electrolytes, glucose, and lipid studies are done to detect abnormalities indicative of endocrine or cardiovascular disease.
- *Intravenous pyelography (IVP)*, *renal ultrasonography*, *renal arteriography*, and *CT* or *MRI* may be done when secondary hypertension is suspected.

Interdisciplinary and nursing care for the patient with secondary hypertension is the same as that for primary hypertension, discussed in the previous section. In addition, the underlying process is treated. See chapters covering specific disorders for more information about treatment measures.

The Patient with Hypertensive Crisis

Some patients with hypertension may, for reasons not clearly understood, develop rapid, significant elevations in systolic and/or diastolic pressures. In a *hypertensive emergency* (or *malignant hypertension*) the systolic pressure is greater than 180 mmHg and the diastolic pressure higher than 120 mmHg. Immediate treatment (within 1 hour) is vital to prevent cardiac, renal, and vascular damage, and reduce morbidity and mortality. Intense cerebral artery spasms help protect the brain from excess pressure; however, cerebral edema often develops. Prolonged severe hypertension damages walls of the arterioles and renal blood vessels, and may lead to intravascular coagulation and acute renal failure.

Patients presenting with a hypertensive emergency may have manifestations such as headache, confusion, swelling of the optic nerve (papilledema), blurred vision, restlessness, and motor and sensory deficits. Manifestations of hypertensive emergencies are listed in the accompanying box.

MANIFESTATIONS of Hypertensive Emergencies

- Rapid onset
- Blurred vision, papilledema
- Systolic pressure > 180 mmHg
- Diastolic pressure > 120 mmHg
- Headache
- Confusion
- Motor and sensory deficits

Most hypertensive emergencies occur when patients suddenly stop taking their medications or their hypertension is poorly controlled. Younger patients (30 to 50 years old), African American men, pregnant women with pre-eclampsia, and people with collagen and/or renal disease also are at higher risk for a hypertensive emergency (Huether & McCance, 2008).

The goal of care in hypertensive emergencies is to reduce the blood pressure by no more than 25% within minutes to 1 hour, then toward 160/100 within 2 to 6 hours. It is important to avoid rapid or excessive blood pressure decreases that may lead to renal, cerebral, or cardiac ischemia (NHLBI, 2004). Blood pressure is monitored frequently (every 5 to 30 minutes) during a

TABLE 32–3 Intravenous Drugs Used to Treat Hypertensive Emergencies

CLASS/DRUG	ONSET	DURATION	NURSING IMPLICATIONS
Vasodilator			
Sodium nitroprusside (Nipride)	seconds	1 to 2 min	■ Effective, easy to titrate ■ May cause nausea, vomiting, muscle twitching, sweating ■ Use with caution in increased intracranial pressure
Nitroglycerin	2 to 5 min	5 to 10 min	■ Used when coronary ischemia accompanies hypertension ■ May cause headache, vomiting ■ Tolerance may develop with prolonged use
Diazoxide (Hyperstat)	1 to 2 min	4 to 24 hr	■ Avoided in patients with coronary artery disease ■ Used with beta-blockers and diuretics ■ Painful if it enters tissues
Fenoldopam (Corlopam)	< 5 min	30 min	■ Use with caution in patients with glaucoma ■ May cause tachycardia, headache, nausea, flushing ■ Do not use concurrently with beta blockers ■ Monitor for heart failure, ischemic heart disease
Hydralazine (Apresoline)	10 to 30 min	2 to 6 hr	■ May be used for hypertension associated with eclampsia ■ Avoided in patients with coronary heart disease ■ May cause tachycardia, flushing, headache, vomiting, angina
Calcium channel blocker			
Nicardipene (Cardene)	5 to 10 min	15 to 30 min; up to 4 hr	■ Use with caution in coronary heart disease ■ Avoid in patients with heart failure ■ May cause tachycardia, headache, flushing, local phlebitis
ACE inhibitor			
Enalaprilat (Vasotec)	15 to 30 min	6 to 12 hr	■ Monitor for hypotension ■ Used in acute left heart failure ■ Avoid in acute myocardial infarction
Adrenergic blockers			
Labetalol (Trandate)	5 to 10 min	3 to 6 hr	■ Avoid in patients with acute heart failure and asthma ■ May cause nausea, vomiting, dizziness ■ Monitor for dyspnea, wheezing, heart block, orthostatic hypotension
Esmolol (Brevibloc)	1 to 2 min	10 to 30 min	■ Avoided in patients with heart failure and asthma ■ May cause nausea ■ Monitor for hypotension, dyspnea, wheezing, heart failure, first degree heart block
Phentolamine (Regitine)	1 to 2 min	10 to 30 min	■ May cause tachycardia, flushing, headache

hypertensive emergency. The BUN, serum creatinine, calcium, and total protein levels are carefully monitored to help determine the prognosis for recovery. Drug treatment for malignant hypertension includes parenteral administration of a rapidly acting antihypertensive, such as the potent vasodilator sodium nitroprusside (Nipride). Other medications that may be used are outlined in the Table 32–3. Management also focuses on treating any underlying or coexisting heart, kidney, and CNS disorders.

Nursing care for the patient with a hypertensive emergency focuses on continuous monitoring of the blood pressure and titrating drugs (administered by intravenous bolus or infusion)

as ordered to achieve desired blood pressure. Avoiding excessive or very rapid blood pressure reductions is as important as achieving the desired blood pressure readings. Reassure the patient and family of the rapid effect of prescribed drugs. Provide psychologic and emotional support as needed. Maintain an attitude of confidence that the treatment will achieve the desired effect. Following resolution of the hypertensive crisis, review causes of the crisis. Teach the patient and family measures to effectively manage hypertension and prevent future hypertensive emergencies.

Disorders of the Aorta and Its Branches

The aorta and its branches may be affected by occlusions, aneurysms, and inflammations. These disorders may be chronic or acute and life threatening (e.g., a thoracic dissection). This section focuses on aneurysms of the aorta and its branches.

The Patient with an Aneurysm

An **aneurysm** is an abnormal dilation of a blood vessel, commonly at a site of a weakness or a tear in the vessel wall. Aneurysms commonly affect the aorta and peripheral arteries because of the high pressure in these vessels. An aneurysm also may develop in the ventricular wall, usually affecting the left ventricle. Most arterial aneurysms are caused by arteriosclerosis or atherosclerosis; trauma also may lead to aneurysm formation.

Arterial aneurysms are most common in men over age 65, with a history of ever smoking (> 100 cigarettes in lifetime), most of whom are asymptomatic at the time of diagnosis. Hypertension is a major contributing factor in the development of some types of aortic aneurysms.

> **FAST FACTS**
> - The incidence of aortic aneurysm is an estimated 5.9 per 100,000 persons per year.
> - Aortic dissection affects an estimated 5 to 30 per 1 million people per year.
> - Although aortic aneurysm and aortic dissection can occur concurrently, this is rare.

Pathophysiology and Manifestations

Aneurysms form due to weakness of the arterial wall. The major structural proteins of the aorta are collagen and elastin. Collagen provides tensile strength of the vessel, preventing excessive dilation. Elastin allows vessel recoil, during which the vessel returns to its original size following systole. This recoil provides continued propulsion of the bolus of blood expelled from the ventricle. Elastin is a primary component of internal elastic lamina, which separates the intimal and medial layers of the aorta, and of the media, the smooth muscle layer of the aorta. Destruction of elastin can lead to abnormal dilation of the vessel; collagen destruction can allow the vessel to rupture.

True aneurysms are caused by slow weakening of the arterial wall due to the long-term, eroding effects of atherosclerosis and

hypertension. True aneurysms affect all three layers of the vessel wall, and most are fusiform and circumferential. *Fusiform aneurysms* are spindle shaped and taper at both ends. *Circumferential* aneurysms involve the entire diameter of the vessel (Figure 32–4 ■). They generally grow slowly but progressively. Their length and diameter vary considerably among patients. A large fusiform aneurysm may affect most of the ascending aorta as well as a large portion of the abdominal aorta.

False aneurysms, also known as traumatic aneurysms, are caused by a traumatic break in the vessel wall rather than weakening of the vessel. They often are *saccular*, shaped like small outpouchings (sacs) on a portion of the vessel wall (Figure 32–5 ■). A *berry aneurysm* is a type of saccular aneurysm. They are often small (less than 2 cm in diameter), caused by congenital weakness in the tunica media of the artery. Berry aneurysms are commonly found in the circle of Willis in the brain.

Dissecting aneurysms are unique, developing when a break or tear in the tunica intima and media allows blood to invade or *dissect* the layers of the vessel wall. The blood usually is contained by the adventitia, forming a saccular or longitudinal aneurysm (Figure 32–6 ■).

Figure 32–4 ■ A magnetic resonance angiogram (MRA) showing a circumferential aneurysm of the lower abdominal aorta.

Figure 32–5 ■ An angiogram showing a saccular (berry) aneurysm in the carotid artery of a 50-year-old man.

Figure 32–6 ■ In an aortic dissection, a tear in the intima and media of the artery allows blood to invade and dissect the wall of the aorta.

Aneurysms affect different segments of the aorta and its branches. Their manifestations generally are due to pressure of the aneurysm on adjacent structures. Table 32–4 summarizes the manifestations and complications of various types of aortic aneurysms.

Thoracic Aortic Aneurysms

Thoracic aortic aneurysms account for about 10% of aortic aneurysms, with an annual incidence of about 6 per 100,000 people. They usually result from weakening of the aortic wall by arteriosclerosis and hypertension. Other causes include trauma, coarctation of the aorta, tertiary syphilis, fungal infections, and Marfan syndrome. The syphilis spirochete can invade and weaken aortic smooth muscle, causing an aneurysm to develop as long as 20 years after the primary infection. Marfan syndrome fragments elastic fibers of the aortic media, weakening the vessel wall. The accompanying box discusses genetic links associated with thoracic aortic aneurysms.

Thoracic aneurysms frequently are asymptomatic. When present, manifestations are caused by the effects of the aneurysm on blood flow (e.g., to the coronary arteries and great vessels of the head and upper body) and pressure placed by distended aorta on surrounding structures. Consequently, manifestations vary by the location, size, and growth rate of the aneurysm. Substernal, neck, or back pain may occur. Pressure on the trachea, esophagus, laryngeal nerve, or superior vena cava may cause dyspnea, stridor, cough, difficult or painful swallowing, hoarseness, edema of the face and neck, and distended neck veins.

Aneurysms of the ascending aorta typically cause angina due to disruption of blood flow into the coronary arteries. Heart failure may develop as a result of disruption of the aortic valve

TABLE 32–4 Manifestations and Complications of Aortic Aneurysms

TYPE OR LOCATION	MANIFESTATIONS	COMPLICATIONS
Thoracic	■ May be asymptomatic ■ Back, neck, or substernal pain ■ Dyspnea, stridor, or brassy cough if pressing on trachea ■ Hoarseness and dysphagia if pressing on esophagus or laryngeal nerve ■ Edema of the face and neck ■ Distended neck veins	■ Ruptured and hemorrhage
Abdominal	■ Pulsating abdominal mass ■ Aortic calcification noted on x-ray ■ Mild to severe midabdominal or lumbar back pain ■ Cool, cyanotic extremities if iliac arteries are involved ■ Claudication (ischemic pain with exercise, relieved by rest)	■ Peripheral emboli to lower extremities ■ Rupture and hemorrhage
Aortic dissection	■ Abrupt, severe, ripping or tearing pain in area of aneurysm ■ Mild or marked hypertension early ■ Weak or absent pulses and blood pressure in upper extremities ■ Syncope	■ Hemorrhage ■ Renal failure ■ MI, heart failure, cardiac tamponade ■ Sepsis ■ Weakness or paralysis of lower extremities

Figure 32–7 ■ An angiogram showing several popliteal aneurysms.

and regurgitation of blood back into the left ventricle. Aneurysms of the aortic arch often cause dysphagia, dyspnea, hoarseness, confusion, and dizziness (due to disrupted cerebral blood flow). Thrombi that form within a thoracic aneurysm can embolize, causing a stroke, renal or mesenteric ischemia, or ischemia of the lower extremities. Aneurysms of the thoracic aorta tend to enlarge progressively and may rupture, causing death (Ramanath, Oh, Sundt, & Eagle, 2009).

Abdominal Aortic Aneurysms

Abdominal aortic aneurysms are associated with arteriosclerosis and hypertension. Increasing age and smoking are believed to contribute as well. Most abdominal aortic aneurysms are found in adults over age 65. The vast majority (over 90%) develop below the renal arteries, usually where the abdominal aorta branches to form the iliac arteries (see Figure 32–4).

Most abdominal aneurysms are asymptomatic, but a pulsating mass in the mid and upper abdomen and a bruit over the mass are found on exam. When pain is present, it may be constant or intermittent, usually felt in the midabdominal region or lower back. Its intensity may range from mild discomfort to severe pain. Pain intensity often correlates with the size and severity of the aneurysm. Severe pain may indicate impending rupture.

Sluggish blood flow within the aneurysm may cause thrombi (blood clots) to form. These can become emboli (circulating clots), traveling to the lower extremities and occluding peripheral arteries. The aneurysm may also rupture, with hemorrhage and hypovolemic shock. The risk of rupture increases as the size of the aneurysm increases; 20% to 40% of aneurysms more than 5 cm in diameter rupture. After acute rupture, the mortality rate is greater than 50%, even when emergency surgery is performed.

Popliteal and Femoral Aneurysms

Most popliteal and femoral aneurysms are due to arteriosclerosis. They are often bilateral and usually affect men.

Popliteal aneurysms may be asymptomatic (Figure 32–7 ■). Manifestations, if any, are due to decreased blood flow to the lower extremity and include **intermittent claudication** (cramping or pain in the leg muscles brought on by exercise and relieved by rest), rest pain, and numbness. A pulsating mass may be palpable in the popliteal fossa (behind the knee).

Thrombosis and embolism are complications; gangrene may result, often necessitating amputation.

A *femoral aneurysm* usually is detected as a pulsating mass in the femoral area. The manifestations are similar to those of popliteal aneurysms, resulting from impaired blood flow. Femoral aneurysms may rupture.

Aortic Dissections

Dissection is a life-threatening emergency caused by a tear in the intima of the aorta with hemorrhage into the media. The hemorrhage dissects or splits the vessel wall, forming a blood-filled channel between its layers. Dissection can occur anywhere along the aorta. *Type A dissection* (also called *proximal dissection*) affects the ascending aorta; *type B dissection* (*distal dissection*) is limited to the descending aorta (see Figure 32–6).

Hypertension is a major predisposing factor for aortic dissection, accounting for 70% of aortic dissections. Cystic medial necrosis (see the Genetic Considerations box) also is a major risk factor. Other risk factors include male gender, advancing age, pregnancy, congenital defects of the aortic valve, coarctation of the aorta, and inflammatory aortitis (Huether & McCance, 2008).

Dissection of the thoracic aortic walls progresses along the length of the vessel, moving both proximally and distally. As the aneurysm expands, pressure may prevent the aortic valve from closing or may occlude the branches of the aorta. Descending aortic dissection may extend into the renal, iliac, or femoral arteries.

The primary symptom of an aortic dissection is sudden, excruciating pain. The pain, often described as a ripping or tearing sensation, is usually over the area of dissection. Thoracic dissections cause chest or back pain. Other symptoms may include syncope, dyspnea, and weakness. The blood pressure may initially be increased, but rapidly falls and is often inaudible as the dissection occludes blood flow. Peripheral pulses are absent for the same reason.

Complications develop if major arteries are affected. Obstruction of the carotid artery causes neurologic symptoms such as weakness or paralysis. The myocardium, kidneys, or

Aortic Aneurysm Animation

bowel may become ischemic or infarct if blood flow to the coronary arteries, renal arteries, or mesenteric artery is affected. Acute aortic regurgitation may develop with dissection of the ascending aorta. With treatment, the long-term prognosis is generally good, although the in-hospital mortality rate following surgery is 15% to 20%.

Interdisciplinary Care

Most aneurysms are asymptomatic, detected through a routine physical examination. Treatment depends on the size of the aneurysm. Small, asymptomatic aneurysms may not be treated or are medically managed; large aneurysms (> 5 cm) at risk for rupture require surgery.

Diagnosis

Diagnostic studies done to establish the diagnosis and determine the size and location of the aneurysm may include the following:

- *Chest x-ray* to visualize thoracic aortic aneurysms.
- *Abdominal ultrasonography* to diagnose abdominal aortic aneurysms. One-time screening of men 65 to 75 who ever smoked is recommended (U.S. Preventative Services Task Force, 2005).
- *Transesophageal echocardiography* to identify the specific location and extent of a thoracic aneurysm and to visualize a dissecting aneurysm.
- *Contrast-enhanced CT* or *MRI* allows precise measurements of aneurysm size.
- *Angiography* uses contrast solution injected into the aorta or involved vessel to visualize the precise size and location of the aneurysm.

Medications

Thoracic aortic aneurysms may be treated with long-term beta-blocker therapy and additional antihypertensive drugs as needed to control heart rate and blood pressure.

Patients with aortic dissection are initially treated with intravenous beta blockers such as propranolol (Inderal), metoprolol (Lopressor), or esmolol (Brevibloc) to reduce the heart rate to about 60 BPM. Sodium nitroprusside (Nipride) infusion is started concurrently to reduce the systolic pressure to 120 mmHg or less. Calcium channel blockers (verapamil and diltiazem) also may be used. Direct vasodilators such as diazoxide (Hyperstat) and hydralazine (Apresoline) are avoided as they may actually worsen the dissection. Constant monitoring of vital signs, hemodynamic pressures (via Swan-Ganz catheter; ∞ see Chapter 30 for more information about hemodynamic pressure monitoring), and urine output are vital to ensure adequate perfusion of vital organs.

Following surgical correction of an aneurysm, anticoagulant therapy may be initiated. Heparin therapy is used initially, with conversion to oral anticoagulation prior to discharge. Many patients are maintained indefinitely on anticoagulant therapy; others may use lifelong, low-dose aspirin therapy to reduce the risk of clot formation.

Surgery

Operative repair of aortic aneurysms is indicated when the aneurysm is symptomatic or expanding rapidly. Thoracic aneurysms of more than 6 cm in diameter are surgically

repaired; asymptomatic abdominal aneurysms greater than 5 cm in diameter may be repaired, depending on the patient's operative risk factors. Type A dissections are repaired as soon as feasible; type B dissections may be surgically repaired, depending on the extent of involvement and risk for rupture.

Endovascular stent grafts (EVSG) are increasingly being used to treat abdominal and thoracic aortic aneurysms. The use of EVSG to treat aortic dissections is in investigational stages. The stent, which consists of a metal sheath covered with polyester fabric or a woven polyester tube, usually is placed percutaneously via the femoral artery. Fluoroscopy is used to guide its placement. Both straight and bifurcated grafts are available. Endovascular stent placement results in a shorter hospital stay and lower treatment cost. EVSG is associated with fewer pulmonary, renal, and cardiovascular complications than open surgical aneurysm repair (Huether & McCance, 2008). This option generally is preferred for patients who have a high surgical risk. The most common complication of endovascular aneurysm repair is persistent perfusion of the aneurysm (endoleak) caused by an ineffective seal at the proximal or distal end of the graft (Way & Doherty, 2003). Regular follow up with abdominal CT scans is necessary to detect this complication, which can develop at any time postoperatively. Because stent grafts are handcrafted to fit the individual, repeated CT scans with contrast media are required preoperatively, increasing the risk for kidney damage and renal failure. On rare occasions, the graft may be malpositioned or may migrate from the desired location.

An open surgical procedure in which the aneurysm is excised and replaced with a synthetic fabric graft is the standard treatment for expanding abdominal aortic aneurysms (Figure 32–8 ■). Although the aneurysm walls may be excised, they usually are left intact and used to cover the graft. Surgical repair of thoracic aneurysms is similar but more complex due to major vessels exiting at the aortic arch. Cardiopulmonary bypass is required if the ascending aorta is involved. The aortic valve also may be replaced during surgery. See the box on page 1038 for nursing care of the patient having surgery on the aorta.

Figure 32–8 ■ Repair of an abdominal aortic aneurysm. The aorta is exposed and clamped between the renal and iliac arteries. Atherosclerotic plaque and thrombotic material is removed. A synthetic graft is used to replace the aneurysm. The aneurysm walls are then sutured around the graft.

NURSING CARE OF THE PATIENT   Having Surgery of the Aorta

PREOPERATIVE CARE

- As time permits, provide routine preoperative care and teaching as outlined in ∞ Chapter 4. *Patients having vascular surgery have similar preoperative nursing care needs to other patients having major abdominal or thoracic surgery. If emergent surgery is required, time for preoperative care and teaching may be limited.*
- Implement measures to reduce fear and anxiety:
  a. Orient to the intensive care unit, if appropriate.
  b. Describe and explain the reason for all equipment and tubes, such as cardiac monitors, ventilators, nasogastric tubes, urinary catheters, intravenous lines and fluids, and intra-arterial lines.
  c. Explain what to expect following surgery (sights, sounds, frequency of taking vital signs, dressings, pain relief measures, communication strategies).
  d. Allow time for questions and expression of fears and concerns.
  These explanations provide a sense of control for the patient and family.
- Monitor for and implement care to reduce the risk of aneurysm rupture (see the following Nursing Diagnoses and Interventions). *Patients with a rapidly expanding or symptomatic aneurysm are at risk for rupture prior to surgical repair.*

POSTOPERATIVE CARE

- Provide routine postoperative care and specific measures as ordered by the healthcare provider. *Patients undergoing aneurysm repair require nursing care similar to that provided to all patients with major thoracic or abdominal surgery, in addition to specific measures related to vascular surgery.*
- Maintain fluid replacement and blood or volume expanders as ordered. Promptly report changes in vital signs, level of consciousness, and urine output. *Hypovolemic shock may develop due to blood loss during surgery, third spacing, inadequate fluid replacement, and/or hemorrhage if graft separation or leakage occurs.*

PRACTICE ALERT

Monitor for and report manifestations of graft leakage:
a. Ecchymoses of the scrotum, perineum, or penis; a new or expanding hematoma
b. Increased abdominal girth
c. Weak or absent peripheral pulses; tachycardia; hypotension
d. Decreased motor function or sensation in the extremities
e. Fall in hemoglobin and hematocrit
f. Increasing abdominal, pelvic, back, or groin pain
g. Decreasing urinary output (less than 30 mL/ hour)
h. Decreasing CVP, pulmonary artery pressure, or pulmonary artery wedge pressure

These manifestations may signal graft leakage and possible hemorrhage. Pain may be due to pressure from an expanding hematoma or bowel ischemia. Decreased renal perfusion causes the glomerular filtration rate and urine output to fall.

- Report manifestations of lower extremity embolism: pain and numbness in lower extremities, decreasing pulses, and pale, cool, or cyanotic skin. *Pulses may be absent for 4 to 12 hours postoperatively due to vasospasm; however, absent pulses with pain, changes in sensation, and a pale, cool extremity are indicative of arterial occlusion.*
- Report manifestations of bowel ischemia or gangrene: abdominal pain and distention, occult or fresh blood in stools, and diarrhea. *Bowel ischemia may result from an embolism or occur as a complication of surgery.*
- Report manifestations of impaired renal function: urine output less than 30 mL per hour, fixed specific gravity, and increasing BUN and serum creatinine levels. *Hypovolemia or clamping of the aorta during surgery may impair renal perfusion, leading to acute renal failure.*
- Report manifestations of spinal cord ischemia: lower extremity weakness or paraplegia. *Impaired spinal cord perfusion may lead to ischemia and impaired function.*

∞ Nursing Care

Assessment

Focused assessment for the patient with a suspected aortic aneurysm includes the following:

- *Health history:* Complaints of chest, back, or abdominal pain; extremity weakness; shortness of breath, cough, difficult or painful swallowing, hoarseness; history of hypertension, coronary heart disease, heart failure, or peripheral vascular disease.
- *Physical examination:* Vital signs including blood pressure in upper and lower extremities; peripheral pulses; skin color and temperature; neck veins; abdominal exam including gentle palpation for masses and auscultation for bruits; neurologic exam including level of consciousness, sensation, and movement of extremities.

Nursing Diagnoses and Interventions

Nursing care for patients with an aneurysm of the aorta or its branches focuses on monitoring and maintaining tissue perfusion, relieving pain, and reducing anxiety. Nursing care usually is acute, precipitated by a complication or surgical repair of the aneurysm.

EVIDENCE FOR NURSING CARE   The Patient with Aortic Aneurysm

Selected resource that nurses may find helpful when planning evidence-based nursing care follows.

- Soat, M. (2009). Aortic aneurysm: Causes, clues, and treatment options. *American Nurse Today, 4*(7), 7–9.

Risk for Ineffective Tissue Perfusion

Patients with aortic aneurysms are at risk for impaired tissue perfusion due to aneurysm rupture with resulting hemorrhage and lack of blood flow to tissues distal to the rupture. In addition, thrombi often form within the aneurysm and may become emboli, obstructing distal arterial blood flow.

> **PRACTICE ALERT**
> Immediately report manifestations of impending rupture, expansion, or dissection of the aneurysm: increased pain, discrepancy between upper and lower extremity blood pressures and peripheral pulses, increased mass size, change in LOC or motor or sensory function, and laboratory results. Rapid expansion may indicate increased risk for rupture, with resulting hemorrhage, shock, and possible death. Elective or planned surgery may rapidly become emergency surgery to prevent complications.

- Implement interventions to reduce the risk of aneurysm rupture:
    a. Maintain bed rest with legs flat.
    b. Maintain a calm environment, implementing measures to reduce psychologic stress.
    c. Prevent straining during defecation and instruct to avoid holding the breath while moving.
    d. Administer beta blockers and antihypertensives as prescribed.

Activity, stress, and the Valsalva maneuver increase blood pressure, increasing the risk of rupture. Elevating or crossing the legs restricts peripheral blood flow and increases pressure in the aorta or iliac arteries. Beta blockers and antihypertensives often are ordered to reduce pressure in the dilated vessel.

  - Report manifestations of arterial thrombosis or embolism: absent peripheral pulses; a pale or cyanotic, cool extremity; severe, diffuse abdominal pain with guarding; or increased groin, lumbar, or lower extremity pain. Sluggish blood flow within the aneurysm often causes thrombi to form. These thrombi can break loose, becoming emboli that can occlude peripheral arteries or arteries to the kidneys or mesentery. *Arterial occlusion may necessitate emergency surgery to restore blood flow and prevent tissue infarct or gangrene.*

- Continuously monitor cardiac rhythm. Report complaints of chest pain or changes in ECG tracing. Administer oxygen as indicated. *Aortic dissection and repair place the patient at significant risk for myocardial infarction (MI), a major cause of postoperative mortality and morbidity (Kasper et al., 2005). Rapid identification and treatment of this complication can reduce the risk of death or long-term adverse effects of MI.*

  - Immediately report changes in mental status or symptoms of peripheral neurologic impairment (weakness, paresthesias, paralysis). The expanding aneurysm or dissection can affect carotid and cerebral blood flow or spinal cord perfusion, leading to neurologic symptoms. *Immediate restoration of blood flow is vital to prevent permanent neurologic deficits.*

Risk for Injury

Potent antihypertensive drugs often are given intravenously to reduce the pressure on an expanding or dissecting aneurysm. Continuous monitoring of infusions and hemodynamic parameters such as arterial pressure, pulmonary pressures, and cardiac output is vital to ensure that adequate tissue perfusion is maintained during infusions of these potent drugs.

- Use an infusion control device for all drug infusions. *These devices prevent accidental or inadvertent changes in the rate of the infusion and dose of the drug.*
- Continuously monitor arterial pressure and hemodynamic parameters as indicated. Promptly report results outside the specified parameters to the healthcare provider. *Many of the drugs used are effective within minutes. Responses vary among individuals, particularly in the older adult, necessitating continuous monitoring.*
- Monitor urine output hourly. Report output less than 30 mL/hr. *The kidneys are very sensitive to reduced perfusion pressure; inadequate renal blood flow can lead to acute renal failure.*

Anxiety

Patients with aortic aneurysms often are highly anxious because of the urgent nature of the disorder. The nurse must manage the anxiety levels of both the patient and family members to effectively address physiologic care needs. Stress reduction also is necessary to help maintain the blood pressure within desired limits.

- Explain all procedures and treatments, using simple and understandable terms. *Simplified explanations are necessary when anxiety levels interfere with learning and understanding.*
- Respond to all questions honestly, using a calm, empathetic, but matter-of-fact manner. *Honesty with the patient and family promotes trust and provides reassurance that the true nature of the situation is not being "hidden" from them.*
- Provide care in a calm, efficient manner. *Using a calm manner even during preparations for emergency surgery reassures the patient and family that although the situation is critical, the staff is prepared to handle things effectively.*
- Spend as much time as possible with the patient. Allow supportive family members to remain with the patient when possible. *The presence of a health professional and supportive family member reassures the patient that he or she is not alone in facing this crisis.*

Community-Based Care

Topics to discuss when preparing patients and their families for home care or care in a community-based setting depend on the treatment plan. Discuss the following topics when surgical repair is not immediately planned and the aneurysm will be monitored.

- Measures to control hypertension, including lifestyle and prescribed drugs
- The benefits of smoking cessation
- Manifestations of increasing aneurysm size or complications to report to the healthcare provider

Following surgery, discuss the following topics in preparing the patient and family for home care.

- Wound care and preventing infection; manifestations of impaired healing or infection to be reported
- Prescribed antihypertensive and anticoagulant medications and their expected and unintended effects
- The importance of adequate rest and nutrition for healing
- Measures to prevent constipation and straining at stool (such as increasing fluid and fiber in the diet)

- The importance of avoiding prolonged sitting, lifting heavy objects, engaging in strenuous exercise, and having sexual intercourse until approved by the healthcare provider (usually 6 to 12 weeks)
- Signs and symptoms of complications to report to the healthcare provider

Provide referrals to a home health agency or community health service as necessary. Referrals are especially important for older adults and their caregivers, who may require additional assistance with the complex care needs.

Disorders of the Peripheral Arteries

Disorders that impair peripheral arterial blood flow may be *acute* (e.g., arterial thrombosis) or *chronic* (e.g., peripheral arteriosclerosis). Chronic occlusive disorders may be due to structural defects of the arterial walls or spasm of affected arteries. Impaired peripheral arterial circulation limits the availability of oxygen and nutrients to the tissues, and can have significant adverse effects. This section focuses on acute and chronic disorders affecting peripheral arteries. The nurse's role in caring for patients with peripheral arterial disorders focuses on maintaining tissue perfusion and educating the patient and family about the disorder and its management.

Physiology Review

Peripheral arteries are the part of the systemic circulation that delivers oxygen and nutrients to the skin and the extremities. Arterial walls have three layers: the intima, which includes the endothelium and a layer of connective tissue and the basement membrane; the media, composed of smooth muscle and elastic fibers; and the adventitia, a thin layer of connective tissue that contains collagen and elastic fibers. The smooth muscle of peripheral arteries controls blood flow as it contracts and relaxes. Contraction narrows the vessel lumen (**vasoconstriction**), whereas smooth muscle relaxation expands the vessel (**vasodilation**). Peripheral arteries become progressively smaller; arterioles are less than 0.5 mm in diameter and are composed primarily of smooth muscle. The arterioles control blood flow through the capillary beds where gas, nutrient, and waste product exchange occurs. Capillary walls are very thin, consisting of a single layer of endothelial cells surrounded by a thin basement membrane.

Blood flows from an area of higher pressure to an area of lower pressure. *Resistance* opposes blood flow. Resistance is created by friction of the blood itself, although the primary determinants of vascular resistance are the diameter and length of the blood vessel. See the physiology review section under "Disorders of Blood Pressure Regulation" for more information about factors that determine vessel resistance.

The Patient with Peripheral Vascular Disease

Arteriosclerosis is the most common chronic arterial disorder, characterized by thickening, loss of elasticity, and calcification of arterial walls. **Atherosclerosis** is a form of arteriosclerosis in which deposits of fat and fibrin obstruct and harden the arteries.

In the peripheral circulation, these pathologic changes impair the blood supply to peripheral tissues, particularly the lower extremities. This is known as **peripheral vascular disease (PVD)**.

Pathophysiology

The pathophysiology of atherosclerosis is detailed in ∞ Chapter 30. Atherosclerotic lesions involve both the intima and the media of the involved arteries. There are three types of PVD: Type 1 (10% to 15% of patients) involving the aorta and iliac arteries; Type 2 (~25% of patients) where the aorta, common and external iliac arteries are involved and Type 3 (~60% to 70% of patients where the aorta, iliac, femoral, popliteal, and tibial arteries are involved (Papadakis & McPhee, 2007). Arteriosclerosis in the abdominal aorta leads to the development of aneurysms as plaque erodes the vessel wall.

Plaque tends to form at arterial bifurcations. The vessel lumen is progressively obstructed, decreasing blood flow to the lower extremities. Tissue hypoxia or anoxia results. With gradual obstruction of the vessel, collateral circulation often develops. However, it is usually not adequate to supply tissue needs, especially when metabolic demand increases (e.g., during exercise). Manifestations typically develop only when the vessel is occluded by 60% or more.

Manifestations and Complications

Pain is the primary symptom of peripheral atherosclerosis. Intermittent claudication, a cramping or aching pain in the calves of the legs, the thighs, and the buttocks that occurs with a predictable level of activity, is characteristic of PVD. The pain is often accompanied by weakness and is relieved by rest.

Rest pain, in contrast, occurs during periods of inactivity. It is often described as a burning sensation in the lower legs. Rest pain increases when the legs are elevated and decreases when the legs are dependent (e.g., hanging over the side of the bed). The legs also may feel cold or numb along with the pain. Sensation is diminished and the muscles may atrophy.

Peripheral pulses may be decreased or absent. A bruit may be heard over large affected arteries, such as the femoral artery and the abdominal aorta. The legs are pale when elevated, but often are dark red (*dependent rubor*) when dependent. The skin often is thin, shiny, and hairless, with discolored areas. Toenails may be thickened. Areas of skin breakdown and ulceration may be evident. Edema may develop with severe PVD. See the Manifestations of peripheral atherosclerosis box.

MANIFESTATIONS of Peripheral Atherosclerosis

- Intermittent claudication
- Rest pain
- Paresthesias (numbness, decreased sensation)
- Diminished or absent peripheral pulses
- Pallor with extremity elevation, dependent rubor when dependent
- Thin, shiny, hairless skin; thickened toenails
- Areas of discoloration or skin breakdown

Complications of peripheral atherosclerosis include gangrene and extremity amputation, rupture of abdominal aortic aneurysms, and possible infection and sepsis.

Incidence and Risk Factors

PVD usually affects people in their 60s and 70s; men are more often affected than women. Deaths attributed to peripheral arterial disease are about the same for Black and White males, but are higher among Black women than White women (AHA 2009).

Risk factors for PVD are similar to those for atherosclerosis and coronary heart disease (∞ see Chapter 30). Diabetes mellitus, hypercholesterolemia, hypertension, cigarette smoking, and high homocystine levels are risk factors for PVD (AHA, 2009).

FAST FACTS
- PVD is a common manifestation of atherosclerosis, particularly in older men.
- PVD interferes with arterial blood flow to the lower extremities, increasing the risk for neuropathy and paresthesias, ulcers that do not heal, necrosis, gangrene, and amputation.
- Regular daily exercise is a primary intervention for all types of peripheral arterial disease to promote development of collateral circulation and maintain tissue perfusion.

Interdisciplinary Care

Management of peripheral vascular disease focuses on slowing the atherosclerotic process and maintaining tissue perfusion.

Diagnosis

Although PVD often can be diagnosed by the history and physical examination, diagnostic tests may be ordered to evaluate its extent. Noninvasive studies often are sufficient.

- *Segmental pressure measurements* use sphygmomanometer cuffs and a Doppler device to compare blood pressures between the upper and lower extremities (normally similar) and within different segments of the affected extremity. In PVD, the BP may be lower in the legs than in the arms.
- *Stress testing* using a treadmill provides functional assessment of limitations. In PVD, pressure at the ankle may decline even further with exercise, confirming the diagnosis. Evaluation for coronary heart disease may be done simultaneously during exercise testing.
- *Doppler ultrasound* uses sound waves reflected off moving red blood cells within a vessel to evaluate blood flow. The

impulses may be translated into an audible signal or a graphic waveform. With significant PVD, the waveform becomes progressively flatter as the transducer is moved distally along the affected vessel. Segmental pressures may be used to locate the site of obstruction.

- *Duplex Doppler ultrasound* combines the audible or graphic Doppler ultrasound with ultrasound imaging to identify arterial or venous abnormalities. Ultrasonic imaging provides views of the affected vessel while Doppler ultrasound evaluates blood flow. *Color-flow Doppler ultrasound (CDU)* provides color images of the vessel and blood flow.
- *Transcutaneous oximetry* evaluates oxygenation of tissues.
- *Angiography* or *magnetic resonance angiography* is done before revascularization procedures to locate and evaluate the extent of arterial obstruction. For angiography, a contrast medium is injected and vessels are visualized using fluoroscopy and x-rays. Magnetic resonance angiography does not require injection of a contrast medium and may replace angiography.

∞ See Chapter 32 for more information on diagnostic testing for PVD.

Medications

Drug treatment of peripheral atherosclerosis is less effective than with coronary heart disease. Medications to inhibit platelet aggregation, such as aspirin or clopidogrel (Plavix) are ordered to reduce the risk of arterial thrombosis. Cilostazol (Pletal), a platelet inhibitor with vasodilator properties, improves claudication. Pentoxifylline (Trental) decreases blood viscosity and increases red blood cell flexibility, increasing blood flow to the microcirculation and tissues of the extremities. Parenteral vasodilator prostaglandins may be given on a long-term basis to decrease pain and facilitate healing in patients with severe limb ischemia (Deglin & Vallerand, 2009).

Treatments

Smoking cessation is vital. Nicotine not only promotes atherosclerosis, but also causes vasospasm, further reducing blood flow to the extremities.

Meticulous foot care is vital to prevent ulceration and infection (Box 32–4). Elastic support hose, which reduce circulation to the skin, are avoided. Elevating the head of the bed on blocks may help relieve rest pain. Regular, progressively strenuous exercise, such as 30 to 45 minutes of walking daily, is important. The patient is taught to rest at the onset of claudication, resuming activity when the pain resolves.

Other measures to slow the process of atherosclerosis, such as controlling diabetes and hypertension, lowering cholesterol levels, and weight loss, also are recommended (∞ see Chapter 30). See the box on page 1042 for care of the older adult.

Revascularization

Revascularization may be performed if symptoms are progressive, severe, or disabling. Other indications for surgery include symptoms that significantly interfere with activities of daily living, rest pain, and pregangrenous or gangrenous lesions. Either nonsurgical revascularization procedures or surgery may be performed.

BOX 32–4 Foot Care for the Patient with Peripheral Atherosclerosis

1. Keep legs and feet clean, dry, and comfortable.
   - Wash legs and feet daily in warm water, using mild soap.
   - Pat dry using a soft towel; be sure to dry between the toes.
   - Apply moisturizing cream to prevent drying.
   - Use powder on the feet and between the toes.
   - Buy shoes in the afternoon (when feet are largest); never buy shoes that are uncomfortable. Be sure toes have adequate room.
   - Wear a clean pair of cotton socks each day.
2. Prevent accidents and injuries to the feet.
   - Always wear shoes or slippers when getting out of bed.
   - Walk on level ground and avoid crowds, if possible.
   - Do not go barefoot.
   - Inspect legs and feet daily; use a mirror to examine backs of legs and bottoms of feet.
   - Have a professional foot care provider trim toenails and care for corns, calluses, ingrown toenails, or athlete's foot.
   - Always check the temperature of the water before stepping into the tub.
   - Do not get the legs or tops of the feet sunburned.
   - Report leg or foot problems (increased pain, cuts, bruises, blistering, redness, or open areas) to your healthcare provider.
3. Improve blood supply to the legs and feet.
   - Do not cross legs.
   - Do not wear garters or knee stockings.
   - Do not swim or wade in cold water.

Nonsurgical procedures include percutaneous transluminal angioplasty (PTA), stent placement, or atherectomy. Techniques may include balloon angioplasty to dilate the narrowed lumen, mechanical atherectomy to remove plaque, or laser or thermal angioplasty to vaporize the occluding material. In either case, a stent typically is placed at the time of PTA to maintain vessel patency. Iliac and femoral-popliteal PTA initially reestablish good blood flow and relieve symptoms in more than 80% of patients. While the 3-year success rate is lower, stent placement improves the duration of symptom relief. ∞ See Chapter 30 for more information about revascularization procedures.

Surgical options include endarterectomy to remove occlusive plaque from the artery and bypass grafts. Knitted Dacron bypass grafts are commonly used. Both immediate and long-term graft patency is better with bypass grafting than with nonsurgical revascularization procedures, but the risk for operative complications such as myocardial infarction, stoke, infection, and peripheral embolization is higher. Nursing care for the patient having revascularization surgery is similar to that provided for patients having surgery of the aorta (see the box on page 1038).

Complementary Therapies

Complementary therapies for peripheral vascular disease include interventions to improve circulation and to reduce stress. A number of complementary therapies may improve peripheral circulation, including aromatherapy with rosemary or vetiver; biofeedback; healing or therapeutic touch and massage; herbals such as ginko, garlic, cayenne, hawthorn, and bilberry; and exercise including yoga. Aromatherapy and yoga also may reduce stress, as can breathing exercises, meditation, and counseling. In

NURSING CARE OF THE OLDER ADULT — Peripheral Vascular Disease

With aging, blood vessels thicken and become less compliant. These changes reduce oxygen delivery to the tissues and impair carbon dioxide and waste product removal from the tissues. When normal effects of aging combine with an increased risk of atherosclerosis, the risk of peripheral vascular disease is high.

The older adult with peripheral vascular disease requires the same care and teaching as other patients. However, visual deficits and osteoarthritis may make foot care more difficult. Long-standing smoking habits are difficult to break. Mobility may be impaired by arthritis or the effects of neurologic disorders. The patient who lives alone may resist walking. Periodic visits by a community or home health nurse may be helpful, as may be encouraging the patient to join a support group for stopping smoking, changing eating habits, and taking part in regular activity.

addition, complementary therapies to reduce atherosclerosis and lower cholesterol levels may slow the progress of PVD. Measures such as a very low-fat or vegetarian diet, including antioxidant nutrients or using vitamin C, vitamin E, or garlic supplements, and traditional Chinese medicine may be useful.

Nursing Care

Health Promotion

Discuss healthy lifestyle habits with community and religious groups, school children (grades K through 12), and through the print media to reduce the incidence and slow the progression of atherosclerosis.

Strongly encourage all patients to avoid smoking in the first place, and to stop all forms of tobacco use. Discuss the adverse effects of smoking and the benefits of quitting. Provide information about dietary recommendations to maintain a healthy weight and optimal cholesterol levels. Discuss the benefits and importance of regular exercise. Finally, encourage patients with cardiovascular risk factors to undergo regular screening for hypertension, diabetes, and hyperlipidemia.

Assessment

Focused assessment related to peripheral atherosclerosis includes the following:

- *Health history:* Complaints of pain, its relationship to exercise or rest, timing, associated symptoms, and relief measures; history of coronary heart disease, peripheral vascular disease, hyperlipidemia, hypertension, or diabetes; current medications; smoking history; usual diet and activity patterns.
- *Physical examination:* Vital signs; strength and equality of peripheral pulses of all extremities; capillary refill; skin color, temperature, hair distribution, presence of any discolorations or lesions; movement and sensation of lower extremities.

Nursing Diagnoses and Interventions

Impaired tissue perfusion is an obvious problem in peripheral atherosclerosis. Acute and chronic pain may interfere with activities of daily living, and ambulation may be limited. The possibility of losing a lower extremity is frightening.

Ineffective Tissue Perfusion: Peripheral

Impaired blood flow to the lower extremities affects gas, nutrient, and waste product exchange between the capillaries and cells. Oxygen and nutrient deprivation impairs cell function and tissue integrity, causing pain and impaired healing. Pain develops with exercise and when extremities are elevated.

■ Assess peripheral pulses, pain, color, temperature, and capillary refill every 4 hours and as needed. Use a Doppler device if pulses are not palpable. Mark pulse locations with an indelible marker. *Assessment data provide a baseline for evaluating the effectiveness of interventions and identifies changes in arterial blood flow.*

■ Position with extremities dependent. *Gravity promotes arterial flow to the dependent extremity, increasing tissue perfusion and relieving pain.*

■ Instruct to avoid smoking. If necessary, obtain an order for a nicotine patch or gum from the healthcare provider. Nicotine is a potent vasoconstrictor that further impairs arterial blood flow. Nicotine patches and gum contain less nicotine than cigarettes, and can help reduce the stress of smoking cessation. *Smoking cessation is a vital component of care.*

■ Discuss the benefits of regular exercise. *Exercise promotes development of collateral circulation to ischemic tissues and slows the process of atherosclerosis.*

■ Use a foot cradle and lightweight blankets, socks, and slippers to keep extremities warm. Avoid electric heating pads or hot water bottles. *Keeping extremities warm conserves heat, prevents vasospasm, and promotes arterial flow. External heating devices are avoided to reduce the risk of burns in the patient with impaired sensation. The foot cradle protects tissues from compression by linens.*

■ Encourage frequent position changes. Instruct to avoid crossing legs or using a pillow under the knees. *Position changes promote blood flow and reduce damage caused by pressure. Leg crossing and excessive flexion of the hip or knee joints can compress partially obstructed arteries and impair blood flow to distal tissues.*

Pain

Impaired blood flow results in tissue ischemia. Metabolism shifts from an efficient aerobic process to an anaerobic process. Lactic acid and metabolic waste products accumulate in tissues, causing pain. Severe and cramping pain generally occurs with exercise early in the disease. Rest initially produces relief, similar to the process of angina (∞ see Chapter 30). As the disease progresses, pain develops with less exercise and often occurs even at rest. Rest pain disrupts sleep, the sense of well-being, and has significant disruptive effects on life roles.

■ Assess pain at least every 4 hours using a standard pain scale more often as needed. *Pain is a subjective experience. Using a standard pain scale allows evaluation of treatment measures in relieving pain and restoring blood flow.*

■ Keep extremities warm. *Cooling leads to vasoconstriction, increasing pain. Warming the extremities promotes vasodilation and improves arterial flow, reducing pain.*

■ Teach pain relief and stress reduction techniques such as relaxation, meditation, and guided imagery. *Pain increases stress. The stress response leads to vasoconstriction, increasing pain.*

Stress reduction techniques, when combined with other measures to promote blood flow, can help reduce pain.

Impaired Skin Integrity

Patients with PVD are at risk for impaired skin integrity as a result of oxygen and nutrient deprivation. Chronic tissue ischemia leads to dry, scaly, and atrophied skin. Pruritus can lead to scratching; minor injuries may go unnoticed due to impaired sensation. Impaired tissue healing can lead to ulceration, infection, and potential gangrene.

■ Assess and document skin condition at least every 8 hours a with each home visit, more frequently as indicated. *Tissue ischemia increases the risk for damage, even with minor trauma such as pressure from poorly fitting shoes or bed linens. Frequent inspection and documentation of skin condition is vital to identify early indicators of impaired skin integrity and reduce the risk of complications such as infection.*

■ Provide meticulous daily skin care, keeping the skin clean and dry. Apply a moisturizing cream to dry or scaly areas. *Intact skin is the body's first defense against bacterial invasion. Ischemic tissues of the injured extremity provide an excellent medium for microorganism growth. Clean, dry, supple skin decreases the risk of breakdown.*

■ Apply a bed cradle. *The bed cradle suspends bed linens over the legs, preventing them from placing pressure on extremities and injured tissues. Minimizing pressure on the tissues promotes capillary blood flow.*

■ Provide an egg crate mattress, flotation pad, sheepskin, or heel protectors. *Ischemic tissues may be damaged by minor trauma such as that created by the shearing forces of skin against bed linens.*

Activity Intolerance

Pain and impaired perfusion of peripheral tissues may limit the patient's ability to engage in desired activities, even impairing self-care.

■ Assist with care activities as needed. *Severe claudication or rest pain may limit activities. Muscle atrophy of affected extremities is common, leading to fatigue and weakness.*

■ Unless contraindicated, encourage gradual increases in duration and intensity of exercise. Teach to rest with extremities dependent when claudication develops, resuming activity after pain has abated. *Gradual increases in the duration and intensity of exercise promote development of collateral circulation, improve exercise tolerance, provide a sense of well-being, and support self-esteem.*

■ Provide diversional activities during periods of prescribed bed rest. Encourage relaxation techniques to reduce muscle tension. *Diversional activities help prevent boredom and stress associated with enforced rest. Relaxation techniques reduce vasoconstriction induced by stress, improving peripheral circulation.*

■ Encourage frequent position changes and active range-of-motion exercises. Encourage self-care to the extent possible. *Position changes relieve pressure on tissues, improving capillary circulation and reducing tissue ischemia. Range-of-motion exercises help prevent muscle atrophy and joint contractures. Self-care supports self-esteem.*

CASE STUDY & NURSING CARE PLAN   A Patient with Peripheral Vascular Disease

William Duffy, aged 69, is retired. His wife convinces him to see his primary care provider for increasing leg pain with walking and other exercise.

ASSESSMENT

Katie Kotson, RN, obtains Mr. Duffy's history before he sees his healthcare provider. He states that he can only walk about a block before the pain in his calves gets so bad that he has to stop and rest. As a result, he has been less and less active, spending most of his time the past few months watching sports on television. He denies rest pain. He was diagnosed with type 2 diabetes about 15 years ago, which he manages with daily glyburide (DiaBeta), an oral hypoglycemic. He also has stable angina, for which he takes atenolol (Tenormin) and an occasional nitroglycerin tablet. His alcohol intake is moderate, averaging 1 to 2 beers per day, and he smokes about a pack of cigarettes per day. He states he tried to quit smoking after developing angina, but "after nearly 50 years of smoking, I think that's impossible!"

Physical exam findings include height 68 inches (173 cm), weight 235 lb (107 kg), BP 168/78, P 66, R 16, T 97.6°F (36.5°C); upper extremities warm and pink, normal hair distribution, pulses strong and equal; lower extremities below knees cool and ruddy when dependent, pale to pink when elevated, skin shiny, scant hair; posterior tibial pulses weak bilaterally; weak pedal pulse on R, unable to palpate on L; 1+ to 2+ edema both feet and ankles.

The healthcare provider finds that Mr. Duffy's systolic blood pressure in his legs is an average of 28 mmHg lower than in his arms. He makes the diagnosis of peripheral atherosclerosis, and schedules Mr. Duffy for an exercise stress test with ankle pressure measurements before and after exercise and a color-flow Doppler ultrasound. Mr. Duffy is to return in 3 weeks after these studies have been completed.

DIAGNOSES

- *Activity Intolerance* related to poor blood flow to lower extremities
- *Ineffective Health Maintenance* related to smoking and lack of information about disease management
- *Risk for Impaired Skin Integrity* related to ischemic tissues of legs and feet
- *Risk for Peripheral Neurovascular Dysfunction* related to impaired peripheral blood flow to lower extremities

EXPECTED OUTCOMES

- Walk for at least 15 minutes three to four times per day, gradually increasing his pace and duration of exercise.
- Relate the benefits of smoking cessation.
- Identify strategies to improve chances for success in stopping smoking.
- Meet with dietitian before next visit to discuss dietary measures to promote weight loss and slow atherosclerosis.

- Verbalize an understanding of appropriate foot care measures.
- Identify measures to prevent inadvertent injury of feet and legs.

PLANNING AND IMPLEMENTATION

- Teach about peripheral atherosclerosis and its relationship to Mr. Duffy's symptoms.
- With Mr. and Mrs. Duffy, plan strategies to start and maintain a program of regular exercise.
- Instruct to warm up slowly, and to stop exercise and rest for 3 minutes (or until pain is relieved) when claudication develops, then resume exercising.
- Discuss the effects of smoking on blood vessels.
- Help Mr. Duffy identify smoking cessation strategies such as support groups, clinics, and nicotine patches.
- Schedule an appointment with the dietitian to develop a low-calorie, low-fat, and low-cholesterol ADA diet that includes preferred foods and considers usual eating patterns.
- Reinforce and supplement previous foot care teaching.
- Discuss effects of impaired circulation on sensation in feet and legs and measures to prevent injury.

EVALUATION

When Mr. Duffy returns to the office 3 weeks later, his diagnosis has been confirmed by the diagnostic studies. The healthcare provider decides to continue conservative therapy, now prescribing atorvastatin (Lipitor) to lower Mr. Duffy's serum cholesterol level, and cilostazol (Pletal) to reduce the risk of thrombosis and improve symptoms of claudication. Mr. Duffy also asks his healthcare provider for a prescription for nicotine patches, saying he is ready to quit smoking, but thinks he needs help to be successful. Mr. and Mrs. Duffy tell Miss Kotson that they are walking before every meal and really enjoying being outside more. They plan to walk in the local shopping mall when the weather gets worse. Mrs. Duffy has bought an American Heart Association cookbook, and is carefully planning their meals. Both Mr. and Mrs. Duffy have lost 5 lb since the previous visit. Mr. Duffy's skin on his legs and feet remains intact, and he identifies the measures he is using to protect his lower extremities from injury.

CRITICAL THINKING IN THE NURSING PROCESS

1. What additional lifestyle changes related to peripheral atherosclerosis might be appropriate to suggest to Mr. Duffy at this time? Why?
2. Explain the relationship between physical exercise and pain in the patient with peripheral atherosclerosis. Compare this relationship to that between exercise and angina.
3. Mr. Duffy uses a beta blocker, atenolol, to prevent angina. Why is this drug not effective in preventing claudication?
4. Develop a nursing care plan for the diagnosis *Imbalanced Nutrition: More than Body Requirements*.

See Evaluating Your Response in Appendix C.

Using NANDA, NIC, and NOC

Linkages between a selected NANDA nursing diagnosis, NIC, and NOC for the patient with peripheral vascular disease are shown in the chart that follows.

Community-Based Care

Discuss the following topics when preparing the patient and family for home and community-based care. See the accompanying Case Study & Nursing Care Plan for additional community-based nursing interventions.

- Smoking cessation strategies and ways to avoid second-hand smoke
- Prescribed medications and anticoagulants, their purpose, doses, desired and adverse effects
- Signs of excess bleeding to report to the healthcare provider
- Skin surveillance and foot care (see Box 32–4)
- Recommended diet and exercise
- Weight loss strategies if appropriate

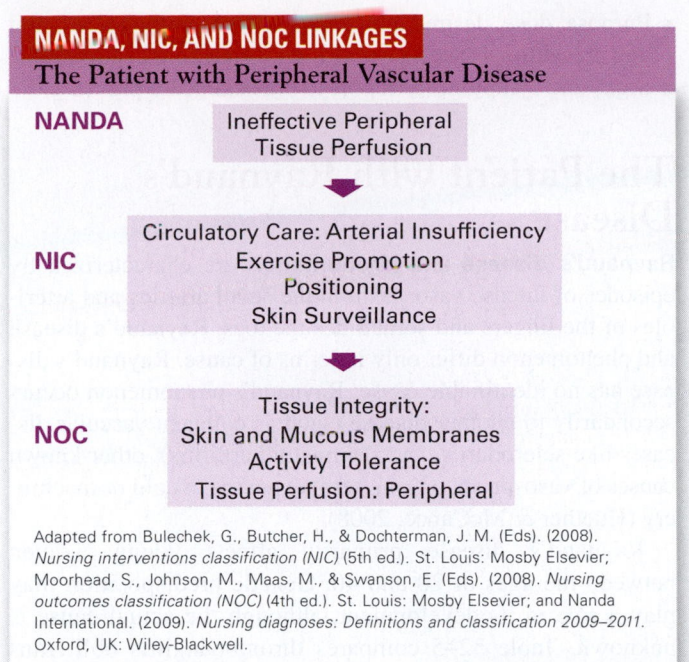

If revascularization or surgery has been performed, include the following topics as appropriate.

- Incision care
- Manifestations of complications (e.g., infection, graft leakage, or thrombosis) to be reported to the healthcare provider
- Activity limitations

Provide referrals to home health services, physical or occupational therapy, and home maintenance assistance services as indicated. Consider resources such as Meals-on-Wheels for patients who are severely limited by their disease.

The Patient with Thromboangiitis Obliterans

Thromboangiitis obliterans (also called *Buerger's disease*) is an occlusive vascular disease in which small and midsize peripheral arteries become inflamed and spastic, causing clots to form. This disease may affect either the upper or lower extremities; it often affects a leg or foot. Its exact etiology is unknown, but there is evidence of significant T cell activation, autoimmunity, and inflammation (Huether & McCance, 2008).

Pathophysiology and Course

Inflammatory cells infiltrate the wall of small and midsize arteries in the feet and possibly the hands. This inflammatory process is accompanied by thrombus formation and vasospasms of arterial segments that impair blood flow. Adjacent veins and nerves also may be affected. As the disease progresses, affected vessels become scarred and fibrotic.

The course of the disease is intermittent with dramatic exacerbations and marked remissions. The disease may remain dormant for periods of weeks, months, or years. As the disease progresses, collateral vessels are more extensively involved. Consequently, subsequent episodes are more intense and prolonged. Prolonged periods of tissue hypoxia increase the risk for tissue ulceration and gangrene.

Manifestations and Complications

Pain in the affected extremities is the primary manifestation of thromboangiitis obliterans. Both claudication, cramping pain in calves and feet or the forearms and hands, and rest pain in the fingers and toes may occur. Sensation is diminished. Eventually, the skin becomes thin and shiny and the nails are thickened and malformed. On examination, the involved digits and/or extremities are pale, cyanotic, or ruddy, and cool or cold to touch. Distal pulses (e.g., the dorsalis pedis, posterior tibial, ulnar, or radial) are either difficult to locate or absent, even with a Doppler device.

Painful ulcers and gangrene may develop in the fingers and toes, as a result of severely impaired blood flow. Amputation may be necessary to remove necrotic tissue.

Incidence and Risk Factors

Thromboangiitis obliterans primarily affects men under age 40 who smoke. Cigarette smoking is the single most significant cause of the disease. The disease is more prevalent in Asians and people of eastern European descent. The incidence of HLA-B5 and 2A9 antigens is higher in people with thromboangiitis obliterans, suggesting a genetic link.

Interdisciplinary Care

Thromboangiitis obliterans usually is diagnosed by the history and physical examination. Doppler studies may be used to locate and determine the extent of the disease. Angiography and magnetic resonance imaging may also be used to evaluate the extent of the disease, but usually are unnecessary.

The one most important component in managing this disease is smoking cessation. While stopping smoking does not cure the disease, it may slow its extension to other vessels. With continued smoking, attacks become increasingly intense and last much longer, significantly increasing the risk for ulcerations and gangrene.

Additional conservative measures are used to prevent vasoconstriction, improve peripheral blood flow, and prevent complications of chronic ischemia. These measures include keeping extremities warm, managing stress, keeping affected extremities in a dependent position, preventing injury to affected tissues, and regular exercise. Walking for 20 or more minutes several times a day is recommended.

There are no specific drugs for thromboangiitis obliterans. A calcium channel blocker such as diltiazem (Cardizem) or verapamil (Isoptin), or pentoxifylline (Trental), which decreases blood viscosity and increases red blood cell flexibility to improve peripheral blood flow, may provide some symptom relief.

Surgical approaches for thromboangiitis obliterans include sympathectomy or arterial bypass graft. Sympathectomy interrupts sympathetic nervous system input to affected vessels, reducing vasoconstriction and spasm. Arterial bypass grafts may be useful when larger vessels are affected by the disease. Amputation of an affected digit or extremity may be necessary if gangrene develops. (∞ See Chapter 39 for more information about amputation.) Only portions of digits or of limbs (e.g., below the knee) may be amputated, to preserve as much healthy tissue as possible.

The prognosis for thromboangiitis obliterans depends significantly on the patient's ability and willingness to stop smoking. With smoking cessation and good foot care, the prognosis for saving the extremities is good, even though no cure is available.

∞ Nursing Care

Health promotion activities to prevent thromboangiitis obliterans focus on preventing smoking, especially in high-risk populations. Nursing assessment and care for patients with this disease is similar to that provided for patients with other arterial occlusive diseases. Nursing care focuses on promoting arterial circulation and preventing prolonged tissue hypoxia. Because inflammatory, spastic episodes may be unpredictable, care focuses on smoking cessation and relieving acute manifestations. In addition, postsurgical care is necessary if surgery has been performed. See the nursing care section for peripheral atherosclerosis as well as nursing care of the postsurgical patient (∞ Chapter 4) and following amputation (∞ Chapter 39).

Community-Based Care

Discuss the following topics when preparing patients with thromboangiitis obliterans and their families for home or community-based care.

- Absolute necessity of smoking cessation
- Foot care
- Protecting affected extremities from injury

- Purpose, dose, desired and adverse effects, interactions, and any precautions associated with prescribed medications
- Signs and symptoms to report to the healthcare provider

The Patient with Raynaud's Disease

Raynaud's disease and **phenomenon** are characterized by episodes of intense vasospasm in the small arteries and arterioles of the fingers and sometimes the toes. Raynaud's disease and phenomenon differ only in terms of cause. Raynaud's disease has no identifiable cause; Raynaud's phenomenon occurs secondarily to another disease (such as collagen vascular diseases like scleroderma and rheumatoid arthritis), other known causes of vasospasm, or long-term exposure to cold or machinery (Huether & McCance, 2008).

Raynaud's disease primarily affects young women between the ages of 20 and 40. Genetic predisposition may play a role in its development, although the actual cause is unknown. Table 32–5 compares thromboangiitis obliterans and Raynaud's disease.

Pathophysiology and Manifestations

Raynaud's disease and phenomenon are characterized by spasms of the small arteries in the digits. The arterial spasms limit arterial blood flow to the fingers and possibly the toes. Initial attacks may involve only the tips of one or two fingers; with disease progression, the entire finger and all fingers may be affected.

TABLE 32–5 Comparison of Raynaud's Disease and Thromboangiitis Obliterans

TOPIC	RAYNAUD'S DISEASE	THROMBOANGIITIS OBLITERANS
Etiology	■ Unknown ■ Possible genetic predisposition	■ Cigarette smoking most probable single cause ■ Possible autoimmune response
Incidence/course of the disease	■ Onset commonly between 15 and 45 years of age ■ Usually affects young women ■ Becomes progressively worse over time	■ Occurs predominantly in men under 40 ■ More common in Asians and people of European heritage ■ Intermittent course with exacerbations and remissions ■ Increase severity and duration of attacks over time
Triggering stimuli	■ Emotional stress ■ Exposure to cold	■ Cigarette smoking
Assessment findings	■ Usually affects hands, sometimes toes ■ Pain becomes more severe and prolonged as disease progresses ■ "Blue-white-red" changes in color of hands with accompanying changes in skin temperature	■ Claudication and pain ■ Numbness or diminished sensation ■ Cool, pale, or cyanotic skin ■ Shiny, thin skin and white, malformed nails in affected extremities ■ Distal pulses difficult to find or absent ■ Trophic changes to nail beds ■ Ulceration and gangrene in later stages ■ Small, red, tender vascular cords in affected extremities
Management	■ Avoid unnecessary cold exposure ■ Emphasize smoking cessation ■ Medications such as calcium channel or alpha adrenergic blockers as indicated ■ Teach stress management	■ Stop smoking (crucial) ■ Regular exercise ■ Protect extremities from cold injury ■ Teach stress management

The manifestations of Raynaud's occur intermittently when spasms develop. Raynaud's disease has been called "the blue-white-red disease," because affected digits initially turn blue as blood flow is reduced due to vasospasm, then white as circulation is more severely limited, and finally very red as the fingers are warmed and the spasm resolves (Figure 32–9 ■). Sensory changes may occur during attacks, including numbness, stiffness, decreased sensation, and aching pain.

The attacks tend to become more frequent and prolonged over time. With repeated attacks (and resultant decrease in oxygenation), the fingertips thicken and the nails become brittle. Ulceration and gangrene are serious complications that rarely occur.

Interdisciplinary Care

Raynaud's disease and phenomenon are primarily diagnosed by the history and physical examination. There are no specific diagnostic tests for these disorders.

Vasodilators may be prescribed to provide symptomatic relief. Low doses of a sustained release calcium channel blocker such as nifedipine (Procardia) or diltiazem (Cardizem) may be prescribed. The α-adrenergic blocker prazosin (Minipress) also may reduce the frequency and severity of attacks. Transdermal nitroglycerine (or longer-acting oral nitrates) helps some patients by decreasing the amount of time necessary for the hands to return to normal following an attack (Papadakis & McPhee, 2007).

Conservative measures are a mainstay of treatment. Patients are instructed to keep their hands warm, wearing gloves when outside in cold weather and kitchen gloves when handling cold items (for instance, when preparing and serving cold foods and cleaning the refrigerator). Measures to avoid injury to the hands are taught. Sometimes attacks can be stopped by swinging the arms back and forth, increasing perfusion pressure in the small arteries by centrifugal force.

Smoking cessation is important. Stress reduction measures such as exercise, relaxation techniques, massage therapy, hobbies, aroma therapy, and counseling are taught or suggested. Additional lifestyle habits that contribute to vascular health are encouraged, such as reducing dietary fat, increasing activity level, and maintaining normal body weight.

✍ Nursing Care

Nursing care for the patient with Raynaud's disease or phenomenon is primarily educative and supportive. Protecting the hands and feet from exposure to cold and trauma is the major teaching topic. Nursing diagnoses and interventions previously outlined for peripheral atherosclerosis also are appropriate for patients with Raynaud's.

Community-Based Care

Reassure patients with Raynaud's phenomenon that most people with the disorder experience only mild, infrequent episodes. Discuss the following topics in preparing the patient for managing the disorder.

- Dress warmly, keeping the trunk and hands warm.
- Avoid unnecessary exposure to cold.
- Stop smoking or do not start.
- Discuss the use, purpose, desired and potential adverse effects of prescribed medications, if any.

The Patient with Acute Arterial Occlusion

A peripheral artery may be acutely occluded by development of a thrombus (blood clot) or by an embolism. Blood flow to tissues supplied by the artery is impaired, resulting in acute tissue ischemia and a risk for necrosis and gangrene.

Pathophysiology

Arterial Thrombosis

A **thrombus** is a blood clot that adheres to the vessel wall. Thrombi tend to develop in areas where intravascular factors stimulate coagulation (e.g., where a vessel lumen is partially obstructed and its wall is damaged and roughened by atherosclerosis). Other disorders, such as infection or inflammation of the vessel wall or pooling of blood (e.g., in an aneurysm) also can prompt coagulation and thrombus formation (Huether & McCance, 2008). A developing thrombus can occlude arterial blood flow through the vessel, leading to ischemia of tissues supplied by that artery. The extent of ischemia depends on the size of the affected artery and the degree of collateral circulation. In gradual processes of arterial occlusion such as atherosclerosis, collateral vessels often develop to compensate for impaired arterial flow. The extent of collateral circulation affects the degree of tissue ischemia distal to the thrombus.

Arterial Embolism

An **embolism** is sudden obstruction of a blood vessel by debris. A thrombus can break loose from the arterial wall to become a **thromboembolus**. Other substances also can become emboli: atherosclerotic plaque, masses of bacteria, cancer cells, amniotic fluid, bone marrow fat, and foreign objects such as air bubbles or broken intravenous catheters. Regardless of cause, an embolus eventually lodges in a vessel that is too small to allow it to pass.

Figure 32–9 ■ Hands of a patient with Raynaud's phenomenon. Note cyanosis of fingers on the right hand and the left thumb and the extreme pallor of the other digits of the left hand.

Arterial emboli often originate in the left side of the heart. They are associated with myocardial infarction, valvular heart disease, left-sided heart failure, atrial fibrillation, or infectious heart diseases. Emboli from the left heart often enter the carotid arteries and become trapped in the cerebral circulation, causing neurologic deficits (∞ see Chapter 42). Thromboemboli that develop in the aorta or peripheral arterial circulation tend to lodge in areas where the arterial lumen is narrowed by atherosclerotic plaque and at arterial bifurcations.

Manifestations

The manifestations of arterial thrombosis and embolism are those of tissue ischemia. Ischemic tissues are painful, pale, and cool or cold. Distal pulses are absent. Paresthesias (numbness and tingling) develop in the extremity. Cyanosis and mottling are common. Paralysis and muscle spasms may develop in the affected extremity. A line of demarcation between normal and ischemic tissue may be seen, particularly with embolism. Tissue below the line is cool or cold, and pale, cyanotic, or mottled. See the Manifestations box.

Arterial occlusion can result in permanent vessel and limb damage. Complete arterial occlusion leads to tissue necrosis and gangrene unless blood flow is promptly restored.

Interdisciplinary Care

Acute arterial occlusions may require emergency treatment to preserve the limb if the obstructed vessel is large or collateral circulation is minimal. If the limb is not in jeopardy, more conservative management may be initiated.

Diagnosis

The diagnosis of acute arterial occlusion often is apparent by the signs and symptoms. *Arteriography* is used to confirm the diagnosis, locate the occlusion, and determine its extent.

Medications

Anticoagulation with intravenous heparin is initiated to prevent further clot propagation and recurrent embolism. Anticoagulation is continued with oral anticoagulants after discharge. See the section on venous thrombosis later in this chapter for more information about anticoagulant therapy.

Arterial thrombosis may be treated with intra-arterial thrombolytic therapy using streptokinase, urokinase, or tissue plasminogen activator (t-PA) (∞ see Chapter 30). Lysis of the thrombus or embolus is achieved in 50% to 80% of the cases

(Papadakis & McPhee, 2007). Local intra-arterial injection of the thrombolytic drug allows use of lower doses and reduces the bleeding risk associated with thrombolytic drugs.

Surgery

Immediate *embolectomy* (within 4 to 6 hours) is the treatment of choice for acute arterial occlusion by an embolus to prevent tissue necrosis and gangrene. When the involved vessel is in an extremity, local anesthesia and a special balloon-tipped catheter known as a Fogarty catheter may be used for high surgical risk patients (Papadakis & McPhee, 2007). An embolus in the mesenteric circulation necessitates emergency laparotomy. The risk of complications and limb loss increases significantly if surgery is delayed by 12 or more hours. Potential major complications include compartment syndrome (∞ see Chapter 39), acute respiratory distress syndrome (∞ Chapter 37), or acute renal failure (∞ Chapter 28).

Arterial thrombosis also may be treated surgically, although the required surgery may be more extensive due to the length of the vessel involved. *Thromboendarterectomy* is done to remove the thrombus and plaque in the artery. An arterial graft may be required. Nursing care for patients who have undergone embolectomy or thrombus removal is discussed in the nursing care section that follows.

∞ Nursing Care

Assessment

Nursing assessment for the patient with an acute arterial occlusion is highly focused due to the emergency nature of the problem.

- *Health history:* Complaints of pain, numbness, tingling, or weakness in the involved extremity; history of atherosclerotic vessel disease, heart disease, or recent invasive procedure (e.g., angiography, percutaneous revascularization procedure).
- *Physical examination:* Vital signs; peripheral pulses in both extremities; color, temperature, sensation, and movement of involved extremity; skin condition; presence of a line of demarcation.

Nursing Diagnoses and Interventions

Nursing care related to acute arterial occlusion focuses on protecting the affected extremity, managing anxiety, and reducing the risk of complications related to anticoagulant therapy.

Ineffective Tissue Perfusion: Peripheral

Protecting ischemic tissue from injury prior to surgery or medical thrombolysis is vital. Following surgery, there is a risk for thrombosis at the graft site or impaired perfusion due to edema of the surgical site.

- Monitor extremity perfusion, comparing affected and unaffected extremities. Assess peripheral pulses (using the Doppler stethoscope as needed), skin temperature and color, capillary refill, movement, and sensation every 1 to 4 hours. Promptly report changes or complaints of increased or unrelieved pain. Propogation of a thrombus can further obstruct

---

MANIFESTATIONS of Acute Arterial Occlusion

- Pain
- Pallor or mottling
- Paresthesias (numbness and tingling)
- Cool or cold skin
- Pulselessness distal to the blockage
- Possible paralysis, weakness, or muscle spasms
- Possible line of demarcation; with pallor, cyanosis, and cooler skin distal to the blockage (especially with arterial embolism)

arterial flow, increasing tissue ischemia. Following surgery, arterial spasms may cause a cyanotic, pulseless extremity; normal color and pulses should return within 12 hours. *A thrombus may form at the surgical site or within a graft, causing tissue ischemia with pain and other manifestations of arterial occlusion. Further measures to restore circulation may be necessary.*

- Maintain intravenous fluids as ordered. *Adequate circulating blood volume is necessary to maintain cardiac output and tissue perfusion.*

- Protect the extremity, keeping it horizontal or lower than the heart. Use a cradle to keep bedclothes off the extremity and sheepskin or foam pad to protect it from hard or abrasive surfaces. Do not apply heat or cold. *Keeping the extremity lower than the heart promotes collateral blood flow. Ischemic tissue is easily damaged by minimal trauma such as shearing by bed linens, or heat or cold application.*

- Following surgery, avoid raising the knee, placing pillows under the knees, or sitting with 90-degree hip flexion. *These activities may impair blood flow through the affected vessel.*

Anxiety

Patients with an acute arterial occlusion often are very anxious. The rapid and intense nature of preoperative activities can be overwhelming, increasing anxiety about the disorder and its outcome. Manifestations of anxiety may include trembling, palpitations, restlessness, dry mouth, helplessness, inability to relax, irritability, forgetfulness, and lack of awareness of surroundings. Nursing measures focus on establishing trust and minimizing the effects of anxiety to decrease surgical risk and improve recovery.

- Spend as much time as possible with the patient. Provide opportunities to verbalize anxiety; offer reassurance and support. Support adaptive coping mechanisms. *The presence of a caring nurse provides a safe environment for expressing fears and anxieties. Coping mechanisms reduce the immediate perceived threat and increase the ability to deal with the situational crisis.*

- Perform required measures in an expedient but calm manner. *Calm, confident performance of treatment measures reassures the patient and family that appropriate care is being given to treat the problem at hand.*

- Assess anxiety level at least every 8 hours, and more often as needed. Intervene as indicated to reduce anxiety. *Assessment helps determine the intensity of anxiety, the patient's ability to control it, and directs interventions to reduce it.*

- Decrease sensory stimuli as much as possible. *Reducing environmental stimuli provides the patient a degree of control over anxiety.*

- Speak slowly and clearly and avoid unnecessary interruptions when listening. Give concise directions, focusing on the present. Involve the patient in simple tasks and decisions to the extent possible. *High levels of anxiety interfere with learning. Keeping interactions focused on the present situation directs the patient's focus and provides reassurance that it is the most important focus of the nurse as well. Providing*

opportunities for self-care and decision making reinforces the patient's importance and power to control the situation.

Altered Protection

Thrombolytic and/or anticoagulant therapy used to dissolve existing clots and prevent further clot formation increase the risk for bleeding. Close monitoring of physical status and laboratory data is vital, as are measures to reduce the risk for injury and bleeding.

> **PRACTICE ALERT**
>
> Assess for and report manifestations of impaired clotting, including excessive incisional bleeding; prolonged oozing from injection sites; bleeding gums, nose bleed, or hematuria; petechiae, bruising, or purpura. Anticoagulants and thrombolytics interfere with the clotting cascade and may cause abnormal bleeding.

- Monitor activated partial thromboplastin time (APTT) during heparin therapy and prothrombin time (PT) or international normalized ratio (INR) during oral anticoagulant therapy. Report values outside desired range. *The APTT, PT, and INR are prolonged by anticoagulant therapy. Values higher than the desired range may indicate an increased risk for bleeding; values below the target may indicate inadequate anticoagulation.*

- Protect from injury: Use side rails or other measures as needed to prevent falls; avoid parenteral injections and other invasive procedures as much as possible; hold firm pressure over injection and intravenous sites for 5 minutes and over arterial punctures for 20 minutes; use a soft toothbrush or sponge for oral care; use an electric razor for shaving. *Minor trauma can lead to extensive bleeding, particularly in the patient who has received a thrombolytic drug.*

Community-Based Care

When preparing the patient and family for home or community-based care related to an acute arterial occlusion, discuss the following topics as indicated.

- Care of the incision
- Manifestations of complications to be reported, including symptoms of infection or occlusion of the graft or artery
- Long-term anticoagulant therapy, including the reason, prescribed dose, follow-up laboratory testing and appointments, interactions with other drugs, and manifestations of excessive bleeding
- Any activity restrictions or dietary modifications
- Lifestyle modifications to slow atherosclerosis and control hypertension
- Measures to promote peripheral circulation and maintain tissue integrity (see the discussion of venous peripheral atherosclerosis that follows)

Refer for home care services (nursing care, physical therapy, housekeeping services) as indicated.

Disorders of Venous Circulation

The two primary categories of venous system disorders are occlusive disorders and those related to ineffective venous blood flow. Impaired venous blood flow can lead to stasis and clotting, as well as tissue changes associated with venous congestion.

Physiology Review

The venous system is a low-pressure system in comparison with the arterial circulation. Veins and venules are thin-walled, distensible vessels. While they contain smooth muscle that allows them to contract or expand, the media (muscle layer) of veins is significantly thinner than that of arteries. The low pressures in the venous system allow it to serve as a reservoir for blood. Stimulation by the sympathetic nervous system causes veins to contract, helping maintain vascular volume. The low pressure venous system relies on skeletal muscle contractions and pressure changes in the abdomen and thorax to facilitate blood return to the heart. Unlike arteries, veins of the extremities contain valves to prevent retrograde blood flow.

The Patient with Venous Thrombosis

Venous thrombosis (also known as *thrombophlebitis*) is a condition in which a blood clot (thrombus) forms on the wall of a vein, accompanied by inflammation of the vein wall and some degree of obstructed venous blood flow.

Venous thrombi are more common than arterial thrombi because of lower pressures and flow within the venous system (Huether & McCance, 2008). Thrombi can form in either superficial or deep veins. **Deep venous thrombosis (DVT)** is a common complication of hospitalization, surgery, and immobilization. Obstetric and orthopedic procedures carry a higher risk for venous thrombosis; it may develop in more than 50% of patients having orthopedic surgery, particularly surgeries involving hip or knee. Other significant risk factors for venous thrombosis include abdominal or thoracic surgery, certain cancers, trauma, pregnancy, and use of oral contraceptives or hormone replacement therapy. See Box 32–5.

Pathophysiology

Three pathologic factors, called *Virchow's triad*, are associated with thrombophlebitis: stasis of blood, vessel damage, and increased blood coagulability. Vessel trauma stimulates the clotting cascade. Platelets aggregate at the site, particularly when venous stasis is present. Platelets and fibrin form the initial clot. Red blood cells are trapped in the fibrin meshwork, and the thrombus propagates (grows) in the direction of blood flow. The inflammatory response is triggered, causing tenderness, swelling, and erythema in the area of the thrombus. Initially the thrombus floats within the vein. Pieces of the thrombus may break loose and travel through the circulation as emboli. Fibroblasts eventually invade the thrombus, scarring the vein wall and destroying venous valves. Although patency of the vein may be restored, valve damage is permanent, affecting directional flow (Papadakis & McPhee, 2007).

Deep Vein Thrombosis

The deep veins of the legs, primarily in the calf, and the pelvis provide the most hospitable environment for venous thrombosis. Approximately 80% of deep vein thromboses begin in the deep veins of the calf, often propagating into the popliteal and femoral veins (Figure 32–10 ■) (Papadakis & McPhee, 2007). DVT usually is asymptomatic; in some patients, a pulmonary embolism may be the first indication.

MANIFESTATIONS When present, the manifestations of DVT are primarily due to the inflammatory process accompanying the thrombus. Calf pain, which may be described as tightness or a dull, aching pain in the affected extremity, particularly upon walking, is the most common symptom. Tenderness, swelling, warmth, and erythema may be noted along the course of involved veins. The affected extremity may be cyanotic and often is edematous. Rarely, a cord may be palpated over the affected vein. A positive Homan's sign (pain in the calf when the foot is dorsiflexed) is an unreliable indicator of DVT. See the Manifestations box for a summary of the manifestations of deep and superficial venous thrombosis.

COMPLICATIONS The major complications of deep vein thrombosis are chronic venous insufficiency (see the next section of this chapter) and pulmonary embolism. Pulmonary embolism occurs when the clot fragments or breaks loose from the vein wall. As the clot travels, it moves through progressively larger veins and into the right side of the heart. From there it enters the pulmonary circulation, where it eventually occludes arterial flow to a portion of the lungs. The result is a mismatch between ventilation (air flow) and perfusion (blood flow) in a portion of the lungs. The effect on gas exchange depends on the size of the embolism and the vessel it occludes. ∞ See Chapter 37 for more information about pulmonary emboli.

BOX 32–5 **Factors Associated with Venous Thrombosis**

- Immobilization: myocardial infarction, heart failure, stroke, postoperative
- Surgery: orthopedic, thoracic, abdominal, genitourinary
- Cancer: pancreatic, lung, ovary, testes, urinary tract, breast, stomach
- Trauma: fractures of the spine, pelvis, femur, tibia; spinal cord injury
- Pregnancy and delivery
- Hormone therapy: oral contraceptives, hormone replacement therapy
- Coagulation disorders

FAST FACTS

- DVT is a common complication of surgery and immobility. It usually develops in the deep veins of the calf (80%).
- Venous stasis (sluggish blood flow), altered blood coagulation, and damage (e.g. inflammation) to blood vessels are precipitating factors for DVT.
- A thrombus or a portion of a thrombus may break loose, traveling through the venous system to the right side of the heart and into the pulmonary circulation, where it ultimately becomes lodged (pulmonary embolus).

(margin text) Deep Vein Thromboembolism (DVT) Animation

Figure 32–10 ■ Common locations of venous thrombosis. *A,* The most common sites of deep vein thrombosis. *B,* DVT extending from the calf to the iliac veins. *C,* superficial venous thrombosis.

Superficial Vein Thrombosis

Venous catheters and infusions are the primary risk factors for superficial venous thrombosis. Superficial vein thrombosis also may develop in conjunction with thromboangiitis obliterans, varicose veins, or deep vein thrombosis. It may develop spontaneously in pregnant women or following delivery. In some cases, superficial venous thrombosis of the long saphenous vein is the earliest sign of an abdominal cancer such as pancreatic cancer (Papadakis & McPhee, 2007).

Superficial vein thrombosis is marked by pain and tenderness at the site of the thrombus. A reddened, warm, tender cord extending along the affected vein can be palpated. The area surrounding the vein may be swollen and red (see the Manifestations box).

Interdisciplinary Care

It is important to differentiate venous thrombosis from other causes of extremity pain, such as cellulitis, muscle strain, contusion, and lymphedema. The history, physical examination, and diagnostic tests are used to establish the diagnosis. Treatment focuses on preventing further clotting or extension of the clot and addressing underlying causes.

Diagnosis

- *Duplex venous ultrasonography* is a noninvasive test used to visualize the vein and measure the velocity of blood flow in the veins. Although the clot often cannot be visualized directly, its presence can be inferred by an inability to compress the vein during the examination.
- *Plethysmography* is a noninvasive test that measures changes in blood flow through the veins. It is often used in conjunction with Doppler ultrasonography. Plethysmography is most valuable in diagnosing thromboses of larger or more superficial veins.
- *Magnetic resonance imaging (MRI)* is another noninvasive means of detecting deep vein thrombosis. It is particularly

MANIFESTATIONS of Venous Thrombosis

DEEP VEIN THROMBOSIS
- Usually asymptomatic
- Dull, aching pain in affected extremity, especially when walking
- Possible tenderness, warmth, erythema along affected vein
- Cyanosis of affected extremity
- Edema of affected extremity

SUPERFICIAL VEIN THROMBOSIS
- Localized pain and tenderness over the affected vein
- Redness and warmth along the course of the vein
- Palpable cordlike structure along the affected vein
- Swelling and redness of surrounding tissue

useful when thrombosis of the vena cavae or pelvic veins is suspected.

- *Ascending contrast venography* uses an injected contrast medium to assess the location and extent of venous thrombosis. Although invasive, expensive, and uncomfortable, contrast venography is the most accurate diagnostic tool for venous thrombosis. It is used when the results of less invasive tests leave the diagnosis unclear (van Leeuwen, Kranpitz, & Smith, 2006).

Prophylaxis

Medications and other measures are used to prevent venous thrombosis when the risk is high. Low-molecular-weight heparins (see the following section) prevent deep vein thrombosis in patients who are undergoing general or orthopedic surgery, experiencing acute medical illness, or on prolonged bed rest. Oral anticoagulation also may be used as a prophylactic measure in patients with fractures or who are undergoing orthopedic surgery.

Elevating the foot of the bed with the knees slightly flexed promotes venous return. Early mobilization and leg exercises such as ankle flexion and extension assist venous flow by muscle compression. Intermittent pneumatic compression devices applied to the legs are effective to prevent DVT. They also are used when anticoagulation is contraindicated due to the increased risk for bleeding. Elastic stockings are used to prevent venous thrombosis as well in patients at risk.

Medications

Anticoagulants to prevent clot propagation and enable the body's own lytic system to dissolve the clot are the mainstay of treatment for venous thrombosis. Thrombolytic drugs such as streptokinase or tissue plasminogen activator (t-PA) may accelerate the process of clot lysis and prevent damage to venous valves. There is, however, no evidence that thrombolytic therapy is more effective in preventing pulmonary embolism in patients with existing DVT than anticoagulants. It also significantly increases the risk for bleeding and hemorrhage.

Nonsteroidal anti-inflammatory agents such as indomethacin (Indocin) or naproxen (Naprosyn) may be ordered to reduce inflammation in the veins and provide symptomatic relief, particularly for patients with superficial vein thrombosis.

ANTICOAGULANTS Anticoagulants are given to prevent clot extension and reduce the risk of subsequent pulmonary embolism. Anticoagulation is initiated with unfractionated heparin or low-molecular-weight (LMW) heparin. Following an initial intravenous bolus of 7,500 to 10,000 units of unfractionated heparin, a continuous heparin infusion of 1000 to 1500 IU per hour is started. The dosage is calculated to maintain the activated partial thromboplastin time (aPTT) at approximately twice the control or normal value. An infusion pump is used to deliver the prescribed dosage. Frequent monitoring of the infusion is an important nursing responsibility. Subcutaneous heparin injections may be used as an alternate to intravenous infusion in some instances.

LMW heparins are increasingly used to prevent and treat venous thrombosis. They do not require the close laboratory monitoring of unfractionated heparins. LMW heparin is administered subcutaneously in fixed doses once or twice daily, allowing the option of outpatient treatment. LMW heparins have additional advantages, in that they are more effective and carry lower risks for bleeding and thrombocytopenia than conventional, unfractionated heparins.

Oral anticoagulation with warfarin may be initiated concurrently with heparin therapy. Overlapping heparin and warfarin therapy for 4 to 5 days is important because the full anticoagulant effect of warfarin is delayed, and it may actually promote clotting during the first few days of therapy (Papadakis & McPhee, 2007). Warfarin doses are adjusted to maintain the international normalized ratio (INR) at 2.0 to 3.0 (Deglin & Vallerand, 2009).

Once this level is achieved, the heparin is discontinued and a maintenance dose of warfarin is prescribed to prevent recurrent thrombosis. Anticoagulation generally is continued for at least 3 months. When DVT is recurrent or risk factors such as altered coagulability or cancer are present, anticoagulant therapy may be prolonged. Regular follow-up is necessary to be sure prothrombin times (INR) remain within the desirable range for anticoagulation. See the Medication Administration box for the nursing implications for anticoagulant therapy.

Treatments

Treatment of venous thrombosis also includes measures to relieve symptoms and reduce inflammation. With superficial vein thrombosis, applying warm, moist compresses over the affected vein, extremity rest, and anti-inflammatory agents usually provide relief of symptoms.

Bed rest may be ordered for deep vein thrombosis. The duration of bed rest typically is determined by the extent of leg edema. The legs are elevated 15 to 20 degrees, with the knees slightly flexed, above the level of the heart to promote venous return and discourage venous pooling. Elastic antiembolism stockings (TEDS) or pneumatic compression devices are also frequently ordered to stimulate the muscle-pumping mechanism that promotes the return of blood to the heart. When permitted, walking is encouraged while avoiding prolonged standing or sitting. Crossing the legs also is avoided, as are tight-fitting garments or stockings that bind.

Surgery

Venous thrombosis usually is effectively treated with conservative measures and anticoagulation. In some cases, however, surgery is required to remove the thrombus, prevent its extension into deep veins, or prevent the effects of embolization.

Venous thrombectomy is done when thrombi lodge in the femoral vein and their removal is necessary to prevent pulmonary embolism or gangrene. Successful thrombus removal rapidly improves venous circulation. The duration of this effect varies.

When venous thrombosis is recurrent and anticoagulant therapy is contraindicated, a filter may be inserted into the vena cava to capture emboli from the pelvis and lower extremities, preventing pulmonary embolism. Several different filters are available (Figure 32–11 ■). The Greenfield filter is widely used for its ability to trap emboli within its apex while maintaining patency of the vena cava. The filter can be inserted under fluoroscopy with local anesthesia. Mortality and morbidity associated with the filter are very low.

MEDICATION ADMINISTRATION Anticoagulant Therapy

HEPARIN

Heparin interferes with the clotting cascade by inhibiting the effects of thrombin and preventing the conversion of fibrinogen to fibrin. This prevents the formation of a stable fibrin clot. At therapeutic levels, heparin prolongs the thrombin time, clotting time, and activated partial thromboplastin time. When given intravenously, its effect is immediate. Given subcutaneously, its onset of action is within 1 hour. When heparin is discontinued, clotting times return to normal within 2 to 6 hours (Deglin & Vallerand, 2009). *Heparin-induced thrombocytopenia (HIT)* is a potential complication of therapy with unfractionated heparin. ∞ See Chapter 33 for more information about HIT and nursing responsibilities in monitoring for this dangerous potential complication.

Nursing Responsibilities

- Assess for history of unexplained or active bleeding. Assess laboratory results for abnormal clotting profile or evidence of active bleeding.
- Give a test dose as indicated to patients with a history of multiple allergies or a history of asthma.
- Administer by deep subcutaneous injection; abdominal sites are preferred. Avoid injecting within 2 inches of the umbilicus. Rotate sites. Do not aspirate prior to injecting or massage after the injection.
- Intravenous solutions may be diluted with dextrose, normal saline, or Ringer's solution. Use an infusion pump.
- Keep protamine sulfate, a heparin antagonist, available to treat excessive bleeding.
- Monitor and report abnormal laboratory results and aPTT values outside the desired range.
- Promptly report evidence of bleeding such as hematemesis, hematuria, bleeding gums, or unexplained abdominal or back pain.

Health Education for the Patient and Family

- Report unusual bleeding or excessive menstrual flow.
- Use an electric razor and a soft-bristle toothbrush; prevent injury by clearing pathways, using a night light, and other measures. Do not consume alcohol.
- Avoid contact sports while on anticoagulant therapy.
- Do not consume large amounts of food rich in vitamin K (yellow and dark green vegetables).
- Do not use aspirin or NSAIDs while on heparin therapy unless advised to do so by your healthcare provider.
- Wear a MedicAlert tag and advise all healthcare providers (including dentists and podiatrists) of therapy.

LOW-MOLECULAR-WEIGHT HEPARINS

Ardeparin (Normiflo)	Enoxaparin (Lovenox)
Dalteparin (Fragmin)	Tinzaparin (Innohep)

LMW heparins are the most bioavailable fraction of heparin. They provide a more precise and predictable anticoagulant effect than unfractionated heparins. Like unfractionated heparin, LMW heparin prevents conversion of prothrombin to thrombin, liberation of thromboplastin from platelets, and formation of a stable clot. LMW heparins cannot be used interchangeably with each other or with unfractionated heparin. Although the risk of heparin-induced thrombocytopenia is significantly lower with LMW heparin, patients who were previously treated with unfractionated heparin may develop HIT when treated with LMW heparin.

Nursing Responsibilities

- Assess for evidence of active bleeding, a history of bleeding disorders or thrombocytopenia, or sensitivity to heparin, sulfites, or pork products.

- Monitor for unusual or masked bleeding. PT and aPTT levels may be within normal levels even in the presence of hemorrhage.
- Administer by deep subcutaneous injection into abdominal wall, thigh, or buttocks. Rotate sites. Do not aspirate or massage.

Health Education for the Patient and Family

- Subcutaneous self-administration technique, timing of doses, and site rotation. Do not rub site after administering to minimize bruising.
- Do not take aspirin, NSAIDs, or other over-the-counter drugs unless recommended by your healthcare provider.
- Promptly report excessive bruising or bleeding, chest pain, difficulty breathing, itching, rash, or swelling to your healthcare provider.
- Keep follow-up appointments as scheduled.

ORAL ANTICOAGULANT

Warfarin (Coumadin)

Warfarin interferes with synthesis of vitamin K-dependent clotting factors by the liver, leading to depletion of these factors. It has no effect on already circulating clotting factors or on existing clots. Warfarin inhibits extension of existing thrombi and the formation of new clots. Its action is cumulative and more prolonged than that of heparin.

Nursing Responsibilities

- Assess laboratory results and history for evidence of abnormal bleeding.
- Multiple drugs affect the metabolism and protein binding of warfarin; note all medications and assess for interactions with warfarin.
- Do not give during pregnancy as warfarin may cause congenital malformations.
- Oral tablets may be crushed and given without regard to meals.
- Dilute intravenous warfarin with supplied diluent; administer within 4 hours by direct intravenous injection at a rate of 25 mg/min.
- Keep vitamin K available to reverse effects of warfarin in the event of excessive bleeding or hemorrhage.
- Monitor PT or INR; report values outside the desired range.

Health Education for the Patient and Family

- Do not take your prescribed dose and notify your healthcare provider immediately if bleeding occurs (hematemesis, bright red or black, tarry feces, hematuria, bleeding gums, excessive bruising, etc.). Report rash or manifestations of hepatitis (dark urine, malaise, yellow skin or sclera).
- Take your warfarin at the same time every day; do not change brands as their effects may differ.
- Menstrual bleeding may be slightly increased; contact your healthcare provider if it increases significantly. Use reliable birth control to prevent pregnancy while taking warfarin. Immediately contact your healthcare provider if you think you may be pregnant.
- Take precautions to prevent injury and bleeding: Use a soft toothbrush and electric razor, wear shoes, and use a night light. Avoid participating in contact sports.
- Do not smoke, use alcohol, or take any over-the-counter drugs unless specifically recommended by your healthcare provider. Notify all healthcare providers, including dentists and podiatrists, of therapy. Wear a MedicAlert tag.
- Obtain lab tests as scheduled and keep all scheduled follow-up appointments.

Figure 32–11 ■ Venal caval filters. *A*, Greenfield filter. *B*, Nitinol filter.

Extensive thrombosis of the saphenous vein may necessitate ligation and division of the saphenous vein where it joins the femoral vein to prevent clot extension into the deep venous system. A vein affected by septic venous thrombosis is excised to control the infection. Antibiotic therapy also is initiated.

∞ Nursing Care

Health Promotion

Prevention of venous thrombosis is an important component of nursing care for all at-risk patients. Position patients to promote venous blood flow from the lower extremities, with the feet elevated and the knees slightly bent. Avoid placing pillows under the knees and positions in which the hips and knees are sharply flexed. Use a recliner chair or foot stool when sitting. Ambulate patients as soon as possible, and maintain a regular schedule of ambulation throughout the day. Teach ankle flexion and extension exercises, and frequently remind patients to perform them. Apply elastic hose and pneumatic compression devices when appropriate. Instruct patients to avoid crossing legs when in bed or sitting. Inquire about possible prophylactic heparin or warfarin therapy for patients undergoing orthopedic surgery or other high-risk procedures. Frequently assess intravenous sites. Change the site and catheter as dictated by agency protocol and if evidence of local inflammation is noted.

Assessment

Assess patients at risk for venous thrombosis for manifestations and risk factors.

- *Health history:* Complaints of leg or calf pain, its duration and characteristics, and the effect of walking on the pain; history of venous thrombosis or other clotting disorders; current medications.
- *Physical examination:* Inspect affected extremity for redness, edema; palpate for tenderness, warmth, cordlike structures; body temperature.
- *Laboratory data:* Clotting studies (APTT, pro time, INR).

See the accompanying Case Study & Nursing Care Plan for an example of an assessment of a patient with deep vein thrombosis.

Nursing Diagnoses and Interventions

In addition to the preventive measures identified earlier, priority nursing diagnoses for the patient with venous thrombosis relate to pain, maintenance of tissue perfusion and integrity, and the potential adverse effects of prescribed treatments.

Pain

The pain associated with venous thrombosis results from inflammation of the involved vein. It may be aggravated by use of the involved extremity. Associated edema and swelling may contribute to discomfort. Measures to reduce the inflammation often help relieve the pain.

- Regularly assess pain location, characteristics, and level using a standardized pain scale. Report increasing pain or changes in its location or characteristics. *Tissue substances released during the inflammatory process can stimulate pain receptors. In addition, localized swelling presses on pain-sensitive structures in the area of the inflammation, contributing to discomfort. As inflammation and swelling are reduced, pain should abate. Continued or increasing pain may indicate extension of the thrombosis. Sudden chest pain may indicate a pulmonary embolism, necessitating immediate intervention.*
- Measure calf and thigh diameter of the affected extremity on admission and daily thereafter. Report increases promptly. *The inflammatory process causes vasodilation and increases vessel permeability, causing edema of the affected extremity. Baseline and subsequent measurements provide a measure of treatment effectiveness.*
- Apply warm, moist heat to affected extremity at least four times daily, using warm, moist compresses or an aqua-K pad. *Moist heat penetrates tissues to a greater depth. Warmth promotes vasodilation, allowing reabsorption of excess fluid into the circulation. Vasodilation also reduces resistance within the affected vessel, reducing pain. As edema subsides, pressure on surrounding tissues is relieved, thereby reducing pain.*

EVIDENCE FOR NURSING CARE — **The Patient with Deep Vein Thrombosis**

Selected resources that nurses may find helpful when planning evidence-based nursing care follow.

- Blondin, M. & Titler, M. G. (2008). Prevention of deep vein thrombosis. University of Iowa Gerontological Nursing Research Center, Research Dissemination Core. Retrieved from http://www.guideline.gov/summary/summary.aspx?doc_id=9266&nbr=004960&string=varicose+AND+veins
- Deep vein thrombosis prevention. (2005). *American Association of Critical-Care Nurses (AACN) Practice Alert.* Retrieved from http://www.aacn.org/WD/Practice/Docs/PracticeAlerts/DVT_Prevention_12-2005.pdf
- Race, T. K. & Collier, P. E. (2007). The hidden risk of deep vein thrombosis—the need for risk factor assessment. *Critical Care Nursing Quarterly.* Practice Perspectives for Universal Problems, *30*(3), 245–54.
- Winslow, E. H., & Brosz, D. L. (2008). Graduated compression stockings in hospitalized postoperative patients: Correctness of usage and size. *The American Journal of Nursing, 108*(9), 40–50.

■ Maintain bed rest as ordered. *Using leg muscles during walking exacerbates the inflammatory process and increases edema. This, in turn, increases venous compression and pain.*

Ineffective Tissue Perfusion: Peripheral

As thrombi develop, they occlude the lumen of the vein and obstruct blood flow. In addition, the accompanying inflammatory response may precipitate vessel spasms, further impairing arterial and venous blood flow and tissue perfusion. Impaired tissue perfusion, in turn, deprives tissues of nutrients and oxygen. As a result, distal tissues of the affected extremity are at risk for ulceration and infection.

■ Assess peripheral pulses, skin integrity, capillary refill times, and color of extremities at least every 8 hours. Report changes promptly. Assessment of both extremities allows comparison of the affected and unaffected limbs. *Weak or absent pulses, impaired capillary refill, or significant color changes in the affected extremity may indicate extension of the thrombus or a possible complication.*

■ Assess the skin of the affected lower leg and foot at least every 8 hours, and more often as indicated. *Frequent assessment is important to rapidly detect early signs of tissue breakdown and implementation of measures to protect vulnerable tissues. Early intervention allows healing and restoration of tissue integrity; allowed to continue, the process can lead to necrosis and potential gangrene.*

■ *Elevate extremities at* all times, keeping knees slightly flexed and legs above the level of the heart. *Elevation of the extremities promotes venous return and reduces peripheral edema. Knee flexion promotes muscle relaxation.*

PRACTICE ALERT

Remove antiembolic stockings or pneumatic compression device for 30 to 60 minutes during daily hygiene. Antiembolic stockings (e.g., TED hose) and pneumatic compression devices exert pressure on the extremity and promote venous return. They can, however, impair perfusion of the dermis. Removing them periodically allows assessment of the underlying tissue and restores perfusion of the dermis, reducing the risk for skin breakdown. Their use may be continued following discharge to reduce the risk of recurrent venous thrombosis.

■ Use mild soaps, solutions, and lotions to clean the affected leg and foot daily. Pat dry after washing, and apply a nonalcohol-based lotion or moisturizing cream. *Daily hygiene with nondrying soaps and solutions removes potential pathogens from the skin surface, and maintains skin integrity and the first line of defense against infection. Caustic or harsh soaps or solutions can dry and crack the skin. Dry, cracked skin permits bacteria and other microorganisms to enter and infect the tissue, potentially leading to ulceration and venous gangrene.*

■ Use an egg crate mattress or sheepskin on the bed as needed. *Egg crate mattresses and sheepskins distribute weight more evenly, preventing excess pressure on affected tissues.*

■ Encourage frequent position changes at least every 2 hours while awake. *Frequent position changes reduce pressure on bony prominences and edematous tissue, reducing the risk of tissue breakdown.*

Ineffective Protection

Anticoagulant therapy interferes with the body's normal clotting mechanisms, increasing the risk for bleeding and hemorrhage.

PRACTICE ALERT

Assess for and promptly report evidence of bleeding, such as petechiae; bruising; bleeding gums; obvious or occult blood in vomitus, stool, or urine; or unexplained back or abdominal pain. Anticoagulants interfere with the ability to form a stable clot and prevent excessive bleeding. Even minor trauma such as tooth brushing or bumping into furniture can result in bleeding.

■ Monitor laboratory results, including the INR (prothrombin time), aPTT, hemoglobin, and hematocrit as indicated. Report values outside the normal or desired range. *Coagulation studies are used to monitor the effect of anticoagulant medications. Values within the desired range prevent further clot development while carrying a low risk for bleeding and hemorrhage. A fall in the hemoglobin and hematocrit may indicate undetected bleeding.*

Impaired Physical Mobility

Although prolonged bed rest rarely is required, it is associated with many problems, including constipation, joint contractures, muscle atrophy, and boredom. Nursing care goals include maintaining joint range of motion, minimizing muscle atrophy, and reducing boredom.

■ Encourage active range-of-motion exercises at least every 8 hours. Provide passive range of motion as needed. *Range-of-motion exercises maintain joint mobility and prevent contractures. Active range of motion (performed by the patient) also helps prevent muscle atrophy and preserve function. While passive range-of-motion exercises do not prevent muscle atrophy, they do maintain joint mobility.*

■ Encourage frequent position changes, deep breathing, and coughing. *Prolonged immobility can lead to impaired airway clearance and respiratory complications, such as atelectasis or pneumonia. Turning, coughing, and deep breathing facilitate expulsion of secretions from the respiratory tract, airway clearance, and alveolar ventilation.*

■ Encourage increased fluid and dietary fiber intake. *Constipation is a frequent complication of immobility due to decreased gastrointestinal motility and loss of abdominal muscle strength. Increasing fluid and fiber intake helps maintain soft, easily expelled stools.*

■ Assist with and encourage ambulation as allowed. *Ambulation promotes venous blood flow, helps maintain muscle tone and joint mobility, and increases the sense of well-being.*

■ Encourage diversional activities such as reading, handiwork or other hobbies, television or video games, and socializing. *Boredom may lead to dozing and inertia, with little physical movement or mental stimulation, increasing the risk for complications of immobility.*

Risk for Ineffective Tissue Perfusion: Cardiopulmonary

A thrombus that forms in the deep veins of the legs or pelvis may break loose or fragment, becoming an embolism. Emboli that originate in the venous system usually become trapped in

CASE STUDY & NURSING CARE PLAN   A Patient with Deep Vein Thrombosis

Mrs. Opal Hipps, aged 75, lives alone with her dog, Chester, in her family home in the suburbs. She retired from her job as a postal clerk 10 years ago and now spends a lot of time reading and watching television. Over the past week she has developed a vague aching pain in her right leg. She ignored the pain until last night when it developed into a much more severe pain in her right calf. She noticed that her right lower leg seemed larger than the left, and it was very tender to the touch. After seeing her healthcare provider and undergoing Doppler ultrasound studies, Mrs. Hipps is admitted to the hospital with the diagnosis of deep vein thrombosis in the right leg. She is placed on bed rest, and intravenous heparin. Michael Cookson, RN, is assigned to admit and care for Mrs. Hipps.

ASSESSMENT

Mr. Cookson notices that Mrs. Hipps was admitted 14 months ago for repair of a fractured femur. Mrs. Hipps says, "This business about a blood clot really has me worried." She also tells Mr. Cookson that she is worried about who will care for her dog while she is in the hospital. Physical findings include height 62 inches (157 cm), weight 149 lb (68 kg), T 99.2 F (37.3°C); vital signs within normal limits otherwise. Her left leg is warm and pink, with strong peripheral pulses and good capillary refill. Her right calf is dark red, very warm, and dry to touch. It is tender to palpation. The right femoral and popliteal pulses are strong, but the pedal and posterior tibial pulses are difficult to locate. The right calf diameter is 0.5 inch (1.27 cm) larger than the left.

DIAGNOSES

- *Pain* related to inflammatory response in affected vein
- *Anxiety* related to unexpected hospitalization and uncertainty about the seriousness of her illness
- *Ineffective Tissue Perfusion: Peripheral* related to decreased venous circulation in the right leg
- *Risk for Impaired Skin Integrity* related to pooling of venous blood in the right leg

EXPECTED OUTCOMES

- Verbalize relief of right leg pain by day of discharge.
- Verbalize reduced anxiety by the second day of her hospitalization.
- Demonstrate reduced right leg diameter by 0.25 inch (0.64 cm) by the fifth day of hospitalization.

- Maintain intact skin in the right foot throughout the hospital stay.

PLANNING AND IMPLEMENTATION

- Elevate legs, maintaining slight knee flexion, while in bed.
- Apply warm, moist compresses to right leg using a 2-hour-on, 2-hour-off schedule around the clock.
- Administer prescribed analgesics and evaluate effectiveness.
- Spend time with Mrs. Hipps to explain venous thrombosis and its treatment.
- Arrange for a friend or neighbor to care for Mrs. Hipps's dog.
- Apply antiembolism stockings as ordered; remove for 30 minutes every 8 hours.
- Monitor laboratory values to assess effect of anticoagulant therapy; report values outside desired range.
- Assist with progressive ambulation when allowed.
- Inspect legs and feet and record findings every 8 hours.

EVALUATION

Seven days after admission, the pain in Mrs. Hipps's right leg has subsided and the diameter of her right calf is equal to her left calf. Mrs. Hipps admits to Mr. Cookson that her fears really relate to a cousin who was hospitalized for a similar problem and had his leg amputated. After talking about her condition and the steps she can take to prevent its recurrence, she is much less anxious. Before discharge, Mr. Cookson reviews instructions for antiembolism stockings, daily walking, warfarin schedule, and scheduled follow-up appointment. Her neighbor, Kate, came to pick her up. As Mr. Cookson was helping Mrs. Hipps into the car, Kate handed her a small brown dog and said, "I took good care of Chester for you, but he's missed you." Mrs. Hipps smiled, and assured Mr. Cookson that she would call the number he provided if she had any questions.

CRITICAL THINKING IN THE NURSING PROCESS

1. Describe the pathophysiologic reasons for the pain in Mrs. Hipps's right leg.
2. How would you respond if Mrs. Hipps tells you she does not have the money to buy the prescribed anticoagulant when she goes home?
3. How would you change your teaching and discharge planning if Mrs. Hipps had difficulty caring for herself?
4. Design a plan of care for Mrs. Hipps for the diagnosis *Activity Intolerance*.

See Evaluating Your Response in Appendix C.

---

the pulmonary circulation (pulmonary embolism). Gas exchange in the affected area is impaired as blood flow ceases or is reduced to an area of the lungs that is well-ventilated (∞ see Chapter 37).

- Frequently assess respiratory status, including rate, depth, ease, and oxygen saturation levels. *A mismatch of ventilation and perfusion can significantly affect gas exchange, leading to rapid, shallow respirations, dyspnea and air hunger, and a fall in oxygen saturation levels.*

> **PRACTICE ALERT**
> Immediately report complaints of chest pain and shortness of breath, anxiety, or a sense of impending doom. The manifestations of pulmonary embolism are similar to those of myocardial infarction. Prompt intervention to restore pulmonary blood flow can reduce the risk of significant adverse effects.

- Initiate oxygen therapy, elevate the head of the bed, and reassure the patient who is experiencing manifestations of pulmonary embolism. *Oxygen therapy and elevating the head of the bed promote ventilation and gas exchange in those alveoli that are well-perfused, helping maintain tissue oxygenation. Reassurance helps reduce anxiety and slow the respiratory rate, promoting greater respiratory depth and alveolar ventilation.*

Using NANDA, NIC, and NOC

Linkages between a selected NANDA nursing diagnosis, NIC, and NOC for the patient with deep venous thrombosis are shown in the chart that follows.

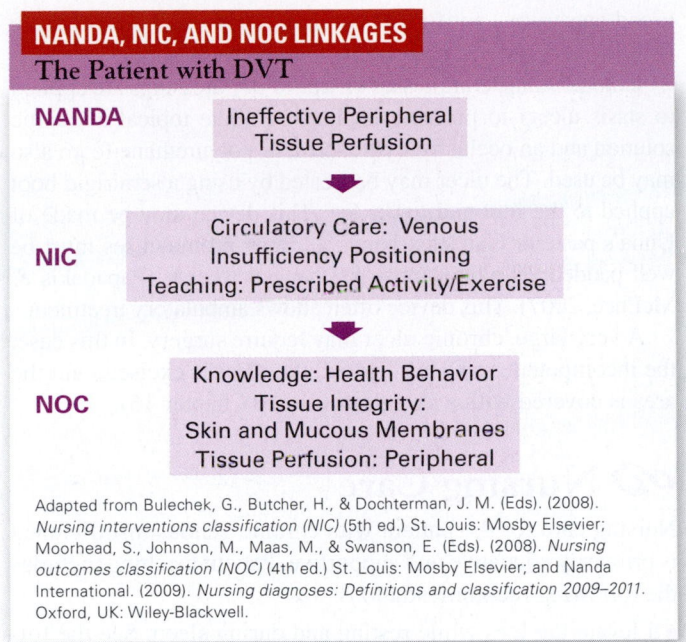

Community-Based Care

Treatment measures for venous thrombosis may be initiated and carried out on an outpatient basis or continued for an extended period of time following hospital discharge. Include the following topics when teaching for home care.

- Explanation of the disease process
- Treatment measures, including laboratory tests and their purposes, medications and adverse effects that should be reported
- Appropriate methods of heat application
- Prescribed activity restrictions
- Measures to prevent future episodes of venous thrombosis
- The importance of follow-up visits and laboratory tests as scheduled

Refer patients for community nursing services for continued assessment and reinforcement of teaching. Provide referrals for assistance with ADLs and home maintenance services as indicated. Consider referral for physical therapy if needed.

The Patient with Chronic Venous Insufficiency

Chronic venous insufficiency is a disorder of inadequate venous return over a prolonged period. Deep vein thrombosis is the most frequent cause of chronic venous insufficiency. Other conditions, such as varicose veins or leg trauma, may contribute; in some instances, it develops without an identified precipitating cause (Huether & McCance, 2008).

Pathophysiology

Following DVT, large veins may remain occluded, increasing the pressure in other veins of the extremity. This increased pressure distends the veins, separating valve leaflets and impairing their ability to close. DVT also damages valve leaflets, causing them to thicken and contract. The result is

impaired unidirectional blood flow and deep vein emptying (Huether & McCance, 2008).

When venous valves are incompetent, the muscle-pumping action produced during activity cannot propel blood back to the heart. Venous blood collects and stagnates in the lower leg (*venous stasis*). Venous pressures in the calf and lower leg increase, particularly during ambulation. This increased pressure impairs arterial circulation to the lower extremities as well. The body's ability to provide sufficient oxygen and nutrients to the cells and remove metabolic waste products diminishes. Eventually, there is so little oxygen and nutrients that cells begin to die. The skin atrophies, and subcutaneous fat deposits necrose. Breakdown of red blood cells in the congested tissues causes brown skin pigmentation. Venous stasis ulcers develop. Congested tissues impair the body's ability to increase the supply of oxygen, nutrients, and metabolic energy to heal the ulcer. As a result, the condition worsens and, over time, the ulcers enlarge. The congested venous circulation also prevents the blood from mounting effective inflammatory and immune responses, significantly increasing the risk for infection in the ulcerated tissue (Huether & McCance, 2008).

Manifestations

Manifestations of chronic venous insufficiency include lower leg edema, itching, and discomfort of the affected extremity that increase with prolonged standing. The extremity is cyanotic. Recurrent stasis ulcers develop (Figure 32–12 ■), usually forming just above the ankle, on the medial or anterior aspect of the leg. They heal poorly, forming scar tissue that breaks down easily. Tissue surrounding the ulcer is shiny, atrophic, and cyanotic, and there is a brownish pigmentation to the skin. Other skin changes may develop as well, such as eczema or stasis dermatitis. Necrosis and fibrosis of subcutaneous tissue cause the affected area of the leg to feel hard and somewhat leathery to the touch, but even the slightest trauma to the area can produce serious tissue breakdown. See the Manifestations box of chronic venous insufficiency. Table 32–6 compares venous and arterial ulcers.

Figure 32–12 ■ Chronic venous insufficiency. Note the discoloration of the ankle and the stasis ulcer.

MANIFESTATIONS of Chronic Venous Insufficiency

- Lower extremity edema that worsens with standing
- Itching, dull leg discomfort or pain that increases with standing
- Thin, shiny, atrophic skin
- Cyanosis and brown skin pigmentation of lower leg and foot
- Possible weeping dermatitis
- Thick, fibrous (hard) subcutaneous tissue
- Recurrent ulcerations of medial or anterior ankle

Interdisciplinary Care

Collaborative care for the patient with venous insufficiency focuses on relieving symptoms, promoting adequate circulation, and healing and preventing tissue damage.

The history and physical examination often establish the diagnosis of chronic venous insufficiency. Because a history of deep vein thrombosis is a major risk factor, careful evaluation of the past medical history and questioning of the patient is important. There are no specific diagnostic tests to confirm the diagnosis of chronic venous insufficiency.

Conservative management of venous insufficiency focuses on reducing edema and treating ulcerations. Prolonged standing or sitting is discouraged. Graduated compression hosiery is ordered for daytime use, and frequent elevation of the legs and feet during the day is recommended. At night, the legs and feet should be elevated above the level of the heart by raising the foot of the mattress.

Treatment of associated stasis dermatitis varies, based on the duration of the condition. Wet compresses of boric acid, buffered aluminum acetate (Burrow's solution), or isotonic saline solution are applied to acute weeping dermatitis four times a day for 1-hour periods. Following the compress, a topical corticosteroid (such as 0.5% hydrocortisone cream) is applied. Bed rest is prescribed during the acute period. Stasis dermatitis that is subsiding or chronic may be treated with a topical corticosteroid, zinc oxide ointment, or a topical

broad-spectrum antifungal cream such as clotrimazole (Lotrimin) cream or miconazole (Monistat) cream.

Isotonic saline compresses or wet-to-dry dressings are applied to stasis ulcers to promote healing. A dilute topical antibiotic solution and an occlusive hydroactive or polyurethane foam also may be used. The ulcer may be treated by using a semirigid boot applied to the foot and lower leg. This device may be made of Unna's paste or Gauzetex bandage. Bony prominences must be well padded. The boot must be changed weekly (Papadakis & McPhee, 2007). This device often allows ambulatory treatment.

A very large, chronic ulcer may require surgery. In this case, the incompetent veins are ligated, the ulcer is excised, and the area is covered with a skin graft (∞ see Chapter 16).

Nursing Care

Nursing care for the patient with chronic venous insufficiency is primarily educative and supportive. Patient teaching includes the following recommendations.

- Elevate the legs while resting and during sleep. See the following box for a nursing research study that suggests the supine position for resting.
- Walk as much as possible, but avoid sitting or standing for long periods of time.
- When sitting, do not cross your legs or allow pressure on the back of the knees (such as sitting on the side of the bed).
- Do not wear anything that pinches your legs (such as knee-high hose, garters, or girdles).
- Wear elastic hose as prescribed. The elastic hose should be tighter over the feet than at the top of the leg. Be sure the tops of the elastic hose do not cut into your legs. Put on the hose after you have had your legs elevated.
- Keep the skin on your feet and legs clean, soft, and dry.
- Follow guidelines in Box 32–4 for care of the legs and feet.

The following nursing diagnoses may apply to the patient with chronic venous insufficiency.

- *Disturbed Body Image* related to edema and stasis ulcers on lower leg

TABLE 32–6 Comparison of Arterial and Venous Leg Ulcers

FACTOR	ARTERIAL ULCERS	VENOUS ULCERS
Location	Toes, feet, shin	Over medial or anterior ankle
Ulcer appearance	Deep, pale	Superficial, pink
Skin appearance	Normal to atrophic	Brown discoloration
	Pallor on elevation	Stasis dermatitis
	Rubor on dependency	Cyanosis on dependency
Skin temperature	Cool	Normal
Edema	Absent or mild	May be significant
Pain	Usually severe	Usually mild
	Intermittent claudication	Aching pain
	Rest pain	
Gangrene	May occur	Does not occur
Pulses	Decreased or absent	Normal

MOVING EVIDENCE INTO ACTION — The Patient with Venous Leg Ulcers

Chronic leg ulcers due to venous insufficiency are a challenge to treat and heal. Oxygen is necessary for tissue repair and to prevent infection; however, peripheral perfusion to deliver oxygen to the tissues is impaired in patients with chronic venous insufficiency. Using measurements of transcutaneous tissue oxygen (TcPO$_2$), a group of nurse researchers evaluated the effects of four different positions and supplemental oxygen on a small group of subjects with venous ulcers (Wipke-Tevis, Stotts, Williams, Froelicher, & Hunt, 2001). Not surprisingly, these researchers found lower extremity resting TcPO$_2$ levels in patients with venous ulcers than in healthy adults. Changes in position resulted in minimal TcPO$_2$ changes in tissue surrounding the ulcer. When supplemental oxygen was given, TcPO$_2$ levels were higher in the supine position than with the legs elevated, sitting, or standing. These results suggest that control of peripheral circulation and tissue oxygenation may be impaired in patients with venous ulcers.

IMPLICATIONS FOR NURSING

The results of this study support advising patients with chronic venous ulcers to stay off their feet and rest in bed as much as possible to promote healing of venous ulcers. Remove compression stockings and devices while the patient is in bed to promote perfusion of subcutaneous tissues and of the region surrounding the ulcer itself. Discuss the effects of position on peripheral tissue perfusion with patients, and encourage frequent rest periods during the day. Consider discussing the option of supplemental oxygen therapy for a patient with delayed ulcer healing with the primary care provider.

CRITICAL THINKING IN PATIENT CARE

1. What is the usual response of blood vessels to changing positions from supine or sitting to standing? How does this compare with the results found here?
2. What is required for tissue healing? What measures can the nurse take to promote tissue healing in a patient with impaired peripheral tissue perfusion?
3. How do the measures used to treat arterial and venous ulcers compare? Explain the rationale for differing treatment measures.

Adapted from Wipke-Tevis, D.D., Stotts, N. A., Williams, D. A., Froelicher, E. S., & Hunt, T. K. (2001). Tissue oxygenation, perfusion, and position in patients with venous leg ulcers. *Nursing Research, 50*(1), 24–32.

- *Ineffective Health Maintenance* related to lack of knowledge about disorder and prescribed treatments
- *Risk for Infection* related to ulcerations
- *Impaired Physical Mobility* related to pain and edema in lower legs
- *Impaired Skin Integrity* related to presence of stasis ulcers
- *Ineffective Tissue Perfusion: Peripheral* related to incompetent venous valves

See other sections of this chapter for specific nursing interventions related to many of these diagnoses. See the accompanying box for nursing care for the older adult with chronic venous stasis.

NURSING CARE OF THE OLDER ADULT — Chronic Venous Stasis

Disorders of venous stasis are common after the fifth decade of life. Aging affects vessels and tissues, increasing the risk for venous insufficiency and varicose veins. In addition, mobility frequently declines with aging, reducing the effect of the muscle pump in promoting venous return.

Regular exercise, walking in particular, is an important part of the treatment plan. Safety when walking is an important issue for older patients. Assess the patient's mobility and stability during ambulation. If appropriate, suggest using a walker and quad-cane as needed. Assist older patients holding jobs that require prolonged standing to identify strategies to minimize standing and incorporate periods of activity into their work.

Following surgery or during treatment for stasis ulcers, older patients may need additional assistance with home care and maintenance. Initiate referral to social services as needed to arrange for home nursing care, meals, assistance with ADLs, and home maintenance services as indicated. In some instances, temporary placement in an extended care facility is necessary until the patient and family can assume care.

The Patient with Varicose Veins

Varicose veins are irregular, tortuous veins with incompetent valves. Varicosities may develop in any veins, and may be called by other names, such as hemorrhoids in the rectum and varices in the esophagus. Varicosities usually affect the veins of the lower extremities; the long saphenous vein is often affected, and they also may develop in the short saphenous vein.

Pathophysiology

Varicose veins are classified as primary (with no involvement of deep veins) or secondary (caused by the obstruction of deep veins). In both cases, long-standing increased venous pressure stretches the vessel wall. This sustained stretching impairs the ability of the venous valves to close, causing them to become incompetent.

The erect position produces a twofold negative effect on the veins. When standing, the leg veins resemble vertical columns and must withstand the full force of venous blood pressure. Prolonged standing, the force of gravity, lack of leg exercise, and incompetent venous valves all weaken the muscle-pumping mechanism, reducing venous blood return to the heart. As standing continues, the amount of blood pooled in the veins increases, further stretching the vessel wall. The venous valves become increasingly incompetent.

Manifestations

Although varicose veins may be asymptomatic, most cause manifestations such as severe aching leg pain, leg fatigue, leg heaviness, itching, or feelings of heat in the legs. The degree of valvular incompetence does not seem to correlate well with the extent of symptoms. The menstrual cycle tends to worsen symptoms, suggesting a possible correlation with hormonal factors in women. Assessment reveals obvious dilated, tortuous veins beneath the

MANIFESTATIONS of Varicose Veins

- Severe, aching pain in the leg
- Leg fatigue, heaviness
- Itching of the affected leg (stasis dermatitis)
- Feelings of warmth in the leg
- Visibly dilated veins
- Thin, discolored skin above the ankles
- Stasis ulcers

skin of the upper and lower leg. If varicose veins are long-standing, the skin above the ankles may be thin and discolored, with a brown pigmentation. See the Manifestations box.

Complications

Complications of varicose veins include venous insufficiency and stasis ulcers. Chronic stasis dermatitis may also develop. Superficial venous thrombosis may develop in varicose veins, especially during and after pregnancy, following surgery, and in patients on estrogen therapy (oral contraceptives or hormone replacement therapy).

Incidence and Risk Factors

Varicose veins affect about 15% of adults. They are more common in women over 35 with an increased risk related to venous stasis during pregnancy. Aging is a risk factor, possibly related to decreased exercise and other factors that contribute to venous stasis. People in occupations that involve prolonged standing (such as beauticians, salespeople, and nurses) also have an increased incidence of varicose veins. Race is a risk factor: Whites are more frequently affected than Blacks. The majority of people with primary varicose veins (those affecting superficial veins) have a family history of the disorder, suggesting a genetic link (Huether & McCance, 2008).

Most varicosities occur in the deep veins of the legs. Contributing causes include obesity, venous thrombosis, congenital arteriovenous malformations, or sustained pressure on abdominal veins (as in pregnancy and/or the presence of abdominal tumors). The effects of gravity, produced by long periods of standing, are a major causative factor.

Interdisciplinary Care

Varicose veins usually can be managed using conservative measures, although surgery may be required if symptoms are severe, when complications develop, or for cosmetic reasons.

Diagnosis

While varicose veins often are diagnosed by the history and physical examination, diagnostic tests may be ordered.

- *Doppler ultrasonography* or *duplex Doppler ultrasound* may be performed to identify specific locations of incompetent valves. This test is particularly useful before surgery to identify valves that allow reflux of blood from the femoral, popliteal, or peripheral deep veins into the superficial veins.
- *Trendelenburg test* may be performed to determine the underlying cause of superficial venous insufficiency. The leg is elevated, then an elastic tourniquet is placed around the distal thigh. The varicosities then are observed as the patient

stands. When valves of the deep veins are incompetent, the veins remain flat on standing; they rapidly distend when the superficial venous valves are the underlying cause.

Treatments

Although there is no real cure, conservative measures are the core of treatment for most patients with uncomplicated varicose veins. These measures often relieve symptoms and prevent complications by improving venous circulation and relieving pressure on venous tissues. Properly fitted graduated compression stockings are commonly prescribed. They compress the veins, propelling blood back to the heart. Compression stockings augment the muscle pumping action of the legs. When worn during times of prolonged standing and in combination with frequent leg elevation, compression stockings often prevent progression of the condition and development of complications.

Regular, daily walking also is important. Prolonged sitting and standing are discouraged, although elevating the legs for specified periods during the day is beneficial. Leg elevation promotes venous return, prevents venous stasis, and decreases leg heaviness and fatigue.

Compression Sclerotherapy

In compression sclerotherapy, a sclerosing solution is injected into the varicose vein and a compression bandage is applied for a period of time. This obliterates the vein. Venous blood is rerouted through healthy vessels whose valves are not compromised. Compression sclerotherapy may be used to treat small, symptomatic varicosities. It may be the primary treatment, or it may be used in conjunction with varicose vein surgery. While compression sclerotherapy may be done for cosmetic reasons, complications such as phlebitis, tissue necrosis, or infection may occur and need to be considered prior to the procedures.

Surgery

Surgical treatment of varicose veins generally is reserved for patients who are very symptomatic, experience recurrent superficial venous thrombosis, and/or develop stasis ulcers. The objective of surgery is to remove the diseased veins. It may be considered for cosmetic reasons.

Surgery usually involves extensive ligation and stripping of the greater and lesser saphenous veins. The evening before surgery, the surgeon marks all incompetent superficial and perforating varicose veins with a permanent ink marker. Under either regional or general anesthesia, the greater saphenous vein is removed and the connected smaller tributaries that have not naturally clotted off are tied off. Multiple small incisions may be made over the varicosities, allowing removal of the affected segments of the vein. Incompetent tributaries that communicate with larger vessels also are ligated. For patients with less extensive disease or patients seeking cosmetic improvement, surgery may involve only the removal of the lesser saphenous vein through an incision in the popliteal fossa.

Postoperative care includes applying pressure bandages for a minimum of 6 weeks, elevating the extremities to minimize postoperative edema, and gradually increasing amounts of ambulation. Sitting and standing are prohibited during the initial recovery period, and are gradually reintroduced as deemed appropriate by the surgeon.

∞ Nursing Care

Health Promotion

Health promotion activities to reduce the incidence of varicose veins include teaching all patients, particularly young women, the benefits of regular exercise continued over the lifetime. Discuss the effect of prolonged sitting or standing on the legs, and encourage the patient whose occupation involves these activities to periodically get up and move or to sit with the legs elevated. Encourage all patients to maintain normal weight for their height.

Assessment

Focused assessment of the patient with varicose veins includes the following:

- *Health history:* Complaints of leg pain, aching, heaviness, or fatigue; ankle swelling; history of venous thrombosis.
- *Physical examination:* Visible, dilated, tortuous superficial veins in lower extremities.

Nursing Diagnoses and Interventions

In planning and providing nursing care for patients with varicose veins, emphasis is placed on the importance of health teaching to manage the symptoms of varicose veins, particularly because there is no cure for the disease. Nursing care for patients who have undergone surgical treatment for varicose veins focuses on assessing and promoting wound healing and preventing infection. Nursing diagnoses may include those related to pain, impaired tissue perfusion and skin integrity, and a risk for impaired neurovascular function.

Chronic Pain

Varicose veins can lead to pooling of venous blood in the lower extremities. Venous congestion can cause a dull ache or feeling of pressure in the legs, particularly after prolonged standing. As venous pressure rises, arterial circulation and delivery of oxygen and nutrients to tissues is impaired. Tissue ischemia contributes to the pain. The pain associated with varicose veins tends to be chronic, developing and progressing gradually over a long period of time.

- Assess pain, including its intensity, duration, and aggravating and relieving factors. *Pain assessment allows collaborative planning with the patient to identify appropriate interventions.*
- Inquire about current measures being used by the patient to manage pain and its effects. Ask about the effectiveness of current management strategies and the desire to change. *Chronic pain management ultimately falls to the patient. Strategies to address the pain must meet the patient's needs.*
- Suggest keeping a diary of pain intensity, timing, precipitating events, and effectiveness of relief measures. *Systematic tracking of pain is an important measure in improving its management.*
- Teach and reinforce nonpharmacologic pain management strategies such as progressive relaxation, imagery, deep breathing, distraction, and meditation. *The effectiveness of such strategies is well-documented. Nonpharmacologic measures provide a variety of options for controlling pain*

while maintaining independence. These measures also can reduce reliance on analgesics.

- Collaborate with the patient to establish a pain control plan. *Collaborative planning for pain management increases the patient's sense of control and reduces powerlessness. This, in turn, enhances the ability to cope with pain and its effects.*
- Regularly evaluate the effectiveness of planned interventions and pain management strategies. *Regular evaluation allows modification of the care plan as needed, as well as providing a measure of disease progression. Increasing or poorly controlled pain may necessitate additional collaborative interventions to manage the disorder.*

Ineffective Tissue Perfusion: Peripheral

Varicose veins and venous stasis impair delivery of nutrients and oxygen to peripheral tissues as elevated venous pressures interfere with blood flow through the capillary beds. Improving venous blood flow reduces venous pressures and promotes arterial flow to peripheral tissues.

- Assess peripheral pulses, capillary refill, skin color and temperature, and extent of edema. *Assessment of arterial flow and tissue perfusion provide baseline and continuing data for evaluating the effectiveness of interventions.*
- Teach application and use of properly fitted elastic graduated compression stockings. *Elastic compression stockings compress the veins, promoting venous return from the lower extremities. During ambulation, the stockings enhance the blood-pumping action of the muscles. Because elastic stockings inhibit blood flow through small superficial vessels, they should be removed at least once each day for at least 30 minutes.*
- Instruct to maintain a program of regular exercise, such as walking for 20 to 30 minutes several times a day. When ambulation is restricted, active range-of-motion exercises help maintain muscle tone, joint mobility, and venous return. *Exercise stimulates circulation and promotes blood flow through the vascular system.*
- Advise to elevate the legs for 15 to 20 minutes several times a day and to sleep with the legs elevated above the level of the heart. *Elevating the legs promotes venous return, reducing tissue congestion and improving arterial circulation. Improved venous return also increases the cardiac output and renal perfusion, promoting elimination of excess fluid and decreasing peripheral edema.*

Risk for Impaired Skin Integrity

Ineffective venous valve function impairs venous return and increases venous pressures. *These increased pressures oppose arterial blood flow and the delivery of oxygen and nutrients to the cells. As a result, tissues are vulnerable to any additional insult, and may break down.*

- Assess lower extremity color, temperature, moisture, and for evidence of pressure or breakdown on admission and at each visit. *Initial and continuing assessment allows timely detection of early signs of skin and tissue breakdown. This, in turn, allows early institution of measures to prevent further tissue damage and promote healing.*
- Teach foot and skin care measures such as daily cleansing with nondrying soap, gentle drying, and lotions to prevent

skin dryness and cracking. *Cleansing removes potentially harmful microorganisms and stimulates circulation. Care is taken to keep the skin moist and supple, promoting its function as the first line of defense against infection.*

■ Discuss the importance of adequate nutrition and fluid intake. *Adequate nutrients are necessary to maintain tissue integrity and promote healing. A diet high in protein, carbohydrates, and vitamins and minerals promotes growth and maintenance of skin cells, provides energy, and helps prevent skin breakdown. Adequate hydration helps maintain the moisture and turgor of skin, reducing the risk of drying and breakdown.*

Risk for Peripheral Neurovascular Dysfunction

Severe varicose veins can lead to chronic venous insufficiency, impaired arterial circulation, and ultimately, disrupted sensation in the affected extremity. Impaired neurologic function increases the patient's risk for injury and infection of the extremity, as minor trauma may go unnoticed.

■ Assess circulation, sensation, and movement of the lower extremities. *Disrupted circulation and venous congestion may interfere with sensory and motor function of the affected extremity. The potential for nerve and muscle involvement is especially high in patients with venous stasis ulcers.*

■ Instruct to report signs of neurovascular dysfunction, such as numbness, coldness, pain, or tingling of an extremity. *Early recognition of neurovascular dysfunction facilitates institution of interventions to prevent complications. Because the* postoperative hospital stay following varicose vein surgery or venous stasis ulcer repair is brief, manifestations of neurovascular dysfunction may initially be detected by the patient. *Careful assessment and prompt reporting helps prevent potential complications such as skin breakdown, infection, and nerve damage.*

■ Teach measures to protect the extremities from injury, such as always wearing shoes or firm slippers, cotton socks to absorb moisture, and testing the temperature of bath water with a thermometer or the upper extremities before stepping in. *Sensation in the lower extremities may be affected by poor circulation, necessitating additional measures to protect the legs and feet from injury.*

Community-Based Care

Most patients with varicose veins provide self-care at home. Include the following topics when preparing the patient and family for home care.

■ Leg elevation and exercise program
■ Application and use of graduated elastic compression stockings
■ Foot and leg care (see Box 32–4)
■ Measures to avoid injury and skin breakdown
■ Symptoms or potential complications to report to the healthcare provider

Provide information about suppliers for elastic stockings and any other required supplies. If venous stasis ulcers have developed, consider referral to home health services for regular assessment of healing and additional teaching.

Disorders of the Lymphatic System

The lymphatic system, which includes the lymphatic vessels and the lymph nodes, is a unique part of the circulatory system. The lymphatic system returns plasma and plasma proteins filtered out of the capillaries from interstitial tissues to the bloodstream. This fluid is called *lymph*. The lymphatic system consists of closed capillaries leading to larger lymphatic venules and lymphatic veins. These vessels contain smooth muscle and one-way valves that help move fluid toward the heart. Lymphatic vessels share the same sheath as arteries and veins; arterial pulsations and skeletal muscle contractions compress the lymphatic vessels to assist in maintaining lymph flow. As lymph moves through the lymphatic system, it is filtered through thousands of bean-shaped lymph nodes clustered along the vessels. Within these nodes, phagocytes remove foreign material from the lymph, preventing it from entering the bloodstream.

The Patient with Lymphadenopathy

Lymphadenopathy, enlarged lymph nodes, may be localized or generalized. Localized lymphadenopathy usually results from an inflammatory process (e.g., streptococcal pharyngitis or an infected wound). The node enlarges as lymphocytes and monocytes proliferate within the node to destroy infectious material. Palpable lymph nodes often develop in response to minor trauma or a localized infection. Generalized lymphadenopathy usually is associated with malignancy or disease. Malignant cells or other abnormal cells invade the node, causing it to enlarge.

Lymphangitis, inflammation of the lymph vessels draining an infected area of the body, is characterized by a red streak along the inflamed vessels, pain, heat, and swelling. Fever and chills also may be present. Local lymph nodes are swollen and tender.

Treatment for lymphadenopathy and lymphangitis focuses on identifying and treating the underlying condition. Elevating the body part and applying heat to inflamed lymphatic vessels help reduce swelling and promote blood flow to the affected area.

The Patient with Lymphedema

Lymphedema may be a primary or a secondary disorder, resulting from inflammation, obstruction, or removal of lymphatic vessels. It is characterized by extremity edema due to accumulation of lymph. *Primary lymphedema* is uncommon, affecting about 1 in 10,000 people. It affects females more frequently than males, and may be associated with a genetic disorder such as Turner syndrome or Kleinfelter syndrome. See the accompanying Genetic Considerations box.

Secondary lymphedema is an acquired condition, resulting from damage, obstruction, or removal of lymphatic vessels. The most common worldwide cause of secondary lymphedema is *filariasis*, infestation of the lymphatic vessels by filaria, a nematode worm. Other important causes of secondary lymphedema

Primary lymphedema develops as a result of agenesis, hypoplasia, or obstruction of lymphatic vessels.
- *Congenital lymphedema* appears shortly after birth; two other forms of lymphedema develop later, one at the time of puberty (*lymphedema praecox*), the other usually after age 35 (*lymphedema tarda*).
- Congenital lymphedema and lymphedema praecox may be inherited as an autosomal dominant trait with variable penetrance.
- Lymphedema also may be inherited (although less commonly) as an autosomal or sex-linked recessive disorder (Kasper et al., 2005).

include recurrent episodes of bacterial lymphangitis, obstruction of lymph vessels by tumors, and surgical or radiation treatment for breast cancer (Kasper et al., 2005).

Pathophysiology and Manifestations

Obstruction of lymph drainage prevents fluid and protein molecules from interstitial tissues from returning to the circulation. The protein molecules increase the osmotic pressure in interstitial tissues, drawing in additional fluid that causes edema in the soft tissues. One or both extremities may be affected.

The edema begins distally, progressing up the limb to involve the entire extremity. Initial edema is soft and pitting; with chronic congestion, subcutaneous tissues become fibrotic, causing thick, rough skin and a woody texture of the limb (*brawny edema*). In contrast, the edema associated with venous disorders is softer, and the skin often is hyperpigmented with evidence of stasis dermatitis. Lymphedema generally is painless, although the limb may feel heavy.

Interdisciplinary Care

Interdisciplinary care for the patient with lymphedema focuses on relieving edema and preventing or treating infection. The disorder may be difficult to treat effectively, and can lead to progressive disability due to the weight and awkwardness of the affected extremity.

Diagnosis

Abdominal or pelvic ultrasound and computed tomography (CT) scans are used to detect obstructing lesions. Magnetic resonance imaging (MRI) can show edema and identify lymph nodes and enlarged lymphatic vessels. More invasive procedures such as lymphangiography and radioactive isotope studies may occasionally be necessary to identify the lymphatic defect causing lymphedema.

- *Lymphangiography* uses injected contrast media to illustrate lymphatic vessels on x-rays. Organic dyes are used to identify a distal lymphatic vessel, and then a contrast medium is injected into the vessel for visualization of the lymphatic system of the limb. In primary lymphedema, lymph vessels are absent or hypoplastic (underdeveloped). In secondary lymphedema, lymph channels often are dilated; it may be possible to determine the level of obstruction.

- *Lymphoscintigraphy* involves injecting a radioactively tagged substance into distal subcutaneous tissues of the extremity, then mapping its flow through the lymphatic system. The pattern of lymph fluid distribution and transport is abnormal in patients with lymphedema.

Treatments

Meticulous skin and foot care is vital to prevent infection in the affected extremity. Shoes should always be worn to reduce the risk of injury. Careful cleansing and use of emollient lotions are recommended to prevent drying of the skin. Exercise is encouraged, as are frequent periods of leg elevation. The foot of the bed is raised by 15 to 20 degrees at night to promote lymph flow. Elastic graduated compression stockings may be ordered for use during the day. In some cases, an intermittent pneumatic compression device to reduce edema may be prescribed for home use.

Antibiotics are given to prevent and treat infection, which can be recurrent and difficult to eradicate. Diuretic therapy may be used intermittently, particularly when primary lymphedema is exacerbated by the menstrual cycle or seasonal variability.

Patients who do not respond to conservative treatment measures or who experience recurrent episodes of cellulitis and lymphangitis may require surgical treatment. Microvascular techniques may be used to create anatomoses between obstructed lymphatic vessels and adjacent veins, providing channels to redirect lymph into the venous system. Successful surgery may improve both extremity function and its cosmetic appearance.

Nursing Care

Nursing care for patients with lymphatic disorders focuses on reducing edema, preventing tissue damage related to the edema, and promoting effective coping with the effect of the disorder on body image and function.

Nursing Diagnoses and Interventions

Nursing diagnoses for the patient with lymphedema may include *Impaired Tissue Integrity*, *Excess Fluid Volume*, and *Disturbed Body Image*.

Impaired Tissue Integrity

Obstructed lymphatic flow leads to fluid congestion of the interstitial spaces of subcutaneous tissue. The resulting edema compresses and damages tissues of the affected extremity. Subcutaneous tissues become fibrotic, reducing their protective functions of shock absorption and insulation. In addition, obstructed lymphatic flow reduces the effectiveness of lymph nodes in filtering and removing foreign material and pathogens from the body. This increases the risk for local tissue infection such as *cellulitis*, a diffuse bacterial infection of the skin. Cellulitis increases the risk for skin and tissue breakdown and, if not effectively treated, can lead to sepsis.

- Frequently inspect the skin of the affected extremity, documenting the condition with each assessment. Promptly report areas of pallor, redness, or apparent inflammation. Breaks in the skin surface allow microbial invasion, and increase the risk for infection. *Prompt identification and treatment of any lesions is vital to prevent further tissue breakdown and infection.*

- Apply well-fitting elastic graduated compression stockings or intermittent pneumatic pressure devices as ordered. *Elastic stockings and/or pneumatic pressure devices oppose the movement of fluid out of capillaries and improve its reabsorption into vascular spaces for transportation back to the heart.*
- Remove elastic stockings and intermittent pressure devices every 8 hours or at each home visit to inspect the underlying skin for evidence of redness, irritation, dryness, or breakdown. *Elastic graduated compression stockings, antiembolic stockings, and pneumatic compression devices compress small vessels nourishing the skin and subcutaneous tissue. Periodic removal not only allows inspection of the underlying skin, but also allows restoration of blood flow to these small vessels and the tissues.*
- Instruct to elevate the extremities while seated and during sleep. *Elevation of the extremities diminishes venous congestion, promotes venous return, facilitates arterial circulation and tissue perfusion, and helps reduce the accumulation of excess fluids in interstitial spaces of the affected extremity.*
- Use preventive skin care devices as indicated. Collected fluid in the affected extremity increases its weight and interferes with regular movement. The increased weight places greater pressure on surfaces of the limb that come in contact with furniture. *Protective devices such as egg crate foam, sheepskin, pillows, or padding help prevent tissue compression, promoting circulation and reducing the risk of skin and tissue breakdown.*
- Keep skin clean and dry, especially in interdigital spaces. Teach skin and foot care to the patient and family. *Clean, dry skin provides the first line of defense against infection. Significant limb edema can interfere with reaching the distal extremity and cleaning interdigital spaces. The dark, moist spaces between the toes are an excellent environment for bacterial growth. Teaching fosters self-care and independence, as well as preparing the patient and family to manage this often chronic condition.*
- Discuss the importance of adhering to the therapeutic regimen. *Lymphedema generally is a chronic condition; effective management requires active patient participation in planning and implementing care to reduce edema and maintain tissue integrity.*

Excess Fluid Volume

In lymphedema, obstruction, destruction, or congenital malformation of lymphatic vessels interferes with the normal circulation of lymphatic fluid. As a result, lymph collects in the subcutaneous tissues of the affected extremity, causing excess fluid volume of that extremity. Some patients may benefit from intermittent diuretic therapy and dietary sodium restriction.

PRACTICE ALERT
Monitor intake and output and/or weight (daily or weekly). Use consistent scales, timing, and clothing for accurate weight measurements. Intake and output records and short-term changes in weight reflect fluid balance. Measures of fluid balance permit evaluation of the effectiveness of interventions such as restricted sodium intake and diuretic therapy.

- Discuss the rationale for restricted sodium intake if ordered. Teach ways to maintain the recommended sodium restriction, and assist to choose foods that are low in sodium. *Sodium causes retention of extracellular water; restricting dietary sodium may help prevent additional fluid accumulation in interstitial spaces.*
- During acute periods, assess the affected extremity daily for increased edema; measure girth of the extremity using consistent technique. *The size of the affected extremity provides a measure of the effectiveness of ordered interventions and progression of the disorder.*

Disturbed Body Image

The disproportionate size of an extremity or extremities due to lymphedema can profoundly affect body image. During early stages of the disease, conservative measures may effectively reduce the edema and size of the affected limb. However, as the disease progresses, conservative measures may become less effective, leading to more permanent disfigurement. Mobility may be impaired, and the patient may develop an increasingly negative self-perception.

- Encourage discussions about usual coping patterns and perception of self. *Knowledge of existing coping patterns and behaviors helps the nurse assess the patient's ability to cope with the current situation. This knowledge is then used to reinforce effective coping mechanisms and help develop more effective coping strategies. This exchange also allows the patient to voice feelings related to actual or perceived changes in body image.*
- Accept the patient's perception of self and of the impact of the changes in appearance. *Nonjudgmental acceptance of the patient's view of self and of the effects of changes in appearance builds trust and promotes rapport. A trusting relationship promotes the patient's ability to take an active role in managing the disorder, participate in healthcare decisions, and adhere to the plan of care. Nonjudgmental listening also promotes mutual respect and demonstrates caring and compassion.*
- Encourage active participation in self-care. Assist with identifying alternative self-care strategies when the extent of edema interferes with performing some aspects of self-care such as trimming toenails or washing feet. *The patient initially may have difficulty viewing or touching the affected body part. Gentle encouragement and support from the nurse helps the patient assume self-care and accept the affected body part. Brainstorming to identify alternative care strategies promotes the patient's independence even when total self-care is not feasible.*

Community-Based Care

When preparing the patient with chronic lymphedema and family to manage the disorder, include the following teaching topics.

- Recommended program of exercise and elevation of the extremity
- Foot and skin care
- Use of elastic graduated compression stockings and/or intermittent pressure devices

- Importance of wearing elastic stockings during the majority of waking hours, removing them once during the daytime and while sleeping
- Measures to prevent infection in the affected extremity, such as wearing gloves while gardening
- Signs and symptoms to report to the healthcare provider (e.g., manifestations of tissue breakdown or infection, increasing edema, or evidence of compromised circulation)

- Use and precautions associated with any prescribed medications
- Sodium-restricted diet if ordered

Provide information about contacts for questions, and make referrals as needed. Evaluate the need for home health, home maintenance assistance, and other services such as physical or occupational therapy.

CHAPTER HIGHLIGHTS

- Essential hypertension, blood pressure of 140/90 or higher with no clearly identified cause, rarely causes symptoms but is a major risk factor for coronary heart disease, heart failure, stroke, and renal insufficiency.
- Prehypertension, a newly identified category, is an average blood pressure of 120–139/80–89. Patients with prehypertension are advised to make lifestyle changes indicated for hypertension (weight loss, exercise, dietary changes, limited alcohol intake, and stress reduction), but generally are not treated with medications unless other risk factors such as diabetes or kidney disease are present.
- Systolic hypertension, an elevated systolic blood pressure without elevation of the diastolic pressure, is common in older adults and contributes to complications such as coronary heart disease and stroke.
- Medications to treat hypertension include diuretics, alpha- and beta-adrenergic blockers, ACE inhibitors and angiotensin II blockers, calcium channel blockers, and vasodilators. A combination of two or more drugs often is required for effective blood pressure control.
- Aneurysms, abnormal dilation of a blood vessel, commonly affect the aorta and the iliac arteries, particularly in older men. A slowly expending abdominal aortic aneurysm that does not produce symptoms or impair flow through the renal arteries may not

be repaired, particularly in an older patient. Percutaneously inserted endovascular splints provide an alternative to surgery for abdominal aortic aneurysms.
- Peripheral vascular disease, obstruction or occlusion of peripheral arteries by atherosclerotic plaque, is common and a leading cause of disability and amputation.
- Smoking cessation and regular daily exercise are key components of treatment for peripheral vascular disorders such as atherosclerosis, thromboangiitis obliterans, and Raynaud's disease.
- Venous thrombosis, particularly of the deep veins of the legs and pelvis, develop as a result of venous stasis, blood vessel damage, and increased coagulability of the blood. The developing clot may fragment or break loose, becoming an embolus that typically lodges in the pulmonary circulation (pulmonary embolus). Chronic venous insufficiency and venous stasis may develop as a result of deep venous thrombosis.
- Prophylactic anticoagulation and mobilization of the patient are the primary preventive measures for venous thrombosis. Monitoring coagulation studies and assessing for evidence of bleeding (overt or covert) are important nursing measures for the patient on anticoagulant therapy.
- Lymphadenopathy (enlarged lymph nodes), lymphangitis (inflammation of the lymph vessels), and lymphedema are the most common disorders affecting the lymph system.

TEST YOURSELF NCLEX-RN® REVIEW

1. A potential blood donor whose blood pressure is found to average 180/106 on two different readings tells the nurse, "I don't understand how it could be so high—I feel just fine." The appropriate response by the nurse is which of the following?
   1. "This is probably just a false reading due to 'white coat syndrome.' Don't worry about it."
   2. "It is unusual that you are not having some symptoms such as severe headaches and nosebleeds."
   3. "High blood pressure often has few or no symptoms; that's why it is called the 'silent killer.'"
   4. "You probably should have your blood pressure rechecked in 3 months or so and then follow up with your primary care provider if it is still high."

2. The nurse teaching a patient about the DASH diet determines that additional teaching is necessary when the patient states which of the following?
   1. "I'm glad I can still eat as much pasta as usual; I was afraid I would have to give up my weekly lasagna."
   2. "It will be a challenge to incorporate all those servings of fruits and vegetables into my diet."
   3. "Having a handful of nuts when the pre-dinner 'munchies' hit is a good idea."
   4. "I will enjoy having frozen yogurt as my bedtime snack on occasion."

3. The nurse teaching a patient about his new prescription for Diovan HCT, a combination angiotensin II receptor blocker and thiazide diuretic, includes which of the following in his instructions? **Select all that apply.**
   1. Use a potassium-based salt substitute to prevent hypokalemia while taking this drug.
   2. Use caution when rising from bed or a chair to prevent dizziness.
   3. Take the drug at bedtime to reduce the risk of falling due to light-headedness.
   4. Report a persistent disruptive cough to your healthcare provider.
   5. You may stop taking this drug once your blood pressure is within the normal range for at least 2 months.

4. A patient is complaining of new onset calf and foot pain. The nurse notes that the leg below the knee is cool, pale, and dorsalis pedis and posterior tibial pulses are absent. The priority nursing intervention is to do which of the following?
   1. Notify the healthcare provider.
   2. Place a cradle over the leg to prevent pressure from bedding.
   3. Position the leg flat, supported in anatomic position.
   4. Prepare to initiate heparin therapy.

5. An 86-year-old patient with a newly diagnosed abdominal aortic aneurysm wonders if he will need surgery to repair the aneurysm, even though he feels fine. The nurse's response is based on the knowledge of which of the following?
   1. The risk of surgical repair is lower than the risk that the aneurysm will rupture.
   2. Opening the abdomen for the surgical procedure greatly increases the risk of rupture.
   3. Surgery is indicated for type A aneurysms.
   4. A percutaneously inserted endovascular stent may be considered because of his age.

6. An expected assessment finding in a patient with peripheral atherosclerosis would be which of the following?
   1. pallor of the legs and feet when dependent
   2. increased hair growth on the affected extremity
   3. higher blood pressure readings in the affected extremity
   4. impaired sensation in the affected extremity

7. All of the following are appropriate home care measures for the patient with peripheral vascular disease. Place them in order of priority.
   1. foot and leg care
   2. smoking cessation
   3. daily inspection of feet and legs
   4. regular daily exercise
   5. weight loss strategies

8. The nurse evaluates her teaching of a patient admitted with deep vein thrombosis as effective when the patient states which of the following?
   1. "I'll use a hard-backed, upright chair when sitting instead of my recliner."
   2. "I'll get my blood drawn as scheduled and notify the doctor if I have any unusual bleeding or bruising."
   3. "I understand why I am not allowed to exercise for the next 6 weeks and will take it easy."
   4. "I'll have my wife buy a low-cholesterol cookbook and we'll make an appointment with the dietician to learn about a low-fat, low-cholesterol diet."

9. A patient with visible varicose veins tells the nurse that she wants to have surgery to remove them, because "my legs ache every evening and they are really ugly!" The most appropriate response would be which of the following?
   1. "Often measures such as elevating your legs and elastic stockings can relieve the discomfort associated with varicose veins."
   2. "Surgery will have a good cosmetic effect, but will not relieve the discomfort associated with varicose veins."
   3. "All varicose veins should be surgically removed to restore adequate blood flow to your legs and prevent gangrene."
   4. "Surgery is never indicated unless the varicose veins are interfering with circulation. Have you tried cosmetic measures to cover them up?"

10. Which of the following nursing interventions is of highest priority for the patient with lymphedema?
    1. Elevate affected extremities at night.
    2. Assist to don elastic compression stockings during the day.
    3. Carefully dry and apply emollient lotion to affected extremities after bathing.
    4. Reinforce the importance of taking prescribed diuretics.

See Test Yourself answers in Appendix C.

Pearson Nursing Student Resources
Find additional review materials at
www.nursing.pearsonhighered.com
Prepare for success with additional NCLEX®-style practice questions, interactive assignments and activities, Web links, animations and videos, and more!

BIBLIOGRAPHY

American Heart Association. (2009). *Heart disease and stroke statistics – 2009 update.* Dallas, TX: American Heart Association.

Applying antiembolism stockings isn't just pulling on socks. (2004). *Nursing, 34*(8), 48–49.

Bulechek, G., Butcher, H., & Dochterman, J. M. (Eds). (2008). *Nursing interventions classification (NIC)* (5th ed.). St. Louis: Mosby Elsevier.

Crowther, M., & McCourt, K. (2005). Venous thromboembolism: A guide to prevention and treatment. *Nurse Practitioner, 30*(8), 26–29, 32–34, 30–45.

Deglin, J. H., & Vallerand, A. H. (2009). *Davis's drug guide for nurses.* Philadelphia: F.A. Davis.

Fontaine, K. L. (2005). *Healing practices: Alternative therapies for nursing* (2nd ed.). Upper Saddle River, NJ: Prentice Hall Health.

Goldhaber, S. Z., McRae, S. J., & Wang, J. (2005). How to use low-molecular-weight heparin to prevent DVT. *Patient Care for the Nurse Practitioner,* April 1, 6.

Huether, S. E. & McCance, K. L. (2008). *Understanding Pathophysiology* (4th ed.). St. Louis: Mosby Elsevier.

McCaffrey, R., Ruknui, P., Hatthakit, U., & Kasetsomboon, P. (2005). The effects of yoga on hypertensive persons in Thailand. *Holistic Nursing Practice, 19*(4), 173–180.

Miller, E. R. III, & Jehn, M. L. (2004). New high blood pressure guidelines create new at-risk classification: Changes in blood pressure classification by JNC 7. *Journal of Cardiovascular Nursing, 19*(6), 367–373.

Moorhead, S., Johnson, M., Maas M., & Swanson, E. (Eds). (2008). *Nursing outcomes classification (NOC)* (4th ed.). St. Louis: Mosby Elsevier.

National Heart, Lung, and Blood Institute. (2003). Facts about the DASH eating plan. NIH Publication No. 06-4082. Retrieved from http://www.nhlbi.nih.gov/health/public/heart/hbp/dash/new_dash.pdf

National Heart, Lung, and Blood Institute. (2005). NHLBI study: High blood pressure not well controlled among older men and women. *NIH News.* Retrieved from http://www.nhlbi.nih.gov/new/press/05-07-26.htm.

National Heart, Lung, and Blood Institute: National High Blood Pressure Education Program. (2004). *The Seventh Report of the Joint National Committee on Prevention, Detection, Evaluation, and Treatment of High Blood Pressure.* Bethesda, MD: National Institutes of Health.

NANDA International. (2009). *Nursing diagnoses: Definitions and classification 2009–2011.* Oxford, UK: Wiley-Blackwell.

Papadakis, M. A. & McPhee, S. J. (2007). *Current Consult Medicine 2007.* New York: McGraw-Hill.

Rice, K. L. (2005). How to measure ankle/brachial index. *Nursing, 35*(1), 56–57.

Ramanath, V. S., Oh, J. K., Sundt, T. M. & Eagle, K. A. (2009). Acute aortic syndromes and thoracic aneurysm. *Mayo Clinic Proceedings 84* (5), 465–481.

Spencer, J. W., & Jacobs, J. J. (2003). *Complementary and alternative medicine: An evidence-based approach* (2nd ed.). St. Louis: Mosby.

U.S. Preventive Services Task Force. (2005). Screening for abdominal aortic aneurysm: Recommendation statement. *The American Journal for Nurse Practitioners, 9*(5), 55–60

Van Leeuwan, A. M., Krapipitz, T. R. & Smith, L. R. (2006). *Davis' Laboratory and Diagnostic Tests* (2nd ed). New York: F.A. Davis.

Way, L. W., & Doherty, G. M. (2003). *Current surgical diagnosis & treatment* (11th ed.). New York: McGraw-Hill.

Wipke-Tevis, D. D., Stotts, N. A., Williams, D. A., Froelicher, E. S., & Hunt, T. K. (2001) Tissue oxygenation, perfusion, and position in patients with venous leg ulcers. *Nursing Research, 50*(1), 24–32.

Wung, S., & Aouizerat, B. E. (2004). Newly mapped gene for thoracic aortic aneurysm and dissection. *Journal of Cardiovascular Nursing, 19*(6), 409–416.

Yucha, C. B., Tsai, P. S., Calderon, K. S., & Tian, L. (2005). Biofeedback-assisted relaxation training for essential hypertension: Who is most likely to benefit? *Journal of Cardiovascular Nursing, 20*(3), 198–205.

CHAPTER 33

Nursing Care of Patients with Hematologic Disorders

LEARNING OUTCOMES

1. Relate the physiology and assessment of the hematologic system and related systems to commonly occurring hematologic disorders.
2. Describe the pathophysiology of common hematologic disorders.
3. Explain nursing implications for medications and other treatments prescribed for hematologic disorders.
4. Discuss indications for and complications of bone marrow or stem cell transplantation, as well as related nursing care.
5. Compare and contrast the pathophysiology, manifestations, and management of bleeding disorders.
6. Describe the major types of leukemia and the most common treatment modalities and nursing interventions.
7. Differentiate Hodgkin's disease from non-Hodgkin's lymphomas.

CLINICAL COMPETENCIES

1. Assess effects of hematologic disorders and prescribed treatments on patients' functional health status.
2. Monitor and document continuing assessment data, including laboratory test results, subjective and objective information, and reporting data outside the normal or expected range.
3. Based on knowledge of pathophysiology, prescribed treatment, and assessed data, identify and prioritize nursing diagnoses for patients with hematologic disorders.
4. Use nursing research and evidence-based practice to identify and implement individualized nursing interventions for the patient with a hematologic disorder.
5. Safely administer prescribed medications and treatments for patients with hematologic disorders.
6. Collaborate with the interdisciplinary care team to plan and provide coordinated, effective care for patients with hematologic disorders.
7. Provide appropriate teaching for patients with hematologic disorders, evaluating learning and the need for continued reinforcement of information.
8. Use continuing assessment data to revise the plan of care as needed to restore, maintain, or promote functional health in the patient with a hematologic disorder.

KEY TERMS

anemia, *1069*
aplastic anemia, *1076*
bone marrow transplant (BMT), *1089*
disseminated intravascular coagulation (DIC), *1112*
hemolytic anemia, *1072*
hemophilia, *1108*

hemostasis, *1105*
iron deficiency anemia, *1071*
leukemia, *1084*
lymphoma, *1095*
multiple myeloma, *1102*
myelodysplastic syndrome, *1081*
pernicious anemia, *1072*

polycythemia, *1083*
sickle cell anemia, *1073*
sickle cell crisis, *1073*
stem cell transplant (SCT), *1090*
thalassemia, *1074*
thrombocytopenia, *1105*

Disorders affecting the blood and blood-forming organs have effects that range from minor disruptions in daily activities to major life-threatening crises. Patients with hematologic disorders need holistic nursing care, including emotional support and care for problems involving major body systems. This chapter focuses on health changes resulting from changes in red cells, white cells, platelets, and clotting factors.

Red Blood Cell Disorders

Red blood cells (RBCs) transport oxygen to body tissues and help return carbon dioxide to the lungs for excretion. Alterations in the number, size, shape, or composition of RBCs affect their ability to effectively carry out these functions.

Anemia, the most common RBC disorder, is an abnormally low RBC count or reduced hemoglobin content. Polycythemia is an abnormally high RBC count.

The Patient with Anemia

Anemia is an abnormally low number of circulating RBCs, low hemoglobin concentration, or both. Decreased numbers of circulating RBCs is the usual cause of anemia. This may result from blood loss, inadequate RBC production, or increased RBC destruction. Insufficient or defective hemoglobin within RBCs contributes to anemia. Depending on its severity, anemia may affect all major organ systems.

> **FAST FACTS**
> - Iron-deficiency anemia, a nutritional anemia, is the most common type of anemia.
> - Blood loss anemia may be either acute, resulting from hemorrhage, or chronic, resulting from chronic blood loss (e.g., menstrual flow, slow gastrointestinal (GI) bleeding).
> - Risk for anemia increases with age. Persons older tan 85 years are two to three times more likely to have anemia compared to other older adults (Lash & Coyer, 2008).

Physiology Review

As blood flows through the pulmonary vascular system, oxygen diffuses from alveoli into capillary blood. The majority of the oxygen binds reversibly with the hemoglobin in RBCs; only about 3% of the oxygen remains in solution in the blood. When the blood reaches the capillaries serving body tissues, oxygen is released from the hemoglobin molecule and diffuses out of the capillary to reach the cells. The amount of oxygen that reaches the tissues depends on a number of factors, including the following:

- Available oxygen in the alveoli
- The diffusing surface and capacity of the lungs
- The number of RBCs and the amount and type of hemoglobin they contain
- The ability of the cardiovascular system to transport blood and oxygen to the tissues

For more information about red blood cells (RBCs), hemoglobin, and their production and function, ∞ see Chapter 29.

Physiology and Manifestations

A number of different pathologic mechanisms can lead to anemia (Box 33–1). Regardless of the cause, every type of anemia reduces the oxygen-carrying capacity of the blood due to a deficiency of RBCs or hemoglobin, leading to tissue hypoxia. The resulting manifestations depend on the severity of the anemia, how quickly it develops, and other factors such as age and health status.

When anemia develops gradually and the RBC reduction is moderate, successful compensatory mechanisms may result in few symptoms except when the oxygen needs of the body increase due to exercise or infection. Symptoms develop as RBCs and hemoglobin levels are further reduced. Pallor of the skin, mucous membranes, conjunctiva, and nail beds develops as a result of blood redistribution to vital organs and lack of hemoglobin (Figure 33–1 ■). As tissue oxygenation decreases, the heart and respiratory rates rise in an attempt to increase cardiac output and tissue perfusion. Tissue hypoxia may cause angina, fatigue, dyspnea on exertion, and night cramps. It also stimulates erythropoietin release; increased erythropoietin activity stimulates RBC production in the bone marrow, and may lead to bone

Figure 33–1 ■ The skin of the patient with anemia appears pale beside that of a person with a normal hemoglobin and hematocrit.

pain. Cerebral hypoxia can lead to headache, dizziness, and dim vision. Heart failure may develop in severe anemia.

With rapid blood loss, blood volume is decreased as well as the oxygen-carrying capacity of the blood. Initial manifestations include tachycardia and tachypnea; the skin may be pale, cool, and clammy as peripheral vessels constrict to maintain blood flow to the heart and brain. With significant blood loss, signs of circulatory shock may occur, including hypotension, tachycardia, decreased level of consciousness, and oliguria. With chronic bleeding, fluid shifts from the interstitial spaces into the vessels, maintaining blood volume. Blood viscosity is reduced, which may result in a systolic heart murmur. See page 1070 for the Multisystem Effects of Anemia feature.

> **BOX 33–1 Pathophysiologic Mechanisms of Anemia**
>
> **Decreased RBC Production**
> - Altered hemoglobin synthesis
>   - Iron deficiency
>   - Thalassemias
>   - Chronic inflammation
> - Altered DNA synthesis
>   - Vitamin B_{12} or folic acid malabsorption or deficiency
> - Bone marrow failure
>   - Aplastic anemia (stem cell dysfunction)
>   - Red cell aplasia
>   - Myeloproliferative leukemias
>   - Cancer metastasis, lymphoma
>   - Chronic infection or inflammation, physical and emotional fatigue
>
> **Increased RBC Loss or Destruction**
> - Acute or chronic blood loss
>   - Hemorrhage or trauma
>   - Chronic gastrointestinal bleeding, menorrhagia
> - Increased hemolysis
>   - Hereditary cell membrane disorders
>   - Defective hemoglobin—Sickle cell anemia or trait
>   - Pyruvate kinase (PK) or G6PD deficiency affecting glycolysis or cell oxidation
>   - Immune mechanisms and disorders (e.g., blood reaction, hypersensitivity responses, autoimmune disorders)
>   - Splenomegaly and hypersplenism
>   - Infection
>   - Erythrocyte trauma (e.g., due to cardiopulmonary bypass, hemolytic uremic syndrome)

MULTISYSTEM EFFECTS OF
Anemia

Neurologic
- Paresthesias[4]
- Proprioception deficits[4]
- Headache[5]
- Fainting[5]
- Forgetfulness[5]
- Pain[6]
- Behavioral disturbances (pica)[3]

Respiratory
- Increased rate
- Dyspnea on exertion

Urinary
- Hemoglobinuria[7]

Cardiovascular
- Tachycardia
- Palpitations
- Systolic murmur
- Ventricular hypertrophy
- Angina

Potential complication
- Heart failure[6]

Gastrointestinal
- Diarrhea[4]
- Anorexia[5]
- Nausea[5]
- Gallstones[6]
- Splenomegaly[1]
- Abdominal pain[6]

Musculoskeletal
- Night cramps[5]
- Bone pain
- Joint pain[6]
- Bone deformity and fractures[1]

Integumentary
- Pallor
  - Skin
  - Mucous membranes
  - Conjunctiva
  - Nail beds
- Jaundice[1]
- Petechiae[2]
- Purpura[2]
- Spoon-shaped nails[3]
- Cheilosis[3]
- Sore, beefy red tongue[4]
- Chronic leg ulcers[6]

Key (symptoms usually caused by a specific form of anemia)
1 Hemolytic anemias
2 Aplastic anemia
3 Iron deficiency anemia
4 Pernicious anemia
5 Vitamin B_{12} anemia
6 Sickle cell anemia
7 G6PD anemia

Anemia is categorized by cause: blood loss, bone marrow suppression, nutritional, and hemolytic. Genetics also plays a role in some anemias. The pathophysiology and specific manifestations of these types of anemias follows.

Blood Loss Anemia

When anemia results from acute or chronic bleeding, RBCs and other blood components (such as iron) are lost from the body. With acute blood loss, circulating volume decreases. As a result, the cardiac output falls. Compensatory mechanisms are activated to maintain the cardiac output: The heart rate increases, and peripheral blood vessels constrict. Vessels in the liver, a blood storage organ, also constrict, increasing circulating volume. Fluid shifts from the interstitial spaces into the vascular compartment to maintain blood volume, diluting the cellular components of the blood and reducing its viscosity. If hemorrhage continues, compensatory mechanisms become less effective, increasing the risk for shock and circulatory failure (∞ see Chapter 11).

In acute blood loss, circulating RBCs are of normal size and shape (*normocytic*). Early in the hemorrhage, the RBC count, hemoglobin, and hematocrit may be normal; as fluid shifts from the interstitial space into the vascular space to maintain circulating volume, the RBC count, hemoglobin, and hematocrit fall. If sufficient iron is available, the number of circulating RBCs and hemoglobin levels return to normal within 3 to 4 weeks after the bleeding episode. Chronic blood loss, on the other hand, depletes iron stores as RBC production attempts to maintain the RBC supply. The resulting RBCs are *microcytic* (small) and *hypochromic* (pale).

Nutritional Anemias

A number of different nutrients are required for normal RBC development (erythropoiesis). Iron is a key nutrient necessary for hemoglobin synthesis. In addition, adequate supplies of protein (and its building blocks, amino acids), vitamins, and other minerals are required. The B vitamins, particularly B_{12} (cobalamin) and folate, play a key role in RBC development. Vitamins C and E also are necessary. Nutritional anemias result from nutrient deficits that affect RBC formation or hemoglobin synthesis. The nutrient deficit may be caused by inadequate diet, malabsorption of the nutrient, or an increased need for the nutrient. The most common types of nutritional anemias are iron deficiency anemia, vitamin B_{12} anemia, and folic acid deficiency anemia. Vitamin B_{12} and folic acid anemias are sometimes called *megaloblastic* anemias, as enlarged nucleated RBCs called megaloblasts are seen in these anemias.

IRON DEFICIENCY ANEMIA **Iron deficiency anemia** is the most common type of anemia. It develops when the supply of iron is inadequate for optimal RBC formation. The body cannot synthesize hemoglobin without iron. Normally, the body efficiently recycles and stores iron, reusing much of the iron contained in RBCs that are removed from circulation due to age or damage. However, small amounts of iron continually are lost in the feces; therefore, adequate iron intake is necessary for normal hemoglobin synthesis and RBC production. Iron deficiency anemia results in fewer numbers of RBCs, microcytic and hypochromic RBCs, as well as malformed RBCs (*poikilocytosis*) (Figure 33–2 ■).

Iron Deficiency Anemia Video

Figure 33–2 ■ A blood smear showing RBCs characteristically seen in iron-deficiency anemia. Note the pale color of the RBCs (hypochromic). Many of the cells also are smaller than normal (microcytic) and misshapen, reducing their oxygen-carrying capacity.

Excessive iron loss due to chronic bleeding is the usual cause of iron deficiency anemia in adults. Menstrual blood loss is the most common cause in adult females. Iron deficiency anemia also may result from inadequate dietary iron intake (less than 1 mg/day), malabsorption syndromes, or the increased iron requirements associated with pregnancy and lactation. Box 33–2 summarizes common causes of iron deficiency anemia.

Iron deficiency anemia is particularly common in older adults. Chronic, occult (hidden) blood loss may occur from slowly bleeding peptic ulcers, GI inflammation, hemorrhoids, and cancer. Inadequate dietary iron intake also contributes to anemia in the older adult. Access to transportation may limit fresh food consumption, a factor contributing to poor iron intake among all adults, especially people with limited or fixed incomes. See the Nursing Care of the Older Adult box on page 1072.

Manifestations   In addition to the general manifestations of anemia described earlier, chronic iron deficiency may lead to brittle, spoon-shaped nails; cheilosis (cracks at the corners of the mouth); a smooth, sore tongue; and *pica* (a craving for unusual substances, such as clay or starch).

BOX 33–2 Causes of Iron Deficiency Anemia

- Dietary deficiencies
  a. Vegetarian diet
  b. Inadequate protein intake
- Decreased absorption
  a. Partial or total gastrectomy
  b. Chronic diarrhea
  c. Malabsorption syndromes
- Increased metabolic requirements
  a. Pregnancy
  b. Lactation
- Blood loss
  a. Gastrointestinal bleeding (especially due to ulcers or chronic aspirin use)
  b. Menstrual losses
- Chronic hemoglobinuria

NURSING CARE OF THE OLDER ADULT   Anemia

Anemia is a significant problem in older adults. When the data from the third National Health and Nutrition Examination Survey (NHANES) 1988–1994 was evaluated, Woodman and colleagues (2005) found that 11% of men and 10.2% of women older than 65 were identified as anemic. The prevalence increased with age, as more than 20% of persons greater than 85 were identified as anemic. The causes were multifactorial, including nutritional deficiencies and chronic illness (i.e., chronic kidney disease), each accounting for about a third of the cases. However, cause in the final third could not be identified. Anemia has been identified as prognostic for loss of mobility and decreased physical function. In older adults, increased risk for mortality and mobility loss are seen even with hemoglobin levels considered low normal. This gives rise to the concern of what is the optimal hemoglobin level in older adults.

BOX 33–3 Causes of Folic Acid Deficiency Anemia

- Inadequate dietary intake
  At risk:
  a. Older adults
  b. Alcoholics
  c. Patients receiving total parenteral nutrition
- Increased metabolic requirements
  At risk:
  a. Pregnant women
  b. Infants and teenagers
  c. Patients undergoing hemodialysis
  d. Patients with forms of hemolytic anemia
- Folic acid malabsorption and impaired metabolism
  a. Celiac sprue
  b. Chemotherapeutic agents, folate antagonists (methotrexate, pentamidine), or anticonvulsants
  c. Alcoholism

VITAMIN B_{12} DEFICIENCY ANEMIA   Vitamin B_{12} is necessary for DNA synthesis and is almost exclusively found in foods derived from animals. Vitamin B_{12} deficiency occurs when inadequate vitamin B_{12} is consumed, or, more commonly, when it is poorly absorbed from the GI tract. Deficiency of this vitamin impairs cell division and maturation of the cell nucleus, especially in rapidly proliferating RBCs. As a result, macrocytic (large), misshapen (oval rather than concave) RBCs with thin membranes are produced. Great numbers of these large, immature RBCs enter the circulation. These cells are fragile, incapable of carrying adequate amounts of oxygen, and have a shortened life span.

Failure to absorb dietary vitamin B_{12} is called **pernicious anemia**. It develops due to lack of *intrinsic factor*, a substance secreted by the gastric mucosa. Intrinsic factor binds with vitamin B_{12} and travels with it to the ileum, where the vitamin is absorbed. In the absence of intrinsic factor, vitamin B_{12} cannot be absorbed into the body.

Vitamin B_{12} deficiency may also result from other malabsorption disorders and dietary factors. Resection of the stomach or ileum, loss of pancreatic secretions, and chronic gastritis can affect vitamin B_{12} absorption. Dietary deficiencies of vitamin B_{12} are rare, usually occurring only among strict vegetarians.

Manifestations   Manifestations of vitamin B_{12} deficiency anemia develop gradually as bodily stores of the vitamin are depleted. Pallor or slight jaundice and weakness develop. In pernicious anemia, a smooth, sore, beefy red tongue and diarrhea may occur. Because vitamin B_{12} is important for neurologic function, *paresthesias* (altered sensations, such as numbness or tingling) in the extremities and problems with *proprioception* (the sense of one's position in space) develop. These manifestations may progress to difficulty maintaining balance due to spinal cord damage. Central nervous system manifestations of relatively short duration (6 months or less) are reversible with treatment, but may be permanent if treatment is delayed (Tierney et al., 2005).

FOLIC ACID DEFICIENCY ANEMIA   Like vitamin B_{12}, folic acid is required for DNA synthesis and normal maturation of RBCs. Folic acid deficiency anemia is characterized by fragile,

megaloblastic (large and immature) cells. Folic acid is found in green leafy vegetables, fruits, cereals, and meats, and is absorbed from the intestines.

Folic acid deficiency anemia due to inadequate intake is more common among people who are chronically undernourished. This includes older adults, alcoholics, and the drug addicted. Alcoholics are especially at risk because alcohol suppresses folate metabolism, which forms folic acid. Increased folic acid requirements also may lead to anemia. Pregnant women are at the greatest risk. Infants and teenagers can develop temporary folic acid deficiencies during periods of rapid growth. Impaired folic acid absorption and metabolism can cause folic acid deficiency anemia. Malabsorption disorders such as celiac sprue (a hereditary GI disorder characterized by inability to metabolize amino acids found in gluten), and certain medications, such as methotrexate and some chemotherapeutic agents, may be implicated. Causes of folic acid deficiency anemia are summarized in Box 33–3.

Manifestations   The manifestations develop gradually as folic acid stores are depleted. Signs and symptoms may include pallor, progressive weakness and fatigue, shortness of breath, and heart palpitations. Manifestations similar to those associated with vitamin B_{12} anemia, such as glossitis, cheilosis, and diarrhea, are common. No neurologic symptoms occur with folic acid deficiency anemia, helping differentiate it from vitamin B_{12} deficiency anemia. These two nutritional anemias do, however, sometimes coexist.

Folic acid deficiency is strongly associated with neural tube defects such as meningomyelocele. The neural tube develops early in the process of fetal development, often before pregnancy is recognized.

Hemolytic Anemias

Hemolytic anemias are characterized by premature destruction (*lysis*) of RBCs. When RBCs break down, iron and other by-products of their destruction remain in the plasma. RBC lysis (hemolysis) may occur within the circulatory system or due to phagocytosis by WBCs such as circulating monocytes and macrophages in the spleen. In response to hemolysis, the hematopoietic activity of bone marrow increases, leading to

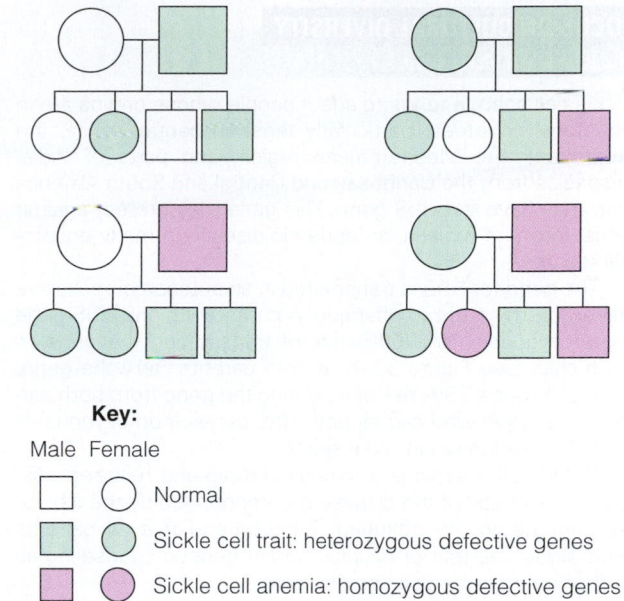

Key:

Male Female

□ ○ Normal

■ ○ Sickle cell trait: heterozygous defective genes

■ ○ Sickle cell anemia: homozygous defective genes

Figure 33–3 ■ Inheritance pattern for sickle cell anemia.

increased reticulocytes (immature RBCs) in circulating blood. Most types of hemolytic anemia are characterized by normocytic and normochromic RBCs.

There are many different causes of hemolytic anemias (Box 33–4). The cause may be *intrinsic*, arising from disorders within the RBC itself, or *extrinsic*, originating outside the RBC. Intrinsic disorders include cell membrane defects, defects in hemoglobin structure and function, and inherited enzyme deficiencies. See the accompanying Focus on Cultural Diversity box for more information about inherited intrinsic RBC disorders associated with hemolytic anemia. Extrinsic causes of hemolytic anemia include drugs, bacterial and other toxins, and trauma. This section discusses sickle cell anemia, thalassemia, acquired hemolytic anemia, and glucose-6-phosphate dehydrogenase anemia.

SICKLE CELL ANEMIA   **Sickle cell anemia** is a hereditary, chronic hemolytic anemia. It is characterized by episodes of *sickling*, during which RBCs become abnormally crescent shaped. The disorder is transmitted as an autosomal recessive genetic defect (Figure 33–3 ■). This defect causes synthesis of an abnormal form of hemoglobin (HbS) within RBCs. Sickle cell anemia can significantly shorten the life span, with most deaths occurring due to infection (Huether & McCance, 2008).

The disease is most common among people of African descent (see the Focus on Cultural Diversity box on page 1074).

BOX 33–4 Causes of Hemolytic Anemia

Intrinsic
- RBC cell-membrane defects
- Hemoglobin structure defects (e.g., sickle cell anemia, thalassemia)
- Inherited enzyme defects (e.g., G6PD deficiency)

Extrinsic
- Drugs, chemicals
- Toxins and venoms
- Bacterial and other infections
- Trauma, burns
- Mechanical damage (prosthetic heart valves)

In the United States, 7% to 13% of Blacks carry the defective gene, having inherited it from one parent (Huether & McCance, 2008). These people have *sickle cell trait*. About 40% of their hemoglobin is HbS. They are likely to remain asymptomatic unless stressed by severe hypoxia. Less than 1% of African Americans are homozygous for the disorder; that is, they have inherited a defective gene from both parents. These people have *sickle cell disease*; nearly all their hemoglobin is HbS. They are at risk for **sickle cell crisis**, severe episodes of fever and intense pain that are the hallmark of this disorder.

The HbS gene changes the structure of the beta chain of the hemoglobin molecule. When hypoxemia develops and HbS is deoxygenated, it crystallizes into rodlike structures. Clusters of these rods form long chains that deform the erythrocyte into a crescent or sickle shape (Figure 33–4 ■). The sickled cells tend to clump together and obstruct capillary blood flow, causing ischemia and possible infarction of surrounding tissue. See the Pathophysiology Illustrated feature on page 1075.

When normal oxygen tension is restored, the sickled RBCs resume their normal shape; that is, they "unsickle." Repeated episodes of sickling and unsickling weaken RBC cell membranes. The weakened RBCs are hemolyzed and removed. Consequently, the normal life span of RBCs is greatly reduced in sickle cell anemia, increasing the demand for RBC production. Conditions likely to trigger sickling include hypoxia, low environmental or body temperature, excessive exercise, anesthesia, dehydration, infections, or acidosis.

Manifestations and Complications   The acute and chronic manifestations of sickle cell anemia arise from episodes of RBC sickling. Sickling causes general manifestations of hemolytic anemia, including pallor, fatigue, jaundice, and irritability. Extensive sickling can precipitate a crisis due to occluded circulation, impaired erythropoiesis, or sequestration of large amounts of blood in the liver or spleen.

A vasoocclusive or thrombotic crisis occurs when sickling develops in the microcirculation. Obstruction of blood flow

Sickle Cell Anemia Video

triggers vasospasm that halts all blood flow in the vessel. Lack of blood flow leads to tissue ischemia and infarction. Vasoocclusive crises are painful and last an average of 4 to 6 days. Infarction of small vessels in the extremities causes painful swelling of the hands and feet; large joints also may be affected. Priapism (persistent, painful erection of the penis) may develop. Abdominal pain may signal infarction of abdominal organs and structures. Infarction may affect bone marrow or lead to aseptic necrosis of affected bones. Stroke may result from cerebral vessel occlusion (Huether & McCance, 2008). Skin ulcers may develop as result of occluded vessels supplying the dermis. Repeated infarcts associated with sickling can affect the structure and function of nearly every organ system. People with sickle cell disease may develop an enlarged spleen and liver, renal insufficiency, gallstones, and other manifestations of organ dysfunction. *Acute chest syndrome*, a symptom complex that includes fever, chest pain, an increasing WBC count, and pulmonary infiltrates, may develop, as well as other pulmonary complications like pneumonia, pulmonary infarction, and pulmonary embolism (De, 2008).

The shortened RBC lifespan and compromised erythropoiesis can lead to profound *aplastic anemia* in sickle cell disease. *Sequestration crises* are marked by pooling of large amounts of blood in the liver and spleen. This sickle cell crisis only occurs in children, but is thought to be the cause of sickle cell disease-related deaths in early childhood (Huether & McCance, 2008).

THALASSEMIA   The **thalassemias** are inherited disorders of hemoglobin synthesis in which either the alpha or beta chains of the hemoglobin molecule are missing or defective. This leads to deficient hemoglobin production and fragile hypochromic, microcytic RBCs called *target cells* because of their distinctive bull's-eye appearance.

Thalassemia usually affects certain populations. People of Mediterranean descent (southern Italy and Greece) are more likely to have beta-defect thalassemias (often called *Cooley's anemia* or Mediterranean anemia). People of Asian ancestry, especially from Thailand, the Philippines, and China, more often have alpha-defect thalassemia. Africans and African Americans may have both alpha- and beta-defect thalassemia. As with sickle cell anemia, only one defective beta chain-forming gene may be present (*beta-thalassemia minor*), causing mild symptoms, or both may be defective (*beta-thalassemia major*), leading to more severe symptoms. Children with thalassemia major rarely reach adulthood, although repeated blood transfusions may extend their life span (Huether & McCance, 2008). Four genes are responsible for alpha chain formation; one, two, three, or all four may be defective. In the latter case (*alpha-thalassemia major*), death is inevitable and usually occurs in utero. Genetic studies and counseling are recommended for people at risk for this illness.

Manifestations and Complications   People with thalassemia minor often are asymptomatic. When manifestations do occur, they include mild to moderate anemia, mild splenomegaly, bronze skin coloring, and bone marrow hyperplasia. The major form of the disease causes severe anemia, heart failure, and liver and spleen enlargement from increased red cell destruction. Fractures of the long bones, ribs, and vertebrae may result from bone marrow expansion and thinning due to increased hematopoiesis. Jaundice may develop due to hemolysis, as well as hepatomegaly and splenomegaly. Accumulation of iron in the heart, liver, and pancreas following repeated transfusions for treatment may eventually cause failure of these organs.

ACQUIRED HEMOLYTIC ANEMIA   *Acquired hemolytic anemia* results from hemolysis due to factors outside of the RBC. Causes of acquired hemolytic anemias include the following:

- Mechanical trauma to RBCs produced by prosthetic heart valves, severe burns, hemodialysis, or radiation
- Autoimmune disorders
- Bacterial or protozoal infection
- Immune-system-mediated responses, such as transfusion reactions
- Drugs, toxins, chemical agents, or venoms

Figure 33–4 ■ Blood smear containing normal red blood cells and sickle cells.

PATHOPHYSIOLOGY ILLUSTRATED
Sickle Cell Anemia

Hemoglobin S and Red Blood Cell Sickling

Sickle cell anemia is caused by an inherited autosomal recessive defect in Hb synthesis. Sickle cell hemoglobin (HbS) differs from normal hemoglobin only in the substitution of the amino acid valine for glutamine in both beta chains of the hemoglobin molecule.

When HbS is oxygenated, it has the same globular shape as normal hemoglobin. However, when HbS off-loads oxygen, it becomes insoluble in intracellular fluid and crystallizes into rodlike structures. Clusters of rods form polymers (long chains) that bend the erythrocyte into the characteristic crescent shape of the sickle cell.

The Sickle Cell Disease Process

Sickle cell disease is characterized by episodes of acute painful crises. Sickling crises are triggered by conditions causing high tissue oxygen demands or that affect cellular pH. As the crisis begins, sickled erythrocytes adhere to capillary walls and to each other, obstructing blood flow and causing cellular hypoxia. The crisis accelerates as tissue hypoxia and acidic metabolic waste products cause further sickling and cell damage.

Sickle cell crises cause microinfarcts in joints and organs, and repeated crises slowly destroy organs and tissues. The spleen and kidneys are especially prone to sickling damage.

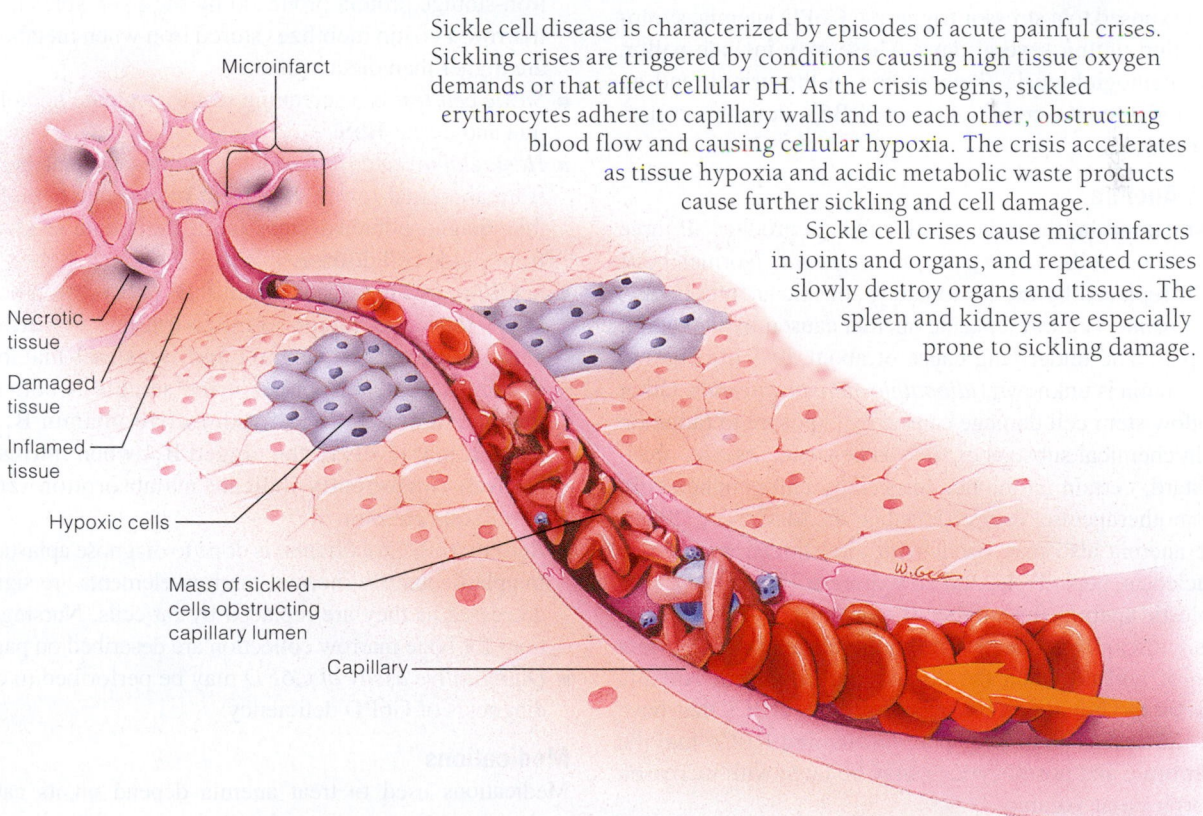

The manifestations of acquired hemolytic anemia depend on the extent of hemolysis and the body's ability to replace destroyed RBCs. The anemia itself often is mild to moderate as erythropoiesis increases to replace the destroyed RBCs. The spleen enlarges as it removes damaged or destroyed RBCs. If the breakdown of heme units exceeds the liver's ability to conjugate and excrete bilirubin, jaundice develops. When the condition is severe, bone marrow expands, and bones may be deformed or may develop pathologic fractures. The severity of generalized manifestations of anemia (tachycardia, pallor, etc.) depends on the degree of anemia and deficiency of tissue oxygenation.

GLUCOSE-6-PHOSPHATE DEHYDROGENASE (G6PD) ANEMIA *Glucose-6-phosphate dehydrogenase (G6PD) anemia* is caused by a hereditary defect in RBC metabolism. It is relatively common in people of African and Mediterranean descent. The defective gene is located on the X chromosome and therefore affects more males than females. There are many variations of this genetic defect.

G6PD is an enzyme that catalyzes glycolysis, the process in which an RBC derives cellular energy. A defect in G6PD action causes direct oxidation of hemoglobin, damaging the RBC. Hemolysis usually occurs only when the affected person is exposed to stressors (e.g., drugs such as aspirin, sulfonamides, or vitamin K derivatives) that increase the metabolic demands on RBCs. The G6PD deficiency impairs the necessary compensatory increase in glucose metabolism and causes cellular damage. Damaged RBCs are destroyed over a period of 7 to 12 days.

When exposed to a stressor triggering G6PD anemia, symptoms develop within several days. These may include pallor, jaundice, hemoglobinuria (hemoglobin in the urine), and an elevated reticulocyte count. As new RBCs develop, counts return to normal.

Aplastic Anemia

In **aplastic anemia**, the bone marrow fails to produce all three types of blood cells, leading to *pancytopenia*. Normal bone marrow is replaced by fat. Fortunately, aplastic anemia is rare. *Fanconi anemia* is a rare aplastic anemia caused by defects of DNA repair. The underlying cause of about 50% of acquired aplastic anemia is unknown (*idiopathic aplastic anemia*). Other cases follow stem cell damage caused by exposure to radiation or certain chemical substances such as benzene, arsenic, nitrogen mustard, certain antibiotics (especially chloramphenicol), and chemotherapeutic drugs (Huether & McCance, 2008). Aplastic anemia also may occur with viral infections such as mononucleosis, hepatitis C, and HIV disease.

In aplastic anemia, the number of stem cells in the bone marrow is significantly reduced. The stem cell pool may be less than 1% of normal when the disease is recognized. Anemia develops as the bone marrow fails to replace RBCs that have reached the end of their life span. Remaining RBCs may be normochromic and normocytic or may be large with increased mean corpuscular volume.

MANIFESTATIONS Manifestations of aplastic anemia vary with the severity of the pancytopenia. Its onset usually is insidious, but may be sudden. Manifestations include fatigue, pallor, progressive weakness, exertional dyspnea, headache, and ultimately tachycardia and heart failure. Platelet deficiency leads to bleeding problems; bleeding gums, excessive bruising, and nose bleeds may be the initial symptoms. A deficiency of WBCs increases the risk of infection, causing manifestations such as sore throat and fever.

Interdisciplinary Care

Ensuring adequate tissue oxygenation is the priority of care in treating anemia. Specific therapy is determined by the underlying cause of the disorder. Usual treatments include medications, dietary modifications, blood replacement, or supportive interventions. Table 33–1 outlines interdisciplinary care measures for selected types of anemia.

Diagnosis

When anemia is suspected, the following laboratory and diagnostic tests may be ordered.

- *Complete blood count (CBC)* is done to determine blood cell counts, hemoglobin, hematocrit, and RBC indices (see Table 32–1). The severity of the anemia, shape, volume, and iron content of the RBCs can help determine the cause of anemia.
- *Iron levels* and *total iron-binding capacity* are performed to detect iron deficiency anemia. A low serum iron concentration and elevated total iron-binding capacity are indicative of iron deficiency anemia.
- *Serum ferritin* is low due to depletion of the total iron reserves available for hemoglobin synthesis. Ferritin is an iron-storage protein produced by the liver, spleen, and bone marrow. Ferritin mobilizes stored iron when metabolic needs are higher than dietary intake.
- *Sickle cell test* is a screening test to evaluate hemolytic anemia and detect HbS.
- *Hemoglobin electrophoresis* separates normal hemoglobin from abnormal forms. It is used to evaluate hemolytic anemia, diagnose thalassemia, and differentiate sickle cell trait from sickle cell disease.
- *Schilling test* measures vitamin B_{12} absorption before and after intrinsic factor administration to differentiate between pernicious anemia and intestinal malabsorption of the vitamin. A 24-hour urine sample is collected following administration of radioactive vitamin B_{12}. Lower than normal levels of the tagged B_{12} when intrinsic factor is given concurrently indicate malabsorption rather than pernicious anemia.
- *Bone marrow examination* is done to diagnose aplastic anemia. In aplastic anemia, normal marrow elements are significantly decreased as they are replaced by fat cells. Nursing implications for bone marrow collection are described on page 890.
- *Quantitative assay of G6PD* may be performed to confirm a diagnosis of G6PD deficiency.

Medications

Medications used to treat anemia depend on its cause. Iron replacement therapy is ordered for iron deficiency anemia. Supplemental iron may be given by mouth or parenterally. Intravenous administration of iron is becoming more common, particularly in patients with an acute deficiency and in anemia associated with chronic GI blood loss, chronic renal failure, and other chronic conditions that increase the need for blood cell production (e.g., cancers). The risk of anaphylaxis is a major concern when iron dextran is given intravenously. Other parenteral iron solutions, including intravenous sodium ferric gluconate (Ferrlecit) and iron sucrose (Venofer), carry a much lower risk of adverse and allergic reactions (Papadakis & McPhee, 2007).

Parenteral vitamin B_{12} is given when malabsorption or lack of intrinsic factor leads to vitamin B_{12} deficiency anemia. Folic acid is ordered for women of childbearing age, pregnant women, and patients with folic acid deficiency or sickle cell anemia to meet the increased demands of the bone marrow. Hydroxyurea,

a drug that promotes fetal hemoglobin production, may be prescribed for patients with sickle cell disease, particularly those with frequent crises or severe disease. Resulting increased levels of fetal hemoglobin interfere with the sickling process and reduce the incidence of painful crises. Nursing implications for patients receiving iron, vitamin B_{12}, and folic acid are found in the Medication Administration box on page 1078.

Erythropoietin may be ordered for patients with low erythropoietin levels (e.g., patients with chronic renal failure) and people with anemia associated with other chronic diseases. Erythropoietin is given subcutaneously, and may be given as often as three times a week in chronic renal failure. Because erythropoietin stimulates RBC production, adequate iron must be present. Patients receiving erythropoietin may require regular intravenous iron therapy as well (Deglin & Vallerand, 2009).

Immunosuppressive therapy with antithymocyte globulin (ATG), corticosteroids, and cyclosporine may be used to treat aplastic anemia. Androgens may stimulate blood cell production in some patients with aplastic anemia. ∞ See Chapter 12 for more information about immunosuppression.

Nutrition

Dietary modifications are recommended for nutritional deficiency anemias, such as iron deficiency anemia, vitamin B_{12} deficiency anemia, or folic acid deficiency anemia. Box 33–5 identifies good sources of dietary iron, vitamin B_{12}, and folic acid.

TABLE 33–1 Interdisciplinary Care Focus for Major Anemias

TYPE OF ANEMIA	INTERDISCIPLINARY CARE
Iron-deficiency anemia	■ Increased dietary intake of iron-rich foods ■ Oral or parenteral iron supplements
Vitamin B_{12} deficiency anemia	■ Increase dietary intake of foods containing vitamin B_{12} (e.g., meats, eggs, and dairy products) ■ Oral or parenteral vitamin B_{12} supplements ■ Parenteral vitamin B_{12} for deficency due to malabsorption or lack of intrinsic factor
Folic acid deficiency anemia	■ Increased dietary intake of foods rich in folic acid (folate) ■ Oral folic acid supplements ■ Folic acid supplements recommended for women who are pregnant or may become pregnant to prevent neural tube defects

Sickle cell anemia	■ Treatment is primarily supportive
	■ Hydroxyurea 10–30 mg/kg per day
	■ Sickle cell crisis:
	  ■ Rest
	  ■ Oxygen therapy to maintain SAO_2
	  ■ Narcotic analgesia
	  ■ Vigorous hydration
	  ■ Treatment of precipitating factors
	■ Acute chest syndrome:
	  ■ Careful hydration; hemodynamic monitoring
	  ■ Oxygen therapy
	  ■ Transfusion
	■ Folic acid supplements
	■ Blood transfusions during surgery or pregnancy as necessary
	■ Genetic counseling recommended

Thalassemia	■ Regular blood transfusions ■ Folic acid supplements ■ Possible splenectomy ■ Genetic counseling
Aplastic anemia	■ Withdrawal of the causative agent, if known ■ Blood transfusions ■ Bone marrow transplant as indicated

---

BOX 33–5 Dietary Sources of Iron, Folic Acid, and Vitamin B_{12}

Iron

Iron in the diet comes from two sources. *Heme iron* makes up about one-half of the iron from animal sources. *Nonheme iron* includes the remaining iron from animal sources and all the iron from plants, legumes, and nuts. Heme iron promotes absorption of nonheme iron from other foods when both forms are consumed at the same time. Absorption of nonheme iron is also enhanced by vitamin C and inhibited by tea and coffee.

Sources of Heme Iron

■ Beef	■ Pork loin
■ Chicken	■ Turkey
■ Egg yolk	■ Veal
■ Clams, oysters	

Sources of Nonheme Iron

■ Bran flakes	■ Dried fruits
■ Brown rice	■ Greens
■ Whole-grain breads	■ Oatmeal
■ Dried beans	

Sources of Folic Acid

■ Green leafy vegetables	■ Asparagus
■ Broccoli	■ Liver
■ Organ meats	■ Milk
■ Eggs	■ Yeast
■ Wheat germ	■ Kidney beans

Sources of Vitamin B_{12}

■ Liver	■ Kidney
■ Fresh shrimp and oysters	■ Meats (muscle)
■ Eggs	■ Cheese
■ Milk	

MEDICATION ADMINISTRATION   Drugs to Treat Anemia

IRON SOURCES

Ferrous sulfate (Feosol, Fer-in-sol)

Ferrous gluconate (Fergon, Ferralet, Fertinic)

Iron dextran injection (Imferon)

Iron polysaccharide

Iron sucrose (Venofer)

Sodium ferric gluconate (Ferrlecit)

Iron preparations are normally taken by mouth and are absorbed from the GI tract. They are given to treat anemias resulting from iron deficiency or blood loss. When absorbed, iron combines with transferrin. This complex then is transported to the bone marrow and incorporated into hemoglobin.

Nursing Responsibilities

- Prior to giving the drug, assess for use of drugs that might interact with iron (e.g., antacids, allopurinol, chloramphenicol, tetracyclines, vitamin E), GI bleeding, and manifestations of anemia.
- Administer iron preparations with orange juice to enhance absorption.
- If using an elixir, give it through a straw to prevent staining the teeth.
- Monitor for manifestations of iron toxicity: nausea, diarrhea, or constipation; symptoms of anaphylactic shock (extreme cases).
- Monitor hemoglobin and reticulocyte counts.
- If the patient is also taking tetracyclines, schedule the dose of iron 2 hours before tetracycline (iron reduces the absorption of tetracycline).
- When administering IM or IV, monitor closely for anaphylaxis.

Health Education for the Patient and Family

- GI side effects may be reduced by taking iron with food (but not milk, which decreases absorption).
- Stools may be dark green or black; this is harmless.
- Increase fluids and fiber in diet to decrease constipation.

VITAMIN B$_{12}$ SOURCES

Cyanocobalamin (Kaybovite [oral], Anacobin [parenteral], Bedoz)

Cyanocobalamin is used to treat vitamin B$_{12}$ deficiencies or malabsorption and pernicious anemia. It is rapidly absorbed when administered orally or by injection, and it is stored in the liver. Intrinsic factor is necessary for absorption from the GI tract.

Nursing Responsibilities

- Do not expose crystalline injection to light.
- Assess for other drugs that might interfere with the therapeutic response: chloramphenicol, cimetidine, colchicine, and timed-release potassium decrease its effectiveness.
- Do not mix cyanocobalamin in a syringe with other medications.
- Administer parenteral doses intramuscularly or deep subcutaneously to decrease local irritation.
- Monitor hemoglobin, RBC counts, reticulocyte counts, and potassium levels.

Health Education for the Patient and Family

- A burning sensation with injection is temporary.
- Avoid alcohol, which interferes with absorption.
- If used to treat pernicious anemia, the medication must be taken for life.

FOLIC ACID SOURCES

Folic acid (Folvite, novofolacid)

Synthetic folic acid is used to treat folic acid deficiency and megaloblastic or macrocytic anemia. It is absorbed from the GI tract and stored in the liver.

Nursing Responsibilities

- Prior to giving the medication, assess for use of drugs that alter its effect: corticosteroids, methotrexate, oral contraceptives, phenytoin, sulfonamides.
- Do not mix folic acid with other medications in the same syringe.
- Monitor for possible hypersensitivity response of skin rash.

Health Education for the Patient and Family

- Large doses of folic acid may cause the urine to become darker yellow.
- Excess alcohol intake increases folic acid requirements.

Blood Transfusion

Blood transfusions may be indicated to treat anemias resulting from major blood loss, such as from trauma or major surgery, and severe anemia regardless of cause. In acute hemorrhage, whole blood may be given to replace both blood cells and volume. A unit of packed RBCs may be given when anemia is severe and the patient demonstrates cardiovascular instability or compromise. Blood transfusions are fully discussed in ∞ Chapter 11.

Complementary Therapies

Complementary healthcare practitioners may recommend specific plant enzymes to treat nutritional anemias. Plant enzymes are believed to aid digestion of proteins, fats, and carbohydrates, facilitating absorption of their nutrients. Therapy is determined by the specific type of anemia. Plant enzymes should not be used alone to treat anemia, and it is important to check for possible interactions with prescribed medications before starting therapy.

∞ Nursing Care

For nursing care specific to the patient with a nutritional anemia, see the accompanying Case Study & Nursing Care Plan.

Health Promotion

Nursing measures to prevent anemia focus on teaching good dietary habits to all patients, regardless of age. Stress the importance of consuming adequate amounts of iron, folate, and the B vitamins. Provide a list of dietary sources of these nutrients. Discuss alternate iron sources with vegetarian patients, and teach them that foods high in vitamin C enhance the absorption of iron from grains, legumes, and other sources. Emphasize the importance of adequate iron intake in women of childbearing age and older adults. Stress the increased need for these nutrients during pregnancy, and discuss strategies to ensure an adequate intake.

Assessment

Assessment data to collect for patients with suspected anemia includes the following:

- *Health history:* Complaints of shortness of breath with activity, fatigue, weakness, dizziness or fainting, palpitations; history of previous anemia, bleeding episodes; menstrual history (if appropriate); medications; chronic diseases; usual diet and patterns of alcohol intake or cigarette smoking.

- *Physical examination:* General appearance, skin color; vital signs including temperature; heart and lung sounds; peripheral pulses, capillary refill; abdominal tenderness; obvious bleeding or bruising.
- *Laboratory data:* CBC, hemoglobin and hematocrit; bone marrow studies; specialized tests (e.g. hemoglobin electrophoresis, Schilling test).

Nursing Diagnoses and Interventions

Anemia affects circulating oxygen levels and tissue oxygenation. Priority nursing diagnoses include *Activity Intolerance*, *Altered Oral Mucous Membranes*, and *Self-Care Deficits*. With acute blood-loss anemia, risk for insufficient cardiac output also is a priority. Patients with sickle cell disease have specific needs related to the effects of the disease on tissue perfusion; see the section on disseminated intravascular coagulation (DIC) later in this chapter for nursing interventions appropriate to ineffective tissue perfusion, associated pain, and maintaining oxygenation.

Activity Intolerance

Anemia causes weakness and shortness of breath on exertion. These symptoms are due to decreased circulating oxygen levels secondary to low hemoglobin levels. Weakness, fatigue, and/or vertigo may occur even during activities of daily living (ADLs), including those associated with self-care, home life, job performance, and social roles.

- Help identify ways to conserve energy when performing necessary or desired activities. *Modifying the approach to a particular activity may reduce cardiorespiratory symptoms and activity-related fatigue. Alternative ways of performing tasks (e.g., sitting when performing hygiene care and kitchen tasks) may reduce oxygen demands. In some cases, assistance from others is necessary to conserve energy and reduce symptoms.*
- Help the patient and family establish priorities for tasks and activities. *Because family members may need to assume responsibility for additional tasks, the plan's success depends on mutually established goals.*

EVIDENCE FOR NURSING CARE **The Patient with Iron-Deficiency Anemia**

Selected resources that nurses may find helpful when planning evidence-based nursing care follow.

- Bowe, D. (2008). IV iron therapy and anemia management in patients on hemodialysis: Benefits of a revised CQI strategy. *Nephrology Nursing Journal, 35*(4). Retrieved from http://www.nursingconsult.com
- Peebles, G. (2008). Intravenous iron administration in a short-stay hospital setting. *Nursing Standard, 22*(48), 35–41.
- Wilson, S. (2008). Challenges in managing anemia in patients returning to dialysis after transplant failure. *Nephrology Nursing Journal, 35*(4), 383–386. Retrieved from http://www.nursingconsult.com

- Assist to develop a schedule of alternating activity and rest periods throughout the day. *Rest periods decrease oxygen needs, reducing strain on the heart and lungs, and allowing restoration of homeostasis before further activities.*
- Encourage 8 to 10 hours of sleep at night. *Rest decreases oxygen demands and increases available energy for morning activities.*
- Monitor vital signs before and after activity. *Vital signs provide a measure of activity tolerance. Increased heart and respiratory rates or a change in blood pressure may indicate intolerance of the activity.*
- Discontinue activity if any of the following occurs:
  a. Complaints of chest pain, breathlessness, or vertigo
  b. Palpitations or tachycardia that does not return to normal within 4 minutes of resting
  c. Bradycardia
  d. Tachypnea or dyspnea
  e. Decreased systolic blood pressure
  These changes may signify cardiac decompensation due to insufficient oxygenation. The intensity, duration, or frequency of the activity needs to be reduced.
- Instruct the patient not to smoke. *Smoking causes vasoconstriction and increases carbon monoxide levels in the blood, interfering with tissue oxygenation.*

Impaired Oral Mucous Membrane

Glossitis and cheilosis may occur with nutritional deficiencies of iron, folate, and vitamin B_{12}. The tongue and lips become very red, and fissures or cracks may form at the corners of the mouth.

- Monitor condition of lips and tongue daily. *Glossitis and cheilosis increase the risk for bleeding and infection and may require medical treatment. Pain and discomfort may interfere with oral intake, further worsening the nutritional deficiency.*
- Use a mouthwash of saline, saltwater, or half-strength peroxide and water to rinse the mouth every 2 to 4 hours. Avoid alcohol-based mouthwashes. *This cleanses and soothes oral mucous membranes. Alcohol-based mouthwashes further irritate and dry oral tissues.*
- Provide frequent oral hygiene (after each meal and at bedtime) with a soft bristle toothbrush or sponge. *Removing food debris from painful fissures promotes comfort. A soft toothbrush reduces irritation or bleeding of oral mucosa. Keeping the oral cavity clean also reduces the risk of infection.*
- Apply a petroleum-based lubricating jelly or ointment to the lips after oral care. *Lubricating ointment helps to retain moisture, facilitate healing, and protect the lips from other drying agents.*
- Instruct to avoid hot, spicy, or acidic foods. *Such foods may further irritate and dry mucous membranes.*
- Encourage soft, cool, bland foods. *Foods that are soothing to the mucous membranes promote comfort and help maintain adequate food and fluid intake. Minimizing oral pain may also promote compliance with oral care routines.*
- Encourage eating four to six small meals daily with high protein and vitamin content. *Small, frequent meals may be better tolerated, increasing intake. Nutrient-rich meals promote healing of the mucous membranes.*

CASE STUDY & NURSING CARE PLAN   A Patient with Folic Acid Deficiency Anemia

Sheri Matthews is a 76-year-old widow who lives alone. She tells Lisa Apana, RN, the nurse in her care provider's office, that she liked to cook when her husband was alive, but preparing an entire meal just for herself seems senseless. She relates that her typical day's menu includes coffee for breakfast; a bologna sandwich and coffee for lunch; and a hot dog or two, a few cookies, and a glass of milk for dinner.

ASSESSMENT

Mrs. Matthews's nursing history includes a 20 lb (9 kg) weight loss since her husband died 8 months ago. She states that she sometimes has heart palpitations and always feels weak. Physical assessment shows T 98.8°F (37.1°C), P 110, R 22, BP 90/52. Skin warm, pale, and dry. Diagnostic tests indicate folic acid deficiency anemia, and Mrs. Matthews is started on an oral folic acid supplement and instructed about foods containing folic acid.

DIAGNOSES

- *Activity Intolerance* related to weakness secondary to decreased tissue oxygenation
- *Imbalanced Nutrition: Less than Body Requirements* related to lack of motivation to cook and understanding of nutritional needs, as manifested by weight loss of 20 lb, and folic acid deficiency
- *Deficient Knowledge* related to lack of information about a well-balanced diet and foods containing folic acid

EXPECTED OUTCOMES

- Verbalize the importance of taking folic acid supplements and eating a balanced diet.
- Gain at least 1 lb (0.45 kg) per week.
- Return to previous level of physical energy.
- Consume a balanced diet, including foods containing folic acid.

PLANNING AND IMPLEMENTATION

- Discuss foods required for a well-balanced diet, as well as dietary sources of folic acid.
- Develop a dietary plan with Mrs. Matthews that includes food preferences and foods that are easy and quick to prepare.
- Discuss the importance of taking the folic acid supplement. Advise to continue taking it even after she begins to feel better.
- Help Mrs. Matthews develop a schedule of activities that provides adequate rest and energy for cooking.

EVALUATION

Mrs. Matthews gained 1 lb (0.45 kg) during the first week of treatment. She has met with a nutritionist and has a better understanding of nutritional needs. She states that she can prepare hot meals when she schedules a rest period before and after lunch. Ms. Apana has provided written and verbal information about the folic acid supplement and diet. Mrs. Matthews verbalizes understanding, stating, "I will continue to take the folic acid until the doctor tells me to stop. I'm beginning to enjoy cooking again, now that I have a reason to cook!" Ms. Apana contacts the local senior services representative to determine if Mrs. Matthews is able to participate in the local Meals on Wheels program.

CRITICAL THINKING IN THE NURSING PROCESS

1. What is the pathophysiologic basis for Mrs. Matthews's abnormal vital signs during her initial assessment?
2. Design a week's menu that includes foods high in folic acid.
3. Why was Mrs. Matthews placed on a folic acid supplement in addition to dietary modifications?
4. Why is the older adult at increased risk for developing folic acid deficiency anemia? Consider physiologic, economic, and social factors.

See Evaluating Your Response in Appendix C.

Risk for Decreased Cardiac Output

Cardiac output may be affected by acute bleeding and volume loss or by heart failure resulting from severe anemia. In addition, impaired tissue oxygenation leads to an increased respiratory rate and dyspnea.

- Monitor vital signs, breath sounds, and apical pulse. *Increased cardiac workload can affect the blood pressure, heart, and respiratory rates. Increased blood flow can lead to heart murmur or abnormal heart sounds such as S_3 or S_4. Tachypnea and dyspnea may affect the depth of respirations, alveolar ventilation, and blood and tissue oxygenation.*
- Assess for pallor, cyanosis, and dependent edema. *Blood is shunted to the vital organs, causing vasoconstriction of skin vessels. This, in addition to lower levels of hemoglobin, cause pallor. Cyanosis, especially of the lips and nail beds, indicates inadequate oxygenation of blood. Dependent edema occurs in response to right ventricular failure.*

PRACTICE ALERT

Report signs of decreased cardiac output to the healthcare provider. Severe anemia can lead to heart failure, necessitating additional treatment.

- Closely monitor for manifestations of anaphylaxis (urticaria, erythema or flushing, edema, wheezing, dyspnea, nausea and vomiting, anxiety) when administering parenteral iron preparations, particularly iron dextran. Immediately notify the healthcare provider, and prepare to administer prescribed drugs such as diphenhydramine (Benadryl) or epinephrine as ordered. Institute cardiopulmonary resuscitation measures as necessary. *Anaphylaxis, a systemic type I hypersensitivity (allergic) reaction, is a risk when administering parenteral iron preparations, iron dextran in particular. Anaphylaxis can lead to severe cardiopulmonary compromise, necessitating emergency measures to preserve life.*

Self-Care Deficit

Energy expenditures for ADLs may cause oxygen demands to exceed supply in the patient with severe anemia.

- Assist with ADLs, such as bathing, grooming, and eating, as needed. *Assistance decreases energy expenditures and tissue requirements for oxygen, reducing cardiac workload.*
- Discuss the importance of rest periods prior to such activities as dressing. *Rest reduces oxygen demand and cardiac workload. The person who is able to perform self-care in ADLs maintains independence, self-esteem, and morale.*

Using NANDA, NIC, and NOC

Linkages between a selected NANDA nursing diagnosis, NIC, and NOC for the patient with anemia are shown in the chart that follows.

Community-Based Care

With the exception of anemia resulting from acute hemorrhage, most patients with anemia are treated in the home and community setting. Include the following topics when preparing the patient and family for home care:

- Nutritional strategies to address deficiencies
- Prescribed medications, vitamins, or mineral supplements and their appropriate use, intended effect, possible adverse effects, and interactions with food or other medications
- Energy conservation strategies
- Other recommended treatment measures and follow-up
- If the anemia is genetically transmitted, such as sickle cell anemia, include inheritance patterns of the disorder, symptoms of crisis, and manifestations to report to the healthcare provider

Provide referrals for counseling to facilitate decisions about pregnancy as indicated. Also refer for nutritional assistance and teaching, home health care, or assistance with self-care and home maintenance activities as indicated. Older adults with nutritional anemias may benefit from community services such as senior meals or Meals on Wheels.

The Patient with Myelodysplastic Syndrome

Myelodysplastic syndrome (MDS) is a group of blood disorders characterized by abnormal-appearing bone marrow and cytopenia (low numbers of circulating blood cells). MDS is not a single disease; at least five variations of the disorder have been identified. Anemia that does not respond to treatment (*refractory anemia*) is a characteristic of most forms of myelodysplasia.

Idiopathic MDS primarily affects older adults; men have a slightly higher incidence of the disorder than women. Risk factors for secondary MDS include exposure to environmental toxins such as cigarette smoke, benzene and radiation, radiation therapy or chemotherapy for cancer treatment, and other anemias such as aplastic anemia or Fanconi's anemia (Kurtin, 2006; National Comprehensive Cancer Network [NCCN], 2009).

Pathophysiology

MDS is a stem cell disorder in which stem cells fail to reproduce and differentiate into the various types of blood cells. The genetic components of stem cells (nuclear DNA and/or mitochondrial DNA) are altered. The bone marrow loses its ability to produce normal blood cells, instead producing abnormal (*dysplastic*) cells. With significant alterations, leukemia (proliferation of abnormal WBCs) may develop in people with MDS.

Manifestations

Anemia is the predominant early manifestation of MDS. The patient may develop symptoms of the anemia with increasing fatigue, weakness, dyspnea, and pallor. In many cases, the disorder is asymptomatic, identified when a routine blood count shows anemia. Splenomegaly may develop, leading to discomfort and a feeling of fullness in the LUQ of the abdomen. Hepatomegaly also may develop, leading to RUQ discomfort. Thrombocytopenia can lead to abnormal bleeding tendencies, and neutropenia increases the risk for infection (Kurtin, 2006; NCCN, 2009).

Interdisciplinary Care

Patients with MDS require long-term supportive care and therapy to maintain their quality of life. Stem cell transplant offers the only real hope for cure in MDS. See the leukemia section later in this chapter for more information about stem cell transplant and associated nursing care.

Diagnosis

- The *CBC* reveals anemia. Although anemia may be the only abnormality of the blood count, the WBC count also may be low, as may be the platelet count. Abnormalities of size and shape may be noted in all blood cells.
- The *bone marrow* often appears normal, although precursor cells may have an abnormal appearance. Increased numbers of myeloblasts (granulocyte precursor cells) may be present in the bone marrow.
- *Serum erythropoietin, vitamin B_{12}, serum iron, total iron binding capacity, ferritin levels*, and *RBC folate levels* are drawn to help guide supportive therapy.

Treatment

Management of MDS is based on the severity of the disease. Several classification systems are available, including the French-American-British (FAB) classification system, the International Prognostic Scoring System (IPSS), and the World Health Organization (WHO) classification system (National Comprehensive Cancer Network [NCCN], 2009). These systems are used to guide therapy for the patient with MDS.

All patients with MDS require monitoring, with regular health-care provider visits and laboratory evaluations. Psychosocial support is provided to assist the patient and family dealing with a chronic, progressive, and ultimately fatal disease.

Patients with MDS may require frequent RBC transfusions to treat the predominant anemia. Each unit of packed RBCs contains 250 to 300 mg of iron. The body is unable to excrete this excess iron, so it accumulates, leading to problems such as endocrine dysfunction, cirrhosis, pericarditis, and heart failure. *Iron chelation therapy* is used to remove excess iron from the body. Desferoxamine (Desferal) is administered by slow intravenous infusion or continuous subcutaneous infusion using an infusion pump to maintain a normal or negative iron balance. This drug is relatively safe, although local skin reactions such as rash and urticaria may develop. An oral form of the drug, deferasirox, is available, but not widely used.

Blood cell growth factors may be administered to stimulate stem cell development in MDS, although the response rate is low. Platelet transfusions are given when bleeding occurs due to low platelet levels. Antibiotic therapy is initiated for bacterial infections (NCCN, 2009). Chemotherapy regimens similar to those employed to treat leukemia may be used, but rarely are effective in treating MDS. Azacitidine (Vidaza), an antileukemic agent that acts on abnormal blood-forming cells in the bone marrow, may be more effective in treating MDS than standard chemotherapy regimens (Demakos & Linebaugh, 2005). As previously noted, stem cell transplant offers the only hope for cure. This high-risk therapy, however, is reserved for higher risk patients. Factors such as age, functional ability, and other existing disease conditions help guide the decision to undergo stem cell transplant (NCCN, 2009).

✍ Nursing Care

Activity intolerance and the need for education about this disorder are the priorities of nursing care for the patient with MDS being managed in a community-based setting. Although neutropenia and thrombocytopenia may accompany the anemia of MDS, these problems are less common. See the section of this chapter on leukemia for additional potential nursing diagnoses and interventions for the patient with MDS (Kurtin, 2006).

Activity Intolerance

The patient with MDS experiences fatigue, weakness, and shortness of breath on exertion related to the lack of RBCs and ineffective oxygen transport. These symptoms may affect the patient's ability to maintain self-care, home life, job performance, and social roles.

- Monitor vital signs, breath sounds, and apical pulse. *Increased cardiac workload due to anemia and impaired oxygen transport can affect the blood pressure, heart, and respiratory rates. Increased blood flow can lead to heart murmur or abnormal heart sounds such as S_3 or S_4. Accumulated iron can lead to pericarditis and a pericardial friction rub.*
- Help identify energy-conserving ways of performing necessary or desired activities. *Alternative ways of performing tasks (e.g., sitting while performing hygiene measures) may reduce oxygen demands and fatigue.*

- Help the patient and family establish priorities for tasks and activities. *Because family members may need to assume responsibility for additional tasks, the plan's success depends on mutually established goals.*
- Suggest planning recreational activities following a transfusion and adjusting activity level between transfusions to match energy and minimize fatigue. *The patient with MDS will have more energy and activity tolerance following a transfusion when RBC counts, hemoglobin, and hematocrit approach normal levels and oxygen transport is optimal.*
- Encourage 8 to 10 hours of sleep at night. *Rest decreases oxygen demands and increases available energy for morning activities.*
- Discontinue activity if any of the following occurs:
  a. Complaints of chest pain, breathlessness, or vertigo
  b. Palpitations or tachycardia that does not return to normal within 4 minutes of resting
  c. Bradycardia
  d. Tachypnea or dyspnea
  e. Decreased systolic blood pressure
  These changes may signify cardiac decompensation due to insufficient oxygenation. The intensity, duration, or frequency of the activity needs to be reduced.
- Instruct the patient not to smoke. *Smoking causes vasoconstriction and increases carbon monoxide levels in the blood, interfering with tissue oxygenation.*

Risk for Ineffective Health Maintenance

MDS is a chronic, usually progressive disorder, requiring active management to maintain functional status and quality of life. Regular visits to the healthcare provider or clinic may be necessary. In addition, the patient or family members may need to learn to administer iron chelation therapy or chemotherapy drugs and measures to prevent complications (NCCN, 2009). The chronic nature of the disorder and the often advanced age of the patient and family caregivers may interfere with effective management of the disorder.

- Assess knowledge of disorder and the related treatments. *Assessment allows identification of knowledge gaps and provides a basis on which to provide additional information. Impaired disease management may be due to lack of knowledge or an inability to learn and perform psychomotor skills, for example, administration of parenteral drug therapy.*
- Provide information about the disorder, its effects, and prescribed medications and treatments. *Individualized instruction is more effective than general, possibly irrelevant information. The patient and caregivers need to be able to identify and manage possible adverse effects of drug therapy, as well as recognize potential complications to be reported to the healthcare provider.*
- Provide emotional support, expressing confidence in the patient's and caregivers' abilities to manage care. *Emotional support helps the patient and family caregivers incorporate the care regimen into their lifestyle.*
- Provide supervised learning and practice opportunities for administering parenteral medications if ordered. *Successful practice sessions instill confidence in the ability to manage care and provide an opportunity for questions and exploring alternatives.*

Community-Based Care

The patient with myelodysplastic syndrome needs information about this chronic and ultimately fatal disease. Provide information about treatment options, including management of the infusion pump if ordered. Discuss the timing of and options for stem cell transplant, and assist the patient to evaluate the potential benefits and risks of this treatment option.

The Patient with Polycythemia

Polycythemia, or *erythrocytosis*, is an excess of RBCs characterized by a hematocrit higher than 55%. The two major types of polycythemia are primary and secondary. A third type of polycythemia, relative polycythemia, results from a fluid volume deficit, not excess RBCs.

FAST FACTS

- *Primary polycythemia (polycythemia vera)* is uncommon.
  - In primary polycythemia, RBC production is increased.
  - Primary polycythemia more commonly affects men of European Jewish ancestry between the ages 40 and 70.
- *Secondary polycythemia (erythrocytosis)* is the most common form of polycythemia.
  - Secondary polycythemia occurs when erythropoietin levels are elevated.
  - It may affect patients of any age or origin.
  - It usually develops in response to hypoxia (living at a high altitude, smoking, or chronic lung disease).
- *Relative polycythemia* occurs due to fluid deficit, not excess RBCs.
  - In relative polycythemia the total RBC count is normal.
  - The hematocrit is elevated because of increased cell concentration.
  - It is corrected by rehydration.

Pathophysiology

Primary Polycythemia

Primary polycythemia, or polycythemia vera (PV), is a neoplastic stem cell disorder characterized by overproduction of RBCs and, to a lesser extent, WBCs and platelets. It is classified as a myeloproliferative disorder. Its cause is unknown. In PV, colonies of endogenous erythroid stem cells develop. These colonies produce RBCs in the absence of erythropoietin, leading to excess RBC production.

MANIFESTATIONS Initially, PV is asymptomatic, and the diagnosis may be made during routine blood tests. Its manifestations are caused by increased blood volume and viscosity. Hypertension is common, and may lead to complaints of headaches, dizziness, and vision and hearing disruptions. Venous stasis causes *plethora*, a ruddy, red color of the face, hands, feet, and mucous membranes. This often is accompanied by severe, painful itching of the fingers and toes. Retinal and cerebral vessels may be engorged. Hypermetabolism develops, causing weight loss and night sweats. Mental status may be altered, leading to drowsiness or delirium.

Thrombosis and hemorrhage are potential complications of PV. Thrombosis may cause transient ischemic attacks, angina, or manifestations of peripheral vascular disease. GI bleeding may occur, and portal hypertension may develop.

Secondary Polycythemia

Secondary polycythemia, or erythrocytosis, is increased numbers of RBCs in response to excess erythropoietin secretion or prolonged hypoxia. Secondary polycythemia is the most common form of polycythemia.

Abnormally high erythropoietin levels can result from kidney disease or erythropoietin-secreting tumors (e.g., renal cell carcinoma). Chronic hypoxia that stimulates erythropoietin release is a more common cause of secondary polycythemia. People living at high altitudes where the atmospheric oxygen pressure is lower develop a degree of polycythemia, as do people with chronic heart or lung disease and smokers. Abnormal hemoglobin that forms tighter bonds with oxygen also may lead to secondary polycythemia.

MANIFESTATIONS The manifestations of secondary polycythemia are similar to those of primary polycythemia. Splenomegaly, however, does not develop. Early symptoms often are overshadowed by the manifestations of the underlying disorder. For the manifestations of polycythemia see the accompanying box.

Interdisciplinary Care

Diagnosis

In PV, serum erythropoietin levels are low. Bone marrow studies show hyperplasia of all hematopoietic elements. With secondary polycythemia, serum erythropoietin levels usually are high, and bone marrow studies show only red stem cell hyperplasia.

Treatments

For secondary polycythemia, treatment focuses on the underlying cause of the disorder. It is a physiologic response in people living at high altitudes, and unless the hematocrit is too high or oxygen saturation levels are low, no treatment is usually necessary. Smokers are urged to quit. Measures to raise oxygen saturation levels and reduce tissue hypoxia often will relieve the polycythemia. Patients with both primary and secondary polycythemia benefit from periodic phlebotomy, removing 300 to 500 mL of blood, to keep blood volume and viscosity within normal levels. For PV, chemotherapeutic agents such as hydroxyurea may be used to suppress marrow function but may increase the risk of developing leukemia (discussed later in this chapter). Pruritus may be relieved by antihistamines, or may require more aggressive treatment with

MANIFESTATIONS of Polycythemia

- Hypertension
- Headache, tinnitus, blurred vision
- Plethora: dark redness of the lips, feet, ears, fingernails, and mucous membranes
- Splenomegaly (polycythemia vera)
- Severe pruritus, extremity pain
- Weight loss, night sweats
- GI bleeding
- Intermittent claudication
- Symptoms from thrombosis within various organs

interferon alpha or other treatments. One 325 mg aspirin tablet daily may be ordered to control thrombosis without increasing the risk of bleeding.

Nursing Care

Preventing polycythemia begins with educating children and adults about the dangers of smoking. Measures to reduce risk factors for cardiovascular disease also may be beneficial.

This chronic condition is managed in community-based settings unless a complication develops. Teach the patient and family the importance of maintaining adequate hydration, increasing fluid intake during hot weather and when exercising. Discuss measures to prevent blood stasis: elevating legs and feet when sitting, using support stockings, and continuing treatment measures. Instruct to report manifestations of thrombosis (leg or calf pain, chest pain, neurologic symptoms) or bleeding (black, tarry stools, vomiting blood or coffee-ground emesis) immediately. Monitor the hematocrit and cell counts throughout treatment.

Examples of nursing diagnoses appropriate for the patient with polycythemia follow:

- *Decisional Conflict Regarding Smoking Cessation* related to addictive effects
- *Pain* related to effects of altered blood flow in distal extremities
- *Risk for Ineffective Tissue Perfusion* related to sluggish blood flow and increased risk for thrombosis

White Blood Cell and Lymphoid Tissue Disorders

Disorders of the WBCs and lymphoid tissue include infectious mononucleosis, the leukemias, multiple myeloma, and malignant lymphomas (Hodgkin's disease and non-Hodgkin's lymphoma). Review the physiology of white blood cells (WBCs) and their function in ∞ Chapter 12.

The Patient with Leukemia

Leukemia (literally, "white blood") is a group of chronic malignant disorders of WBCs and WBC precursors. In leukemia, the usual ratio of red to white blood cells is reversed. Leukemias are characterized by replacement of bone marrow by malignant immature WBCs, abnormal immature circulating WBCs, and infiltration of these cells into the liver, spleen, and lymph nodes throughout the body.

Physiology Review

WBCs are the most diverse of the cellular components of the blood. They arise from three different precursor cells: myeloblasts, which further differentiate into the granular leukocytes (granulocytes), neutrophils, eosinophils, and basophils; monoblasts, which mature into circulating monocytes, and ultimately into macrophages; and lymphoblasts, which become lymphocytes and mature in lymphoid tissue to B cells and T cells.

As a whole, the primary function of WBCs is to help maintain the body's immune defenses. Neutrophils, the most numerous WBCs in circulation, are active phagocytes, the first cells to arrive to injured tissue. Monocytes and macrophages also are phagocytic cells that dispose of foreign and waste material from tissues. Eosinophils and basophils are more specialized. Eosinophils are primarily involved in allergic responses and parasitic infections. Basophils are actively involved in the inflammatory response, releasing substances such as histamine and heparin into inflamed tissues. Lymphocytes, the smallest of the WBCs, are an integral part of the immune system. B cells are part of the humoral immune response, producing antibodies to specific antigens. T cells are part of the cell-mediated immune response. For more information about the inflammatory and immune responses, ∞ see Chapter 13. The normal WBC count and differential is presented in Table 33–2.

Pathophysiology

Leukemia begins with malignant transformation of a single stem cell. Leukemic cells proliferate slowly, but do not differentiate normally. They have a prolonged life span and accumulate in the bone marrow. As they accumulate, they compete with the proliferation of normal cells. Leukemic cells do not function as mature WBCs, and are ineffective in the inflammatory and immune processes. Leukemic cells replace normal hematopoietic elements in the marrow. Because erythrocyte- and platelet-producing cells are crowded out, severe anemia, splenomegaly, and bleeding difficulties result.

Leukemic cells leave the bone marrow and travel through the circulatory system, infiltrating other body tissues such as the central nervous system, testes, skin, GI tract, and the lymph nodes, liver, and spleen. Death usually is due to internal hemorrhage and infections.

Manifestations

The general manifestations of leukemia (regardless of type) result from anemia, infection, and bleeding. These include pallor, fatigue, tachycardia, malaise, lethargy, and dyspnea on exertion. Infection may cause fever, night sweats, oral ulcerations, and frequent or recurrent respiratory, urinary, integumentary, or other infections. Increased bleeding due to thrombocytopenia leads to bruising, petechiae, bleeding gums, and bleeding within specific organs and tissues. See the Multisystem Effects of Leukemia feature on page 1085.

TABLE 33–2 Normal White Blood Cell Count and Differential

LABORATORY TEST	VALUE
WBC count	5000–10,000/mm^3
Differential WBC count	
Neutrophils	60–70% or 3000–7000/mm^3
Eosinophils	1–3% or 50–400/mm^3
Basophils	0.3–0.5% or 25–200/mm^3
Lymphocytes	20–30% or 1000–4000/mm^3
Monocytes	3–8% or 100–600/mm^3

MULTISYSTEM EFFECTS OF
Leukemia

Neurologic
- Headache
- Altered LOC
- Cranial nerve impairment

Potential complications
- Subarachnoid hemorrhage
- Retinal hemorrhage
- Seizures, coma

Respiratory
- Dyspnea on exertion
- Pharyngitis, sore throat
- Frequent respiratory infections

Potential complication
- Pulmonary bleeding

Gastrointestinal
- Anorexia, nausea
- Oral ulcerations, infection
- Bleeding gums
- Gingival hyperplasia
  (gum overgrowth)
- Abdominal pain
- Hepatomegaly
- Occult GI bleeding

Urinary
- Urinary tract infection
- Hematuria

Potential complication
- Renal insufficiency or failure

Musculoskeletal
- Weakness
- Bone tenderness, pain
- Joint pain

Metabolic Processes
- Malaise, lethargy
- Heat intolerance
- Diaphoresis
- Chills, fever
- Night sweats
- Weight loss

Cardiovascular
- Tachycardia, palpitations
- Orthostatic hypotension
- Heart murmurs
- Hematomas
- Edema

Potential complications
- Hemorrhage
- Thrombophlebitis

Hematologic
- Anemia
- Thrombocytopenia
- Leukopenia
- Bleeding (epistaxis)
- Splenomegaly

Potential complication
- DIC

Immunologic
- Frequent or recurrent infections
- Lymphadenopathy

Potential complications
- Abscesses
- Septicemia

Integumentary
- Skin and mucous membrane pallor
- Petechiae
- Bruising, purpura
- Ulcerations
- *Chloromas* (skin infiltrations near
  bony prominences)

Other manifestations result from leukemic cell infiltration, increased metabolism, and increased leukocyte destruction. Infiltration of the liver, spleen, lymph nodes, and bone marrow causes pain and tissue swelling in the involved areas. Meningeal infiltration may cause manifestations of increased intracranial pressure, such as headache, altered level of consciousness, cranial nerve impairment, nausea, and vomiting. Infiltration of the kidneys may affect renal function, with decreased urine output and increased blood urea nitrogen and creatinine. Increased metabolism causes heat intolerance, weight loss, dyspnea on exertion, and tachycardia. Destruction of large numbers of WBCs releases substantial amounts of uric acid into the circulation; uric acid crystals may obstruct renal tubules, causing renal insufficiency.

Without treatment, leukemia is invariably fatal, usually due to complications of leukemic cell infiltration of bone marrow or vital organs. With treatment, prognosis varies. The overall 5-year survival rate is 46%. Survival rates differ by type of leukemia: People with acute myeloid leukemia have a 20% 5-year survival rate, whereas the rate is 73% for people with chronic lymphocytic leukemia (American Cancer Society, 2008). The types, pathology, manifestations, and treatment for the major leukemias are outlined in Table 33–3.

Incidence and Risk Factors

Although leukemia is often thought of as a childhood disease, it is diagnosed 10 times more often in adults than in children. An estimated 34,810 new cases of leukemia occur annually; slightly more than half are acute leukemia and less than half are chronic leukemia. In 2008, the American Cancer Society (2008) estimated that 44,270 were diagnosed with leukemia and more than 21,000 people died of leukemia. The highest incidence of leukemia is found in the United States, Canada, Sweden, and New Zealand (Huether & McCance, 2008).

Although the cause of most leukemias is unknown, certain risk factors have been identified. Men are affected more frequently than are women. People with certain genetic disorders such as Down syndrome have a higher incidence of leukemia.

Environmental risk factors play a role as well. Risk factors for myeloid leukemia include cigarette smoking and chemicals such as benzene (present in cigarette smoke and gasoline). Exposure to ionizing radiation increases the risk for several types of leukemia. Patients who have undergone treatment for cancer have an increased risk. The human T-cell leukemia/lymphoma virus-1, a retrovirus, is known to cause certain leukemias and lymphomas (ACS, 2005).

Classifications

Leukemias are classified by their acuity and by the predominant cell type involved. The *acute* leukemias are characterized by an acute onset, rapid disease progression, and immature or undifferentiated blast cells. *Chronic* leukemias, on the other hand, have a gradual onset, prolonged course, and abnormal mature-appearing cells. *Lymphocytic* (or *lymphoblastic*) leukemias involve immature lymphocytes and their precursor cells in the bone marrow. Lymphocytic leukemias infiltrate the spleen, lymph nodes, CNS, and other tissues. *Myeloid* (also called *myelogenous*, *myelocytic*, or *myeloblastic*) leukemias involve myeloid stem cells in the bone marrow, interfering with the maturation of all types of blood cells, including granulocytes, RBCs, and thrombocytes (Huether & McCance, 2008). Acute lymphoblastic leukemia is the most common type of leukemia in children. In adults, acute myeloid leukemia and chronic lymphocytic leukemia are the most common types (Huether & McCance, 2008). In summary, the general types of leukemia are as follows:

- Acute lymphocytic (lymphoblastic) leukemia (ALL)
- Chronic lymphocytic leukemia (CLL)
- Acute myeloid (myeloblastic) leukemia (AML)
- Chronic myeloid (myelogenous) leukemia (CML)

This general system of classifying leukemias does not differentiate subtypes of acute leukemias. The FAB system for classifying acute leukemias further differentiates acute leukemias by the predominant cell involved and the degree of cell differentiation (Table 33–4).

TABLE 33–3 Major Types of Leukemia

CLASSIFICATION	CHARACTERISTICS	MANIFESTATIONS	TREATMENT
Acute lymphoblastic leukemia (ALL)	Primarily affects children and young adults; leukemic cells may infiltrate CNS	Recurrent infections; bleeding; pallor, bone pain, weight loss, sore throat, fatigue, night sweats, weakness	Chemotherapy; bone marrow transplant (BMT), or stem cell transplant (SCT)
Chronic lymphocytic leukemia (CLL)	Primarily affects older adults; insidious onset and slow, chronic course	Fatigue; exercise intolerance; lymphadenopathy and splenomegaly; recurrent infections, pallor, edema, thrombophlebitis	Often requires no treatment; chemotherapy; BMT
Acute myeloid leukemia (AML)	Common in older adults, may affect children and young adults. Strongly associated with toxins, genetic disorders, and treatment of other cancers	Fatigue, weakness, fever; anemia; headache, bone and joint pain; abnormal bleeding and bruising; recurrent infection; lymphadenopathy, splenomegaly, and hepatomegaly	Chemotherapy; SCT
Chronic myeloid leukemia (CML)	Primarily affects adults; early course slow and stable, progressing to aggressive phase in 3 to 4 years	Early: weakness, fatigue, dyspnea on exertion; possible splenomegaly Later: fever, weight loss, night sweats	Interferon-α; chemotherapy with imatinib mesylate (Gleevac), SCT

TABLE 33–4 FAB Classification of Acute Leukemia

TYPE	CLASS	PREDOMINANT CELLS	PROGNOSIS
Acute Lymphocytic Leukemia (ALL)	L_1	Immature lymphoblasts	> 90 remission rate in children
	L_2	Mature lymphoblasts	Relapse common after 2 or more years of remission
Acute Myeloid Leukemia	M_0	Undifferentiated cells	Poor
	M_1	Immature myeloblasts	Good; complete response in 65 or more
	M_2	Mature myeloblasts	Good for 2 or more years of remission
	M_3	Promyelocytes	Good in adults
	M_4	Myelocytes and monocytes	Poorest in adults
	M_5	Poorly or well-differentiated monocytes	Poor
	M_6	Predominant erythroblasts	Variable
	M_7	Megakaryocytes	

Acute Myeloid Leukemia

Acute myeloid leukemia (AML) is characterized by uncontrolled proliferation of myeloblasts (the precursors of granulocytes) and hyperplasia of the bone marrow and spleen (Figure 33–5 ■). AML accounts for 80% of acute leukemia cases in adults. Treatment induces complete remission in 66% of patients, although only about 30% to 40% achieve cure or long-term remission (Huether & McCance, 2008).

The manifestations of AML result from neutropenia and thrombocytopenia. Decreased neutrophils lead to recurrent severe infections, such as pneumonia, septicemia, abscesses, and mucous membrane ulceration. The manifestations of thrombocytopenia include petechiae, purpura, ecchymoses (bruising), epistaxis (nosebleeds), hematomas, hematuria, and GI bleeding. Bone infarctions or subperiosteal infiltrates of leukemic cells may cause bone pain. Anemia is a late manifestation, causing fatigue, headaches, pallor, and dyspnea on exertion. Death usually results from infection or hemorrhage.

Bone marrow aspiration shows a proliferation of immature WBCs. The CBC shows thrombocytopenia and normocytic, normochromic anemia.

Figure 33–5 ■ A blood smear from the bone marrow of a patient with acute myeloid leukemia. Note the abnormally large number of myelocyte WBCs (stained purple) among the small RBCs.

Chronic Myeloid Leukemia

Chronic myeloid leukemia (CML) is characterized by abnormal proliferation of all bone marrow elements. This type of leukemia constitutes approximately 15% of adult leukemias. It affects men more frequently than women. The onset of CML typically is between ages 30 or 40 and 50, although it is seen in children and adolescents as well (Huether & McCance, 2008).

CML is usually associated with a chromosome abnormality called the Philadelphia chromosome, a balanced translocation of chromosome 22 to chromosome 9 (Figure 33–6 ■). The fusion gene produced by this translocation, known as *bcr/abl*, is an *oncogene* capable of initiating a malignancy. Very large doses of ionizing radiation also may induce CML in some patients (Papadakis & McPhee, 2007).

People with CML are often asymptomatic in the early stages and, in fact, are often diagnosed when a routine blood test reveals abnormal cell counts. Anemia causes weakness, fatigue, and dyspnea on exertion. The spleen often is enlarged,

Figure 33–6 ■ The Philadelphia chromosome. Note the chromosomes of pairs 9 and 22. In each instance, the left-hand chromosome of the pair is normal, whereas an exchange of material between chromosomes has made the right-hand chromosome 9 larger and the right-hand chromosome 22 smaller. In stem cells within the bone marrow, the chromosome 22 defect leads to chronic myeloid leukemia.

causing abdominal discomfort. Within 3 to 4 years, disease progresses to a more aggressive phase. Rapid cell proliferation and hypermetabolism cause fatigue, weight loss, sweating, and heat intolerance. The spleen enlarges, leading to a sensation of abdominal fullness and discomfort. Platelet function is affected in this stage, leading to bleeding and increased bruising. Finally, the disease evolves to acute leukemia, with blast cell proliferation. This stage, known as the *terminal blast crisis phase*, is characterized by significant constitutional manifestations, splenomegaly, and infiltration of leukemic cells into the skin, lymph nodes, bones, and central nervous system (Huether & McCance, 2008). Survival following the onset of this final stage averages only 2 to 4 months.

Acute Lymphocytic Leukemia

Acute lymphocytic leukemia (ALL) is the most common type of leukemia in children and young adults. In adults, ALL is rarely seen until late middle age, and then its incidence increases with aging. Genetic factors may play a role in its development, particularly the *bcr/abl* translocation also implicated in CML.

Most (80%) cases of ALL result from malignant transformation of B cells, with the remaining 20% arising from T cells. The malignant cells resemble immature lymphocytes (*lymphoblasts*); however, they do not mature or function effectively to maintain immunity. These lymphoblasts accumulate in the bone marrow, lymph nodes, and spleen, as well as in circulating blood. Some types of lymphoma (discussed later in this chapter) are thought to represent a later stage of the same disease.

The onset of ALL is usually rapid. Lymphoblasts proliferating in bone marrow and peripheral tissues crowd the growth of normal cells (Figure 33–7 ■). Normal hematopoiesis is suppressed, leading to thrombocytopenia, leukopenia, and anemia. Manifestations of infections, bleeding, and anemia develop. Bone pain resulting from rapid generation of marrow elements, lymphadenopathy, and liver enlargement are also common. Infiltration of the central nervous system causes headaches, visual disturbances, vomiting, and seizures.

The CBC shows an elevated WBC count with increased lymphocytes on the differential. RBC and platelet counts are

Figure 33–7 ■ A blood smear from the bone marrow of a patient with acute lymphocytic leukemia. Note the abnormally large number of lymphocytes (stained purple) crowding the bone marrow. As a result, normal production of RBCs, functional WBCs, and platelets is suppressed.

decreased. Bone marrow studies reveal a hypercellular marrow with growth of lymphoblasts. Combination chemotherapy produces complete remission in 80% to 90% of adults with ALL.

Chronic Lymphocytic Leukemia

Chronic lymphocytic leukemia (CLL) is characterized by proliferation and accumulation of small, abnormal, mature lymphocytes in the bone marrow, peripheral blood, and body tissues. The abnormal cells are usually B-lymphocytes that are unable to produce adequate antibodies to maintain normal immune function. Only about 5% of CLL involves T cells (Noonan, 2007). CLL occurs more commonly in adults, especially in older adults (median age 65). CLL is the least common type of the major leukemias.

CLL has a slow onset and is often diagnosed during a routine physical examination. If symptoms are present, they usually include vague complaints of weakness or malaise. Possible clinical findings include anemia, infection, and enlarged lymph nodes, spleen, and liver. As in other leukemias, bone marrow hyperplasia is present. Erythrocyte and platelet counts are reduced. Leukocyte counts may either be elevated or reduced, but abnormal cells are always present. In CLL, years may elapse before treatment is required. Survival of this disease averages approximately 7 years.

Interdisciplinary Care

Treatment for leukemia focuses on achieving remission or cure and relieving symptoms. The methods of treatment may include chemotherapy, radiation therapy, and bone marrow or stem cell transplantation. Cure is more often achieved in children with acute leukemia than in adults, although long-term remissions (disease-free periods with no signs or symptoms) often can be achieved.

Diagnosis

The following diagnostic tests are ordered when leukemia is suspected:

- *CBC* with differential is done to evaluate cell counts, hemoglobin and hematocrit levels, and the number, distribution, and morphology (size and shape) of WBCs.
- *Platelets* are measured to identify possible thrombocytopenia secondary to the leukemia and the risk of bleeding.
- *Bone marrow examination* provides information about cells within the marrow, the type of erythropoiesis, and the maturity of erythropoietic and leukopoietic cells.

Table 33–5 outlines usual diagnostic test results in the various forms of leukemia.

Chemotherapy

Single agent or combination chemotherapy is the treatment of choice for most types of leukemia, with the goal of eradicating leukemic cells and producing remission. Table 33–6 outlines typical chemotherapy regimens for different types of leukemia. Combination chemotherapy reduces drug resistance and toxicity, and interrupts cell growth at various stages of the cell cycle, producing complimentary effect of the drugs used. Cancer treatment with chemotherapy is discussed in detail in ∞ Chapter 14.

Chemotherapy for leukemia generally is divided into the induction phase and postremission therapy. During *induction*,

TABLE 33–5 Diagnostic Findings by Type of Leukemia

TEST	AML	CML	ALL	CLL
RBC count	Low	Low	Low	Low
Hemoglobin	Low	Low	Low	Low
Hematocrit	Low	Low	Low	Low
Platelet count	Very low	High early, low late	Low	Low
WBC count	Varies	Increased	Varies	Increased
Myeloblasts	Present			
Neutrophils	Decreased	Increased	Decreased	
Lymphocytes		Normal		Normal
Monocytes		Normal/low		Increased
Blasts	Present	Present (crisis)	Present	
Bone marrow	Hypercellular		Hypercellular	
Myeloblasts	Present			
Lymphoblasts			Present	
Lymphocytes				Present

drug doses are high to eradicate leukemic cells from the bone marrow. These high doses often also damage stem cells and interfere with production of normal blood cells. Circulating mature blood cells are not affected because they are no longer dividing. The degree of bone marrow suppression is influenced by a number of factors, including age, nutritional status, concurrent chronic diseases such as impaired liver or renal function, the drug and drug dose, and prior treatment.

Colony-stimulating factors (CSFs), also called hematopoietic growth factors, often are administered to "rescue" the bone marrow following induction chemotherapy. CSFs are cytokines that regulate the growth and differentiation of blood cells. Factors that support neutrophil maturation, *granulocyte-macrophage CSF (GM-CSF)* and *granulocyte CSF (G-CSF)*, are commonly used. Bone pain is a common side effect of therapy with these agents. Patients also may experience fevers, chills, anorexia, muscle aches, and lethargy (Deglin & Vallerand, 2009).

Once remission has been achieved, postremission chemotherapy is continued to eradicate any additional leukemic cells, prevent relapse, and prolong survival. A single chemotherapeutic agent, combination therapy, or bone marrow transplant may be used for postremission treatment.

Radiation Therapy
Radiation therapy damages cellular DNA. While the cell continues to function, it cannot divide and multiply. Cells that divide rapidly, such as bone marrow and cancer cells (radiosensitive cells), respond quickly to radiation therapy. Although normal cells are affected, they are better able to recover from the damage caused by the radiation than are cancer cells. The types of delivery, effects, and toxicities of radiation are discussed in greater detail in ∞ Chapter 14.

Bone Marrow Transplant
Bone marrow transplant (BMT) is the treatment of choice for some types of leukemia. BMT often is used in conjunction with or following chemotherapy or radiation. There are two major categories of BMT: In allogeneic BMT, the bone marrow of a healthy donor is infused into the patient with the illness; in autologous BMT, the patient is infused with his or her own bone marrow.

ALLOGENEIC BMT   *Allogeneic BMT* uses bone marrow cells from a donor (often from a sibling with closely matched tissue antigens; closely matched unrelated donors also may be used). Prior to allogeneic BMT, high doses of chemotherapy and/or total body irradiation are used to destroy leukemic cells in the

TABLE 33–6 Chemotherapeutic Regimens Used to Treat Leukemia

Acute myeloid leukemia	■ Cytarabine (Cytoxan, an alkylating agent) *with* daunorubicin (Cerubidine, an antitumor antibiotic), or idarubicin (Idamycin, an antitumor antibiotic) ■ All-*trans* retinoic acid (ATRA) added for patients with promyelocytic leukemia
Chronic myeloid leukemia	■ Imatinib mesylate (Gleevec), a bcr/abl tyrosine kinase (enzyme) inhibitor ■ Hydroxyurea (a DNA inhibitor) *or* homoharringtonine (HHT, a plant alkaloid) if imatinib not tolerated
Acute lymphocytic leukemia	■ Dau norubicin (Cerubidine, an antitumor antibiotic) *with* vincristine (Oncovin, a plant alkaloid) *with* prednisone *with* asparaginase (Elspar)
Chronic lymphocytic leukemia	■ Fludarabine (Fludara, an antimetabolite) *or* chlorambucil (Chloromycetin, an antitumor antibiotic) ■ Cyclophosphamide (Cytoxan, an alkylating agent), vincristine, and prednisone ■ Cyclophosphamide, doxorubicin (Adriamycin, an antitumor antibiotic), vincristine, and prednisone

Figure 33–8 ■ Allogenic bone marrow transplant. Bone marrow from the donor is aspirated, then filtered and infused into the recipient.

bone marrow. The donor's bone marrow is aspirated (Figure 33–8 ■) and infused through a central venous line into the recipient. Prior to BMT and reestablishment of bone marrow function, the patient is critically ill and at significant risk for infection and bleeding due to depletion of WBCs and platelets.

AUTOLOGOUS BMT *Autologous BMT* uses the patient's own bone marrow to restore bone marrow function after chemotherapy or radiation. This procedure is often called *bone marrow rescue*. In autologous BMT, about 1 L of bone marrow is aspirated (usually from the iliac crests) during a period of disease remission. The bone marrow is then frozen and stored for use after treatment. If relapse occurs, lethal doses of chemotherapy or radiation are given to destroy the immune system and malignant cells, and to prepare space in the bone marrow for new cells. The filtered bone marrow is then thawed and infused intravenously through a central line. The infused marrow cells slowly become a part of the patient's bone marrow, the neutrophil count increases, and normal hematopoiesis takes place.

As in allogeneic BMT, the patient is critically ill during the period of bone marrow destruction and immunosuppression. The patient is hospitalized in a private room for 6 to 8 weeks or more. Potential complications include malnutrition, infection, and bleeding.

Stem Cell Transplant

Allogeneic **stem cell transplant (SCT)** is an alternative to bone marrow transplant. SCT results in complete and sustained replacement of the recipient's blood cell lines (WBCs, RBCs, and platelets) with cells derived from the donor stem cells.

Donors must have tissue that is closely matched with that of the recipient. Prior to harvesting, hematopoietic growth factors, including G-CSF and GM-CSF, are administered to the donor for 4 to 5 days. This increases the concentration of stem cells

in peripheral blood, allowing it to be used for the transplant instead of bone marrow. Peripheral blood is removed and white cells are separated from the plasma, then administered via a large central venous catheter. Large concentrations of stem cells also are present in umbilical cord blood. This may be stored and used in some cases (Papadakis & McPhee, 2007).

The recipient undergoes similar treatment prior to SCT as for BMT. The risks for infection and other complications, as well as graft-versus-host disease, are similar.

GRAFT-VERSUS-HOST DISEASE Allogeneic BMT or SCT may precipitate *graft-versus-host disease (GVHD)*, which develops in up to 60% of all patients receiving an allogeneic BMT or SCT. In GVHD, immune cells of the donated bone marrow identify the recipient's body tissue as foreign. Consequently, T lymphocytes in the donated marrow attack the liver, skin, and GI tract, causing skin rashes progressing to desquamation (loss of skin), diarrhea, GI bleeding, and liver damage. *Acute GVHD* develops within days or weeks of the transplant and is usually marked by a pruritic, maculopapular rash that begins on the palms and soles of the feet, and may extend over the entire body. Vaso-occlusive disease of the liver affects up to 25% of allogenic bone marrow transplant recipients, with jaundice and elevated liver function tests (Porth, 2005). *Chronic GVHD* develops later, 100 or more days after the transplant, affecting 20% to 50% of patients who survive 6 months or more following allogenic BMT or SCT. It may follow acute GVHD or develop in patients with no prior symptoms. GVHD is treated with antibiotics and steroids; immunosuppressant drugs such as thalidomide and immunotoxin (Xomazyme) may be used if necessary.

Biologic Therapy

Cytokines such as interferons and interleukins are biologic agents that may be used to treat some leukemias. These agents modify the body's response to cancer cells; in some cases they are cytotoxic as well. Interferons are a complex group of messenger proteins normally produced in response to antigens such as viruses (∞ see Chapter 12). They have multiple effects, including moderating immune function and inhibiting abnormal cell proliferation and growth. Interferon-α may be used to treat some leukemias, particularly CML. Side effects commonly associated with interferon therapy include flulike symptoms, persistent fatigue and lethargy, weight loss, and muscle and joint pain.

Complementary Therapies

Although many complementary and alternative medicine therapies have been purported to treat cancer in general, at this time none have been shown to have sustained benefit in treating leukemia. Clinical trials have demonstrated the efficacy of both coping skills training (relaxation and imagery) and hypnosis to significantly reduce oral discomfort associated with leukemia and its treatment.

∞ Nursing Care

For nursing care specific to the patient undergoing diagnostic testing for leukemia, see the accompanying Case Study & Nursing Care Plan.

Health Promotion

Health promotion activities related to leukemia include teaching about leukemia risk factors, particularly those that can be controlled. Discuss the potential dangers of exposure to ionizing radiation and certain chemicals such as benzene. Encourage all patients to avoid smoking cigarettes. Discuss genetic counseling with patients at high risk for having a child with Down syndrome (over age 35).

Assessment

Focused assessment data related to leukemia includes the following:

- *Health history:* Complaints of fatigue, weakness, dyspnea on exertion, frequent infections, sore throat, night sweats, bleeding gums, or nose bleeds; recent weight loss; exposure to ionizing radiation (multiple x-rays, residence near a site of radiation or atomic testing) or chemicals (occupational); prior treatment for cancer; history of an immune disorder.
- *Physical examination:* Skin and mucous membranes for bruising, purpura, petechiae, ulcers or lesions; pallor; vital signs including orthostatic vitals; heart and lung sounds; abdominal examination; stool for occult blood.
- *Laboratory tests:* Blood count with differential; bone marrow studies.

Nursing Diagnoses and Interventions

When caring for the patient with leukemia, the nurse considers the chronic and life-threatening nature of the disease as well as the effects of treatment. See the Moving Evidence into Action box on the following page. Priority nursing problems may include *Risk for Infection, Imbalanced Nutrition, Impaired Oral Mucous Membranes, Impaired Protection (Bleeding),* and *Grieving.*

EVIDENCE FOR NURSING CARE — The Patient with Bone Marrow Transplant

Selected resources that nurses may find helpful when planning evidence-based nursing care follow.

- Schmit-Pokorny, K. (2009). Expanding indications for stem cell transplantation. *Seminars in Oncology Nursing, 25*(2), 105–114. Retrieved from http://www.nursingconsult.com
- Shelburne, N., & Bevans, M. (2009). Non-myeloablative allogeneic hematopoietic stem cell transplantation. *Seminars in Oncology Nursing, 25*(2), 120–128. Retrieved from http://www.nursingconsult.com

Risk for Infection

Changes in WBC function impair the immune and inflammatory responses in leukemia, increasing the risk for infection. WBCs may be immature and ineffective, or, in some cases, deficient. Chemotherapy or radiation therapy further depresses bone marrow function, and increases the risk for infection.

- Promptly report manifestations of infection: fever, chills, throat pain, cough, chest pain, burning on urination, purulent drainage, and itching and burning in vaginal or rectal areas. *Prompt reporting allows timely intervention to prevent overwhelming infection and sepsis.*
- Institute infection protection measures.
  a. Maintain protective isolation as indicated.
  b. Ensure meticulous hand hygiene among all people in contact with the patient.
  c. Assist as needed with appropriate hygiene measures.
  d. Restrict visitors with colds, flu, or infections.
  e. Provide oral hygiene after every meal.

MOVING EVIDENCE INTO ACTION — Patients with Acute Leukemia and Lymphoma

Patients with acute leukemia and malignant lymphoma experience a number of distressing manifestations of their disease, including malaise and fatigue, fever, night sweats, infections, and possible hemorrhage. Treatments such as radiation therapy and chemotherapy often have numerous adverse effects as well, including anorexia and nausea, stomatitis, lethargy, malaise, and fatigue. In these studies, patients in remission from acute leukemia or malignant lymphoma were surveyed regarding physical problems, their view of help they received and who was of most help during treatment, and the impact of the disease and treatment on their current life (Persson, Hallberg, & Ohlsson, 1997; Persson & Hallberg, 2004).

Patients identified energy loss and nutritional problems as being most troublesome during disease treatment. In general, patients with more physical problems were less satisfied with the nursing care they received, suggesting that nurses were less effective in meeting the needs of the sickest patients. Patients continued to experience reduced psychological and sexual energy and a significant need for intimate help and counseling during remission. While family relationships improved, work and finances were negatively impacted by their disease.

IMPLICATIONS FOR NURSING

This study points out the need for nurses to actively focus their care on the physical problems experienced during treatment, especially energy loss and nutritional problems. Overwhelming fatigue interferes with the patient's ability to provide self-care, but its effects may not be readily apparent to nurses. The long-term effects of reduced psychological and sexual energy, as well as continued susceptibility to infections, indicate a need for continued follow-up care, teaching, and possibly referral to counseling services.

CRITICAL THINKING IN PATIENT CARE

1. Explain the physiologic responses to malignancies and cancer treatments that cause fatigue, malaise, and nutritional problems.
2. Patients undergoing treatment for leukemia, malignant lymphoma, and other cancers may have few outward manifestations of their disease or responses to treatment. Discuss how this apparent well-being may affect the nurses' perception of care needs.
3. How may continued problems of fatigue and lack of psychologic and sexual energy affect family relations?
4. Develop a nursing care plan for a patient with acute leukemia to address the problem: *Ineffective Sexuality Patterns related to fatigue and lack of energy.*

Adapted from Persson, L., & Hallberg, I. R. (2004). Lived experience of survivors of leukemia or malignant lymphoma. *Cancer Nursing, 27*(4), 303–s313 and Persson, L., Hallberg, I. R., & Ohlsson, O. (1997). Survivors of acute leukemia and highly malignant lymphoma—retrospective views of daily life problems during treatment and when in remission. *Journal of Advanced Nursing, 25*(1), 68–78.

f. Avoid invasive procedures when possible, including injections, intravenous catheters, catheterizations, and rectal and vaginal procedures. When necessary, use strict aseptic technique for all invasive procedures and monitor carefully for infection.

These precautions minimize exposure to bacterial, viral, and fungal pathogens. Infection is the major cause of death in patients with leukemia. Mucous membranes are especially susceptible to breakdown and infection as a result of tissue damage from chemotherapy or radiation.

- Monitor vital signs including temperature and oxygen saturation every 4 hours. Report temperature spikes with chilling, tachypnea, tachycardia, restlessness, change in PaO_2, and hypotension. *The inflammatory response may be impaired in leukemia, masking signs of infection until sepsis develops, indicated by manifestations such as those listed.*

- Monitor neutrophil levels (measured in cubic millimeters) for relative risk for infection:

  2000 to 2500: no risk
  1000 to 2000: minimal risk
  500 to 1000: moderate risk
  Below 500: severe risk
  Neutrophils are the first line of defense against infection. As levels decrease, the risk for infection increases.

- Explain infection precautions and restrictions and their rationale; explain that these measures are usually temporary. *Patient and family understanding increases compliance and lowers the risk of infection.*

Imbalanced Nutrition: Less than Body Requirements

The patient with leukemia may have difficulty meeting nutritional needs due to increased metabolism, fatigue, loss of appetite from radiation, nausea and vomiting from chemotherapy, or painful oral mucous membranes that make chewing and swallowing difficult and/or painful.

- Weigh regularly and evaluate weight loss over time to determine degree of malnutrition. A weight loss of 10% to 20% may indicate malnutrition. *A minimum intake of nutrients is necessary for health and tissue repair; cancer increases metabolic needs over this basal requirement. Weight loss occurs when metabolic requirements are not met. Both the disease process and its treatment can interfere with nutrient intake.*

- Address causative or contributing factors to inadequate food and fluid intake.

  a. Provide mouth care before and after meals; use a soft toothbrush or sponges as necessary.
  b. Provide liquids with different textures and tastes.
  c. Increase liquid intake with meals.
  d. Reduce intake of milk and milk products, which makes mucus more tenacious.
  e. Assist to a sitting position for eating.
  f. Ensure that the environment is clean and odor-free.
  g. Provide medications for pain or nausea 30 minutes before meals, if prescribed.
  h. Provide rest periods before meals.
  i. Offer small, frequent meals including low-fat, high kcal foods throughout the day.
  j. Provide commercial supplements, such as Ensure.

k. Avoid painful or unpleasant procedures immediately before or after meals.
l. Suggest measures to improve food tolerance, such as eating dry foods when arising, consuming salty foods if allowed, and avoiding very sweet, rich, or greasy foods.

Anorexia, nausea and vomiting, diarrhea, stomatitis, taste changes, and dysphagia often make eating difficult during cancer treatment when good nutrition is most important. Maintaining nutritional status decreases morbidity and mortality by preventing weight loss, improving the response to treatment, minimizing adverse effects, and improving quality of life. Small, frequent meals are often better tolerated, especially high-protein, high-kcal foods.

Impaired Oral Mucous Membrane

Stomatitis, inflammation and ulceration of the oral mucous membrane, is common in leukemia. Chemotherapy can further impair the integrity of constantly dividing oral tissues.

- Inspect the buccal region, gums, sublingual area, and the throat daily for swelling or lesions. Ask about oral pain or burning. *Breakdown of the oral mucous membrane increases the risk of infection and bleeding, causes pain and discomfort with eating and swallowing, and may cause swelling that interferes with the airway.*

- Culture any oral lesions. *Herpes simplex virus and* Candida *(yeast) are more common in patients with neutropenia. Herpes lesions are usually red, raised, fluid-filled blisters;* Candida *causes a white coating and patches of white plaque.*

- Assist with mouth care and oral rinses with saline or a solution of hydrogen peroxide and water (1:1 or 1:3 hydrogen peroxide and water) every 2 to 4 hours. Apply petroleum jelly to the lips to prevent dryness and cracking. *These measures help prevent infection and increase comfort.*

- Encourage use of soft-bristle toothbrush or sponge to clean teeth and gums. *Toothbrushes with hard bristles may abrade inflamed mucosa, causing bleeding and increasing the risk of infection.*

- Administer medications as ordered to treat infection or relieve pain. *Topical antifungal agents such as nystatin may be prescribed to treat* Candida *infections. Topical anesthetics such as lidocaine may be prescribed to relieve comfort and facilitate good oral care.*

- Instruct to avoid alcohol-based mouthwashes, citrus fruit juices, spicy foods, very hot or very cold foods, alcohol, and crusty foods. Suggest bland, cool foods and cool liquids at least every 2 hours. *Avoiding mucosa-traumatizing foods and liquids increases comfort; bland, cool foods and liquids cause the least pain. Intake of adequate fluids is necessary to prevent dehydration.*

Ineffective Protection

Bleeding is the second most common cause of leukemia deaths. As platelet counts decrease, the risk of bleeding increases (see the section later in this chapter on thrombocytopenia). Tumor lysis syndrome also is a risk in patients with leukemia who are undergoing their initial treatment with chemotherapy. Tumor lysis syndrome develops when a large number of malignant cells are destroyed by treatment with chemotherapy or radiation. The resultant byproducts of cell lysis can overwhelm the body's ability to effectively eliminate them, leading to hyperkalemia, hyperphosphatemia with secondary hypocalcemia, and hyperuricemia (Cantril & Haylock, 2004).

- Assess vital signs every 4 hours and body systems every shift for bleeding.
  a. Skin and mucous membranes for petechiae, ecchymoses, and purpura
  b. Gums, nasal membranes, and conjunctiva for bleeding
  c. Vomitus, stool, and urine for visible or occult blood
  d. Vaginal bleeding
  e. Prolonged bleeding from puncture sites
  f. Neurologic changes such as headache, visual changes, altered mentation, decreased level of consciousness, seizures
  g. Abdomen for complaints of epigastric pain, diminished bowel sounds, increasing abdominal girth, rigidity, or guarding
  Early identification of bleeding helps prevent significant blood loss and potential shock. Internal hemorrhage may lead to tachycardia, hypotension, pallor, and diaphoresis. Bleeding into the lungs may cause dyspnea; bleeding into the abdomen causes increased girth, pain, and guarding. Intracranial bleeding affects mental status and level of consciousness.

- Avoid invasive procedures such as rectal temperatures and suppositories, vaginal douches, suppositories, tampons, urinary catheterization, and parenteral injections if possible. Diagnostic procedures such as biopsy or lumbar puncture should not be done if the platelet count is less than 50,000. *Invasive procedures can cause tissue trauma and bleeding. Procedures that use large-bore needles should be delayed until the platelet count is increased.*

- Apply pressure to injection sites for 3 to 5 minutes, and to arterial punctures for 15 to 20 minutes. *Pressure prevents prolonged bleeding by prompting hemostasis and clot formation.*

- Instruct to avoid forcefully blowing or picking the nose, forceful coughing or sneezing, and straining to have a bowel movement. *These activities can damage mucous membranes, increasing the risk for bleeding.*

- Monitor and promptly report abnormal blood levels of electrolytes, uric acid, urea nitrogen, and creatinine, or manifestations of tumor lysis syndrome. *Significant alterations in electrolyte levels can lead to complications such as cardiac dysrhythmias, muscle weakness or tetany, parethesias, and mental status changes. Excess uric acid can compromise renal function, and lead to metabolic acidosis and gout.*

- Maintain adequate hydration and administer prescribed medications such as allopurinol and diuretics as ordered. *Hydration is vital to maintain renal function and promote elimination of tumor lysis byproducts. Allopurinol reduces the risk of uric acid crystallization in the kidneys and other tissues (Deglin & Vallerand, 2009).*

Anticipatory Grieving

The diagnosis of cancer and a potentially life-threatening illness causes actual or perceived losses, such as loss of function, independence, normal appearance, friends, self-esteem, and self. Grieving is the emotional response to those losses. The adaptive process of mourning a loss and resolving grief is called grief work; grief work cannot begin until a loss is acknowledged. ∞ See Chapter 5 for a detailed discussion of grief and loss.

- Discuss roles of the patient and family and ways in which they managed stressful situations in the past. Assess coping strategies and their effectiveness. Help identify sources of strength and support. Discuss changing roles resulting from leukemia diagnosis, and its effect on spiritual, social, and economic status, and usual lifestyle. Evaluate cultural or ethnic factors that affect grief reactions. *Grieving is a normal response to a real or potential loss that begins at the time of diagnosis. The timing, duration, and intensity of grief and responses to grief may differ among family members. Share information on diagnosis, role change, and physical loss among all family members to build the foundation for mutual understanding and trust.*

- Use therapeutic communication skills to facilitate open discussion of losses and provide permission to grieve. *Encouraging discussion of the meaning of the loss helps decrease some of the anxiety associated with loss. This in turn allows the patient and family to examine the current situation and compare it with past situations that they have coped with successfully.*

- Provide information about agencies that may help in resolving grief, and make referrals as indicated. Consider self-help groups, cancer support groups, and bereavement groups. *Participating in support groups with others who are anticipating or experiencing a similar loss can decrease feelings of isolation.*

Using NANDA, NIC, and NOC

Linkages between a selected NANDA nursing diagnosis, NIC, and NOC for the patient with leukemia are shown in the chart that follows.

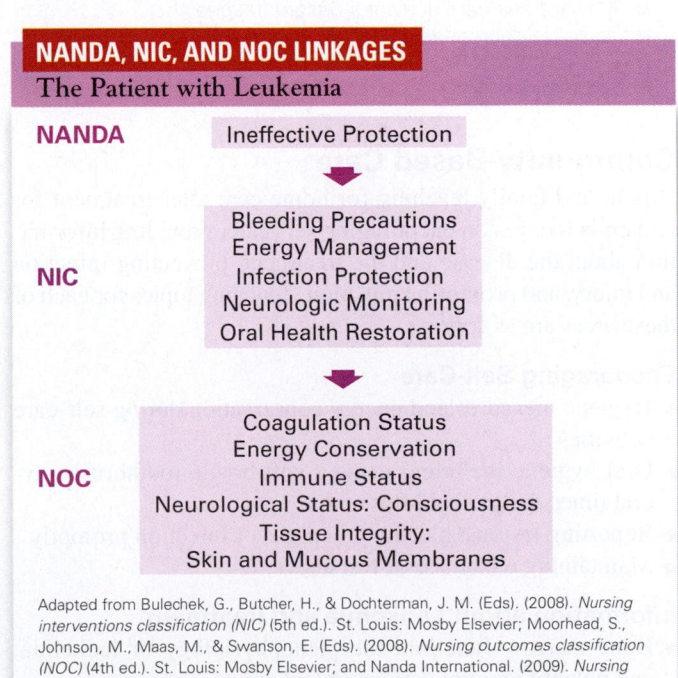

NANDA, NIC, AND NOC LINKAGES
The Patient with Leukemia

NANDA

Ineffective Protection

NIC

Bleeding Precautions
Energy Management
Infection Protection
Neurologic Monitoring
Oral Health Restoration

NOC

Coagulation Status
Energy Conservation
Immune Status
Neurological Status: Consciousness
Tissue Integrity:
Skin and Mucous Membranes

Adapted from Bulechek, G., Butcher, H., & Dochterman, J. M. (Eds). (2008). *Nursing interventions classification (NIC)* (5th ed.). St. Louis: Mosby Elsevier; Moorhead, S., Johnson, M., Maas, M., & Swanson, E. (Eds). (2008). *Nursing outcomes classification (NOC)* (4th ed.). St. Louis: Mosby Elsevier; and Nanda International. (2009). *Nursing diagnoses: Definitions and classification 2009–2011.* Oxford, UK: Wiley-Blackwell.

CASE STUDY & NURSING CARE PLAN   A Patient with Acute Myelocytic Leukemia

Catherine Cole is a 37-year-old secretary who lives with her husband, Ray, and teenaged daughter, Amy, in an apartment in a large metropolitan area. About 2 months ago, Mrs. Cole began to tire easily and experience night sweats several times a week. She also noted that she was pale, bruised easily, and was having heavier menstrual periods. Blood tests ordered by her primary care provider are abnormal. She is admitted for a bone marrow biopsy.

ASSESSMENT

Mary Losapio, RN, obtains a nursing history and physical assessment for Mrs. Cole. Mrs. Cole tells her, "I'm so tired, and I have these bruises all over me. I'm so afraid of the results of the bone marrow examination. I don't know what we will do if I have cancer." Mrs. Cole clutches her husband's hand and then begins to cry. Physical assessment data include height 64 inches (156 cm), weight 106 lb (48.1 kg); vital signs T 100°F, P 102, R 22, BP 130/82. Numerous petechiae scattered over trunk and arms; ecchymoses noted on lower right arm and right calf. Oral mucosa is red, with several small ulcerations in buccal areas.

Blood count shows reduced RBCs, hemoglobin, and hematocrit levels. The WBC is high, with myeloblasts seen on differential. The platelet count is very low. A tentative diagnosis of acute myelogenous leukemia is made.

DIAGNOSES

- *Risk for Infection* related to altered WBC production and immune function
- *Ineffective Protection* related to reduced platelet count and risk for bleeding
- *Impaired Oral Mucous Membrane* secondary to anemia and reduced platelets
- *Fatigue* related to anemia
- *Anxiety* related to fear of leukemia diagnosis

EXPECTED OUTCOMES

- Remain free of infection.
- Experience no significant bleeding.
- Have intact oral mucous membranes.
- Manage self-care activities despite fatigue.
- Verbalize decreased anxiety.

PLANNING AND IMPLEMENTATION

- Place in a private room.
- Limit visitors to immediate family for the present.
- Instruct all staff, the family, and patient to carefully wash hands. Post a sign over the washbasin in the room as a reminder.
- Record vital signs every 4 hours.
- Avoid invasive procedures unless absolutely necessary.
- Monitor for bleeding every 4 hours, including skin, oral mucosa, abdominal assessment, body fluids, and menstrual pad count.
- Instruct to perform oral hygiene every 2 to 4 hours, using a soft-bristle toothbrush.
- Ask the dietitian to work with Mrs. Cole to identify preferred foods. Instruct to avoid foods that may damage oral mucosa, such as very hot, very cold, or highly acidic or spicy foods.
- Provide for periods of rest alternating with activity.
- Teach about the bone marrow biopsy. Allow time for questions and to verbalize fears.
- Refer to the oncology nurse specialist for further teaching and support.

EVALUATION

The bone marrow biopsy confirms the diagnosis of acute myelogenous leukemia. Mrs. Cole is very upset, but calms as the healthcare provider and the oncology nurse discuss treatment plans and the possibility of remission. She decides to have outpatient chemotherapy. During her hospital stay, Mrs. Cole remained free of infection or further bleeding. She tells Ms. Losapio that her mouth feels better, although it is still painful. During routine assessment, Mrs. Cole remarks, "You know, I was so scared when I came here, but I think I am a little less so now. Sometimes not knowing what is wrong is worse than knowing."

CRITICAL THINKING IN THE NURSING PROCESS

1. Describe how alterations in WBCs can increase a person's susceptibility to infection.
2. List sources of potential infection for the hospitalized patient.
3. What is the rationale for having the patient do her own oral and physical hygiene?
4. Outline a teaching plan for this patient and her family for home care to prevent infection.
5. Develop a care plan for Mrs. Cole for the nursing diagnosis *Activity Intolerance*.

See Evaluating Your Response in Appendix C.

Community-Based Care

Patient and family teaching for home care after treatment for leukemia focuses on encouraging self-care, providing information about the disease and the treatment, preventing infection and injury, and promoting nutrition. Teaching topics for each of these areas are as follows.

Encouraging Self-Care

- Hygiene measures and energy conservation during self-care activities
- Oral hygiene including using a soft-bristle toothbrush several times daily; avoid flossing
- Reporting lesions, bleeding, or signs of infection promptly
- Maintaining a balance of rest and activity

Information about Leukemia and Treatment

- Bone marrow function, the pathophysiology of leukemia, and potential complications of leukemia
- Prognosis for the specific type of leukemia

- Treatment measures such as chemotherapy, radiation, bone marrow or stem cell transplant, their purpose and effects, where treatment is available, and potential adverse effects or risks
- Community, regional, and national resources for people with leukemia

Preventing Infection and Injury

- Hand hygiene and other measures to reduce exposure to pathogens such as avoiding people who are ill and avoiding crowds
- Avoiding foodborne illnesses by washing fruits and vegetables, proper food storage
- Dental hygiene measures
- Avoiding immunizations
- Manifestations to report: fever, chills, burning on urination, foul-smelling urine, vaginal or rectal discharge, skin lesions
- Avoiding contact sports or strenuous exercise if platelet count is low

- Using an electric razor for shaving, avoiding rectal or vaginal suppositories, vaginal tampons, or enemas
- Increasing dietary fiber and using a bulk-forming laxative as needed to prevent straining
- Avoiding over-the-counter or prescription drugs that interfere with platelet function (see Box 33–7 on page 1108)
- The importance of reporting any bleeding (nosebleeds, rectal bleeding, vomiting blood, excessive menstrual periods, blood in the urine, bleeding gums, bruises, or collections of blood under the skin) or changes in behavior to the healthcare provider

Promoting Nutrition

- Eating several small, low-fat, high-calorie meals and drinking five to eight glasses of water daily
- Reporting continued weight loss, loss of appetite, or inability to eat for 24 hours
- Discussing dietary needs with the dietitian

Assistance with physical care, finances, and transportation may be required following discharge. Refer the patient and family to social services, support groups, home care services as needed, and other agencies that can provide needed services (such as local chapters of the American Cancer Society, which can provide hospital beds and transportation for outpatient cancer treatment).

The Patient with Malignant Lymphoma

Lymphomas are malignancies of lymphoid tissue. They are characterized by the proliferation of lymphocytes, histiocytes (resident monocytes or macrophages), and their precursors or derivatives. Lymphomas are closely related to lymphocytic leukemias. Some experts consider them to be different forms or stages of the same disease processes.

Although there are many types of malignant lymphoid cells, at this time lymphomas commonly are identified as Hodgkin's disease or non-Hodgkin's lymphoma (Noonan, 2007).

Pathophysiology

Hodgkin's Disease

Hodgkin's disease is a lymphatic cancer, occurring most often in people between the ages of 15 and 35 or over age 50. It is somewhat more common in men than women. Approximately 8270 new cases of Hodgkin's disease were diagnosed in 2008 (ACS, 2008). The exact cause of Hodgkin's disease is unknown, but both Epstein-Barr virus (EBV) infection and genetic factors appear to play a role in its development. Hodgkin's disease is one of the most curable cancers. While as many as 60% to 90% of people with localized disease achieve cure with a normal life span, there may be an increased risk for a second cancer occurrence throughout life (Leahy, 2008).

Hodgkin's disease develops in a single lymph node or chain of nodes, spreading to adjoining nodes. Involved lymph nodes contain *Reed-Sternberg cells* (malignant cells) surrounded by host inflammatory cells. These malignant cells secrete inflammatory mediator substances, attracting inflammatory cells to the tumor site. They may invade almost any tissue in the body. The spleen often is involved; as the disease progresses, the

liver, lungs, digestive tract, and CNS may be affected (Huether & McCance, 2008). Rapid proliferation of abnormal lymphocytes impairs the immune response, especially cell-mediated immune responses. Infections are common.

Hodgkin's disease is classified as classic Hodgkin's disease or as nodular lymphocyte-predominant Hodgkin's disease. The classic form of the disease accounts for 95% of all cases; nodular lymphocyte-predominant Hodgkin's is rare. Classic Hodgkin's can be further divided into four subtypes by cells identified within the tumor, but the subtype does not affect the prognosis (Noonan, 2007).

MANIFESTATIONS The most common symptom of Hodgkin's disease is one or more painlessly enlarged lymph nodes, usually in the cervical or subclavicular region. Systemic manifestations such as persistent fever, night sweats, fatigue, and weight loss are associated with a poorer prognosis for the disease. Late symptoms such as malaise, pruritus, and anemia indicate spread of the disease (Porth, 2005). The spleen may be enlarged, and other organ systems such as the lungs and GI tract are occasionally involved.

Non-Hodgkin's Lymphoma

Non-Hodgkin's lymphoma is a diverse group of lymphoid tissue malignancies that do not contain Reed-Sternberg cells. Non-Hodgkin's lymphomas tend to arise in peripheral lymph nodes and spread early to tissues throughout the body. Non-Hodgkin's lymphoma is more common than Hodgkin's disease, affecting an estimated 56,390 people annually and causing about 19,160 deaths in 2008 (ACS, 2008). Older adults are more often affected, and it occurs more frequently in men than in women. Like Hodgkin's disease, its cause is unknown, although both genetic and environmental factors (e.g., viral infections such as EBV, HTLV-1 and HTLV-2, and HIV) are thought to play a role.

As in most malignancies, non-Hodgkin's lymphoma begins as a single transformed cell; it may arise from T cells, B cells, or tissue macrophages (histiocytes). The primary types of non-Hodgkin's lymphoma are identified in Table 33–7. Although non-Hodgkin's lymphoma usually arises in a lymph node, it can originate in any lymphoid tissue. It tends to spread early and unpredictably to other lymphoid tissues and organs. Extranodal spread may involve the nasopharynx, GI tract, bone, CNS, thyroid, testes, and soft tissue.

The prognosis for non-Hodgkin's lymphoma ranges from excellent to poor, depending on the identified cell type and grade of differentiation. Low grade tumors (better differentiated) tend to be less aggressive and more curable. Higher grade tumors often are disseminated at the time of diagnosis, and have a poorer prognosis (Noonan, 2007; Papadakis & McPhee, 2007).

MANIFESTATIONS The early manifestations of non-Hodgkin's lymphoma are similar to those for Hodgkin's disease. Painless lymphadenopathy may be localized or widespread (Figure 33–9 ■). Systemic manifestations such as fever, night sweats, fatigue, and weight loss may be present, but are less common in non-Hodgkin's lymphoma. Organ system involvement may cause symptoms such as abdominal pain, nausea, and vomiting. Headaches, peripheral or cranial

TABLE 33–7 Subtypes of Non-Hodgkin's Lymphoma

SUBTYPE	INCIDENCE	COURSE AND PROGNOSIS
B-Cell Lymphomas		
Diffuse large B-cell lymphomas	Most common adult type (40%–50% of adult lymphomas) More common in males Incidence increases with aging	Aggressive tumor 45%–50% cure rate
Follicular lymphoma	Accounts for 40% of adult lymphomas, rare in children Incidence increases with aging	Bone marrow frequently involved Course slow, indolent; 72% 5-year survival
Extranodal marginal zone lymphoma (MALT lymphoma)	Accounts for about 5% of adult lymphomas, rare in children Incidence increases with aging More common in Italy	Presents with tumors outside lymphatic system: GI tract, lung, thyroid, urinary tract, skin, CNS Slow, indolent course; 74% 5-year survival
Mantle cell lymphoma	Accounts for 3% to 4% of adult lymphomas, rare in children Predominantly affects older men (74%)	Aggressive, difficult to cure 27% 5-year survival
Burkitt lymphoma	Rare in adults (< 1% of lymphomas), more common in children (~ 30% NHL)	Rapidly progressive but responds well to therapy 45% 5-year survival
T-Cell Lymphoma		
Precursor T-cell lymphoblastic leukemia/lymphoma	More common in children and young adults More common in males than females	Can present either as ALL or lymphoma Aggressive disease; 26% 5-year survival
Peripheral T-cell lymphoma	Most common T-cell lymphoma in adults	Often presents as disseminated disease 25% 5-year survival
Mycosis fungoides/ cutaneous T-cell lymphoma	Onset typically during mid-50s; more common in African Americans	Cutaneous lymphoma Slow course, progressing from patchy skin lesions to plaque to cutaneous tumors

nerve symptoms, altered mental status, or seizures may signal CNS involvement.

The manifestations and clinical features of Hodgkin's disease and non-Hodgkin's lymphoma are compared in Table 33–8.

Course

In both Hodgkin's disease and non-Hodgkin's lymphoma, the stage of the disease, the presence of systemic manifestations, and factors such as age help determine the prognosis. The prognosis is good when the disease is localized to one or two node regions. Factors such as anemia, thrombocytopenia, and older age reduce the likelihood of disease cure.

Incidence and Risk Factors

Malignant lymphomas are the seventh leading cause of cancer deaths in the United States. Approximately 74,340 new cases of lymphoma were diagnosed in 2008, and 20,510 deaths were attributed to the disease. The incidence of non-Hodgkin's lymphoma has nearly doubled since 1970, but currently has stabilized, primarily due to a fall in its incidence related to HIV infection and AIDS. The incidence of Hodgkin's disease has significantly declined since 1990 (ACS, 2008).

While the cause of lymphoma is unknown, some risk factors have been identified. See the accompanying Genetic Considerations box for information about identified genetic links for lymphoma development. Immunosuppression due to drug therapy following organ transplant or to HIV disease increases the risk for non-Hodgkin's lymphoma. Infectious agents such as human T-cell leukemia/lymphoma virus-1 (HTLV-1) and the Epstein-Barr virus (EBV) also have been identified as risk factors. Others may include occupational herbicide or chemical exposure (ACS, 2008).

Interdisciplinary Care

Chemotherapy and radiation therapy, either alone or in combination, are the primary treatments for Hodgkin's disease and non-Hodgkin's lymphoma. Use of monoclonal antibodies to target lymphoma cells, and bone marrow and peripheral stem cell transplants are under investigation for treating lymphomas

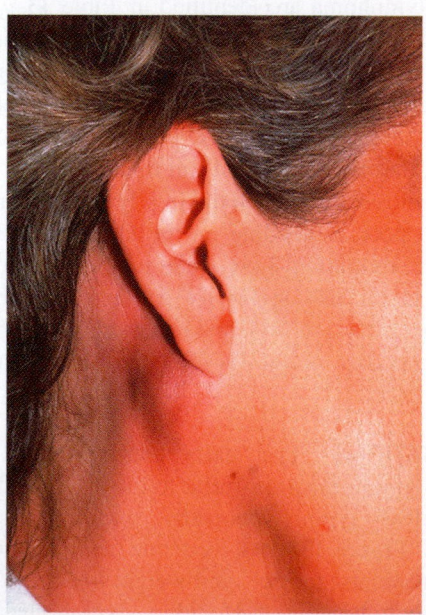

Figure 33–9 ■ Cervical lymphadenopathy in a patient with lymphoma of the neck.

TABLE 33–8 Features and Manifestations of Hodgkin's Disease and Non-Hodgkin's Lymphoma

FEATURE OR MANIFESTATION	HODGKIN'S DISEASE	NON-HODGKIN'S LYMPHOMA
Lymphadenopathy	Localized to a single node or chain, often cervical, subclavicular, or mediastinal	Multiple peripheral nodes, nodes of the mesentery often involved
Spread	Orderly and continuous	Diffuse and unpredictable
Extranodal involvement	Rare	Early and common
Bone marrow involvement	Uncommon	Common
Fever, night sweats, weight loss	Common	Uncommon until disease is extensive
Other manifestations	Fatigue, pruritus, splenomegaly; anemia, neutrophilia	Abdominal pain, nausea, vomiting; dyspnea, cough; CNS symptoms; lymphocytopenia

as well. See the previous section on treatment of leukemia for more information about these transplants.

Diagnosis
The following diagnostic tests may be ordered for lymphomas.

- *CBC* often shows a mild normochromic, normocytic anemia in Hodgkin's disease; other findings in Hodgkin's disease may include leukocytosis with high neutrophil and eosinophil counts, and an elevated sed rate. In non-Hodgkin's lymphoma, the CBC typically remains normal until late in the disease, when pancytopenia may develop.
- An erythrocyte sedimentation rate (ESR) is done to identify possible inflammatory causes of lymph node enlargement.
- *Chemistry studies* of major organ function (including liver function tests and renal function studies) are performed to identify possible organ involvement. Serum LDH levels and *protein electrophoresis* also may be done when Hodgkin's disease is suspected.
- *Chest x-ray* is done to identify possible enlarged mediastinal lymph nodes and pulmonary involvement.
- *CT scans* of the chest, abdomen, and pelvis are performed to identify abnormal or enlarged nodes.
- *PET or gallium scans* may be performed in diagnosing the disease, as well as to evaluate the effectiveness of treatment.
- *Biopsy* of the largest, most central enlarged lymph node and of the bone marrow is done to establish the diagnosis for

GENETIC CONSIDERATIONS
Focus on Lymphoma

Although specific genetic alterations have not been identified for all types of lymphoma, recurring genetic abnormalities associated with lymphomas point to a genetic link in disease development. Three distinct genetic abnormalities have been identified in non-Hodgkin's lymphomas: gross chromosomal changes such as translocations; rearrangements of specific genes; and altered expression of specific oncogenes (over-expression, underexpression, or mutation). Consistent genetic changes are associated with some lymphomas; in other cases, several genetic abnormalities may be seen. Hodgkin's disease is unique from other lymphomas in that no specific genetic abnormalities have been identified (Kasper et al., 2005). For more information about genetics and disease, ∞ see Chapter 8.

both Hodgkin's disease and non-Hodgkin's lymphoma. The presence of Reed-Sternberg cells confirms the diagnosis of Hodgkin's disease.

Staging
Staging is used to determine the extent of the disease and appropriate treatment. The Ann Arbor Staging System is used to assess the extent and severity of lymphomas. The stages are as follows:

Stage I: involvement of a single lymph node region or lymphoid structure (e.g., spleen, thymus, lymphoid tonsillar tissue)

Stage II: involvement of two or more lymph node regions on the same side of the diaphragm

Stage III: involvement of lymph node regions or structures on both sides of the diaphragm
- III_1: limited to upper abdomen (spleen, splenic, celiac, or portal nodes)
- III_2: involvement of lower abdominal nodes (para-aortic, iliac, or mesenteric)

Stage IV: involvement of an extranodal site (not proximal or contiguous with an involved node) such as the liver, lung or pleura, bone or bone marrow, or skin

The presence or absence of systemic symptoms is indicated by either an A (no systemic symptoms) or B (systemic symptoms of fever, night sweats, weight loss).

Chemotherapy
Combination chemotherapy is used to treat both Hodgkin's disease and non-Hodgkin's lymphoma. In both cases, chemotherapy often is followed by radiation therapy to involved lymph node regions. The choice of drug combination depends on the stage of the disease as well as the patient's age and general condition. Combination regimens used in the United States include CHOP (cyclophosphamide, doxorubicin, vincristine, and prednisone), ABVD (doxorubicin, bleomycin, vinblastine, and dacarbazine), MOPP (nitrogen mustard, vincristine, procarbazine, and prednisone), and ChlVPP (chlorambucil, vinblastine, procarbazine, and prednisone). These regimens also may be combined in alternating months to reduce the adverse effects and improve tumor cell kill. More than 75% of patients with Hodgkin's disease who do not have systemic symptoms achieve complete remission with treatment. The prognosis for patients

with non-Hodgkin's lymphoma varies by the type and stage of the disease. For more information about nursing care of the patient receiving combination chemotherapy, ∞ see Chapter 14.

Immunotherapy

Rituximab (Rituxan) is a monoclonal antibody used to destroy the CD20 antigen in B lymphocytes. This destruction results in cellular death of the lymphoma cell. It can be used alone or with cyclophosphamide, vincristine, and prednisone (CVP). The patient should be closely monitored for tumor lysis syndrome (see later in chapter). It is recommended that patients be premedicated with diphenhydramine and acetaminophen. It should be used cautiously in patients with known cardiac disorders (Deglin & Vallerand, 2009; Noonan, 2007).

Radiation Therapy

Radiation therapy may be the primary treatment for early-stage Hodgkin's disease, although early chemotherapy is becoming more common. In later stages and in non-Hodgkin's lymphoma it usually is combined with chemotherapy. Many lymphomas are highly responsive to radiation. The involved lymph node region is treated, with careful shielding to protect unaffected areas and minimize the extent of radiation burn and normal cell destruction (Figure 33–10 ■). If the disease is advanced, total nodal irradiation may be done. ∞ See Chapter 14 for nursing care of the patient receiving radiation therapy.

Stem Cell Transplant

Autologous peripheral blood stem cell transplant (PBSCT) is a treatment option for patients who experience remission of malignant lymphoma. Autologous PBSCT uses the patient's own stem cells to restore bone marrow function after chemotherapy or radiation. In autologous PBSCT, stem cells are obtained from peripheral blood following chemotherapy and treatment with colony-stimulating factors to promote development of normal blood cells. The blood containing these normal stem cells is then frozen and stored for use after treatment. If relapse occurs, lethal doses of chemotherapy or radiation are given to destroy the immune system and malignant cells. The blood is then thawed and infused intravenously through a peripheral line. The infused stem cells become a part of the patient's bone marrow and normal hematopoiesis takes place.

The patient is critically ill during the period of bone marrow destruction and immunosuppression. He or she is hospitalized in a private room for 6 to 8 weeks or more. See the accompanying Moving Evidence into Action box for discussion of fatigue related to autologous PBSCT.

Complications of Treatment

Both chemotherapy and radiation therapy may have long-term effects. Permanent sterility is common, especially in older adults. Bone marrow depression can lead to immunosuppression, anemia, and bleeding. Secondary cancers and cardiac injury are the most serious late adverse effects of treatment. Chemotherapy regimens using the MOPP or a related protocol carry a risk of acute leukemia. Cancers such as breast or lung cancer may develop 10 or more years after thoracic radiation. Thoracic radiation also increases the risk for coronary heart disease and hypothyroidism (Kasper et al., 2005).

Local, or involved field (IF) irradiation

Extended field (EF) irradiation

Mantle field irradiation

Inverted-Y field irradiation

Figure 33–10 ■ Patterns of radiation therapy used to treat lymphoma based on the location and extent of the disease.

∞ Nursing Care

Assessment and priority nursing care for the patient with lymphoma follows. See also the Case Study & Nursing Care Plan at the end of this section for application of nursing care strategies for a specific patient with Hodgkin's disease.

Assessment

Focused assessment of the patient with Hodgkin's disease or non-Hodgkin's lymphoma includes the following:

- *Nursing history:* Complaints of enlarged lymph node(s), fever, night sweats, weight loss, fatigue or general malaise, abdominal pain, respiratory symptoms, numbness or tingling of extremities, visual changes, or changes in mentation; history of infectious mononucleosis, HIV disease, or other immunosuppressive disorders.
- *Physical examination:* Mental status exam; inspect and palpate lymph nodes (cervical, subclavicular, axillary, and inguinal) for enlargement, tenderness; heart and lung sounds; abdominal examination for tenderness, masses, liver or spleen enlargement.

MOVING EVIDENCE INTO ACTION   Patient Undergoing Stem Cell Transplant

Fatigue and depression are common adverse effects of chemotherapy and radiation therapy in patients undergoing cancer treatment. Fatigue is prevalent, affecting 80% to 100% of people undergoing standard chemotherapy and often leading to lost work time and difficulty maintaining functional roles within the family and society. This study (El-Banna, Berger, Farr, Foxall, Friesth, & Schreiner, 2004) sought to describe patterns of fatigue and depression and their relationship to one another among patients undergoing autologous PBSCT. Three time periods during therapy were selected for evaluation: prior to the initiation of chemotherapy, during chemotherapy just prior to transplant, and following the transplant. The setting for this study allowed transplant patients to reside in a hotel-like suite with a designated caregiver (family member or friend).

This study revealed that, among study participants, total fatigue and all its identified dimensions (behavioral, cognitive/mood, sensory, and affective) increased sharply at the time of the transplant, peaking at 7 days post-transplant. Depression followed the same pattern as fatigue, peaking at post-transplant day 7. Peak depression scores were indicative of major depression using the tool employed in this study.

IMPLICATIONS FOR NURSING
This study suggests that nurses should assess for fatigue and depression in patients following stem cell transplant. Nursing measures to help conserve the patient's energy are appropriate to manage fatigue. Early detection and intervention for fatigue may actually reduce the intensity of fatigue at its peak. Nurses can use this information to prepare patients for common symptom patterns following SCT, thus reducing anxiety and concern that their condition may be declining rather than improving after SCT. Additionally, assessment tools to measure fatigue and depression among patients undergoing SCT should be incorporated into nursing care.

CRITICAL THINKING IN PATIENT CARE
1. The average age of participants (N = 27) in this study was 49 years (range 19 to 71 years); 56% were male, 44% female. Does this sample reflect the demographic of patients with malignant lymphoma and those undergoing autologous PBSCT? How can information about the sample be used to guide application of study findings to the general population of patients undergoing this treatment? To older adults? To adolescents and young adults?
2. In this study, participants resided in a hotel-like setting with a family member or friend who participated in care. How might you expect the results to differ had the patient been unable to closely interact with a caregiver of their own choosing?
3. Can the results of this study be applied when caring for patients undergoing allogenic BMT or SCT? Why or why not?

Adapted from El-Banna, M. M., Berger, A. M., Farr, L., Foxall, M. J., Friesth, B., & Schreiner. E. (2004). Fatigue and depression in patients with lymphoma undergoing autologous peripheral blood stem cell transplantation. *Oncology Nursing Forum, 31*(5), 937–944.

- *Diagnostic studies:* CBC, hemoglobin and hematocrit, ESR; serum chemistry results; x-ray, scan, and biopsy results.

Nursing Diagnoses and Interventions
Nursing care of the patient with malignant lymphoma involves both physical and emotional support during diagnosis and treatment. Common nursing care problems include impaired protection due to bone marrow suppression, fatigue, nausea, and altered body image. See the nursing care section for leukemia for specific nursing interventions for *Ineffective Protection*.

Fatigue
General malaise and fatigue may accompany malignant lymphoma and are side effects of chemotherapy. In addition, the physical and psychologic stress of dealing with a chronic, debilitating disease and its treatment may cause fatigue.

- Inquire about feelings of malaise (a vague feeling of body weakness or discomfort) and fatigue (a pervasive, drained feeling that cannot be eliminated). *Both malaise and fatigue are subjective experiences with physiologic, situational, and psychologic components.*
- Encourage verbalization of feelings about the impact of the disease and fatigue on lifestyle. *Discussion of feelings helps the patient clarify values and may assist in identifying priorities.*
- Encourage enjoyable but quiet activities, such as reading, listening to music, or hobbies. *Enjoyable activities help decrease feelings of fatigue. Quiet activities conserve energy while yielding a sense of accomplishment.*

- Encourage to establish priorities and include rest periods or naps when scheduling daily activities. *This provides a sense of control over activities and helps maintain self-esteem. Scheduled rest periods help restore energy and decrease fatigue.*
- Encourage delegation of some responsibilities to family members. *Delegation helps maintain the patient's involvement and role in family decisions and responsibilities, while conserving energy for those activities identified as high priority by the patient.*
- Identify and encourage the patient to use energy-saving equipment. *Performing tasks with less exertion and in less time helps conserve energy.*
- Encourage a diet high in carbohydrates and fluids. *A high-carbohydrate diet helps maintain muscle glycogen stores. A liberal fluid intake promotes excretion of metabolic by-products that may contribute to malaise and fatigue.*

Nausea
The effects of malignant lymphoma and its treatment with chemotherapy and/or radiation therapy can contribute to nausea and interfere with nutritional status. Nausea, a sensation of abdominal fullness, and fear of vomiting often limit food intake. See also the nursing diagnosis *Imbalanced Nutrition* in the section on leukemia for additional interventions.

- Assess precipitating factors for nausea and/or vomiting, the frequency of vomiting, and relief measures used by the patient. *Careful assessment allows development of interventions tailored to the patient's situation and needs.*

- Teach measures to prevent or relieve nausea and vomiting.
  a. Eat soda crackers and suck on hard candy.
  b. Eat soft, bland foods that are cold or at room temperature.
  c. Avoid unpleasant odors, and get fresh air.
  d. Eat prior to but not immediately before chemotherapy.
  e. Use distraction or progressive muscle relaxation when nauseated.
  f. If vomiting occurs, gradually resume oral intake with frequent sips of clear liquids or ice, progressing to bland foods.

Crackers and hard candy often relieve queasiness, whereas hot, spicy, sweet, or strong smelling foods may increase nausea. Alternative nausea relief measures may be effective.

- Provide small feedings of high-kcal, high-protein foods and fluids. *This increases nutritional intake.*
- Assist with oral care, general hygiene, and environmental control of temperature, appearance, and odors. *These measures enhance appetite.*
- Identify and provide preferred foods. *This promotes nutritional intake.*
- Assist to a sitting position during and immediately after meals. *The sitting position helps decrease early feelings of fullness.*

Disturbed Body Image

The diagnosis of cancer is often devastating to the sense of trust in and the perception of one's body. Radiation and chemotherapy lead to changes in appearance and body function (e.g., hair loss, reduced libido, and infertility), further altering body image. Reactions to this diagnosis vary and may include refusal to look in a mirror, refusal to discuss the effects of the disease or treatment, unwillingness to participate in rehabilitation, inappropriate treatment decisions, increasing dependence on others or refusal to provide self-care, hostility, withdrawal, and signs of grieving.

- Assess perception of body image through subjective information such as
  - what the patient likes most and least about his or her body,
  - pre-illness perception of sick or disabled people,
  - current understanding of health and limitations imposed by illness or treatment, and
  - feelings about the illness and its effect on perception of self and others.

Body image is one's mental idea or picture of the body. It is based on past and present experiences and includes components of one's actual body and emotional responses to that body. Body image changes constantly. There is often a time lag between an actual body change and the changed body image; during this time, the diagnosis, teaching, and treatment may be rejected.

- Discuss the risk for and measures to cope with alopecia. Suggest wearing wigs, scarves, hats, or caps. Teach proper scalp care using baby shampoo or mild soap, a soft brush, sunscreen, and mineral oil to reduce itching. If eyelashes and eyebrows are lost, teach eye protection, such as wearing eyeglasses and caps with wide brims. *Chemotherapeutic agents attack rapidly dividing cells such as those responsible for hair growth. Hair loss usually begins 1 to 2 weeks after initiation of chemotherapy, with maximum loss 1 to 2 months later. Alopecia may range from thinning to total hair loss. Regrowth depends on the treatment schedule and doses; however, it usually begins 2 to 3 months after treatment ends. New hair may be softer, curlier, and slightly different in color. Teaching and emotional support help the patient anticipate hair loss, discuss its potential effect on body image, and learn self-care techniques.*

- Discuss available resources for financial assistance with purchase of wigs, including local American Cancer Society chapters and insurance plans. *A well-matched wig (or one the color the patient has always wished for!) can help maintain a positive body image.*

Sexual Dysfunction

Sexual dysfunction may result from the malignancy and the effects of radiation and chemotherapy. Reproductive tissues are made of rapidly dividing cells, and cancer treatment may cause temporary or permanent sterility, changes in menstruation, and changes in libido.

- Encourage discussion of actual or potential sexual dysfunction or sterility with the patient and significant other. *Patients may be reluctant to discuss this unintended effect of treatment unless encouraged.*
- Assess knowledge, provide information, and clarify misconceptions. Discuss realistic measures for coping (e.g., sperm banking prior to chemotherapy or radiation therapy). *Patients and their partners may be unclear about expected effects on sexuality, reproduction, and the permanency of these effects.*
- Refer for counseling as indicated. *Sexual counseling can help the patient and partner develop alternative strategies for expressing their sexuality.*

Risk for Impaired Skin Integrity

Malignant lymphomas may cause significant pruritus and drenching night sweats. As a result, skin integrity may be impaired. In addition, radiation therapy can cause superficial burns, which also may affect skin integrity.

- Frequently assess skin, especially in areas undergoing radiation. *Early identification of lesions allows timely treatment and can prevent further disruption of this important line of defense against infection.*
- Provide and teach measures to promote comfort and relieve itching: Use cool water and a mild soap to bathe; blot (rather than rub) dry skin; apply plain cornstarch or non-perfumed lotion or powder to the skin unless contraindicated; use lightweight blankets and clothing; maintain adequate humidity and a cool room temperature; wash bedding and clothes in mild detergent, and put them through second rinse cycle. *Pruritus is aggravated by excessive warmth, excessive dryness, rough fabrics, fatigue, and stress. Lotions and some powders may be contraindicated during radiation therapy.*

Albin Quito, aged 28, is the nurse manager of a thoracic intensive care unit in a large teaching hospital. Lately he has been more tired than usual, often wakes up at night covered with sweat, and just does not feel well. He had thought that his symptoms were due to a viral illness and his busy work schedule. However, yesterday morning Mr. Quito noticed a large swollen area on the right side of his neck. He made an appointment with his primary health provider who found a large cervical lymph node. A biopsy of the node and a CT scan of the chest were scheduled.

ASSESSMENT

David Herzog, the nurse in charge of the outpatient clinic, obtains a nursing history and assessment on Mr. Quito. His physical examination is essentially normal, with the exception of the enlarged node, which is not tender to palpation. When Mr. Quito is weighed, he tells Mr. Herzog that he has lost 7 lb (3.2 kg) in the past 2 months. In reviewing the results of the blood studies, Mr. Herzog notes mild anemia and an increased neutrophil count. The lymph node biopsy shows Reed-Sternberg cells. The clinic healthcare provider and Mr. Herzog tell Mr. Quito that the findings indicate stage 1-B Hodgkin's disease but that the prognosis is very good. The healthcare provider recommends a short course of combination chemotherapy followed by radiation therapy to involved sites.

DIAGNOSES

- *Anxiety* related to the diagnosis of Hodgkin's disease and effects of treatment on job performance
- *Risk for Infection* related to potential bone marrow depression due to chemotherapy
- *Fatigue* related to effects of cancer, chemotherapy, and radiation therapy

EXPECTED OUTCOMES

- Verbalize reduced anxiety.
- Remain free of infection.
- Identify and use methods to preserve energy.

PLANNING AND IMPLEMENTATION

- Encourage to consider a leave of absence from work during course of treatment.
- Discuss joining a support group for people with cancer.
- Provide information about the illness, combination chemotherapy, and radiation therapy.
- Reinforce knowledge of actions to decrease the risk of infection.
- Discuss ways to decrease fatigue and maintain energy:
  - Take a 1- to 2-hour nap once or twice a day.
  - Avoid overexertion during weekends and time off.
  - Maintain a well-balanced diet.

EVALUATION

When Mr. Quito returns the following week to begin chemotherapy, he brings his friend Nancy to meet Mr. Herzog and asks him to discuss his treatment with her. Mr. Quito says, "I am still really scared, but being able to talk about this with Nancy will help a lot." Mr. Quito has made arrangements to take a 4-month leave from work, with the understanding that his job will be held for him. He states that he will have some problems with money but is working them out. He also says he feels that taking a nap is silly but that he will rest to maintain his energy level. Mr. Quito and Nancy express confidence that he will be cured and say they plan to be active members of the cancer support group—even after recovery.

CRITICAL THINKING IN THE NURSING PROCESS

1. Discuss the rationale for treating Hodgkin's disease with chemotherapy and radiation.
2. Design a teaching plan to help Mr. Quito prevent infection while he is at home.
3. What effect does the diagnosis of cancer have on the developmental tasks of a young adult?
4. Develop a care plan for Mr. Quito for the diagnosis *Ineffective Role Performance*.

See Evaluating Your Response in Appendix C.

Using NANDA, NIC, and NOC

Linkages between a selected NANDA nursing diagnosis, NIC, and NOC for the patient with malignant lymphoma are shown in the chart that follows.

Community-Based Care

When teaching the patient and family about home care, include the following topics in addition to those previously identified for specific nursing diagnoses.

- Information about the illness, planned treatment, and anticipated side effects of treatment
- Skin care and measures to relieve itching and protect areas of radiation
- Symptoms to report to the healthcare provider, including those of vertebral compression (decreased sensation or strength in lower extremities)
- Use of analgesics and alternative relief strategies for abdominal pain and peripheral neuropathies
- Respiratory care if mediastinal nodes are enlarged or lungs or pleurae are involved
- Planning ADLs to ensure adequate rest and exercise
- Measures to relieve nausea and maintain adequate nutrition

Refer patients and family members to the local chapter of the American Cancer Society for information, assistance, and

NANDA, NIC, AND NOC LINKAGES
The Patient with Malignant Lymphoma

NANDA — Sexual Dysfunction

NIC — Active Listening / Coping Enhancement / Emotional Support / Sexual Counseling

NOC — Body Image / Psychosocial Adjustment: Life Change / Self-Esteem / Sexual Functioning

Adapted from Bulechek, G., Butcher, H., & Dochterman, J. M. (Eds). (2008). *Nursing interventions classification (NIC)* (5th ed.). St. Louis: Mosby Elsevier; Moorhead, S., Johnson, M., Maas, M., & Swanson, E. (Eds). (2008). *Nursing outcomes classification (NOC)* (4th ed.). St. Louis: Mosby Elsevier; and Nanda International. (2009). *Nursing diagnoses: Definitions and classification 2009–2011.* Oxford, UK: Wiley-Blackwell.

counseling. A list of state and local agencies that offer information about malignant lymphoma and financial assistance can be obtained from the Leukemia Society of America.

The Patient with Multiple Myeloma

Multiple myeloma is a malignancy in which plasma cells multiply uncontrollably and infiltrate the bone marrow, lymph nodes, spleen, and other tissues. *Plasma cells* are B-cell lymphocytes that develop to produce antibodies (immunoglobulin).

Pathophysiology

Malignant plasma cells arise from one clone (*monoclonal*) of B cells that produce abnormally large amounts of a particular immunoglobulin called the *M protein*. This abnormal protein interferes with normal antibody production and impairs the humoral immune response. It also increases blood viscosity and may damage kidney tubules. As myeloma cells proliferate, they replace the bone marrow and infiltrate the bone itself. Cortical bone is progressively destroyed by tumor growth and enzymes produced by myeloma cells. These enzymes facilitate bone destruction, its infiltration by tumor cells, development of new blood vessels to sustain the tumor, and growth of myeloma cells (Huether & McCance, 2008). Affected bones (primarily the vertebrae, ribs, skull, pelvis, femur, clavicle, and scapula) are weakened and may break without trauma (*pathologic fracture*). With disease progression, malignant cells spread via the bloodstream to invade other organs (Figure 33–11 ■).

Figure 33–11 ■ An illustration of the progress of multiple myeloma in an African American male. Abnormal plasma cells proliferate uncontrollably, gradually replacing bone marrow and infiltrating bone itself. As the disease progresses, these cells spread to other organs via the bloodstream.

Manifestations

The disease develops slowly, with up to 30% of patients diagnosed during evaluation for unrelated problems, and is known for being difficult to diagnose (Dvorak, 2006). Manifestations of multiple myeloma are due to its effects on the bone and the impaired immune response due to M protein production. Bone pain is the most common presenting symptom. With progression of the disease, the pain may increase in severity and become more localized. Rapid bone destruction releases calcium from the bone, leading to hypercalcemia and manifestations of neurologic dysfunction, such as lethargy, confusion, and weakness.

As functional antibody formation decreases and the humoral immune response is suppressed, recurrent infections develop. Cell-mediated immunity remains intact. *Bence Jones proteins* are found in the urine in multiple myeloma. These proteins are toxic to the renal tubules, and may lead to renal failure with azotemia and uremia (∞ see Chapter 28 for more information about renal failure).

About 15% of patients with multiple myeloma die within 3 months of the diagnosis. More frequently, the disease course is chronic, progressing more rapidly with each relapse after remission. The acute terminal stage of the disease is marked by pancytopenia and widespread organ infiltration by myeloma cells (Huether & McCance, 2008).

Incidence and Risk Factors

The incidence of multiple myeloma is increasing slightly, with an estimated 19,920 cases diagnosed and 10,620 deaths due to the disease in 2008 (ACS, 2008). It affects Blacks nearly twice as often as Whites, and men slightly more frequently than women. The incidence of multiple myeloma increases with age, rarely occurring before age 40 (Dvorak, 2006; Huether & McCance, 2008)). Its cause is unknown. Possible contributing factors include genetic alterations, radiation exposure, oncogenic virus, inflammatory stimuli, and chronic antigenic stimulation. The risk for developing multiple myeloma is higher in people of lower socioeconomic status. This increased risk may relate to environmental factors such as poor housing, occupational hazards, poor nutritional status, and other physical and psychosocial stressors such as exposure to infectious agents (Dvorak, 2006).

Interdisciplinary Care

Diagnosis and Staging

Diagnostic tests for multiple myeloma include the following:

- *X-rays* and other radiologic studies of the bone may reveal multiple punched-out lesions.
- *Bone marrow examination* shows an abnormal number of immature plasma cells.
- *CBC* shows moderate to severe anemia, and the ESR usually is elevated.
- *Protein electrophoresis* shows a spike of one type of antibody, usually IgG.
- *Serum calcium, creatinine, uric acid,* and *BUN* levels often are elevated.
- *Urinalysis* shows Bence Jones protein in the urine.
- *Biopsy* of myeloma lesions confirms the diagnosis of multiple myeloma.

Staging of multiple myeloma is based on the hemoglobin and serum calcium levels, the amount of abnormal protein present, and the degree of bone involvement.

Treatment

There is no cure for multiple myeloma. In some patients, active observation is indicated, as the disease may continue with a slow, *indolent* (sluggish, not developing or progressing) course for many years (Dvorak, 2006). When indicated by disease stage or progression, standard treatment includes induction chemotherapy followed by stem cell transplant and maintenance chemotherapy to control progression of the disease. Supportive care is provided to reduce complications of the disease and their effects.

Combination chemotherapy with an alkylating agent (melphalan [Alkeran], cyclophosphamide [Cytoxan], or chlorambucil [Chloromycetin]) and prednisone administered for 4 to 7 days every 4 to 6 weeks is commonly used. Chemotherapy typically reduces bone pain, hypercalcemia, anemia, and the number of infections. Novel therapies that include immunomodulatory drugs lenalidomide (Revlimid) and thalidomide (Thalomid) and the proteasome inhibitor bortezomib (Velcade) contribute to improved survival rates and better response rates when compared to conventional chemotherapy (Miceli et al., 2008). Localized radiation therapy may be used to treat painful bone lesions. High-dose chemotherapy followed by peripheral allogenic stem cell transplant may be more effective in achieving cure, but is associated with a high mortality rate. When autologous SCT is used, granulocyte colony-stimulating factor is administered prior to harvesting and preserving peripheral stem cells for collection, preservation, and transplant.

Supportive care may include treatment of hypercalcemia with hydration, possible biphosphonate therapy to reduce bone loss (∞ see Chapter 40), and calcium, vitamin D, and fluoride supplements to support bone structure. Plasma exchange therapy (plasmapheresis) to remove circulating M proteins is used as needed to treat acute renal failure. Infections are treated promptly when they develop.

∞ Nursing Care

Assessment

Focused assessment data for the patient with multiple myeloma includes the following:

- *Health history:* Complaints of back or bone pain, onset, duration, and intensity; complaints of weakness, fatigue, anorexia; history of frequent or recurrent infections; neurologic symptoms such as numbness and tingling or clumsiness.
- *Physical examination:* Level of consciousness and mental status; mobility, gait; localized tenderness or pain, bony crepitus with movement or palpation; movement and sensation in extremities.

Nursing Diagnoses and Interventions

Nursing care of the patient with multiple myeloma focuses on problems of chronic pain, impaired mobility, and the risk for injury. Risk for infection is a major nursing care focus; see the previous section on leukemia for specific interventions to reduce this risk. Other nursing care needs are similar to those of patients with other cancers and chronic pain. ∞ See Chapters 9 and 14 for additional specific nursing interventions for these problems.

Chronic Pain

Patients with multiple myeloma typically experience chronic back pain and deep bone pain as myeloma cells saturate the bone marrow and invade the bone structure. Pathologic fractures are a common and reoccurring problem.

- Assess pain, including intensity (use a standard pain scale), onset, duration, precipitating factors, and effective relief measures. *Identifying the intensity, causes, and precipitating factors of pain helps determine and evaluate effective pain relief measures.*
- Determine position of greatest comfort, and assist as needed into this position. *The patient is best able to identify positions that minimize pain, but may need assistance with repositioning.*
- Support position with pillows. *Bony prominences may be painful due to infiltrates. Pillows can help relieve pressure on these prominences, thus reducing pain.*
- Provide uninterrupted rest periods. *Adequate rest facilitates pain relief and improves pain tolerance.*
- Teach adjunctive pain relief strategies such as relaxation or guided imagery. *A combination of pharmacologic and nonpharmacologic methods provides better management of chronic pain, especially bone pain.*
- Teach effective analgesic use, including the family in instruction. *Analgesics are most effective when taken before pain becomes severe. Patients and their families may be reluctant to use prescription analgesics on a regular basis.*
- Report unrelieved pain to the healthcare provider. *A different analgesic or addition of an adjunctive medication such as a nonsteroidal anti-inflammatory drug (NSAID) may be needed to effectively control pain.*

Impaired Physical Mobility

Painful bony infiltrates and pathologic fractures may limit mobility. A brace or splint may be used to protect extremities or support the back. In addition, persistent weakness associated with the cancer and anemia may limit the patient's ability to participate in usual activities.

- Assist to change position at least every 2 hours. *Assistance with repositioning is necessary due to weakness. Frequent repositioning improves comfort and reduces the risk for impaired skin and tissue integrity.*

> **PRACTICE ALERT**
> Gently support extremities during repositioning. Weakened extremities due to infiltration of bone by myeloma cells and muscle atrophy from lack of use increase the risk for pathologic fractures.

- Provide a trapeze to assist in repositioning. *A trapeze provides better leverage, allowing the patient to assist with repositioning and providing a degree of independence. The ability to participate in self-care improves self-esteem.*

Risk for Injury

The bone involvement of multiple myeloma places the patient at high risk for pathologic and traumatic fractures. Pathologic fractures can occur with simple activities such as turning or reaching for an item. The spine usually is affected; the ribs and bones of the extremities also may be at risk for fracture.

- Place needed items close at hand. *Straining to reach objects increases the risk of falling or sustaining other injury.*
- Provide safety measures to prevent falls from bed: Place the bed in a low position, use side rails as indicated, and place the call bell within reach. *Safety measures help prevent accidental injury. A secure environment minimizes risk and helps prevent falls.*
- Provide shoes with nonskid soles, a clear pathway, adequate lighting, and a level surface free of scatter rugs or other hazards when ambulating. Provide a walker as needed for support and security. *Weightbearing exercise promotes bone repair. Safety measures, such as an unobstructed pathway and a firm walking surface, help prevent falls.*

Community-Based Care

When teaching patients and their families for home care, include the following topics:

- Strategies for home maintenance management
- Signs and symptoms of complications to be reported to the healthcare provider (e.g., symptoms of vertebral and extremity fractures)
- Manifestations of infection to report: fever and chills; increased malaise, fatigue, or weakness; cough with or without sputum; sore throat; dysuria, nocturia, frequency, urgency, or malodorous urine

Provide referrals for home health and home maintenance services, physical or occupational therapy, social services, and hospice care as appropriate.

The Patient with Neutropenia

Leukopenia is a decrease in the total circulating WBC count. Although any type of WBC may be affected, neutrophils, which make up the majority of WBCs, are affected most often. *Neutropenia* is a decrease in circulating neutrophils, usually less than 1500 cells/μm. Neutropenia may be either congenital or acquired, developing secondarily to prolonged infection, hematologic disorders, starvation, or autoimmune disorders (such as rheumatoid arthritis). Chemotherapy and other drugs can suppress the bone marrow. Neutropenia develops in approximately half of patients undergoing chemotherapy to treat cancer (Miceli et al., 2008). *Agranulocytosis* is severe neutropenia, with less than 200 cells/μm. Numbers of other granulocytes also are reduced. It is usually due to impaired leukocyte formation in the bone marrow or increased cell destruction in circulating blood. Agranulocytosis significantly increases the risk for infection. *Aplastic anemia* affects production of all blood cells, resulting in anemia, thrombocytopenia, and agranulocytosis.

Pathophysiology and Manifestations

Neutrophils are an integral component of the immune response. They are phagocytes, drawn to and activated by infection and inflammation to engulf and degrade invading microorganisms. Their lifespan in peripheral blood is short, less than 1 day. When *granulopoiesis* (the development and maturation of granulocytes) in the bone marrow is suppressed, the number of circulating neutrophils falls rapidly. As a result, the body's ability to defend itself against infection is significantly reduced.

The manifestations of neutropenia reflect the resulting impaired immunity and inflammatory response. Opportunistic bacterial, fungal, and protozoal infections develop, commonly affecting the respiratory tract and mucosa of the mouth, GI tract, and vagina. Malaise, chills, and fever with extreme weakness and fatigue are common manifestations.

Interdisciplinary Care

The diagnosis of neutropenia is made based on the patient's manifestations, risk factors and the CBC. The total WBC is low, often less than 1000/mm^3.

Hematopoietic growth factors such as GM-CSF are administered to stimulate granulocyte maturation and differentiation. Infections are treated with antibiotic therapy. Protective isolation procedures may be initiated to prevent exposure to pathogens. When neutropenia is related to chemotherapy, cancer treatment often must be halted, at least temporarily, to allow the bone marrow to recover.

Nursing Care

The primary nursing care focus is early identification of neutropenia and protecting the patient from infection. The WBC count is monitored on a regular basis, and any decline reported to the healthcare provider. Protective isolation may be indicated, including restricting the number of visitors and people with apparent illness. See Risk for Infection in the earlier section on leukemia for specific nursing interventions for the patient with neutropenia.

The Patient with Infectious Mononucleosis

Infectious mononucleosis is characterized by invasion of B cells in the oropharyngeal lymphoid tissues by the Epstein-Barr virus (EBV). This disease is usually benign and self-limiting. It often affects young adults between the ages of 15 and 30. Although many children are infected with EBV, symptomatic infectious mononucleosis is uncommon in early childhood. The virus is present in saliva, which appears to be the primary mode of transmission. As a result, infectious mononucleosis is often called the "kissing disease."

EBV also is associated with some cancers, including Burkitt's lymphoma and Hodgkin's disease, B-cell lymphoma, and nasopharyngeal carcinoma (Noonan, 2006).

Pathophysiology and Manifestations

When the virus enters the body, unaffected B cells produce antibodies against the virus, and T cells directly attack the virus. Infected B cells are destroyed as the virus replicates. The proliferation of B and T cells, as well as the removal of dead and damaged leukocytes, is responsible for the swelling of lymphoid tissues.

The incubation period for infectious mononucleosis is 4 to 8 weeks. Its onset is insidious, with headache, malaise, and fatigue. Fever, sore throat, and cervical lymphadenopathy (lymph node enlargement and pain) lasting 1 to 3 weeks is common. Symptom severity varies from person to person. Lymph node involvement may be generalized; about 50% of

people with infectious mononucleosis develop an enlarged spleen (splenomegaly).

Interdisciplinary Care

Laboratory findings include increased lymphocytes and monocytes, with about 20% of the cells atypical in form. Early in the infection, the WBC count usually is normal or low, but by the second week it increases and remains elevated for 4 to 8 weeks. Platelet counts are often low during the illness.

Recovery occurs in 2 to 3 weeks; however, debility and lethargy may last for up to 3 months. The treatment includes bed rest and analgesic agents to alleviate the symptoms. Nursing care is primarily educational to prevent further spread of the disease.

Platelet and Coagulation Disorders

Platelet and coagulation disorders affect **hemostasis**, control of bleeding. Hemostasis maintains a relatively steady state of blood volume, blood pressure, and blood flow through injured vessels.

Bleeding disorders result from deficient platelets, disruption of the clotting cascade, or a combination of factors.

The Patient with Thrombocytopenia

Thrombocytopenia is a platelet count of less than 100,000 per milliliter of blood. It can lead to abnormal bleeding. A continuing decline in circulating platelets to less than 20,000/mL can lead to spontaneous bleeding and hemorrhage from minor trauma (Figure 33–12 ■). Bleeding due to platelet deficiency usually occurs in small vessels, causing manifestations such as *petechiae* and *purpura*. The mucous membranes of the nose, mouth, GI tract, and vagina often bleed. Serious and potentially fatal bleeding occurs when the platelet count is less than 10,000/mL.

Thrombocytopenia results from one of three mechanisms: decreased production, increased sequestration in the spleen, or

accelerated destruction. Primary thrombocytopenia that leads to increased platelet destruction is discussed next. Secondary thrombocytopenia may be caused by aplastic anemia, bone marrow malignancy, infection, radiation therapy, or drug therapy (Box 33–6). Heparin therapy is the most common drug-induced thrombocytopenia; it is included in the discussion that follows. Platelet sequestration usually is due to an enlarged spleen. Up to 80% of platelets may be removed from circulation with significant splenomegaly (Huether & McCance, 2008). Finally, thrombocytopenia may result from premature platelet destruction associated with disseminated intravascular coagulation (DIC).

Physiology Review

Effective control of bleeding requires a series of complex interactions between the damaged tissue and blood vessel, platelets, clotting factors, and processes to dissolve clots once bleeding has been controlled. Platelets are formed in the bone marrow under control of thrombopoietin, a protein produced by the

Figure 33–12 ■ Significant ecchymosis of the eyelid associated with minor trauma in a patient with thrombocytopenia.

BOX 33–6 Selected Causes of Secondary Thrombocytopenia

Diseases
- Vitamin-B_{12} anemia
- Folic acid anemia
- Aplastic anemia
- Leukemia
- Alcoholism
- DIC
- Infectious mononucleosis
- Viral infections
- HIV disease

Drugs
- Thiazide diuretics
- Aspirin
- Ibuprofen
- Indomethacin
- Naproxen
- Sulfonamides
- Phenytoin
- Cimetidine
- Digoxin
- Furosemide
- Heparin
- Morphine

Treatments
- Radiation therapy
- Chemotherapy
- Massive transfusion of stored blood

liver, kidney, smooth muscle, and bone marrow. Platelets are attracted to the damaged vessel wall, where they aggregate and release mediators that activate the clotting process. ∞ See Chapter 29 for a more complete discussion about platelets, clotting, and hemostasis.

Pathophysiology

The two types of primary thrombocytopenia are immune thrombocytopenic purpura and thrombotic thrombocytopenic purpura.

Immune Thrombocytopenic Purpura

Immune thrombocytopenic purpura (ITP), also known as *idiopathic thrombocytopenic purpura*, is an autoimmune disorder in which platelet destruction is accelerated. In ITP, proteins on the platelet cell membrane stimulate autoantibody production, usually IgG antibodies. These autoantibodies adhere to the platelet membrane. Although the platelets function normally, the spleen reacts to them as being foreign and destroys the altered platelets after only 1 to 3 days of circulation.

MANIFESTATIONS The manifestations of ITP are due to bleeding from small vessels and mucous membranes. Petechiae and purpura develop, often on the anterior chest, arms, neck, and oral mucous membranes. Bruising also may be apparent. As bleeding progresses, epistaxis (nosebleed), hematuria, excess menstrual bleeding, and bleeding gums occur. Spontaneous intracranial bleeding is rare but does occur. Associated symptoms include weight loss, fever, and headache.

INCIDENCE AND COURSE Acute ITP affects people of any age following a viral illness (Papadakis & McPhee, 2007). Acute ITP typically lasts only 1 to 2 months, resolving without long-term consequences. In its chronic form, ITP typically affects adults between the ages of 20 and 50; women are affected more often than men. Its onset is insidious. Chronic (or adult) ITP often occurs in people with other immune-associated disorders such as systemic lupus erythematosus or HIV disease (Papadakis & McPhee, 2007).

Thrombotic Thrombocytopenic Purpura

Thrombotic thrombocytopenic purpura (TTP) is a rare disorder in which thrombi occlude arterioles and capillaries of the microcirculation. Many organs are affected, including the heart, kidneys, and brain. The incidence of TTP is increasing (Huether & McCance, 2008). Its cause is unknown. Platelet aggregation is a key feature of the disorder. As RBCs circulate through partially occluded vessels, they fragment, leading to hemolytic anemia (Porth, 2002).

MANIFESTATIONS TTP may be acute, the more common and severe form, or chronic. Acute idiopathic TTP may be fatal within months if untreated. The manifestations of TTP include purpura and petechiae, and neurologic symptoms such as headache, seizures, and altered consciousness.

Heparin-Induced Thrombocytopenia

Heparin-induced thrombocytopenia (HIT) develops as a result of an abnormal response to heparin therapy. Unfractionated heparin carries a greater potential to precipitate HIT; it can, however, develop in patients receiving low-molecular weight

heparin who have previously been treated with unfractionated heparin. ∞ See Chapter 32 for further discussion of heparin therapy and the forms of heparin.

Heparin is a protein that occurs naturally in human tissues and inflammatory cells. It can react directly with platelets, causing them to agglutinate (clump), and be removed from circulation by phagocytosis. This form of HIT, called type I HIT, typically causes mild thrombocytopenia. The more severe form, type II HIT, results from an immune reaction to heparin. In type II HIT, heparin forms an immune complex with a platelet protein known as platelet factor 4 (PF4). This complex acts as a foreign antigen in some patients, stimulating antibody production. The antibody binds with the heparin-PF4 complex, and these antibody-heparin-PF4 complexes subsequently bind with circulating platelets, causing them to aggregate. As affected platelets aggregate, they are removed from circulation, leading to thrombocytopenia. In addition, small pieces of platelets can break loose, stimulating the clotting cascade and the development of thrombosis (clotting). The thrombocytopenia and the thrombosis can be reversed by prompt withdrawal of heparin therapy (Papadakis & McPhee, 2007).

MANIFESTATIONS Despite thrombocytopenia, bleeding is usually a manifestation of HIT, probably because of the increased tendency to form clots. The patient may develop manifestations of an arterial thrombosis (severe pain, paresthesias, pallor and cool skin temperature, and pulselessness distal to the arterial occlusion) or of venous thrombosis (edema, redness, and warmth of the affected area). On rare occasion, an intravenous bolus of unfractionated heparin can precipitate an acute inflammatory response with manifestations that may mimic an acute pulmonary embolism—fever, chills, hypertension, tachycardia, dyspnea, chest pain, and cardiopulmonary arrest.

Interdisciplinary Care

The diagnosis of thrombocytopenia is based on history, manifestations, and diagnostic test results. Management focuses on treating or removing any causative factors and treating the platelet deficiency.

Diagnosis

The following diagnostic tests are used to identify thrombocytopenia.

- *CBC with platelet count* is done to evaluate blood cell counts, hemoglobin, and hematocrit.
- *Antinuclear antibodies (ANA)* are measured to assess for autoantibodies and identify possible contributing disorders such as systemic lupus erythematosus.
- *Serologic studies* for hepatitis viruses, cytomegalovirus (CMV), Epstein-Barr virus, toxoplasma, and HIV may be done. Serologic testing also may be performed when HIT is suspected.
- *Bone marrow examination* evaluates for aplastic anemia and megakaryocyte production.

Medications

Oral glucocorticoids, such as prednisone, are prescribed to suppress the autoimmune response. Many patients who respond to glucocorticoid treatment relapse when the drug is withdrawn, however. Immunosuppressive drugs such as azathioprine, cyclophosphamide, and cyclosporine may be used.

Prompt withdrawal of heparin therapy is vital when HIT is the cause of thrombocytopenia. All sources of heparin are removed, including heparin used to flush intravenous or other catheters and heparin-coated catheters. A non-heparin anticoagulant such as lepirudin (Refludan) or argatroban may be substituted. Lepirudin is a thrombin inhibitor. It is a recombinant form of hirudin, originally isolated from the salivary glands of leeches. Its primary adverse effect is bleeding; as a protein, it also can stimulate antibody development, resulting in rare instances of anaphylaxis. Argatroban is a synthetic direct thrombin inhibitor with a short half-life. It clears quickly when the infusion is discontinued, an advantage if excessive bleeding develops or invasive procedures must be performed (Deglin & Vallerand, 2009).

Treatments

Platelet transfusions may be required to treat acute bleeding due to thrombocytopenia. Platelets are prepared from fresh whole blood; one unit contains 30 to 60 mL of platelet concentrate. The expected increase in platelets after one unit is infused is 10,000/mL. *Plasmapheresis*, or *plasma exchange therapy*, is the primary treatment for acute thrombotic thrombocytopenic purpura. The patient's plasma is removed and replaced with fresh frozen plasma to remove autoantibodies, immune complexes, and toxins.

Surgery

A *splenectomy* (surgical removal of the spleen) is the treatment of choice if the patient with ITP relapses when glucocorticoids are discontinued. The spleen is the site of platelet destruction and antibody production. This surgery often cures the disorder, although relapse may occur years after splenectomy.

♒ Nursing Care

Assessment

- *Health history:* Complaints of bruising with minor or no trauma, bleeding gums, nosebleed, heavy or prolonged menstrual periods; black, tarry, or bloody stools; hematemesis, headache, fever, or neurologic symptoms; recent weight loss; recent viral or other illness; current and recent medications; exposure to toxins; previous exposure to heparin.
- *Physical examination:* Skin and mucous membranes for color, temperature, petechiae, purpura, or bruises; vital signs; weight; mental status and level of consciousness; heart and breath sounds; abdominal exam; body fluids for occult blood.
- *Laboratory data:* CBC, hemoglobin and hematocrit, platelet count; serologic and ANA test results; bone marrow examination results.

Nursing Diagnoses and Interventions

Inadequate platelets impair hemostasis, placing the patient at risk for bleeding. Bleeding gums, an early sign of the disorder, affects oral mucous membrane integrity as well.

Ineffective Protection

Bleeding is a serious complication associated with thrombocytopenia. As platelet counts (measured in cubic millimeters) decrease, the risk of bleeding increases: The risk is minimal with counts greater than 50,000 mm^3; moderate when the count is between 20,000 and 50,000 mm^3; and significant when the count falls below 20,000 mm^3.

- Monitor vital signs, heart and breath sounds every 4 hours. Frequently assess for other manifestations of bleeding:
  a. Skin and mucous membranes for petechiae, ecchymoses, and hematoma formation
  b. Gums, nasal membranes, and conjunctiva for bleeding
  c. Overt or occult blood in emesis, urine, or stool
  d. Vaginal bleeding
  e. Prolonged bleeding from puncture sites
  f. Neurologic changes: headache, visual changes, altered mental status, decreasing level of consciousness, seizures
  g. Abdominal: epigastric pain, absence of bowel sounds, increasing abdominal girth, abdominal guarding or rigidity
  Early identification of bleeding is important to prevent serious blood loss and shock.

> **PRACTICE ALERT**
> Avoid invasive procedures such as rectal temperatures, urinary catheterization, and parenteral injections to the extent possible. Diagnostic procedures such as biopsy or lumbar puncture should be avoided if the platelet count is less than 50,000 mm^3. Invasive procedures can cause tissue trauma and bleeding. Procedures that use large-bore needles should be delayed until the platelet count is increased.

- Apply pressure to puncture sites for 3 to 5 minutes; apply pressure to arterial blood gas sites for 15 to 20 minutes. *Pressure promotes hemostasis and clot formation.*
- Instruct to avoid forcefully blowing the nose or picking crusts from the nose, straining to have a bowel movement, and forceful coughing or sneezing. *These activities increase the risk of external and internal bleeding.*

Impaired Oral Mucous Membranes

Thrombocytopenia frequently leads to bleeding of the gums and oral mucosa. As a result, risk for infection and impaired nutrition increases.

- Frequently assess the mouth for bleeding. Inquire about oral pain or tenderness. *Breakdown of oral mucous membranes increases the risk of infection and bleeding, and causes discomfort with eating.*
- Encourage use of a soft-bristle toothbrush or sponge to clean teeth and gums. *Hard bristles may abrade oral mucosa, causing bleeding and increasing the risk of infection.*
- Instruct to rinse the mouth with saline every 2 to 4 hours. Apply petroleum jelly to lips as needed to prevent dryness and cracking. *Saline mouth rinses and petroleum jelly help maintain oral tissue integrity and promote cleansing and healing.*
- Instruct to avoid alcohol-based mouthwashes, very hot foods, alcohol, and crusty foods. Teach to drink cool liquids at least every 2 hours. *Avoiding foods and liquids that traumatize oral mucosa increases comfort; fluid intake prevents dehydration and helps maintain mucous membrane integrity.*

BOX 33–7 Medications That May Interfere with Platelet Function

Over-the-Counter Medications

- Aspirin and salicylates, including the following:
  - Alka-Seltzer
  - Bufferin
  - Doan's Pills
  - Ecotrin
  - Excedrin
  - Midol
  - Pepto-Bismol
  - Vanquish
- NSAIDS such as the following:
  - Advil
  - Aleve
  - Nuprin
  - Pamprin IB

Prescription Medications

- Aspirin-containing analgesics
- Chemotherapy drugs
- Antibiotics such as penicillin
- Carbamazepine (Tegretol)
- Colchicine
- Dipyridamole (Persantine)
- Gold salts
- Heparin
- Quinine derivatives
- Sulfonamides
- Thiazide diuretics

Community-Based Care

In the adult, ITP often is a chronic disorder that the patient and family must learn to manage. Secondary thrombocytopenia may be either acute or chronic. Discuss the following topics when preparing the patient and family for home care:

- Nature of the disorder, its usual course, and the treatment plan
- Use and desired and potential adverse effects of prescribed medications
- Risks and benefits of surgery or treatments such as plasma replacement therapy
- The importance of follow-up tests and visits for care
- Measures to reduce the risk of bleeding: safety measures such as a soft-bristle toothbrush, electric razor, avoidance of contact sports and hazardous activities, and avoidance of medications that further interfere with platelet function (Box 33–7)

Refer for home health or other community services (e.g., housekeeping, shopping) as indicated.

The Patient with Hemophilia

Hemophilia is a group of hereditary clotting factor disorders that lead to persistent and sometimes severe bleeding (see the accompanying Genetic Considerations box). Although often considered a disease of children, hemophilia may be diagnosed in adults. Deficiencies of three clotting factors, VIII, IX, and XI, account for 90% to 95% of the bleeding disorders collectively called hemophilia (Huether & McCance, 2008).

Physiology Review

When tissue injury occurs, platelets collect at the site, adhering to the damaged vessel wall (the platelet plug). Activation of the clotting cascade, a sequential process of interactive reactions of clotting factors, is vital to form a stable clot. Clotting factors are plasma proteins primarily produced by the liver. A number of these factors require the presence of vitamin K for synthesis and activation. Once the clot has been formed and stabilized, it

GENETIC CONSIDERATIONS
Focus on Hemophilia

The incidence and pattern of inheritance for the forms of hemophilia differs.

- Hemophilia A occurs in about one in 10,000 male births, transmitted on the X chromosome: Each male offspring has a 50% risk of inheriting the defective gene; each female offspring has a 50% risk of becoming a carrier.
- Hemophilia B occurs in about one in 100,000 male births, transmitted on the X chromosome.
- Von Willebrand's disease affects about 1 in 100 to 500 people, usually inherited as an autosomal dominant trait: Offspring of an affected person have a 50% risk of inheriting the trait and the disorder.
- Factor XI deficiency inherited as an autosomal recessive trait: Each offspring of a carrier and an unaffected individual has as 50% risk of inheriting the trait; each offspring of two carriers has a 50% risk of being a carrier and a 25% risk of having the disorder. This deficiency is common in Ashkenazi Jews.

begins to retract, pulling together the edges of the damaged blood vessel to initiate the healing process.

Pathophysiology

Hemophilia A (or *classic hemophilia*) is the most common type of hemophilia, caused by deficiency or dysfunction of clotting factor VIII. It is transmitted as an X-linked recessive disorder from mothers to sons (Figure 33–13 ■). The genetic defect of hemophilia A on the X chromosome may cause deficient factor VIII production or a defective form of the protein. When the concentration of the clotting factor is 5% to 35% of normal, the disease is *mild*. Bleeding is infrequent, and usually associated with trauma. Concentrations of 1% to 5% of normal result in *moderate* disease. Again, bleeding usually occurs secondarily to trauma. *Severe* hemophilia occurs when concentrations are less than 1% of normal. Bleeding is frequent, often occurring without trauma (Huether & McCance, 2008).

Hemophilia B (also called *Christmas disease*), accounts for about 15% of cases, and is caused by a deficiency in factor IX. Despite the difference in clotting factor deficits, hemophilia A and B are clinically identical.

Von Willebrand's disease, often considered as a type of hemophilia, is the most common hereditary bleeding disorder (Huether & McCance, 2008). It is caused by a deficit of or

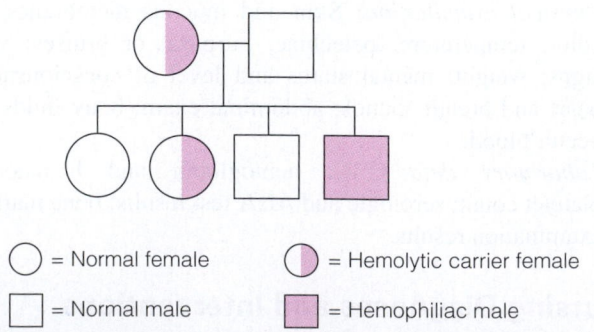

= Normal female   = Hemolytic carrier female

= Normal male   = Hemophiliac male

Figure 33–13 ■ The inheritance pattern of hemophilia A and B. Both are transmitted as X-linked recessive disorders. Females may be carriers, but only males develop these disorders.

defective von Willebrand (vW) factor, a protein that mediates platelet adhesion (Tierney et al., 2005). Reduced levels of factor VIII often also are present, because vW factor carries factor VIII. This clotting disorder affects men and women equally. Bleeding associated with von Willebrand's disease rarely is severe. It often is diagnosed when prolonged bleeding follows surgery or a dental extraction.

Factor XI deficiency (or *hemophilia C*) is usually a mild disorder, identified when postoperative bleeding is prolonged. A comparison of the types of hemophilia is found in Table 33–9.

People with hemophilia form a platelet plug at the site of bleeding, but the clotting factor deficit impairs formation of a stable fibrin clot. The effect of vW factor deficiency is somewhat different, in that platelet aggregation at the site of injury is impaired. In either case, prolonged or extensive bleeding may result. Often bleeding occurs in response to injury or as a result of surgery. However, a severe clotting factor deficit can lead to spontaneous bleeding into the joints (*hemarthrosis*), deep tissues, and central nervous system. Hemarthrosis often causes joint deformity and disability, usually of the elbows, hips, knees, and ankles.

Manifestations

The following are manifestations of hemophilia:

- Hemarthrosis
- Easy bruising and cutaneous hematoma formation with minor trauma (e.g., an injection)
- Bleeding from the gums and prolonged bleeding following minor injuries or cuts
- GI bleeding, with hematemesis (vomiting blood), occult blood in the stools, gastric pain, or abdominal pain
- Spontaneous hematuria or epistaxis (nosebleed)
- Pain or paralysis due to the pressure of hematomas on nerves

Intracranial hemorrhage is a potentially life-threatening manifestation of hemophilia.

Interdisciplinary Care

Treatment of hemophilia focuses on preventing and/or treating bleeding, primarily by replacing deficient clotting factors. Specific treatment depends on the severity of the disorder and the specific factor deficiency. Care may be complicated by hepatitis or HIV disease in people with hemophilia treated with clotting factor concentrates prepared from multiple units of donated blood. Today, routine testing of all blood, improved blood donor

screening, and current methods of treating hemophilia have significantly reduced the risk for these bloodborne diseases.

Diagnosis

The following laboratory tests may be ordered.

- *Serum platelet levels* are measured and are usually normal.
- *Coagulation studies* such as APTT, bleeding time, and prothrombin time are used to screen for hemophilia when abnormal bleeding occurs. APTT is increased in all types of hemophilia. Prothrombin time is unaffected in these disorders but may be measured to rule out other disorders. Bleeding time is prolonged in von Willebrand's disease but normal in hemophilia A and B.
- *Factor assays* are performed; factor VIII is decreased in hemophilia A and often in von Willebrand's disease, factor IX is decreased in hemophilia B, and factor XI in hemophilia C.
- *Amniocentesis* or *chorionic villus sampling* are used to identify the genetic defect of hemophilia when there is a known family history of the disease.

Medications

Deficient clotting factors are replaced regularly, as a prophylactic measure before surgery and dental procedures, and to control bleeding. Clotting factors may be given as fresh-frozen plasma, cryoprecipitates, or concentrates. Factor levels are measured on a regular basis to determine whether the treatment is adequate. Clotting factors are often self-administered and may be taken either on a regular or intermittent schedule.

Fresh-frozen plasma replaces all clotting factors (including both factor VIII and factor IX) except platelets. When the cause of bleeding is not yet determined, fresh-frozen plasma may be administered intravenously until a definitive diagnosis is made.

Hemophilia A is usually treated with either heat-treated factor VIII concentrate (heat treating reduces the risk of transmitting disease) or recombinant factor VIII. Although recombinant factor VIII, produced using recombinant DNA technology, eliminates the risk of viral disease transmission, its use is limited by cost. The dose of factor VIII is determined by the severity of the deficit and the presence or prospect of active bleeding (e.g., planned surgery).

Desmopressin acetate (DDAVP, Stimate) may be given to people with mild hemophilia A or von Willebrand's disease prior to minor surgeries. This drug causes release of factor VIII and will raise blood levels by two- or threefold for several hours, reducing the risk of bleeding and the need for clotting factor concentrate (Deglin & Vallerand, 2009).

TABLE 33–9 Types of Hemophilia

TYPE/NAME	DEFICIENCY	CHARACTERISTICS	TREATMENT
Hemophilia A (Classic hemophilia)	Factor VIII	Transmitted by females; occurs primarily in males; bleeding time normal; coagulation time prolonged.	Factor VIII concentrate or cryoprecipitate
Hemophilia B	Factor IX	Transmitted by females; occurs primarily in males; bleeding time normal; coagulation time prolonged.	Factor IX (Christmas disease concentrate)
Von Willebrand's disease	vW Factor VIII	Occurs in both females and males; bleeding time and coagulation time are both prolonged.	Cryoprecipitate and DDAVP
Factor XI deficiency	Factor XI	Occurs in both males and females; the activated partial thromboplastin time is prolonged.	Fresh frozen plasma

Factor IX concentrate (administered intravenously) is used to treat hemophilia B. Because factor IX concentrates also contain a number of other proteins, there is risk of thrombosis with recurrent use. They are used judiciously, only when needed. Products produced by recombinant technology or that are monoclonally purified carry a lower risk of stimulating thrombus formation (Deglin & Vallerand, 2009). Fresh-frozen plasma replaces factor XI and is used when necessary. It may be given daily until the risk for bleeding decreases.

Factor VIII concentrates contain functional vW factor, and may be used to treat von Willebrand's disease. Aspirin is avoided in all types of hemophilia.

EVIDENCE FOR NURSING CARE — The Patient with Hemophilia

Selected resources that nurses may find helpful when planning evidence-based nursing care follow.

- Cook, L. S. (2009). Learning about blood component therapy. *Nursing2009, 39*(4), 30–33.
- Mitchell, J. (2008). Haemophilia and inhibitors. 1: Diagnosis and treatment. *Nursing Times, 104*(26), 26–27.
- Mitchell J. (2008). Haemophilia and inhibitors. 2: Surgical management. *Nursing Times, 104*(27), 28–29.

∞ Nursing Care

Although primary responsibility for care falls to the patient and family, nursing care presents challenges. For additional assessment and nursing care strategies, see the accompanying Case Study & Nursing Care Plan.

Health Promotion

Encourage patients with a family history of hemophilia or bleeding disorders to seek genetic counseling during their family planning process. Although tests are available for the hemophilia gene, the technology to correct the disorder in utero does not yet exist. ∞ See Chapter 8.

Assessment

While severe hemophilia usually is diagnosed in childhood, milder cases may not be identified until surgery, invasive dental work, or a traumatic injury causes extensive or prolonged bleeding. Focused assessment related to hemophilia includes the following:

- *Health history:* Previous bleeding episodes with or without trauma; history of easy bruising, hematomas, epistaxis, bleeding gums, hematuria, vomiting blood, or joint pain; aspirin use; family history of hemophilia or bleeding disorders.
- *Physical examination:* Vital signs; bruising or bleeding of skin or mucous membranes; mental status; abdominal assessment; presence of joint deformity, decreased range of motion
- *Diagnostic studies:* CBC including hemoglobin, hematocrit, and platelet count; clotting factor assays; tests for occult blood (urine, stool, emesis); x-ray and scan results for evidence of bleeding.

Nursing Diagnoses and Interventions

Impaired blood clotting, the need for continuing care and disease management, and the risk for genetic transmission of hemophilia are priority problems for the patient with hemophilia.

Ineffective Protection

The inability to form stable clots and stem bleeding from injured blood vessels creates a significant risk for the patient with hemophilia. Nursing care measures focus on preventing injury and protecting the skin from damage.

- Monitor for signs of bleeding, including hematomas, ecchymoses, and purpura, as well as surface oozing or bleeding. Check emesis and stool for occult blood. *Bleeding may occur in cutaneous tissues as well as internal organs. Bleeding in the upper GI tract may not be readily apparent in the stool.*
- Notify the healthcare provider of any apparent bleeding. *Prompt intervention with administration of clotting factor concentrate decreases the risk of hemorrhage and subsequent hypovolemia.*
- Avoid intramuscular injections, rectal temperatures, and enemas. *These can pose a risk of tissue and vascular trauma, which can precipitate bleeding.*
- Use safety measures in personal care. For example, use an electric razor rather than a razor blade to shave. *Use of an electric razor minimizes the opportunity to develop superficial cuts that may result in bleeding.*
- If bleeding occurs, control blood loss using gentle pressure, ice, or a topical hemostatic agent, such as absorbable gelatin sponge, microfibrillar collagen hemostat, or topical thrombin. *Direct pressure occludes bleeding vessels. Ice, a vasoconstrictor, may facilitate bleeding control, as do topical hemostatic agents.*
- Instruct to avoid activities that increase the risk of trauma, including contact sports, physical exertion associated with job performance, and to eliminate safety hazards in the home. *Depending on the severity of the clotting factor deficit, even minor trauma can lead to serious bleeding episodes. Safer activities such as noncontact sports (e.g., swimming, golf) and occupations that do not require physical labor may be substituted.*

Risk for Ineffective Health Maintenance

Hemophilia is a chronic disorder, requiring active management to prevent and control bleeding and complications. Frequent visits to the healthcare provider or clinic may be necessary. In addition, the patient may need to learn to self-administer clotting factors and measures to prevent complications. The lifelong nature of the disorder may interfere with compliance, especially during early adulthood.

- Assess knowledge of disorder and the related treatments. *Assessment allows identification of knowledge gaps and provides a basis on which to provide additional information. Impaired disease management may be due to lack of knowledge or a conscious decision not to follow the recommendations of the healthcare provider.*
- Provide information about the bleeding disorder and prescribed medications and treatments. *Individualized instruction is more effective than general, possibly irrelevant information.*

CASE STUDY & NURSING CARE PLAN   A Patient with Hemophilia

Jermiel Cruise is a 20-year-old student at the community college. He is admitted to the emergency department with a nosebleed that began when he fell during a touch football game. It has continued to bleed for over an hour.

ASSESSMENT

Mr. Cruise states that he has hemophilia and realizes that playing contact sports "is probably a dumb thing to do." He adds that he has not had any recent bleeding episodes. An ice bag and manual pressure are applied in the emergency department. The healthcare provider orders factor VIII concentrate to be administered. Physical assessment findings are T 97.2°F (36.2°C), BP 118/64, R 18. Skin pale but warm. Laboratory tests reveal a prolonged APTT and a normal bleeding time and PT. Following treatment, Mr. Cruise's bleeding subsides.

DIAGNOSES

- *Risk for Aspiration* related to uncontrolled nosebleed
- *Noncompliance* with activity recommendations
- *Ineffective Protection* related to lack of clotting factor VIII

EXPECTED OUTCOMES

- Exhibit no further signs of bleeding.
- Maintain vital signs within his usual range.
- Maintain an open airway.
- Identify sports and recreation activities in which he can safely participate.
- Verbalize self-care measures to control bleeding.

PLANNING AND IMPLEMENTATION

- Monitor vital signs and for further signs of bleeding.
- Assess airway and auscultate breath sounds.
- Review emergency measures to help stop bleeding.
- Reiterate the importance of seeking prompt medical attention if bleeding should occur.
- Advise regarding the importance of wearing a MedicAlert bracelet identifying him as a hemophiliac.
- Discuss alternative noncontact sports and recreational activities.

EVALUATION

On discharge, Mr. Cruise has no further signs of bleeding, shock, or aspiration. He is able to verbalize methods to help stop local bleeding and the importance of seeking medical attention promptly when bleeding continues. Mr. Cruise agrees to stop at a local drug store on the way home to order a MedicAlert bracelet. In addition, Mr. Cruise verbalizes an understanding of the importance of avoiding contact sports and has identified swimming and golf as alternative leisure activities that he might enjoy.

CRITICAL THINKING IN THE NURSING PROCESS

1. What is the pathophysiologic basis for the bleeding that occurs in hemophilia A and B?
2. What was Mr. Cruise's priority nursing diagnosis? Why?
3. Why is family planning a special consideration with a patient who has hemophilia?
4. Outline a plan to teach the family of a patient diagnosed with hemophilia how to administer an intravenous infusion.
5. Develop a care plan for Mr. Cruise for the nursing diagnosis *Impaired Social Interaction*. Consider Mr. Cruise's age and developmental level in creating the plan.

See Evaluating Your Response in Appendix C.

- Provide emotional support, expressing confidence in the patient's self-care abilities. *Emotional support helps the patient incorporate the care regimen into his or her lifestyle.*
- Provide supervised learning and practice opportunities for administering clotting factors and topical hemostatic agents. *Successful practice sessions instill confidence in the ability to manage care and provide an opportunity for questions and exploring alternatives.*

Using NANDA, NIC, and NOC

Links between NANDA nursing diagnoses, NIC, and NOC are represented by the linkages box summarizing care of the patient with hemophilia are shown in the chart that follows.

Community-Based Care

Discuss the following topics when preparing the patient with a bleeding disorder and the family for home care.

- Recognizing the manifestations of internal bleeding: pallor, weakness, restlessness, headache, disorientation, pain, swelling. These manifestations require emergency medical care and should be reported immediately.
- Applying cold packs and immobilizing the joint for 24 to 48 hours if hemarthrosis occurs.
- Using analgesics for pain; avoiding prescription and over-the-counter drugs containing aspirin.

- Ensuring a safe home environment (e.g., padding sharp edges of furniture, using transition lighting or a night light; avoiding scatter rugs, and wearing protective gloves when working in the house or yard).
- Using safe grooming practices such as electric razors.

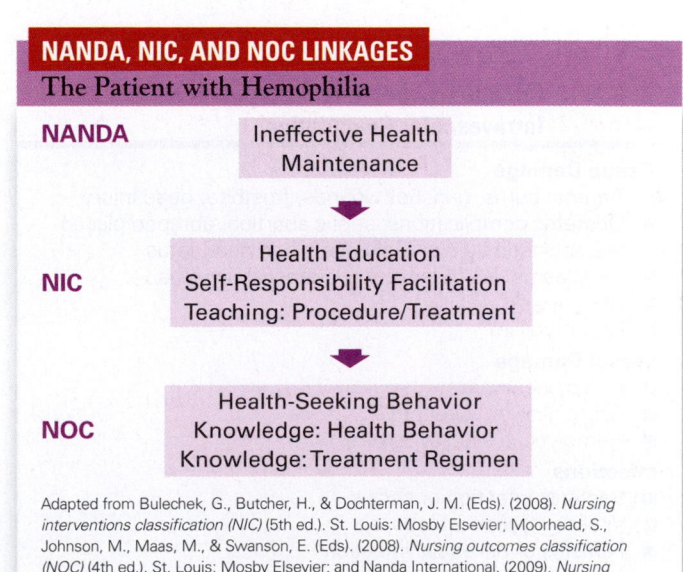

NANDA, NIC, AND NOC LINKAGES
The Patient with Hemophilia

NANDA → Ineffective Health Maintenance

NIC → Health Education / Self-Responsibility Facilitation / Teaching: Procedure/Treatment

NOC → Health-Seeking Behavior / Knowledge: Health Behavior / Knowledge: Treatment Regimen

Adapted from Bulechek, G., Butcher, H., & Dochterman, J. M. (Eds). (2008). *Nursing interventions classification (NIC)* (5th ed.). St. Louis: Mosby Elsevier; Moorhead, S., Johnson, M., Maas, M., & Swanson, E. (Eds). (2008). *Nursing outcomes classification (NOC)* (4th ed.). St. Louis: Mosby Elsevier; and Nanda International. (2009). *Nursing diagnoses: Definitions and classification 2009–2011.* Oxford, UK: Wiley-Blackwell.

- Wearing a MedicAlert bracelet in case of accident.
- Practicing good dental hygiene to decrease potential tooth decay and extractions. If dental procedures are necessary, discuss the need for prophylactic factor administration with the dentist and healthcare provider.
- Following safer-sex practices.
- Preparing and administering intravenous medications.

Refer the patient and family to a local hemophilia or bleeding disorders support group. Provide contact information for national organizations and information clearinghouses, such as the National Hemophilia Foundation.

The Patient with Disseminated Intravascular Coagulation

Disseminated intravascular coagulation (DIC) is a disruption of hemostasis characterized by widespread intravascular clotting and bleeding. It may be acute and life threatening or relatively mild. DIC is a clinical syndrome that develops as a complication of a wide variety of other disorders (Box 33–8). Sepsis is the most common cause of DIC. Gram-negative and gram-positive bacteria as well as viruses, fungi, and protozoal infections may lead to DIC (Huether & McCance, 2008).

Pathophysiology

DIC is triggered by endothelial damage, release of tissue factors into the circulation, or inappropriate activation of the clotting cascade by an endotoxin. Both the intrinsic and the extrinsic clotting cascade may be activated, although the extrinsic cascade usually is the one activated. Extensive thrombin entering the systemic circulation overwhelms natural anticoagulants, leading to unrestricted clot formation (Huether & McCance, 2008). Clotting

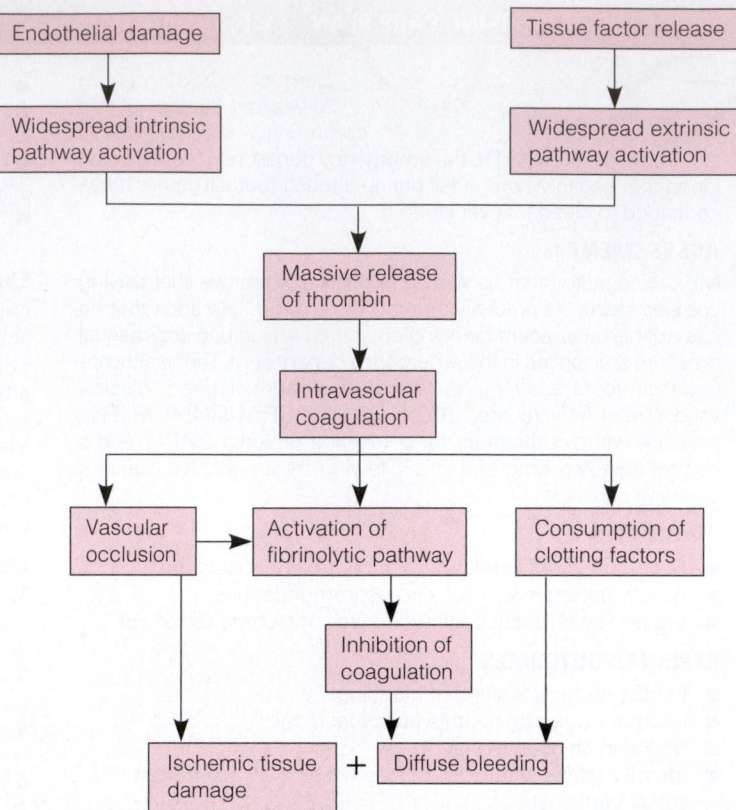

Figure 33–14 ■ Disseminated intravascular coagulation (DIC). Endothelial cell injury or release of tissue factors activate the intrinsic or extrinsic clotting pathway (or both). As a result, numerous microthrombi form throughout the vasculature, causing ischemic tissue damage. Simultaneously, rapid consumption of clotting factors and activation of fibrinolytic mechanisms trigger widespread bleeding.

may be localized to an individual organ, or widespread with deposition of small thrombi and emboli throughout the microvasculature (Kasper et al., 2005). The widespread clotting consumes clotting factors (prothrombin, platelets, factor V, and factor VIII in particular) and activates fibrinolytic processes with anticoagulant production. As a result, hemorrhage occurs (Figure 33–14 ■).

The sequence of DIC follows:

1. Endothelial damage, tissue factors, or toxins stimulate the clotting cascade.
2. Excess thrombin within the circulation overwhelms naturally occurring anticoagulants.
3. Widespread clotting occurs within the microvasculature.
4. Thrombi and emboli impair tissue perfusion, leading to ischemia, infarction, and necrosis.
5. Clotting factors and platelets are consumed faster than they can be replaced.
6. Clotting activates fibrinolytic processes that begin to break down clots.
7. Fibrin degradation products (*FDPs*, potent anticoagulants) are released, contributing to bleeding.
8. Clotting factors are depleted, the ability to form clots is lost, and hemorrhage occurs.

BOX 33–8 Conditions That May Precipitate Disseminated Intravascular Coagulation

Tissue Damage
- Trauma: burns, gunshot wounds, frostbite, head injury
- Obstetric complications: septic abortion, abruptio placentae, amniotic fluid embolus, retained dead fetus
- Neoplasms: acute leukemia, adenocarcinomas
- Hemolysis
- Fat embolism

Vessel Damage
- Aortic aneurysm
- Acute glomerulonephritis
- Hemolytic uremic syndrome

Infections
- Bacterial infection or sepsis
- Viral or mycotic infections
- Parasitic or rickettsial infection

Manifestations

The manifestations of DIC result from both clotting and bleeding, although bleeding is more obvious, especially in acute DIC. Bleeding ranges from oozing blood following an injection to frank hemorrhage from every body orifice (see the accompanying Manifestations box). Chronic DIC may be asymptomatic, or may present with peripheral cyanosis, thrombosis, and pregangrenous changes in the fingers and toes, nose, and genitalia (Papadakis & McPhee, 2007).

Interdisciplinary Care

Treatment of DIC is directed toward treating the underlying disorder and preventing further bleeding or massive thrombosis. Treatment stabilizes the patient, reduces complications, and allows recovery to occur; it does not cure DIC (Papadakis & McPhee, 2007).

Diagnosis

Diagnostic tests are used to confirm the diagnosis of DIC and evaluate the risk for hemorrhage.

- *CBC* and *platelet count* are used to evaluate the hemoglobin, hematocrit, and number of circulating platelets. *Schistocytes*, fragmented RBCs, may be noted due to cell trapping and damage within fibrin thrombi. The platelet count is decreased.
- *Coagulation studies* show prolonged *prothrombin time (PT)*, *partial thromboplastin time (PTT)*, and *thrombin time*, and a low *fibrinogen level* due to depletion of clotting factors. The fibrinogen level helps predict bleeding in DIC: As it falls, the risk of bleeding increases (Van Leeuwen, Kranpitz, & Smith, 2006).
- *Fibrin degradation products (FDPs)* or *fibrin split products (FSPs)* are increased due to the fibrinolysis that occurs with DIC.

Treatments

When bleeding is the major manifestation of DIC, fresh frozen plasma and platelet concentrates are given to restore clotting factors and platelets. Heparin, although controversial, may be administered. Heparin interferes with the clotting cascade and may prevent further clotting factor consumption due to uncontrolled thrombosis. It is used when bleeding is not controlled by plasma and platelets, as well as when the patient has manifestations of thrombotic problems such as acrocyanosis and

possible gangrene. Long-term heparin therapy (administered by injection or continuous infusion using a portable pump) may be necessary for patients with chronic DIC.

Nursing Care

Assessment

Nurses can be instrumental in identifying early manifestations of DIC, facilitating timely intervention. Focused nursing assessment for DIC includes the following:

- *Health history:* Recent abortion (spontaneous or therapeutic) or current pregnancy; presence of a known malignant tumor; history of abnormal bleeding episodes or a hematologic disorder.
- *Physical examination:* Bleeding from puncture wounds (e.g., injections), IV sites, incisions; hematuria, obvious or occult blood in emesis or stool, epistaxis, other abnormal bleeding; vital signs; heart and breath sounds; abdominal assessment including girth, contour, bowel sounds, tenderness or guarding to palpation; color, temperature, skin condition of hands, feet, and digits; petechiae or purpura of skin, mucous membranes.
- *Diagnostic studies:* CBC with hemoglobin, hematocrit; platelet count; coagulation studies; evaluations of organ system function (e.g., liver and renal function tests); CT scans of the head and abdomen.

Nursing Diagnoses and Interventions

Patients with acute DIC often are critically ill, with multiple nursing care needs. Priority nursing diagnoses discussed in this section focus on impaired tissue perfusion and gas exchange, pain, and fear. Septic shock may precipitate DIC; hemorrhagic shock may occur as a complication of DIC. ∞ See Chapter 11 for nursing diagnoses and interventions related to these problems.

Ineffective Tissue Perfusion

Thrombi and emboli forming throughout the microcirculation affect the perfusion of multiple organs and tissues. Additionally, bleeding due to clotting factor consumption affects cardiac output and blood flow to these tissues.

- Assess extremity pulses, warmth, and capillary refill. Monitor level of consciousness (LOC) and mental status. *Monitoring central and peripheral tissue perfusion facilitates early treatment of impaired perfusion.*

PRACTICE ALERT

Promptly report complaints of chest pain, changes in mental status, LOC, tissue perfusion, respirations, GI function, and urinary output. Chest pain or respiratory changes (tachypnea, dyspnea, orthopnea) may be due to angina, pulmonary embolism, or bleeding into lung tissue. Changes in mentation or LOC can indicate cerebral ischemia. A painful, pale, and cold extremity with no or diminished pulses indicates arterial occlusion. Prompt intervention is critical to save the extremity. Acute abdominal pain, decreased bowel sounds, and GI bleeding may indicate mesenteric occlusion, a surgical emergency. Decreased urine output may signify renal artery thrombosis; renal failure may develop.

- Carefully reposition at least every 2 hours. *Position changes facilitate circulation and tissue perfusion, as well as provide an opportunity to assess for purpura, pallor, and bleeding.*
- Discourage crossing the legs, and do not elevate the knees on the bed or with a pillow. *These positions may impair arterial and venous flow to the lower legs and feet, increasing vascular stasis and the risk for thrombosis.*
- Minimize use of tape on the skin, using binders, nonadhesive dressings, and other devices as needed. *Preventing skin trauma reduces the risk for bleeding and potential infection.*

Impaired Gas Exchange

Microclots in the pulmonary vasculature are likely to interfere with gas exchange in the patient with DIC.

- Monitor oxygen saturation continuously. Administer oxygen as ordered. *Oxygen saturation levels are a noninvasive means of assessing gas exchange. Supplemental oxygen promotes gas exchange and reduces cardiac work, relieving dyspnea.*

> **PRACTICE ALERT**
> Monitor arterial blood gas results; report abnormal results to the healthcare provider. Low PaO_2 and rising $PaCO_2$ levels indicate impaired gas exchange and may signify the need for additional treatment.

- Place in Fowler's or high-Fowler's position as tolerated. *Elevating the head of the bed improves diaphragmatic excursion and alveolar ventilation.*
- Maintain bed rest. *Bed rest reduces oxygen demands and cardiac work.*
- Encourage deep breathing and effective coughing. *Increased respiratory depth and clearance of secretions from airways improves alveolar ventilation and oxygenation.*
- Cautious nasotracheal suctioning may be instituted if cough is ineffective or an endotracheal tube is in place. *Removal of secretions facilitates ventilation and oxygenation. However, care must be used to minimize suction-induced hypoxia and airway trauma.*
- Administer analgesics and antianxiety drugs as needed to control pain and anxiety. Provide reassurance and comfort measures. *Pain and anxiety increase the respiratory rate and decrease the depth of respirations, reducing effective ventilation and gas exchange.*

Pain

Both the underlying cause of DIC and tissue ischemia from microvascular clots can cause pain. Identifying the etiology of pain is important to identify potential complications or harmful effects of DIC and to institute effective treatment.

- Use a standard pain scale chart to evaluate and monitor pain and analgesic effectiveness. *Monitoring pain and response to medication facilitates development of an appropriate and effective treatment plan.*

> **PRACTICE ALERT**
> Notify the healthcare provider promptly of new or a sudden increase in pain, especially when accompanied by changes in assessment findings. New or increased complaints of pain may signify increased circulatory impairment and ischemic changes in tissues such as the heart, bowel, or extremities. Circulation to a painful, pale or cyanotic, or cold extremity may be occluded by an arterial clot. Prompt intervention is necessary to save the extremity. Acute abdominal pain may signify mesenteric occlusion, a surgical emergency. Anginal pain may indicate occlusion of coronary arteries.

- Handle extremities gently. *Gentle handling reduces the risk of further injury to and pain in ischemic tissues.*
- Apply cool compresses to painful joints. *Application of cold decreases pain through the gate-control mechanism, inhibiting the dorsal horn of the spinal cord and reducing the sensation of pain.*

> **PRACTICE ALERT**
> Continuously monitor effects of analgesics and mental and respiratory status. Analgesics may mask manifestations of neurologic impairment due to thromboembolism, and may depress the respiratory center, further impairing gas exchange. Judicious analgesic administration with careful monitoring is vital to safely provide effective pain relief.

Fear

The underlying serious illness and a complication such as DIC results in an uncertain prognosis, often accompanied by fear.

- Encourage the patient and family to verbalize concerns. *This helps the patient and family identify their concerns and frame questions.*
- Answer questions truthfully. *Providing honest answers is vital to developing a therapeutic nurse–patient relationship. Accurate responses allow the patient and family to set priorities as they plan for an uncertain future.*
- Help the patient and family identify coping strategies to manage this significant situational stressor. *Implementing past effective coping methods may provide the skills to manage the current crisis.*
- Provide emotional support. *The presence of a caring nurse helps reduce the fear and anxiety associated with a crisis.*
- Maintain a calm environment. *A calm environment provides reassurance that the situation is in control, reduces anxiety, and promotes rest.*
- Respond promptly when the patient calls for help. *Prompt responses to expressed needs helps develop a trusting relationship and a sense of security that assistance is readily available.*
- Teach relaxation techniques. *Relaxation techniques can reduce muscle tension and other signs of anxiety. Gaining control over physical responses can help the patient gain a sense of control over the situation.*

Community-Based Care

Although the immediate crisis of acute DIC is resolved prior to discharge, the patient may have some continuing effects of the disorder, such as impaired tissue integrity of distal extremities. Teach the patient and family about specific care needs, such as foot care or dressing changes. Provide instruction about any continuing medications and follow-up care.

Patients with chronic DIC may require continuing heparin therapy, using either intermittent subcutaneous injections or a portable infusion pump. Teach the patient and family members how to administer the injection or manage the infusion pump. Provide a referral to home health care or a home intravenous management service for assistance. Discuss the manifestations of excessive bleeding or recurrent clotting that need to be reported to the healthcare provider.

CHAPTER HIGHLIGHTS

- Anemia is the most common disorder of the red blood cells; nutritional deficiencies are the most common causes of anemia. Its manifestations relate to the function of RBCs and hemoglobin, transporting oxygen to the cells: fatigue, increased respiratory and heart rates, shortness of breath with activity, and pallor.
- Genetically transmitted disorders such as sickle cell disease and thalassemia can cause significant anemia and associated problems in affected populations. These patients require teaching and episodic acute care for crises such as vaso-occlusive crisis in sickle cell disease.
- Nursing care related to anemia is primarily educational to prepare the patient for effective self-care, including diet, prescribed medications, and measures to prevent sickling episodes (for patients with sickle cell disease).
- Leukemia and lymphomas are the primary disorders of white blood cells and lymphoid tissues.
- Manifestations of the leukemias reflect the altered ability of abnormal WBCs to perform effective immune surveillance and crowding of the bone marrow and other organs by rapidly proliferating cells. Frequent sore throats, increased risk for infection, and manifestations of anemia and thrombocytopenia are seen, as well as an enlarged spleen and abdominal pain.
- Four major subgroups of leukemia are identified: acute and chronic myeloid leukemias, and acute and chronic lymphocytic (or lymphoblastic) leukemias. The primary population affected differs for each of these leukemias, as does their course.
- Genetic alterations and certain viruses are linked to the development of leukemia, as are exposure to chemotherapy drugs, environmental toxins, and ionizing radiation.
- Lymphocytic leukemias and lymphomas are closely related disorders.
- Nursing care for patients with leukemia and lymphoma focuses on reducing the risk for infection and bleeding, managing the effects of chemotherapy and radiation therapy, and, in some cases, caring for patients before and after bone marrow or stem cell transplant.
- The major risks associated with bone marrow and stem cell transplant are infection prior to and immediately following the transplant and graft-versus-host disease, a potentially fatal condition. A pruritic rash and desquamation of the palms and soles; abdominal pain, nausea, and diarrhea; and jaundice and elevated liver enzymes are common early manifestations of GVHD.
- The treatment of and nursing care for patients with lymphomas (including Hodgkin's disease and non-Hodgkin's lymphoma) is similar to that provided for patients with leukemia.
- Multiple myeloma is a malignancy of plasma cells, B lymphocytes that produce antibodies. Circulating M proteins and Bence Jones proteins in the urine are seen in multiple myeloma. The usual presenting manifestation is bone pain. Pathologic fractures and hypercalcemia are common complications of multiple myeloma as bone is destroyed.
- Bleeding and clotting disorders can result from either inadequate platelets (thrombocytopenia) or disruption of the clotting mechanisms (hemophilia, disseminated intravascular coagulation). Petechiae and purpura are common manifestations of bleeding/clotting disorders.
- Hemophilias are genetically transmitted disorders. Hemophilia A and B are transmitted on the X chromosome (sex-linked) from mother to son. Von Willbrand's disease, the most common bleeding disorder, is transmitted as an autosomal dominant disorder and affects men and women equally.
- Hemophilias are treated by replacement of the missing clotting factor and measures to prevent injury and bleeding.
- Disseminated intravascular coagulation is a disorder of widespread microvascular clotting. It commonly is precipitated by sepsis, but also may occur with conditions such as major trauma, malignancy, or as an obstetric emergency.
- In DIC platelets and clotting factors are consumed by the abnormal clotting processes, leading the manifestations of bleeding, including frank hemorrhage, hematuria, oozing blood from parenteral and intravenous injection sites, and GI bleeding. Blood flow to organs and tissues is compromised by clot formation, leading to manifestations such as cyanosis of extremities, abdominal pain, renal failure, and changes in mental status and level of consciousness. Nursing care is supportive, focusing on administering prescribed treatments and monitoring and supporting cardiovascular, respiratory, and renal function.

TEST YOURSELF NCLEX-RN® REVIEW

1. In assessing a female patient with moderate anemia, the nurse would expect to find which of the following?
   1. hematocrit 45%
   2. pulse rate 140
   3. complains of shortness of breath with exercise
   4. WBC 14,000/µL

2. The nurse following a patient after gastric resection observes carefully for evidence of nutritional deficiency anemia related to malabsorption, including which of the following?
   1. numbness and tingling of extremities
   2. steatorrhea
   3. dark yellow or bronze skin color
   4. bone pain

3. Which of the following nursing diagnoses would be of highest priority for the patient hospitalized for a bone marrow transplant to treat relapse of acute myelocytic leukemia?
   1. *Disturbed Body Image*
   2. *Ineffective Protection*
   3. *Anxiety*
   4. *Imbalanced Nutrition: Less than Body Requirements*

4. The nurse caring for a patient with acute myeloid leukemia plans which of the following nursing interventions during hospitalization? **Select all that apply.**
   1. Place in a private room.
   2. Implement airborne infection control precautions.
   3. Assist with oral hygiene after meals.
   4. Monitor rectal temperature q4h.
   5. Request soft, bland diet.

5. A patient with non-Hodgkin's lymphoma tells the nurse, "I might as well give up on dating. No woman will want me now." What is the most appropriate response?
   1. "It sounds like you are concerned about the effects of this disease and the proposed treatment plan."
   2. "Don't worry. Malignant lymphomas are very treatable when caught in an early state of the disease."
   3. "Well, you may never be able to have children all right, but there are other ways to have a satisfying relationship with a woman."
   4. "Lots of women find bald men attractive; besides, your hair may grow back soft and curly."

6. The nurse caring for a patient with lymphoma who is being started on the CHOP chemotherapy regimen understands that chemotherapy drugs are used in combination to do which of the following?
   1. Target malignant cells in different organs.
   2. Prevent the development of adverse effects.
   3. Target different phases of the cell cycle.
   4. Support growth and development of normal cells.

7. A patient with multiple myeloma calls the home health nurse complaining of severe back pain of new onset. The appropriate response by the nurse is to do which of the following?
   1. Reassure the patient that bone pain is expected with this disease.
   2. Inquire about the patient's use of NSAIDs and analgesics to manage pain.
   3. Suggest use of a back brace to reduce pain.
   4. Notify the healthcare provider of the onset of new pain.

8. The nurse observes reddish-purple spots and areas of purple bruising on a newly admitted patient. Which laboratory results support this assessment finding?
   1. hematocrit 28%
   2. platelets $60 \times 10^3/mm^3$
   3. INR 4.0
   4. WBC 4,500/mm^3

9. A patient whose husband has hemophilia asks if her newborn baby girl could have the disease. The nurse's response is based on which of the following?
   1. The most common forms of hemophilia are transmitted as sex-linked recessive disorders; her daughter is at risk for carrying the defective gene.
   2. Because hemophilia is a sex-linked recessive disorder carried on the Y chromosome, her daughter has no risk of having or carrying the disease.
   3. Hemophilia is an autosomal dominant disorder; therefore, her daughter has a 50% chance of having the disorder.
   4. Although hemophilia is genetically transmitted, its pattern of inheritance is unknown, and her daughter will need to be tested for the defective gene.

10. The nurse administering platelets to a patient with disseminated intravascular coagulation (DIC) understands that the intended effect of this treatment is to do which of the following?
    1. Replace specific clotting factors.
    2. Promote intravascular clotting.
    3. Restore tissue oxygenation.
    4. Replace depleted platelets.

See Test Yourself answers in Appendix C.

Pearson Nursing Student Resources
Find additional review materials at
www.nursing.pearsonhighered.com
Prepare for success with additional NCLEX®-style practice questions, interactive assignments and activities, Web links, animations and videos, and more!

BIBLIOGRAPHY

American Cancer Society. (2008). *Cancer facts and figures 2008.* Atlanta: Author.

Armand, P., & Antin, J. H. (2007). Allogeneic stem cell transplantation for aplastic anemia. *Biology of Blood and Marrow Transplantation 13,* 505–516.

Bulechek, G., Butcher, H., & Dochterman, J. M. (Eds). (2008). *Nursing interventions classification (NIC)* (5th ed.). St. Louis: Mosby Elsevier.

Calzone, K. A., Lea, D. H., & Masny A. (2006). Non-Hodgkin's lymphoma as an exemplar of the effects of genetics and genomics. *Journal of Nursing Scholarship, 38*(4), 335–343.

Coleman, E. A., Coon, S. K., Kennedy, R. L., Lockhart, K. D., Stewart, C. B., Anaissie, E. J., et al. (2008). Effects of exercise in combination with Epoetin alfa during high-dose chemotherapy and autologous peripheral blood stem cell transplantation for multiple myeloma. *Oncology Nursing Forum, 35*(3), E53–E61.

Coyer, S. M., & Lash, A. A. (2008). Pathophysiology of anemia and nursing care implications. *MEDSURG Nursing 17*(2), 77–91.

De, D. (2008). Acute nursing care and management of patients with sickle cell. *British Journal of Nursing, 17*(13), 818–823.

Deglin, J. H., & Vallerand, A. H. (2009). *Davis' Drug Guide* (10th ed.). Philadelphia: F.A. Davis.

Demakos, E. P., & Linebaugh, J. A. (2005). Advances in myelodysplastic syndrome: Nursing implications of azacitidine. *Clinical Journal of Oncology Nursing, 9*(4), 417–423.

Dvorak, C. (2006). Common complaints, difficult diagnosis: Multiple myeloma. *Journal of the American Academy of Nurse Practitioners,18,* 190–194.

El-Banna, M. M., Berger, A. M., Farr, L., Foxall, M. J., Friesth, B., & Schreiner. E. (2004). Fatigue and depression in patients with lymphoma undergoing autologous peripheral blood stem cell transplantation. *Oncology Nursing Forum, 31*(5), 937–944.

Elphee, E. E. (2008). Understanding the concept of uncertainty in patients with indolent lymphoma. *Oncology Nursing Forum, 35*(3), 449–454.

Faiman, B. (2007). Clinical updates and nursing considerations for patients with multiple myeloma. *Clinical Journal of Oncology Nursing, 11*(6), 831–840.

Huether, S. E. & McCance, K. L. (2008). *Understanding pathophysiology* (4th ed.). St. Louis: Mosby Elsevier.

Kurtin, S. E. (2006). Advances in the management of low- to intermediate-risk myelodysplastic syndrome: Integrating the national comprehensive cancer network guidelines. *Clinical Journal of Oncology Nursing, 10*(2), 197–208.

Lash, A. A., & Coyer, S. M. (2008). Anemia in older adults. *MEDSURG Nursing 17*(5), 298–304.

Leahy, Y. (2008). Second cancers in survivors of Hodgkin lymphoma: Risks and recommendations. *Clinical Journal of Oncology Nursing, 12*(3), 437–442.

Liebenguth, P., & Temple, S. V. (2006). Radioimmunotherapy for non-Hodgkin's lymphoma. *Seminars in Oncology Nursing, 22*(4), 257–266.

Long, J. M. (2007). Treatment approaches and nursing applications for non-Hodgkin lymphoma. *Clinical Journal of Oncology Nursing, 11*(1), 13–21.

McCann, S. A. (2007). Cutaneous T-cell lymphoma: Overview and nursing perspectives. *Nursing Clinics of North America, 42,* 421–455.

Miceli, T., Colson, K., Gavino, M., Lilleby, K., & IMF Nurse Leadership Board. (2008). Myelosuppression associated with novel therapies in patients with multiple myeloma: Consensus statement of the IMF nurse leadership board. *Clinical Journal of Oncology Nursing, 12*(3), 13–19.

Moorhead, S., Johnson, M., Maas, M., & Swanson, E. (Eds). (2008). *Nursing outcomes classification (NOC)* (4th ed.). St. Louis: Mosby Elsevier.

NANDA International. (2009). *Nursing diagnoses: Definitions and classification 2009–2011.* Oxford, UK: Wiley-Blackwell.

National Comprehensive Cancer Network. (2009). *Clinical practice guidelines in oncology. Myelodysplastic syndromes* (V.2). Retrieved from www.nccn.org/professionals/physician_gls/PDF/mds.pdf

National Heart, Lung, and Blood Institute, National Institutes of Health. (2009). *Morbidity & mortality: 2009 chart book of cardiovascular, lung, and blood diseases.* Bethesda, MD: Author.

Noonan, K. (2007). Introduction to B-cell disorders. *Clinical Journal of Oncology Nursing, 11*(1), 3–12.

Papadakis, M. A. & McPhee, S. J. (2007). *Current Consult Medicine 2007.* New York: McGraw-Hill.

Persson, L., & Hallberg, I. R. (2004). Lived experience of survivors of leukemia or malignant lymphoma. *Cancer Nursing, 27*(4), 303–313.

Persson, L., Hallberg, I. R., & Ohlsson, O. (1997). Survivors of acute leukemia and highly malignant lymphoma—retrospective views of daily life problems during treatment and when in remission. *Journal of Advanced Nursing, 25*(1), 68–78.

Thomas, C. M., Coleman, H. R., & Taub, L-F. M. (2007). A case study of an older adult with severe anemia refusing blood transfusion. *Journal of the American Academy of Nurse Practitioners, 19,* 43–48.

Van Leeuwen, A. M., Kranpitz, T. R., Smith, L. S. (2006). *Davis' laboratory and diagnostic tests* (2nd ed.). Philadelphia: F.A. Davis.

Woodman R., Ferrucci L., & Guralnik, J. (2005). Anemia in older adults. *Current Opinion in Hematology, 21*(2), 123–128.

Wright, K. (2009). Barriers to effective pain management in sickle cell disease. *British Journal of Nursing, 18*(3), 158–161.

Functional Health Pattern: Activity-Exercise Patterns

Think about patients with altered cardiac function for whom you have cared in your clinical experiences.

- What were the patients' major pathophysiologic conditions (medical diagnoses) (e.g., myocardial infarction, heart failure, valvular heart disease, anemia, polycythemia, leukemia, malignant lymphoma, multiple myeloma, neutropenia, infectious mononucleosis, thrombocytopenia, hemophilia, disseminated intravascular coagulation, hypertension, aneurysm, peripheral vascular disease thromboangiitis obliterans, Raynaud's disease, acute arterial occlusion, venous thrombosis, chronic venous insufficiency, varicose veins, lymphadenopathy, or lymphedema)?

- What kinds of manifestations did each of these patients have? Were these manifestations similar or different?

- How did each of these patients respond to activities such as talking, eating, completing activities of daily living (ADLs), moving from bed to chair or bathroom, or ambulating? Did the patients' heart rates increase or decrease? How about their respiratory rates and effort? Did any of your patients become light-headed or develop chest pain during activity? Did their oxygen saturation levels remain stable or drop during activity? Did these patients exercise regularly? Did leg pain occur with activities such as walking, or also during rest? Did their ankles swell at the end of the day, after sitting for prolonged periods, or after sleeping at night? Did the patients have leg cramps that awakened them at night? Did temperature or the position of their body affect their symptoms? Did the patients have any pain, burning, numbness or tingling in the hands and fingers or feet and toes? Did the patients have any changes in skin color or temperature, texture of hair, ulcers or skin irritations, varicose veins, or edema? Did the patients notice any swelling in the glands in the neck after an infection? Did the patients notice increased fatigue or weakness? Did the patients have a history of other illnesses, surgeries, or environmental exposures? What medications did your patients take? Did your patients drink alcohol or smoke?

The Activity-Exercise Pattern Functional Health Pattern includes disorders that result in insufficient physiologic energy to carry out ADLs. The heart functions as a pump to deliver fuel for energy production to the cells. Blood is the exchange medium between the external environment and the body's cells. With each heart beat, the heart ejects blood through a closed system of blood vessels that transport oxygenated blood to all body organs and tissues and then returns deoxygenated blood to the heart for reoxygenation by the lungs. The functions of blood include transporting oxygen; nutrients; hormones and metabolic wastes; protecting against invasion of pathogens; maintaining blood coagulation; and regulating fluids, electrolytes, acids, bases, and body temperature. The lymphatic system is also a vascular system that helps to maintain sufficient blood volume by picking up excess tissue fluid (lymph) and returning it to the bloodstream.

Cardiac disorders affect the heart's pumping ability in two primary ways:

- The heart muscle is directly damaged by ischemic processes (e.g., coronary heart disease), inflammatory responses (e.g.,

rheumatic carditis, endocarditis), or a primary cardiac muscle disorder (cardiomyopathy)

- Excessive cardiac work (e.g., resulting from hypertension, valve disorders, or congenital defects), prompts compensatory mechanism to meet cellular needs for fuel; over time, these compensatory mechanisms damage the heart muscle

When the cardiac pump fails, less fuel is delivered to the cells and energy production falls. This in turn affects the patient's ability to exercise and maintain ADLs, leading to manifestations such as the following:

- **Fatigue** (*decreased oxygen and glucose delivery to cells leads to decreased ATP production*)

- **Shortness of breath, dyspnea** (*decreased cardiac output leads to decreased pulmonary blood flow, which leads to carbon dioxide retention stimulating the respiratory center; decreased cellular oxygen causes a shift to anaerobic cellular metabolism, which causes increased production of nonvolatile acids and stimulation of the respiratory center*)

- **Tachycardia** (*decreased stroke volume leads to decreased cardiac output, which leads to catecholamine release, increased heart rate and contractility, and increased cardiac work*)

Disorders that interfere with peripheral blood flow and lymphatic flow include constriction, obstruction, inflammation, and vasospasm. Sufficient blood volume, blood cells, blood and lymph flow, and oxygen are required to carry out ADLs. Activity-exercise patterns are affected by peripheral tissue perfusion and perceived health status in two primary ways:

- Factors affected by too few cells: anemia (e.g., blood loss, nutritional, hemolytic), leukopenia (e.g., neutropenia, autoimmune disorders), thrombocytopenia (e.g., aplastic anemia, thrombocytopenic purpura, disseminated intravascular coagulation)

- Factors affected by too many cells: polycythemia (e.g., polycythemia vera or secondary polycythemia), leukocytosis (e.g., leukemia), lymphocytosis (malignant lymphoma, multiple myeloma)

The hematopoietic system is the blood-forming system that includes the bone marrow tissues where blood cells are formed and the lymphoid tissues of the lymph nodes where white blood cells mature and circulate. Disorders affecting blood and blood-forming organs, peripheral blood flow, and lymphatic fluid flow lead to disorders of blood pressure regulation, peripheral artery function, aortic structure, venous circulation, and lymphatic circulation. These disorders disturb a patient's perceived pattern of activity-exercise patterns, which affects how health is managed, leading to manifestations such as the following:

- **Edema** (*obstruction of blood vessels or lymphatic circulation causes buildup of fluid, resulting in swelling*)

- **Bleeding** (*deficiency in platelets and clotting factors affect homeostasis, resulting in inability to clot*)

CLINICAL SCENARIO

Directions: *Read the following clinical scenarios and answer the questions that follow. To complete this exercise successfully, you will utilize not only knowledge of the content in this unit but also principles related to priority setting and maintaining patient safety.*

You have been assigned to work with the following four patients for the 0700 shift on a cardiac telemetry unit. Significant data obtained during report is as follows:

- Betty Williams, aged 62, was admitted with acute anterior MI and had successful fibrinolytic therapy 3 days ago. Significant history includes type 2 diabetes, angina, hypertension, and a history of smoking (1.5 to 2 packs per day for 45 years). Her CCU course was uneventful. Current vital signs are T 98.9°F, P 76, R 16, BP 148/88. Cardiac monitor shows normal sinus rhythm with no ectopy. She has been pain free since her nitroglycerin drip was titrated off in the CCU 2 days ago. Lung sounds are clear.
- Arnold Markus, aged 71, was admitted with acute heart failure 2 days ago, treated and stabilized in the CCU, and transferred to the cardiac telemetry unit. Current vital signs

are T 98.4°F, P 88, R 18, BP 112/74. Cardiac monitor shows normal sinus rhythm with new isolated premature ventricular contractions (PVCs). Lung sounds are clear in upper lobes with crackles in the left bases, and he was able to sleep intermittently during the night using two pillows.
- Theresa Cartwright, a 34-year-old mother of four young children, was admitted for anticoagulant therapy after developing a deep vein thrombosis after a fall down the steps and hitting her calf. She was started on heparin yesterday and needs blood drawn for an activated partial thromboplastin time (aPTT) to determine her morning dose of heparin.
- Scott Jacoby is a 25-year-old with Down's syndrome. He was admitted yesterday with an upper respiratory infection. Upon assessment he was pale, had a temperature of 101°F, a heart rate of 100, respiratory rate of 30 with dyspnea on exertion, blood pressure of 118/86, and multiple bruises and petechiae on his arms and legs. He is scheduled for a bone marrow examination this morning.

Priority nursing diagnoses within the Activity-Exercise Pattern that may be appropriate for patients with cardiac disease include the following:

- *Decreased Cardiac Output* as evidenced by increased heart rate, fatigue, shortness of breath, decreased urine output, impaired mental processing, and decreased level of consciousness
- *Activity Intolerance* as evidenced by prolonged heart rate increases following activity, shortness of breath with exercise, activity-related chest pain, and fatigue
- *Ineffective Tissue Perfusion* as evidenced by changes in skin color and temperature, lack of hair growth, skin irritations, or ulcers
- *Risk for Peripheral Neurovascular Dysfunction* as evidenced by numbness and tingling in extremities, extremity pain, and cool and pale color to extremities
- *Fatigue* as evidenced by inability to consume a full meal without resting, frequent napping or dozing, expressions of tiredness, and weakness

Nursing diagnoses from other functional health patterns often are of high priority for the patient with heart disease because the physiologic responses to these problems increase cardiac work:

- *Acute Pain* (Cognitive-Perceptual)
- *Anxiety* (Coping-Stress-Tolerance)
- *Impaired Tissue Integrity* (Nutritional-Metabolic)

Question

1. What did you do to help your patients manage their activity needs without increasing their cardiac workload? What safety measures did you take to protect your patients with peripheral vascular or hematologic disorders?

Questions

Priority Setting

1. In what order would you visit these patients after report?
   A. _____
   B. _____
   C. _____
   D. _____

Health Promotion

1. In preparing discharge teaching for Mr. Markus, what information about a low sodium diet should the nurse include?
2. What health promotion topics should be included in teaching for Mrs. Williams?
3. What health promotion topics should the nurse discuss with Ms. Cartwright?

Nursing Process

1. What top priority nursing diagnoses would you choose for each of the patients presented earlier? Explain the rationale for your choices.

	Nursing Diagnosis	Rationale
Betty Williams		
Arnold Markus		
Theresa Cartwright		
Scott Jacoby		

2. You are completing a beginning-of-shift assessment with Mr. Markus. Which of the following items would take priority?
   A. rhythm strip analysis
   B. lung sounds
   C. oxygen saturation
   D. heart sounds

3. The charge nurse tells you that the monitor at the nurse's station shows that Mr. Markus is having an increase in PVCs. You would be most concerned after reviewing a rhythm strip if the PVC had which of the following characteristics?
   A. had a frequency of 4 per minute
   B. could be felt by the patient
   C. was unifocal in morphology
   D. fell on the T wave of the preceding beat

4. Ms. Williams rings the call bell and tells you that she is having pressure in her chest. On assessment, she rates it as a 5. Which of the following nursing actions should take priority?
   A. Obtain a full symptom assessment.
   B. Administer a prn nitroglycerine tablet SL.
   C. Call for an electrocardiogram.
   D. Notify the physician.

5. Which is the most important for you to report when caring for Mr. Jacoby?
   A. constipation and straining with bowel movements
   B. fever and burning on urination
   C. weight loss and decreased appetite
   D. dyspnea and shortness of breath with exercising

6. When Mrs. Cartwright is placed on warfarin (Coumadin) therapy, which laboratory studies would you expect to draw? **Select all that apply.**
   A. activated partial thromboplastin time (aPTT)
   B. international normalized ratio (INR)
   C. partial thromboplastin time (PTT)
   D. complete blood cell count (CBC)
   E. white blood cell count (WBC)
   F. prothrombin time (PT)

Communication

1. Mrs. Cartwright needs further teaching regarding anticoagulant therapy when she makes which statement?
   A. "It takes four to five days of heparin and Coumadin to reach a good effect from the drugs."
   B. "I need to continue to have blood drawn to watch my drug levels as long as I am taking these drugs."
   C. "I cannot continue to take birth control pills while I am taking these drugs."
   D. "I need to take the medication at the same time every day for the drug to be effective."

2. Ms. Williams asks how this heart attack will affect her active life. How will you answer?

Delegation

1. For each patient, what assessment data and nursing interventions can be delegated to a nursing assistant?

Related Questions

1. Considering the mitral valve replacement surgery, the nurse would be most concerned about possible risks to

medication therapy if the patient had a history of which of the following disorders?
   A. glaucoma
   B. gout
   C. duodenal ulcer
   D. osteoarthritis

2. Which nursing diagnosis has the highest priority for the patient with varicose veins?
   A. body image disturbance
   B. impaired tissue perfusion
   C. activity intolerance
   D. risk for infection

3. Which is a priority teaching instruction for the patient with a history of Raynaud's disease?
   A. Enter a cease smoking program.
   B. Reduce dietary fats and carbohydrates.
   C. Wear gloves and socks in cold weather.
   D. Begin an exercise program.

4. A prescription for the calcium channel blocker diltiazem (Cardizem) is ordered for the patient with hypertension. With which of the following will the nurse instruct the patient regarding administration of the medication?
   A. Limit fluids to decrease the development of peripheral edema.
   B. Notify the physician for a pulse less than 60 beats per minute.
   C. Increase fiber in the diet, as diarrhea may be a side effect.
   D. Report tachycardia and increase in blood pressure.

5. A patient with history of hemophilia fell and cut his leg while hiking in the woods. Which intervention should the patient perform until help arrives?
   A. Apply a tourniquet above the cut.
   B. Splint the leg to prevent movement.
   C. Apply pressure to the femoral artery.
   D. Apply direct pressure over the cut.

CASE STUDY: Grace Schmidt

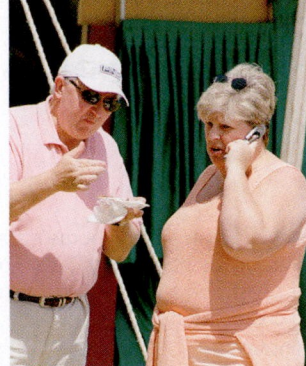

Grace Schmidt is a 49-year-old female who works as a teaching assistant at an elementary school. She comes to the medical clinic complaining of a throbbing headache and dizziness. Her height and weight are obtained at 5'6" and 245 pounds. Upon assessment her vital signs are pulse 100, respirations 16, blood pressure lying 180/115, sitting 170/110, and standing 165/105. Her skin is cool and dry. Her capillary refill is 4 seconds. She denies smoking, drinks an occasional glass of wine, and does not participate in a regular exercise program. She states that her job can be stressful at times. Nutrition assessment indicates a diet high in fats and sodium. She denies any family history of hypertension or heart disease. She is married and has a daughter and son who live in the same town.

Due to the high blood pressure readings, a medical diagnosis of hypertension is determined. The pathophysiology of hypertension is that excessive sympathetic nervous system stimulation overstimulates adrenergic receptors, resulting in vasoconstriction and increased cardiac output. Systemic venous resistance increases due to high levels of angiotensin II resulting from the release of renin, which is involved in the renin–angiotensin–aldosterone system. Atrial natriuretic and other chemical mediators cause sodium and water retention, which increases blood volume and also cause vasoconstriction. Excess insulin causes sodium retention, increased sympathetic nervous system activity, hypertrophy of vascular smooth muscle, and changes in ion transport across cell membranes contributing to hypertension. The resulting increased blood volume, increased systemic vascular resistance, increased cardiac output, and vasoconstriction cause hypertension. The manifestations of hypertension are initially asymptomatic. When manifestations begin to appear, they begin with a headache usually in the back of the head and neck. Other manifestations are nocturia, confusion, nausea and vomiting, visual disturbances, and papilledema. Complications of hypertension are related to accelerated atherosclerosis, which results in an increased risk for coronary heart disease and increased risk for stroke. Other complications are hypertensive encephalopathy, dysrhythmias, myocardial infarction, heart failure, nephrosclerosis, renal insufficiency, and chronic renal failure.

Based on Mrs. Schmidt's assessment, blood pressure readings, and weight, a nursing diagnosis of *Ineffective Health Maintenance* is appropriate for planning nursing care.

- Excess SNS stimulation → vasoconstriction and ↑ cardiac output → ↑ BP
- Altered renin-angiotensin-aldosterone system function → ↑ SVR, Na+ and water retention → ↑ BP
- Imbalanced chemical mediators → ↑ SVR, Na+ and water retention → ↑ BP
- Insulin resistance and hyperinsulinemia → Na+ retention, ↑ SNS activity, vascular smooth muscle hypertrophy, changes in cell membrane transport → sustained HTN

affects

Mrs. G.S.
49 y.o. female
Hypertension

leads to

assess

- Height 5' 6", weight 245 lb
- BP 180/115 lying, 170/110 sitting, and 165/105 standing
- Skin cool and dry, capillary refill 4 sec.
- C/o throbbing headache, dizziness
- Denies smoking, drinks wine on occasion; diet high in fat and sodium
- No regular exercise, states job is stressful at times
- Denies family history of hypertension or heart disease

generates

- Imbalanced Nutrition: More than Body Requirements
- Deficient Knowledge: Diet and Exercise
- Readiness for Enhanced Therapeutic Regimen Management
- Acute Pain

generate nursing diagnosis

prioritized to

Ineffective Health Maintenance

expected outcomes

- Verbalizes understanding of prescribed medications and their desired effects
- Consumes a nutritionally sound diet low in fat, sodium, and calories
- Loses 1-2 lb per week
- Engages in aerobic exercise 5 + days/wk, gradually increasing duration and intensity
- Identifies stress-reducing techniques
- BP 140/85 or lower

evaluate

Two weeks after initial visit:
- BP 136/86
- Wt 239 lb
- Denies headache
- States she is eating more whole grains, fruits and vegetables, and fewer high-fat foods
- Walking 1-1.5 miles in 30 minutes "most days"
- States she still experiences stress at work, but exercise during lunch hour and breaks helps relieve tension

Interdisciplinary Interventions
- Provide verbal and written instructions about medications.
- Monitor blood pressures and laboratory results on a continuing basis, reporting abnormal results or negative trends.

Independent Interventions
- Refer to dietitian for diet planning and teaching.
- Provide information about and referral to weight loss programs and support groups such as Weight Watchers.
- Refer to cardiac rehab program for exercise evaluation, teaching, and support.
- Discuss stress-reduction techniques; provide referrals as desired (e.g., herbalist, licensed massage therapist, counselor).

Activity:

1. After reviewing the concept map, is there anything you would change to make it more understandable?

2. Go to the Pearson Nursing Student Resources for this book at www.nursing.pearsonhighered.com to write a concept map based on hypertension complicated by chronic kidney disease.

UNIT 9

Responses to Altered
Respiratory Function

LEARNING OUTCOMES

1. Describe the anatomy, physiology, and functions of the respiratory system.
2. Compare and contrast factors affecting respiration.
3. Identify specific topics for consideration during a health history interview of the patient with health problems involving the respiratory system.
4. Give examples of genetic disorders of the respiratory system.
5. Describe normal variations in assessment findings for the older adult.
6. Identify abnormal findings that may indicate alterations in respiratory function.

CLINICAL COMPETENCIES

1. Conduct and document a health history for patients having or at risk for alterations in the respiratory system.
2. Conduct and document a physical assessment of respiratory structures and functions.
3. Monitor the results of diagnostic tests and report abnormal findings.

EQUIPMENT NEEDED

- Tongue blade
- Penlight
- Nasal speculum
- Metric ruler
- Marking pen
- Stethoscope with diaphragm

KEY TERMS

apnea, 1135
atelectasis, 1135
bradypnea, 1135
crackles, 1138

friction rub, 1138
lung compliance, 1128
oxyhemoglobin, 1128
surfactant, 1128

tachypnea, 1135
tidal volume (TV), 1127
vital capacity (VC), 1127
wheezes, 1138

The respiratory system provides oxygen to cells and eliminates carbon dioxide, formed as a waste product of cellular metabolism. The events in this process, called respiration, are ventilation (the movement of air into and out of the lungs), perfusion (the flow of blood through the capillary system surrounding the lungs) and diffusion (the process of gas exchange between the blood and the alveoli of the lungs). The movement of respiratory muscles is controlled by the nervous system and respiratory rate is adjusted to match body requirements during various activities.

Anatomy, Physiology, and Functions of the Respiratory System

The respiratory system functions as a whole, but is divided in this chapter into the upper respiratory system and the lower respiratory system for discussion purposes.

The Upper Respiratory System

The upper respiratory system, composed of the conducting airways (nose, mouth and pharynx, larynx, and trachea) serves as a passageway for air moving into the lungs and for carbon dioxide moving out to the external environment (Figure 34–1 ■). As air moves through these structures, it is cleaned, filtered, humidified, and warmed.

The Nose and Sinuses

The nose, the external opening of the respiratory system, is given structure by the nasal, frontal, and maxillary bones as well as plates of hyaline cartilage. The nostrils (also called the external nares) are two cavities within the nose, separated by the nasal septum. Nasal hairs filter the air as it enters the nares and secreted mucus not only traps dust and bacteria but also contains lysozyme, an enzyme that destroys bacteria as they enter the nose. As mucus and debris accumulate, mucosal ciliated cells move it toward the pharynx, where it is swallowed. The mucosa is highly vascular, warming air that moves across

Superior turbinate
Middle turbinate
Inferior turbinate
External nares
Hard palate
Soft palate
Tongue
Epiglottis
Thyroid cartilage of larynx
Cricoid cartilage
Trachea

Internal nares
Adenoids
Auditory tube opening
Nasopharynx
Uvula
Tonsils
Oropharynx
Laryngopharynx
Esophagus

Figure 34–1 ■ The upper respiratory system.

its surface. The nasal cavity is surrounded by paranasal sinuses (Figure 34–2 ■), located in the frontal, sphenoid, ethmoid, and maxillary bones. Sinuses lighten the skull, assist in speech, and produce mucus that drains into the nasal cavities to help trap debris. The mouth is an alternate airway, used if the nasal passages are plugged or a large intake of air is needed (for example, during strenuous exercise) (Porth, 2007).

The Pharynx

The pharynx, a funnel-shaped passageway about 5 inches (13 cm) long, extends from the base of the skull to the level of the C6 vertebra. The pharynx serves as a passageway for both air and food. It is divided into three regions: the nasopharynx, the oropharynx, and the laryngopharynx.

The nasopharynx serves only as a passageway for air. Masses of lymphoid tissue (the tonsils and adenoids), located in the mucosa high in the posterior wall trap and destroy infectious agents entering with the air. The eustachian tubes also open into the nasopharynx, connecting it with the middle ear. The

oropharynx lies behind the oral cavity and extends from the soft palate to the level of the hyoid bone. It serves as a passageway for both air and food. An upward rise of the soft palate prevents food from entering the nasopharynx during swallowing. The laryngopharynx, extending from the hyoid bone to the larynx, serves as a passageway for both food and air.

The Larynx

The larynx is about 2 inches (5 cm) long. It provides an airway, routes air and food into the proper passageway, and contains the vocal cords. As long as air is moving through the larynx, its inlet is open; however, the inlet closes during swallowing. The larynx is framed by the thyroid, the cricoid, and the epiglottis cartilages. The thyroid cartilage is formed by the fusion of two cartilages; the fusion point is visible as the Adam's apple. The cricoid cartilage lies below the thyroid cartilage. The epiglottis normally projects upward to the base of the tongue; however, during swallowing, the larynx moves upward and the epiglottis tips to cover the opening to the larynx. If anything other than air enters the larynx, a cough reflex expels the foreign substance before it can enter the lungs. This protective reflex does not work if the person is unconscious.

The Trachea

The trachea begins at the inferior larynx and descends anteriorly to the esophagus to enter the mediastinum, where it divides to become the right and left primary bronchi of the lungs. The trachea is about 4 to 5 inches (12 to 15 cm) long and 1 inch (2.5 cm) in diameter. The mucosa lining the trachea contains seromucous glands that produce thick mucus. Dust and debris in inspired air are trapped in this mucus, moved toward the throat by the cilia, and then either swallowed or coughed out through the mouth.

Frontal sinuses
Ethmoid sinuses
Sphenoid sinus
Maxillary sinuses

Frontal view

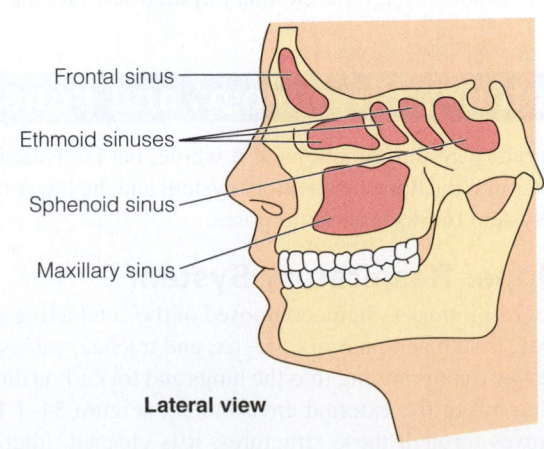

Frontal sinus
Ethmoid sinuses
Sphenoid sinus
Maxillary sinus

Lateral view

Figure 34–2 ■ Sinuses, frontal and lateral views.

Trachea

Apex of lung

Parietal pleura

Lung

Rib

Pleural cavity

Intercostal muscle

Visceral pleura

Right upper lobe

Horizontal fissure

Right middle lobe

Oblique fissure

Right lower lobe

Heart
(in mediastinum)

Left upper lobe

Cardiac notch

Oblique fissure

Left lower lobe

Base of lung

Diaphragm

Figure 34–3 ■ The lower respiratory system, showing the location of the lungs, the mediastinum, and layers of visceral and parietal pleura.

The Lower Respiratory System

The lower respiratory system includes the lungs, the bronchi, and the bronchioles (Figure 34–3 ■ and Figure 34–4 ■).

The Lungs

The center of the thoracic cavity is filled by the mediastinum, which contains the heart, great blood vessels, bronchi, trachea, and esophagus. The mediastinum is flanked on either side by the lungs (see Figure 34–3). Each lung is suspended in its own pleural cavity, with the anterior, lateral, and posterior lung surfaces lying close to the ribs. The hilus, on the mediastinal surface of each lung, is where blood vessels of the pulmonary

and circulatory systems and the primary bronchus enter and exit the lungs. The apex of each lung lies just below the clavicle and the base of each lung rests on the diaphragm. The lungs are elastic connective tissue, called stroma, and are soft and spongy. The two lungs differ in size and shape. The left lung is smaller and has two lobes, whereas the right lung has three lobes.

The vascular system of the lungs consists of the pulmonary arteries, which deliver blood to the lungs for oxygenation, and the pulmonary veins, which deliver oxygenated blood to the heart. Within the lungs, the pulmonary arteries branch into a pulmonary capillary network that surrounds the alveoli. Lung tissue receives its blood supply from the bronchial arteries and drains by the bronchial and pulmonary veins.

The Pleura

The pleura is a double-layered membrane that covers the lungs and the inside of the thoracic cavities (see Figure 34–3). The parietal pleura lines the thoracic wall and mediastinum. It is continuous with the visceral pleura, which covers the external lung surfaces. The pleura produces pleural fluid, a lubricating, serous fluid that allows the lungs to move

Terminal
bronchiole

Respiratory
bronchioles

Alveolar
duct

Alveoli

Figure 34–4 ■ Respiratory bronchi, bronchioles, alveolar ducts, and alveoli.

Figure 34–5 ■ *A*, Anterior rib cage, showing intercostal spaces. *B*, Posterior rib cage.

easily over the thoracic wall during breathing. The structure of the pleura creates a slightly negative pressure in the pleural space (which is actually a potential rather than an actual space), necessary for lung function.

The Bronchi and Alveoli
The trachea divides into right and left primary bronchi; the right primary bronchus is shorter, wider, and situated more vertically (making aspiration of foreign bodies into the right primary bronchus more likely). The point where the trachea divides is innervated with sensory neurons; activities such as tracheal suctioning may induce coughing and bronchospasm from stimulation of these neurons. The bronchi subdivide into smaller bronchi, and then into smaller bronchioles, ending in the terminal bronchioles, which are extremely small (see Figure 34–4). These branching passageways collectively are called the bronchial tree. From the terminal bronchioles, air moves into air sacs, which further branch into alveolar ducts that lead to alveolar sacs and then to the tiny alveoli. During inspiration, air enters the lungs through the primary bronchus and then moves through the increasingly smaller passageways of the lungs to the alveoli, where oxygen and carbon dioxide exchange occurs.

Alveoli cluster around the alveolar sacs, which open into a common chamber called the atrium. The adult lung has approximately 300 million alveoli, providing an enormous surface for gas exchange (Porth, 2007). The walls of alveoli are a single layer of squamous epithelial cells over a very thin basement membrane. The external surface of the alveoli are covered with pulmonary capillaries. The alveolar and capillary walls form the respiratory membrane. Gas exchange across the respiratory membrane occurs by simple diffusion. The alveolar walls also contain cells that secrete a surfactant-containing fluid, necessary for maintaining a moist surface and reducing the surface tension of the alveolar fluid to help prevent collapse of the lungs.

The Rib Cage and Intercostal Muscles
The lungs are protected by the bones of the rib cage and the intercostal muscles. There are 12 pairs of ribs, which all articulate with the thoracic vertebrae (Figure 34–5 ■). The sternum has three parts: the manubrium, the body, and the xiphoid process. The spaces between the ribs are called the intercostal spaces. Each intercostal space is named for the rib immediately above it (e.g., the space between the third and fourth ribs is designated as the third intercostal space). The intercostal muscles between the ribs, along with the diaphragm, are called the inspiratory muscles.

Factors Affecting Respiration
Many factors affect respiration. Those discussed here include changes in volume and capacity; air pressures; oxygen, carbon dioxide, and hydrogen ion concentrations in the blood; airway resistance, lung compliance and elasticity; and alveolar surface tension.

Respiratory Volume and Capacity
Pulmonary function tests measure respiratory volumes and capacities, and are described and illustrated in Box 34–1.

Air Pressures
Ventilation has two phases: inspiration, during which air flows into the lungs; and expiration, during which gases flow out of the lungs. The two phases make up a single breath, and normally occur from 12 to 20 times each minute. A single inspiration lasts for about 1 to 1.5 seconds, whereas an expiration lasts for about 2 to 3 seconds.

During inspiration, the diaphragm contracts and flattens to increase the vertical diameter of the thoracic cavity (Figure 34–6 ■). The external intercostal muscles contract, elevating the rib cage and moving the sternum forward to expand the lateral and anteroposterior diameter of the thoracic cavity, decreasing intrapleural pressure. The lungs stretch and the intrapulmonary volume increases, decreasing intrapulmonary pressure slightly below atmospheric pressure. Air rushes into the lungs as a result of this pressure gradient until the intrapulmonary and atmospheric pressures equalize. In contrast, expiration is primarily a passive process that occurs as a result of the elasticity of the lungs (Figure 34–7 ■). The inspiratory muscles relax, the diaphragm rises, the ribs descend, and the lungs recoil. Both the thoracic and intrapulmonary pressures increase, compressing the alveoli.

Ventilation depends on volume changes within the thoracic cavity. A change in the volume of air in the thoracic cavity leads

BOX 34–1 Pulmonary Function Tests

Pulmonary function tests (PFTs) are performed in a pulmonary function laboratory. After preparing the patient, a nose clip is applied and the patient breathes into a spirometer or body plethysmograph, a device for measuring and recording lung volume in liters versus time in seconds. The patient is instructed how to breathe for specific tests: for example, to inhale as deeply as possible and then exhale to the maximal extent possible. Using measured lung volumes, respiratory capacities are calculated to assess pulmonary status. The specific values determined by PFT and illustrated in the figure include the following.

■ *Total lung capacity (TLC)* is the total volume of the lungs at their maximum inflation. Four values are used to calculate TLC, with normal values for a healthy adult in parentheses.

  a. **Tidal Volume (TV)**, the volume inhaled and exhaled with normal quiet breathing (500 mL)

  b. *Inspiratory reserve volume (IRV)*, the maximum amount that can be inhaled over and above a normal inspiration (2000 mL–3100 mL)

  c. *Expiratory reserve volume (ERV)*, the maximum amount that can be exhaled following a normal exhalation (1000 mL)

  d. *Residual volume (RV)*, the amount of air remaining in the lungs after maximal exhalation (1100 mL)

■ **Vital capacity (VC)** is the total amount of air that can be exhaled after a maximal inspiration. It is calculated by adding together the IRV, TV, and the ERV (4500 mL).

■ *Inspiratory capacity* is the total amount of air that can be inhaled following a normal quiet exhalation. It is calculated by adding the TV and IRV.

■ *Functional residual capacity (FRC)* is the volume of air left in the lungs after a normal exhalation. The ERV and RV are added to determine the FRC.

■ *Forced expiratory volume (FEV_1)* is the amount of air that can be exhaled in 1 second.

■ *Forced vital capacity (FVC)* is the amount of air that can be exhaled forcefully and rapidly after maximum air intake.

■ *Minute volume (MV)* is the total amount or volume of air breathed in 1 minute.

to a change in the air pressure within the cavity. Because gases always flow along their pressure gradients, a change in pressure results in gases flowing into or out of the lungs to equalize the pressure. The pressures normally present in the thoracic cavity are the intrapulmonary pressure and the intrapleural pressure.

The intrapulmonary pressure, within the alveoli of the lungs, rises and falls constantly as a result of inhalation and exhalation. The intrapleural pressure, within the pleural space, also rises and falls with inhalation and exhalation, but it is always less than (or negative to) the intrapulmonary pressure. Intrapulmonary and

Figure 34–6 ■ Respiratory inspiration: lateral and anterior views. Note the volume expansion of the thorax as the diaphragm flattens.

Figure 34–7 ■ Respiratory expiration: lateral and anterior views.

intrapleural pressures are necessary not only to expand and contract the lungs, but also to prevent their collapse. The intrapulmonary pressure rises to a level greater than atmospheric pressure, and gases flow out of the lungs.

Oxygen, Carbon Dioxide, and Hydrogen Ion Concentrations

The rate and depth of respirations are controlled by respiratory centers in the medulla oblongata and pons of the brain and by chemoreceptors located in the medulla and in the carotid and aortic bodies. The centers and chemoreceptors respond to changes in the concentration of oxygen, carbon dioxide, and hydrogen ions in arterial blood. For example, when carbon dioxide concentration increases or the pH decreases, the respiratory rate increases. This process is further described in ∞ Chapter 10.

Airway Resistance, Lung Compliance, and Elasticity

Respiratory passageway resistance, lung compliance, and lung elasticity also affect respiration. Respiratory passageway resistance is created by the friction encountered as gases move along the respiratory passageways, by constriction of the passageways (especially the larger bronchioles), by accumulations of mucus or infectious material, and by tumors. As resistance increases, gas flow decreases. **Lung compliance** is the distensibility of the lungs. It depends on the elasticity of the lung tissue and the flexibility of the rib cage. Compliance is decreased by factors that decrease the elasticity of the lungs, block the respiratory passageways, or interfere with movement of the rib cage. Lung elasticity is essential for lung distention during inspiration and lung recoil during expiration. Decreased elasticity from disease such as emphysema impairs respiration.

Alveolar Surface Tension

A liquid film, primarily composed of water, covers the alveolar walls. At any gas–liquid boundary, the molecules of liquid are more strongly attracted to each other than to gas molecules. This produces a state of tension, called surface tension that draws the liquid molecules even more closely together. The water content of the alveolar film compacts the alveoli and aids

in the lungs' recoil during expiration. **Surfactant**, a lipoprotein produced by the alveolar cells, interferes with this adhesiveness of the water molecules, reducing surface tension, and helping expand the lungs.

Oxygen and Carbon Dioxide Transport

The alveolar and capillary structures of the lungs allow oxygen to be restored to the arterial blood and carbon dioxide to be removed from the venous blood. The blood carries both oxygen and carbon dioxide as dissolved gases and in chemical combination with hemoglobin. In addition, carbon dioxide is changed to and transported as bicarbonate. When arterial blood gases are measured in the practice setting, they are given values that reflect the partial pressure of the gas in the alveoli (PO_2= partial pressure of oxygen, PCO_2= partial pressure of carbon dioxide). Arterial blood gases are used for clinical measurement as they reflect the gas exchange function of the alveoli (venous blood reflects the metabolic demands of the tissues) (Porth & Matfin, 2009). Normally, the PO_2 of arterial blood is greater than 80mmHg and the PCO_2 of arterial blood ranges from 35 to 45 mmHg. The arterial blood gases reflect the partial pressure of the gas in the alveoli, increasing and decreasing as the alveolar pressure increases and decreases.

Oxygen Transport and Unloading

In the alveoli, oxygen moves to the pulmonary capillaries as a dissolved gas, moving down a concentration gradient. Oxygen is carried in the blood either dissolved or bound to hemoglobin. As oxygen is relatively insoluble in solution, its ability to bind with hemoglobin is essential. Approximately 98% to 99% of oxygen is transported in the blood combined with hemoglobin as **oxyhemoglobin**; the remaining 1% to 2% is carried in the dissolved state (Porth & Matfin, 2009).

Each hemoglobin molecule is made of four polypeptide chains, with each chain bound to an iron-containing heme group. The iron groups are the binding sites for oxygen; each hemoglobin molecule can form a loose and reversible bond with four molecules of oxygen. Oxygen binding is rapid and its affinity to hemoglobin is affected by temperature, blood pH, PO_2, PCO_2, and serum concentration of 2,3-DPG. These factors interact to ensure adequate delivery of oxygen to the cells.

- Under normal conditions, the hemoglobin in arterial blood is almost fully saturated at a PO_2 of 70 mmHg. As arterial blood flows through the capillaries, oxygen is unloaded, so that the oxygen saturation of hemoglobin in venous blood is 75%.
- The affinity of oxygen and hemoglobin decreases as the temperature of body tissues increases above normal. As a result, less oxygen binds with hemoglobin, and oxygen unloading increases. Conversely, as the body is chilled, oxygen unloading decreases.
- The oxygen-hemoglobin bond is weakened by increased hydrogen ion concentrations. As blood becomes more acidotic, oxygen unloading to the tissues increases. The same process occurs when the partial pressure of carbon dioxide increases because this decreases the pH (acid–base balance is discussed in ∞ Chapter 10).
- The organic chemical 2,3-DPG is formed in red blood cells and increases the release of oxygen from hemoglobin by binding to it during times of increased metabolism (as when body temperature increases). This binding alters the structure of hemoglobin to facilitate oxygen unloading.

When the blood reaches the capillary level, it is critical that oxygen be able to dissociate from hemoglobin as only dissolved oxygen that is not bound to hemoglobin is able to pass through the capillary wall, diffuse through the cell membrane, and be available for use in cell metabolism. The relation between the oxygen carried in combination with hemoglobin and the PO_2 of the blood can be illustrated in the oxygen-hemoglobin dissociation curve, which demonstrates the release of oxygen from hemoglobin at the tissue capillaries. (See Figure 34–8 ■.)

Carbon Dioxide Transport

Active cells produce about 200 mL of carbon dioxide each minute; this amount is exactly the same as that excreted by the lungs each minute. Excretion of carbon dioxide from the body requires transport by the blood from the cells to the lungs. Carbon dioxide is transported in three forms: as bicarbonate ions in the plasma (the largest amount is in this form), dissolved in plasma, and bound to hemoglobin.

The amount of carbon dioxide transported in the blood is strongly influenced by the oxygenation of the blood. When the PO_2 decreases, with a corresponding decrease in oxygen saturation, increased amounts of carbon dioxide can be carried in the blood. Carbon dioxide entering the systemic circulation from the cells causes more oxygen to dissociate from hemoglobin, in turn allowing more carbon dioxide to combine with hemoglobin and more bicarbonate ions to be generated. This situation is reversed in the pulmonary circulation, where the uptake of oxygen facilitates the release of carbon dioxide.

Assessing Respiratory Function

Function of the respiratory system is assessed by findings from diagnostic tests, a health assessment interview to collect subjective data, and a physical assessment to collect objective data.

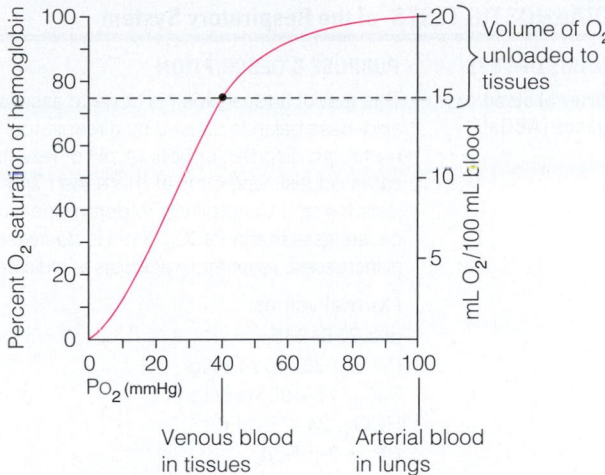

Figure 34–8 ■ Oxygen-hemoglobin dissociation curve. The percent O_2 saturation of hemoglobin and total blood oxygen volume are shown for different oxygen partial pressures (PO_2). Arterial blood in the lungs is almost completely saturated. During one pass through the body, about 25% of hemoglobin-bound oxygen is unloaded to the tissues. Thus, venous blood is still about 75% saturated with oxygen. The steep portion of the curve shows that hemoglobin readily off-loads or on-loads oxygen at PO_2 levels below about 50 mmHg.

Diagnostic Tests

The results of diagnostic tests of respiratory function are used to support the diagnosis of a specific disease, to provide information to identify or modify the appropriate medications or therapy used to treat the disease, and to help nurses monitor the patient's responses to treatment and nursing care interventions. Diagnostic tests to assess the structures and functions of the respiratory system are described in the Diagnostic Tests table. More information is included in the discussion of specific disorders in ∞ Chapters 35, 36 and 37.

Regardless of the type of diagnostic test, the nurse is responsible for explaining the procedure and any special preparation needed, assessing for medication use that may affect the outcome of the tests, supporting the patient during the examination as necessary, ensuring the consent form is signed (if necessary), documenting the procedures as appropriate, and monitoring the results of the tests.

Genetic Considerations

When conducting a health assessment interview and a physical assessment, it is important for the nurse to consider genetic influences on health of the adult. During the health assessment interview, ask about family members with health problems affecting respiratory function. In addition, ask about a family history of emphysema, asthma, cystic fibrosis, or lung cancer. During the physical assessment, assess for any manifestations that might indicate a genetic disorder (see the Genetic Considerations box on page 1133). If data are found to indicate genetic risk factors or alterations, ask about genetic testing and refer for appropriate genetic counseling and evaluation. ∞ Chapter 8 provides further information about genetics in medical-surgical nursing.

DIAGNOSTIC TESTS of the Respiratory System

NAME OF TEST	PURPOSE & DESCRIPTION	RELATED NURSING INTERVENTIONS
Arterial blood gases (ABGs)	This test of arterial blood is done to assess alterations in acid–base balance caused by a respiratory disorder, a metabolic disorder, or both. A pH of less than 7.35 indicates acidosis and a pH of more than 7.45 indicates alkalosis (∞ see Chapter 10). To determine a respiratory cause, assess the $PaCO_2$: If pH is decreased and $PaCO_2$ is increased, respiratory acidosis is indicated. Normal values: pH: 7.35–7.45 $PaCO_2$: 35–45 mmHg PaO_2: 75–100 mmHg HCO_3: 24–28 mEq/L BE: ± 2 mEq/L	Arterial blood is collected in a heparinized needle and syringe. Notify the person collecting the blood sample if the patient is taking anticoagulants or aspirin, or has a clotting problem. The sample is placed on an ice-water bag and taken immediately to the lab. If patient is receiving oxygen indicate the type, flow rate, administration device, and patient's temperature on lab slip. Apply pressure to puncture site for 5 minutes or longer if needed (for example, taking anticoagulants or streptokinase). Do not collect blood from the same arm used for an IV infusion.
Biopsy of the lung	A biopsy of the lung is done to obtain tissue to differentiate benign from malignant tumors of the lungs. The biopsy may be done during a bronchoscopy, or by surgical procedure.	Same as bronchoscopy or the same as a thoracotomy (incision through the chest wall) if a surgical biopsy is performed.
Bronchoscopy	A bronchoscopy is the direct visualization of the larynx, trachea, and bronchi through a bronchoscope to identify lesions, remove foreign bodies and secretions, obtain tissue for biopsy, and improve tracheobronchial drainage (Figure 34–9 ■). The bronchoscope (in most cases, a fiber optic scope) is passed through the nose or mouth and into the trachea. During the test, a catheter brush or biopsy forceps can be passed to obtain secretions or tissue for examination for cancer. The test is done in the hospital, and may be done at the bedside, in a special procedure room, or in the surgical suite.	Assess for pregnancy and hypersensitivity to anesthetics, antibiotics, iodine, or contract dyes; if present, notify the physician. Tell the patient not to eat or drink fluids for 8 to 12 hours before the test. Remove dentures, contact lenses, and jewelry. Assess and record vital signs. Administer ordered premedications. After the procedure, assess for complications (laryngeal edema, bronchospasm, pneumothorax, cardiac dysrhythmias, and bleeding). Monitor for manifestations of respiratory difficulty (dyspnea, decreased breath sounds, decreased O_2 saturation) and hemoptysis (bloody sputum). Assess if the gag reflex is present before beginning food or fluids. Instruct the patient not to smoke for 6 to 8 hours after the procedure as smoking may cause coughing and start bleeding. Tell the patient it is normal to have some blood-tinged sputum, hoarseness and/or a sore throat, but to notify the physician of any bleeding, pain, or respiratory difficulty.

Figure 34–9 ■ Fiberoptic bronchoscopy.

| Chest x-ray | Chest x-rays are used to identify abnormalities in chest structure and lung tissue, for diagnosis of diseases and injuries of the lungs, and to monitor treatment. | No special preparation is needed. |

DIAGNOSTIC TESTS of the Respiratory System (continued)

NAME OF TEST	PURPOSE & DESCRIPTION	RELATED NURSING INTERVENTIONS
CT Scan of the thorax	CT of the thorax may be performed when x-rays do not show some areas well, such as the pleura and mediastinum. It is also done to differentiate pathologic conditions (such as tumors, abscesses, and aortic aneurysms), to identify pleural effusion and enlarged lymph nodes, and to monitor treatment. Images are shown in cross-section.	If contrast dye is used, inform patient to not take oral food or fluids for 4 hours before the test; if dye is not used there are no food or fluid restrictions. Assess for allergies to iodine (for example, to shellfish or previous procedures) and if present, notify the physician; medications such as diphenhydramine (Benadryl) and ranitidine (Zantac) may be given one hour before the procedure. Assess medications: Oral hypoglycemic agents are contraindicated for use with iodinated contrast. Instruct the patient to increase oral fluid intake after the examination.
Magnetic resonance imaging (MRI) of the thorax	An MRI of the thorax is used to diagnose alterations in lung tissue more difficult to visualize by CT scan and to identify abnormal masses and fluid accumulation.	Inform patient of need to lie still during the examination. Assess for any metallic implants (such as pacemakers, clips on brain aneurysms, body piercing, tattoos, shrapnel). If present, notify imaging physician. Remove transdermal medication patches (both OTC and prescribed) unless otherwise ordered (FDA, 2009). Replace the patch following the procedure. Tell the patient to inform the staff about the patch when making the appointment and when completing the admission information. Ask if patient is pregnant; if so the test is not performed. Ask about claustrophobia; if it is a problem request the patient to ask for a relaxing medication to take prior to the MRI.
Pulmonary angiography (angiogram)	This test, conducted in the hospital setting, is done to identify pulmonary emboli, tumors, aneurysms, vascular changes associated with emphysema, and pulmonary circulation. A catheter is inserted into the brachial or femoral artery, threaded into the pulmonary artery and dye is injected. ECG leads are applied to the chest for cardiac monitoring. Images of the lungs are taken.	Assess for hypersensitivity to iodine, seafood, or previous procedures using contrast dye. Take and record baseline vital signs. After the procedure, apply pressure to the injection site for 5 to 10 minutes (or until bleeding has stopped). Enforce bed rest for 12 to 24 hours as ordered. Monitor vital signs, injection site and peripheral pulses distal to the site after the test. Tell patient that coughing is a common occurrence after this test.
Pulmonary ventilation scan (V/Q scan)	This test is performed with two nuclear scans to measure breathing (ventilation) and circulation (perfusion) in all parts of the lungs. A ventilation scan is performed by scanning the lungs as the patient inhales radioactive gas. A perfusion scan is performed by injecting radioactive albumin into a vein and scanning the lungs. A decreased uptake of radioisotope during the perfusion scan indicates a blood flow problem, such as from a pulmonary embolus or pneumonitis. A decreased uptake of gas during the ventilation scan may indicate airway obstruction, pneumonia, or chronic pulmonary obstructive disease (COPD).	Tell the patient to remove all jewelry from the neck and chest.
Pulse oximetry	This noninvasive test is used to evaluate or monitor oxygen saturation of the blood. A device that uses infrared light is attached to an extremity (most commonly the finger, but can also be used on the toe, earlobe, or nose) and light is passed through the tissues or reflected off bony structures. Normal value: 90%–100%	Assess for factors that may alter findings, including faulty placement, movement, dark skin color, and acrylic nails. Light may affect the readings; the area of application should be shielded from external light sources.
Positron emission tomography (PET)	This relatively noninvasive test, when used to examine the lungs, is performed to identify lung nodules (cancers). The patient is given a radioactive substance and cross-sectional images are displayed on a computer.	Tell the patient that no alcohol, coffee, or tobacco is allowed for 24 hours prior to the test. Encourage increased fluid intake post-test to help eliminate the radioactive material.

(continued)

DIAGNOSTIC TESTS of the Respiratory System (continued)

NAME OF TEST	PURPOSE & DESCRIPTION	RELATED NURSING INTERVENTIONS
Sputum Studies ■ Culture and sensitivity ■ Acid-fast smear and culture ■ Cytology	Culture and sensitivity of a single sputum specimen is done to diagnose bacterial infections, identify the most effective antibiotic, and evaluate treatment. Sputum is examined for presence of acid-fast bacillus, specifically tuberculosis. A series of three early morning sputum specimens is used. Sputum is examined for presence of abnormal (malignant) cells. A single sputum specimen is collected in a special container of fixative solution.	Instruct the patient to collect the specimen early in the morning. Explain that the sputum should come from deep in the lungs; take two or three deep breaths, and then cough the specimen into a sterile container. Sputum specimens may also be obtained by a respiratory therapist or during bronchoscopy (described earlier) if the patient is unable to provide a specimen.
Thoracentesis	A thoracentesis is done to obtain a specimen of pleural fluid for diagnosis (and used as a procedure to remove pleural fluid or instill medication). A large-bore needle is inserted through the chest wall and into the pleural space. Following the procedure, a chest x-ray is taken to check for a pneumothorax.	Nursing care of the patient having a thoracentesis is provided in ∞ Chapter 36.

PROCEDURE 34–1   Obtaining a Sputum Specimen

GATHER SUPPLIES
■ Sterile sputum container, specimen cup, or mucous trap
■ Mouth care supplies
■ Sterile suction kit, if necessary
■ Gloves

BEFORE THE PROCEDURE

If the sputum specimen is to establish the initial diagnosis, obtain the specimen before starting oxygen and/or antibiotic therapy. Antibiotics reduce the bacterial count, making it difficult to identify the infecting organism. Oxygen therapy dries mucous membranes, making it more difficult to obtain a specimen. Unless otherwise instructed, obtain the specimen early in the morning, just after awakening. Respiratory secretions tend to pool during sleep; it is easier to obtain a specimen before normal coughing and daily activity has cleared them.

Provide for privacy, and explain the procedure. Emphasize the importance of coughing deeply to obtain sputum from the lower respiratory tract, avoiding expectoration of saliva. Increasing fluid intake prior to obtaining the specimen can help liquefy secretions, making them easier to expectorate.

DURING THE PROCEDURE

1. Use standard precautions.

2. Provide for mouth care prior to obtaining the specimen to reduce contamination by oral flora.

3. Instruct to cough deeply several times, expectorating mucus into the container.

4. Close the container securely.

5. Label the container with name and other identifying data, time and date, and any special conditions, such as antibiotic or oxygen therapy. Enclose specimen container in a clean plastic bag, and take to the laboratory or refrigerate as ordered to preserve the specimen.

6. To obtain a specimen by suctioning do the following:
   ■ Provide mouth care.
   ■ Obtain a sterile mucous trap. Using aseptic technique, attach the trap to the suction apparatus between the suction catheter and tubing.
   ■ Preoxygenate for suctioning as needed.
   ■ Perform tracheal suctioning using aseptic technique via either the nasotracheal route, endotracheal tube, or tracheostomy. Lubricate the catheter with sterile normal saline. Apply no suction as the catheter is being inserted into the trachea; apply suction for no longer than 10 seconds while withdrawing the catheter.
   ■ Detach the mucous trap, close, and label. Clear the suction catheter and tubing with normal saline after removing the mucus trap. Dispose of equipment appropriately.

7. A sputum specimen also may be obtained during bronchoscopy procedure.

AFTER THE PROCEDURE

Provide mouth care as needed. Teach the importance of completing all ordered antibiotic prescriptions to ensure complete eradication of microorganisms. Document the time and date that the specimen was obtained; and note color, consistency, and odor of sputum.

Health Assessment Interview

A health assessment interview to determine problems with respiratory structure and function may be conducted during a health screening, may focus on a chief complaint (such as shortness of breath), or may be part of a total health assessment. If the patient has a problem with respiratory function, analyze its onset, characteristics, course, severity, precipitating and relieving factors, and any associated symptoms, noting the timing and circumstances. For example, ask the patient the following:

- Describe the problems you are having with your breathing. Is your breathing more difficult if you lie flat? Is it painful to breathe in or out?
- When did you first notice that your cough was becoming a problem? Do you cough up mucus? What color is the mucus?
- Have you had nosebleeds in the past?

During the interview, carefully observe the patient for difficulty in breathing, pausing to breathe in the middle of a sentence, hoarseness, changes in voice quality, and cough. Ask about present health status, medical history, family health history, and risk factors for illness. To determine present health status, ask about pain in the nose, throat, or chest. Information about cough includes what type of cough (for example: dry, constant, worse at night, painful), when it occurs, and how it is relieved. The patient should describe any sputum associated with the cough. Is the patient experiencing any dyspnea (difficult or labored breathing)? How is the dyspnea associated with activity levels and time of day? Is the patient having chest pain? How is this related to activity and time of day? Note the severity, type, and location of the pain. Explore problems with swallowing, smelling, or taste. Also ask about nosebleeds and nasal or sinus stuffiness or pain, and about current medication use, aerosols or inhalants, and oxygen use.

Document past medical history by asking questions about a history of allergies, asthma, bronchitis, emphysema, pneumonia, tuberculosis, or congestive heart failure. Other questions include a history of surgery or trauma to the respiratory structures and a history of other chronic illnesses such as cancer, kidney disease, and heart disease. If the patient has a health problem involving the respiratory system, ask about medications used to relieve nasal congestion, cough, dyspnea, or chest pain. Document a family history of allergies, tuberculosis, emphysema, and cancer.

The patient's personal lifestyle, environment, and occupation may provide clues to risk factors for actual or potential health problems. Question the patient about a history of smoking and/or

---

GENETIC CONSIDERATIONS
Examples of Respiratory Disorders

- Deficiency of alpha₁-antitrypsin (a protein that protects the body from damage by its immune cells) is caused by a mutation of a gene located on chromosome 14. Deficiency of this protein leaves the lung susceptible to emphysema.
- Asthma, a disease that affects more than 5% of the population, is an inheritable disease with a number of responsible genes. (There are also other causes of asthma.)
- Cystic fibrosis is the most common fatal genetic disease in the United States today. All gene defects result in defective transport of chloride and sodium by epithelial cells. As a result, the amount of sodium chloride is increased in body secretions. Thick mucus is produced that clogs the lungs, leads to infection, and blocks pancreatic enzymes from reaching the intestines to digest food.
- A familial history of lung cancer increases the risk of developing lung cancer, and small-cell lung cancer has a definite genetic component. In addition, researchers have found that lung cancer patients who never smoked are more likely than smokers to have one of two genetic mutations linked to the disease.

---

exposure to environmental chemicals (including smog), dust, vapors, animals, coal dust, asbestos, fumes, or pollens. Other risk factors include a sedentary lifestyle and obesity. Also ask the patient about use of alcohol and substances that are injected (such as heroin) or inhaled (such as cocaine or marijuana).

Interview questions categorized by functional health patterns follow on page 1134.

Physical Assessment

Physical assessment of the respiratory system may be performed either as part of a total assessment, or alone for a patient with known or suspected problems. The techniques used to assess the respiratory system are inspection, palpation, percussion, and auscultation. In addition, note the patient's level of consciousness, restlessness, and anxiety level, and assess the color of the lips and nail beds. Normal age-related findings for the older adult are summarized in the Nursing Care of the Older Adult box.

The room should be warm and well-lighted. Ask the patient to remove all clothing above the waist; give women a gown to wear during the examination. Conduct the examination with the patient in the sitting position. Prior to the examination, collect all necessary equipment and explain the techniques to the patient to decrease anxiety.

NURSING CARE OF THE OLDER ADULT Age-Related Changes in the Respiratory System

AGE-RELATED CHANGE

- ↓ elastic recoil of lungs during expiration because of less elastic collagen and elastin.
- Calcification of the costal cartilage and weakening of the intercostal muscles.
- Loss of skeletal muscle strength in the thorax and diaphragm. Flattening of the diaphragm.
- Alveoli are less elastic, more fibrotic, and have fewer functional capillaries.
- Cough is less effective.
- PO_2 reduces as much as 15% by age 80.

SIGNIFICANCE

The older adult often has an increased anterior-posterior chest diameter, with kyphosis and barrel chest. There is a reduction in vital capacity and an increase in residual volume, with decreased effectiveness in coughing up phlegm or sputum. All of these changes greatly increase the risk of respiratory infections (such as pneumonia), especially if the person becomes immobile. They also mean that respiratory infections are more difficult to treat.

FUNCTIONAL HEALTH PATTERN INTERVIEW Respiratory System

Functional Health Pattern	Interview Questions and Leading Statements
Health Perception-Health Management	■ Describe any respiratory problems (such as allergies, asthma, bronchitis, frequent cold, pneumonia, tuberculosis, emphysema), injuries or surgery of the nose, throat, or lungs you have had. ■ If you had such problems, how were they treated (for example, medications, surgery, breathing treatments, oxygen, environmental control of allergens, other)? ■ Do you use oxygen for your respiratory problem? If so, how and when do you use it and at what flow rate? ■ Do you now or have you ever smoked tobacco? If so, what type, how long, and how much? If you no longer smoke, when did you quit? ■ Do you notice more respiratory problems at certain times of the year? Explain. ■ Do you do anything to decrease environmental irritants in your home or at work? Describe if so. ■ When was your last chest x-ray and TB skin test? What were the results of those tests? ■ Do you have annual flu shots? Have you had a pneumonia shot (if over age 65)? ■ Do certain foods, pollens, dust, or animals seem to increase your difficulty breathing? Explain. ■ Do you work or do hobbies in an area where you are exposed to paints, glues, dust, pollen, fumes, or chemicals that might irritate your respiratory system? If so, describe.
Nutritional-Metabolic	■ Describe your usual 24-hour intake of food and fluids. ■ Has your appetite been affected by your respiratory problem? Is it difficult for you to eat because of your breathing problems? Explain. ■ Has there been a recent change in your weight? Explain.
Elimination	■ Has having this health problem made it more difficult for you to have a bowel movement? ■ *For women:* Have you had difficulty controlling your urine when you cough?
Activity-Exercise	■ Describe your usual activities in a 24-hour period. ■ What type of exercise do you usually do? Has this changed, and if so, how? ■ Has your ability to care for yourself changed with this respiratory problem? Explain. ■ Has your energy level decreased since you have had this problem with breathing? If so, how has it affected your daily life? ■ How many flights of stairs can you climb before you become short of breath? ■ Do certain activities make you very tired? Explain. ■ Are your activities interrupted by frequent coughing? Explain. ■ Do you cough up phlegm or sputum? If so, describe its amount, color, odor, and the presence of blood.
Sleep-Rest	■ Does having this problem interfere with your ability to rest and sleep? Explain. ■ How many pillows do you use at night to breathe more easily? Has this changed? ■ Do you ever wake up coughing?
Cognitive-Perceptual	■ Do you have any pain in your sinuses, nose, chest, with breathing? If so, using a scale from 0 to 10, with 10 being the most severe pain, how would your rate that pain? Describe where and when you have the pain, how often you have it, what makes it worse, and what you do to relieve it. ■ Are there times when you feel anxious, restless, apprehensive, confused, or faint? Describe what you do if you have these feelings. ■ Tell me about the medications, inhalers, or oxygen prescribed for your respiratory problem? Show me how you use your inhaler.
Self-Perception-Self-Concept	■ How does having this condition make you feel about yourself?
Role-Relationships	■ How has having this condition affected your relationships with others? ■ Has having this condition interfered with your ability to work? Explain. ■ Is there a history of lung disease in your family? Explain.
Sexuality-Reproductive	■ Has this condition interfered with your usual sexual activity?
Coping-Stress-Tolerance	■ Has having this condition created stress for you? If so, does your breathing seem to be more difficult when you are stressed? ■ Have you experienced any kind of stress that makes the condition worse? Explain. ■ Describe what you do when you feel stressed.
Value-Belief	■ Describe how specific relationships or activities help you cope with this problem. ■ Describe specific cultural beliefs or practices that affect how you care for and feel about this problem. ■ Is there anything interfering with your spiritual beliefs, needs, or practices during your illness? What can I or another caregiver do to help you with your spiritual needs? ■ Are there any specific treatments (such as being on a machine that breathes for you) that you would not use to treat this problem?

Respiratory Assessments

Technique/Normal Findings	Abnormal Findings

Nasal Assessment

Inspect the nose for changes in size, shape, or color. *The nose should be midline in the face, of the same color as the face, and the nares should be symmetric.*

- The nose may be asymmetrical as a result of previous surgery or trauma.
- The skin around the nostrils may be red and swollen in allergies or upper respiratory infections.

Inspect the nasal cavity. Use an otoscope with a broad, short speculum. Gently insert the speculum into each of the nares and assess the condition of the mucous membranes and the turbinates. *The septum should be midline with pink mucosa and without drainage.*

- The septum may be deviated.
- Perforation of the septum may occur with chronic cocaine abuse.
- Red mucosa indicates infection.
- Purulent drainage indicates nasal or sinus infection.
- Allergies may be indicated by watery nasal drainage, pale turbinates, and polyps on the turbinates.

Assess ability to smell (cranial nerve I, olfactory). Ask the patient to breathe through one nostril while pressing the other one closed. Ask the patient to close his or her eyes. Place a substance with an aromatic odor under the patient's nose (use ground coffee or alcohol) and ask the patient to identify the odor. Test each nostril separately. *This test is usually done only if the patient has problems with the sense of smell, but the patient should be able to distinguish different odors.*

- Changes in the ability to smell may be the result of damage to the olfactory nerve or to chronic inflammation of the nose.
- Zinc deficiency may cause a loss of the sense of smell.

Sinus Assessment

Palpate the frontal and maxillary sinuses. *The sinuses should not be tender to palpation.*

- Frontal and maxillary sinuses are tender to palpation with allergies or sinus infections.

Thoracic Assessment

Assess respiratory rate. *The normal respiratory rate is 12 to 20 breaths per minute.*

- **Tachypnea** (rapid respiratory rate) is seen in **atelectasis** (collapse of lung tissue following obstruction of the bronchus or bronchioles), pneumonia, asthma, pleural effusion, pneumothorax, congestive heart failure, anxiety, and in response to pain.
- Damage to the brainstem from a stroke or head injury may result in either tachypnea or **bradypnea** (low respiratory rate).
- Bradypnea is seen with some circulatory disorders, lung disorders, and as a side effect of some medications.
- **Apnea**, cessation of breathing lasting from a few seconds to a few minutes, may occur following a stroke or head trauma, as a side effect of some medications, or following airway obstruction.

Inspect the anteroposterior diameter of the chest. The anteroposterior diameter of the chest should be less than the transverse diameter. *Normal ratio is 1:2.*

- The anteroposterior diameter is equal to the transverse diameter in barrel chest, which typically occurs with emphysema.

Inspect for intercostal retraction or bulging. *There should be no retraction or bulging.*

- Retraction of intercostal spaces may be seen in asthma.
- Bulging of intercostal spaces may be seen in pneumothorax.

Technique/Normal Findings	Abnormal Findings
Inspect and palpate for chest expansion. Place your hands with the fingers spread apart palm down on the patient's posterolateral chest. Gently press the skin between your thumbs (Figure 34–10 ■). Ask the patient to breathe deeply. As the patient inhales, watch your hands for symmetry of movement. *Chest expansion should be bilaterally symmetric, with the examiner's hands moving 5 to 10 cm apart.*	■ Thoracic expansion is decreased on the affected side in atelectasis, pneumonia, pneumothorax, and pleural effusion. ■ Bilateral chest expansion is decreased in emphysema.

Figure 34–10 ■ Palpating for chest expansion.

Gently palpate the location and position of the trachea. *The trachea should be midline.*	■ The trachea shifts to the unaffected side in pleural effusion and pneumothorax and shifts to the affected side in atelectasis.
Percuss the lungs for dullness over shoulder apices and over anterior, posterior, and lateral intercostal spaces (Figure 34–11 ■). *The normal percussion tone over normal lung tissue is resonance.*	■ Dullness is heard in patients with atelectasis, lobar pneumonia, and pleural effusion. ■ Hyperresonance is heard in those with chronic asthma, emphysema, and pneumothorax.

Figure 34–11 ■ Sequence for lung percussion.

Technique/Normal Findings

Percuss the posterior chest for diaphragmatic excursion. Systematic percussion of the posterior chest from a level of lung resonance to the level of diaphragmatic dullness reveals diaphragmatic excursion, a measurement of the level of the diaphragm. First percuss downward over the posterior thorax while the patient exhales fully and holds the breath. Mark the spot at which the sound changes from resonant to dull. Then ask the patient to inhale and hold the breath while you percuss downward again to note the descent of the diaphragm. Again mark the spot where the sound changes. Measure the difference. *Diaphragmatic excursion normally varies from about 3 to 5 cm (Figure 34–12 ■).*

Abnormal Findings

■ Diaphragmatic excursion is decreased in emphysema, ascites, on the affected side in pleural effusion, and in pneumothorax.
■ A high level of dullness or a lack of excursion may indicate atelectasis or pleural effusion.

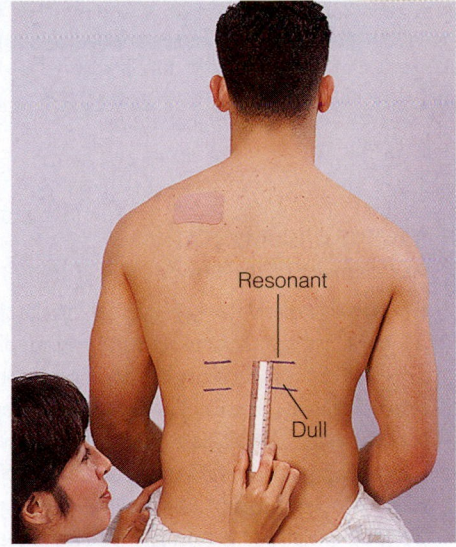

Figure 34–12 ■ Measuring diaphragmatic excursion.

Breath Sound Assessment

Auscultate the lungs for breath sounds with the diaphragm of the stethoscope by having the patient take slow deep breaths through the mouth. Listen over anterior, posterior, and lateral intercostal spaces (Figure 34–13 ■). *The three different types of normal breath sounds are vesicular, bronchovesicular, and bronchial (Table 34–1).*

■ Bronchial breath sounds (expiration > inspiration) and bronchovesicular breath sounds (inspiration = expiration) are heard over lungs filled with fluid or solid tissue.
■ Breath sounds are decreased or diminished over atelectasis, emphysema, asthma, pleural effusion, and pneumothorax.
■ Breath sounds are increased over lobar pneumonia.
■ Breath sounds are absent over collapsed lung, surgical removal of lung, pleural effusion, and primary bronchus obstruction.

Figure 34–13 ■ Sequence for lung auscultation.

TABLE 34–1 Normal Breath Sounds

TYPE OF BREATH SOUND	CHARACTERISTICS
Vesicular	■ Soft, low-pitched, gentle sounds ■ Heard over all areas of the lungs except the major bronchi ■ Have a 3:1 ratio for inspiration and expiration, with inspiration lasting longer than expiration
Bronchovesicular	■ Medium pitch and intensity of sounds ■ Have a 1:1 ratio, with inspiration and expiration being equal in duration ■ Heard anteriorly over the primary bronchus on each side of the sternum, and posteriorly between the scapulae
Bronchial	■ Loud, high-pitched sounds ■ Gap between inspiration and expiration ■ Have a 2:3 ratio for inspiration and expiration, with expiration longer than inspiration ■ Heard over the manubrium

Technique/Normal Findings	Abnormal Findings
Auscultate for crackles, wheezes, and friction rubs. If crackles or wheezes are heard, ask the patient to cough and note if adventitious sound is cleared. *Normally, there are no crackles, wheezes, or friction rubs.*	■ **Crackles** (short, discrete, crackling or bubbling sounds) may be noted in pneumonia, bronchitis, and congestive heart failure. ■ **Wheezes** (continuous, musical sounds) may be heard in patients with bronchitis, emphysema, and asthma. ■ A **friction rub** is a loud, dry, creaking sound that indicates pleural inflammation.

SAMPLE DOCUMENTATION
Assessment of the Lungs

57-year-old male, history of smoking 2 packs cigarettes/day for 37 years; continues to smoke despite previous discussions. Works as a dry-wall installer. No family history of cancer or TB. States he has trouble breathing, especially at night. Often sleeps on a recliner "to breathe better." Complains of a cough, but denies sputum production. Diagnosed 3 years ago with emphysema. Color of face is dusky red. Fingernails pink. Respirations 30, unlabored, regular (R varies from 26 to 32 on visits to the clinic). Thoracic assessment = intercostal bulging, barrel chest, diminished lung sounds bilaterally in lower lobes. Crackles present in upper lobes, not cleared by coughing. Discussed possible use of low-flow nasal oxygen at night to help with breathing; will check with primary provider.

TEST YOURSELF NCLEX-RN® REVIEW

1. A nurse is assessing breath sounds. Where would he place the diaphragm of the stethoscope to listen to the apex of the left lungs?
   1. in the mediastinum
   2. resting on the diaphragm
   3. within the parietal pleura
   4. just below the clavicle

2. What factor is implicated in an increased risk of developing lung cancer?
   1. childhood obesity
   2. a family history of asthma
   3. a family history of lung cancer
   4. frequent upper respiratory infections

3. Prior to providing care for a patient the nurse reviews the previous day's vitals signs and notes that bronchovesicular breath sounds have been documented. What would the nurse do next?
   1. request a respiratory therapy treatment
   2. notify the physician
   3. document the inability to hear breath sounds
   4. take and record vital signs as usual

4. What process is initiated between oxygen and hemoglobin as the temperature of body tissues increases?
   1. Oxygen unloading is enhanced.
   2. Oxygen unloading is inhibited.
   3. Respiratory rate decreases.
   4. Lung compliance increases.

5. A nurse is teaching a patient about a thoracentesis. How would she best describe this procedure?
   1. "You will be asleep when they make the incision."
   2. "Fluid will be drawn off the area around your lung."
   3. "It involves lying very still in a large, noisy machine."
   4. "The doctor will be able to see inside your lung."

6. Which of the following questions should be included in a respiratory assessment to identify health problems?
   1. "Tell me how much you exercise each day."
   2. "Has anyone in your family had a stroke or heart attack?"
   3. "What did the doctor recommend for your emphysema?"
   4. "Do your children have trouble breathing at night?"

7. While auscultating a patient's breath sounds, the nurse notes continuous musical sounds. These are documented as which of the following?
   1. murmurs
   2. wheezes
   3. crackles
   4. rales

8. A patient has had a lung removed. What type of breath sound would a nurse expect to assess over the affected side?
   1. resonance
   2. crackles
   3. bronchovesicular
   4. absent

9. What would the nurse ask the patient to do when auscultating the lungs?
1. "Hold your breath."
2. "Repeat the number 99 several times."
3. "Take slow deep breaths through your mouth."
4. "Breathe in and out through your nose."

10. While assessing a patient with a left pneumothorax the nurse notes decreased diaphragmatic excursion on the left. What would the nurse do next?
1. Notify the physician immediately.
2. Document the assessment.
3. Repeat the assessment several times.
4. Tell the patient to hold his or her breath.

See Test Yourself answers in Appendix C.

Pearson Nursing Student Resources

Find additional review materials at
www.nursing.pearsonhighered.com

Prepare for success with additional NCLEX®-style practice questions, interactive assignments and activities, Web links, animations and videos, and more!

BIBLIOGRAPHY

Armstrong, J., & Mitchell, E. (2008). Comprehensive nursing assessment in the care of older people. *Nursing Older People, (20)*1, 36–40.

Bickley, L., & Szilagyi, P. (2007). *Bates' guide to physical examination and history taking* (9th ed.). Philadelphia: Lippincott.

Considine, J. (2005). The role of nurses in preventing adverse events related to respiratory dysfunction: Literature review. *Journal of Advanced Nursing, 49*(6), 624–633.

Considine, J., Botti, M., & Shane, T. (2005). Effect of a self-directed learning package on emergency nurses' knowledge of assessment of oxygenation and use of supplemental oxygen. *Nursing & Health Sciences, 7*(3), 199–208.

Eliopoulos, E. (2005). *Gerontological nursing* (6th ed.). Philadelphia: Lippincott Williams & Wilkins.

Hogan, J. (2006). Why don't nurses monitor the respiratory rate of patients? *British Journal of Nursing, 15*(9), 489–492.

Kee, J. (2009). *Prentice Hall handbook of laboratory & diagnostic tests with nursing implications* (6th ed.) Upper Saddle River, NJ: Prentice Hall.

Kennedy, S. (2007). Detecting changes in the respiratory status of ward patients. *Nursing Standard, 21*(49), 42–46.

MacDonald, S., Yates, J., Lance, R., Giganti, N., & Cheppurko, D. (2005). Are you asking the right admission questions when assessing dyspnea? *Heart & Lung, 34*(4), 260–269.

National Institute of Health. (2008). *Genes and disease: Respiratory diseases*. Retrieved from http://www.ncbi.nlm.nih.gov/books/bookres.fegi/gnd/pdf.html

Porth, C. (2007). Essentials of *Pathophysiology: Concepts of altered health states* (2nd ed.) Philadelphia: Lippincott Williams & Wilkins.

Porth, C. & Matfin, G. (2009). *Pathophysiology: Concepts of altered health states.* (8th ed.). Philadelphia: Lippincott Williams & Wilkins.

Pulse oximetry. (2008). *Nursing, 38*(9), 42–44.

Swiderski, D., & Byrum, D. (2007). Strictly clinical: Are you an ABG ace? *American Nurse Today, 2*(4), 18–21.

Take a look inside the lungs with bronchoscopy. (2007). *Nursing Made Incredibly Easy, 5*(2), 11–12.

Weber, J., & Kelley, J. (2009). *Health assessment in nursing* (4th ed.). Philadelphia: Lippincott Williams & Wilkins.

35 Nursing Care of Patients with Upper Respiratory Disorders

LEARNING OUTCOMES

1. Relate anatomy and physiology of the upper respiratory tract to commonly occurring disorders and risk factors for these disorders.

2. Describe the pathophysiology of common upper respiratory tract disorders, relating their manifestations to the pathophysiologic process.

3. Discuss nursing implications for medications and other interdisciplinary care measures to treat upper respiratory disorders.

4. Describe surgical procedures used to treat upper respiratory disorders and their implications for patient care and recovery.

5. Identify health promotion actitivities related to reducing the incidence of upper respiratory disorders, describing the appropriate population and setting for implementing identified measures.

6. Discuss treatment options for oral and laryngeal cancers with their implications for the patient's body image and functional health.

CLINICAL COMPETENCIES

1. Assess functional health status of patients with upper respiratory disorders, using data to identify and prioritize holistic nursing care needs.

2. Use nursing research and evidence-based practice to plan and implement nursing care for patients with upper respiratory disorders.

3. Provide safe and effective nursing care for patients having surgery involving the upper respiratory system and/or with a tracheostomy.

4. Safely administer medications and prescribed treatments for patients with disorders of the upper respiratory tract.

5. Provide appropriate teaching for the patient and family affected by upper respiratory tract disorders.

6. Evaluate the effectiveness of care, reassessing and modifying the plan of care as needed to achieve desired patient outcomes.

KEY TERMS

coryza, 1141
epistaxis, 1155
influenza, 1143
laryngectomy, 1166

laryngitis, 1153
pertussis, 1154
pharyngitis, 1150
rhinitis, 1140

rhinoplasty, 1158
sinusitis, 1147
sleep apnea, 1162
tonsillitis, 1150

Upper respiratory disorders may affect the nose, paranasal sinuses, tonsils, adenoids, larynx, and pharynx, including nasopharynx and oropharynx. Upper respiratory disorders may be minor, such as the common cold. However, a patent upper airway is necessary for effective breathing. Acute and even life-threatening problems develop when upper airway patency is affected (e.g., by laryngeal edema). Upper respiratory disorders can affect breathing, communication, eating, swallowing, and body image. When breathing is compromised because of swelling, bleeding, or accumulation of secretions, fear and anxiety develop.

Nursing care focuses on maintaining the airway, managing pain and symptoms, promoting effective communication, and providing psychologic support for the patient and family. Prior to proceding with this chapter, review the anatomy and physiology, diagnostic tests, and assessment of the upper respiratory system in ∞ Chapter 34 as needed.

Infectious or Inflammatory Disorders

Constant exposure of the upper respiratory tract to the environment makes it vulnerable to a variety of infectious and inflammatory conditions. Although most upper respiratory infections and inflammations are minor, complications may result. In the frail older adult, the risk of serious problems following an upper respiratory infection can be significant.

Rhinitis, inflammation of the nasal cavities, is the most common upper respiratory disorder. Rhinitis may be either acute or chronic. *Acute viral rhinitis*, or the common cold, is discussed next. Chronic rhinitis includes allergic, vasomotor, and atrophic rhinitis. *Allergic rhinitis*, or hay fever, results from a sensitivity reaction to allergens such as plant pollens. It tends to occur seasonally but can be perennial. The etiology of *vasomotor rhinitis* is unknown. Although its manifestations are similar to those of allergic rhinitis, it is not linked to allergens. *Atrophic rhinitis* is characterized by changes in the mucous membrane of the nasal cavities.

The Patient with Viral Upper Respiratory Infection

Viral upper respiratory infections (URIs or the common cold) are the most common respiratory tract infections and are among the most common human diseases. URIs are highly contagious and are prevalent in schools and work environments. The incidence of acute URI peaks during September and late January, coinciding with the opening of schools, as well as toward the end of April. Most adults experience two to four colds each year (Huether & McCance, 2008).

FAST FACTS

- Rhinoviruses are the most common cause of viral URI.
- Colds due to rhinovirus are more common in early fall and late spring.
- More than 100 different serotypes of rhinovirus have been identified.
- Parainfluenza viruses, respiratory synctial viruses (RSV), coronaviruses, and adenoviruses also can cause URI.
- Colds due to RSV, coronavirus, and adenovirus peak in winter and spring (Huether & McCance, 2008).

Pathophysiology

More than 200 strains of virus cause URI, including rhinoviruses, adenoviruses, parainfluenza viruses, coronaviruses, and respiratory syncytial virus (see the section that follows for more information about respiratory synctial virus). Occasionally, more than one virus may be present. Viruses causing acute URI spread by aerosolized droplet nuclei during sneezing or coughing or by direct contact. The virus usually spreads when the hands and fingers pick it up from contaminated surfaces and carry it to the eyes and mucous membranes of the susceptible host. Infected patients are highly contagious, shedding virus for a few days prior to and after the appearance of symptoms. Although immunity is produced to the individual virus strain, the number of viruses causing URI ensures that most people continue to experience colds throughout their lifetime.

Viscous mucus secretions in the upper respiratory tract trap invading organisms, preventing contamination of more vulnerable areas. Cells of the upper respiratory tract are infected when the virus attaches to receptors on the cell. Local immunologic defenses, such as secretory IgA antibodies in respiratory secretions, then attempt to inactivate the antigen, producing a local inflammatory response. The mucous membranes of the nasal passages swell and become hyperemic and

engorged. Mucus-secreting glands become hyperactive. These responses to the virus produce the typical manifestations of viral URI.

Manifestations and Complications

Acute viral upper respiratory infection often presents as the common cold. Nasal mucous membranes appear red (*erythematous*) and *boggy* (swollen). Swollen mucous membranes, local vasodilation, and secretions cause nasal congestion. Clear, watery secretions lead to **coryza**, profuse nasal discharge. Sneezing and coughing are common. Sore throat is common, and may be the initial symptom. Systemic manifestations of acute viral URI infrequently include low-grade fever, headache, malaise, and muscle aches. Symptoms generally last for a few days up to 2 weeks. Although acute viral URI is typically mild and self-limited, its effects on the immune defenses of the upper respiratory tract can increase the risk for more serious bacterial infections, such as sinusitis or otitis media.

Interdisciplinary Care

Because most acute viral upper respiratory infections are self-limiting, self-care is appropriate and encouraged. Medical treatment is usually required only when complications such as sinusitis or otitis media develop.

Diagnosis of acute viral URI is usually based on the history and physical examination. Diagnostic testing may be indicated if a complication such as bacterial infection is suspected. A white blood count (WBC) is generally not needed but may be ordered to assess for leukocytosis (an elevated WBC) if there are complications. Cultures of purulent discharge may also be obtained.

Treatment is symptomatic. Adequate rest, maintaining fluid intake, and avoiding chilling help relieve systemic symptoms such as fever, malaise, and muscle ache. Instruct patients to cover the mouth and nose with tissue when coughing or sneezing, and to dispose of soiled tissues properly. Additionally, avoiding crowds helps prevent spread of the infection to others.

Medications

Medications may be recommended to shorten the duration of the illness and relieve symptoms. Mild decongestants or over-the-counter antihistamines may help relieve coryza and nasal congestion. Nasal sprays such as phenylephrine (Neo-Synephrine) rapidly relieve nasal congestion, but may lead to dependence and rebound congestion if used for more than a few days at a time. Warm saltwater gargles, throat lozenges, or mild analgesics may be used for sore throat. Although no specific antiviral therapy has been shown to be effective in shortening the duration of a URI, experimental vaccines to prevent acute viral URI are in developmental stages (National Institute of Allergy and Infectious Diseases, 2009). For the nursing implications of decongestants and common antihistamines see the accompanying box.

Complementary Therapies

Complementary therapies are appropriate for treating most acute viral URI. Herbal remedies such as Echinacea and garlic may have antiviral and antibiotic effects (Fontaine, 2005). Echinacea also is thought to stimulate the immune system, improving the body's response to infection. Taken at the first sign of infection,

MEDICATION ADMINISTRATION   Decongestants and Antihistamines

DECONGESTANTS

Phenylephrine (Neo-Synephrine, others)

Phenylpropanolamine (Comtrex, Ornade, Triaminic, others)

Pseudoephedrine (Sudafed, Actifed, others)

Decongestants promote vasoconstriction, reducing the inflammation and edema of nasal mucosa and relieving nasal congestion. They are very effective when applied topically (by nasal spray) because of their rapid onset of action. However, the duration of effect is short, followed by vasodilation and rebound congestion. Because of their rapid effect and short duration, these preparations are habit-forming. Chronic use may lead to *rhinitis medicamentosa*, a rebound phenomenon of drug-induced nasal irritation and inflammation.

Nursing Responsibilities

■ Assess for contraindications, such as hypertension or chronic heart disease. These drugs stimulate the sympathetic nervous system, increasing peripheral vascular resistance, blood pressure, and heart rate.

■ Evaluate medication regimen for potential interactions such as antihypertensive medications and monoamine oxidase (MAO) inhibitors.

Health Education for the Patient and Family

■ Do not use more than the recommended dose.

■ Check with the healthcare provider before taking decongestants if you are taking any prescription medications or are being treated for high blood pressure or heart disease.

■ Use nasal sprays for no more than 3 to 5 days.

■ Increase fluid intake to relieve mouth dryness.

■ These drugs may cause nervousness, shakiness, or difficulty sleeping. Stop the drug if these effects occur.

■ In some states, drugs containing pseudoephedrine may require a prescription or be kept behind the counter to reduce its use in preparing methamphetamine.

ANTIHISTAMINES

Brompheniramine (Dimetane, others)

Chlorpheniramine (Chlor-Trimeton, others)

Clesmastine (Tavist)

Dexchlorpheniramine (Dexchlor, others)

Diphenhydramine (Benadryl, others)

Triprolidine (Actidil, Myidil)

Nonsedating

Cetirizine (Zyrtec)

Fexofenadine (Allegra)

Loratadine (Claritin)

Antihistamines are widely available with and without a prescription. They are frequently combined with decongestants in over-the-counter cold and allergy preparations. Antihistamines relieve the systemic effects of histamine and dry respiratory secretions through an anticholinergic effect. Most antihistamines cause drowsiness; nonsedating forms are less likely to interfere with alertness. Diphenhydramine is used in numerous over-the-counter sleep aids as well as in cold and allergy preparations.

Nursing Responsibilities

■ Before administering or recommending these drugs, assess for possible contraindications, including the following:
  ■ Acute asthma or lower respiratory disease that may be aggravated by drying of secretions
  ■ Hypersensitivity to antihistamines
  ■ Glaucoma (increased intraocular pressure)
  ■ Impaired gastrointestinal motility or obstruction
  ■ Prostatic hypertrophy or other urinary tract obstruction
  ■ Heart disease

■ For patients who must remain alert while on antihistamine therapy, recommend nonsedating forms.

Health Education for the Patient and Family

■ Do not drive or operate machinery while taking over-the-counter or prescription forms of antihistamines known to be sedating.

■ Stop the drug and notify your doctor immediately if you develop confusion, excessive sedation, chest tightness, wheezing, bleeding, or easy bruising while taking antihistamines.

■ Do not use alcohol or other CNS depressants while taking antihistamines.

■ Hard candy, gum, ice chips, and liquids help relieve mouth dryness caused by antihistamines.

Echinacea may reduce the duration and symptoms, although clinical trials have shown no consistent benefit. The recommended dose of Echinacea varies, depending on the part of the plant used in the preparation. It should not be used for longer than 2 weeks. It is contraindicated for use during pregnancy and lactation, and in people who have an autoimmune disease such as rheumatoid arthritis.

Dietary supplements such as vitamin C and zinc also are promoted as measures to reduce the severity and duration of URI. Again, however, no consistent benefit is demonstrated in clinical trials (National Center for Complementary and Alternative Medicine [NCCAM], 2009). Although selected studies have shown a beneficial effect of zinc gluconate lozenges to reduce the duration of an induced URI, no such benefit was found when zinc was compared with placebo to treat naturally occuring URI (NCCAM, 2009).

Aromatherapy with essential oils such as basil, cedarwood, eucalyptus, frankincense, lavender, marjoram, peppermint, or rosemary can reduce congestion, and promote comfort and recovery. Teach patients that these essential oils are to be used only for inhalation, not for internal consumption. Acupuncture and acupressure have been shown to be effective in treating URI in adults, particularly when combined with use of Chinese herbs. Their beneficial effect is most likely related to stimulation of the immune response by accupuncture and accupressure.

✍ Nursing Care

Health Promotion

Patients can limit their incidence of acute viral URI by frequent handwashing and avoiding exposure to crowds. Maintaining good general health and stress-reducing activities support the immune system and help prevent acute viral URI. Teach the patient that becoming chilled or going out in the rain does not cause colds and that URI are more likely to occur during periods of physical or psychologic stress.

Community-Based Care

The primary nursing role in caring for patients with acute viral URI is educational. Self-care is appropriate for most patients unless the problem is recurrent or a complication occurs. Acute viral URI may interfere with work and recreational activities. Unless limited by symptoms, normal daily activities and roles usually can be maintained. Additional rest during the acute phase of illness is recommended. Additional fluid intake and a well-balanced diet help support the immune response, hastening recovery.

Include the following topics in teaching for home care:

- Using disposable tissues to cover the mouth and nose while coughing or sneezing to reduce airborne spread of the virus.
- Blowing the nose with both nostrils open to prevent infected matter from being forced into the eustachian tubes.
- Washing hands frequently, especially after coughing or sneezing, to limit viral transmission.
- Using over-the-counter preparations for symptomatic relief; precautions related to the sedating effects of antihistamines.
- Limiting use of nasal decongestants to every 4 hours for only a few days at a time to prevent rebound effect.

The Patient with Respiratory Syncytial Virus (RSV)

Respiratory syncytial virus (RSV) is a common virus that is the primary cause of respiratory illnesses in young children and the majority of lower respiratory disease in infants. Older children and adults also are commonly and repetitively infected by RSV, but the disease is milder, usually presenting as a common cold. However, the elderly and people who are immunocompromised may develop severe pneumonitis when exposed to RSV. RSV is transmitted in much the same way as other URI: via contaminated hands or objects and by coarse droplets spread by coughing and sneezing. The incubation period is 4 to 6 days.

In adults, the manifestations of RSV are those of other common URIs, including rhinorrhea, sore throat, and cough. Headache, malaise, and low-grade fever may occur. In older adults, RSV may present as lower respiratory infection with fever or pneumonia (Huether & McCance, 2008). While the illness also presents as URI in infants, it is more likely to progress to pneumonia, bronchiolitis, and tracheobronchiolitis in this population.

Treatment for adults with upper respiratory RSV is symptomatic (see the preceding section on URI). When the lower respiratory tract is involved, hydration and other measures to mobilize respiratory secretions are important. Intubation and mechanical ventilation may be necessary if hypoxia develops. Aerosolized ribavirin (Virazole, and antiviral drug) may be prescribed for older adults and immunocompromised patients with RSV pneumonia.

Nursing care is supportive. The focus of nursing care for the adult with URI manifestations of RSV is on teaching for self-care, identification of complications such as pneumonia, sinusitis, and prevention of viral spread. When lower respiratory symptoms are present, nursing care is similar to that provided for patients with pneumonia (∞ see Chapter 37).

The Patient with Influenza

Influenza, or *flu*, is a highly contagious viral respiratory disease characterized by coryza, fever, cough, and systemic symptoms such as headache and malaise. Influenza usually occurs in epidemics or pandemics, although sporadic cases do occur. Localized outbreaks of influenza usually occur about every 1 to 3 years. Global epidemics (pandemics) are less frequent, developing every 10 to 15 years until the past two decades. A recently identified strain of avian (bird) influenza has raised concerns about a potential future pandemic. This strain of influenza virus has not yet demonstrated the ability to spread between humans; however, concerns are that it will mutate to allow person-to-person spread. This viral strain has a mortality rate of greater than 50% in people who have been infected due to close association with infected birds. See Box 35–1 for more information about avian influenza.

Although influenza tends to be mild and self-limited in healthy adults, older adults and people with chronic heart or pulmonary disease have a high incidence of complications (such as pneumonia) and a higher risk for mortality related to the disease and its complications (World Health Organization, 2009). See the accompanying Nursing Care of the Older Adult box.

Pathophysiology

Influenza virus is transmitted by airborne droplet and direct contact. Three major strains of the virus have been identified as influenza A virus, influenza B virus, and influenza C virus. Influenza A is responsible for most infections and the most severe outbreaks of influenza. This is primarily due to its ability to alter its surface antigens, bypassing previously developed immune defenses to the virus. New strains of influenza virus are named according to the strain, geographic origin, and year the strain was identified (e.g., A/Taiwan/89). Surface antigens of the specific virus may be used to further differentiate influenza A viruses. Outbreaks of influenza B virus are generally less extensive and less severe than those caused by influenza A virus. Illness associated with influenza C virus is mild and often goes unrecognized.

In 2009, the emergence of a novel influenza A virus (H1N1) influenza led to the World Health Organization (WHO) classifying its spread as a pandemic (phase 6) in June 2009. Isolated

NURSING CARE OF THE OLDER ADULT　　**Seasonal Influenza**

Seasonal influenza is a significant problem in older adults leading to increased morbidity and mortality compared to other age groups. One question remains as to when the best time is for older adults to receive their yearly influenza vaccine. A study by Lee and colleagues (2009) found that immunizations provided in the month of October were most cost effective in reducing healthcare utilization. The authors report that vaccines delivered through the end of February are cost effective, but to a lesser level than those delivered prior to the flu season.

From Lee, B. Y, Tai, H. J., Bailey, R. R. & Smith K. J. (2009). Timing of influenza vaccination for older adults (65 years and older). *Cell (online)*. Retrieved September 26, 2009, from http://www.cell.com/

BOX 35–1 Focus on Avian Influenza

Influenza viruses are common in nature, found in wild birds such as ducks and shore birds. While these birds carry the virus, they usually are not harmed by it. Movement of the virus into domesticated flocks of ducks and chickens can not only devastate populations of these birds, but can also spread the virus to other domestic animals such as pigs.

Avian influenza is caused by a type A influenza virus identified as H5N1. Type A influenza viruses are subclassified by two proteins found one the surface of the virus, hemagglutinin (HA) and neuraminidase (NA). HA allows the virus to attach to a cell and initiate an infection, while NA allows the virus to exit the host cell after replicating. Currently, there are only three known subtypes of influenza A circulating among humans (H1N1, H1N2, and H3N2). The H5N1 virus, which is particularly virulent and spread by migratory birds, raises fears of a potential human pandemic should it evolve to become transmissible from human to human.

Influenza viruses are very changeable, undergoing small, continuous changes as well as occasional large and abrupt changes. *Antigenic drift* is the term for small changes that occur continuously as a virus makes copies of itself. These changes help the virus elude the immune system, and necessitate the production of new vaccines every year. Sudden, dramatic changes occur when two different strains of influenza virus (for example, avian influenza and human influenza) infect the same cell and exchange genetic material. These changes, called *antigenic shift*, create a new subtype of the virus to which people have little or no immunity.

As of June 2009, the World Health Organization identified the novel A type virus, H1N1, as a pandemic (WHO, 2009). As with most reported cases of avian influenza A have occurred in previously healthy children and young adults often with an underlying chronic illness.

Symptoms of avian influenza include typical flulike manifestations such as fever, cough, sore throat, and myalgias. In addition, affected people may develop eye infections, pneumonia, and respiratory distress, including acute respiratory distress syndrome (ARDS; ∞ see Chapter 37 for more information about ARDS and its manifestations).

No vaccine to protect against the H5N1 virus has yet been developed for commercial use. Measures are being taken, however, to develop prepandemic vaccines based on current strains of H5N1 influenza virus, to increase the capacity for vaccine production in the United States, and to research new types of vaccines. Some currently available antiviral medications may effectively treat avian influenza, however, the virus implicated in deaths in Southeast Asia was found to be resistant to amantadine and rimantadine, two commonly used drugs to treat influenza (WHO, 2009).

A severe pandemic of H1N1 or avian influenza could disrupt all aspects of life, not only causing severe illness and death, but also overwhelming the healthcare system, impacting social services, and causing significant economic loss. Advance preparations such as those currently being undertaken by the World Health Organization and the United States and other countries can reduce the impact of a pandemic.

---

cases in Europe were found to be resistant to oseltamivir (Tamiflu), but most in the Untied States are sensitive to Tamiflu. The impact of this virus is evolving (WHO, 2009).

FAST FACTS

- Type A influenza viruses are found in birds, pigs, whales, and humans.
- Type A influenza is believed to have caused three pandemics in 1918, 1957, and 1968.
- Type B influenza viruses are commonly found among humans, and often are responsible for influenza outbreaks but not pandemics.
- Type C influenza viruses, found in humans, pigs, and dogs, typically cause mild respiratory infections (NIAID, 2008).

The incubation period for influenza is short, only 18 to 72 hours. The virus infects the respiratory epithelium. It rapidly replicates in infected cells and is released to infect neighboring cells. Inflammation leads to necrosis and shedding of serous and ciliated cells of the respiratory tract. This allows extracellular fluid to escape, producing rhinorrhea. With recovery, serous cells are replaced more rapidly than ciliated cells, leading to continued cough and coryza. Systemic manifestations of influenza likely are caused by release of inflammatory mediators such as tumor necrosis factor α, interleukin α, and interleukin 6 (Huether & McCance, 2008). The humoral and cell-mediated immune responses are activated by influenza infection, and are supplemented by other local and systemic responses (such as interferons).

Manifestations

Infection with influenza virus produces one of three syndromes: uncomplicated nasopharyngeal inflammation, viral upper respiratory infection followed by bacterial infection, or viral pneumonia. The onset is rapid; profound malaise may develop in a matter of minutes.

Manifestations of influenza include abrupt onset of chills and fever, malaise, muscle aches, and headache. Respiratory manifestations include dry, nonproductive cough, sore throat, substernal burning and coryza (see the accompanying box). Acute symptoms subside within 2 to 3 days, although fever may last as long as a week. The cough may be severe and productive. Along with fatigue and weakness, the cough can persist for days or several weeks.

Complications

The respiratory epithelial necrosis caused by influenza increases the risk for secondary bacterial infections. Sinusitis and otitis media are frequent complications of influenza. Tracheobronchitis, inflammation of the trachea and bronchi,

MANIFESTATIONS of Influenza

RESPIRATORY MANIFESTATIONS	SYSTEMIC MANIFESTATIONS
■ Coryza	■ Fever and chills
■ Cough, initially dry	■ Malaise
■ Substernal burning	■ Muscle aches
■ Sore throat becoming productive	■ Fatigue

may develop. While tracheobronchitis is not a serious health risk, its manifestations may persist for up to 3 weeks.

Influenza is clearly linked to an increased risk for pneumonia, particularly in older adults. Changes in respiratory function associated with aging, including decreased effectiveness of cough and increased residual lung volume, pose little risk in the healthy older adult but greatly increase the risk for pneumonia associated with influenza. Primary influenza viral pneumonia, while uncommon, is a serious complication that may be fatal. It typically develops within 48 hours of the onset of influenza, often in patients with preexisting heart valve or pulmonary disease. Influenza pneumonia progresses rapidly and can cause hypoxemia and death within a few days. Secondary bacterial pneumonia is more likely to occur in older at-risk adults but also may affect otherwise healthy adults. It usually presents as a relapse of influenza, with a productive cough and evidence of pneumonia on the chest x-ray. ∞ See Chapter 37 for more information about pneumonia.

Other respiratory complications of influenza include exacerbation of chronic obstructive pulmonary disease (COPD), chronic bronchitis, or asthma. Sinusitis (discussed later in this chapter) also may develop.

Reye's syndrome is a rare but potentially fatal complication of influenza. Although it is more likely to affect children, it also has been identified in older adults. It is most often associated with influenza B virus. Reye's syndrome develops within 2 to 3 weeks after the onset of influenza. It has a 30% mortality rate. Hepatic failure and encephalopathy develop rapidly in patients with Reye's syndrome.

While uncommon, other potential complications of influenza include myositis (inflammation of skeletal muscles), myocarditis (inflammation of the heart muscle), and central nervous system disorders such as encephalitis and Guillain-Barré syndrome.

Interdisciplinary Care

Preventing community outbreaks and protecting vulnerable populations (e.g., older adults and people with chronic diseases) are the primary focus for interdisciplinary care related to influenza. Medical treatment of influenza focuses on establishing the diagnosis, providing symptomatic relief, and preventing complications.

Prevention

Preventing influenza by immunizing at-risk populations is an important aspect of care. Immunization with polyvalent (containing antigens of several viral strains) influenza virus vaccine is about 85% effective in preventing influenza infection for several months to a year (Fiore et al., 2008). Annual immunization is recommended for all children (6 months to 18 years) and all adults who want it, at-risk patients, including people over the age of 50, residents of nursing homes, adults and children with chronic cardiopulmonary disorders (e.g., asthma) or chronic metabolic diseases such as diabetes, and healthcare workers who have frequent contact with high-risk patients. Additionally, family members of at-risk patients should be vaccinated to reduce the patient's risk of exposure. The vaccine is given in the fall, prior to the annual winter outbreak. Live attenuated vaccine, administered by internasal spray, is available for healthy people under age 50 (CDC, 2009).

Diagnosis

The diagnosis of influenza is based on history, clinical findings, and knowledge of an influenza outbreak in the community. A chest x-ray and white blood cell (WBC) count may be done to rule out complications such as pneumonia. The WBC is commonly decreased in viral infections such as influenza; bacterial infections usually cause increased WBCs.

Medications

Yearly immunization with influenza vaccine is the single most important measure to prevent or minimize symptoms of influenza. Although the vaccine is readily available and inexpensive, only about 30% of at-risk patients are vaccinated each year. Many may fear a reaction from the vaccine, although the vaccines are highly purified and reactions are rare. About 5% of people experience mild symptoms of low-grade fever, malaise, or myalgia for up to 24 hours after vaccination. Because the vaccine is produced in eggs, it should not be given to people who are allergic to egg protein. Serious adverse reactions to influenza vaccine are rare. Guillain-Barré syndrome, an acute neurologic disorder characterized by muscle weakness and distal sensory loss, has been associated with certain batches of vaccine.

Amantadine (Symmetrel) or rimantadine (Flumadine) may be used for prophylaxis in unvaccinated people who are exposed to the virus. If the drug is given before or within 48 hours of exposure, it inhibits viral shedding and prevents or decreases the symptoms of influenza. If possible, unvaccinated people should receive the vaccine along with the antiviral drug. The drug is continued for several weeks or for the duration of the influenza outbreak. Some strains of type A influenza virus have been found to be resistant to amantadine and rimantadine, potentially limiting their effectiveness in preventing or treating an influenza outbreak.

Amantadine, rimantadine, and the antiviral drugs zanamivir (Relenza), oseltamivir (Tamiflu) (about 90% resistance to Influenza A last year, 2008–2009, but H1N1 is sensitive), and ribavirin (Virazole) also may be used to reduce the duration and severity of flu symptoms. Both zanamivir and ribavirin are administered by inhalation; the other drugs are given orally. Zanamivir can precipitate bronchospasm in patients with a history of asthma or chronic obstructive pulmonary disease (COPD), and is not recommended for use in these patients (Deglin & Vallerand, 2009). ∞ See Chapter 12 for nursing implications for antiviral drugs.

Over-the-counter analgesics such as aspirin, acetaminophen, or NSAIDs provide symptomatic relief of fever and muscle ache. Antitussives and mucolytics may decrease cough, promoting rest. Antibiotics are not indicated unless secondary bacterial infection occurs.

∞ Nursing Care

Health Promotion

Stress the importance of yearly influenza vaccination for everyone, unless contraindicated, especially patients in the high risk groups and their families. Teach about spread of the disease, including not going to work or school if sick and measures to reduce the risk of contracting influenza, such as handwashing, avoiding crowds, and avoiding people who are ill.

Assessment

Unless there is a known outbreak of influenza in the community, it can be difficult to differentiate the manifestations of influenza from those of other URI.

- *Health history:* Known exposure to virus; current symptoms, their onset and duration; presence of dyspnea, chest pain, productive cough, facial pain, or pressure in sinus areas; current medications, history of influenza vaccine; chronic diseases such as heart disease, chronic obstructive pulmonary disease (COPD), or diabetes; smokers and alcoholics; institutionalized, communal living such as college dormitories; known medication allergies.
- *Physical examination:* General appearance; vital signs including temperature; skin color; lung sounds; abdominal exam; ear, nose and throat examination.
- *Diagnostic tests:* Inflenza tests (nasal swabs, nasal aspirates), but usually not WBC, throat and sputum cultures, and chest x-ray unless suspect for evidence of bacterial infection or pneumonia.

Nursing Diagnoses and Interventions

Although the symptoms of influenza are distressing, most people with the illness provide self-care and do not contact a healthcare provider. Recommendations to rest in bed during the acute phase of the illness and limit activities until recovery are appropriate for influenza.

Severe disease or complications of influenza may necessitate hospitalization for respiratory support and management. For these patients, nursing care focuses on maintaining airway clearance, breathing patterns, and adequate rest.

Ineffective Breathing Pattern

Muscle aches, malaise, and elevated temperature may increase the respiratory rate and alter the depth of respirations, decreasing effective alveolar ventilation. Shallow respirations also increase the risk of *atelectasis*, lack of ventilation in an area of lung.

> **PRACTICE ALERT**
> Monitor respiratory rate and pattern. Tachypnea and/or rapid, shallow respirations may impair effective alveolar ventilation and gas exchange.

- Pace activities to provide for periods of rest. *Tachypnea increases the work of breathing, causing fatigue; fatigue, in turn, can further impair ventilation and reduce the effectiveness of coughing.*
- Elevate the head of the bed. *The upright position promotes drainage of nasal secretions, improves lung excursion, and reduces the work of breathing by lowering the diaphragm, which moves abdominal contents downward creating less resistance to diaphragmatic excursion, and slightly decreasing venous return.*

Ineffective Airway Clearance

Swelling and congestion of mucous membranes, extracellular fluid exudate, and impaired ciliary action due to cell damage increase the risk of impaired airway clearance in influenza. The older adult is at particular risk because of normally reduced ciliary activity and increased lung compliance.

> **PRACTICE ALERT**
> Monitor the effectiveness of cough and ability to remove airway secretions. Fatigue and general malaise may impair the ability to cough effectively and mobilize secretions.

- Maintain adequate hydration. Assess mucous membranes and skin turgor for evidence of dehydration. *Fever, increased mucous membrane secretions and decreased oral fluid intake may lead to dehydration and increased viscosity of secretions. Thick, viscous secretions are more difficult to expectorate.*
- Increase the humidity of inspired air with a bedside humidifier. *Increasing the water content of inhaled air helps loosen thick secretions and soothe mucous membranes.*
- Teach effective cough techniques. Administer analgesics as ordered. *The huff cough is effective to maintain open airways and spares energy (∞ see Chapter 37 for patient teaching of this technique). Relieving muscle ache increases the ability to cough effectively.*

Disturbed Sleep Pattern

Airway congestion, fever, malaise, muscle aches, and persistent cough may interfere with the ability to rest, increasing fatigue and prolonging recovery.

- Assess sleep patterns using subjective and objective information. *The patient may appear to be sleeping but not achieving normal sleep patterns because of influenza symptoms. Both subjective and objective data are important to accurately assess sleep.*
- Provide antipyretic and analgesic medications at or shortly before bedtime. *These drugs promote comfort by reducing fever and relieving muscle aches.*

> **PRACTICE ALERT**
> If necessary, request a cough suppressant for nighttime use. Cough suppressants are not recommended during the day because coughing promotes airway clearance. They may, however, be necessary at night to allow rest.

Risk for Infection

Infection control measures are recommended to prevent person-to-person transmission of influenza and control influenza outbreaks in healthcare facilities.

- Use standard precautions and encourage all staff and visitors to frequently wash hands. *Hand hygiene is a primary infection control measure for infections transmitted via respiratory secretions.*
- Instruct patients and visitors to control respiratory secretions by using tissues, and to maintain a distance of at least 3 feet from others when coughing or sneezing. Provide masks for patients and visitors who are coughing or sneezing. *Limiting*

EVIDENCE FOR NURSING CARE — The Patient with Influenza (includes H1N1)

Selected resources that nurses may find helpful when planning evidence-based nursing care follow.

- Bautista, E., Hayden, F. G., Chotpitayasunondh, T., Kawaoka, Y., Codeco, C. T., Mardel, S. et al. (2009). WHO guidelines for pharmacological management of pandemic (H1N1) 2009 influenza and other influenza viruses. World Health Organization (WHO) Global Alert and Response. Retrieved from http://www.who.int/csr/resources/publications/swineflu/h1n1_use_antivirals_20090820/en/index.html
- Brewer, K. (2009). Environment, health, & safety. *American Nurse Today, 4*(9), 56.
- Munro, C. L., & Morris, P. E. (2009). Seasonal influenza: Protect your patients by protecting yourself. *American Journal of Critical Care, 18*(5), 396–398.
- Snow, M. (2009). Updates and recommendations about the seasonal influenza vaccine. *Nursing2009, 39*(10), 61–62.
- Use of influenza A (H1N1) 2009 monovalent vaccine. (2009) Recommendations of the Advisory Committee on Immunization Practices (ACIP). Retrieved from http://www.cdc.gov/mmwr/preview/mmwrhtml/rr58e0821a1.htm

the spread of aerosolized secretions by covering the nose and mouth and maintaining distance from other people can reduce the spread of the disease to vulnerable populations.

- Use droplet precautions for patients with suspected or confirmed influenza: private room, masks for caregivers and visitors, and mask the patient when transporting within the facility. *These measures limit the spread of respiratory secretions.*

Using NANDA, NIC, and NOC

Linkages between a selected NANDA nursing diagnosis, NIC, and NOC for the patient with influenza are shown in the chart that follows.

NANDA, NIC, AND NOC LINKAGES
The Patient with Influenza

NANDA	Ineffective Breathing Pattern
	▼
NIC	Cough Enhancement Respiratory Monitoring Vital Signs Monitoring
	▼
NOC	Respiratory Status: Airway Patency Vital Signs

Adapted from Bulechek, G., Butcher, H., & Dochterman, J. M. (Eds). (2008). *Nursing interventions classification (NIC)* (5th ed.). St. Louis: Mosby Elsevier; Moorhead, S., Johnson, M., Maas, M., & Swanson, E. (Eds). (2008). *Nursing outcomes classification (NOC)* (4th ed.). St. Louis: Mosby Elsevier; and NANDA International. (2009). *Nursing diagnoses: Definitions and classification. 2009–2011.* Oxford, UK: Wiley-Blackwell.

Community-Based Care

Encourage appropriate self-care for patients with influenza. Discuss the following topics related to home care:

- Increase rest during the acute, febrile phase of the illness.
- Increase fluid intake (to greater than normal level) even if anorexic.
- Use over-the-counter medications at safe and effective dose and frequency for symptom relief.
- Employ hygiene measures such as using disposable tissues and frequent hand hygiene to reduce spread of the disease.
- Know manifestations of potential complications of influenza to report to the primary care provider.

The Patient with Sinusitis

Sinusitis is inflammation of the mucous membranes of one or more of the sinuses (see Figure 34–2). Sinusitis is a common condition that usually follows an upper respiratory infection such as acute viral upper respiratory infection or influenza. Common causative organisms include viruses, streptococci, *S. pneumoniae*, *Haemophilus influenzae*, and staphylococci. The risk of sinusitis is higher when the immune system is suppressed by immunosuppressive drugs or HIV infection. Sinusitis is common and difficult to treat in people who have AIDS.

Physiology Review

The sinuses (or *paranasal sinuses*) are air-filled cavities in the facial bones that open into the turbinates of the nasal cavity. They are lined with ciliated mucous membranes that help move fluid and microorganisms out of the sinuses into the nasal cavity. The sinuses normally are sterile. Air within the sinuses has a lower oxygen content than inspired air.

Pathophysiology

Sinusitis develops when nasal mucous membranes swell or other disorders (such as polyps or tumors) obstruct sinus openings, impairing drainage. Mucus secretions collect in the sinus cavity, serving as a medium for viral or bacterial growth. The nasal and sinus mucous membranes are continuous; therefore, pathogens generally spread to the sinuses via the opening into the nasal turbinates. The inflammatory response provoked by pathogen invasion draws serum and leukocytes to the area to combat the infection, increasing swelling and pressure.

Any process that impairs drainage from the sinuses may precipitate sinusitis. These include nasal polyps, deviated septum, rhinitis, tooth abscess, or swimming or diving trauma. In hospitalized patients, sinusitis may develop following prolonged nasotracheal intubation. Usually more than one sinus is infected. The frontal and maxillary sinuses are usually involved in adults.

Sinusitis may be acute or chronic. Chronic sinusitis results when acute sinusitis is untreated, inadequately treated, or there are recurrent episodes or other factors that prevent sinus drainage. With continued infection, bacteria can become isolated, producing chronic inflammation. Over time, mucous membranes become thickened. Fungal infections may cause chronic infections, especially in immunosuppressed patients.

Other factors that may contribute to chronic sinusitis are smoking, allergies, and habitual use of nasal sprays or inhalants.

Manifestations and Complications

The patient with acute sinusitis often looks sick. Manifestations of sinusitis include pain and tenderness across the infected sinuses, headache, fever, and malaise. The pain usually increases with leaning forward. When the maxillary sinuses are involved, pain and pressure are felt over the cheek. The pain may be referred to the upper teeth. Frontal sinusitis causes pain and tenderness across the lower forehead. Infection of the ethmoid sinus produces retro-orbital pain and pain over the high lateral aspect of the nose. Sphenoid sinusitis, the rarest form, may cause pain in the occiput, vertex, or middle of the head. Symptoms often worsen for 3 to 4 hours after awakening and then become less severe in the afternoon and evening as secretions drain. The intensity and location of headache pain may change as sinuses drain. In acute sinusitis, the pain is usually constant and severe. In chronic sinusitis, the pain is described as dull and may be constant or intermittent.

Other symptoms include nasal congestion, purulent nasal discharge, and bad breath. The nasal mucous membrane is red and swollen. Purulent drainage may be noted at the opening to the middle turbinate. This may be the only sign of chronic sinusitis. Swallowed secretions from post nasal drip irritate and inflame the throat, and may cause nausea or vomiting.

Complications develop when the infection spreads to surrounding structures (Box 35–2). These include periorbital abscess, or cellulitis, cavernous sinus thrombosis, meningitis, brain abscess, or sepsis. Eustachian tube edema may lead to temporary hearing loss.

Interdisciplinary Care

Treatment of sinusitis focuses on restoring drainage of obstructed sinuses, controlling infection, relieving pain, and preventing complications.

Diagnosis

The diagnosis of acute sinusitis usually can be made using the history and physical exam. Diagnostic studies such as CT scan or less frequently, sinus x-rays generally are done only when sinusitis is persistent, chronic, or recurrent. ∞ See Chapter 34 for more information about diagnostic studies and their nursing implications.

- *Sinus x-rays* are used infrequently. Sinuses are normally translucent because they are filled with air; affected sinuses appear cloudy or opaque. A visible air-fluid level or thickening of the sinus mucosa may be seen in infected sinuses.

BOX 35–2 Potential Complications of Sinusitis

Local Complications	Intracranial Complications
■ Orbital cellulitis	■ Meningitis
■ Subperiosteal abscess	■ Epidural abscess
■ Orbital abscess	■ Subdural abscess
■ Cavernous sinus thrombosis	■ Brain abscess
■ Mucocele	■ Venous sinus thrombosis
■ Osteomyelitis	

- *CT scan* is a more sensitive indicator of acute and chronic sinusitis and often is performed without preceding x-rays.
- *Magnetic resonance imaging (MRI)* may be ordered if malignancy of the sinus is suspected.

Medications

Antibiotic therapy directed at the usual organisms causing sinusitis typically is prescribed if the symptoms have lasted for more than 7 days. Amoxicillin (possibly combined with clavulanate [Augmentin]), trimethoprim-sulfamethoxazole (Bactrim, Septra), cefuroxime (Ceftin), cefaclor (Ceclor), ciprofloxacin (Cipro), or clarithromycin (Biaxin) are commonly used antibiotics for sinusitis. Antibiotic therapy is continued for 10 to 14 days; occasionally a longer course is prescribed to prevent relapse. If the sinusitis does not respond to treatment with oral antibiotics, hospitalization and intravenous antibiotic therapy may be required. ∞ See Chapter 12 for nursing care related to antibiotic therapy.

Topical steroids (such as fluticasone) and decongestants (in the form of nasal sprays) or oral decongestants such as pseudoephedrine or phenylephrine are also prescribed to reduce mucosal edema and promote sinus drainage. Antihistamines may decrease nasal congestion and facilitate sinus drainage, but they also tend to increase the viscosity of secretions and hinder drainage. For this reason, they may not be as effective as decongestants. Saline nose drops or sprays promote sinus drainage, as does inhalation of warm steam.

> **PRACTICE ALERT**
> To administer topical drugs, the patient's head is tilted backward and to the side on which the drops are to be instilled. The patient may need to remain in position for 5 minutes to allow the drops to reach the posterior nares.

Systemic mucolytic agents such as guaifenesin may be useful to liquefy secretions, promoting sinus drainage. Aerobic exercise also promotes mucous flow and may be recommended.

Surgery

Patients who do not respond to pharmacologic measures and who experience persistent facial pain, headache, or nasal congestion may require *endoscopic sinus surgery*. Detailed evaluation of the sinuses by CT scan is done prior to surgery. Under local or general anesthesia, a fiberoptic nasal endoscope is inserted to visualize the sinus opening. If obstruction is present, it can be removed, restoring patency and drainage. This surgery is most effective for local disease, recurrent acute sinusitis, and for removing anatomic obstructions (Way & Doherty, 2003). Patients who have endoscopic sinus surgery usually do not require nasal packing postoperatively. Instead, frequent nasal cleaning and irrigation with normal saline are performed. The patient is instructed to sneeze with the mouth open and avoid blowing the nose, lifting, or straining for a week following surgery.

Antral irrigation can be done in the healthcare provider's office under local anesthesia. A 16-gauge needle is inserted under the inferior turbinate of the nose into the maxillary sinus on the affected side. Saline solution is instilled to irrigate the area

Figure 35–1 ■ Incision to access ethmoid and frontal sinuses. Resulting scar is nearly invisible in folds of the eye.

and wash out the sinus of purulent exudate. The patient is seated with the head forward and mouth open to allow drainage of the solution through the nose and mouth. A culture of the exudate may be obtained to determine appropriate antibiotic therapy.

The *Caldwell-Luc procedure* may be necessary if endoscopic sinus surgery is unsuccessful. It is performed under local or general anesthesia. An incision is made under the upper lip into the maxillary sinus, and diseased mucous membrane and periosteum are removed. An opening between the maxillary sinus and lateral nasal wall, a "nasal antral window," is created to increase aeration of the sinus and promote drainage into the nasal cavity. The area is packed with gauze for 24 to 48 hours postoperatively. The gauze packing obstructs nasal breathing while it is in place. As the maxillary sinus heals, exposed bone is covered by mucosa. The upper lip and teeth may be numb for several months after the procedure because of nerve trauma. Chewing may be impaired on the affected side. Only liquids are given for the first 24 hours, followed by a soft diet. The patient is instructed to avoid wearing dentures and the Valsalva maneuver (no blowing the nose, coughing, or straining at stool) for about 2 weeks after the packing has been removed to prevent bleeding.

In *external sphenoethmoidectomy,* an incision along the side of the nose from the middle of the eyebrow is used to open and remove diseased tissue from the sphenoid or ethmoid sinuses (Figure 35–1 ■). Nasal polyps may also be removed using this approach. Nasal packing is inserted, and an eye pressure patch is applied to decrease periorbital edema. Care is similar to that following the Caldwell-Luc procedure.

Complementary Therapies

Complementary therapies may help relieve symptoms of sinusitis and promote comfort. The use of high volume, low pressure nasal irrigation has expanded beyond postoperative management. It has been shown to be more effective in managing sinusitis symptoms than nasal sprays (Pynnonen, Mukerji, Kim, Adams & Terrell, 2007). Nasal irrigation systems such as the Nasa-flo® neti-pot (NeilMed Products, Inc.) are widely available over the counter. Aromatherapy using herbs such as basil, marjoram, or eucalyptus in a vaporizor or on a handkerchief; herbal teas made from goldenseal, yarrow, or coltsfoot; hot or cold compresses or steam inhalation; and accupressure may be employed (National Cancer Institute, 2009a).

♋ Nursing Care

Health Promotion

Measures to prevent sinusitis are those that promote nasal drainage: encouraging increased fluid intake, judicious use of nasal decongestants as needed, and treating any obstructive process (e.g., with nsasl steroid spray). Encourage patients with URI to blow their nose with both nares open. Advise patients that use of saline nasal sprays can help maintain patency of the opening to the sinuses, promoting drainage and reducing the risk of obstruction and infection.

Assessment

Focused assessment of the patient with suspected sinusitis includes the following:

- *Health history:* Complaints of frontal or periorbital headache, cheek, teeth, or ear pain; timing of pain and changes in intensity over course of the day; nasal discharge or postnasal drip; other symptoms like tenderness over the cheeks; previous sinus infections or trauma; current medications, known medication and environmental allergies (allergic rhinitis).
- *Physical examination:* General appearance, vital signs including temperature; inspect nasal and pharyngeal mucous membranes; percuss sinuses for tenderness.
- *Diagnostic tests:* CT of the sinuses, and infrequently sinus x-rays WBC and differential, cultures of sinus drainage.

Nursing Diagnoses and Interventions

The patient with sinusitis is often acutely uncomfortable. Obstructed and congested sinuses cause pain and pressure that increase with position changes and leaning forward. Treatment usually is community based, making education the key nursing role. When the patient is hospitalized for intravenous antibiotic therapy or sinus surgery, *Pain* and *Imbalanced Nutrition* are priority nursing diagnoses.

Pain

Although sinus surgery is relatively minor, both the incision and postoperative swelling can cause discomfort. Nasal packing, if used, contributes to the discomfort.

- Assess pain using a standardized pain scale. Administer analgesics as ordered. *Relief of pain promotes a feeling of well-being and enhances recovery.*
- Apply ice packs to the nose. *Cold compresses reduce swelling, control bleeding, and provide local analgesia.*
- Elevate the head of the bed to Fowler's or high-Fowler's position for 24 to 48 hours after surgery. *Elevating the operative site minimizes tissue swelling and promotes comfort.*

Imbalanced Nutrition: Less than Body Requirements

Postoperatively, the sense of smell, an appetite stimulus, is diminished by nasal packing. Mouth discomfort from the incision and numbness of the upper teeth also may impact appetite and eating.

- Provide clear liquid diet progressing to soft foods as tolerated. High-calorie dietary supplements may be used. *A progressive diet is used to assess the ability to swallow without choking and allay fears. Foods high in calories and nutritional value provide for metabolic and healing requirements.*
- Monitor intake, output, and weight. *This information allows assessment of overall fluid balance and the adequacy of dietary intake.*
- Elevate the head of the bed during meals. *The upright position facilitates swallowing and minimizes risk of aspiration.*

Community-Based Care

Teaching for patients with sinusitis and their families focuses on following through with appropriate treatment and promoting comfort. Discuss the following topics when preparing for home care:

- The importance of completing the entire course of prescribed antibiotics to achieve cure and prevent the development of antibiotic-resistant bacteria. Assist in developing a schedule that helps ensure all doses are taken.
- Measures to prevent superinfections (such as vaginitis or oral thrush) during the prolonged course of treatment (e.g., consume 8 oz of yogurt containing live bacterial cultures daily while on antibiotics).
- Use systemic or topical decongestants to promote sinus drainage.
- Maintain a liberal fluid intake to reduce the viscosity of mucous drainage.
- Use a humidifier or steam inhalation to promote sinus drainage.
- Sleep with the head of the bed elevated to a 45-degree angle and on the unaffected side to promote drainage of affected sinuses.
- Application of a warm, moist pack to the area of pain and tenderness to promote comfort.
- Notify the healthcare provider if symptoms do not improve with treatment or if signs of a complication develop, such as increased pain, and redness and swelling on the side of the nose or around the eyes.
- Postoperative instructions to prevent bleeding, such as avoiding blowing the nose for 7 to 10 days and avoiding strenuous activity such as heavy lifting for about 2 weeks.
- Use saline nasal sprays or nasal irrigation postoperatively to keep the nasal mucosa moist.

The Patient with Pharyngitis or Tonsillitis

Pharyngitis, acute inflammation of the pharynx, is one of the most commonly identified clinical problems. Although it is usually viral in origin, pharyngitis may also be caused by bacterial infection. *Group A beta-hemolytic streptococcus (GABHS)* (strep throat) is the most common cause of bacterial pharyngitis. Other bacteria that may cause pharyngitis include *Neisseria gonorrheae*, a gram-negative diplococcus that is sexually transmitted, *Mycoplasma*, and *Chlamydia trachomatis*. Pharyngitis may also be a result of postnasal drip from allergic rhinitis or as a result of gastroesophageal reflux into the throat.

Tonsillitis is acute inflammation of the palatine tonsils. Although it is sometimes viral in origin, tonsillitis is usually due to streptococcal infection. The incidence of streptococcal infections is greatest between late fall and spring, especially in cold climates. Viral tonsillitis may occur in epidemics in people living in crowded conditions, such as military recruits.

Pathophysiology and Manifestations

Pharyngitis and tonsillitis are contagious and spread by droplet nuclei. Incubation varies from a few hours to several days, depending on the organism. Viral infections are communicable for 2 to 3 days. Symptoms usually resolve within 3 to 10 days after onset.

Viral pharyngitis may be attributed to the same viruses causing the common cold, rhinovirus, coronavirus, or parainfluenza virus. Pharyngitis caused by adenovirus, influenza virus, or Epstein-Barr virus (associated with infectious mononucleosis) may be particularly severe.

Acute pharyngitis causes pain and fever. The pain may vary from a scratchy sore throat to one so painful that swallowing is difficult. Streptococcal pharyngitis is usually marked by an abrupt onset, with fever of 101° F (38.3° C) or higher, severe sore throat with dysphagia, headache, malaise, and often arthralgias and myalgias and the absence of a cough. Anterior lymph nodes are often enlarged and tender. Exudate (pus) may be seen on the pharynx and tonsils (Figure 35–2 ■). In contrast, the onset of viral pharyngitis is often gradual, with manifestations of low-grade fever, sore throat, mild hoarseness, headache, and rhinorrhea. The pharyngeal membranes appear mildly red with vascular congestion. Infectious mononucleosis, caused by the Epstein-Barr virus, often presents as acute pharyngitis, with visible patches of exudate on the pharynx or tonsils (Domino et al., 2010). The cervical lymph nodes are enlarged and tender as well. See the accompanying box for the manifestations of pharyngitis and tonsillitis.

In tonsillitis, the tonsils appear bright red and edematous. White exudate may be present on the tonsils; pressing on a tonsil may produce purulent drainage The uvula may also be reddened and swollen. The tonsillar lymph nodes are usually tender and enlarged.

The patient with tonsillitis complains of a sore throat, difficulty swallowing, general malaise, fever, and otalgia (pain referred to the ear). Manifestations are often more severe in adolescents and adults than in children. Infection may extend via the eustachian tubes to cause acute otitis media. This may lead to further damage such as spontaneous rupture of the eardrums and mastoiditis. ∞ See Chapter 46 for more information about otitis media.

Complications

Although GABHS pharyngitis may be mild and indistinguishable from viral pharyngitis by its signs and symptoms, it can lead to significant complications such as abscess, scarlet fever, toxic shock syndrome, rheumatic fever, or acute poststreptococcal

Figure 35–2 ■ The appearance of the oral pharynx and tonsils in acute pharyngitis and tonsillitis.

MANIFESTATIONS of Pharyngitis and Tonsillitis

LOCAL
- Sore throat
- Possible dysphagia and otalgia
- Tender, swollen anterior cervical lymph nodes
- Hoarse voice
- Red, swollen pharyngeal mucous membranes and/or tonsils
- Possible visible exudate on pharyngeal membranes and/or tonsils

GENERAL
- Fever
- General malaise
- Arthralgia, myalgia

glomerulonephritis. GABHS is treated with antibitotics to prevent these sequelae. *Peritonsillar abscess*, or *quinsy*, is a potential complication of tonsillitis. It usually results from group A beta-hemolytic streptococcus infection extending from the tonsils to the surrounding tissue. The abscess causes pus formation behind the tonsil with marked swelling and asymmetric deviation of the uvula. The degree of swelling may make it difficult to swallow anything other than liquids. The patient may exhibit thickening of the voice, drooling, and a tonic contraction of the muscles of mastication, called trismus.

Rare (1% to 3%) but serious complications of group A beta hemolytic streptococcal pharyngitis and tonsillitis include acute glomerulonephritis and rheumatic fever, abnormal immune responses to the infection. Acute glomerulonephritis generally presents with sudden onset of hematuria, proteinuria, and less commonly, hypertension and edema within 7 to 10 days after the acute infection. Rheumatic fever typically presents 3 to 5 weeks after acute infection with fever, painful or swollen joints, rash, and heart murmur. Other complications of bacterial infection include sinusitis, otitis media, mastoiditis, and cervical adenitis.

Interdisciplinary Care

Both viral and bacterial pharyngitis are usually self-limited diseases. However, because of the risk for serious complications associated with GABHS sore throat, an effort is usually made to identify this pathogen and treat only this pharyngitis with antibiotics.

- *Throat swab* is obtained and examined for streptococcus antigen using the latex agglutination (LA) antigen test or enzyme immunoassay (ELISA) testing. These tests allow rapid identification of the antigen (in as little as 10 minutes for the LA test) but are not highly sensitive. When the test is positive, treatment for strep throat is initiated. If the test is negative, the swab is cultured to ensure that streptococcus organisms are not present. Even throat cultures are not always accurate, with approximately 10% false negative and 20% false positive results. ∞ See Chapter 34 for nursing care related to obtaining a throat swab.
- *Complete blood count (CBC)* may be done on severely ill patients or to rule out other causes of pharyngitis. The WBC count is usually normal or low in viral infections and elevated in bacterial infections.

Antipyretics and mild analgesics such as aspirin or acetaminophen provide symptomatic relief for throat pain and associated myalgias. Penicillin is the drug of choice for group A streptococci. Erythromycin, amoxicillin, or cefuroxime (Ceftin, Kefurox) may be used if the patient is allergic to penicillin. Antibiotic therapy is continued for at least 10 days. The patient is no longer contagious after 24 hours of antibiotic therapy.

A peritonsillar abscess is drained by needle aspiration or by incision and drainage. The area is first sprayed with a topical anesthetic such as cetacaine and then injected with a local anesthetic. The sitting position is preferred for the procedure, because it enables expectoration of blood and pus. (See the accompanying Case Study & Nursing Care Plan for nursing care of the patient with a peritonsillar abscess.) Tonsillectomy is done either immediately or 6 weeks after incision and drainage of peritonsillar abscess.

Tonsillectomy (surgical removal of the tonsils) is indicated for recurrent or chronic infections that have not responded to antibiotic therapy, hypertrophy of the tonsils with risk of airway obstruction, peritonsillar abscess, repeated attacks of purulent otitis media, and tonsil malignancy. Adenoid tissue usually is removed at the same time. Bleeding is the most significant postoperative complication of tonsillectomy, and may develop up to two weeks following the surgery.

Nursing Care

Because of the risk of significant complications associated with GABHS pharyngitis, encourage all patients with symptoms that persist for several days or that include fever, lymphadenopathy, and myalgias to seek evaluation and treatment.

Home care is appropriate for acute uncomplicated pharyngitis. Treatment focuses on adequate rest and relief of symptoms. A liquid or soft diet is useful when swallowing is difficult. Increased fluid intake is encouraged, especially when febrile. Warm saline gargles, moist inhalations, and application of an ice collar are soothing to the sore throat.

Following tonsillectomy, ensure a patent airway by placing the patient in semi-Fowler's position with the head turned to the side to allow secretions to drain from the mouth and pharynx. Keep the airway in place until the gag and swallowing reflexes have returned. Apply an ice collar to reduce swelling and pain. Notify the surgeon immediately if excessive bleeding or hemorrhage occurs. If there is no bleeding, allow water and cracked ice as desired. Warm saline mouthwashes are helpful in managing thick oral secretions following tonsillectomy. A liquid or semiliquid diet is recommended for several days.

Community-Based Care

Discuss the following topics when preparing the patient for home care.

- The importance of completing the full 10 days of antibiotic therapy if prescribed
- Using warm saline gargles or throat lozenges for symptomatic relief
- Signs and symptoms of possible complications of GABHS streptococcal infection such as glomerulonephritis or rheumatic fever

Patient Monica Wunderman, aged 27, was recently treated for tonsillitis caused by infection by group A streptococcus. She presents to the emergency department 10 days later appearing acutely ill. She states that her throat is so sore that she has difficulty swallowing even liquids. Ms. Ironhorse, the ED nurse, completes an assessment of Ms. Wunderman.

ASSESSMENT

Findings include T 102°F (38.8°C). An acutely swollen and reddened area of the soft palate is noted in her mouth, half occluding the orifice from the mouth into the pharynx. Yellow exudate is present. CBC reveals an elevated WBC of 16,000/mm³. A diagnosis of peritonsillar abscess is made. Needle aspiration of the abscess is performed.

DIAGNOSIS

- *Acute Pain* related to swelling
- *Risk for Ineffective Airway Clearance* related to pain and swelling
- *Deficient Fluid Volume* related to fever and difficulty in swallowing fluids

EXPECTED OUTCOMES

- Have minimal or no pain.
- Maintain a patent airway as demonstrated by normal respiratory rate and rhythm.
- Maintain optimal fluid intake as evidenced by consumption of fluids and semiliquid foods, moist mucous membranes, normal skin turgor, and normal temperature.

PLANNING AND IMPLEMENTATION

- Teach that ice-cold fluids may be easier to swallow than hot or room-temperature beverages and may provide a local analgesic effect.
- Advise to avoid citrus juices, hot or spicy foods, and rough-textured foods for 1 week.
- Teach pain management strategies such as applying an ice collar as desired and gargling with warm saline or mouthwash solution every 1 to 2 hours for the first 24 to 48 hours after aspiration of the abscess.
- Instruct to take medications (antibiotics) as prescribed.

EVALUATION

When Ms. Ironhorse contacts Ms. Wunderman by telephone 2 days after her visit to the emergency department, she reports complete relief of symptoms. She is afebrile, taking fluids without difficulty, and has had no difficulty breathing. She has not experienced any pain.

CRITICAL THINKING IN THE NURSING PROCESS

1. Describe common symptoms of infectious or inflammatory diseases of the upper airway and discuss methods of symptom relief.
2. Describe common pharmacologic interventions for these disorders.
3. What themes of nursing diagnoses emerge for these patients?

See Evaluating Your Response in Appendix C.

- Monitoring temperature in the morning and evening until well to ensure that the infection has not spread to deeper tissues
- Proper use and disposal of tissues and frequent hand hygiene to prevent spreading the infection to others

For the patient who has had a peritonsillar abscess drainage or tonsillectomy, provide the following instructions.

- Postoperative mouth and throat care
- Avoiding use of aspirin for 2 weeks to reduce the risk of postoperative bleeding
- Manifestations of bleeding to report to the healthcare provider (delayed hemorrhage may occur for up to 1 week post surgery)

The Patient with a Laryngeal Infection

The larynx, located between the upper airways and the lungs, protects the lower respiratory tract from inhaled substances other than air, and allows speech. The larynx includes the epiglottis, which covers the larynx during swallowing, and the glottis, or vocal cords. Either portion of the larynx may become inflamed.

Epiglottitis

Epiglottitis, inflammation of the epiglottis, is an uncommon disorder that presents as a medical emergency. *H. influenzae* infection is the most common cause of epiglottitis. Epiglottitis is a rapidly progressive cellulitis that begins between the base of the tongue and the epiglottis. The epiglottis itself becomes swollen and inflamed; swelling of adjacent tissues pushes the epiglottis posteriorly. This swelling and edema threatens the airway. Adults usually present with a 1 to 2 day history of sore throat, *odynophagia* (painful swallowing), dyspnea, and possibly drooling and stridor.

Using a tongue blade to view the oropharynx is avoided; this may precipitate laryngospasm and airway obstruction. The epiglottis is visualized using a flexible fiberoptic laryngoscope to establish the diagnosis. The epiglottis appears red, swollen, and edematous. Nasotracheal intubation may be required to ensure airway patency. The patient is admitted to a critical care unit and intravenous antibiotic therapy is initiated. Ceftriaxone (Rocephin), cefuroxime (Ceftin), or ampicillin/sulbactam (Unasyn) may be prescribed. If allergic to penicillin, a combination of clindamycin (Cleocin) and either trimethoprim-sulfamthoxazole (TMP-SMZ) or ciprofloxacin (Cipro) may be used. Dexamethasone, a systemic corticosteroid, is also given to suppress the inflammatory response and rapidly reduce swelling of the epiglottis.

Nursing care for the patient with acute epiglottitis focuses on monitoring and maintaining airway patency. Monitor oxygen saturation continuously. Observe closely for signs of airway obstruction, including nasal flaring, restlessness, stridor, use of accessory muscles, and decreased oxygen saturation measurements. If the patient is not intubated, supplies for emergency intubation should be kept in the unit. Epiglottitis is frightening for both the patient and the nurse. Maintaining a calm, reassuring manner is an essential nursing role.

Laryngitis

Laryngitis, inflammation of the larynx, is a common disorder that may occur alone or in conjunction with other upper respiratory infections. It is commonly associated with viral URI such as influenza. It may also occur with bronchitis, pneumonia, other respiratory infections or due to a tumor or polyp on the vocal cord. Excessive use of the voice, sudden changes in temperature or exposure to dust, irritating fumes, smoke, or other pollutants can also cause acute or chronic laryngitis. It is more common in the winter and in colder climates. Persistnet laryngitis after the URI resolution or removal of the irtiyant should be evaluated to rule out malignancy.

In laryngitis, the mucous membrane lining the larynx becomes inflamed; the vocal cords also may become edematous. The primary symptom of laryngitis is a change in the voice. Hoarseness or *aphonia*, complete loss of the voice, may occur. The throat is often sore and scratchy, and a dry, harsh cough may be present.

There is no specific treatment for viral laryngitis. Any identified precipitating factors such as overuse of the voice and exposure to irritants should be eliminated. Voice rest is advised, as is abstinence from tobacco and alcohol, which are chemical irritants. Treatment may also include inhaling steam or spraying the throat with antiseptic solutions. Identifying and eliminating irritants is helpful to prevent future attacks.

Impaired verbal communication is the priority nursing problem for patients with laryngitis. The meaning of messages is conveyed not only by the words used, but also by the tone and loudness of voice. Instruct to rest the voice as much as possible. Encourage speaking in short sentences or using alternate methods of communication, such as writing. Resting the voice hastens recovery and decreases throat discomfort. Advise to use soothing throat lozenges, sprays, or other comfort measures such as gargling with a warm antiseptic solution. Help identify potential irritants, such as fumes, chemicals, or cold temperature, to prevent future bouts of laryngitis.

The Patient with Diphtheria

Diphtheria is an acute, contagious disease caused by *Corynebacterium diphtheriae*, a small aerobic pathogen. This disease, which primarily affects adults, is uncommon in the United States. Waning immunity due to lack of periodic booster immunizations is the primary risk factor for diphtheria in the United States.

The disease is spread through droplet nuclei and by contamination of articles such as eating utensils. Asymptomatic carriers can be a factor in spreading this infection. People who have recovered from diphtheria can harbor bacteria in their throats for up to 4 weeks. Diphtheria is easily spread in areas where sanitation is poor, living conditions are crowded, and access to health care is limited. Immunization is readily available, and infants and children are usually immunized against diphtheria, pertussis, and tetanus concurrently.

Pathophysiology and Manifestations

C. diphtheriae infects the mucous membranes of the respiratory tract and can invade skin lesions. The tonsils and pharynx are common sites of infection. Toxins released by the organism inflame mucosal surfaces of the pharynx. Exudate from inflamed tissues forms a thick, grayish, rubbery pseudomembrane over the posterior pharynx and sometimes into the trachea. This pseudomembrane adheres to inflamed, eroded surfaces and interferes with eating, drinking, and breathing. The airway may be obstructed, necessitating tracheostomy to maintain respirations. The toxins damage the heart and central nervous system and may cause myocarditis and paralysis of cranial or peripheral nerves.

Patients with diphtheria develop fever, malaise, sore throat, and malodorous breath. In severe cases, the neck may be warm and swollen because of lymphadenopathy. Isolated patches of gray or white exudate grow and extend to form a gray membrane that becomes progressively thicker. Dislodging the membrane often causes bleeding. Symptoms of airway obstruction, such as stridor and cyanosis, can develop quickly.

Interdisciplinary Care

Collaborative care goals for diphtheria are to prevent its transmission, treat the infection, neutralize toxins, and provide respiratory support. The diagnosis is confirmed by a throat culture. Gram-stain or immunofluorescent antibody stains may also be used.

Strict isolation procedures are instituted, and all contacts are screened and immunized. Booster shots are given to people who were immunized 5 or more years previously. Unimmunized contacts are treated with immunization and antibiotics.

Diphtheria antitoxin is given to neutralize free toxin and prevent further toxin production. It is delivered via IV over one hour or IM. Diphtheria antitoxin is produced in horses; a skin test for sensitivity to horse serum should precede immunization as about 7% of the population is sensitive to it (Domino et al., 2010). Anaphylaxis is a risk during antitoxin therapy; epinephrine must be readily available. Antibiotics such as penicillin or erythromycin are administered to eliminate the organism.

◯ Nursing Care

Patients with diphtheria require intensive nursing care. The patient is placed on bed rest and monitored closely for airway obstruction, cardiac manifestations, and CNS complications. Nutrition and fluid balance may be affected by difficulty swallowing. Upright positioning can promote fluid intake during the acute phase of the disease. Equipment for suction, emergency intubation, and tracheostomy are kept at the bedside.

> **PRACTICE ALERT**
> Diphtheria is a reportable disease. Immediately contact the local health department and the Centers for Disease Control and Prevention of all suspected and confirmed cases.

Preventing further cases of diphtheria is a nursing responsibility. Symptomatic patients are isolated and treated until two negative throat cultures are obtained. Nasopharyngeal and throat cultures are also obtained from all close contacts. Asymptomatic disease carriers are confined to home until at least 3 days of antibiotic therapy have been completed. All contacts, including hospital personnel, receive tetanus and diphtheria toxoids (Td).

The Patient with Pertussis

Pertussis, or *whooping cough*, is a highly contagious acute upper respiratory infection caused by the bacterium *Bordetella pertussis*. Although it is thought to be a childhood disease that has been virtually eliminated by aggressive immunization of infants, pertussis still occurs in North America. Up to 45% of people affected by pertussis are adolescents and adults. Adults are thought to be an important reservoir for this disease (Domino et al., 2010).

Pathophysiology

B. pertussis is a gram-negative rod that is spread by respiratory droplets. The bacteria attach to ciliated epithelial cells of the nasopharynx, multiplying and invading respiratory tissues. The damage and effects of pertussis are not due to the infection itself, but to toxins produced by the bacteria. These toxins damage the mucosa and paralyze the cilia. As a result, clearance of respiratory secretions is impaired, increasing the risk for pneumonia. The toxins also prompt an inflammatory response and inhibit immune defenses.

Although immunization does not appear to confer lifetime immunity, the disease tends to be milder in adolescents, adults, and people who have been immunized. These infected individuals can, however, transmit the disease to other susceptible people, including unimmunized or underimmunized infants (Huether & McCance, 2008).

Young infants have the highest risk for complications of the disease, such as pneumonia and neurologic complications. Neurologic complications are thought to result from hypoxia due to prolonged paroxysms of coughing. Complications in adolescents and adults may occur as a result of increased intrathoracic pressure during prolonged coughing spells. These may include pneumothorax, weight loss, inguinal hernia, rib fracture, and *cough syncope* (fainting due to hypoxia) (Domino et al., 2010).

Manifestations

Classic pertussis follows a predictable pattern, with typical upper respiratory infection symptoms (coryza, sneezing, low-grade fever, and mild cough) beginning 7 to 10 days after exposure. After 1 to 2 weeks, the cough becomes more frequent, occurring in paroxysms or bursts of rapid coughs, often ending

---

MANIFESTATIONS of Pertussis

CLASSIC
- Catarrhal phase: coryza, malaise, low-grade fever, sneezing, cough
- Paroxysmal phase: frequent spasms of sometimes violent coughing, worse at night; characteristic whoop on inspiration following cough paroxysm; vomiting, fatigue, weight loss resulting from severe cough
- Convalescent phase: gradually decreasing frequency and severity of coughing episodes

ATYPICAL (OFTEN SEEN IN ADOLESCENTS AND ADULTS)
- Severe, prolonged cough that may not be paroxysmal; whoop uncommon
- Vomiting with cough
- Cough at night

---

with an audible whoop caused by rapid inspiration. This whoop is less common in adolescents and adults, often delaying diagnosis. Vomiting commonly follows an episode of coughing. Coughing paroxysms vary in frequency from several per hour to 5 to 10 per day, interfering with eating and sleep. This stage of the disease, called the *paroxysmal stage*, usually lasts no more than 6 weeks, after which coughing becomes less severe and gradually resolves over a period of up to 3 months.

In adolescents and adults, pertussis is suspected when an upper respiratory infection produces a cough that persists longer than 7 days, is accompanied by vomiting, and is worse at night. See the Manifestations box.

Interdisciplinary Care

Active immunization with pertussis vaccine is the primary preventive strategy for pertussis. Acellular pertussis vaccines that are effective, but produce fewer adverse reactions than traditional whole-cell vaccines, are available and preferred for immunization.

The diagnosis of pertussis is established by culture of nasopharyngeal secretions. However, nasopharyngeal secretions may remain positive for the organism for only about 3 weeks after the onset of symptoms, so blood tests for antibodies to the organism may be necessary to confirm the diagnosis. Lymphocytosis (elevated lymphocyte count) may be present.

Erythromycin is the antibiotic of choice to eradicate *B. pertussis* infection. Trimethoprim-sulfamethoxazole (TMP-SMZ) may be used as an alternate to erythromycin. Hospitalization rarely is required for adults, although children and infants with severe disease often are hospitalized to prevent complications such as neurologic effects of hypoxia and malnutrition. Respiratory isolation is instituted for 5 days after antibiotic therapy is started. Prophylactic erythromycin or TMP-SMZ is prescribed for all in the household and close contacts of the infected patient.

∞ Nursing Care

Nurses are instrumental in promoting effective immunization of all infants and young children against pertussis. Education is a key nursing role related to immunization, as significant controversy currently exists about potential long-term adverse consequences of the vaccine. Recommend that all parents request acellular vaccine due to its lower risk of adverse effects.

Recommend nasopharyngeal culture for patients complaining of persistent cough, especially when the cough is accompanied by vomiting or significantly worse at night, or if other members of the household or close contacts have a similar illness.

PRACTICE ALERT
Pertussis is a reportable communicable disease. Report all probable and confirmed cases to the local health department and Centers for Disease Control and Surveillance.

Education is a primary nursing role related to pertussis. Adult patients usually remain in the community for treatment. Teach respiratory isolation measures to be used until the disease is no longer communicable to others. Discuss ways to control respiratory secretions, and the importance of disposing of tissues and secretions personally to prevent exposure of others. Stress the importance of prophylactic treatment for all household and close contacts. Discuss measures to maintain fluid and nutrient intake, and use of a cough suppressant at night to promote rest. Encourage increased fluid intake to promote expectoration of respiratory secretions. Teach about the prescribed antibiotic, including its potential adverse effects and measures to reduce them, such as taking erythromycin with meals to prevent gastric upset. Contact the local county health department for follow-up of contacts and compliance with prescribed treatment. Due to resurgence of pertussis among children, adults are recommended to obtain tetanus/diptheria/pertussis (Tdap) to boost immunity.

PRACTICE ALERT
Adults should receive a diphtheria vaccine booster immunization every 10 years (usually given in combination with tetanus vaccine (Immunization Action Center, 2008).

Upper Respiratory Trauma or Obstruction

Obstruction of the upper airway due to trauma (fracture of the nasal septum or the larynx), bleeding (e.g. epistaxis), or a tumor is not only frightening for the patient, but it also may interfere with the ability to breathe.

The Patient with Epistaxis

The nose has a rich blood supply, receiving major arterial vessels from both the internal and external carotid artery systems. **Epistaxis**, a nosebleed, may be precipitated by a number of factors. Trauma (picking the nose or blunt trauma) can cause epistaxis, as can drying of nasal mucous membranes, infection, substance abuse (e.g., cocaine), arteriosclerosis, or hypertension. Epistaxis may also indicate a bleeding disorder related to acute leukemia, thrombocytopenia, aplastic anemia, or severe liver disease. Additionally, treatment with an anticoagulant or antiplatelet drug may cause a nosebleed. In adults, men more frequently have nosebleeds than women.

Pathophysiology and Manifestations

Ninety percent of all nosebleeds arise in the anterior nasal septum from Kiesselbach's area, a rich vascular plexus. Because of their location, these vessels are susceptible to trauma from nose picking, drying, and infection. Posterior epistaxis more often develops secondarily to systemic disorders such as blood dyscrasias, hypertension, or diabetes. In posterior epistaxis, bleeding is from the terminal branches of the sphenopalatine and internal maxillary arteries. Posterior epistaxis tends to be more severe and occurs more frequently in the older adult.

Anterior nosebleeds usually produce obvious bleeding from the nares, as well as bleeding into the posterior nasal and oral pharynx. The bleeding from a posterior nosebleed may be less apparent, with most of the blood draining into the posterior nasopharynx and swallowed by the patient. Nausea and vomiting may occur due to swallowed blood.

Interdisciplinary Care

The goal of treatment for epistaxis is to identify and control the source of bleeding.

Anterior bleeding can usually be managed by simple first-aid measures, such as applying pressure (pinching the nose toward the septum) for 5 to 10 minutes and applying ice packs to the nose and forehead to cause vasoconstriction. The patient is placed in a sitting position to decrease blood flow to the head and reduce venous pressure. Leaning forward reduces drainage of blood backward into the nasopharynx and decreases swallowing of blood. The patient is instructed to spit out the blood to help estimate the amount of bleeding and to prevent nausea and vomiting as a result of swallowed blood.

If applying pressure does not control the bleeding, medications, nasal packing, or surgery may be necessary.

Medications

Topical vasoconstrictors such as cocaine (0.5%), phenylephrine (Neo-Synephrine) (1:1000), or adrenaline (1:1000) may be used to control anterior bleeding. These medications may be applied by nasal spray or on a cotton swab held against the bleeding site. Chemical cauterization of the bleeding vessel may be done using agents such as silver nitrate or Gelfoam. A topical anesthetic such as tetracaine, lidocaine, or cocaine may be used prior to nasal packing. If posterior nasal packing is required, prophylactic antibiotic therapy is initiated to prevent sinusitis or possible toxic shock syndrome.

Nasal Packing

If bleeding cannot be controlled with pressure and local medications, a nasal tampon (a soft balloon filled with air) may be used to apply direct pressure to the bleeding vessel or the nasal cavity may be packed with 0.25-inch petroleum gauze. For an anterior pack, several feet of packing are placed carefully and systematically along the floor of the nasal cavity and then into the vault of the nose. Anterior nasal packs are usually left in place for 24 to 72 hours. If epistaxis is caused by a bleeding disorder, the packing may be left in place for 4 to 5 days while the disorder is treated.

Posterior nosebleeds are more difficult to control, requiring both anterior and posterior packing (Figure 35–3 ■). Posterior packs are usually left in place for 2 to 5 days. A loose anterior nasal pack may also be inserted. Posterior nasal packing is very uncomfortable, and can cause respiratory and cardiovascular complications. Hypoxemia is common; supplementary oxygen is administered. Endotracheal intubation may be necessary to maintain adequate ventilation and gas exchange. Narcotic analgesics are prescribed to manage the discomfort. Hypertension, dysrhythmias, and even acute myocardial infarction may occur in patients with severe cardiovascular

disease. Toxic shock syndrome is another potential complication of posterior nasal packing. The pack may occlude the eustachian tube and sinus openings, resulting in ear discomfort, possible otitis media, or sinusitis. Oral and nasal dryness can be minimized by use of a high-humidity face tent. Nursing care of the patient with nasal packing is outlined in the accompanying box.

A Foley catheter or inflatable nasal balloons may be used as an alternative to posterior nasal packing for effective tamponade. The catheter or nasal balloon is inserted through the nose into the nasopharynx, inflated, and left in place for 2 to 3 days.

Surgery

Chemical or surgical cautery procedures may be used to sclerose involved vessels in the anterior aspect of the nose. The resulting scab must be left undisturbed until the mucosa has healed, or further bleeding may occur.

Surgical procedures to control bleeding are often preferred to posterior nasal packing for posterior bleeding. The bleeding vessel may be cauterized using an endoscopic approach. In some cases, surgery is required to occlude the internal maxillary artery by ligation (tying off) or embolization. These procedures may be done under either conscious sedation and local anesthesia or general anesthesia. Facial paralysis, paresthesias, facial pain, and dental injury are potential complications (Way & Doherty, 2003).

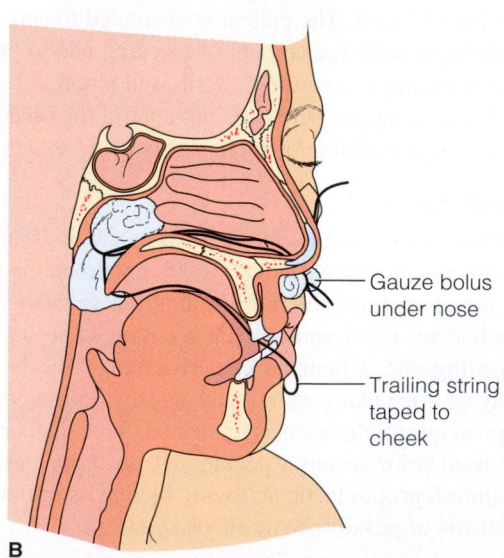

A

B

Gauze bolus under nose

Trailing string taped to cheek

Figure 35–3 ■ Posterior nasal packing. *A,* A rubber catheter is inserted through the nose and out the mouth and attached to the packing. *B,* The catheter is withdrawn through the nose to position the packing in the posterior nasopharynx. Ties exiting through the nose and mouth are used to stabilize the packing in position and remove it when it is no longer needed.

NURSING CARE OF THE PATIENT
with Nasal Packing

- Continuously monitor oxygen saturation. Administer supplementary oxygen as ordered. *Posterior nasal packing causes hypoxemia. Supplemental oxygen is given to maintain tissue oxygenation.*
- Frequently monitor vital signs and respiratory rate or pattern. *Posterior nasal packing increases the risk for respiratory and cardiovascular complications. Tachycardia and tachypnea may be early signs of cardiac or respiratory compromise.*
- Inspect the mouth and oropharynx. Notify the healthcare provider if the packing is seen in the oropharynx. *Misplacement of nasal packing can obstruct the upper airway.*
- Elevate the head of the bed. *Elevating the head of the bed facilitates ventilation.*
- Encourage deep, slow breathing through the mouth. Provide psychologic support, reassurance, and teaching. *Inability to breathe through the nose causes anxiety and fear.*
- Check for blood at the back of the throat and frequent swallowing. *Visible blood or frequent swallowing could indicate posterior bleeding.*
- Report hematemesis. *Bleeding from the posterior portion of the nose often drains down the nasopharynx and is swallowed. Hematemesis may indicate continued bleeding.*
- Apply cold compresses to nose. *An ice or cold compress decreases pain and promotes vasoconstriction, decreasing bleeding and swelling.*
- Provide for rest. *Rest reduces the metabolic demands and oxygen consumption.*
- Ensure adequate oral fluid intake. *Fluid intake helps maintain fluid balance and decreases dryness of oral mucous membranes because of mouth breathing.*
- Provide frequent oral hygiene. Use a bedside humidifier. *These measures reduce drying of oral mucous membranes and promote comfort.*

Nursing Care

Assessment

Nursing assessment of the patient with a nosebleed focuses on the immediate problem and possible underlying conditions.

- *Health history:* Duration of current bleed; any identified precipitating factors such as trauma; history of prior nosebleeds; current medications; chronic conditions such as hypertension, bleeding disorders, etc.
- *Physical examination:* Estimated amount of bleeding; presence of blood in oropharynx; vital signs; evidence of facial or nasal trauma.
- *Laboratory data:* Hemoglobin, hematocrit, platelets, and WBC as indicated; oxygen saturation; tests of organ function such as liver function tests (bilirubin, AST, ALT, LDH) or kidney function tests (serum creatinine, BUN).

Nursing Diagnoses and Interventions

Nosebleeds can be frightening, particularly when they occur without preceding trauma. Nurses provide care for patients with epistaxis in outpatient and emergency settings, and may care for hospitalized patients with nasal packing. Support, reassurance, and education are important nursing roles related to epistaxis. Priority nursing diagnoses include *Anxiety* and *Risk for Aspiration.*

Anxiety

The amount of blood lost in a nosebleed can be frightening. The sensation of blood draining down the throat and inability to breathe through the nose contribute to anxiety. Spontaneous epistaxis may lead to fear of a major health problem such as high blood pressure.

> **PRACTICE ALERT**
> Maintain an attitude of calm reassurance. By remaining calm and confident, the nurse reassures the patient that the nosebleed is not a life-threatening event.

- Instruct the patient to pinch the nares together at the bridge of the nose. *Most nosebleeds are anterior in origin; direct pressure usually stops the bleeding. Having the patient place pressure on the nose provides a focus and helps restore a sense of control, reducing anxiety.*
- Encourage slow, deep breathing through the mouth. *Controlled mouth breathing maintains lung ventilation and reduces anxiety.*
- Provide a basin and tissues; encourage the patient to expectorate blood, not swallow it. *These measures give the patient greater control and reduce the fear of choking on blood.*

> **PRACTICE ALERT**
> Assess the patient with nasal packing frequently for adequate oxygenation. Maintain supplemental oxygen as ordered. Cerebral hypoxia produces a sense of apprehension and fear.

Risk for Aspiration

Anxiety and blood draining into the nasopharynx increase the risk for aspiration of blood into the trachea. When nasal packing is in place, the patient is unable to breathe through the nose, increasing the risk of aspiration when food or fluids are consumed.

> **PRACTICE ALERT**
> Position upright with the head forward. Provide a basin for expectorating blood. These measures minimize the amount of blood draining down the nasopharynx and swallowed, reducing the risk of aspiration and minimizing nausea from swallowed blood. Vomiting of swallowed blood increases the risk of aspiration.

- Apply ice or a cold compress to the nose. *Cold causes vasoconstriction, reducing bleeding.*

> **PRACTICE ALERT**
> Position the patient with nasal packing with the head elevated and on the side when asleep. This position reduces the risk of aspiration of oral secretions.

Community-Based Care

Following an episode of epistaxis, teaching for home care focuses on measures to prevent further bleeding. Include the following teaching topics.

- Avoid strenuous exercise for several days or weeks, depending on the severity of the nosebleed and its treatment.
- Do not blow the nose or engage in activities such as heavy lifting or bending that could increase pressure and dislodge the crust; sneeze with the mouth open to avoid increasing pressure in nasal vessels.
- For an anterior nose bleed, use petroleum jelly, a watersoluble lubricant, or bacitracin ointment to lubricate nasal mucosa and reduce the risk of spontaneous bleeding.
- Use a humidifier or vaporizer to minimize dryness of the mucous membranes.
- Do not forcefully blow the nose or pick the nose.
- For spontaneous nose bleed, seek medical evaluation for any possible underlying problem, such as hypertension or a bleeding disorder.

The Patient with Nasal Trauma or Surgery

The nose is the most commonly broken bone of the face. A nasal fracture (broken nose) usually is caused by a sports injury or trauma related to violence or motor vehicle crashes. The nasal septum normally divides the nose into two equal parts. Deviation of the septum can result from nasal trauma. Soft tissue trauma commonly accompanies nasal fracture.

Pathophysiology and Manifestations

One or both sides of the nose may be broken. A *unilateral fracture* involves only one side of the nose. It causes little displacement or cosmetic deformity. It is usually not serious, but septal deviation and swelling can obstruct the airway. *Bilateral fractures* are more common, with depression or displacement of both nasal bones to one side. The nose appears flattened or deviated with an S or C configuration. *Complex fractures* may also involve the septum, ascending processes of the maxilla, and frontal bones of the face.

Soft-tissue trauma commonly accompanies nasal fracture. Mucous membrane tears cause epistaxis. Soft-tissue hematomas (black eye) are also frequent. Swelling develops rapidly following the injury and may obscure the fracture. Boney crepitus may be felt on gentle palpation. Septal hematoma may develop, increasing the risk for infection. The manifestations of nasal fracture are listed in the Manifestations box.

Complications

Potential complications of nasal fracture include septal hematoma and abscess formation, septal perforation or deviation, and cerebrospinal fluid (CSF) leakage. Septal hematoma can lead to complete and bilateral nasal obstruction. If undrained, hematoma increases the risk of staphylococcal abscess, which can lead to necrosis of septal cartilage and *saddle nose deformity.*

Septal deviation causes varying degrees of nasal obstruction. The septal cartilage bulges or deviates to one side, partially or totally obstructing the nares. Mild deviation is generally asymptomatic. Partial obstruction of air flow through one side may cause noisy breathing while awake and snoring during sleep. Major deviations can cause pain because of sinus obstruction or infection. They may also cause nosebleeds due to dryness of the nasal mucosa. Occasionally, the defect is severe enough to cause cosmetic deformity. Perforations are usually not serious and do not usually require repair unless obstruction or external deformity occur.

Fractures of other facial bones may accompany a broken nose, particularly when facial trauma is severe. Fractures in the nasoethmoidal or frontal region can disrupt the dura, causing CSF leakage or rhinorrhea. CSF rhinorrhea is suspected when watery nasal drainage tests positive for glucose.

Interdisciplinary Care

The major treatment goals for nasal fractures are to maintain a patent airway and prevent deformity. Respirations are closely monitored.

Diagnosis

Head and facial x-rays are done to identify the fracture and assess for other facial fractures. The intranasal cavity is examined using a nasal speculum to rule out septal hematoma. If a CSF leak is suspected, a CT scan is done. A radiopaque substance or fluorescein dye may be instilled into the intrathecal or lumbar subarachnoid space to identify the site of leakage.

Treatments

Ideally, the fracture is reduced early, before significant edema develops. Nasal fractures heal rapidly. Simple reduction may be done in the emergency department with local anesthesia. An external splint may be applied for 7 to 10 days to maintain

MANIFESTATIONS of Nasal Fracture

- Epistaxis
- Deformity or displacement to one side
- Crepitus
- Periorbital edema and ecchymosis
- Nasal bridge instability

proper alignment until healing occurs. The splint is padded to prevent skin breakdown. Ice may be gently applied to the face and nose to control edema and bleeding. Nasal packing may be used to control epistaxis.

Surgery

Complex nasal fractures, nasal septal deviation, or persistent CSF leakage may require surgical repair or realignment of nasal bones. Rhinoplasty with concurrent septoplasty is the most common procedure used to repair nasal fracture or a deviated nasal septum.

Rhinoplasty is surgical reconstruction of the nose. It is done to relieve airway obstruction and repair visible deformity of the nose following fracture. If edema is excessive after nasal fracture, surgery is delayed for 7 to 10 days to allow swelling to subside. Using an intranasal incision, the nasal skin is lifted and the framework of the nose reshaped by removing, rearranging, or augmenting bone or cartilage. The skin is then repositioned over the reconstructed frame. Prosthetic implants may help reshape the nose. Either local or general anesthesia may be used; hospitalization is often unnecessary. Following surgery, nasal packing is left in place for up to 72 hours to minimize bleeding and provide tissue support. A temporary plastic splint molded to the shape of the nose is removed in 3 to 5 days. The splint protects the reshaped nose and helps to control swelling. Most swelling and bruising subside within 10 to 14 days; normal sensation returns within several months following surgery. Rhinoplasty generally has few complications.

Either a septoplasty or a submucous resection (SMR) may be done under local anesthesia to correct a deviated septum. *Septoplasty* involves incising one side of the septum, elevating the mucous membrane, and removing or straightening the deviated portion of septal cartilage. In a *submucous resection*, bone and cartilage are removed. In both procedures, packing is applied to both sides of the nose to prevent bleeding and to keep the septal mucosa in midline position.

Small defects in the cribriform plate, fovea ethmoidalis, or sphenoid sinus associated with persistent CSF leakage may require endoscopic repair. Either a tissue graft or fibrin glue may be used to repair the defect. The graft or glue is held in place with an absorbable packing. Large defects may require craniotomy for repair.

✑ Nursing Care

Health Promotion

Teach all people, children and adolescents in particular, about the importance of wearing helmets and facial protectors when participating in high-risk sports such as football, hockey, and baseball catching. Promote the use of seatbelts with shoulder harness and airbags in vehicles to reduce the risk of facial injury in motor vehicle crashes.

Assessment

Focused nursing assessment for the patient with a suspected nasal fracture includes the following:

- *Health history:* Nature and circumstances of the injury; pain; ability to breathe through the nose; complications from prior head injury.

■ *Physical examination:* Evident trauma, swelling, ecchymosis, or deformity of the nose; vital signs, respiratory rate and ease; gently palpate nose and facial bones for crepitus; inspect oropharynx for drainage; test nasal discharge for glucose.

Nursing Diagnoses and Interventions

Nursing care for patients with nasal fracture focuses on controlling pain, bleeding, and swelling. Airway management is a priority. Most nasal fractures are managed on an outpatient basis, and education is a vital nursing function. See the accompanying Case Study & Nursing Care Plan for additional nursing diagnoses and interventions for the patient with nasal trauma.

Ineffective Airway Clearance

Immediately following nasal trauma and fracture, the airway is at risk for obstruction by bleeding and edema. Deformity resulting from inappropriate fracture position during healing also can impair nasal airway clearance. This is a consideration when inserting nasogastric tubes or suctioning patients with septal deviation.

> **PRACTICE ALERT**
> Monitor airway patency. Edema and bleeding may obstruct the airway, causing signs of respiratory distress such as tachypnea, dyspnea, shortness of breath, tachycardia, and use of accessory muscles.

■ Monitor cough effectiveness and ability to clear airway secretions. *Pain, edema, and nasal bleeding may impair the ability to cough effectively.*

> **PRACTICE ALERT**
> Have suction equipment available. Airway patency is a priority; oropharyngeal suctioning may be necessary to remove secretions and maintain a clear airway. Suctioning of the nasopharynx is avoided to prevent additional tissue trauma.

■ Maintain adequate hydration. Assess mucous membranes and skin turgor for evidence of dehydration. *Decreased oral fluid intake may lead to dehydration and thick, viscous secretions that are more difficult to expectorate.*

■ Assess patency of both nares before inserting a nasogastric tube or feeding tube. If airflow is obstructed through one side, insert the tube through the unobstructed nare. Carefully monitor respiratory status following tube insertion. *The nasogastric tube is inserted through the unobstructed nare to avoid mucosal trauma; however, a large gastric tube may interfere with nasal breathing, necessitating close monitoring.*

Risk for Infection

The patient with a nasal fracture is at increased risk for infection. The nasal mucosa is a natural barrier to infection, and trauma increases the risk for invasion by pathogens. Septal hematoma can lead to abscess formation and staphylococcal infection. A CSF leak indicates disruption of the dura, increasing the risk of ascending infection and meningitis.

> **PRACTICE ALERT**
> Test watery, clear fluid dripping from the ear or nose for glucose. CSF will test positive for glucose on a Dextrostrip.

■ Avoid suctioning if possible. *Suctioning catheters could introduce microorganisms and cause additional trauma to tissues.*

■ Monitor vital signs every 4 hours. *A rise in temperature may indicate infection.*

■ Administer antibiotics as ordered. *Antibiotics may be prescribed to prevent abscess formation, and, if CSF leakage is present, to prevent meningitis.*

Using NANDA, NIC, and NOC

Linkages between a selected NANDA nursing diagnosis, NIC, and NOC for the patient with nasal trauma are shown in the chart that follows.

Community-Based Care

Provide the following teaching when preparing the patient with a nasal fracture for home care.

■ Elevate the head of the bed with blocks and apply ice or cold packs to the nose for 20 minutes four times a day to reduce swelling.

■ Swelling usually subsides in several days; bruising may persist for several weeks.

■ It is difficult to determine the final cosmetic outcome until swelling has subsided.

■ If indicated by delayed fracture reduction or malformation, discuss rhinoplasty and its potential benefits.

If CSF leakage is present, also include the following instructions.

■ Rest in bed with the head of the bed elevated to 30 to 45 degrees.

■ Restrict fluid intake as ordered and take the prescribed diuretic to reduce intracranial pressure and CSF leakage.

■ Distribute allowed fluids throughout the day.

■ List name, purpose, effects, and precautions for any prescribed medication.

■ Avoid straining, blowing the nose, sneezing, or vigorous coughing until allowed by the healthcare provider.

NANDA, NIC, AND NOC LINKAGES
The Patient with Nasal Trauma

NANDA	Ineffective Airway Clearance
NIC	Airway Management
Positioning
Respiratory Monitoring
NOC	Aspiration Control
Respiratory Status:
Airway Patency

Adapted from Bulechek, G., Butcher, H., & Dochterman, J. M. (Eds). (2008). *Nursing interventions classification (NIC)* (5th ed.). St. Louis: Mosby Elsevier; Moorhead, S., Johnson, M., Maas, M., & Swanson, E. (Eds). (2008). *Nursing outcomes classification (NOC)* (4th ed.). St. Louis: Mosby Elsevier; and NANDA International. (2009). *Nursing diagnoses: Definitions and classification 2009–2011.* Oxford, UK: Wiley-Blackwell.

CASE STUDY & NURSING CARE PLAN   A Patient with Nasal Trauma

Patient Clifton Kavanaugh is a 36-year-old mailman who broke his nose when he was hit in the face by a baseball. He is admitted to the emergency department accompanied by a friend.

ASSESSMENT

Mr. Kavanaugh presents with obvious deformity of the nose. It is swollen, bloody, and deviated to one side. The nose is bleeding slightly. Mr. Kavanaugh rates the pain as a 6 on a scale of 1 to 10. Vital signs are BP 132/70, P 120 and regular, R 22, T 98.6°F (37°C) axillary.

Mr. Kavanaugh is breathing through his mouth and holding an ice compress to his nose. Boney crepitus and edema are felt on palpation. There is no evidence of CSF leak from either nose or ears. X-ray confirms a nasal fracture.

DIAGNOSES

- *Acute Pain* related to nasal fracture
- *Ineffective Breathing Pattern* related to nasal swelling and bleeding
- *Anxiety* related to pain and need for emergency care
- *Disturbed Body Image* related to nasal deformity

EXPECTED OUTCOMES

- Verbalize relief of pain.
- Maintain a patent airway and normalize his breathing pattern.
- Demonstrate reduced anxiety.
- Express concerns about potential body image change.

PLANNING AND IMPLEMENTATION

- Administer analgesics as ordered.
- Apply ice compress to nose.
- Inspect oropharynx for evidence of bleeding.
- Encourage deep, slow breathing through the mouth.
- Provide oral hygiene.
- Discuss concerns regarding injury.
- Assist with nasal splint application.

EVALUATION

Following treatment, Mr. Kavanaugh reports his pain has decreased to a level of 2 on a scale of 1 to 10. He appears more relaxed, no longer grimacing and with a relaxed posture. His respirations are easy at 18. The nasal splint is intact. Mr. Kavanaugh is able to look in a mirror and state with a laugh, "I look like a raccoon." He is admitted to the hospital for rhinoplasty.

CRITICAL THINKING IN THE NURSING PROCESS

1. A patient in the emergency department with nasal trauma becomes extremely panicky because of blood draining down his throat. How would you intervene to reduce this patient's anxiety without using nasal suction? Why is it important to avoid suctioning the nasopharynx in the patient with nasal trauma?
2. Develop a plan of care for the patient with a leak of CSF from a nasal fracture.
3. Compare immediate versus delayed rhinoplasty for the patient with nasal fracture.

See Evaluating Your Response in Appendix C.

- Immediately report manifestations of infection, including stiff neck, headache, and fever to the healthcare provider.

Following rhinoplasty or septoplasty, provide the following instructions.

- Apply ice packs to the nose to relieve discomfort and reduce swelling.
- Elevate the head of the bed on blocks to decrease local edema.
- Do not blow the nose for 48 hours after the packing is removed to prevent bleeding.
- Vigorous coughing or straining at stool may cause bleeding and should be avoided.
- Clean teeth and mouth frequently and increase fluid intake to decrease oral dryness due to mouth breathing.
- Bruising around the eyes and nose will last for several days.

The Patient with Laryngeal Obstruction or Trauma

The larynx is the narrowest portion of the upper airway. As such, it is at risk for obstruction. Laryngeal obstruction is a life-threatening emergency. Blows to the neck or other traumatic injuries may damage the larynx, interfering with its patency and function.

Pathophysiology and Manifestations

Laryngeal Obstruction

The larynx may be partially or fully obstructed by aspirated food or foreign objects, or by laryngospasm or edema due to inflammation, injury, anaphylaxis, or a tumor. Anything that occludes the larynx can obstruct the airway. The most common cause of obstruction in adults is ingested meat that lodges in the airway (the so-called *café coronary*). Risk factors for food aspiration include ingesting large boluses of food and chewing them insufficiently, consuming excess alcohol, and wearing dentures. A foreign body in the larynx causes pain, laryngospasm, dyspnea, and inspiratory stridor. Aspirated foreign bodies may pass through the larynx into the trachea and lungs, causing pneumonitis.

Laryngospasm occurs due to repeated or traumatic intubation attempts, chemical irritation, or hypocalcemia. An acute type I hypersensitivity response may cause anaphylaxis with release of inflammatory mediators leading to angioedema of upper airways and severe laryngeal edema.

The most common manifestations of laryngeal obstruction are coughing, choking, gagging, obvious difficulty breathing with use of accessory muscles, and inspiratory stridor. As the airway is obstructed, signs of asphyxia become apparent. Respirations are labored and noisy with wheezing and stridor. Cyanosis may develop. Respiratory arrest and death may result without prompt treatment.

Laryngeal Trauma

Trauma to the larynx can occur in motor vehicle crashes or assaults (e.g., blows to the neck or attempted strangulation). The larynx also may be traumatized during endotracheal intubation or tracheotomy. Trauma may fracture thyroid and/or cricoid cartilage, resulting in loss of airway patency. Soft-tissue injuries can cause swelling that further impairs the airway. Manifestations of laryngeal trauma may include subcutaneous emphysema or crepitus, voice change, dysphagia and pain with swallowing, inspiratory stridor, hemoptysis, and cough.

Interdisciplinary Care

The treatment goal is to maintain an open airway. If airway obstruction is partial and the patient is able to cough and move air in and out of the lungs, radiologic and laryngoscopic examination may be done to locate the foreign body. An endotracheal tube may be inserted to maintain airflow through the larynx in spasm or an edematous larynx. For anaphylaxis, epinephrine may be administered to reduce laryngeal edema and relieve obstruction.

When airway obstruction due to a foreign body is complete, the Heimlich maneuver is performed immediately to clear the obstruction. For the conscious person, the rescuer wraps his or her arms around the victim from behind, places one fist between the umbilicus and xiphoid process, covers the fist with the other hand and forcefully thrusts the hands upward (Figure 35–4A ■). For the unconscious victim, the rescuer straddles the victim's thighs and delivers thrusts upward and inward on the upper abdomen (Figure 35–4B). These moves are continued until the obstruction is relieved or more definitive care can be given. Endotracheal intubation may be attempted. If intubation is unsuccessful, an immediate cricothyrotomy or tracheotomy must be performed to open the airway.

CT scan is used to identify laryngeal fractures; however, emergency treatment may be required prior to diagnosis to ensure airway patency and preserve life. Soft-tissue injuries may be managed conservatively with bedside humidifier, intravenous fluids, antibiotics, and corticosteroids to reduce edema. More severe injuries require endotracheal intubation or immediate tracheostomy. Nursing care related to caring for the patient with a tracheostomy is presented later in this chapter. ∞ See Chapter 37 for more information about endotracheal intubation and nursing care for the intubated patient.

> **PRACTICE ALERT**
> The priority of nursing care in laryngeal obstruction or trauma is restoring a patent airway to prevent cerebral anoxia and death. Laryngeal obstruction and trauma are medical emergencies requiring immediate intervention.

✑ Nursing Care

Closely monitor patients at risk for laryngeal obstruction (e.g., following neck trauma, newly extubated patients, and people receiving medications with a high risk of anaphylaxis, such as intravenous antibiotics or radiologic dyes) for manifestations of obstruction, including dyspnea, nasal flaring, tachypnea, anxiety, wheezing, and stridor. Suction the airway as needed; small aspirated foreign bodies might possibly be removed by suctioning. If obstruction is complete, initiate a cardiopulmonary arrest procedure and perform the Heimlich maneuver until the obstruction is relieved or the emergency response team arrives. Prepare to assist with emergency intubation or tracheotomy as needed. Provide emotional support, reassurance, and teaching for the patient and family to reduce anxiety.

Community-Based Care

Health promotion and teaching for home care focus on preventing laryngeal obstruction and early intervention techniques. Everyone should be aware of the risk factors for adult aspiration. Caution patients who wear dentures to take small bites, chewing each bite carefully before swallowing. Discuss the relationship between excess alcohol intake and food aspiration. Participate in promoting training of the general public in CPR and the Heimlich maneuver. The more people who are adequately trained in emergency procedures, the more likely it is that emergency procedures will be initiated in a timely manner. Patients with a known risk for anaphylaxis, such as people with a previous anaphylactic response and those allergic to bee venom,

A

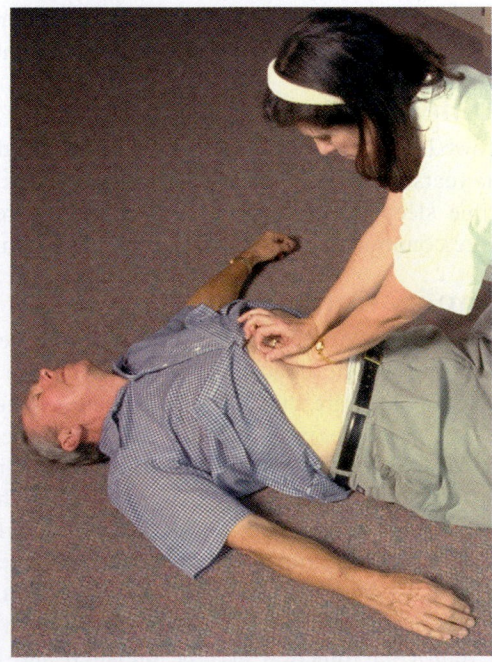

B

Figure 35–4 ■ Administering abdominal thrusts (the Heimlich maneuver) to *A*, a conscious victim, and *B*, an unconscious victim.

should wear a MedicAlert tag and carry a bee-sting kit to allow early intervention to prevent severe laryngeal edema and spasm.

The Patient with Obstructive Sleep Apnea

Sleep apnea, intermittent absence of airflow through the mouth and nose during sleep, is a serious and potentially life-threatening disorder. It affects at least 2% of middle-aged women and 4% of middle-aged men. Sleep apnea is a leading cause of excessive daytime sleepiness, and may contribute to other problems such as poor work performance and motor vehicle crashes (Weaver, 2008a, 2008b, Huether & McCance, 2008). Recent studies have linked sleep apnea with an increased risk for hypertension, ischemic heart disease, and exaccerbation of heart failure (Huether & McCance, 2008).

Types of sleep apnea include obstructive and central. In *obstructive sleep apnea*, the more common type, the respiratory drive remains intact, but airflow ceases due to occlusion of the oropharyngeal airway. *Central sleep apnea* is a rare neurologic disorder that involves transient impairment of the neurologic drive to respiratory muscles.

Pathophysiology

During sleep, skeletal muscle tone decreases (except the diaphragm). The most significant decrease occurs during rapid eye movement (REM) sleep (Weaver, 2008b; Huether & McCance, 2008). Loss of normal pharyngeal muscle tone permits the pharynx to collapse during inspiration as pressure within the airways becomes negative in relation to atmospheric pressure. The tongue is also pulled against the posterior pharyngeal wall by gravity during sleep, causing further obstruction. Obesity or skeletal or soft-tissue changes that decrease inspiratory tone, such as a relatively large tongue in a relatively small oropharynx, contribute to the problem. Airflow obstruction causes the oxygen saturation, PO_2, and pH to fall, and the PCO_2 to rise. This progressive asphyxia causes brief arousal from sleep, which restores airway patency and airflow. Sleep can be severely fragmented as these episodes may occur hundreds of times each night.

Manifestations

Narrowed upper airways produce loud snoring during sleep, often years before obstructive sleep apnea occurs. Excessive daytime sleepiness, headache, irritability, and restless sleep also are common manifestations. See the following box.

Complications

Recurrent episodes of apnea and arousal during sleep have secondary physiologic effects. Sleep fragmentation and loss of slow-wave sleep are thought to contribute to neurologic and behavior problems such as excessive daytime sleepiness, impaired intellect, memory loss, and personality changes. Recurrent nocturnal asphyxia and negative intrathoracic pressure due to airway obstruction increase the workload of the heart. People with coronary heart disease may develop myocardial ischemia and angina. Dysrhythmias such as significant bradycardia and dangerous tachydysrhythmias may develop. Left ventricular function may be impaired and heart failure may occur. Systemic blood pressure remains high during sleep

---

MANIFESTATIONS of Obstructive Sleep Apnea

- Loud, cyclic snoring
- Periods of apnea lasting 15 to 120 seconds during sleep
- Gasping or choking during sleep
- Restlessness, thrashing during sleep
- Daytime fatigue and sleepiness
- Morning headache
- Personality changes, depression
- Intellectual impairment
- Impotence
- Hypertension

---

and may contribute to systemic hypertension that affects more than 50% of people with obstructive sleep apnea (Weaver, 2008b). Pulmonary hypertension also may develop. Sudden cardiac death is believed to be a potential fatal complication of obstructive sleep apnea.

Obstructive sleep apnea is a common condition in people who are morbidly obese. When these patients undergo gastric bypass surgery to treat their obesity, sleep apnea places them at significant risk for postoperative respiratory complications. Not only does the obesity interfere with chest movement and ventilation, it increases metabolic demands and carbon monoxide production. Anesthetic and analgesics used during surgery and in the postoperative period can lead to hypoxemia due to muscle relaxation and depression of the respiratory drive (Deutzer, 2005).

Risk Factors

In addition to male gender, risk factors for obstructive sleep apnea include increasing age and obesity. Large neck circumference (> 17 inches in men and > 16 inches in women) also is a known risk factor for obstructive sleep apnea (Weaver, 2008b; Huether & McCance, 2008). Use of alcohol and other central nervous system depressants may contribute to sleep apnea.

Interdisciplinary Care

The goal of care for obstructive sleep apnea is to restore airflow and prevent the adverse effects of the disorder. Sustained weight loss may cure obstructive sleep apnea.

Diagnosis

The diagnosis of obstructive sleep apnea is based on *polysomnography*, an overnight sleep study. Several variables are recorded during the study, including the following:

- Electroencephalogram and measurements of ocular activity and muscle tone
- Recordings of ventilatory activity and airflow
- Continuous arterial oxygen saturation readings
- Heart rate

Transcutaneous arterial PCO_2 readings also may be monitored during the study. Because sleep studies are time consuming and expensive, overnight monitoring of oxygen saturation by pulse oximetry may be used to confirm the diagnosis of sleep apnea when symptoms indicate a high probability of the disorder (Weaver, 2008b). Nursing implications for pulmonary function studies and pulse oximetry

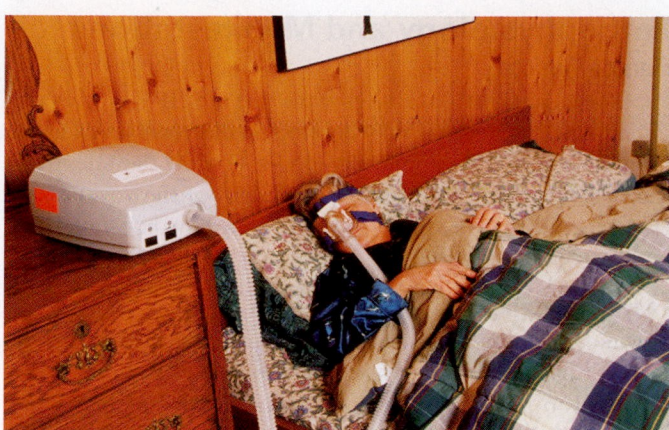

Figure 35–5 ■ A patient using a nasal mask and CPAP to treat sleep apnea.

are presented in ∞ Chapter 34. ∞ See Chapter 41 for more information about electroencephalography.

Treatments

Mild to moderate obstructive sleep apnea may be treated by weight reduction, alcohol abstinence, improving nasal patency, and avoiding the supine position for sleep. Although weight reduction often cures the disorder, maintaining optimal weight is difficult. Oral appliances designed to keep the mandible and tongue forward also may be prescribed.

Nasal continuous positive airway pressure (CPAP) is the treatment of choice for obstructive sleep apnea. Positive pressure generated by an air compressor and administered through a tight-fitting nasal mask (Figure 35–5 ■) splints the pharyngeal airway, preventing collapse and obstruction. With proper training, this device is well-tolerated by the patient. Nasal airways can become dry and irritated with CPAP, so in-line humidifier or a room humidifier is recommended. A newer device, the BiPaP ventilator, delivers higher pressures during inhalation and lower pressures during expiration, providing less resistance to exhaling.

Surgery

Tonsillectomy and adenoidectomy may relieve upper airway obstruction in some patients. Excision of obstructive tissue from the soft palate, uvula, and posterior lateral pharyngeal wall may be accomplished by *uvulopalatopharyngoplasty* (*UPPP*).

Although only about 50% of these surgeries are successful in treating sleep apnea, UPPP is useful in selected cases. In severe cases, tracheostomy may also be performed to bypass the area of obstruction.

∞ Nursing Care

Obstructive sleep apnea usually is treated in the home. Nursing care focuses on teaching the patient and family about equipment use and strategies to decrease contributing factors such as obesity and alcohol intake. The following nursing diagnoses are appropriate for patients with sleep apnea.

- *Disturbed Sleep Pattern* related to repeated apneic episodes
- *Fatigue* related to interrupted sleep patterns
- *Ineffective Breathing Pattern* related to obstruction of upper airway during sleep
- *Impaired Gas Exchange* related to altered lung ventilation during obstructive episodes
- *Risk for Injury* related to daytime somnolence and altered judgment
- *Risk for Sexual Dysfunction* related to impotence resulting from sleep apnea

Community-Based Care

Effective sleep apnea management depends on the patient's willingness to participate in care. Provide teaching about the following topics.

- Relationship between obesity and sleep apnea
- Plans, resources, and referrals as needed for weight loss (e.g., programs such as Weight Watchers to provide additional support)
- Relationship of alcohol and sedatives to sleep apnea; referral to an alcohol treatment program or Alcoholics Anonymous as indicated
- How to use CPAP if ordered
- The importance of using CPAP continuously at night
- Measures to reduce airway dryness, including supplemental humidity and an adequate fluid intake to maintain moist mucous membranes

If a support group for people with sleep apnea syndrome is available in the local area, refer the patient and family to the group.

Upper Respiratory Tumors

Although tumors of the upper respiratory tract are relatively uncommon, they have the potential to impair the upper airways and interfere with breathing and ventilation of the lungs. Of the upper respiratory tract structures, the larynx is affected by abnormal growths most often.

The Patient with Nasal Polyps

Nasal polyps are benign grapelike growths of the mucous membrane lining the nose. These benign tumors can interfere with air movement through nasal passages or obstruct sinus openings, leading to sinusitis. They usually affect people who have chronic allergic rhinitis or asthma.

Pathophysiology and Manifestations

Chronic irritation and swelling of the mucous membranes from allergic rhinitis may cause slow polyp formation. Polyps form in areas of dependent mucous membrane, presenting as pale, edematous masses covered with mucous membrane. They are usually bilateral and have a stemlike base, making them fairly moveable. Polyps can continue to enlarge, eventually becoming larger than a grape. Polyps may be asymptomatic, although large polyps may cause nasal obstruction, rhinorrhea, and loss of sense of smell. Sinusitis may develop because sinus drainage is obstructed. The voice may have a nasal tone. Asthmatics who have nasal polyps may have an associated aspirin allergy of which they are not aware.

Interdisciplinary Care

When polyps occur in conjunction with an acute upper respiratory infection, they may regress spontaneously with resolution of the infection. When symptomatic, polyps may be managed with topical corticosteroid nasal sprays or low-dose oral corticosteroids to shrink the edematous polyps and manage allergic symptoms. However, polyps continue to enlarge when corticosteroid therapy is discontinued.

Surgery may be required to restore normal breathing. Surgical removal of polyps (*polypectomy*) often is done in the healthcare provider's office under local anesthesia. A wire snare is used to clip the polyps from their stemlike base. Nasal packing is inserted to control bleeding after removal. Alternatively, laser surgery may be used to remove polyps. Healing is more rapid following laser intervention, and the risk of bleeding is reduced. Because polyps tend to recur, repeated surgeries may be necessary.

✎ Nursing Care

Teaching about home care following polypectomy is the primary nursing responsibility for the patient with nasal polyps. Provide postoperative care instructions, and discuss measures to reduce the risk of bleeding.

a. Apply ice or cold compresses to the nose to decrease swelling, promote comfort, and prevent bleeding.
b. Avoid blowing the nose for 24 to 48 hours after nasal packing is removed.
c. Avoid straining at stool, vigorous coughing, and strenuous exercise.

Discuss manifestations of possible bleeding, such as frequent swallowing or visible blood at the back of the throat. Swallowed blood may cause nausea and vomiting. Encourage the patient to rest for 2 to 3 days after surgery to reduce the risk of bleeding. Instruct to increase fluid intake and clean mouth frequently to reduce oral dryness associated with mouth breathing while nasal packing is in place.

The Patient with a Laryngeal Tumor

Laryngeal tumors may be either benign or malignant. Benign tumors of the larynx include papillomas, nodules, and polyps. People who chronically shout, project, or vocalize in an abnormally high or low tone, abusing their voice, are at risk for developing benign laryngeal tumors. In adults, vocal cord nodules are often referred to as "singer's nodules"; cheerleaders and public speakers may also develop them. Voice abuse also contributes to the development of vocal cord polyps, as does cigarette smoking and chronic irritation from industrial pollutants.

FAST FACTS
- Malignancy, or cancer of the larynx is uncommon and is often curable if detected early.
- An estimated 3660 people died from laryngeal cancer in 2009; and 12,290 new cases were diagnosed (National Cancer Institute [NCI], 2009b).

Pathophysiology and Manifestations
Benign Tumors
Papillomas are small, warty growths that are HPV viral in origin. Polyps and nodules may develop on the vocal cords of the larynx as a result of voice abuse (Figure 35–6 ■). Nodules often foccur as paired lesions on the free edges of the vocal cords. Hoarseness and a breathy voice quality are manifestations of benign vocal cord tumors.

Laryngeal Cancer
Squamous cell carcinoma is the most common malignancy of the larynx. Changes in the laryngeal mucosa occur over time as it is subjected to noxious irritants such as cigarette smoke. White, patchy, precancerous lesions known as *leukoplakia* appear. Red, velvety patches, called *erythroplakia*, are thought to represent a later stage of carcinoma development. The initial cancerous lesion, carcinoma in situ (CIS), is superficial. Malignant cells replace the lining layer, but do not invade into deeper tissues. Untreated, most CIS lesions develop into squamous cell cancer (NCI, 2009). Laryngeal cancer spreads by both direct invasion of surrounding tissues and by metastasis. It may metastasize to the lungs; however, metastases of other cancers to the larynx are rare.

Laryngeal cancer may develop in any of the three areas of the larynx—the glottis, the supraglottis, and the subglottis. Manifestations vary according to site of the lesion.

Lesions of the true vocal cords or glottis account for nearly 60% of all laryngeal cancers. Fortunately, these cancers tend to be well-differentiated and slow growing. Metastasis occurs late in the course of the disease because of a limited lymphatic supply. The usual symptom of glottic cancer is hoarseness, or a change in the voice because the tumor prevents complete closure of the vocal cords during speech.

Approximately 35% of laryngeal cancers develop in the supraglottic area, which includes the epiglottis, aryepiglottic folds, arytenoid muscles and cartilage, and false vocal cords (Figure 35–7 ■). Lymphatic supply to this region of the larynx is rich; tumors often invade locally and metastasize early. Symptoms often do not develop until the tumor is relatively large, delaying diagnosis. Manifestations of supraglottic cancer include painful swallowing, sore throat, or a feeling of a lump in the throat. Later manifestations include dyspnea, foul breath, and pain that radiates to the ear.

Figure 35–6 ■ Laryngoscopy showing a polyp on the left vocal cord.

Figure 35–7 ■ Cancer of the larynx and epiglottis.

Subglottic tumors (below the vocal cords) are the least common, accounting for the remaining 5% of laryngeal tumors. They often are asymptomatic until the enlarging tumor obstructs the airway. Common manifestations of laryngeal cancer are listed in the box on this page.

Risk Factors

Men are affected more than 4 times as often as women. Cancer of the larynx usually develops between age 50 and 70. Tobacco use is the major risk factor for laryngeal cancer: The risk of developing laryngeal cancer is significantly greater in smokers (cigarette, pip, or cigar) than in nonsmokers. Alcohol consumption is a significant cofactor in increasing the risk. When combined with smoking, the risk increases synergistically and significantly, perhaps as much as 100 times (NCI, 2009). Other risk factors include poor nutrition, human papillomavirus (HPV) infection, exposure to asbestos and other occupational pollutants, and race (laryngeal cancer is more common in African Americans than among Whites).

Interdisciplinary Care

Benign laryngeal tumors may resolve with correction of the underlying problem, such as voice training with a speech therapist or smoking cessation. Treatment of laryngeal malignancy varies with the extent of the cancer. Early diagnosis and

treatment are important: 80% to 95% of early stage tumors can be cured, whereas 50% to 80% of people with advanced laryngeal cancer die of the disease.

Diagnosis
- *Direct* or *indirect laryngoscopy* is used for initial evaluation when laryngeal cancer is suspected. A fiberoptic laryngoscope is used for direct laryngoscopy; mirrors are used to visualize the larynx in indirect laryngoscopy.
- *Biopsy* is obtained from suspicious lesions to examine the cells. Biopsy is usually obtained under general anesthesia or conscious sedation. Tissue may be obtained via endoscopy or by fine needle aspiration of the mass.
- *Imaging studies* such as CT scan, MRI, and chest x-ray are obtained to evaluate the size of the mass, possible extension into deeper tissues, involvement of lymph nodes, and possible metastasis to the lungs. A barium swallow may be done to evaluate the effects of the tumor on swallowing. A PET scan also may be done (possibly in conjunction with CT scan) to detect tumor metastasis.

Treatments
An inhaled steroid spray may be used for vocal cord polyps. In some cases, surgical excision of benign nodules or polyps is required. This usually is performed via laryngoscopy, using microforceps or a laser. A biopsy of the tumor is done to rule out malignancy.

Laryngeal cancer treatment is determined by *staging* the cancer. Information such as tumor size and location (T), number of involved lymph nodes (N), and presence or absence of metastases (M) is combined to assign a stage, designated by Roman numerals I to IV. Table 35–1 outlines laryngeal cancer stages.

RADIATION THERAPY Radiation therapy is often the treatment of choice for early laryngeal cancer. Radiation disrupts the DNA of the cell, causing it to die. External radiation commonly is used; brachytherapy, implants of iridium seeds placed into hollow plastic needles that are inserted directly into or near

---

MANIFESTATIONS of Laryngeal Cancer

- Hoarseness
- Change in the voice
- Painful swallowing
- Dyspnea
- Foul breath
- Palpable lump in neck
- Earache

TABLE 35–1 Staging of Laryngeal Tumors	
Stage 0	■ Carcinoma *in situ* ■ No lymph node involvement or metastasis
Stage I	■ Tumor confined to site of origin with normal vocal cord mobility ■ No lymph node involvement or metastasis
Stage II	■ Tumor involves adjacent tissues ■ No lymph node involvement or metastasis
Stage III	■ Tumor confined to larynx with fixation of vocal cords; immediately surrounding supraglottic tissues may be involved ■ No lymph node involvement or a single positive node on the side of the tumor ■ No metastasis
Stage IV	■ Massive tumor that extends beyond boundaries of larynx to involve surrounding tissues ■ Single or multiple lymph nodes may be involved ■ Distant metastasis may be present

the tumor site during surgery to deliver radiation, is less frequently used for laryngeal or hypopharyngeal cancer. Radiation therapy is extremely effective for treating glottic cancer, with cure rates equal to those achieved by surgery. Radiation therapy preserves the voice, although the tone or timber of the voice may be affected.

Radiation therapy may be used in combination with chemotherapy (*chemoradiotherapy*) to treat more advanced laryngeal cancers. Nearly two-thirds of patients with locally invasive cancers can avoid total laryngectomy when treated with combination radiation and chemotherapy. Survival rates are equal to those achieved with total laryngectomy (Domino et al., 2010).

Radiation therapy also may be used in conjunction with surgery to destroy any remaining cancerous cells, or as a palliative treatment for advanced tumors. ∞ See Chapter 14 for more information about radiation therapy and its nursing implications.

CHEMOTHERAPY Chemotherapy is used in combination with radiation therapy as the primary treatment for some laryngeal cancers. It also is used to treat distant metastasis and for palliation when the tumor is unresectable. The most commonly used chemotherapy drugs to treat laryngeal cancer are cisplatin (Platinol) and 5-fluorouracil (5-FU). Other drugs that may be used include methotrexate (Mexate), bleomycin sulfate (Blenoxane), and carboplatin (Paraplatin). A multiple-drug treatment regimen may be employed to maximize therapeutic effects. ∞ See Chapter 13 for the nursing implications for chemotherapy.

Surgery

The type of surgery used to treat laryngeal cancer is based on site, size, and invasiveness of the tumor into the larynx and surrounding tissues. The goals of surgery are to remove the malignancy, maintain airway patency, and achieve optimal cosmetic appearance.

Carcinoma in situ, vocal cord polyps, and early vocal cord cancers may be removed by laser during a laryngoscopy procedure. The cure rate for early tumors using this method is excellent. This surgery may be performed on an outpatient basis. The degree of trauma to the vocal cords varies, depending on the size of the lesion. The voice is preserved, but total voice rest with whispering only may be ordered for a week or more following surgery. In some cases, a temporary tracheostomy may be done at the time of surgery to ensure that swelling does not interfere with airway patency. Once the tracheostomy tube is removed and the opening is closed, the patient can eat, speak, and breathe normally.

Laryngectomy, removal of the larynx, may be necessary. A *partial laryngectomy* (hemilaryngectomy, vertical partial laryngectomy) may be used for tumors localized to a portion of the larynx with limited extension beyond the larynx. In a partial laryngectomy, 50% or more of the larynx is removed. The voice generally is well-preserved, although it may be changed by the surgery. A tracheostomy tube may be inserted for early postoperative airway management. It is usually removed in 5 to 7 days as postoperative swelling subsides, and the stoma is allowed to close. Normal speaking, breathing, and swallowing are restored. If the epiglottis has been removed, careful monitoring for aspiration is necessary. Enteral tube feedings or parenteral

nutrition may be required for several weeks after surgery. Swallowing techniques to prevent aspiration are taught.

A *total laryngectomy* is required for cancers that extend beyond the vocal cords. The entire larynx is removed, along with the epiglottis, thyroid cartilage, several tracheal rings, and the hyoid bone. Because the trachea and the esophagus are permanently separated by this surgery (Figure 35–8 ■), there is no risk of aspiration during swallowing. Normal speech is lost, and a permanent tracheostomy is created in a total laryngectomy. The tracheostomy tube inserted during surgery may be left in place for several weeks and then removed, leaving a natural stoma, or it may be left in place permanently. See page 1167 for nursing care of the patient having a total laryngectomy. Procedure 35–1 on page 1168 outlines tracheostomy care.

If cervical lymph nodes are involved but there is no evidence of distal metastasis, *radical* or *modified neck dissection* may be performed along with total laryngectomy. In a radical neck dissection, all soft tissue from the lower edge of the mandible down to the clavicle is removed, including cervical lymph nodes, the sternocleidomastoid muscle, internal jugular vein, cranial nerve XI (spinal accessory), and submaxillary salivary gland. Extensive tissue dissection can result in significant deformity. Skin grafts or flaps may be used to close the wound. Hemovac drains are placed in the wound to prevent hematoma and extensive edema formation. After surgery, the patient may have difficulty lifting and turning the head because

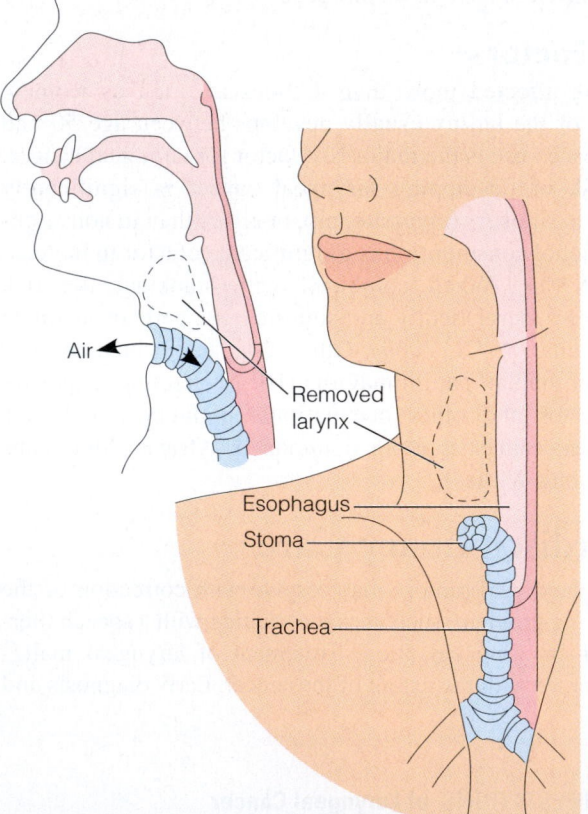

Figure 35–8 ■ Following a total laryngectomy, the patient has a permanent tracheostomy. No connection between the trachea and esophagus remains.

NURSING CARE OF THE PATIENT Having a Total Laryngectomy

PREOPERATIVE CARE

- Assess knowledge and understanding of the diagnosis and proposed surgery. Clarify information and reinforce previous teaching as needed. *A clear understanding by the patient and family of the purpose, anticipated benefits, and consequences of total laryngectomy prior to surgery is vital to promote postoperative recovery.*
- Provide routine preoperative care and teaching as explained in ∞ Chapter 4.
- Assess anxiety levels of the patient and family related to the diagnosis and proposed surgery. *High levels of anxiety interfere with learning and the ability to cooperate in care. Interventions to reduce anxiety may be required prior to teaching and providing preoperative instructions.*
- Without increasing fear, emphasize that total laryngectomy results in a loss of speech and that the patient will breathe through a permanent stoma in the neck. *Although patients and family members may verbalize an understanding of the loss of speech following surgery, they may believe that verbal communication will still be possible through the stoma.*
- Establish a means of communicating postoperatively, using a magic slate, alphabet board, eye or hand signals, or other strategies. *Learning techniques for communicating preoperatively decreases the patient's and family's postoperative anxiety. Long-term speech rehabilitation measures, such as the tracheoesophageal puncture are not appropriate for use in the immediate postoperative period.*
- Point out that surgery will affect the sense of taste and smell, and eating in the initial postoperative period. Reassure that nutritional and fluid needs will be met with intravenous or enteral feedings until eating can be resumed. *The patient may not be prepared for the effect of surgery on taste and smell, and therefore the enjoyment of food.*
- If possible and desired by the patient and family, arrange a visit by a postlaryngectomy patient who effectively uses an alternate form of verbal communication. *The patient and family may feel more comfortable expressing their fears and asking questions of someone who has gone through the same experience they are facing.*

POSTOPERATIVE CARE

- Provide routine postoperative nursing care and monitoring as explained in ∞ Chapter 4.

- Frequently monitor airway patency and respiratory status, including respiratory rate and pattern, lung sounds, oxygen saturation. *Excessive or retained respiratory secretions can impair gas exchange, increase the work of breathing, and lead to complications such as pneumonia.*
- Encourage deep breathing and coughing. *Deep breathing helps ensure adequate ventilation of lower airways; coughing helps to move secretions out of airways.*
- Elevate the head of the bed. *The upright position promotes effective ventilation of the lungs, and reduces edema and swelling of the neck.*
- Maintain humidification of inspired gases. *With a tracheostomy, humidification of inspired air in the upper airways is lost. Humidified air helps maintain moist mucous membranes and secretions, promoting secretion removal by coughing or suctioning.*
- Maintain an adequate fluid intake (intravenously, enteral, and oral when allowed). *Adequate hydration keeps secretions liquid and mucous membranes moist.*
- Suction via tracheostomy using sterile technique as needed. *Surgery, impaired nutrition, and the effects of radiation therapy may cause fatigue and a weak cough effort. Suctioning may be necessary to clear secretions and maintain airway patency.*
- Provide tracheostomy care as needed. See Procedure 35–1. *Periodic cleaning of the tracheostomy tube is necessary to remove accumulated secretions and maintain airway patency.*
- Teach to protect the stoma from particulate matter in the air with a gauze square or other stoma protector. *Permanent tracheostomy results in loss of the protective mechanisms of the upper airway that prevent foreign material from entering the lungs.*
- Instruct to support the head when moving in bed. *Additional head support reduces the strain on tissues in the operative area.*
- Place the call light within easy reach at all times; answer the call light promptly. *The patient who is unable to speak needs reassurance that help is within reach at all times.*
- Encourage family members to remain present when possible. *Supportive family presence helps reassure the patient that he or she will not be left alone or helpless.*
- Spend as much time as possible with the patient. When leaving the room, specify the time when you will return. *These measures help establish trust and relieve anxiety.*

---

of muscle loss. Resection of the spinal accessory nerve causes shoulder drop on the affected side. In a modified neck dissection, neck contents are removed, with the exception of the sternocleidomastoid muscle, internal jugular vein, and spinal accessory nerve.

A gastrostomy also may be performed to maintain nutrition in the patient with laryngeal or hypopharyngeal cancer. ∞ See Chapter 23 for more information about caring for the patient with a gastrostomy tube.

Speech Rehabilitation

Various techniques may be used to restore speech after total laryngectomy. *Tracheoesophageal puncture (TEP)* is the usual method used to restore speech. A small fistula is created

between the posterior tracheal wall and the anterior esophagus. A small, one-way shunt valve is fitted into the fistula (Figure 35–9 ■). Occluding the tracheostomy stoma with a finger forces exhaled air through the valve into the esophagus and hypopharynx, creating vibration and sound. The muscles of speech are used to form words. The one-way valve prevents aspiration from the esophagus into the trachea. An external tracheostoma valve may be used to avoid using the hand to occlude the stoma. This device covers the entire tracheal stoma and closes during exhalation, forcing air directly into the voice prosthesis. Not all postlaryngectomy patients are candidates for this device, because its use requires motivation and manual dexterity.

PROCEDURE 35–1 Providing Tracheostomy Care

GATHER SUPPLIES
- Tracheostomy cleaning kit
- Sterile suction catheter and glove kit
- Sterile disposable replacement inner cannula, if appropriate
- Cleaning solutions, e.g., hydrogen peroxide and sterile normal saline
- Sterile 4 × 4 gauze dressings (not cotton-filled) or precut dressing
- Sterile cotton-tipped applicators
- Single-use tracheostomy tube holder or cotton twill ties
- Scissors
- Clean exam gloves

BEFORE THE PROCEDURE
Provide for privacy. Explain the procedure. Provide for a means of communication (e.g., eye blinking or raising a finger to indicate distress). If condition permits, provide a pencil and paper or magic slate for questions. Place in semi-Fowler's or Fowler's position to facilitate lung ventilation. Assess lung sounds; suction the tracheostomy using sterile technique as needed.

PROCEDURE
- Use standard precautions.
- Wearing a clean disposable glove, remove the tracheostomy dressing. Dispose of the glove and dressing.
- Open sterile supplies, pouring hydrogen peroxide and normal saline into separate containers. Don sterile gloves.
- Using sterile applicators or gauze dressings moistened with normal saline, clean around the incision, using each applicator or gauze dressing only once. Hydrogen peroxide may be used to remove crusted secretions; thoroughly rinse the area with gauze moistened with normal saline afterward to prevent skin irritation from hydrogen peroxide.
- If the tracheostomy tube has an inner cannula that can be removed for disposal or cleaning, remove the tube and set it aside for disposal or place it in the hydrogen peroxide. Cleanse the flange of the outer cannula in the same manner as the incision.
- Clean reusable inner cannulas using a small brush, pipe cleaners (provided in the tracheostomy care kit), or cotton-tipped applicators.
- Rinse the inner cannula thoroughly in normal saline. Tap it gently against the inner aspect of the sterile bowl to remove excess liquid.
- Suction the outer cannula using sterile technique.
- Replace the inner cannula (using a new disposable cannula or the cleaned cannula) into the tracheostomy tube.
- Replace the dressing, using either a commercially prepared tracheostomy dressing or an opened gauze 4 × 4 refolded into a V shape (see the accompanying figure). Do not cut the dressing or use a cotton-filled dressing to prevent aspiration of foreign material into the respiratory tract.
- Apply a clean tracheostomy holder or clean ties using either the one- or two-strip method.
  One-Strip Method
  a. Cut a length of twill tape 2.5 times the length needed to go around the patient's neck from one tube flange to the other.
  b. Thread one end of the tape through one flange of the tracheostomy tube. Bring the other end around the back of the patient's neck, then thread it through the other flange and back around the back of the neck to meet the first end. Tie the loose ends securely using a square knot and allowing one or two fingers' breadth of slack between the tie and the patient's neck.
  Two-Strip Method
  a. Cut a length of twill tape about 1.5 times the distance from flange to flange under the patient's neck. Divide this into two unequal pieces (approximately 1/3, 2/3).
  b. Make a small slit approximately 2 to 3 cm from one end of each piece. Thread the end of the tape with the slit through the flange, then thread the other end of the tape through the slit to secure it. Repeat with the other portion of tape.
  c. Position the longer tape behind the patient's neck and tie the free ends of tape securely, using a square knot and allowing a small amount of slack as before.
- *Once the clean ties are secured, remove the old ties.*
- *Pad the knot to reduce skin irritation.*

Steps of folding a gauze 4 × 4 into a tracheostomy dressing.

AFTER THE PROCEDURE
Assess breathing and tolerance of the procedure. Dispose of supplies and used solutions. Wash hands. Chart the procedure and any observations made during the procedure such as amount, color, and consistency of sputum and appearance of the incision.

Figure 35–9 ■ The tracheoesophageal prosthesis (TEP) allows diversion of air from the trachea through a one-way valve into the esophagus and oropharynx, producing speech when the tracheostomy stoma is occluded. The one-way valve prevents food from entering the trachea.

Esophageal speech uses swallowed air to create sound and form words as it is expelled in a controlled belch. The pharyngoesophageal segment vibrates with the belch, creating sound. Muscles of the mouth and tongue are used to control the sound and form words. This form of speech takes practice, and fluent speech may not be restored.

Several speech generators (electrolarynx) are available. One type is held to the neck and creates vibrations that are transmitted to the neck and into the mouth (Figure 35–10A ■). The transmitted vibrations are formed into words using the normal muscles of speech. Another device delivers a tone into the mouth via a plastic tube inserted into the corner of the mouth (Figure 35–10B). The lips, tongue, and mouth muscles are used to form the sound into words.

✎ Nursing Care

Nurses can be instrumental in early identification and treatment of laryngeal disorders by emphasizing the need for patients with new chronic hoarseness to seek treatment.

Health Promotion

Health promotion activities to prevent laryngeal cancer focus on preventing smoking and chewing tobacco among children, adolescents, and young adults, and promoting smoking cessation in people who do smoke. Activities to promote abstinence or moderate alcohol use also are beneficial in reducing a significant risk factor for laryngeal cancer.

Assessment

Nurses can be instrumental in identifying early signs of laryngeal cancer, facilitating early diagnosis and treatment.

- *Health history:* Current symptoms, including voice change, difficulty swallowing, throat pain, weight loss; risk factors such as voice abuse (e.g. shouting), family history of cancer, occupational exposures (e.g. chemical inhalation); smoking, use of alcohol and amount.
- *Physical examination:* Voice character; general appearance and apparent state of health, weight loss; swallowing ability; visible or palpable mass in neck.

Nursing Diagnoses and Interventions

Nursing care for the patient with a benign tumor of the larynx focuses on maintaining a patent airway and teaching about the disorder and strategies to prevent its recurrence. The patient with laryngeal cancer has multiple nursing care needs. The risk for impaired verbal communication is significant. Dysphagia

Figure 35–10 ■ Speech generators. *A,* The patient holds the vibrating tip of the speech generator against the throat, using the mouth to form words. *B,* A plastic handpiece of the generator is held in the corner of the mouth. The audible tone produced by the generator is formed into words.

may interfere with swallowing and nutrition. Nutrition also may be impaired by radiation, chemotherapy, and surgery. Changes in body image may be due to weight loss due to increased metabolic demands of the malignancy. The diagnosis of cancer is frightening for most patients, no matter what the potential for cure is with treatment. See the Case Study & Nursing Care Plan that follows for additional nursing diagnoses and interventions.

Risk for Impaired Airway Clearance

Following resection of a benign or malignant vocal cord nodule, local tissue edema may interfere with airway patency.

> **PRACTICE ALERT**
> During the immediate postoperative period, closely monitor for signs of airway obstruction, such as labored breathing or inspiratory stridor. The larynx is the narrowest portion of the upper airways. Tissue edema following surgery can further restrict the airway, interfering with lung ventilation and gas exchange.

- Apply cold packs to the neck as ordered or indicated. *Cold application constricts local blood vessels and reduces edema development.*
- Withhold food and fluids until the cough and gag reflexes have returned. *Local anesthesia used during removal of benign tumors and nodules impairs the cough and gag reflexes, increasing the risk for aspiration.*

Impaired Verbal Communication

Treatment of laryngeal cancer often alters the quality of the voice, results in short-term restriction on speaking, or, in the case of total laryngectomy, causes loss of the voice. The patient ultimately determines treatment choices for laryngeal cancer; some choose to forgo laryngectomy to avoid voice loss when the chance for long-term success and cancer cure is minimal.

- Prior to surgery, assess for additional obstacles to communication. *Communication may be impaired by hearing loss, illiteracy, or weakness associated with the disease process, altering the ability to use alternative communication strategies.*
- Assess the importance of verbal communication to self-concept, occupation, and lifestyle. *Many factors influence adaptation to the loss of normal verbal communication. If the ability to speak is central to an occupation (e.g., elementary school teacher, singer) or self-concept (e.g., a politician or attorney), adapting to a total laryngectomy may be difficult. For these patients, laryngectomy may mean a loss of employment or career.*

> **PRACTICE ALERT**
> Prior to surgery, introduce nonverbal communication strategies such as pencil and paper, magic slate, or an alphabet board. Encourage the patient to practice using each method and to choose the most acceptable one. Having the patient determine a means of communication prior to surgery helps to alleviate anxiety and increases the sense of control.

- Arrange consultation with a speech therapist about alternate forms of oral communication prior to surgery if possible. *Determining a means of communicating on a continuing basis prior to surgery helps to relieve fear of inability to communicate and may guide the choice of a surgical procedure.*

> **PRACTICE ALERT**
> After surgery, assess frequently. Place the call bell at hand. The presence of a caring nurse helps to decrease anxiety and promotes communication. Knowing that help is readily available enhances feelings of security and decreases anxiety.

- Reinforce teaching about alternative communication strategies. *Anxiety or information overload may impair the ability to retain information; reinforcement facilitates learning.*
- Maintain a positive attitude about postoperative communication, but do not promote unrealistic expectations. *Not all patients are able to use all alternative methods of verbal communication after the laryngectomy. Some patients remain nonverbal.*
- If desired, arrange a visit by a rehabilitated laryngectomy patient who has mastered an alternative form of verbal communication and has a positive attitude about rehabilitation. *Many patients and their families find that they are better able to communicate their fears with someone who has gone through the same experience they are facing.*

See the accompanying Moving Evidence into Action box for more information about assistive devices for use in the early postoperative period.

Impaired Swallowing

Disruption of laryngeal structures by the tumor itself or due to radiation or surgery can impair the swallowing mechanism. Additionally, even when a total laryngectomy has been performed and a connection between the oropharynx and trachea no longer exists, swallowing may cause fear of choking.

- Maintain intravenous fluids and enteral feedings or parenteral nutrition until adequate food and fluids can be ingested orally. *It is important to maintain nutritional and fluid balance until normal eating can be resumed.*
- Postoperatively, initiate oral intake with soft foods, not liquids. *Soft foods are easier than liquids to handle and swallow initially. As recovery progresses, thickened liquids can be swallowed, progressing to liquids, and, eventually, a normal diet.*
- Following total laryngectomy, reassure that choking is not possible, because there is no connection between the esophagus and trachea. *Patients often fear that swallowing will result in choking and they will be unable to cough effectively.*
- Instruct to initiate a swallow by placing a small amount of food on the back of the tongue, flex the head forward, and then think "swallow." *Swallowing is no longer an automatic function and needs to be relearned.*

> **PRACTICE ALERT**
> Provide for privacy during initial attempts at eating. Eating in the presence of others may cause embarrassment until confidence in eating is regained. Privacy also reduces distractions, allowing concentration on swallowing.

Imbalanced Nutrition: Less than Body Requirements

Large laryngeal tumors often place pressure on the esophagus and may cause dysphagia (difficulty swallowing) or odynophagia (painful swallowing). In either case, difficulty eating may

MOVING EVIDENCE INTO ACTION | The Patient Undergoing Laryngectomy

Communication methods and content among patients who had undergone surgery for head or neck cancer were evaluated in this pilot study of the use of electronic speech-generating devices (SGDs) (Happ, Roesch, & Kagan, 2005). The researchers also looked at the quality (ease and patient satisfaction) of communications among study participants, as well as barriers to SGD use and the effect of patient factors such as age and illness severity on communications. All study participants were alert and able to write legibly; the majority had at least some experience using a computer. While 60% of study participants were found to be able to use SGDs with minimal assistance and instruction, the devices were used in only 17% of observed communications; writing and nonverbal communications were used the majority of the time. Barriers seen that reduce/prevent use of the devices included placement of the device out of the patient's reach, mechanical malfunctions, and impatience of caregivers with the time required for typed communications. Patients expressed frustration with the lack of a standard keyboard and with the impersonality of the computerized voice. Overall, the devices were found to be useful as one of several methods of communication used by the patient.

IMPLICATIONS FOR NURSING

Speech-generating devices can facilitate communication for selected patients, particularly when the content of the message is complex. Training of patients, caregivers, and family members is necessary for effective use of these devices, however. Preoperatively, patients scheduled for laryngectomy should be instructed in communication methods to use after surgery, including use of gestures, written messages (including predeveloped messages, such as "I am in pain."), and use of any assistive communication devices.

CRITICAL THINKING IN PATIENT CARE

1. In this study, SGDs often were found out of the patient's reach. What planning should the nurse do to help ensure that assistive communication devices are accessible to the patient?
2. Patients in this study were literate and many had at least some experience using computers. Do you think results of the study would differ if the study population had less education, was illiterate, or had minimal English language proficiency? Why or why not?
3. Develop a teaching plan for a preoperative laryngectomy patient using the nursing diagnosis *Deficient Knowledge: Postoperative Communication Strategies.*

From Happ, M. B., Roesch, T. K., & Kagan, S. H. (2005). Patient communication following head and neck cancer surgery: A pilot study using electornic speech-generative devices. *Oncology Nursing Forum, 32*(6), 1179–1187.

ultimately impair nutrition. Additionally, cancer often produces a hypermetabolic state, increasing calorie requirements. If surgery is performed, difficulty swallowing and a fear of aspiration in the early postoperative period also interfere with eating. Enteral or parenteral feedings are usually needed initially to meet nutritional status. After a total laryngectomy, the senses of taste and smell are disrupted. Although the sense of taste may be partially recovered, patients may complain that eating no longer is pleasurable.

- Assess nutritional status using height and weight charts, reported weight loss, and anthropometric measurements such as skinfolds. *Thorough assessment of nutritional status is important in planning to meet current and anticipated calorie needs.*

PRACTICE ALERT
Monitor food and fluid intake and urinary output. Pain or fatigue, rather than a sensation of fullness, may prompt the decision to stop eating, resulting in inadequate intake.

- Evaluate current and preferred eating habits and foods, as well as understanding of nutrition. *This evaluation provides additional information about nutrition as well as a basis for future planning.*

PRACTICE ALERT
Weigh daily. Daily weight is an accurate measure of both fluid balance and nutritional status.

- Refer to a dietitian for further evaluation, planning, and education. *A professional can identify nutritional needs and help plan a diet that will meet them.*

- *Refer to a swallowing therapist (specialized speech therapist) for additional resources to improve nutritional intake.*
- Encourage experimentation with foods of different textures and temperatures. *Very cold foods or foods of a soft texture may be easier to swallow.*
- Encourage frequent, small meals rather than three large meals per day. *Frequent, small quantities of food improve overall intake when dysphagia, odynophagia, or fatigue interfere with nutrition.*
- Recommend liquid supplements such as Ensure when calorie needs are not being met. Provide information about where to obtain nutritional supplements. *Liquid dietary supplements provide balanced nutrition as well as additional calories and are an effective way of increasing intake. They are available without prescription in major supermarkets.*
- Provide mouth care before meals and supplemental feedings. Provide a topical anesthetic such as viscous lidocaine before eating for stomatitis or esophagitis related to radiation or chemotherapy. *The tumor or its treatment may cause bad breath or a foul taste in the mouth, which suppresses appetite. Inflamed mucosa may make eating uncomfortable. A topical anesthetic may relieve this discomfort and thus promote food intake.*
- Provide an antiemetic 30 minutes before eating as needed to relieve nausea. *Nausea interferes with food intake. An antiemetic can relieve nausea and make eating possible.*
- Suggest enteral (tube) feedings via nasogastric or gastrostomy tube if the patient is unable to consume enough food to maintain weight and nutritional status. *Both cancer and surgery increase calorie needs. Supplemental enteral feedings may be necessary to prevent catabolism and to promote healing and recovery.*

- Instruct to perform mouth rinses before initiating feeding postoperatively. *Rinsing helps clean the mouth and also practice in using tongue and cheek muscles to control fluid in the mouth.*
- Refer to a physical or speech therapist for swallowing rehabilitation following laryngectomy. *Because surgery changes the relationship of the trachea, esophagus, and oropharynx, swallowing needs to be relearned before eating.*
- Reinforce swallowing instructions. *Reinforcement promotes learning.*

Anticipatory Grieving

The patient with laryngeal cancer faces not only the diagnosis of cancer, which is often perceived as a death sentence, but also the prospect of mutilating surgery. If laryngectomy is necessary, the patient grieves the loss of both a body part and an important function, speech, a vital aspect of social interaction and interpersonal relationships and often necessary for one's career. It also enables people to express their needs when they cannot meet them alone. The loss of speech, therefore, is a major loss. In addition, the tracheal stoma changes the manner in which the patient breathes. If radical neck dissection is required, loss of neck musculature and function also alters body image and self-concept.

- Provide opportunities for expressing feelings of grief, anger, or fear about the diagnosis of cancer, the impending surgery, and the anticipated loss of speech. *The patient with laryngeal cancer needs the opportunity (and may need permission) to grieve anticipated losses. A cancer diagnosis may precipitate grieving for unfulfilled plans and expectations, even though a cure may be anticipated. Laryngectomy causes a major change in body image, with loss of a vital body part and creation of a stoma. The patient also grieves the loss of speech. This loss can have a significant impact on occupation and social interaction.*

- Help the patient and family discuss the potential impact of the loss on family structure and function. *Discussion helps family members understand each other's feelings and support one another.*
- Refer for psychologic or spiritual counseling as appropriate. *Counseling and spiritual guidance can help the patient and family deal with the diagnosis and proposed treatment, and help prevent a sense of defeat and hopelessness.*

- Help identify additional resources, such as coping strategies that have been successfully used in the past to deal with crises. *This exercise helps the patient and family identify strengths they can use to deal with the present situation.*

Using NANDA, NIC, and NOC

Linkages between a selected NANDA diagnosis, NIC, and NOC for the patient with laryngeal cancer are shown in the chart that follows.

Community-Based Care

Teaching for the patient with a benign laryngeal tumor emphasizes management of contributing factors. Stress the importance of not yelling or screaming. Refer patients, particularly singers, to a speech therapist for voice training. Emphasize the need to keep the voice within its normal range to reduce vocal cord stress. Encourage smoking cessation, particularly if the patient is also a singer. Discuss the relationship of industrial or occupational pollutants to laryngeal tumors and help explore ways of reducing pollutant exposure.

Teaching the patient and family about laryngeal cancer, treatment options, and home care related to those treatments is an important nursing responsibility. Include the following topics when teaching.

- Clarification of treatment options, including risks and benefits.
- Importance of early intervention to reduce the risk of local spread and metastasis.
- If a total laryngectomy is proposed, options for communication after surgery, including the pros and cons of each:
  a. The tracheoesophageal puncture device requires some manual dexterity to manipulate.
  b. Only about 30% of patients are able to master esophageal speech.
  c. A trial of the speech generator prior to surgery may reduce frustration in learning to use it postoperatively.

NANDA, NIC, AND NOC LINKAGES
The Patient with Laryngeal Cancer

NANDA   Impaired Verbal Communication

⬇

NIC   Communication Enhancement: Speech Deficit
Anxiety Reduction
Aspiration Precautions
Support System Enhancement

⬇

NOC   Communication
Communication: Expressive
Coping
Aspiration Prevention

Adapted from Bulechek, G., Butcher, H., & Dochterman, J. M. (Eds). (2008). *Nursing interventions classification (NIC)* (5th ed.). St. Louis: Mosby Elsevier; Moorhead, S., Johnson, M., Maas, M., & Swanson, E. (Eds). (2008). *Nursing outcomes classification (NOC)* (4th ed.). St. Louis: Mosby Elsevier; and NANDA International. (2009). *Nursing diagnoses: Definitions and classification 2009–2011.* Oxford, UK: Wiley-Blackwell.

CASE STUDY & NURSING CARE PLAN   A Patient with Total Laryngectomy

David Tom is a 61-year-old accountant who is divorced and has two adult children. He has smoked two packs of cigarettes daily since high school, and usually has three or four cocktails each evening. After several months of persistent sore throat and hoarseness, Mr. Tom was diagnosed with cancer of the larynx. He has been admitted to the surgical care unit from the ICU 2 days post total laryngectomy.

ASSESSMENT

Mr. Tom's vital signs are stable: BP 146/84, P 92 and regular, R 18, T 98°F (36.7°C) axillary. A tracheostomy tube is sutured in place, and he is receiving humidified oxygen at 28% per tracheostomy collar. Pulse oximetry is 94%. He is receiving continuous tube feeding per nasogastric feeding tube. Two Hemovac wound drains are present in the right neck area. A moderate amount of edema is noted in the right facial and submandibular area. Mr. Tom is ambulatory within the room.

DIAGNOSES

- *Risk for Ineffective Airway Clearance* related to postoperative edema
- *Risk for Ineffective Breathing Pattern* related to pain and anxiety
- *Disturbed Body Image* related to total laryngectomy and presence of tracheostomy stoma
- *Impaired Verbal Communication* related to total laryngectomy
- *Pain* related to surgical procedure
- *Risk for Imbalanced Nutrition: Less than Body Requirements* related to difficulty eating after surgery

EXPECTED OUTCOMES

- Maintain clear airways and lung sounds.
- Maintain oxygen saturation level greater than 92%.
- Demonstrate interest in providing incision and stoma care.
- Accept information about potential communication strategies.
- Communicate effective pain management.
- Maintain appropriate body weight, intake, and output.

PLANNING AND IMPLEMENTATION

- Assess respiratory status including rate, pattern, lung sounds, and cough effectiveness at least every 4 hours.
- Monitor quantity, color, and odor of secretions.
- Assess vital signs and pain at least every 4 hours. Administer analgesics as ordered.
- Schedule time to sit with Mr. Tom and discuss his concerns and feelings at least three times per day.
- Provide written information as requested.
- Monitor intake, output, and daily weight.
- Arrange dietary consultation to determine caloric requirements.

EVALUATION

Mr. Tom reports in writing that his pain is adequately controlled. His respiratory status is stable with clear breath sounds throughout and an oxygen saturation of 94%. He is afebrile. Mr. Tom is tolerating tube feedings well and expresses a desire to begin eating. The dietitian has visited and assisted in planning to begin oral feedings. Intake and output are stable, as is his weight. Mr. Tom has been receptive to receiving information about follow-up care and exploration of various modalities of speech.

CRITICAL THINKING IN THE NURSING PROCESS

1. Compare and contrast advantages and disadvantages of various methods to allow speech following total laryngectomy.
2. Develop a plan of care for Mr. Tom for the nursing diagnosis *Disturbed Body Image*.
3. Discuss nursing interventions to provide wound care for the patient with laryngectomy and radical neck dissection.
4. List strategies to optimize ventilation.

See Evaluating Your Response in Appendix C.

- Care related to radiation therapy, including skin and mouth care, management of secretions (∞ see Chapter 14 for more information about radiation therapy and its effects).
- Strategies and resources for smoking cessation and alcohol abstinence.
- Ways to achieve and maintain optimal nutrition.
- Tracheostomy stoma care and preventing respiratory infection. Provide opportunities to practice and redemonstrate techniques. Clean technique (rather than sterile) is used; the tracheostomy tube may not be needed once the stoma is fully healed. Discuss these additional measures.
  a. Using a humidifier or vaporizer to add humidity to inspired air.
  b. Increasing fluid intake to maintain mucosal moisture and loosen secretions.
  c. Shielding the stoma with a stoma guard, such as a gauze square on a tie around the neck, to prevent particulate matter from entering the lower respiratory tract.
  d. Promptly removing secretions from skin surrounding the stoma to prevent irritation and skin breakdown.
  e. Water sports are contraindicated with a permanent tracheostomy; there is no restriction on other activities although lifting may be more difficult because of inability to hold the breath (the Valsalva maneuver).
  f. Showering and bathing (without submerging the neck or head) are allowed; protect the stoma with a cupped hand or washcloth.
- Manifestations of potential complications of laryngectomy to be reported to the healthcare provider, including loss of hearing or facial expression due to auditory or facial nerve injury, or shoulder drop due to damage to the spinal accessory nerve.

The patient and family need emotional and motivational support through this trying time. Refer to local support groups such as a laryngectomy club or lost cord club. If the patient and family are having difficulty adjusting to the diagnosis of cancer and the effects of treatment, provide referral to counseling.

CHAPTER HIGHLIGHTS

■ Upper respiratory infections (the common cold) are caused by a multitude of different viruses. Most are mild, self-limiting infections, appropriate for self-care; some viruses, however, such as RSV can cause serious lower respiratory illness in the very young or very old.

■ Three different strains of influenza virus are identified; type A causes most outbreaks of influenza. Because this disease increases the risk of pneumonia in older adults, people with chronic diseases, and people who are immunocompromised, annual immunization is important for these populations and their caregivers. The H1N1 virus pandemic was identified in 2009 and its impact is evolving.

■ Influenza is differentiated from URI primarily by the presence of systemic manifestations, the duration and degree of fever, and the presence of persistent cough.

■ Pharyngitis (sore throat) may be either viral or bacterial in origin; manifestations are similar. Patients with persistent or severe symptoms that include fever, enlarged lymph nodes, and myalgias should be evaluated to rule our GABHS pharyngitis, which can have significant complications such as rheumatic fever or poststreptococcal glomerulonephritis.

■ The incidence of pertussis, a highly contagious reportable disease, is increasing due to waning immunity, decreased rates of childhood pertussis immunizations, and improved identification of the infection among adults. In adults, it is often recognized by prolonged and persistent coughing spells. Pertussis is treated in community settings with antibiotic therapy (usually erythromycin or sulfamethoxazole-trimethoprim [SMZ-TMP]).

■ Epistaxis (nosebleed) and nasal fracture are relatively common, and pose a risk only when airway clearance is impaired. Emergency care for epistaxis includes pinching the nares or bridge of the nose, sitting upright leaning forward, and applying ice to the nose. When nasal packing is required to control bleeding, close monitoring of respiratory status (respiratory rate and effort, oxygen saturation) is critical.

■ Persistent voice hoarseness is the primary manifestation of laryngeal cancer. When identified and treated early, the rate of cure for laryngeal cancer is high. Some laryngeal tumors, however, have few manifestations until advanced. They may be treated by radiation therapy, chemotherapy, or surgery (laryngectomy and neck dissection).

■ Following total laryngectomy, a permanent tracheostomy is created and the upper trachea and esophagus are separated, preventing aspiration when feedings are resumed. A tracheoesophageal puncture (TEP) may be created to allow verbal communication following total laryngectomy.

TEST YOURSELF NCLEX-RN® REVIEW

1. A patient with hypertension asks the nurse what he can do to relieve the symptoms of an acute URI. The nurse recommends that he do which of the following?
   1. Ask his healthcare provider for an antibiotic prescription.
   2. Use an over-the-counter decongestant such as pseudoephedrine to relieve symptoms.
   3. Take 1000 mg of vitamin C and use zinc lozenges on a regular basis.
   4. Use an over-the-counter nasal spray for no more than three days to relieve congestion.

2. Which of the following health promotion activities planned by a nurse working with a group of community-dwelling senior citizens would be most likely to prevent influenza and pneumonia?
   1. indoor exercise programs during winter months
   2. influenza vaccine clinics at the senior center
   3. teaching effective handwashing
   4. advising seniors to avoid crowds

3. In teaching a patient with bacterial sinusitis about home care, the nurse stresses the importance of which of the following?
   1. completing the antibiotic prescription as ordered
   2. sleeping with the head of the bed elevated to 45 degrees
   3. using a humidifier to promote sinus drainage
   4. maintaining a liberal fluid intake to help liquify secretions

4. Which of the following nursing interventions for the patient with posterior nasal packing is of highest priority?
   1. Elevate the head of the bed.
   2. Apply cold compresses to the nose.
   3. Maintain oxygen therapy.
   4. Provide frequent oral hygiene.

5. A patient in the emergency department following facial trauma complains that his nose "just keeps dripping." The drainage appears like watery blood. The most appropriate nursing action would be to do which of the following?
   1. Provide a box of tissues.
   2. Reassure the patient that this is expected with a nasal fracture.
   3. Suction the nasopharynx.
   4. Obtain a specimen for glucose testing.

6. Expected findings in a patient with obstructive sleep apnea would include which of the following? **Select all that apply.**
   1. confusion and signs of dementia
   2. enlarged tongue
   3. complaints of daytime sleepiness
   4. decreased oxygen saturation levels while awake
   5. elevated blood pressure
   6. complaints of morning headache

7. The nurse in a healthcare provider's office notes that a regular patient's voice is hoarse, a change from previous visits. The most appropriate question to ask the patient would be which of the following?
   1. "How long has your voice been hoarse?"
   2. "Do you smoke?"
   3. "Do you have a sore throat?"
   4. "Would you like a prescription for throat lozenges?"

8. The nurse evaluates his teaching as effective when a patient with stage 1 laryngeal cancer states which of the following?
   1. "I'm glad I don't have to worry about treating this cancer now because it is so early."
   2. "I hate to think about eventually losing the ability to speak, but I'd rather treat it aggressively than lose my life to cancer."
   3. "I'm glad this was diagnosed early, when it can be treated with radiation so I won't lose my voice."
   4. "Thank goodness this type of cancer usually doesn't spread anywhere else."

9. Place the following nursing interventions for the patient who has undergone total laryngectomy and radical neck dissection in order of priority.
   1. arrange consultation with speech therapist
   2. provide small, frequent meals
   3. encourage to express feelings regaring loss of voice
   4. suction via tracheostomy as needed
   5. instruct to support head when moving

10. When providing tracheostomy care, the nurse does which of the following?
    1. cuts the dressing using sterile scissors
    2. secures clean ties before removing soiled ones
    3. uses clean technique to cleanse the outer cannula
    4. cleanses the incision with an iodine-based antiseptic

See Test Yourself answers in Appendix C.

Pearson Nursing Student Resources
Find additional review materials at
www.nursing.pearsonhighered.com
Prepare for success with additional NCLEX®-style practice questions, interactive assignments and activities, Web links, animations and videos, and more!

BIBLIOGRAPHY

Alper, B. S. (2005). Evidence-based medicine. Antiviral resistance in influenza may be increasing. *Clinical Advisor for Nurse Practitioners, 8*(12), 125.

Alper, B. S. (2005). Evidence-based medicine. Ginseng may reduce incidence of upper respiratory infection in adults. *Clinical Advisor for Nurse Practitioners, 8*(12), 126, 128.

American Cancer Society. (2009). *Cancer facts and figures 2009.* Atlanta: Author.

American Cancer Society. (2009). *Laryngeal and hypopharyngeal cancer.* Retrieved from http://www.cancer.org/docroot/CRI/CRI_2_1x.asp?rnav=criov&dt=23

Antic N. A., Buchan, C., Esterman, A., Hensley, M., Naughton, M. T., Rowland, S. et al. (2009). A randomized controlled trial of nurse-led care for symptomatic moderate–severe cbstructive sleep apnea. *American Journal of Respiratory and Critical Care Medicine 179,* 501–508.

Bulechek, G., Butcher, H., & Dochterman, J. M. (Eds). (2008). *Nursing interventions classification (NIC)* (5th ed.). St. Louis: Mosby Elsevier.

Campbell, S. (2007). Speaking up after laryngectomy. *Nursing 37*(8), 8.

Centers for Disease Control and Prevention. (2008). Infection control guidance for the prevention and control of influenza in health-care facilities. Atlanta: Author.

Centers for Disease Control and Prevention. (2009). H1N1 flu (swine flu). Retrieved from http://www.cdc.gov/h1n1flu/

Chasens, E. R., Pack, A. I., Maislin, G., Dinges, D. F., & Weaver, T. E. (2005). Claustrophobia and adherence to CPAP treatment. *Western Journal of Nursing Research, 27*(3), 307–321.

Chasens, E. R., Sereika, S. M., Weaver, T. E. & Umlauf, M. G. (2007). Daytime sleepiness, exercise, and physical function in older adults. *Journal of Sleep Research, 16,* 60–65.

Curry, K. (2007). Pertussis: A reemerging threat. *Journal for Nurse Practitioners 3*(2), 97–100.

Davey, M. J. (2003). Understanding obstructive sleep apnoea. *Nursing Times, 99*(22), 26–27.

deCastro, A. B. (2005). Health and safety. Preventing exposure to influenza: Steps health care workers can take. *American Journal of Nursing, 105*(1), 112.

Deglin, J. H., & Vallerand, A. H. (2009). *Davis' Drug Guide* (10th ed.) Philadelphia: F.A. Davis.

Desbiens, N. A. (2005). A 5-year experience with influenza prevention and containment in a program of all-inclusive care for elderly adults. *American Journal of Infection Control, 33*(4), 238–242.

Deutzer, J. (2005). Potential complications of obstructive sleep apnea in patients undergoing gastric bypass surgery. *Critical Care Nursing Quarterly, 28*(3), 293–299.

Dochterman, J., & Bulechek, G. (2004). *Nursing Interventions Classification (NIC)* (4th ed.). St. Louis: Mosby

Domino, F. J., Baldor, R. A., Golding, J., Grimes, J., & Taylor, J. S. (2010). *The 5-minute clinical consult* (18th ed.). Philadelphia: Lippincott, Williams & Wilkins.

Ecklund, M. M. (2004). Caring for the bariatric patient with obstructive sleep apnea. *Critical Care Nursing Clinics of North America, 16*(3), 311–317.

Edington-Winn, M., & Wright, K. (2005). Clinical update. Tracheostomy: A guide to nursing care. *Australian Nursing Journal, 13*(5), 17–20.

Fiore, A. E., Shay, D. K., Haber P., et al. (2008). Prevention and control of influenza. Recommendations of the Advisory Committee on Immunization Practices (ACIP). *MMWR 57*(RR-7),1–59.

Fontaine, K. L. (2005). *Healing practices: Alternative therapies for nursing* (2nd ed.). Upper Saddle River, NJ: Prentice Hall Health.

Goldrick, B. A. (2004). Emerging infections. Influenza 2004–2005: What's new with the flu. *American Journal of Nursing, 104*(10), 34–36.

Happ, M. B., Roesch, T. K., & Kagan, S. H. (2005). Patient communication following head and neck cancer surgery: A pilot study using electornic speech-generative devices. *Oncology Nursing Forum, 32*(6), 1179–1187.

Holman, M. L. (2005). Obstructive sleep apnea syndrome: implications for primary care. *Nurse Practitioner, 30*(9), 38–45.

Huether, S. E. & McCance, K. L. (2008). *Understanding Pathophysiology* (4th ed.). St. Louis: Mosby Elsevier.

Immunization Action Center. (2008). Summary of recommendations for adult immunization. Retrieved from http://www.immunize.org/catg.d/p2011.pdf

Jull, A. (2003). Review: Specific signs and symptoms can help practitioners to diagnose acute purulent sinusitis in general practice. *Evidence-Based Nursing, 6*(1), 24.

Larsson, M., Hedelin, B., Johansson, I., & Athlin, E. (2005). Eating problems and weight loss for patients with head and neck cancer: A chart review from diagnosis until one year after treatment. *Cancer Nursing, 28*(6), 425–35.

Lee, B. Y, Tai, H. J., Bailey, R. R. & Smith K. J. (2009). Timing of influenza vaccination for older adults (65 years and older). *Cell (online)* Retrieved September 26, 2009, from http://www.cell.com/

McErlane, K., & Pence, C. (2004). Action stat. Epistaxis. *Nursing, 34*(8), 88.

Merritt, S. L., & Johnson, J. (2004). Beats & breath. Obstructive sleep apnea-hypopnea syndrome: Nurses may detect a problem often overlooked by other providers. *American Journal of Nursing, 104*(7), 49–52.

Moorhead, S., Johnson, M., Maas, M., & Swanson, S. (Eds). (2008). *Nursing outcomes classification (NOC)* (4th ed.). St. Louis: Mosby Elsevier.

NANDA International. (2009). *Nursing diagnoses: Definitions and classification 2009–2011.* Oxford, UK: Wiley-Blackwell.

National Cancer Institute. (2009a). Aromatherapy and essential oils. Retrieved from http://www.cancer.gov/cancertopics/pdq/cam/aromatherapy/patient

National Cancer Institute. (2009b). Laryngeal cancer treatment: General information. Retrieved from http://www.cancer.gov/cancertopics/pdq/treatment/laryngeal/healthprofessional/page2

National Center for Complementary and Alternative Medicine (NCCAM). (2005). Echinacea. Retrieved from http://nccam.nih.gov/health/echinacea/

National Institute of Allergy and Infectious Diseases (NIAID). (2009). Flu (influenza) 2009 H1N1 (swine), seasonal, avian (bird), pandemic. Retrieved from www3.niaid.nih.gov/topics/flu/

National Institute of Allergy and Infectious Diseases. (2009). Vaccine research center. Retrieved from http://www3.niaid.nih.gov/about/organization/vrc/

Novel Swine-Origin Influenza A (H1N1) Virus Investigation Team. (2009). Emergence of a novel swine-origin influenza A (H1N1) virus in humans. *New England Journal of Medicine 360*(25), 2605–2615

Papadakis, M. A. & McPhee, S. J. (2007). *Current Consult Medicine 2007.* New York: McGraw-Hill.

Pynnonen, M. A., Mukerji, S. S., Kim H. M., Adams, M. E., & Terrell, J. E. (2007). Nasal saline for chronic sinonasal symptoms: A randomized controlled trial. *Archives of Otolaryngology and Head and Neck Surgery 133*(11), 1115–1120.

Roman, M. (2005). Clinical "how to." Tracheostomy tubes. *MEDSURG Nursing, 14*(2), 143–145.

Schweon, S., & Mangan, D. (2003). Don't underestimate group A strep. *RN, 66*(8), 28–33.

Sheff, K. B. (2006). Avian influenza: Poised to launch a pandemic? *Nursing, 36*(1), 51–53.

St. John, R. E. (2004). Contemporary issues in adult tracheostomy management. *Critical Care Nursing Clinics of North America, 16*(3), 413–430.

Stafanski, A. M. (2005). Obstructive sleep apnea: A primary care approach. *American Journal for Nurse Practitioners, 9*(10), 21–24, 27–28.

Van Leeuwen, A. M., Kranpitz, T. R., Smith, L. S. (2006). *Davis' Laboratory and Diagnostic Tests* (2nd ed.) Philadelphia: F.A. Davis.

Weaver, T. E. (2008a). Impaired Sleep. In Geiger-Bronsky (Ed.), *Respiratory Nursing Society Core Curriculum.* Philadelphia, PA: Lippincott Publishing Company.

Weaver, T. E. (2008b). Sleep Apnea. In Geiger-Bronsky (Ed.), *Respiratory Nursing Society Core Curriculum.* Philadelphia, PA: Lippincott Publishing Co.

Wilkinson, J. M. (2005). *Nursing diagnosis handbook with NIC interventions and NOC outcomes* (8th ed.). Upper Saddle River, NJ: Prentice Hall Health.

World Health Organization (WHO). (2009). Avian influenza guidelines, recommendations, descriptions. Retrieved from www.who.int/csr/disease/avian_influenza/guidelinestopics/en/index.html

CHAPTER 36

Nursing Care of Patients with Ventilation Disorders

LEARNING OUTCOMES

1. Relate the pathophysiology and manifestations of lower respiratory infections and inflammation, lung cancer, chest wall disorders, and trauma to the ability to maintain effective ventilation and respiration (gas exchange).

2. Compare and contrast the etiology, risk factors, and vulnerable populations for lower respiratory infections, lung cancer, chest wall disorders, and trauma.

3. Describe interdisciplinary care and the nursing role in health promotion and caring for patients with lower respiratory infections, lung cancer, chest wall disorders, and trauma.

4. Discuss surgery and other invasive procedures used to treat lung cancer, chest wall disorders, and trauma, and nursing responsibilities in caring for patients undergoing these procedures.

5. Describe the nursing implications for medications used to treat respiratory disorders and oxygen therapy.

CLINICAL COMPETENCIES

1. Assess functional health status and the effects of lower respiratory and chest wall disorders on ventilation and gas exchange.

2. Use assessed data and knowledge of the effects of the disorder and prescribed treatment to identify priority nursing diagnoses and plan care for patients with lower respiratory disorders.

3. Use the nursing process and evidence-based nursing research to plan and implement individualized nursing care, including measures to promote ventilation and gas exchange for patients with lower respiratory disorders.

4. Plan and provide appropriate teaching for health promotion among vulnerable populations and to prepare patients and families for community-based care.

5. Evaluate the effectiveness of nursing interventions and teaching, revising strategies and teaching plans as needed.

6. Knowledgably and safely coordinate interdisciplinary care and administer prescribed medications and treatments for patients with lower respiratory disorders.

KEY TERMS

asphyxiation, *1215*
bronchitis, *1177*
cyanosis, *1176*
dyspnea, *1176*
empyema, *1179*
flail chest, *1212*

hemoptysis, *1176*
hemothorax, *1211*
hypoxemia, *1185*
lung abscess, *1190*
pleural effusion, *1205*
pleuritis, *1205*

pneumonia, *1177*
pneumothorax, *1207*
severe acute respiratory syndrome (SARS), *1188*
thoracentesis, *1206*
tuberculosis (TB), *1191*

Disorders affecting the lower respiratory system (below the larynx), pleural cavity, and chest wall can affect the ability to effectively move air into and out of the lungs (ventilation) and the exchange of oxygen and carbon dioxide across the alveolar-capillary membrane (respiration). The disorders discussed in this chapter—respiratory infections and inflammation, trauma and disorders of the chest wall or pleural cavity, and neoplasms of the lung—all affect the ability to maintain clear and patent airways and ventilate the lungs. While these disorders can also affect gas exchange, nursing care for patients with these disorders generally focuses on maintaining airway patency and an effective

breathing pattern. Disorders that primarily affect gas exchange are discussed in ∞ Chapter 37.

The lower respiratory and chest wall disorders discussed in this chapter and ∞ Chapter 37 have both local and systemic effects. Local effects include cough, excess mucus production, shortness of breath or **dyspnea** (difficult or labored breathing), **hemoptysis** (bloody sputum), and chest pain. Systemic effects may include fever, anorexia and malaise, **cyanosis** (gray to blue or purple skin color caused by deoxygenated hemoglobin), and other manifestations of impaired gas exchange. Before continuing, review the anatomy, physiology, and assessment of the lower respiratory system in ∞ Chapter 34.

Infections and Inflammatory Disorders

Infections and inflammation of the lower respiratory system are common. The respiratory tree is constantly exposed to the environment as air moves into and out of the lower respiratory tract. In addition, the oropharynx is colonized by huge numbers of microorganisms that may be aspirated into the bronchial tree. Both anatomic and physiologic defenses help maintain the sterility of the lower respiratory tract. When these defenses are impaired, the risk for infection increases. For example, drugs, alcohol, or neuromuscular disease may suppress the cough reflex, and the influenza virus can leave the respiratory epithelium vulnerable to bacterial infection. Even in healthy people, microorganisms and other foreign material occasionally enter the bronchial tree and lung parenchyma.

The Patient with Acute Bronchitis

Bronchitis, inflammation of the bronchi, may be either an acute or a chronic condition. Acute bronchitis is relatively common in adults. Impaired immune defenses and cigarette smoking increase the risk for acute bronchitis. In otherwise healthy adults, it typically follows a viral upper respiratory infection. Chronic bronchitis is a component of chronic obstructive pulmonary disease (COPD) and is discussed in ∞ Chapter 37.

Pathophysiology and Manifestations

Infectious bronchitis can be caused by either viruses or bacteria that damage the respiratory mucosa. In healthy adults, bacterial bronchitis generally only occurs as a complication of viral infection. Inhalation of toxic gases or chemicals can lead to inflammatory bronchitis.

The inflammatory response to infection or tissue damage from inhaled substances causes capillary dilation and edema of the mucosal lining of the bronchi. Inflammatory cells infiltrate the affected mucosa, leading to exudate formation and increased mucus production. Ciliated epithelium is damaged by the inflammatory response and ciliary function is impaired. The immune response of lymphocytes and tissue macrophages is inhibited by some viruses and mycobacteria, increasing the risk for bacterial infection. Mucosal irritation and increased mucus production initiate the cough reflex. The respiratory tract may become hyperirritable for an extended period of time, leading to paroxysms of coughing and bronchospasm.

Acute bronchitis is typically heralded by a nonproductive cough that later becomes productive. The cough often occurs in paroxysms, and may be aggravated by cold, dry, or dusty air. Chest pain, often substernal, is common. Other manifestations include moderate fever and general malaise.

Interdisciplinary Care

The diagnosis of acute bronchitis typically is based on the history and clinical presentation. A chest x-ray may be ordered to rule out pneumonia, because the presenting manifestations can be similar. Other diagnostic testing is rarely indicated. Treatment is symptomatic and includes rest, increased fluid intake, and the use of aspirin or acetaminophen to relieve fever and malaise. Many healthcare providers prescribe a broad-spectrum antibiotic such as erythromycin or penicillin, because approximately 50% of acute bronchitis is bacterial in origin. An expectorant cough medication is recommended for use during the day and a cough suppressant for night to facilitate rest.

✍ Nursing Care

Nursing interventions for patients with acute bronchitis are primarily educational. Include the following teaching topics:

- Increase fluid intake to keep mucus thin and meet increased needs related to fever.
- Use over-the-counter analgesics and cough preparations containing dextromethorphan for symptom relief.
- Be aware of the use and effects of any prescribed medications.
- Understand the importance of smoking cessation (as appropriate).

The Patient with Pneumonia

Inflammation of the lung parenchyma (the respiratory bronchioles and alveoli) is known as **pneumonia**. Despite significant advances in antibiotic therapy, pneumonia remains the eighth leading cause of death in the United States, and the leading cause of death from infectious disease (CDC, 2009a). In 2006, more than 656,326 deaths in the United States were attributed to pneumonia and influenza (CDC, 2009a). Its incidence and mortality are highest in older adults and people with debilitating diseases. Pneumonia currently accounts for about 10% of adult hospital admissions in the United States.

> **FAST FACTS**
> - The age-adjusted death rate for influenza and pneumonia per 100,000 population declined from 53.7 in 1960 to 22.8 in 2006.
> - Overall, men have a higher death rate attributed to influenza and pneumonia than women, with a ratio of 1.4 to 1.0.
> - The differences in death rates attributed to influenza and pneumonia among different races and ethnicity are relatively small; Asian/Pacific Islanders have the lowest rate at 20.5 per 100,000, and Black/African Americans have the highest rate at 24.3 per 100,000 (ALA, 2009).

Pneumonia may be either infectious or noninfectious. Bacteria, viruses, fungi, protozoa, and other microbes can lead to infectious pneumonia. Noninfectious causes include aspiration of gastric contents and inhalation of toxic or irritating gases. Infectious pneumonias often are classified as community acquired, nosocomial (hospital acquired), or opportunistic. Different organisms are implicated in each of these classifications (Table 36–1). The most common causative organism for community-acquired pneumonia is *Streptococcus pneumoniae* (also called pneumococcus), a gram-positive bacterium. This organism causes about 66% of cases of community-acquired pneumonia leading to hospital admission. *Mycoplasma pneumoniae*, *Chlamydia pneumoniae*, *Haemophilus influenzae*, and the influenza virus are also leading causes of community-acquired pneumonia

TABLE 36–1 Common Organisms Causing Pneumonia in Adults

COMMUNITY ACQUIRED	HOSPITAL ACQUIRED	OPPORTUNISTIC
■ *Streptococcus pneumoniae*	■ *Staphylococcus aureus*	■ *Pneumocystis carinii*
■ *Mycoplasma pneumoniae*	■ *Pseudomonas aeruginosa*	■ *Mycobacterium tuberculosis*
■ *Haemophilus influenzae*	■ *Klebsiella pneumoniae*	■ Cytomegalovirus (CMV)
■ *Influenza virus*	■ *Escherichia coli*	■ Atypical mycobacteria
■ *Chlamydia pneumoniae*		■ Fungi
■ *Legionella pneumophila*		

(Papadakis & McPhee, 2007). *Staphylococcus aureus* and gram-negative bacteria such as *Klebsiella pneumoniae*, *Pseudomonas aeruginosa*, and enteric bacilli, including *Escherichia coli*, are often implicated as nosocomial causes of pneumonia. Organisms such as *Pneumonocystis* generally cause infections only in immunocompromised people (opportunistic infections).

Physiology Review

The lower respiratory tract normally is sterile. A number of defense mechanisms help maintain this sterile environment. Infectious particles trapped by the mucous membranes of the nose are removed by sneezing, while those deposited in the nasopharynx usually are swallowed or expectorated. Reflex closure of the epiglottis and the branching bronchial tree present anatomic barriers to entry of microorganisms and other possible contaminants. The cilia and mucus that line the respiratory tract and the cough reflex serve to trap and eliminate foreign matter that enters the lower respiratory tract. Organisms that make it past these barriers usually are rapidly phagocytized in the alveolus by resident macrophages, then attacked by the inflammatory and immune defenses of the body. Aging impairs these immune responses, increasing the risk for pneumonia (see the accompanying box).

Pathophysiology

The most common means of entry of pathogens into the lung is aspiration of oropharyngeal secretions containing microbes. Microorganisms also may be inhaled after having been released when an infected person coughs, sneezes, or talks. Contaminated aerosolized water also may be inhaled, an important means of spread for viral and some other types of pneumonia. Finally, bacteria may spread to the lungs through the bloodstream from infection elsewhere in the body. Host defenses must be overwhelmed either by the number of organisms or their *virulence* (disease-causing ability) in order for an infection to develop.

When the invading microorganisms colonize the alveoli, an inflammatory and immune response is initiated. The antigen–antibody response and endotoxins released by some organisms damage bronchial and alveolar mucous membranes, causing inflammation with vascular congestion and edema. Infectious debris and exudate can fill alveoli, interfering with ventilation and gas exchange (Figure 36–1 ■). Pneumonia may develop in four distinct patterns: lobar pneumonia, bronchopneumonia, interstitial pneumonia, and miliary pneumonia (Table 36–2).

The pathologic process, anatomic location, and manifestations of pneumonias vary according to the infective organism.

Acute Bacterial Pneumonia

Of the bacterial pneumonias, the pathogenesis of pneumococcal (*Streptococcus pneumoniae*) pneumonia is best understood (Figure 36–2 ■). These bacteria reside in the upper respiratory tract of up to 70% of adults. They may be spread by direct person-to-person contact via droplets. In many cases, infection results from aspiration of resident bacteria. In the lower respiratory tract, the inflammatory response initiated by these organisms causes alveolar edema and the formation of exudate. As alveoli and respiratory bronchioles fill with serous exudate, blood cells, fibrin, and bacteria, *consolidation* (solidification) of lung tissue occurs. The lower lobes of the lungs are usually

NURSING CARE OF THE OLDER ADULT Pneumonia

Several changes associated with aging and disease affect respiratory function and airway clearance. The number of cilia decreases, and the cough weakens. Gag and cough reflexes diminish. The older adult is at greater risk for dehydration, leading to thick, viscous mucus that is difficult to expectorate. Immune function declines with aging. These factors increase the risk of pulmonary infection and reduce the older adult's ability to respond effectively to infectious processes.

Other factors also may increase the risk for and severity of lower respiratory infections in the older adult: immobility, smoking history, surgical procedures, use of multiple medications, malnutrition, and such diseases as chronic obstructive pulmonary disease (COPD) and heart disease.

Figure 36–1 ■ In pneumonia, the inflammatory response causes fluid to accumulate in the alveoli and edema to form as alveolar capillaries dilate and allow fluid to leak into interstitial tissues.

TABLE 36–2 Patterns of Lung Involvement in Pneumonia

PATTERN OF INVOLVEMENT	DESCRIPTION
Lobar pneumonia	Typically involves an entire lobe of a lung. Early in the process, when the immune response is minimal, bacteria spread throughout the affected lobe by rapid accumulation of edema fluid. As the immune and inflammatory responses develop, RBCs and neutrophils, damaged epithelial cells, and fibrin accumulate in the alveoli. Purulent exudate containing neurophils and macrophages forms. As alveoli and respiratory bronchioles fill with exudate, blood cells, fibrin, and bacteria, *consolidation* (solidification) of lung tissue occurs. Finally, the process resolves as ezymes destroy the exudate and residual debris is reabsorbed, phagocytized, or coughed out.
Bronchopneumona	Usually involves dependent portions of lung tissue, characterized by patchy consolidation. Exudate tends to remain primarily in the bronchi and bronchioles, with less edema and congestion of the alveoli than in lobar pneumonia.
Interstitial pneumonia	The inflammatory process primarily involves the interstitium: the alveolar walls and connective tissue supporting the bronchial tree. Involvement may be patchy or diffuse as lymphocytes, macrophages, and plasma cells infiltrate the alveolar septa. While alveoli typically do not contain significant exudates, protein-rich hyaline membranes may line the alveoli, interfering with gas exchange.
Miliary pneumonia	In miliary pneumonia, numerous discrete inflammatory lesions develop as a result of spread of the pathogen to the lungs via the bloodstream. Miliary pneumonia is primarily seen in people who are severely immunocompromised. As a result, the immune response is poor and damage to pleural tissue may be significant.

affected because of gravity. Consolidation of a large portion of an entire lung lobe is known as *lobar pneumonia*. This is the typical pattern for pneumococcal pneumonia. *Bronchopneumonia* is patchy consolidation involving several lobules. Other bacterial pneumonias often present with the patchy involvement of bronchopneumonia; pneumococcal pneumonia may also follow this pattern. The process resolves when macrophages predominate, digesting and removing inflammatory exudate from the infected lung.

MANIFESTATIONS   The presentation of bacterial pneumonia is usually acute, with rapid onset of shaking chills, (rigors) fever, and cough productive of rust-colored or purulent sputum. Chest aching or *pleuritic pain* (sharp localized chest pain that increases with breathing and coughing) is common. Limited breath sounds and fine crackles or rales are heard over the affected area of lung. A pleural friction rub may be audible. If the involved area is large and gas exchange is impaired, dyspnea and cyanosis may be noted.

A more insidious onset with low-grade fever, cough, and scattered crackles is more typical of bronchopneumonia. Dyspnea is less commonly seen. The older adult or debilitated patient may have atypical manifestations of pneumonia, with little cough, scant sputum, and minimal evidence of respiratory distress. Fever, tachypnea, and altered mentation or agitation may be the primary presenting symptoms.

COMPLICATIONS   Pneumococcal pneumonia typically resolves uneventfully; normal lung structure is restored on completion of the process. Local extension of the infection to involve the pleura (*pleuritis*) is the most common complication. Pneumonias caused by *Staphylococcus aureus* and gram-negative bacteria often cause extensive parenchymal damage with necrosis, lung abscess, and empyema or pleural effusion. Progressive destruction of lung tissue and functional impairment is a possible consequence of *Klebsiella* pneumonia.

A *lung abscess* is a local area of necrosis and pus formation within the lung itself. They are relatively uncommon. The manifestations of lung abscess develop slowly, and include weight loss, malaise, night sweats, fever, and a productive cough. Sputum is foul smelling and tasting. Rupture of the abscess into a larger airway is heralded by production of copious amounts of purulent sputum.

Empyema is accumulation of purulent exudate in the pleural cavity. It is identified by chest x-ray or CT scan. Thoracentesis may be done or a chest tube inserted to remove purulent exudates. (Nursing care of the patient undergoing thoracentesis or with a chest tube is discussed later in this chapter.) Bacteremia can spread the infection to other tissues, leading to meningitis, endocarditis, or peritonitis, and increasing the risk of mortality.

Legionnaires' Disease

Legionnaires' disease is a form of bronchopneumonia caused by *Legionella pneumophila*, a gram-negative bacterium widely found in water, particularly warm standing water. Legionnaires'

Figure 36–2 ■ The pathogenesis of pneumococcal pneumonia.

disease occurs sporadically and in outbreaks, such as that which occurred at an American Legion convention in 1976, when the disease was first recognized. Contaminated water-cooled air-conditioning systems and other water sources have been implicated in its spread.

Smokers, older adults, and people with chronic diseases or impaired immune defenses are most susceptible to Legionnaires' disease. Symptoms develop gradually, beginning 2 to 10 days after exposure. Dry cough, dyspnea, general malaise, chills and fever, headache, confusion, anorexia and diarrhea, myalgias, and arthralgias are common manifestations. Consolidation of lung tissue is patchy or lobar. The mortality rate in Legionnaires' disease is reported to be 25%; however, this may be low due to lack of reporting of the disease. Mortality with nosocomial infections is about 50% (Domino et al., 2009; Papadakis & McPhee, 2007).

Primary Atypical Pneumonia

Pneumonia caused by *Mycoplasma pneumoniae* is generally classified as *primary atypical pneumonia* because its presentation and course significantly differ from other bacterial pneumonias. Mycoplasma infection often causes pharyngitis or bronchitis. When pneumonia develops, patchy inflammatory changes in the alveolar septum and interstitial tissue of the lung occur. Alveolar exudate and consolidation of lung tissue are not features of atypical pneumonia.

Young adults—college students and military recruits in particular—are the primary affected population. Primary atypical pneumonia is highly contagious. Its manifestations resemble those of viral pneumonia; systemic manifestations of fever, headache, myalgias, and arthralgias often predominate. The cough associated with atypical pneumonia is dry, hacking, and nonproductive. Because of the typically mild nature and predominant systemic manifestations, mycoplasmal and viral pneumonia are often referred to as "walking pneumonias."

Viral Pneumonia

Approximately 10% of pneumonias in adults are viral. Influenza and adenovirus are the most common organisms; however, the incidence of cytomegalovirus (CMV) pneumonia is increasing in immunocompromised people. Other viruses such as herpes viruses and measles virus also may cause viral

pneumonia. As in primary atypical pneumonia, lung involvement in viral pneumonia is limited to the alveolar septum and interstitial spaces.

Viral pneumonia is typically a mild disease that often affects older adults and people with chronic conditions. It usually occurs in community epidemics. Flulike symptoms of headache, fever, fatigue, malaise, and muscle aching are common, along with a dry cough.

Pneumocystis Pneumonia

People with acquired immune deficiency syndrome (AIDS) and others with significant immunocompromise are at risk for developing an opportunistic pneumonia caused by *Pneumocystis jiroveci*, a common parasite found worldwide. Immunity to *Pneumocystis* is nearly universal, except in immunocompromised people. Opportunistic infection may develop in people treated with immunosuppressive or cytotoxic drugs for cancer or organ transplant and in people with genetic or acquired immunodeficiency. *Pneumocystis* pneumonia can be seen in up to 80% of AIDS patients who do not receive prophylaxis (Papadakis & McPhee, 2007).

Infection with *Pneumocystis* produces patchy involvement throughout the lungs, causing affected alveoli to thicken, become edematous, and fill with foamy, protein-rich fluid. Gas exchange is severely impaired as the disease progresses. *Pneumocystis* pneumonia (PCP) has an abrupt onset with fever, tachypnea and shortness of breath, and a dry, nonproductive cough. Respiratory distress can be significant, with intercostal retractions and cyanosis.

Table 36–3 compares the manifestations of infectious pneumonias.

Aspiration Pneumonia

Aspiration of gastric contents into the lungs results in a chemical and bacterial pneumonia known as *aspiration pneumonia*. Major risk factors for aspiration pneumonia include emergency surgery or obstetric procedures, depressed cough and gag reflexes, and impaired swallowing. Older surgical patients are at significant risk. Enteral nutrition by either nasogastric or gastric tube also increases the risk for aspiration pneumonia. Vomiting is not always apparent; silent regurgitation of gastric contents may occur when

TABLE 36–3 Manifestations of Infectious Pneumonias

TYPE	ONSET	RESPIRATORY MANIFESTATIONS	SYSTEMIC MANIFESTATIONS
Pneumococcal or lobar pneumonia	Abrupt	Cough productive of purulent or rust-colored sputum; pleuritic or aching chest pain; decreased breath sounds and crackles over affected area; possible dyspnea and cyanosis	Chills and fever
Bronchopneumonia	Gradual	Cough, scattered crackles; minimal dyspnea and respiratory distress	Low-grade fever
Legionnaires' disease	Gradual	Dry cough; dyspnea	Chills and fever; general malaise; headache; confusion; anorexia and diarrhea; myalgias and arthralgias
Primary atypical pneumonia	Gradual	Dry, hacking, nonproductive cough	Fever, headache, myalgias, and arthralgias predominate
Viral pneumonia	Sudden or gradual	Dry cough	Flulike symptoms
Pneumocystis pneumonia	Abrupt	Dry cough; tachypnea and shortness of breath; significant respiratory distress	Fever

the level of consciousness is decreased. Measures to reduce the risk for aspiration pneumonia include minimizing the use of pre-operative medications, promoting anesthetic elimination from the body, and preventing nausea and gastric distention.

The low pH of gastric contents causes a severe inflammatory response when aspirated into the respiratory tract. Pulmonary edema and respiratory failure may result. Common complications of aspiration pneumonia include abscesses, bronchiectasis (chronic dilation of the bronchi and bronchioles), and gangrene of pulmonary tissue.

Interdisciplinary Care

Prevention is a key component in managing pneumonia. Identifying vulnerable populations and instituting preventive strategies are measures to reduce the mortality and morbidity associated with pneumonia. With early identification of the infecting organism, appropriate treatment, and support of respiratory function, most patients recover uneventfully. However, pneumonia remains a serious disease with significant mortality, especially in aged and debilitated populations.

Diagnosis

The history and physical examination, along with diagnostic testing are used to establish the diagnosis, determine the extent of lung involvement, and identify the causative organism. ∞ See Chapter 34 for more information about the following tests and their nursing implications:

- *Chest x-ray* is obtained to determine the extent and pattern of lung involvement. Fluid, infiltrates, consolidated lung tissue, and atelectasis (areas of alveolar collapse) appear as densities on the film. The *CT scan* provides a more detailed image of pulmonary tissue and may be used when the chest x-ray is not diagnostic.
- *Sputum gram stain* rapidly identifies the infecting organisms as gram-positive or gram-negative bacteria. Antibiotic therapy can then be directed at the predominant type of organism until culture and sensitivity results are obtained.

- *Sputum culture and sensitivity* is ordered to identify the infecting organism and determine the most effective antibiotic therapy. When obtaining sputum for culture, it is important to obtain secretions from the lower respiratory tract, not the mouth and nasal passages. See Procedure 34–1.
- *Complete blood count (CBC) with white blood cell (WBC) differential* shows an elevated WBC ($11,000/mm^3$ or higher) with increased circulating immature leukocytes (a left shift) in response to the infectious process. WBC changes are minimal in viral and other pneumonias.
- *Serology* testing, blood tests to detect antibodies to respiratory pathogens, may be used to identify the infecting organism when blood and sputum cultures are negative.
- *Pulse oximetry*, a noninvasive method of measuring arterial oxygen saturation, is ordered to continuously monitor gas exchange. The SaO_2 normally is 95% or higher. An SaO_2 of less than 95% may indicate impaired alveolar gas exchange.
- *Arterial blood gases (ABGs)* may be ordered to evaluate gas exchange. Respiratory secretions or pleuritic pain can interfere with alveolar ventilation. Alveolar inflammation can interfere with gas exchange across the alveolar-capillary membrane, especially if exudate or consolidation is present. An arterial oxygen tension (PO_2) of less than 75 to 80 mmHg indicates impaired gas exchange or alveolar ventilation. ∞ See Chapters 10 and 34 for more information about gas transport, arterial blood gases, and normal or expected values.
- *Fiberoptic bronchoscopy* may be done to obtain a sputum specimen or remove secretions from the bronchial tree (Figure 34–4). Nursing responsibilities related to bronchoscopy are summarized in the box on page 1130.

Immunization

Vaccines offer some degree of protection against the most common bacterial and viral pneumonias.

Pneumococcal vaccine, made of antigens from 23 types of pneumococcus, usually imparts lifetime immunity with a single dose. The vaccine is recommended for people who have a high risk of adverse outcome from bacterial pneumonias: people over

TABLE 36–4 Antibiotic Therapy for Selected Pneumonias

CAUSATIVE ORGANISM	ANTIBIOTIC OF CHOICE	ALTERNATIVE ANTIBIOTICS
Streptococcus pneumoniae	Penicillin G; amoxicillin	Erythromycin, cephalosporins, doxycycline, fluoroquinolones, clindamycin, vancomycin, TMP-SMZ*, linezolid
Haemophilus influenzae	Second- or third-generation cephalospornins, doxycycline, azithromycin, TMP-SMZ*	Fluoroquinolones, clarithromycin
Staphylococcus aureus	Penicillinase-resistant penicillin (e.g., nafcillin); vancomycin for methicillin-resistant organisms	Cephalosporins, vancomycin, clindamycin; ciprofloxacin, fluoroquinolones, TMP-SMZ*
Mycoplasma pneumoniae	Erythromycin, doxycycline	Clarithromycin, azithromycin, fluoroquinolones
Klebsiella pneumoniae	Third-generation cephalosporin (with aminogly-coside if severe); methronidazole	Aztreonam, imipenem-cilastatin, fluoroquinolones
Legionella pneumophila	Macrolide + rifampin; fluoroquinolones	TMP-SMZ*, doxycycline + rifampin
Pneumocystis	TMP-SMZ*, pentamidine + prednisone	Dapsone + trimethoprim, clindamycin + primaquine, trimetrexate + folinic acid
Chlamydia pneumoniae	Doxycycline	Macrolide, fluoroquinolones

*Trimethoprim-sulfamethoxazole

age 65; those with chronic cardiac or respiratory conditions, diabetes mellitus, alcoholism, or other chronic diseases; and immunocompromised people. A one-time revaccination is recommended for selected populations, including people over age 65 who were immunized more than 5 years previously and before age 65, people with chronic renal failure or immunosuppressive conditions (e.g., malignancy), and people receiving chemotherapy with selected agents (CDC, 2005).

Influenza vaccine is also recommended for high-risk populations. The predominant strain of influenza virus varies from year to year. A new vaccine formulation is prepared yearly, incorporating antigens of the influenza strains predicted to be the most prevalent for the upcoming flu season (typically the winter months). Vulnerable populations for whom yearly vaccine is recommended include those listed earlier as well as healthcare workers and residents of long-term care facilities. The vaccine contains egg protein, and is not recommended for people who have a severe allergy to eggs or who have previously experienced a severe hypersensitivity response to the vaccine.

Medications

Medications used to treat pneumonia may include antibiotics to eradicate the infection and bronchodilators to reduce bronchospasm and improve ventilation.

Initial antibiotic therapy is based on the results of sputum Gram stain and the pattern of lung involvement shown on the chest x-ray. Considerations such as the presence of cardiovascular disease or residence in a long-term care facility also are considered in the initial antibiotic choice. Typically, a broad-spectrum antibiotic such as a macrolide (e.g., clarithromycin, azithromycin, or erythromycin), a penicillin or a second- or third-generation cephalosporin, or a fluoroquinolone (e.g., ciprofloxacin) is ordered until the results of sputum culture and sensitivity tests are available. Table 36–4 lists commonly prescribed antibiotics for selected pneumonias; nursing implications for selected antibiotics are summarized on pages 298–300 of ∞ Chapter 12.

When an inflammatory response to the infection causes bronchospasm and constriction, bronchodilators may be ordered to improve ventilation and reduce hypoxia. Bronchodilators generally belong to one of two major groups: the sympathomimetic drugs, such as albuterol sulfate (Proventil) and metaproterenol (Alupent); or the methylxanthines, such as theophylline and aminophylline. Use of these drugs and related nursing implications are discussed in detail in the section on asthma.

An agent to "break up" mucus or reduce its viscosity may be prescribed. Acetylcysteine (Mucomyst), potassium iodide, and guaifenesin (a common ingredient in expectorant cough syrups), help to liquefy mucus, making it easier to expectorate. For many patients, however, increasing fluid intake is an effective means of liquefying mucus.

Treatments

When mucous secretions are thick and viscous, increasing fluid intake to 2500 to 3000 mL per day helps liquefy secretions, making them easier to cough up and expectorate. If the patient is unable to maintain an adequate oral intake, intravenous fluids and nutrition may be required.

Incentive spirometry may be used to promote deep breathing, coughing, and clearance of respiratory secretions. Endotracheal

suctioning may be required if the cough is ineffective. This invasive technique is discussed in the section describing nursing care for the patient with acute respiratory failure in ∞ Chapter 37. On occasion, bronchoscopy is used to perform pulmonary toilet and remove secretions.

A

B

C

Figure 36–3 ■ Low-flow oxygen delivery devices. *A*, Nasal cannula. *B*, Simple face mask. *C*, Nonrebreather mask.

OXYGEN THERAPY Oxygen therapy may be indicated for the patient who is tachypneic or hypoxemic.

Inflammation of the alveolar-capillary membrane interferes with diffusion of gases across the membrane. Diffusion is affected by several other factors, including the partial pressure of gases on each side of the membrane. Increasing the percentage of inspired oxygen above that of room air (21%) increases the partial pressure of oxygen in the alveoli and enhances its diffusion into the capillaries. Supplemental oxygen therefore improves oxygenation of the blood and tissues in patients with pneumonia.

Depending on the degree of hypoxia, oxygen may be administered by either a low-flow or high-flow system. Low-flow systems include the nasal cannula, simple face mask, partial rebreathing mask, and nonrebreathing mask (Figure 36–3 ■). A nasal cannula can deliver 24% to 45% oxygen concentrations with flow rates of 2 to 6 L/min. The nasal cannula is comfortable and does not interfere with eating or talking. A simple face mask delivers 40% to 60% oxygen concentrations with flow rates of 5 to 8 L/min. Up to 100% oxygen can be delivered by the nonrebreather mask, the highest concentration possible without mechanical ventilation. When the amount of oxygen delivered must be precisely regulated, a high-flow system such as a Venturi mask is used (Figure 36–4 ■). The Venturi mask regulates the ratio of oxygen to room air, allowing precise regulation of the oxygen percentage delivered, from 24% to 50%. High flow oxygen can also be delivered via nasal cannula (Vapotherm). In these

Figure 36–4 ■ Venturi mask, a high-flow oxygen delivery system.

methods, oxygen and warmed normal saline are aresolized. Flow at 15L/min provides up to 90% FiO_2 while 10L/min provides 65% FiO_2. Severe hypoxia may necessitate intubation and mechanical ventilation. Endotracheal intubation and methods of mechanical ventilation are discussed in ∞ Chapter 37.

CHEST PHYSIOTHERAPY Chest physiotherapy, including percussion, vibration, and postural drainage, may be prescribed to reduce lung consolidation and prevent atelectasis. *Percussion* is performed by rhythmically striking or clapping the chest wall with cupped hands (Figure 36–5A ■), using rapid

A

B

Figure 36–5 ■ *A*, Percussing (clapping) the upper posterior chest. Notice the cupped position of the nurse's hands. *B*, Vibrating the upper posterior chest.

wrist flexion and extension. Cupping traps air between the palm and the patient's skin, setting up vibrations through the chest wall that loosen respiratory secretions. The trapped air also provides a cushion, preventing injury. When performed correctly, percussion produces a hollow, popping sound. Percussion may also be done using a mechanical percussion cup, vibration modes on certain hospital beds, or via a vest or chest wrap. The breasts, sternum, spinal column, and kidney regions are avoided during percussion.

Vibration facilitates secretion movement into larger airways. It usually is combined with percussion, although it may be used when percussion is contraindicated or poorly tolerated. Vibration is performed by repeatedly tensing the arm and hand muscles while maintaining firm but gentle pressure over the affected area with the flat of the hand (Figure 36–5B).

Percussion and vibration are done in conjunction with *postural drainage*, which uses gravity to facilitate removal of

secretions from a particular lung segment. The patient is positioned with the segment to be drained superior to or above the trachea or mainstem bronchus. Drainage of all lung segments requires a variety of positions (Figure 36–6 ■); rarely do all segments require drainage. Bronchodilators or nebulizer treatments are administered as ordered prior to postural drainage. It is best to perform postural drainage before meals to avoid nausea and vomiting.

Complementary Therapies

Although complementary therapies do not replace conventional treatment for pneumonia, they often promote comfort and speed recovery. The herb Echinacea is widely used to stimulate immune function and treat upper respiratory infections (URIs). Because viral URIs often precede pneumonia, it may be helpful in preventing pneumonia. Recent research, however, shows mixed results for the effectiveness of Echinacea in reducing the duration and severity of URI (NCCAM, 2005). Goldenseal, which often is sold in combination with Echinacea, is used to treat bacterial, fungal, and protozoal infections of the mucous membranes of the respiratory tract.

Advise patients inquiring about the use of Chinese herbal remedies to reduce pneumonia symptoms to determine if any recommended product contains ma hung or ephedra and to avoid such products, as ephedra is banned in the United States.

Figure 36–6 ■ Positions for postural drainage. *A*, Left and right anterior apical. *B*, Left and right posterior apical. *C*, Left and right anterior upper. *D*, Right middle lobe. *E*, Superior lower lobes. *F*, Left and right lower posterior. *G*, Left lower lateral. *H*, Right lower lateral.

∽ Nursing Care

Health Promotion

Health promotion activities focus on pneumonia prevention. Make patients in high-risk groups aware of the benefits of immunizations against influenza and pneumococcal pneumonia. A single dose of pneumococcus vaccine usually produces immunity to most strains of pneumococcal pneumonia, although repeat doses may be needed for older adults and people who are immunosuppressed. (Pneumococcusal vaccine is contraindicated for people receiving immunosuppressive therapy.) Annual influenza vaccine helps prevent pneumonia because pneumonia often occurs as a sequela to influenza.

> **PRACTICE ALERT**
> Inquire about allergic responses to eggs or previous influenza vaccinations prior to administering influenza vaccine. A significant hypersensitivity response may occur in patients who are allergic to egg protein.

Additional measures to screen for and detect pneumonia in older adults are appropriate. Frequent pulmonary assessment and aggressive interventions help prevent problems. Restoring and maintaining mobility improves ventilation and helps mobilize secretions. Promoting adequate fluid intake liquefies secretions, making them easier to expectorate.

Assessment

Focused assessment of the patient with pneumonia includes the following:

- *Health history:* Current symptoms and their duration; presence of shortness of breath or difficulty breathing, chest pain and its relationship to breathing; cough, productive or nonproductive, color, consistency of sputum; other symptoms; recent upper respiratory or other acute illness; chronic diseases such as diabetes, chronic lung disease, or heart disease; current medications; medication allergies.
- *Physical examination:* Presentation, apparent distress, level of consciousness; vital signs including temperature; skin color, temperature; respiratory excursion, use of accessory muscles of respiration; lung sounds.
- *Diagnostic tests:* WBC with differential, sputum gram stain, culture and sensitivity, chest x-ray or CT scan.

Nursing Diagnoses and Interventions

Patients with lower respiratory disorders such as pneumonia may have multiple nursing care needs, depending on the severity of the illness. Alveolar ventilation and the process of alveolar respiration can be affected by inflammation and secretions. **Hypoxemia**, low levels of oxygen in the blood, and tissue hypoxia may result. Nursing care focuses on supporting optimal respiratory function and promoting rest to reduce metabolic and oxygen needs. Priority nursing diagnoses include *Ineffective Airway Clearance*, *Ineffective Breathing Pattern*, and *Activity Intolerance*.

Ineffective Airway Clearance

The inflammatory response to infection causes tissue edema and exudate formation. In the lungs, the inflammatory response can narrow and potentially obstruct bronchial passages and alveoli. Assessment findings supporting this nursing diagnosis include adventitious breath sounds such as crackles (rales), rhonchi, and wheezes; dyspnea and tachypnea; coughing; and indicators of hypoxia such as cyanosis, reduced SaO_2 levels, anxiety, and apprehension.

- Assess respiratory status, including vital signs, breath sounds, SaO_2, and skin color at least every 4 hours. *Early identification of respiratory compromise allows intervention before tissue hypoxia is significant.*
- Assess cough and sputum (amount, color, consistency, and possible odor). *Assessment of the cough and nature of sputum produced allow evaluation of the effectiveness of respiratory clearance and the response to therapy.*
- Monitor arterial blood gas results; report increasing hypoxemia and other abnormal results to the healthcare provider. *Blood gas changes may be an early indicator of impaired gas exchange due to airway narrowing or obstruction.*
- Place in Fowler's or high-Fowler's position. Encourage frequent position changes and ambulation as allowed. *The upright position promotes lung expansion; position changes and ambulation facilitate the movement of secretions.*
- Assist to cough, deep breathe, and use assistive devices. Provide endotracheal suctioning using aseptic technique as ordered. *Coughing, deep breathing, and suctioning help clear airways.*
- Provide a fluid intake of at least 2500 to 3000 mL per day. *A liberal fluid intake helps liquefy secretions, facilitating their clearance.*
- Work with the healthcare provider and respiratory therapist to provide pulmonary hygiene measures, such asincentive spirometer, postural drainage, percussion, and vibration. *These techniques help mobilize and clear secretions.*
- Administer prescribed medications as ordered, and monitor their effects. *If the infecting organism is resistant to the prescribed antibiotic, little improvement may be seen with treatment. Bronchodilators help maintain open airways but may have adverse effects such as anxiety and restlessness.*

Ineffective Breathing Pattern

Pleural inflammation often accompanies pneumonia, causing sharp localized pain that increases with deep breathing, coughing, and movement, which can lead to rapid and shallow breathing. Distal airways and alveoli may not expand optimally with each breath, increasing the risk for atelectasis and decreasing gas exchange. Fatigue from the increased work of breathing is an additional problem in pneumonia. This, too, can lead to decreased lung inflation and an ineffective breathing pattern.

> **PRACTICE ALERT**
> Assess respiratory rate, depth, and lung sounds at least every 4 hours. Tachypnea and diminished or adventitious breath sounds may be early indicators of respiratory compromise.

- Provide for rest periods. *Rest reduces metabolic demands, fatigue, and the work of breathing, promoting a more effective breathing pattern.*
- Assess for pleuritic discomfort. Provide analgesics as ordered. *Adequate pain relief minimizes splinting and promotes adequate ventilation.*

■ Provide reassurance during periods of respiratory distress. *Hypoxia and respiratory distress produce high levels of anxiety, which tends to further increase tachypnea and fatigue and decrease ventilation.*

■ Administer oxygen as ordered. *Oxygen therapy increases the alveolar oxygen concentration and facilitates its diffusion across the alveolar-capillary membrane, reducing hypoxia and anxiety.*

■ Teach slow abdominal breathing. *This breathing pattern promotes lung expansion.*

■ Teach use of relaxation techniques, such as visualization and meditation. *These techniques help reduce anxiety and slow the breathing pattern.*

Activity Intolerance

Impaired airway clearance and gas exchange interfere with oxygen delivery to body cells and tissues. At the same time, the infectious process and the body's response to it increase metabolic demands on the cells. The net result of this imbalance between oxygen delivery and oxygen demand is a lack of physiologic energy to maintain normal daily activities.

■ Assess activity tolerance, noting any increase in pulse, respirations, dyspnea, diaphoresis, or cyanosis. *These assessment findings may indicate limited or impaired activity tolerance.*

> **PRACTICE ALERT**
> Activity intolerance may be an early sign of cardiorespiratory compromise, particularly in the older adult or patient with pre-existing heart disease. New or worsening manifestations of activity intolerance should be reported to the healthcare provider.

■ Assist with self-care activities, such as bathing. *Assistance with ADLs reduces energy demands.*

■ Schedule activities, planning for rest periods. *Rest periods minimize fatigue and improve activity tolerance.*

■ Provide assistive devices, such as an overhead trapeze. *These assistive devices facilitate movement and reduce energy demands.*

■ Enlist the family's help to minimize stress and anxiety levels. *Stress and anxiety increase metabolic demands and can decrease activity tolerance.*

■ Perform active or passive ROM exercises. *Exercises help maintain muscle tone and joint mobility, and prevent contractures if bed rest is prolonged.*

■ Provide emotional support and reassurance that strength and energy will return to normal when the infectious process has resolved and the balance of oxygen supply and demand is restored. *The patient may be concerned that activity intolerance will continue to be a problem after the acute infection is resolved.*

Using NANDA, NIC, and NOC

Linkages between a selected NANDA nursing diagnosis, NIC, and NOC for the patient with pneumonia are shown in the chart that follows.

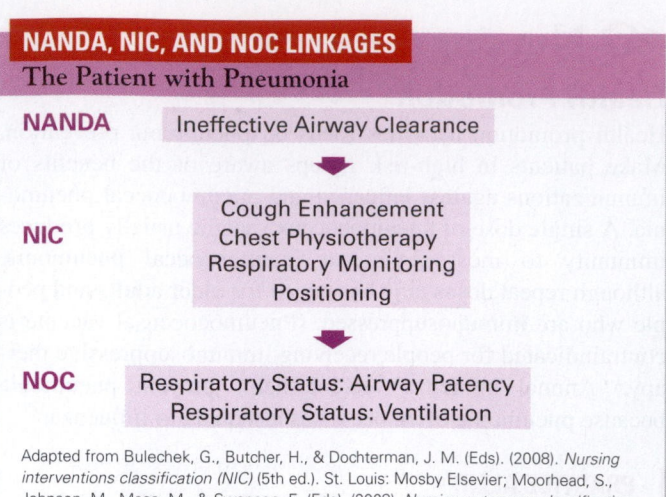

NANDA, NIC, AND NOC LINKAGES
The Patient with Pneumonia

NANDA — Ineffective Airway Clearance

NIC — Cough Enhancement
Chest Physiotherapy
Respiratory Monitoring
Positioning

NOC — Respiratory Status: Airway Patency
Respiratory Status: Ventilation

Adapted from Bulechek, G., Butcher, H., & Dochterman, J. M. (Eds). (2008). *Nursing interventions classification (NIC)* (5th ed.). St. Louis: Mosby Elsevier; Moorhead, S., Johnson, M., Maas, M., & Swanson, E. (Eds). (2008). *Nursing outcomes classification (NOC)* (4th ed.). St. Louis: Mosby Elsevier; and NANDA International. (2009). *Nursing diagnoses: Definitions and classification 2009–2011.* Oxford, UK: Wiley-Blackwell.

Community-Based Care

Patients with pneumonia usually are treated in the community, unless their respiratory status is significantly compromised (e.g., altered mental status, tachypnea, tachycardia, hypotension, hypo- or hyperthermia, and altered blood gases) or risk factors such as advanced age and/or coexisting heart, kidney, or liver disease are present.

EVIDENCE FOR NURSING CARE **The Patient with Pneumonia**

Selected resources that nurses may find helpful when planning evidence-based nursing care follow.

■ Cason, C. L., Tyner, T. Saunders, S., & Broome, L. (2007). Nurses' implementation of guidelines for ventilator-associated pneumonia from the centers for disease control and prevention. *American Journal of Critical Care, 16*(1), 28–36.

■ Fowler, S. B. (2008). Community-acquired pneumonia: Follow the guidelines to better outcomes. *American Nurse Today, 3*(9), 26–30.

■ Grap, M. J. (2009). Not-so-trivial pursuit: Mechanical ventilation risk reduction. *American Journal of Critical Care, 18*(4), 299–309.

■ Mandell, L. A., Wunderink, R. G., Anzueto, A., Bartlett, J. G., Campbell, G D., Dean, N. C., et al. (2007). Infectious Diseases Society of America/American Thoracic Society consensus guidelines on the management of community-acquired pneumonia in adults. *Clinical Infectious Diseases, 44*(Suppl 2), S27–S72. Retrieved from http://www.guideline.gov/summary/summary.aspx?doc_id=10560&nbr=005516&string=empyema

■ Munro, C. L., Grap, M. J., Jones, D. J., McClish, D. K. & Sessler, C. N. (2009). Chlorhexidine, toothbrushing, and preventing ventilator-associated pneumonia in critically ill adults. *American Journal of Critical Care, 18*(5), 428–437.

■ Ventilator assisted pneumonia. (2008). *American Association of Critical-Care Nurses (AACN) Practice Alert.* Retrieved from http://www.aacn.org/WD/Practice/Content/practicealerts.pcms?menu=Practice

CASE STUDY & NURSING CARE PLAN A Patient with Pneumonia

Mary O'Neal is a 35-year-old executive assistant and a part-time college student. On returning home from class one evening, she begins to chill. She alternates between chills and sweats all night. Staying home from work, she remains in bed most of the next day. Her fever continues, and she develops a cough and dull aching chest pain. When the cough becomes productive of rust-colored sputum the following day, she seeks medical treatment from her family doctor.

ASSESSMENT

Debby Kowalski, RN, the family practice clinic nurse, admits Mrs. O'Neal to the clinic and obtains the nursing assessment. Mrs. O'Neal denies any previous history of respiratory diseases "other than the usual colds, flu, and such." She also denies any history of smoking or medication allergies. She says her symptoms began abruptly with the onset of the chills. She describes her chest pain as a dull ache that was initially substernal but now is localized in her lower lateral right chest. The pain increases with deep breathing, coughing, and moving. Her cough is increasing in frequency and severity, and her sputum appears rusty brown. Her vital signs are BP 116/74, P 104 and regular, R 26, T 101.8°F (38.7°C). Skin warm and flushed, with no evidence of cyanosis. Respirations shallow, unlabored; respiratory excursion equal. Diminished breath sounds in bases bilaterally, crackles noted in right posterior and lateral base. Faint pleural rub heard at right midaxillary line.

A STAT CBC shows a WBC of 18,900/mm³; differential shows increased numbers of neutrophils and immature WBCs (bands). Ms. Kowalski has Mrs. O'Neal rinse with an antiseptic mouthwash and collect a sputum specimen for culture and Gram stain prior to seeing the healthcare provider.

The healthcare provider orders a chest x-ray after examining Mrs. O'Neal. Based on her history, examination, and the chest x-ray, he makes the diagnosis of acute bacterial pneumonia, probably pneumococcal. He prescribes oral penicillin V, 500 mg every 6 hours for 10 days. He asks Mrs. O'Neal to return for a follow-up appointment in 10 days and refers her back to Ms. Kowalski for appropriate teaching.

DIAGNOSIS

- *Ineffective Breathing Pattern* related to pleuritic chest pain
- *Hyperthermia* related to inflammatory process
- *Deficient Knowledge* related to diagnosis of pneumonia and its treatment

EXPECTED OUTCOMES

- Maintain normal pulmonary function.
- Describe measures to minimize elevations in body temperature.
- Identify a schedule for taking her medication that will facilitate compliance with the regimen.

- Describe manifestations that should be reported to the healthcare provider.

PLANNING AND IMPLEMENTATION

- Assess knowledge and understanding of pneumonia and its effects.
- Assist to develop a medication schedule that coordinates with normal daily routine.
- Teach about the following:
  a. Importance of avoiding use of a cough suppressant except at night to facilitate rest
  b. Ways to increase fluid intake to reduce fever and maintain thin mucus for easy expectoration
  c. Beneficial effects of rest, especially during the acute phase of her illness
  d. Safe use of aspirin and acetaminophen to reduce fever
  e. Importance of taking all prescribed medication doses as scheduled
  f. Common side effects of penicillin V and their management
  g. Early manifestations of penicillin allergy that necessitate stopping the medication and notifying the healthcare provider
  h. Signs of complications of pneumonia or worsening pneumonia to report

EVALUATION

The sputum culture confirms *S. pneumoniae* as the cause of Mrs. O'Neal's pneumonia. When she returns for her follow-up appointment, she reports that she began to feel better after 2 days on the penicillin and returned to work the following Monday. Her examination reveals good breath sounds throughout with no adventitious sounds.

CRITICAL THINKING IN THE NURSING PROCESS

1. Do any of the factors identified in the case study increase Mrs. O'Neal's risk for acute bacterial pneumonia?
2. Mrs. O'Neal's WBC differential showed increased neutrophil and band counts. Describe the reason for and effect of this change.
3. Even though Mrs. O'Neal has no history of medication allergies, anaphylactic shock remains a potential risk. Describe the sequence of events leading to anaphylactic shock, its initial symptoms, and immediate nursing interventions.
4. Had Mrs. O'Neal required hospitalization to treat her acute pneumonia, interruption of her usual activities and responsibilities could lead to anxiety. Develop a care plan for this situation, using the nursing diagnosis *Altered Role Performance* related to hospitalization.

See Evaluating Your Response in Appendix C.

Discuss the following topics when preparing the patient and family for home care:

- The importance of completing the prescribed medication regimen as ordered; potential drug side effects and their management, including manifestations that necessitate stopping the drug and notifying the healthcare provider
- Recommendations for limiting activities and increasing rest
- Maintaining adequate fluid intake to keep mucus thin for easier expectoration
- Ways to maintain adequate nutritional intake, such as small, frequent, well-balanced meals
- The importance of avoiding smoking or exposure to second-hand smoke to prevent further irritation of the lungs

- Manifestations to report to the healthcare provider, such as increasing shortness of breath, difficulty breathing, increased fever, fatigue, headache, sleepiness, or confusion
- The importance of keeping all follow-up appointments to ensure disease cure

The accompanying Case Study & Nursing Care Plan provides further nursing interventions for patients treated in the community.

Patients with respiratory compromise or who are elderly or debilitated may require home care assistance to remain at home. Provide referrals to home intravenous services, home health nursing services, and home maintenance services as indicated. Community services such as Meals on Wheels can provide support to reduce the energy demands of meal preparation.

The Patient with Severe Acute Respiratory Syndrome

Severe acute respiratory syndrome (SARS) is a lower respiratory illness of unknown etiology first described in people in Asia in February 2003. Cases were identified in patients in North America, South America, Europe, and Asia before the outbreak was contained (Centers for Disease Control and Prevention [CDC], 2009d). The primary population affected by SARS is previously healthy adults aged 25 to 70 years.

Pathophysiology

The infective agent responsible for SARS is a coronavirus not previously identified in humans. This virus appears to spread primarily by contact with respiratory secretions. Other potential sources of the infection are through direct contact with an infected person or contaminated object, and exposure of the eyes or mucous membranes to respiratory secretions (CDC, 2009d). Contact with contaminated water or sewage may transmit the disease, suggesting a fecal–oral transmission as well.

The virus infects cells of the respiratory tract, leading to surface necrosis and sloughing of pneumoncytes in the alveolar spaces and formation of hyaline membranes (a fibrin and protein "film," that interferes with gas exchange within the alveoli). The alveolar damage is accompanied by inflammation of interstitial pulmonary tissues with infiltration by lymphocytes and monocyts. The virus also is found in the blood, urine, and feces.

Manifestations and Complications

The incubation period for SARS is generally 2 to 7 days, although it may be as long as 10 days in some people. Fever higher than 100.4°F (38°C) is typically the initial manifestation of the disease. The high fever may be accompanied by chills, headache, malaise, and muscle aches. After 1 to 2 days, respiratory manifestations of SARS develop, including nonproductive cough, shortness of breath, dyspnea, and possible hypoxemia. Respiratory symptoms may worsen, progressing to respiratory distress, during the second week of the illness.

While the majority of people with SARS recover, up to 20% of affected patients require intubation and mechanical ventilation (∞ see Chapter 37). Acute respiratory distress syndrome (ARDS) or multiorgan dysfunction (∞ see Chapter 11) may develop. The overall mortality rate for SARS is about 11%. The disease is less severe in children than in adults (Fishman et al., 2009).

Interdisciplinary Care

Prompt identification of SARS, infection control measures, and reporting of the disease are vital to control this potentially fatal disease. Healthcare providers and public health personnel should report cases of SARS to state and local health departments.

Diagnosis

Diagnostic testing for SARS may include the following:

- *Serology tests* (including ELISA or immunofluorescence tests) for antibodies to the coronavirus may performed, but often are undetectable during the acute stage of the illness.
- *Reverse-transcriptase PCR (RT-PCR)* testing of respiratory and blood samples provides a rapid mechanism for identifying the virus, but only about 33% of early samples are positive.
- *Chest x-ray* may be normal or show interstitial infiltrates in a focal or generalized patchy pattern. In late stages of SARS, consolidation may be evident.
- *Pulse oximetry (oxygen saturation)* often shows hypoxemia in the respiratory phase of the illness.
- *Complete blood count (CBC)* often demonstrates a low lymphocyte count early in the disease. Leukopenia and thrombocytopenia may develop at the peak of the respiratory illness.
- *Creatinine phosphokinase (CPK or CK)*, *ALT*, and *AST* levels may be markedly increased in SARS.
- *Sputum specimen* is obtained. Gram stain and culture are performed on the specimen to rule out other causes of pneumonia.
- *Blood culture* may be done to identify possible bacteremia.

Medications

At this time, no medications have been shown to be consistently effective in treating SARS. Antibiotic and/or antiviral therapy targeted at community-acquired forms of pneumonia may be administered if the diagnosis is unclear.

Infection Control

Because healthcare workers are at risk for developing SARS after caring for infected patients, infection control precautions should be immediately instituted when SARS is suspected. Standard precautions (see Appendix A) are implemented along with contact and airborne precautions. The CDC (2009d) recommends hand hygiene, gown, gloves, eye protection, and an N95 respirator to prevent transmission of SARS in healthcare settings.

When patients with SARS are managed in the community, they are advised to remain home for 10 days after the fever has resolved and until respiratory symptoms are absent or minimal. Members of the household are advised to wash hands frequently or use alcohol-based hand rubs. The patient is advised to cover the mouth and nose with tissue when coughing or sneezing and to wear a surgical mask during close contact with uninfected people. Sharing of utensils, towels, and bedding should be avoided. Routine cleaning (e.g., washing with soap and hot water) is adequate to disinfect objects and no special precautions are necessary for disposing of waste.

Treatments

Care of the patient with SARS is supportive. Oxygen may be administered to treat hypoxemia. Intubation and mechanical ventilation may be required if respiratory failure or acute respiratory distress syndrome (ARDS) develops.

∞ Nursing Care

Nursing care of the patient with SARS focuses on preventing spread of the disease to others and providing respiratory support.

Health Promotion

Use respiratory and contact infection control precautions in addition to standard precautions when caring for all patients with suspected SARS to prevent spread of the disease to healthcare workers or other patients.

Assessment

Focused assessment data for the patient with suspected SARS include the following. For a more complete respiratory assessment, ∞ see Chapter 34.

- *Health history:* Current symptoms, including fever, malaise, shortness of breath, and cough; onset of symptoms; recent international travel or exposure to a person known to have SARS.
- *Physical assessment:* Vital signs including temperature; respiratory status, including respiratory rate, depth, and effort; presence of cough; adventitious lung sounds.

Nursing Diagnoses and Interventions

The patient with SARS poses a risk for spread of the infection to healthcare workers and others. In addition, while many people with this disease experience only mild symptoms and recover fully and uneventfully, others develop severe respiratory distress and may require significant respiratory support. Gas exchange may be impaired, leading to significant hypoxemia. In addition to the nursing diagnoses discussed in the previous section on pneumonia, *Impaired Gas Exchange* and *Risk for Infection* are priority nursing diagnoses.

Impaired Gas Exchange

SARS causes hypoxemia of varying degrees in affected patients. Significant hypoxemia may necessitate intubation and mechanical ventilation to support cellular function until recovery occurs.

- Monitor vital signs, color, oxygen saturation, and arterial blood gases. Assess for manifestations such as anxiety or apprehension, restlessness, confusion or lethargy, or complaints of headache. *These assessment data alert the nurse and care providers to potential hypoxemia or hypercapnia due to impaired gas exchange.*

> **PRACTICE ALERT**
> Promptly report signs of respiratory distress, including tachypnea, tachycardia, nasal flaring, use of accessory muscles, intercostal retractions, cyanosis, increasing restlessness, anxiety, or decreased level of consciousness. These may be early manifestations of respiratory failure and inability to maintain ventilatory effort.

- Promptly report worsening arterial blood gases and oxygen saturation levels. *Close assessment of these values allows timely intervention as needed.*
- Maintain oxygen therapy and mechanical ventilation as ordered. Hyperoxygenate prior to suctioning. *Oxygen and mechanical ventilation support alveolar gas exchange. Hyperoxygenation prior to suctioning reduces the degree of hypoxemia that occurs during suctioning.*
- Place in Fowler's or high Fowler's position. *Sitting positions decrease pressure on the diaphragm and chest, improving lung ventilation and decreasing the work of breathing.*
- Minimize activities and energy expenditures by assisting with ADLs, spacing procedures and activities, and allowing uninterrupted rest periods. *Rest is vital to reduce oxygen and energy demands.*

> **PRACTICE ALERT**
> Avoid sedatives and respiratory depressant drugs unless mechanically ventilated. These medications can further depress the respiratory drive, worsening respiratory failure.

- If intubation and mechanical ventilation is necessary, explain the procedure and its purpose to the patient and family, providing reassurance that this *temporary* measure improves oxygenation and reduces the work of breathing. Alert that talking is not possible while the endotracheal tube is in place, and establish a means of communication. *Thorough explanation is important to relieve anxiety.*

See the section in ∞ Chapter 37 on respiratory failure for more information about caring for a patient who is intubated and mechanically ventilated.

Risk for Infection

The spread of SARS is a risk both in the healthcare facility and the community in which the patient resides. Respiratory and contract precautions are recommended to prevent the spread of SARS via respiratory secretions or contact with the virus.

- Place the patient in a private room with airflow control that prevents air within the room from circulating into the hallway or other rooms. A negative flow room in which air is diluted by at least six fresh-air exchanges per hour is recommended. *A negative flow room and multiple fresh-air exchanges dilute the concentration of virus within the room and prevent its spread to adjacent areas.*
- Use standard precautions and respiratory and contact isolation techniques as recommended by the CDC, including wearing respirators, gowns, and eye protection when caring for patients with SARS. *These measures are important to prevent the spread of SARS to others.*
- Discuss the reasons for and importance of respiratory and contact isolation procedures during treatment. *Maintenance of infection control precautions during and immediately following the febrile and respiratory phases of SARS is vital to prevent its spread to healthcare workers and the community.*
- Place a mask on the patient when transporting to other parts of the facility for diagnostic or treatment procedures. *Covering the patient's nose and mouth during transport minimizes air contamination and the risk to visitors and personnel.*
- Inform all personnel having contact with the patient of the diagnosis. *This allows personnel to take appropriate precautions.*
- Assist visitors to mask prior to entering the room. *Providing visitors with appropriate masks or respirators reduces their risk of infection.*
- Teach the patient how to limit transmitting the disease to others:
  a. Always cough and expectorate into tissues.
  b. Dispose of tissues properly, placing them in a closed bag.
  c. Wear a mask if sneezing or unable to control respiratory secretions.
  d. Do not share eating utensils, towels, bedding, or other objects with others, as this disease may also be spread by contact with contaminated objects.

Teaching appropriate precautions helps prevent the spread of SARS to others while allowing as much freedom from restraints as possible.

Community-Based Care

Many patients with SARS experience only mild symptoms and are appropriately cared for in the community. Teaching about home care and infection control precautions is vital to prevent spread of this disease to the community. Include the following topics when teaching for home care:

■ The disease, its origin, and how it is spread
■ Manifestations of impaired respiratory status to report to the healthcare provider
■ Preventing spread of the disease to others:
  1. Cover the mouth and nose with tissues when coughing or sneezing. Personally dispose of tissues in a paper bag or the garbage. Wear a surgical mask during close contact with other members of the household.
  2. Limit interactions outside the home; do not go to work, school, or other public areas until you have been free of fever for 10 days and your respiratory symptoms are resolving.
  3. Remind all members of the household to wash hands (or use an alcohol-based hand sanitizer) frequently, particularly after direct contact with body fluids.
  4. Do not share eating utensils, towels, or bedding with others. These items can be cleaned with soap and hot water between uses. Clean contaminated surfaces with a household disinfectant.
■ Monitoring uninfected members of the household for signs of the illness (Instruct to report fever or respiratory symptoms to the healthcare provider.)

The Patient with Lung Abscess

A **lung abscess** is a localized area of lung destruction or necrosis and pus formation. The most common cause of lung abscess is aspiration and resulting pneumonia. Risk factors, therefore, are those for aspiration: decreased level of consciousness due to anesthesia, injury or disease of the central nervous system, seizure, excessive sedation, or alcohol abuse; swallowing disorders; dental caries; and debilitation secondary to cancer or chronic disease. Lung abscess also may occur as a complication of some types of pneumonia, including those due to *Staphylococcus aureus*, *Klebsiella*, and *Legionella*.

Pathophysiology and Manifestations

A lung abscess forms after lung tissue becomes consolidated (i.e., after alveoli become filled with fluid, pus, and microorganisms). In up to 89% of patients, anaerobic organisms are identified. Consolidated tissue becomes necrotic. This necrotic process can spread to involve the entire bronchopulmonary segment and progress proximally until it ruptures into a bronchus. With rupture, the contents of the abscess empty into the bronchus, leaving a cavity filled with air and fluid, a process known as *cavitation*. If purulent material from the abscess is not expectorated, the infection may spread, leading to diffuse pneumonia or a syndrome similar to acute respiratory distress syndrome (ARDS, discussed in ∞ Chapter 37).

Manifestations of lung abscess typically develop about 2 weeks after the precipitating event (aspiration, pneumonia, and so on). Their onset may be either acute or insidious. Early symptoms are those of pneumonia: productive cough, chills and fever, pleuritic chest pain, malaise, and anorexia. The temperature may be significantly elevated, 103°F (39.4°C) or higher. When the abscess ruptures, the patient may expectorate large amounts of foul-smelling, purulent, and possibly blood-streaked sputum. Breath sounds are diminished, and crackles may be noted in the region of the abscess. A dull percussion tone is also present.

Interdisciplinary Care

The diagnosis of lung abscess usually is based on the history and presentation. The CBC may indicate leukocytosis. Sputum culture may not show the organism involved unless rupture occurs. Chest x-ray shows a thick-walled, solitary cavity with surrounding consolidation, although differentiating lung abscess from consolidation can be difficult until cavitation occurs.

Lung abscess is treated with antibiotic therapy, usually intravenous clindamycin (Cleocin), amoxicillin-clavulanate (Augmentin), or penicillin (Papadakis & McPhee, 2007). Antibiotic therapy should be continued until the chest radiograph improves, usually at least one month. Postural drainage may be ordered to relieve obstruction and promote drainage. In some cases, bronchoscopy is used to drain the abscess. If the pleural space becomes involved, a chest tube (*tube thoracostomy*) may be used to drain the abscess. See the section on pneumothorax for further discussion of chest tubes.

∾ Nursing Care

Although most patients with lung abscess recover fully with appropriate antibiotic treatment, rupture and drainage of the abscess into a bronchus is a frightening experience. Nursing care needs of the patient relate primarily to maintaining a patent airway and adequate gas exchange. The following nursing diagnoses may be appropriate for the patient with lung abscess:

■ *Risk for Ineffective Airway Clearance* related to large amounts of purulent drainage in bronchi
■ *Impaired Gas Exchange* related to necrotic and consolidated lung tissue
■ *Hyperthermia* related to infectious process
■ *Anxiety* related to copious amounts of purulent sputum

Patient and family teaching focuses on the importance of completing the prescribed antibiotic therapy. Most lung abscesses are successfully treated with antibiotics; however, treatment may last up to 1 month or more. Emphasize the importance of completing the entire course of therapy to eliminate the infecting organisms. Teach about the medication, including the name, dose, and desired and adverse effects. Stress the need to contact the healthcare provider if symptoms do not improve or if they become worse. Infection from lung abscess can spread not only to lung and pleural tissue but systemically, causing sepsis. If postural drainage is ordered, teach the patient and family how to perform this procedure. When procedures such as bronchoscopy or thoracostomy are performed to drain the abscess, provide preoperative teaching and instruction on postoperative care.

The Patient with Tuberculosis

Tuberculosis (TB) is a chronic, recurrent infectious disease that usually affects the lungs, although any organ can be affected. Caused by *Mycobacterium tuberculosis*, TB is uncommon in the United States, especially among young adults of European descent.

M. tuberculosis is a relatively slow-growing, slender, rod-shaped, acid-fast organism with a waxy outer capsule, which increases its resistance to destruction. Although the lungs are usually infected, TB can involve other organs as well. It is transmitted by *droplet nuclei*, airborne droplets produced when an infected person coughs, sneezes, speaks, or sings. The tiny droplets can remain suspended in air for several hours. Infection may develop when a susceptible host breathes in air containing droplet nuclei and the contaminated particle eludes the normal defenses of the upper respiratory tract to reach the alveoli.

Pathophysiology
Pulmonary Tuberculosis
Minute droplet nuclei containing one to three bacilli that elude upper airway defense systems to enter the lungs implant in an alveolus or respiratory bronchiole, usually in an upper lobe. As the bacteria multiply, they cause a local inflammatory response. The inflammatory response brings neutrophils and macrophages to the site. These phagocytic cells surround and engulf the bacilli, isolating them and preventing their spread. *M. tb* continues to slowly multiply; some enter the lymphatic system to stimulate a cellular-mediated immune response (∞ see Chapter 12 to review immune responses). Neutrophils and macrophages isolate the bacteria but cannot destroy them. A granulomatous lesion called a *tubercle*, a sealed-off colony of bacilli, is formed. Within the tubercle, infected tissue dies, forming a cheeselike center, a process called *caseation necrosis*.

If the immune response is adequate, scar tissue develops around the tubercle, and the bacilli remain encapsulated. These lesions eventually calcify and are visible on x-ray. The patient, while infected by *M. tb*, does not develop TB disease. If the immune response is inadequate to contain the bacilli, the disease of TB can develop. Occasionally, the infection can progress, leading to extensive destruction of lung tissue. In *primary tuberculosis*, granulomatous tissue may erode into a bronchus or into a blood vessel, allowing the disease to spread throughout the lung or other organs. This severe form of TB is uncommon in adults (Fishman et al., 2008; Huether & McCance, 2008).

A previously healed TB lesion may be reactivated. *Reactivation tuberculosis* occurs when the immune system is suppressed due to age, disease, or use of immunosuppressive drugs. The extent of lung disease can vary from small lesions to extensive cavitation of lung tissue. Tubercles rupture, spreading bacilli into the airways to form satellite lesions and produce tuberculosis pneumonia. Without treatment, massive lung involvement can lead to death, or a more chronic process

of tubercle formation and cavitation may result. People with chronic disease continue to spread *M. tb* into the environment, potentially infecting others. The Pathophysiology Illustrated feature on pages 1192–1193 illustrates the pathogenesis of TB.

Patients with HIV disease are at high risk for developing active TB, due to primary infection or reactivation. HIV infection suppresses cellular immunity, which is vital to limiting the replication and spread of *M. tb*.

Manifestations and Complications
The initial infection causes few symptoms and typically goes unnoticed until the tuberculin test becomes positive or calcified lesions are seen on chest x-ray. Manifestations of primary progressive or reactivation TB often develop insidiously and are initially nonspecific (see the following Manifestations box). Fatigue, weight loss, anorexia, low-grade afternoon fever, and night sweats are common. A dry cough develops, which later becomes productive of purulent and/or blood-tinged sputum. It is often at this stage that the patient seeks medical attention.

Tuberculosis empyema and bronchopleural fistula are the most serious complications of pulmonary TB. When a TB lesion ruptures, bacilli may contaminate the pleural space. Rupture also may allow air to enter the pleural space from the lung, causing pneumothorax.

Extrapulmonary Tuberculosis
When primary disease or reactivation allows live bacilli to enter the bronchi, the disease may spread through the blood and lymph system to other organs. These distant disease metastases may produce an active lesion, or they may become dormant and reactivate at a later time. Extrapulmonary TB is especially prevalent in people with HIV disease.

MILIARY TUBERCULOSIS *Miliary tuberculosis* results from hematogenous spread (through the blood) of the bacilli throughout the body. Miliary tuberculosis causes chills and fever, weakness, malaise, and progressive dyspnea. Multiple lesions evenly distributed throughout the lungs are noted on x-ray. The sputum rarely contains organisms. The bone marrow is usually involved, causing anemia, thrombocytopenia, and leukocytosis. Without appropriate treatment, the prognosis is poor.

GENITOURINARY TUBERCULOSIS The kidney and genitourinary tract are common extrapulmonary sites for TB. The organism spreads to the kidney through the blood, initiating an inflammatory process similar to that which occurs in the lungs. Reactivation can occur years after the original infection. As the lesion then enlarges and caseates, a large portion of the renal parenchyma is destroyed. The infection then can spread to rest

PATHOPHYSIOLOGY ILLUSTRATED
The Pathogenesis of Tuberculosis

Alveolus

Alveolar duct

Pulmonary arteriole

Terminal bronchiole

Pulmonary venule

M. tuberculosis, a rod-shaped aerobic bacterium, is spread via droplet nuclei from an infected person to a susceptible host. Droplet nuclei are tiny droplets of respiratory secretions spread via coughing, sneezing, or speaking. When dried, they can remain suspended in air for several hours. Most inhaled bacilli are trapped in the upper airways; those reaching distal airways implant in the respiratory bronchioles and alveoli. Rarely, these tubercule bacilli multiply unchecked to cause primary tuberculosis. In most cases, activated alveolar macrophages ingest the bacilli. The bacilli may be destroyed; however, unique characteristics of the tuberculosis bacillus resist its destruction by the macrophage. The bacilli multiply within the macrophage, eventually killing the macrophage.

Alveolar macrophages

Tubercle bacillus

Infiltrating macrophage (not activated)

Pulmonary capillary

Infiltrating neutrophils

Bronchiole

Ingested tubercle bacillus

Early tubercle

Neutrophil

The dead macrophages lyse, releasing various chemotaxic factors into the bloodstream. Neutrophils and non-activated macrophages are attracted to the site. These phagocytic cells ingest the tubercule bacilli released from the lysed macrophages.

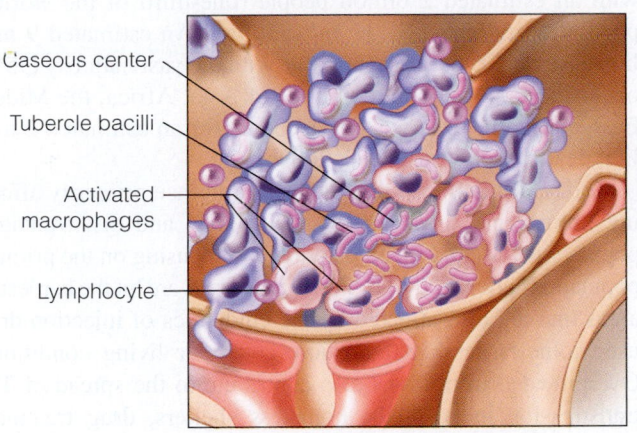

Caseous center

Tubercle bacilli

Activated macrophages

Lymphocyte

After several weeks, a delayed hypersensitivity response to bacterial antigens destroys many of the macrophages. Concurrently, a cell-mediated immune response activates additional macrophages, which ingest and destroy the bacilli. The lysed macrophages and bacilli are surrounded by a mass of live, activated macrophages and lymphocytes. Scar (granulomatous) tissue forms, encapsulating the primary lesion. Most lesions calcify and are visible on x-ray. These lesions may remain dormant for a year or more (in some cases, many years) before being reactivated to produce secondary or reactivation tuberculosis.

When the immune and macrophage-activating responses are weakened by age or disease (e.g., HIV disease), the tuberculosis bacilli continue to multiply within the lesion. The caseous material at the center of the lesion liquefies, and the lesion grows.

Outer scar tissue layer of mature tubercle

Tubercle bacilli

Tuberculous cavity

Rupture of bronchiole wall

Rupture of capillary wall

The enlarging lesion damages surrounding bronchial walls and blood vessels. Granulomatous tissue surrounding the lesion can erode into a bronchus, forming an air-filling cavity. Within this cavity, the bacilli multiply, spreading into the airways and the environment via infected sputum. Bacilli multiply, spreading into the airways and the environment via infected sputum. Bacilli also spread via the blood and within macrophages to regional lymph nodes, and from there to many organs and tissues. Resulting extrapulmonary lesions evolve in the same sequence as pulmonary lesions.

MANIFESTATIONS of Pulmonary Tuberculosis

- Fatigue
- Weight loss
- Anorexia
- Low-grade afternoon fever and night sweats
- Cough: initially dry, later productive of purulent and/or blood-tinged sputum

of the urinary tract, including the ureters and bladder. Scarring and strictures commonly result. In men, the prostate, seminal vesicles, and epididymis may be involved. In women, TB may affect the fallopian tubes and ovaries.

Manifestations of genitourinary tuberculosis develop insidiously. Symptoms of a urinary tract infection, including malaise, dysuria, hematuria, and pyuria, develop. Flank pain may be present. Men may develop manifestations of epididymitis or prostatitis: perineal, sacral, or scrotal pain and tenderness; difficulty voiding; and fever. Women may have manifestations of pelvic inflammatory disease, impaired fertility, or ectopic pregnancy.

TUBERCULOSIS MENINGITIS Tuberculosis meningitis results when TB spreads to the subarachnoid space. In the United States, this complication most often affects older adults, usually from reactivation of latent disease. Manifestations develop gradually, with listlessness, irritability, anorexia, and fever. Headache and behavior changes are common early symptoms in the older adult. As the disease progresses, the headache increases in intensity, vomiting develops, and the level of consciousness decreases. Convulsions and coma may follow. Without appropriate treatment, neurologic effects may become permanent.

SKELETAL TUBERCULOSIS TB of the bones and joints is most likely to occur during childhood, when bone epiphyses are open and their blood supply is rich. The organisms spread via the blood to vertebrae, the ends of long bones, and joints. Immune and inflammatory processes isolate the bacilli, and the disease often becomes evident years or decades later.

Tuberculous spondylitis usually involves the thoracic vertebrae, eroding vertebral bodies and causing them to collapse. Significant kyphosis develops, and the spinal cord may be compressed. The large, weight-bearing joints (hips and knees) are most often affected by tuberculous arthritis, although other joints may be affected, particularly if they have been previously damaged. The involved joint is painful, warm, and tender.

Incidence and Prevalence

The incidence of TB fell steadily until the mid-1980s, thanks to improved sanitation, surveillance, and treatment of people with active disease. The late 1980s and early 1990s saw a resurgence of the disease, attributed primarily to the HIV/AIDS epidemic, the emergence of multiple-drug-resistant (MDR) strains of TB, and social factors such as immigration, poverty, homelessness, and drug abuse. Today, the TB rates have been dropping since 1993; however, the rate of decline has lessened since 2000. There were 12,898 cases of TB reported in the United States in 2008, the lowest number recorded since national reporting

began in 1953 (CDC, 2009c). This decline can be attributed to TB-control programs that emphasize promptly identifying new cases and initiating and completing appropriate therapy.

Worldwide, TB continues to be a significant health problem, with an estimated 2 billion people (one-third of the world's population) infected by *M. tuberculosis*. An estimated 9 million cases of TB develop annually, with the vast majority (95%) occurring in developing countries of Asia, Africa, the Middle East, and Latin America. TB accounts for an estimated 2 million deaths each year (CDC, 2009c).

Today, TB in the United States is a disease primarily affecting immigrants, those infected with HIV, and disadvantaged populations. See the accompanying box focusing on the primary populations affected by TB. Poor urban areas are hit the hardest—areas that are also affected by the epidemics of injection drug use, homelessness, malnutrition, and poor living conditions. Overcrowded institutions also contribute to the spread of TB; transmission in hospitals, homeless shelters, drug treatment centers, prisons, and residential facilities has been documented. People with altered immune function, including older adults (see the box on page 1195) and people with AIDS are at particular risk for TB. Some strains of *M. tb* have become resistant to the first line drugs used to treat the disease (isoniazid and rifampin), with the number of multidrug-resistant (MDR TB) cases of TB increasing by 13.3% between 2004 and 2005 (CDC, 2009c). In 2006, the World Health Organization added the category of extensively drug resistant (XDR TB) to describe the rare TB case that is resistant to the first line TB drugs as well as at least one of the second line TB drugs (kanamycin, capreomycin, or amikacin) and at least one drug in the quinilone antibiotic sub-class (World Health Organziation, 2008).

FAST FACTS

- World-wide, approximately 39% of identified *M. tuberculosis* strains are MDR, demonstrating resistance to at least isoniazid and rifampin.
- Of MDR TB strains identified worldwide, 7% are XDR. XDR TB is resistant to isoniazid and rifampin, as well as at least three of the six main classes of second-line TB drugs (CDC, 2009c).
- The prevalence of MDR and XDR TB in the United States is lower, with 1.6% of cases reported from 1993 through 2004 identified as MDR. Of these, 4.1% were resistant to three or more classes of antituberculosis drugs, qualifying as XDR TB (CDC, 2009c; WHO, 2008).

Risk Factors

The risk for infection by *M. tb* is affected by characteristics of the infectious person, the extent of air contamination, duration of exposure, and susceptibility of the host. The number of microbes in the sputum, frequency and force of coughing, and behaviors such as covering the mouth when coughing affect the production of droplet nuclei. In a small, closed, or poorly ventilated space, droplet nuclei become more concentrated, increasing the risk of exposure. Prolonged contact, such as living in the same household, increases the risk. Less-than-optimal immune function, a problem for people in lower socioeconomic groups, injection drug users, the homeless, alcoholics, and people with HIV infection, increases the susceptibility of the host. See the box on page 1195.

NURSING CARE OF THE OLDER ADULT **Tuberculosis**

The prevalence of active TB is significantly higher among older Caucasian adults in the United States than it is in young adults (Kasper, 2005). Of cases among older adults, approximately 90% occur due to reactivation of the dormant bacterium. Older adults are at increased risk for reactivation TB due to age-related decreases in cell-mediated immunity. Chronic illnesses, poor nutrition, gastrectomy, alcoholism, or the long-term use of steroids and immunosuppressive agents may also reactivate dormant TB lesions.

Presenting symptoms of TB in the older adult are often vague, including coughing, weight loss, anorexia, or periodic fevers. These signs and symptoms should not be dismissed as a normal part of aging.

Residents of nursing homes are at increased risk for acquiring TB because of group living. Yearly tuberculin skin testing with purified protein derivative (PPD) is often required by state health departments. If the initial test is negative, a repeat PPD in 1 to 2 weeks is recommended. This improves sensitivity to the test so that silent cases of TB are not missed. A chest x-ray and sputum culture for acid-fast bacilli are obtained if the PPD is positive.

Successful treatment for TB includes taking at least two drugs for at least 6 to 9 months to totally eradicate the organism. Older adults usually do not develop drug-resistant forms of TB because they acquired the disease prior to emergence of drug-resistant strains.

ASSESSING FOR HOME CARE

Community-dwelling older adults are susceptible to TB as well as those in care facilities. The older adult with respiratory symptoms often is treated presumptively for pneumonia, without a sputum smear and Gram stain. Older adults living in the community may not have had a tuberculin test or chest x-ray for many years.

Assess risk factors for TB:

- General health and nutritional status, including intake of specific nutrients such as vitamin D (lack of vitamin D is associated with a higher risk of developing active TB)
- Presence of a chronic disease such as silicosis, diabetes, alcoholism, or HIV infection; past history of a gastrectomy
- Past history of a positive tuberculin test that now has converted to negative
- Medications such as corticosteroids or other immunosuppressive drugs
  Assess living and social situation:
- Natural light and ventilation in the home
- Access to clean water, cooking facilities, grocery stores, and other services
- Possible exposure to infected people, for example, sharing a household with someone with active TB, crowded living facilities, homelessness, frequent participation in senior activities, volunteer work in residential care facilities or other institutional settings
- Access to health care

TB is typically treated in the community; hospitalization or institutionalization rarely is necessary or desirable. For the older adult being treated for active TB in the community, assess the following:

- Knowledge and understanding of the disease and the prescribed treatment regimen
- Mental status and ability to follow prescribed regimen and precautions to avoid exposing others to the disease
- Transportation and ability to access healthcare services on a regular basis
- Financial resources to complete treatment and follow-up care
- Need for home health or social services to ensure adequate treatment

TEACHING FOR HOME CARE

Teaching focuses on improving the older adult's ability to self-manage the disease and treatment. Teach about TB and how it is spread. Emphasize the importance of taking all medications as prescribed and complying with follow-up appointments and testing. Discuss the importance of the following:

- Using disposable tissues to contain respiratory secretions, especially during the first 2 weeks of treatment when the disease may be transmitted to others
- Avoiding exposure to crowds or people with infectious diseases
- Eating a well-balanced diet with adequate nutrients
- Getting adequate rest, sleep, and exercise to maintain good general health
- Ensuring that housemates or others having frequent contact with the patient are tested and receive prophylactic treatment if indicated

Teach about possible side effects of the prescribed medications and the importance of reporting these to healthcare providers:

- Peripheral neuropathy (numbness, tingling, or a burning sensation of the extremities) may occur with isoniazid (INH). Pyridoxine (vitamin B_6) often is prescribed to prevent this adverse effect.
- Both INH and rifampin may cause hepatitis. Avoid alcohol while taking these drugs, and report any manifestations such as nausea and anorexia, jaundice, a change in urine or stool color, or pain in the upper right quadrant.
- Rifampin may cause an orange-red coloration of saliva and urine.
- Streptomycin can affect hearing and balance; promptly report any changes, as they may be irreversible.
- Ethambutol may affect red-green color discrimination and visual acuity. Use caution when driving or walking in unfamiliar areas and promptly report any vision changes.

FOCUS ON CULTURAL DIVERSITY
Tuberculosis

- The TB case rate for foreign-born U.S. residents is 8.7 times higher than that for people born in the United States (CDC, 2006b).
- Asians and Pacific Islanders living in the United States have the highest case rates, nearly 20 times higher than that for Whites.
- Case rates for Blacks and Hispanics in the United States are 7 to 8 times that for Whites.

Interdisciplinary Care

TB was a major public health concern earlier in this century, before the development of effective sanitation measures and drug treatment. Developing drug-resistant strains, susceptibility of people with HIV disease, and inadequate access to healthcare for high-risk populations contribute to the continuing significance of TB as a significant public health threat. Interdisciplinary care, therefore, focuses on the following:

- Early detection
- Accurate diagnosis

- Effective disease treatment
- Preventing TB spread to others

Hospitalization is rarely required to treat TB. With appropriate treatment, patients become noninfective to others fairly rapidly. However, a patient with active TB may be admitted for a concurrent problem or a complication of the disease. Nurses and other healthcare workers are at risk for exposure if the disease has not yet been diagnosed. When a patient with TB is institutionalized, maintain respiratory isolation to minimize the risk of infection to other patients and to the healthcare workers.

Noncompliance with prescribed treatment is a major problem in treating active TB: The patient can continue transmitting the disease to others, and drug-resistant strains of bacteria can develop when treatment is incomplete. TB must be reported to local and state public health departments; contacts are identified and examined. People who share living or work environments with the patient are tested and receive prophylactic treatment. Continuing contact with patients who have active TB is vital to ensure effective cure.

Screening

The tuberculin test is used to screen for TB infection. A cellular, or delayed hypersensitivity, response to *M. tuberculosis* develops within 3 to 10 weeks after the infection. Injecting a small amount of *purified protein derivative (PPD)* of tuberculin any time thereafter activates this response, attracting macrophages to the area and causing a pronounced local inflammatory response. The amount of induration surrounding the injection site is used to determine infection (see Table 36–5 and Figure 36–7 ■). It is important to remember that a positive response indicates that infection and a cellular (T-cell)

Figure 36–7 ■ *A,* Intradermal injection for tuberculin testing. *B,* The injection causes a local inflammatory response (wheal). *C,* Measurement of induration following tuberculin testing.

response have developed; however, it does not mean that active disease is present or that the patient is infectious to others.

Several methods are currently available for tuberculin testing:

- *Intradermal PPD (Mantoux) test:* 0.1 mL of PPD (5 tuberculin units, or TU) is injected intradermally into the dorsal aspect of the forearm. This test is read within 48 to 72 hours, the peak reaction period, and recorded as the diameter of induration (raised area, not erythema) in millimeters.
- *Multiple-puncture (tine) test:* A multiple-puncture device is used to introduce tuberculin into the skin. This test is less accurate than other testing methods. A vesicular reaction is considered positive; any other reaction must be confirmed using a Mantoux test.

Although it is impractical and unnecessary to screen the entire population, the CDC recommends screening people in the following risk groups:

- People with or at high risk for HIV infection
- Close contacts of people who have or are suspected of having infectious TB
- People with medical risk factors, such as silicosis, chronic malabsorption, end-stage renal failure, diabetes mellitus, immunosuppression, and hematologic and other malignancies
- People born in countries with a high prevalence of TB
- Medically underserved low-income populations, including racial and ethnic minorities
- Alcoholics and injection drug users

(Left margin: Tuberculosis Video)

TABLE 36–5 Interpreting Tuberculin Test Results

AREA OF INDURATION	SIGNIFICANCE
Less than 5 mm	Negative response; does not rule out infection.
5 to 9 mm	Positive for people who - are in close contact with a patient with infective TB. - have an abnormal chest x-ray. - have HIV infection or are immunocompromised. - have an organ transplant. Negative for all others.
10 to 15 mm	Positive for people who have other risk factors: - Birth in a high-incidence country - African American, Hispanic, Asian American in poverty areas - Injection drug use - Residence in a long-term care facility, correctional institution, residential care setting, homeless shelter - Medical risk factors (e.g., malnutrition, diabetes, others)
Greater than 15 mm	Positive for all people

■ Residents and staff of long-term residential facilities, such as long-term care facilities, correctional institutions, and mental health facilities

False-negative responses are common in people who are immunosuppressed. A two-step procedure may be necessary to elicit a positive response. If the first test elicits a negative response, a second PPD test is given 1 week later. If the second test also is negative, the patient either is free of infection or is *anergic* (unable to react to common antigens). This two-step procedure is recommended for long-term care residents and workers.

Diagnosis

A positive tuberculin test alone does not indicate active disease. Sputum tests for the bacillus and chest x-rays are routinely used to diagnose and evaluate active disease. A series of three consecutive early-morning sputum specimens is typically examined for bacilli. Use special procedures or personal protective devices when obtaining sputum specimens. If possible, collect specimens in a room equipped with airflow control devices, ultraviolet light, or both. Alternatively, have the patient step outside to collect the specimen. Wear a mask capable of filtering droplet nuclei when collecting sputum specimens. Aerosol therapy, percussion, and postural drainage may help the patient produce sputum. Occasionally, tracheal suctioning, bronchoscopy, or gastric lavage may be necessary to obtain a specimen. See the box on page 1130 for nursing care related to bronchoscopy.

■ *Sputum smear* is microscopically examined for *acid-fast bacilli*. M. tuberculosis resists decolorizing chemicals after staining. This property is called "acid-fast." The acid-fast smear provides a rapid indicator of the tubercle bacillus.
■ *Sputum culture* positive for *M. tuberculosis* provides the definitive diagnosis. However, *M. tuberculosis* is slow growing, requiring 4 to 8 weeks before it can be detected using traditional culture techniques. Automated radiometric culture systems (such as Bactec) allow detection of *M. tuberculosis* in several days.
■ Once the organism is detected, *sensitivity testing* is performed to identify appropriate drug therapy.
■ *Polymerase chain reaction (PCR)* permits rapid detection of DNA from *M. tuberculosis*.
■ *Chest x-ray* is ordered to diagnose and evaluate TB. Typical findings in pulmonary TB include dense lesions in the apical and posterior segments of the upper lobe and possible cavity formation.

Prior to initiating antituberculosis drug therapy, several additional diagnostic tests should be done to establish baseline data for monitoring potential adverse effects of the drugs.

■ *Liver function tests* are obtained prior to treatment with isoniazid (INH) as this drug is hepatotoxic.
■ A thorough *vision examination* is done prior to treatment with ethambutol, a commonly used antituberculosis medication. Optic neuritis is a potential adverse effect of this drug. Periodic eye examinations are scheduled during the course of therapy.
■ *Audiometric testing* is performed before streptomycin therapy is initiated. Ototoxicity is a significant adverse effect of streptomycin and other aminoglycoside antibiotics. Hearing also is evaluated periodically during the course of therapy to detect any hearing loss.

Medications

Chemotherapeutic medications are used both to prevent and treat TB infection. Goals of the pharmacologic treatment of TB are to do the following:

■ Make the disease noncommunicable to others.
■ Reduce symptoms of the disease.
■ Effect a cure in the shortest possible time.

Prophylactic treatment is used to prevent active TB. Patients with a recent skin test conversion from negative to positive are often started on prophylactic therapy, especially when other risk factors are present. Prophylactic therapy also is used for people in close household contact with a person whose sputum is positive for bacilli. Single-drug therapy is effective for prophylactic treatment, whereas treatment of active disease always involves two or more chemotherapeutic medications. For adults, isoniazid (INH), 300 mg per day for a period of 6 to 12 months, is commonly used to prevent active TB.

When isoniazid prophylaxis is contraindicated, bacilli Calmette-Guérin (BCG) vaccine may be prescribed. This vaccine is widely used in developing countries. BCG is made from an attenuated strain of *M. bovis*, a closely related bacillus that causes TB in cattle. In the United States, BCG vaccine is recommended only for infants, children, and healthcare workers with a negative tuberculin test who are repeatedly exposed to untreated or ineffectively treated people with active disease. After vaccination with BCG, a positive reaction to tuberculin testing is common. Periodic chest x-rays may be required for screening purposes.

The tuberculosis bacillus mutates readily to drug-resistant forms when only one anti-infective agent is used. Active disease is always treated with concurrent use of at least two antibacterial medications to which the organism is sensitive. The primary antituberculosis drugs can prevent development of resistance because all act by different mechanisms. However, the organism is protected within the tubercle, and 6 or more months of treatment is necessary to eradicate it.

Newly diagnosed TB is typically treated with an initial regimen of four oral antitubercular drugs, isoniazid (INH), rifampin, and pyrazinamide, and ethambutol daily (or several times per week on a decreasing schedule of frequency) for the first 2 months of treatment. This initial regimen is followed by at least 4 additional months of therapy with isoniazid and rifampin, given daily, twice per week, or weekly. In the presence of HIV infection, treatment is continued for at least 9 months. The most common antituberculosis drugs are outlined in Table 36–6; their nursing implications are outlined in the following Medication Administration box.

If a drug-resistant strain is suspected, therapy is tailored to the resistance. In some cases, four or more anti-infective drugs may be used.

Antitubercular medications have many adverse and toxic effects. Close monitoring during therapy is necessary. Most have some degree of, or risk for, hepatotoxicity. For this reason, patients should avoid using alcohol and other drugs (such as acetaminophen) or chemicals that can damage the liver. Baseline liver and renal function studies are done prior to initiating therapy. Audiometric testing also may be done before

TABLE 36–6 Antituberculosis Medications

DRUG AND DOSAGE	ADVERSE EFFECTS	NURSING IMPLICATIONS
Isoniazid (INH), oral: 300 mg daily or 900 mg one, two, or three times weekly	Peripheral neuropathy Hepatitis	Administer pyridoxine (vitamin B$_6$) concurrently. Monitor liver function studies (AST and ALT); avoid other hepatotoxins.
Rifampin (RMP), oral: 600 mg daily or two or three times weekly	Hepatitis Flulike syndrome; fever Colors body fluids—including sweat, urine, saliva, tears, and cerebrospinal fluid (CSF)—orange-red	As for INH. Do not miss or skip doses; flulike syndrome and fever occur when drug is resumed. Contact lenses may become discolored and should not be worn.
Pyrazinamide (PZA), oral: 1 g to 2 g daily; or 2 g to 4 g twice weekly	Hyperuricemia Hepatotoxicity	Monitor uric acid levels. Monitor AST and ALT; avoid other hepatotoxins.
Ethambutol (EMB), oral: 800 mg to 1600 mg daily; or 2 g to 4 g twice weekly	Optic neuritis	Monitor red-green color discrimination and visual acuity.
Streptomycin (SM), intramuscular: 15 mg/kg, up to 1 g daily; or 25 to 30 mg/kg twice weekly	Ototoxicity, vertigo Nephrotoxicity	Have periodic audiometric examinations conducted. Monitor renal function studies, including BUN and serum creatinine.

treatment is started, because several commonly used medications can affect hearing. Regular visits to a healthcare provider are necessary to evaluate regularly for adverse effects. Although none of these drugs have been proved to be teratogenic, potential adverse effects on the fetus are weighed against the benefit to the mother before they are prescribed during pregnancy.

Compliance with the prescribed regimen also is evaluated during follow-up visits. The urine can be examined for color changes characteristic of rifampin and tested for metabolites of INH. When compliance is a problem, medications are administered under direct supervision. Twice-weekly therapy is more cost-effective in this instance, with a public health nurse watching the patient take and swallow the prescribed medication.

Repeat sputum specimens and chest x-rays are used to evaluate the effectiveness of therapy. In most cases, sputum cultures for *M. tuberculosis* are negative within 2 months of therapy; virtually all patients have negative sputum cultures within 3 months. If cultures remain positive at 3 months and beyond, treatment failure and drug resistance are suspected. In this case, cultures of the organism are tested for susceptibility to antitubercular agents, and two or three previously unused drugs are added to the treatment regimen (Fishman et al., 2008).

With adherence to prescribed treatment, virtually all patients should have negative sputum cultures for *M. tuberculosis* within 3 months. The relapse rate for current treatment regimens is less than 5%. The principal cause of treatment failure is noncompliance (Papadakis & McPhee, 2007).

♋ Nursing Care

Health Promotion

TB today presents a greater threat to public health than it does to individuals. Nurses play a key role in maintaining public health. Education and TB screening are major nursing strategies to prevent TB. See the accompanying Moving Evidence into Action box regarding TB screening for a homeless population.

Public health teaching includes increasing awareness of TB as a reemerging threat. Teach patients in all settings how to reduce the spread of TB by covering their mouths when coughing or sneezing and disposing of sputum appropriately. The benefit of screening programs to identify infected (though not necessarily infective) people also needs to be included in public health education.

The best TB prevention is early diagnosis of infections and appropriate treatment to achieve cure. BCG vaccine is recommended for infants born in countries where TB is prevalent, but is not widely used in the United States. It may be administered to healthcare workers in settings where the risk of infection with MDR strains of *M. tb* is high despite rigorous infection control measures (Papadakis & McPhee, 2007).

The primary preventive strategy used in the United States is treating people with latent TB infection demonstrated by a positive tuberculin test. A 9- to 10-month course of treatment with isoniazid reduces the risk of active TB by 90% or more (Papadakis & McPhee, 2007). Isoniazid also is prescribed prophylactically for people with HIV infection who have been exposed to TB.

Assessment

Focused assessment for the patient with suspected TB includes the following:

- *Health history:* Complaints of fatigue, weight loss, night sweats, difficulty breathing, cough (productive or nonproductive), bloody sputum, or chest pain; known exposure to TB; most recent tuberculin test and results; living circumstances; alcohol and other recreational drug use.
- *Physical examination:* Vital signs including temperature; general appearance; respiratory rate and lung sounds.
- *Diagnostic tests:* Tuberculin test results, presence of acid-fast bacilli in sputum, chest x-ray.

Nursing Diagnoses and Interventions

Nursing care related to TB focuses primarily on infection control and compliance with prescribed treatment. See the accompanying Case Study & Nursing Care Plan on page 1202.

ISONIAZID (INH, LANIAZID, NYDRAZID)

Isoniazid is the drug of choice for TB prophylaxis and a first-line drug for treating active disease. It is effective against both intracellular and extracellular organisms. Isoniazid is used alone as a prophylactic medication and in combination with rifampin, ethambutol, or both. A fixed-dose combination form with 150 mg of INH and 300 mg of rifampin (Rifamate) is available as well.

Nursing Responsibilities

- Administer on an empty stomach 1 hour before or 2 hours after meals for maximal effect if tolerated; may be given with meals to reduce gastrointestinal effects.
- Monitor for adverse effects.
  a. Numbness and tingling of the extremities (most likely to occur in malnourished, alcoholic, or diabetic patients)
  b. Hepatotoxicity, as evidenced by abnormal liver function studies and scleral jaundice
  c. Hypersensitivity reactions, such as rash, drug fever, or evidence of anemia, bruising, bleeding, or infection related to agranulocytosis
- Isoniazid interferes with the metabolism of diazepam (Valium), phenytoin (Dilantin), and carbamazepine. Doses of these drugs may need to be reduced to prevent toxicity.

Health Education for the Patient and Family

- Take the medication as prescribed for the entire treatment period to prevent incomplete eradication of the bacteria and development of resistant strains.
- Take the medication on an empty stomach. If nausea and vomiting occur, take with meals.
- If anorexia, nausea, vomiting, and jaundice (yellowing of the skin and the whites of the eyes) develop, notify your doctor immediately.
- Take pyridoxine as prescribed to prevent peripheral neuropathy.
- Avoid alcohol and other agents that may be harmful to the liver.
- Notify your doctor if you develop signs of an allergic reaction, such as rash, fever, easy bruising, bleeding gums, or fatigue.
- Use measures to prevent pregnancy while taking INH; this drug may be harmful to the developing fetus.

RIFAMPIN (RIFADIN, RIMACTANE)

Rifampin is commonly used in combination with INH and other antitubercular drugs. It is relatively low in toxicity, although it can cause hepatitis, a flulike immune response, and, rarely, renal failure. Rifampin stimulates the microsomal enzymes of the liver, increasing the rate of metabolism of many drugs and decreasing their effectiveness.

Nursing Responsibilities

- Administer on an empty stomach.
- Monitor CBC, liver function studies, and renal function studies for evidence of toxicity.
- Rifampin reduces the effect of oral contraceptives, quinidine, corticosteroids, warfarin, methadone, digoxin, and hypoglycemics. Monitor for the effectiveness of these drugs.

Patient and Family Teaching

- Rifampin causes body fluids, including sweat, urine, saliva, and tears, to turn red-orange. This is not harmful. Avoid wearing soft contact lenses because they may be permanently stained.
- Aspirin may interfere with rifampin absorption and should not be taken concurrently.
- Fever, flulike symptoms, excessive fatigue, sore throat, or unusual bleeding may indicate an adverse reaction to the drug and should be reported to your doctor.

PYRAZINAMIDE (TEBRAZID)

Pyrazinamide typically is given with INH and rifampin for the first 2 months of TB treatment. Concurrent use of pyrazinamide allows a shorter course of therapy. As with many of the antitubercular agents, pyrazinamide is toxic to the liver. Its other principal adverse effect is hyperuricemia. Gout, however, rarely develops.

Nursing Responsibilities

- Administer with meals to reduce gastrointestinal side effects.
- Monitor liver function studies and serum uric acid levels. Notify the healthcare provider if changes are noted.

Health Education for the Patient and Family

- Notify your doctor if you develop loss of appetite, nausea, vomiting, jaundice, or symptoms of gout (a painful, red, hot, swollen joint, often the great toe or elbow).
- While taking this drug, avoid using alcohol or other substances that may be harmful to the liver.

ETHAMBUTOL (MYAMBUTOL)

Ethambutol is added to the initial treatment regimen or substituted for INH when an INH-resistant strain of TB is suspected. Ethambutol is a bacteriostatic drug that reduces the development of resistance to the bactericidal first-line agents. Its principal toxic effect is optic neuritis; fortunately, this is reversible. Early signs of optic neuritis include decreased visual acuity and loss of red-green discrimination. This drug may be safe for use in pregnancy.

Nursing Responsibilities

- Record a baseline visual examination prior to therapy. Schedule periodic eye exams during the course of treatment.
- Administer with meals to reduce gastrointestinal side effects.
- Monitor liver and renal function studies and neurologic status while taking this drug. Notify the healthcare provider of abnormal findings or significant changes.

Health Education for the Patient and Family

- Monitor vision daily by reading newspapers and looking at the same blue object (using usual corrective lenses, if appropriate). Notify your doctor if changes in vision or color perception occur.

STREPTOMYCIN

An aminoglycoside antibiotic, streptomycin is highly effective in treating most mycobacterial infection. Resistance may develop if it is used alone. There are two primary drawbacks to streptomycin: (1) It must be administered parenterally because it is not absorbed in the gastrointestinal tract, and (2) it has toxic effects on the kidneys and ears.

Nursing Responsibilities

- Administer by deep intramuscular injection into a large muscle mass, rotating sites to minimize tissue trauma.
- Monitor urine output, weight, and renal function studies (including BUN and serum creatinine) to detect early signs of nephrotoxicity. Report significant changes to the healthcare provider.
- Maintain fluid intake at 2000 to 3000 mL per day to minimize the concentration of drug in the kidney tubules.
- Assess hearing and balance frequently. Have audiometric testing performed as indicated.

Health Education for the Patient and Family

- Maintain a daily fluid intake of at least 2.5 to 3 quarts.
- Weigh yourself on the same scale at least twice a week; report any significant weight gain to your doctor.
- Notify your doctor if hearing acuity decreases, ringing or buzzing sensations in the ear develop, or dizziness occurs.

Risk for Tuberculosis

Homeless people and those living in homeless shelters have several identified risk factors for TB: high incidence of drug and alcohol abuse, lowered immune status, and crowded living conditions. Access to and participation in TB screening, however, often is problematic. This study (Swigart & Kolb, 2004) identified factors contributing to homeless persons' decisions to participate in free TB screening. Contrary to the beliefs of may healthcare providers, many homeless people chose to participate in the screening out of a desire to maintain good health and a recognition that homelessness and shelter life increased their risk of developing TB. The desire to maintain good health was particularly noted as a reason among those participants in early recovery from drug or alcohol addiction. Other major factors cited for participating included a history of lung problems, a desire to identify possible problems related to smoking, and encouragement by shelter personnel. Fear of the results and a desire "not to be bothered" had negative effects on participation. Women with children were least likely to participate in screening in this study, citing fear of being identified as ill, which could result in loss of child custody.

IMPLICATIONS FOR NURSING

Outreach to homeless populations for health services, while difficult, has personal and public health benefits. The homeless often lack access to preventive and health promotion services, instead interacting with healthcare providers only intermittently when urgent care is needed. This study suggests, however, that a portion of this population desires to maintain good health and is receptive when screening and health promotion services are accessible. Shelter personnel were instrumental in getting many of the study participants to the screening. Recruiting the support of these workers can improve resident participation. Regularly scheduling a nurse in a shelter can allow trust to develop, also improving participation in health promotion activities. This may be a particularly important strategy in shelters for women with children—bringing services to the residents to reduce the fear of being perceived as unable to care for dependent children.

CRITICAL THINKING

1. What factors contribute to the perception of many healthcare providers that homeless people and shlter residents do not care about maintaining good health?
2. The participants in this study were screened for their ability to understand English and to read or hear and comprehend the interview and process. How might the healthcare team need to alter their approach to reach homeless people with mental illness that affects thinking and cognition?
3. Design a TB screening program using a multidisciplinary team to reach a specific population. Identify members of the team and discuss your rationale for their inclusion on the team.

From Swigart, V., & Kolb, R. (2004). Homeless persons' decisions to accept or reject public health disease detection services. *Public Health Nursing, 21*(2), 162–170.

Deficient Knowledge

Adequate knowledge and information are necessary to manage the disease and prevent its transmission to others. The patient needs to understand reasons for prolonged drug therapy and the importance of complying with treatment and follow-up. Antituberculosis drugs are relatively toxic. The patient needs to know how to minimize toxicity.

- Assess knowledge about the disease process; identify misperceptions and emotional reactions. *Teaching based on previous learning enhances understanding and retention of information.*
- Assess ability and interest in learning, developmental level, and obstacles to learning. *Assessment allows presentation of information in a manner tailored to the learning needs and style of the patient, promoting learning.*
- Identify support systems, and include significant others in teaching. *A knowledgeable significant other provides reinforcement of learning, confirmation of understanding, and encouragement for the patient. Including significant others also reduces the risk of inadvertent sabotage of the treatment plan.*

The Patient with Tuberculosis

Selected resource that nurses may find helpful when planning evidence-based nursing care follows.

- Knechel, N. A. (2009). Tuberculosis: Pathophysiology, clinical features, and diagnosis. *Critical Care Nurse, 29*(2), 34–43.

- Establish a relationship of mutual trust with the patient and significant others. *An atmosphere of trust increases receptiveness to teaching and learning.*
- Develop mutually acceptable learning goals with the patient and significant other. *Working together to identify learning needs and establish goals increases the patient's "ownership" and interest in the process.*
- Select appropriate teaching strategies, using learning aids such as literature and visual materials that are appropriate for age, level of education, and intellect. *Teaching tailored to the patient is more effective and results in better learning.*
- Teach about TB and the prescribed treatment, including the following:
  a. Nature of the disease and its spread
  b. Purpose of treatment and follow-up procedures
  c. Measures to prevent spreading the disease to others
  d. Importance of maintaining good general health by eating a well-balanced, high-protein, high-carbohydrate diet; balancing exercise with rest; and avoiding crowds and people with upper respiratory infections
  e. Names, doses, purposes, and adverse effects of prescribed medications
  f. Importance of avoiding alcohol and other substances that may damage the liver while taking chemotherapeutic drugs
  g. Fluid intake needs of 2.5 to 3.0 quarts of fluid per day
  h. Manifestations to report to the healthcare provider: chest pain, hemoptysis, difficulty breathing; anorexia, nausea, or vomiting; yellow tint to skin or sclera; sudden weight gain, swollen feet, ankles, legs, or hands; hearing loss, tinnitus, or vertigo; change in vision or difficulty discriminating colors

TB is a chronic disease requiring lengthy treatment with antitubercular medications. A good understanding of the disease, its treatment, and potential adverse effects of therapy prepares the patient to manage care.

- Document teaching and level of understanding. Reinforce teaching and learning as needed. *Teaching is not complete until the patient can demonstrate learning of the information.*

Ineffective Therapeutic Regimen Management

The populations at highest risk for developing active TB—the homeless and members of lower socioeconomic groups—are also at high risk for being unable to manage its complex treatment regimen. Three or more costly medications that may have unpleasant or even dangerous side effects are prescribed. Frequent medical follow-up is required. Infectious diseases such as TB carry a stigma that may lead to denial of the disease or its seriousness. Alcoholics and IV drug users need to withdraw from their addiction to be successful in treating the disease. The patient with HIV infection faces a potentially fatal disease and costly treatment that may well override concerns about TB management.

- Assess self-care abilities and support systems. *Assessment is used to help determine the patient's ability to follow the prescribed regimen.*
- Assess knowledge and understanding of the disease, its complications, treatment, and risks to others. Provide additional teaching and reinforcement as indicated. *Lack of understanding is a barrier to compliance with and management of the treatment regimen.*
- Work collaboratively to identify barriers or obstacles to managing the prescribed treatment. *Working collaboratively with the patient and other members of the healthcare team provides insight for overcoming identified barriers to effective treatment.*
- Assist the patient, significant others (if available), and healthcare team members to develop a plan for managing the prescribed regimen. *Including the patient in developing a plan to manage care increases the sense of control and ownership and helps ensure that personal, cultural, and lifestyle factors are considered. This increases the likelihood of compliance.*
- Provide verbal and written instructions that are clear and appropriate for level of literacy, knowledge, and understanding. *Clearly written directions provide support and reinforcement for the patient.*
- Provide active intervention for homeless people, including shelter placement or other housing and ongoing follow-up by easily accessed healthcare providers (clinics and public health workers in the neighborhood that do not present transportation or access problems, either real or perceived). *Simple referral will not ensure compliance, especially among disenfranchised populations. Active intervention is needed to help ensure treatment compliance.*
- Refer patients who are unlikely to comply with the treatment regimen to the public health department for management and follow-up. *Because TB presents a significant public health risk, public health follow-up is essential. In some cases, it is necessary for nurses to administer medications, observing the patient swallow all pills.*

Risk for Infection

The spread of TB is a risk in any facility housing many people. It is especially high in residential care facilities for older patients and for people with AIDS. The increasing incidence of TB among homeless people and members of lower socioeconomic groups increases the risk in hospitals, emergency departments, and public and urgent care clinics. Respiratory precautions are necessary to prevent the spread of TB via microscopic airborne droplets to other patients and to healthcare workers.

- Place the patient in a private room with airflow control that prevents air within the room from circulating into the hallway or other rooms. A negative flow room in which air is diluted by at least six fresh-air exchanges per hour is recommended. *A negative flow room and multiple fresh-air exchanges dilute the concentration of droplet nuclei within the room and prevent their spread to adjacent areas.*
- Use standard precautions and TB isolation techniques as recommended by the CDC, including wearing masks and gowns when caring for patients who do not reliably cover the mouth when coughing. *These measures are important to prevent the spread of TB to others.*
- Discuss the reasons for and importance of respiratory isolation procedures during initial hospitalization. When treatment is provided as an outpatient, instruct to avoid crowds and close physical contact and maintain ventilation in living facilities, particularly during the first 3 weeks of treatment. *These measures help protect others during initial treatment, when sputum is still likely to contain significant numbers of bacilli.*

> **PRACTICE ALERT**
> Use personal protective devices to reduce the risk of transmission during patient care. The Occupational Safety and Health Administration (OSHA) requires use of a HEPA-filtered respirator for protection against occupational exposure to TB. Surgical masks are ineffective to filter droplet nuclei, necessitating the use of protective devices capable of filtering bacteria and particles smaller than 1 micron.

- Place a mask on the patient when transporting to other parts of the facility for diagnostic or treatment procedures. *Covering the patient's nose and mouth during transport minimizes air contamination and the risk to visitors and personnel.*
- Inform all personnel having contact with the patient of the diagnosis. *This allows personnel to take appropriate precautions.*
- Assist visitors to mask prior to entering the room. *Providing visitors with appropriate masks or respirators reduces their risk of infection.*
- Teach the patient how to limit transmitting the disease to others:
  a. Always cough and expectorate into tissues.
  b. Dispose of tissues properly, placing them in a closed bag.
  c. Wear a mask if you are sneezing or unable to control respiratory secretions.
  d. The disease is not spread by touching inanimate objects, so no special precautions are required for eating utensils, clothing, books, or other objects used.

  Teaching appropriate precautions helps prevent the spread of TB to others while allowing as much freedom from restraints as possible.

CASE STUDY & NURSING CARE PLAN   A Patient with Tuberculosis

Harry Facée, aged 53, arrives at a metropolitan public health clinic complaining of aching chest pain that has lasted for the past few days. He also says that his sputum is bloody. He is afraid he might have lung cancer, so he came in to see a doctor.

ASSESSMENT

Raj Kamil, RN, the public health nurse at the clinic, obtains an admission history and physical examination of Mr. Facée. Mr. Kamil notes that Mr. Facée is a homeless person who has lived on the streets and in various shelters for the past "10 years or so." He usually prefers to sleep outdoors, taking refuge in shelters only during very cold or very wet weather. He has a small disability income, but usually scrounges for food or eats with other homeless people at soup kitchens. Mr. Facée states that he has had a cough for a long time, which has become worse recently. It is now productive, especially in the mornings. He also admits that he has recently been waking up drenched with sweat in the middle of the night and is more tired than usual.

Although Mr. Facée's clothes are tattered, he is fairly clean. He answers questions appropriately and intelligently. Mr. Kamil does not detect any odor of alcohol on his breath. He is very thin, almost emaciated. Mr. Facée's vital signs are BP 152/86, P 92, R 20, and T 100.2°F (37.8°C).

Suspecting tuberculosis, Mr. Kamil obtains a sputum specimen for Gram stain and culture, administers a tuberculin test, and sends Mr. Facée for a chest x-ray before he sees the clinic healthcare provider. Although the chest x-ray is inconclusive, the Gram stain is positive for acid-fast bacilli. The diagnosis of probable active pulmonary tuberculosis is made. The healthcare provider prescribes isoniazid, 300 mg orally; rifampin, 600 mg orally; and pyrazinamide, 1500 mg orally daily for 2 months, to be followed by twice weekly isoniazid 900 mg orally and rifampin 600 mg orally. The healthcare provider also orders weekly sputum cultures for the first month.

DIAGNOSES

- *Ineffective Health Maintenance* related to homelessness
- *Risk for Noncompliance with Prescribed Treatment* related to lack of understanding and resources
- *Imbalanced Nutrition: Less than Body Requirements* related to increased metabolic needs associated with infection
- *Risk for Disturbed Sensory Perception: Kinesthetic* related to effects of isoniazid therapy

EXPECTED OUTCOMES

- Keep all follow-up appointments as scheduled.
- Verbalize an understanding of his disease and its treatment.

- Follow the prescribed plan of care.
- Demonstrate measures to prevent spread of the organism to others.
- Gain 1 to 2 lb of weight per week.
- Promptly report symptoms of peripheral neuropathy, including numbness, tingling, or burning sensations.

PLANNING AND IMPLEMENTATION

- Teach about tuberculosis, and provide a patient education pamphlet about the disease.
- Instruct about the prescribed medications, potential adverse effects, and the importance of completing the entire prescribed regimen.
- Emphasize the importance of continued follow-up.
- Teach and demonstrate sputum and droplet control measures.
- Escort to the local incentive shelter program for directly observed medical therapy and meals.
- Identify verbally and in writing manifestations to report to the healthcare provider.

EVALUATION

Mr. Kamil successfully enrolls Mr. Facée in the local incentive shelter program. In this program, a healthcare worker administers Mr. Facée's medications daily, watching him swallow them. He is assigned a small individual room and can eat three daily meals at the shelter. He still prefers to sleep outside when the weather permits, but he complies with the requirement for supervised medication administration because he "likes the food there." Always a clean person, Mr. Facée is able to demonstrate appropriate sputum control measures and practices them faithfully. The sputum culture done after 2 months of treatment is negative for tubercle bacilli, and his chest x-ray indicates no disease progression.

CRITICAL THINKING IN THE NURSING PROCESS

1. Many homeless people have schizophrenia or other mental diseases. How would you adapt the care plan for a homeless schizophrenic patient with active tuberculosis?
2. Mr. Kamil was fortunate in having access to an incentive shelter with healthcare workers to supervise medication compliance. Identify available resources in your area for homeless patients infected with tuberculosis.
3. Develop a care plan for the nursing diagnosis *Ineffective Airway Clearance* related to mucopurulent sputum and weak cough.

See Evaluating Your Response in Appendix C.

- Teach how to collect sputum specimens. If necessary, have the patient step outside to collect a sputum specimen. *This minimizes the risk of exposure to healthcare personnel and provides for rapid dilution of any droplet nuclei produced and their exposure to ultraviolet light (which kills the bacteria).*
- Teach the importance of complying with prescribed treatment for the entire course of therapy. *Completion of the entire treatment regimen is important to reduce the risk of relapse and creation of drug-resistant organisms.*

Using NANDA, NIC, and NOC

Linkages between a selected NANDA nursing diagnosis, NIC, and NOC for the patient with tuberculosis are shown in the chart that follows.

Community-Based Care

Most patients with TB are managed in community settings; few require institutionalization. The accompanying Case Study & Nursing Care Plan presents community-based nursing care for a patient with TB. In addition to the teaching topics and strategies identified earlier, discuss the following topics when preparing the patient and significant others for home care.

- Importance of screening close contacts for infection and possibly prophylactic treatment
- Effect, dose, and timing for all medications, and potential side effects and their management
- Importance of long-term therapy in eradicating the disease
- Principles of good nutrition, dietary guidelines for a patient with TB, and other measures to help maintain good health, such as balancing rest with exercise

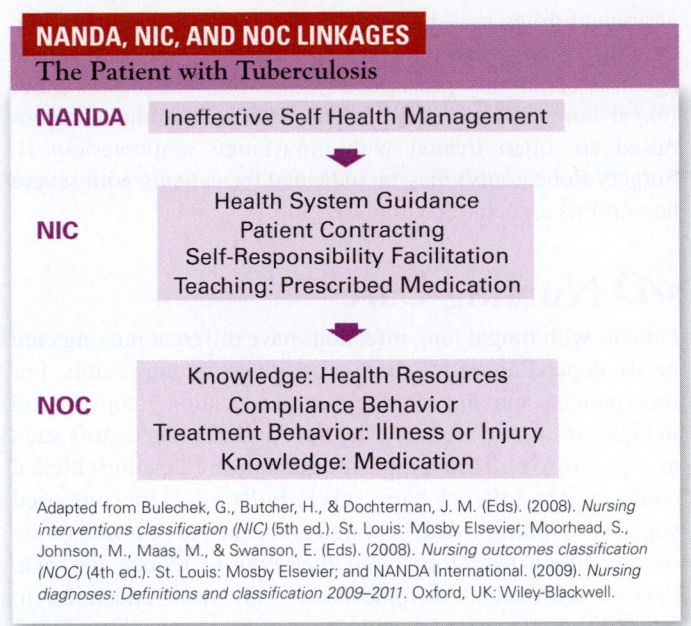

- Signs and symptoms of complications to report to the health-care provider

  Provide referrals as appropriate:

- Smoking cessation clinics or support groups
- Alcohol treatment facilities, Alcoholics Anonymous, other treatment programs or support groups
- Drug treatment facilities, Narcotics Anonymous, other out-patient or inpatient treatment programs or support groups
- Low-cost community clinics and incentive programs for people with TB
- Counseling, support groups, and other community resources that provide additional assistance and support

The Patient with Inhalation Anthrax

Inhalation anthrax is a potential threat in the United States. This disease rarely affects humans in nature, even though both wild and domestic animals can be infected. However, *Bacillus anthracis*, the spore-forming rod responsible for causing anthrax, has been identified as an agent likely to be used as a biologic weapon. Anthrax spores can be aerosolized so they remain suspended in the air, allowing them to be inhaled into the lungs. Person-to-person transmission does not occur.

Inhalation anthrax causes initial flulike symptoms, including malaise, dry cough, and fever. This is followed by an abrupt onset of severe dyspnea, stridor, and cyanosis. Lymph nodes in the mediastinum and thorax become inflamed and enlarged. Septic shock and/or meningitis may develop. Untreated, death results from hemorrhagic thoracic lymphadenitis and hemorrhagic mediastinitis. Even with treatment, inhalation anthrax has a 45% mortality rate (CDC, 2009e).

Blood cultures and chest x-ray are used to diagnose inhalation anthrax. However, because death can quickly result from the disease, people who are known or suspected to have been exposed to anthrax spores often are treated prophylactically. Ciprofloxacin (Cipro) is used to both prevent and treat inhalation anthrax.

Doxycycline (Vibramycin) is an alternative to ciprofloxacin. Although an anthrax vaccine exists, its use at this time is considered experimental (CDC, 2009e). See the section on bioterrorism in ∞ Chapter 7 for more information about anthrax and the section of this chapter on respiratory failure for nursing care measures for the patient with inhalation anthrax.

The Patient with a Fungal Infection

Fungal spores are endemic, present in the air everyone breathes. Normal respiratory defense mechanisms allow few of these spores to reach the lungs. If they reach the lungs, pulmonary macrophages and neutrophils efficiently remove them in most people. When they do cause infection, it is typically mild and self-limiting. Most fungi are opportunistic, able to cause infection only in people who are immunocompromised. For this reason, patients with AIDS, renal failure, leukemia, burns, or chronic diseases, as well as people receiving corticosteroids or immunosuppressants, are particularly susceptible to fungal diseases.

Many fungal lung diseases have a geographic distribution pattern. Histoplasmosis and blastomycosis are more common in the southeastern, mid-Atlantic, and central states. California, Arizona, and western Texas are the primary sites for coccidioidomycosis, also known as San Joaquin valley fever (Papadakis & McPhee, 2007).

The course and manifestations of fungal lung diseases resemble those of TB. Lung lesions are slow to develop, and symptoms are mild. The fungus can disseminate from the lung to other organs.

Pathophysiology

Histoplasmosis

Histoplasmosis, an infectious disease caused by *Histoplasma capsulatum*, is the most common fungal lung infection in the United States. The organism is found in the soil and is linked to exposure to bird droppings and bats. Infection occurs when the spores are inhaled and reach the alveoli. Most infections develop into *latent asymptomatic disease*, much like TB, or *primary acute histoplasmosis*, a mild, self-limiting influenza-like illness. Initial chest x-rays are nonspecific; later ones show areas of calcification. *Chronic progressive disease*, usually seen in older adults, typically is limited to the lung but may involve any organ. Progressive lung changes and cavitation occur, with increasing dyspnea and eventual disabling pulmonary disease.

Regional lymph vessels spread the organism from the lungs to other parts of the body, much like the process that occurs in TB. In the healthy host, normal immune responses inactivate and remove the organism. In the immunocompromised host, however, macrophages remove the fungi but are unable to destroy them, resulting in *disseminated histoplasmosis*. This type of histoplasmosis is often fatal. Manifestations of fever, dyspnea, cough, weight loss, and muscle wasting are usual. Ulcerations of the mouth and oropharynx may be present, and the liver and spleen are enlarged.

Coccidioidomycosis

Coccidioidomycosis is an infectious disease caused by the fungus *Coccidioides immitis*. This mold grows in the soil of the arid Southwest, Mexico, and Central and South America. When inhaled, the fungus typically causes an acute, self-limiting pulmonary infection that often is asymptomatic and goes unrecognized. If manifestations do occur, they resemble those of influenza, with malaise, fever, body aches, and cough. Pleuritic pain, skin rash, and arthritis of the knees and ankles also may develop. Disseminated disease, which may affect the lymph nodes, meninges, spleen, liver, kidney, skin, and adrenal glands, is rare in immunocompetent people. When it does occur, the mortality rate is high. Meningitis is the usual cause of death.

Blastomycosis

The fungus *Blastomyces dermatitidis* causes the infectious disease blastomycosis. It occurs primarily in the south central and midwestern regions of the United States and in Canada. Men are affected more frequently than women. The lungs are the primary site for the disease, although it may spread to involve the skin, bones, genitourinary system, and, rarely, the central nervous system. Pulmonary symptoms include fever, dyspnea, pleuritic chest pain, and cough, which may become productive of bloody or purulent sputum. If untreated, the disseminated disease is slowly progressive and ultimately fatal.

Paracoccidioidomycosis

The fungus *Paracoccidioides brasiliensis* causes paracocciodioidomycosis. It is also known as Brazilian blastomycosis or Lutz-Spendore-Almeida disease. As with blastomycosis, it often enters through the lungs but can spread to the lymph nodes and bone. It can occur in immunocompetent persons, often with onset in childhood. The pulmonary presentation includes lobar pneumonia or pleurisy that continues past the ninth day. Sulfa drugs and anti-fungals are used to eradicate the disease (Restrepo et al., 2008).

Aspergillosis

Aspergillus spores are common in the environment, but rarely cause disease except in the immunocompromised. When they do cause infection, *Aspergillus* species invade blood vessels and produce hyphae that branch at acute angles, frequently causing venous or arterial thrombosis. In the lungs, aspergillosis can cause an acute, diffuse, self-limited pneumonitis. The manifestations of pulmonary aspergillosis include dyspnea, nonproductive cough, pleuritic chest pain, chills, and fever. If the organism invades a pulmonary blood vessel, hemoptysis or massive pulmonary hemorrhage can occur. In patients with underlying lung disease, balls of *Aspergillus* hyphae may form within cysts or cavities, usually in the upper lobes of the lung. Symptoms often are milder and more insidious in onset, with fever, weight loss, night sweats, and cough (Fishman et al., 2008).

Interdisciplinary Care

Most fungal lung infections can be diagnosed by microscopic examination of a sputum specimen for the fungus. (∞ See Chapter 34 for nursing responsibilities related to collecting a sputum specimen.) Blood cultures also may be done, as well as cultures of cerebrospinal fluid if indicated. Chest x-ray may show typical changes in lung tissue or widening of the mediastinum, depending on the infecting organism.

Acute pulmonary histoplasmosis and acute pulmonary coccidioidomycosis usually resolve without treatment, although antifungal drugs may be given to shorten the disease course. Oral itraconazole (Sporanox), a broad-spectrum antifungal agent, is commonly prescribed to treat histoplasmosis. Other fungal lung diseases and patients who are immunocompromised are often treated with intravenous amphotericin B. Surgery (lobectomy) may be indicated for patients with severe hemoptysis associated with aspergillosis.

∞ Nursing Care

Patients with fungal lung infections have different nursing care needs, depending on the disease and their immune status. For most patients, nursing care focuses on education. People living in high-prevalence areas or who have specific risk factors such as exposure to bird droppings (for example, by cleaning chicken coops, pigeon lofts, or barns where birds roost), decomposed vegetation, rotting wood, or stored grain need to be aware of the risk, common symptoms, and measures to reduce the risk. Patients with latent histoplasmosis may need education to maintain good general health to prevent reactivation. Teach patients receiving antifungal drugs about the specific drug, its intended and adverse effects, the duration of therapy, and symptoms to report to the healthcare provider. Include teaching about any specific precautions such as drug or food interactions. Itraconazole interacts with many medications; verify the safety of concurrent usage with all other prescribed drugs. Its use is contraindicated during pregnancy and lactation; emphasize the importance of effective birth control and of notifying the healthcare provider immediately if pregnancy occurs. Amphotericin B is a toxic drug. Administer the initial intravenous dose slowly after premedicating with an antihistamine and antiemetic as ordered to manage its adverse effects. Monitor carefully during infusion and therapy for changes in vital signs, hydration, nutrition, weight, or urine output.

EVIDENCE FOR NURSING CARE | **The Patient with Hemoptysis**

Selected resources that nurses may find helpful when planning evidence-based nursing care follow.

- Clifton, S. (2009). Bronchoscopy assisting—2007 revision & update. American Association of Respiratory Care. *Respiratory Care 52*(1), 74–80. Retrieved from http://www.guideline.gov/summary/summary.aspx?doc_id=10668&nbr=005573&string=hemoptysis

- Jensen, P. A., Lambert, L. A., Iademarco, M. F., Ridzon, R., & Bennett, D. I. (2005). Guidelines for preventing the transmission of *Mycobacterium tuberculosis* in healthcare settings, 2005. Centers for Disease Control and Prevention. *MMWR Recommendations and Reports, 54*(17), 1–141. Retrieved from http://www.guideline.gov/summary/summary.aspx?doc_id=8532&nbr=004748&string=hemoptysis

- Kvale, P. A., Selecky, P. A., & Prakash, U. B. S. (2009). Palliative care in lung cancer: ACCP evidence-based clinical practice guidelines (2nd ed.). *Chest, 132*(3 Suppl), 368S–403S. Retrieved from http://www.guideline.gov/summary/summary.aspx?doc_id=11422&nbr=005941&string=hemoptysis

Disorders of the Pleura

The *pleura* is a thin membrane with two layers: the visceral pleura, which overlies the lung surface, and the parietal pleura, which lines the inner chest wall. Between the layers of pleura is a potential space, the *pleural cavity*, which contains a thin layer of serous fluid. As the thoracic cavity expands during inspiration, the pressure in this space becomes negative in relation to atmospheric and alveolar pressure. The expansible lung is drawn out, and air rushes into the alveoli. When the pleura is inflamed or affected by disease or injury, air or fluid can collect in the pleural cavity, restricting lung expansion, air movement, and ventilation.

The Patient with Pleuritis

Pleuritis (*pleurisy*), inflammation of the pleura, irritates sensory fibers of the parietal pleura, causing characteristic pain. Pleural inflammation usually occurs secondarily to another process, such as a viral respiratory illness, pneumonia, or rib injury.

The onset of pleuritis is typically abrupt. The pain is unilateral and well localized; it is usually sharp or stabbing in nature. Pain may be referred to the neck or the shoulder. Deep breathing, coughing, and movement aggravate the pain. Respirations are rapid and shallow, and chest wall movement is limited on the affected side. Breath sounds are diminished, and a pleural friction rub may be heard over the site.

The diagnosis of pleuritis is based on its manifestations. Chest x-ray and ECG may be ordered to rule out other causes of chest pain. Treatment for pleuritis is symptomatic. Analgesics and NSAIDs, indomethacin (Indocin) in particular, help relieve the pain. Codeine may be ordered, both to relieve pain and to suppress the cough.

Nursing care for the patient with pleuritis is directed toward promoting comfort, including administration of NSAIDs and analgesics. Positioning and splinting the chest while coughing also are helpful. Although wrapping the chest with 6-inch-wide elastic bandages may help relieve pain, this may excessively restrict chest motion, increasing the risk of impaired airway clearance.

Teach the patient and family that pleuritis is generally self-limited and of short duration. Discuss symptoms to report to the healthcare provider: increased fever, productive cough, difficulty breathing, or shortness of breath. Provide information about prescription and nonprescription NSAIDs and analgesics, including the drug ordered, how to use it, and its desired and possible adverse effects.

The Patient with a Pleural Effusion

The pleural space normally contains only about 10 to 20 mL of serous fluid. **Pleural effusion** is collection of excess fluid in the pleural space. Pleural effusions result from either systemic or local disease. Systemic disorders that may lead to pleural effusion include heart failure, liver or renal disease, and connective tissue disorders, such as rheumatoid arthritis and systemic lupus erythematosus. Pneumonia, atelectasis, TB, lung cancer, and trauma are local conditions that may cause pleural effusion.

Pathophysiology and Manifestations

Excess pleural fluid may be either *transudate*, formed when capillary pressure is high or plasma proteins are low, or *exudate*, the result of increased capillary permeability. Heart failure is the most common precipitating factor in transudate formation; it also may accompany renal failure, nephrosis, liver failure, and malignancy. Exudate, a protein-rich fluid, is seen with inflammatory processes such as infections, systemic inflammation (e.g., rheumatoid arthritis or systemic lupus erythematosus), pulmonary infarction (leading to tissue necrosis and an inflammatory response), and malignancy (Huether & McCance, 2008). Other pleural fluid collections include *empyema*, pus in the pleural cavity; *hemothorax*, the presence of blood in the cavity; *hemorrhagic pleural effusion*, a mixture of blood and pleural fluid; and *chylothorax*, a collection of lymph in the pleural space. In adults, chylothorax may result from thoracic surgery or placement of a central catheter in one of the great veins (Huether & McCance, 2008).

A large pleural effusion compresses adjacent lung tissue. This causes the characteristic manifestation of dyspnea. Pain may develop, although with inflammatory processes pleuritic pain often is relieved by formation of an effusion, as the fluid reduces friction between inflamed visceral and parietal pleura. Breath sounds are diminished or absent, and a dull percussion tone is heard over the affected area. Chest wall movement may be limited.

Interdisciplinary Care

Chest x-ray often provides the first evidence of a pleural effusion. Because fluid typically collects in dependent regions, it is seen at the base of the affected lung on an upright chest x-ray, and along the lateral wall when the patient is positioned on the

Pleural effusion

Figure 36–8 ■ Thoracentesis. With the patient seated, a needle is inserted between the ribs into the pleural space to withdraw accumulated fluid.

NURSING CARE OF THE PATIENT | Undergoing a Thoracentesis

PREPROCEDURE CARE

- Verify a signed informed consent for the procedure. *This invasive procedure requires informed consent.*
- Assess knowledge and understanding of the procedure and its purpose; provide additional information as needed. *An informed patient will be less apprehensive and more able to cooperate during the thoracentesis.*
- Preprocedure fasting or sedation is not required. *Only local anesthesia is used in this procedure, and the gag and cough reflexes remain intact.*
- Administer a cough suppressant if indicated. *Movement and coughing during the procedure may cause inadvertent damage to the lung or pleura.*
- Obtain a thoracentesis tray, sterile gloves, injectable lidocaine, povidone-iodine or chlorhexidine, dressing supplies, and an extra overbed table or mayo stand. *These supplies are used by the healthcare provider performing the procedure.*
- Position the patient upright, leaning forward with arms and head supported on an anchored overbed table. *This position spreads the ribs, enlarging the intercostal space for needle insertion.*
- Inform the patient that although local anesthesia prevents pain as the needle is inserted, a sensation of pressure may be felt. *A pressure sensation occurs as the needle punctures the parietal pleura to enter the pleural space.*

POSTPROCEDURE CARE

- Monitor pulse, color, oxygen saturation, and other signs during thoracentesis. *These are indicators of physiologic tolerance of the procedure.*
- Apply a dressing over the puncture site, and position on the unaffected side for 1 hour. *This allows the pleural puncture to heal.*
- Label obtained specimen with name, date, source, and diagnosis; send specimen to the laboratory for analysis. *Fluid obtained during thoracentesis may be examined for abnormal cells, bacteria, and other substances to determine the cause of the pleural effusion.*
- During the first several hours after thoracentesis, frequently assess and document vital signs; oxygen saturation; respiratory status, including respiratory excursion, lung sounds, cough, or hemoptysis; and puncture site for bleeding or crepitus. *Frequent assessment is important to detect possible complications of thoracentesis, such as pneumothorax.*
- Obtain a chest x-ray. *Chest x-ray is ordered to detect possible pneumothorax.*
- Normal activities generally can be resumed after 1 hour if no evidence of pneumothorax or other complication is present. *The puncture wound of thoracentesis heals rapidly.*

affected side. CT scans and ultrasonography also are used to localize and differentiate pleural effusions.

Thoracentesis

If the cause of pleural effusion is not apparent, a thoracentesis may be done. **Thoracentesis** is an invasive procedure in which fluid (or occasionally air) is removed from the pleural space with a needle. Aspirated fluid is analyzed for appearance, cell counts, protein and glucose content, the presence of enzymes such as LDH and amylase, abnormal cells, and culture.

When pleural effusion is significant and interferes with respirations, thoracentesis is the treatment of choice to remove the fluid (Figure 36–8 ■). Thoracentesis may be performed at the bedside, in a procedure room, or in an outpatient setting. Local anesthesia is used, and the procedure requires less than 30 minutes to complete. Percussion, auscultation, radiography, or ultrasonography are used to locate the effusion and needle insertion site. The amount of fluid removed is limited to 1200 to 1500 mL at one time to reduce the risk of cardiovascular collapse from rapid removal of too much fluid. Pneumothorax is a possible complication of thoracentesis if the visceral pleura is punctured or a closed drainage system not maintained during the procedure. Nursing care for the patient undergoing a thoracentesis is outlined in the accompanying box.

Treatments

Because pleural effusion usually occurs secondarily to another disease or disorder, medical management also focuses on treating the underlying condition to prevent further fluid accumulation. An empyema may require repeated drainage, as well as high doses of parenteral antibiotics. Occasionally, thoracotomy and surgical excision may be necessary. See the box above for nursing care of the patient undergoing thoracic

surgery. Recurrent pleural effusions, often due to cancer, may be prevented by instilling an irritant, such as doxycycline, bleomycin, or talc, into the pleural space to cause adhesion of the parietal and visceral pleura (*pleurodesis*). Water-seal chest tube drainage is often employed for hemothorax.

✎ Nursing Care

Nursing care for the patient with a pleural effusion is directed toward supporting respiratory function and assisting with procedures to evacuate collected fluid. With a large pleural effusion and partial lung collapse, impaired gas exchange and activity intolerance are high-priority nursing problems. Risk for impaired gas exchange is also a priority problem during the initial period following thoracentesis.

Teaching for home care focuses on symptoms of recurrent effusion or complications following a thoracentesis to report to the healthcare provider: increasing dyspnea or shortness of breath, cough, and hemoptysis. Pleuritic pain may be an early

EVIDENCE FOR NURSING CARE | **The Patient with Pleural Effusion**

Selected resources that nurses may find helpful when planning evidence-based nursing care follow.

- DiSalvo, W. M., Joyce, M. M., Tyson, L. B., Culkin, A. E., & Mackay, K. (2008). Putting evidence into practice: Evidence-based interventions for cancer-related dyspnea. *Clinical Journal of Oncology Nursing, 12*(2), 341–352.
- Held-Warmkessel, J., & Schiech, L. (2008). Caring for a patient with malignant pleural effusion. *Nursing2008, 38*(11), 43–47.

sign of effusion and also should be reported. Further teaching about an underlying condition also may be necessary; for example, the patient with heart failure may need teaching about a salt-restricted diet.

The Patient with Pneumothorax

Accumulation of air in the pleural space is called **pneumothorax**. Pneumothorax can occur spontaneously, without apparent cause, as a complication of preexisting lung disease, as a result of blunt or penetrating trauma to the chest, or from an iatrogenic cause (e.g., following thoracentesis).

Pathophysiology

Pressure in the pleural space is normally negative in relation to atmospheric pressure. This negative pressure is vital to the process of breathing. Contraction of the diaphragm and the intercostal muscles enlarges the thoracic space. Negative intrapleural pressure draws the lung outward, increasing its volume so air rushes in to fill the expanded lung space.

When either the visceral or parietal pleura is breached, air enters the pleural space, equalizing this pressure. Lung expansion is impaired, and the natural recoil tendency of the lung causes it to collapse to a greater or lesser extent, depending on the size and rapidity of air accumulation. Table 36–7 illustrates the classifications of pneumothorax.

Spontaneous Pneumothorax

Spontaneous pneumothorax develops when an air-filled bleb, or blister, on the lung surface ruptures. Rupture allows air from the airways to enter the pleural space. Air accumulates until pressures are equalized or until collapse of the involved lung section seals the leak. Spontaneous pneumothorax may be either *primary* (*simple*) or *secondary* (*complicated*).

Primary pneumothorax affects previously healthy people, usually tall, slender men between ages 16 and 24 (Noppin & DeKeukeleire, 2008). The cause of primary pneumothorax is unknown. Risk factors include smoking and familial factors. Air-filled blebs tend to form in the apices of the lungs. This is considered to be a benign condition, although recurrences are common. Certain activities also increase the risk of spontaneous pneumothorax, such as high altitude flying and rapid decompression during scuba diving.

Secondary pneumothorax, generally caused by overdistention and rupture of an alveolus, is more serious and potentially life threatening. It develops in patients with underlying lung disease, usually COPD. Middle-aged and older adults are primarily affected. Secondary pneumothorax also may be associated with asthma, cystic fibrosis, pulmonary fibrosis, tuberculosis, acute respiratory distress syndrome (ARDS), and other lung diseases. Rarely, a form of secondary pneumothorax called *catamenial pneumothorax* can develop in affected women within 24 to 48 hours of the onset of menstrual flow.

Manifestations

The manifestations of spontaneous pneumothorax depend on the size of pneumothorax, extent of lung collapse, and any underlying lung disease. Typically, pleuritic chest pain and shortness of breath begin abruptly, often while at rest. The respiratory and heart rates increase as gas exchange is affected. Chest wall movement may be asymmetrical, with less movement on the affected side than the unaffected side. The affected side is hyperresonant to percussion, and breath sounds may be diminished or absent. Hypoxemia may develop, although normal mechanisms that shunt blood flow to the unaffected lung often maintain normal oxygen saturation levels. Hypoxemia is more pronounced in secondary pneumothorax.

Traumatic Pneumothorax

Blunt or penetrating trauma of the chest wall and pleura can cause pneumothorax. Blunt trauma, for example, due to a motor vehicle crash, fall, or during cardiopulmonary resuscitation (CPR), can lead to a *closed pneumothorax*. Fractured ribs penetrating the pleura are the leading cause of pneumothorax due to blunt trauma (Yamamoto, Schroeder, & Beliveau, 2005). Fracture of the trachea and a ruptured bronchus or esophagus also may result from blunt trauma, leading to closed pneumothorax.

Open pneumothorax (*sucking chest wound*) results from penetrating chest trauma such as a stab wound, gunshot wound, or impalement injury. With open pneumothorax, air moves freely between the pleural space and the atmosphere through the wound. Pressure on the affected side equalizes with the atmosphere, and the lung collapses rapidly. The result is significant hypoventilation.

Iatrogenic pneumothorax may result from puncture or laceration of the visceral pleura during central-line placement, thoracentesis, or lung biopsy. During bronchoscopy, bronchi or lung tissue can be disrupted. Alveoli can become overdistended and rupture during anesthesia, resuscitation procedures, or mechanical ventilation.

MANIFESTATIONS   With traumatic pneumothorax, manifestations of pain and dyspnea may be masked or missed due to other injuries. Tachypnea and tachycardia may be attributed to the primary injury. Focused assessment for evidence of pneumothorax is vital. Chest wall movement on the affected side is diminished, and breath sounds are absent. If a penetrating wound is present, air may be heard and felt moving through it with respiratory efforts. Hemothorax frequently accompanies traumatic pneumothorax. The manifestations of iatrogenic pneumothorax are similar to those of spontaneous pneumothorax.

Tension Pneumothorax

Tension pneumothorax develops when injury to the chest wall or lungs allows air to enter the pleural space but prevents it from escaping. Pressure within the pleural space becomes positive in relation to atmospheric pressure as air rapidly accumulates with each breath. The lung on the affected side collapses, and pressure on the mediastinum shifts thoracic organs to the unaffected side of the chest, placing pressure on the opposite lung as well. Ventilation is severely compromised, and venous return to the heart is impaired. Tension pneumothorax is a medical emergency requiring immediate intervention to preserve respiration and cardiac output.

TABLE 36–7 Types of Pneumothorax

TYPE	PATHOPHYSIOLOGY	MANIFESTATIONS
Spontaneous 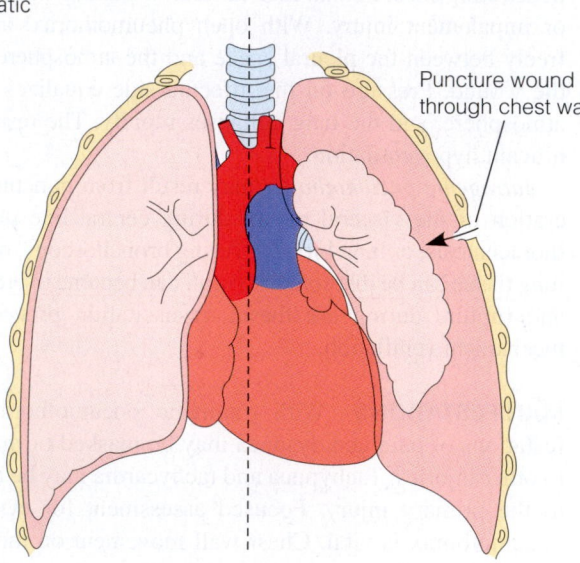	Rupture of a bleb on the lung surface allows air to enter pleural space from airways. ■ *Primary pneumothorax* affects previously healthy people. ■ *Secondary pneumothorax* affects people with preexisting lung disease (e.g., COPD).	■ Abrupt onset ■ Pleuritic chest pain ■ Dyspnea, shortness of breath ■ Tachypnea, tachycardia ■ Unequal lung excursion ■ Decreased breath sounds and hyperresonant percussion tone on affected side
Traumatic	Trauma to the chest wall or pleura disrupts the pleural membrane. ■ *Open* occurs with penetrating chest trauma that allows air from the environment to enter the pleural space. ■ *Closed* occurs with blunt trauma that allows air from the lung to enter the pleural space. ■ *Iatrogenic* involves laceration of visceral pleura during a procedure such as thoracentesis or central-line insertion.	■ Pain ■ Dyspnea ■ Tachypnea, tachycardia ■ Decreased respiratory excursion ■ Absent breath sounds in affected area ■ Air movement through an open wound
Tension 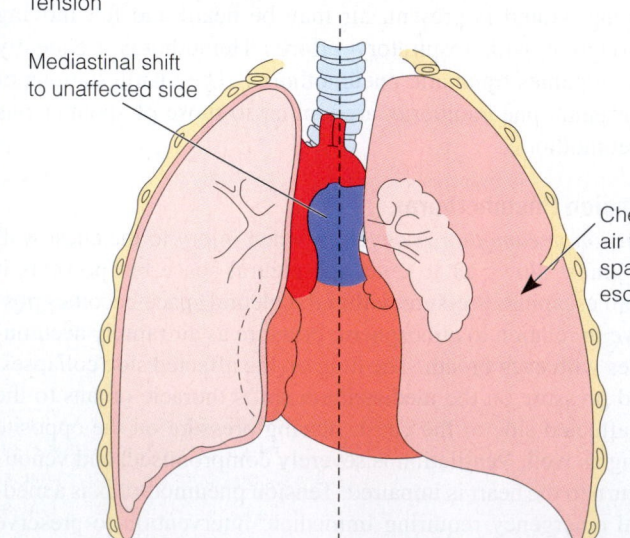	Air enters pleural space through chest wall or from airways but is unable to escape, resulting in rapid accumulation. Lung on affected side collapses. As intrapleural pressure increases, heart, great vessels, trachea, and esophagus shift toward the unaffected side.	■ Hypotension, shock ■ Distended neck veins ■ Severe dyspnea ■ Tachypnea, tachycardia ■ Decreased respiratory excursion ■ Absent breath sounds on affected side ■ Tracheal deviation toward unaffected side

Figure labels (Spontaneous): Normal lung; Pleural space

Figure labels (Traumatic): Puncture wound through chest wall

Figure labels (Tension): Mediastinal shift to unaffected side; Chest wound allows air to enter pleural space but prevents escape.

NURSING CARE OF THE PATIENT with Chest Tubes

PREPROCEDURE CARE

- Ensure a signed informed consent for chest tube insertion. *This invasive procedure requires informed consent.*
- Provide additional information as indicated. Explain that local anesthesia will be used but that pressure may be felt as the trocar is inserted. Reassure that breathing will be easier once the chest tube is in place and the lung re-expands. *The patient may be extremely dyspneic and anxious and may need reassurance that this invasive procedure will provide relief.*
- Gather all needed supplies, including thoracostomy tray, injectable lidocaine, sterile gloves, chest tube drainage system, sterile water, and a large sterile catheter-tipped syringe to use as a funnel for filling water-seal and suction chambers. *These supplies are used during the insertion procedure to establish a water-seal drainage system.*
- Position as indicated for the procedure. *Either an upright position (as for thoracentesis) or side-lying position may be used, depending on the site of the pneumothorax.*
- Assist with chest tube insertion as needed. The procedure may be performed in a procedure room, in the surgical suite, or at the bedside. *Although chest tube insertion is a relatively simple procedure, nursing assistance is necessary to support the patient and rapidly establish a closed drainage system.*

POSTPROCEDURE CARE

- Assess respiratory status at least every 4 hours. *Frequent assessment is necessary to monitor respiratory status and the effect of chest tube.*
- Maintain a closed system. Tape all connections, and secure the chest tube to the chest wall. *These measures are important*

to prevent inadvertent tube removal or disruption of the system integrity.
- Keep the collection apparatus below the level of the chest. *Pleural fluid drains into the collection apparatus by gravity flow.*
- Check tubes frequently for kinks or loops. *These could interfere with drainage.*
- Check the water seal frequently. The water level should fluctuate with respiratory effort. If it does not, the system may not be patent or intact. Periodic air bubbles in the water-seal chamber are normal and indicate that trapped air is being removed from the chest. *Frequent assessment of the system is important to ensure appropriate functioning*
- Measure drainage every 8 hours, marking the level on the drainage chamber. Report drainage that is cloudy, in excess of 70 mL per hour, or red, warm, and free flowing. *Red, free-flowing drainage indicates hemorrhage; cloudiness may indicate an infection.*
- Periodically assess water level in the suction control chamber, adding water as necessary. *Adequate water in the suction control chamber prevents excess suction from being placed on delicate pleural tissue*
- Assist with frequent position changes and sitting and ambulation as allowed. *Chest tubes should not prevent performance of allowed activities. Care is needed to prevent inadvertent disconnection or removal of the tubes.*
- When the chest tube is removed, immediately apply a sterile occlusive petroleum jelly dressing. *An occlusive dressing prevents air from reentering the pleural space through the chest wound.*

MANIFESTATIONS In addition to manifestations of pneumothorax, hypotension and distended neck veins are evident as venous return and cardiac output are affected. The trachea is displaced toward the unaffected side as a result of the mediastinal shift. Signs of shock may be present. ∞ See Chapter 11 for the manifestations and treatment of shock.

Interdisciplinary Care

Treatment for pneumothorax depends on the severity of the problem. A small simple pneumothorax may require no treatment other than monitoring with serial x-rays. Air is absorbed from the pleural space, allowing most small pneumothoraces to resolve spontaneously. A large pneumothorax or significant symptoms usually requires treatment with *thoracostomy*, or the placement of chest tubes. Surgical intervention may be necessary to prevent recurrent spontaneous pneumothorax.

Diagnosis

Oxygen saturation measurements are obtained to evaluate the effect of pneumothorax on gas exchange. ABGs may be obtained to further assess gas exchange.

The chest x-ray is an effective diagnostic tool for pneumothorax. In tension pneumothorax, air is evident on the affected side, and mediastinal structures are shifted toward the opposite or unaffected side.

Treatments

CHEST TUBES The treatment of choice for significant pneumothorax is placement of a closed-chest catheter to allow the lung to re-expand. When a tube is placed in the pleural cavity to remove air or fluid, it must be sealed to prevent air from also entering the tube and, in essence, creating an open pneumothorax. Chest tubes are sealed with a Heimlich (one-way) valve (Figure 36–9 ■) or connected to a closed drainage system with a "water seal." The valve or water seal prevent air from entering the chest cavity during inspiration and allow air to escape during expiration. Applying a low level of suction to the system helps to reestablish negative pressure in the pleural space, allowing the lung to re-expand.

A number of closed-drainage chest tube systems are available. Most are self-contained disposable systems (Figure 36–10 ■). Drainage from the chest tube is collected in the first collection chamber. This sealed chamber is connected to a water-seal chamber, which is in turn connected to the suction-control chamber. Nursing care of the patient with chest tubes is discussed in the accompanying box.

A large-bore needle or plastic intravenous catheter may be

Figure 36–9 ■ The Heimlich one-way valve allows air to escape from the pleural space, helping re-establish negative pressure and allowing the lung to re-expand.

Connect to external suction source

Connect to chest tube

Atmosphere vent

Suction control chamber

Water seal chamber

Collection chamber

Figure 36–10 ■ A closed-chest drainage system.

inserted through the chest wall as emergency treatment of a tension pneumothorax. This allows air to escape from the affected side, relieving pressure on mediastinal structures and the opposite lung.

PLEURODESIS   Although controversial, *pleurodesis*, or creation of adhesions between the parietal and visceral pleura, may be used to prevent recurrent pneumothorax. This procedure involves instilling a chemical agent such as doxycycline into the pleural space. The subsequent inflammatory response creates scar tissue and adhesions between the pleural layers. This procedure reduces the recurrence rate to as low as 2% but can make subsequent surgery more difficult.

Surgery

The risk for recurrence of spontaneous pneumothorax increases with each attack. Patients at high risk for recurrent pneumothorax may have surgery to reduce the risk of future ruptures. A thoracotomy is done to excise or oversew blebs (usually at the apices of the lungs). The overlying pleura is then roughened or irritated to induce scarring and adhesion to the surface of the lung. In some cases, the parietal pleura may be partially excised. These procedures can be done using video-assisted thoracoscopic surgery (VATS), a minimally invasive surgical technique (Fishman et al., 2008).

∞ Nursing Care

Health Promotion

Health promotion activities to prevent spontaneous and traumatic pneumothorax primarily involve health teaching. Initiate and participate in programs to prevent smoking among children and teenagers. Teach safe behaviors such as always wearing a

seat beat in an automobile, driving safely, and using precautions to prevent falls when working or recreating in high places.

Assessment

The patient with pneumothorax may be in acute respiratory distress, necessitating rapid and focused assessment.

- *Health history:* Current symptoms and their duration; precipitating factors or activities if known; previous episodes of pneumothorax; smoking history; chronic pulmonary diseases such as COPD.
- *Physical assessment:* General appearance and degree of apparent respiratory distress; evidence of chest trauma; vital signs, oxygen saturation, skin color, level of consciousness; respiratory excursion, percussion tone, and breath sounds anterior and posterior chest; neck vein inspection, position of trachea; peripheral pulses.
- *Diagnostic tests:* Chest x-ray, arterial blood gases.

Nursing Diagnoses and Interventions

Maintaining or restoring adequate alveolar ventilation and gas exchange is of highest priority for the patient with a pneumothorax. Chest tubes may interfere with physical mobility, contributing to a high risk for injury.

Impaired Gas Exchange

Loss of negative pressure in the pleural cavity and the resulting collapse of lung tissue can cause poor chest expansion and loss of alveolar ventilation. As the pneumothorax is removed or reabsorbed, ventilation and gas exchange improve.

- Assess and document vital signs and respiratory status, including rate, depth, lung sounds, and oxygen saturation at least every 4 hours. *Frequent assessment is important to monitor the adequacy of respirations and lung expansion.*

> **PRACTICE ALERT**
> Evaluate chest wall movement, position of the trachea, and neck veins frequently. Early identification of tension pneumothorax and appropriate interventions are vital to preserve cardiorespiratory function.

- Place in Fowler's or high-Fowler's position. *This position facilitates lung expansion.*
- Administer oxygen as ordered. *Supplemental oxygen is given to improve oxygenation of the blood and tissues.*

> **PRACTICE ALERT**
> Provide emotional support, particularly in early stages and during chest tube insertion. Dyspnea and hypoxemia can cause extreme anxiety and apprehension, impairing the ability to cooperate with procedures.

- Assess chest tube, system function, and drainage at least every 2 hours. *The system must remain patent and intact to function effectively.*
- Provide for rest. *Adequate rest is important to conserve energy and reduce oxygen demand.*

Risk for Injury

Pain and the presence of chest tubes can reduce the perceived ability to ambulate and provide self-care. Moderate activity is encouraged unless respiratory function is significantly impaired. Caution is taken to maintain integrity of the chest tube system. If the tube is inadvertently pulled out or system integrity is disrupted, the pneumothorax may increase or infection may develop.

> **PRACTICE ALERT**
> Avoid placing tension on chest tubes during positioning, ambulation, and care activities. The chest tubes are minimally secured to the chest wall and can be dislodged if tension is placed on them.

- Secure a loop of drainage tubing to the sheet or gown. *Looping the drainage tubing prevents direct pressure on the chest tube itself.*
- When turning to the affected side, ensure that neither the chest tube nor drainage tubing is kinked or occluded under the patient. *This maintains patency of the system.*
- Teach the patient how to ambulate with the drainage system, keeping the system lower than the chest. In most cases, suction can be discontinued during ambulation. *Ambulation facilitates lung ventilation and expansion. Drainage systems are portable to allow ambulation while chest tubes are in place. Keeping the drainage system lower than the chest promotes drainage and prevents reflux.*
- Observe insertion site when changing chest tube dressings for redness, swelling, pain, or drainage. Report any signs of infection, including fever, to the healthcare provider. *Interruption of skin integrity by chest tube insertion increases the risk for infection.*
- Ensure all tubing connections are taped per hospital policy or provider preference. If a connection does come loose, reconnect it as soon as possible. *A closed, sealed system is vital to prevent air from entering the pleural space and an open pneumothorax.*

> **PRACTICE ALERT**
> Seal the wound of an open pneumothorax or from inadvertent tube removal as soon as possible with a sterile occlusive dressing, such as gauze impregnated with petroleum jelly. If a sterile dressing is not available, other occlusive material such as foil or plastic wrap can be used. Tape the dressing on three sides only. An occlusive dressing taped on three sides prevents the development of a tension pneumothorax by inhibiting air from entering the wound during inhalation but allowing it to escape during exhalation.

Community-Based Care

Patients who have experienced spontaneous pneumothorax need education about their future risk. After a single episode of spontaneous pneumothorax, the risk of recurrence is 40% to 50%. This risk increases with subsequent episodes. Stress the importance of quitting smoking to reduce the risk. Other activities that can precipitate recurrent episodes include mountain climbing or those involving exposure to high altitudes, flying in unpressurized aircraft, and scuba diving (Papadakis & McPhee, 2007). The client may be advised to avoid contact sports.

Following a pneumothorax, instruct the patient to gradually increase exercise and activity to previous levels. Stress the importance of follow-up care and monitoring. Discuss manifestations to report to the healthcare provider: upper respiratory infections; fever, cough, or difficulty breathing; sudden, sharp chest pain; or redness, pain, swelling, tenderness, or drainage from the chest tube puncture wound.

The Patient with Hemothorax

Hemothorax, or blood in the pleural space, usually occurs as a result of chest trauma, surgery, or diagnostic procedures. Hemothorax develops in about 25% of patients with chest trauma, usually due to laceration of the lung, an intercostals vessel, or the internal mammary artery. If a major thoracic vessel is disrupted, hemorrhage can be massive (Azfar, Lippmann, Mundathaje, & Khaleeq, 2008). Tumors, pulmonary infarction, and infections such as TB also can cause hemothorax. When blood collects in the pleural space, pressure on the affected lung impairs ventilation and gas exchange. With significant hemorrhage, a risk of shock exists.

Hemothorax causes symptoms similar to those of pneumothorax or pleural effusion. Lung sounds are diminished, and a dull percussion tone is noted over the collected blood, typically at the base of the lung. Chest x-ray is used to confirm the diagnosis of hemothorax.

Thoracentesis or thoracostomy with chest tube drainage is used to remove blood from the pleural space. With significant hemorrhage (e.g., due to trauma or surgery), the blood may be collected for subsequent autotransfusion. Blood for autotransfusion should be collected and reinfused within 4 hours. Strict aseptic technique is used in collecting the blood. It is collected through a gross particulate filter into a container primed with anticoagulant and reinfused when the container is full or when transfusion is necessary. Air is removed from the blood container prior to reinfusion and a filter used to eliminate debris, such as degenerating blood cells, fat particles, and fibrin.

Priority nursing care for the patient with hemothorax focuses on assessing and maintaining adequate respiratory function and cardiac output. The priority of care depends on the rate and extent of hemothorax. In a large, slow-developing hemothorax, ventilatory status may be affected significantly. In this instance, *Impaired Gas Exchange* and *Ineffective Breathing Pattern* are priority nursing diagnoses (Perrin, 2009). When hemothorax develops rapidly and hemorrhage is significant, additional priority nursing diagnoses include *Decreased Cardiac Output* and *Risk for Deficient Fluid Volume.*

When preparing the patient for home care following a hemothorax, discuss the importance of avoiding smoking and preventing respiratory infection. Include symptoms to report to the healthcare provider. If trauma or infection caused the hemothorax, discuss measures to prevent future trauma and continuing treatment for the infection as indicated.

Trauma of the Chest or Lung

Chest injury is a leading cause of death from trauma. It is commonly associated with motor vehicle crashes, violent crime, and falls. Chest injuries can range from mild, such as a simple rib fracture, to severe and fatal. Traumatic injury to the chest may involve both the chest wall and underlying thoracic structures, including the lungs, heart, great vessels, and esophagus. Chest and lung injury can result from several different mechanisms: penetrating trauma, such as a stab or gunshot wound; blunt trauma, such as a fall, motor vehicle crash, vehicle-pedestrian impact, or crush injury; or inhalation injury, such as smoke inhalation or near drowning.

Rapid and continuing assessment of the airway, breathing, and circulation (ABCs) is vital in chest or lung injuries. Chest trauma can disrupt any or all of these functions. Chest injuries that may be life threatening include airway obstruction, tension pneumothorax, open pneumothorax, massive hemothorax, and flail chest with pulmonary contusion.

The Patient with a Thoracic Injury

Thoracic injuries may be minor and have little effect on respiratory status, for example, simple rib fracture in a previously healthy patient. When pain or chest wall instability impair breathing or the underlying lung tissue is damaged, the risk is more significant. Thoracic trauma usually is caused by motor vehicle crashes or falls.

Pathophysiology and Manifestations

Acceleration-deceleration injury and direct mechanisms of injury (e.g., crush injuries) are the most common mechanisms of thoracic injuries. Acceleration-deceleration injuries are caused by a rapid change in velocity as occurs in a motor vehicle crash or fall. The body stops suddenly, but the tissues and organs within the chest cavity continue to move forward until they impact with the chest wall. Injuries sustained can be significant, depending on the velocity (speed) of the vehicle or body at the point of impact, the surface with which the body impacts, and individual characteristics (e.g., size and bone structure).

Rib Fracture

Simple rib fracture, usually involving a single rib, is the most common chest wall injury. Rib fracture generally is tolerated well and heals rapidly in a young, previously healthy person. In an older adult or person with preexisting lung disease, however, a fractured rib may lead to significant complications, such as pneumonia, atelectasis, and, potentially, respiratory failure. Displaced fractured ribs can penetrate the pleura, leading to pneumothorax and possible hemothorax. Fractures of certain ribs are more frequently associated with underlying tissue damage. Intrathoracic vessels may be damaged or torn with fractures of the first and second ribs. Fractures of the seventh through tenth ribs may cause liver or spleen injuries.

Rib fracture causes pain on inspiration and coughing. This leads to voluntary splinting, with rapid, shallow respirations and inhibited cough. Bruising may be seen over the fracture, and crepitus may be palpated with respiratory movement. Breath sounds are diminished, especially in the bases, due to splinting. If pneumothorax develops, chest wall movement on the affected side may be reduced, and breath sounds absent or significantly diminished. A hyperresonant percussion tone usually is noted. Hemothorax also causes diminished or absent breath sounds on the affected side, with a dull percussion note.

Flail Chest

Multiple rib fractures may impair chest wall stability and normal chest wall function. When two or more consecutive ribs are fractured in multiple places, a free-floating segment of the chest wall, or **flail chest**, results. Physiologic function of the chest wall is impaired as the flail segment is sucked inward during inhalation and moves outward with exhalation. This is known as *paradoxic movement* (Figure 36–11 ■).

Flail chest can significantly affect ventilation, and consequently, gas exchange. Lung expansion is impaired and the work of breathing increases. Flail chest is frequently associated with underlying pulmonary contusion, which may lead to respiratory failure.

Flail chest causes dyspnea and pain, especially on inspiration. Paradoxic chest movement is evident with inspection. Chest expansion is unequal, and palpable crepitus is present. Breath sounds are diminished, and crackles may be heard on auscultation.

Pulmonary Contusion

Pulmonary contusion, or lung tissue injury, is frequently associated with flail chest and other blunt chest trauma. It may occur unilaterally or bilaterally. Pulmonary contusion often results from abrupt chest compression followed by sudden decompression, as can occur with a motor vehicle accident (MVA), significant fall, or crush injury. Alveoli and pulmonary arterioles rupture, causing intra-alveolar hemorrhage and interstitial and bronchial edema. The resulting inflammatory response increases capillary permeability, leading to edema that may be localized to the damaged lung tissue or more generalized. Inflammation and edema impair the production of surfactant within the alveoli, decreasing compliance. Pulmonary vascular resistance increases and blood flow decreases. Airway obstruction, atelectasis, and impaired gas diffusion result. Associated chest wall injury impairs the ability to clear secretions effectively, and the work of breathing is significantly increased.

Manifestations of pulmonary contusion may not be apparent until 12 to 24 hours after the injury. Increasing shortness of breath, restlessness, apprehension, and chest pain are early signs. Copious sputum, which may be blood tinged, is present. Later manifestations include tachycardia, tachypnea, dyspnea, and cyanosis. Even with appropriate treatment, pulmonary contusion can lead to acute respiratory distress and potential death.

Interdisciplinary Care

Chest x-ray is used to identify most chest wall injuries. Rib fractures are evident on x-ray. Pulmonary contusion may show as initial patchy opacifications progressing to diffuse opacification, or

Flail (free floating) segment

A Fracture pattern of flail chest

B Inspiration

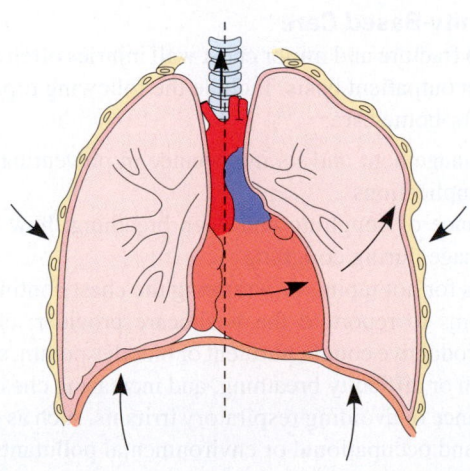

C Expiration

Figure 36–11 ■ Flail chest with paradoxical movement.

"white-out." Changes in oxygen saturation and arterial blood gases depend on the degree to which ventilation and gas exchange are affected by the injury.

Simple rib fractures typically heal uneventfully. Providing adequate analgesia to promote breathing, coughing, and movement is the primary intervention. With multiple rib fractures, an intercostal nerve block may be used to ensure adequate ventilation. Rib belts, binders, and taping to stabilize the rib cage are not recommended, because they may interfere with ventilation and lead to atelectasis. Even with simple rib fracture, older patients and patients with preexisting lung disease require close monitoring to prevent and detect atelectasis, pneumonia, and other complications.

Intercostal nerve blocks or continuous epidural analgesia may be employed to manage the pain associated with flail chest. For a small flail chest, analgesia combined with supplemental oxygen therapy may be adequate. In some cases, internal or external fixation of the flail segment may be done.

The preferred treatment for flail chest is intubation and mechanical ventilation. Positive-pressure ventilation provides support and stabilization of the flail segment and improves ventilation and gas exchange. The work of breathing is decreased and healing improved.

Patients with pulmonary contusion often are critically ill, requiring intensive care management. Treatment is supportive, directed at maintaining adequate ventilation and alveolar gas exchange. Endotracheal intubation and mechanical ventilation are necessary in most cases. Repeated bronchoscopy may be done to remove secretions and cellular debris, preventing atelectasis. Although adequate hydration is necessary to prevent shock, overhydration can increase pulmonary edema. Pulmonary arterial pressure monitoring with a Swan-Ganz catheter and frequent arterial blood gas measurement is required for optimal fluid replacement and management of ventilatory support. ∞ See Chapter 31 for more information about pulmonary artery pressure monitoring, and ∞ Chapter 37 for nursing care of the patient who is intubated and ventilated.

Unilateral pulmonary contusion may present a unique management problem. Mechanical ventilation with positive end-expiratory pressure (PEEP) to maintain open alveoli and adequate gas exchange can damage the unaffected lung. Intubation with a double-lumen endotracheal tube that permits independent ventilation of each lung may be used.

∞ Nursing Care

Health Promotion
Encourage the use of seat belts, shoulder harness, and supplemental restraint systems such as air bags to significantly reduce the incidence of thoracic injury associated with motor vehicle crashes. Discuss the importance of appropriate protective equipment and gear for people engaging in potentially hazardous activities such as contact sports, mountain climbing, and occupations such as roofing or house painting.

Assessment
The nursing assessment of the patient with a thoracic injury may need to be rapid and focused.

- *Health history:* Pain, difficulty breathing; circumstances of the injury, including position in the motor vehicle, use of restraints, speed and type of impact; distance of a fall, surface and position on impact; history of chronic lung or heart disease; smoking history.

- *Physical examination:* Airway, breathing, circulation; level of consciousness; color, vital signs; respiratory rate, depth, ease; symmetry of chest movement; lung sounds and percussion tone; presence of bruising, crepitus, or paradoxical chest movement.

Nursing Diagnoses and Interventions

Chest wall trauma can interfere with adequate chest expansion and alveolar ventilation. When a pulmonary contusion is also present, gas exchange is affected as well. Priorities for nursing management include controlling pain, ensuring adequate ventilation, and promoting gas exchange.

Acute Pain

With many thoracic injuries, pain interferes with lung expansion and coughing, leading to such complications as pneumonia and atelectasis. Adequate pain management is a key component of medical and nursing management for these patients.

- Frequently assess pain, using a standard pain scale and objective data. *Increased respiratory rate, shallow respirations, diminished breath sounds, and reluctance to move and cough may indicate inadequate pain control in a thoracic injury.*
- Administer analgesics by patient-controlled analgesia or on a schedule to maintain pain control. *Analgesics are more effective when pain is not allowed to become intense.*

> **PRACTICE ALERT**
> Assess for possible respiratory depression due to narcotic analgesia. Respiratory depression can further compromise ventilation in the patient with thoracic injury.

- Notify the healthcare provider if pain relief is inadequate or excess sedation and respiratory depression occur. *An intercostal nerve block may be done to reduce the need for narcotic analgesia. Assess for bleeding and adequate ventilation following a nerve block.*

Ineffective Airway Clearance

Aggressive respiratory hygiene may be necessary to maintain open airways and adequate ventilation.

- Assess lung sounds and respiratory rate, depth, and effort frequently. Encourage to cough, deep breathe, and change position every 1 to 2 hours, and use the incentive spirometer. *Frequent assessment and measures to maintain airway patency are vital to prevent complications in the patient with thoracic injury.*
- Teach how to splint the affected area with a blanket or pillow when coughing. *Splinting reduces movement and discomfort of the affected area.*
- Suction airway as indicated. Work with respiratory therapy to maintain optimal mechanical ventilation. Secure the endotracheal tube to maintain appropriate position and lung ventilation. *Endotracheal tube security is particularly important when a double-lumen endotracheal tube is in place, because malposition can occlude one main bronchus and prevent ventilation of the affected lung.*
- Elevate the head of the bed. *Elevating the head of the bed facilitates lung expansion and reduces the work of breathing.*

> **PRACTICE ALERT**
> Promptly report to the healthcare provider signs of complications, such as diminished breath sounds, increasing crackles (rales) or rhonchi, dull or hyperresonant percussion tones, unequal chest movement, hemoptysis, chills or fever, or changes in vital signs. Prompt intervention for complications is vital to promote healing and recovery.

Impaired Gas Exchange

Impaired gas exchange is of particular concern in pulmonary contusion. Alveolar damage and pulmonary edema can significantly impair oxygenation of the blood and removal of carbon dioxide.

- Monitor vital signs, color, oxygen saturation, and arterial blood gases. Assess for manifestations such as anxiety or apprehension, restlessness, confusion or lethargy, or complaints of headache. *These assessment data alert the nurse and care providers to potential hypoxemia or hypercapnia due to impaired gas exchange.*
- Maintain oxygen therapy and mechanical ventilation as ordered. Hyperoxygenate prior to suctioning. *Oxygen and mechanical ventilation support alveolar gas exchange. Hyperoxygenation prior to suctioning reduces the degree of hypoxemia that occurs during suctioning.*
- Monitor intake and output, weigh daily, and monitor central venous pressure and pulmonary artery pressure as ordered. Maintain any ordered fluid restriction. *Fluid volume status is monitored to reduce the effects of pulmonary edema on lung tissues.*
- Maintain bed rest or activity restriction as ordered. Space activities to allow periods of uninterrupted rest. *Rest reduces the metabolic rate and oxygen consumption.*

Community-Based Care

Simple rib fracture and minor chest wall injuries often are managed on an outpatient basis. Include the following topics when teaching for home care:

- Pain management and its importance in preventing respiratory complications
- Importance of coughing and deep breathing; how to splint the rib cage during coughing
- Reasons for not taping or wrapping the chest continuously
- Symptoms to report to the healthcare provider: chills and fever, productive cough, purulent or bloody sputum, shortness of breath or difficulty breathing, and increasing chest pain
- Importance of avoiding respiratory irritants, such as cigarette smoke and occupational or environmental pollutants

Significant pulmonary contusion can result in long-term respiratory insufficiency. Discuss activity modifications and occupational changes with the patient and family as indicated. Refer to home care services such as respiratory therapy and home health if needed.

The Patient with Inhalation Injury

The internal environment of the lungs normally is protected from noxious substances by respiratory defense mechanisms. If these defenses are breached, inhaled agents, such as gases, fumes, toxins, and water, can cause internal trauma to the lungs.

Pathophysiology and Manifestations

Smoke Inhalation

Pulmonary injury due to inhalation of hot air, toxic gases, or particulate matter is the leading cause of death in burn injury (Perrin, 2009). Smoke inhalation affects up to one-third of patients admitted to burn units. Smoke inhalation can significantly affect normal respiratory function through three different mechanisms:

- Thermal damage to the airways, leading to impaired ventilation
- Carbon monoxide or cyanide poisoning, resulting in tissue hypoxia
- Chemical damage to the lung from noxious gases, which can impair gas exchange

Smoke inhalation is suspected whenever a burn occurs in a closed space; if there are burns to the face or upper torso or singed nasal hairs; if sputum contains ash-like material; and when manifestations such as dyspnea, wheezing, rales, or rhonchi develop.

The lower airways of the lungs typically are protected from thermal damage by cooling of the inhaled gases in the upper airway and laryngeal spasm. Upper airway obstruction due to tissue edema and laryngeal spasm can occur quickly, however, resulting in **asphyxiation**, or oxygen deprivation, without lung damage. Steam inhalation can cause thermal damage to tissues of the lower respiratory tract.

Inhalation of carbon monoxide or cyanide gas poses an immediate threat to life. Carbon monoxide is a colorless, odorless gas produced in a fire. It binds readily with hemoglobin. The affinity of carbon monoxide for hemoglobin is 200 to 250 times stronger than that of oxygen. Hemoglobin bound to carbon monoxide reduces the oxygen-carrying capacity of blood and oxygen delivery to cells of the body. Carbon monoxide poisoning is suspected if the burn occurred in a closed space, if there is evidence of inhalation injury, or if dyspnea develops.

The manifestations of carbon monoxide poisoning depend on the level of carboxyhemoglobin saturation. When hemoglobin is 10% to 20% saturated with carbon monoxide, symptoms include headache, dizziness, dyspnea, and nausea. A characteristic "cherry-red" skin color and mucous membranes may be seen. With increasing levels, confusion, visual disturbances, irritability, hallucinations, hypotension, seizures, and coma develop. Permanent neurologic deficit can occur in survivors of severe acute carbon monoxide poisoning.

Many other toxic chemicals may be present in smoke, especially in a house fire or industrial plant fire. Hydrogen cyanide can be lethal when inhaled. Inhalation of toxic chemicals causes bronchospasm and edema of the airways and alveoli. Acute respiratory distress syndrome may develop within 1 to 2 days. Sloughing of damaged mucosa leads to airway obstruction and atelectasis. Pneumonia is common following smoke inhalation.

Near-Drowning

Drowning is a leading preventable cause of accidental death in the United States. Approximately 5500 people die of drowning every year in the United States. Alcohol ingestion is a factor in about 25% of adult drowning deaths. Other circumstances that may contribute to drowning and near-drowning include excessive fatigue, a sudden acute condition such as seizure or myocardial infarction, and head or spinal cord injury associated with diving (Papadakis & McPhee, 2007).

Asphyxiation and aspiration are the primary problems associated with drowning and near-drowning. About 10% of victims do not aspirate water; instead, laryngeal spasm causes asphyxia. This is known as "dry drowning." In most cases, however, asphyxia and hypoxemia are the result of fluid aspiration. The effects of hypoxemia occur rapidly; loss of consciousness can occur within 3 to 5 minutes after total immersion. Circulatory impairment, brain injury, and brain death can occur within 5 to 10 minutes. Immersion in very cold water and the *dive reflex*, a protective mechanism that slows the heartbeat, constricts peripheral vessels, and shunts blood to the brain and heart, may prolong survival.

Water aspiration can cause delayed death from near-drowning. Respiratory and systemic effects differ, depending on whether freshwater or saltwater has been aspirated. Freshwater is hypotonic; when aspirated, it is rapidly absorbed from the alveoli, leading to hypervolemia and hemodilution. Hemolysis occurs as blood cells are subjected to a hypotonic environment, and serum electrolytes are diluted. Electrolyte imbalances can cause cardiac dysrhythmias and death. Hemolysis can lead to acute tubular necrosis and acute renal failure. Aspiration of freshwater impairs pulmonary surfactant and damages the alveolar-capillary membrane. Respiratory failure can result.

Nearly the opposite effects occur with saltwater aspiration. As a hypertonic fluid, saltwater draws fluid into the alveoli, resulting in hypovolemia and hemoconcentration. Hemolysis is insignificant, and small elevations in serum sodium and chloride levels rarely cause life-threatening effects. With either type of near-drowning episode, inhaled microorganisms and debris can lead to pneumonia. The pathophysiologic changes associated with freshwater and saltwater near-drowning are illustrated in Figure 36–12.

Manifestations of near-drowning may include altered level of consciousness, restlessness, and apprehension. The patient may complain of headache or chest pain. Other signs include vomiting, possible cyanosis, apnea, tachypnea, and wheezing. If pulmonary edema is present, pink froth may be visible in

Figure 36–12 ■ The pathogenesis of near-drowning, freshwater and saltwater.

the mouth and nose. Other manifestations include tachycardia, dysrhythmias, hypotension, shock, and cardiac arrest. Hypothermia may be present.

The near-drowning victim who never loses consciousness or is conscious on admission to the emergency department has a good prognosis for recovery. The prognosis is less optimistic when neurologic damage has occurred.

Interdisciplinary Care

With inhalation injuries, the most effective treatment is prevention. A working smoke detector (with functioning batteries) could prevent the majority of deaths from smoke inhalation occurring in the home. The line, "A smoke detector was found, but the batteries had been removed," is all too familiar in news reports of fire-related deaths.

To prevent drowning, life preservers and flotation vests or jackets should be worn on the body, not stored in the hold of the boat. These devices are designed to keep the head above water. Even accomplished swimmers should never enter the water alone in unguarded areas. Just as alcohol and driving do not mix, neither do alcohol and boating or other water sports.

The second most important line of defense against death or permanent injury from inhalation injuries is removing the victim from the area of the fire or water and administering effective cardiopulmonary resuscitation. In many cases, immediate restoration of effective breathing and circulation is key to preserving life. Hypoxemia progresses rapidly until breathing is restored; reversal of tissue hypoxia depends on adequate circulation. In both smoke inhalation and near drowning, intubation may be necessary to establish an airway. Oxygen is administered as soon as possible. Attempts to drain water from the lungs of the near-drowning victim waste time and are generally ineffective in restoring alveolar ventilation. External cardiac defibrillation may be necessary to reestablish an effective cardiac rhythm and circulation. When the victim is hypothermic, resuscitation measures are continued until the core body temperature reaches approximately 90°F (32°C). The basic rule in hypothermia is that the patient is not declared dead until the body has been rewarmed and life signs remain absent.

Diagnosis

When inhalation injury is known or suspected, the following diagnostic tests may be done:

- *ABGs* are drawn to evaluate gas exchange and the degree of hypoxemia. Combined respiratory and metabolic acidosis may be apparent. With effective ventilation and supplemental oxygen, acidosis may reverse quickly. With carbon monoxide poisoning, arterial PO_2 may be normal, but oxyhemoglobin saturation is less than normal.
- *Carboxyhemoglobin levels* are drawn in suspected carbon monoxide poisoning. Normal levels are less than 5% in nonsmokers and less than 10% in smokers. Higher levels indicate carbon monoxide poisoning. Levels less than 20% are considered mild poisoning; between 20% and 40% is moderate poisoning; and 40% to 60% is severe poisoning. Levels higher than 60% are generally fatal.
- *Serum electrolytes* and *osmolality levels* vary in near-drowning, depending on the type of water aspirated. In freshwater

drowning, serum electrolyte levels and osmolality may be significantly reduced. With saltwater drowning, serum sodium and chloride may be somewhat high, and osmolality is increased because of hypovolemia.

- *Chest x-ray* is done, but may not show changes until 12 or more hours after the insult. Evidence of acute respiratory distress syndrome may be seen 24 to 48 hours after inhalation injury.
- *Bronchoscopy* may be ordered to inspect damaged lung tissue, particularly with smoke inhalation and possible thermal injury.

Treatments

Treatment of inhalation injury is generally supportive. Endotracheal intubation and mechanical ventilation often are required to maintain the airway and provide adequate alveolar ventilation and oxygenation. All patients with inhalation injury require supplemental oxygen, even when intubation and ventilation are not required. *Hyperbaric oxygen therapy*, the delivery of 100% oxygen at increased atmospheric pressure, may be used to treat carbon monoxide poisoning. This treatment carries some risks, such as oxygen toxicity and potential trauma to lung tissues, sinuses, and ears due to the increased pressures.

Other treatment measures may include bronchodilator therapy to manage bronchospasm. Bronchodilators can be administered by aerosol inhalation or intravenous infusion. Coughing and suctioning is important to remove secretions and debris. Chest physiotherapy with percussion and postural drainage may be performed.

Intravenous fluids may be ordered; if significant hemolysis has occurred, packed red blood cells may be given to improve the oxygen-carrying capacity of the blood. Fluid therapy is monitored carefully, using pulmonary artery or central venous pressures to reduce the risk of pulmonary edema.

With near-drowning victims, measures such as inducing hypothermia or barbiturate-induced coma and administering corticosteroids and osmotic diuretics may be employed to help prevent neurologic damage. Careful monitoring for complications such as pneumonia and acute respiratory distress syndrome is vital throughout the course of treatment. Respiratory status, vital signs, and other data are frequently assessed to identify complications and allow early intervention.

Nursing Care

Health Promotion

Prevention of inhalation injuries is an important nursing responsibility. Teach everyone the value of a working smoke detector, especially in the sleeping areas of the house. Encourage families to develop an escape plan in case of fire and to use fire drills to rehearse getting out of the house. Smoldering cigarettes are a leading cause of house fires; help patients develop a plan to stop smoking. Teach people to drop and roll should clothing catch fire. (Flames rise, increasing the risk of respiratory injury when upright.)

Learning to swim safely is important to prevent drowning. Teach patients never to swim alone, when fatigued, or immediately following a meal. Remind patients that knowing how to swim will not prevent drowning in very cold water or in large bodies of water, such as lakes, rivers, or the ocean. Instruct to always wear flotation devices while boating, water-skiing, surfing, or wind-surfing. Wet suits help prevent hypothermia during activities in very cold water. Advise covering or fencing swimming pools, hot tubs, and ponds to prevent inadvertent entry and drowning.

A population well trained in effective, safe cardiopulmonary resuscitation (CPR) provides the best second line of defense against inhalation injury. Rapid restoration of breathing is essential to prevent hypoxia and brain damage. Encourage all people to be trained and regularly update CPR skills. Work with communities to increase the number of trained people. Refer patients to local chapters of the American Red Cross or American Heart Association for classes.

Assessment

Inhalation injuries may be a medical emergency, necessitating focused and timely nursing assessment.

- *Health history:* Circumstances of the injury, including duration of exposure to smoke or time under water, explosion or fire in a closed area, type and temperature of water immersed in; resuscitation measures used; allergies, and current medical problems.
- *Physical examination:* Airway, breathing, circulation; level of consciousness; color, oxygen saturation level; vital signs; heart and lung sounds; urine output; evidence of burns or soot around nares or mouth.
- *Diagnostic tests:* Carboxyhemoglobin levels, serum electrolytes and osmolality; arterial blood gases; chest x-ray.

Nursing Diagnoses and Interventions

Nursing care priorities for the patient with an inhalation injury are determined by the type of injury or tissue damage. Airway clearance is a major concern in all inhalation injuries, as is impaired gas exchange. Tissue hypoxia also can be a significant problem.

Ineffective Airway Clearance

Nursing measures to maintain an adequate airway begin with careful and frequent assessment of respiratory status, including rate, depth, and effort as well as breath sounds. Note amount, color, and consistency of sputum. Assist to cough frequently; suction the intubated patient as needed to remove secretions. Elevate the head of the bed to facilitate alveolar ventilation unless otherwise ordered. Stabilize endotracheal tube with tape and ties to prevent displacement into a mainstem bronchus, which could lead to ventilation of only one lung. Report changes in the character of secretions that may indicate complications: pink, frothy sputum suggesting pulmonary edema, or purulent

sputum suggestive of pneumonia. Administer bronchodilators as ordered. Perform percussion and postural drainage as ordered.

Impaired Gas Exchange

Support gas exchange by administering supplemental oxygen, with or without mechanical ventilation. Frequently assess oxygen saturation, skin color, and mental status. Decreasing level of consciousness may be an early sign of hypoxemia. Monitor exhaled carbon dioxide, arterial blood gases, and pulmonary artery pressures as ordered and indicated. Report changes to the healthcare provider. Maintain oxygen flow rates as ordered. Provide frequent mouth care to reduce the discomfort of dry mucous membranes and prevent tissue breakdown. Work with respiratory therapy to maintain effective oxygen delivery with mechanical ventilation. Administer sedation as required. Maintain fluid restriction if ordered.

Ineffective Tissue Perfusion: Cerebral

Impaired cerebral tissue perfusion is a priority problem, especially with near-drowning. Hypoxia and possible hypervolemia can lead to cerebral edema and increased intracranial pressure (IICP), further impairing blood flow. Monitor vital signs and neurologic status frequently. A change in level of consciousness or behavior is typically the earliest sign of IICP. Changes noted on an intracranial pressure monitor also provide early evidence of IICP. Increasing systolic blood pressure and pulse pressure and slowed heart rate are late signs. Other manifestations may include pupillary changes and decreasing muscle strength. Report changes promptly to the healthcare provider. Elevate the head of the bed and keep the head in neutral position to promote drainage from the cranial vault. Maintain effective ventilation and oxygenation; hypercapnia and hypoxemia increase cerebral edema. Administer sedation, osmotic diuretics, or corticosteroids as ordered to reduce cerebral edema. Maintain fluid restriction. Space activities and promote rest to reduce metabolic demands.

Community-Based Care

Teach patients who do not require hospitalization for inhalation injury about symptoms that may indicate a complication and should be reported to the healthcare provider: increasing dyspnea, cough productive of purulent or pink frothy mucus, confusion, or other changes. Manifestations of respiratory damage may not be apparent for 24 to 48 hours following the injury.

Significant hypoxia due to near-drowning or carbon monoxide poisoning may cause permanent neurologic effects. Work with the family to develop communication techniques and identify remaining strengths. Help the family identify future care needs and means for meeting them, such as home health, personal care aides, or long-term care facilities. Provide social services and support group referrals.

Lung Cancer

The Patient with Lung Cancer

Lung cancer is the leading cause of cancer deaths in the United States, accounting for 31% of all cancer deaths. In 2009, about 219,440 people died from lung cancer in the United States; an estimated 159,390 new cases were diagnosed in that same year (ACS, 2009). It is a major health

problem with a grim prognosis: Most people with lung cancer die within 1 year of the initial diagnosis.

Pathophysiology

Lung cancer develops as damaged bronchial epithelial cells mutate over time to become neoplastic. The genetic abnormality commonly seen is on chromosome 3, with loss of genetic material. Alterations of tumor suppressor genes also are seen in some types of lung cancer.

The vast majority of primary lung lesions are *bronchogenic carcinoma*, tumors of the airway epithelium. These tumors are further differentiated by cell type: small-cell carcinoma, adenocarcinoma, squamous cell carcinoma, and large-cell carcinoma. For clinical purposes, the latter three cell types frequently are classified together as non-small-cell carcinomas. *Small-cell carcinomas*, which account for approximately 25% of lung cancers, grow rapidly and spread early. These tumors have paraneoplastic properties; that is, they produce manifestations at sites that are not directly affected by the tumor. Small-cell lung carcinomas can synthesize bioactive products and hormones such as adrenocorticotropic hormones (ACTH), antidiuretic hormone (ADH), a parathormone-like hormone, and gastrin-releasing peptide. *Non-small-cell carcinoma* accounts for about 75% of

lung cancers. Each cell type differs in its incidence, presentation, and manner of spread. Table 36–8 outlines the incidence and unique characteristics of each cell type.

Bronchogenic cancer, regardless of cell type, tends to be aggressive, locally invasive, and have widespread metastatic lesions. Tumors begin as mucosal lesions that grow to form masses that obstruct the bronchi or invade adjacent lung tissue. All types frequently spread via the lymph system to nodes and other organs such as the brain, bones, and liver.

Manifestations

The manifestations of lung cancer are related to the location and spread of the tumor. Patients may present with symptoms related to the primary tumor, manifestations of metastatic disease, or with systemic symptoms. Initial symptoms often are attributed to smoking or chronic bronchitis. Chronic cough is common, as is

TABLE 36–8 Comparison of Lung Cancer Cell Types

	CELL TYPE AND PREVALENCE	PRESENTATION AND ASSOCIATED MANIFESTATIONS	SPREAD
	Small-cell (oat cell) carcinoma 20% to 25% of all lung cancers	Central lesion with hilar mass common, early mediastinal involvement, no cavitation; SIADH, Cushing's syndrome, thrombophlebitis	Aggressive tumor; more than 40% of patients have distant metastasis at time of presentation
	Adenocarcinoma 20% to 40% of all lung cancers	Peripheral mass involving bronchi; few local symptoms; hypertrophic pulmonary osteoarthropathy	Early metastasis to central nervous system, skeleton, and adrenal glands
	Squamous cell carcinoma 30% to 32% of all lung cancers	Central lesion located in large bronchi; patient presents with cough, dyspnea, atelectasis, and wheezing; hypercalcemia common	Spreads by local invasion
	Large-cell carcinoma 10% to 15% of all lung cancers	Usually, peripheral lesion that is larger than that associated with adenocarcinoma and tends to cavitate; gynecomastia, thrombophlebitis	Early metastasis

hemoptysis. Wheezing and shortness of breath occur as a result of airway obstruction. Dull, aching chest pain occurs as the tumor spreads to the mediastinum; pleuritic pain occurs when the pleura is invaded. Hoarseness and/or dysphagia indicates pressure of the tumor on the trachea or esophagus.

Systemic and paraneoplastic manifestations of lung cancer include weight loss, anorexia, fatigue, and weakness; bone pain, tenderness, and swelling; clubbing of the fingers and toes; and various endocrine, neuromuscular, cardiovascular, and hematologic symptoms. See the Multisystem Effects of Lung Cancer illustration on page 1220.

Confusion, impaired gait and balance, headache, and personality changes may indicate brain metastasis. Bone metastases cause bone pain, pathologic fractures, and possible spinal cord compression, as well as thrombocytopenia and anemia if bone marrow is invaded. When the liver is affected, symptoms of liver dysfunction and biliary obstruction—including jaundice, anorexia, and upper right quadrant pain—are evident.

Complications and Course

Superior vena cava syndrome, partial or complete obstruction of the superior vena cava, is a potential complication of lung cancer, particularly when the tumor involves the superior mediastinum or the mediastinal lymph nodes. Obstructed venous flow from the head and neck produce the symptoms of superior vena cava syndrome (edema of the neck and face, headache, dizziness, vision disturbances, and syncope), and may develop acutely or more gradually. Veins of the upper chest and neck are dilated; flushing occurs, followed by cyanosis. Cerebral edema may affect the level of consciousness; laryngeal edema may impair respirations.

Paraneoplastic syndromes commonly associated with lung cancer include syndrome of inappropriate ADH secretion (SIADH) with fluid retention, hyponatremia, edema, Cushing's syndrome (∞ see Chapter 18) related to abnormal ACTH production, and hypercalcemia. Lung tumors also may produce procoagulation factors, increasing the risk for venous thrombosis, pulmonary embolism, and thrombotic endocarditis. In lung cancer, neuromuscular symptoms such as muscle weakness and wasting of the limbs may be the first indication of the disease (Huether & McCance, 2008).

At the time of diagnosis, cancer of the lung typically is well advanced, with distant metastasis present in 39% of patients and regional lymph node involvement in another 37%. The prognosis is generally poor: The overall 5-year survival rate is only 15% (ACS, 2009).

Incidence and Risk Factors

The incidence of lung cancer varies from state to state and among nations. It increases with age, occurring most commonly in patients over age 50. Family clusters of lung cancer suggest a genetic predisposition; however, exposure to tobacco smoke may be necessary for expression of the trait. Cigarette smoke, which contains 43 known chemical carcinogens and cancer promoters, is clearly the most significant cause of lung cancer (ACS, 2009). More than 80% of lung cancer cases are related to smoking, and the disease is 23 times more common in male smokers than male nonsmokers. There is a dose–response relationship between smoking and lung cancer; the more the person smokes and the longer the person smokes, the greater the risk. Even former smokers who have abstained for a number of years have a higher risk of developing lung cancer than nonsmokers. Exposure to ionizing radiation and inhaled irritants, asbestos in particular, is also recognized as a risk factor for lung cancer (Huether & McCance, 2008). Exposure to radon, a radioactive gas, also is identified as a lung cancer risk factor (ACS, 2009). Radon forms as radium, an element present in the earth's crust, disintegrates. Radon tends to accumulate in closed spaces where air circulation in poor, such as caves, mines, and energy-efficient houses.

> **FAST FACTS**
> - In the United States, the incidence of lung cancer is second to prostate cancer in men and breast cancer in women.
> - Lung cancer is, however, the leading cause of cancer deaths in the United States, responsible for 31% of cancer deaths in men and 27% of cancer deaths in women.
> - Lung cancer kills more women than breast, cervical, uterine, and ovarian cancers combined.
> - Tobacco use and exposure to cigarette smoke are the leading risk factors for lung cancer.

Interdisciplinary Care

Because lung cancer typically is advanced when diagnosed and the prognosis generally is poor, prevention of the disease must be a primary goal for all healthcare providers. With 80% of lung cancer related to cigarette smoking, reducing tobacco use can have a significant impact on the death rate from lung cancer—a far greater impact than advances in treatment.

Establishing an accurate diagnosis is the first step in treating lung cancer. Treatment decisions are based on the tumor location, type of cancer cell, staging of the tumor, and the patient's ability to tolerate treatment. Lung cancer is staged by the tumor size, location, degree of invasion of the primary tumor, and the presence of metastatic disease. Lung cancer staging is summarized in Table 36–9. Surgery is the treatment of choice for most forms of lung cancer.

Diagnosis

- *Chest x-ray* usually provides the first evidence of lung cancer. It is particularly reliable as a diagnostic tool when compared with previous chest x-ray. In high-risk populations, the chest x-ray may be used as a screening tool for lung cancer.
- *Sputum specimen* is sent for *cytologic examination* to establish the diagnosis of lung cancer. The sputum sample is collected on arising in the morning. If malignant cells are found in the sputum, more expensive and invasive examinations may be unnecessary. However, a sputum sample negative for malignant cells does not rule out lung cancer; it may simply indicate that the tumor is not shedding cells into mucous secretions.
- *Bronchoscopy* is frequently done to visualize and obtain tissue for biopsy from the tumor. When a tumor mass or suspicious tissue is identified visually, a cable-activated instrument is used to obtain a biopsy specimen. If the tumor cannot be seen, the airways may be flushed with a saline solution (bronchial washing) to obtain cells for cytologic examination.

MULTISYSTEM EFFECTS OF
Lung Cancer

Respiratory
- Cough
- Hemoptysis
- Wheezing and dyspnea
- Chest pain, dull or pleuritic
- Hoarseness and dysphagia
- Pleural effusion

Cardiovascular
- Compression of the superior vena cava

Gastrointestinal
- Anorexia

Metabolic Processes
- Weight loss
- Fever

Paraneoplastic Syndromes

Endocrine System
- Hypercalcemia
- Hyperphosphatemia
- Cushing's syndrome
- Syndrome of inappropriate antidiuretic hormone (SIADH) with water retention and hyponatremia

Cardiovascular System
- Thrombophlebitis
- Endocarditis

Hematologic Effects
- Anemia
- Disseminated intravascular coagulation (DIC)
- Eosinophilia

Connective Tissue
- Osteoarthropathy with clubbing and periosteal inflammation

Neuromuscular Effects
- Peripheral neuropathy
- Cerebellar degeneration
- Myasthenia-like muscle weakness

TABLE 36–9 Lung Cancer Staging

	PRIMARY TUMOR (T-STAGE)	REGIONAL LYMPH NODES (N)	DISTANT METASTASIS (M)
Stage 0	T_0—No evidence of primary tumor T_X—Malignant cells in bronchopulmonary secretions, but no tumor visualized		M_X—Presence of distant metastasis cannot be assessed
Stage I	T_1S—Carcinoma *in situ* T_1—Tumor that is 3 cm diameter or less, with no evidence of invasion	N_0—No regional lymph node metastasis	M_0—No distant metastasis
Stage II	T_2—Tumor that is greater than 3 cm diameter, or invades visceral pleura, or has associated atelectasis or pneumonitis	N_1—Metastasis or direct extension to peribronchial or ipsilateral hilar nodes	
Stage III	T_3—Tumor with direct extension into an adjacent structure, or any tumor with associated pleural effusion or atelectasis or pneumonitis of entire lung	N_2—Metastasis to ipsilateral mediastinal or subcarinal nodes	
Stage IV	T_4—Tumor that invades mediastinum or involves the heart, great vessels, trachea, esophagus, vertebral body, or carina; presence of malignant pleural effusion	N_3—Metastasis to contralateral mediastinal, scalene, or supraclavicular nodes	M_1—Distant metastasis present

Nursing care of the patient undergoing a bronchoscopy is included in the box on page 1130 of ∞ Chapter 34.

- *CT scan* is used to evaluate and localize tumors, particularly tumors in the lung parenchyma and pleura. It also is done prior to needle biopsy to localize the tumor. CT scanning can also detect distant tumor metastasis and evaluate tumor response to treatment.
- Cells or tissue for *cytologic examination and biopsy* may be obtained by aspirating fluid from a pleural effusion, percutaneous needle biopsy, and lymph node biopsy. These procedures may be done in an outpatient or a surgical setting.
- *CBC, liver function studies*, and *serum electrolytes* including calcium are obtained to evaluate for evidence of metastatic disease or paraneoplastic syndromes.
- *Tuberculin test (PPD)* is performed to rule out tuberculosis as the cause of symptoms and abnormalities seen on chest x-ray.
- *Pulmonary function tests (PFTs)* and *aterial blood gases* may be performed prior to the initiation of treatment if the patient has manifestations of respiratory insufficiency (e.g., dyspnea, activity intolerance, low oxygen saturation levels).

∞ See Chapter 34 for nursing care related to commonly used diagnostic tests for lung cancer.

Medications

Combination chemotherapy (often combined with radiation therapy and/or surgery) is the treatment of choice for small-cell lung cancer because of its rapid growth, dissemination, and sensitivity to cytotoxic drugs. Used in combination, chemotherapeutic drugs allow tumor cells to be attacked at different parts of the cell cycle and in different ways, increasing the effectiveness of therapy. Fifty percent of patients with tumors at early stages achieve complete tumor remission with combination chemotherapy. When a complete tumor response is achieved in the first few cycles of chemotherapy, the chances for long-term survival are much greater.

Combination chemotherapy is used also as an adjunct to surgery or radiation therapy for other types of lung cancer. It may be used to reduce the size of advanced local tumors prior to surgery, and to lengthen survival when distant metastases are present. ∞ See Chapter 14 for further discussion of chemotherapy.

Bronchodilators may be prescribed to reduce airway obstruction. Analgesics and pain management strategies are vital when the cancer is advanced. ∞ See Chapter 9 for more information about postoperative and cancer pain management.

Surgery

Surgery offers the only real chance for a cure in non-small-cell lung cancer. Unfortunately, most tumors are inoperable or only partially resectable at the time of diagnosis. The 5-year survival rate following curative surgery in patients with resectable tumors is about 30%, with most patients succumbing to metastatic disease within 5 years (Papadakis & McPhee, 2007). The type of surgery performed depends on the location and size of the tumor, as well as the patient's pulmonary and general health. The goal of surgery is to remove all involved tissue while preserving as much functional lung as possible. Table 36–10 outlines various surgical procedures used to treat lung cancer. Nursing care for the patient having lung surgery is outlined in the box on page 1222.

Radiation Therapy

Radiation therapy is used alone or in combination with surgery or chemotherapy for lung cancer. The treatment goal may be either cure or symptom relief (palliative). Prior to surgery, radiation therapy is used to "debulk" tumors. When cancer has spread by direct extension to other thoracic structures and surgery is not feasible, radiation therapy may be the treatment of choice. It also may be used to relieve manifestations such as cough, hemoptysis, pain due to bone metastasis, and dyspnea from bronchial obstruction. Complications of lung cancer, such as superior vena cava syndrome, may be treated with radiation.

TABLE 36–10 Types of Lung Surgery for Lung Cancer

PROCEDURE	DESCRIPTION	USED FOR
Laser bronchoscopy	Bronchoscopy-guided laser used to resect tumor	Tumors localized in a main bronchus
Mediastinoscopy	Visualization of the mediastinum using an endoscope passed through a suprasternal incision	Evaluation and biopsy of a mediastinal tumor and lymph nodes
Thoracotomy	Incision into the chest wall	Access the lung and thoracic cavity for surgery
Wedge resection	Removal of a small section (wedge) of peripheral lung tissue	Small, peripheral lung tumors
Segmental resection	Removal of an individual bronchovascular segment of a lobe	Peripheral lung tumor with no evidence of extension to the chest wall or metastasis
Sleeve resection (bronchoplastic reconstruction)	Resection of a section of a major bronchus with reconstruction of remaining normal bronchus	Small lesion of a major bronchus
Lobectomy	Removal of a single lung lobe	Tumors confined to a single lobe
Pneumonectomy	Removal of an entire lung	Tumor widespread throughout the lung, involving the main bronchus, or fixed to the hilum

NURSING CARE OF THE PATIENT Undergoing Lung Surgery

PREOPERATIVE CARE

- Provide routine preoperative nursing care as outlined in ∞ Chapter 4.
- Note any history of smoking, respiratory and cardiac diseases, and other chronic conditions in the nursing history. *These factors may affect the response to surgery and the risk for postoperative complications.*
- Provide emotional and psychologic support for the patient and family. *In addition to facing surgery, the patient may be adjusting to a new diagnosis of cancer and the possibility that surgical intervention will be only partially successful.*
- Instruct about postoperative procedures, including respiratory therapy, breathing exercises, and coughing techniques. Allow practice time. *Learning will be easier in the preoperative period, when pain and analgesia are not affecting mental function.*
- If the patient will return from surgery with an endotracheal tube and mechanical ventilation, establish a means of communication using hand or eye signals or a magic slate. *Establishing a means of communication prior to surgery reduces postoperative anxiety at being unable to speak.*
- If the patient will return to ICU, introduce the patient and family to the unit and any machines, such as ventilators and monitors, that will be used. *The knowledge that this is an expected part of surgical recovery reduces the patient's and family's postoperative anxiety.*

POSTOPERATIVE CARE

- Assess and provide routine postoperative care as outlined in ∞ Chapter 4.
- Assess for adequate pain control, and provide analgesics as needed. *Incisional pain commonly causes altered breathing patterns in the patient who has undergone lung surgery.*
- Frequently assess respiratory status, including color, oxygen saturation, respiratory rate and depth, chest expansion, lung sounds, percussion tone, and arterial blood gases. *Maintaining adequate ventilation and gas exchange postoperatively is vital to reduce mortality and morbidity.*

Gas exchange may be impaired by complications of lung surgery, including pneumothorax, atelectasis, bronchospasm, pulmonary embolus, bronchopleural fistula, and acute respiratory distress syndrome (ARDS).

- Assist with effective coughing techniques, postural drainage, and incentive spirometry. Perform endotracheal suctioning as needed while intubated. *Surgical manipulation and anesthesia can increase the mucous production, leading to airway obstruction. Aggressive pulmonary hygiene is important to prevent this complication.*
- Monitor and maintain effective mechanical ventilation. *This is vital to ensure adequate ventilation and gas exchange in the early postoperative period.*
- Maintain patent chest tubes and a closed drainage system. Monitor chest tube output every hour initially, then every 2 to 4 or 8 hours as indicated. Notify the healthcare provider if chest tube output exceeds 70 mL per hour and/or is bright red, warm, and free flowing. *Maintaining a patent, intact chest drainage system is vital to reestablish negative pressure within the chest cavity and re-expansion of the lungs. Increased amounts of warm, free-flowing blood indicate intrathoracic hemorrhage that may necessitate surgical intervention.*
- Assess for signs of infection involving the incision or chest tube site(s). Use strict aseptic technique in caring for incisions and invasive monitoring devices. *The postoperative patient is at risk for incisional infections, empyema in the chest cavity, and pneumonia.*
- Assist with turning and to ambulate as soon as possible. *Early mobility is important to prevent possible complications, such as pneumonia or pulmonary embolus.*
- Assess and maintain nutritional status. Initiate enteral or parenteral nutrition early if intubation and mechanical ventilation will be required for an extended period. Provide frequent small feedings once extubated. *Maintaining nutritional status promotes wound healing and prevents negative nitrogen balance. Frequent small feedings reduce the fatigue associated with eating.*

NURSING CARE OF THE PATIENT | Receiving Radiation Therapy

Although radiation therapy is well controlled and specifically directed toward the tumor cells, some normal cells are also damaged in the process of treatment. Nursing care and patient teaching help the patient cope with uncomfortable side effects associated with radiation therapy.

Nursing Responsibilities

- Monitor for potential complications:
  a. Radiation pneumonitis—dyspnea on exertion, dry cough, fever
  b. Pericarditis—chest pain, pericardial friction rub; muffled heart sounds, paradoxical pulse, ECG abnormalities (Notify the healthcare provider if symptoms develop.)
  c. Esophagitis—pain, sore throat, difficulty swallowing
- Encourage adequate fluid intake to liquefy respiratory secretions.
- Provide local analgesics and local anesthetics such as viscous lidocaine as ordered to relieve dysphagia and sore throat.
- Offer small frequent meals of soft, cool foods and liquids to maintain nutritional status.

Patient and Family Teaching

- If dyspnea or pneumonitis develop, teach positioning, pursed-lip techniques, and relaxation exercises to facilitate breathing.
- Reassure that pneumonitis is generally a self-limiting process and should resolve when the course of radio-therapy is completed.
- Teach the manifestations of pericarditis, which may develop during treatment or up to 1 year after its completion. Chest pain or pressure, rapid heartbeat, and fever may signal pericarditis; increasing fatigue, dyspnea, and lightheadedness can indicate a chronic process with pericardial effusion and possible cardiac tamponade.
- Instruct to eliminate hot, spicy, or acidic foods from the diet if esophagitis is a problem. Alcohol and tobacco should also be avoided.
- Adequate rest and nutrition are important to alleviate the symptoms of radiation fatigue, which is common in patients receiving radiation therapy for lung cancer. The fatigue is generally temporary.

Radiation therapy may be delivered by external beam to the primary tumor site or by intraluminal radiation, or brachytherapy. Radiation therapy and related nursing care is discussed further in ∞ Chapter 14. Specific nursing measures for the patient undergoing radiation therapy for lung cancer are outlined in the accompanying Nursing Care box.

Complementary Therapies

Research indicates that a significant number of patients diagnosed with lung cancer use complementary and alternative medicine (CAM). In a systematic review of CAM in lung cancer, between 10% and more than 60% of cancer patients use at least one form of CAM (Cassileth et al., 2007). The CAM remedies used included herbal medicines, medicinal teas, homeopathy, animal extracts, and spiritual therapies. While these therapies may be safe when used alone, the potential for interactions with conventional medical treatment must be considered. Inquire of patients about their use of complementary and alternative therapies, and inform members of the healthcare team when present.

∞ Nursing Care

Health Promotion

The incidence of lung cancer is decreasing as the use of tobacco products declines. Teach people of all ages, particularly children and teenagers, about the link between cigarette smoking and lung cancer. Not smoking and avoiding exposure to secondhand smoke is the primary preventive measure for lung cancer. In addition, explain the risk of lung cancer to patients with occupational risk factors, exposure to asbestos products in particular.

Assessment

Nursing assessment related to lung cancer focuses on identifying risk factors for the disease, early manifestations of lung cancer, and respiratory function in the patient undergoing treatment.

- *Health history:* Current symptoms, including chronic cough, shortness of breath, blood-tinged sputum; systemic manifestations such as recent weight loss, fatigue, anorexia, bone pain; smoking history; occupational exposure to carcinogens; chronic diseases such as COPD.
- *Physical examination:* General appearance; skin color, evidence of clubbing; weight and height; vital signs; respiratory rate, depth, excursion; lung sounds to percussion and auscultation.
- *Laboratory tests and diagnostic studies:* CBC and coagulation studies, serum electrolytes and osmolality, liver and renal function studies; chest x-ray and CT scan results; arterial blood gases and oxygen saturation levels.

Nursing Diagnoses and Interventions

The patient with lung cancer is facing invasive treatments with undesirable side effects, possibly surgery, and typically a poor prognosis for long-term survival. Nursing care needs are diverse, related to respiratory status, the cancer itself and possible metastases, and the treatment plan. Priority nursing diagnoses related to respiratory function include *Ineffective Breathing Pattern* and *Activity Intolerance.* Pain and anticipatory grieving also are likely to be high-priority problems. See the accompanying Case Study & Nursing Care Plan on page 1225.

Ineffective Breathing Pattern

Breathing pattern and ventilation may be affected by the tumor itself or by treatment of the tumor. Thoracic surgery increases the risk due to the incision and disruption of the muscles of respiration. Maintaining effective lung ventilation is particularly important postoperatively to re-expand remaining lung tissue and prevent surgical complications.

- Assess and document respiratory rate, depth, and lung sounds at least every 4 hours; evaluate more frequently in the immediate postoperative period or as indicated by condition. *Early detection of signs of respiratory compromise or adventitious lung sounds is vital for effective intervention.*

- Frequently assess and document pain level (using a standard pain scale); provide analgesics as needed. *Pain and attempting to avoid chest movement to prevent additional pain can lead to rapid, shallow respirations and ineffective ventilation.*
- Elevate the head of the bed to 60 degrees. *Elevating the head of the bed reduces pressure on the diaphragm and permits optimal lung expansion.*
- Assist to turn, cough, and deep breathe and use incentive spirometry. Help splint the chest with a pillow or blanket when coughing. *These measures promote airway clearance.*
- Suction airway as needed. *Suctioning may be required to remove secretions that the patient is unable to cough up and expectorate.*

- Provide chest physiotherapy with percussion and postural drainage as needed or ordered. *Percussion and postural drainage help maintain airway patency and effective respirations.*
- If mechanical ventilation is instituted, work with respiratory therapy and use analgesia or sedation as needed to synchronize respirations with the ventilator. *Coordination of the patient's respiratory effort with ventilator-delivered breaths is important for fully effective mechanical ventilation.*
- Provide reassurance and emotional support. *These measures help relieve anxiety and promote an effective breathing pattern.*

Activity Intolerance

Both resectional lung surgery and inoperable lung cancer reduce the amount of functional lung tissue and surface area for gas diffusion. This can lead to activity intolerance if the oxygen supply is insufficient to meet the body's oxygen demand.

- Plan rest periods between activities and procedures. *Rest periods reduce oxygen demands and fatigue.*
- Assist the postoperative patient to increase activities gradually. *Increasing activity levels gradually improves exercise tolerance.*
- Teach measures to conserve energy while performing ADLs, such as sitting while showering and dressing and wearing slip-on shoes. *These energy-conserving measures reduce oxygen demand and allow the patient to remain independent as long as possible.*
- Keep frequently used objects within easy reach. *This helps conserve energy.*
- Administer oxygen as prescribed. Teach the patient and family about home oxygen use if appropriate. *Supplemental oxygen can help improve activity and exercise tolerance.*
- Encourage maintenance of physical activity to tolerance. *Maintaining activity levels to the degree possible improves physical and emotional well-being.*
- Allow family members to provide assistance as needed. *This helps the patient conserve energy and allows the family to retain a sense of usefulness.*

Pain

Pain is a priority problem in both the postoperative period as well as in the terminal stages of cancer. Poorly managed pain prolongs recovery from surgery. In the terminal cancer patient, chronic and acute pain must be managed effectively to allow a peaceful death.

- Assess and document pain using a standardized pain scale and objective data. *Pain is a subjective experience, best evaluated by the patient. Changes in vital signs, guarded movement, or unwillingness to move may indicate unreported pain.*
- Provide analgesics as needed to maintain comfort. *Postoperative recovery and restoration of function is facilitated by adequate pain management.*
- For cancer pain, maintain an around-the-clock medication schedule using narcotic, nonsteroidal anti-inflammatory drugs, and other medications as ordered. *Addiction is not a concern in terminal cancer; providing adequate pain relief that does not allow "breakthrough" pain is important.*
- Provide or assist with comfort measures, such as massage, positioning, distraction, and relaxation techniques. *These techniques promote relaxation and enhance pain relief.*
- Assist the patient and family to plan and engage in activities that distract from pain such as reading, watching television, and engaging in social interactions. *Distraction helps the patient focus away from the pain.*
- Spend as much time with the patient as possible; allow family members to remain with the patient. *Physical presence of the nurse and family provides emotional support for the patient.*

Anticipatory Grieving

Because lung cancer often is advanced when diagnosed, the patient faces the very real prospect of dying from the disease. Grieving for the anticipated loss of life is a normal response as the patient and family begin to adapt to the diagnosis. Nursing care goals are to promote expression of feelings and thoughts about the loss, and to help the patient and family initiate grief work, make decisions, and use appropriate resources and coping mechanisms to deal with the loss.

- Spend time with the patient and family. *Time is necessary to develop a trusting, therapeutic relationship.*
- Answer questions honestly; do not deny the probable outcome of the disease. *Honesty reinforces reality and provides a sense of control over decisions to be made.*
- Encourage the patient and family to express their feelings, fears, and concerns. *Open expression of feelings helps to promote understanding and acceptance.*

CASE STUDY & NURSING CARE PLAN   A Patient with Lung Cancer

After coughing up bloody sputum one morning, James Mueller, a 68-year-old retired millworker, sees his healthcare provider. A chest x-ray shows a suspicious density in the central portion of his right lung. Mr. Mueller is admitted to the hospital the following Monday for diagnostic tests.

ASSESSMENT

Anita Sarros, RN, admits Mr. Mueller to the oncology unit and obtains a nursing history. Mr. Mueller is married and has three grown children. He worked in a local paper mill for 35 years before retiring at age 62. He describes himself as "pretty healthy," except for a chronic smoker's cough. He started smoking as a young man in the army. He has a 50 pack-year smoking history, having smoked a pack a day for 50 years, since age 18. Mr. Mueller says he briefly quit smoking following a small heart attack 3 years ago, but started again after 4 months. On further questioning, Mr. Mueller says his cough has been productive for the past few months, especially in the morning, and that he is shorter of breath than usual with activity.

Mr. Mueller's examination data includes BP 162/86, P 78 and regular, R 20, and T 98.4°F (36.9°C). Color good, skin warm and dry. Inspiratory and expiratory wheezes noted in right chest but good breath sounds throughout. No other abnormal findings are noted on examination. The healthcare provider orders early-morning sputum specimens times 3 days for cytologic examination and schedules a CT scan of the chest the morning after admission.

Mr. Mueller's CBC shows mild anemia, but remaining routine laboratory tests are essentially normal. Sputum cytology is positive for small-cell bronchogenic cancer. The CT scan shows a central mass approximately 4 cm in diameter with involved mediastinal and subclavicular lymph nodes. A small mass is also noted on the lumbar spine. After conferring with his healthcare provider and an oncologist, Mr. Mueller decides to undergo a trial course of chemotherapy.

DIAGNOSES

- *Ineffective Airway Clearance* related to tumor mass
- *Risk for Imbalanced Nutrition: Less than Body Requirements* related to effects of chemotherapy
- *Risk for Compromised Family Coping* related to new diagnosis of lung cancer
- *Deficient Knowledge* about lung cancer and aids to smoking cessation

EXPECTED OUTCOMES

- Maintain a patent airway.
- Maintain current weight.
- Express feelings and concerns about the effect of cancer on the family unit.
- Participate in care.
- Contact appropriate support groups.
- Verbalize an understanding of the disease, its treatment, and prognosis.
- Develop a plan to stop smoking.

PLANNING AND IMPLEMENTATION

- Teach coughing, deep breathing, and hydration measures to facilitate airway clearance
- Discuss symptoms to report to the healthcare provider: increased dyspnea or hemoptysis, severe stridor or wheezing, chest pain.
- Discuss measures to relieve nausea associated with chemotherapy, including premedication with a prescribed antiemetic.
- Have dietitian consult with Mr. and Mrs. Mueller to develop a diet plan for maintaining ideal weight.
- Discuss possible effects of lung cancer with Mr. and Mrs. Mueller.
- Encourage Mr. and Mrs. Mueller to call a family conference to discuss the disease with their children and grandchildren.
- Evaluate family members' knowledge and understanding of lung cancer, correcting misinformation and teaching as needed.
- Have an American Cancer Society volunteer contact the family.
- Refer to local cancer support group.
- Refer to home health department for follow-up and further teaching.
- Work with Mr. Mueller to develop a plan to stop smoking.
- Ask the healthcare provider for a prescription for nicotine patches or gum for Mr. Mueller.

Make Mr. Mueller aware of decisions that will need to be made regarding end of life issues. Encourage him to discuss his wishes with family if he is able.

EVALUATION

Mr. Mueller had his first chemotherapy treatment in the hospital and was discharged 4 days after admission. After 3 months of chemotherapy, his tumor shows little regression, and a liver scan reveals further metastasis. He and his wife decide to stop chemotherapy, a decision with which the children reluctantly agree. Mr. and Mrs. Mueller are referred to hospice services. With the help of hospice nurses and volunteers, Mr. Mueller is able to remain at home. His pain is managed initially with oral MS Contin, a sustained-release form of morphine sulfate, and later with an intravenous morphine infusion. Mr. Mueller dies at home with his family at his side 9 months after his diagnosis of lung cancer.

CRITICAL THINKING IN THE NURSING PROCESS

1. The oncologist prescribed a chemotherapy regimen of cyclophosphamide, doxorubicin, and vincristine. Describe how each of these drugs works against cancer cells, and discuss the rationale for using this combination.
2. Develop a care plan to deal with the specific side effects for the treatment regimen given in question 1.
3. Mr. Mueller had small-cell (oat cell) cancer. How would his presentation and treatment differ if the diagnosis had been non-small-cell adenocarcinoma, stage $T_2N_2M_0$?

See Evaluating Your Response in Appendix C.

- Assist with understanding the grieving process and acceptance of feelings as normal. *Feelings of guilt, anger, or depression may cause the patient to withdraw from others. Explanation of the grieving process enhances understanding and ability to cope.*
- Help identify strengths and coping measures that have been used effectively in the past. Provide positive reinforcement for effective coping behavior. *Past effective coping measures can help the patient and family deal with the present situation and regain a sense of control.*

- Help the patient and family make decisions regarding treatment and care. *This also is important to give them a sense of control.*
- Encourage use of other support systems, such as spiritual and social groups. Refer the patient and family to support groups, social support services, and hospice care as indicated. Provide American Cancer Society literature and information as appropriate. *These support systems provide emotional support and help the patient and family cope with the diagnosis.*

- Discuss advance directives (the living will) and power of attorney for health care with the patient and family. *These documents give the patient and family a sense of control over medical care provided if the patient is no longer able to express his or her own wishes.*

Using NANDA, NIC, and NOC

Linkages between a selected NANDA nursing diagnosis, NIC, and NOC for the patient with lung cancer are shown in the chart that follows.

Community-Based Care

A primary teaching need to prepare the patient and family affected by lung cancer for home care is information about the disease itself, expected prognosis, and planned treatment strategies. Provide honest information; do not promote false hope. Include the following additional topics in teaching for home care:

- Importance of quitting smoking, especially if surgery has been performed (The patient with lung cancer may have difficulty recognizing the need to stop smoking. Include information about the effects of nicotine and the tars in cigarette smoke on healing and already compromised lung tissue.)
- Planned treatments such as chemotherapy or radiation therapy, including expected effects and usual side effects of each
- Strategies to cope with noxious effects of radiation or chemotherapy
- Activities and exercises to improve strength and regain function for the postoperative patient
- The need to continue coughing and deep-breathing exercises at home

- Symptoms to report to the healthcare provider: fever, increasing or continued shortness of breath, cough, increased or purulent sputum, redness, pain, swelling, or incisional drainage
- Use of prescribed medications, including desired and potential side effects and interactions with other drugs or foods
- Use of analgesics and other pain relief measures for postoperative or cancer pain
- Information about hospice services, home health, local cancer support groups for patients and caregivers, and American Cancer Society services

Refer the patient and family for home health services including nursing care, assistance with ADLs, respiratory care, and respite care as needed.

NANDA, NIC, AND NOC LINKAGES
The Patient with Lung Cancer

NANDA	Ineffective Coping
NIC	Coping Enhancement Decision-Making Support Support System Enhancement
NOC	Coping Decision Making Social Support

Adapted from Bulechek, G., Butcher, H., & Dochterman, J. M. (Eds). (2008). *Nursing interventions classification (NIC)* (5th ed.). St. Louis: Mosby Elsevier; Moorhead, S., Johnson, M., Maas, M., & Swanson, E. (Eds). (2008). *Nursing outcomes classification (NOC)* (4th ed.). St. Louis: Mosby Elsevier; and NANDA International. (2009). *Nursing diagnoses:. Definitions and classification 2009–2011*. Oxford, UK: Wilely-Blackwell.

CHAPTER HIGHLIGHTS

- Pneumonia, inflammation of the respiratory bronchioles and alveoli, usually is bacterial in origin. Different organisms commonly are found in hospital-acquired pneumonia than in community acquired pneumonia. Nursing care focuses on promoting airway clearance, supporting effective gas exchange, and promoting rest.
- Infection control measures, including standard, airborne, and contract precautions, are vital to prevent the spread of viral severe acute respiratory syndrome (SARS).
- Tuberculosis affects many people worldwide; in the United States, the primary affected populations are immigrants, people with compromised immunity, and people living in crowded or unsanitary conditions.
- The tuberculin test (PPD) detects a cellular immune response to *M. tb*, indicating infection, but not necessarily active disease.
- Effective tuberculosis treatment is a public health concern, requiring therapy and compliance monitoring, contact follow-up, and assessment for adverse treatment effects.

- Fungal lung infections tend to have a geographic pattern of distribution. People with compromised immune status are more likely to be affected. Their manifestations resemble those of pneumonia or tuberculosis.
- Disorders of the pleura, such as pleural effusion and pneumothorax, can affect lung expansion, ventilation, and gas exchange when significant.
- Tension pneumothorax develops when air enters the pleural space but is unable to escape, collapsing the lung on the affected side and placing pressure on the unaffected lung and mediastinum. Ventilation, gas exchange, venous return, and cardiac output can be significantly affected.
- Trauma may affect the chest wall (rib fracture, flail chest), the surface of the lungs (pulmonary contusion), or the airways and alveoli (smoke inhalation and near-drowning). Flail chest and pulmonary contusion often occur concurrently; hemothorax also frequently develops with chest trauma. Chest trauma (chest wall or airways) can endanger effective ventilation and gas exchange.

- Lung cancer, the leading cause of cancer deaths, typically is advanced when diagnosed. Surgery, radiation therapy, and chemotherapy are used to treat lung cancer, often in combination.

- Superior vena cava syndrome (impaired venous drainage from the head and neck) and paraneoplastic syndromes (abnormal hormone production, fluid and electrolyte imbalance, and altered clotting with possible venous thrombosis and pulmonary emboli) may complicate lung cancer.

TEST YOURSELF NCLEX-RN® REVIEW

1. Admitting orders for a patient with acute bacterial pneumonia include an intravenous antibiotic every 8 hours, oxygen per nasal cannula at 5 L/min, continuous pulse oximetry monitoring, bedrest with bathroom privileges and chair at bedside as desired, diet as tolerated, sputum specimen for C&S, CBC, urinalysis, and chemistry panel. Which order should the nurse carry out first?
   1. Start the oxygen per nasal cannula.
   2. Insert an intravenous catheter and start the prescribed antibiotic.
   3. Provide a dinner tray to the patient.
   4. Obtain the sputum specimen.

2. When assessing a patient with bacterial pneumonia, the nurse notes that the patient's overall skin tone is somewhat grey and there is a bluish tinge around the patient's lips. The nurse should do which of the following? (Place the following in the correct order of priority.)
   1. Start oxygen.
   2. Assess breath sounds.
   3. Notify the healthcare provider.
   4. Raise the head of the bed.
   5. Obtain oxygen saturation level.

3. The nurse evaluating a tuberculin test result 72 hours after it was administered notes an area of induration 9 m in diameter. What additional information would indicate to the nurse that this is a positive result?
   1. The patient resides in a long-term care facility.
   2. The patient was born in Southeast Asia.
   3. The patient has HIV disease.
   4. The patient is an injection drug user.

4. The nurse teaching a patient taking prophylactic daily isonizid (INH) following tuberculin test conversion includes which of the following in the instructions?
   1. This drug turns your urine red-orange. This is harmless.
   2. Report numbness and tingling of your extremities to your doctor.
   3. You will need to have periodic eye examinations during treatment.
   4. Do not use aspirin while taking this drug, as abnormal bleeding may occur.

5. Which of the following statements made by a patient with a new diagnosis of lung cancer would indicate that the nurse's teaching has been effective?
   1. "Well, since I'm going to die anyway, I may as well go home, put my affairs in order, and spend the rest of my time in the easy chair."
   2. "I understand that because the cancer has already spread I will be undergoing aggressive cancer treatment for the next several years to beat this thing."
   3. "Even though I can't undo the damage caused by cigarette smoking, I will try to quit to prevent further damage to my lungs."
   4. "Having the 'big C' is very scary; I'm just glad it is one of the more curable forms of cancer."

6. The nurse caring for a patient following a lobectomy notes 100 mL of red drainage in the chest drainage container since checking it 30 minutes previously. The nurse should do which of the following? **Select all that apply.**
   1. Empty the chest-tube drainage system.
   2. Note the finding and re-evaluate drainage in 30 minutes.
   3. Notify the surgeon.
   4. Assess vital signs and level of consciousness.
   5. Apply pressure to the chest tube insertion site.

7. The nurse caring for a patient having a thoracentesis appropriately assists the patient to do which of the following?
   1. Sit upright leaning forward during the procedure.
   2. Breathe deeply as the needle is inserted.
   3. Remain on quiet bedrest for 4 hours following the procedure.
   4. Cough as the fluid is withdrawn.

8. The nurse teaches a patient being discharged from the emergency department with a diagnosis of fractured rib to do which of the following?
   1. Avoid using pain medications to prevent respiratory depression.
   2. Use elastic roller bandages (ACE wraps) to stabilize the chest wall and promote comfort.
   3. Remain on bed rest for a week to allow the fracture to stabilize.
   4. Use a small pillow to splint the area when coughing.

9. Which of the following assessment findings of a patient with smoke inhalation does the nurse find of greatest concern?
   1. ash-like material in the sputum
   2. respiratory rate of 36
   3. skin and mucous membranes pink
   4. fine crackles in bilateral bases

10. Which of the following nursing diagnoses does the nurse identify as of highest priority for a patient with tension pneumothorax?
    1. *Decreased Cardiac Output*
    2. *Ineffective Breathing Pattern*
    3. *Acute Pain*
    4. *Risk for Aspiration*

See Test Yourself answers in Appendix C.

BIBLIOGRAPHY

Ailinger, R. L., Armstrong, R., Nguyen, N., & Lasus, H. (2004). Latino immigrants' knowledge of tuberculosis. *Public Health Nursing, 21*(6), 519–523.

Alberts, W. M. (2007). Diagnosis and management of lung cancer executive summary: ACCP Evidence-based clinical practice guidelines (2nd ed.). *Chest, 132*(3), 1S–19S.

American Lung Association. (2009). Influenza and Pneumonia. *Lung Disease Data*. Retrieved from http://www.lungusa.org

American Thoracic Society, CDC, & Infectious Diseases Society of America. (2003). Treatment of tuberculosis. *American Journal of Respiratory and Critical Care Medicine, 167*, 603–662.

Azfar, H., Lippmann, M., Mundathaje, U., & Khaleeq, E. (2008). Spontaneous hemothorax, a comprehensive review. *American Journal of Respiratory and Critical Care Medicine, 134*, 1056–1065.

Barry, R. M. (2004). Penetrating chest wounds. *RN, 67*(5), 36, 42.

Bulechek, G., Butcher, H., & Dochterman, J. M. (Eds.). (2008). *Nursing interventions classification (NIC)* (5th ed.). St. Louis: Mosby Elsevier.

Cassileth, B. R., Deng, G. E., Gomez, J. E., Johnstone, P. A. S., Kumar, N., & Vickers, A. J. (2007). Complementary therapies and integrative oncology in lung cancer; ACCP evidence-based clinical practice guidelines (2nd ed). *Chest, 132*, 340S–354S.

Cava, M. A., Fay, K. E., Beanlands, H. J., McCay, E. A., & Wignall, R. (2005). Risk perception and compliance with quarantine during the SARS outbreak. *Journal of Nursing Scholarship, 37*(4), 343–347.

Centers for Disease Control and Prevention (CDC). (2009a). Deaths: Final Report, 2006. *National Vital Statistics Reports, 57*(14). Hyattsville, MD: National Center for Health Statistics. DHHS Pub. No. 2009-1120.

Centers for Disease Control and Prevention (CDC). (2009b). *Pneumococcal vaccine*. Retrieved from http://www.cdc.gov/vaccines/vpd-vac/pneumo/default.htm

Centers for Disease Control and Prevention (CDC). (2009c). Trends in tuberculosis—United States, 2008. *MMWR, 55*(11), 305–308.

Centers for Disease Control and Prevention (CDC). (2009d). *Severe Acute Respiratory Syndrome (SARS)*. Retrieved from http://www.cdc.gov/ncidod/sars/

Centers for Disease Control and Prevention (CDC). (2009e). *Anthrax*. Retrieved from http://www.cdc.gov/nczved/dfbmd/disease_listing/anthrax_gi.html

Coleman, P. R. (2004). Pneumonia in the long-term care setting: Etiology, management and prevention. *Journal of Gerontological Nursing, 30*(4), 14–23, 54–55.

Deglin, J. H., & Vallerand, A. H. (2009). *Davis' drug guide* (10th ed.). Philadelphia: F.A. Davis.

Dick, J., Lewin, S., Rose, E., Zwarenstein, M., & van der Walt, H. (2004). Changing professional practice in tuberculosis care: An educational intervention. *Journal of Advanced Nursing, 48*(5), 434–442.

Domino, F. J., Baldor, R. A., Golding, J., Grimes, J., & Taylor, J. S. (2010). *The 5-minute clinical consult* (18th ed.). Philadelphia: Lippincott, Williams & Wilkins.

Fishman, A. P., Elias, J. A., Fishman, J. A., Grippi, M. A., Senior, S. M., & Pack, A. J. (2008). *Fishman's pulmonary diseases and disorders* (4th ed.). New York: McGraw-Hill Co.

Gift, A. G., Jablonski, A., Stommel, M., & Given, C. W. (2004). Symptom clusters in elderly patients with lung cancer. *Oncology Nursing Forum, 31*(2), 203–210.

Grap, M. J., Munro, C. L., Hummel, R. S. III, Elswick, R. K., McKinney, J. L., & Sessler, C. N. (2005). Effect of backrest elevation on the development of ventilator-associated pneumonia. *American Journal of Critical Care, 14*(4), 325–333.

Huether, S. E., & McCance, K. L. (2008). *Understanding Pathophysiology* (4th ed.). St. Louis: Mosby Elsevier.

Jantarakupt, P., & Porock, D. (2005). Dyspnea management in lung cancer: Applying the evidence from chronic obstructive pulmonary disease. *Oncology Nursing Forum, 32*(4), 785–797.

Ladd, E. (2005). The use of antibiotics for viral upper respiratory tract infections: An analysis of nurse practitioner and physician prescribing practices in ambulatory care, 1997–2001. *Journal of the American Academy of Nurse Practitioners, 17*(10), 416–424.

Lakasing, E., & Tester, M. (2006). How to manage lung cancer in primary care. *Practice Nursing, 17*(1), 35–39.

Leonard, M. K., Osterhlot, D., Kourbatova, E. V., Del Rio, C., Wand, W., & Blumberg, H. M. (2005). How many sputum specimens are necessary to diagnoses pulmonary tuberculosis? *American Journal of Infection Control, 33*(1), 58–61.

Montgomery, S. S., Burke, E. M., Wissman, S. A., Feldman, D. S., & Leier, C. V. (2005). Natural course of large spontaneous pneumothorax. *Heart & Lung, 34*(5), 332–334.

Moorhead, S., Johnson, M., Maas, M., & Swanson, E. (Eds). (2008). *Nursing outcomes classification (NOC)* (4th ed.). St. Louis: Mosby Elsevier.

NANDA International. (2009). *Nursing diagnoses: Definitions and classification 2009–2011*. Oxford, UK: Wilely-Blackwell.

National Center for Complementary and Alternative Medicine (NCCAM). (2005). Herbs at a glance. Echinacea. Retrieved from www1228.nccam.nih.gov/health/echinacea/

Noppen, M., & DeKeukelerie, T. (2008). Pneumothorax. *Respiration, 76*(2), 121–127.

Nyamathi, A., Berg, J., Jones, T., & Leake, B. (2005). Predictors of perceived health status of tuberculosis-infected homeless. *Western Journal of Nursing Research, 27*(7), 896–914.

Papadakis, M. A., & McPhee, S. J. (2007). *Current Consult Medicine 2007*. New York: McGraw-Hill.

Perrin, K. O. (2009). *Understanding the essentials of critical care nursing. Critical Care Nursing*. Upper Saddle River, NJ: Pearson Prentice-Hall.

Pruitt, B., & Jacobs, M. (2006). Best-practice interventions: How can you prevent ventilator-associated pneumonia? *Nursing, 36*(2), 36–42.

Restrepo, A., Benard, G., deCastro, C. C., Aqudelo, C. A., Tobon, A. M. (2008). Pulmonary paracoccidioidomycosis. *Seminars in Respiratory and Critical Care Medicine, 29*(2), 182–197.

Ross, J. L. (2005). Near drowning. *RN, 68*(7), 36, 42.

Ryan, B. (2005). Pneumothorax: Assessment and diagnostic testing. *Journal of Cardiovascular Nursing, 20*(4), 251–253.

Sarna, L., Brown, J. K., Cooley, M. E., Williams, R. D., Chernecky, C., Padilla, G., & Danao, L. L. (2005). Quality of life and meaning of illness in women with lung cancer. *Oncology Nursing Forum, 32*(1), E9–E19.

Swigart, V., & Kolb, R. (2004). Homeless persons' decisions to accept or reject public health disease detection services. *Public Health Nursing, 21*(2), 162–170.

Todd, B. (2005). Emerging infections. Legionella pneumonia: Many cases of Legionnaire disease go unreported or unrecognized. *American Journal of Nursing, 105*(11), 35–36, 38.

Tseng, H., Chen, T., & Chou, S. (2005). SARS: Key factors in crisis management. *Journal of Nursing Research, 13*(1), 58–64.

Van Leeuwen, A. M., Kranpitz, T. R., Smith, L. S. (2006). *Davis' laboratory and diagnostic tests* (2nd ed.). Philadelphia: F.A. Davis.

Wilkinson, J. M. (2005). *Nursing diagnosis handbook* (8th ed.). Upper Saddle River, NJ: Prentice Hall.

Williams. V. G. (2006). Tuberculosis: Clinical features, diagnosis and management. *Nursing Standard, 20*(22), 49–53.

Willis, D., VanSickle, D. Van Riper, S., & Valerio, C. (2005). Pneumonia: Bringing JCAHO and CMS to the bedside. *American Journal of Nursing, 105*(3), 72A, 72C–D.

Withy, K., & Alper, B. S. (2005). Stat consult. Acute bronchitis. *Clinical Advisor for Nurse Practitioners, 8*(1), 73–74, 77.

Woods, A., & Hathaway, L. (2004). Treating community-acquired pneumonia. *Nurse Practitioner, 29*(6), 11.

World Health Organization. (2008). *Anti-tuberculosis drug resistance in the world Report no. 4*. Geneva: Author. Retrieved from http://www.who.int/tb/publications/mdr_surveillance/en/index.html

Yamamoto, L., Schroeder, C., Morley, D., & Beliveau, C. (2005). Thoracic trauma: The deadly dozen. *Cricial Care Nursing Quarterly, 28*(1), 22–40.

Nursing Care of Patients with Gas Exchange Disorders

LEARNING OUTCOMES

1. Relate the pathophysiology and manifestations of obstructive, pulmonary vascular, and critical respiratory disorders to their effects on ventilation and respiration (gas exchange).

2. Compare and contrast the etiology, risk factors, and vulnerable populations for disorders affecting ventilation and gas exchange within the lungs.

3. Describe interdisciplinary care and the nursing role in health promotion and caring for patients with disorders that affect the ability to ventilate the lungs and exchange gases with the environment.

4. Discuss interdisciplinary interventions to provide airway and ventilatory support for the patient with respiratory failure, and nursing responsibilities in caring for patients with airway and ventilatory support.

5. Describe the nursing implications for medications used to promote ventilation and gas exchange.

CLINICAL COMPETENCIES

1. Assess functional health status of patients with disorders affecting ventilation and gas exchange.

2. Use assessed data and knowledge of the effects of the disorder and prescribed treatment to identify priority nursing diagnoses and plan care for patients with disorders affecting ventilation and gas exchange.

3. Use the nursing process and evidence-based nursing research to plan and implement individualized nursing care for patients, including measures to promote ventilation and gas exchange.

4. Plan and provide appropriate teaching for health promotion among vulnerable populations and to prepare patients and families for community-based care.

5. Evaluate the effectiveness of nursing interventions and teaching, revising strategies and teaching plans as needed.

6. Knowledgably and safely coordinate interdisciplinary care and administer prescribed medications and treatments for patients with disorders affecting ventilation and gas exchange.

KEY TERMS

acute respiratory distress syndrome (ARDS), *1273*
asthma, *1230*
atelectasis, *1252*
bronchiectasis, *1252*
chronic bronchitis, *1239*

chronic obstructive pulmonary disease (COPD), *1239*
cor pulmonale, *1261*
cystic fibrosis (CF), *1249*
emphysema, *1239*
pulmonary embolism, *1255*

pulmonary hypertension, *1260*
respiratory failure, *1262*
sarcoidosis, *1255*
status asthmaticus, *1231*
weaning, *1268*

Normal function of the lower respiratory system depends on several organ systems: the central nervous system, which stimulates and controls breathing; chemoreceptors in the brain, aortic arch, and carotid bodies, which monitor the pH and oxygen content of blood; the heart and circulatory system, which provide for blood supply and gas exchange; the musculoskeletal system, which provides an intact thoracic cavity capable of expanding and contracting; and the lungs and bronchial tree, which allow air movement and gas exchange. Impaired function of any of these systems affects ventilation and respiration. As a result, tissues may become *hypoxic*, with inadequate oxygen to support metabolic activity.

Although some of the disorders discussed in this chapter can affect ventilation (air movement into and out of the airways and alveoli), all can have significant effects on gas exchange. The mechanisms by which they affect gas exchange differ:

- In reactive airway disease (asthma) and obstructive disorders, air trapping reduces the amount of oxygen available to drive gas exchange.
- Interstitial lung disorders affect the ability of the lungs to expand and the work of breathing, again, reducing alveolar oxygenation and gas exchange.
- Pulmonary vascular disorders affect blood flow to the lungs or a portion of the lungs, reducing gas exchange through their effects on perfusion of the lungs.
- Respiratory failure is the ultimate consequence of impaired gas exchange; the lungs cannot adequately oxygenate the blood or eliminate carbon dioxide.

With a few exceptions, the disorders discussed in this chapter are relatively common, chronic lung diseases.

Disorders of other body systems, such as neurologic disorders (e.g., head injury, spinal cord trauma or disorders, amotropic lateral sclerosis [ALS], myasthenia gravis) also can affect gas exchange through their effects on the central or peripheral nervous systems. These disorders and their effects on the respiratory system are discussed in subsequent chapters of this text.

Aging affects pulmonary ventilation and gas exchange as well. The number of alveoli decrease, and emphysematous changes (senile emphysema) reduce the surface area for gas exchange. Alveoli become less elastic, causing increased air trapping and dead space. For most older adults who remain active, these changes have minimal effect on exercise tolerance and activities of daily living (ADLs). When combined with lung disease, however, age-related pulmonary changes increase the patient's risk for developing respiratory failure.

Reactive Airway Disorders

In reactive airway disorders, the airways narrow in response to a stimulus. Airway narrowing limits airflow both into and out of the alveoli. Limited airflow increases the work of breathing and the residual volume of the lungs as air is trapped distal to narrowed airways. Inspired air mixes with an abnormally large volume of residual air, effectively reducing the amount of oxygen available in the alveoli. Decreased alveolar ventilation further reduces oxygen available for exchange.

The Patient with Asthma

Asthma is a chronic inflammatory disorder of the airways characterized by recurrent episodes of wheezing, breathlessness, chest tightness, and coughing. Inflammation causes increased responsiveness of the airways to multiple stimuli. The widespread airflow obstruction that occurs during acute episodes usually reverses either spontaneously or with treatment. While most episodes of asthma "attacks" are relatively brief, some patients with asthma may experience longer episodes with some degree of airway impairment daily. In rare cases, an acute episode of asthma is so severe that respiratory failure and death results.

Physiology Review

Airways within the lungs contain crisscrossing strips of smooth muscle that control their diameter. This muscle is innervated by the autonomic nervous system. Parasympathetic (cholinergic) stimulation leads to bronchoconstriction, or narrowing of the airways. Sympathetic stimulation through β_2-adrenergic receptors causes bronchodilation, or expansion of the airways. Slight bronchoconstriction normally predominates. However, when increased airflow is necessary (e.g., during exercise), the parasympathetic system is inhibited, and stimulation of the sympathetic system causes bronchodilation. Inflammatory mediators (such as histamine) released during an antigen-antibody response act directly on bronchial smooth muscle to produce bronchoconstriction.

Pathophysiology

In asthma, the airways are in a persistent state of inflammation. During symptom-free periods, airway inflammation in asthma is subacute or quiet. Even during these periods, however, inflammatory cells such as eosinophils, neutrophils, and lymphocytes may be found in airway tissues and edema may be present. An acute inflammatory response, during which resident inflammatory cells interact with inflammatory mediators, cytokines, and additional infiltrating inflammatory cells, may be triggered by a variety of factors. Common triggers for an acute asthma attack include exposure to allergens, respiratory tract infection, exercise, inhaled irritants, and emotional upsets

Attack Triggers

Childhood asthma (which may continue into adulthood) is most often linked to inhalation of allergens such as pollen, animal dander, or household dust. Patients with allergic asthma often have a history of other allergies. Environmental pollutants, such as tobacco smoke and irritant gases (e.g., sulfur dioxide, nitrogen dioxide, and ozone), can provoke asthma. Exposure to secondhand smoke as a child is associated with a higher risk for and increased severity of asthma. Agents found in the workplace, such as noxious fumes and gases, chemicals, and dusts, may cause occupational asthma.

Respiratory infections, viral in particular, are a common internal stimulus for an asthmatic attack. Exercise-induced asthma attacks also are common, affecting 40% to 90% of people with bronchial asthma (Huether & McCance, 2008). Loss of heat or water from the bronchial surface may contribute to exercise-induced asthma. Exercising in cold, dry air increases the risk of an asthma attack in susceptible people.

Emotional stress is a significant etiologic factor for attacks in as many as half of patients with asthma. Common pharmacologic triggers include aspirin and other NSAIDs, beta blockers, and sulfites (which are used as preservatives in wine, beer, fresh fruits, and salad).

Asthma Video

Responses

When a trigger such as inhalation of an allergen or irritant occurs, an *acute* or *early response* develops in the hyperreactive airways predisposed to bronchospasm. Sensitized mast cells in the bronchial mucosa release inflammatory mediators such as histamine, prostaglandins, and leukotrienes. Resident and infiltrating inflammatory cells also produce inflammatory mediators such as cytokines, bradykinin, and growth factors. These mediators stimulate parasympathetic receptors and bronchial smooth muscle to produce bronchoconstriction. They also increase capillary permeability, which allows plasma to escape and leads to mucosal edema. Mucus production is stimulated; excess mucus collects in the narrowed airways.

The attack is prolonged by the *late phase response*, which develops 4 to 12 hours after exposure to the trigger. Inflammatory cells such as basophils and eosinophils are activated, which damage airway epithelium, produce mucosal edema, impair mucociliary clearance, and produce or prolong bronchoconstriction. The degree of hyperreactivity depends on the extent of inflammation. Together, bronchoconstriction, edema and inflammation, and mucous secretion narrow the airway. Airway resistance increases, limiting airflow, and increasing the work of breathing (Figure 37–1 ■).

Limited expiratory airflow traps air distal to the spastic, narrowed airways. Trapped air mixes with inspired air in the alveoli, reducing its oxygen tension and gas exchange across the alveolar-capillary membrane. Distended alveoli compress alveolar capillaries, reducing blood flow and further affecting gas exchange. As a result, hypoxemia develops. Hypoxemia and increased lung volume due to trapping stimulate the respiratory rate. Hyperventilation causes the $PaCO_2$ to fall, leading to respiratory alkalosis. (∞ See Chapter 10 for more information about acid–base imbalances.)

To summarize, in an acute asthma attack, inflammatory mediators are released from sensitized airways followed by activation of inflammatory cells. These events lead to bronchoconstriction, airway edema, and impaired mucociliary clearance. Airway narrowing limits airflow and increases the work of breathing; trapped air mixes with inhaled air, impairing gas exchange.

Manifestations and Complications

An asthma attack is characterized by a subjective sensation of chest tightness, cough, dyspnea, and wheezing (see the accompanying box). The onset of symptoms may be either abrupt or insidious, and an attack may subside rapidly or persist for hours or days. A sense of chest constriction and nonproductive cough are common early manifestations of an attack. During an attack, tachycardia, tachypnea, and prolonged expiration are common. Diffuse wheezing is heard on auscultation. With more severe attacks, use of accessory muscles of respiration, intercostal retractions, loud wheezing, and distant breath sounds may be noted. Fatigue, anxiety, apprehension, and severe dyspnea that allows speaking only one or two words between breaths, may occur with persistent severe episodes. The onset of respiratory failure is marked by inaudible breath sounds with reduced wheezing and an ineffective cough. Without careful assessment, this apparent relief of symptoms can be misinterpreted as an improvement.

The frequency of attacks and severity of symptoms vary greatly from person to person. Although some people have infrequent, mild episodes, others have nearly continuous manifestations of cough, dyspnea on exertion, and wheezing with periodic severe exacerbations (Table 37–1).

Status asthmaticus is severe, prolonged asthma that does not respond to routine treatment. Without aggressive therapy, status asthmaticus can lead to respiratory failure with hypoxemia, hypercapnia, and acidosis. Endotracheal intubation, mechanical ventilation, and aggressive drug treatment may be necessary to sustain life.

In addition to acute respiratory failure, other complications associated with acute asthma include dehydration, respiratory infection, atelectasis, pneumothorax, and cor pulmonale.

Cough-Variant Asthma

Asthma is one of the three most common causes of chronic cough (the other two being postnasal drip and gastroesophageal reflux [GERD]) (Fishman et al., 2008). Cough can be initiated by either upper airway irritants (e.g., postnasal drip or GERD) or by inflammation or constriction of the lower airways. Most commonly, cough associated with asthma is accompanied by classic asthma symptoms such as chest constriction, dyspnea, and wheezing. Patients with *cough-variant asthma*, however, have persistent cough without wheezing or dyspnea, often delaying diagnosis. These patients do have significant airway inflammation and demonstrate the pathophysiologic features of asthma.

Figure 37–1 ■ The pathogenesis of an acute episode of asthma.

MANIFESTATIONS of Acute Asthma

- Chest tightness
- Cough
- Dyspnea
- Wheezing
- Tachypnea and tachycardia
- Anxiety and apprehension

TABLE 37–1 Classification of Asthma Severity

CLASSIFICATION	SYMPTOM FREQUENCY	NIGHTTIME SYMPTOMS
Mild intermittent	■ No more than twice a week ■ Brief attacks (hours to days) of varied intensity ■ Asymptomatic and normal peak expiratory flow (PEF) rate between attacks	No more than twice a month
Mild persistent	■ More than twice a week but less than once a day ■ Exacerbations may affect activity	More than twice a month
Moderate persistent	■ Daily symptoms ■ Daily short-acting bronchodilator use ■ Exacerbations affect activity ■ Exacerbations more than twice a week; may last for days	More than once a week
Severe persistent	■ Continual symptoms ■ Limited physical activity ■ Frequent exacerbations	Frequent

Note: Adapted from National Education and Prevention Program. (1997). Expert panel report 2: Guidelines for the diagnosis and management of asthma, Publication No. 97-4051. Bethesda, MD: National Institutes of Health.

Incidence and Risk Factors

In the United States, approximately 16.2 million adults had asthma in 2007. Asthma is a serious disease, causing about 3,613 deaths in the United States in 2006 (CDC, 2009).

FAST FACTS

- Asthma is more common in children (9.1%) than adults; 7.3% of adults are affected (CDC, 2009).
- Across races, the mortality rate associated with asthma is higher in women than in men.
- The asthma mortality rate of Blacks is nearly three times that of Whites and is higher than that of Hispanics and other ethnic groups.
- Deaths due to asthma are rare in children and increase with age, particularly in middle and late adulthood and old age (CDC, 2009).

A number of risk factors can be identified for asthma, although many patients develop the disease in the absence of known risk factors. Allergies play a strong role in childhood asthma, although less so in adults. There is a strong genetic component to the disease, although a specific pattern of inheritance has not been identified. Multiple regions on several chromosomes appear to contribute to asthma-related factors such as airway hyper-reactivity and high IgE levels (Fishman et al., 2008). Environmental factors, including air pollution and occupational exposure to industrial compounds, may contribute. Respiratory viruses such as rhinovirus and influenza can precipitate asthma attacks. Other contributory factors include exercise (particularly in cold air) and emotional stress.

Interdisciplinary Care

The diagnosis of asthma is based primarily on the history and manifestations. Treatment goals are twofold. Daily management focuses on controlling symptoms and preventing acute attacks. During an acute attack, therapy is directed toward restoring airway patency and alveolar ventilation.

Diagnosis

Diagnostic tests are used to determine the degree of airway involvement during and between acute episodes and identify causative factors such as allergens. ∞ See Chapter 34 for more information about and the nursing care related to these diagnostic tests.

- *Pulmonary function tests (PFTs)* are used to evaluate the degree of airway obstruction. Pulmonary function testing done before and after use of an aerosolized bronchodilator helps determine the reversibility of airway obstruction. Airway reversibility is a cardinal sign seen on pulmonary function testing in asthma. The residual volume (RV) of the lungs may be increased and vital capacity decreased or normal even during periods of remission. The forced expiratory volume (FEV_1) and peak expiratory flow rate (PEFR), commonly referred to as "peak flow," are the most valuable pulmonary function studies to evaluate the severity of an asthma attack and the effectiveness of treatment measures. See Box 34–1.
- *Challenge or bronchial provocation testing* uses an inhaled substance such as methacholine or histamine with PFTs to confirm the diagnosis of asthma by detecting airway hyperresponsiveness.
- *ABGs* are drawn during an acute attack to evaluate oxygenation, carbon dioxide elimination, and acid–base status. ABGs initially show hypoxemia with a low PO_2, and mild respiratory alkalosis with an elevated pH and low PCO_2 due to tachypnea. Severe airflow obstruction causes significant hypoxemia and respiratory acidosis (pH less than 7.35 and PCO_2 greater than 45 mmHg), indicative of respiratory failure and the need for mechanical ventilation. ∞ See Chapter 10 for more information about arterial blood gases and their interpretation.
- *Skin testing* may be done to identify specific allergens if an allergic trigger is suspected for asthma attacks. ∞ See Chapter 36 for more information about skin testing.

Disease Monitoring

Peak expiratory flow rate (PEFR) is used on a day-to-day basis to evaluate the severity of bronchial hyperresponsiveness. Small, inexpensive meters to measure PEFR are available.

Readings taken at varying times of day over several weeks are used to establish the patient's personal best or normal PEFR. This value is then used to evaluate the severity of airway obstruction. Traffic signal colors are used for simplicity: *green* (80% to 100% of personal best) indicates asthma that is under control; *yellow* (50% to 80%) is caution, indicating a need for further medication or treatment; and *red* (50% or less) signals an immediate need for a bronchodilator and medical treatment if the level does not immediately return to the yellow range (Fishman et al., 2008; Huether & McCance, 2008).

Preventive Measures

Asthma attacks often can be prevented by avoiding allergens and environmental triggers. Modifying the home environment by controlling dust, removing carpets, covering mattresses and pillows to reduce dust mite populations, and installing air filtering systems may be useful. Pets may need to be removed from the household. Eliminating all tobacco smoke in the home is vital. Wearing a mask that retains humidity and warm air while exercising in cold weather may help prevent attacks of exercise-induced asthma. Early treatment of respiratory infections is vital to prevent asthma exacerbations.

Medications

Medications are used to prevent and control asthma symptoms, reduce the frequency and severity of exacerbations, and reverse airway obstruction. Drugs used for long-term control of asthma are taken daily to maintain control of the disease. The primary drugs in this group are anti-inflammatory agents, long-acting bronchodilators, and leukotriene modifiers. Quick-relief medications provide prompt relief of bronchoconstriction and airflow obstruction with associated wheezing, cough, and chest tightness. Short-acting adrenergic stimulants (rapid-acting bronchodilators), anticholinergic drugs, and methylxanthines fall into this category.

A stepwise approach for managing asthma is recommended. This approach is based on the severity of disease (see Tables 37–1 and 37–2). For all patients, a short-acting inhaled beta-2 agonist is recommended for quick relief of acute symptoms. Up to 3 treatments at 20 minute intervals or a single nebulizer treatment may be used as needed. Strategies for long-term control may need to be modified if a short-acting bronchodilator is needed more than twice a week (NHLBI, 2007).

Many of the drugs used for continued asthma management and relief of an acute attack can be administered by a metered-dose inhaler (MDI), dry powder inhaler (DPI), or nebulizer. The advantages of administering medications locally by inhalation include rapid onset and reduced systemic effects of the drugs. In an MDI, a chemical propellant is used to deliver the medication when the canister is depressed. DPI, in contrast, contain no propellant. Instead, the medication is released by inhaling rapidly through the mouthpiece. Box 37–1 outlines patient teaching for use of an MDI or DPI.

BRONCHODILATORS Most asthmatics need bronchodilator therapy to control their symptoms. Inhalation of nebulized medication is the preferred means of administration. The primary bronchodilators used include adrenergic stimulants, anticholinergic agents, and methylxanthines. These drugs often are administered in combination with an anti-inflammatory agent.

Adrenergic stimulants (beta-2 agonists) affect receptors on smooth muscle cells of the respiratory tract, causing smooth muscle relaxation and bronchodilation. Long-acting adrenergic stimulants such as inhaled salmeterol and oral sustained-release albuterol are used in conjunction with anti-inflammatory drugs to control symptoms, but are not appropriate to treat an acute episode of asthma. Inhaled short-acting beta-adrenergic agonists such as albuterol, bitolterol, pirbuterol, and terbutaline, administered by MDI or DPI, are the treatment of choice for quick relief. They act within minutes, but their duration generally is short, lasting only 4 to 6 hours. Tachycardia and muscle tremors, common side effects of adrenergic agonists, are minimal with inhalation therapy.

Anticholinergic medications prevent bronchoconstriction by blocking parasympathetic input to bronchial smooth muscle. Ipratropium bromide, an anticholinergic drug administered by MDI or hand held nebulizer, is useful when asthma symptoms are poorly controlled by adrenergic stimulants alone. Anticholinergic drugs act more slowly than adrenergic stimulants, requiring up to 60 to 90 minutes to achieve maximal effect.

Theophylline is a methylxanthine used as adjunctive treatment for asthma. It relaxes bronchial smooth muscle and may

TABLE 37–2 Stepwise Approach to Asthma Management for Adults

STEP/DISEASE SEVERITY	PREFERRED TREATMENT	ALTERNATE OR AS NEEDED TREATMENT
Step 1 Mild Intermittent	No daily medication needed	Systemic corticosteroids for severe exacerbations
Step 2 Mild Persistent	Low-dose inhaled corticosteroids	Cromolyn, leukotriene modifier, nedocromil, or sustained release theophylline
Step 3 Moderated Persistent	Low-to-moderate dose inhaled corticosteroids *and* long-acting inhaled beta-2 agonist	Increase inhaled corticosteroid dose *or* combine inhaled corticosteroid with leukotriene modifier or theophylline
Step 4 Severe Persistent	High-dose inhaled corticosteroid *and* long-acting inhaled beta-2 agonist	Add systemic corticosteroid

Note: Adapted from National Education and Prevention Program. (2007). Expert panel report 3: Guidelines for the diagnosis and management of asthma, update on selected topics 2007, Publication No. 08-5846. Bethesda, MD: National Institutes of Health.

BOX 37–1   Patient Teaching: Using a Metered-Dose Inhaler or Dry Powder Inhaler

Metered-Dose Inhaler

- Firmly insert a charged metered-dose inhaler (MDI) canister into the mouthpiece unit or spacer (if used).
- Remove mouthpiece cap. Shake canister vigorously for 3 to 5 seconds.
- Exhale slowly and completely.
- Holding the canister upside down, place the mouthpiece in the mouth, closing lips around it, if a spacer is being used. When no spacer is used, hold the mouthpiece directly in front of the mouth.
- Press and hold the canister down while inhaling deeply and slowly for 3 to 5 seconds (see accompanying figure).
- Hold breath for 10 seconds, release pressure on the container, remove from mouth, and exhale. Wait 20 to 30 seconds before repeating the procedure for a second puff.
- Rinse the mouth after using the inhaler to minimize systemic absorption and drying the mucous membranes.
- Rinse the inhaler mouthpiece and spacer after use; store in a clean location.

Dry Powder Inhaler

- Keep the inhaler and medication in a clean, dry location. Do not refrigerate or store in a humid place (for example, the bathroom).
- Remove the cap and hold the inhaler upright. Inspect to be sure that the mechanism is clean and the mouthpiece is clear.
- If necessary, load the dose into the inhaler following manufacturer's directions.
- Hold the inhaler level with the mouthpiece end facing down.
- Breathe slowly and completely. Tilt your head back slightly.
- Place the mouthpiece in your mouth with your teeth over the mouthpiece. Seal your lips around the mouthpiece. Do not block the inhaler with your tongue.

- Breathe in rapidly and deeply through your mouth over 2 to 3 seconds to activate the flow of medication.
- Remove the inhaler from your mouth and hold your breath for 10 seconds.
- Exhale slowly through pursed lips to allow the medication to enter distal airways. Never exhale into the inhaler mouthpiece to prevent clogging.
- Rinse your mouth or brush your teeth after using the inhaler to avoid a bad taste from the medication and to prevent a yeast infection (if a corticosteroid medication is being used).
- Store the inhaler in a clean, sealed plastic bag; do not wash the inhaler unless so directed by the manufacturer. The mouthpiece should be cleaned weekly using a dry cloth.

also inhibit the release of chemical mediators of the inflammatory response. Monitoring of serum theophylline levels is necessary because of wide individual variations in metabolism and elimination of the drug and its toxic effects. Serum levels of 10 to 20 μg/mL or lower are recommended. Theophylline may be used as a long-term bronchodilator, given once or twice daily. A related drug, aminophylline, may be administered intravenously to treat an acute, severe exacerbation of the disease.

ANTI-INFLAMMATORY AGENTS   Corticosteroids and two nonsteroidal anti-inflammatory agents, cromolyn sodium and nedocromil, are used to suppress airway inflammation and reduce asthma symptoms.

Corticosteroids block the late response to inhaled allergens and reduce bronchial hyperresponsiveness. The preferred route of administration is by MDI or DPI to minimize systemic absorption and reduce the adverse effects of prolonged steroid use (cushingoid effects). For a severe acute attack, corticosteroids may be given systemically to alleviate symptoms and induce remission.

Cromolyn sodium and nedocromil are used to prevent acute episodes of asthma. They reduce airway hyperreactivity and inhibit the release of mediator substances. These drugs are used for long-term control of asthma, not quick relief. They have a wide margin of safety and few side effects.

LEUKOTRIENE MODIFIERS   Leukotriene modifiers montelukast (Singulair), zafirlukast (Accolate), and zileuton (Zyflo Filmtab) are oral medications that reduce the inflammatory

response in asthma. They appear to improve lung function, diminish symptoms, and reduce the need for short-acting bronchodilators. These drugs affect the metabolism and excretion of other medications such as warfarin and theophylline and may cause liver toxicity.

Nursing implications for medications used to treat asthma are outlined on pages 1235–1236.

Complementary Therapies

A number of herbal preparations and other complementary therapies have been shown to be helpful in treating asthma. Dietary therapies, environmental medicine, and nutritional supplements are the complementary therapies most widely recommended by healthcare professionals for asthma. Nutritional and dietary therapies may include elimination of certain foods or food additives (e.g., sulfite) from the diet, often in the absence of a documented food allergy or relationship between consumption and the onset of asthma symptoms. Although the evidence is inconsistent, some studies suggest that increasing intake of ascorbic acid, an antioxidant, zinc, and magnesium may help alleviate manifestations of asthma. People with mild asthma may benefit from addition of omega-3 polyunsaturated fatty acids to the diet, experiencing less severe and fewer acute attacks.

Herbal preparations may include atropa belladonna (the natural form of atropine) or ephedra (also called ma huang), an herb that contains ephedrine. These herbals have effects similar to those of drugs used to treat asthma, and should not be used in combination with sympathetic stimulants or anticholinergic

MEDICATION ADMINISTRATION Asthma

ADRENERGIC STIMULANTS
Epinephrine

Isoproterenol (Isuprel)

Metaproterenol (Alupent, Metaprel)

Terbutaline (Brethaire, Brethine)

Isoetharine (Bronkosol, Bronkometer)

Albuterol (Proventil, Ventolin)

Bitolterol (Tornalate)

Pirbuterol (Maxair)

Salmeterol (Serevent)

Formoterol (Foradil)

Combined Forms: albuterol/ipratropium (Combivent); salmeterol/fluticasone (Advair)

Adrenergic stimulants affect sympathetic receptors in the respiratory tract. Administered by metered-dose inhalers or dry powder inhalers, these drugs are the treatment of choice for acute bronchial asthma. Nearly all of the drugs in this class (epinephrine and isoproterenol being the exceptions) selectively activate beta-2 receptors at the doses typically used to treat asthma. Beta-2 receptor activation results in smooth muscle relaxation and bronchodilation. Formoterol and salmeterol are highly selective to beta-2 receptors, resulting in fewer adverse effects. Formoterol and salmeterol have been shown to increase the risk of serious asthma exacerbations and death, however. The Food and Drug Administration recommends using these drugs only when the disease cannot be adequately controlled with other medications.

Oral forms of adrenergic agonists may be used for prophylaxis but are not effective in treating an acute attack because of their slow onset. When administered orally or parenterally, their effect on sympathetic nervous system receptors can produce undesirable side effects such as nervousness, irritability, tachycardia, and cardiac dysrhythmias.

Nursing Responsibilities
- Use with caution in patients with hypertension, cardiovascular disease, dysrhythmias, hyperthyroidism, or diabetes.
- When given to a patient who is hypoxemic and acidotic, these drugs may cause potentially dangerous cardiac stimulation.
- When given by MDI wait 1 to 2 minutes between puffs to allow airways to dilate, permitting the second dose to reach distal airways.
- Observe for desired effect of reduced dyspnea and wheezing. Central nervous system stimulation (anxiety, irritability, and insomnia) and tremor are common side effects.

Health Education for Patient and Family
- Use the prescribed inhaler or nebulizer as directed.
- If you are taking a bronchodilator along with another medication by inhalation, use the bronchodilator first to open airways and enhance the effectiveness of the second medication.
- Rinse the mouth after using inhalers to reduce systemic absorption of the medication.
- Keep a log to track your bronchodilator use. If the drug becomes less effective, or if you need a higher dosage or more frequent doses than prescribed, contact your physician.
- Report palpitations, irregular pulse, and other side effects to the physician.

METHYLXANTHINES
Theophylline (Bronkotabs, Quibron, Slo-Phyllin Theolair, Theo-Dur, others)

Aminophylline (Somophyllin)

The methylxanthines are central nervous system stimulants chemically related to caffeine. These drugs produce bronchodilation through relaxation of bronchial smooth muscle. As CNS stimulants, they produce adverse effects such as nervousness, insomnia, and tremors. When administered in large doses, convulsions may result.

Once the drugs of choice for preventing and treating asthma attacks, they are now are used primarily to prevent nocturnal asthma in affected adult patients. Theophylline has a narrow margin of safety and high potential for toxicity. Because the metabolism and excretion of theophylline vary significantly from person to person—affected by such factors as age, smoking, genetic factors, alcoholism, and other chronic diseases—monitoring of serum levels is vital.

Nursing Responsibilities
- The therapeutic blood level for theophylline is 10 to 20 μg/mL.
- Monitor for manifestations of toxicity. Anorexia, nausea, vomiting, restlessness, insomnia, cardiac dysrhythmias, and seizures are early manifestations. Other manifestations include epigastric pain, hematemesis, diarrhea, headache, irritability, muscle twitching, palpitations, tachycardia, flushing, and circulatory failure.
- Administer with meals or a full glass of water or milk to minimize gastric irritation.
- Monitor the effect closely when administering concurrently with other medications such as barbiturates, anticonvulsants, thyroid hormone, beta blockers, bronchodilators, and others.
- Aminophylline is incompatible with many other intravenous drugs. Use a separate line or flush the line with normal saline before and after administering any other preparation.

Health Education for Patient and Family
- Oral methylxanthines are ineffective to treat an acute asthma attack; do not delay other treatment by using these drugs.
- Check with the physician before taking any over-the-counter medications or other prescription drugs while on theophylline.
- Do not smoke while using this drug.
- Report adverse effects to the physician.

ANTICHOLINERGICS
Atropine

Ipratropium bromide (Atrovent)

Tiotropium bromide (Spiriva)

Combination Products: albuterol/ipratropium (Combivent)

Anticholinergics are potent bronchodilators, blocking muscarinic receptors of the parasympathetic nervous system. Activation of muscarinic receptors produces smooth muscle contraction and bronchoconstriction; blockade of these receptors facilitates smooth muscle relaxation and bronchodilation. Atropine is used infrequently because of its tendency to dry secretions of the mucous membranes and other side effects. Ipratropium and tiotropium bromide are available as inhalers and have fewer side effects than atropine.

(continued)

MEDICATION ADMINISTRATION   Asthma (continued)

Nursing Responsibilities

- Assess for possible contraindications to the drug, including hypersensitivity, glaucoma, prostatic hypertrophy, or bladder-neck obstruction.
- Assess for desired and/or adverse effects: improving or worsening symptoms; nausea, vomiting, abdominal cramping, anxiety, dizziness; headache.
- Provide ice chips, fluids, or hard candy to relieve dry mouth.

Health Education for Patient and Family

- To prevent overdose, take no more than the prescribed number of doses per day.
- If the drug becomes less effective over time, notify the physician; an adjustment in dosage may be needed.

CORTICOSTEROIDS

Beclomethasone dipropionate (Vanceril, Beclovent)

Triamcinolone acetonide (Azmacort)

Flunisolide (AeroBid)

Fluticasone propionate (Flovent)

Dexamethasone sodium phosphate (Decadron Phosphate Respihaler)

Combination Products: salmeterol/fluticasone (Advair)

The anti-inflammatory effect of corticosteroids helps both prevent and treat acute episodes. Corticosteroids are used to reduce the frequency and severity of asthma attacks and allow reduced dosages of other drugs. The beneficial effects of corticosteroids for asthma result from their ability to decrease the synthesis and release of inflammatory mediators (such as histamine and leukotrienes), reduce inflammatory cell activation and infiltration, and decrease airway edema. Corticosteroids also decrease mucus production in the airways and increase the number and receptivity of beta-2 receptors (Deglin & Vallerand, 2009). The cushingoid side effects of corticosteroids, always a major concern with their use, are minimized when they are inhaled. Note that the combination product salmeterol/fluticasone is associated with an increased risk of serious asthma exacerbations and death. It is a second-line drug, recommended for use only when asthma is inadequately controlled using other preparations.

Nursing Responsibilities

- Administer inhaler doses after bronchodilators to facilitate transit of the medication to distal airways.
- Assess for common side effects: sore throat; hoarseness; and oropharyngeal or laryngeal *Candida albicans* infection.
- Administer antifungal medications or gargles as ordered.

Health Education for Patient and Family

- Rinse the mouth after using the inhaler and maintain good oral hygiene to reduce the risk of fungal infections.
- These medications should not be used to alleviate the symptoms of an acute attack.
- Several weeks of continued therapy may be required before a beneficial effect is noticed.
- Notify the physician if you develop weight gain, fluid retention, muscle weakness, redistribution of fat, or mood changes.

MAST CELL STABILIZERS

Cromolyn sodium (Intal, Nasalcrom)

Nedocromil (Tilade)

Cromolyn sodium and nedocromil inhibit inflammatory cells in the airway, blocking early and late responses to inhaled antigens. Both drugs also prevent bronchoconstriction in response to inhaling cold air. These drugs act primarily by stabilizing the cytoplasmic membrane of mast cells, preventing the cells from releasing inflammatory mediators such as histamine (Deglin & Vallerand, 2009). These drugs are used only for preventing asthma attacks, not to treat an acute attack. They are administered by metered-dose inhaler, and have a wide margin of safety. Patients using nedocromil may complain of an unpleasant taste.

Nursing Responsibilities

- Evaluate for potential adverse effects of wheezing and bronchoconstriction.

Health Education for Patient and Family

- Gargling or sipping water can decrease the throat irritation associated with nebulizer treatment.
- Use appropriate technique. Inhale deeply with head tipped back to open airways, hold breath, and then exhale. Repeat until all of the drug has been inhaled.
- These drugs are used only to prevent asthma attacks; they are not effective in treating an acute attack.
- Several weeks may be required before a beneficial effect is noted.

LEUKOTRIENE MODIFIERS

Montelukast (Singulair)

Zafirlukast (Accolate)

Zileuton (Zyflo)

Leukotriene modifiers interfere with the inflammatory process in the airways by suppressing the effects of leukotrienes, a group of inflammatory mediators. Leukotrienes are powerful bronchoconstrictors and vasodilators; blocking their synthesis or their receptors improves airflow, decreases symptoms, and reduces the need for short-acting bronchodilators. They are used for maintenance therapy in adults and children over the age of 12 as an alternative to inhaled corticosteroid therapy. They are not used to treat an acute attack.

Nursing Responsibilities

- Administer at least 1 hour before or 2 hours after meals.
- These drugs inhibit some liver enzymes, affecting the metabolism of warfarin and possibly terfenadine and theophylline. Monitor prothrombin times and theophylline blood levels.
- Monitor liver enzymes, as these drugs may be toxic to the liver.

Health Education for Patient and Family

- Take the drugs as prescribed on an empty stomach.
- Notify the physician if a change in color of stools or urine is noted or if jaundice develops.

---

preparations. Because of the dangers associated with its use, sale of herbal products containing ephedra has been banned. Advise patients inquiring about the use of Chinese herbal remedies to treat asthma to inquire if any recommended product contains ma hung or ephedra, and to avoid such products. Capsaicin also may relieve acute asthma symptoms. Other herbal preparations include quercetin and grape seed extract. Refer patients

interested in using natural preparations to a qualified herbalist, and emphasize the importance of talking to the physician before using these preparations along with conventional treatment.

In addition to herbals, other complementary therapies such as biofeedback, yoga, breathing techniques, acupuncture, homeopathy, and massage have been found to alleviate or help control asthma symptoms.

✍ Nursing Care

Nurses encounter patients with asthma both in the acute care setting during an acute exacerbation and as outpatients or in homes. The priority nursing care needs differ with each setting.

Health Promotion

Although specific measures to prevent asthma have not yet been identified, the link between parental smoking and childhood asthma is strong. Discuss this link with young people and families with children. Encourage all patients to not start smoking, and if they do smoke, to quit. Provide referrals to smoking cessation clinics, help groups, or a care provider for nicotine patches as needed to facilitate quitting. Additional evidence suggests that early exposure to certain infectious diseases and to other children and limited use of antibiotics reduces the risk for developing asthma (NHLBI, 2007).

Assessment

Assessment of the patient experiencing an acute asthma attack must be very focused and timely.

- *Health history:* Current symptoms, including chest tightness, shortness of breath, dyspnea; duration of current attack; measures used to relieve symptoms and their effect; identified precipitating factors for the attack; frequency of attacks; current medications; known allergies.
- *Physical examination:* Apparent level of distress; color; vital signs; respiratory rate and excursion, breath sounds throughout lung fields; apical pulse.
- *Diagnostic tests:* Forced expiratory volume, peak expiratory flow rate; arterial blood gases.

Nursing Diagnoses and Interventions

An acute asthma attack causes fear as breathing becomes increasingly difficult and hypoxemia develops. Anxiety in turn tends to increase the severity and manifestations of the attack. Priority nursing care needs during an acute attack focus on improving airway clearance and reducing fear and anxiety. Teaching about prevention of future attacks and home management must be postponed until adequate ventilation is restored.

Ineffective Airway Clearance

Bronchospasm and bronchoconstriction, increased mucus secretion, and airway edema narrow the airways and impair airflow during an acute attack of asthma. Both inspiratory and expiratory volume are affected, decreasing the oxygen available at the alveolus for the process of respiration. Narrowed air

EVIDENCE FOR NURSING CARE — The Patient with Asthma

Selected resources that nurses may find helpful when planning evidence-based nursing care follow.

- Bateman, E. D., Bousquet, J., FitzGerald, M., Haahtela, T., O'Byrne, P., Ohta, K. et al. (2008). Global strategy for asthma management and prevention. Bethesda (MD): Global Initiative for Asthma (GINA). Retrieved from http://www.ginasthma.com/
- Lawes, R. (2009). Putting the squeeze on asthma. *Nursing2009, 39*(3); 56hn1-4.

passages increase the work of breathing, increasing the metabolic rate and tissue demand for oxygen.

> **PRACTICE ALERT**
> Frequently assess respiratory status (at least every 1 to 2 hours): respiratory rate and depth, chest movement or excursion, breath sounds, and peak expiratory flow rate. Respiratory status can change rapidly during an acute asthma attack and its treatment. Decreasing PEFRs indicate worsening airflow restriction. Slowed, shallow respirations with significantly diminished breath sounds and decreased wheezing may indicate exhaustion and impending respiratory failure. Immediate intervention is necessary.

- Monitor skin color and temperature and level of consciousness. *Cyanosis, cool clammy skin, and changes in level of consciousness (agitation, lethargy, or confusion) indicate worsening hypoxia.*
- Assess arterial blood gas results and pulse oximetry readings; notify the physician of abnormal values or changes in status. *These values provide information about gas exchange and the adequacy of alveolar ventilation. A fall in oxygen saturation levels is an early indicator of impaired gas exchange.*

> **PRACTICE ALERT**
> Assess cough effort and sputum for color, consistency, and amount. Ineffective cough may also signal impending respiratory failure.

- Place in Fowler's, high-Fowler's, or orthopneic (with head and arms supported on the overbed table) position to facilitate breathing and lung expansion. *These positions reduce the work of breathing and increase lung expansion, especially of basilar areas.*
- Administer oxygen as ordered. If a mask is used, monitor closely for feelings of claustrophobia or suffocation. *Supplemental oxygen reduces hypoxemia. Although the mask is a very effective oxygen delivery system, it may increase anxiety.*
- Administer nebulizer treatments and provide humidification as ordered. *Nebulizer treatments are used to administer bronchodilators and other medications; humidity helps loosen secretions.*
- Initiate or assist with chest physiotherapy, including percussion and postural drainage. *Percussion and postural drainage facilitate the movement of secretions and airway clearance.*
- Increase fluid intake. *Increasing fluids helps keep secretions thin.*
- Provide endotracheal suctioning as needed. *Endotracheal suctioning may be necessary to remove secretions and improve ventilation if the patient is unable to clear secretions by coughing.*

Ineffective Breathing Pattern

The physiologic changes in lung ventilation that occur during an acute asthma attack impair both lung expansion and emptying. Anxiety caused by hypoxia and dyspnea compounds the problem by increasing the respiratory rate. Collaborative and nursing interventions can help restore a more normal breathing pattern and adequate lung ventilation.

- Monitor vital signs and laboratory results. *Tachypnea, tachycardia, an elevated blood pressure, and increasing hypoxemia and hypercapnia are signs of compromised respiratory status.*
- Assist with ADLs as needed. *This conserves energy and reduces fatigue.*
- Provide rest periods between scheduled activities and treatments. *Scheduled rest is important to prevent fatigue and reduce oxygen demands.*
- Teach and assist to use techniques to control breathing pattern:
  a. Pursed-lip breathing
  b. Abdominal breathing
  c. Relaxation techniques including visualization, meditation, and others
  Pursed-lip breathing helps keep airways open by maintaining positive pressure, and abdominal breathing improves lung expansion. Relaxation techniques reduce anxiety and its effect on the respiratory rate.
- Administer medications, including bronchodilators and anti-inflammatory drugs, as ordered. Monitor for desired and possible adverse effects. *Medications are used to improve airway status and facilitate breathing.*

Anxiety

Acute exacerbations of asthma can produce significant anxiety. Fear of being unable to breathe and feelings of suffocation associated with acute asthma are significant. Financial or other concerns may cause the patient to want to avoid hospitalization. Increasingly frequent and severe episodes may cause fear for the future. Hypoxia contributes to anxiety as well, stimulating the sympathetic nervous system and the fight-or-flight response.

- Assess level of anxiety. *Interventions for severe anxiety or panic differ from those for mild or moderate anxiety.*
- Assist to identify coping skills that have been successful in the past. *Successful coping helps the patient regain control of the situation, reducing anxiety.*

- Listen actively to concerns; do not deny or negate the fear of dying or of being unable to breathe. *Active listening promotes trust and helps the patient express concerns.*

- Include the patient in care planning and decisions as appropriate, without making excessive demands. *Participating in decision making increases the patient's sense of control. Because high levels of anxiety interfere with the ability to make decisions, it is important to avoid placing demands on the patient that may further increase the level of anxiety.*
- Reduce excessive environmental stimuli, and maintain a calm demeanor. *This promotes rest.*
- Allow supportive family members to remain with the patient. *Significant others provide additional support and can help reduce anxiety.*
- Assist to use relaxation techniques, such as guided imagery, muscle relaxation, and meditation. *These techniques help restore psychologic balance and reduce sympathetic stimulation and responses.*

Ineffective Therapeutic Regimen Management

Once acute asthma is under control and effective respirations have been reestablished, it is important to help the patient identify contributing factors to the attack. This helps the patient prevent future episodes.

- Assess level of understanding about asthma and the prescribed treatment regimen. Provide additional information and teaching as indicated. *Assessment helps to identify and clarify misperceptions and difficulties with disease management.*
- Discuss the patient's perception of the illness and its effect on his or her lifestyle. *Open discussion can help identify conflicts between lifestyle and the treatment regimen.*

- Assist the patient and significant others to identify problems or difficulties integrating the treatment regimen into their lifestyle. *Asthma and its management may necessitate lifestyle modifications to prevent acute exacerbations. This can significantly impact family members, for example, eliminating cigarette smoking or pets from the household, removing carpets, or daily damp-dusting to remove dust mites.*
- Assess knowledge and understanding of prescribed medications and use of over-the-counter preparations. *This is important to determine misperceptions or possible misuse of medications.*
- Provide verbal and written instructions. *Written instructions reinforce teaching and allow future reference.*
- Refer to counseling, support groups, or self-help organizations. *Counseling, support groups, and self-help organizations can help the patient and family adapt to living with asthma and the treatment regimen.*

Community-Based Care

Asthma is a chronic disease that is best managed by the patient with assistance from medical personnel. Teaching for home care focuses on promoting the highest level of wellness and preventing and managing acute episodes and exacerbations of the disease. Topics to include in teaching are as follows:

- Suggestions for lifestyle changes to avoid specific triggers for asthma attacks:
  - Warm up slowly before exercising in cold weather; wear a special mask or scarf to retain air warmth and humidity while exercising.
  - Substitute indoor exercises during cold, dry weather.
  - Reduce the risk for respiratory infections (e.g., adequate rest, good nutrition, and stress management to maintain immune function, yearly influenza vaccines and immunization against pneumococcal pneumonia).
  - Use techniques to reduce or manage physical and psychologic stress.
- Using PEFR meter to monitor airway status; how to manage the disease based on results
- Using prescribed medications, including the following:
  - Name, frequency, dose, and desired effect
  - Potential adverse effects and their management, including effects to report to the physician
  - Potential interactions with other drugs (including over-the-counter herbal preparations) or foods
  - If tolerance is a potential risk, how to identify it and steps to take

Provide referrals to local or regional resources for further teaching and support as needed. Consider the need for home health services, home respiratory care services, and others as needed.

The Patient with Chronic Obstructive Pulmonary Disease

Patients with chronic airflow obstruction due to chronic bronchitis and/or emphysema are said to have **chronic obstructive pulmonary disease (COPD)**.

Pathophysiology

COPD is characterized by slowly progressive obstruction of the airways. The disease is one of periodic exacerbations, often related to respiratory infection, with increased symptoms of dyspnea and sputum production. Unlike acute processes in which lung tissues recover, airways and lung parenchyma do not return to normal following an exacerbation; instead, they demonstrate progressive destructive changes.

Although one or the other may predominate, COPD typically includes components of both chronic bronchitis and emphysema, two distinctly different processes. Small airways disease, narrowing of small bronchioles, is also part of the COPD complex.

Through different mechanisms, these processes cause airways to narrow, resistance to airflow to increase, and expiration to become slow or difficult (Figure 37–2 ■). The result is a mismatch between alveolar ventilation and blood flow or perfusion, leading to impaired gas exchange.

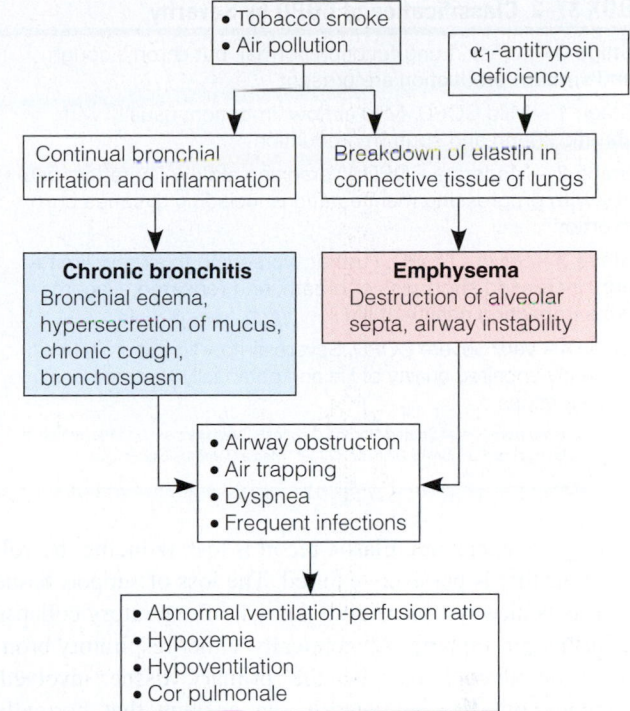

Figure 37–2 ■ The pathogenesis of chronic obstructive pulmonary disease.

Chronic Bronchitis

Chronic bronchitis is a disorder of excessive bronchial mucus secretion. It is characterized by a productive cough lasting 3 or more months in 2 consecutive years (Huether & McCance, 2008). Cigarette smoke is the major factor implicated in the development of chronic bronchitis.

Inhaled irritants lead to a chronic inflammatory process with vasodilation, congestion, and edema of the bronchial mucosa. Goblet cells increase in size and number, and mucous glands enlarge. Thick, tenacious mucus is produced in increased amounts. Changes in bronchial squamous cells impair the ability to clear mucus (Fishman et al., 2008). Narrowed airways and excess secretions obstruct airflow; expiration is affected first, then inspiration. Because ciliary function is impaired, normal defense mechanisms are unable to clear the mucus and any inhaled pathogens. Recurrent infection is common in chronic bronchitis. An imbalance between ventilation and perfusion leads to hypoxemia, hypercapnia, and pulmonary hypertension. Pulmonary hypertension often leads to right-sided heart failure.

Emphysema

Emphysema is characterized by destruction of the walls of the alveoli, with resulting enlargement of abnormal air spaces. As in chronic bronchitis, cigarette smoking is strongly implicated as a causative factor in most cases of emphysema. Macrophages from the alveoli (air sacs) and CD-8 T lymphocytes increase and destroy lung tissue. Cytokines also play a role in the inflammation. Additionally anti-proteinases, which protect lung tissue become inactivated, leading to reductions in lung repair. This results in alveolar wall destruction. Alveolar wall destruction causes alveoli and air spaces to enlarge with loss of corresponding portions of the pulmonary capillary bed. As a result, the surface area for alveolar-capillary diffusion is reduced, affecting gas exchange. Elastic recoil is lost, reducing the volume of air that is passively expired. The loss of support tissue also affects airways, increasing the risk of expiratory collapse and further air trapping. Anatomically, either respiratory bronchioles or alveoli may be the primary tissue involved. Deficiency of alpha$_1$-antitrypsin, an enzyme that normally inhibits the activity of proteolytic enzymes and tissue destruction in the lungs, contributes to the development of emphysema, especially when combined with exposure to cigarette smoke.

To summarize, COPD is a progressive, nonreversible process of airway narrowing and loss of supporting tissue. Three separate processes typically are involved:

- Chronic bronchitis with persistent airway edema, excessive mucus production, and impaired airway clearance
- Emphysema with loss of alveolar walls, capillary bed, and airway support tissue resulting in airway collapse and reductions in gas exchange
- Small airways disease with bronchoconstriction

The result of these processes and their combined effects is increased work of breathing, impaired expiration with air trapping, and impaired gas exchange.

Manifestations

The clinical presentation of COPD varies from simple chronic bronchitis without disability to chronic respiratory failure and severe disability. Box 37–2 outlines the classifications of COPD severity. Manifestations are typically absent or minor early in the disease. When the patient finally seeks care, productive cough, dyspnea, and exercise intolerance often have been present for as long as 10 years. The cough typically occurs in the mornings and often is attributed to "smoker's cough." Initially, dyspnea occurs only on extreme exertion; as the disease progresses, activity tolerance spirals downward. Patients abandon activity to avoid dyspnea, leading to further deconditioning. This results in a patient so deconditioned that dyspnea occurs with light activity or even at rest. The clinical features and manifestations of COPD are summarized in Table 37–3.

Manifestations of chronic bronchitis are a cough productive of copious amounts (at least 1/2 cup/day) of thick, tenacious sputum, cyanosis, and evidence of right-sided heart failure, including distended neck veins, edema, liver engorgement, and an enlarged heart. Adventitious sounds, including loud rhonchi and possible wheezes, are prominent on auscultation.

Emphysema is insidious in onset. Dyspnea is the initial symptom. Initially occurring only with exertion, dyspnea may progress to become severe even at rest. Cough is minimal or absent. Air trapping and hyperinflation increase the anterior-posterior chest diameter, causing *barrel chest*. The patient often is thin, tachypneic, uses accessory muscles of respiration and often assumes a position of sitting and leaning forward (Figure 37–3 ■). The expiratory phase of the respiratory cycle is prolonged. On auscultation, breath sounds are diminished, and the percussion tone is hyperresonant.

Incidence and Risk Factors

In 2007, approximately 11.3 million Americans were affected by COPD (CDC, 2009). It is more common among Whites than Blacks and affects men more frequently than women. It is the fourth leading cause of death in the United States. The death rate from COPD continues to rise among Black and American

TABLE 37–3 Clinical Features and Manifestations of COPD

	FEATURE	CHRONIC BRONCHITIS	EMPHYSEMA
History	Onset	After age 35; recurrent respiratory infections	After age 50; insidious progressive dyspnea
	Smoking	Usual	Usual
	Cough	Persistent, productive of copious mucopurulent sputum	Absent or mild with scant clear sputum, if any
Physical Examination	Appearance	Often obese; edematous and cyanotic; distended neck veins and other symptoms of right-sided heart failure	Usually thin and cachectic; barrel chest; prominent accessory muscles of respiration
	Chest	Adventitious sounds with wheezing and rhonchi; normal percussion note	Distant or diminished breath sounds; hyper-resonant percussion note
Other Features	Blood gases	Hypercapnia and hypoxemia; respiratory acidosis	Normal or mild hypoxemia; normal pH
	Pulmonary function studies	Normal or decreased total lung capacity; moderately increased residual volume	Increased total lung capacity; markedly increased residual volume
	Pulmonary hypertension	May be severe	Only when advanced

Figure 37–3 ■ Typical appearance of a patient with emphysema. Note the patient's anxious expression and assumption of the tripod position, leaning forward with the hands on the knees.

Indian males, and females of all ethnic groups; the death rate is stable in Whites, Hispanics, and Asians. In the year 2006, COPD and other chronic obstructive lung diseases accounted for over 120,000 deaths (CDC, 2009). In addition, COPD morbidity is significant. In people under age 65, COPD is second only to heart disease as a cause of disability, resulting in an estimated 250 million lost work hours yearly.

FAST FACTS

- Since 2001, the number of deaths due to COPD in women has exceeded men.
- Chronic bronchitis was diagnosed in 7.6 million Americans in 2007.
- Females are now more than twice as likely to be diagnosed with chronic bronchitis as males.
- Approximately 3.7 million Americans have emphysema.
- While more men than women have emphysema, its prevalence is increasing in women and decreasing in men.

(Data from CDC, 2009).

Obstructive lung disease typically affects middle-aged and older adults. Cigarette smoking is clearly implicated as the primary cause of COPD. Even though COPD develops in a minority of smokers, smokers are 12 to 13 times more likely to die from COPD than nonsmokers (Fishman et al., 2008). Cigarette smoke and the irritants it contains impair ciliary movement, inhibit the function of alveolar macrophages, and cause mucus-secreting glands to hypertrophy. Smoking also produces emphysema or airway destruction and constricts smooth muscle, increasing airway resistance. Other contributing factors include air pollution, occupational exposure to noxious dusts and gases, airway infection, and familial and genetic factors (see the accompanying Genetic Considerations box).

Interdisciplinary Care

Although COPD can be prevented in most people, it cannot be cured. Smoking abstinence is the only certain way to prevent COPD and to slow its progression. To a certain extent, airway

---

GENETIC CONSIDERATIONS
Chronic Obstructive Pulmonary Disease

Severe α_1 antitrypsin (α_1AT or ATT) deficiency, present in about 1% to 2% of patients with COPD, is a proven risk factor for COPD. Normal α_1AT levels are associated with the common M allele. Two other alleles, the S allele and the Z allele, lead to reduced α_1AT levels. An estimated 25 million Americans carry a single gene associated with α_1AT deficiency and can pass that gene on to their offspring. People who inherit two Z alleles or one Z allele and one null allele have severe α_1AT deficiency. Approximately 1 in 3000 people in the United States inherit severe α_1AT deficiency (Fishman et al., 2008). An estimated 100,000 people in the United States have emphysema related to α_1AT deficiency. Although studies suggest additional genetic factors in the development of COPD, at this time none have been proven (Fishman et al., 2008).

---

obstruction can be reversed and disability minimized early in the disease. Treatment generally focuses on relieving symptoms, minimizing obstruction, and slowing disability.

Diagnosis

Diagnostic tests are used to help establish the diagnosis of chronic obstructive pulmonary disease and identify the predominant component, emphysema or chronic bronchitis. These procedures also are used to assess respiratory status and monitor treatment effectiveness. ∞ See Chapter 34 for more information about these diagnostic procedures and related nursing care.

- *Pulmonary function testing* is performed to establish the diagnosis and evaluate the extent and progress of COPD (see Box 35–1). Results are based on calculated norms for each person by age, height, sex, and weight; note these as well as all current medications on the requisition. In COPD, the total lung capacity and residual volume typically are increased. The forced expiratory volume (FEV_1) and forced vital capacity (FVC) are decreased due to narrowed airways and resistance to airflow.
- *Ventilation-perfusion scanning* may be performed to determine the extent of ventilation/perfusion mismatch—that is, the extent to which lung tissue is ventilated but not perfused (dead space), or perfused but inadequately ventilated (physiologic shunting) (Figure 37–4 ■). A radioisotope is injected or inhaled to illustrate areas of shunting and absent capillaries.
- *Serum alpha₁-antitrypsin levels* may be drawn to screen for deficiency, particularly in patients with a family history of obstructive airway disease, those with an early onset, women, and nonsmokers. Normal adult serum alpha₁-antitrypsin levels range from 80 to 260 mg/dL. Fasting is not required prior to this test.
- *Arterial blood gases (ABGs)* are drawn to evaluate gas exchange, particularly during acute exacerbations of COPD. Patients with predominant emphysema often have mild hypoxemia and normal or low carbon dioxide tension. Respiratory alkalosis may be present due to an increased respiratory rate. Predominant chronic bronchitis and airway obstruction may cause marked hypoxemia and hypercapnia with respiratory acidosis. Oxygen saturation levels are low due to marked hypoxemia. ∞ See Chapter 10 page 223 for steps to interpret ABGs.

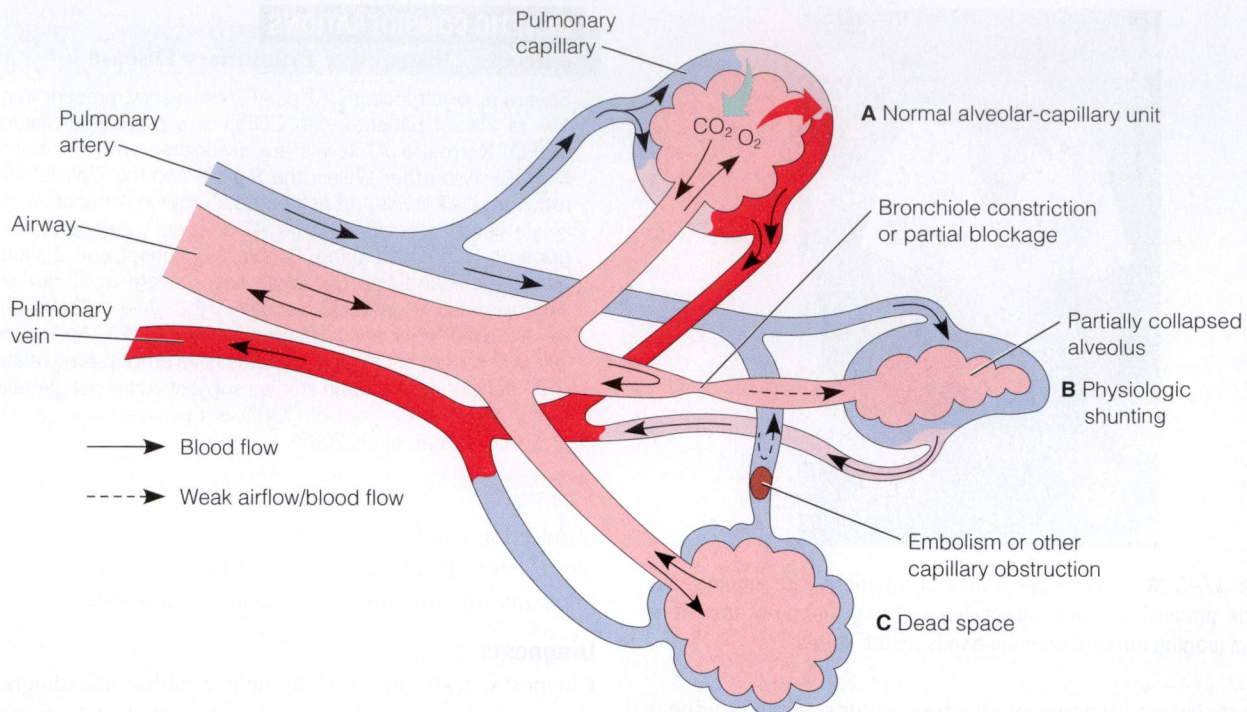

Figure 37–4 ■ Ventilation-perfusion relationships. *A,* Normal alveolar-capillary unit with an ideal match of ventilation and blood flow. Maximum gas exchange occurs between alveolus and blood. *B,* Physiologic shunting: A unit with adequate perfusion but inadequate ventilation. *C,* Dead space: A unit with adequate ventilation but inadequate perfusion. In the latter two cases, gas exchange is impaired.

PRACTICE ALERT

Hypercapnia (elevated $PaCO_2$ levels) often is chronic in patients with COPD (CO_2 retainers). In these patients, administering oxygen can actually increase the $PaCO_2$, leading to somnolence and acute respiratory failure. While oxygen is the drug of choice for treating patients with COPD, close monitoring is necessary during oxygen therapy.

- *Pulse oximetry* is used to monitor oxygen saturation of the blood. Marked airway obstruction and hypoxemia often causes oxygen saturation levels less than 95%. Pulse oximetry may be continuously monitored to assess the need for supplemental oxygen.
- *Exhaled carbon dioxide (capnogram or ETCO$_2$)* may be measured in ventilated patients to evaluate alveolar ventilation. The normal ETCO$_2$ reading is 35 to 45 mmHg; it is elevated when ventilation is inadequate, and decreased when pulmonary perfusion is impaired. ETCO$_2$ monitoring can reduce the frequency of ABG determinations.
- *CBC with WBC differential* often shows increased RBCs and hematocrit (erythrocytosis) as chronic hypoxia stimulates increased erythropoiesis to increase the oxygen-carrying capacity of the blood. *Polycythemia*, increased numbers of all blood cells, may be evident. Increased WBC count and a higher percentage of immature WBCs (bands) are often indicative of bacterial infection.
- *Chest x-ray* may show flattening of the diaphragm due to hyperinflation and evidence of pulmonary infection if present.

Smoking Cessation

Smoking cessation can not only prevent COPD from developing, but also can improve lung function once the disease has been diagnosed. Forced expiratory volume (FEV$_1$) improves, and survival is prolonged, largely due to lower rates of lung cancer and heart disease. Sustained quitting is difficult; only 6% of smokers succeed in long-term abstinence from smoking. Use of nicotine patches or gum and an antidepressant such as bupropion (Wellbutrin, Zyban) or varenicline (Chantix) improve the chances of success (Fiore et al., 2008).

Medications

Immunization against pneumococcal pneumonia and yearly influenza vaccine are recommended to reduce the risk of respiratory infections. A broad-spectrum antibiotic is prescribed if infection is suspected. Recent studies indicate that patients with purulent sputum and increased dyspnea will likely benefit from antibiotic therapy, even if no other signs of infection are present. Prophylactic antibiotics may be ordered for patients who experience four or more disease exacerbations per year (Fishman et al., 2008).

Bronchodilators improve airflow and reduce air trapping in COPD, resulting in improved dyspnea and exercise tolerance. Bronchodilators may be given by metered-dose inhaler (MDI), dry powder inhaler (DPI), by nebulizer, or orally. Oral administration may promote adherence, but is associated with much higher rates of adverse effects. A spacer or holding chamber may facilitate effective use of an MDI. Ipratropium bromide, an anticholinergic agent administered by MDI, is frequently prescribed. It has a longer duration of action than the short-acting

β_2-adrenergic stimulant bronchodilators and few side effects. Salmeterol, a longer-acting β_2 agonist, may be used in combination therapy. Oral theophylline, a methylxanthine, is a weak bronchodilator and has a narrow therapeutic range, but often is prescribed for its other effects. Theophylline stimulates the respiratory drive, strengthens diaphragmatic contractions, and improves cardiac output. As a result, dyspnea, exercise tolerance, and quality of life improve for the patient with COPD. Bronchodilators are discussed in further detail in the section on asthma, and their nursing implications are outlined in the box on pages 1235–1236.

Corticosteroid therapy may be used when asthma is a major component of COPD. It also improves symptoms and exercise tolerance, and may reduce the severity of exacerbations and the need for hospitalization. Oral corticosteroids, such as prednisone, are used initially. If a beneficial response occurs, the amount is reduced to the lowest effective dose. Every other day dosing or administration by inhaler is preferred to minimize steroid side effects, such as cushingoid effects and an increased risk for osteoporosis and vertebral fractures.

Alpha$_1$-antitrypsin (α_1AT) replacement therapy is available for patients with emphysema due to a genetic deficiency of the enzyme. Although expensive and inconvenient (α_1AT is administered weekly by intravenous infusion), it has been shown to reduce the rate of airflow decline and mortality.

Treatments

In addition to refraining from smoking, exposure to other airway irritants and allergens should be avoided. The patient should remain indoors during periods of significant air pollution to prevent exacerbations of the disease. Air filtering systems or air conditioning may be useful.

Pulmonary hygiene measures, including hydration, effective cough, percussion, and postural drainage, are used to improve clearance of airway secretions. Maintaining adequate systemic hydration is essential to keep secretions thin. Forceful coughing is often less effective than leaning forward and repeatedly "huffing," with relaxed breathing between huffs. Percussion and postural drainage may be necessary if the patient is unable to clear secretions by usual means. Cough suppressants and sedatives generally are avoided as they may cause retention of secretions.

While optimal medical management is helpful it cannot reverse the pathologic changes of COPD. Pulmonary rehabilitation (PR) teaches patients how to manage their symptoms and attain their maximum level of functioning. PR includes exercise, education, and psychological support. PR is most commonly delivered in the outpatient setting with exercise sessions of 30 to 90 minutes, 3 to 5 times per week. While PR doesn't change lung function, improvements in exercise and functional capacity and quality of life is seen. It is important that both lower and upper extremity exercise be used to promote activity tolerance during activities of daily living. See the accompanying Moving Evidence into Action feature.

Breathing exercises are used to slow the respiratory rate and relieve accessory muscle fatigue. Pursed-lip breathing slows the respiratory rate and helps maintain open airways during exhalation by keeping positive pressure in the airways. Abdominal breathing relieves the work of accessory muscles of respiration.

Oxygen

Long-term oxygen therapy is used for severe and progressive hypoxemia. Oxygen therapy improves exercise tolerance, mental functioning, and quality of life in advanced COPD. It also reduces the rate of hospitalization and increases length of survival. Oxygen may be used intermittently, at night, or continuously. For severely hypoxemic patients, the greatest benefit is seen with continuous oxygen. Home oxygen may be supplied as liquid oxygen, compressed gas cylinders, or oxygen concentrators. Patients may be provided a combination of delivery systems to promote mobility outside of the home (i.e., oxygen concentrator and compressed gas).

MOVING EVIDENCE INTO ACTION   The Patient with COPD

Exercise-induced dynamic hyperinflation is believed to be a significant factor in reduced activity tolerance in patients with COPD. This development is especially an important consideration in pulmonary rehabilitation exercise.

A study by Collins and colleagues (2008) evaluated the impact of a ventilation-feedback intervention + exercise vs. exercise alone or ventilation-feedback alone. The ventilation-feedback intervention used a computer interface with the patient to provide a visual representation of breathing pattern. This visual representation was used to assist the patients to modify their breathing pattern, thereby reducing dynamic hyperinflation. This randomized controlled trial found that combination of ventilation-feedback plus exercise-training decreased exercise-induced dynamic hyperinflation and increased exercise duration more than ventilation-feedback alone.

IMPLICATIONS FOR NURSING

This study and others support a program of regular physical activity to maintain functional status and reduce symptom progression. Additionally, this study suggests the importance

of developing and testing innovative interventions to can reduce dynamic hyperinflation, thereby improving exercise duration.

CRITICAL THINKING IN NURSING

1. Consider other populations for whom regular exercise is recommended (e.g., patients who are overweight, patients with heart failure). What strategies have been shown to reduce symptoms during exercise in these groups? How could these strategies be adapted for patients with COPD?

2. Use the physiologic and psychologic effects of regular exercise to explain its correlation with improved symptoms in the patient with COPD.

3. Consider the age of most patients with COPD. What other physical or psychosocial factors commonly limit physical activity in this population? How can you use this information in designing an appropriate exercise program?

An acute exacerbation of COPD may necessitate oxygenation and inspiratory positive-pressure assistance with a face mask or intubation and mechanical ventilation. Oxygen administered without intubation and mechanical ventilation requires caution: Administering oxygen to patients with chronic elevated carbon dioxide levels in the blood can actually increase the $PaCO_2$, leading to increased somnolence and even respiratory failure. Close monitoring of level of consciousness and arterial blood gases during oxygen therapy is vital (Fishman et al., 2004; Global Obstructive Lung Disease Initiative [GOLD], 2009).

Surgery

When medical therapy is no longer effective, lung transplantation may be an option. Both single and bilateral transplants have been performed successfully, with a 2-year survival rate of 75%. Lung reduction surgery is an experimental surgical intervention for advanced diffuse emphysema and lung hyperinflation. The procedure reduces the overall volume of the lung, reshapes it, and improves elastic recoil. As a result, pulmonary function and exercise tolerance improve and dyspnea is reduced. See the box on page 1222 of ∞ Chapter 36 for nursing care of the patient undergoing lung surgery. Special nursing care considerations related to lung or heart-lung transplant are summarized in Box 37–3.

Complementary Therapies

Complementary therapies may be useful to help manage symptoms of COPD. Dietary measures such as minimizing intake of dairy products and salt may help reduce mucous production and to keep mucus more liquefied. Be sure to recommend measures to replace the protein and calcium in dairy products to help maintain nutritional balance.

Herbal teas made with peppermint and yarrow, coltsfoot, or comfrey may act as expectorants to help relieve chest congestion. Licorice root, which may be taken in several forms, also has expectorant and anti-inflammatory effects that may be beneficial. Licorice root can, however, cause toxicity when used for extended periods of time (Spencer & Jacobs, 2003). Refer patients to a qualified herbalist for treatment.

Acupuncture may help the patient with smoking cessation, and also has been used to treat asthma and other respiratory conditions. Hypnotherapy and guided imagery are used to assist with smoking cessation. These techniques also can help the patient control anxiety and breathing patterns. Refer patients to a trained professional. Nurses, physicians, psychologists, counselors, social workers, and others can take professional training in hypnotherapy and guided imagery (Fontaine, 2005).

∞ Nursing Care

Health Promotion

Not smoking is the best preventive measure for chronic obstructive pulmonary disease. Even in patients with COPD, smoking cessation improves lung function and increases survival. Educate all patients, including preschool and school-age children, about the risks of smoking. See Box 37–4.

Assessment

Focused assessment for the patient with chronic obstructive pulmonary disease includes the following:

- *Health history:* Current symptoms, including cough, sputum production, shortness of breath or dyspnea, activity tolerance; frequency of respiratory infections and most recent

---

BOX 37–3 Nursing Considerations Related to Lung Transplant

While immediate postoperative care for patients undergoing lung or heart lung transplant is provided by specially trained interdisciplinary teams in transplant centers, increased survival following transplant means that these patients increasingly are seen in community-based settings, nontransplant hospitals, and on general nursing care units. An understanding of common posttransplant complications and care needs of the posttransplant patient facilitates appropriate nursing care.

Common Posttransplant Complications

In the early posttransplant period, the most common complications relate to the surgical procedure itself or to rejection of the transplanted organ(s).

Rejection. Acute organ rejection can occur at any time following the transplant. An acute change in FEV1 and FVC on home spirometry often is the first indication of acute rejection. Other manifestations of rejection include fever, shortness of breath, and an elevated WBC. Because these manifestations are similar to those of infection, the patient is instructed to return to the transplant clinic or center for a transbronchial biopsy. Acute rejection is treated with increased corticosteroids and adjustment of the immunosuppressive regimen (∞ see Chapter 13). Chronic rejection is less amenable to therapy, ultimately necessitating retransplant.

Infection. Prevention of infection is vital in lung transplant patients. The patient is encouraged to reduce his or her risk of infection by avoiding contact with people who have an infectious disease (e.g., URI, shingles, diseases of childhood). Prophylactic trimethoprim-sulfamethoxazole (TMP-SMZ) is administered weekly to prevent *Pneumocystis* pneumonia (∞ see Chapter 36).

Bacterial endocarditis prophylaxis also is provided as needed (∞ see Chapter 31). The posttransplant patient may not have typical manifestations of infection due to immunosuppression. Any vague symptoms with or without fever or leukocytosis are investigated. Recurrent viral infections such as CMV have been associated with chronic rejection, so are aggressively treated with antiviral therapy. Treatment of other infections is targetted to the infectious organism.

Nursing Considerations for the Posttransplant Patient

Reverse isolation procedures are not necessary unless the neutrophil count is very low (< 500/mm^3). Use good hand hygiene and standard precautions at all times, and aseptic technique for dressing changes, IV starts and site care, and other invasive procedures (such as urinary catheterization). Do not allow caregivers or visitors with URI to have contact with the patient; a mask may be provided for short visits if contact is unavoidable. Skin surveillance and care is vital following transplant. Intact skin reduces the risk of infection; however, corticosteroid therapy increases the risk for skin tears and breakdown.

The effect of all medications on immunosuppressive therapy and the transplanted organ(s) should be carefully investigated prior to administration. Some antibiotics and other drugs can affect blood levels of immunosuppressants.

Particular attention must be paid to pulmonary hygiene. Denervation of the transplanted lung eliminates the usual cough stimuli. Regularly scheduled coughing and deep breathing, and the use of vibration, percussion, and postural drainage are important to prevent acculation of secretions.

BOX 37–4 Cigarette Smoking and Tobacco Use

The use of tobacco reaches back to early civilizations, when it was used in religious ceremonies and as an offering of friendship. At one time, tobacco was thought to have medicinal qualities effective against all common diseases. Widespread use of tobacco among the male population of the industrialized world began during World War I.

Tobacco is now recognized as the leading cause of preventable illness in the world. Diseases directly related to tobacco use are responsible for the deaths of more than 438,000 Americans every year. Smoking will lead to the deaths of about half of all regular cigarette smokers (ALA, 2006). In spite of this knowledge, aggressive marketing of the product continues, and its worldwide use is increasing, especially in underdeveloped countries.

The link between tobacco use and lung cancer was reported as early as 1912. In 1987, lung cancer became the leading cause of cancer-related death in the United States among both men and women.

Cigarette smoke contains over 4,800 (69 of which are known to cause cancer) chemicals, including nicotine (Fiore et al., 2008). Nicotine is a highly addictive psychoactive substance that is relatively cheap and readily available. It produces euphoria, which acts as a positive reinforcer for continued use. In North American society, tobacco is more acceptable than many other dependency-producing drugs.

Tar is the particulate matter in cigarette smoke that is responsible for most of its carcinogenic and pathologic effects on the lungs. Smoke also paralyzes the cilia, reducing their ability to remove tars from contact with the respiratory epithelium. The risk for cancer and other lung diseases is dose related, affected by the age at which smoking began, the number of cigarettes smoked per day, and the number of years smoked. Smoking cessation reduces the risks associated with tobacco use. For some, such as the risk of coronary heart disease, quitting smoking yields rapid benefits. For others, the degree of risk reduction is less immediate, but still significant.

Nurses need to do more than simply advise patients to quit smoking and talk about the risks of smoking. Nurses can take an active role in smoking cessation. Identify smoking habits, smoking-related illnesses, and previous efforts to quit. Work with the patient to identify barriers and obstacles to quitting. Educate about the addictive nature of nicotine, and explain the manifestations of nicotine withdrawal (anxiety, irritability, headache, and disturbed sleep). Develop a plan with the patient that specifies a target date to quit and includes ways to deal with obstacles to quitting, withdrawal symptoms, and the temptation to resume smoking. Offer self-help material at an appropriate reading level. Refer to a counselor, physician, self-help group, or smoking cessation clinic. If a relapse occurs, accept it as a normal part of rehabilitation from any addictive substance. Continue to provide support and encouragement, helping the patient avoid further relapses.

Nurses can be especially effective in primary prevention of cigarette smoking and the diseases associated with it. Just as tobacco companies direct advertising at women and teens, nurses can target these populations and younger children for programs to prevent smoking. In addition, nurses need to become active in reducing minors' access to tobacco products, especially cigarettes and chewing tobacco (often the first product used by teens).

Nursing diagnoses that may be appropriate related to smoking include the following:

- *Ineffective Health Maintenance* related to tobacco use
- *Decisional Conflict* related to tobacco use
- *Ineffective Denial* related to acknowledgment of substance abuse and dependence

episode; previous diagnosis of emphysema, chronic bronchitis, or asthma; current medications; smoking history (in pack years—packs per day times number of years smoked), history of exposure to secondhand smoke, occupational or other pollutants.

- *Physical examination:* General appearance, weight for height, mental status; vital signs including temperature; skin color and temperature; anterior-posterior: lateral chest diameter, use of accessory muscles, nasal flaring or pursed-lip breathing; respiratory excursion and diaphragmatic excursion; percussion tone; breath sounds throughout; neck veins, apical pulse and heart sounds, peripheral pulses, edema.
- *Diagnostic tests:* Forced vital capacity (FVC) and forced expiratory volume in one second (FEV_1), arterial blood gases, hematocrit.

Nursing Diagnoses and Interventions

Patients with chronic obstructive pulmonary disease, whether hospitalized or in the community, have multiple nursing care needs. Because of the obstructive nature of the disease, airway clearance is a high priority. Nutritional deficit is common, particularly when emphysema is predominant. Because this chronic disease affects all functional health patterns, psychosocial issues are also of concern in planning nursing care. In addition to the nursing diagnoses presented here, see the Case Study & Nursing Care Plan that follows.

Ineffective Airway Clearance

Both chronic bronchitis and emphysema affect the ability to maintain open airways. In chronic bronchitis, copious amounts of thick, tenacious mucus are produced. Ciliary action is impaired, making it difficult to clear mucus from the airways. The loss of supporting tissue caused by emphysema increases the risk for airway collapse. In both cases, air is trapped distally, and less oxygen is available to the alveoli for diffusion. Normal respiratory defense mechanisms are impaired, and mucus-plugged airways provide an ideal environment for bacterial growth. Respiratory infection further impairs airway clearance and is often the cause of an acute exacerbation.

- Assess respiratory status every 1 to 2 hours or as indicated. Assess rate and pattern; cough and secretions (color, amount, consistency, and odor); and breath sounds, both normal and adventitious. *Frequent assessment is vital to monitor current status and response to treatment. Adventitious sounds should decrease with effective intervention. Diminished or absent breath sounds may indicate increasing airway obstruction and possible atelectasis.*

PRACTICE ALERT
Promptly report changes in oxygen saturation, skin color, or mental status. A drop in oxygen saturation levels, increasing cyanosis, or altered level of consciousness indicate hypoxemia, possibly related to airway obstruction.

The Patient with COPD

Selected resources that nurses may find helpful when planning evidence-based nursing care follow.

■ Bauldoff, G. S. (2009). When breathing is a burden: How to help patients with COPD. *American Nurse Today, 4*(9), 17–21.
■ Daly, M. L. (2009). Stopping a COPD flare-up. *American Nurse Today, 4*(8), 40.
■ Global Initiative for Chronic Obstructive Lung Disease (GOLD). (2008). Global strategy for the diagnosis, management, and prevention of chronic obstructive pulmonary disease. Bethesda (MD): Global Initiative for Chronic Obstructive Lung Disease (GOLD). Retrieved from http://www.goldcopd.com/

■ Monitor arterial blood gas results. *Increasing hypoxemia, hypercapnia, and respiratory acidosis may indicate increasing airway obstruction.*

■ Weigh daily, monitor intake and output, and assess mucous membranes and skin turgor. *Dehydration causes respiratory secretions to become thicker, more tenacious, and difficult to expectorate; fluid overload can further compromise respiratory status.*

■ Encourage a fluid intake of at least 2000 to 2500 mL per day unless contraindicated. *Adequate fluid intake helps keep mucous secretions thin.*

■ Place in Fowler's, high-Fowler's, or orthopneic position; encourage movement and activity to tolerance. *Upright positions improve ventilation and reduce the work of breathing. Activity helps mobilize secretions and prevent them from pooling.*

■ Assist with coughing and deep breathing at least every 2 hours while awake. Position seated upright, leaning forward during coughing. *The upright position promotes chest expansion, increasing the effectiveness of coughing and reducing the work involved.*

■ Provide tissues and a paper bag to dispose of expectorated sputum. *This important infection control measure reduces the spread of respiratory organisms to other people.*

■ Refer to a respiratory therapist, and assist with or perform percussion and postural drainage as needed. *Percussion helps loosen secretions in airways; postural drainage facilitates movement of these secretions out of the respiratory tract.*

■ Provide rest periods between treatments and procedures. *The patient with COPD fatigues easily; adequate rest is important to conserve energy and reduce fatigue.*

■ Administer expectorant and bronchodilator medications as ordered. Correlate timing with respiratory treatments. *Using expectorants and bronchodilators prior to coughing, percussion, and postural drainage increases their effectiveness in clearing airways.*

■ Provide supplemental oxygen as ordered. *Supplemental oxygen helps maintain adequate blood and tissue oxygenation.*

Imbalanced Nutrition: Less than Body Requirements

With advanced COPD, minimal activity, including eating, can cause fatigue and dyspnea. The patient may be unable to consume a full meal without resting. At the same time, the increased work of breathing (8 to 10 times that of normal) increases metabolic demands, and more calories are required. The patient may appear cachectic (thin and wasted). Poor nutritional status further impairs immune function and increases the risk of a complicating infection.

■ Assess nutritional status, including diet history, weight for height (use reference tables of desired weights), and anthropometric (skinfold) measurements. *It is important to differentiate nutritional status from body type rather than assume a nutritional impairment.*

■ Observe and document food intake, including types, amounts, and caloric intake. *This information can provide direction for supplementation, if needed.*

■ Monitor laboratory values, including serum albumin, prealbumin and electrolyte levels. *These values provide information about the adequacy of nutritional intake, including protein.*

■ Consult with a dietitian to plan meals and nutritional supplements that meet caloric needs. *More concentrated sources of high-energy foods may be required to maintain caloric intake without excess fatigue. A diet high in proteins and fats without excess carbohydrates is recommended to minimize carbon dioxide production during metabolism (carbohydrates are metabolized to form CO_2 and water).*

■ Provide frequent, small feedings with between-meal supplements. *Frequent, small meals help maintain intake and reduce fatigue associated with eating.*

■ Place seated or in high-Fowler's position for meals. *An upright position promotes lung expansion and reduces dyspnea.*

■ Assist to choose preferred foods from the menu; encourage family members to bring food from home if allowed. *Providing preferred foods encourages eating.*

■ Keep snacks at the bedside. *Snacks provide additional caloric intake.*

■ Provide mouth care prior to meals. *This helps enhance the appetite.*

■ If unable to maintain oral intake, consult with the physician about enteral or parenteral feedings. *Maintenance of caloric and nutrient intake is vital to prevent catabolism.*

Compromised Family Coping

Chronic illness affects the entire family structure. Roles and relationships change; additional demands are placed on the family. Family members may become over protective of the patient. Conversely, family members may blame the patient for causing the illness or have distorted perceptions about it, even denying its existence. In the most severe cases, they may refuse to assist or participate in care. The patient may develop an attitude of helplessness or dependence or may demonstrate anger, hostility, or aggression.

- Assess interactions between patient and family. *Assessment helps identify desired and potential destructive behaviors.*
- Assess the effect of the illness on the family. *Assessment of family interactions, roles, and relationships assists in planning appropriate interventions.*
- Help the patient and family identify strengths for coping with the situation. *Identifying personal and family strengths helps the family regain a sense of control.*
- Provide information and teaching about COPD. *Education helps the family gain an understanding of the patient's condition and needs.*
- Encourage expression of feelings. Avoid judging feelings expressed or family members as "good" or "bad," "right" or "wrong." *It is important that the nurse remain objective to maintain the therapeutic relationship.*
- Help family members recognize behaviors and attitudes that may hinder effective treatment, such as continuing to smoke in the house. *Family members may be unaware of the effect of their behavior on the patient's ability to change habits and cope with a disabling disease.*
- Encourage family members to participate in care. *This helps develop skills for use at home.*
- Initiate a care conference involving the patient, family, and healthcare team members from a variety of disciplines. *A wide range of perspectives and areas of expertise aids in problem solving and facilitates communication.*
- If dysfunctional family relationships interfere with measures to enhance coping, advocate for the patient, reaffirming his or her right to make decisions. *Dysfunctional family relationships are not likely to change simply because of illness. The nurse can better meet the patient's needs by accepting his or her limitations in dealing with family members.*
- Refer the patient and family to support groups and pulmonary rehabilitation programs, as available. *Support groups and structured rehabilitation programs enhance coping abilities.*
- Arrange a social services consultation. *This can help the patient and family identify care and support service needs.*
- Refer community agencies or services such as home health, homemaker services, or Meals on Wheels as appropriate. *Agencies or community services can provide additional support beyond the family's means or capability.*

Decisional Conflict: Smoking

Smoking is more than a habit; it is an addiction. The patient who must quit is facing a significant loss, not only of nicotine but also of a lifestyle. Although the patient may fully comprehend the consequences of continuing to smoke, the decision to give up a part of his or her life is not easy. This fear may be expressed in such concerns as "I'll gain weight," or "What will I do with my hands?" In addition to providing practical information, a plan, and assistance with nicotine withdrawal, the nurse must support the patient's decision-making process to comply with an order to stop smoking.

- Assess knowledge and understanding of the choices involved and possible consequences of each. *The decision to quit smoking ultimately belongs to the patient. He or she needs a full understanding of the consequences of quitting or continuing to smoke.*
- Acknowledge concerns, values, and beliefs; listen nonjudgmentally. *The nurse needs to avoid imposing his or her values and beliefs about smoking on the patient.*
- Spend time with the patient, encouraging expression of feelings. *This demonstrates acceptance of the patient and his or her right to make the decision.*
- Help plan a course of action for quitting smoking and adapt it as necessary. *When the patient develops the plan, he or she has more ownership in it and interest in making it work.*
- Demonstrate respect for decisions and the right to choose. *Respect supports self-esteem and the ability to cope.*
- Provide referral to a counselor or other professional as needed. *Counselors or other people trained to assist with smoking cessation can help with decision making.*

Using NANDA, NIC, and NOC

Linkages between a selected NANDA nursing diagnosis, NIC, and NOC for the patient with COPD are shown in the chart that follows.

Community-Based Care

As with any chronic disease, the patient and family will have primary responsibility for disease management. Teaching is vital to promote optimal health and slow disease progression. Teaching for home care focuses on effective coughing and breathing techniques (Box 37–5), preventing exacerbations, and managing prescribed therapies.

In addition, include the following topics when teaching for home care:

- Maintaining adequate fluid intake, at least 2.0 to 2.5 quarts of fluid daily
- Avoiding respiratory irritants, including cigarette smoke, both primary and secondary, other smoke sources, dust, aerosol sprays, air pollution, and very cold dry air
- Preventing exposure to infection, especially upper respiratory infections

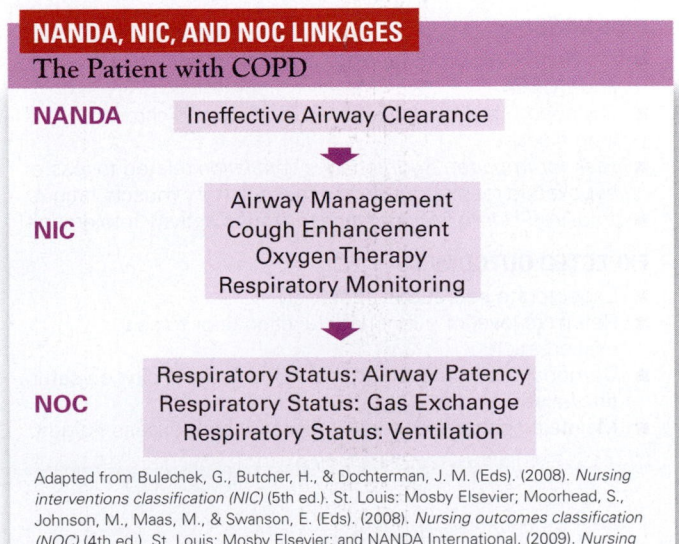

NANDA, NIC, AND NOC LINKAGES
The Patient with COPD

NANDA — Ineffective Airway Clearance

NIC — Airway Management / Cough Enhancement / Oxygen Therapy / Respiratory Monitoring

NOC — Respiratory Status: Airway Patency / Respiratory Status: Gas Exchange / Respiratory Status: Ventilation

Adapted from Bulechek, G., Butcher, H., & Dochterman, J. M. (Eds). (2008). *Nursing interventions classification (NIC)* (5th ed.). St. Louis: Mosby Elsevier; Moorhead, S., Johnson, M., Maas, M., & Swanson, E. (Eds). (2008). *Nursing outcomes classification (NOC)* (4th ed.). St. Louis: Mosby Elsevier; and NANDA International. (2009). *Nursing diagnoses: Definitions and classification 2009–2011.* Oxford, UK: Wilely-Blackwell.

CASE STUDY & NURSING CARE PLAN   A Patient with COPD

Anna Mercurio, known as "Happy" to all her friends, is an 83-year-old widow who lives with her two adult sons. Over the past 15 years, Mrs. Mercurio has become increasingly short of breath while gardening and walking, two of her favorite activities. She also has developed a chronic cough that is particularly bad in the mornings. Ten years ago, her family physician told her that she had emphysema. She is admitted to the hospital with possible pneumonia and acute exacerbation of COPD.

ASSESSMENT

Jeff Harris, RN, admits Mrs. Mercurio to the medical unit. In the nursing history, Mr. Harris notes that she denies ever smoking, but says that her husband and two sons have been smokers "for practically their whole lives." She says she lived an active life before developing lung disease, but now her breathing and cough have progressed so that she now must rest after just a few minutes of housework or other activity. Her cough is productive of moderate to large amounts of sputum, particularly in the mornings. She developed increasing shortness of breath and sputum 2 days ago; this morning, she could not complete her morning activities without resting, so she contacted her doctor.

On physical examination, Mr. Harris notes the following: skin very warm and dry, color dusky. Pauses frequently while speaking to breathe. Respiratory rate 36, fairly shallow; coughs frequently, producing large amounts of thick, tenacious green sputum. Other vital signs: P 115 and irregular, BP 186/60, T 102.4°F (39°C). Appears very thin; weight 96 lb (43.6 kg), height 63 inches (160 cm). Anteroposterior: lateral chest diameter approximately 1:1 indicating barrel chest; moderate kyphosis noted. Chest hyperresonant to percussion. Auscultation reveals distant breath sounds with scattered wheezes and rhonchi throughout lung fields. Chest x-ray shows flattening of diaphragm, slight cardiac enlargement, prominent vascular and bronchial markings, and patchy infiltrates. Initial laboratory work reveals moderate erythrocytosis, leukocytosis, and low serum albumin. Arterial blood gas results: pH 7.19; PO_2 54 mmHg; PCO_2 59 mmHg; HCO_3^- 30 mg/dL, and O_2 saturation 88%. Admitting orders include sputum specimen for culture; intravenous penicillin G, 2 million units every 4 hours; albuterol/ipratropium (Combivent) inhaler, two puffs every 6 hours; salmeterol/fluticasone (Advair) dry powder inhaler, twice a day; bed rest with bathroom privileges; oxygen per nasal cannula at 2 L continuously; and regular diet.

DIAGNOSES

- *Ineffective Airway Clearance* related to pneumonia and COPD
- *Impaired Gas Exchange* related to acute and chronic lung disease
- *Risk for Impaired Spontaneous Ventilation* related to loss of hypoxemic respiratory drive and respiratory muscle fatigue
- *Impaired Home Maintenance* related to activity intolerance

EXPECTED OUTCOMES

- Expectorate secretions effectively.
- Return to level of pulmonary function prior to acute exacerbation.
- Demonstrate improved arterial blood gas and oxygen saturation values.
- Maintain spontaneous respirations without excess fatigue.

- Verbalize willingness to allow sons or a housekeeper to assist with daily household tasks.

PLANNING AND IMPLEMENTATION

- Assess respiratory status and level of consciousness every 1 to 2 hours until stable, then at least every 4 hours.
- Closely monitor response to oxygen therapy, including skin color, oxygen saturation, sputum consistency, and respiratory drive.
- Increase fluid intake to at least 2500 mL per day and provide bedside humidifier.
- Elevate head of bed to at least 30 degrees at all times.
- Teach "huff" coughing technique.
- Administer medications as ordered; providing ipratropium inhaler before beclomethasone inhaler. Provide mouth care after inhalers.
- Contact respiratory therapy for percussion and postural drainage following inhaler treatments.
- Provide for uninterrupted rest periods following treatments and procedures.
- Meet with Mrs. Mercurio and her sons to develop a post discharge care plan.
- Refer to home health department for nursing follow-up.
- Refer to social services for possible assistance with home maintenance.

EVALUATION

After the first day in the hospital, Mrs. Mercurio's condition begins to improve slowly. On discharge 6 days later, she is able to provide self-care with less fatigue and dyspnea. She is using oxygen at night only, admitting that it is just for security. Although a few scattered wheezes and rhonchi are still present in her lungs, Mrs. Mercurio's sputum is thinner, white, and easily expectorated. She will continue taking oral penicillin V for an additional 10 days at home. She will also continue using the Advair and Combivent inhalers as prescribed at home. Although Mrs. Mercurio's sons admit they will probably never be able to quit smoking, they have agreed to smoke only in the garage or outside. A home health nurse will initially evaluate Mrs. Mercurio's progress three times weekly. Arrangements have been made for a housekeeper to come twice a week for cleaning and laundry. Mrs. Mercurio is glad to be returning home and grateful for the arrangements that have been made.

CRITICAL THINKING IN THE NURSING PROCESS

1. Mrs. Mercurio has never been a smoker but had long-term exposure to secondhand smoke. How does secondhand smoke contribute to lung diseases in adults and children?
2. Mr. Harris's nursing care plan included the nursing diagnosis, *Risk for Impaired Spontaneous Ventilation* related to loss of hypoxemic respiratory drive and respiratory muscle fatigue. Identify the normal physiologic events that stimulate breathing, and describe how these differ for the patient with chronic hypoxemia and hypercapnia.
3. The patient with an acute exacerbation of COPD is at risk for respiratory failure. What changes in Mrs. Mercurio's assessment findings could indicate this complication?
4. Develop a nursing care plan for Mrs. Mercurio for the nursing diagnosis, *Deficient Diversional Activities* related to inability to continue preferred activities.

See Evaluating Your Response in Appendix C.

BOX 37–5 Patient Teaching: Effective Coughing and Breathing Techniques

Pursed-lip and diaphragmatic breathing techniques help minimize air trapping and fatigue. Pursed-lip breathing helps maintain open airways by maintaining positive pressures longer during exhalation. Teach the patient to do the following:

1. Inhale through the nose with the mouth closed.
2. Exhale slowly through pursed lips, as though whistling or blowing out a candle, making exhalation twice as long as inhalation.

Diaphragmatic or abdominal breathing helps conserve energy by using the larger and more efficient muscles of respiration. Teach the patient to do the following:

1. Place one hand on the abdomen, the other on the chest.
2. Inhale, concentrating on pushing the abdominal hand outward while the chest hand remains still.
3. Exhale slowly, while the abdominal hand moves inward and the chest hand remains still.

Repeat these exercises as often as necessary until the techniques become incorporated into normal breathing.

Several different coughing techniques may be useful. For controlled cough technique, teach the patient to do the following:

1. Following prescribed bronchodilator treatment, inhale deeply, and hold breath briefly.
2. Cough twice, the first time to loosen mucus, the second to expel secretions.
3. Inhale by sniffing to prevent mucus from moving back into deep airways.
4. Rest. Avoid prolonged coughing to prevent fatigue and hypoxemia.

For huff coughing, teach the patient to do the following:

1. Inhale deeply while leaning forward.
2. Exhale sharply with a "huff" sound, to help keep airways open while mobilizing secretions.

- Importance of pneumococcal vaccine and annual influenza immunization
- Prescribed exercise program, maintaining ADLs, and balancing rest and exercise
- Maintaining nutrient intake (e.g., eating small frequent meals and using nutritional supplements to provide adequate calories)
- Ways of reducing sodium intake if prescribed
- Identifying early signs of an infection or exacerbation and the importance of seeking medical attention for the following: fever, increased sputum production, purulent (green or yellow) sputum, upper respiratory infection, increased shortness of breath or difficulty breathing, decreased activity tolerance or appetite, increased need for oxygen
- Prescribed medications, including purpose, proper use, and expected effects
- Avoiding use of over-the-counter medications unless approved by the physician
- Other prescribed therapies, such as use of home oxygen, percussion, postural drainage, and nebulizer treatments
- Use, cleaning, and maintenance of any required special equipment
- Importance of wearing an identification band and carrying a list of medications at all times in case of an emergency

Provide referrals to home care services such as home health, assistance with ADLs as needed, home maintenance services, respiratory therapy and home oxygen services, and other agencies such as Meals on Wheels and senior services as indicated.

The Patient with Cystic Fibrosis

Cystic fibrosis (CF) is an autosomal recessive disorder that affects epithelial cells of the respiratory, gastrointestinal, and reproductive tracts and leads to abnormal exocrine gland secretions (see the accompanying box). Although it can affect many organ systems, CF is particularly damaging to the lungs, leading to COPD in childhood and early adulthood. Respiratory manifestations of CF are the usual cause of morbidity and death from this disease. The gastrointestinal tract also is affected significantly; exocrine pancreatic insufficiency is characteristic of CF. Abnormally high sweat electrolytes also occur in CF.

Pathophysiology

The CFTR protein is involved in membrane transport of chloride and sodium in cells lining the ducts of exocrine glands (sweat glands, pancreas, liver, and reproductive systems). The genetic abnormality of CF leads to a lack or abnormality of this protein, with resulting abnormal electrolyte transport across epithelial cell membranes. Defective chloride transport causes more water and sodium reabsorption than normal. Secretions in affected organs become thick and viscous, obstructing glands and ducts. This obstruction causes dilation of secretory glands and damage to exocrine tissue. The hallmark pathophysiologic effects of CF include the following:

- Excess mucus production in the respiratory tract with impaired ability to clear secretions and progressive COPD
- Pancreatic enzyme deficiency and impaired digestion
- Abnormal elevation of sodium and chloride concentrations in sweat

GENETIC CONSIDERATIONS
Cystic Fibrosis

The gene responsible for cystic fibrosis is at a single locus on the long arm of chromosome 7. This gene codes for a protein known as the *cystic fibrosis transmembrane conductance regulator* (CFTR). Over 1,000 mutations of this gene have been identified. The most common mutation, identified as Δ F508, accounts for about 66% of cystic fibrosis (Aronson & Marquis, 2004). Cystic fibrosis is an autosomal recessive disorder: It is not transmitted as a sex-linked trait, and the normal gene is dominant. People with one abnormal gene do not have the disorder but can transmit this abnormal gene to their offspring. When a child inherits an abnormal gene from both parents, the disorder is seen. Genetic screening of family members of a CF patient can detect 70% to 75% of carriers of the CF gene. Screening for the CF gene is not recommended for the general population.

In the lungs, viscous mucus plugs small airways and impairs mucociliary clearance, leading to atelectasis, infection, bronchiectasis, and dilation of distal airways. Lower respiratory infections with *Staphylococcus aureus* and *Pseudomonas* are common (Huether & McCance, 2008). Acute and chronic damage to lung parenchyma causes tissue loss and extensive scarring and fibrosis. The upper lobes are involved to a greater extent than the lower lobes. Severe airway obstruction and chronic hypoxemia lead to pulmonary hypertension, right ventricular hypertrophy, and eventual cor pulmonale. Death usually results from a combination of cardiovascular changes and respiratory failure.

Pancreatic insufficiency is a frequent component of CF. It can range from slight pancreatic dysfunction to complete absence of function due to obstruction of pancreatic ducts with thick mucus and degenerative and fibrotic changes. Pancreatic insufficiency and impaired enzyme secretion leads to impaired digestion and absorption of proteins, carbohydrates, and fats.

About 8% of patients with CF develop diabetes mellitus (Huether & McCance, 2008). Liver failure is another potential complication of the disease (McCance & Huether, 2002). Because the genetic defect also affects cells of the reproductive tract, males with CF usually are sterile. While females may have difficulty conceiving, pregnancies usually are carried to term (Papadakis & McPhee, 2007).

Manifestations

Manifestations of CF in a young adult include a history of chronic lung disease. Recurrent pneumonia, exercise intolerance, and chronic cough are typical. Other pulmonary manifestations include *clubbing* of the fingers and toes (Figure 37–5 ■), increased anteroposterior chest diameter (barrel chest), hyperresonant percussion tone, and basilar crackles on auscultation. Distended neck veins, ascites, and peripheral edema accompany right-sided heart failure. Abdominal pain and *steatorrhea* (excess fat in the stools, causing frequent, bulky, foul-smelling stool) commonly result from associated pancreatic insufficiency. Growth and development are often retarded, resulting in small stature.

Figure 37–5 ■ Clubbing of fingers caused by chronic hypoxemia.
Source: John Radcliffe Hospital/Science Photo Library/Photo Researchers, Inc.

Incidence and Prevalence

CF is the most common lethal genetic disease in Caucasian Americans, affecting about 1 in 2500 live births. It is less common in African Americans and rare in Asians. About 5% of Caucasians in the United States carry the CF trait. Although the manifestations of CF usually develop in childhood, about 7% of patients with CF are diagnosed as adults. Adults now make up just over one-third of the CF population in the United States, with about 13% surviving into their 30s (Papadakis & McPhee, 2007).

Interdisciplinary Care

The treatment plan for cystic fibrosis is multidisciplinary, with the goals of preventing or treating respiratory complications and maintaining adequate nutrition. Psychosocial care is vital, as is genetic and occupational counseling.

Diagnosis

Although evidence of lung disease and pancreatic insufficiency suggest CF, analysis of Cl⁻ concentration in sweat is used to confirm the diagnosis. In CF, the Cl⁻ concentration is > 70 meq/L. Pilocarpine (a parasympathomimetic agent) and a small electric current are used to increase sweat production on the forearm. Absorbent paper or gauze is used to collect the sweat for analysis.

ABGs and oxygen saturation levels show hypoxemia. Pulmonary function studies reveal reduced air flow, reduced forced vital capacity (see Box 34–1 on page 1127), and reduced total lung capacity. Alveolar-capillary diffusion also is typically reduced.

Medications

Immunization against respiratory infections is vital to promote optimal health. Yearly influenza vaccine is recommended, along with measles and pertussis boosters as needed.

Bronchodilator inhalers may be used to control airways constriction. Acute pulmonary infections are treated with appropriate antibiotic therapy as determined by sputum culture and sensitivity tests. A prolonged treatment course or multiple antibiotics may be required to eradicate pulmonary infections. Antibiotics may be administered by several routes, including inhalation, to achieve the desired concentration in large airways (Aronson & Marquis, 2004). Dornase alfa, recombinant human DNase, breaks down the excess DNA in the sputum of patients with CF, decreasing its viscosity and making it easier to clear. Dornase alfa, administered by aerosol, reduces the frequency of hospitalizations and the need for antibiotics for some patients.

Treatments

Chest physiotherapy with percussion and postural drainage is used to promote airway clearance. Newer airway clearance techniques include the use of the "huff" cough technique with specified breathing cycles or patterns. In one technique, a valved mask or mouthpiece is used to maintain positive expiratory pressure (PEP) for approximately 20 breaths, followed by 3 to 5 "huff" coughs. This cycle is repeated for a total of 20 minutes. The autogenic drainage technique, a form of biofeedback, involves controlled breathing at specific lung volumes and patterns to facilitate the movement of mucus into larger airways, where it can be cleared with the "huff" cough. Oscillating positive expiratory pressure uses a flutter valve device, which looks like a fat pipe, contains a steel ball within an inner cone. The weight of the ball provides intermittent PEP, which vibrates airway walls to loosen secretions (Cystic Fibrosis Foundation [CFF], 2009).

Oxygen therapy may be required for hypoxemia. A liberal fluid intake helps reduce the viscosity of mucus secretions. A diet high in protein, fat, and calories may be necessary to maintain weight. Vitamins and minerals are supplemented to counteract excess losses in the sweat and stools. Enteral or parenteral nutrition may be required during acute exacerbations of the disease.

Surgery

Lung transplantation currently offers the only definitive treatment for CF, but is not considered a "cure"—the patient "trades" CF for the lifelong management of transplanted organs. Lung transplantation lengthens life span and improves quality of life. In CF, double lung transplant is indicated. Single-lung transplant is contraindicated due to the chronic infection in the lungs. Because the donor lungs do not have the CF gene, they do not develop the pathophysiologic changes of CF. Although the other defects characteristic of CF remain, these can be managed with pharmacologic therapy.

🙢 Nursing Care

Nursing care for the patient with cystic fibrosis is much the same as that for any chronic obstructive lung disease. Promoting airway clearance is the priority of nursing care. The genetic component of the disease and the patient's age are important considerations. Adults with CF are just entering their productive years and face a life span that is likely to be shortened significantly. Females who do conceive face the prospect of transmitting the defective gene to their offspring.

Ineffective Airway Clearance

Bronchial hygiene measures, including vibration, percussion, and postural drainage are the mainstay of treatment for patients with CF.

- Assess respiratory status, including vital signs, breath sounds, SaO₂, and skin color at least every 4 hours. *Early identification of respiratory compromise allows intervention before tissue hypoxia is significant.*
- Assess cough and sputum (amount, color, consistency, and possible odor). *Assessment of the cough and nature of sputum produced allow evaluation of the effectiveness of respiratory clearance and the response to therapy.*
- Monitor arterial blood gas results; report increasing hypoxemia and other abnormal results to the physician. *Blood gas changes may be an early indicator of impaired gas exchange due to airway obstruction.*
- Place in Fowler's or high-Fowler's position. Encourage frequent position changes and ambulation as allowed. *The upright position promotes lung expansion; position changes and ambulation facilitate the movement of secretions.*
- Assist to cough, deep breathe, and use assistive devices. Provide endotracheal suctioning using aseptic technique as

ordered. *Coughing, deep breathing, and suctioning help clear airways.*
- Provide a fluid intake of at least 2500 to 3000 mL per day. *A liberal fluid intake helps liquefy secretions, facilitating their clearance.*
- Work with the physician and respiratory therapist to provide pulmonary hygiene measures, such as postural drainage, percussion, and vibration. *These techniques help mobilize and clear secretions.*
- Administer prescribed medications as ordered, and monitor their effects. *If the infecting organism is resistant to the prescribed antibiotic, little improvement may be seen with treatment. Bronchodilators help maintain open airways but may have adverse effects such as anxiety and restlessness.*

Anticipatory Grieving

The patient with CF and family members face the knowledge that lifespan is likely to be short: The median survival is 36.8 years (CFF, 2009).

- Spend time with the patient and family. *Time is necessary to develop a trusting, therapeutic relationship.*
- Answer questions honestly; do not deny the probable outcome of the disease. *Honesty reinforces reality and provides a sense of control over decisions to be made.*
- Encourage the patient and family to express their feelings, fears, and concerns. *Open expression of feelings helps to promote understanding and acceptance.*
- Assist with understanding the grieving process and acceptance of feelings as normal. *Feelings of guilt, anger, or depression may cause the patient to withdraw from others. Explanation of the grieving process enhances understanding and ability to cope.*
- Help the patient and family make decisions regarding treatment and care. *This also is important to give them a sense of control.*
- Encourage use of other support systems, such as spiritual and social groups. Refer the patient and family to support groups, social support services, and hospice care as indicated. *These support systems provide emotional support and help the patient and family cope with the diagnosis.*
- Discuss advance directives (the living will) and power of attorney for health care with the patient and family. *These documents give the patient and family a sense of control over medical care provided if the patient is no longer able to express his or her own wishes.*

Community-Based Care

Education of the patient and family affected by cystic fibrosis is essential to maintaining optimal health. The adult whose disease was diagnosed in infancy or childhood has grown up with the disease and often has a much greater knowledge level than many caregivers. However, when the initial diagnosis is made as an adolescent or young adult, teaching needs are significant. Include the following topics when teaching for home care:

- Respiratory care techniques, including percussion, postural drainage, and controlled cough techniques
- Specific breathing and coughing exercises and procedures

- The importance of avoiding respiratory irritants, such as cigarette smoke, air pollution, and occupational dusts and gases
- Measures to prevent respiratory infection, such as maintaining immunizations and optimal general health, and avoiding exposure to large crowds and infected people.

Refer to a dietitian for planning and teaching to maintain adequate nutrition and minimize gastrointestinal symptoms. Referral to community agencies and support groups is also helpful.

Discuss the genetic transmission of cystic fibrosis and refer for counseling and possible genetic testing. Help the patient and family sort through the impact of the disease on future pregnancies and generations. Remember that the possibility of CF may present an ethical dilemma regarding future pregnancies. Provide support as needed.

The Patient with Atelectasis

Atelectasis is not a disease but a condition associated with many respiratory disorders. It is a state of partial or total lung collapse and airlessness. It may be acute or chronic. The most common cause of atelectasis is obstruction of the bronchus ventilating a segment of lung tissue. The affected segment may be small or an entire lobe. Other causes include compression of the lung by pneumothorax, pleural effusion, or tumor; or loss of pulmonary surfactant and inability to maintain open alveoli.

The manifestations of atelectasis depend on its size. Diminished breath sounds over the affected area may be the only sign of a small atelectasis. If a large lung segment is affected, manifestations may include tachycardia, tachypnea, dyspnea, cyanosis, and other signs of hypoxemia. Chest expansion may be reduced and breath sounds absent on the affected side. Fever and other manifestations of infection may be present.

Chest x-ray shows an area of airless lung. CT scan may help determine the cause of atelectasis.

The primary therapy for atelectasis is prevention. High-risk patients, such as those with COPD, smokers undergoing surgery, and people on prolonged bed rest or mechanical ventilation, should have vigorous chest physiotherapy to maintain open airways. Frequently assess respiratory status, including rate, breath sounds, and spirometry readings for early detection and treatment.

When atelectasis develops, treatment focuses on the underlying cause. Vigorous coughing and chest therapy may relieve obstruction by a mucus plug. Bronchoscopy may be necessary to remove the obstruction. Antibiotic therapy is ordered to treat infectious causes.

Nursing care to prevent and treat atelectasis is directed toward airway clearance. Position the patient with atelectasis on the unaffected side to promote gravity drainage of affected segment. Encourage frequent position changes, ambulation, coughing, and deep breathing. Unless contraindicated, encourage fluids to help liquefy secretions. Teach the patient at high risk for developing atelectasis about pulmonary care measures, fluid intake, and preventing pulmonary infections.

The Patient with Bronchiectasis

Bronchiectasis is characterized by permanent abnormal dilation of one or more large bronchi and destruction of bronchial walls. Infection often is present. The destructive process of bronchiectasis is initiated by inflammation, usually due to recurrent airways infection. About half of all cases of bronchiectasis are related to cystic fibrosis. Other causes include infections, such as severe pneumonia, tuberculosis, or fungal infections; lung abscess; exposure to toxic gases; abnormal lung or immunologic defenses; and localized airway obstruction due to a foreign body or tumor. Inflammation and airway obstruction are common to all these processes. Bronchial walls become weakened and dilated as a result, leading to pooling of secretions and further infection and inflammation.

A chronic cough productive of large amounts of mucopurulent sputum is characteristic. Other manifestations of bronchiectasis include hemoptysis, recurrent pneumonia, wheezing and shortness of breath, malnutrition, right-sided heart failure, and cor pulmonale.

Collaborative care for bronchiectasis focuses on maintaining optimal pulmonary function and preventing progression of the disorder. The diagnosis is typically based on the history and physical examination. Chest x-ray and CT scan may be ordered to help confirm the diagnosis and determine the extent of lung damage.

Antibiotics are prescribed at the first indication of infection and may also be used prophylactically. Inhaled bronchodilators may be ordered. Chest physiotherapy is a vital component of continuing care for bronchiectasis. Percussion and postural drainage help mobilize secretions. Oxygen may be prescribed. Bronchoscopy may be used to clear retained secretions or obstruction or to evaluate hemoptysis. If lung destruction is localized and unresponsive to conservative management, surgical lung resection may be necessary.

Nursing care of the patient with bronchiectasis is similar to that for patients with other obstructive lung diseases. Airway clearance is a primary problem, as is ineffective breathing pattern. Other applicable nursing diagnoses may include *Impaired Gas Exchange*, *Imbalanced Nutrition: Less than Body Requirements*, and *Self-Care Deficit*.

Interstitial Lung Disease

There are more than 130 pulmonary disorders that are considered interstitial lung diseases (ILD). These damage the interstitial or connective tissue of the lung. Occupational lung diseases, sarcoidosis, and rheumatological diseases such as scleroderma or systemic lupus erythematosus can result in ILD. Toxic drugs and radiation also cause interstitial damage. Table 37–4 identifies common causes of interstitial lung disorders.

These disorders may be acute or insidious. Their rate of progression varies from person to person, as does the degree of disability they produce.

TABLE 37–4 Selected Causes of Interstitial Lung Disorders

CAUSE	EXAMPLES
Inorganic dusts	Silica (silicosis), asbestos (asbestosis), coal (coal workers' pneumoconioses), talc (talcosis)
Organic dusts	Cotton (byssinosis), sugar cane (bagassosis), moldy hay (farmer's lung)
Drugs	Antineoplastic agents, antibiotics, gold salts, phenytoin
Radiation	External radiation or inhaled radioactive materials
Infections	Widespread TB or fungal infections, viral or *Pneumocystis carinii* pneumonia
Poisons and noxious gases	Paraquat, nitrogen dioxide, chlorine, ammonia, sulfur dioxide
Systemic diseases	Uremia, pulmonary edema
Unknown causes	Sarcoidosis, idiopathic pulmonary fibrosis, connective tissue disorders

The Patient with an Occupational Lung Disease

Occupational lung diseases are a diverse group of disorders directly related to inhalation of noxious substances in the work environment. There are two major classifications of occupational lung diseases:

- *Pneumoconioses*, chronic fibrotic lung diseases caused by inhalation of inorganic dusts and particulate matter. These include silicosis, coal workers' pneumoconiosis, and asbestosis.
- *Hypersensitivity pneumonitis*, allergic pulmonary diseases caused by exposure to inhaled organic dusts. These include farmers' lung, hot tub lung, and pigeon-breeders' lung.

FAST FACTS

- In the United States, occupational illnesses and injuries account for more than $45.8 billion in direct and $229 billion in indirect costs per year.
- The National Institute of Allergy and Infectious Diseases estimate that poorly ventilated office space aids in the transmission of pneumonia to 3 million persons per year (ALA, 2009).

Physiology Review

Lung tissue contains elastin and collagen fibers. Elastin fibers are easily stretched, facilitating lung expansion. Collagen fibers, in contrast, resist stretching. This increases the work of breathing. Both elastin and collagen affect lung compliance, or the ease with which the lungs are inflated. Other factors affecting compliance include the water content of lung tissue and surface tension (Huether & McCance, 2008).

Pathophysiology and Manifestations

When a noxious substance is inhaled, the response to that substance depends on the following:

- The size of particulates
- Its nature (organic or inorganic)
- Where it deposits in the respiratory tract
- The susceptibility of the individual

Relatively large particles, larger than 6 microns, are too big to reach lower airways and often are deposited in the nose.

Smaller particles can be carried with inspired air into the alveoli. Normal lung defenses, including alveolar macrophages, lymph channels, and the mucociliary escalator, attempt to remove particulate matter from the alveoli. Cigarette smoking, alcohol ingestion, or hypersensitivity reactions can impair these defenses.

The inhaled substance damages alveolar epithelium, leading to an inflammatory process of the alveoli and interstitial tissue of the lung. The inflammatory response produces further damage, and abnormal fibrotic (scar) tissue replaces the elastin fibers of normal lung tissue. As a result, the lungs become stiff and noncompliant. Lung volumes decrease, the work of breathing increases, and alveolar-capillary diffusion is impaired, leading to hypoxemia.

Asbestosis

Inhalation of asbestos fibers is a common cause of occupational lung disease. *Asbestosis* is a diffuse interstitial fibrotic disease involving the terminal airways, alveoli, and pleurae. Exposure to asbestos fibers occurs during mining, milling, manufacturing, and application of asbestos products. Although symptoms may not become apparent until 20 years after exposure, they tend to progress, even when further exposure has been halted. Asbestosis is also associated with an increased risk of bronchogenic carcinoma, especially in cigarette smokers. Mesothelioma, a rare cancer of the pleural membrane, is also associated with asbestos exposure. The period between asbestos exposure and tumor development in mesothelioma is long, ranging from 20 to 30 years (Fishman et al., 2008). People exposed to asbestos prior to imposition of strict environmental controls may only now be developing manifestations of this disease.

The manifestations of asbestosis include exertional dyspnea, exercise intolerance, and inspiratory crackles. Diffuse, small, irregular, or linear opacities appear on chest x-ray, primarily in the lower lobes. As the disease progresses, respiratory failure and marked hypoxemia may develop.

Silicosis

Inhalation of silica dust by hard-rock miners, foundry workers, sandblasters, pottery makers, and granite cutters can lead to *silicosis*, a nodular pulmonary fibrosis. Silicosis affects 1.2 to 3 million workers in the United States. Although generally associated with long-term exposure to silica, it can develop in as little as 10 months of intense exposure (Fishman et al., 2008). In silicosis, macrophages are destroyed as they engulf silica particles, releasing substances that damage lung tissue and lead to fibrosis and scarring.

Simple silicosis is asymptomatic with no demonstrable respiratory impairment. Complicated silicosis, in contrast, is characterized by large conglomerate densities in the upper lungs. These patients may be severely dyspneic and have a productive cough. Pulmonary function testing shows both restrictive and obstructive changes. Increasing size of conglomerate masses can lead to severe disability, cor pulmonale, and death.

Coal Worker's Pneumoconiosis

Ingestion of coal dust by alveolar macrophages causes "coal macules" to form, leading to *coal worker's pneumoconiosis*, or *black lung disease*. This occupational lung disease affects 12% of all miners, with a higher incidence in the eastern United States than in the West (Fishman et al., 2008). Coal macules appear on chest x-ray as diffuse, small opacities primarily affecting the upper lungs.

Simple coal worker's pneumoconiosis (CWP) generally is asymptomatic. A small percentage of patients (1% to 2%) develop progressive massive fibrosis, which destroys the pulmonary vascular bed and airways of the upper lungs. This progressive form of the disease causes symptoms similar to those of complicated silicosis.

Hypersensitivity Pneumonitis

Workers exposed to organic dusts and gases may develop *hypersensitivity pneumonitis*, an allergic pulmonary disease affecting the airways and alveoli. Byssinosis (resulting from cotton dust exposure), bagassosis (due to exposure to moldy sugar cane fiber), farmer's lung, and bird-fancier's lung are examples of hypersensitivity pneumonitis.

Either acute or subacute illness can occur. Acute illness occurs 4 to 8 hours after exposure and is heralded by sudden onset of malaise, chills and fever, dyspnea, cough, and nausea. The subacute syndrome is characterized by an insidious onset of chronic cough, progressive dyspnea, anorexia, and weight loss. Diffuse fibrosis occurs after repeated exposure to the organic material, leading to respiratory insufficiency.

Interdisciplinary Care

Prevention is a key strategy for all occupational lung diseases. Containing dust and wearing personal protective devices that limit the amount of inhaled particles are essential for people who work in industries with known risks.

Chest x-ray, pulmonary function studies, bronchoscopy, and possibly lung biopsy are used to establish the diagnosis of pneumoconioses. Characteristic patterns are seen for each disorder on x-ray. Pulmonary function testing shows restrictive impairment of lung ventilation, with reduced vital capacity and reduced total lung capacity. The diffusing capacity of the lungs is also decreased. Blood gas analysis reveals hypoxemia, especially with exercise. Bronchoscopy may be performed to obtain tissue for biopsy. Specialized lung scans may be used to determine the extent of fibrosis.

Eliminating further exposure to the offending agent is an important part of disease management. There is no specific

therapy. Anti-inflammatory drugs, such as corticosteroids, may reduce the inflammatory response and slow the progression of the disease. Preventing exposure to other damaging substances such as cigarette smoke and pollution is vital. Pneumococcal vaccine and annual influenza immunizations are recommended to reduce the risk of lower respiratory infections. Other care is supportive, similar to that for COPD.

Nursing Care

Health Promotion

Teaching about the dangers of occupational lung diseases and ways to reduce their risk needs to begin early, before the disease develops. Nurses in industrial and public health settings can begin by recognizing potential dangers and teaching workers about measures to reduce dust in their work area and the use of personal protective devices such as masks. Nurses working with affected families have an excellent opportunity to begin educating children about the risks associated with the occupation.

Nursing Diagnoses and Interventions

Nursing care for patients with occupational lung diseases is similar to that for patients with COPD. Activity intolerance is a high-priority problem for many patients. Severe dyspnea can significantly interfere with ADLs. Nursing measures to reduce energy expenditures and provide for rest are essential. Caregiver role strain, either actual or potential, must be considered when the patient with severe disability is being cared for at home.

Both patient and family coping may be compromised. Many of these diseases develop after 20 to 30 years of exposure to the hazardous material. Patients who entered the industry following high school may develop evidence of disease in their 40s and face the possibility of changing their occupation or developing significant disability. The resulting role strain affects all members of the family.

Other nursing diagnoses to consider for the patient with an occupational lung disease follow:

- *Ineffective Breathing Pattern* related to restrictive lung disease
- *Anticipatory Grieving* related to potential loss of employment and income
- *Low Self-Esteem: Situational* related to change of occupation

Community-Based Care

The affected patient and family need teaching in preparation for home care, including the following:

- Prevention of further lung damage, e.g., avoiding cigarette smoke and heavy air pollution
- Recommendations for pneumococcal and annual influenza immunizations; yearly tuberculin testing for patients with silicosis
- Pulmonary hygiene measures, such as liberal fluid intake, coughing, and deep-breathing exercises
- Use and care of oxygen therapy equipment if required
- Use and effects of any prescribed or recommended over-the-counter medications

The Patient with Sarcoidosis

Sarcoidosis is a chronic, multisystem disease characterized by an exaggerated cellular immune response in involved tissues. This abnormal immune response leads to granuloma formation in the lungs, lymph nodes, liver, eyes, skin, and other organs. Its cause is unknown. Sarcoidosis primarily affects young adults between the ages of 20 and 40. In the United States, the incidence is highest in African Americans. Women are affected at a slightly higher rate than men (Fishman et al., 2008).

In sarcoidosis, multiple granulomas form; these lesions may resolve spontaneously or proceed to fibrosis. The lungs are affected in about 90% of patients with sarcoidosis. Sarcoidosis has a low mortality rate—less than 3%—but a relatively high rate (approximately 10%) of serious disability from ocular, respiratory, or other organ damage. Pulmonary hemorrhage and cardiac and respiratory failure from pulmonary fibrosis are the leading causes of death from sarcoidosis.

The manifestations of sarcoidosis vary, depending on the organ system affected. It may be asymptomatic, diagnosed by characteristic findings on routine chest x-ray. Symptoms may be insidious, with anorexia, fatigue, weight loss, fever, dyspnea, arthralgias, and myalgias. Skin lesions, uveitis, lymphadenopathy, hepatomegaly, or other manifestations may also develop.

Leukopenia, eosinophilia, and an elevated erythrocyte sedimentation rate (ESR) typically are noted in sarcoidosis. The chest x-ray helps to determine the extent of pulmonary involvement. Biopsy of a granulomatous lesion may be required to confirm the diagnosis. Pulmonary function tests reveal decreased compliance and impaired diffusing capacity.

Sarcoidosis often resolves spontaneously, therefore treatment is indicated only when symptoms are severe or disabling. Corticosteroid therapy is prescribed to suppress the inflammatory process when indicated. Relapse frequently occurs when corticosteroids are discontinued. Other anti-inflammatory or immune-modifier medications may also be used, including chloroquine, indomethacin, azathioprine, and methotrexate.

Nursing care for patients with sarcoidosis is directed by involved organ systems and related manifestations. Respiratory care is supportive and includes avoiding respiratory irritants and maintaining adequate ventilation. Refer for smoking cessation assistance as needed.

Teach patients with limited symptoms about the disease and symptoms to report to a healthcare provider, including shortness of breath, tearing and eye inflammation, chest pain or irregular pulse, skin lesions, and swollen and painful joints. If corticosteroid therapy is prescribed, teach the importance of taking the drug as prescribed and not stopping it abruptly. Include information about managing the side effects of corticosteroids by limiting sodium and increasing potassium in the diet, taking the medication with food or milk to minimize gastric irritation, and identifying early signs of infection.

Pulmonary Vascular Disorders

The cardiovascular and respiratory systems are closely interrelated. As blood flows through the capillary network of the pulmonary vascular system, oxygen diffuses into it, and carbon dioxide diffuses out. An effective match of alveolar ventilation and capillary perfusion is essential to maintain this process and, ultimately, tissue oxygenation and function of all organ systems. Both vascular and alveolar changes can alter gas exchange. Arteriosclerotic changes in pulmonary vasculature reduce blood flow to the alveolus. Nearly all lower respiratory system disorders potentially can affect ventilation. Many also have a secondary effect on lung perfusion, because breakdown or fibrosis of alveolar walls destroys the capillary network as well. This section focuses on primary disorders of the pulmonary vascular system.

The Patient with Pulmonary Embolism

A **pulmonary embolism** (or *thromboembolism*) is obstruction of blood flow in part of the pulmonary vascular system by an embolus. Thromboemboli, or blood clots, that develop in the venous system (deep venous thrombosis or DVT) or right side of the heart are the most frequent cause of pulmonary embolism. Other sources of emboli include tumors that have invaded venous circulation, fat or bone marrow entering the circulation due to fracture or other trauma, amniotic fluid released into the circulation during childbirth, and intravenous injection of air or other foreign substances.

Pulmonary embolism is a medical emergency. Fifty percent of deaths from pulmonary embolism occur within the first two hours following embolization. In many cases, DVT has not been recognized or treated; often embolization also goes undetected. Prevention is the most effective treatment strategy for pulmonary embolism.

Physiology Review

The right heart receives deoxygenated blood from the systemic venous circulation. The entire output of the right ventricle enters the pulmonary circulation via the pulmonary artery. This artery branches into successively smaller arteries, arterioles, and capillaries of the pulmonary vascular system. Each alveolus of the lungs is surrounded by a meshwork of capillaries. Oxygen and carbon dioxide readily diffuse across the alveolar-capillary membrane, driven by a concentration gradient. The partial pressure of oxygen in the alveolus is greater than in the capillary, therefore it diffuses into the blood. Carbon dioxide diffuses from the capillaries into the alveoli, driven by the higher pressure of dissolved carbon dioxide in venous blood.

A match between blood flow through the pulmonary vascular system (perfusion) and lung ventilation is necessary for effective *respiration* (gas exchange) (see Figure 37–4). Local factors regulate ventilation and perfusion to maintain this match. A low alveolar PO_2 constricts alveolar capillaries, directing blood flow to better ventilated areas of the lung. High alveolar PCO_2 levels cause local bronchodilation, increasing airflow and eliminating excess carbon dioxide.

Pathophysiology

Thrombi affecting only the deep veins of the calf rarely embolize to the pulmonary circulation. However, thrombi often propagate proximally to the popliteal and iliofemoral veins. From there, they may break loose to become an embolus. As vessels of the venous system become progressively larger, the embolus moves freely until it enters the pulmonary arterial system with its progressively smaller vessels leading to the pulmonary capillary beds (Figure 37–6 ■).

The impact of a pulmonary embolus depends on the extent to which pulmonary blood flow is obstructed, the size of the embolus, its nature, and secondary effects of the obstruction. The effects can range widely:

- Occlusion of a large pulmonary artery with sudden death. Gas exchange is significantly reduced or prevented, and cardiac output falls dramatically as blood fails to move through the pulmonary vascular system and return to the left heart.
- Lung tissue infarction due to occlusion of a significant portion of pulmonary blood flow. Fewer than 10% of pulmonary emboli result in pulmonary infarction.
- Obstruction of a small segment of the pulmonary circulation with no permanent lung injury.
- Chronic or recurrent small emboli which may be multiple.

Obstruction of pulmonary blood flow by an embolus affects both perfusion and ventilation. Neurohumoral reflexes triggered by obstruction cause vasoconstriction, increasing pulmonary vascular resistance. In severe cases, this can lead to pulmonary hypertension and right ventricular heart failure. Systemically, hypotension and a drop in cardiac output may develop. Bronchoconstriction occurs in the affected area of lung. Dead space (areas of the lung that are ventilated but not perfused) increases. Alveolar surfactant decreases, increasing the risk for atelectasis.

If infarction does not occur, the fibrinolytic system (∞ see Chapter 30) ultimately dissolves the clot, and pulmonary function returns to normal. Infarcted tissue becomes scarred and fibrotic.

Fat emboli are the most common nonthrombotic pulmonary emboli. A fat embolism usually occurs after fracture of long bone (typically the femur) releases bone marrow fat into the circulation. Adipose tissue or liver trauma may also lead to fat emboli.

Manifestations

The manifestations of pulmonary embolism depend on its size and location. Small emboli may be asymptomatic. Manifestations usually develop abruptly, over a period of minutes. The most common symptoms are dyspnea and pleuritic chest pain. Anxiety, a sense of impending doom, and cough are also common. See the accompanying box. Diaphoresis and hemoptysis may develop. Massive pulmonary embolus can cause syncope and cyanosis. On examination, tachycardia and tachypnea are noted. Crackles may be heard on auscultation of the chest, and a cardiac gallop (S_3 and possibly S_4) may be noted. A low-grade fever may develop. It is difficult to differentiate pulmonary embolism from myocardial infarction or pneumonia by manifestations.

Characteristic manifestations of fat emboli include sudden onset of cardiopulmonary and neurologic symptoms: dyspnea, tachypnea, tachycardia, confusion, delirium, and decreased level of consciousness. Petechiae often develop on the chest and arms.

Incidence and Risk Factors

Pulmonary embolism causes an estimated 60,000 deaths annually, occurring in more than 600,000 patients per year (Fishman et al., 2008). Although many substances can become emboli, thrombus arising from the deep veins of the legs is the leading cause of pulmonary embolism. *Deep venous thrombosis (DVT)* develops in approximately 5 million people per year in the United States. The risk factors for pulmonary embolus are those for DVT: stasis of venous blood flow, vessel wall damage, and altered blood coagulation.

Prolonged immobility; trauma, including hip and femur fractures; surgery (orthopedic, pelvic, and gynecologic surgery

Figure 37–6 ■ A thromboembolism lodged in a pulmonary vessel.
Source: Steve Oh. M.S., Phototake, NYC.

MANIFESTATIONS of Pulmonary Embolism

COMMON	LESS COMMON
■ Dyspnea and shortness of breath	■ Diaphoresis
■ Chest pain	■ Hemoptysis
■ Anxiety and apprehension	■ Syncope
■ Cough	■ Cyanosis
■ Tachycardia and tachypnea	■ S_3 and/or S_4 gallop
■ Crackles (rales)	
■ Low-grade fever	

in particular); myocardial infarction and heart failure; obesity; and advanced age are risk factors for DVT. Women who use oral contraceptives or estrogen therapy are at risk, as are women during pregnancy and childbirth. ∞ See Chapter 35 for more information about DVT.

Interdisciplinary Care

Because deep venous thrombosis may not be identified until pulmonary embolism occurs, prevention is the primary goal in treating pulmonary embolism. Prophylactic anticoagulation can be used to prevent the development of DVT. Early ambulation of medical and surgical patients is an effective means of preventing venous stasis and reducing the incidence of pulmonary embolism. External pneumatic compression of the legs is also effective for patients undergoing neurosurgery, urologic surgery, or major surgery of the hip or knee, or when anticoagulant therapy is contraindicated. Other preventive measures include elevating the legs and active and passive leg exercises.

When pulmonary embolism occurs, treatment is supportive. Oxygen therapy is initiated, and analgesics may be ordered to relieve severe pleuritic pain and anxiety. Pulmonary artery and wedge pressures may be monitored with a balloon (Swan-Ganz) catheter. While cardiac outputs also may be assessed, this is rarely performed in this population. Cardiac rhythm is monitored to detect dysrhythmias.

Diagnosis

The studies performed to identify DVT differ from those used to diagnose a pulmonary embolism. ∞ See Chapter 32 for diagnostic studies for venous thrombosis.

- *Plasma D-dimer levels* are highly specific to the presence of a thrombus. D-dimer is a fragment of fibrin formed during lysis of a blood clot; elevated blood levels indicate thrombus formation and lysis (e.g., DVT and pulmonary embolism).
- *Chest CT with contrast* is the principle test used to diagnose pulmonary embolism. Chest CT effectively shows large, central PE; newer generation scanners also can detect peripheral emboli.
- *Lung scans*, including perfusion and ventilation scans, may be used. In a perfusion lung scan, radiotagged albumin is injected intravenously and distributed in the lungs by the pulmonary blood flow. The lungs are then scanned for distribution of the isotope. An area of lung in which the isotope is undetectable is suggestive of occluded blood flow and pulmonary embolism. For a ventilation scan, a radiotagged gas is inhaled and the lungs are scanned for gas distribution. Combined perfusion and ventilation scans allow identification of areas of the lungs that are ventilated but not perfused, a characteristic of pulmonary embolism.
- *Pulmonary angiography* is the definitive test for pulmonary embolism when other, less invasive tests are inconclusive. It is possible to detect very small emboli with angiography. A contrast medium injected into the pulmonary arteries illustrates the pulmonary vascular system on x-ray.
- *Chest x-ray* often shows pulmonary infiltration and occasionally pleural effusion.
- *Electrocardiogram (ECG)* is ordered to rule out acute myocardial infarction as the cause of symptoms. ECG findings commonly associated with pulmonary embolism include tachycardia and nonspecific T wave changes.
- *ABGs* usually show hypoxemia (PO_2 less than 80 mmHg), and often respiratory alkalosis (pH > 7.45, PCO_2 < 38 mmHg) due to tachypnea and hyperventilation.
- *Exhaled carbon dioxide ($ETCO_2$)* may be measured to evaluate alveolar perfusion. The normal $ETCO_2$ reading is 35 to 45 mmHg; it is decreased when pulmonary perfusion is impaired.
- *Coagulation studies* are ordered to monitor the response to therapy. The *activated partial thromboplastin time (aPTT or PTT)* is used to assess the intrinsic clotting pathway and the response to heparin therapy. Desired levels with anticoagulant therapy are 1.5 to 2 times the control value. The risk of recurrent thromboembolism is high at lower levels; the risk of bleeding increases at higher levels. The *International Normalized Ratio (INR)* is used to assess the extrinsic clotting system and oral anticoagulation with warfarin (Coumadin). The goal of anticoagulant therapy is to achieve a therapeutic range of 2.0 to 3.0.

Medications

Anticoagulant therapy is the standard treatment to prevent pulmonary emboli. It is often instituted in high-risk patients who have no evidence of pulmonary embolism, to prevent possible devastating effects. In the patient with DVT or a pulmonary embolus, anticoagulants are administered to prevent further clotting and embolization. ∞ See Chapter 34 for more information about anticoagulant therapy to prevent and treat DVT. ∞ See Chapter 32 for the Medication Administration box on pages 1052 and 1053 for the nursing implications for anticoagulant therapy.

For pulmonary embolus, heparin therapy is initiated with an intravenous bolus of 5000 to 10,000 units of heparin, followed by continuous infusion at the rate of 1000 to 1500 units per hour. The aPTT or PTT is monitored frequently until stabilized. Heparin therapy is typically continued for about 5 days or until oral anticoagulant therapy has become fully effective. ∞ See Chapter 32 for further information on low-molecular-weight heparin.

Oral anticoagulant therapy with warfarin sodium (Coumadin) is initiated at the same time as heparin. Warfarin alters the synthesis of vitamin K-dependent clotting factors and requires 5 to 7 days to be fully effective. Anticoagulant therapy is continued for 2 to 3 months when few risk factors for thromboemboli exist; long-term therapy is used when chronic disorders that increase the risk of thromboemboli are present.

Bleeding is a risk associated with anticoagulant therapy. Although major hemorrhage is uncommon, it occurs in approximately 5% of patients receiving intravenous heparin. Cardiac, hepatic, and renal disease increase the risk of significant bleeding, as does age over 60 years. Protamine, a protein that combines with heparin to inactivate it, is used to stop its anticoagulant effect if major bleeding occurs. Vitamin K is given to treat bleeding associated with Coumadin therapy.

Thrombolytic therapy may be used to treat massive pulmonary embolus and hypotension. Streptokinase, urokinase, or tissue plasminogen activator (t-PA) are used to *lyse* (disintegrate) the embolus, restore pulmonary blood flow, and reduce pulmonary artery and right heart pressures. Although thrombolytic therapy may not reduce mortality associated with pulmonary embolus, it may reduce the incidence of pulmonary hypertension, which develops 3 to 5 years after an embolism. Thrombolysis significantly increases the risk of bleeding, particularly cerebral bleeding. Contraindications to thrombolysis include intracranial disease, recent stroke, active bleeding or a bleeding disorder, pregnancy, severe hypertension, and recent surgery or trauma. Because of the increased risk of hemorrhage, invasive procedures are avoided after thrombolysis. ∞ See Chapter 30 for further discussion of thrombolytic therapy and its nursing implications.

Surgery

When anticoagulant therapy fails to prevent recurrent emboli, an umbrella-like filter may be inserted into the inferior vena cava to trap large emboli while allowing continued blood flow (see Figure 32–11A). The filter usually is inserted percutaneously, via either the femoral or jugular vein.

∞ Nursing Care

Health Promotion

Nurses are key in preventing pulmonary embolism. Encouraging patients to ambulate after surgery or illness, applying compression stockings or pneumatic compression devices, teaching and encouraging leg exercises, discouraging the use of pillows under the knees—all these measures help prevent DVT and subsequent pulmonary emboli.

Teach patients to reduce the risks associated with long periods of immobility, stopping every 1 to 2 hours during long automobile trips for a brief stretch and walk, getting up every hour or so and doing leg exercises while seated during long flights, and avoiding crossing the legs to prevent venous stasis and pooling. Regular exercise such as walking also reduces the risk of DVT. Instruct patients who stand for long periods to use well-fitted elastic stockings, being careful to avoid hose that bind around the knee or thigh.

Assessment

Because pulmonary embolus can be a medical emergency, assessment may be very focused. In other instances, when emboli are small and not life threatening, a more extensive nursing assessment may be done.

- *Health history:* Chest pain, shortness of breath, other symptoms, including onset, severity, precipitating factors; history of recent surgery, venous thrombosis, or other risk factor such as childbirth or malignancy; current medications.
- *Physical examination:* Level of consciousness, presence of respirations and pulse; color, skin temperature, and moisture; vital signs including apical pulse and temperature; breath sounds and heart sounds; oxygen saturation level; neck vein distention, peripheral edema.
- *Diagnostic tests:* Plasma D-dimer levels, coagulation studies; chest x-ray and other imaging studies; oxygen saturation and ABGs; ECG.

Nursing Diagnoses and Interventions

A large pulmonary embolus can cause a significant mismatch between pulmonary ventilation and circulation. Impaired gas exchange is a priority problem and focus for interventions.

Cardiac output may be significantly affected by obstructed pulmonary blood flow. Thrombolytic and anticoagulant therapy affect the clotting process, increasing the risk for bleeding. Anxiety accompanies pulmonary embolism almost universally.

Impaired Gas Exchange

Pulmonary embolism results in areas of the lung that are ventilated but not perfused; they receive no capillary blood flow. If the embolus is large and a major segment of the lung is unperfused, gas exchange is significantly affected. Nursing interventions are directed toward compensating for impaired gas exchange.

- Frequently assess respiratory status, including rate, depth, effort, lung sounds, and oxygen saturation. *Impaired ventilation will further compromise gas exchange and worsen hypoxemia. Oxygen saturation can be monitored continuously and noninvasively to evaluate gas exchange.*

> **PRACTICE ALERT**
> Monitor and record level of consciousness, mental status, and skin color. Hypoxemia often causes confusion and agitation; hypercapnia may reduce level of consciousness. Cyanosis indicates significant hypoxemia.

- Place in Fowler's or high-Fowler's position, with the lower extremities dependent. *This position facilitates maximal lung expansion and reduces venous return to the right side of the heart, lowering pressures in the pulmonary vascular system.*

> **PRACTICE ALERT**
> Start oxygen per nasal cannula or mask. Obtain a physician's order if one has not been written. Supplemental oxygen increases alveolar and arterial oxygenation. Oxygen is a drug and must be prescribed by the physician. It may, however, be initiated by the nurse in an emergency to prevent tissue hypoxia.

- Monitor arterial blood gas results, reporting abnormal findings as indicated. *ABGs are used to assess gas exchange and tissue oxygenation. An arterial line may be inserted for monitoring arterial pressure and arterial blood sampling.*
- Maintain bed rest. *Bed rest reduces metabolic demands and tissue needs for oxygen.*

Decreased Cardiac Output

The impact of a large pulmonary embolus on hemodynamic status can be significant. Pressures in the pulmonary vascular system and right heart increase; blood return to the left heart and cardiac output may significantly decrease. Nursing interventions focus on preserving an adequate blood pressure and organ function until cardiopulmonary status stabilizes. A central line for hemodynamic monitoring may be instituted (∞ see Chapter 30 for nursing care related to hemodynamic monitoring).

> **PRACTICE ALERT**
> Assess and record vital signs and cardiopulmonary status every 15 to 30 minutes initially, then every 2 to 4 hours as condition stabilizes. Frequent assessment facilitates timely interventions to maintain cardiovascular status and preserve organ function.

- Auscultate heart sounds every 2 to 4 hours, reporting any abnormalities. *Sounds such as an S$_3$ or S$_4$ gallop may indicate cardiac compromise.*

PRACTICE ALERT
Record intake and output hourly. Decreased urinary output often is an early indicator of decreased cardiac output. Maintaining renal perfusion is vital to preserve renal function and prevent acute renal failure.

- Assess skin color and temperature. *These assessments monitor tissue perfusion.*
- Monitor cardiac rhythm. *A drop in cardiac output and other hemodynamic alterations resulting from pulmonary embolism can precipitate dysrhythmias. Dysrhythmias, in turn, can further impair cardiac output.*
- Administer vasopressors and other medications as ordered. Carefully monitor the response to prescribed medications. *Drugs may be prescribed to maintain adequate arterial pressure and tissue perfusion. Potent drugs such as vasopressors require careful monitoring for desired and adverse effects.*
- Monitor pulmonary artery pressures, neck vein distension, and peripheral edema. Report findings as indicated. *Right-sided heart failure is a potential complication of pulmonary embolism because of increased pulmonary artery pressures.*
- Maintain intravenous and arterial access sites as well as central lines. *The patient may be in unstable and critical condition, potentially needing immediate interventions to maintain life.*

PRACTICE ALERT
Provide frequent skin care. Impaired tissue perfusion and oxygenation increase the risk of skin and tissue breakdown.

- Instruct to report chest pain or other symptoms. *Decreased cardiac output and an increased workload due to pulmonary hypertension may cause anginal pain.*

Ineffective Protection

Thrombolytics and anticoagulant therapy impair normal clotting mechanisms, increasing the risk for bleeding and hemorrhage. This risk is particularly acute during the first 24 to 48 hours following thrombolytic drug administration.

- Assess frequently for overt and covert signs of bleeding: bleeding gums; hematuria; obvious or occult blood in stool or vomitus; incisional bleeding, bleeding or bruising of injection sites or with minor trauma; joint pain or immobility; abdominal or flank pain. *Careful monitoring is necessary to identify early signs of abnormal bleeding and prevent potential hemorrhage.*

PRACTICE ALERT
Promptly report changes in neurologic status. Although cerebral bleeding is not evident externally, changes in level of consciousness and other neurologic signs suggest it and should be reported immediately.

- Report coagulation study results outside the desired range for anticoagulant therapy. *Levels less than the target range may indicate an increased risk for further clot development and*

pulmonary emboli; levels above the target range indicate an increased risk for bleeding.

- Keep protamine sulfate available for heparin therapy and vitamin K available for warfarin (Coumadin) therapy. *Bleeding or hemorrhage due to excess anticoagulant may require antidote administration to rapidly reverse anticoagulant effects.*
- Assess medication regimen for possible drug interactions that could potentiate or inhibit anticoagulant effects. *Drug interactions can increase the risk for hemorrhage or further embolus formation.*
- Avoid invasive procedures, injections, and venous punctures when possible, particularly during and following thrombolytic therapy. *Invasive procedures increase the risk of tissue trauma and bleeding.*
- Maintain firm pressure on injection and venipuncture sites. Maintain pressure for 30 minutes following arterial puncture. *Firm pressure reduces the risk for bleeding into the tissues.*

PRACTICE ALERT
Use an infusion device to administer heparin infusion. Using an infusion pump or device helps prevent administration of excess medication.

- Maintain adequate fluid intake. Administer stool softeners as ordered. *These measures help prevent constipation and straining, which may precipitate bleeding of hemorrhoids.*

Anxiety

Pulmonary embolism is a physiologic and psychologic threat to safety and integrity. It is a major physiologic stressor, eliciting a strong neuroendocrine stress response. The feeling of suffocation and inability to catch one's breath that accompanies a pulmonary embolus is also a strong psychologic stressor. Fear, anxiety, and apprehension are common responses.

- Assess anxiety level. *Appropriate interventions are determined by the level of anxiety.*

PRACTICE ALERT
Provide reassurance and emotional support, listening to fears. Do not negate the fear of dying, but reassure that treatment usually restores effective respiratory function. The fear of death is very real and must not be discounted; however, it is important to provide reassurance to alleviate excess anxiety.

- Remain with the patient as much as possible. *The presence of a caring nurse helps reduce fear.*
- Explain procedures and treatments, using short, simple sentences. *Providing clearly understood, simple instructions reduces fear of the unknown.*
- Reduce environmental stimuli, and use a calm, reassuring manner. *These measures help reduce anxiety (for both the nurse and the patient).*
- Allow supportive family members to remain with the patient as much as possible. *Calm, supportive family members provide further reassurance.*
- Administer morphine sulfate as ordered. *Morphine is given to reduce pain and anxiety.*

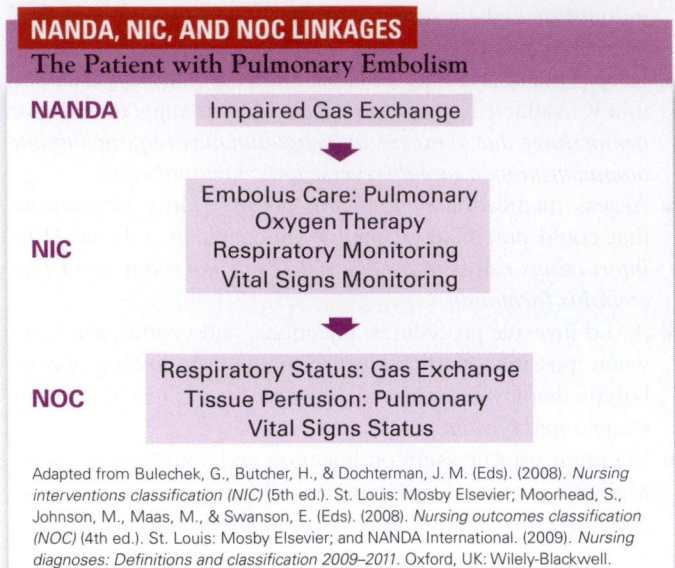

NANDA, NIC, AND NOC LINKAGES
The Patient with Pulmonary Embolism

NANDA   Impaired Gas Exchange

NIC   Embolus Care: Pulmonary
Oxygen Therapy
Respiratory Monitoring
Vital Signs Monitoring

NOC   Respiratory Status: Gas Exchange
Tissue Perfusion: Pulmonary
Vital Signs Status

Adapted from Bulechek, G., Butcher, H., & Dochterman, J. M. (Eds). (2008). *Nursing interventions classification (NIC)* (5th ed.). St. Louis: Mosby Elsevier; Moorhead, S., Johnson, M., Maas, M., & Swanson, E. (Eds). (2008). *Nursing outcomes classification (NOC)* (4th ed.). St. Louis: Mosby Elsevier; and NANDA International. (2009). *Nursing diagnoses: Definitions and classification 2009–2011.* Oxford, UK: Wiley-Blackwell.

Using NANDA, NIC, and NOC

Linkages between a selected NANDA nursing diagnosis, NIC, and NOC for the patient with pulmonary embolism are shown in the accompanying chart.

Community-Based Care

Discuss the following topics when preparing the patient with pulmonary embolism and family members for home care.

- Use of prescribed anticoagulant, including drug interactions, scheduled laboratory testing, and manifestations of bleeding to report to the primary care provider
- Using a soft toothbrush and electric razor to reduce the risk of bleeding
- Avoiding aspirin (unless prescribed) and other over-the-counter medications without approval by the physician
- Importance of wearing a MedicAlert tag for anticoagulant use
- Health promotion measures to reduce the risk of recurrent pulmonary embolism
- Symptoms of recurrent pulmonary embolism, such as sudden chest pain, shortness of breath, and possibly bloody sputum

The Patient with Pulmonary Hypertension

The pulmonary vascular system is normally a high-flow, low-pressure, low-resistance system that can accommodate large increases in blood flow when necessary (e.g., during exercise). The normal mean arterial pressure in the pulmonary system is 12 to 15 mmHg (25 to 28 systolic/8 diastolic). **Pulmonary hypertension** (PHTN) is abnormal elevation of the pulmonary arterial pressure.

Pathophysiology

Pulmonary hypertension can develop as a primary disorder, but can also occur secondarily to another condition. In both instances, changes in the pulmonary artery lead to abnormal

growth and remodeling of pulmonary vessels. Smooth muscle cells and fibroblasts proliferate, leading to abnormal vasoconstriction and fibrosis of pulmonary vessels. Once initiated, pulmonary vascular changes are progressive and nonreversible. Vasoconstrictive substances such as endothelin 1 and thromboxane A2 are produced in excess, while the production of vasodilating substances such as nitric oxide is reduced. This further contributes to vasoconstriction and increased pulmonary artery pressures. Thromboxane A2 also stimulates platelet aggregation, promoting clot formation in pulmonary vessels. The development of plexiform lesions are also a hallmark of PHTN. Inflammation may contribute to progression of the disease. Vasoconstriction and increased pressures in the pulmonary system increase the workload of the right ventricle, ultimately leading to right ventricular failure (Bauldoff, Housten-Harris, & Nunley, 2008).

Primary Pulmonary Hypertension

Primary pulmonary hypertension is an uncommon disorder without an identified cause. It occurs in both familial and sporadic patterns. In the 50% of persons with the familial form, the bone morphogenetic protein receptor (BMPR2) a gene transmitted in an autosomal dominant pattern, affects the walls of pulmonary arteries, leading to abnormal vessel growth and remodeling This gene is located at chromosomal region 2q32. Presence of the mutation carries a 10% to 20% risk of developing PAH over the lifetime (Bauldoff, Housten-Harris, & Nunley, 2008). Primary pulmonary hypertension affects primarily women in their 30s or 40s.

> **FAST FACTS**
> - An estimated 500 to 1000 new cases of primary pulmonary hypertension are diagnosed annually primarily in women between 20 and 40 years (American Heart Association, 2009).
> - Median survival after being diagnosed with primary pulmonary hypertension is 3 years without effective treatment, but this has increased with new treatment modalities (Bauldoff, Housten-Harris & Nunley, 2008).

Secondary Pulmonary Hypertension

Secondary pulmonary hypertension is more common than primary. HIV infection and collagen diseases such as scleroderma and lupus may lead to secondary pulmonary hypertension. However, its usual cause is reduced size of the pulmonary vascular bed, which may be due to vasoconstriction or widespread vessel destruction or obstruction. Hypoxemia is a potent pulmonary vasoconstrictor and a common initiating factor in pulmonary hypertension. Chronic lung diseases, sleep apnea, and hypoventilation due to obesity or neuromuscular disease can lead to hypoxemia. Alveolar wall destruction associated with emphysema leads to loss of pulmonary capillaries. Large or multiple pulmonary emboli may cause significant vessel obstruction. Other factors such as left ventricular failure or mitral stenosis also can lead to elevated pulmonary pressures. Once initiated, pulmonary hypertension becomes self-sustaining, as pulmonary vessels undergo changes that further narrow the pulmonary bed.

Manifestations

The manifestations of pulmonary hypertension are progressive dyspnea, fatigue, angina, and syncope with exertion. In secondary pulmonary hypertension, the signs and symptoms often are masked by those of the underlying disease. Dull, retrosternal chest pain may occur in addition to the manifestations of the primary disease. Primary pulmonary hypertension is a progressive disorder that generally causes a steady decline to death within 3 to 4 years.

Complications

Cor pulmonale is a condition of right ventricular hypertrophy and failure resulting from long-standing pulmonary hypertension. Chronic obstructive pulmonary disease is the most common cause of cor pulmonale.

The manifestations of cor pulmonale are those of the underlying pulmonary disorder and right-sided heart failure. Chronic productive cough, progressive dyspnea, and wheezing are common. With right-sided heart failure, peripheral edema and distended neck veins are seen. Skin is warm, moist, and both ruddy and cyanotic because of increased numbers of RBCs and hypoxemia.

Interdisciplinary Care

The CBC commonly shows *polycythemia*, increased numbers of red blood cells. ABGs and oxygen saturation measurements reveal hypoxemia. The chest x-ray shows right heart enlargement and dilation of central pulmonary arteries. Typical ECG changes are those of right ventricular hypertrophy. An echocardiogram may be done to identify cardiac changes occurring either as a cause or result of pulmonary hypertension. Doppler ultrasonography is a noninvasive means of estimating pulmonary artery pressure, but cardiac catheterization may be required for definitive diagnosis. The info is in ∞ Chapter 30 page 929 for Nursing Care of the patient having PCR.

Treatment for pulmonary hypertension focuses on slowing the course of the disease, preventing thrombus formation, and reducing pulmonary vasoconstriction. Oxygen is administered to reduce hypoxemia and improve activity tolerance. If polycythemia is present, phlebotomy is performed to reduce the viscosity of the blood.

The calcium channel blockers nifedipine (Procardia) or diltiazem (Cardizem) may be given to reduce pulmonary vascular resistance and improve cardiac output. Short-acting direct vasodilators such as intravenous epoprostenol (Flolan) or treprostinil (Remodulin), or oral bosentan (Tracleer) may be used for patients who do not respond to calcium channel blockers. An oral anticoagulant (coumadin) is given to prevent clotting (Bauldoff, Housten-Harris, & Nunley, 2008).

Bilateral lung or heart lung transplant is the most effective long-term treatment for primary pulmonary hypertension. When cor pulmonale is present, salt and water restrictions as well as diuretic therapy are added to the previously mentioned regimen to manage the right-sided heart failure.

ꙮ Nursing Care

Nursing care for the patient with pulmonary hypertension or cor pulmonale is largely supportive. The focus is toward the underlying lung disease. Impaired gas exchange due to contraction of the pulmonary vascular system is a significant problem that causes many secondary problems, such as activity intolerance, anxiety, fatigue, and others. Nursing interventions for impaired gas exchange are directed toward maintaining adequate alveolar ventilation, oxygenation, and perfusion. The following measures may be included.

- Monitoring breath sounds, respiratory rate, skin color, and use of accessory muscles
- Positioning for optimal lung expansion
- Coughing, deep breathing, and chest physiotherapy
- Administering prescribed vasodilators

It is important to assess fatigue and dyspnea with activities and to plan frequent rest periods. Assist with self-care as needed to conserve energy.

With primary pulmonary hypertension, *Anticipatory grieving* and *Hopelessness* are additional potential nursing diagnoses. When cor pulmonale is present, *Decreased Cardiac Output*, *Excess Fluid Volume*, and *Ineffective Individual Coping* must be considered.

Community-Based Care

Most care for these chronic conditions is provided in the home and community settings. Teaching is directed both at the underlying lung disease, if present, and the resulting hypertensive process. Refer to the section on COPD for teaching related to this disease, the most frequent underlying cause of cor pulmonale.

In addition, provide teaching about the following topics for the patient and family.

- Disease process, its management, and the prognosis
- Manifestations or changes in condition to report to the physician, such as a change in activity tolerance, increased edema, and signs of respiratory infection or exacerbation
- Importance of planned rest periods between activities and measures to conserve energy, such as using a shower chair
- Importance of not smoking due to its irritant and vasoconstrictive effects
- Prescribed medications, including their use and effects

EVIDENCE FOR NURSING CARE The Patient with Pulmonary Hypertension

Selected resources that nurses may find helpful when planning evidence-based nursing care follow.

- Galiè, N., Simonneau, G., Torbicki, A., Barst, R., Dartevelle, P., Haworth, S. et al. (2004). Guidelines on diagnosis and treatment of pulmonary arterial hypertension. The Task Force on Diagnosis and Treatment of Pulmonary Arterial Hypertension of the European Society of Cardiology. *European Heart Journal 25*(24), 2243–2278. Retrieved from http://eurheartj.oxfordjournals.org/content/25/24/2243.full.pdf+html
- McLaughlin, V. V., Archer, S. L., Badesch, D. B., Barst, R. J., Farber, H. W., Lindner, J. R. et al. (2009). ACCF/AHA 2009 Expert consensus document on pulmonary hypertension: A report of the American college of cardiology foundation task force on expert consensus documents and the American heart association: Developed in collaboration with the American college of chest physicians, American thoracic society, Inc., and the pulmonary hypertension association. *Circulation 119*: 2250–2294. http://www.circ.ahajournals.org

Respiratory Failure

Many of the conditions discussed in this chapter and in ∞ Chapter 36, from pneumonia to acute respiratory distress syndrome (ARDS), can lead to respiratory failure. In **respiratory failure**, the lungs are unable to oxygenate the blood and remove carbon dioxide adequately to meet the body's needs, even at rest.

The Patient with Acute Respiratory Failure

Respiratory failure is not a disease but a consequence of severe respiratory dysfunction. It is often defined by arterial blood gas values. An arterial oxygen level (PO_2) of less than 50 to 60 mmHg and an arterial carbon dioxide level (PCO_2) of greater than 50 mmHg are generally accepted as indicators of respiratory failure. However, patients with advanced COPD may be alert and functional with blood gas values that would indicate respiratory failure in someone whose respiratory function was previously normal. In patients with COPD, respiratory failure is indicated by an acute drop in blood oxygen levels along with increased carbon dioxide levels.

Respiratory failure can result from inadequate alveolar ventilation (hypoventilation), impaired gas exchange, or a significant ventilation-perfusion mismatch. COPD is the most common cause of respiratory failure. Other lung diseases, chest injury, inhalation trauma, neuromuscular disorders, and cardiac conditions can also lead to respiratory failure. Selected causes of acute respiratory failure are identified in Table 37–5.

Pathophysiology

Respiratory failure may be characterized by primary hypoxemia or a combination of hypoxemia and hypercapnia (Figure 37–7 ■). In hypoxemic respiratory failure, PO_2 is significantly reduced, whereas PCO_2 remains normal or is low due to stimulation of the respiratory center and tachypnea. Impaired diffusion across the alveolar-capillary membrane, and a ventilation-perfusion mismatch can cause a drop in arterial oxygen levels that is more rapid than the rise in carbon dioxide. Metabolic acidosis results from tissue hypoxia. The increased work of breathing can eventually lead to respiratory muscle fatigue and hypoventilation.

Hypoventilation, or reduced movement of air into and out of the lung, causes carbon dioxide retention. With significant hypoventilation, the carbon dioxide level in the blood rises rapidly, leading to respiratory acidosis. Hypoxemia develops more slowly, and responds readily to administration of oxygen unless gas exchange also is impaired.

In summary, hypoxemia without a corresponding rise in carbon dioxide levels indicates a failure of oxygenation; hypoxemia with hypercapnia is the result of lung hypoventilation.

Manifestations and Course

The manifestations of respiratory failure are caused by hypoxemia and hypercapnia, as well as the underlying disease process. Hypoxemia causes dyspnea and neurologic symptoms such as restlessness, apprehension, impaired judgment, and motor impairment. Tachycardia and hypertension develop as the cardiac output increases in an effort to bring more oxygen to the tissues. Cyanosis is present. As hypoxemia progresses, dysrhythmias, hypotension, and decreased cardiac output may develop.

Increased carbon dioxide levels depress CNS function and cause vasodilation. Dyspnea and headache are early signs. Other manifestations include peripheral and conjunctival vasodilation, papilledema, neuromuscular irritability, and decreased level of consciousness. As hypercapnia worsens, the respiratory center may be depressed, reducing dyspnea and slowing respirations. Increased carbon dioxide and hydrogen ion concentrations no longer stimulate the respiratory center; hypoxemia provides the primary active breathing stimulus. Administering oxygen without ventilatory support may further reduce the drive to breathe, leading to respiratory arrest.

The prognosis for acute respiratory failure varies, depending on the underlying disease process. Respiratory failure resulting from uncomplicated drug overdose generally resolves quickly without long-term effects. When respiratory failure results from underlying lung disease, the course may be prolonged and the outcome less favorable.

TABLE 37–5 Selected Causes of Respiratory Failure

TYPE OF DYSFUNCTION	EXAMPLES
Impaired ventilation:	
■ Airway obstruction	Laryngospasm, foreign body aspiration, airway edema
■ Respiratory disease	Asthma, COPD
■ Neurologic causes	Spinal cord injury, poliomyelitis, Guillain-Barré syndrome, drug overdose, stroke
■ Chest wall injury	Flail chest, pneumothorax
Impaired diffusion:	
■ Alveolar disorders	Pneumonia, pneumonitis, COPD
■ Pulmonary edema	Heart failure, acute respiratory distress syndrome (ARDS), near-drowning
Ventilation-perfusion mismatch	Pulmonary embolism

FAST FACTS

Among adults requiring mechanical ventilation for acute respiratory failure the following results:
■ An estimated 62% survive to be weaned from the ventilator.
■ Only 43% survive to be discharged from the hospital.
■ About 30% remain alive at 1 year after discharge (Papadakis & McPhee, 2007).

Interdisciplinary Care

Treatment of respiratory failure focuses on correcting the underlying cause or disease, supporting ventilation, and correcting hypoxemia and hypercapnia. Care related to disorders that can precipitate respiratory failure is discussed in the sections specific to each disorder.

Figure 37–7 ■ Causes and manifestations of respiratory failure.

Diagnosis

Exhaled carbon dioxide and arterial blood gases are used to diagnose and monitor treatment of respiratory failure.

- *Exhaled carbon dioxide (ETCO$_2$)* is used to evaluate alveolar ventilation. The normal ETCO$_2$ is 35 to 45 mmHg; it is elevated when ventilation is inadequate, and decreased when pulmonary perfusion is impaired.
- *Arterial blood gases* also are used to evaluate alveolar ventilation and gas exchange. With hypoxemic respiratory failure, the PCO$_2$ may be normal, 35 to 45 mmHg, or even low due to tachypnea. A pH of less than 7.35 and low bicarbonate levels indicate metabolic acidosis, typical of hypoxemic respiratory failure.

In respiratory failure due to hypoventilation, the PCO$_2$ is elevated, usually greater than 50 mmHg. The pH is low due to respiratory acidosis. Acidosis develops rapidly in hypoxemia and hypercapnia because of increased acid production (metabolic) and decreased acid elimination (respiratory).

Medications

Drugs used in treating respiratory failure depend on the underlying cause of the failure and the need for intubation and mechanical ventilation.

Beta-adrenergic (sympathomimetic) or anticholinergic medications may be administered by inhalation to promote bronchodilation. If mechanical ventilation is required, the drugs may be given by nebulizer attached to the ventilator. Methylxanthine bronchodilators (theophylline derivatives) may be given intravenously. See the table on page 1235 and the asthma section of this chapter for more information about bronchodilators and their nursing implications. Corticosteroids, administered by inhalation or intravenously, may be ordered to reduce airway edema. Antibiotics are given to treat any underlying infection.

Sedation and analgesia often are required during mechanical ventilation to decrease pain and anxiety. Benzodiazepines such as diazepam (Valium), lorazepam (Ativan), or midazolam (Versed) may be used for sedation and to inhibit the respiratory drive. Intravenous morphine or fentanyl provide analgesia and also inhibit the respiratory drive, allowing more effective mechanical ventilation. Occasionally, the patient's respiratory drive competes with the ventilator despite sedation, decreasing its effectiveness and increasing the work of breathing. A neuromuscular blocking agent in combination with sedation may be necessary to induce paralysis and suppress the ability to breathe. Nursing implications of neuromuscular blockers are described in the Medication Administration box on page 1264.

Oxygen Therapy

Oxygen is administered to reverse hypoxemia in acute respiratory failure. In general, the goal is to achieve an oxygen saturation of 90% or greater without oxygen toxicity. A PO$_2$ of about 60 mmHg usually is adequate to meet the oxygen needs of body tissues. Higher levels do not significantly increase oxygen saturation and may lead to hypoventilation in patients with chronic hypercapnia. As little as 1 to 3 L of oxygen per nasal cannula or 28% oxygen per Venturi mask may correct hypoxemia in advanced COPD. Oxygen concentrations of 40% to 60% may be required when diffusion is impaired (e.g., in pneumonia or acute respiratory distress syndrome). High concentrations are used only for short periods to avoid oxygen toxicity. Both the oxygen concentration and duration of therapy contribute to oxygen toxicity. Continued high oxygen concentrations impair the synthesis of surfactant, reducing lung compliance (ease of inflation). Acute respiratory distress syndrome or absorption atelectasis may develop.

When respiratory failure is caused by hypoventilation or usual oxygen delivery systems do not correct hypoxemia, a tight-fitting mask to maintain *continuous positive airway pressure (CPAP)* may be used. CPAP increases lung volume, opening previously closed alveoli, improving ventilation of under ventilated alveoli, and improving ventilation-perfusion relationships.

Airway Management

If the upper airway is obstructed or positive pressure mechanical ventilation is necessary to correct hypoxemia and hypercapnia, an endotracheal tube that extends from the mouth or nose into the trachea is inserted (Figure 37–8 ■). To maintain positive pressure ventilation, the tube is cuffed with an air-filled or foam sac just above the end of the tube. When the cuff is inflated, it obstructs the upper airway, preventing air from escaping back into the nose or mouth. Excess pressure of the cuff can cause tissue ischemia and necrosis of the trachea. To minimize this risk, high-volume, low-pressure ("floppy") cuffs are used. Tubes with low-pressure cuffs may be left in place for 3 to 4 weeks.

A tracheostomy may be performed if long-term ventilatory support is required. Although a tracheostomy is more comfortable and easier to secure in place, complications such as

NONDEPOLARIZING NEUROMUSCULAR BLOCKERS

Rocuronium (Zemuron)

Pancuronium bromide (Pavulon)

Atracurium besylate (Tracrium)

Cisatracurium (Nimbex)

Nondepolarizing neuromuscular blockers competitively block the action of acetylcholine (ACh) at skeletal muscle receptors, preventing muscle depolarization and contraction. Complete muscle paralysis is achieved within minutes. Facial muscles are affected first, followed by muscles of the limbs, neck, and trunk. The muscles of respiration (the diaphragm and intercostal muscles) are least sensitive to the effects of neuromuscular blockers and are paralyzed last. When the drug is discontinued or an antagonist is given, respiratory function is recovered first as the muscle groups recover in reverse order.

Nursing Responsibilities

- Prior to administering, assess endotracheal tube placement and ensure effective mechanical ventilator function. The risk of hypoxemia and organ damage is significant if respiratory muscles are paralyzed without adequate ventilatory support in place.

- Administer the drug by slow intravenous injection and/or intravenous infusion as prescribed.
- Keep an acetylcholinesterase (AChE) inhibitor such as neostigmine (Prostigmin) available at the bedside to rapidly reverse neuromuscular effects if needed.
- Administer morphine sulfate, diazepam (Valium), or other anti-anxiety agent or sedative as ordered. Neuromuscular blockers provide no sedation or pain relief; muscle paralysis produces extreme anxiety.
- Instill artificial tears every 2 to 4 hours.
- Suction oral cavity as needed to remove saliva.
- *Never* turn off ventilator alarms when administering neuromuscular blockers. Should the tubing become disconnected or plugged, the patient is unable to breathe independently or call for help.
- Treat the patient as though awake and alert. Although unable to respond, mental function is unaffected.

Health Education for the Patient and Family

- Reassure that the ability to move and communicate will return when the drug is discontinued.
- Teach the family about the effects of the drug and the reason for its use. Explain that the patient can hear and understand what is going on.

---

cuff necrosis and increased risk of infection are associated with tracheostomy as well as endotracheal intubation. Table 37–6 compares the advantages, disadvantages, and possible complications of endotracheal tubes and tracheostomy.

When the patient is able to maintain effective respirations and ventilatory support is no longer required, the endotracheal tube is removed (*extubation*). Gag, cough, and swallow reflexes must be intact to prevent aspiration. After oxygenation and suctioning, the cuff is deflated and the tube removed. Humidified oxygen is provided immediately following removal. Close observation for respiratory distress is vital following extubation. Inspiratory stridor within the first 24 hours indicates laryngeal edema, which may necessitate reintubation. Sore throat and a hoarse voice are common after extubation. Oral intake is reinitiated slowly, with careful assessment of swallowing.

Figure 37–8 ■ Nasal endotracheal (nasotracheal) intubation.

Trachea

Cuff

Mechanical Ventilation

Mechanical ventilation is indicated when alveolar ventilation is inadequate to maintain blood oxygen and carbon dioxide levels. Specific indications for mechanical ventilation include the following:

- Apnea or acute ventilatory failure
- Hypoxemia unresponsive to oxygen therapy alone
- Increased work of breathing with progressive patient fatigue

The most common indicators for ventilation support is actual or potential respiratory muscle fatigue (Fishman et al., 2008). Drug overdose, neural disorders, chest wall injury, and airway problems such as severe asthma or COPD can lead to acute ventilatory failure. Disorders that affect alveolar-capillary diffusion, such as pulmonary contusion, pneumonia, and ARDS, may necessitate mechanical ventilation to attain adequate oxygenation. Positive pressure ventilation increases lung volume, helps redistribute fluid from the alveolar to the interstitial space, and helps reduce the oxygen demand caused by increased work of breathing.

TYPES OF VENTILATORS Two broad general classifications of mechanical ventilators are available. Negative-pressure ventilators create negative (subatmospheric) pressure externally to draw the chest outward and air into the lungs, mimicking spontaneous breathing. The iron lung, cuirass ventilator, and PulmoWrap are examples of negative-pressure ventilators. Negative pressure ventilators primarily are used by patients with neuromuscular disorders (e.g., post-polio syndrome, amyotrophic lateral sclerosis) that interfere with the ability to maintain adequate ventilation. They also may be used by patients who primarily require ventilator support during sleep.

TABLE 37–6 A Comparison of Endotracheal Tubes and Tracheostomy

	ADVANTAGES	DISADVANTAGES	POTENTIAL COMPLICATIONS
Oral endotracheal tube	■ More easily inserted ■ Larger tube can be used, facilitating work of breathing, suctioning	■ More difficult to secure ■ Can be obstructed by biting ■ Communication and mouth care more difficult ■ Increased risk of lower respiratory infection	■ Obstruction or displacement ■ Pressure necrosis of lip ■ Tracheoesophageal fistula
Nasal endotracheal tube	■ More easily secured and stabilized ■ Well-tolerated by patient ■ Facilitate communication and oral hygiene	■ Necessitate smaller tube, which may impede removal of secretions ■ Increased risk of lower respiratory infection	■ Obstruction or displacement ■ Pressure necrosis of nares ■ Obstruction of sinus drainage, possible sinusitis ■ Tracheoesophageal fistula
Tracheostomy	■ Easily secured and stabilized ■ Enable swallowing, speech, and oral hygiene ■ Avoid upper airway complications	■ Require surgical incision ■ Increased risk of lower respiratory infection	■ Hemorrhage due to incision or vessel erosion by tube ■ Wound infection ■ Subcutaneous emphysema ■ Tracheoesophageal fistula ■ Tracheal infarction and stenosis

Positive-pressure ventilators are more commonly used, especially in treating acute respiratory failure (Figure 37–9 ■). These ventilators push air into the lungs, rather than drawing it in like negative-pressure ventilators. Either invasive ventilation using an endotracheal tube or tracheostomy or noninvasive positive-pressure ventilation may be used. Increasingly, noninvasive techniques, which use a nasal or face mask, nasal plugs, or an oral mouthpiece are used (Fishman et al., 2008).

Several variables are used to trigger, cycle, and limit airflow with positive-pressure ventilators. The *trigger* prompts the ventilator to deliver a breath. The patient's inspiratory effort triggers *ventilator-assisted breaths. Ventilator-controlled breaths* usually are triggered by a preset time interval (e.g., a breath is delivered every 5 seconds for a rate of 12 breaths per minute).

A

B

Figure 37–9 ■ *A,* Positive-pressure ventilator and *B,* the control panel used to set the mode, rate, limits, and percentage of oxygen.

The ventilator *cycle*, or duration of inspiration, can be limited by volume, pressure, flow, or time. *Volume-cycled ventilators* deliver air until a preset volume is delivered. *Pressure-cycled ventilators* cycle off when a preset pressure is achieved within the airways. *Flow-cycled ventilators* are cycled by a preset inspiratory flow rate, and *time-cycled ventilators* deliver air for a set time interval. Airflow delivered by the ventilator also can be limited by factors such as airway pressure (e.g., a volume-cycled ventilator can be set to immediately stop inspiratory flow if airway pressure exceeds a preset value).

MODES OF VENTILATION

A number of different *modes* or patterns of ventilation may be used with positive-pressure ventilators. The mode determines whether a breath is initiated by the patient or the ventilator and the pattern of airway support provided by the ventilator. Continuous positive airway pressure, bi-level airway pressure support, assist-control mode ventilation, synchronized intermittent mandatory ventilation, positive end-expiratory pressure, pressure support ventilation, and pressure-control ventilation are common modes and adjuncts of ventilation in use today (Table 37–7).

Noninvasive ventilation (NIV) provides ventilator support using a tight-fitting facemask, thus avoiding intubation. Its primary use is to support patients with obstructive sleep apnea, neuromuscular disease, or impending respiratory failure (e.g., advanced COPD). NIV also may be used for patients in respiratory failure who refuse intubation. The degree of success varies, primarily limited by patient intolerance due to the physical and psychologic discomfort of wearing a mask when dyspneic (Fishman et al., 2008). NIV tends to be more successful in patients without significant underlying lung disease (e.g., respiratory failure related to neuromuscular disease).

Continuous positive airway pressure (CPAP) applies positive pressure to the airways of a spontaneously breathing patient. CPAP may be used with either endotracheal intubation or a tight-fitting face mask. All breathing is spontaneous (patient triggered) and pressure controlled. CPAP is used to help maintain open airways and alveoli, decreasing the work of breathing. *BiPAP* provide inspiratory positive airway pressure as well as airway support during expiration. BiPAP ventilation is primarily used at night with a tight-fitting mask (nasal, facial, or oral). Bi-level ventilation is a ventilator mode with high PEEP and low PEEP. Three modes of ventilation can be used with BiPAP: spontaneous breathing (S); timed mode (T), in which pressure supported breaths are delivered at a predetermined rate; and spontaneous/timed (S/T), in which the ventilator switches to timed mode if spontaneous breathing falls below a preset rate (Fishman et al., 2008). *Assist-control mode ventilation (ACMV or AC)* is frequently used to initiate mechanical ventilation and when the patient is at risk for respiratory arrest (e.g., overdose or head injury). Assisted breaths are triggered by inspiratory effort; however, if the respiratory rate falls below a preset number (e.g., 14 per minute), ventilator-controlled breaths are delivered. All breaths, assisted and controlled, are delivered at a specific tidal volume or pressure and inspiratory flow rate.

Synchronized intermittent mandatory ventilation (SIMV) allows the patient to breathe spontaneously, without ventilator assistance, between delivered ventilator breaths. Mandatory or ventilator-controlled breaths are delivered at a preset rate, volume, and/or pressure, coordinated with the patient's inspiratory efforts. This mode of ventilation is used to support ventilation, to exercise respiratory muscles between ventilator-assisted breaths and during the weaning process (Fishman et al., 2008).

Positive end-expiratory pressure (PEEP) requires intubation and can be applied to any of the previously described ventilator modes. With PEEP, a positive pressure is maintained in the airways during exhalation and between breaths. Keeping alveoli open between breaths improves ventilation-perfusion relationships and diffusion across the alveolar-capillary membrane. This reduces hypoxemia and allows use of lower percentages of inspired oxygen. PEEP is particularly useful for treating ARDS.

In *pressure support ventilation (PSV)*, ventilator-assisted breaths are delivered when the patient initiates an inspiratory effort. The cycle is flow limited; inspiration is terminated when inspiratory airflow falls below a preset rate. This mode decreases the work of breathing. It can be used in combination with SIMV when the respiratory drive is depressed. Ventilatory support can be gradually withdrawn during weaning.

Pressure-control ventilation (PCV), in contrast, controls pressure within the airways to reduce the risk of airway trauma (e.g., following thoracic surgery). Ventilation is time triggered and time cycled, but pressure is limited. The ventilator maintains a preset airway pressure throughout inspiration. Because all breaths are controlled by the ventilator, heavy sedation may be required to prevent competition between inspiratory effort and ventilator control.

Independent lung ventilation, provides separate ventilation for each lung. Indications include unilateral lung disease. It can be used post-lung transplantation to address pulmonary pressure differences between the native lung and allograft. It requires a double-lumen endotracheal tube, two ventilators. Patients may require heavy sedation.

High frequency ventilation provides small gas volumes delivered at a rapid rate. It is indicated in patients who are hemodynamically unstable and intolerant of conventional MV. Use requires sedation and possibly pharmacologic paralysis (Perrin, 2009).

VENTILATOR SETTINGS

In addition to choosing the mode of ventilation, other parameters are set to meet individual patient needs when positive-pressure ventilation is used (Table 37–8).

For most adult patients, the rate is initially set between 12 and 15 breaths per minute. With ACMV or SIMV, the patient's respiratory rate often is higher than the ventilator setting due to spontaneous breathing. Exhaled carbon dioxide ($ETCO_2$) or the PCO_2 may be used to determine the rate. A PCO_2 less than 35 mmHg indicates hyperventilation and respiratory alkalosis; the set rate is reduced. A PCO_2 above 45 mmHg or an $ETCO_2$ greater than 45 mmHg indicates hypoventilation and a need to increase the rate.

The tidal volume setting controls the amount of gas delivered with each ventilator breath. The normal adult tidal volume at rest is about 7 mL/kg of body weight, or 400 to 550 mL. The tidal volume delivered by mechanical ventilation is slightly higher (500 to 750 mL) to compensate for tubing dead space. Higher tidal volumes can cause lung tissue trauma.

TABLE 37–7 Modes of Positive-Pressure Ventilator Operation

MODE	DESCRIPTION	PATTERN
Spontaneous breathing	Patient has full control of rate, tidal volume, pressures.	
Assist-control mode ventilation (ACMV)	Patient can trigger ventilator to deliver breaths at preset volume or pressure and inspiratory flow rate; breaths will be delivered at preset rate if patient does not initiate.	
Synchronized intermittent mandatory ventilation (SIMV)	Mandatory breaths delivered by ventilator are synchronized with patient's inspiratory effort.	
Continuous positive airway pressure (CPAP)	Positive pressure is maintained in airways; all breaths are spontaneous.	
Positive end-expiratory pressure (PEEP)	Used in conjunction with other ventilator modes; positive airway pressure is maintained throughout respiratory cycle.	
Pressure support ventilation (PSV)	Pressurized inspiratory flow supports the patient's inspiratory effort, decreasing the work of breathing.	

TABLE 37–8 Ventilator Settings

PARAMETER	DESCRIPTION
Rate (f)	Number of ventilator-delivered breaths per minute: usually 12 to 15 in adults using ACMV, may be lower in SIMV
Tidal volume (V_t)	Amount of gas delivered with each ventilator breath: usually 8 to 10 mL/kg of body weight
Oxygen concentration (FIO_2)	Percentage of oxygen delivered with ventilator breaths: can be set between 21% (room air) and 100%
I:E ratio	Duration of inspiration to expiration: usually 1:2 to 1:1.5
Flow rate	Speed at which air is delivered
Sensitivity	Effort required by patient to initiate a ventilator-assisted breath
Pressure limit	Maximal pressure within airways that will terminate a ventilator breath

The percentage of oxygen delivered with ventilator breaths is adjusted to maintain the oxygen saturation and PO_2 within acceptable ranges. Because prolonged delivery of high oxygen concentrations increases the risk of oxygen toxicity and pulmonary fibrosis, the FIO_2 is set at the lowest possible level for adequate tissue oxygenation. For most patients, the goal is to maintain an oxygen saturation greater than 90%. Lower oxygen saturation levels may be appropriate for patients with longstanding COPD.

COMPLICATIONS Although endotracheal intubation and mechanical ventilation can be life-saving in respiratory failure, they are not without risk. Improper endotracheal tube placement or advancement of the tube into a mainstem bronchus can result in ventilation of one lung only. The inflated lung becomes overdistended and traumatized, and the uninflated lung develops atelectasis. In noninvasive ventilation, associated complications include gastric dilation, aspiration, facial skin necrosis, drying of the eyes and mucous membranes, stress and claustrophobia (Fishman et al., 2008).

Nosocomial Pneumonia Infection is a significant risk associated with intubation and mechanical ventilation. Normal upper respiratory tract defense mechanisms are bypassed, with loss of air humidification and trapping of pathogens. Oral secretions and gastric contents can enter the respiratory tree through the open epiglottis. Frequent, meticulous oral hygiene is vital in preventing ventilator-associated pneumonia. Often the cough reflex is inhibited or impaired by the underlying disease process and the continued presence of the endotracheal tube. Even when strict asepsis is used for suctioning and other respiratory procedures, the lower airways are contaminated within 24 hours of intubation. Secretions often become thick and tenacious, increasing the risk of atelectasis.

Barotrauma Barotrauma (also called *volutrauma*) is lung injury due to alveolar over distention. Both the volume of delivered gas and the pressures under which it is delivered can contribute to barotraumas. As a result, overdistended alveoli rupture, allowing air to escape into the pulmonary interstitial spaces and the mediastinum, pleural space, and other tissues. Subcutaneous emphysema, pneumothorax, and pneumomediastinum are possible results of barotrauma. *Subcutaneous emphysema,* or air in the subcutaneous tissue, causes tissue swelling of the chest, neck, and face. A "crackling" or air-bubble-popping sensation is felt on palpation of subcutaneous emphysema. Swelling may be massive. Once the cause is corrected, the air is gradually reabsorbed over weeks.

Pneumothorax is identified by signs of unequal chest expansion, a sudden loss or significant decrease in breath sounds on the affected side, and a hyperresonant percussion tone. Rapid chest tube insertion is necessary to prevent tension pneumothorax and cardiovascular compromise. *Pneumomediastinum* is the presence of air in the mediastinum, the space between the lungs that contains the heart, great vessels, trachea, and esophagus. Air in the mediastinal space can interfere with the function of all these organs and lead to such complications as pneumopericardium (air in the pericardial sac). Pneumomediastinum may have few manifestations, but the chest x-ray shows widening of the mediastinal space.

Cardiovascular Effects Positive-pressure ventilation increases intrathoracic pressure, which can interfere with venous return to the heart and ventricular filling. As a result, cardiac output falls. Use of PEEP increases the effects of mechanical ventilation on cardiac output. The decreased cardiac output can affect liver and kidney function secondarily.

Gastrointestinal Effects Gastrointestinal complications are commonly associated with prolonged mechanical ventilation. Stress ulcers (erosive gastritis) may develop, leading to painless gastrointestinal hemorrhage. Histamine H_2-receptor blockers or sucralfate are often used to prevent stress ulcers. Air leaks around the endotracheal tube can cause gastric distention; a nasogastric tube often is inserted to prevent vomiting. Sedation and other medications used during mechanical ventilation can slow intestinal motility, leading to constipation.

WEANING The process of removing ventilator support and reestablishing spontaneous, independent respirations is called **weaning**. Weaning begins only after the underlying process causing respiratory failure has been corrected or stabilized. The process and time required for weaning depend on factors such as preexisting lung condition, duration of mechanical ventilation, and the patient's general condition, both physical and psychologic. In all cases, the vital signs, respiratory rate, extent of dyspnea, blood gases, and clinical status are used to evaluate weaning and its progress.

Following a brief period of mechanical ventilation, T-piece or CPAP may be used for weaning. In T-piece weaning, the ventilator is removed for brief periods during which oxygen is delivered using a T-piece (Figure 37–10 ■). The duration of periods off the ventilator is gradually increased until the patient can maintain adequate independent respirations for several hours. Vital signs, oxygen saturation, $ETCO_2$, and PO_2 are carefully monitored during the process. The patient is placed back on the ventilator at previous settings if signs of respiratory distress develop. When mechanical ventilation is no longer needed, the endotracheal tube is removed. CPAP weaning follows a

Figure 37–10 ■ A T-piece, or "blow-by" unit, for weaning from mechanical ventilation.

similar process, with trials of spontaneous breathing supported by the ventilator in CPAP mode.

SIMV and PSV are used for weaning when the duration of mechanical ventilation has been longer and reconditioning of respiratory muscles is needed. When SIMV is used, the number of mandatory ventilator-assisted breaths is gradually decreased as ABGs, ETCO$_2$, and the respiratory rate are monitored. When the patient is able to tolerate SIMV at 4 breaths per minute without rest periods of greater ventilatory support, CPAP or T-piece weaning is attempted prior to extubation (Fishman et al., 2008).

Weaning is the primary use for pressure-support ventilation (PSV). Initially, PSV is set slightly below peak inspiratory pressures required during volume-cycled ventilation. Pressure support levels are gradually decreased, often in a cyclic pattern of periods of minimal support alternating with higher support to recondition respiratory muscles. When the PSV level is just enough to overcome endotracheal tube resistance, support is discontinued and the patient is extubated (Fishman et al., 2008).

Terminal Weaning   When an illness is terminal or irreversible with a poor prognosis, terminal weaning may be requested by the patient or family. *Terminal weaning* is the gradual withdrawal of mechanical ventilation when survival without assisted ventilation is not expected. Unlike weaning when recovery is expected, which usually occurs in an intensive care unit (ICU), the patient is moved to a quiet medical-surgical or hospice room or even home prior to initiating terminal weaning. Family members are encouraged to remain with the patient throughout the process. If possible, decisions about sedation and analgesia prior to and during weaning are made with the patient, as are decisions about hydration and nutritional support following weaning. Ventilator support is withdrawn using the same modes described earlier (SIMV, PSV). Analgesia and sedation are given to promote comfort during weaning.

Nutrition and Fluids

Attention also must be paid to fluid and electrolyte status and adequate nutrition. Mechanical ventilation promotes sodium and water retention due to its effects on cardiac output. Renal perfusion is decreased, stimulating the renin-angiotensin-aldosterone system to retain sodium and water. A Swan-Ganz catheter is often inserted to monitor pulmonary artery pressures and cardiac output. An arterial line allows repeated blood gas

analysis and continuous arterial pressure monitoring. Serum electrolytes are drawn frequently, and intake, output, and daily weight are carefully monitored.

Enteral or parenteral nutrition are provided during mechanical ventilation, because the endotracheal tube prohibits eating. A nasogastric, gastrostomy, or jejunostomy feeding tube is placed for enteral nutrition. A jejunostomy tube may be used to reduce the risk of regurgitation and aspiration.

Nursing Care

Health Promotion

Education is a primary strategy to prevent respiratory failure. Teach all patients and the public about the risks of smoking, water safety, the value of a working smoke detector, and measures to prevent smoke inhalation in a fire. Discuss the importance of pneumococcal vaccine and annual influenza immunizations for people who are at high risk, including those over age 65 and people with chronic diseases. Teach patients with spinal cord injury or neuromuscular disease to use effective breathing and coughing techniques to maintain airway patency. Work with patients addicted to narcotic drugs to attain and maintain drug-free status. Teach patients with COPD about measures to reduce their risk of respiratory infection and symptoms to report to the physician.

Assessment

Focused assessment data related to respiratory failure includes the following:

- *Health history:*   Current manifestations, their duration, and identified precipitating factors (may need to be obtained from family members if mental status is affected); history of previous episodes; chronic diseases such as COPD, occupational lung disease; current medications.
- *Physical examination:*   Level of consciousness, mental status; vital signs; color and oxygen saturation; respiratory assessment including rate and depth, use of accessory muscles, respiratory excursion, auscultation; cardiovascular assessment including heart rate and sounds, neck vein distention, peripheral pulses, evidence of clubbing.
- *Diagnostic tests:*   ABGs, chest x-ray, pulmonary artery pressure and wedge pressure readings, cardiac output.

Nursing Diagnoses and Interventions

Patients in respiratory failure are often unstable and critically ill. They require both intensive medical care and intensive nursing care. Priority nursing needs relate to maintaining ventilation and a patent airway. Perhaps less obvious, but no less critical, nursing care needs relate to preventing injury and managing anxiety.

Impaired Spontaneous Ventilation

In acute respiratory failure, fatigue from the work of breathing may impair the ability to maintain adequate ventilation. This is a concern both prior to initiation of mechanical ventilation and during the weaning process.

- Assess and document respiratory rate, vital signs, and oxygen saturation every 15 to 30 minutes. *Close monitoring is vital to detect early signs of increasing respiratory distress and inability to sustain adequate breathing.*

- Chronic obstructive pulmonary disease (COPD) is a long-term process of progressive lung dysfunction. COPD involves two different disease processes: chronic bronchitis, characterized by airways edema and excessive mucus production, and emphysema, characterized by destruction of supporting tissue with enlargement of respiratory bronchioles and alveolar spaces and loss of surface area for gas exchange.
- Smoking and exposure to tobacco smoke is the single greatest risk factor for COPD. A small percentage of cases result from an inherited deficiency of alpha1-antitripsin, an enzyme that inhibits lung tissue destruction. Although smoking cessation does not reverse COPD, it does slow the progress of the disease.
- Cystic fibrosis, inherited as an autosomal recessive disorder, causes thick, viscous secretions in affected organs, primarily the lungs, pancreas, sweat glands, and reproductive tract. In the lungs, small airway clearance is impaired, leading to atelectasis, bronchiectasis, infection, and dilation of distal airways with air trapping and impaired gas exchange. Chest physiotherapy and early treatment of respiratory infections are key components of disease management. Ultimately, lung or heart-lung transplant may be required.
- Occupational lung diseases, pneumoconiosis and hypersensitivity pneumonitis, damage interstitial tissues of the lungs, leading to fibrosis and scarring that causes the lungs to become stiff and noncompliant. Lung volumes decrease, the work of breathing increases, and gas diffusion is impaired. Most occupational lung diseases are progressive and nonreversible. Interdisciplinary care is similar to that provided for patients with COPD.
- Pulmonary vascular disorders affect blood flow through the pulmonary vascular system and gas exchange. Pulmonary embolism, obstruction of pulmonary blood flow, is a potentially critical condition usually resulting from deep venous thrombosis. Sudden onset of chest pain and dyspnea with changes in hemodynamic status are possible manifestations of pulmonary embolism. Prevention through early ambulation, lower extremity exercises, and sequential compression devices is the most effective treatment for pulmonary embolism.

- In primary and secondary forms of pulmonary hypertension, constriction of pulmonary vessels and remodeling of the pulmonary vascular bed increase pressure in the pulmonary system and right heart, ultimately leading to right-sided heart failure (cor pulmonale). Treatment focuses on slowing disease progression through oxygen therapy, administration of vasodilators and anticoagulants, and supporting patient function.
- Hypoventilation, impaired gas exchange and significant ventilation-perfusion mismatch (e.g. pulmonary embolism) can lead to respiratory failure. Hypoventilation leads to hypoxemia and hyercapnia, whereas in impaired gas exchange or ventilation-perfusion mismatch, hypoxemia predominates.
- The manifestations of respiratory failure relate directly to the effects of hypoxemia (dyspnea, restlessness, apprehension, impaired judgment, motor impairment, tachycardia, hyper- or hypotension, and cyanosis) and hypercapnia (dyspnea, headache, peripheral and conjunctival vasodilation, papilledema, neuromuscular irritability, and decreased LOC).
- Respiratory support often is required, using positive pressure ventilators. Variables of mechanical ventilation include the mode or cycle of ventilation, the flow rate and amount, pressures delivered, and the oxygen concentration. Either invasive or noninvasive techniques may be used.
- Complications of mechanical ventilation include lung and mucous membrane trauma and infection, reduced cardiac output, gastric dilation, impaired communication, and stress.
- ARDS is noncardiac pulmonary edema caused by a diffuse inflammatory response with increased pulmonary capillary permeability leading to interstitial and alveolar edema and impaired gas exchange. As the process continues, lung compliance decreases, increasing the work of breathing, and atelectalsis and consolidation of lung tissue develop. Respiratory failure with refractory hypoxemia result.
- Mechanical ventilation and measures to support physiologic function are the primary treatments for ARDS. The mortality rate, however, remains high at about 40%.

TEST YOURSELF NCLEX-RN® REVIEW

1. All of the following nursing diagnoses are appropriate for a patient with an acute asthma attack. Which is of highest priority?
   1. *Anxiety* related to difficulty breathing
   2. *Ineffective Airway Clearance* related to bronchoconstriction and increased mucous production
   3. *Ineffective Breathing Pattern* related to anxiety
   4. *Ineffective Health Maintenance* related of lack of knowledge about attack triggers and appropriate use of medications
2. The nurse caring for a patient with asthma notices that the patient's respirations have slowed and he is no longer coughing. Breath sounds are diminished throughout his lung fields and absent in the bases. The nurse should do which of the following?
   1. Notify the healthcare provider.
   2. Allow the patient to rest undisturbed.
   3. Obtain a chest x-ray.
   4. Ask family members to leave.
3. When teaching use of a metered dose inhaler (MDI), the nurse instructs her patient to do which of the following?
   1. Take quick shallow breaths in rapid succession while holding the canister down.
   2. Use the inhaler containing the anti-inflammatory drug first, then the bronchodilator.
   3. Use the anti-inflammatory drug as needed to treat acute episodes of wheezing.
   4. Rinse the mouth after using the inhaler to reduce systemic absorption of the drug.

4. Which of the following would be an expected assessment finding in a patient admitted with chronic obstructive airway disease?
   1. AP chest diameter equal to or greater than lateral chest diameter
   2. mental confusion and lethargy
   3. three+ pitting edema of ankles and lower legs
   4. oxygen saturation readings of 85% or less
5. An appropriate goal for a patient admitted with an acute exacerbation of COPD would be which of the following?
   1. Will verbalize self-care measures to regain lost lung function.
   2. Arterial blood gases will be within normal limits by discharge.
   3. Will maintain SaO_2 of 90% or higher.
   4. Will identify strategies to help reduce number of cigarettes smoked per day.
6. Which of the following statements best represents a nurse's understanding of use of supplemental oxygen in patients with COPD?
   1. Because oxygen is flammable, the patient should not smoke.
   2. Oxygen is used only at night for patients with COPD.
   3. Oxygen is never used for patients with COPD as they may become dependent on it.
   4. The patient needs to be closely monitored for signs of respiratory depression.

7. The home care nurse working with a patient who has cystic fibrosis specifically directs the home care aide to report which of the following? **Select all that apply.**
   1. thick, tenacious, milky, and white sputum
   2. fever
   3. bulky, fatty stools
   4. difficulty clearing mucus secretions
   5. increasing shortness of breath and fatigue

8. A patient in skeletal traction suddenly develops right-sided chest pain and shortness of breath. The nurse should do which of the following?
   1. Check for Homan's sign.
   2. Start oxygen per nasal cannula.
   3. Administer the prescribed analgesic.
   4. Elevate the head of the bed to 45 degrees.

9. The nurse caring for a patient with COPD recognizes which of the following as an early sign of possible respiratory failure?
   1. restlessness and tachypnea
   2. deep coma
   3. hypotension and tachycardia
   4. decreased urine output

10. The nurse caring for a patient undergoing mechanical ventilation for acute respiratory failure plans and implements which of the following measures to help maintain effective alveolar ventilation?
    1. Keeps the patient in supine position.
    2. Increases the tidal volume on the ventilator.
    3. Maintains ordered oxygen concentration.
    4. Performs endotracheal suctioning as indicated.

See Test Yourself answers in Appendix C.

Pearson Nursing Student Resources

Find additional review materials at
www.nursing.pearsonhighered.com

Prepare for success with additional NCLEX®-style practice questions, interactive assignments and activities, Web links, animations and videos, and more!

BIBLIOGRAPHY

American Heart Association. (2009). *Primary or unexplained pulmonary hypertension.* Retrieved from http://www .americanheart.org/presenter.jhtml?identifier=4752

American Lung Association (ALA). (2009). Occupational lung diseases. Retrieved from http://www.lungusa.org/assets/documents/publications/solddc-chapters/occupational.pdf

Bauldoff, G. S., Housten-Harris, T., & Nunley, D. R. (2008). Cardiovascular consequences of pulmonary hypertension. *Nursing Clinics of North America 43,* 17–36.

Belza, B., Steele, B. G., Hunziker, J., Lakshminaryan, S., Holt, L., & Buchner, D. M. (2001). Correlates of physical activity in chronic obstructive pulmonary disease. *Nursing Research, 50*(4), 195–202.

Bulechek, G., Butcher, H., & Dochterman, J. M. (Eds). (2008). *Nursing interventions classification (NIC)* (5th ed.). St. Louis: Mosby Elsevier

Burns, S. M. (2005). Mechanical ventilation of patients with acute respiratory distress syndrome and patients requiring weaning: The evidence guiding practice. *Critical Care Nurse, 25*(4), 14–16, 18, 20–24.

Burns, S. M. (2004). The science of weaning: When and how? *Critical Care Nursing Clinics of North America, 16*(3), 379–386.

Cardin, T., & Marinelli, A. (2004). Pulmonary embolism. *Critical Care Nursing Quarterly, 27*(4), 310–324.

Caroci, A. D. S., & Lareau, S. C. (2005). Descriptors of dyspnea by patients with chronic obstructive pulmonary disease versus congestive heart failure. *Heart & Lung,* 33(2), 102–110.

Centers for Disease Control and Prevention [CDC]. (2009). *Fast facts: Asthma.* Retrieved from http://www.cdc.gov/nchs/fastats/asthma.htm

Charlebois, D. (2005). Early recognition of pulmonary embolism: The key to lowering mortality. *Journal of Cardiovascular Nursing, 20*(4), 254–259.

Chlan, L. L, Engeland, W. C., Anthony, A. & Guttormson, J. (2007). Influence of music on the stress response in patients receiving mechanical ventilatory support: A pilot study. *American Journal of Critical Care,* 16, 141–145.

Chlan, L. (2009). A review of the evidence for music intervention to manage anxiety in critically ill patients receiving mechanical ventilatory support. *Archives of Psychiatric Nursing* 23(2), 177–179.

Collins, E. G., Langbein, W. E., Fehr, L, O'Connell, S., Jelinek, C., Hagarty, E., Edwards, L., Reda, D., Tobin, M. J., & Laghi, F. (2008). Can ventilation-feedback training augment exercise tolerance in patients with COPD? *American Journal of Respiratory and Critical Care Medicine,* 177, 844–852.

Cystic Fibrosis Foundation. (2009). Home page. Retrieved from http://www.cff.org/

Deglin, J. H., & Vallerand, A. H. (2009). *Davis' Drug Guide* (10th ed.). Philadelphia: F.A. Davis.

Domino, F. J., Baldor, R. A., Golding, J., Grimes, J., & Taylor, J. S. (2010). *The 5-minute clinical consult* (18th ed.). Philadelphia: Lippincott, Williams & Wilkins.

Esmond, G., Butler, M., & McCormack, A. M. (2006). Comparison of hospital and home intravenous antibiotic therapy in adults with *cystic fibrosis. Journal of Clinical Nursing, 15*(1), 52–60.

Fiore, M. C., Jaen C. R., Baker, T. B., Bailey, W. C., Benowitz, N. L., Curry, S. J. et al. (2008). *Treating tobacco use and dependence: 2008 update.* US Public Health Service. Retrieved from http://www.surgeon-general.gov/tobacco/treating_tobacco_use08.pdf

Fishman, A. P., Elias, J. A., Fishman, J. A., Grippi, M. A., Senior, S. M., & Pack, A. J. (2008). *Fishman's pulmonary Diseases and Disorders* (4th ed.). New York: McGraw-Hill Co.

Global Lung Disease Initiative [GOLD]. (2008). *Global strategy for the diagnosis, management and prevention of chronic obstructive pulmonary disease.* Media Communications Inc. Retrieved from http://www.goldcopd.org/

Gelinas, C., Fortier, M., Viens, C., Fillion, L., & Puntillo, K. (2004). Pain assessment and management in critically ill intubated patients: A retrospective study. *American Journal of Critical Care,* 13(2), 126–135.

Grossman, S., & Grossman, L. C. (2005). Pulmonary care. Pathophysiology of cystic fibrosis: Implications for critical care nurses. *Critical Care Nurse, 25*(4), 46–51.

Huether, S. E. & McCance, K. L. (2008). *Understanding Pathophysiology* (4th ed.). St. Louis: Mosby Elsevier.

Jacobs, M. (2005). Ease the stress of managing ARDS. *Nursing Made Incredibly Easy! 3*(1), 6–15, 17–18.

Kane, C., & Galanes, S. (2004). Adult respiratory distress syndrome. *Critical Care Nursing Quarterly, 27*(4), 325–335.

Kapella, M. C., Larson, J. L., Patel, M. K., Covey, M. K., & Berry, J. K. (2006). Subjective fatigue, influencing variables, and consequences in chronic obstructive pulmonary disease. *Nursing Research,* 55(1), 10–17.

Khan, N. U. A., & Novahed, A. (2005). Pulmonary embolism and cardiac enzymes. *Heart & Lung,* 34(2), 142–146.

Lindgren, V. A., & Ames, N. J. (2005). Caring for patients on mechanical ventilation: What research indicates is best practice. *American Journal of Nursing,* 105(5), 50–61.

Markou, N. K., Myrianthefs, P. M., & Baltopoulos, G. J. (2004). Respiratory failure: An overview. *Critical Care Nursing Quarterly,* 27(4), 353–379.

Moorhead, S., Johnson, M., Maas, M., & Swanson, E. (Eds). (2008). *Nursing outcomes classification (NOC)* (4th ed.). St. Louis: Mosby Elsevier.

Mukherjee, R., & Burge, P. S. (2006). Occupational asthma. *Practice Nursing, 17*(2), 77–80.

NANDA International. (2009). *Nursing diagnoses. Definitions and classification 2009–2011.* Oxford, UK: Wilely-Blackwell.

National Center of Health Statistics [NCHS]. (2009). *Health, United States, 2008 with chartbook.* Hyattsville, MD: Author.

National Heart, Lung, and Blood Institute. (2007). National education and prevention program expert panel report 3: Guidelines for the diagnosis and management of asthma. Bethesda, MD: Author. NIH Publication No. 08-5846.

National Heart, Lung, and Blood Institute. (2009). What is ARDS? Retrieved from http://www.nhlbi.nih.gov/health/dci/Diseases/Ards/Ards_WhatIs.html

O'Leary-Kelley, C. M., Puntillo, K. A., Barr, J., Stotts, N., & Douglas, M. K. (2005). Nutritional adequacy in patients receiving mechanical ventilation who are fed enterally. *American Journal of Critical Care,* 14(3), 222–231.

Papadakis, M. A. & McPhee, S. J. (2007). *Current consult medicine 2007.* New York: McGraw-Hill.

Perrin, K. O. (2009). *Understanding the essentials of critical care nursing.* Upper Saddle River, NJ: Pearson Prentice-Hall.

Smyth, M. (2005). Acute respiratory failure, part 1. Failure in oxygenation. *American Journal of Nursing,* 105(5), Critical Care Extra, 72GG-72JJ, 72MM, 7200.

Smyth, M. (2005). Acute respiratory failure, part 2. Failure of ventilation: Exploring the other cause of acute respiratory failure. *American Journal of Nursing,* 105(6), Critical Care Extra 72AA-72DD.

Tang, B. M., Crait, J. C., Eslick, G. D., Seppelt, I. & McLean, A. S. (2009). Use of corticosteroids in acute lung injury and acute respiratory distress syndrome: A systematic review and meta-analysis. *Critical Care Medicine,* 37, 1594–1603.

Van Leeuwen, A. M., Kranpitz, T. R., Smith, L. S. (2006). *Davis' laboratory and diagnostic tests* (2nd ed.). Philadelphia: F.A. Davis.

Yang, J. C. (2005). Prevention and treatment of deep vein thrombosis and pulmonary embolism in critically ill patients. *Critical Care Nursing Quarterly,* 28(1), 72–29.

Yang, P. S., & Chen, C. H. (2005). Exercise stage and processes of change in patients with chronic obstructive pulmonary disease. *Journal of Nursing Research,* 13(2), 97–104.

Building Clinical Competence
Responses to Altered Respiratory Function

Functional Health Pattern: Activity-Exercise Patterns

Think about patients with altered activity-exercise patterns for whom you have cared in your clinical experiences.

- What were their major medical diagnoses (e.g., viral respiratory infection, sinusitis, pharyngitis, laryngeal infection, diphtheria, pertussis, respiratory trauma or obstruction, epistaxis, obstructive sleep apnea, upper respiratory tumors, bacterial respiratory infection, severe acute respiratory syndrome, lung abscess, tuberculosis, inhalation anthrax, fungal infections, lung cancer, pleuritis, pleural effusion, pneumothorax, hemothorax, inhalation injury, asthma, chronic obstructive pulmonary disease, cystic fibrosis, atelectasis, occupational lung disease, sarcoidosis, pulmonary embolism, pulmonary hypertension, respiratory failure, acute respiratory distress syndrome)?

- What kinds of manifestations did each of these patients have? Were these manifestations similar or different?

- How did the patients' healthcare behaviors interfere with their health status? Were the patients having difficulty breathing or shortness of breath? Was the breathing difficulty associated with activity levels? Was breathing more difficult when your patients were lying down? How many pillows did the patient's use at night to sleep more easily? Was breathing painful? Did your patients have a cough? Was the cough productive or nonproductive? What color or odor was the sputum? Have your patients had nosebleeds? Did your patients smoke, become exposed to second-hand smoking, or exposed to environmental chemicals? Did your patients have any medical history of respiratory disorders? Were your patients taking any medications for respiratory disorders? Did your patients use oxygen? Have your patients had a chest x-ray and a tuberculosis skin test?

The Activity-Exercise Functional Health Pattern includes disorders that result in insufficient physiologic energy to carry out activities of daily living. The respiratory system provides the cells of the body with oxygen and eliminates carbon dioxide with each respiration. The upper respiratory system is the passageway for air entering the lungs and carbon dioxide leaving the lungs. It also cleans, humidifies, and warms the entering air. The lower respiratory system is the area of exchange of oxygen and carbon dioxide in the bronchi and lungs. Activity-Exercise Functional Health Patterns are affected by the amount of gas exchange in the respiratory system and by perceived health status in two primary ways:

- Factors affecting respiration: infectious or inflammatory disorders (e.g., influenza, sinusitis, laryngitis, pertussis), respiratory trauma or obstruction (e.g., epistaxis, obstructive sleep apnea), or tumors (e.g., nasal polyps, cancer)

- Factors affecting ventilation: infections or inflammatory disorders (e.g., bronchitis, pneumonia, acute respiratory syndrome, tuberculosis), pleura disorders (e.g., pleural effusion, pneumothorax),

trauma (e.g., flail chest, pulmonary contusion), inhalation injury (e.g., smoke inhalation, near-drowning), obstructive disorders (e.g., asthma, COPD, cystic fibrosis), pulmonary vascular disorders (e.g., pulmonary embolism), or respiratory failure (e.g., acute respiratory distress syndrome)

A patent airway is necessary for effective respirations and ventilation. Upper respiratory disorders affect breathing, communication, and the patient's body image. Lower respiratory system disorders affect the ability to move air into and out of the lungs (ventilation) and the exchange of oxygen and carbon dioxide across the alveolar-capillary membrane (respiration). Therefore, respiratory disorders affect the ability to clear the airways, ventilate the lungs, and exchange gases. Respiratory disorders disturb a patient's perceived pattern of activity-exercise functional health patterns, which affects how health is managed, leading to manifestations such as the following:

- **Rhinorrhea** (*Allergens cause the release of chemicals from white blood cells in the nasal mucosa, which causes blood vessels to dilate and capillaries to leak, resulting in nasal mucosa edema and watery discharge from the nose.*)

- **Cyanosis** (*Decreased oxygen intake causes deoxygenated hemoglobin resulting in gray to blue or purple color of the skin and mucous membranes.*)

- **Wheezing** (*Bronchospasms, inflammation, or obstruction of the airway causes flow of air through a narrowed airway, resulting in high-pitched or low-pitched musical respirations.*)

Priority nursing diagnoses within the Activity-Exercise Functional Health Pattern that may be appropriate for patients include the following:

- *Ineffective Breathing Pattern* as evidenced by shortness of breath, dyspnea, orthopnea, retractions, nasal flaring, and altered chest excursion

- *Ineffective Airway Clearance* as evidenced by ineffective cough, diminished or abnormal breath sounds, cyanosis, and restlessness

- *Impaired Spontaneous Ventilation* as evidenced by dyspnea, use of accessory muscles, tachycardia, and apprehension

- *Impaired Gas Exchange* as evidenced by cyanosis, abnormal respiratory rate and rhythm, nasal flaring, tachycardia, diaphoresis, and confusion

Two nursing diagnoses from other functional health patterns often are of high priority for the patient with altered respiratory function:

- *Disturbed Sleep Pattern* (Sleep-Rest Functional Health Pattern)

- *Ineffective Therapeutic Regimen Management* (Health Perception-Health Management Functional Health Pattern)

Question

1. What did you do to facilitate breathing in your patients with respiratory disorders?

CLINICAL SCENARIO

Directions: *Read the following clinical scenarios and answer the questions that follow. To complete this exercise successfully, you will use not only knowledge of the content in this unit, but also principles related to priority setting and maintaining patient safety.*

You have been assigned to work with the following four patients for the 0700 shift on a respiratory medical-surgical unit. Significant data obtained during report is as follows:

- Jack Holt, a 65-year-old male, is admitted to the nursing unit with bacterial pneumonia. Vital signs are temperature 101°F, pulse 94, respirations 30. He is complaining of chest pain with breathing and has a productive cough of rusty-colored sputum. His pulse oximeter is reading 90% in room air.
- Maggie Sawyer is an 82-year-old female who is ready to be discharged today back to the nursing home. She is hospitalized for treatment for a deep vein thrombosis and chronic obstructive pulmonary disease (COPD). Suddenly she complains of difficulty breathing, chest pain, coughing, restlessness, and a feeling that she is going to die.
- James Mohr, a 25-year-old male, was transferred from ICU yesterday after being treated for head, neck, and chest injuries and has a tracheostomy from a motor vehicle accident. His vital signs were stable at the last assessment. He begins coughing and puts on his call light for assistance.
- Amy Campbell, a 30-year-old female, is being treated after having a severe asthma attack. Her current vital signs are temperature 99°F, pulse 64, respirations 26, and blood pressure 124/84. She has inspiratory and expiratory wheezing. Her O_2 Sat reading is 94% on 4L O_2 via nasal cannula.

Questions

Priority Setting

1. In what order would you visit these patients after report? What is the rationale for your choice.

   A. _____

   B. _____

   C. _____

   D. _____

Health Promotion

1. In planning care for Ms. Sawyer, what will you teach about nutrition for optimal respiratory function?

2. In planning care for Ms. Campbell, what will you teach her to help decrease anxiety during an asthma attack?

Nursing Process

1. What priority nursing diagnoses would you choose for each of the patients presented previously? Give the rationale for your choices.

	Nursing Diagnosis	Rationale
Jack Holt		
Maggie Sawyer		
James Mohr		
Amy Campbell		

2. Mr. Holt's bacterial pneumonia is spread by droplet infection. When using standard precautions, which equipment is necessary to prevent spread of the infection?

   A. Wear a gown when bathing the patient.

   B. Wear gown and gloves when touching the patient.

   C. Wear a mask and gloves when suctioning the patient.

   D. Wear a cap to keep hair from touching the patient.

3. If Mr. Holt is receiving percussion and vibration with postural drainage for left lower lobe pneumonia, which position most facilitates removal of secretions?

   A. semi-Fowler's position with arms elevated

   B. right Sim's position with head in Trendelenberg

   C. high-Fowler's position leaning on a bedside tray

   D. left Sim's position with head flat

4. Upon discharge, the nurse teaches Mrs. Sawyer ways to prevent having another pulmonary embolism. Which intervention is appropriate for preventing pulmonary embolism?

   A. Use pillows under the knees when in bed.

   B. Apply knee high elastic stockings when ambulating.

   C. Exercise the legs vigorously to encourage blood flow.

   D. Stop every one to two hours to stretch legs when traveling.

5. Mr. Mohr will be discharged with a tracheostomy. Which should the nurse teach the patient about tracheostomies?

   A. The tracheostomy will not interfere with lifting when returning to work.

   B. Water skiing is allowed but swimming in a pool or lake is not allowed.

   C. Showering is allowed as long as the tracheostomy is covered with a washcloth.

   D. A small amount of alcohol is allowed but smoking is not allowed.

6. Amy Campbell is instructed in the proper administration of medications for asthma. In what order is she instructed to take her medications?

   A. atrovent, cromolyn, and albuterol

   B. albuterol, atrovent, and cromolyn

   C. cromolyn, atrovent, and albuterol

   D. albuterol, cromolyn, and atrovent

Communication

1. If Ms. Campbell asks if she will have to "put up with breathing problems for the rest of her life," how will you answer her?

Delegation

1. What data collection and interventions can be delegated to a nursing assistant for each patient?

   A. _____

   B. _____

   C. _____

   D. _____

Content-Specific Questions

1. When a patient with an inhalation injury is admitted to the emergency department, which laboratory studies would you expect to obtain?
   A. arterial blood gases, carboxyhemoglobin levels, electrolytes
   B. sputum cultures and sensitivity, serology testing, sputum gram stain
   C. methemoglobin levels, venous blood gases, white blood cell count
   D. complete blood cell count, oxygen saturation, sputum specimen

2. Arterial blood gases results are ordered on a patient with acute respiratory distress. The results are pH 7.22, pO_2-50 mm Hg, pCO_2-58mm Hg, HCO_3 29-mEq/l. Which is the interpretation of these results?
   A. respiratory acidosis
   B. respiratory alkalosis
   C. metabolic acidosis
   D. metabolic alkalosis

3. Corticosteroids are ordered to decrease the inflammatory process of asthma. The patient understands how to take corticosteroids when the patient makes which comment?
   A. "Corticosteroids have very few side effects to worry about."
   B. "I understand that I can not stop taking the medication abruptly."
   C. "I can stop taking the corticosteroids as soon as I feel better."
   D. "I can take an over-the-counter medication if I develop a cold."

4. Which are early manifestations of pulmonary tuberculosis?
   A. tachypnea, tachycardia, activity intolerance
   B. bradypnea, foul-smelling sputum, weight gain
   C. blood-tinged sputum, high-grade fever, fatigue
   D. low-grade fever, night sweats, dry cough

5. The older adult is prone to respiratory problems due to which age-related changes in the respiratory system? **Select all that apply.**
   A. loss of skeletal muscle strength in the thorax
   B. increased elastic recoil of lungs during expiration
   C. alveoli are less elastic and more fibrotic
   D. decrease in residual volume of lung
   E. decreased effectiveness of coughing

CASE STUDY: Gladys Hamer

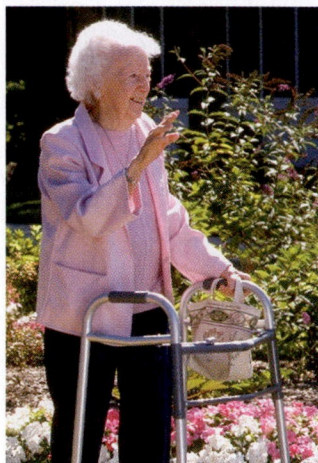

Gladys Hamer is an 83-year-old female who is seen in the emergency department with complaints of shortness of breath. Her vital signs are temperature 98.4°F, pulse 115 and irregular, respirations 35 and shallow. Her height is 63" and weight is 96 pounds. On assessment, her skin is very dry and warm. Her color is dusky. Scattered wheezes and rhonchi are heard throughout all lung fields. Her chest is hyperresonant to percussion. A pulse oximeter is applied and the O_2 Sat reading is 88%. Mrs. Hamer has a past medical history of emphysema for 10 years, complaints of shortness of breath on exertion, and has a productive chronic cough of thick greyish sputum. Her spouse passed away 5 years ago and she has lived with her two adult sons since then.

Blood is drawn for arterial blood gases and results are pH = 7.19, pO_2 = 54 mm Hg, pCO_2 = 55 mm Hg, HCO_3 = 30 mEq/l. These results indicate respiratory acidosis. Based on her current assessment, arterial blood gas results, and past medical history, a medical diagnosis of chronic obstructive pulmonary disease (COPD) is determined. COPD is a slowly progressive obstruction of the airways. The disease is one of periodic exacerbations with increased dyspnea and sputum production, leading to progressive destructive changes in the pulmonary system. The pathophysiology of emphysema is characterized by destruction of the walls of the alveoli, resulting in enlargement of abnormal air spaces. Deficiency of $alpha_1$-antitrypsin enzyme also leads to tissue destruction. Inflammatory cells that collect in the distal airway tissues lead to destruction of elastic fibers in the bronchioles and alveolar ducts. This destruction causes alveoli and air spaces to enlarge with loss of corresponding portions of the pulmonary capillary bed. The surface area for alveolar-capillary diffusion is reduced and elastic recoil is lost. The amount of air expired is reduced. This results in a mismatch between alveolar ventilation and blood flow or perfusion, leading to impaired gas exchange and further air trapping. Manifestations of COPD due to emphysema are dyspnea, tachypnea, exercise intolerance, thin and cachectic, barrel chest, prominent accessory muscles of respiration, distant or diminished breath sounds, and hyperresonant tone to percussion. Complications of COPD are severe airflow limitation that impairs quality of life and life-threatening exacerbations. When medical therapy is no longer effective, lung transplantation may be necessary to maintain life.

When planning nursing care for Mrs. Hamer, the nursing diagnosis of *Impaired Gas Exchange* related to acute and chronic lung disease is appropriate for implementing nursing interventions.

Inflammatory cells in distal airways → destruction of elastic fibers → enlargement of alveoli and air spaces, loss of pulmonary capillaries → loss of surface area for gas exchange → reduced gas diffusion; loss of elastic recoil, airway collapse → air trapping and increased residual lung volume → reduced oxygen tension in alveoli → impaired gas exchange

affects

Mrs. H.
83 y.o. female
COPD

leads to

assess

- C/o shortness of breath, fever.
- PMH emphysema X 10 yrs, exertional dyspnea, chronic cough productive of thick greyish sputum
- T 102.4°F, P 115 irreg, R 35 shallow.
- Ht 63" Wt 96 lbs.
- Skin very dry and warm, color dusky.
- Scattered wheezes and rhonchi throughout all lung fields.
- Chest hyperresonant to percussion.
- O2 sat 88%, ABGs: pH 7.19, PO2 54 mmHg, PCO2 55 mmHg, HCO3 30 mEq/l.

generates

- Ineffective Breathing Pattern as evidenced by rapid, shallow respirations
- Imbalanced Nutrition: Less than Body Requirements as evidenced by wt less than recommended for ht.
- Hyperthermia as evidenced by elevated temperature, warm, dry skin

generate nursing diagnosis   *prioritized to*

Impaired Gas Exchange

expected outcomes

- O2 sat 92% or higher
- Vital signs within normal limits for client
- Breathing improves
- Lung sounds are clear
- Consumes adequate fluids and calories without dyspnea
- Identifies measures to reduce risk of respiratory infections

evaluate

Six days after admission:
- T 99.2°F, P 93, R 22
- Skin warm, dry, and pink
- Scattered crackles in lung bases
- Consuming 100% of meals without dyspnea or fatigue
- O2 Sat 93% on supplemental oxygen, 90% on room air
- Pneumococcal and influenza vaccines administered

Interdisciplinary Interventions
- Administer supplemental oxygen at 2 L/nasal cannula as ordered.
- Encourage fluids to at least 2500 mL/day
- Administer intravenous fluids and antibiotics as ordered.
- Provide six small feedings per day, encouraging rest before and after meals.

Independent Interventions
- Teach huff cough and abdominal breathing techniques.
- Encourage to obtain pneumococcal pneumonia and influenza vaccines.
- Teach measures to reduce risk of respiratory infection: avoid contact with ill people and crowds, maintain good general health.

Activity:

1. After reviewing the concept map, is there anything you would change to make it more understandable?

2. Go to the Pearson Nursing Student Resources for this book at www.nursing.pearsonhighered.com to write a concept map using the nursing diagnosis of *Imbalanced Nutrition: Less than Body Requirements*.

See answers and hints in Appendix C.

Technique/Normal Findings	Abnormal Findings
Perform McMurray's test. While reclining, ask the patient to turn the flexed knee toward the center of the body. Stabilize the knee with one hand, and apply pressure on the lower leg with the other hand (Figure 38–12 ■). *There should be no pain or clicking.*	■ Pain, locking (inability to fully extend the knee), or a popping sound may indicate an injury to a meniscus, a disk of cartilaginous tissue in the knee.

Figure 38–12 ■ McMurray's test.

Perform the Thomas test. Ask the patient to lie down and extend one leg while bringing the knee of the opposite leg to the chest (Figure 38–13 ■). *The extended leg should not rise off the table.*	■ A hip flexion contracture will cause the extended leg to rise off the table.

Figure 38–13 ■ Thomas test for hip contracture.

SAMPLE DOCUMENTATION
Assessment of the Musculoskeletal System

58-year-old Hispanic male, employed as a roofer, comes to the orthopedic clinic for evaluation of chronic knee pain. Patient states, "The pain in my knees is worse when I get up in the morning and when I carry something heavy at work." Posture erect, gait even without obvious limp. Bones of lower extremities appear equal in size and shape bilaterally. No swelling noted, bulge test negative for fluid around knee. Crepitus heard in both knees during flexion and extension. ROM in both knees slightly decreased. No obvious decrease in muscle mass. Patient states knee pain during ROM is a 3 on a 1 to 10 scale. Referred to clinic physician for further evaluation, including x-rays of both knees.

TEST YOURSELF NCLEX-RN® REVIEW

1. A patient has an epiphyseal fracture. Based on this information, what classification of bone is involved?
   1. irregular
   2. flat
   3. long
   4. short

2. The nurse is asking a patient to move an extremity away from the body midline. What is being assessed?
   1. abduction
   2. adduction
   3. extension
   4. flexion

3. A patient with gout asks a nurse, "Why is my blood being examined for uric acid?" What would be the most accurate response?
   1. "A uric acid test is done to see if your gout medication is effective."
   2. "A uric acid test is done to diagnose rheumatoid arthritis."
   3. "Do you have a family history of muscle or bone disease?"
   4. "Tell me how you got that big bruise on your hip."

4. What age woman would be most likely to have a bone density examination?
   1. teenager
   2. woman in her 20s
   3. woman in her 30s
   4. woman in her 60s

5. With aging, bone mass and calcium absorption decrease. What risk is increased as a result?
   1. obesity
   2. weakness
   3. fractures
   4. deformity

6. What would a nurse ask a patient to do in order to assess facial muscle strength?
   1. "Close your eyes tightly."
   2. "Stick out your tongue."
   3. "Bend your head forward."
   4. "Open your eyes widely."

7. A nurse is documenting a grating sound when a joint is moved. What term would be used?
   1. crackles
   2. arthritis
   3. synovitis
   4. crepitation

8. While conducting the ballottement test, a nurse notes that the patella rebounds against her fingers. What does this finding indicate?
   1. deformity of the elbow
   2. infection of the metatarsals
   3. fluid in the knee joint
   4. crepitus in the hip joint

9. During the physical assessment of a young adult, the nurse notes a lateral, S-shaped curve of the spine. What is the name of this condition?
   1. lordosis
   2. scoliosis
   3. kyphosis
   4. musclosis

10. What are the most common manifestations of musculoskeletal disorders?
    1. pain and limited mobility
    2. swelling and exaggerated reflexes
    3. cyanosis and decreased pulses
    4. pallor and decreased ROM

See Test Yourself answers in Appendix C.

Pearson Nursing Student Resources

Find additional review materials at
www.nursing.pearsonhighered.com

Prepare for success with additional NCLEX®-style practice questions, interactive assignments and activities, Web links, animations and videos, and more!

BIBLIOGRAPHY

Armstrong, J., & Mitchell, E. (2008). Comprehensive nursing assessment in the care of older people. *Nursing Older People, (20)*1, 36–38.

Assessment of a limb in a cast. (2003). *Nursing Times, 99*(31), 27.

Bickley, L., & Szilagyi, P. (2005). *Bates' guide to physical examination and history taking* (9th ed.). Philadelphia: Lippincott.

Burrow, J., & McLarnon, N. (2004). Foot assessment: Recognizing potential problems. *Nursing & Residential Care, 6*(2), 68–71.

Cole, E. (2004). Assessment and management of the trauma patient. *Nursing Standard, 18*(41), 45–52, 54.

Della-Giustina, D., & Nolan, R. (2004). Evaluation and management of low back pain. *Emergency Medicine, 36*(7), 20–26, 27–28.

Eliopoulos, E. (2005). *Gerontological nursing* (6th ed.). Philadelphia: Lippincott Williams & Wilkins.

Kee, J. (2009). *Prentice Hall handbook of laboratory & diagnostic tests with nursing implications* (6th ed). Upper Saddle River, NJ: Prentice Hall.

National Institute of Health. (2008). *Genes and disease: Muscle and bone.* Retrieved from http://www.ncbi.nlm.nih.gov/books/bookres.fegi/gnd/pdf.html

Porth, C. (2007). *Essentials of pathophysiology: Concepts of altered health states* (2nd ed.). Philadelphia: Lippincott Williams & Wilkins.

Porth, C., & Matfin, G. (2009). *Pathophysiology: Concepts of altered health states* (8th ed.). Philadelphia: Lippincott Williams & Wilkins.

Weber, J., & Kelley, J. (2009). *Health assessment in nursing* (4th ed.). Philadelphia: Lippincott Williams & Wilkins.

CHAPTER 39

Nursing Care of Patients with Musculoskeletal Trauma

LEARNING OUTCOMES

1. Compare and contrast the causes, risk factors, pathophysiology, manifestations, interdisciplinary care, and nursing care of contusions, strains, sprains, joint dislocations, and fractures.
2. Describe the pathophysiology, interdisciplinary care, and nursing care for repetitive use injuries: carpal tunnel syndrome, bursitis, and epicondylitis.
3. Describe the stages of bone healing.
4. Explain the pathophysiology, manifestations, and related treatment for complications of bone fractures: compartment syndrome, fat embolism syndrome, deep venous thrombosis, infection, delayed union and nonunion, and complex regional pain syndrome.
5. Discuss the purposes and related nursing interventions for casts, fixation devices, traction, and stump care.
6. Explain the causes, levels, types, and potential complications (infection, delayed healing, chronic stump pain, phantom pain, and contractures) of an amputation.

CLINICAL COMPETENCIES

1. Assess functional health status of patients with musculoskeletal injuries, and recognize, monitor, document, and report abnormal or unexpected findings.
2. Use evidence-based research to plan and implement nursing care for patients who have experienced musculoskeletal trauma.
3. Determine priority nursing diagnoses, based on assessed data, to plan and implement individualized nursing interventions for patients with musculoskeletal injuries.
4. Provide skilled care for patients with a cast, fixation device, traction, or amputation, maintaining patient and caregiver safety at all times.
5. Coordinate and integrate interdisciplinary care into care of patients with musculoskeletal trauma.
6. Provide teaching appropriate for prevention and self-care of traumatic injuries of the musculoskeletal system.
7. Revise plan of care as needed to provide effective interventions to promote, maintain, or restore functional health status to patients with traumatic injuries of the musculoskeletal system.

KEY TERMS

amputation, *1328*
compartment syndrome, *1310*
contracture, *1330*
contusion, *1305*

dislocation, *1306*
fat embolism syndrome (FES), *1311*
flail chest, *1321*
fracture, *1309*

phantom limb pain, *1330*
sprain, *1305*
strain, *1305*
subluxation, *1306*

Musculoskeletal trauma is an injury to muscle, bone, or soft tissue that results from excessive external force. The external force transmits more kinetic energy than the tissue can absorb, and injury results. The severity of the trauma depends not only on the amount of force but also on the location of the impact, because different parts of the body can withstand different amounts of force. A wide variety of external forces can cause trauma, and the force involved can vary in severity (e.g., a step off the curb, a fall, being tackled in a football game, and a motor vehicle crash). ∞ See Chapter 11 for a detailed discussion of the results of different forces and types of injury from trauma.

Traumatic musculoskeletal injuries include blunt tissue trauma, alterations in tendons and ligaments, and fractures of bones. Various forces that cause musculoskeletal trauma are typical for a specific environment, activity, or age group. For example, motorcycle crashes resulting in fractures of the distal tibia, midshaft femur, and radius are common in young men.

Sports injuries, resulting from either overuse or acute trauma, are seen more often in adolescents and young adults. Falls are the most common cause of injury in people aged 65 or older, with fractures of the vertebrae, proximal humerus, and hip seen most often (Porth & Matfin, 2009). Regardless of the cause, the injury may require rehabilitation and temporary or permanent changes in lifestyle.

Musculoskeletal trauma can result in mild or severe injuries. A patient may experience a soft tissue injury, a fracture, and/or a complete amputation. In addition, trauma to one part of the musculoskeletal system often produces dysfunction in adjacent structures. For example, a fracture of the femur prevents the adjacent muscles from abducting and adducting. Nursing care helps minimize the effects of trauma, prevents complications, and hastens restoration of function. This chapter discusses fractures, amputations, soft tissue injuries, dislocations, and repetitive use injuries.

Traumatic Injuries of the Muscles, Ligaments, and Joints

The Patient with a Contusion, Strain, or Sprain

Contusions, strains, and sprains are among the most commonly reported injuries. They account for about 50% of work-related injuries, with lower back injuries being the most commonly reported occupational injury. However, many sprains and strains are not work related and often are not reported. The lower back and cervical region of the spine are the most common sites for muscle strains; the ankle is the most commonly sprained joint, usually caused by forced inversion of the foot.

Pathophysiology and Manifestations

A **contusion**, the least serious form of musculoskeletal injury, is bleeding into soft tissue that results from a blunt force, such as a kick or striking a body part against a hard object. The skin remains intact, but small blood vessels rupture and bleed into soft tissues. A contusion with a large amount of bleeding is referred to as a hematoma. The manifestations of a contusion include swelling and discoloration of the skin. The blood in the soft tissue initially results in a purple and blue color commonly referred to as a *bruise*. As the blood begins to reabsorb, the area involved becomes brown and then yellow until it disappears.

A **strain** is a stretching injury to a muscle or a muscle-tendon unit caused by mechanical overloading. A muscle that is forced to extend past its elasticity will develop microscopic tears. Lifting heavy objects without bending the knees, or a sudden acceleration-deceleration, as in a motor vehicle crash, can cause strains. Common sites for a muscle strain are the lower back and the hamstring muscle in the back of the thigh. The manifestations of a strain include pain, limited motion, muscle spasms, swelling, and possible muscle weakness. Severe strains that partially or completely tear the muscle or tendon can be disabling with significant bleeding, swelling, and bruising around the muscle.

A **sprain** is a stretch and/or tear of one or more ligaments surrounding a joint. Forces going in opposite directions cause the ligament to overstretch and/or tear. The ligaments may be partially or completely torn. Although any joint may be involved, sprains of the ankle and knee are most common, with more than

25,000 people spraining an ankle each day in the United States (National Institute of Arthritis and Musculoskeletal and Skin Diseases [NIAMS], 2009). Manifestations include loss of the functional ability of the joint, a feeling of a "pop" or tear, discoloration, pain, and rapid swelling. Motion increases the joint pain. The intensity of the manifestations depends on the severity of the sprain. Grades of sprain severity are presented in Table 39–1.

Interdisciplinary Care

The goal of the initial stage of treating soft tissue trauma is to reduce swelling and pain. Patients should follow a regimen of rest, ice, compression, and elevation for the first 24 to 48 hours (see Table 39–2).

> **MEMORY CUE**
> Use the acronym RICE to remember initial measures to treat a musculoskeletal injury:
> **R**est
> **I**ce
> **C**ompression
> **E**levation

When soft tissue trauma occurs, x-rays are taken to rule out fracture, and magnetic resonance imaging (MRI) may be done to determine the extent of tissue damage. Nonsteroidal anti-inflammatory drugs (NSAIDs) are used to reduce pain, swelling, and inflammation associated with the injury.

Ankle sprains may be immobilized with a cast or splint, with no limitations on weight bearing. A knee injury often requires a knee immobilizer. If an upper extremity is injured, a sling is provided. Surgery to repair the torn ligaments, muscle, or tendons may be required for severe sprains or strains. Physical therapy may be recommended for rehabilitation. Time required for healing depends on the severity of the injury; for example, a mild ankle sprain may require up to 3 to 6 weeks of rehabilitation, whereas a severe sprain may require up to 8 to 12 months to return to full activities (NIAMS, 2009).

TABLE 39–1 Grades of Sprain Severity

GRADE	DESCRIPTION	MANIFESTATIONS
Grade 1 (mild)	Overstretching or minimal tear of ligaments with no joint instability	■ Mild pain, swelling, tenderness ■ Little or no bruising ■ Minimal or no loss of joint function or ability to bear weight
Grade 2 (moderate)	Partial tear of the ligament	■ Moderate pain, bruising, and swelling ■ Mild to moderate joint instability, functional disability ■ Weight bearing difficult
Grade 3 (severe)	Complete tear or rupture of the ligament	■ Severe pain, swelling, and bruising ■ Significant functional loss and joint instability ■ Inability to bear weight

TABLE 39–2 RICE Therapy for Musculoskeletal Injuries

ACTION	PATIENT AND FAMILY EDUCATION
Rest	■ Decrease regular activities of daily living and exercise as needed. ■ Limit weight bearing on the injured extremity for 48 hours. ■ If you use a cane or crutch to avoid weight bearing, use it on the uninjured side so you can lean away from and relieve weight on the injured leg.
Ice	■ To avoid cold injury or frostbite, apply an ice pack to the injured area for no more than 20 minutes at a time, four to eight times a day. ■ An ice bag, cold pack, plastic bag filled with crushed ice and wrapped in a towel, or a bag of frozen peas may be used.
Compression	■ Loosen the compression bandage if you experience numbness, tingling, or swelling distal to the injury, or if the distal extremity becomes cool or cyanotic (bluish-grey). ■ Examples of compression bandages include Ace wraps, special boots, air casts, and splints.
Elevation	■ Keep the injured extremity elevated on a pillow above heart level to help reduce swelling and pain.

∞ Nursing Care

The nursing care of each patient is individualized. A strain or sprain may not be as devastating to an attorney as it is to a professional athlete; therefore, the nurse should determine what the injury means to the particular patient.

Nursing Diagnoses and Interventions

Nursing diagnoses focus on providing information about self-care to decrease pain and return physical mobility to preinjury levels.

Acute Pain

The pain that results from soft tissue trauma is due primarily to the injury to the muscle or ligament and secondarily to bleeding and edema at the injury site.

■ Teach the patient to use RICE (rest, ice, compression, elevation) therapy to care for the injury. *The interventions included in RICE therapy allow the injured muscle, ligament or tendon to heal (rest), cause vasoconstriction and reduce pain (ice), decrease edema formation and pain (compression), and promote venous return to decrease edema and pain (elevation).*

Impaired Physical Mobility

Pain causes the patient to avoid using or bearing weight with the injured extremity. Always observe the patient's use of assistive devices; if the device is inappropriate, the patient can face a greater risk of falling. Also consider that the device may be appropriate, but the patient may not be using it correctly or safely. As a person ages, muscle mass in the upper extremities declines. As a result, the older patient with a sprained ankle may not be able to use crutches, because crutches require that the person distribute body weight along the upper extremities. Therefore, older patients may find a walker more useful.

■ Teach the correct use of crutches, walkers, canes, or slings if prescribed. *Use of the correct technique increases safety and encourages use of these devices.*

■ Encourage follow-up care. *Severe sprains may require further evaluation to determine if surgical intervention is indicated.*

The Patient with Joint Trauma

The synovial joints of the upper and lower extremities can be subjected to injury from trauma as a result of recreational activities or accidents.

Pathophysiology and Manifestations

Joint trauma affects the joint structure itself or the soft tissues supporting the joint.

Rotator Cuff Injuries

The shoulder joint is particularly vulnerable to injuries because of a combination of factors, including its wide range of motion, its complexity as a joint, and its exposed position. Most shoulder problems result from rotator cuff injuries. The rotator cuff is the group of muscles that control arm movement. Rotator cuff disorders include tendinitis, bursitis, and partial and complete muscle tears. These injuries can be acute or may result from repetitive use injury or degenerative changes of the involved tissues.

Manifestations of rotator cuff damage include shoulder pain, which may be worse at night or when lying on the involved shoulder. Range of motion, abduction and flexion in particular often is limited.

Knee Injuries

The knee is vulnerable to ligament tears, meniscal injury, and patellar dislocation. These injuries frequently are associated with sports activities that lead to falls or abnormal twisting of the knee joint. The menisci are two C-shaped plates of cartilage within each knee joint. A tear of the medial meniscus is a common knee injury. The patella, or knee cap, can become partially or completely dislocated.

The patient with a knee injury often relates a history of an acute injury, with immediate pain, a tearing or popping sensation, or the knee "giving out." Swelling of the affected joint may develop immediately or over several hours after the injury.

Joint Dislocation

A **dislocation** is an injury in which the ends of bones are displaced out of their normal position and joint articulation is lost. Dislocations usually follow trauma such as a fall or blow. They commonly occur during contact sports such as football or from falls resulting from activities such as skiing. Pathologic dislocations result from disease of the joint, including infection, rheumatoid arthritis, paralysis, and neuromuscular diseases.

Although dislocations may occur in any joint, they occur most frequently in the shoulder and acromioclavicular joints. A **subluxation** is a partial dislocation in which the bones of the joint remain in partial contact.

Dislocation causes pain, deformity, and limited motion of the affected joint.

Interdisciplinary Care

Care of the patient with a joint injury focuses on relieving pain, managing or correcting the resulting disorder, and preventing complications. The history and physical often are sufficient to identify joint trauma. Specific examination maneuvers may be performed. X-rays of the affected joint are obtained; an MRI also may be performed.

Treatment

Treatment is dictated by the type of injury. A dislocation is usually *reduced* (bone ends realigned) using manual traction. If closed reduction fails, surgery may be necessary to realign the joint and prevent complications such as neurovascular injury.

Dislocations of the shoulder joint usually can be managed with closed reduction and a limited period of post-reduction immobilization. A dislocated hip requires immediate reduction to prevent necrosis of the femoral head and injury to the sciatic and femoral nerves. After reduction, the patient is placed on bed rest for several days or even weeks. If a hip dislocation is accompanied by a fracture, the patient will undergo surgery to increase mobility, decrease complications, and rapidly stabilize the joint.

Treatment for rotator cuff injuries usually is conservative, including joint rest, NSAIDs, moist heat, and, for persistent problems, physical therapy. Some patients require surgery to repair a torn rotator cuff.

Joint rest, with compression, ice, elevation, and restricted weight bearing, are initially prescribed for knee injuries. Physical therapy is ordered during rehabilitation. Patients with recurrent pain, swelling, or injuries may require surgery to repair the joint damage.

✍ Nursing Care

Nursing care of the patient with joint trauma is individualized to the cause of injury and the age of the patient. It is important to teach patients to seek immediate medical attention for a joint dislocation, to splint the joint to prevent further damage, and to put ice on the injured joint.

Assessment

- *Health history:* History of trauma, including circumstances of injury if known; pain, including location, character, timing, and activities or movements that aggravate or relieve it; history of prior musculoskeletal injuries; chronic illnesses; medications.
- *Physical assessment:* Compare the position, color, size, and temperature of the affected joint to the corresponding unaffected joint. Palpate for tenderness, crepitus, temperature, and swelling. Instruct the patient or assist to move the joint through its normal range of motion, stopping and noting where pain is experienced. Do not move the affected joint beyond that point. When a joint dislocation is suspected, assess color, temperature, pulses, movement, and sensation of the limb distal to the affected joint.

Nursing Diagnoses and Interventions

Nursing diagnoses focus on relieving pain and preventing complications.

Risk for Injury

The patient with a dislocation requires frequent assessments to ensure that neurovascular compromise does not develop.

- Monitor neurovascular status by assessing the 5 "P's": pain, pulses, pallor, paralysis, and paresthesia. *Neurovascular compromise is indicated by increased pain, decreased or absent pulses, pale skin with decreased capillary refill, inability to move a body part or extremity, and changes in sensation (such as "pins and needles" sensations, or loss of sense of sharp/dull touch).*
- Maintain immobilization as ordered after reduction. *Immobilization prevents the joint from dislocating again.*

Acute Pain

- Encourage use of an appropriate splint or joint immobilizer. *Splinting maintains joint alignment and reduces pain and inflammation.*
- Teach safe application of ice or heat to the affected joint as indicated. *Ice causes vasoconstriction and numbs the tender area; heat decreases swelling by increasing venous return. Inappropriately applied, both ice and heat can damage tissues.*
- Instruct about using NSAIDs as ordered. *Taken on a regular basis (not as needed for pain), NSAIDs decrease swelling and inflammation, reducing pain.*
- Teach use of assistive devices such as a sling, crutches, or cane to reduce stress on the affected joint or minimize weight bearing. *When used appropriately, assistive devices help minimize use of and stress on the affected joint, promoting joint rest and healing. When used inappropriately, these assistive devices can increase the risk of further injury or damage.*

Impaired Physical Mobility

- Refer to physical therapy for appropriate exercises. *The physical therapist can teach exercises to strengthen supportive joint tissues and maintain joint mobility.*
- Suggest occupational therapy. *Occupational therapy can help the patient learn new ways to perform tasks to prevent recurring symptoms.*

Community-Based Care

Teach about the specific joint injury or disorder and its causes and treatments. Joint injuries often tend to be recurring for patients actively participating in contact sports and other vigorous physical activities. Prolonged immobilization (for several weeks after the injury) and aggressive rehabilitation following the initial injury can reduce the risk of recurrent problems. The following topics should be addressed in preparing the patient for community-based care:

- Importance of complying with the prescribed length of immobilization
- Skin care and ways to prevent skin-to-skin contact, particularly in the axillary area

- Prescribed rehabilitation exercises to strengthen muscles and other supportive structures in the affected joint, decreasing the risk of future trauma
- Alternatives to activities that precipitate recurrent trauma
- Instructions or referrals to physical therapy if needed for further teaching about using assistive devices
- Referrals to physical and occupational therapy and home health services as needed

The Patient with a Repetitive Use Injury

Repeatedly twisting and turning the wrist, pronating and supinating the forearm, kneeling, or raising arms over the head can result in repetitive use injuries. Patients with repetitive use injuries pose a challenge to the healthcare team. Often these patients appear puzzled as they relate a history of manifestations that have worsened over time. They deny abrupt trauma and often worry about the ability to return to work. Repetitive use injuries are common. The number of worker's compensation claims for these types of injuries is steadily growing, with the increase believed to be a result of technology advances in the workplace.

Pathophysiology

Common repetitive use injuries include carpal tunnel syndrome, bursitis, and epicondylitis.

Carpal Tunnel Syndrome

The carpal tunnel is a canal through which flexor tendons and the median nerve pass from the wrist to the hand. The syndrome develops from narrowing of the tunnel and irritation of the median nerve. Carpal tunnel syndrome involves compression of the median nerve as a result of inflammation and swelling of the synovial lining of the tendon sheaths. The patient complains of numbness and tingling of the thumb, index finger, and lateral ventral surface of the middle finger. The patient may also complain of pain in this area that interferes with sleep and is alleviated by shaking or massaging the hand and fingers. The affected hand may become weak and the patient may be unable to hold utensils or perform activities that require precision.

Carpal tunnel syndrome is one of the three most common work-related injuries. The incidence is believed to be related directly to the number of people using computers. The incidence of carpal tunnel syndrome is higher in women, especially postmenopausal women.

Bursitis

Bursitis is an inflammation of a bursa. A bursa is an enclosed sac found between muscles, tendons, and bony prominences. The bursae that commonly become inflamed are in the shoulder, hip, knee, and elbow. Constant friction between the bursa and the musculoskeletal tissue around it causes irritation, edema, and inflammation. Manifestations develop as the sac becomes engorged. The area around the sac is tender, and extension and flexion of the joint near the bursa produce pain. The inflamed bursa is hot, red, and edematous. The patient guards the joint to decrease pain and may point to the area of the bursa when identifying joint tenderness.

Epicondylitis

Epicondylitis is the inflammation of the tendon at its point of origin into the humerus. Epicondylitis is also referred to as *tennis elbow* or *golfer's elbow*. The exact pathophysiology of epicondylitis is unknown. Current theories attribute inflammation of the tendon to microvascular trauma. Tears, bleeding, and edema are thought to cause avascularization (lack of blood supply) and calcification of the tendon. Manifestations of epicondylitis include point tenderness, pain radiating down the dorsal surface of the forearm, and a history of repetitive use.

Interdisciplinary Care

Medical management of repetitive use disorders focuses on relieving pain and increasing mobility. Once the diagnosis is made, treatment can range from conservative measures, such as rest, medications, and physical therapy, to aggressive measures such as surgery.

Diagnosis

Carpal tunnel syndrome is diagnosed by the patient's history and physical examination. The history may reveal an occupation that involves areas such as computer work, jackhammer operation, mechanical work, or gymnastics. History of a radial bone fracture or rheumatoid arthritis also increases the risk of carpal tunnel syndrome. Tests specific for carpal tunnel include the Phalen's test (∞ see Chapter 38). Ultrasound or magnetic resonance imaging (MRI), electromyography (EMG), and nerve conduction studies may be done to confirm the diagnosis. Bursitis and epicondylitis are diagnosed by history and physical examination.

Medications

The patient with a repetitive use injury usually receives NSAIDs. Narcotics also may be administered for acute flare-ups and severe pain. For the patient who has epicondylitis or carpal tunnel syndrome, corticosteroids may be injected into the joint.

Treatments

Initial treatment for repetitive use injuries is conservative, followed, if necessary, by surgery.

CONSERVATIVE MANAGEMENT   The first steps in the care of all repetitive use injuries are to immobilize and rest the involved joint. The joint may be splinted, and ice may be applied (as described in Table 39–2) in the first 24 to 48 hours to decrease pain and inflammation. Ice application may be followed by heat application every 4 hours.

SURGERY   Surgery is usually reserved for the patient who does not obtain relief with conservative treatment. Surgery for carpal tunnel syndrome includes resection of the carpal ligament to enlarge the tunnel. In epicondylitis and bursitis, calcified deposits may be removed from the area surrounding the tendon or bursa.

✍ Nursing Care

The nursing care of a patient with a repetitive use injury focuses on relieving pain, teaching about the disease process and treatment, and improving physical mobility.

Nursing Diagnoses and Interventions

Acute Pain

Swelling and nerve inflammation cause pain in the patient with a repetitive use injury.

- Ask the patient to rate the pain on a scale of 0 to 10 (with 10 being the most severe pain) before and after any intervention. *This facilitates objective assessment of the effectiveness of the chosen pain relief strategy.*
- Encourage the use of immobilizers. *Splinting maintains joint alignment and prevents pain due to movement of inflamed tissues.*
- Teach the patient to apply ice and/or heat as prescribed. *Ice causes vasoconstriction and decreases the pooling of blood in the inflamed area. Ice may also numb the tender area. Heat decreases swelling by increasing venous return.*
- Encourage use of NSAIDs as prescribed. *NSAIDs decrease swelling by inhibiting prostaglandins and interrupting the inflammatory process.*
- Explain why treatment should not be abruptly discontinued. *Abrupt discontinuation of treatment may cause reinflammation of the injured area.*

Impaired Physical Mobility

Joint pain and swelling can limit range of motion of the affected joint.

- Suggest interventions to alleviate pain (such as using an immobilizer and taking pain medications). *If the joint is pain free, the patient will be more likely to take an active role in therapy.*
- Refer to a physical therapist for exercises. *The physical therapist can assist the patient with exercise to prevent joint stiffness.*
- Suggest consultation with an occupational therapist. *Occupational therapy can help the patient learn new ways to perform tasks to prevent recurring symptoms.*

Community-Based Care

Address the following topics for home care:

- Causes of and treatments for repetitive use injury.
- Rehabilitation to allow the patient to return to a state of independence.
- Ways to avoid unnecessary exposure to the activities that increase risk of redeveloping the injury. Suggest evaluation of the patient's work environment by an environmental risk manager who can prescribe measures to reduce the risk of repetitive use injuries. Wrist supports or an ergonomic keyboard may be useful for the patient who uses a computer extensively. Appropriate desk and chair height also are important in maintaining the correct anatomic position while working.
- Information about sources for braces or other assistive devices.

Traumatic Injuries of Bones

The Patient with a Fracture

A **fracture** is any break in the continuity of a bone. Fractures vary in severity according to the location and the type of fracture. Although fractures occur in all age groups, they are more common in people who have sustained trauma and in older patients.

Pathophysiology

Any of the 206 bones in the body can be fractured. A fracture occurs when the bone is subjected to more kinetic energy than it can absorb. Fractures may result from a direct blow, a crushing force (compression), a sudden twisting motion (torsion), a severe muscle contraction, or disease that has weakened the bone (called a *stress* or *pathologic fracture*). Two basic mechanisms produce fractures: direct force and indirect force. With direct force, the kinetic energy is applied at or near the site of the fracture. The bone cannot withstand the force. With indirect force, the kinetic energy is transmitted from the point of impact to a site where the bone is weaker. The fracture occurs at the weaker point.

Fractures in adults are classified in the following ways:

- If the skin is intact, the fracture is considered a *closed (simple) fracture*. If the skin integrity is interrupted, the fracture is considered an *open (compound) fracture* (Figure 39–1 ■). An open fracture allows bacteria to enter the injured area and increases the risk of complications.
- *Complete* fractures involve the entire width of the bone (Figure 39–2 ■), whereas *incomplete* fractures involve only a part of the width of the bone.

- The fracture line may be *oblique* (at an angle to the bone) or *spiral* (curves around the bone). An *avulsed* fracture occurs when the fracture pulls bone and other tissues away from the point of attachment. Fractures may also be described as *comminuted* (the bone breaks in many pieces), *compressed* (the bone is crushed), *impacted* (the broken bone ends are forced into each other), or *depressed* (the broken bone is forced inward).

Figure 39–1 ■ *A,* An open fracture. *B,* A closed fracture.

Hip Fracture Animation

Figure 39–2 ■ Types of fractures. *A*, A complete fracture. *B*, An incomplete (Greenstick) fracture. *C*, An oblique fracture. *D*, A comminuted fracture.

- A *stable* (nondisplaced) fracture is one in which the bones maintain their anatomic alignment. An *unstable* (displaced) fracture occurs when the bones move out of correct anatomic alignment. If a fracture is displaced, immediate interventions are required to prevent further damage to soft tissue, muscle, and bone.

    Fractures may also be classified by point of reference on the bone, such as midshaft, middle third, and distal third. The point of reference may also be specific, such as intra-articular or diaphyseal.

Fracture Healing

Fracture healing progresses over four phases: hematoma formation, fibrocartilaginous callus formation, bony callus formation, and remodeling. (See the Pathophysiology Illustrated feature on pages 1312–1313.) When a bone fractures, bleeding and tissue damage at the site of the fracture initiate an inflammatory response. A hematoma forms between the fractured bone ends and around the bone surfaces. The fractured bone surfaces and fragments are deprived of oxygen and nutrients, leading to localized cellular necrosis, which heightens the inflammatory response and release of inflammatory mediators. These chemicals in turn cause vasodilation and edema. Fibroblasts, lymphocytes, and macrophages migrate to the fracture site, and fibroblasts within the hematoma form a fibrin meshwork. Lymphocytes and macrophages wall off the area, localizing and containing the inflammation.

    Within 48 hours, fibroblasts and new capillaries growing into the fracture form granulation tissue that gradually replaces the hematoma. Phagocytes remove cell debris. Osteoblasts (bone-forming cells) migrate to the fracture site, where they

Repair of a Fracture Animation

build a web of collagen fibers from both sides of the fractured bone. Chondroblasts lay down patches of cartilage as a base for bone growth. This fibrocartilaginous callus connects bone fragments, splinting the fracture and maintaining bone alignment. It cannot yet, however, support weight bearing.

    The third stage of fracture healing, bony callus formation, begins 3 to 4 weeks after the injury and continues for 2 to 3 months. Osteoblasts continue to form collagen fibers and bone matrix, which are gradually mineralized with calcium and mineral salts. Osteoclasts migrate to the repair site to remove damaged and excess bone in the callus. Fibrocartilaginous callus is gradually replaced with spongy bone. This process progresses from the outer surface of the bone toward the fracture site.

    In the final phase of healing, remodeling, excess callus is removed and new bone is laid down along the fracture line. As the bone heals and again is subjected to the mechanical stress of everyday use, osteoblasts and osteoclasts remodel the repair site along the lines of force. Spongy bone is replaced by compact bone, and the remodeled area closely resembles the original, unbroken bone.

    The age, physical condition of the patient, and the type of fracture influence healing. Other factors, both local and systemic, also influence bone healing either positively or negatively (Box 39–1). Healing time varies with the individual. An uncomplicated fracture of the arm or foot can heal in 6 to 8 weeks. A fractured vertebra will take at least 12 weeks to heal. Healing of a fractured hip may take from 12 to 16 weeks.

Manifestations

Fractures are often accompanied by soft tissue injuries that involve muscles, arteries, veins, nerves, or skin. The degree of soft tissue involvement depends on the amount of energy or force transmitted to the area. Fracture manifestations and their causes are outlined in the Pathophysiology Linkage box on page 1311.

Complications

Complications of musculoskeletal trauma include pressure from edema and hemorrhage, development of fat emboli, deep venous thrombosis, infection, impaired healing, or disruption of neural transmission.

Compartment Syndrome

Muscles, nerves, and blood vessels of the extremities are enclosed by a fibrous membrane or fascia. The fascia, which is nonexpendable, supports these tissues. **Compartment syndrome** occurs when pressure within this confined space constricts and entraps the structures within it. Acute compartment syndrome

BOX 39–1 Factors Influencing Bone Healing

Positive Factors

Local
- Immobilization
- Timely correction of displacement
- Application of ice
- Electrical stimulation

Systemic
- Adequate amounts of growth hormone, vitamin D, and calcium
- Adequate blood supply
- Absence of infection or diseases
- Younger age
- Moderate activity level prior to injury

Negative Factors

Local
- Delay in correction of displacement
- Open fracture (increases risk of infection)
- Presence of foreign body at fracture site

Systemic
- Immunocompromised status
- Decreased circulation (as in diabetes or peripheral vascular disease)
- Malnutrition
- Osteoporosis
- Advanced age

MANIFESTATIONS of Compartment Syndrome

EARLY MANIFESTATIONS
- Pain
- Normal or decreased peripheral pulse

LATER MANIFESTATIONS
- Cyanosis
- Tingling, loss of sensation (paresthesias)
- Weakness (paresis)
- Severe pain, especially when the extremity is passively flexed

may result from hemorrhage and edema within the compartment following a fracture or from a crush injury, or from external compression of the limb by a cast that is too tight.

Compression of nerves within the compartment causes severe pain, paresthesias (burning, tingling, or loss of sensation), and diminished reflexes. Entrapment of the blood vessels limits tissue perfusion, beginning a cycle of events that may result in the loss of the limb. Inadequate oxygen supply causes cellular acidosis, which intensifies as cellular energy requirements are met through anaerobic metabolism. The capillaries inside the compartment dilate in an attempt to increase the supply of blood and oxygen. Additional blood and oxygen are not available, and plasma proteins leak out into the interstitial tissues. The interstitial tissue then pulls fluid in to balance the protein load. As a result, edema within the compartment increases. The edema

causes further compression of the vascular network, and the cycle continues. Uninterrupted, this cycle threatens the patient's limb and increases the risk of sepsis. Acute renal failure also is a risk if pressure is unrelieved, as the breakdown of muscle cells releases myoglobin, a protein toxic to the kidney tubules.

Compartment syndrome usually develops within the first 48 hours of injury, when edema is at its peak. Manifestations of compartment syndrome are listed in the box above. It is important to note that arterial pulses may remain normal, even when pressure within the compartment is high enough to significantly impair tissue perfusion.

If compartment syndrome develops, interventions to alleviate pressure are implemented. Restrictive dressings are removed or a tight-fitting cast is split. *Fasciotomy*, surgical incision of the muscle fascia to relieve pressure within the compartment, may be necessary. After a fasciotomy, the incision is left open, leading to a potential infection risk.

Volkmann's contracture, an uncommon complication of elbow or forearm fractures, can result from unresolved compartment syndrome. Arterial blood flow decreases, leading to ischemia, degeneration, and contracture of forearm muscles. The severity of Volkmann contracture varies from mild, limited to wrist flexors, to severe, affecting both flexor and extensor muscles of the forearm (Kare, 2008).

Fat Embolism Syndrome

Fat emboli occur when fat globules lodge in the pulmonary vascular bed or peripheral circulation. **Fat embolism syndrome (FES)** is characterized by neurologic dysfunction, pulmonary insufficiency, and a petechial rash on the chest, axilla, and

PATHOPHYSIOLOGY LINKAGE   Manifestations of Fractures

MANIFESTATION	PATHOPHYSIOLOGY
Deformity	Abnormal position of bones secondary to fracture and muscles pulling on fractured bone
Swelling	Edema from localization of serous fluid and bleeding
Pain/tenderness	Muscle spasm, direct tissue trauma, nerve pressure, movement of fractured bone
Numbness	Nerve damage or nerve entrapment
Guarding	Pain
Crepitus	Grating of bones or entrance of air in an open fracture. Note: Do not manipulate the extremity to elicit crepitus; doing so may cause additional damage.
Hypovolemic shock	Blood loss or associated injuries
Muscle spasms	Muscle contraction near the fracture
Ecchymosis	Extravasation of blood into the subcutaneous tissue

PATHOPHYSIOLOGY ILLUSTRATED
Bone Healing

Osteon — Lamellae

Blood vessel in central canal

Blood vessel in perforating canal

Compact bone

Trabecular bone

Periosteum

Hematoma in fracture

Periosteum   Capillary   Endosteum

Fibrin

Bone fragment

Osteocyte

1. Bone Injury

When a bone fractures, blood vessels within the bone and surrounding soft tissues tear and begin to bleed, forming a hematoma. Necrotic bone tissue adjacent to the fracture causes an intense inflammatory response characterized by vasodilation, exudate formation, and white cell migration to the fracture site.

2. Fibrocartilaginous Callus Formation

Clotting factors within the hematoma form a fibrin meshwork. Within 48 hours, fibroblasts and new capillaries growing into the fracture form granulation tissue that gradually replaces the hematoma. Phagocytes begin to remove cell debris.

Osteoblasts, bone-forming cells, proliferate and migrate into the fracture site, forming a fibrocartilaginous callus. The osteoblasts build a web of collagen fibers from both sides of the fracture site that eventually unites to connect bone fragments, thus splinting the bone. Chondroblasts lay down patches of cartilage that provide a base for bone growth.

Phagocyte

Osteoblast

Fibroblast

Collagen

Chondroblast

Cartilage

4. Bone Remodeling

Osteoblasts continue to form new woven bone, which is in turn organized into the lamellar structures of compact bone. Osteoclasts resorb excess callus as it is replaced by mature bone.

As the bone heals and is subjected to the mechanical stress of everyday use, osteoblasts and osteoclasts respond by remodeling the repair site along the lines of force. This ensures that the repaired section of bone eventually resembles the structure of the uninjured part.

Osteoclast   New compact bone

3. Bony Callus Formation

Osteoblasts continue to proliferate and synthesize collagen fibers and bone matrix, which are gradually mineralized with calcium and mineral salts to form a spongy mass of woven bone. The trabeculae of woven bone bridge the fracture. Osteoclasts migrate to the repair site and begin removing excess bone in the callus. Bony callus formation usually continues for 2 to 3 months.

Bone forming in callus

Woven bone

Osteoblasts

upper arms. Long bone fractures and other major trauma are the principal risk factors for fat emboli; hip replacement surgery also poses a risk for FES.

When a bone is fractured, pressure within the bone marrow rises and exceeds capillary pressure; as a result, fat globules leave the bone marrow and enter the bloodstream. Another contributing factor may be the stress-induced release of catecholamine, which causes the rapid mobilization of fatty acids. Once the fat globules are released, they combine with platelets and travel to the brain, lungs, kidneys, and other organs, occluding small blood vessels and causing tissue ischemia.

Manifestations usually develop within a few hours to a week after injury. The manifestations result from the occlusion of the blood supply and the presence of fatty acids. Altered cerebral blood flow causes confusion and changes in level of consciousness. Pulmonary circulation may be disrupted, and free fatty acids damage the alveolar-capillary membrane. Pulmonary edema, impaired surfactant production, and atelectasis can result in significant respiratory insufficiency and manifestations of acute respiratory distress syndrome (∞ see Chapter 37). Fat droplets activate the clotting cascade, causing thrombocytopenia. Petechiae (pin-sized purplish spots that do not blanch with pressure) appearing on the skin, soft palate, and conjunctiva are thought to result from either microvascular clotting or the accompanying thrombocytopenia.

Early stabilization of long bone fractures is preventive for FES. Prompt identification and treatment of the syndrome are necessary to maintain adequate pulmonary function. In severe cases, the patient may require intubation and mechanical ventilation to prevent hypoxemia. Fluid balance is closely monitored. Corticosteroids may be administered to decrease the inflammatory response of lung tissues, stabilize lipid membranes, and reduce bronchospasm (Porth & Matfin, 2009).

Deep Venous Thrombosis

Pulmonary embolism resulting from deep venous thrombosis is the leading preventable cause of hospital deaths (Maynard & Stein, 2008). *Deep venous thrombosis (DVT)* is a condition in which a blood clot forms along the intimal lining of a large vein, accompanied by inflammation of the vein wall. Risk factors for DVT are (1) venous stasis, or decreased blood flow; (2) injury to blood vessel walls; and (3) altered blood coagulation (Table 39–3). Trauma to the vein stimulates the clotting cascade. Platelets aggregate (clump together) at the site, forming the thrombus. Fibrin, white blood cells (WBCs), and red blood cells (RBCs) begin to cling to the thrombus, and the inflammatory response is initiated. The tail of the clot or the entire thrombus may dislodge and become an embolus, ultimately lodging in the pulmonary circulation. Up to 50% of patients with hip fracture experience venous thromboemboli. If the thrombus remains in the vein, venous insufficiency may result from scarring and valve damage.

Although DVT often is asymptomatic, it may cause swelling, pain, tenderness, or cramping of the affected extremity. Doppler ultrasonography, a noninvasive diagnostic test that uses sound waves to form an image on a computer screen, commonly is used to identify DVT. In some cases, MRI or a venogram may be required for diagnosis.

TABLE 39–3 Risk Factors for Deep Venous Thrombosis

RISK FACTOR	IMPLICATIONS FOR FRACTURES
Decreased blood flow	Muscle contractions facilitating venous flow may be impaired by immobility or stabilization of the fracture (e.g., with a cast or fixation device).
Injury to blood vessel wall	May occur as a direct result of trauma or from surgical manipulation.
Altered blood coagulation	The body's attempt to maintain homeostasis leads to increased production of platelets and clotting factors.

The best treatment for DVT is prevention. Early immobilization of the fracture and early ambulation of the patient are imperative. Prophylactic anticoagulation is beneficial. Antiembolism stockings and compression boots increase venous return and prevent venous stasis. For more information about preventing and treating DVT, ∞ see Chapter 32.

Infection

Infection is more likely to occur in an open fracture than a closed fracture, but any complication that decreases blood supply increases the risk of infection. Infection may result from contamination at the time of injury or during surgery. *Pseudomonas*, *Staphylococcus*, or *Clostridium* organisms may invade the wound or bone. *Clostridium* infection is particularly serious because it may lead to severe gas gangrene and cellulitis, but any infection may delay healing and result in osteomyelitis, infection within the bone that can lead to tissue death and necrosis. (∞ See Chapter 40 for a discussion of osteomyelitis.)

Delayed Union and Nonunion

Delayed healing can affect any fracture, but it most commonly affects the long bones: the humerus, femur, or tibia (Tosounidis et al., 2009). *Delayed union* is the prolonged healing of bones beyond the usual time period. Both injury-related factors (the type and location of facture and accompanying soft tissue injury) and systemic factors (age, general health, immune status, chronic diseases, and smoking) can affect healing, Delayed union is diagnosed by means of serial x-ray studies. It is important to note that x-ray findings may lag 1 to 2 weeks behind the healing process; for example, a patient may be completely healed by week 13, but this fact may not be apparent on the x-ray until week 14.

Delayed union may lead to nonunion, which can cause persistent pain and movement at the fracture site. Nonunion may require surgical interventions, such as internal fixation and bone grafting. If infection is present, the bones are surgically debrided. Electrical or ultrasonic stimulation of the fracture site may be effective to promote healing. Biologic agents such as growth hormone or parathyroid hormone may be given to stimulate bone growth (Tosounidis et al., 2009).

Complex Regional Pain Syndrome

Complex regional pain syndrome (CRPS, also called reflex sympathetic dystrophy) may occur after musculoskeletal or nerve trauma. Female gender and older age are risk factors for CRPS (Stevermer & Ewigman, 2008). It causes extremity pain that is severe, diffuse, and burning. Initially the affected extremity appears inflamed and edematous, later becoming cool and pale. Muscle wasting, skin and nail changes, and bone abnormalities can develop. In CRPS, it appears that pain receptors in the affected extremity become sensitized to catecholamines, neurotransmitters associated with sympathetic nervous system activity. Its cause is unclear; it may be related to central or peripheral nervous system damage, or a disrupted healing or immune process. Diagnosis is made by the patient's history and physical examination. X-rays may demonstrate spotty osteoporosis, and bone scans may reveal increased uptake of radionuclide. Treatment with a sympathetic nervous system blocking agent often alleviates the manifestations.

Interdisciplinary Care

A fracture requires treatment to stabilize the fractured bone(s), maintain bone alignment, prevent complications, and restore function. The diagnosis of a fracture is primarily based on physical examination and x-rays.

Emergency Care

Emergency care of the patient with a fracture includes immobilizing the fracture, maintaining tissue perfusion, and preventing infection. In the case of serious trauma, the cervical spine is immobilized and normal body alignment is maintained. Once the patient is in a secure location, he or she is assessed for instability or deformity of the bone. If any deformity or instability is detected, the extremity is immobilized. Open wounds are covered with sterile dressings, and bleeding is controlled with a pressure dressing. The extremities are assessed for the presence and equality of pulses, movement, and sensation. The joint above and below the deformity is immobilized.

The fracture is splinted to maintain normal anatomic alignment and prevent the fracture from dislocating. Splinting relieves pain and prevents further damage to the arteries, nerves, and bones. Pulses, movement, and sensation are reevaluated after splinting.

Diagnosis

Diagnosis of a fracture usually is confirmed by radiographic tests. X-rays and bone scans are used to identify fractures (Figure 39–3 ■). Blood chemistry studies, complete blood count (CBC), and coagulation studies may be used to assess blood loss, renal function, muscle breakdown, and the risk of excessive bleeding or clotting. Diagnostic tests are described in ∞ Chapter 38.

Medications

Most patients with a fracture initially require analgesia to relieve pain. In the case of multiple fractures or fractures of large bones, opioids are administered initially. NSAIDs are prescribed to decrease inflammation and supplement analgesia. Pain management for the patient with a fracture is described in Box 39–2.

Antibiotics may be administered prophylactically, particularly to patients with open or complex fractures. Anticoagulants may be prescribed to prevent DVT, particularly if surgery or prolonged immobilization is necessary. Stool softeners may be given to decrease the risk of constipation secondary to narcotics and immobility. Patients who have sustained trauma are often placed on antiulcer medications or antacids.

Treatments

Before the fractured bone is stabilized for healing, the fracture is *reduced* or restored to its normal alignment. In *closed reduction*, the bone is repositioned using external manipulation. Local or regional anesthesia or conscious sedation usually is given before closed reduction. The fracture is then immobilized with a splint, cast, or traction. An x-ray may be done to verify proper position, and pulses, movement, and sensation are assessed distal to the fracture. An *open reduction* is done in surgery. The bone is exposed and realigned; nails or screws may be used to maintain its position.

TRACTION Muscle spasms usually accompany fractures and may pull bones out of alignment. Traction applies a straightening or pulling force to return or maintain the fractured bones in normal anatomic position. Types of traction are as follows:

- *Manual traction* is applied by physically pulling on the extremity. Manual traction often is used to reduce a fracture or dislocation (Figure 39–4A ■).
- *Skin traction* (also called straight traction) is used to control muscle spasms and to immobilize a part of the body during transport or before surgery, with traction exerting its grabbing and pulling force through the patient's skin (Figure 39–4B). Skin traction is noninvasive and is relatively comfortable for the patient. The most common type of skin traction is Buck's traction, used to immobilize the leg before surgery to repair a hip or proximal femur fracture. Buck's traction uses traction tape or a foam boot applied to the lower leg and attached to a free-hanging weight to immobilize the leg.

Figure 39–3 ■ X-ray of an oblique fracture of the femur.

Source: Charles Stewart and Associates.

BOX 39–2 Pain Management for the Patient with a Fracture

The patient who has had musculoskeletal trauma experiences pain from many different causes:

- Disruption of the continuity of the bone
- Damage to ligaments and tendons
- Swelling of tissues around the trauma site
- Muscle spasms
- Tissue ischemia from swelling inside a cast, splint, or the muscle fascia sheath
- Hematoma formation
- Pressure over bony prominences from casts or splints.

The pain is often severe and may be described as sharp, aching, or burning. Carefully assess any complaint of pain, including the location, character, and duration of pain. Nursing interventions for acute pain due to fracture include the following:

1. Administer prescribed analgesics, including NSAIDs and opioid analgesics. For serious fractures or following orthopedic surgery, patient-controlled analgesia (PCA) or epidural analgesia may be used. Administer NSAIDs and analgesics at regular intervals for the first 24 to 48 hours, then instruct the patient to request or take the medication before the pain is severe. Reassure the patient that addiction does not result from taking medications to relieve fracture or surgical pain. Most patients require only oral analgesics by the third or fourth day after orthopedic surgery.
2. Elevate the involved extremity, and apply cold (if prescribed) to help decrease swelling.
3. Monitor and drain accumulated fluids in any drainage devices to ensure patency, reduce swelling, and decrease the possibility of hematoma formation.
4. Encourage the patient to wiggle fingers or toes on an extremity in a cast or traction to improve venous return and decrease edema.
5. Assist the patient to frequently change positions to relieve pressure and use pillows to provide support.
6. Teach the patient adjunctive pain management techniques, such as relaxation and guided imagery.
7. Notify the physician of severe or unrelieved pain, which may indicate a serious complication such as compartment syndrome or neurovascular impairment.

A

B

C

D

Figure 39–4 ■ Traction is applying a pulling force to restore or maintain bone alignment for fracture healing. *A*, Manual traction is applied to restore or maintain alignment during emergency treatment of a fracture. *B*, Skin traction (also called straight traction), such as is shown here, is often used to temporarily maintain alignment. *C*, Balanced suspension traction is commonly used for fractures of the femur. *D*, Skeletal traction, in which the pulling force is applied directly to the bone, may be used to treat fractures of the spine.

- *Balanced suspension traction* involves more than one force of pull to raise and support the injured extremity off the bed and maintain its alignment (Figure 39–4C). Balanced suspension traction increases mobility while maintaining bone position. It also makes it easier to change linen and perform back care.
- In *skeletal traction*, the pulling force is applied directly through pins inserted into the bone (Figure 39–4 D). Local, spinal, or general anesthetic is provided during pin placement. One or more pulling forces may be applied with skeletal traction. Skeletal traction allows more weight to be used to maintain the proper anatomic alignment. The risk of infection is greater, however, and it may cause more discomfort. The weights used for skeletal traction are not removed by the nurse. Nursing interventions for patients in traction are described in Box 39–3.

Figure 39–5 ■ Padding to protect the skin is applied under the cast.

CASTS A cast is a rigid device applied to immobilize the injured bones and promote healing. The cast immobilizes the joint above and the joint below the fractured bone so that the bone will not move during healing. A fracture is first reduced manually and a cast is then applied. Casts are applied on patients who have relatively stable fractures.

The cast, which may be composed of plaster or fiberglass, is applied over a thin cushion of padding and molded to the normal contour of the body (Figure 39–5 ■). The cast must be allowed to dry before any pressure is applied to it; simply palpating a wet cast with the fingertips will leave dents that may cause pressure ulcers. A plaster cast may require up to 48 hours to dry, whereas a fiberglass cast dries within an hour. The type of cast applied is determined by the location of the fracture (Figure 39–6 ■). Nursing care of the patient with a cast is discussed in the box on page 1318. During follow-up appointments, the physician may x-ray the bone to assess alignment and healing, and possibly remove the cast for skin assessment.

SURGERY Surgery is indicated for a fracture that requires direct visualization and repair, a fracture with common long-term complications, or a fracture that is severely comminuted and threatens vascular supply.

The simplest type of surgery is application of an external fixator device. An external fixator consists of a frame connected to pins that are inserted perpendicular to the long axis of the bone (Figure 39–7 ■). The number of pins inserted varies with the type and site of the fracture; in general, the same number of pins is inserted above and below the fracture line. The pins require care similar to that provided for skeletal traction pins. The patient is monitored for infection, and frequent neurovascular assessment is performed. The fixator increases independence while maintaining immobilization.

Internal fixation is accomplished through a surgical procedure called an *open reduction and internal fixation (ORIF)*. In this procedure, the fracture is reduced (placed in correct anatomic alignment) and nails, screws, plates, or pins are

---

BOX 39–3 Nursing Interventions for Patients in Traction

- Maintain the pulling force and direction of the traction:
  a. In most instances, the patient's weight provides countertraction.
  b. Center the patient on the bed; maintain body alignment with the direction of pull.
  c. Do not wedge the patient's foot or place it flush with the footboard of the bed.
  d. Ensure that weights hang freely and do not touch the floor.
  e. Ensure that nothing is lying on or obstructing the ropes.
  f. Do not allow the knots at the end of the rope to come into contact with the pulley.
- Perform neurovascular assessments frequently.
- Assess for common complications of immobility, including pressure ulcer formation, renal calculi, deep venous thrombosis, pneumonia, paralytic ileus, and loss of appetite.
- If a problem is detected, assist in repositioning. Stabilize the fracture site during repositioning.

- Teach the patient and family about the type and purpose of the traction.
- For skin traction:
  a. Frequently assess skin, bony prominences, and pressure points for evidence of pressure, shearing, or pending breakdown.
  b. Protect pressure sites with padding and protective dressings as indicated.
  c. Remove weights only if intermittent traction has been ordered to alleviate muscle spasm.
- For skeletal traction:
  a. Never remove the weights.
  b. Frequently assess pin insertion sites and provide pin site care per policy.
  c. Report signs of infection at the pin sites, such as redness, drainage, and increased tenderness.

Figure 39–6 ■ A short arm cast that also immobilizes the thumb is used to stabilize a wrist fracture.

Figure 39–7 ■ In external fixation, pins are placed through the bone above and below the fracture site to immobilize the bone. External fixation rods hold the pins in place.

inserted to hold the bones in place (Figure 39–8 ■). Open fractures of the extremities are most commonly repaired in this way. Hip fractures in older patients are frequently repaired with ORIF to prevent complications and to allow early rehabilitation. Interventions for postoperative nursing care are presented in Box 39–4.

ELECTRICAL BONE STIMULATION Electrical bone stimulation is the application of an electrical current at the fracture site. It is a painless method of treating fractures that are not healing appropriately. The electrical stress increases the migration of osteoblasts and osteoclasts to the fracture site. Mineral deposition increases, promoting bone healing. Electrical bone stimulation can be accomplished invasively or noninvasively (Figure 39–9 ■). In invasive stimulation, the surgeon inserts a cathode and a lead wire at the fracture site. The lead wire is attached to an internal or external generator, which delivers electricity to the cathode 24 hours a day. In noninvasive inductive stimulation, a treatment coil encircles the cast or skin directly over the fracture site. The coil is attached to an external generator that runs on batteries. The electricity goes through the skin to the fracture site. The time period for external stimulation can vary from 3 to 10 hours per day. The patient may be taught to self-administer noninvasive electrical stimulation. Electrical bone stimulation is contraindicated in the

---

NURSING CARE OF THE PATIENT
with a Cast

Nursing Interventions
- Perform frequent neurovascular assessments.
- Palpate the cast for "hot spots" that may indicate the presence of underlying infection.
- Promptly report increased or severe pain; changes in neurovascular status; or a hot spot or drainage on the cast.

Health Education for the Patient and Family
- The cast dries from the inside out; do not use a blow dryer to speed drying; do not cover the cast while it is drying.
- A sensation of warmth during drying is normal.
- Do not put anything into the cast.
- Keep the cast clean and dry; use plastic wrap as needed to protect it.
- If the cast is made of fiberglass, dry it with a blow dryer on the cool setting if it becomes wet.
- Notify your doctor immediately if you develop increased pain, coolness, changes in color, increased swelling, and/or loss of sensation.
- Use a blow dryer on the cool setting to relieve itching by blowing cool air into the cast.
- A sling may be used to distribute the weight of the cast evenly around the neck. Do not roll the sling; this can impair circulation to the neck.
- If crutches are used, arrange for physical therapist to teach correct crutch walking.
- When the cast is removed, an oscillating cast saw will be used. It is noisy and you will feel its vibration, but a guard prevents it from penetrating past the depth of the cast, so it will not cut the skin.

Figure 39–8 ■ Internal fixation hardware is entirely within the body. *A*, Fixation of a short oblique fracture using a plate and screws above and below the fracture. *B*, Fixation of a long oblique fracture using screws through the fracture site. *C*, Fixation of a segmental fracture using a medullary nail.

presence of infection and for upper extremities if the patient has a pacemaker.

Fractures of Specific Bones or Bony Areas

Causes, manifestations, complications, treatment, and selected nursing interventions are described for the following fractures: skull, face, spine, clavicle, humerus, elbow, radius/ulna, wrist/hand, ribs, pelvis, femur, hip, tibia/fibula, and ankle/foot.

Fracture of the Skull

A skull fracture may result from either a fall or a direct blow. The patient must be assessed for neurologic changes and any loss of consciousness must be documented. A complete neurologic assessment is conducted: level of consciousness (LOC) and orientation to person, place, and time, pupillary reaction to light, movement and strength of all extremities, and complaints of nausea and vomiting are noted. A displaced skull fracture, which is referred to as depressed, may press on the brain and cause neurologic damage. Brain injuries related to skull fractures are discussed in ∞ Chapter 42.

BOX 39–4 Nursing Interventions for Patients with Internal Fixation

- Frequently assess type, location, and severity of pain. Report pain that is increasing in severity, unexpected, or unrelieved by prescribed analgesia.
- Perform neurovascular assessments frequently, promptly reporting any change in pulses, color, temperature, capillary refill, movement, or sensation of the affected extremity.
- Assess the following:
  a. Amount, color, odor of drainage on dressing and in wound drain device (e.g., Hemovac, Jackson-Pratt)
  b. Bowel sounds
  c. Lung sounds
- Administer medications, such as analgesics and antibiotics, per physician's orders.
- In hip fractures, place an abductor pillow between patient's legs to prevent dislocation of the hip joint.
- Arrange for physical and occupational therapy, as ordered.
- Assist with weight-bearing program, if ordered.
- Encourage early mobilization, coughing, and deep breathing, as appropriate to help prevent complications.

Fracture of the Face

Fracture of the facial bones may result from a direct blow. The patient presents with hematomas, pain, edema, and bony deformity. Nondisplaced fractures are monitored to ensure the airway is not compromised. The patient is observed for any neurologic deficits. Severely displaced or multiple facial fractures are treated with ORIF with wires or plates.

Nursing care focuses on maintaining the airway by helping the patient clear secretions from the oropharynx. The nurse monitors the patient's breathing for increased effort or tachypnea and notifies the physician immediately if these findings are noted. Pain is treated with analgesics, and body image disturbances are addressed. If the patient asks to see his or her face, the nurse should plan to stay with the patient and answer questions while the patient looks in a mirror.

Fracture of the Spine

The spine can be injured in many ways, including sports injuries, falls, and motor vehicle crashes. Cervical and lumbar fractures occur most commonly, but the thoracic and sacral spine also can be fractured. The most severe complication of spine fracture is injury to the spinal cord (discussed in ∞ Chapter 43). A displaced or unstable fracture of the vertebrae may apply pressure on the spinal cord. This pressure on the spinal cord may result in ischemia and permanent paralysis.

A nondisplaced cervical spinal fracture may be treated with a cervical collar or a halo immobilizing brace (see Figure 39–4). The displaced cervical fracture is reduced by manual or skeletal traction and, eventually, application of a brace and/or surgical stabilization of the bones with plates and screws. Immobilization after a spinal fracture may last as long as 6 months.

Figure 39–9 ■ External electrical bone growth stimulator.
Courtesy of Orthologic, Inc.

Fracture of the Clavicle

A fracture of the clavicle commonly results from a direct blow or a fall. The most common location is midclavicular. A person with a midclavicular fracture typically assumes a protective slumping position to immobilize the arm and prevent shoulder movement. A less common fracture occurs along the distal third of the clavicle. This type of fracture may be associated with ligament damage. Injuries to the clavicle may be associated with skull or cervical fractures. Displaced clavicular fractures may damage subclavian vessels, leading to hemorrhage, or the lung, with resulting pneumothorax. Injury to the brachial plexus may result in numbness and decreased movement of the arm on the affected side. Malunion of a clavicular fracture can result in asymmetry of the shoulders.

A deformity may be observed or palpated along the clavicle. The fractured bone is immobilized in normal anatomic position by applying a clavicular strap, or via surgical repair.

Fracture of the Humerus

The severity of humerus fractures and appropriate treatment is determined by the location of the fracture, the presence of displacement, and the presence of neurovascular compromise. Treatment focuses on immobilizing the fractured bone in normal anatomic position. Common complications of humeral fracture include nerve and ligament damage, frozen or stiff joints, and malunion. Early interventions may prevent permanent damage.

Fractures of the proximal humerus are common in older adults. A simple nondisplaced fracture of the proximal humerus (near the humeral head) with a normal neurovascular assessment can be safely treated with immobilization. A more complicated displaced fracture of the proximal humerus with bone fragmentation requires surgical intervention. The risk for impaired range of motion (ROM) of the shoulder increases with fracture severity and soft tissue damage. Rehabilitative measures focus on increasing ROM.

The humerus may also fracture along the shaft, usually as a result of direct trauma. If the humeral shaft fracture is simple and nondisplaced, a hanging arm cast is applied. This cast maintains alignment of the fracture by using the pulling force of gravity; therefore, the patient is instructed not to rest the cast on anything to alleviate the weight. If the patient is on bed rest, a hanging arm cast is not applied, because the arm would not be able to hang freely. Instead, the fracture is immobilized with external skeletal traction. This traction places the injured arm in an upright position over the face, and weights are hung off the distal portion of the humerus. Nursing interventions for patients with fractures of the humerus are presented in Box 39–5.

Fracture of the Elbow

The most common location of an elbow fracture is the distal humerus. Elbow fractures usually result from a fall or direct blow to the elbow. The patient guards the injured extremity, holding the arm rigidly in a flexed position or an extended position. Because the radius, ulna, or humerus may be involved in the elbow fracture, all three bones must be visualized by x-ray.

Complications of an elbow fracture include nerve or artery damage and hemarthrosis, a collection of blood in the elbow joint. The most serious complication of an elbow fracture is Volkmann's contracture, which results from arterial occlusion

---

BOX 39–5 Nursing Interventions for Patients with Fractures of the Humerus

- Perform neurovascular assessments frequently.
- Administer prescribed medications to alleviate pain.
- Encourage exercises for patients with a hanging cast:
   a. Finger exercises: Move each finger of the affected arm through complete range of motion.
   b. Pendulum shoulder exercises: Dangle the affected arm at the side, and move it forward and backward about 30 degrees in each direction.
- Instruct the patient and family in cast care and sling application, neurovascular assessments, exercises, prescribed pain medications, and manifestations of complications.
- If patient is admitted to the hospital, provide preoperative teaching.

---

and muscle ischemia. The patient complains of forearm pain, impaired sensation, and loss of motor function. Rapid interventions are aimed at relieving pressure on the brachial artery and nerve and preventing muscle atrophy.

Nondisplaced elbow fractures are treated by immobilizing the fracture with a posterior splint or cast. The displaced fracture is first reduced and then immobilized. Nursing interventions focus on alleviating pain, maintaining immobilization, and educating the patient in neurovascular assessments.

Fracture of the Radius and/or Ulna

Fractures of the radius and ulna may result from either indirect injury, such as twisting or pulling on the arm, or direct injury, such as that resulting from a fall. The usual treatment of radius fractures depends on the location. The proximal radial head may be fractured from a fall on an outstretched hand. Blood commonly collects in the elbow joint and must be aspirated. If the fracture is nondisplaced, a sling is applied. A displaced fracture is surgically repaired and posterior plaster splint is applied. The patient avoids movement for the first week and then initiates movement gradually.

When both bones are broken, the fracture is usually displaced. The patient complains of pain and cannot supinate the hand (turn the palm up). A nondisplaced fracture is casted for about 6 weeks, followed by application of a shorter cast or a brace for 6 more weeks. Displaced fractures are surgically repaired with ORIF. After the surgery, a cast is applied, and the patient is encouraged to exercise the fingers.

Complications after a radius and/or ulnar fracture include compartment syndrome, delayed healing, and decreased wrist and finger movement. After surgery, the patient also has an increased risk of infection. Nursing interventions focus on alleviating pain, maintaining immobilization, and educating patients in neurovascular assessments, the importance of elevation, and the need to inform the physician of changes in sensation or an increase in pain.

Fractures in the Wrist and Hand

Wrist fractures often result from a fall onto an outstretched hand or onto the back of the hand. A common type of wrist fracture is *Colles' fracture*, in which the distal radius fractures after a fall onto an outstretched hand. The patient with a wrist fracture presents with a bony deformity, pain, numbness, weakness, and decreased ROM of the fingers. The capillary refill and sensation of the hand must be assessed.

The hand is composed of many bones. Most commonly, the metacarpals and phalanges are involved in a hand fracture. The injuring mechanism varies from striking an object with a closed fist to closing a hand in a door. The patient presents with complaints of pain, edema, and decreased ROM.

Comparative x-rays of both the injured and uninjured wrist and hand may be obtained to identify the fracture. Complications of wrist and hand fractures are compartment syndrome, nerve damage, ligament damage, and delayed union. A wrist fracture is commonly treated with closed reduction, cast application, and elevation of the injured extremity. A hand fracture is splinted and elevated.

Nursing interventions focus on alleviating pain and teaching the patient about neurovascular assessments, the importance of elevation, and how to exercise the fingers to prevent stiffness. If the dominant hand is injured, the patient may require assistance in performing activities of daily living (ADLs).

Fracture of the Ribs

Rib fractures commonly result from blunt chest trauma. The location of the fracture and involvement of underlying organs determine the severity of the injury. Fractures of the first through third ribs may damage the subclavian artery or vein. Fractures of the lower ribs may cause spleen and liver injuries.

The patient typically presents with a history of recent chest trauma and complaints of pain along the lateral portion of the rib. Palpation of the rib reveals a bony deformity and increases pain. Deep inspiration also increases pain. The skin over the fracture site may be ecchymotic (bruised).

Flail chest results from the fracture of two or more adjacent ribs in two or more places and the formation of a free-floating segment that moves in the opposite direction of the rib cage. The bony instability impairs respirations. Treatment is aimed at stabilizing the flail segment and supporting respirations.

Potential complications of rib fractures include pulmonary contusion, pneumothorax, and/or hemothorax. The fractured rib may pierce the lung and injure it. The lower ribs may pierce the liver or spleen, resulting in intra-abdominal bleeding. Pneumonia may also develop from ineffective clearing of respiratory secretions.

A simple rib fracture is treated with pain medication and instructions for coughing, deep breathing, and splinting. The patient is also instructed to return to the emergency room if shortness of breath develops. Nursing interventions focus on alleviating pain and teaching the patient about splinting. Because deep inspiration increases pain, patients frequently avoid it. The patient may be instructed to splint the injured rib with the hand or a pillow and take deep breaths and cough to decrease the chance of developing pneumonia and/or atelectasis. Incentive spirometry is encouraged.

Fracture of the Pelvis

Pelvic fractures are often caused by trauma, such as a fall or an automobile crash. Pelvic fracture may result from a fall from standing position in the older adult. Hemorrhage with significant blood loss and damage to organs contained within the pelvis (e.g., the bladder, urethra, reproductive organs, and bowel) are significant risks associated with pelvic fracture. Trauma to extra-pelvic organs such as the kidneys is common.

The patient with a pelvic fracture presents with pain in the back or hip area. A single fracture in the pelvis is treated conservatively with analgesia and activity limitation. Log rolling increases patient comfort.

A pelvic sling is used to stabilize unstable pelvic fractures pending surgical reduction and fixation. If necessary, an external fixator may be applied to stabilize the pelvis.

Nursing care focuses on alleviating discomfort, maintaining immobilization, and identifying potential complications. The nurse monitors for increased heart rate, decreased blood pressure, and decreasing hemoglobin levels. Any blood in the urine should be reported to the physician; this may indicate kidney, bladder, or urethral damage. Urethral catheterization is avoided until bladder and urethral trauma has been ruled out.

Fracture of the Shaft of the Femur

A large amount of force, such as from motor vehicle crashes, falls, or acts of violence, is required to fracture the shaft of the femur. Patients with femoral shaft fractures often have associated multiple traumas. A fracture of the femoral shaft is manifested by an edematous, deformed, painful thigh. The patient is unable to move the hip or knee. Initial assessment focuses on the circulation and sensation present in the affected extremity. Pedal pulses and capillary refill in the affected extremity are compared to the unaffected extremity. Complications of a femoral shaft fracture include hypovolemia due to blood loss (which may be as great as 1.0 to 1.5 L), fat embolism, dislocation of the hip or knee, muscle atrophy, and ligament damage.

Treatment of fractures of the shaft of the femur initially includes skeletal traction to separate the bony fragments and reduce and immobilize the fracture. Depending on the location and severity of the fracture, traction may be followed by either external or internal fixation. Strength in the affected extremity is maintained through gluteal and quadricep exercises. ROM exercises for unaffected extremities are critical in preparation for ambulation. Although full weight bearing is usually restricted until x-rays demonstrate bone union, the patient may be allowed to carry out non-weight-bearing activities with an assistive device.

The nurse assesses pulses in the extremity and compares them bilaterally. Sensation is evaluated by asking whether the patient can feel touch and discriminate sharp from dull objects. Nursing interventions include providing pain medication, providing reassurance and decreasing anxiety, and assisting with exercises of the lower legs, feet, and toes.

Fracture of the Hip

A hip fracture refers to a fracture of the femur at the head, neck, or trochanteric regions (Figure 39–10 ■). Hip fractures are classified as intracapsular or extracapsular. *Intracapsular fractures* involve the head or neck of the femur; *extracapsular fractures* involve the trochanteric region. The majority of hip fractures involve the neck or trochanteric regions. The femoral head and neck lie within the joint capsule and are not covered in periosteum; thus, they do not have a large blood supply. Fractures at this location usually fragment, further decreasing blood supply and increasing the risk of nonunion and avascular necrosis. The trochanteric region is covered in periosteum and therefore has more blood supply than the head or neck.

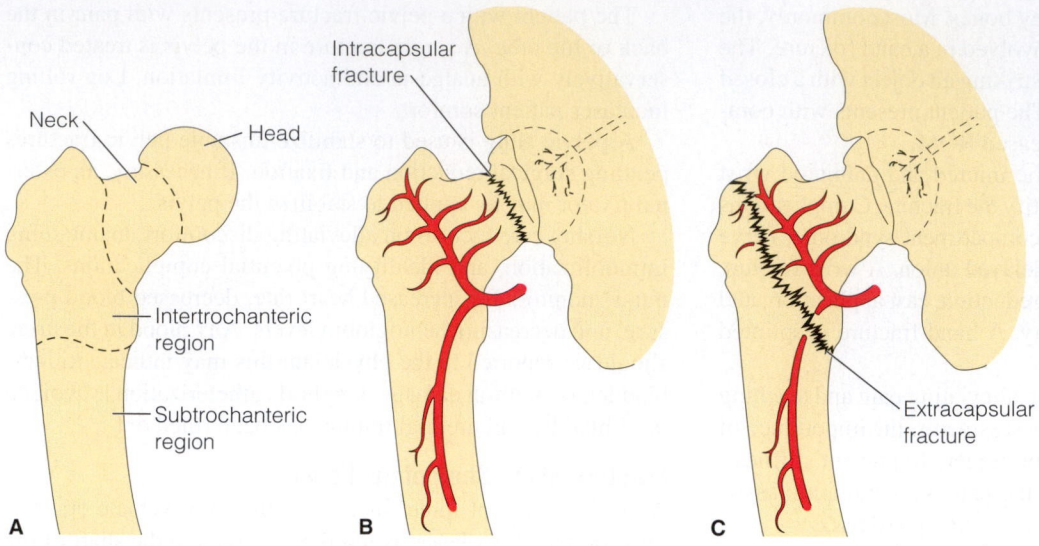

Figure 39–10 ■ Regions where hip fractures may occur. *A*, The head of the femur, the neck of the femur, and the trochanteric regions of the femur. *B*, Intracapsular fractures occur across the head or neck of the femur. *C*, Extracapsular fractures occur across the trochanteric regions. Note how both intracapsular and extracapsular fractures disrupt the blood supply to the bone.

Hip fractures result from falls and are the most common injury in the older population, requiring hospitalization of more than 320,000 older adults each year in the United States. They result in serious health problems and increase the risk of dying in people 65 years or older (Centers for Disease Control and Prevention, [CDC], 2008). By the year 2040, the number of hip fractures is expected to exceed 500,000, which reflects society's increasing older population. Factors contributing to falls include problems with gait and balance, neurologic and musculoskeletal impairments, dementia, psychoactive medications, and visual impairments. Modifiable risk factors, identified through research, include lower body weakness, problems with walking and balance, and taking four or more medications or any psychoactive medications. See the accompanying Moving Evidence into Action box for evidence-based fall prevention for older adults.

FAST FACTS

Hip Fracture in Older Adults

- More than one-third of all adults over the age of 65 fall each year. Of those, White men have the highest fall-related death rates, followed by White women, Black men, and Black women.
- Older adults most often fracture the hip from falls; in contrast, motor vehicle crashes are the most common cause in young and middle adults.
- The risk for a fractured hip increases with each decade of life, especially in White postmenopausal women, who have the highest incidence of osteoporosis. Women have about 80% of all hip fractures. Women who smoke are at greater risk, because smoking reduces bone density among menopausal women.
- Complications are related both to the fracture and to the resulting treatment. Only a small number of patients regain their previous mobility, while about 20% require nursing home care.
- Half of all older adults hospitalized for a hip fracture cannot return home or live independently after the fracture.

Data from CDC (2009).

Hip fractures are common in older adults as a result of decreases in bone mass and the increased tendency to fall. Whether the femur breaks spontaneously and causes the fall or whether the fall causes the fracture is not always clear; regardless of the cause of the fracture, rapid interventions are required to prevent bone necrosis. Assessment findings commonly associated with a hip fracture are pain, inability to walk, and shortening and external rotation of the affected lower extremity. Rarely, the fracture dislocates posteriorly; if that occurs, the extremity may internally rotate. However, some patients with a hip fracture have only vague pain in the buttocks, knees, thighs, groin, or back, and their ability to walk is unaffected. If the fracture is not visible on x-ray, a bone scan or MRI may be done to confirm the presence of the fracture.

A hip fracture may be treated with traction to decrease muscle spasms, followed by surgery; or surgery may be performed immediately or within the first 24 hours. The goal of surgery is to reduce and stabilize the fracture, thereby increasing mobility, decreasing pain, and preventing complications. Surgery usually consists of ORIF of the fracture. Fixation is accomplished by securing the femur in place with pins, screws, nails, or plates (Figure 39–11*A* and *B* ■). An ORIF works well for fractures in the trochanteric area. Fractures of the femoral neck frequently disrupt blood supply to the femoral head. If blood supply is disrupted, the surgeon will replace the femoral head with a prosthesis (Figure 39–11*C*). If the acetabulum has been damaged, the surgeon may insert a metal cup. Replacement of either the femoral head or the acetabulum with a prosthesis is called a *hemiarthroplasty*. Replacement of both the femoral head and the acetabulum is a *total hip arthroplasty (THA)*, discussed in ⬗ Chapter 40.

Nursing care for a patient with a hip fracture focuses on maintaining skin integrity, preventing infection, alleviating pain, maintaining circulation to the injured extremity, and increasing mobility. This is discussed in more detail in the following nursing care section.

Fracture of the Tibia and/or Fibula

Fractures of the lower extremities often result from a fall on a flexed foot, a direct blow, or a twisting motion. The patient presents with edema, pain, bony deformity, and a hematoma at the level of injury.

Circulation and sensation are assessed to rule out common complications of the fracture, including damage to the peroneal nerve or tibial artery, compartment syndrome, hemarthroses,

MOVING EVIDENCE INTO ACTION   Preventing Falls in Hospitalized Older Adults

Evidence-based clinical guidelines for specific patient care interventions, such as fall prevention, should be based on research. The recommendations provided by the Hartford Institute for Geriatric Nursing are made based on published research. Falls are identified as a geriatric syndrome with identifiable risk factors and precipitating causes. Assessment for fall risk includes intrinsic factors such as age (particularly over 75 years), chronic conditions (e.g., dementia, arthritis, or diabetes), use of an assistive device, visual impairment, and use of high-risk medications. Regular assessment of the patient care environment for factors such as spills, lighting, grab bars, and equipment repair is recommended. Care planning to prevent falls is individualized to identified risks, and involves an integrated, multidisciplinary team.

IMPLICATIONS FOR NURSING

Although advancing age is a fall risk factor, it is only one of many. Nurses need to evaluate each patient as an individual, assessing and planning care to address those fall risk factors that can be changed. Use of standardized environmental checklists to identify extrinsic risk factors and standardized or empirically tested fall risk tools to evaluate intrinsic risk factors is recommended.

CRITICAL THINKING IN PATIENT CARE

1. Several intrinsic risk factors for falls, including age, medications, and chronic diseases, are identified here. List at least five additional intrinsic risk factors common among older adults for which you should assess.
2. This practice guideline notes that falls among hospitalized older adults occur most frequently on medicine and neurology units. What intrinsic and extrinsic factors contribute to place patients on these units at greater risk for falling?
3. Use of physical restraints is identified as a fall risk factor. Identify three alternatives to using physical restraints in a confused older adult.

Data from Gray-Micelli, D. (2008). Want to know more. Falls. Nursing standard of practice protocol: Fall prevention. Retrieved from www.consultgerirn.org/topics/falls/want_to_know_more

and ligament damage. An inability to point the toe on the affected side upward may indicate peroneal nerve damage. Absence of the dorsalis pedis pulse on the affected side may indicate tibial artery damage. Potential manifestations of compartment syndrome include pain on passive movement and paresthesias. An edematous knee may indicate a collection of blood in the knee joint. Ligament damage may be present if the patient cannot move the knee and/or ankle.

If the fracture is closed, a closed reduction and casting are frequently performed. A long leg cast that allows for partial weight bearing is used. Partial weight bearing usually is allowed within 10 days of the fracture. A short leg cast will be applied in 3 to 4 weeks. If the fracture is open, either external fixation or ORIF will be performed. After surgery, a cast may be applied, and weight bearing begins according to the physician's orders, usually in about 6 weeks.

Nursing care is designed to increase comfort, monitor neurovascular status, and prevent complications. The nurse instructs the patient in cast care, on the use of assistive devices, how to perform neurovascular assessment, and when to follow up with the physician.

Fracture in the Ankle and Foot

The patient with an ankle fracture presents with pain, limited ROM, hematoma, edema, and difficulty ambulating. Most ankle fractures are treated by closed reduction and casting. Open fractures are treated by surgical intervention and splinting.

The patient with a foot fracture presents with similar symptoms; however, ROM of the ankle is not usually affected. Most foot fractures are nondisplaced and treated with closed reduction and casting. More severe displaced foot fractures may require surgery and the placement of wires to maintain reduction of the fracture.

Nursing care focuses on increasing comfort, increasing mobility, and educating the patient. Analgesia is given for pain. The extremity should be elevated, and ice can be applied. The patient is taught cast care, neurovascular assessment, and crutch walking.

Nursing Care

In planning and implementing nursing care for the patient with fractures, the nurse should consider the patient's response to the traumatic experience. Although each patient has individual needs, nursing care commonly focuses on associated acute pain, impaired physical mobility, and the risks for impaired tissue perfusion and neurovascular compromise.

Health Promotion

Trauma prevention can save lives. Many communities are educating people of all ages, from grade-schoolers to older adults, in trauma prevention. Young adults face a high risk of sustaining trauma. They need to be taught the importance of safety equipment—such as automobile seat belts, bicycle and motorized vehicle helmets, football pads, proper footwear, protective eyewear, and hard hats—in preventing or decreasing the severity of injury from trauma. Older adults should

Figure 39–11 ■ Surgical fixation of hip fractures. *A* and *B*, A surgical nail or screw used to stabilize an intertrochanteric fracture. *C*, Use of a hip prosthesis (artificial hip) to replace a damaged femoral head.

have regular screenings for osteoporosis (with a bone density test), activity levels, cognitive and affective disorders, vision impairments, and risk for falls. Older adults can reduce their risk of falling by increasing lower body strength and balance through regular physical activity, and by asking their healthcare provider or pharmacist to review their medications. Educational programs about workplace and farm safety, including information about ergonomic principles, can also help prevent musculoskeletal injuries.

Having a regular exercise program and avoiding obesity are important factors in maintaining good bone health in all adults. An adequate intake of calcium is essential to ensure proper growth, development, and maintenance of strong bones throughout life. It is important that women ensure good bone health prior to menopause, because the loss of estrogen during and after menopause decreases calcium use and increases the risk of osteoporosis. Strong bones are formed by calcium intake and weight-bearing exercise, both of which are equally important in the postmenopausal woman.

Older patients are at higher risk for musculoskeletal trauma due to falls. For these patients, home assessments must be performed and potential hazards removed. Specific teaching topics for preventing falls in older adults are outlined in the accompanying Meeting Individualized Needs box below.

Assessment

Collect the following data through the health history and physical examination (∞ see Chapter 38).

- *Health history:* Age, history of traumatic event, history of prior musculoskeletal injuries, chronic illnesses, medications (ask the older adult specifically about anticoagulants and calcium supplements).
- *Physical assessment:* Pain with movement, pulses, edema, skin color and temperature, deformity, range of motion, touch. The 5 P's of neurovascular assessment, as follows, are included in both the initial assessment and ongoing focused assessments:
  - *Pain.* Assess pain in the injured extremity by asking the patient to grade it on a scale of 0 to 10, with 10 as the most severe pain.

- *Pulses.* Assess distal pulses beginning with the unaffected extremity. Compare the quality of pulses in the affected extremity to those of the unaffected extremity.
- *Pallor.* Observe for pallor and skin color in the injured extremity. Paleness and coolness may indicate arterial compromise, whereas warmth and a bluish tinge may indicate venous blood pooling. Assess capillary refill, comparing the affected and unaffected extremities.
- *Paralysis/Paresis.* Assess ability to move body parts distal to the fracture site. Inability to move indicates paralysis. Loss of muscle strength (weakness) when moving is paresis. A finding of limited range of motion may lead to early recognition of problems such as nerve damage and paralysis.
- *Paresthesia.* Ask the patient if any change in sensation such as burning, numbness, prickly feeling, or stinging (all these are paresthesias) has occurred. Assess sensation distal to the injury, including ability to discriminate sharp and dull touch and two-point discrimination.

Nursing Diagnoses and Interventions

Nursing care for patients with fractures ranges from teaching for home care following treatment in the emergency or urgent care department (such as manual reduction and cast application) to providing interventions to maintain health and decrease the risk of complications in patients with complex or multiple fractures. Teaching is also necessary for caregivers of the older adult who is discharged home or to a long-term care or rehabilitation facility following a fracture. A Case Study & Nursing Care Plan for a patient with hip fracture is included on page 1327.

Acute Pain

Pain is caused by soft tissue damage and is compounded by muscle spasms and swelling.

- Monitor vital signs. *Some analgesics decrease respiratory effort and blood pressure.*
- Ask the patient to rate the pain on a scale of 0 to 10 (with 10 as the most severe pain) before and after any intervention. *This facilitates objective assessment of the effectiveness of the chosen pain relief strategy. Pain that increases in*

MEETING INDIVIDUALIZED NEEDS   **Teaching Older Adults to Prevent Falls**

- Begin a regular exercise program; lack of exercise leads to weakness and an increased chance of falling. Exercises that improve balance and coordination (such as yoga or tai chi) are the most helpful.
- Make your home safer:
  - Remove any items in your pathway, including from stairs, to avoid tripping.
  - Remove small throw rugs or use double-sided tape to keep rugs from slipping.
  - Place frequently used items within easy reach to avoid use of a step stool.
  - Install grab bars next to your toilet and in the tub or shower.
  - Use nonslip mats in the bathtub and on shower floors.

- Improve lighting, using lamp shades or frosted bulbs to reduce glare. Install nightlights in hallways and bathroom.
- Install handrails and lights in all staircases.
- Wear shoes that give good support and have thin, nonslip soles. Avoid wearing slippers and athletic shoes with deep treads.
- Ask your healthcare provider to review your medications, including prescriptions and over-the-counter medications. Some medications or a combination of medications may cause dizziness or drowsiness, leading to falls.
- Have your vision checked by an eye doctor. Your glasses may no longer have the correct prescription, or you may have developed an eye condition such as cataracts or glaucoma that limits your vision.

intensity or remains unrelieved with analgesics can indicate compartment syndrome.

- For the patient with a hip fracture, apply Buck's traction per physician's orders. Keep the traction weights hanging freely. *Buck's traction immobilizes the fracture and decreases pain and additional trauma.*

> **PRACTICE ALERT**
> Do not let weights lie on the bed or the floor. The weights can be removed long enough to move the patient up or down in bed to ensure freely hanging weights.

- Move the patient gently and slowly. *Gentle moving helps prevent the development of severe muscle spasms.*
- Elevate the injured extremity above the level of the heart. *Elevating the extremity promotes venous return and decreases edema, which decreases pain.*
- Encourage distraction or other adjunctive methods of pain relief, such as deep breathing and relaxation. *Distraction, deep breathing, and relaxation help decrease the focus on the pain and may lessen the intensity of pain.*
- Administer NSAIDs and pain medications as prescribed. For home care, explain the importance of taking pain medications before the pain is severe. *Analgesics alleviate pain by stimulating opiate receptor sites. NSAIDs mediate inflammation as well as providing an analgesic effect.*

> **PRACTICE ALERT**
> In the case of fracture in an extremity, supporting the extremity above and below the fracture can also decrease pain and muscle spasms.

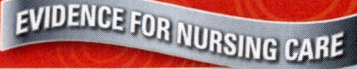

EVIDENCE FOR NURSING CARE — The Patient with Fracture

Selected resources that nurses may find helpful when planning evidence-based nursing care follow.

- Avenell, A., & Handoll, H. (2010). Nutritional supplementation for hip fracture aftercare in older people. *Cochrane Database of Systematic Reviews*, (1).
- Crilly, R., Hillier, L., Mason, M., Gutmanis, I., & Cox, L. (2010). Prevention of hip fractures in long-term care: relevance of community-derived data. *Journal of the American Geriatrics Society, 58*(4), 738–745.
- Egol, K., & Strauss, E. (2009). Perioperative considerations in geriatric patients with hip fracture: What is the evidence? *Journal of Orthopaedic Trauma, 23*(6), 386–394.
- Eid, T., & Bucknall, T. (2008). Documenting and implementing evidence-based post-operative pain management in older patients with hip fractures. *Journal of Orthopaedic Nursing, 12*(2), 90–98.
- Handoll, H., Cameron, I., Mak, J., & Finnegan, T. (2009). Multidisciplinary rehabilitation for older people with hip fractures. *Cochrane Database of Systematic Reviews*, (4).
- Morrison, R., Flanagan, S., Fischberg, D., Cintron, A., & Siu, A. (2009). A novel interdisciplinary analgesic program reduces pain and improves function in older adults after orthopedic surgery. *Journal of the American Geriatrics Society, 57*(1), 1–10.

Risk for Peripheral Neurovascular Dysfunction

In the patient with a fracture, compartment syndrome or deep venous thrombosis can impair circulation and, in turn, tissue perfusion. Furthermore, peripheral nerves may be damaged as a result of the initial trauma, during movement of the affected extremity, or as a consequence of compartment syndrome.

- Support the injured extremity above and below the fracture site when moving the patient. *Supporting the injured extremity above and below the fracture site helps prevent displacement of bony fragments and decreases the risk of further nerve damage.*
- Assess the 5 P's every 1 to 2 hours. Report abnormal findings immediately. *Unrelenting pain, pallor, diminished distal pulses, paresthesias, and paresis are strong indicators of compartment syndrome.*

> **PRACTICE ALERT**
> Pulses may remain strong, even in the presence of compartment syndrome.

- Assess nail beds for capillary refill. If nails are too thick or discolored, assess the skin around the nail. *Delayed capillary refill may indicate decreased tissue perfusion.*
- Monitor the extremity for edema and swelling. *Excessive swelling and hematoma formation can compromise circulation.*
- Assess for deep, throbbing, unrelenting pain. *Pain that is not relieved by analgesics may indicate neurovascular compromise.*
- Assess the ability to differentiate between sharp and dull touch and the presence of paresthesias and paralysis every 1 to 2 hours. *Paresthesias develop as a result of pressure on nerves and may indicate compartment syndrome.*

> **PRACTICE ALERT**
> Paralysis is a late sign of nerve entrapment and requires that the physician be notified immediately.

- Monitor the tightness of the cast. *Edema can cause the cast to become tight; a tight-fitting cast may lead to compartment syndrome or paralysis.*
- If the cast is tight, be prepared to assist the physician with bivalving (Figure 39–12 ■). *Bivalving, the process of splitting the cast down both sides, alleviates pressure on the injured extremity.*
- If compartment syndrome is suspected, assist the physician in measuring compartment pressure. Normal compartment pressure is 10 to 20 mmHg. *Compartment pressure greater than 30 mmHg indicates compartment syndrome.*
- Unless contraindicated, elevate the injured extremity above the level of the heart. *Elevating the extremity increases venous return and decreases edema. It may be contraindicated, however, if compartment syndrome develops, as elevation may further reduce arterial flow to the extremity.*
- Administer anticoagulant per physician's order. *Prophylactic anticoagulation decreases the risk of clot formation.*

Figure 39–12 ■ Bivalving is the process of splitting the cast down both sides to alleviate pressure on or allow visualization of the extremity.

Risk for Infection

An open fracture carries significant risk for wound contamination and subsequent infection. The patient who undergoes surgical repair will have a postoperative wound. Any break in skin integrity must be monitored for infection. Wound healing in orthopedic patients is affected by the cause of the wound as well as the therapies used to repair musculoskeletal structures. It is important for nurses to understand normal wound healing processes, characteristics of musculoskeletal wounds, contamination, and drainage, and potential complications to plan for and implement appropriate interventions.

■ For patients with skeletal pins, follow established guidelines for skeletal pin site care. *Pins or wires attached to traction, casts, or external fixators stabilize a segment of bone so optimal healing can occur.*
■ Monitor vital signs and lab reports of WBCs. *Increases in pulse rate, respiratory rate, temperature, and WBCs may indicate infection.*
■ Use sterile technique for dressing changes. *The initial postoperative dressing will be changed by the surgeon. The nurse must change all subsequent dressings without introducing organisms into the operative site.*
■ Assess the wound for size, color, and the presence of any drainage. *Redness, swelling, and purulent drainage indicate infection.*
■ Administer antibiotics per physician's orders. *Prophylactic antibiotic administration inhibits bacterial reproduction and thereby helps prevent skin flora from entering the wound. In the case of "dirty wounds," such as those occurring from vehicular crashes, antibiotics are routinely administered.*

Impaired Physical Mobility

The patient who has experienced a fracture requires immobilization of the fractured bone(s). Immobilization alters normal gait and mobility. The patient will need to use assistive devices such as crutches, canes, slings, or walkers.

■ Teach or assist patient with ROM exercises of the unaffected limbs. *ROM exercises help prevent muscle atrophy and maintain strength and joint function. Flexion and extension exercises prevent the development of foot drop, wrist drop, or frozen joints.*
■ Teach isometric exercises, and encourage the patient to perform them every 4 hours. *Isometric exercises help prevent muscle atrophy and force synovial fluid and nutrients into the cartilage.*
■ Encourage ambulation when able; provide assistance as necessary. *Ambulation maintains and improves circulation, helps prevent muscle atrophy, and helps maintain bowel function.*

> **SAFETY ALERT**
> Teach and observe the patient's use of assistive devices (such as canes, crutches, walkers, slings) in conjunction with the physical therapist. Proper use of devices is necessary for safe ambulation and helps prevent the loss of joint function secondary to complications and falls.

■ Turn the patient on bed rest every 2 hours. If the patient is in traction, teach the patient to shift his or her weight every hour. *Turning and shifting weight increase circulation and help prevent skin breakdown.*

Using NANDA, NIC, and NOC

Linkages between a selected NANDA nursing diagnosis, NIC, and NOC for the patient with a compound fracture are shown in the chart that follows.

Community-Based Care

Patient and family teaching focuses on individualized needs. The type of fracture and its location determine how much teaching the patient and family will require. For example, a patient who has a simple nondisplaced tibial fracture may need to be

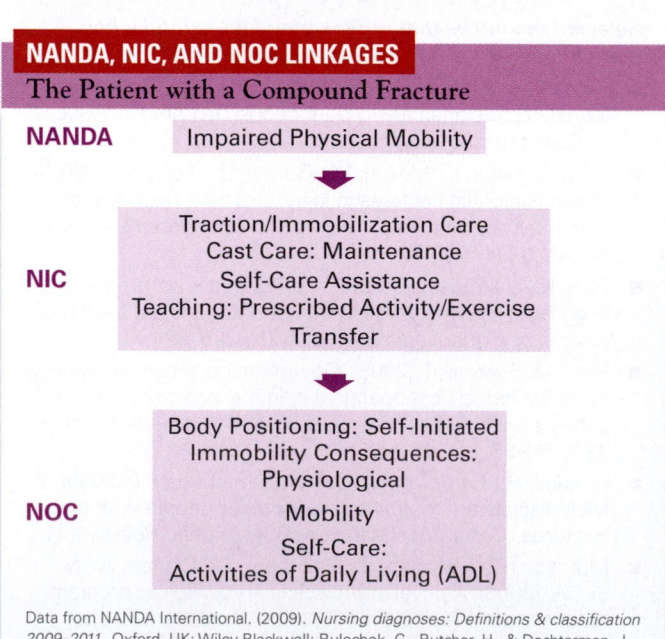

NANDA, NIC, AND NOC LINKAGES
The Patient with a Compound Fracture

NANDA Impaired Physical Mobility

NIC
Traction/Immobilization Care
Cast Care: Maintenance
Self-Care Assistance
Teaching: Prescribed Activity/Exercise
Transfer

NOC
Body Positioning: Self-Initiated
Immobility Consequences:
Physiological
Mobility
Self-Care:
Activities of Daily Living (ADL)

Data from NANDA International. (2009). *Nursing diagnoses: Definitions & classification 2009–2011.*, Oxford, UK: Wiley-Blackwell; Bulechek, G., Butcher, H., & Dochterman, J. (Eds.). (2008). *Nursing interventions classification (NIC)* (5th ed.). St. Louis, MO: Mosby; and Moorhead, S., Johnson, M., Maas, M., & Swanson, E. (Eds.). (2008). *Nursing outcomes classification (NOC)* (4th ed.). St. Louis, MO: Mosby.

CASE STUDY & NURSING CARE PLAN A Patient with a Hip Fracture

Stella Carbolito is a 74-year-old Italian American with a history of osteoporosis. She is a widow and lives alone in a two-story row home. Mrs. Carbolito is retired and depends on a pension check and social security for her income. She takes pride in making all her own food from scratch.

While walking to the market one day, Mrs. Carbolito falls and fractures her left hip. She is transported by ambulance to the nearest hospital emergency department.

ASSESSMENT

During the initial assessment at the emergency department, abnormal findings are that Mrs. Carbolito's left leg is shorter than her right leg and is externally rotated. Distal pulses are present and bilaterally strong; both legs are warm. Mrs. Carbolito complains of severe pain but states that no numbness or burning is present. She is able to wiggle the toes on her left leg and has full movement of her right leg. Initial vital signs are as follows: T 98.0°F (36.6°C), P 100, R 18, BP 120/58. Diagnostic tests include CBC, blood chemistry, and x-ray studies of the left hip and pelvis. The CBC reveals a hemoglobin of 11.0 g/dL and a normal WBC count. Blood chemistry findings are within normal limits. The x-ray reveals a fracture of the left femoral neck. Mrs. Carbolito is admitted to the hospital with an order for 10 lb of straight leg traction. An open reduction and internal fixation (ORIF) is planned for the following day.

DIAGNOSES

- *Acute Pain* related to fractured left femoral neck and muscle spasms
- *Impaired Physical Mobility* related to bed rest and fractured left femoral neck
- *Risk for Ineffective Peripheral Tissue Perfusion* related to unstable bones and swelling
- *Risk for Disturbed Sensory Perception: Tactile* related to the risk of nerve impairment

EXPECTED OUTCOMES

- Verbalize a decrease in pain.
- Verbalize the purpose of traction and surgery.
- Maintain normal neurovascular status.
- Demonstrate postoperative exercises.

PLANNING AND IMPLEMENTATION

- Assess pain on a scale of 0 to 10 before and after implementing measures to reduce pain.
- Administer analgesics per the physician's order.
- Perform neurovascular assessment every 2 to 4 hours, and document findings.
- Apply straight leg traction per physician's order.
- Encourage deep breathing and relaxation techniques.
- Teach the purpose of traction and surgery.
- Teach the purpose of and the procedure for performing isometric and flexion/extension exercises.

EVALUATION

Three days after surgery, Mrs. Carbolito is out of bed and in a chair. She verbalizes a decrease in pain. There have been no abnormal neurovascular assessments. She is able to independently perform isometric and flexion/extension exercises in both lower extremities. Discharge planning includes referrals for home care. A home health nurse will visit, and the social worker at the hospital has ordered a trapeze for her bed, an elevated toilet seat, an elevated cushion for her chair, and a walker.

CRITICAL THINKING IN THE NURSING PROCESS

1. What factors placed Mrs. Carbolito at risk for a hip fracture?
2. Mrs. Carbolito says, "I don't understand why they had to put that heavy thing on my leg before I went to surgery to get my hip fixed." What would you tell her? What preoperative factors might have decreased teaching effectiveness?
3. Describe how each of the following, if manifested by Mrs. Carbolito, would increase her risk for postoperative complications: urinary incontinence, weight more than 20% under normal for her height, chronic constipation. What nursing diagnoses and interventions would you include in her plan of care to decrease the risk?

See Evaluating Your Response in Appendix C.

---

taught only cast care and crutch walking. An older patient who has sustained a hip fracture and requires surgical intervention, by contrast, has a wider array of teaching needs, including the use of an abduction pillow, proper bending, and proper sitting. Address the following topics for home care of the patient who has fractured a hip:

- Encourage independence in ADLs:
  - Explain that the patient should sit only on high chairs to prevent excess flexion of the hip; an elevated toilet seat can be added to a regular toilet seat.
  - Encourage the patient and family to equip the shower with a hand rail to aid stability and prevent falls.
  - If a walker is needed, teach the patient its proper use: Do not carry the walker, but lift it, advance it, and then take two steps, or use a rolling walker.
  - If a cane is needed, instruct the patient to use it on the affected side.
- Stress the importance of well-balanced meals, and explain all prescribed medications.

Patients who have experienced a fracture or who have had orthopedic surgery often have a cast and require an extended period of immobilization or limited activities. Address the following topics for home care:

- Do not scratch under a cast with a sharp object; use a blow dryer on the cool setting to relieve itching.
- Do not get a plaster cast wet.
- Follow the physician's order for weight bearing.
- Physical therapy departments or offices often can evaluate the home environment for safety and suggest modifications as needed. Physical therapists also teach crutch walking, limited weight bearing, transferring, and other activities.
- Home care agencies can teach wound care and provide ongoing monitoring of wound healing.
- Local medical equipment and supply sources rent or sell durable equipment such as crutches, walkers, wheelchairs, overhead trapeze units, shower chairs, elevated toilet seats, grab bars, and bedside commodes. Slings or braces may be purchased through medical equipment dealers.
- Local pharmacies are good resources for dressing supplies such as antiseptic solutions or ointments, dressings, and tape.
- Fitness equipment suppliers may be able to provide rehabilitation equipment such as hand or ankle weights for strengthening exercises.

Amputation Video

The Patient with an Amputation

An **amputation** is the partial or total removal of an extremity. Amputation may be the result of an acute process, such as a traumatic event, or a chronic condition, such as peripheral vascular disease or diabetes mellitus. Regardless of the cause, an amputation is devastating to the patient.

FAST FACTS

Amputation

- It is estimated that 1.7 million people with amputations live in the United States, and that 134,000 new amputations occur each year.
- In the United States, the most common cause of lower extremity amputations is vascular disease (82%). Men and Blacks have the greatest risk of undergoing lower extremity amputation due to vascular disease.
- Trauma is the second leading cause of amputation in the United States. Upper extremity amputations account for more than 68% of traumatic amputations. Men have a significantly higher risk of traumatic amputation than women.
- Cancer-related amputations affect men and women equally; cancer-related lower extremity amputations are more common than are upper extremity amputations.

Data from National Limb Loss Information Center (2009).

The loss of all or part of an extremity has a significant physical and psychosocial effect on the patient and family. Adaptation may take a long time and require much effort. Interdisciplinary health care is always important, but is especially necessary to meet the patient's physical, spiritual, cultural, and emotional needs after an unexpected or planned amputation.

Causes of Amputation

Peripheral vascular disease (PVD) is the major cause of amputation of the lower extremities (∞ see Chapter 32). Common risk factors for the development of PVD include hypertension, diabetes, smoking, and hyperlipidemia. Peripheral neuropathy also places the person with diabetes at risk for amputation. In peripheral neuropathy, loss of sensation frequently leads to unrecognized injury and infection. Untreated infection may lead to gangrene and the need for amputation. These risks are discussed in ∞ Chapter 20.

The incidence of traumatic amputations is highest among young men. Most amputations in this group result from motor vehicle crashes or accidents involving machinery at work. Combat-related trauma also accounts for a significant number of traumatic amputations in young adults. The patient presents to the trauma center with an injury that may be life threatening; significant loss of blood and tissue may have already occurred, and shock may develop. (∞ See Chapter 11 for a discussion of shock and trauma.) Other traumatic events that may necessitate an amputation are frostbite, burns, or electrocution.

Amputations result from or are necessitated by interruption in blood flow, either acute or chronic. In acute trauma situations, the limb is partially or completely severed, and tissue death ensues. However, replantation of fingers, small body parts, and entire limbs has been successful. In chronic disease processes,

circulation is impaired, venous pooling begins, proteins leak into the interstitium, and edema develops. Edema increases the risk of injury and further decreases circulation. Stasis ulcers develop and readily become infected because impaired healing and altered immune processes allow bacteria to proliferate. The presence of progressive infection further compromises circulation and ultimately leads to gangrene (tissue death), which requires amputation.

Levels of Amputation

The level of amputation is determined by local and systemic factors. Local factors include ischemia and gangrene; system factors include cardiovascular status, renal function, and severity of diabetes mellitus. The goals are to alleviate symptoms, to maintain healthy tissue, and to increase functional outcome. When possible, the joints are preserved because they allow greater function of the extremity. Figure 39–13 ■ illustrates common sites of amputation.

Types of Amputation

Amputations may be open (*guillotine*) or closed (*flap*). Open amputations are performed when infection is present. The wound is not closed but remains open to drain. When infection is no longer present, surgery is performed to close the wound. In closed amputations, the wound is closed with a flap of skin that is sutured in place over the stump. Terms used to refer to amputations are defined in Table 39–4.

Amputation Site Healing

For the prosthesis to fit well, the amputation site must heal properly. To promote healing, a rigid or compression dressing is applied to prevent infection and minimize edema. A rigid dressing is made by placing a cast on the stump and molding the stump to fit a prosthesis. A soft compression dressing is applied when frequent wound checks are necessary. When this

---

TABLE 39–4 Amputation Terms

TERM	MEANING
Arm	Amputation of a portion of the arm, either above or below the elbow
Disarticulation	Amputation through a joint
Forequarter	Removal of the entire arm and disarticulation of the shoulder
Closed (flap)	Amputation in which a flap of skin is formed to cover the end of the wound
Open (guillotine)	Perpendicular cutting of the extremity in which the wound is left open; used when infection is present
Leg	Amputation below the knee (BK)
Thigh	Amputation above the knee (AK)
Finger or toe	Amputation of one or all of the fingers or toes
Syme	Modified disarticulation of the ankle
Foot	Amputation of part of the foot and toes

Figure 39–13 ■ Common sites of amputation. *A,* The upper extremities. *B,* The lower extremities. The surgeon determines the level of amputation based on blood supply and tissue condition.

type of dressing is used, a splint is sometimes applied to help mold the extremity to fit the prosthesis. After the wound is dressed, the patient is encouraged to toughen the stump skin by pushing it into first soft and then harder surfaces. The stump is wrapped in an Ace bandage to allow a conical shape to form and to prevent edema. The bandage is applied from the distal to the proximal extremity (Figure 39–14 ■).

Figure 39–14 ■ Stump dressings increase venous return, decrease edema, and help shape the stump for a prosthesis. With an above-knee amputation, a figure-eight bandage is started by bringing the bandage down over the stump and back up around the hips.

Complications

Complications that may occur after an amputation include infection, delayed healing, chronic stump pain and phantom pain, and contractures.

Infection

Generally, the patient who suffers a traumatic amputation has a greater risk of infection than the person who has a planned amputation. However, even planned amputations carry a risk of infection. The patient who is older, has diabetes mellitus, or suffers peripheral neurovascular compromise is at a particularly high risk for infection. Infection may present itself locally or systemically. Local manifestations of infection include drainage, odor, redness, and increased discomfort at the suture line. Systemic manifestations include fever, an increased heart rate, a decrease in blood pressure, chills, and positive wound or blood cultures.

Delayed Healing

If infection is present or if the circulation remains compromised, delayed healing (occurring at a slower rate than expected) will result. In older patients, other preexisting conditions can increase the risk of delayed healing. In patients of any age, electrolyte imbalances can contribute to delayed healing processes, as can a diet that lacks the proper nutrients to meet the body's increased metabolic demands during healing. Smoking compromises healing by causing vasoconstriction and decreasing blood flow to the stump. Deep venous thrombosis and compromised venous return, which may result from prolonged immobilization, are other potential factors. Decreased cardiac output decreases blood flow and thus also delays healing.

Chronic Stump Pain and Phantom Limb Pain

Chronic stump pain is the result of neuroma formation, causing severe burning pain. Interventions to relieve this pain include medications, nerve blocks, transcutaneous electrical nerve stimulation (TENS), and surgical stump reconstruction. **Phantom limb pain** is not the same as phantom limb sensation. A majority of amputees experience phantom limb sensation (sensations such as tingling, numbness, cramping, or itching in the phantom foot or hand) early in the postoperative period. It is often self-limited, but may last for decades in some patients. When phantom limb sensation is painful, it is referred to as phantom limb pain. Phantom limb pain more frequently affects people who had pain in the amputated limb prior to its removal than those who did not. Several theories for phantom limb pain have been developed. These include regeneration of severed peripheral nerves and abnormal impulses generated by spinal cord neurons that no longer receive normal sensory input from the body (Porth & Matfin, 2009). Treatments include pain management, TENS, and a variety of surgical procedures. The management of phantom limb pain is difficult for both patients and healthcare professionals. Patients with phantom limb pain often benefit from referral to a pain clinic for a comprehensive pain management program.

Contractures

A **contracture** is an abnormal flexion and fixation of a joint caused by muscle atrophy and shortening. Contracture of the joint above the amputation is a common complication. The patient needs to be taught to extend the joint and to perform muscle-strengthening exercises. The patient with an above-the-knee amputation should lie prone for periods throughout the day. The patient with a below-the-knee amputation should elevate the stump, keeping the knee extended. A knee immobilizer may be used to help maintain joint extension (Department of Veterans Affairs, 2007). The same principles apply to the upper extremities. All joints should receive either active or passive ROM exercises every 2 to 4 hours. A trapeze frame should be added to the bed to encourage the patient to change position every 2 hours. The patient who has an upper extremity amputation should exercise both shoulders. Postural exercises can help prevent the patient from hunching over secondary to the loss of weight on the affected side. The patient with an above-the-knee amputation should not sit for prolonged periods of time; prolonged sitting can lead to hip contracture.

Interdisciplinary Care

Interdisciplinary care is essential for the patient who has sustained an amputation. Physical therapy and occupational retraining are necessary, and the patient may also benefit from the presence of clergy. The entire healthcare team must view both the positive and the negative effects of amputation; that is, they must see amputation as a means to increase the patient's independence and to relieve symptoms. The patient should be able to become familiar with the members of the healthcare team and their roles; this allows the patient greater control over his or her care and rehabilitation and promotes independence.

Diagnosis

Preoperatively, the patient has routine laboratory and diagnostic tests (∞ see Chapter 4 for care of the patient having surgery). Preoperative tests, including Doppler flowmetry, segmental blood pressure determination, transcutaneous partial pressure oxygen readings, and angiography are performed to assess the circulation present in the limb at different levels and to determine the level of viable tissue. Postoperative tests include CBC to monitor for hemorrhage, WBC count to monitor for infection, blood chemistries to evaluate electrolytes and fluid balance, and a vascular Doppler ultrasonography if a DVT is suspected.

Medications

Medications are used to manage pain, prevent or treat infection, and as needed to maintain cardiac output and tissue perfusion. Postoperatively, the patient resumes any routinely prescribed medications and in addition may receive antibiotics and analgesics. Steroids may be administered to decrease swelling. A histamine H_2 antagonist may also be ordered to decrease the risk of peptic ulcer formation. Stool softeners may be administered to prevent constipation.

Prosthesis

The type of prosthesis selected for the patient with an amputation depends on the level of the amputation as well as the patient's occupation and lifestyle. Each prosthesis is based on a detailed prosthetic prescription and is custom made for the patient. Most are made of plastic and foam materials. Many factors influence the patient's use of the prosthesis, including the status of the remaining limb, cognitive status, cardiovascular status, preoperative activity level, and motivation to use the prosthesis.

Patients with a lower extremity amputation are often fitted with early walking aids. Pneumatic devices that fit over the stump are used in the immediate postoperative period to allow early ambulation, decrease postoperative swelling, and improve morale. Patients may begin weight bearing as soon as 2 weeks after surgery. Patients with upper extremity amputations may be fitted for a prosthesis immediately after surgery. Rehabilitation of the patient with an amputation is a team effort, involving the patient, nurse, physician, physical therapist, occupational therapist, social worker, prosthetist, and vocational counselor.

∞ Nursing Care

Health Promotion

The goals of health promotion activities focus on preventing the progression of chronic diseases such as PVD and diabetes mellitus, and on safety. Patients with PVD from any cause need education about foot care and early recognition of decreased circulation. Education within both urban and rural populations should provide knowledge about working safely with lawn care equipment as well as farm and occupational machinery.

In addition, it is important that the public know what to do if a traumatic amputation occurs in the home, community, or workplace. Preserving life is the first priority: First ensure that the patient can breathe; administer CPR as necessary, and control bleeding with direct pressure. The following guidelines may help preserve the amputated part until it can be surgically reattached:

- Keep the person in a supine position with the legs elevated.
- Apply firm pressure to the bleeding area, using a towel or article of clothing.
- Wrap the amputated part in a clean cloth. If possible, soak the cloth in saline (such as contact lens solution).
- Put the amputated part in a plastic bag and put the bag on ice. Do not let the amputated part come into direct contact with the ice or water.
- Send the amputated part to the emergency department with the injured person, and be sure the emergency personnel know what it is.

Assessment

Collect the following data through the health history and physical examination. Further focused assessments are described in the following nursing interventions sections.

- *Health history:* Mechanism of injury, current and past health problems, pain, occupation, ADLs, changes in sensation in the feet, cultural and/or religious guidelines for handling the amputated part.
- *Physical examination:* Bilateral neurovascular status of the extremities, bilateral capillary refill time, skin over the lower extremities (discoloration, edema, ulcerations, hair, gangrene).

Nursing Diagnoses and Interventions

The goals of nursing care for a person with an amputation are to relieve pain, promote healing, prevent complications, support the patient and family during the process of grieving and adaptation to alterations in body image, and restore mobility. Care is individualized, and the circumstances that led to the amputation (e.g., traumatic injury or disease) also must be

EVIDENCE FOR NURSING CARE — **The Patient with Amputation**

Selected resources that nurses may find helpful when planning evidence-based nursing care follow.

- Department of Veterans Affairs, Department of Defense. (2007). *VA/DoD clinical practice guideline for rehabilitation of lower amputation.* Washington (DC): Department of Veterans Affairs, Department of Defense. Retrieved from www.guideline.gov
- Gailey, R., Allen, K., Castles, J., Kucharik, J., & Roeder, M. (2008). Review of secondary physical conditions associated with lower-limb amputation and long-term prosthesis use. *Journal of Rehabilitation Research & Development, 45*(1), 15–29.
- Lyon, K. (2008). The case for evidence in wound care: investigating advanced treatment modalities in healing chronic diabetic lower extremity wounds. *Journal of Wound, Ostomy & Continence Nursing, 35*(6), 585–590.
- van Twillert, S., Postema, K., Geertzen, J., Hemminga, T., & Lettinga, A. (2009). Improving rehabilitation treatment in a local setting: A case study of prosthetic rehabilitation. *Clinical Rehabilitation, 23*(10), 938–947.

addressed. See the accompanying Case Study & Nursing Care Plan on page 1332. Applying rehabilitation principles to nursing care is also important.

Acute Pain

Pain from the surgical procedure can be compounded by muscle spasms, swelling, and phantom limb pain.

- Ask the patient to rate the pain on a scale of 0 to 10 (with 10 as the most severe pain) before and after any intervention. *This facilitates objective assessment of the effectiveness of the chosen pain relief strategy. Pain that increases in intensity or remains unrelieved with analgesics can indicate compartment syndrome.*
- Splint and support the injured area. *Splinting prevents additional injury by immobilizing the stump and decreasing edema while molding the stump for a good prosthetic fit.*
- Unless contraindicated, elevate the stump on a pillow for the first 24 hours after surgery. *Elevating the stump promotes venous return and decreases edema, which will decrease pain.*

> **PRACTICE ALERT**
> Elevating the stump for long periods after the immediate postoperative period increases the risk for hip contractures.

- Move and turn the patient gently and slowly. *Gentle moving and turning prevents the development of severe muscle spasms.*
- Administer pain medications as prescribed. A PCA pump may be ordered by the physician. *Analgesics alleviate pain by stimulating opiate receptor sites. PCA pumps increase patient control over and allow early relief of pain before it intensifies.*
- Encourage deep breathing and relaxation exercises. *These techniques increase the effectiveness of analgesics and modify the pain experience.*
- Reposition patient every 2 hours; turn from side to side and onto abdomen. *Repositioning alleviates pressure from one area and distributes it throughout the body and helps prevent cramping of muscles.*

> **PRACTICE ALERT**
> Lying prone prevents hip contracture.

Risk for Infection

The patient who has an amputation is at risk for wound infection. Early recognition of infection can lead to early treatment and prevent wound dehiscence.

- Assess the wound for redness, drainage, temperature, edema, and suture line approximation. *Redness is normal in the immediate postoperative period; if it persists, however, it can indicate infection. A hot area that is palpated over the incision or increased drainage may also indicate infection.*
- Take the patient's temperature every 4 hours. *Increased body temperature may indicate infection.*
- Monitor WBC count. *The WBC count rises in the presence of infection.*
- Use aseptic technique to change the wound dressing. *Aseptic technique prevents the contamination of the wound with bacteria.*

CASE STUDY & NURSING CARE PLAN   A Patient with a Below-the-Knee Amputation

John Rocke is a 45-year-old divorcee with no children. He has a history of type 1 diabetes mellitus and poor control of blood glucose levels. Mr. Rocke is unemployed and currently receives unemployment compensation. He lives alone in a second-floor apartment. Mr. Rocke had developed gangrene in the foot and failed to seek prompt medical attention; as a result, a left below-the-knee amputation was necessary.

Mr. Rocke is in his second postoperative day and his vital signs are stable. The stump is splinted and has a soft dressing. The wound is approximating well without signs of infection. He has not performed ROM exercises or turning since his surgery, complaining of severe pain. When the nurse goes into the room, he yells, "Get out! I don't want anyone to see me like this." No one has visited him since his hospitalization. He is tolerating an 1800-kcal diabetic diet and is using a urinal independently. He has an order for morphine, 10 mg IM every 3 to 4 hours prn for pain, and cefazolin (Ancef), 1 g IV every 8 hours. He is on blood glucose coverage with regular insulin subcutaneously.

ASSESSMENT

Jane Simmons, RN, has just come on duty. She notes that the patient is upset and angry. Mr. Rocke will not let anyone enter the room to give him medication or assess his vital signs.

DIAGNOSES

- *Disturbed Body Image* related to amputation of left lower leg
- *Complicated Grieving* related to anger and loss of left lower leg
- *Situational Low Self-Esteem* related to appearance
- *Ineffective Self-Health Management* related to refusal of care
- *Acute Pain* related to surgery

EXPECTED OUTCOMES

- Verbalize his feelings about the amputation.
- Allow the staff to monitor his vital signs and administer medications.
- Be allowed to control his pain with a PCA pump.
- Verbalize a decrease in pain.
- Verbalize the importance of turning.
- Turn every 2 hours.

PLANNING AND IMPLEMENTATION

- Encourage verbalization of feelings.
- Actively listen to the patient.
- Offer to arrange a visit with a fellow amputee.
- Ask the physician if the patient can be placed on a PCA pump.
- Teach the patient the importance of turning every 2 hours to prevent contractures.
- Encourage turning and lying prone.
- Teach the importance of antibiotics in preventing and treating infection.

EVALUATION

One week after his surgery, Mr. Rocke is actively participating in his care. He has apologized for his behavior and has explained to Ms. Simmons that he was angry about the loss of his leg. He states, "I thought I knew what to expect but I didn't."

CRITICAL THINKING IN THE NURSING PROCESS

1. Once Mr. Rocke is ready to assist with his stump care, how would you proceed? Would you give him full responsibility for care and dressings, or would you gradually increase his participation? Why?
2. What factors in Mr. Rocke's home environment and medical history may make self-care more difficult? Do you expect Mr. Rocke to follow up on care after his discharge? Why or why not?
3. Mr. Rocke states, "Why should I exercise this leg—it was already cut off!" How would you respond? What is the purpose of exercising the stump?

See Evaluating Your Response in Appendix C.

- Administer antibiotics as ordered. *Antibiotics inhibit bacterial cell replication and help prevent or eradicate infection.*
- Teach the patient stump-wrapping techniques. *Correctly wrapping the stump from the distal to proximal extremity increases venous return and prevents pooling of fluid, thereby reducing the chance of infection.*

Risk for Impaired Skin Integrity

Stump care is essential, not only in the postoperative healing period, but also throughout life with a prosthesis. A variety of skin problems may be caused by a prosthesis, including epidermoid cysts, abrasions, blisters, and hair follicle infections. The patient must be taught stump care prior to discharge.

- Each day, preferably at night, wash the stump with soap and warm water and dry thoroughly. Inspect the stump for redness, irritation, or abrasions. *It is essential to maintain intact skin to ensure successful use of the prosthesis.*
- Massage the end of the stump, beginning 3 weeks after surgery. *Massage helps desensitize the remaining part of the*

limb and prevents scar tissue formation. If the skin adheres to the underlying tissue, it will tear when stressed by wearing a prosthesis.

- Expose any open areas of skin on the remaining part of the limb for 1 hour four times a day. *Air exposure promotes healing.*
- Change stump socks and elastic wraps each day. Wash these in mild soap and water, and allow to completely dry before using again. *Stump socks and elastic wraps must be kept clean and dry to prevent skin breakdown.*

Risk for Complicated Grieving

The patient who has lost an extremity is at risk for complicated grieving. Denial of the need for surgery and the inability to discuss feelings compound this risk.

- Encourage verbalization of feelings, using open-ended questions. *Asking open-ended questions allows the patient to discuss feelings and communicates the listener's willingness to listen.*

- Actively listen and maintain eye contact. *Active listening and eye contact communicate respect for what the patient is expressing.*
- Reflect on the patient's feelings. *Reflection statements such as "You seem angry" allow the patient to recognize feelings and perhaps develop a plan for resolution.*
- Allow the patient to have unlimited visiting hours, if possible. *Unlimited visiting hours allow increased social support.*
- If desired by the patient, provide spiritual support by encouraging activities such as visits from a spiritual leader, prayer, and meditation. *These activities often provide support during the grieving process.*

Disturbed Body Image

Although amputation is a reconstructive surgery, the patient's body image will be disturbed. Risk for body image disturbance is higher in young trauma patients, in whom body image is a particularly important component of self-image.

- Encourage verbalization of feelings. *This allows the patient to communicate concerns and fears and lets the patient know the nurse is willing to listen.*
- Allow the patient to wear clothing from home. *Familiar clothing provides emotional comfort and helps the patient retain a sense of his or her own identity.*
- Encourage the patient to look at the stump. *Looking at and touching the stump helps the patient face his or her fear of the unknown and move from denial to acceptance.*
- Encourage the patient to care for the stump. *Active participation in care increases self-esteem and independence.*
- Offer to have a fellow amputee visit the patient. *A support person who has experienced the same change gives the patient the hope that he or she can regain independence.*
- Encourage active participation in rehabilitation. *Active participation in rehabilitation increases independence and mobility.*

Impaired Physical Mobility

If time allows, the patient should begin strengthening muscles preoperatively. If the amputation is the result of an emergency, exercises begin within 24 to 48 hours of surgery. The return of independent mobility boosts self-esteem and promotes adaptation to amputation.

- Perform ROM exercises on all joints. *ROM exercises help prevent the development of joint contractures that limit mobility.*
- Maintain postoperative stump shrinkage devices. These may be elastic bandages, shrinker socks, an elastic stockinette, or a rigid plaster cast. *Postoperative dressings decrease edema and shape the stump for prosthetic wear.*
- Turn and reposition the patient every 2 hours. *The patient with a lower extremity amputation should lie prone every 4 hours. Repositioning increases blood flow to muscles, forces synovial fluid into joints, and helps prevent contractures.*
- Reinforce teaching by the physical therapist in crutch walking or the use of assistive devices. *These devices increase mobility by balancing the patient and facilitating ambulation.*
- Encourage active participation in physical therapy. *Physical therapy will fatigue the patient in the early stage of healing. Encouragement may increase the patient's participation in the physical therapy regimen and thereby increase activity tolerance.*

Using NANDA, NIC, and NOC

Linkages between a selected NANDA nursing diagnosis, NIC, and NOC for the patient with an amputation are shown in the chart that follows.

Community-Based Care

Patient and family teaching includes stump care, prosthesis fitting and care, medications, assistive devices, exercises, rehabilitation, counseling, support services, and follow-up appointments. The depth of teaching depends on the cause and site of the amputation and the needs of the patient. See the Meeting Individualized Needs box on page 1334.

Holistic nursing care is especially important for the older patient with an amputation. The normal aging process decreases renal and liver function; hence, medications have longer half-lives. Altered circulation prolongs wound healing, and slowing of reflexes and alterations in gait may disrupt balance. A walker may be more appropriate than crutches, because older patients have less strength in the upper extremities. Safety issues, such as decreasing the risk for recurrent falls, must be addressed. The nurse should also assess the patient's need for in-home assistance and make appropriate referrals to visiting nurses and home health aides.

In addition, suggest the following resources:

- The Amputee Coalition of America
- Amputee Resource Foundation of America

NANDA, NIC, AND NOC LINKAGES
The Patient with an Amputation

NANDA — Disturbed Body Image

NIC — Amputation Care / Grief Work Facilitation / Coping Enhancement / Body Image Enhancement

NOC — Adaptation to Physical Disability / Grief Resolution / Body Image

Data from NANDA International. (2009). *Nursing diagnoses: Definitions & classification 2009–2011.* Oxford, UK: Wiley-Blackwell; Bulechek, G., Butcher, H., & Dochterman, J. (Eds.). (2008). *Nursing interventions classification (NIC)* (5th ed.). St. Louis, MO: Mosby; and Moorhead, S., Johnson, M., Maas, M., & Swanson, E. (Eds.). (2008). *Nursing outcomes classification (NOC)* (4th ed.). St. Louis, MO: Mosby.

MEETING INDIVIDUALIZED NEEDS   **The Patient with an Amputation**

Amputation of a limb has significant long-term consequences for the patient. The patient will grieve the loss of a body part and must adjust to a new self-image. The patient's ability to perform normal ADLs and to maintain his or her usual family and social roles may be significantly affected, at least initially. Depending on the patient's occupation, job performance may be affected, necessitating a change of career.

The nurse may be responsible for involving multiple members of the healthcare team in the patient's care and rehabilitation and coordinating their activities. Following an amputation, the patient may need the services of any or all of the following:

- Social services to help with rehabilitative and financial arrangements
- Physical therapists to teach ambulation techniques, and to provide deep heat or massage
- Occupational therapists to assist the patient in developing adaptive techniques to deal with the loss of a limb
- Prosthetists to develop a prosthesis for the missing limb that will meet the patient's needs for ADLs and other activities
- Home health services for nursing care such as assessments and wound care
- Support group services to assist in adapting to the body image change and effects of amputation on ADLs

ASSESSING FOR HOME CARE

Preparing the amputee for home care includes a careful assessment of the patient, the family, available support services and the home for possible barriers to the patient's safety and independence.

Assess the patient's acceptance of the amputation and knowledge base about care needs, any activity restrictions or special needs, and resources for home care. Discuss home management—who is responsible for household activities such as cleaning and cooking. Inquire about arrangements that have been made for home care activities and ADLs. Evaluate the patient's use of prescription and nonprescription medications, paying particular attention to possible interactions and drugs

that may affect the patient's balance, mental alertness, or appetite. Ask about social habits, such as cigarette smoking, alcohol use, or other drug use, that may affect healing or the patient's ability to provide self-care.

Assess the patient's home environment for possible safety hazards or barriers to ambulation, such as the following:

- Scatter rugs
- Stairs between living areas of the house
- Presence of grab bars to facilitate toileting and bathing
- Access to clean water and other needs for wound care

TEACHING FOR HOME CARE

The new amputee needs a great deal of teaching to learn to adapt to loss of a limb, whether it is an upper or lower extremity that has been lost. Because the patient must be ready to learn before teaching can be effective, use therapeutic communication techniques to encourage the patient to verbalize feelings about the amputation and its effects. Use active listening and teach the patient ways to reduce anxiety and deal with feelings of helplessness and loss. Encourage the patient to participate in care of the stump to build self-esteem and reinforce teaching. Include the following in teaching for home care:

- Teach the patient to wrap the stump appropriately in preparation for fitting the prosthesis.
- Discuss positioning of the stump. Contractures are a particular problem for patients with an above-knee amputation, and can interfere with ability to effectively use a prosthesis.
- Teach the patient how to perform stump exercises to maintain joint mobility and muscle tone of the affected limb.
- Encourage the patient to resume physical activities as soon as possible. This improves the patient's health and well-being, as well as the patient's self-esteem.
- Discuss household modifications to promote independence, such as grab bars in the bathroom, faucets with single-handle controls for water flow and temperature, and handheld shower heads and shower chairs for bathing.

CHAPTER HIGHLIGHTS

- The most commonly reported musculoskeletal injuries are contusions, strains, and sprains. Immediate treatment includes RICE (rest, ice, compression, elevation) therapy.
- Trauma to the joints may damage soft tissue, cartilage, or even lead to dislocation of the joint. Nursing assessments include monitoring neurovascular status by assessing for increased pain, decreased or absent pulses, pale skin, inability to move a body part or extremity, and changes in sensation.
- Repetitive use injuries, especially common in the workplace, include carpal tunnel syndrome, bursitis, and epicondylitis.
- Any of the 206 bones of the body may sustain a fracture. Fractures are closed or simple (skin is intact) or open or compound (skin

integrity is interrupted); open fractures are at risk for infection. Other fracture descriptors include oblique or spiral, avulsed, comminuted, compressed, impacted, or depressed.

- Fractures heal through four phases: hematoma, fibrocartilaginous callus, bony callus, and remodeling. Healing is influenced by the age and physical condition of the patient and by the type of fracture.
- Fracture complications include compartment syndrome, fat embolism syndrome, deep venous thrombosis, infection, delayed union and nonunion, and complex regional pain syndrome.
- Fractures are treated with surgery, traction, and/or casts to stabilize the fractured bone, maintain bone immobilization, prevent complications, and restore function.

- Fractures of the hip are most often sustained by older adult women, and are usually the result of a fall. They are the most common injury in the older population, resulting in the greatest number of deaths and most serious health problems of all fractures for people aged 65 years and older.
- Nursing care for the patient with a fracture focuses on interventions for acute pain, risk for peripheral vascular dysfunction, risk for infection, impaired physical mobility, and risk for disturbed tactile sensory perception.
- An amputation is the partial or total removal of an extremity. This loss has a significant physical and psychosocial effect on the patient and on the family. The most common cause for amputation

of a lower extremity is peripheral vascular disease. Trauma is the most common cause for upper extremity amputation.
- Complications that may follow an amputation include infection, delayed healing, chronic stump pain, phantom pain, and contractures. Stump care is necessary to prevent complications and to prepare the stump for a prosthesis.
- Nursing care for the patient with an amputation is provided as part of the interdisciplinary team, and is focused on a return to functional health, with interventions to meet needs for acute pain, impaired skin integrity, grieving, disturbed body image, and impaired physical mobility.

TEST YOURSELF NCLEX-RN® REVIEW

1. You are teaching a young adult how to provide self-care for a sprained ankle. You explain that the reason for applying ice immediately after the injury is based on the principle that ice does which of the following?
   1. increases the diameter of blood vessels
   2. decreases the diameter of blood vessels
   3. is helpful in increasing white blood cells
   4. lowers the blood pressure and pulse

2. A patient with a compound, open fracture has been admitted to the emergency department and is scheduled for immediate surgery. Which of the following nursing diagnoses would be most appropriate in the immediate postoperative period?
   1. *Risk for Post-Trauma Syndrome*
   2. *Impaired Transfer Ability*
   3. *Risk for Infection*
   4. *Risk for Falls*

3. While providing care to an older woman with a cast on her left lower arm (from below the elbow to above the fingers), you perform a neurovascular assessment. Which of the following assessments indicates a possible complication?
   1. slightly edematous fingers
   2. warm, pink skin above the cast
   3. pale, cold fingers
   4. pain rating of 2 on a 0 to 10 scale

4. Which of the following minerals is essential to bone healing?
   1. potassium
   2. magnesium
   3. sodium
   4. calcium

5. You are assessing a young man with a newly applied longleg cast. He complains of extreme pain in his leg, and his toes are cyanotic and lack sensation. What is your priority intervention?
   1. Document the assessments carefully and accurately.
   2. Notify the healthcare provider who applied the cast.
   3. Elevate the leg on at least three pillows.
   4. Apply an ice bag over the painful area.

6. Your assigned patient has been diagnosed with DVT of the left lower extremity. What body system would require very careful monitoring?
   1. hematologic
   2. respiratory
   3. digestive
   4. renal

7. Although nursing diagnoses are always individualized, what is one nursing diagnosis common to all musculoskeletal injuries?
   1. *Disturbed Body Image*
   2. *Acute Pain*
   3. *Chronic Pain*
   4. *Risk for Infection*

8. At what position would you place the remaining extremity following a below-the-knee amputation during the first 24 hours after surgery?
   1. elevated above the level of the heart
   2. lower than the rest of the body
   3. crossed over the intact extremity
   4. level with the rest of the body

9. The day following a below-the-knee amputation, your patient tells you that he feels as though his toes are cramping in the amputated foot. What is this experience called?
   1. chronic stump pain
   2. contractures
   3. attention-seeking
   4. phantom limb pain

10. Your husband is cutting wood with a circular saw. He suddenly screams that he has cut off his finger. What would you do with the amputated finger?
    1. Don't worry about it; the important thing is to get him to the hospital.
    2. Put it in a storage bag filled with warm water.
    3. Tape it to his hand so the emergency personnel will know where it is.
    4. Wrap it in a towel, put it in a plastic bag, and lay it on ice.

See Test Yourself answers in Appendix C.

Pearson Nursing Student Resources

Find additional review materials at
www.nursing.pearsonhighered.com

Prepare for success with additional NCLEX®-style practice questions, interactive assignments and activities, Web links, animations and videos, and more!

BIBLIOGRAPHY

Bulechek, G., Butcher, H., & Dochterman, J. (Eds.). (2008). *Nursing interventions classification (NIC)* (5th ed.). St. Louis, MO: Mosby.

Centers for Disease Control and Prevention. (2009 July 29). Falls among older adults: An overview. Retrieved from www.cdc.gov/HomeandRecreationalSafety/Falls/adultfalls.html

Christofi, T., Kallis, A., Raptis, D., Rowland, M., & Ryan, J. (2007). Management of shoulder dislocations. *Trauma 2007, 9,* 39–46.

Deakin, D., & Porter, K. (2009). Traumatic hip dislocation in adults. *Trauma 2009, 11,* 189–197.

Department of Veterans Affairs, Department of Defense. (2007). *VA/DoD clinical practice guideline for rehabilitation of lower amputation.* Washington, DC: Author.

Drozd, M., Miles, S., & Davies, J. (2009 May). Essential practice in casting. *Emergency Nurse, 17*(2), 18–19.

Drozd, M., Miles, S., & Davies, J. (2009 June). Casting: Complications and after care. *Emergency Nurse, 17*(3), 26–27.

Gray-Micelli, D. (2008 January). Falls. Nursing standard of practice protocol: Fall prevention. Retrieved from www.consultgerirn.org/topics/falls/want_to_know_more

Healy, A., & Tai, N. (2009). Traumatic amputation – a contemporary approach. *Trauma 2009, 11,* 177–187.

Holmes, S., & Brown, S. (2005). Skeletal pin site care. National Association of Orthopaedic Nurses guidelines for orthopaedic nursing. *Orthopaedic Nursing, 24*(2), 99–108.

Kare, J. (2008 August). *Volkmann contracture.* Retrieved from www.emedicine.medscape.com

Maynard G., & Stein J. (2008). *Preventing hospital-acquired venous thromboembolism: A guide for effective quality improvement.* Prepared by the Society of Hospital Medicine. AHRQ Publication No. 08-0075. Rockville, MD: Agency for Healthcare Research and Quality.

Mayo Clinic. (2006). *Dislocation; first aid.* Retrieved from http://health/first-aid-dislocation/FA0009www.mayoclinic.com

McPhee, S., Papadakis, M., & Tierney, L. (Eds.). (2008). *Current medical diagnosis & treatment* (47th ed.). New York, NY: McGraw Hill.

Mechem, C. (2008 August 11). Fracture, Pelvic. Retrieved from www.emedicine.medscapte.com

Moorhead, S., Johnson, M., Maas, M., & Swanson, E. (Eds.). (2008). *Nursing outcomes classification (NOC)* (4th ed.). St. Louis, MO: Mosby.

NANDA International. (2009). *Nursing diagnoses: Definitions & classification 2009–2011.* Oxford, UK: Wiley Blackwell.

National Center for Injury Prevention and Control. (2006). *Falls and hip fractures among older adults.* Retrieved from http://www.cdc.gov/ncipc/factsheets/falls.htm

National Institute of Arthritis and Musculoskeletal and Skin Diseases. (2009). *Questions and answers about sprains and strains.* Retrieved from http://www.niams.nih.gov/Health_Info/Sprains_Strains

National Limb Loss Information Center. (2009). Amputation statistics by cause: Limb loss in the United States. Retrieved from www.amputee-coalition.org/fact_sheets/amp_stats_cause.html

Norvell, J., & Steele, M. (2009). Carpal tunnel syndrome. Retrieved from www.emedicine.medscape.com

Piazzini, D., Aprile, I., Ferrara, P., Bertolini, C., Tonali, P., Maggi, L., et al. (2007). A systematic review of conservative treatment of carpal tunnel syndrome. *Clinical Rehavilitation 2007, 21,* 299–314.

Porth, C., & Matfin, G. (2009). *Pathophysiology: Concepts of altered health states* (8th ed.). Philadelphia: Lippincott.

Siddle, L. (2004). The challenge and management of phantom limb pain after amputation. *British Journal of Nursing, 13*(11), 664–667.

Stevermer, J., & Ewigman, B. (2008 February). Give vitamin C to avert lingering pain after fracture. *The Journal of Family Practice, 57*(2), 86–89.

Taylor, S., Kalbaugh, C., Cass, A., Buzzell, N., Daly, C., Cull, D., et al. (2008 July). "Successful outcome" after below-knee amputation: An objective definition and influence of clinical variables. *The American Surgeon, 74,* 607–613.

Theivendran, K., McBryde, C., & Massoud, S. (2008). Scapula fractures: A review. *Trauma 2008, 10,* 25–33.

Tosounidis, T., Kontakis, G., Nikolaou, V., Papathanassopoulos, A., & Giannoudis, P. (2009). Fracture healing and bone repair: An update. *Trauma 2009, 11,* 145–156.

Volkmann's ischemic contracture. (2008 July 29). Retrieved from www.nlm.nih.gov/medlineplus

Westerman, R., & Porter, K. (2007). Ankle fractures in adults: An overview. *Trauma 2007, 9,* 267–272.

Wilkinson, J., & Ahern, N. (2009). *Prentice Hall nursing diagnosis handbook* (9th ed.). Upper Saddle River, NJ: Prentice Hall.

Wilson, B., Shannon, M., Shields, K., & Stang, C. (2008). *Prentice Hall nurse's drug guide 2008.* Upper Saddle River, NJ: Prentice Hall.

Youssef, B., Youssef, S., Ansara, S., & Porter, K. (2008). Fractures of the distal humerus. *Trauma 2008, 10,* 125–132.

Nursing Care of Patients with Musculoskeletal Disorders

LEARNING OUTCOMES

1. Explain the etiology, pathophysiology, manifestations, complications, interdisciplinary care, and nursing care of patients with musculoskeletal disorders.
2. Compare and contrast the pathophysiology, manifestations, diagnosis, and management of osteoporosis, osteoarthritis, Paget's disease, and rheumatoid arthritis.
3. Discuss the purposes, nursing implications, and health education for the patient and family for medications used to prevent and treat specific musculoskeletal disorders.
4. Describe the surgical procedures used to treat patients with arthritis.

CLINICAL COMPETENCIES

1. Assess functional status of patients with musculoskeletal disorders, and recognize, monitor, document, and report abnormal or unanticipated manifestations.
2. Use evidence-based research and practice guidelines to plan and provide safe and effective individualized care for patients with musculoskeletal disorders.
3. Determine priority nursing diagnoses, based on assessed data, to select and implement patient-centered nursing interventions for patients with musculoskeletal disorders.
4. Administer medications used to treat musculoskeletal disorders knowledgeably and safely, monitoring for desired and adverse effects of prescribed medications.
5. Provide skilled care of patients having a surgical debridement for osteomyelitis and a total joint replacement.
6. Integrate and coordinate interdisciplinary care into care of patients with musculoskeletal disorders.
7. Provide teaching appropriate for community-based care of patients with musculoskeletal disorders.
8. Revise plan of care as needed to provide effective interventions to promote, maintain, or restore functional health status to patients with musculoskeletal disorders.

KEY TERMS

arthritis, *1337*	osteoarthritis (OA), *1353*	rheumatoid arthritis (RA), *1363*
arthroplasty, *1356*	osteomyelitis, *1381*	systemic lupus erythematosus
arthroscopy, *1355*	osteoporosis, *1338*	(SLE), *1374*
fibromyalgia, *1391*	rheumatic disorders, *1337*	tophi, *1347*
gout, *1347*		

Various metabolic, degenerative, autoimmune, inflammatory, infectious, neoplastic, connective tissue, and structural disorders may affect the musculoskeletal system. Many of these diseases have significant physical, psychosocial, and financial consequences. When these problems occur, patients experience a variety of individualized responses to their altered health status. Nursing care is directed toward meeting physiologic needs, providing education, and ensuring psychologic support for the patient and family.

Arthritis refers to inflammation of the joints, while **rheumatic disorders** refer to diseases of the muscles and bones as well as the joints. These diseases affect not only the joints but also the connective tissues of the body. The various types of arthritis are discussed in this chapter in different sections, depending on the primary etiology of the disorder. Arthritis and other rheumatic disorders are widespread, affecting about 46 million (nearly 1 in 5) adults in the United States (Centers for Disease Control and Prevention [CDC], 2010). Arthritic disorders are a leading cause of disability; however, their very prevalence may lead the public and healthcare professionals to treat them as normal aging processes or discount the validity of the pain and disability experienced by the person with arthritis.

There are more than 100 different types of arthritis, but the most common are osteoarthritis, rheumatoid arthritis, fibromyalgia, and gout (CDC, 2008). The etiology of rheumatic disorders often is not clear; in many cases, the pathophysiologic processes involved are complex and poorly understood. Many are primary disorders; others occur as secondary processes associated with another disease. The wear and tear of aging, autoimmune processes, metabolic disorders, genetic factors, and infection are also implicated as causative factors in some forms of rheumatic disease.

Metabolic Disorders

Metabolic bone and joint disorders arise from disrupted metabolic processes or impaired elimination of metabolic wastes. Metabolic bone disorders originate in the bone remodeling process, which normally involves a sequence of bone reabsorption and formation. Trabecular (spongy) bone, the honeycomb-like interior portion of bone, has a significantly higher turnover rate than cortical (compact) bone. Adults replace existing bone every 4 months through reabsorption of old bone by osteoclasts and formation of new bone by osteoblasts (Porth & Matfin, 2009). Ideally, the amount of new bone formed is equal to the amount of bone resorbed. Metabolic bone disorders may result from a variety of factors, including aging, calcium and phosphate imbalances, genetics, and changes in levels of hormones. Gout, a metabolic joint disorder, results from altered uric acid metabolism and elimination.

The Patient with Osteoporosis

Osteoporosis, literally defined as "porous bones," is a metabolic bone disorder characterized by loss of bone mass, increased bone fragility, and an increased risk of fractures. The reduced bone mass is caused by an imbalance of the processes that influence bone growth and maintenance. Although osteoporosis may result from an endocrine disorder or malignancy, it is most often associated with aging.

The National Osteoporosis Foundation (2008) has found that osteoporosis is a health threat for an estimated 44 million Americans; 10 million people have osteoporosis and 34 million have low bone mass, increasing their risk for the disease. Although osteoporosis can occur at any age and in both men and women, 80% of those with osteoporosis are women. One in two women and one in four men over age 50 will have an osteoporosis-related fracture in his or her remaining lifetime.

Risk Factors

The risk of developing osteoporosis depends on how much bone mass is achieved between ages 25 and 35, and how much is lost later. Certain diseases, lifestyle habits, and ethnic backgrounds increase the risk of developing osteoporosis

*(side text, rotated)* Osteoporosis Video

(see the accompanying Focus on Cultural Diversity box). Different variables affect one's risk of osteoporosis—some can be modified and others cannot. The risk factors are summarized in Box 40–1.

Nonmodifiable Risk Factors

Both men and women are susceptible to osteoporosis as they age, because the activity of osteoblasts and osteoclasts diminishes. Women have a significantly higher risk for manifestations and complications of osteoporosis because their peak bone mass is 10% to 15% less than that of men. In addition, age-related bone loss begins earlier and proceeds more rapidly in women, beginning in their 30s and accelerating before menopause. Estrogen in women and testosterone in men appear to help prevent bone loss; decreasing levels of these hormones associated with aging contribute to bone loss. Age-related bone loss in men occurs 15 to 20 years later than in women and at a slower rate.

European Americans and Asians are at a higher risk for osteoporosis than African Americans, who have greater bone density (bone mass positively correlates with the amount of skin pigmentation). Patients who have an endocrine disorder such as hyperthyroidism, hyperparathyroidism, Cushing's syndrome, or diabetes mellitus are at high risk for osteoporosis. These disorders affect the metabolism, in turn affecting nutritional status and bone mineralization. Malabsorption disorders such as celiac disease, pancreatic disorders, and inflammatory bowel disease affect calcium absorption and increase the risk for osteoporosis.

Modifiable Risk Factors

Modifiable risk factors include behaviors that place a person at risk for developing osteoporosis, as well as physical changes such as menopause whose contribution to osteoporosis can be modified by preventive strategies. Calcium deficiency is an important modifiable risk factor contributing to osteoporosis. Calcium is an essential mineral in the process of bone formation and other significant body functions. When dietary intake of calcium is insufficient, the body compensates by removing calcium from the skeleton, weakening bone tissue. Acidosis, which may result from a high-protein diet, contributes to osteoporosis in two ways. Calcium is withdrawn from the bone as

---

FOCUS ON CULTURAL DIVERSITY
The Patient with Osteoporosis

- Significant risk is reported for people of all ethnic backgrounds, but the highest percentage of cases is in non-Hispanic and Asian women aged 50 or older, with 20% estimated to have osteoporosis, and 52% estimated to have low bone mass. Ten percent of Hispanic women aged 50 or older are affected with 49% estimated to have low bone mass.
- Non-Hispanic Black women over the age of 50 have a lower incidence, with an estimated 5% having osteoporosis and 35% low bone mass.
- In men aged 50 and older, 7% of non-Hispanic White and Asian men have osteoporosis, compared with 4% of non-Hispanic Black men, and 3% of Hispanic men.

Source: National Osteoporosis Foundation. (2008). *Fast Facts.*

BOX 40–1 Risk Factors for Osteoporosis

Nonmodifiable
- Older age
- A family history of osteoporosis
- History of fracture in a first-degree relative
- Being female, especially Caucasian or Asian
- Being thin and/or having a small frame

Modifiable
- Low estrogen levels in women (amenorrhea, menopause)
- Low testosterone levels in men
- Dietary: low lifetime calcium intake, vitamin D deficiency
- Medication use: corticosteroids, some anticonvulsants
- Lifestyle: inactivity, cigarette smoking, excess alcohol use

the kidneys attempt to buffer the excess acid. Acidosis also may directly stimulate osteoclast function. A high intake of diet soda containing significant phosphate also can deplete calcium stores.

In women, estrogen levels affect osteoporosis risk. Estrogen promotes the activity of osteoblasts, increasing new bone formation. In addition, estrogen enhances calcium absorption and stimulates the thyroid gland to secrete calcitonin, a hormone that suppresses osteoclast activity and increases osteoblast activity. With menopause and decreasing estrogen levels, bone loss accelerates in women. Premature osteoporosis is increasing in female athletes, who have a greater incidence of eating disorders and amenorrhea. Poor nutrition and intense physical training can result in a deficient production of estrogen. Decreased estrogen, combined with a lack of calcium and vitamin D, results in a loss of bone density (Porth & Matfin, 2009).

Both cigarette smoking and excess alcohol intake are risk factors for osteoporosis. Smoking decreases the blood supply to bones. Nicotine slows the production of osteoblasts and impairs the absorption of calcium, contributing to decreased bone density. Alcohol has a direct toxic effect on osteoblast activity, suppressing bone formation during periods of alcohol intoxication. In addition, heavy alcohol use may be associated with nutritional deficiencies that contribute to osteoporosis. Interestingly, moderate alcohol consumption in postmenopausal women actually may increase bone mineral content, possibly by increasing levels of estrogen and calcitonin.

Sedentary lifestyle is another modifiable risk factor that can cause osteoporosis. Weight-bearing exercise, such as walking, influences bone metabolism in several ways. The stress of this type of exercise increases blood flow to bones, which brings growth-producing nutrients to the cells. Walking increases osteoblast growth and activity.

Prolonged use of medications that increase calcium excretion, such as aluminum-containing antacids and anticonvulsants, increase the risk of developing osteoporosis. Recent research has also shown a positive correlation between long-term use of proton pump inhibitors (such as omeprazole [Prilosec]) and osteoporosis-related fracture (Targownik et al., 2008). Heparin therapy increases bone resorption, and its prolonged use is associated with osteoporosis. Antiretroviral therapy for people with AIDS or HIV infection may cause decreased bone density and osteoporosis (Porth & Matfin, 2009).

Anyone who takes a glucocorticoid medication for more than 3 months is at risk for glucocorticoid-induced osteoporosis. These medications, often prescribed to manage rheumatic diseases, include prednisone (Deltasone, Orasone), prednisolone (Prelone), dexamethasone (Decadron, Hexadrol), and cortisone (Cortisone Acetate). These drugs can directly affect bone cells, slowing the rate of bone formation. They also interfere with how the body uses calcium and affect levels of sex hormones, leading to bone loss. The resulting problems, such as an increased possibility of fractures, can be prevented by taking a daily regimen of calcium supplements with vitamin D (American College of Rheumatology [ACR], 2008).

> **MEMORY CUE**
> **Osteoporosis Risk Factors**
> **ACCESS**
>
> **A**lcohol
> **C**orticosteroid
> **C**alcium low
> **E**strogen low
> **S**moking
> **S**edentary lifestyle

Pathophysiology

Although the exact pathophysiology of osteoporosis is unclear, it is known to involve an imbalance of the activity of osteoblasts that form new bone and osteoclasts that resorb bone. Until adulthood when peak bone mass is reached, bone formation occurs more rapidly than does reabsorption. After peak bone mass is achieved at about age 30, however, resorption exceeds formation and slightly more bone is lost than is gained (about 0.7% per year). This loss is accelerated if the diet is deficient in vitamin D and calcium. In women, bone loss further increases after menopause (with loss of estrogen), then slows but does not stop at about age 60. While testosterone levels in men decline with aging, this is a more gradual process and associated bone loss occurs more slowly.

The rate of bone loss varies both among individuals and at different skeletal sites. The spine, which is 66% to 75% trabecular bone, may show significant osteoporotic changes before bones such as the forearm or wrist, which are predominantly cortical bone (DiPiro, 2008). *Postmenopausal osteoporosis* primarily affects bones such as vertebral bodies. Accelerated bone loss at one site magnifies the imbalance of bone resorption and formation. Cortical bone becomes more porous with increased remodeling activity. When coupled with changes to internal bone structure, this reduces the biomechanical strength of long bones and increases the risk for fracture (Fauci et al., 2008). *Senile osteoporosis*, associated with aging, tends to affect cortical bone (Porth & Matfin, 2009).

Manifestations

The most common manifestations of osteoporosis are loss of height, progressive curvature of the spine, low back pain, and fractures of the forearm, spine, or hip. Osteoporosis is often called the "silent disease," because bone loss occurs without symptoms.

The loss of height occurs as vertebral bodies collapse. Acute episodes generally are painful, with radiation of the pain around the flank into the abdomen. Vertebral collapse can occur with little or no stress; minimal movements such as bending, lifting, or jumping may precipitate the pain. In some patients, vertebral collapse may occur slowly, accompanied by little discomfort. Along with loss of height, characteristic dorsal kyphosis and cervical lordosis develop, accounting for the "dowager's hump" often associated with aging. The abdomen tends to protrude and knees and hips flex as the body attempts to maintain its center of gravity (Figure 40–1 ■).

Height
5'6"
5'3"
5'
4'9"
4'6"
4'3"

Age   40   60   70

Figure 40–1 ■ Spinal changes caused by osteoporosis. As the condition progresses, height can be reduced by as much as 7 inches.

Complications

Fractures are the most common complication of osteoporosis, with the disease being responsible for an estimated 2 million fractures each year. These include 547,000 vertebral compression fractures, 297,000 hip fractures, 397,000 wrist fractures, 135,000 pelvic fractures, and 675,000 fractures at other sites (National Osteoporosis Foundation, 2008). There may be no obvious manifestations of osteoporosis until fractures occur.

Some fractures are spontaneous; others may result from everyday activities. While wrist fractures have not been shown to increase disability or mortality, persistent pain may restrict the patient's activities or interfere with activities of daily living (ADLs). Hip and vertebral fractures, by contrast, are associated with a significant increased risk for death and disability.

Interdisciplinary Care

Care of the patient with osteoporosis focuses on early identification of risk, stopping or slowing the process, alleviating symptoms, and preventing complications. Proper nutrition and exercise are important components of treatment. The American College of Physicians' Clinical Guidelines (Qaseem et al., 2008) strongly recommend pharmacologic treatment of patients who have known osteoporosis and those who have had a fracture due to fragile bone.

Diagnosis

Bone mineral density (BMD) tests are used to estimate skeletal mass or density in patients at risk for osteoporosis. A loss of more than 1 to 1.5 inches in height (> 2.5 to 3.8 cm), significant dorsal kyphosis, or back pain also indicate a need for BMD testing.

Dual-energy x-ray absorptiometry (DXA) measures bone density in the lumbar spine or hip and is considered to be highly accurate. Ultrasound transmits painless sound waves through the heel of the foot to measure bone density. This 1-minute test is not as sensitive as DXA, but is accurate enough for screening purposes. CT scanning of the spine, hip, forearm, or tibia also may be used to evaluate BMD. It is more costly, however, and exposes the patient to more radiation. These tests are described in ∞ Chapter 38.

Laboratory tests such as a complete blood count (CBC), serum and urine calcium, and liver and renal function studies may be done to rule out other causes of bone loss. Serum 25(OH) D measures total body vitamin D levels, and may be ordered for

TABLE 40–1 Differential Features of Osteoporosis, Osteomalacia, and Paget's Disease

DIFFERENTIATING FEATURES	OSTEOPOROSIS	OSTEOMALACIA	PAGET'S DISEASE
Pathophysiology	Bone resorption outpaces bone formation	Inadequate mineralization of bone matrix	Excessive osteoclastic activity and formation of poor-quality bone
Calcium level (serum)	Normal	Low or normal	Normal or elevated (especially in immobilized patients)
Phosphate level (serum)	Normal	Low or normal	Normal
Parathyroid hormone level (serum)	Normal	High or normal	Normal
Alkaline phosphatase level (serum)	Normal	Elevated	Increased; not a reliable test for patients who have liver disease or are pregnant
Hydroxyproline (urine)	Not applicable	Not applicable	Increased
Radiographic findings	Osteopenia, fractures	Decreased bone density, radiolucent bands known as Looser's zones, or pseudofractures	"Punched-out" appearance of bone, increase in bone thickness, linear fractures, mosaic pattern of bone matrix

patients at risk for deficiencies, for example, older adults with minimal sun exposure. Biochemical markers of bone turnover, including serum bone-specific alkaline phosphatase, osteocalcin, and others may be used to monitor treatment response (Fauci et al., 2008). A comparison of laboratory tests for metabolic bone diseases is outlined in Table 40–1.

Medications

An adequate intake of calcium and vitamin D is critical to prevent and treat osteoporosis. Studies indicate that the majority of children and adults in the United States do not ingest adequate calcium in the diet (DiPiro, 2008). See Table 40–2 for recommended calcium and vitamin D intakes for adults. ∞ See Chapter 10 for a list of foods high in calcium and nursing responsibilities related to administering calcium supplements.

Bisphosphonates are the current drugs of choice for preventing and treating osteoporosis. Bisphosphonates are potent

TABLE 40–2 Recommended Adult Intake of Calcium and Vitamin D

AGES	ELEMENTAL CALCIUM (mg)	VITAMIN D (UNITS)
19 to 50 years	1000	200
51 to 70 years	1200	400
> 70 years	1200	600

inhibitors of bone resorption that preserve bone mass and increase bone density in the hip and vertebrae. Alendronate, risedronate, and oral ibandronate are approved for preventing and treating postmenopausal osteoporosis. Alendronate and risedronate also may be prescribed for men and to prevent or treat glucocorticoid-induced osteoporosis. The nursing implications

---

MEDICATION ADMINISTRATION The Patient with Osteoporosis

BISPHOSPHONATES

Alendronate (Fosamax)   Etidronate (Didronel)

Ibandronate (Boniva)   Pamidronate (Aredia)

Risedronate (Actonel)   Tiludronate (Skelid)

Zoledronate (Zometa)

The bisphosphonates inhibit bone resorption, increasing the mineral density of bones and reducing the incidence of fractures. They are used both in the prevention and treatment of osteoporosis. When used for Paget's disease, bisphosphonates slow the accelerated bone turnover associated with this disease.

Nursing Responsibilities
- Administer oral forms with water 30 minutes before food or other medications.
- Do not give foods high in calcium, vitamins with mineral supplements, or antacids within 2 hours of administering oral bisphosphonates.
- Instruct the patient to avoid lying down for 30 to 60 minutes after taking the drug.
- Assess renal function studies before initiating therapy; alendronate is not recommended for use in patients with renal insufficiency.
- Dilute the prescribed dose of intravenous preparations and administer by slow intravenous injection or infusion as recommended. Do not add to calcium-containing solutions such as Ringer's or lactated Ringer's solutions.
- Monitor the IV site for signs of thrombophlebitis.
- Assess the patient for signs of electrolyte imbalance or other adverse responses such as a drug fever.

Health Education for the Patient and Family
- Take the medication as directed with clear water only. Consuming other beverages or food within 30 minutes of taking the drug may interfere with its absorption and effectiveness.
- Do not lie down until after you have eaten as the drug can irritate the esophagus.
- Report symptoms such as new or worsening heartburn, difficult or painful swallowing, or jaw pain to your primary care provider.
- Fever with or without chills and flu like symptoms may occur while receiving intravenous bisphosphonates; this will subside without treatment.
- Report any abnormal symptoms such as tingling around the mouth or numbness and tingling of the fingers or toes, which may indicate an imbalance of electrolytes in the blood.

- Take calcium and vitamin D supplements as instructed by your primary care provider.
- Response to these medications is gradual, and continues for months after the drug is stopped.

CALCITONIN

Calcitonin-salmon injection, synthetic

Calcimar

Miacalcin (injection or nasal spray)

In postmenopausal osteoporosis, calcitonin prevents further bone loss and increases bone mass if the patient consumes adequate amounts of calcium and vitamin D. Calcitonin may be used in postmenopausal women who cannot or will not take estrogen.

Nursing Responsibilities
- Calcitonin is protein in nature; both the parenteral and nasal spray forms may cause an anaphylactic-type allergic response. Observe the patient for 20 minutes after administration; have appropriate emergency equipment and drugs available to treat anaphylaxis.
- Alternate nostrils daily when administering calcitonin nasal spray.
- Review medical history for conditions that contraindicate use of calcitonin products: hypersensitivity to salmon calcitonin and lactation (calcitonin is secreted in breast milk and may inhibit lactation).
- Observe for side effects: nausea and vomiting, anorexia, mild transient flushing of the palms of the hands and the soles of the feet, and urinary frequency.
- Teach the patient the proper technique for handling and injecting the drug at home.

Health Education for the Patient and Family
- Take the medication in the evening to minimize side effects.
- Warm nasal spray to room temperature before using.
- Rhinitis (runny nose) is the most common side effect with calcitonin nasal spray. Other possible side effects include sores, itching, or other nasal symptoms. Report nosebleeds to your primary care provider.
- Nausea and vomiting may occur during initial stages of therapy; they disappear as treatment continues.
- While taking the medication, be sure to consume adequate amounts of calcium and vitamin D.

of bisphosphonates are found in the Medication Administration box on page 1341. Adverse effects such as heartburn, difficulty swallowing, and gastric upset may limit long-term adherence to bisphosphonate therapy. The FDA recently approved a new drug, denosumab (Prolia), for treating postmenopausal osteoporosis in women. This drug has a different mechanism of action, blocking the formation of osteoclasts, the cells that break down bone. It is administered by subcutaneous injection every 6 months. Its long-term safety is not yet known.

Estrogen replacement therapy reduces bone loss, increases bone density in the spine and hip, and reduces the risk of fractures in postmenopausal women. It is particularly recommended for women who have undergone surgical menopause before age 50, and often is prescribed for women with other osteoporosis risk factors. Estrogen therapy alone is associated with an increased risk of endometrial cancer, so it usually is prescribed in combination with progestin (hormone replacement therapy or HRT). The choice of using HRT to prevent osteoporosis is one that must be made between the woman and her healthcare provider.

Raloxifene (Evista) and tamoxifen (Nolvadex, Tamofen) are selective estrogen receptor modulators (SERMs) that prevent bone loss by mimicking estrogen's beneficial effects on bone density in postmenopausal women. SERMs do not have the risks of estrogen and have the added benefit of reducing the risk for invasive breast cancer. Hot flashes are a common side effect, and these drugs should not be taken by women with a history of blood clots.

Calcitonin (Miacalcin) is a hormone that increases bone formation and decreases bone resorption. Calcitonin increases spinal bone density and reduces the risk of compression fractures; it may reduce the risk of hip fracture as well. Calcitonin usually is prescribed as a nasal spray, although it also is available in parenteral form. Because calcitonin is a protein, it can precipitate anaphylactic-type allergic responses. Teriparatide (Forteo) is a synthetic parathyroid hormone, administered subcutaneously to stimulate new bone formation and mass. It is used to decrease the risk of bone fracture from osteoporosis in postmenopausal women and in men with high risk for fracture (DiPiro, 2008).

℅ Nursing Care

Osteoporosis is both preventable and treatable; therefore, nursing care focuses primarily on planning and implementing interventions to prevent the disease, its manifestations, and the resulting injuries. An important aspect of preventing osteoporosis is educating patients under age 35. See the Case Study & Nursing Care Plan for a patient with osteoporosis on page 1344.

Health Promotion

Health promotion activities to prevent or slow osteoporosis focus on calcium intake, exercise, and health-related behaviors.

Nutrition

For patients of all ages, stress the importance of maintaining a daily calcium intake that meets National Institutes of Health (NIH) recommendations (see Table 40–2). This is particularly important for adolescent girls and young adult women who may avoid eating many high-calcium foods such as dairy products

because of concerns about weight. Optimal calcium intake before ages 30 to 35 probably increases peak bone mass. Emphasize that low-fat (or nonfat) dairy products also contain calcium, although some fat in the product may enhance calcium absorption.

Milk and milk products are the best sources of calcium. The lactose in milk facilitates calcium absorption as well. Other food sources of calcium include sardines, clams, oysters, and salmon, as well as dark green, leafy vegetables such as broccoli, collard greens, bok choy, and spinach. For patients who avoid dairy products because of lactose intolerance or a vegetarian diet, suggest alternate sources.

Calcium supplements are available in many forms. Most supplements (including Tums) provide calcium carbonate in the range of 200 to 600 mg per tablet. Other forms of calcium, including citrate, gluconate, and lactate, generally provide a lower amount of elemental calcium per tablet. A combination of calcium with vitamin D is recommended, particularly for older adults who may have a vitamin D deficiency that impairs their ability to absorb and use calcium.

Exercise

Teach patients the importance of physical activity and weight-bearing exercises in preventing and slowing bone loss and reducing fall risk (NOF, 2008). Suggest that patients participate in regular exercise such as walking, stair climbing, or tai chi for at least 20 minutes five or more times a week. Inform patients that swimming and pool aerobic exercises are not as beneficial for maintaining bone density because of the lack of weight-bearing activity.

Healthy Behaviors

Behaviors that help prevent osteoporosis include not smoking, avoiding excessive alcohol intake, and limiting caffeine intake to two or three cups of coffee each day.

Assessment

Collect the following data through the health history and physical examination (℅ see Chapter 38):

- *Health history:* Age, risk factors, history of fractures, smoking history, alcohol intake, medications, usual diet, menstrual history including menopause, usual exercise/activity level, low back pain.
- *Physical examination:* Height, spinal curves.

Nursing Diagnoses and Interventions

Nursing care of patients who have osteoporosis focuses on teaching about the disease process, helping maintain physical mobility and nutrition, and solving problems associated with pain and injury.

Readiness for Enhanced Self Health Management

At multiple points in the patient's lifetime, nurses can provide vital information that will help patients use self-care strategies to reduce their risk of developing osteoporosis:

- Assess the patient's health habits, including diet, exercise, smoking, and alcohol use. *The risk of developing osteoporosis in later life is affected by such things as diet, regular participation in weight-bearing exercise, and personal habits such as smoking and alcohol consumption.*

EVIDENCE FOR NURSING CARE — The Patient with Osteoporosis

Selected resources that nurses may find helpful when planning evidence-based nursing care follow.

- Bonner, S. M. (2009). Getting to the root of your patient's back pain. *Nursing2009, 39*(7), 36–41.
- Institute for Clinical Systems Improvement (ICSI). (2008 September). *Diagnosis and treatment of osteoporosis.* Bloomington, MN: Institute for Clinical Systems Improvement (ICSI). Retrieved from http://www.guideline .gov/summary/summary.aspx?doc_id=13190&nbr=006738&string=osteoporosis
- Kaiser Permanente Care Management Institute. (2008 November). *Osteoporosis/fracture prevention clinical practice guidelines.* Oakland, CA: Kaiser Permanente Care Management Institute. Retrieved from http://www .guideline.gov/summary/summary.aspx?doc_id=13967&nbr =007057&string=osteoporosis
- Kulie, T., Groff, A., Redmer, J., Hounshell, J., & Schrager, S. (2009). Vitamin D: An evidence-based review. *Journal of the American Board of Family Medicine, 22*(6), 698–706.
- Lim, L., Hoeksema, L., Sherin, K., ACPM Prevention Practice Committee. (2009 April). Screening for osteoporosis in the adult U.S. population: ACPM position statement on preventive practice. *American Journal of Preventive Medicine, 36*(4), 366–375. Retrieved from http://www.guideline.gov/summary/summary.aspx?ss=15 &doc_id=15270&nbr=007503&string=osteoporosis
- Voda, S. C. (2009). Help older men bone up on osteoporosis. *Nursing2009, 39*(12), 66–67.

- Teach women and men of all ages the importance of maintaining an adequate calcium intake. Provide a list of calcium-rich foods, and discuss the use of calcium supplements with patients who do not consume adequate dietary calcium. *Calcium needs vary during the course of a lifetime; however, many patients never consume adequate amounts of calcium. This affects their peak bone mass and the rate of bone loss with aging. Calcium in foods is more completely absorbed than that supplied by calcium supplements.*
- Discuss the importance of maintaining a regular schedule of weight-bearing exercise, either through an exercise program or regular physical activity. *Weight-bearing exercise promotes osteoblast activity, helping maintain bone strength and integrity.*
- Refer patients to smoking-cessation programs and alcohol treatment programs as appropriate. *Smoking interferes with estrogen's protective effects on bones, promoting bone loss. Excess alcohol intake affects the nutritional status of the patient, increasing the risk of calcium and vitamin D deficiency.*
- Refer patients with significant risk factors for osteoporosis to primary care providers or clinics for bone-density evaluation. *Early identification and treatment of osteoporotic changes in bones can reduce the risk and possible long-term consequences of falls and fractures.*

Risk for Injury

Falls that would result in little or no injury in the healthy adult may cause fractures in the patient with osteoporosis. Even normal movements such as twisting, bending, lifting, or rising from bed can precipitate a vertebral fracture.

- Implement safety precautions as necessary for the patient who is hospitalized or in a long-term care facility. Maintain the bed in low position; use side rails if indicated to prevent the patient from getting up alone; provide nighttime lighting to toilet facilities. *Most falls are preventable, particularly in hospitals and long-term care facilities.*
- Avoid using restraints (if hospitalized or a resident in a long-term care facility) if at all possible. *Restraints may actually increase the patient's risk of falling and increase the risk of injury associated with a fall.*

> **SAFETY ALERT**
> Patients may fracture osteoporotic bones when pulling against restraints.

- Teach patients who are able to participate in weight-bearing exercises to perform exercises at least three times a week for a sustained period of 30 to 40 minutes. The mechanical force of weight-bearing exercises promotes bone growth. *Bones weaken and demineralize without exercise. Walking is an easy, low-impact form of exercise. Swimming (including walking on the bottom of the pool) does not provide the needed weight-bearing activity.*
- Encourage older adults to use assistive devices to maintain independence in ADLs. *Walking sticks, canes, and other assistive devices encourage patient independence and support activities that promote bone growth.*
- Teach older patients about safety and fall precautions. *An assessment of the patient's home for safety and fall risks may reduce the risk of fractures and, in turn, the cost of hospitalization and potential disability and/or death.*

Readiness for Enhanced Nutrition

Most Americans do not maintain their recommended daily intake of calcium. Patients must therefore be made aware of the relationship between an adequate calcium intake and maintaining strong bones.

- Teach adolescents, pregnant or lactating women, and adults through age 50 to eat foods high in calcium and to maintain a daily calcium intake of 1000 mg. *The NIH recommends a daily calcium intake of 1000 mg per day for all adults until age 50 years.*
- Encourage older adults and postmenopausal women to maintain a calcium intake of 1200 mg daily, either through diet or a calcium supplement. *Calcium needs for older adults and postmenopausal women are higher than for young adults.*
- Teach patients taking calcium supplements the importance of taking the medication at the proper time and the side effects that may occur. *Free hydrochloric acid is needed for calcium absorption. Calcium carbonate supplement (e.g., Tums) should be taken 30 to 60 minutes before meals to allow adequate absorption. Calcium citrate supplements should be taken with meals to prevent gastrointestinal (GI) distress.*

> **PRACTICE ALERT**
> Calcium supplements should be taken in divided doses (two to three times daily) for improved distribution.

Nancy Bauer is a 53-year-old schoolteacher. She has been married for 36 years and has two children. Mrs. Bauer is 65 inches tall. She has smoked one pack of cigarettes a day for 30 years and drinks one to two glasses of wine with dinner each evening. She does not routinely exercise. Mrs. Bauer has had symptoms of menopause for 8 years, including hot flashes in the early years and mood swings of late. She has never been on hormone replacement therapy.

Mrs. Bauer is currently seeking medical advice for continuous low back pain. The pain is not relieved with an over-the-counter (OTC) analgesic, and she frequently wakes up during the night because of the pain. She is diagnosed with osteoporosis.

ASSESSMENT

The nurse practitioner notes that Mrs. Bauer's vital signs are within normal limits. She has full range of motion of all extremities and is able to stand and bend over, but she reports discomfort when returning to the upright position. Mrs. Bauer has a slightly pronounced "hump" on her upper back and is 1 inch shorter than her stated height on admission. Her muscle strength is symmetric and strong.

DIAGNOSIS

- *Acute Pain* of the lower spine related to vertebral compression
- *Readiness for Enhanced Knowledge* related to osteoporosis and treatment to prevent further damage
- *Imbalanced Nutrition: Less than Body Requirements* related to inadequate intake of calcium
- *Risk for Injury* related to effects of change in bone structure secondary to osteoporosis

EXPECTED OUTCOMES

- Verbalize a decrease in back pain.
- Be able to describe ways to treat her osteoporosis and prevent further complications.
- Verbalize an understanding of the current research and treatment regarding osteoporosis.
- Verbalize how stopping smoking can help prevent further progression of osteoporosis.
- Seek consultation for supplements and medications to prevent further bone loss.

- Design a program of physical activity to prevent complications of osteoporosis.
- Verbalize safety precautions to prevent fractures due to falls.

PLANNING AND IMPLEMENTATION

- Teach back strengthening exercises.
- Refer to an osteoporosis support group, if available.
- Provide realistic, yet optimistic, feedback about loss of height and bone integrity and the potential outcomes of treatment.
- Assess current knowledge base, and correct misconceptions regarding treatment of osteoporosis.
- Provide current educational literature regarding treatment of osteoporosis.
- Instruct in dietary and calcium supplements that help prevent effects of osteoporosis.
- Discuss physical exercises that help prevent complications due to osteoporosis.
- Review safety and fall precautions, and provide literature regarding how to create a safe home environment.

EVALUATION

On her return visit 6 months later, Mrs. Bauer reports that she feels much better. She is no longer irritable and does not experience mood swings, because she has been taking her prescribed hormone replacements for 6 months. She is eating products rich in calcium and taking a daily supplement of calcium with vitamin D. Mrs. Bauer has reduced her wine intake to one glass in the evening and now drinks decaffeinated coffee and tea. She also states that since she stopped smoking, she has been walking 30 to 45 minutes every day.

CRITICAL THINKING IN THE NURSING PROCESS

1. What is the rationale for stopping smoking and limiting caffeine and alcohol intake in the treatment of osteoporosis?
2. What foods would you encourage for patients at high risk for osteoporosis whose serum cholesterol and LDL/HDL ratios indicate a high risk for cardiovascular disease?
3. What physical activities would you consider beneficial in helping to prevent the effects of osteoporosis in the female patient who is wheelchair bound or has limited mobility?
4. Develop a care plan for Mrs. Bauer for the nursing diagnosis *Risk for Trauma*.

See Evaluating Your Response in Appendix C.

Acute Pain

Advanced stages of osteoporosis can result in pain and immobilization. Acute pain usually results from a complicating fracture, especially a compression fracture of the vertebrae.

- Suggest anti-inflammatory pain medications for treatment of both acute and chronic phases of pain. Patients should be instructed in the amount and frequency as noted on the manufacturer's labels. *Continuous administration of ibuprofen or other nonsteroidal anti-inflammatory drugs (NSAIDs) can be useful to provide relief from pain, but patients must be cautioned not to exceed dosage recommendations.*

PRACTICE ALERT
Teach patients on long-term anti-inflammatory medications to watch for bright red bleeding from the stomach (in vomitus) or dark black bowel movements.

- Suggest the application of heat to relieve pain. *A heating pad may offer temporary pain relief. To avoid the "rebound effect," the heat should be removed every 20 to 30 minutes.*

Using NANDA, NIC, and NOC

Linkages between a selected NANDA nursing diagnosis, NIC, and NOC for the patient with osteoporosis are shown in the chart that follows.

Community-Based Care

The patient who has osteoporosis needs education on safety and preventing falls. In addition to home safety, outdoor safety is important, too. Patients should be taught to use assistive devices for added stability, to wear rubber-soled shoes for traction, to walk on the grass when sidewalks are slippery, and to sprinkle salt or cat litter on icy sidewalks in the winter.

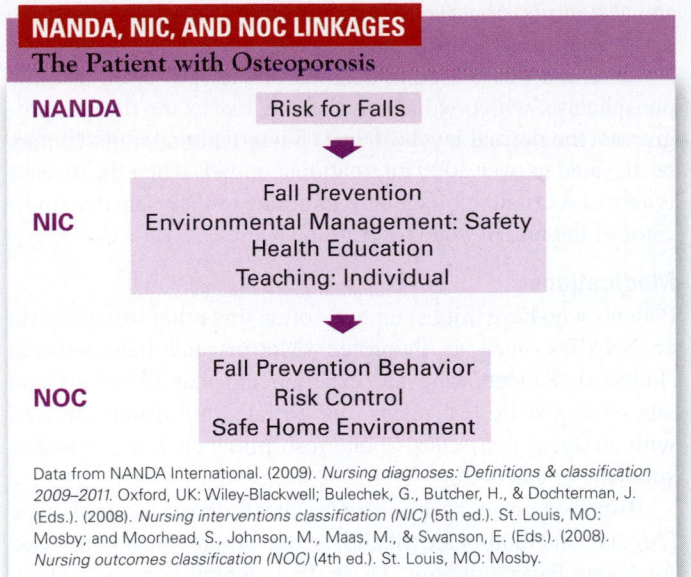

Address the following topics when discussing home care:

- Resources for medical supplies and assistive devices
- Diet, exercise, and medications
- Pain management
- Maintaining good posture to help prevent stress on the spine
- Helpful resources:
  - National Osteoporosis Foundation
  - Osteoporosis and Related Bone Diseases National Resource Center (NIH)
  - National Women's Health Resource Center
  - Older Women's League
  - American College of Rheumatology

The Patient with Paget's Disease of Bone

Paget's disease of bone, also called osteitis deformans, is a progressive metabolic skeletal disorder that results from localized excessive metabolic activity in bone, with excessive bone resorption followed by excessive bone formation. This chronic remodeling results in the affected bones being larger and softer, causing bone pain, arthritis, obvious skeletal deformities, and fractures. The disorder affects bones of the axial skeleton, especially the femur, pelvis, vertebrae, and skull. The disease may affect one bone or multiple bones. It is the second most common bone disease in the United States.

The cause is unknown; however, it appears that both genetic and environmental factors play a role in its development. A reported 15% to 25% of patients report a family history of Paget's disease. Viral particles have been found in osteoclasts of people with Paget's disease, suggesting that viral infection plays a role in its development (Fauci et al., 2008; Porth & Matfin, 2009).

Paget's disease occurs in both men and women, affecting 1.5% to 8% of the population over the age of 50 in many countries. It is less common in people of Asian, Indian, and Scandinavian descent (Paget Foundation, 2007).

Pathophysiology

In Paget's disease, the number, size, and activity of osteoclasts increase significantly, resulting in excessive osteoclastic bone resorption and hyperemia in affected segments of bone. This initial phase of hyperactive bone resorption is followed by very active bone formation. In this phase, normal laminar bone is replaced by haphazard or disorganized bone. This bone is not as structurally sound as normal bone, and can bow and fracture more easily. During this phase, normal bone marrow may be replaced by fibrous connective tissue. When the excessive bone cell activity decreases in the third or "burned out" phase of the disease, the newly formed bone becomes hard and brittle. This brittleness may lead to fractures. Multiple areas of the skeleton may be affected by Paget's disease, often in different phases at various sites (Fauci et al., 2008).

Manifestations

Most patients with Paget's disease are asymptomatic for years, and the disease often is discovered when typical changes are seen on an incidental x-ray (Figure 40–2 ■). Manifestations are often vague and depend on the specific area involved (see the box on page 1346). The most common manifestation is localized pain of the long bones, spine, pelvis, and cranium. The pain is described as a mild to moderate deep ache that is aggravated by pressure and weight bearing. It is more noticeable at night or when the patient is resting. The pain usually is due to metabolic bone activity, secondary degenerative osteoarthritis, fractures, or nerve impingement. Because of the increase in blood flow to pagetic bone, flushing and warmth of the overlying skin may be apparent.

Figure 40–2 ■ An x-ray of a leg bone affected by Paget's disease. Note how the bone is misshapen, curved, and has a "punched out" appearance.

MANIFESTATIONS of Paget's Disease

MUSCULOSKELETAL EFFECTS
- Pain (in the long bones of lower extremities or joints), headache (with skull involvement)
- Deformity (enlargement of skull, bowing of lower extremities, and deformity of elbows and knees)
- Pathologic fractures (upper femur, pelvis)
- Compression fractures
- Collapse of the vertebrae, resulting in kyphosis and loss of height
- Muscle weakness

NEUROLOGIC EFFECTS
- Hearing loss
- Spinal cord injuries
- Dementia
- Pain from spinal stenosis
- Bladder and/or bowel dysfunction

CARDIOVASCULAR EFFECTS
- Heart failure

METABOLIC EFFECTS
- Symptoms of hypercalcemia in immobilized patients
- Hypercalciuria and renal calculi
- Increased skin temperature over affected bone

Complications

Potential complications of Paget's disease are as follows:

- Nerve palsy syndromes from involvement of the upper extremities
- Pathologic fractures from loss of bone structure
- Neurologic complications from compression of the brain when the skull is involved
- Compression of the spinal cord from affected cervical vertebrae causing quadriplegia
- Cardiovascular disease, including high-output heart failure, resulting from increased vascularity of the affected bones
- Osteogenic sarcoma, seen in 5% to 10% of people with severe disease (Porth & Matfin, 2009)

Interdisciplinary Care

Care of the patient with Paget's disease focuses on relieving pain, suppressing active disease, and preventing or minimizing the effects of complications. Many patients with Paget's disease are asymptomatic and do not require treatment. For more severely affected patients, pharmacologic agents are usually effective. Rarely, surgery may be required.

Diagnosis

Many of the diagnostic tests that are useful for the diagnosis of osteoporosis are equally useful for patients with Paget's disease (see Table 40–1). These include x-rays and bone scans to illustrate localized areas of demineralization in the early stages, seen as "punched-out" areas that lend a coarse, irregular appearance to the bone (see Figure 40–2). In the later phase, x-rays show enlargement of the bones, tiny cracks in the long bones, and/or bowing of the weight-bearing bones. Computed tomography (CT) scans and magnetic resonance imaging (MRI) help identify possible causes of pain, including degenerative problems,

spinal stenosis, or nerve root impingement. Diagnostic tests are described in ∞ Chapter 38.

Laboratory tests used in diagnosis include a serum alkaline phosphatase, which will show a steady rise as the disease progresses; the normal level (30 to 115 international units/L) may be elevated to over 3000 international units/L when the disease is active. A urinary collagen pyridinoline test is a sensitive indicator of the rate of bone resorption.

Medications

Patients who have mild symptoms often find relief using aspirin or NSAIDs, such as ibuprofen (Motrin) and indomethacin (Indocin). Patients who are experiencing manifestations and whose diagnostic test results are elevated are usually treated with an agent that retards bone resorption, such as a bisphosphonate or calcitonin.

Bisphosphonates such as alendronate (Fosamax), pamidronate (Aredia), and tiludronate (Skelid) are the primary treatments used for severe Paget's disease. These drugs inhibit bone resorption, possibly by attaching to the surface of the calcium/phosphate phase of bone and inhibiting osteoclast activity. They are safe and usually are well tolerated by the patient. Bone pain is relieved, and the incidence of pathologic fractures is reduced. Cardiac and vascular manifestations of the disease also improve. Alendronate and several other bisphosphonates are available for oral administration. Oral preparations are poorly absorbed from the GI tract, and may cause gastric or esophageal irritation. They should be given with a full glass of water on an empty stomach, at least 30 minutes before other medications or food. Pamidronate is given as an intravenous infusion in D_5W or normal saline. It is given for 3 successive days, generally promoting a rapid response with reduced urinary excretion of hydroxyproline and pyridinium and a fall in alkaline phosphatase. Intravenous pamidronate may cause flulike symptoms, but these generally are brief. Intravenous zoledronate (Zometa) also is approved for treating Paget's disease; one 5 mg infusion of this drug produces a prolonged response (up to a year) in most patients (Fauci et al., 2008). Calcium and vitamin D supplements also are prescribed for patients receiving bisphosphonates. After bisphosphonate treatment, patients often experience remission of symptoms for a year or more. See the Medication Administration box on page 1341 for nursing implications for bisphosphonates.

Calcitonin inhibits osteoclastic resorption of bone. It also works as an analgesic for bone pain. Calcitonin may be derived from salmon (fish) and human. Salmon calcitonin (Calcimar) is generally preferred because it is effective, inexpensive, and widely available. Human calcitonin (Cibacalcin) is derived from human thyroid glands, which makes it more expensive and difficult to obtain. The parenteral form of calcitonin is used in treating Paget's disease. (Refer to the Medication Administration Box on page 1341 for nursing implications.)

Surgery

Surgical interventions may be necessary for patients with Paget's disease, such as repairing a complete fracture through pagetic bone, realigning a knee through tibial osteotomy to decrease pain, or replacing a hip and/or knee for osteoarthritis. Excessive operative bleeding is a risk in Paget's disease due to increased vascularity of affected bone. Pretreatment with a potent bisphosphonate reduces disease activity prior to surgery and decreases the risk of excessive operative blood loss (Paget Foundation, 2007).

Nursing Care

Nursing Diagnoses and Interventions

The nursing interventions for the patient with Paget's disease focus on pain control, prevention of injury or fractures, and education regarding the disease process and prescribed therapies.

Chronic Pain

The most common manifestation of Paget's disease is bone pain. This usually is the manifestation that prompts the patient to seek health care.

- Assess the location and extent of the pain to determine the bone areas involved. *Bone pain in Paget's disease may be poorly localized and described as "aching and deep."*
- Teach the patient to take NSAIDs on a regular basis as prescribed. Acetaminophen may be taken as needed for pain (Paget Foundation, 2007). *Pain is most noticeable at night or when the patient is resting. The pain can become evident when it is aggravated by pressure and weight bearing.*
- Ensure correct placement of prescribed brace or corset. The patient may be required to wear a light brace or corset to relieve back pain and provide support when assuming an upright position. *The patient may need instruction in the correct application of the device and in the evaluation of pressure areas that may result from wearing the device.*
- Suggest referral for heat therapy and massage. *Heat therapy and massage can alleviate mild discomfort. Care should be taken when applying massage over areas prone to pathologic fractures.*

Impaired Physical Mobility

Patients with Paget's disease need to maintain or improve mobility so that they can perform necessary self-care activities and prevent complications of immobility.

- Provide an assistive device for use when ambulating. *During the active phase of Paget's disease, the patient is prone to fractures. Bone deformities, activity intolerance, fear of falling, and pain are all factors that may make the patient more prone to falls. An assistive device can provide both physical and psychologic support during ambulation, permit the patient to ambulate further, and provide a device for resting during ambulation.*
- Teach good body mechanics. *The patient with bone deformities should avoid activities that require lifting and twisting.*

> **PRACTICE ALERT**
> Activities as seemingly simple as lifting a heavy box may result in a fracture in the patient with Paget's disease.

- Reinforce information about exercise protocols and activity regimens. *Exercise and activity protocols should be planned carefully to prevent injury and to minimize fatigue.*

Community-Based Care

A diagnosis of Paget's disease can be frightening for the patient and family. It is important that they understand that this is a treatable disease, and that many manifestations of the disease will be relieved with treatment. Inform the patient that remissions of the disease often last for a year or more after effective treatment. The Paget Foundation should be suggested as a resource. Discuss the following topics:

- The importance of following the prescribed treatment regimen and keeping scheduled follow-up appointments
- Because it may take several weeks to notice a response to treatment, the importance of continuing therapy during this time and after a response is obtained
- If bisphosphonates such as alendronate or pamidronate are ordered, the importance of taking supplemental calcium to prevent low blood calcium levels
- The importance of remaining active
- Safety in the home and outdoor environment to prevent falls
- The need to report to the primary care provider any sudden pain or disability, even if no trauma has occurred, because pathologic fractures are possible.

The Patient with Gout

Gout is a metabolic disorder characterized by an acute inflammatory arthritis triggered by crystallization of urate within the joints. It develops in response to the overproduction or underexcretion of uric acid, resulting in high levels of uric acid in the blood (hyperuricemia) and in other body fluids, including synovial fluid. This typically progressive disorder is characterized by deposits of urates (insoluble precipitates) in joints and connective tissues of the body. Gout typically has an abrupt onset, usually at night, and often involves the first metatarsophalangeal joint (great toe). The initial acute attack is usually followed by a period of months or years without manifestations. As the disease progresses, urates are deposited in various other connective tissues. Deposits in the synovial fluids cause acute inflammation of the joint (*gouty arthritis*). Over time, urate deposits in subcutaneous tissues cause the formation of small white nodules called **tophi**. Deposits of crystals in the kidneys can form urate kidney stones and result in kidney failure.

Gout affects an estimated 3 million Americans annually; over 6 million have been affected by the disorder at some point (Choi, 2009). Gout occurs more often in men, usually after age 40. In women, attacks of gout are rarely seen until after menopause. The incidence and prevalence of gout are increasing (Terkeltaub, 2009).

A number of risk factors for gout have been identified (Box 40–2). Of these, male gender and aging cannot be modified; the others can be. Consumption of a diet rich in meat and seafood is associated with a higher risk of developing gout, whereas total protein intake and consumption of purine-rich vegetables have not been shown to contribute to its development (Terkeltaub, 2009). While alcohol intake has long been known to increase the risk for hyperuricemia and gout, recent studies have shown that consumption of soft drinks sweetened with sugar or fructose (corn syrup) also increases the risk for

BOX 40–2 Risk Factors for Gout

- Male gender
- Age
- Diet: higher consumption of meat and seafood
- Alcohol intake, beer in particular
- Consumption of sugar- or fructose-sweetened soft drinks
- Obesity
- Medications: diuretics, aspirin

gout in men. Obesity and metabolic syndrome (abdominal obesity, hyperlipidemia, hypertension, and insulin resistance) are strongly correlated with hyperuricemia and gout (Choi, 2009).

Pathophysiology

Uric acid is the breakdown product of purine metabolism. Normally, a balance exists between its production and excretion, with approximately two-thirds of the amount produced each day excreted by the kidneys and the rest in the feces. The serum uric acid level is normally maintained between 3.5 and 7.0 mg/dL in men and 2.8 and 6.8 mg/dL in women. At levels greater than 7.0 mg/dL, the serum is saturated with urate, the ionized form of uric acid. As the concentration increases, plasma becomes supersaturated, creating a risk for formation of monosodium urate crystals. Most of the time, hyperuricemia results from underexcretion of uric acid by the kidneys; overproduction accounts for hyperuricemia in only about 10% of individuals (Terkeltaub, 2009). In hyperuricemia, increased urate levels are present in other extracellular fluids, including synovial fluid, as well as in plasma. Synovial fluid, however, is a poorer solvent for urate than plasma, increasing the risk for urate crystal formation (Porth & Matfin, 2009). Monosodium urate crystals may form in the synovial fluid or in the synovial membrane, cartilage, or other joint connective tissues. Crystals tend to form in peripheral tissues of the body, where lower temperatures reduce the solubility of the uric acid. They may also form in connective tissue and the kidneys. These crystals stimulate and continue the inflammatory process, during which neutrophils respond by ingesting the crystals. The neutrophils release their phagolysosomes, causing tissue damage, which perpetuates the inflammation. Ultimately, the inflammatory process destroys joint cartilage and underlying bone (Porth & Matfin, 2009).

Manifestations

The manifestations of gout typically develop in four stages: asymptomatic hyperuricemia, acute gouty arthritis, asymptomatic intervals between acute episodes, and advanced gout. See the Manifestations box on page 1349.

Asymptomatic Hyperuricemia

The first stage is asymptomatic hyperuricemia, with serum levels averaging 9 to 10 mg/dL. Most people with hyperuricemia do not progress to further stages of the disease.

Acute Gouty Arthritis

The second stage is acute gouty arthritis. The acute attack (called a "flare"), usually affecting a single joint, occurs unexpectedly, often beginning at night. It may be triggered by trauma, alcohol ingestion, dietary excess, or a stressor such as surgery. The affected joint becomes red, hot, swollen, and exquisitely painful and tender.

Approximately 50% of initial attacks of acute gouty arthritis occur in the metatarsophalangeal joint of the great toe. Other sites for acute attacks include the instep of the foot, ankles, heels, knees, wrists, fingers, and elbows. The pain, often intense, peaks within several hours and may be accompanied by fever and an elevated white blood cell (WBC) count and sedimentation rate. The affected joints are swollen, and the skin over the joint is warm and dusky red (Figure 40–3 ■).

Acute attacks of gouty arthritis last from several hours to up to 10 days and typically subside spontaneously. There are no long-lasting sequelae, and the patient enters the third stage, an asymptomatic period called intercritical gout. The intercritical period may last up to 10 years; however, approximately 60% of people experience a recurrent attack within 1 year. Successive attacks tend to last longer, occur with increasing frequency, involve more than one joint, and resolve less completely than the initial attack.

Advanced Gout

Advanced or chronic gout occurs when hyperuricemia is not treated. The urate pool expands, and monosodium urate crystal deposits (tophi) develop in cartilage, synovial membranes, tendons, and soft tissues. They are seen most often in the helix of the ear, in tissues surrounding joints and bursae (especially around the elbows and knees), along tendons of the fingers or ankles, and on ulnar surfaces of the forearms. The skin over tophi may ulcerate, exuding chalky material containing inflammatory cells and urate crystals. Tophi can also develop in the tissues of the heart and spinal epidura. Although tophi themselves are not painful, they may restrict joint movement and cause pain and deformities of the affected joints. Tophi may also compress nerves and erode and drain through the skin.

Figure 40–3 ■ Acute gouty arthritis affecting the distal interphalangeal joints of an elderly woman.

ACUTE GOUTY ARTHRITIS
- Usually monoarticular, affecting metatarsophalangeal joint of great toe, instep, ankle, knee, wrist, or elbow
- Acute pain
- Red, hot, swollen, and tender joint
- Fever, chills, malaise
- Elevated WBC and sedimentation rate

ADVANCED GOUT
- Tophi evident on joints, bursae, tendon sheaths, pressure points, helix of ear
- Joint stiffness, limited ROM, and deformity
- Ulceration of tophi with chalky discharge

Complications

Kidney disease may occur in patients with untreated gout, particularly when hypertension is also present. Urate crystals are deposited in renal interstitial tissue. Uric acid crystals also form in the collecting tubules, renal pelvis, and ureter, forming stones. The stones can range in size from a grain of sand to a massive structure filling the spaces of the kidney. Uric acid stones can potentially obstruct urine flow and lead to acute renal failure.

Interdisciplinary Care

The classic presentation of acute gouty arthritis is so distinctive that the diagnosis can often be based on the patient's history and physical examination. Treatment is directed toward terminating an acute attack, preventing recurrent attacks, and reversing or preventing complications resulting from crystal deposition in tissues and formation of uric acid kidney stones. Lifestyle changes such as weight loss, reduced intake of purine-rich foods, and limited alcohol intake are important to reduce serum uric acid levels. Because of the association between hyperuricemia, hypertension, and the metabolic syndrome, patients with asymptomatic hyperuricemia and gout should undergo cardiovascular risk factor screening (Terkeltaub, 2009).

Diagnosis

Diagnostic testing is performed to establish an accurate diagnosis and direct long-term therapy. Diagnostic tests are described in ∞ Chapter 38.

Serum uric acid is nearly always elevated (usually above 7.5 mg/dL) in patients with gout, but may actually be low or within the normal range during an acute attack (Fauci et al., 2008). The WBC count shows significant elevation, reaching levels as high as 20,000/mm³ during an acute attack. Eosinophil sedimentation rate (ESR or sed rate) is elevated during an acute attack from the acute inflammatory process that accompanies deposits of urate crystals in a joint. Serum creatinine is obtained to evaluate kidney function. In addition, a 24-hour urine specimen is analyzed to determine uric acid production and excretion, and analysis of fluid aspirated from the acutely inflamed joint or material aspirated from a tophus shows typical needle-shaped urate crystals, providing the definitive diagnosis of gout.

Medications

Medications are used to terminate an acute attack, prevent further attacks, and reduce serum uric acid levels to prevent long-term sequelae of the disease. It is important to treat the acute attack of gouty arthritis before initiating treatment to reduce serum uric acid levels, because an abrupt decrease in serum uric acid may lead to further acute manifestations. Pharmacologic therapy is a mainstay of treatment in achieving these goals.

ACUTE ATTACK NSAIDs are the treatment of choice for most patients experiencing an acute attack of gout. Indomethacin (Indocin) is the most frequently used NSAID for acute gout, although others are equally effective. Other NSAIDs that may be prescribed include ibuprofen (Motrin), naproxen (Naprosyn, Anaprox), tolmetin sodium (Tolectin), piroxicam (Feldene), and sulindac (Clinoril). Although extremely effective, NSAIDs are contraindicated for patients with active peptic ulcer disease, impaired renal function, or a history of hypersensitivity reactions to the drugs. As with other anti-inflammatory drugs, patients should be aware of possible risks and follow recommended doses carefully.

Colchicine may be used to terminate an acute attack. Joint pain begins to diminish within 12 hours of the initiation of treatment and disappears within 2 days. Colchicine apparently acts by interrupting the cycle of urate crystal deposition and inflammation in an acute attack of gout. It has no anti-inflammatory effect in other forms of arthritis, and its use is limited to gout. The use of colchicine is limited by significant side effects. When administered orally, many patients develop abdominal cramping, diarrhea, nausea, or vomiting. It is contraindicated for patients who have significant GI, renal, hepatic, or cardiac disease.

Corticosteroids may be prescribed for the patient with acute gouty arthritis for whom NSAIDs are contraindicated. If possible, the intra-articular route is preferred for monoarticular arthritis to avoid the multiple systemic effects of steroid therapy. When gout is polyarticular, corticosteroids may be administered either orally or intravenously.

PROPHYLACTIC THERAPY In patients at high risk for future attacks of acute gout, prophylactic therapy with colchicine may be initiated. Prophylaxis is particularly useful during the first 1 to 2 years of treatment with antihyperuricemic agents. Although colchicine does not affect the serum uric acid directly, it reduces the frequency of attacks by preventing crystal deposition within the joint. The doses required to achieve this effect are small, and few side effects are associated with therapy.

Treatment to reduce serum uric acid levels is typically initiated for patients with recurring gout, tophi, or renal damage. Asymptomatic hyperuricemic patients require no treatment. Allopurinol (Zyloprim) is the drug of choice for lowering serum urate levels (Terkeltaub, 2009). Allopurinol is a xanthine oxidase inhibitor that lowers plasma uric acid levels and facilitates the mobilization of tophi. Because of its effectiveness in lowering serum uric acid levels, it may trigger an attack of acute gout. Although its primary action occurs through reduction of uric acid production, it is indicated for patients with impaired uric acid excretion as well as those who produce excessive amounts.

MEDICATION ADMINISTRATION **The Patient with Gout**

ALLOPURINOL (ALLOPRIN, ZYLOPRIM, OTHERS)

Allopurinol acts on purine metabolism, reducing the production of uric acid and decreasing serum and urinary concentrations of uric acid. It is used for patients with manifestations of primary or secondary gout, including acute attacks, tophi, joint destruction, urinary stones, and nephropathy. It is not indicated for use in the treatment of asymptomatic hyperuricemia.

Nursing Responsibilities
- Monitor intake and output and increase fluid intake to approximately 3 L/day.
- Monitor for desired effect of decreased serum uric acid levels, and for adverse effects such as nausea, diarrhea, and rash.
- Assess BUN and creatinine levels prior to the initiation of and during treatment with allopurinol. Report signs of impaired renal function such as an elevated BUN and creatinine, decreased urine output, and dilute or frothy urine to the physician.
- Administer with meals to minimize gastric distress.
- Monitor CBC periodically because allopurinol therapy may cause bone marrow depression.
- In patients receiving warfarin concurrently, monitor prothrombin times and be alert to evidence of bleeding, because allopurinol prolongs the half-life of warfarin.
- Monitor patients receiving chlorpropamide, cyclophosphamide, hydantoin, theophylline, vidarabine, or ACE inhibitors concurrently for increased drug effects.
- Discontinue the drug and notify the physician immediately if the patient develops a rash. Rash and hypersensitivity responses occur more frequently in patients receiving ampicillin, amoxicillin, or thiazide diuretics.

Health Education for the Patient and Family
- Stop taking the drug and report any skin rash, painful urination, blood in the urine, eye irritation, or swelling of the lips or mouth to the physician immediately.
- Take the medication after meals to minimize gastric distress.
- Drink 3 to 4 quarts of fluid daily to maintain a urinary output greater than 2 L/day.
- Acute gouty attacks may occur during the initial stages of allopurinol therapy; continue therapy prescribed for attacks (such as colchicine) to minimize acute episodes.
- Do not take a double dose of medication if you miss a dose.

COLCHICINE

Colchicine is used to prevent recurrent episodes of the disease. Colchicine does not alter serum uric acid levels, but appears to interrupt the cycle of urate crystal deposition and inflammatory response. It is given once or twice daily by mouth. Colchicine is also available as a fixed-dose combination with a uricosuric agent, probenecid (Benemid). Plain colchicine may, on rare occasion, be used to treat an acute attack of gout; combination therapy is employed to prevent further attacks.

Nursing Responsibilities
- Assess for possible contraindications to colchicine therapy, including serious GI, renal, hepatic, or cardiac disease.
- Administer oral colchicine on an empty stomach to facilitate absorption.

- Evaluate for adverse effects, including abdominal cramping, nausea, vomiting, and diarrhea, and report promptly because these side effects may necessitate discontinuation of the drug.

Health Education for the Patient and Family
- Drink 3 to 4 quarts of liquid per day.
- Report adverse responses, including GI problems, fatigue, bleeding, easy bruising, or recurrent infections, to the physician.
- Do not drink alcohol.

URICOSURIC DRUGS

Probenecid (Benemid)

Sulfinpyrazone (Anturane)

Probenecid is a uricosuric drug that inhibits the tubular reabsorption of urate, promoting the excretion of uric acid and decreasing serum uric acid levels. Sulfinpyrazone is a uricosuric drug that potentiates the renal excretion of uric acid, reducing serum uric acid levels. It is used to prevent recurrent attacks of acute gouty arthritis and treat chronic gout.

Nursing Responsibilities
- Assess for prior hypersensitivity responses to this drug.
- Administer after meals or with milk to minimize gastric distress.
- Increase fluid intake to at least 3 L/day to prevent the formation of uric acid kidney calculi.
- Administer sodium bicarbonate or potassium citrate as ordered to maintain an alkaline urine.
- Do not administer aspirin to patients receiving probenecid because salicylates interfere with the action of the drug.
- Monitor patients receiving the following drugs concurrently with probenecid for increased or toxic effects: penicillin and related antibiotics, indomethacin, acetaminophen, naproxen, ketoprofen, meclofenamate, lorazepam, and rifampin.
- Monitor for possible adverse effects of probenecid, including headache, dizziness, hepatic necrosis, nausea and vomiting, renal colic, bone marrow depression, anaphylaxis, fever, hives, and pruritus.
- Administer sulfinpyrazone with meals or antacid to minimize gastric distress.
- Monitor patients taking sulfinpyrazone with other sulfa drugs for increased or toxic effects; monitor for hypoglycemia in patients receiving insulin or oral hypoglycemics concurrently, and monitor for bleeding or increased anticoagulant effect in patients receiving warfarin concurrently.
- Assess for contraindications to therapy with sulfinpyrazone, including active peptic ulcer disease, a history of hypersensitivity to phenylbutazone or other pyrazoles, or blood dyscrasias.

Health Education for the Patient and Family
- Do not take aspirin or products containing aspirin while taking probenecid. Use acetaminophen for relief of mild pain.
- Drink at least 3 quarts of fluids per day to minimize the risk of kidney stone formation.
- Take sulfinpyrazone with meals to minimize gastric distress, and report epigastric pain, nausea, or black stools to the physician promptly.

Clinical trials of a selective xanthine oxidase inhibitor, febuxostat, are currently underway. This drug may be particularly helpful for patients with impaired renal or liver function who are unable to take allopurinol (Terkeltaub, 2009).

Uricosuric drugs block the tubular reabsorption of uric acid, promoting its excretion and reducing serum levels. Uricosuric agents are primarily used for patients who do not eliminate uric acid adequately or who cannot tolerate allopurinol. These drugs reduce the frequency of acute attacks, particularly when administered with colchicine. Probenecid (Benemid) and sulfinpyrazone (Aprazone, Anturane, Zynol) are the primary uricosuric drugs employed.

The nursing implications for medications used to treat gout are included in the Medication Administration box.

Complementary and Alternative Therapy

A variety of nutritional and herbal supplements may be used to help prevent gout or decrease the onset of manifestations. These include the following:

- Vitamin E and selenium may decrease tissue inflammation.
- Amino acids (alanine, aspartic acid, glutamic acid, and glycine) increase the ability of the kidneys to excrete uric acid.
- Dark reddish-blue berries (such as cherries and blackberries) are good sources of flavonoids, which help lower uric acid levels, decrease inflammation, and prevent or repair joint tissue damage.
- Acupuncture can provide pain relief.

Treatments

Treatments for gout, in addition to medications, include dietary management and rest.

NUTRITION   Dietary purines contribute only slightly to uric acid levels in the body, and no specific diet may be recommended. If a low-purine diet is recommended, the patient should be taught that high purine foods such as meats and seafood are associated with hyperuricemia, whereas purine-rich vegetables like spinach, asparagus, cauliflower, and mushrooms generally are not. The obese patient is advised to lose weight, but fasting is contraindicated for patients with gout. Alcohol intake and specific foods that tend to precipitate attacks are avoided.

A liberal fluid intake to maintain a daily urinary output of 2000 mL or more is recommended to increase urate excretion and reduce the risk of urinary stone formation. Urinary alkalinizing agents, such as sodium bicarbonate or potassium citrate, may be prescribed as well to minimize the risk of uric acid stones. It is important to monitor patients receiving these preparations carefully for signs of fluid and electrolyte or acid–base imbalances.

REST   During an acute attack of gouty arthritis, rest of the involved joint(s) is prescribed. The affected joint may be elevated and ice packs applied for comfort.

✍ Nursing Care

Patients with gout provide self-care at home. Teaching focuses on self-management of pain and altered mobility.

Nursing Diagnoses and Interventions

Pain is a primary focus for nursing interventions in the patient experiencing an acute attack of gout. The patient's mobility is also impaired during an acute attack, both because of pain and prescribed activity limitations.

Acute Pain

The pain associated with an attack of acute gouty arthritis is intense and accompanied by exquisite tenderness of the affected joint. Measures to alleviate the pain are vital in the initial period until anti-inflammatory medications become effective and the acute inflammatory response is relieved. The following are important in teaching about pain relief:

- Position the affected joint for comfort. Elevate the joint or extremity (usually the foot) on a pillow, maintaining alignment. *Elevation and normal body alignment facilitate blood return from the affected joint, alleviating some of the edema.*

- Protect the affected joint from pressure, placing a foot cradle on the bed to keep bed covers off the foot. *A foot cradle keeps bed linens from applying pressure on the affected joint.*
- Take anti-inflammatory and antigout medications as prescribed. In the initial period, colchicine may be given several times a day. *These medications reduce the acute inflammatory response, gradually relieving discomfort. Taking the medications around the clock is important to attain and maintain a therapeutic blood level.*

> **PRACTICE ALERT**
> The affected joints are so painful that even the weight of a sheet can be unbearable.

- Take analgesics as prescribed. Avoid aspirin. *Supplemental analgesia may be necessary in the acute period until the inflammatory response is mediated. Aspirin interferes with the action of some anti-inflammatory drugs.*
- Maintain joint rest. *It is important to immobilize the affected joint and promote rest to prevent exacerbation of joint inflammation.*

Community-Based Care

Discuss the following topics with the patient:

- *The disease and its manifestations.* Tell the patient that initial attacks cause no permanent damage but that recurrent attacks can lead to permanent damage and joint destruction. Discuss other potential effects of continued hyperuricemia, including tophaceous deposits in subcutaneous and other connective tissues. Discuss the potential for kidney damage and kidney stones.
- *The rationale for and use of prescribed medication.* Stress the need to continue the medication until the physician discontinues it, even though the patient is free of manifestations of gout. Tell the patient to avoid drugs that increase uric acid blood levels: hydrochlorothiazide (HydroDIURIL), cyclosporine (Neoral, Sandimmune), furosemide (Lasix), and high doses of aspirin. Patients who need to reduce their risk of heart attacks may safely take one baby aspirin each day.
- *The importance of a high intake of fluids each day and avoiding the use of alcohol.*

The Patient with Osteomalacia

Osteomalacia, often referred to as adult rickets, is a metabolic bone disorder characterized by inadequate or delayed mineralization of bone matrix in mature compact and spongy bone, resulting in softening of bones. Bone mineralization requires adequate calcium and phosphate ions in extracellular fluid. When either of these ions is insufficient due to (1) inadequate calcium intake or decreased calcium absorption from the intestines, or (2) increased renal losses or decreased intestinal absorption of phosphate, the bone matrix is not mineralized and cannot sustain weight bearing. Marked deformities of weight-bearing bone and pathologic fractures occur. Vitamin D deficiency is the most common cause of osteomalacia; hypophosphatemia also can lead to osteomalacia, which can be corrected with treatment.

Osteomalacia has been rare in the United States because many foods are fortified with vitamin D, but its incidence is increasing among older adults and people who have limited sun exposure. It is a significant health problem in cultures whose diets tend to be deficient in calcium and vitamin D. Women in northern China, Japan, and northern India have a higher incidence of the disorder (Porth & Matfin, 2009).

The major risk factors for vitamin D deficiency are a diet low in vitamin D, inadequate sun exposure, impaired intestinal absorption of fats (vitamin D is a fat-soluble vitamin), liver or kidney disorders that interfere with the metabolism of vitamin D to its active forms, and certain drugs (Box 40–3). Race plays a role; for unknown reasons, Black people have lower levels of vitamin D than White people (Moore & Kiebzak, 2007).

Hypophosphatemia can result from insufficient dietary intake, excessive losses through the urine or stool, or a shift into the cells. Alcohol abuse is the most common cause of hypophosphatemia, because of related dietary deficiencies, vomiting, antacid use, and increased renal excretion of phosphate. Ingesting large amounts of nonabsorbable antacids increases phosphate losses in the stool. Several acquired and genetic disorders cause increased losses of phosphate in the urine.

Pathophysiology

The two main causes of osteomalacia are (1) insufficient calcium absorption in the intestine due to a lack of calcium intake or vitamin D deficiency, and (2) increased losses of phosphorus through the urine (Porth & Matfin, 2009). In its natural form, vitamin D is obtained from certain foods and ultraviolet radiation of the sun. Vitamin D maintains adequate serum levels of calcium and phosphate for normal mineralization of the bone. Vitamin D deficiency or resistance to its action disrupts the normal mineralization of the bone, causing softening of the bone.

Vitamin D is inactive when it is absorbed from the intestine or synthesized from exposure to ultraviolet light. For vitamin D

to become active, a two-step process must occur. Vitamin D (and its metabolites) is transported in the blood to the liver, where it is converted to calcidiol. Calcidiol is then transported to the kidney and transformed to an active form, calcitriol.

The active form of vitamin D is needed for optimal absorption of calcium and phosphorus from the intestine. Calcium and phosphorus are transported in the blood to the bones for normal mineralization. If there is a lack of vitamin D, calcium and phosphorus are not absorbed from the intestine, and serum calcium and phosphorus levels therefore fall. A deficiency in these minerals in turn activates the parathyroid glands, with loss of calcium and phosphorus from bone. The continued loss of calcium and phosphate in the bone disrupts bone mineralization.

Impaired bone mineralization causes abnormalities in both spongy and compact bone. The osteoid (the soft, noncalcified part of the matrix) continues to be produced but is not mineralized. This abnormal buildup of demineralized bone leads to gross deformities of the long bones, spine, pelvis, and skull, because the bone is soft and unable to bear the weight and stress of body movement.

Manifestations

Muscle fatigue and weakness, manifestations of vitamin D deficiency, may be noted before overt manifestations of osteomalacia are seen. The manifestations of osteomalacia include bone pain and tenderness (see the following box). As the disease progresses, fractures occur. In contrast to osteoporosis, osteomalacia is not associated with a significant occurrence of hip fractures. Instead, pathologic fractures occur in the commonly weakened areas (e.g., distal radius and proximal femur).

Interdisciplinary Care

Osteomalacia may be difficult to differentiate from osteoporosis because the manifestations are very similar; however, once the specific cause is determined, appropriate therapy will correct the disorder.

Diagnosis

A history of inadequate dietary intake, renal failure, or some malabsorption states may suggest osteomalacia. Diagnostic tests are described in ∞ Chapter 38. Table 40–1 compares the diagnostic findings of osteomalacia with those of osteoporosis and Paget's disease. X-rays demonstrate the effects of generalized bone demineralization: trabecular bone loss, cyst formation, compression fractures, bowing and bending deformities of the long bones, and osteoid deposits, particularly in the vertebral bodies and pelvis.

Laboratory tests include serum calcium, parathyroid hormone, and alkaline phosphatase levels. Calcium may be normal or low, depending on the cause of the disease. Calcium levels may be reduced when calcium absorption is impaired or in severe vitamin D deficiency. Secondary hypoparathyroidism may shift calcium from the bone into extracellular fluid, maintaining a normal serum calcium level. Parathyroid hormone is frequently elevated as a compensatory response to hypocalcemia in renal failure or vitamin D deficiency. Alkaline phosphatase usually is elevated.

BOX 40–3 Causes of Osteomalacia

Vitamin D Deficiency
- Inadequate dietary intake
- Lack of sun exposure
- Malabsorption: gastric bypass, small-bowel disorders, gallbladder disease, chronic pancreatic insufficiency
- Renal or liver disorders
- Drug effects: isoniazid, rifampin, anticonvulsants

Phosphate Depletion
- Inadequate intake
- Impaired absorption due to chronic antacid use
- Impaired renal tubular reabsorption due to either acquired or genetic disorders

Systemic Acidosis
- Renal tubular acidosis
- Ureterosigmoidostomy
- Fanconi's syndrome

Bone Mineralization Inhibitors
- Hypophosphatasia
- Sodium fluoride or disodium etidronate (Didronel)
- Aluminum intoxication

Chronic Renal Failure
Calcium Malabsorption

MANIFESTATIONS of Osteomalacia

- Bone pain: May be vague and generalized at first, becoming more intense with activity as the disease progresses; occurs most frequently in the pelvis; long bones of the extremities, spine, and ribs
- Muscle weakness: May be an early sign of vitamin D deficiency
- Difficulty changing from lying to sitting position and sitting to standing position
- Waddling gait: May be due to pain and muscle weakness
- Dorsal kyphosis: May occur in severe cases
- Pathologic fractures

Medications

Therapeutic management of osteomalacia usually involves administration of calcium and vitamin D (800 IU daily) supplements. Patients in whom metabolic activation of vitamin D is impaired may require a metabolite of the vitamin that does not require activation (Fauci et al., 2008). Phosphate supplements may be indicated. Radiologic evidence of healing often is apparent within weeks of initiating therapy.

✍ Nursing Care

Managing the patient with osteomalacia includes assessing the patient's current dietary intake of vitamin D, calcium, and phosphorus and exposure to ultraviolet light. It also includes managing patient responses to bone pain and tenderness, fractures, and muscle weakness.

Teaching is important, not only for the patient with osteomalacia, but also for people at risk for developing the disease. When milk and other dairy products began to be fortified with vitamin D, the incidence of childhood rickets decreased dramatically. Now many patients are unaware of the importance of vitamin D, calcium, and phosphorus to bone health.

Older adults as a group are at high risk for osteomalacia because of dietary deficiencies, age-related intestinal malabsorption, and possible physical mobility limitations that restrict their exposure to sunlight. Teach older adults about the importance of maintaining an adequate intake of milk and other dairy products that are not only rich in calcium and phosphorus, but also are fortified with vitamin D. Few other food sources provide enough vitamin D to meet recommended levels. Cod liver oil may be used as a supplement because it contains significant amounts of vitamin D. Supplements are not recommended, however, for patients who get adequate vitamin D through dietary sources and sun exposure, because this fat-soluble vitamin may become toxic at very high levels. Instruct patients who are taking supplements to report to their primary care provider symptoms such as anorexia, nausea and vomiting, frequent urination, muscle weakness, and constipation that may be indicative of hypervitaminosis D.

Teach the patient with osteomalacia about safety measures to prevent falls. Discuss the importance of eliminating scatter rugs and clutter from living areas to prevent tripping. Teach the patient to place a night-light in hallways and the bathroom to prevent falls associated with nighttime toileting. Suggest installing grab bars in the shower and tub and next to the toilet for safety.

Teach patients with bone pain and muscle weakness to use assistive devices such as walkers, canes, or crutches when ambulating. Provide referrals to physical therapy for teaching patients how to safely use these devices. Encourage patients to participate in a supervised exercise program such as water aerobics or tai chi to improve muscle strength and balance.

Degenerative Disorders

Degenerative joint disorders, osteoarthritis in particular, are among the most common causes of pain and disability in older adults. Muscular dystrophy, a degenerative muscle disorder, affects significantly fewer people but can have devastating effects. Regardless of cause, degenerative disorders of the joints and muscles can lead to impaired mobility and chronic pain. These problems may in turn cause disability, especially in the performance of ADLs.

The Patient with Osteoarthritis

Osteoarthritis (OA) (also labeled *degenerative joint disease*) is the most commonly occurring of all forms of arthritis, and a leading cause of pain and disability in older adults (CDC, 2008). This disease is characterized by progressive loss of joint cartilage, synovitis (inflammation of the synovium lining the joint), joint pain, stiffness, and loss of joint motion (Porth & Matfin, 2009). OA may be idiopathic (without known cause) or secondary (associated with known risk factors), although it may be difficult to differentiate between primary and secondary OA. OA affects more than 27 million Americans; it is uncommon in adults under age 40 and prevalent in older adults, with half of those 65 years and older reporting doctor-diagnosed arthritis (Arthritis Foundation, 2008; CDC, 2008). While nearly all older adults have x-ray evidence of OA, many have no symptoms of the disorder (Fauci et al., 2008). Men are affected more than women at an earlier age, but the rate of OA in women exceeds men by the middle adult years. The joints most affected are in the hand, neck, lower back, hip, and knee. Men are more likely than women to have hip OA, whereas postmenopausal women more often have hand OA. Racial and ethnic effects on the prevalence and effects of OA as reported by the CDC (2007) are outlined in the following box.

Osteoarthritis Video

FOCUS ON CULTURAL DIVERSITY
The Patient with Osteoarthritis

- Blacks are more likely to have diagnosed arthritis than non-Hispanic Whites.
- More Blacks and Hispanics report arthritis-related activity limitations than Whites.
- Arthritis is more likely to limit activity in people with a lower educational level, who are obese, or who are physically inactive.

While x-ray evidence of OA of the hand is extremely prevalent, most patients have few symptoms. The knee is the joint most frequently affected by symptomatic OA, followed by the hand and the hip (Fauci et al., 2008).

Risk Factors

Increasing age is the primary risk factor for OA. Its incidence and prevalence increase significantly with age. Joint cartilage thins with aging, and is less able to respond to joint loading than cartilage in younger adults. Age-related decreases of muscle strength and ligament stretching, as well as slowed sensory input reduce protection of the joints from injury, further increasing the risk of OA with aging (Fauci et al., 2008). Genetics play a role: A strong genetic linkage has been identified for OA of the hand and the hip. The role of genetics in knee OA is less clear.

Excessive weight contributes to the development of OA, especially in the hip and knee. Increasing body weight significantly increases the load placed on the knees during walking. An increased risk for OA of the hands suggests there also may be a metabolic risk factor associated with obesity. Inactivity is another risk factor. Moderate recreational exercise has been shown to both decrease the chance of developing OA and the progression of manifestations when OA is present. Repetitive joint use, however, also increases the risk for OA. People involved in occupations that require regular bending of the knee or hips or carrying heavy loads have increased risk for hip, knee, or spine OA. Textile mill workers have a higher rate of OA involving the interphalangeal joints. People involved in strenuous, repetitive exercise (such as participating in sports) have an increased risk of developing OA, particularly of the hip or knee.

Pathophysiology

The cartilage that lines joints provides a smooth surface, so that the bones of the joint glide over one another without friction, and it distributes the load from one bone to the next, dissipating the mechanical stress that occurs with joint loading. This cartilage normally contains more than 70% water. More than 90% of its dry weight is collagen, which provides strength, and proteoglycans, which provide elasticity and stiffness to compression. Cartilage cells, the chondrocytes, nest in this meshwork of collagen and proteoglycans. Chondrocytes regularly break down worn joint cartilage and synthesize the components to replace it. Normal articular cartilage exudes some of its water with compression, providing lubrication for joint surfaces. This water is reabsorbed during relaxation of the joint.

In OA, proteoglycans and collagen are lost from the cartilage as a result of enzymatic degradation. The water content of the cartilage increases as the collagen matrix is destroyed. With the loss of proteoglycans and collagen fibers, the cartilage becomes yellow or brownish gray and loses its tensile strength. Surface ulcerations occur, and fissures develop in deeper layers of the cartilage. Eventually, large areas of articular cartilage are lost, and underlying bone is exposed. The bone thickens in exposed areas, reducing its ability to absorb energy in joint loading. Cysts can also develop in the bone as synovial fluid leaks through damaged cartilage. Cartilage-coated *osteophytes* (bony outgrowths often called "joint mice") change the anatomy of the joint. As these spurs or projections enlarge,

small pieces may break off, leading to mild synovitis (inflammation of the synovial membrane).

Manifestations

The onset of OA is usually gradual and insidious, and the course slowly progressive. Pain and stiffness in one or more joints (usually weight bearing) are the first manifestations of OA. The pain is localized to the affected joints and may be described as a deep ache. It typically is associated with use or motion of the joint and relieved by rest, although it may become persistent as the disease progresses. Pain at night may be accompanied by paresthesias (numbness, tingling). Pain may also be referred to other parts of the body; for example, OA of the lumbosacral spine may cause severe pain along the path of the sciatic nerve. Following periods of immobility, such as sleeping all night or after a long automobile ride, involved joints may stiffen. Usually only a few minutes of activity are necessary to relieve the stiffness. Range of motion (ROM) of the joint decreases as the disease progresses, and grating or crepitus may be noted during movement. Bony overgrowth may cause joint enlargement (Figure 40–4 ■), and flexion contractures may occur because of joint instability. In OA, enlarged joints are characteristically bony-hard and cool on palpation. Manifestations specific to affected joints are outlined in the box on page 1355.

The presentation of OA in older patients is similar to that in younger adults. However, in this population, the risk of debilitation because of OA is greater, and the disease may progress faster. In addition, pain, stiffness, and limited ROM increase the risk of falls and fractures in the older adult.

Interdisciplinary Care

The primary treatment goals for the patient with osteoarthritis are to (1) control discomfort, (2) improve or maintain joint function and mobility, and (3) reduce or prevent physical disability (Altman, Kuritzky, & Ruoff, 2009).

Diagnosis

The diagnosis of OA is generally based on the patient's history, physical examination, and x-rays of affected joints. Diagnostic tests are described in ∞ Chapter 38.

Figure 40–4 ■ Typical interphalangeal joint changes associated with osteoarthritis.

Source: L. Samsuri/Custom Medical Stock Photo.

MANIFESTATIONS of Osteoarthritis

AFFECTED SITE	MANIFESTATIONS
Interphalangeal joints	■ *Heberden's nodes*—bony enlarge-ments of distal interphalangeal (DIP) joints ■ *Bouchard's nodes*—bony enlargement of proximal interphalangeal (PIP) joints
First carpometacarpal	■ Swelling, tenderness at base of thumb ■ Crepitus with movement ■ "Squared" appearance of joint
Spine	■ Localized pain and stiffness ■ Muscle spasm ■ Limited range of motion ■ Nerve root compression with radicular pain and motor weakness
Hips	■ Pain referred to inguinal area, buttock, thigh, or knee ■ Loss of internal rotation ■ Limited extension, adduction, and flexion
Knees	■ Pain and bony enlargement ■ Effusions ■ Crepitus ■ Instability and deformity with advanced disease ■ Flexion contracture may develop

Characteristic changes of OA are visible in x-ray studies of affected joints. Initially, irregular joint space narrowing is seen. Progressive changes include increased density of subchondral (under cartilage) bone, osteophyte formation at the joint periphery, and the formation of cysts in the bone. In some cases, MRI may be done to determine the extent of joint damage. Examination of synovial fluid from involved joints can help rule out other types of arthritis (e.g., inflammatory arthritis, gout).

Medications

The pain of OA often can be managed through the use of mild analgesics such as acetaminophen. Acetaminophen (Tylenol) is generally preferred for long-term use because it has fewer toxic side effects. NSAIDs such as ibuprofen (Motrin), naproxen (Aleve), or ketoprofen (Orudis KT) are prescribed to relieve the pain and stiffness associated with OA of the hip or knee. Osteoarthritis Research Society International (OARSI) guidelines specify, however, that NSAIDs are to be given at the lowest effective dose and are not to be considered long-term treatment (Gutierrez, 2008). A selective COX-2 inhibitor (celecoxib or Celebrex) may be ordered for patients with a history of GI bleeding or who do not tolerate other NSAIDs. ∞ See Chapter 9 and the section on rheumatoid arthritis that follows for more information about these drugs.

Strong evidence also supports the use of topical NSAIDs (e.g., diclofenac topical gel [Pennsaid]) and capsaicin (Capzasin, Zostrix) for relief of OA pain (Gutierrez, 2008). These drugs have the advantage of minimizing systemic adverse effects. The patient should be taught to keep the medications away from the eyes, nose, mouth, or any open skin, and not to bandage or apply heat to the treated area. The products should be used no more than three or four times a day and discontinued

immediately if severe irritation occurs. Up to two weeks of regular use may be necessary for full effect (DiPiro, 2008).

Potent anti-inflammatory medications, such as systemic corticosteroids, are seldom prescribed for patients with OA, although intra-articular corticosteroid injections may be used. With intra-articular injections, a long-acting corticosteroid medication, often mixed with a local anesthetic such as lidocaine, is injected directly into the joint space of the affected joints. Although this procedure may provide marked pain relief, it can hasten the rate of cartilage breakdown if performed more frequently than every 4 to 6 months. Intra-articular hyaluronic acid (HA) is an option for patients with OA of the knee joint. HA is a component of synovial fluid; it also appears to have anti-inflammatory effects. It is given in a series of three or five weekly intra-articular injections, and may be effective for as long as 6 months following completion of the series (DiPiro, 2008).

Prescription analgesics such as tramadol or an opioid analgesic may be necessary for patients with advanced OA and moderate to severe pain. ∞ See Chapter 9 for more information about these drugs.

Treatments

Conservative measures, including regular exercise and weight loss as indicated, are primary components of the treatment plan for OA.

The goals of OA treatment are to relieve pain and maintain as much normal joint function as possible. Conservative treatment may include any or all of the following:

■ ROM exercises, muscle strengthening exercises, aerobic exercises. Walking, quadriceps strengthening exercises, yoga, tai chi, and water-based exercises are recommended (Blackham, Garry, Cummings, & Russell, 2008).
■ Heat and ice.
■ A balance between exercise and rest.
■ Use of a cane, crutches, or a walker as needed.
■ Weight loss, if indicated.

Surgery

Surgical procedures can provide dramatic results for patients with significant chronic pain and loss of joint function. Although elective surgical procedures are frequently avoided in the older adult, even older patients can benefit significantly if they do not have a chronic medical condition that contraindicates surgery.

Arthroscopy

An **arthroscopy** is a surgical procedure in which an arthroscope (a thin tube that is lighted and has a camera in one end) is inserted into a joint. It may be done to diagnose the type of arthritis or to perform debridement by smoothing rough cartilage and flushing out the joint to remove debris. Although arthroscopic debridement and lavage of involved joints have been used, arthroscopy has not proven effective in the treatment of knee OA (Gutierrez, 2008). It may be useful to remove large pieces of debris or repair a torn cartilage.

Osteotomy

An *osteotomy*, an incision into or transection of the bone, may be performed to realign an affected joint, particularly when significant bony overgrowth or osteophyte formation has occurred. This procedure may also be used to shift the joint load toward areas of less severely damaged cartilage. Although osteotomy does not halt the process of OA, it may have a beneficial effect on joint function and pain, delaying the need for a joint replacement by several years.

Joint Arthroplasty

A joint **arthroplasty** is the reconstruction or replacement of a joint. Arthroplasty is usually indicated when the patient has severely restricted joint mobility and pain at rest. Pain is virtually eliminated, and the function of the joint is generally improved. Arthroplasty may involve partial joint replacement or reshaping of the bones of a joint. For most patients with OA, both surfaces of the affected joint are replaced with prosthetic parts in a procedure known as a *total joint replacement*. Joints that may be replaced include the hip, knee, shoulder, elbow, ankle, wrist, and joints of the fingers and toes.

In a total joint replacement, some or all of the synovium, cartilage, and bone on both sides of the joint are removed. A metallic prosthesis is inserted to replace one joint surface (generally the load-end or distal portion of a weight-bearing joint). The other joint surface is replaced by a silicone-lined ceramic or plastic prosthesis.

Most prosthetic joints are uncemented, that is, made of porous ceramic and metal components inserted so that they fit tightly into existing bone. The implant is secured by new bone growth into the prosthesis, a process that requires approximately 6 weeks. Although a longer non-weight-bearing period is necessary initially until the prosthesis is fixed in place by the bony growth, the implant appears to have a longer useful life span than cemented prostheses. In a cemented joint replacement, methyl methacrylate (a pliable polymer that hardens to hold the prosthesis in place) is used to secure the prosthesis to existing bone. Although the patient is able to resume normal activities more rapidly following a cemented joint replacement, methyl methacrylate initiates an inflammatory response, and the joint eventually loosens.

- In a *total hip replacement*, the articular surfaces of the acetabulum and femoral head are replaced. The entire head of the femur and part of the femoral neck are removed and replaced with a prosthesis (Figure 40–5 ■). The acetabulum

Figure 40–5 ■ Total hip prosthesis.

is remodeled, and a prosthesis of high-molecular-weight polyethylene is inserted. The success rate for total hip replacement is reported to be greater than 90%. Approximately 233,000 total hip replacements are done each year in the United States; most are for treatment of OA (CDC, 2008). Most hip replacements last 10 to 15 years, after which a second joint replacement, called a revision, can be performed. Potential problems associated with a total hip replacement include blood clots in leg veins, dislocation within the prosthesis, loosening of joint components from surrounding bone, and infection. If recurrent or ineffectively treated, these complications may necessitate removal of the prosthesis, resulting in severe shortening of the extremity and an unstable hip joint.

- *Total knee replacement* is performed if the patient has intractable pain and x-ray films show evidence of arthritis of the knee. More than 450,000 knee replacements are performed in the United States each year (CDC, 2008). Several prosthetic devices involving removal of varying amounts of bone are available for knee joint replacement (Figure 40–6 ■). The femoral side of the joint is replaced with a metallic surface, and the tibial side with

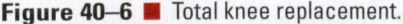
Figure 40–6 ■ Total knee replacement.

polyethylene. More than 80% of patients obtain significant or total relief of pain with a total knee replacement. They must, however, engage in a vigorous program of rehabilitation to achieve the best results. Joint failure is more common with knee replacement than with a total hip replacement. Loosened joint components, often on the tibial side, are the most common cause of failure. The possible complications following a total knee replacement are the same as for a total hip replacement.

- *Total shoulder replacement* is indicated for unremitting pain and marked limitation of ROM because of arthritic involvement of both the humeral and glenoid joint surfaces of the shoulder. The joint is immobilized in a sling or abduction splint for 2 to 3 weeks following arthroplasty. Dislocation, loosening of the prosthesis, and infection are potential problems associated with total shoulder replacement.
- *Total elbow replacement* involves replacement of the humeral and ulnar surfaces of the elbow joint with a metal and polyethylene prosthesis. Pain and disabling stiffness of the joint are indications for an elbow arthroplasty. Complications, including dislocation, fracture, tricep weakness, loosening, and infection, occur frequently.

Infection is the major complication associated with total joint replacement. Not only does infection interfere with healing and prolong recovery, but it may also necessitate removal of the prosthesis and may lead to loss of joint function. Other potential complications include circulatory impairment to the affected limb, thromboembolism, nerve damage, and dislocation of the joint.

Nursing care for the patient undergoing total joint replacement is outlined in the box beginning on page 1358. Refer to ∞ Chapter 4 for further discussion of care for the patient undergoing surgery. The Moving Evidence into Action box provides evidence nurses can use in planning and providing individualized care for patients undergoing joint replacement surgery.

PHYSICAL THERAPY AND REHABILITATION Recovery from all types of joint replacement requires postoperative physical therapy, focusing on building strength and regaining joint flexibility. Rehabilitation begins in the hospital, most often the day following surgery, and may be continued during home care. Recovery from a hip replacement is 80% complete in 4 weeks and 100% complete in 6 months. Recovery from a knee replacement is 80% complete in 4 weeks and 100% complete after 1 year. During rehabilitation, the patient must follow a regimen of exercise, rest, and medication (Flynn & Johnson, 2005).

COMPLEMENTARY AND ALTERNATIVE THERAPIES The following complementary therapies are examples of those that may be used by people with OA to relieve pain and stiffness. These same therapies are also used by people with rheumatoid arthritis.

- Biomagnetic therapy.
- Acupuncture. Studies have demonstrated a beneficial effect of acupuncture for OA of the shoulder and the knee (Lathia, Jung, & Chen, 2009; McPhee et al., 2008).
- Eliminating nightshade foods such as potatoes, tomatoes, peppers, eggplant, tobacco.
- Taking nutritional supplements, such as glucosamine, chondroitin, boron, zinc, copper, selenium, manganese, flavonoids, and/or SAM-e. The evidence supporting use of glucosamine and chondroitin is mixed. Analysis of multiple studies shows these agents may be helpful to reduce pain for some people with mild-to-moderate OA of the knee (Seed, Dunican, & Lynch, 2009).
- Herbal therapy.
- Massage therapy.
- Osteopathic manipulation.
- Vitamin therapy.
- Yoga.

MOVING EVIDENCE INTO ACTION The Patient Having Joint Replacement Surgery

Two recent studies by nurses in Sweden (Gustafsson, Ponzer, Heikkilä, & Ekman, 2007) and the United States (Jacobson, Myerscough, DeLambo, Fleming, Huddleston, Bright et al., 2008) provide insight into the experience of patients undergoing hip or knee replacement surgery. In both studies, patients describe an extended period of increasing pain and disability, letting go of previous activities, and learning to live with a now unreliable body. The decision to undergo surgery was difficult and often delayed; however, when made, patients began to dream of becoming as able-bodied as previously (Gustafsson et al., 2007). Most patients related being unprepared for the period of recovery after surgery. While postoperative pain was anticipated and the need for rehabilitation cognitively understood, patients expressed surprise at their inability to provide self-care, the fatigue experienced, and the difficulty regaining mobility.

IMPLICATIONS FOR NURSING
Joint replacement surgery has become very common. Healthcare providers, including nurses, therefore may not always understand the anxiety experienced by patients preoperatively or the need for psychologic as well as physical support postoperatively. These studies demonstrate the need for teaching that includes not only usual postoperative information, but also what to expect in terms of functional recovery. Patients expressed the desire to have

someone of whom they could ask questions rather than simply being provided with written information. Many would have appreciated the ability to talk with other patients who previously underwent joint replacement surgery. Nursing care should include strategies to support the patient's physical and psychosocial recovery in their care. Pain management is critical and continues beyond the immediate postoperative period. So too is providing information about and support during the expected process of recovery and rehabilitation.

CRITICAL THINKING IN PATIENT CARE
1. Many patients reported delaying the decision to undergo joint replacement despite increasing pain and disability. How can nurses provide support for the patient and family during this period of decision making?
2. Postoperatively, many patients expressed surprise about initially feeling very helpless and the amount of time and work required for full recovery and rehabilitation. What do you think healthcare providers can or should do to better prepare patients preoperatively?
3. Design a strategy to support patients considering joint replacement surgery during the pre- and postoperative periods. Include a mechanism to evaluate the effectiveness of your planned intervention(s).

NURSING CARE OF THE PATIENT   Having Total Joint Replacement

PREOPERATIVE CARE

■ Assess the patient's knowledge and understanding of the planned operative procedure. Provide further explanations and clarification as needed. *It is important that the patient have a clear and realistic understanding of the surgical procedure and expected results. Knowledge decreases anxiety and increases the patient's ability to assist with postoperative care procedures.*

■ Obtain a health history and physical assessment, including ROM of the affected joints. *This information not only allows nurses to tailor care to the needs of the individual but also serves as a baseline for comparison of postoperative assessment data.*

■ Explain necessary postoperative activity restrictions. Teach how to use the overhead trapeze for changing positions. *The patient who learns and practices moving techniques before surgery can use them more effectively in the postoperative period.*

■ Provide or reinforce teaching of postoperative exercises specific to the joint on which surgery is to be performed. *Exercises are prescribed postoperatively to (a) strengthen muscles providing joint stability and support, (b) prevent muscle atrophy and joint contractures, and (c) prevent venous stasis and possible thromboembolism.*

■ Teach respiratory hygiene procedures such as the use of incentive spirometry, coughing, and deep breathing. *Adequate respiratory hygiene is imperative for all patients undergoing joint replacement to prevent respiratory complications associated with immobility and the effects of anesthesia. In addition, many patients undergoing total joint replacement are elderly and may have reduced mucociliary clearance.*

■ Discuss postoperative pain control, including use of patient-controlled analgesia (PCA) or epidural infusion as appropriate. *It is important for the patient to understand the purpose and use of postoperative pain control measures to allow early mobility and reduce complications associated with immobility.*

■ Teach or provide prescribed preoperative skin preparation such as shower, shampoo, and skin scrub with antibacterial solution. *These measures help reduce transient bacteria that may be introduced into the surgical site.*

■ Administer intravenous antibiotic as ordered. *Antibiotic therapy is initiated before or during surgery and continued postoperatively to further reduce the risk of infection.*

POSTOPERATIVE CARE

■ Monitor vital signs, including temperature and level of consciousness, every 4 hours or more frequently as indicated. Report significant changes or unanticipated findings to the physician. *These routine assessments provide information about the patient's cardiovascular status and can give early indications of complications such as excessive bleeding, fluid volume deficit, and infection.*

■ Perform neurovascular checks (color, temperature, pulses and capillary refill, movement, and sensation) on the affected limb hourly for the first 12 to 24 hours, then every 2 to 4 hours. Report abnormal findings to the physician immediately. *Surgery can disrupt the blood supply to or innervation of the affected extremity. If so, rapid intervention is important to preserve the function of the extremity.*

■ Monitor incisional bleeding by emptying and recording suction drainage every 4 hours and assessing the dressing frequently. *Significant blood loss can occur with a total joint replacement, particularly a total hip replacement.*

■ Reinforce the dressing as needed. *The dressing is usually changed 24 to 48 hours after surgery but may need reinforcement if excess bleeding occurs.*

■ Maintain intravenous infusion and accurate intake and output records during the initial postoperative period. *The patient is at risk for fluid volume deficit in the initial postoperative period because of blood and fluid loss during surgery, as well as the effects of the anesthetic.*

■ Maintain bed rest and prescribed position of the affected extremity using a sling, abduction splint, brace, immobilizer, or other prescribed device. *Proper positioning of the affected extremity is vital in the initial postoperative period so that the joint prosthesis does not become dislocated or displaced.*

■ Help the patient shift position at least every 2 hours while on bed rest. *Shifting of position helps prevent pressure ulcers and other complications of immobility.*

■ Remind the patient to use the incentive spirometer, to cough, and to breathe deeply at least every 2 hours. *These measures are important to prevent respiratory complications such as pneumonia.*

■ Assess the patient's level of comfort frequently. Maintain PCA, epidural infusion, or other prescribed analgesia to promote comfort. *Adequate pain management promotes healing and mobility.*

■ Help the patient get out of bed as soon as allowed. Teach and reinforce the use of techniques to prevent weight bearing on the affected extremity, such as the overhead trapeze, pivot turning, and toe touch. *Early mobility prevents complications such as pneumonia and thromboembolism, but appropriate techniques must be used to prevent injury to the operative site.*

■ Initiate physical therapy and exercises as prescribed for the specific joint replaced, such as quadriceps setting, leg raising, and passive and active ROM exercises. *These exercises help prevent muscle atrophy and thromboembolism and strengthen the muscles of the affected extremity so that it can support the prosthetic joint.*

■ Use sequential compression devices or antiembolism stockings as prescribed. *These help prevent thromboembolism and pulmonary embolus for the patient who must remain immobile following surgery.*

■ For the patient with a total hip replacement, prevent hip flexion of greater than 90 degrees or adduction of the affected leg. Provide a seat riser for the toilet or commode. *These measures prevent dislocation of the joint.*

■ Assess the patient with a total hip replacement for signs of prosthesis dislocation, including pain in the affected hip or shortening and internal rotation of the affected leg.

■ For the patient with a total knee replacement, use a continuous passive range-of-motion (CPM) device or ROM exercises as prescribed. *Dislocation is not a problem with a knee replacement, and more emphasis is placed on ROM exercises in the early postoperative period.*

■ Maintain fluid intake and encourage a high-fiber diet. Administer stool softeners or rectal suppositories as needed. *Immobility and analgesia contribute to the potential problem of constipation; these measures help maintain regular fecal elimination.*

■ Encourage consumption of a well-balanced diet with adequate protein. *Adequate nutrition promotes tissue healing.*

(continued)

NURSING CARE OF THE PATIENT **Having Total Joint Replacement** (continued)

- Teach or reinforce postdischarge exercises and activity restrictions. Emphasize the importance of scheduled follow-up physician visits. *Patients are discharged from the acute care facility before healing is complete. Exercises are prescribed and activities are resumed gradually to protect the integrity of the joint replacement and prevent contractures.*

- For those patients needing additional direct care after discharge, arrange placement in a long-term care or rehabilitation facility. *Activity restrictions may preclude discharge to home for some patients.*
- Make referrals as needed to home health agencies and physical therapy. *Patients often require home health care for both nursing care needs and continued physical therapy following discharge from acute or long-term care.*

Nursing Care

OA is a chronic process for which there is no cure. The focus of nursing care for the patient with OA is providing comfort, helping maintain mobility and ADLs, teaching, and assisting with adaptations to maintain life roles. A Case Study & Nursing Care Plan for a patient with OA is found on page 1361.

Health Promotion

Although OA cannot be prevented, maintaining a normal weight and having a program of regular, moderate exercise will reduce risk factors. Glucosamine and chondroitin are nutritional supplements for OA that are increasingly popular and have been found to be of benefit in reducing manifestations. Patients should discuss these supplements with their healthcare provider before using them.

Assessment

Collect the following data through the health history and physical examination (∞ see Chapter 38):

- *Health history:* Family history of OA, occupation, recreational activities, joint pain and stiffness, ability to carry out ADLs and self-care activities.
- *Physical assessment:* Height/weight; gait; joints: symmetry, size, shape, color, appearance, temperature, pain, crepitus, range of motion, Heberden's nodes, Bouchard's nodes.

Nursing Diagnoses and Interventions

The priority nursing interventions for patients with OA are directed toward managing chronic pain, facilitating physical mobility, and improving ability to provide self-care.

Chronic Pain

Pain is a primary manifestation of OA. As joint tissues degenerate and changes in joint structure occur, the amount of discomfort generally increases. The pain associated with OA increases with activity and tends to be relieved with rest. Nonpharmacologic comfort measures are appropriate, with mild analgesics used to supplement these as needed.

- Monitor the level of pain, including intensity, location, quality, and aggravating and relieving factors. *Accurate assessment of pain provides a basis for evaluation of the effect of interventions.*
- Teach patients to take prescribed analgesic or anti-inflammatory medication as directed. *Analgesics reduce the perception of pain and may decrease muscle spasm as well.*

Anti-inflammatory medication may be ordered to decrease local inflammatory response in affected joints. Regularly scheduled doses of analgesic or NSAIDs may be prescribed to prevent severe pain, muscle spasm, or inflammation.

- Encourage rest of painful joints. *The pain of OA is often relieved by joint rest.*
- Suggest applying heat to painful joints using the shower, a tub or sitz bath, warm packs, hot wax baths, heated gloves, or diathermy, which uses high-frequency electrical currents to generate heat. *Heat application reduces accompanying muscle spasm, relieving pain. Moist heat penetrates deeper than dry heat; diathermy delivers heat directly to lesions in deeper body tissues.*
- Emphasize the importance of proper posture and good body mechanics for walking, sitting, lifting, and moving. *Good body mechanics and posture reduce stress on affected joints.*

 EVIDENCE FOR NURSING CARE **The Patient with Osteoarthritis**

Selected resources that nurses may find helpful when planning evidence-based nursing care follow.

- Antman, E. M., Bennett, J. S., Daugherty, A., Furberg, C., Roberts, H., & Taubert, K. A. (2007, March). Use of nonsteroidal anti-inflammatory drugs: An update for clinicians. A scientific statement from the American Heart Association. *Circulation, 115*(12),1634–1642. Retrieved from http://www.guideline.gov/
- Finnish Medical Society Duodecim. (2007 October). Physical activity in the prevention, treatment and rehabilitation of diseases. In: *EBM Guidelines. Evidence-Based Medicine* [Internet]. Helsinki, Finland: Wiley Interscience. John Wiley & Sons. Retrieved from http://www.guideline.gov/
- Gray-Micelli, D. (2008). *Falls. Nursing standard of practice protocol: Fall prevention.* New York, NY: Hartford Institute for Geriatric Nursing, New York University College of Nursing. Retrieved from http://consultgerirn.org/topics/falls/want_to_know_more
- Michigan Quality Improvement Consortium. (2009 August). *Medical management of adults with osteoarthritis.* Southfield, MI: Michigan Quality Improvement Consortium. Retrieved from http://www.guideline.gov/
- National Collaborating Centre for Chronic Conditions. (2008, February). *Osteoarthritis. The care and management of osteoarthritis in adults.* London, UK: National Institute for Health and Clinical Excellence (NICE). Retrieved from http://www.guideline.gov/

- Encourage the overweight patient to reduce weight. *Excess weight places abnormal stress on joints, particularly the knees.*
- Encourage the use of nonpharmacologic pain relief measures such as progressive relaxation, meditation, visualization, and distraction. *These adjunctive pain relief measures can reduce the patient's reliance on analgesics and increase comfort.*

Impaired Physical Mobility

As intra-articular cartilage degenerates and joint structures are altered, the patient with OA experiences pain, stiffness, and decreased ROM in affected joints. When the spine, large weight-bearing joints of the hips and knees, or the ankles and feet are affected, physical mobility can be significantly reduced.

- Assess the ROM of affected joints. *Assessing joint mobility is important as a basis for planning appropriate interventions.*
- Perform a functional mobility assessment, evaluating gait, ability to sit and rise from sitting position, ability to step into and out of the tub or shower, and negotiation of stairs. *The functional assessment provides vital data about the patient's ability to maintain ADLs.*
- Teach active and passive ROM exercises as well as isometric, progressive resistance, and low-impact aerobic exercises. *Active ROM exercises help maintain muscle tone and mobility of affected joints and prevent contractures. Isometric and progressive resistance exercises improve muscle tone and strength; aerobic exercise improves endurance and cardiovascular fitness.*

> **PRACTICE ALERT**
> The older woman with OA may be more willing to take part in weight-bearing exercises if she does so as part of a group or organized activity.

Readiness for Enhanced Self-Care

Just as OA of the lower extremities can reduce the patient's mobility, OA of the upper extremities (the wrist, hand, and finger joints in particular) can significantly interfere with performance of ADLs such as cooking and brushing the hair. When the lower extremities are affected, bathing and toileting can be difficult.

- Perform a functional assessment of the upper and lower extremities. For upper extremities, assess the ability to touch the back of the head, and to hold and use small items such as eating utensils. *The functional assessment provides important data about the patient's ability to provide self-care.*
- Assess the home setting to determine the need for assistive devices such as handrails, grab bars, walk-in shower stall, or shower chair and handheld showerhead. *Many assistive devices are relatively easy and inexpensive to obtain and can significantly improve the patient's independence while maintaining safety in performing ADLs.*
- Assist in obtaining other assistive devices such as long-handled shoehorns, zipper grabbers, long-handled tongs or grippers for retrieving items from the floor, jar openers, and special eating utensils. *These devices can prolong independence in performing ADLs.*

Using NANDA, NIC, and NOC

Linkages between a selected NANDA nursing diagnosis, NIC, and NOC for the patient with OA are shown in the chart that follows.

Community-Based Care

Because of the chronicity of OA, patients and their families need appropriate teaching to manage the disease and its consequences effectively. Much of the teaching focus is on preservation of joint function and mobility. Discuss the following topics:

- Safeguard against hazards to safe mobility, such as scatter rugs. Encourage installation of safety devices such as handrails and grab bars.
- Understand the disease process and its chronic degenerative nature.
- Learn exercise techniques, including ROM, isometric, postural, stretching, and strengthening to maintain healthy cartilage, preserve ROM, and develop supportive muscles and tendons. A walking program is beneficial for patients with OA of the knee.
- Do not overuse or stress affected joints with heavy lifting, excessive stair climbing or bending, or other repetitive actions.
- Sit in a straight chair without slumping, avoid soft chairs or recliners, and sleep on a firm mattress or use a bed board.
- Use pain relief measures including prescribed or OTC analgesic medications and nonpharmacologic pain relief measures such as heat, rest, massage, relaxation, and meditation.

For the patient who has had a total joint replacement, discuss the following:

- Use and weight bearing of the affected limb
- Appropriate environmental modifications, such as an overhead trapeze for getting out of bed, elevated toilet seats, and types of chairs to use and avoid when sitting
- Prescribed exercises
- Use of assistive devices for ambulation, such as crutches or a walker

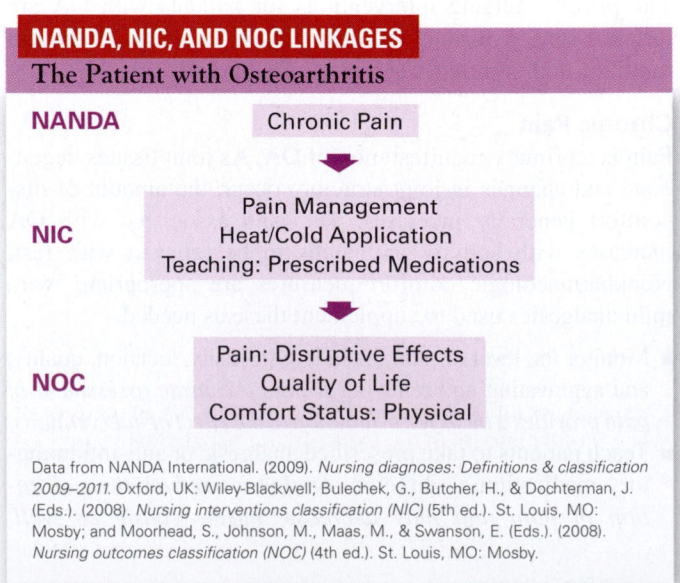

NANDA, NIC, AND NOC LINKAGES
The Patient with Osteoarthritis

NANDA Chronic Pain

NIC Pain Management / Heat/Cold Application / Teaching: Prescribed Medications

NOC Pain: Disruptive Effects / Quality of Life / Comfort Status: Physical

Data from NANDA International. (2009). *Nursing diagnoses: Definitions & classification 2009–2011.* Oxford, UK: Wiley-Blackwell; Bulechek, G., Butcher, H., & Dochterman, J. (Eds.). (2008). *Nursing interventions classification (NIC)* (5th ed.). St. Louis, MO: Mosby; and Moorhead, S., Johnson, M., Maas, M., & Swanson, E. (Eds.). (2008). *Nursing outcomes classification (NOC)* (4th ed.). St. Louis, MO: Mosby.

CASE STUDY & NURSING CARE PLAN   A Patient with Osteoarthritis

Robert Cerulli is a 72-year-old retired commercial fisherman who has experienced arthritic pain in his hips for the past 10 to 15 years. During the past year, the pain in his right hip has become severe, prompting him to seek medical attention. Significant degenerative changes in both hip joints are noted on x-ray films. The physician recommends a total replacement of the right hip, and total replacement of the left hip to follow in 6 to 12 months. Mr. Cerulli has preoperative teaching and tests the afternoon prior to his surgery, scheduled for 0800 the following morning.

ASSESSMENT

Christie Phlaugh, RN, completes a health history and examination of Mr. Cerulli on admission. Reviewing his medical record, she notes that Mr. Cerulli has mild Parkinson's disease and is taking carbidopa/levodopa (Sinemet 25-100) four times a day to control his symptoms. No other chronic medical conditions have been reported. Mr. Cerulli says he has been essentially healthy his entire life. He has no known allergies to medications, has never smoked, and consumes only small amounts of alcohol.

On examination of Mr. Cerulli, Ms. Phlaugh notes that he is alert and oriented. His vital signs are BP 116/64, P 68 regular, R 18, T 97.4°F (36.3°C) PO. Peripheral pulses are strong and equal in the upper extremities, and slightly weaker but equal in the lower extremities. His feet are cool to touch but have immediate capillary refill. He has full ROM of his shoulders, elbows, and wrists. The ROM of both hips is significantly restricted. Hip flexion beyond 90 degrees prompts pain on both sides. Both flexion and extension of the knees are limited slightly. Mr. Cerulli walks with a limp, favoring his right hip, and has a shuffling gait.

Preoperative laboratory studies including CBC, coagulation studies, chemistry panel, and urinalysis show a serum creatinine of 1.7 mg/dL and BUN of 30 mg/dL, with no other abnormal values noted. His ECG and chest x-ray show no apparent pathologies. Cefazolin (Ancef) 500 mg is to be administered intravenously at 0600 prior to surgery, and Mr. Cerulli is to shower and shampoo with antibacterial soap at bedtime. The physical therapist meets with Mr. Cerulli to evaluate his mobility and begin teaching him about postoperative weight-bearing restrictions.

DIAGNOSES (POSTOPERATIVE)

- *Acute Pain* related to surgical incision
- *Impaired Physical Mobility* related to activity and weight-bearing restrictions
- *Risk for Infection* related to disruption in skin integrity
- *Risk for Ineffective Peripheral Tissue Perfusion, Right Leg* related to vascular disruption and edema

EXPECTED OUTCOMES

- Maintain an adequate level of comfort postoperatively as demonstrated by the following:
  - The ability to move easily within restrictions
  - Compliance with instructions to cough and breathe deeply
  - Verbal expressions of comfort
- Remain free of adverse consequences of immobility such as pneumonia, pressure areas, thromboembolism, or contracture.
- Remain free of infection.

- Maintain adequate perfusion of affected leg.
- Remain free of injury postoperatively.

PLANNING AND IMPLEMENTATION

- Assess pain at least hourly during first 24 to 48 hours postoperatively, and as needed thereafter.
- Instruct in the use of PCA and monitor its effectiveness.
- Help change position at least every 2 hours; encourage the use of the overhead trapeze to shift positions frequently.
- Maintain sequential compression device and antiembolic stocking as ordered; remove for 1 hour daily.
- Encourage the use of the incentive spirometer hourly for first 24 hours, then at least every 2 hours while awake.
- Assist out of bed three times a day after the first 24 hours.
- Maintain abduction of the right hip with pillows.
- Perform passive ROM exercises of unaffected extremities every shift.
- Encourage frequent quadriceps-setting exercises and plantar and dorsiflexion of feet.
- Assess the surgical site frequently; report signs of excess bleeding or inflammation.
- Monitor temperature every 4 hours.
- Assess pulses, color, movement, and sensation of right foot hourly for the first 24 hours, then every 2 hours for 24 hours, then every 4 hours.

EVALUATION

Mr. Cerulli returns to the orthopedic unit from the postanesthesia care unit. He becomes confused and disoriented during the first 36 hours after surgery, but his orientation and thought processes gradually clear. His family has stayed with him, and he has not experienced injury or other adverse consequences from his confusion. Otherwise, Mr. Cerulli has had an uneventful postoperative recovery. Six days after surgery, he is transferred to an extended care rehabilitation facility for further therapy until he is able to ambulate with partial weight bearing on his affected leg. He returns home 5 weeks after surgery, able to use a walker for ambulation. Arrangements are made for an overbed trapeze, elevated toilet seat, and shower chair in his home. A home health nurse and physical therapist visit Mr. and Mrs. Cerulli weekly for a month following his discharge. During this time he gradually resumes full weight bearing. Mr. Cerulli expresses pleasure with the relief of his hip pain and says he has no fear of having his left hip replaced in the future.

CRITICAL THINKING IN THE NURSING PROCESS

1. Mr. Cerulli's preoperative laboratory work showed a modest elevation in his serum creatinine and BUN. What do these studies indicate? How might these changes affect nursing responsibilities related to medication administration for Mr. Cerulli?
2. Mr. Cerulli became confused postoperatively. What factors in his history might have alerted the nurses to this possibility? How might anesthesia and postoperative analgesics have contributed to his confusion?
3. Develop a care plan for Mr. Cerulli using the nursing diagnosis *Acute Confusion*.

See Evaluating Your Response in Appendix C.

- Possible complications, including signs of infection or dislocation, and the need to notify the physician promptly if these occur.

Make referrals to home care, physical or occupational therapy, or other community agencies as indicated, and suggest the following resources:

- National Institute of Arthritis and Musculoskeletal and Skin Diseases
- Arthritis Foundation
- American College of Rheumatology
- Moss Rehab Resource Net

The Patient with Muscular Dystrophy

Muscular dystrophy (MD) is a group of inherited muscle diseases that cause progressive muscle degeneration and wasting. The differences in the types of MD relate to the genetic pattern of transmission, the age at onset, the gender affected, the muscles involved, and the rate at which the disease progresses. These factors are summarized in Table 40–3. In the majority of cases of MD, there is a positive family history.

The most common form of MD, Duchenne muscular dystrophy (DMD), is inherited as a recessive single gene defect on the X chromosome (a sex-linked recessive disorder), and is transmitted from the mother to male children. This disorder affects males exclusively and occurs in 1 of 3500 live male births. It can be recognized as early as the 12th week of pregnancy by DNA analysis of chorionic villi sample. DNA analysis also can be used to identify female relatives who may carry the defective gene (Porth & Matfin, 2009). Manifestations of DMD appear in early childhood, with progressive muscle weakness ultimately leading to death from respiratory and cardiac muscle involvement by the late teens or early adulthood.

Other types of MD have an onset at any age, and a slow progression with a normal life span.

Pathophysiology

Although the underlying genetic defect and cellular pathology differ among the muscular dystrophies, all are primary diseases characterized by progressive necrosis of muscle tissue. Fat and connective tissue replace muscle fibers, increasing size of the muscle while causing progressive weakness. Muscle weakness has an insidious onset but is relentlessly progressive (Porth & Matfin, 2009). DMD, the best understood of the muscular dystrophies, results from mutation of the gene that codes for dystrophin, a protein necessary for stability of the sarcolemma. Instability leads to membrane tears, muscle necrosis, and a continuous process of repair, regeneration, and muscle fibrosis. Ultimately, there is almost complete loss of muscle fibers (Fauci et al., 2008; Porth & Matfin, 2009).

Manifestations

All forms of MD exhibit manifestations of muscle weakness. The specific muscles involved depend on the type of MD. As the disease progresses, the person develops difficulty with ambulation and eventually becomes wheelchair-bound and finally bed-bound. Cardiac abnormalities, endocrine abnormalities, and mental retardation may also occur.

Interdisciplinary Care

Because there is no cure or specific treatment for MD, care focuses on preserving and promoting mobility. An interdisciplinary approach involving many members of the healthcare team is necessary to meet the physical and psychologic needs of these patients and their families. Diagnosis and classification of the muscular dystrophies are most often based on the manifestations and the pattern of muscle involvement. Biochemical examination, muscle biopsy, and electromyography confirm the diagnosis. Diagnostic tests are described in ∞ Chapter 38.

Tests include measuring creatine kinase (CK-MM, the isoenzyme found in skeletal muscle) which is elevated in the patient with suspected MD; performing a muscle biopsy to identify fibrous connective tissue and fatty deposits that displace functional muscle fibers; and conducting an electromyogram (EMG), which will show a decrease in amplitude in MD.

TABLE 40–3 Types of Muscular Dystrophy

TYPE	SEX AND AGE AT ONSET	CLINICAL MANIFESTATIONS	PROGRESSION
Duchenne	Males Ages 3 to 5	Weakness of pelvic and shoulder girdles Waddling gait Toe walking Lordosis Cardiac abnormalities Low IQ in 50% of cases	Rapid; patient usually confined to wheelchair by age 15; death occurs by age 20
Myotonic	Males and females Any age	Weakness and atrophy of facial muscles Muscle weakness of distal extremities Cardiac abnormalities Endocrine abnormalities Mental retardation (common)	Slow; death usually occurs in early 50s
Becker	Males Ages 5 to 20	Weakness of pelvic and shoulder girdles Cardiac involvement, possible heart failure	Slow; patient usually confined to wheelchair at 25 years after onset; life span into 30s to 50s
Facioscapulohumeral	Males and females Ages 10 to 20	Weakness of face and shoulder girdles Eventual involvement of abdominal, feet, and pelvic muscles	Slow; normal life span
Limb-girdle	Males and females Ages 15 to 40	Weakness of shoulder and pelvic girdles	Extremely variable; usually slow

∂ Nursing Care

Nursing care for a patient with MD focuses on promoting independence and mobility and providing psychologic support for both the patient and family. A holistic approach is essential in planning and implementing care.

Nursing Diagnoses and Interventions

Self-Care Deficit

The progressive muscle weakness that is associated with MD impairs the patient's ability to perform self-care.

- Provide patients and family with supportive care during the progress of the disease. *The goal of treatment is to prolong each functional stage and delay or prevent deformity. When transition from ambulation to a wheelchair occurs, depression and grief may occur.*
- Promote independence. Encourage tasks that can be accomplished rather than letting the patient struggle with tasks that

may prove frustrating. *All forms of MD result in progressive muscle weakness. Management of the disease is directed toward keeping the patient as functional as possible while preventing any deformities.*

Community-Based Care

Teaching the patient with MD focuses on maintaining function and independence and preventing deformities. Teach prescribed exercises such as stretching and counterposturing exercises. For the patient with braces, discuss skin care and ways to prevent irritation under the brace. Because the patient may have weakness involving muscles of respiration, teach the patient how to prevent respiratory infections, such as avoiding crowds during flu season and being immunized against pneumococcal pneumonia and influenza. Provide information about support services and organizations such as the Muscular Dystrophy Association.

Autoimmune and Inflammatory Disorders

Autoimmune and inflammatory disorders of the musculoskeletal system are chronic systemic rheumatic disorders, characterized by diffuse inflammatory lesions and degenerative changes in connective tissues. The disorders have similar clinical features and may affect many of the same structures and organs.

The Patient with Rheumatoid Arthritis

Rheumatoid arthritis (RA) is a chronic systemic autoimmune disease that causes inflammation of connective tissue, primarily in the joints. Its course and severity are variable, and the range of manifestations is broad. Manifestations of RA may be minimal, with mild inflammation of only a few joints and little structural damage, or relentlessly progressive, with multiple inflamed joints and marked deformity. Most patients exhibit a pattern of symmetric involvement of multiple peripheral joints and periods of remission and exacerbation.

> **FAST FACTS**
> **RA**
> - RA is found worldwide, affecting 0.3% to 2% of the total population and all races.
> - RA affects three times as many women as men.
> - The onset of RA occurs most frequently between the ages of 30 and 50 years (Fauci et al., 2008; Porth & Matfin, 2009).

RA is less common than osteoarthritis: An estimated 27 million adults in the United States are affected by OA, whereas about 1.3 million have RA (CDC, 2008). It is important to establish an accurate diagnosis because the management of these disorders differs significantly. Clinical features distinguishing RA from OA are listed in Table 40–4.

The cause of RA is unknown. Genetic factors are believed to play a role in its development, likely in combination with environmental factors. It is speculated that an infectious agent, such as mycoplasma, Epstein-Barr virus, or another virus may play a role in initiating the abnormal immune responses present in RA.

TABLE 40–4 Comparison of the Manifestations of Rheumatoid Arthritis and Osteoarthritis

FEATURE	RHEUMATOID ARTHRITIS	OSTEOARTHRITIS
Onset	Usually insidious, may be abrupt	Insidious
Course	Generally progressive, characterized by remissions and exacerbations	Slowly progressive
Pain and stiffness	Predominant on arising, lasting > 1 hour; also occurs after prolonged inactivity	Pain with activity; stiffness following periods of immobility generally relieved within minutes
Affected joints	■ Appear red, hot, swollen; "boggy" and tender to palpation; decreased ROM, weakness ■ Multiple joints affected in symmetric pattern; PIP, MCP, wrists, knees, ankles, and toes often involved	■ Affected joints may appear swollen; cool and bony hard on palpation; decreased ROM ■ One or several joints affected including hips, knees, lumbar and cervical spine, PIP and DIP, and 1st MTP joint
Systemic manifestations	Fatigue, weakness, anorexia, weight loss, fever; rheumatoid nodules; anemia	Fatigue

Several studies have found that heavy smokers are at increased risk for developing RA. It is known that the incidence of RA has decreased during the past 40 years, supporting the theory that environmental factors may change and either promote or protect against RA (CDC, 2007; Flynn & Johnson, 2005).

The course of RA is variable and fluctuating. Remissions are most likely to occur in the first year of the disease. About 10% of people with RA go into long-term remission within 1 year; and another 50% to 60% go into remission within 2 years (Flynn & Johnson, 2005). The rate at which joint deformities develop is not constant. RA contributes to disability; about 50% of patients experience work disability within 10 years. Life expectancy is shortened in people with RA, largely due to an increased risk for infection, GI bleeding, and cardiovascular disease (Fauci et al., 2008).

Pathophysiology

It is believed that exposure to an unidentified antigen (e.g., a virus) causes an aberrant immune response in a genetically susceptible host. As a result, normal antibodies (immunoglobulins) become autoantibodies and attack host tissues. These transformed antibodies, usually present in people with RA, are called *rheumatoid factors (RFs)*. The self-produced antibodies bind with their target antigens in blood and synovial membranes, forming immune complexes (∞ see Chapter 13 for further information about autoimmune processes). Complement is activated by the immune complexes, prompting an inflammatory response in synovial tissue.

Leukocytes are attracted to the synovial membrane from the circulation, where neutrophils and macrophages ingest the immune complexes and release enzymes that degrade synovial tissue and articular cartilage. Activation of B and T lymphocytes results in increased production of rheumatoid factors and enzymes that increase and continue the inflammatory process.

The synovial membrane is damaged by the inflammatory and immune processes. It swells from infiltration of the leukocytes and thickens as cells proliferate and abnormally enlarge. Prostaglandins promote vasodilation, and synovial cells and tissue become hyperactive. New blood vessels grow to support synovial hyperplasia, forming a vascular granulation tissue called *pannus*.

The joint damage that occurs in RA is the result of at least three processes:

- Inflammatory pannus spreads to cover joint cartilage and produces enzymes such as collagenase and other proteases that promote tissue damage.
- Cytokines, especially interleukin-1 (IL-1) and tumor necrosis factor alpha (TNF-α), activate chondrocytes to attack joint cartilage.
- These cytokines, along with IL-6, also activate osteoclasts, leading to resorption and demineralization of underlying bone.

Circulating immune complexes and the cytokines IL-1, TNF, and IL-6 account for the systemic features of RA as well, including malaise, fatigue, and vasculitis.

Joint Manifestations

The onset of RA is typically insidious, although it may be acute, precipitated by a stressor such as infection, surgery, or trauma. Joint manifestations are often preceded by systemic manifestations of inflammation, including fatigue, anorexia, weight loss, and nonspecific aching and stiffness. Patients report joint swelling with associated stiffness, warmth, tenderness, and pain. The pattern of joint involvement is typically polyarticular (involving multiple joints) and symmetric. The proximal interphalangeal (PIP) and metacarpophalangeal (MCP) joints of the fingers, the wrists, the knees, the ankles, and the toes are most frequently involved, although RA can affect any joint. Stiffness is most pronounced in the morning, lasting more than 1 hour. It may also occur with prolonged rest during the day and may be more severe following strenuous activity. Swollen, inflamed joints feel "boggy" or sponge-like on palpation because of synovial edema. ROM is limited in affected joints, and weakness may be evident.

The persistent inflammation of RA causes deformities of the joint itself and supporting structures such as ligaments, tendons, and muscles (Figure 40–7 ■). As the joint is destroyed, ligaments, tendons, and the joint capsule are weakened or destroyed. Joint cartilage and bone are also destroyed. Weakening or destruction of these supporting structures results in lack of opposition to muscle pull, causing deformity.

Characteristic changes in the hands and fingers include ulnar deviation of the fingers and subluxation at the MCP joints. *Swan-neck deformity* is characterized by hyperextension of the PIP joint with compensatory flexion of the distal interphalangeal (DIP) joints (Figure 40–8 ■). A flexion deformity of the PIP joints with extension of the DIP joint is called a *boutonnière deformity*. The ability to effect a pinch is limited by hyperextension of the interphalangeal joint and flexion of the MCP joint of the thumb.

Wrist involvement is nearly universal, leading to limited movement, deformity, and carpal tunnel syndrome. Inflammation of the elbows often causes flexion contracture.

The knees are frequently affected in RA, with visible swelling often obliterating normal contours. Instability of the knee joint along with quadriceps atrophy, contractures, and valgus (knock-knee) deformities can lead to significant disability.

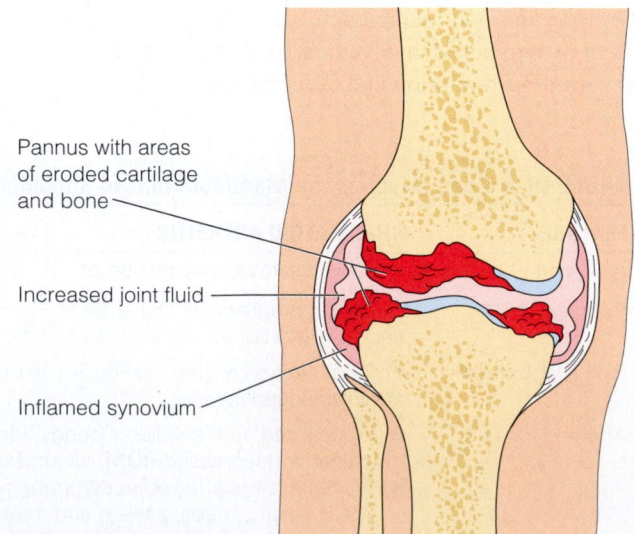

Pannus with areas of eroded cartilage and bone

Increased joint fluid

Inflamed synovium

Figure 40–7 ■ Joint inflammation and destruction in rheumatoid arthritis. Note synovial inflammation with pannus formation and the erosion of cartilage and underlying bone.

Swan neck deformity   Ulnar Deviation

Figure 40–8 ■ Typical hand deformities associated with rheumatoid arthritis.

Ambulation may be limited by pain and deformities when the ankles and feet are involved. Typical deformities of the feet and toes include subluxation, hallux valgus (deviation of the great toe toward the other digits of the foot), lateral deviation of the toes, and cock-up toes (interphalangeal joint hyperextension).

Spinal involvement is usually limited to the cervical vertebrae. Neck pain is common, and neurologic complications can occur.

Extra-Articular Manifestations

RA is a systemic disease with a variety of extra-articular manifestations. These are seen particularly in patients with high levels of circulating rheumatoid factor. Fatigue, weakness, anorexia, weight loss, and low-grade fever are common when the disease is active. Anemia resistant to iron therapy frequently affects patients with RA. Skeletal muscle atrophy is common, usually most apparent in the musculature around affected joints.

Rheumatoid nodules may develop, usually in subcutaneous tissue in areas subject to pressure: on the forearm, olecranon bursa, over the MCP joints, and on the toes. Rheumatoid nodules are granulomatous lesions that are firm and either movable or fixed. They may also be found in viscera, including the heart, lungs, intestinal tract, and dura.

Other possible extra-articular manifestations of RA include pleural effusion, vasculitis, pericarditis, and splenomegaly (enlargement of the spleen). See the Multisystem Effects of Rheumatoid Arthritis feature on page 1366.

People with rheumatoid arthritis have an increased risk of developing cardiovascular disease (CVD). In turn, CVD increases the risk of myocardial infarction, stroke, and death; in fact, RA is associated with a 30% increase in cardiovascular mortality. This increased risk for CVD in patients with RA is likely due to the systemic inflammation of RA. The systemic effects of RA also are thought to be responsible, at least in part, for an increased risk for infection and for developing lymphoma (Bergman. 2009).

Rheumatoid Arthritis in the Older Adult

Older adults are not immune from developing RA; its incidence continues to increase after age 60. Although some older adults may develop relatively mild, self-limited RA, those with elevated RA titers may experience a more aggressive disease course, with persistent disease activity, more systemic manifestations, and more rapid joint destruction (Fauci et al., 2008).

Interdisciplinary Care

The diagnosis of RA is based on the patient's history, physical assessment, and diagnostic tests. Diagnostic criteria developed by the American Rheumatism Association are used as well (Box 40–4). At least four of seven criteria must be present to establish the diagnosis.

Once the diagnosis of RA has been established, the goals of therapy are to relieve pain, reduce inflammation, slow or stop joint damage, and improve well-being and ability to function. No cure currently exists for RA; the goal of treatment is to relieve its manifestations. An interdisciplinary approach is used, with a balance of rest, exercise, physical therapy, and suppression of the inflammatory processes.

Because a cure is not available and traditional therapies are not always fully effective, the patient with RA is vulnerable to quackery. Many nontraditional treatments, including diets, topical preparations, vaccines, hormones, plant extracts, and copper bracelets, have been put forth. These treatments are often costly, and none has been shown to be effective.

Diagnosis

Diagnostic tests are used to help establish the diagnosis of RA. Testing is also used to rule out other forms of arthritis and connective tissue disorders. Diagnostic tests are described in ∞ Chapter 38.

Laboratory tests are used to measure rheumatoid factors, C-reactive protein levels, and the ESR, which is typically elevated. The anti-CCP blood test, which detects antibodies to cyclic citrullinated peptide (CCP) provides a more specific marker for RA. Anti-CCP and rheumatoid factor may be present in only about 50% of patients with early disease, however. A complete blood count (CBC) is done to identify anemia.

Synovial fluid examination will demonstrate changes associated with inflammation, including increased turbidity (cloudiness), decreased viscosity, and increased protein and WBC levels. X-rays of affected joints are the most specific

---

BOX 40–4 Diagnostic Criteria for Rheumatoid Arthritis

- Morning stiffness lasting for at least 1 hour and persisting for at least 6 weeks
- Arthritis with swelling or effusion of three or more joints persisting for at least 6 weeks
- Arthritis of wrist, MCP, or PIP joints persisting for at least 6 weeks
- Symmetric arthritis with simultaneous involvement of corresponding joints on both sides of the body
- Rheumatoid nodules
- Positive serum rheumatoid factor
- Characteristic radiologic changes of rheumatoid arthritis noted in hands and wrists

symptoms and the chronic but treatable nature of this disease is important (Huynh et al., 2008). Teach patients about the disorder, and reassure them that its course is not progressive and it does not cause crippling or deformity. Provide verbal and written instructions about the use of heat, exercise, stress-reduction techniques, and prescribed medications to relieve manifestations. In addition, suggest the following resources:

- Fibromyalgia Network
- National Fibromyalgia Association
- Arthritis Foundation
- National Institute of Arthritis and Musculoskeletal and Skin Diseases

Structural Disorders

Structural disorders of the musculoskeletal system most commonly affect the spine. The disorders discussed in this section are spinal deformities, low back pain, and common foot disorders.

The Patient with Spinal Deformity

Scoliosis and kyphosis are the two most common deformities of the spinal column. *Scoliosis* is a lateral curvature of the spine. *Kyphosis* is excessive angulation of the normal posterior curve of the thoracic spine (Figure 40–14 ■).

An estimated 600,000 people in the United States are affected by scoliosis. It usually is diagnosed in adolescence. Although the incidence is equal between genders, females are eight times more likely to require treatment for significant curvature (National Scoliosis Foundation, 2009). Idiopathic scoliosis is the most common form of the disorder, accounting for approximately 85% of cases. Congenital and neuromuscular disorders such as cerebral palsy, poliomyelitis, and MD account for the rest (Porth & Matfin, 2009).

Pathophysiology

Detailed discussions of the causes and treatment of scoliosis and kyphosis in younger patients can be found in pediatric nursing textbooks. This discussion focuses on the nursing care of adults with these disorders. The manifestations of scoliosis and kyphosis are listed in the box on page 1393.

Scoliosis

Scoliosis is classified as *postural* when the small curve corrects with bending, and *structural* when the curve does not correct with bending (Porth & Matfin, 2009). Most patients requiring treatment have structural scoliosis, a curve caused by a fixed deformity.

The lateral curve that occurs in scoliosis is usually evident in the thoracic, lumbar, or thoracolumbar regions of the spine. A right thoracic curve is the most common. The vertebral bodies in these spinal regions can be rotated as well as curved to one side or the other. Curves greater than 40 degrees are considered severe (Porth & Matfin, 2009).

A   Normal spine   Scoliosis   B   Normal spine   Kyphosis

Figure 40–14 ■ Common deformities of the spinal column: *A,* Scoliosis is a lateral curvature of the spine. *B,* Kyphosis is an exaggerated posterior curvature of the thoracic spine.

MANIFESTATIONS of Scoliosis and Kyphosis

SCOLIOSIS
- Asymmetry of shoulders, scapulae, waist creases
- Prominence of the thoracic ribs or paravertebral muscles on forward bend
- Lateral curvature and vertebral rotation on postero-anterior x-ray film

SEVERE SCOLIOSIS
- Back pain
- Shortness of breath
- Anorexia, nausea

KYPHOSIS
- Posterior rounding at the thoracic level
- Kyphotic curve of over 45 degrees on x-ray film

As scoliosis emerges, the soft tissues (muscles and ligaments) shorten on the concave side of the curvature. Over time, progressive deformities of the vertebral column and ribs develop, causing one-sided compression of the vertebral bodies. The degree of compression and twisting varies according to the location of each vertebra within the curved portion of the spine.

Scoliosis is usually first noted by the deformity it causes, such as one shoulder that is higher than the other, a prominent hip, or a projecting scapula. Pain is present in severe cases, usually in the lumbar region. Pain also may be caused by pressure on the ribs or the crest of the ilium. Shortness of breath may result from diminished chest expansion, and GI disturbances may occur because of crowding of the abdominal organs.

Kyphosis

Like scoliosis, kyphosis is classified as postural or structural. Postural kyphosis is caused by a slumping posture. Structural kyphosis may result from congenital malformations or pediatric disorders such as rickets or poliomyelitis. However, kyphosis also may occur during adulthood from vertebral tuberculosis and Paget's disease or from metabolic disorders such as osteoporosis and osteomalacia. The condition can also result from the surgical removal or radiation of intervertebral disks for the treatment of spinal cord tumors or cysts.

The manifestations of kyphosis include moderate back pain and increased curvature of the thoracic spine as viewed from the side ("hunchback"). Impaired mobility and respiratory problems may occur in cases of severe curvature.

Interdisciplinary Care

Diagnosis of scoliosis and kyphosis is important to prevent severe spinal deformity in the adult. The patient stands with the arms relaxed and hanging freely at the sides while the examiner evaluates him or her from both the back and the front for symmetry of the shoulders, scapulae, waist creases, and the length of the arms. The patient then bends forward, and the examiner observes for prominence of the thoracic ribs or vertebral muscles. The patient is then viewed from the side while the screener looks for increased thoracic rounding or lumbar swayback.

Diagnosis

Upright posteroanterior and lateral x-rays are used to confirm the diagnosis of curvature of the spine. For the patient with scoliosis, the degree of curvature is measured by determining the amount of lateral deviation to the left or right. For the patient with kyphosis, anteroposterior and lateral views typically reveal wedging of the vertebrae.

Treatments

Scoliosis and kyphosis may be treated conservatively or with surgery.

CONSERVATIVE TREATMENT Braces can be used to prevent progression of scoliosis and kyphosis in younger patients whose skeletons have not yet matured. Bracing is the treatment of choice for adolescents with curves of 20 or 25 to 30 degrees. Unfortunately, this approach is ineffective in the adult patient. Conservative treatment for adults with scoliosis and kyphosis may include weight reduction, active and passive exercises, and the use of braces for support.

SURGERY The use of surgery to correct spinal deformities depends on factors such as the degree of curvature and the patient's overall physical, emotional, and neurologic status. Even with surgery, it is not possible to correct the abnormal curvature completely. The surgical procedure involves attaching metal reinforcing rods to the vertebrae, and is usually performed using an anterior approach, although more severe curvature may require both an anterior and a posterior approach. The types of straightening devices used most frequently use bilateral rods with wire hooks or screws that stabilize the spine and correct the deformity.

Nursing Care

Nursing Diagnoses and Interventions

Nursing interventions focus on minimizing the risk for injury and neurologic impairment.

Risk for Injury

Patients with spinal deformities are at risk for injury from several sources, including structural aspects of bracing both before and after surgical intervention, dislocation of hooks and rods resulting from improper alignment or movement of the back, and changes in body position after prolonged immobilization.

- Assess the environment for safety hazards. *The patient needs to learn to use handrails on stairways and take precautions when walking on slippery surfaces or areas with throw rugs.*

> **PRACTICE ALERT**
> Some braces do not allow the patient to flex or hyperextend the spinal column.

- Teach the patient ways to reduce irritation of skin surfaces beneath the brace: wearing a smooth cotton t-shirt or cotton tube under the brace at all times, changing undergarments at least once daily, and washing them with a mild soap. Undergarments should be changed more frequently in warmer weather. *The patient wearing a brace is especially prone to skin breakdown and must take precautions to prevent it.*

- Teach the patient to loosen the brace during meals and for the first 30 minutes after each meal. *Patients have difficulty eating if the brace is tight. Loosening the brace during and after each meal will allow adequate nutritional intake and promote comfort.*
- Teach patients how to apply the brace, and explain ambulatory restrictions. *Patients requiring a brace need to learn how to apply the brace prior to ambulating. Ambulation is frequently restricted to walking rather than sitting for long periods.*
- Turn patients who have undergone spinal surgery by using the log-rolling technique. Patients require a position change at least every 2 hours. *The use of a turn sheet and sufficient assistance allow the nurse to maintain the patient's proper body alignment during the turning procedure.*
- Use a fracture bedpan following surgery. *The fracture bedpan provides minimal misalignment of spine and is more comfortable.*

Risk for Peripheral Neurovascular Dysfunction

Surgical procedures can lead to neurologic impairment in the patient with a spinal deformity.

- Monitor the movement and sensation of lower extremities every 2 hours for the first 8 hours then every shift and as needed. *Neurologic assessment related to sensation and movement of the lower extremities is necessary because the surgical procedure is in close proximity to spinal nerves. Swelling of the surgical site can impinge on the spinal nerves and cause a loss of sensation and movement.*

Community-Based Care

Patients with structural scoliosis or kyphosis need reassurance that the condition was not caused by poor posture. If a brace is prescribed to relieve pain and other symptoms associated with the disorder, provide verbal and written instructions for wearing the brace, such as the number of hours per day it is to be worn and activity restrictions to follow when wearing or not wearing the brace. Teach the patient how to protect and care for skin under the brace.

Surgical patients need postoperative teaching regarding site care and activities. Patients who have spinal surgery often are allowed to ambulate fairly soon after surgery, but sitting may be restricted because of the stresses it places on the spine. Instruct the patient to notify the physician if numbness, tingling, pain, or weakness of an extremity develops after surgery.

Discuss the importance of not smoking and of avoiding respiratory infections for patients with scoliosis or kyphosis that restricts respiratory excursion. Encourage these patients to obtain pneumococcal pneumonia and influenza immunizations.

The Patient with Low Back Pain

Acute or chronic low back pain involves the lumbar, lumbosacral, or sacroiliac areas of the back. In most cases, low back pain is due to strains in the muscles and tendons of the back caused by abnormal stress or overuse. Low back pain caused by degenerative disk disease and herniated vertebral disks is covered in ∞ Chapter 43.

Pathophysiology

The pathophysiology of back pain varies with its many causes (Box 40–6). In general, the five causes and types of back pain are as follows:

- Local pain is caused by compression or irritation of sensory nerves. Fractures, strains, and sprains are common causes of local pain; tumors also may press on pain-sensitive structures.
- Referred pain may originate from abdominal or pelvic viscera.
- Pain of spinal origin, that is, pain associated with pathology of the spine such as disk disease or arthritis, may be referred to other structures such as the buttocks, groin, or legs.
- Radicular back pain is sharp, radiating from the back to the leg along a nerve root. This pain may be aggravated by movements such as coughing, sneezing, or sitting.
- Muscle spasm pain is associated with many spine disorders, although its origin may be unclear. This type of back pain is dull and may be accompanied by abnormal posture and taut spinal muscles.

Manifestations

Patients with low back pain report pain ranging from mild discomfort lasting a few hours to chronic debilitating pain. Acute pain is usually caused when the patient participates in an activity that is not usually pursued, such as unusual lifting or bending, playing an active sport, or shoveling snow. Manifestations are presented in the following box.

Interdisciplinary Care

Care of the patient with low back pain focuses on relieving pain, correcting the condition if possible, preventing complications, and educating the patient.

BOX 40–6 Factors Associated with Back Pain

Mechanical Injury or Trauma
- Muscle strain or spasm
- Compression fracture
- Lumbar disk disease

Degenerative Disorders
- Spondylosis
- Spinal stenosis
- Osteoarthritis

Systemic Disorders
- Osteomyelitis
- Osteoporosis or osteomalacia
- Neoplasms, primary or metastatic

Referred Pain
- Gastrointestinal disorders
- Genitourinary disorders
- Gynecologic disorders
- Abdominal aortic aneurysm
- Hip pathology

Other
- Fibromyalgia
- Psychiatric syndromes
- Chronic anxiety
- Depression

MANIFESTATIONS of Low Back Pain

ALTERATIONS IN GAIT AND FLEXION
- Walking in a stiff, flexed state
- Inability to bend at waist
- Limp, which may indicate impairment of the sciatic nerve

NEUROLOGIC INVOLVEMENT
- When tested for light and deep touch with a pin and cotton ball, may feel sensations in both limbs but experience a stronger sensation in the unaffected side
- Loss of both bowel and bladder control due to involvement of the sacral nerve

PAIN
- Pain in the affected leg when walking on heel or toes
- Continuous, knifelike localized pain in muscles close to the affected disk
- Pain that radiates down posterior of leg
- Sharp, burning pain in the posterior thigh or calf
- Pain in middle of buttock
- Tenderness when muscle close to the affected disk is palpated
- Severe pain with straight leg-raising maneuver

Diagnosis

The choice of diagnostic tests for the patient with low back pain depends on the suspected diagnoses, clinical findings, and history. Current guidelines for care recommend that radiography, CT scans, and MRI be used only with clinical signs of a potentially serious underlying condition. Diagnostic testing may be considered if pain and other manifestations continue to limit the patient after 4 weeks of conservative treatment. Diagnostic tests are described in ∞ Chapter 38.

Medications

The medications of choice for low back pain include NSAIDs and analgesics. NSAIDs block prostaglandin production and reduce inflammation, thus relieving the pain. Muscle relaxants, such as cyclobenzaprine (Flexeril), methocarbamol (Robaxin), or carisoprodol (Soma), may be used, but little evidence supports their efficacy.

Epidural steroid injections may be used to help reduce intense, intractable pain. A steroid solution is injected into the epidural space, which helps decrease the swelling and inflammation of the spinal nerves.

Conservative Treatment

The majority of patients with acute low back pain need only a short-term treatment regimen. Limited rest, combined with appropriate exercise and education, is often the primary method of treatment. There is no evidence that activity is harmful or aggravating to the source of pain. In fact, activity promotes bone and muscle strength and may increase endorphin levels. Therefore, active rehabilitation helps to restore function and reduce pain.

Pain may be relieved by an ice bag or heating pad applied to the back. Exercise programs are helpful provided that the patient begins gradually and increases activity gradually as the recovery process continues. Physical therapy procedures include diathermy (deep heat therapy), ultrasonography, hydrotherapy, and transcutaneous electrical nerve stimulation (TENS) units. These therapies reduce the muscle spasms and

pain temporarily. They are frequently used in combination with exercise to provide early mobilization for the patient.

Complementary and alternative medicine strategies for low back pain include chiropractic, acupuncture, and massage.

Nursing Care

Nursing care of the patient with low back pain focuses on relieving the pain. In addition, most patients have very little understanding of the anatomy of the spine, the reasons for the pain, the choices for treatment, and the importance of self-management. Therefore, education is another essential aspect of treating low back pain.

Health Promotion

Recommendations for preventing back pain from the National Institute of Neurological Disorders and Stroke include the following:

- Have a regular exercise program.
- Stretch before working in the yard, jogging, and playing sports.
- Quit smoking.
- Lose weight, if needed.
- Maintain a correct posture.
- Use supportive seats when driving.
- Lift by bending at the knees rather than at the waist.
- Reduce emotional stress that causes muscle tension.

In industrial and work settings, nurses should be alert for situations that increase the risk of back pain and injury. Office workers should have chairs with appropriate seat height and length and back support. Modifications of work space or machinery may be necessary for industrial workers to avoid excess stresses on back muscles. Finally, it is important to remember that back pain is a leading cause of lost work time for nurses themselves. Remind coworkers to use good body mechanics and to seek help when lifting or moving patients.

Nursing Diagnoses and Interventions

Nursing interventions for the patient with low back pain are based on problems with acute pain, deficient knowledge, and risk for impaired adjustment.

Acute Pain

Muscle spasms and inflammation are among the contributing factors of low back pain.

- Teach the patient appropriate comfort measures. *Patients with low back pain have discomfort due to muscle spasms and/or inflammation due to nerve compression, surgery, or irritation from a brace.*
- Instruct the patient to take NSAIDs or analgesics on a routine schedule rather than as needed. *Maintaining a constant blood level of the NSAIDs or analgesics reduces inflammation and provides continuous pain relief.*

Readiness for Enhanced Knowledge

The patient with low back pain requires information regarding treatment modalities.

- Encourage patients to stay active. *There is little scientific evidence to show that bed rest is beneficial, but there is ample evidence about the adverse effects of bed rest. Staying in bed*

EVIDENCE FOR NURSING CARE | The Patient with Low Back Pain

Selected resources that nurses may find helpful when planning evidence-based nursing care follow.

■ Bonner, S. M. (2009). Getting to the root of your patient's back pain. *Nursing2009, 39*(7), 36–41.

■ Chou, R., Qaseem, A., Snow V., Casey, D., Cross, J. T. Jr., Shekelle, P., et al., Clinical Efficacy Assessment Subcommittee of the American College of Physicians, American College of Physicians, American Pain Society Low Back Pain Guidelines Panel. (2007 October 2). Diagnosis and treatment of low back pain: A joint clinical practice guideline from the American College of Physicians and the American Pain Society. *Annals of Internal Medicine, 147*(7), 478–491.

■ Institute for Clinical Systems Improvement (ICSI). (2008 November). *Adult low back pain.* Bloomington, MN: Institute for Clinical Systems Improvement (ICSI).

■ Manchikanti, L., Boswell, M. V., Singh, V., Benyamin, R. M., Fellows, B., Abdi, S., et al. (2009). Comprehensive evidence-based guidelines for interventional techniques in the management of chronic spinal pain. *Pain Physician, 12*, 699–802.

for more than one to two days can actually increase pain, and cause joint stiffness and muscle weakness.

■ Teach the patient about the "rebound phenomenon" of prolonged heat or ice therapy. *Ice remaining on the skin longer than 15 minutes or heat longer than 30 minutes causes a reverse effect known as the rebound phenomenon. For example, heat produces maximum vasodilation in 20 to 30 minutes. Continuation of the application beyond 30 to 45 minutes causes tissue congestion, and the blood vessels constrict. Likewise, with cold application, maximum vasoconstriction occurs when the skin reaches a temperature of 60°F (15°C). Prolonged cold can create a drop in temperature, at which time vasodilation occurs.*

■ Provide instructions about appropriate back exercises such as partial sit-ups with the knees bent and knee-chest exercises to stretch hamstrings and spinal muscles. Each exercise should be done 5 times and gradually increased to 10 times. Advise the patient to discontinue any exercise that is painful and to seek professional advice before continuing the exercise. *Repetition of prescribed back exercises, such as the pelvic tilt, partial sit-ups, and back rolls, will strengthen the muscles that protect the spine and thus prevent back strain.*

Readiness for Enhanced Self Health Management
The need for lifestyle changes may lead to impaired adjustment in people with back pain.

■ Teach the use of appropriate body mechanics in lifting and reaching. The patient should be instructed to plan the lift, keep the object being lifted close to the body, and avoid twisting when lifting. Encourage the patient to obtain help when lifting. *An item is considered excessively heavy if it equals 35% of the lifter's body weight.*

■ Instruct the patient to modify the workplace or environment to minimize stress to the lower back. *Lumbar supports in chairs, adjustment of chair or table height, and rubber floor mats help prevent back strain or injury.*

■ Encourage obese patients to lose weight. *The trunk of the body must carry excess weight when the patient is obese. Obese people are farther away from the objects they lift because of their greater abdominal girth. They may also have more difficulty squatting to lift. The greater the distance between an object and the patient's center of gravity, the higher the risk for straining the lower back.*

Community-Based Care
Back pain is a common problem in the United States and other industrialized countries. Nurses can have an effect on this significant problem by teaching health practices to prevent back injury to patients of all ages. Teach patients how to safely lift, bend, and turn when engaging in physical activity. Stress the importance of using large muscle groups of the legs to lift rather than bending and lifting with the smaller muscles of the back. Teach other aspects of good body mechanics, including posture, sleeping on a firm mattress, and sitting in chairs that provide good support. Discuss the positive effect of maintaining optimal body weight and good physical fitness.

The Patient with a Common Foot Disorder
Hallux valgus, hammertoe, and Morton's neuroma are common foot disorders that cause pain or difficulty in walking. All three disorders may be caused by wearing poorly fitting or confining shoes. These disorders are more prevalent among women.

Pathophysiology
Hallux Valgus
Hallux valgus, commonly called a *bunion*, is the enlargement and lateral displacement of the first metatarsal (the great toe) (Figure 40–15 ■). Hallux valgus develops when chronic pressure against the great toe causes the connective tissue in the sole of the foot to lengthen so that the stabilizing action of the great toe is gradually lost. The toe bends laterally away from the midline of the body, and the metatarsophalangeal joint (MTP) is exposed to friction during walking and becomes enlarged. As the deformity progresses, calluses form over the metatarsal head, and bursitis develops in the MTP. In severe cases, the lateral displacement of the great toe may approach

Bunion

Figure 40–15 ■ Hallux valgus (bunion).

70 to 90 degrees, and the second toe may be forced upward, causing hammertoe. Although bunions may be a congenital disorder, most are caused by wearing pointed, narrow-toed shoes or high heels.

Hallux valgus is obvious on physical examination of the foot. The patient may report an inability to fit into shoes. Often, the patient may report joint pain or pain around calluses. In advanced or severe cases, the first metatarsal joint may have limited ROM, particularly in dorsiflexion, and crepitus (crackling or popping) may occur during joint movement.

Hammertoe

Hammertoe (claw toe) is the dorsiflexion of the first phalanx with accompanying plantar flexion of the second and third phalanges. The condition may affect any toe, but the second toe is most commonly affected. Patients initially experience mild inflammation of the synovial membranes of the involved joints. As the deformity progresses, the dorsiflexed joint rubs against the overlying shoe, causing painful corns to develop.

Morton's Neuroma

Morton's neuroma is a tumorlike mass formed within the neurovascular bundle of the intermetatarsal spaces (Figure 40–16 ■). The neuromas usually occur in only one foot, most frequently in the third web space. Like other common foot disorders, Morton's neuroma usually is caused by wearing tight, confining shoes. The condition develops when repeated compression of the toes causes irritation and scarring of tissues surrounding the plantar digital nerve. The affected nerve becomes inflamed and swells. After repeated episodes of inflammation, the nerve fibers become fibrotic, and a neuroma forms.

Manifestations include a burning pain at the web space of the affected foot that radiates into the tips of the involved toes. Weight bearing usually worsens any symptoms; removing the shoe and massaging the foot often relieves the pain. The neuroma may present as a palpable mass between the affected toes. The area over the neuroma usually is tender.

Figure 40–16 ■ Morton's neuroma.

Interdisciplinary Care

Care of the patient with common foot disorders such as hallux valgus, hammertoe, and Morton's neuroma focuses on relieving pain, correcting the structural deformity, and preventing reoccurrence. In most cases, all three conditions are diagnosed by inspection. X-ray films of the affected foot are taken if the need for surgery arises.

Conservative treatment for common foot disorders usually involves the use of corrective shoes. Orthotic devices that cushion and stretch the affected joints may be placed within shoes or between the patient's toes. For Morton's neuroma, metatarsal pads are used to spread the patient's toes and decompress the affected nerve. Analgesics may be prescribed to relieve pain and inflammation. In severe cases, corticosteroid drugs may be injected into the affected joints or surrounding tissue to relieve acute inflammation.

Surgery is reserved for patients with intractable toe deformities or pain. Hallux valgus is treated with bunionectomy; ligaments are lengthened or shortened as needed, and pins are drilled into place so the toe remains in position. Similarly, the correction of hammertoe also involves straightening the affected toe and inserting pins to retain the correction. A cast may be applied over the foot following surgery to correct toe deformities. Surgery for Morton's neuroma causes loss of sensation to a portion of the foot because removing the neuroma involves cutting out a portion of the plantar nerve.

℘ Nursing Care

Nursing care for patients with these foot deformities focuses on the same areas because the conservative treatment and preoperative and postoperative interventions are similar.

Nursing Diagnoses and Interventions

Pain relief, prevention of infection, and patient education are important priorities for the nursing care of patients with foot disorders.

Chronic Pain

In the patient with a foot deformity, constant pressure of footwear over the involved joint can cause pain.

- Instruct patients to wear corrective footwear to assist in the conservative treatment of foot problems. *Pain related to foot problems can result from footwear that does not provide proper toe room; in addition, heels higher than 1 inch can cause constant flexion and hyperextension problems. In some instances, the patient must purchase special shoes or orthotics to ensure correct fit and relief of symptoms.*
- Suggest purchasing appropriate pads to wear over painful bunions, calluses/corns, and the ball of the foot. *Protective pads are manufactured for specific foot problems; these include bunion pads, corn pads, and metatarsal pads.*
- Instruct patients to remove pads and inspect the skin every other day. Patients who have difficulty reaching or observing the involved foot should ask another person to do the inspection for them. *It is especially important to emphasize the need for inspection to patients who have experienced loss of sensation of the feet due to such disorders as diabetes and chronic peripheral vascular disease.*

Risk for Infection

Like all surgeries, foot surgery carries a risk of infection. This risk may be increased because of impaired peripheral circulation and exposure of the feet to the environment.

- Teach patients proper care and cleaning of exposed pins implanted during the surgical procedure. *Pins inserted into soft tissue of the toes and bones are prone to becoming infected and can potentially result in osteomyelitis.*
- Teach patients how to keep pins and casts dry while bathing or ambulating in inclement weather. Patients must wear a plastic bag over the cast or pins when bathing or walking in rain or snow. *When casts or pins are exposed in water, infection may result.*

Community-Based Care

For patients in all age groups, teach the importance of well-fitting footwear. Discuss the long-term effects of wearing high-heeled shoes with constricting toes with women in particular. Suggest alternatives for stylish footwear, and encourage patients to wear supportive and nonrestrictive footwear at all times. Discuss the possible effects of bunions on balance, and talk about safety measures to prevent falls and injury. Teach patients techniques to relieve pressure on affected joints.

CHAPTER HIGHLIGHTS

- Metabolic bone disorders begin in the bone remodeling process, and may result from aging, calcium and phosphate imbalances, genetics, and changes in hormone levels. The disorders include osteoporosis, Paget's disease, gout, and osteomalacia.
- Osteoporosis is a major health problem in the United States, with fractures being the most common complication. Health promotion activities to prevent development of the disease include a calcium-rich diet, weight-bearing exercise, and a healthy lifestyle.
- Gout is characterized by hyperuricemia and urate crystal formation in the joint synovium. Attacks of the disease typically begin with an acutely painful inflammation of the first joint of the great toe, although other joints such as the knee or elbow may be affected.
- Degenerative musculoskeletal disorders include osteoarthritis (OA) and muscular dystrophy (MD). OA is the most commonly occurring of all forms of arthritis, and a leading cause of pain and disability in older adults. The disease is characterized by loss of cartilage in articulating joints and hypertrophy of bone at the articular margins. Pain and inflammation are most often conservatively managed with NSAIDs.
- Significant pain and disability not controlled with NSAIDs, exercise, and physical therapy may necessitate total joint replacement.
- Autoimmune and inflammatory disorders of the musculoskeletal system include rheumatoid arthritis (RA), ankylosing spondylitis (AS), reactive arthritis (ReA), systemic lupus erythematosus (SLE), polymyositis, and Lyme disease.
- Although the cause of RA is unknown, it is believed to be a combination of genetic and environmental factors. RA is a systemic disease, affecting one or many joints with the risk for severe contractures and deformity, and also causing fatigue, weakness,

anorexia, weight loss, and fever. The primary objectives of treatment and care are to reduce pain and inflammation, preserve function, and prevent deformity.
- SLE is a chronic inflammatory connective tissue disease, affecting almost all body systems, including the musculoskeletal system. Skin lesions are a common manifestation, exhibited by a characteristic rash on the face. The patient with SLE is at increased risk for infection.
- Lyme disease is caused by the spirochete *Borrelia burgdorferi*, carried and transmitted primarily by ticks. The disease can be treated effectively with antibiotics.
- Osteomyelitis and septic arthritis are infectious musculoskeletal disorders. Osteomyelitis may be the result of a bloodborne pathogen, a contiguous infection, or a complication of vascular insufficiency. Septic arthritis is a medical emergency, requiring immediate treatment to preserve joint function.
- Bone tumors may be benign or malignant, primary or metastatic. The primary manifestations of a bone tumor are pain, a mass, and impaired function. Nursing care is directed toward teaching to prevent injury and interventions to relieve pain.
- Systemic sclerosis is a chronic disease characterized by the formation of excess connective tissue and diffuse fibrosis of the skin and internal organs. It may be either localized or generalized. Other connective musculoskeletal disorders are Sjögren's syndrome and fibromyalgia.
- Structural musculoskeletal disorders affecting the spine are manifested by scoliosis, kyphosis, and low back pain. Those commonly affecting the feet are hallux valgus, hammertoe, and Morton's neuroma.

TEST YOURSELF NCLEX-RN® REVIEW

1. Although all of the following nursing diagnoses are important when planning care for the patient with osteoporosis, which is most significant in terms of long-term disability?
   1. *Chronic Pain*
   2. *Risk for Falls*
   3. *Activity Intolerance*
   4. *Acute Pain*

2. You are preparing a teaching plan for a woman with osteoarthritis. Which group of medications should you prepare to discuss?
   1. opioids
   2. antibiotics
   3. hormones
   4. NSAIDs

3. You are monitoring the laboratory reports for a patient with an acute attack of gout. Which of the following measurements would you expect to be increased?
    1. hematocrit
    2. uric acid
    3. alkaline phosphatase
    4. creatinine

4. What is a potential complication of both osteoporosis and osteomalacia?
    1. infection
    2. blood clots
    3. fractures
    4. contractures

5. You are assessing a woman who has come to an orthopedic clinic complaining of knee pain. Which of the following assessments you made would indicate an increased risk for osteoarthritis?
    1. being overweight by 30 pounds
    2. having a history of falls
    3. eating a diet high in calcium
    4. walking 30 minutes each day

6. A postoperative nursing care plan for a patient who has had a total knee replacement includes monitoring vital signs and laboratory results. The rationale for these interventions is to do which of the following?
    1. Teach the patient the importance of these assessments.
    2. Promote rapport between the patient and the health-care providers.
    3. Ensure adequate circulation to the involved extremity.
    4. Prevent the progression of infection.

7. When comparing osteoarthritis and rheumatoid arthritis, what assessment finding would be different in the patient with rheumatoid arthritis?
    1. Health history includes weight loss and fever.
    2. Abnormal joint findings are limited to the hands.
    3. Stiffness is relieved by activity.
    4. Heberden's nodes are located on the finger joints.

8. *Ineffective Protection* is an appropriate nursing diagnosis for the patient with SLE. What would be your most important intervention for the hospitalized patient?
    1. Monitor laboratory findings.
    2. Provide appropriate skin care.
    3. Practice careful hand hygiene.
    4. Administer prescribed medications.

9. How is the causative organism for Lyme disease spread?
    1. through the bite of an infected mosquito
    2. by brief contact with an infected tick
    3. primarily by droplets from infected people
    4. by an infected tick embedded for > 24 hours

10. Of the different types of arthritis, which one is considered a medical emergency, requiring immediate diagnosis and treatment?
    1. osteoarthritis
    2. septic arthritis
    3. reactive arthritis
    4. gouty arthritis

See Test Yourself answers in Appendix C.

Pearson Nursing Student Resources
Find additional review materials at
www.nursing.pearsonhighered.com
Prepare for success with additional NCLEX®-style practice questions, interactive assignments and activities, Web links, animations and videos, and more!

BIBLIOGRAPHY

Altman, R., Kuritzky, L., & Ruoff, G. (2009 February). Improving long-term management of osteoarthritis: Strategies for primary care physicians. *The Journal of Family Practice, 58*(2 Suppl.), S17–S24.

American College of Rheumatology. (2008a). *Glucocorticoid-induced osteoporosis.* Retrieved from http://www.rheumatology.org/public/factsheets/diseases_and_conditions/gi-osteoporosis.asp

American College of Rheumatology. (2008b). *Lyme disease.* Retrieved from http://www.rheumatology.org/public/factsheets/

Barclay, L., Vega, C., & Martin, B. (2008 February 28). New guidelines issued for management of hip and knee osteoarthritis. *Medscape Medical News.* Retrieved from www.medscape.com

Bergman, M. (Ed.). (2008). Rheumatoid arthritis: Ongoing management and clinical assessment. *Practicing Clinicians Exchange, 2008 PCE Updates in Rheumatology, 2*(1), 1–11.

Bergman, M. (Ed.). (2009). Looking beyond joint damage in rheumatoid arthritis: Managing extra-articular manifestations and comorbidities. *Practicing Clinicians Exchange, 2009 PCE Updates in Rheumatology, 2*(3), 1–11.

Bingham, C. (2009 June 30). Advances in rheumatology nursing care: Basic immunology and its relationship to rheumatoid arthritis and treatment. *Medscape CME.* Retrieved from www.cme.medscape.com

Blackham, J., Garry, J., Cummings, D., & Russell, R. (2008 July). Does regular exercise reduce the pain and stiffness of osteoarthritis? *The Journal of Family Practice, 57*(7), 476–477.

Bratton, R., Whiteside, J., Hovan, M., Engle, R., & Edwards, F. (2008 May). Diagnosis and treatment of Lyme disease. *Mayo Clinic Proceedings, 83*(5), 566–571.

Brown, A., & Murata, P. (2009 May 22). Sustained benefits seen with combination drug therapy for rheumatoid arthritis. Reuters Health Information, 2009. Retrieved from www.cme.medscape.com

Bulechek, G., Butcher, H., & Dochterman, J. (2008). *Nursing interventions classification (NIC)* (5th ed.). St. Louis, MO: Mosby.

Cancro, M., D'Cruz, D., & Khamashta, M. (2009 May). The role of B lymphocyte stimulator (BLyS) in systemic lupus erythematosus. *The Journal of Clinical Investigation, 119*(5), 1066–1073.

Centers for Disease Control and Prevention (CDC). (2007 January 26). Errata: Vol. 55, No. 40 (Prevalence of doctor-diagnosed arthritis and arthritis-attributable activity limitation – United States, 2003-2005.). *MMWR, 56*(03), 55. Retrieved from www.cdc.gov/mmwr

Centers for Disease Control and Prevention (CDC). (2007 June). *Data and statistics. Racial/ethnic differences.* Retrieved from www.cdc.gov/arthritis/data_statistics

Centers for Disease Control and Prevention (CDC). (2008 June). *Data and statistics. Arthritis related statistics.* Retrieved from www.cdc.gov/arthritis/data_statistics

Centers for Disease Control and Prevention (CDC). (2010). *Estimates for specific forms of arthritis.* Retrieved from www.cdc.gov/Features/dsArthritis/

Centers for Disease Control and Prevention (CDC). (2010). *Arthritis: Meeting the challenge. At a glance 2010.* Retrieved from http://www.cdc.gov/chronicdisease/resources/publications/AAG/arthritis.htm

Choi, H. (2009 August 25). *Complexities of gout: Comorbidities cause or effect?* Retrieved from www.cme.medscape.com

Crosby, J. (2009 July). Osteoarthritis: Managing without surgery. *The Journal of Family Practice, 58*(7), 354–361.

Dell, D. (2007, February). Getting to the point about fibromyalgia. *Nursing, 37*(2), 61–64.

DiPiro, J., Talbert, R., Yee, G., Matzke, G., Wells, B., & Posey, L. (2008). *Pharmacotherapy: A pathophysiologic approach* (7th ed.). New York, NY: McGraw Hill.

Fauci, A., Braunwald, E., Kasper, D., Hauser, S., Longo, D., Jameson, J., et al. (2008). *Harrison's principles of internal medicine* (17th ed.). New York, NY: McGraw Hill.

Flynn, J., & Johnson, T. (2005). *The Johns Hopkins white papers: Arthritis.* Baltimore, MD: Johns Hopkins Medicine.

Gibofsky, A. (2009 June 18). Latest evidence on biologic therapy for RA: Weighing the risks and benefits. *Medscape.* Retrieved from www.cme.medscape.com

Goldenberg, D. (2010 May 28). Comprehensive assessment of fibromyalgia and overlapping conditions. *MedscapeCMA Rheumatology.* Retrieved from http://cme.medscape.com/viewarticle/722159/

Gustafsson, B., Ponzer, S., Heikkilä, K., & Ekman, S. (2007). The lived body and the perioperative period in replacement surgery: Older people's experiences. *JAN: Journal of Advanced Nursing, 2007,* 20–28.

Gutierrez, G. (2008 October). Managing osteoarthritis: What's best for your patient? *The Journal of Family Practice, 57*(10), 644–650.

Harvard Women's Health Watch. (2009 October). Study shows that a new type of osteoporosis drug reduces fracture risk. Retrieved from www.health.harvard.edu

Huynh, C., Yanni, L., & Morgan, L. (2008). Fibromyalgia: Diagnosis and management for the primary healthcare provider. *Journal of Women's Health, 17*(8), 1379–1387.

Ioannidis, G., Papaioannou, A., Hopman, W., Akhtar-Danesh, N., Anastassiades, T., Pickard, L., et al., (2009 September 1). Relation between fractures and mortality: Results from the Canadian Multicentre Osteoporosis Study. *CMAJ: Canadian Medical Association Journal, 181*(5), 265–271.

Jacobson, A., Myerscough, R., DeLambo, K., Fleming, E., Huddleston, A., Bright, N., et al. (2008 May). Patients' perspectives on total knee replacement. *American Journal of Nursing, 108*(5), 54–63.

Jimenez, S., Cronin, P., Koenig, A., & O'Brien, M. (2008 October 14). Scleroderma. *Emedicine.* Retrieved from www.emedicine.medscape.com

Kee, J. (2009). *Handbook of laboratory and diagnostic tests with nursing implications* (6th ed.). Upper Saddle River, NJ: Prentice Hall.

Kennel, K., & Drake, M. (2009 July). Adverse effects of bisphosphonates: Implications for osteoporosis management. *Mayo Clinic Proceedings, 84*(7), 632–638.

Lathia, A., Jung, S., & Chen, L. (2009 June). Efficacy of acupuncture as a treatment for chronic shoulder pain. *Journal of Alternative & Complementary Medicine, 15*(6), 613–618.

Mayo Clinic. (2008). *Paget's disease of bone.* Retrieved from www.mayoclinic.com/pagets-disease-of-bone

McPhee, S., Papadakis, M., & Tierney, L., Jr. (Eds.). (2008). *Current medical diagnosis & treatment* (47th ed.). New York, NY: McGraw Hill.

Meyerhoff, J. (2009 July 24). Lyme disease. *Emedicine.* Retrieved from www.emdicine.medscape.com

Moore, N., & Kiebzak, G. (2007). Suboptimal vitamin D status is a highly prevalent but treatable condition in both hospitalized patients and the general population. *Journal of the American Academy of Nurse Practitioners, 19*(2007), 642–651.

Moorhead, S., Johnson, M., Maas, M., & Swanson, E. (2008). *Nursing outcomes classification (NOC)* (4th ed.). St. Louis, MO: Mosby.

MossRehab Resource Net. (2009). *Arthritis fact sheet.* Retrieved from http://www.mossresourcenet.org/arthritis/htm

Muscular Dystrophy Association (MDA). (2001). *Facts about muscular dystrophy (MD).* Available at www.mda.org

NANDA International. (2009). *Nursing diagnoses: Definitions & classification 2009–2011.* Oxford, UK: Wiley-Blackwell.

Napoli, M. (2009 April). The marketing of osteoporosis. *American Journal of Nursing, 109*(4), 58–61.

National Institute of Arthritis and Musculoskeletal and Skin Diseases (NIAMS). (2009a). Fibromyalgia. Retrieved from www.niams.nih.gov/Health_Info/Fibromyalgia

National Institute of Arthritis and Musculoskeletal and Skin Diseases (NIAMS). (2008). Scoliosis. Retrieved from www.niams.nih.gov/Health_Info/Scoliosis

National Institute of Arthritis and Musculoskeletal and Skin Diseases (NIAMS). (2009b). *Handout on health: Systemic lupus erythematosus.* Retrieved from www.niams.nih.gov/Health_Info/lupus/

National Institutes of Health Osteoporosis and Related Bone Diseases – National Resource Center. (2007). *Osteoporosis overview.* Retrieved from www.niams.nih.gov/bone

National Institutes of Health Osteoporosis and Related Bone Diseases – National Resource Center. (2008). *Facts a new patient needs to know about Paget's disease of bone.* Retrieved from www.niams.nih.gov/bone

National Osteoporosis Foundation. (2008). *Clinician's guide to prevention and treatment of osteoporosis.* Washington, DC: Author.

National Osteoporosis Foundation. (2008). *Fast facts.* Retrieved from http://www.nof.org/osteoporosis/diseasefacts.htm

National Scoliosis Foundation. (2009). Information and Support. Retrieved from www.scoliosis.org/info.php

Paget Foundation. (2007). *A nurse's guide to the management of Paget's disease of bone.* Retrieved from www.paget.org

Porth, C., & Matfin, G. (2009). *Pathophysiology: Concepts of altered health states* (8th ed.). Philadelphia: Lippincott.

Qaseem, A., Snow, V., Shekelle, P., Hopkins, R., Jr., Forciea, M., & Owens, D. (2008 September). Pharmacologic treatment of low bone density or osteoporosis to prevent fractures: A clinical practice guideline from the American College of Physicians. *Annals of Internal Medicine, 149*(6), 404–415.

Rao, S., Gendreau, J., & Kranzier, J. (2008 March 6). Understanding the fibromyalgia syndrome. *Medscape.* Retrieved from www.medscape.com

Saag, K., Teng, G., Patkar, N., Anuntiyo, J., Finney, C., Curtis, J., et al. (2008 June 15). American College of Rheumatology 2008 recommendations for the use of nonbiologic and biologic disease modifying antirheumatic drugs in rheumatoid arthritis. *Arthritis & Rheumatism, 59*(6), 762–784.

Scleroderma Foundation. (2009). *What is scleroderma?* Retrieved from http://scleroderma.org/medical/overview.shtm

Seed, S., Dunican, K., & Lynch, A. (2009 May). Osteoarthritis: A review of treatment options. *Formulary, 44,* 143–151.

Shaikh, S. (2007). Ankylosing spondylitis: Recent breakthroughs in diagnosis and treatment. *Journal of the Canadian Chiropractic Association 2007, 51*(4), 249–260.

Spondylitis Association of America. (2009). *Ankylosing spondylitis.* Retrieved from www.spondylitis.org/about/as.aspx

Spondylitis Association of America. (2009). *Reactive arthritis.* Retrieved from www.spondylitis.org/about/reative.aspx

Targownik, L., Lix, L., Metge, C., Prior, H., Leung, S., & Leslie, W. (2008 August 12). Use of proton pump inhibitors and risk of osteoporosis-related fractures. *CMAJ: Canadian Medical Association Journal, 179*(4), 319–326.

Terkeltaub, R. (2009 April 27). *Management of gout: An up-to-date perspective.* Retrieved from www.cme.medscape.com

What are the best treatments for fibromyalgia? (2008 July). *The Journal of Family Medicine, 57*(7), 440.

Wilkinson, J., & Ahern, N. (2009). *Prentice Hall nursing diagnosis handbook* (9th ed.). Upper Saddle River, NJ: Prentice Hall.

Wilson, B., Shannon, M., Shields, K., & Stang, C. (2008). *Prentice Hall nurse's drug guide 2008.* Upper Saddle River, NJ: Prentice Hall.

Functional Health Pattern: Activity-Exercise

Think about patients with altered activity-exercise patterns for whom you have cared in your clinical experiences.

■ Did a musculoskeletal condition discussed in this unit affect the patient's activity and exercise? Was this the patient's primary or secondary reason for seeking care? What kinds of manifestations did each of these patients have? How were these manifestations similar or different?

■ How did the patients' musculoskeletal condition affect their health status and abilities to maintain ADLs, roles, and responsibilities? Did the patients take any medications or herbal supplements for musculoskeletal disorders? If so, did the patients experience adverse drug effects or interactions as a result? Did the patients exercise regularly? Did the patients need assistive devices to move around?

The Activity-Exercise Pattern describes the patient's patterns of exercise, activity, leisure and recreation. Injury to or disorders of the musculoskeletal system often affect the patient's mobility, and, in turn, patterns of activity and exercise.

The tissues and structures of the musculoskeletal system perform many functions, including support, protection, and movement. The bones form the body's internal structure, provide support for soft tissues, protect vital internal organs from injury, and store minerals and serve as a site for hematopoiesis (blood cell formation). The bones and joints of the skeleton and the skeletal muscles work together to allow both gross, simple movements and fine, complex movements. Musculoskeletal disorders often have manifestations such as the following:

■ **Pain** (*tissue damage stimulates sensory nerve endings, which release chemical mediators such as bradykinin and histamine, resulting in transmission of pain sensation to brain and nerve fibers*).

■ **Limited mobility** (*disease or injury affect movement of muscles and joints, resulting in reduction or restriction of range of motion to a body part*).

■ **Swelling** (*inflammation or infection causes release of chemical mediators, increased capillary permeability, and proteins leaking into the interstitium, resulting in edema*).

Priority nursing diagnoses within the Activity-Exercise Pattern that may be appropriate for patients include the following:

■ *Risk for Disuse Syndrome* as evidenced by splinting or guarding of the affected part.

■ *Impaired Physical Mobility* evidenced by limited ROM, pain with movement or weight-bearing.

■ *Risk for Peripheral Neurovascular Dysfunction* as evidenced by pain, pallor, diminished pulses, paralysis, and paresthesia.

■ *Self-Care Deficit* as evidenced by difficulty completing ADLs.

Nursing diagnoses from other health patterns often are of high priority for the patient with altered musculoskeletal function:

■ *Acute and/or Chronic Pain* (Cognitive-Perceptual Pattern)

■ *Impaired Skin Integrity* (Nutritional-Metabolic Pattern)

■ *Impaired Home Maintenance* (Health-Perception-Health-Management Pattern)

Question

1. What teaching should you provide to help your patients with musculoskeletal disorders maintain their usual or desired roles and activities?

Questions

Refer to the Clinical Scenario on the next page in order to answer the following questions.

Priority Setting

1. In what order would you visit these patients after report?
   A. _____
   B. _____
   C. _____
   D. _____

Health Promotion

1. When Ms. Stevens is ready for discharge, what foods will you recommend she eat to promote healing?

2. Will you recommend the same diet for Mr. Rivera as for Ms. Stevens? If yes, why? If no, what will you recommend for him? What is your rationale for this decision?

Nursing Process

1. What priority nursing diagnoses would you choose for each of the patients presented earlier? Explain the rationale for your choices.

	Nursing Diagnosis	Rationale
Jesse Drummond		
Joyce Stevens		
José Rivera		
Kim Wong		

2. After the amputation wound is dressed, which is Mr. Drummond taught to do to toughen the stump?
   A. Dangle the stump for 20 minutes every hour while awake.
   B. Push the stump into soft and then harder surfaces.
   C. Elevate the stump on two pillows, keeping the knee straight.
   D. Apply prosthesis over the compression dressing.

3. Ms. Wong's laboratory results are hematocrit of 28%, hemoglobin of 8 g/dL, white blood cell count of 4,000/mm³, platelet count of 98,000/mL, eosinophil sedimentation rate of 100 mm/hr, positive anti-DNA antibodies. Which diagnosis should the nurse anticipate based on these lab values?
   A. Patient has systemic lupus erythematosus.
   B. Patient has rheumatoid arthritis.
   C. Patient has ankylosing spondylitis.
   D. Patient has polymyositis.

CLINICAL SCENARIO

Directions: *Read the following clinical scenarios and answer the questions that follow. To complete this exercise successfully, you will use not only knowledge of the content in this unit, but also principles related to priority setting and maintaining patient safety.*

You have been assigned to work with the following four patients for the 0700 shift on an orthopedic unit. Significant data obtained during report is as follows:

■ Jesse Drummond is a 70-year-old African American diabetic patient who is 3 days postoperative with bilateral below-the-knee amputations. Vital signs are temperature 99°F, pulse 88, respirations 24, and blood pressure 150/92. He is complaining of feeling pain in his feet.

■ Joyce Stevens is an 84-year-old who is 2 days postoperative for hip replacement surgery. Her vital signs are temperature 99.6°F, pulse 100, respirations 30 and shallow, blood pressure 110/86. She is confused when spoken to.

Petechiae are noted on her arms and legs. She is complaining of difficulty breathing.

■ José Rivera, a 21-year-old, admitted with osteomyelitis of the upper right leg following a gunshot wound to the leg. Vital signs are temperature 102.6°F, pulse 98, respirations 22, blood pressure 138/80. He is scheduled for surgical debridement of the wound this morning. He is complaining of pain and requesting pain medication.

■ Kim Wong is a 30-year-old who is admitted with symptoms of painful and swollen joints, muscle pain, pale and cyanotic fingers and toes, and edema of the legs and periorbital areas. Her vital signs are temperature 100.6°F, pulse 78, respirations 16, blood pressure 108/72. She is complaining of extreme fatigue. She is to have blood drawn for complete blood count (CBC), anti-DNA antibody testing, and serum complement levels.

---

4. Which actions by the nurse are appropriate when caring for Mr. Rivera with osteomyelitis?
   A. Place the patient in a private room and use gloves and gown with wound care and good hand hygiene.
   B. Place the patient in a semi-private room with another infected patient and use isolation precautions for both patients.
   C. Place the patient near the nurse's station and use standard precautions when caring for the patient.
   D. Place the patient at the end of the hall away from other patients to prevent spread of infection and teach the patient to use good hand hygiene.

Communication

1. Mr. Drummond states, "If I knew my legs would hurt so bad after they were cut off, I would not have had the surgery. Will they ever quit hurting?" How will you answer his question?

2. Ms. Wong states, "If I have lupus, how will the doctor cure it?" How will you answer her question?

Delegation

1. What data collection and interventions can be delegated to a nursing assistant for each patient?
   A. _____
   B. _____
   C. _____

Content-Specific Questions

1. To prevent hip contractures in the patient with an above-the-knee amputation, which does the nurse instruct the patient in?
   A. Lie supine for periods throughout the day.
   B. Elevate the stump above the level of the heart.
   C. Perform active ROM exercises every 8 hours.
   D. Do not sit for prolonged periods of time.

2. The nurse explains to the patient with gout that a low-purine diet is recommended. The patient understands a low-purine diet when which meal plan is ordered?
   A. ham and asparagus casserole
   B. chicken and dumplings
   C. chili and spinach salad
   D. shrimp and scallop pasta

3. Patients who have autoimmune diseases such as systemic lupus erythematosus are at increased risk for developing which disease?
   A. chronic renal failure
   B. hypertension
   C. liver insufficiency
   D. coronary heart disease

4. A prescription for ibuprofen (Advil) is given upon discharge to the patient with rheumatoid arthritis. Which toxic effects of the medication does the nurse instruct the patient in?
   A. diarrhea, nausea, and vomiting
   B. blurred vision, tinnitus, and headache
   C. gastric irritation, ulceration, and bleeding
   D. dizziness, dry mouth, and abdominal cramps

5. When performing a neurovascular assessment on a postoperative orthopedic patient, which are included in the initial and focused assessments? **Select all that apply.**
   A. pain
   B. paroxysm
   C. pallor
   D. pulses
   E. paresis
   F. pallesthesia
   G. paresthesia

6. Which patient is at greatest risk for developing osteoporosis?
   A. menopausal, Caucasian woman who smokes one pack of cigarettes a day
   B. menopausal, African American woman who is a diabetic and has hypertension
   C. premenopausal, underweight Asian woman who is allergic to dairy products
   D. premenopausal, obese African American woman who has a sedentary lifestyle

7. An elderly patient sprained an ankle when tripping on an uneven sidewalk. Which is the most appropriate initial intervention for the patient with a sprained ankle?
   A. Use a walker when ambulating.
   B. Take anti-inflammatory and pain medications to reduce ankle pain.
   C. Follow a regimen of rest, ice, compression, and elevation.
   D. Immobilize the ankle with an air splint.

CASE STUDY: William Cole

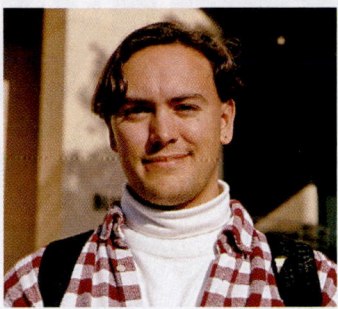

William Cole is a 24-year-old Caucasian male admitted with a compound fracture of the left femur following a four-wheeler accident in which he was thrown from the vehicle. He slid approximately 50 feet down the hill until his fall was stopped when his foot became tangled in some brush. Upon admission, his vital signs were temperature 99.8°F, pulse 100 and thready, respirations 24, and blood pressure 116/70. His height is 74" and weight is 198 pounds. Assessment revealed an open fracture of the left leg with bleeding and edema around the open site. He complains of pain and numbness of the leg. His left leg is pale and cool to touch with a capillary refill of 4 seconds. Distal pulses are difficult to palpate. Multiple lacerations and abrasions are noted on his left trunk and arm. He states he does not have any medical problems and has not seen a doctor in the past 5 years. He is employed and lives in an apartment with two friends.

Blood is drawn for a baseline compete blood count (CBC) and urine is obtained for a urinalysis. An intravenous line is started in the right arm with lactated Ringer's running at 150 mL/hr. He is given a tetanus toxoid immunization and morphine sulfate for pain. X-rays are done of the left leg, left arm, and abdomen. The wounds are cleansed with an antibacterial solution and antibiotic ointment is applied. An open reduction of the left leg fracture is performed, and he has been placed in skeletal traction to immobilize the fracture.

The pathophysiology of a femur fracture is a large amount of force applied to the shaft of the femur, which results in a breaking of the bone. In an open fracture, skin integrity is broken with possible protrusion of bone fragments. Manifestations of a femur fracture are edema and deformed and painful thigh. The patient is unable to move the hip or knee. Popliteal and pedal pulses are difficult to palpate. Capillary refill time is increased. Pallor and coolness indicate arterial compromise. Sensations to the leg may be burning, numbness, prickly feeling, or stinging. Complications of a femur fracture are hypovolemia, fat embolism, dislocation of the hip or knee, muscle atrophy, and ligament damage.

Skeletal traction applies a pulling force through placement of pins into the bone. One or more pulling forces may be applied to maintain alignment of the fracture. The disadvantages of skeletal traction are increased anxiety, increased risk of infection, and increased discomfort.

When planning nursing care for Mr. Cole, the nursing diagnosis of *Impaired Physical Mobility* related to fracture of femur with applied skeletal traction is appropriate for implementing nursing interventions.

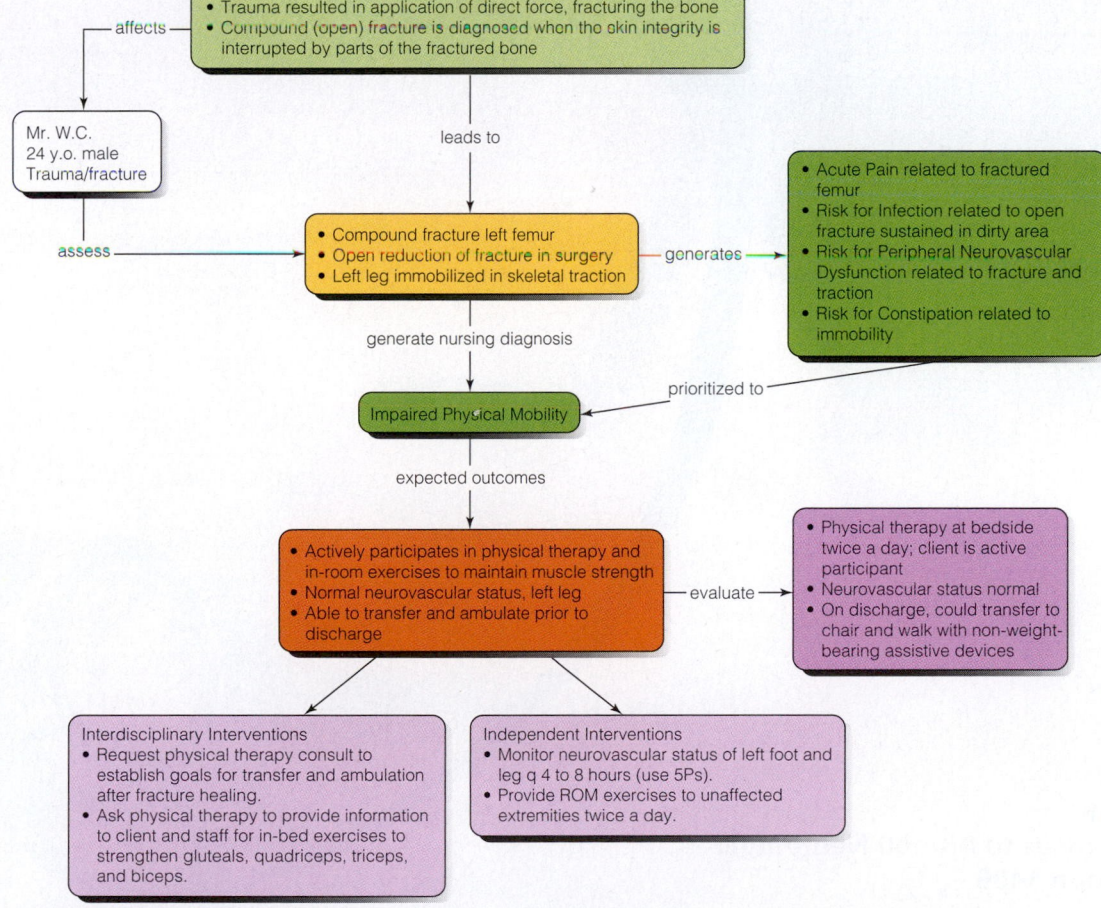

Activity:

1. After review of the concept map, is there anything you would change to make it more understandable?

2. Go to the Pearson Nursing Student Resources for this book at www.nursing.pearsonhighered.com to write a concept map based on a different nursing diagnosis.

   See answers and hints in Appendix C.

Cognitive-Perceptual Pattern

PART V

Functional Health Patterns with Related Nursing Diagnoses

HEALTH PERCEPTION HEALTH MANAGEMENT

- Perceived health status
- Perceived health management
- Health care behaviors: health promotion and illness prevention activities, medical treatments, follow-up care

VALUE-BELIEF

- Values, goals, or beliefs (including spirituality) that guide choices or decisions
- Perceived conflicts in values, beliefs, or expectations that are health related

COPING-STRESS-TOLERANCE

- Capacity to resist challenges to self-integrity
- Methods of handling stress
- Support systems
- Perceived ability to control and manage situations

NUTRITIONAL-METABOLIC

- Daily consumption of food and fluids
- Favorite foods
- Use of dietary supplements
- Skin lesions and ability to heal
- Condition of the integument
- Weight, height, temperature

PART V
Cognitive-Perceptual Patten: Examples of Related NANDA Nursing Diagnoses

- Acute Confusion
- Acute Pain
- Autonomic Dysreflexia
- Caregiver Role Strain
- Chronic Confusion
- Chronic Pain
- Decisional Conflict
- Decreased Intracranial Adaptive Capacity
- Disturbed Body Image
- Disturbed Personality Identity
- Disturbed Sensory Perception
- Disturbed Thought Processes
- Impaired Environmental Interpretation Syndrome
- Impaired Memory
- Impaired Verbal Communication
- Peripheral Neurovascular Dysfunction
- Risk for Falls
- Risk for Poisoning
- Post-Traumatic Response
- Risk for Ineffective Cerebral Tissue Perfusion
- Risk for Post-Traumatic Syndrome
- Wandering
- Unilateral Neglect

SEXUALITY-REPRODUCTIVE

- Satisfaction with sexuality or sexual relationships
- Reproductive pattern
- Female menstrual and perimeno-pausal history

ELIMINATION

- Patterns of bowel and urinary excretion
- Perceived regularity or irregularity of elimination
- Use of laxatives or routines
- Changes in time, modes, quality or quantity of excretions
- Use of devices for control

ROLE-RELATIONSHIP

- Perception of major roles, relationships, and responsibilities in current life situation
- Satisfaction with or disturbances in roles and relationships

ACTIVITY-EXERCISE

- Patterns of personally relevant exercise, activity, leisure, and recreation
- ADLs which require energy expenditure
- Factors that interfere with the desired pattern (e.g., illness or injury)

SELF-PERCEPTION– SELF-CONCEPT

- Attitudes about self
- Perceived abilities, worth, self-image, emotions
- Body posture and movement, eye contact, voice and speech patterns

SLEEP-REST

- Patterns of sleep and rest/relaxation in a 24-hr period
- Perceptions of quality and quantity of sleep and rest
- Use of sleep aids and routines

COGNITIVE-PERCEPTUAL

- Adequacy of vision, hearing, taste, touch, smell
- Pain perception and management
- Language, judgment, memory, decisions

UNIT 11 Responses to Altered Neurologic Function

Assessing the Nervous System

LEARNING OUTCOMES

1. Describe the anatomy, physiology, and functions of the nervous system.
2. Explain manifestations of impairment of neurologic function.
3. Give examples of genetic disorders of the nervous system.
4. Describe normal variations in assessment findings for the older adult.
5. Identify specific topics for consideration during a health history assessment interview of the patient with neurologic disorders.
6. Explain techniques for assessment of neurologic function.
7. Identify abnormal findings that may indicate alterations in nervous system function.

CLINICAL COMPETENCIES

1. Conduct and document a health history for patients having or at risk for alterations in the neurologic system.
2. Conduct and document a physical assessment of neurologic structures and functions.
3. Perform specific neurologic assessments for patients with suspected meningeal irritation and for disoriented or comatose patients.
4. Monitor the results of diagnostic tests and report abnormal findings.

EQUIPMENT NEEDED

- Cotton balls
- Safety pin
- Tongue depressor
- Tuning fork
- Reflex hammer
- Pencil and paper
- Penlight
- Printed materials
- Substances to test the senses of smell and taste

KEY TERMS

anosmia, *1422*
aphasia, *1421*
ataxia, *1425*
decerebrate posturing, *1427*
decorticate posturing, *1427*
diaphoresis, *1414*

dysarthria, *1421*
dysphagia, *1423*
dysphonia, *1421*
fasciculations, *1424*
flaccidity, *1425*

kinesthesia, *1424*
nystagmus, *1422*
ptosis, *1422*
spasticity, *1425*
tremors, *1425*

The nervous system regulates and integrates all body functions, muscle movements, senses, mental abilities, and emotions. It collects information from the internal and external environments as sensory input, processes and interprets the input, and initiates and coordinates responses that are manifested as motor or sensory output. Alterations in structure and/or function of the nervous system have the potential to affect a wide variety of human functions, including activity and exercise, comfort, cardiovascular and respiratory function, elimination, and sexuality. Changes in appearance and abilities for self-care further increase the risk for alterations in self-concept and relationships.

Anatomy, Physiology, and Functions of the Nervous System

The nervous system is divided into two regions: the central nervous system (CNS), which consists of the brain and spinal cord, and the peripheral nervous system (PNS), which consists of the cranial nerves, the spinal nerves, and the autonomic nervous system.

Nerve Cells, Action Potentials, and Neurotransmitters

The highly integrated CNS and PNS consist of just two types of cells: neurons, which receive impulses and send them on to other cells, and neuroglia, which protect and nourish the neurons.

Neurons

Each neuron consists of a dendrite, a cell body, and an axon (Figure 41–1 ■). The dendrite is a short projection from the cell body that conducts impulses toward the cell body. Cell bodies, most of which are located within the CNS, are clustered in ganglia or nuclei. The cell bodies and dendrites comprise what is often called the gray matter of the CNS. The axon, a long process, conducts impulses away from the cell body. Many axons are covered with a myelin sheath, a white lipid substance. It is interrupted at intervals in unmyelinated areas called nodes of Ranvier, which allow movement of ions between the axon and the extracellular fluid. The myelin sheath serves to increase the speed of nerve impulse conduction in axons and is essential for the survival of larger nerve processes. Myelinated nerve fibers comprise the white matter of the brain and spinal cord.

Action Potentials

Action potentials are impulses (movements of electrical charge along an axon membrane) that allow neurons to communicate with other neurons and body cells. They are initiated by stimuli and propagated by the rapid movement of charged ions through the cell membrane. When a neuron reaches a certain level of stimulation, an electrical impulse is generated and conducted along the length of its axon. The movement of impulses to and from the CNS is made possible by afferent and efferent neurons. Afferent, or sensory, neurons have receptors in skin, muscles, and other organs and relay impulses to the CNS. Efferent, or motor, neurons transmit impulses from the CNS to cause some type of action.

Nerve impulses occur when a stimulus reaches a point great enough to generate a change in electrical charge across the cell membrane of a neuron. A neuron that is not involved in impulse conduction is in a resting, or polarized, state, in which the number of positive ions in the fluid outside of the cell membrane is greater than in the fluid within the cell. The chief regulators of membrane potential are sodium and potassium: Sodium is the major positive ion in the extracellular fluid, and potassium is the major positive ion in the intracellular fluid. In response to an electrical stimulus, the cell membrane becomes permeable

Figure 41–1 ■ A typical neuron.

to sodium, which moves into the cell. This changes the polarity of the cell membrane, and the neuron is said to depolarize. This event stimulates an action potential (a nerve impulse) to travel down the axon. When the charges and ions return to their original resting state, the neuron is repolarized. The events in an action potential are as follows:

1. Initially, sodium permeability increases. As the membrane is depolarized, sodium channels open and sodium rushes into the cell to a point of depolarization (the inside of the cell becomes less negative in comparison to the outside of the cell).
2. This is followed by a decrease in sodium permeability, lasting only about 1 millisecond. The sodium gates close and the sodium influx stops.
3. The final event is an increase in potassium permeability. The potassium gates open, potassium rushes out of the cell, and the cell interior becomes progressively less positive. The membrane potential moves back to its resting state and is repolarized.

The action potential is generated only at the point of the stimulus; but once generated, it is propagated along the entire length of the axon regardless of whether the stimulus continues. Conduction of the impulse is rapid in myelinated fibers, with the action potential "jumping" from one node of Ranvier to the next. The conduction of the impulse is slower in unmyelinated fibers.

Neurotransmitters

Neurotransmitters are the chemical messengers of the nervous system. When the action potential reaches the end of the axon at the presynaptic terminal, a neurotransmitter is released and travels across the synaptic cleft to bind with receptors in the postsynaptic neuron dendrite or cell body. The neurotransmitter may either be inhibitory or excitatory. The excitatory neurotransmitter is almost always acetylcholine (ACh), which is rapidly degraded by the enzyme acetylcholinesterase. Nerves that transmit impulses through the release of ACh are called *cholinergic*. Receptors that bind ACh are found in the viscera, skeletal muscle cells, and the adrenal medulla (where they stimulate the release of epinephrine). The effect of ACh binding may be either to stimulate or to inhibit a response.

Norepinephrine (NE), which may be either excitatory or inhibitory, is another major neurotransmitter. Nerves that transmit impulses through the release of NE are called *adrenergic*. Receptors that bind NE are found in the heart, lungs, kidneys, blood vessels, and all target organs stimulated by the sympathetic division except the heart. Adrenergic receptors are further divided into alpha and beta types. Alpha-adrenergic receptors help control such varied functions as arterial vasoconstriction and pupil dilation. Beta-adrenergic fibers may be either Beta$_1$- or Beta$_2$- receptors. Beta$_1$-receptors are found in the heart, where they regulate the rate and force of contraction. Beta$_2$-receptors are found in receptor cells of the lungs, arteries, liver, and uterus; they help regulate bronchial diameter, arterial diameter, and glycogenesis. Generally, binding of NE to alpha-receptors stimulates a response, whereas binding to beta-receptors inhibits a response.

Other neurotransmitters include gamma aminobutyric acid (GABA), which inhibits CNS function; dopamine, which may be inhibitory or excitatory and helps control fine movement and emotions; and serotonin, which is usually inhibitory and controls sleep, hunger, and behavior and also affects consciousness.

The Central Nervous System

The central nervous system (CNS) consists of the brain and spinal cord, highly evolved clusters of neurons that act to accept, interconnect, interpret, and generate a response to nerve impulses originating throughout the body.

The Brain

The brain is the control center of the nervous system and also generates thoughts, emotions, and speech. The brain has four major regions: the cerebrum, the diencephalon, the brainstem, and the cerebellum (Figure 41–2 ■). The general functions of these regions are summarized in Table 41–1.

The two hemispheres of the cerebrum account for almost 60% of brain weight. The surface of the cerebrum is folded into elevated ridges of tissue called gyri, which are separated by shallow grooves (sulci) and deep grooves (fissures). The longitudinal fissure separates the hemispheres, and the transverse fissure separates the cerebrum from the cerebellum. In addition, each cerebral hemisphere is divided into frontal, parietal, temporal, and occipital lobes (Figure 41–3 ■). The cerebral hemispheres are connected by a thick band of nerve fibers called the corpus callosum, which allows communication between the two hemispheres. Each hemisphere receives sensory and motor impulses from the opposite side of the body. Most people have a more highly developed left hemisphere, which is responsible for the control of language. The right hemisphere has greater control over nonverbal perceptual functions.

The cerebral cortex is the outer surface of the cerebrum. It consists of neuron cell bodies, unmyelinated fibers, neuroglia,

TABLE 41–1 General Functions of the Four Regions of the Brain

REGION	FUNCTIONS
Cerebrum	Interprets sensory input.
	Controls skeletal muscle activity.
	Processes intellect and emotions.
	Contains skills memory.
Diencephalon	Conducts sensory and motor impulses.
	Regulates autonomic nervous system.
	Regulates and produces hormones.
	Mediates emotional responses.
Brainstem	Serves as conduction pathway.
	Serves as site of decussation of tracts.
	Contains respiratory nuclei.
	Helps regulate skeletal muscles.
Cerebellum	Processes information.
	Provides information necessary for balance, posture, and coordinated muscle movement.

and blood vessels. The functions of the different lobes of the cerebrum and the specific areas of the cerebral cortex are shown in Figure 41–3 and listed in Table 41–2.

The diencephalon is embedded in the cerebrum superior to the brainstem. It consists of the thalamus, hypothalamus, and epithalamus. The thalamus begins to process sensory impulses before they ascend to the cerebral cortex. It serves as a sorting, processing, and relay station for input into the cortical region. The hypothalamus, located inferior to the thalamus, regulates temperature, water metabolism, appetite, emotional expressions, part of the sleep–wake cycle, and thirst. The epithalamus forms the dorsal part of the diencephalon and includes the pineal body, which is part of the endocrine system that affects growth and development.

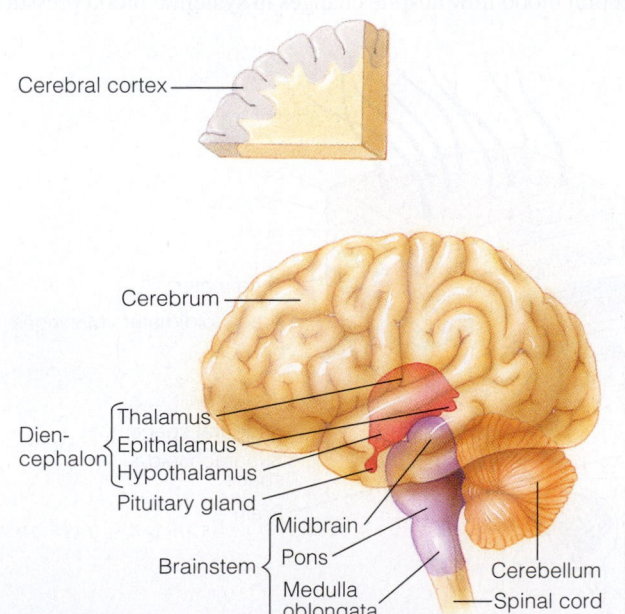

Figure 41–2 ■ The four major regions of the brain.

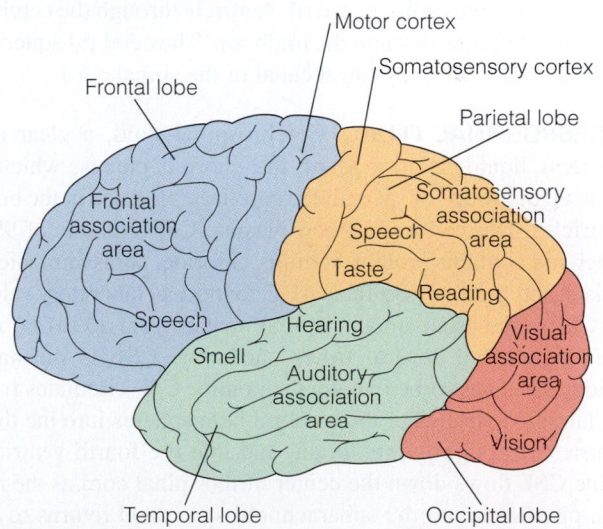

Figure 41–3 ■ Lobes of the cerebrum and functional areas of the cerebral cortex.

TABLE 41–2 Functions of Lobes of the Cerebrum and Areas of the Cerebral Cortex

AREA	FUNCTIONS
Parietal lobe (somatic sensory area of cerebral cortex)	Promotes recognition of pain, coldness, and light touch. The left side receives input from the right side of the body, and vice versa.
Occipital lobe	Receives and interprets visual stimuli.
Temporal lobe	Receives and interprets olfactory and auditory stimuli.
Frontal lobe	Controls movements of voluntary muscles.
Primary motor area	Facilitates voluntary movement of skeletal muscles.
Speech area	Promotes understanding of spoken and written words.
Motor speech area (Broca's area)	Promotes vocalization of words.

TABLE 41–3 Normal Laboratory Values for Cerebrospinal Fluid

COMPONENT	NORMAL VALUE
Appearance	Clear and colorless
pH	7.35
Specific gravity	1.007
WBCs	0–8 mm^3
Protein	15–45 mg/dL
Glucose	40–80 mg/dL
Chloride	118–132 mEq/L
Pressure	<200 mmH$_2$O

BRAINSTEM The brainstem consists of the midbrain, pons, and medulla oblongata. The midbrain is a center for auditory and visual reflexes and functions as a nerve pathway between the cerebral hemispheres and lower brain. The pons is located just below the midbrain. It consists mostly of fiber tracts, but it also contains nuclei that control respiration. The medulla oblongata, located at the base of the brainstem, is continuous with the superior portion of the spinal cord. Nuclei of the medulla oblongata play an important role in controlling cardiac rate, blood pressure, respiration, and swallowing.

The cerebellum is connected to the midbrain, pons, and medulla. Its functions include coordinating skeletal muscle activity, maintaining balance, and controlling fine movements.

VENTRICLES The brain contains four ventricles, which are chambers filled with cerebrospinal fluid (CSF). They are linked by ducts that allow the CSF to circulate. One lateral ventricle is located within each hemisphere. These communicate with the third ventricle through the foramen of Monro. The third ventricle communicates with the fourth ventricle through the cerebral aqueduct that runs through the midbrain. The cerebral aqueduct is continuous with the central canal of the spinal cord.

CEREBROSPINAL FLUID Cerebrospinal fluid, a clear and colorless liquid, is formed by the choroid plexus, which is made up of groups of specialized capillaries located in the brain ventricles. Derived from blood plasma, CSF consists of 99% water and contains protein, sodium, chloride, potassium, bicarbonate, and glucose (see Table 41–3 for normal laboratory values for CSF). The usual amount of CSF ranges from 80 to 200 mL and is replaced several times each day. CSF is normally produced and absorbed in equal amounts. CSF circulates from the lateral ventricles of the cerebral hemispheres into the third ventricle, through the midbrain, and into the fourth ventricle. Some CSF flows down the center of the spinal cord as the rest of it circulates into the subarachnoid space and returns to the blood through the arachnoid villi. CSF forms a cushion for the brain tissue, protects the brain and spinal cord from trauma, helps provide nourishment for the brain, and removes waste products of cerebrospinal cellular metabolism.

Meninges The brain and spinal cord are covered and protected by three connective tissue membranes called meninges. The meninges form divisions within the skull, enclose venous sinuses, and contain CSF. The meninges have three layers (Figure 41–4 ■). The outermost double layer, the dura mater, is attached to the inner surface of the skull. The middle layer is the arachnoid mater, which encloses the entire CNS and forms the subarachnoid space that contains CSF. The innermost layer, the pia mater, clings to the brain, spinal cord, and segmental nerves and is filled with small blood vessels.

CEREBRAL CIRCULATION AND THE BLOOD–BRAIN BARRIER The brain receives about 750 mL of blood each minute and uses 20% of the body's total oxygen uptake. The large amount of oxygen is necessary for metabolism of glucose, which is the brain's sole source of energy. Blood flow to the brain is mostly controlled by autoregulatory or local mechanisms that respond to the brain's metabolic needs. Autoregulation is the ability of the brain to maintain constant cerebral blood flow despite changes in systemic blood pressure.

Figure 41–4 ■ Anatomy of the meninges.

At least three metabolic factors affect cerebral blood flow: carbon dioxide, hydrogen ion, and oxygen concentrations. Of these, increased carbon dioxide is the major stimulus for vasodilatation with resultant increased cerebral blood flow.

The anterior part of the brain is supplied with blood by the two internal carotid arteries, and the posterior part of the brain is supplied with blood by the vertebral arteries. The internal carotid artery branches into further arteries: the ophthalmic, posterior communicating, anterior choroidal, anterior cerebral, and middle cerebral. The brainstem and cerebellum receive their blood supply from the basilar artery. These major arteries are connected by small anterior and posterior communicating arteries, which form a circle of connected blood vessels called the circle of Willis (Figure 41–5 ■). This circle serves as a protective device, providing alternative routes for brain tissues to receive their blood supply.

The capillaries in the brain have low permeability because the cells that compose their walls join at very tight junctions and are surrounded by a basement membrane and by the processes of astrocytes in the brain. This blood–brain barrier allows lipids, glucose, some amino acids, water, carbon dioxide, and oxygen to pass through it, thus maintaining a controlled environment. Substances such as urea, creatinine, proteins, some toxins, and most antibiotics cannot pass this barrier and enter brain tissue. However, injury to or infection of the brain may cause increased permeability of the blood–brain barrier, altering concentrations of proteins, water, and electrolytes.

THE LIMBIC SYSTEM AND THE RETICULAR FORMATION
The limbic system and the reticular formation are functional brain systems. These systems, made of networks of neurons, communicate across areas of the brain.

The limbic system consists of structures that form a ring of tissue in the medial side of each hemisphere, surrounding the upper portion of the brainstem and corpus callosum. The limbic system integrates and modulates input to make up the affective part of the brain, providing emotional and behavioral responses to environmental stimuli.

The reticular formation is located through the central core of the medulla oblongata, pons, and midbrain. This system has widespread connections throughout the brain and relays sensory input from all body systems to all levels of the brain. The reticular formation includes the reticular activating system (RAS). The RAS is a stimulating system for the cerebral cortex, keeping it alert and responsive to incoming sensory stimuli while filtering out repetitive or unwanted stimuli. The sleep center inhibits activity of the RAS, and drugs and alcohol may depress it. Other parts of the reticular formation include motor nuclei that help maintain muscle tone and coordinated movements through interconnections with spinal nerves, and the vasomotor and cardiovascular regulatory centers, which are part of autonomic regulation of the cardiovascular system.

The Spinal Cord
The spinal cord, protected by the vertebrae, the meninges, and CSF, extends from the medulla to the level of the first lumbar vertebra (Figure 41–6 ■). It serves as a center for conducting messages to and from the brain and as a reflex center. The spinal cord is about 17 inches (42 cm) long and 0.75 inch (1.8 cm) thick. The gray matter of the cord is on the inside, and the white matter is on the outside (the reverse of the arrangement in the brain).

The spinal cord is surrounded by 33 vertebrae: 7 cervical, 12 thoracic, 5 lumbar, 5 sacral, and 4 fused vertebrae that form the coccyx. Each vertebra consists of a body and a vertebral arch formed by projections from the body. This arch encloses a space called the vertebral foramen. The vertebral foramina of all the vertebrae form the vertebral canal through which the spinal cord passes. Intervertebral foramina are spaces between the vertebrae through which spinal nerve roots pass as they exit the vertebral column. Intervertebral disks are located between each of the movable vertebrae. Each disk is made of a thick capsule surrounding a gelatinous core called the nucleus pulposus. Ligaments that provide mobility and protection surround the vertebral column.

FUNCTIONS OF THE SPINAL CORD AND SPINAL ROOTS
Messages to and from the brain are conducted via ascending (sensory) pathways and descending (motor) pathways (Figure 41–7 ■). The major ascending tracts are the lateral and anterior spinothalamic tracts, which carry sensations for pain, temperature, and crude touch; and the posterior tracts, which carry sensations for fine touch, position, and vibration. The pyramidal tracts are descending tracts consisting of fibers that originate in the motor cortex of the brain and travel to the brainstem and then down the spinal cord. They mediate voluntary purposeful movements and stimulate certain muscular actions while inhibiting others. They also carry fibers that

Anterior

Frontal lobe

Optic chiasma

Middle cerebral artery
Internal carotid
Pituitary gland

Temporal lobe

Pons

Occipital lobe

Circle of Willis:
• Anterior cerebral artery
• Anterior communicating arteries
• Posterior communicating artery
• Posterior cerebral artery

Basilar artery

Vertebral artery
Cerebellum

Posterior

Figure 41–5 ■ Major arteries serving the brain and the Circle of Willis.

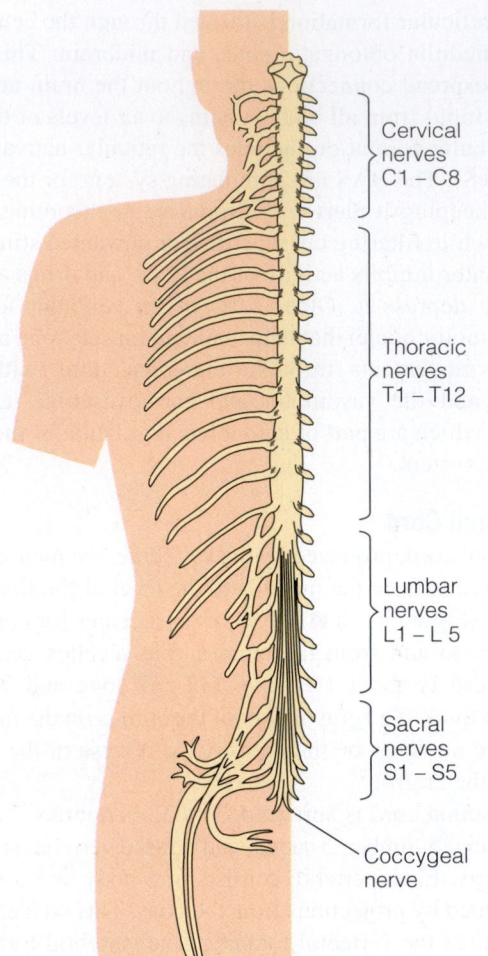

Figure 41–6 ■ Distribution of spinal nerves.

inhibit muscle tone. The extrapyramidal tracts include the pathways between the cerebral cortex, basal ganglia, brainstem, and spinal cord outside the pyramidal tract. They maintain muscle tone and gross body movements.

UPPER AND LOWER MOTOR NEURONS Upper motor neurons carry impulses from the cerebral cortex to the anterior gray column of the spinal cord. Damage to upper motor neurons results

in increased muscle tone, decreased muscle strength, decreased coordination, and hyperactive reflexes. Lower motor neurons begin in the anterior gray column of the spinal cord and end in the muscle. Damage to lower motor neurons results in decreased muscle tone, muscle atrophy, fasciculations, and loss of reflexes.

The Peripheral Nervous System

The peripheral nervous system (PNS) links the CNS with the rest of the body. It is responsible for receiving and transmitting information from and about the external environment. The PNS consists of nerves, ganglia (groups of nerve cells), and sensory receptors located outside—or peripheral to—the brain and spinal cord. The PNS is divided into a sensory (afferent) division and a motor (efferent) division. Most nerves of the PNS contain fibers for both divisions and all are classified regionally as either spinal nerves or cranial nerves.

Spinal Nerves

The 31 pairs of spinal nerves (see Figure 41–6) are named by their location: cervical 8 pairs, thoracic 12 pairs, lumbar 5 pairs, sacral 5 pairs, and coccygeal 1 pair. Spinal nerves exit the vertebral column through intervertebral foramina to travel to the body regions they serve. The spinal cord does not reach the end of the vertebral column; as a result, the lumbar and sacral nerve roots travel inferiorly through the vertebral canal for some distance before exiting the vertebral column through their associated intervertebral foramina. This collection of descending nerve roots is called the cauda equina.

Each spinal nerve contains both sensory and motor fibers. The sensory fibers are located in the dorsal root, and their cell bodies are located within the dorsal root ganglion. The motor fibers are located in the ventral root, and their cell bodies are located within the spinal cord. The dorsal and ventral roots merge outside the vertebral canal just past the dorsal root ganglion, forming a spinal nerve. Each spinal nerve further divides into branches called rami. An area of skin innervated by cutaneous branches of a single spinal nerve is called a dermatome. The dorsal roots of the spinal nerves carry sensations from these specific dermatomes. Dermatomes provide anatomic landmarks that are useful for locating neurologic lesions (Figure 41–8 ■).

Figure 41–7 ■ Ascending and descending tracts of the spinal cord.

Figure 41–8 ■ *A,* Anterior and *B,* posterior dermatomes of the body.

Cranial Nerves

Twelve pairs of cranial nerves originate in the forebrain and brainstem (Figure 41–9 ■). The vagus nerve extends into the ventral body cavity, but the other 11 pairs innervate only head and neck regions. Although most are mixed nerves, three pairs (olfactory, optic, and acoustic) are solely sensory. The cranial nerves and their related functions are listed in Table 41–4.

Reflexes

A reflex is a rapid, involuntary, predictable motor response to a stimulus. Reflexes are categorized as either somatic or autonomic. Somatic reflexes result in skeletal muscle contraction. Autonomic reflexes activate cardiac muscle, smooth muscle, and glands. A reflex occurs over a pathway called a reflex arc.

The essential components of a reflex arc are a receptor, a sensory neuron to carry afferent impulses to the CNS, an integration center in the spinal cord or brain, a motor neuron to carry efferent impulses, and an effector (the tissue that responds by contracting or secreting) (Figure 41–10 ■).

Somatic reflexes mediated by the spinal cord are called spinal reflexes. Many spinal reflexes occur without impulses traveling to and from the brain, with the cord serving as the integration center. Deep tendon reflexes (DTRs) occur in response to muscle contraction and cause muscle relaxation and lengthening. DTRs depend on intact sensory and motor nerve roots, functional synapses in the spinal cord, a functional neuromuscular junction, and a competent muscle. Thus, an abnormal DTR could indicate a variety of health problems, including a lesion of a spinal nerve. Flexor, or withdrawal,

reflexes are caused by actual or perceived painful stimuli and result in withdrawal of the part of the body that is threatened. Superficial responses result from gentle stimulation of the skin. These responses depend on functional upper motor pathways and an intact reflex arc.

The Autonomic Nervous System

The autonomic nervous system (ANS) is a division of the PNS that regulates the internal environment of the body. It is also called the general visceral motor system, because it consists of motor neurons that innervate the body's viscera. Whereas skeletal muscle activity and reflexes are regulated by a division of the PNS called the somatic nervous system, the ANS regulates the activity of cardiac muscle, smooth muscle, and glands. The ANS is primarily controlled by the reticular formation in the brainstem. Stimulation of centers in the medulla initiates reflexes that regulate cardiac rate, blood vessel diameter, and gastrointestinal function.

The ANS has sympathetic and parasympathetic divisions. Although fibers from both divisions affect the same structures, the actions of the two divisions are opposite in effect, and they serve to counterbalance each other. The major neurotransmitters for impulse transmission in the ANS are norepinephrine and acetylcholine.

Sympathetic Division

Norepinephrine is the primary neurotransmitter of the sympathetic division. The sympathetic division of the ANS prepares the body to handle situations that are perceived as harmful or

Figure 41–9 ■ Cranial nerves.

stressful and to participate in strenuous activity. Cell bodies for this division arise in the lateral horns of the spinal cord in the area from T1 through L2. The fibers separate after leaving the cord and form a chain of ganglia that extends from the neck to the pelvis. Long fibers then extend to the organs that are supplied by the sympathetic division. Stimulation of the sympathetic division can exert the following effects on target organs or tissues:

- Dilated pupils
- Inhibited secretions
- Copious production of sweat (**diaphoresis**)
- Increased rate and force of heartbeat
- Vasodilation of the coronary arteries
- Dilation of the bronchioles

Figure 41–10 ■ A typical reflex arc of a spinal nerve. In the two-neuron reflex arc, the stimulus is transferred from the sensory neuron directly to the motor neuron at the point of synapse in the spinal cord.

- Decreased digestion
- Increased release of glucose by the liver
- Decreased urine output
- Vasoconstriction of arteries
- Vasoconstriction of abdominal and skin blood vessels
- Increased blood clotting
- Increased metabolic rate
- Increased mental alertness

Parasympathetic Division

Acetylcholine is the primary neurotransmitter of the parasympathetic division. The parasympathetic division of the ANS operates during nonstressful situations. Cell bodies for this division are located in the brainstem (for the cranial nerves) and in the lateral gray matter of S2 through S4. Other than the fibers supplying the cranial nerves III, VII, IX, and X, the fibers are carried by the vagus nerve to body tissues, thoracic organs, and visceral organs. Stimulation of the parasympathetic division of the ANS produces the following effects:

- Constriction of pupils
- Stimulation of glandular secretions
- Decreased heart rate
- Vasoconstriction of coronary arteries
- Constriction of the bronchioles
- Increased peristalsis and secretion of gastrointestinal fluid

Assessing Neurologic Function

Structures and functions of the neurologic system are assessed by findings from diagnostic tests, a health assessment interview to collect subjective data, and a physical assessment to collect objective data.

TABLE 41–4 Cranial Nerves

NAME	FUNCTION
I Olfactory	Sense of smell
II Optic	Vision
III Oculomotor	Eyeball movement
	Raising of upper eyelid
	Constriction of pupil
	Proprioception
IV Trochlear	Eyeball movement
V Trigeminal	Sensation of the upper scalp, upper eyelid, nose, nasal cavity, cornea, and lacrimal gland
	Sensation of the palate, upper teeth, cheek, top lip, lower eyelid, and scalp Sensation of the tongue, lower teeth, chin, and temporal scalp
	Chewing
VI Abducens	Lateral movement of the eyeball
VII Facial	Movement of facial muscles
	Secretions of lacrimal, nasal, submandibular, and sublingual glands
	Sensation of taste
VIII Acoustic	Sense of equilibrium
	Sense of hearing
IX Glossopharyngeal	Swallowing
	Gag reflex
	Secretions of parotid salivary gland
	Sense of taste
	Touch, pressure, and pain from pharynx and posterior tongue
	Pressure from carotid arteries
	Receptors to regulate blood pressure
X Vagus	Swallowing
	Regulation of cardiac rate
	Regulation of respirations
	Digestion
	Sensation from thoracic and abdominal organs
	Proprioception
	Sense of taste
XI Accessory	Movement of head and neck
	Proprioception
XII Hypoglossal	Movement of tongue for speech and swallowing

Diagnostic Tests

The results of diagnostic tests of neurologic structure and function are used to support the diagnosis of a specific injury or disease, to provide information to identify or modify the appropriate medications or therapy used to treat the disease, and to help nurses monitor the patient's responses to treatment and nursing care interventions. Diagnostic tests to assess the structures and functions of the neurologic system are described in the table beginning on 1416 to 1418. More information is included in the discussion of specific injuries or diseases in ∞ Chapters 42, 43, and 44.

Regardless of the type of diagnostic test, the nurse is responsible for explaining the procedure and any special preparation needed, assessing for medication use that may affect the outcome of the tests, ensuring the consent form is signed (if necessary) supporting the patient during the examination as necessary, documenting the procedures as appropriate, and monitoring the results of the tests. The nurse is also responsible for post-procedure care and patient teaching for self-care at home.

Genetic Considerations

When conducting a health assessment interview and a physical assessment, it is important to consider genetic influences on the health of the adult. Several neurologic diseases that directly affect the nervous system have a genetic component; some are due to mutation of a single gene while others have a more complex method of inheritance. During the health assessment interview, ask about family members with health problems affecting neurologic structure or function. In addition, ask about a family history of problems with muscular coordination, Parkinson's disease, narcolepsy, tremor, seizures, Alzheimer's disease, multiple sclerosis, or amyotrophic lateral sclerosis (ALS). During the physical assessment, assess for any manifestations that might indicate a genetic disorder (see the box on page 1419). If data are found to indicate genetic risk factors or alterations, ask about genetic testing and refer for appropriate genetic counseling and evaluation. ∞ Chapter 8 provides further information about genetics in medical-surgical nursing.

Health Assessment Interview

A health assessment to determine problems with neurologic structure and/or function may be conducted during a health screening, may focus on a chief complaint (such as headaches), or may be part of a total health assessment. Health problems affecting the neurologic system may manifest as problems with musculoskeletal function and an assessment of both systems may be necessary. If the patient's level of consciousness is altered, the nurse may need to rely on family members for information. The patient's level of consciousness may be assessed by using the Glasgow Coma Scale (Table 41–5).

If the patient has problems with neurologic structure or function, analyze its onset, characteristics, course, severity, precipitating and relieving factors, and any associated symptoms, noting the time and circumstances. For example, ask the patient the following:

- Describe the location and intensity of the pain you have experienced in your left leg. Is it made worse by coughing, sneezing, or walking?
- When did you first notice that you were having numbness in your fingers?
- Describe the difficulty you have when you try to walk.

DIAGNOSTIC TESTS of the Neurologic System

NAME OF TEST	PURPOSE & DESCRIPTION	RELATED NURSING INTERVENTIONS
Carotid Duplex Study Transcranial Doppler Study	A carotid duplex study evaluates the velocity of blood flow through the carotid arteries and identifies occlusive disease. Sound waves produced by the blood flow are used to produce an image. A transcranial Doppler study follows the same procedure, but is used to evaluate intracranial blood vessels.	No special preparation is needed.
Cerebral Angiogram	A cerebral angiogram is the definitive diagnostic procedure for aneurysms, arteriovenous malformations, blood vessel patency and stenosis, thrombosis, vasospasm, aneurysm, and space-occupying lesions (such as tumors or hematomas). It may be performed either as part of a surgical procedure or with local anesthesia. In radiology, a contrast medium is injected and films are taken at various time intervals.	Tell the patient not to eat or drink fluids 8 hours prior to the procedure. Assess for history of allergy to iodine, seafood, or previous contrast dye; if present, notify physician. After the procedure, vital signs are monitored, and fluids are forced to clear the contrast medium. Bed rest is maintained for 12 to 24 hours. Monitor for manifestations of a transient ischemic attack (weakness or numbness in an extremity, confusion, slurred speech) and delayed allergic reaction to the contrast dye (itching, rash, tachycardia, dyspnea, hypotension).
Computed tomography (CT) scan—brain, spine	A CT scan of the brain is used to identify intracerebral hemorrhage, tumors, cysts, aneurysms, edema, ischemia, atrophy, and tissue necrosis. It may also be used to evaluate a shift in intracranial contents and differentiate type of stroke. CT scans of the spine are primarily done to assess bony abnormalities. The tests involve computer assisted x-rays of several levels of cross sections of the body part being examined; they may be done with or without contrast.	If a contrast dye is used, tell the patient to not to eat or drink liquids for 8 hours prior to the test, or if the test is in the afternoon to not eat or drink fluids after a liquid breakfast. Assess medications; if a iodinated contrast is used, oral hypoglycemic agents are contraindicated. Ask the patient to remove hairpins, clips, and jewelry, and dentures if contrast dye is used. Explain to the patient that when a brain scan is done, the head is positioned in a cradle and a strap is applied snugly around the head during the test (the test last from 5 to 10 minutes). After a scan with contrast, monitor for and report signs of a delayed allergic reaction, such as rash, itching, headache, or vomiting.
Electroencephalogram (EEG) Magnetoencephalogram (MEG)	An EEG is used to measure the electrical activity of the brain to diagnose brain disease and brain death. Electrodes are applied to the scalp with skin clips and a graphic picture is obtained (similar to an ECG of the heart). An MEG detects magnetic fields generated by activity of neurons and can identify the area of the brain affected by a stroke, brain disorders or trauma, or seizures.	Assess medications and tell the patient not to take prescribed medications or liquids that may stimulate or depress brain waves as ordered (usually for 24 to 48 hours) before the test. These include anticonvulsants, tranquilizers, depressants, and caffeine-containing foods and beverages (e.g., coffee, tea, colas, alcohol, and chocolate). Instruct the patient to wash his or her hair the night before the procedure, but to not use oil or hair spray on the hair. After the test, acetone may be used to remove the paste from the patient's head.
Electromyogram (EMG)	An EMG measures the electrical activity of skeletal muscles at rest and during contraction; and so is useful in diagnosing neuromuscular diseases. Needle electrodes are inserted into skeletal muscle (as on the legs) and electrical activity can be heard, viewed on an oscilloscope, and recorded on graph paper. Normally, there is no electrical activity at rest.	Tell patient not to drink fluids containing caffeine or to smoke for 3 hours before the test. Assess medications: If approved by healthcare provider, patient should not take medications such as muscle relaxants, anticholinergics, and cholinergics. If serum enzymes are ordered (such as SGOT, CPK, or LDH) the specimen should be drawn before an EMG or 5 to 10 days after the test.
Evoked Potentials	This test measures nerve conduction along pathways to evaluate evoked potential of muscle contractions. It is used to diagnose and evaluate neuromuscular diseases and identify nerve damage. Transcutaneous or percutaneous electrodes are applied to the skin and provide recordings.	No special preparation is needed.

DIAGNOSTIC TESTS of the Neurologic System (continued)

NAME OF TEST	PURPOSE & DESCRIPTION	RELATED NURSING INTERVENTIONS
Lumbar Puncture (LP)	An LP is used to measure CSF pressure and to obtain a sample of CSF to use in diagnosis of multiple sclerosis, or increased intracranial pressure from meningitis, subarachnoid hemorrhage, brain tumor, brain abscess, encephalitis, and viral infections. A needle is inserted in L3–L4 or L4–L5 and fluid is aspirated.	Ask the patient to void. Assess and document vital signs. Collect sterile lumbar puncture tray, an antiseptic solution, a local anesthetic, sterile gloves, and tape. Label the test tubes 1, 2, and 3. Place the patient on his/her side in the fetal position with back bowed, head flexed on the chest, and the knees drawn up to the abdomen. Assist the healthcare provider with the procedure. Following the LP, assess and document vital signs at specified intervals. Monitor for changes in neurologic status (fever, hypertension, irritability, lower extremity numbness or tingling, nonreactive pupils). Administer ordered analgesic for headache. Instruct the patient to lie flat in bed in the prone or supine position for 4 to 8 hours. Monitor the puncture site for leakage of cerebrospinal fluid or hematoma formation. Encourage increased intake of fluids (up to 3000 mL in 24 hours).
Magnetic Resonance Imaging (MRI) Functional MRI, Magnetic Resonance Angiography (MRA), Magnetic Resonance Spectroscopy (MRS)	An MRI is done to identify and monitor conditions of the brain and spinal cord, including stroke, tumors, trauma, seizures, and multiple sclerosis. It uses magnetic energy to provide images, and a Gadolinium contrast media may be used to enhance visualization. A functional MRI is done to evaluate metabolic or blood flow responses of the brain to specific tasks, such as activity and rest. An MRA can provide information about the blood vessels of the brain and identify vascular lesions. It uses the signals from blood vessels to reconstruct only those vessels with blood flow. An MRS uses a scanner to confirm the presence of Alzheimer's disease, determine the extent of head injury from trauma or stroke, and identify the causes of coma.	Assess for any metallic implants (such as clips on brain aneurysms, pacemaker, body piercing, tattoos, and shrapnel). If present, notify physician. Remove transdermal medication patches (both OTC and prescribed) unless otherwise ordered (FDA, 2009). Replace the patch following the procedure. Tell the patient to inform the staff about the patch when making the appointment and when completing the admission information. Ask if patient is pregnant; if so the test is not performed. Ask about claustrophobia, if a problem exists, request patient to ask the referring physician for a relaxing medication prior to the MRI. If the patient is very claustrophobic, obese, or confused, an open MRI may be used.
Myelogram	A myelogram is used to identify lesions of the spinal cord, such as tumors or herniated intervertebral disk. A lumbar puncture is done, a contrast medium is injected into the subarachnoid space, and x-rays are taken.	Instruct the patient to drink additional fluids the day before the test, and then to stop all food and fluids for 4 hours prior to the test. Assess medications: antipsychotics, antidepressants, and anticoagulants may be withheld for several days before the procedure, depending on physician orders. Tell the patient not to smoke the day before the test. Assess for history of allergy to iodine, seafood, or previous contrast dye; if present, notify physician. Ask the patient to void immediately before the test. After the procedure, position the patient in a supine position with the head slightly elevated for several hours. Encourage oral fluid intake. Monitor for and notify the physician of a fever, excessive nausea and vomiting, a severe headache, or a stiff neck. Take and record vital signs as specified. Monitor lumbar insertion site for CSF leakage or hematoma. Monitor neurologic status and ensure patient voids within 8 hours. Encourage increased oral fluids. Administer prescribed analgesic for headache.

(continued)

DIAGNOSTIC TESTS of the Neurologic System (continued)

NAME OF TEST	PURPOSE & DESCRIPTION	RELATED NURSING INTERVENTIONS
Positron Emission Tomography (PET) Single-Photon Emission Computed Tomography (SPECT)	When used to study the brain, a PET can assess normal brain function and cerebral blood flow and volume; it can differentiate different types of dementia; and it can identify stages of brain tumors. A substance containing a radionuclide is given by gas or by injection and cross sections of tissue are detected and displayed by computer. A SPECT is similar to a PET, but uses different substances. It can be used to diagnose strokes, brain tumors, and seizure disorders.	Tell the patient not to drink coffee or alcohol or smoke for 24 hours before the test. Assess glucose levels pretest. Post-test, encourage oral fluids to facilitate excretion of the radioactive substance.
X-rays of skull and spine	Standard x-rays of the skull and spine are done to identify fractures, displacement of vertebrae, spinal curves, and tissue displacement (as by tumors).	No special preparation is needed.

Questions about present health status include information about numbness, tingling sensations, tremors, problems with coordination or balance, or loss of movement in any part of the body. Ask the patient about difficulty with speaking, seeing, hearing, tasting, or detecting odors. In addition, elicit information about memory, feeling state (such as anxiety or depression), recent changes in sleep patterns, ability to perform self-care and activities of daily living, sexual activity, and weight. If the patient is taking prescribed medications, over-the-counter medications, or herbal supplements, ask about the type and purpose, as well as the frequency and duration of use.

Ask about any past history of seizures, fainting, dizziness, headaches, and any trauma, tumors, or surgery of the brain,

GENETIC CONSIDERATIONS
Examples of Neurologic Disorders

- One risk factor for Parkinson's disease is a positive family history of the disease. This neurodegenerative disease is manifested by tremor, muscular stiffness, and difficulty with balance and walking.
- Although multiple sclerosis (MS) is not directly inherited, genetic factors may influence a predisposition to MS within families as well as the severity and course of the disease.
- Narcolepsy, a sleep disorder, has a familial connection.
- Huntington's disease (HD) is an inherited degenerative disorder that results in degeneration of neurons in certain areas of the brain. A child of a parent with HD has a 50-50 chance of inheriting the gene for the disease.
- Friedreich's ataxia is a rare inherited disease that causes a progressive loss of voluntary muscle coordination and enlargement of the heart.
- Essential tremor, as a primary disorder, affects as many as 3 to 4 million people. In more than half of cases, essential tremor is inherited as an autosomal dominant trait, meaning that children of an individual with the disease have a 50% chance of also developing the disorder.
- Epilepsy is one of the most common neurologic diseases, characterized by abnormal cell firing in the brain that causes recurring seizures. A genetic predisposition is found in many cases.
- Charcot-Marie-Tooth syndrome is the most common inherited peripheral neuropathy in the world, characterized by a slowly progressive degeneration of the muscles of the foot, lower leg, hand, and forearm.
- Alzheimer's disease (AD) is a leading cause of death in adults, increasing in incidence with age and more common in women. AD tends to run in families, with mutations in four genes believed to be responsible for the disease.
- Amyotrophic lateral sclerosis (ALS) is a neurologic disease that causes progressive degeneration of motor neurons in the brain and spinal cord, resulting in paralysis and death. Chromosome abnormalities have been linked to familial ALS.
- Although Tay-Sachs disease is most often considered a disease of children, there is a chronic adult form that causes neuron dysfunction and psychosis.

NURSING CARE OF THE OLDER ADULT   **Age-Related Changes in the Neurologic System**

AGE-RELATED CHANGE	SIGNIFICANCE
■ ◆ number of brain cells, cerebral blood flow, and metabolism.	Delayed response to multiple stimuli and slower reflexes; may need additional time to process and respond to verbal stimuli.
■ Slower nerve conduction velocity.	
■ Slower retrieval of information from long-term memory.	There is some age-related forgetfulness, which can be improved by using memory aids such as making lists.
■ Slower response to changes in balance.	May contribute to increased risk for falls.
■ May exhibit less readiness to learn and depend on prior experiences to solve problems.	Learning new skills or knowledge is improved when they are related to previously learned information and when limits are set on times for learning (for example, no more than 30 minutes at one time).
■ Is more easily distracted and has a decrease in the ability to maintain attention.	

spinal cord, or nerves. Discuss illnesses that may cause neurologic manifestations, including cardiac disease, strokes, pernicious anemia, sinus infections, liver disease, and/or renal failure. Also ask the patient about family history of neurologic health problems, diabetes mellitus, hypertension, seizures, or mental health problems.

Question the patient about occupational hazards, such as exposure to toxic chemicals or materials, use of protective headgear, and the amount of time spent performing repetitive motions (e.g., data entry and assembly). Ask questions about self-care to assess the patient's diet and use of tobacco, drugs, or alcohol, and ask whether the patient wears a helmet when riding a bike or motorcycle or participating in contact sports or if seat belts are used when driving a vehicle.

Interview questions categorized by functional health patterns are listed in the Functional Health Pattern Interview table on page 1420.

Physical Assessment

Physical assessment begins when the nurse first meets the patient and makes an overall evaluation of the patient's mental and physical status. The mental status examination is conducted with both the nurse and the patient seated. The rest of the neurologic examination may be performed with the patient either sitting or standing. A thorough neurologic examination is discussed here, but in most instances, the nurse will conduct a focused assessment specific to the patient's health status.

The neurologic system is assessed through inspection, palpation, and percussion (with a reflex hammer). When conducting the mental status and cognitive portions of the examination, be aware that fatigue or illness may alter findings. Provide rest periods for the patient as needed. When interpreting findings, consider the patient's age, educational background, and cultural orientation. Normal age-related findings for the older adult are summarized in the Nursing Care of the Older Adult box.

The assessment should take place in a private, comfortable setting. Ask the patient to remove outer clothing, shoes, and stockings. Provide a gown for the patient to wear. It is important to explain that the neurologic examination is lengthy and may consist of questions and requests that seem strange to the patient. Explain the rationale for each part of the examination.

A brief version of this physical assessment, often referred to as a *neuro check*, may be performed in a shorter time period when a patient requires frequent ongoing assessments of neurologic status (Box 41–1).

BOX 41–1 Abbreviated Neurologic Assessment (Neuro Check)

1. Assess level of consciousness (response to auditory and/or tactile stimulus).
2. Obtain vital signs (BP, P, R).
3. Check pupillary response to light.
4. Assess strength of hand grip and movement of extremities bilaterally.
5. Determine ability to sense touch/pain in extremities.

FUNCTIONAL HEALTH PATTERN INTERVIEW   The Neurologic System

Functional Health Pattern	Interview Questions and Leading Statements
Health Perception–Health Management	■ Have you ever had a surgery, injury, or illness of the neurologic system (for example, head or spine), such as seizures, stroke, tumor, or meningitis? If so, describe the problem and how it was treated. ■ Do you have high blood pressure? If so, how is it treated? ■ Have you ever had problems with the ability to move body parts? Describe. ■ Would you say you think clearly? If not, how and when did the change occur? ■ Are you having any problems with the ability to see, hear, taste, or smell? Explain. ■ Have you ever had any diagnostic tests for a neurologic problem, such as an MRI or spinal tap? If so, what were the results? ■ Do you take medications for seizures, headaches, or other neurologic problems? If so, what are they and how often do you take them? ■ Do you now or have you ever smoked, used street drugs, or drank alcohol? If so, what type, how much, and for how long? ■ Where were you born and raised as a child?
Nutritional-Metabolic	■ Describe your usual food and fluid intake for a 24-hour period. ■ Have you noticed any problems with chewing or swallowing your food? ■ Do you have trouble with coughing when you eat or drink?
Elimination	■ Has there been any change in your urinary or bowel elimination? If so, describe the change. ■ Do you use laxatives, suppositories, or enemas to assist with bowel elimination? If so, what type and how often? ■ Are you able to go to the bathroom without assistance? If not, describe your usual routine.
Activity-Exercise	■ Describe your usual activities in a 24-hour period. ■ Do you have any problems with balance, coordination, or walking? Do you use any assistive device when you walk, such as a cane or walker? ■ Have you noticed any weakness in your arms or legs? If so, describe. ■ Are you able to move all of your body parts? If not, explain. ■ Do you trip or fall easily? ■ Have you experienced any shakiness or tremors? Where? ■ If you have seizures, what type do you have? Can you tell when they are going to happen? Does anything specific make you have a seizure? How do you feel after the seizure is over?
Sleep-Rest	■ Does this health problem interfere with your ability to sleep and rest? If so, how? ■ Do you take any medication to help you sleep? If so, what? ■ Describe your energy level. Do rest and sleep restore your energy?
Cognitive-Perceptual	■ Describe any headaches you experience, including frequency, type, location, and precipitating/relieving factors. ■ Do you ever feel dizzy or have you fainted? Do you ever feel the room is spinning? Explain. ■ Do you ever experience any numbness, burning, or tingling sensations? If so, where and when? ■ Do you have any visual problems, such as double vision, blurring, or blind spots? ■ Do you have any problems with hearing? Explain. ■ Has there been any change in your ability to taste or smell? If so, explain. ■ Do you have any difficulty remembering things? If so, describe what you do.
Self-Perception-Self-Concept	■ How does having this condition make you feel about yourself?
Role-Relationships	■ How has having this condition affected your relationships with others? ■ Has having this condition interfered with your ability to work? Explain. ■ Has anyone in your family had problems with neurologic disease? Explain.
Sexuality-Reproductive	■ Has this condition interfered with your usual sexual activity?
Coping-Stress-Tolerance	■ Has having this condition created stress for you? If so, does your health problem seem to be more difficult when you are stressed? ■ Have you experienced any kind of stress that makes the condition worse? Explain. ■ Describe what you do when you feel stressed.
Value-Belief	■ Describe how specific relationships or activities help you cope with this problem. ■ Describe specific cultural beliefs or practices that affect how you care for and feel about this problem. ■ Is there anything interfering with your spiritual beliefs, needs, or practices during your illness? What can I or another caregiver do to help you with your spiritual needs? ■ Are there any specific treatments that you would not use to treat this problem?

Neurologic Assessments

Technique/Normal Findings	Abnormal Findings

Mental Status Assessment

Assess appearance, including dress, hygiene, grooming, gait, and posture. *The patient should be appropriately dressed and clean, with normal gait and posture.*

- Unilateral neglect (inattention to one side of body) may occur with some strokes. Poor hygiene and grooming may be seen in patients with dementing disorders.
- Abnormal gait and posture may be seen in transient ischemic attacks (TIAs), strokes, and Parkinson's disease.

Assess behavior, including actions and affect, content and quality of speech, and level of consciousness (LOC). Use the Glasgow Coma Scale (see Table 41–5) to document findings. *A score of 15 on the Glasgow Coma Scale indicates the patient is alert and oriented.*

- Emotional swings or changes in personality may be observed in patients who have had a stroke.
- The face appears masklike (very little expressive movement of facial muscles) in patients with Parkinson's disease.
- Apathy is seen in dementing disorders.
- **Aphasia** (defective or absent language function) may occur in TIAs and strokes. Aphasias are seen with damage to the left cerebral cortex. Aphasias are more often seen with strokes of the left hemisphere than the right hemisphere.
- **Dysphonia** (change in the tone of the voice) is common in strokes. Dysphonia is seen with paralysis of the vocal cords (cranial nerve X).
- **Dysarthria** (difficulty speaking) is seen with lesions of upper and lower motor neurons, the cerebellum, and the extrapyramidal tract.
- Damage to the brainstem and/or cerebral cortex may alter LOC.
- Drowsiness and decreased LOC may be associated with brain trauma, infections, TIAs, stroke, and brain tumors.
- Level of consciousness, ranging from confusion to coma, is usually altered with a stroke.

TABLE 41–5 Glasgow Coma Scale

ASSESSMENT	RESPONSE	SCORE
Eyes open (Record C if eyes are closed by swelling.)	Spontaneously	4
	To speech	3
	To pain	2
	No response	1
Best motor response (Record best upper arm response.)	Obeys commands	6
	Localizes pain	5
	Flexion-withdrawal	4
	Abnormal flexion	3
	Abnormal extension	2
	No response	1
Best verbal response (Record T if an endotracheal or tracheostomy tube is in place.)	Oriented	5
	Confused	4
	Inappropriate words	3
	Incomprehensible sounds	2
	No response	1
Total Score:		*

*A higher score indicates a higher level of functioning.

Technique/Normal Findings	Abnormal Findings

Assess cognitive function.

Note orientation to time, place, and person.

Note attention span and recent and remote memory.

Ask the patient to do the following:
1. Repeat five to seven numbers.
2. Recall three items after 5 minutes.
3. Recall his or her address, break-fast, or birthday.

Assess thought processes (both content and perceptions) by noting responses to questions.

Note ability to understand what is said and to express thoughts.

Note ability to make logical and safe judgments. *The patient should be oriented to time, place, and person; demonstrate attention and ability to remember recent and past events; respond appropriately to questions; and be able to make judgments.*

- Disorientation to time and place may occur in patients with stroke of the right cerebral hemisphere.
- Memory deficits are often seen in patients with a stroke.
- Perceptual deficits may be seen in strokes. These same deficits may occur following brain trauma and in dementing disorders.
- Impaired cognition is often noted with strokes, cerebral trauma, and brain tumors.

Cranial Nerve Assessments

Test CN I (olfactory).

Note patient's ability to smell scents (e.g., soap, coffee) with each nostril. This test is usually done only if a problem with the ability to smell is reported. *Sense of smell should be equal in both nostrils.*

- **Anosmia** (an inability to smell) may be seen with lesions of the frontal lobe and may also occur with impaired blood flow to the middle cerebral artery.

Test CN II (optic).

Assess vision in each eye with Snellen chart (∞ see Chapter 45 for guidelines). *Based on previous ability to see and use of visual aids, patient should be able to see with both eyes.*

- Blindness in one eye may be seen with strokes or with TIAs. Impaired vision or blindness in one side of both eyes (homonymous hemianopia) is associated with stroke.
- Impaired vision may be seen with strokes and brain tumors.
- Blindness or double vision may be noted with stroke and TIAs.
- Diplopia (double vision) may occur in multiple sclerosis.

Test CN III, IV, and VI (oculomotor, trochlear, and abducens).

Assess extraocular movements by asking the patient to follow your finger as you write an *H* in the air (∞ see Chapter 45).

Assess PERRL ("pupils equally round and reactive to light") by covering one eye at a time and shining a bright light directly into the uncovered eye. (use a penlight or the oph-thalmoscope.) ∞ See Chapter 45 for more detailed assessment guidelines. *Extraocular movements should be present bilaterally, and pupils should be equally round and reactive to light.*

- **Nystagmus** (involuntary eye movement) may be seen with strokes.
- Constricted pupils are associated with impaired blood flow from a stroke, or medications/drug use.

Assess for **ptosis** (drooping eyelids). *Eyelids should not droop.*

- Ptosis (also called Horner syndrome) occurs with strokes, myasthenia gravis, and palsy of CN III.

Technique/Normal Findings	Abnormal Findings
Test CN V (trigeminal). Assess ability to feel light, dull, and sharp sensations on the face. With the patient's eyes closed, check whether sensation is the same on both sides of the face. Stroke the cheek with a wisp of cotton for light touch, with a closed safety pin for dull touch, and with a tongue depressor for sharp touch. If the sharp point of a safety pin is used to assess sharp touch, be sure to avoid scratching the surface of the skin, and discard the pin after it is used. Assess the corneal reflex by touching the corneal surface with a wisp of cotton. The reflex may be absent or decreased in patients who wear contact lenses. *Ability to feel light, dull, and sharp sensations should be intact. Normally the patient blinks.*	■ Changes in facial sensations are noted with impaired blood flow to the carotid artery. ■ Decreased sensations to the face and cornea on the same side of the body, as well as numbness of the lip and mouth, occur with strokes. ■ Loss of facial sensation or contraction of the masseter and temporal muscles is seen with lesions of CN V. ■ Severe facial pain is seen with trigeminal neuralgia (tic douloureux). ■ The corneal reflex may be impaired with lesions of CN V or VII.
Test CN VII (facial). Assess ability to taste sweet, sour, and salt on the anterior two-thirds of the tongue by asking the patient to stick out the tongue and applying a salty, sweet, or sour substance. Assess ability to frown, show teeth, blow out cheeks, raise eyebrows, smile, and close eyes tightly. *Patient should be able to taste sweet, sour, and salt should be intact. Should be able to frown, show teeth, blow out cheeks, raise eyebrows, smile, and close eyes tightly. Muscle movement should be equal bilaterally.*	■ Loss of ability to taste may occur with brain tumors or with nerve impairment. ■ Asymmetry or decreased movement of facial muscles is noted with lesions of the upper and lower motor neurons. ■ Paralysis of the lower motor neurons from injury to CN VII results in the inability to close eyes, a flat nasolabial fold, paralysis of lower face, and inability to wrinkle forehead. ■ Paralysis of the upper motor neurons from a stroke results in weakness of eyelids and paralysis of lower face. ■ Pain, paralysis, and sagging of facial muscles is seen on the affected side in Bell's palsy.
Test CN VIII (acoustic). Assess ability to hear the ticking of a watch and whispered and spoken words (∞ see Chapter 45). *Patient should be able to hear with both ears.*	■ Decreased hearing or deafness may occur with strokes and/or tumors of CN VIII.
Test CN IX and X (glossopharyngeal and vagus). If gag reflex is intact, observe patient swallowing a small drink of water. Observe for a symmetrical rise of the soft palate and uvula as the patient says "ah." Assess gag reflex by touching back of patient's throat with tongue depressor. *Patient should have intact gag reflex.* Assess ability to taste salty, sweet, and sour substances on the posterior third of the tongue (see previous description). *Patient should be able to swallow without difficulty, have symmetrical rise of the soft palate, and taste appropriately.*	■ **Dysphagia** (difficulty swallowing) is common with impaired blood flow to the brain. ■ Unilateral loss of the gag reflex occurs with lesions of CN IX and X.

Technique/Normal Findings	**Abnormal Findings**
Test CN XI (spinal accessory). Assess the patient's ability to shrug the shoulders and turn head against resistance: Ask the patient to turn the head to one side against the resistance of your hand; ask the patient to shrug the shoulders while you exert downward pressure. Observe symmetry, strength, and size of muscles. *Patient should be able to shrug shoulders and turn head against resistance.*	■ Muscle weakness is noted with lower motor neuron disease. Contralateral hemiparesis is seen with strokes.
Test CN XII (hypoglossal). Assess the patient's ability to stick out the tongue and move the tongue from side to side against resistance of a tongue depressor. *Patient should be able to stick out tongue, and move it from side to side against resistance.*	■ Atrophy and **fasciculations** (twitches) of the tongue are seen in lower motor neuron disease. The tongue may deviate toward involved side of the body.
Sensory Function Assessments	
Assess abilty to feel touch. Touch both sides of various parts of the body (the chest, abdomen, arms, and legs) with one or more of the following: ■ Cotton wisp ■ Sharp object ■ Dull object ■ Vibrating tuning fork placed on bony prominences *Patient can differentiate between soft and sharp, and can feel vibrations appropriately.*	■ Decreased sensation of pain occurs with injury to the spinothalamic tract. ■ Decreased vibratory sensations are seen with injuries to the posterior column tract. ■ Transient numbness of face, arm, or hand is seen with TIAs. ■ Sensory loss on one side of the body is seen with lesions of higher pathways to the spinal cord. ■ Bilateral sensory loss is seen in polyneuropathy (a disease in which multiple peripheral nerves are affected, such as Guillain-Barré syndrome or diabetes mellitus). Sensations are impaired with strokes, brain tumors, and spinal cord trauma or compression.
Assess sense of position (**kinesthesia**). Move the patient's finger or big toe up or down. Ask the patient to describe the movement. *Patient can accurately describe position of finger or toe when moved up or down.*	■ Lesions of the posterior column of the spinal cord may affect sense of position.
Assess ability to discriminate fine touch. Ask the patient to identify the following: 1. Object in hand, such as a coin or key (tests stereognosis) 2. Number written on hand (tests graphesthesia) (Figure 41–11 ■) 3. Two points of simultaneous pinpricks on the hand (tests two-point discrimination) (Figure 41–12 ■) 4. Where he or she is being touched (tests localization) 5. How many sensations are felt when touched simultaneously on both sides of the body (tests extinction) *Patient can identify and discriminate fine touch.*	■ Inability to discriminate fine touch (stereognosis, graphesthesia, two points, point localization, and extinction) may occur with injury to the posterior columns or sensory cortex.

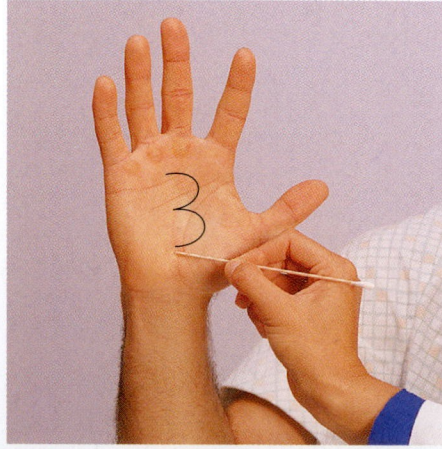

Figure 41–11 ■ Testing graphesthesia.

Figure 41–12 ■ Testing two-point discrimination.

6.

7.

8.

| **Technique/Normal Findings** | **Abnormal Findings** |

Motor Function Assessments

Assess bilateral symmetry and size of muscles.

Assess for **tremors** (rhythmic movements) and fasciculations (irregular movements). Observe movements as patient is at rest (not making a purposeful movement) and with activity (making a purposeful movement, such as reaching for a glass of water). *Muscles are bilaterally symmetrical and of equal size. Tremors or fasciculations are not present.*

- Atrophy of muscles is seen with disease of the lower motor neurons.
- Tremors that occur with activity are seen in multiple sclerosis and diseases of the cerebellar system.
- Tremors that occur at rest and disappear with movement are common in Parkinson's disease.
- Fasciculations occur in disease or trauma to the lower motor neurons, as a side effect of medications, in fever, in sodium deficiency, and in uremia.

Assess muscle tone. *Muscle tone is appropriate.*

- Muscle tone is decreased (**flaccidity**) in disease or trauma of the lower motor neurons and early stroke.
- Muscle tone is increased (**spasticity**) in disease of the corticospinal motor tract.
- Muscles are rigid in disease of the extrapyramidal motor tract.
- Muscles move in small, regular jerky movements (cogwheel rigidity) in Parkinson's disease.

Assess bilateral muscle strength and movement.

Ask the patient to do the following:
1. Squeeze your hands.
2. Push feet against the resistance of your hands.
3. Raise both legs off the bed.

∞ *See Chapter 38 for a scale to grade muscle strength. Muscle strength and movement are bilaterally equal and strong.*

- Weakness of the arms, legs, or hands is often seen with TIAs.
- Hemiplegia (paralysis of one-half of the body vertically) is noted with strokes.
- Flaccid paralysis is noted with strokes.
- Paralysis or decreased movement is seen in multiple sclerosis and myasthenia gravis.
- There is total loss of motor function below the level of injury in complete spinal cord transection and in injuries to the anterior portion of the spinal cord.
- Spasticity of muscles may occur as a result of incomplete spinal cord injuries.

Cerebellar Function Assessments

Assess the gait. Ask the patient to walk normally, then in a heel-to-toe fashion, then on toes, and finally on heels. *Patient has appropriate gait, and can walk heel-to-toe, on toes, and on heels.*

Perform Romberg's test: Ask the patient to stand with the feet together and eyes closed. (Stand close to patient to prevent falling). *There should be minimal swaying for up to 20 seconds.*

- **Ataxia** is a lack of coordination and a clumsiness of movements, with staggering, wide-based, and unbalanced gait. Ataxia is often seen with strokes and cerebellar tumors. Swaying and falling are seen in cerebellar ataxia. Inability to walk on toes, then heels, may indicate disease of the upper motor neurons.
- Spastic hemiparesis is often associated with strokes or upper motor neuron disease. The patient walks with one leg stiffly dragging while the other leg circles out and forward. One arm is held flexed and close to the side.
- Steppage gait is noted with disease of the lower motor neurons. The patient drags or lifts the foot high, then slaps the foot onto the floor. The patient cannot walk on the heels.
- Sensory ataxia may be associated with polyneuropathy or damage to the posterior columns. The patient walks on the heels before bringing down the toes and the feet are held wide apart. Gait worsens with the eyes closed.
- Parkinsonian gait is often seen in Parkinson's disease. The patient stoops over while walking and shuffles the feet. The arms are held close to the side.
- A positive Romberg's test may be seen in cerebellar ataxia.

Assess coordination.

Observe ability to pat knees, alternating front and back of hands and increasing speed. Observe ability to touch each finger of one hand to the thumb. Observe ability to touch the nose, then one of your fingers, then the nose again.

Observe ability to run each heel down each shin, while in a supine position (Figure 41–13 ■). *Patient demonstrates coordinated movements.*

- Ataxic movements are apparent in cerebellar disease.

Figure 41–13 ■ Heel-to-shin test.

who are unresponsive to medical management, who have a unilateral focus, and who have impaired quality of life from seizures. The goal of surgery is to reduce the patient's uncontrollable seizures. General postoperative care for the patient with intracranial surgery follows the nursing management guidelines outlined later in the chapter. Another surgical option in clinical trials, the Responsive Neurostimulator System, uses electrodes implanted in the brain that are stimulated by low-level electrical current to suppress a seizure.

Vagal Nerve Stimulation Therapy

This therapy is designed to send regular small pulses of electrical energy to the brain via the vagus nerve. A flat, round battery (about the size of a silver dollar) is implanted in the chest wall, and electrodes are threaded under the skin and wound around the vagus nerve in the neck. The battery is programmed to deliver a few seconds of electrical energy every few seconds. The therapy does not stop the seizures, but rather reduces the number and improves the patient's quality of life.

✏ Nursing Care

Nursing care is described for patients with a seizure disorder, but the care of the person during a seizure is the same no matter the cause. See the Case Study & Nursing Care Plan for a patient with seizures on page 1448.

Health Promotion

Health promotion activities for the patient with seizures focus on teaching to reduce the incidence of seizure activity and to promote safety. Stress the following:

- Stress the importance of follow-up care, of keeping medical appointments, and of continuing to take AEDs as prescribed even when no seizures are experienced.

- Review any state and local laws that apply to people with seizure disorders. Driving a motor vehicle is usually prohibited for 6 months to 2 years after a seizure episode. Usually, a driver's license can be reinstated or obtained after a seizure-free period and a letter from the healthcare provider.
- Know drug interactions with other prescribed drugs, over-the-counter (OTC) drugs, street drugs, and alcohol.
- Teach family members first aid for a seizure: Cushion the head, loosen anything tight around the neck, turn on the side, do not hold down.
- Teach family members to call for medical assistance if the seizures lasts for more than 5 minutes, recovery is slow, a second seizure occurs, there is difficulty breathing after recovery, or if there are signs of injury (such as bleeding from the mouth).

Assessment

Collect the following data through the health history and physical examination:

- *Health history:* Past seizures; age when the first seizure occurred, most recent seizure, factors precipitating a seizure, any warning signs (aura), prophylactic anticonvulsant therapy, and specific concerns the patient may have about the seizures.
- *Physical assessment:* Important data used in determining an accurate diagnosis describes manifestations obtained from nursing assessments before, during, and after a seizure. (Table 42–3 lists nursing assessments with rationale.)

Nursing Diagnoses and Interventions

Nursing care of patients with seizures focuses on providing care during and immediately after the seizure and on patient/family teaching. The patient with seizures has a wide variety of responses to actual or potential changes in health status; interventions discussed in this section focus on facilitating physical and psychologic comfort and safety.

TABLE 42–3 Nursing Assessments Before, During, and After a Seizure

ASSESSMENT	RATIONALE
What was the patient's level of consciousness? If consciousness was lost, at what point?	Indicates area of brain involved and type of seizure.
What was the patient doing just before the attack?	May suggest precipitating factors.
In what part of the body did the seizure start?	May indicate the site of seizure activity in the brain tissue; for example, if jerking movements were first observed in the right hand, the seizure focus may be in the left motor cortex.
Was there an epileptic cry?	Usually indicates the tonic stage of a generalized tonic-clonic seizure.
Were any automatisms such as eyelid fluttering, chewing, lip smacking, or swallowing observed?	Often seen in complex, partial, and absence seizures.
How long did movements last? Did the location or character change (tonic to clonic)? Did movements involve both sides of the body or just one?	Indicates areas in which focal activity originated.
Did the head and/or eyes turn to one side and, if so, which side?	Helps localize the focus of the seizure. During the seizure, the head and eyes typically will turn away from the side of the epileptogenic focus.
Were there changes in pupillary reactions?	Indicates involvement of the autonomic nervous system.
If the patient fell, was the head hit?	Skull x-ray studies may be needed to rule out subdural hematoma or fracture.
Was there foaming or frothing from the mouth?	Usually indicates a tonic-clonic seizure.
Was there urinary or bowel incontinence?	Usually indicates a tonic-clonic seizure.

EVIDENCE FOR NURSING CARE The Patient with Seizures

Selected resources that nurses may find helpful when planning evidence-based nursing care follow.

- Roberts, R., Farrugia, M. E., Bevan, S., Brodie, M., Caldwell, E., et al. (2010). (1) Diagnosis and management of epilepsy in adults. A national clinical guideline. (2) Diagnosis and management of epilepsy in adults. Update to printed guideline. *National Guideline Clearinghouse.* Retrieved from http://www.guideline.gov/summary/summary.aspx?doc_id=5694&nbr=003832&string=seizures
- Larrson, R. L., & Larsson, S. B. (2009). Epilepsy patients' conceptions of epilepsy as a phenomenon. *Journal of Neuroscience Nursing, 41*(4), 201–210.
- Tocco, S. (2009). Phenytoin: Keep patients in the range and out of danger. *American Nurse Today, 4*(1), 12–13.

Risk for Ineffective Airway Clearance

During a seizure, the tongue may fall back and obstruct the airway, the gag reflex may be depressed, and secretions may pool at the back of the throat. These may put the patient at risk for an obstructed airway. Most seizures occur in the home or community; therefore, teach these interventions to the patient's family:

- Provide interventions to maintain a patent airway:
  - Loosen clothing around the neck.
  - Turn on the side.
  - Do not force anything into the mouth.
  - If prescribed and available, administer oxygen by mask. *Although it was at one time believed that it was necessary to place a padded tongue blade in the patient's mouth during a seizure, this is no longer recommended; an improperly placed tongue blade can obstruct the airway. Turning the patient on the side allows secretions to drain from the mouth.*
- Teach family members or significant others how to care for the patient during a seizure to prevent airway obstruction. *Family members are often the only people present to provide this emergency intervention.*

Anxiety

The patient with a seizure disorder is understandably anxious about the future, with questions about ability to go to school, work, have a family, and drive a car. Feelings of embarrassment about having a seizure in public and rejection by others are common and also increase the patient's anxiety.

- Provide support by explaining that concerns are normal. *It is important to be sensitive to the effect of seizures on the patient's self-concept and body image; alterations in these areas not only increase anxiety but also cause withdrawal from socialization with others. Demonstrating acceptance of the patient's concerns allows further discussion.*
- Help identify safe leisure activities. *Worrying about being hurt if a seizure occurs may cause withdrawal from social activities that are pleasurable.*
- Provide information about sources and support groups. *Sharing information with other people with similar health problems allows for a more realistic viewpoint; accurate information can clear up misconceptions that cause anxiety.*

- Provide accurate information about hiring practices and legal limitations on driving or operating heavy or dangerous machinery. *Accurate information decreases anxiety about the unknown. The Americans with Disabilities Act prohibits discrimination; however, there are legal limitations on driving until the person is proven free of seizures.*

Readiness for Enhanced Knowledge

Women with epilepsy require specific knowledge related to their menstrual cycle, contraception, and childbearing.

- Encourage discussion with the woman's healthcare provider about the increased probability of seizures at the time of menses. *Medications to prevent seizures may require dosage adjustments and avoidance of other triggers is important.*
- Discuss the effects of AEDS. *AEDs decrease the effectiveness of oral contraceptives (decreased effectiveness is indicated by breakthrough bleeding); other forms of birth control (such as intrauterine devices) may be necessary. In addition, some AEDs can cause birth defects if pregnancy does occur.*

Using NANDA, NIC, and NOC

Linkages between a selected NANDA nursing diagnosis, NIC, and NOC for the patient with a seizure disorder are shown in the chart that follows.

Community-Based Care

Teaching follows a systematic assessment of the needs of both the patient and family. Include family members so that they can learn seizure management, including the care and observations necessary before and during a seizure. Stress the importance of safety and keeping the airway patent during a seizure.

Help both the patient and family adjust to a diagnosis of epilepsy. Address the following topics:

- The importance of wearing a Medic-Alert band or carrying a medical alert card at all times
- Avoiding alcoholic beverages and limiting coffee intake

NANDA, NIC, AND NOC LINKAGES
The Patient with Seizures

NANDA — Risk for Falls

NIC — Fall Prevention
Environmental Management: Safety
Seizure Precautions
Surveillance: Safety

NOC — Fall Prevention Behavior
Knowledge: Fall Prevention
Seizure Control

Adapted from Bulechek, G., Butcher, H., & Dochterman, J. M. (Eds). (2008). *Nursing interventions classification (NIC)* (5th ed.). St. Louis: Mosby Elsevier, 326, 343, 630, 704; NANDA International. (2009). *Nursing diagnoses: Definitions and classifications 2009–2011.* Oxford, UK: Wiley-Blackwell; and Moorhead, S., Johnson, M., Maas, M., & Swanson, E. (Eds). (2008). *Nursing outcomes classification (NOC)* (4th ed.). St. Louis: Mosby Elsevier, 346, 618.

CASE STUDY & NURSING CARE PLAN   A Patient with a Seizure Disorder

Janet Carlson is a 19-year-old college student who lives with her parents and one younger sister. Although Janet had seizures while she was in grade school, they have been controlled with medication. However, she had a tonic-clonic seizure yesterday and immediately made an appointment with her family physician. She is currently taking phenytoin (Dilantin) 300 mg/day as a maintenance medication to prevent seizures.

ASSESSMENT

Evita Farias, RN, completes a health history for Ms. Carlson. During the history, she tells Ms. Farias that she has been under stress because of difficulties in completing her course requirements this semester. She has not been sleeping as many hours per night, and sometimes she forgets to take her medication. Janet's serum phenytoin level is 8 mg/mL. Therapeutic level is 10 to 20 mg/mL.

DIAGNOSES

- *Risk for Injury* related to recurrence of generalized tonic-clonic seizure activity and low serum phenytoin levels
- *Deficient Knowledge* of activities that may trigger seizure occurrence, the effect of stress on seizures, and medication information

EXPECTED OUTCOMES

- Verbalize precipitating and triggering factors related to the onset of seizures.
- Verbalize the relationship between emotional and physical stress and seizures.
- Verbalize the importance of taking AEDs.

PLANNING AND IMPLEMENTATION

- Teach patient and her family the following:
  - Current information about seizures
  - Care during and after a seizure
  - Medication protocols
  - Factors and activities that can trigger seizures
  - The importance of follow-up care
- Refer patient and her family to a local epilepsy support group.
- Recommend that she purchase and wear a Medic-Alert bracelet.

EVALUATION

Ms. Carlson is instructed to continue taking Dilantin 300 mg/day. She states the importance of nutrition, rest, and measures to reduce stress. She also discusses the importance of maintaining the proper blood levels of her medication, stating that too little or too much of the medication could cause problems. Ms. Carlson recognizes that the seizures had recurred during a busy time in school during which she had forgotten to take her medication. She is now wearing a Medic-Alert bracelet. Ms. Farias provides the Carlsons with the telephone number of the Epilepsy Foundation of America.

CRITICAL THINKING IN THE NURSING PROCESS

1. If you were Ms. Carlson's nurse, would your teaching differ if she were living alone? If so, how?
2. Ms. Carlson tells you that although she knows she should not drive a car, she often drives her friend to work. How would you approach this problem?
3. Ms. Carlson states that "it's embarrassing to wear a Medic-Alert bracelet." How would you respond, and what recommendation(s) would you make?

See Evaluating Your Response in Appendix C.

- Taking showers versus tub baths, because of safety issues during a generalized seizure
- Factors that may trigger a seizure, and paying attention to an aura if one occurs
- Helpful resources, including the American Epilepsy Society and the Epilepsy Foundation

The Patient with a Stroke

A **stroke** (cerebral vascular accident [CVA], or brain attack), is an emergency condition in which neurologic deficits result from a sudden decrease in blood flow to a localized area of the brain. Strokes may be ischemic (when blood supply to a part of the brain is suddenly interrupted by a thrombus, embolus, or blood vessel stenosis), or hemorrhagic (when a blood vessel ruptures, spilling blood into spaces surrounding neurons). The neurologic deficits caused by ischemia and the resultant necrosis of cells in the brain vary according to the area of the brain involved, the size of the affected area, and the length of time blood flow is decreased or stopped. A major loss of blood supply to the brain can cause severe disability or death. When the duration of decreased blood flow is short and the anatomic area involved is small, the person may not be aware that damage has been done.

Incidence and Prevalence

On average, someone in the United States has a stroke every 45 seconds and dies of a stroke every 3 minutes. Stroke is the third leading cause of death and the leading cause of adult disability in North America, where almost 800,000 people suffer a stroke each year. Of those, 160,000 die and many patients who survive are left with some type of functional impairment (National Stroke Association, 2009). The risk doubles for every decade after age 55, and two-thirds of all strokes occur in people over the age of 65. As the population of baby boomers reach and exceeds this age, stroke will be even more significant to healthcare providers.

Risk Factors

Certain diseases, lifestyle habits, and ethnic backgrounds increase the risk of a stroke. Risk factors include hypertension, sickle cell anemia, atrial fibrillation, diabetes mellitus, hyperlipidemia, sleep apnea, smoking, and substance and alcohol abuse. Other risk factors include a previous stroke or transient ischemia attack (TIA or "little stroke"), family history of stroke, obesity, a sedentary lifestyle, and recent viral and bacterial infections. Risk factors specific to women are oral contraceptive use, pregnancy, childbirth, menopause, migraine headaches with aura, autoimmune disorders (such as diabetes and lupus), hormone replacement therapy, and clotting disorders. Blacks have almost twice the risk of having a stroke as do Whites. Hispanics have a higher incidence of ischemic stroke at an earlier age and also have a higher incidence of intracerebral hemorrhage and subarachnoid hemorrhage (American Stroke Association, 2009).

Risk factors are classified as unmodifiable (age, gender, race, and heredity) and modifiable (all disease and lifestyle risks).

Modifiable risk factors can be altered by prevention. The National Institute of Neurological Disorders and Stroke (2009) recommends the following preventive measures for the most important treatable conditions that increase the risk of stroke:

- Hypertension: *Treat it*. Eat a balanced diet, maintain a healthy weight, and exercise to reduce blood pressure.
- Cigarette Smoking: *Quit it*. Medical help is availble.
- Heart Disease: *Manage it*. Healthcare providers can treat heart disease and prescribe medications to help prevent the formation of clots. For those over the age of 50, discuss aspirin therapy with your provider.
- Diabetes: *Control it*. Treatment can delay complicaitons that increase the risk of stroke.
- TIAs: *Seek help*. TIAs should never be ignored and can be treated.

Pathophysiology

The brain, which makes up only 2% of total body weight, receives approximately 20% of the cardiac output each minute (about 750 mL) and accounts for 20% of the body's oxygen consumption. Cerebral blood flow, especially in the deep cerebral vessels, is largely self-regulated by the brain to meet metabolic needs. This self-regulation (also called autoregulation) allows the brain to maintain a constant blood flow despite changes in systemic blood pressure. However, autoregulation is not effective when systemic blood pressure falls below 50 mmHg or rises above 160 mmHg. In the latter case, the increased systemic pressure causes an increase in cerebral blood flow with resultant overdistention of cerebral vessels. Cerebral blood flow also increases in response to increased carbon dioxide concentrations, increased hydrogen ion concentrations, and decreased oxygen concentrations.

When blood flow to and oxygenation of cerebral neurons are decreased or interrupted from a stroke, pathophysiologic changes at the cellular level take place in 4 to 5 minutes. Each minute during a stroke, 2 million brain cells die. The changes that take place are the result of a chain of chemical reactions called the ischemic cascade (National Stroke Association, 2009). This process occurs in three stages: primary cell death, secondary cell death, and inflammation and immune response.

Primary cell death begins as blood supply is cut off to a part of the brain, resulting in ischemia in the core area of involved brain tissue. Anoxia and lack of nutrients to the cells affect the mitochondria of the cells, essentially depriving the cells of their energy source. As the mitochondria break down, they release oxygen-free radicals (such as glutamate) into the cytoplasm, destroying other intercellular structures. Cell membrane channels open, allowing calcium, sodium, and potassium to enter the cells. At the same time, the affected cells release excitatory amino acids into the intracellular spaces. Homeostasis is lost and water enters the cell (called cytoxic edema) to the point that the cells burst and quickly become infarcted and necrotic. This process begins in 4 to 5 minutes and may last as long as 2 to 3 hours.

Secondary cell death ensues from exposure to excessive amounts of glutamate, nitric oxide, free radicals, and excitatory amino acids released from necrotic cells. These cells, surrounding the area of initial damage, have only enough blood supply to remain alive for a few hours. If blood supply is restored to these cells within 2 to 3 hours, some cells can live and become functional. The area of living cells in and around the area of dead and necrotic cells is called the penumbra.

As secondary cell death is taking place, the body's immune system does further damage through an inflammatory reaction mediated by the vascular system. The initial damage attracts leukocytes to the damaged area; these white cells penetrate the endothelial wall, move through the blood-brain barrier, and invade the substance of the brain, causing further injury and cell death. Monocytes and macrophages release inflammatory chemicals (cytokines, interleukins, and tissue necrosis factor) at the site of injury to inhibit the release of natural tissue plasminogen activator and inactivate anti-clotting factors. These effects make it more difficult for the body to dissolve a clot.

A stroke is characterized by a gradual or rapid onset of neurologic deficits due to compromised cerebral blood flow. The neurologic deficits that occur as a result of a stroke can often be used to identify its location. Because the motor pathways cross at the junction of the medulla and spinal cord (decussation), strokes lead to loss or impairment of sensorimotor functions on the side of the body *opposite* the side of the brain that is damaged. This effect, known as a **contralateral deficit**, means that a stroke in the right hemisphere of the brain is manifested by deficits in the left side of the body (and vice versa).

Ischemic Stroke

This type of stroke accounts for 87% of all strokes (Hickey, 2009). The blockage may result from a blood clot (either as a thrombus or an emboli), or from stenosis of a vessel resulting from a buildup of plaque. Plaque may cause stenosis in large blood vessels or small blood vessels. Large vessel blockage usually is the result of thrombi. Small vessel strokes are small to very small infarcts in the deep, noncortical areas of the brain or the brainstem. Cardiogenic embolic strokes are caused by a blood clot (most commonly from atrial fibrillation) moving through cerebral blood vessels until the vessel is too small to allow further movement.

TRANSIENT ISCHEMIC ATTACK A **transient ischemic attack (TIA)**, sometimes called a mini-stroke, is a brief period of localized cerebral ischemia that causes neurologic deficits lasting for less than 24 hours (Hickey, 2009), or as defined by Porth and Matfin (2009), "a deficit lasting less than 1 hour and being a zone of penumbra without central infarction" (p. 1320). TIAs are often warning signals of an ischemic thrombotic stroke. One or many TIAs may precede a stroke, with the time between the TIA and a stroke ranging from hours to months. The etiology of TIA includes inflammatory artery disorders, sickle cell anemia, atherosclerotic changes in carotid and cerebral arteries, thrombosis, and emboli. Neurologic manifestations of a TIA vary according to the location and size of the cerebral vessel involved and have a sudden onset. Commonly occurring deficits include contralateral numbness or weakness of the leg, hand, forearm, and corner of the mouth, aphasia, and visual disturbances such as blurring. The patient may also experience a visual disturbance called

Thrombotic Stroke Animation

amaurosis fugax (a fleeting blindness of one eye, described as a shade coming down over vision in the affected eye).

LARGE VESSEL (THROMBOTIC) STROKE   A thrombotic stroke is caused by occlusion of a large cerebral vessel by a thrombus (blood clot). Thrombotic strokes most often occur in older people who are resting or sleeping. The blood pressure is lower during sleep, so there is less pressure to push the blood through an already narrowed arterial lumen, and ischemia may result.

Thrombi tend to form in large arteries that bifurcate and have narrowed lumens as a result of deposits of atherosclerotic plaque. The plaque involves the intima of the arteries, causing the internal elastic lamina to become thin and frayed with exposure of underlying connective tissue. This structural change causes platelets to adhere to the rough surface and release the enzyme adenosine diphosphate. This enzyme initiates the clotting sequence, and a thrombus forms. A thrombus may remain in place and continue to enlarge, completely occluding the lumen of the vessel, or a part of it may break off and become an embolus. These strokes commonly affect a single cerebral artery supplying the cerebral cortex, causing aphasia, neglect syndrome, and/or visual field defects.

SMALL VESSEL STROKE (LACUNAR INFARCT)   Thrombotic strokes affecting the smaller cerebral vessels are called lacunar (small vessel) strokes, because the infarcted areas slough off, leaving a small cavity or "lake" in the brain tissue. They occur in the deeper parts of the brain or the brain stem from occlusion of small branches of large cerebral arteries; most often the middle cerebral and posterior cerebral arteries. Manifestations include motor hemiplegia, sensory hemiplegia, and dysarthria.

CARDIOGENIC EMBOLIC STROKE   A cardiogenic embolic stroke results when a blood clot from atrial fibrillation, ventricular thrombi, myocardial infarction, congestive heart disease, or atherosclerotic plaque (and other sources) enters the circulatory system and becomes lodged in a cerebral vessel too narrow to permit further movement. The blood vessel is then occluded. The most frequent sites of cerebral emboli are at bifurcations of vessels, particularly those of the middle cerebral artery (Hickey, 2009).

Hemorrhagic Stroke

A hemorrhagic stroke, or intracranial hemorrhage, occurs when a cerebral blood vessel ruptures. There are two types of hemorrhagic strokes: intracerebral hemorrhage and subarachnoid hemorrhage. An intracerebral hemorrhage often occurs in older adults with sustained increase in systolic-diastolic blood pressure. A subarachnoid hemorrhage is commonly seen in younger people. Intracranial hemorrhage usually occurs suddenly, often when the affected person is engaged in some activity. Although hypertension is the most common cause, a variety of factors may contribute to a hemorrhagic stroke, including rupture of a brittle plaque-encrusted artery wall, ruptured intracranial aneurysms, trauma, erosion of blood vessels by tumors, arteriovenous malformations, anticoagulant therapy, and blood disorders. Of all forms of stroke, this form is most

often fatal. (Hemorrhagic strokes that result from ruptured cerebral aneurysm or an arteriovenous malformation are discussed in the next sections of the chapter.)

As a result of rupture of the blood vessel, blood enters the brain tissue, the cerebral ventricles, or the subarachnoid space, compressing adjacent tissues and causing blood vessel spasm and cerebral edema. Blood in the ventricles or subarachnoid space irritates the meninges and brain tissue, causing an inflammatory reaction and impairing absorption and circulation of cerebrospinal fluid (CSF). The onset of manifestations from a hemorrhagic stroke is rapid. Manifestations depend on the location of the hemorrhage, but may include vomiting, headache, seizures, hemiplegia, and loss of consciousness. Pressure on brain tissue from IICP may cause coma and death.

Manifestations

Manifestations of a stroke vary according to the cerebral artery involved and the area of the brain affected. Women with stroke are more likely to report nontraditional manifestations (especially disorientation, confusion, or loss of consciousness) than men (International Stroke Conference, 2009). Manifestations are always sudden in onset, focal, and usually one sided. The various deficits associated with involvement of a specific cerebral artery are collectively referred to as stroke syndromes, although the deficits often overlap, as shown in the following Manifestations box.

Complications

Typical complications include sensoriperceptual deficits, cognitive and behavioral changes, communication disorders, motor deficits, and elimination disorders. These may be transient or permanent, depending on the degree of ischemia and necrosis as well as time of treatment. As a result of the neurologic deficits,

---

MANIFESTATIONS of a Stroke by Involved Cerebral Vessel

INTERNAL CAROTID ARTERY
- Contralateral paralysis of the arm, leg, and face
- Contralateral sensory deficits of the arm, leg, and face
- If the dominant hemisphere is involved: aphasia
- If the nondominant hemisphere is involved: apraxia, agnosia, unilateral neglect
- Homonymous hemianopia (see Figure 42–5 ■)

MIDDLE CEREBRAL ARTERY
- Drowsiness, stupor, coma
- Contralateral hemiplegia of the arm and face
- Contralateral sensory deficits of the arm and face
- Global aphasia (if dominant hemisphere involved)
- Homonymous hemianopia

ANTERIOR CEREBRAL ARTERY
- Contralateral weakness or paralysis of the foot and leg
- Contralateral sensory loss of the toes, foot, and leg
- Loss of ability to make decisions or act voluntarily
- Urinary incontinence

VERTEBRAL ARTERY
- Pain in face, nose, or eye
- Numbness and weakness of the face on involved side
- Problems with gait
- Dysphagia

MANIFESTATIONS AND COMPLICATIONS of Stroke by Body System

INTEGUMENT
- Decubitus ulcers

NEUROLOGIC
- Hyperthermia
- Neglect syndrome
- Seizures
- Agnosia
- Communication deficits: expressive aphasia, receptive aphasia, global aphasia, agraphia
- Visual deficits: homonymous hemianopia, diplopia, decreased acuity
- Cognitive changes: memory loss, short attention span, distractibility, poor judgment, poor problem solving, disorientation
- Behavioral changes: emotional lability, loss of social inhibitions, fear, hostility, anger, depression
- IICP
- Alterations in consciousness
- Sensory loss to touch, pain, heat, cold, pressure

RESPIRATORY
- Respiratory center damage
- Airway obstruction
- Decreased ability to cough

GASTROINTESTINAL
- Dysphagia
- Constipation, stool impaction

GENITOURINARY
- Incontinence, frequency, urgency
- Urinary retention
- Renal calculi

MUSCULOSKELETAL
- Hemiplegia
- Contractures
- Bony ankylosis
- Disuse atrophy
- Dysarthria

the patient with a stroke has complications that involve many different body systems (see the accompanying Manifestations box). The disabilities resulting from a stroke often cause serious alterations in functional health status.

Sensoriperceptual Deficits

A stroke may involve pathologic changes in neurologic pathways that alter the ability to integrate, interpret, and attend to sensory data. The patient may experience deficits in vision, hearing, equilibrium, taste, and sense of smell. The ability to perceive vibration, pain, warmth, cold, and pressure may be impaired, as may proprioception (the body's sense of its position). The loss of these sensory abilities increases the risk for injury. Deficits may include the following:

- **Hemianopia:** the loss of half of the visual field of one or both eyes; when the same half is missing in each eye, the condition is called homonymous hemianopia (Figure 42–5).

Key: ○ Normal vision
      ● Blind area

Figure 42–5 ■ Abnormal visual fields. *A,* Normal left field of vision with loss of vision in right field. *B,* Loss of vision in temporal half of both fields (bitemporal hemianopia). *C,* Loss of vision in nasal field of right eye and temporal field of left eye (homonymous hemianopia).

- **Agnosia:** the inability to recognize one or more subjects that were previously familiar; agnosia may be visual, tactile, or auditory.
- **Apraxia:** the inability to carry out some motor pattern (e.g., drawing a figure, getting dressed) even when strength and coordination are adequate.

Another form of sensory-perceptual deficit is the **neglect syndrome** (or unilateral neglect), in which the patient has a disorder of attention. In this syndrome, the person cannot integrate and use perceptions from the affected side of the body or from the environment on the affected side, and ignores that part. In severe cases, the patient may even deny the paralysis. This deficit is more common following a stroke of the right hemisphere where damage to the parietal lobe (a center for mediation of directed attention) results in perceptual deficits.

Pain and discomfort may accompany a stroke, with the patient experiencing acute pain, numbness, or strange sensations. Although not common, damage to the thalamus may cause central stroke pain or central pain syndrome (CPS). The pain in this syndrome includes hot and cold, burning, tingling, and sharp stabbing pain, most often in the extremities. It is worsened by movement and temperature changes. The painful sensations are not relieved by pain medications, nor are there any specific treatments.

Cognitive and Behavioral Changes

A change in consciousness, ranging from mild confusion to coma, is a common manifestation of a stroke. It may result from tissue damage following ischemia or hemorrhage involving either the carotid or vertebral arteries. Altered consciousness may also be the result of cerebral edema or IICP.

Behavioral changes include emotional lability (in which the patient may laugh or cry inappropriately), loss of self-control (manifested by behavior such as swearing or refusing to wear clothing), and decreased tolerance for stress (resulting in anger or depression). Intellectual changes may include memory loss, decreased attention span, poor judgment, and an inability to think abstractly.

Communication Disorders

Communication is a complex process, involving motor functions, speech, language, memory, reasoning, and emotions. Communication disorders are usually the result of a stroke affecting the dominant hemisphere. The left hemisphere is dominant in about 95% of right-handed people and 70% of left-handed people (Porth & Matfin, 2009). Many different impairments may occur, and most are partial. Disorders of communication affect both speech (the mechanical act of articulating language through the spoken word) and language (the vocal or written formulation of ideas to communicate thoughts and feelings). Language involves oral and written expression and auditory and reading comprehension. Among these disorders are the following:

- **Aphasia**: the inability to use or understand language; aphasia may be expressive, receptive, or mixed (global).
- *Expressive aphasia:* a motor speech problem in which one can understand what is being said but can respond verbally only in short phrases; also called Broca's aphasia.
- *Receptive aphasia:* a sensory speech problem in which one cannot understand the spoken (and often written) word. Speech may be fluent but with inappropriate content; also called Wernicke's aphasia.
- *Mixed or global aphasia:* language dysfunction in both understanding and expression.
- *Dysarthria:* any disturbance in muscular control of speech.

Motor Deficits

Body movement results from a complex interaction between the brain, spinal cord, and peripheral nerves. The motor areas of the cerebral cortex, the basal ganglia, and the cerebellum initiate voluntary movement by sending messages to the spinal cord, which then transmits the messages to the peripheral nerves. A stroke may interrupt the CNS component of this relay system and produce effects in the contralateral side ranging from mild weakness to severe limitation of any kind of movement.

Depending on the area of the brain involved, strokes may cause weakness, paralysis, and/or spasticity. The deficits include the following:

- **Hemiplegia**: paralysis of the left or right half of the body (Figure 42–6 ■).
- **Hemiparesis**: weakness of the left or right half of the body.
- *Flaccidity:* absence of muscle tone (hypotonia).
- *Spasticity:* increased muscle tone (hypertonia), usually with some degree of weakness. The flexor muscles are usually more strongly affected in the upper extremities, and the extensor muscles are more strongly affected in the lower extremities.

When the corticospinal tract is involved, the affected arm and leg almost always are initially flaccid and then become spastic within 6 to 8 weeks. Spasticity often causes characteristic body positioning: adduction of the shoulder, pronation of the forearm, flexion of the fingers, and extension of the hip and knee. There is often foot drop, outward rotation of the leg, and dependent edema in the involved extremities.

The motor deficits may result in altered mobility, further impairing body function. The complications of immobility involve multiple body systems and include orthostatic hypotension,

Figure 42–6 ■ Types of paralysis. *A*, Quadriplegia is complete or partial paralysis of the upper extremities and complete paralysis of the lower part of the body. *B*, Hemiplegia is paralysis of one-half of the body when it is divided along the median sagittal plane. *C*, Paraplegia is paralysis of the lower part of the body.

increased thrombus formation, decreased cardiac output, impaired respiratory function, osteoporosis, formation of renal calculi, contractures, and decubitus ulcer formation.

Elimination Disorders

Disorders of bladder and bowel elimination are common. A stroke may cause partial loss of the sensations that trigger bladder elimination, resulting in urinary frequency, urgency, or incontinence. Control of urination may be altered as a result of cognitive deficits. Changes in bowel elimination are common, resulting from changes in LOC, immobility, and dehydration.

Interdisciplinary Care

The type of treatment a patient with a stroke receives depends on the stage of the disease. In general there are three treatment stages: stroke prevention, acute care immediately after a stroke, and rehabilitation after a stroke. The patient with an acute stroke may receive medical and/or surgical treatment. The focus in the acute care phase is on diagnosing the type and cause of the stroke, supporting cerebral circulation, and controlling or preventing further deficits. The goals of stroke care are to minimize brain injury and maximize patient recovery. The focus of acute care has shifted from "the nearest hospital" to certified stroke centers (if possible) where patients with a stroke can be provided appropriate care from entrance to the emergency department to discharge following rehabilitation.

Diagnosis

Diagnosis begins with a complete history and careful physical assessment, including a thorough neurologic examination. The time of the onset of stroke manifestations is a critical part of assessment. The National Institute of Health (NIH) Stroke Scale (2003) is a clinical evaluation tool widely used to assess neurologic outcome and degree of recovery. Part of the scale is illustrated in Table 42–4. The tool measures LOC, vision, facial paralysis, motor abilities, ataxia, sensation, language, and

TABLE 42–4 NIH Stroke Scale: Assessment of Level of Consciousness

INSTRUCTIONS	SCALE DEFINITION	SCORE
1a. Level of Consciousness: The investigator must choose a response, even if a full evaluation is prevented by such obstacles as an endotracheal tube, language barrier, orotracheal trauma/bandages. A 3 is scored only if the patient makes no movement (other than reflexive posturing) in response to noxious stimulation.	0 = Alert, keenly responsive. 1 = Not alert, but arousable by minor stimulation to obey, answer, or respond. 2 = Not alert, requires repeated stimulation to attend, or is obtunded and requires strong or painful stimulation to make movements (not stereotyped). 3 = Responds only with reflex motor or autonomic effects or totally unresponsive, flaccid, movements are dysreflexic.	_____
1b. LOC Questions: The patient is asked the month and his or her age. The answer must be correct. There is no partial credit for being close. Aphasic and stuporous patients who do not comprehend the questions will score 2. Patients unable to speak because of endotracheal intubation, orotracheal trauma, severe dysarthria from any cause, language barrier, or any other problem not secondary to aphasia are given a 1. It is important that only the initial answer be graded and that the examiner not "help" the patient with verbal or nonverbal cues.	0 = Answers both questions correctly. 1 = Answers one question correctly. 2 = Answers neither question correctly.	_____
1c. LOC Commands: The patient is asked to open and close the eyes and then to grip and release the non-paretic hand. Substitute another one-step command if the hands cannot be used. Credit is given if an unequivocal attempt is made but not completed due to weakness. If the patient does not respond to command the task should be demonstrated to him or her (pantomime) and score the results (i.e., follows none, one, or two commands). Patients with trauma, amputation, or other physical impediments should be given suitable one-step commands. Only the first attempt is scored.	0 = Performs both tasks correctly. 1 = Performs one task correctly. 2 = Performs neither task correctly.	_____

*Note: A lower score indicates better function.

attention. The entire scale may be accessed at the website for the National Institute of Neurological Disorders and Stroke.

Imaging tests are used to identify an increased risk for a stroke or to identify pathophysiologic changes after a stroke has occurred. Computed tomography (CT) is the first imaging technique used to demonstrate the presence of hemorrhage, tumors, aneurysm, ischemia, edema, and tissue necrosis. A CT scan can also demonstrate a shift in intracranial contents and is useful in distinguishing the type of stroke (e.g., a hemorrhagic stroke results in an increase in density). Cerebral infarctions usually are visible with a CT scan 6 to 8 hours post stroke; hemorrhage is visible immediately. Other imaging tests that may be used for diagnosis include a cerebral arteriogram, a transcranial ultrasound Doppler, an MRI, an MRA, a PET, and a SPECT (∞ see Chapter 41). A perfusion- and diffusion-weighted imaging (DWI) test can be used to identify cerebral ischemia immediately after onset of the stroke and also identify areas of possibly reversible damage (the penumbra). In addition to imaging tests, a blood test has recently been approved to screen for recurrent stroke risk. The PLAC test scans the blood for high levels of lipoprotein-associated phospholipase A2 (Lp-Pla2), found to be more common in people who have had strokes.

A lumbar puncture may be performed to obtain CSF for examination if there is no danger of IICP. An ischemic stroke may elevate CSF pressure; after a hemorrhagic stroke blood may be seen in the CSF.

Medications

Medications are administered to prevent a stroke in patients with TIAs or a previous stroke, and to treat the patient during the acute phase of a stroke. Treatment for IICP was discussed in a previous section of the chapter.

PREVENTION Antiplatelet agents are often used to treat patients with TIAs or who have had a previous stroke. Platelets are concentrated in high blood flow arteries, where they adhere to endothelial tissue damaged by atherosclerosis and occlude the vessel. The drugs used to prevent clot formation and blood vessel occlusion include aspirin, clopidogrel (Plavix), dipyridamole (Persantine), and ticlopidine (Ticlid). Daily low-dose aspirin reduces TIA occurrence and stroke risk by interfering with platelet aggregation. Ticlopidine (Ticlid) is a platelet-aggregation inhibitor that has shown reduction in thrombotic stroke risk.

ACUTE STROKE Medications are used to treat the patient during the acute phase of an ischemic stroke to prevent further thrombosis formation, increase cerebral blood flow, and protect cerebral neurons. The type of medication used varies according to the type of stroke.

Fibrinolytic therapy, using a tissue plasminogen activator such as recombinant tissue-type plasminogen activator alteplase (tPA), sometimes given concurrently with an anticoagulant, is used to treat ischemic stroke. The drug converts plasminogen to plasmin, resulting in fibrinolysis of the clot. To be effective, it must be given IV within 3 hours of the onset of manifestations, after confirming (with a CT scan) that the patient has not had a hemorrhagic stroke (McPhee et al., 2008). However, a European study found that tPA administered between 3 and 4.5 hours after the onset of manifestations significantly improved clinical outcomes, although it also increased the risk of intracranial hemorrhage (Hacke, Kaste, Bluhmki et al., 2008). Antithrombotic drugs, which inhibit the platelet phase of clot formation, have been used as a preventive measure for patients at risk for ischemic stroke. Both aspirin and dipyridamole have been used for this purpose. These drugs are sometimes also used in combination with other drugs during acute treatment. Antiplatelet agents are contraindicated in patients with a hemorrhagic stroke.

Anticoagulant drug therapy (discussed in ∞ Chapter 30) may be ordered for an ischemic stroke. The most commonly used anticoagulants are warfarin (Coumadin), heparin, and enoxaparin (Lovenox). Anticoagulants do not dissolve an existing clot but rather prevent further extension of the clot and formation of new clots. Sodium heparin may be given subcutaneously or by continuous IV drip, or warfarin sodium (Coumadin) may be given orally. It is recommended that the use of antifactor Xa be used to monitor blood coagulation (Hickey, 2009).

SAFETY ALERT
Anticoagulants are never administered to a patient with a hemorrhagic stroke.

Management of hypertension is controversial but if the patient is eligible for fibrinolytic therapy, blood pressure control is essential to decrease the risk of bleeding. If the blood pressure is sustained at systolic levels > 185 mmHg systolic or diastolic levels > 110 diastolic, the patient cannot be treated with IV tPA (McPhee et al., 2008).

Treatments
The treatments used in the management of a stroke include surgery and rehabilitation.

SURGERY   Surgery may be performed to prevent the occurrence of a stroke, to restore blood flow when a stroke has already occurred, or to repair vascular damage or malformations. In

people who have had TIAs or are in danger of having another stroke, a carotid endarterectomy at the carotid artery bifurcation may be performed to remove atherosclerotic plaque (Figure 42–7 ■). Nursing care for the patient in the initial postoperative period following a carotid endarterectomy is described in the following box.

When an occluded or stenotic vessel is not directly accessible, an extracranial-intracranial bypass may be performed through bypass of the internal carotid, middle cerebral, or vertebral arteries. The procedure reestablishes blood flow to the affected area of the brain. A carotid angioplasty with stenting is an option for treating cerebral stenosis. During the procedure an angioplasty balloon catheter is inserted through an artery in the patient's arm or leg. Under fluoroscopy, the catheter is advanced to the area of carotid artery stenosis and a small filter is inserted to catch any clots or pieces of debris that might break loose. The balloon is then inflated to widen the artery, followed by insertion of a permanent stent in the area of the angioplasty.

NURSING CARE OF THE PATIENT
Having a Carotid Endarterectomy

POSTOPERATIVE CARE
- Position on the unoperated side and either maintain a flat position or elevate the head of the bed 30 degrees as prescribed. Maintain head and neck alignment and avoid rotating, flexing, or hyperextending head. *Pressure on the wound is undesirable. Elevating the head decreases edema in the operative site. Maintaining head and neck alignment prevents additional tension or pressure on the operative side.*
- Support the head when changing position. Teach to support the head with the hands when able to move about. *Supporting the head helps prevent stress on the operative site (which may cause bleeding and hematoma formation); it also helps reduce stress on the suture line.*
- Assess respirations and oxygen saturation.
  a. *Hemorrhage.* Assess the dressing and the area under the neck and shoulders for drainage. Assess for increased pulse and decreased blood pressure. *The most common cause of respiratory problems is pressure on the trachea from a hematoma formation.*
  b. *Respiratory distress.* Assess respiratory rate, rhythm, depth, and effort. Observe for restlessness. Keep a tracheostomy tray at the bedside. *Respiratory distress may result from edema and hematoma formation, which may compress the trachea.*
  c. *Cranial nerve impairment.* Observe and record any facial drooping, tongue deviation, hoarseness, dysphagia, or loss of facial sensation. *Cranial nerves may be stretched during surgery, leading to temporary deficits in cranial nerve function.*
  d. *Hypertension or hypotension.* Take and record blood pressure at least hourly. Report any changes immediately and implement orders for medications to treat hypertension or hypotension. *About one-half of all patients having a carotid endarterectomy develop unstable blood pressure related to surgical denervation of the carotid sinus. Uncontrolled hypertension may precipitate a stroke. The most common problem is hypotension, possibly related to stimulation of the carotid body baroreceptors, which are exposed during surgery. Hypotension may result in myocardial ischemia.*

Figure 42–7 ■ Carotid endarterectomy. *A*, The occluded area is clamped off and an incision is made in the artery. *B*, Plaque is removed from the inner layer of the artery. *C*, To restore blood flow through the artery, the artery is sutured, or a graft is completed.

Other treatments include suctioning the clot out of the artery or threading a wire through the clot and pulling it out. A non-invasive method of improving recovery from a stroke, called noninvasive transcranial direct current stimulation (TDCS) has been shown to improve motor outcomes and is under study.

REHABILITATION Various types of interdisciplinary therapy are necessary for post stroke rehabilitation. These are most often provided in a setting dedicated to rehabilitation. Patients are frequently transferred to these settings for post stroke care for several weeks before being discharged to home. Listed next are the types and goals of therapies used:

- Physical therapy may help prevent contractures and improve muscle strength and coordination. Physical therapists teach exercises to enable the patient to relearn how to walk, sit, lie down, and change from one type of movement to another.
- Occupational therapy provides assistive devices and a plan for regaining lost motor skills that greatly improve quality of life after a stroke. These skills include eating, drinking, bathing, cooking, reading, writing, and toileting.
- Speech therapy is provided to help the patient improve swallowing as well as how to relearn language and communication skills.

Nursing Care

Even though many people who have a stroke have full recovery, a substantial number are left with disabilities that affect their physical, emotional, interpersonal, and family status. The required nursing care is often complex and multidimensional, requiring consideration of continuity of care for patients in acute care settings, long-term care settings, rehabilitation centers, and the home.

Nurses caring for patients who have had a stroke require knowledge and skill to meet patient and family needs during both the acute and the rehabilitative phases of care. The patient may have multiple losses: loss of mobility, ability to provide self-care, communications, concept of self, and interpersonal or intimate relationships with others. Holistic, individualized nursing care is essential in all settings and focuses on promoting the achievement of maximum potential and quality of life.

The patient's family is often faced with many changes. The young to middle-aged adult with a family member who has had a stroke may be faced with economic difficulties and social isolation. The middle-aged adult family member may become the caretaker for an older parent. An older adult may not be able to care for a spouse and may have to accept long-term care placement. In addition, the older adult who has no family may have to struggle alone to regain the ability to function independently. Although not all of these problems are amenable to nursing solutions, the nurse is most often the healthcare provider who assesses and identifies the needs of each individual and provides information and referrals to patients and families to help meet those needs.

Because a stroke has the potential to cause many different health problems, a wide variety of nursing diagnoses may be appropriate. It is important to remember that each person will be affected differently, depending on the degree of ischemia and the area of the brain involved. Nursing diagnoses discussed in this section focus on problems with cerebral tissue perfusion (specific to nursing care during the acute phase), physical mobility, self-care, communication, sensory-perceptual deficits, bowel and urine elimination, and swallowing (specific to prevention of complications and rehabilitation). In addition, many of the nursing diagnoses and interventions provided for the patient with alterations in consciousness, IICP, and seizures may be appropriate. A Case Study & Nursing Care Plan for a patient with a stroke is found on page 1459.

Health Promotion

Health promotion activities focus on stroke prevention, especially for those people with known risk factors. More lives are saved by preventing strokes than by treating them. It is important to discuss, as appropriate, the importance of stopping smoking and drug use with patients of all ages. Maintaining a normal weight through diet and exercise can help reduce obesity, which increases the risk of hypertension and type 2 diabetes mellitus (both in turn increase the risk of a stroke). Cholesterol levels should be screened regularly to monitor for hyperlipidemia. Regular health care to monitor for and treat cardiovascular disorders and to detect and treat infections such as infective endocarditis is important.

It is also important to increase public awareness of the signs of a TIA or stroke and of the need to call 911 or to seek care immediately if warning signs or symptoms occur. There are several public awareness campaigns that are useful. The symptoms listed next are those publicized by the National Institute of Neurogical Disorders and Symptoms (2008). The Fast Facts box provides clues to recognizing a stroke from the National Stroke Association. In addition, The Stroke Collaborative (2008) provides methods of recognizing a stroke in its campaign called "Give me 5 for stroke" that provides stroke indicators for a person's walk, talk, reach, vision, and feel (available at the organization's website).

- Sudden weakness or numbness of the face, arm, or leg, especially on one side of the body
- Sudden confusion, trouble speaking or understanding speech
- Sudden trouble walking, dizziness, loss of balance or coordination
- Sudden trouble with vision in one or both eyes
- Sudden severe headache without a cause

FAST FACTS
How to detect stroke symptoms and act F.A.S.T.

F = Face	Ask the person to smile. Does one side of the face droop?
A = Arm	Ask the person to raise both arms. Does one arm drift downward?
S = Speech	Ask the person to repeat a simple sentence. Does the speech sound blurred or strange?
T = Time	If you observe any of these symptoms, it is time to call 911 or get to the nearest stroke center or hospital.

(National Stroke Association, 2009.)

Assessment

The following data are collected through the health history and physical examination (∞ see Chapter 41). Further focused assessments are described with nursing interventions. If the patient is a woman, she has risks for stroke that are different than a man and should be asked questions specific to her gender (see the following Meeting Individualized Needs box).

- *Health history:* Risk factors, previous stroke, drug use (prescribed, over-the-counter, street drugs), smoking history, when manifestations began, severity of manifestations, presence of incontinence, family support system, advance directives or medical power of attorney.
- *Physical assessment:* Stroke scale, level of consciousness, vital signs, motor strength, coordination, communication, cranial nerves, sensory function, skin integrity, mobility status.

Nursing Diagnoses and Interventions

Depending on the severity of the stroke, the patient may be admitted to the intensive care unit. Regardless of the hospital setting, the nurse provides interventions to maintain functional status and prevent complications.

Risk for Ineffective Tissue Perfusion: Cerebral

The initial assessment and care of the patient admitted for intensive care focuses on identifying changes that may indicate altered cerebral perfusion. The patient's airway, breathing, circulation, and neurologic status are monitored and interventions are provided to maintain cerebral perfusion.

- Monitor respiratory status, oxygen saturation, and airway patency. Auscultate pulmonary sounds and monitor respiratory rate and results of studies of arterial blood gases.
- Suction as necessary, using care to suction no longer than 10 seconds at any one time, using sterile technique.
- Place in a side-lying position.
- Administer oxygen as prescribed.

  The patient may be unconscious and breathing may be impaired. Suctioning removes secretions that obstruct air flow, but also decreases O_2, increases CO_2, and partially obstructs the airway. Suctioning for longer than 10 seconds at a time may increase intracranial pressure (Hickey, 2009). Respiratory complications develop rapidly, as manifested by crackles and wheezes, rapid respirations, and respiratory acidosis. The administration of oxygen decreases the risk for hypoxia and hypercapnia, which can increase cerebral ischemia and intracranial pressure.

EVIDENCE FOR NURSING CARE — The Patient with a Stroke

Selected resources that nurses may find helpful when planning evidence-based nursing care follow.

- Barber, A., Beer, C., Beilby, J., Bernhardt, J., Bladin, C., Booth, B., et al. (2008). Prevention and management of complications. In: Clinical guidelines for acute stroke management. *National Guideline Clearinghouse.* Retrieved from http://www.guideline.gov/summary/summary.aspx?doc_id=12931&nbr=006645&string=DVT
- Kenner, C., Godfrey, C., Lamb, M., Patusky, K., & Williams, J. (2009). The psychosocial spiritual experience of elderly individuals recovering from stroke. *The Joanna Briggs Institute, Best Practice.* Retrieved from http://www.joannabriggs.edu.au/pdf/BPISEng_13_6.pdf
- Summers, D., Leonard, A., Wentworth, D., Saver, J. L., Simpson, J., Spilker, J. A., et al. (2009). Comprehensive overview of nursing and interdisciplinary care of the acute ischemic stroke patient: A scientific statement from the American Heart Association. *Stroke.* Retrieved from http://stroke.ahajournals.org/DOI: 10.1161/STROKEAHA.109.192362
- Ostwald, S. K., Davis, S., Hersch, G., Kelley, C., & Godman, K. M. (2008). Evidence-based educational guidelines for stroke survivors after discharge home. *Journal of Neuroscience Nursing, 40*(3), 173–179, 191.

PRACTICE ALERT

Positioning the patient on the side allows secretions to drain out of the mouth, helping to prevent aspiration.

- Monitor mental status and LOC: restlessness, drowsiness, lethargy, inability to follow commands, unresponsiveness. *Changes in mental status and LOC are often initial manifestations of IICP.*
- Assess for pain, headache, decreased muscle strength, sluggish pupillary reflexes, absent gag or swallowing reflexes, hemiplegia, Babinski's sign, and decerebrate or decorticate posturing. *Frequent monitoring of neurologic status is necessary to detect changes. Alterations in mental status, LOC, movement, strength, and reflexes indicate IICP, the major cause of death in the acute phase of a stroke.*
- Continuously monitor cardiac status, observing for dysrhythmias. *A stroke may cause cardiac dysrhythmias, including bradycardia, PVCs, tachycardia, and AV block. Characteristic*

MEETING INDIVIDUALIZED NEEDS — **Risk Factors for Stroke in Women**

Some risk factors for stroke apply only to women, most specifically pregnancy, childbirth, and menopause. These risks are the result of fluctuations in hormones that occur at different stages of life. However, other risks are also more common for women, and information should be collected during a health history. For accurate assessment, ask the following questions, depending on the woman's age:

- How many pregnancies have you had?
- Have you had a miscarriage? If so, how many?

- How many births have you had? When was your last delivery?
- When was your last menstrual period?
- Do you take any type of hormone replacement therapy?
- Do you take birth control pills?
- Do you have migraine headaches? If so, do you have an aura?
- Have you ever been diagnosed with diabetes or lupus?
- Have you ever been diagnosed with a clotting disorder? Have you ever had a clot in your leg?

ECG changes include a shortened PR interval, peaked T waves, and a depressed ST segment.

- Monitor body temperature and maintain temperature at less than 37°C at all times during acute care. *In a large meta-analysis, fever was consistently found to be associated with worse outcomes in patients with stroke (Greer, Funk, Ouzounelli, & Utman, 2008).*
- Maintain accurate intake and output records; measure urinary output via a Foley catheter. *A stroke may damage the pituitary gland, resulting in diabetes insipidus and the possibility of dehydration from greatly increased urinary output. If a Foley catheter is inserted, follow strict guidelines to prevent infection and for securing the catheter (Securing the indwelling catheter, 2008).*

> **PRACTICE ALERT**
> Diabetes insipidus is indicated by a large output of dilute urine; dehydration is indicated by scanty amounts of dark, concentrated urine.

- Monitor for seizures. Pad the side rails, and administer prescribed AEDs. *Seizures may be the result of cerebral tissue damage or IICP. Padded side rails prevent injury if a seizure occurs. AEDs prevent or treat seizures.*

Impaired Physical Mobility

The goals of care for patients with impaired mobility are to maintain and improve functional abilities (by maintaining normal function and alignment, preventing edema of extremities, and reducing spasticity) and to prevent complications.

- Encourage active ROM exercises for unaffected extremities and perform passive ROM exercises for affected extremities every 4 hours during day and evening shifts and once during the night shift. Support the joint during passive ROM exercises. *Active ROM exercises maintain or improve muscle strength and endurance, and help to maintain cardiopulmonary function. Passive ROM exercises do not strengthen muscles but do help maintain joint flexibility.*

> **PRACTICE ALERT**
> Both active and passive exercises increase venous return, decreasing the risk of thrombophlebitis.

- Turn every 2 hours around the clock, following a posted schedule for side-to-side and supine-to-prone position changes (verify prone positioning with the physician). Maintain body alignment and support extremities in proper position with pillows. *Turning on a regular basis, accompanied by proper positioning, maintains joint function, alleviates pressure on bony prominences that can lead to skin breakdown, decreases dependent edema in hands and feet, and lessens the risk of complications resulting from immobility.*

> **PRACTICE ALERT**
> When lying on the affected side, patients may be restless because they do not have normal sensation and feel as if they may fall.

- Monitor the lower extremities each shift for manifestations of thrombophlebitis. Assess for increased warmth and redness in calves; measure the circumference of the calves and thighs. Provide care for sequential compression stockings (per agency protocol), if prescribed. *Patients on bed rest (especially those with loss of muscle strength and tone) are particularly prone to the development of deep venous thrombosis. Promptly report manifestations of thrombophlebitis.*
- Collaborate with the physical therapist as the patient gains mobility, using consistent techniques to move the patient from the bed to the wheelchair and to help the patient ambulate. *The use of consistent techniques facilitates rehabilitation.*

Self-Care Deficit (Bathing, Dressing, Feeding, and/or Toileting)

The patient who has had a stroke may have a self-care deficit as a result of impaired mobility or mental confusion. It is important for patients to perform as much of their own physical care and grooming as possible to promote functional ability, increase independence, decrease feelings of powerlessness, and improve self-esteem. Before establishing a plan to increase self-care, determine which hand was dominant before the stroke. If the patient's dominant side is affected, self-care will be more difficult.

- Screen for executive cognitive dysfunction (abstract thought, actions planned and taken toward a goal, adaptation to the unexpected). *Executive cognitive dysfunction can more reliably predict loss of autonomy than memory impairment can. This assessment (see further information at the Lippincott's Nursing Center website) is essential to helping a patient remain as safe and independent as possible (Kennedy & Smith, 2008).*
- Encourage use of the unaffected arm to bathe, brush teeth, comb hair, dress, and eat. *Use of the unaffected arm promotes functional ability and independence.*
- Teach the patient to put on clothing by first dressing the affected extremities and then dressing the unaffected extremities. *This technique facilitates self-dressing with minimal assistance.*
- Collaborate with the occupational therapist in scheduling times for training for upper extremity functioning necessary for activities of daily living (ADLs). Encourage the use of assistive devices (if required) for eating, physical hygiene, and dressing. *Following a regular schedule in daily routines promotes learning. The use of assistive devices promotes independence and decreases feelings of powerlessness. Optimal grooming facilitates positive self-concept.*

Impaired Verbal Communication

The patient who loses communication abilities requires intensive speech therapy and emotional support. It is important to determine the specific nature of the impairment when planning interventions and helping family members understand specific problems. Although the speech therapist is usually most involved with speech rehabilitation, nurses must plan interventions to meet communication needs during all phases of care. Use the following guidelines:

- Approach and treat the patient as an adult.
- Do not assume that the patient who does not respond verbally cannot hear. Do not use a raised voice when addressing the patient.

- Allow adequate time for the patient to respond.
- Face the patient and speak slowly.
- When you do not understand the patient's speech, be honest and say so.
- Use short, simple statements and questions.
  Accepting the patient and providing dignity and respect enhances the nurse–patient relationship. Allowing adequate response time and using short verbal statements or questions while facing the patient motivates the patient to communicate and decreases frustration.
- Accept frustration and anger as a normal reaction to the loss of function. *Anger represents the patient's frustration at the inability to control the loss of function.*
- Try alternate methods of communication, including writing tablets, flash cards, and computerized talking boards. *Patients unable to communicate verbally may use other methods effectively.*

Impaired Urinary Elimination and Risk for Constipation

Both urinary and bowel elimination may be altered because of neurologic deficits, impaired mobility, cognitive impairment, communication deficits, or preexisting problems (especially if the patient is an older adult). Other causes include changes in food and fluid intake and side effects of medications. Urinary incontinence or retention and constipation, fecal incontinence, and fecal impaction are the usual manifestations.

- Assess for urinary frequency, urgency, incontinence, nocturia, and voiding in small amounts. In addition, assess the patient's ability to respond to the need to void, the ability to use the call light, and the ability to use toileting equipment. Use established guidelines to assess and manage patients with urinary incontinence (Dowling-Castronovo & Gradway, 2008).

> **PRACTICE ALERT**
> Voiding small amounts of urine frequently may be a manifestation of a bladder dysfunction. Assess for a distended bladder.

- Encourage bladder training by having patient void on schedule, such as every 2 hours, rather than in response to the urge to void.
- Teach Kegel exercises. To perform Kegel exercises, the patient contracts the perineal muscles as though stopping urination, holds the contraction for 5 seconds, and then releases.
- Use positive reinforcement (verbal praise) for successful management of urinary elimination.
  Voiding every 2 hours or on schedule promotes bladder tone and urine storage. Kegel exercises increase pubococcygeal muscle tone and bladder control, decreasing incontinence. Positive reinforcement can be a useful part of the teaching program.
- Discuss prestroke bowel habits, as well as the pattern of bowel elimination since the stroke.
- If the patient is able to swallow without difficulty, encourage fluids (up to 2000 mL per day) and a high-fiber diet.
- Increase physical activity as tolerated.

- Assist in using the toilet facilities at the same time each day (based on usual patterns of bowel elimination), ensuring privacy and having the patient sit in an upright position if at all possible.
- Administer prescribed stool softeners if the patient is following a bowel elimination routine or is not drinking sufficient fluids.
  Increased fluids, fiber, and activity stimulate intestinal motility. Establishing a regular daily time for bowel movements in the upright position and in privacy promotes normal bowel elimination. Stool softeners help prevent the formation of hard stool that is more difficult to expel.

Impaired Swallowing

A stroke may impair the ability to swallow. Weakness or lack of coordination of the tongue, attention deficits, and deficits involving the swallowing reflex all play a role. Dysphagia (difficulty swallowing) may result in choking, drooling, aspiration, or regurgitation. Nursing care focuses on maintaining safety by preventing aspiration and on ensuring adequate nutrition.

- Monitor results of swallowing studies (often conducted by a physical therapist) prior to providing oral food and fluids.
- When eating, do the following to avoid aspiration and ensure safety.
  - Position in upright sitting position with neck slightly flexed.
  - Order puréed or soft food. Liquids should be of the same consistency as honey.
  - Feed or teach patient to eat by putting food behind the front teeth on the unaffected side of the mouth and tilting the head slightly backward. Teach to swallow one bite at a time.
  - Assess for coughing with eating or drinking.
  - Have suction equipment available at the bedside in case of choking or aspiration.
  Sitting upright with the head and neck first slightly flexed and then tilted back helps the patient swallow. The patient can usually swallow puréed or soft foods more easily than liquid or solid foods. Using the unaffected side of the mouth helps prevent food from collecting in the mouth and makes swallowing safer; in addition, food is less likely to fall out of the mouth.

> **PRACTICE ALERT**
> After eating, check the mouth for "pocketing" of food, especially in the affected cheek.

- Monitor lung sounds. *Coarse lung sounds heard in the right upper and/or lower lobes may indicate aspiration as the right bronchus is the first division of the bronchi and where the majority of aspirations occur.*
- Minimize distractions and, if necessary, give step-by-step instructions for eating. *Distractions increase the risk of aspiration. Complex activities are easier to perform when broken down into small steps.*

Using NANDA, NIC, and NOC

Linkages between a selected NANDA nursing diagnosis, NIC, and NOC for the patient with a stroke are shown in the chart that follows.

CASE STUDY & NURSING CARE PLAN   A Patient with a Stroke

Orville Boren is a 63-year-old African American who had a stroke due to a right cerebral thrombosis 1 week ago. He is a history instructor at the local community college. His hobbies are wood carving and gardening. Mr. Boren is also an active member of his church. For the past 2 years, Mr. Boren has been taking medication for hypertension, but his wife Emily reports that he often forgets to take it and that his blood pressure was high at his last physical examination. Mrs. Boren tells the staff that she has never had to worry about her husband's health before and that she wants to learn everything she can to care for him at home. However, she says that her husband was always the one to make the decisions and pay the bills. Mrs. Boren adds that all the children, grandchildren, neighbors, and family pastor want to see Mr. Boren back at home as soon as possible.

ASSESSMENT

Carol Merck, RN, the nurse assigned to Mr. Boren, completes a health history and physical assessment, with Mrs. Boren providing information for the history. Mrs. Boren reports that her husband did have several spells of dizziness and blurred vision the week before his stroke, but they lasted only a few minutes and he believed them to be due to "old age and working out in the sun." On the morning of admission, Mr. Boren woke up and could not move his left arm or leg; he also could not speak sensibly. Mrs. Boren called 911, and an ambulance took her husband to the hospital.

Physical assessment findings include the following: Mr. Boren is drowsy but responds to verbal stimuli. Although he does not respond verbally, he can nod his head to indicate "yes" when asked questions. Flaccid paralysis is present in his left arm and left leg, with no response noted to touch in those extremities (he is left handed). Visual fields are decreased in a pattern consistent with homonymous hemianopia. A CT scan, negative on admission; is repeated on the day after admission and confirms the medical diagnosis of a right-brain stroke due to a thrombus of the middle cerebral artery.

Mr. Boren's medical treatment includes heparin sodium administered by continuous intravenous drip, with clotting studies to be performed every 4 hours and the dose adjusted accordingly.

DIAGNOSES

- *Feeding Self-Care Deficit* related to loss of the ability to use the left hand and arm
- *Impaired Physical Mobility* related to neurologic deficits causing left hemiplegia
- *Risk for Impaired Skin Integrity* related to inability to change position
- *Sensory Perception Disturbed: Visual* related to changes in visual fields
- *Impaired Verbal Communication* related to cerebral injury

EXPECTED OUTCOMES

- Learn to use his right hand to feed himself.
- Participate in exercises necessary to maintain muscle strength and tone.
- Maintain skin integrity.
- Indicate understanding that visual fields may improve in a few weeks.
- Practice and implement speech therapy activities while at the same time using alternative methods of communication.

PLANNING AND IMPLEMENTATION

- Arrange mealtimes so that he is sitting up by the window in a clean and private environment.
- Provide adaptive devices (silverware with thick handles and nonslip plates).
- Encourage Mrs. Boren to visit at mealtimes, to assist with meals, and periodically to bring a favorite food from home.
- Provide passive ROM exercises for his left arm and leg; schedule active ROM exercises for his right extremities as well as quadriceps and gluteal sets every 4 hours during waking hours.
- Keep his skin clean and dry at all times.
- Establish and maintain a regular schedule for turning when he is in bed.
- Place objects (e.g., call bell, tissues) on unaffected side and approach him from that side.
- Support attempts to communicate verbally; when he is not understood, he prefers to use a large marker and tablet.

EVALUATION

Mr. Boren is discharged to his home with home health visits ordered for physical therapy, occupational therapy, speech therapy, and skilled nursing care. During the first 2 months after discharge, Martha Grimes, RN, the home health nurse, visits Mr. and Mrs. Boren at home. At the end of 2 months, Mr. Boren is using his right hand to feed himself. He has regained partial use of his left arm and leg and is using a walker to move around the house and yard; he is even able to work in his flower garden. His skin has remained intact, and his vision is back to normal. He is slowly relearning speech; this has been the most difficult change for him to accept. Once he writes on his tablet, "I think God has forgotten me."

CRITICAL THINKING IN THE NURSING PROCESS

1. Hypertension is sometimes referred to as "the silent killer." Provide justifications for this statement.
2. The functional changes Mr. Boren has experienced may make a return to teaching difficult. What other uses of his knowledge and abilities might you suggest?
3. What would be your reply if, after you had completed passive ROM on Mr. Boren's left arm, he wrote, "I just ignore that part of my body—it doesn't work anyway"?

See Evaluating Your Response in Appendix C.

Community-Based Care

Throughout the rehabilitation process, it is important not only to encourage self-care as much as possible but also to involve family members in the plan of care. Stress that ADLs may take twice as long as they did before the stroke. Emphasize that physical function may continue to improve for up to 3 months, and speech may continue to improve for even longer. Address the following topics in preparing the patient and family for community-based care:

- Physical care, medications, physical therapy, occupational therapy, speech therapy.
- Home environment conducive to using equipment (such as a wheelchair or walker) and equipment modifications (e.g., a raised toilet seat, grab bars in the bathroom, a bath chair, a vise lid opener, a long-handled shoehorn).

- Home health services.
- Community resources, such as Meals on Wheels, senior centers, eldercare, large-print telephone dials, stroke clubs, Lifeline (emergency alerting systems through a local hospital or agency). Financial assistance may be available within the community for housekeeping and personal care assistance.
- Helpful organizational resources include the American Heart Association, the National Stroke Association, Stroke Clubs International, and The National Institute of Neurological Disorders and Stroke.

The Patient with an Intracranial Aneurysm

An *intracranial aneurysm* is a saccular outpouching of a cerebral artery that occurs at the site of a weakness in the vessel wall. It is believed to be the result of a congenital defect in a cerebral vessel wall. A ruptured cerebral aneurysm is the most common cause of a hemorrhagic stroke. Seen most often in adults over the age of 50, a ruptured intracranial aneurysm often results in death or severe disability in those who survive (Porth & Matfin, 2009).

Pathophysiology

Intracranial aneurysms tend to occur at the bifurcations in the circle of Willis. Intracranial aneurysms often enlarge over time, making the vessel wall thin and increasing the probability of rupture. There are several types, but most are small saccular aneurysm called berry aneurysms (small berry-like projections). Rupture of these aneurysms results in bleeding into the subarachnoid space (causing a subarachnoid hemmorhage).

Manifestations

The manifestations of a ruptured intracranial aneurysm (and subsequent subarachnoid hemorrhage) include a sudden, explosive headache and neck pain; nausea and vomiting; a stiff neck and photophobia (due to meningeal irritation); cranial nerve deficits; and stroke syndrome. Hypertension and cardiac dysrhythmias may occur from the massive release of catecholamines triggered by the subarachnoid hemorrhage. Fibrin and platelets seal off the bleeding point, but the escaped blood forms a clot that irritates the brain tissue. The resulting inflammatory response causes cerebral edema, and both the edema and the hemorrhage increase intracranial pressure. The pituitary gland is in close proximity to the circle of Willis and is often affected secondary to edema and irritation, with resulting diabetes insipidus and hyponatremia.

Complications

The major complications of a ruptured intracranial aneurysm are rebleeding and vasospasm. Hypothalamic dysfunction, hydrocephalus, and seizures are also potential complications. The greatest risk for rebleeding is within the first two weeks after the initial rupture, although it may occur at any time following the initial occurance. Approximately 70% of patients who have rebleeding will die (Hickey, 2009). Cerebral vasospasm is a common but dangerous complication that is associated with a large number of deaths and disability. A cerebral vasospasm narrows the lumen of one or more cerebral vessels, causing ischemia and infarction of brain tissue supplied by the affected vessels. It occurs in blood vessels surrounded by thick blood clots, and is thought to be the result of the release of ET-1, a potent vasoconstrictor of cerebral arteries (Hickey, 2009). The manifestations vary according to the degree of spasm and the area of brain affected. Regional alterations may cause focal deficits (such as hemiplegia), whereas global alterations cause loss of consciousness.

Interdisciplinary Care

The care of the patient with a ruptured intracranial aneurysm includes determining the location of the aneurysm, treating the manifestations of the hemorrhage, and preventing rebleeding and vasospasm. Interventions using radiology, angiography, and a variety of procedures may be used to prevent aneurysm rupture or to stop the bleeding. Surgery is usually the treatment of choice to repair the bleeding artery.

Diagnosis

The diagnostic tests conducted to identify the site and extent of a ruptured intracranial aneurysm, as well as rebleeding, are a CT scan, a spiral computed tomography angiogram (CTA), and bilateral carotid and vertebral cerebral angiograms. A CT is used to initially detect the hemorrhage, and a CTA can rapidly identify the arterial anatomy. Angiograms provide visualization of all four major cerebral vessels and their branches, providing early diagnosis and treatment. A lumbar puncture will reveal blood-tinged spinal fluid.

Medications

Calcium channel blockers, such as nimodipine (Nimotop), are used to improve neurologic deficits due to vasospasm following subarachnoid hemorrhage from ruptured intracranial aneurysms. Administered orally or by feeding tube (never IV), it has been found to enhance collateral blood flow and improve outcomes (Hickey, 2009; McPhee et al., 2008).

Other medications that may be prescribed include anticonvulsants, such as phenytoin (Dilantin), to prevent seizures if the patient has IICP; analgesics for headache; antacids and H2-receptor antagonist (such as ranitidine [Xanax]) to prevent gastric irritation; and stool softeners to prevent constipation and straining with a bowel movement (which increases intracranial pressure and blood pressure and may cause rebleeding).

Procedures Used to Treat Aneurysm

Treatments for an intracranial aneurysm are performed either to prevent rupture or to isolate the vessel to prevent further bleeding. Patients with good neurologic status may have surgery soon after the rupture. In patients with significant neurologic deficits, surgery may be delayed until they are more stable and less at risk for vasospasm; however, the trend is toward surgery as soon as possible.

Several different types of procedures are used to repair a ruptured intracranial aneurysm or to prevent the rupture of an existing large aneurysm. The neck of the aneurysm may be clipped with a metal clip to prevent entry of blood into the aneurysm. Endovascular techniques that may be used include balloon embolization and platinum coil electrothrombosis.

✎ Nursing Care

Nursing care is planned and implemented for the patient with a ruptured intracranial aneurysm to prevent rebleeding as well as to meet needs resulting from neurologic deficits. Appropriate nursing diagnoses and interventions are described earlier in the chapter in the discussion of nursing care for the patient with a stroke. The priority interventions in the acute care stage of a ruptured intracranial aneurysm focus on ineffective cerebral tissue perfusion.

The Patient with an Arteriovenous Malformation

An arteriovenous (AV) malformation is a congenital intracranial lesion, formed by a tangled collection of dilated arteries and veins that allows blood to flow directly from the arterial into the venous system, bypassing the normal capillary network. Most AV malformations (90%) are located in the cerebral hemispheres; the remainder are found in the cerebellum and brainstem.

Rupture of vessels in the malformations account for 2% of all strokes. Patients with this condition develop manifestations before 40 years of age; it affects men and women equally (Porth & Matfin, 2009). The manifestations are the result of spontaneous bleeding from the lesion into the subarachnoid space or brain tissue.

Pathophysiology

AV malformations, believed to arise from failure of development of the capillary network in the embryo, displace rather than encompass normal brain tissue. The pathophysiologic effects of an AV malformation are the result of the shunting of blood from the arterial to the venous system and of altered perfusion of cerebral tissue near the malformation. The

shunting of arterial blood directly into the venous system within the malformation transfers the higher arterial pressure directly into the lower pressure venous system. This increased pressure is likely to cause spontaneous bleeding or progressive expansion and rupture of a blood vessel. Altered cerebral perfusion results when blood flow through a large, high-flow malformation is diverted from the normal cerebral circulation, causing tissue ischemia of the area surrounding the malformation. This is sometimes called a vascular "steal" phenomenon.

AV malformations range in size from very small to very large. Large malformations are usually initially manifested by seizure activity. In contrast, the manifestations of a small malformation are more often due to a hemorrhage that causes neurologic deficits. In both instances, the patient may have recurrent headaches that do not respond to treatment.

Interdisciplinary Care

AV malformations are diagnosed with the same diagnostic tests used to diagnose an intracranial aneurysm. Treatment is by surgical excision, vascular occlusion, and radiosurgery. When the malformation is excised or obstructed, blood flow is no longer shunted, and cerebral perfusion improves.

✎ Nursing Care

Nursing care depends on the condition of the malformation. If hemorrhage has not occurred, teach the patient to avoid activities that raise blood pressure or could cause injury. The patient is usually given medications to control blood pressure and prevent seizures. If the malformation ruptures and causes an intracranial hemorrhage, nursing care is the same as for the patient who has had a stroke.

The Patient with a Traumatic Brain Injury

Traumatic brain injury (TBI) (also called craniocerebral trauma) refers to any injury of the scalp, skull (cranium or facial bones), or brain. TBI is a leading cause of death and disability in the United States. The National Head Injury Foundation defines TBI as a traumatic insult to the brain capable of causing physical, intellectual, emotional, social, and vocational changes. A TBI may be classified as a penetrating (or open) head injury (when an object pierces the skull and enters the brain) or a closed head injury (the head suddenly and violently hits an object but the object does not break through the skull). Damage to the brain may be focal (confined to one area) or diffuse (involving more than one area of the brain). TBI may cause problems with cognition, movement, sensation, and emotions. Even mild brain injuries, if repeated over an extended period of time, can result in cumulative neurologic and cognitive deficits. TBI is a major public health problem, especially among males ages 15 to 24 and among both men and women 75 years of age or older (NINDS, 2008c). People ages 75 and older have the highest rates of TBI-related hospitalizations and death (CDC, 2008).

FAST FACTS
TBI

- 1.4 million people have a TBI each year; of those, 230,000 are hospitalized and survive.
- Each year, 50,000 people die of TBI.
- An estimated 5.3 million Americans are living with disabilities from TBI.
- Blasts are the leading cause of TBI among military personnel in war zones; veterans advocates believe 150,000 to 300,000 Iraq veterans have suffered TBI.

(Brain Trauma Organization, 2007; Coyle & Martin, 2007; NINDS. 2008c)

According to the NINDS (2008c), more than 50% of all TBIs in adults under the age of 75 are the result of crashes involving cars, motorcycles, bicycles, and pedestrians. TBIs in adults over the age of 75 are the result of falls. Other causes include violence and sports injuries. At least half of all TBIs involve alcohol or other drug use. The cause often determines the outcome; 91% of TBI from firearms (two-thirds of which may involve suicides) result in death, while 11% of TBIs from falls result in death.

Specific damage following craniocerebral injuries is related to the mechanism of the injury (how it occurs), the nature of the injury (type), and the location of the injury (where it occurs).

Head injuries may occur through several mechanisms:

- Contact phenomena injury is sustained when the head is struck by a moving object, such as a swinging bat. It includes local effects such as scalp lacerations and/or skull fractures and intracerebral contusions, lacerations, hematoma, and hemorrhage.
- Acceleration-deceleration injury (linear injuries) occurs when the head hits an object and the brain "rebounds" within the skull (Figure 42–8 ■). The brain is injured at the point of impact (the coup) and on the opposite side of the impact (the contrecoup). Strain on cerebral tissue produce injury by compression, tension, or shearing. This type of injury is responsible for acute subdural hematoma and diffuse axonal injury.
- Rotational injury occurs when the brain rotates within the skull and hits bony buttresses in the cranial vault; these injuries are more severe than those from linear injuries.

Contrecoup

Coup

Figure 42–8 ■ Coup-contrecoup head injury. Following the initial injury (coup), the brain rebounds within the skull and sustains additional injury (contrecoup) in the opposite part of the brain.

Types of craniocerebral trauma include injuries to the skull, injuries to the brain (including concussion and contusion), and intracranial hematomas and hemorrhage. Brain injury can result either from the direct effects of the trauma on brain tissue or from secondary responses to trauma, such as cerebral edema, hematoma, or IICP.

Focal or Diffuse Traumatic Brain Injury

The brain is protected from injury by enclosure in the bones of the skull and the cushioning effects of cerebral spinal fluid. Metabolic stability is maintained by a variety of mechanisms, including the blood-brain barrier and autoregulation of blood supply. However, damage to the brain can occur from the direct effects of trauma as well as from injury from ischemia, cerebral edema, IICP, hypoxia, and infection. These mechanisms of injury are often interrelated.

Pathophysiology

Brain injury results from both primary and secondary mechanisms. Primary injury results from the impact. A blow to the head, even with no break in the skull, can cause serious and diffuse brain injury. Injury to axons disrupts oligodendroglia, and direct mechanical disruption is caused by debris and leakage.

Secondary injury is the progression of the initial injury resulting from events that affect perfusion and oxygenation of brain cells. The theories of cause and mechanisms of secondary injury are summarized here. They include the effects of hypoxia, ischemia, and inflammation. Hypoxia interferes with the delivery of oxygen; ischemia interferes with the delivery of oxygen and glucose and with the removal of metabolic wastes. The consequences of cerebral ischemia include increased cellular permeability to sodium (cytotoxic edema), and release of free fatty acids and lactic acidosis. The release of excitatory amino acids (such as glutamate and aspartate) causes an influx of calcium with changes in electrophysiology. The inflammatory process begins immediately, resulting in the release of cytokines. It is unknown if these cytokines are protective or injurious, but it is known that inflammatory mediators such as tumor necrosis factor increase with TBI and are associated with cerebral edema, disruption of the blood-brain barrier, and death of neurons (Hickey, 2009; Porth & Matfin, 2009).

Acute brain injury affects all body systems as well as the central nervous system. Systemic effects of acute brain injury are listed in Table 42–5.

Focal Brain Injuries

Focal brain injuries are specific brain lesions confined to one area of the brain. They include contusions and hemorrhage/hematomas. The force of an impact produces contusions from direct contact with the inside of the skull that in turn may cause epidural hemorrhage and subdural and intracerebral hematomas. The mechanisms of injury are damage to the brain at the point of the impact and the rebound effect. The damaged area is surrounded by edema, contributing to IICP. Infarction and necrosis, multiple hemorrhages, and edema are found within the contused areas.

TABLE 42–5 Systemic Effects of Acute Brain Injury

CAUSE	EFFECT
■ Stimulation of the sympathetic nervous system, which stimulates the adrenal cortex and medulla to increase glucocorticoid and mineralocorticoid levels	■ Increased metabolism of carbohydrates, fats, and proteins ■ Retention of sodium and water
■ Stimulation of the sympathetic nervous system, increasing the serum catecholamine levels	■ Hypertension ■ EEG changes ■ Dysrhythmias (bradycardia, sinus tachycardia)
■ Altered release of ADH from the posterior pituitary	■ Retention of water or diuresis and diabetes insipidus
■ Neurogenic pulmonary dysfunction	■ Abnormal respiratory patterns ■ Reduced residual capacity with retention of CO_2, vasodilation, and increased ICP ■ Pulmonary edema
■ Stress response to trauma	■ Hyperglycemia
■ Increased platelet, plasma fibrinogen, and thromboplastin levels	■ Decreased clotting and prothrombin times ■ Vascular occlusion ■ Disseminated intravascular coagulation ■ Anemia
■ Immunosuppression	■ Infection
■ Decreased gastric motility and increased gastric acidity	■ Gastritis ■ Gastric ulcers

Intracranial hemorrhage can result directly from the trauma or from shearing forces on cerebral arteries and veins that occur with acceleration–deceleration. Depending on the site and rate of bleeding, manifestations may appear immediately or may not become evident for hours or even weeks. Intracranial hemorrhages and the hematomas they cause place pressure on surrounding structures, causing manifestations of an expanding focal lesion. They also cause IICP, leading to altered levels of consciousness and potential herniation syndromes. Intracranial hematomas are classified by their location as epidural, subdural, or intracerebral. Table 42–6 compares the frequency, locations, common sites, precipitating factors, and manifestations of intracranial hematomas; Figure 42–9 ■ illustrates their locations.

Figure 42–9 ■ Three types of hematomas: epidural hematoma, subdural hematoma, and intracerebral hematoma.

CONTUSION A cerebral contusion is a bruise of the surface of the brain, typically accompanied by small, diffuse venous hemorrhages. Both white and gray matter may have a bruised, discolored appearance. Contusions (and other focal brain injuries) occur when the brain strikes the inner skull, often with a coup (point of impact) lesion and a contrecoup lesion on the opposite side of the brain. Contusions occur most frequently near bony prominences of the skull. Cerebral edema can follow contusion, resulting in IICP. Contusions; small, diffuse venous hemorrhages; and brain swelling are at their peak 12 to 24 hours after injury.

Manifestations of the contusion depend on the size and location of the brain injury. An initial loss of consciousness occurs; LOC may remain altered, and behavior changes such as combativeness may persist for an extended period. Full consciousness may be regained extremely slowly, and residual deficits may persist; in some patients, full LOC never really returns. Focal effects of the contusion may cause loss of reflexes, hemiparesis (muscular weakness of one-half of the body), or abnormal posturing. Manifestations of IICP may occur if cerebral edema develops. Regaining full LOC may take an extended period of time and residual deficits may persist.

EPIDURAL HEMATOMA An **epidural hematoma** (also called an extradural hematoma) develops in the potential space between the dura and the skull, which normally adhere to one another. As the blood collects, the expanding hematoma pulls the dura away from the skull. Epidural hematomas affect young to middle-aged adults more frequently than older adults, because the dura becomes more tightly attached to the skull with aging.

Epidural hematomas usually result from a skull fracture that tears an artery, often the middle meningeal artery. Because

TABLE 42–6   Comparison of Intracranial Hematomas

TYPE/FREQUENCY	LOCATION/COMMON SITE	PRECIPITATING FACTORS	MANIFESTATIONS
Epidural Hematoma 2% to 6% of all types of head injuries	Located in the space between the skull and the dura mater **Common site:** the temporal bone (over the middle meningeal artery)	Skull fractures Contusion	Momentary loss of consciousness followed by a lucid period lasting from a few hours to 1 to 2 days Rapid deterioration in level of consciousness (drowsiness to confusion to coma) Seizures Headache Hemiparesis (may be ipsilateral or contralateral) Fixed dilated ipsilateral pupil Rise in blood pressure with decreases in pulse and respirations indicates a rapidly increasing hematoma
Subdural Hematoma Approximately 29% of all types of head injuries	Located in the space below the dural surface (between the dura and arachnoid and pia mater layers of meninges) **Common site:** may occur any place in cranium	Closed head injury Acceleration–deceleration injury Cerebral atrophy (seen in older adults) Chronic alcoholism Use of anticoagulants Contusion	Acute: ■ Headache ■ Drowsiness ■ Agitation ■ Slowed thinking ■ Confusion Subacute: ■ Same as those of acute subdural hematoma but develop more slowly Chronic: ■ Manifestations may not appear until weeks to months after injury ■ Confusion, slowed thinking, drowsiness
Intracerebral Hematoma 14% to 15% of all types of head injuries	Located directly in the brain tissue **Common site:** frontal or temporal region	Gunshot wounds Depressed bone fractures Stab injury Long history of systemic hypertension Contusions	Headache Deteriorating consciousness to deep coma Hemiplegia on contralateral side Dilated pupil on the side of the clot

epidural hematomas are arterial in origin, they tend to develop rapidly. The patient may lose consciousness with the initial injury and then have a brief lucid period before the LOC rapidly declines from drowsiness to coma as the hematoma expands, compressing brain tissue. Other manifestations include headache; vomiting; a fixed, dilated pupil on the same side (ipsilateral) as the hematoma; contralateral (opposite side) hemiparesis or hemiplegia; and possible seizures. Because epidural hematomas usually develop rapidly, timely intervention is vital to prevent significant increases in ICP and herniation.

SUBDURAL HEMATOMA   **Subdural hematomas**, in which a localized mass of blood collects between the dura mater and the arachnoid mater, are more common than epidural hematomas. Acute subdural hematomas are usually located at the top of the head, and develop within 48 hours of the initial head injury. Although a lucid period may occur, the patient commonly develops drowsiness, confusion, and enlargement of the ipsilateral pupil within minutes or hours of the injury. If responsive, the patient may complain of a unilateral headache. Hemiparesis and respiratory pattern changes may occur.

Chronic subdural hematomas develop over weeks or months. The chronic type is seen most often in older adults and people who have some brain atrophy with subsequent enlarged epidural space. Chronic subdural hematomas are often associated with relatively minor trauma such as a fall or may occur spontaneously in the older adult or in patients with bleeding disorders. Manifestations of the hematoma develop slowly and may be mistaken for the onset of dementia in the older adult. Slowed thinking, confusion, drowsiness, or lethargy are common early manifestations. Other manifestations include headache, dilation and sluggishness of the ipsilateral pupil, and possible seizures.

INTRACEREBRAL HEMATOMA   Intracerebral hematomas may be single or multiple, and are associated with contusions. They may occur in any location but usually are found in the frontal or temporal lobes. They may result from closed head trauma, particularly contusion or shearing of small blood vessels deep within the hemispheres. Intracerebral hematomas can also accompany other types of head trauma such as lacerations. Older adults are particularly vulnerable to intracerebral hemorrhage because cerebral blood vessels are more fragile and easily torn. The manifestations of intracerebral hematoma vary according to the location of the hematoma. Headache may develop, along with decreasing LOC, hemiplegia, and dilation of the ipsilateral pupil. The expanding clot increases intracranial pressure, and herniation may occur.

Diffuse Cerebral Injury

A diffuse cerebral injury (concussion and diffuse axonal injury) affects the entire brain and is caused by a shaking motion, with twisting movement (rotational injury) as the primary mechanism of injury. Shearing stresses on brain tissue cause axonal damage from shearing, tearing, or stretching of nerve fibers. The most serious axonal injuries are located farthest from the brainstem, with the frontal and temporal axonal tracts being most vulnerable to injury. Physical deficits include spastic paralysis, peripheral nerve injury, swallowing disorders, visual and hearing impairments, and taste and smell disorders. Damage to axons decreases the speed of information processing and responding and disrupts attention, resulting in serious cognitive and affective impairments. Cognitive deficits that may result include disorientation and confusion, short attention span, problems with memory and learning, perceptual problems, and poor judgment. Possible behavioral deficits include agitation, impulsivity, depression, and social withdrawal.

Initially, the damage involves tearing of axons, blood vessels, and brain tissue (visible only by electron microscope). The number of damaged axons progressively increases, with pathology involving the nuclei and axons. The damaged axons, which resemble sausage links, regress into round balls called retraction balls (visible with light microscopy). After several weeks, the retraction balls are replaced by clusters of microglia. In the final phase, astrocytosis (equivalent to scarring) occurs at the site of axonal damage, accompanied by demyelination of long axon tracts.

MILD CONCUSSION   The word **concussion** means violent shaking. A concussion involves temporary axonal disturbances. It is defined as a momentary interruption of brain function. A concussion is associated with an immediate, brief loss of consciousness on impact. Altered consciousness may last only seconds or persist for several hours. Amnesia for events immediately preceding (antegrade amnesia) and following (retrograde amnesia) the injury is common. Other manifestations of concussion are listed in the accompanying box.

CLASSIC CEREBRAL CONCUSSION   A classic cerebral concussion involves diffuse cerebral disconnection from the brainstem RAS. An immediate loss of consciousness occurs, lasting less than 6 hours. Both retrograde and antegrade amnesia occur, and cerebral contusions may be present. In a severe concussion, a brief seizure and respiratory arrest may occur; transient pallor, bradycardia, and hypotension may accompany loss of consciousness. Patients may develop postconcussion syndrome with persistent headache, dizziness, irritability, insomnia, impaired memory and concentration, and learning problems. Postconcussion syndrome may last for several weeks or, rarely, up to a year.

MANIFESTATIONS of Concussion

- Immediate loss of consciousness (lasting usually no longer than 5 minutes)
- Amnesia for events surrounding injury
- Headache
- Drowsiness, confusion, dizziness
- Visual disturbances (diplopia, blurred vision)
- Possible brief seizure activity with transient apnea, bradycardia, pallor, and hypotension

POSTCONCUSSION SYNDROME

- Persistent headache
- Dizziness
- Irritability and insomnia
- Impaired memory and concentration, learning problems

DIFFUSE AXONAL INJURY   Diffuse axonal injury (DAI) is a brain injury in which a high-speed acceleration–deceleration injury, typically associated with motor vehicle crashes, causes widespread disruption of axons in the white matter. Focal lesions may be found in the corpus callosum, midbrain, and brainstem. An immediate loss of consciousness occurs. DAI accounts for approximately 50% of primary brain injuries and accounts for 35% of deaths from all TBIs (Hickey, 2009).

DAIs may range from mild to severe. In mild DAI, coma lasts 6 to 24 hours, and cognitive, psychologic, and sensorimotor deficits may persist. In moderate DAI, injury and impairment is spread throughout the cerebral cortex and diencephalon. There is axonal tearing, coma lasting more than 24 hours, and often incomplete recovery. In severe DAI, axonal injury occurs in both cerebral hemispheres, the diencephalon, and the brainstem. Immediate autonomic dysfunction occurs, and IICP is manifested. Profound cognitive and sensorimotor deficits occur, involving movement, verbal and written communication, ability to learn and reason, and ability to modulate behavior.

Interdisciplinary Care

The patient with a brain injury may receive medical and/or surgical treatment. Although patients with a mild concussion may be assessed and sent home for recovery, most people who have a TBI require intensive care at a trauma center. Evidence-based guidelines for medical care have been established by the Brain Trauma Foundation in the document *Guidelines for the Management of Severe Traumatic Brain Injury* (2007b) and are updated periodically. A summary of the immediate care of the patient with a TBI follows:

- *Concussion:* Following a concussion, the patient may be observed for 1 to 2 hours in the emergency department (ED), and then discharged home with instructions for further observation to detect manifestations of secondary injury. If the loss of consciousness extended more than 2 minutes, the patient may be admitted to the hospital for observation.
- *Acute TBI:* Recognition and management of acute TBI with transport to an ED is essential to patient outcomes. Morbidity and mortality increase with hypotension (systolic pressure less than 90 mmHg) and hypoxia (PaO_2 less than 60 mmHg), so fluids are given to support a mean systolic arterial blood pressure at more than 90 mmHg. The fluid of choice for IV

fluids is hypertonic saline because it reduces IICP (Hickey, 2009). Assessment of the patient's airway, breathing, and circulation (ABCs), with management of dysfunction, is necessary to decrease the secondary effects of the brain injury. An intracranial pressure monitor probe may be inserted to assess ICP and monitor therapy to reduce cerebral edema and maintain cerebral perfusion. Osmotic diuretics such as mannitol also may be administered to reduce cerebral edema. Adequate oxygenation is vital to maintain cerebral metabolism; carbon dioxide is a potent vasodilator, and increased levels may contribute to cerebral edema and IICP.

On admission to the ICU from the ED, the patient may be placed on a special bed and connected to various monitoring devices. Invasive lines are inserted, including a central venous pressure (CVP) catheter, arterial line, pulmonary catheter, ventriculostomy, ICP monitor, and perhaps a retrograde jugular catheter. In most instances, an endotracheal tube is inserted and connected to a mechanical ventilator, cardiac monitoring is initiated, bilateral sequential pressure boots are applied, pulse oximetry is started, and a rectal temperature probe is inserted. Laboratory values are monitored for changes to ensure early detection of cerebral hypoxia and impending ischemia to prevent secondary brain injury.

Diagnosis

Diagnostic testing may be done to monitor hemodynamic status and detect conditions that may contribute to cerebral edema. Radiologic examinations include skull x-rays (to identify skull fractures and assess penetrating objects) and CT scan or MRI to detect contusions and lacerations associated with diffuse axonal injury. ABGs are analyzed, with particular attention to oxygen and carbon dioxide levels.

Managing IICP

IICP is managed to reestablish equilibrium of the intracranial contents and prevent secondary brain damage. Treatments include airway management, hyperventilation (used if signs of herniation appear), fluid resuscitation, positioning, temperature regulation, and medications. Medications other than those previously discussed include a category of drugs called neuroprotectants. These drugs are used to treat or alter some of the pathologic pathways that occur in ischemia, and must be administered within a short time of the injury to be effective. Classifications of the drugs include lipid peroxidase inhibitors, free radical scavengers, receptor antagonists, calcium channel blockers, and gangliosides.

Surgery

Small subdural hematomas can frequently be reabsorbed and may be treated conservatively with close observation and supportive care. However, the treatment of choice for epidural hematomas and large acute subdural hematomas is surgical evacuation of the clot. This can often be performed through burr holes made into the skull (Figure 42–10 ■). In an epidural hematoma, the bleeding vessel can also be ligated during this procedure, preventing further bleeding. Rebleeding may occur following evacuation of an acute subdural hematoma in older adults and patients with chronic alcoholism. A craniotomy is

Figure 42–10 ■ Possible location of Burr holes.

necessary to evacuate chronic subdural hematomas because the hematoma tends to solidify, making it difficult or impossible to remove through burr holes. Surgery is less successful in treating intracerebral hematomas because of widespread tissue damage. Supportive care to manage intracranial pressure and prevent complications is provided.

෴ Nursing Care

In addition to the nursing care discussed in this section, a Case Study & Nursing Care Plan for a patient with a subdural hematoma is found on page 1468.

Health Promotion

The best way to treat any injury is to prevent it from happening. Public education must continue to stress the importance of safe driving, the dangers of driving under the influence of alcohol or drugs, and the necessity of wearing seat belts and cycle helmets. Legislation has mandated such motor vehicle changes as seat belts, child safety seats, air bags, use of headsets with cell phones, and prohibition of texting while driving. Other behaviors that can reduce the morbidity and mortality associated with TBI are following gun safety rules, promoting farm safety, and teaching older adults about safety (such as preventing falls) in the home.

Assessment

Collect the following data through the health history and physical examination (∞ see Chapter 41):

- *Health history:* A history of the injury is helpful in understanding the nature of the craniocerebral trauma; knowledge about loss of consciousness assists the nurse in planning care. However, most patients with severe TBI will not be able to communicate (either from the injury itself or from intubation).

- *Physical examination:* Neurologic assessment, including pupils, LOC, Glasgow Coma Scale (a finding of 3 to 8 denotes severe TBI as defined by the Brain Trauma Foundation), brainstem reflexes (cornea, cough, gag, extraocular movements), spontaneous movement; response to pain; vital signs; skull and face (deformity, lacerations, bruising, bleeding); movement of extremities, other injuries.

Nursing Diagnoses and Interventions

Nursing care of the patient in the acute care phase initially focuses on maintaining an effective airway and breathing pattern. Nursing care is also directed toward continuous assessment and monitoring of neurologic function as well as other body systems. This close monitoring provides early recognition and treatment of problems and complications, and initiation of aggressive forms of therapy that may be needed.

Many nursing diagnoses associated with traumatic brain injury correspond with those outlined previously for the patient with altered LOC, IICP, and seizures. Specific nursing diagnoses discussed in this section focus on problems with intracranial adaptive capacity, airway clearance, and breathing patterns.

Decreased Intracranial Adaptive Capacity

The patient with a traumatic brain injury has or is at high risk for IICP. As the mechanisms that normally compensate for changes in intracranial pressure are compromised, intracranial pressure increases in disproportional response to a variety of stimuli. (See the discussion earlier in the chapter for other nursing diagnoses and interventions for the patient with IICP.)

- Monitor for manifestations of IICP, including eye opening response, motor response, and verbal response. *These responses evaluate the ability to integrate commands with conscious and involuntary movement.*

EVIDENCE FOR NURSING CARE — The Patient with Traumatic Brain Injury

Selected resources that nurses may find helpful when planning evidence-based nursing care follow.

- Carson, S., Davis-O'Reilly, C., Drexel, P., Fu, R., Norris, S., Pappas, M., et al. (2007). Guidelines for the management of severe traumatic brain injury. Brain oxygen monitoring and thresholds. *National Guideline Clearinghouse.* Retrieved from http://www.guideline.gov/summary/summary.aspx?ss=15&doc_id=10998&nbr=5778
- Knuth, T., Letarte, P. B., Ling, G., Moores, L. E., Rhee, P., Tauber, D., et al. (2008). Guidelines for the field management of combat-related head trauma. Treatment: fluid resuscitation. *National Guideline Clearinghouse.* Retrieved from http://www.guideline.gov/summary/summary.aspx?doc_id=11007&nbr=005787&string=hypovolemia
- Marks, J. P., & Daggett, L. M. (2006). A critical pathway for meeting the needs of families of patients with severe traumatic brain injury. *Journal of Neuroscience Nursing, 38*(2), 84–89.
- Bay, E., Sikorskii, A, & Saint-Arnault, D. (2009). Sex differences in depressive symptoms and their correlates after mild-to-moderate traumatic brain injury. *Journal of Neuroscience Nursing, 41*(6), 298–309.

- Monitor for changes in vital signs: bradycardia or tachycardia, varying breathing patterns, hypertension, and/or widening pulse pressure. Vital signs vary depending on the site of impairment. *Cushing's triad (bradycardia, increased systolic blood pressure, and increased pulse pressure) indicates brainstem ischemia leading to cerebral herniation.*
- Monitor for vomiting, headache, lethargy, restlessness, purposeless movements, and changes in mentation. *These manifestations may be early indicators of intracranial pressure changes.*
- Monitor temperature and initiate hypothermia treatment as prescribed. *Impaired hypothalamic function can interfere with temperature regulation. Hyperthermia may increase ICP.*
- Monitor fluid status: Regularly compare intake and output (a urinary catheter is inserted to assess renal perfusion), review serum osmolality, and use infusion pump to administer IV fluids (if prescribed). *Osmotic diuretics, if used to treat cerebral edema, may cause hypotension and decreased cardiac output.*

> **PRACTICE ALERT**
> Overhydration from rapid infusion of IV fluids may cause or further increase IICP.

Ineffective Airway Clearance

The primary objective in the care of any trauma patient is maintaining a patent airway to prevent hypoxia. However, in the initial acute care phase, the risk of cervical vertebral fractures and spinal cord injury may complicate the process of establishing a patent airway. In addition, other multisystem injuries may complicate the interpretation of vital signs. In general, all unconscious people with a head injury should be intubated with an endotracheal tube to prevent aspiration. Patients with head trauma may also require a tracheostomy to provide an airway and be placed on a ventilator.

- Monitor neurologic manifestations on a regular schedule. *Changes in neurologic manifestations may indicate IICP, with the risk of further depression of the respiratory system and respiratory arrest.*
- Maintain head and neck in neutral alignment, immobilized until injury is determined. *Head rotation and neck flexion are associated with IICP, decreased jugular venous outflow, and localized changes in cerebral blood flow. Immobilization prevents spinal cord injury in suspected or actual fractures of the cervical spine; spinal cord injury at this level would further impair respiratory function.*
- Clear the nose and mouth of mucus and blood. *This helps maintain patency of the upper airway.*
- Suction the airway as needed, limiting suctioning time to no more than 10 seconds at one time. Do not suction the nasal passages until a dural tear has been ruled out. *Suctioning is usually necessary to maintain a patent airway.*

Ineffective Breathing Pattern

The patient with a traumatic brain injury and hematoma is at high risk for ineffective breathing pattern related to IICP. If ICP increases dramatically, tentorial herniation may occur, leading to sudden respiratory arrest.

CASE STUDY & NURSING CARE PLAN   The Patient with a Subdural Hematoma

Wong Lee is a 50-year-old tug boat mechanic who is married and has three sons.

Although Mr. Lee has been through rehabilitation twice for alcoholism, he has not been able to quit drinking. His physician has explained the physical consequences and the possible interaction between alcohol and the anticoagulant Mr. Lee is taking for chronic atrial fibrillation. While attending a family reunion, during which he eats a large meal and drinks several beers, Mr. Lee joins a game of softball. Mrs. Lee is concerned that Mr. Lee has consumed too much alcohol to play ball in the heat, but Mr. Lee is adamant and states that he wants to pitch. During the end of the second inning, the batter hits a ball that strikes Mr. Lee in the head. Mr. Lee stumbles and drops to the ground, holding his head. He does not lose consciousness and gets up on his own. His sons and wife try to persuade him to go to the hospital, but Mr. Lee insists he feels fine.

Two weeks later, after an evening of consuming several mixed drinks, Mr. Lee develops a headache. He attributes the headache to a hangover, but instead of improving the next day, the headache becomes steadily worse. He becomes confused and disoriented. His wife, concerned that his drinking is increasing again, calls the physician, who admits Mr. Lee to the detoxification center at the local hospital. A CT scan is performed. The diagnosis of a subdural hematoma is made, and Mr. Lee is transferred to the neurosurgical unit.

ASSESSMENT

When Saundra Knight, the nurse on the neurosurgical unit, enters the room, she notices that Mr. Lee is sitting in bed, laughing and giddy. As she begins to talk to Mr. Lee, he states, "Don't ask me anything—I can't think. My headache is getting worse." Over the next few hours, the giddiness subsides, and Mr. Lee becomes drowsy. Ms. Knight reports a Glasgow Coma Scale score of 11. An ICP monitor is inserted and reveals IICP. Mr. Lee is scheduled to have burr holes and hematoma evacuation that afternoon.

DIAGNOSES
- *Risk for Ineffective Breathing Pattern* related to pressure on respiratory center by intracranial hematoma
- *Ineffective Cerebral Tissue Perfusion* related to IICP secondary to cerebral edema

EXPECTED OUTCOMES
- Maintain a respiratory rate and rhythm within normal limits.
- Maintain adequate cerebral perfusion, as evidenced by stable vital signs, stable neurologic status, and no decrease in level of consciousness.

PLANNING AND IMPLEMENTATION
- Perform neurologic assessment every 2 hours or as needed.
- Monitor vital signs every 2 hours or as needed.
- Explain to the family the procedure for intracranial surgery.

EVALUATION
The first day postoperatively, Mr. Lee begins breathing on his own without ventilatory support. His respiratory rate and rhythm are within normal limits, with no signs of abnormal breath sounds. The ICP monitor readings are appropriate, and Mr. Lee shows significant improvement in level of consciousness, with a Glasgow Coma Scale score of 15. Mr. Lee continues to improve and is discharged to home 5 days after surgery.

CRITICAL THINKING IN THE NURSING PROCESS
1. Describe the similarities and differences between Mr. Lee's disorder and the manifestations of other types of intracranial hematomas.
2. Mr. Lee kept trying to pull out his ICP line. You know he should not be restrained, because pulling against restraints increases restlessness and increases intracranial pressure. What would you do?
3. Write a care plan for Mr. Lee for the nursing diagnosis *Acute Confusion*.

See Evaluating Your Response in Appendix C.

- Monitor the respiratory pattern for rate, depth, and rhythm every 2 hours or as needed if the patient is not on a ventilator. Assess breath sounds, presence of cyanosis, restlessness, and use of accessory respiratory muscles. Monitor pulse oximetry and blood gas levels. *Head injuries may cause alterations in respirations. An increased respiratory rate may indicate hypoxia. A decrease in respiratory rate may be the result of depression of the medullary respiratory center.*

PRACTICE ALERT
In general, an initial increase in intracranial pressure causes respirations to slow; as the pressure continues to increase, respirations become rapid.

- Monitor ICP readings. Continuous measurement of ICP is used to diagnose and monitor IICP. *As ICP increases, herniation may occur, leading to respiratory arrest and death.*
- If the patient is not intubated, prepare for oxygen administration and/or tracheal intubation if respiratory distress occurs. *Supplying oxygen prevents hypoxia until a hematoma can be evacuated, relieving pressure on the respiratory center.*
- Prepare for cranial surgery if deteriorating respiratory pattern and neurologic changes are noted. *Surgical intervention*

usually consists of placing several burr holes in the skull or performing a craniotomy to remove the hematoma. (Intracranial surgery is discussed later in the chapter.) However, the cerebral edema and IICP may cause death even if surgery is performed.

Using NANDA, NIC, and NOC
Linkages between a selected NANDA nursing diagnosis, NIC, and NOC for the patient with an acute brain injury are shown in the chart that follows.

Community-Based Care
Inform the patient and family that a postconcussion syndrome sometimes occurs. If the patient experiences persistent headaches and dizziness, is uncharacteristically emotional, seems overly tired, or has difficulty paying attention or remembering, the healthcare provider should be notified. Explain that these manifestations may persist for some time. Rehabilitation may help the patient compensate for memory impairment and attention deficits.

Patients who survive an acute brain injury will require long-term physical care and rehabilitation. Although recovery is highly individualized, many patients who regain consciousness

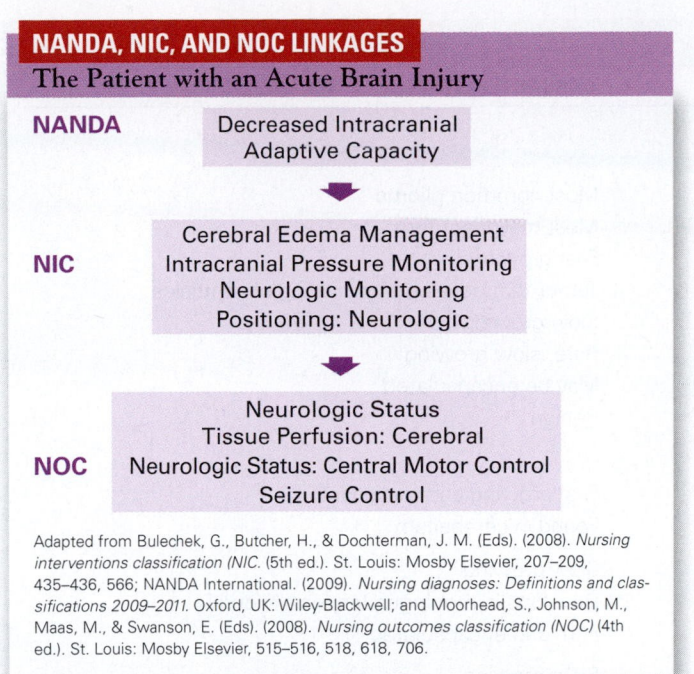

NANDA, NIC, AND NOC LINKAGES
The Patient with an Acute Brain Injury

NANDA
Decreased Intracranial Adaptive Capacity

NIC
Cerebral Edema Management
Intracranial Pressure Monitoring
Neurologic Monitoring
Positioning: Neurologic

NOC
Neurologic Status
Tissue Perfusion: Cerebral
Neurologic Status: Central Motor Control
Seizure Control

Adapted from Bulechek, G., Butcher, H., & Dochterman, J. M. (Eds). (2008). *Nursing interventions classification (NIC.* (5th ed.). St. Louis: Mosby Elsevier, 207–209, 435–436, 566; NANDA International. (2009). *Nursing diagnoses: Definitions and classifications 2009–2011.* Oxford, UK: Wiley-Blackwell; and Moorhead, S., Johnson, M., Maas, M., & Swanson, E. (Eds). (2008). *Nursing outcomes classification (NOC)* (4th ed.). St. Louis: Mosby Elsevier, 515–516, 518, 618, 706.

require life-long care; others remain in a coma or vegetative state. The family members often expect the patient to recover fully after the coma subsides, and they need information about the real possibility of residual deficits in self-care, emotional responses, cognition, communication, and movement. Topics that should be addressed for home care include the following:

- The need to encourage self-care and independence as much as possible
- Information to enhance recovery (CDC, 2006):
  - Get lots of rest. Don't rush back to work or school.
  - Avoid anything that could cause another blow or jolt to the head.
  - Consult with physician about when it will be safe to drive a car, ride a bike, or use heavy equipment (reaction time is often slower after a TBI).
  - Take only prescribed drugs and don't drink alcohol.
  - Write things down if you are having problems remembering.
  - If the injury was severe, therapy may be needed to learn lost skills, such as speaking, walking, or reading.
- Safety issues
- Equipment needs, such as a wheelchair and hospital bed
- Vocational counseling and services
- Referral to community resources and support groups
- Helpful resources: National Head Injury Foundation, Brain Injury Association of America, Brain Trauma Foundation, and the International Center for Individuals with Disabilities

The Patient with a Brain Tumor

Brain tumors are growths of abnormal cells in brain tissue, meninges, the pituitary gland, or blood vessels. Brain tumors may be benign or malignant, primary or secondary (metastatic), and intracerebral or extracerebral. Regardless of type or location, brain tumors are potentially lethal as they grow within a closed cranial vault and displace or impinge on CNS structures. ∞ Chapter 14 provides information about cancer in adults.

Incidence and Prevalence

It is estimated that almost 22,000 new cases of primary malignant brain tumors are diagnosed annually in the United States, and approximately 13,000 people die each year (National Cancer Institute, 2008). Even more brain tumors are the result of metastasis of cancer in other parts of the body, with an estimated incidence of 80,000 per year (Hickey, 2009).

The cause of many brain tumors is largely unknown. The brain itself is relatively protected from cancer-causing chemicals that are inhaled or eaten, including cigarette smoke. DNA mutations may affect oncogenes (speed up cell division) or tumor suppressor genes (slow cell division or cause cell death) so that the risk for or actual abnormal cell growth occurs. These mutations may be genetic or may occur as cells continually divide, die, and are replaced. Research is ongoing in this area.

Pathophysiology

Brain tumors may be classified as benign or malignant, based on the tissue type and characteristics of the cells. The use of the term benign may be misleading. A tumor that is benign by histologic examination but is surgically inaccessible may continue to grow and expand, increasing intracranial pressure and causing neurologic deficits, herniation, and finally death. In discussions of brain tumors, the term malignant is used to describe the lack of cell differentiation and the invasive nature of the tumor.

Brain tumors also may be classified as primary or metastatic, depending on their origin (Table 42–7). Primary tumors of CNS tissue arise from the cells and structures that are found within the brain, for example, neurons and neuroglia. The primary intracranial tumors that originate in the skull cavity but not from brain tissue itself arise from the supporting structures, including the meninges, pituitary gland, and pineal gland. Primary brain tumors rarely metastasize outside the CNS. Metastatic brain tumors originate from structures outside the brain, such as the lungs (most common origination), breasts, and prostate gland.

Focal disturbances from both primary and metastatic tumors take place when there is compression of brain tissue, tumor infiltration, or direct invasion of brain parenchyma with destruction of neural tissue, altered blood flow, and brain edema. Vasogenic edema occurs as the tumor grows and compresses adjacent tissue. Increased capillary permeability allows plasma to seep into the extracellular space and between the layers of the myelin sheath, altering electrical potential and impairing cell activity. Venous obstruction and edema due to breakdown of the blood–brain barrier by substances released by the tumor cells increase intracranial volume and intracranial pressure.

Manifestations

Manifestations can develop as a result of the growth of the tumor, while others are related to the location of the lesion (see the following box). Some of the more common manifestations include changes in cognition or consciousness, a headache that is usually worse in the morning, seizures, and vomiting. Compression of brain tissue and the invasion of the brain tumor into the cerebral tissue may lead to changes typically seen with cerebral edema and IICP (described earlier in the chapter). Cerebral blood supply may diminish as the tumor compresses blood vessels. Shifts in brain tissue can occur, leading to brain herniation syndromes and, if untreated, death.

TABLE 42–7 Classification of Primary Brain Tumors

TUMOR TYPE	TUMOR NAME	CHARACTERISTICS
Primary Tumors		
Intracerebral tumors Originate from neuroglia and invade brain tissue Most common type of brain tumor	Glioma ■ Astrocytoma ■ Glioblastoma multiforme ■ Ependymoma ■ Oligodendroglioma ■ Astroblastoma	Most common glioma Most malignant form Fast growing Tumor that develops from lining of ventricles Slow growing Rare, slow growing May be encapsulated Benign
Extracerebral Tumors		
Tumors arising from the supporting structures of the nervous system	Medulloblastoma	Fast growing and malignant Found in cerebellum
	Meningioma	Slow growing Develops in meninges (especially dura) Firm and encapsulated
	Acoustic neuroma (neurofibromatosis)	Slow growing Benign Originates from Schwann cells of the cranial nerve XIII May also affect cranial nerves V, VII, IX, and X Genetic origin due to autosomal dominant mendelian trait Firm, encapsulated lesions attached to nerve
Congenital (developmental) Tumors	Hemangioblastoma	Vascular tumor Slow growing
	Craniopharyngioma	Solid or cystic tumor Compresses pituitary gland Presses on the third ventricle and may cause blockage of cerebrospinal fluid (CSF)
Pituitary Adenomas	Chromophobic	Account for most pituitary tumors Nonsecreting tumor Slow growing
	Eosinophilic	Secreting tumors that produce growth hormone
	Basophilic	Secreting tumors that produce adrenocortico-tropic hormone Fast growing

Interdisciplinary Care

Treatment for a brain tumor may involve chemotherapy, radiation therapy, surgery, or any combination of these as discussed in ∞Chapter 14. Several variables are considered when selecting the appropriate treatment modality: the size and location of the tumor, the type of tumor, related symptoms (such as neurologic deficits), and the patient's overall condition.

Diagnosis

A thorough history and physical is conducted, with abnormal findings from an examination of the fundus of the eye, visual fields, neurologic assessment, and EEG used to identify a possible tumor. An MRI with gadolinium enhancement, the test of choice, can locate the tumor and define its size, shape, extent to which normal anatomy is distorted, and the degree of any associated cerebral edema. Arteriograms may show stretching or displacement of cerebral vessels by the tumor, as well as the presence of tumor vascularity. Endocrine studies are conducted if a pituitary tumor is suspected. (∞See Chapters 18 and 41 for further information about diagnostic tests of the endocrine and neurologic systems.)

Chemotherapy

The use of chemotherapy to treat brain tumors has been limited by the blood-brain barrier. Various methods are used to overcome the barrier. An intraventricular method of medication administration uses an Ommaya reservoir that is surgically implanted into a lateral ventricle of the brain (Figure 42–11 ■). Convection-enhanced delivery (CED) is the continuous injection of chemotherapy (as a fluid) directly to the tumor site through a catheter with positive pressure (in this case, the blood-brain barrier keeps the chemotherapy inside the brain). Biodegradable anhydrous wafers, which are impregnated with

MANIFESTATIONS of Brain Tumors by Location

LOBE	MANIFESTATIONS
Frontal Lobe Tumors	■ Inappropriate behavior ■ Recent memory loss ■ Personality changes ■ Headache ■ Inability to concentrate ■ Expressive aphasia ■ Impaired judgment ■ Motor dysfunctions
Parietal Lobe Tumors	■ Sensory deficits: paresthesia, loss of two-point discrimination, visual field deficits
Temporal Lobe Tumors	■ Psychomotor seizures
Occipital Lobe Tumors	■ Visual disturbances
Cerebellum Tumors	■ Disturbances in coordination and equilibrium
Pituitary Tumors	■ Endocrine dysfunction ■ Visual deficits ■ Headache

the chemotherapeutic drug may be implanted into the tumor at the time of surgery as another option.

An oral chemotherapeutic medication, temozolomide (Temodar), is used for palliative therapy for glioblastoma. Research is ongoing to develop agents that will specifically target genetic features and molecular profiles of a tumor (Porth & Matfin, 2009).

Surgery

Surgery is the preferred treatment of primary tumors, to remove the tumor if possible, to reduce the size of the tumor, or for symptom relief (palliation). The type of procedure, the surgical approach, and the timing of surgery (emergency versus planned procedure) influence the overall nursing management of the patient having intracranial surgery.

Some of the more common intracranial neurosurgical procedures follow:

■ *Burr hole:* A hole made in the skull with a special drill. The hole may facilitate the evacuation of an extracerebral clot, or a series of holes may be made in preparation for craniotomy (see Figure 42–10).
■ *Craniotomy:* A surgical opening into the cranial cavity (Figure 42–12 ■). A series of burr holes are made and the bone between the holes is cut with a special saw called a craniotome. The tumor is excised, and the bone flap is returned to the opening. A craniotomy may also be performed to repair defects associated with traumatic head injuries or to repair a cerebral aneurysm. In some cases, the patient is awake during the surgery, as described in the Moving Evidence into Action box on page 1472.
■ *Craniectomy:* An excision of a portion of the skull and complete removal of the bone flap. This procedure may be done to provide decompression after cerebral edema. Pressure on the brain structures is lessened by providing space for expansion.
■ *Cranioplasty:* Plastic repair to the skull in which synthetic material is inserted to replace the cranial bone that was removed. This procedure may be performed after a large craniectomy. The plastic repair restores the contour and integrity of the cranium.

Radiation Therapy

Radiation therapy may be administered alone or as adjunctive therapy with surgery. Radiation is often the treatment of choice for surgically inaccessible tumors; it may also be used to decrease the size of a tumor prior to surgery. Tumors that were not completely excised by surgery may also be treated with radiation.

Figure 42–11 ■ Ommaya reservoir for medication administration.

Figure 42–12 ■ In a craniotomy, a portion of the skull and overlying scalp is removed to allow access to the brain.

MOVING EVIDENCE INTO ACTION   Patients Undergoing an Awake Craniotomy

Brain mapping is a procedure conducted to identify the functional areas of the brain that control language and motor abilities. The patient is awake during the surgery, and a hand-held probe is used to stimulate areas of the brain. The areas stimulated become temporarily inactivated (as evidenced by asking the patient to speak or move), so that the surgeon knows which areas to avoid when removing a brain tumor. This study (Palese, Skrap, Fachin, Visioli, & Zannini, 2008) examined the experiences of patients in term of their feelings, what they think about, and how they approach this type of surgery without an anesthetic.

Findings from the study illustrated the complexity of the experience and the effect on the patient. Preoperatively, the patients felt a part of the decision making about being awake during the surgery, needed strong emotional support, kept busy to remain distracted, and avoided thinking about how they would handle the surgery itself. During the surgery, patients concentrated on doing what they were asked to do and having their senses (especially hearing) play the strongest role. After the surgery, the patients tested their ability to speak and move to ensure they had returned to normal, felt tired, and were surprised that no typical postoperative complications (e.g., nausea, pain) occurred.

IMPLICATIONS FOR NURSING

There is very little in the literature about nursing care of patients who are awake during surgery. This study identified initial information about the experience, providing a base for the development of guidelines for preoperative, intraoperative, and postoperative nursing interventions. Certainly, having surgery for a brain tumor, having a malignancy, and knowing one will be awake during the procedure are each traumatic, but when combined they can easily be overwhelming. Nursing care before the surgery must focus on meeting the emotional needs of the patient as well as providing interventions (such as active listening and focused discussions) to relieve anxiety and fear. Because hearing the surgeon explain what was being done was very important to the patients, it is important that the nurse discuss this aspect with the physician.

CRITICAL THINKING IN PATIENT CARE

1. Provide examples of leading statements you might use to discuss awake surgery with a patient.
2. In this study, patients wanted to see their family members immediate after surgery to reassure themselves that they were back to normal. Very few hospitals allow visitors in the recovery area. What process would you use to change this general rule? How would you handle the same request from other patients if the rule were changed for this population?
3. Considering the surgery, describe the immediate postoperative care necessary. What would be the priority assessments?

Source: Palese, A., Skrap, M., Fachin, M., Visiolik, S., & Zannini, L. (2008). The experience of patients undergoing awake craniotomy: In the patients' own words. A qualitative study. *Cancer Nursing, 31*(2), 166–172.

Specialty Procedures

Technologic advances—including the development of special instruments, the use of stereotaxic techniques for localizing a specific target, and the use of the laser beam—have greatly advanced neurosurgical practice. Microsurgery involves an operating microscope with microinstruments and supportive illumination equipment. Using stereotaxic techniques to precisely locate a specific target point allows for location of discrete areas of the brain that control specific functions and exact locations of deep brain lesions. The use of a laser beam for excision of a tumor results in less damage to surrounding tissue and less postoperative swelling. The gamma knife, which is not actually a knife but a heavily shielded helmet, is capable of destroying deep and otherwise inaccessible lesions in a single treatment session (Porth & Matfin, 2009). Research is being conducted on other methods of treating brain tumors, including hyperthermia and duplicating the immune response.

✎ Nursing Care

The nursing care of the patient with a brain tumor includes support during the diagnostic period and specific management as directed by the selected treatment. The foundation for care is data from the health history and physical assessment, which includes identifying neurologic deficits. Many of the alterations in health commonly experienced by the patient with a brain tumor have been discussed throughout this chapter, including altered level of consciousness, IICP, and seizures. The patient will require intensive care in the immediate postoperative period. In addition to the nursing care described in this section, see the Case Study & Nursing Care Plan for a patient with a brain tumor on page 1474.

Nursing Diagnoses and Interventions

This section of the chapter focuses on nursing interventions for the patient who has intracranial surgery. The nursing diagnoses discussed are anxiety, risk for infection, ineffective protection, acute pain, and low self-esteem.

Anxiety

The diagnosis of a brain tumor brings anxiety and feelings of uncertainty about the future. Both the patient and family members are likely to be apprehensive and require education and emotional support.

- Explain routine medical procedures, including blood work and radiologic studies. *Baseline laboratory and radiologic studies are needed to ensure that the patient has no other preexisting medical condition. Explaining the procedures and assisting the patient through this process help decrease anxiety.*
- Reinforce, clarify, and repeat information. *Both patient and family may have limited understanding of the scheduled diagnostic tests, procedures, and treatment modalities. The patient may be confused or have altered thought processes as a result of the tumor. Information may need to be repeated or reexplained.*
- Encourage patient and family to verbalize feelings, questions, and fears; provide realistic information appropriate to their level of understanding. *Verbalization helps reduce anxiety and fear.*
- Review patient and family strengths and effective coping skills. *Personal strengths, support systems, and coping skills can aid in the development of appropriate strategies to reduce anxiety.*
- Arrange for a member of the clergy to visit if desired. *Faith in a higher being is often a strong source of strength and support.*

- Provide preoperative teaching, including the following information:
  - Type of anesthesia and surgery
  - Time surgery will begin and expected length of procedure and recovery room stay
  - Where the patient will be taken after surgery (CCU, ICU) (If possible, show the patient and family the CCU or ICU and introduce them to the nurse who will be in charge of care after the surgery.)
  - Where family can wait during and following surgery
  - Appearance of the patient after surgery, which may include swollen, bruised eyelids and other facial features; a large dressing covering the head; a partially or fully shaved head; and a tracheostomy or endotracheal tube
  - Behavior of the patient after surgery, which will differ depending on the site of surgery, although cognitive and behavioral changes are common
  Information about what to expect reduces anxiety.
- Allow time for patient and family to be together. *Patients and families need quiet time together to support each other and prepare emotionally for surgery.*

Risk for Infection

The patient who has had intracranial surgery is at risk for infection from multiple invasive lines, the scalp wound, and the risk of introduction of bacteria into the operative area. The nurse provides interventions to monitor for and prevent infection.

- Monitor for leakage of CSF: Presence of glucose in clear drainage from ears, nose, or wound; constant swallowing; statements of "something dripping down the back of my throat." *These manifestations indicate an opening in the dura, which provides an avenue for an ascending infection.*
- Provide interventions to prevent contamination of area leaking CSF, if appropriate:
  - If leaking from the nose: Keep head of bed elevated 20 degrees unless contraindicated; do not suction nasally; do not clean nose; tell patient not to put finger in nose; do not insert packing.
  - If leaking from the ear: Position patient on side of leakage unless contraindicated; do not clean ear; tell patient not to put finger in ear; do not insert packing.
  - Place a sterile dressing over the area of drainage and change as soon as it becomes damp.
  Leakage of CSF indicates a break in the dura and increases the risk of an ascending infection. Surgery may be necessary to repair the break; however, the leak usually heals spontaneously in about 1 week.
- Monitor for and report manifestations of infection:
  - Take and record temperature on a regular basis.
  - Assess IV insertion sites for redness, swelling, drainage, and pain.
  - Assess scalp wound for redness, swelling, bulging, drainage, and pain.
  - Assess for manifestations of meningitis: fever and chills, increasing headache, neck stiffness, positive Kernig's or Brudzinski sign, photophobia.
  - Monitor laboratory reports for increased WBC count.
  Intact skin is the first line of defense against infection. Any break in the skin increases the risk of infection. Intracranial

surgery increases the risk of meningitis, with infectious agents ascending into the brain.
- Implement interventions to prevent infection:
  - Use strict aseptic technique when changing dressings and when caring for wound drains and ICP monitor lines.
  - Keep the patient's hands away from drains and dressings; use mitten restraints if necessary.
  - Administer prescribed antibiotics.
  Sterile technique decreases the risk of introducing infection into a wound. Antibiotics are usually prescribed prophylactically to prevent infection.

Ineffective Protection

The patient who has intracranial surgery does not have normal human defenses against changes in intracranial pressure and is also at risk from cerebral edema, IICP (with seizures) and a shift of intracerebral contents. In addition, the surgery may cause cerebral bleeding or hematoma formation. Assessments and interventions for IICP and seizures were described earlier in the chapter. If a shunt has been inserted, the following applies:

- For internal shunts: Avoid pressure on the shunt, reservoir, or tubing. Pump the shunt only if prescribed.
- For external shunts: Avoid kinks in tubing, and maintain the drainage collecting device and patient's head at the prescribed levels.

Acute Pain

The patient who has intracranial surgery has a headache as a result of either compression or displacement of brain tissue or from IICP.

- Assess the location, duration, and intensity of the pain, using a scale of 0 (no pain) to 10 (worst pain) in the patient who can verbally communicate. *The patient is the best source of information about pain.*
- Implement interventions to reduce the pain:
  - Raise the head of the bed slightly.
  - Reduce noise and bright lights in the room.
  - If allowed, loosen head dressing.
  - Administer narcotic analgesics with caution.
  Nonpharmacologic measures and medications may be used to reduce IICP and headache.

PRACTICE ALERT
Narcotic analgesics mask changes in eye signs and depress respirations.

Situational Low Self-Esteem

The patient who has intracranial surgery has many alterations that affect self-esteem and body image. Physical changes include a loss of hair on the scalp, swelling and bruising in the eyelids and face, and perhaps an indentation in the skull. The patient must depend on others to meet basic needs. There are often long-term neurologic deficits, affecting areas such as speech, vision, and motor abilities, which require changes in roles and relationships.

- Assess for verbal and nonverbal manifestations of negative self-esteem: denial of changes, preoccupation with changes, refusal to look in the mirror, withdrawal from family and friends, expressions of grief and loss. *Low self-esteem can be initiated by stressful situations and changes in body image.*

CASE STUDY & NURSING CARE PLAN   The Patient with a Brain Tumor

Claire Lange is a 42-year-old television announcer. During one night's broadcast, she confuses several major news items so badly that her co-anchor tries to correct her. Ms. Lange responds angrily that she does not need any help and then rises and storms off the set. As she leaves the camera area, she limps noticeably and appears to drag her left leg. The show's producer asks her what is wrong; she screams that nothing is wrong—she simply has another headache. He follows her to her dressing room and inquires about her headaches. She tells him that they come and go but have been getting worse lately. He then asks her if she has injured her left leg; she responds that the leg was weak because she was tired. As the producer leaves the dressing room, Ms. Lange begins to shake and collapses on the floor. The producer recognizes that she is having a seizure and calls for an ambulance.

Ms. Lange is admitted to the neurology floor of the local hospital for evaluation. A CT scan, MRI, and EEG are completed and identify an intracranial mass. A biopsy of the mass is positive for malignant cells. A glioma in the frontal lobe is identified, and surgery is scheduled for that week.

ASSESSMENT

When Clara Rosetti, RN, enters Ms. Lange's room, she sees Ms. Lange looking at her shoulder-length hair in the mirror. Ms. Lange tells Ms. Rosetti that she has never in her life worn her hair any shorter, and "Now you're going to cut it all off!" She paces the room and makes the statement, "I guess the hair isn't really important if I survive this situation." She also says that she has a headache.

DIAGNOSES

■ *Acute Pain* (headache) related to tumor and increase in intracranial pressure
■ *Disturbed Body Image* related to upcoming hair loss and cranial incision
■ *Anxiety* related to unknown future following surgery

EXPECTED OUTCOMES

■ Verbalize the causes of pain.
■ Verbalize an understanding of the changes in body appearance that are associated with the scheduled intracranial surgery

(e.g., shaving of the head prior to surgery, cranial incision, facial swelling postoperatively).
■ Identify measures that will help minimize the effect of the hair loss.
■ Verbalize a reduction in anxiety.

PLANNING AND IMPLEMENTATION

■ Assess level of discomfort using a rating scale of 0 to 10.
■ Provide a quiet, nonstimulating environment.
■ Position the patient for comfort, keeping the head of the bed elevated to promote venous drainage.
■ Assess level of consciousness for potential increases in ICP.
■ Encourage to verbalize feelings about the surgery.
■ Suggest measures that may help minimize the hair loss, such as the use of turbans, scarves, hats, and wigs.
■ Suggest relaxation techniques to decrease anxiety.

EVALUATION

By the time of surgery, Ms. Lange has recognized the relationship between the brain tumor and the headache. She states that lying in a flat position and coughing increase the headache. The head of the bed is kept at a 30- to 42-degree angle. Daily activities are spaced to provide periods of rest. Ms. Lange demonstrates no significant changes in level of consciousness. She has talked about the effect of the loss of her hair and television responsibilities. Ms. Lange has learned that the hair preparation would be done in surgery and that the hair would be saved for her. She states she has already consulted her hair stylist and that "scarves and turbans are on the way."

CRITICAL THINKING IN THE NURSING PROCESS

1. Outline interventions to decrease intracranial pressure both before and after surgery.
2. When making your initial assessments on the morning of surgery, you find that Ms. Lange has a decreased pulse and increased blood pressure. She tells you her headache is worse and suddenly vomits. What do you do now?
3. Ms. Lange asks you to be sure that she has absolutely no visitors after surgery, because she knows how ugly she will look. How would you respond?
4. Design a plan of care for Ms. Lange for the nursing diagnosis of *Powerlessness*.

See Evaluating Your Response in Appendix C.

■ Provide interventions to improve self-concept:
  ■ Limit negative self-assessment.
  ■ Help focus on positive areas of life.
  ■ Help identify sources of support and strength.
  ■ Help identify and use helpful coping methods.
  ■ Encourage significant others to visit.
  ■ Encourage independence in self-care.
  Self-esteem is derived from one's own perceptions of competence and from the responses of others. When one's self-concept and self-ideal are congruent, self-esteem is enhanced.

Using NANDA, NIC, and NOC

Linkages between a selected NANDA nursing diagnosis, NIC, and NOC for the patient with a brain tumor are shown in the accompanying chart.

Community-Based Care

The effect of the possible outcomes following the surgery often produces fear in both patient and family, interfering with their ability to retain information. The patient may have cognitive or

NANDA, NIC, AND NOC LINKAGES
The Patient with a Brain Tumor

NANDA   Powerlessness

⬇

NIC   Self-Esteem Enhancement
Self-Responsibility Facilitation
Emotional Support

⬇

NOC   Self-Esteem, Situational Low
Health Beliefs: Perceived Control
Health Beliefs: Perceived Resources
Social Support
Hope

Adapted from Bulechek, G., Butcher, H., & Dochterman, J. M. (Eds). (2008). *Nursing interventions classification* (NIC) (5th ed.). St. Louis: Mosby Elsevier, 314, 641–642, 646; NANDA International. (2009). *Nursing diagnoses: Definitions and classifications 2009–2011.* Oxford, UK: Wiley-Blackwell; and Moorhead, S., Johnson, M., Maas, M., & Swanson, E. (Eds). (2008). *Nursing outcomes classification* (NOC) (4th ed St. Louis: Mosby Elsevier, 380, 381, 390, 603–604, 809.

neurologic deficits that interfere with learning. Family members must be assessed for their ability to cope with the stress of the surgery. Information may have to be repeated several times.

Patients and their families who have experienced intracranial surgery require emotional support. The process of recovery is often extended and may involve adaptation to changes in body image and management of any motor or sensory deficits. If family members are willing, they may begin to assist with ADLs while the patient is in the hospital, such as assisting with personal hygiene and meals. Patients should also be encouraged to take an active role in their own care. Discharge planning includes a discussion of the following topics: medication information; wound care; the use of wigs, turbans, hats, or colorful scarves; and the importance of follow-up visits. In addition, emphasize the importance of reporting manifestations such as stiff neck, increasing headache, elevated temperature, new motor or sensory deficits, vision changes, or seizures.

Provide information about the overall treatment plan, management of deficits and/or disabilities, and future needs. Specific teaching topics are as follows:

- Safety measures for motor deficits, sensory deficits, lack of coordination, seizures, and cognitive deficits
- Comfort measures for nausea, vomiting, and pain
- Measures for communication if aphasia is present
- Measures to improve vision if visual deficits are present
- How to buy wigs and hairpieces
- Referrals to support groups and community resources
- Helpful resources: American Cancer Society, American Brain Tumor Association, National Brain Tumor Foundation, Brain Tumor Society

The Patient with a Headache

Headache, one of the most frequent manifestations of a health problem is pain within the cranial vault. Headaches may occur as a result of benign or pathologic conditions, intracranial or extracranial conditions, diseases of other body systems, stress, musculoskeletal tension, or a combination of these factors. Most tension headaches are mild, transient, and relieved by a mild analgesic. However, some headaches are chronic, intense, and recurrent. Manifestations of headache vary according to the cause, type, and precipitating symptoms.

Pathophysiology

The bones of the skull and the brain tissue lack pain-sensitive nerve fibers, but selected structures within and surrounding the cranial vault are sensitive to pain. There are many different types of headaches, and headaches may be primary or secondary to many other illnesses and injuries. This discussion focuses on migraine headache and cluster headache.

Migraine Headache

Migraine headache is a recurring primary headache, often initiated by a triggering event and usually accompanied by a neurologic dysfunction. It affects about 20 million people in the United States and is more common in women than in men. The headaches have a familial association, and are thought to be inherited as an autosomal dominant trait. Migraine headaches may occur daily or as infrequently as once a year.

The two most common types of migraine headaches are migraine without an aura (occurring in about 85% of cases) and classic migraine with aura (Porth & Matfin, 2009). In a migraine with aura, some type of sensory manifestation (such as visual disturbances) occurs prior to the manifestations. The manifestations, except for the aura, are the same for both types. The exact causes of migraine are not fully understood, but there is a relationship between serotonin and migraine headaches. It is thought that cerebral blood vessels narrow and reduce blood flow, followed by vasodilation, swelling, and pain.

A variety of factors are believed to trigger the onset of a migraine headache. Rapid changes in blood glucose levels, stress, emotional excitement, fatigue, alcohol intake, stimuli such as bright lights, and food high in tyramine or other vasoactive substances (e.g., aged cheese, nuts, chocolate, and alcoholic beverages) have been associated with migraine attacks. Hypertension and fever may make the disorder worse. The menstrual cycle is a trigger for many women.

In a migraine headache, the pain is unilateral and throbbing, but can become bilateral as the headache continues. Physical activity or even moving the head can intensify pain. Chills, nausea and vomiting, fatigue, and sensitivity to light, sound, or odor are often present. Other manifestations may include blurred vision, anorexia, hunger, diarrhea, abdominal cramping, facial pallor, sweating, and stiffness or tenderness of the neck. The headache lasts 4 to 72 hours and then gradually subsides. The patient may be acutely ill and is often extremely irritable. The sensory organs often become hypersensitive, and the patient withdraws from sound and light. The scalp is tender. After the headache, the headache area is sensitive to touch, and a deep aching is present. The patient is exhausted.

Cluster Headache

A cluster headache is an extremely severe, unilateral, burning pain located behind or around the eyes. It is predominantly experienced by men between the ages of 20 and 40 years. The headaches occur in groups or "clusters" of one to eight each day for several weeks or months, followed by remission lasting months to years (Hickey, 2009). The physiologic mechanism underlying cluster headaches is not well understood, but involves a vascular disorder, a disturbance of serotonergic mechanisms, a sympathetic defect, or dysregulation of the hypothalamus. The headaches often occur in the spring and fall and then disappear for an extended period. Triggers for cluster headaches are individualized and include alcohol intake, certain foods, smoking, high altitude, and sleep cycle disturbances.

Although the headache may occur at any time, it typically begins 2 to 3 hours after falling asleep, awakens the person, and then lasts from 15 minutes to 3 hours. Intense unilateral pain around or behind one eye is accompanied by rhinorrhea, lacrimation, flushing, sweating, facial edema, and possible miosis or ptosis on the affected side. The same side of the head is involved in each cluster of attacks.

Interdisciplinary Care

Therapeutic management of migraine and cluster headache includes a combination of patient teaching, medications, and measures to control contributing factors.

Diagnosis

Diagnosis and treatment are based on history, identifying triggering or precipitating events, and the type of headache. A thorough history and physical examination are integral parts of the assessment. Neurodiagnostic testing may be done to rule out a structural disease process. Testing may include a brain scan, MRI, x-ray studies of the skull and cervical spine, EEG, or lumbar puncture for CSF if inflammation is suspected. Serum metabolic screens and hypersensitivity testing also may be performed if systemic problems are suspected.

Medications

The management of migraine and cluster headaches includes administering medications to prevent pain (prophylactic therapy) as well as drugs to stop (or abort) a headache in progress. The patient with frequent migraine headaches is a candidate for prophylactic therapy. When the manifestations of migraine are recognized early, medications may be used to abort or limit the severity and duration of the headache. Drug categories used to treat migraine headaches, followed by examples, include beta blockers (propranolol, [Inderol]), tricylcic antidepressants (amitriptyline [Endep]), ergotalkaloids (methysergide [Sansert]), selective serotonin re-uptake inhibitors (SSRIs) (paroxetine [Paxil]), and calcium channel antagonists (verapamil [Canlan]).

Sumatriptan (Imitrex) is available in oral, nasal spray, or subcutaneous injection forms. It binds with serotonin$_1$ receptors and is rapidly effective. Zolmitriptan (Zomig), a sersotinin 5-HT$_1$ receptor agonist, is administered orally or by nasal spray and is effective in the treatment of acute headache. Once a migraine is in progress, a narcotic analgesic such as codeine or meperidine (Demerol) may be required. Antiemetics may be prescribed to control nausea and vomiting.

BOX 42–2 Suggestions to Decrease Incidence of Migraine Headaches

- Wake up at the same time every morning.
- Eat your meals and exercise on a regular schedule.
- No smoking or caffeine after 3 PM
- No artificial sweeteners or MSG.
- Reduce or eliminate red wine, cheese, alcohol, chocolate, and caffeine.
- Practice relaxation techniques, such as yoga, mediation, or biofeedback.

Many of the same medications used to treat migraine headaches are used to treat cluster headaches. Medications such as ergotamine tartrate may be given in suppository form at bedtime to prevent headache during the episodic attacks. Patients may find that inhaling 100% oxygen at 7 L/min for 15 minutes at the onset of an attack relieves their headache. Preventive treatment includes calcium channel blockers, lithium carbonate, topiramate, and baclofen. Intranasal lidocaine may be effective. Deep-brain surgical neurostimulation is an experimental approach that is having some success in eliminating cluster headaches (Porth & Matfin, 2009).

Nursing Care

The primary response of the patient requiring nursing interventions is teaching for self-care at home. Provide suggestions for strategies to control the pain (see Box 42–2). In addition, suggest the patient keep a diary of duration, onset, location, relation to menstruation or food intake, and precipitating triggers. Referrals for methods of stress reduction may be necessary for patients with long-term or migraine headaches.

CHAPTER HIGHLIGHTS

- Altered level of consciousness (LOC) is a common response to intracranial disorders, and is an early manifestation of deterioration of the function of the cerebral hemispheres. The alteration in cerebral function occurs in a sequential pattern, with characteristic changes in LOC, respiratory patterns, pupillary and oculomotor responses, and motor function. Coma states include persistent vegetative state and locked-in syndrome.
- Increased intracranial pressure (IICP) is a sustained elevated pressure (greater than 10 mmHg) within the cranial cavity. IICP may result from cerebral edema, hydrocephalus, head trauma, tumors, abscesses, inflammation, hemorrhage, or stroke.
- The manifestations of IICP include a decreasing LOC, abnormal motor weakness and responses, altered vision, altered vital signs, headache, papilledema, and projectile vomiting. If untreated, IICP causes a displacement (herniation) of cerebral tissue, and herniation of the cerebellum through the tentorium, followed by herniation of the brainstem through the foramen magnum. This is a lethal complication of IICP because it puts pressure on the vital centers in the medulla. IICP is primarily managed with osmotic diuretics and monitored with continuous intracranial pressure monitors.

- A seizure is a single event of abnormal electrical discharge. Epilepsy is a chronic seizure disorder of abnormal, recurring, excessive, and self-terminating electrical discharges from neurons. Seizures are categorized into those that affect only a part of the brain (partial seizures) and those that affect all of the brain (generalized). The most common type of seizure in adults is a tonic-clonic generalized seizure.
- A stroke is a condition in which neurologic deficits result from a sudden decrease in blood flow to a localized area of the brain. Strokes may be ischemic or hemorrhagic. Ischemic strokes result from a blockage of a cerebral artery by formation of a blood clot or by a clot or foreign substance (such as fat or bacteria) lodging in a blood vessel; they include transient ischemic attacks, thrombotic strokes, or embolic strokes. Hemorrhagic strokes occur when a cerebral blood vessel ruptures.
- Depending on the size and location of cerebral tissue damage, strokes may cause cognitive and behavior changes, sensory-perceptual deficits, language disorders, and motor deficits. Treatment of an ischemic stroke with fibrinolytic therapy within 3 hours of the onset of manifestations may reverse damage to cerebral neurons.

- Nursing care is directed toward both prevention of a stroke through community-based educational programs and interventions to promote recovery and decrease complications.
- Intracerebral hemorrhage may follow rupture of an intracranial aneurysm or arteriovenous malformation. Intracranial aneurysms occur at the site of a weakness in a cerebral blood vessel, while AV malformations are a tangled collection of dilated arteries and veins.
- Traumatic brain injury (TBI) refers to any injury of the scalp, skull, or brain, and is a leading cause of death and disability. TBIs include focal or diffuse brain injury. An acute brain injury affects all body systems, and carries the risk of secondary injury to the brain from hypoxia and ischemia.
- An epidural hematoma develops in the potential space between the dura and the skull. A subdural hematoma collects between the dura mater and the arachnoid mater. Diffuse brain injuries include contusions, concussions, and diffuse axonal injury. Patients with an acute TBI must have immediate transport and treatment in an ED, followed by care in an ICU. They will require long-term physical care and rehabilitation.
- Brain tumors are growths within the cranium, including on or in brain tissue, the meninges, the pituitary gland, or blood vessels. Brain tumors may be benign or malignant, primary or metastatic, and intracerebral or extracerebral. Regardless of the type or location, brain tumors are potentially lethal because they displace or impinge on CNS structures within a closed bony system.
- Headaches, a common type of intracranial pain, are categorized as tension, migraine, and cluster. A classic migraine is characterized by an aura; a common migraine does not have an aura.

TEST YOURSELF NCLEX-RN® REVIEW

1. Which of the following pathophysiologic events results in irregular respiratory patterns as LOC decreases?
   1. pressure on the meninges
   2. reflexive motor responses
   3. loss of the oculocephalic reflex
   4. brainstem responses to changes in $PaCO_2$
2. The unconscious patient has depressed or absent gag and swallowing reflexes. Which nursing diagnosis would be appropriate?
   1. *Decreased Intracranial Adaptive Capacity*
   2. *Risk for Aspiration*
   3. *Imbalanced Nutrition: Less than Body Requirements*
   4. *Ineffective Breathing Pattern*
3. What is the rationale for the use of osmotic diuretics to treat IICP?
   1. Hyperthermia increases the cerebral metabolic rate and exacerbates IICP.
   2. Increased blood osmolality draws edematous fluid into the vascular system.
   3. Patients with ICP are at increased risk for gastrointestinal hemorrhage.
   4. Brain injury and IICP often cause seizures.
4. The nurse is monitoring the neurologic status of a patient in a coma. Which of the following commands would be most accurate in identifying changes in mental status?
   1. "Tell me your name."
   2. "Look at this light when I shine it in your eyes."
   3. "Squeeze my hand."
   4. "Are you having trouble breathing?"
5. On admission to the ED, a patient who has altered LOC has a variety of laboratory tests to facilitate the diagnosis of the etiology of the condition. Which tests would likely be performed? **Select all that apply.**
   1. blood glucose
   2. serum electrolytes
   3. blood and urine toxicology
   4. urine for WBCs
   5. spinal fluid osmolarity
6. Of the following diagnostic tests, which one is the most accurate indicator of hydration status in the patient with altered LOC?
   1. CBC
   2. urinalysis
   3. serum osmolality
   4. blood culture
7. Which of the following manifestations would alert the nurse to the possibility that a patient has had a TIA?
   1. sudden severe pain over the left eye
   2. numbness and tingling in the corner of the mouth
   3. complete paralysis of the right arm and leg
   4. loss of sensation and reflexes in both legs
8. Although all of the following are risk factors for a stroke, which one is the greatest risk?
   1. hypertension
   2. heart disease
   3. diabetes
   4. high cholesterol levels
9. A nurse is providing care for a patient who has had an acute ischemic stroke of a left cerebral vessel. The chart includes the information that the patient has contralateral deficits. What does this mean?
   1. Both sides of the body are involved.
   2. The patient will have neurologic deficits on the left side of the body.
   3. The patient will have neurologic deficits on the right side of the body.
   4. Deficits will be present below the level of the stroke.
10. What is the rationale for administration of a tissue plasminogen activator within the first 3 hours of a thrombotic stroke?
    1. to reduce the risk of vasospasm
    2. to decrease the risk of infection
    3. to increase platelet aggregation
    4. to cause fibrinolysis of the clot

See Test Yourself answers in Appendix C.

Pearson Nursing Student Resources

Find additional review materials at
www.nursing.pearsonhighered.com

Prepare for success with additional NCLEX®-style practice questions, interactive assignments and activities, Web links, animations and videos, and more!

BIBLIOGRAPHY

American Brain Tumor Association. (2008). *Facts and statistics, 2008*. Retrieved from http://www.abta.org

American Cancer Society (ACS). (2008). *Detailed guide: Brain/CNS tumors in adults*. Retrieved from http://www.cancer.org

American Heart Association. (2009). *African Americans and Cardiovascular Disease—Statistics- 2009 update*. Retrieved from http://www.strokeassociation.org

American Heart Association Stroke Council Panel. (2007). Guidelines for the early management of adults with ischemic stroke. *Stroke, 38*, 1655–1711.

Baggaley, S. (2007). Could your headache really be a migraine? *American Nurse Today, 2*(12), 35–36.

Barker, E. (2008). *Neuroscience nursing: A spectrum of care* (3rd ed.). St. Louis: Mosby Elsevier.

Bauer, D. (2008). Caring for a patient who has suffered a cerebrovascular accident. *Medsurg Nursing, 17*(3), 204–205.

Brain Trauma Foundation. (2007a). *Facts about TBI in the USA*. Retrieved from http://www.braintrauma.org/site/PageServer?pagename=TBI_Facts

Brain Trauma Foundation. (2007b). *Guidelines for the management of severe traumatic head injury*. New York: The Brain Trauma Foundation.

Bulechek, G., Butcher, H., & Dochterman, J. (Eds.). (2008). *Nursing interventions classification (NIC)* (5th ed.). St. Louis: Mosby Elsevier.

Centers for Disease Control and Prevention (CDC). (2008). *Help seniors live better, longer: Prevent brain injury*. Retrieved from http://www.cdc.gov/BrainInjurySeniors

Cleveland Clinic. (2007). Hope for epilepsy patients. *Cleveland Clinic Magazine, 4*(2), 39.

Coyle, M., & Martin, E. (2007). Reflecting on a self-care process in the home setting for traumatic brain injury survivors. *Journal of Neuroscience Nursing, 39*(5), 274–277.

Don't let your head explode over increased ICP. (2007). *Nursing Made Incredibly Easy, 5*(2), 21–25.

Dowling-Castronovo, A., & Bradway, C. (2008). *Nursing standard of practice protocol: Urinary Incontinence (UI) in older adults admitted to acute care (with evidence-based content)*. The Hartford Institute for Geriatric Nursing. Retrieved from http://consultgerirn.org

Epilepsy Foundation. (n.d.). *About epilepsy: Epilepsy and seizure statistics*. Retrieved from http://www.epilepsyfoundation.org/about/statistics.cfm

Fagley, M. (2007). Taking charge of seizures. *Nursing, 37*(9), 42–44.

FDA adds suicide warning to epilepsy drugs. (2008). Health News. The Associated Press, Tuesday, December 16.

Greer, D., Funk, S., Reaven, N., Ouzounelli, M., & Uman, G. (2008). Impact of fever on outcome in patients with stroke and neurologic injury: A comprehensive meta-analysis. *Stroke, 39*(11), 3029–3035.

Hacke, W., Kaste, M., Bluhmki, E., Brozman, M., Ddvalos, A., et al. (2008). Thrombolysis with alteplase 3 to 4.5 hours after acute ischemic stroke. *The New England Journal of Medicine, 359*(13), 1317–1329.

Hickey, J. V. (2009). *The clinical practice of neurological and neurosurgical nursing* (6th ed.). Philadelphia: Lippincott Williams & Wilkins.

Hinkle, J., & Guanci, M. (2007). Acute ischemic stroke review. *Journal of Neuroscience Nursing, 39*(5), 285–293, 310.

International Stroke Conference. (2009). Women with stroke, TIA, more likely than men to report mental status change. Presented February 19, 2009. Abstract 82.

Kee, J. (2009). *Prentice Hall handbook of laboratory and diagnostic tests with nursing implications* (6th ed.). Upper Saddle River, NJ: Pearson Prentice Hall.

Kennedy, G., & Smyth, C. (2008). Screening older adults for executive dysfunction. *American Journal of Nursing, 108*(12), 62–70.

McPhee, S., Papadakis, M., & Tierney, L. (Eds.). (2008). *Current medical diagnosis & treatment* (47th ed.). New York: McGraw-Hill Lange.

Medscape Medical News. (2008). *Falls in the elderly a major cause of TBI death, injury*. Retrieved from http://www.medscape.com/viewarticle/576553

Moorhead, S., Johnson, M., Maas, M., & Swanson, E. (2008). *Nursing outcomes classification (NOC)* (4th ed.). St. Louis: Mosby Elsevier.

NANDA International. (2009). *Nursing diagnoses: Definitions & classification 2009–20011*. Oxford: Wiley-Blackwell.

National Cancer Institute. (2009). *Adult brain tumors treatment*. Retrieved from http://www.cancer.gov

National Institute of Neurological Disorders and Stroke (NINDS). (2009a). *NINDS brain and spinal tumors information page*. Retrieved from http://www.ninds.nih.gov/disorders/brainandspinaltumors/brainandspinaltumors.htm

National Institute of Neurological Disorders and Stroke (2009b). *Stroke: Hope through research*. Retrieved from http://ninds.nih.gov/disorders/stroke/detail_stroke.htm

National Institute of Neurological Disorders and Stroke. (2008a). *Seizures and Epilepsy: Hope through research*. Retrieved from http://www.ninds.nih.gov/disorders/epilepsy/epilepsy.htm

National Institute of Neurological Disorders and Stroke. (2008b). *Stroke risk factors and symptoms*. Retrieved from http://www.ninds.nih.gov/disorders/stroke/stroke_bookmark.htm

National Institute of Neurological Disorders and Stroke. (2008c). *Traumatic brain injury: Hope through research*. Retrieved from http://www.ninds.nih.gov/disorders/tbi/detail_tbi.htm

National Stroke Association. (2009). *Stroke facts*. Retrieved from www.stroke.org

Ostwald, S., Davis, S., Hersch, G., Kelley, C., & Godwin, K. (2008). Evidence-based educational guidelines for stroke survivors after discharge home. *Journal of Neuroscience Nursing, 40*(3), 173–179, 191.

Palese, A., Skrap, M., Fachin, M., Visiolik S., & Zannini, L. (2008). The experience of patients undergoing awake craniotomy: In the patients' own words. A qualitative study. *Cancer Nursing, 31*(2), 166–172.

Petchprapai, N., & Winkelman, C. (2007). Mild traumatic brain injury: Determinants and subsequent quality of life. A review of the literature. *Journal of Neuroscience Nursing, 39*(5), 260–72.

Porth, C. M., & Matfin, G. (2009). *Pathophysiology: Concepts of altered health states* (8th ed.). Philadelphia: Lippincott Williams & Wilkins.

Rank, W. (2008). Interrupting status epilepticus. *Nursing, 38*(10), 56cc1–56cc3.

Ryan, D. (2009). Caring for patients with traumatic brain injuries: Are you up to the challenge? *American Nurse Today, 4*(80), 18–23.

Securing the indwelling catheter. (2008). *American Journal of Nursing, 108*(12), 44–50.

Stiver, S., & Manley, G. (2008). Prehospital management of traumatic brain injury. *Neurosurgical Focus, 25*(4), E5.

The Stroke Collaborative. (2008). Give me 5 for stroke. Retrieved from http://www.giveme5forstroke.org

U.S. Food and Drug Administration (FDA). (2008). *FDA alert: Information for healthcare professionals. Suicidality and antieleptic drugs*. Retrieved from http://www.fda.gov/cder/drug/InfoSheets/HCP/antiepilepticsHCP.htm

Vacca, V. (2007). Epidural hemorrhage and hematoma. *Nursing, 37*(7), 72.

Wagner, K., Johnson, K., & Kidd, P. (2006). *High acuity nursing* (4th ed.). Upper Saddle River, NJ: Pearson Prentice Hall.

Wilson, B., Shannon, M., & Shields, K. (2009). *Prentice Hall nurse's drug guide 2009*. Upper Saddle River, NJ: Pearson Prentice Hall.

Nursing Care of Patients with Spinal Cord Disorders and CNS Infections

LEARNING OUTCOMES

1. Explain the pathophysiology, manifestations, complications, interdisciplinary care, and nursing care of patients with spinal cord injury, herniated intervertebral disk, spinal cord tumor, and CNS infections.
2. Compare and contrast the pathophysiologic effects of injuries and tumors of the spinal cord by level of injury.
3. Discuss the purposes, nursing implications, and health education of the patient and family for medications used to treat spinal cord injury and CNS infections.
4. Explain the methods used to stabilize and immobilize spinal cord injuries.
5. Describe the surgical procedures used to treat spinal cord disorders.

CLINICAL COMPETENCIES

1. Assess the functional health status of patients with spinal cord disorders and CNS infections, and monitor, document, and report abnormal manifestations.
2. Use assessed data, patient values, clinical expertise, and evidence to determine priority nursing diagnoses and select and implement individualized nursing interventions.
3. Adapt individual and cultural values and variations as well as expressed needs and preferences into the plan of care for patients with spinal cord disorders and CNS infections.
4. Administer oral and injectable medications used to treat spinal cord disorders and CNS infections knowledgeably and safely.
5. Provide appropriate and safe care to patients having a carotid endarterectomy, halo fixation, and a posterior laminectomy.
6. Effectively communicate with and function within the interdisciplinary team to plan and provide care.
7. Provide teaching to facilitate self-catheterization, self-care of a ruptured intervertebral disk, and community-based self-care of disabilities resulting from spinal cord disorders and CNS infections.
8. Use evidence-based research to prevent ventilator-associated pneumonia in patients in the neurologic ICU.
9. Revise plan of care as needed to provide effective interventions to promote, maintain, or restore functional health status to patients with spinal cord disorders and CNS infections.

KEY TERMS

autonomic dysreflexia, *1483*
botulism, *1506*
Creutzfeldt-Jakob disease (CJD), *1504*
deformation, *1480*
encephalitis, *1499*
meningitis, *1498*

paraplegia, *1481*
paresthesia, *1492*
postpoliomyelitis syndrome, *1505*
quadriplegia, *1481*
rabies, *1505*

radiculopathy, *1492*
sciatica, *1492*
spinal cord injury (SCI), *1480*
spinal shock, *1481*
tetanus, *1503*

The health problems discussed in this chapter result from disorders of the spinal cord and infections of the central nervous system (CNS). Patients with these disorders experience a wide variety of neurologic deficits that affect functional health patterns. They often also require treatment and care for both acute and long-term health problems.

Nursing care for patients with these disorders is tailored to meet the needs of the patient and is individualized by the patient's responses to alterations in structure and function. The disabilities and long-term effects from spinal cord disorders, spinal cord injuries, and CNS infections have the potential to cause loss and grief, not only in the patient but also in the family of the patient. ∞ Chapter 5 provides information about

patient responses to loss and nursing interventions to help promote coping and reduce grieving.

The Patient with a Spinal Cord Injury

Nursing care of patients with a spinal cord injury takes place from acute care through ongoing rehabilitation in a variety of settings. Although priorities may change depending on the patient and setting, care focuses on maximizing functional health status to preserve quality of life. The nurse provides care and also collaborates with other members of the interdisciplinary team in meeting this goal.

Spinal Cord Injury Animation

A **spinal cord injury (SCI)** involves damage to the neural elements of the spinal cord. Because the spinal cord contains the tracts that connect sensory afferent neurons and lower motor neurons with centers in the brain, both sensory and motor functions are often involved. The major causes of SCI are contusion, compression, laceration, transection, hemorrhage, damage to blood vessels that supply the spinal cord, and damage to blood vessels in the spinal cord (Hickey, 2009). If vertebrae are fractured and ligaments are torn, both fractures and tears can damage the cord and spinal nerves and make the spinal column unstable. Injury to blood vessels supplying the cord can cause permanent damage. This discussion focuses on traumatic injuries, but the information is also applicable to congenital deformities, primary or metastatic tumors, ischemia and infarction, and bone disease with pathologic fractures of the vertebrae.

> **FAST FACTS**
> **SCI**
> - Approximately 12,000 people have an SCI each year.
> - An estimated 87% of all people with SCIs live at home.
> - Although SCIs occur in people of all ages, they are most often seen in young men.
> - Most of the injuries are due to motor vehicle crashes, followed by falls, acts of violence, and sports injuries.
>
> (National Spinal Cord Injury Statistical Center, 2010)

Pathophysiology

The spinal cord provides a two-way pathway for the conduction of impulses and information to and from the brain and the body, serves as a major reflex center, and (through its attached spinal nerves) is involved in the sensory and motor innervation of the entire body below the head. It consists of an outer region of white matter and an inner region of gray matter. The gray matter comprises the central canal of the cord, the posterior horns, the anterior horns, and the lateral horns. It is divided into a sensory half (dorsally) and a motor half (ventrally) and innervates somatic and visceral regions of the body. The white matter consists of tracts or pathways that convey information. The ascending (sensory) pathways carry information about proprioception, fine touch, discrimination, pain, temperature, deep pressure, and touch. The descending (motor) pathways carry information about movement. The pyramidal tracts control skilled voluntary movements (such as writing). The extrapyramidal tracts (all tracts other than the pyramidal tracts) bring about all other body movements.

Most spinal cord injuries involve damage to the vertebrae and supporting ligaments as well as the spinal cord itself. Damage to these structures may in turn damage the spinal cord. The pathophysiology of SCI involves primary and secondary injury. When the spinal cord is injured, the irreversible neurologic primary injury causes microscopic hemorrhages in the gray matter of the cord and edema of the white matter of the cord that leads to necrosis of neural tissue. These initial pathologic changes are followed by the secondary injury, with mechanisms that increase the area of injury. Neuronal injury leads to loss of reflexes below the level of injury. The hemorrhages extend, eventually involving the entire gray matter. Microcirculation to the cord is impaired by edema and hemorrhage. The injured tissue releases norepinephrine, serotonin, dopamine, and histamine; these vasoactive substances cause vasospasm and further decrease microcirculation, with resulting ischemia. Proteolytic and lipolytic enzymes from injured neurons are released, causing further swelling, demyelination, and necrosis in spinal cord neural tissue (Porth & Matfin, 2009).

When ischemia is prolonged, necrosis of both gray and white matter begins within a few hours, and within 24 hours the function of nerves passing through the injured area is lost. Although circulation returns to the white matter of the cord in about 24 hours, decreased circulation in the gray matter continues. Because edema extends the level of injury for two cord segments above and below the affected level, the extent of injury cannot be determined for up to 1 week.

Tissue repair occurs over a period of 3 to 4 weeks. Phagocytes enter the area in 36 to 48 hours after the initial injury. Neurons degenerate and are removed by microphages in the first 10 days after the injury. Red blood cells (RBCs) disintegrate, and the hemorrhages are reabsorbed. Eventually the area of injury is replaced by acellular collagenous tissue, and the meninges thicken.

Forces Resulting in SCI

SCIs are the result of the application of excessive force to the spinal column. The most common cause of abnormal spinal column movements are acceleration and deceleration (forces that are applied to the body, for example, in automobile crashes and falls). Acceleration occurs when external force is applied in a rear-end collision; the upper torso and head are forced backward and then forward. Deceleration occurs in a head-on collision; the external force is applied from the front. The head and body move forward until they meet a stationary object and then are forced backward. The alteration of the spinal cord and soft tissues caused by these abnormal movements is called **deformation**. The following forces and movements (Figure 43–1 ■) may cause a variety of spinal cord injuries, with the extent of injury depending on the amount and direction of motion, and the rate of application of force:

- *Hyperflexion*, or forcible forward bending, may compress vertebral bodies and disrupt ligaments and intervertebral disks.
- *Hyperextension*, or forcible backward bending, often disrupts ligaments and causes vertebral fractures. A whiplash injury is a less severe form of hyperextension, with injury to soft tissues but no vertebral or spinal cord damage.
- *Axial loading*, a form of compression, is the application of vertical force to the spinal column (for instance, by falling and landing on the feet or buttocks or by diving into shallow water).
- *Excessive rotation*, in which the head is excessively turned, may tear ligaments, fracture articular surfaces, and cause compression fractures.

The spinal cord may be penetrated by bullets and other foreign objects (e.g., sharp objects used as weapons, shrapnel from explosions). Penetrating injuries may cause vertebral fractures, blood vessel damage, tear ligaments and muscles, or cut through a part or all of the spinal cord. Complete severing of the cord is rare.

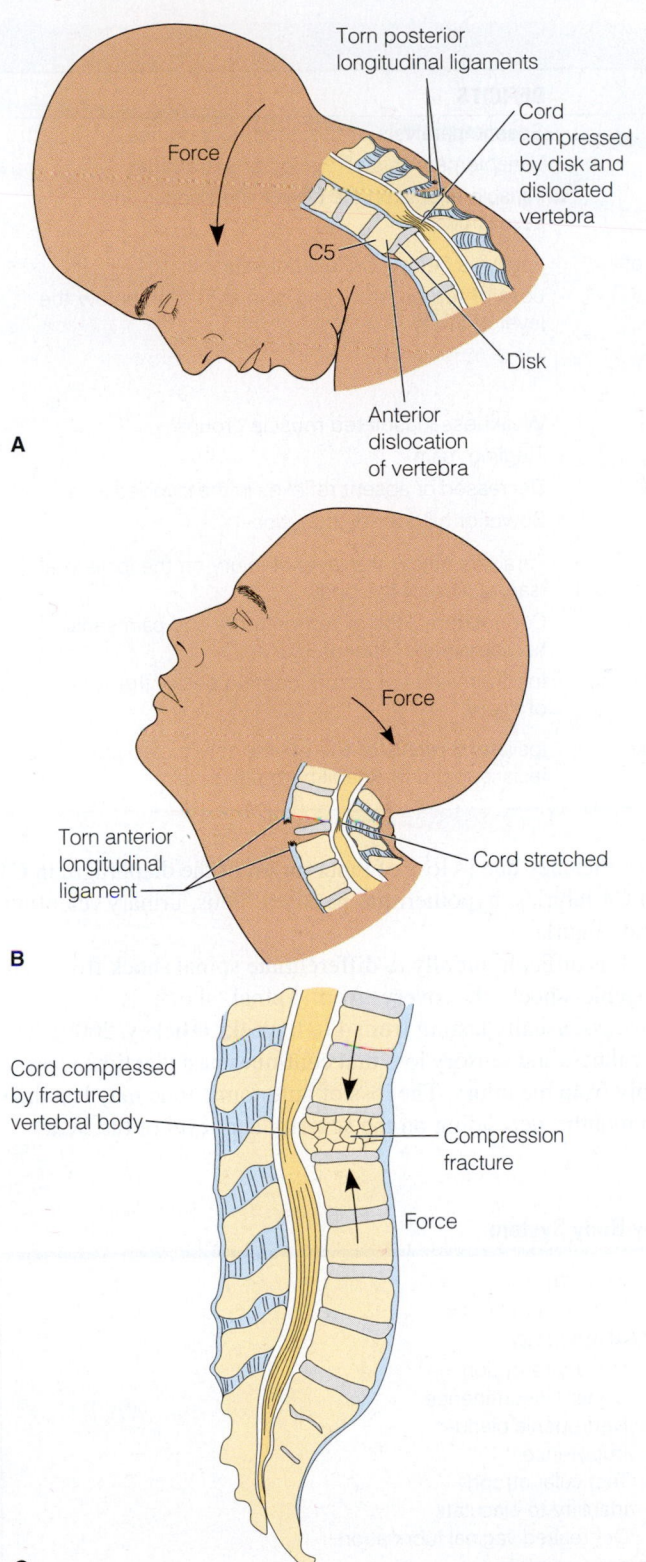

Figure 43–1 ■ Spinal cord injury mechanisms. *A*, Hyperflexion. *B*, Hyperextension. *C*, Axial loading, a form of compression.

Sites of Pathology

The injury is identified by vertebral level. For example, a C6 spinal cord injury is at the sixth cervical vertebra. The most frequent sites of injury of the cord are at the first, second, and fourth to sixth cervical vertebrae (C1, C2, C4 to C6); and the eleventh thoracic to second lumbar vertebrae (T11 to L2). Because the cervical spine has a wider range of movement than the rest of the spine, the cervical portion is more likely to be affected by externally applied forces. In addition, the cord fills most of the vertebral canal in the cervical and lumbar regions and thus is more easily injured. Damage to the vertebrae and ligaments causes the spinal column to become unstable, increasing the possibility of compression or stretching of the spinal cord with any further movement.

Classification of SCI

SCIs are further classified according to the amount of cord involvement. **Quadriplegia** (also called tetraplegia) occurs with damage to the neural structures in the cervical area of the cord, resulting in loss or impairment of motor and/or sensory function in the arms, trunk, legs, and pelvic organs. **Paraplegia** occurs with damage to the neural structures in the thoracic, lumbar, or sacral area of the cord, resulting is loss or impairment of motor and/or sensory function in the trunk, legs, and pelvic organs. Function of the arms is spared; the other losses depend on the level of injury.

In a complete SCI, the motor and sensory neural pathways are completely interrupted (transected), resulting in total loss of motor and sensory function below the level of the injury. However, "complete" does not necessarily mean the spinal cord has been severed. In an incomplete SCI, the motor and sensory pathways are only partially interrupted, with variable loss of function below the level of injury. Incomplete spinal cord injuries are further classified into syndromes as outlined in Table 43–1. Both complete and incomplete injuries can occur in paraplegia and quadriplegia. The alterations in function that occur as the result of a spinal cord injury vary greatly depending on the amount of tissue damage and the level of injury.

Manifestations

The spinal cord, the vertebrae, the intervertebral disks, the spinal nerves, the ligaments, and the surrounding soft tissue structures are in such close anatomic proximity that any condition or injury affecting one structure may well affect any one or all of the other structures. Injuries of the spinal cord have the potential to affect movement, perception, sensation, sexual function, and elimination. Manifestations and complications of SCI by body system are listed in the box on page 1482.

Spinal shock is the temporary loss of reflex function (called areflexia) below the level of injury at the cervical and upper thoracic spinal cord. As a result of the injury, sympathetic function is interrupted and parasympathetic function is unopposed. This condition is characterized by flaccid paralysis, loss of skin reflexes and deep tendon reflexes, and loss of all sensations below the level of injury. There is loss of urinary bladder tone, intestinal peristalsis, perspiration, and vasomotor tone. Additionally, the autonomic dysfunction results in hypotension, bradycardia (50 to 70 beats/minute), warm skin, and body temperature that responds to the immediate environment (Hickey, 2009). The pathophysiology of the characteristic manifestations of spinal shock is described in the Pathophysiology Linkage box on page 1483. This response begins immediately after complete transection of the spinal cord, when connections between the brain and the spinal cord are interrupted and the

TABLE 43–1 Incomplete Spinal Cord Injury Syndromes

TYPE	CAUSE	LOCATION	DEFICITS
Central cord syndrome	Cord transection Hyperextension	Cervical	Spastic paralysis of the upper extremities Variable paralysis of the lower extremities Variable effects on the bowel, the bladder, and sexual function
Anterior syndrome	Damage to the anterior spinal artery Infarction of the anterior spinal artery Hyperflexion	Anterior two-thirds of the cord	Paralysis below the level of injury Loss of temperature and pain sensation below the level of injury
Posterior syndrome	Vertebral dislocation Herniated disk Compression	Nerve roots	Weakness in isolated muscle groups Tingling, pain Decreased or absent reflexes in the involved area Bowel or bladder dysfunction
Brown-Séquard syndrome	Penetrating trauma	Hemisection of the anterior and posterior cord	Paralysis below the level of injury on the ipsilateral (same) side of the body Contralateral loss of temperature and pain sensation below the level of injury Ipsilateral loss of proprioception below the level of injury
Homer's syndrome	Incomplete cord transection	Cervical sympathetic nerves	Ipsilateral ptosis of the eyelid, constricted pupil, and facial anhidrosis (inability to perspire)

cord does not function at all. The response also occurs (although in varying degrees) after partial transection as well as after spinal cord contusions, compression, and ischemia.

A person with a cervical or upper thoracic SCI may also have neurogenic shock, resulting in cardiovascular changes. These changes are due to the inability of higher centers in the brainstem to modulate reflexes. As a result, vascular beds below the level of injury dilate, and the cardiac accelerator reflex is suppressed. The patient experiences hypotension and bradycardia. Other manifestations may include respiratory

insufficiency due to loss of innervation of the diaphragm in C1 to C4 injuries, hypothermia, paralytic ileus, urinary retention, and oliguria.

It is difficult initially to differentiate spinal shock from neurogenic shock. Recovery from spinal shock is a gradual process, usually lasting from 4 to 6 weeks (Hickey, 2009). The weakness and sensory loss that continues past that time is probably from the injury. The loss of autonomic tone may last days to months, depending on the severity and level of the SCI.

MANIFESTATIONS AND COMPLICATIONS of Spinal Cord Injury by Body System

INTEGUMENT
- Decubitus (pressure) ulcers

NEUROLOGIC
- Pain
- Areflexia
- Hypotonia
- Autonomic dysreflexia

CARDIOVASCULAR
- Spinal shock
- Paroxysmal hypertension
- Orthostatic hypotension
- Cardiac dysrhythmias
- Decreased venous return
- Hypercalcemia

RESPIRATORY
- Limited chest expansion
- Decreased cough reflex
- Decreased vital capacity

GASTROINTESTINAL
- Stress ulcers
- Paralytic ileus

- Stool impaction
- Stool incontinence

GENITOURINARY
- Urinary retention
- Urinary incontinence
- Neurogenic bladder
- Impotence
- Testicular atrophy
- Inability to ejaculate
- Decreased vaginal lubrication

MUSCULOSKELETAL
- Joint contractures
- Bone demineralization
- Osteoporosis
- Muscle spasms
- Muscle atrophy
- Pathologic fractures
- Paraplegia
- Quadriplegia

PATHOPHYSIOLOGY LINKAGE Spinal Shock

MANIFESTATIONS	RELATED PATHOPHYSIOLOGY
Decreased peripheral vascular resistance with decreased peripheral vascular tone and vasodilatation	Loss of sympathetic input to the blood vessels of the peripheral system and the heart; unopposed vagal tone.
Bradycardia	Suppression of the cardiac accelerator reflex and vasodilatation.
Hypotension	Loss of autonomic vasoconstrictor reflexes and vascular tone.
Flaccid paralysis	Lower motor neuron injury at or below T12.
Bowel and bladder dysfunction	Lower motor neuron injury at or below T12.
Inability to regulate body temperature and lack of perspiration	Communication between thermoregulatory center in the hypothalamus and sympathetic effector responses below the level of injury is lost, causing loss of ability to conserve or dissipate heat (as by perspiring).
Loss of sensation	Interrupted impulses to the brain.

Complications

The complications of an SCI involve many different body systems and often result in permanent disability and loss of functional health status. The complications include but are not limited to upper and lower motor neuron deficits, paraplegia and quadriplegia, and autonomic dysreflexia. Other complications, depending on the level and severity of the injury, are ineffective respirations; altered skin integrity; increased risk of thrombosis; and alterations in bowel elimination, urinary elimination, and sexual patterns.

Upper and Lower Motor Neuron Deficits

Motor neurons are functional units that carry motor impulses. Injuries to the spinal cord are often classified as either upper motor neuron lesions or lower motor neuron lesions. The upper motor neurons (located in the cerebral cortex, thalamus, brainstem, and corticospinal and corticobulbar tracts) are responsible for voluntary movement. When these motor pathways are interrupted, the patient experiences spastic paralysis and hyperreflexia and may be unable to carry out skilled movement.

Lower motor neurons (located in the anterior horn of the spinal cord, the motor nuclei of the brainstem, and the axons that reach the motor end plate of skeletal muscles) are responsible for innervation and contraction of skeletal muscles. Interruption of lower motor neurons results in muscle flaccidity and extensive muscle atrophy, with loss of both voluntary and involuntary movement. If only some of the motor neurons supplying a muscle are affected, the patient experiences partial paralysis; if all motor neurons to a muscle are affected, the patient experiences complete paralysis and hyporeflexia.

Paraplegia and Quadriplegia

Two common neurologic deficits resulting from an SCI are paraplegia and quadriplegia, described earlier and illustrated in the previous chapter (Figure 42–6 on page 1452).

Autonomic Dysreflexia

Autonomic dysreflexia (also called autonomic hyperreflexia) is an exaggerated sympathetic response that occurs in patients with SCIs at or above the T6 level. This response, which is seen only after recovery from spinal shock, occurs as a result of a lack of control of the autonomic nervous system by higher centers. When stimuli are unable to ascend the cord, mass reflex stimulation of the sympathetic nerves below the level of the injured cord area occurs, triggering massive vasoconstriction. In response, the vagus nerve causes bradycardia and vasodilation above the level of injury. If untreated, autonomic dysreflexia is potentially fatal.

Autonomic dysreflexia is triggered by stimuli that would normally cause abdominal discomfort, by stimulation of pain receptors, and by visceral contractions. Causes include a full bladder (the most common cause) resulting from a blocked urinary catheter, fecal impaction, bladder infections or stones, intrauterine contractions, pressure ulcers or ingrown toenails, dressing changes, and surgical procedures.

The manifestations include pounding headache, bradycardia, and hypertension (with readings as high as 240/120). As baroreceptor function and parasympathetic control of heart rate travel via the cranial nerves, these responses remain intact (Porth & Matfin, 2009). Continued hypertension produces a baroreflex-mediated vagal slowing of the heart and bradycardia. There is also a baroreceptor-mediated vasodilation, with warm, flushed skin and profuse sweating above the level of injury and pale, cold, and dry skin below it (Porth & Matfin, 2009). Dysreflexia is a neurologic emergency and requires immediate treatment.

Interdisciplinary Care

The patient with an acute SCI requires emergency assessment and care and medications; the patient may also require immobilization and surgery. The patient is first assessed and stabilized at the scene of the accident, initially treated in the ED, and then admitted to the hospital intensive care unit. Management requires an interdisciplinary team and is complex; SCI affects every body system and function.

Emergency Care

The danger of death from SCI is greatest when there is damage to or transection of the upper cervical region. When the injury is at the C1 to C4 level, respiratory paralysis is common, and the patient who survives requires ventilator assistance to breathe. Injuries below C4 may increase the risk of respiratory failure if edema ascends the cord. It is of critical importance not to complicate the initial injury by allowing the fractured vertebrae to damage the cord further during transport to the hospital. Although at one time injuries to the high cervical cord were

Spinal Injury Immobilization Video

almost always fatal, advances in trauma care have greatly improved the survival rate.

All people who have sustained trauma to the head or spine, or who are unconscious, should be treated as though they have a spinal cord injury. Prehospital management includes rapid assessment of the ABCs (airway, breathing, circulation), immobilizing and stabilizing the head and neck, removing the person from the site of injury, stabilizing other life-threatening injuries, and rapidly transporting the person by ambulance or helicopter to the appropriate facility (a trauma center, if available). Guidelines for emergency care are as follows:

- Do not flex, extend, or rotate the neck.
- Immobilize the neck, using rolled towels or blankets, or apply a cervical collar before moving the patient onto a backboard.
- Secure the head by placing a belt or tape across the forehead and securing it to the stretcher.
- Maintain the patient in the supine position.
- Transfer directly from the stretcher with backboard still in place to the type of bed that will be used in the hospital.

Assessment findings at the scene of the accident or in the emergency room vary according to the level of injury. The assessment findings common to the level of injury are outlined in Box 43–1. Manifestations of spinal shock (described earlier) are also assessed.

The patient in the ED with a suspected or identified SCI is also treated for respiratory problems, paralytic ileus, atonic bladder, and cardiovascular alterations. Respiratory distress in the patient with a cervical-level injury is treated by placing the patient on a ventilator. Oxygen is administered to the patient with a thoracic-level injury. Paralytic ileus (obstruction of the intestines due to lack of peristalsis) is common in patients with an SCI and is treated by the insertion of a nasogastric tube with connection to suction. To prevent overdistention of an atonic bladder, an indwelling catheter is inserted and connected to dependent drainage. Cardiovascular status is assessed on a continuous basis by inserting invasive monitoring devices, such as a Swan-Ganz catheter, and attaching the patient to a cardiac monitor, or by arterial monitoring to identify hypotension and to draw arterial blood gases (ABGs).

If used, high-dose steroid protocol using methylprednisolone (Medrol) must be implemented within 8 hours of the injury to improve neurologic recovery. Clinical research indicates that the use of this adrenocorticosteroid is effective in preventing secondary spinal cord damage from edema and ischemia. However, this treatment is controversial as it also increases the risk of serious complications (Barker, 2008; Porth & Matfin, 2009).

BOX 43–1 Assessment Findings in Acute SCI

Cervical Injury
- Paralysis or weakness of extremities
- Respiratory distress manifested by changes in ABG studies, cyanosis, flaring of the nostrils, use of accessory muscles of respiration, and restlessness
- Pulse rate below 60 and systolic BP below 80
- Decreased peristalsis

Thoracic and Lumbar Injury
- Paralysis or weakness of extremities

Diagnosis
Diagnostic tests are ordered to identify the level and extent of injury, and to detect any complications. The tests include x-rays of the spine, CT or MRI of the spine, and somatosensory-evoked potential studies to locate the level of spinal cord injury by stimulating peripheral nerves and measuring response times. ABGs are measured to establish a baseline or to identify problems due to respiratory insufficiency. A trauma screen (blood type and cross-match, blood alcohol level, urine drug screen, and pregnancy test for women up to age 45) is conducted in the ED.

Fluids
IV fluids of D51/2 NS are administered. Potassium and multivitamins may be added to the IV fluids. If the patient becomes hypotensive in the early stage of treatment, IV crystalloid solutions are administered to increase blood pressure. Fluid resuscitation of the trauma patient is described in ∞ Chapter 11.

Medications
The pharmacologic treatment of the patient with SCI is primarily symptomatic. It is directed toward decreasing edema from the injury, treating hypotension and bradycardia, relieving pain, treating spasticity, and maintaining bowel function.

- Corticosteroids may be used to decrease or control inflammation and edema of the cord.
- Vasopressors are used in the immediate acute care phase to treat bradycardia or hypotension due to spinal and neurogenic shock. Examples of drugs are dopamine (Intropin) to treat hypotension in neurogenic shock and dobutamine (Dobutrex) to support cardiac function. Atropine should be available at the bedside to treat bradycardia.
- Antispasmodics (baclofen [Lioresal], diazepam [Valium], and dantrolene [Dantrium]) may be used to treat spasticity in patients with spinal cord injury.
- Antiemetics may be administered to prevent vomiting.
- Analgesics such as nonsteroidal anti-inflammatory drugs (NSAIDs) and narcotics are administered to reduce pain.
- Proton pump inhibitors, such as omeprazole (Prilosec), rabeprazole (AcipHex), or pantoprazole (Protonix), are often administered to prevent stress-related gastric ulcers, a common complication in SCI.
- Unless contraindicated, anticoagulants (heparin or warfarin) may be given to prevent thrombophlebitis.
- Stool softeners may be administered as part of a bowel training program.

Treatments
The treatments used in the management of an SCI include surgery, stabilization, and immobilization.

SURGERY Early surgical treatment may be necessary if there is evidence of compression of the spinal cord by bone fragments or a hematoma. Surgery may also be done to stabilize and support the spine. However, many patients are treated with stabilization devices and do not require surgery. Surgeries that may be performed include a decompression laminectomy, a spinal fusion, and insertion of metal rods. Surgeries of the spine are discussed later in the chapter.

STABILIZATION AND IMMOBILIZATION As a result of one or more dislocations or fractures of the cervical vertebrae, the patient with an SCI may be immobilized in some type of traction or external fixation device to stabilize the vertebral column and prevent further damage to the cord (Figure 43–4 ■). Traction may also be used to stabilize the spinal column for patients who are not yet in a condition to have surgery or who have severe bleeding and edema of the injured cord. The physician applies the traction or fixation device; the nurse is responsible for assessments and interventions following the application.

Although used less frequently today, various devices provide cervical traction. For example, Gardner-Wells tongs may be used (Figure 43–3 ■). In this type of traction, the physician applies pins to the skull, approximately 1 cm above each ear, and weights are attached to the device.

The halo external fixation device is often used to provide stabilization if there is no significant involvement of the ligaments (Figure 43–2 ■). It is most often used to provide stability for fractures of the cervical and high thoracic

Figure 43–3 ■ Cervical traction may be applied by several methods, including Gardner-Wells tongs.

vertebrae without cord damage. This device allows greater mobility, self-care, and participation in rehabilitation programs. The device is secured with four pins inserted into the skull, two in the frontal bone and two in the occipital bone. The halo ring is then attached to a rigid plastic vest lined with sheepskin. Nursing interventions for the patient using a halo fixation device are described in the box on page 1486.

Research to Improve SCI Mangement

An SCI is costly in terms of human life, human function, and healthcare costs. For the patient with a high cervical injury, improving the ability of even one spinal segment to function may make an enormous difference in quality of life. Research is currently conducted on neurons of the spinal cord, stimulators to improve muscle function, and equipment to aid activities of daily living (ADLs) (National Institute of Neurological Disorders, 2009b).

Scientists are focusing on methods of advancing our knowledge of spinal cord repair, including protecting surviving neurons from further damage, replacing damaged neurons, stimulating the

Figure 43–2 ■ The halo external fixation device.

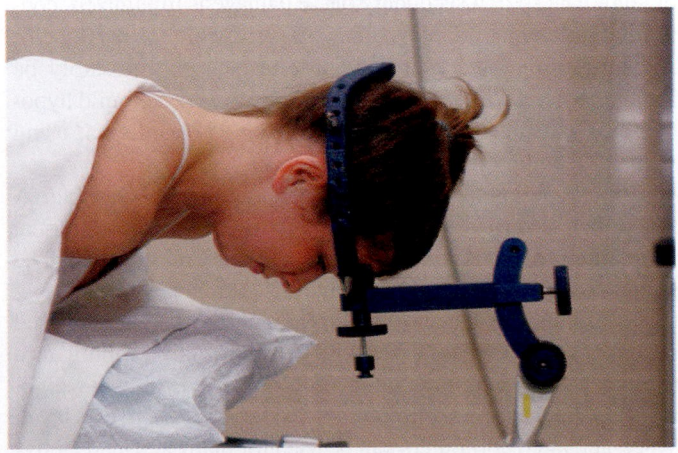

Figure 43–4 ■ Traction device.

NURSING CARE OF THE PATIENT
in Halo Fixation

- Maintain integrity of the halo external fixation device.
  a. Inspect pins and traction bars for tightness; report loosened pins to physician.
  b. Tape the appropriate wrench to the head of the bed for emergency intervention.
  c. Never use the halo ring to lift or reposition the patient.
  Loosening of the apparatus poses the risk of further damage to the cord. It is the responsibility of the nurse to maintain the integrity of the apparatus and the safety of the patient.
- Assess muscle function and skin sensation every 1 hour in the acute phase and every 4 hours thereafter.
  a. Assess motor function on a scale of 0 to 5, with 0 being no evidence of muscle contraction and 5 being normal muscle strength with full range of motion (ROM).
  b. Assess sensation by comparing touch and pain, moving from impaired to normal areas, and testing both the right and left sides of the body.
  Monitoring muscle function and skin sensation allows early identification of potential neurologic deficits.
- Monitor pin sites each shift and follow hospital policy for pin care daily for the first 48 to 72 hours, and then weekly. General guidelines include the following (Holmes & Brown, 2005):
  a. Assess pin sites for redness, edema, odor, and drainage.
  b. Clean each pin site with a sterile applicator dipped in a sterile solution (such as sterile chlorhexidine solution, 2 mg/mL) using one applicator per stroke in a circular motion, moving away from the pin. Remove crusts.
  c. Apply a topical antibiotic and cover with sterile 2-inch split gauze squares.
  Organisms can enter the body through the pin-insertion site and crusts; assessments and care are provided to detect signs of and prevent infection.
- Maintain skin integrity.
  a. Turn the immobile patient every 2 hours.
  b. Inspect the skin around edges of the vest every 4 hours.
  c. Change the sheepskin liner when it is soiled and at least once each week.
  These interventions prevent skin injury and irritation.

regrowth of axons and correctly targeting their connections, and retraining neural circuits to restore body functions. Basic research is ongoing about areas such as decreasing or blocking the action of glutamate so that secondary nerve damage is minimized, controlling inflammation, preventing self-destruction of nerve cells, and promoting regeneration. These effects may possibly be initiated by medications, cooling the body to a state of mild hypothermia, transplanting cell grafts into the damaged area, using stem cells, and promoting axonal growth.

Clinical research to improve rehabilitation in ongoing. A functional electrical stimulation (FES) system uses electrical stimulators to encourage functional walking and gripping. The stimulators must be implanted and the computer interface system is still limited. Devices implanted in the brain might be used to send a signal to a computer that in turn signals a robotic arm to move. New technologies include improved, lighter-weight wheelchairs; some can climb stairs and lift a person to eye-level. Voice-activated computers can be used for many self-care activities, including banking, dialing a phone, reading, and dressing.

Nursing Care

The patient with an SCI has complex needs during both the acute phase and the rehabilitative phase that involve all members of the healthcare team. Because these injuries are more common in younger patients, consideration of lifelong effects on both the patient and the family is essential. The nurse coordinates patient care and develops and implements a care plan that is individualized to each patient and family. The focus of the plan is to prevent the secondary complications of immobility and altered body functions, to promote self-care, and to educate the patient and family. A Case Study & Nursing Care Plan for a patient with an SCI is found on page 1490.

Health Promotion

Health promotion for SCI primarily involves preventing injuries. Nurses can provide valuable information in the community and in the workplace to prevent SCI. Programs that focus on wearing seat belts and using approved infant seats and child booster chairs in automobiles can do much to help decrease the number of SCIs each year. Educational programs that promote workplace safety and farm safety should include information about how to prevent falls and how to use heavy equipment safely.

Assessment

The following data are collected through the health history and physical examination (∞ see Chapter 41). Further focused assessments are described with nursing interventions in the next section.

- *Health history:* Time, location, and type of event causing injury; location, duration, quality, and intensity of pain; dyspnea; sensation; paresthesia.
- *Physical examination:* Vital signs, motor strength, movement, spinal reflexes, bowel sounds, bladder distention, level of consciousness.

Nursing Diagnoses and Interventions

Because an SCI has many possible effects, many nursing diagnoses may be appropriate. Nursing diagnoses discussed in this section focus on problems with physical mobility, respirations, dysreflexia, bowel and bladder elimination, sexual dysfunction, and self-esteem.

Impaired Physical Mobility

After the initial period of spinal shock and areflexia, the patient regains spinal reflex activity and muscle tone that is not under the control of higher centers. Patients with injuries above the level of T12 experience involuntary spastic movements of skeletal muscles. These movements reach a peak about 2 years after the injury and then gradually subside (Porth & Matfin, 2009). Spasms impair the ability to carry out activities of daily life and work. If present, paraplegia or quadriplegia increases the potential for impaired skin integrity, thrombophlebitis, and contractures.

The goals of care for patients with impaired mobility related to a spinal cord injury are to reduce the effects of spasticity and to prevent complications involving the skin, the cardiovascular system, and joint function.

- Perform passive ROM exercises for all extremities at least twice a day. Identify stimuli that cause spastic movements

EVIDENCE FOR NURSING CARE — The Patient with Spinal Cord Injury

Selected resources that nurses may find helpful when planning evidence-based nursing care follow.

- Groen, D., Biddle, A. K., Fahey, V., Gardiner, Jr., G. A., Hull, R., Lee, M. Y., et al. (2008). Prevention of thromboembolism in spinal cord injury. *National Guideline Clearinghouse.* Retrieved from http://www.guideline.gov
- King, R. B., Biddle, A. K., Braunschweig, C., Chen, D., Cowell, F., Dingus, C. M., et al. (2005). Neurogenic bowel management in adults with spinal cord injury. *National Guideline Clearinghouse.* Retrieved from www.guideline.gov
- Parsons, K. C., Buhrer, R., Burns, S. P., Butt, L., Jimenez, F., Kirshblum, S., et al. (2005). Respiratory management following spinal cord injury: A clinical practice guideline for healthcare professionals. *National Guideline Clearinghouse.* Retrieved from www.guideline.gov

and either avoid the stimuli (such as certain exercises) or teach the patient to expect the movements. *ROM exercises help prevent contractures and stretch spastic muscles, promoting rehabilitation.*

- Maintain skin integrity by turning every 2 hours, assessing pressure points at least once each shift, and using a special bed if necessary. The patient may be placed on a regular or special bed, such as a kinetic bed. *Immobility compresses soft tissues and promotes the development of decubitus ulcers. The lack of sensory warning mechanisms and of voluntary motor control of skin dermatomes further increases the risk for altered skin integrity. Special beds allow movement or turning while keeping the spinal column in alignment.*
- Assess the lower extremities each shift for manifestations of deep vein thrombosis (DVT). Observe for redness, swelling, and increased heat; measure thigh and calf circumference daily. If antiembolic stockings or sequential compression devices are ordered, remove for 30 to 60 minutes each shift and assess for skin impairment and provide skin care. *Patients with neurologic deficits are at high risk for deep venous thrombosis as a result of immobility, vasomotor dysfunction, and decreased venous return with venous stasis, especially during the first 2 to 3 weeks after injury. Thigh-high graduated compression stockings and/or sequential compression boots help prevent pooling of blood in the lower extremities and increase venous return, lessening the risk for venous stasis and thrombus formation. Nurses must ensure the stockings are properly sized and used (Winslow & Brosz, 2008).*

Impaired Gas Exchange

Injuries at the level of C3 to C5 affect the diaphragm, innervated by the phrenic nerve; the intercostals are affected at the level of T1 through T7; and at T6 to T12 the abdominal muscles (necessary for exhalation) are denervated, compromising respiratory function. In addition, because the abdominal muscles are paralyzed, the patient cannot expel secretions by coughing, increasing the risk of pneumonia. Patients with cord injuries at C3 or above have paralysis of the respiratory muscles and cannot breathe without a ventilator (see the Moving Evidence into Action box for related nursing care).

- Monitor vital capacity and respiratory effectiveness, assessing for tachycardia, restlessness, PaO_2 less than 60 mmHg, $PaCO_2$ greater than 50 mmHg, and vital capacity less than 1 L. *Patients with cervical cord injuries frequently require ventilatory support; injuries at other levels may reduce deep breathing, vital capacity, and the ability to expel secretions by coughing.*

MOVING EVIDENCE INTO ACTION — Reducing Incidence of Ventilator-Associated Pneumonia

Ventilator-associated pneumonia (VAP) is a preventable secondary complication from intubation and mechanical support. Mechanically intubated patients in neurologic ICUs are at increased risk of VAP from factors such as a decreased level of consciousness; dry, open mouth; and aspiration of secretions. This randomized, controlled study was conducted by Fields (2008) to support the premise that oral care, including tooth brushing, would further support the recommendations by the Institute of Healthcare Improvement's VAP prevention protocol (elevating the head of the bed 30 degrees, using sequential compression devices or anticoagulation, administering histamine blockers, practicing hand hygiene, initiating early mobilization, and interrupting sedation daily to evaluate neurologic status). In addition to these recommendations, an oral care procedure was instituted for the intervention group. Oral care consisted of brushing the patient's teeth, tongue, and hard palate with a suction toothbrush and toothpaste for at least 1 minute three times a day, followed by swabbing the same area with a Toothette for 1 minute, and then applying moisturizing ointment to the lips every 4 hours. In addition, a full oral assessment was performed every 12 hours. As a result of these nursing interventions, the rate of VAP dropped significantly. This study changed nursing practice and saved lives.

IMPLICATIONS FOR NURSING

Although studies have been conducted to determine if oral care and preventing VAP are related, the role of tooth brushing largely has been ignored. This study demonstrated that timed, consistent oral care can almost totally reduce the incidence of VAP in ICU patients who are mechanically intubated. As such, the study provides evidence on which to base nursing practice to prevent complications, and also demonstrates the cost effectiveness of a simple nursing intervention.

CRITICAL THINKING IN PATIENT CARE

1. One major problem for the researcher was the failure of nurses to document the oral care. How do you think this could have been avoided?
2. Instituting a new protocol is often difficult. How could you use this study to recommend the oral care described in this article?
3. This study was designed for a specific population. How do you think it could be adapted to prevent respiratory problems in patients who are not mechanically ventilated, but are comatose, demented, quadriplegic, or very old?

Source: Fields, S. B. (2008). Oral care intervention to reduce incidence of ventilator-associated pneumonia in the neurologic intensive care unit. *Journal of Neuroscience Nursing, 40*(5), 291–298.

- Monitor for signs of ascending edema of the spinal cord, including difficulty in swallowing or coughing, respiratory stridor, use of accessory muscles of respiration, bradycardia, and increasing motor and sensory loss. Report these manifestations immediately. *Hemorrhage and edema can further impair respiratory function. Patients with injuries above C7 may need a tracheostomy in addition to mechanical ventilation.*

Ineffective Breathing Pattern

The impairments of respiratory function described in the previous nursing diagnoses also affect breathing patterns. In patients with injury at higher levels, assisted ventilation and a tracheostomy are often necessary; when the injury is at lower levels, the patient's ability to take a deep breath and cough is diminished. The goal of nursing interventions is to maintain normal respiratory rate (12 to 20 breaths per minute) and to prevent pulmonary complications such as atelectasis and pneumonia.

- Assess respiratory rate, rhythm, and depth every 4 hours (or more frequently if needed). Auscultate breath sounds as a part of respiratory assessment. *Injury to the cord in the cervical or thoracic regions can decrease respiratory function and increase the risk for respiratory problems.*
- Monitor results of oxygen saturation with pulse oximetry and ABG studies. *ABG studies provide information about gas exchange; decreasing pH, oxygen, and oxygen saturation levels, and increasing carbon dioxide levels signal respiratory acidosis.*
- Administer supplemental oxygen as prescribed. *Oxygen saturation must be maintained at 100% with supplemental oxygen to prevent hypoxemia and secondary SCI in all acute SCI patients.*
- Help the patient turn, cough, and deep breathe at least every 2 hours. *Paralysis of intercostal or abdominal muscles decreases the ability to expel secretions by coughing; retained secretions increase the risk for pneumonia. The inability to breathe deeply may result in atelectasis.*
- Increase fluids given by mouth to 3000 mL per day (if oral intake is approved), according to patient preference for type of liquids and predicated on the patient's ability to swallow. *Increased fluid intake thins secretions, which can more easily be expelled and expectorated.*

Autonomic Dysreflexia

Autonomic dysreflexia is an emergency that requires immediate assessment and intervention to prevent complications of extremely high blood pressure (loss of consciousness, seizure, and even death).

- Elevate the head of the patient's bed and remove compression stockings or boots. *These measures increase pooling of blood in the lower extremities and decrease venous return, thus decreasing blood pressure.*
- Assess blood pressure every 2 to 3 minutes while at the same time assessing for stimuli that initiated the response (such as a full bladder, impacted stool, or skin pressure). *The most serious*

danger in dysreflexia is elevated blood pressure, which could precipitate a stroke, myocardial infarction, dysrhythmias, or seizures. If the patient has a Foley catheter, ensure that there are no kinks in the tubing. If the patient does not have a Foley catheter, drain the bladder with a straight catheter. If manifestations persist, assess for a fecal impaction. If an impaction is present, insert Nupercaine cream into the anus, wait 10 minutes, and manually remove the impaction.

- If blood pressure remains dangerously elevated, the physician may prescribe intravenous administration of diazoxide (Hyperstat). Other medications that may be used include nifedipine (Procardia) and hydralazine (Apresoline). *Diazoxide is an antihypertensive drug used in emergency situations to lower blood pressure in adults with dangerously high readings. Nifedipine and hydralazine are peripheral vasodilators that are administered to decrease the elevated blood pressure.*

Impaired Urinary Elimination and Constipation

Depending on the level of the injury, the patient with an SCI may have alterations in bowel and bladder function. Patients with injuries to the cord at or above the S2 to S4 levels will have a neurogenic bladder, with deficits in control of micturition. Voluntary and involuntary bowel control is affected in the patient with a lower motor neuron injury. Both bowel and bladder retraining are possible; if not, some form of assisted elimination is necessary. Although an indwelling catheter may be used in the acute phase of care, the goal is to reestablish a catheter-free state.

- Monitor for manifestations of a full bladder. *Overdistention stretches the bladder and can lead to backflow of urine into the ureters and kidney; stasis of urine in an incompletely emptied bladder increases the risk for infection.*

- Teach how to use trigger voiding techniques prior to straight catheterization. These techniques include stroking the inner thigh, pulling the pubic hair, tapping on the abdomen over the bladder, and (in females) pouring warm water over the vulva. *These trigger voiding techniques stimulate parasympathetic nerve fibers to cause reflex activity and may facilitate voiding.*
- Teach self-catheterization to patients who will be able to carry out the procedure alone or with minimal assistance (Procedure 43–1). *Straight catheterization at regular intervals is part of bladder training because periodic distention and relaxation of the muscles of the bladder promote reflex bladder activity. In addition, self-care fosters independence.*
- Monitor residual urine throughout the bladder retraining program. *A residual urine amount of less than 80 mL after a triggered voiding is considered satisfactory.*

PROCEDURE 43–1 Patient Self-Catheterization

Self-catheterization on an intermittent basis (usually a part of self-care at home) is a clean rather than a sterile procedure. The hands should be washed before and after the procedure, and the urinary meatus should be cleaned by washing with soap and water.

FEMALE SELF-CATHETERIZATION

■ Attempt to void. If urine is not of sufficient quantity (at least 100 mL) or if you cannot void at all, do self-catheterization. *A large amount of residual urine means that more frequent catheterizations (every 4 to 6 hours) are necessary.*

■ While sitting on the wheelchair or the commode, locate the urethra. Visualize the urethra by looking in a mirror, or palpate the urethra with a fingertip. *Visualization or palpation of the meatus is necessary for proper catheter insertion.*

■ Lubricate the meatus with a water-soluble lubricant. *Lubrication facilitates the insertion of the catheter and reduces trauma to tissues.*

■ Take a deep breath and insert the catheter tip 2 to 3 inches or until urine flows. *The catheter enters the bladder more easily when the sphincter is relaxed. The deep breath relaxes the sphincter. The female urethra is 1½ to 2½ inches long.*

■ Hold the catheter securely and allow urine to drain until the flow stops. *Withdrawing and reinserting the catheter increase the risk of infection.*

■ Withdraw the catheter and wash it with soap and water. Store the catheter in a clean container. *The catheter can be reused until it is too soft or too hard to be directed into and through the urinary meatus. Clean rather than sterile technique is usually used for self-catheterization at home.*

MALE SELF-CATHETERIZATION

■ Attempt to void. If urine is not of sufficient quantity (e.g., less than 100 mL) or if you cannot void at all, do self-catheterization. *A large amount of residual urine means that more frequent catheterizations (every 4 to 6 hours) are necessary.*

■ Sit either on the commode or in the wheelchair. Hold the penis with slight upward tension and extend it to its full length. *Extending the penis straightens the urethra.*

■ Lubricate the catheter from the tip to about 6 inches downward. *Lubrication is especially important for male catheterization because of the length of the urethra.*

■ Take a deep breath and insert the catheter 6 to 7 inches or until urine flows. *The catheter enters the bladder more easily when the sphincter is relaxed. The deep breath relaxes the sphincter. The male urethra is about 6 inches long.*

■ Hold the catheter securely and allow urine to drain until flow has stopped. *Withdrawing and reinserting the catheter increase the risk of infection.*

■ Withdraw the catheter and wash it with soap and water. Store the catheter in a clean container. *The catheter can be reused until it is too soft or too hard to be directed into and through the urethra. Clean rather than sterile technique is usually used for self-catheterization at home.*

■ Monitor for elimination of frequent, small, liquid, foul-smelling stools. *Injuries to the sacral cord elements or higher often results in loss of the defecation reflex. Even if peristalsis is present, the ability to have a bowel movement is impaired by loss of this reflex. Fecal impactions are an ongoing problem, and are manifested by this type of bowel elimination.*

■ Institute a bowel retraining program as follows:
  ■ Assess usual patterns of bowel elimination to establish best times for individualized program.
  ■ Maintain a high-fluid, high-fiber diet.
  ■ Use stool softeners as prescribed; rectal suppositories and enemas may be used 30 minutes after meals to stimulate stronger peristalsis and facilitate evacuation.
  ■ Maintain upright position if at all possible and ensure privacy.
  ■ If patient is unable to evacuate, digital stimulation or manual removal on a regular basis may be the most effective long-term management.

  A bowel retraining program to regulate the bowel through reflex activity may be instituted in patients with upper motor neuron injuries. The patient with a lower motor neuron injury loses the defecation reflex, and bowel retraining is more difficult (if not impossible).

Sexual Dysfunction

Sexual intercourse is often still possible for the patient with an SCI. In men, the general rule is that the higher the level of injury the greater the potential to have reflexogenic erections, although ejaculation or orgasm may not occur, and fertility is usually lower as a result of a lack of temperature control of the testes. However, ejaculation may be stimulated and the sperm used to inseminate the patient's partner, so that fatherhood is a possibility. Men who have sacral-level injuries do not have reflexogenic erections but may have psychogenic erections. They are also more likely to remain fertile.

Women with SCI generally do not have sensation during sexual intercourse, but pregnancy is possible. However, pregnant women with an SCI are at increased risk for autonomic dysreflexia during labor and delivery. Birth control options should be discussed prior to discharge from the acute care setting.

A patient with an SCI may be deeply concerned about alterations in sexual function. These concerns may lead to lowered self-esteem, altered self-image, or changes in feelings about being an attractive and desirable person. Assess concerns and provide a climate that is receptive to discussion about sexuality. Examples of objectives for sexual counseling for the patient with an SCI are that the patient will understand how the injury has altered sexual functioning, will be aware of alternative ways of achieving sexual pleasure, and will have a positive self-concept and body image.

■ Include data about sexuality when obtaining the nursing history and database. *Sexuality is a private matter for most people, and the patient may not discuss it unless the nurse introduces the topic.*

■ Provide accurate information about the effect of the SCI on sexual function. *Accurate information gives the patient a realistic picture of how the injury will affect sexuality.*

■ Initiate a discussion with the patient and partner of alternative means of gaining sexual satisfaction; these include the use of vibrators, and oral–genital and manual stimulation.

CASE STUDY & NURSING CARE PLAN   A Patient with an SCI

Jim Valdez, a 19-year-old college sophomore, is admitted to the hospital by ambulance following an automobile crash. His family (father, mother, and sister) live 100 miles away and cannot visit often, although they are very concerned. On admission to the hospital, a CT scan of the spine shows a fracture and partial laceration of the cord at the C7 level. Mr. Valdez is in halo traction. One night, he tells the nurse, "I wish I had just died when I got hurt. I don't think I can stand to live like this."

ASSESSMENT

When Mr. Valdez is admitted to the intensive care unit, he has flaccid paralysis involving all extremities. He has no sensation below the clavicle or in portions of his arms and legs. His bladder is distended and bowel sounds are absent. Other assessment findings include BP 90/56, P 50, T 97°F (36.1°C), arterial blood gases pH 7.4, PaO_2 96, $PaCO_2$ 37, SaO_2 96%. Oxygen per nasal cannula is given at 2 L/min, and halo traction is applied. A Foley catheter is inserted into his bladder, and a nasogastric tube is inserted and attached to low-pressure continuous suction.

After 3 days, Mr. Valdez is moved from the intensive care unit to the neurosurgical unit for continuing care and planning for transfer to a rehabilitation hospital in his home town. His vital signs have stabilized and are normal for his age; respirations and oxygenation are normal. Other neurologic assessments remain the same.

DIAGNOSES

- *Impaired Physical Mobility* related to paralysis of lower and upper extremities
- *Bowel Incontinence* related to lack of voluntary sphincter control
- *Complicated Grieving* related to denial of loss

EXPECTED OUTCOMES

- Be actively involved in exercise programs.
- Have a soft, formed stool every second or third day.
- Verbally express his grief to parents and staff.

PLANNING AND IMPLEMENTATION

- Conduct passive exercises on all extremities four times a day.
- Provide progressive mobilization by initially raising the head of the bed 90 degrees (repeat two to three times during the first day of movement); if blood pressure remains normal, dangle for 5 minutes before transferring him to a chair.
- His usual time for a bowel movement is after breakfast; schedule retraining program for that time.
- Encourage a diet high in fiber and fluids. Likes whole-wheat bread, orange juice, and cola; does not like water.
- Promote grief work by providing time to express feelings. Explain to the family that his denial and anger are part of the grieving process.
- Determine food likes and dislikes and order preferred foods from the menu. Encourage his friends to bring in his favorite foods periodically.
- Take and record weight every third day, using the bed scales.

EVALUATION

By the time Mr. Valdez is transferred to the rehabilitation hospital he is looking forward to learning how to use special equipment and getting his own motorized wheelchair. He is able to sit up in a chair without dizziness or hypotension. The use of ordered stool softeners combined with a high-fiber diet and fluid intake of 2000 to 3000 mL per day has maintained bowel elimination. Mr. Valdez and his parents have spent 3 hours talking about their feelings related to the accident and the future. Although the discussion is emotionally difficult, all three say they now feel much better. Mr. Valdez still has episodes of angry outbursts and tears, but he is more optimistic about what can be done and believes he can finish college. He selects foods from the menu each day and eats most of his meals, but he especially enjoys the times his friends bring in pizza or hamburgers.

CRITICAL THINKING IN THE NURSING PROCESS

1. Considering Mr. Valdez's age and developmental level, do you think his emotional responses to his injury were appropriate?
2. Issues of sexuality are obviously important for the patient with a spinal cord injury. How would you approach Mr. Valdez about this topic?
3. What would be your response as a male or female nurse if Mr. Valdez would allow only male nurses to provide care?
4. Outline a teaching program to help Mr. Valdez meet long-term urinary elimination needs.

See Evaluating Your Response in Appendix C.

Alternatives to intercourse can meet sexual needs and help maintain the relationship with a significant other.

- Refer for sexual counseling, if appropriate, or to local support groups where questions can be answered by others with similar experiences. *Knowing that others have had similar experiences can decrease social isolation and provide a means of learning alternative methods of sexual functioning.*

Situational and Chronic Low Self-Esteem

An SCI is the result of sudden trauma. Within moments, a formerly independent, fully functioning individual is suddenly unable to move and faces enormous adjustments in social, economic, and personal roles and relationships. Body image, self-esteem, and role performance are all affected by the damage. As a result, the patient often demonstrates behaviors that may be difficult for the nurse to handle: depression, denial, and anger are seen in the period immediately after the injury. In addition to these responses, the young adult patient may act out by making sexually overt statements.

- Encourage talking about all aspects of physical function and care. *Talking provides a safe outlet for fears and frustrations and also increases self-awareness. Acceptance of self facilitates rehabilitation.*
- Encourage self-care and independent decision making. *Participating in self-care can promote positive coping; making decisions decreases feelings of powerlessness.*
- Help identify strategies to increase independence in desired roles; include both short- and long-term goals. Discuss assistive devices (such as hand-operated automobiles). *Identifying strategies to increase independence in the future fosters a positive self-concept and motivates the patient to achieve rehabilitation goals.*
- Include family members and important others in discussions. *The realization that others do care and will continue to provide support is important in fostering positive self-regard.*
- Refer the patient and family to support groups or for psychologic counseling. *Adjustment to change is more likely when the patient and family seek peer and professional assistance.*

Using NANDA, NIC, and NOC

Linkages between a selected NANDA nursing diagnosis, NIC, and NOC for the patient with an SCI are shown in the chart that follows.

Community-Based Care

Rehabilitation of the patient with an SCI is an ongoing process that moves from intensive care through intermediate care to rehabilitation and then community-based and home care. Nursing interventions are necessary at all points in the process to prevent the complications of altered physical mobility and body functions and to teach the patient and family measures that promote independence in self-care.

Discharge planning should be addressed even in the initial plan of care while the patient is in the critical care setting. Advance planning ensures continuity of care when the patient leaves the hospital setting.

The following should be included in teaching the patient and family about care at home.

- Self-care activities (ADLs, exercises, bowel and bladder programs, skin care)
- Mobility (use of assistive devices: wheelchair, crutches, special automobiles)
- Preparation of the home environment
  - If the patient is in a wheelchair, will steps, stairs, doors, or carpeted floors present physical barriers?
  - If a special bed is necessary, have arrangements been made, and is it in the home?
- Psychologic support
- Independent activities
- Community resources, such as Lifeline (emergency alerting systems through a local hospital or agency), support groups, career centers for job retraining, counseling
- Coping skills for patient and caregiver

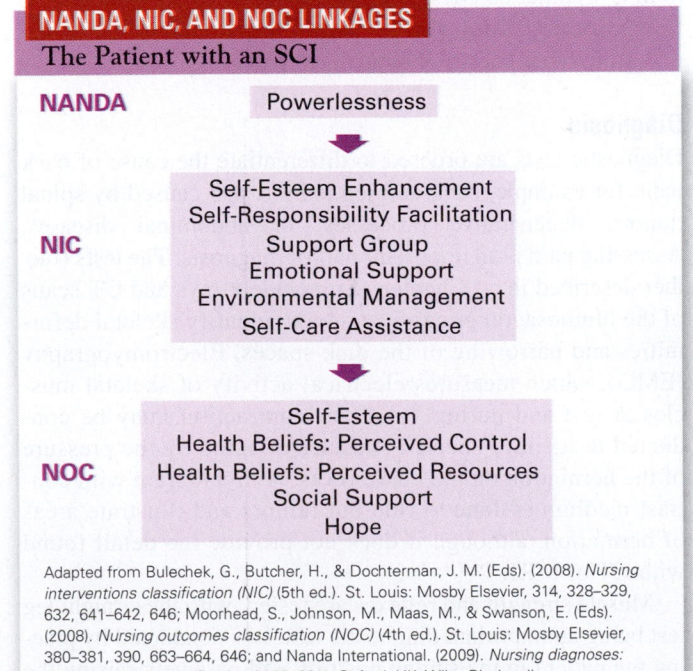

NANDA, NIC, AND NOC LINKAGES

The Patient with an SCI

NANDA — Powerlessness

↓

NIC
Self-Esteem Enhancement
Self-Responsibility Facilitation
Support Group
Emotional Support
Environmental Management
Self-Care Assistance

↓

NOC
Self-Esteem
Health Beliefs: Perceived Control
Health Beliefs: Perceived Resources
Social Support
Hope

Adapted from Bulechek, G., Butcher, H., & Dochterman, J. M. (Eds). (2008). *Nursing interventions classification (NIC)* (5th ed.). St. Louis: Mosby Elsevier, 314, 328–329, 632, 641–642, 646; Moorhead, S., Johnson, M., Maas, M., & Swanson, E. (Eds). (2008). *Nursing outcomes classification (NOC)* (4th ed.). St. Louis: Mosby Elsevier, 380–381, 390, 663–664, 646; and Nanda International. (2009). *Nursing diagnoses: Definitions and classification 2009–2011.* Oxford, UK: Wiley-Blackwell.

- Referral to a home health agency and physical therapist for the patient who is returning home
- Helpful resources:
  - American Spine Injury Association
  - The National Spinal Cord Injury Association
  - American Paralysis Association
  - Christopher and Dana Reeve Paralysis Foundation
  - Paralyzed Veterans of America

The Patient with a Herniated Intervertebral Disk

A herniated intervertebral disk (also called a ruptured disk, herniated nucleus pulposus, or "slipped disk") is a rupture of the cartilage surrounding the intervertebral disk with protrusion of the nucleus pulposus (Figure 43–5 ■). This disorder is the most common cause of low back pain, a common problem estimated to affect as many as two-thirds of people at some point in their lifetimes (Porth & Matfin, 2009).

FAST FACTS

Herniated Intervertebral Disks
- Herniated intervertebral disks are more common in men than women.
- Most patients are between the ages of 30 and 50.
- The majority of herniated disks occur in the lumbar region (L4 or L5 to S1); when disks herniate in the cervical region, they most commonly do so at C6 to C7.
- Multiple herniations are not common, occurring in only about 10% of all patients.

(Hickey, 2009)

Pathophysiology

The intervertebral disks, located between the vertebral bodies, are made of an inner nucleus pulposus and an outer collar (the annulus fibrosus). The disks allow the spine to absorb compression by acting as shock absorbers. A herniated intervertebral disk occurs when the nucleus pulposus protrudes through a weakened or torn annulus fibrosus of an intervertebral disk (see Figure 43–5 ■). This protrusion may occur anywhere along the vertebral column, but herniation of thoracic disks is uncommon.

Figure 43–5 ■ A herniated intervertebral disk. The herniated nucleus pulposus is applying pressure against the nerve root.

MANIFESTATIONS of a Ruptured Intervertebral Disk

L4 TO L5 LEVEL (AFFECTS FIFTH LUMBAR NERVE ROOT)
- Pain in hip, lower back, posterolateral thigh, anterior leg, dorsal surface of foot, great toe
- Muscle spasms in affected areas
- Paresthesia over lateral leg and web of great toe
- Foot drop (rare)
- Decreased or absent ankle reflex
- Cauda equina syndrome (with complete nerve root compression): bowel and bladder incontinence, paralysis of lower extremities

L5 TO S1 LEVEL (AFFECTS FIRST SACRAL NERVE ROOT)
- Pain in midgluteal region, posterior thigh, calf to heel, plantar surface of the foot to the fourth and fifth toes
- Paresthesias in posterior calf and lateral heel, foot, and toes
- Difficulty walking on toes

C5 TO C6 LEVEL (AFFECTS SIXTH CERVICAL NERVE ROOT)
- Pain in neck, shoulder, anterior upper arm, radial area of forearm, thumb
- Paresthesia of forearm, thumb, forefinger, and lateral arm
- Decreased biceps and supinator reflex
- Triceps reflex normal to hyperactive

A herniated intervertebral disk may result from trauma, degenerative disorders of the spine, or aging. The protrusion may occur spontaneously or as a result of trauma, such as lifting heavy objects while in the flexed position, or falling on the buttocks or back. It may also result from degenerative diseases, such as osteoarthritis, and aging. Aging causes degeneration in the annulus fibrosus and the posterior longitudinal ligaments, and the vertebrae and disks are less able to respond to movement and are more easily injured.

Rupture of the disk most often allows herniation of the nucleus pulposus in a posterolateral direction, with compression of the associated nerve root. The resulting pressure on adjacent spinal nerves causes characteristic manifestations, which vary with the location and the amount of protruding disk material (see the box on this page). Occasionally the herniation is central rather than posterolateral, with pressure on the spinal cord.

The herniation may be abrupt or gradual. Lifting incorrectly or suddenly twisting the spine can cause rupture with immediate intense pain and muscle spasms. Gradual herniation is the result of degenerative changes, osteoarthritis, or ankylosis spondylitis. Patients with a gradual herniation have a slow onset of pain and neurologic deficits. Both motor and sensory manifestations occur, and are localized to the area of the body innervated by the nerve root. The manifestations may be described as **radiculopathy** (a condition in which one or more nerves, especially nerve roots, do not function normally), and/or **paresthesia** (an abnormal sensation of the skin, such as numbness, burning, or pricking).

Lumbar Disk Manifestations

The classic manifestation of a ruptured lumbar disk is recurrent episodes of pain in the lower back. The pain typically radiates across the buttock and down the posterior leg. **Sciatica** is a term used to describe lumbar back pain that radiates down the posterior leg to the ankle and is increased by sneezing or coughing (the result of pressure on nerve roots L4, L5, S1, S2, or S3, which give rise to the sciatic nerve). The patient feels pain when lifting one leg while dorsiflexing the foot of that leg. Sciatica pain varies in intensity, ranging from mildly uncomfortable to excruciating. It is aggravated by a variety of positions and activities, including sitting, straining, coughing, sneezing, climbing stairs, walking, and riding in a car. Prolonged sitting and climbing stairs are especially painful.

Other manifestations include postural deformity, motor deficits, sensory deficits, and changes in reflexes. When standing, the patient typically has a slight forward tilt to the trunk, scoliosis of the lumbar spine, slight flexion of the hip and knee on the affected side, and paravertebral muscle spasms. Motor deficits include weakness and some patients may experience problems with sexual function and urinary elimination. Sensory deficits include paresthesias and numbness. Knee and ankle reflexes are decreased or absent.

Cervical Disk Manifestations

Most (70% to 75%) of cervical herniations are the result of degeneration; other causes include trauma, such as a whiplash injury (Hickey, 2009). Cervical disks that herniate laterally cause radicular pain in the shoulder, neck, and arm and paresthesias along the dermatome of the compressed nerve root. Other manifestations of lateral cervical herniation include muscle spasms and stiff neck and decreased or absent arm reflexes. Central cervical herniations result in a dull, intermittent pain; however, the patient may also experience lower extremity weakness, unsteady gait, muscle spasms, urinary elimination problems, altered sexual function, and hyperactive lower extremity reflexes. A cervical herniation due to acute trauma may be manifested by immediate weakness of the extremity, or if severe, by paralysis.

Interdisciplinary Care

Considerations for the patient with a ruptured intervertebral disk include identifying the location of herniation and determining whether conservative treatment or surgery is indicated. Diagnostic tests may also be performed to identify herniated disk from other causes of acute back pain.

Diagnosis

Diagnostic tests are ordered to differentiate the cause of back pain; for example, back and leg pain is also caused by spinal tumors, degenerative processes, or abdominal diseases. Assessing pain is an important part of diagnosis. The tests (further described in ∞ Chapter 41) include x-rays and CT scans of the lumbosacral or cervical area to identify skeletal deformities and narrowing of the disk spaces. Electromyography (EMG), which measures electrical activity of skeletal muscles at rest and during voluntary contraction, may be conducted to identify specific muscles affected by the pressure of the herniation on the nerve roots. A myelogram with contrast medium is done to rule out tumors and illustrate areas of herniation, although it does not provide the detail found with CT or MRI.

Muscle strength and reflexes are tested, with the straight leg test being an important diagnostic test. It is conducted by placing the patient in the supine position and passively raising the leg, or by having the patient sit on a table and slowly extending

NURSING CARE OF THE PATIENT | Having a Posterior Laminectomy

PREOPERATIVE TEACHING

- Demonstrate and ask for a return demonstration of logrolling; explain that it will be done by the nurses for the first day or two, and then the patient can do it alone. *To ensure healing, the spinal column must remain in alignment when turning and moving.*
- Explain the importance of taking pain medications regularly and of asking for them before the pain is severe. Include information about the possibility of the pain being much the same after surgery. *Pain is easier to control if medications are taken before the pain is severe. Pain may be the same for a period of time following surgery for a herniated intervertebral disk because edema due to surgery irritates and compresses the nerve roots.*
- Demonstrate the use of a fracture bedpan and ask the patient to practice its use. *The patient usually must remain flat in bed for a period of time following surgery. A fracture bedpan is more comfortable for patients who must lie flat.*
- Explain the need to eat while lying flat. *This position prevents flexion of the spine.*
- Demonstrate and ask for a return demonstration of deep breathing, the use of the incentive spirometer, and leg exercises. *These measures prevent respiratory and circulatory complications.*

POSTOPERATIVE CARE

- Maintain a position that minimizes stress on the surgical wound. For patients with cervical laminectomy do the following:
  a. Elevate the head of the bed slightly.
  b. Position a small pillow under the neck.
  c. Maintain the position of the cervical collar.
  For patients with lumbar laminectomy do the following:
  a. Keep the bed flat or elevate the head of the bed slightly.
  b. Place a small pillow under the head.
  c. Place a small pillow under the knees, or use a pillow to support the upper leg when the patient lies on one side.
  These positions minimize stress on the surgical wound and suture line. A cervical collar provides stability and prevents flexing or twisting the neck.
- Turn every 2 hours, using the logrolling technique. Teach the patient not to use the side rails to change position. Maintain proper body alignment in all positions. *The patient's body is turned as a single unit (usually with a turning sheet) to avoid movement of the operative area. Pulling on the side rails puts stress on the operative area and may also cause misalignment of the vertebral column.*
- Monitor for signs of nerve root compression.
  a. Cervical laminectomy: Assess hand grips and arm strength, ability to move the fingers, and ability to detect touch.
  b. Lumbar laminectomy: Assess leg strength, ability to wiggle the toes, and ability to detect touch.
  Compare bilateral findings. Report muscle weakness or sensory impairment to the physician immediately. *Loss of motor and sensory function may indicate nerve root compression.*
- Assess for hematoma formation as manifested by severe incisional pain that is not relieved by analgesics and decreased motor function. Report these findings immediately. *A hematoma may form at the surgical site. If untreated, it may cause irreversible neurologic deficits including paraplegia and bowel/bladder dysfunctions (Hickey, 2003).*
- Assess for leakage of cerebrospinal fluid (CSF). Assess the dressing for increased moisture. Check the sheets for wetness when the patient is lying supine; check for clear liquid running down the back when the patient is sitting or standing. Gently palpate the sides of the wound to detect a bulge. Use

a Dextrostix strip to assess any leakage for the presence of glucose, a positive indicator of CSF. *Although uncommon, leakage of CSF greatly increases the risk for infection of the wound and of the meninges.*

- Assess for nerve root injury. Assess the ability to dorsiflex the foot (lumbar laminectomy) and the grip strength (cervical laminectomy). Assess the patient who has had a cervical laminectomy for hoarseness. Report hoarseness and further assess ability to swallow. *Nerve root compression may cause permanent damage, resulting in footdrop (in lumbar laminectomy patients) and hand weakness (in cervical laminectomy patients). Damage to the laryngeal nerve may cause permanent hoarseness. Impaired ability to swallow puts the patient at risk for aspiration.*
- Assess for urinary retention. The patient should void within 8 hours after surgery. If the physician allows, let males stand to void. Compare intake and output for each 8-hour period. Use a bladder scanner to identify urinary retention or residual urine. *All patients who have received a general anesthetic are at risk for urinary retention. The patient who has had a lumbar laminectomy may have even more difficulty voiding as a result of stimulation of sympathetic nerves during surgery.*
- Assess for pain using a scale from 0 (no pain) to 10 (severe pain). Administer prescribed analgesics on a regular basis, or teach how to use patient-controlled analgesia (PCA), if prescribed. Discuss concerns about pain that is unrelieved by surgery. *Compression of the nerve root over time results in edema and inflammation. Because of surgery-induced edema, the patient is likely to experience either the same pain or perhaps more severe pain in the period immediately after surgery. This pain usually persists for several weeks after surgery. In addition, many patients who have had a lumbar laminectomy have muscle spasms in the lower back, abdomen, and thighs for the first few days after surgery.*
- Assess for infection by taking and recording vital signs at least every 4 hours; report increased body temperature. Assess the wound and dressing for signs of infection: increased redness, drainage, pain, and pus. Use sterile technique to change dressings. *The surgical patient is always at risk for infection; the patient with a laminectomy is also at risk for arachnoiditis. This inflammation of the arachnoid layer of the spinal meninges results from wound infection or contamination during surgery and may cause the formation of painful adhesions.*
- Encourage deep breathing and the use of the incentive spirometer every 2 hours; coughing may be discouraged. *Anesthesia and immobility depress respiratory function. Coughing may be discouraged because it can disrupt healing tissues, especially in patients having a cervical laminectomy.*
- Increase mobility as prescribed. (The time frame for ambulation is prescribed by the physician; the routine here is representative.) Patients often sit on the side of the bed and dangle their legs the evening after surgery or the first day thereafter. Many patients ambulate the first postoperative day. To help the patient out of bed, first elevate the head of the bed. Then bring the patient's legs over the side of the bed at the same time that the upper body moves into the upright position. Patients should not ambulate without assistance until they are no longer dizzy or weak. *Early ambulation increases respiratory and circulatory function and decreases the risk of thrombophlebitis of the lower extremities. The vertebral column should remain in alignment while the patient sits and stands. Safety must be considered throughout care.*

the knee with both hip and knee flexed at a 90-degree angle. This movement places traction on the nerve root, which increases the pain if the nerve root is inflamed.

Medications

The patient with a ruptured intervertebral disk is treated with medications to relieve pain and reduce swelling and muscle spasms. Pain is usually managed with NSAIDs (∞ see Chapter 9). Muscle spasms are treated with muscle relaxants.

Treatments

A ruptured intervertebral disk may be treated conservatively or with surgery.

CONSERVATIVE TREATMENT A ruptured intervertebral disk is usually managed conservatively unless the patient is experiencing severe neurologic deficits. The goals of treatment are pain relief and healing of the involved disk by fibrosis. Conservative treatment is usually prescribed for 2 to 6 weeks. If the patient continues to have pain after that time, surgery may be considered. The treatment regimen depends on the severity of the manifestations. Decreasing activity level with bed rest is no longer recommended; in many cases, the patient is advised to continue with normal activities while taking prescribed medications for pain, inflammation, and muscle spasms.

Medications used to treat back pain include nonnarcotic analgesics, anti-inflammatory drugs such as the NSAIDs, muscle relaxants, and sedative-tranquilizers.

SURGERY Surgery is indicated for patients who do not respond to conservative management or have serious neurologic deficits. Several surgical interventions are used to treat a ruptured intervertebral disk. The type of surgery chosen depends on the location of the disk and the stability of the spinal column.

- A laminectomy, the type of surgery most often performed, is the removal of a part of the vertebral lamina. The surgery is done to relieve pressure on the nerves. It is often combined with removal of the protruding nucleus pulposus (nucleotomy). Nursing care for the patient having a laminectomy is discussed in the box on page 1493. A diskectomy is the removal of the nucleus pulposus of an intervertebral disk. Diskectomy may be performed alone or in conjunction with a laminectomy.
- Spinal fusion is the insertion of a wedge-shaped piece of bone or bone chips between the vertebrae to stabilize them. The bone is usually taken from a patient donor site, such as the iliac crest. A spinal fusion may also be performed through a spinal implant with a device called a BAK (a hollow titanium cylinder with holes), which is packed with grafted bone from a donor site and placed in the space where a disk is removed. Although not appropriate for all patients requiring a spinal fusion, this does facilitate a short hospital stay and convalescence.
- Foraminotomy is an enlargement of the opening between the disk and the facet joint to remove bony overgrowth compressing the nerve. The location and size of the incision vary according to the surgeon's preference and the location and size of the ruptured disk. The posterior approach is taken for lumbar surgery. Either the posterior or the anterior approach may be taken for cervical disks.

- Intradiscal electrothermal therapy (IDET) uses thermal energy to treat pain from a bulging spinal disk. A special needle is inserted into the disk and heated to a high temperature. The heat thickens and seals the disk wall and decreases bulging of the disk.
- A microdiskectomy, in which microsurgical techniques are used, is performed through a very small incision. This type of surgery decreases the possibility of trauma to surrounding structures during surgery and allows early postoperative mobility and a short hospital stay.

✍ Nursing Care

Nursing care for the patient with a ruptured intervertebral disk may be provided through information in community and work settings, during conservative treatment, and during pre- and postoperative treatment. The pain of the ruptured disk is often discouraging and debilitating, and may well affect the patient's ability to work.

Health Promotion

Proper body mechanics may help prevent the occurrence of a ruptured intervertebral disk. Teaching the proper method of lifting and moving heavy objects should begin when children enter school. This information should also be given to all workers (including nurses) who have lifting as part of their responsibilities. The guidelines for proper body mechanics are as follows:

- Begin activities by spreading the feet apart to broaden the base of support.
- Use large muscles of the arms to lift and the legs to push when lifting.
- Work as closely as possible to the object that is to be lifted or moved.
- Slide, roll, push, or pull an object rather than lift it.
- When lifting, bend the knees and lift up over your center of gravity.
- When lifting, use a back support belt.

Assessment

The following data are collected through the health history and physical examination (∞ see Chapter 41).

- *Health history:* Type of employment, risk factors, pain (location, duration, intensity).
- *Physical assessment:* Muscle strength and coordination, sensation, reflexes.

Nursing Diagnosis and Interventions

Nursing care for patients with a herniated intervertebral disk focuses largely on pain management, both during conservative management and after surgery.

Acute Pain

Patients with a ruptured intervertebral disk experience acute back and leg pain. Acute pain may be related to preoperative muscle spasms or nerve root compression. After surgery, the patient may have pain at the site of the incision and in the surgical area.

- Assess the degree of pain on a 0 to 10 scale (10 being greatest pain) and identify contributing and relieving factors. *Pain is a subjective experience. The nurse needs to assess it thoroughly before initiating interventions.*

- Use a firm mattress or place a board under the mattress. *A firm bed supports the spinal column and muscles.*
- Teach the patient to avoid turning or twisting the spinal column and to assume positions that decrease stress on the vertebral column (e.g., when in the supine position, flex the hips slightly). A small pillow may be placed under the knees (for patients with a herniated lumbar disk) or under the neck (for patients with a herniated cervical disk). *Correct body positions can decrease intradisk pressure.*
- Provide analgesic medications around the clock. *Intense pain can increase muscle spasms; maintaining serum levels of analgesics often prevents severe pain.*

Chronic Pain

The patient with a ruptured intervertebral disk often has pain for an extended period of time. Despite conservative treatment or previous surgery, pain may be ongoing or intermittent. If previous surgery has not relieved the pain, the patient may be depressed or angry. Caring for a patient with chronic pain is frustrating, and the patient is often regarded as difficult.

- Treat the patient's reports of pain with respect. *The patient is the person experiencing the pain and is thus the expert about it.*
- Do not refer to the patient as being addicted to pain medication. *All types of pain medications may be used legitimately to manage pain.*

> **PRACTICE ALERT**
> Although the patient may develop tolerance to a narcotic analgesic, tolerance does not imply addiction.

- Monitor the patient carefully for any changes in condition. *Significant changes in the patient's condition may go unrecognized when pain is present for a prolonged period of time.*
- Maintain written plans of care for pain management that are individualized and ensure continuity of care. *When the patient makes several visits (for instance, to an emergency department or a pain clinic), written records help caregivers determine what is effective in managing pain and what is not.*
- Teach the patient alternative methods of pain management. *Consider the patient's coping style when recommending methods. Patients who have a passive coping style are often better able to manage pain by depending on others, taking medications, and resting. Patients with an active coping style are probably better able to manage pain by learning self-management methods, taking part in activities, and staying busy.*
- Develop effective methods of improving rest and sleep. Problems with rest and sleep make pain management more difficult. *Sleeping poorly at night contributes to decreased motivation, confused thinking, depression, and muscle aches.*
- Refer the patient to a physical therapist for an exercise program, if appropriate. *The patient needs to know exactly what*

exercises to do, how many repetitions are recommended, for how long, and how often. The patient should not exercise to the point of causing increased pain.

- Assess the need for referrals (and make them if necessary) for the patient who is depressed or anxious. *Anxiety and depression often are a part of long-term chronic pain, making pain management more difficult. Suggest that referrals for help with the frustration (rather than "depression") may make a significant difference in the patient's ability to manage pain.*

Constipation

The patient with a ruptured intervertebral disk often has problems with constipation because of reduced mobility. Nursing interventions to alleviate and prevent constipation are important because straining to have a bowel movement can increase intradisk pressure, thus increasing pain.

- Assess the patient's usual bowel routine, including diet, fluid intake, and the use of laxatives or enemas. *Effective interventions are based on individualized needs.*

> **PRACTICE ALERT**
> People who use laxatives or enemas for long periods of time may be dependent on them to have a bowel movement.

- Encourage a fluid intake of 2500 to 3000 mL per day unless contraindicated by the presence of renal or cardiac disease. *Adequate fluid intake facilitates the passage of feces.*
- Increase fiber and bulk in the diet. If the patient is unable to tolerate increased fiber, consult with the physician about the use of stool softeners or bulk-forming agents. *Bulk and fiber promote regularity by retaining water in the large intestine.*

Community-Based Care

It is the nurse's responsibility to teach the patient and family about chronic pain control, including specific interventions to alleviate pain. The nurse's role may be that of advocate and creative problem solver (see the following Meeting Individualized Needs box). The following topics should be addressed:

- Often the goal is to control pain so that the patient can perform normal ADLs, rather than to reach a pain-free state.
- Nonpharmacologic methods of pain management include relaxation techniques, guided imagery, distraction, hypnosis, and music. Joining a support group may be an effective intervention in coping with and managing pain.
- Patients may be referred to a physical therapist for education about body mechanics and back-strengthening exercises. Nurses should have the patient demonstrate the exercises to reinforce teaching.

The Patient with a Spinal Cord Tumor

Spinal cord tumors may be benign or malignant, primary or metastatic. Tumors of the spinal cord are seen equally in men and in women, and they most often occur between the ages of 20 and 60. They are rarely seen in the older adult.

MEETING INDIVIDUALIZED NEEDS   Teaching the Patient with a Ruptured Intervertebral Disk

- Sleep on a firm mattress; use a bed board if necessary.
- When lying in the supine position, flex the knees to approximately a 45-degree angle with a small pillow and use a small pillow under the head.
- Avoid any activities that flex the spine, such as bending or lifting, and do not twist the back.
- Follow a diet to maintain body weight or to lose weight if needed.
- Follow the prescribed exercise program; for example, do the following:
  a. Lie flat on your back on the floor. Tighten your abdominal and buttock muscles and tilt your pelvis forward so that your lower back is flat on the floor (this is called a *pelvic tilt*). Hold the position for 3 seconds and repeat for the prescribed number of times.
  b. Lying on the back on a firm surface, press the feet to the floor, tighten the abdominal muscles, and lift the upper

half of the body off the floor. Hold the position for 3 seconds, and repeat as prescribed.
  c. Lying on your back on a firm surface, bring your knees up to the chest. Put your hands around your knees and raise the buttocks off the floor. Repeat as prescribed.
  d. Sit upright on the floor or a firm surface. Keep one leg straight and bend the other knee. Reach for the toes of the straightened leg. Switch legs. Repeat as prescribed.
  e. Stand upright. Squat down, flexing the hips and knees. Straighten your back. Stand upright by straightening the knees. Repeat as prescribed.
- Wear flat-heeled shoes that provide good support.
- Use proper lifting techniques. For instance, squat and use your thigh muscles to lift an object from the floor, and spread your feet to get a wide base of support when you lift while you are standing.

Classification

Tumors of the spinal cord are classified as either primary or secondary (metastatic). Primary tumors are rare and have an unknown cause. They may arise at any level of the spinal column, with the majority being thoracic. Most spinal cord tumors are metastatic. Metastatic tumors occur in approximately 20% of all patients with cancer (Hickey, 2009) and are most commonly the result of malignancies of the lung, breast, prostate, colon, kidney, or uterus.

Spinal cord tumors may also be classified by anatomic location as either intramedullary or extramedullary tumors. Intramedullary tumors arise from within the neural tissues of the spinal cord; those that occur most frequently are ependymomas and gliomas. Extramedullary tumors, the most common type, arise from tissues outside the spinal cord, with commonly occurring tumors including neurofibromas, meningiomas, sarcomas, chordomas, and vascular tumors. Extramedullary tumors are further categorized as intradural (arising from the nerve roots or meninges within the subarachnoid space) or extradural (arising from epidural tissue or the vertebrae outside the dura). Extradual tumors are the most comon location for metastatic cancer. Both primary and metastatic intradural tumors can invove the cerebrospinal fluid, called leptomeningeal disease (LMD).

Pathophysiology

Depending on their anatomic location, spinal cord tumors result in pathologic changes as a result of compression, invasion, or ischemia secondary to arterial or venous obstruction. Extramedullary tumors (whether benign or malignant) alter normal function through compression of the spinal cord, with destruction of white matter and eventual filling of the space around the spinal cord. Cord compression interferes with normal blood flow and membrane potentials, altering afferent and efferent motor, sensory, and reflex impulses. Compression of the spinal cord also causes edema, which can ascend the cord and cause further neurologic deficits. Intramedullary tumors both compress and invade. As the tumor grows within the cord, the cord also enlarges and distorts the white matter.

The vertebral column is the most common site in the bony skeleton for cancer metastasis. Metastatic tumors can involve the vertebrae, grow through the vertebral foramina, or directly affect the dura, spinal fluid, or spinal cord. The lesion, as it grows, causes epidural compression of the cord or spinal nerves. Most tumors (70%) are thoracic, and multiple spinal levels may be involved (Porth, 2009).

Manifestations

The manifestations of a spinal cord tumor depend on the anatomic location, level of occurrence, type of tumor, and spinal nerves involved. General manifestations of a spinal cord tumor include pain, motor and sensory deficits, changes in

MANIFESTATIONS of Spinal Cord Tumors

CERVICAL CORD TUMORS
- Ipsilateral arm motor involvement, followed by ipsilateral and contralateral leg involvement, followed by contralateral arm involvement
- Paresis of the arms and legs
- Stiffness of the neck
- Paraplegia
- Pain in the shoulders and arms
- Hyperactive reflexes

THORACIC CORD TUMORS
- Paresis and spasticity of one leg, followed by paresis and spasticity of the other leg
- Pain in the back and chest
- Positive Babinski reflex
- Bowel and bladder dysfunction
- Sexual dysfunction

LUMBOSACRAL CORD TUMORS
- Paresis and spasticity of one leg, followed by paresis and spasticity of the other leg
- Pain in the lower back, radiating to the legs and perineal area
- Loss of sensation in the legs
- Bowel and bladder dysfunction
- Sexual dysfunction
- Decreased or absent ankle and knee reflexes

bowel and/or bladder elimination, and changes in sexual function. Specific manifestations by anatomic level are outlined in the box on page 1496.

Pain is often the first manifestation of a spinal cord tumor. It is caused by compression of the spinal cord, tension on the spinal nerves, or tumor attachment to the proximal dura (the covering of the spinal cord). The pain may be either localized or radicular. Localized pain is felt when pressure is applied over the spinous process of the involved area; this type of pain often accompanies metastatic tumors involving the vertebrae. Radicular pain is felt along the course of a nerve as a result of compression, irritation, or tension of a nerve root. The pain is often made worse by any activity that causes intraspinal pressure, such as sneezing or coughing.

Motor manifestations resulting from a spinal cord tumor include paresis and paralysis below the level of the tumor, spasticity, and hyperactive reflexes. The Babinski reflex may be positive. These deficits are the result of involvement of the corticospinal tracts.

Many different sensory manifestations may occur, depending on the location and level of the tumor. Lateral tumor growth and compression affect the lateral spinothalamic tracts, causing pain, numbness, tingling, and coldness. If the tumor involves the posterior columns, the senses of vibration and proprioception of body parts are affected.

Bladder and bowel elimination and sexual function are often affected. Bowel elimination deficits include constipation that may progress to paralytic ileus. Initial bladder elimination deficits include frequency, urgency, and difficulty voiding. The deficits may progress to urinary retention and a neurogenic bladder. The male patient may be impotent.

Syringomyelia is a complication of some spinal cord tumors. In this condition, a fluid-filled cystic cavity forms in the central intramedullary gray matter. This syndrome causes pain, motor weakness, and spasticity.

Interdisciplinary Care

The medical management of the patient with a spinal cord tumor focuses first on diagnosis. Treatment depends on the type of tumor, its location, and the patient's condition.

Diagnosis

The patient with a spinal cord tumor undergoes many of the same diagnostic tests as does the patient with a ruptured intervertebral disk. The tests used to identify the tumor include x-rays, CT scans, MRI, and myelogram (∞ see Chapter 41). A lumbar puncture of the patient with a spinal cord tumor will demonstrate CSF that is commonly xanthochromic (having a yellow color), has increased protein, has few to no cells, and clots immediately (this cluster of findings is called Froin's syndrome). A biopsy may be done to identify the tumor type.

Medications

The patient with a spinal cord tumor is given medications to relieve pain and control edema. If the pain is severe and the result of a metastatic tumor, an epidural catheter may be inserted for narcotic analgesic administration. Pain management for patients with a spinal cord tumor is provided by narcotic analgesics (∞ see Chapter 9). Steroids, such as dexamethasone (Decadron), are administered to control edema of the cord.

Surgery

Intramedullary and intradural tumors are surgically excised when possible. Advances in microsurgical techniques and laser surgery have increased the possibility of tumor excision. Metastatic tumors may be partially excised to reduce cord compression; rapidly growing metastatic lesions may require surgical decompression to preserve motor, bowel, or bladder function. The surgical excision is made through a laminectomy. The patient with a tumor involving more than two vertebrae often has a spinal fusion and may also have rods inserted to stabilize the spinal column.

Radiosurgery

An advanced device called the CyberKnife may be used for some patients. This is a painless, noninvasive treatment that delivers high doses of precisely targeted radiation to destroy tumors while minimizing damage to healthy tissue. The device is controlled by a flexible robotic arm, making it possible to treat the spine and spinal cord (areas that cannot be treated with other radiosurgery techniques).

Radiation Therapy

Radiation therapy is used to treat metastatic spinal cord tumors for several different reasons. It may be used on an emergency basis to treat the patient with rapidly progressing neurologic deficits. It may be used to reduce pain. Radiation may also be used following surgical excision of as much tumor mass as possible.

Radiation of the spinal cord may cause the development of radiation-induced myelopathy. This complication of radiation exposure occurs over time, with manifestations of a *Brown-Séquard syndrome* (weakness or paralysis on one side of the body and loss of sensation on the opposite side) developing 12 to 15 months after therapy. The manifestations may progress to paraplegia, sensory loss, and loss of bowel and bladder control (Hickey, 2009).

∞ Nursing Care

Nursing care for the patient with a spinal cord tumor is individualized to the type of tumor and the type of treatment. The patient with a benign tumor that is removed by surgery has different healthcare needs than the patient with a metastatic tumor, even though they may have similar neurologic deficits. The patient with a spinal cord tumor (regardless of type) requires nursing care to monitor for neurologic changes, to provide pain management, and to manage motor and sensory deficits in order to preserve quality of life.

The assessments and nursing interventions for the patient with a spinal cord tumor are much the same as those described for the patient with an SCI or who is undergoing surgery for a ruptured intervertebral disk. Following surgical treatment, the patient may be transferred to a rehabilitation center or go home for the recovery period. Referrals for home care, occupational therapy, and physical therapy often help the patient

Lumbar Puncture Video

regain functional abilities. Teach family members how to move the patient in the bed and from the bed to a chair. Also teach them how to provide physical care, care for any appliances (such as an indwelling catheter), and prevent or treat constipation.

The Patient with a Central Nervous System Infection

The CNS, including the brain, spinal cord, meninges, neural tissues, and blood vessels, may be directly affected by bacteria, viruses, fungi, protozoans, and rickettsiae. The CNS may also be affected by toxins from bacterial infections. In general, organisms enter the brain in two ways: through the bloodstream by spreading from infections of adjacent or nearby structures (such as sinusitis, otitis media, or pneumonia) and crossing the blood–brain barrier or by direct invasion through a skull fracture or bullet hole. The incidence of pathogenic infections of the CNS increased with the onset of AIDS. Patients who are HIV positive may have CNS infections caused by toxoplasmosis, cryptococcus, tuberculosis, herpes simplex, cytomegalovirus (CMV), or a polyoma virus.

Pathophysiology

When pathogens enter the CNS and the meninges, an infection and inflammatory process results. The pathology of CNS infections includes the invading pathogens, the infection, the subsequent inflammation, and an increase in intracranial pressure (IICP) that may result from the inflammatory processes. Both the pathogenic damage and the IICP may result in brain damage and life-threatening complications.

Meningitis

Meningitis is a pyogenic (purulent) infection that involves the pia mater, the arachnoid, and the subarachnoid space, including the cerebrospinal fluid. The infection spreads rapidly throughout the CNS because of the circulation of CSF around the brain and spinal cord. Meningitis may be acute or chronic, and it may be bacterial, viral, fungal, or parasitic in origin. There are two types of acute infectious meningitis: acute purulent meningitis (usually bacterial) and acute lymphocytic meningitis (usually viral).

The organism responsible for meningitis must overcome nonspecific and specific host defense mechanisms to invade and replicate in the CSF. These defenses include the skin barrier, the blood–brain barrier, the nonspecific inflammatory response, and the immune response. Host response to the particular pathogen is responsible for the manifestations of meningitis. The organisms that initiate the host response in meningitis demonstrate an affinity for the nervous system. They colonize and invade the nasopharyngeal mucosa, survive intravascularly, and penetrate the CNS if the blood–brain barrier is damaged, as can happen during surgery, the inflammatory response, or cerebral edema.

Infection of the CSF and meninges causes an inflammatory response in the pia, arachnoid, and CSF. Because the meninges and subarachnoid space are continuous around the brain, spinal cord, and optic nerves, the infection and inflammatory response are always cerebrospinal, involving both the brain and the spinal cord. Inflamed blood vessels in the area leak fluids as cell permeability increases. Purulent exudate infiltrates cranial nerve sheaths and blocks the choroid plexus and subarachnoid villi. IICP occurs as brain tissue responds to the pathogen. With IICP, cerebral perfusion decreases and cerebral autoregulation is lost.

BACTERIAL MENINGITIS The causative organisms of bacterial meningitis include *Neisseria meningitis*, meningococcus, *Streptococcus pneumoniae*, *Haemophilus influenzae*, and *Escherichia coli*. Most cases of meningitis are caused by the pneumococcus or the meningococcus. The incidence of meningitis from *H. influenzae* has been greatly reduced because of vaccination against the organism. Epidemics of meningococcal meningitis occur in populations who live in close contact, such as military recruits and students living in college dormitories. Risk factors include head trauma with a basal skull fracture, otitis media, mastoiditis, sinusitis, neurosurgery, systemic sepsis, or immunocompromise. Even when appropriate antibiotics are used, the mortality rate for adults remains at approximately 21% (Porth & Matfin, 2009).

Once the pathogen enters the CNS, it or its toxic products (free radicals) initiate an inflammatory response in the meninges, CSF, and ventricles. Meningeal vessels become engorged, and their permeability increases. Phagocytic white blood cells (WBCs) migrate into the subarachnoid space, forming a purulent exudate that thickens and clouds the CSF and interferes with its flow. Rapid exudate formation causes further inflammation and edema of meningeal cells. Blood vessel engorgement, exudate formation, impaired CSF flow, and cellular edema cause the intracranial pressure to increase.

Manifestations The patient with bacterial meningitis typically presents with fever and chills, severe headache, back and abdominal pain, and nausea and vomiting. (The older adult may not have a high fever, but may instead exhibit confusion.) Meningeal irritation causes nuchal rigidity (stiff neck), positive Brudzinski sign (flexion of the neck that causes the hip and knee to flex), and positive Kernig's sign (inability to extend the knee while the hip is flexed at a 90-degree angle). Photophobia is present; the patient may also experience diplopia. With

MANIFESTATIONS of Bacterial Meningitis

- Restlessness, agitation, and irritability
- Severe headache
- Signs of meningeal irritation:
  a. Nuchal rigidity
  b. Positive Brudzinski sign
  c. Positive Kernig's sign
- Chills and high fever
- Confusion, altered LOC
- Photophobia (aversion to light), diplopia (double vision)
- Seizures
- Signs of IICP (widened pulse pressure and bradycardia, respiratory irregularity, decreased LOC, headache, and vomiting)
- Petechial rash or ecchymosis (in meningococcal meningitis)

meningococcal meningitis, a rapidly spreading petechial rash involving the skin and mucous membranes or large ecchymotic areas (especially on the lower parts of the body) are characteristic. The patient may also have IICP, manifested by decreased LOC, seizures, changes in vital signs and respiratory pattern, and papilledema (∞ see Chapter 42 for information about IICP). The manifestations of bacterial meningitis are listed in the box on the previous page.

Complications   The arachnoid layer may have fibrotic changes and formation of scar tissue from the infection. Adhesions and effusions can develop, interfering with the normal circulation of CSF. Complications of bacterial meningitis include cranial nerve damage and hydrocephalus. Cranial nerve VIII, the auditory nerve, is frequently affected, with resulting nerve deafness.

VIRAL MENINGITIS   Acute viral meningitis, also called *aseptic meningitis*, is a less severe disease than bacterial meningitis. It can be caused by numerous viruses, such as herpes simplex virus (HSV), herpes zoster, Epstein-Barr virus, cytomegalovirus (CMV), or West Nile virus. Although viral infection also triggers the inflammatory response, the course of the disease is benign and of short duration. Recovery is uneventful.

Manifestations   The manifestations of viral meningitis are similar to those of bacterial meningitis, although usually milder. The patient may have a mild flulike illness prior to the onset of meningitis. Headache is intense and is accompanied by malaise,

nausea, vomiting, and lethargy. Photophobia may be present. The patient generally remains oriented, although possibly drowsy. Temperature is mildly elevated. Neck stiffness, positive Brudzinski sign, and positive Kernig's sign are usually present.

Encephalitis

Encephalitis is a generalized infection of the parenchyma of the brain or spinal cord. It is almost always caused by a virus, but it may also be caused by bacteria, fungi, and other organisms. See Table 43–2 for a list of the most common causes of encephalitis.

VIRAL ENCEPHALITIS   Viruses depend on living tissue for reproduction and become highly destructive when they invade brain tissue. The inflammatory response extends over the cerebral cortex, the white matter, and the meninges, with degeneration of the neurons. The pathology of encephalitis includes local necrotizing hemorrhage, which ultimately becomes generalized, with prominent edema. There is progressive degeneration of nerve cell bodies. The inflammatory response in encephalitis does not cause exudate formation as it does in meningitis. Certain viruses show a propensity for specific areas of the brain (e.g., herpes simplex virus involves frontal and temporal lobes). The virus gains access to the CNS via the bloodstream or along peripheral or cranial nerves, or it may already be present in the meninges in the patient with meningitis.

The manifestations of viral encephalitis vary, depending on the organism and area of the brain affected. Usual manifestations are similar to those of meningitis, including fever, headache,

TABLE 43–2 Causes of Encephalitis

CAUSE	COMMENTS
Arboviruses	Transmitted most often by bites from mosquitoes.
	Bites from mosquitoes occur in middle to late summer.
	Most common types are St. Louis, eastern and western equine encephalitis, and West Nile encephalitis.
	May destroy major parts of the lobe or hemisphere.
	Two-thirds of patients who develop eastern equine encephalitis either die or develop severe residual disabilities (e.g., seizures, blindness, deafness, speech disorders, or mental retardation).
	The incubation is 5 to 15 days.
	Mortality rates associated with arboviruses are higher than those associated with enteroviruses.
Enteroviruses, such as echovirus, coxsacievirus, poliovirus, paramyxovirus (the virus that causes mumps), and varicella-zoster (the virus that causes chickenpox)	Infection occurs more frequently in summer (except infection by the mumps virus, which occurs more frequently in early winter).
	Some degree of protection can be afforded by immunization against measles, mumps, and poliomyelitis.
	Mortality rates are lower than those associated with herpes simplex type 1 virus.
Herpes simplex type 1 virus	Most common nonepidemic encephalitis in North America.
	Can occur any time of year and throughout the world.
	Has an affinity for the frontal and temporal lobes.
	Prognosis is grave but not hopeless: Mortality rate can be as high as 40%, and patient may die within 2 weeks.
Amebic meningoencephalitis due to infection by Naegleria and Acanthamoeba protozoa	Both protozoa are found in warm freshwater.
	Enter the nasal mucosa of people swimming in ponds or lakes.
	May also be found in soil and decaying vegetation.
	Incidence of infection is increasing in North America.
Exogenous poisoning	May occur after ingestion of lead or arsenic or inhalation of carbon monoxide.

seizures, stiff neck, and altered LOC. The patient may be disoriented, agitated and restless, or lethargic and drowsy. As the disease progresses, the LOC deteriorates, and the patient may become comatose.

ARBOVIRUS ENCEPHALITIS The arboviruses are arthropod-borne (mosquito and tick) agents that infect humans. They include many different types, including western equine encephalitis, St. Louis encephalitis, and West Nile encephalitis. Adults are most often infected with St. Louis encephalitis, with older adults affected more often. The most common arboviral encephalitis in the United States is West Nile encephalitis; this infection has become endemic in the United States.

The arthropod-borne agents cause widespread degeneration of nerve cells, and edema and necrosis with or without hemorrhage occur. IICP may develop. Manifestations include fever, malaise, sore throat, nausea and vomiting, stiff neck, tremors, paralysis of extremities, exaggerated deep tendon reflexes, seizures, and altered LOC.

Brain Abscess

A brain abscess is an infection with a collection of purulent material within the brain tissue. Approximately 80% are found in the cerebrum and 20% are cerebellar.

The causes of a brain abscess include open trauma and neurosurgery; infections of the mastoid, middle ear, nasal cavity, or nasal sinuses; metastatic spread from distant foci (such as heart, lungs, skin, abscessed teeth, and dirty needles); and arising from other associated areas of infection. The immunocompromised are at increased risk for abscesses. The most common pathogens causing the abscess are streptococci, staphylococci, and bacteroids. Yeast and fungi may also cause brain abscess.

A brain abscess results from the presence of microorganisms in the brain tissue. If the abscess is encapsulated, it has the ability to enlarge and behave as a space-occupying lesion within the cranium. This predisposes the patient not only to the systemic effects of the inflammatory process but also to the serious consequences of IICP. Occasionally, the abscess does not become encapsulated; instead, it spreads through the brain tissue to the subarachnoid space and ventricular system.

Initially, the patient exhibits the general symptoms associated with an acute infectious process, such as chills, fever, malaise, and anorexia. Because brain abscess generally forms after infection, the patient may consider these signs to be an exacerbation of that illness. The patient may experience seizures, altered LOC, and manifestations of IICP. As the abscess enlarges, specific symptoms are related to location; for example, the patient with a frontal lobe abscess may have contralateral hemiparesis, expressive aphasia, focal seizures, and frontal headache.

Interdisciplinary Care

Both meningitis and encephalitis can be fatal if they are not promptly diagnosed and treated. Even with treatment, CNS damage can cause serious neurologic deficits. Bacterial meningitis is a medical emergency and must be treated with appropriate antibiotics and supportive interventions. The treatment for viral meningitis and encephalitis are primarily symptomatic. Brain abscesses are treated with antibiotics; if this is not effective, the abscess may be drained or surgically removed.

Diagnosis

The diagnosis of bacterial or viral meningitis is based on manifestations and diagnostic test results. Gram stain and culture of the CSF are used to determine if a bacterial infection is present and to identify the specific infectious agent. Counterimmunoelectrophoresis (CIE) is a laboratory test that may be ordered to determine the presence of viruses or protozoa. Polymerase chain reaction techniques may be used to detect viral DNA or RNA in spinal fluid. CT scan will show an area of increased contrast surrounding a low-density core with brain abscess.

Lumbar puncture with examination of the CSF is the definitive diagnostic measure for bacterial meningitis. Data that indicate bacterial meningitis include turbid, cloudy fluid; a markedly increased WBC count and protein content; and a decreased glucose content. The opening pressure on the lumbar puncture is elevated. In contrast, the patient with encephalitis may have a normal CSF analysis and pressure or may have some lymphocytes. The patient with a brain abscess will have a markedly elevated pressure with elevated protein content and elevated WBC count. Glucose content is normal. (Because a lumbar puncture in the presence of a space-occupying lesion can result in brain herniation and death, a CT scan is performed first if neurologic findings support such a lesion.)

Medications

Immediate intravenous administration of a broad-spectrum antibiotic that crosses the blood–brain barrier into the subarachnoid space is instituted in cases of bacterial meningitis. Once culture reports identify the causative organism, drug therapy with a high dose of one or more specific antibiotics IV is continued for 2 weeks. The penicillin (such as ampicillin) and cephalosporin (such as rifampin [Rifadin]) antibiotics are preferred. If resistant strains of bacteria are identified, vancomycin (Vancocin) may be administered. However, as the bacteria are killed, the toxins they release increase production of inflammatory cytokines, which are potentially lethal. Steroids such as dexamethasone (Decadron) are often given with the antibiotics to suppress inflammation. Universal precautions are used for CSF as well as blood.

Treatment for encephalitis consists of administering specific medications and preventing complications. Fungal meningitis is treated with antifungal agents, such as amphotericin-B (Amphotec), flucytosine (Ancobon), and fluconazole (Diflucan). Viral encephalitis is treated with intravenous acyclovir (Zovirax) or vidarabine (Vira-A).

Antibiotic therapy is the primary treatment for brain abscess. A combination of broad-spectrum antibiotics is used if the infecting organism is unknown.

Anticonvulsant medications such as phenytoin (Dilantin) are often prescribed to prevent or control seizure activity. Antipyretic and analgesic medications may provide symptomatic relief; however, analgesics that have a depressant effect on the CNS (such as opiates) are avoided to prevent masking of early manifestations of deteriorating level of consciousness (LOC). The patient initially may require antiemetics to control nausea and vomiting. Fluid and electrolyte status is maintained through intravenous fluid replacement until the patient is able to resume oral intake.

Surgery

Surgical drainage of an encapsulated abscess may be necessary. The decision to perform surgery is based on the patient's general condition, the stage of abscess development, and the site of the abscess.

∞ Nursing Care

Central nervous system infections are serious illnesses, with potentially life-threatening effects and complications. Nursing assessments and interventions are critical in identifying changes in the patient's neurologic status and preventing complications from IICP. In addition to the nursing care described in this section, a Case Study & Nursing Care Plan for a patient with bacterial meningitis is found on page 1502.

Health Promotion

As with many other intracranial injuries and disorders, educational activities to promote health by preventing meningitis and encephalitis are important nursing interventions. The following information to reduce risk should be provided:

- Vaccinations for meningococcal meningitis are recommended by the Centers for Disease Control (CDC) (2008) and are often required for military recruits and college students. The CDC also recommends the vaccine for anyone traveling to a part of the world where meningococcal disease is common (i.e., parts of Africa), anyone with an immune system disorder, and people who might have been exposed to meningitis. Two vaccines are available: meningococcal conjugate vaccine (MCV4) for adults through age 55 and meningococcal polysaccharide vaccine (MPSV4) for adults over age 55.
- Adults over the age of 65 years should receive the pneumococcal vaccine.
- Wash hands with soap and water before and after contact with a person who may be infected with meningitis or encephalitis and after using the bathroom.
- Do not share food, drinking glasses, eating utensils, tissues, towels, lipstick, or cigarettes.
- Mosquito control with repellants, insecticides, and protective clothing; destruction of the insect larvae and elimination of breeding places, such as pools of stagnant water; and community mosquito control programs can help prevent meningitis and encephalitis.
- Prompt diagnosis and treatment of infections of the head, neck, and respiratory system, or of manifestations of meningitis is very important.

Assessment

Collect the following data through the health history and physical examination (∞ see Chapter 41). Further focused assessments are described with nursing interventions next.

- *Health history:* Risk factors (place of residence, exposure to someone with meningitis or encephalitis, concurrent infections, other illnesses, travel), when manifestations began, severity of manifestations, current nausea, headache and stiff neck, seizures.
- *Physical examination:* Glasgow Coma Scale, level of consciousness, vital signs, motor function, pupillary check,

EVIDENCE FOR NURSING CARE — The Patient with Meningitis

Selected resources that nurses may find helpful when planning evidence-based nursing care follow.

- Chaudhuri, A., Martin, P. M., Kennedy, P., Seaton, R. A., Portegies, P., & Bojar, M (2009). EFNS guideline on the management of community-acquired bacterial meningitis. Report of an EFNS Task Force on acute bacterial meningitis in older children and adults. Retrieved from www.guideline.gov
- Gjini, A. B., Stuart, J. M., Cartwright, K., Cohen, J., Jacobs, M., Nichols, T., et al. (2006). Quality of in-hospital care for adults with acute bacterial meningitis: A national retrospective survey. Retrieved from http://qjmed.oxfordjournals.org/cgi/content/full/99/11/761doi:10.1093/qjmed/hcl111

cranial nerves, neck ROM, Brudzinski sign, Kernig's sign, skin (rash, petechiae, purpura), muscle movement and strength, speech.

Nursing Diagnoses and Interventions

In planning and implementing nursing care for the patient with a CNS infection, the prognosis may depend on the supportive care given. The patient is often very ill, and the combination of fever, dehydration, and IICP may predispose him or her to seizures. Airway obstruction, respiratory arrest, or cardiac dysrhythmias may occur. Nursing diagnoses and interventions discussed in ∞ Chapter 42 for the patient with an altered LOC, IICP, and seizures are also appropriate for the patient with a CNS infection. Nursing interventions in this section focus on ineffective protection and risk for fluid volume deficit.

Ineffective Protection

Patients with CNS infections are less able to protect themselves against insults from both internal and external sources. The effects of the infection, inflammation and resulting pathophysiologic processes may include pain, fever, altered LOC, seizures, IICP, and cranial nerve dysfunction. In addition, pathophysiologic effects on the brain may lead to permanent neurologic deficits, such as loss of motor function or dementia.

- Monitor neurologic status on a regular basis. *Many complications are evidenced by changes in neurologic manifestations.*
- Monitor vital signs, including temperature, on a regular basis. *The patient often has a high temperature throughout the illness, ranging from 101°F (38°C) to 105°F (40.5°C).*

> **PRACTICE ALERT**
> Hyperthermia may result from IICP, while an increased temperature can also increase ICP.

- Monitor levels of consciousness. Assess levels of orientation, memory, attention span, and response to stimuli. *Early in the infection, the patient often has problems with memory and orientation. There may be problems with following commands, restlessness, irritability, and combativeness. As the illness progresses, the LOC decreases to lethargy and finally into deep coma.*

CASE STUDY & NURSING CARE PLAN   A Patient with Bacterial Meningitis

Monty Cook is a 22-year-old musician who plays in a local rock band. He is unmarried and lives with his parents. He is known by everyone in the community as a quiet, low-key, easygoing person and an excellent guitar player. During a performance 2 days ago, he had difficulty playing his guitar, complaining of bright stage lights blazing in his eyes. When he tried to keep his head down to prevent the lights from hurting his eyes, he noticed his neck was very stiff. After the performance, one of the newest members of the band remarked that it certainly was not their best performance. Monty responded angrily that maybe the new members of the group needed more practice. Then he stomped out and went home to bed.

He wakes at 4:00 AM with a severe headache, sweating, and chills; his temperature is 102°F, and he cannot bend his neck without severe pain. His mother recognizes that he is agitated and irritable, which is uncharacteristic. Frightened, she rushes him to the hospital emergency room. A lumbar puncture performed in the emergency room reveals turbid, cloudy fluid; a markedly increased WBC count; and protein with a decreased glucose content. Bacterial meningitis is the medical diagnosis. Mr. Cook is admitted to the hospital for treatment and care.

ASSESSMENT

When the nurse, Aisha Aldi, enters Mr. Cook's isolation room, she sees him thrashing about in the bed, talking incoherently, and becoming more agitated. On assessment, Ms. Aldi notes dry mucous membranes, cracked lips, and small petechiae over the upper torso and abdomen. Mr. Cook's temperature is 104°F. Kernig's sign is positive. Intravenous broad-spectrum antibiotics are prescribed and initiated. After the first 2 hours of care, Ms. Aldi notes a decrease in Mr. Cook's level of consciousness.

DIAGNOSES

- *Hyperthermia* related to infection and abnormal temperature regulation by hypothalamus
- *Disturbed Thought Processes* related to intracranial infection
- *Ineffective Protection* related to progression of illness

EXPECTED OUTCOMES

- Have a decrease in body temperature.
- Become less restless and agitated.
- Remain free of injury.

PLANNING AND IMPLEMENTATION

- Monitor vital signs every 2 hours.
- Provide sponge baths if temperature continues to rise.
- Provide a quiet, nonstimulating environment with the shades drawn.
- Provide oral care every 4 hours.
- Measure and compare intake and output every 2 hours.
- Perform neurologic assessments every 2 to 4 hours.
- Monitor for and report seizure activity and decreasing level of consciousness.
- Keep bed in low position with side rails elevated.
- Administer prescribed intravenous antibiotics.

EVALUATION

After 4 days of antibiotic therapy, Mr. Cook's temperature has returned to near normal. Ms. Aldi notes that he has begun opening his eyes and visually tracking her as she moves about the room. Mr. Cook responds to a request to squeeze Ms. Aldi's fingers and after several hours asks her what had happened. On day 5, Mr. Cook states that he feels better and his headache is gone. He ask for sips of juice and begins urinating regularly. Seven days after admission, Mr. Cook is discharged and is able to go home with his mother. He has some weakness in his legs, but otherwise has no evidence of neurologic deficits.

CRITICAL THINKING IN THE NURSING PROCESS

1. What strategies should the nurse use to decrease the environmental stimuli for Mr. Cook, and what is the rationale for doing these?
2. If you were caring for Mr. Cook in the initial phase of the illness and he became combative, what would you do?
3. Develop a plan of care for Mr. Cook for the nursing diagnosis *Acute Pain.* Consider the effect of narcotics on respiratory function in designing the plan.

See Evaluating Your Response in Appendix C.

- Monitor for manifestations of seizure activity, and institute seizure precautions:
  - Monitor twitching of hands or face and tonic-clonic movements.
  - Have an oral airway and suction equipment readily available.
  - Pad side rails, maintain bed in low position, and keep side rails up.
    Irritation of the cerebral cortex secondary to meningeal inflammation may cause seizures. Careful monitoring and seizure precautions are necessary to prevent injury.
- Monitor for manifestations of cranial nerve damage; monitor extraocular movements, facial movement, dizziness, ability to hear, double vision, drooping upper eyelids (ptosis), and pupillary changes. *Cranial nerve dysfunction may result from inflammation or vascular changes in the brain.*
- Monitor for manifestations of IICP: decreased pulse, increased blood pressure, widening pulse pressure, respiratory changes, and vomiting. *IICP results from infectious or inflammatory exudate, cerebral edema, and hydrocephalus.*

- Administer prescribed medications and fluids *Antiepileptics are prescribed to prevent or control seizures, and antibiotics are prescribed to eradicate the bacteria. Mannitol may be prescribed to reduce IICP. IV fluids are administered to replace fluids lost through vomiting and diaphoresis.*

Risk for Imbalanced Fluid Volume

The patient is at risk for fluid volume deficit related to increased metabolic rate and diaphoresis.

- Monitor for presence, or worsening, of fluid volume deficit.
  - Measure and compare intake and output every 2 to 4 hours.
  - Monitor daily body weights.
  - Monitor skin turgor and condition of mucous membranes and tongue.
  - Monitor urine amount, color, and odor.
  - Monitor BUN:creatinine ratio.
    The elastic property of the skin depends partially on interstitial fluid volume. If there is a fluid volume deficit, skin flattens more slowly after a pinch is released. Mucous membranes and tongue are dry, urine output is decreased, urine is dark in color and concentrated with a strong odor,

urine specific gravity is greater than 1.020, and BUN will rise out of proportion to serum creatinine.

PRACTICE ALERT
A weight loss of 1 lb represents a fluid loss of approximately 500 mL.

- When administering fluids, either orally or parenterally, consider concurrent illnesses. *Patients with IICP or renal failure require complex management. ∞ See Chapter 10 for a further discussion of fluid volume deficit.*

Using NANDA, NIC, and NOC

Linkages between a selected NANDA nursing diagnosis, NIC, and NOC for the patient with a CNS infection are shown in the accompanying chart.

The Patient with Tetanus

Tetanus, more commonly called lockjaw, is a disorder caused by a neurotoxin elaborated by *Clostridium tetani*. This anaerobic bacillus lives in the soil. Spores of the bacillus enter the body through open wounds contaminated with dirt, street dust, or feces (animal or human). The wounds may result from punctures, scratches or abrasions, bee stings, abortions, surgery, trauma, burns, or IV drug use. Incidence is highest among people who have never been immunized, older adults whose immunity has been lost, and women. Death, more common in older adults, occurs in over 10% to 20% of all cases (CDC, 2007a). Contaminated lesions of the head and face are more dangerous than those in other parts of the body.

When the spores of *C. tetani* enter the open wound, they germinate and produce a toxin called tetanospasmin. The incubation period averages 8 to 12 days but can range from 5 days to 15 weeks (McPhee et al., 2008). The toxins are absorbed by the peripheral nerves and carried to the spinal cord, where they block the action of inhibitory enzymes at spinal synapses and interfere with transmission of neuromuscular impulses. As a result, even minor stimuli cause uncontrolled muscle spasms.

The manifestations begin with pain at the site of the infection. The infected person has stiffness of the jaw and neck and dysphagia. There is often profuse perspiration and drooling from increased salivation. As the infection progresses, the person experiences hyperreflexia, spasms of the jaw muscles (trismus) or facial muscles, and rigidity and spasms of the abdominal, neck, and back muscles. Generalized tonic seizures are caused by even minor stimuli, and the person assumes a typical opisthotonic position during the seizures: The head is retracted, the back is arched, and the feet are extended. The muscle spasms are painful. The person may be unable to breathe from spasms of the glottis and respiratory muscles. Despite these physical effects, the patient has no change in mental status.

The complications of tetanus include urinary retention and airway obstruction from the spasms. Cardiac and respiratory failure are late, life-threatening complications.

Interdisciplinary Care

There are no specific diagnostic tests for tetanus; diagnosis is based on manifestations. Tetanus is completely preventable by active immunization. Immunization for children includes tetanus toxoid, administered as part of the diphtheria-pertussis-tetanus (DPT) immunization series. In adults, immunization is obtained by administering tetanus toxoid as two doses 4 to 6 weeks apart, with a third dose in 6 to 12 months. All individuals should have a booster dose every 10 years throughout life or at the time of a major injury if the last booster dose was given more than 5 years prior to the injury (CDC, 2009).

If a wound is contaminated or if the person's immunization status is uncertain, passive immunization with tetanus immune globulin is administered. Active immunization with tetanus toxoid is begun at the same time. The wound is carefully and thoroughly debrided and antibiotics administered.

The patient with tetanus requires intensive care in an area of minimal stimulation. Penicillin is administered to help destroy the toxin-producing organism. Muscle spasms and seizures are controlled by chlorpromazine (Thorazine) or diazepam (Valium), often combined with a sedative. Anticoagulants may be prescribed to prevent venous thrombosis. In severe cases, seizures and spasms are controlled with paralysis by a curare-like medication, and airway obstruction is managed by mechanical ventilation.

⌒ Nursing Care

Nursing care for the patient with tetanus is intensive and focuses on assessments and interventions to promote safety, prevent injury, maintain nutrition, and maintain pulmonary and cardiovascular function. The patient usually requires in-hospital care for 2 to 5 weeks. The nursing care plan commonly includes the following:

- Place in a quiet, darkened room to decrease stimuli that cause muscle spasms and seizures.
- Provide only necessary physical care, and do so during periods of maximal sedation to decrease tactile stimulation that causes muscle spasms.

- Maintain oxygenation through mechanical ventilator and frequent suctioning of secretions.
- Maintain intravenous access for the administration of fluids and medications.
- Administer prescribed antibiotics, anticonvulsants, and sedatives. In the case of cardiovascular complications, administer prescribed beta-adrenergic blocking agents such as propranolol (Inderal).
- Provide adequate nutrition through prescribed nutritional support, such as total parenteral nutrition.
- Monitor respiratory and cardiovascular status and provide immediate interventions for respiratory or cardiovascular failure.
- Monitor fluid and electrolyte status. Ensure adequate fluid intake to maintain hydration and urinary output.
- Monitor urinary output, which should be maintained at 1.5 to 2 L per day.
- Monitor for the hazards of immobility, including constipation, pneumonia, deep venous thrombosis, and pressure ulcers.

Health Promotion

Tetanus is a preventable disorder, and nurses have a major role in promoting immunizations for all children and for educating adults about the need for booster doses. The older population is especially at risk for never having been immunized or for letting immunizations lapse. Information for this age group can be provided through activities such as community health fairs and programs at senior citizen groups.

It is also necessary to teach the proper care of wounds. All wounds, no matter how small, should be thoroughly washed with soap and water. All foreign material should be carefully flushed out or removed from a wound, and medical care should be sought for wounds that are more extensive or contaminated.

The Patient with Creutzfeldt-Jakob Disease

Classic **Creutzfeldt-Jakob disease (CJD)** (also called spongiform encephalopathy) is a rapidly progressive, degenerative, neurologic disease that causes brain degeneration without inflammation. The disease is not transmissible and is progressively fatal. The causative agent is believed to be an abnormal form of a cellular glycoprotein known as the prion protein. Transmission of the agent is by direct contamination with infected neural tissue, such as during eye and brain surgery. The disease occurs worldwide, but clusters occur in several areas, more often in England, Chile, and Italy. CJD affects adults over the age of 50 years.

A different form of the disease, called new variant CJD (vCJD) is also a rare, degenerative, fatal brain disorder, but is not the same as the classic form of CJD. New variant CJD, referred to as "mad-cow disease," is believed to result from consumption of cattle products contaminated with bovine spongiform encephalopathy (BSE). This form primarily affects young adults. Because the illness is fatal and is associated with infected cattle, severe restrictions have been placed on the importation of cattle, sheep, and goats and on products from these animals

from countries in which BSE is known to exist. Creutzfeldt-Jakob disease is characterized by degeneration of the gray matter of the brain. The spongiform degeneration (involving the formation of tiny holes and resembling a sponge) produces severe dementia, myoclonus (muscle contractions), and characteristic changes in brain waves. On autopsy or biopsy of brain tissue, the brain shows loss of neurons and a proliferation of astrocytes (indicating destruction of nearby neurons).

The disease has characteristic stages and manifestations. The onset is characterized by memory changes, an exaggerated startle reflex, sleep disturbances, and nervousness. The person then experiences rapid deterioration in motor, sensory, and language function. Tremors, hyperreflexia, rigidity, and a positive Babinski reflex are often present, and confusion progresses to dementia in almost all cases. Patients in the terminal state are comatose and exhibit decorticate and decerebrate posturing. The median duration of illness for CJD is 4 to 5 months; the median duration of illness for vCJD is 13 to 14 months (CDC, 2007b).

No specific treatment is available to stop or slow the progression of CJD. Collaborative interventions focus on the disease's manifestations. The disease is diagnosed by a thorough neurologic examination, specific EEG changes, and a CT scan. However, the final diagnosis of CJD can be made only by postmortem examination. It is often difficult to differentiate this disease from Alzheimer's disease, especially in the early stages.

The nurse may identify the manifestations of Creutzfeldt-Jakob disease when conducting a health history and total physical assessment. Include questions about familial history, cultural and geographic risk, and high-risk occupations or procedures in the history. Assessment of mental function, reflexes, and cranial nerve function may provide information to assist in diagnosis.

Nursing care focuses on maximizing comfort, preventing injury, preventing transmission, and providing support. The following guidelines are useful in designing the plan of care:

- Although comfort is difficult to assess in patients with impaired cognitive function, interventions that provide a quiet environment and analgesia are important.
- Communication is essential, even if the patient is unable to respond.
- Institute seizure precautions, and pad side rails.
- Provide skin care, changes in position, and pressure-relief mattresses to decrease the risk of pressure ulcers, venous stasis, and pneumonia.
- Use standard precautions for blood and body fluids when providing care. Disinfect surfaces with a solution of 5% bleach. Sterilize contaminated equipment by autoclave, or soak in 5% bleach solution for 1 hour. Label all specimens as biohazardous. Teach staff members and family members guidelines for care, including careful hand hygiene. However, it is not necessary to place the patient in isolation.
- Provide time for family members to verbalize grief and loss, which may be manifested as anger and frustration with the healthcare system.
- Provide information to family members about all procedures and the plan of care.
- Refer family members to sources of support, such as social services and the appropriate clergy.

The Patient with Postpoliomyelitis Syndrome

Postpoliomyelitis syndrome is a complication of a previous infection by the poliomyelitis virus. This disease was epidemic in the 1940s and 1950s, but has largely been eradicated through immunization with oral live trivalent virus vaccine. However, it is thought that nearly 25% to 50% of the estimated 440,000 people in the United States who had the disease are reexperiencing manifestations of the acute illness (NINDS, 2008). These people have struggled for years to rehabilitate themselves and lead productive lives. Now, having reached retirement age, they are again experiencing manifestations that may be physically and psychologically incapacitating.

In the initial infection, the poliomyelitis virus destroyed some of the motor cells of the anterior horn cells of the spinal cord, causing neuromuscular effects that ranged from mild to severe flaccid paralysis and atrophy. The primary cause of death was respiratory arrest. Manifestations of reoccurance of the disease may occur years later, with new weakness in both previously affected and unaffected muscles. The manifestations include progressive muscle weakness, fatigue, and pain. As the syndrome progresses, the patient may experience muscle atrophy and scoliosis.

The cause of postpoliomyelitis syndrome is not known. The new weakness of muscles is believed to be due to degeneration of individual nerve terminals in the motor units that remain after the initial illness. Over time, nerve terminals malfunction and permanent weakness occurs.

Postpoliomyelitis syndrome is diagnosed by a previous history of polio and manifestations that persist for at least 1 year. Diagnostic studies of nerve conduction, muscle strength, and pulmonary function determine current physical status. Treatment addresses the manifestations and often involves physical therapy and pulmonary rehabilitation programs.

The patient with postpoliomyelitis syndrome faces the challenge of unexpected physical changes. Patients are often anxious about how others will react or what the future holds. Respiratory dysfunction may result in the need for oxygen. Muscular weakness and decreased pulmonary function may make walking difficult, if not impossible. ADLs, independent self-care, and careers are threatened.

Many patients have not fully recovered psychologically from having polio and may respond to a recurrence of manifestations with denial and disbelief. Older patients may not know they had polio as children. Nurses are responsible for assessing and identifying the manifestations of postpoliomyelitis syndrome. It is essential to question middle to older adults about a past history of polio when conducting the health history and to ask specific questions about manifestations that the patient may be experiencing. The nurse individualizes teaching to meet the physical and psychosocial needs of the patient and family. Provide candid explanations, and teach the patient how to prevent fatigue, promote optimal respiratory function, meet self-care needs, modify ADLs, and maintain safety. Follow-up care with nurses, physicians, physical therapists, respiratory therapists, and counselors is indicated. Referral to a support group can make a positive difference in the patient's and family's ability to cope with the disorder.

The Patient with Rabies

Rabies is a viral infection of the CNS transmitted by infected saliva that enters the human body through a bite or an open wound. If untreated, rabies is fatal; however, the number of deaths from rabies is 1 to 2 per year. The rabies virus is carried by both wild and domestic animals, including bats, skunks, foxes, raccoons, cats, and dogs. Currently, more than 90% of all animal cases reported to the CDC are in wildlife, with the primary rabies hosts being wild carnivores and bats (CDC, 2007c). After an incubation period that usually lasts from 3 to 7 weeks, the virus travels to the brain of the infected animal via the nerves. It multiplies and migrates to the salivary glands. Saliva and brain tissue are considered infectious materials; blood, urine, and feces are not considered infectious and do not require postexposure prophylaxis.

The patient with rabies usually has a history of an animal bite but may also become infected through an abrasion or open wound that is exposed to the infected saliva. The virus spreads from the wound to local muscle cells and then invades the peripheral nerves. It eventually travels to the CNS.

The manifestations occur in stages. During the initial, or prodromal, stage, the site of the wound is painful and then exhibits various paresthesias. The infected person is anxious, irritable, and depressed. General manifestations of infection (such as headache, loss of appetite, and sore throat) may appear. The person may also have increased sensitivity to light and sounds, and the skin is especially sensitive to changes in temperature. The prodromal stage is followed by an excitement stage. The infected person has periods of excitement that alternate with periods of quiet. Attempts to drink cause such painful laryngospasms that the person refuses to drink (a phenomenon called hydrophobia). Large amounts of thick, tenacious mucus are present. The patient experiences convulsions, muscle spasms, and periods of apnea. If untreated, death occurs approximately 7 days from the onset of manifestations and is usually due to respiratory failure.

Animals that bite are kept under observation, if possible, for 7 to 10 days to detect rabies manifestations. Sick animals should be euthanized and their brains examined for presence of the rabies virus, which is detected by fluorescent antibody testing. The blood of an infected person can also be tested with the same diagnostic study to demonstrate the presence of rabies antibodies.

Nursing care for patients with rabies is provided in an intensive care unit, with the patient in a quiet, darkened room to decrease stimulation as much as possible. The patient requires interventions to maintain the airway, maintain oxygenation, and control seizures. Standard precautions are essential, because the rabies virus is present in the saliva of the patient. If an open wound of a healthcare provider is contaminated with infected saliva, the provider must receive postexposure immunizations.

Patient and family teaching focuses on the importance of immunizing pets, providing proper care of wounds, seeking immediate medical attention for animal bites, and obtaining treatment after any suspicious bite. Because the untreated disease is almost always fatal, the best intervention is prevention. Preventive activities follow:

- Immunize household dogs and cats; immunize people who are exposed to animals.
- Local treatment of animal bites and scratches:
  - Carefully and thoroughly clean and flush wounds with soap and water to remove the saliva and dilute the viral exposure.
  - Immediately take the person with the bite for emergency treatment.
- Following exposure, rabies immune globulin (RIG) is administered once for passive immunization. Up to 50% of the globulin is infiltrated around the wound, and the rest is administered intramuscularly. At the same time, an inactivated human diploid cell vaccine (HDCV) is administered intramuscularly, beginning on the day of exposure and on days 3, 7, 14, and 28 after exposure (McPhee et al., 2005). RIG and HDCV should never be given in the same syringe or at the same site. Local and mild systemic reactions include itching, tenderness, headaches, muscle aches, and nausea.

The Patient with Botulism

Botulism is food poisoning caused by ingestion of food contaminated with a toxin produced by the bacillus *Clostridium botulinum*. This anaerobic spore-forming bacillus is found in the soil. Most cases of botulism occur from eating improperly canned or cooked foods, especially home-canned vegetables and fruits, smoked meats, and vacuum-packed fish. The mortality rate is high if the disease is untreated.

The toxins liberated by *C. botulinum* are absorbed by the gastrointestinal tract and bound to nerve tissues. They block the release of acetylcholine from nerve endings and thus cause respiratory paralysis due to paralysis of skeletal muscles.

Manifestations appear 12 to 36 hours after ingestion of the contaminated food. They usually begin with visual disturbances such as diplopia, loss of accommodation, and fixed, dilated pupils. Ptosis is often present. Gastrointestinal manifestations include nausea and vomiting, diarrhea, dysphagia, and dry mouth. Involvement of the larynx is manifested by dystonia (impaired muscle tone). Paralysis of all muscle groups progresses throughout the body, with respiratory paralysis causing death.

Infection with the *Clostridium* toxin is verified by laboratory analysis of the serum and stool and of suspected food, if possible. If botulism is suspected, the state health department and the CDC should be notified for assistance with laboratory assays and procuring botulism antitoxin. All people who may have eaten the contaminated food must be located and observed. Any toxins in the gastrointestinal system are removed by cathartics, enemas, and gastric lavage. The patient with respiratory paralysis is placed on a mechanical ventilator and may require a tracheostomy. Botulism antitoxin is administered to eradicate toxins in the circulation. Nutritional support is often provided with total parenteral nutrition. Intravenous fluids are administered to prevent dehydration and renal failure. If ventilation can be maintained, the patient often recovers without further neurologic deficits.

The patient with botulism is hospitalized, and interventions focus on monitoring for respiratory failure and providing ventilatory assistance if necessary. Ongoing assessments are also made for manifestations of paralytic ileus and urinary retention. The patient will be NPO until able to swallow and breathe; therefore, hydration and nutritional status are monitored. Teach the patient and family that fatigue and weakness may persist for up to a year. During this time, the patient may need to modify ADLs and take rest periods throughout the day.

Education of the public to prevent botulism is important. Address the following topics at health fairs and community programs:

- Home-canned foods must be processed in a pressure cooker rather than in boiling water because the organism is difficult to kill.
- Do not eat home-processed foods that have a change in color, are soft, contain gas bubbles, or have a bad odor.
- Always heat both home-processed and commercial foods at temperatures over 248°F (120°C) or boil for 10 minutes before tasting or eating them.
- Discard home-processed or commercially canned or bottled foods with defective seals.
- Discard commercially prepared canned foods that are damaged or have bulging sides or leaking contents.

CHAPTER HIGHLIGHTS

- Spinal cord injuries are almost always the result of trauma, with the major risk factors being age (young adults), gender (male), and alcohol or drug abuse. The causes of injury to the spinal cord include direct trauma to the cord, vertebral fractures, torn ligaments, and damage to spinal cord blood vessels. The cord may be contused, lacerated, or transected.
- In a complete SCI, the motor and sensory pathways in the spinal cord are completely interrupted (*transected*), resulting in total loss of motor and sensory function below the level of the injury. In an incomplete SCI, the motor and sensory pathways are only partially interrupted, resulting in variable loss of function below the level of injury. Injuries of the spinal cord have the potential to affect movement, perception, sensation, sexual function, and elimination.
- Spinal shock is the temporary loss of all reflexes (areflexia) below the level of injury. Manifestations of spinal shock include bradycardia, hypotension, and flaccid paralysis.
- Autonomic dysreflexia is an exaggerated sympathetic response in patients with an SCI at or above the T6 level. Triggered by noxious stimuli (such as a blocked urinary catheter or a fecal impaction),

this condition results in extreme hypertension and, if untreated, may cause seizures, stroke, or a myocardial infarction.

- Rehabilitation of the patient with an SCI is an ongoing process from intensive care to home care. Nursing interventions are necessary in all settings to promote independence in self-care.

- A herniated intervertebral disk is a rupture of the cartilage surrounding the intervertebral disk with protrusion of the nucleus pulposus. The major manifestation of lumbar disks is lower back and sciatic pain on the affected side. Cervical disks cause pain in the shoulder, neck, and arm. A variety of medications, treatments, and surgical procedures are available for the patient.

- Spinal cord tumors may be benign or malignant, primary or metastatic. Depending on their size and location, they cause pathologic changes in spinal cord function through compression, invasion, or ischemia.

- CNS infections may be caused by bacteria, bacterial toxins, viruses, fungi, protozoans, and rickettsiae. Organisms may enter the CNS through the bloodstream or by direct invasion. The major CNS infections are meningitis and encephalitis. CNS infections are treated with broad-spectrum antibiotics or antifungal agents.

- CNS infections resulting from neurotoxins or viral damage include tetanus, Creutzfeldt-Jakob disease, postpoliomyelitis syndrome, rabies, and botulism. Community-based health education can provide information and also prevent illness in the case of rabies, tetanus, and botulism.

TEST YOURSELF NCLEX-RN® REVIEW

1. A patient is admitted to the emergency department following an automobile crash. An SCI at the cervical level is identified. What intervention will be done to facilitate respirations?
   1. No treatments are necessary.
   2. Oxygen per nasal cannula will be administered.
   3. The patient will be placed on a ventilator.
   4. The head of the bed will be elevated.

2. Many different medications may be given to the patient with an acute SCI. Which of the following may be administered? **Select all that apply.**
   1. corticosteroids
   2. vasopressors
   3. antibiotics
   4. analgesics
   5. antihistamines

3. What is the primary pathophysiologic process of spinal shock?
   1. temporary loss of reflex function below the level of injury
   2. loss of control of cardiovascular mechanisms
   3. exaggerated sympathetic response
   4. damage to the lower motor neurons

4. A patient has manifestations of autonomic dysreflexia. Which of these assessments would indicate a possible cause for this condition?
   1. hypertension
   2. kinked catheter tubing
   3. respiratory wheezes and stridor
   4. diarrhea

5. An industrial nurse is conducting a class to teach methods to prevent back pain. What should be included? **Select all that apply.**
   1. Spread the feet apart to broaden the base of support.
   2. Bend from the waist to lift articles from the floor.
   3. Use large leg muscles to push when lifting.
   4. Always lift articles rather than rolling or pushing them.
   5. Work as closely as possible to the object to be moved.

6. A nurse is assessing a postoperative patient who has had a posterior cervical laminectomy for manifestations of spinal cord compression. How would this assessment be conducted?
   1. Ask the patient to wiggle his or her toes.
   2. Ask the patient to grip the nurse's hands.
   3. Use a reflex hammer to assess Babinski's reflex.
   4. Use a stethoscope to auscultate heart sounds.

7. A nurse is establishing a nursing care plan for a patient with a metastatic spinal cord tumor. What nursing diagnosis would have priority?
   1. acute pain
   2. risk for constipation
   3. impaired transfer ability
   4. risk for shock

8. Of the following, which group is most at risk for bacterial meningitis?
   1. older adults
   2. pregnant women
   3. college students
   4. low-income adults

9. A nurse is conducting a class on the prevention of CNS infections through community services. What topic might be included in the discussion?
   1. sanitation services
   2. garbage pickup
   3. mosquito spraying
   4. washing fruits and vegetables

10. How can the nurse prevent tetanus?
    1. Teach safe food preparation techniques.
    2. Promote immunizations for adults and children.
    3. Demonstrate proper disposal of soiled dressings.
    4. Promote immunization of household pets.

See Test Yourself answers in Appendix C.

Pearson Nursing Student Resources

Find additional review materials at
www.nursing.pearsonhighered.com

Prepare for success with additional NCLEX®-style practice questions, interactive assignments and activities, Web links, animations and videos, and more!

BIBLIOGRAPHY

American Academy of Physical Medicine and Rehabilitation. (2009). *Advances made in treatment of spinal cord injuries.* Retrieved from http://www.aapmr.org/condtreat/injuries/sciadvance.htm

American Association of Neuroscience Nurses. (2006). *Lumbar spine surgery. A guide to preoperative and postoperative patient care.* Retrieved from http://www.aann.org/guidelines.html

Barker, E. (2008). *Neuroscience nursing: A spectrum of care* (3rd ed.). St. Louis: Mosby Elsevier.

Brillhart, B. (2005). A study of spirituality and life satisfaction among persons with spinal cord injury. *Rehabilitation Nursing, 30*(1), 31–34.

Bulechek, G., Butcher, H., & Dochterman, J. (Eds.). (2008). *Nursing interventions classification (NIC)* (5th ed.). St. Louis: Mosby Elsevier.

Centers for Disease Control and Prevention [CDC]. (2007a). *Tetanus disease; vaccines & immunizations.* Retrieved from http://www.cdc.gov/vaccines/vpd-vac/tetanus/default.htm

Centers for Disease Control and Prevention [CDC]. (2007b). *vCJD (Variant Creutzfeldt-Jakob Disease).* Retrieved from http://www.cdc.gov/nicdod/dvrd/vcjd/index.htm

Centers for Disease Control and Prevention [CDC]. (2007c). *About rabies.* Retrieved from http://www.cdc.gov/print.do?url-http%3A//www.cdc.gov/rabies/about.html

Centers for Disease Control and Prevention [CDC]. (2008a). *Botulism.* Retrieved from http://www.cdc.gov/nczved/DFBMD/disease_listing/botulism_gi.html

Centers for Disease Control and Prevention [CDC]. (2008b). *Meningococcal vaccines: What you need to know.* CDC Vaccine Information Statement (Interim).

Centers for Disease Control and Prevention [CDC]. (2009 January 9). Recommended adult immunization schedule—United States. *MMWR, 57*(53).

Fields, L. B. (2008). Oral care intervention to reduce incidence of ventilator-associated pneumonia in the neurologic intensive care unit. *Journal of Neuroscience Nursing, 40*(5), 291–298.

Fisher, V. (2004). Manual evacuation can be vital. *Nursing Standard, 18*(34), 30.

Hickey, J. V. (2009). *The clinical practice of neurological and neurosurgical nursing* (6th ed.). Philadelphia: Lippincott Williams & Wilkins.

Holmes, S., & Brown, S. (2005). Skeletal site pin care: National Association of Orthopaedic Nurses guidelines for orthopaedic nursing. *Orthopaedic Nursing, 24*(2), 99–107.

Kee, J. (2009). *Prentice Hall handbook of laboratory and diagnostic tests with nursing implications* (6th ed.). Upper Saddle River, NJ: Pearson Prentice Hall.

Laws, R. (2007). Uncovering the layers of meningitis. *Nursing Made Incredibly Easy, 5*(4), 26–36.

Matthews, C., Miller, L., & Mott, M. (2007). Getting ahead of acute meningitis & encephalitis. *Nursing, 37*(11), 37–42.

McPhee, S., Papadakis, M, & Tierney, L. (Eds.). (2008). *Current medical diagnosis & treatment* (47th ed.). New York: McGraw-Hill Lange.

Moorhead, S., Johnson, M., Maas, M., & Swanson, E. (2008). *Nursing outcomes classification (NOC)* (4th ed.). St. Louis: Mosby Elsevier.

NANDA International. (2009). *Nursing diagnoses: Definitions & classification 2009–20011.* Oxford: Wiley-Blackwell.

National Institute of Neurological Disorders and Strokes [NINDS]. (2007). *Meningitis and encephalitis information page.* Retrieved from http://www.ninds.nih.gov/disorders/encephalitis_meningitis/encephalitis_meningitis.htm

National Institute of Neurological Disorders and Stroke [NINDS] (2009a). *NINDS brain and spinal tumors information page.* Retrieved from http://www.ninds.nih.gov/disorders/brainandspinaltumors/brainandspinaltumors.htm

National Institute of Neurological Disorders and Stroke [NINDS]. (2009b). *Spinal cord injury: Hope through research.* Retrieved from http://www.ninds.nih.gov/disorders/sci.detail_sci.htm

National Spinal Cord Injury Association Resource Center. (2008). *Post-polio syndrome fact sheet.* Retrieved from http://www.ninds.nih.gov/disorders/post_polio/detail_post_polio.htm

National Spinal Cord Injury Statistical Center, Birmingham, Alabama. (2010). *Spinal cord injury facts and figures at a glance.* Available at NSCISC@uab.edu

Porth, C. M., & Matfin, G. (2009). *Pathophysiology: Concepts of altered health states* (8th ed.). Philadelphia: Lippincott Williams & Wilkins.

Securing the indwelling catheter. (2008). *American Journal of Nursing, 108*(12), 44–50.

Sherwood, P., Crago, E., Spiro, R., & Okonkwo, D. (2007). Cervical spine injuries: Preserving function, improving outcomes. *American Nurse Today, 2*(9), 26–29.

Tocco, S. (2009). Recognizing spinal cord compression. *American Nurse Today, 4*(2), 33.

UCSF Medical Center. (2008). *Spinal cord tumors.* Retrieved from http://www.ucsfhealth.org/adult/medical_services/cancer/brainconditions/spinal_cord_tumors

Vacca, V. (2007). Action stat. Autonomic dysreflexia. *Nursing, 37*(9), 72.

Wagner, K., Johnson, K., & Kidd, P. (2006). *High acuity nursing* (4th ed.). Upper Saddle River, NJ: Pearson Prentice Hall.

Wilson, B., Shannon, M., & Shields, K. (2009). *Prentice Hall nurse's drug guide 2009.* Upper Saddle River, NJ: Pearson Prentice Hall.

Winslow, E., & Brosz, D. (2008). Graduated compression stockings in hospitalized postoperative patients. Correctness of usage and size. *American Journal of Nursing, 108*(9), 40–50.

Nursing Care of Patients with Neurologic Disorders

LEARNING OUTCOMES

1. Identify risk factors for degenerative neurologic, peripheral nervous system (PNS), and cranial nerve disorders.
2. Explain the pathophysiology, manifestations, complications, interdisciplinary care, and nursing care of patients with degenerative neurologic disorders (dementia, Alzheimer's disease, multiple sclerosis, Parkinson's disease, Huntington's disease, amyotrophic lateral sclerosis), PNS disorders (myasthenia gravis, Guillian-Barré syndrome), and cranial nerve disorders (trigeminal neuralgia, Bell's palsy).
3. Compare and contrast the manifestations of the progressive stages of Alzheimer's disease.
4. Discuss the purposes, nursing implications, and health education for the patient and family for medications used to treat Alzheimer's disease, multiple sclerosis, Parkinson's disease, and myasthenia gravis.
5. Describe the procedures (thymectomy, percutaneous rhizotomy, plasmapheresis) used to treat selected neurologic disorders.

CLINICAL COMPETENCIES

1. Assess functional status of patients with neurologic disorders, and monitor, document, and report abnormal manifestations.
2. Use evidence-based research to design nursing interventions specific to the needs of aging patients with multiple sclerosis.
3. Use assessed data, patient values, clinical expertise, and evidence to determine priority nursing diagnoses and select and implement nursing interventions.
4. Administer oral and injectable medications used to treat Alzheimer's disease, multiple sclerosis, Parkinson's disease, and myasthenia gravis accurately and safely.
5. Provide competent care to patients having a thymectomy, percutaneous rhizotomy, or plasmapheresis.
6. Effectively communicate with and function within the interdisciplinary team to plan and provide care of patients with neurologic disorders.
7. Provide appropriate teaching to facilitate safety, communications, and community-based self-care for acute and chronic healthcare needs resulting from neurologic disorders.
8. Adapt individual and cultural values and variations as well as expressed needs and preferences into the plan of care.
9. Revise plan of care as needed to provide effective interventions to promote, maintain, or restore functional health status to patients with neurologic disorders.

KEY TERMS

Alzheimer's disease (AD), *1510*
amyotrophic lateral sclerosis (ALS), *1536*
Bell's palsy, *1547*
dementia, *1510*

Guillain-Barré syndrome (GBS), *1543*
Huntington's disease, *1533*
multiple sclerosis (MS), *1518*
myasthenia gravis (MG), *1538*

neuralgia, *1545*
Parkinson's disease (PD), *1526*
trigeminal neuralgia (TN), *1545*

This chapter discusses degenerative neurologic disorders, PNS disorders, and cranial nerve disorders. For many of the disorders, care is based on similar nursing diagnoses. To avoid repeating those diagnoses and interventions for each disorder, they have been divided among the nursing care discussions as appropriate.

Degenerative Neurologic Disorders

Degenerative neurologic disorders affect the central nervous system (CNS) and the peripheral nerves. By progressively disrupting cognitive processes or motor functions, disorders such as Alzheimer's disease, Parkinson's disease, and multiple sclerosis strike at the core of an individual's sense of personal autonomy and well-being and can be psychologically and emotionally devastating to family members and caregivers.

Ongoing medical research into degenerative neurologic disorders offers an increasing measure of hope to patients and their families. The discovery of genetic or biochemical markers associated with some of these disorders is leading to the development of effective screening and diagnostic methods. In addition, new drugs may make it possible to halt the progression of the disorders in some patients, transforming the disorders into

Alzheimer's Disease Video

manageable conditions. This chapter begins with a discussion of dementia, which is not a specific disease, but rather a collection of manifestations that are caused by a variety of disorders that affect the brain.

Dementia

Dementia (literally meaning "deprived of mind") is cognitive decline caused by any disorder that permanently damages areas of the brain necessary for memory and learning. The hallmark of dementia is impairment of both short- and long-term memory, with resultant deficits in abstract thinking, impaired judgment, problem solving, and/or changes in personality (Porth & Matfin, 2009). Impairments of cognitive function are usually accompanied by deterioration in emotional control, social behavior, and motivation. People with dementia may also have agitation, delusions, and hallucinations. All forms of dementia result from death of neurons and/or the loss of communication among the cells. Although the exact cause is not always known, many forms of dementia are characterized by abnormal structures in the brain called inclusions, and there is clearly a genetic component in the development of some types of dementia. It is important to remember that although the incidence of dementia increases with aging, it is not a normal component of aging.

To be diagnosed with dementia, the following criteria must be met:

- It must include decline in memory and at least one of the following cognitive abilities:

  1. Ability to generate coherent speech or understand spoken or written language
  2. Ability to recognize or identify objects, assuming intact sensory function
  3. Ability to execute motor activities, assuming intact motor abilities, sensory function, and comprehension of the required task
  4. Ability to think abstractly, make sound judgments, and carry out complex tasks

- The decline in cognitive abilities must be severe enough to interfere with daily life (Alzheimer's Association, 2009).

Although exact numbers are difficult to determine, it is estimated that, in the United States, as many as 4.5 million people have dementia, and of those 60% to 80% have Alzheimer's disease (AD) (Porth & Matfin, 2009). Literally millions of people in every country across the world have some type of dementia in what is often called a worldwide epidemic. To illustrate the soaring incidence rate worldwide, AD occurred in 10% of people over the age of 85 in the 1960s whereas it currently occurs in 50% of those over the age of 85 (Anderson, 2009).

Many different diseases and conditions may cause dementia, including Alzheimer's disease, vascular dementia, Parkinson's disease, normal pressure hydrocephalus, Creutzfeldt-Jakob disease, metabolic disorders, medications, poisoning, and anoxia. Even though the actual cause of all dementias may not be known, factors that increase the risk of developing one or more kinds of dementia have been identified. These risk factors include aging, a family history of a disease that causes dementia, smoking and alcohol use, atherosclerosis, high cholesterol and plasma homocysteine levels, diabetes mellitus, and Down syndrome.

The Patient with Alzheimer's Disease

Alzheimer's disease (AD) (also called dementia of Alzheimer type [DAT] or senile disease complex) is a form of dementia characterized by progressive, irreversible deterioration of general intellectual functioning. AD occurs in middle or late life and is the most common cause of dementia. It affects almost twice as many women as men, but this is believed to be the result of women living relatively longer than men. People with AD die an average of 4 to 6 years after diagnosis, but the disease duration varies from 3 to 20 years (Alzheimer's Association, 2007).

Although the exact cause is unknown, it appears that AD develops from the interaction of multiple factors. Age is the major risk factor, but other risk factors include head trauma, inflammatory factors, and oxidative stress. In addition, risk factors being evaluated include low educational level, lack of mental stimulation, migraines, and heavy smoking and alcohol consumption. People who develop AD under age 65 are said to have early-onset AD; those who develop AD after age 65 have late-onset AD. A small percentage of AD is caused by a genetic variation and is characterized by an early onset—sometimes affecting people as young as 30. Research into the genetics of early-onset AD has identified mutations of at least three genes: APP gene on chromosome 21, PSI gene on chromosome 14, and PS2 on chromosome 1. The ApoE gene on chromosome 19 increases the risk for the development of late-onset AD and lowers the age of onset, but it is not yet known how this occurs.

Memory loss is usually the first sign of Alzheimer's disease. Memory deficits are initially subtle and family members and friends may not suspect a problem until the disease progresses and manifestations become more noticeable. Family members and patients with AD may also deny the manifestations and hide deficits until the person exhibits unsafe or extremely unusual behavior. Progression of the disease varies, but the course is one of deteriorating cognition and judgment with eventual physical decline and total inability to perform activities of daily living (ADLs). With the loss of the ability to perform even the most basic ADLs, the burden of meeting the patient's needs shifts to the caregiver.

FAST FACTS
Alzheimer's Disease
- Scientists estimate that more than 5.3 million people have AD.
- AD is the sixth leading cause of death in the United States.
- A new case of AD is diagnosed every 70 seconds.
- The lifetime risk for AD for those living to age 55 is 17% in women and 9% in men.
- Of the 78 million baby boomers alive today, 10 million are projected to have AD in their lifetime.
- 9.9 million unpaid caregivers take care of people with AD.

Source: Alzheimer's Foundation, 2009; Jeffrey, 2008; NINDS, 2009a.

Pathophysiology

Characteristic findings in the brains of AD patients are loss of nerve cells and the presence of neuritic plaques, neurofibrillary tangles, and amyloid angiopathy (Figure 44–1 ■). These changes are clearly illustrated by the Alzheimer's Association in *Inside the Brain: An Interactive Tour* that explains how the brain works and

Figure 44–1 ■ Neuron with neurofibrillary tangles seen in Alzheimer's disease.

how AD affects it. Several theories are proposed for the cause of AD. The theories include the amyloid hypothesis (AD is the result of an accumulation of beta-amyloid in plaques), the tau hypothesis (AD is the result of tau protein dysfunction), and the vascular hypothesis (many AD patients also have vascular dementia; the result of cardiovascular and cerebrovascular disease causing endothelial damage). Making diagnosis more difficult is that some people have these same pathophysiologic changes, but do not develop AD.

Neuritic plaques are groups of nerve cells (and especially the terminal axons) that degenerate and clump around an amyloid core as plaques, found in the spaces between the neurons of the brain. These plaques, which develop first in areas used for memory and cognition, disrupt transmission of nerve impulses. The plaques consist primarily of insoluble deposits of beta-amyloid, a protein fragment from a larger protein called amyloid precursor protein, mixed with other neurons and non-nerve cells. It is believed by many scientists that beta-amyloid is the critical component in the development of AD (Porth & Matfin, 2009).

Neurofibrillary tangles, found in the cytoplasm of abnormal neurons, are composed of fibrous proteins wound around each other in a helical way. The fibrous proteins contain tau, also a protein. Tau normally holds together the microtubules, which guide nutrients and molecules to the end of the axon. Because tau no longer maintains the transport system, communication is lost between neurons. Death of neurons may follow, contributing to the development of dementia.

Blood flow to the affected areas of the brain is decreased. The brain atrophies, and corresponding enlargement of ventricles and sulci is evident (Figure 44–2 ■). As AD progresses, more areas of the brain are affected. Neuronal and neurotransmitter losses (especially of choline acetyltransferase, necessary for the synthesis of acetylcholine, a neurotransmitter associated with memory) are correlated with the number of neuritic plaques and the severity of AD.

AD is characterized by atrophy of the cortical area of the brain and loss of neurons, especially in the parietal and temporal lobes. With significant atrophy and loss of brain tissue, the ventricles enlarge (a form of hydrocephalus). Several structural and chemical changes in the brain occur with AD, especially in the hippocampus and the frontal and temporal lobes of the cerebral cortex. As AD destroys neurons in the hippocampus and related structures, short-term memory fails and the ability to perform easy and familiar tasks declines. The effect of AD on neurons in the cerebral cortex is loss of language skills and judgment. Emotional outbursts and behavior changes (such as wandering and agitation) begin to occur and become more frequent as the disease progresses. Eventually, other areas of the brain are affected; all affected areas begin to atrophy, and the person becomes totally helpless and unresponsive.

Stages and Manifestations

Alzheimer's disease is classified into seven stages based on the patient's manifestations and abilities by the Alzheimer's Association (2007), as outlined next. It is important to note that the progression of AD varies for each individual and may not precisely follow these stages.

Stage 1: No Cognitive Impairment
Memory problems are not experienced nor evident to others.

Figure 44–2 ■ Changes in neuroanatomy associated with Alzheimer's disease. Note areas of cortical atrophy, narrowing of the gyri, enlargement of sulci, and ventricular dilation.

Courtesy of Churchill Livingstone.

Stage 2: Very Mild Decline

People find themselves having memory lapses, forgetting familiar names, or losing everyday objects such as keys and glasses. These memory problems are not evident to others nor are they detectable during a medical examination.

Stage 3: Mild Cognitive Decline

Early-stage AD may be diagnosed in some, but not all, people with AD in this stage. Family and friends begin to notice problems and the deficits may be measured or detected during a medical examination. Common problems include trouble finding words or names, decreased ability to remember names when introduced to new people, retaining little information when reading a passage, decreased ability to plan or organize, losing or misplacing valuable objects, and having performance issues in social and work setting that are noticable to others.

Stage 4: Moderate Cognitive Decline

A careful medical interview will identify deficiencies in knowledge of recent events, impaired ability to perform challenging mental arithmetic (such as counting backward from 100 by 7s), decreased capacity to perform complex tasks (such as buying groceries or paying bills), and a reduced memory for personal history. The person often appears subdued and withdrawn, especially in social or mentally challenging situations.

State 5: Moderately Severe Cognitive Decline

Major deficits in memory and a decline in cognitive function emerge. Some assistance with ADLs becomes essential, but the person can usually eat and use the toilet. People with AD in this stage do usually retain knowledge about themselves, and know their name and the names of family members. Problems include inability to recall current address or telephone number; confusion about where they are as well as the date, day of the week, or season; and trouble with less challenging mental arithmetic (such as counting backward by 4s from 40).

Stage 6: Severe Cognitive Decline

This stage is characterized by worsening memory, emergence of personality changes, and the need for extensive help for ADLs. There is loss of most awareness of recent experiences and events as well as of the surroundings. The person generally knows his or her own name, but has problems recalling most personal history. People with AD in this stage do sometimes forget the names of family members, but they can usually distinguish familiar from unfamiliar faces. Without supervision they may, for example, put pajamas over daytime clothing or shoes on wrong feet. They need help with details of toileting (flushing, wiping, disposing of tissue) and are increasingly incontinent of urine or feces. There is disruption of their normal sleep/waking cycle. They tend to wander and get lost. Significant personality and behavior changes occur, such as suspiciousness and delusions, hallucinations, or compulsive/repetitive behavior (such as hand wringing or tissue shredding).

Stage 7: Very Severe Cognitive Decline

This is the final stage. The person loses the ability to respond to his or her environment, the ability to speak, and the ability to control movement. Some words or phrases may be spoken, but they are not recognizable. Total care is needed for eating and toileting (there is general incontinence). The ability to walk without assistance is lost first, followed by the ability to sit without support, the ability to smile, and the ability to hold up the head. Reflexes become abnormal, muscles grow rigid, and swallowing is impaired. There are many possible causes of death as the person with AD reaches the final stage. The affected person is at increased risk for aspiration pneumonia from impaired swallowing. Loss of neurons impairs sensations such as hunger or thirst, leading to complications of malnutrition or dehydraton. Infections can result in sepsis.

Interdisciplinary Care

There is no cure for AD, and the main objective of care is to provide an environment that matches the patient's functional abilities. Nurses, physicians, physical therapists, and social workers collaborate with the patient's family to provide the least restrictive environment in which the patient can safely function.

Diagnosis

There is no specific diagnostic test for AD. The only definitive method of diagnosis is postmortem examination of brain tissue. AD is diagnosed by ruling out causes for the patient's manifestations. An extensive workup is especially important, because the dementia may be due to a reversible or treatable condition. For example, an older patient's misuse of medications can lead to overdosing and resulting confusion. Other conditions that may be considered are depression, infection, hypothyroidism, dehydration, heart disease, stroke, and chronic obstructive respiratory disease. Mental status is assessed with tests such as the Folstein Mini Mental Status Examination (measures orientation, registration, attention, calculation, recall, and language) and the Alzheimer's Disease Assessment Scale (assesses memory, speech, language, depression, psychosis, and vegetative manifestations). A simple test is the clock drawing test (requires the patient to draw a clock), often used to track cognitive changes over time (Holcomb, 2008).

A diagnosis of AD requires the documented presence of dementia established by clinical examination and the results of a mental status test, onset between age 40 and 90 years (most often after age 65), and absence of systemic or brain disorders that could cause deficits in memory and cognition (Alzheimer's Association, 2009).

Medications

There is no cure for AD, but the medications listed in the Medication Administration box are effective in slowing the progression of the disease. Other medications are prescribed for manifestations such as sleep disturbances and agitation. Guidelines for pharmacologic treatment of AD recommend that decisions should be based on a drug's potential adverse side effects, ease of use, and cost (Cassels & Murata, 2008).

Depression often accompanies AD and is treated with the appropriate medication. Antihistamines and tricyclic antidepressants that have high anticholinergic activity are usually avoided because they can increase AD manifestations. Occasionally patients with AD require tranquilizers such as thioridazine (Mellaril) or haloperidol (Haldol) to manage severe agitation. However, antipsychotic drugs commonly used to treat AD may double the risk of dying within a few years, and the FDA (2008) has ordered this information be included in all prescribing information.

MEDICATION ADMINISTRATION   **The Patient with Alzheimer's Disease**

ACETYLCHOLINESTERASE INHIBITORS (AChEIs)

Tacrine hydrochloride (Cognex)

Donepezil hydrochloride (Aricept)

Rivastigmine tartrate (Exelon)

In the early stages of AD, the pathologic changes in neurons result in a deficiency of acetylcholine (a key neurotransmitter involved in cognitive functioning). Cholinesterase inhibitors slow the breakdown of acetylcholine release by the remaining intact neurons. In addition, rivastigmine tartrate inhibits the G_1 form of acetylcholinesterase (found in higher levels in the brain of patients with AD), so less acetylcholine is degraded. The drugs are used to improve memory in mild to moderate AD dementia.

Nursing Responsibilities
- Administer tacrine hydrochloride 1 hour before meals, if possible.
- Administer donepezil hydrochloride at bedtime.
- Administer rivastigmine tartrate (both capsules and liquid) with food. Liquid form may be administered undiluted or mixed with water, juice, or soda. Stir to completely dissolve. The rivastigmine patch is applied once every 24 hours at the same time of day, using the upper chest, upper or lower back, or upper arm.
- Monitor for jaundice, increased bilirubin levels, and other signs of liver involvement, such as rising serum amino-transferase (AST, ALT) levels. Therapy is usually

decreased when the enzyme level exceeds four times normal limits and is discontinued when the level reaches five times normal.
- Observe for GI bleeding and gastric pain.
- Monitor for cholinergic-related problems: bladder outlet obstruction, seizures, and slowed cardiac rate.
- Assist with ambulation because dizziness is a common side effect.
- Monitor glycemic control in patients with diabetes.
- Assess for improvement in AD symptoms, especially in reasoning, memory, and ADLs.

N-methyl-D-aspartate (NMDA)

Memantine (Namenda)

This drug binds to NMDA receptor-operated cation channels, slowing death of neurons. It temporarily delays more severe AD manifestations.

Health Education for the Patient and Family
- Notify the physician promptly if jaundice, seizures, slowed heart rate, GI bleeding, or difficulty urinating occurs.
- Follow directions for times and instructions about administration of specific medication.
- Follow your healthcare provider's recommendation for periodic EEG, blood tests, and urine tests.
- These medications do not cure AD, and will at some point become ineffective as the disease progresses.

Alternative and Complementary Therapy

Alternative and complementary therapies have been used in treating the manifestations of AD. Ginkgo and vitamin E were thought at one time to prevent memory loss, but this is no longer true (DeKosky et al., 2008; Johnson, 2008). Other therapies include the following:

- Huperzine A, a traditional Chinese medicine, which acts as an acetylcholinesterase inhibitor
- Coenzyme Q10, an antioxidant that naturally occurs in the body
- Supplements, such as zinc, selenium, and evening primrose oil
- Therapies involving massage, art, music, sound, and dance

∽ Nursing Care

Patients with AD often require intensive, supportive nursing interventions directed at the physical and psychosocial responses to illness. Equally important, the nurse can facilitate the long-term support of these patients by providing teaching and referrals to follow-up care in the community. A Case Study & Nursing Care Plan for a patient with AD is found on page 1517.

Health Promotion

The public needs to be aware of the warning signs of AD, and seek medical care when they are observed. The 10 warning signs of AD are memory loss, difficulty performing familiar tasks, problems with language, disorientation to time and place, poor or decreased judgment, problems with abstract thinking, misplacing things, changes in mood or behavior, changes in personality, and loss of initiative (Alzheimer's Association, 2009).

Although there is no proven way to prevent AD, recommendations have been made to delay the onset of manifestations.

These include staying active mentally, physically, and socially. Activities such as walking each day, reading the newspaper, visiting the library, or writing a letter are important in maintaining cognitive ability in old age. Other recommendations hold true for health in general: Eat a healthy diet (with an emphasis on fruits, vegetables, and fiber), control cardiovascular and diabetes mellitus risk factors (weight, smoking, blood pressure, and cholesterol), and avoid head injuries (by wearing seat belts and helmets and avoiding falls). Many older adults experience mild problems with memory, but do not have AD.

Health promotion for the patient with AD focuses on maintaining functional abilities and safety. If the patient will be cared for at home, address safety considerations (see the Meeting Individualized Needs box) as well as the caregivers' abilities to meet the patient's basic needs, such as maintaining hygiene and other ADLs. Adapt nursing interventions and teaching to the patient's stage of AD. Nurses also promote caregiver health; information about caregiver support systems and respite care should be provided.

Assessment

Collect the following data through the health history and physical examination (∞ see Chapter 41). Further focused assessments are described with nursing interventions that follow.

- *Health history:* Family member/caregiver support, living arrangements, ability to carry out ADLs, drug use, work history (e.g., exposure to metals), previous history of multiple strokes, brain injury or brain infection, family history of dementia, sleep pattern, changes in cognition and memory, ability to communicate, changes in behavior.
- *Physical assessment:* Height/weight, orientation, abstract reasoning, mental status.

EVIDENCE FOR NURSING CARE   **The Patient with Alzheimer's Disease**

Selected resources that nurses may find helpful when planning evidence-based nursing care follow.

- Dementia care practice recommendations for assisted living residences and nursing homes: Phase 3 end-of-life care. (2009). *Alzheimer's Association - Disease Specific Society.* Retrieved from http://www.guideline.gov
- Elliott, A. F., & Horgas, A. L. (2009). Effects of an analgesic trial in reducing pain behaviors in community-dwelling older adults with dementia. *Nursing Research, 58*(2), 140–145.
- Futrell, M., Melillo, K. D., & Remington, R. (2008). Evidence-based practice guideline. Wandering. Retrieved from www.guideline.gov
- Miller, C. A. (2008). Communication difficulties in hospitalized older adults with dementia. *The American Journal of Nursing, 108*(3), 58–66.

Nursing Diagnoses and Interventions

During the early stage of AD, nursing care focuses on helping the patient make minor adaptations to his or her environment. As the patient becomes progressively unable to manage self-care tasks, more adaptations are required. Equally important, the caregiver needs much support—both physical and psychosocial—as the patient becomes increasingly dependent.

Impaired Memory

Impaired memory is an appropriate nursing diagnosis in stage 3 AD. At this stage, techniques to help with the memory loss should be included in teaching for both the patient and the caregiver.

- Suggest complementary therapies, such as meditation, massage, or exercise. *These activities can help reduce stress; stress can aggravate memory loss.*
- Suggest using a calendar, keeping lists of reminders, or asking someone else to remind of appointments and events. *Written or verbal reminders are helpful if memory is impaired.*
- Recommend using a medication box labeled with days and times. *A medication box is a good way to remember to take medications.*
- If treatment or professional care of the person with AD is necessary, provide information to the healthcare staff about the person's memory problems. For further information, see Bradway & Hirschman (2008), *Working with Families of Hospitalized Older Adults with Dementia.* Although developed for the acute care setting, much of the information is equally useful for long-term care patients. The tool may be accessed online at the Hartford Institute for Geriatric Nursing or the consultGeriRN website. A video demonstrating the use of the included form is available at Lippincott's Nursing Center (search for A301). *Families provide much of the care and support of older adults living with dementia. Family caregivers are an important source of information and should be regarded as an integral part of the healthcare team.*

PRACTICE ALERT
It may be necessary to teach the caregiver how to refill the medication box, or to stress the importance of spot checking if the patient fills it.

- Provide continuity in nursing staff. *This not only promotes consistency of care for the patient but also allows the nurse to determine more accurately changes in the patient's condition.*
- Repeat explanations simply and as needed to decrease anxiety. *Loss of short-term memory leads to loss of a point of reference; eventually, AD patients think they are experiencing everything for the first time.*

Anxiety

Managing the AD patient's behaviors associated with anxiety, restlessness, and confusion is a major challenge confronting nurses and caregivers. Frequently, patients are relatively calm in the morning hours, only to experience increasing periods of agitation in the afternoon and evening hours. The AD patient may even wake from the night's sleep with confusion, fearfulness, or panic attacks.

- Monitor for early behaviors of fatigue and agitation. *Early assessment of problems results in prompt intervention to promote rest or to remove the patient from the situation causing anxiety.*
- Remove from situations that are causing increased anxiety, such as noisy activities involving large groups. *High-stimulus situations may increase anxious feelings and agitation.*
- Keep daily routine as consistent as possible. *Providing a structured day enhances feelings of familiarity and decreases stress.*
- Schedule rest periods or quiet times throughout the day. *Fatigue contributes to anxiety and lowers the ability to tolerate stress.*
- Provide quiet activities, such as listening to favorite music, in the afternoon or early evening. *Quiet activities may help decrease sundowning.*
- If confusion and agitation persist or escalate, assess for physical causes such as decreased oxygenation, infections, fatigue, constipation, and electrolyte imbalance. *Physical factors can increase agitation in patients with AD.*
- Use therapeutic touch or gentle hand massage. *These activities induce relaxation and have a calming effect.*

Hopelessness

As the patient and family recognize the effect of AD on their lives, they may feel a sense of hopelessness. They may not have the coping skills to deal effectively with the diagnosis and anticipated problems. The increasingly degenerative, irreversible nature of the disorder tends to diminish hope; only the ability to adapt to the many problems can restore it.

- Assess the patient's and family's response to the diagnosis and understanding of AD; encourage expression of feelings. *Understanding the patient's and family's perspective enables the nurse to dispel myths about AD.*
- Provide realistic information about the disorder; provide information at the patient's and family's level of understanding. *Patient and family may need to have separate sessions. Factual information provides a foundation for decision making.*
- Avoid criticizing or judging expressed feelings. *An environment accepting of the expression of real feelings promotes both further expression of feelings and willingness to discuss other issues.*

- Support positive family bonds and enhance communication among family members; promote mutual positive regard. *Strong family relationships can provide direction for living and convey a willingness to share the burden.*
- Encourage the patient to make as many decisions as possible. *Self-determination enhances a feeling of control over a situation and may give a sense of hope.*
- Encourage the patient and family to seek spiritual guidance that previously inspired hope. *The patient's church is a legitimate support system. Belief in God can inspire hope beyond present circumstances.*

Caregiver Role Strain

Most caregivers of patients with AD are spouses or other family members. Because AD is a chronic and eventually debilitating disorder, caregivers may feel overwhelmed by

their responsibilities. The caregiving spouse faces not only the responsibility for the patient's multiple physical demands but also economic and psychosocial stressors. An area that must be discussed is the ability and safety of the patient in driving an automobile. Although it may be necessary, the loss of independence represented by the loss of the ability to drive may further trigger anxiety and anger. Fear of the future, loss of income, loss of companionship and a mate—combined with fatigue—make the caregiver vulnerable. Caregivers may become physically and mentally exhausted and socially isolated because of the overwhelming responsibilities of providing total care to the incapacitated family member. Although most families prefer to keep the person with AD at home as long as possible, most people with the disease eventually need more assistance than

---

 Safety Interventions for the Patient with Alzheimer's Disease

DECREASING THE RISK OF FALLS

The risk for falls in patients with AD may be evaluated by the Hendrich II Fall Model (Hendrich, 2007; Gray-Miceli, 2007). Although designed originally to be used with patients in the acute care setting, most of the information is equally as useful for home-care or long-term care patients. The tool may be accessed online at the Hartford Institute for Geriatric Nursing or the consultGeriRN website. A video demonstrating its use is available at the Hartford website.

- Assess usual environment for hazards, such as throw rugs, electrical cords, and slick floors.
- Observe areas of special concern, such as the bathroom, kitchen, and stairs, and modify as needed; for example, provide skid proof surfaces, and mark stairs to show depth.
- Evaluate muscle strength and gait; consult a physical therapist to plan exercises to increase strength and balance.
- Check shoes for fit and support.
- Inquire about alcohol use and medications that affect balance or cause mobility problems; for example, antihypertensive agents can cause dizziness with position changes.
- Use night-lights and increase daytime lighting in dark areas, such as hallways.
- Keep traffic areas free from clutter.

DECREASING INJURIES RELATED TO COGNITIVE IMPAIRMENTS

- Secure items that may be mistakenly ingested, such as cleaning preparations and house plants.
- Modify potentially unsafe areas, such as unenclosed porches.
- Provide double lock systems to outside doors and doors to rooms that are off-limits.
- Protect from fire hazards; for example, make matches and cigarettes inaccessible.
- Fence the yard with a locked gate to prevent wandering. (For further information, see the publication by Rowe (2008), *Wandering in Hospitalized Older Adults.* Although developed for patients with dementia in the acute care setting, much of the information is equally useful for home care and long-term care patients.
- Modify the controls on the oven and stove.
- Adjust the water heater to a safe temperature.

GENERAL SAFETY CONSIDERATIONS

- Plan a calling system for emergencies; have children call at about the same time every day as a check.
- Ensure that the cognitively impaired family member has no

access to objects in the home such as knives and guns.
- If safety is a concern (such as turning on the stove and forgetting it), suggest using alternatives such as a microwave. Program emergency numbers into the telephone. Ask patient to consider a Life-Line telephone program. *These measures can increase safety.*
- Suggest using cues, such as an alarm on a watch or a pocket computer, to trigger actions at designated times. *Cues are often helpful when memory loss is a problem.*

DECREASING INJURIES FROM CHRONIC CONFUSION

Patients with AD often have memory deficits that make functioning in a nonstructured environment difficult. Many of the nursing interventions for this diagnosis need to be modified over time as the patient continues to lose cognitive function.

- Label rooms, drawers, and other items as needed. *Visual cues promote the highest possible degree of independence for the patient.*
- Remove potential hazards (such as sharp knives or potentially harmful liquids or chemicals) from the environment. *Ensuring safety is a critical factor in providing care.*
- Keep environmental stimuli to a minimum: Decrease noise levels; speak in a calm, low voice; and take an unhurried approach. *Minimizing sensory input and maintaining a calm manner may decrease anxiety.*
- Begin each interaction by identifying self and calling patient by name. See Box 44–1 for other communication techniques. *These techniques provide information for the patient with memory loss.*
- Limit questions to those that require a simple yes or no response. *Questions need to be appropriate to the patient's ability as decision making and verbal skills decline.*
- Orient to the environment, person, and time as able; place large, easy-to-read calendars and clocks in the patient's line of vision. Make references to the season or day of the week when conversing with the patient. *Orient the patient according to his or her level of ability; orienting to precise time may not be possible in the later stages of AD.*
- Provide boundaries by placing red or yellow tape on the floor. *Boundaries help the patient stay within safe areas.*

PRACTICE ALERT
Red and yellow are more easily seen by older adults.

BOX 44–1 Communicating with the Patient with Alzheimer's Disease

- Face the patient and talk directly to him or her; call the patient by name.
- When first approaching the patient, identify yourself.
- Use simple sentences and words with few syllables.
- Speak in a calm, low voice.
- Ask one question at a time. Use questions that require only a yes or no response.
- Keep nonverbal communication relaxed and parallel to the verbal communication.
- Avoid giving the impression of being in a hurry; try to have a relaxed approach.
- Observe for anxiety—wringing hands, pacing, darting eye movements—and alter your approach to decrease anxiety.
- Avoid arguing with patients; do not insist on orienting patient to reality; the patient's point of reference may not be based in reality.
- Give plenty of time for the patient with AD to process what you are trying to say; do not expect patients to perform skills beyond their abilities.
- Repeat explanations in simple terms.

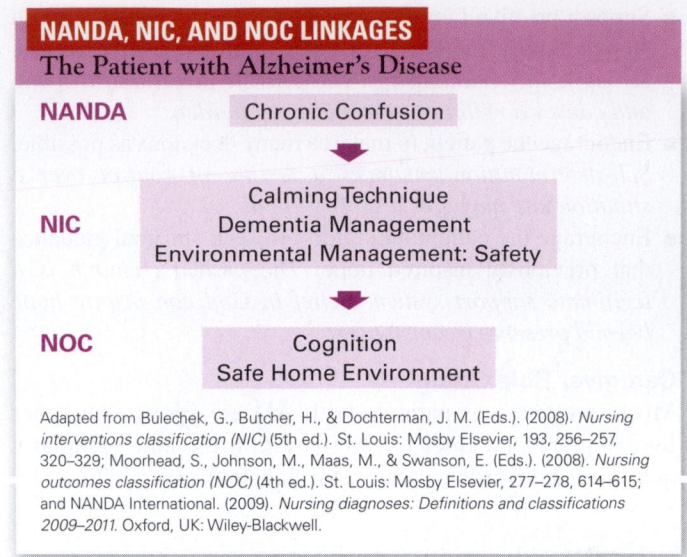

NANDA, NIC, AND NOC LINKAGES
The Patient with Alzheimer's Disease

Adapted from Bulechek, G., Butcher, H., & Dochterman, J. M. (Eds.). (2008). *Nursing interventions classification (NIC)* (5th ed.). St. Louis: Mosby Elsevier, 193, 256–257, 320–329; Moorhead, S., Johnson, M., Maas, M., & Swanson, E. (Eds.). (2008). *Nursing outcomes classification (NOC)* (4th ed.). St. Louis: Mosby Elsevier, 277–278, 614–615; and NANDA International. (2009). *Nursing diagnoses: Definitions and classifications 2009–2011.* Oxford, UK: Wiley-Blackwell.

family members can provide, and must move to a facility for professional care. The topic of caregiving is so important that an entire issue of *The American Journal of Nursing* (2008, 108, 9 supplement) titled *State of the Science: Professional Partners Supporting Family Caregivers* has been published. The supplement may be viewed online at Lippincott's Nursing Center.

- Teach the caregivers self-care techniques, such as taking rest periods and avoiding fatigue. *Fatigue adds to stress and potentially leads to poor decision making.*
- Have the caregivers list and regularly take part in physical activities they enjoy, such as walking or swimming. *Regular physical exercise decreases stress.*
- Refer the caregivers to local AD support groups. Suggest books pertinent to the subject. *Explicit suggestions in locating support systems and providing specific information promotes coping.*
- Refer the caregivers to Meals on Wheels, home health, respite care, and other community services. *Community agencies can relieve some of the daily care burdens, thus providing time for other activities. Programs that support caregivers have been shown to delay nursing home placement.*
- Ensure the family knows that hospice care is available during the end stages of AD. *Hospice services can support the family during this difficult time.*

Using NANDA, NIC, and NOC

Linkages between a selected NANDA nursing diagnosis, NIC, and NOC for the patient with Alzheimer's Disease are shown in the chart that follows.

Community-Based Care

Family caregiving takes an enormous toll on mental, physical, emotional, and financial resources. Family members see a former fully functioning and independent loved one become progressively more impaired and dependent on others for total care. The patient with AD drains time and energy, leading to high rates of depression, symptoms of "burnout," and frequent illnesses in the caregiver. The stress

may even cause them to become physically abusive to the patient (Holcomb, 2008).

Teaching for patients and families centers initially on explaining the disorder and exploring available support systems. Anticipate the need to re-explain the disorder and its consequences because patients and families may be in shock or denial during the initial period of the disease. In addition to explaining the anticipated changes with AD, suggest practical solutions to identified problems. It is important to evaluate both the patient and caregivers; interventions must be appropriate for the family's situation and resources. Maintaining the least restrictive environment that promotes safety for the patient is a major goal of teaching. Using memory cues, such as labeling drawers to indicate the specific types of clothing and labeling rooms, can help orient the patient and foster independence. Consistency in the environment and daily routine is an essential part of care. Emphasizing realistic expectations means adjusting care and communication techniques to the patient's level of ability.

Address the following topics for home care of the patient and for the caregiver:

- Support groups and peer counseling are helpful in handling caregiver stress.
- A person with AD who is confused or agitated is not comfortable and is usually frightened.
- Plan care that matches the person's level of coping, using a consistent routine.
- Provide regular rest periods to decrease the patient's stress and fatigue (these do not increase nighttime wandering).
- Plan care for the caregiver. Periodic adult day care or respite care during the initial stages, with plans for increasing assistance to meet the patient's daily needs as the disease progresses, may be sufficient. Referrals to the appropriate agency for long-term care, including skilled nursing facilities, may be indicated. Family members may need help adjusting to the idea of extended care but may be relieved to relinquish the physical care needs.
- Suggest the following resources: Alzheimer's Association, Alzheimer's Disease and Related Disorders Association, Alzheimer's Disease Education and Referral Center, and the National Institute of Neurological Disorders and Stroke.

Arthur and Ruth Joste, both aged 73, have been married for 47 years; he is a retired history teacher, and she has been a homemaker. They have four children; two live in the same town, and two live out of state. Arthur has noticed that he is having problems remembering friends' names and phone numbers; his wife has been asking him if he is driving in the correct direction when they go shopping.

Mrs. Joste has severe osteoarthritis and is unable to lift heavy objects or perform all but light housekeeping tasks. For about 18 months, Mrs. Joste has been aware of her husband's progressive cognitive decline, including forgetting current news from last night's newspaper, miscalculating checkbook balances, neglecting his hygiene needs, and confusing their children's and grandchildren's names. The Jostes are referred to a neurologist for evaluation.

ASSESSMENT

Martha Spital, RN, assesses Mr. Joste at the neurologist's office. She notes that he is unable to recall his home address without prompting, to name the correct date (although he does know the day of the week), to subtract serial 7s more than twice, and to recall two of three objects. He is alert to his surroundings. Mrs. Joste states that the problems seem to be getting worse with time and that she has had to "cover up" mistakes for her husband. Mr. Joste seems easily agitated, and his wife reports that his sleep habits are "jumbled"; he has long periods of wakefulness in the nighttime hours.

Following a thorough evaluation and diagnostic testing to rule out other possible disorders, the neurologist tells the couple that Mr. Joste has probable dementia of the Alzheimer's type. Both have feared this diagnosis; they want to know how they can be sure that Mr. Joste has this disease and what they can do to prevent further decline. Both are obviously much saddened, and they verbalize their feelings of being overwhelmed. The Jostes intend to remain in their home "for as long as we can."

DIAGNOSES

- *Chronic Confusion* related to deterioration of brain function and dementia
- *Self-Care Deficits* related to forgetfulness and declining physical abilities
- *Risk for Injury* related to decreased orientation
- *Disturbed Sleep Pattern* related to time disorientation
- *Caregiver Role Strain* (wife) related to need to care for self and husband

EXPECTED OUTCOMES

- Remain free of injury.
- Navigate home environment with modifications as needed.
- Participate in grooming and hygiene activities with prompting and supervision.
- Obtain a minimum of 7 uninterrupted hours of sleep a night.
- Mrs. Joste will participate in a minimum of two out-of-home activities a week.

PLANNING AND IMPLEMENTATION

The home health nurse, Erick Montane, RN, makes a home visit to evaluate the environment, assess available support, and determine needs. He meets two of the Jostes' children, Dawn and Jay, who live in the same community and are willing to participate as much as possible in providing care and modifying the home.

Mr. Montane discusses the importance of establishing and maintaining a consistent daily routine. He emphasizes the importance of matching activities to Mr. Joste's mental abilities to avoid frustration and increased agitation. Mr. Montane recommends labeling drawers with their contents, such as Mr. Joste's sock drawer. Labeling rooms may eventually be necessary.

Because his inability to comprehend and process information distresses and agitates Mr. Joste, Mr. Montane teaches the family to modify their communications to fit Mr. Joste's cognitive ability, such

as using simple, direct statements and directions. Mr. Montane also recommends that family members keep background noise to a minimum because this may be a source of confusion.

After assessing the home, Mr. Montane makes the following recommendations about safety:

- Remove throw rugs from hallways, and tack down any remaining carpets.
- Secure the kitchen, bathroom, and workshop cabinets as well as the controls on the oven and stove.
- Modify the doors so that negotiating locks requires a two-step system of unlocking, such as with a deadbolt and a key.
- Provide extra lighting in dark areas, especially a night-light in the bathroom.

Mr. Montane explains that Mrs. Joste will need assistance with housekeeping as Mr. Joste continues to decline. Mr. Montane provides referrals to community services, including Meals on Wheels, which can supply a daily meal. He also suggests that the Jostes obtain the services of a home health aide to provide daily hygiene care. Most of the remaining home maintenance needs can be met with the children's help.

Mr. and Mrs. Joste and the two children attend the weekly local support group meetings for Alzheimer's disease and related disorders for approximately 3 months; thereafter, Mrs. Joste attends with her daughter.

EVALUATION

Six months after the initial home visit and family planning session, Mr. Joste assesses as follows:

- Has not had a fall, burn, or other injury.
- Has periods of confusion when outside his home, but 90% of the time is oriented to place when at home.
- Has attended several support group meetings until 3 months ago. Currently, his wife attends weekly, and a daughter occasionally accompanies her. She has continued to participate in their church and maintains contact with a few friends. She is finding it harder to leave her husband unattended for even a few minutes.
- Is able to clean and dress himself with prompting; he is not able to choose his own clothing. If hygiene articles are "set up" (e.g., if the toothpaste is placed on the toothbrush), he remembers to perform the hygiene activity. The children have been replacing buttons and zippers with Velcro closures on his clothing.
- Sleeps an average of 6 hours a night with a 30-minute nap in the afternoon; this pattern is consistent with his previous sleep pattern.
- Has seemed to be more easily agitated for the past month. He wanders from room to room, apparently looking for something. These behaviors are worse in the evening and on cloudy days. Mrs. Joste sadly acknowledges her progressive inability to care for her husband.

CRITICAL THINKING IN THE NURSING PROCESS

1. Develop a tool to teach safety needs for the patient and family with Alzheimer's disease.
2. List five interventions to decrease agitation in cognitively impaired older adults; give three additional examples of activities suited to an older adult with AD who has osteoarthritis.
3. You are caring for a patient in stage 5 Alzheimer's disease. She is 65 inches (165 cm) tall and weighs 132 lb (59.9 kg); she has lost 3 lb within the past month. The patient has difficulty focusing on eating and is easily agitated. Describe your plan for ensuring that she has adequate nutrition. (A suggested resource is the Edinburgh Feeding Evaluation in Dementia Scale [2008]. The tool may be accessed at the Hartford Institute for Geriatric Nursing or the ConsultGeriRN website. A video demonstrating its use is available at the Lippincott website; search for A281.)

See Evaluating Your Response in Appendix C.

The Patient with Multiple Sclerosis

Multiple sclerosis (MS) is a chronic demyelinating disease of the CNS (brain, optic nerves, and spinal cord). The disease ranges from relatively mild to totally disabling. The manifestations of MS vary according to the area of the nervous system affected. The initial onset may be followed by a total remission, making diagnosis difficult. In many patients, MS is characterized by periods of exacerbation, when manifestations are highly pronounced, followed by periods of remission, when manifestations are not obvious. The end result is progression of the disease with increasing loss of function.

The onset of MS is usually between 20 and 40 years of age, but the disease has been diagnosed in individuals as young as 2 years and as old as 75 years. MS is the most prevalent CNS demyelinating disorder, and is a leading cause of neurologic disability in young adults. Although all races are affected, MS is primarily a disease of people of northern European ancestry. The risk of developing MS is 15-fold greater when MS is also present in a first-degree relative, and even higher in monozygotic twins. Those with the human leukocyte antigen HLA-DR2 haplotype are especially at risk, although the reason is unknown (Porth & Matfin, 2009).

FAST FACTS
Multiple Sclerosis
- Approximately 400,000 people in the United States have MS; the incidence is approximately 1 to 2 million worldwide.
- Women are affected two times more often than men.
- The disease is more prevalent in colder northern latitudes, such as the northern Atlantic states, the Great Lakes region, and the Pacific Northwest.

Source: Hickey, 2009; NINDS, 2009b; Porth & Matfin, 2009.

Pathophysiology

MS is believed to occur as a result of an autoimmune response in a genetically susceptible person. The target antigen has not been identified, but is suggested to be an immune response to a protein in the CNS. As with other demyelinating disorders, MS is characterized by inflammation and selective destruction of CNS myelin (Porth & Matfin, 2009).

Myelin sheaths are fatty, segmented wrappings that normally protect and insulate nerve fibers and increase the speed of transmission of nerve impulses. In multiple sclerosis, these myelin sheaths of the white matter of the spinal cord, brain, and optic nerve are destroyed in patches, called plaques, along the axon (see Pathophysiology Illustrated on pages 1520–1521). The demyelination of nerve fibers slows and distorts the conduction of nerve impulses and sometimes results in the total absence or distortion of impulse transmission. The neurons affected by MS are located in the spinal cord, brainstem, cerebral and cerebellar areas, and the optic nerve. The peripheral nerves are not affected.

Plaques typically are scattered through the white matter of the CNS, although they may extend into adjacent gray matter. Early manifestations are the result of inflammatory edema in and around the plaque and partial demyelination. These manifestations typically disappear within weeks after the initial episode. With progression of the disease, the demyelination and plaque formation result in scarring of glia (gliosis) and degeneration of axons. MS develops in two stages. In the first stage there is sequential development of small inflammatory lesions, during the second stage these lesions extend and consolidate as gliosis and demyelination occurs. It is unknown whether the inflammatory process is directed against the myelin or against oligodendrocytes that produce myelin. Evidence suggests that remyelination can occur in the CNS if the disease process is stopped before the oligodendrocytes are destroyed (Porth & Matfin, 2009).

There are four possible courses of MS: relapsing-remitting (characterized by periodic remission and exacerbation of manifestations) primary progressive (almost continuous neurologic deterioration from onset of manifestations), secondary progressive (gradual deterioration with or without relapses), and progressive-relapsing (gradual progression of neurologic deterioration with super-imposed relapses). Most individuals with MS present with the relapsing-remitting type.

Manifestations

The manifestations of MS (listed in the box on page 1519) vary according to the areas destroyed by demyelination and the affected body system (see Multisystem Effects of Multiple Sclerosis on page 1522). The most common manifestations are sensory loss, visual deficits, weakness, paresthesias, ataxia, and vertigo. In many patients, the initial manifestation involves blurred or double vision (diplopia), red-green color distortion, or even blindness in one eye (NINDS, 2009b). Fatigue is one of the most disabling manifestations, and affects almost all patients with MS. The manifestations (individualized to each patient) typically last for several days or weeks and then completely or partially resolve. After a period of relatively normal function, manifestations reappear.

Interdisciplinary Care

Management of the patient with MS varies according to the severity of the manifestations. The focus is on retaining the optimal level of functioning possible, given the degree of disability. Rehabilitation—physical, occupational/vocational, and psychosocial—is a cornerstone of an interdisciplinary approach to treatment. During exacerbations, the focus of interventions shifts to controlling manifestations and quickly returning to remission.

Diagnosis

A diagnosis of MS requires that the patient have one of the following: (1) two or more exacerbations separated by 1 month or more and lasting more than 24 hours, followed by recovery; (2) a history of repeated exacerbations and remissions with or without complete recovery, followed by progressively more severe manifestations lasting for 6 months or more; or (3) slowly increasing manifestations for at least 6 months.

Diagnostic tests (∞ described in Chapter 41) vary with the presenting complaints. Magnetic resonance imaging (MRI) with findings of lesions is the most definitive test available; however, it is only one of several laboratory and diagnostic tests that may be performed when establishing the diagnosis. Cerebrospinal fluid (CSF) analysis reveals an increased number of T lymphocytes that are reactive with antigens, indicating the presence of an immune response. The majority of patients with MS have elevated levels of immunoglobulin G (IgG) in the CSF. A CT scan of the brain may reveal atrophy and white matter lesions.

Medications

Medications slow the progression of MS and decrease the number of attacks. (See the Medication Administration box on page 1523.) Medications are used for a variety of reasons, including to treat manifestations, to modify the course of the disease, or to interrupt the progression of the disease.

The medications used during an exacerbation are aimed at decreasing inflammation to inhibit manifestations and induce remission. A combination of adrenal corticosteroid hormone (ACTH) and glucocorticoids is often used to decrease inflammation and suppress the immune system. Immunosuppressive agents, including azathioprine (Imuran) and cyclophosphamide (Cytoxan), are also used. Interferon and glatiramer acetate are used to reduce exacerbations in patients with relapsing-remitting MS. Interferon alpha, beta, and gamma (Roferon-A, Intron A, Wellferon, Infergen, Avonex or Rebif, Betaseron, Actimmune) enhance immune function, while glatiramer acetate (Copaxone) stimulates parts of the myelin basic protein to reduce the relapse rate of MS. Both drugs are given by injection and are usually well-tolerated. Natalizumab (Tysabri) is given to patients with relapsing forms of MS to delay physical disability and reduce the frequency of exacerbations. An oral form of the drug cladribine (Leustatin) (an anticancer drug) to treat relapsing forms of MS is in clinical trials and expected to gain FDA approval.

Other medications treat the manifestations of MS. Anticholinergics are administered for bladder spasticity; cholinergics are given if the patient has a problem with urinary retention related to flaccid bladder. Fatigue may be treated with amantadine (Symmetrel), pemoline (Cylert) and an experimental drug, aminopyridine.

Surgery

Surgery may be indicated for patients who experience severe spasticity and deformity. However, physical therapy can prevent most severe problems. Foot drop from severe plantar flexion can be relieved with an Achilles tenotomy, a surgical procedure in which the Achilles tendon is transected.

Nutrition and Fluids

Patients with MS may be overweight because of their inability to ambulate; depression may contribute to the problem because people who are depressed tend to eat more. Ideally, the patient should maintain a weight as close as possible to that recommended for the patient's height and body type.

As MS progresses, the patient's ability to prepare food and eat may be compromised. Changes in muscle tone, tremor, weakness, and ataxia all contribute to nutritional problems. Dysphagia also is a common problem. The diet must be adapted to accommodate changes in the patient's ability to chew and swallow.

Rehabilitation

Physical and rehabilitative therapies are tailored to the patient's level of functioning. The long-term goal is to enable the patient to retain as much independence as possible. One major intervention is to maintain and increase existing muscle strength.

Spasticity is managed with stretching exercises, gait training, and braces, splints, or other assistive devices. To maintain balance, the patient is encouraged to widen the base of support by standing with the feet slightly further apart. Walkers and canes may be weighted to provide support and balance for the ataxic patient.

An interdisciplinary approach to rehabilitation will provide supportive services: speech therapy for problems with phonation, occupational therapy to maintain strength in the upper extremities and carry out ADLs, and occupational counseling. Referrals to a urologist are indicated for problems with urinary incontinence, urinary tract infections, retention, and impotence. Consultation with a respiratory therapist may be needed if the patient develops chronic respiratory infections from inability to cough, move secretions, or breathe deeply, especially with increased debilitation.

MANIFESTATIONS of Multiple Sclerosis

- Visual deficits, with visual blurring, fogginess, or haziness; diplopia, impaired color perception, decreased central visual acuity, area of diminished vision in the visual fields, acquired color vision deficit (especially to red and green), and an altered pupillary reaction to light
- Brainstem lesions (cranial nerves III to XII) with nystagmus, dysarthria, deafness, vertigo, vomiting, tinnitus, facial weakness, decreased sensation, diplopia, and eye pain; and cognitive dysfunctions involving concentration, short-term memory, word finding, and planning
- Mood alterations are manifested as depression more often than euphoria
- Weakness and/or numbness in one or both extremities (most often the legs)
- Upper motor neuron involvement is manifested by stiffness, slowness, weakness (spastic paresis)
- Bladder dysfunctions include urgency, hesitancy, and incontinence
- Bowel dysfunction is most often seen as constipation
- Sexual dysfunction

PATHOPHYSIOLOGY ILLUSTRATED
Multiple Sclerosis

Neuron
Oligodendrocyte
Microglial cell
Astrocyte
Venule
Myelin sheath
Axon (Node of Ranvier)

Normal Anatomy of the Central Nervous System

The central nervous system (CNS) is composed of several cell types arranged in a dense, interconnected lattice. The basic functional cell of the CNS is the *neuron*, which transmits electrochemical impulses. Dendrites, thin projections extending from the neuron body, receive impulses that are passed down the neuronal axon for transmission to other cells. Myelin, a lipid-protein substance, surrounds the axons, insulating them and speeding nerve impulse transmission.

Neurons are surrounded by a network of cells:

- *Astrocytes* support neurons and connnect them to surrounding capillaries and venules.
- *Microglia* are motile phagocytic cells.
- *Oligodendrocytes* wrap concentric layers of myelin around nearby axons.

Acute Attack

Multiple sclerosis (MS) is a demyelinating disease in which axonal myelin in the central nervous system is eroded, destroyed, and replaced by scar tissue.

An autoimmune process apparently triggered by genetic and environmental factors is believed to cause inflammation of venules in the CNS. This disrupts the blood–brain barrier, allowing lymphocytes to enter CNS tissue. These lymphocytes proliferate and produce IgG, an antibody that attacks and damages myelin and causes the release of inflammatory chemicals and edema. As the inflammation subsides, the myelin regenerates and manifestations of the disease subside.

Damaging substances released from macrophages and lymphocytes
Microglial cell ingesting myelin fragment
Macrophage
Inflamed myelin sheath
Lymphocyte

Chronic Lesion

After repeated inflammatory attacks, myelin is irreparably damaged. Segments of axons become totally demyelinated and may degenerate. Astrocytes proliferate in damaged regions of the CNS (a process called *gliosis*), forming plaques. The plaques are scattered throughout the CNS, appearing as gray or pinkish lesions. The relapsing-remitting character of MS and the scattered areas of damage within the CNS account for the variable nature of MS manifestations.

Abnormal Nerve Impulse Transmission

In an undamaged neuron, nerve impulses travel down the axon by "leaping" from one node of Ranvier to the next, thus greatly increasing the speed of impulse transmission. When nerve impulses travel down an axon damaged by MS, they are significantly slowed and weakened as they pass across the surface of demyelinated areas. Impulses may be blocked entirely when axons degenerate. The weakening or interruption of the transmission of nerve impulses and plaque formation within the CNS cause the manifestations of MS, including extremity weakness, paresthesias, visual disturbances, bladder dysfunction, and vertigo.

MULTISYSTEM EFFECTS OF
Multiple Sclerosis

Neurologic
- Emotional lability (euphoria or depression)
- Forgetfulness
- Apathy
- Scanning speech
- Impaired judgment
- Irritability

Potential Complications
- Convulsive seizures
- Dementia

Sensory

Visual
- Blurred vision
- Diplopia
- Nystagmus
- Visual field defects (blind spots)
- Eye pain

Auditory
- Vertigo
- Nausea

Tactile (especially hands or legs)
- Numbness
- Paresthesias (tingling, burning sensation)
- Diminished sense of temperature
- Pain with spasms
- Loss of proprioception

Potential Complication
Visual
- Blindness

Respiratory
- Diminished cough reflex

Potential Complication
- Respiratory infections

Urinary
- Hesitancy
- Frequency
- Retention
- Reflex bladder emptying

Potential Complications
- Recurring UTIs
- Incontinence

Gastrointestinal
Oral/esophageal
- Difficulty chewing
- Dysphagia

Upper/lower GI
- Decreased or absent sphincter control
- Bowel incontinence
- Constipation

Musculoskeletal
- Fatigue
- Limb weakness
- Ataxic movements (shaky, irregular, uncoordinated)
- Intention tremors
- Spasticity
- Muscular atrophy
- Dragging of foot and foot drop
- Dysarthria with slurred speech

Reproductive
- Impotence (male)
- Loss of genital sensation

MEDICATION ADMINISTRATION   The Patient with Multiple Sclerosis

IMMUNOMODULATORS

Interferon beta-1a (Avonex) (administered IM one time a week)

Interferon beta-1a (Rebif) (administered subcutaneously three times a week)

Interferon beta-1b (Betaseron) (administered subcutaneously every other day)

Glatiramer acetate (Copaxone, Copolymer-1) (administered subcutaneously daily)

Natalizumab (Tysabri) (administered IV monthly)

Interferon beta-la, interferon beta-1b, and glatiramer acetate are administered to patients with relapsing-remitting MS to prolong the time of onset to disability. Their use is based on the assumption that MS is an immunologically mediated disease. Interferon beta-1b produces a decrease in the MS lesions in some patients. Some patients, however, develop a decrease in the absolute neutrophil count and increases in the levels of liver enzymes. Anxiety, confusion, and depression with suicidal tendencies also have been reported. Other adverse reactions include pain, inflammation, hypersensitivity at the injection site, and generalized flulike manifestations. Some women experience menstrual disorders. Pregnant women should not take these medications. Natalizumab (Tysabri) has strict treatment guidelines, and can only be administered in infusion centers with monitoring by specially trained physicians.

Nursing Responsibilities

- Assess baseline parameters to evaluate drug side effects: psychologic profile, liver function tests, and CBC with differential.
- Monitor CBC and liver function tests every 3 months or as prescribed.
- Assess injection site and report ulceration promptly (pain and redness are common reactions).
- Evaluate patient's baseline neurologic, sensory, and motor function. Monitor changes in condition and function.
- Report if patient is pregnant or breast-feeding.

Health Education for the Patient and Family

- These drugs may cause depression and thoughts of suicide; report these feelings immediately to the physician.
- Administer medication within 3 hours of reconstitution. Rotate injection sites, and avoid any areas that are red or show other skin reactions.
- Seek follow-up care to monitor neurologic changes, CBC, and liver function.
- Avoid prolonged exposure to sunlight.
- Flulike manifestations may occur within hours to days after an injection.

ADRENOCORTICOSTEROID THERAPY

Adrenocorticotropic hormone (ACTH) (Acthar)

Prednisone (Deltasone, Meticorten, Orasone)

Methylprednisolone (Medrol, Solu-Medrol)

Adrenalcorticosteroids are used both to sustain a remission and to treat exacerbations of MS. ACTH is usually given to induce a remission. It is administered intravenously for 1 week and may be followed by oral prednisone therapy. Another protocol involves administering ACTH intravenously for 3 days followed by intramuscular injections every 12 hours for 1 week (Hickey, 2003). The drugs are given to suppress the immune system, implicated in the etiology of MS. If the drug is used long term the usual steroid precautions are indicated, such as monitoring for glucose intolerance, osteoporosis, and cataract formation. The drugs are used with caution in pregnant and lactating women.

MUSCLE RELAXANTS

Baclofen (Lioresal)

Dantrolene (Dantrium)

Diazepam (Valium)

Muscle relaxants are given to patients with MS to relieve muscle spasms. Baclofen and diazepam act by suppressing CNS reflexes that regulate muscle activity; neither drug affects muscle strength. Baclofen therapy should be discontinued over 1 to 2 weeks; sudden withdrawal may cause seizures and paranoid ideation. In contrast to diazepam and baclofen, dantrolene acts directly on skeletal muscles, and it may affect muscle strength. Dantrolene may cause hepatotoxicity and should not be administered when hepatitis or cirrhosis is present.

Nursing Responsibilities

- Evaluate baseline muscle strength and spasticity, ROM, and dexterity.
- Maintain safety or fall precautions; dizziness and drowsiness are common side effects.
- For the patient taking dantrolene, monitor liver function tests (enzymes and bilirubin) for signs of hepatotoxicity.

Health Education for the Patient and Family

- These drugs may cause sedative effects. Take appropriate safety measures (e.g., avoid driving).
- Avoid CNS depressants (antihistamines, alcohol); they can increase the sedative effects of the medication.
- Continue follow-up care; if you are taking dantrolene, for example, liver function will need to be monitored.
- If you are taking baclofen, do not suddenly stop the medication.
- Increase fiber and fluids in the diet to prevent constipation.
- Change positions slowly to minimize dizziness and other effects of orthostatic hypotension.

IMMUNOSUPPRESSANTS

Azathioprine (Imuran)

Cyclophosphamide (Cytoxan)

Immunosuppressants are given to patients with MS because of the autoimmune component of the disease. Both medications can cause bone marrow suppression and increase the risk of cancer. Azathioprine may produce hepatitis. Toxic effects of cyclophosphamide include hemorrhagic cystitis, sterility, and stomatitis.

Nursing Responsibilities

- Monitor baseline parameters: CBC with platelet count and differential, urinalysis, liver function tests, hepatitis profile.
- Assess for anemia: fatigue, lethargy, pallor.
- Watch for bleeding.
- Protect against and observe for subtle signs of infection.

Health Education for the Patient and Family

- Report infection, bleeding, and anemia immediately.
- Drink at least 2 L (2 quarts) of fluid a day, and observe urine for blood.
- Report jaundice immediately.
- Check oral cavity daily for changes or ulcers.
- Avoid becoming pregnant while taking these drugs.
- Obtain follow-up care, including frequent blood tests.

✍ Nursing Care

Because the disease most often affects young adults, the psychosocial and economic effect can be devastating. People with MS have to make adjustments to the body image changes while simultaneously adapting to the altered relationships and decreased earnings usually encountered with the disease. A once-healthy spouse becomes wheelchair bound; a person once independent may eventually become dependent for even the most basic ADLs. The unpredictable course of MS is a challenge for long-term planning. A Case Study & Nursing Care Plan for the patient with MS is given on page 1526.

Health Promotion

Following an overview of the disorder, the patient needs to understand how to prevent fatigue and exacerbations. Teach the patient to avoid stress, extremes of cold and heat, high humidity, physical overexertion, and infections, as these may trigger a relapse of manifestations. Because the woman in the postpartum period has a 20% to 40% greater risk for relapse in the first 6 months (Stachowiak, 2008), counseling about this risk is indicated. However, pregnancy itself seems to be protective against relapse. Also, address preventive measures to avoid risk of respiratory and urinary tract infections.

Assessment

Collect the following data through the health history and physical examination (∞ see Chapter 41):

- *Health history:* History of childhood viral illnesses, geographical residence as a child, exposure to physical or emotional stressors (pregnancy/delivery, extremes of heat), medications, symptom onset, severity of manifestations.
- *Physical assessment:* Affect, mood, speech, eye movements, gait, tremors, vision and hearing, reflexes, muscle strength and movement, sensation. Assess for the Lhermitte's sign: an electrical shock-like tingling down the back, trunk, arms, and legs produced when the neck is flexed (the sign is positive in MS).

Nursing Diagnoses and Interventions

Interventions for the patient with MS vary with the acuity of exacerbations and the presenting problems. Many nursing diagnoses relate to the inability to perform ADLs, for example, *Self-Care Deficit* and *Impaired Home Maintenance*. Others reflect problems with musculoskeletal changes or altered nerve conduction, for example, *Impaired Physical Mobility, Ineffective Breathing Pattern, Constipation*, and *Functional Urinary Incontinence*. The nursing diagnoses discussed in this section are *Fatigue* and *Self-Care Deficit*.

Fatigue

Fatigue is experienced by almost all patients with MS. Fatigue in the patient with MS may be both primary and secondary. Primary fatigue is caused by the disease itself; secondary fatigue is the result of some of the pathophysiologic consequences of the disease. It is experienced both mentally and physically. Fatigue affects every aspect of the MS patient's life: the ability to remain independent and perform self-care, sexual function, mobility, airway clearance, and ultimately self-concept and coping. A great deal of teaching is needed to help the patient and

EVIDENCE FOR NURSING CARE **The Patient with Multiple Sclerosis**

Selected resources that nurses may find helpful when planning evidence-based nursing care follow.

- Broughton, S., Davies-Smith, A., Ingham, J., Johnson, M., Jones, C., Keen, J. et al. (2009). Multiple sclerosis. National clinical guideline for diagnosis and management in primary and secondary care. Retrieved from www.guideline.gov
- Newland, P. K., Wipke-Tevis, D. D., Williams, D. A., Rantz, M. J., & Petroski, G. F. (2005). The impact of pain on outcomes in long-term care residents with and without multiple sclerosis. *Journal of the American Geriatrics Society, 53,* 1490–1496.
- Schmit-Pokorny, K. (2009). Expanding indications for stem cell transplantation. *Seminars in Oncology Nursing, 25*(2), 105–114. Retrieved from http://www.nursingconsult.com

family understand fatigue and how to adapt. Patients and families need assistance managing fatigue in a society in which energy is highly valued.

- Assess degree of fatigue and identify contributing factors. The Fatigue Impact Scale may be used to assess the effect of fatigue on ADLs (Dittner, Wessley, & Brown, 2004). *Fatigue is a subjective experience that needs to be evaluated thoroughly before planning can begin.*
- Arrange daily activities to include rest periods. In this form of energy conservation, more strenuous activities are carried out in the morning, with regular rest periods between activities (Johnson, 2008). *Rest is essential to manage feelings of fatigue; periods of relaxation may help replenish energy reserves.*

> **PRACTICE ALERT**
> It is important to remember that the fatigue from chronic illnesses such as MS is very different from being "tired," and that rest and sleep may not result in improvement.

- Ask the patient to consider which activities are really necessary and to set priorities. *Prioritizing activities promotes independence and self-control.*
- Suggest performing tasks in the morning hours. *Biorhythm studies indicate that people usually have greater energy reserves in the morning hours and diminished reserves in the afternoon.*
- Advise to avoid temperature extremes, such as hot showers or exposure to cold. *Maintaining a relatively constant body temperature may avoid exacerbation of the disorder. Heat can delay impulse transmission across demyelinated nerves, which contributes to fatigue.*
- Provide interventions to relieve pain (a fairly common manifestation of MS). *Pain can increase fatigue; fatigue can increase the experience of pain. In one study, women with relapsing-remitting MS were found to have more pain than healthy women (Newland, 2008).*
- Refer to the appropriate professionals to manage fatigue: stress management groups, support groups, occupational or physical therapist, as indicated. *Support groups and therapy can facilitate self-management and improve coping.*

MOVING EVIDENCE INTO ACTION — Aging Patients with Multiple Sclerosis

MS is a chronic debilitating disease, but it does not reduce life expectancy. Most patients are diagnosed with the disease as young to middle adults, and they must learn how to live with the disease for the rest of their lives. However, little research has been published regarding the experiences and health-related concerns of people aging with MS. This study by Finlayson and colleagues (2004) was conducted to initiate dialogue about the role of nurses in addressing those concerns. The study subjects perceived two major differences between their experience of aging with MS and that of people aging without MS: having less freedom (not being able to travel, restriction of social activities, physical accessibility of buildings, and financial limitations) and needing more assistance (with housework, shopping, hygiene, cooking, getting to places).

IMPLICATIONS FOR NURSING

The findings of this study support the need for nurses to include consideration of issues of daily living for patients with chronic disabilities, including MS. Nurses have the knowledge and ability to include information in patient teaching that facilitate quality of life, coping with disability, and symptom management. By working closely with members of the interdisciplinary health team, nurses select and implement appropriate interventions to enable patients with MS to age in place, and to continue to be active and involved members of the family and community as they age.

CRITICAL THINKING IN PATIENT CARE

1. How would your teaching differ for the following patients with MS?
   a. A 45-year-old woman, married, with family who lives nearby
   b. A 70-year-old woman, widowed, no family living
   c. A man who has been a farmer all his life and lives in an isolated rural area
   d. A man who has always lived in an urban area with access to public transportation
2. You are making a home visit to an older woman who has had MS for 30 years. She tells you, "I never leave my condo anymore because I just can't control my urine and I'm so afraid I will have an accident." What can you do to help her resolve this problem?
3. Design a plan of care focused on the nursing diagnosis *Fatigue* for a 73-year-old man who is living independently but says, "Some days I am just too tired to even cook anything to eat."

Source: Finlayson, M., Van Denend, T., & Hudson, E. (2004). Aging with multiple sclerosis. *Journal of Neuroscience Nursing, 36*(5), 245–251, 259.

Self-Care Deficits

Patients with MS may need assistance with bathing, toileting, dressing, grooming, and feeding. The help needed can range from minimal guidance to total dependence. The patient's ability to perform self-care activities is the gauge by which family members and caregivers need to adjust assistance. Self-care encompasses both the decisions about care and the provision of care; most patients are capable of making decisions even after physical limitations prevent physical self-care. The need to maintain self-determination cannot be overemphasized and must be incorporated into each intervention. As the patient with MS ages, there may be even more need for teaching to provide self-care, as described in the Moving Evidence into Action box.

- Assess the extent of the patient's self-care deficit; refer to other health team members for assessment as appropriate. For example, refer to a speech pathologist to assess swallowing and gag reflex, if indicated. *An accurate assessment is crucial to individualizing interventions.*
- Suggest adaptive devices, such as arm or wrist braces, as needed. *Meeting hygiene needs and feeding self are essential for positive self-concept, self-esteem, and socialization.*
- Teach to use assistive devices, such as plate guards, to modify consistency of foods, and to eat when energy level is better. If unable to buy and prepare meals, provide referral to Meals on Wheels. *Proper nutrition is basic to health; adapting utensils and foods can facilitate meeting nutritional needs.*
- Teach interventions related to altered bowel and bladder function: fluid intake of at least 2000 mL daily, bowel routine as indicated to prevent constipation, and self-catheterization skills as necessary. *Maintaining optimal bowel and bladder function decreases the risk of urinary tract infection and bowel impaction.*

Using NANDA, NIC, and NOC

Linkages between a selected NANDA nursing diagnosis, NIC, and NOC for the patient with Multiple Sclerosis are shown in the chart that follows.

Community-Based Care

The inconsistent and erratic nature of MS can make teaching for self-care difficult. Initial teaching focuses on a realistic explanation of MS. Referral to a support group early in the course of

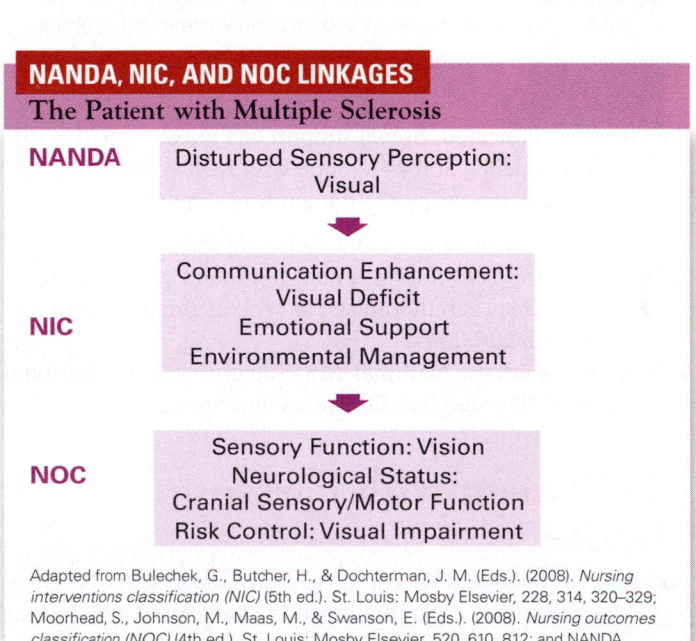

NANDA, NIC, AND NOC LINKAGES
The Patient with Multiple Sclerosis

NANDA — Disturbed Sensory Perception: Visual

NIC — Communication Enhancement: Visual Deficit / Emotional Support / Environmental Management

NOC — Sensory Function: Vision / Neurological Status: Cranial Sensory/Motor Function / Risk Control: Visual Impairment

Adapted from Bulechek, G., Butcher, H., & Dochterman, J. M. (Eds.). (2008). *Nursing interventions classification (NIC)* (5th ed.). St. Louis: Mosby Elsevier, 228, 314, 320–329; Moorhead, S., Johnson, M., Maas, M., & Swanson, E. (Eds.). (2008). *Nursing outcomes classification (NOC)* (4th ed.). St. Louis: Mosby Elsevier, 520, 610, 812; and NANDA International. (2009). *Nursing diagnoses: Definitions and classification 2009–2011.* Oxford, UK: Wiley-Blackwell.

CLINICAL SCENARIO

Directions: *Read the clinical scenarios below and answer the questions that follow. To complete this exercise successfully, you will use not only knowledge of the content in this unit, but also principles related to priority setting and maintaining patient safety.*

You have been assigned to care for the following patients on a neurologic hospital unit. Significant data obtained during report are as follows:

- Louie Hemandez is a 74-year-old male who was admitted from the emergency department to the neurologic unit last night. Mr. Hernandez was found by family in his home. He was unable to speak or move the right side of his body and continues to experience paralysis on the right side in both his arm and leg. He is aphasic with facial drooping but is able to nod his head to communicate. Mr. Hemandez has a known history of hypertension, CHF, and type 2 diabetes controlled by oral hypoglycemic medications. He has smoked a package of cigarettes a day for 40 years. BP is now 140/105, P 98, R 24. Lungs reported to have crackles. A swallowing evaluation has been ordered to be done today.

- Jane Thomas is a 56-year-old female. She was admitted 4 days ago and underwent a lumbar laminectomy. She was able to ambulate with assistance on day 2 after surgery and now reports no dizziness on ambulation. Her leg strength has progressively increased since surgery. She has equal sensation and is able to wriggle her toes on both feet. Pain is controlled at the patient's desired level of 2 to 3 on a scale of 1 to 10 with oral medications.

- Cesar Phillips is a 39-year-old male, admitted 4 days ago after experiencing paralysis and severe headache at work. He has been diagnosed with stroke following MRI. He has a history of smoking one package of cigarettes per day and hypertension. His wife reported that he had stopped taking his blood pressure medication due to the side effects of impotence. Mr. Phillips is awake and alert, but has exhibited impulsive behavior and dysphagia. He has difficulty remembering words and neglects the left side of his body in ADLs. BP had been 130/85 at the beginning of last shift, but has increased to 170/119. He received an additional blood pressure medication 1.5 hours ago.

- Tonya Walton is a 29-year-old female. She was involved in a car crash 12 hours before her admission 5 days earlier. She developed a headache, drowsiness, confusion, and pupil enlargement several hours after the crash. Following an MRI, Ms. Walton underwent intracranial surgery to evacuate a subdural hematoma. She was been complaining of a headache that has increased in intensity from 2 to 6 on a scale of 1 to 10 on the previous shift. She received two Tylenol ES tabs 1 hour ago. BP was 140–150 systolic and 90–100 diastolic for most of the shift. Her BP at the time the Tylenol was administered was 175/115. She has not experienced any changes in her neuro assessment except for the increasing headache and blood pressure elevation.

Questions

Priority Setting

1. In what order would you visit these patients after report?
   - A. _____
   - B. _____
   - C. _____
   - D. _____

Health Promotion

1. Before she is discharged, what instruction should be given to Ms. Thomas regarding lifting and moving objects?

2. What instruction should be given to Mr. Hernandez and Mr. Phillips about stop-smoking programs?

Nursing Process

1. After completing Mr. Hernandez's beginning-of-shift baseline assessment, what assessment would be your next priority?
   - A. rhythm strip interpretation
   - B. intake and output
   - C. heart sounds
   - D. level of pain

2. You are completing the beginning-of-shift assessment for Ms. Walton. What changes would best indicate that the plan initiated by the previous shift was effective?
   - A. Ms. Walton has no neurologic changes or deterioration.
   - B. Ms. Walton's BP is 142/94.
   - C. Ms. Walton's pain level is now 1–2.
   - D. Ms. Walton's dressing is dry and intact.

3. You are completing the beginning-of-shift assessment for Mr. Phillips. What changes would indicate that the plan initiated by the previous shift was effective?
   - A. Mr. Phillips no longer has a craving for cigarettes.
   - B. Mr. Phillips' respiratory rate is 18–20.
   - C. Mr. Phillips' LOP is now 1–2.
   - D. Mr. Phillips' blood pressure has decreased to 145/90.

4. What are the top two education priorities for Jane Thomas as you plan for discharge? **Select all that apply.**
   - A. appropriate exercise
   - B. pain management
   - C. weight control
   - D. incision care
   - E. importance of rest

5. You review lab reports for Jane Thomas. You are most interested in the results for which of the following studies? **Select all that apply.**
   - A. white blood cell count
   - B. red blood cell indices
   - C. serum sodium
   - D. hemoglobin
   - E. hematocrit
   - F. osteocalcin
   - G. prealbumin

6. If you reevaluated Ms. Walton and her headache pain had not decreased, what should be your next priority?
   A. Reposition Ms. Walton on her left side with the head of the bed flat.
   B. Call the physician about patient report of increasing headache.
   C. Decrease stimuli in the room by darkening the room and limiting noise.
   D. Check the prn orders to evaluate if a stronger pain medication has been ordered.

Communication

1. Mr. Phillips' wife says her husband seems too young to have a stroke. She asks what caused his symptoms. How will you answer her?

2. Mr. Hernandez's daughter asks if he will have to go to a nursing home? How will you answer her?

Delegation

1. For each patient, what assessment data and nursing interventions can be delegated to a nursing assistant?

Content-Specific Questions

1. If you were planning an effective team meeting with all disciplines that should be collaborating to provide care and a discharge plan for a patient who had a stroke, which six disciplines should be represented any why?

2. Would the same six disciplines need to be represented if the patient had a C4-C5 spinal cord injury? Why or why not?

CASE STUDY: Leticia Hays

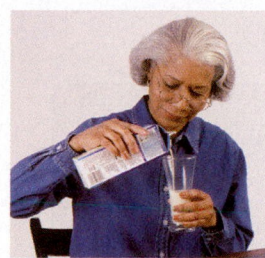

Leticia Hays is a 69-year-old African American female. She was admitted 2 days earlier after being diagnosed with a stroke. She lives with her husband of 52 years and her 14-year-old grandson. Her grandson found her lying on the kitchen floor when he got home from school. When he asked her what had happened, she was unable to say words that were clear or understandable. He tried to help her stand up, but was unable to because she was extremely weak in her left side. He called 911 and an ambulance transported her to the emergency department. Her blood pressure when the ambulance arrived was 220/125, P 105, R 24 and she was very anxious and spoke garbled words loudly at the paramedics. She was diagnosed with acute stroke after evaluation at the hospital and was admitted for treatment. Ms. Hayes has a history of hypertension and type 2 diabetes. She recently stopped taking her blood pressure medication because it made her feel "tired."

The pathophysiology of a stroke is dependent on location of the causative factor, size of tissue affected, and time of loss of cellular perfusion and oxygenation. Cerebral neuron cellular metabolism is severely affected within 4 to 5 minute of compromised perfusion. Compromised cellular metabolism leads to glucose, glycogen, and adenosine triphosphate depletion and sodium-potassium pump failure. Wherever sodium goes, water follows. When the sodium-potassium pump fails, the sodium in the cell draws water into the cell, resulting in edema. Additionally, cerebral vessel walls also swell, further compromising blood and oxygen supply. Severe or prolonged ischemia leads to cellular death. The manifestations of a stroke include, but are not limited to, motor deficits, elimination disorders, sensory-perceptual deficits, communication disorders, and behavioral changes. The manifestations are always sudden in onset, focal, and usually unilateral. Typically, a stroke is manifested by weakness of the face, arm, and leg; loss of vision in one eye; speech and swallowing problems; and difficulties with balance. There are many different complications of a stroke, including IICP, coma, death, chronic long-term confusion, and intellectual changes.

The nursing diagnosis of *Ineffective Tissue Perfusion: Cerebral* is appropriate for implementing care for Ms. Hays.

Ms. H.
69 y.o. female
Stroke

affects

• Cellular perfusion and oxygenation of area of brain decreased or stopped
• Ischemia of cerebral neurons leads to cellular death

• History of hypertension and type 2 diabetes
• Not taking antihypertensives
• BP 220/125, P 105
• Left side weakness
• Garbled speech
• Confused

generates →

• Impaired Verbal Communication related to effects of stroke
• Self-Care Deficits related to left-sided weakness and confusion
• Impaired Physical Mobility related to left-sided weakness
• Risk for Impaired Swallowing related to neurologic deficits from stroke

generate nursing diagnosis

prioritized to

Ineffective Tissue Perfusion: Cerebral

expected outcomes

• Actively participates in rehabilitation, including physical therapy, speech therapy, and occupational therapy
• Demonstrates improved ability to think, speak, carry out self-care, and ambulate
• Verbalizes necessity of taking prescribed medications
• Transfers to rehabilitation facility when health status improves

evaluate →

• PT, OT and ST initiated twice daily
• Speech is much improved and understandable
• Alert and oriented to person, place and time
• Able to feed self and walking with the assistance of a walker and another person
• Verbalized need for medications
• Transferred to rehabilitation facility for further care

Interdisciplinary Interventions
• Request referrals to physical therapy, speech therapy, and occupational therapy.
• Apply nasal oxygen as prescribed.
• Administer prescribed hypoglycemic and antihypertensive medications.

Independent Interventions
• Schedule nursing activities for care around rehabilitation times.
• Monitor neurologic status, including orientation, LOC, and reflexes.
• Monitor pulse oximetry levels.
• When appropriate, discuss effects and side effects of medications as well as risks of not taking them.
• Discuss future transfer to rehabilitation facility with family members.

Activity:

1. After reviewing the concept map, is there anything you would change to make it more understandable?

2. Go to the Pearson Nursing Student Resources for this book at www.nursing.pearsonhighered.com to write a concept map based on a nursing diagnosis of *Impaired Swallowing*.

See answers and hints in Appendix C.

Responses to Altered **Visual** and **Auditory** **Function**

Assessing the **Eye** and **Ear**

LEARNING OUTCOMES

1. Describe the anatomy, physiology, and functions of the eye and the ear.
2. Identify specific topics for consideration during a health history interview of the patient with health problems involving the eye or ear.
3. Give examples of genetic disorders in vision and hearing.
4. Describe normal variations in assessment findings for the older adult.
5. Identify abnormal findings that may indicate impairment in the function of the eye and the ear.

CLINICAL COMPETENCIES

1. Conduct and document a health history for patients having or at risk for alterations in the structure or functions of the eye and ear.
2. Conduct and document a physical assessment of the structure and functions of the eye and ear.
3. Monitor the results of diagnostic tests and report abnormal findings.

EQUIPMENT NEEDED

- Visual acuity charts
- Opaque eye cover
- Pen
- Penlight
- Cotton-tipped applicator
- Ophthalmoscope
- Otoscope
- Tuning fork

KEY TERMS

accommodation, *1560*
cerumen, *1567*
convergence, *1560*
corneal reflex, *1557*

hyperopia, *1564*
myopia, *1564*
nystagmus, *1564*
presbyopia, *1564*

ptosis, *1565*
pupillary light reflex, *1557*
refraction, *1559*

The eyes and ears provide pathways for visual and auditory stimuli to reach the brain. In addition, specialized structures within the ear help maintain position sense and equilibrium.

Deficits in vision and hearing may limit self-care, mobility, safety, independence, communication, and relationships with others.

Anatomy, Physiology, and Functions of the Eyes

The eyes are complex structures, containing 70% of the sensory receptors of the body. Each eye is a sphere measuring about 1 inch (2.5 cm) in diameter, surrounded and protected by a bony orbit and cushions of fat. The primary functions of the eyes are to encode the patterns of light from the environment through photoreceptors and to carry the coded information from the eyes to the brain. The brain gives meaning to the coded information, allowing us to make sense of what we see.

Extraocular Structures

Although the extraocular structures of the eye are outside the eyeball, they are vital to its protection. These structures are the eyebrows, eyelids, eyelashes, conjunctiva, lacrimal apparatus, and extrinsic eye muscles (Figure 45–1 ■).

The eyebrows shade the eyes. The eyelashes, short hairs that project from the top and bottom borders of the eyelids, protect the eye from foreign bodies, regulate the entry of light into the

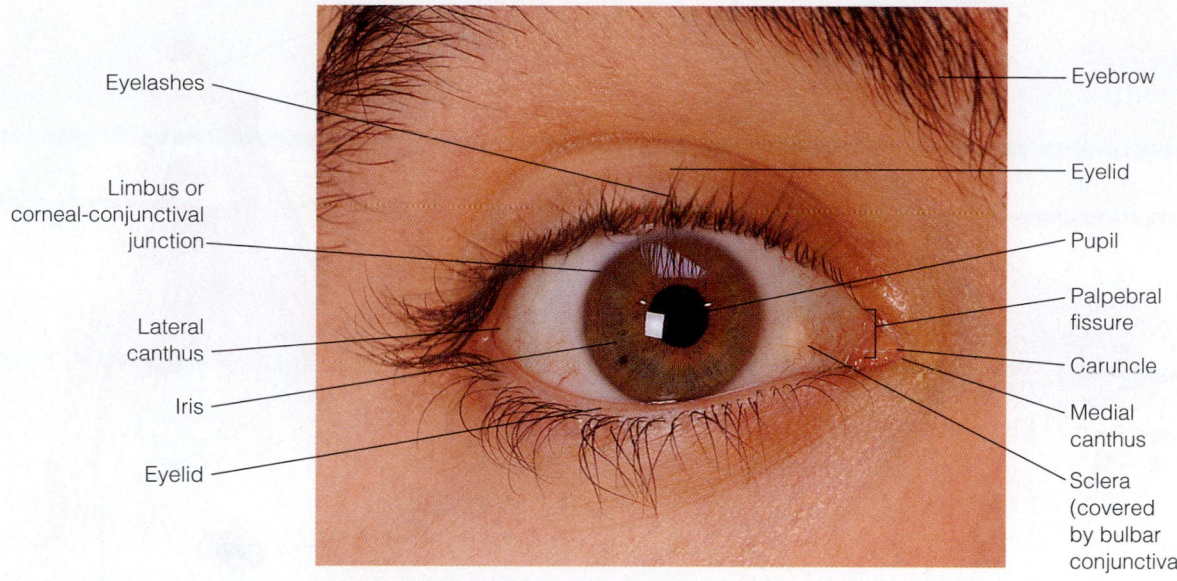

Figure 45–1 ■ Accessory and external structures of the eye.
Source: Todd Buck.

eye, and distribute tears by blinking. An unexpected touch to the eyelashes initiates the blinking reflex to protect the eyes from foreign objects. The conjunctiva is a thin, transparent mucous membrane that lines the inner surfaces of the eyelids and also folds over the anterior surface of the eyeball, lubricating the eyes. The palpebral conjunctiva lines the upper and lower eyelids, whereas the bulbar conjunctiva loosely covers the anterior sclera (the white part of the eye). The lacrimal apparatus is composed of the lacrimal gland, the puncta, the lacrimal sac, and the nasolacrimal duct. Together, these structures secrete, distribute, and drain tears to cleanse and moisten the eye's surface.

The six extrinsic eye muscles control movement of the eye, allowing it to follow a moving object and move precisely. The muscles also help maintain the shape of the eyeball. The cranial nerves control the extrinsic muscles (Figure 45–2 ■).

Intraocular Structures

The intraocular structures transmit visual images and maintain homeostasis of the inner eye. Those in the anterior portion of each eyeball are the sclera and the cornea (forming the outermost coat of the eye, called the fibrous tunic), the iris, the pupil, and the anterior cavity (Figure 45–3 ■).

Sclera and Cornea

The white sclera lines the outside of the eyeball and protects and gives shape to the eyeball. The sclera gives way to the cornea over the iris and pupil. The cornea is transparent, avascular, and sensitive to touch. It forms a window that allows light to enter the eye and is a part of its light-bending apparatus. When the cornea is touched, the eyelids blink (the **corneal reflex**) and tears are secreted.

Iris

The iris is a disc of muscle surrounding the pupil and lying between the cornea and the lens. The iris gives the eye its color and regulates light entry by controlling the size of the pupil. The pupil is the dark center of the eye through which light enters. The pupil constricts when bright light enters the eye and when it is used for near vision; it dilates when light conditions are dim and when the eye is used for far vision. In response to intense light, the pupil constricts rapidly in the **pupillary light reflex**.

Aqueous Fluid

The anterior cavity is made of the anterior chamber (the space between the cornea and the iris) and the posterior chamber (the space between the iris and the lens). The anterior cavity is filled with aqueous humor. Aqueous humor, a clear fluid, is constantly formed and drained to maintain a relatively constant intraocular pressure. The canal of Schlemm, a network of channels that circles the eye in the angle at the junction of the sclera and the cornea, is the drainage system for fluid moving between the anterior and posterior chambers. Aqueous humor provides nutrients and oxygen to the cornea and the lens.

Internal Chamber

The intraocular structures that lie in the internal chamber of the eye are the lens, the posterior cavity and vitreous humor, the ciliary body, the uvea, and the retina.

The lens is a biconvex, avascular, transparent structure located directly behind the pupil. It can change shape to focus and refract light onto the retina. The posterior cavity lies behind the lens. It is filled with a clear gelatinous substance, the vitreous humor, which supports the posterior surface of the lens, maintains the position of the retina, and transmits light. The

Name	Controlling cranial nerve	Action
Lateral rectus	VI (abducens)	Moves eye laterally
Medial rectus	III (oculomotor)	Moves eye medially
Superior rectus	III (oculomotor)	Elevates eye or rolls it superiorly
Inferior rectus	III (oculomotor)	Depresses eye or rolls it inferiorly
Inferior oblique	III (oculomotor)	Elevates eye and turns it laterally
Superior oblique	IV (trochlear)	Depresses eye and turns it laterally

Figure 45–2 ■ Extraocular muscles. *A,* Lateral view of the right eye. *B,* Superior view of the right eye. *C,* Innervation of the extraocular muscles by the cranial nerves.

uvea, also called the vascular tunic, is the middle layer of the eyeball. This pigmented layer has three components: the iris, ciliary body, and choroid. The ciliary body encircles the lens, and along with the iris, regulates the amount of light reaching the retina by controlling the shape of the lens. Most of the uvea is made up of the choroid.

The retina is the innermost lining of the eyeball. It has an outer pigmented layer and an inner neural layer. The outer layer, next to the choroid, serves as the link between visual stimuli and the brain. The transparent inner layer is made up of millions of light receptors in structures called rods and cones. Rods enable vision in dim light as well as peripheral vision. Cones enable vision in bright light and the perception of color. The optic disc, a cream-colored round or oval area within the retina, is the point at which the optic nerve enters the eye. The slight depression in the center of the optic disc is called the physiologic cup. The macula, located laterally to the optic disc, primarily contains cones. The fovea centralis is a slight depression in the center of the macula that contains only cones and is a main receptor of detailed color vision.

The Visual Pathway

The optic nerves are cranial nerves formed of the axons of ganglion cells. The two optic nerves meet at the optic chiasma, just anterior to the pituitary gland in the brain. At the optic chiasma, axons from the medial half of each retina cross to the opposite side to form pairs of axons from each eye. These pairs continue as the left and right optic tracts (Figure 45–4 ■). The crossing of the axons results in each optic tract carrying information from both eyes. The left optic tract carries visual information from the lateral half of the retina of the left eye and the medial half of the retina of the right eye, whereas the right optic tract carries visual information from the lateral half of

Figure 45–3 ■ Internal structures of the eye.

the retina of the right eye and the medial half of the retina of the left eye.

The ganglion cell axons in the optic tracts travel to the thalamus and synapse with neurons, forming pathways called optic radiations. The optic radiations terminate in the visual cortex of the occipital lobe, where the nerve impulses that originated in the retina are interpreted. The visual fields of each eye overlap considerably, and each eye sees a slightly different view. Because of this overlap and the crossing of the axons, information from both eyes reaches each side of the visual cortex, which then fuses the information into one image. This fusion of images accounts for the ability to perceive depth; however, depth perception depends on visual input from two eyes that both focus well.

Refraction

Refraction is the bending of light rays as they pass from one medium to another medium of different optical density. As light rays pass through the eye, they are refracted at several points: as they enter the cornea, as they leave the cornea and enter the aqueous humor, as they enter the lens, and as they leave the lens and enter the vitreous humor. At the lens, the

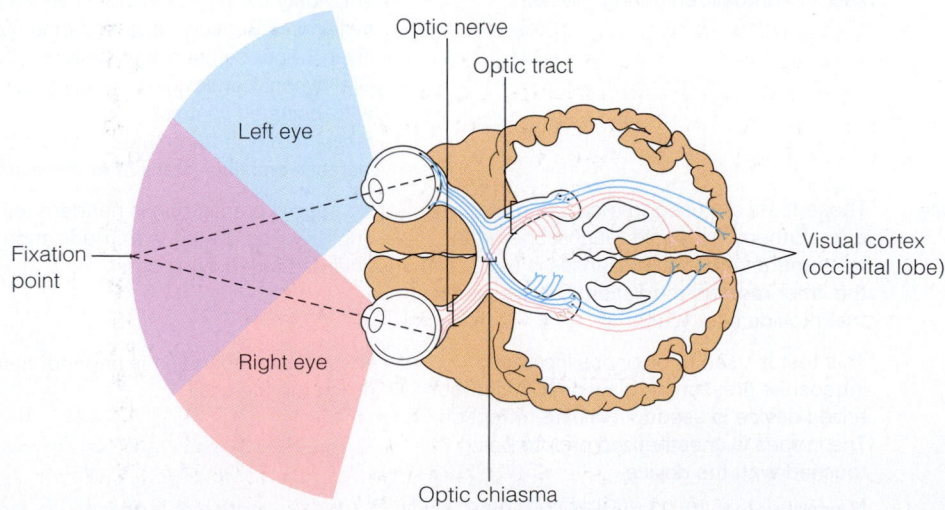

Figure 45–4 ■ The visual fields of the eye and the visual pathways to the brain.

light is bent so that it converges at a single point on the retina. This focusing of the image is called **accommodation**. Because the lens is convex, the image projected onto the retina (the real image) is upside down and reversed from left to right. This real image is coded as electric signals that are sent to the brain. The brain decodes the image so that the person perceives it as it occurs in space.

The eyes are best adapted to see distant objects. Both eyes fix on the same distant image and do not require any change in accommodation. For people with emmetropic (normal) vision, the distance from the viewed object at which the eyes require no accommodation is 20 ft (6 m). This point is called the far point of vision. To focus for near vision, the eyes must instantly contract the ciliary muscles to accommodate the lens, constrict the pupils, and converge the eyeballs. The contraction reduces the tension on the lens capsule so that it bulges outward to increase the curvature. This change in shape also achieves a shorter focal length, another requirement for focusing close images on the retina. The closest point on which a person can focus is called the near point of vision; in young adults with normal vision this is usually 8 to 10 inches (20 to 25 cm). Pupillary constriction helps eliminate most of the divergent light rays and sharpens focus. **Convergence** (the medial rotation of the eyeballs so that each is directed toward the viewed object) allows the focusing of the image on the retinal fovea of each eye.

Assessing the Eyes

Structures and functions of the eyes are assessed by findings from diagnostic tests, a health assessment interview to collect subjective data, and a physical assessment to collect objective data.

GENETIC CONSIDERATIONS
Examples of Eye Disorders

- Glaucoma is a term used for a group of diseases that damage the optic nerve and cause blindness. The diseases are primarily the result of increased intraocular pressure (IOP) on the optic nerve.
- Gyrate atrophy of the choroid and retina is a genetic disorder resulting in progressive vision loss, with total blindness occurring between ages 40 and 60.
- Best disease is a familial disorder found most often in Caucasians who originated in Europe. The disease causes gradual loss of vision, beginning during the teenage years.

Diagnostic Tests

The results of diagnostic tests of the structure and functions of the eyes are used to support the diagnosis of a specific injury, disease, or vision problem; to provide information to identify or modify the appropriate medications or assistive devices used to treat the disease or problem; and to help nurses monitor the patient's responses to treatment and nursing care interventions. Diagnostic tests of the eye, especially for vision testing, are most often conducted in a healthcare provider's office. Diagnostic tests to assess the structure and functions of the eyes are described in the following Diagnostic Tests table on this page. More information is included in the discussion of specific injuries or diseases in ∞ Chapter 46.

Regardless of the type of diagnostic test, the nurse is responsible for explaining the procedure and any special preparation needed, for assessing any medication use that might affect the outcome of the tests, for supporting the patient during the

DIAGNOSTIC TESTS of the Eye

NAME OF TEST	PURPOSE & DESCRIPTION	RELATED NURSING INTERVENTIONS
Computed tomography (CT) scan of the eye	Radiologic examination used to identify foreign objects or tumors within the eyeball or orbit. The head is positioned in a cradle and a wide strap is applied around the head to keep it immobilized during the test.	Tell the patient to remove all hairpins, clips, and earrings before the test. If a contrast dye is used, dentures must also be removed. Assess for allergies to iodine (for example, to shellfish or previous procedures) and if present, notify the physician; medications such as diphenhydramine (Benadryl) and ranitidine (Zantac) may be given 1 hour before the procedure. Assess medications: Oral hypoglycemic agents are contraindicated for use with iodinated contrast. Inform the patient that the test takes from 5 to 10 minutes. Instruct the patient to increase oral fluid intake after the examination.
Refraction, retinoscopy, refractometry	These tests are used to measure refractive error. Either a handheld retinoscope or an instrument with multiple lenses is used; with the latter method the patient chooses lenses that provide best vision.	No special preparation is needed; tell the patient that pupils will be dilated with medication and may be enlarged for several hours.
Tonometry	This test is used to diagnose increased intraocular pressure in glaucoma. A computerized device is used to evaluate refraction. The cornea is anesthetized prior to being touched with the device. Normal value: 10–22 mmHg.	No special preparation is needed. Instruct the patient not to rub the eyes.

FUNCTIONAL HEALTH PATTERN INTERVIEW   The Eye

Functional Health Pattern	Interview Questions and Leading Statements
Health Perception-Health Management	■ Describe your vision. Rate it on a scale of 1 to 10, with 10 being excellent vision. Is it the same in both eyes? If not, which eye is better? ■ Describe your current vision problems. How have these been treated? ■ What eye medications do you use? What type and how often? ■ Have you ever had eye surgery? Describe. ■ Describe the type of corrective lens that you use. Are you satisfied with this appliance? How do you care for it? ■ Describe how you care for your eyes each day. ■ Do you wear sunglasses when you are outside? ■ When was your last eye examination? Have you been tested for glaucoma?
Nutritional-Metabolic	■ Do you have any redness, swelling, watering, or dryness of your eyes?
Activity-Exercise	■ Does your vision problem interfere with your usual activities of daily living? Explain. ■ Do you wear protective goggles when you take part in activities that increase the risk of injury to your eyes (such as at work or when operating machinery at home)?
Sleep-Rest	■ Does your eye problem interfere with your ability to rest or sleep (for example, from pain)? If so, what do you do?
Cognitive-Perceptual	■ Do you have any difficulty focusing on objects? If so, do you have more difficulty with near objects or far objects? ■ Is your vision blurry? Do you see halos around lights? Do you see flashes of light or "floaters"? Do you see double? ■ Do you have pain in or around your eyes? If so, describe its location, intensity, what makes it worse, and how long it lasts. How do you treat it?
Self-Perception-Self-Concept	■ Has this problem with your eyes affected how you feel about yourself?
Role-Relationships	■ How has having this condition affected your relationships with others? ■ Has having this condition interfered with your ability to work? Explain. ■ Has anyone in your family had problems with eye disease? Explain.
Sexuality-Reproductive	■ Has this condition interfered with your usual sexual activity?
Coping-Stress-Tolerance	■ Has having this condition created stress for you? If so, describe. ■ Have you experienced any kind of stress that makes the condition worse? Explain. ■ Describe what you do when you feel stressed.
Value-Belief	■ Describe how specific relationships or activities help you cope with this problem. ■ Describe specific cultural beliefs or practices that affect how you care for and feel about this problem. ■ Is there anything interfering with your spiritual beliefs, needs, or practices during your illness? What can I or another caregiver do to help you with your spiritual needs? ■ Are there any specific treatments that you would not use to treat this problem?

examination as necessary, for ensuring the consent form is signed (if required), and for monitoring the results of the tests. The nurse is also responsible for postprocedure care and patient teaching for self-care at home.

Genetic Considerations

When conducting a health assessment interview and a physical assessment, it is important for the nurse to consider genetic influences on health of the adult. Several diseases of the eyes have a genetic component. During the health assessment interview, ask about a family history of glaucoma or blindness.

During the physical assessment, assess for any manifestations that might indicate a genetic disorder (see the preceding Genetic Considerations box). If data are found to indicate genetic risk factors or alterations, ask about genetic testing and refer for appropriate genetic counseling and evaluation. ∞ Chapter 8 provides further information about genetics in medical-surgical nursing.

Health Assessment Interview

A health assessment interview to determine problems with the eyes may be conducted during a health screening, may focus on a chief complaint (such as blurred vision or an eye infection), or may be part of a total health assessment. If the patient has a health problem involving one or both eyes, analyze its onset, characteristics and course, severity, precipitating and relieving factors, and any associated symptoms, noting the timing and circumstances. For example, you may ask the patient the following:

- Describe the type of pain you experience in your eyes. When did it begin? How long does it last?
- Have you noticed rings of color around streetlights at night?
- When did you first notice having difficulty reading the paper?

Throughout the interview, be alert to nonverbal behaviors (such as squinting or abnormal eye movements) that suggest problems with eye function. Explore problems such as watery, irritated eyes or changes in vision. Assess the patient's use of corrective eyewear and care of eyeglasses or contact lenses. If the patient uses eye medications, ask about the type and purpose as well as the frequency and duration of use. When taking the history, find out about eye trauma, surgery, or infections, as well as the date and results of the last eye examination. In addition, ask the patient about a medical history of diabetes, hypertension, thyroid disorders, glaucoma, cataracts, and eye infections. Include questions about a family history of nearsightedness or

farsightedness, cancer of the retina, color blindness, and any other eye or vision disorders.

Collect information about environmental or work exposure to irritating chemicals, participation in sports or hobbies that pose the risk of eye injury, and the use of protective eyewear during dangerous activities, such as sawing wood or using a grass trimmer.

Interview questions categorized by functional health patterns are listed on page 1561.

Physical Assessment of the Eyes

Physical assessment of the eyes and of visual acuity may be performed as part of a total assessment or separately for patients with known or suspected problems of the eyes. The eyes and vision are primarily assessed through inspection of external structures and assessment of visual fields and visual acuity, extraocular muscle function, and internal structures. Palpation (e.g., of a blocked lacrimal duct) may be used if a problem is identified. Prior to the examination, explain the techniques to the patient to decrease anxiety. The patient may sit or stand during the assessment. Normal age-related findings for the older adult are summarized in the Nursing Care of the Older Adult box.

 Age-Related Changes in the Eye

AGE-RELATED CHANGE	SIGNIFICANCE
The lens: ■ ⬇ elasticity, decreasing focus and accommodation for near vision (presbyopia). ■ ⬆ density and size, making lens more stiff and opaque. ■ Yellowing of the lens and changes in the retina affect color perception.	Most older adults require corrective lenses to accommodate close and detailed work. Increased opacity leads to the development of cataracts. As cataracts develop, they increase sensitivity to glare and interfere with night vision.
The cornea: ■ Fat may be deposited around the periphery and throughout the cornea. ■ ⬇ corneal sensitivity.	A partial or complete white circle may form around the cornea (arcus senilis). Lipid deposits in the cornea cause vision to be blurred. Decreased sensitivity increases the risk of injury to the eye.
The pupil: ■ ⬇ size and responsiveness to light pupil; sphincter hardens.	Increased light perception threshold and difficulty seeing in dim light or at night means increased light is needed to see adequately.
The retina and visual pathways: ■ Visual fields narrow. ■ Photoreceptor cells are lost. ■ Rods work less effectively. ■ Macular degeneration is a risk. ■ Depth perception is distorted. ■ Adaptation to dark and light takes longer.	Peripheral vision is decreased and central vision may be lost from macular degeneration. Increased risk of falls as a result of changes in depth perception and adaptation to changes in light. Vision progressively declines with age.
The lacrimal apparatus: ■ ⬇ reabsorption of intraocular fluid. ■ ⬇ production of tears.	Increased risk of developing glaucoma, and eyes feel and look dry.
The posterior cavity: ■ Debris and condensation become visible. ■ Vitreous body may pull away from the retina.	Vision is blurred and distorted, and "floaters" are often seen by the older person.

Assessing Visual Fields

Visual fields are tested to assess the functioning of the mac-ula and peripheral vision. The visual fields of the examiner (which must be normal to perform this assessment) are used as the standard. To measure visual fields, sit directly opposite the patient at a distance of 18 to 24 inches. Ask the patient to cover one eye with the opaque cover while you cover your own eye opposite to the patient (for example, if the patient covers the right eye, you cover your left eye). Ask the patient to look directly at you. Move the penlight from the periphery toward the center from right to left, above and below, and from the middle of each of these directions. Both you and the patient should see the penlight enter the field of vision at the same time if the examiner has normal peripheral vision. Visual fields may also be tested with an instrument called a perimeter.

The central visual field may be assessed with an Amsler grid (Figure 45–5 ■). The most basic form has black lines on a white grid, forming squares (boxes) that measure 5 mm. There is a black dot in the center of the grid. The Amsler grid is useful for identifying early changes in vision from macular

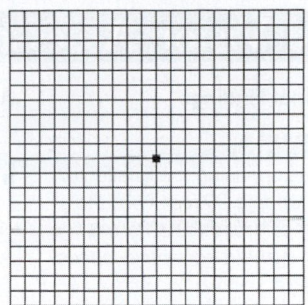

Figure 45–5 ■ The Amsler grid.

degeneration and diabetes mellitus. To use the Amsler grid, ask the patient to hold the grid at normal reading distance (about 12 to 14 inches), cover one eye, and stare at the cen-ter dot. Ask the patient if any of the lines look crooked or bent, if any of the boxes are different in size or shape, and if any of the lines are wavy, missing, blurry, or discolored. Repeat with the other eye. The test should be conducted before the pupils are dilated, and the patient should be wear-ing corrective lenses.

Eye and Vision Assessments

Vision Assessment

Visual acuity is assessed with an eye chart such as the Snellen chart or the E chart for testing distance vision and the Rosenbaum chart for testing near vision. The Snellen chart contains rows of letters in various sizes, with standardized numbers at the end of each row. The number at the end of the row indicates the visual acuity of a patient who can read the row at a distance of 20 feet. (If the patient is unable to read or does not read English, you can use the E chart to test visual acuity.) The top number at the end of the row is always 20, representing the distance between the patient and the chart. The bottom number is the distance (in feet) at which a person with normal vision can read the line. A person with normal vision can read the row marked 20/20. To conduct the assessment,

ask the person to stand 20 feet from the chart in a well-lit area. Ask the patient to cover one eye with an opaque cover (Figure 45–6 ■). Then ask the patient to read each row of let-ters, moving from largest letters to the smallest ones that the patient can see. Measure visual acuity in the other eye in the same way, and then assess visual acuity while the patient has both eyes uncovered. The patient who wears corrective lenses may be tested with and without the lenses.

The Rosenbaum chart is held at a distance of from 12 to 14 inches from the eyes, with visual acuity measured in the same manner as with the Snellen chart (Figure 45–7 ■). A gross estimate of near vision may also be assessed by asking the person to read from a magazine or newspaper.

Figure 45–6 ■ Testing distant vision using the Snellen eye chart.

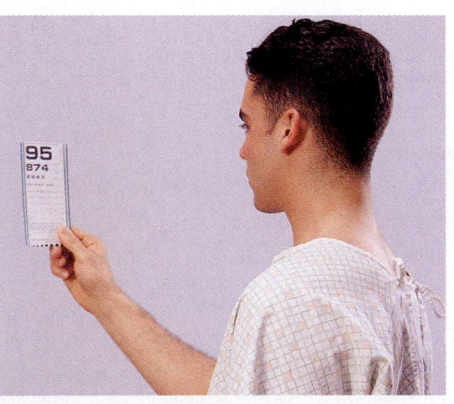

Figure 45–7 ■ Testing near vision using Rosenbaum eye chart.

Eye and Vision Assessments

Technique/Normal Findings	Abnormal Findings

Vision Assessment

Assess distant vision, using the Snellen or E chart. *When standing 20 feet from the chart, the patient can read the smallest line of letters with or without corrective lenses (recorded as 20/20).*

- Changes in distant vision are most commonly the result of **myopia** (nearsightedness). For example, a reading of 20/100 indicates impaired distance vision. A person has to stand 20 feet from the chart to read a line that a person with normal vision could read 100 feet from the chart.

Assess near vision, using a Rosenbaum chart or a card with newsprint held 12 to 14 inches from the patient's eyes. *Normal near visual acuity is 14/14 with or without corrective lenses.*

- Changes in near vision, especially in patients over age 45, can indicate **presbyopia**, impaired near vision resulting from a loss of elasticity of the lens related to aging. In younger patients, this condition is referred to as **hyperopia** (farsightedness).

Eye Movement Assessment

Assess the cardinal fields of vision to gain information about extraocular eye movements. Ask the patient to follow a pen or your finger while keeping the head stationary. Move the pen or your finger through the six fields one at a time, returning to the central starting point before proceeding to the next field (Figure 45–8 ■). *The eyes should move through each field without involuntary movements.*

- Failure of one or both eyes to follow the object in any given direction may indicate extraocular muscle weakness or cranial nerve dysfunction.
- An involuntary rhythmic movement of the eyes, **nystagmus**, is associated with neurologic disorders and the use of some medications.

1 Penlight is to nurse's extreme left. 4 Penlight is to nurse's extreme right.

2 Penlight is left and up. 5 Penlight is right and up.

3 Penlight is left and down. 6 Penlight is right and down.

Figure 45–8 ■ The six cardinal fields of vision.

The cover–uncover test is a test for strabismus, a weakening of a muscle that causes one eye to deviate from the other when the person is focusing on an object. To conduct the test, hold a pen or your finger about 1 foot from the eyes and ask the person to focus on that object. Cover one of the patient's eyes and note any movement in the uncovered eye; as you remove the cover, assess for movement in the eye that was just uncovered. Repeat the procedure with the other eye. *The uncovered eye should remain fixed straight ahead. The covered eye should remain fixed straight ahead after being uncovered.*

Assess convergence. Ask the patient to follow an object as you move it toward the patient's eyes. *Normally both eyes converge toward the center.*

- Failure of the eyes to converge equally on an approaching object may indicate a neuromuscular disorder or improper eye alignment.

Assess the corneal light reflex. Direct a light source onto the bridge of the nose from 12 to 15 inches. *Observe for equal reflection of the light from each eye.*

- Reflections of the light from different sites on the eyes reveal improper alignment.

Pupillary Assessment

Observe pupil size and equality. *Pupils should be of equal size, 3 to 5 mm.*

- Pupils that are unequal in size may indicate a serious neurologic problem, such as increased intracranial pressure.

Assess direct and consensual pupil response. Ask the patient to look straight ahead. Shine a light obliquely into one eye at a time. Observe for constriction of the pupil in the illuminated eye. Test both eyes. To test consensual pupil response, again shine a light obliquely into one eye at a time as the patient looks straight ahead. Observe constriction of the pupil in the opposite eye. *The normal direct and consensual pupillary response is constriction.*

- Failure of the pupils to respond to light may indicate degeneration of the retina or destruction of the optic nerve.
- A patient who has one dilated and unresponsive pupil may have paralysis of the oculomotor nerve.
- Some eye medications may cause unequal dilation, constriction, or inequality of pupil size. Morphine and narcotic drugs may cause small, unresponsive pupils, and anticholinergic drugs such as atropine may cause dilated, unresponsive pupils.

Technique/Normal Findings	Abnormal Findings
Test for accommodation. Hold an object at a distance of a few feet from the patient. The pupils should dilate. Ask the patient to follow the object as you bring it to within a few inches of his or her nose. *The pupils should constrict and converge as they change focus to follow the object.*	■ Failure of accommodation along with lack of pupil response to light may signal a neurologic problem. ■ Lack of response to light with appropriate response to accommodation is often seen in patients with diabetes.

External Eye Assessment

Inspect the eyelids. *Eyelids should be the color of the patient's facial skin, without redness, discharge, or drooping. The sclera should not be visible.*	■ Unusual redness or discharge may indicate an inflammatory state due to trauma, allergies, or infection. ■ Drooping of one eyelid, called **ptosis**, may be the result of a stroke, indicate a neuromuscular disorder, or be congenital (Figure 45–9 ■). ■ Unusual widening of the lids may be due to exophthalmos (protrusion of the eyeball). Exophthalmos is often associated with hyperthyroid conditions. ■ Yellow plaques noted on or near the lid margins are referred to as xanthelasma and may indicate high lipid levels. ■ An acute localized inflammation of a hair follicle is known as a hordeolum (sty) and is generally caused by staphylococcal organisms. ■ A chalazion is an infection or retention cyst of the meibomian glands.

Figure 45–9 ■ Ptosis.
Source: Leonard Lessen/Peter Arnold, Inc.
Source: Custom Medical Stock Photo, Inc.

Inspect the puncta. *The puncta should be free of redness or discharge.*	■ Unusual redness or discharge from the puncta may indicate an inflammation due to trauma, infection, or allergies.
Inspect the bulbar and palpebral conjunctiva. *The conjunctiva should be clear, moist, and smooth. The upper and lower palpebral conjunctiva should be clear, without redness or swelling.*	■ Increased erythema or the presence of exudate may indicate acute conjunctivitis. ■ A cobblestone appearance is often associated with allergies. ■ A fold in the conjunctiva, called a pterygium, may be seen as a clouded area that extends over the cornea. This is an abnormal growth of the bulbar conjunctiva, usually seen on the nasal side of the cornea. It may interfere with vision if it covers the pupil.
Inspect the sclera. *The sclera is white in people of European descent; people with darker skin normally have yellow sclera.*	■ Unusual redness may indicate an inflammatory state as a result of trauma, allergies, or infection. ■ Yellow discoloration of the sclera in patients with fair skin may be seen in conditions involving the liver, such as hepatitis. ■ Bright red areas in the sclera are often subconjunctival hemorrhages and may indicate trauma or bleeding disorders. They may also occur spontaneously.
Inspect the cornea. *The cornea is normally transparent.*	■ Dullness, opacities, or irregularities of the cornea may be abnormal. ■ Corneal arcus is a thin, grayish-white arc seen toward the edge of the cornea. It is normal in older adults.
Assess corneal sensitivity. Lightly touch a wisp of cotton to the patient's cornea. *This action should cause a corneal reflex (blinking the eye).*	■ Failure of the corneal reflex may indicate a neurologic disorder.
Inspect the iris. *The iris is normally round, flat, and evenly colored.*	■ Lack of clarity of the iris may indicate a cloudiness of the cornea. ■ Constriction of the pupil accompanied by pain and circumcorneal redness indicates acute iritis.

Internal Eye Assessment

Assess internal structures of the eye by using the ophthalmoscope, an instrument that allows visualization of the lens, the vitreous humor, and the retina. Box 45–1 provides guidelines for using the ophthalmoscope.

BOX 45–1 Guidelines for Using the Ophthalmoscope

The ophthalmoscope has a head and a handle (see the figure below). The head contains a focus wheel (also called a lens selector dial) located on the side, lenses of varying magnification, and an opening through which the eye structures are visualized. The focus wheel adjusts the lens refraction, which is measured in diopters. The diopter measurements range from 0 to +40 when the lens is rotated clockwise, and from 0 to –25 when the lens is rotated counterclockwise. By moving the focus wheel, the examiner can converge or diverge light rays to visualize the retina. The handle usually contains batteries that can be recharged. *Note:* Assessing the internal eye with the ophthalmoscope is a skill that takes practice.

Before the examination, explain the procedure to the patient. Assemble the ophthalmoscope. Wash your hands and wear disposable gloves if the patient has any drainage from the eyes. Darken the room (to allow the pupils of the patient to dilate) and ask the patient to look straight ahead, focusing on a fixed point such as an object on the wall. Hold the ophthalmoscope in one hand, resting the index finger on the focus wheel (see the figure at right).

1. Turn on the ophthalmoscope light, and set the focus wheel to 0 diopters. Hold the ophthalmoscope in your right hand with your index finger on the focus wheel. Standing in front of the patient, position yourself at a 15-degree angle to the patient's line of vision.
2. Hold the opening of the ophthalmoscope up to your right eye and direct the light toward the patient's right eye from a distance of about 12 inches.
3. As the beam of light falls on the patient's pupil, observe for the red reflex, which appears as a sharply outlined orange glow from within the pupil. This glow is the reflection of the light from the retina.
4. Move closer to the patient, turning the focus wheel clockwise toward the positive numbers as needed to maintain clear focus.
5. Examine the lens and the vitreous body, both of which should be clear.
6. Gradually rotate the focus wheel counterclockwise toward the negative numbers as needed, focusing on a structure of the retina (such as the disc or a blood vessel). Turn the focus wheel until the image is clear. Examine the structures of the retina as follows:
   a. The optic disc (see the accompanying figure). Assess for size, shape, color, distinct margins, and the physiologic cup. The disc is round to slightly oval and about 1.5 mm in diameter. It has a yellow to pink color that is lighter than the retina itself. The margins should be sharp and clear. The physiologic cup is a small depression that occupies about one-third of the optic disc, lying temporal to the center of the disc.
   b. The vessels of the retina. Assess for color, arteriolar light reflex, ratio of arterioles to veins, and arteriovenous crossings. The arterioles are red, brighter than

Technique for holding an opthalmoscope.

the veins, and about one-fourth smaller. The arterioles normally have a narrow light reflex from the center of each vessel; veins do not have this light reflex. The ratio of arterioles to veins is usually 2:3 or 4:5. The vessels normally cross and become smaller toward the periphery.
   c. The retinal background. Assess color and changes in color. The retina is normally reddish orange and regular in color.
   d. The macula. Assess size and color. To assess the macula, ask the patient to look directly into the ophthalmoscope light. The macula is temporal to the optic disc, appears slightly darker than the retina, and has no visible vessels. The fovea centralis may be seen as a bright spot of light. Because looking directly into the light causes some discomfort, conduct this portion of the examination last. The macula is often difficult to visualize.
7. Using the same technique, examine the left eye.

An ophthalmoscope.

Blood vessels

Optic disc

Macula

Fovea centralis

The optic disc.

Technique/Normal Findings	Abnormal Findings
Inspect for the red reflex. *The red reflex should be clearly visible.*	■ Absence of a red reflex often indicates improper position of the ophthalmoscope, but also may indicate total opacity of the pupil by a cataract or a hemorrhage into the vitreous humor.
Inspect the lens and vitreous body. *The lens should be clear.*	■ A cataract is an opacity of the lens, often seen as a dark shadow on ophthalmoscopic examination. It may be due to aging, trauma, diabetes, or a congenital defect.
Inspect the retina. *There should be no visible hemorrhages, exudate, or white patches.*	■ Areas of hemorrhage, exudate, and white patches may be a result of diabetes or long-standing hypertension.
Inspect the optic disc. *The optic disc should be round to oval in shape with clear, well-defined borders.*	■ Loss of definition of the optic disc, as well as an increase in the size of the physiologic cup, is seen in papilledema from increased intracranial pressure.
Inspect the blood vessels of the retina. *The retinal blood vessels should be distinct.*	■ Glaucoma often results in displacement of blood vessels from the center of the optic disc due to increased intraocular pressure. ■ Hypertension may cause a narrowing of the vein where an arteriole crosses over. ■ Engorged veins may occur with diabetes, atherosclerosis, and blood disorders.
Inspect the retinal background. *The retina should be a consistent red-orange color, becoming lighter around the optic disc.*	■ Variations in color or a pale color overall may indicate disease. ■ Absence of the fovea centralis is common in older patients. It may indicate macular degeneration, a cause of loss of central vision.
Inspect the macula. *The macula should be visible on the temporal side of the optic disc.*	
Palpate over the lacrimal glands, puncta, and nasolacrimal duct. (Wear gloves if you see any drainage.) *There should be no tenderness, drainage, or excessive tearing.*	■ Tenderness over any of these areas or drainage from the puncta may indicate an infectious process. ■ Excessive tearing may indicate a blockage of the nasolacrimal duct.

Anatomy, Physiology, and Functions of the Ears

As a sensory organ, the ears have two primary functions: hearing and maintaining equilibrium. Anatomically, each ear is divided into three areas: the external ear, the middle ear, and the inner ear (Figure 45–10 ■). All three are involved in hearing, but only the inner ear is involved in equilibrium.

The External Ear

The external ear consists of the auricle (or pinna), the external auditory canal, and the tympanic membrane. The auricles contain sebaceous and sweat glands and sometimes hair. Each auricle has a rim (the helix) and a lobe. The auricle serves to direct sound waves into the ear. The external auditory canal, which is about 1 inch (2.5 cm) long, extends from the auricle to the tympanic membrane. The canal is lined with skin that contains hair, sebaceous glands, and ceruminous glands. The external auditory canal serves as a resonator for the range of sound waves typical of human speech and increases the pressure that sound waves in this frequency range place on the tympanic membrane. The canal's ceruminous glands secrete a yellow to brown waxy substance called **cerumen**. Cerumen traps foreign bodies; it also has bacteriostatic properties, protecting the tympanic membrane and the middle ear from infections. The tympanic membrane lies between the external ear and the middle ear. It is a thin, semitransparent, fibrous structure covered with skin on the external side and mucosa on the inner side. The

membrane vibrates as sound waves strike it; these vibrations are transferred as sound waves to the middle ear.

The Middle Ear

The middle ear is an air-filled cavity in the temporal bone. The middle ear contains three auditory ossicles: the malleus, the incus, and the stapes. These bones extend across the middle ear to the tympanic membrane. The medial side of the middle ear is a bony wall containing two membrane-covered openings: the oval window and the round window. The posterior wall of the middle ear contains the mastoid antrum. This cavity communicates with the mastoid sinuses, which help the middle ear adjust to changes in pressure. It also opens into the eustachian tube, which connects with the nasopharynx. The eustachian tube helps to equalize the air pressure in the middle ear by opening briefly in response to differences between middle ear pressure and atmospheric pressure. The mucous membrane lining the middle ear is continuous with the mucous membranes lining the throat.

The malleus attaches to the tympanic membrane and articulates with the incus, which in turn articulates with the stapes. The stapes fits into the oval window. When the tympanic membrane vibrates, the vibrations are conducted across the middle ear to the oval window by the ossicles. The vibrations then set in motion the fluids of the inner ear, which in turn stimulate the

Figure 45–10 ■ Structures of the external ear, middle ear, and inner ear.

Source: Todd Buck.

hearing receptors. Two small muscles attached to the ossicles contract reflexively in response to sudden loud noises, decreasing the vibrations and protecting the inner ear.

The Inner Ear

The inner ear, also called the labyrinth, is a maze of bony chambers located deep within the temporal bone, just behind the eye socket. The labyrinth is further divided into two parts: the bony labyrinth, a system of open channels that houses the second part, the membranous labyrinth. The bony labyrinth is filled with a fluid called perilymph, which bathes the membranous labyrinth. Within the chambers of the membranous labyrinth is a fluid called endolymph.

The bony labyrinth has three regions: the vestibule, the semicircular canals, and the cochlea. The vestibule is the central portion of the inner ear, one side of which is a bony wall containing the oval window. Two sacs within the vestibule (the saccule and the utricle) join the vestibule with the cochlea and the semicircular canals. The saccule and the utricle contain receptors for equilibrium that respond to changes in gravity and changes in position of the head. The three semicircular canals each project into a different plane (anterior, posterior, and lateral). Each canal contains a semicircular duct that communicates with the utricle of the vestibule. Each duct has an enlarged area at one end containing an equilibrium receptor that responds to angular movements of the head.

The cochlea is a tiny bony chamber that houses the organ of Corti, the receptor organ for hearing. The organ of Corti is a series of sensory hair cells, arranged in a single row of inner hair cells and three rows of outer hair cells. The hair cells are innervated by sensory fibers from cranial nerve VIII. The organ of Corti is supported in the cochlea by the flexible basilar membrane, which has fibers of varying lengths that respond to different sound wave frequencies.

Sound Conduction

Hearing is the perception and interpretation of sound. Sound is produced when the molecules of a medium are compressed, resulting in a pressure disturbance evidenced as a sound wave. The intensity or loudness of sound is determined by the amplitude (height) of the sound wave, with greater amplitudes causing louder sounds. The frequency of the sound wave in vibrations per second determines the pitch or tone of the sound, with higher frequencies resulting in higher sounds. The human ear is most sensitive to sound waves with frequencies between 1000 and 4000 cycles per second, but can detect sound waves with frequencies between 20 and 20,000 cycles per second.

Sound waves enter the external auditory canal and cause the tympanic membrane to vibrate at the same frequency. The ossicles not only transmit the motion of the tympanic membrane to the oval window but also amplify the energy of the sound wave. As the stapes moves against the oval window, the perilymph in the vestibule is set in motion. The increased pressure of the perilymph is transmitted to fibers of the basilar membrane and then to the organ of Corti. The up-and-down movements of the fibers of the basilar membrane pull the hair cells in the organ of Corti, which in turn generates action potentials that are transmitted to cranial nerve VIII and then to the brain for interpretation.

Several brainstem auditory nuclei transmit impulses to the cerebral cortex. Fibers from each ear cross, with each auditory cortex receiving impulses from both ears. Auditory processing is so finely tuned that a wide variety of sounds of different pitch and loudness can be heard at any one time. In addition, the source of the sound can be localized.

Equilibrium

The inner ear also provides information about the position of the head. This information is used to coordinate body movements so that equilibrium and balance are maintained. The types of equilibrium are static balance (affected by changes in the position of the head) and dynamic balance (affected by the movement of the head).

Receptors called maculae in the vestibule detect changes in the position of the head. Maculae are groups of hair cells that have protrusions covered with a gelatinous substance. Embedded in this gelatinous substance are tiny particles of calcium carbonate called otoliths (ear stones), which make the gelatin heavier than the endolymph that fills the membranous labyrinth. As a result, when the head is in the upright position, gravity causes the gelatinous substance to bear down on the hair cells. When the position of the head changes, the force on the hair cells also changes, bending them and altering the pattern of stimulation of the neurons. Thus, a different pattern of nerve impulses is transmitted to the brain, where stimulation of the motor centers initiates actions that coordinate various body movements according to the position of the head.

The receptor for dynamic equilibrium is in the crista, a crest in the membrane lining the ampulla of each semicircular canal. The cristae are stimulated by rotatory head movement (acceleration and deceleration) as a result of changes in the flow of endolymph and of movement of hair cells in the maculae. The direction of endolymph and hair cell movement is always opposite to the motion of the body.

Assessing the Ears

The structure and functions of the ears are assessed by findings from diagnostic tests, a health assessment interview to collect subjective data, and a physical assessment to collect objective data.

Diagnostic Tests

The results of diagnostic tests of the structure and functions of the ears are used to support the diagnosis of a specific injury, disease, or hearing problem; to provide information to identify or modify the appropriate medications or assistive devices used to treat the disease or problem; and to help nurses monitor the patient's responses to treatment and nursing care interventions. Diagnostic tests of the ear, especially for hearing, are most often conducted in a healthcare provider's office. Diagnostic

DIAGNOSTIC TESTS of Ear Disorders

NAME OF TEST	PURPOSE & DESCRIPTION	RELATED NURSING INTERVENTIONS
Audiometry	Audiometry is used to evaluate and diagnose conductive and sensorineural hearing loss. Patient sits in soundproof room and responds by raising a hand when sounds are heard.	No special preparation is needed.
Auditory evoked potential (AEP)	This test is used to identify electrical activity of the auditory nerve. Electrodes are placed on various areas of the ear and on the forehead and a graphic recording is made.	No special preparation is needed.
Auditory brainstem response (ABR)	An ABR measures the electrical activity of the auditory pathway from inner ear to brain to diagnose brainstem pathology, stroke, and acoustic neuroma.	No special preparation is needed.
Caloric test	A caloric test is used to assess vestibular system function. Cold or warm water is used to irrigate the ear canals one at a time and the patient is observed for nystagmus (repeated abnormal movements of the eyes). Normally, the nystagmus occurs opposite to the ear being irrigated. If no nystagmus occurs, the patient needs further testing for brain lesions.	Assess patient for use of alcohol, central nervous system depressants, and barbiturates. These chemicals may alter the test results.

tests to assess the structure and functions of the ears are described in the Diagnostic Tests table. More information is included in the discussion of specific injuries or diseases in ∞ Chapter 46.

Regardless of the type of diagnostic test, the nurse is responsible for explaining the procedure and any special preparation needed, for assessing for any medication use that might affect the outcome of the tests, for supporting the patient during the examination as necessary, for ensuring the consent form is signed (if necessary), for documenting the procedures as appropriate, and for monitoring the results of the tests.

Genetic Considerations

When conducting a health assessment interview and a physical assessment, it is important for the nurse to consider genetic influences on health of the adult. Several diseases of the ears have a genetic component. During the health assessment interview, ask about a family history of congenital deafness, deafness associated with a thyroid goiter, or tumors of the auditory nerve.

During the physical assessment, assess for any manifestations that might indicate a genetic disorder (see the accompanying Genetic Considerations box on this page). If data are found to indicate genetic risk factors or alterations, ask about genetic testing and refer for appropriate genetic counseling and evaluation. ∞ Chapter 8 provides further information about genetics in medical-surgical nursing.

Health Assessment Interview

The health history assessment to collect subjective data about the ears and hearing may be part of a health screening, may focus on a chief complaint (such as hearing problems or pain in the ear), or may be part of a total health assessment. If the patient has a problem involving one or both ears, analyze its onset, characteristics and course, severity, precipitating and relieving factors, and any associated symptoms, noting the timing and circumstances. For example, you may ask the following questions:

- Have you noticed any difficulty hearing high-pitched sounds, low-pitched sounds, or both?
- When did you first notice the ringing in your ears?
- Is your workplace very noisy? If so, do you wear protective ear equipment at work?

Throughout the examination, be alert to nonverbal behaviors (such as inappropriate answers or requests to repeat statements) that suggest problems with ear function. Explore changes in hearing, ringing in the ears (tinnitus), ear pain, drainage from the ears, or the use of hearing aids. When taking the history, ask about trauma, surgery, or infections of the ear as well as the date of the last ear examination. In addition, ask the patient about a medical history of infectious diseases, such as meningitis or mumps, as well as the use of medications that may affect hearing. Because ear problems tend to run in families, ask about a family history of hearing loss, ear problems, or diseases that could result in such problems. If the patient has a hearing aid, ascertain the type and assess measures for its care.

 Age-Related Changes in the Ear

AGE-RELATED CHANGE	SIGNIFICANCE
The inner ear:	
- Loss of hair cells, �](blood supply, less flexible basilar membrane, degeneration of spiral ganglion cells, and ➤production of endolymph result in progressive hearing loss with age (presbycusis). - High-frequency sounds are lost; middle and low-frequency sounds may also be lost or decreased. - Vestibular structures degenerate, organ of Corti and cochlea atrophy.	Older adults may require hearing aids to hear well. With loss of high frequency sounds, speech may be distorted, contributing to a risk for problems with communication. Degeneration and atrophy of inner ear structures concerned with balance and equilibrium increase the risk for falls.
The middle ear:	
- Muscles and ligaments weaken and stiffen, decreasing the acoustic reflex.	Sounds made from one's own body and speech are louder and may further interfere with hearing, speech, and communications.
The external ear:	
- Cerumen has a higher keratin content, contributing to increased cerumen in the ear canal.	Accumulated cerumen may impair hearing.

FUNCTIONAL HEALTH PATTERN INTERVIEW   The Ear

Functional Health Pattern	Interview Questions and Leading Statements
Health Perception-Health Management	■ Describe your hearing. Rate it on a scale of 1 to 10, with 10 being excellent hearing. Is it the same in both ears? If not, which ear is better? ■ Describe your current hearing problems. How have these been treated? ■ Do you use ear medications? What type and how often? ■ Have you ever had ear surgery? Describe. ■ Describe the type of hearing aid that you use. Are you satisfied with this appliance? How do you care for it? ■ Describe how you care for your ears each day. ■ When was your last ear examination? Have you ever had your hearing tested? ■ Do you listen to loud music? Do you use ear phones when you listen to loud music?
Nutritional-Metabolic	■ Do you have any swelling or tenderness in the ears or drainage from the ears?
Activity-Exercise	■ Does your hearing problem interfere with your usual activities of daily living? Explain. ■ Do you wear protective earplugs when you take part in activities that increase the risk of injury to your ears (such as at work or when operating machinery at home)?
Sleep-Rest	■ Does your ear problem interfere with your ability to rest or sleep (for example, from pain)? If so, what do you do?
Cognitive-Perceptual	■ Do you have pain in or around your ears? Have you ever had ringing in your ears? If so, describe its location, intensity, what makes it worse, and how long it lasts. How do you treat it? ■ Do you have difficulty hearing conversations, either in person or on the telephone? Do you have trouble hearing the television? Do you have difficulty hearing when you are in crowds or there is background noise? ■ Have you noticed your hearing is different in each ear? ■ Do you have buzzing, ringing, or crackling noises in one or both ears? Explain. ■ Do you ever feel dizzy?
Self-Perception-Self-Concept	■ Has this problem with your ears affected how you feel about yourself?
Role-Relationships	■ How has having this condition affected your relationships with others? ■ Has having this condition interfered with your ability to work? Explain. ■ Has anyone in your family had problems with ear disease? Explain.
Sexuality-Reproductive	■ Has this condition interfered with your usual sexual activity?
Coping-Stress-Tolerance	■ Has having this condition created stress for you? Describe if so. ■ Have you experienced any kind of stress that makes the condition worse? Explain. ■ Describe what you do when you feel stressed.
Value-Belief	■ Describe how specific relationships or activities help you cope with this problem. ■ Describe specific cultural beliefs or practices that affect how you care for and feel about this problem. ■ Is there anything interfering with your spiritual beliefs, needs, or practices during your illness? What can I or another caregiver do to help you with your spiritual needs? ■ Are there any specific treatments that you would not use to treat this problem?

Interview questions categorized by functional health patterns are found in the Functional Health Pattern table.

Physical Assessment of the Ears and Hearing

Physical assessment of the ears and hearing may be performed as part of a total health assessment or separately for patients with known or suspected problems with the ears. The ears and hearing are assessed primarily through inspection of external structures, the external auditory canal, and the tympanic membrane. Disorders of the middle ear may be identified with tympanometry. Hearing acuity is assessed by voice tests and tuning fork tests. The external structures may be palpated. Normal age-related findings for the older adult are summarized in the Nursing Care of the Older Adult box.

The patient should be sitting, and the examiner's head should be level with the head of the patient. Prior to the assessment, collect all necessary equipment and explain the techniques to the patient to decrease anxiety. The auditory canal and tympanic membrane are inspected with the otoscope. Guidelines for use of the otoscope are listed in Box 45–2.

BOX 45–2 Guidelines for Using the Otoscope

The otoscope has a handle that contains batteries for the light and various specula that fit onto the handle (see the accompanying figure). This instrument is used to inspect the auditory canal and the tympanic membrane.

Before the examination, explain the procedure to the patient. Assemble the otoscope, using the largest speculum that will fit into the patient's auditory canal without discomfort. Wash your hands; wear disposable gloves if the patient has any drainage from the ears. Turn on the otoscope light. Ask the patient to tip the head slightly toward the shoulder opposite the ear being examined. When the patient is in this position, the auditory canal is aligned with the speculum.

1. Hold the handle of the otoscope in your dominant hand. If the patient is restless, hold the otoscope handle upward, resting the hand against the patient's head. If the patient is cooperative, hold the handle downward.
2. For adult patients, grasp the superior portion of the auricle and pull up, out, and back to straighten the auditory canal (see the accompanying figure).
3. Insert the speculum into the ear and advance it gently. Assess the walls of the auditory canal while advancing the speculum, inspecting for color, obstructions, hair growth, and cerumen. Old cerumen is very dark and may obstruct visualization of part or all of the tympanic membrane.
4. Move the otoscope so that you can see the tympanic membrane. You may need to realign the auditory canal by gently continuing to pull up and back on the auricle. A normal membrane is semitransparent, allowing visualization of a portion of the auditory ossicles. The concave nature of the tympanic membrane and its oblique position in the auditory canal account for the triangular light reflex (cone of light) seen on otoscopic examination.
5. Note the color and surface of the membrane. The normal tympanic membrane is pearly gray, shiny, and semitransparent. The surface should be continuous, intact, and either flat or concave.
6. Identify the landmarks on the tympanic membrane (see the accompanying figure):
   a. The cone of light, located over the anteroinferior quadrant
   b. The malleus, pars tensa, annulus, pars flaccida, and malleolar folds
7. Assess movement of the tympanic membrane. If the auditory tube is patent, the membrane moves in and out when air is injected (or when the patient performs the Valsalva maneuver).

8. Gently withdraw the speculum. If the speculum is soiled with drainage or cerumen, use a clean speculum for the other ear.
9. Using the same technique, examine the other ear.

Technique for using an otoscope.

Structures of the tympanic membrane visible through otoscope.

An otoscope.

Ear and Hearing Assessments

Hearing Assessment

Tuning forks are used to determine whether a hearing loss is conductive or perceptive (sensorineural). Hold the tuning fork at the base and make it ring softly by stroking the prongs or by lightly tapping them on the heel of the opposite hand. The vibrating tuning fork emits sound waves of a particular frequency, measured in hertz (Hz). Tuning forks with a frequency of 512 to 1024 Hz are preferred for auditory evaluation, because that range corresponds to the range of normal speech.

Technique/Normal Findings	Abnormal Findings
Perform the Weber test. Place the base of a vibrating tuning fork on the midline vertex of the patient's head (Figure 45–11 ■). Ask whether the patient hears the sound equally in both ears or better in one than the other. *Sound is normally heard equally in both ears.*	■ Sound heard in, or lateralized to, one ear indicates either a conductive loss in that ear or a sensorineural loss in the other ear. The sound will be louder on the impaired side with a conductive hearing loss. The sound will be softer on the impaired side with a sensorineural hearing loss. Conductive losses may be due to a buildup of cerumen, an infection such as otitis media, or perforation of the eardrum.

Figure 45–11 ■ Performing the Weber test with a tuning fork.

Perform the Rinne test. Place the base of a vibrating tuning fork on the patient's mastoid bone. Ask the patient to indicate when the sound is no longer heard. When the patient does so, quickly reposition the tuning fork in front of the patient's ear close to the ear canal. Ask whether the patient can hear the sound. If the patient says yes, ask the patient to indicate when the sound is no longer heard. Repeat over the opposite mastoid bone (Figure 45–12 ■). *The patient with no conductive hearing loss will hear the sound twice as long by air conduction as by bone conduction.*	■ Bone conduction is greater than air conduction in the ear with a conductive loss. The normal pattern is AC > BC (air conduction greater than bone conduction).

Figure 45–12 ■ Performing the Rinne test with a tuning fork.

Perform the whisper test. Ask the patient to occlude one ear with a finger. Stand 1 to 2 feet away from the patient, on the side of the unoccluded ear. Softly whisper numbers and ask the patient to repeat them. Repeat the procedure, having the patient occlude the other ear. Note whether you need to raise your voice or to stand closer to make the patient hear you. *The patient with no hearing loss will hear your whispered voice.*	■ This test provides a rough estimate of hearing loss.

Technique/Normal Findings	Abnormal Findings

A tympanogram may be used to measure the pressure of the middle ear and observe the tympanic membrane's response to waves of pressure. Insert the device into the ear canal. Ask the patient not to speak, move, swallow, or jump when hearing a sound. Tell the patient he or she will hear a loud tone as the measurements are taken. Repeat for the other ear. *The normal pressure inside the middle ear is a 100 daPa (a very small amount).*

■ Abnormal findings may include fluid in the middle ear, a perforated eardrum, impacted earwax, or a tumor of the middle ear.

External Ear Assessment

Inspect the auricle. *External ears are normally bilaterally equal in size, of equal color with the patient's face, and without redness or lesions.*

■ Unusual redness or drainage may indicate an inflammatory response to infection or trauma.
■ Scales or skin lesions around the rim of the auricle may indicate skin cancer.
■ Small, raised lesions on the rim of the ear are known as tophi and indicate gout.

Inspect the external auditory canal with the otoscope. *Canal walls should be pink and smooth without lesions.* People with darker skin tend to have darker cerumen. *Cerumen is normally present in small, odorless amounts.*

■ Unusual redness, lesions, or purulent drainage may indicate an infection.
■ Cerumen varies in color and texture, but hardened, dry, or foul-smelling cerumen may indicate an infection or an impaction of cerumen that requires removal.

Inspect the tympanic membrane. *The tympanic membrane should be pearly gray, shiny, and translucent without bulging or retraction.*

■ White, opaque areas on the tympanic membrane are often scars from previous perforations (Figure 45–13 ■).
■ Inconsistent texture and color may be due to scarring from previous perforations caused by infection, allergies, or trauma.
■ Bulging membranes are indicated by a loss of bony landmarks and a distorted light reflex. Such bulges may be the result of otitis media or malfunctioning auditory tubes.

Figure 45–13 ■ Scarring of the tympanic membrane.
Source: Professor Tony Wright, Institute of Laryngology and Otology/SPL/Photo Researchers, Inc.

■ Retracted tympanic membranes are indicated by accentuated bony landmarks and a distorted light reflex. Such retraction is often due to an obstructed auditory tube.

Palpate the auricles and over each mastoid process. *There should be no pain or swelling on palpation.*

■ Tenderness, swelling, or nodules may indicate inflammation of the external auditory canal or mastoiditis.

SAMPLE DOCUMENTATION

Assessment of the Ear

22-year-old male with complaints of "having some problems hearing these days." States he often listens to music in his car "as loud as it will go" and uses ear phones at home so he does not bother other family members. Ears are normally placed bilaterally; skin smooth without lesions. Small amount of dark brown cerumen present in ear canals. Tympanic membranes gray and shiny. No bulging or retraction noted. Whisper test: Unable to repeat back words spoken by examiner. Weber's test: Sound lateralized to left ear. Rinne test: BC ≥ AC. No tenderness noted when mastoids palpated. Referred to ear clinic for further evaluation.

TEST YOURSELF NCLEX-RN® REVIEW

1. During an eye assessment, a nurse touches the part of the eye covering the iris and pupil. What normal patient response would be expected?
   1. excess tearing
   2. blinking of eyelids
   3. bilateral nystagmus
   4. pupil dilates

2. The nurse is conducting a health history. Which of the following statements would indicate a patient has presbyopia?
   1. "I just am having so much trouble hearing music."
   2. "I can't seem to remember anything these days."
   3. "I think I have a lot of earwax in my ears."
   4. "My arms just don't seem long enough to read."

3. What equipment would the nurse use to test sound conduction during an assessment of the ear?
   1. ophthalmoscope
   2. tuning fork
   3. otoscope
   4. penlight

4. What physiologic process occurs when light enters the lens of the eye?
   1. accommodation
   2. convergence
   3. pupillary reflex
   4. hyperopia

5. What would the nurse tell or ask a patient before a test of refraction is done?
   1. "This test is uncomfortable, but it doesn't take long."
   2. "You will be blindfolded during the test."
   3. "Are you allergic to seafood?"
   4. "Your pupils will be dilated for several hours."

6. What function, in addition to hearing, is provided by the inner ear?
   1. coordinates visual pathways
   2. integrates efferent neuron messages
   3. provides information about head position
   4. maintains middle ear structure and function

7. Why would a nurse use the Snellen eye chart during vision assessment?
   1. to test distant vision
   2. to test near vision
   3. to determine visual fields
   4. to examine convergence

8. Of the following ear assessments, which one is a rough estimate of the ability to hear?
   1. whisper test
   2. Rinne test
   3. Weber test
   4. audiometry

9. What is a high-priority risk for the older adult with age-related changes in the vestibular structures of the ear?
   1. infection
   2. falls
   3. medication errors
   4. food intolerance

10. Which criterion is important to accurately assess visual fields?
    1. Patient must wear corrective lenses.
    2. Patient must have no less than 20/30 vision.
    3. Examiner must not wear glasses.
    4. Examiner must have normal visual field.

See Test Yourself answers in Appendix C.

Pearson Nursing Student Resources

Find additional review materials at
www.nursing.pearsonhighered.com
Prepare for success with additional NCLEX®-style practice questions, interactive assignments and activities, Web links, animations and videos, and more!

BIBLIOGRAPHY

Armstrong, J., & Mitchell, E. (2008). Comprehensive nursing assessment in the care of older people. *Nursing Older People, (20)*1, 36–40.

Bickley, L., & Szilagyi, P. (2007). *Bates' guide to physical examination and history taking* (9th ed.). Philadelphia: Lippincott.

Demers, K. (2007). Hearing screening in older adults: A brief hearing loss screener. *Best Practices in Nursing Care to Older Adults. The Hartford Institute for Geriatric Nursing, Issue 12*. Retrieved from www.hartfordign.org

Eliopoulos, E. (2009). *Gerontological nursing* (7th ed.). Philadelphia: Lippincott Williams & Wilkins.

Katlinowski, M. A. (2008). "Eye" dentifying vision impairment in the geriatric patient. *Geriatric Nursing, 29*(2), 125–132.

Kee, J. (2009). *Prentice Hall handbook of laboratory & diagnostic tests with nursing implications* (6th ed.). Upper Saddle River, NJ: Prentice Hall.

Keeping an eye on abnormalities. (2008). *Nursing, 38*(1), 48–49.

National Institute of Health. (2008). *Genes and disease: Diseases of the eye; ear, nose, & throat*. Retrieved from http://www.ncbi.nlm.nih.gov/books/bookres.fegi/gnd/pdf.html

Visualizing the eye. Optical coherence tomography. (2007). *Cleveland Clinic Magazine, 4*(2), 28.

Weber, J., & Kelley, J. (2009). *Health assessment in nursing* (4th ed.). Philadelphia: Lippincott.

Whiteside, M., Wallhagen, M., & Pettengill, E. (2006). Sensory impairment in older adults: Part 2: Vision loss. *American Journal of Nursing, 106*(11), 52–61.

CHAPTER 46

Nursing Care of Patients with Eye and Ear Disorders

LEARNING OUTCOMES

1. Relate knowledge of normal anatomy, physiology, and sensory functions of the eye and ear to the effects of disorders of these organs on the cognitive/perceptual health pattern.
2. Describe the pathophysiology of commonly occurring disorders of the eyes and ears, relating their manifestations to the pathophysiologic process.
3. Explain the risk factors for selected disorders of the eyes and ears, identifying the nursing implications for these risk factors.
4. Identify diagnostic tests used for specific eye and ear disorders.
5. Discuss the effects of and nursing implications for medications prescribed to treat eye and ear disorders.
6. Describe surgical and other invasive procedures used to treat eye and ear disorders, identifying their implications for nursing care.
7. Discuss the nurse's role in caring for patients with impaired vision or hearing loss.

CLINICAL COMPETENCIES

1. Assess vision, hearing, functional health, and safety of patients with eye and ear disorders.
2. Using assessed data, determine priority nursing diagnoses and interventions for patients with eye and ear disorders.
3. Collaborate and coordinate with other members of the healthcare team to provide safe, effective care for patients with eye and ear disorders.
4. Plan and implement appropriate and individualized evidence-based nursing interventions and teaching for the patient with an eye or ear disorder.
5. Safely and effectively administer eye and ear medications and prescribed treatments.
6. Provide appropriate care and teaching for the patient having eye or ear surgery.
7. Evaluate the effectiveness of nursing care provided for patients with eye and ear disorders, revising plan of care as indicated.

KEY TERMS

astigmatism, *1581*
cataract, *1588*
conjunctivitis, *1577*
diabetic retinopathy, *1599*
enucleation, *1602*
glaucoma, *1591*
hyperopia, *1581*

hyphema, *1587*
macular degeneration, *1598*
Ménière's disease, *1611*
myopia, *1581*
myringotomy, *1607*
nystagmus, *1611*
otitis media, *1606*

presbycusis, *1614*
ptosis, *1602*
tinnitus, *1603*
tympanoplasty, *1608*
vertigo, *1606*

Vision and hearing provide the primary means of input for much of what we know about the world. The ability to receive and organize information orients us to our surroundings. These senses allow us to communicate easily, gain access to information, and derive pleasure from the sights and sounds of the world around us.

This chapter discusses conditions affecting vision and hearing as the result of eye and ear disorders. Nursing care focuses on patients with vision and hearing deficits that can result from the disorders presented.

Eye Disorders

Any portion of the eye and its protective structures may be affected by an acute or chronic condition. While many eye disorders are minor and have little or no effect on vision, others can and often do result in vision impairment. Disorders and diseases of the outer, visible portion of the eye often cause discomfort and may have cosmetic effects. With appropriate treatment, vision impairment often can be prevented or reversed. Disorders of the cornea present the greatest risk to vision in this group. The patient who has had eye surgery or minor trauma may have either temporary or permanent visual impairment. Disorders affecting the internal structures or the function of the eye are more likely to have adverse effects on vision. These disorders are more likely to affect adults over the age of 40, and older adults in particular. More than 3.6 million adults in the United States have some degree of visual impairment (Prevent Blindness America, 2008).

FAST FACTS

Among adults aged 40 and older in the United States:
- Nearly 3.6 million or 2.8% of the population are classified as blind or low vision.
- The prevalence of impaired vision and blindness increases significantly after age 75.
- Refractory errors, including myopia (nearsightedness) and hyperopia (farsightedness), are the most common causes of impaired vision.
- Other common conditions affecting the vision of middle and older adults, in order of prevalence, are as follows:
  1. Cataracts—17.2%
  2. Macular degeneration—7.6%
  3. Diabetic retinopathy—3.4%
  4. Glaucoma—1.9%

Source: All data from Prevent Blindness America. (2008). *Vision problems in the U.S.* Retrieved from www.preventblindness.net/site/DocServer/VPUS_2008_update.pdf?docID=1561

Although disorders that commonly affect vision often cannot be prevented or cured, some can be controlled and vision corrected to normal or near normal. Regardless of the real threat a disorder poses to vision, the patient may experience anxiety related to a perceived threat. The box on page 1578 discusses major causes of significantly impaired vision and nursing care for the patient who is blind. These principles of nursing care may apply to patients with many of the disorders discussed in this chapter.

The Patient with Conjunctivitis

The conjunctiva—the thin, transparent membrane that covers the anterior surface of the eye and lines the inner surfaces of the eyelids—is vulnerable to inflammation and infection because of its constant exposure to the environment. **Conjunctivitis**, inflammation of the conjunctiva, is the most common eye disease. Its usual cause is a bacterial or viral infection. These infections can be transmitted to the eye by direct contact (e.g., hands, tissues, towels). Allergens, chemical irritants, and exposure to radiant energy such as ultraviolet light from the sun or tanning devices can also lead to this common condition. Its severity can range from mild irritation with redness and tearing to conjunctival edema, hemorrhage, or a severe necrotizing process with tissue destruction.

Pathophysiology and Manifestations

Acute Conjunctivitis

Infectious conjunctivitis may be bacterial, viral, or fungal in origin. Bacterial conjunctivitis, also known as "pink eye," is highly contagious, and often is caused by *Staphylococcus* or *Haemophilus.* Adenovirus infection is the leading cause of conjunctivitis in adults. Systemic infections that may affect the eyes include herpes simplex and other viral infections. Contact with genital secretions infected with *Gonococcus* can cause gonococcal conjunctivitis, a medical emergency that can lead to corneal perforation.

Redness and itching of the affected eye are common manifestations of acute conjunctivitis (Figure 46–1 ■). The patient may also complain of a scratchy, burning, or gritty sensation. Pain is not common; however, photophobia may occur. Tearing and discharge accompany the inflammatory process. The discharge may be watery, purulent, or mucoid, depending on the cause of conjunctivitis. The patient may have associated manifestations such as pharyngitis, fever, malaise, and swollen preauricular lymph nodes.

Trachoma

Trachoma, a chronic conjunctivitis caused by *Chlamydia trachomatis*, is a significant preventable cause of blindness worldwide. Trachoma is endemic in sub-Saharan Africa, the Middle East, and parts of Asia. In the United States, it can be found in Native Americans of the Southwest, but less frequently than in endemic regions. Trachoma is contagious, transmitted primarily by close personal contact (eye-to-eye, hand-to-eye) or by fomites such as towels, handkerchiefs, and flies. Certain forms of trachoma are transmitted during delivery when the newborn

Figure 46–1 ■ The appearance of an eye with conjunctivitis.
Source: Centers for Disease Control and Prevention (CDC).

Visual impairment exists on a continuum from blindness to decreased visual acuity that can be corrected with refractive lenses to normal or near normal. *Visual impairment* is defined as 20/40 vision in the better eye, even with corrective lenses. The legal definition of *blindness* is visual acuity no better than 20/200 in the better eye with optimal correction, or a visual field of less than 20 degrees in diameter (compared to the normal of 180 degrees) (Prevent Blindness America, 2008). Total blindness usually indicates that the patient has no light perception at all. In practical terms, a person with a visual deficit sufficient to need assistive devices or aid from other people for normal activities of daily living is considered blind.

Ten to twelve million people in the United States have a visual impairment that cannot be corrected. More than 900,000 Americans are legally blind and an additional 2.3 million are visually impaired (National Eye Institute [NEI], 2004). In the United States, blindness affects more Blacks than Whites and Hispanics, whereas more Hispanics are visually impaired (Prevent Blindness America, 2008). Worldwide, between 30 and 40 million people have visual impairment significant enough to be considered blind.

Although blindness often can be prevented or cured, it remains a significant problem worldwide because of lack of access to care, fear of surgery or treatment, poor sanitation and nutrition, and ignorance of need. In the United States, cataracts, age-related macular degeneration, glaucoma, and diabetic retinopathy remain significant causes of blindness in adults.

NURSING CARE

Blind people need to cope not only with the loss of a major sense but often also with societal attitudes that make them feel inferior, helpless, and inadequate. The idea of losing the ability to see is uniformly feared, leaving sighted people often unable to understand the magnitude and impact of the loss in those who have experienced it. Because of this fear and confusion, sighted people are unsure of what the blind expect from them.

The adjustment of the person who is born blind and raised to become an independent member of society differs from that of the person who has been sighted and becomes blind. The person who has been blind from birth has developed numerous adaptive strategies that the newly blind person has yet to learn.

Although adaptation may be easier for the patient who experiences a gradual loss of vision than for someone with an abrupt loss, both must grieve the lost sense. The blind patient needs to grieve the lost body part as well as the loss of mobility, self-sufficiency, perhaps economic security, and, to a certain extent, contact with reality as it has been perceived. The patient's self-concept and self-esteem are threatened. Anger, denial, remorse, and self-pity are not uncommon in the initial period following loss of sight. Interpersonal relationships and roles are affected. Communication patterns change with the loss of the ability to perceive many nonverbal cues. Expressions of sexuality may be impaired.

Acceptance of the change from sighted to blind is characterized by releasing the hope that vision will be regained. Self-esteem increases as the patient attempts and masters activities of self-sufficiency such as completing activities of daily living (ADLs), cooking, and becoming mobile outside the known home environment.

Health professionals often confuse the role of the blind person with the role of the patient, seeing the person as helpless, dependent, and lacking in personal identity and control. Although nurses need to take blindness into account in planning care and maintaining patient safety, it is vital to give the blind patient the same respect and decision-making power that all patients deserve. Nurses who have dealt with their own emotions and responses to vision loss are better prepared to help the patient adapt.

Nurses can foster independence in the hospitalized patient with a significant vision deficit by doing the following:

- Orient to the environment verbally and physically. Describe the room using a central point such as the bed. Lead the patient around the room, identifying chairs, sink, bathroom, and other landmarks. Be sure that objects such as chairs, personal items, and clothing remain in the same place unless moved by the patient. Leave doors either fully open or closed as the patient wishes, but, to preserve safety, do not leave doors partially open. Keep the room and hallways free of clutter.
- Use verbal communication freely. Describe activities going on around the patient. Introduce yourself as you enter the room and let the patient know when you are leaving.
- Provide other sensory stimuli such as radio and television as desired by the patient.
- Orient to food trays by using the face of a clock to describe the position of food items on the plate and tray (unless the patient has always been blind and cannot visualize a clock face).
- When assisting with ambulation, allow the patient to hold your arm as you walk slightly ahead. Do not hold the patient's arm. Verbally describe the environment, such as "There will be two steps up five feet ahead."
- Do not hesitate to ask what assistance the patient desires.

For the patient with a new loss of sight, refer to available services. Counseling can help the patient cope with and eventually adapt to the loss of sight. People who are blind can receive mobility training, assistance with relearning self-care activities, education in the use of Braille to communicate, and vocational and other forms of rehabilitation. Local, state, and national agencies such as the American Foundation for the Blind, National Braille Association, and National Federation for the Blind coordinate services for the blind. Many assistive devices are available, including guide or pilot dogs, computer services, talking books and tape players, and low-vision aids.

---

is exposed to contaminated genital secretions of the mother (Fauci et al., 2008).

Early manifestations of trachoma include redness, eyelid edema, tearing, and photophobia. Small conjunctival follicles develop on the upper lids. The inflammation also causes superficial corneal vascularization and infiltration with granulation tissue. Scarring of the conjunctival lining of the lid causes entropion (Figure 46–2 ■). The lashes then abrade the cornea, eventually causing ulceration and scarring. The scarred cornea is opaque, resulting in loss of vision.

Interdisciplinary Care

Management of the patient with conjunctivitis focuses on establishing an accurate diagnosis and prompt treatment.

Diagnosis

Accurate diagnosis of conjunctivitis is especially important because other potentially vision-threatening conditions, such as acute uveitis or acute angle-closure glaucoma, can also

Figure 46–2 ■ Entropion.

Source: Science Photo Library/Photo Researchers, Inc.

cause a red eye (Table 46–1). Diagnostic procedures may include the following:

- *Culture and sensitivity* of exudates to determine presence of an infection and identify the infecting organism
- *Fluorescein stain* with slit-lamp examination to identify possible corneal ulcerations or abrasions, which appear green with staining
- *Conjunctival scrapings* are examined microscopically or cultured to identify the organisms

Additional laboratory testing such as blood counts or antibody titers may be used to identify underlying infectious or autoimmune processes.

Medications

Conjunctivitis is treated with antibiotic, antiviral, or anti-inflammatory drugs as appropriate. Topical anti-infectives applied as either eyedrops or ointment may include erythromycin, gentamicin, penicillin, bacitracin, sulfacetamide sodium, amphotericin B, or idoxuridine. For severe infections or cellulitis, anti-infectives may be administered by subconjunctival injection or systemic intravenous infusion. Antihistamines are used to minimize symptoms of conjunctivitis when an allergic response underlies the inflammatory process.

Complementary Therapies

Frequent eye irrigations may be ordered to remove the copious purulent discharge associated with conjunctivitis. Soaking the lids with warm saline compresses prior to cleansing promotes comfort and facilitates the removal of crusts and exudate in conjunctivitis.

ℳ Nursing Care

The nursing role in treating conjunctivitis is primarily one of education to prevent the disorder and to prevent its spread when it does occur.

Health Promotion

Education is a vital strategy for preventing conjunctivitis. Teach all patients about proper eye care, including the importance of not sharing towels, makeup, or contact lenses, and avoiding rubbing or scratching the eyes. Instruct to avoid using old eye makeup, which can cause eye infections. Teach contact lens users appropriate care (Box 46–1). Emphasize the need to follow cleaning instructions precisely to avoid bacterial contamination of lenses. If the eyes become red, irritated, or develop discharge, instruct the patient to avoid wearing contact lenses until the inflammatory process has cleared.

Assessment

- *Health history:* Presence of redness, discomfort, tearing, photophobia, and drainage; symptom onset; care measures; use of contact lenses; exposure to "pink eye" or recent travel; allergies; previous history of conjunctivitis; presence of any chronic diseases.
- *Physical assessment:* Visual acuity; inspect eyelids, conjunctiva, sclera, and cornea; vital signs including temperature.

Nursing Diagnoses and Interventions

Nursing care focuses primarily on preventing complications from the disorder. The priority nursing diagnoses include risk for infection and risk of altered vision.

Risk for Infection

Acute conjunctivitis is highly contagious. While most patients experience no more than discomfort from the disease, the infection carries a risk for scarring and damage to the delicate cornea of the eye. Preventing the spread of this infection is a vital nursing role.

- Teach to wash hands thoroughly before instilling eye medications. Instruct to avoid touching or rubbing the eyes.

TABLE 46–1 Possible Causes of Acute Red Eye

	ACUTE CONJUNCTIVITIS	CORNEAL TRAUMA OR INFECTION	ACUTE UVEITIS	ACUTE ANGLE CLOSURE GLAUCOMA
Incidence	Very common	Common	Common	Rare
Pain	Mild	Moderate to severe	Moderate	Severe
Vision	Normal	Blurred	Blurred	Markedly blurred
Discharge	May be copious	Watery, may be purulent	None	None
Conjunctival erythema	Diffuse	Primarily around cornea	Primarily around cornea	Primarily around cornea
Cornea	Clear	Depends on cause	Usually clear	Cloudy
Pupils	Normal size, response to light	Normal size, response to light	Small, minimal response to light	Moderately dilated, fixed

BOX 46–1 Contact Lens Care

- Wash hands thoroughly before handling contact lenses.
- Keep storage case clean.
- Remove lenses before sleep, cleaning and storing as recommended by manufacturer.
- Use cleaning and wetting solutions recommended by eye care professional or lens manufacturer. Do not use water or home-made solutions for wetting or cleaning lenses.
- If eye redness, tearing, vision loss, or pain occurs, remove lenses and contact eye care professional as soon as possible.
- Do not share contact lenses or allow another person to "try on" lenses.

Advise to use a new, clean cotton-tipped swab or cotton ball for cleaning each eye. *Hand hygiene is the single most important measure to prevent transmission of infection to the eye. Touching or rubbing the eyes increases the risk of infection and corneal trauma. Using a new swab or cotton ball prevents cross-contamination between eyes.*

- Teach to instill prescribed eyedrops as ordered. *Prescribed medications reduce inflammation and eliminate infection.*
- Discuss the importance of avoiding contact lens use until the infectious process has cleared and of completing the prescribed treatment. *Use of contact lenses in the inflamed eyes can lead to further damage and impair healing.*

Risk for Disturbed Sensory Perception: Visual

Conjunctivitis can potentially disrupt the integrity or clarity of the cornea. Because of its vital role in focusing light on the retina, corneal damage can impair visual acuity.

- Assess vision with and without corrective lenses. *Assessment provides a baseline to evaluate possible changes in vision resulting from the infection.*
- Instruct to avoid activities requiring high visual acuity until the infection has cleared. *The inflammatory process, edema of the conjunctiva, and local antibiotic applications can decrease visual acuity and cloud vision.*
- Instruct to use dark sunglasses with appropriate UV protection when out of doors, even on cloudy days. *Photophobia, a common manifestation of conjunctivitis, causes eye pain with increased light intensity.*

EVIDENCE FOR NURSING CARE | The Patient with Conjunctivitis

Selected resources that nurses may find helpful when planning evidence-based nursing care follow.

- American Academy of Ophthalmology Cornea/External Disease Panel, Preferred Practice Patterns Committee. (2008). *Conjunctivitis.* San Francisco, CA: American Academy of Ophthalmology (AAO).
- University of Texas, School of Nursing, Family Nurse Practitioner Program. (2005 May). *Guidelines for the treatment and management of acute bacterial conjunctivitis in children and adults.* Austin, TX: University of Texas, School of Nursing.

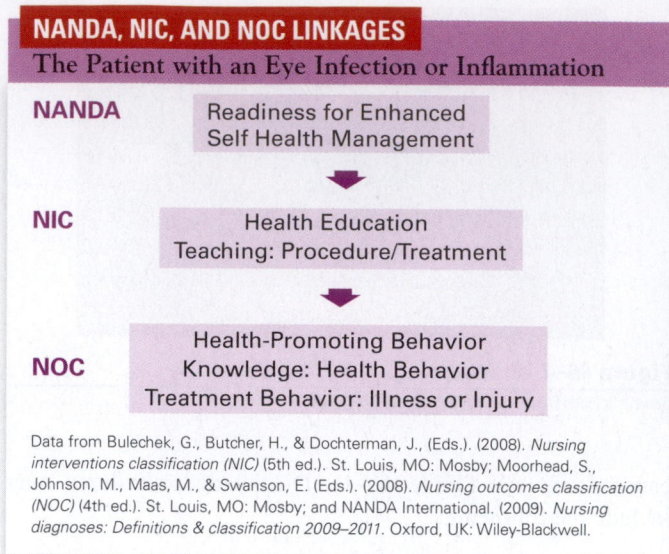

NANDA, NIC, AND NOC LINKAGES
The Patient with an Eye Infection or Inflammation

NANDA — Readiness for Enhanced Self Health Management

NIC — Health Education
Teaching: Procedure/Treatment

NOC — Health-Promoting Behavior
Knowledge: Health Behavior
Treatment Behavior: Illness or Injury

Data from Bulechek, G., Butcher, H., & Dochterman, J., (Eds.). (2008). *Nursing interventions classification (NIC)* (5th ed.). St. Louis, MO: Mosby; Moorhead, S., Johnson, M., Maas, M., & Swanson, E. (Eds.). (2008). *Nursing outcomes classification (NOC)* (4th ed.). St. Louis, MO: Mosby; and NANDA International. (2009). *Nursing diagnoses: Definitions & classification 2009–2011.* Oxford, UK: Wiley-Blackwell.

Using NANDA, NIC, and NOC

Linkages between a selected NANDA nursing diagnosis, NIC, and NOC for the patient with an eye infection or inflammation are shown in the accompanying chart.

Community-Based Care

Patients with conjunctivitis typically are managed in the community, reinforcing the need for effective teaching for home care. Emphasize to the family ways to prevent transmission of infection. If the patient is unable to administer eye medications, involve the family in teaching. Include the following topics:

- Safety and medical asepsis when cleansing the eye
- Instillation of prescribed eyedrops and ointments
- Comfort measures such as reducing lighting intensity and wearing sunglasses
- Avoidance of activities such as excessive reading while eye is inflamed

The Patient with a Corneal Disorder

The clear cornea allows light rays to enter the eye and transmits images onto the retina. It helps to focus light on the retina and protects the internal eye structures. The cornea can be affected by a variety of disorders, including infection and trauma. While the cornea heals quickly after minor injuries or abrasions, injury to its deeper layers can delay healing or result in scarring.

Physiology Review

The cornea has three major layers: the outermost epithelium, which consists of five or six layers of cells that are constantly being renewed; the stroma, which makes up 90% of corneal tissue; and the single-cell thickness endothelium adjacent to the aqueous humor of the anterior chamber. The cornea is avascular tissue; the central cornea is dependent on atmospheric oxygen to meet its metabolic needs. Because there is no blood supply, immune defenses have difficulty fending off infections of the cornea.

Pathophysiology and Manifestations

Light enters the eye through the normally clear cornea. As light passes through the curved cornea, it is bent or *refracted* onto the lens, which then focuses the light on sensory cells of the retina. A change in the curvature of the cornea or in its clarity affects the ability of the eye to clearly focus; as a result, vision is distorted or blurred. Refractive errors such as nearsightedness, farsightedness, and astigmatism are common. Corneal scarring or ulceration are two major causes of blindness worldwide.

Refractive Errors

Refractive errors are the most common problem affecting visual acuity; they result from an abnormal curvature of the cornea or an altered shape of the eyeball. People with *emmetropia* (normal vision) see near and far objects clearly because light rays focus directly on the retina. In **myopia** (nearsightedness) the curvature of the cornea is excessive or the eyeball is elongated, causing the image to focus in front of the retina instead of on it. Objects in close range are seen clearly and those at a distance are blurred. The eyeball is too short in **hyperopia** (farsightedness), causing the image to focus behind the retina. People with this condition see objects clearer at a distance than those close to them.

> **FAST FACTS**
> - The prevalence of myopia decreases with aging, from an estimated 36.4% of Americans ages 40 to 49 affected (15.5 million) to 17.5% of people ages 80 and older (1.6 million).
> - In contrast, the prevalence of hyperopia increases with aging, affecting an estimated 3.1% of Americans ages 40 to 49 (1.5 million) and 23.6% of people ages 80 and older (2.2 million) (NEI, 2008).

Astigmatism develops due to an irregular or abnormal curvature of the cornea. Instead of the round, even curvature of the normal cornea, the cornea curves more in one direction than the other in astigmatism, resembling the back of a spoon. As a result, light rays focus on more than one area of the retina, distorting both near and distance vision.

Keratitis

Keratitis is inflammation of the cornea. When the inflammatory process involves both the conjunctiva and the cornea, the term *keratoconjunctivitis* may be used. Keratitis may be caused by infection, hypersensitivity reactions, ischemia, tearing defects, trauma, and impaired innervation of the cornea. Scarring that occurs as a result of keratitis is a leading cause of blindness worldwide (Porth & Matfin, 2009).

Keratitis is described as either nonulcerative or ulcerative. In *nonulcerative keratitis*, all layers of corneal epithelium are affected, but remain intact. Viral infections, tuberculosis, and autoimmune disorders such as lupus erythematosus may cause nonulcerative keratitis. *Ulcerative keratitis*, in contrast, affects the epithelium and stroma of the cornea, leading to tissue destruction and ulceration. Bacterial conjunctivitis (e.g., *Staphylococcus, S. pneumoniae, Chlamydia*) may lead to ulcerative keratitis.

Keratitis commonly causes tearing, discomfort ranging from a gritty sensation in the eye to severe pain, decreased visual acuity, and *blepharospasm* (spasm of the eyelid and inability to open the eye). A discharge may be present, especially if the conjunctiva is also inflamed. Corneal ulceration may be visible on direct examination.

Corneal Ulcer

A *corneal ulcer*, local necrosis of the cornea, may be caused by infection, exposure trauma, or the misuse of contact lenses. A frequent cause is bacterial infection following trauma or contact lens overuse. Herpes viruses, including herpes simplex and herpes zoster, are a leading cause of ulcerative corneal disease. Corneal ulcers may also complicate bacterial conjunctivitis, trachoma, gonorrhea, and other acute infections. Patients who are immunosuppressed because of disease or drug therapy are at particular risk for developing corneal ulcers due to infection.

In corneal ulceration, a portion of the epithelium and/or stroma is destroyed. Ulcers may be superficial or deep, penetrating underlying layers and posing a risk of perforation. Fibrous tissue may form during healing, resulting in scarring and opacity of the cornea. Perforation can lead to infection of deeper eye structures or extrusion of eye contents. Partial or total vision loss may result.

Corneal Dystrophies

A corneal dystrophy is accumulation of cloudy material in part or parts of the normally clear cornea, potentially affecting visual acuity. Corneal dystrophies typically are inherited disorders that progress gradually and affect both eyes. *Keratoconus*, progressive thinning of the cornea, is the most common corneal dystrophy. It typically affects teenagers and young adults. In keratoconus, the center of the cornea thins and bulges outward, affecting the shape of the cornea and its ability to focus light on the lens of the eye. In most cases, the thinning stabilizes over time; up to 20% of patients, however, eventually require corneal transplant (NEI, 2009a).

Interdisciplinary Care

Management of the patient with a disorder of the cornea focuses on establishing an accurate diagnosis and prompt treatment to reduce the risk of permanent vision deficit. The history and physical assessment are key in diagnosing these disorders.

Although many eye disorders can be treated in the community, the patient with a severe corneal infection or ulcer may require hospitalization. Corneal ulcers are medical emergencies, requiring prompt referral to an ophthalmologist for treatment. Pressure dressings may be applied to both eyes for comfort and to reduce the risk of perforation and loss of eye contents.

Diagnosis

Visual acuity is tested on all patients presenting with refractory or corneal disorders. ∞ See Chapter 45 for more information about testing visual acuity. The following tests may be ordered to identify the cause and extent of eye infections or inflammations:

- *Fluorescein stain* with slit-lamp examination allows visualization of any corneal ulcerations or abrasions, which appear green with staining.

■ *Conjunctival* or *ulcer scrapings* are examined microscopically or cultured to identify the organisms.

Additional laboratory testing such as blood counts or antibody titers may be used to identify any underlying infectious or autoimmune processes.

Medication

Infectious processes are treated with antibiotic or antiviral therapy as appropriate. Topical anti-infectives applied as either eyedrops or ointment may include erythromycin, gentamicin, penicillin, bacitracin, sulfacetamide sodium, amphotericin B, or idoxuridine. For severe infections, central ulcers, or cellulitis, anti-infectives may be administered by subconjunctival injection and/or systemic intravenous infusion. Corticosteroids may be prescribed for keratitis related to systemic inflammatory disorders or trauma; however, it is important to avoid their use with local infections to avoid suppressing the immune and inflammatory responses.

Corrective Lenses

Corrective lenses, either in the form of eyeglasses or contact lenses, generally are prescribed to restore visual acuity for patients with refractive errors such as myopia, hyperopia, and astigmatism. Specially fitted contact lenses to reduce vision distortion are ordered for patients with keratoconus. Because contact lenses are a risk factor for corneal infection and ulcers, teaching appropriate care is vital (see Box 46–1).

Surgery

LASER EYE SURGERY Laser eye surgery is commonly performed to correct refractive errors such as myopia, hyperopia, and astigmatism. In these surgeries, a laser is used to permanently change the shape of the cornea. In most cases, the need to use corrective lenses is reduced or eliminated. Several surgical procedures are available:

■ Laser *in situ* keratomileusis (LASIK)
■ Photorefractive keratectomy (PRK)
■ Laser epithelial keratomileusis (LASEK)
■ Laser thermokeratoplasty (LTK)

These procedures reshape the cornea using laser technology to remove a thin layer of epithelial cells or to shrink and reshape the cornea. Candidates for laser vision-correction surgery should be in good health and must have adequate corneal thickness such that perforation is not a risk.

Following surgery, patients may experience a temporary loss of contrast sharpness (images do not appear as crisp as with corrective lenses), over- or undercorrection of visual acuity, dry eyes, or temporarily decreased night vision with halos, glare, and starbursts. Diffuse lamellar keratitis (DLK) is a rare complication of surgery that, while treatable, can lead to vision impairment if not identified and treated early.

Phototherapeutic keratectomy (PTK) provides an alternative to corneal transplant in treating corneal dystrophies, scars, and some infections. In this procedure, diseased corneal tissue is vaporized and surface irregularities are corrected with little trauma to surrounding tissue. Healing occurs rapidly.

CORNEAL TRANSPLANT Once the cornea has become scarred and opaque, no treatment can restore its clarity. The first successful corneal transplant (or *keratoplasty*), replacement of diseased cornea by healthy corneal tissue from a donor, was performed in 1906. Current corneal transplant procedures have a success rate of approximately 80% (NEI, 2009a).

Corneas are harvested from the cadavers of uninfected adults who were under the age of 65 and who died as a result of acute trauma or illness. After harvesting, the cornea can be stored in a tissue-culture medium for up to 4 weeks before being used as a graft. Corneal transplantation is usually an elective surgery, although emergency transplantation may be required for perforation of the cornea.

Corneal transplant may be either lamellar or penetrating. In a lamellar keratoplasty, the superficial layer of cornea is removed and replaced with a graft. The anterior chamber remains intact. In a penetrating keratoplasty, a button or full thickness of cornea is removed and replaced by donor tissue (Figure 46–3 ■). The graft is then sutured in place using suture finer than human hair and a continuous or interrupted stitch. Because the cornea is avascular, these sutures remain in place for up to a year to ensure healing.

Most corneal transplants do not require hospitalization. The eye is patched for 24 hours following surgery. Narcotic analgesia

A

B

Figure 46–3 ■ Corneal transplant. *A,* The diseased, opaque cornea. *B,* The diseased cornea is removed and a corneal graft is sutured in place using material finer than a human hair.

Source: Custom Medical Stock Photo, Inc.

may be required initially because the cornea is extremely sensitive. Corticosteroid eyedrops are ordered to reduce the inflammatory response and prevent edema of the graft. Antibiotic drops may be prescribed to prevent infection.

The risk of transplant rejection is low. Because the cornea is avascular, there is little exposure of the transplanted corneal tissue to the host's immune defenses (Porth & Matfin, 2009). Research suggests that matching of blood type (not tissue type, as is required for major organ transplants) between the donor and the transplant recipient may reduce the risk of transplant rejection (NEI, 2009a). When rejection does occur, it occurs within 3 weeks of the transplant, beginning with inflammation at the edge of the grafted tissue and spreading to involve the entire graft.

See the box on page 1585 for nursing care of the patient having eye surgery.

∾ Nursing Care

The nursing role in caring for patients with corneal disorders may involve direct care, but more often focuses on prevention and education. Nurses working in clinics and outpatient surgical settings care for patients undergoing corneal transplant and surgeries to correct refractive errors.

Health Promotion

Education is a vital strategy for preventing many corneal disorders. Teach all patients about proper eye care, including the importance of not sharing towels and makeup and avoiding rubbing or scratching the eyes as well as preventing trauma and infection. Teach contact lens users appropriate care and cleaning techniques. Stress the importance of periodic removal of lenses, even extended-wear lenses. In general, lenses should be removed at night, even though manufacturers may claim it is safe to wear them while sleeping. Emphasize the need to follow cleaning instructions precisely to avoid bacterial contamination of lenses and possible corneal infection. If the patient experiences a corneal abrasion or keratitis, instruct the patient to avoid wearing contact lenses until the cornea has healed completely.

Assessment

Collect the following data through health history and physical examination (∾ see Chapter 45). Additional focused assessments are described with the interventions that follow.

- *Health history:* Risk factors; presence of redness, discomfort, tearing, photophobia, edema, and drainage; symptom onset; presence of pain, effect on vision.
- *Physical assessment:* Visual acuity; inspect external eye, including conjunctiva, sclera, and cornea; extraocular movements.

Nursing Diagnoses and Interventions

Nursing care focuses primarily on preventing complications and promoting healing. The priority nursing diagnoses for patients with corneal disorders include risk of altered vision, pain, and risk for injury.

Risk for Disturbed Sensory Perception: Visual

Disorders affecting the cornea may disrupt its integrity or clarity. Because the cornea plays a vital role in focusing light on the retina, corneal damage can affect vision, impairing visual acuity and even causing legal blindness.

- Assess vision with and without corrective lenses. *Assessment provides a baseline to evaluate possible vision changes resulting from the disorder or treatment.*
- Instruct about thorough hand hygiene before inserting or removing contact lenses or instilling any eye medications. Teach to avoid touching or rubbing the eyes. Instruct to use a new, clean cotton-tipped swab or cotton ball for cleaning each eye. *Hand hygiene is the single most important measure to prevent transmission of infection to the eye. Touching or rubbing the eyes increases the risk of infection and corneal trauma. Using a new swab or cotton ball prevents cross-contamination between eyes.*
- Emphasize the importance of proper care of contact lenses specific to the type of lens used. *Patients who wear hard contact lenses must remove them daily because the central cornea needs exposure to atmospheric oxygen. Although soft and extended-wear lenses allow the cornea to "breathe," improper cleaning carries a major risk for infection.*
- Teach the importance of using eye protection when engaging in potentially dangerous activities. *Trauma increases the risk of infection and scarring of the cornea.*
- If corneal perforation is suspected, place the patient in the supine position, close the eye, and cover it with a dry, sterile dressing. Notify the physician immediately. *Corneal perforation may occur without warning in patients with corneal ulcers. It places the patient at risk for loss of eye contents. Emergency measures are taken to reduce intraocular pressure and maintain eye integrity to preserve vision.*

> **PRACTICE ALERT**
> Suspect corneal perforation with complaints of sudden, severe eye pain and photophobia.

Acute Pain

The cornea of the eye is extremely sensitive; therefore, corneal disorders frequently cause significant pain. Pain, in turn, increases the stress response and interferes with rest, potentially impairing healing.

- Assess pain, using verbal and nonverbal cues. *Pain is a subjective experience and can be evaluated only by the patient's response and in terms of its effect on the patient.*
- Administer prescribed analgesia routinely in the first 12 to 24 hours after corneal surgery. *Routine administration of analgesics prevents pain from reaching a level of severity at which it becomes difficult to relieve.*
- Patch both eyes if necessary. *Patching both eyes reduces eye movement and irritation of the affected eye.*
- Teach to apply warm compresses to reduce inflammation and pain. *Warm compresses for 15 minutes, three to four times a day, promote comfort for patients with keratitis or corneal injury.*
- Instruct to use dark sunglasses with appropriate UV protection when out of doors, even on cloudy days. *True photophobia,*

often associated with corneal disorders, causes eye pain with increased light intensity.

■ Teach to instill prescribed eyedrops as ordered. *Prescribed medications may reduce inflammation and eliminate infection, reducing discomfort.*

Risk for Injury

The patient who has undergone corneal transplantation has an increased risk for injury for several reasons. The eye on which surgery was performed is patched for 24 hours after surgery, changing depth perception and increasing the risk for falls. Increased intraocular pressure or trauma to the eye may damage the graft, resulting in graft rejection.

■ Instruct to call for help before getting up or ambulating after surgery. Ensure access to the call light. *It may take time for the patient to adjust to changes in depth perception caused by the eye patch. Assistance helps prevent falls that may not only injure the patient but also traumatize the operative site.*

■ Encourage to deep breathe and use the incentive spirometer to promote lung expansion. *These important postoperative measures help prevent pulmonary complications. Coughing is avoided because it increases intraocular pressure.*

■ Teach how to apply an eye shield at night after the eye patch is removed. *An eye shield may be recommended at night to prevent inadvertent rubbing or trauma to the eye during sleep.*

■ Instruct not to rub or scratch the eye. *Rubbing or scratching may disrupt suture lines or damage the grafted tissue.*

■ Reinforce the importance of using eye protection during hazardous activities. *Following a corneal transplant, the patient has the same risk of eye injury as other people who perform hazardous activities.*

> **PRACTICE ALERT**
> Administer prescribed antiemetics and stool softeners post-operatively to prevent vomiting and straining at stool, activities that increase intraocular pressure, damaging suture lines.

Community-Based Care

Following treatment, teach patients to manage these conditions at home. Emphasize to the family ways to prevent transmission of infection. If the patient is unable to administer eye medications or to perform other eye care techniques, involve the family in the teaching session. The following topics should be included:

■ Safety and medical asepsis when cleansing the eye
■ Instillation of prescribed eyedrops and ointments
■ Application of an eye patch and where to obtain supplies
■ Avoidance of activities such as excessive reading while eye is inflamed
■ Follow-up appointments after corneal transplant surgery
■ Signs of graft rejection
■ Avoidance of activities that increase intraocular pressure such as straining, coughing, sneezing, bending over, lifting heavy objects
■ Helpful resources:
  ■ National Eye Institute
  ■ Lighthouse National Center for Vision and Aging

The Patient with a Disorder Affecting the Eyelids

The eyelids and eyelashes are constantly exposed to the environment as they protect the eye from damage. When these structures are inflamed, deformed, or their function is impaired, it affects both appearance and their protective functions.

Pathophysiology and Manifestations

The most common disorder affecting the eyelids is *marginal blepharitis*, an inflammation of the glands and lash follicles on the margins of the eyelids. This inflammatory disorder can be caused by a staphylococcal infection or it may be seborrheic in origin; commonly, both types are present. Seborrheic blepharitis is usually associated with seborrhea (dandruff) of the scalp or eyebrows. Irritation, burning, and itching of eyelid margins are common manifestations of blepharitis. The eye appears red rimmed with mucous discharge, and there is crusting or scaling of lid margins. Lid margins may ulcerate, resulting in a loss of eyelashes.

Infection of one or more of the sebaceous glands of the eyelid may cause a hordeolum (sty). Hordeolum is a staphylococcal abscess that may occur on either the external or internal margin of the lid (Figure 46–4 ■). An external hordeolum is characterized initially by acute pain at the lid margin and redness. A small tender raised area is visible. The patient may also experience photophobia, tearing, and the sensation of a foreign body in the affected eye. Internal hordeola are seen on the conjunctival side of the lid and may have more severe manifestations.

Chronic inflammation of a meibomian gland may lead to formation of a chalazion, a granulomatous cyst or nodule of the lid (Figure 46–5 ■). It presents as a hard swelling on the lid, and surrounding conjunctival tissue is reddened. Chalazion may also follow a hordeolum that was inadequately treated. Unlike a hordeolum, a chalazion is painless. It may slowly increase in size and eventually require removal, but most resolve within several months. A lid lesion that ulcerates or does not heal may indicate basal or squamous cell carcinoma and should be further investigated (Fauci et al., 2008).

Figure 46–4 ■ Hordeolum.
Source: Science Photo Library/Photo Researchers, Inc.

NURSING CARE OF THE PATIENT Having Eye Surgery

PREOPERATIVE CARE

- Review ∞ Chapter 4 for routine preoperative care.
- Assess visual acuity of the nonoperative eye prior to surgery. *The patient with limited vision in the nonoperative eye may need additional attention and ADL assistance postoperatively to ensure safety.*
- Assess the patient's support systems and the possible effect of impaired vision on lifestyle and ability to perform ADLs in the postoperative period. *Safety measures such as installing handrails and removing throw rugs from the home can help promote mobility and safety, especially if the patient has limited vision in the unaffected eye.*
- Teach measures to prevent eye injury postoperatively: avoid vomiting, straining at stool, coughing, sneezing, lifting more than 5 lb, and bending over at the waist. *These activities temporarily increase intraocular pressure and may lead to postoperative complications.*
- Remove all eye makeup and contact lenses or glasses prior to surgery. Store corrective lenses in a safe place, and make them readily available to the patient on return from surgery. *Maintaining visual acuity in the unaffected eye helps reduce fear and maintain safety.*
- Administer preoperative medications and eyedrops or ointments as prescribed. *Mydriatic (pupil-dilating) or cycloplegic (ciliary-paralytic) drops and drops to lower intraocular pressure may be prescribed preoperatively.*

POSTOPERATIVE CARE

- Review ∞ Chapter 4 for routine postoperative care.
- Assess eye dressing for bleeding or drainage following surgery. *Bleeding or drainage may indicate a surgical complication.*
- Maintain the eye patch or shield in place. *The eye patch or shield helps prevent inadvertent injury to the operative site.*
- Place in semi-Fowler's or Fowler's position on the unaffected side. *Elevating the head of the bed and lying on the unaffected side reduce intraocular pressure in the affected eye.*
- Remind the patient to avoid coughing, sneezing, or straining as needed. *These activities increase intraocular pressure.*
- Assess and medicate as necessary for complaints of pain, aching, or a scratchy sensation in affected eye. Immediately report complaints of sudden, sharp eye pain to the physician. *An abrupt increase in or onset of eye pain may indicate hemorrhage or other ocular emergency requiring immediate intervention to preserve sight.*

- Assess for potential complications:
  a. Pain in or drainage from the affected eye
  b. Hemorrhage with blood in the anterior chamber of the eye
  c. Flashes of light, floaters, or the sensation of a curtain being drawn over the eye (indicators of retinal detachment)
  d. Cloudy appearance to the cornea (corneal edema)
  Evidence of complications or unusual complaints should be reported to the physician at once. Early intervention is often necessary to preserve sight.
- Approach the patient on the unaffected side. *This approach facilitates eye contact and communication.*
- Place personal articles and the call light within easy reach. *These measures prevent stretching and straining by the patient.*
- Administer antibiotic, anti-inflammatory, and other systemic and topical eye medications as prescribed. *Medications are prescribed to prevent infection or inflammation of the operative site, maintain pupil constriction, and control intraocular pressure.*
- Administer antiemetic medication as needed. *It is important to prevent vomiting to maintain normal intraocular pressures.*

Health Education for the Patient and Family

- Teach the patient and family about home care:
  a. How to instill eyedrops
  b. The name, dosage, schedule, duration, purpose, and side effects of medications
  c. How and when to use the eye patch and eye shield
  d. The importance of avoiding scratching, rubbing, touching, or squeezing the affected eye
  e. Measures to avoid constipation and straining
  f. Activity limitations, if ordered
  g. Symptoms to report, including eye pain or pressure, redness or cloudiness, drainage, decreased vision, floaters or flashes of light, or halos around bright objects
  h. The need to wear sunglasses with side shields when outdoors to reduce photophobia
- Remind the patient that vision may not stabilize for several weeks following eye surgery. New corrective lenses, if necessary, are not prescribed until vision has stabilized. *Patients may be alarmed that vision seems worse after surgery than before and need reassurance that visual acuity usually improves with time and healing of the affected eye.*
- Emphasize the importance of keeping recommended follow-up appointments. Provide referral to a community home health agency for assistance with home care after discharge as needed.

Figure 46–5 ■ Chalazion.

Source: Science Photo Library/Photo Researchers, Inc.

Entropion, inversion of the lid margin (see Figure 46–2), may be associated with the normal aging process (senile entropion) or result from an infectious process such as trachoma. Entropion can lead to corneal irritation and, potentially, scarring as the lashes rub on the conjunctiva and cornea during blinking and sleep. *Ectropion,* or eversion of the lid margin, occurs primarily as an effect of aging (Figure 46–6 ■). Other conditions may also lead to ectropion, including facial nerve paralysis or palsy (Bell's palsy), scarring, or infection. With ectropion, the eye does not close effectively, increasing the risk for drying and damage to conjunctival membrane and the cornea. Both entropion and ectropion have cosmetic effects as well, altering the appearance of the eye and face.

Figure 46–6 ■ Ectropion.
Source: Science Photo Library/Photo Researchers, Inc.

Interdisciplinary Care

Disorders affecting the eyelids typically are managed in the community. Diagnosis is typically made through the history and physical examination. Diagnostic tests are rarely required except to identify corneal or conjunctival damage resulting from the condition.

Topical antibiotics (eyedrops or ointments) may be prescribed for the patient with hordeolum and to treat infection resulting from irritation of the eye by a deformed lid. Careful cleansing of the lid margins using a "no-tears" baby shampoo is often recommended for marginal blepharitis. Soaking the lids with warm saline compresses prior to cleansing facilitates the removal of crusts and exudate in blepharitis. Local heat applications may be used to treat hordeolum or chalazion; excision and drainage may be required if this is not effective. In entropion or ectropion, surgery may be performed to correct the defect, reduce the risk of damage to the eye, and improve cosmetic appearance.

∞ Nursing Care

The nursing role focuses on education and comfort measures. Teach patients about appropriate eye care, including avoiding rubbing or scratching the eyes. Discuss the importance of not using old eye makeup, which can cause lid infections. Instruct to wash hands well before cleansing the eyelids or instilling any eye medications. Instruct to use a new, clean cotton-tipped swab or cotton ball for cleaning each eye. Teach to instill prescribed eyedrops and apply ointments as ordered. If the patient is unable to administer eye medications, involve the family in teaching. Teach to apply warm compresses to reduce inflammation and discomfort.

The Patient with Eye Trauma

More than 2 million eye injuries occur each year. Many eye injuries are minor, but without timely and appropriate intervention, even a minor injury can threaten vision. For this reason, all eye injuries should be considered medical emergencies requiring immediate evaluation and intervention.

Pathophysiology and Manifestations

Any part of the eye, especially the exposed parts, may be affected by trauma. Foreign bodies, abrasions, and lacerations are the most common types of eye injury. Traumatic injury may also be due to a burn, penetrating objects, or blunt force.

Corneal Abrasion

Corneal abrasion is disruption of the superficial epithelium of the cornea. Objects commonly causing corneal abrasion include contact lenses, eyelashes, small foreign bodies such as dust and dirt, and fingernails. Drying of the eye surface and chemical irritants may also result in a corneal abrasion.

Superficial abrasions of the cornea are extremely painful but generally heal rapidly without complication or scarring. Photophobia and tearing are commonly present. When the stroma is damaged by a deep abrasion or laceration, there is an increased risk of infection, slowed healing, and scar formation.

Burns

The outer surface of the eye may be subjected to burns caused by heat, radiation, or explosion, but chemical burns are the most common. Either acid or alkaline substances may burn the eye. Ammonia, products that contain lye (such as oven and drain cleaners), and acids from car batteries or other sources are often implicated in eye injuries. Burns caused by alkaline substances are particularly serious because tiny particles of the chemical may remain in the conjunctival sac, causing progressive damage. Acid causes rapid damage to the eye, but generally causes less serious burns than alkaline substances.

Explosions and flash burn injuries pose the greatest risk for thermal burns of the eye. Ultraviolet rays can also cause corneal damage ranging in severity from mild to extensive. Depending on the source of the ultraviolet light, these burns may be known by various names such as snowblindness, welder's arc burn, or flash burn.

In addition to giving a history of face and eye contact with a caustic substance or other burning agent, the patient complains of eye pain and decreased vision. Eyelids are often swollen. Burns may also affect the face or lids. The appearance of the eye may vary, depending on the type of burn. The conjunctiva is reddened and edematous; sloughing may be seen, particularly with chemical burns. The cornea often appears cloudy or hazy, and ulcerations may be evident.

Penetrating Trauma

Perforation of the eye occurs from a variety of causes. Metal flakes or other particles produced by high-speed drilling or grinding, glass shards, or other substances may penetrate the eye. Gunshots (including BBs), arrows, and knives can penetrate the eye. In a penetrating injury, the layers of the eye spontaneously reapproximate after entry of a sharp-pointed object or small missile into the globe. These injuries may not be readily apparent with inspection of the eye. In a perforating injury, the layers of the eye do not spontaneously reapproximate, resulting in rupture of the globe and potential loss of ocular contents (Doherty, 2009).

Penetrating injuries may be hidden because of tissue swelling or missed when the patient has other significant injuries that command attention. When the eyelid is lacerated or has a puncture wound, inspection of the underlying eye tissue for possible damage is vital. Eye perforations cause pain, partial or complete loss of vision, and possibly bleeding or extrusion of eye contents.

Blunt Trauma

Sports injuries are a common cause of blunt trauma to the eye: It may be struck with a ball (baseball, tennis, racquetball, and handball are frequently implicated) or injured in contact sports such as basketball, football, boxing, or wrestling. Motor vehicle crashes, falls, and physical assault are examples of other causes of blunt eye trauma.

Blunt trauma may lead to a minor eye injury such as lid ecchymosis (black eye) or subconjunctival hemorrhage, caused by rupture of a blood vessel in the conjunctiva. A well-defined bright area of erythema appears under the conjunctiva. No pain or discomfort is associated with the hemorrhage and no treatment is necessary. The blood typically reabsorbs within 2 to 3 weeks.

Hyphema, bleeding into the anterior chamber of the eye, is a potential result of blunt eye trauma. When the highly vascular uveal tract of the eye is disrupted by blunt force, hemorrhage may result, filling the anterior chamber. The patient complains of eye pain, decreased visual acuity, and seeing a reddish tint. Blood is visible in the anterior chamber.

An orbital blowout fracture is another potential result of blunt eye trauma. Although any part of the eye orbit may be fractured, the ethmoid bone on the orbital floor is the most likely site. Orbital contents, including fat, muscles, and the eye itself, may herniate through the fracture into the underlying maxillary sinus. The patient complains of diplopia (double vision), pain with upward movement of the affected eye, and decreased sensation on the affected cheek. The eye appears sunken (enophthalmos) and has limited movement on examination.

Interdisciplinary Care

When trauma to the eye is known or suspected, a thorough examination is conducted to determine the type and extent of the injury. Unless immediate treatment is indicated, as with a chemical burn, vision is evaluated initially. If the patient normally wears corrective lenses, vision assessment is performed while glasses are worn. Eye movement is evaluated unless a penetrating object is present, and the lid and eye are inspected for lacerations. Inspection is performed using strong light and magnification with a headband loupe or slit lamp. Topical anesthesia may be used prior to inspection if eye pain and photophobia make eye opening difficult. Fluorescein staining can help identify foreign bodies and abrasions. Any conjunctival or anterior chamber hemorrhage is noted, as is the presence or absence of the red reflex. Ophthalmoscopic examination is used to detect hemorrhage or trauma to the interior chamber.

Facial x-rays and CT scans are used to identify orbital fractures or foreign bodies within the globe. Ultrasonography may be employed to detect a detached retina or vitreous hemorrhage.

Foreign bodies are removed using irrigation, a sterile cotton-tipped applicator, or a sterile needle or other instrument. Antibiotic ointment—erythromycin or sulfacetamide sodium—is applied after their removal. In patients with corneal abrasions and large foreign bodies in the eye, an eye patch is applied firmly after the antibiotic application to keep the eye closed for approximately 24 hours.

The immediate priority of care for patients with chemical burns is flushing the affected eye with copious amounts of fluid (Figure 46–7 ■). Normal saline is preferred; however, water may be used if saline is not available. A special contact lens irrigating unit (Morgan lens) or a bottle of irrigant with intravenous tubing held to flush all eye surfaces may be useful. The eyelid is everted to identify and remove material from the conjunctival sac. A topical anesthetic, such as tetracaine drops, helps relieve pain, making inspection and irrigation easier. During irrigation, fluid is directed from the inner canthus of the eye to the outer or lateral canthus. Tipping the patient's head slightly to the affected side prevents contamination of the unaffected eye. Irrigation is continued until the pH of the eye is normal (in the range of 7.2 to 7.4). Following irrigation, a topical antibiotic ointment such as gentamicin ophthalmic is applied.

Penetrating wounds of the eye generally require surgical intervention by an ophthalmic surgeon. Immediate care focuses on relieving pain and protecting the eye from further injury. To prevent loss of intraocular contents, do not place pressure on the eye itself, but gently cover with sterile gauze or an eye pad. If a foreign body is embedded in or sticking out of the eye, no attempt is made to remove it. The object should be immobilized and the eye protected with a metal eye shield until an ophthalmologist can see the patient. A paper cup or other protective device may be used if the object is too large to use an eye shield. Patching the unaffected eye as well decreases ocular movement. Pain is managed using narcotic analgesics such as morphine. The patient may also require sedation (e.g., diazepam) and antiemetic medications to prevent vomiting.

Figure 46–7 ■ A nurse uses sterile normal saline to flush the eye of a patient with a suspected chemical burn.

Antibiotics such as intravenous cefazolin (Ancef) or gentamicin (Garamycin) are prescribed to prevent infection.

Interventions for the patient with blunt trauma to the eye include placing the patient on bed rest in semi-Fowler's position and protecting the eye from further injury with an eye shield. The unaffected eye is also patched to minimize eye movement. A carbonic anhydrase inhibitor such as acetazolamide (Diamox) or dichlorphenamide (Daranide) may be prescribed to reduce intraocular pressure.

Nursing Care

The nursing role involves educating people about the prevention of eye injuries and providing direct care to patients with eye injuries.

Health Promotion

Teaching related to eye injuries focuses on prevention and first-aid measures. Teaching individuals and groups how to prevent eye injuries is an important nursing role, especially for people involved in hazardous occupations and activities. Teach employees and participants in high-risk sports or activities how and when to use eye protection devices. Stress the importance of using seat belts and air bags to prevent eye injury in automobile crashes. Instruct patients to immediately flush the eye with copious amounts of water if a chemical splash occurs. Loose, visible foreign bodies can be removed using a clean, moistened cotton-tipped swab. If an abrasion, penetrating, or blunt injury is suspected, the eye should be covered loosely with sterile gauze and medical attention sought immediately. Instruct patients not to remove objects that penetrate the eye.

Nursing Diagnoses and Interventions

Ocular injuries require immediate interventions simultaneously with assessment and accurate history collection. The time, type, and extent of injury and the circumstances under which it occurred are determined. In addition, ask about pre-existing visual problems.

Impaired Tissue Integrity: Ocular

All types of eye trauma pose the risk of violating the integrity of the eye, threatening vision. The goals of nursing care, therefore, are preserving vision and the integrity of the eye, and preventing further damage.

- Assess vision in each eye and both eyes, with and without corrective lenses, on entry into the emergency department or primary care setting. *An initial assessment provides valuable information about the effect of the injury on the patient's vision and a baseline for future comparisons.*
- Inspect eye(s) carefully for evidence of foreign bodies, burns, penetrating injury, or blunt trauma. Note if lacerations, burns, or other trauma are evident in tissues surrounding the eye. *Eye trauma may be hidden by other injuries and, as a result, remain untreated.*
- If a burn or foreign body is present, anesthetic drops may be instilled and the eye irrigated either before or after the physician evaluates the patient. *Blepharism and eye pain

may impair assessment of the injured eye. Irrigation to remove the chemical is of higher priority than assessment of the eye.
- Loose foreign bodies may be removed using a moist, sterile, cotton-tipped applicator. *Prompt removal of foreign bodies may prevent corneal abrasion.*
- For a severe or penetrating injury, promote rest and stabilize the injured eye by applying an eye pad or gauze dressing loosely over both the affected and unaffected eye. Stabilize any penetrating object if possible. *These measures reduce eye movement and can help preserve the patient's vision.*
- Following treatment, apply eyedrops or ointment as prescribed and apply an eye pad or shield if ordered. *An eye pad is applied to the affected eye to reduce pain and photophobia and to promote healing.*

Community-Based Care

Following an injury, discuss the following topics with the patient and family:

- Prescribed medications and possible adverse effects
- Strategies to prevent further trauma
- Application of the eye pad or shield
- Avoidance of activities that increase intraocular pressure
- Importance of activity restrictions

The Patient with Uveitis

The middle vascular layer of the eye, including the choroid, the ciliary body, and the iris, is known as the uvea and uveal tract. *Uveitis* is inflammation of all or part of this vascular layer. *Iritis*, inflammation of the iris only, occurs more commonly than uveitis.

Uveitis is usually a disease limited to the eye; it may be idiopathic or caused by an autoimmune process, infection, parasitic disease, or trauma. Many cases can be linked to a systemic disease, often an arthritic or autoimmune disorder such as ankylosing spondylitis, Reiter's syndrome, rheumatoid arthritis, or sarcoidosis (∞ see Chapter 40). Uveitis has also been linked with tuberculosis and syphilis (Fauci et al., 2008). Manifestations of uveitis include pupillary constriction and erythema around the limbus. The patient may complain of severe eye pain and photophobia, as well as blurred vision.

Immunosuppressive therapy may be used to suppress the inflammatory response in patients with severe uveitis. Atropine may also be prescribed for associated inflammation of the iris. The patient may require analgesics such as acetaminophen and/or codeine for pain management. Nursing care is supportive, focusing on promotion of comfort and teaching about the disorder and its management.

The Patient with Cataracts

A **cataract** is an opacification (clouding) of the lens of the eye. This opacification can significantly interfere with light transmission to the retina and the ability to perceive images clearly.

Incidence and Risk Factors

Cataracts are a common and significant cause of visual deficits, affecting more than 22 million people over age 40 in the United States. By age 80, over half of the population is affected. In many cases, however, cataracts do not significantly impair vision. Cataracts affect slightly more women than men, and more Whites than people of other ethnicities. More than a million cataract removal surgeries are performed annually in the United States, costing an estimated 3.4 billion Medicare dollars (Prevent Blindness America, 2008).

FAST FACTS

The prevalence of cataracts in the United States increases rapidly with aging:

- 2.5% (just over 1 million) of adults ages 40 to 49 are affected.
- This increases to more than 2 million (or 6.8%) of those ages 50 to 59, and nearly doubles to over 4 million or 20% of adults ages 60 to 69.
- 68.3% of adults age 80 and older (over 6 million) are affected by cataract (NEI, 2008).

Age is the greatest single risk factor for cataract. Genetics may contribute to the risk, although the link is unclear. Environmental and lifestyle factors play a role: Long-term exposure to sunlight (UV-B rays) contributes; cigarette smoking and heavy alcohol consumption are associated with earlier cataract development. Although senile cataracts are by far the most common, cataracts also may be congenital or acquired in origin. Eye trauma, including injury to the lens capsule by a foreign body, blunt trauma, or exposure to heat or radiation, can precipitate cataract formation. Diabetes mellitus is associated with earlier development of cataracts, especially when the blood glucose level is not carefully controlled at or near normal levels. Certain drugs such as systemic or inhaled corticosteroids, chlorpromazine (Thorazine), and busulfan (Myleran) also prompt the formation of cataracts.

MEMORY CUE

To remember risk factors for cataracts, use the following mnemonic:

CATARACt:
Congenital
Aging
Toxicity (steroids, etc)
Accidents
Radiation (sunlight)
Altered metabolism (diabetes mellitus)
Cigarette smoking

Pathophysiology

The majority of cataracts are senile cataracts, formed as a result of the aging process. As the lens ages, its fibers and proteins change and degenerate. The proteins clump, clouding the lens and reducing light transmission to the retina. This process generally begins at the periphery of the lens, gradually spreading to involve the central portion. As the cataract continues to develop, the entire lens may become opaque. When only a portion of the lens is affected, the cataract is called immature. A mature cataract is opacity of the entire lens. In addition to clouding, the lens may discolor over time, affecting the ability to accurately discriminate colors.

Manifestations

Cataracts tend to occur bilaterally unless related to eye trauma. Fortunately, they tend to develop at different rates, and one cataract generally matures more rapidly than the other. As a cataract interferes with light transmission through the lens, visual acuity decreases, affecting both close and distance vision (Figure 46–8 ■). Light rays are scattered as they pass through the lens, causing complaints of glare. Glare affects the ability to adjust between light and dark environments. Color discrimination is impaired, particularly in the blue to purple range. When the cataract is mature, the pupil may appear cloudy gray or white rather than black.

Interdisciplinary Care

The diagnosis of a cataract is made based on the history and eye examination. Ophthalmoscopic examination confirms the diagnosis by identifying the location and extent of a cataract. As the cataract matures, ophthalmoscopy reveals a dark area instead of the red reflex.

Surgery

Surgical removal is the only treatment used at this time for cataracts; no medical treatment is available to prevent or treat them. If the patient presents with bilateral cataracts, surgery is only performed on one eye at a time. If an intraocular lens (an

Figure 46–8 ■ A scene as viewed by a patient with cataracts.

Source: Courtesy of National Eye Institute, National Institutes of Health.

artificial lens to replace the diseased lens of the eye) is to be implanted during surgery, the corneal curvature and antero-posterior diameter of the eye are measured prior to surgery to determine the lens power needed for the intraocular lens implant.

Surgical removal of the cataract and lens is indicated when the cataract has developed to the point that vision and activities of daily living are affected. A mature cataract may also be removed when it causes a secondary condition such as glaucoma or uveitis.

Cataract surgery is usually done on an outpatient basis, using local anesthesia. If general anesthesia is required, the patient may be hospitalized overnight. Extracapsular extraction, in which the anterior capsule, nucleus, and cortex of the lens are removed leaving the posterior capsule intact, is the procedure of choice (Figure 46–9 ■). Using an operating microscope, the surgeon makes a small incision at the edge of the cornea and extracts the lens via emulsification and aspiration. In this technique, ultrasound vibrations are used to break the lens material into fragments (phacoemulsification), which are then suctioned out of the eye (Porth & Matfin, 2009). The remaining capsule supports the lens implant and protects the retina.

After removal of the lens, a polymethylmethacrylate (PMMA or Plexiglas) or silicone intraocular lens is implanted to replace the light-focusing functions of the diseased lens. This implant rapidly restores binocular vision and depth perception. Following extracapsular lens removal, the intraocular lens is positioned in the posterior capsule behind the iris (see Figure 46–9). Currently available intraocular lenses allow for correction of refractive disorders of distance vision or astigmatism, often allowing the patient to no longer rely on corrective lenses for visual acuity (Goldman, Kiffel, & Weinstock, 2009). These specialized lenses are not always appropriate however. The patient with a preexisting refractive error may continue to require corrective lenses and often needs a prescriptive change after surgery.

Complications of cataract surgery are unusual and occur in less than 1% of the surgeries. Loss of vitreous humor, corneal edema, increased intraocular pressure, hemorrhage, inflammation or infection, retinal detachment, and displacement of the implanted lens are potential complications. Some patients may develop opacification of the remaining posterior capsule. Vision can be restored using laser capsulotomy (creating an opening for light to pass through the opacified capsule) or surgical incision into the posterior capsule to allow light to reach the retina (Fauci et al., 2008; Doherty, 2009).

✍ Nursing Care

Health Promotion

Advise all patients about the importance of protecting the eyes from UVB rays by wearing eye protection during activities such as welding and sunglasses with UVB protection when out of doors. Discuss the link between heavy smoking and cataract development. Provide anti-tobacco use education for young people and resources to stop smoking for people who do smoke.

Assessment

- *Health history:* Effect of vision changes on lifestyle and activities (e.g., ability to read, watch television, participate in work and recreational activities); history of smoking, diabetes, use of prescription drugs associated with increased risk of cataract.
- *Physical examination:* General health; visual acuity (using corrective lenses and Snellen chart) in each eye; presence of red reflex.

Nursing Diagnoses and Interventions

The patient with cataracts has few physical care nursing needs. Patient advocacy, psychologic and emotional support, and teaching/learning needs are typically of higher priority for

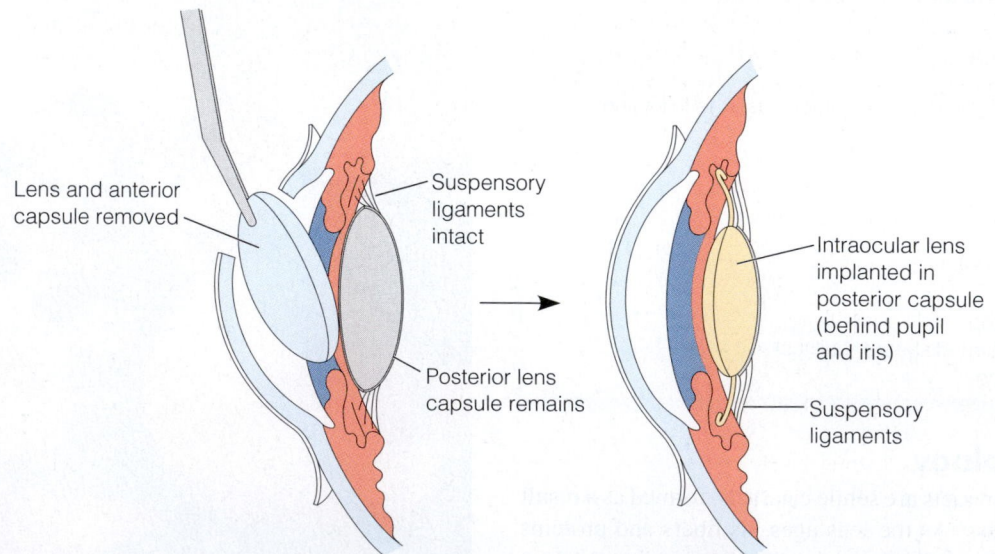

Figure 46–9 ■ Extracapsular cataract extraction with removal of the lens and anterior capsule, leaving the posterior capsule intact. The intraocular lens is implanted within posterior capsule.

Lens and anterior capsule removed

Suspensory ligaments intact

Posterior lens capsule remains

Intraocular lens implanted in posterior capsule (behind pupil and iris)

Suspensory ligaments

these patients. Review nursing care of the patient having eye surgery as outlined in the box on page 1585.

Decisional Conflict: Cataract Removal

With the initial diagnosis of cataract, the nurse often becomes an important information resource for the patient.

- Explain the nonemergent nature of the condition and help the patient determine the extent to which the cataract is affecting daily life. *This helps the patient decide when to proceed with surgery. Providing information about cataracts and their surgical removal also assists with decision making.*
- Attend to verbalized concerns about surgery and its outcome. Address questions factually and completely. *Fear of blindness is second only to fear of cancer for many patients. Careful listening, teaching, and a caring, understanding attitude can help the patient deal with this fear prior to surgery.*

Readiness for Enhanced Self-Health Management

- Assess for factors that may interfere with the patient's ability to provide self-care postoperatively. *A chronic condition such as arthritis that may affect the ability to administer eyedrops may indicate the need to include a family member in teaching.*
- Assess for other care needs that may be impacted by vision changes in the early postoperative period. *Other care needs, such as insulin injections, may suggest the need for home health or nursing care postoperatively.*

Community-Based Care

With the initial diagnosis, teaching focuses on the disorder, indications for surgery, and vision restoration following cataract removal. Teaching adaptive strategies to deal with effects of the cataract on vision and depth perception are also useful. When surgery is scheduled, provide pre- and postoperative teaching, including a significant other in teaching sessions. Reinforce the following information with written instructions:

- Initial limitations such as avoiding lifting, strenuous activity, sleeping on operative side, or getting water in the eye
- Importance of not rubbing or scratching the eye
- Prescribed medications and side effects
- Importance of follow-up appointments
- Manifestations of postoperative complications such as eye pain, decreased visual acuity or other change in vision, headache, nausea, or itching and redness of the affected eye
- Instillation of eyedrops, and application of eye shield (for nighttime use)
- Anticipated vision changes as appropriate

The Patient with Glaucoma

Glaucoma is a condition characterized by optic neuropathy with gradual loss of peripheral vision and, usually, increased intraocular pressure of the eye. Glaucoma is a silent thief of vision. The patient typically experiences no manifestations other than narrowing of the visual field, which occurs so gradually that it often goes unnoticed until late in the disease process.

Incidence and Risk Factors

Glaucoma affects about 2.2 million people over the age of 40 in the United States; it remains undetected in approximately 25% of these cases. Glaucoma is a leading cause of blindness worldwide and the leading cause of blindness among African Americans. Age and race are the primary identified risk factors; it is more common in Blacks and Hispanics than in Whites (Prevent Blindness America, 2008).

Glaucoma is usually a primary condition without an identified cause. Primary glaucoma is most common in adults over the age of 60, but may be a congenital condition in infants and children. Secondary glaucoma can develop as a result of infection or inflammation of the eye, cataract, tumor, hemorrhage, or eye trauma.

Pathophysiology

Aqueous humor, a thick fluid, occupies both the anterior and posterior chambers of the eye. The normal intraocular pressure of approximately 12 to 15 mmHg is maintained by a balance between the production of aqueous humor in the ciliary body, its flow through the pupil from the posterior to the anterior chamber of the eye, and its outflow or absorption through the trabecular meshwork and canal of Schlemm (see Figure 45–3). When this balance is disrupted, usually because of a decrease in the outflow or absorption of aqueous humor, the intraocular pressure increases. Although the exact relationship is unclear, it appears that increased intraocular pressure injures the optic nerve. Axons in the periphery of the optic disc are damaged first. As optic fibers are destroyed, the rim of the optic disc shrinks, and the normal depression in its center (the *optic cup*) becomes larger and deeper (called optic "cupping"). These changes to the optic disc are visible before visual field changes can be detected (Porth & Matfin, 2009). As the disease progresses, there is a painless, progressive narrowing of the visual field (Figure 46–10 ■) and eventual blindness. Vision loss is often significant before the patient seeks treatment and glaucoma is diagnosed.

Primary glaucoma in adults has two major forms: open-angle glaucoma and angle-closure glaucoma. Both terms refer to the angle formed at the point where the iris meets the cornea

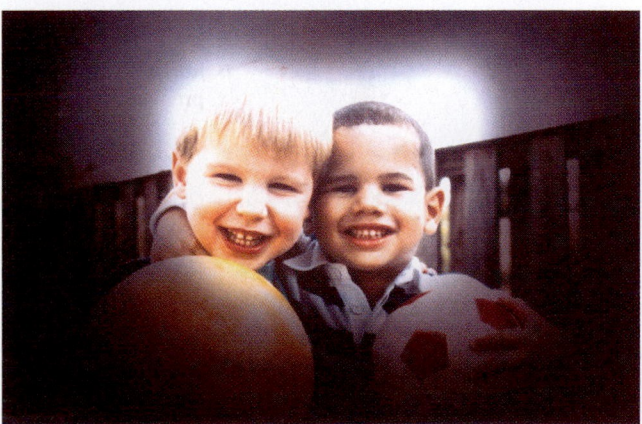

Figure 46–10 ■ Narrowing of visual fields typical of untreated glaucoma.
Source: Courtesy of National Eye Institute, National Institutes of Health.

Glaucoma or Blind Patient Video

in the eye's anterior chamber (Figure 46–11 ■). Forms of primary glaucoma are compared in Table 46–2.

Open-Angle Glaucoma

Open-angle glaucoma, often called chronic simple glaucoma, is the most common form in adults, accounting for approximately 90% of all glaucoma. Its cause is unknown; it is thought to have a hereditary component, but no clear inheritance pattern can be identified. Open-angle glaucoma occurs more frequently and at an earlier age in African Americans than in Whites (McPhee et al., 2008).

In open-angle glaucoma, the anterior chamber angle between the iris and cornea is normal (Figure 46–11A), hence the term *open angle*. However, the flow of aqueous humor through the trabecular meshwork and into the canal of Schlemm is relatively obstructed; the cause of this obstruction is unknown. Restricted outflow leads to an increased amount of fluid in the eye and increased intraocular pressure. Open-angle glaucoma tends to be a chronic, gradually progressive disease. The trabecular meshwork increasingly inhibits the outflow of aqueous humor, and the intraocular pressure gradually

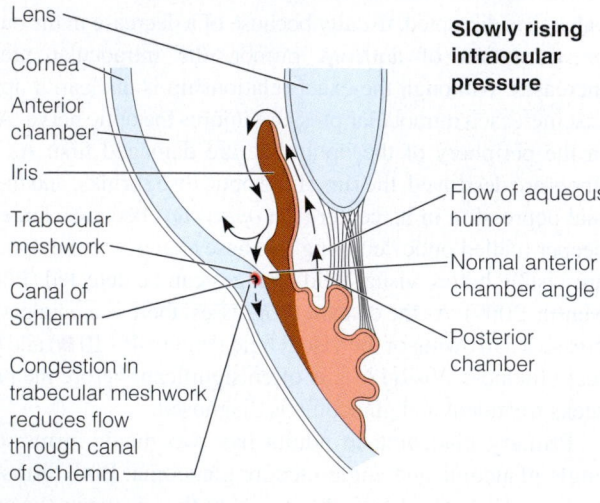

Lens
Cornea
Anterior chamber
Iris
Trabecular meshwork
Canal of Schlemm
Congestion in trabecular meshwork reduces flow through canal of Schlemm

Slowly rising intraocular pressure

Flow of aqueous humor
Normal anterior chamber angle
Posterior chamber

A

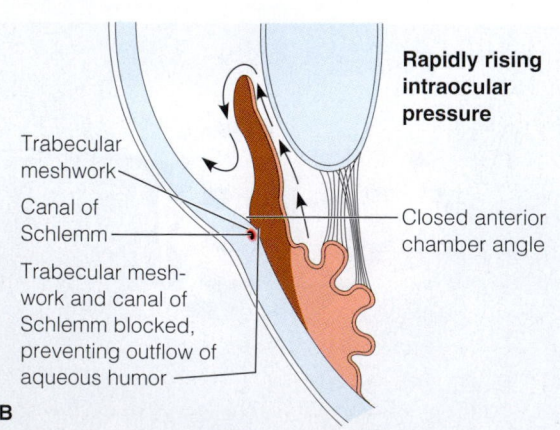

Trabecular meshwork
Canal of Schlemm
Trabecular meshwork and canal of Schlemm blocked, preventing outflow of aqueous humor

Rapidly rising intraocular pressure

Closed anterior chamber angle

B

Figure 46–11 ■ Forms of primary adult glaucoma. *A,* In chronic open-angle glaucoma, the anterior chamber angle remains open, but drainage of aqueous humor through the canal of Schlemm is impaired. *B,* In acute angle-closure glaucoma, the angle of the iris and anterior chamber narrows, obstructing the outflow of aqueous humor.

increases. The result is neuronal ischemia and optic nerve degeneration, leading to gradual loss of vision.

Open-angle glaucoma typically affects both eyes, although the pressures and progression may not be symmetric.

MANIFESTATIONS   Open-angle glaucoma is painless, with gradual loss of visual fields. This loss of peripheral vision generally occurs so gradually that the patient is often unaware of it and only when it is detected through a comprehensive vision examination is it found. Intraocular pressure usually, but not always, is elevated (Fauci et al., 2008).

Angle-Closure Glaucoma

Acute angle-closure (also called narrow-angle or closed-angle) glaucoma is the other, less common form of primary glaucoma in adults. It accounts for approximately 5% to 10% of all cases of glaucoma (Porth & Matfin, 2009). Approximately 1% of people over the age of 35 have narrowed anterior chamber angles; the incidence is higher in older adults and in people of Far Eastern, Asian, or Inuit (Alaska native) ancestry (Porth & Matfin, 2009).

Narrowing of the anterior chamber angle (see Figure 46–11A for an illustration of the normal anterior chamber angle) occurs because of corneal flattening or bulging of the iris into the anterior chamber. When the lens thickens during accommodation or the iris thickens during pupil dilation, this angle can close completely. Closure of the angle blocks the outflow of aqueous humor through the trabecular meshwork and canal of Schlemm, and the intraocular pressure rises abruptly (Figure 46–11B). This abrupt increase in intraocular pressure damages the neurons of the retina and the optic nerve, leading to a rapid and permanent loss of vision if not treated promptly.

Episodes of angle-closure glaucoma are typically unilateral. However, a history of angle-closure glaucoma of one eye increases the risk that it will occur in the other eye.

Because of the effect of pupil dilation on aqueous outflow in angle-closure glaucoma, episodes often occur in association with darkness, emotional upset, or other factors that cause the pupil to dilate. Patients may have intermittent episodes lasting several hours before having a more typical prolonged attack of angle-closure glaucoma. For patients with a history of the condition, it is vital to avoid medications such as atropine and other anticholinergics, which have a mydriatic or pupil-dilating effect.

MANIFESTATIONS   Symptoms such as severe eye and face pain, general malaise, nausea and vomiting, seeing colored halos around lights, and an abrupt decrease in visual acuity are associated with acute episodes of angle-closure glaucoma. The conjunctiva of the affected eye may be reddened and the cornea clouded with corneal edema. The pupil may be fixed (nonreactive to light) at midpoint. Some patients may experience periodic mild attacks, usually in the evening, with eye discomfort, impaired vision, and colored rings around lights (Plester, 2008).

Interdisciplinary Care

Although glaucoma cannot be predicted, prevented, or cured, in most cases it can be controlled and vision preserved if diagnosed early. Because the most prevalent type of glaucoma, open-angle glaucoma, has few symptoms, routine eye examinations are

TABLE 46–2 A Comparison of Open-Angle and Angle-Closure Glaucoma

	OPEN-ANGLE GLAUCOMA	ANGLE-CLOSURE GLAUCOMA
Incidence	▪ Common ▪ Accounts for 90% of all cases of glaucoma	▪ Uncommon
Risk Factors	▪ Over age 35 ▪ Genetic link ▪ African American ancestry	▪ Narrow anterior chamber angle ▪ Aging ▪ Asian ancestry
Pathophysiology	▪ Impaired aqueous outflow through the canal of Schlemm ▪ Cause unknown ▪ Gradual, consistent increase in intraocular pressure ▪ Usually bilateral	▪ Pupil dilation or lens accommodation causes already narrowed angle to close, blocking aqueous outflow ▪ Rapid rise in intraocular pressure ▪ Usually unilateral
Manifestations	▪ No initial manifestations ▪ Frequent lens changes in glasses ▪ Impaired dark adaptation ▪ Halos around lights ▪ Gradual reduction of visual fields with preservation of central vision until late in the disease ▪ Mild to severe increased intraocular pressure	▪ Abrupt onset of eye pain, headache ▪ Decreased visual acuity ▪ Nausea and vomiting ▪ Reddened conjunctiva ▪ Cloudy cornea ▪ Fixed pupil ▪ Rapid, significant increase in intraocular pressure
Management	▪ Topical medications such as beta-blockers, adrenergics, prostaglandin analogs ▪ Carbonic anhydrase inhibitors ▪ Laser trabeculoplasty, trabeculectomy	▪ Topical miotics or beta-blockers ▪ Systemic osmotic agents, carbonic anhydrase inhibitors ▪ Laser iridotomy or peripheral iridectomy

recommended for early detection. Measurement of intraocular pressure, funduscopy to assess the optic disc, and visual field testing are used for diagnosis and monitoring of treatment effectiveness.

Diagnosis

The following diagnostic studies are used to detect and evaluate for the presence, severity, type, and effects of glaucoma.

■ *Tonometry* indirectly measures intraocular pressure (Figure 46–12 ▪). Contact or noncontact tonometry may be used. Routine tonometry screening is recommended for all people over the age of 60. A single elevated pressure reading does not warrant a diagnosis of glaucoma; variations in

intraocular pressure occur throughout the day. ∞ See Chapter 45 for more information about tonometry and related nursing care.
■ *Funduscopy* (visual inspection of the optic fundus using an ophthalmoscope) identifies pallor and an increase in the size and depth of the optic cup on the optic disc. These changes are significant for diagnosing glaucoma.
■ *Gonioscopy* uses a gonioscope to measure the depth of the anterior chamber. This test differentiates open-angle from angle-closure glaucoma.
■ *Visual field testing* (Figure 46–13 ▪) identifies the degree of central visual field narrowing and peripheral vision loss. The patient with glaucoma may retain 20/20 central vision even though there is severe peripheral vision loss.

Medications

Although medications cannot cure glaucoma, many patients with open-angle glaucoma can control intraocular pressure and preserve vision indefinitely with medications. Medications are used alone or in combination with the timing and dosage individually determined by pressure measurements. The primary pharmacologic agents used to treat glaucoma are topical beta-adrenergic blocking agents, adrenergics (mydriatics), prostaglandin analogs, or carbonic anhydrase inhibitors. An oral carbonic anhydrase inhibitor also may be used.

Prostaglandin analogs such as latanoprost (Xalatan) are generally the drugs of choice for treating chronic glaucoma as they can be administered daily and have a low adverse effect rate. These drugs increase aqueous outflow. Although they have fewer systemic effects, these drugs may cause conjunctival hyperemia and permanent changes in the color of the iris and eyebrows.

Figure 46–12 ▪ An eye professional uses a tonometer to indirectly measure the intraocular pressure of a patient's eye.

Source: Courtesy of National Eye Institute, National Institutes of Health.

Figure 46–13 ■ Visual field testing. Peripheral vision or visual fields are assessed by testing the patient's ability to detect an object brought into the line of vision from the periphery. The patient's peripheral vision is compared to the nurse examiner's. Each eye is tested separately.

Topical beta-adrenergic blocking agents decrease the production of aqueous humor in the ciliary body. Beta-adrenergic blockers can be used once or twice a day, depending on the drug and dosage form. When administering beta-blockers or teaching about their use, it is important to remember that ophthalmic preparations can produce systemic effects, including bronchospasm, bradycardia, and heart failure.

The adrenergic agonist brimonidine may be prescribed along with a beta-blocker or if beta-blockers are contraindicated (e.g., in a patient with heart failure, asthma, or COPD). Another adrenergic agonist, apraclonidine, may be prescribed when other drugs do not sufficiently reduce intraocular pressure, but adverse effects make it inappropriate for long-term use (McPhee et al., 2008).

Dorzolamide (Trusopt), a carbonic anhydrase inhibitor, decreases the production of aqueous humor and reduces intraocular pressure. It is used with other drugs to control pressures and in patients for whom beta-blockers are contraindicated because of heart failure or reactive airway disease (asthma). Acetazolamide (Diamox), a systemic carbonic anhydrase inhibitor, also may be used for some patients.

Nursing implications for the medications used to control chronic glaucoma are outlined in the Medication Administration box on page 1595.

In acute angle-closure glaucoma, diuretics may be administered intravenously to achieve a rapid decrease in intraocular pressure prior to surgical intervention. Both the carbonic anhydrase inhibitor acetazolamide and osmotic diuretics, such as mannitol, are used. Fast-acting miotic drops, such as pilocarpine, are also administered to constrict the pupil and draw the iris away from the angle and from the canal of Schlemm. Prostaglandin analogs, beta-blockers, and adrenergic agents also may be given by topical application (Fauci et al., 2008).

Surgery

Surgical intervention is indicated for patients with acute angle-closure glaucoma and for patients with chronic open-angle glaucoma that is not effectively controlled by medication.

Surgical management of chronic open-angle glaucoma involves improving the drainage of aqueous humor from the anterior chamber of the eye. Trabeculoplasty and trabeculectomy filtration surgery are the most commonly used procedures.

In a *laser trabeculoplasty,* an argon laser is aimed through a gonioscope to create multiple laser burns spaced evenly around the trabecular meshwork. As the burns heal, the scars they create cause tension, stretching and opening the meshwork. This noninvasive technique is the treatment of choice because it requires no incision and can be performed as an outpatient procedure.

Trabeculectomy is a type of filtration surgery in which a permanent fistula is created to drain aqueous humor from the anterior chamber of the eye. A portion of trabecular meshwork is removed, and a flap of sclera is left unsutured to create a channel or fistula between the anterior chamber and the subconjunctival space. Aqueous humor is able to drain into the space under the conjunctiva, where it can be absorbed into the systemic circulation. A trabeculectomy is usually performed under general anesthesia and requires hospitalization.

If these procedures are not fully effective, either photocoagulation using an argon laser (heat) or cyclocryotherapy using a probe to freeze tissue may be employed to destroy portions of the ciliary body. This tissue destruction reduces the production of aqueous humor, subsequently reducing intraocular pressure. Another surgical procedure involves insertion of a glaucoma drainage device that regulates the outflow of aqueous humor.

Surgical procedures used in the treatment of acute angle-closure glaucoma include gonioplasty, laser iridotomy, and peripheral iridectomy. Because of the high risk for a future attack of angle-closure glaucoma in the unaffected eye, these procedures are often performed prophylactically.

In *gonioplasty*, the healing and scarring of microscopic lesions created at the periphery of the iris draw the iris away from the cornea, widening the anterior chamber. This widening of the chamber increases the angle and opens drainage channels for aqueous humor.

Laser iridotomy is a noninvasive procedure using a laser to create multiple small perforations in the iris of the eye. These perforations allow aqueous humor to drain from the posterior chamber to the anterior chamber and out through the trabecular meshwork and the canal of Schlemm. During an *iridectomy,* a small segment of the iris is removed to facilitate the flow of aqueous humor between the posterior and anterior chambers and to open the anterior chamber angle.

MEDICATION ADMINISTRATION   The Patient with Glaucoma

ADRENERGIC AGONISTS (MYDRIATICS)

Brimonidine (Alphagan)

Apraclonidine

Adrenergic agonists dilate the pupil, reduce the production of aqueous humor, and increase its absorption, effectively reducing intraocular pressure in open-angle glaucoma.

Nursing Responsibilities

- Assess the patient for contraindications and adverse reactions to adrenergic agonists, including acute angle-closure glaucoma, hypertension, cardiac dysrhythmias, and coronary heart disease.
- Assess for central nervous system side effects of anxiety, nervousness, and muscle tremors. If these side effects are severe, notify the physician.
- Assess for a hypersensitivity reaction, including itching, lid edema, and discharge from the eyes. Notify the physician if you notice these signs.

Health Education for the Patient and Family

- Report any change in visual acuity or eye pain. (Eye pain may indicate an attack of angle-closure glaucoma and must be reported to the physician immediately.)
- Avoid over-the-counter sinus and cold medications containing pseudoephedrine and phenylephrine. They may accentuate the side effects of this drug.

BETA-ADRENERGIC BLOCKERS

Betaxolol (Betoptic)

Carteolol (Cartrol, Ocupress)

Levobunolol (Betagan)

Metipranolol (OptiPranolol)

Timolol (Timoptic)

Selected beta-adrenergic blockers reduce intraocular pressure by decreasing the production of aqueous humor. Because beta-blockers do not affect pupil size and lens accommodation, they do not have the adverse effects on visual acuity that adrenergic agonists do. Their systemic effects, however, may limit their usefulness for certain patients.

Nursing Responsibilities

- Assess the patient for allergies or contraindications to beta-blocker therapy, including asthma, chronic obstructive pulmonary disease (COPD), heart block, and heart failure.
- Maintain pressure over the lacrimal sac after administration to prevent systemic absorption.
- Assess for side effects such as bradycardia, hypotension, and depression.
- Teach about the drug, its dose, administration, desired effects, and side effects.

Health Education for the Patient and Family

- After instilling the eyedrops, put pressure on the lacrimal sac, at the corner of the eye near the bridge of the nose, to keep the drug from entering your system.
- Your vision may be blurred during the initial period of therapy, but it will improve as you continue to use the drug.
- Report adverse effects, including worsening vision, difficulty breathing, reduced exercise tolerance, and sweating or flushing, to the physician.

CARBONIC ANHYDRASE INHIBITORS

Dorzolamide (Trusopt)

Brinzolamide (Azopt)

Acetazolamide (Diamox)

The carbonic anhydrate inhibitors lower intraocular pressure and are used primarily as adjunctive therapy. Dorzolamide and brinzolamide are administered as eyedrops, whereas acetazolamide may given PO, IM, or IV.

Nursing Responsibilities

- Assess for allergies or other contraindications to the use of carbonic anhydrase inhibitors, including known allergy to sulfa, or severe renal or hepatic disease.
- Monitor for increased drug interactions of amphetamines, procainamide, quinidine, tricyclic antidepressants, and ephedrine and pseudoephedrine.
- Assess daily weight, intake and output, serum electrolytes, and vital signs in patients taking oral or parenteral carbonic anhydrase inhibitors.
- Administer PO in the morning to prevent sleep disruption because of the diuretic effect.
- If used with another topical ophthalmic, administer 10 minutes apart.
- Teach the patient about the drug, its dose, administration, desired effects, and side effects.

Health Education for the Patient and Family

- For oral medications, maintain a fluid intake of 2 to 3 L per day and rise slowly from lying or sitting positions because you may feel dizzy when you first stand (orthostatic hypotension).
- For topical medications, notify the physician if you have prolonged eye irritation.

PROSTAGLANDIN ANALOGS

Bimatoprost (Lumigan)

Latanoprost (Xalatan)

Travoprost (Travatan)

The prostaglandin analog drugs relax the ciliary muscle, improving the outflow of aqueous humor and reducing intraocular pressure. These drugs have the advantage of requiring only a single daily dose. They do, however, have some adverse effects such as blurred vision and stinging, and, when used long term, cause permanent darkening of the iris of the eye and eyebrows, increased growth of eyelashes, and conjunctival hyperemia (redness).

Nursing Responsibilities

- Assess and note eye color, presence of inflammation, exudates, or pain.
- Note vital signs and most recent liver function test results because these may be altered by the drug.

Health Education for the Patient and Family

- Use once daily at bedtime as directed. This drug may blur vision; use at bedtime minimizes associated safety risks.
- Remove contact lenses before administering this drug.
- Minor eye discomfort, including burning and tearing, may occur with this drug. Notify your doctor if adverse effects are severe or intolerable.
- This drug may cause darkening of your iris, the skin around the eyes, and the eyebrows, as well as increased growth of the eyelashes. These color changes are permanent but will not progress if the drug is discontinued by your doctor.

∽ Nursing Care

When planning and providing nursing care for the patient with glaucoma, both the specific form of the disease and its actual or potential effects on the patient's vision, lifestyle, safety, and psychosocial well-being must be considered. In the hospitalized patient, glaucoma is typically a concurrent diagnosis rather than the primary reason for seeking care, unless the diagnosis is acute angle-closure glaucoma. For additional nursing activities for the patient with glaucoma, see the accompanying Case Study & Nursing Care Plan.

Health Promotion

Although glaucoma cannot be prevented, its severity and potentially deleterious permanent effects can be limited with early visual screening. The nurse assumes an important role in educating the public about the risk factors for glaucoma such as increased age, and the higher incidence in African Americans and Asians. All people over the age of 40 are encouraged to receive an eye examination every 2 to 4 years, including tonometry screening. Those with a predominant family history should be evaluated more frequently, every 1 to 2 years. After the age of 65, yearly ophthalmologic examinations are recommended.

Assessment

Collect the following data through a health history and physical examination (∞ see Chapter 45).

- *Health history:* Family history; presence of altered vision, halos, and excessive tearing; sudden, severe eye pain; use of corrective lenses; most recent eye examination.
- *Physical examination:* Distant and near vision, peripheral fields, retina for optic nerve cupping.

Nursing Diagnoses and Interventions

Nursing care planning focuses on problems associated with the temporary or permanent visual impairment, the resultant increased risk for injury, and the psychosocial problems of anxiety and coping.

Disturbed Sensory Perception: Visual

Whether glaucoma and resulting impaired vision is the patient's primary problem or a preexisting condition in a patient with another disorder, it must be a primary consideration in nursing care planning.

EVIDENCE FOR NURSING CARE — **The Patient with Glaucoma**

Selected resources that nurses may find helpful when planning evidence-based nursing care follow.

- National Collaborating Center for Acute Care. (2009, April). *Glaucoma. Diagnosis and management of chronic open angle glaucoma and ocular hypertension.* London, UK: National Institute for Health and Clinical Excellence (NICE).
- U.S. Preventive Services Task Force. (2009). Clinical guidelines. Screening for impaired visual acuity in older adults: U.S. Preventive Services Task Force recommendation statement. *Annals of Internal Medicine, 151,* 37–43.

- Address by name and identify yourself with each interaction. Orient to time, place, person, and situation as indicated. State the purpose of your visit. *The patient with impaired vision must rely on input from the other senses. A lack of visual cues increases the importance of verbal ones. For example, the patient with impaired vision cannot see the nurse checking an intravenous infusion and needs a verbal explanation of who is in the room and why. When the patient's normal daily routine is disrupted by illness or hospitalization, additional sensory input such as a radio, television, and explanations of the routine and activities are useful to maintain the patient's orientation.*

- Provide any visual aids that are routinely used. Keep them close, making sure that the patient knows where they are and can reach them easily. *Easy access encourages the patient to use these items and enhances the ability to provide self-care.*

- Orient to the environment. Explain the location of the call bell, personal items, and the furniture in the room. If able, tour patient's room, including the bathroom and sink. *Patients with visual impairments are usually very capable of providing self-care in a known environment.*

- Provide other tools or items that can help compensate for diminished vision:
  a. Bright, nonglare lighting
  b. Books, magazines, and instructions in large print
  c. Books on tape
  d. Telephones with oversize pushbuttons
  e. A clock with numbers and hands that can be felt

- Assist with meals by doing the following:
  a. Reading menu selections and marking choices.
  b. Describing the position of foods on a meal tray according to the clock system, for example, "On the plate, the peas are at 9 o'clock, the mashed potatoes at 1 o'clock, and the chicken breast at 6 o'clock. The milk glass is at 2 o'clock on the tray above the plate, and coffee is at 11 o'clock."
  c. Placing the utensils in a readily accessible position.
  d. Removing lids from containers, buttering the bread, and cutting meat, as needed.
  e. If the visual impairment is new or temporary, the patient may need feeding or continued assistance during the meal.
  Providing assistance during eating is important to maintain the patient's nutritional status. The patient may be ashamed of needing help or embarrassed to request it and may respond by not eating or by claiming not to be hungry.

- Assist with mobility and ambulation as needed:
  a. Have the patient hold your arm or elbow, and walk slightly ahead as a guide. Do not hold the patient's arm or elbow.
  b. Describe the surroundings and progress as you proceed. Warn in advance of potential hazards, turns, and steps.
  c. Teach to feel the chair, bed, or commode with the hands and the back of the legs before sitting.
  These measures help ensure the patient's safety while providing for mobility and helping prevent complications associated with immobility.

- If the vision loss is unilateral and recent, provide instructions related to unilateral vision loss and change in depth perception:
  a. Caution about the loss of depth perception and teach safety precautions, such as reaching slowly for objects and using visual cues as to distance, especially when driving.

b. Teach to scan, turning the head fully toward the affected side to identify potential hazards and looking up and down to compensate for the loss of depth perception. *The patient with a unilateral vision loss is often unaware of its effect on peripheral vision and depth perception.*

Risk for Injury

Whether the patient is experiencing a sudden loss of vision due to acute angle-closure glaucoma or significant visual impairment due to inadequately managed chronic glaucoma, both are at an increased risk for injury. Patients who have had surgical interventions for glaucoma are at even greater risk.

■ Assess ability to perform ADLs. *Patients may be reluctant to request assistance, believing that they should be able to perform these familiar tasks. Careful assessment and provision of needed assistance help prevent injury and maintain the patient's self-esteem.*

■ Notify housekeeping and place a sign on the patient's door to alert all personnel not to change the arrangement of the patient's room. *The patient with impaired vision is at high risk for falling when in an unfamiliar environment. It is important to maintain a safe, familiar room when the patient is hospitalized.*

■ Raise two or three side rails on the patient's bed. *Raised rails remind patients to ask for assistance before ambulating in an unfamiliar environment.*

■ Discuss possible adaptations in the home to help the patient remain as independent as possible and prevent falls or other injuries. *Often minor changes in the home environment, such as removing scatter rugs and small items of furniture, allow the patient to navigate safely in this already familiar environment.*

> **SAFETY ALERT**
> Keep traffic areas free of clutter to reduce the risk for injury in patients with impaired vision.

Anxiety

The actual or potential loss of sight threatens the patient's self-concept, role functioning, patterns of interaction, and, potentially, environment. The patient with impaired vision who functions well in a familiar environment will feel anxious in the unfamiliar setting of a hospital or care facility.

■ Assess for verbal and nonverbal indications of level of anxiety and for normal coping mechanisms. Repeated expressions of concern or denial that the vision change will affect the patient's life indicate anxiety. Nonverbal indicators include tension, difficulty concentrating or thinking, restlessness, poor eye contact, and changes in vocalization (rapid speech, voice quivering). Physical indicators include tachycardia, dilated pupils, cool and clammy skin, and tremors. *The patient may not recognize this feeling as anxiety. Identifying and acknowledging the anxiety state can help the patient recognize and deal with it.*

■ Encourage to verbalize fears, anger, and feelings of anxiety. *Verbalizing helps externalize the anxiety and allows fears to be addressed.*

■ Discuss perception of the eye condition and its effects on lifestyle and roles. *Discussion provides an opportunity to correct misperceptions and introduce alternative activities and assistive devices for patients with visual impairments.*

■ Introduce yourself when entering the room, explain all procedures fully before and as they are being performed, and use touch to convey proximity and caring. *The patient with impaired vision must rely on the other senses to make up for the loss of sight. Because the patient cannot see what you are doing, complete explanations of even simple tasks such as refilling a water glass help to relieve anxiety.*

■ Identify coping strategies that have been useful in the past and adapt these strategies to the present situation. *Previously successful coping strategies may be employed to increase the patient's sense of control.*

Using NANDA, NIC, and NOC

Linkages between a selected NANDA nursing diagnosis, NIC, and NOC for the patient with glaucoma are shown in the chart that follows.

Community-Based Care

Patients with glaucoma require teaching about lifetime strategies for managing the disease at home. They need to understand the importance of lifelong therapy to control the disease and prevent blindness. If a permanent visual impairment has resulted, the patient needs information on achieving the maximum possible independence while maintaining safety. The following topics should be discussed with the patient and family:

■ Prescribed medications, including proper way to instill eyedrops

■ Importance of not taking certain prescription and over-the-counter medications without consulting a physician

■ Periodic eye examinations with intraocular pressure measurement

■ Risks, warning signs, and management of acute angle-closure glaucoma

■ Possible surgical options

■ Community resources, such as Visually Impaired Society, local library, and transportation services

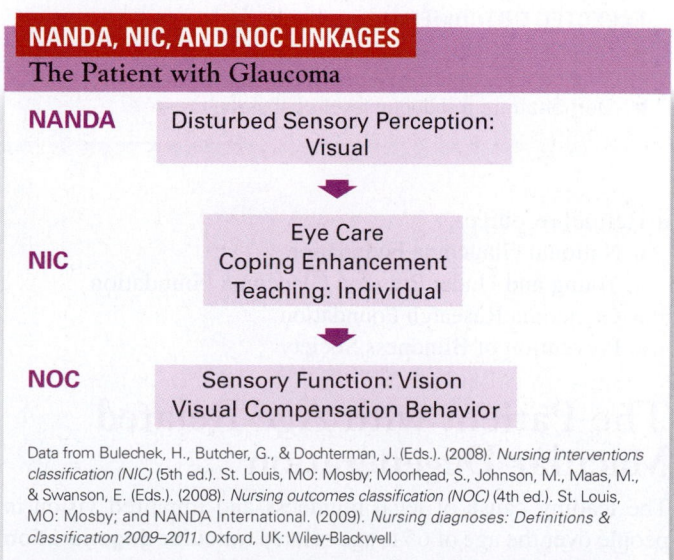

NANDA, NIC, AND NOC LINKAGES
The Patient with Glaucoma

NANDA	Disturbed Sensory Perception: Visual
NIC	Eye Care Coping Enhancement Teaching: Individual
NOC	Sensory Function: Vision Visual Compensation Behavior

Data from Bulechek, H., Butcher, G., & Dochterman, J. (Eds.). (2008). *Nursing interventions classification (NIC)* (5th ed.). St. Louis, MO: Mosby; Moorhead, S., Johnson, M., Maas, M., & Swanson, E. (Eds.). (2008). *Nursing outcomes classification (NOC)* (4th ed.). St. Louis, MO: Mosby; and NANDA International. (2009). *Nursing diagnoses: Definitions & classification 2009–2011.* Oxford, UK: Wiley-Blackwell.

Lila Rainey is an 80-year-old widow who lives alone in the house she and her late husband built 50 years ago. She has worn glasses for nearsightedness since she was a young girl, and now wears bifocals to correct her near vision as well. She was diagnosed 4 years ago with chronic open-angle glaucoma, for which she takes timolol maleate (Timoptic) 0.5%. Recently she has noticed difficulty reading and watching television despite a new lens prescription. She has stopped driving at night because the glare of oncoming headlights makes it difficult for her to see. Mrs. Rainey's ophthalmologist has told her that she has cataracts but that they do not need to come out until they bother her. Although her glaucoma is still controlled with timolol maleate 0.5%, one drop in each eye twice a day, her intraocular pressure measurements have been gradually increasing. Mrs. Rainey has taken 325 mg of aspirin daily since a transient ischemic attack 8 years ago. She is being admitted to the outpatient surgery unit for a cataract removal and intraocular lens implant in her right eye.

ASSESSMENT

Mrs. Rainey is admitted to the eye surgery unit by Susan Schafer, RN. In her assessment, Ms. Schafer finds Mrs. Rainey to be alert and oriented, though apprehensive about her upcoming surgery. Assessment findings include BP 134/72, P 86, R 18. Mrs. Rainey's neurologic, respiratory, cardiovascular, and abdominal assessments are essentially normal. Her pupils are round and equal, and react briskly to light and accommodation. Her conjunctivae are pink; sclera and corneas are clear. Using the ophthalmoscope, Ms. Schafer notes that the red reflex in Mrs. Rainey's right eye is diminished. Ophthalmic examination shows visual acuity of 20/150 OD (right eye) and 20/50 OS (left eye) with corrective lenses. Her intraocular pressures are 21 mmHg OD and 17 mmHg OS. On funduscopic exam, no disease of the blood vessels, retina, macula, or disc is found. Ms. Schafer reviews the operative procedure with Mrs. Rainey, answering her questions and telling her what to expect after surgery. Following preoperative protocols, Mrs. Rainey is prepared and transported to surgery.

DIAGNOSES

- *Disturbed Sensory Perception: Visual* related to myopia and lens extraction
- *Anxiety* related to anticipated surgery
- *Readiness for Enhanced Knowledge* related to postoperative care

EXPECTED OUTCOMES

- Regain sufficient visual acuity to maintain ADLs, including reading and watching television for enjoyment.
- Demonstrate a reduced level of anxiety.

- Demonstrate the procedure for instilling eyedrops postoperatively.
- Demonstrate knowledge of the home care she will require after surgery, signs of complications, and actions to take if complications occur.

PLANNING AND IMPLEMENTATION

- Provide a safe environment, placing the call light and personal care items within easy reach.
- Encourage Mrs. Rainey to express her fears about surgery and its potential effect on vision.
- Explain all procedures related to surgery and recovery.
- Instruct her to avoid rubbing the eye, shutting the eyelids tightly, lifting, or straining to have a bowel movement. Teach her to wear glasses during the day and an eye shield at night to prevent injury to the surgical site.
- Explain and demonstrate the procedure for administering eyedrops.
- Provide verbal and written instructions about postoperative care, including a schedule of follow-up examinations, potential complications, and actions to take in response.

EVALUATION

Mrs. Rainey is discharged the morning after her surgery. She is visibly relieved when the eye patch is removed because her vision in the operated eye is better than before surgery, even without her glasses. She is able to relate the recommended activity restrictions. Mrs. Rainey administers her own eyedrops before discharge and relates an understanding of the prescribed postoperative care and safety precautions. Mrs. Rainey's daughter plans to visit her mother two to three times a week to help with laundry and vacuuming until Mrs. Rainey is able to resume all her household activities. Mrs. Rainey says that she won't "be so scared when I need my other eye done." She understands the chronic nature of her glaucoma and says that her vision is too important for her to neglect her timolol drops and routine eye exams.

CRITICAL THINKING IN THE NURSING PROCESS

1. Why did it become more difficult to control Mrs. Rainey's intraocular pressure as her cataract matured?
2. Identify medications that are commonly prescribed following cataract surgery. What are the risks of interactions between these medications and Mrs. Rainey's timolol drops?
3. Develop a care plan for the nursing diagnosis *Bathing Self-Care Deficit,* related to visual impairment and instructions to avoid getting water in the eye.

See Evaluating Your Response in Appendix C.

- Helpful resources:
  - National Glaucoma Foundation
  - Young and Under Pressure Glaucoma Foundation
  - Glaucoma Research Foundation
  - Prevention of Blindness Society

The Patient with Age-Related Macular Degeneration

The leading cause of legal blindness and impaired vision in people over the age of 65 is age-related **macular degeneration** (AMD) (Prevent Blindness America, 2008).

Although the exact cause of AMD is unknown, factors associated with it include aging, female gender, smoking, race, and genetic factors. Whites and Hispanics have a significantly higher risk of developing AMD than Blacks or people of Asian ancestry. Recent evidence suggests that inflammation plays a role in the development of AMD (Fauci et al., 2008). Evidence suggests that the risk for developing AMD may be reduced by consumption of omega-3 fatty acids in fish and vegetables high in lutein and zeaxanthin (carotenoids found in vegetables such as spinach, kale, and broccoli) (Kaufman, 2009; Linus Pauling Institute, 2009).

Pathophysiology

The macula is the area of the retina that provides sharp central vision, receiving light from the center of the visual field. Two forms of age-related macular degeneration are identified, a nonexudative (dry) form and an exudative (wet) form. Although both are progressive disorders, their manifestations and management differ.

Nonexudative, or dry, *macular degeneration* is the more common form of AMD. It is a gradual process that begins with accumulation of deposits called *drusen* beneath the pigment epithelium of the retina. Over time, these deposits enlarge and become more numerous. The pigment epithelium detaches in small areas and becomes atrophic, interfering with sensory function of the macula. Vision loss typically is not significant, and the disorder progresses slowly. There is, however, a risk that the disorder will progress to an exudative stage of the disease.

Exudative macular degeneration is characterized by the formation of new, weak blood vessels in the potential space between the choroid (vascular layer of the eye) and the retina (neurosensory layer). These new vessels are prone to leak, elevating the retina from the choroid and distorting vision. Although exudative macular degeneration typically is a gradual process, bleeding can lead to acute vision loss in some cases. With significant or repeated bleeding episodes, scar tissue forms, and central vision is permanently lost (Fauci et al., 2008).

Manifestations

When the macula is damaged, central vision becomes blurred and distorted, but peripheral vision remains intact. Distortion of vision in one eye is a common initial manifestation; straight lines appear wavy or distorted. With the loss of central vision, activities that require close central vision, such as reading and sewing, are particularly affected (Figure 46–14 ■).

Figure 46–14 ■ Loss of central vision with advanced age-related macular degeneration.

Source: Courtesy of National Eye Institute, National Institutes of Health.

Interdisciplinary Care

AMD is diagnosed through vision and retinal examination. The Amsler grid (see Figure 45–5) may be used to identify distortion of central vision caused by AMD. If treatment for wet AMD is planned, a *fluorescein angiogram* may be done. Pictures are taken as the dye passes through the blood vessels of the retina, allowing detection of leaks.

In its early or intermediate stages, the progress of dry AMD can be slowed through the use of high-dose antioxidants and zinc. Research demonstrated a benefit when vitamin C, vitamin E, beta-carotene (vitamin A), zinc, and copper were administered daily (Kaufman, 2009).

Wet AMD is treated with laser surgery or photodynamic therapy. Although these treatments do not cure the disease, they may slow the rate of vision loss. In laser surgery, fragile blood vessels are destroyed, preventing bleeding. There is a risk, however, of damage to surrounding healthy tissue, some vision loss, and continued growth of new vessels. In photodynamic therapy, verteporfin, a drug that tends to adhere to the surface of new blood vessels, is injected systemically. Light is then shined into the affected eye, activating the drug and destroying new blood vessels. This treatment is relatively fast and painless, but does require avoidance of exposure to direct sunlight or bright indoor light for 5 days following treatment (NEI, 2009b).

Large-print books and magazines, the use of a magnifying glass, and high-intensity lighting can help the patient to cope with the reduced vision of macular degeneration.

✍ Nursing Care

Nurses should be alert for patients demonstrating new and rapid onset manifestations of macular degeneration and promptly refer these patients for ophthalmologic evaluation. Early intervention may preserve a greater degree of vision and slow the progress of the disease. For patients with slowly progressive manifestations, the nursing focus is on helping the patient and family members adapt to the gradual decline in vision by recommending visual aids and other coping strategies. Patient education materials should be in a large-print format.

The Patient with Diabetic Retinopathy

Diabetic retinopathy is a vascular disorder affecting the capillaries of the retina. The capillaries become sclerotic and lose their ability to transport sufficient oxygen and nutrients to the retina.

FAST FACTS

■ In the United States, diabetic retinopathy is the leading cause of new blindness in people ages 20 to 74.

■ People with diabetes are 25 times more likely to become legally blind than people unaffected by the disease (Fauci et al., 2008).

■ The Los Angeles Latino Eye Study projects that nearly half of Hispanic/Latino adults with diabetes have diabetic retinopathy (National Eye Institute, 2004, updated 2008).

The risk of developing diabetic retinopathy is related to the duration of the diabetes and the degree of glycemic control. Hypertension also is a risk factor (Fauci et al., 2008). Retinopathy is seen in both type 1 and type 2 diabetes. Nursing care of the patient with diabetes is discussed in ∞ Chapter 20.

Pathophysiology and Manifestations

Diabetic retinopathy progresses through four stages: (1) mild *nonproliferative* or background retinopathy, (2) moderate nonproliferative retinopathy, (3) severe nonproliferative retinopathy, and (4) *proliferative* retinopathy. Nonproliferative retinopathy is typically the initial form seen. The venous capillaries of the eye dilate and develop microaneurysms that may then leak, causing retinal edema, or they may rupture, causing small hemorrhages into the retina. On ophthalmoscopic examination, yellow exudates, cotton-wool patches indicative of retinal ischemia, and red-dot hemorrhages are observed (Figure 46–15 ■). When the peripheral retina is involved, the patient may experience few symptoms other than light glare. Edema of the macula or a large hemorrhage may cause vision loss.

Diabetic retinopathy may progress to the proliferative form. This disease is marked by large areas of retinal ischemia and the formation of new blood vessels (neovascularization) spreading over the inner surface of the retina and into the vitreous body. These vessels are fine and fragile, making them permeable and easily ruptured. Blood and blood protein leakage contribute to retinal edema, and hemorrhage into the vitreous body may occur. The vessels gradually become fibrous and firmly attached to the vitreous body, increasing the risk of retinal detachment.

Interdisciplinary Care

Patients with diabetes should be examined yearly by an ophthalmologist. The development of any new visual manifestations is an additional indication for prompt ophthalmologic examination and possibly retinal angiography. Strict control of blood glucose levels and blood pressure are important preventive measures, and may slow the progression of retinopathy as well (Fauci et al., 2008).

Figure 46–15 ■ Appearance of the ocular fundus in diabetic retinopathy.
Source: Courtesy of National Eye Institute, National Institutes of Health.

Laser photocoagulation is used to treat both the nonproliferative and proliferative forms of diabetic retinopathy. Leaking microaneurysms are sealed and proliferating vessels destroyed, reducing the risk of hemorrhage, retinal edema, and retinal detachment. This treatment also slows the progress of aneurysms and new vessel formation; however, it does not cure the disorder. Patients with severe proliferative retinopathy may undergo vitrectomy to remove vitreous hemorrhage or treat associated retinal detachments (McPhee et al., 2008). Although conclusive research is lacking, the diabetic patient with retinopathy may be advised to avoid physical activity associated with the Valsalva maneuver (e.g., weight training) (Fauci et al., 2008).

✑ Nursing Care

As with many other eye disorders, the nursing care focus for diabetic retinopathy is primarily educational. The newly diagnosed diabetic patient needs to understand the importance of regular eye examinations beginning approximately 5 years after the onset of type 1 diabetes and at the time of diagnosis of type 2 diabetes. Changes of diabetic retinopathy may already be present when type 2 diabetes is diagnosed.

Teach the patient to report promptly any new visual manifestation, including blurred vision; black spots (floaters), cobwebs, or flashing lights in the visual field; or a sudden loss of vision in one or both eyes. Emphasize to the patient that careful blood glucose control may help prevent diabetic retinopathy from developing; it may also slow its progress. The patient's blood pressure should also be maintained within normal limits to prevent further damage to retinal vessels. Although diabetic retinopathy cannot be halted or cured, its progress can be slowed with aggressive management. Much of the burden for this management falls on the patient, increasing the importance of good teaching.

The Patient with a Retinal Detachment

The retina contains the photoreceptors of the eye, which allow the perception of light and initial processing of images and stimuli for transmission to the optic center of the brain. Disruption of this neural layer of the eye by trauma or disease interferes with light perception and image transmission, potentially resulting in blindness.

Both primary eye conditions and systemic diseases can affect the retina and interfere with vision. Retinal tears or detachments can occur either spontaneously or as a result of trauma.

Pathophysiology and Manifestations

Separation of the retina or sensory portion of the eye from the choroid, the pigmented vascular layer, is known as a *retinal detachment*. Although retinal detachment may be precipitated by trauma, it usually occurs spontaneously. The vitreous humor normally adheres to the retina at the optic disc, the macula, and the periphery of the eye. With aging, the vitreous humor shrinks and may pull the retina away from the choroid. Aging therefore is a common risk factor, as are myopia and aphakia, absence of the lens (e.g., following lens removal for cataracts) (McPhee et al., 2008; Porth & Matfin, 2009).

The retina may actually tear and fold back on itself, or the retina may remain intact but no longer adhere to the choroid. A break or tear in the retina allows fluid from the vitreous cavity to enter the defect. This, along with fluid that escapes from choroid vessels, the pull of gravity, and traction exerted by the vitreous humor, separates the retina from the choroid. The detached area may rapidly increase in size, increasing loss of vision. Unless contact between the retina and choroid is reestablished, the neurons of the retina become ischemic and die, causing permanent vision loss. For this reason, retinal detachment is a true medical emergency, requiring prompt ophthalmologic referral and treatment.

When the retina detaches, the patient experiences floaters, or "spots," and lines or flashes of light in the visual field. Often the patient describes the sensation of having a curtain drawn across the vision, much like a curtain being drawn over a window. The area of the visual field affected is directly related to the area of detachment. For example, because light rays cross as they pass through the lens, a retinal tear in the superior portion of the eye results in a deficit in the lower part of the visual field. The patient feels no pain, and the eye appears normal to visual inspection. Common manifestations of retinal detachment are listed in the accompanying box.

Interdisciplinary Care

Retinal detachment is a medical emergency; prompt treatment is necessary to preserve vision. The manifestations and examination of the ocular fundus by ophthalmoscopy establish the diagnosis of retinal detachment. Early diagnosis and intervention are vital. If the condition is left untreated, the detached portion will become necrotic because of separation from the vascular supply of the choroid. The result is permanent blindness in that portion of the eye. If an ophthalmologist is not readily available, the patient's head is positioned so that gravity pulls the detached portion of the retina into closer contact with the choroid.

Interventions are directed toward bringing the retina and choroid back into contact and reestablishing the blood and nutrient supply to the retina. Either cryotherapy, using a supercooled probe, or laser photocoagulation may be used to create an area of inflammation and adhesion to "weld" the layers together.

A surgical procedure called scleral buckling also may be used. In this procedure, an indentation or fold is created in the sclera, bringing the choroid into contact with the retina. Contact is maintained with a local implant on the sclera or an encircling strap or "buckle." Air may also be injected into the vitreous cavity, a procedure called pneumatic retinopexy. The patient is positioned so that the air bubble pushes the detached portion of the retina into contact with the choroid.

With a retinal tear, it may be necessary to use surgical instruments to manipulate the detached section of retina into place. Air or a liquid is then injected into the vitreous to maintain retinal contact with the choroid, or laser therapy is used to create a bond.

MANIFESTATIONS of Retinal Detachment

- Floaters: irregular, dark lines or spots in the field of vision
- Flashes of light
- Blurred vision
- Progressive deterioration of vision
- Sensation of a curtain or veil being drawn across the field of vision
- If the macula is involved, loss of central vision

Nursing Care

The nursing focus for the patient with a detached retina is on early identification and treatment. Because early intervention is vital to preserve the patient's sight, nurses must recognize early manifestations of retinal detachment and intervene appropriately to obtain definitive treatment for the patient. Retinal detachment can be successfully treated on an outpatient basis, often in an ophthalmologist's office. For these patients, the nursing focus is on education.

Ineffective Tissue Perfusion: Retinal

Restoring contact between the retina and choroid is a priority of nursing and medical care for the patient with retinal detachment. Vitreous humor may leak through a retinal tear, and fluid exudate may collect behind the tear, causing further detachment. If the macula is detached, central vision is lost, and the prognosis for full vision restoration is poorer.

> **PRACTICE ALERT**
> Carefully assess anyone who complains of a sudden rapid loss of vision because these are often medical emergencies.

- Assess for other manifestations of eye disease. *Retinal detachment is painless and has no outward manifestations. The patient with a red eye or cloudy cornea may be experiencing acute angle-closure glaucoma rather than retinal detachment.*
- Notify physician and the ophthalmologist immediately. *Immediate medical intervention is required in patients with retinal detachment to preserve vision.*
- Position so the area of detachment is inferior. For instance, for a superior temporal retinal detachment of the right eye (with corresponding vision loss in the inferior medial visual field of that eye), place supine with the head turned to the right. *Correct positioning allows the contents of the posterior portion of the eye to place pressure on the detached area, bringing the retina in closer contact with the choroid.*

Anxiety

Retinal detachment causes a rapid decline in vision in the affected eye, often occurring spontaneously and without pain. Unless previous episodes have occurred, the patient usually does not know what is causing the problem. Anxiety and fear of complete vision loss are common, expected reactions.

- Maintain a calm, confident attitude while carrying out priority interventions. *Administering care in a calm although urgent manner helps reassure the patient that the problem is treatable and that appropriate measures are being taken.*

- Reassure that most retinal detachments are successfully treated, usually on an outpatient basis. *Reassurance can help allay the patient's fear of permanent vision loss.*
- For spontaneous detachments, assure the patient that he or she did not cause the detachment to occur. *The patient may believe that the detachment is related to a specific activity and feel guilty for "causing" this loss of vision.*
- Explain all procedures fully, including the reason for positioning. *Explanations facilitate understanding and help relieve anxiety in unfamiliar settings.*
- Allow supportive family members or friends to remain with the patient as much as possible. *Additional support helps lower the patient's anxiety level.*

Community-Based Care

Teaching for the patient undergoing surgical repair of retinal detachment is similar to that for patients experiencing other types of eye surgery (see page 1585). If the retina remains detached, provide instructions about the change in peripheral vision or other visual fields and changes in depth perception.

Discuss the following topics with the patient and family to prepare for home care:

- Limitations on positioning the head before or following repair
- Activity restrictions such as no bending or straining at stool
- Use of eye shield
- Early manifestations and the importance of seeking immediate treatment
- Follow-up treatment with the ophthalmologist

The Patient with Retinitis Pigmentosa

Retinitis pigmentosa is a hereditary degenerative disease characterized by retinal atrophy and loss of retinal function progressing from the periphery to the central region of the retina. It is inherited as an autosomal dominant, autosomal recessive, or X-linked trait and may be associated with other genetic defects (Fauci et al., 2008; Porth & Matfin, 2009).

In retinitis pigmentosa, the genetic defect appears to cause production of an unstable form of rhodopsin, the receptor protein of rod cells in the retina. Rod cells degenerate, initially at the periphery of the retina. The areas of degeneration and cell death slowly expand, causing vision to narrow. Central vision is finally lost as well.

The initial manifestation of retinitis pigmentosa, difficulty with night vision, is often noted during childhood. As the disease progresses, there is slow loss of visual fields, photophobia, and disrupted color vision. The progression to tunnel vision and blindness is gradual; the patient may be totally blind by age 40.

Currently, there is no effective treatment for retinitis pigmentosa. Research into the role that defective rhodopsin plays in the disease holds future promise for the development of therapy that may at least slow its progress.

Patients with retinitis pigmentosa may benefit from low vision aids, much like those for the patient with macular degeneration. Additionally, information about the disease and its progress is vital so the patient can plan for the eventual total loss of sight. Patients with retinitis pigmentosa should be referred for genetic counseling prior to starting a family to determine the risk of transmitting the disease to their children.

The Patient with HIV Infection

More than 50% of people infected with the human immunodeficiency virus (HIV) develop an infectious or noninfectious ocular condition, generally as a late manifestation of the disease (Fauci et al., 2008).

HIV retinopathy, seen as cotton-wool spots around the optic nerve, is the most common noninfectious ophthalmic lesion in AIDS. Cotton-wool spots indicate areas of retinal ischemia. Microaneurysms and dot-, blot-, or flame-shaped hemorrhages may also be seen in HIV retinopathy.

Neoplasms common in the patient with AIDS can also affect the eye. Kaposi's sarcoma may affect the external surface or anterior segment of the eye or the eyelids. Kaposi's lesions vary in color (red, brown, or purple) and in size, shape, and location. Conjunctival lesions resemble a benign subconjunctival hemorrhage. Kaposi's lesions of the lid may cause **ptosis** (drooping of the lid) and abnormal lid function. Vision or eye position and movement may be affected by the tumor or by the effect of increased intracranial pressure on the cranial nerves.

The most serious and frequent opportunistic eye infection associated with HIV infection is cytomegalovirus (CMV) retinitis. CMV retinitis generally develops when CD4 cell counts drop below 50/μL. Initially unilateral, CMV retinitis commonly progresses to become bilateral because of the systemic nature of the infection. CMV invades the retina of the eye directly, producing exudate and cotton-wool spots, hemorrhage, cell death, and necrosis. Visual field deficits develop and can progress to eventual blindness.

Corneal ulcers from opportunistic bacterial, fungal, protozoal, or viral infections are also associated with HIV infection. Toxoplasmic and fungal retinal infections may occur.

The patient with an HIV-associated eye disorder may complain of a change in visual acuity, blurring, floaters, or gaps in the field of vision. Extensive retinal damage may cause retinal detachment and symptoms of flashing lights, multiple floaters, and a loss of vision. Because the observed changes in the retina are nonspecific, it is important for the examining physician to know that the patient is HIV positive in order to make an accurate diagnosis.

In addition to the general treatment of HIV infection with retroviral medications, specific therapies may be directed toward the ocular manifestations of the disease. CMV retinitis is commonly treated with the antivirals ganciclovir (Cytovene) and foscarnet sodium (Foscavir).

Although treatment of ocular Kaposi's sarcoma is usually not indicated, conjunctival lesions may be excised for comfort or cosmetic reasons. Lid lesions may be treated with radiation or intralesional chemotherapy.

The Patient with an Enucleation

Occasionally surgical removal of an eye is necessary because of trauma, infection, glaucoma, intractable pain, or malignancy. This procedure is known as **enucleation**.

PROCEDURE 46-1 Removing and Reinserting a Prosthetic Eye

GATHER SUPPLIES
- Gloves
- Clean basin or plastic denture cup
- Sterile normal saline or soap and water for cleaning the prosthesis
- Gauze squares or cotton cloth for cleaning the socket
- A bulb syringe for irrigation if necessary

BEFORE THE PROCEDURE
Most patients who have an artificial eye provide self-care and require little assistance. However, it may be necessary for the nurse to remove an eye prosthesis from the unconscious or debilitated patient. Before proceeding, explain the procedure and provide for privacy.

PROCEDURE
1. Follow standard precautions.
2. Wash the hands and put on clean exam gloves.
3. To remove the prosthesis, do one of the following:
   - Pull down the lower lid and gently exert outward and upward pressure on the lower edge of the prosthesis. This pressure usually causes the prosthesis to slip out.
   - Pull down the lower lid and apply a moistened suction cup to the prosthesis by squeezing the device. Twist gently to remove the prosthesis from the socket.
4. Wash the prosthesis using mild soap and water or normal saline. Rinse thoroughly. Do not use abrasives or chemicals for cleaning.
5. If the prosthesis is not immediately replaced in the eye socket, store it in a clearly labeled plastic container lined with a soft cloth or gauze squares. Avoid scratching or damaging the prosthesis. Store it in a safe place to prevent loss.

6. If irrigation of the eye socket is ordered, have the patient lean over a sink or basin if possible, or position on the affected side with a clean emesis basin to hold the irrigant as it flows out of the socket. Gently hold the lids open and irrigate the socket using a bulb syringe and clean warm water.
7. Reinsert the prosthesis.
   a. Moisten the prosthesis with warm normal saline or water.
   b. Gently hold the lids open. Insert the upper edge of the prosthesis under the upper lid first, then the lower edge under the lower lid using slight pressure.
   c. If a suction device is used, attach it to the cleaned prosthesis over the pupil. Holding the lids open, insert the prosthesis using the above procedure, then remove the suction cup by squeezing it gently and exerting slight pressure on the edge of the cup with the lower lid.

AFTER THE PROCEDURE
Ensure that the patient is comfortable. Chart the procedure and any abnormal findings, such as drainage or inflammation.

Enucleation is performed under local or general anesthesia. After the globe is removed, the conjunctiva and eye muscles are sutured to a round implant inserted into the orbit to maintain its shape. A pressure dressing is left in place for 24 to 46 hours. The patient is permitted out of bed on the day of surgery. Hemorrhage and infection are the most commonly seen complications.

Postoperative nursing care includes teaching, psychologic support, and observation for potential complications. The patient may be instructed to apply warm compresses and instill antibiotic ointment or drops postoperatively.

Within 1 week, a temporary prosthesis called a conformer is fitted into the empty socket. The permanent prosthesis is individually designed to closely resemble the patient's other eye. The prosthesis can be fitted 1 to 2 months after surgery. Often it is difficult to discern which eye is functional and which is the prosthesis. Procedure 46–1 outlines the proper way to remove and reinsert an eye prosthesis when the patient is unable to do so.

Ear Disorders

For a person to hear, sound waves must enter the external auditory meatus and travel through the ear canal to vibrate the tympanic membrane and bony structures of the middle ear, which in turn activate the receptors of the cochlea. Trauma or disease involving any portion of this pathway can affect hearing. **Tinnitus**, the perception of sound such as ringing, buzzing, or roaring in the ears, is another potential result of problems affecting the auditory system.

Disorders of the external ear, including the auricle, auditory meatus, and ear canal, can affect the conduction of sound waves and hearing. Obstruction of the external auditory canal or damage to the tympanic membrane, which separates the outer from the middle ear, may lead to conductive hearing loss. Infection or inflammation, trauma, and obstruction of the ear canal with cerumen (wax) or a foreign body are the most common conditions affecting the external ear.

Disorders of the middle ear may be either acute or chronic. Unless these disorders are treated promptly and effectively, damage and scarring of middle ear structures can result in a permanent conductive hearing loss. Infectious or inflammatory disorders such as otitis media and mastoiditis are the most common conditions affecting the middle ear. Otosclerosis, a genetic condition, may also affect the structures of the middle ear.

The Patient with Otitis Externa

Otitis externa is inflammation of the ear canal. Commonly known as *swimmer's ear*, it is most prevalent in people who spend significant time in the water. Competitive athletes, including swimmers, divers, and surfers, are particularly prone to otitis externa. Wearing a hearing aid or ear plugs, which hold moisture in the ear canal, is an additional risk factor. Although *Pseudomonas aeruginosa* or other bacterial infection is the most common cause, external otitis may also be due to fungal infection, mechanical trauma (such as cleaning the ear with a toothpick), or a local hypersensitivity reaction.

Pathophysiology and Manifestations

Disruption of the normal environment within the external auditory canal typically precedes the inflammatory process. Retained moisture, cleaning, or drying of the ear canal remove the protective layer of cerumen, an acidic, water-repellent substance with antimicrobial properties. Its removal leaves the skin of the ear canal vulnerable to invasion and infection. For surfers, the presence of *exostoses*, bony growths in the ear canals resulting from prolonged exposure to cold, predisposes to impaction and retained moisture within the canal.

The patient with otitis externa often complains of a feeling of fullness in the ear. Ear pain typically is present and may be severe. The pain of otitis externa can be differentiated from that associated with otitis media by manipulation of the auricle. In external otitis, this maneuver increases the pain, whereas the patient with otitis media experiences no change in pain perception. Odorless watery or purulent drainage may be present. The ear canal appears inflamed and edematous on examination.

Interdisciplinary Care

Management of the patient with an external ear disorder focuses on restoring the normal balance of the external ear and canal and teaching the patient how to prevent future problems.

For otitis externa, the following steps are recommended in treatment:

- Thorough cleansing of the ear canal, particularly if drainage or debris is present
- Treatment of the infection with local antibiotics; if cellulitis is present, systemic antibiotics may be necessary
- Medication to relieve the pain and itching
- Teaching to prevent future episodes of swimmer's ear

A topical antibiotic is often prescribed for the treatment of otitis externa. A topical corticosteroid may be ordered in combination with the antibiotic to provide immediate relief of the pain, swelling, and itching. Polymyxin B-neomycin-hydrocortisone (Cortisporin Otic) is a typical combination preparation used to treat external otitis; these antibiotics are effective against *Pseudomonas*. It is important to identify known sensitivity to any of the drugs in this preparation prior to initiating therapy. Patients who are sensitive to neomycin may develop dermatitis, in which case the drug must be stopped. Other preparations such as 1% tolnaftate solution (Tinactin) may be prescribed for a fungal infection of the ear canal.

℘ Nursing Care

External otitis can cause severe pain and discomfort. Although the disorder is rarely serious enough to require hospitalization, the nurse teaches the patient about the disorder, comfort measures, and prevention of future episodes.

Nursing Diagnoses and Interventions

Impaired Tissue Integrity

External otitis may result from attempts to clean the ear canal with a toothpick, cotton-tipped applicator, or other implement that damages the skin, allowing an infectious organism to invade the tissue. Even if the canal is not damaged by attempts to clean it, the cleaning process often interrupts normal mechanisms, causing cerumen and debris to collect in the canal. This collected debris, in turn, tends to trap water within the canal, causing maceration of the skin.

- Inform that ear canals rarely need cleansing beyond washing of the external meatus with soap and water. Teach patients of all ages not to clean ear canals with any implement. *"Cleaning" increases the risk of tissue damage and impairs the normal mechanism that clears the canal of accumulated cerumen and debris.*
- Teach patient (and, if necessary, a family member) how to instill prescribed eardrops:
  a. Wash the hands.
  b. Warm the medication briefly by holding the container in the hand or placing it in a pocket for approximately 5 minutes before instilling the drops. *Warming the medication promotes comfort.*
  c. Lie on the unaffected side; if sitting, tilt the head toward the unaffected side. *This position allows gravity to assist in moving the medication to the inner portion of the ear canal.*
  d. Partially fill the ear dropper with medication.
  e. Using the nondominant hand, straighten the ear canal by pulling the pinna of the ear up and back. *Straightening helps the medication travel along the length of the canal.*
  f. Administer the prescribed number of drops into the ear canal. *It is important that the full amount of prescribed medication be administered to penetrate the length of the canal and achieve full effectiveness.*
  g. Remain in the side-lying position for approximately 5 minutes after the instillation of drops. *This position allows the medication to penetrate into deeper portions of the canal and prevents it from running out when the head is moved upright.*
  h. Loosely place a small piece of cotton in the auditory meatus for 15 to 20 minutes. *The cotton helps keep the medication in the canal.*
- Teach to avoid getting water in the affected ear until it is fully healed. Cotton balls may be used while showering to prevent water from entering the ear canal. The patient should refrain from water sports and activities until approved by the primary care provider. *Retained moisture in the ear canal can further impair skin integrity, increasing inflammation.*

- Stay out of the water until the acute inflammatory process is completely resolved. Ideally, allow 7 to 10 days before resuming water activities.
- Take precautions to keep the ear canal dry while in the water:
  a. Use silicone earplugs, which can keep water out of the ear without reducing hearing significantly.
  b. Wear a tight-fitting swim cap or wet suit hood, especially in cold ocean water. Although these do not prevent water from entering the ear, they protect the ear from the cold and possibly slow the formation of bony growths in the ears. They also protect the ear from sand and other water debris.
- Immediately after swimming, dry the ear canal. Allow water to drain by tilting the head and jumping to shake water out of the ear. Dry the outer ear with a towel, then use a hair dryer on the lowest setting several inches from the ear to dry the canal.
- Do not insert cotton swabs or other objects into the ear canal to dry it. This removes the protective layer of cerumen and may damage the skin of the canal, increasing the risk of bacterial infection. In addition, if debris such as sand is present, the swab may actually push debris further into the canal, forming an impacted mass.
- Use a drying agent in the ear canal after swimming. A 2% acetic acid solution or 2% boric acid in ethyl alcohol is effective in drying the canal and restoring its normal acidic environment.
- If it is necessary to remove impacted debris from the ear canal, irrigate the ear with warm tap water. A bulb syringe available over the counter or a 20-mL syringe attached to a short Teflon intravenous catheter (with the needle removed) is effective. With the head tilted toward the affected side, direct a stream of warm water toward the upper wall of the ear canal, allowing the water to run out into a bowl or sink. Repeated instillations may be necessary to break up and flush out impacted wax and debris.

Community-Based Care

The patient is ultimately responsible for carrying out the prescribed treatment regimen in external otitis and for implementing measures to prevent future episodes. Teaching is vital. Provide verbal and written instructions on use of the prescribed medications. Teach the patient care measures to prevent recurrent episodes especially important in swimmers, divers, and surfers (Box 46–2).

Cellulitis of the surrounding tissue is a possible complication of external otitis. Instruct the patient to report to the primary care provider any increase in pain, swelling, or redness of surrounding tissues; fever; or other manifestations of infection such as malaise or increased fatigue.

The Patient with Impacted Cerumen or a Foreign Body

The external auditory canal can be obstructed by cerumen or foreign bodies. The curved shape and narrow lumen of the canal make it particularly vulnerable to obstruction.

Pathophysiology and Manifestations

As cerumen dries, it moves down and out of the ear canal. In some individuals it tends to accumulate, narrowing the canal. Aging is a risk factor for impaction because less cerumen is produced and it is harder and drier. The accumulation of cerumen is often aggravated by attempting to remove it using cotton-tipped swabs or hairpins, which pack it more deeply into the ear canal.

A variety of objects become foreign bodies in the ear canal. In adults, implements used to clean the ear canal may break and become lodged. Insects also may enter the ear canal and be unable to exit.

When the ear canal becomes occluded with either cerumen or a foreign body, the patient experiences a conductive hearing loss in the affected ear. Manifestations include a sensation of fullness, along with tinnitus and coughing due to stimulation of the vagal nerve. The foreign body or impacted cerumen may be visualized on otoscopy. Impacted cerumen appears as a yellow, brown, or black mass in the canal.

Interdisciplinary Care

Treatment focuses on clearing the canal. If there is no evidence of tympanic membrane perforation, irrigation of the canal is often the initial therapy.

Impacted wax, objects, or insects may require physical removal using an ear curet, forceps, or right-angle hook inserted via an otoscope and ear speculum. Mineral oil or topical lidocaine drops are used to immobilize or kill insects prior to their removal from the ear. When an organic foreign body such as a bean or an insect is suspected, water should not be instilled into the ear canal, because it may cause the object to swell, making its removal more difficult. Smooth, round objects present the biggest challenge to remove from the ear canal. Suction applied using a piece of soft intravenous tubing may be effective.

Nursing Care

Nurses are often involved in identifying and relieving obstructions of the ear canal, especially in outpatient and community settings. Any patient with evidence of a new conductive hearing loss or complaints of discomfort and fullness in one ear should be evaluated for possible obstruction. Inability to visualize the tympanic membrane or observation of a dark, shiny mass obstructing the canal may indicate a need for an irrigation or other procedure to clear the canal. It is important to determine that the tympanic membrane is intact before irrigating; assessment by a physician or advanced practitioner may be necessary if a ruptured membrane is suspected.

Because obstruction of the ear canal with cerumen or a foreign body is generally preventable, teaching is a key component of nursing care. Patients need to know appropriate care measures for the external ear. Although the ear canal rarely needs cleaning, the patient prone to cerumen impaction needs teaching about the use of mineral oil or commercial products to soften wax and of irrigation to remove it. All patients should understand the importance of not inserting anything smaller than a finger wrapped with a washcloth into the ear canal to avoid trauma to the canal or eardrum. Stress the risk of impacting cerumen against the tympanic membrane when using cotton-tipped swabs to clean the ear canal. Additionally, the swab may break and lodge in the canal. If eardrops have been prescribed, teach the patient and a family member how to instill them.

The Patient with Otitis Media

Otitis media, inflammation or infection of the middle ear, primarily affects infants and young children but may also occur in adults. The tympanic membrane, which separates the middle ear from the external auditory canal, protects the middle ear from the external environment. The eustachian (auditory) tube connects the middle ear with the nasopharynx to help equalize the pressure in the middle ear with the atmospheric pressure. Unfortunately, this connecting tube also provides a route by which infectious organisms enter the middle ear from the nose and throat, causing otitis media, the most common disease of the middle ear.

Pathophysiology

There are two primary forms of otitis media: (1) serous and (2) acute. Both forms are associated with upper respiratory infection and eustachian tube dysfunction. The eustachian tube is narrow and flat, normally opening only during yawning and swallowing. Allergies or upper respiratory tract infections can cause edema of the tube lining, impairing its function. Air within the middle ear is trapped and gradually absorbed, creating negative pressure in this space.

Serous Otitis Media

Serous otitis media (also called *otitis media with effusion*) occurs when the eustachian tube is obstructed for a prolonged time, impairing air pressure equalization in the middle ear. Air within the middle ear space is gradually absorbed; the tube obstruction prevents more air from entering the middle ear. The resulting negative pressure in the middle ear causes sterile serous fluid to move from the capillaries into the space, forming a sterile effusion of the middle ear.

Upper respiratory infection or allergies such as hay fever predispose the patient to serous otitis media. In addition, patients with narrowed or edematous eustachian tubes may also be subject to barotrauma. In these patients, the middle ear cannot adapt to rapid changes in barometric pressure such as those that occur during air travel or underwater diving. Barotrauma tends to occur during descent in an airplane because negative pressure within the middle ear causes the eustachian tube to collapse and lock. However, underwater diving places even greater stress on the eustachian tube and middle ear (McPhee et al., 2008).

MANIFESTATIONS Typical manifestations of serous otitis media include decreased hearing in the affected ear and complaints of "snapping" or "popping" in the ear. On examination, the tympanic membrane demonstrates decreased mobility and may appear retracted or bulging. Fluid or air bubbles are often visible behind the drum (Figure 46–16 ■). Severe pressure differences such as those occurring with barotrauma may cause

Figure 46–16 ■ The appearance of the tympanic membrane in serous otitis media.
Source: Kevin Kavanagh, MD.

acute pain, hemorrhage into the middle ear, rupture of the tympanic membrane, or even rupture of the round window with sensory hearing loss and severe **vertigo** (a sensation of whirling or rotation). *Hemotympanum*, bleeding into or behind the tympanic membrane, may be observed on otoscopic examination.

Acute Otitis Media

The eustachian tube also provides a route for the entry of pathogens into the normally sterile middle ear, resulting in acute otitis media. Acute otitis media typically follows an upper respiratory infection. Edema of the eustachian tube impairs drainage of the middle ear, causing mucus and serous fluid to accumulate. This fluid is an excellent environment for the growth of bacteria, which may enter from the oronasopharynx via the eustachian tube. Although a viral upper respiratory infection may predispose the patient to a middle ear infection, the bacteria *Streptococcus pneumoniae*, *Haemophilus influenzae*, and *Streptococcus pyogenes* account for most cases of otitis media in adults. Invasion and colonization of the middle ear by bacteria and the resultant migration of white blood cells cause pus formation. Accumulated pus can increase middle ear pressure sufficiently to rupture the tympanic membrane. The bacterial infection may also migrate internally, causing mastoiditis, brain abscess, or bacterial meningitis. A more common complication of otitis media is a persistent conductive hearing loss, which typically resolves when the middle ear effusion clears.

MANIFESTATIONS The patient with acute otitis media experiences mild to severe pain in the affected ear. The patient's temperature is often elevated. Diminished hearing, dizziness, vertigo, and tinnitus are common associated complaints. Pus within the mastoid air cells often causes mastoid tenderness in acute otitis media. On otoscopic examination, the tympanic membrane appears red and inflamed or dull and bulging (Figure 46–17 ■). Decreased movement of the membrane is demonstrated by tympanometry or air insufflation. Spontaneous rupture of the tympanic membrane releases a purulent discharge.

Figure 46–17 ■ A red, bulging tympanic membrane of acute otitis media.

Source: Janet Hayes/Medical Images, Inc.

Interdisciplinary Care

The diagnosis of otitis media is usually based on the history and the physical examination. The tympanic membrane can be visualized and its mobility evaluated using a pneumatic otoscope that allows a puff of air to be instilled into the ear canal. Generally, the tympanic membrane moves slightly when air is instilled or the patient performs the Valsalva maneuver. Less movement is seen in patients with eustachian tube dysfunction and acute otitis media with effusion.

Diagnosis

■ *Impedance audiometry*, also known as tympanometry, is an accurate diagnostic test for otitis media with effusion. A continuous tone is delivered to the tympanic membrane by an audiometer with a sealed probe tip. Compliance of the tympanic membrane and middle ear is measured by recording energy reflected from the membrane surface. With middle ear effusion, compliance is reduced.

■ A *complete blood count (CBC)* may be done to assess for an elevated WBC count and increased numbers of immature cells indicative of acute bacterial infection.

■ If the tympanic membrane has ruptured or a tympanocentesis or myringotomy is performed, drainage is cultured to determine the infecting organism.

Medications

When eustachian tube dysfunction and serous otitis media do not spontaneously resolve or lead to hearing loss, a short course of an anti-inflammatory drug (e.g., oral prednisone for 7 days) is prescribed to reduce mucosal edema of the tube and improve its patency. Although a decongestant or antihistamine may be used, there is little evidence of their effectiveness in treating serous otitis media. ∞ See Chapter 13 for the nursing implications of corticosteroid medications.

The patient with eustachian tube dysfunction may be taught to autoinflate the middle ear by performing the Valsalva maneuver or by forcefully exhaling against closed nostrils. Additionally, the patient is advised to avoid air travel and underwater diving.

Acute otitis media often resolves spontaneously, making "watchful waiting" a valid option in normally healthy patients (Fauci et al., 2008). However, it usually is treated with antibiotic therapy, especially amoxicillin, trimethoprim-sulfamethoxazole, cefaclor, or azithromycin for 5 to 10 days. This course of treatment is long enough to ensure eradication of the infective organism, yet short enough to reduce the incidence of bacterial resistance. (∞ See Chapter 12 for further discussion of antibiotics.) Symptomatic relief may be provided by analgesics, antipyretics, antihistamines, and local application of heat.

Surgery

Myringotomy (an incision of the tympanic membrane) or tympanocentesis may be performed to relieve excess pressure in the middle ear and prevent spontaneous rupture of the eardrum. To perform a tympanocentesis, the physician inserts a 20-gauge spinal needle through the inferior portion of the tympanic membrane, allowing aspiration of fluid and pus from the middle ear to relieve pressure and, if necessary, obtain a specimen for culture. Myringotomy may be performed to relieve severe pain or when complications of acute otitis media, such as mastoiditis, are present. As soon as the pressure is released, pain subsides and hearing improves.

Patients who do not respond to antibiotic therapy may require myringotomy with insertion of ventilation (tympanostomy) tubes. Small tubes are inserted into the inferior portion of the tympanic membrane, providing for ventilation and drainage of the middle ear during healing. The tube is eventually extruded from the ear, and the tympanic membrane heals. While the tube is in place, it is important to avoid getting any water in the ear canal because it may then enter the middle ear space.

∞ Nursing Care

Patients with otitis media are commonly treated in outpatient and community settings. The nursing role is primarily one of support and education.

Health Promotion

Health promotion for otitis media focuses on educating patients about the importance of seeking medical care for prolonged, severe ear pain with or without drainage combined with an upper respiratory tract infection. Untreated or repeated attacks of otitis media can progress to a chronic form of otitis media, acute mastoiditis, or eardrum perforation.

Assessment

Collect assessment data through a health history and physical examination (∞ Chapter 45).

■ *Health history:* Recent upper respiratory infection; presence, intensity, and nature of pain in affected ear; sense of fullness or pressure in the ear; change in hearing; snapping or popping sensation in the affected ear; presence of vertigo.

■ *Physical examination:* Temperature; hearing test; inspect tympanic membrane.

Nursing Diagnosis and Interventions

Pain can be a significant problem for patients with otitis media, as can the risk of damage to delicate tissues of the middle ear by the infectious and inflammatory processes.

Acute Pain

Tissue edema, effusion of the middle ear, and the inflammatory response can affect the pain-sensitive tissues of the middle ear in otitis media, causing acute discomfort. This discomfort is increased by pressure changes, such as those that occur during air travel or underwater diving.

- Assess pain for severity, quality, and location. *A thorough assessment is important to determine the source of the pain. The pain of otitis media, unlike that of external otitis, is not aggravated by movement of the external ear.*
- Encourage the use of mild analgesics such as aspirin or acetaminophen every 4 hours as needed to relieve pain and fever. *These nonprescription medications are effective in reducing the perception of pain. Aspirin also has anti-inflammatory properties that may help relieve the inflammation of the ear.*
- Advise to apply heat to the affected side unless contraindicated. *Heat dilates blood vessels, promoting the reabsorption of fluid and reducing swelling.*
- Instruct to avoid air travel, rapid changes in elevation, or diving. *A rapid change in barometric pressure can increase the patient's pain significantly.*
- Instruct to report promptly an abrupt relief of pain to the primary care provider. *Pain that subsides abruptly may indicate spontaneous perforation of the tympanic membrane with relief of pressure within the middle ear.*

Community-Based Care

The patient who has otitis media needs teaching about the disorder, its causes and prevention, and any specific treatment recommended or prescribed. Discuss the following topics with the patient and family:

- Antibiotic therapy and potential side effects
- Importance of completing all ordered doses
- Follow-up examinations in 2 to 4 weeks
- Avoidance of swimming, diving, or submerging the head while bathing if ventilation tubes are in place.

If surgical intervention is necessary, teach the patient and family members about the surgery and postoperative care. Provide instruction about any special postoperative precautions, such as avoiding water in the ear canals or avoiding sudden changes in air pressure.

The Patient with Acute Mastoiditis

The mastoid process is a portion of the temporal bone of the skull lying adjacent to the middle ear. It is full of air cavities called mastoid air cells or mastoid sinuses. The infection of acute otitis media generally extends into the mastoid air cells; effective treatment of acute otitis media eliminates the infection from the mastoid cells as well. When treatment is ineffective, pus remains in the mastoid air cells, and acute *mastoiditis*, bacterial infection of the mastoid process, may develop.

The incidence of acute mastoiditis is low in the United States and in other countries in which the use of antibiotics to treat acute otitis media is similar to that of the United States. Its incidence is higher in countries where antibiotics are less likely to be prescribed for acute otitis media (Fauci et al., 2008).

Pathophysiology and Complications

In acute mastoiditis, the bony septa between mastoid air cells are destroyed and cells coalesce to form large spaces. Portions of the mastoid process are eroded. With chronic infection, an abscess may form, or bony sclerosis of the mastoid may result. Acute mastoiditis increases the risk of meningitis because only a very thin bony plate separates mastoid air cells from the brain. Fortunately, this complication is rare since the advent of effective antibiotic therapy for treating otitis media.

Manifestations

Manifestations of acute mastoiditis usually develop approximately 2 to 3 weeks after an episode of acute otitis media and include recurrent earache and hearing loss on the affected side. The pain is persistent and throbbing; tenderness is present over the mastoid process (behind the ear). It may also be red and inflamed. Swelling of the process can cause the auricle of the ear to protrude more than normal. Fever may be accompanied by tinnitus and headache. Profuse drainage from the affected ear may be noted.

Interdisciplinary Care

In addition to the manifestations of acute mastoiditis, loss of septa between mastoid air cells may be noted on radiologic examination. Acute mastoiditis is treated aggressively with antibiotic therapy. Intravenous ticarcillin-clavulanate (Timentin) and gentamicin may be used initially, with therapy tailored to the specific organism once culture results are obtained. Antibiotics are continued for at least 14 days. Infections that do not respond to medical therapy or that pose a high risk of spreading to the brain may necessitate *mastoidectomy*, surgical removal of the infected mastoid air cells, bone, and pus, and inspection of the underlying dura for possible abscess. The extent of tissue destruction determines the extent of surgery required. In a modified mastoidectomy, as much tissue is preserved as possible to avoid disruption of hearing. A radical mastoidectomy involves removal of middle ear structures including the incus and malleus as well as the diseased portions of the mastoid process. Unless reconstruction is performed at the time of surgery, this surgery results in conductive hearing loss. **Tympanoplasty**, surgical reconstruction of the middle ear, can restore or preserve hearing.

∽ Nursing Care

Prevention is the primary focus of collaborative and nursing care related to mastoiditis. Adequate, effective antibiotic treatment of acute otitis media prevents mastoiditis in nearly all instances.

Following surgical intervention, carefully assess the wound and drainage for evidence of infection or other complications. The patient's hearing may be temporarily or permanently affected, depending on the extent of the surgery. If the patient has impaired hearing in the unaffected ear as well, develop a means of communication with the patient prior to surgery. If the hearing is preserved in the unaffected ear, position the patient with that ear toward the door. Speak slowly and clearly; do not shout or speak unusually loudly. Be sure that family and staff know about the patient's hearing loss and use appropriate communication techniques. Assist the patient with ambulation initially, because dizziness and vertigo are not unusual following surgery. Nursing care of the patient having ear surgery is discussed in the accompanying box.

Community-Based Care

When teaching about acute mastoiditis, stress the importance of complying with the prescribed antibiotic therapy and recommendations for follow-up. Instruct the patient and family to report any adverse reactions to the primary care provider so that therapy can be adjusted. Teach the patient and family how to change the surgical dressing using aseptic technique. Provide referrals to appropriate community agencies for the patient with a new hearing loss resulting from mastoiditis or its treatment.

The Patient with Chronic Otitis Media

Chronic otitis media involves permanent perforation of the tympanic membrane, with or without recurrent pus formation. Changes in the mucosa and bony structures (ossicles) of the middle ear often accompany chronic otitis media. It usually is the result of recurrent acute otitis media and eustachian tube dysfunction, but may also result from trauma or other diseases.

Marginal perforations, which usually occur in the posterior-superior portion of the tympanic membrane, are associated with more complications than central perforations. With marginal perforations, squamous epithelium may migrate from the ear canal into the middle ear, where it begins to desquamate and accumulate, forming a *cholesteatoma* (a cyst or mass filled with epithelial cell debris). Its incidence is highest in children and young adults. The desquamating epithelium continues to accumulate and remains infected, producing collagenases (enzymes) that destroy adjacent bone. The inflammatory process impairs the blood supply to the stapes, causing its destruction and conductive hearing loss. Cholesteatomas are benign and slow-growing tumors, which can enlarge to fill the entire middle ear. Untreated, the cholesteatoma can progressively destroy the ossicles and erode into the inner ear, causing profound hearing loss.

NURSING CARE OF THE PATIENT | Having Ear Surgery

PREOPERATIVE CARE
- ∞ Review Chapter 4 for routine preoperative care.
- Assess hearing or verify documentation of preoperative hearing assessment. *These data are important in evaluating the results of the surgical procedure.*
- Establish a means of communication to be used after surgery. *Hearing may be impaired after surgery.*
- Explain that blowing of the nose, coughing, and sneezing are restricted postoperatively to prevent pressure changes in the middle ear and potential disruption of the surgical site. Keeping the mouth open during a cough or sneeze minimizes pressure changes in the middle ear. *Providing teaching and the opportunity to practice before surgery promotes cooperation in the postoperative period.*

POSTOPERATIVE CARE
- ∞ Review Chapter 4 for routine postoperative care.
- Assess for bleeding or drainage from the affected ear. *Infection and hemorrhage are possible complications.*
- Administer antiemetics as ordered to prevent vomiting. *Vomiting may increase the pressure in the middle ear, disrupting the surgical site.*
- Elevate the head of bed and position the patient on the unaffected side. *This position minimizes the pressure in the middle ear.*
- Assess for vertigo or dizziness, especially with ambulation or movement in bed. Avoid unnecessary movements such as turning. Take measures to ensure safety during ambulation. *Surgery on the ear may disrupt equilibrium, increasing the risk of falling.*
- Assess hearing postoperatively. Stand on the unaffected side to communicate and use other measures such as written

messages as needed for effective communication with the patient with impaired hearing. Reassure the patient that decreased hearing acuity immediately after surgery is expected. *Hearing improvement, if an expected result of the ear surgery, typically does not occur until earplugs are removed and edema and drainage at the operative site have resolved. If no reconstruction of the middle ear is done or the cochlea is involved, permanent hearing loss in the affected ear may be an expected result.*
- Remind to avoid coughing, sneezing, or blowing the nose. *These increase pressure in the middle ear.*

Health Education for the Patient and Family
- Provide instructions for home care:
  a. To prevent contamination of the ear canal, avoid showers, shampooing, and immersing the head until the physician says you can do so.
  b. Keep the outer earplug clean and dry, changing it as needed. Do not remove inner ear dressing until instructed to do so by the physician.
  c. Avoid blowing the nose; if you need to cough or sneeze, keep the mouth open.
  d. Do not swim or dive without physician approval. Check with your doctor regarding air travel.
  e. Meclizine hydrochloride (Antivert) or other antiemetic/antihistamine medication may be necessary for up to 1 month following surgery.
  f. Fever, bleeding, increased drainage, increased dizziness, or decreased hearing after discharge may indicate a complication. Notify the physician if any of these occur.

Systemic antibiotics are prescribed for exacerbations of purulent otitis media. Tympanic membrane perforation is repaired with a tympanoplasty to restore sound conduction and the integrity of the middle ear. A cholesteatoma may require delicate surgery for its removal. If at all possible, radical mastoidectomy with removal of the tympanic membrane, ossicles, and tumor is avoided.

As with other complications of acute otitis media, a priority of nursing care is prevention of chronic otitis media and cholesteatoma. Patients with chronic otitis media need to understand various treatment options and their risks and benefits, as well as the long-term risk of not treating a perforated tympanic membrane. They are also taught how to instill eardrops, to clean the external auditory meatus, and to not irrigate the ear when the tympanic membrane is perforated or if they think it might be.

If surgical treatment of chronic otitis media will affect the patient's hearing, include this information in preoperative teaching. Teach the patient and family how to use alternative means of communication if this will be necessary postoperatively. When an assistive device is ordered, teach the patient and a family member about its use.

The Patient with Otosclerosis

Otosclerosis is a common cause of conductive hearing loss. Abnormal bone formation in the osseous labyrinth of the temporal bone causes the footplate of the stapes to become fixed or immobile in the oval window. The result is a conductive hearing loss.

Otosclerosis is a hereditary disorder with an autosomal dominant pattern of inheritance. It occurs most commonly in Caucasians and in females. The progressive hearing loss typically begins in adolescence or early adulthood and seems to be accelerated by pregnancy. Although both ears are affected, the rate of hearing loss is asymmetric. Because bone conduction of sound is retained, the patient may be able to use the telephone but have difficulty conversing in person. Tinnitus may also be associated with otosclerosis.

On examination, a reddish or pinkish-orange tympanic membrane may be noted because of increased vascularity of the middle ear. The Rinne test (∞ Chapter 45) shows bone sound conduction to be equal to or greater than air conduction, an abnormal finding.

Patients with otosclerosis may choose conservative treatment, relying on a hearing aid to improve their ability to hear and interact with others. Sodium fluoride may be prescribed to slow bone resorption and overgrowth. Surgical treatment involves a stapedectomy and middle ear reconstruction or a stapedotomy. A *stapedectomy* is a microsurgical technique for removing the diseased stapes. A metallic prosthesis is then inserted, with one end connected to the incus and the other inserted into the oval window. *Stapedotomy* involves creation of a small hole in the footplate of the stapes and insertion of a wire or platinum ribbon prosthesis. An argon, KTP, or CO_2 laser may be used for surgery. Surgery usually restores hearing for the patient with otosclerosis.

Education and referral of the patient to appropriate community agencies are important nursing care priorities for the patient with otosclerosis. For the patient who chooses surgical treatment, nursing care is similar to that for other patients undergoing ear surgery. The following nursing diagnoses may be appropriate:

- *Risk for Injury* related to hearing loss or postoperative vertigo
- *Disturbed Sensory Perception: Auditory* related to bony sclerosis of the stapes
- *Impaired Verbal Communication* related to hearing loss
- *Anxiety* related to concern about transmission of a genetic disorder to children

The Patient with an Inner Ear Disorder

Disorders affecting the inner ear are much less common than disorders of the outer or middle ear. Inner ear disorders affect equilibrium and may also affect sensorineural hearing, the perception of sound. Labyrinthitis and Ménière's disease are the most common diseases of the inner ear. Vertigo may be a disorder of the inner ear itself or a manifestation of other disorders.

Pathophysiology and Manifestations

The inner ear (also called the labyrinth) contains the cochlea and the semicircular canals. The hair cells and neurons that allow sound perception and transmission to the auditory center of the brain are in the cochlea. The semicircular canals filled with endolymph are the primary organs involved in maintaining equilibrium. Disruption of this portion of the ear by an inflammatory process or excess endolymph not only affects balance but may also result in permanent hearing loss.

Vertigo

Normally, the integration of input from the labyrinths, eyes, muscles, joints, and neural centers maintains balance and posture. This input and integration can be affected by disorders of the labyrinth, vestibular nerve or nuclei, eyes, cerebellum, brainstem, or cerebral cortex, causing vertigo. Vertigo, the sensation of movement when there is none, is a disorder of equilibrium. The sensation of whirling, rotation, or movement is described as either subjective or objective.

Patients with subjective vertigo report the sensation of being in motion in a stable environment. This is not always a sense of spinning; the patient may have a sense of tumbling or falling forward or backward. The sensation is reversed in objective vertigo; patients report a sensation of stability in a moving environment. This motion may be perceived as the room spinning around the patient or the ground rocking beneath the patient's feet. Dizziness, which may be mistaken for vertigo, is a sensation of unsteadiness, lack of balance, light-headedness, or movement within the head. The person who is dizzy does not have the rotational sensation felt with vertigo.

Vertigo may be disabling, resulting in falls, injury, and difficulty walking. Attacks of vertigo are often accompanied by nausea and vomiting, nystagmus, and autonomic symptoms such as pallor, sweating, hypotension, and salivation.

Labyrinthitis

Labyrinthitis, also called otitis interna, is inflammation of the inner ear. It is an uncommon disorder, because the bony protection of the membranous labyrinth makes it difficult for organisms to enter the inner ear. However, bacteria, viruses, and other organisms may enter and infect the inner ear through the oval window during acute otitis media, through the cochlear aqueduct during meningitis, or through the blood. Viral labyrinthitis is suspected when the patient has a sudden onset of symptoms after an upper respiratory infection or when there is no evidence of concurrent otitis media. Labyrinthitis also may result from an autoimmune process of unknown etiology.

MANIFESTATIONS Inflammation of the labyrinth typically causes vertigo, sensorineural hearing deficit, and **nystagmus** (rapid involuntary eye movements).

Vertigo is the hallmark manifestation of inner ear disorders. The vertigo of labyrinthitis is severe and often accompanied by nausea and vomiting. Any movement can aggravate the vertigo, and falling is a significant risk if the patient attempts to stand. Vertigo lasts days to weeks in labyrinthitis, making patient education a vital component of care.

Hearing loss in the ear affected by labyrinthitis may be temporary or permanent. If inflammation destroys tissue of the membranous labyrinth, the hearing loss may be complete and permanent.

The involuntary rhythmic eye movements of nystagmus may not be present in all patients with labyrinthitis. When present, the eye movement is typically horizontal. Applying positive or negative pressure to the tympanic membrane of the affected ear may stimulate nystagmus, as will caloric testing (irrigating the ear canal with warm or cool water). Although nystagmus may also be a symptom of brainstem or cerebellar dysfunction, vertigo and hearing loss are not typically associated with those disorders.

Ménière's Disease

Ménière's disease, also known as endolymphatic hydrops, is a chronic disorder characterized by recurrent attacks of vertigo with tinnitus and a progressive unilateral hearing loss. This disorder affects men and women equally, with adults between the ages of 35 and 60 at highest risk. The cause of Ménière's disease is unclear, although the most common form of the disease is thought to result from viral injury to the fluid transport system of the inner ear. Other factors that may increase the risk for Ménière's disease include trauma, bacterial infections such as syphilis, autoimmune processes, and vascular disorders (Copstead & Banasik, 2010; Porth & Matfin, 2009). A family history of the disease increases risk, suggesting a possible genetic link in some patients.

Ménière's disease results from an excess of endolymph, the fluid in the membranous labyrinth of the inner ear. Although the precise pathophysiologic mechanism leading to accumulation of endolymph is unclear, it is thought to result from impaired filtration and excretion of the fluid by the endolymphatic sac (Porth & Matfin, 2009). Excessive pressure resulting from the increased fluid volume causes neural organs of the cochlea to degenerate.

COURSE AND MANIFESTATIONS The onset of Ménière's disease may be gradual or sudden. It is characterized by recurrent attacks of vertigo, gradual loss of hearing, and tinnitus. Attacks may be preceded by a feeling of fullness in the ears, and a roaring or ringing sensation. The sensorineural hearing loss and tinnitus are usually unilateral but can become bilateral. Attacks of severe rotary vertigo occur abruptly and often unpredictably, lasting from minutes to hours. An attack may be linked to increased sodium intake, stress, allergies, vasoconstriction, or premenstrual fluid retention. As the disease continues, hearing loss progresses and the vertigo can be severe enough to cause immobility, nausea, and vomiting. Attacks are often accompanied by hypotension, sweating, and nystagmus.

Interdisciplinary Care

The manifestations associated with inner ear disorders are similar, making testing necessary to establish a diagnosis. Once the diagnosis is determined, collaborative care is directed toward managing symptoms and preventing permanent hearing loss. Patients with labyrinthitis or an acute attack of Ménière's disease may require hospitalization to manage the vertigo and its effects.

Diagnosis

The following diagnostic studies may be ordered:

- *Caloric testing (electronystagmography)* evaluates the vestibulo-ocular reflex by identifying eye movements (nystagmus) in response to caloric testing. In patients with impaired vestibular function, the normal nystagmus response is blunted or absent. This portion of the test is contraindicated in patients who have a perforated tympanic membrane.
- *Rinne* and *Weber tests* of hearing (∞ Chapter 45) show decreased air and bone conduction on the affected side if a sensorineural hearing loss is present. In Ménière's disease, audiology shows sensorineural hearing loss involving the low tones.
- *X-rays* and *CT scans* of the petrous bones are used to evaluate the internal auditory canal. In patients with Ménière's disease, the vestibular aqueducts may be shorter and straighter than normal.
- *Glycerol test* is conducted by giving the patient oral glycerol to decrease fluid pressure in the inner ear. An acute temporary hearing improvement is considered diagnostic for Ménière's disease.

Medications

In Ménière's disease, a diuretic such as acetazolamide (Diamox) or hydrochlorothiazide may be prescribed to reduce endolymphatic pressure. A central nervous system depressant such as diazepam (Valium) or lorazepam (Ativan) may halt an attack of vertigo. Parenteral droperidol (Inapsine) provides both a sedative and antiemetic effect, making it a useful drug for acute attacks. Antivertigo/antiemetic medications such as meclizine (Antivert), prochlorperazine (Compazine), or hydroxyzine hydrochloride (Vistaril) are prescribed to reduce the whirling sensation and nausea. Intratympanic gentamicin, injected through the tympanic membrane into the middle ear, has been shown to be effective in reducing the vertigo of Ménière's disease. The gentamicin damages vestibular hair cells, effectively reducing attacks of vertigo while causing less hearing loss than traditional surgical approaches (De Beer, Stokroos, & Kingma, 2007).

Treatments

Bed rest in a quiet, darkened room with minimal sensory stimuli and minimal movement provides the most comfort for the patient experiencing an acute attack of vertigo.

Between acute attacks, management of the patient with Ménière's disease is directed at preventing future attacks and preserving hearing. A low-sodium diet helps reduce labyrinthine pressure. A very low salt diet (1 gm) may be prescribed if moderate sodium restriction is ineffective in controlling attacks. Patients should avoid tobacco, which causes vasoconstriction and can precipitate an attack, along with alcohol and caffeine.

Surgery

When episodes of vertigo are not controlled through medical interventions, surgery may be necessary. Surgical *endolymphatic decompression* relieves the excess pressure in the labyrinth; a shunt is then inserted between the membranous labyrinth and the subarachnoid space to drain excess fluid away from the labyrinths and maintain lower pressure. This procedure preserves hearing for most patients. Vertigo is relieved in approximately 70% of patients, but about half of patients undergoing this procedure continue to experience sensations of fullness and tinnitus.

Destruction of a portion of the acoustic nerve is an alternative to shunting procedures. In a *vestibular neurectomy*, the portion of cranial nerve VIII that controls balance and sensations of vertigo is severed. This procedure relieves vertigo for up to 90% of patients. Although there is a risk of damage to the cochlear portion of the nerve and resultant hearing loss, for most patients hearing loss stabilizes after neurectomy, even improving for some.

The surgery of last resort for Ménière's disease is a *labyrinthectomy*. The labyrinth is completely removed, destroying cochlear function. This procedure is used only when hearing loss is nearly complete and vertigo is persistent. Although labyrinthectomy relieves vertigo in nearly all cases, the patient may remain unsteady and have continued problems with balance.

After surgery on the inner ear, the patient is positioned to minimize ear pressure and vertigo. Movement is restricted, and assistance is provided when the patient gets up. Antiemetics and antivertigo medications are used to manage symptoms resulting from disruption of the inner ear. Complications include infection and leakage of cerebrospinal fluid.

♫ Nursing Care

The patient with an inner ear disorder has multiple nursing care needs related to the manifestations of the disorder.

Health Promotion

Health promotion focuses on identifying patients with potential inner ear disorders. Persistent episodes of dizziness, ringing in the ears, balance problems, or loss of hearing should be reported to a healthcare provider. Patients diagnosed early may have a lower risk for injury and can be taught strategies for maintaining as near normal as possible their work and social life.

Assessment

In addition to the following, assess the older patient for other medical causes of imbalance and dizziness, such as neurologic dysfunction, musculoskeletal and cardiovascular disorders, and endocrine problems.

- *Health history:* Medication use; presence of vertigo, tinnitus, nausea and vomiting, and hearing loss; balance problems; frequency and duration of symptoms, precipitating factors for an attack.
- *Physical examination:* Vital signs, general health; hearing, nystagmus, balance.

Nursing Diagnoses and Interventions

The risk for trauma in patients with inner ear disorders is great. Attacks of vertigo may occur without warning and can be so severe that the patient is unable to remain upright. If frequent attacks are accompanied by nausea, nutrition may be compromised. Constant or intermittent tinnitus can interfere with sleep and rest. Finally, because nearly all inner ear disorders are associated with some degree of hearing loss, which may be progressive, the patient has significant psychosocial needs.

Risk for Trauma

Because of the unpredictable nature of attacks, the patient with vertigo due to an inner ear disorder needs to learn strategies for dealing with an acute episode. Because vertigo tends to be chronic except in acute labyrinthitis, the emphasis is on helping the patient develop strategies to reduce the frequency of attacks and the risk of injury.

- Monitor for vertigo, nystagmus, nausea, vomiting, and hearing loss. *Monitoring is important to determine the severity of impairment, the duration of attacks, and the patient's ability to predict an impending attack.*
- Instruct to not get up without assistance during episodes of vertigo. *During attacks of vertigo, assistance reduces the risk of falling.*

> **SAFETY ALERT**
> During an acute attack of vertigo, keep on bed rest with the side rails raised and the call light readily accessible.

- Teach to avoid sudden head movements or position changes. *Sudden movement may precipitate an attack of vertigo.*
- Administer prescribed medications as ordered, including antiemetics, diuretics, and sedatives. *These medications may reduce the frequency, severity, and duration of vertigo attacks.*
- Instruct to take the prescribed medication and lie down in a quiet, darkened room when an impending attack is sensed. *These measures help protect the patient from injury and may shorten the duration and reduce the severity of the attack.*
- Advise to pull to the side of the road and wait for the symptoms to subside if an attack occurs while driving. *Perception and judgment necessary for safe driving may be impaired*

during an acute attack; pulling off the road is vital to protect the safety of the patient and others.

■ Discuss the effect of unilateral hearing loss on the ability to identify the direction of sounds. To ensure safety, encourage the patient to use other senses (e.g., when crossing the street). *Just as depth perception changes when vision is lost in one eye, sound perception and differentiation of direction change when hearing is lost unilaterally.*

Disturbed Sleep Pattern

The tinnitus often associated with inner ear disorders may be loud and continuous, interfering with the patient's ability to concentrate, relax, and sleep. It may be perceived as a continuous high-pitched whine, buzzing, ringing, or a humming sound. In some patients, it may have a pulsatile quality.

■ Refer for a complete hearing and ear examination if one has not been done. *Although most tinnitus is associated with hearing loss, often due to noise exposure, it may also be associated with treatable conditions such as impacted cerumen, hypertension, cerebrovascular disorders, and other conditions.*

■ Discuss options for masking tinnitus to promote concentration and sleep:
  ■ Ambient noise from a radio or sound system
  ■ Masking device or white-noise machine
  ■ Hearing aid that produces a tone to mask the tinnitus
  ■ Hearing aid that amplifies ambient sound
  These techniques or devices help mask the subjective perception of tinnitus, allowing the patient to focus on something other than the sound.

■ Discuss the possible risks and benefits of medications to treat tinnitus. *Many medications have been used to treat tinnitus; oral antidepressants such as nortriptyline (Aventyl, Pamelor) taken at bedtime have been shown to be most effective.*

Using NANDA, NIC, and NOC

Linkages between a selected NANDA nursing diagnosis, NIC, and NOC for the patient with an inner ear disorder are shown in the chart that follows.

NANDA, NIC, AND NOC LINKAGES
The Patient with an Inner Ear Disorder

NANDA | Disturbed Sensory Perception: Auditory

▼

NIC | Communication Enhancement: Hearing Deficit
Environmental Management: Safety

▼

NOC | Hearing Compensation Behavior
Sensory Function: Hearing
Safety Behavior: Fall Prevention

Data from Bulechek, G., Butcher, H., & Dochterman, J. (Eds.). (2008). *Nursing interventions classification (NIC)* (5th ed.). St. Louis, MO: Mosby; Moorhead, S., Johnson, M., Mass, M., & Swanson, E. (Eds.). (2008). *Nursing outcomes classification (NOC)* (4th ed.). St. Louis, MO: Mosby; and NANDA International. (2009). *Nursing diagnoses: Definition & classification 2009–2011.* Oxford, UK: Wiley-Blackwell.

Community-Based Care

Because disorders of the inner ear disrupt balance, safety is a primary focus of teaching. Assist the patient to identify possible hazards in the home environment. Discuss the following points during the teaching session:

■ Change positions slowly, especially when ambulating.
■ Turn the whole body rather than just the head.
■ Sit down immediately with the onset of vertigo and lie down if possible.
■ Take prescribed antiemetic and antivertigo medications.
■ Wear Medic-Alert identification.
■ If appropriate, discuss the surgical procedure, the immediate postoperative period, and the long-term effects of the surgery.
■ Discuss alternative communication techniques as needed.
■ Suggest the following resources:
  ■ Better Hearing Institute
  ■ Self-Help for Hard of Hearing People

The Patient with an Acoustic Neuroma

An acoustic neuroma or schwannoma is a benign tumor of cranial nerve VIII. It typically occurs in adults between the ages of 40 and 50. Acoustic neuromas are common, developing in about 1 in 100,000 people annually (National Institute on Deafness and Other Communication Disorders [NIDCD], 2008).

These tumors usually occur in the internal auditory meatus, compressing the auditory nerve where it exits the skull to the inner ear. Both the vestibular and cochlear branches are affected; however, the tumor arises from the vestibular division of the auditory nerve twice as often. If allowed to grow, the tumor eventually destroys the labyrinth, including the cochlea and vestibular apparatus. As the tumor expands, it erodes the wall of the internal auditory meatus. The tumor may eventually impinge on the inferior cerebellar artery, which provides blood to the lateral pons and medulla, the brainstem, and the cerebellum. An obstructive hydrocephalus can also occur. Cranial nerves VII (facial) and V (trigeminal) are often affected by the expanding tumor; the tumor frequently wraps around the facial nerve.

Early manifestations of an acoustic neuroma are those associated with disorders of the inner ear: tinnitus, unilateral hearing loss, and nystagmus. Dizziness or vertigo may occur. As the tumor expands and occupies increasing amounts of space in the closed cranium, the patient experiences neurologic signs related to the area of the brain affected.

The presence of the tumor can generally be identified on CT or MRI scans. X-ray films of the petrous pyramid of the temporal bone may show erosion caused by the tumor.

The treatment of choice for an acoustic neuroma is surgical excision. In surgery, every effort is made to preserve this nerve and its function as well as other cranial nerves that may be affected. Small tumors of the vestibular division of the acoustic nerve may be excised using microsurgical techniques; hearing can often be preserved. A translabyrinthine approach provides good access to the tumor and allows the facial nerve to be preserved. However, this approach destroys hearing in the affected ear, and it is usually used only when the tumor is large or little effective hearing remains in the affected ear. Larger tumors require craniotomy for removal; facial nerve paralysis is a common result of surgery.

Postoperative nursing care focuses on preserving cerebral function. Position the patient to minimize cerebral edema and monitor frequently for signs of increased intracranial pressure. Because the gag reflex may be affected, assess the patient carefully before food and fluids are allowed by mouth. Speech therapy is often prescribed for the patient after surgery. Because deficits may not resolve for a long time after surgery, education and support are vital components of nursing care for the patient. (∞ See Chapter 42 for care of the patient undergoing craniotomy.)

Geriatric Sensations Video

The Patient with Hearing Loss

Hearing loss is a significant problem, affecting an estimated 17% of adults in the United States. The problem of hearing loss is particularly significant in older adults, affecting about 30% of people between the ages of 65 and 74, and more than 47% of those over age 75 (NIDCD, 2010). As many as 70% of nursing home residents have impaired hearing.

Hearing loss impairs the ability to communicate in a world filled with sound and hearing individuals. A hearing deficit can be partial or total, congenital or acquired. It may affect one or both ears. In some types of hearing loss, the ability to perceive sound at specific frequencies is lost. In others, hearing is diminished across all frequencies.

Patients with hearing loss often display signs that caregivers can recognize. The voice volume of the patient with impaired hearing frequently increases, and the patient positions the head with the better ear toward the speaker. The patient frequently may ask people to repeat what they have said or respond inappropriately to questions or statements. A question may elicit a blank look if the patient has not heard or understood its content.

Pathophysiology and Manifestations

Lesions in the outer ear, middle ear, inner ear, or central auditory pathways can result in hearing loss. The process of aging also can affect the structures of the ear and hearing. Hearing loss is classified as conductive, sensorineural, or mixed, depending on what portion of the auditory system is affected. Profound deafness is often a congenital condition.

Conductive Hearing Loss

Anything that disrupts the transmission of sound from the external auditory meatus to the inner ear results in a conductive hearing loss. The most common cause of conductive hearing loss is obstruction of the external ear canal. Impacted cerumen, edema of the canal lining, stenosis, and neoplasms all may lead to canal obstruction. Other causes of conductive loss include a perforated tympanic membrane, disruption or fixation of the ossicles of the middle ear, fluid, scarring, or tumors of the middle ear.

With conductive hearing loss, there is an equal loss of hearing at all sound frequencies. If the level of sound is greater than

the threshold for hearing, speech discrimination is good. Because of this, the patient with a conductive hearing loss benefits from amplification by a hearing aid.

Sensorineural Hearing Loss

Disorders that affect the inner ear, the auditory nerve, or the auditory pathways of the brain may lead to a sensorineural hearing loss. In this type of hearing loss, sound waves are effectively transmitted to the inner ear. In the inner ear, however, lost or damaged receptor cells, changes in the cochlear apparatus, or auditory nerve abnormalities decrease or distort the ability to receive and interpret stimuli.

A significant cause of sensorineural hearing deficit is damage to the hair cells of the organ of Corti. In the United States, noise exposure is the major cause, resulting in high-frequency hearing loss in about 26 million Americans between ages 20 and 69 (NIDCD, 2010). Damage may result from either loud impulse noise (e.g., an explosion) or loud continuous noise (e.g., machinery). Exposure to a high level of noise (e.g., standing close to the stage or speakers at a rock concert) on an intermittent or continuing basis damages the hair and supporting cells of the organ of Corti. Ototoxic drugs also damage the hair cells; when combined with high noise levels, the damage is greater and resultant hearing loss more profound. Ototoxic drugs include aspirin, furosemide (Lasix), aminoglycosides, streptomycin, vancomycin (Vancocin), antimalarial drugs, and chemotherapy such as cisplatin (Platinol). Other potential causes of sensory hearing loss include prenatal exposure to rubella, viral infections, meningitis, trauma, Ménière's disease, and aging.

Tumors such as acoustic neuromas, vascular disorders, demyelinating or degenerative diseases, infections (bacterial meningitis in particular), or trauma may affect the central auditory pathways and produce a neural hearing loss.

Sensorineural hearing losses typically affect the ability to hear high-frequency tones more than low-frequency tones. This loss makes speech discrimination difficult, especially in a noisy environment. Hearing aids are often not useful, because they amplify both speech and background noise. The increased sound intensity may actually cause discomfort for the patient.

Presbycusis

With aging, the hair cells of the cochlea degenerate, producing a progressive sensorineural hearing loss. In **presbycusis**, gradual hearing loss associated with aging, hearing acuity begins to decrease in early adulthood and progresses as long as the individual lives. Higher pitched tones and conversational speech are lost initially. Hearing aids and other amplification devices are useful for most patients with presbycusis.

Because the hearing loss of presbycusis is gradual, the patient and family may not realize the extent of the deficit. The individual with a hearing impairment may be described as unsociable or paranoid. The family may worry that the person is becoming increasingly forgetful, absentminded, or perhaps "senile." Depression, confusion, inattentiveness, tension, and negativism have been noted in older adults with hearing impairments. Functional problems such as poor general health, reduced mobility, and impaired interpersonal communication are also associated with hearing loss. Caregivers need to be alert for signs of impaired hearing such as cupping an ear, difficulty understanding verbal communication when the person cannot see the speaker's face, difficulty following conversation in a large group, and withdrawal from social activities.

Tinnitus

Tinnitus is the perception of sound or noise in the ears without stimulus from the environment. The sound may be steady, intermittent, or pulsatile and is often described as a buzzing, roaring, or ringing.

Tinnitus is usually associated with hearing loss (conductive or sensorineural); however, the mechanism producing the sound is poorly understood. It is often an early symptom of noise-induced hearing damage and drug-related ototoxicity. Tinnitus is especially associated with salicylate, quinine, or quinidine toxicity. Other etiologies include obstruction of the auditory meatus, presbycusis, middle or inner ear inflammations and infections, otosclerosis, and Ménière's disease. Most tinnitus, however, is chronic and has no pathologic importance.

Tinnitus that is intermittent or slight enough to be masked by environmental sounds is often well-tolerated. When it is loud, continuous, and not responsive to treatment, tinnitus can be a significant stressor. It can interfere with activities of daily living, sleep, and rest.

Interdisciplinary Care

The best treatment for hearing loss is prevention. Patients need to know the risk for hearing damage and how to prevent it. Awareness of the effects of noise exposure, especially when combined with the ototoxic effects of aspirin or other drugs, is important to prevent sensorineural hearing loss.

Diagnosis

Hearing evaluation includes gross tests of hearing (such as the whisper test), the Rinne and Weber tests, and audiometry.

- *Rinne* and *Weber tests* compare air and bone sound conduction. When bone conduction of sound is better than air conduction, the hearing deficit is a conductive loss. The Rinne test can identify even mild conductive hearing losses. If both air and bone conduction are impaired, a sensorineural loss is indicated (∞ Chapter 45).
- *Audiometry* identifies the type and pattern of hearing loss. Specific sound frequencies are presented to each ear by either air or bone conduction.
- *Speech audiometry* identifies the intensity at which speech can be recognized and interpreted. *Speech discrimination* evaluates the ability to discriminate among various speech sounds.
- *Tympanometry* is an indirect measurement of the compliance and impedance of the middle ear to sound transmission. The external auditory meatus is subjected to neutral, positive, and negative air pressure while the resultant sound energy flow is monitored.
- *Acoustic reflex testing* uses a tone presented at various intensities to evaluate movement of the structures of the middle ear.

Amplification

A hearing aid or other amplification device can help many patients with hearing deficits. These assistive devices do nothing to prevent, minimize, or treat the hearing loss itself. They amplify the sound presented to the hearing apparatus of the ear, which may bring the level of sound above the hearing threshold, allowing more accurate perception and interpretation of its meaning. When sound perception is distorted, a hearing aid may be less helpful, because it simply amplifies the distorted sound.

Unfortunately, less than one-fifth of older patients with a hearing deficit have or use a hearing aid. Denial of the deficit, other health problems, poor visual acuity, decreased manual dexterity, and cost all contribute to this low usage. Hearing aids must be individually prescribed by an audiologist. Proper design, proper fit, and regular maintenance are necessary for their effectiveness.

All hearing aids include a microphone, amplifier, speaker, earpiece, and volume control. Many include an option to turn off the microphone when using the telephone, others can be adjusted for the patient's pattern of hearing loss. Hearing aids are available in a variety of styles, each with advantages and disadvantages:

- Canal hearing aids (in-the-canal and completely-in-canal) are the least noticeable style, fitting in the ear canal. They are appropriate for mild to moderately severe hearing loss. These small and unobtrusive devices allow use of the telephone and can be worn during exercise. Because of their small size, the patient must have good manual dexterity to insert, clean, and change the batteries on canal hearing aids (Figure 46–18 ■). For this reason, older patients or patients with impaired dexterity may be unable to use them.
- The in-ear style of hearing aid fits into the external ear and is used for mild to severe hearing loss (Figure 46–19 ■). Its larger size makes manipulation somewhat easier, although it

Figure 46–18 ■ A person holds a tiny, completely-in-canal hearing aid.

Figure 46–19 ■ An in-ear hearing aid fits inconspicuously in the outer ear. The small dial is a volume control. The plastic flap is the lid of the battery case.

Source: Photo Researchers, Inc.

still may be difficult for less dexterous individuals. A greater degree of amplification is possible with the in-ear aid. Many have a toggle switch for telephone usage.

■ The behind-ear hearing aid allows finer adjustment of the level of amplification and is easier for the patient to manipulate (Figure 46–20 ■). It can be used by patients with mild to profound hearing loss. For the patient who wears glasses, this style can be modified, with all components fitting into the temple of the eyeglasses.

■ Patients with profound hearing loss may require a body hearing aid. The microphone and amplifier of this aid are contained in a pocket-sized case that the patient clips onto clothing, slips into a pocket, or carries in a harness. The receiver is attached by a cord to the case and clips onto the ear mold, which delivers the sound to the ear canal.

Figure 46–20 ■ A woman wearing a behind-ear hearing aid.

With both the in-canal and in-ear style, cleaning is important. Small portals may become plugged with cerumen, interfering with sound transmission.

For the patient who does not have a hearing aid, an *assistive listening device*, or "pocket talker," with a microphone and MP3 player type earpieces, is useful. Pocket talkers are available over the counter or through an audiologist and are relatively inexpensive. The earpiece requires no special fitting, and the external microphone allows the patient to focus on the desired sound rather than simply amplifying all sounds. Assistive listening devices may also be used in conjunction with a hearing aid.

Patients with tinnitus may find a white-noise masking device helpful to promote concentration and rest. These devices conduct a pleasant sound to the affected ear, allowing the patient to block out the abnormal sound.

Surgery

Reconstructive surgeries of the middle ear, such as a stapedectomy or tympanoplasty, may help restore hearing with a conductive hearing loss. Stapedectomy is the removal and replacement of the stapes. This procedure is used to treat hearing loss related to otosclerosis.

In a tympanoplasty, the structures of the middle ear are reconstructed to improve conductive hearing deficits. Chronic otitis media with necrosis and scarring of the middle ear is a common indication for this type of surgery.

For the patient with a sensorineural hearing loss, a *cochlear implant* may be the only hope for restoring sound perception. The cochlear implant consists of a microphone, speech processor, transmitter, receiver/stimulator, and electrodes (Figure 46–21 ■). Its function is more similar to the way the ear normally receives and processes sounds than it is to a hearing aid. The microphone picks up sounds, sending them to the speech processor, which selects and processes useful sounds. The transmitter and receiver/stimulator receive signals from the speech processor, convert them to electrical impulses, and send these impulses to the electrodes for transmission to the brain.

Cochlear implants provide sound perception but not normal hearing. The patient is able to recognize warning sounds such as automobiles, sirens, telephones, and doors opening or closing. The implants also receive stimuli to alert them to incoming communication so they can focus on the person speaking. Many patients learn to interpret perceived sounds as words, especially when the hearing loss is acquired as an adult.

✑ Nursing Care

In planning and implementing nursing care for the patient with a hearing deficit the type and extent of hearing loss, the patient's adaptation to the loss, and the availability of assistive hearing devices are considered, as well as the patient's ability and willingness to use assistive devices.

Health Promotion

Healthcare personnel can be instrumental in the early identification of hearing loss (see the accompanying Moving Evidence into Action box) and in preventing hearing loss through education. It

Transmitter

Receiver/Stimulator

Electrode

Microphone

Speech processor worn on body

Figure 46–21 ■ A cochlear implant for hearing loss.

is important to promote environmental noise control and the use of ear protection. The Occupational Safety and Health Administration requires ear protection for work environments that consistently exceed 85 decibels. Teaching for primary prevention focuses on the following:

■ Care of the ears and ear canals, including cleaning and treatment of infection
■ Not placing hard objects into the ear canal

■ Use of plugs to protect the ears during swimming or diving
■ Avoiding intermittent or frequent exposure to loud noise
■ Monitoring for side effects with ototoxic medications
■ Hearing evaluation when hearing difficulty is present

Assessment

■ *Health history:* Perceived ability to hear; effect of hearing loss on function and lifestyle; risk factors such as use of ototoxic medications; upper respiratory tract or frequent ear infection; noise exposure; presence of vertigo, tinnitus, unsteadiness, or imbalance.
■ *Physical examination:* Apparent perception of normal speech; inspection of external ear, tympanic membrane; whisper, Rinne, and Weber tests; tests of balance and cranial nerve function.

Nursing Diagnoses and Interventions

This section focuses on the problems of having a hearing deficit, impaired communication, and social isolation for the patient who is hearing impaired.

Disturbed Sensory Perception: Auditory

Whether the patient's hearing deficit is partial or total, impaired sound perception is the primary problem. The patient needs to understand what causes the deficit and what to expect for the future. Nursing interventions focus on maximizing available hearing and preventing further deterioration to the extent possible.

■ Encourage to talk about the hearing loss and its effect on activities of daily living. *Hearing loss affects each individual in a different way. The patient may be denying the extent of the deficit or grieving the loss. Listening and providing support encourage the patient to develop coping strategies.*
■ Provide information about the type of hearing loss. Refer to an audiologist for evaluation of the hearing loss and possible exploration of amplification devices. *With improved understanding of the deficit, the patient can plan ways to compensate.*

MOVING EVIDENCE INTO ACTION   **Hearing Loss**

Hearing loss is recognized as a significant problem, affecting more than 30% of older adults. Hearing loss can lead to negative outcomes such as isolation, depression, and possibly declining cognition. Despite these widely recognized statistics and consequences, nurse researchers found that 85% of study participants with documented hearing loss and clear recall reported that their primary care provider had never proactively asked about or screened for hearing loss (Wallhagen & Pettengill, 2008). Furthermore, some participants reported lack of concern or affirmative action when asking the physician about their perceived hearing loss.

IMPLICATIONS FOR NURSING
This study suggests that hearing loss among older adults is underaddressed and even discounted by many healthcare providers. Nurses are in a position to overcome this healthcare disparity and promote health by initiating hearing screening and providing information about hearing loss and its treatment. Initial screening can be as simple as asking the patient about hearing loss or difficulty hearing. It is important to avoid

assuming that a patient with hearing loss has undergone hearing evaluation and chosen to "live with it." Including screening for hearing loss as a regular part of nursing assessment of older adults can prevent or reduce negative effects of untreated hearing loss (Wallhagen & Pettengill, 2008).

CRITICAL THINKING IN PATIENT CARE
1. Several participants in this study reported that their concerns about hearing loss were discounted by the primary care provider with statements such as "it was just normal for me to lose my hearing a little bit." Identify more appropriate possible responses to a patient's concerns about hearing loss.
2. Depression and cognitive decline are identified as potential negative outcomes of untreated hearing loss. How does hearing loss contribute to these problems in the older adult?
3. A patient who admits to "some" hearing loss is reluctant to undergo a hearing screening. How would you approach the patient to identify and address his or her concerns?

EVIDENCE FOR NURSING CARE — **The Patient with Impaired Hearing**

Selected resources that nurses may find helpful when planning evidence-based nursing care follow.

■ Adams-Wendling, L. & Pimple, C. (2007 June). *Nursing management of hearing impairment in nursing facility residents.* Iowa City, IA: University of Iowa Gerontological Nursing Interventions Research Center, Research Dissemination Core. Retrieved from www.guideline.gov

■ Grue, E. V., Kirkevold, M., & Ranhoff, A. H. (2009). Prevalence of vision, hearing, and combined vision and hearing impairments in patients with hip fractures. *Journal of Clinical Nursing, 18*(21), 3037–49.

■ University of Texas, School of Nursing, Family Nurse Practitioner Program. (2007 May). *Evaluation and management of obstructing cerumen.* Austin, TX: University of Texas, School of Nursing.

■ Replace batteries in hearing aids regularly and as needed. *Hearing aid batteries last approximately 1 week. If a battery is old or has been improperly stored, the life may be reduced further.*

■ If the hearing aid has a toggle switch for microphone/ telephone, be sure it is in the appropriate position. *This ensures proper amplification with the hearing aid.*

> **PRACTICE ALERT**
> Check hearing aids for patency, cleaning out cerumen as necessary.

Impaired Verbal Communication

A hearing deficit impairs the patient's ability to receive and interpret verbal communication. A hearing loss affects the patient's ability to follow conversations, use the telephone, and enjoy television or other forms of entertainment.

■ Use the following techniques to improve communication:
   a. Wave the hand or tap the shoulder before beginning to speak.
   b. If the patient wears corrective lenses, ensure that they are clean, and encourage the patient to wear them.
   c. When speaking, face your patient and keep your hands away from your face.
   d. Keep your face in full light.
   e. Reduce the noise in the environment before speaking.
   f. Use a low voice pitch with normal loudness.
   g. Use short sentences and pause at the end of each sentence.
   h. Speak at a normal rate, and do not overarticulate.
   i. Use facial expressions or gestures.
   j. Provide a magic slate for written communication.

Individuals with hearing impairments often lip-read, making good visibility of the speaker's face necessary. Excessive environmental noise interferes with the ability to perceive the message. Higher tones are typically lost with presbycusis and other types of hearing loss. Using short sentences and pausing give the patient time to interpret the message. Overarticulating makes it more difficult to follow the flow and to lip-read. Nonverbal cues and written messages enhance the patient's understanding.

■ Be sure hearing aid is properly placed, is turned on, and has fresh batteries. *The patient may not be aware that the hearing aid is not functioning well.*

■ Do not place intravenous catheters in the dominant hand. *The patient may need to use that hand to write.*

■ Rephrase sentences when there is difficulty understanding. *Hearing losses may affect different sound tones, making some words more difficult to comprehend. Using alternative words and phrases may increase the patient's ability to perceive the message.*

■ Repeat important information. *The nurse makes sure that the patient understands the information.*

■ Inform other staff about the patient's hearing deficit and effective strategies for communication. *Consistent use of effective strategies for communication decreases the patient's frustration.*

Social Isolation

The patient with impaired hearing often becomes socially isolated. This isolation may be self-imposed because of difficulty communicating, especially in a group. Often, however, the isolation comes about gradually and without intention. The patient finds social settings such as family dinners or community gatherings increasingly difficult. Friends and family become frustrated trying to communicate with someone who has a hearing impairment, and invitations to participate in social activities dwindle.

■ Identify the extent and cause of the social isolation. Help to differentiate the reality of the isolation and its cause from the patient's perception of isolation. *Patients with impaired hearing may be unaware that they are isolated. Identifying factors that contribute to isolation may provide the needed impetus to remedy the hearing loss. Patients may also experience paranoid thinking as a result of impaired communication and believe that friends and family have purposely begun to avoid interactions.*

■ Encourage to interact with friends and family on a one-to-one basis in quiet settings. *Patients with impaired hearing are more successful in understanding conversations that take place in small groups and quiet settings.*

■ Treat with dignity and remind friends and family that a hearing deficit does not indicate loss of mental faculties. *Inappropriate responses due to a hearing deficit can cause others to perceive the patient as "stupid" or demented.*

■ Involve in activities that do not require acute hearing, such as checkers and chess. *The patient has an opportunity to interact socially without the stress of straining to hear.*

■ Obtain a pocket talker or encourage the patient and family to do so.

■ Refer the patient to an audiologist for evaluation and possible hearing-aid fitting.

■ Refer to resources such as support groups and senior citizen centers. *These groups provide new social outlets.*

Using NANDA, NIC, and NOC

Linkages between a selected NANDA nursing diagnosis, NIC, and NOC for the patient with a hearing deficit are shown in the chart that follows.

NANDA, NIC, AND NOC LINKAGES
The Patient with a Hearing Deficit

NANDA   Impaired Verbal Communication

NIC   Communication Enhancement:
Hearing Deficit
Socialization Enhancement

NOC   Communication: Receptive
Hearing Compensation Behavior
Social Involvement

Data from Bulechek, G., Butcher, H., & Dochterman, J. (Eds.). (2008). *Nursing interventions classification (NIC)* (5th ed.). St. Louis, MO: Mosby; Moorhead, S., Johnson, M., Maas, M., & Swanson, E. (Eds.). (2008). *Nursing outcomes classification (NOC)* (4th ed.). St. Louis, MO: Mosby; and NANDA International. (2009). *Nursing diagnoses: Definitions & classification 2009–2011.* Oxford, UK: Wiley-Blackwell.

Community-Based Care

Teaching for home and community-based care for the patient with hearing loss focuses on managing the deficit and developing coping strategies. Referral to an audiologist for evaluation of the deficit and the usefulness of a hearing aid may be appropriate. In addition, discuss the following topics as appropriate for each patient:

- Use, care, and maintenance of a hearing aid
- Strategies for coping with the hearing deficit
- Voicing a preference for individual visits and small group interactions rather than large social functions
- Helpful resources include the following:
  - American Academy of Audiology
  - American Speech-Language-Hearing Association
  - House Ear Institute
  - National Institute on Deafness and Other Communication Disorders
  - National Deaf Education Center
  - Self-Help for Hard of Hearing People

CHAPTER HIGHLIGHTS

- Structures of the external eye are vulnerable to trauma and infection. While usually minor, these problems can cause significant pain, scarring and clouding of the cornea, and loss or impairment of vision.
- Cataracts, glaucoma, age-related macular degeneration, and diabetic retinopathy are leading causes of visual impairment in the United States. While these conditions cannot, in most cases, be prevented, they often can be treated or their progress slowed, preserving vision.
- Age, smoking, diabetes, radiation (sun exposure), and long-term use of certain drugs are risk factors for cataract development. Removal of the clouded lens with insertion of an intraocular lens is the treatment of choice for cataracts. Surgery is elective, performed only when the cataract significantly impairs the ability to maintain ADLs and recreational activities.
- Glaucoma is progressive loss of visual fields associated with increased intraocular pressure and impaired aqueous humor drainage. Open-angle or chronic glaucoma, the predominant form of the disorder, can be controlled using medications and, as needed, laser surgery to promote aqueous humor drainage.
- Angle-closure glaucoma is a medical emergency requiring immediate treatment to lower intraocular pressure to preserve vision. Angle-closure glaucoma usually affects only one eye; however, the patient is at risk for future attacks affecting the other eye.
- Age-related macular degeneration, a leading cause of blindness, cannot be effectively treated, although its progress may be slowed or halted through use of high-dose antioxidant vitamins and zinc if it is identified early. Macular degeneration affects the macula, the area of high-acuity central vision.

- Diabetic retinopathy eventually affects nearly all people with diabetes. It is a disease of the small blood vessels of the retina, leading to formation of aneurysms, retinal ischemia, and growth of fragile new vessels (neovascularization) that easily rupture leading to hemorrhage. It is treated with laser surgery to seal fragile vessels.
- Otitis media is related to eustachian tube dysfunction, with impaired pressure equalization of the middle ear. Otitis media may be either serous (sterile) or infectious. Both cause acute discomfort with diminished hearing, snapping, popping, and possible vertigo and systemic symptoms. The risk of complications, including rupture of the tympanic membrane, damage to structures of the middle ear, and spread of infection to surrounding tissues, is greater with acute otitis media.
- Potential complications of acute otitis media include mastoiditis, chronic otitis media with tympanic membrane perforation, and cholesteatoma formation. Hearing loss in the affected ear is a possibility with these disorders. The primary treatment is prevention through adequate treatment of acute otitis media.
- The primary manifestations of disorders of the inner ear are vertigo and possible hearing loss. Severe vertigo can interfere with safety, nutrition, and the patient's ability to maintain ADLs and life roles.
- The two major types of hearing loss are conductive and sensorineural. Presbycusis, hearing loss associated with aging, is a type of sensorineural hearing loss. Hearing loss may be accompanied by tinnitus, the perception of sound without an environmental stimulus. Amplification devices (hearing aids) are the primary treatment for hearing loss.

TEST YOURSELF NCLEX-RN® REVIEW

1. A nurse is working with a group of residents in a long-term care facility. All of the residents have moderate to severe hearing or vision impairment. Which of the following does the nurse identify as the highest priority of care?
   1. preventing sensory deprivation
   2. encouraging social interaction
   3. promoting family relationships
   4. maintaining resident safety

2. The nurse teaching a patient with newly diagnosed glaucoma emphasizes which of the following instructions?
   1. turning the head side to side to compensate for impaired peripheral vision
   2. using the prescribed eyedrops as directed on a continuing basis
   3. contacting the physician if further decline in vision is noticed
   4. avoiding coughing, sneezing, or straining to have a bowel movement

3. A patient with glaucoma has a history of heart failure. Which medication should the nurse discuss with the physician before administering it?
   1. brimonidine (Alphagan)
   2. dorzolamide (Trusopt)
   3. timolol (Timoptic)
   4. latanoprost (Xalatan)

4. A patient with Ménière's disease experiences frequent attacks of vertigo and tinnitus. Of the following teaching points, which one has the highest priority for this patient?
   1. Follow a low-sodium diet.
   2. Stop smoking.
   3. Take prescribed antiemetic medications.
   4. Sit down when an attack develops.

5. On a patient's return from cataract surgery, the nurse in the ambulatory surgery recovery unit does which of the following?
   1. places the patient in semi-Fowler's position
   2. positions the patient on the affected side
   3. places the patient in a private room
   4. ensures the patient is in proximity to the nurses' station

6. A patient calls her primary care provider's office with complaints of bright flashing lights to the side of her vision. Which is the most appropriate response by the nurse?
   1. Recommend that she lie down until the sensation has passed.
   2. Advise her to make an appointment to have her blood pressure checked.
   3. Initiate immediate referral to an ophthalmologist.
   4. Reassure her that this is not unusual and should resolve without treatment.

7. A patient presents at the urgent care clinic with complaints of right ear pain. Which of the following should be included in physical assessment of this patient? **Select all that apply.**
   1. vital signs with temperature
   2. inspection of the oral pharynx
   3. manipulation of the ear pinna
   4. palpation of cervical lymph nodes
   5. inspection of the ear canal and tympanic membrane

8. An elderly resident in an assisted living facility complains to the nurse that his head "feels stuffy" and he has ringing in his ears. How should the nurse respond?
   1. Make an appointment with the resident's primary care physician.
   2. Refer the patient for evaluation by a local audiologist.
   3. Provide nonprescription eardrops for daily use.
   4. Inspect the ear canals for patency.

9. The nurse caring for a patient with a severe hearing deficit identifies which of the following as an appropriate goal toward improving the patient's social interactions?
   1. Will plan to have dinner with one or two friends weekly.
   2. Will participate in senior center communal lunches at least twice per week.
   3. Will engage in activities such as card tournaments and dancing.
   4. Will attend religious services of choice.

10. When assessing a patient, the nurse notes absence of the red reflex in the patient's right eye. On questioning, the patient responds, "Oh yes, my doctor told me I have cataracts. When do you think I should have them removed?" How should the nurse respond?
    1. "It appears that the right eye is due for surgery."
    2. "Are you having difficulty reading or doing activities you enjoy?"
    3. "Are you starting to experience pain in your right eye or frequent headaches?"
    4. "Cataracts can be removed any time that it is convenient for you."

See Test Yourself answers in Appendix C.

Pearson Nursing Student Resources

Find additional review materials at
www.nursing.pearsonhighered.com

Prepare for success with additional NCLEX®-style practice questions, interactive assignments and activities, Web links, animations and videos, and more!

BIBLIOGRAPHY

Alper, B. S. (2005a). Evidence-based medicine. Lowering intraocular pressure delays visual-field loss in glaucoma. *Clinical Advisor for Nurse Practitioners, 8*(12), 128.

Alper, B. S. (2005b). Evidence-based medicine. Lowering intraocular pressure may prevent glaucoma. *Clinical Advisor for Nurse Practitioners, 8*(12), 128.

American Academy of Ophthalmology Retina/Vitreous Panel, Preferred Practice Patterns Committee. (2008). *Diabetic retinopathy.* San Francisco, CA: American Academy of Ophthalmology (AAO). Retrieved from www.guideline.gov/summary/summary.aspx?doc_id=13502

Bulechek, G., Butcher, H., & Dochterman, J. (Eds.). (2008). *Nursing interventions classification (NIC)* (5th ed.). St. Louis, MO: Mosby.

Chou, R., Dana, T., & Bougatsos, C. (2009). Clinical guidelines. Screening older adults for impaired visual acuity: A review of the evidence for the U.S. Preventive Services Task Force. *Annals of Internal Medicine, 151,* 44–58.

Copstead, L. E., & Banasik, J. L. (2010). *Pathophysiology* (4th ed.). Philadelphia: W. B. Saunders.

Davies, S., & de Guzman, A. (2004). Ear drops containing steroids were better than acetic acid for otitis externa. *Evidence-Based Nursing, 7*(2), 43.

De Beer, L., Stokroos, R., & Kingma, H. (2007). Intratympanic gentamicin therapy for intractable Ménière's disease. *Acta Oto-Laryngologica, 127,* 605–612.

Doherty, G. (2009). *Current surgical diagnosis & treatment* (13th ed.). New York, NY: McGraw-Hill.

Fauci, A., Kasper, D., Braunwald, E., Hauser, S., Longo, D., Jameson, J., et al. (Eds.). (2008). *Harrison's principles of internal medicine* (17th ed.). New York, NY: McGraw-Hill.

Fontaine, K. L. (2005). *Healing practices: Alternative therapies for nursing* (2nd ed.). Upper Saddle River, NJ: Prentice Hall Health.

Goldman, H., Kiffel, S., & Weinstock, F. (2009, May). Cataract surgery and the primary care practitioner. *Geriatrics, 64*(5), 19–26.

Kaufman, S. (2009, March). Developments in age-related macular degeneration: Diagnosis and treatment. *Geriatrics, 64*(3), 16–19.

Lighthouse International. (2009). *Prevalence of vision impairment.* Retrieved from www.lighthouse.org

Lin, A., Orengo-Nania, S., & Braun, U. (2009, July). Management of chronic open-angle glaucoma in the aging US population. *Geriatrics, 64*(7), 20–28.

Linus Pauling Institute. (2009). *Micronutrient information center. Carotinoids.* Retrieved from http://lpi.oregonstate.edu/infocenter/phytochemicals/carotenoids/#armd

McPhee, S., Papadakis, M., & Tierney, L., (Eds.). (2008). *Current medical diagnosis & treatment* (47th ed.). New York, NY: McGraw Hill.

Moorhead, S., Johnson, M., Maas, M., & Swanson, E. (Eds.). (2008). *Nursing outcomes classification (NOC)* (4th ed.). St. Louis, MO: Mosby

National Eye Institutes, National Institutes of Health. (2009b). *Age-related macular degeneration.* Retrieved from http://www.nei.nih.gov/health/maculardegen/armd_facts.asp#1d

National Eye Institutes, National Institutes of Health. (2009c). *Facts about cataract.* Retrieved from www.nei.nih.gov/health/cataract/cataract_facts.asp

National Eye Institutes, National Institutes of Health. (2009d). *Facts about diabetic retinopathy.* Retrieved from www.nei.nih.gov/health/diabetic/retinopathy.asp

National Eye Institutes, National Institutes of Health. (2009e). *Facts about glaucoma.* Retrieved from www.nei.nih.gov/health/glaucoma/glaucoma_facts.asp

National Eye Institutes, National Institutes of Health. (2009f). *Facts about retinal detachment.* Retrieved from www.nei.nih.gov/health/retinaldetach/retinaldetach.asp

National Eye Institutes, National Institutes of Health. (2009a). *Facts about the cornea and corneal disease.* Retrieved from www.nei.nih.gov/health/cornealdisease/

National Eye Institutes, National Institutes of Health. (2008a). *Statement on the prevalence of diabetic retinopathy and age-related macular degeneration amon Hispanic/Latino Americans.* Retrieved from www.nei.nih.gov/news/statements/latinostudy.asp

National Eye Institutes, National Institutes of Health. (2008b). *Statistics and data.* Retrieved from http://www.nei.nih.gov/eyedata/pbd_tables.asp

National Guideline Clearinghouse. (2005). *Contact lens care.* Retrieved from http://www.guideline.gov

National Institute on Deafness and Other Communication Disorders, National Institutes of Health. (2009a). *Cochlear implants.* Retrieved from www.nidcd.nih.gov/health/hearing/coch.asp

National Institute on Deafness and Other Communication Disorders, National Institutes of Health. (2007). *Hearing aids.* Retrieved from http://www.nidcd.nih.gov/health/hearing/hearingaid.asp

National Institute on Deafness and Other Communication Disorders, National Institutes of Health. (2008). *Noise-induced hearing loss.* Retrieved from http://www.nidcd.nih.gov/health/hearing/noise.asp

National Institute on Deafness and Other Communication Disorders, National Institutes of Health. (2002). *Presbycusis.* Retrieved from http://www.nidcd.nih.gov/health/hearing/presbycusis.asp

National Institute on Deafness and Other Communication Disorders, National Institutes of Health. (2010). *Quick statistics.* Retrieved from www.nidcd.nih.gov/health/statistics/quick.htm

Plester, G. (2008, November 7). Glaucoma: Avoiding preventable loss of sight. *Practice Nurse, 36*(8), 27030.

Porth, C., & Matfin, G. (2009). *Pathophysiology: Concepts of altered health states* (8th ed.). Philadelphia, PA: Lippincott.

Postema, R., Kingma, C., Wit, H., Albers, F., & Van Der Laan, B. (2008). Intratympanic gentamicin therapy for control of vertigo in unilateral Ménière's disease: A prospective, double-blind, randomized, placebo-controlled trial. *Acta Oto-Laryngologicia, 128,* 876–880.

Prevent Blindness America, & National Eye Institute, National Institutes of Health. (2008). *Vision problems in the U.S.: Prevalence of adult vision impairment and age-related eye disease in America.* Retrieved from http://www.preventblindness.net/site/DocServer/VPUS_2008_update.pdf?docID=1561

Rhone, M., & Basu, A. (2008). Phytochemical and age-related eye diseases. *Nutrition Reviews, 66*(8), 465–472.

Rothrock, J. C. (2007). *Alexander's care of the patient in surgery* (13th ed.). St. Louis, MO: Mosby.

Rowe, S., MacLean, C., & Shekelle, P. (2004). Preventing visual loss from chronic eye disease in primary care: Scientific review. *JAMA, 291*(12), 1487–1496.

Ryskulova, A., Turczyn, K., Makuc, D., Cotch, M., Klein, R., & Janiszewski, R. (2008, March). Self-reported age-related eye diseases and visual impairment in the United States: Results of the 2002 National Health Interview Survey. *American Journal of Public Health, 98*(3), 454–461.

U.S. Preventive Services Task Force. (2005). Screening for glaucoma: Recommendation statement. *American Journal for Nurse Practitioners, 9*(9), 49–50, 52–55.

U.S. Preventive Services Task Force. (2009). Clinical guidelines. Screening for impaired visual acuity in older adults: U.S. Preventive Services Task Force recommendation statement. *Annals of Internal Medicine, 151,* 37–43.

Wallhagen, M., & Pettengill, E. (2008). Hearing impairment: Significant but underassessed in primary care settings. *Journal of Gerontological Nursing, 34*(2), 36–42.

Warren, E. (2008, May). Vertigo. *Practice Nurse, 35*(10), 36–41.

Wilkinson, J., & Ahern, N. (2009). *Nursing diagnosis handbook* (9th ed.). Upper Saddle River, NJ: Prentice Hall.

Watkinson, S. (2005). Visual impairment in older people: The nurse's role. *Nursing Standard, 19*(17), 45–52, 54–55.

Building Clinical Competence
Responses to Altered Visual and
Auditory Function

Functional Health Pattern: Cognitive-Perceptual

Think about patients with altered vision or hearing for whom you have cared in your clinical experiences.

- What were their major medical diagnoses? Was the vision or hearing deficit the primary diagnosis or a secondary one? Did the patient use an assistive or corrective device such as corrective lenses or a hearing aid?

- Was the loss of vision or hearing age-related, disease-related, or a consequence of treatment (iatrogenic)?

- How did the patients' vision or hearing loss affect their health status and ability to manage their own health?

The Cognitive-Perceptual Health Pattern includes adequacy of vision and hearing. The eyes and ears provide pathways for visual and auditory stimuli to reach the brain. These stimuli allow us to interpret and interact with our environment. Deficits in vision and hearing may limit self-care, mobility, independence, communication, and relationships with others.

Vision and hearing disorders disturb the patient's cognitive-perceptual health pattern, and may cause manifestations such as the following:

- **Loss of visual acuity** (*disruption of normal structures of the eye impairs transmission of light rays to photoreceptors in the retina or from photoreceptors to the brain, leading to impaired visual perception or clarity*)

- **Pain** (*tissue edema and purulent drainage due to inflammation, leading to acute discomfort of involved tissue*)

- **Vertigo** (*sensations of movement, such as whirling or falling, that are caused by disturbance in inner ear, result in loss of equilibrium*)

The senses of vision and hearing allow the patient to communicate, to gain access to information, and to derive pleasure from sights and sounds in the environment. Priority nursing diagnoses within the Cognitive-Perceptual Health Pattern that may be appropriate for patients with deficits affecting these senses include the following:

- *Disturbed Sensory Perception* as evidenced by blurred vision, seeing black spots or floaters, seeing halos, difficulty hearing, altered sense of balance

- *Impaired Verbal Communication* as evidenced by difficulty comprehending and maintaining communication, inability to articulate speech, absence of eye contact

- *Risk for Acute Confusion* as evidenced by inability to identify potential environmental dangers, use of visual aids or hearing aids

Two nursing diagnoses from other health patterns often are of high priority for the patient with altered visual and/or auditory function:

- *Anxiety* (Coping-Stress-Tolerance Pattern)

- *Ineffective Health Maintenance* (Health Perception-Health Management Pattern)

Questions

1. What measures should you implement to maintain a safe environment for your patient with visual impairment?

2. What communication techniques should you use with your patient who is hearing impaired?

CLINICAL SCENARIO

Directions: *Read the clinical scenarios below and answer the questions that follow. To complete this exercise successfully, you will use not only knowledge of the content in this unit, but also principles related to priority setting and maintaining patient safety.*

You have been assigned to work with the following four patients for the 0700 shift on a medical-surgical unit. Significant data obtained during report is as follows:

■ Andrew Hardy, a 50-year-old type I diabetic with a blood glucose of 600 and hypertension, is a new admission during the night shift. Upon assessment the patient reveals that he has been seeing black spot floaters and flashing lights at times. He is now complaining of blurred vision.

■ Gladys Harvey is an 84-year-old who had right eye cataract surgery yesterday. Her vital signs have been stable since surgery. She has begun complaining of itching and slight discomfort in the right eye.

■ Georgia Stanley is a 45-year-old admitted with complaints of feeling like she is spinning or falling and ringing and a fullness feeling in her left ear. Her vital signs are temperature 98.6°F, pulse 78, respirations 16, and blood pressure 102/68. She is diaphoretic and complains of nausea. She is scheduled for x-rays and a CT scan of her head at 0800.

■ Kenneth Koch, a 30-year-old, is a postoperative patient who had a right ear tympanoplasty yesterday because of hearing loss due to chronic otitis media. Vital signs are temperature 99.6°F, pulse 90, respirations 20, and blood pressure 136/86. The patient is requesting pain medication for ear pain. Pain is rated as 9 out of 10 on a scale of 10 being the highest.

Questions

Priority Setting

1. In what order would you visit these patients after report?
   A. _____
   B. _____
   C. _____
   D. _____

Health Promotion

1. What strategies should Ms. Stanley be taught for maintaining near normal social and work life?

2. What instruction should Mr. Hardy be given about controlling his risk factors for vision loss?

3. Which is the appropriate primary prevention to teach Mr. Koch to prevent hearing loss?
   A. Cleanse the ear with ear swabs to prevent earwax buildup.
   B. Avoid getting water in the ears when showering.
   C. Monitor for ringing in the ears when taking acetaminophen (Tylenol).
   D. Wear ear protectors when exposed to loud noises.

Nursing Process

1. What top priority nursing diagnosis would you choose for each of the patients presented previously? What is the rationale for your choices?

	Nursing Diagnosis	Rationale
Andrew Hardy		
Gladys Harvey		
Georgia Stanley		
Kenneth Koch		

2. Which treatment should the nurse anticipate when caring for a patient such as Mr. Hardy who has symptoms diabetic retinopathy?
   A. scleral buckling
   B. enucleation
   C. photorefractive keratectomy
   D. laser photocoagulation

3. After cataract surgery, Ms. Harvey is placed in which position to reduce intraocular pressure?
   A. Sims' position on the unaffected side
   B. semi-Fowler's position on the unaffected side
   C. supine with the head elevated 10 degrees
   D. prone position on the affected side

4. A low-sodium diet is ordered for Ms. Stanley with Ménière's disease. The patient understands this diet when she picks which meal plan?
   A. hot dog on a roll with ketchup and mustard
   B. ham and cheese sandwich with potato salad
   C. grilled chicken sandwich with lettuce and tomato
   D. hamburger on a roll with potato chips

5. When evaluating for Ménière's disease, which diagnostic studies would you expect to be ordered? **Select all that apply.**
   A. caloric testing
   B. Rinne and Weber tests
   C. troponins
   D. complete blood cell count
   E. glycerol test
   F. blood glucose test

6. After Ms. Harvey's eye surgery, which teaching measures does the nurse instruct the patient in?
   A. Avoid lifting more than 15 pounds.
   B. Avoid coughing or sneezing.
   C. Lie on the affected side.
   D. Remove the eye patch when sleeping.

1. Which techniques may improve communication with the patient who is hearing impaired? **Select all that apply.**

   A. Speak loudly to enhance hearing.

   B. Speak at a normal rate and avoid over articulating.

   C. Stand in front of a window so patient can see the face.

   D. Face the patient to enhance lip-reading.

   E. Turn down the television or radio.

   F. Use short sentences and pause frequently.

Delegation

1. For each patient, what assessment data and nursing interventions can be delegated to a CNA?

Content-Specific Questions

1. Which assessment data would be most indicative of hyphema, a potential result of blunt eye trauma?

   A. eye pain, decreased visual acuity, seeing a reddish tint

   B. hypertension, headache, facial pain

   C. white eye reflex, pressure and blindness in affected eye

   D. double vision, sunken eye, limited eye movement

2. A prescription for gentamicin (Garamycin) is ordered for a patient with conjunctivitis. The nurse understands that a serious adverse effect of aminoglycosides is which effect?

   A. damage to the eighth cranial nerve resulting in hearing loss

   B. vasodilation leading to migraine headaches

   C. leg pain caused by thromboembolism

   D. stomach irritation leading to gastric ulcers

3. Which is the correct way to instill ear drops in the adult patient with otitis media?

   A. Have patient hang head over side of bed, pull pinna of the ear straight up, instill ear drops, and have patient turn to instill drops to other ear.

   B. Have patient tilt head toward unaffected side, pull pinna of the ear down and back, instill ear drops, and have patient remain for 3 minutes.

   C. Have patient lie on unaffected side, pull the pinna of the ear up and back, instill ear drops, and have patient remain still for 5 minutes.

   D. Have patient lie in Sims' position on unaffected side, pull the pinna of the ear up and back, instill ear drops, and have the patient turn to other side after 1 minute.

CASE STUDY: Reggie Madison

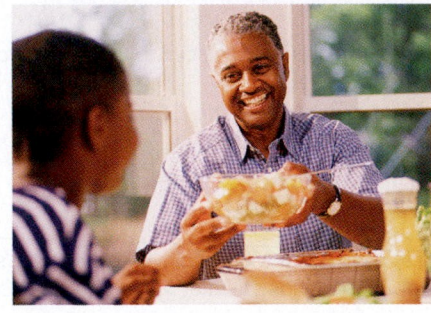

Reggie Madison is a 65-year-old African American male who is seen in the eye clinic with complaints of decreasing peripheral vision in both eyes. He states he has not had any recent eye infections or eye injuries. He denies pain in the eyes. Vital signs are temperature 98.8°F, pulse 84, respirations 16, blood pressure 168/88. His height is 5'8" and weight is 200 pounds. His medical history indicates that he has hypertension and type 2 diabetes. He is taking hydrochlorothiazide, captopril, and glyburide. He states that he is on a 2000 calorie diabetic diet but he is often noncompliant with the diet. He sees his medical doctor about once a year but has not had an eye exam in about 10 years. He is married with five grown children and six grandchildren. Mr. Madison states he does not know if there is any family history of glaucoma as his father died of a heart attack at age 50 and his mother died of cancer at 60 years of age.

The ophthalmologist performs a tonometry, which indicates an increase in intraocular pressure. A funduscopic examination indicates pallor and an increase in the size and depth of the optic cup on the optic disk. Visual field testing indicates significant peripheral vision loss. The results of these tests indicate a diagnosis of glaucoma. A gonioscopy is performed to measure the depth of the anterior chamber to differentiate a medical diagnosis of open-angle glaucoma.

In open-angle glaucoma the fluid balance in the eye is disrupted. Obstructed flow of aqueous humor through the trabecular meshwork and into the canal of Schlemm increases the amount of fluid in the eye causing increased intraocular pressure. The increased intraocular pressure is thought to cause neuronal ischemia and injure the optic nerve. As optic fibers are destroyed, the rim of the optic disc shrinks. The normal depression in the center becomes larger and deeper. As the disease progresses, there is a painless, progressive narrowing of the visual field. The patient experiences gradual loss of peripheral vision without pain.

Based on the medical diagnosis of open-angle glaucoma and the patient's decreased peripheral vision, the nursing diagnosis of *Disturbed Sensory Perception: Visual* is appropriate for planning care for Mr. Madison.

- Obstruction of aqueous humor flow into canal of Schlemm → increased aqueous fluid in eye → increased intraocular pressure
- Increased intraocular pressure → neuronal ischemia → damage to and destruction of optic fibers in the periphery of the optic disc → painless, progressive loss of peripheral vision with narrowing of the visual field and eventual blindness

affects

Mr. R.M,
65 y.o. male
Open-angle glaucoma

leads to

assess →

- 5' 8" tall, 200 lbs.
- T 98.8°F, P 84, R 16
- BP 168/88
- C/o decreased peripheral vision
- History of hypertension, type 2 diabetes
- No known family history of glaucoma
- Current medications: hydrochlorothiazide, captopril, glyburide
- Intraocular pressure 32 mmHg OD, 29 mmHg OS
- Visual field testing reveals significant loss of peripheral vision

generates

- Risk for Injury r/t loss of vision as evidenced by decreased peripheral visual fields
- Impaired Home Maintenance r/t impaired vision as evidenced by decreased peripheral vision
- Anxiety r/t perceived threat of loss of sight as evidenced by restlessness, poor eye contact, verbalized fears

generate nursing diagnosis

prioritized to

Disturbed Sensory Perception: Visual

expected outcomes

- Vital signs stable
- Verbalizes understanding of prescribed medications, their administration and side effects
- Able to effectively and appropriately instill eye medications
- Verbalizes understanding of need for continuing follow-up care
- Able to verbalize safety precautions and compensatory measures related to decreased peripheral vision

evaluate →

Follow-up visit 6 weeks later:
- No further loss of peripheral vision, intraocular pressure 15 mmHg OD and 13 mmHg OS
- Using eye drops as ordered without adverse effects
- Returns for follow-up examinations as instructed.
- No accidents or injury due to decreased peripheral vision

Interdisciplinary Interventions
- Assess and record vital signs.
- Teach how to instill eye medications as prescribed.
- Discuss use and side effects of prescribed medications.

Independent Interventions
- Provide psychological support to decrease anxiety.
- Teach safety measures and techniques to compensate for loss of peripheral vision.
- Discuss possible restrictions such as avoiding sports in which peripheral vision is vital (e.g. contact sports).

Activity:

1. After reviewing the concept map, is there anything you would change to make it more understandable?

2. Review Mr. Madison's history. What additional risk factors for visual impairment does he have? Go to the Pearson Nursing Student Resources for this book at www.nursing.pearsonhighered.com to write a concept map identifying a major risk factor, appropriate nursing diagnoses, and interventions to address the highest priority nursing diagnosis.

See answers and hints in Appendix C.

Sexuality-Reproductive Pattern

PART VI

Functional Health Patterns with Related Nursing Diagnoses

HEALTH PERCEPTION HEALTH MANAGEMENT

- Perceived health status
- Perceived health management
- Health care behaviors: health promotion and illness prevention activities, medical treatments, follow-up care

VALUE-BELIEF

- Values, goals, or beliefs (including spirituality) that guide choices or decisions
- Perceived conflicts in values, beliefs, or expectations that are health related

COPING-STRESS-TOLERANCE

- Capacity to resist challenges to self-integrity
- Methods of handling stress
- Support systems
- Perceived ability to control and manage situations

NUTRITIONAL-METABOLIC

- Daily consumption of food and fluids
- Favorite foods
- Use of dietary supplements
- Skin lesions and ability to heal
- Condition of the integument
- Weight, height, temperature

PART VI

Sexuality-Reproductive Pattern: Examples of Related NANDA Diagnoses

- Anxiety
- Fear
- Disturbed Body Image
- Grieving
- Impaired Tissue Integrity
- Impaired Urinary Elimination
- Ineffective Sexuality Patterns
- Infection
- Sexual Dysfunction
- Risk for Bleeding
- Risk Prone Behavior

SEXUALITY-REPRODUCTIVE

- Satisfaction with sexuality or sexual relationships
- Reproductive pattern
- Female menstrual and perimeno-pausal history

ELIMINATION

- Patterns of bowel and urinary excretion
- Perceived regularity or irregularity of elimination
- Use of laxatives or routines
- Changes in time, modes, quality or quantity of excretions
- Use of devices for control

ROLE-RELATIONSHIP

- Perception of major roles, relationships, and responsibilities in current life situation
- Satisfaction with or disturbances in roles and relationships

ACTIVITY-EXERCISE

- Patterns of personally relevant exercise, activity, leisure, and recreation
- ADLs which require energy expenditure
- Factors that interfere with the desired pattern (e.g., illness or injury)

SELF-PERCEPTION– SELF-CONCEPT

- Attitudes about self
- Perceived abilities, worth, self-image, emotions
- Body posture and movement, eye contact, voice and speech patterns

SLEEP-REST

- Patterns of sleep and rest/relaxation in a 24-hr period
- Perceptions of quality and quantity of sleep and rest
- Use of sleep aids and routines

COGNITIVE-PERCEPTUAL

- Adequacy of vision, hearing, taste, touch, smell
- Pain perception and management
- Language, judgment, memory, decisions

UNIT 13

Responses to Altered
Reproductive Function

Assessing the **Male** and **Female** Reproductive Systems

LEARNING OUTCOMES

1. Describe the anatomy, physiology, and functions of the male and female reproductive systems, including the breasts.
2. Identify specific topics for consideration during a health history interview of the patient with health problems of the reproductive system and breasts.
3. Give examples of genetic disorders of the male and female reproductive system and breasts.
4. Describe normal variations in reproductive assessment findings for the older adult.
5. Identify manifestations of impairment in the male and female reproductive system and breasts.

CLINICAL COMPETENCIES

1. Conduct and document a health history for men and women having or at risk for alterations of the reproductive system and breasts.
2. Conduct and document a physical assessment of male and female reproductive system and breasts.
3. Monitor the results of diagnostic tests and report abnormal findings.

EQUIPMENT NEEDED

- Disposable gloves
- Water-soluble lubricant
- A good light source
- Sterile cotton swabs (for culture)
- Culture media (for culture)
- A spatula, cotton swab or endocervical brush, slides, and cytologic fixative (for Pap smear)
- Vaginal speculum of appropriate size

KEY TERMS

androgens, *1630*	gynecomastia, *1634*	phimosis, *1634*
anorgasmia, *1641*	impotence, *1632*	progesterone, *1637*
dyspareunia, *1641*	menstrual cycle, *1637*	semen, *1630*
estrogens, *1637*	menstruation, *1636*	testosterone, *1630*

The reproductive organs in men and women share the functions of enabling sexual pleasure and reproduction. The reproductive organs, in conjunction with the neuroendocrine system, produce hormones important in biologic development and sexual behavior. Parts of the reproductive organs in men enclose and are integral to the function of the urinary system.

The assessment of the reproductive system may be difficult for both the nurse and the patient and requires sensitivity on the part of the nurse when asking questions about topics that the patient may be hesitant to talk about. Skill in conducting physical examinations of an area of the body usually considered private is also required.

Anatomy, Physiology, and Functions of the Male Reproductive System

The male reproductive system consists of the paired testes, the scrotum, ducts, glands, and penis (Figure 47–1 ■). The breasts are also part of the male reproductive system.

The Breasts

The male breast is comprised primarily of an areola (circular pigmented area) and a small nipple. These lie over a thin disk of undeveloped breast tissue that may not be overtly different from surrounding tissue. Approximately one in three men have a firm area of breast tissue 2 cm or larger; the limits of normal size of this area have not been established (Bickley & Szilagyi, 2007).

The Penis

The penis is the genital organ that encloses the urethra. It is homologous to the clitoris of the female. The penis is composed of a shaft and a tip called the glans, which is covered in

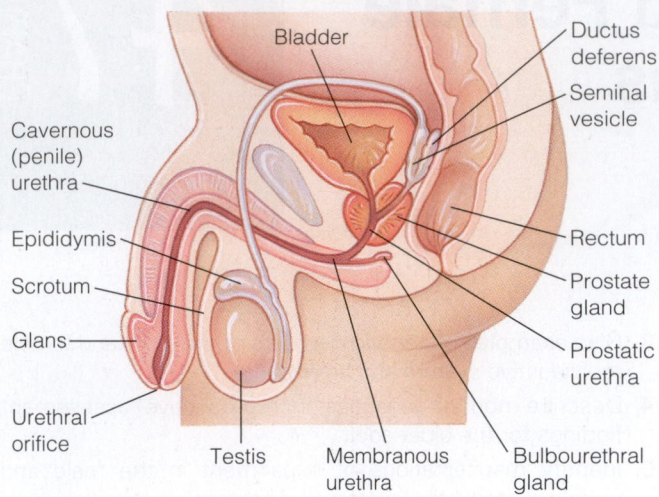

Bladder
Ductus deferens
Seminal vesicle
Cavernous (penile) urethra
Epididymis
Scrotum
Glans
Urethral orifice
Rectum
Prostate gland
Prostatic urethra
Testis
Membranous urethra
Bulbourethral gland

Figure 47–1 ■ The male reproductive system.

the uncircumcised man by the foreskin (or prepuce). Erection of the penis occurs when erectile tissue is filled with blood in response to a reflex that triggers the parasympathetic nervous system to stimulate arteriolar vasodilation. The erection reflex may be initiated by touch, pressure, sights, sounds, smells, or thoughts of a sexual encounter. After ejaculation, the arterioles vasoconstrict, and the penis becomes flaccid.

The Scrotum

The scrotum hangs at the base of the penis, anterior to the anus, and regulates the temperature of the testes. The optimum temperature for sperm production is about 2 to 3 degrees below body temperature. When the testicular temperature is too low, the scrotum contracts to bring the testes up against the body. When the testicular temperature is too high, the scrotum relaxes to allow the testes to lie further away from the body.

The Testes

The testes develop in the abdominal cavity of the fetus and then descend through the inguinal canal into the scrotum. They are homologous to the female's ovaries. These paired organs are each about 1.5 inches (4 cm) long and 1 inch (2.5 cm) in diameter. Each testis is divided into 250 to 300 lobules, with each lobule containing one to four seminiferous tubules. The testes produce sperm and testosterone. The seminiferous tubules are responsible for sperm production. Leydig's cells (or interstitial cells) lie in the connective tissue surrounding the seminiferous tubules and produce testosterone.

The Ducts and Semen

The seminiferous tubules lead into the efferent ducts and become the rete testis. From the rete testis, 10,000 to 20,000 efferent ducts join the epididymis, a long coiled tube that lies over the outer surface of each testis. The epididymis is the final area for the storage and maturation of sperm. When a man is sexually excited, the epididymis contracts to propel the sperm through the vas deferens to the ampulla, where the sperm are stored until ejaculation.

The seminal vesicles produce most of the volume of seminal fluid. Seminal fluid is also made of secretions from the accessory sex organs, the epididymis, the prostate gland, and Cowper's glands. Seminal fluid nourishes the sperm, provides bulk, and increases its alkalinity. An alkaline pH is essential to mobilize the sperm and ensure fertilization of the ova. Sperm mixed with this fluid is called **semen**. Each seminal vesicle joins its corresponding vas deferens to form an ejaculatory duct, which enters the prostatic urethra. During ejaculation, seminal fluid mixes with sperm at the ejaculatory duct and enters the urethra for expulsion. The total amount of semen ejaculated is 2 to 4 mL, although the amount varies. The total ejaculate of a healthy male contains from 20 to 150 million sperm per mL (WebMD, 2007).

The Prostate Gland

The prostate gland is about the size of a walnut. It encircles the urethra just below the urinary bladder and is surrounded by smooth muscle. Secretions of the prostate gland make up about one-third of the volume of the semen. These secretions enter the urethra through several ducts during ejaculation.

Male Sex Hormones

The male sex hormones are called **androgens**. Most androgens are produced in the testes, although the adrenal cortex also produces a small amount. **Testosterone**, the primary androgen produced by the testes, is essential for the development and maintenance of sexual organs and secondary sex characteristics, and for spermatogenesis. It also promotes metabolism, growth of muscles and bone, and libido (sexual desire).

Assessing the Male Reproductive System

The structures and functions of the male reproductive system are assessed by findings from diagnostic tests, a health assessment interview to collect subjective data, and a physical assessment to collect objective data.

Diagnostic Tests

The results of diagnostic tests of the structures and functions of the male reproductive system are used to support the diagnosis of a specific sexual problem, injury, or disease; to provide information to identify or modify the appropriate medications or treatments used to treat the disease; and to help nurses monitor the man's responses to treatment and nursing interventions. Diagnostic tests used to assess the male reproductive system are described in the Diagnostic Tests table. More information is included in the discussion of specific health problems or diseases in ∞ Chapter 48.

Regardless of the type of diagnostic test, the nurse is responsible for explaining the procedure and any special preparation needed, for assessing any medication use that might affect the outcome of the tests, for supporting the man during the examination as necessary, for ensuring the consent form is signed (if required), and for monitoring the results of the tests. The nurse is also responsible for postprocedure care and patient teaching for self-care at home.

DIAGNOSTIC TESTS of the Male Reproductive System

NAME OF TEST	PURPOSE & DESCRIPTION	RELATED NURSING INTERVENTIONS
Biopsy of the prostate	A biopsy of the prostate is conducted to help determine the cause of an elevated PSA and to diagnose cancer if a lump is found in the prostate. Various routes may be used to insert a biopsy needle into the prostate, through the rectum (transrectal), through the urethra (transurethral), or through the perineum. A transrectal ultrasound (TRUS) is often used to guide the placement of the needle during the procedure. The biopsy may be done in a physician's office, in an out-patient surgery unit or clinic, or in a hospital operating room.	Assess for a history of bleeding problems, allergies to medications, and if taking any anticoagulant medications (such as warfarin [Coumadin], heparin, enoxaparin [Lovenox], aspirin, or NSAIDs). If the biopsy is done with a local anesthetic, no other preparation is needed. If the biopsy is done transrectally, the patient may need an enema before the procedure. If the biopsy is done with general anesthesia, tell the patient he will be unable to eat or drink fluids for 8 to 12 hours before the procedure, and that he will be given antibiotics. After the biopsy, advise the man to avoid strenuous activity for 4 hours. Explain that there may be some discomfort in the biopsy area for 1 to 2 days, there may be some blood in the urine or from the rectum, and semen may appear dark. Following a transurethral biopsy, a urinary catheter may remain in place for a few hours after the procedure. Excess bleeding, pain, inability to urinate, or signs of infection should be reported to the physician.
Gonorrhea culture	A culture is performed to evaluate for gonorrhea. A swab is used to collect a sample of discharge from the infected area (urethra, penis, anus, or throat), smeared on a slide, and a Gram stain is conducted to identify the organism (*N. gonorrheae*). A urine sample is used in some tests.	No special preparation is needed. If test is positive, request referral to an STD testing center or clinic and emphasize need for treatment to eradicate the infection.
Prostate specific antigen (PSA)	A blood test used to screen for prostate cancer and to monitor treatment of prostate cancer. Routine prostate screening with a PSA for men over the age of 75 is no longer recommended. **Normal value:** 0–4.0 ng/ml	Inform the patient that transient increases in PSA occur following prostate palpation or rectal examinations; these procedures as well as prostate surgery should not be scheduled for 3 days before the TSA is done.
Prostate ultrasound	This test is conducted to identify testicular torsion or masses, and to evaluate prostate enlargement. Uses high-frequency sound waves, passed through tissues of various densities, to produce a visual graphic of tissue being examined.	Tell the patient to administer a Fleets enema about 1 hour before the procedure (if ordered). Ask the patient to void and remove clothing from the waist down prior to the procedure.
Semen analysis	Done to assess volume, motility and sperm count, and percent of abnormal sperm. **Normal values:** Volume: 2–5 mL Sperm count: >20 million/mL Motility: 60% motile % normal sperm: 60%	The patient is asked to bring in a fresh specimen (usually in a condom) within 2 hours of ejaculation.
Syphilis Screening Tests ■ Venereal Disease Research Laboratory (VDRL) ■ Rapid plasma reagin (RPR) ■ Fluorescent treponemal antibody absorption (FTA-ABS)	These blood tests are conducted to screen for syphilis. Positive findings can be made within 1 to 2 weeks after primary lesion appears or 1 to 4 months after the initial infection. The FTA-ABS test is considered the most accurate, and is often used if findings from the VDRL or RPR are questionable.	No special preparation is needed. If test is positive, request referral to an STI testing center or clinic and emphasize need for treatment to eradicate the infection.

Genetic Considerations

When conducting a health assessment interview and a physical assessment, it is important for the nurse to consider genetic influences on health of the adult. Several diseases of the male reproductive system have a genetic component. During the health assessment interview, it is especially important to ask about a family history of testicular or prostate cancer. During the physical assessment, assess for any manifestations that might indicate a genetic disorder (see the accompanying Genetic Considerations box on this page). If data are found to indicate genetic risk factors or alterations, ask about genetic testing and refer for appropriate genetic counseling and evaluation. ∞ Chapter 8 provides further information about genetics in medical-surgical nursing.

Health Assessment Interview

A health assessment interview to determine problems with the male reproductive system may be conducted during a health screening, may focus on a chief complaint (such as a discharge from the penis), or may be part of a total health assessment. Men may be embarrassed to discuss health problems or concerns involving their reproductive organs; it is important for the nurse to ask questions in a nonthreatening, matter-of-fact manner. Consider the psychologic, social, and cultural factors that affect sexuality and sexual activity. Use words that the man can understand, and do not be embarrassed or offended by the words he uses. The man may perceive the interview as less threatening if the discussion begins with more general questions and then progresses to specific questions, and if questions are asked in a way that gives him permission to describe behaviors and manifestations. For example, rather than asking a man if he has difficulty achieving or maintaining an erection, ask him to describe any changes he has noticed in his erections.

If the man has a health problem, analyze its onset, characteristics and course, severity, precipitating and relieving factors, and any associated symptoms, noting the timing and circumstances. For example, you may ask the man the following questions:

- When did you first notice that you were having difficulty urinating?
- Did you use a different brand of condoms before you noticed the rash on your penis?
- Describe the changes that occurred in your ability to have an erection after you started taking medicine for high blood pressure.

In questioning the man about past medical history, ask about chronic illnesses such as diabetes, chronic renal failure, cardiovascular disease, multiple sclerosis, spinal cord tumors or trauma, or thyroid disease. The effects of these illnesses as well as the treatment of the illnesses may cause **impotence** (inability to achieve or maintain an erection). The following drugs may cause erectile dysfunction: antihypertensives, antidepressants, antispasmodics, beta blockers, tranquilizers, sedatives, and histamine$_2$-receptor antagonists. Psychosocial stressors also may contribute to impotence.

If the man was born to a woman treated during pregnancy with diethylstilbestrol (DES), a drug used in the 1940s and 1950s to prevent miscarriage, he may have congenital deformities of the urinary tract as well as decreased semen levels. If the man had mumps as a child, sterility is possible. The risk for testicular cancer is greatest in men who have a history of an undescended testicle, an inguinal hernia, testicular swelling with mumps, a history of maternal use of DES or oral contraceptives, and a family history of testicular cancer.

Explore the lifestyle and social history of the man; the use of alcohol, cigarettes, or street drugs may affect sexual function. Unprotected sexual intercourse increases the potential for sexually transmitted infections (STIs) including HIV infection. Ask about sexual preference. Sexual intercourse with same-sex partners further increases the risk for HIV infection. Other questions about sexuality may include number of sexual partners; history of premature ejaculation, impotence, or other sexual problems; any history of sexual trauma; use of condoms or other contraceptives; and current level of sexual satisfaction.

Interview questions categorized by functional health patterns are listed in the Functional Health Pattern Interview table on page 1633.

Physical Assessment

Physical assessment of the male reproductive system may be performed as part of a total assessment or separately for men with known or suspected problems. If conducted as part of a total physical assessment, this is usually the final system to be assessed. Problems of the male reproductive system may

---

NURSING CARE OF THE OLDER ADULT — **Age-Related Changes in the Male Reproductive System**

AGE-RELATED CHANGE	SIGNIFICANCE
Prostate Gland	
• A significant number of older men have some degree of benign prostatic hyperplasia.	Although aging does not cause prostate cancer, its incidence does increase with age.
Penis, Testes, and Scrotum	
• Epithelial tissue and mucosa of seminal vesicles are thinner and have reduced capacity to hold fluid.	Although men may father children throughout life, the sperm count is reduced in some men. Changes in the vascular system of the penis may
• Sclerosis of penile arteries and veins may occur.	mean the aging man takes longer to achieve an erection and ejaculation, or may be impotent.

FUNCTIONAL HEALTH PATTERN INTERVIEW The Male Reproductive System

Functional Health Pattern	Interview Questions and Leading Statements
Health Perception-Health Management	■ Have you ever had problems with your reproductive organs (penis, testicles, prostate gland)? Explain. If so, how was the problem treated? ■ Have you ever had surgery on your reproductive organs? If so, what type, when, and what was the outcome? ■ Have you ever noticed any pain or swelling in your breasts? Explain. ■ Do you practice testicular self-examination? How often? ■ Do you smoke? If so, how much and for how long?
Nutritional-Metabolic	■ Describe your usual intake of food and fluids in a 24-hour period.
Elimination	■ Do you now or have you ever had a discharge from your penis? If so, describe the color, odor, consistency, amount, and frequency. ■ Have you ever had any bleeding from your penis? Explain. ■ Have you noticed any change in your urination, such as burning, frequency, urgency, difficulty starting the stream, size of the stream, dribbling, or getting up frequently at night? Explain.
Activity-Exercise	■ Describe your usual activity in a 24-hour period. ■ Do you participate in sports or heavy lifting? If so, do you wear a protective cup or athletic support?
Sleep-Rest	■ Describe the quality of your rest and sleep.
Cognitive-Perceptual	■ Describe any pain you have had in the groin area, testicles, penis, or scrotum. Where is it? Do you experience it in other parts of your body? How long does it last? What makes it worse or relieves it? ■ Has there been a change in the condition or color of the skin on your scrotum or penis? Explain.
Self-Perception-Self-Concept	■ Has this problem affected how you feel about yourself as a man? If so, how? ■ Do you feel that your needs for intimacy and affection are being met?
Role-Relationships	■ Has having this condition affected your relationships with others? ■ Has having this condition interfered with your ability to work? Explain. ■ Has anyone in your family had problems with prostate cancer?
Sexuality-Reproductive	■ Are you currently in a sexual relationship? If so, has having this problem interfered with your usual sexual activity? ■ How long have you been with your current partner? ■ Have you had any other partners during this time? ■ What is your sexual preference? ■ Are you satisfied with your current level of sexual functioning? If no, explain. ■ Have you ever had any problem with achieving or maintaining an erection or ejaculation? What do you think caused it? ■ Do you use any medications to facilitate your sexual ability? Describe. ■ Do you use condoms every time you have sexual contact?
Coping-Stress-Tolerance	■ Has having this condition created stress for you? If so, does your health problem seem to be more difficult when you are stressed? ■ Have you experienced any kind of stress that makes the condition worse? Explain. ■ Describe what you do when you feel stressed.
Value-Belief	■ Describe how specific relationships or activities help you cope with this problem. ■ Describe specific cultural beliefs or practices that affect how you care for and feel about this problem. ■ Is there anything interfering with your spiritual beliefs, needs, or practices during your illness? What can I or another caregiver do to help you with your spiritual needs? ■ Are there any specific treatments that you would not use to treat this problem?

involve the urinary system, making an assessment of both systems important (∞ see Chapter 26 for assessment of the urinary system). The nurse must feel comfortable with the examination of patients of the opposite gender; if either the nurse or the patient is not comfortable, a nurse of the same gender should be asked to conduct this part of the assessment. Normal age-related findings for the older man are summarized in the Nursing Care of the Older Adult Box.

The male reproductive system is assessed by inspection and palpation. Explain the procedures for the examination thoroughly and in a matter-of-fact way to decrease anxiety and embarrassment. If the man is unfamiliar with his internal genitalia, charts may be used to demonstrate the parts that will be examined. Ask the man to empty his bladder (to be more comfortable during the examination), remove his clothing, and put on a gown or drape. The assessment may be done with the man sitting or standing. Expose only those body parts being examined to preserve modesty. Ensure that the examining room is warm and private. Put on gloves before beginning and wear them throughout the examination.

Male Reproductive System Assessments

Technique/Normal Findings	Abnormal Findings

Breast and Lymph Node Assessment

Inspect and palpate both breasts, including areola and nipple. *Breast tissue should not be swollen, tender, or enlarged (although soft, fatty, and enlarged breast tissue does occur with obesity in men).*

- A smooth, firm, mobile, tender disk of breast tissue behind the areola indicates **gynecomastia**, abnormal enlargement of the breast(s) in men. Gynecomastia requires additional investigation to determine the cause.
- A hard, irregular nodule in the nipple area suggests carcinoma.

Palpate the axillary and supraclavicular lymph nodes. *Lymph nodes should not be palpable.*

- Enlarged axillary nodes are common with infections of the hand or arm but may be caused by cancer.
- Enlarged supraclavicular nodes may indicate metastasis.

External Genitalia Assessment

Inspect and palpate the inguinal and femoral area for bulges. Ask the man to bear down or cough as you palpate (Figure 47–2 ■). *There should be no bulging with coughing or bearing down.*

- A bulge that increases with coughing or straining suggests a hernia.

Figure 47–2 ■ Palpating the male inguinal area for bulges.

Inspect the penis. If the man is uncircumcised, retract the foreskin or ask him to do so. *When nonerect, the penis is normally soft, flaccid, and nontender. The foreskin should be without lesions, of color equal with the penis, and should retract easily. The glans is normally free of lesions.*

- **Phimosis** (tightness of prepuce that prevents retraction of foreskin) may be congenital or due to recurrent balanoposthitis (generalized infection of glans penis and prepuce).
- Narrow or inflamed foreskin can cause paraphimosis, retraction of the foreskin that causes painful swelling of the glans.
- Balanitis (inflammation of the glans) is associated with bacterial or fungal infections.
- Ulcers, vesicles, or warts suggest a sexually transmitted infection.
- Nodules or sores seen in uncircumcised men may be cancer.

Inspect the external urinary meatus. Press the glans between the thumb and forefinger (Figure 47–3 ■). Replace the foreskin if appropriate. *The external urinary meatus is normally in the center of the glans, without redness or discharge.*

- Erythema or discharge indicates inflammatory disease. Further assessment is required.

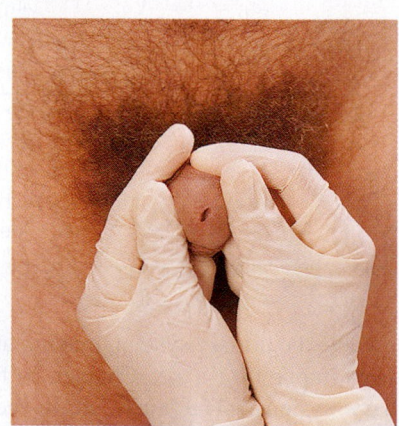

Figure 47–3 ■ Inspecting the external urinary meatus of the male.

Inspect the skin on the shaft of the penis. *The skin on the shaft of the penis should be free of redness or lesions.*

- Excoriation or inflammation suggests lice or scabies.

Palpate the shaft of the penis. *The shaft of the penis should not be tender.*

- Induration with tenderness along the ventral surface suggests urethral stricture with inflammation.

Technique/Normal Findings	Abnormal Findings
Inspect the scrotum. Further assess any swelling in the scrotum using trans-illumination: Darken the room and place a lighted flashlight against the skin of the scrotum. *The normal scrotum and epididymis appear as dark masses with regular borders.*	■ A unilateral or bilateral poorly developed scrotum suggests cryptorchidism (failure of one or both testes to descend into the scrotum). ■ Swelling of the scrotum may indicate indirect inguinal hernia, hydrocele (accumulation of fluid in the scrotum), or scrotal edema. Swellings containing serous fluid will transilluminate. Swellings containing blood or tissue will not transilluminate.
Palpate each testis and epididymis. *The testes should not be tender or swollen.*	■ Tender, painful scrotal swelling occurs in acute epididymitis, acute orchitis, torsion of the spermatic cord, and strangulated hernia. ■ A painless nodule in the testis is associated with testicular cancer.

Prostate Assessment

The prostate gland is assessed by digital rectal examination (DRE). (See ∞ Chapter 21 [Figure 21–20] for the technique used to palpate the prostrate through the rectal wall.) This assessment is usually conducted by a physician or advanced practice nurse.

With a gloved index finger, palpate the posterior rectal wall for the rounded, two-lobed structure of the posterior prostate. *The prostate is normally nontender, with two lateral lobes that are divided, smooth, and about 2.5 cm long.*	■ Enlargement (1-cm protrusion into the rectum) with obliteration of the median sulcus suggests benign prostatic hypertrophy. ■ Enlargement with asymmetry and tenderness suggests prostatitis. ■ A hard irregular nodule is suspicious of carcinoma.

Anatomy, Physiology, and Functions of the Female Reproductive System

The female reproductive system consists of the external genitalia (mons pubis, labia, clitoris, vaginal and urethral openings, and glands) and the internal organs (vagina, cervix, uterus, fallopian tubes, and ovaries). The breasts are a part of women's reproductive organs. In women, the urethra and urinary meatus are separated from the reproductive organs; however, they are so close to each other that a health problem with one often affects the other.

The Breasts

The breasts (or mammary glands) are located between the third and seventh ribs on the anterior chest wall. They are supported by the pectoral muscles and are richly supplied with nerves, blood, and lymph (Figure 47–4 ■). A pigmented area called the areola is located slightly below the center of each breast and contains sebaceous glands and a nipple. The nipple is usually protrusive and becomes erect in response to cold and stimulation. The breasts produce milk for the infant following delivery.

The breasts are made of adipose tissue, fibrous connective tissue, and glandular tissue. Cooper's ligaments support the breast and extend from the outer breast tissue to the nipple, dividing the breast into 15 to 25 lobes. Each lobe is made of alveolar glands connected by ducts that open to the nipple.

The External Genitalia

The external genitalia collectively are called the vulva. They include the mons pubis, the labia, the clitoris, the vaginal and urethral openings, and glands (Figure 47–5 ■).

The mons pubis is a pad of adipose (fat) tissue covered with skin and hair that lies anterior to the symphysis pubis. The labia are divided into two structures. The labia majora, outermost folds of skin and adipose tissue covered with hair, begin at the base of the mons pubis and end at the anus. The labia minora, usually light pink and hairless, are located between the clitoris and the base of the vagina, and are enclosed by the labia majora.

The vestibule (the area between the labia), contains the openings for the vagina and the urethra as well as the Bartholin's and Skene's glands. Prior to menopause Bartholin's and Skene's glands secrete lubricating fluid during the sexual response cycle. The clitoris is an erectile organ analogous to the penis in the male. Like the penis, it is highly sensitive and distends during sexual arousal. The vaginal opening, called the

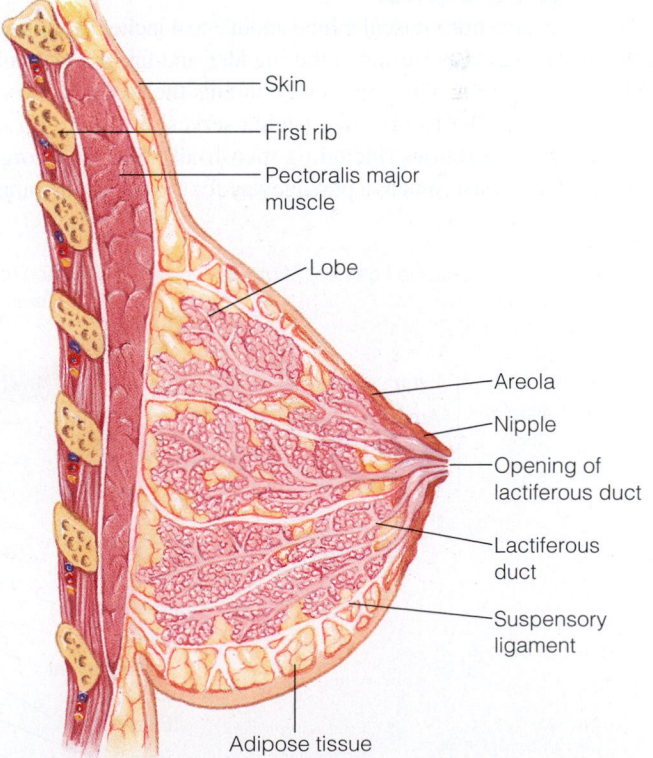

Figure 47–4 ■ Structure of the female breast.

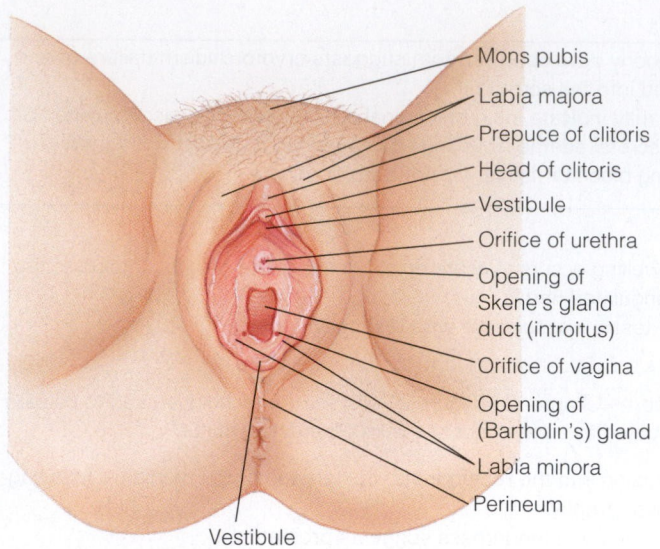

Figure 47–5 ■ The external organs of the female reproductive system.

introitus, is the opening between the internal and the external genitals. Prior to the first intercourse or trauma, the introitus is surrounded by a connective tissue membrane called the hymen.

The Internal Organs

The vagina, cervix, uterus, fallopian tubes, and ovaries are the internal organs of the female reproductive system (Figure 47–6 ■). The ovaries are the primary reproductive organs in women and also produce female sex hormones. The vagina, uterus, and fallopian tubes serve as accessory ducts for the ovaries and a developing fetus.

The Vagina and Cervix

The vagina is a fibromuscular tube about 3 to 4 inches (8 to 10 cm) in length located posterior to the bladder and urethra and anterior to the rectum. The upper end contains the uterine cervix in an area called the fornix. The vagina serves as a route for the excretion of secretions (including menstrual fluid), as an organ of sexual response, and as a passageway for the birth of an infant.

The walls of the vagina are usually moist and maintain a pH ranging from 3.8 to 4.2. This pH is bacteriostatic and is maintained by the action of the hormone estrogen and normal vaginal flora. Estrogen stimulates the growth of vaginal mucosal cells so that they thicken and have increased glycogen content. The glycogen is fermented to lactic acid by Döderlein's bacilli (lactobacilli that normally inhabit the vagina), slightly acidifying the vaginal fluid. The cervix projects into the vagina and forms a pathway between the uterus and the vagina. The cervix is a firm structure, protected by mucus that changes consistency and quantity during the menstrual cycle and during pregnancy.

The Uterus

The uterus is a hollow pear-shaped muscular organ with thick walls located between the bladder and the rectum. It has three parts: the fundus, the body, and the cervix. It is supported in the abdominal cavity by the broad ligaments, the round ligaments, the uterosacral ligaments, and the transverse cervical ligaments. The uterus receives the fertilized ovum and provides a site for growth and development of the fetus.

The uterine wall has three layers. The perimetrium is the outer serous layer that merges with the peritoneum. The myometrium is the middle layer and makes up most of the uterine wall. This layer has muscle fibers that run in various directions, allowing contractions during **menstruation** (the periodic shedding of the uterine lining in a woman of childbearing age who is not pregnant) or childbirth, and expansion as the fetus grows. The endometrium lines the uterus; its outermost layer is shed during menstruation.

The Fallopian Tubes

The fallopian tubes are thin cylindrical structures about 4 inches (10 cm) long and 2.5 inches (1 cm) in diameter. They are attached to the uterus on one end and are supported by the broad ligaments. The lateral ends of the fallopian tubes are open and made of projections called fimbriae that drape over the ovary. The fimbriae pick up the ovum after it is discharged from the ovary. The fallopian tubes are made of smooth muscle and are lined with ciliated, mucous-producing epithelial cells. The movement of the cilia and contractions of the smooth muscle

Figure 47–6 ■ The internal organs of the female reproductive system.

move the ovum through the tubes toward the uterus. Fertilization of the ovum by the sperm usually occurs in the outer portion of a fallopian tube.

The Ovaries

The ovaries are flat, almond-shaped structures located on either side of the uterus below the ends of the fallopian tubes. They are homologous to the male's testes. The ovaries store the female germ cells (ova) and produce the female hormones estrogen and progesterone. A woman's total number of ova is present at her birth.

Female Sex Hormones

The ovaries produce estrogens, progesterone, and androgens in a cyclic pattern. **Estrogens** are steroid hormones that occur naturally in three forms: estrone (E_1), estradiol (E_2), and estriol (E_3). Estradiol is the most potent and is the form secreted in greatest amount by the ovaries. Estrogens are essential for the development and maintenance of secondary sex characteristics; and in conjunction with other hormones, they stimulate the female reproductive organs to prepare for growth of a fetus. Estrogens are responsible for the normal structure of skin and blood vessels. They also decrease the rate of bone resorption, promote increased high-density lipoproteins, reduce cholesterol levels, and enhance the clotting of blood. Estrogens also promote the retention of sodium and water.

Progesterone primarily affects the development of breast glandular tissue and the endometrium. During pregnancy, progesterone relaxes smooth muscle to decrease uterine contractions. It also increases body temperature. Androgens are responsible for normal hair growth patterns at puberty and may also have metabolic effects.

The Menstrual Cycle

The **menstrual cycle** begins with the menstrual phase, lasting from days 1 to 5. The inner endometrial (functionalis) layer detaches and is expelled as menstrual fluid (fluid and blood) for 3 to 5 days. As the maturing follicle begins to produce estrogen (days 6 to 14), the proliferative phase begins. In response, the functionalis layer is repaired and thickens, while spiral arteries increase in number and tubular glands form. Cervical mucus changes to a thin, crystalline substance, forming channels to help the sperm move up into the uterus.

The final phase, lasting from days 14 to 28, is the secretory phase. As the corpus luteum produces progesterone, the rising levels act on the endometrium, causing increased vascularity, changing the inner layer to secretory mucosa, stimulating the secretion of glycogen into the uterine cavity, and causing the cervical mucus again to become thick and block the internal os. If fertilization does not occur, hormone levels fall. Spasm of the spiral arteries causes hypoxia of the endometrial cells, which begin to degenerate and slough off as menstrual fluid.

Assessing the Female Reproductive System

The structures and functions of the female reproductive system are assessed by findings from diagnostic tests, a health assessment interview to collect subjective data, and a physical assessment to collect objective data. Information from the health assessment interview is used to individualize the questions that are asked; for example, the postmenopausal woman would not be asked specific questions about her menstrual cycle, but it would be important to ask about vaginal dryness. Sample documentation of an assessment of the female reproductive system is included following the physical assessment section.

Diagnostic Tests

The results of diagnostic tests of the structures and functions of the female reproductive system are used to monitor the health of female reproductive structures; to support the diagnosis of a specific sexual problem, injury, or disease; to provide information to identify or modify the appropriate medications or treatments used to treat the disease; and to help nurses monitor the woman's responses to treatment and nursing care interventions. Diagnostic tests to assess the female reproductive system are described in the Diagnostic Tests table on pages 1638–1641. More information is included in the discussion of specific health problems or diseases in ∞ Chapter 49.

Regardless of the type of diagnostic test, the nurse is responsible for explaining the procedure and any special preparation needed, for assessing any medication use that might affect the outcome of the tests, for supporting the woman during the examination as necessary, for ensuring the consent form is signed (if appropriate), for documenting the procedures as appropriate, and for monitoring the results of the tests. The nurse is also responsible for postprocedure care and patient teaching for self-care at home.

Genetic Considerations

When conducting a health assessment interview and a physical assessment, it is important for the nurse to consider genetic influences on health of the adult. Several diseases of the female reproductive system have a genetic component. During the health assessment interview, it is especially important to ask about a family history of ovarian or breast cancer. During the physical assessment, assess for any manifestations that might indicate a genetic disorder (see the accompanying box). If data are found to indicate genetic risk factors or alterations, ask about genetic testing and refer for appropriate genetic counseling and evaluation. ∞ Chapter 8 provides further information about genetics in medical-surgical nursing.

GENETIC CONSIDERATIONS
Examples of Female Reproductive System Disorders

- There is a clear genetic link for some of the cases of both breast and ovarian cancer. Two breast cancer susceptibility genes have been identified: BRCA1 and BRCA2. If a woman has either of these genes, she is at increased risk for having breast or ovarian cancer at some point in her life.
- A family history of endometrial, colon, or breast cancer increases a woman's risk for endometrial cancer.
- Turner syndrome is a disorder in a female caused by complete or partial absence of one of the two X chromosomes. The disorder is characterized by short stature and the lack of sexual development at puberty. Other physical effects include a webbed neck, heart defects, and kidney abnormalities.

DIAGNOSTIC TESTS of the Female Reproductive System

NAME OF TEST	PURPOSE & DESCRIPTION	RELATED NURSING INTERVENTIONS
Breast biopsy ■ Fine-needle aspiration ■ Core needle biopsy ■ Vacuum-assisted mammotome ■ Large core surgical biopsy ■ Open surgical biopsy	■ A fine-needle aspiration is conducted to withdraw fluid from cysts, and may be used to sample cells from masses in the breast. A 22- to 25-gauge needle is used to collect five to six samples of fluid or cells. ■ A core needle biopsy is conducted to obtain a sample of tissue from a solid mass or calcium deposits in the breast. A 10-, 11-, or 12-gauge needle is used to collect five to six tissue samples. ■ A vacuum-assisted mammotome is primarily used to evaluate calcifications. An 11- or 14-gauge needle is inserted through a small (1/4-inch) incision and 8 to 10 samples are removed. ■ A large core surgical biopsy is performed to evaluate breast masses or calcification identified with a mammogram but nonpalpable. An incision is made and a 5- to 20-mm cylinder of breast tissue (about the size of a wine cork) is removed. ■ An open surgical biopsy is performed to evaluate breast masses, hard-to-reach lesions, multiple lesions, and masses with calcifications. A 1.5- to 2-inch incision is made and a golf ball size (or larger) area of tissue is removed.	Explain that, depending on the physician, some procedures may be performed with or without a local anesthetic. Explain that a local anesthetic is used, but no stitches are required for a fine-needle aspiration, a core needle biopsy, or mammotome. Explain that a local anesthetic will be administered and stitches will be used to close the incision for a large-core biopsy. Explain that a general anesthetic is usually used and that the incision will require stitches and leave a scar for an open surgical biopsy. For all types, wearing a bra, applying ice packs, and mild analgesics decrease discomfort postprocedure.
Breast cancer genetic testing (BRAC-1, BRAC-2)	This blood test is used to identify a predisposition to breast and ovarian cancers by mutations of the genes BRAC-1 and BRAC-2. The genetic defect is passed to children by both the male and female parents.	Food and fluids are not restricted. Suggest the patient have genetic counseling, regardless of the test outcome.
Breast ultrasound	This examination uses high-frequency sound waves passing through tissues to detect masses in the breast. It may be performed if lesions are identified in a mammogram.	Tell the woman not to apply ointment, body powder or underarm deodorant prior to the test, or if present, to wash it off.
Chlamydia Screening	This test is performed to screen for or diagnose chlamydial infections. A swab of cells from the infected area is taken and either smeared on a slide and analyzed or cultured. Although usually taken from the urethra, vagina, or cervix, cultures may also be taken from the throat and rectum.	Assess if the woman is pregnant or has enlargement of inguinal lymph nodes. Withhold antibiotics (if prescribed) until after obtaining the specimen. Instruct not to douche before the examination. If the test is positive, emphasize need for treatment to eradicate the infection.
Colposcopy	A colposcopy may be done if a Pap test detects cell changes. The procedure, done in the health provider's office, uses a small binocular microscope to visualize the cervix. Acetic acid is applied to the cervix and abnormal cells turn white. A biopsy of the cervix and/or cryosurgery (freezing) of abnormal cells may be done during the procedure.	Instruct the woman to abstain from douching and intercourse for 48 hours prior to the examination. Assess for pregnancy, which may alter the procedure. Postprocedure: Tell the woman there may be slight vaginal bleeding for several days after the procedure, to abstain from vaginal intercourse for 1 to 2 days, and to take NSAIDs for discomfort or cramping.

DIAGNOSTIC TESTS of the Female Reproductive System (continued)

NAME OF TEST	PURPOSE & DESCRIPTION	RELATED NURSING INTERVENTIONS
Conization, loop electrosurgical excision of transformation zone (LEETZ), cervical biopsy	A conization, LEETZ, or biopsy is performed to remove cervical tissue for evaluation (most often for cervical cancer) or to treat cervical abnormalities. An area of tissue surrounding the cervical os is removed. The procedure is usually done on an out-patient basis or surgery center.	Explain that the procedure requires general anesthesia and that from 1 to 4 hours will be spent in the recovery room after the procedure before going home. Postoperative self-care includes rest for 2 to 3 days. Explain that minor vaginal bleeding and discharge are expected for several days after the procedures and spotting may continue for about 3 weeks; perineal pads (not tampons) should be used. Sexual intercourse and douching should be avoided until all vaginal discharge stops. Notify physician if increased bleeding or signs of infection (pain, foul-smelling discharge, fever) occur.
Cultures for Bacteria, Candidae (yeast), or Trichomonas	A culture is performed to identify vaginal organisms or blood cells. A specimen of vaginal discharge is obtained with a swab, placed in solution, and examined under the microscope immediately after it is collected (referred to as a wet-mount).	Request the patient not douche before the examination.
Endometrial biopsy	An endometrial biopsy is performed to identify endometrial hyperplasia or endometrial cancer. The cervix is cleaned and tissue is obtained transcervically from the endometrium either by curettage or vacuum aspiration.	Explain that the procedure is briefly painful, and causes vaginal bleeding for a few days. Advise to use perineal pads, and avoid tampons and sexual intercourse while bleeding.
Gonorrhea culture	A culture is performed to evaluate for gonorrhea. A swab is used to collect a sample of discharge from the infected area (cervix, urethra, anus, or throat), smeared on a slide, and a Gram stain is conducted to identify the organism (*N. gonorrhoeae*). A urine sample is used in some tests.	Instruct not to douche before the examination. If the test is positive, request referral to an STI testing center or clinic and emphasize need for treatment to eradicate the infection.
HPV test (HPV DNA test, genital human papilloma test)	An HPV test is used as a screening tool for human papillomavirus (HPV) in women after the age of 30. It is usually conducted in conjunction with a pelvic examination and Pap smear. A finding of "low-grade changes" on the Pap smear with HPV indicates the likely presence of HPV and the need for further testing. A positive test for HPV indicates the presence of a high risk for cancer type of HPV, but does not specify which type is present.	Explain that the test should be done during a time when the woman is not menstruating, and that she should not douche, use tampons, or use vaginal medications for at least 48 hours prior to the examination. Ask the woman to void prior to the examination. Explain that following the test there may be a small amount of vaginal bleeding or gray-green discharge; a panty liner may be used to avoid spotting clothing. Instruct her not to have intercourse until the healthcare provider says it is safe to do so.
Hysterosalpingogram	This test is conducted to diagnose causes of infertility and abnormalities of the uterus or fallopian tubes. A contrast medium is instilled through the cervix, through the uterus, and out the fallopian tubes while x-rays are taken. The test should be done on the seventh to the ninth day after the end of the menstrual period.	Assess for pregnancy, vaginal bleeding, or acute infection (all would contraindicate the test). Assess for allergy to seafood (iodine) or previous contrast media. A cleansing enema and douche may be ordered prior to the test. Inform the woman that there may be some bloody discharge for 3 to 4 days after the test; if it continues after that time, she should notify her healthcare provider.

(continued)

DIAGNOSTIC TESTS of the Female Reproductive System (continued)

NAME OF TEST	PURPOSE & DESCRIPTION	RELATED NURSING INTERVENTIONS
Laparoscopy	This examination is conducted to visualize the organs in the peritoneal cavity (uterus, fallopian tubes, ovaries); to withdraw fluid for analysis; and to perform a tubal ligation. A fiber-optic scope is inserted through small abdominal incisions and carbon dioxide is inserted into the peritoneal cavity for better visualization. It is performed in an ambulatory surgery center. A microlaparoscopy uses much smaller instruments and is considered only minimally invasive, resulting in less postprocedure discomfort.	Instruct the woman not to smoke, eat, or drink fluids after midnight the day of the procedure. Depending on protocol, the woman may be asked to take laxatives and/or enemas to empty the bowel. Ask the woman to shower or bathe and remove nail polish and make-up the evening before the procedure. Ask the woman to void prior to the examination and explain that a general anesthetic will be used. Following the procedure, the woman remains in the recovery room for about 1 hour, and remains in the treatment center for 3 to 4 hours. After voiding, the woman is discharged home. After the procedure, the woman will have medications for pain, and may experience watery, pink-tinged drainage from the small abdominal incisions (the drainage usually lasts less than 48 hours). Explain that shoulder pain is common after the procedure (referred pain from the retained carbon dioxide gas); that some vaginal bleeding may occur and the woman should use a perineal pad; and to report excess bleeding, pain, or signs of infection to the physician.
LEEP (loop electrosurgical excision procedure)	This procedure, conducted in the physician's office, is done if a Pap smear indicates abnormal cervical cells or cervical dysplasia. A thin wire electrode that transmits a painless electrical current is used to cut away the affected cervical tissue. The tissue is sent to the lab for further examination.	The patient should ask the physician about taking an OTC pain medication prior to the examination. Following the procedure, explain that the patient should not use tampons, douche, lift heavy objects, have sexual intercourse for the recommended length of time, and that she should take showers (not tub baths). The physician should be called for bleeding heavier than a normal period, severe pain, heavy vaginal discharge, or strong vaginal odor.
Mammogram Recommendations from some groups are that women over the age of 50 have this examination every 2 years; the American Cancer Society recommends annual examinations for women starting at age 40. Women should discuss this difference with their healthcare provider.	Used to detect tumors in the breast. Breasts are flattened in the mammography machine and low-dose x-rays are taken.	Ask the woman if she is pregnant; if so, the test is contraindicated. Tell the woman not to apply ointment, body powder, or underarm deodorant prior to the test, or if present, to wash it off.
Papanicolaou smear (Pap test)	This test is conducted to diagnose malignant and premalignant lesions of the cervix; assess the effects of hormone replacement; identify viral, bacterial, fungal, and parasitic conditions; and to evaluate response to chemotherapy or radiation therapy to the cervix. Cells are obtained during a pelvic examination with a wooden spatula, a cotton swab, or an endocervical brush. The sample collected may be smeared on a glass slide or put into a special liquid preservative and then the cells in suspension are processed onto a slide. The cells are then stained and examined.	Explain that the test should be done during a time when the woman is not menstruating, and that she should not have intercourse, douche, or use vaginal medications for at least 24 hours, and preferably 48 hours prior to the examination. Ask about menstrual history, including any menstrual problems, last menstrual period, bleeding, and flow. Ask about vaginal discharge and vaginal itching. Assess medication use; digitalis preparations, tetracycline, and female hormones can change the cellular structure (Kee, 2009). Ask the woman to void prior to the examination.
Syphilis (dark-field examination)	See the Male Diagnostic Tests table.	

DIAGNOSTIC TESTS of the Female Reproductive System (continued)

NAME OF TEST	PURPOSE & DESCRIPTION	RELATED NURSING INTERVENTIONS
Syphilis screening tests ■ Venereal Disease Research Laboratory (VDRL) ■ Rapid plasma reagin (RPR) ■ Fluorescent treponemal antibody absorption (FTA-ABS)	See the Male Diagnostic Tests table.	
Ultrasound (abdominal, vaginal)	An ultrasound is used to detect the presence of space-occupying lesions, such as fibroid tumors, cysts, abscesses, and neoplasms. The abdomen is coated with transducing gel, and a graphic visualization is made. For a vaginal ultrasound, a transducer is covered with a condom or vinyl glove coated with transducer gel and then introduced into the vagina.	Explain the need to increase intake of fluids and tell the woman not to void until the test is completed to ensure a full bladder (this lifts the pelvic organs higher in the abdomen and improves visualization).

Health Assessment Interview

A health assessment interview to determine problems with the female reproductive system may be conducted during a health screening, may focus on a chief complaint (such as severe menstrual cramping), or may be part of a total health assessment. Women may be embarrassed to discuss health problems or concerns involving their reproductive organs; it is important for the nurse to ask questions in a nonthreatening, matter-of-fact manner. Consider the psychologic, social, and cultural factors that affect sexuality and sexual activity. Use words that the woman can understand, and do not be embarrassed or offended by the words she uses. The woman may perceive the interview as less threatening if the discussion begins with more general questions and then progresses to specific questions, and if questions are asked in a way that gives the woman permission to describe behaviors and manifestations. For example, first ask a female patient about menstrual and childbirth histories before asking questions about STIs.

The focused interview for the female reproductive system is usually extensive. However, the questions may in many instances be tailored to the specific health problem of the woman. As with the assessment of other body systems, analyze and document the onset of the problem, its duration, frequency, precipitating and relieving factors, any associated symptoms, treatment, self-care, and outcome. For example, ask the woman the following questions:

■ Have you noticed vaginal bleeding after intercourse?
■ Does over-the-counter medication relieve the vaginal itching and discharge?
■ Have you had any fever or abdominal pain with this vaginal infection?

Ask about menstrual history, sexual history, obstetric history, use of contraceptives, use of medications, and reproductive system examinations. Assess the use of condoms during intercourse; unprotected sexual intercourse increases the risk of STIs, including HIV infection. Ask about smoking; a history of smoking increases the risk of circulatory problems in the woman taking oral contraceptives and increases the risk for cancer of the cervix.

Chronic illnesses may affect the function of the female reproductive system. Diabetes mellitus increases the risk of vaginal infections and vaginal dryness, both of which interfere with sexual pleasure. Chronic heavy menstrual flow may result in anemia. Thyroid and adrenal disorders may affect secondary sex characteristics, the menstrual cycle, and the ability to become pregnant.

Obtaining any family history of cancer is important. The risk for endometrial cancer is higher in women with a family history of endometrial, breast, or colon cancer; the risk for ovarian cancer is higher in women with a family history of ovarian or breast cancer; and the risk for breast cancer is higher in women with a family history of breast cancer. Exposure to DES *in utero* increases the risk of cancer of the cervix and vagina. Exposure to asbestos poses a risk of cancer of the ovary. The risk for breast cancer is also greater if the woman has a history of fibrocystic disease.

Carefully explore any history of vaginal bleeding and vaginal discharge. Ask about the onset of vaginal bleeding, any related factors, the color (pink, red, dark red, brown), the character (thin, watery, presence of mucus, size and number of clots), the amount (spotting, how many pads or tampons in a specific amount of time), and relationship to menstrual cycle. Regarding vaginal discharge, ask about the onset, color (white, green, gray), character (thin, thick, curdlike), odor, itching, and rash.

Questions about sexuality may include sexual preference, number of sexual partners; history of **anorgasmia** (absence of orgasm), **dyspareunia** (painful intercourse), or other problems with intercourse; history of sexual trauma; use of condoms or other contraceptives; and current level of sexual satisfaction.

Interview questions categorized by functional health patterns are listed in the Functional Health Pattern Interview table on pages 1642–1643.

FUNCTIONAL HEALTH PATTERN INTERVIEW   The Female Reproductive System

Functional Health Pattern	Interview Questions and Leading Statements
Health Perception-Health Management	■ Have you ever had problems with your reproductive organs (ovaries, tubes, uterus, vagina) or with menstruation or menopause? Explain. If so, how was this problem treated? ■ If appropriate: Do you routinely take any prescribed or herbal medications for symptoms of menopause? If so, what and when do you take it? Did you ever take hormone replacement therapy for menopausal symptoms? If so, what type and how long? ■ Do you practice breast self-examination? When and how often do you do this? ■ Have you noticed any lumps in your breasts or discharge from your nipples? If so, describe. ■ Have you ever had a breast examination or mammogram? When was your last one? How often do you have these? ■ When was your last gynecologic examination? Pap smear? How often do you have these done? ■ Do you use birth control? If so, what do you use? ■ What do you do to provide self-care if you have mood swings or menstrual cramps? ■ Have you ever had a sexually transmitted infection or an infection of the reproductive organs? What was it? How was it treated? ■ Do you use douches? If so, what type and how often? ■ Do you smoke? If so, how much and for how long?
Nutritional-Metabolic	■ Do you notice a change in your appetite right before your menstrual period? ■ Have you gained weight recently? If so, why do think this happened? ■ Describe your usual food intake for a 24-hour period.
Elimination	■ When was your last menstrual period? ■ At what age did you start/end having menstrual periods? ■ Describe the length, amount of flow, and clotting with your menstrual periods. Do you ever have bleeding between your menstrual periods? If so, describe the type and amount. ■ Describe any unusual vaginal discharge you have had (color, consistency, odor, itching, or rash). ■ Have you noticed any changes in urination (frequency, urgency, burning)? ■ Have you noticed changes in bowel elimination during your menstrual periods?
Activity-Exercise	■ Describe your usual activities of daily living. ■ Have you noticed any change in activity or energy during your menstrual period? ■ Have you noticed any change in activity or energy since menopause (if applicable)? If so, how?
Sleep-Rest	■ How long do you sleep at night? ■ Do night sweats wake you? ■ Do menstrual cramps ever wake you at night?
Cognitive-Perceptual	■ Do you have pain or other symptoms (such as headache, mood swings, irritability, bloating, constipation, diarrhea, and/or breast tenderness) before your menstrual period? Describe. What do you do about this? ■ Do you have cramping before or during your menstrual period? Describe the type of cramping, how long it lasts, and what you do to be more comfortable. ■ Do you ever have vaginal itching, pain, burning, or dryness? If so, is it affected by sexual intercourse? Does dryness interfere with intercourse?
Self-Perception-Self-Concept	■ Has this problem affected how you feel about yourself as a woman? ■ Do you believe your needs for intimacy and affection are being met? Explain.
Role-Relationships	■ How has having this condition affected your relationships with others? ■ Has having this condition interfered with your ability to work? Explain. ■ Has anyone in your family had problems with breast or ovarian cancer? Explain.
Sexuality-Reproductive	■ Are you currently in a sexual relationship? If so, has this condition interfered with your usual sexual activity? How long have you been with your current partner? Have you had any other partners during this time? ■ What is your sexual preference? ■ Has having this problem affected your relationship with your spouse or sexual partner? ■ Have you ever been pregnant? How many times? Have you ever had a miscarriage? ■ Do you practice birth control? If so, what do you use? ■ Do you ensure that your partner of the opposite gender uses a condom every time you have intercourse? ■ Do you use a vaginal condom?
Coping-Stress-Tolerance	■ Has having this condition created stress for you? If so, does your health problem seem to be more difficult when you are stressed? ■ Have you experienced any kind of stress that makes the condition worse? Explain. ■ Describe what you do when you feel stressed.

FUNCTIONAL HEALTH PATTERN INTERVIEW The Female Reproductive System (continued)

Functional Health Pattern	Interview Questions and Leading Statements
Value-Belief	■ Describe how specific relationships or activities help you cope with this problem.
	■ Describe specific cultural beliefs or practices that affect how you care for and feel about this problem.
	■ Is there anything interfering with your spiritual beliefs, needs, or practices during your illness? What can I or another caregiver do to help you with your spiritual needs?
	■ Are there any specific treatments that you would not use to treat this problem?

Physical Assessment

Physical assessment of the female reproductive system usually is conducted as part of a scheduled screening (e.g., for an annual Pap smear) or for a specific reproductive health problem. If conducted as part of a total physical assessment, this is usually the final system to be assessed. The nurse must feel comfortable with the examination of patients of the opposite gender; if either the nurse or the patient is not comfortable, or if cultural beliefs prohibit examination by a nurse of the opposite gender, a nurse of the same gender should be asked to conduct this part of the assessment.

The female reproductive system is assessed by inspection and palpation. Ask the woman to void before having the examination. Prior to the examination, collect all necessary equipment and explain the techniques to the woman to decrease anxiety. Put on disposable gloves before beginning the examination and wear them throughout the examination. Ask the woman to remove her clothing and put on a gown. Ensure that the examining room is private and warm.

The female reproductive system is assessed by inspection and palpation. Explain the procedures for the examination thoroughly and in a matter-of-fact way to decrease anxiety and embarrassment. If the woman is unfamiliar with her reproductive organs, charts may be used to demonstrate the parts that will be examined. Carefully explain the procedure for the examination, and show the speculum to the woman. The assessment may be done with the woman in the sitting or supine position to examine the breasts and in the lithotomy position to assess the external genitalia and internal organs. Expose only those body parts being examined to preserve modesty. Normal age-related findings for the older woman are summarized in the Nursing Care of the Older Adult feature.

The examination usually begins with examination of the breasts with the woman in the sitting and supine positions. The nurse then helps the woman move to the lithotomy position on the examining table, with the feet in the stirrups and the buttocks even with the foot of the table. Older or frail women may not be able to tolerate this position. In this case, the woman is examined in the supine position. Although the entire examination is described here, the internal examination is conducted only by a nurse with advanced practice in the procedure. However, nurses are often asked to assist with the examination and should be able to explain the examination to a woman.

NURSING CARE OF THE OLDER ADULT   **Age-Related Changes in the Female Reproductive System**

AGE-RELATED CHANGE	SIGNIFICANCE
Breasts	
■ Atrophy, with sagging of breast tissue	Although aging does not cause breast cancer, the incidence rises in older women; age-related changes may make finding tumors more difficult.
■ Linear strands may appear from shrinkage and fibrotic changes	
External Genitalia	
■ Labia flatten, and vulvar adipose tissue and hair decrease.	Vagina is more easily irritated, increasing the risk of vaginal infections.
■ ↓ collagen and adipose tissues in the vaginal canal, resulting in loss of rugae, and shortening and narrowing of vaginal canal.	
■ ↓ vaginal lubrication; epithelium becomes thinner and avascular.	Lubricants are necessary for comfortable intercourse.
■ More alkaline pH of vagina.	
■ Cervix becomes smaller.	
Internal Organs	
■ Uterus shrinks.	With the completion of menopause, the menstrual cycles end and the woman is infertile. Weakening of the pelvic floor muscles may contribute to involuntary incontinence with increased intra-abdominal pressure (as with coughing and sneezing). Skin is dry and thin.
■ Fallopian tubes shrink and shorten.	
■ Ovaries are smaller and thicker.	
■ With menopause, hormone production of estrogen decreases.	
■ Loss of estrogen may cause pelvic floor muscles to weaken.	
■ Loss of estrogen causes changes throughout the body, including loss of skin tone (wrinkling) and growth of facial hair.	

Female Reproductive System Assessments

Technique/Normal Findings	Abnormal Findings

Breast Assessment

Inspect both breasts simultaneously with the woman seated in the following positions: arms at sides, arms overhead, hands pressed on hips, leaning forward. Inspect breast size, symmetry, contour, skin color, texture, venous patterns, and lesions. Lift the breasts, and inspect the lower and lateral aspects. *Breasts normally vary in size and shape, and one breast may normally be larger than the other. Color should be consistent with the skin tone and texture smooth. There should be no redness, swelling, prominent veins, or lesions.*

- Retractions, dimpling, and abnormal contours suggest lesions, and should be further evaluated for malignancy.
- Thickened, dimpled skin with enlarged pores (called peau d'orange, orange peel, or pig skin) and unilateral venous patterns are associated with malignancy.
- Redness may be seen with infection or carcinoma.

Inspect the areolae and nipples. *The color of the areolae should be consistent with the woman's skin color (ranging from dark pink to dark brown), and Montgomery tubercles may be present. The nipples should be equal bilaterally in size, centrally located in each breast, and free of lesions or discharge. Nipples are usually everted, but may normally be inverted or flat.*

- Peau d'orange may be noted first in the areola.
- Recent unilateral inversion of the nipple or asymmetry in the directions in which the nipples point suggests cancer.

Palpate both breasts, axillae, and supraclavicular areas. Figure 47–7 ■ illustrates a possible pattern for breast palpation. Various palpation patterns may be used as long as every part of each breast is palpated, including the axillary tail (also called tail of Spence), which is the breast tissue that extends from the upper outer quadrant toward and into the axillae. Ask the woman to assume a supine position with a small pillow under the shoulder and the arm over the head, and repeat the systematic palpation sequence. Describe identified masses by location, size, shape, consistency, tenderness, mobility, and delineation of borders. *Breasts should feel smooth, firm, and elastic, without palpable masses. Prior to the menstrual cycle, there may be increased nodularity and tenderness.*

- Tenderness may be related to premenstrual fullness, fibrocystic disease, or inflammation.
- Nodules in the tail of the breast may be enlarged lymph nodes.
- Hard, irregular, fixed unilateral masses that are poorly delineated suggest carcinoma.
- Bilateral, single or multiple, round, mobile, well-delineated masses are consistent with fibrocystic breast disease or fibroadenoma.
- Swelling, tenderness, erythema, and heat may be seen with mastitis.

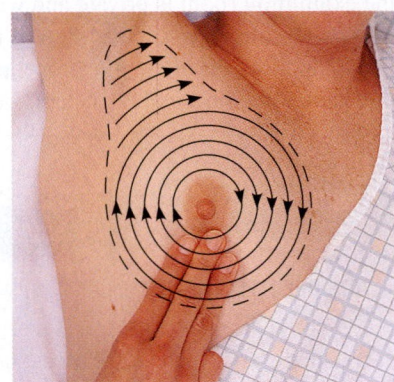

Figure 47–7 ■ Possible pattern for palpation of the breast.

Palpate the nipple then compress it between the thumb and index finger. Note the color of any discharge. *Nipples should be firm and elastic, normally without discharge (although some women normally have a clear discharge, and a milky substance may be expressed during pregnancy and lactation).*

- Loss of nipple elasticity is seen in cancer.
- Bloody or serous discharge is associated with intraductal papilloma.
- Milky discharge not due to prior pregnancy and found on both sides suggests galactorrhea (lactation not associated with pregnancy or nursing), which is sometimes associated with a pituitary tumor.
- Unilateral discharge from one or two ducts can be seen in fibrocystic breast disease, intraductal papilloma, or carcinoma.

Technique/Normal Findings	Abnormal Findings

Axillary Assessment

Inspect and palpate the axillae. *There should be no redness, irritation, lesions, or enlarged lymph nodes on palpation.*

- Rash may be due to allergy or other causes.
- Signs of inflammation and infection may be due to infection of the sweat glands.
- Palpate all sections of both axillae for palpable nodes (Figure 47–8 ■).
- Enlarged axillary nodes are most often due to infection of the hand or arm but can be caused by malignancy.
- Enlarged supraclavicular nodes are associated with lymphatic metastases from abdominal or thoracic carcinoma.

Figure 47–8 ■ Palpating the axillary lymph nodes.

External Genitalia Assessment

Help the woman to the lithotomy position with the knees flexed and separated.

Inspect and palpate the labia majora. *The labia majora should be equal in size and free of lesions or bulging.*

- Excoriation, rashes, or lesions suggest inflammatory or infective processes.
- Bulging of the labia that increases with straining suggests a hernia.
- Varicosities may be present on the labia.

Inspect the labia minora. Separate the labia majora for better visualization. *The labia minora should be symmetrical, dark pink and moist, without redness or lesions.*

- Inflammation, irritation, excoriation, or caking of discharge in tissue folds suggests vaginal infection or poor hygiene.
- Ulcers or vesicles may be manifestations of sexually transmitted infection.

Palpate the inside of the labia minora between thumb and forefinger. *There should be no nodules, ulcers, or lesions.*

- Small, firm, round cystic nodules in labia suggest sebaceous cysts.
- Wartlike lesions suggest condylomata acuminata (genital warts).
- Firm, painless ulcers suggest chancre of primary syphilis.
- Shallow, painful ulcers suggest herpes infection.
- Ulcerated or red raised lesions in older women suggest vulvar carcinoma.

Inspect the clitoris. *The clitoris is normally not enlarged.*

- Enlargement may be a symptom of a masculinizing condition.

Inspect the vaginal opening. *There should be no swelling, discoloration, lacerations, discharge, or lesions visible in the vaginal opening.*

- Swelling, discoloration, or lacerations may be caused by trauma.
- Discharge or lesions may be symptoms of infection.
- Fissures or fistulas may be related to injury, infection, growth of a malignancy, or trauma.

Palpate Skene's glands. Using the index finger, "milk" Skene's glands on both sides and over the urethra and inspect for possible discharge (Figure 47–9 ■). *There should be no discharge or tenderness present.*

- Discharge from Skene's glands and/or tenderness suggests infection.

Urethra

Skene's gland

Vagina

Bladder

Rectum

Figure 47–9 ■ Palpating Skene's glands.

Technique/Normal Findings	Abnormal Findings
Palpate Bartholin's glands at the posterior labia majora (Figure 47–10 ■). *There should be no masses, redness, swelling, or tenderness on palpation.*	■ A nontender mass in the posterolateral portion of the labia majora is indicative of a Bartholin's cyst. ■ Swelling, redness, or tenderness, especially if unilateral, may indicate abscess of Bartholin's glands.

Bartholin's gland

Figure 47–10 ■ Palpating Bartholin's glands.

Inspect the vaginal orifice for bulging and urinary incontinence. Ask the woman to strain or "bear down." *No bulging should be visible with straining.*	■ Bulging of the anterior vaginal wall and urinary incontinence suggest a cystocele. ■ Bulging of the posterior wall suggests a rectocele. ■ Protrusion of the cervix or uterus into the vagina indicates uterine prolapse.
Inspect and palpate the perineum. *The perineum should be free of redness or lesions. Episiotomy scars are a normal finding.*	■ Inflammation, lesions, and growths may be seen in infections or cancer. ■ Fistulas may be the result of injury, trauma, infection, or growth of a malignancy.

Vaginal and Cervical Assessment

This assessment is primarily conducted by a physician or an advanced practice nurse.

Use a vaginal speculum to inspect the vaginal walls and cervix. See the guidelines in Box 47–1. *The vaginal opening varies, depending on age, sexual history, and vaginal births. Vaginal mucosa is normally pink and moist, without discharge or odor. There should be no bulging or loss of urine. The cervix is normally smooth and pink, without lesions and has a consistency similar to the tip of the nose.*	■ Bluish color of the cervix and vaginal mucosa may be a sign of pregnancy. ■ A pale cervix is associated with anemia. ■ A cervix to the right or left of the midline may indicate a pelvic mass, uterine adhesions, or pregnancy. ■ Projection of the cervix more than 3 cm into the vaginal canal may indicate a pelvic or uterine mass. ■ Transverse or star-shaped cervical lacerations reflect trauma causing tearing of the cervix. ■ An enlarged cervix is associated with infection. ■ Nabothian cysts (small, white, or yellow raised, round areas on the cervix) are considered normal but may become infected. ■ Cervical polyps may be cervical or endometrial in origin.
Palpate the cervix, uterus, and ovaries. See the guidelines in Box 47–2. *The cervix can be moved slightly without discomfort. The uterus is normally at the level of the pubis, moves freely, and is nontender. The ovaries (about the size of a walnut) are firm, smooth, mobile, and slightly tender on palpation. The ovaries are not usually palpable 3 to 5 years after menopause. A small amount of clear drainage is normal.*	■ The uterus may be retroverted (tilted backward) or retroflexed (angled backward). ■ Pain on movement of the cervix during manual examination suggests pelvic inflammatory disease (PID). ■ Softening of the uterine isthmus (Hegar's sign), softening of the cervix (Goodell's sign), and uterine enlargement may be objective signs of pregnancy. ■ Firm, irregular nodules that vary greatly with size and are continuous with the uterine surface are likely to be myomas (fibroids). ■ Unilateral or bilateral smooth, compressible adnexal masses are found in ovarian tumors. ■ Profuse menstrual bleeding is seen with endometrial polyps, dysfunctional uterine bleeding (DUB), and use of an intrauterine device. ■ Irregular bleeding may be associated with endometrial polyps, DUB, uterine or cervical carcinoma, or oral contraceptives. ■ Postmenopausal bleeding is seen with endometrial hyperplasia, estrogen therapy, and endometrial cancer.

BOX 47–1 Guidelines for Intravaginal Assessment and Use of the Vaginal Speculum

The size of the speculum that is used for an internal examination of the female reproductive system depends on the age of the woman and size of the vagina. Two types of specula are available. The Graves speculum, used most often for examinations of adult women, is available in lengths of 3½ to 5 inches and widths of ¾ to 1½ inches. The Pederson speculum, which is narrower, may be used to examine adolescents or adult woman who are virgins, who have never had a baby, or who are postmenopausal with vaginal atrophy. The speculum should be warm. If cultures or smears are to be obtained, neither water nor gel should be used to warm or to lubricate the speculum.

If cells are to be taken for cytologic studies, the patient should not douche, use vaginal medications, or take a tub bath for 24 hours before the examination. Finally, the examination is usually deferred if the patient is menstruating or has a vaginal infection. The general procedure is as follows:

1. Place the index and middle finger of one hand into the vagina, just inside the introitus, and press the fingers toward the rectum. Hold the speculum in the other hand.
2. Ask the patient to bear down, and insert the closed blades of the speculum into the vagina at an oblique angle until the ends of the blades reach the fingertips (see the accompanying figure). Withdraw the fingers and rotate the speculum to a transverse position.
3. Continue to insert the speculum until it reaches the end of the vagina. Depress the lever of the speculum to open the blades. If the cervix is not in full view, try closing the blades, withdrawing the speculum about halfway, and inserting it again at a more downward angle. When the cervix is in full view, fix the depressed lever to an open position.
4. Inspect the cervix. The normal cervix is pink and midline. Assess color, position, size, projection into the vagina, surface and shape, and any discharge.

If a Pap smear to collect cervical cells for cytologic studies is done, the following procedure may be used:

1. To collect cells from the vaginal pool, roll a sterile cotton-tipped applicator on the vaginal wall below the cervix. Paint the smear on the slide, and spray the slide with fixative.
2. To collect endocervical cells, place the groove of the spatula snugly against the cervical os, and rotate it 360 degrees. In a single stroke, spread the material from both sides of the spatula on a slide, and immediately spray with fixative.

If cultures are to be done, take a specimen from the vagina and/or cervix with a sterile, cotton-tipped applicator, and then either spread the specimen on a culture plate or place it in a culture container. Follow institutional protocols for preparing specimens for vaginal infections from suspected organisms.

At the end of the examination, loosen the lever control and slowly withdraw the speculum, closing the blades slowly and rotating the speculum while observing all areas of the vaginal wall. Assess the color of the mucosa and the color and appearance of any discharge.

BOX 47–2 Guidelines for Bimanual Pelvic Examination

The bimanual pelvic examination is done to palpate the cervix, uterus, and ovaries. The examiner's hand that will be used intravaginally is held with the index and middle fingers extended, the thumb abducted, and the fourth and fifth fingers folded on the palm of the hand. The extended fingers are lubricated. The general procedure is as follows:

1. Spread the labia with the thumb and finger of the opposite hand and insert the lubricated fingers into the vagina with the palm upward.
2. Place the opposite hand on the abdomen; it is used to press on the abdomen and gently move the internal genitals toward the intravaginal fingers (see the accompanying figure).
3. Ask the patient to take deep breaths to relax the abdominal wall.
4. Palpate the cervix, assessing size, contour, position, surface, consistency, tenderness, and mobility. The cervix should be freely movable and nontender.
5. Palpate the uterus by pressing downward on the abdomen while placing the intravaginal fingers in the anterior fornix and gently lifting against the abdominal hand. Assess the size, shape, surface, consistency, position, mobility, and tenderness of the uterus. The normal uterus is freely movable and nontender.
6. Palpate the adnexal areas, which surround the uterus and contain the fallopian tubes and ovaries. Because these

structures are small, palpation may not be possible. If the ovaries are palpable, they should be smooth and firm. The normal ovary is sensitive to touch, firm, and highly movable.

7. Withdraw the fingers. Provide tissues for the patient's use in wiping the genital area.

SAMPLE DOCUMENTATION

Assessment of the Female Reproductive System

A 32-year-old female, first visit to health department for problems with "burning and pain in my crotch area" and "It really hurts to urinate." Also states she had unprotected sex on a date about 2 weeks ago. Oral temperature 101°F. Vaginal examination findings of vesicles and red ulcerations on labia majora and vaginal mucosa. Inguinal lymph nodes enlarged and tender to palpation. Culture of discharge from ulcerations sent to lab.

TEST YOURSELF NCLEX-RN® REVIEW

1. When assessing the breasts of an obese man, the nurse may notice what common physical change?
   1. phimosis
   2. enlarged axillary lymph nodes
   3. gynecomastia
   4. absent areola

2. What female structure is analogous to the penis in the male?
   1. ovaries
   2. labia majora
   3. labia minora
   4. clitoris

3. A nurse is assessing a 65-year-old man. He says, "I don't understand how having prostate problems can cause me to urinate all the time." What would you say to begin your explanation?
   1. "The prostate gland presses on the bladder."
   2. "The prostate gland surrounds your urethra."
   3. "Your kidneys respond to prostate enlargement."
   4. "The prostate glands sit on top of the kidneys."

4. What blood test may be an indicator of prostate cancer?
   1. PSA
   2. VDRL
   3. CBC
   4. WBC

5. A nurse is conducing a health history for a young man. What question would be appropriate to identify his health perception-health management?
   1. "Do you practice testicular self-examination?"
   2. "Are you currently in a sexual relationship?
   3. "Have you ever noticed blood in your urine?"
   4. "Have you experienced dribbling of urine?"

6. The loss of estrogen production following menopause may increase the risk for cardiovascular disease from what substance?
   1. uric acid
   2. glucose
   3. cholesterol
   4. testosterone

7. Cessation of menstruation in young women is a normal response to what biologic event?
   1. implantation of an embryo
   2. onset of menopause
   3. onset of puberty
   4. beginning spermatogenesis

8. Which of the following diagnostic tests may be used to detect cervical cancer?
   1. colposcopy
   2. mammogram
   3. blood culture
   4. Pap smear

9. A nurse is assessing a woman's breasts. What assessment technique is primarily used to determine abnormalities of the breast?
   1. inspection
   2. auscultation
   3. palpation
   4. percussion

10. A 72-year-old woman tells you she is suddenly having menstrual periods. What would you tell her?
    1. "This is perfectly normal, even at your age."
    2. "You need to see your doctor, because you should not be having these."
    3. "Do you still have sexual activity?"
    4. "Do you have menstrual cramps with the periods?"

See Test Yourself answers in Appendix C.

BIBLIOGRAPHY

Armstrong, J., & Mitchell, E. (2008). Comprehensive nursing assessment in the care of older people. *Nursing Older People, (20)* 1, 36–40.

Bickley, L., & Szilagyi, P. (2007). *Bates' guide to physical examination and history taking* (9th ed.). Philadelphia: Lippincott.

Breslin, T., & Finestone, S. (2007). What patients need to know about breast biopsies. *Medscape Hematology-Oncology.* Retrieved from http://www.medscape.com/viewarticle/567831?src=mp

D'Amico, D., & Barbarito, C. (2007). *Health & physical assessment in nursing.* Upper Saddle River, NJ: Pearson Prentice Hall.

Eliopoulos, E. (2005). *Gerontological nursing* (6th ed.). Philadelphia: Lippincott Williams & Wilkins.

Hubert, J., & Bergin, D. (2008). Imaging the female pelvis: When should MRI be considered? *Applied Radiology, 37*(1), 9–24.

Kee, J. (2009). *Prentice Hall handbook of laboratory & diagnostic tests with nursing implications.* (6th ed.). Upper Saddle River, NJ: Pearson Prentice Hall.

Knight, D. (2004). Health care screening for men who have sex with men. *American Family Physician, 69*(9), 2147–2156.

Koren, M., & Hertz, J. (2007). Older women's breast screening behaviors: What nurses need to know. *MEDSURG Nursing, 16*(2), 80–86.

Locovara, J., & Ray, J. (2007). Deciphering the diagnostics of breast cancer. *MEDSURG Nursing, 16*(6), 391–400.

Linn, M., Gall, R., & Maradieque, A. (2007). Prostate-specific antigen screening: Friend or foe? *Urologic Nursing, 27*(6), 481–489.

Mick, J. (2007). Sexuality assessment: 10 strategies for improvement. *Clinical Journal of Oncology, 11*(5), 67 1–5.

National Institute of Health. (2008). *Genes and Disease: Male-Specific Diseases; Female-Specific Diseases.* Retrieved from http://www.ncbi.nlm.nih.gov/books/bookres.fegi/gnd/pdf.html

Porth, C. (2007). Essentials of *Pathophysiology: Concepts of altered health states* (2nd ed.). Philadelphia: Lippincott Williams & Wilkins.

Porth, C., & Matfin, G. (2009). *Pathophysiology: Concepts of altered health states.* (8th ed.). Lippincott Williams & Wilkins.

Quallich, S. (2008). Disorders of the male genitalia. *Urologic Nursing, 28*(2), 132–133.

Quallich, S. (2005). Male infertility. *Urologic Nursing, 25*(5), 378, 391.

Unber, J. (2004). How to assess and treat erectile dysfunction. *Emergency Medicine, 36*(1), 28–30, 33–37.

Wallace, M. (2007). Sexuality assessment for older adults. *Best practices in nursing care to older adults. Hartford Institute for Geriatric Nursing, 10.* Retrieved from www.hartfordign.org

Weber, J., & Kelley, J. (2009). *Health assessment in nursing* (4th ed.). Philadelphia: Lippincott Williams & Wilkins.

WebMD, Healthwise. (2007). *Semen analysis.* Retrieved from http://www.webmd.com/infertility-and-reproduction/guide/semen-analysis?page=2

Nursing Care of Men with Reproductive System and Breast Disorders

LEARNING OUTCOMES

1. Explain the pathophysiology, manifestations, complications, interdisciplinary care, and nursing care of disorders of the male reproductive system, including disorders of sexual function, the penis, the testes and scrotum, the prostate gland, and the breast.

2. Compare and contrast the risk factors for cancer of the penis, testes, and prostate gland.

3. Discuss the purposes, nursing implications, and health education for medications and treatments used to treat disorders of sexual function, the penis, the testes and scrotum, the prostate gland, and the breast.

4. Describe the various surgical procedures used to treat disorders of the male reproductive system.

CLINICAL COMPETENCIES

1. Assess the functional health status of men with reproductive system and breast disorders and monitor, document, and report abnormal manifestations.

2. Use evidence-based research to provide appropriate pre- and postoperative teaching to men having a laporoscopic radical prostatectomy.

3. Use assessed data, patient values, clinical expertise, and evidence to determine priority nursing diagnoses and select and implement individualized nursing interventions.

4. Administer, and/or teach patients how to administer, medications used to treat disorders of the male reproductive system knowledgeably and safely.

5. Provide safe and knowledgeable care to men having prostate surgery.

6. Effectively communicate with and function within the interdisciplinary team to plan and provide patient care.

7. Adapt individual and cultural values and variations as well as expressed needs and preferences into the plan of care.

8. Revise plan of care as needed to provide effective interventions to promote, maintain, or restore functional health status to men with disorders of the reproductive system and breast.

KEY TERMS

benign prostatic hyperplasia (BPH), *1660*
epididymitis, *1656*
erectile dysfunction (ED), *1650*
gynecomastia, *1673*
hydrocele, *1655*
impotence, *1650*

libido, *1650*
orchitis, *1656*
phimosis, *1654*
premature ejaculation, *1654*
priapism, *1654*
prostatitis, *1659*

retrograde ejaculation, *1654*
spermatocele, *1656*
testicular torsion, *1657*
varicocele, *1656*

Men are subject to various disorders of the penis, scrotum and testes, prostate gland, and breast. These disorders may be inflammatory, structural, benign, or malignant. Young men are at increased risk for testicular cancer. As men age, both benign and malignant conditions of the prostate gland become common. Many of the disorders pose significant risk to the man's fertility and sexual and urinary function, and some are life threatening. This chapter discusses disorders of the male reproductive system, including disorders of sexual expression and the male breast. Because many of the treatments and disorders of the male reproductive system have the potential to affect erection and ejaculation, these problems are discussed first.

Disorders of Male Sexual Function

The Man with Erectile Dysfunction

Erectile dysfunction (ED) is the inability of the male to attain and maintain an erection sufficient to permit satisfactory sexual intercourse. **Impotence**, a term often used synonymously with erectile dysfunction, may involve a total inability to achieve erection, an inconsistent ability to achieve erection, or the ability to sustain only brief erections. ED has many possible causes (Table 48–1), and may or may not be associated with a loss of **libido** (sexual desire).

TABLE 48–1 Causes of Erectile Dysfunction

MAJOR PATHOLOGIC CAUSES		MAJOR IATROGENIC CAUSES	
		MEDICATIONS	PROCEDURES AND INFECTIONS
Neurogenic	*Arterial*	*Antihypertensives*	*Surgery*
Spinal cord injury	Atherosclerosis	Hydrochlorothiazide	Coronary artery bypass
Stroke	Hypertension	Spironolactone	Pelvic lymphadenectomy
Parkinson's disease	Aortic aneurysm	Methyldopa	Radical prostatectomy
Multiple sclerosis	Sickle cell anemia	Clonidine	Radical cystectomy
Endocrinologic	*Mechanical*	Prazosin	Abdominal perineal resection
Diabetes mellitus	Decreased penile distensibility	Propranolol	Sympathectomy
Hypogonadism	Congenital disorders	Reserpine	Aortic aneurysm repair
Hypothyroidism	Morbid obesity	*Psychotropic Agents*	Transplant surgeries
Inflammatory	Hydrocele	Phenothiazines	*Other*
Prostatitis	Hip or pelvic fractures	Butyrophenones	Severe nosocomial infection
Cystitis	*Psychogenic*	Tricyclic antidepressants	Radiation therapy to pelvis
Activity Intolerance	Depression	MAO inhibitors	
Pulmonary problems	Stress	Diazepam	
Anemias	Fatigue	Chlordiazepoxide	
Myocardial infarction	Fear of failure	*Endocrinologic Agents*	
Congestive heart failure	*Compulsive Food Disorders*	LHRH agonists	
Hepatic diseases	Compulsive overeating	Estrogen compounds	
Renal failure	Anorexia nervosa	Progesterone	
Substance Dependency	Bulimia	*Other*	
Alcohol		Antiparkinsonian agents	
Marijuana		Anticholinergic agents	
Narcotics		Immunosuppressive agents	
Sedatives		Antihistamines	
Tobacco			

The incidence of ED is difficult to estimate because many affected men may not report the disorder. It is estimated that as many as 30 million men in the United States have ED, and most are older than age 65 (National Kidney and Urologic Disease Information Clearinghouse [NKUDIC], 2009). The incidence of the problem increases rapidly after age 50. Most problems with erection are the result of a disease (with a three times greater incidence in men with diabetes mellitus), injury, or chemical substances (such as prescribed medications, alcohol, nicotine, cocaine, or marijuana) that affect nerve conduction, hormone levels, or decrease blood flow in the penis (Cleveland Clinic, 2008). Clinical studies have also found a correlation between obesity and ED; a 30% higher risk has been found in men with a BMI greater than 28.7 kg/m^2 (Pasquali, Patton, & Gambineri, 2008). ED also occurs more often in men who smoke. Because impotence most often occurs in aging men, the discussion of pathophysiology focuses on this age group.

Pathophysiology

Age-related changes in sexual function involve cellular and tissue changes in the penis, decreased sensory activity, hypogonadism, and the effects of chronic illness. In the penis, a change from elastic collagen to a more rigid collagen results in decreased distensibility (a less rigid erection). This, in turn, interferes with the veno-occlusive mechanism, which prevents blood from "leaking" out of the penis into the general vasculature prematurely. Problems with this mechanism result in incomplete erections. Vibrotactile sensation over the skin of the penis declines with age: some older men require longer stimulation to achieve an erection. Hypogonadism, common in aging men, results in decreased testosterone levels. There may be a relationship between lower androgen levels and erectile function.

Many illnesses affect erectile function. Damage to arteries, smooth muscles, and fibrous tissues are the most common causes of impotence. Diseases such as diabetes, kidney disease, chronic alcoholism, atherosclerosis, and vascular disease are responsible for organic ED. Innervation and blood flow to the penis may be damaged from disease processes such as Parkinson's disease and also during prostate surgery. Given the effects of aging on the vasculature of the penis, the increased incidence of chronic illness, and the multiple medications and treatments required to manage those illnesses, it is not surprising that many older men have problems with ED.

Interdisciplinary Care

The management of men with ED is growing in importance and scale because the population as a whole is aging, with the incidence increasing proportionately. Another factor is the positive change in the willingness of men and their partners to discuss sexual concerns. Although sexuality is still a very sensitive and private area for most people, the knowledge that help is available is causing men to seek answers. Many older men are coming to believe that loss of erectile function is not an inevitable part of aging.

Diagnosis

The diagnostic tests that may be ordered include laboratory studies, penile monitoring, and penile blood flow. Blood chemistry, complete blood count, lipid profile, urinalysis, testosterone, prolactin, thyroxin, and prostate specific antigen (PSA) levels are measured to identify possible cardiovascular, metabolic, and endocrine problems that may be causing the dysfunction. Nocturnal penile tumescence and rigidity (NPTR) monitoring helps differentiate between psychogenic and organic causes. NPTR can be performed in a sleep laboratory, although home testing with portable devices is an alternative. The number and quality of erections occurring during REM sleep can be determined. Cavernosometry and cavernosography of the corpora are used to evaluate arterial inflow and venous outflow of blood in the penis.

Medications

ED can be treated with medications taken orally, injected directly into the penis, or inserted into the urethra at the tip of the penis.

- *Oral medications:* The oral medications used to treat ED include sildenafil citrate (Viagra), vardenafil hydrochloride (Levitra), or tadalafil (Cialis). Viagra and Levitra are taken an hour before sexual activity and enhance the effects of nitrous oxide to facilitate relaxation of the smooth muscle in the penis during sexual stimulation to increase blood flow. Both drugs should be taken no more than once a day, and should not be taken by men who are also taking nitrate-based medications as this may result in severe hypotension or serious cardiac side effects. It is recommended that patients taking alpha-blockers to treat hypertension and prostate enlargement should only use these drugs if the base line blood pressure is at least 90/60, other treatments have been unsuccessful, and the patient is monitored closely by a physician (Reffelmann & Kloner, 2006). Cialis is a selective phosphodiesterase type 5 inhibitor that allows smooth muscle relaxation to facilitate inflow of blood into the penis. Different forms of Cialis allow a single dose as a sustained release medication that lasts for 36 hours or as a daily low-dose medication. In either case, an erection only occurs with sexual stimulation. Cialis should not be taken if the man is also taking nitrates, alpha-blockers, erythromycin or rifampicin (antibiotics), ketoconazole or itraconazole (antifungals), or protease inhibitors (for HIV). Men taking any of these medications should be told to call their healthcare provider for erections lasting more than 4 hours.

- *Injectable medications:* Hormone replacement therapy with testosterone injections or topical patches may be used for men with documented androgen deficiency and who do not have prostate cancer. Injectable medications, including papaverine and prostaglandin E injections, may be used. When injected directly into the penis, papaverine relaxes the arterioles and smooth muscles of the cavernosum, thus inducing tumescence (swelling). An erection usually develops that lasts from 30 minutes to 4 hours. Prostaglandin E functions much as papaverine does, but has fewer side effects. One problem with this treatment is its mode of delivery. There is a high attrition rate, and patients report dissatisfaction with lack of spontaneity, loss of interest in sex, physical limitations, cost, and, occasionally, pain. Alprostadil (Caverject) is another injectable medication that may be used to treat ED. It may be injected into the penis or placed in the urethra as a minisuppository.

Mechanical Devices

The vacuum constriction device (VCD) is a frequently prescribed mechanical device for ED. The VCD draws blood into the penis with a vacuum, trapping it there with a constricting band at the base of the penis. After the device is removed for intercourse, a single small band, often called an O-ring, is left at the base of the penis to maintain the erection. If the man can attain an erection but cannot maintain it, then an O-ring alone can be used.

Surgery

Surgical treatment for ED involves either revascularization procedures or implantation of prosthetic devices. Venous or arterial procedures are generally not successful. The result is often temporary because the underlying cause of the vascular insufficiency is usually not corrected. Implantation of penile prostheses is now common (Figure 48–1 ■). Men are generally satisfied with their prostheses, and they rank the inflatable type highest. Partners are also more likely to report satisfaction with the penile implant, although not to the same degree as patients. Some partners report that the implanted penis is harder than a normal erect penis and therefore causes pain. Also, the man can have intercourse for a prolonged period of time, and some partners do not find prolonged penetration enjoyable. Patient and partner teaching is necessary to ensure proper use of and satisfaction with the device. Counseling by a sex therapist may be needed to facilitate adaptation to the implant.

Lifestyle Changes

Depending upon the cause of the ED, changes in lifestyle may improve the condition or decrease the progression of the problem. Smoking cessation, eating a healthy diet, and regular exercise may improve overall health and cardiovascular functioning. If the man is overweight a weight loss program as well as avoidance of alcohol and practicing stress reducing activities may be beneficial.

A Semirigid

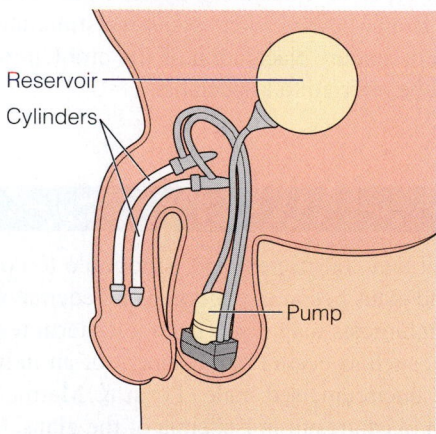

Reservoir
Cylinder
Pump

B Self-contained

Reservoir
Cylinders
Pump

C Inflatable

Figure 48–1 ■ Types of penile implants. *A,* With semirigid rods implanted in the corpora cavernosa, the penis is always in a state of semi-erection, which may not be acceptable to the man. *B,* With a self-contained penile implant, the penis remains flaccid until the man compresses a pump at the head of the penis, which transfers fluid from a reservoir to a cylinder within the penis to achieve an erection. The man presses a release valve to return the fluid to the reservoir. *C,* With an inflatable penile implant, the penis remains flaccid until the man compresses a pump in the scrotum, which transfers fluid from an abdominal reservoir to cylinders in the corpora cavernosa to achieve an erection. Pressing a release valve returns the fluid to the reservoir.

✍ Nursing Care

Nurses in any healthcare setting may encounter men with ED, either through routine examinations or through assessment of patients' conditions and treatments that may incidentally cause ED. Nurses employed in clinics, operating rooms, and surgical units with urologic services commonly encounter men being treated for ED. Nurses in a variety of settings, including long-term care, encounter men who have had surgical interventions, such as penile implants.

Nursing Diagnoses and Interventions

Because nurses often complete a patient's health history, they are most likely to discover problems of ED (see the Functional Health Pattern Interview guide in ∞ Chapter 47 for appropriate questions to elicit information). Once a problem is known, nurses are involved in providing information and emotional support, and referring patients to physicians or counselors. Although there are many possible nursing diagnoses, this section focuses on nursing care related to sexual dysfunction and self-esteem.

Sexual Dysfunction

Many men who lose erectile function are not aware of the cause. Not knowing causes anxiety and increased risk for depression. Often the man blames the loss on unrelated factors, such as age, a medication for an illness, a dangerous illness, or his sexual partner. Other medications (such as those used to treat hypertension, known to have ED as a side effect) may not be taken as prescribed if the man believes this is the cause of the ED.

- Assess for risk factors for ED. Be especially alert to men who have recently begun medications or had recent surgeries that could cause ED. *Awareness of risk factors helps the nurse prioritize care, although nurses must remember that almost all aging men have at least one risk factor for ED.*
- Assess for sexual dysfunction. Men have shown increasing willingness to discuss sexual concerns and expect nurses to be aware of the physiologic effects of their disease and side effects of treatment on all aspects of their health. *If a problem exists, information obtained in a sexual assessment guides the nurse in deciding if the next step should be patient teaching, referral, or both.*
- Conduct a detailed assessment of current sexual practices. *It is essential for healthcare providers to understand the patient and partner's sexual pattern in order to provide appropriate, individualized care.*
- Discuss previous methods of coping with ED. *Awareness of coping strategies can provide insight for the nurse and guide teaching.*
- Provide information about treatment options. *The man needs to know the details of the intervention, the chances for success, and the possible complications.*
- Encourage discussion of condition with partner. *It is not uncommon for men to withdraw from their partners, causing strain on the relationship and adding to the feelings of anxiety.*

> **PRACTICE ALERT**
> Many men will not volunteer information about sexual function unless asked, but then are open about concerns and appreciate being asked.

Situational Low Self-Esteem

The man with ED often believes himself to be "less than a man." In addition, the insertion of a penile implant with a semi-rigid prosthesis may result in disturbances in body image related to changes in sexual activity as well as the appearance and embarrassment of a permanent semi-erection.

- Collect data during the health history, in a nonjudgmental manner, about physiologic function, other chronic illnesses, and feelings about sexual inadequacy. *This information is necessary to establish the database for individualized interventions.*

- If the man has had a penile implant, teach him and his partner how to use the pump, including how to inflate and deflate the device. Suggest he practice inflation and deflation during the postoperative period. Suggest wearing snug-fitting underwear with the penis placed in an upright position on the abdomen and loose trousers. Provide information about length of healing, and that sexual activity may resume within 6 to 8 weeks following surgery. *Practicing use of the pump will maintain the pump position and promote tissue growth around the implant. The type of clothing worn can improve the ability to conceal a semirigid prosthesis and decrease embarrassment. Recovery from surgery is necessary before resuming sexual activity.*

Community-Based Care

Many nurses find that men with ED and their partners have lived in isolation with the problem for many years. The partner may even be unaware of the problem, believing that the man is seeing someone else or that the man has lost his attraction to the partner. The man may have kept his problem a secret because an intense feeling of shame makes him unable to admit that he cannot perform sexually. Many men greet the information about the high incidence of ED with a sense of relief that they are not alone in having this problem. All men and their partners need to be aware of support services available to them. Referral sources include the Sexual Function Health Council, the American Urological Association, and the American Association of Sex Educators, Counselors, and Therapists.

The Man with Ejaculatory Dysfunction

There are many types of ejaculatory dysfunction. **Retrograde ejaculation** (seminal fluid discharged into the bladder) may develop in aging men but is usually related to surgery of the prostate or for testicular cancer. **Premature ejaculation** is the most common form of sexual dysfunction in men and is usually psychogenic in origin, but some studies suggest alterations in serotonin regulation affect sexual function (Mercado, Kimmer, & Holman, 2008). Comorbidities such as diabetes can cause the problem as well. Delayed ejaculation can be related to aging changes, such as decreased vibrotactile sensation over the penis or decreased libido secondary to hypogonadism. Delayed ejaculation and inability to ejaculate at all may be caused by certain medications, such as antihypertensives, antidepressants, anxiolytics, and narcotics.

Among these problems, premature ejaculation has proved most responsive to medical management. Medications such as selective serotonin reuptake inhibitors (SSRIs), tricyclic antidepressants, and topical anesthetics are often prescribed. The man can also experiment with ways to decrease sensitivity (such as wearing condoms). Using relaxation and guided imagery can delay orgasm. Mechanical devices, such as constrictive rings around the base of the penis, can help the man delay ejaculation and sustain an erection.

Nursing care focuses on assessment of the problem and teaching for all types of ejaculatory dysfunction. The man's partner can be taught how to avoid excessive stimulation that would result in premature ejaculation. If the problem persists, the man should be referred to a specialist.

Disorders of the Penis

The Man with Phimosis or Priapism

Two less common disorders of the penis are phimosis and priapism. Although uncommon, these disorders can cause problems with urination and sexual activity. In some cases, they are considered a medical emergency because decreased blood flow to the penis may result in tissue ischemia and necrosis.

Pathophysiology

Phimosis is constriction of the foreskin in uncircumcised men so that it cannot be retracted over the glans penis. Phimosis may be congenital, or it may be related to chronic infections under the foreskin, which lead to adhesions. The major problem with this condition is that it prevents adequate hygiene, which in turn may increase the risk of cancer of the penis. Phimosis also may interfere with urinary elimination and intercourse. In a related disorder, called paraphimosis, the foreskin is tight and constricted, and is not able to cover the glans penis. The glans becomes engorged and edematous, and is painful. Paraphimosis may result from long-term retraction of the foreskin, such as occurs in placement of an indwelling catheter in the uncircumcised male (Porth & Matfin, 2009). The tight foreskin can result in ischemia of the glans.

Priapism is an involuntary, sustained, painful erection that is not associated with sexual arousal. The prolonged erection may result in ischemia and fibrosis of the erectile tissue with high risk of subsequent impotence (Porth, 2007). The disorder, classified as either primary or secondary, is caused by impaired blood flow in the corpora cavernosa. Primary priapism results from conditions such as tumors, infection, or trauma. Secondary priapism is caused by blood disorders (e.g., leukemia, sickle cell anemia, and thrombocytopenia), neurologic disorders (e.g., spinal cord injury or stroke), renal failure, and some medications (e.g., papaverine, alcohol, marijuana, psychotropic drugs). Men who use intracavernous injection therapy or medications for ED are at risk for priapism.

Interdisciplinary Care

Severe phimosis or paraphimosis may require surgical circumcision. If infection is present, the appropriate antibiotic is administered.

Treatment of priapism includes iced saline enemas, intravenous ketamine (Ketalar) administration to induce anesthesia, and spinal anesthesia. Blood may be aspirated from the corpus through the dorsal glans, followed by catheterization and pressure dressings to maintain decompression. If necessary, more aggressive surgery to create vascular shunts to maintain blood flow is performed. When priapism is prolonged, it increases the risk of subsequent ED.

∞ Nursing Care

Nursing care for priapism focuses on assessing the penis, monitoring urinary output, and providing pain control. Assessment of the penis includes inspection for degree of erection and changes in color due to ischemia, and palpation of the penis for firmness and degree of rigidity. Monitor urine output, assessing for oliguria or signs of acute urinary retention. Pain is treated with analgesics.

The man usually has moderate to severe anxiety related to pain, the treatment, and the threat to his sexual function. The treatment may sound bizarre and painful, especially since the area is already extremely sensitive. The man may be acutely embarrassed by the erection and needs reassurance that the nurse understands that the erection is not within his control.

The Man with Cancer of the Penis

Cancer of the penis is a rare cancer in North America, occurring in approximately 1300 men per year (American Cancer Society [ACS], 2009b). Age is a factor, as the greatest incidence is in men aged 60 and above. The cause is unknown. It is lower in populations in which routine circumcision is practiced, although the correlation between circumcision and this cancer is unclear. Phimosis and poor genital hygiene are risk factors, as are human papillomavirus HPV and HIV infections. Ultraviolet radiation exposure (such as that used to treat psoriasis) also may play a role (Porth & Matfin, 2009).

Pathophysiology

Squamous cell carcinoma accounts for 95% of all penile cancers (Porth & Matfin, 2009). The tumor usually develops as a nodular or wartlike growth or a red velvety lesion on the glans or foreskin. (Squamous cell carcinoma is illustrated in ∞ Chapter 16). The tumors tend to grow slowly. Penile cancer spreads to the superficial or deep inguinal nodes, and very late in the disease may spread to the bone, liver, or lungs. If the lesion is treated before inguinal node involvement, chances for a cure are good. Most of these lesions are painless but there may be significant ulceration and bleeding. Purulent, foul-smelling discharge may be evident under the foreskin. Occasionally, men with penile cancer may present with enlarged inguinal lymph nodes.

Interdisciplinary Care

Cancer of the penis is diagnosed by a biopsy of the lesion, including any suspicious inguinal lymph nodes. The cancer is staged according to the size of the tumor, extent of invasion, status of inguinal lymph nodes, and presence or absence of distant metastasis. Small, localized lesions may be treated with fluorouracil cream, external-beam radiation, laser therapy, or surgical excision. Larger lesions with superficial or deep infiltration of penile structures require partial or total amputation of the penis. Chemotherapy (∞ discussed in Chapter 14) may be administered to men with distant metastasis.

∞ Nursing Care

Education can help prevent this disease or provide early detection and cure. Teach men about genital hygiene (including retraction of the foreskin if uncircumcised and washing the glans penis while bathing or showering), the risks of unprotected sex, and the importance of using condoms. Instruct men to shield their genitals when having ultraviolet light therapy or using tanning salons. Discuss the importance of seeking prompt treatment for any lesion or abnormal drainage noted on the penis.

If the man has a penile amputation (penectomy), nurses can help in coping with the problems of a shortened or absent penis, including the potentially devastating effect on body image and self-concept. If a total penectomy is performed, the surgeon creates a perineal urethrostomy, preserving urinary continence. However, the man must void in the sitting position, reinforcing the feeling of loss. Dribbling of urine after voiding may be a problem for a few weeks. The man should be taught to perform careful perineal hygiene following surgery, using mild soap and water. Sitz baths may be helpful to relieve pain and to promote healing. If an inguinal lymph node dissection is performed, the man may experience persistent lymphedema of the lower extremities.

Radiation therapy may affect skin integrity and possibly cause irritation and stricture of the urethra. Radiation prior to surgery may impede incision healing. It is important to assess skin integrity and the man's ability to void. Leakage of urine from dribbling or catheters could also further irritate sensitive tissues.

Disorders of the Testis and Scrotum

The Man with a Benign Scrotal Mass

Most scrotal masses are benign and can be managed in a manner that is satisfactory to the patient. The most common benign scrotal masses are hydroceles, spermatoceles, and varicoceles (Figure 48–2 ■).

Pathophysiology

A **hydrocele**, the most common cause of scrotal swelling, is a collection of fluid within the tunica vaginalis. The swelling ranges from slightly larger than the testicle to larger than a grapefruit. Hydroceles may occur secondary to trauma, infection, or a tumor. The cause of chronic hydrocele in men over the age of 40 years is an imbalance between production and reabsorption of fluid

Fluid-filled mass in scrotum

Hydrocele

Cystic mass on epididymis

Spermatocele

Dilation of pampiniform venous complex

Varicocele

Figure 48–2 ■ Common disorders of the scrotum. Hydroceles and spermatoceles do not usually require treatment unless they become large and cause pain. Varicoceles are usually treated to prevent infertility.

within the layers of the scrotum. A hydrocele may be differentiated from a solid mass by transillumination or ultrasound of the scrotum. If the hydrocele becomes large enough to cause embarrassment or significant pain, the fluid is aspirated and an agent is injected into the scrotal sac to sclerose the tunica vaginalis. Hydroceles are not associated with infertility.

A **spermatocele** is a mobile, usually painless mass that forms when efferent ducts in the epididymis dilate and form a cyst. It is thought to result from leakage of sperm due to trauma or infection. Treatment is usually not necessary. Spermatoceles are not associated with infertility.

A **varicocele** is an abnormal dilation of a vein within the spermatic cord. It is caused by incompetent or congenitally missing valves that allow blood to pool in the spermatic cord veins. The dilated vein forms a soft mass that may be painful. Most varicoceles occur on the left side. A major concern with this condition is that it can decrease blood flow through the testis, interfere with spermatogenesis, and cause infertility. Varicoceles can be felt by scrotal palpation and most often disappear when the man is in the supine position. Sonography is also frequently used for diagnosis. If infertility is a concern, the spermatic vein may be ligated or occluded with a sclerosing agent or balloon catheter. If the varicocele is small and infertility is not a concern, a scrotal support is recommended.

∾ Nursing Care

Nursing care focuses on reducing anxiety and teaching about comfort measures. Almost all men are aware of the possible pain associated with scrotal manipulation. They need information and reassurance about pain management if surgical treatment is necessary. External bleeding is minimal after surgery; however, some men do develop scrotal hematomas, manifested by scrotal edema and a purple discoloration.

The Man with Epididymitis

Epididymitis is an infection or inflammation of the epididymis, the structure that lies along the posterior border of the testis. This disorder is more often seen in sexually active men who are less than 35 years of age.

Sexually transmitted urethritis caused by *C. trachomatis* or *N. gonorrhoeae* is the usual precipitating factor for epididymitis in younger men. Men who practice unprotected anal intercourse may acquire sexually transmitted epididymitis from *E. coli, H. influenzae, Cryptococcus,* or tuberculosis. In men older than age 35, epididymitis is often associated with a urinary tract infection or prostatitis. Chemical epididymitis is associated with an inflammatory response to the reflux of urine into the ejaculatory ducts from urethral strictures, congenital structural anomalies, or increased abdominal pressure from excessive heavy lifting. This type is usually self-limiting and does not require treatment.

Infectious epididymis spreads by ascending the vas deferens from an already infected urethra or bladder. Early manifestations include pain and local edema, which can progress to erythema and edema of the entire scrotum, especially on the side of the involved epididymis. Complications of the disorder include abscess formation, infarction of the testis, and infertility.

Interdisciplinary Care

The infection is diagnosed with a specimen culture from a urethral swab or epididymal aspiration. Severe epididymitis may be treated with intravenous antibiotics and hospitalization. Less acute forms of the disease are treated with outpatient antibiotic therapy. The man's sexual partner should be treated with antibiotics if the causative organism is sexually transmitted.

∾ Nursing Care

Nursing care involves symptomatic relief and teaching. Ice packs and a scrotal support may be applied to the scrotum to relieve pain. Ensure the man knows that complete resolution of the infection may take weeks to months, and that treatment should continue until the infection is gone. Provide information about the possibility of infertility, because the man may wish to seek evaluation for this problem at a later date. Instruction on sexually transmitted infection prevention may also be necessary if the epididymitis is caused from a sexually transmitted organism.

The Man with Orchitis

Orchitis is an acute inflammation or infection of the testes. It most commonly occurs from an extension of a genitourinary infection or as a complication of a systemic illness. Infection may reach the testes through the vas deferens and the lymphatic and vascular channels. Trauma, including vasectomy and other scrotal surgeries, may cause inflammation of the testes.

The most common systemic infectious cause of orchitis in postpubertal men is mumps. Other causes include scarlet fever or pneumonia. The manifestations have a sudden onset, usually within 3 to 4 days after the swelling of the parotid glands. Manifestations include a high fever, increased WBCs, and unilateral or bilateral scrotal redness, swelling, and pain. If both testes are involved, permanent sterility may result, but this is rare (Porth, 2007).

Interdisciplinary Care

Treatment is supportive and symptomatic, including antibiotic therapy if urine cultures are positive. Bed rest, scrotal support and elevation, hot or cold compresses, and analgesics for pain are prescribed. If a hydrocele occurs, it is aspirated. Nursing care is similar to that of the patient with epididymitis and other scrotal disorders.

The Man with Testicular Torsion

Testicular torsion, twisting of the spermatic cord resulting in sudden onset of scrotal swelling, pain, and nausea and vomiting is a potential medical emergency. The condition occurs most often between birth and age 20, but can occur at any age. Testicular torsion may occur spontaneously, or it may follow trauma or physical exertion. The torsion of the arteries and veins decreases or stops testicular circulation with resultant vascular engorgement and ischemia.

Testicular torsion is usually diagnosed by history and physical examination. It may be confused with epididymitis but is much more serious in nature, so accurate assessment and diagnosis is imperative for successful outcome of the patient. Testicular scanning may be used to determine if blood flow to the testicle is reduced, or a prostate ultrasound may be done to identify masses or torsion. Surgical treatment, which involves detorsion of the testicle and fixation to the scrotum, must begin as quickly as possible. If the testicle is necrotic or has sustained significant damage, an orchiectomy (surgical removal of a testes) is performed.

The Man with Testicular Cancer

Testicular cancer accounts for only 1% of all cancers in men; however, it is the most common cancer in men between the ages of 15 and 40 and can occur from infancy through old age. Annually, more than 8000 new cases are diagnosed (American Cancer Society, 2009). Although the cause is unknown, White American men are five times more likely to develop testicular cancer than are men from other races (see the Focus on Cultural Diversity box). The incidence of testicular cancer has increased over the last several decades but survival from testicular cancer has improved dramatically as a result of treatment with effective combination chemotherapy. Testicular cancer is considered to be one of the most curable cancers, with almost 140,000 men who have survived the disease living in the United States (American Cancer Society, 2009a).

The cause of testicular cancer is unknown, but both congenital and acquired factors have been associated with tumor development. About 5% develop in a man with a history of undescended testicle (cryptorchidism). Testicular cancer is more common on the right side (Newton et al., 2009).

Risk Factors

Risk factors for testicular cancer follow:

- Age
- Cryptorchidism (undescended testicle)
- A family history of testicular cancer
- Cancer of the other testicle
- Other risk factors under investigation include occupational risks, presence of multiple atypical nevi, HIV infection, cancer *in situ*, and age (20% occur between the ages of 20 and 54) (ACS, 2009a)

Pathophysiology

Approximately 95% of testicular malignancies are germ cell tumors (Porth & Matfin, 2009). Germ cell tumors are classified, depending on their origin and ability to differentiate, as seminomas and nonseminomas. Seminomas are the most common type, and are believed to arise from the seminiferous epithelium of the testes. Nonseminomas contain more than one cell type; they include embryonal carcinoma, teratoma, choriocarcinoma, and yolk cell carcinoma. Testicular cancer may also arise from specialized cells of the gonadal stroma. These tumors are named for the cells from which they originate: Leydig cell, Sertoli cell, granulosa cell, and theca cell tumors.

Manifestations

The first sign of testicular cancer may be a slight, painless enlargement of one testicle. The man may also have an abdominal ache and a feeling of heaviness in the scrotum. Local spread of the cancer to the epididymis or spermatic cord is inhibited by the outer covering of the testicles, the tunica albuginea. Therefore, spread by lymphatic and vascular channels to other organs often causes distant disease before large masses develop in the scrotum. Lymphatic dissemination usually leads to disease in retroperitoneal lymph nodes, whereas vascular dissemination can lead to metastasis in the lungs, bone, or liver. Bilateral testicular cancer is unusual. Manifestations of testicular cancer are summarized in the following box. Manifestations of metastasis include lower extremity edema, back pain, cough, hemoptysis, or dizziness. HCG-producing tumors may cause breast enlargement (gynecomastia).

FOCUS ON CULTURAL DIVERSITY
Risk for Testicular Cancer

- White American men have about a five times greater risk of testicular cancer than do Black American men.
- White American men have more than three times the risk of Asian American and American Indian men.
- Hispanic men have a risk between that of Asians and non-Hispanic Whites.

Source: American Cancer Society, 2009a.

MANIFESTATIONS of Testicular Cancer

COMMON
- Painless swelling on one testicle

METASTATIC SYMPTOMS
- Neck mass
- Respiratory symptoms
- Gastrointestinal disturbance
- Lumbar back pain

OCCASIONAL
- Dull ache in pelvis or scrotum
- Painless nodule on one testicle

UNCOMMON
- Acute pain in scrotum

RARE
- Infertility
- Gynecomastia

Interdisciplinary Care

Care focuses on diagnosis, elimination of the cancer, and prevention or treatment of metastasis. Once testicular cancer is suspected, the man undergoes a number of screening tests to help identify the disease and its stage. If the disease is confined to the testicle, it is classified as stage I. Stage II disease is limited to the testicle and regional lymph nodes. Stage III disease involves metastasis above the diaphragm or extensive visceral involvement. Often, the man does not undergo biopsy before the beginning of treatment, but instead receives a definitive diagnosis after orchiectomy. Most men treated for testicular cancer will live a normal life span.

Diagnosis

Diagnosis may be made by various laboratory tests. Serum studies are done to identify tumor markers. Germ cell tumors produce biochemical markers such as human chorionic gonadotropin (hCG) and alpha-fetoprotein (AFP) that can be measured using radioimmunoassay techniques. Elevated levels provide strong evidence of testicular cancer. These markers are also measured after surgery to help determine the presence of residual disease that remains undetected by other means. Persistent elevation may indicate the need for further therapy. Serum lactate dehydrogenase (LDH) levels are elevated in testicular cancer, and may be significantly elevated when metastatic disease is present. The LDH is a less specific indicator of testicular cancer than the hCG and AFP.

Medications

Progress in chemotherapy to treat testicular cancer is one of the chief reasons why curative rates are as high as 95% (Feldman, Bosl, Sheinfeld, & Motzer, 2008). The patient with advanced disease receives platinum-based combination chemotherapy Chemotherapy is discussed in ∞ Chapter 14.

Surgery

Radical orchiectomy, which removes the affected testicle and spermatic cord is the treatment used in all forms and stages of testicular cancer. A modified retroperitoneal lymph node dissection that preserves the nerves necessary for ejaculation often is performed at the same time.

Radiation Therapy

Radiation therapy is used for stage I seminoma to treat cancer in the retroperitoneal lymph nodes, the most frequent site for distant metastasis. The man may experience temporary diarrhea, nausea, or a decline in bone marrow function, such as thrombocytopenia or leukopenia. These problems are usually mild and respond well to symptomatic treatment or time. Damage to the contralateral testicle is minimized by careful shielding. Pretreatment and posttreatment analysis of sperm number and function is necessary. The most common long-term complication is dyspepsia or ulcer disease. Radiation therapy is discussed in ∞ Chapter 14.

∞ Nursing Care

Health Promotion

Unfortunately, most men who develop testicular cancer do not have overt risk factors. Therefore, beginning at the age of 15, all men should perform monthly testicular self-examination, as described in Box 48–1.

(margin, left side) Testicular Cancer Video

Nursing Diagnoses and Interventions

Nursing care of the man with testicular cancer is complex. The nurse must consider the reactions to the diagnosis, the change in body image accompanying treatment, and sexual and reproductive issues. Although chances of a cure are excellent, the long-term effect on quality of life may be extensive, requiring a change in life goals.

Deficient Knowledge

The nurse often initiates and reinforces teaching about what to expect after radical orchiectomy. The man's knowledge about surgery is assessed, and postoperative routines such as early ambulation are explained (∞ see Chapter 4).

- Explain pain control methods. In addition to the usual analgesics used to control postoperative incisional pain, ice bags may be applied to the scrotum. A scrotal support provides relief, especially when the patient ambulates. *Surgery results in incisional pain, and the scrotum is tender and slightly swollen.*
- Teach the manifestations of complications. The incision is closed with Steri-Strips or staples, and, although rare, wound dehiscence is possible. If the incision gapes open, or if there is bleeding beyond slight oozing after 24 hours, the man should call the surgeon. Another rare complication is a hematoma in the scrotum caused by bleeding from the spermatic cord stump. Rapid onset of scrotal edema is a sign of this problem. *Because the man is usually discharged early, complications may not become apparent until he is at home.*

Ineffective Sexuality Pattern

The effect of testicular cancer and its treatment on sexual and reproductive function is varied. If the man has a retroperitoneal lymph node dissection, severing of the sympathetic plexus may result in retrograde ejaculation or failure to

---

BOX 48–1 Testicular Self-Examination

- Examine your testicles when you are taking a warm shower or bath, or just after if you prefer to use a mirror to compare size.
- The scrotum, testicles, and hands should be soapy to allow easy manipulation of the tissue.
- Gently roll each testicle between the thumb and fingers of each hand. If one testicle is substantially larger than the other, or if you feel any hard lumps, consult your physician immediately.
- Normal scrotal contents may be confusing. Just above and behind the testicle is the epididymis. It feels soft and tender overall, although parts of it may be rather firm. This is normal. The spermatic cord, a small, round, movable tube, extends up from the epididymis. It feels firm and smooth. Of greatest concern is any hard lump felt directly on the testicle, even if it is painless.
- Choose a day of each month on which to examine yourself. Most men choose an easy day to remember, such as the first or last day of the month. Star this day on your calendar to help you remember.

EVIDENCE FOR NURSING CARE | The Patient with Testicular Cancer

Selected resources that nurses may find helpful when planning evidence-based nursing care follow.

- Barlow, D., Brimblecombe, P., Brown, C., Duckitt, K., Dunlop, J., Hartshorne, G., et al. (2004). Fertility: Assessment and treatment for people with fertility problems. *National Guideline Clearinghouse.* Retrieved from www.guideline.gov
- Gates, T. J., Beelen, M. J., & Hershey, C. L. (2008). Cancer screening in men. *Nursing Clinics of North America, 43*(2), 283–306.
- Gleason, A. M. (2006). Racial disparities in testicular cancer: Impact on health promotion. *Journal of Transcultural Nursing, 17*(1), 58–64.
- McCullagh, J., Lewis G., & Warlow, C. (2005). Promoting awareness and practice of testicular self-examination. *Nursing Standard, 19*(51), 41–49.

ejaculate. Infertility may be caused by ejaculation disorders, surgery, chemotherapy, or radiation therapy.

- Assess the man's prediagnosis sexual function. To assess this area, the nurse must establish an atmosphere of openness and permission to discuss sexual concerns. After the initial shock of the diagnosis, men report intense concern about sexual and reproductive issues, which can be relieved only by information. *Knowledge of the man's usual sexual function is used to guide teaching.*
- Discuss the possibility of preserving sperm in a bank prior to treatment. *This option may help relieve the man's fears about his ability to father children in the future, but must be completed prior to initiating treatment with surgery, chemotherapy, or radiation therapy.*
- Help with coping with feelings about altered sexual function and appearance. Explain that testicular implants can be inserted to preserve appearance. *Many patients, regardless of whether they are in a significant relationship, deeply grieve the loss of the ability to father children. It is important to maintain body image despite disfiguring surgery.*

Community-Based Care

Families need to be included in teaching for a variety of reasons. If the man is of reproductive age, his partner will have significant anxiety and will require information. For a young single man, parents need information about the effect on sexual function and are often very involved in postoperative care. The man needs the support of the people he loves, and knowledgeable loved ones can give effective support.

Provide teaching and reinforcement of the need for follow-up, especially if the retroperitoneal lymph nodes were not surgically explored. For men with a risk for recurrence, surveillance with periodic physical examinations, chest x-ray films, tumor markers, and CT scans of the retroperitoneal nodes could continue for a minimum of 5 years and possibly 10 years after orchiectomy. Studies have found that men treated with chemotherapy are at an increased risk of developing cardiovascular disease and secondary malignancies. Men receiving both chemotherapy and radiation have an even higher rate of secondary malignancies. Educating men on the need to remain proactive in their health care throughout their lifetime is important (Feldman et al., 2008).

Disorders of the Prostate Gland

The Man with Prostatitis

Prostatitis is a term used to refer to different types of inflammatory disorders of the prostate gland. Chronic prostatis/chronic pelvic pain syndrome (CP/CPPS), previously known as prostatodynia, is a condition in which the patient experiences the symptoms of prostatitis but shows no evidence of inflammation or infection. Manifestations of prostatitis and prostatodynia are summarized in the box on the next page.

Pathophysiology and Manifestations

The National Institutes of Health have defined four types of prostatitis: acute bacterial prostatitis, chronic bacterial prostatitis, chronic prostatitis/pelvic pain syndrome, and asymptomatic inflammatory prostatitis. Men with asymptomatic inflammatory prostatitis have no subjective manifestations, but are diagnosed when a biopsy or prostatic fluid examination is conducted.

Acute Bacterial Prostatitis

Acute bacterial prostatitis is most often caused by an ascending infection from the urethra or reflux of infected urine into the ducts of the prostate gland. The organism most often responsible for the infection is *E. coli*; other causative organisms include *Pseudomonas*, *Klebsiella*, and *Chlamydia*.

Manifestations of acute bacterial prostatitis include fever, malaise, muscle and joint pain, painful ejaculation, urinary frequency and urgency, dysuria, and urethral discharge. The man often experiences dull, aching pain in the perineum, and/or pain in the prostate gland, rectum, or lower back. On rectal examination, the prostate is enlarged and painful.

Chronic Bacterial Prostatitis

Men with chronic bacterial prostatitis often present with a history of recurrent urinary tract infections. The causative organisms are most often *E. coli*, *Proteus*, or *Klebsiella*. Calculi may form in the prostate and contribute to the chronicity of the problem.

The manifestations of chronic bacterial prostatitis include urinary frequency and urgency, dysuria, low back pain, and perineal discomfort. Epididymitis may be associated with the prostatitis.

Chronic Prostatitis/Chronic Pelvic Pain Syndrome (CP/CPPS)

This type of prostatitis is both the most common and the least understood of the syndromes (NKUDIC, 2008). It is being questioned whether the disorder has anything to do with the prostate gland or whether other etiologies such as pelvic wall pain or dysfunction of the pelvic floor musculature are the cause of the symptoms. This is primarily the reason the disorder is now named chronic pelvic pain syndrome (Turner, Ciol, Von Korff, Yung-wen, & Berger, 2006). The two types (inflammatory and noninflammatory) are based on the presence or absence of white blood cells in the prostatic fluid.

- *Inflammatory prostatitis* is believed to be an autoimmune disorder, but the actual cause is unknown. Men with this type of prostatitis have low back pain; urinary manifestations; pain in the penis, testicles, scrotum, lower back, and rectum; decreased libido; and painful ejaculations. They do not have bacteria in their urine, but do have abnormal inflammatory cells in prostatic secretions.
- *Noninflammatory prostatitis* has manifestations similar to those of inflammatory prostatitis, but no evidence of urinary or prostatic infection or inflammation can be found. The cause is not known, but is believed to be the result of a problem outside the prostate gland, such as obstruction of the bladder neck.

Interdisciplinary Care

Diagnosis

It is often difficult to diagnose prostatitis. Urine and prostatic secretion examination and cultures are obtained to determine the presence and type of blood cells and bacteria. X-ray studies and ultrasound to visualize pelvic structures also may be useful.

Medications

Bacterial prostatitis is treated with appropriate antibiotics. Men with the chronic form must take antibiotics for up to 4 months, and may still relapse as soon as the antibiotic is discontinued. Nonbacterial prostatitis and CP/CPPS do not usually respond satisfactorily to drug therapy, although relief from symptoms is possible. Nonsteroidal anti-inflammatory drugs are useful for pain, and anticholinergics may reduce voiding symptoms. Muscle relaxants and alpha-adrenergic blocking agents are also prescribed, depending upon symptom severity. Stress reducing

MANIFESTATIONS of Prostatitis

ACUTE BACTERIAL PROSTATITIS
- Onset (may be abrupt): obstruction, irritation, or pain upon voiding; frequency; and urgency
- Positive cultures of infectious organism
- Nonurinary symptoms: chills, fever, low back and pelvic floor pain

CHRONIC BACTERIAL PROSTATITIS
- Urinary symptoms sometimes similar to those of the acute form, except less sudden, less dramatic, or even absent
- Positive cultures of causative organism not always obtainable

CHRONIC PROSTATITIS
- Perineal, suprapubic, low back, or genital pain
- Irritation upon voiding
- Postejaculatory pain
- Negative cultures of organisms

CHRONIC PROSTATIS/CHRONIC PELVIC PAIN SYNDROME
- Pelvic, low back, or perineal pain
- Irritation or obstruction upon voiding
- No evidence of inflammation in the prostate
- No urinary tract infection
- Normal prostatic secretions
- Pain when sitting

activities, warm baths, and avoidance of sitting when pain is most severe have been reported to assist in pain reduction. Some men also state that increasing sexual activity causes a reduction in symptoms (Turner et al., 2006).

Nursing Care

Teaching plans for the man with prostatitis focus on symptom management. Men with acute and chronic bacterial prostatitis should be taught to increase fluid intake to around 3 L daily and to void often. These measures help decrease irritation when voiding. Increasing fiber intake to promote regular bowel movements helps ease the pain associated with defecation. Local heat, such as sitz baths, may be helpful to relieve pain and irritation. It is important to teach the man to finish the course of antibiotic therapy. Men with CP/CPPS need to know that the condition is not contagious (Mayo Clinic, 2007). Referral sources for information include the National Kidney and Urologic Diseases Information Clearinghouse, the American Foundation for Urologic Disease, and the Prostatitis Foundation.

The Man with Benign Prostatic Hyperplasia

Benign prostatic hyperplasia (BPH), an age-related, nonmalignant enlargement of the prostate gland, is a common disorder of the aging male. Benign hyperplasia (increased number of cells) begins at 40 to 45 years of age and continues slowly through the rest of life. It is estimated that more than one-half of all men over age 60 have BPH (Porth, 2007). The problem that brings men to a healthcare provider is the associated urinary dysfunction.

Risk Factors

Although the exact cause of BPH is unknown, risk factors include age, family history, race, and a diet high in meat and fats.

Pathophysiology

The two necessary preconditions for BPH are age of 48 or greater and the presence of testes. Men who are castrated before puberty do not develop BPH. The androgen that mediates prostatic growth at all ages is dihydrotestosterone (DHT), which is formed in the prostate from testosterone. Although androgen levels decrease in aging men, the aging prostate appears to become more sensitive to available DHT. Estrogen, produced in small amounts in men, appears to sensitize the prostate gland to the effects of DHT. Increasing estrogen levels associated with aging or a relative increase in estrogen related to testosterone levels may contribute to prostatic hyperplasia.

BPH begins as small nodules in the periurethral glands, which are the inner layers of the prostate. The prostate enlarges through formation and growth of nodules (hyperplasia) and enlargement of glandular cells (hypertrophy). Enlargement occurs in an inward fashion, gradually compressing the urethra and resulting in the urologic symptoms associated with BPH. These changes occur over a long period of time. The pathophysiologic effects result from a combination of factors, including urethral resistance to the effects of BPH, intravesical pressure during voiding, detrusor muscle strength, neurologic functioning, and general physical health.

Manifestations

The expanding prostatic tissue compresses the urethra (Figure 48–3 ■) and causes partial or complete obstruction of the outflow of urine from the urinary bladder. The detrusor muscles hypertrophy to compensate for increased resistance to urinary flow; however, eventually decreased bladder compliance and bladder instability occur. As a result, the man with BPH has manifestations from urinary obstruction and a decrease in bladder contractibility and compliance. Urinary retention may become chronic, resulting in overflow incontinence with any increase in intra-abdominal pressure. There is little correlation between the size of the prostate gland and the urinary manifestations. The linkage of the manifestations of BPH with the related pathophysiology are summarized in the following Pathophysiology Linkage box.

Complications

Unless the enlarging mass is reduced, multiple complications may occur. As urine is retained in the bladder, increasing bladder distention occurs. Diverticula (outpouchings) on the bladder wall result from the distention. The distention may also obstruct the ureters. Infection, more common in retained urine and in diverticula, may ascend from the bladder to the kidneys. Hydroureter, hydronephrosis, and renal insufficiency are possible complications (∞ see Chapter 28).

Interdisciplinary Care

Care of men with BPH focuses on diagnosing the disorder, correcting or minimizing the urinary obstruction, and preventing or treating complications. There is no way to reverse BPH. Treatment is often determined by the severity of the manifestations and the presence of complications. Mild cases are often monitored over time, and may remain stable or improve.

Diagnosis

It is important for clinicians to determine the actual cause of manifestations, differentiating them from those of infections, stones, urinary strictures, cancer of the prostate or bladder, and side effects of certain medications such as antihistamines and decongestants. A diagnosis of BPH involves both physical examination and laboratory tests. A digital rectal examination (DRE) is done to examine the external surface of the prostate; in BPH it is asymmetrical and enlarged. Examination of the creatinine levels of the blood is conducted to assess for kidney damage.

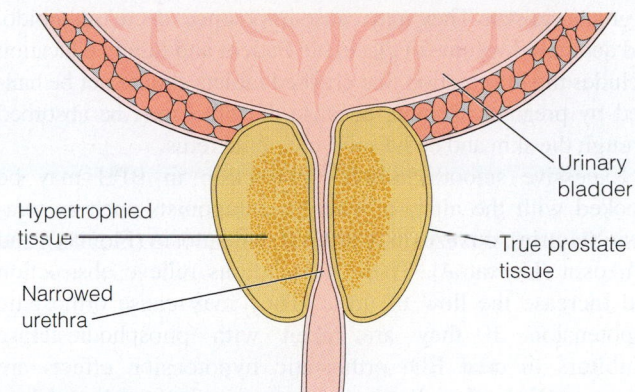

Figure 48–3 ■ Benign prostatic hyperplasia.

The urine is examined for WBCs, RBCs, and bacteria. Urinary function is assessed by measuring residual urine (amount of urine remaining in the bladder after voiding) with ultrasonography or postvoiding catheterization (more than 100 mL is considered high), and through uroflowmetry, which measures urine flow rate; normal is greater than 14 mL/sec. A finding of less than 10 mL/sec indicates obstruction.

Prostate-specific antigen (PSA) levels are obtained to rule out prostate cancer. PSA is a glycoprotein produced only in the cytoplasm of benign and malignant prostate cells; the serum level corresponds with the volume of both benign and malignant prostate tissue. Further information is provided in the next section under diagnosis of prostate cancer.

In addition, the man's own subjective experiences with BPH are included in the diagnosis and treatment. For example, the International Prostate Symptom Score and the American Urologic Association BPH Symptom Score questionnaires use scales of 0 (not at all) to 5 (almost always) to collect data about areas such as feeling as though the bladder did not empty with urinating, need to urinate within 2 hours after urinating, starting and stopping the stream several times while urinating, and straining to urinate. These questionnaires also ask how many times during the night the man gets up to urinate and how the man feels about having the disorder.

Medications

Treatment with medications is based on two considerations: The hyperplastic tissue is androgen dependent, and smooth muscle contraction within the prostate can exacerbate urinary obstruction. The first consideration is usually addressed by treatment for mild prostate enlargement with finasteride (Proscar) or dutasteride (Avodart), antiandrogen agents that inhibit the conversion of testosterone to DHT and cause the enlarged prostate to shrink in size. These are usually only effective if the prostate is 40 mL

PATHOPHYSIOLOGY LINKAGE Benign Prostatic Hyperplasia

MANIFESTATIONS	RELATED PATHOPHYSIOLOGY
Urinary frequency, increased time to begin voiding, small urinary stream	As a result of the anatomic placement of the prostate at the bladder neck, an increase in the size of the prostate compresses the urethra and outflow of urine.
Dribbling of urine, time required to void increases, urgency, nocturia	Compression of the urethra and retention of urine in the bladder, coupled with impaired bladder contractibility and a decrease in bladder compliance.

or greater in size. They may cause impotence, decreased libido, and decreased volume of ejaculate. Patient and family education includes the information that crushed tablets should not be handled by pregnant women, because the drug may be absorbed through the skin and be harmful to a male fetus.

Excessive smooth muscle contraction in BPH may be blocked with the alpha-adrenergic antagonists such as terazosin (Hytrin), doxazosin (Cardura), tamsulosin (Flomax), and alfuzosin (Uroxatral). These medications relieve obstruction and increase the flow of urine. They may cause orthostatic hypotension. If they are taken with phosphodiesterase inhibitors to treat ED, orthostatic hypotension effects are increased. Federal studies found that using finasteride and doxazosin together is more effective than using each alone to relieve manifestations and prevent the progression of BPH, but medication side effects are increased as well as the costs of the medication (McPhee, Papdakis, & Tierney, 2008). Patient and family teaching includes advice about making position changes slowly to avoid dizziness and accidental falls, how to take and record blood pressure, and to check with the healthcare provider before taking any medication for coughs, colds, or allergies (because these over-the-counter [OTC] medications may contain an adrenergic agent).

Surgery

Men who have urinary retention, recurrent urinary tract infection, hematuria, bladder stones, or renal insufficiency secondary to BPH are candidates for surgical intervention. Surgical treatment may be performed by minimally invasive surgery or through transurethral surgery, open surgery, or by laser surgery.

MINIMALLY INVASIVE SURGERY   Because medications are not effective for all men, a number of procedures have been developed to relieve the manifestations of BPH that are less invasive than traditional surgery.

Microwaves are used to heat and destroy excess prostate tissue in a procedure called transurethral microwave thermotherapy. During the procedure, a cooling system protects the urinary tract. The procedure takes about an hour and can be performed on an outpatient basis. Although microwave procedures do not cure BPH, they do reduce urinary manifestations. The procedures do not cause impotence or incontinence.

The transurethral needle ablation (TUNA) system uses low-level radio frequency through twin needles to burn away a region of the enlarged prostate. Shields protect the urethra. TUNA improves the flow of urine through the urethra. It does not cause impotence or incontinence.

TRANSURETHRAL SURGERY   A transurethral resection of the prostate (TURP) is the surgical procedure used most often. Obstructing prostate tissue is removed using the wire loop of a resectoscope and electrocautery, inserted through the urethra (Figure 48–4 ■). No external incision is necessary. During the procedure the surgeon uses the resectoscope to remove obstructing tissue one piece at a time. The tissue is flushed into the bladder with fluid and then flushed out at the end of the operation. This surgery has potential risks, however, including postoperative hemorrhage or clot retention, inability to void,

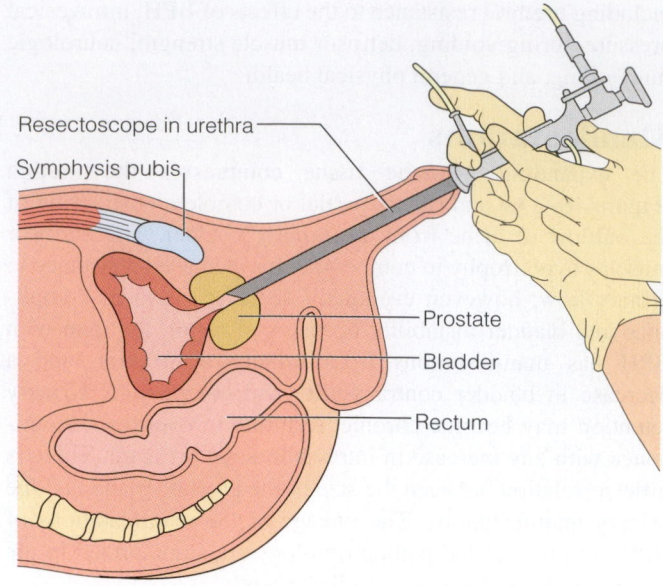

A   Transurethral resection of the prostate

B   Retropubic prostatectomy

Figure 48–4 ■ *A,* In a transurethral resection of the prostate, a resectoscope inserted through the urethra is used to remove excess prostate tissue. *B,* In a retropubic prostatectomy, prostate tissue is removed through an abdominal incision.

and urinary tract infection. Other possible complications are incontinence, impotence, and retrograde ejaculation.

In the transurethral incision of the prostate (TUIP) procedure, small incisions are made in the smooth muscle where the prostate is attached to the bladder. The gland is split to reduce pressure on the urethra. No tissue is removed, so this procedure is most appropriate for men with smaller prostate glands. TUIP can be done on an outpatient basis, and has the additional advantage of less risk of postoperative retrograde ejaculation than is associated with TURP or other prostatectomy procedures.

OPEN SURGERY   When the prostate gland is very large, an open prostatectomy may be used. These procedures are discussed in the section on prostate cancer that follows. Nursing care for the patient having prostate surgery is outlined in the box on page 1663.

NURSING CARE OF THE PATIENT Having a Prostatectomy

PREOPERATIVE CARE

- Assess the man's and family's knowledge about the surgery *Some men are confused about the surgical approach because there are several quite different methods.*
- Inform the man that he will have a urinary catheter when he returns from surgery, and he may have a drain(s) in his incision. He also will be wearing antiembolic stockings or sequential pneumatic compression stockings. *This knowledge can reduce anxiety postoperatively and increase cooperation with postoperative care.*
- Ensure that a signed consent form is in the chart and that all other preoperative tasks outlined in ∞ Chapter 4 are done.
- Bowel preparation with a 2% neomycin enema may be ordered. *This cleanses the bowel if a perineal approach will be used.*
- Communicate willingness to address any concerns of anxiety *Men may be anxious about the outcome of their surgery and potential long-term effects of the surgery on their sexuality. When a prostatectomy is performed for prostate cancer, additional fears include the extent of the cancer and surgery, chances for cure, and possible end-of-life issues.*

POSTOPERATIVE CARE

- Maintain the usual postoperative assessments (∞ see Chapter 4) and follow aseptic techniques in urinary drainage and irrigation care. Monitor vital signs closely for the first 24 hours and regularly thereafter. *The man who has had prostate surgery is at risk for hemorrhage and infection. Vital sign changes may be early manifestations of complications.*
- Maintain accurate intake and output records, including amounts of irrigating solution used. Frequently assess patency of any catheters and drains. Monitor color and character of urine. *Catheters may become occluded by blood clots or kinks, interfering with urinary drainage and increasing the risk of hemorrhage.*
- Assess and manage pain. *The man may have at least three types of pain: incisional pain, bladder spasms, and abdominal cramps due to intestinal gas. Analgesics and nonsteroidal anti-inflammatory drugs (NSAIDs) are administered on a routine and prn basis to control incisional pain. Bladder spasms may be accompanied by strong urges to void and urine leakage around the catheter. Belladonna and opium (B&O) suppositories may be used to relieve bladder spasms.*
- Maintain antiembolic stockings or sequential compression stockings as prescribed, following agency protocol for assessments and times of removal. Assist with leg exercises and ambulation as ordered. *The man who has had prostate surgery is at risk for developing thromboemboli; these are important preventive measures.*
- Encourage the man to maintain a liberal fluid intake of 2 to 3 L a day. *Increased fluids reduce burning on urination after catheter removal and the risk of urinary tract infection.*

THE MAN WITH A TRANSURETHRAL RESECTION OF THE PROSTATE (TURP)

- For the first 24 to 48 hours, monitor for hemorrhage, evidenced by frankly bloody urinary output, presence of large blood clots, decreased urinary output, increasing bladder spasms, decreased hemoglobin and hematocrit, tachycardia, and hypotension. Notify the physician if any of these manifestations occur. *Postoperative hemorrhage may be either arterial or venous, and may be precipitated by movement, bladder spasms, or an obstructed urinary drainage system.*

- Instruct the man with a three-way indwelling catheter with traction to keep the leg straight while the traction is applied. *A No. 18- to 22-Fr three-way catheter with a 30- to 45-mL balloon usually is inserted following a TURP. The inflated balloon is pulled down into the prostatic fossa and the catheter tubing is pulled down and secured to the man's leg with a urinary catheter attachment device to apply pressure against the operative site, preventing bleeding.*
- Explain that the presence of a urinary catheter will cause the sensation of needing to void, but it is important not to strain to try to void around the catheter or when having a bowel movement. Explain that bladder spasms, experienced as lower abdominal pressure or pain and a desire to urinate, may occur. Ensure that the man understands that this is an expected sensation, and that medications can help alleviate this discomfort. *Pressure on the urethra by the large catheter and on the internal sphincter by the catheter's balloon stimulate the micturition reflex. Straining to void or to have a bowel movement may stimulate bladder spasms and increase pain; it also may increase the risk for bleeding. Administer pain medications at regular intervals.*
- If the man has a continuous bladder irrigation (CBI), assess the catheter and the drainage tubing at regular intervals. Maintain the rate of flow of irrigating fluid to keep the output light pink or colorless. Assess the urinary output every 1 to 2 hours for color, consistency amount, and presence of blood clots; assess for bladder spasms. *CBI is used to prevent the formation of blood clots, which could obstruct urinary output. Bladder distention resulting from output obstruction increases the risk of bleeding. Irrigating fluids are continuously infused and drained at a rate to keep urine light pink or colorless. Urine that is frankly bloody, contains many blood clots, or is decreased in amount, as well as bladder spasms, are indicators of obstruction and bleeding.*
- Assess for fluid volume excess and hyponatremia, called TURP syndrome, which is manifested by hyponatremia, decreased hematocrit, hypertension, bradycardia, nausea, and confusion. If these manifestations occur, notify the physician. *TURP syndrome results from the absorption of irrigating fluids during and after surgery. Untreated, it may result in dysrhythmias, seizures, or both.*
- If the man does not have CBI, follow agency procedure and physician orders for irrigating the indwelling catheter (usually when the urine is frankly bloody or has numerous larger blood clots, or when bladder spasms increase). In most instances, using sterile technique, the catheter is gently irrigated with 50 mL of sterile irrigating solution at a time, until the obstruction is relieved or the urine is clear. Ensure equal input and output of irrigating fluid. *Intermittent irrigation may be used to prevent obstruction of urinary drainage.*
- Following catheter removal, assess the amount, color, and consistency of urine. Explain that the man may experience burning on urination, that dribbling after urination is a common experience, and that the urine may contain small blood clots after catheter removal. *The CBI and catheter usually are removed in the 24 to 48 hours following surgery. Urinary control may be improved by teaching the man to start and stop the urine stream several times during each voiding and by practicing Kegel exercises. Regaining full control may take up to 1 year.*

(continued)

NURSING CARE OF THE PATIENT Having a Prostatectomy (continued)

THE MAN WITH A RETROPUBIC PROSTATECTOMY

- Assess the abdominal incision for the presence of urine. *Because the bladder is not entered during a retropubic prostatectomy, no urine should be found on the dressing.*
- Assess the abdominal incision for increased or purulent drainage, and the man for an increased temperature and pain. *These manifestations indicate the presence of infection.*

THE MAN WITH A SUPRAPUBIC PROSTATECTOMY

- Assess urinary output from both the suprapubic and the urethral catheters. *The man with a suprapubic prostatectomy often has two separate closed drainage systems: one from the suprapubic incision and one from a urethral catheter.*
- Assess the abdominal dressing for urinary drainage, and change saturated dressings frequently. Consult with a skin care specialist if necessary. *Urine is highly irritating to the skin.*
- Following removal of the urethral catheter (usually 2 to 4 days after surgery) and based on physician orders, clamp the suprapubic catheter and encourage the man to void. Assess residual urine by unclamping the suprapubic

catheter and measuring urinary output after voiding. *If residual urine is 75 mL or less with several voidings, the suprapubic catheter is removed.*

THE MAN WITH A PERINEAL PROSTATECTOMY

- Assess perineal incision for drainage and manifestations of infection. *Location of the incision in the perineum increases the risk of infection.*
- Do not take rectal temperatures or administer enemas. *Insertion of a thermometer or enema tubing into the rectum may precipitate bleeding.*
- Use a T-binder or padded scrotal support to hold the dressing in place. Following removal of the dressing and perineal sutures, heat lamps or sitz baths may be used. *The location of the dressing makes application difficult: Heat lamps or sitz baths provide heat and promote healing.*
- Teach the man to perform perineal irrigations with sterile normal saline as ordered and after each bowel movement. *Because of the proximity of the incision to the anus, special wound care is necessary to prevent infection.*

LASER SURGERY In laser surgery, the surgeon uses a cystoscope to pass the YAG laser fiber through the urethra into the prostate and then vaporizes obstructing prostate tissue with several short bursts of energy. An advantage of laser surgery is decreased blood loss and a more rapid recovery time. However, this method may not be as effective for larger prostates.

Other Treatments

Other treatments for BPH include minimally invasive procedures such as balloon urethroplasty and placement of intraurethral stents to maintain patency of the urethra. Balloon urethroplasty is a simple procedure in which a balloon-tipped catheter is inserted into the narrowed portion of the urethra and inflated. Inflation of the balloon widens the urethra, relieving obstruction. These procedures can be done as outpatient surgery. Transurethral needle ablation devices use heat produced by radiofrequency waves to destroy prostate tissue. This technique is performed for men with large prostates who are not good candidates for more invasive surgical procedures.

Alternative and Complementary Therapies

Phytotherapy is the use of plants or plant extracts for medical treatment. Several plant extracts have been used for years in Europe to treat BPH and are being used more often in the United States. The phytotherapy used includes saw palmetto berry; the bark of *Pygeum africanum*; the roots of *Echinacea, purpurea,* and *Hypoxis rooperi*; and the leaves of the trembling poplar. The mechanisms of action of these extracts is unknown. There are men who report effectiveness in relieving manifestations but recent studies have revealed no significant reduction in symptoms or growth of the prostate when used (McPhee et al., 2008).

☙ Nursing Care

Most men are unsure of the function of the prostate gland and even the prostate's exact location, though its relationship to sexual and urinary function is at least generally known. This

lack of knowledge, coupled with the growing number of treatment options, is confusing to many men. There are many similarities between the nursing care of men with BPH and that of men with prostate cancer (see the section that follows).

Nursing Diagnoses and Interventions

This section provides interventions related to deficient knowledge, urinary retention, risk for infection, and risk for imbalanced fluid volume.

Deficient Knowledge

- Explain the anatomy and physiology of the prostate gland, as well as normal changes that occur with aging. *Men must know about their bodies in order to make accurate decisions about treatment.*
- Discuss treatment options, including information about effects on erectile function, ejaculation, and fertility. Counsel the man to discuss specific concerns with his urologist. *Many different treatment options are available; the choice should be a mutual decision between the man, his partner, and the urologist.*
- Discuss effects of prostate surgery, including urinary retention and urinary incontinence. *These common transient postoperative effects are related to the surgical procedure and the postoperative indwelling catheter.*
- Explain to the man having a TURP that a catheter will be placed into the bladder, with the tubing taped to his inner thigh, and that irrigation fluid may be infusing into and out of the catheter for the first 36 to 72 hours following surgery. *The catheter and irrigation are necessary to remove blood clots from the bladder and allow drainage of urine. Gentle traction is applied to the catheter to apply pressure to the operative site (prostatic fossa) and prevent excessive bleeding.*
- Explain that, following removal of the catheter, he will most likely have urinary frequency and urgency. He may also experience dribbling of urine after voiding. Stress the importance of increasing oral fluid intake and regular Kegel exercises.

Urinary manifestations are related to the surgical procedure and the indwelling catheter. Increased fluid intake helps decrease dysuria. Kegel exercises strengthen periurethral muscles and decrease postvoiding urine leakage.

Urinary Retention

- Teach the manifestations of acute urinary retention: dysuria, overflow incontinence, bladder pain and distention, no urine output. *Acute urinary retention is a potential complication of BPH, requiring immediate medical attention.*

- Teach that the risk of developing urinary retention increases when the man with BPH takes OTC decongestant medications, or prescription medications such as antidepressants, anticholinergics, calcium channel blockers, antipsychotics, and medications to treat Parkinson's disease. *OTC decongestants may contain alpha-adrenergic agonists that increase smooth muscle tone of the prostate, bladder neck, and proximal urethra. The prescribed medications may relax detrusor muscle contractions. Both actions may increase the risk of urinary retention (Nettina, 2006).*

- Suggest avoiding intake of large volumes of liquid at any one time. *A single intake of a large volume of liquid results in rapid bladder filling and increases the risk of urinary retention.*

- Teach how to use the double-voiding technique: Urinate, then sit on the toilet for 3 to 5 minutes, then urinate again. *This technique may relieve mild to moderate urinary retention.*

PRACTICE ALERT

In addition to avoiding a large amount of fluids at one time, it is also important to teach the man to limit liquids that stimulate voiding, such as coffee and alcoholic beverages.

Risk for Infection

- Monitor WBC and vital signs. *Infection is indicated by an increase in WBCs, body temperature, and pulse rate.*

TABLE 48–2 Urine Characteristics after Prostatectomy with Related Nursing Implications

URINE COLOR	NURSING IMPLICATIONS
Light red to red	Normal day of surgery and first postoperative day
Very dark red	May indicate increased venous bleeding or inadequate dilution. Catheter at risk for occlusion. Increase flow rate of irrigant. If urine does not clear, notify physician.
Bright red	May indicate arterial bleeding. Increase flow rate of irrigant, monitor vital signs, and notify physician.
Contains blood clots	Occasional blood clot normal. If clots are frequent, catheter may become obstructed. Increase flow rate of irrigant.
Clear to light pink	Normal throughout hospitalization.

- Maintain sterile procedures when changing irrigation fluids and emptying Foley catheter draining bag. *Sterile procedures are necessary to prevent infection.*

Risk for Imbalanced Fluid Volume

A prostatectomy increases the risk for imbalanced fluid volume as a result of excessive bleeding from the operative site (prostatic fossa) as well as absorption of irrigating fluid. Report manifestations indicating hypovolemic shock, excess bleeding, and/or TURP syndrome immediately.

- Monitor pulse and blood pressure. *Manifestations of hypovolemic shock include an increasing pulse and a decreasing blood pressure.*

- Monitor color of drainage in urinary drainage bag (Table 48–2). *The appearance of urine and irrigation fluid in the urinary*

 Discharge Instructions after Prostate Surgery

ACTIVITY
The healing period lasts from 4 to 8 weeks. Avoid strenuous activity and heavy lifting. Do not drive for 2 weeks, except for short rides. Do not take long walks; take stairs slowly and carefully. Continue exercises that you did in the hospital to prevent blood clots in the legs. You can take showers; avoid tub baths while the catheter is in place.

BLEEDING
Bleeding can occur any time after surgery. It is fairly common after a bowel movement, coughing, or increased exercise. If you notice blood in the urine, increase fluids and rest until the urine is clear. If heavy bleeding plugs the channel, call the care provider immediately. Avoid aspirin and NSAIDs for at least 2 weeks.

BOWEL MOVEMENTS
Keep bowel movements regular and soft to avoid pressure on the prostate area. Drink fruit juices, increase fiber in the diet, and take mild laxatives or stool softeners if needed.

DIET
Resume your normal diet. Increase fluids to 10 glasses (8 oz) daily. Avoid alcohol unless otherwise approved by your physician.

SEXUAL INTERCOURSE
Do not have sex for 6 weeks after surgery to avoid bleeding. You may still have erections even with the catheter in place. When you resume sex, ejaculate may flow back into the bladder, if so you will expel little or no semen when having an orgasm.

URINATION
After your catheter is removed, you may experience some burning, stinging, or leakage for several weeks, and you may pass small blood clots occasionally. These symptoms will disappear as the area heals. It is best to use pads to control leakage. Kegal exercises can help gain urinary control.

WORK
If work is not strenuous you may return in 4 weeks; otherwise, wait 6 to 8 weeks.

Please Call Immediately If the Following Occurs:
- You are unable to urinate.
- Bleeding is not controlled by fluids and rest, or is excessive.
- You have chills and fever or severe abdominal pain.
- Your scrotum becomes swollen and tender.
- You have pain in one calf, chest pain, or difficulty breathing.

drainage bag is an excellent indicator of bleeding after a prostatectomy.

- Monitor for manifestations of transurethral resection (TURP) syndrome: nausea and vomiting, confusion, hypertension, bradycardia, and visual disturbances. *The absorption of isotonic bladder irrigating fluids during and after surgery may cause this hypervolemic, hyponatremic state. Treatment includes diuresis and, in severe cases, hypertonic saline administration (McPhee et al., 2008).*

Community-Based Care

Depending on the man's choice of treatment, the procedure may be performed on an outpatient basis. The man having a TURP, although hospitalized for the surgery, may be discharged within 2 days after surgery if there are no complications. Discharge instructions after prostate surgery are provided in the Meeting Individualized Needs box on the previous page. Home care often involves care of an indwelling urinary catheter. Teaching how to care for the catheter and drainage bag includes the following information:

- Change from the daytime leg drainage bag to a larger night drainage bag. A larger bag suspended from the bed frame at night permits gravity drainage of urine and prevents reflux of urine back into the bladder.
- Avoid strapping the leg bag on too tightly, which can decrease venous return and increase risk for thrombophlebitis and embolic complications such as pulmonary emboli.
- Place a soft cloth between the leg bag and thigh to decrease friction and absorb dampness under the bag, reducing the risk of skin irritation.
- Empty the leg bag every 3 to 4 hours during waking hours to prevent overfilling.
- Promptly report any unexpected changes in urine color, consistency, or odor, hematuria, evidence of frank bleeding, or large blood clots, as well as a lack of or significant decrease in urine output to the urologist.

The Man with Prostate Cancer

Cancer of the prostate is the most common type of cancer among men and the second leading cause of death in North America (ACS, 2009b). It is thought to be a disease of older men, but there is histological evidence of the disease in around 30% of men in their 50s. This increases to 70% in men in their 80s (NIH, 2008). It is estimated that each year, more than 234,000 men will be diagnosed with prostate cancer; approximately 27,000 will die of it. Even though the death rates resulting from prostate cancer are decreasing, this cancer poses major health concerns for older men and implications for health care. Improved screening in the aging population is resulting in increasing numbers of men diagnosed and treated at earlier ages. With improved overall health and longevity of people on a whole, many men in this age group are remaining physically and sexually active. A diagnosis of prostate cancer not only elicits feelings of anxiety related to possible loss of life but can also reflect the possible loss of sexual function (Ramon & Denis, 2007).

FOCUS ON CULTURAL DIVERSITY
Risk and Incidence of Prostate Cancer

- Prostate cancer occurs more often in Black men than in men of other races.
- Blacks are more likely to be diagnosed later and to die of prostate cancer, with a mortality rate more than double that of other racial and ethnic groups.
- Asians and Native Americans have the lowest incidence of prostate cancer.

Source: American Cancer Society, 2009d.

Prostate cancer is usually curable if detected early. When the cancer is confined to the prostate at diagnosis, the 5-year survival rate is 100%. Even when the cancer has spread regionally, approximately 95% of patients are alive after 5 years and 91% reach 10 years (ASCO, 2007). Many men are found to have prostate cancer on autopsy; usually the cancer has produced no manifestations or complications. If, however, the cancer has metastasized outcomes are less positive and debilitation and death are a great possibility.

Risk Factors

In addition to age, race is a significant risk factor for prostate cancer, although the cause is unknown (see the accompanying Focus on Cultural Diversity box). Other risk factors being investigated are as follows:

- Genetic and hereditary factors, with risk increased in men who have a family history of the disease. A father or brother having prostate cancer doubles a man's chances of developing it in his lifetime (Newton et al., 2009)
- Having a vasectomy, believed to increase the levels of circulating free testosterone
- Dietary factors, including a diet high in animal fat and excessive supplemental vitamin A

Pathophysiology

The prostate gland consists primarily of glandular epithelial cells. The exact etiology of prostate cancer is unknown, although androgens are believed to have a role in its development. Almost all primary prostate cancers are adenocarcinomas, and they develop in the peripheral zones of the prostate gland. This location increases the risk of local spread to the prostatic capsule. Despite its proximity to the rectum, metastasis to the bowel is uncommon because a tough sheet of fascia acts as an effective physical barrier.

As the tumor enlarges, it may compress the urethra, obstructing urinary flow. The tumor may metastasize and involve the seminal vesicles or bladder by direct extension. Metastasis by lymph and venous channels is common.

Manifestations

Men with early-stage prostate cancer are often asymptomatic. Pain from metastasis to bones may be the initial manifestation noted. Urinary manifestations depend on the size and location of the tumor and the stage of the malignancy. They are often

MANIFESTATIONS of Prostate Cancer

GENITOURINARY
- Dysuria
- Frequency of urination
- Reduction in urinary stream
- Nocturia
- Hematuria
- Abnormal prostate on digital rectal examination

MUSCULOSKELETAL
- Bone or joint pain
- Migratory bone pain
- Back pain

NEUROLOGIC
- Nerve pain
- Bilateral lower extremity weakness
- Bowel or bladder dysfunction
- Muscle spasms

SYSTEMIC
- Weight loss
- Fatigue

much like manifestations of BPH: urgency, frequency, hesitancy, dysuria, and nocturia. The man may also notice hematuria or blood in the ejaculate (Porth & Matfin, 2009). Manifestations of prostate cancer are summarized in the accompanying box.

Complications

Death usually occurs secondary to debility caused by multiple sites of skeletal metastasis, especially to the vertebrae. The spinal cord may be compressed by tumors or by fractures of the spine, resulting in the possible loss of mobility and bowel and bladder function. Tumors may eventually involve bone marrow, resulting in severe anemias and impaired immune function.

Interdisciplinary Care

Care of the man with prostate cancer focuses on diagnosis, elimination or containment of the cancer, and prevention or treatment of complications. There are currently no clinical strategies to prevent the development of prostate cancer. Therefore, education

and early detection remains the major emphasis for control of this disease.

Diagnosis

Although an increasing number of patients are now diagnosed with asymptomatic prostate cancer, many patients with prostate cancer have either locally advanced cancer or distant metastasis at the time of diagnosis. The definitive diagnosis can be made only by biopsy (prostate biopsy is discussed in ∞ Chapter 47); however, other tests may suggest the presence of prostate cancer.

A digital rectal examination (DRE) will find the prostate gland nodular and fixed in prostate cancer. Prostate-specific antigen (PSA) levels are used to diagnose and stage prostate cancer, and to monitor response to treatment. Levels depend on age, and there is no specific normal or abnormal level. An increase over time is more significant than one reading. The PSA test is used with a DRE to help detect prostate cancer in men age 48 or older, and is also used to monitor effects of treatment. (However, a PSA is no longer recommended for men after the age of 75.)

Transrectal ultrasonography (TRUS) may be used when the DRE is abnormal or if the PSA is elevated. In this test, a small probe is inserted in the rectum. The probe gives off sound waves that make a picture of the prostate on a video screen. Guided by this picture, the physician inserts a narrow needle through the rectal wall into the prostate gland, and the needle removes a sample of tissue for examination. Other tests that may be ordered include a urinalysis or cystoscopy. Bone scan, MRI, or CT scans may be performed to determine the presence of tumor metastasis.

Grade and stage help to determine prognosis and guide treatment decisions. Grade (cancer cell differentiation) is determined by the pathologist. Prostate cancer is staged with a variety of tests. Table 48–3 outlines treatment options according to the stage of the cancer.

TABLE 48–3 Prostate Cancer Staging and Treatment

STAGE	DESCRIPTION	TREATMENT
I	Confined to prostate, nonpalpable, focal involvement; well differentiated	Observation and follow-up Interstitial or external-beam radiation therapy Prostatectomy
II	Confined to prostate, palpable, involves one or both lobes; poorly differentiated	Careful observation in selected patients Prostatectomy Interstitial or external-beam radiation therapy Ultrasound-guided percutaneous cryosurgery
III	Extension of the tumor outside the prostate capsule, possible seminal vesicle involvement	External-beam radiation therapy Interstitial radiation Radical prostatectomy Adjunctive hormone therapy Palliative surgery (TURP)
IV	Extension of the tumor into surrounding tissues; lymph node involvement or distant metastasis	Hormone therapy External-beam radiation therapy Palliative treatment with radiation therapy and/or TURP Radical prostatectomy with orchiectomy Chemotherapy

Research for Prevention

Research trials are underway to determine if the drug Sipuleucel-T will be effective in treating prostate cancer. This drug is mixed with the patient's immune cells and returned to the body to attack the tumor. Further studies are being performed and researchers are hopeful that this drug could improve outcomes (McBride, 2007). There is also evidence that finasteride (Proscar) may reduce the incidence of the disease but does not stop the progression of established tumors. There have not been recommendations for use as a preventative drug, as there is controversy over how to monitor for prostate cancer in men receiving this drug. Finasteride may alter PSA results, which could lead to increased prostate biopsies. The side effects of Finasteride (used to treat erectile dysfunction and loss of libido) also are concerning as a preventative medication (deVere & White, 2007; National Cancer Institute, 2008).

Treatments

The treatment of prostate cancer is complex and depends on the grade and stage of the cancer as well as the age, general health, and preference of the patient. In some cases, for example, when the patient with a slow-growing tumor is elderly or has a limited life expectancy, watchful waiting is the treatment of choice. Treatments for prostate cancer include surgery, radiation therapy, and hormone manipulation.

Medications

Androgen deprivation therapy is used to treat advanced prostate cancer. Many cells in the growing tumor are androgen dependent and either cease to grow or die if deprived of androgens. Unfortunately, other cancer cells thrive without androgen and are unaffected by therapy to reduce circulating androgens. Therefore, the effects of hormone manipulations vary from complete but temporary regression of the tumor to no response at all. Strategies to induce androgen deprivation vary from orchiectomy to oral administration of hormonal agents. In addition, new drugs are being developed that block the effects of male hormones, and research is being conducted to demonstrate what mix of hormones is best and at what time in the perioperative period they are most effective. The Food and Drug Administration recently approved Degarelix, which decreases levels of the hormone testosterone. Degarelix was noted to be more effective, as it decreases levels more quickly than older drugs of its type (Smart, 2009). Hormonal therapy may also be used in conjunction with radiation therapy.

The FDA has also approved the Provenge vaccine to treat advanced prostate cancer that has spread to other places in the body and does not respond to hormone therapy. The medication uses the body's own immune system cells to attack the cancer. Although called a vaccine, it is used to treat rather than prevent the cancer.

SURGERY   Surgery for prostate cancer includes several types of prostatectomies. For very early disease in older men, cure may be achieved with a simple prostatectomy (such as TURP), discussed in the section on benign prostate hyperplasia. Following the surgery men usually experience erectile dysfunction for at least the first 3 months and return of sexual activity may take up

TABLE 48–4 Potential Complications Related to Radical Prostatectomy and Radiation Therapy

RADICAL PROSTATECTOMY	RADIATION THERAPY
Erectile dysfunction	Erectile dysfunction*
Urethral stricture	Urethral stricture
Fistula/rectal injury	Rectal/anal stricture*
Urinary incontinence	Cystitis
Surgical/anesthetic risk	Diarrhea
	Proctitis
	Rectal ulcer
	Bowel obstruction*
	Urinary incontinence

*Delayed complications; may appear months or years after completion of therapy.

to 2 years. Incontinence can also be a problem following prostatectomy surgery. Refer to Table 48–4.

- *Radical prostatectomy* involves removal of the prostate, prostate capsule, seminal vesicles, and a portion of the bladder neck. In a laparoscopic radical prostatectomy (LRP), small incisions are made in the abdomen and a laparoscope is inserted and used to remove the prostate. Some surgeons do this from an area other than the operating room by using a robotic interface. See the Moving Evidence into Action box for information about the experiences of men following laparoscopic surgery.

The most common radical prostatectomy techniques are the following:

- *Retropubic prostatectomy* is currently the favored method and is being combined with nerve-sparing techniques to improve erectile dysfunction problems. This form of surgery allows adequate control of bleeding, visualization of the prostate bed and bladder neck, and access to pelvic lymph nodes (Ramon & Denis, 2007).
- *Perineal prostatectomy* is often preferred for older men or those who are poor surgical risks. This approach requires less time, involves less bleeding and pain, and results in shorter hospital stays. A disadvantage to this approach is that lymph nodes cannot be accessed and require additional incisions to obtain.
- *Suprapubic prostatectomy* is rarely used, usually when problems with the bladder are expected. Control of bleeding is more difficult because the surgical approach is through the bladder.

For patients with stage III, locally advanced (beyond the prostatic capsule) cancer, surgery is controversial because of the likelihood of hidden lymph node metastasis and relapse. TURP is not performed as curative therapy but may be used to relieve urinary obstruction for men with advanced disease (stage III or IV).

Surgical intervention is now available for men with urinary sphincter insufficiency, which is the major cause of incontinence after prostatectomy. An artificial urinary sphincter is

MOVING EVIDENCE INTO ACTION — Improving Pre- and Postoperative Teaching

Laparoscopic radical surgery for prostate cancer is less invasive than open retropubic prostatectomy but is increasingly performed. The surgery itself has been associated with decreased blood loss during surgery, less pain following surgery, and fewer days in the hospital. However, men who have a laparoscopic radical prostatectomy may not be prepared for the level of postoperative pain they experience based on their expectations of a less invasive surgery. In addition, although the benefits and functional outcomes of laparoscopic surgery to remove prostate cancer appear equal to those of open surgery, there is a need for improved pre- and postoperative teaching for this group of men. This study by Milne, Spiers, and Moore (2007) was conducted to explore what men experience following laparoscopic radical prostatectomy and how adequately their pre- and postoperative needs are being met.

IMPLICATIONS FOR NURSING

Although the men who were subjects in the study had actively sought information about the surgery, they were not prepared for the intensity of pain (from early ambulation, gas pains, bowel movements, and/ bladder spasms) or the incontinence they experienced after surgery. Erectile dysfunction was a major concern, but most did not know where to go to seek help. Nurses should discuss the surgery and identify the expectations of the man prior to surgery. Meeting another man who has had this type of surgery is especially helpful. Following the procedure, discussions about urinary incontinence and sexual dysfunction should be initiated and written information about available community resources should be provided.

CRITICAL THINKING IN PATIENT CARE

1. You are caring for a 75-year-old man who has had a laparoscopic radical prostatectomy for prostate cancer. His wife tells you they have always had an active sex life and she hopes this surgery will not change that. What would you say to her?

2. Would the nursing diagnosis *Risk for Infection* be appropriate for a man following a radical laparoscopic prostatectomy? If so, what type of interventions would you suggest during discharge teaching to reduce this risk?

3. If you were developing a list of community resources for men following prostate surgery for cancer, what would you include? How would your list vary for the following situations?
   - A 64-year-old man with a wife and four married children who all live close
   - A 77-year-old man who lives alone and has no family
   - A 90-year-old man who will go to an assisted living facility after discharge from the hospital

surgically implanted (Figure 48–5 ■). To be eligible, the man must be able to manipulate the pump placed in the scrotum and have adequate cognitive function to know when a problem with the appliance occurs.

RADIATION THERAPY Radiation therapy may be used as a primary treatment for prostate cancer. Long-term problems of impotence and urinary incontinence occur less frequently, and survival rates often are comparable. Radiation may be delivered either by external beam or interstitial implants of radioactive seeds of iodine, gold, palladium, or iridium (brachytherapy). Interstitial radiation has a lower risk of impotence and rectal damage than external-beam radiation. ∞ See Chapter 14 for nursing care of the patient receiving radiation therapy.

Radiation therapy has a palliative role for patients with metastatic prostate cancer, reducing the size of bone metastasis, controlling pain, and restoring function, such as continence or the ability to ambulate for patients with spinal cord compression.

Table 48–5 compares surgical and hormone therapies and the advantages and disadvantages of each.

TABLE 48–5 Surgical and Hormone* Therapy in the Management of Advanced Prostate Cancer

TREATMENT	ADVANTAGES	DISADVANTAGES
Orchiectomy	Inexpensive Immediate effect; i.e., men report diminished pain from metastasis in the recovery room	Body image problems due to loss of testicles
Estrogen compounds (diethylstilbestrol)	Inexpensive Effects reversible	Increased risk of cardiovascular problems More likely to cause gynecomastia, hypertrophy of breast tissue
Luteinizing hormone-releasing hormone agonist (LHRH) (leuprolide)	Effects reversible No cardiovascular risk Monthly administration	Very expensive Subcutaneous injection route Slow onset: up to 4 weeks
Steroidal antiandrogens (megestrol [Megace])	Effects reversible No cardiovascular risk Inexpensive	May not drop testosterone levels sufficiently Weight gain
Nonsteroidal antiandrogens (flutamide; often used in conjunction with LHRH)	Does not alter circulating androgens Blocks some side effects of LHRH May be effective if other methods fail	Very expensive

*All hormonal manipulations have the potential disadvantage of loss of libido, erectile dysfunction, hot flashes, and gynecomastia.

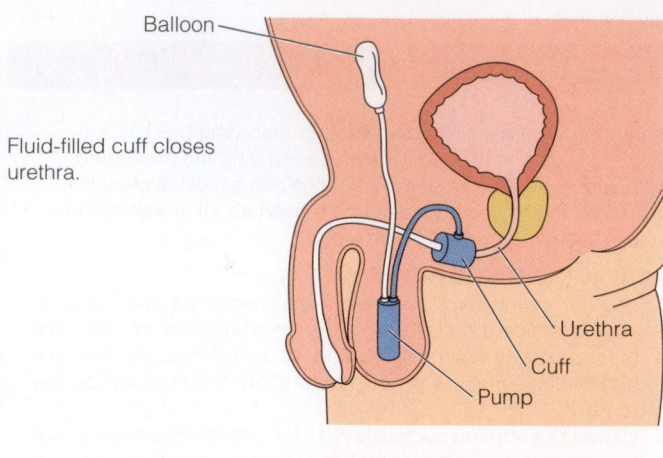

Balloon

Fluid-filled cuff closes urethra.

Urethra
Cuff
Pump

To void, bladder pump is squeezed, drawing fluid from cuff to balloon. Urine drains through open urethra.

After voiding, fluid drains back to cuff, closing urethra.

Figure 48–5 ■ Method of operation of an artificial urinary sphincter.

∞ Nursing Care

Nurses plan and provide interventions to help prevent prostate cancer and to facilitate a return to functional health status. Interventions may range from teaching to using knowledge and skill in physical care following a radical prostatectomy. A Case Study & Nursing Care Plan for a man having a radical prostatectomy is found on page 1672.

Health Promotion

Nurses are in a unique position to increase public awareness about early detection of prostate cancer. Every encounter with men and their families—in clinics, hospital units, or in the home—is an opportunity to provide information about early detection and

identify needs. Several studies have shown a positive correlation between increased awareness of and participation in prostate cancer screening procedures. The American Cancer Society has free pamphlets about early detection of prostate cancer, which are useful in educating the public.

One risk factor that can be easily changed is diet. Men should know that they can lower their risk of prostate cancer by eating less red meat and fat. They should include fruits and vegetables as recommended in the new food pyramid; tomatoes, pink grapefruit, and watermelon are high in lycopenes that help prevent damage to DNA and may help lower prostate cancer risk. Men should be informed of the genetic predisposition in the development of prostate cancer.

All men should be given information about the limitations and benefits of testing for early detection and of treatment so they can make an informed decision. Men at high risk (men of African descent and those with a first-degree relative diagnosed at a younger age) should begin testing at age 45. The National Cancer Institute (2007) recommends that the PSA test and DRE should be offered each year, beginning at age 48, to all men with a life expectancy of at least 10 years. The U.S. Preventative Task Force, however, now recommends that men 75 or over not be screened for prostate cancer as the benefit of treating the cancer if detected, outweighs the benefits. This recommendation has caused some controversy. Opponents are concerned with having an age attached to the recommendation as there are men at age 75 who may have a longer life expectancy than 10 years and some men younger than 75 may have lower life expectancies (Chustecka, Lie, Scudder, & Martin, 2008).

Assessment

Collect the following data through the health history and physical examination (∞ see Chapter 47). Note that a digital rectal examination is an advanced nursing assessment.

- *Health history:* Risk factors, urinary elimination patterns and manifestations, hematuria, pain.
- *Physical assessment:* DRE to assess prostate size, symmetry, firmness, and nodules.

Nursing Diagnoses and Interventions

The nursing care of men with prostate cancer must be holistic, sensitive, and individualized. The nursing diagnoses discussed for the man with BPH may also be appropriate. This section focuses on problems with urinary incontinence, sexual function, and pain.

Urinary Incontinence (Reflex, Stress, Total)

Urinary incontinence is a disturbing complication following treatment for prostate cancer. Both radical prostatectomy and external-beam radiation therapy can cause incontinence, ranging from a drop or two when the patient lifts a heavy object (stress incontinence) to no control at all. Older men may experience urge incontinence, the involuntary passage of urine soon after a strong sense of urgency to void. Total and unpredictable loss of urine is classified as total incontinence. The man's reaction to incontinence may be severe even if the incontinence is not great. Many men have significant anxiety at the prospect of an incontinent episode in public, because they feel shame and often guilt about the loss of control.

- Assess the degree of incontinence and its effects on lifestyle. *The nurse needs to determine previous urinary patterns and the type of incontinence currently being experienced to plan appropriate interventions.*
- Teach Kegel exercises to help restore continence. *Pelvic muscle or Kegel exercises can often either eliminate or improve stress incontinence.*
- Teach methods to control dampness and odor from stress incontinence as follows:
  - Do not attempt to prevent accidental voiding by restricting fluids. *Not only will the man continue to have incontinent episodes, but also his urine will become concentrated, exacerbating the problem with odor.*
  - Manage occasional episodes (one to three small-volume accidents per day) with absorbent pads worn inside the underwear and changed as needed. Most pads are made with a polymer gel that controls odor. *Appropriate measures help promote good hygiene, decrease anxiety, and increase comfort.*
- Refer to physical therapy or a continence specialist for additional measures to promote continence. *Special exercises, restricting some types of fluid, and other measures such as bladder training can help the patient deal with incontinence.*
- Explore options such as an external collection device (external catheter or Texas catheter) for the man with total incontinence. *This device may improve the man's self-esteem and allow resumption of social activities.*
- Encourage verbalizing feelings about the impact of incontinence on quality of life. *The degree of incontinence does not necessarily correlate with the perceived level of suffering. Listening to these concerns with sensitivity can help the man work through these feelings and may allow him to move toward a healthy adaptation to his disability.*

Sexual Dysfunction

Surgical treatment for prostate cancer may cause ED and changes in ejaculatory function. Hormone therapy for advanced prostate cancer lowers libido and may also cause ED. The diagnosis of cancer and body image changes caused by hormone therapy may lower self-esteem, which in turn can diminish sexual desire and willingness to interact sexually with a partner. Many older men are active sexually and fully capable of sustaining an erection. They are likely to fear the effect of treatment on their sexual health. They may allow this concern to guide their decision about the treatment course, or they may refuse all therapy because of this fear. Reactions vary greatly, and the nurse must maintain a nonjudgmental approach to education and support. It is also important to assess the spouse/partner's sexuality concerns as this will ultimately affect the man's decisions and well-being.

- Assess the man's pretreatment sexual function. *Knowledge of previous sexual function is necessary to plan appropriate interventions.*
- Teach the man about the actual or potential effects of therapy on sexual function. *The incidence of ED varies with different therapies for prostate cancer.*
- Provide an opportunity for the man and his partner to discuss implications of and concerns about the diagnosis and treatment of sexual function. *The treatments for prostate cancer often affect the physiology of erection. The man and his partner need support and counseling during the period of adjustment.*
- Discuss medical and surgical treatments for ED (see the first section of this chapter). *Many men are as devastated by the loss of erectile function as they are by the diagnosis of cancer. Information about achieving erection and maintaining sexual intimacy is essential to quality of life.*
- Refer for sexual counseling as appropriate. *The man and his partner may require therapy beyond that provided by nurses.*

> **PRACTICE ALERT**
> A therapeutic approach to assessing how the man feels is to use an opening statement such as "Some men are very concerned about the effects of (type of treatment) on their ability to have an erection. Tell me how you feel about it."

Acute Pain/Chronic Pain

There are many causes of pain in men with advanced prostate cancer. It is not unusual for a patient to have three or four distinct pains simultaneously, all from different sources. The most common cause of pain is metastasis to the spinal column, usually the thoracic spine. Other sources of pain include fractures, lymphedema of the lower extremities, and muscle spasms. Because most men with prostate cancer are over the age of 65, many also have pain associated with preexisting conditions, such as osteoarthritis, unrelated to the cancer.

- Assess the intensity, location, and quality of the pain. *A cardinal rule of successful pain management is the importance of reducing or eliminating the cause of pain. Appropriate interventions are based on a careful assessment of the patient's pain.*
- Provide optimal pain relief with prescribed analgesics. *It is important that the man and his family understand that pain medications should be used on a regular basis to maintain comfort and should not be delayed until pain is severe.*
- Teach the man and his family noninvasive methods of pain control. *Various modalities can be successful in alleviating pain or reducing its perception, thus enhancing the comfort of the patient (∞ see Chapter 9).*

> **EVIDENCE FOR NURSING CARE** **The Patient with Prostate Cancer**
>
> *Selected resources that nurses may find helpful when planning evidence-based nursing care follow.*
> - Harrington, J. M., & Badger, T. A. (2009). Body image and quality of life in men with prostate cancer. *Cancer Nursing, 32*(2), E1–E7.
> - King, C. R. (2006). Patient-driven, evidence-based treatment for breast, lung, and prostate cancer. *Oncology Nursing Society, 21*(8), S33–S34.
> - Rustøen, T., Gaardsrud, T., Leegaard, M., & Wahl, A. K. (2009). Nursing pain management—A qualitative interview study of patients with pain, hospitalized for cancer treatment. *Pain Management Nursing, 10*(1), 48–55.

CASE STUDY & NURSING CARE PLAN   A Man with Prostate Cancer

William Turner, a 71-year-old African American, lives with his wife in a small retirement community in Florida. His wife had a stroke 2 years ago, and Mr. Turner does all the cooking and housework. He has been in good health for most of his life, having only "a small touch" of osteoarthritis in his knees and hands. He has noticed a gradual onset of urinary urgency and frequency over the past 2 years, but has never had incontinence. During a routine checkup, the nurse practitioner at the local health clinic performs a digital rectal examination and palpates a hard nodule on the surface of Mr. Turner's prostate. After his PSA is found to be elevated, he is referred to a urologist, who diagnoses prostate cancer. Mr. Turner chooses to have surgery, and a radical retropubic prostatectomy and lymph node dissection are performed. The lymph nodes are negative for metastasis. Following surgery, his recovery is uncomplicated. However, the nurse caring for Mr. Turner is concerned about his ability to care for his indwelling catheter because of his arthritis and his wife's physical disabilities from the stroke. The nurse makes a referral to a home health agency to ensure Mr. Turner can manage his care at home. An initial home health assessment is scheduled for the day after Mr. Turner is discharged from the hospital.

ASSESSMENT

The home health nurse notes that the house is clean and neat. Mr. Turner is dressed, but still wearing his night urinary drainage bag, even though it is 1300. Mr. Turner tells the nurse that his main problem is going to get groceries, because he is embarrassed to be seen with the drainage bag. He says he has not been able to remove the drainage bag and attach the leg bag because of his arthritis. Physical assessment findings include the pelvic incision to be healing without signs of infection. There is no tenderness in his calves, chest pain, or shortness of breath. The urine is yellow, without odor. Mr. Turner does state that he sees no need for the pelvic exercises since he is no longer in the hospital. He also expresses the belief that he is cured of cancer and questions the need for follow-up care.

DIAGNOSES

- *Risk for Stress Urinary Incontinence* related to surgical procedure
- *Ineffective Health Maintenance* related to inability to care for the urinary drainage system, not understanding

need for postoperative exercises, and questions about follow-up care

EXPECTED OUTCOMES

- Regain urinary continence after catheter removal.
- Change the urinary drainage bag with the appropriate assistance.
- Verbalize the rationale for performing postoperative exercise.
- Verbalize the need for continued follow-up care.

PLANNING AND IMPLEMENTATION

- Discuss the possibility of stress incontinence after the catheter is removed.
- Reinforce the need for Kegel exercises while the catheter is still in place.
- Explore Mr. Turner's support system to identify people who could assist him with catheter care, and arrange a teaching session with them.
- Teach Mr. Turner the importance of follow-up care, relating the care to the history of the disease.

EVALUATION

Good friends from Mr. Turner's church have assisted him with care of his drainage bag, and have reminded him to do his Kegel exercises several times a day while the catheter is in place. When the catheter is removed, Mr. Turner has only a small amount of leaking of urine after voiding. He understands that it may take several weeks for this to resolve. Efforts to help him understand the need for continued medical care are less successful. Mr. Turner continues to state that he is cured, his wife needs him, and he sees no need to go back to the doctor.

CRITICAL THINKING IN THE NURSING PROCESS

1. Outline a teaching plan for Mr. Turner for the risk for altered skin integrity related to urinary incontinence.
2. As a result of Mr. Turner's refusal to have ongoing medical care, he might be labeled as noncompliant. Would you make this nursing diagnosis? Why or why not?
3. If you were the home health nurse making a home visit and found that Mr. Turner had no urinary drainage for 16 hours, what assessments would you make? How would you handle this problem?

See Evaluating Your Response in Appendix C.

Using NANDA, NIC, and NOC

Linkages between a selected NANDA nursing diagnosis, NIC, and NOC for the patient with surgical treatment for prostate cancer are shown in the accompanying chart.

Community-Based Care

Depending on the type of treatment, the following topics should be addressed in preparing the patient and his family for home care:

- For the man having a surgical procedure: manifestations of infection and excessive bleeding, catheter care, wound care, pain management
- For the man receiving radiation therapy:
  - Danger of radiation damage to others (sleep in a room alone for a week; avoid close contact with pregnant women, infants, and children)
  - Condom use during sexual contact (ejaculate may be discolored, distressing sexual partner)

NANDA, NIC, AND NOC LINKAGES
The Man Having Surgery for Prostate Cancer

NANDA   Impaired Urinary Elimination

NIC
Urinary Elimination Management
Bladder Irrigation
Fluid Management
Tube Care: Urinary
Infection Control

NOC   Urinary Elimination
Risk Control

Adapted from Bulechek, G., Butcher, H., & Dochterman, J. M. (Eds). (2008). *Nursing interventions classification (NIC)* (5th ed.). St. Louis: Mosby Elsevier, 170, 368, 428–431, 772, 790; and Moorhead, S., Johnson, M., Maas, M., & Swanson, E. (Eds). (2008). *Nursing outcomes classification (NOC)* (4th ed.). St. Louis: Mosby Elsevier, 586–587, 600–601, 715–716; and NANDA International. (2009). *Nursing diagnoses: Definitions and classification 2009–2011.* Oxford, UK: Wiley-Blackwell.

- The importance of keeping appointments with healthcare providers and having yearly PSA and rectal examinations
- If appropriate, community services, such as support groups, home health nurses, and hospice

- Helpful resources:
  - American Cancer Society
  - American Urological Association
  - National Cancer Institute

Male Breast Disorders

The Man with Gynecomastia

Gynecomastia, the abnormal enlargement of the male breast, is thought to result from a high ratio of estradiol to testosterone. It is common during puberty, affecting one breast in as many as 48% of adolescent males, but usually resolves within 1 to 2 years (Fitzgerald, 2007). Any condition that increases estrogen activity or decreases testosterone production can contribute to gynecomastia. Conditions that increase estrogen activity include obesity, testicular tumors, liver disease, and adrenal carcinoma; conditions that decrease testosterone production include chronic illness such as tuberculosis or Hodgkin's disease, injury, and orchitis. Drugs such as digitalis, opiates, and chemotherapeutic agents are also associated with gynecomastia. Gynecomastia after adolescence is usually bilateral. If it is unilateral, biopsy may be necessary to rule out breast cancer.

No treatment is necessary for the transient gynecomastia of puberty. If the condition becomes chronic, however, creating psychologic discomfort, surgery may be necessary to remove the subcutaneous breast tissue. When related to an underlying disorder, treatment of that disorder is required. In severe cases, tamoxifen is given to decrease estrogen activity.

Nursing care for the patient with gynecomastia includes education about the cause and treatment of the condition, and emotional support for the psychosocial implications of this feminizing condition.

The Man with Breast Cancer

Although male breast cancer is rare, accounting for about 1% of all breast cancer cases, it is as serious to the men who have it as it is to the women. About 1900 men in the United States are estimated to be diagnosed with breast cancer each year, accounting for more than 400 deaths (ACS, 2009b). The etiology of male breast cancer is unclear; hormonal, genetic, and perhaps environmental factors appear to be important.

Male breast cancer is clinically and histologically similar to female breast cancer, although lobular cancer is rare in males. Most tumors are estrogen-receptor positive. Because many men believe that breast cancer is only a woman's disease, they often delay seeking medical attention for manifestations and thus may present with advanced disease.

Treatment of male breast cancer is much like the treatment of female breast cancer, beginning with lumpectomy or mastectomy, node dissection, and staging to determine the therapeutic options. Radiation, chemotherapy, and hormonal therapy (usually tamoxifen) are the conventional adjuncts to surgery. Castration (surgical removal of the testes) was previously used but current treatments consist of anti-androgen therapy resulting in tumor regression and prolonging life (Mayo Clinic, 2008).

Nursing care for the man with breast cancer is essentially the same as for the woman with breast cancer (∞ see Chapter 49). The nurse has an opportunity to help the man and his family cope with the psychosocial effects of having breast cancer. He may feel embarrassment or shame about his condition as well as fear about the life-threatening nature of the disease. His family may share those feelings. By listening with understanding and empathy, the nurse can help the patient and family resolve their feelings and move toward healing.

CHAPTER HIGHLIGHTS

- Disorders of male sexual function include erectile dysfunction (ED) and ejaculatory dysfunction. Many different illnesses, medications, and surgical procedures may affect male sexual function. Treatments include medications, mechanical devices, and surgical procedures. It is important for nurses to initiate a discussion of sexual concerns during assessments and to recognize that many male reproductive treatments and surgeries may result in sexual dysfunction.
- Phimosis and priapism are disorders of the penis that can cause problems with urination and sexual activity and may in some cases be considered medical emergencies. The risk of cancer of the penis, although rare, is increased by phimosis, poor genital hygiene, and viral HPV and HIV infections.

- Benign scrotal masses include hydrocele, spermatocele, and varicocele. Epididymitis may be associated with a urinary tract infection, prostatitis, urethral strictures, or a sexually transmitted infection.
- The testes may be infected (orchitis), twisted (testicular torsion), or develop cancer. Testicular cancer is the most common cancer in men between the ages of 15 and 40. Monthly testicular self-examination is critical to early detection and treatment of cancer.
- The prostate gland may be inflamed or infected (prostatitis), enlarged (benign prostatic hyperplasia [BPH]), or may develop cancer. BPH is a common disorder of the aging male that causes problems with urination as the enlarging prostate gland constricts

the urethra. Treatments include medications and various types of surgery, depending on the size of the prostate and the age and health status of the man.
- Cancer of the prostate is the most common type of cancer and the second leading cause of death in American men. When diagnosed

early, prostate cancer is curable. Diagnosis is often based on an increasing level of PSA and an abnormal DRE. The cancer is treated with surgery, radiation, or hormonal manipulation.
- The male breast may become enlarged (gynecomastia) or develop cancer.

TEST YOURSELF NCLEX-RN® REVIEW

1. A nurse is conducting a health history. Which of the following statements would most likely elicit information about sexual concerns?
   1. "Following your prostate surgery, when did you first notice you had problems with sexual intercourse?"
   2. "Why do you think you should be sexually active at your age?"
   3. "Do you miss having sex?"
   4. "Tell me about your experience with sexual function since you developed prostate enlargement."

2. A nurse is conducting a health teaching session for young men. What topic would be appropriate to reduce the risk of cancer of the penis?
   1. wearing a condom during sexual intercourse
   2. retracting the foreskin of the penis when showering
   3. avoiding tight pants and very hot showers
   4. maintaining a regular testicular self-examination schedule

3. What disease of the male reproductive system is a risk if a man also has a sexually transmitted infection (such as gonorrhea)?
   1. epididymitis
   2. hydrocele
   3. erectile dysfunction
   4. gynecomastia

4. Which of the following statements is true of testicular cancer?
   1. The incidence increases with age.
   2. It occurs most between ages 15 and 40.
   3. It rarely occurs in brothers.
   4. Severe pain is the initial manifestation.

5. A nurse is teaching a man with chronic prostatitis how to care for himself at home. What simple measures can be used to decrease discomfort?
   1. Take cold showers and restrict oral fluids.
   2. Wear a scrotal support and take anti-inflammatory drugs.
   3. Increase oral fluid intake to 3 L/day and void often.
   4. Increase fiber intake and avoid sexual activity.

6. What diagnostic tests are used to differentiate BPH from prostate cancer? **Select all that apply.**
   1. pelvic ultrasound
   2. digital rectal examination
   3. blood chemistry
   4. PSA level
   5. sperm count

7. The enlarging prostate in BPH typically is manifested by assessment of problems with which of the following?
   1. bowel elimination
   2. urinary elimination
   3. peripheral vascular function
   4. skin integrity

8. A nurse is caring for a man who has returned to the unit from the recovery room following a TURP. His urinary drainage bag is filled with dark red fluid with obvious clots. He is having painful bladder spasms. What would the nurse do first?
   1. Assess his intake and output since surgery.
   2. Administer pain medication in the form of a B&O suppository.
   3. Report your assessments to his urologist.
   4. Nothing, because these manifestations are expected following a TURP.

9. What cancer is the most common malignancy in American men?
   1. prostate cancer
   2. testicular cancer
   3. lung cancer
   4. colon cancer

10. What nutritional information should a nurse include in a community program to reduce the risk of prostate cancer?
   1. Increase fiber intake.
   2. Decrease lycopene intake.
   3. Avoid foods high in sodium.
   4. Decrease red meat and fat intake.

See Test Yourself answers in Appendix C.

Pearson Nursing Student Resources
Find additional review materials at
www.nursing.pearsonhighered.com
Prepare for success with additional NCLEX®-style practice questions, interactive assignments and activities, Web links, animations and videos, and more!

BIBLIOGRAPHY

Adis Data Information. (2008). *Determine the cause of premature ejaculation before initiating psychological and/or off label pharmacological treatment. Drugs & Therapy Perspectives, 24*(1), 9–12.

American Cancer Society (ACS). (2009a). *Overview: Testicular cancer. What causes testicular cancer.* Retrieved from http://www.cancer.org/docroot/CRI/content/CRI_2_2_2X_

American Cancer Society (ACS). (2009b). *Cancer facts & figures 2009.* Atlanta: Author. Retrieved from http://www.cancer.org/downloads/STT/500809web.pdf

American Cancer Society (ACS). (2009d). What are the risk factors for prostate cancer? Retrieved from http://www.cancer.org/docroot/CRI/content/CRI_2_4_2X_What_are_the_risk_factors_for...

American Urologic Association (2006). *Management of BPH.* Retrieved from http://www.auanet.org/guidelines/bph.cfm

American Society of Clinical Oncology (ASCO). (2007). *Prostate cancer.* Retrieved from http://www.cancer.net/prostate

Barclay, L. (2009). ACP issues guidelines for treatment of erectile dysfunction. *Medscape Medical News.* Retrieved from http://www.medscape.com/viewarticle/710946?src=nlcrb&usv=87128CN

Blanco-Yarosh, M. (2007). Penile cancer: An overview. *Urologic Nursing, 27*(4), 286–290.

Bulechek, G., Butcher, H., & Dochterman, J. M. (2008). *Nursing interventions classification* (5th ed.). St. Louis: Mosby Elsevier.

Centers for Disease Control and Prevention. (2007). *Prostate cancer.* Retrieved from http://www.cdc.gov/cancer/prostate/index.htm

Chustecka, Z., Lie, D., Scudder, L., & Martin, B. (2008). *USPSTF recommends against prostate cancer screening in men 75 years or older.* Retrieved from http://www.medscape.com/viewarticle/578591_print

Cleveland Clinic (2008a). *Erectile dysfunction overview.* Retrieved from http://my.clevelandclinic.org/disorders/Erectile_Disorder_impotence/hic_Erectile_Dysfunction_Overview.aspx

Cleveland Clinic. (2008b). *Medications that may cause erectile dysfunction.* Retrieved from http://my.clevelandclinic.org/disorders/Erectile_Disorder_impotence/hic_Medications_That_May_Cause_Erectile_Dysfunction.aspx

Darst, E. (2007). Sexuality and prostatectomy: Nursing assessment and intervention. *Urologic Nursing, 27*(6), 534–541.

Davidson, J., & Chutka, D. (2008). Benign prostatic hyperplasia: Treat or wait? Questionnaire with "bother score" can help you decide. *Journal of Family Practice, 57*(7), 454–463.

de Vere White, R. (2007). Finasteride for chemoprevention of prostate cancer: Why has it not been embraced? *Journal of Clinical Oncology, 25*(21), 2999–3000.

DiMeo, P. (2006). Psychosocial and relationship issues in men with erectile dysfunction. *Urologic Nursing, 26*(6), 442–446.

Dorey, G. (2007). A clinical overview of the treatment of post-prostatectomy incontinence. *British Journal of Nursing, 16*(19), 1194–1199.

Edwards, J. (2008). Diagnosis and management of benign prostatic hyperplasia. *American Family Physician, 77*(10), 1403–1410.

Feldman, D., Bosl, G., Sheinfeld, J., & Motzer, R. (2008). Medical treatment of advanced testicular cancer. *The Journal of the American Medical Association 299*(6), 672–684.

Fischbach, F., & Dunning, M. (2009). *A manual of laboratory and diagnostic tests* (8th ed.). Philadelphia: Wolters Kluwer.

Lee, S., Liong, M., Yuen, K., Liong, Y., & Krieger, J. (2007). Chronic prostatitis/chronic pelvic pain syndrome: Role of alpha blocker therapy. *Urologia Internationalis, 78,* 97–105.

Liechty, A., & Quallich, S. (2008). Teaching a patient to successfully operate a penile prosthesis. *Urologic Nursing, 28*(2), 106–108.

Ludwig, C. (2007). Understanding benign prostatic hyperplasia. *MEDSURG Nursing, 16*(5), 340–341.

Matthews, P. (2007). Hormone ablation therapy: Lightening the load for today's prostate cancer patient. *Urologic Nursing, (27)* Supplement, 3–10.

Mayo Clinic. (2007). *Prostatitis.* Retrieved from http://www.mayoclinic.com/health/prostatitis/DS00341

Mayo Clinic. (2008). *Male breast cancer.* Retrieved from http://www.mayoclinic.com/health/male-breast-cancer/DS00661/DSECTION=treatments-and-drugs

Mercado, M., Kimmer, S., Holman, J., & Wanserski, G. (2008). What's the best drug treatment for premature ejaculation? *The Journal of Family Practice, 57*(3), 192–194.

McBride, D. (2007). Immune-boosting prostate cancer vaccine endorsed by FDA advisors. *Oncology Nursing Society (ONS) Connect.* Retrieved from http://www.ons.org/publications/journals/connect/pdf/2207.pdf

McCorkle, R., Siefert, M., Dowd, M., Robinson, J., & Pickett, M. (2007). Effects of advanced practice nursing on patient and spouse depressive symptoms, sexual function, and marital interaction after radical prostatectomy. *Urologic Nursing, 27*(1), 65–77.

McPhee, S., & Papadakis, M., & Tierney, L. (Eds.). (2008). *Current medical diagnosis & treatment* (47th ed.). New York: Lange Medical Books/McGraw Hill.

Mercado, M., Kimmer, S., & Holman, J. (2008). What's the best drug treatment for premature ejaculation? *The Journal of Family Practice, 57*(3), 192–194.

Milne, J., Spiers, J., & Moore, K. (2007). Men's experiences following laparoscopic radical prostatectomy: A qualitative descriptive study. *International Journal of Nursing Studies, 45*(5), 765–774.

Moorhead, S., Johnson, M., Maas, M., & Swanson, E. (2008). *Nursing outcomes classification (NOC)* (4th ed.). St. Louis: Mosby Elsevier.

NANDA International. (2009). *Nursing diagnoses: Definitions & classification 2009–2011.* Oxford, UK: Wiley-Blackwell.

National Cancer Institute. (2008). *Prostate cancer prevention (PDQ).* Retrieved from http://www.cancer.gov/cancertopics/pdq/prevention/prostate/HealthProfessional/page1

National Kidney and Urologic Diseases Information Clearinghouse (NKUDIC). (2009). *Erectile dysfunction.* Retrieved from http://kidney.niddk.nih.gov/kudiseases/pubs/ED/index.htm

National Kidney and Urologic Diseases Information Clearinghouse (NKUDIC). (2008). *Prostatitis: Disorders of the prostate.* Retrieved from http://kidney.niddk.nih.gov/kudiseases/pubs/prostatitis/index.htm

Newton, S., Hickey, M. & Marrs, J. (2009). *Mosby's oncology nursing advisor: A comprehensive guide to clinical practice.* St. Louis: Mosby Elsevier.

Pasquali, R., Patton, L., & Gambineri, A. (2008). Obesity and infertility. *Current Opinion in Internal Medicine, 7*(1), 23–28.

Porth, C. M. (2007). *Essentials of pathophysiology: Concepts of altered health states* (2nd ed.). Philadelphia: Lippincott Williams & Wilkins.

Porth, C. M., & Matfin, G. (2009). *Pathophysiology: Concepts of altered health states* (8th ed.). Philadelphia: Lippincott Williams & Wilkins.

Ramon, J., & Denis, L., (Eds.). (2007). *Prostate cancer.* Heidelberg: Springer.

Shaw, J. (2008) Diagnosis and treatment of testicular cancer. *American Family Physician, 77*(4), 469–474.

Smart, M. (2009). Oncology update. *Oncology Nursing Forum, 36*(3), 362–363.

Strief, D. (2007). An overview of prostate cancer: Diagnosis and treatment. *Urologic Nursing, 27*(6), 475–479.

Summers, A. (2008). Practice makes perfect: Testicular torsion. *Emergency Nurse, 16*(1) 22–23.

Tubaro, A., De Nunzio, C., & Miano, R. (2007). Transurethral needle ablation of the prostate. *Current Opinion in Urology, 17*(7), 7–11.

Turner, J., Ciol, M., Von Korff, M., Yung-wen, L., & Berger, R. (2006). Men with pelvic pain: Perceived helpfulness of medical and self-management strategies. *Clinical Journal of Pain, 22*(1), 19–24.

Wallace, M. (2008). How to try this: Assessment of sexual health in older adults. *American Journal of Nursing, 108*(7), 52–60.

Wilson, B., Shannon, M., & Stang, C. (2010). *Pearson's nurse's drug guide 2010.* Upper Saddle River, NJ: Pearson Prentice Hall.

Nursing Care of **Women** with **Reproductive System** and **Breast Disorders**

LEARNING OUTCOMES

1. Explain the pathophysiology, manifestations, complications, interdisciplinary care, and nursing care of disorders of female sexual function, menstrual disorders, structural disorders, reproductive tissue disorders, and breast disorders.

2. Describe the physiologic process of the perimenopause.

3. Compare and contrast the incidence, risk factors, pathophysiology, manifestations, diagnosis, treatment, and nursing care for cancer of the cervix, endometrium, ovary, vulva, and breast.

4. Explain the purposes, nursing implications, and health education for women and their families for cancer screening, medications, and treatments for disorders of the reproductive system and breast.

5. Discuss alternative and complementary therapies used by women to relieve manifestations associated with menopause and menstrual disorders.

6. Describe the surgical procedures used to treat female reproductive system and breast disorders.

CLINICAL COMPETENCIES

1. Assess functional status of women with reproductive system and breast disorders, and monitor, document, and report abnormal manifestations.

2. Use evidence-based research to design interventions to promote early diagnosis and treatment of African American women with breast cancer.

3. Use assessed data, patient values, clinical expertise and evidence to determine priority nursing diagnoses and select and implement individualized nursing interventions.

4. Administer medications used to treat female reproductive system and breast disorders knowledgeably and safely.

5. Provide individualized care for the woman having a D&C, laparoscopy, hysterectomy, mastectomy, and breast reconstruction.

6. Effectively communicate with and function within the interdisciplinary team to plan and provide care.

7. Provide teaching appropriate for community-based self-care of female reproductive and breast disorders.

8. Adapt individual and cultural values and variations as well as expressed needs and preferences into the plan of care as needed.

9. Revise plan of care as needed to provide effective interventions to promote, maintain, or restore functional health status to women with reproductive system and breast disorders.

KEY TERMS

amenorrhea, *1684*
anorgasmia, *1677*
dysfunctional uterine bleeding (DUB), *1684*
dysmenorrhea, *1683*

dyspareunia, *1677*
endometriosis, *1692*
fibrocystic changes (FCC), *1702*
leiomyoma, *1691*
lymphedema, *1706*

menopause, *1677*
menorrhagia, *1684*
metrorrhagia, *1684*
premenstrual syndrome (PMS), *1681*

Disorders of the female reproductive system range from menstrual cramps to life-threatening diseases such as cancer. Many of these disorders can occur at any point in a woman's adult life. They may affect her ability to bear children, her sexuality, and her sense of well-being as a woman. Women who experience reproductive system changes and disorders require a holistic approach to meet their physical, emotional, and educational needs. Because the ability to reproduce affects self-esteem, feelings of femininity, and general health, both sensitivity and understanding from caregivers are essential. Providing a medical and family history and undergoing diagnostic tests often require women to disclose personal, intimate information and have invasive procedures, which they may

find embarrassing and uncomfortable. When providing care, nurses must consider the woman within the context of her culture, socioeconomic and educational level, sexual orientation, and lifestyle.

This chapter discusses female perimenopause, sexual function, menstrual disorders, structural disorders, disorders of reproductive tissues, and disorders of the breast. Sexually transmitted infections (STIs), including vaginal infections and pelvic inflammatory disease, are discussed in ∞ Chapter 50. Many of the disorders discussed in this chapter result in actual or potential health problems requiring nursing care based on similar nursing diagnoses. To avoid repeating those diagnoses and interventions for each disorder, they have been divided among the nursing care discussions as appropriate. Treatment of cancer with chemotherapy and radiation is discussed in ∞ Chapter 14. Disorders of female sexual function may result from the physical or emotional effects of the disorders discussed in this chapter and thus are discussed first.

Disorders of Female Sexual Function

The female body maintains the capacity for sexual activity for all of her life. In a typical sexual event, two physiologic sexual responses occur: vasocongestion and myotonia. Sexual stimulation results in vasocongestion of the blood vessels surrounding the vagina, causing engorgement, increased lubrication, and genital swelling and enlargement. Arousal, or myotonia, increases muscular tension, resulting in voluntary and involuntary muscle contraction.

The sexual response cycle has four phases: excitement, plateau, orgasm, and resolution. These phases always occur in the same sequence; however, the duration of each phase may vary. Sexual arousal typically ends in orgasm (climax), but sometimes fails to do so. A refractory period, or period in which the sexual organs are incapable of responding to stimulus, does not occur in the female. Multiple orgasms are physically possible in all women.

Although nurses may not conduct sexual counseling, they should be able to obtain a sexual history without embarrassment, discuss sexual concerns with women, and make appropriate referrals.

Pathophysiology

Disorders of sexual function include dyspareunia, inhibited sexual desire, and orgasmic dysfunction.

Dyspareunia

The woman with **dyspareunia** (pain during intercourse) may find it difficult to express her feelings to her partner. This condition may manifest itself as decreased desire or inhibited orgasm. Physical conditions, such as imperforate hymen, vaginal scarring, or vaginismus, may cause dyspareunia. Vaginismus is a rare condition in which the vaginal muscles at the introitus contract so tightly that an erect penis cannot be inserted. The muscle contraction without penetration may be painful for the woman. An early traumatic event, such as sexual abuse, fear of men, or rape, may contribute to this disorder. However, it is estimated that most dyspareunia is psychogenic in origin. The woman develops an anxiety–fear–guilt cycle in which negative thoughts become associated with the act of vaginal penetration, initiating a conditioned involuntary reflex. Other sexual activity may be pleasurable.

Inhibited Sexual Desire

Inhibited sexual desire may be a result of pathophysiologic processes or may be psychogenic in origin. Often, inhibited sexual desire is rooted deeply in childhood teaching or experiences that may be too painful to recall. Cultural and religious values can also affect the processing of sexual stimuli. Fear of pregnancy or STIs and depression also contribute to decreased libido.

Orgasmic Dysfunction

Inhibited female orgasm (**anorgasmia**) is a relatively common sexual problem among women. Primary anorgasmia, occurring in 10% to 15% of women, exists when a woman has never experienced an orgasm during the waking state, either through self-stimulation or intercourse. Secondary anorgasmia exists when a woman who previously experienced at least one orgasm in the past is no longer able to do so. Surveys suggest that one-third to one-half of all women are dissatisfied with how often they reach orgasm (Medline Plus, 2008). Organic causes of anorgasmia include the presence of disease that results in general debilitation or that affects the sexual response cycle, and the use of drugs that depress the central nervous system (CNS).

Interdisciplinary Care

Although there is not currently a female version of Viagra, there are are medications being tested to treat female sexual-desire problems. These include Flibanserin, now in a clinical trial, and three topical agents: Zestra (a topical fluid), Alista cream, and LibiGel (a topically applied testosterone product) (Barclay, 2008).

✍ Nursing Care

Nursing care focuses on identifying the type of sexual dysfunction with a thorough history, including the onset, duration, frequency, and context or situation in which the problem occurs. Questioning the woman about medication use is important as many drugs can contribute to sexual dysfunction. Antidepressants, especially selective serotonin reuptake inhibitors (SSRIs), often prescribed for premenstrual symptoms, contribute to lack of libido and delayed or absent orgasm (Frank, Mistretta, & Will, 2008). The woman's partner should be included in discussions when possible.

Teach the woman and her partner about varied normal sexual responses. The goal is to increase self-awareness and understanding of communication and their relationship to sexual desire. Explain the differences in the behaviors that men and women consider sexually stimulating. Sex therapists may provide training in autostimulation techniques (masturbation) after inhibitions against this practice are discussed. Group therapy may be encouraged to help the woman discuss her problem and to decrease the sense of isolation it gives her.

The Perimenopausal Woman

Menopause ("change of life") is a normal physiologic process as a woman ages. It is included here because it increases the risk of disorders of various aspects of women's health. In the United States, most women stop menstruating between 48 and 55 years of age (Porth & Matfin, 2009). Menopause is the permanent cessation of menses as a result of aging, surgical removal of the ovaries, or chemotherapy (this discussion focuses on natural menopause). The climacteric, or perimenopausal, period denotes the time during which reproductive function gradually ceases. For most women, the perimenopausal period lasts several years. It begins with a decline in the production of the hormone estrogen, includes the permanent cessation of menstruation due to loss of ovarian function, and extends for 1 year after the final menstrual period, at which time a woman is said to be postmenopausal. The average woman will live one-third of her life after menopause.

Many women welcome the freedom from monthly menstrual periods and have relatively minor physical effects from the estrogen depletion. However, the hormonal changes that occur can be accompanied by side effects (discussed later in this section). Early menopause (before the age of 40) can be familial, occur in women who smoke, or occur in women who have received chemotherapy drugs. Some studies suggest that women who never gave birth go through menopause at an earlier age (NAMS, 2007). Certain health risks increase after menopause, including heart disease, osteoporosis, macular degeneration, and breast cancer.

The Physiology of Menopause

The menopausal period marks the natural biologic end of reproductive ability. Surgical menopause occurs when the ovaries are removed in premenopausal women, dramatically reducing the production of estrogen and progestins. Chemical menopause often occurs during cancer chemotherapy, when cytotoxic drugs arrest ovarian function.

As ovarian function decreases, the production of estradiol (E_2), the most biologically active estrogen, decreases and is ultimately replaced by estrone as the major ovarian estrogen. Estrone is produced in small amounts and has only about one-tenth the biologic activity of estradiol. With decreased ovarian function, the second ovarian hormone, progesterone, which is produced during the luteal phase of the menstrual cycle, also is markedly reduced.

Manifestations

As estrogen decreases, various tissues are affected. There is a decrease in breast tissue, body hair, skin elasticity, and subcutaneous fat. The ovaries and uterus become smaller, and the cervix and vagina also decrease in size and become pale in color. These changes may result in problems with vaginal dryness, dyspareunia (painful intercourse), urinary stress incontinence, urinary tract infections (UTIs), and vaginitis. Vasomotor instability may cause hot flashes, palpitations, dizziness, and headaches. Other problems resulting from vasomotor instability include insomnia, frequent awakening, and perspiration (night sweats). The woman may experience irritability and have problems with memory during the transition (National Institute on Aging, 2008).

Long-term estrogen deprivation results in an imbalance in bone remodeling and osteoporosis, leading to fractures and kyphosis. The risk for cardiovascular diseases increases in response to an increase in atherosclerosis (from an increase in the LDL-to-HDL cholesterol ratio). Manifestations of the perimenopausal period are listed in the accompanying Manifestations box. These manifestations vary widely. Some women experience severe symptoms, others experience moderate symptoms, and some women experience few or no symptoms.

Interdisciplinary Care

Care of the woman experiencing menopausal symptoms focuses on relieving symptoms and minimizing postmenopausal health risks.

MANIFESTATIONS of the Perimenopausal Period

- Menstrual cycles become erratic. Menstrual flow varies widely in amount and duration and eventually ceases.
- Vaginal, vulval, and urethral tissues begin to atrophy.
- Vaginal pH rises, predisposing the woman to vaginal infections.
- Vaginal lubrication decreases, and vaginal rugae decrease in number. This may result in dyspareunia, injury, and fungal infections.
- Vasomotor instability due to a decrease in estrogen may result in hot flashes and night sweats. A hot flash starts in the chest and moves upward toward the face and may last from seconds to several minutes.
- Psychologic symptoms may include moodiness, nervousness, insomnia, headaches, irritability, anxiety, inability to concentrate, and depression.

Diagnosis

As estrogen secretion diminishes, levels of follicle-stimulating hormone (FSH) and luteinizing hormone (LH) rise and remain elevated. A woman who has not menstruated for 1 full year or who has an increased FSH blood level is considered menopausal (Porth & Matfin, 2009).

Medications

Although controversial, menopause hormone therapy (HRT) may be prescribed to alleviate severe manifestations of menopause, but only for a limited amount of time and only after a woman has been provided with known risks. HRT may include estrogen alone for women who have had a hysterectomy, or a combination of estrogen and progestin. The addition of progestin stimulates monthly shedding of the interuterine lining, decreasing the risk of uterine cancer. HRT relieves hot flashes and night sweats and decreases problems of vaginal dryness and urogenital tissue atrophy, which can lead to painful intercourse and urinary incontinence. Long-term HRT may increase the risk for breast cancer, ovarian cancer, stroke, heart attacks, and venous thrombosis (McPhee, Tierney, & Papadakis, 2008). However, women who have had a hysterectomy and take estrogen alone do not have an increased risk of breast cancer (Mayo Clinic, 2008).

Selective estrogen receptor modulators (SERMs) such as raloxifene (Evista) and triphenylethylene (Tamoxifen) bind to estrogen receptors and exert site-specific effects in different target tissues. Tamoxifen and toremifene (a derivative of tamoxifen) have a beneficial effect on bone mineral density and serum lipids and decrease the risk of invasive breast cancer in women at high risk. They also provide an alternative to HRT for preventing osteoporosis.

Antidepressants may be prescribed as an off-label use for hot flashes and irritability. The selective serotonin reuptake inhibitors (SSRIs) promote increased use of serotonin (a neurotransmitter) to in turn affect heat regulation in the body. Examples include fluoxetine (Prozac), paroxetine (Paxil), and veniafaxine (Effexor). Possible side effects include headache, nausea, insomnia, anorexia, nightmares, diarrhea, and hypertension. Women over the age of 50 have an increased risk of bone fracture. Women should be told to discuss these medications with their physician prior to beginning or stopping use (WebMD, 2008).

Alternative and Complementary Therapies

As a result of the controversy surrounding the use of HRT, non-traditional or alternative therapies have become more popular. For example, phytoestrogens are estrogen-like substances found in some cereals, vegetables, legumes (including soy in tofu, tempeh, soymilk, and soy nuts) and herbs. Caution is recommended when using herbal therapies regarding the purity of the products and use in conjunction with traditional medications as adverse effects may occur. Healthcare professionals need to assess for the use of these therapies as some plant products may be harmful when combined with other drugs. The following complementary therapies are examples of those used by menopausal women to reduce associated discomforts (NCCAM, 2008; Mayo Clinic, 2007a; Cleveland Clinic, 2008):

- Acupuncture
- Biofeedback
- Massage
- Herbs: *Cimcifuga racemosa* (black cohosh), Vitex agnus castii (chaste tree), *Rehmannia*, ginseng, Kava, dong quai, golden seal, flaxseed, valerian, and evening primrose
- Meditation and yoga

✎ Nursing Care

Nursing care during and after the menopausal period focuses on minimizing the symptoms associated with hormonal changes; reducing the risk of cardiovascular disease, cancer, and osteoporosis; and educating the woman about lifestyle changes important to health and well-being.

Health Promotion

The American Cancer Society recommends a cancer-related checkup every year after the age of 40. This checkup includes examination for cancers of the thyroid, ovaries, lymph nodes, oral cavity, and skin. Other important checkups include screening for cervical, breast, and colorectal cancer. Health counseling should also include information about alcohol and tobacco use, sun exposure, diet and nutrition, exercise, risk factors, sexual practices (although pregnancy is not possible after menopause, the woman may still be at risk for STIs), and environmental and occupational exposures. It is important to discuss the benefits of rest and exercise, as well as a diet that includes fruits, vegetables, and fiber. In addition, suggest the following resources for further information: the National Institute on Aging, the North American Menopause Society, the Association of Reproductive Health Professionals, the Women's Health Initiative, and the National Women's Health Information Center.

Assessment

Collect the following data through the health history and physical examination. When assessing the older woman, be aware of normal changes with aging, as outlined in ∞ Chapter 47.

- *Health history:* Problems with urinary frequency, urgency, or incontinence; menstrual history; sexual history; dyspareunia; use of alcohol, nicotine, and drugs; medications, sleep patterns, hot flashes, night sweats, changes in emotional responses.

- *Physical assessment:* Height and weight, posture, vital signs, breast examination, pelvic examination, abdominal assessment.

Nursing Diagnoses and Interventions

Although each nursing care plan must be individualized, interventions often focus on problems with lack of information, sexuality, self-esteem, and a disturbed body image.

Deficient Knowledge

Because menopausal manifestations vary widely, it is difficult to predict their effect on an individual woman. However, the well-informed woman is better prepared to deal with whatever symptoms she experiences.

- Discuss physiologic manifestations, such as hot flashes and night sweats. *The underlying cause of hot flashes is not known. Recent studies correlate the increased chance of vasomotor symptoms in women who have higher percentages of body fat (Porth, 2007; Kaunitz, 2008). Many physiologic effects of menopause are amenable to nonpharmacologic methods of relief, such as lifestyle changes.*
- Provide information about dietary recommendations. The recommended daily intake of calcium for women over 50 is 1200 mg. *Some women need to use calcium supplements or calcium-containing antacid tablets to meet this requirement.*
- Emphasize the importance of weight-bearing exercise. *Weight-bearing exercise reduces the rate of bone loss, helps maintain optimum weight, and reduces cardiovascular risk.*
- Provide information about the benefits and risks of HRT. Not every woman will need or want it. *Every woman needs to understand both the risks and the benefits before deciding whether to use HRT.*
- Encourage the woman to obtain yearly mammograms, clinical breast examinations, and Pap tests, and to be familiar with the tissues and consistency of their breasts. The option of doing breast self-examination (BSE) should be discussed with the woman's healthcare provider and/or may be a personal choice. *The increased risk for cancer of the breast and pelvic reproductive organs makes healthcare provider screening during and after menopause even more important. There are benefits and limitations to BSE: the American Cancer Society (ACS)(2008) states that it is acceptable for women to choose or not choose to do BSE, but all women should be familiar with their own breasts in order to recognize abnormalities. If a woman chooses to do BSE, specific guidelines ("How to Perform a Breast Self-Exam") are published by the ACS based on an extensive review of the medical literature and input from an expert advisory panel.*

Risk for Sexual Dysfunction

Vaginal dryness and atrophy can interfere with sexual expression and satisfaction (see the Nursing Care of the Older Adult box). Suggesting measures to help the woman and her partner cope with these changes can enable them to continue or resume a mutually satisfying sexual relationship.

- Encourage expression of feelings and concerns about how menopause is changing her sex life, if appropriate. *Midlife and older women may not be comfortable in discussing their intimate sexual behavior.*

- Explain that as women age, it may take longer for vaginal lubrication and orgasm to occur. This information is important to prevent the woman from believing something is wrong with her, or her partner believing he or she is no longer interesting or sexually exciting. Suggest ways to increase vaginal lubrication, such as spending more time in foreplay and/or using water-soluble gels (e.g., Replens) or a vaginal HRT cream for vaginal lubrication. *A more leisurely approach to sexual activity can be mutually gratifying for both the woman and her partner. Use of water-soluble gels and vaginal HRT cream can prevent vaginal pain and irritation and improve the quality of the sexual experience.*

> **PRACTICE ALERT**
> Plant estrogens, found in food such as brown rice, corn, green beans, lemon and orange peels, and tofu, are mildly estrogenic and may improve vaginal dryness.

Situational Low Self-Esteem

Each woman responds to the aging process in her own way, and most women have coping skills that adequately equip them to deal with the gradual changes associated with aging. Among the factors that may provoke a self-esteem disturbance are the loss of youth, a sense of emptiness as children leave home, and the need to redefine one's self-concept and roles as parenting becomes less important. Women who place a high value on their physical attractiveness may experience a painful psychologic response to the physical changes of menopause.

- Encourage expression of fears and concerns related to changes in interpersonal and family functions. *Many women associate aging with "uselessness" and unattractiveness.*
- Suggest volunteer activities or employment for the woman who has extra time. *This enables the woman to feel that she is still a contributing member of society. Volunteering for* activities involving young people can help reduce anxiety about the loss of reproductive ability or any late regrets about not having had children.
- Discuss the importance of a healthy lifestyle in maintaining physical attractiveness. Identify risk factors and high-risk behaviors. *Lifestyle habits and behaviors affect many body systems and physical appearance. For example, cigarette smoking and overexposure to the sun make the skin age faster, contributing to wrinkles. Active women who exercise and eat a well-balanced diet look and feel better.*

Disturbed Body Image

As women progress through the perimenopausal period, changes in appearance and the loss of childbearing ability may combine to make the woman feel "old, ugly, and useless." Although this is far from the truth, it nevertheless is the perception of many women. The physical changes the woman often experiences include growth of facial hair, excessive perspiration and flushing of the face, and weight gain.

- Encourage the woman to describe her perceptions of her own body. *This information is necessary to obtain data to establish an individualized plan of care.*
- Encourage verbalization of feelings of concern, anger, anxiety, loss, and fear over body changes. *Expressing these emotions can facilitate the grieving process and acceptance of change.*
- Stress that certain physical characteristics of a person cannot be changed; emphasize the importance of learning to recognize and appreciate one's own special strengths. *These help the woman gain acceptance and a realistic appraisal of self.*
- Refer, as appropriate, for dietary management, exercise, stress management, and cosmetic assistance (e.g., for aggravating facial hair). *These actions increase wellness and a positive sense of self.*

NURSING CARE OF THE OLDER ADULT — Sexual Function in the Aging Woman

Myths, taboos, and stereotypes held by society may foster the belief that older women are no longer interested in expressing their sexuality. Two commonly held myths are that menopause is the death of a woman's sexuality and that hysterectomy results in the inability to function sexually. Loss of sexual function is not an inevitable result of aging, although physical changes related to aging do affect the female sexual response. These physical changes, along with chronic conditions common in aging women, may alter a woman's sexual function. In addition, some medications used to treat the chronic conditions associated with aging can also alter the sexual response. It is the role of the nurse to educate women about the myths and misinformation about changes in sexual functioning and to provide information about ways to achieve optimal sexual health.

PHYSIOLOGIC CHANGES

Changes in aging women's sexual function often begin in the perimenopausal period as estrogen levels decrease. Estrogen-sensitive cells are found throughout the central nervous system and the cardiovascular system. These cells are involved in the female sexual response. With menopause comes a decrease in the levels of estradiol, which affects nerve transmission and the response in the peripheral vascular system. As a result, the timing and degree of vasocongestion during the sexual response are affected. The capacity for vasocongestion decreases during the plateau phase, as does muscle tension. In the orgasmic phase, the contractions are fewer and less intense. During the resolution phase, vasocongestion subsides more quickly.

NURSING CARE

The nurse's role in assisting aging women to reach optimal sexual functioning centers on teaching them about the physiologic and psychologic changes associated with menopause. In addition, the nurse should instruct the woman in how the effects of chronic illness and the medications used to treat these illnesses affect sexual functioning. The woman should be taught the importance of maintaining a healthy lifestyle, which includes a balanced diet, weight-bearing and aerobic exercises, stress management, and routine health examinations.

For problems related to vaginal dryness and dyspareunia, the nurse can recommend water-soluble vaginal lubricants or vaginal gels before intercourse. Intercourse on a regular basis and estrogen replacement therapy can also be suggested for these problems. Women who experience joint pain or other musculoskeletal pain due to conditions such as arthritis can benefit from instruction in how to adapt positions for intercourse.

Menstrual Disorders

Monthly menstruation normally involves some minor discomfort, including breast tenderness, a feeling of heaviness and congestion in the pelvic area, uterine cramping, and lower backache. Many women, however, experience more serious effects, both physiologic and psychologic. This section discusses premenstrual syndrome, dysmenorrhea, and abnormal uterine bleeding.

The Woman with Premenstrual Syndrome

Premenstrual syndrome (PMS) is a complex of manifestations (e.g., mood swings, breast tenderness, fatigue, irritability, food cravings, and depression) that are limited to 3 to 14 days before menstruation and relieved by the onset of menses. It is estimated that 20%–50% of all adult women experience moderate to severe symptoms and 5% have severe symptoms (Pearlstein & Steiner, 2008). For a small number of women, PMS is so disabling that it is called by the psychiatric label of premenstrual dysphoric disorder (PMDD).

The syndrome is seen less frequently during the teens and 20s, reaching a peak in women in their mid-30s. Major life stressors, age greater than 30, and depression are risk factors associated with PMS. Premenstrual syndrome can be a factor in absenteeism at school or work, decreased productivity, interpersonal relationship difficulties, and lifestyle disruption.

Pathophysiology

Although the pathophysiology of PMS is not clearly understood, it is believed that hormonal changes such as altered estrogen–progesterone ratios, increased prolactin levels, and rising aldosterone levels during the luteal phase of the menstrual cycle contribute to the problem. Increased production of aldosterone results in sodium retention and edema. Decreased levels of monoamine oxidase in the brain are associated with depression, and reduced levels of serotonin can lead to mood swings.

Manifestations

Manifestations of PMS occur during the luteal phase of the menstrual cycle (7 to 10 days prior to the onset of the menstrual flow), abating when the menstrual flow begins. The Multisystem Effects of PMS are shown on page 1682. Although PMS may produce a variety of physiologic and psychologic manifestations, the exact nature of these manifestations and their intensity are individualized for each woman with this disorder. The manifestations may even differ from month to month in the same woman.

Interdisciplinary Care

If no organic cause can be identified, the goals of care are to relieve manifestations and to help develop self-care patterns that will help the woman anticipate and cope more effectively with future episodes of PMS. There are no definitive diagnostic tests for PMS; instead, the regular recurrence of manifestations preceding the onset of menses for at least 3 months leads to a diagnosis. The treatment of PMS integrates this self-monitored record of manifestations, regular exercise, avoiding caffeine, and a diet low in simple sugars and high in lean proteins (Porth & Matfin, 2009). Although many different medications, vitamins, and herbal supplements have been used to treat the manifestations of PMS, the most promising appears to be the use of SSRIs.

Medications

If the manifestations of PMS are severe or incapacitating, ovulation may be suppressed by the use of gonadotropin-releasing hormone (GnRH) agonists, oral contraceptives, or danazol (an anabolic steroid). Progesterone and antiprostaglandin agents such as nonsteroidal anti-inflammatory drugs (NSAIDs) may help relieve cramping. Diuretics may be prescribed to relieve bloating. SSRIs such as fluoxetine (Prozac), sertraline (Zoloft), and paroxetine (Paxil) may be used to manage mood and some physical manifestations of PMS.

Alternative and Complementary Therapies

The woman with PMS may find diet, exercise, relaxation, and stress management helpful.

- A diet high in complex carbohydrates with limited salt, simple sugars, and alcohol is recommended to minimize reactive hypoglycemia, which can contribute to the manifestations of PMS. Limiting salt intake can assist with fluid retention. Caffeine is restricted to reduce irritability.
- Reduced sodium intake helps minimize fluid retention. Increased intake of calcium (1200 mg per day), magnesium (200 mg per day), vitamin B_6 (50 to 100 mg per day), and vitamin E (400 international units per day) may be helpful (Mayo Clinic, 2007b).
- Herbal remedies include black cohosh, ginger, bilberry, chaste berry, red clover, thunder god vine, and evening primrose oil. Natural progesterone creams, derived from wild yams and soybeans, relieve manifestations in some women (Mayo Clinic, 2007b; National Institutes of Health, 2008). Discussion about these alternative therapies with the healthcare provider is recommended.
- Exercise is beneficial, but adequate rest also is necessary.
- Techniques for relaxation and stress management include deep abdominal breathing, meditation, muscle relaxation, and guided imagery.

✍ Nursing Care

Nursing Diagnoses and Interventions

Nursing care for the woman with PMS focuses on relieving manifestations. Most women experiencing PMS require interventions to manage pain and enhance coping.

Acute Pain

The woman with PMS may have pain from headache (including migraine), menstrual cramps, excessive fluid retention, breast swelling, joint and muscle pain, and backache.

MULTISYSTEM EFFECTS OF PMS

Neurologic
- Syncope
- Vertigo
- Dizziness
- Paresthesia
- Headache
- Inability to concentrate
- Depression
- Irritability
- Anxiety
- Mood swings
- Anger
- Aggressive behavior

Sensory
- Conjunctivitis
- Visual disturbances

Cardiovascular
- Bruising
- Palpitations

Integumentary
- Acne
- Herpes recurrence
- Urticaria

Metabolic Processes
- Breast tenderness
- Edema
- Transient weight gain
- Food cravings

Urinary
- Cystitis
- Oliguria

Gastrointestinal
- Constipation
- Nausea
- Vomiting

Musculoskeletal
- Backache
- Pelvic stiffness

Immune System
- ↑ Susceptibility to infection
- Asthma
- ↑ Allergic reactions

- Teach effective pharmacologic and nonpharmacologic self-care measures to relieve pain: application of heat, relaxation techniques (such as breathing exercises, imagery techniques, or meditation), and exercise. *Heat relieves muscle spasms and dilates blood vessels, increasing blood supply to the pelvis and uterine muscles. Relaxation and exercise aid the release of naturally produced pain relievers called endorphins.*
- Review daily activities and suggest ways to balance rest periods and activity. *During rest periods, energy and oxygen requirements decrease, increasing the amount of energy and oxygen available to muscles.*
- Review manifestations and, if possible, correlate these with dietary patterns and activity levels. Encourage the woman to keep a diary of PMS manifestations. *Maintaining a diary of PMS manifestations, activity, and foods eaten can provide data to identify modifiable causes of discomfort.*
- If appropriate, suggest sexual activity as a way to lessen menstrual cramps. *Orgasm may help relieve dysmenorrhea.*

Ineffective Coping

Many women experience wide mood swings during episodes of PMS, sometimes exhibiting self-destructive or aggressive behaviors toward others. These mood swings can interfere with a woman's ability to manage her responsibilities at home or at work.

- Encourage the woman to keep a journal of her menstrual cycle and to document her mood changes in the 7 to 10 days prior to menstruation. *Recognizing the signs and timing of PMS is the first step in developing methods to cope with the problem.*
- Explore possible ways to rearrange or reschedule activities when experiencing PMS. *Planning ahead enables the woman to assume more control and promotes coping methods.*
- Explore what, if any, self-care measures have helped cope with mood alterations in the past. *Encourage healthful coping mechanisms, such as relaxation techniques and exercise. Some women may rely on alcohol or other drugs during PMS, which only exacerbate the manifestations.*

The Woman with Dysmenorrhea

Dysmenorrhea (pain or discomfort associated with menstruation) is estimated to occur in 46% to 95% of menstruating women (Emedicine, 2006). Primary dysmenorrhea is most often seen in girls who have just begun menstruating, becoming less severe after the mid-20s or giving birth. Secondary dysmenorrhea most commonly is seen when a woman is in her 20s and 30s, beginning after years of relatively painless menstrual periods.

Pathophysiology

In primary dysmenorrhea, prostaglandins are released from sloughing endometrial cells, causing myometrial contraction and vasoconstriction. As the muscles contract, uterine circulation is compromised, resulting in uterine ischemia and pain. These contractions can range from mild cramping to severe muscle spasms. Psychologic factors, such as anxiety and tension, may contribute

to dysmenorrhea. Secondary dysmenorrhea is related to underlying pathologic conditions that involve scarring or injury to the reproductive tract. Endometriosis, fibroid tumors, chronic pelvic inflammatory disease, endometrial polyps, and use of an intrauterine device (IUD) use may result in painful menses.

Manifestations

Manifestations of primary dysmenorrhea (see the accompanying Manifestations box) may be severe enough to disrupt activities of daily living, work activities, school attendance, and sexual function.

Interdisciplinary Care

Care of the woman with menstrual pain focuses on identifying the underlying cause, reestablishing functional capacity, and managing pain. A careful history and physical assessment are performed to rule out any underlying organic cause of dysmenorrhea. If no organic cause is found, the diagnosis is primary dysmenorrhea.

Diagnosis

Various diagnostic tests are performed to identify structural abnormalities, hormonal imbalances, and pathologic conditions that could cause menstrual pain. Diagnostic tests are described in ∞ Chapter 47.

Diagnosis is made based on findings from a pelvic examination and diagnostic procedures, including a Papanicolaou (Pap) smear and cervical and vaginal cultures, ultrasound of the pelvis and vagina, and CT scan or MRI to detect structural abnormalities, malignancy, or infections. Laboratory tests used to assess possible causes of dysmenorrhea include FSH and LH levels to assess pituitary function, progesterone and estradiol levels to assess ovarian function, and thyroid function tests.

Laparoscopy is used to diagnose structural defects and blockages caused by scarring, endometriosis, tumors, and cysts (Figure 49–1 ■). See the box on page 1684 for nursing care of the woman having a laparoscopy. A dilation and curettage (D&C) of the uterus may be performed to obtain tissue for evaluation or to relieve dysmenorrhea and heavy menstrual bleeding. (This procedure is discussed later in this chapter.)

Medications

Dysmenorrhea may be treated with analgesics, prostaglandin inhibitors such as NSAIDs, or oral contraceptives (see the Medication Administration box on page 1685).

MANIFESTATIONS of Primary Dysmenorrhea

- Abdominal pain beginning with onset of menses and lasting 12 to 48 hours
- Pain radiating to lower back and thighs
- Headache
- Nausea
- Vomiting
- Diarrhea
- Fatigue
- Breast tenderness

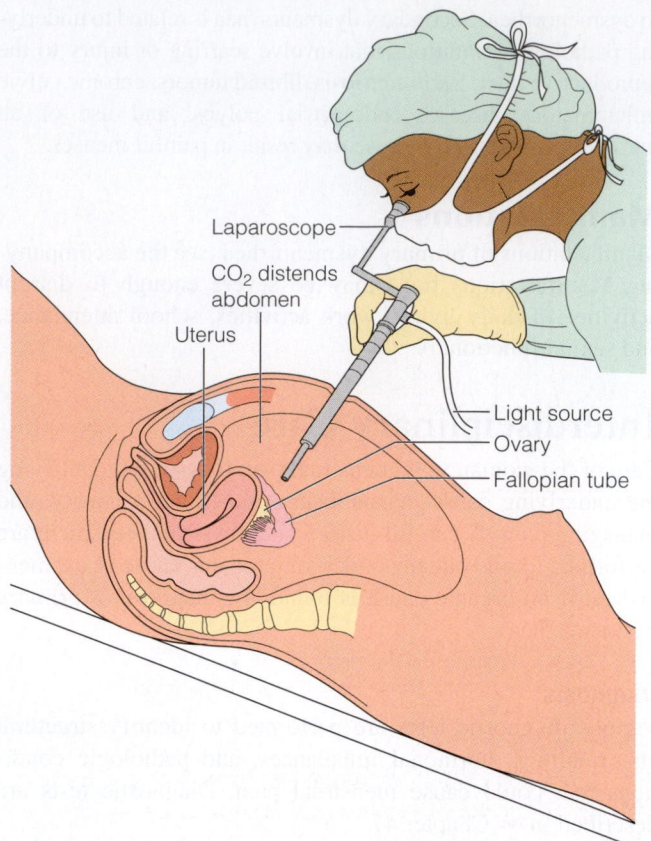

Laparoscope
CO₂ distends abdomen
Uterus
Light source
Ovary
Fallopian tube

Figure 49–1 ■ Laparoscopy. In this surgical procedure, a flexible, lighted instrument (laparoscope) is inserted through a periumbilical incision. Laparoscopy allows visualization of the pelvic cavity.

NURSING CARE OF THE PATIENT
Having a Laparoscopy

PREOPERATIVE CARE
- Instruct the woman to empty the bladder prior to the surgical procedure.
- Explain to the woman that referred shoulder pain or expulsion of gas through the vagina may occur postoperatively. *During the procedure, the woman's abdomen is insufflated with carbon dioxide gas to distend it and facilitate visualization of the pelvic organs. The surgical table is then tilted so that the intestines will fall away from the pelvic organs. Some carbon dioxide gas may remain in the abdomen after the procedure.*
- Explain that pain should be minimal. Instruct the woman to report excessive pain to the nurse or physician at once. *Excessive pain signals infection or other postoperative complication.*

POSTOPERATIVE CARE
- Apply a perineal pad. Teach the woman proper perineal hygiene, emphasizing the need to change pads at least every 4 hours. *Proper perineal hygiene reduces the risk of postoperative infection.*
- Ask the woman to keep a pad count. Minor bleeding is normal; excessive bleeding may indicate hemorrhage. *A pad count of more than one per hour is an indication of blood loss and should be reported to the healthcare provider.*

Nursing Care

Nursing care for the woman with primary dysmenorrhea focuses on controlling manifestations and providing education about the normal physiology of the menstrual cycle and self-care measures. Care of the woman with secondary dysmenorrhea varies according to the underlying cause and is discussed in this chapter within sections on specific disorders. Nursing interventions previously described for the woman with PMS are also appropriate for the woman with dysmenorrhea.

The Woman with Dysfunctional Uterine Bleeding

Dysfunctional uterine bleeding (DUB) refers to vaginal bleeding that is usually painless but abnormal in amount, duration, or time of occurrence. A number of factors may predispose a woman to DUB. These factors include stress, extreme weight changes, use of oral contraceptive agents or IUDs, and peritmenopausal status. Dysfunctional uterine bleeding is usually related to hormonal imbalances or pelvic neoplasms, either benign or malignant. DUB, depending on cause, may occur in women from early to late adulthood.

Pathophysiology

The types of DUB include amenorrhea, oligomenorrhea, menorrhagia, metrorrhagia, and postmenopausal bleeding.

- **Amenorrhea** is the absence of menstruation. Primary amenorrhea, absence of menarche by age 16, or by age 14 if secondary sex characteristics fail to develop, may be caused by structural abnormalities, hormonal imbalances, polycystic ovary disease, or an imperforate hymen. Because a certain percentage of body fat is required for menstruation to occur, anorexia nervosa, bulimia, or excessive athletic training can also cause primary amenorrhea. Secondary amenorrhea, absence of menses for at least 6 months in a previously menstruating female, may also be caused by anorexia nervosa, excessive athletic activity or training, or a large weight loss. Other causes include hormonal imbalances and ovarian tumors. Normal (physiologic) secondary amenorrhea occurs during pregnancy, breast-feeding, and menopause.
- Oligomenorrhea (scant menses) usually is related to hormonal imbalances.
- **Menorrhagia** (excessive or prolonged menstruation) may result from thyroid disorders, endometriosis, pelvic inflammatory disease, functional ovarian cysts, or uterine fibroids or polyps. Clotting disorders and anticoagulant medications also can cause menorrhagia. A single heavy or long menses is not in itself a cause for concern; however, repetitive long or heavy menses can lead to hemorrhage, excessive blood loss, fatigue, and anemia.
- **Metrorrhagia** (bleeding between menstrual periods) may be caused by hormonal imbalances, pelvic inflammatory disease, cervical or uterine polyps, uterine fibroids, or cervical or uterine cancer. Because cancer is a possible cause of metrorrhagia, early evaluation and treatment are extremely important. Mittelschmerz (midcycle mild abdominal pain

MEDICATION ADMINISTRATION The Woman with Dysmenorrhea

EXAMPLES OF ORAL CONTRACEPTIVES

Norethindrone and ethinyl estradiol (Brevicon, Norinyl)

Norgestrel and ethinyl estradiol (Ovral)

Oral contraceptives inhibit ovulation and help reduce cramping and bleeding. Side effects of oral contraceptives include breast tenderness, weight gain, nausea, midcycle bleeding, mood swings, depression, chloasma (skin discoloration) on the face and chest, hypertension, vascular complications, vaginal candidiasis, migraines, and glucose intolerance. Oral contraceptives are contraindicated in women with personal or family history of breast cancer in first-degree relatives, hypertension, history of stroke or transient ischemic attack (TIA), smoking, history of estrogendependent cancer, pregnancy, liver disease, or thrombophlebitis.

Nursing Responsibilities
- Assess the patient for potential contraindications to drug therapy.

Health Education for the Patient and Family
- Take the drug as prescribed until the physician indicates otherwise or until side effects prevent you from continuing to take them.
- If you are taking oral contraceptives, be sure to take them at the same time every day.
- Report to the physician suspected pregnancy and any side effects such as nausea, rash, drowsiness, stomach pain, ringing in the ears, tenderness in the calf of the leg, and shortness of breath.
- Do not smoke while taking oral contraceptives.

associated with ovulation) occurs in many women and is not considered metrorrhagia.

- Postmenopausal bleeding may be caused by cervical polyps, endometrial polyps, endometrial hyperplasia, or uterine cancer. The possibility of cancer makes early evaluation and treatment essential.

Hormonal imbalances, especially progesterone deficiency with relative estrogen excess, result in endometrial hyperplasia. Estrogen stimulates endometrial proliferation. However, without the support provided by progesterone, sloughing occurs, resulting in vaginal bleeding that may be irregular, prolonged, or profuse. Defects in the follicular phase shorten the proliferative phase of the menstrual cycle, resulting in spotting and breakthrough bleeding. Defects during the luteal phase result in excessive amount or duration of flow due to persistence of the corpus luteum. This leads to a deficiency of progesterone, resulting in vaginal bleeding. Anovulation (absence of ovulation) is associated with both estrogen and progesterone deficiencies. Emotional upsets or stress can cause hormonal imbalances and thus affect menstruation. Pelvic cancers, discussed later, also cause abnormal bleeding.

Interdisciplinary Care

The care of the woman with DUB focuses on identifying and treating the underlying disease. A careful history and physical examination are performed. Abdominal and pelvic examinations are performed to rule out abdominal masses. The woman may need to keep a menstrual history and basal body temperature chart for several months to determine whether ovulation is occurring.

Diagnosis

A variety of diagnostic tests are used to diagnose the cause of DUB. Diagnostic tests are discussed in ∞ Chapter 47, and include a Pap test to rule out or identify cervical carcinoma, a pelvic ultrasound to identify luteal cysts or ovarian tumors, and an endometrial biopsy to obtain endometrial tissue for histologic examination.

Laboratory studies may include a complete blood count (CBC) to rule out a systemic disease, coagulant factors, PT and

PTT to rule out clotting disorders, thyroid function studies, serum progesterone levels, and endocrine studies to evaluate pituitary and adrenal function (thyroid and pituitary dysfunction may be manifested by menstrual irregularities).

Medications

For many women, hormonal agents can correct menstrual irregularities. For anovulatory DUB, oral contraceptives may be prescribed for 3 to 6 months or a levonorgestrel-releasing intrauterine device (IUD) may be used. Progesterone or medroxyprogesterone also may be prescribed to regulate uterine bleeding. Ovulatory DUB may be treated with progestins during the luteal phase. Oral iron supplements may be prescribed to replace iron lost through menstrual bleeding.

Surgery

Surgical intervention emphasizes the least invasive method that proves effective relief, beginning with a therapeutic D&C, then endometrial ablation, and, lastly, hysterectomy.

THERAPEUTIC D&C In a therapeutic D&C, the cervical canal is dilated and the uterine wall is scraped. D&C is used to diagnose and treat DUB and other disorders of the female reproductive system. It may be performed to correct excessive or prolonged bleeding. D&C is contraindicated in any woman who has been taking anticoagulant drugs or whose condition precludes the use of regional or general anesthesia. Postoperative nursing care of the woman having a D&C is described in the Nursing Care box on page 1686.

ENDOMETRIAL ABLATION In an endometrial ablation, the endometrial layer of the uterus is destroyed by using a laser, thermal balloon, or electrocautery. It is performed in women who do not respond to pharmacologic management or D&C. This procedure usually produces amenorrhea but there are cases where menstrual flow returns. A woman going through endometrial ablation should understand that she should use contraception, as fertilization may occur from tissue that may not have been totally destroyed. If pregnancy does occur there may be major complications (American Society for Reproductive Medicine, 2008).

Having a Dilation and Curettage (D&C)

■ Monitor circulation and sensation in the legs, and avoid compression of the popliteal area. *The lithotomy position requires the woman's legs to be elevated in stirrups, which can impair circulation.*

■ Instruct the woman to use perineal pads and avoid tampons for 2 weeks. *This reduces the risk of infection and allows tissues to heal.*

■ Explain that the onset of the next menstrual period may be delayed. *The surgical procedure removes the endometrial lining.*

■ Explain that intercourse should be avoided until after the postoperative checkup and after vaginal discharge has stopped. *This precaution reduces the risk of infection.*

■ Instruct the woman to rest for several days after surgery, avoid heavy lifting, and report any bleeding that is bright red or exceeds that of a normal menstrual period. *Vigorous activity, lifting, or straining interferes with healing and may cause hemorrhage.*

HYSTERECTOMY   Hysterectomy (surgical removal of the uterus) may be performed when medical management of bleeding disorders is unsuccessful or cancer is present, particularly if the woman no longer wishes to have children. Approximately 600,000 hysterectomies are performed each year in the United States, and an estimated 20 million women have had a hysterectomy (Centers for Disease Control and Prevention, 2008d). In premenopausal women the ovaries are usually left in place; in postmenopausal women a total hysterectomy, or panhysterectomy, may be performed; this procedure involves removal of the uterus, fallopian tubes, and ovaries.

Hysterectomy may involve either an abdominal or a vaginal approach. The choice depends on the underlying disorder, the need to explore the abdominal cavity, and the preference of the surgeon and woman. When a hysterectomy is performed, the woman is hospitalized for 1 to 3 days and requires a recovery period of from 4 to 6 weeks for an abdominal hysterectomy and from 1 to 2 weeks for a vaginal and laparoscopic hysterectomy.

Postoperative nursing care of the woman undergoing a hysterectomy is described in the Nursing Care box below.

Abdominal hysterectomy is performed when a preexisting abdominal scar is present, when adhesions are thought to be present, or when a large operating field is necessary. For example, the woman with endometriosis is more likely to have an abdominal hysterectomy because endometrial tissue implants that may be present on other abdominal organs need to be removed. The surgical incision may be either longitudinal, made in the midline from umbilicus to pubis, or a Pfannenstiel incision, also known as the bikini cut. Vaginal hysterectomy, removal of the uterus through the vagina, is desirable when the

Having a Hysterectomy

■ Monitor vital signs every 4 hours, auscultate lungs every shift, and measure intake and output. *These data are important indicators of hemodynamic status and complications.*

■ Assess pain on a regular schedule, using a 1 (none) to 10 (severe) scale. Administer analgesics as prescribed. Splint incision if present to facilitate moving, coughing, and deep breathing. Assist with ambulation as prescribed. *Postoperative pain results from the surgery itself, as well as from gas pains prior to the return of peristalsis. Splinting the incision decreases pain from moving, turning, and deep breathing. Ambulation assists in the return of peristalsis.*

■ Monitor for hemorrhage by keeping a perineal pad count and assessing abdominal dressing. Instruct the woman on how to conduct these assessments and to report abnormal findings to the surgeon. *As most women are discharged to home in 1 or 2 days, the woman's knowledge of possible hemorrhage is important.*

■ Monitor voiding after surgery or after removal of a Foley catheter. *Voiding difficulty may occur after surgery or after the removal of a Foley catheter inserted prior to or during surgery. If the woman has not voided within 8 hours, notify the surgeon.*

■ Instruct the woman about the manifestations of infection: increased or a change in color or odor of drainage from the incision or perineal pads, general malaise, fever. If any of these occur, the woman should notify the surgeon. Discuss action of prescribed antibiotics and need to continue them until they are gone. *Early discharge mandates providing information about the risk for infection.*

■ Explain the rationale for antiembolic or compression stockings and encourage leg exercises. Discuss manifestations of deep vein thrombosis (leg pain, redness, localized heat and swelling) and pulmonary embolism (cough, difficulty breathing, rapid heart beat, chest pain) with importance of notifying the physician immediately if these occur. Instruct to avoid prolonged sitting in a chair that puts pressure behind the knees or sitting with legs crossed. *Positioning during surgery as well as postoperative edema and inactivity increase the risk for deep vein thrombosis, which in turn may break loose and travel to the lungs.*

■ After an abdominal hysterectomy, instruct to restrict physical activity for 4 to 6 weeks. Heavy lifting, stair climbing, douching, tampons, and sexual intercourse should be avoided. The woman should shower, avoiding tub baths, until bleeding has ceased. *Infection and hemorrhage are the greatest postoperative risks; restricting activities and preventing the introduction of any foreign material into the vagina helps reduce these risks.*

■ Explain that appetite may be depressed and bowel elimination may be sluggish. *These are aftereffects of general anesthesia, handling of the bowel during surgery, and loss of muscle tone in the bowel while empty.*

■ Encourage the woman to express feelings that may signal a negative self-concept. Correct any misconceptions. *Some women believe that hysterectomy means weight gain and the end of sexual activity.*

■ Provide information about continuing to have regular gynecologic screenings. *If the cervix has not been removed, regular Pap tests should continue. Pelvic examination should continue regardless of removal of the cervix.*

uterus has descended into the vagina or if the urinary bladder or rectum have prolapsed into the vagina. Vaginal hysterectomy leaves no visible abdominal scar. A laparoscopy-assisted vaginal hysterectomy (LAVH) or a laparoscopic supracervical hysterectomy (LSH) are minimally invasive options to an open procedure. The recovery time following these procedures is often only 1 to 2 weeks.

✍ Nursing Care

DUB usually causes the woman anxiety. Her self image, sexuality, or reproductive capacity may be threatened, and she may fear the possibility of cancer. She may be embarrassed to discuss her menstrual history, sexual history, and hygiene practices.

Nursing Diagnoses and Interventions

Interventions for the woman with DUB commonly address problems with anxiety and sexual function.

Anxiety

The anxiety associated with abnormal uterine bleeding can be intense. Until the cause of the bleeding is identified and has been addressed, the woman may fear cancer or other life-threatening conditions.

- Discuss the results of tests and examinations with the woman. *This allows for open exchange of information.*
- Provide information about the causes, treatments, risks, long-term effects of treatments, and prognosis. *This allows the woman to assume responsibility for her own health and become involved in her own treatment plan.*
- Evaluate coping strategies and psychosocial support systems. Teach coping strategies if indicated. *The possibility of surgery or cancer represents a crisis for the woman and her support system. Support groups can provide assistance for the woman through crisis intervention.*

Sexual Dysfunction

The woman with DUB may be unwilling to express herself sexually, particularly if bleeding is frequent or heavy. Additionally, fatigue may prevent her from participating in sexual activity.

- Offer information about engaging in sexual activity during menstruation. Explain that conception is possible during this time and that orgasm may help relieve symptoms. *Some women mistakenly believe that birth control measures are unnecessary during menstruation. Orgasm causes a release of tension and vascular congestion and frequently provides at least temporary relief of symptoms.*
- Provide an opportunity for the expression of concerns related to alterations in lifestyle and sexual functioning. *Some women have had a prolonged period of sexual abstinence related to DUB. Allowing women to verbalize concerns can assist them in working collaboratively with the healthcare provider to minimize the impact of illness and optimize function.*
- Encourage frequent rest periods. *This conserves energy and may allow sexual activities to resume.*
- Provide information about alternative methods of sexual expression. *Methods of sexual expression other than vaginal intercourse may satisfy the needs of both partners.*

> **PRACTICE ALERT**
> If the nurse is not comfortable with frank discussions about sexual activities, referral is indicated.

Community-Based Care

Provide support, appropriate reassurance, and information to help the woman and her family better understand her disorder and the therapeutic interventions indicated. Teaching also includes self-care measures that help minimize the effects of DUB on the daily functioning of the woman. The following topics should be included:

- Administration and side effects of prescribed medications, including iron.
- The need to maintain a balanced diet, increasing iron-rich foods such as eggs, beans, liver, beef, and shrimp. (Inform the woman that while orange juice may improve the absorption of iron, foods high in calcium and oxalic acid, such as spinach, may reduce its absorption.)
- Importance of maintaining a fluid intake of 2000 to 3000 mL a day.
- The need to immediately report recurring episodes of DUB, particularly in postmenopausal women, to the healthcare provider.

Structural Disorders

Structural disorders of the female reproductive system include displacement disorders and fistulas. Structural disorders may occur in women of any age.

The Woman with a Uterine Displacement

The uterus may be displaced within the pelvic cavity or may descend into the vaginal canal. Displacement of the uterus within the pelvic cavity is classified according to the direction of the displacement, as illustrated in Figure 49–2 ■.

Prolapse of the uterus into the vaginal canal can vary from mild to complete prolapse outside of the body. First-degree prolapse involves a descent of less than half the uterine corpus into the vagina. Second-degree prolapse involves the descent of the entire uterus into the vaginal canal so that the cervix is at the introitus to the vagina. Third-degree prolapse, or procidentia, is complete prolapse of the uterus outside the body, with inversion of the vaginal canal (Figure 49–3 ■). Prolapse of the uterus is often accompanied by cystocele (herniation of the bladder into the vagina) or rectocele (herniation of the rectum into the vagina).

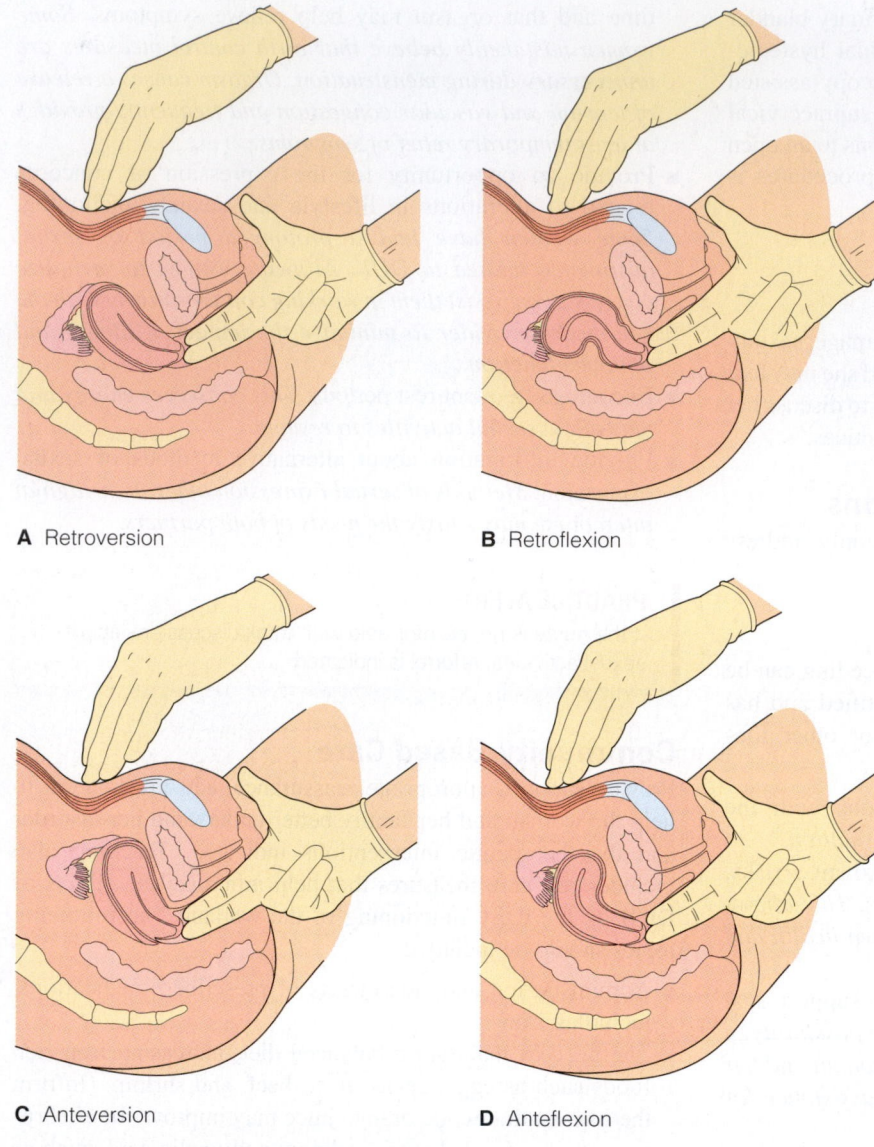

A Retroversion

B Retroflexion

C Anteversion

D Anteflexion

Figure 49–2 ■ Displacements of the uterus within the uterine cavity. *A*, Retroversion is a backward tilting. *B*, Retroflexion is a backward bending. *C*, Anteversion is a forward tilting. *D*, Anteflexion is a forward bending.

Pathophysiology

Displacement or prolapse of the uterus, bladder, or rectum can be a congenital or an acquired condition. Congenital tilting or flexion of the uterus is rare. More commonly, tilting or flexion disorders in which the uterus remains within the pelvic cavity are related to the scarring and inflammation of pelvic inflammatory disease, endometriosis, pregnancy, and tumors.

Downward displacement of the pelvic organs into the vagina results from weakened pelvic musculature, usually attributable to stretching of the supporting ligaments and muscles during pregnancy and childbirth. Unrepaired lacerations from childbirth, rapid deliveries, multiple pregnancies, congenital weakness, or loss of elasticity and muscle tone with aging may contribute to these disorders.

Manifestations

The manifestations of displacement disorders are listed in the accompanying box.

Interdisciplinary Care

Interdisciplinary care focuses on identifying the cause of the structural disorder, correcting or minimizing the condition, relieving pain, preventing or treating infection, and supporting and educating the woman.

A careful history and physical examination are performed. Diagnosis of uterine displacement is made after physical examination. If herniation of the rectum or bladder is suspected, the woman is asked to bear down or cough during the examination so the prolapse can be palpated and any leakage of urine or feces visualized. A history of infections, multiple pregnancies in rapid succession, and rapid labors support this diagnosis.

Treatment may include Kegel exercises to strengthen weakened pelvic muscles. Kegel exercises can be useful in the early stages of downward displacement. These exercises are discussed in ∞ Chapter 27.

Surgery

Several surgical procedures are used to repair structural disorders. For women presenting with a cystocele, anterior colporrhaphy (repair of the cystocele) is the most common procedure. The anterior repair shortens the pelvic muscles, providing tighter support for the bladder. The Marshall-Marchetti-Krantz procedure involves resuspension of the urinary bladder in correct anatomic position. A rectocele is repaired with a posterior colporrhaphy, which shortens the pelvic muscles, providing a tighter support for the rectum. A prolapsed uterus may be surgically repositioned and the supporting muscles shortened to provide greater support. In postmenopausal women or women with procidentia, hysterectomy is the preferred treatment.

MANIFESTATIONS **of Displacement Disorders**

UTERINE DISPLACEMENT WITHIN THE PELVIC CAVITY
- Dysmenorrhea
- Dyspareunia
- Backache
- Infertility

UTERINE PROLAPSE
- Backache
- Bearing-down sensation
- Constipation
- Urinary incontinence
- Hemorrhoids
- Dyspareunia

CYTOCELE/RECTOCELE
- Bearing-down sensation
- Constipation
- Fecal incontinence
- Hemorrhoids
- Urinary incontinence

Figure 49–3 ■ Prolapse of the uterus can vary from mild to complete. In third-degree uterine prolapse, or procidentia, the uterus prolapses completely outside the body, with inversion of the vagina.

Source: M. English/Custom Medical Stock Photo.

Pessary

When surgery is contraindicated, a pessary (a removable device) may be inserted into the vagina to provide temporary support for the uterus or bladder. At regular intervals, the pessary is removed, cleaned, and reinserted.

✍ Nursing Care

Nursing care focuses on education about the disorder, proposed treatments, and self-care measures for relief of symptoms.

Nursing Diagnoses and Interventions

Nursing interventions for the woman with a displacement disorder address problems with urinary incontinence and anxiety.

Stress Incontinence

Relaxation of the pelvic floor can lead to stress incontinence. This can prove both troublesome and embarrassing and can increase the incidence of urinary tract infection.

- Teach Kegel exercises. *These exercises strengthen perineal muscle tone, minimize urinary leakage, and minimize descent of the bladder and rectum into the vagina. In postmenopausal women, estrogen supplements also can improve muscle tone in the perineal area.*
- Suggest the use of perineal pads (ranging from thin panty liners to full-thickness incontinence pads) or special underwear (such as Depends) to absorb urine leakage. *Using pads or undergarments often allows the woman to once again take part in her usual social activities.*
- Explain perineal care and proper use of perineal pads. *Cleansing the perineum from front to back and applying and removing perineal pads the same way minimizes cross infection from the anus to the vaginal and urethral openings.*

Incontinence pads need to be changed frequently to minimize surface bacterial counts.

- Suggest reducing or eliminating caffeine intake. *Reducing caffeine intake can reduce urinary frequency and urgency.*
- Stress the importance of cleaning the perineal area. *Urine is very irritating to the skin.*

Anxiety

Anxiety is common among women with a displacement disorder. Many women have only a cursory understanding of their reproductive anatomy. This lack of knowledge often compounds the anxiety. The nurse can use drawings and models to explain structural disorders and treatment options available.

- Encourage questions from the woman and her partner. *This helps assess the level of understanding so that teaching can be more effective.*
- Explain that the relief from discomfort and fatigue may positively influence sexual expression, and reassure the woman that the capacity for orgasm will not be affected. *Many women and their partners have major concerns about the effects of the disorder and its treatment on their sex life and capacity for sexual pleasure.*
- Explore coping mechanisms that have been previously successful. *This can help relieve anxiety and boost self-esteem.*

Community-Based Care

If surgery is the treatment of choice, teaching centers on what to expect in the preoperative and postoperative periods. If medical treatment is used initially, teaching focuses on measures to relieve the manifestations, such as Kegel exercises, use of incontinence pads, or the use, care, and insertion of a pessary. Because obesity is a risk factor associated with relaxation of the pelvic and abdominal muscles, dietary counseling may be indicated. Preoperatively, a diet high in fiber may alleviate constipation, a particular concern during the postoperative period.

The Woman with a Vaginal Fistula

A fistula is an abnormal opening or passage between two organs or spaces that are normally separated or an abnormal passage to the outside of the body. Vaginal fistulas may be vesicovaginal or rectovaginal. A vesicovaginal fistula is an abnormal opening between the urinary bladder and the vagina, leading to incontinent leakage of urine through the vagina. A rectovaginal fistula (less common) is an abnormal opening between the rectum and vagina, causing incontinent leakage of stool or flatus through the vagina.

Fistulas may develop as a complication of childbirth, gynecologic or urologic surgery, or radiation therapy for gynecologic cancer. Cancer of the bladder is sometimes involved. The woman with a vaginal fistula often presents with a complaint of involuntary leakage of urine or flatus and symptoms of infection.

Interdisciplinary Care

Fistulas are usually diagnosed by pelvic examination. Diagnosis of a vesicovaginal fistula can be made by instilling dye into the urinary bladder through a catheter and observing the vagina for leakage. If no leakage is detected, a tampon or vaginal pack is inserted into the vagina, and the woman is asked to ambulate. If an abnormal opening is present, the tampon will absorb the dye. Dye may also be injected intravenously because it is excreted by the kidneys. Urine and vaginal cultures may be performed to rule out infections. Antibiotics are administered if infection is present.

A small vaginal fistula may resolve spontaneously. Otherwise, surgery is performed after inflammation has subsided, often a period of several months. Rarely, in the presence of a large, highly inflamed rectovaginal fistula, a temporary colostomy is performed, allowing inflammation and irritation to subside (∞ see Chapter 24).

Nursing Care

Nursing care for the woman with repair of a vaginal fistula is similar to that for the woman with a displacement disorder. Teaching is an important component of nursing care. Stress the importance of careful perineal cleansing to reduce irritation and prevent further tissue breakdown. Suggest perineal irrigation or sitz baths for cleansing. Perineal pads or special underwear may be used to absorb urine or fecal drainage. For the woman with a rectovaginal fistula, provide information about avoiding gas-forming foods to minimize embarrassment from odor.

Disorders of Female Reproductive Tissue

Both benign and malignant tissue disorders affect the female reproductive system. Benign tumors and cysts include Bartholin's gland cysts, cervical polyps, endometrial cysts and polyps, ovarian cysts, and uterine leiomyomas (fibroids). Endometriosis is a condition in which endometrial tissue implants outside the uterus in various locations in the pelvic cavity. Malignant tumors of reproductive tissue include cervical cancer, endometrial cancer, ovarian cancer, and vulvar cancer.

The Woman with Cysts or Polyps

A cyst is a fluid-filled sac. A polyp is a highly vascular solid tumor attached by a pedicle or stem. Cysts or polyps of the female reproductive system can occur in the vulva, cervix, endometrium, or ovaries; depending on the type, they may occur at any age.

Pathophysiology

Following are different types of female reproductive tissue cysts and polyps:

- *Bartholin's gland cysts* are the most common cystic disorder of the vulva. These cysts are caused by the infection or obstruction of Bartholin's gland.
- *Cervical polyps* tend to occur in women over age 40 who have borne several children and have a history of using oral contraceptives. It is possible that cervical polyps develop from endocervical hyperplasia. The polyp develops at the vaginal end of the cervix, has a stem, and is highly vascular.
- *Endometrial cysts and polyps* are caused by endometrial overgrowth and are often filled with old blood (the dark color leads to the label "chocolate cysts"). Endometrial cysts are the result of endometrial implants on the ovary and are associated with endometriosis. Endometrial polyps, in contrast, are intrauterine overgrowths, similar to cervical polyps, and usually have a stalk.
- *Ovarian cysts* are classified as follicular cysts and corpus luteum cysts. Follicular cysts develop as a result of failure of the mature follicle to rupture or failure of an immature follicle to reabsorb fluid after ovulation. Corpus luteum cysts develop as a result of increased hormone secretion by the corpus luteum after ovulation. Most functional cysts regress spontaneously within two or three menstrual cycles.

- *Polycystic ovarian syndrome* (POS, also known as Stein-Leventhal syndrome) is an endocrine disorder characterized by an excess of androgens and a long-term lack of ovulation. The exact cause is unknown. As a part of the disease, as many as 8 to 10 cysts form in the ovaries from a failure to release ovum. Manifestations include amenorrhea or irregular menses, hirsutism, obesity, acne, hypertension, sleep apnea, and infertility. Women with POS often have insulin resistance and are at increased risk for type 2 diabetes, as well as heart disease, breast cancer, and endometrial cancer.

Manifestations and Complications

The causes and manifestations of benign cysts and polyps of the female reproductive system are presented in Table 49–1. Complications associated with these disorders include infection, rupture, infertility, hemorrhage, and recurrence.

Interdisciplinary Care

Care focuses on identifying and correcting the disorder and preventing its recurrence. A health history and physical examination are performed. Examination of the reproductive tract reveals the presence of most cysts and polyps. The menstrual history may include menstrual irregularities.

Diagnosis

Diagnostic tests that may be used to diagnose cysts and polyps of the female reproductive system (and to eliminate the diagnosis of cancer) include a Pap smear, an endometrial biopsy, a laparoscopy to visualize ovarian cysts, an ultrasound or x-ray to differentiate cysts from solid tumors, and/or a pregnancy test when luteal cysts are suspected. Laboratory analysis will demonstrate elevated LH and testosterone levels, as well as a reverse in FSH/LH in the woman with polycystic ovary syndrome (POS).

Medications

Antibiotics are used to treat infection or abscess, and oral contraceptives are used to promote regression of functional ovarian cysts. Clomiphene (Clomid, Serophene) may be prescribed to stimulate ovulation in the woman with POS who wishes to become pregnant. Dexamethasone (Decadron) suppresses ACTH and adrenal androgens, and may be added to increase the likelihood of ovulation.

TABLE 49–1 Benign Cysts and Polyps of the Female Reproductive System

SITE	TYPE	ETIOLOGIC ORIGIN	MANIFESTATIONS
Ovary	Functional cysts	Ovulation—include follicular cysts and corpus luteum cysts	May resolve spontaneously; can cause pain, menstrual irregularity, or amenorrhea
	Polycystic ovarian syndrome	Unknown; possible hypothalamic-pituitary dysfunction	Hirsutism, obesity; amenorrhea or irregular menses; hyperinsulinemia; infertility
Vulva	Bartholin's cysts	Obstruction or infection of Bartholin's gland	Pain, redness, perineal mass, dyspareunia
Endometrium	Chocolate cysts	Endometrial overgrowth; filled with old blood	
	Endometrial polyps	Unknown	Bleeding between periods
Cervix	Cervical polyps	Unknown	Bleeding after intercourse or after activities involving heavy lifting

Surgery

Cervical polyps are visible through a vaginal speculum and usually are removed with a clamp. A transcervical approach is used to remove endometrial cysts or polyps. The specimen is sent to the laboratory for evaluation, and chemical or electrical cauterization may be applied after cyst removal. For Bartholin's gland cysts and any abscesses, the lesion is incised and drained, and a drainage device is left in place. Follicular cysts may be punctured through laser surgery, or a wedge resection of the ovary may be performed to restore ovulation. Rarely, oophorectomy (removal of the ovary) is performed if ovarian cysts are very large.

✪ Nursing Care

Nursing care focuses on relieving pain and preventing recurrence and complications. Address the following topics for self-care at home:

- The condition, its treatment, and measures to relieve pain.
- The importance of keeping follow-up appointments.
- Manifestations of infection (for postsurgical care) and the need to notify the physician should they occur.
- If cervical polypectomy is performed, advise use of external pads for 1 week. The woman should be able to recognize that saturating more than one pad in an hour indicates the need for immediate follow-up.
- The importance of long-term follow-up care for the woman with POS.

The Woman with Leiomyoma

Leiomyomas (fibroids) are benign tumors that originate from smooth muscle of the uterus. They are the most common form of pelvic tumor, believed to occur in one of every four or five women older than 35 years of age. Fibroids are seen more often and grow more rapidly in Black women than they do in White women (Porth & Matfin, 2009).

Pathophysiology

The actual cause of fibroid tumors is not clearly understood, but there is a strong association with estrogen stimulation. Fibroid tumors usually develop in the uterine corpus, and may be intramural, subserous, or submucous (Figure 49–4 ■).

Intramural fibroid tumors (the most common type) are embedded in the myometrium. They usually present as an enlargement of the uterus. Subserous fibroid tumors lie beneath the serous lining of the uterus and project into the peritoneal cavity. They may become pedunculated (on a stem) and displace or compress other tissues, such as the ureter or bladder. Submucous fibroid tumors lie beneath the endometrial lining of the uterus. They displace endometrial tissue and are more likely to cause bleeding, infection, and necrosis than the other types.

Manifestations

Small tumors may be asymptomatic. The rate of growth varies, but they may increase in size during pregnancy or with use of oral contraceptives or HRT. Large fibroid tumors can crowd other organs, leading to pelvic pressure, pain, dysmenorrhea, menorrhagia, and fatigue. Depending on the location of the tumor, constipation and urinary urgency and frequency may occur.

Figure 49–4 ■ Types of uterine fibroid tumors (leiomyomas). Intramural fibroid tumors lie within the uterine wall. Subserous fibroid tumors lie beneath the serous lining of the uterus and project into the peritoneum. Submucous fibroid tumors lie beneath the endometrial lining of the uterus.

Interdisciplinary Care

Treatment of the woman with uterine fibroids depends on the size and location of the tumors, the severity of the manifestations, and her age and childbearing status. Most fibroids grow as a woman ages, then shrink after menopause. Tests used to diagnose uterine fibroids may include an ultrasound to differentiate leiomyoma from endometriosis and a laparoscopy to visualize subserosal leiomyomas. In asymptomatic women who wish to bear children, the fibroid tumors are monitored for growth.

Medications

There are no medications to permanently shrink fibroids. Heavy vaginal bleeding may be decreased by using birth control pills. Medications that stop ovarian production of estrogen and progesterone (hormones necessary for fibroid growth), may provide termpory decrease in manifestations. Injectable leuprolide acetate (Lupron) and nasal spray fluocinolone (Synaral) decrease bleeding and shrink the fibroids, but the tumors grow again when the medications are stopped. Long-term use of these medications is limited because of their side effects (hot flashes, vaginal dryness, and headaches) and significant risk of bone loss if treatment continues 6 months or more.

Surgery

Myomectomy, removal of the tumor without removing the entire uterus, is the surgical procedure of choice for young women who wish to retain reproductive capability. Laparoscopic laser technique is used for many women. A hysterectomy is performed if tumors are large, and if bleeding or other problems continue in perimenopausal women. A nonsurgical method of treatment is a uterine fibroid embolization. In this procedure, a catheter is guided through the femoral artery to the uterus, where tiny particles are injected into the artery supplying the fibroid to cut off the fibroid's blood supply. This procedure requires only an overnight hospital stay with a return to normal activities in 1 week.

ᨠ Nursing Care

If surgery is deferred, teaching emphasizes the importance of regular follow-up assessments to monitor tumor growth. If a hysterectomy is performed, teaching emphasizes appropriate preoperative and postoperative care. Dietary modifications to increase iron intake, prevent constipation, and promote healing are important.

The Woman with Endometriosis

Endometriosis is a condition in which multiple, small, usually benign implantations of endometrial tissue develop most commonly in the pelvic cavity, but also possibly in other areas of the body, such as the lungs. Endometriosis affects from 10% to 15% of women of childbearing age and is more common in women who postpone childbearing. Risk factors for endometriosis include early menarche, regular periods with a cycle of less than 27 days, menses lasting more than 7 days, heavier flow, increased menstrual pain, and a history of the condition in first-degree female relatives (Porth & Matfin, 2009).

Pathophysiology

The cause of endometriosis is unclear, but several theories have been proposed. The metaplasia theory asserts that endometrial tissue develops from embryonic epithelial cells as a result of hormonal or inflammatory changes. The theory of retrograde menstruation suggests that menstrual tissue backs up through the fallopian tubes during menses, implants on various pelvic structures, and survives. The transplantation theory asserts that endometrial implants spread via lymphatic or vascular routes.

The abnormally located endometrial tissue responds to cyclic ovarian hormone stimulation, and bleeding at the time of menstruation occurs at the sites of implantation. Scarring, inflammation, and adhesions may develop. Endometriosis is a slowly progressive disease, responsive to ovarian hormone stimulation. Thus, the implants regress during pregnancy and atrophy at menopause unless the woman is receiving HRT. Because progressive scarring may interfere with the ability to conceive, women with significant endometriosis are encouraged to have children early if they wish to do so.

Manifestations

Manifestations of endometriosis are summarized in the accompanying box.

Interdisciplinary Care

Endometriosis may be difficult to diagnose, but a history of dysmenorrhea, dyspareunia, and infertility strongly suggests this diagnosis. Interventions depend on the severity of symptoms, the extent of the disease, and the woman's age and desire for childbearing. Treatment goals focus on pain management and restoring fertility.

Diagnosis

Diagnostic tests are ordered to rule out other medical conditions and identify the endometrial implants. The tests include a pelvic ultrasound and laparoscopy (∞ see Chapter 47) as well as a CBC with differential to rule out pelvic abscesses and infectious processes. A low hemoglobin and hematocrit may be noted if menorrhagia accompanies endometriosis or tissue implants bleed significantly during menses.

Medications

A variety of medications may be used to decrease bleeding in and enlargement of the endometrial implants. Hormone therapy may include oral contraceptives. GnRH agonist therapy

---

MANIFESTATIONS of Endometriosis

- Heavy, throbbing pain of the lower abdomen and pelvis, radiating down the thighs and around the back. (The degree of pain, however, is not indicative of the severity of the disease.) Pain can begin 2 to 3 days prior to menses and last for several days.
- Feeling of rectal pressure and discomfort when having a bowel movement.
- Dyspareunia.
- Dysfunctional uterine bleeding.
- Infertility.

(GnRG-a) is used to lower estrogen, initiating a menopause-like state to shrink implants and reduce pain in most women. Oral or injectable progestin (such as Depo-Provera) increases progesterone levels similar to pregnancy, stopping ovulation and lowering estrogen to reduce the size of implants and relieve pain. Danazol, an anabolic steroid, suppresses release of FSH and LH by the pituitary to interrupt the cause of atrophy and involution of both normal and ectopic endometrial tissue. However, danazol may increase the risk of ovarian cancer and has masculinizing side effects. Aromatase inhibitors (aromatase, a protein responsible for producing estrogen, is found in the ovary, skin, adipose tissue, and ectopic endometrial tissue) used in combination with hormone therapy such as birth control pills or progestin have been shown to reduce pain and reoccurrence of endometrial growths. Long-term use of aromatase inhibitors may cause bone loss. Further information about these drugs is provided in the later discussion of hormone therapy used to treat endometrial cancer.

Surgery

Surgical interventions include laparoscopy with laser ablation (excision or removal) of endometrial implants or a total hysterectomy.

∞ Nursing Care

Nursing care includes providing pain relief, providing education about the condition and the treatment options, and helping the woman cope with treatment outcomes. The severity of the disease and its manifestations are not necessarily related. Advanced disease may exhibit few manifestations, whereas early disease may be quite painful. A Case Study & Nursing Care Plan for a woman with endometriosis is found on page 1694.

Nursing Diagnoses and Interventions

Interventions for pain, discussed previously, are also appropriate for the woman with endometriosis. A priority diagnosis for the young woman with this disorder is anxiety related to the risk for loss of reproductive function.

Anxiety

Anxiety about the unsure prognosis related to infertility is a particular problem for young women who plan to have a family in the future.

- Encourage expression of fears and anxiety about infertility, and answer questions honestly. *Knowledge helps relieve anxiety and fear.*
- Provide information on fertility awareness methods, including measurement of basal body temperature and other techniques for recognizing ovulation. *Understanding these techniques helps the woman and her partner optimize the conditions for conception.*

Using NANDA, NIC, and NOC

Linkages between a selected NANDA nursing diagnosis, NIC, and NOC for the patient with endometriosis are shown in the chart that follows.

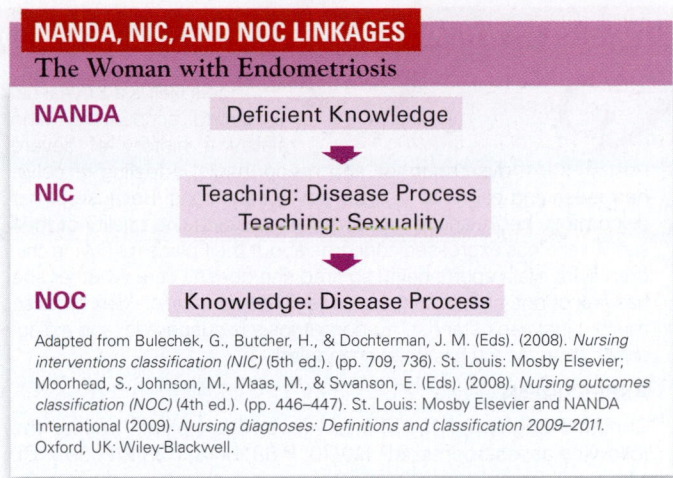

NANDA, NIC, AND NOC LINKAGES
The Woman with Endometriosis

NANDA	Deficient Knowledge
NIC	Teaching: Disease Process / Teaching: Sexuality
NOC	Knowledge: Disease Process

Adapted from Bulechek, G., Butcher, H., & Dochterman, J. M. (Eds). (2008). *Nursing interventions classification (NIC)* (5th ed.). (pp. 709, 736). St. Louis: Mosby Elsevier; Moorhead, S., Johnson, M., Maas, M., & Swanson, E. (Eds). (2008). *Nursing outcomes classification (NOC)* (4th ed.). (pp. 446–447). St. Louis: Mosby Elsevier and NANDA International (2009). *Nursing diagnoses: Definitions and classification 2009–2011.* Oxford, UK: Wiley-Blackwell.

Community-Based Care

Explain the cause of the disorder and the various treatment options, including their side effects. Discuss fertility awareness methods and the risks and benefits of long-term use of oral contraceptives. Stress the importance of exercise, smoking cessation, and weight control. If surgical treatment is chosen, provide preoperative and postoperative teaching.

The Woman with Cervical Cancer

Cancer of the cervix is the second most common cancer in women worldwide, and the 14th most common in women in the United States. The incidence is higher in Black women than in White women. Effective screening for cervical cancer with the Pap smear test and treatment of an existing malignancy have reduced the death rate during the last 30 years. Failure to have the recommended screenings and compliance with follow up care after colposcopic procedures has been identified as a leading reason for development of the disease.

Cervical Cancer Video

FAST FACTS
Cervical Cancer

- The American Cancer Society estimates that there will be more than 11,000 newly diagnosed cases and slightly more than 4000 deaths from cervical cancer each year.
- Cervical cancer is most often diagnosed women between the ages of 20 and 50; however, about 20% of women diagnosed with cervical cancer are over 65 (making regular Pap tests essential at any age).
- Cervical cancer occurs most often in Hispanic women; the rate is almost twice that of non-Hispanic White women.

(American Cancer Society, 2009a; 2009c)

Risk Factors

Risk factors for cervical cancer include infection of the external genitalia and anus with HPV, first intercourse before 16 years of age, multiple sex partners or male partners with multiple sex partners, a history of STIs, and infection with HIV. Infection with HPV is the most important risk factor for cancer of the cervix. Other risk factors include smoking and poor nutritional status, obesity, multiple pregnancies, long-term use of birth control pills, family history of cervical cancer, and exposure to diethylstilbestrol (DES) *in utero*.

Angela Hall is a 31-year-old married accountant, who relates a history of severe dysmenorrhea and menorrhagia, a feeling of pelvic heaviness and pain that radiates down her thighs. Because of her discomfort, her husband has complained about the quality of their sex life and has expressed concerns about their plans for having children. Mrs. Hall reports being so tired she doesn't care whether she has sex or not, and, in fact, would really prefer not to: "Sex hurts so much, I just can't stand it." Endometriosis is suspected, and a diagnostic laparoscopy has been scheduled.

ASSESSMENT

Christine Brigham, RN, NP, interviews Mrs. Hall and makes the following assessments: BP 110/70, P 68, R 18, T 98.2°F (36.7°C). Mrs. Hall's weight is 130 lb (59 kg) and within normal limits for her height. Review of laboratory findings indicate a hemoglobin level of 9.8 g/dL (normal range: 12 to 16 g/dL) and a hematocrit of 33.1% (normal range: 35% to 45%). Physical examination reveals pelvic tenderness on manipulation of the cervix, and small masses that are palpable on abdominal/pelvic examination.

DIAGNOSES

- *Chronic Pain* related to endometrial pelvic implants
- *Anxiety* related to effect of endometriosis on fertility
- *Deficient Knowledge* related to diagnosis and treatment options
- *Ineffective Sexuality Pattern* related to the manifestations of endometriosis

EXPECTED OUTCOMES

- Develop effective self-care measures to deal with the pain and discomfort.
- Verbalize decreased anxiety.
- Demonstrate understanding of the disease and treatment options.
- Verbalize an improvement in sexual functioning and a decrease in interpersonal stress between herself and her husband.

PLANNING AND IMPLEMENTATION

- Identify the location, type, duration, and history of the pain.
- Recommend analgesics and heat therapy.
- Provide information on biofeedback, relaxation, and imagery to lessen pain.
- Discuss with Mr. and Mrs. Hall the causes of endometriosis and its manifestations.
- Encourage the Halls to discuss their feelings about the effect of the disease on their sex life, lifestyle, and fertility.
- Refer the couple to the local mental health center if appropriate.

EVALUATION

Two years after the initiation of treatment, Mr. and Mrs. Hall have become parents of a baby girl. Mrs. Hall states that the discomfort and other manifestations of endometriosis have eased. Relaxation and imagery have effectively minimized her pain and brought about improvement in her function as wife, mother, and sexual partner. Counseling has improved the interpersonal and sexual relations between the Halls. Dietary management has improved her anemia, although the menorrhagia persists. The Halls are trying to have a second child, understanding the advantages of rapid succession of pregnancies. They will be followed in the nursing clinic and referred to an infertility clinic if conception does not occur within 1 year.

CRITICAL THINKING IN THE NURSING PROCESS

1. Explain the pathophysiologic basis for Mrs. Hall's anemia.
2. How would you handle the situation if Mr. and Mrs. Hall were extremely uncomfortable and embarrassed about discussing their sexual problems?
3. Develop a plan of care for Mrs. Hall for the nursing diagnosis *Situational Low Self-Esteem* related to the manifestations of endometriosis.

See Evaluating Your Response in Appendix C.

Pathophysiology

Most cervical cancers are squamous cell carcinomas that begin as neoplasia in the cervical epithelium. Precancerous dysplasia (cervical intraepithelial neoplasia [CIN], cervical carcinoma *in situ*) is estimated to occur in one of eight women before the age of 20 and is often associated with HPV infection. Studies have also found a strong association with reproductive infections with *Chlamydia trachomatis*. (These infections are discussed in ∞ Chapter 50.) The precursor lesions may spontaneously regress, persist, or progress and undergo malignant change. A very small percent become invasive (Porth & Matfin, 2009). Systems of grading of dysplastic changes in the cervix use the term cervical intraepithelial neoplasia (CIN) or the Bethesda system (Table 49–2). Carcinoma *in situ* is localized; invasive cancer spreads to deeper layers.

TABLE 49–2 Classification Systems for Pap Smears

DYSPLASIA/NEOPLASIA	CIN (CERVICAL INTRAEPITHELIAL NEOPLASIA)	BETHESDA SYSTEM	NUMERICAL
Benign	Benign	■ Normal	1
Benign with inflammation	Benign with inflammation	■ Normal ■ Atypical squamous cells of undetermined significance (ASCUS)	2
Moderate dysplasia	CIN I	■ Low-grade squamous intraepithelial lesion (SIL)	3
Severe dysplasia	CIN II	■ High-grade SIL	3
Carcinoma *in situ*	CIN III	■ High-grade SIL	4
Invasive cancer	Invasive cancer	■ Invasive cancer	5

Cervical cancer spreads by direct invasion of accessory structures, including the vaginal wall, pelvic wall, bladder, and rectum. Although metastasis is most frequently confined to the pelvic area, distant metastasis may occur through the lymphatic system.

Manifestations

Preinvasive cancer is limited to the cervix and rarely causes manifestations. Invasive cancer causes vaginal bleeding after intercourse or between menstrual periods and a bloody or brown vaginal discharge that increases as the cancer progresses. These changes are subtle, and may be more readily noticed by the postmenopausal woman. Manifestations of advanced disease include referred pain in the back or thighs, hematuria, bloody stools, anemia, and weight loss.

Interdisciplinary Care

The goals of treatment are to eradicate the cancer and minimize complications and metastasis. The type of treatment depends on the degree of malignant change, the size and location of the lesion, and the extent of metastasis.

Diagnosis

Tests used to diagnose cervical cancer include a Pap smear, colposcopy, and cervical biopsy (∞ see Chapter 47 for further information about these procedures). A loop diathermy technique (loop electrosurgical excision procedure [LEEP]) allows simultaneous diagnosis and treatment of dysplastic lesions found on colposcopy. This procedure is performed in the health provider's office, using a wire for both cutting and coagulation during excision of the dysplastic region of the cervix. An MRI or CT of the pelvis, abdomen, or bones may be performed to evaluate the spread of the tumor.

Medications

Chemotherapy is used for tumors not responsive to other therapy, tumors that cannot be removed, or as adjunct therapy if metastasis has occurred (∞ see Chapter 14).

Surgery

When combined with colposcopy, laser surgery is a viable treatment method if the cancer is limited to the cervical epithelium. Cryosurgery, which involves the use of a probe to freeze tissue, causing necrosis and sloughing, is also used for noninvasive lesions. Conization (Figure 49–5 ■) is performed to treat microinvasive carcinoma when colposcopy cannot define the limits of the invasion. For invasive lesions, hysterectomy or radical hysterectomy (removal of the uterus, fallopian tubes, lymph nodes, and ovaries) is performed.

A pelvic exenteration, the removal of all pelvic contents, including the bowel, vagina, and bladder, may be performed if the cancer recurs without involvement of the lymphatic system. An anterior exenteration is the removal of the uterus, ovaries, fallopian tubes, vagina, bladder, urethra, and lymphatic vessels and nodes. An ileal conduit is created for excretion of urine (∞ see Chapter 28). A posterior exenteration is the removal of the uterus, ovaries, fallopian tubes, bowel, and rectum. A

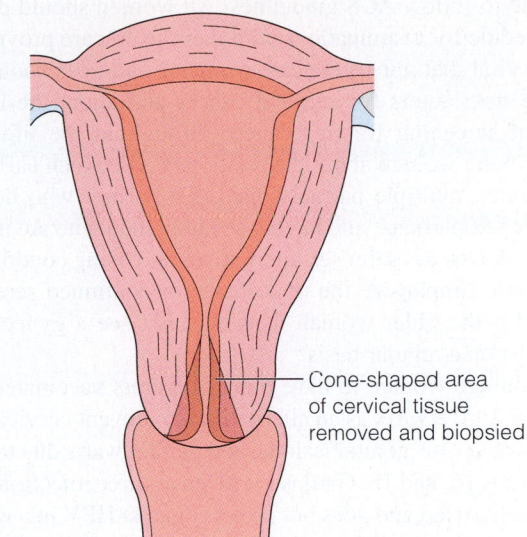

Cone-shaped area of cervical tissue removed and biopsied

Figure 49–5 ■ Conization, the surgical removal of a cone-shaped section of the cervix, is used to treat microinvasive carcinoma of the cervix.

colostomy is created for excretion of feces (∞ see Chapter 24). This is an extensive procedure with many possible complications, and it requires a lengthy recovering period

Radiation Therapy

Radiation therapy is used to treat invasive cervical cancer. External radiation beam therapy and intracavitary cesium irradiation can be used. Radiation is discussed in ∞ Chapter 14.

∞ Nursing Care

Nursing care involves helping the woman cope with the physical and psychologic effects of a potentially life-threatening illness, providing information needed to make informed decisions, and minimizing the adverse effects of therapy. Pain relief measures are important, as is grief work on the part of the woman and family. The woman should be encouraged to perform self-care activities and resume normal everyday activities and sexual functioning to the extent possible. A Case Study & Nursing Care Plan for a woman with cervical cancer is found on page 1697.

Health Promotion

The ACS (2009b) recommends that a woman should begin annual screening for cervical cancer with the Pap test about 3 years after she begins having vaginal intercourse, but no later than 21 years of age. The most recent guidelines from the American College of Obstetricians and Gynecologists say that most women in their 20s can have Pap tests every 2 years instead of annually. Cervical cancer screening with HPV DNA tests and Pap tests may be performed every 3 years for the woman over age 30. Women 70 years of age and older who have had three or more normal Pap smears in the last 10 years may choose to stop cervical cancer screening. Screening for women who have had a total hysterectomy (including the cervix) is not recommended unless the surgery was done as a treatment for cancer. Women who have a hysterectomy without removal of the cervix should continue to follow ACS guidelines. All women should discuss the schedule for examinations with their healthcare provider.

It is vital that nurses educate women of all ages about controlling risk factors for cervical cancer and about the importance of screening for this cancer throughout the life span. Teach young women about the relationship between early sexual activity, multiple partners, having a partner who has had multiple sex partners, and having sex with men who are not circumcised. Discuss safer sex alternatives and using condoms for protection. Emphasize the importance of continued screening exams for the older woman who may not see a gynecologic specialist on a regular basis.

Encourage women to have their daughters vaccinated with Gardasil (or Cervarix as an alternative) to prevent cervical cancer, precancerous genital lesions, and genital warts due to HPV types 6, 11, 16, and 18. Gardasil is given as three injections over a 6-month period and does not protect against HPV in a woman already infected. For this reason, a federal advisory panel is recommending that the vaccine be routinely given to girls ages 11 and 12 and catch-up vaccines to girls aged 13 to 18. Evidence is inconclusive regarding vaccination for all women aged 19 to 26. Women and parents of pre-teen and teenage girls should discuss risks and benefits with their physicians (ACS, 2009b). There has been controversy around the issue of vaccination for a sexually transmitted disease even though it prevents cancer. Many parents fear if they permit vaccination they are promoting premarital sex. Educating parents about the risks and the progression of HPV is important to insure girls are permitted to receive the vaccination. Legislation to mandate vaccination for HPV is pending in many states. Nurses should become familiar with and advocate for health-related legislation.

Assessment

Collect the following data through a health history and physical examination (∞ see Chapter 47):

- *Health history:* History of STIs, sexual history, partner's sexual history, family history of cervical cancer, vaginal bleeding or discharge, smoking history, maternal treatment with DES.
- *Physical assessment:* Pelvic examination, abdomen, lymph glands.

EVIDENCE FOR NURSING CARE | **The Patient with Cervical Cancer**

Selected resources that nurses may find helpful when planning evidence-based nursing care follow.

- Clemmens, D. A., Knafl, K., Lev, E. L., & McCorkle, R. (2008). Cervical cancer: Patterns of long-term survival. *Oncology Nursing Forum, 35*(6), 897–903.
- Lindsey, K., Decristofaro, C., & James, J. (2009). Anal pap smears: Should we be doing them? *Journal of the American Academy of Nurse Practitioners, 21*(8), 437–443.
- Siddiqui, N., Allam, M., Beattie, G., Connor, R., Cruickshank, M., Downs, F., et al. (2008). Management of cervical cancer. *National Guideline Clearinghouse.* Retrieved from http://www.guideline.gov/summary/summary.aspx?doc_id=12110&nbr=006233&string=lymphedema

Nursing Diagnoses and Interventions

This section discusses nursing interventions for the woman who has been diagnosed with cervical cancer and requires surgical and/or radiation treatment. Other nursing diagnoses and interventions that may be appropriate for the woman with cervical cancer are discussed in the sections discussing other female reproductive system cancers.

Fear

Many people believe that cancer equals death; however, this is no longer true in many cases, especially with early diagnosis. For cervical cancer that is diagnosed at an early stage, the 5-year survival rate is about 71% (ACS, 2009b).

- Explain that many women with cervical cancer survive for 5 years or more and that the earlier the cancer is detected, the better the prognosis. *This gives the woman hope, an essential ingredient in recovery.*
- Allow adequate time for the woman and her partner to express their concerns and to ask questions. *Unexpressed feelings and fears and lack of understanding may cause the woman to view the situation as worse than it is.*
- Refer to a cancer counselor or support group for additional information. *Cancer survivors who visit patients in the hospital provide proof that people can survive the diagnosis and treatment of cancer and lead normal, productive lives.*

Impaired Tissue Integrity

Surgery interrupts the integrity of the skin surface, providing a potential portal of invasion for bacteria. Radiation therapy causes an inflammatory response in the skin and mucous membranes within the field of radiation, creating further risk of tissue reaction and breakdown.

- Teach wound and skin care, particularly if pelvic exenteration is performed. Irrigations with saline or solutions of saline and hydrogen peroxide are performed at intervals, with dry heat applied thereafter to dry the area. *Open and damaged tissue increases the risk for infection. Meticulous skin and wound care is necessary to prevent infection and further tissue destruction.*
- If appropriate, teach stoma care, and care for the skin surrounding the stoma. (These procedures are discussed in ∞ Chapters 24 and 28.) *Urine and stool are irritating to the skin. Without proper care, the skin surrounding the stoma can become excoriated.*
- Apply non-oil-based lotions to skin surface. This may minimize itching and help maintain integrity. *Oil-based lotions are not recommended for tissue undergoing radiation.*
- Instruct the woman not to remove the markings used to localize the radiation beam to the target area. *Markings are used in future radiation treatments.*
- Monitor for evidence of fistula formation, and teach the woman to do the same. *Fistula formation is a potential complication of radiation to the pelvic or abdominal cavities. Vaginal fistulas may form between the vagina and the bladder or rectum. Fistulas may also develop between the bladder and rectum, resulting in the expulsion of stool in the urine or loss of urine through the anus.*

CASE STUDY & NURSING CARE PLAN   A Woman with Cervical Cancer

Anna Eliza Gillam is a 45-year-old divorced mother of four children ranging in age from 16 to 23. She was married at age 18 and had several sexual partners prior to her marriage. She has had three sexual partners since her marriage ended. Last year she was treated with cryosurgery for venereal warts. The Pap smear taken 2 weeks ago showed atypical cells, and she has come in for a repeat test.

ASSESSMENT

Judy Davis, RN, FNP, the admitting nurse, interviews Ms. Gillam and records the following assessment findings: BP 130/80, P 72, R 18, T 99.2°F (37.3°C). Ms. Gillam weighs 142 lb (64.5 kg). Examination of the cervix reveals a large necrotic lesion at the 7 o'clock position. She has reduced her smoking to fewer than 10 cigarettes per day, and she does not drink alcohol.

Ms. Gillam is extremely fearful and anxious and has told no one about her abnormal Pap smear. She reveals that she has had back pain radiating down her thighs for several months and a foul vaginal discharge that increases after intercourse. Until 2 weeks ago, she had not had a Pap smear for 5 years. Ms. Davis performs the repeat Pap smear, which is positive for squamous cell carcinoma of the cervix. A CT scan and lymphangiography are scheduled. Laparoscopy shows the disease to be widespread in the pelvic cavity.

DIAGNOSES

- *Decisional Conflict* related to treatment options
- *Acute Pain* related to metastasis and surgery
- *Risk for Impaired Skin Integrity* related to radiation
- *Fear* related to diagnosis of cervical cancer
- *Grieving* related to potential loss of life

EXPECTED OUTCOMES

- Gain knowledge to make informed decisions about treatment options.
- Develop strategies for pain control.
- Maintain skin and tissue integrity during radiation treatment.
- Express her feelings about the fear of cancer and death.
- Develop effective coping strategies for dealing with life-threatening illness and pain.

PLANNING AND IMPLEMENTATION

- Discuss treatment alternatives, including the prognosis with each option.
- Administer pain medications as prescribed.
- Inspect skin surfaces daily before and after radiation therapy.
- Provide information on biofeedback training and relaxation techniques for control of moderate pain.
- Assess for and assist with referrals for spiritual counseling as this has been shown to improve coping with life-altering cancer.
- Refer to a local cancer support group so that she can interact with cancer survivors.
- Refer Ms. Gillam to a social worker in preparation for her altered level of functioning.

EVALUATION

Ms. Gillam has begun radiation therapy following pelvic exenteration. She controls her pain with relaxation and imagery techniques, requiring only occasional analgesics. She uses a water-based lotion to soothe the skin surface and is careful not to remove the skin markings. She seems optimistic and has quit smoking. She and her family have continued to attend the cancer support group meetings. Ms. Gillam is planning for the future and has talked with her family about what it means to live with cancer.

CRITICAL THINKING IN THE NURSING PROCESS

1. Compare and contrast your teaching plan for health promotion interventions to decrease the risks of cervical cancer for a young woman of 17 and an older woman of 70. Would they differ and, if so, how?
2. Develop a teaching plan to help Ms. Gillam cope with the effects of radiation.
3. During a home visit, Ms. Gillam tells the nurse that she has been so tired since beginning radiation treatments that all she can do is sit in her chair. Design a plan of care for the nursing diagnosis *Fatigue*.

See Evaluating Your Response in Appendix C.

Using NANDA, NIC, and NOC

Linkages between a selected NANDA nursing diagnosis, NIC, and NOC for the patient with cervical cancer are shown in the chart that follows.

NANDA, NIC, AND NOC LINKAGES
The Woman with Cervical Cancer

NANDA	Risk for Infection

NIC	Infection Control Surgical Precautions Chemotherapy Management

NOC	Infection Risk

Adapted from Bulechek, G., Butcher, H., & Dochterman, J. M. (Eds). (2008). *Nursing interventions classification (NIC)* (5th ed.). (pp. 213-214, 428–431, 694). St. Louis: Mosby Elsevier; Moorhead, S., Johnson, M., Maas, M., & Swanson, E. (Eds). (2008).(p. 782). *Nursing outcomes classification (NOC)* (4th ed.). St. Louis: Mosby Elsevier; and NANDA International. (2009). *Nursing diagnoses: Definitions and classification 2009–2011.* Oxford, UK: Wilely-Blackwell.

Community-Based Care

Teaching varies according to the stage of the cancer and the treatment selected. Provide information concerning radiation, chemotherapy, or surgery, as indicated. Preoperative teaching focuses on postoperative expectations, including management of urinary or fecal diversion, if indicated. Help the woman and family recognize signs of infection and understand the importance of follow-up care. In addition, suggest the following resources: the American Cancer Society, the National Cancer Institute, and the Women's Cancer Network.

The Woman with Endometrial Cancer

Endometrial cancer is the most frequently diagnosed pelvic cancer in the United States. The ACS (2009a) estimates that each year more than 42,000 women are diagnosed with endometrial cancer, and more than 7800 women die annually from this disease. Most endometrial cancer is diagnosed in older women, with more than half of the cases diagnosed in women between the ages of 55 and 74. The incidence of endometrial cancer is higher in White women, but Black women are more likely to die from it. The overall 5-year survival rate is about 83%, but if found and treated early in the disease, that rate increases to over 95% (ACS, 2009c).

Risk Factors

Significant risk factors for endometrial cancer are prolonged estrogen stimulation and obesity. Recent studies report that obesity was a factor in 70% of early stage endometrial diagnoses (Sorosky, 2008). Other factors that increase risk are anovulatory menstrual cycles, increased number of menstrual cycles during one's lifetime, a high fat diet, having cancer of the breast or ovary, prior radiation therapy of the pelvic region, atypical endometrial hyperplasia, decreasing ovarian function (as from menopause), estrogen-secreting tumors, and unopposed estrogen (e.g., estrogen therapy without progesterone) (ACS, 2009c). Medical conditions that may alter estrogen metabolism and increase the risk of endometrial cancer are diabetes mellitus, hypertension, and polycystic ovary disease (Porth & Matfin, 2009). Tamoxifen, a drug that blocks estrogen receptor sites and is used to treat breast cancer, has a weak estrogenic effect on the endometrium, and is also a risk factor. Endometrial cancer is the most commonly inherited gynecologic cancer. A family history of hereditary nonpolyposis colon cancer (HNPCC) may mean that a woman has an inherited mutation that is a mismatch of repair genes, and has a 40%–60% risk of developing endometrial cancer (ACS, 2009c). The risk for endometrial cancer is decreased by using birth control pills, using an intrauterine device (IUDs) without hormones to prevent pregnancy and having multiple pregnancies.

Pathophysiology

Most endometrial malignancies are adenocarcinomas that are slow to grow and metastasize. These cancers develop in the glandular cells or endometrial lining of the uterus (the same tissue that is shed each month during a normal menstrual period). Endometrial hyperplasia (excessive growth) is a precursor of endometrial cancer. A second and much less common type of tumor is not estrogen driven, and occurs primarily in older menopausal women. These tumors are associated with endometrial atrophy and have a poorer prognosis (Porth & Matfin, 2009).

Tumor growth usually begins in the fundus, invades the vascular myometrium, and spreads throughout the female reproductive tract. Metastasis occurs by means of the lymphatic system, through the fallopian tubes to the peritoneal cavity, and to the rest of the body via the bloodstream. Target areas for metastasis include the lungs, liver, and bone. The International Federation of Gynecology and Obstetrics (FIGO) classification of endometrial cancer is outlined in Table 49–3.

Manifestations

The major manifestation of endometrial hyperplasia or overt endometrial cancer is abnormal, painless vaginal bleeding. In menstruating women, this bleeding is manifested as menorrhagia or metrorrhagia. In postmenopausal women, any bleeding is abnormal. Later manifestations include pelvic cramping, bleeding after intercourse, and lower abdominal pressure. In advanced disease, lymph node enlargement, pleural effusion, abdominal masses, and ascites may be present.

TABLE 49–3 FIGO Staging Classification for Endometrial Cancer

STAGE	DESCRIPTION
I	Tumor limited to endometrium or myometrium
II	Endocervical glandular involvement or invasion of cervical stroma
III	Metastasis or invasion of serosa, adnexa, vagina, and pelvic or para-aortic lymph nodes
IV	Tumor invasion of bladder or bowel mucosa; distant metastases

Interdisciplinary Care

The goals of care for the woman with endometrial cancer are to eradicate the cancer and minimize complications and metastasis. Following diagnosis, there are four basic types of treatment for endometrial cancer: surgery, radiation therapy, hormonal therapy, and chemotherapy.

Diagnosis

Tests used to diagnose cancer of the endometrium include a transvaginal ultrasound, used to determine endometrial thickening, which may indicate hypertrophy or malignant changes, or an endometrial biopsy or a D&C to provide tissue for a definitive diagnosis (∞ see Chapter 47 for further information). Other tests to determine the extent of the disease include chest x-ray, cystoscopy and intravenous pyelogram (IVP) to examine the urinary system, proctoscopy (to assess the rectum), tests to look for cancer cells and tissue changes (CT scan, PET, MRI), bone scans to look for metastasis, CBC (to identify anemia from bleeding), and a CA 125 blood test (a substance that is released into the blood stream by many, but not all, endometrial and ovarian cancers).

Surgery

After the diagnosis is confirmed, a total abdominal hysterectomy and bilateral salpingo-oophorectomy is performed for stage I cancer. A radical hysterectomy with node dissection is performed if the disease is stage II or beyond.

Radiation Therapy

Treatment with external and internal radiation may be performed as a preoperative measure or as adjuvant treatment in advanced cases.

Hormone Therapy

Hormone therapy uses hormones or hormone blocking drugs. They include the following:

- Progestins are progesterone-like drugs. Those used most commonly are medroxyprogesterone acetate (Provera, given by injection or orally) and megestrol acetate (Megace, given orally). These slow the growth of cancer cells. Side effects include hot flashes, night sweats, and weight gain. The drugs increase blood glucose levels in women with diabetes, and may rarely cause serious blood clots.
- Tamoxifen is an anti-estrogen drug also often used to treat breast cancer. It is useful against endometrial cancer as it prevents estrogens from stimulating growth of cancer cells. It does not cause bone loss, but can cause hot flashes and

vaginal dryness; there is additionally an increased risk for serious blood clots in the legs.

- Gonadotropin-releasing hormone agonists lower estrogen levels. Examples are goserelin (Zoladex) and leuprolide (Lupron). These drugs are injected every 1 to 3 months. Side effects are menopausal manifestations, and with long term use, osteoporosis.
- Aromatase inhibitors stop estrogen from being formed to lower estrogen levels. Examples include letrozole (Femara), anastrozole (Arimidex), and exemestane (Aromasin). Often used to treat breast cancer, these drugs are also believed to be helpful in treating endometrial cancer. They may be taken for years, may cause osteoporosis, and are still being studied.

Chemotherapy

A combination of drugs may be used to treat endometrial cancer, including doxorubicin (Adriamycin), cisplatin, carboplatin, and paclitaxel (Taxol) (ACS, 2009c). Two or more drugs are often combined for treatment. Chemotherapy is discussed in detail in ∞ Chapter 14.

Nursing Care

Health Promotion

All perimenopausal and postmenopausal women need annual pelvic examinations. The ACS recommends that at the time of menopause all women be informed of the risks and manifestations of endometrial cancer and strongly encouraged to report any unexpected bleeding or spotting to their healthcare provider. Those in high-risk groups are advised to have endometrial biopsies every 2 years, beginning at age 35. In addition, control of diseases such as diabetes mellitus and hypertension decrease the risk of endometrial hyperplasia.

Assessment

Collect the following data through a health history and physical examination (∞ see Chapter 47):

- *Health history:* Abnormal vaginal bleeding, menstrual history, use of estrogen (without progesterone) to treat menopausal symptoms, breast cancer treated with tamoxifen, childbearing status, presence of chronic illnesses, family history of hereditary nonpolyposis colon cancer.
- *Physical assessment:* Height and weight, pelvic examination, abdomen, lymph glands.

Nursing Diagnoses and Interventions

Nursing care involves helping the woman cope with the physical and psychologic effects of a potentially life-threatening illness, make informed decisions, and minimize the adverse effects of therapy. Pain relief is a key component of care, as is grief work on the part of the woman and family. Encourage the woman to perform self-care and resume normal activities of daily living.

Acute Pain

A total abdominal hysterectomy can result in severe and prolonged pain, not only from the surgical incision but also from the manipulation of internal organs during surgery. Abdominal viscera are highly vascular and easily bruised by handling.

- Administer analgesics as ordered. *Analgesics provide pain relief and promote early ambulation.*
- Encourage ambulation. *Ambulation facilitates the expulsion of flatus, which can cause distention as well as discomfort.*
- Apply heat to the abdomen, and recommend that the woman use a heating pad at home. *Heat dilates blood vessels, increasing blood supply to the pelvis, decreasing pain.*

Disturbed Body Image

For many women, the side effects of cancer treatment can be almost as difficult and painful as the disease itself. Although side effects of the different therapies vary among individuals, the woman's body image and quality of life are always affected. Such side effects as alopecia (hair loss), nausea, vomiting, fatigue, diarrhea, stomatitis, and surgical scarring disturb body image.

- Review the side effects of the treatment regimen proposed, and assist the woman to develop a plan to deal with these effects. *This promotes a sense of control.*
- Remind the woman and family that side effects are usually manageable and may be temporary. *Over-the-counter agents can be used to alleviate stomatitis. Frequent rest periods can relieve fatigue. Medications can be prescribed for nausea, vomiting, and diarrhea.*

Ineffective Sexuality Pattern

Altered sexuality may result from a feeling of unattractiveness, fatigue, or pain and discomfort. The woman's partner may fear that sexual activity will be harmful.

- Encourage expression of feelings about the effect of cancer on their lives and sexual relationship. *Verbalizing feelings helps relieve stress and maximizes relaxation.*
- Suggest that the couple explore alternative sexual positions and coordinate sexual activity with rest periods and times that are relatively free from pain. *This creates a more favorable environment for satisfying sexual activity.*

Community-Based Care

The American Cancer Society recommends that, at the time of menopause, all women should be told about the risks and manifestations of endometrial cancer. They should be strongly encouraged to report any unexpected bleeding to their healthcare provider. Women with or at risk for hereditary nonpolyposis colon cancer should be offered annual screening for endometrial cancer with endometrial biopsy beginning at age 35.

Provide information about the specific treatment and prognosis. Explain the expected side effects of treatment used (∞ see Chapter 14). Pain control measures are also an essential part of the teaching plan (∞ see Chapter 9). The resources listed for the woman with cervical cancer are also appropriate for the woman with endometrial cancer.

The Woman with Ovarian Cancer

Ovarian cancer is the fourth most common gynecologic cancer in women in the United States. Approximately 21,500 women are diagnosed with ovarian cancer and an estimated 14,600 deaths result each year (ACS, 2009a). The cancer primarily develops in older women, with about two/thirds of the cases diagnosed in women aged 55 or older. Ovarian cancer is more common in White women than in other races (ACS, 2009d).

Risk Factors

Ten percent of cases of ovarian cancer have two or more first or second-degree relatives who have had the disease. Other types of inherited risks are genetic mutations such as those in BRCAI and BRCAII (breast and ovarian cancer) and Lynch syndrome (colorectal cancer). Women with a Lynch syndrome mutation have a 10% higher risk of developing ovarian cancer (Newton, et al., 2009; Lee-May, et al., 2007).

Risk factors also include increasing age, having no children or giving birth after age 35, early menarche and late menopause, infertility drugs, obesity, eating a high fat diet, and a personal history of breast cancer. There is also a possibility that polycystic ovarian disease and hormone replacement therapy after menopause may place a woman at risk. Protective factors include long-term contraceptive use, a low-fat diet, having a child before the age of 25, tubal ligation, breast-feeding, and hysterectomy (ACS, 2009d; Bohenkamp, LeBaron, & Yoder, 2007).

Pathophysiology

There are several types of ovarian cancers: epithelial tumors, germ cell tumors, and gonadal stromal tumors. Most ovarian cancers are epithelial tumors, originating from the surface epithelium of the ovary. Ovarian cancer usually spreads by local shedding of cancer cells into the peritoneal cavity and by direct invasion of the bowel and bladder. Cancer cells in peritoneal fluid can implant in the intestines, bladder, and mesentery. Tumor cells also spread through the lymph and blood to such organs as the liver, and across the diaphragm to involve the lungs. Both pelvic and para-aortic lymph nodes may be involved and tumor cells can block lymphatic drainage from the abdomen, resulting in ascites. Staging for ovarian cancer is based on surgical and histologic evaluation (Table 49–4).

Manifestations

In early stages, ovarian cancer generally causes no warning signs or manifestations. When manifestations do develop, they are often vague and mild, such as feeling full quickly, abdominal bloating, urinary urgency and/or frequency, and pelvic or abdominal pain. Other manifestations include fatigue, back pain, pain during intercourse, constipation, and menstrual changes in women prior to menopause. Abnormal vaginal bleeding may occur if the endometrium is stimulated by a hormone-secreting tumor or if the tumor erodes the vaginal wall. An enlarged abdomen with ascites signals later stage disease.

TABLE 49–4 FIGO Staging Classification for Ovarian Cancer

STAGE	DESCRIPTION
I	Growth limited to the ovaries
II	Growth involving one or both ovaries with pelvic extension
III	Tumor involving one or both ovaries, with peritoneal implants outside the pelvis or positive retroperitoneal or inguinal nodes
IV	Growth involving one or both ovaries with distant metastasis

Complications

The complications of advanced ovarian cancer, with related assessments and treatment, are outlined in Table 49–5.

Interdisciplinary Care

As with other malignancies, care of the woman with ovarian cancer involves surgery to determine the stage of the tumor and to remove as much of the tumor as possible. Unfortunately, because there are no specific early manifestations, the disease may be well advanced prior to diagnosis. In younger women, an ovarian mass may be monitored for several menstrual cycles, but any ovarian mass must immediately be investigated in a postmenopausal woman. The treatment involves three modalities: surgery, chemotherapy, and radiation therapy.

Diagnosis

Tests used in the diagnosis of ovarian cancer may include transvaginal or abdominal ultrasound, a CT scan of the abdomen and pelvis, an MRI of the abdomen, a PET scan, a laparoscopy, a colonoscopy, and/or an ovarian biopsy (∞ see Chapter 47 for further information about diagnostic tests). The blood test most useful is a CA-125 antigen level. CA-125 is a tumor marker that is highly specific and elevated in epithelial ovarian cancer. Research is ongoing to develop a blood test to specifically identify ovarian cancer.

Surgery

In young women with stage I disease who wish to have children, treatment may be limited to removal of one ovary. Usually, however, total hysterectomy with bilateral salpingo-oophorectomy (removal of the ovaries and fallopian tubes) is performed. Depending on the stage of the cancer and the woman's general state of health, surgery is combined with chemotherapy and radiation therapy.

Chemotherapy

Combination chemotherapy, discussed in ∞ Chapter 14, is primarily used following surgery.

Radiation Therapy

Radiation therapy using external-beam or intracavitary implants is performed for palliative purposes only and is directed at shrinking the tumor at selected sites.

EVIDENCE FOR NURSING CARE — The Patient with Ovarian Cancer

Selected resources that nurses may find helpful when planning evidence-based nursing care follow.

- Hamilton, R., Williams, J. K., Skirton, H., & Bowers, B. J. (2009). Living with genetic test results for hereditary breast and ovarian cancer. *Journal of Nursing Scholarship, 41*(3), 276–283.
- Hereditary breast and ovarian cancer syndrome. (2009). *American College of Obstetricians and Gynecologists (ACOG) Committee on Practice Bulletins – Gynecology.* Retrieved from http://www.guideline.gov/summary/summary.aspx?view_id=1&doc_id=14336
- Mor, P., & Oberle, K. (2008). Ethical issues related to BRCA gene testing in Orthodox Jewish women. *Nursing Ethics, 15*(4), 512–522.

TABLE 49–5 Complications of Advanced Ovarian Cancer

COMPLICATION	ASSESSMENTS	TREATMENT
Ascites (accumulation of fluid in the abdominal cavity; a form of third spacing)	■ Abdominal distention ■ Shiny abdominal skin ■ Dullness on percussion of dependent areas ■ Dyspnea, constipation ■ Abdominal pain	Paracentesis (removing fluid from the abdomen)
Intestinal obstruction	■ Abdominal distention ■ Abdominal pain ■ Projectile vomiting ■ Constipation ■ Hyperactive bowel sounds	Nasogastric tube insertion, NPO
Deep venous thrombosis	■ Leg edema ■ Leg pain ■ Redness, warmth	Anticoagulants
Lymphedema (leg)	■ Edema of leg ■ Decreased range of motion ■ Tight, shiny skin on leg	Skin care, range-of-motion exercises, massage or physical therapy, compression bandaging

Nursing Care

Although individualized to each woman, nursing care is essentially the same as nursing care for women with other gynecologic cancers. However, research (Lockwood-Rayermann, Donovan, Rambo, & Chien-Wen, 2009) findings support the need for education, as awareness of ovarian cancer manifestations and risk factors in the general population is low. The side effects of treatment of cancer and generally poor prognosis diminish the woman's quality of life and involve major psychosocial implications (∞ see Chapter 14).

Community-Based Care

Address the following topics in preparing the woman and her family for self-care:

■ If a positive family history of breast, ovarian, or colon cancer exists, stress the importance of obtaining regular pelvic examinations. Inform women in this risk group that annual screening with transvaginal ultrasound and CA-125 measurements may be recommended.
■ It is crucial not to ignore manifestations such as indigestion, nausea, or urinary frequency, because these seemingly unrelated manifestations may be early signs of ovarian tumors. Emphasize that ovarian cancer may be asymptomatic in early stages.
■ Discuss treatment options and their side effects and provide information on ways to minimize or manage side effects.
■ Refer to hospice services when appropriate. The resources suggested for the woman with cervical cancer are also appropriate for the woman with ovarian cancer.

The Woman with Cancer of the Vulva

Cancer of the vulva is a relatively rare malignancy, accounting for about 0.6% of all female cancers. It occurs most often in women over 50 years of age, with half of all cases being in women over age 70 (ACS, 2009e). The prognosis of vulvar carcinoma depends on the degree of invasion, general health status of the woman, presence of chronic diseases, and ability to withstand treatment.

The cause of vulvar cancer is unknown, but there is evidence to associate it with STIs, particularly HPV. Nearly 85% of malignant and premalignant cervical and vulvar lesions have been found to contain HPV DNA, HPV structural antigens, or both. Herpes simplex type 2 (HSV2) infection and with a history of leukoplakia (a precancerous lesion on the vulvar mucous membranes characterized by raised white patches) have also been associated with vulvar cancer. Other risk factors include smoking, HIV, precancerous lesions (vulvar intraepithelial neoplasia [VIN]), other genital cancers, and presence of melanoma or other atypical moles.

Most vulvar cancers are epidermoid or squamous cell carcinomas. The primary site is usually the labia majora, but vulvar cancer is also found on the labia minora, clitoris, vestibule, and occasionally in multiple locations. Metastasis occurs by direct extension into the vagina, perineal skin, anus, and urethra. The cancer also spreads through the lymphatic system via the superficial and deep inguinal and femoral nodes, and to the pelvic lymph nodes.

The manifestations of vulvar cancer include pruritus, wart-like growths, patchy changes in color or density of the vulva, vaginal bleeding, dysuria, or changes in a mole on the vulva. Inguinal lymph nodes may be enlarged. If lesions are present, they are biopsied. Imiquimod, which is an immune response modifier used in the treatment of HPV warts, has recently shown positive results in reducing neoplasia; however, surgical resection is the usual treatment (van Seters et al., 2008). If lymph nodes are involved, radiation therapy is used postoperatively. Chemotherapy is reserved for distant metastases.

Nursing care is similar to that for the woman with endometrial cancer. The woman fears death as the ultimate outcome as well as the possible pain and suffering that surgery and other treatments may cause. Radical surgery represents a great loss to women of all ages.

Disorders of the Breast

Mammography Video

Breast disorders are common conditions that primarily affect women (disorders of the male breast are discussed in ∞ Chapter 48). When a woman discovers a breast lump, her first response is often fear: of breast cancer, of losing her breast, and perhaps of losing her life. Because American society views the breast as a significant component of feminine beauty, any problem that threatens the breast often strikes at the core of a woman's self-image.

Nurses play a critical role in the care of women experiencing breast disorders by providing education, support, and advocacy. Part of the nurse's role is educating women about normal breast tissue, common benign breast disorders, screening recommendations, and risk factors for breast cancer.

The Woman with a Benign Breast Disorder

Benign changes in a woman's breast tissue often correspond to hormonal changes of the menstrual cycle. Breast tissue also changes in response to nutritional, physical, and environmental stimuli. Benign breast disorders include fibrocystic breast changes, fibroadenomas, intraductal papillomas, duct ectasia, fat necrosis, and mastitis (Table 49–6).

Pathophysiology

Fibrocystic Changes

Fibrocystic changes (FCC) (fibrocystic breast disease) is the physiologic nodularity and breast tenderness that increases and decreases with the menstrual cycle. An estimated 50% to 80%

of all women experience some of these changes, which include fibrosis, epithelial proliferation, and cyst formation. FCC is most common in women 30 to 50 years of age, and is rare in postmenopausal women who are not taking hormone replacement (Porth & Matfin, 2009).

FCC includes many different lesions and breast changes. The more common nonproliferative form does not increase the risk for breast cancer. The proliferative form, accompanied by giant cysts and proliferative epithelial lesions, does increase the risk for breast cancer.

Nonproliferative changes may be cystic or fibrous. Cystic change refers to the dilation of ducts in the subareolar, lobular, or lobe areas. Cysts often go unnoticed unless pain and tenderness is associated with menses. Fibrous changes are infrequent but can occur during the menstrual years. A firm, palpable mass, 2 to 3 cm in size, is typically located in the upper outer breast quadrant following an inflammatory response to ductal irritation.

Manifestations

Women with fibrocystic changes experience bilateral or unilateral pain or tenderness in the upper, outer quadrants of their breasts, and report that their breasts feel particularly thick and lumpy the week prior to menses. Nipple discharge may be present. Pain is due to edema of the connective tissue of the breast, dilation of the ducts, and some inflammatory response; some women report an increase in breast size. Multiple, mobile cysts may form, usually in both breasts (Figure 49–6 ■). Fluid aspirated from these cysts ranges in color from milky white to

---

TABLE 49–6 Summary of Common Breast Disorders

CONDITION	AGE	PAIN	NIPPLE DISCHARGE	LOCATION	CONSISTENCY AND MOBILITY	DIAGNOSIS AND TREATMENT
Duct ectasia	35 to 55 years; median age 40	Burning around nipple	Sticky, multicolored; usually bilateral	No specific location	Retroareolar mass with advanced disease	Open biopsy; local excision of diseased portion of breast
Fibroadenoma	15 to 39 years; median age 20	No	No	No specific location	Mobile, firm, smooth, well-delineated mass	Mammography, surgical or needle biopsy; excision of the tumor
Fibrocystic changes (FCC)	20 to 49 years; median age 30 (may subside with menopause)	Yes	May occur	Upper outer quadrant	Bilateral multiple lumps influenced by the menstrual cycle	Needle aspiration; observation; biopsy if there is an unresolved mass or mammographic changes
Intraductal papilloma	35 to 55 years; median age 40	Yes	Serous or sanguineous; usually unilateral from one duct	No specific location	Usually soft, poorly delineated mass	Pap smear of nipple discharge; biopsy; wedge resection
Mastitis, acute	Childbearing years	Tenderness, pain	No	No specific location	Generalized redness of overlying skin	Antibiotic therapy; incision and drainage if mastitis progresses to an abscess
Mastitis, chronic	Any age	Tenderness, pain; headache; high fever	No	No specific location	Generalized redness and swelling	Antibiotics, usually penicillin
Fat necrosis	Any age	Tenderness	No	No specific location	Firm, irregular, palpable	Surgical biopsy to rule out cancer

Figure 49–6 ■ Fibrocystic breast changes.

yellow, brown, or green. If the fluid is tinged with blood, there is reason to suspect malignancy.

Intraductal Disorders

An intraductal papilloma is a tiny, wartlike growth on the inside of the peripheral mammary duct that causes discharge from the nipple. The discharge may be clear and sticky or bloody. When more than one of these growths is present, the condition is called intraductal papillomatosis. This condition is most common in women in their 30s and 40s. The lesion must be investigated to rule out malignancy.

Mammary duct ectasia (plasma cell mastitis) is a palpable lumpiness found beneath the areola. Duct ectasia involves periductal inflammation, dilation of the ductal system, and accumulation of fluid and dead cells that block the involved ducts. The condition usually occurs in perimenopausal women and is difficult to differentiate from cancer.

Manifestations of mammary duct ectasia include sticky, thick nipple discharge with burning and itching around the nipple, and inflammation. The discharge may be green, greenish brown, or bloody. Nipple retraction often is associated with duct ectasia in postmenopausal women.

Interdisciplinary Care

Diagnosis of FCC is based on complete history, physical examination, and imaging studies. A biopsy may be required for diagnosis.

Analysis of nipple discharge, mammography, and possibly ductography may be used to diagnose ductal disorders. The affected duct is excised in an open biopsy procedure. The treatment is usually symptomatic. Cyst aspiration may relieve pain, and also allows examination of fluid to confirm the cystic nature of the disease. A well-fitting brassiere that provides good support worn day and night helps relieve discomfort. Some women report that eliminating xanthines (found in coffee, tea, cola, and chocolate) from the diet decreases symptoms. Aspirin, mild analgesics, local heat or cold, and vitamin E may help relieve breast pain. Hormone therapy is controversial because of the benign nature of the disease and potential adverse effects of therapy. Danazol, a synthetic androgen, may be prescribed for women with severe pain.

ʊ Nursing Care

When a woman presents with a breast mass, nursing responsibilities include taking a careful health history and facilitating follow-up care. If a palpable mass is present, it is important to ask how long the lesion has been present and whether the

woman has noticed any pain associated with the mass, any change in its size, and any changes in association with the menstrual cycle.

In many cases, definitive diagnosis of the breast disorder requires surgical biopsy to rule out cancer. During the diagnostic process, the nurse can provide emotional support and education about diagnostic and therapeutic procedures, self-care and comfort measures, and resources to help the woman cope with the experience. Nursing care for the woman is similar to that for any patient with an open biopsy. It also is important to reassure the woman that these disorders are not breast cancer.

The Woman with Breast Cancer

Breast cancer is the unregulated growth of abnormal cells in breast tissue. Breast cancer is the most commonly occurring cancer in women and the second leading cause of death in women in the United States. The ACS (2009a) estimates that more than 194,000 women will be diagnosed with breast cancer each year, and approximately 40,600 women will die from it annually. In addition, more than 62,000 women will be diagnosed with cancer *in situ*. However, the incidence of breast cancer has decreased, primarily the result of findings from the Women's Health Initiative study, published in 2002, that indicate that use of HRT increased the risk of breast cancer and heart disease with a subsequent drop in hormone therapy to treat menopausal symptoms. There are racial differences in the incidence and mortality of breast cancer (see the following Focus on Cultural Diversity box).

Risk Factors

Of the various kinds of risk factors for breast cancer, some can be changed and some cannot. Those that cannot be changed are the following (ACS, 2009e):

- *Age and gender.*   Women are 100 times more likely to have breast cancer than are men, with the risk increasing with age. Two out of three invasive breast cancers are found in women aged 55 and older. See the Nursing Care of the Older Adult box on page 1704.
- *Genetic risk factors.*   Approximately 5% to 10% of breast cancers are believed to be hereditary changes resulting directly from genetic mutations from a parent (see the discussion in the pathophysiology section).
- *Family history of breast cancer.*   Relatives from either the maternal or paternal side of the family. Having a first-degree

> **Breast Cancer Video** (sidebar)

relative (mother, sister, or daughter) with breast cancer approximately doubles the risk, and having two first-degree relatives increases it fivefold. Having a male family member with breast cancer also poses an increased risk.

- *Dense breast tissue.* Dense breast tissue (seen on a mammogram) has more glandular tissue and less fatty tissue, increasing the risk for the development of breast cancer.
- *Personal history of breast cancer.* A woman with cancer in one breast has a three- to fourfold increase in risk for developing a new cancer in the other breast or in a different part of the same breast.
- *Previous chest irradiation.* Radiation of the chest as a child or young woman for other cancer (such as Hodgkin's disease) significantly increases the risk. The risk is greatest in women who had irradiation during adolescent breast development.
- *Menstrual history.* Women who begin menstruating before the age of 12 or who have menopause after the age of 55 are at a slightly higher risk, probably the result of a higher lifetime exposure to estrogen and progesterone.

Lifestyle-related factors and increased breast cancer risk include recent use of oral contraceptives, not having children or having them after the age of 30, long-term use of HRT, not breast-feeding, drinking alcohol (especially two to five drinks daily), being overweight and obese (especially after menopause), and physical inactivity. Lower risk factors for breast cancer include breast-feeding, moderate or vigorous physical activity, and maintaining a healthy body weight.

Pathophysiology

Possible causes of breast cancer include environmental, hormonal, reproductive, and hereditary factors. Two breast cancer susceptibility genes have been identified: BRCA1 on chromosome 17 and BRCA2 on chromosome 13. These genes may be responsible for the approximately 10% of women with hereditary breast cancer, with genetic mutations causing up to 80% of breast cancer in women younger than 50 years of age. A woman with identified mutations in BRCA1 (known to be involved in tumor suppression) has a lifetime risk of 56% to 85% for breast cancer and also has an increased risk for ovarian cancer (Porth & Matfin, 2009). Newest research has found that a family history of breast cancer is the greatest risk, even when the abnormal genes are not present. Changes in other genes that also might lead to inherited breast cancer are the ATM gene (normally helps repair damaged DNA), CHEK2 gene (risk is greatly increased if mutated and there is a strong family history of breast cancer), p53 gene (a tumor suppressor gene), and PTEN gene (normally helps regulate cell growth).

Cancer of the breast begins as a single transformed cell and is hormone dependent. Cancers of the breast are classified as noninvasive (*in situ*) or invasive, depending on the penetration of the tumor into surrounding tissue. Breast cancer may remain a noninvasive disease, or an invasive disease without metastasis, for long periods of time.

Breast cancer may be categorized as carcinoma of the mammary ducts, carcinoma of mammary lobules, or sarcoma of the breast. Most breast cancers are adenocarcinomas and appear to arise in the terminal section of the breast ductal tissue. There are many histologic types of breast cancer, and only examples are described here. The most common type is infiltrating ductal carcinoma. Two atypical types of breast cancer are inflammatory carcinoma and Paget's disease. Inflammatory carcinoma of the breast, a systemic disease, is the most malignant form of breast cancer. Edema with dimpling of the skin that results in the skin looking like the peel of an orange (peau d'orange) is usually present. Paget's disease is a rare type of breast cancer involving infiltration of the nipple epithelium.

Breast cancer can metastasize to other sites through the bloodstream or lymphatic system. The common sites of metastasis of breast cancer are bone, brain, lung, liver, skin, and lymph nodes. The staging of the breast cancer (Table 49–7) provides important information for making decisions about treatment options and is also used as a basis for prognosis.

NURSING CARE OF THE OLDER ADULT   **Older Women with Breast Cancer**

- Although the incidence of breast cancer is increasing among premenopausal women, it is still primarily a disease of older women. However, the needs of older women with breast cancer have been inadequately addressed in the professional literature and in the popular media.
- Women between the ages of 50 and 65 are the group most likely to benefit from annual screening mammography, yet many women in this age group have never had a mammogram. Reasons for lack of compliance with recommendations vary but reports cite costs of co-pays, indirect costs of obtaining a mammogram even if the mammogram is free, a lack of emphasis on obtaining mammograms by health practitioners and campaigns, and women just not thinking about the need (CDC, 2007; McBride, 2008; Rubin, 2007). Promotional campaigns for mammography send a confusing message by showing images of women in their 20s and 30s for whom mammography is largely ineffective, rather than women in older age groups who are more likely to benefit from mammography.
- For too long, mastectomy was perceived as the only treatment option open to most older women with breast cancer, even those with early-stage disease. Slowly that perception is changing as breast-conservation treatment gains greater acceptance. The choice of surgical treatment, particularly for older women, is highly individual. Many older women wish to preserve their breasts.
- Although older women with breast cancer may experience coexisting chronic illnesses and impaired physical function, research suggests that they show lower levels of emotional distress than younger women. However, the need for services such as personal care, shopping, housekeeping, and transportation may increase as the ages of the woman and the caregiver increase.

TABLE 49–7 Staging of Breast Cancer

STAGE	TUMOR	NODE	METASTASIS
0	Tis-Carcinoma *in situ* or Paget's disease of the nipple	N0-No regional lymph node metastasis	M0-No evidence of distant metastasis
I	T1-Tumor no larger than 2 cm	N0	M0
IIA	T0-No evidence of primary tumor	N1-Metastasis to movable ipsilateral	M0
	T1	axillary nodes	
	T2-Tumor no larger than 5 cm	N0	M0
IIB	T2	N1	M0
	T3-Tumor larger than 5 cm	N0	M0
IIIA	T0	N2-Metastasis to ipsilateral fixed	M0
	T1	axillary nodes	
	T2		
	T3	N1	M0
		N2	M0
IIIB	T4-Tumor of any size with direct extension to chest wall or skin	Any N	M0
	Any T	N3-Metastasis to ipsilateral internal mammary lymph nodes	M0
IV	Any T	N0 and N1	M1-Distant metastasis

Manifestations

The manifestations of breast cancer may include a nontender lump in the breast (most often in the upper outer quadrant, the area with the most glandular tissue), abnormal nipple discharge, a rash around the nipple area, nipple retraction, dimpling of the skin, or a change in the position of the nipple (see the accompanying Manifestations box on this page). There may also be nipple pain, scaliness, ulceration, skin irritation, or discharge. Breast cancer is usually painless, but some women report a burning or stinging sensation. Many women with breast cancer have no manifestations, and their tumors are detected by mammography. However, many breast cancers are found by the women themselves or by their partners.

Interdisciplinary Care

Diagnosis of breast cancer begins with detection, either detection of asymptomatic lesions discovered through screening or symptomatic lesions discovered by the woman. Any palpable mass requires evaluation. Once the diagnosis is made, a number of treatment options are available. The choice of treatment depends on several factors, such as the stage of the cancer, the age of the woman, and the woman's preferences.

MANIFESTATIONS of Breast Cancer

- Breast mass or thickening
- Unusual lump in the underarm or above the collarbone
- Persistent skin rash near the nipple area
- Flaking or eruption near the nipple
- Dimpling, pulling, or retraction in an area of the breast
- Nipple discharge
- Change in nipple position
- Burning, stinging, or pricking sensation

Diagnosis

Early detection of breast cancer is possible with clinical breast examination (CBE) and mammogram (∞ see Chapter 47 for further information). Mammography can detect breast tumors 2 years before they reach palpable size; most of these tumors have been present for 8 to 10 years. In addition, an MRI or PET scan of the breast may be used to further identify breast tumors.

Other diagnostic tests include a percutaneous needle biopsy to define a cystic mass or fibrocystic changes and provide specimens for cytologic examination, and a breast biopsy. In aspiration biopsy or fine-needle aspiration biopsy, a needle is used to remove cells or fluid from the breast lesion (Figures 49–7A and B ∎). The types of breast biopsy and related nursing care are described in ∞ Chapter 47. In many facilities, fine-needle aspiration biopsies are performed using a stereotactic biopsy device; mammography and a computer are used to guide the needle.

Medications

In addition to the hormone therapy described later, biphosphonates may be used to help strengthen and reduce the risk of fractures in bones weakened by metastatic breast cancer and may help prevent thinning of bone resulting from treatment with aromatase inhibitors or from early menopause as a side effect of chemotherapy. Examples include pamidronate (Aredia) and zoledronic acid (Zometa). Biphosphonates have many side effects, including flulike manifestations and bone pain. A rare side effect is damage to the mandible, leading to loss of teeth or bone infection. All patients taking biphosphonates should practice good oral hygiene and have regular dental check-ups to help prevent this effect.

A Aspiration biopsy   **B** Excisional biopsy

Figure 49–7 ■ Types of breast biopsy. *A,* In an aspiration biopsy, a needle is used to aspirate fluid or tissue from the breast. *B,* In an excisional biopsy, tissue from the breast lesion is removed surgically.

Surgery

The different types of surgeries used to treat breast cancer are outlined in Table 49–8 and illustrated in Figure 49–8 ■. The type of surgery used depends on the size of the tumor, the woman's age, the type of tumor, and the choice made by the woman after discussing benefits and risks with the surgeon.

Axillary node dissection is generally performed during surgery for all invasive breast carcinoma to stage the tumor. Because this surgery can cause **lymphedema** (accumulation of fluid in the soft tissues caused by removal of lymph channels) in the arm on the operated side, nerve damage, and adhesions, and because of the role of the lymph nodes in immune system function, nonsurgical methods of detecting lymph node involvement are being used. Sentinel node biopsy prior to a node dissection is conducted by injecting a radioactive

substance or dye into the region of the tumor. The dye is carried to the first (sentinel) lymph node to receive lymph from the tumor and would therefore be the node most likely to contain cancer cells if the cancer had metastasized. If the sentinel node is positive, more nodes are removed. If it is negative, further node evaluation is usually not indicated.

After a mastectomy (for all types except a lumpectomy), some women may choose to have their breast reconstructed. They report that surgical reconstruction of the breast simplifies their lives and restores a sense of body integrity. Other women choose to use a removable breast prosthesis, and some women are comfortable without reconstruction or a prosthesis. Breast reconstruction may be performed at the time of the mastectomy or at any time thereafter, depending on the woman's preference. A number of procedures may be used for the breast reconstruction

TABLE 49–8 / Surgical Methods of Treating Breast Cancer

METHOD	TYPE	CONSIDERATIONS
Surgery	Breast Conserving Surgery ■ Lumpectomy ■ Partial (segmental) mastectomy or quadrantectomy	■ Lumpectomy removes only the breast lump and a surrounding margin of tissue (see Figure 49–8*A*). Radiation is usually given after a lumpectomy. ■ A partial mastectomy or quadrantectomy removes more tissue than a lumpectomy; a quadrantectomy removes one-fourth of the breast. Radiation usually follows these surgeries. ■ Both breast conserving surgeries are as effective as a mastectomy for stage I or stage II breast cancer. ■ Radiation may be omitted for women over 70 with a small tumor that is hormone receptor-positive, who are getting hormone therapy, and who have no lymph node involvement. ■ Side effects of the surgeries can include pain, temporary swelling, risk for bleeding and wound infection, and hard scar formation.
	Mastectomy (See the Nursing Care of the woman having a mastectomy box on page 1708.)	■ A simple or total mastectomy removes the entire breast, but not axillary lymph nodes or muscles under the breast. ■ A modified radical mastectomy removes the entire breast and some of the axillary lymph nodes (see Figure 49–8*B*). ■ A skin-saving mastectomy, used for smaller tumors, leaves most over the skin over the breast (except the nipple and areola). ■ A radical mastectomy (not done much today) removes the entire breast, axillary lymph nodes, and pectoral muscles under the breast. ■ Side effects of these surgeries include postoperative pain, change in the shape of the breast, wound infection, hematoma formation, and seroma (buildup of clear fluid in the wound). If axillary lymph nodes are removed, the main long-term side effect in about one in four women is lymphedema of the arm.

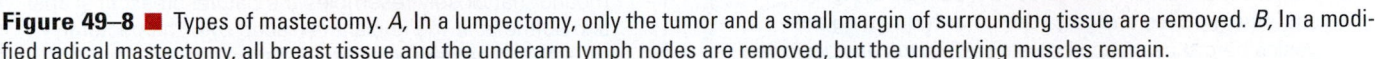

Figure 49–8 ■ Types of mastectomy. *A,* In a lumpectomy, only the tumor and a small margin of surrounding tissue are removed. *B,* In a modified radical mastectomy, all breast tissue and the underarm lymph nodes are removed, but the underlying muscles remain.

(Figure 49–9 ■). These include placement of a submuscular implant, the use of a tissue expander followed by an implant, the transposition of muscle and blood supply from the abdomen or back, or using (most often) the transverse rectus abdominis myocutaneous (TRAM) free tissue flap. Information about breast reconstruction surgery is summarized in Box 49–1 on page 1708.

Radiation Therapy

Radiation therapy is typically used following breast cancer surgery to destroy any remaining cancer cells that could cause recurrence or metastasis. If a tumor is unusually large, radiation may be used to shrink the tumor prior to surgery. Radiation therapy is most commonly used in combination with lumpectomy for early stage (I or II) breast cancer. Palliative radiation therapy is also used to treat chest wall recurrences and some bone metastases to help control pain and prevent fractures. Radiation therapy is administered by means of an external-beam or tissue implants (∞ see Chapter 14).

Intraoperative radiotherapy is provided by a single, concentrated dose of radiation. During surgery, a probe is inserted into the cavity created by the lumpectomy and radiation equivalent to 6 weeks of doses is emitted for about 25 minutes. If this proves successful, the treatment could make lumpectomy available to more women and prevent the woman from having 6 weeks of daily radiation treatments following surgery. Another method being researched is using higher doses of radiation over a shorter period of time following lumpectomy (called accelerated breast irradiation). This method has shown favorable results in cancer treatment while at the same time limiting the cost and time constraints placed on women compared with traditional radiation treatments.

In brachytherapy (internal radiation), radioactive seeds or pellets are placed directly into the breast tissue next to the tumor. It is often used as a means of increasing radiation therapy. Intracavity brachytherapy consists of inserting a small balloon attached to a small tube (that protrudes through the surgical site) into the cavity left by a lumpectomy. The balloon is filled with saline and a source of radioactivity is placed into the balloon and then removed. After five days of treatment, the balloon is removed. Interstitial brachytherapy is performed by inserting several small catheters into the breast around the lumpectomy. Radioactive pellets are inserted through the catheters for short period of time each day and then removed. Clinical trials are being conducted to determine if these therapies might be used as the only source of radiation for women having a lumpectomy.

Chemotherapy

Chemotherapy has become the standard of care for the majority of breast cancer cases with axillary node involvement. In late metastatic disease, chemotherapy becomes the primary treatment to prolong the woman's life. Chemotherapy is discussed

    A Implant   **B** Latissimus dorsi musculocutaneous flap

Figure 49–9 ■ Types of breast reconstruction surgeries. *A,* A breast implant is inserted under the pectoris muscle. *B,* Autogenous procedures transfer a flap of skin, muscle, and fat from the donor site on the woman's body to the mastectomy site. The most frequently used donor muscle sites are the latissimus dorsi and the rectus abdominis (the TRAM flap).

NURSING CARE OF THE PATIENT
Having a Mastectomy

- Encourage deep breathing exercises and use of incentive spirometry every 4 hours. *Deep-breathing exercises are important because after general anesthesia, it is difficult for air to reach the lungs, particularly with the restrictive surgical dressing that decreases chest expansion.*
- Monitor drainage from wound. *A suction apparatus may be placed in the wound to allow drainage of excess body fluids that accumulate when the lymph nodes are removed. This device is usually removed 3 to 5 days after surgery.*
- Administer, as ordered, intravenous fluids and antibiotics. *An IV line may be in place for fluid replacement and antibiotics to reduce the risk of postoperative infection.*
- Instruct the woman how to control pain by using the patient-controlled analgesia device or requesting analgesics before pain becomes severe. *Taking analgesics as needed facilitates deep breathing and movements during physical therapy interventions.*
- Monitor the dressing for bleeding. *Careful assessment for bleeding and of vital signs is important in preventing hemorrhage.*
- Instruct the woman about the following to decrease anxiety, promote healing, and decrease postoperative risks:
  - Numbness or feelings of "pins and needles" in the axillary area are common.
  - Lying on one's back or on the side not operated on helps fluid drain from the site.
  - Moving the arm on the operated side helps regain mobility; specific exercises will be prescribed for increasing mobility after the incisions have healed.
  - Use caution when lifting heavy objects with the arm on the operated side.
  - Be careful about injury and infection on the affected side; wear rubber gloves when washing dishes, garden gloves when working outside. Request that caregivers do not perform blood pressures or venipunctures on the operative side to reduce the risk of injury and infection.
  - Feelings of anxiety, sadness, and fear of looking at the incision are normal; mastectomy means abrupt change in body image. It is normal to mourn the loss of a breast and to fear the loss of one's life after a cancer diagnosis.
  - Sexual intimacy can be affected by mastectomy; it often helps to be able to discuss potential sexual problems with one's partner, with a counselor, or with a breast cancer support group.

BOX 49–1 Breast Reconstruction Information

- Controversy exists about the health effects of silicone. While there is no conclusive evidence that silicone implants induce cancer or autoimmune disease, they are associated with hardening and pain due to contracture of the capsule around the implant. The implant may rupture, releasing silicone gel, or infection may occur. Saline-filled breast implants may be an alternative.
- Reconstruction can be done immediately after a mastectomy, or at any time later on. Some surgeons believe that delayed reconstruction offers better cosmetic results.
- Reconstructive surgery can create a natural looking breast that makes clothes fit better. Since it has no nerve endings the reconstructed breast has no feeling or sensations.
- If a simple mastectomy is done, an implant approximately the same size as the other breast is placed under the pectoral muscle on the operative side. This creates a breast mound that closely resembles the natural breast in shape and softness. If the implant is placed over the pectoral muscle, a high degree of firmness may occur.
- With a simple mastectomy or modified radical mastectomy, a tissue expander may be used to replace the breast. The tissue expander is placed under the pectoral muscle and gradually expanded with saline injections every 2 to 3 weeks to stretch the overlying skin and create a pocket. After a period of time, usually 1 to 2 months, the tissue expander is exchanged for a saline implant.
- With more extensive surgery such as radical mastectomy, a flap of skin, fat, or muscle is transferred from a donor site to the operative area. A new nipple may be created by using tissue from the opposite nipple or from the inner thigh.
- Reconstructive surgery may require multiple surgeries, including all the risks associated with anesthesia. As the complexity of the procedures increases, so does the risk of complications such as infection.
- To decrease the risk of a fibrous capsule forming around the implant, it is important to perform breast massage as instructed.

Hormone Therapy

Tamoxifen citrate (Nolvadex) and toremifene (Fareston) are oral medications that block estrogen activity. They are used to treat advanced breast cancer, as an adjuvant for early-stage breast cancer, and as a preventive treatment for women at high risk of developing breast cancer. Nursing implications for tamoxifen are presented in the Medication Administration box on page 1709. Tamoxifen can be used to treat metastatic breast cancer, and if taken for 5 years following surgery, can reduce the risk of cancer reoccurrence by about half (ACS, 2009e). Toremifene (Fareston) is mainly used to treat postmenopausal women with advanced cancers. Fulvestrant (Faslodex) is a drug that eliminates estrogen receptors. Given by injection once a month, it is currently only approved for postmenopausal women with advanced cancer that no longer responds to tamoxifen or toremifene.

Immunotherapy, using trastuzumab (Herceptin), is used to stop the growth of breast tumors that express the HER2/neu receptor (which binds an epidermal growth factor that contributes to cancer cell growth) on their cell surface. This drug is a recombinant DNA-derived monoclonal antibody that binds to the receptor, inhibiting tumor cell proliferation. It is given intravenously either once a week or as a larger dose every 3 weeks. Side effects include fever and chills, weakness, nausea, vomiting, cough, diarrhea, and headache. A more serious

in ∞ Chapter 14. Neoadjuvant chemotherapy is chemotherapy given before surgery; it can shrink large tumors so they are small enough to be removed by a lumpectomy instead of a mastectomy. Adjuvant (additional) systemic therapy following primary treatment for early-stage breast cancer refers to the administration of chemotherapy and other pharmacologic agents after surgery. This type of therapy has been widely studied; its use reduces the rates of recurrence and death from breast cancer. For example, Femara (an aromatase inhibitor) has reduced the risk of recurrence after surgery (in some cases more effectively than tamoxifen).

MEDICATION ADMINISTRATION   Tamoxifen

TAMOXIFEN (NOLVADEX)

Tamoxifen is the most widely prescribed breast cancer drug, commonly given to prevent recurrence of estrogen-positive breast cancer in postmenopausal women. It inhibits tumor growth by blocking the estrogen receptor sites of cancer cells. Tamoxifen increases a woman's risk of developing endometrial cancer, deep venous thrombosis (DVT), and pulmonary embolism.

Nursing Responsibilities

- Assess for potential contraindications to therapy.
- Assess liver function tests; tamoxifen may interfere with liver function.

Health Education for the Patient and Family

- If in childbearing years, use a nonhormonal, barrier form of contraception; tamoxifen has adverse effects on the developing fetus.
- Take the drug as prescribed until the physician indicates otherwise.
- Side effects such as hot flashes, vaginal dryness, irregular periods, and weight gain are commonly experienced by women taking tamoxifen.
- Do not smoke while taking tamoxifen; smoking further increases the risk of DVT.
- Promptly report any abnormal vaginal bleeding (nonmenstrual bleeding, bleeding after menopause) to your primary care provider.

possible side effect is cardiac damage, leading to congestive heart failure. Other drugs that are used include lapatinib (Tykerb), an oral drug that also targets the HER2 protein.

The aromotase inhibitors stop the production of estrogen in postmenopausal women by blocking the enzyme aromatase (which turns androgen into small amounts of estrogen in the body). The drugs, in oral form, are anastrozole (Arimidex), exemestane (Aromasin), and letrozole (Femara). In comparison of aromatase inhibitors with tamoxifen in treating early-stage, hormone-receptor-positive breast cancer in postmenopausal women, most physicians recommend that an aromatase inhibitor is the best hormone therapy to start with as it has more benefits and fewer serious side effects (Breastcancer.org, 2009).

⚕ Nursing Care

Breast cancer is not one disease entity, but many, depending on the affected breast tissue, the tissue's estrogen dependency, and the age of the person at onset. The psychosocial effect of breast cancer extends beyond the fear and threat of death. The diagnosis may transform the woman's sense of self and lead to reintegration or negotiation of family relationships. A Case Study & Nursing Care Plan for a woman with breast cancer is found on page 1714.

Health Promotion

Although controversy exists about the ability of screening mammography to improve mortality rates for women under 50, the ACS recommends an annual mammogram and CBE by a healthcare professional beginning at age 40 and CBE at least every 3 years for women in their 20s and 30s (recommendations by other agencies are described in ∞ Chapter 47). A screening MRI is recommended for women with an approximately 20% to 25% or greater lifetime risk of breast cancer, including women with a strong family history of breast or ovarian cancer and women who were treated for Hodgkin's disease with radiation. As with any screening examination, decisions about timing should be made by the woman after discussion with her healthcare provider.

Breast self-examination (BSE) is recommended as an optional measure by the ACS, but its use is supported by other

cancer-related organizations as well as by many physicians. Information on how to perform BSE is included in Box 49–2 to enable nurses to provide teaching as prescribed or requested. Premenopausal women should perform BSE 7 to 10 days from the first day of their menstrual period, because hormonal changes increase breast tenderness and lumpiness prior to menses. Postmenopausal women should choose one date of the month (for example, the first day of the month) for BSE.

Educational messages about breast cancer screening need to be culturally sensitive to the intended audience. Media campaigns promoting mammography often show young White women, an approach that has proved ineffective among women

BOX 49–2 Breast Self-Examination (BSE)

- Lie down on your back and place your right arm behind your head. (BSE should be done while lying down because this position spreads breast tissue evenly over the chest wall, making it easier to feel all the breast tissue.)
- Use the finger pads of the middle fingers on your left hand to feel for lumps in the right breast. Use overlapping dime-sized circular motions of the finger pads to feel the breast tissue.
- Use three different levels of pressure to feel all the breast tissue. Light pressure is needed to feel the tissue closest to the skin, medium pressure to feel a little deeper, and firm pressure to feel the tissue closest to the chest and ribs. A firm ridge in the lower curve of each breast is normal. Use each pressure level to feel the breast tissue before moving on to the next spot.
- Move around the breast in an up and down pattern starting at an imaginary line drawn straight down your side from the underarm and moving across the breast to the middle of the chest bone (sternum, breastbone). Be sure to check the entire breast area before going down until you feel only ribs and up to the neck or collar bone.
- Repeat the exam on your left breast, using the finger pads of your right hand.
- Stand in front of the mirror with your hands pressing firmly down on your hips. Look at your breasts for any changes in size, shape, contour, or dimpling.
- Examine your underarm while sitting or standing and with your arm only slightly raised.
- If you find any changes, see your healthcare provider as soon as possible.

of color (see the accompanying Moving Evidence into Action box), although cancer screening is increasing in this population. By working with women of different races and cultures, nurses can help make breast cancer education more meaningful to women in these groups.

Assessment

Collect the following data through the health history and physical examination (∞ see Chapter 47). Further focused assessments are described with nursing interventions.

- *Health history:* Family history of breast cancer, breast changes, nipple discharge, use of HRT, previous diagnostic tests and treatment for cancer, menstrual history, pregnancies, alcohol intake, physical activity, dietary history.
- *Physical assessment:* Height and weight, breasts, axillary lymph glands.

Nursing Diagnoses and Interventions

Although each woman has individual needs, nursing diagnoses prior to surgery are concerned with anxiety, decisional conflict, grief, risk for infection, risk for injury, and disturbed body image over the loss of a breast. Because the typical hospital stay is short, usually from 1 to 3 days, preoperative teaching is done on an outpatient basis.

Anxiety

A woman of any age with breast cancer is often anxious about the diagnosis, the surgery, the outcome of surgery if nodal involvement is found, and the possible changes in sexual and family relationships. Studies show that young women with breast cancer, a growing population, are particularly vulnerable for anxiety and other psychosocial effects, as are their spouses and their children. Young women with breast cancer often have a more aggressive disease and a lower survival rate when compared with older women with breast cancer (Shaha & Bauer-Wu, 2009).

- Provide opportunities to express thoughts and feelings. In this process, the woman can name her fears. *Once the fears are named, the nurse may simply listen, educate, or dispel fears that stem from lack of understanding.*

EVIDENCE FOR NURSING CARE   **The Patient with Breast Cancer**

Selected resources that nurses may find helpful when planning evidence-based nursing care follow.

- Andersen, B. L., Yang, H-C., Farrar, W. B., Golden-Kreutz, D. M., Emery, C. F., Thornton, L. M., et al. (2008). Psychologic intervention improves survival for breast cancer patients. *Cancer, 113*(12), 3450–3458. Retrieved from http://www3 .interscience.wiley.com/cgi-bin/fulltext/121511810/PDFSTART
- Chung, L., Cimprich, B., Janz, N., & Mills-Wisneski, S. (2009). Breast cancer survivorship program: Testing for cross-cultural relevance. *Cancer Nursing, 32*(3), 236–245.
- Hereditary breast and ovarian cancer syndrome. (2009). *American College of Obstetricians and Gynecologists (ACOG) Committee on Practice Bulletins – Gynecology.* Retrieved from http://www.guideline.gov/summary/ summary.aspx?view_id=1&doc_id=14336
- Meneses, K. D., & McNees, M. P. (2007). Upper extremity lymphedema after treatment for breast cancer: A review of the literature. *Ostomy Wound Management, 53*(5), 16–29. Retrieved from http://www.o-wm.com/article/7258

- Discuss with the woman her knowledge of breast cancer. *Assessing the woman's knowledge of breast cancer helps the nurse plan more effective teaching.*
- Encourage discussion relating to immediate concerns about resuming her life at home and the changes she must make. *Anticipatory guidance can help her plan for and cope with changes in her life and relationships.*
- Explain the surgical procedure, including information about preoperative medications, anesthesia, and recovery. *Knowing what to expect helps to decrease anxiety.*
- Explain that it is normal to have decreased sensation in the surgical area. *Severed or damaged nerves reduce sensation.*

Decisional Conflict

The woman with breast cancer must make life-changing decisions about treatment within a relatively brief and highly stressful time. Her age, menopausal status, and stage of cancer

---

MOVING EVIDENCE INTO ACTION   **Improving the Diagnosis and Treatment of Black Women with Breast Cancer**

Despite efforts to improve both the diagnosis and treatment of women with breast cancer, Black women die more often from breast cancer than other groups of women. It is believed that this statistic is the result of Black women's advanced stage of disease at diagnosis, primarily due to a delay in seeking treatment. Bradley (2005) conducted a study to examine the variables affecting delay in seeking treatment as well as the possible effects of worry about breast cancer manifestations in Black women that might delay seeking treatment. The researcher found that, although delay in some women does exist, one cannot assume that all Black women delay seeking treatment. The researcher recommended that the relationship between worry and delaying treatment for breast cancer in Black women be further studied.

IMPLICATIONS FOR NURSING

Nurses must consider multiple factors when considering what may or may not influence Black women to delay seeking diagnosis and treatment for breast cancer, including biologic

characteristics and intra- and intercultural differences and similarities, as well as perceptions and health beliefs. It is important that nurses do not assume that a delay in seeking care exists, but rather make assessments and design interventions based on consideration of both individual and group cultural differences.

CRITICAL THINKING IN PATIENT CARE

1. What barriers to breast cancer screening in women of all races can you identify? Do you think these barriers differ based on culture, race, or socioeconomic level? Why or why not?
2. Are there barriers to breast cancer screening that might be unique to Black women? To Hispanic women? To Asian American women?
3. What type of questions would you include in a health assessment to identify women who may be worried about breast cancer, but have not sought diagnosis?

are only some of the factors that affect her decisions. Culture, values, lifestyle, socioeconomic status, and self-esteem also are considered.

■ Provide an opportunity for the woman to ask questions; answer questions as simply and directly as possible. Make eye contact and pay attention to body language. *During this time, the woman can process information and make informed decisions.*

■ Focus on immediate concerns, and provide up-to-date written material for the woman to review. *Written material provides easy reference to information not processed immediately because of anxiety and stress.*

■ Listen to the woman in a nonjudgmental manner during her decision-making process. *Nonjudgmental, empathic listening helps the woman process information and make informed decisions. Only she knows the context of her life.*

■ If the woman wishes, provide opportunities for her to meet with other women who have had breast cancer surgery. *Not all women are ready to meet others in their situation, but opening the door to this resource is appropriate. The woman may choose to talk with these women after the surgery.*

■ Facilitate a team approach with the surgeon, anesthesiologist, oncologist, plastic surgeon, and other health professionals. *Being the woman's advocate during this time of anxiety and decision making reduces the stress of coordinating multiple healthcare provider schedules.*

Grieving

Breast surgery, even a lumpectomy, alters the appearance of the breast. This loss of appearance, as well as the diagnosis of cancer, is expressed through grief.

■ Listen attentively to expressions of grief and watch for nonverbal cues (failure to make eye contact, crying, silence). *Not all women will express grief clearly; sometimes unspoken grief is the most painful. Grief is relieved only when expressed in a nonthreatening environment.*

■ Allow time to interact and do not rush interactions. *Taking time to be with the woman communicates caring.*

■ Explain that it is normal to have periods of depression, anger, and denial after breast surgery. *All these feelings are appropriate expressions of grief.*

■ If the woman wishes to do so, involve the partner in helping the woman cope with her grief. *Remember that the partner may also be grieving. Not all women want to share their grief, and not all partners are interested and supportive.*

Risk for Infection

Like any surgical patient, the woman who has breast surgery is at risk for infection. Removal of lymph nodes and the presence of a draining wound increase the risk.

■ Assess the surgical dressings for bleeding, drainage, color, and odor every 4 hours for 24 hours and document your findings. Circle any visible bleeding and drainage on the dressing as a baseline for subsequent assessment. *Excessive bleeding or drainage signals postoperative complications that may require emergency attention.*

■ Observe the incision and IV sites for pain, redness, swelling, and drainage. Assess the drainage system for patency and adequate suction; note the color and amount of drainage.

Careful observation for any signs of infection is essential because the woman's immune system is compromised. IV catheters should be placed on the uninvolved side only.

■ Change dressings and IV tubing using aseptic technique. *Moist dressings and intravenous tubing provide sites for bacterial growth. Routine dressing and IV tubing changes using aseptic technique reduce the risk for infection.*

■ Encourage a protein-rich diet. Discuss the woman's nutritional status with the dietitian and request a consultation for the woman. *Adequate nutrition promotes healing and boosts the immune system.*

■ Teach the woman how to care for the drainage system, if present (clean the site, empty the device, and record the amount, color, and type of drainage). *The woman is often discharged prior to removal of the drainage system and dressings and needs teaching to provide self-care.*

■ At discharge, teach the woman to watch for and report to her healthcare provider the manifestations of infection: fever, redness or hardness at the surgical site, or purulent drainage. *Any of these manifestations should be reported to the physician/surgeon. Knowing the signs and symptoms of infection prepares the woman to seek prompt treatment if infection occurs.*

■ Explain that she may experience scaling, flaking, dryness, itching, rash, or dry desquamation of the skin, particularly after radiation therapy. *Impaired skin integrity increases the risk of infection.*

■ Tell the woman to avoid deodorants and talcum powder on the affected side until the incision is completely healed. *These substances may irritate the skin and impede healing.*

Impaired Tissue Integrity

Removal of the axillary lymph nodes puts the woman at risk for lymphedema (LE), a complication that involves an abnormal accumulation of lymph in the arm, shoulder, breast, or thoracic area. It is estimated that this complication affects as many as half of all breast cancer survivors. This complication may develop at any time for years following a mastectomy, but usually develops within three years of the surgery (Fu, Ridner, & Armer, 2009a).

■ Assess/monitor for manifestations of LE: swelling in the affected area (usually the hand and arm), pain, fatigue, and changes in sensations (such as heaviness, numbness or burning) in the affected area. Assess skin color, temperature, texture, scars, or lesions. Ask about tighter rings. Measure the affected extremity (5 cm and 10 cm above and below the olecranon process) on a regular basis and record findings. *When an obstruction to the flow of lymphatic fluid develops, large proteins filter through the lymph vessels and accumulate in an area distal to the obstruction; fluid accumulates, causing tissue and skin changes. Accurate assessments are necessary to identify new-onset LE and to monitor already present LE for progression or improvement.*

■ When obtaining blood pressure, blood draws, and starting IVs, use the nonsurgical side. *Compression of the arm on the surgical side may increase the risk of developing LE; if skin integrity is compromised, the risk for infection increases.*

- Following surgery and while sleeping, elevate the affected arm higher than the shoulder on a pillow, but do not abduct it; the hand should be higher than the elbow. *Elevating the arm permits drainage, prevents swelling, and promotes circulation.*
- Instruct the woman to report any manifestations of infection, including increased swelling, pain, heat, and redness in the affected area; as well as fever and generalized malaise. *Infection may involve cellulitis or lymphangitis, requiring medical treatment with antibiotics. Infection may also precipitate or worsen existing LE.*
- Explain about measures to control and/or reduce swelling and refer to a certified LE therapist: compression bandaging, manual lymph drainage, exercises, wearing a LE sleeve. *These life-long measures can often control and even reduce the swelling of LE.*
- Teach the woman the following guidelines for care of the affected area *to prevent progression or onset of LE and to prevent infection in the affected area (Fu, Ridner, & Armer, 2009b; Marrs, 2007):*
  - Avoid injury from very hot water, popping grease when cooking, and playing sports such as golf.
  - Avoid tight clothing, jewelery, and elastic bands on the affected extremity.
  - Avoid carrying a purse or briefcase on the affected side.
  - Keep skin and nails clean and well cared for.
  - Use cream or lotion to keep the skin moist.
  - Treat small cuts with an antibiotic cream.
  - Use a thimble when sewing or doing handwork.
  - Wear gloves when gardening.

Disturbed Body Image

Breast surgery can change the woman's body image. The surgical changes may be compounded by weight gain and other side effects of chemotherapy or hormone therapy. Self-esteem also affects adjustment to a changed body image.

- Assess how the woman views her body. Discuss with the woman what image of herself she had prior to surgery. *Self-image is related to self-esteem. Discuss whether her self-image has changed.*
- Explain that redness and swelling in the scar will fade with time. *The knowledge that the scar will fade may give the woman a more realistic view of the changes.*
- Include the partner and family if possible when discussing the plan of care and activities of daily living (ADLs). Request consultation with a psychologist or other professional if the woman is interested. *Discussion with the partner and family can facilitate the woman's emotional healing process.*
- Offer pamphlets and suggest books and videos that might increase knowledge about what lies ahead. *Knowing what to expect can help the woman cope.*
- Encourage the woman to look at her incision when she feels ready; often the reality is not as frightening as the woman had imagined. Explain that it is normal to be afraid to look. *Reassurance that her behavior is normal decreases anxiety.*
- If the woman is interested in breast reconstruction, provide written material and encourage her to talk with a plastic surgeon and with women who have had reconstruction. *It is important for the woman to be fully informed about available options to make an informed decision.*

Using NANDA, NIC, and NOC

Linkages between a selected NANDA nursing diagnosis, NIC, and NOC for the woman with breast cancer are shown in the chart that follows.

Community-Based Care

The woman with breast cancer and her family have much to learn to provide self-care at home. Address the following topics in preparation for home care:

- Manifestations of infection and the need to report any that occur to her healthcare provider.
- The importance of ADLs, such as eating, combing her hair, and washing her face.
- Postmastectomy exercises (see examples in Figure 49–10 ■) and lymphedema care as approved by the healthcare provider and physical/occupational/LE therapist.
- The need for adequate rest and emotional support.
- Participation in a breast cancer support group and online information services and bulletin boards for sources of education and support.
- Prosthesis management, if this option is chosen. (A temporary lightweight prosthesis may be worn immediately after the drains and sutures have been removed from the surgical site. Because prostheses are expensive, a permanent one should not be purchased until the wound has completely healed. Prostheses are available at medical stores and many larger department stores. Most private and government insurance policies pay for the first prosthesis.)
- Helpful resources include Reach to Recovery, the American Cancer Society, the National Breast Cancer Coalition, and the National Lymphedema Network.

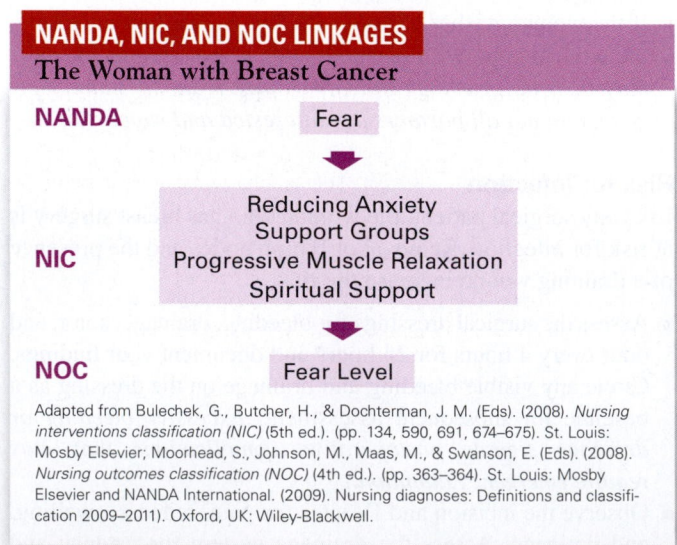

NANDA, NIC, AND NOC LINKAGES
The Woman with Breast Cancer

NANDA Fear

NIC Reducing Anxiety
Support Groups
Progressive Muscle Relaxation
Spiritual Support

NOC Fear Level

Adapted from Bulechek, G., Butcher, H., & Dochterman, J. M. (Eds). (2008). *Nursing interventions classification (NIC)* (5th ed.). (pp. 134, 590, 691, 674–675). St. Louis: Mosby Elsevier; Moorhead, S., Johnson, M., Maas, M., & Swanson, E. (Eds). (2008). *Nursing outcomes classification (NOC)* (4th ed.). (pp. 363–364). St. Louis: Mosby Elsevier and NANDA International. (2009). Nursing diagnoses: Definitions and classification 2009–2011). Oxford, UK: Wiley-Blackwell.

Figure 49–10 ■ Examples of postmastectomy exercises. *A,* Wall climbing: Stand facing wall with toes 6 to 12 inches from wall. Bend elbows and place palms against wall at shoulder level. Gradually move both hands up the wall parallel to each other until incisional pulling or pain occurs. (Mark that spot on wall to measure progress.) Work hands down to shoulder level. Move closer to wall as height of reach improves. *B,* Overhead pulley: Using operated arm, toss 6-foot rope over shower curtain rod (or over top of a door that has a nail in the top to hold the rope in place for the exercise). Grasp one end of rope in each hand. Slowly raise operated arm as far as comfortable by pulling down on the rope on opposite side. Keep raised arm close to your head. Reverse to raise unoperated arm by lowering the operated arm. Repeat. *C,* Rope turning: Tie rope to door handle. Hold rope in hand of operated side. Back away from door until arm is extended away from body, parallel to floor. Swing rope in as wide a circle as possible. Increase size of circle as mobility returns. *D,* Arm swings: Stand with feet 8 inches apart. Bend forward from waist, allowing arms to hang toward floor. Swing both arms up to sides to reach shoulder level. Swing back to center, then cross arms at center. Do not bend elbows. If possible, do this and other exercises in front of mirror to ensure even posture and correct motion.

CASE STUDY & NURSING CARE PLAN   A Woman with Breast Cancer

Rachel Clemments is a 42-year-old mother of two: Sarah, aged 12, and Jennifer, aged 18. Because of a family history of breast cancer, she has been closely monitored (annual mammograms and clinical breast examination, monthly BSE, a needle aspiration biopsy with negative findings) for 4 years prior to her diagnosis. Mrs. Clemments discovers a lump in her left breast while taking a shower. An incisional biopsy reveals invasive lobular carcinoma in the left breast. Mrs. Clemments is debating whether to have reconstructive breast surgery. One of her greatest concerns is how her illness will affect her ability to support and care for her daughters. The breast cancer diagnosis seems part of the family legacy. She wonders, "When will it happen to Jennifer? To Sarah?"

ASSESSMENT

During the history, Laura Nelson, RN, the nurse admitting Mrs. Clemments, learns that her mother, two of her aunts, and one sister had been diagnosed with breast cancer. Her mother and one of the aunts died before age 45. Physical assessment findings include T 98.5°F (37.0°C), BP 110/62, P 65, R 14. Her weight is 120 lb (54 kg); she is 66 inches (168 cm) tall. Modified radical mastectomy is performed; histologic examination shows a 3-cm tumor; axillary node dissection shows that 4 of 16 lymph nodes are positive.

DIAGNOSES

- *Risk for Infection* related to surgical incision
- *Acute Pain* related to surgery
- *Disturbed Body Image* related to loss of breast
- *Decisional Conflict* about treatment, related to concerns about risks and benefits
- *Fear* related to disease process/prognosis

EXPECTED OUTCOMES

- Remain free of infection.
- Experience minimal pain or discomfort during her recovery.
- Maintain a positive body image, regardless of her decision about reconstruction.
- Evaluate the treatment options in relation to personal values and decide on a course of action.
- Identify the sources of her fear and demonstrate behaviors that may reduce fears.

PLANNING AND IMPLEMENTATION

- Teach her about hand hygiene and wound care.
- Assess her pain tolerance and administer analgesics as prescribed.

- Teach her to use caution when moving the arm on the operated side, to avoid lifting heavy objects, and to wear gloves when gardening.
- Encourage her to discuss her thoughts and feelings about her body changes.
- Suggest that she talk with a Reach to Recovery volunteer about her thoughts and feelings.
- Assess her interest in spiritual/religious support and refer if appropriate.
- Discuss the use of a temporary prosthesis and later the fitting of a permanent prosthesis (6 to 8 weeks after surgery), the need to be fitted by an experienced person, and insurance reimbursement for the prosthesis.
- Discuss the possibility of attending a breast cancer support group where she can draw on the experiences of other women who have undergone mastectomy, chemotherapy, or radiation.
- Encourage her to verbalize her fears about her own prognosis and about her daughters' future risk of breast cancer; assess the need/interest for referral to psychologic counseling.

EVALUATION

At discharge, Mrs. Clemments has no signs of physical complications and is looking forward to being at home with her daughters as temporary caregivers. Mrs. Clemments met with a Reach to Recovery volunteer, who brought her a temporary prosthesis and booklets about postmastectomy exercises, chemotherapy, and breast reconstruction. The volunteer also referred her to a local cancer support group. Mrs. Clemments has talked about her concerns related to breast reconstruction. "I want to avoid anything that would increase the risk of complications. The possibility of recurrence and my fear for my daughters' future health are more than enough to worry about."

CRITICAL THINKING IN THE NURSING PROCESS

1. What role could genetic counseling play in helping Mrs. Clemments and her daughters better understand the daughters' risk of breast cancer?
2. Describe the types of mastectomies and their implications for nursing care.
3. What medications might help minimize the side effects of chemotherapy?
4. Develop a plan of care for Mrs. Clemments for the nursing diagnosis *Disturbed Sleep Pattern*.

See Evaluating Your Response in Appendix C.

CHAPTER HIGHLIGHTS

- Disorders of female sexual function include dyspareunia, inhibited sexual desire, and orgasmic dysfunction. Nurses should be able to obtain a sexual history, discuss sexual concerns, and make appropriate referrals without embarrassment.
- Menopause, a normal physiologic event in the life span of a woman, is the permanent cessation of menses. Loss of estrogen results in widespread tissue changes and increases the risk for osteoporosis, fractures, and cardiovascular disease.

- Menstrual disorders encompass PMS, dysmenorrhea, and abnormal uterine bleeding. Nursing interventions are focused on teaching about good health practices and interventions to relieve manifestations. Interdisciplinary care includes a therapeutic D&C and hysterectomy.
- Uterine displacement and vaginal fistulas are structural disorders. Uterine displacements may be treated surgically or with a pessary, and may include teaching Kegel exercises to minimize

urinary leakage. Fistulas may spontaneously resolve if small, or may be surgically repaired.

■ There are both benign and malignant disorders of female reproductive tissue, including cysts or polyps, leiomyomas, endometriosis, and cancers of the cervix, endometrium, ovaries, and vulva.

■ Leiomyomas (fibroids) are benign tumors that originate from smooth muscle of the uterus. Treatment depends on the size and location of the tumors. Both leiomyomas and endometrial implants (benign implants of endometrial tissue in the pelvic cavity) may interfere with the ability to have a child and are reduced in size after menopause.

■ Cervical cancer is a common female reproductive system cancer, but the incidence and mortality has been greatly reduced with the Pap smear for early diagnosis. The major risk for cervical cancer is cervical infection with HPV.

■ Endometrial cancer is the most frequently diagnosed pelvic cancer in the United States. The major manifestation is abnormal, painless vaginal bleeding (menorrhagia or metrorrhagia in menstruating women). Postmenopausal women should have annual pelvic examinations and report any unexpected vaginal bleeding to their healthcare provider.

■ Ovarian cancer increases in incidence with aging; it is seen most often in women over age 65. In early stages, there are generally no warning signs.

■ Benign breast disorders in women include fibrocystic changes and intraductal disorders. Both treatment and nursing care are primarily symptomatic.

■ Breast cancer is the most commonly occurring cancer in women and the second leading cause of death in women in the United States. A strong genetic link has been identified, as have a large number of risk factors. Early diagnosis is possible with breast self-examination, clinical breast examination, and mammograms. Treatment includes surgery (such as lumpectomy or one of several types of mastectomy), radiation therapy, hormone therapy, and chemotherapy. Both combination therapies and immunotherapy are proving to be effective in suppressing tumor growth and facilitating longer life. Among other problems, mastectomy and radiation therapy interfere with lymph drainage on the affected side, leading to lymphedema of the arm.

■ Appropriate preoperative nursing diagnoses for the woman with breast cancer include anxiety and fear, decisional conflict, and grieving. Following surgery, interventions focus on risk for infection, altered tissue perfusion, pain, and disturbed body image.

TEST YOURSELF NCLEX-RN® REVIEW

1. During a health assessment at a local clinic, a woman in her 50s tells the nurse that she is having some pain with intercourse. The nurse is uncomfortable discussing this topic with her. What would he say?
   1. "I know this can be a problem; please discuss it with your physician."
   2. "I don't know anything about that; please ask someone else."
   3. "Do you normally enjoy sexual activity?"
   4. "What do you think is causing your problem?"

2. Long-term estrogen deprivation results in an increased risk for physical disorders. What are these? **Select all that apply.**
   1. colon cancer
   2. osteoporosis
   3. cardiovascular disease
   4. fractures
   5. cervical cancer

3. A nurse is conducting an educational seminar for postmenopausal women. When discussing calcium intake, what amount (in mg) per day is recommended?_____ mg

4. An intervention for the woman with a uterine displacement disorder is to teach Kegel exercises. These exercises may help reduce which of the following?
   1. stress incontinence
   2. menorrhagia
   3. vaginal discharge
   4. retroversion

5. Which of the following topics would a nurse include in a health-promotion seminar to reduce the risk of cervical cancer?
   1. weight loss
   2. safer sex methods
   3. yearly mammograms
   4. a diet high in iron

6. When discussing dietary guidelines with a woman with PMS a nurse recommends a reduced sodium intake. What is the rationale for this recommendation?
   1. Sodium increases reactive hypoglycemia, increasing physical manifestations.
   2. Sodium increases thirst, thereby facilitating increased oral fluid intake.
   3. In and of itself, sodium is not harmful but it may increase cancer risk.
   4. Sodium restriction helps minimize fluid retention.

7. What happens to endometrial implantations after menopause?
   1. They tend to become malignant.
   2. They tend to atrophy and disappear.
   3. The number of implants increases.
   4. Each implant enlarges.

8. A nurse is designing a teaching plan for home care for a woman who had an abdominal hysterectomy. What interventions should be included? **Select all that apply.**
   1. Restrict heavy lifting for 4 to 6 weeks.
   2. Take tub baths until bleeding has stopped.
   3. Report an increase in temperature or severe pain.
   4. Take regular rest periods.
   5. Avoid coughing and deep breathing at home.

9. Of the following women, which one would be most at risk for breast cancer?
   1. aged 23, two children
   2. aged 33, never pregnant
   3. aged 45, very thin
   4. aged 64, positive family history

10. A nurse is caring for a woman who is scheduled to have a mastectomy for breast cancer. The woman is crying. What might be an appropriate nursing diagnosis?
    1. *Disturbed Body Image*
    2. *Fatigue*
    3. *Grieving*
    4. *Risk for Injury*

See Test Yourself answers in Appendix C.

EVIDENCE FOR NURSING CARE | **The Patient with Syphilis**

Selected resources that nurses may find helpful when planning evidence-based nursing care follow.

- Kingston, M, French, P, Goh, B, Goold, P, Higgins, S, et al., Syphilis Guidelines Revision Group 2008, Clinical Effectiveness Group. (2008 November). UK National guidelines on the management of syphilis 2008. *International Journal of STD AIDS, 19*(11), 729–40.
- New York State Department of Health. (2009, January). *Syphilis*. New York, NY: New York State Department of Health.
- U.S. Preventive Services Task Force. (2009 May 19). Screening for syphilis infection in pregnancy: U.S. Preventive Services Task Force reaffirmation recommendation statement. *Annals of Internal Medicine, 150*(10), 705–9.

- Emphasize that syphilis can be effectively treated, preventing the serious complications of late-stage disease. *This information provides a sense of control and helps decrease anxiety.*
- Teach the pregnant patient that taking medications as directed and returning each month for follow-up testing will help ensure the well-being of her baby. *Knowing that treatment can reduce the risk to her baby relieves anxiety and possibly increases compliance.*

Situational Low Self-Esteem

Living with any chronic disease can be damaging to a person's self-esteem. However, the patient with syphilis needs additional support to cope with the stigma of this kind of infection. Unfortunately, the populations most affected by STIs often lack family and other social support networks.

- Create an environment where the patient feels respected and safe to discuss questions and concerns about the disease and its effect on his or her life. *Being treated with respect helps enhance self-esteem.*
- Provide privacy and confidentiality. *Patients are often embarrassed to discuss the intimate details of their sex lives.*
- Let patients know that the nurse and other healthcare providers care about them and the successful treatment of their disease. *Feeling valued enhances self-esteem.*

Community-Based Care

Education is an essential part of nursing care for the patient with any STI, and syphilis is no exception. The nurse emphasizes that untreated syphilis is a chronic disease that can be spread to others even though no symptoms are evident. Address the following topics:

- Taking all prescribed medication
- Referring sexual partners for evaluation and treatment
- Abstaining from all sexual contact as recommended by CDC guidelines
- Using a condom to avoid transmitting or contracting infections in the future
- The need for follow-up testing (at 3 and 6 months for patients with primary or secondary syphilis, and at 6 and 12 months

for those with late-stage disease). If patients are HIV positive, follow-up visits are recommended 1, 2, 3, 6, 9, and 12 months after treatment.

The Patient with Pelvic Inflammatory Disease

Pelvic inflammatory disease (PID) is a term used to describe infection of the pelvic organs, including the fallopian tubes (*salpingitis*), ovaries (*oophoritis*), cervix (*cervicitis*), endometrium (*endometritis*), pelvic peritoneum, and the pelvic vascular system. PID can be caused by one or more infectious agents, including *Neisseria gonorrhoeae*, *Chlamydia trachomatis*, *Haemophilus influenzae*, and enteric Gram-negative rods. *N. gonorrhoeae* and *C. trachomatis* are responsible for most PID; dual infection with both agents is common.

PID is not a reportable disease in the United States; however, it is estimated that about 1 million women experience PID each year. As a result of the infection, more than 100,000 women become infertile and a large proportion of the ectopic pregnancies occurring each year are the result of PID (CDC, 2007). The disease may also cause pelvic abscesses and chronic abdominal pain.

Sexually active women ages 16 to 24 years are most at risk. Risk factors include a history of sexually transmitted infection (especially gonorrhea and chlamydia), bacterial vaginosis, multiple sexual partners, douching, and previous PID. Barrier contraceptive devices such as condoms reduce the risk of PID.

The prognosis depends on the number of episodes, promptness of treatment, and modification of risk-taking behaviors. Prevention includes educating women, especially young women, regarding the causes and transmission of infection and methods of self-protection, such as avoiding unprotected sexual activity.

Pathophysiology

Pelvic inflammatory disease is usually polymicrobial (caused by more than one microbe) in origin, with gonorrhea and chlamydia being common causative organisms. Pathogenic organisms ascend from the vagina via the endocervical canal to the fallopian tubes and ovaries. The endocervical canal is slightly dilated during menstruation, allowing bacteria to enter the uterus. Once in the reproductive tract, the organisms rapidly multiply and ascend to the fallopian tubes and ovaries. The infection can extend beyond the reproductive tract to involve the peritoneum (peritonitis or peritoneal abscess) or other abdominal organs.

Manifestations

Manifestations of PID include fever, purulent vaginal discharge, abnormal bleeding, lower abdominal or back pain, dyspareunia, and painful cervical movement. However, the manifestations may be so mild that the infection is not recognized.

Complications

Complications include pelvic abscess, infertility, ectopic pregnancy, chronic pelvic pain, pelvic adhesions, and chronic pelvic pain. Abscess formation is common.

Interdisciplinary Care

The goals of treatment are to eliminate the infection and prevent complications and recurrence. The physical examination may reveal abdominal, adnexal, and cervical pain.

Diagnosis

Tests used in the diagnosis of PID may include a CBC with differential, which will show a markedly elevated WBC, and an increased sedimentation rate. If a laparoscopy or laparotomy is done, it may reveal inflammation, edema, or hyperemia of the fallopian tubes, or tubal discharge and, possibly, generalized pelvic involvement, abscesses, and scarring.

Medications

Combination antibiotic therapy with at least two broad-spectrum antibiotics administered IV or orally is the typical treatment for PID. If PID is not acute, outpatient antibiotic therapy is prescribed. In acute cases, however, the patient may be hospitalized. Analgesics are given, and antibiotics and fluids are administered intravenously. Commonly prescribed antibiotics include parental cefoxitin (Mefoxin), or clindamycin (Cleocin), plus gentamicin (Garamycin) or doxycycline (Vibramycin). Nursing implications for antibiotics are discussed in ∞ Chapter 12.

Surgery

Surgery may be performed to drain an abscess or treat a life-threatening complication such as rupture of a fallopian tube or abscess.

✍ Nursing Care

The goals of nursing care are to treat the infection and to prevent complications, such as scarring and infertility. The patient who is hospitalized maintains bed rest in the semi-Fowler's position to promote drainage and to localize the infectious process in the pelvic cavity.

Nursing Diagnoses and Interventions

Nursing diagnoses that apply to the patient with PID include a risk for injury and deficient knowledge.

Risk for Injury

PID can have severe, even life-threatening, complications. Scarring of fallopian tubes can lead to ectopic pregnancy or pelvic abscess. Infertility is a common complication, as are recurrent or chronic PID, chronic abdominal pain, pelvic adhesions, premature hysterectomy, and depression. The woman who has severe infection and manifestations may be hospitalized for treatment.

- Administer antibiotic therapy as ordered, and monitor closely for adverse effects. *Antibiotics used in acute PID are potent agents; some can have serious side effects.*
- Practice thorough hand hygiene and strict adherence to standard precautions when handling perineal pads and linens. Appropriate disinfection of bedpans, toilet seats, linens, and utensils is also important. *These practices help avoid disseminating the infection to others.*

Readiness for Enhanced Knowledge

PID is most common in young women, who often do not understand their own anatomy and physiology or sexually transmitted infections. Diagnosis and treatment of PID offer an opportunity to increase that understanding, thereby preventing complications and recurrent infection.

- Explain how infection is spread and what measures to take to prevent future infection. *Understanding can improve compliance with treatment regimens and perhaps change high-risk behavior.*
- Explain the need to complete the treatment regimen and the importance of follow-up visits. If the patient or partner fails to take all of the medication as prescribed, the infection may not be completely cured. *Noncompliance and recurrence are common, particularly if follow-up appointments are not kept.*
- Teach proper perineal care, especially wiping from front to back. *This reduces transmission of fecal organisms to reproductive tissues and reduces the incidence of urinary tract infections.*
- Caution the patient about using tampons. Instruct the patient to change tampons or pads at least every 4 hours. *Menstrual flow and other discharges provide a favorable environment for microorganisms to multiply.*
- Provide information about safer sex practices and family planning. Instruct the patient to remove diaphragms within 6 hours after use. IUDs are contraindicated. Latex condoms offer the most effective protection against infection. *These measures help prevent recurrence of infection.*
- Teach the patient to report any unusual vaginal discharge or odor to the healthcare provider. *Treatment is most effective early in the disease process.*

Community-Based Care

Provide general information related to sexually transmitted infections. Teach measures to eradicate the infection and prevent recurrence, and help the patient deal with the physical and psychosocial implications of treatment, including possible infertility. Inform the patient that the patency of the fallopian tubes can be evaluated after several menstrual cycles; this delay allows for complete resolution of the inflammatory process.

CHAPTER HIGHLIGHTS

- Sexually transmitted infections (STIs) are infections transmitted by sexual contact, including vaginal, oral, and anal intercourse. STIs affect women more than men, and are more common in people who have multiple sex partners, abuse drugs, and are of lower socioeconomic status.

- STIs can coexist in the same person and can be transmitted by either heterosexual or homosexual sexual contact. Effective treatment mandates that both sex partners be treated. Most STIs can be prevented by using latex condoms.

- Genital herpes, caused by an infection with an HSV virus, is a commonly occurring STI in teens and young adults. There is no cure and treatment is primarily symptomatic. Nursing care is directed toward relieving the pain of the lesions, mitigating sexual dysfunction, and relieving anxiety.

- Genital warts, caused by the human papilloma virus (HPV), are a chronic, incurable STI. They are manifested by warts of various forms, or may be present without manifestations. Infection with HPV poses a major risk for cervical cancer, as well as other neoplasms of the reproductive system. A vaccine against the virus is recommended for adolescent girls and young women.

- Urogenital infections include vaginal infections (bacterial vaginosis, candidiasis, and trichomoniasis), chlamydia, gonorrhea, syphilis, and pelvic inflammatory disease (PID).

- Chlamydia, occurring most in young adults under age 25, is a bacterial infection that can spread to the uterus and fallopian tubes in women, causing PID, infertility, and ectopic pregnancy. Untreated chlamydia in men may result in epididymitis, prostatitis, sterility, and Reiter's syndrome.

- Gonorrhea (caused by a bacteria) and syphilis (caused by a spirochete) affect both men and women, and may infect the newborn as it moves through the birth canal in an untreated woman. Syphilis, if untreated, exists in the body in three stages, with the third stage lasting up to 50 years. Both of these STIs are treated with antibiotics. Nursing care focuses on education, preventing injury from complications, relieving anxiety, and supporting self-esteem.

- PID is an infection of the female pelvic organs, and may be caused by one or more infectious agents. Sexually active young women between the ages of 16 and 24 are most at risk. The prognosis depends on the number of episodes, promptness of treatment, and modification of risk-taking behaviors. The goals of nursing care are to treat the infection and prevent complications.

TEST YOURSELF NCLEX-RN® REVIEW

1. Which population is most often affected by STIs?
   1. men
   2. women
   3. adolescent males
   4. older adults

2. Which of the following statements would indicate a patient understands teaching to treat an STI?
   1. "My sex partner and I must both take medications."
   2. "I know I can never have sex again."
   3. "I will douche after every sexual encounter with my partner."
   4. "My sex partner does not have an infection, so won't need medications."

3. You are teaching a male patient information about using condoms to prevent STI. What topics would you include? **Select all that apply.**
   1. Use a new condom with each sex act.
   2. Ensure a small amount of air in the tip.
   3. Use oil-based lubricants, such as petroleum jelly.
   4. Handle carefully to ensure no damage.
   5. Withdraw when the penis is erect.

4. You are assessing a young male. He has both blisters and ulcerations on the shaft of his penis. What is his most likely medical diagnosis?
   1. chlamydia
   2. gonorrhea
   3. genital warts
   4. genital herpes

5. Of the following statements about genital warts, which one is *not* true?
   1. The infection is caused by a yeast organism.
   2. The infection can be spread by any type of intercourse.
   3. The infection may be transmitted to the fetus.
   4. The infection cannot be cured.

6. You are counseling a young woman with an HPV genital infection. What screening test would you recommend she have every year?
   1. breast exam and mammogram
   2. stool for occult blood
   3. CBC to detect anemia and infection
   4. pelvic exam and Pap smear

7. Which of the following manifestations would most commonly be elicited during a health history for a woman with a vaginal infection?
   1. pain
   2. itching
   3. nausea
   4. diarrhea

8. You are teaching a woman with an STI who has severe genital discomfort. What is one simple recommendation that may relieve the discomfort?
   1. Wear nylon panty hose.
   2. Cut fingernails short.
   3. Wear cotton underwear.
   4. Have sex more frequently.

9. The infective organism responsible for gonorrhea *initially* targets what body parts?
   1. male urethra and female cervix
   2. female vulva and vagina
   3. male prostate
   4. male and female external genitalia

10. Which of the following would you teach a patient about syphilis?
    1. Syphilis is caused by a virus.
    2. Syphilis is a local genital infection.
    3. Syphilis is a systemic infection.
    4. Syphilis has no effect on the developing fetus.

See Test Yourself answers in Appendix C.

Pearson Nursing Student Resources
Find additional review materials at
www.nursing.pearsonhighered.com
Prepare for success with additional NCLEX®-style practice questions,
interactive assignments and activities, Web links, animations and
videos, and more!

BIBLIOGRAPHY

Akinsanya-Beysolow, I., & Wolfe, C. (2009, August). Update: Vaccines for women, adolescence through adulthood. *Journal of Women's Health, 18*(8), 1101–1108.

American Social Health Association. (2006). *STD/STI: Statistics Fast facts*. Retrieved from http://www.ashastd.org/learn/learn_statistics.cfm

Campos-Outcalt, D. (2009, March). CDC recommendations expand vaccine indications. *Journal of Family Practice, 58*(3), 146–148.

Casper, M., & Carpenter, L. (2008, September). Sex, drugs, and politics: The HPV vaccine for cervical cancer. *Sociology of Health & Illness, 30*(6), 886–899.

Centers for Disease Control and Prevention. (2006a). Treatment guidelines for sexually transmitted diseases. Retrieved from http://www.cdc.gov/std/treatment.htm

Centers for Disease Control and Prevention. (2006b). *Expedited partner therapy in the management of sexually transmitted diseases*. Atlanta, GA: US Department of Health and Human Services.

Centers for Disease Control and Prevention. (2007). *CDC Fact Sheet (Bacterial vaginosis, Chlamydia, genital herpes, genital HPV, gonorrhea, LGV, trichomoniasis)*. Retrieved from http://www.cdc.gov/std.htm

Centers for Disease Control and Prevention. (2008). *Sexually Transmitted Disease Surveillance, 2007.* Atlanta, GA: U.S. Department of Health and Human Services.

Centers for Disease Control and Prevention. (2009a). QuickStats: Percentage of Adults Aged 20–29 Years with Genital Herpes* Infection, by Race/Ethnicity'—National Health and Nutrition Examination Survey, United States, 1988–1994, 1999–2002, and 2003–2006. *MMWR, 58*(07), 173.

Centers for Disease Control and Prevention. (2009b). *Recommended Adult Immunization Schedule United States—2009*. Retrieved from www.cdc.gov/vaccines/recs/schedules/downloads/adult/2009/adult-schedule-bw.pdf

Dariotis, J., Sonenstein, F., Gates, G., Capps, R., Astone, N., Pleck, J., et al. (2008, December). Changes in sexual risk behavior as young men transition to adulthood. *Perspectives on Sexual & Reproductive Health, 40*(4), 218–225.

Edwards, M. (2008, December 12). Genital warts and genital herpes: A public health perspective. *Practice Nurse, 36*(10), 20–23.

Fauci, A., Braunwald, E., Kasper, D., Hauser, S., Longo, D., Jameson, J., et al. (Eds.). (2008). *Harrison's Principles of Internal Medicine* (17th ed.). New York, NY: McGraw Hill.

Getting treatment to partners: The expedited partner therapy option. (2009, February). *Journal of Family Practice, 58*(2), 80.

Hoff, J. (2008, June). Genital herpes in older women: A silent epidemic. *Journal of the American Academy of Nurse Practitioners, 20*(6), 291–294.

Huang, C. (2008, June). Human papillomavirus and vaccination. *Mayo Clinic Proceedings, 83*(6), 701–707.

Laughon, K., Gielen, A., Campbell, J., Burke, J., McDonnell, K., & O'Campo, P. (2007). The relationships among sexually transmitted infection, depression, and lifetime violence in a sample of predominantly African American women. *Research in Nursing & Health, 30,* 413–428.

McPhee, S., Papadakis, M., & Tierney, L. (Eds.). (2008). *Current medical diagnosis & treatment* (47th ed.). New York, NY: McGraw Hill.

NANDA International. (2009). *Nursing diagnoses: Definitions and classification 2009–2011.* Oxford, UK: Wiley Blackwell.

Porth, C., & Matfin, G. (2009). *Pathophysiology: Concepts of altered health states* (8th ed.). Philadelphia, PA: Lippincott.

Sandfort, J., & Pleasant, A. (2009, September/October). Knowledge, attitudes, and informational behaviors of college students in regard to the human papillomavirus. *Journal of American College Health, 58*(2), 141–149.

Screening pregnant women for bacterial vaginosis: U.S. Preventive Services Task Force recommendations. (2008, February 5). *Annals of Internal Medicine, 148*(3), I30.

Screening pregnant women for syphilis infection: U.S. Preventive Services Task Force recommendation. (2009, May 19). *Annals of Internal Medicine, 150*(10), I40.

Wasik, M., & Kachlic, M. (2009, March). A review of common sexually transmitted diseases. *Formulary, 44*(3), 78–85.

Workowski, K., Berman, S., & Douglas, J. (2008, April 15). Emerging antimicrobial resistance to *Neisseria gonorrhoeae*: Urgent need to strengthen prevention strategies. *Annals of Internal Medicine, 148*(8), 606–W124.

Wilson, B., Shannon, M., Shields, K., & Stang, C. (2008). *Nurse's drug guide 2008.* Upper Saddle River, NJ: Prentice Hall.

Functional Health Pattern: Sexuality-Reproductive

Think about patients with altered patterns of sexuality and reproduction for whom you have cared in your clinical experiences.

- Was this alteration in sexuality or reproduction due to a problem affecting the genitourinary or reproductive system or secondary to another condition (e.g., impotence secondary to liver or kidney failure)?

- What kinds of manifestations did your patient(s) have? Were these manifestations similar or different?

- How were the patients' sexuality or ability to reproduce affected? Were they willing to talk about the problem, or did your patients appear reluctant to discuss the problem and related concerns? Did the patients express any cultural beliefs or practices regarding the reproductive system?

The Sexuality-Reproductive Health Pattern includes patterns of satisfaction or dissatisfaction with sexuality and sexual relationships, reproductive patterns, male prostate history, and female menstrual and perimenopausal history. The male and female reproductive organs produce hormones important in biological development and sexual behavior. The male reproductive system consists of the paired testes, scrotum, ducts, glands, penis, and breasts. The female reproductive system consists of the external genitalia such as mons pubis, labia, clitoris, vaginal and urethral openings, glands, and breasts. The female reproductive system also consists of internal organs, such as the cervix, uterus, fallopian tubes, and ovaries. Parts of the male and female reproductive organs also enclose and/or are integral to the function of the urinary system.

Disorders affecting men may be inflammatory, structural, benign, or malignant. Many of the disorders pose significant risk to fertility, sexual function, and urinary function. Many disorders of the male reproductive system and their treatments have the potential to affect erection and ejaculation. As men age, benign and malignant conditions of the prostate gland become common. A man's perceived pattern of sexuality and reproduction may be affected by manifestations such as the following:

- **Erectile dysfunction** (*aging, illness, injury or medications cause a decrease in blood flow to the penis, resulting in inability to attain or maintain an erection*)

- **Urinary dribbling, frequency, retention** (*enlargement of the prostate gland compresses the urethra, impairing the ability to initiate micturition and completely empty the urinary bladder*)

Female disorders range from the discomfort of menstrual cramps to life-threatening diseases such as cancer. Many of these diseases can occur at any point in the woman's adult life. The disorders may affect the ability to bear children, sexuality and sexual function, and the sense of well-being as a woman. A woman's perceived pattern of sexuality and reproduction may be affected by manifestations such as the following:

- **Dysmenorrhea** (*excessive production of prostaglandins stimulates uterine muscle fibers to contract, which compromises uterine blood flow, resulting in uterine ischemia and pain*)

- **Premenstrual syndrome** (*hormonal changes involving estrogen, progesterone, prolactin, and aldosterone along with neurotransmitter changes involving monoamine oxidase and serotonin cause manifestations prior to the beginning of the menstrual period, resulting in mood swings, breast tenderness, fatigue, irritability, food cravings, and depression*)

Patients who experience reproductive system changes and disorders require a holistic approach to meet their physical, emotional, and educational needs. Priority nursing diagnoses within the Sexuality-Reproductive Health Pattern that may be appropriate for patients include the following:

- *Sexual Dysfunction* as evidenced by impotence, erectile dysfunction, dyspareunia, vaginismus, or inability or alterations in achieving desired sexual satisfaction.

- *Ineffective Sexuality Patterns* evidenced by difficulties or limitations in sexual behaviors, changes in sexual activities, and expression of loss.

Two nursing diagnoses from other functional health patterns often are of high priority for the patient with altered reproductive function:

- *Disturbed Body Image* (Self-Perception-Self-Concept Health Pattern)

- *Powerlessness* (Coping-Stress-Tolerance Health Pattern)

Questions

1. Many patients are very uncomfortable talking about their sexual functioning. What can you do to ease their discomfort and facilitate communication? Would the same techniques work for both male and female patients? Does the patient's age affect his or her comfort level?

CLINICAL SCENARIO

Directions: *Read the clinical scenarios and answer the questions that follow. To complete this exercise successfully, you will use not only knowledge of the content in this unit, but also principles related to priority setting and maintaining patient safety.*

You have been assigned to work with the following four patients for the 0700 shift on a medical-surgical unit. Significant data obtained during report is as follows:

- Wendy Torrell, 53 years old, had an abdominal hysterectomy yesterday afternoon. She has a history of CVA and stopped taking the prescribed Plavix 24 hours before surgery. Postoperatively she developed intra-abdominal bleeding, which was controlled by abdominal pressure and ice. She is to have 2 units of whole blood this morning. Vital signs are temperature 98.2°F, pulse 110, respirations 20, blood pressure 88/54.

- Barney Green, 76 years old, is 3 days postoperative for transurethral resection of the prostate (TURP). Vital signs are temperature 98.7°F, pulse 82, respirations 16, blood pressure 158/82. His urinary catheter was removed at 0600. He is complaining of dribbling of urine after attempting to void.

- Tara Morris is a 21 year old newly admitted from the emergency department with complaints of severe lower abdominal pain, purulent vaginal discharge, and cervical pain on pelvic exam. Her vital signs are temperature 102.6°F, pulse 88, respirations 20, and blood pressure 110/70. She is to be started on ceftriaxone (Rocephin) and gentamicin (Garamycin) IV as soon as possible.

- Regina Perkins, 36 years old, has a history of uterine fibroids. She had a uterine fibroid embolization yesterday. Her vital signs have remained stable throughout the night. Her discharge is written and she is in a hurry to be discharged so her husband can get to work.

Questions

Priority Setting

1. In what order would you visit these patients after report?
   A. _____
   B. _____
   C. _____
   D. _____

Health Promotion

1. When Ms. Torrell is ready for discharge, what specific foods will you encourage her to eat to increase her iron level?

2. What teaching regarding safer sex practices will you provide for Ms. Morris?

Nursing Process

1. What top priority nursing diagnosis would you choose for each of the patients presented earlier? What is the rationale for your choices?

	Nursing Diagnosis	Rationale
Wendy Torrell		
Barney Green		
Tara Morris		
Regina Perkins		

2. Ms. Torrell asks the purpose of the abdominal binder.
   A. The abdominal binder will hold the abdominal muscles together until healing occurs.
   B. The abdominal binder put pressure on the leaking blood vessels, stopping the internal bleeding.
   C. The abdominal binder is routinely used on all patients after abdominal surgery.
   D. The abdominal binder is used on all obese patients.

3. Mr. Green suddenly develops nausea and vomiting, blood pressure is 170/100, pulse is 58, and he becomes confused. What do you suspect is the cause of these symptoms?
   A. allergy reaction to the bladder irrigating fluid solution
   B. anxiety reaction to having prostate surgery
   C. absorption of isotonic bladder irrigating fluids
   D. hypovolemic shock complication of the surgery

4. Which is most important to teach Ms. Morris about pelvic inflammatory disease?
   A. Take all medication as prescribed.
   B. Wipe from front to back after urinating.
   C. Use latex condoms when having sex.
   D. Change tampons or pads every 4 hours.

5. Prior to surgery, Ms. Perkins's hematocrit was 34% and hemoglobin was 10 g/dL. She was instructed to increase iron foods in her diet. Which foods are high in iron?
   A. beef, eggs, brown rice
   B. green, leafy vegetables, chicken
   C. fish, broccoli, kidney beans
   D. liver, cheese, asparagus

Communication

1. Ms. Morris asks if she will be able to have children when the infection is gone. How will you respond?

2. Mr. Green asks if he will be able to urinate normally, or if he will always dribble and have to wear adult diapers. How will you respond?

Delegation

1. For each patient, what assessment data and nursing interventions can be delegated to a nursing assistant?

Content-Specific Questions

1. Which is a priority nursing diagnosis for a young female patient with endometriosis?
   A. *Acute Pain* related to menstrual periods
   B. *Deficient Knowledge* related to complications of endometriosis
   C. *Decisional Conflict* related to treatment plan options
   D. *Anxiety* related to risk for loss of reproductive function

2. A prescription for tadalafil (Cialis) is ordered for the patient with erectile dysfunction. The patient indicates understanding of teaching instructions when he makes which statement?
   A. "I will take Cialis to just before intercourse to increase my sex drive."
   B. "I will consult with the doctor before taking other medications."
   C. "I can take a second pill the same day if the first one doesn't work."
   D. "This pill will relieve all of my sex problems."

3. Which laboratory studies would you expect to draw to diagnose syphilis? **Select all that apply.**
   A. VDRL
   B. gram stain
   C. RPR
   D. DFA
   E. tissue culture
   F. FTA-ABS

4. Which instructions should be taught to the patient who is receiving radiation therapy for prostate cancer?
   A. Eat more red meat to maintain protein for healing.
   B. Avoid close contact with pregnant women, infants, and children.
   C. Avoid sexual contact to prevent stress from dysfunction.
   D. Sleep alone for the first night after radiation therapy.

5. Which symptom would be most significant when assessing a patient with possible cervical cancer?
   A. vaginal discharge
   B. weight loss
   C. pain in back and thighs
   D. vaginal bleeding

6. A sexually active woman is being treated for gonorrhea. Which method of birth control does the nurse tell her is safest to use?
   A. oral contraceptives
   B. intrauterine device
   C. condom
   D. estrogen patch

CASE STUDY: Eva Gibson

Eva Gibson is 43-years-old, married with two children, whose mammogram revealed a mass in the left breast. She does have a family history of breast cancer in her mother and a maternal aunt. She is admitted to outpatient surgery for an incisional biopsy with results of invasive lobular carcinoma. An MRI indicates that chest muscles have been infiltrated with cancer. She is admitted to the hospital and a modified radical mastectomy on the left side is performed. Postoperatively, she is admitted to the chemotherapy unit. Vital signs are temperature 98.5°F, pulse 65, respirations 14, and blood pressure 110/68. She is 66" in height and weighs 120 pounds. She has a dressing on the left chest that is dry and intact and a JP drain in place for wound suction. Her left arm is elevated on two pillows. The decision has been made to start radiation and chemotherapy treatments as soon as possible.

Breast cancer develops as a mutation of breast tissue cells related to hormones and mutations of tumor suppressor genes. Abnormal cell growth occurs. Cancer cells produce an angiogenesis factor that stimulates blood vessels to grow into the tumor. Cancer cells invade the blood vessels and travel through the bloodstream or through the lymphatic system to other sites. Manifestations of breast cancer may include a nontender lump in the breast, abnormal nipple discharge, rash around the nipple area, nipple retraction, edema, dimpling of the skin, or change in position of the nipple. Some women report a burning or stinging sensation in the breast or nipple pain. Complications of breast cancer are metastasis to bone, brain, lung, liver, skin, and lymph nodes and death.

The nursing diagnosis of *Impaired Tissue Integrity* is appropriate for planning care for Mrs. Gibson.

- Breast tissue cells mutate and grow abnormally
- Cancer cells produce a factor that stimulates growth of blood vessels into tumor
- Cancer cells metastasize

affects

leads to

Mrs. E. G.
43 y.o. female
Breast cancer

assess

- Diagnosis of left breast cancer
- Surgical procedure to remove cancer with thoracic incision and JP drain
- Scheduled to have further treatment with radiation and chemotherapy

generates

- Acute Pain related to surgical incision
- Disturbed Body Image related to loss of breast
- Grieving related to diagnosis of cancer
- Anxiety related to concerns about care of children and husband

generate nursing diagnosis

prioritized to

Impaired Tissue Integrity

expected outcomes

- Vital signs will remain within normal limits
- WBC findings remain within normal limits
- Incision progressively heals without manifestations of infection
- Consumes increased protein and vitamins

evaluate

- Vital signs and WBC remained within normal limits
- Incision healed without evidence of infection
- Verbalized importance of increasing protein in diet

Interdisciplinary Interventions
- Monitor results of lab data and report abnormal findings to surgeon.
- Administer prescribed antibiotics.

Independent Interventions
- Wash hands before and after each nursing care activity.
- Monitor vital signs (especially T) every 4 to 8 hours.
- Assess incision each day.
- Assess color and amount of drainage on dressing and from JP drain at the end of each shift.
- Use sterile procedures to change dressing and empty JP drain.
- Discuss importance of diet in wound healing and during treatment for cancer.

Activity:

1. After reviewing the case study and concept map, how would you prioritize the identified nursing diagnoses and nursing interventions?

2. Go to the Pearson Nursing Student Resources for this book at www.nursing.pearsonhighered.com to write a concept map identifying priority nursing diagnoses and interventions to address common adverse effects of planned chemotherapy and radiation therapy.

   See answers and hints in Appendix C.

Appendix A: Standard Precautions

Standard precautions are designed to reduce the risk of transmission of microorganisms from both recognized and unrecognized sources of infection. They are the primary strategies for preventing nosocomial infections within institutions, and are important to protect healthcare workers as well. Standard precautions apply to (1) blood; (2) all body fluids, secretions, and excretions except sweat, regardless of whether or not they contain visible blood; (3) nonintact skin; and (4) mucous membranes. Standard precautions are applied to all patients receiving care in any healthcare setting, regardless of their diagnosis or presumed infection status. Although these precautions are specifically designed for healthcare settings, they also may be implemented in providing home care or in other community-based care settings.

Hand Hygiene

- Avoid unnecessary touching of surfaces in the patient-care area.
- Perform hand hygiene (a) after touching blood, body fluids, secretions, excretions, and contaminated items, whether or not gloves are worn; (b) immediately after removing gloves, even if gloves appear to be intact; (c) between contacts with patients; and (d) when otherwise indicated to prevent transfer of organisms to other patients. You may need to wash your hands between tasks and procedures on the same patient to prevent cross-contaminating different body sites.
- Use soap and warm water for hand hygiene when hands are visibly dirty or contaminated with blood, other body fluids, or material containing body proteins.
- If hands are not visibly soiled, use an alcohol-based hand rub for routinely decontaminating hands in all other situations.

Personal Protective Equipment

Gloves

- Wear clean, nonsterile gloves when touching blood, body fluids, secretions, excretions, and contaminated items.
- Put on clean gloves just before touching mucous membranes and nonintact skin.
- Change your gloves between tasks and procedures on the same patient after contacting material that may contain a high concentration of microorganisms.
- Wear gloves for all invasive procedures such as performing venipuncture or other vascular or surgical procedures.
- Wear gloves if you have cuts, scratches, or other breaks in the skin.
- Remove gloves promptly after use, before touching noncontaminated items and surfaces, and before going to another patient; perform hand hygiene immediately after removing gloves.

Mask, Eye Protection, Face Shield

Wear a mask and eye protection or a face shield to protect mucous membranes of your eyes, nose, and mouth during procedures and patient-care activities that are likely to generate splashes or sprays of blood, body fluids, secretions, or excretions (including suctioning of the respiratory tract or endotracheal intubation). Wear a surgical mask when assisting with lumbar puncture or when material is injected into the spinal canal or subdural space.

Gown

Wear a gown (clean, disposable) to protect your skin and prevent soiling of clothing during procedures and patient-care activities that are likely to generate splashes or sprays of blood, body fluids, secretions, or excretions. Remove soiled gowns promptly, washing your hands immediately after gown removal.

Respiratory Hygiene/Cough Etiquette

Implement measures to control respiratory secretions of patients (and people accompanying them) with manifestations of a respiratory infection on entry into the healthcare setting:

- Post signs alerting patients to cover their mouths/noses when coughing or sneezing, use and dispose of tissues, and perform hand hygiene after contacting respiratory secretions.
- Provide tissues and no-touch receptacles (e.g., a waste container with a foot pedal) for tissue disposal.
- Provide instructions and resources (e.g., alcohol-based hand rub dispensers) for hand hygiene in or near patient waiting areas.
- As appropriate, offer masks to coughing patients, and encourage them to sit at least 3 feet away from other patients in the waiting area.

Environmental Control

Follow hospital procedures for routine care, cleaning, and disinfecting environmental surfaces, beds, bed rails, bedside equipment, and other frequently touched surfaces.

Equipment

Handle used patient-care equipment that is soiled with blood, body fluids, secretions, and excretions in a way that prevents exposing your skin and mucous membranes, contaminating your clothing, and transferring microorganisms to other patients or environments. Ensure that reusable equipment is cleaned and appropriately reprocessed before using for the care of another patient.

Linen

Handle and transport linens soiled with blood, body fluids, secretions, and excretions in a manner that prevents exposing your skin and mucous membranes, contaminating your clothing, and transferring microorganisms to other patients and environments. Place soiled linen in leakage-resistant bags at the location where it is used.

Occupational Health and Bloodborne Pathogens

- Take care to prevent injuries when using needles, scalpels, and other sharps; when handling sharp instruments after procedures; when cleaning used instruments; and when disposing of used needles.
- Never recap used needles, manipulate them using both hands, or handle them in a manner that directs the point of a needle toward any part of your body. If it is necessary to protect the needle prior to disposal, use a one-handed "scoop" technique or mechanical device to hold the needle sheath.
- Do not remove used needles from disposable syringes by hand; do not bend, break, or otherwise manipulate used needles by hand.
- Place used disposable syringes and needles, scalpel blades, and other sharp items in appropriate puncture-resistant containers located as close as practical to the area in which the items were used.
- Place reusable syringes and needles in a puncture-resistant container for transport to the reprocessing area.
- Use mouthpieces, resuscitation bags, or other ventilation devices as an alternative to mouth-to-mouth resuscitation methods whenever possible.

Safe Injection Practices

When using needles, cannulas that replace needles, and intravenous delivery systems do the following:

- Use aseptic technique to avoid contaminating sterile equipment.

- Needles, cannulas, and syringes are single-use items; never use the same syringe, needle, or cannula for more than one patient (even if used to enter or connect to a patient's IV fluid or administration set).
- Use intravenous fluid infusion and administration sets for one patient only and appropriately discard after using.
- Use single-dose vials of parenteral medications whenever possible; do not use the same single-dose vial for more than one patient or combine left-over contents with that from another vial.
- Use a sterile syringe and needle or cannula to access multiple-dose vials if necessary to use; do not store the vial in the patient-care area and discard if sterility is compromised or questionable.

Patient Placement

Place patients who contaminate the environment or who do not (or are not expected to) assist in maintaining appropriate hygiene or environmental control (e.g., an ambulatory, confused patient with fecal incontinence) in a private room.

Source: Centers for Disease Control and Prevention. (2007). *Standard Precautions. Excerpt from Guideline for Isolation Precautions: Preventing Transmission of Infectious Agents in Healthcare Settings 2007.* Atlanta: Public Health Service, U.S. Department of Health and Human Services, Centers for Disease Control and Prevention. Retrieved from www.cdc.gov/ncidod/dhqp/gl_isolation_standard.html#

Appendix B: 2009–2011 NANDA-Approved Nursing Diagnoses

Activity Intolerance
Activity Intolerance, Risk for
Activity Planning, Ineffective
Airway Clearance, Ineffective
Anxiety
Anxiety, Death
Aspiration, Risk for
Attachment, Risk for Impaired
Autonomic Dysreflexia
Autonomic Dysreflexia, Risk for
Bleeding, Risk for
Blood Glucose Level, Risk for Unstable
Body Image, Disturbed
Body Temperature: Imbalanced, Risk for
Bowel Incontinence
Breastfeeding, Effective
Breastfeeding, Ineffective
Breastfeeding, Interrupted
Breathing Pattern, Ineffective
Cardiac Output, Decreased
Caregiver Role Strain
Caregiver Role Strain, Risk for
Childbearing Process, Readiness for Enhanced
Comfort, Impaired
Comfort, Readiness for Enhanced
Communication, Impaired Verbal
Communication, Readiness for Enhanced
Confusion, Acute
Confusion, Acute, Risk for
Confusion, Chronic
Constipation
Constipation, Perceived
Constipation, Risk for
Contamination
Contamination, Risk for
Coping: Community, Ineffective
Coping: Community, Readiness for Enhanced
Coping, Defensive
Coping: Family, Compromised
Coping: Family, Disabled
Coping: Family, Readiness for Enhanced
Coping, Ineffective
Coping, Readiness for Enhanced
Decisional Conflict
Decision Making, Readiness for Enhanced
Denial, Ineffective
Dentition, Impaired
Development: Delayed, Risk for
Diarrhea
Disuse Syndrome, Risk for
Diversional Activity, Deficient
Electrolyte Imbalance, Risk for

Energy Field, Disturbed
Environmental Interpretation Syndrome, Impaired
Failure to Thrive, Adult
Falls, Risk for
Family Processes, Dysfunctional
Family Processes, Interrupted
Family Processes, Readiness for Enhanced
Fatigue
Fear
Fluid Balance, Readiness for Enhanced
Fluid Volume, Deficient
Fluid Volume, Deficient, Risk for
Fluid Volume, Excess
Fluid Volume, Imbalanced, Risk for
Gas Exchange, Impaired
Gastrointestinal Motility, Dysfunctional
Gastrointestinal Motility, Dysfunctional, Risk for
Grieving
Grieving, Complicated
Grieving, Risk for Complicated
Growth, Disproportionate, Risk for
Growth and Development, Delayed
Health Behavior, Risk-Prone
Health Maintenance, Ineffective
Health Management, Ineffective Self
Health Management, Readiness for Enhanced Self
Health-Seeking Behaviors (Specify)
Home Maintenance, Impaired
Hope, Readiness for Enhanced
Hopelessness
Human Dignity, Risk for Compromised
Hyperthermia
Hypothermia
Immunization Status, Readiness for Enhanced
Infant Behavior, Disorganized
Infant Behavior, Disorganized, Risk for
Infant Behavior, Organized, Readiness for Enhanced
Infant Feeding Pattern, Ineffective
Infection, Risk for
Injury, Risk for
Insomnia
Intracranial Adaptive Capacity, Decreased
Jaundice, Neonatal
Knowledge, Deficient
Knowledge, Readiness for Enhanced
Latex Allergy Response
Latex Allergy Response, Risk for
Liver Function, Impaired, Risk for
Loneliness, Risk for
Maternal/Fetal Dyad, Risk for Disturbed

Memory, Impaired
Mobility: Bed, Impaired
Mobility: Physical, Impaired
Mobility: Wheelchair, Impaired
Moral Distress
Nausea
Neglect, Self
Neglect, Unilateral
Neurovascular Dysfunction: Peripheral, Risk for
Noncompliance (Specify)
Nutrition, Imbalanced: Less than Body Requirements
Nutrition, Imbalanced: More than Body Requirements
Nutrition, Imbalanced: More than Body Requirements, Risk for
Nutrition, Readiness for Enhanced
Oral Mucous Membrane, Impaired
Pain, Acute
Pain, Chronic
Parenting, Impaired
Parenting, Readiness for Enhanced
Parenting, Risk for Impaired
Perfusion, Decreased Cardiac Tissue, Risk for
Perfusion, Ineffective Cerebral Tissue, Risk for
Perfusion, Ineffective Gastrointestinal, Risk for
Perfusion, Ineffective Peripheral Tissue
Perfusion, Ineffective Renal, Risk for
Perioperative Positioning Injury, Risk for
Personal Identity, Disturbed
Poisoning, Risk for
Post-Trauma Syndrome
Post-Trauma Syndrome, Risk for
Power, Readiness for Enhanced
Powerlessness
Powerlessness, Risk for
Protection, Ineffective
Rape-Trauma Syndrome
Relationship, Readiness for Enhanced
Religiosity, Impaired
Religiosity, Readiness for Enhanced
Religiosity, Risk for Impaired
Relocation Stress Syndrome
Relocation Stress Syndrome, Risk for
Resilience, Impaired Individual
Resilience, Risk for Compromised
Resilience, Readiness for Enhanced
Role Conflict, Parental
Role Performance, Ineffective
Sedentary Lifestyle
Self-Care, Readiness for Enhanced

Self-Care Deficit: Bathing
Self-Care Deficit: Dressing
Self-Care Deficit: Feeding
Self-Care Deficit: Toileting
Self-Concept, Readiness for Enhanced
Self-Esteem, Chronic Low
Self-Esteem, Situational Low
Self-Esteem, Risk for Situational Low
Self-Mutilation
Self-Mutilation, Risk for
Sensory Perception, Disturbed (Specify:
    Auditory, Gustatory, Kinesthetic,
    Olfactory, Tactile, Visual)
Sexual Dysfunction
Sexuality Pattern, Ineffective
Shock, Risk for
Skin Integrity, Impaired
Skin Integrity, Risk for Impaired
Sleep, Readiness for Enhanced
Sleep Deprivation

Sleep Pattern, Disturbed
Social Interaction, Impaired
Social Isolation
Sorrow, Chronic
Spiritual Distress
Spiritual Distress, Risk for
Spiritual Well-Being, Readiness for
    Enhanced
Spontaneous Ventilation, Impaired
Stress Overload
Sudden Infant Death Syndrome, Risk for
Suffocation, Risk for
Suicide, Risk for
Surgical Recovery, Delayed
Swallowing, Impaired
Therapeutic Regimen Management:
    Ineffective Family
Thermoregulation, Ineffective
Tissue Integrity, Impaired
Transfer Ability, Impaired

Trauma, Risk for
Trauma, Vascular, Risk for
Urinary Elimination, Impaired
Urinary Elimination, Readiness for
    Enhanced
Urinary Incontinence, Functional
Urinary Incontinence, Overflow
Urinary Incontinence, Reflex
Urinary Incontinence, Stress
Urinary Incontinence, Urge
Urinary Retention
Weaning Response, Dysfunctional
Violence: Other-Directed, Risk for
Violence: Self-Directed, Risk for
Walking, Impaired
Wandering

Source: NANDA International. (2009).
Nursing diagnoses: Definitions and classification 2009–2011. Oxford, UK: Wiley-Blackwell. Used with permission.

Appendix C: Test Yourself, End of Unit, and Evaluate Your Response Answers

Test Yourself Answers

Chapter 1: Medical-Surgical Nursing in the Twenty-first Century

1. **Answer: 2 Rationale:** This is done in order to standardize the different healthcare professions nationally and develop guidelines of practice.

2. **Answer: 4 Rationale:** Critical thinking is needed in order to perform nursing assessments, prioritize patient care, evaluate treatment and education needs, and address any potential safety issues.

3. **Answer: 1 Rationale:** The patient is an integral part of developing a care plan. It is very important to include the patient in order to establish individualized goals to best meet the needs of the patient. Nurses develop a partnership with the patient when initiating the plan of care.

4. **Answer: 2, 1, 5, 4, 3 Rationale:** Assessment is the first step to determine the needs of the patient. Based on this information, individualized goals and outcomes can be established. Next, the planning stage determines what is necessary to meet the expected outcomes. These expected outcomes should be short-term and realistic, and should be adjusted as necessary. Implementation follows, which is when the plan is put into action. The final step is evaluation. The plan is evaluated to determine the degree of success of the individualized goals and outcomes. The outcomes may be met, partially met, or not met. This is the time when it may be necessary to change the plan and outcomes in order to best meet the patient's needs. The patient should be involved in each step of the nursing process.

5. **Answer: 3 Rationale:** Although there are many layers of care involved in nursing, the foundation for all aspects of nursing is the knowledge base. Without a strong knowledge base, nurses would not be able to develop clinical competency or practice, or provide holistic care.

6. **Answer: 4 Rationale:** The educator role is the most important function for nurses when developing and providing health information to patients.

7. **Answer: 1 Rationale:** Situations involving a difference of opinion between patients and healthcare providers may arise. The nurse plays an integral part in these situations by assisting and supporting the patient's decision making through advocacy.

8. **Answer: 2 Rationale:** When a nurse is responsible for assignments and determining appropriate work activities for other members of the nursing team, this is a leadership or manager role. This role can be formal or informal.

9. **Answer: 2 Rationale:** Critical pathways are developed to address general standards of care and outcomes for a specific patient population. This often helps to simplify the nursing process, but the nurse still must individualize the plan for the patient.

10. **Answer: 3 Rationale:** The nurse is ultimately responsible for the vital signs performed by unlicensed personnel. If there is any question regarding the readings, it is the nurse's responsibility to evaluate the results, repeat anything in question, and inform the provider as necessary.

Chapter 2: Health and Illness in Adults

1. **Answer: 4 Rationale:** Many patients have underlying disease processes, and daily medications are necessary to assist in maintaining good health. Thus, the definition of wellness is actively practicing healthy behaviors, rather than the absence of disease or illness.

2. **Answer: 1, 2, 4, 5 Rationale:** Genetic makeup can predispose patients for many different chronic illnesses or diseases. Cognitive abilities can affect the understanding, or lack of understanding, a patient has regarding how to maintain wellness. Age can affect health as many chronic illnesses become more problematic with age. Age can also affect cognitive abilities and affect other senses necessary to maintain wellness, such as hearing, sight, smell, and taste. Race can also be a factor of health, as many chronic illnesses are more prevalent in particular races and can also be more difficult to manage, such as hypertension in the Black population.

3. **Answer: 2 Rationale:** Sickle cell disease is an autosomal recessive disease that is primarily found in patients of African descent.

4. **Answer: 1 Rationale:** Practicing safer sex is the only choice with a focus on prevention.

5. **Answer: 2 Rationale:** Assuming the sick role is when you take on the responsibility of calling to explain your illness and you do not go to class as a result.

6. **Answer: 4 Rationale:** A congenital illness is a disorder that a person is born with, often as a result of a physiological imperfection.

7. **Answer: 2 Rationale:** The most important factor when referring to a chronic illness is that it lasts for a lifetime. Although manifestations may wax and wane, and remissions may occur, the underlying disease still exists.

8. **Answer: 1 Rationale:** Although Mr. Jones is at risk for multiple illnesses, the system at greatest risk is the cardiovascular system. He has many risk factors for cardiovascular disease including age, overweight, smoking, and sedentary lifestyle.

9. **Answer: 2 Rationale:** Accident prevention in the home is a very important topic to present to senior citizens. This population is at greatest risk for falls and injury in the home due to sensory problems including vision loss, unsteady gait, loss of sensation to hot and cold, and loss of sense of smell and taste to identify spoiled food.

10. **Answer: 3, 4 Rationale:** Recognizing that dying is a part of living is part of adjusting to aging and recognizing the bodily changes that occur as a result of aging. Coping with loss is part of the grieving process that the widowed spouse must endure as the result of death of a loved one.

Chapter 3: Community and Home-Based Care of Adults

1. **Answer: 3 Rationale:** The focus of community-based nursing care is to provide direct care to individuals and their families with acute or chronic health problems.

2. **Answer: 1 Rationale:** Access to healthcare services may be more challenging for rural residents due to transportation issues. Urban residents often have easier access to public transportation to obtain healthcare services.

3. **Answer: 1 Rationale:** Assessment questions related to transportation, financial, personal, physical, and emotional assistance can help the nurse determine the person's social support system.

4. **Answer: 4 Rationale:** Respite care provides assistance to full-time caregivers and helps relieve some of the stress associated with this huge responsibility.

5. **Answer: 1, 3, 4, 5 Rationale:** All four of these individuals can potentially benefit from home-care services.

6. **Answer: 4 Rationale:** The role of advocate occurs when the nurse explores, informs, supports, and affirms the choices of a patient. These activities include advanced directives, living wills, and durable power of attorney for health care.

7. **Answer: 1, 3, 4 Rationale:** Overloaded extension cords, several throw rugs, cluttered floor space, and expired medications are all environmental threats to safety.

8. **Answer: 2 Rationale:** It is important to determine the priorities of needs from the patient and family perspective before establishing a plan of rehabilitative care.

9. **Answer: 2 Rationale:** Health teaching about the importance of effective hand hygiene, the use of gloves, proper handling of linens, disposal of wastes, and the practice of standard precautions can help to control infection in the home.

10. **Answer: 4 Rationale:** Only interventions identified on the treatment plan are covered by private insurance, Medicare, or Medicaid; therefore, treatment plans are a requirement for reimbursement.

Unit 1 Building Clinical Competence: Dimensions of Medical-Surgical Nursing
Functional Health Pattern: Health Perception-Health Management

Functional Health Patterns
Hint: Ask patients to tell you how they feel and why they think they feel this way.

Priority Setting
1.
   A. The distance and travel time between patients.
   B. The estimated time for each visit.
   C. Tom Smith needs IV antibiotics at 0930.
   Rationale: An absolute plan cannot be addressed without knowing more about the setting. Because all patients are relatively stable, who is seen first is not critical. The nurse should plan a route that would allow adequate time for each visit. Mr. Smith's visit will take at least 90 minutes because IV vancomycin takes a minimum of 60 minutes to infuse. Thirty minutes will be allowed for set up and clean up of the infusion. The dressing can be changed while the antibiotic is infusing. The route should be planned to avoid back-tracking (if possible) to be most efficient and cost effective.

Health Promotion
1. An important part of primary prevention is to provide patient teaching related to his or her primary diagnosis. What primary prevention interventions will you talk to each patient about? The following are examples of answers to this question. Other answers are also possible.
   A. Cora Swank: Ms. Swank should have instruction in adequate fiber and fluids in her diet and daily activity. *Rationale: These primary prevention interventions will help with bowel function as well as regaining strength following surgery, facilitating healing and maintaining optimum health.*

   B. Tom Smith: Mr. Smith should be encouraged to wear appropriate safety equipment during high-risk activities such as riding motorcycles. Appropriate safety equipment includes helmet, gloves, long sleeves, long pants, and boots. *Rationale: Proper use of safety equipment can prevent head injury and decrease the chance of soft tissue damage during an accident.*

   C. Marguerite Garcia: Mrs. Garcia should be encouraged to talk with family members or friends daily. If she fails to contact these people daily, they should be responsible to physically check on her to be sure she is OK. *Rationale: Elderly patients living alone are at risk for falls and injury. A responsible person(s) should be in contact with them daily. Should the elderly patient fail to make contact, someone must physically check on the patient's well-being.*

   D. Sebastian Huian: Mr. Huian should be encouraged to stop smoking and provided with information about local stop-smoking programs. *Rationale: Evidence shows smoking contributes to hypertension and stroke. By stopping smoking Mr. Huian can lower his risk for further strokes. His left-sided weakness could also pose a fire risk if he should drop the lit cigarette.*

2. C. *Rationale: Tertiary level of prevention includes providing training to a patient to become productive to society within the limitation of the patient's abilities. Primary level of prevention is developing a healthy lifestyle to prevent illness, such as maintaining a balanced diet and stopping smoking. Secondary level of prevention is screening for and treating illnesses.*

Nursing Process
1.
   A. Cora Swank: Assess abdominal incision for healing. Assess skin around the ostomy, and the intactness of the ostomy appliance. Assess the amount, color, and consistency of stool. Assess pain control. *Rationale: Ms. Swank is a postoperative patient and it is important to assess the amount of healing.*

   B. Tom Smith: Assess the leg wound for healing, amount and type of drainage, and intactness of wound dressing. Assess pain management. Assess condition of the IV site and the patency of the IV needle. *Rationale: It is important for the nurse to evaluate the effectiveness of treatment by assessing the condition of the wound. The patency and condition of an IV must be determined before administration of any medication. Infection and slow healing of injuries can result in chronic pain, which must be evaluated.*

   C. Marguerite Garcia: Besides obtaining a blood pressure and blood glucose, assess heart and lung sounds. Assess the feet and lower legs for the condition of the skin, normal sensation, pulses, and the presence of swelling. *Rationale: Hypertension and congestive heart failure can cause irregular pulse, moist lung sounds, and swelling and decreased circulation in the feet. Diabetes can cause peripheral nerve damage.*

   D. Sebastian Huian: Assess vital signs, a neurological status including the degree of left-sided weakness, and Sebastian's functional abilities for self-care. *Because Mr. Huian was just discharged from rehabilitation and this is the first time the home health nurse is responsible for his care, it is important to obtain a baseline of his neurological and functional status.*

2. Each patient could have more than one nursing diagnosis. The following is not all-inclusive.

	Nursing Diagnosis	Rationale
Cora Swank	*Actue Pain* related to recent surgery *Risk for Impaired Skin Integrity* related to recent surgery and colostomy	*Patient is 10 days post-op. While pain should be less, mild to moderate analgesics may be required.* *Skin irritation can occur at operative site and around the colostomy appliance.*
Tom Smith	*Acute Pain* related to left leg injury and infection	*Even though the leg injury was some time ago, healing has not taken place. In this situation acute pain can become chronic in nature.*
	Impaired Skin Integrity related to wound infection	*There is an obviously infected wound.*
Marguerite Garcia	*Risk for Knowledge Deficit* related to hypertension and type II diabetes *Risk for Noncompliance* of self-administration of medication	*The scenario implies that Mrs. Garcia may not be taking her medication as prescribed. It is important for the nurse to assess her and determine the need for information or other interventions.*
Sebastian Huian	*Risk for Self-Care Deficit*: bathing/ hygiene, dressing/grooming, feeding, toileting	*Because of Mr. Huian's recent CVA and discharge from rehabilitation, he is at risk for self-care deficit in the home environment.*

3. A, C, E. *Rationale: The patient is more likely to follow the plan of care when the nurse has established an atmosphere of trust and has rapport with the patient. To develop a plan of care, the nurse needs to assess the environment to determine the patient's safety needs and to obtain the patient's input into the goals to be accomplished.*

4. Ask Mrs. Garcia to plan a menu for a week and then determine if she has selected low sodium foods. *Rationale: The best way to determine a patient's understanding of teaching is to have him or her repeat the information or demonstrate his or her knowledge.*

Communication

1. Report your assessment findings and the plan for home care that was established with the patient and family. *Rationale: It is important to communicate assessment findings and plan of care to provide a baseline for evaluating patient progress.*

Delegation

1. A home health aid can take Mrs. Garcia's blood pressure, blood glucose, and observe Mrs. Garcia taking her medication. If Mrs. Garcia takes her medication when the home health aid is not present, the aid can report the medication is or is not in the medication container. *Rationale: Home health aids can be taught to take all vital signs and obtain capillary blood glucose values. In*

most cases, home health aids can remind patients to take their medication and can assist them in opening containers. Home health aids cannot evaluate the effectiveness of medication.

Nursing Ethics

1. The nurse should explain that dating the patient is not allowed. *Rationale: It is not ethical to date a patient or to give him or her the impression that a personal relationship will occur in the future. Once the nurse–patient relationship is no longer established, and the nurse does not have a professional responsibility to provide nursing care, a personal relationship could be established.*

Concept Map

Hint: A concept map is one way to visualize the relationships between nursing diagnosis. Be creative in diagramming these relationships. It will be helpful to review Meeting Health Needs of Adults in Chapter 2 as you develop your concept map for Risk-Prone Health Behavior.

Chapter 4: Nursing Care of Patients Having Surgery

1. **Answer: 2 Rationale:** The nurse's primary responsibility to informed consent is serving as a witness to the patient signature on the consent form.
2. **Answer: 2 Rationale:** When patients are discharged soon after surgery, they need increased information about complications so they will recognize abnormal manifestations as early as possible and report these to the healthcare provider.
3. **Answer: 3 Rationale:** Nonsteroidal anti-inflammatory drugs (NSAIDs) potentiate analgesia and reduce inflammation caused from surgery.
4. **Answer: 4 Rationale:** Creatinine levels specifically reflect renal clearance. When creatinine is increased above normal levels, renal impairment needs to be considered.
5. **Answer: 3 Rationale:** Redness or swelling in the calf may be a manifestation of DVT in the circulatory system distal to the surgery.
6. **Answer: 3 Rationale:** All orders must be cancelled when the patient is admitted to surgery and must be re-ordered following surgery.
7. **Answer: 4 Rationale:** Anesthetic agents cause paralysis and block sympathetic nervous system control. This blocks manifestations of hypoglycemia and could prevent recognition of the condition.
8. **Answer: 3 Rationale:** Administering analgesics on a regular schedule in the immediate postoperative period enhances pain control.
9. **Answer: 4 Rationale:** Remaining in a fixed position for a long period of time impairs circulation, which increases the risk of pressure ulcers; joint stiffness develops from lack of flexion so that pain occurs when the joint is flexed.
10. **Answer: 4 Rationale:** Hypothermia is associated with bleeding from the surgical site and increases cardiac ischemia, which in turn increases the risk of cardiac mortality.

Chapter 5: Nursing Care of Patients Experiencing Loss, Grief, and Death

1. **Answer: 3 Rationale:** Only the person experiencing loss can evaluate his or her experiences. This is highly individualized and cannot be judged by others.
2. **Answer: 1 Rationale:** Anger is a common response to the diagnosis of a terminal illness.
3. **Answer: 2 Rationale:** A strong support system of friends and family is extremely important in helping one through the grieving process and to cope with loss.
4. **Answer: 1 Rationale:** Culture dictates the rituals of mourning, providing a pathway to express the loss.

5. **Answer: 2 Rationale:** A living will expresses the exact wishes of a patient regarding expectations for medical care. It addresses what the patient is willing to or not willing to endure to sustain life.

6. **Answer: 3 Rationale:** Hospice care, representing a model of care rather than a location for care, is for patients suffering from terminal illnesses.

7. **Answer: 4 Rationale:** The nurse would respect the patient's wishes and withhold pain medications.

8. **Answer: 1 Rationale:** It is thought that the sense of hearing is the last sense to go before death occurs.

9. **Answer: 3 Rationale:** It is important to continue to manage pain at all times of life, especially in end-of-life care.

10. **Answer: 2 Rationale:** The open-ended statement of acknowledging to the woman "This must be a difficult time for you" provides an opportunity for her to express her feelings as she recognizes the nurse's willingness to listen.

Chapter 6: Nursing Care of Patients with Problems of Substance Abuse

1. **Answer: 2 Rationale:** A blood alcohol level (BAL) greater than 0.08% is considered legal intoxication in most states.

2. **Answer: 1 Rationale:** Open-ended questions about drug or alcohol use should be asked in a nonthreatening, nonjudgmental, matter-of-fact manner (for example, beginning with how, what, and andandand and when).

3. **Answer: 4 Rationale:** Thiamine replacement is typically ordered for patients with chronic alcoholism, which can lead to thiamine deficiency and neurological impairments.

4. **Answer: 3 Rationale:** All CNS depressants (including alcohol, benzodiazepines, and barbiturates) have a potentially dangerous progress of withdrawal. Severe withdrawal or delirium tremens is a medical emergency.

5. **Answer: 3 Rationale:** Disulfiram is a form of aversion therapy that prevents the breakdown of alcohol, causing physical illness if taken while drinking alcohol.

6. **Answer: 3 Rationale:** Patients who receive care from an impaired nurse may complain of ineffective pain control and may report they did not receive medications while that nurse was on duty.

7. **Answer: 2 Rationale:** The smoking rates for women have steadily increased and it is now the leading known cause of preventable death and disease among women.

8. **Answer: 4 Rationale:** It is recommended that patients wear a medic alert bracelet while on naltrexone (ReVia).

9. **Answer: 1 Rationale:** A realistic goal for substance abusers is the identification of healthy coping mechanisms, relaxation, and stress reduction techniques to decrease the risks of substance abuse.

10. **Answer: 3 Rationale:** *Ineffective Denial* is the best choice. Patients need assistance to recognize and change maladaptive behaviors related to substance abuse.

Chapter 7: Nursing Care of Patients Experiencing Disasters

1. **Answer: 3 Rationale:** Although emergencies can typically be handled by available emergency services, disasters involve multiple services and agencies working together.

2. **Answer: 3 Rationale:** Nurses are an integral part in assisting with disasters. However, they do not serve in a leadership role in the command center. Their role is in assisting with triage and in meeting the emergency healthcare needs of those injured or involved in the disaster.

3. **Answer: 4 Rationale:** Reverse triage is necessary when there are limited resources to care for multiple people injured in a disaster. This is so the majority of people can be helped with the resources currently available.

4. **Answer: 3 Rationale:** It is important to recognize that a patient whose primary language is not English may not read in his or her primary language. This can create a significant problem when providing health education. It is important to have someone translate all information to the patient and have the patient explain what has been taught in order to ensure proper understanding of the information.

5. **Answer: 3 Rationale:** PPE should lessen the likelihood of occupational injury and/or illness, but proper precautions also must be taken to ensure safety. This can be as simple as proper hand hygiene after removing gloves, or following isolation guidelines.

6. **Answer: 2 Rationale:** Decontamination cannot begin in the hot zone as this is the area of greatest contamination. It is important to decontaminate the area outside of the hot zone to prevent its spread.

7. **Answer: 1 Rationale:** A dirty bomb is a bomb that carries a radiological signature and can cause contamination and radiation poisoning.

8. **Answer: 2 Rationale:** Radiation sickness is the direct result of exposure to ionizing radiation, which causes cellular mutation. This condition must be treated rapidly or death may result as the cells continue to mutate and die.

9. **Answer: 3 Rationale:** Older adults have individual needs. Some may be more independent than others regarding the degree of support needed in emergencies, whereas others may require multiple resources and support in an evacuation.

10. **Answer: 4 Rationale:** Nurses often are so involved in caring for others they tend to neglect themselves. In disaster situations, nurses may also suffer from loss while caring for others. As a result the nurse may feel overwhelmed and be as traumatized as those for whom he or she is caring.

Unit 2 Building Clinical Competence: Alterations in Patterns of Health
Functional Health Pattern: Health Perception-Health Management

Functional Health Patterns
Hint: There are many ways we increase the patient's comfort without realizing we are doing so.

Priority Setting
1.
   A. John Linzer should be seen first. Even with a DNR order, Mr. Linzer and his family need support during the dying process. If death is not imminent, the nurse may be able to leave the room after providing reassurance and instruction.
   B. Peter Black should be seen second. Numbness in the legs can be a sign of an undetected nerve injury that must be assessed and diagnosed rapidly to prevent permanent damage.
   C. Paul Goetz should be seen third. He is exhibiting signs of alcohol withdrawal and needs assessment and medication to alleviate the symptoms. A sitter should be designated to stay with Mr. Goetz to ensure his safety.
   D. Mary Black should be seen last. Her condition is the most stable and surgery is not scheduled for several hours.

Health Promotion
1. To facilitate healing of a fracture, Mrs. Black should have increased calories, protein, calcium, and vitamin D.
2. C. *Rationale: This meal plan contains the necessary nutrients with the fewest empty calories.*

Nursing Process

1.

A. Peter Black: A complete neurological assessment is needed with emphasis on the lower extremities. All abrasions and lacerations should be assessed for bleeding and signs of infection.

B. Mary Black: Assess the left ankle for pain and bruising. All abrasions and ecchymotic areas should be assessed for bleeding.

C. John Linzer: Assess for signs of impending death, including level of consciousness, mottling, and respiratory pattern.

D. Paul Goetz: Assess for continued signs of alcohol withdrawal including combativeness, orientation, hallucinations, diaphoresis, and nausea.

2.

	Nursing Diagnosis	Rationale
Peter Black	*Risk for Neurovascular Dysfunction* related to injury	*Mr. Black's most urgent problem is recent numbness in his legs.*
Mary Black	*Anxiety* related to hospitalization of children and upcoming surgery	*Mrs. Black's physical status is stable. She is requesting to see her children before surgery.*
John Linzer	*Death Anxiety* related to terminal illness	*Even when the patient and family have had time to prepare for death, anxiety is common in the final hours.*
Paul Goetz	*Disturbed Sensory Perception (Visual)* related to alcohol withdrawal	*Mr. Goetz is seeing spiders and exhibiting other symptoms of alcohol withdrawal.*

3.

A. Administer pain medications as ordered. *Rationale: Maintaining comfort is a high priority for all patients.*

B. Turn every 1 to 2 hours. *Rationale: Repositioning adds comfort to the bed-fast patient.*

C. Provide hygiene, oral care every 1 hour, peri-care following each incontinence, and bed bath daily. *Rationale: Often the patient breathes through the mouth in the last stage of life. Hygiene care is essential to comfort.*

D. Provide oral liquids as tolerates. *Rationale: As long as swallowing is intact, oral fluids prevent dehydration and add comfort.*

E. Establish therapeutic communication. Encourage patient to share feelings with family members. *Rationale: The dying patient may need to communicate final wishes, thoughts, and feelings with friends and family.*

4. D. *Rationale: Use a nonjudgmental approach to develop a trusting nurse–patient relationship to be able to spend time with the patient to discuss his feelings, fears, and anxieties.*

5. Ativan (lorazepam) is a benzodiazepine anxiolytic agent that produces calmness. Mr. Goetz should be evaluated for a decrease in anxiety, agitation, and hallucinations.

6. B. *Rationale: Frequent coughing helps to remove anesthetic agents from the lungs to prevent pneumonia.*

Communication

1. Report the results of your neuro assessment including time symptoms began, the location of the numbness, and any other abnormal findings.

2. Give a brief report to the pediatric nurse regarding Mr. and Mrs. Black's condition, the change in Mr. Black's neurological status, and Mrs. Black's upcoming surgery. *Rationale: The pediatric nurse needs information about both Mr. and Mrs. Black's condition in order to be supportive of the Black children. Other family members may be needed to make decisions regarding the children's health care if the parents are unable to make informed decisions because of their own health status.*

Delegation

1.

A. Peter Black: Obtaining vital signs and performing basic ADLs can be delegated to the nursing assistant. Mr. Black should not get out of bed; therefore, a urinal should be provided. Until specifically ordered by the physician, he should be kept NPO, so frequent oral care may be necessary.

B. Mary Black: Besides obtaining vital signs, the nursing assistant can assist with elimination. Mrs. Black's ankle needs to remain immobile, so she will need assistance with transferring to the commode or a wheelchair if she is allowed to visit her children on the pediatric unit.

C. John Linzer: Vital signs and physical care including hygiene, turning, and positioning can be delegated.

D. Paul Goetz: Safety is an important factor for Mr. Goetz. A nursing assistant can be delegated to be a sitter in the room at all times. The nursing assistant can also obtain vital signs and assist with ADLs.

Nursing Ethics

1. Paul Goetz asks you to bring him some beer. He says, "You can smuggle it in and no one will know." How will you respond? "No, Paul, I cannot bring you a beer. I know you feel you need alcohol. Even though I cannot provide it for you, I can give you the prescribed medication that will help you get through the detoxification. I can also be sure the counselor sees you as soon as possible." *Rationale: It is not ethical to provide alcohol to the chemically dependent patient. However, in order to maintain a therapeutic relationship, the nurse should offer prescribed medication and psychological support.*

2. D. *Rationale: Nurses must first know how to take care of themselves in a disaster in order to be able to assist others.*

Concept Map

Hint: Changing the shapes of the boxes or adding color can further demonstrate the interconnectedness of the concepts. For the second part of this activity, you may find it helpful to review Chapter 5 and Box 1-5.

Chapter 8: Genetic Implications of Adult Health Nursing

1. Answer: 2 Rationale: In an autosomal dominant condition, you only need one of the genotypes to have the condition. An autosomal dominant condition is not a sex-linked disease and is not found on the x or y chromosomes.

2. Answer: 1, 3 Rationale: Fabry disease is an x-linked genetic disorder. Since the male provides the y chromosome to a male offspring, the male cannot pass on this disease to male offspring. The female can pass this disorder on. Also, which grandmother (maternal or fraternal) is not stated, and if the grandmother was not affected, she could be a carrier since her brother had the disease.

3. Answer: 4 Rationale: It is a nurse's responsibility to explain what is involved in genetic testing. It is not the nurse's responsibility to discuss potential outcomes, as this is the responsibility of the genetic counselor.

4. Answer: 4 Rationale: Mitochondrial mutations are only passed from the mother. This is because mitochondria are primarily found in ova and not sperm. This is considered a matrilineal pattern of inheritance. An affected female will pass the condition on to her children; however, an affected male will not.

5. **Answer: 2 Rationale:** Performing a family history assessment helps the nurse know what is important to focus on regarding health promotion and maintenance when planning prophylactic screening and treatment.

6. **Answer: 2 Rationale:** Retention of information decreases during times of high stress, such as being diagnosed with a genetic disorder.

7. **Answer: 1, 2, 4 Rationale:** Most genetic specialists will complete chromosomal studies and provide information about the condition; this information will in turn facilitate decision making.

8. **Answer: 1, 2, 4 Rationale:** Minor physical anomalies are simply visual. However, an atrial-septal health defect is a functional defect, which can impair activity and cause severe complications as the patient gets older.

9. **Answer: 3 Rationale:** A family history for mutation of the MLH/MSH2 gene greatly increases the risk for colon cancer.

10. **Answer: 4 Rationale:** GINA is a federal law designed to protect consumers from discrimination by employers and health insurance companies based on genetic information.

Chapter 9: Nursing Care of Patients in Pain

1. **Answer: 2 Rationale:** Chronic pain is defined as pain that has persisted for 6 or more months. Low back pain is the most common cause of chronic pain.

2. **Answer: 4 Rationale:** Initial or "fast" pain is sharp and well-defined as the stimulus is transmitted along myelinated A delta fibers to the thalamus and cerebral cortex. The smaller unmyelinated C fibers transmit the stimulus more slowly, producing a second or "slow" pain, which is less well-localized, dull, and throbbing.

3. **Answer: 1, 2, 5 Rationale:** NSAIDs are more effective when taken on a scheduled basis rather than PRN. These drugs, when effective (particularly for musculoskeletal pain), can cause gastrointestinal bleeding and hypertension, necessitating regular follow-up.

4. **Answer: 1 Rationale:** Transdermal patches of opioid are slowly absorbed, reaching a therapeutic level 12 to 72 hours after application. The drug can accumulate in the body tissues, leading to a toxic level accompanied by manifestations such as sleepiness or respiratory difficulty.

5. **Answer: 3 Rationale:** The quality of the pain is assessed through descriptive statements such as sharp, burning, stabbing, dull, etc.

6. **Answer: 3 Rationale:** Pain is objective; the patient provides the most accurate information about its intensity.

7. **Answer: 2 Rationale:** Constipation is a common side effect of opioids narcotics, especially when used on a regular basis.

8. **Answer: 1 Rationale:** Research has shown that patients with moderate cognitive impairment can use a pain scale to indicate the intensity of pain. The faces pain scale may be more accurate and effective in the cognitively impaired adult.

9. **Answer: 3 Rationale:** The combination of glucosamine and chondroitin has been shown to reduce pain in patients with moderate to severe knee pain.

10. **Answer: 1 Rationale:** Rigorous physical activity such as running prompts the release of endorphins (natural opioids-like substances). Endorphins bind with opioids receptors in the CNS, inhibiting the transmission of pain signals.

Chapter 10: Nursing Care of Patients with Altered Fluid, Electrolyte, and Acid–Base Balance

1. **Answer: 1 Rationale:** Ringer's solution is an isotonic, balanced electrolyte solution that can expand plasma volume and help restore electrolyte balance.

2. **Answer: 4 Rationale:** In fluid volume deficit, there is less volume in the vascular system, which decreases venous return and cardiac output, leading to manifestations of dizziness, orthostatic hypotension, and flat neck veins. The heart rate increases and the blood pressure falls.

3. **Answer: 1, 3, 4 Rationale:** Frequent neurological checks are necessary as hypernatremia draws water out of brain cells, causing them to shrink. As the brain shrinks, tension is placed on cerebral vessels, which may cause them to tear and bleed. Hypernatremia affects mental status and brain function (including orientation to time, place, and person), as can rapid correction of hypernatremia. Fluid replacement is the primary treatment for hypernatremia. Maintaining intravenous access is necessary for administration of fluids and possible emergency medications.

4. **Answer: 2 Rationale:** Hypokalemia affects nerve impulse transmission, including the transmission of cardiac impulses. The patient may develop ECG changes and atrial or ventricular dysrhythmias.

5. **Answer: 4 Rationale:** Calcium should be taken with a full glass of water to allow maximum absorption.

6. **Answer: 1 Rationale:** A positive Chvostek's sign indicates increased neuromuscular excitability, commonly associated with both hypomagnesemia and hypocalcemia. Additional manifestations of hypomagnesemia include confusion, hallucinations, and possible psychoses. Administration of magnesium sulfate helps restore magnesium balance and neuromuscular function.

7. **Answer: 1 Rationale:** The pH is indicative of acidosis (less than 7.35), and the bicarbonate level is low (less than 22 mEq/L), indicating bicarbonate deficit as cause of the acidosis. In addition, the $PaCO_2$ is low (less than 35 mmHg), indicating respiratory compensation for the excess acid.

8. **Answer: 1, 3, 5 Rationale:** The slow respiratory rate leads to inadequate alveolar ventilation. As a result, carbon dioxide is not effectively eliminated from the blood, causing it to accumulate. This increases carbonic acid levels, leading to respiratory acidosis, as indicated by the low pH and high $PaCO_2$. Excess carbon dioxide causes vasodilation, leading to warm, flushed skin, particularly in acute respiratory acidosis.

9. **Answer: 2 Rationale:** Gastric suctioning removes highly acidic gastric secretions, increasing the risk of metabolic alkalosis.

10. **Answer: 3 Rationale:** The patient is demonstrating classic manifestations of respiratory alkalosis, a potential complication of mechanical ventilation when the rate or volume of ventilations are too high. Arterial blood gases provide the data necessary to confirm and treat this problem.

Chapter 11: Nursing Care of Patients Experiencing Trauma and Shock

1. **Answer: 4 Rationale:** Although all of the choices can be sources of injury or death in adults of all ages, motor vehicle crashes remain the leading cause of injury.

2. **Answer: 1 Rationale:** Airway obstruction is the first and foremost risk to assess for, as this represents the ABCs of life support: A = airway, B = breathing, C = circulation. A patent airway must be the number one priority for survival.

3. **Answer: 2 Rationale:** Assessing airway patency is the first step in the ABCs of life support in any setting.

4. **Answer: 3 Rationale:** The priority assessment, regardless of setting, is airway patency.
5. **Answer: 2 Rationale:** The endotoxins released from bacteria in septic shock stimulate the release of vasoactive proteins causing peripheral vasodilation and decreased peripheral resistance.
6. **Answer: 1 Rationale:** Direct pressure to the wound is the best method to manage uncontrolled bleeding.
7. **Answer: 1 Rationale:** Trauma is defined as injury to human tissues from the transfer of energy.
8. **Answer: 3 Rationale:** A transfusion reaction is a risk from a blood transfusion.
9. **Answer: 2 Rationale:** Widespread vasodilation can cause distributive shock as the blood pressure drops dangerously due to the very low peripheral vascular resistance.
10. **Answer: 1 Rationale:** Ultimately there is a systemic imbalance between oxygen supply and demand.

Chapter 12: Nursing Care of Patients with Infections
1. **Answer: 3 Rationale:** Acquired passive immunity is the result of a gamma globulin infusion following exposure to hepatitis A. This type of immunity is short-lived and usually lasts only about 4 weeks.
2. **Answer: 3 Rationale:** If a culture and sensitivity is ordered, obtain it before beginning treatment so the anti-infective medication does not alter the ability to identify the causative organisms.
3. **Answer: 4 Rationale:** Although the exact mechanism of action is unknown, aspirin inhibits prostaglandin synthesis.
4. **Answer: 1 Rationale:** Increased banded neutrophils is a response to bacterial infection. This is called a "shift to the left."
5. **Answer: 2 Rationale:** Contact precautions, wearing gloves and gowns for direct contact.
6. **Answer: 1 Rationale:** The T cells of the immune system adapt to kill intracellular organisms.
7. **Answer: 1 Rationale:** Thrombocytosis is best explained as increased platelets.
8. **Answer: 4 Rationale:** When there is a nursing diagnosis of *Risk for Infection*, it can pertain to the patient, caregivers, or other patients. It addresses the possibility that the patient cannot fight infection, the staff is potentially at risk for developing an infection from the infected patient, or the other patients are at risk for becoming infected from the infected patient.
9. **Answer: 4 Rationale:** When administering antibiotics, the nurse must be aware of potential hypersensitivity reactions. It is important to monitor for any hypersensitivities in addition to providing education about the infection, antibiotic, and any potential side effects of treatment.
10. **Answer: 3 Rationale:** Wearing gloves, gowns, and goggles when coming in contact with contaminated body fluids is considered to be a standard procedure.

Chapter 13: Nursing Care of Patients with Altered Immunity
1. **Answer: 4 Rationale:** Anaphylaxis is the most severe form of type 1 IgE reactions. When an allergen is introduced for which there is circulating IgE specific to the allergen a cascade leading to anaphylaxis is initiated.
2. **Answer: 1 Rationale:** This type of rejection episode is the most common and most treatable.
3. **Answer: 3 Rationale:** These manifestations are indicative of a respiratory infection caused by PCP.
4. **Answer: 4 Rationale:** When a patient tests positive for HIV, this means that antibodies to the AIDS virus are present in the blood. HIV does not equal AIDS.

5. **Answer: 2 Rationale:** As Retrovir can cause bone marrow suppression, leukopenia can be an adverse reaction of Retrovir.
6. **Answer: 2 Rationale:** Of all of the choices available, the allergen prick testing has the lowest risk of anaphylaxis because there is the smallest amount of allergen entering the bloodstream.
7. **Answer: 2 Rationale:** When hypersensitivity is suspected it is important to avoid any further exposure to the potential cause. The best way to do this is by replacing all tubing and attaching a new line primed with NS.
8. **Answer: 2 Rationale:** Protease inhibitors and nucleoside analogs are associated with serious metabolic problems such as diabetes mellitus.
9. **Answer: 4 Rationale:** The priority when initiating or changing HIV drug therapy regimens is the patient's willingness to adhere to the drug regimen. Since the side effects can be difficult and challenging to overcome, many patients are not willing to continue with their therapy.
10. **Answer: 4 Rationale:** Antithymocyte globulin (ATC) is used to induce immunosuppression immediately following a transplant. Its purpose is to bind with the peripheral lymphocytes and mononuclear cells to remove them from circulation and prevent them from being able to reject the new organ.

Chapter 14: Nursing Care of Patients with Cancer
1. **Answer: 3 Rationale:** Metastasis occurs when cells from a primary tumor site travel through the lymphatic system or bloodstream to find a secondary target.
2. **Answer: 1 Rationale:** Encouraging the patient to express his feelings about the cancer diagnosis is the most valuable and powerful intervention that could be offered.
3. **Answer: 3 Rationale:** It is important not to rub or scratch the treated skin areas, as this can cause irritation to the surface of the skin as well as breaks in the skin. Rubbing may also wipe off the ink markings, which are important landmarks to ensure that the radiation treatments are directed to the correct location.
4. **Answer: 2 Rationale:** Providing an antiemetic prior to chemotherapy is an excellent preventative treatment to prevent nausea and vomiting following chemotherapy.
5. **Answer: 3 Rationale:** Although all of these choices can be a result of chemotherapy, the one that is directly affected with bone marrow suppression is a low platelet count of 50,000.
6. **Answer: 3 Rationale:** Chemotherapy is not cell type specific. It simply targets cells that are rapidly dividing, which can be both cancer cells and healthy cells. It is important to understand that the destruction of normal cells can cause other manifestations such as mucositis, hair loss, and bone marrow suppression.
7. **Answer: 1 Rationale:** External radiation therapy is when the radiation is initiated outside of the body, directed towards the patient, and is set to deliver to a certain depth for a specified period of time. This exposure is meant to destroy the cancer cells the radiation comes into direct contact with.
8. **Answer: 2 Rationale:** Tumor lysis syndrome can cause high levels of uric acid. Patients are often treated with allopurinol to help excrete the uric acid in the urine.
9. **Answer: 3 Rationale:** The S phase is when DNA replication occurs. This is when the cell is beginning mitosis and the chromosomes multiply from 23 to 46. They then migrate toward each axis in preparation for division of the cell.
10. **Answer: 1 Rationale:** Oncogenes, genes that stimulate cell growth, require something to activate them in order to cause this reaction.

Unit 3 Building Clinical Competence: Pathophysiology and Patterns of Health
Functional Health Pattern: Health Perception-Health Management

Functional Health Patterns
Hint: **There are many nonpharmacologic or complementary therapies the nurse can initiate without a physician's order.**

Priority Setting

A. Allen Barber should be seen second. *Rationale: Post-op pain of 8/10 on day 4 is very unusual and could indicate beginning dehiscence.*

B. Tamra Sanders should be seen first. *Rationale: Severe chest pain and shortness of breath could indicate life-threatening change in conditions.*

C. Mia Windham should be seen third. *Rationale: Bloody diarrhea can lead to severe dehydration, hemorrhage, and shock, but there is no indication that Ms. Windham is in immediate danger.*

D. Harry Anderson should be seen fourth. *Rationale: Harry's confusion can result in his calling for help. While he should be checked on to determine his safety, a CAN could be assigned to stay with him.*

Health Promotion

1. B. *Rationale: A high-protein and high-kilocalorie diet provides necessary nutrients to meet metabolic and tissue healing needs. High fiber can increase intestinal motility and cause diarrhea, further increasing weight loss. High vitamins can cause vitamin overdose.*

2. Allen Barber should be taught to manage his diabetes to maintain blood glucose levels within normal ranges. *Rationale: Wound healing is facilitated by normal glucose levels.*

Nursing Process

1.

A. Allen Barber: Pain scale, direct visualization of surgical wound, and abdominal sounds. *Rationale: It appears the surgical wound is infected, which delays healing. This wound infection could result in intestinal complications and wound dehiscence.*

B. Tamra Sanders: Heart and lung sounds, oxygen saturation. Rationale: Sickle cells can obstruct circulation to any organ. Ms. Sanders's symptoms could indicate a blockage in circulation to the heart or lungs or both, which could be life–threatening.

C. Mia Windham: Abdominal sounds, further incidence of bloody diarrhea, skin condition on hands and feet, location and description of rash. *Rationale: Ms. Windham must be assessed for worsening signs of tissue rejection.*

D. Harry Anderson: Neuro assessment including pupils, clearness of speech, strength in arms and legs, and changes in levels of confusion. Observe for signs of seizure activity. *Rationale: HIV/AIDS affects the nervous system. The nurse must observe for signs of worsening of Harry's condition.*

2.

	Nursing Diagnosis	Rationale
Allen Barber	*High Risk for Impaired Skin Integrity* as evidenced by worsening inflammation at surgical site	*Worsening inflammation indicates an infectious process that can result in wound dehiscence.*
Tamra Sanders	*Impaired Gas Exchange* as evidenced by chest pain and shortness of breath	*Maintaining breathing and circulation is always the highest priority.*
Mia Windham	*Ineffective Management of Therapeutic Regimen* as evidenced by signs of tissues rejection	*Ms. Windham received a bone marrow transplant in treatment of leukemia. It appears her body is rejecting the transplanted tissue.*
Harry Anderson	*Altered Health Maintenance* as evidenced by increased confusion and risk for seizure activity	*As AIDS progresses, Mr. Anderson will have increased difficulty in maintaining his health status.*

3. Tamra Sanders should be placed in semi-fowlers to high fowlers position. *Rationale: Sitting in an upright position causes the abdominal contents to move away from the diaphragm and eases inhalation.*

4. B. *Rationale: Use saline for wound cleansing. Soap and harsh cleansers like povidone-iodine or hydrogen peroxide cause drying and tissue damage.*

5. A. *Rational: Diarrhea increases bicarbonate loss, resulting in metabolic acidosis.*

6. A. *Rationale: White blood cell count indicates extent of inflammatory process, erythrocyte sedimentation rate detects inflammation, and C-reactive protein indicates presence of inflammatory process.*

Communication

1. The doctor must be told about the amount of bloody diarrhea Ms. Windham has had in the last 24 hours, the amount of pain she is experiencing, any change in the rash on her extremities, and any new symptoms. *Rationale: The doctor must be kept up-to-date on Ms. Windham's symptoms of tissue rejection.*

2. C. *Rationale: A child born to carrier parents has a 25% chance of inheriting sickle cell anemia.*

3. Determine Ms. Sanders's level of cognitive development and communicate with her in developmentally appropriate terms. *Rationale: People with Down's syndrome have a wide variety of cognitive abilities. It is important communicate in developmentally appropriate terms, not age appropriate terms.*

Delegation

1.

A. Allen Barber: Delegate vital signs, obtaining blood glucose levels and assistance with ADLs including hygiene, elimination, and ambulation. Rationale: Obtaining vital signs and BG values can be safely delegated to a trained nursing assistant. A 4-day postoperative patient should be able to provide much of his own care, but would need some assistance that could be provided by unlicensed personnel.

B. Tamra Sanders: Delegate vital signs, ADLs, and a sitter. Rationale: Ms. Sanders may need a sitter due to Down's syndrome and chest pain with shortness of breath. While the nursing assistant cannot assess changes in her condition, he or she can summon help and initiate CPR if necessary.

C. Mia Windham: Delegate vital signs, ADLs, and I&O. Rationale: The nursing assistant is able to record intake and output and notify the RN of further bloody diarrhea.

D. Harry Anderson: Delegate vital signs, ADLs, and sitter. Rationale: Due to Mr. Anderson's confusion and risk of seizure activity, a sitter may be necessary to maintain patient safety.

Related Questions

1. D. *Rationale: Supine position with legs elevated increases venous return. Trendelenburg causes abdominal organs to press against the diaphragm, compromising respirations.*

2. D. *Rationale: Notify the physician if WBCs fall below 4000 and platelets fall below 75,000 prior to administering any cytotoxic agents due to being at risk for developing infections.*

3. D. *Rationale: A severe anaphylactic reaction may be treated with 1:100,000 concentration of epinephrine intravenously.*

4. Flushed face, burning sensation along a vein, dyspnea, hypotension, lumbar pain, fever. *Rationale: Clumping of RBCs blocks blood vessels, decreasing circulation to vital organs. Hemolysis of RBCs causes a release of hemoglobin into blood that can block renal circulation.*

5. A, D, E. *Rationale: Maintain a diet low in fat and high in fiber as well as increasing vegetables and fruits in the diet. Increase intake of vitamins E, C, and beta-carotene and omega-3 oils. Limit charcoal grilled meats.*

Concept Map

Hint: Providing care to enable the patient to manage his or her health needs involves providing verbal as well as written information. The patient must be able to verbalize understanding of the information. For the second part of this activity, consider the factors underlying Mr. Blount's breathing pattern in developing your concept map.

Chapter 15: Assessing the Integumentary System

1. **Answer: 2 Rationale:** The layer that has the most glands and hair follicles located in it is the dermis.

2. **Answer: 3 Rationale:** Melanin is the pigment found in skin that is responsible for tanning.

3. **Answer: 1, 2 Rationale:** Inspection is the first assessment technique to check the skin surface. The next assessment step is to palpate any areas of the skin that appear abnormal in order to get a better understanding of depth and size of any lesions.

4. **Answer: 1 Rationale:** Erythema often occurs as a result of increased body temperature. This occurs when the capillaries in the skin dilate to release some of the heat caused from the increased body temperature.

5. **Answer: 3 Rationale:** Often new soap can cause skin irritation and itching. It is important to determine if there is anything that has changed to cause this irritation. This is the easiest variable to assess.

6. **Answer: 1 Rationale:** A decreased skin turgor is a sign of dehydration.

7. **Answer: 4 Rationale:** Edema begins in the distal extremities. The best place to assess for this is the ankle/foot area.

8. **Answer: 4 Rationale:** Lichenification is a condition in which the skin cells multiply, causing what appears to be thickened and calloused skin. The skin often has a rough and leathery appearance to it.

9. **Answer: 4 Rationale:** Angiomas are a common finding in older patients.

10. **Answer: 3 Rationale:** Head lice deposit and attach small white eggs to the hair shaft.

11. **Answer: 4 Rationale:** A family history increases the risk for skin cancer.

Chapter 16: Nursing Care of Patients with Integumentary Disorders

1. **Answer: 3 Rationale:** The best way to help moisturize the skin is to apply a moisturizing agent after bathing.

2. **Answer: 1 Rationale:** Nevi are the skin lesions that can become malignant and need to be monitored for any change.

3. **Answer: 4 Rationale:** Psoriasis causes abnormal growth and division of epidermal cells, causing keratosis. The use of ultraviolet light therapy helps to slow down this cellular division, which decreases the lesions and keratosis associated with psoriasis.

4. **Answer: 2 Rationale:** Actinic keratosis is a premalignant skin lesion, with the risk of developing into a malignancy.

5. **Answer: 4 Rationale:** A linear pattern of painful vesicles indicates shingles, a varicella infection. The virus remains along a nerve from a previous infection with chickenpox.

6. **Answer: 2 Rationale:** Anyone can have lice. Major infestations often occur in areas where many people are in close proximity, especially in the public school setting.

7. **Answer: 1 Rationale:** People with fair skin, blond hair, and freckles are at increased risk for nonmelanoma skin cancers.

8. **Answer: 1 Rationale:** A change in the color or size of a nevus is cause for concern when evaluating for the possibility of melanoma.

9. **Answer: 2 Rationale:** Skin tears may occur as a result of the shearing force of pulling a patient up in bed. Prevention includes lifting, rather than pulling the patient up in bed.

10. **Answer: 3 Rationale:** Dermabrasion is a skin treatment that helps to reduce the appearance of acne scarring and other skin imperfections.

Chapter 17: Nursing Care of Patients with Burns

1. **Answer: 3 Rationale:** In the emergent phase of burn management, it is important to monitor electrolyte levels frequently. Initially the patient is at risk for fluid and electrolyte imbalances, especially for decreased serum potassium levels. This can cause an increased risk for arrhythmias.

2. **Answer: 4 Rationale:** A full thickness burn is not painful, as the nerves have also been affected from the burn. In this situation, pain is not a good sign. It tells the nurse that the depth of the burn goes beyond the nerves. Superficial partial thickness, and deep partial thickness burns will still be very painful to the patient, as the nerves remain intact or exposed.

3. **Answer: 4 Rationale:** The larger the surface area of the burn and the deeper the burn, the more at risk the patient is for burn shock. A high-voltage electrical accident will cause a deeper burn and since this scenario explains that > 50% of the body is affected, this places the patient at the highest risk.

4. **Answer: 2 Rationale:** Silvadene cream can cause neutropenia. It is important for the nurse to monitor the patient's WBC count daily to assess for any changes, which could indicate neutropenia. Although this is the most important intervention, it is also important to keep the patient as comfortable as possible. Premedicating is definitely not a bad idea, as burn dressing changes can be very painful and the Silvadene will help debride the burn.

5. **Answer: 2 Rationale:** The Parkland Formula uses lactated Ringer's solution, administered at 4 mL $\times$ kg $\times$ % TBSA burn, with 50% of the total volume infused in the first 8 hours, and the remaining 50% over the next 16 hours. This would be $4 \times 70 \times 50\% = 14,000 \times 50\% = 7000$.

6. **Answer: 1 Rationale:** Urine output is the most sensitive indicator of fluid resuscitation success. A decrease in urine output is seen in dehydration and a recovery from dehydration is seen with an increase in urine output.

7. **Answer: 4 Rationale:** A decreased left radial pulse is cause for alarm in this type and location of burn. This can be the first symptom seen in compartment syndrome and is a surgical emergency.

8. **Answer: 2 Rationale:** The "rule of nines" is a method of quickly estimating the percentage of TBSA affected by a burn injury. It is most useful in emergency situations but is not accurate for estimating TBSA in adults who are short, obese, or very thin. Anterior trunk = 18%, perineum = 1%, left arm = 9%. These are added together to equal 28%.

9. **Answer: 1, 3, 5, 6 Rationale:** Teaching injury prevention is a very important job in nursing. Burns are a common injury in the home. It is important to help older adults understand ways to help prevent burns. Wearing close-fitting clothing when cooking can help prevent shirtsleeves or scarves from catching on fire. The water temperature of the water heater should not be set above 120°F. This can help prevent burns from water scalding. Installing antiscald devices can also help prevent water burns. As older adults often have decreased olfactory senses, having a neighbor routinely check for the odor of gas can help prevent fires.

10. **Answer: 3 Rationale:** A 15% carbon monoxide level would cause only mild manifestations of dizziness at this stage. Later stages with higher levels will cause the remaining manifestations of the skin color change, drowsiness, and hypotension.

Unit 4 Building Clinical Competence: Responses to Altered Integumentary Structure and Function

Functional Health Pattern: Nutritional-Metabolic

Functional Health Patterns

Hint: Besides contacting the dietitian, the nurse can encourage intake of food and fluids by providing small frequent amounts of the patient's choice of food and drink.

Priority Setting

1.
   A. Mrs. Carter should be seen first. *Rationale: She may need pain medications and should not have to wait for pain relief.*
   B. Mr. Johnson should be seen second. *Rationale: It is important to have him ready for surgery on time at 0800. The nursing assistant can obtain vital signs and help him with urinary elimination while you are seeing Mrs. Carter.*
   C. Mr. Jenkins should be seen third. *Rationale: If new lesions are appearing, they should be assessed and documented, but this is not urgent.*
   D. Mr. Ugandi should be seen last. *Rationale: Discharge is anticipated and teaching should begin as soon as possible, but the other patients' needs are higher priority at this time.*

Health Promotion

1. A. *Rationale: Foods high in protein, such as eggs, milk, and meat, are required for tissue growth and maintenance. Foods high in iron, such as meat, poultry, and eggs, are required for increased red blood cell production and preventing anemia.*
2. D. *Rationale: A cool environment will decrease itching, and light cotton clothing will decrease pain from material rubbing on lesions.*

Nursing Process

1.

	Nursing Diagnosis	Rationale
Mr. Johnson	*Anxiety* related to upcoming surgery	*Even though Mr. Johnson has had previous surgeries and should know what to expect, each surgery carries risks that cause anxiety.*
Mrs. Carter	*Pain* in R. leg related to cellulitis	Because of the number of pain receptors in the skin, cellulitis is very painful.
Mr. Jenkins	*Hopelessness*	Mr. Jenkins is concerned that new lesions are forming, which is out of his control.
Mr. Ugandi	*Knowledge Deficit* related to home care of Toxic Epidermal Necrolysis	Mr. Ugandi has a chronic, progressive disease (AIDS) and is being discharged to continue healing from Toxic Epidermal Necrolysis. He needs instruction in self-care within any limitations of AIDS.

2. *18%. Rationale: Arms are 4.5% each, and anterior trunk is 9% for a total burn area of 18%.*
3. A. *Rationale: Clinical manifestations of infection of the dermis and subcutaneous tissue are redness, swelling, and pain.*
4. C. *Rationale: Hypersensitivity reactions to mafenide acetate include pruritus, edema, facial edema, and urticaria.*

Communication

1. "Mr. Jenkins, I know this is very difficult for you and sometimes you might feel that dying would be better than the burning pain you are experiencing. I'm sorry, but because there is no cure for herpes zoster, the sores can come back. There are some medications you can take that decrease the chance of them recurring. I'll have your doctor talk with you about them. Is there anything else you want to talk about? *Rationale: Honest, direct answers to questions are preferred. At age 86, Mr. Jenkins may be telling you that he is feeling hopeless and may give up. It is important to keep communication lines open.*

Delegation

1. What data collection and interventions can be delegated to a nursing assistant for each patient?
   A. Mr. Johnson: Vital signs, assistance with elimination, transfer to stretcher/transport to surgery, preparing room for his return from surgery.
   B. Mrs. Carter: Vital signs, hygiene, nutrition, turning/activity.
   C. Mrs. Jenkins: Vital signs, hygiene, nutrition, turning/activity. Remind the nursing assistant of contact precautions to prevent spread of infection.
   D. Mr. Ugandi: Vital signs, hygiene, nutrition, turning/activity. Remind the nursing assistant of standard precautions to prevent spread of infection.

Content-Specific Questions

1. A, C, D, E. *Rationale: Burn injuries cause the body to increase energy expenditure and to utilize nutrients for healing.*
2. D. *Rationale: Burns destroy the protective layer of the skin; therefore, due to losses through an open wound, fluid and electrolyte imbalances occur.*
3. B. *Rationale: A quadriplegic is unable to reposition him- or herself without assistance, which places the patient at high risk for pressure ulcers.*
4. A, C, E. *Rationale: These preventative measures are ways to prevent overexposure to the UVA rays of the sun that cause sunburns.*
5. B. *Rationale: Morphine causes respiratory depression. Respiratory rate below 12 is depressed and may require intervention.*

Concept Map
Hint: The differences in distribution of fat and fluid between male and female patients can be significant. Electric burns cause tissue destruction at the point of entry and point of exit as well as internal tissue between those points. The concept map must reflect this tissue damage and related nursing diagnoses.

Chapter 18: Assessing the Endocrine System

1. **Answer: 2 Rationale:** ADH (antidiuretic hormone) causes the distal tubules of the kidneys to reabsorb water, which would decrease the urine output.
2. **Answer: 3 Rationale:** A low calcium level may be tested by the Trousseau's sign. A positive test causes the fingers and hand to contract on the arm where a blood pressure cuff is inflated.
3. **Answer: 1 Rationale:** Excessive amounts of glucocorticoids cause manifestations of immunosuppression with depression of the inflammatory response and inhibition of the effectiveness of the immune system.
4. **Answer: 3 Rationale:** When assessing the endocrine system, it is important to look for manifestations of diabetes. One of the first manifestations is polydipsia, which is increased thirst.
5. **Answer: 2 Rationale:** The thyroid gland is assessed for the size and consistency to assess for goiters, enlargement, or nodules.
6. **Answer: 2 Rationale:** Assess for Chvostek's sign by tapping a finger in front of the ear, at the angle of the jaw. A positive sign causes facial grimacing with repeated contractions of the facial muscle.
7. **Answer: 4 Rationale:** A TSH (thyroid-stimulating hormone) level is the most accurate indicator of thyroid function.
8. **Answer: 3 Rationale:** Thyroid nodules are a normal finding in the older adult.
9. **Answer: 2 Rationale:** Rough, dry skin is often found in patients with hypothyroidism.
10. **Answer: 4 Rationale:** Increased deep tendon reflexes are seen in hyperthyroidism.

Chapter 19: Nursing Care of Patients with Endocrine Disorders

1. **Answer: 1 Rationale:** A self-generated antibody attaches to TSH receptors in the thyroid and results in increased TH production.
2. **Answer: 3 Rationale:** The thyroid gland takes up iodine in any form (including radioactive iodine) and concentrates it within the gland, decreasing the number of cells that produce TH.
3. **Answer: 3 Rationale:** This is a compensatory but ineffective effort to produce more TH by enlarging the gland itself.
4. **Answer: 4 Rationale:** Cushing's syndrome is the result of excessive cortisone; in this case a side effect of cortisone administration.
5. **Answer: 2 Rationale:** Patients with Addison's disease are often stressed by infection or trauma; additional doses of steroids may be needed to prevent crisis. Therefore, patients are urged to carry injectable cortisone and a syringe at all times.
6. **Answer: 2 Rationale:** As blood volume expands, neurons become edematous and irritability occurs.
7. **Answer: 2 Rationale:** Patients with this disorder are at risk for pathological fractures of the bones because of the decreased density of the bone.
8. **Answer: 3 Rationale:** Increased serum calcium decreases neuromuscular excitability, which decreases bowel motility.
9. **Answer: 4 Rationale:** Patients with Addison's disease have decreased cortisone but compensatory mechanisms increase ACTH, which causes skin to appear deeply suntanned or bronzed.

10. **Answer: 1 Rationale:** With a sudden stoppage of steroids, the adrenal cortex cannot recuperate rapidly enough to increase production because it has been suppressed with exogenous steroids.

Chapter 20: Nursing Care of Patients with Diabetes Mellitus

1. **Answer: 1 Rationale:** Ninety-five percent of patients diagnosed with type 1 DM have genetic markers indicating increased susceptibility for the development of type 1 DM.
2. **Answer: 3 Rationale:** A deficit of insulin increases the liver's production of ketone bodies and increased release of free fatty acids. Bicarbonate production is decreased and acid buffering is impaired, resulting in metabolic acidosis.
3. **Answer: 4 Rationale:** Caloric need decreases with aging; unless dietary intake also decreases (and exercise increases), weight gain ensues. Obesity is a risk factor for the development of type 2 DM.
4. **Answer: 3 Rationale:** Changes in sensation, such as numbness or tingling, support this diagnosis.
5. **Answer: 3 Rationale:** Visual inspection of the feet each day is important in preventing more serious complications.
6. **Answer: 3 Rationale:** Since it is clear, Lantus (glargine) could be confused with regular insulin. Regular insulin is short acting in 4 to 6 hours and Lantus is long acting in 24 to 28 hours.
7. **Answer: 3 Rationale:** Only regular insulin can safely be administered intravenously for diabetic ketoacidosis.
8. **Answer: 3 Rationale:** Levels of Hgb A1C greater than 6.5% demonstrate elevated or erratic glucose control over time and support a diagnosis of DM.
9. **Answer: 3 Rationale:** No intermediate- or long-acting insulin is given the day of surgery since dietary intake postoperatively is uncertain. IV glucose (5%) and regular insulin in equally divided doses will compensate for the increase in serum glucose until the patient is eating and drinking normally.
10. **Answer: 4 Rationale:** Insulin is absorbed more rapidly when injected subcutaneously in the abdomen.

Unit 5 Building Clinical Competence: Responses to Altered Endocrine Function

Functional Health Pattern: Nutritional-Metabolic

Functional Health Patterns
Hint: Many endocrine disorders affect metabolism and therefore the patient's need for nutrients. The patient's nutritional intake may be more than or less than body requirements.

Priority Setting
1.
   A. Mrs. Rant should be seen first. *Rationale: Relieving pain is a high priority, especially when the patient's blood pressure is elevated.*
   B. Mr. Blew should be seen second. *Rationale: The effectiveness of admission treatment of his extremely high blood glucose should be determined.*
   C. Mr. Rite should be seen third. *Rationale: While he has been stable, he is exhibiting signs of increased intracranial pressure and must be assessed.*
   D. Mrs. Fox can be seen last. *Rationale: Her vital signs are stable and she is waiting for labs to be drawn.*

Health Promotion
1. Teach Mr. Blew to provide foot care including inspecting his feet daily using a mirror, wearing well-fitting shoes/slippers at all times, caring for his nails, and reporting sores or red skin to his healthcare provider. He should be taught to monitor is blood glucose.

2. A. *Rationale: Hyperparathyroidism is excess in serum calcium levels. Increased fluids and decreased calcium and vitamin A & D supplements are the appropriate treatment.*

Nursing Process
1.

	Nursing Diagnosis	Rationale
Mr. Blew	*Knowledge Deficit* related to self-care of diabetes mellitus, including signs of hyperglycemia, hypoglycemia, and treatment	*A patient with severe hyperglycemia has many nursing diagnoses, the priority is to teach symptoms of worsening condition so the patient can report appropriately to the nurse.*
Mrs. Rant	*Pain* related to renal calculi	*Passing renal calculi causes severe flank pain.*
Mrs. Fox	*Potential for Self-Care Deficit* related to age and depressed condition on admission	*Ability to care for self must be evaluated prior to discharge.*
Mr. Rite	*Risk for Impaired Thought Processes* including cognitive, voluntary, and involuntary control	*The patient is exhibiting signs on increased intracranial pressure, which can rapidly become worse and threaten his life.*

2. B. *Rationale: Signs and symptoms of hypoglycemia are tachycardia, hypotension, and shakiness.*
3. C. *Rationale: Three to six days after a closed head injury, the patient may develop diabetes insipidus due to increased intracranial pressure.*
4. B. *Rationale: The patient must take a pulse prior to taking the medication; a pulse > 100 must be reported to the doctor.*
5. A, B, E, F. *Rationale: Laboratory tests used to monitor diabetes management are fasting blood glucose levels, glycosylated hemoglobin, abnormal electrolyte levels indicating DKA or HHS, and cholesterol levels to monitor for increased risk of cardiovascular impairments.*

Communication
1. C. *Rationale: Fast-acting carbohydrates, such as juice or milk may be administered to raise the blood glucose level.*
2. "I don't know at this time if that will be necessary. We will be assessing Mrs. Fox's ability to care for herself. We will also get information from the doctor. I will have the discharge coordinator contact you to discuss these issues." *Rationale: It is important that elderly patients be given time to improve following a major health event. An evaluation of their ability to care for themselves is necessary as a part of discharge planning.*

Delegation
1. The nurse can delegate the following tasks to a nursing assistant. *Rationale: All tasks must be within the legal scope of practice for the nursing assistant and the facility policy.*
A. Mr. Blew: vital signs, blood glucose
B. Mrs. Rant: vital signs, strain all urine for stones
C. Mrs. Fox: vital signs, assisting with ADLs with instruction for patient to be as independent as possible
D. Mr. Rite: vital signs

Related Questions
1. A. *Rationale: Clinical manifestations of hyperthyroidism are increased perspiration (diaphoresis), diarrhea from increased gastrointestinal motility, and weight loss with increased appetite.*

2. D. *Rationale: Hemorrhage or edema may compress the trachea causing respiratory distress.*
3. A. *Rationale: Classic clinical manifestations of metabolic syndrome are hypertension, abdominal obesity, and blood glucose > 110 mg/dL.*
4. A. *Rationale: Electrolyte imbalances with untreated Cushing's syndrome are hypernatremia, hypokalemia, and hyperglycemia.*

Concept Map
Hint: More details can add to understanding and consistent care. Review information in Chapter 20 regarding type 2 diabetes and the long-term complications of diabetes to assist in developing your concept map for Mr. Gregg's risk for neurovascular dysfunction.

Chapter 21: Assessing the Gastrointestinal System
1. Answer: 2 Rationale: Proteins derived from animal foods (meats, fish, poultry, cheese, eggs, yogurt, and milk) are complete.
2. Answer: 2 Rationale: Vitamin K is an essential element for blood clotting and, without sufficient levels, bleeding can occur.
3. Answer: 4 Rationale: An elevated amylase indicates that the pancreatic enzymes, released during acute pancreatic inflammation, are digesting their own tissues.
4. Answer: 1 Rationale: The condition of the patient's teeth, possible difficulty for her to chew comfortably, and her dry mouth because of decreased production of saliva in the older adult may cause a nutritional deficit because she will tend to eat food that is easier to chew and swallow.
5. Answer: 4 Rationale: In patient with ascites of the liver of more than 500 mL, a method of determining fluid presence is palpating dullness in the abdomen in the supine position and then on the right side. The presence of dullness moving in these two positions indicates ascites with shifting dullness pattern.
6. Answer: 3 Rationale: Internal hemorrhoids occur with impaired venous return during evacuation of stool or increased abdominal pressure in pregnancy causing distension of veins of the anus.
7. Answer: 4 Rationale: A patient with an ostomy should have questions answered about the consistency of the stool. This information may indicate location of the opening within the intestinal tract and demonstrate how the bowel is functioning.
8. Answer: 4 Rationale: A stool specimen will supply the opportunity to directly exam the feces and detect presence of intestinal parasites.
9. Answer: 2 Rationale: Polyps have been documented as increased risk factors for developing cancer; therefore, removal is indicated to prevent neoplastic cell development.
10. Answer: 4 Rationale: Colon cancer is often an inherited disorder; knowledge of family history is important.

Chapter 22: Nursing Care of Patients with Nutritional Disorders
1. Answer: 3 Rationale: The lack of regular exercise in daily life means less expenditure of energy; therefore, nutrients are stored as fat. Research has shown that adopted children's weight is related to their biological parents. "Fast foods" are a contributing factor.
2. Answer: 2 Rationale: This response informs the patient of the calorie–pound relationship and involves the patient in the planning strategies to improve and maintain weight loss.
3. Answer: 1 Rationale: Recent weight loss is the most prevalent finding in protein-calorie malnutrition. Skinfold thickness is decreased and the patient demonstrates lethargy and drowsiness.

4. **Answer: 3 Rationale:** Small-bore feeding tubes displace easily. Accurate placement is evaluated by aspirating contents and checking the pH. In the stomach the pH is < 4.

5. **Answer: 4 Rationale:** An identified contributing factor to anorexia is family pressure. Family therapy commonly is an important part of the interdisciplinary treatment plan.

6. **Answer: 2 Rationale:** A BMI greater than 25 and central obesity as indicated by a waist–hip ratio of 1 or greater are associated with a higher risk for hypertension, elevated lipid levels, heart disease, and stroke. These conditions have the greatest effect on health over time.

7. **Answer: 4, 5 Rationale:** Because this drug causes dry mouth and potential for constipation, fluids are important to maintain function. The drug is intended to be taken along with a restricted calorie diet for weight loss.

8. **Answer: 1, 2, 4, 5 Rationale:** There are many contributing factors that influence nutrition in the home-bound older adult such as inability to shop for nutritional foods, and the ability to afford and to prepare nutritional food. There are also psychosocial issues of depression and loneliness since eating is a social affair; this could well influence the amount and proportion of caloric intake. Arranging for food to be brought to the patient and for the patient to be transported to a senior center for a meal may solve the weight loss issue and no further interventions may be necessary. Referral to the primary care provider is necessary.

9. **Answer: 4 Rationale:** Beginning oral intake of nutrients as soon as possible after surgery is the best way to prevent malnutrition.

10. **Answer: 1 Rationale:** One of the postoperative complications with gastric bypass surgery is an anastomotic leak causing peritonitis. These manifestations could be related to this condition and the surgeon needs to be notified.

Chapter 23: Nursing Care of Patients with Upper Gastrointestinal Disorders

1. **Answer: 4 Rationale:** The use of tobacco and drinking alcohol are the two primary risk factors for oral cancers.

2. **Answer: 2, 5 Rationale:** Placing the head of the bed on blocks and avoiding lying down for at least 3 hours after eating will help prevent backflow of gastric content into the esophagus by decreasing the pressure on the lower esophageal sphincter.

3. **Answer: 1 Rationale:** The most common contributing factor to acute stress gastritis is the interruption of the integrity of the gastric lining by gastric irritants such as aspirin and/or NSAIDs. A period of gastric rest, followed by a slow progression to regular dietary intake is advised.

4. **Answer: 4 Rationale:** A peptic ulcer is an interruption of the integrity of the gastric lining; perforation is the most lethal complication of this process. It produces inflammation, infection, and possibly shock.

5. **Answer: 3 Rationale:** Frequent small meals with solid foods or liquids, not both, are effective in controlling the hyperosmolar problem of dumping syndrome.

6. **Answer: 2 Rationale:** Bright bleeding from the mouth could indicate perforation of the esophageal wall or vessel rupture by invasion of a tumor.

7. **Answer: 1 Rationale:** These manifestations indicate a possible hypersensitivity response to the antibiotics. Anaphylaxis could occur, so this is an emergency situation.

8. **Answer: 3 Rationale:** The discomfort of stomatitis is aggravated by eating; viscous lidocaine to reduce mouth pain is important to promote nutrition.

9. **Answer: 3 Rationale:** Maintaining patency of the nasogastric tube following gastric surgery is vital to prevent pressure gastric distension and pressure on the suture line. Irrigating gently with

NS, if ordered, is the appropriate action. If unable to open tube, notify surgeon.

10. **Answer: 3, 4, 5 Rationale:** Severe pain may be a manifestation of perforation of the ulcer. Oral food and fluids are withheld to prevent vomiting and prepare for possible surgery. The patient is placed in Fowler's position to localize drainage to the pelvic area, and the physician is notified to ensure prompt diagnosis and treatment.

Chapter 24: Nursing Care of Patients with Bowel Disorders

1. **Answer: 2 Rationale:** The nurse should first assess the number, frequency, and water content of stools to support the diagnosis of diarrhea and estimate fluid and electrolyte loss.

2. **Answer: 3 Rationale:** Appendectomy, often performed on an emergency basis, is the usual treatment for appendicitis. Withholding food and fluids are the most appropriate measures in preparing the patient for surgery.

3. **Answer: 1 Rationale:** Sulfasalazine makes the patient susceptible to sunburn so a sunscreen should be used while outside.

4. **Answer: 4 Rationale:** Steatorrhea is a manifestation of malabsorption, and may relate to celiac disease. Exposure to foods containing gluten may trigger manifestations such as these.

5. **Answer: 2 Rationale:** The recommendation for patient health with this familial history of cancer is to monitor for polyps and tumors early through annual digital examinations and periodic colonoscopy. Research has proven a direct genetic link of polyps and cancer development (20%).

6. **Answer: 4, 5, 6 Rationale:** The documentation and frequent measuring of nasogastric output will help maintain vascular volume with replacement of fluids, and the color will indicate if drainage is normal. Measuring abdominal girth will assist in determining if increased intestinal distension is occurring.

7. **Answer: 4 Rationale:** It is most important to maintain the patency of the nasogastric tube to remove gastric secretions and air that may apply pressure to the anastomosis site and cause failure of the suture line. Keeping the stomach decompressed is important to prevent vomiting that could also cause damage to the anastomosis site.

8. **Answer: 2 Rationale:** Raspberry seeds can cause obstruction to the diverticular opening and set up the environment to initiate diverticulitis.

9. **Answer: 1, 3, 5, 6 Rationale:** Fresh fruits and vegetables, whole wheat bread, and bran cereal supply roughage and fiber in the diet that can assist in the evacuation of fecal material and lessen the possibility of developing diverticulum, the incidence of which is high in this age group. Adequate liquid is important to prevent hard, formed stools that are difficult to pass. Taking daily laxatives can decrease the normal bowel reflexes. Colace can be administered safely either in the morning or at nighttime.

10. **Answer: 2 Rationale:** Gastrointestinal decompression removes gastric juices, reducing the amount of accumulated fluid and gas proximal to the obstruction and the risk for bowel ischemia and necrosis.

Chapter 25: Nursing Care of Patients with Gallbladder, Liver, and Pancreatic Disorders

1. **Answer: 1 Rationale:** Right upper quadrant pain following ingestion of a fatty meal is the typical manifestation experienced by patients with cholelithiasis. Chills, fever, nausea, and vomiting may indicate an infection and contraindicate surgery at this time.

2. **Answer: 1, 4 Rationale:** Acute cholecystitis usually develops from a stone obstructing the cystic duct, preventing release of bile from the gallbladder. High fatty foods like gravies and peanut butter stimulate contraction of the obstructed gallbladder,

causing pain. The patient should be instructed to call the physician if severe abdominal pain and a fever are experienced

3. **Answer: 3 Rationale:** Hepatitis A is transmitted by oral-fecal route from an infected person handling food, water, or fish, or through direct contact without washing hands before handling food or after using the bathroom.

4. **Answer: 4 Rationale:** Hepatitis C is transmitted through contact with blood or body fluids.

5. **Answer: 2 Rationale:** The hepatitis A virus can be transmitted before manifestations of the disease (including jaundice) develop; therefore, it is important to identify people who have had direct contact with the newly diagnosed patient.

6. **Answer: 2 Rationale:** Maintaining a patent airway is of highest priority. Placing the patient in Fowler's position may prevent aspiration of blood and should be the primary action.

7. **Answer: 3 Rationale:** It is important to empty the bladder prior to the paracentesis to make sure the bladder is not punctured during the procedure.

8. **Answer: 1 Rationale:** The nurse should assess bowel sounds and palpate for tenderness since spontaneous bacterial infection can develop with ascites, producing fever and worsening encephalopathy.

9. **Answer: 3 Rationale:** In women, the most common contributing factor to development of acute pancreatitis is a gallstone obstructing the duct.

10. **Answer: 4 Rationale:** Maintaining a patent nasogastric tube is vital to prevent accumulation of gastric secretions and pressure on the anastomoses created in Whipple's procedure.

Unit 6 Building Clinical Competence: Responses to Altered Gastrointestinal Function
Functional Health Pattern: Nutritional-Metabolic

Functional Health Patterns
Hint: Even small suggestions to change life style can have a big impact on the patient's health status. Identify what communication you used to answer these questions.

Priority Setting
1.
   A. Thomas Jones should be seen first. *Rationale: Mr. Jones is becoming anxious and irritable, which are signs of DTs from alcohol withdrawal. He needs to be evaluated and treated.*
   B. Paul Bruner should be assessed second. *Rationale: Mr. Bruner is scheduled for surgery and enemas must be given with time to expel the fluid. Assessment must be done before the enemas are given.*
   C. Tonya Cooper should be seed third. *Rationale: Ms. Cooper needs assistance to use the bedpan. Her orthostatic blood pressure is too low for it to be safe to get her out of bed.*
   D. Grace Freeman should be assessed fourth. *Rationale: While the colostomy bag needs to be changed, it is not harmful to leave it for a few minutes. Changing the bag is an optimal time for patient teaching, which will take some time.*

Health Promotion
1.
   A. Thomas Jones: Discuss alcohol treatment, stop-smoking programs, and ways to prevent injury and infection.
   B. Tonya Cooper: Discuss the need for increased fluids and prevention of falls that might occur due to weakness and fainting.

C. Paul Bruner: Discuss the need for progressive activity to prevent pneumonia and DVT; following surgery he will need a balanced diet, high in protein, to promote healing.
   D. Grace Freeman: Discuss the need for daily activity to promote bowel elimination.

2. B, C, D. *Rationale: Liquids soften the stool, exercise increases gastric motility, and bulk-forming laxatives create bulk and draw water into the intestines, which soften the stool, preventing constipation.*

3. A. *Rationale: The most common initial clinical manifestation is rectal bleeding due to impaired integrity of the rectal tissue.*

Nursing Process
1. A, C, D, E. *Rationale: On admission a baseline for the extent of blood loss and life impairment must be determined.*
2.

	Nursing Diagnosis	Rationale
Thomas Jones	*High Risk for Noncompliance: medical management of cirrhosis*	*Patients with advanced cirrhosis and alcoholism find it difficult to change long-standing behavior.*
Tonya Cooper	*Fluid Volume Deficit*	*Ms. Cooper has such severe fluid volume deficit that she has developed orthostatic hypotension.*
Paul Bruner	*Reactive Depression related to abdominal mass and upcoming surgery*	*At 86 years of age, many people lack the mental energy to overcome major medical issues and become depressed.*
Grace Freeman	*Impaired Skin Integrity*	*The colostomy has altered the integrity of the skin. The application of the bag can also further impair the skin.*

3. C. *Rationale: Blood in the stomach can prevent locating the source of the bleeding. Flushing the stomach with cold saline can slow bleeding as well as rinse the blood from the stomach.*

4. The teaching plan should include types of appliances, how to remove and apply the appliance, how to remove flatus from the appliance, skin inspection, and skin care. Also include contact information for professional support and local ostomy support groups.

Communication
1. B. *Rationale: Rewarding good behavior helps to develop a positive self-concept. Monitoring daily food intake provides data of balanced nutrients where weight gain does not.*

2. "We are concerned for you because your blood pressure is so low you can go into shock and die. It is your life, but we care about you and don't want you hurting yourself." *Rationale: The nurse must be honest with the patient and express concern and caring for the patient's welfare.*

3. The nurse should respond with, "I understand your concerns. Have you discussed your feelings with your daughter and the doctor? I can have them come and talk with you before the surgery if you would like." *Rationale: The nurse must respond to the patient's wishes. It is important to facilitate communication between Mr. Bruner, his daughter, and the surgeon.*

Delegation

1. For each patient, vital signs and assisting with ADLs can be delegated. The nursing assistant may need to stay with Mr. Jones or Ms. Cooper to prevent them from hurting themselves. The nursing assistant can help get Ms. Green ready for surgery but cannot administer medication.

2. Tell the nursing assistant assisting Ms. Cooper with her meals to stay with her and prevent her from stimulating vomiting for at least one hour after she eats.

Content-Specific Questions

1. The nurse will need to complete an incident report form and be seen by the hospital infection control department. Blood should be drawn to establish a baseline in case the nurse becomes Hepatitis B positive. Facility policy should be followed.

2. D. *Rationale: Gluten is found in wheat, rye, barley, and oats. Patients on a gluten-free diet can have corn.*

3. B. *Rationale: In metabolic acidosis, pH is decreased below 7.35, pCO2 is decreased below 35 mmHg, and Bicarbonate is decreased below 22 mmEq/L.*

4. C. *Rationale: Instruct the patient to administer a bowel preparation the evening before to cleanse the intestines prior to the procedure.*

5. B. *Rationale: The usual clinical manifestations of large bowel obstruction are constipation and colicky abdominal pain.*

Concept Map

Hint: In identifying the priority nursing diagnosis, look at the circumstances and time frame of the patient's illness and weight loss. You may find it helpful to review Chapter 10 as you consider this question and develop a concept map for the nursing diagnosis of *Deficient Fluid Volume.*

Chapter 26: Assessing the Renal System

1. **Answer: 4 Rationale:** Leakage of urine is not a normal manifestation in women of any age.

2. **Answer: 4 Rationale:** ADH is increased to limit the excretion of water in the urine to maintain fluid balance.

3. **Answer: 3 Rationale:** Creatinine clearance is a test that determines the filtering ability of the glomeruli and the blood circulation to them. If the clearance is decreased, the glomeruli are damaged or the circulation is slowed.

4. **Answer: 3 Rationale:** The prostate surrounds the male urethra at the base of the bladder.

5. **Answer: 2 Rationale:** Nocturia is defined as two or more voidings during the night.

6. **Answer: 1 Rationale:** The contrast media used in IVPs cause some adverse reactions in patients that are allergic to iodine or products containing iodine. Shellfish contain iodine.

7. **Answer: 3 Rationale:** Collecting a urine specimen allows the examiner to assess the urine for color, odor, and clarity before the exam.

8. **Answer: 1 Rationale:** Anesthetic agents used during surgery may cause problems with initiating voiding. Palpation will determine if the bladder is distended.

9. **Answer: 4 Rationale:** Bladder cancer is believed to result from genetic and environmental factors.

10. **Answer: 2 Rationale:** Skin turgor is the best assessment technique to determine hydration of patients.

Chapter 27: Nursing Care of Patients with Urinary Tract Disorders

1. **Answer: 2 Rationale:** The form of birth control, especially for those using a diaphragm and spermicidal gel, can alter the vaginal flora and increase the risk of UTIs. The reoccurrence time factor of the UTI is too long to be a failure to complete antibiotic treatment the first time.

2. **Answer: 1, 3, 4 Rationale:** The nurse needs to inform the patient that a urine culture in 10 days is done to ensure antibiotic therapy was effective. In a perimenopausal woman vaginal cream may maintain tissue integrity to prevent bacterial colonization of perineal tissues; instructions on cleansing may prevent further infections.

3. **Answer: 4 Rationale:** Increasing fluid intake to 3000 mL per day will produce enough urine to prevent stone-forming salts from concentrating sufficiently to precipitate.

4. **Answer: 3 Rationale:** These are manifestations of renal colic and possible ureteral obstruction. Prompt diagnosis and treatment is vital to prevent hydroureter and hydronephrosis should the ureter be completely obstructed.

5. **Answer: 1 Rationale:** Bladder cancer is two times more prevalent in smokers than nonsmokers.

6. **Answer: 2 Rationale:** Painless hematuria is the usual presenting manifestation of bladder cancers and should be evaluated quickly for best outcome.

7. **Answer: 3 Rationale:** The patient with a newly created continent ileal diversion will have to demonstrate self-catheterization since this is the only way to empty the continent ileal diversion. There is no collection device in this surgical procedure.

8. **Answer: 3 Rationale:** Stress incontinence should not be viewed as a normal result of aging, but as a treatable problem. Pelvic floor muscle exercises strengthen perineal muscles, increasing urinary sphincter control, and will reduce the incidence of incontinence.

9. **Answer: 1 Rationale:** Inability to retain urine long enough to reach the toilet following perception of the need to urinate is characteristic of urge incontinence. Caffeine and artificial sweeteners are bladder irritants, causing instability of the detrusor muscle and aggravating manifestations. Restricting intake of fluids containing these substances in the evening reduces nocturia.

10. **Answer: 4 Rationale:** Catheterizing the patient every 3 to 4 hours with a straight catheter prevents overdistension of the bladder and the increased risk for infection associated with an indwelling catheter.

Chapter 28: Nursing Care of Patients with Kidney Disorders

1. **Answer: 2 Rationale:** The GFR tends to decrease with aging, decreasing drug excretion and increasing the risk for toxicity. Administering smaller doses less frequently reduces the risk, but the patient needs continued monitoring for manifestations of digoxin toxicity.

2. **Answer: 3 Rationale:** The adult form of polycystic kidney disease (PKD) is transmitted in an autosomal dominant pattern. Each child has a 50% chance of inheriting the disease.

3. **Answer: 2 Rationale:** The most common cause of acute glomerulonephritis is an abnormal immune response to beta-hemolytic streptococcus A infection, usually strep throat.

4. **Answer: 1 Rationale:** Soy or animal proteins are complete proteins necessary for growth and tissue maintenance. Complete proteins are preferred when total protein intake is restricted, as in acute glomerulonephritis.

5. **Answer: 4 Rationale:** Postoperatively, it is important to monitor separately all drainage device volumes to determine function of each catheter or drain and prevent hydronephrosis.

6. **Answer: 1 Rationale:** Ischemia is the most common cause of acute renal failure (ARF); therefore, maintaining fluid volume, cardiac output, and renal output are the highest priority nursing interventions to prevent renal failure.

7. **Answer: 3 Rationale:** Nephrotoxic drugs, including over-the-counter products, can produce further damage to the kidney cells and should be avoided.
8. **Answer: 1, 3 Rationale:** Weight and orthostatic vital signs are indicators of fluid volume status and electrolyte balance. Laboratory tests are monitored to evaluate the effects of treatment.
9. **Answer: 2 Rationale:** The patient's ability to state advantages and disadvantages of renal replacement therapies indicates understanding of treatment options and the ability to make informed decisions on treatment. Patients may be able to live independently or with the assistance of a part-time caregiver.
10. **Answer: 4 Rationale:** Cloudy urine could be a manifestation of an infection. Prompt treatment is vital to preserve integrity of the transplanted organ in an immunosuppressed patient.

Unit 7 Building Clinical Competence: Responses to Altered Urinary Elimination

Functional Health Pattern: Elimination

Functional Health Patterns
Hint: Be creative in identifying possible interventions.

Priority Setting
1.
   A. Joseph Rouse should be seen first. *Rationale: He has severe pain; tachycardia; and cool, pale, clammy skin following surgery. These can indicate early shock and must be evaluated and reported to the primary care provider.*
   B. Philip Jones should be seen second. *Rationale: Abdominal pain associated with being unable to void could indicate internal bleeding or blockage of the urinary system. These issues must be evaluated and reported to the primary care provider.*
   C. Agnes Smith can be seen third. *Rationale: While Mrs. Smith seems to be stable, if she is confused she may not be able to summon help if needed.*
   D. Angela Baldwin can be seen last. *Rationale: Nephritis can become life threatening and her health status must be evaluated; however, she is able to summon help if needed.*

Health Promotion
1. Agnes Smith should be taught to drink plenty of fluids and to provide perineal care several times daily.
2. Joseph Rouse should be taught to drink adequate fluids and to limit foods high in calcium and oxalate.
3. Angela Baldwin should be taught to limit fluids, and to follow the sodium and protein restrictions prescribed by the primary care provider.

Nursing Process
1.

	Nursing Diagnosis	Rationale
Phillip Jones	*Urinary Retention* related to kidney trauma	*Swelling from trauma can cause urinary retention.*
Agnes Smith	*Urinary Incontinence* related to urinary infection	*Patients with UTI can develop urge incontinence. The incontinent patient is also more at risk for UTI.*
Joseph Rouse	*Pain* related to kidney surgery	*Severe pain can be a sign of postoperative complication of internal bleeding.*

| Angela Baldwin | *Fluid Volume Excess* related to nephritis associated with SLE | *Without normal kidney function, fluid volume excess develops, putting stress on the heart and other internal organs.* |

2. B. *Rationale: Draining urine in 500 mL increments may prevent a vasovagal response from draining the bladder too rapidly.*
3. A. *Rationale: With kidney trauma, the nursing actions are to monitor for level of consciousness, vital signs, skin color and temperature, and urine output for possible signs of shock. Signs of shock, such as hypotension, tachycardia, tachypnea, cool and pale skin, and altered level of consciousness may be present.*
4. A. *Rationale: Urine output of less than 30 mL is a sign of decreased renal and cardiac output. It needs to be reported to the physician promptly.*

Communication
1. A. *Rationale: Three-day medications therapy with trimethoprim-sulfamethoxazole (Bactrim) is the recommended treatment for uncomplicated cystitis.*
2. The nurse should respond, "It seems that the urinary complications you are having are associated with the lupus. Let's ask the doctor to discuss this with you when she comes in this morning." *Rationale: By acknowledging that the urinary symptoms might be associated with the lupus the nurse shows honesty. Because the nurse cannot diagnose medical problems, referring the patient to the primary care provider is appropriate.*

Delegation
1. For each patient, the nursing assistant can obtain vital signs, record intake and output, and provide ADLs.

Content-Specific Questions
1. C. *Rationale: Pyridium turns the urine and other body secretions a red or orange.*
2. D. *Rationale: Foods high in purines are organ meats and those moderate in purines are beef, chicken, pork. The patient on a low-purine diet needs to decrease eating these types of foods.*
3. B. *Rationale: Hematuria, proteinuria, and hypertension are the classic early manifestations of glomerulonephritis.*
4. B, C, F. *Rationale: Decreased cervicovaginal antibodies, sexual intercourse, short urethra, and aging in women are risk factors for urinary tract infections. Circumcision is a protective mechanism in men. Any patient is at risk when urinary catheter is inserted.*
5. B. *Rationale: Weight changes are a more accurate indicator of fluid volume status than intake and output, restricting fluids, and monitoring labs for BUS and creatinine.*
6. C. *Rationale: The most reliable diagnostic procedure for glomerular disorders is kidney biopsy. It determines the type of glomerulonephritis, the prognosis, and appropriate treatment.*

Concept Map
Hint: Note that in the evaluation section of the concept map provided, Mr. Jenkins has undergone hemodialysis and is preparing for placement of a peritoneal dialysis catheter. Review the section on renal replacement therapies for nursing care and patient teaching related to peritoneal dialysis.

Chapter 29: Assessing the Cardiovascular and Lymphatic Systems
1. **Answer: 3 Rationale:** Hemorrhage would decrease the total volume of blood and venous return, which would decrease stroke volume and likewise cardiac output.

2. **Answer: 3 Rationale:** Since pain is subjective, a numerical rating scale assesses what is the patient's perception of pain intensity.

3. **Answer: 1 Rationale:** This is the location of the apex of the heart and can be assessed at left midclavicular, fifth intercostal space on most patients.

4. **Answer: 2 Rationale:** Bradycardia is defined as a pulse rate < 60 beats per minute.

5. **Answer: 3 Rationale:** Fatigue would indicate that the body's tissues are not receiving adequate oxygenation. O_2 is carried by the hemoglobin molecule on the RBC; if RBC numbers are very low there are insufficient numbers to carry adequate oxygen to meet demands.

6. **Answer: 2 Rationale:** Platelet plug formation is the first step in clotting. If the count is low, fewer platelets are available for clotting; therefore, with tissue injury, platelets are not available and bruising occurs.

7. **Answer: 1 Rationale:** The thickness of the blood will affect the ability of the blood to flow through the vessels, thus increasing the peripheral vascular resistance (PVR).

8. **Answer: 2 Rationale:** Auscultating with the bell of the stethoscope will identify soft sounds such as the carotid arteries and identify any bruits.

9. **Answer: 3 Rationale:** A murmuring or blowing sound is the definition of a bruit.

10. **Answer: 4 Rationale:** Notify the physician immediately; these manifestations indicate a severe decrease in perfusion to the leg, and cells are dying from lack of blood flow.

Chapter 30: Nursing Care of Patients with Coronary Heart Disease

1. **Answer: 3 Rationale:** Stopping smoking decreases the risk of coronary heart disease by 50%.

2. **Answer: 1 Rationale:** These manifestations could indicate myopathy, a serious potential complication of statin drugs that needs to be reported promptly.

3. **Answer: 2 Rationale:** Stable angina is predictable and it is associated with increased activity and relieved by rest and nitrates.

4. **Answer: 4 Rationale:** Reestablishing coronary blood flow and cardiac tissue perfusion within 20 to 45 minutes is imperative to minimize damage to the myocardium.

5. **Answer: 2 Rationale:** The cardiac catheter used to insert the stent is usually inserted via the femoral artery, a large, high-pressure vessel. The leg is maintained in extension for a prescribed period after the procedure to reduce the risk of bleeding, hematoma formation, or clot formation at the insertion site.

6. **Answer: 4 Rationale:** Relieving pain in AMI decreases sympathetic nervous system stimulation and cardiac work. Pain relief is of highest priority, although the other goals also are appropriate for the patient with AMI.

7. **Answer: 1 Rationale:** Fibrinolytic therapy, administered to restore myocardial perfusion, disrupts the clotting cascade and can lead to potentially serious bleeding. Establishing bleeding precautions is vital to preserve physiologic integrity.

8. **Answer: 3 Rationale:** A CK of 320 U/L, four times the normal level, is indicative of muscle tissue damage; in the patient with acute chest pain it often indicates acute myocardial infarction.

9. **Answer: 2 Rationale:** Mobitz type II AV block often is associated with a large anterior MI and a high mortality rate. Pacemaker therapy may be necessary to maintain effective ventricular contractions and cardiac output.

10. **Answer: 1 Rationale:** Sinus bradycardia may be well-tolerated in some patients. Assessment is important before treating. However, if decreased mental status and hypotension is present, intervention is necessary.

Chapter 31: Nursing Care of Patients with Cardiac Disorders

1. **Answer: 1 Rationale:** Normal ejection fraction is 60%; an ejection fraction of 25% indicates severe impairment of ventricular function.

2. **Answer: 3 Rationale:** Interdisciplinary treatment goals for the patient with heart failure are to reduce the cardiac workload and improve pump effectiveness. Loss of excess fluid, as indicated by weight loss, reduces cardiac work. The drop in heart rate and reduced pulmonary vascular congestion are indicative of improved cardiac pump.

3. **Answer: 2, 4, 5 Rationale:** In left ventricular failure, the cardiac output falls and pressure in the pulmonary vascular system increases. This leads to fatigue, increasing dyspnea, and crackles in the lung bases.

4. **Answer: 4 Rationale:** Calibrating and leveling the system during each shift ensures accuracy and consistency of measurements.

5. **Answer: 2 Rationale:** Morphine is given intravenously to relieve anxiety; it also is a venous vasodilator, reducing venous return and cardiac work.

6. **Answer: 1 Rationale:** A pericardial friction rub, a grating sound, is a characteristic sign of pericarditis so it is expected, but should be documented in the patient's record.

7. **Answer: 4 Rationale:** Effective treatment for acute infective endocarditis requires long-term intravenous antibiotic therapy to eliminate the infecting organisms.

8. **Answer: 3 Rationale:** The murmur of mitral valve stenosis would be heard during diastole (when blood is flowing through the stenotic valve from the atrium to the ventricle) at the apex of the heart.

9. **Answer: 2 Rationale:** Anticoagulant therapy to prevent clot formation is necessary following insertion of a mechanical valve.

10. **Answer: 1 Rationale:** In hypertrophic cardiomyopathy, manifestations may not develop until the demand for oxygen increases, such as with athletes during activity, causing sudden death due to a ventricular dysrhythmia. This type of cardiomyopathy is not a filling problem but rather an obstruction to ejection of blood to the body to meet oxygen demand.

Chapter 32: Nursing Care of Patients with Vascular and Lymphatic Disorders

1. **Answer: 3 Rationale:** Hypertension generally is asymptomatic.

2. **Answer: 1 Rationale:** While lasagna made with whole-grain pasta, low-fat cheese, and vegetables or lean meats would be allowed, this answer demonstrates the need for additional teaching.

3. **Answer: 2, 4 Rationale:** First-dose hypotension and orthostatic hypotension are potential adverse effects of this drug, as is persistent cough.

4. **Answer: 1 Rationale:** These manifestations indicate a possible arterial occlusion. This is an emergency; immediate intervention is necessary to preserve the extremity.

5. **Answer: 4 Rationale:** Endovascular approach on an 86-year-old patient would mean less surgical risk and faster recovery.

6. **Answer: 4 Rationale:** Patients with peripheral atherosclerosis may have paresthesias and decreased hair on the affected extremity.

7. **Answer: 2, 3, 1, 4, 5 Rationale:** First, smoking cessation, because nicotine causes vasoconstriction, further decreasing blood flow; next, daily skin inspections looking for breaks in integrity to prevent infections; third, maintaining feet by regular cleansing, cotton socks, and protecting feet by wearing shoes; fourth, regular daily exercise to develop collateral circulation; and fifth, weight loss if necessary to keep patient mobile.

8. **Answer: 2 Rationale:** Anticoagulant therapy will be continued after discharge; understanding the importance of follow-up care and monitoring for adverse effects is vital.
9. **Answer: 1 Rationale:** Elevating the legs and wearing elastic stockings may relieve the discomfort associated with varicose veins.
10. **Answer: 3 Rationale:** Careful skin and foot care is a high priority to prevent skin breakdown and potential infection.

Chapter 33: Nursing Care of Patients with Hematologic Disorders

1. **Answer: 3 Rationale:** Red blood cells and the hemoglobin they contain carry oxygen to the tissues; in anemia, the oxygen-carrying capacity of blood is reduced, leading to exertional dyspnea.
2. **Answer: 1 Rationale:** During gastric resection, intrinsic factor production may decrease, leading to vitamin B_{12} deficiency anemia with associated neurologic deficits such as numbness and tingling of extremities.
3. **Answer: 2 Rationale:** Prior to bone marrow transplant, chemotherapy or total body irradiation is used to destroy leukemic cells in the bone marrow. Normal blood cells also are destroyed, causing significant risk for infection and bleeding.
4. **Answer: 1, 3, 5 Rationale:** AML causes both neutropenia and thrombocytopenia, with resulting increased risk for infection and bleeding. A private room and oral hygiene help reduce infection risk, and a soft, bland diet reduces trauma to oral mucosal membranes.
5. **Answer: 1 Rationale:** The correct response is open-ended and allows the patient to state more specifically what he is concerned about.
6. **Answer: 3 Rationale:** Multiple-drug chemotherapy regimes are effective at different phases of the cell cycle, allowing lower doses of individual drugs to decrease adverse effects and produce more effective tumor destruction.
7. **Answer: 4 Rationale:** A new onset of severe pain may signal a pathological fracture and needs to be reported.
8. **Answer: 2 Rationale:** A platelet count of $60,000/mm^3$ is significantly low (normal $150,000–450,000/mm^3$), increasing the risk of bleeding and bruising with minor trauma.
9. **Answer: 1 Rationale:** The most common form of classic hemophilia is transmitted as an x-linked recessive disorder passed from mother to son; therefore, the daughter may be a carrier.
10. **Answer: 4 Rationale:** A platelet infusion replaces those platelets used in the abnormal clotting process of DIC.

Unit 8 Clinical Competencies: Responses to Altered Cardiac Function

Functional Health Pattern: Activity-Exercise Patterns

Functional Health Patterns

Hint: Think about the timing of ADLs and other necessary treatments. Think about safety measures while the patient is in the hospital as well as at home.

Priority Setting

1.
    A. Scott Jacoby should be seen first. *Rationale: Mr. Jacoby needs to be ready for the bone marrow biopsy this morning. The degree of his mental abilities is unclear. The patient with Down's syndrome often needs simple instruction and reassurance.*
    B. Arnold Markus should be seen second. *Rationale: Mr. Markus has started having isolated PVCs and crackles in the lower lobes of the lungs. These signs can indicate a worsening of the CHF, which needs to be evaluated.*

C. Theresa Cartwright can be seen third. *Rationale: Mrs. Cartwright can summon help if needed. Treatment has been initiated, but the Heparin IV must be monitored.*
D. Betty Williams should be seen last. *Rationale: Mrs. Williams's vital signs and heart rhythm are stable.*

Health Promotion

1. Mr. Markus should be taught to eat a low-sodium diet to help prevent water retention. He should avoid obviously salty foods, limit the use of salt during cooking, and refrain from adding salt at the table.
2. Mrs. Williams should be taught to manage her type 2 diabetes, to stop smoking, and to control her hypertension. She should be given the resources (professional resources and support groups) she needs. She should be encouraged to eat a healthy diet and engage in exercise as recommended by her healthcare provider.
3. The nurse should discuss dietary restriction because of anticoagulant therapy. Not massaging or deeply rubbing the legs, wearing anti-embolitic stockings, and taking care to prevent trauma should also be discussed.

Nursing Process

1.

	Nursing Diagnosis	Rationale
Betty Williams	*Risk for Activity Intolerance* related to MI	*A weakened heart may not be able to sustain a high level of activity. Mrs. Williams should increase activity gradually.*
Arnold Markus	*Decreased Cardiac Output*	*Mr. Markus's heart is weak and unable to pump effectively.*
Theresa Cartwright	*Anxiety* related to unexpected hospitalization and uncertainty about the seriousness of her illness	*Mrs. Cartwright is a mother of young children who need her at home.*
Scott Jacoby	*High Risk for Infection* related to upper respiratory infection and possible pathology of the bone marrow	*Mr. Jacoby currently has an infection and has symptoms of bone marrow pathology (possible leukemia). This puts him at greater risk for further infection.*

2. C. *Rationale: While fluid in the lungs will alter lung sounds, oxygen saturation levels indicate the ability of the lungs to function and the heart to circulate the blood.*
3. D. *Rationale: A PVC falling on the T wave of the previous beat can cause the life-threatening dysrhythmia ventricular fibrillation.*
4. A. *Rationale: Assessment should be completed before initiating interventions. A full symptom assessment should be completed before administering the prescribed nitroglycerine tablet.*
5. B. *Rationale: Fever and burning on urination would indicate a urinary tract infection. Mr. Jacoby is at risk for infection, so these symptoms are significant.*

6. B, F. *Rationale: Prothrombin time (PT) and International Normalized Ration (INR) are monitored to determine the dosage levels of warfarin therapy.*

Communication

1. C. *Rationale: Mrs. Cartwright needs to continue to take birth control pills to prevent pregnancy, as Coumadin is a teratogenic drug.*

2. You should explain that her heart has been weakened by the heart attack, but with time it can heal and strengthen. It will be important for her to follow the doctor's instructions.

Delegation

1.

A. Mrs. Williams: The nursing assistant can obtain vital signs and assist with a bed bath unless the doctor has ordered a warm shower. Mrs. Williams will also need blood glucose values obtained.

B. Mr. Markus: The nursing assistant can obtain vital signs and assist with a warm shower and ambulation.

C. Mrs. Cartwright: The nursing assistant can obtain vital signs. Since Mrs. Cartwright will be on bedrest, she will need assistance with all ADLs.

D. Mr. Jacoby: The nursing assistant can obtain vital signs, assist with ADLs, and assist with preparation for bone marrow biopsy. The nursing assistant may accompany the patient to the procedure if support is needed.

Related Questions

1. C. *Rationale: The patient with a mitral valve replacement will be prescribed long-term anticoagulant therapy. Patients with a history of duodenal ulcer are at increased risk of intestinal bleeding and must be monitored closely.*

2. B. *Rationale: Venous stasis impairs delivery of nutrients and oxygen to peripheral tissues.*

3. C. *Rationale: Keep fingers and toes warm to prevent spasms of the small arteries in the digits.*

4. B. *Rationale: Cardizem may cause bradycardia. Notify the physician if the heart rate is less than 60 beats per minute.*

5. D. *Rationale: Use enough direct pressure to control bleeding. Pressure on the femoral artery or a tourniquet will occlude the blood vessels and decrease tissue perfusion, and should only be used as a last resort to save a life.*

Concept Map

Hint: Review Unit 7 to determine the impact of chronic kidney disease on hypertension. The concept map for Unit 8 (this one) would reflect both disorders.

Chapter 34: Assessing the Respiratory System

1. Answer: 4 Rationale: The apex or top of the lungs is located just below the clavicle.

2. Answer: 3 Rationale: A family history of lung cancer is a risk factor for developing lung cancer.

3. Answer: 4 Rationale: Bronchovesicular breath sounds are normal; the nurse would take and record the vital signs as usual.

4. Answer: 1 Rationale: As the body temperature rises the bond between oxygen and hemoglobin decreases so less oxygen binds and unloading is enhanced.

5. Answer: 2 Rationale: Thoracentesis is the removal of fluid around the lung.

6. Answer: 3 Rationale: Information about illness management is important in identifying health problems.

7. Answer: 2 Rationale: Wheezes are continuous musical sounds heard in the chest.

8. Answer: 4 Rationale: If the patient had a lung removed, breath sounds would be absent from that side because without air movement no sound would be generated.

9. Answer: 3 Rationale: While auscultating the lungs, the patient should take slow deep breaths to allow adequate time for air to go into and out of the lungs. Breathing through the mouth amplifies the sound, making it easier to hear.

10. Answer: 2 Rationale: Decreased diaphragmatic movement on the left side should be documented; it is an expected outcome with pneumothorax on the left since air movement and diaphragm movement would be decreased.

Chapter 35: Nursing Care of Patients with Upper Respiratory Disorders

1. Answer: 4 Rationale: Over-the-counter nasal spray is the best choice to relieve URI manifestations in the patient with hypertension, since its effects are local, not systemic. The duration of use is limited to prevent rebound.

2. Answer: 2 Rationale: Yearly influenza vaccinations are the most effective way of preventing flu and pneumonia in this group.

3. Answer: 1 Rationale: Completion of the antibiotic medication is the most important in order to cure the bacterial infection and prevent reoccurrence.

4. Answer: 3 Rationale: Posterior nasal packing obstructs the nares and may compromise oxygenation. Oxygenation has the highest priority.

5. Answer: 4 Rationale: Fracture of other facial bones may accompany nasal fracture, damaging the dura and causing spinal fluid leak. A positive glucose indicates the presence of spinal fluid.

6. Answer: 3, 5, 6 Rationale: The manifestations of sleep apnea include daytime sleepiness, elevated BP, and complaints of morning headache.

7. Answer: 1 Rationale: Persistent voice hoarseness may be the first sign of a laryngeal tumor, necessitating follow-up diagnostic testing.

8. Answer: 3 Rationale: With stage I laryngeal cancer, radiation can cure the cancer, and preserve the voice. This cancer does metastasize to other areas.

9. Answer: 4, 5, 2, 1, 3 Rationale: Maintaining airway patency is of highest priority. The head may need additional support because of the removal of neck muscles. Frequent, small meals help meet metabolic needs; swallowing may be difficult and the effort may produce fatigue. Regaining speech will require practice and assistance from a speech therapist. Loss of the voice will result in grieving; encouraging expression of feelings can facilitate gradual acceptance of the loss.

10. Answer: 2 Rationale: When providing tracheostomy care, the nurse secures clean ties before removing soiled ones to prevent accidental dislodgement of the tube.

Chapter 36: Nursing Care of Patients with Ventilation Disorders

1. Answer: 4 Rationale: Unless oxygenation is compromised by the inflammatory process, the sputum specimen is obtained first.

2. Answer: 1, 4, 5, 2, 3 Rationale: Overall gray skin color and bluish tinge to lips indicate hypoxemia; supplemental oxygen is highest priority. Second, raise the head of the bed to promote chest expansion and alveolar ventilation. Assessment of oxygen saturation and breath sounds provide important information to be provided to the physician.

3. Answer: 3 Rationale: A 9 mm induration is a positive result in a patient with HIV disease.

4. **Answer: 2 Rationale:** When teaching a patient who is taking INH, the nurse needs to include information on adverse effects such as numbness and tingling of extremities to the doctor.

5. **Answer: 3 Rationale:** Smoking cessation is important with the diagnosis of lung cancer to prevent further damage from the chemicals in the cigarettes.

6. **Answer: 3, 4 Rationale:** Chest tube drainage that is red, free-flowing, and exceeds 70mL/hour indicates hemorrhage and must be reported. Vital signs and level of consciousness are measured to evaluate cardiac output and hemodynamic stability.

7. **Answer: 1 Rationale:** The patient having a thoracentesis needs to sit upright, leaning forward during the procedure to spread the rib cage for easier placement of the needle.

8. **Answer: 4 Rationale:** A patient with a fractured rib would be urged to use a small pillow to splint the area when coughing to reduce the movement of rib cage and pain.

9. **Answer: 2 Rationale:** A respiratory rate of 36 indicates respiratory distress, and is of greatest concern.

10. **Answer: 1 Rationale:** Tension pneumothorax displaces structures in the mediastinum, including the great vessels. Cardiac output may be severely compromised, resulting in inadequate oxygen delivery and nutrients to cells and tissues.

Chapter 37: Nursing Care of Patients with Gas Exchange Disorders

1. **Answer: 2 Rationale:** Ineffective airway clearance is the highest priority because it impairs alveolar ventilation and the exchange of oxygen and carbon dioxide at the capillaries, decreasing the blood and tissue oxygen levels.

2. **Answer: 1 Rationale:** The physician needs to be informed because this indicates increasing fatigue and impending respiratory failure.

3. **Answer: 3 Rationale:** The patient should be taught to use the anti-inflammatory drug as needed to treat acute episodes of wheezing.

4. **Answer: 1 Rationale:** Development of a barrel chest due to air trapping is an expected finding in COPD.

5. **Answer: 3 Rationale:** During an acute exacerbation of COPD, keeping the SaO_2 above 90% is an appropriate goal.

6. **Answer: 4 Rationale:** In some patients with COPD, decreased arterial oxygen concentrations drive respirations. Administered O_2 may decrease the drive to breathe; however, many patients with COPD require supplemental oxygen.

7. **Answer: 1, 2, 4, 5 Rationale:** Thick, tenacious, milky white sputum and fever indicate possible infection. Difficulty coughing up mucus and increased shortness of breath and fatigue indicate potential early manifestations of respiratory failure.

8. **Answer: 2 Rationale:** These manifestations may indicate pulmonary embolism. Oxygen is administered to support gas exchange and tissue oxygenation.

9. **Answer: 1 Rationale:** Restlessness and tachypnea are early signs of respiratory failure caused by hypoxemia and stimulation of the respiratory center.

10. **Answer: 4 Rationale:** Patent airways are necessary to maintain effective alveolar ventilation and gas exchange.

Unit 9 Building Clinical Competence: Responses to Altered Respiratory Function
Functional Health Pattern: Activity-Exercise Patterns

Functional Health Patterns
Hint: To facilitate breathing the nurse must not only think about positioning, but also how to maintain a patent airway and facilitate oxygen/carbon dioxide exchange.

Priority Setting
1.
   A. James Mohr should be seen first. *Rationale: Mr. Mohr has been coughing, and because of the tracheostomy he may be unable to clear his airway. Immediate suctioning is needed to open the airway.*
   B. Maggie Sawyer should be seen second. *Rationale: Ms. Sawyer could be having a pulmonary embolism, which can be life-threatening.*
   C. Jack Holt should be seen third. *Rationale: Mr. Holt's vital signs are elevated and he is experiencing pain with breathing. He may need medication for pain.*
   D. Amy Campbell should be seen last. *Rationale: While Ms. Campbell is wheezing, her vital signs and oxygen saturation level appear the most stable.*

Health Promotion
1. Patients with COPD need high-calorie, high-protein diets without excessive carbohydrates, which can increase levels of carbon dioxide, adding stress to the lungs.
2. Allow family members or significant others to remain with the patient while maintaining a quiet environment. Assist with guided imagery, relaxation techniques, and gentle massage, and administer medication as needed.

Nursing Process
1.

	Nursing Diagnosis	Rationale
Jack Holt	*Pain in Chest* related to breathing difficulty and frequent cough	*Chest pain caused by frequent coughing can diminish coughing effort, which results in mucus remaining in lungs.*
Maggie Sawyer	*Impaired Gas Exchange* as evidenced by sudden onset of difficulty breathing, chest pain, coughing, restlessness, and a feeling that she is going to die	*Ms. Sawyer's history of deep vein thrombosis can result in pulmonary embolism (PE). PE blocks blood to the alveoli, resulting in impaired gas exchange.*
James Mohr	*Ineffective Airway Clearance* related to trauma and tracheostomy	*A tracheostomy tube irritates the trachea, causing increased mucus and cough. The tube can become obstructed with mucus.*
Amy Campbell	*Ineffective Airway Clearance* as evidenced by wheezing	*Bronchospasm that occurs during an asthma attack obstructs the air flow into and out of the lungs.*

2. C. *Rationale: Wearing a mask is standard precaution for a patient with a droplet infection.*
3. B. *Rationale: The patient is positioned with the area to be drained above the trachea or mainstem bronchus. Head down allows gravity to facilitate drainage of secretions.*
4. D. *Rationale: Stretching the legs and walking every 1 to 2 hours when traveling will reduce the risk of pulmonary embolism. Hose that bind around the knee and use of pillows can contribute to deep vein thrombus formation and subsequently pulmonary embolism.*

5. C. *Rationale: Showering and bathing are allowed as long as the tracheostomy is protected from the flow of water.*

6. B. *Rationale: Short-acting bronchodilators are used first to dilate the bronchi quickly (albuterol), followed by longer-acting bronchodilators (atrovent), and lastly preventative medications (cromolyn).*

Communication

1. "Chronic asthma is a life-long disease, but with treatment it can be controlled. Most patients lead a very productive life."

Delegation

1. What data collection and interventions can be delegated to a nursing assistant for each patient?

   A. Jack Holt: The nursing assistant can obtain vital signs and oxygen saturation, and assist with ADLs. Frequent oral care, disposing of contaminated tissues, and supplying clean ones is needed.

   B. Maggie Sawyer: The nursing assistant can obtain vital signs and oxygen saturation, assist with ADLs, assist with set up of oxygen, and stay with the patient in case further assistance is needed.

   C. James Mohr: The nursing assistant can obtain vital signs and oxygen saturation, and assist with ADLs. He or she should call the RN immediately if the patient coughs productively and indicates the airway is becoming blocked.

   D. Amy Campbell: The nursing assistant can obtain vital signs and oxygen saturation, and assist with ADLs. He or she should notify the RN immediately if the patient develops severe respiratory distress. Adjusting the oxygen is not a nursing assistant function.

Content-Specific Questions

1. A. *Rationale: Arterial blood gases are drawn to evaluate gas exchange and hypoxemia. Carboxyhemoglobin levels determine carbon monoxide poisoning. Electrolytes are drawn if water aspiration is a possibility.*

2. A. *Rationale: A pH of less than 7.35 indicates acidosis. A pCO_2 greater than 45 mmHG indicates a respiratory problem. These results indicate respiratory acidosis.*

3. B. *Rationale: Corticosteroids have to be weaned off due to adrenal atrophy caused by taking them.*

4. D. *Rationale: Early signs of pulmonary tuberculosis are fatigue, weight loss, anorexia, low-grade afternoon fever, night sweats, and a dry cough. Purulent and/or blood-tinged sputum are later manifestations.*

5. A, C, E. *Rationale: Age-related changes in the older adults are decreased elastic recoil of lungs, loss of skeletal muscle strength, less elastic and more fibrotic alveoli, increases in residual volume, and decreased effectiveness of coughing.*

Concept Map

Hint: As you plan interventions to address Mrs. Hamer's nutritional status, consider the impact of her chronic lung disease on her oxygenation needs, nutrition/fluid needs, and ADLs.

Chapter 38: Assessing the Musculoskeletal System

1. **Answer: 3 Rationale:** Long bones have two broad ends that are called epiphyses.

2. **Answer: 1 Rationale:** *Abduction* is the term for moving an extremity away from the midline of the body.

3. **Answer: 1 Rationale:** Patients with gout have increased serum uric acid and if medication for treating gout is effective the serum level of uric acid should be decreased.

4. **Answer: 4 Rationale:** Women in their 60s are usually post-menopausal, and are at risk for decreased bone density as well as for fractures due to osteoporosis.

5. **Answer: 3 Rationale:** With decreased bone mass and decreased calcium absorption, the bones become brittle and at risk for fractures.

6. **Answer: 2 Rationale:** When assessing facial muscle strength the nurse would ask the patient to stick out his or her tongue.

7. **Answer: 4 Rationale:** Crepitation is a grating sound as the joint moves.

8. **Answer: 3 Rationale:** The ballottement test is used to assess for fluid in the knee joint.

9. **Answer: 2 Rationale:** Scoliosis is the term used to describe a lateral curve in the spine.

10. **Answer: 1 Rationale:** Pain and limited mobility are the most common manifestations of musculoskeletal disorders.

Chapter 39: Nursing Care of Patients with Musculoskeletal Trauma

1. **Answer: 2 Rationale:** Ice used on a sprained ankle immediately after injury will cause vasoconstriction of the blood vessels to decrease edema and pain.

2. **Answer: 3 Rationale:** A compound fracture means bone has broken the skin, which is the first line of defense against bacterial invasion.

3. **Answer: 3 Rationale:** Pale, cold fingers of an older woman with a cast could indicate decreased circulation to the hand.

4. **Answer: 4 Rationale:** Calcium deposits in the fracture site allow callus to begin to form as healing occurs.

5. **Answer: 2 Rationale:** Cyanosis and lack of sensation in the toes indicates decreased circulation and pressure on nerves; if this is not relieved soon permanent damage could occur.

6. **Answer: 2 Rationale:** Patients with deep vein thrombosis of the lower extremity require careful monitoring of the respiratory system for complications of emboli.

7. **Answer: 2 Rationale:** Patients who have suffered musculoskeletal injuries have soft tissue damage, muscle spasm, and swelling causing acute pain.

8. **Answer: 1 Rationale:** During the first 24 hours after amputation the remaining extremity is elevated above the level of the heart to promote venous return and decrease swelling.

9. **Answer: 4 Rationale:** Phantom limb pain is experienced by a majority of amputees, especially in the early postoperative period.

10. **Answer: 4 Rationale:** The amputated finger should be wrapped in a clean cloth, put in a plastic bag, and placed on ice (although not directly on ice, which could cause tissue frostbite) to preserve tissue. This will preserve the amputated finger so that it can be surgically reattached.

Chapter 40: Nursing Care of Patients with Musculoskeletal Disorders

1. **Answer: 2 Rationale:** *Risk for Falls* is the most significant nursing diagnosis in terms of long-term disability because falls may cause fractures in the patient with osteoporosis.

2. **Answer: 4 Rationale:** Most patients with osteoarthritis use NSAIDs for control of discomfort from disease.

3. **Answer: 2 Rationale:** Patients with gout have increased serum levels of uric acid.

4. **Answer: 3 Rationale:** In patients with osteoporosis and osteomalacia, fractures are a potential complication because of lack of calcium intake and vitamin D intake.

5. **Answer: 1 Rationale:** Being overweight by 30 pounds is indicative of an increased risk for osteoarthritis, especially in the joints of the legs.

6. **Answer: 3 Rationale:** By monitoring vital signs, hemoglobin, and hematocrit, the nurse can determine early if the fluid volume is deficient (caused by excessive bleeding), or if blood supply to an extremity is compromised.

7. **Answer: 1 Rationale:** Fever and weight loss are found in patients with rheumatoid arthritis.

8. **Answer: 3 Rationale:** In the nursing diagnosis *Ineffective Protection*, the most important intervention for the patient with SLE would be to practice careful hand hygiene, as SLE patients are at risk for opportunistic and severe infection.

9. **Answer: 4 Rationale:** Most cases of Lyme disease occur when an infected tick remains embedded for at least 24 hours.

10. **Answer: 2 Rationale:** Septic arthritis is a medical emergency; if not diagnosed quickly and treatment begun, destruction of the affected joint may occur.

Unit 10 Building Clinical Competence: Responses to Altered Musculoskeletal Function
Functional Health Pattern: Activity-Exercise Patterns

Functional Health Patterns
Hint: Because protecting the patient from falling is a top priority, the nurse uses many basic techniques to protect the patient when ambulating, but also turning, positioning, and transferring.

Priority Setting
1.
   A. Joyce Stevens should be seen first. *Rationale: Petechiae, difficulty breathing, and confusion can be signs of life-threatening pulmonary embolism that must be evaluated immediately.*
   B. Jesse Drummond should be seen second. *Rationale: While phantom pain is common following an amputation, Mr. Drummond had a bilateral amputation, which increases his anxiety and pain. The nurse needs to assess the stumps to determine if complications are also adding to the pain level.*
   C. José Rivera should be seen third. *Rationale: Mr. Rivera may need pain medication. The upcoming surgery may be causing anxiety, which increases pain.*
   D. Kim Wong should be seen last. *Rationale: Her vital signs do not indicate immediate concern, and results from the blood tests are needed to determine the cause of the symptoms.*

Health Promotion
1. Ms. Stevens should be taught to eat a diet high in protein to promote healing and high in calcium to strengthen bones. If she is prescribed anticoagulant medication, she may need to limit her intake of food high in vitamin K.
2. Yes. He needs high protein to heal and high calcium to strengthen his weakened bones.

Nursing Process
1.

	Nursing Diagnosis	Rationale
Jesse Drummond	*Impaired Physical Mobility* related to bilateral amputation	*Mr. Drummond had both legs amputated. He will be wheelchair bound unless he is able to get prosthetic legs.*
Joyce Stevens	*Ineffective Breathing Pattern*	*Ms. Stevens is exhibiting signs of pulmonary embolism, a life-threatening complication.*
José Rivera	*Altered Tissue Perfusion* related to surgery, gun shot wound, and osteomyelitis	*The circulation to the tissue of the upper leg was damaged by the gun shot. Subsequent infection impairs circulation further.*
Kim Wong	*Altered Tissue Perfusion*	*The symptoms of swollen joints, pain, and cyanotic digits indicates lack of circulation.*

2. B. *Rationale: Pushing the stump against soft and then harder surfaces will help toughen the skin.*
3. A. *Rationale: Anti-DNA antibodies are a specific indicator of systemic lupus erythematosus. Patients also have anemia, leukopenia, thrombocytopenia, and elevated eosinophil sedimentation rate.*
4. A. *Rationale: Place the patient in a private room and use standard precautions with good hand hygiene to prevent spread of the infection.*

Communication
1. "Mr. Drummond, I am sorry your legs hurt. What you are describe is called phantom pain and is very common immediately after amputation. Generally the pain eases as healing occurs. I will get you some medication. When your doctor gets here, I will have him talk with you more about your pain."
2. "Ms. Wong, I know it is hard for you to wait for the results of your tests, but until we have them, the doctor cannot determine if you have lupus or not. Once a diagnosis is made the options for treatment can be discussed with you. I will have the doctor talk with you as soon as possible."

Delegation
1.
   A. Jesse Drummond: The nursing assistant can obtain vital signs and help with all ADLs.
   B. Joyce Stevens: The nursing assistant can obtain vital signs, help with all ADLs, and help with the hip exerciser as directed and supervised by the RN.
   C. José Rivera: The nursing assistant can obtain vital signs, help transfer the patient to surgery, and set up the post-op room for his return.
   D. Kim Wong: The nursing assistant can obtain vital signs and help with all ADLs.

Content-Specific Questions
1. D. *Rationale: The patient with an above-the-knee amputation should not sit for prolonged periods of time, as prolonged sitting can lead to hip contracture.*
2. B. *Rationale: Meats, seafood, beans, spinach, asparagus are high-purine foods.*
3. D. *Rationale: Patients with autoimmune diseases are at increased risk of coronary heart disease such as myocardial infarction.*
4. C. *Rationale: The most toxic effects of NSAIDS are gastric irritation, ulceration, and bleeding.*
5. A, C, D, E, G. *Rationale: The 5 Ps of a neurovascular assessment are pain, pulses, pallor, paresis, and paresthesia.*

6. A. *Rationale: Smoking reduces bone density in menopausal women, making them at risk for osteoporosis.*
7. C. *Rationale: All answers are correct but the most important is to follow a regimen of rest, ice, compression, and elevation for 24 to 48 hours to reduce swelling and pain.*

Concept Map
Hint: Are there other Independent Interventions that can help this patient with impaired physical mobility? Which other identified nursing diagnosis would you identify as of highest priority during the first 48 hours after admission? Five days after the accident?

Chapter 41: Assessing the Nervous System

1. **Answer: 4 Rationale:** The blood-brain barrier controls the environment within by allowing oxygen, carbon dioxide, lipids, glucose, and water into the capillaries but preventing entry of urea, creatinine, toxins, proteins, and antibiotics.
2. **Answer: 3 Rationale:** The lower motor neurons maintain muscle tone and reflexes; any damage could result in loss of reflexes.
3. **Answer: 3 Rationale:** Cerebrospinal fluid (CSF) cushions the brain tissue and spinal cord, protects them from trauma, provides nourishment to the brain, and removes waste products.
4. **Answer: 1 Rationale:** The posterior spinal roots contain cells that discriminate fine touch sensations such as dull and sharp; therefore, damage to these roots would mean the patient would be unable to detect dull or sharp sensation.
5. **Answer: 1 Rationale:** The sympathetic division of the ANS has the purpose of preparing the body to handle stressful events, such as a near auto crash, by increasing heart rate, force of contraction, vasodilation of coronary arteries, and increased mental alertness.
6. **Answer: 2 Rationale:** Auscultation is not used in assessing the neurologic system.
7. **Answer: 1 Rationale:** A cotton ball and a safety pin would be used to assess sensations of light, dull, and sharp on the face.
8. **Answer: 4 Rationale:** In patients who are unconscious the corneal reflex is absent, so when the cornea is touched with a wisp of cotton, the patient does not blink.
9. **Answer: 3 Rationale:** A tongue depressor is used on the posterior section of the tongue to illicit a gag reflex, testing cranial nerve IX.
10. **Answer: 2 Rationale:** In decorticate posturing the upper arms are close to the body; the elbows, wrists, and fingers are flexed; and the legs are extended with internal rotation.

Chapter 42: Nursing Care of Patients with Intracranial Disorders

1. **Answer: 4 Rationale:** Normally the RAS and cerebral hemispheres control respirations with a regular pattern; however, when they are damaged, the lower brainstem responds to changes in $PaCO_2$, resulting in irregular respiratory patterns.
2. **Answer: 2 Rationale:** The unconscious patient with impaired gag or swallowing reflexes would be at risk for aspiration since saliva and any fluids taken by mouth could not be swallowed normally.
3. **Answer: 2 Rationale:** Osmotic diuretics increase the osmolality of blood by excreting water and leaving solutes; as a result, the water in the brain would is drawn into the vascular space.
4. **Answer: 3 Rationale:** Motor responses to a direct stimuli such as "squeeze my hand" are the best way to identify changes in mental status.
5. **Answer: 1, 2, 3 Rationale:** A patient with an altered LOC would probably have blood glucose to check for hypoglycemia, electrolytes to check for metabolic disturbances (especially sodium), and toxicology to test for drug or alcohol toxicity.

6. **Answer: 3 Rationale:** Serum osmolality would assess water and solute balance in the blood, indicating the hydration status of the patient.
7. **Answer: 2 Rationale:** Numbness and tingling in the corner of the patient's mouth that disappears within minutes or hours is a manifestation of temporary occlusion of the middle cerebral artery.
8. **Answer: 1 Rationale:** Hypertension is the greatest risk factor for a stroke because sustained systolic and diastolic pressure damage cerebral blood vessels.
9. **Answer: 3 Rationale:** The motor pathways of the nervous system cross at the medulla and spinal cord, meaning damage to the left cerebral vessel will demonstrate neurologic deficits on the right side, an effect called contralateral.
10. **Answer: 4 Rationale:** Tissue plasminogen activator is given within the first 3 hours of the ischemic stroke to cause fibrinolysis of the clot.

Chapter 43: Nursing Care of Patients with Spinal Cord Disorders and CNS Infections

1. **Answer: 3 Rationale:** SCI at the C1-C4 level produces respiratory paralysis and the patient will be unable to breathe on his or her own, so a ventilator will be necessary to maintain respiratory function.
2. **Answer: 1, 2, 4 Rationale:** Corticosteroids will be used to decrease cord edema. Vasopressors will be used to treat bradycardia or hypotension from spinal shock. Analgesics will be used to control pain.
3. **Answer: 1 Rationale:** In a patient with spinal cord injury no impulses are transmitted between the brain and spinal cord and the cord does not function at all, producing spinal shock that may last from minutes to weeks or months.
4. **Answer: 2 Rationale:** Autonomic dysreflexia can be caused by kinked catheter tubing that allows the bladder to become full, triggering massive vasoconstriction below the injury site and producing the manifestations of this process. The other answers will not cause autonomic dysreflexia.
5. **Answer: 1, 3, 5 Rationale:** In teaching prevention of back injuries the nurse would incorporate principles of proper body mechanics, which are spread feet apart, use large leg muscles, and work as close to the object as possible. Bending from the waist to lift rather than sometimes rolling or pushing will contribute to back injuries.
6. **Answer: 2 Rationale:** Monitor for signs of nerve root compression by assessing hand grips and arm strength, ability to move the fingers, and ability to detect touch.
7. **Answer: 1 Rationale:** The patient with a spinal cord tumor (regardless of type) requires nursing interventions to provide management of acute pain.
8. **Answer: 3 Rationale:** Young adults living in close proximity (such as college students living in a dormitory) are at a greater risk of contracting bacterial meningitis.
9. **Answer: 3 Rationale:** Mosquito control with repellants, insecticides, and protective clothing; destruction of the insect larvae and elimination of breeding places, such as pools of stagnant water; and community mosquito control programs can help prevent meningitis and encephalitis.
10. **Answer: 2 Rationale:** Tetanus is completely preventable by active immunization.

Chapter 44: Nursing Care of Patients with Neurologic Disorders

1. **Answer: 1, 2 Rationale:** Dementia is a general term used to describe the outcome of the death of neurons, and the cognitive and behavioral manifestations of AD.

2. **Answer: 3 Rationale:** Memory deficits are usually the first indication of AD. They are subtle and may not be noticed by friends and family until the patient exhibits unsafe behaviors.

3. **Answer: 1 Rationale:** *Fatigue* affects all patients with MS regardless of type or severity.

4. **Answer: 3 Rationale:** Interferons are used to reduce exacerbations in patients with multiple sclerosis and enhance immune function.

5. **Answer: 4 Rationale:** When teaching a young adult with MS it is important to stress avoidance of extremes of heat and cold since maintaining a constant body temperature will decrease exacerbations of manifestations, and heat slows down transmission of nerve impulses.

6. **Answer: 2 Rationale:** Parkinson's disease manifestations appear when the brain cells no longer produce enough dopamine to inhibit acetylcholine; this results in uncoordinated motor movement.

7. **Answer: 3 Rationale:** With the gait changes, balance problems, and possible orthostatic hypotension, patients with PD are at increased risk for falls. This safety issue needs to be addressed with the caregivers.

8. **Answer: 4 Rationale:** Antiglutamate is the drug classification used to treat ALS because it prevents the release of glutamic acid and protects against toxicity of neurons.

9. **Answer: 3 Rationale:** When teaching patients about Bell's palsy, the nurse needs to tell the patient that one side of the face will not move normally since the affected nerve supplies the muscles that produce expression on one side of the face.

10. **Answer: 1 Rationale:** Riluzole (Rilutek) is administered without food at the same time each day.

Unit 11 Building Clinical Competence: Responses to Altered Neurologic Function
Functional Health Pattern: Cognitive-Perceptual

Functional Health Patterns
Hint: Because neurological disorders can affect many aspects of the patient's ability to function independently, there are numerous things the nurse must assist with to maintain patient safety.

Priority Setting
1.
   A. Cesar Phillips should be seen first. *Rationale: BP 170/110 before medication 1.5 hours ago. The effectiveness of this treatment must be evaluated.*
   B. Louie Hernandez should be seen second. *Rationale: Mr. Hernandez may have swallowing difficulty and therefore may have difficulty keeping his airway clear. Aphasia may prevent him from summoning help if needed. Frequent observation is needed.*
   C. Tonya Walton should be seen second. *Rationale: The increasing head pain can indicate complications after neurosurgery and must be evaluated.*
   D. Jane Thomas should be seen last. *Rationale: Ms. Thomas is the most stable and has no urgent needs.*

Health Promotion
1. Ms. Thomas should be taught not to lift or move anything over 10 pounds until her surgeon approves. Once healing is complete, she must lift by using her legs, not her back. *Rationale: Lifting can traumatize the incision and prevent adequate healing. Using the back to lift heavy objects can cause further injury to lumbar discs.*
2. Both Mr. Hernandez and Mr. Phillips have been smokers for a long time. They should be informed that smoking increases blood pressure, which can lead to stroke. They should be provided with

information on local stop-smoking programs. *Rationale: Research shows that smoking increases the risk of hypertension, strokes, and heart disease. Many stop-smoking programs are effective.*

Nursing Process
1. B. *Rationale: Heart sounds and pain assessment are part of a beginning-of-shift baseline assessment. Because Mr. Hernandez may be having difficulty swallowing, assessing fluid balance is important.*
2. C. *Rationale: The previous nurse gave Ms. Walton Tylenol ES for a headache of 6 on a scale of 1 to 10. You should evaluate the effectiveness of this medication by determining the current pain level on the same 1 to 10 scale.*
3. D. *Rationale: Mr. Phillips was given an antihypertensive medication 1.5 hours ago. Because his blood pressure was 170/110 when the medication was given, a blood pressure of 145/90 would indicate that the medication was effective.*
4. A, B, D, E. *Rationale: All of these are topics that should be discussed before discharge. There is no indication that Ms. Thomas is overweight.*
5. A, D, E. *Rationale: White blood cell count would indicate the presence of infection. Hematocrit and hemoglobin would indicate fluid balance and hemostasis. These are priorities after any surgery.*
6. B. *Rationale: Increased headache that is not controlled with medication indicates increased intracranial pressure and must be reported to the physician.*

Communication
1. Explain to Mrs. Phillips that the MRI indicated that a stroke has caused her husband's symptoms. Acknowledge that strokes are more common in older people, but that Mr. Phillips is at risk because of his uncontrolled hypertension and smoking. *Rationale: Mrs. Phillips is grieving the loss of her husband's function and needs accurate information and reassurance.*
2. Explain that it is too early to determine how much permanent neurologic deficits Mr. Hernandez will have. Explain that Mr. Hernandez's rehabilitation will be evaluated frequently and plans will be discussed with her at that time. *Rationale: Over time, rehabilitation can be effective in restoring neurologic function. The amount of permanent neurologic deficit cannot be determined until this time.*

Delegation
1.
   A. Mr. Hernandez: The nursing assistant can obtain vital signs and assist with ADLs. Instruct him or her not to provide oral intake until swallowing evaluation is obtained.
   B. Ms. Thomas: The nursing assistant can obtain vital signs and assist with ADLs. Remind the him or her to assist the patient to log roll to prevent twisting of the lumbar spine.
   C. Mr. Phillips: The nursing assistant can obtain vital sings and assist with ADLs. Mr. Phillips should remain in bed and will need assistance to turn every 2 hours.
   D. Ms. Walton: The nursing assistant can obtain vital signs and assist with ADLs. Ms. Walton should remain in bed, and will need assistance turning every 2 hours.

Content-Specific Questions
1. The disciplines the nurse should include in a discharge planning meeting would be Medicine, Physical Therapy, Occupational Therapy, Speech Therapy, Dietitian, and Social Work. The patient and/or a family member should also be included. These disciplines can provide valuable input for planning rehabilitation services.

2. Yes, with the exception that speech therapy would not be necessary because the patient with cervical injury can still speak. Respiratory therapy would be a valuable addition because the patient may experience respiratory distress and have difficulty clearing the airway.

Concept Map

Hint: When planning care for the patient with impaired swallowing, consider not only independent nursing interventions, but also patient, family, and caregiver teaching as well as appropriate referrals.

Chapter 45: Assessing the Eye and Ear

1. **Answer: 2 Rationale:** When the cornea is touched the patient will blink as a mechanism to protect it from foreign objects.
2. **Answer: 4 Rationale:** Presbyopia develops in older adults as the lens of the eye looses its ability to adjust, requiring the patient to hold papers farther away in order to focus and read.
3. **Answer: 2 Rationale:** Tuning forks are used to assess if hearing loss is conductive or sensorineural.
4. **Answer: 1 Rationale:** As the light enters the lens, the rays bend and are focused on a single point on the retina; this focusing is called accommodation.
5. **Answer: 4 Rationale:** Patients having a test of refraction will have the pupil dilated to examine the internal eye structures.
6. **Answer: 3 Rationale:** Receptors within the inner ear maintain equilibrium by responding to changes in head position in order to coordinate body movements and balance.
7. **Answer: 1 Rationale:** The Snellen eye chart measures the patient's ability to read letters at a standard distance of twenty feet. The patient reads the smallest line possible, and the numbers on the side indicate visual acuity, for example, 20/20, 20/30.
8. **Answer: 1 Rationale:** The examiner can whisper a word 1 or 2 feet behind the patient, asking the patient to repeat the word; this may provide a rough estimate of hearing acuity.
9. **Answer: 2 Rationale:** The vestibular structures maintain balance. As the person ages this function may decrease and the patient may be at risk for falling.
10. **Answer: 4 Rationale:** The examiner must have a normal visual field when assessing the visual field of a patient because the examiner's field becomes the standard or norm. If the examiner does not have normal visual field then the results of this part of the exam will be inaccurate.

Chapter 46: Nursing Care of Patients with Eye and Ear Disorders

1. **Answer: 4 Rationale:** The highest priority for residents with moderate to severe hearing or vision impairment is safety.
2. **Answer: 2 Rationale:** In teaching a patient with newly diagnosed glaucoma, the nurse emphasizes the importance of taking eye drops as prescribed on a continuing basis to control intraocular pressure and prevent vision loss.
3. **Answer: 3 Rationale:** Timolol is a beta adrenergic blocker that can decrease myocardial contractility and impair cardiac function in the patient with heart failure.
4. **Answer: 4 Rationale:** The highest priority for a patient with repeated attacks of vertigo and tinnitus is maintenance of safety. Sitting when an attack occurs reduces the risk of injury from falling.
5. **Answer: 1 Rationale:** Following eye surgery, patients are placed in semi-Fowler's or Fowler's position to reduce intraocular pressure and edema.

6. **Answer: 3 Rationale:** Immediate referral to an ophthalmologist is necessary because the manifestations suggest a detached retina. Immediate treatment is necessary to optimize sight restoration.
7. **Answer: 1, 2, 3, 4, 5 Rationale:** All the assessments should be included because each provides information about infection and possible location in the ear.
8. **Answer: 4 Rationale:** Aging is a risk factor for cerumen impaction because there is less and it is harder and drier. The nurse should inspect the ear canal for patency.
9. **Answer: 1 Rationale:** One-on-one social interactions in a quiet environment facilitate effective communication for the patient with a severe hearing deficit.
10. **Answer: 2 Rationale:** Cataract removal is elective surgery, generally performed only when visual impairment interferes with activities of daily living.

Unit 12 Building Clinical Competence: Responses to Altered Visual and Auditory Function
Functional Health Pattern: Cognitive-Perceptual Pattern

Functional Health Patterns

Hint: When the patient cannot see clearly, the nurse must be diligent to maintain a safe environment including helping others to be aware of safety measures. The nurse can use a variety of communication techniques when working with hearing impaired patients. If written communication is used, the nurse must be sure the patient can read and write.

Priority Setting
1.
   A. Kenneth Koch should be seen first. *Rationale: Mr. Koch is having severe pain and needs to be assessed and medicated.*
   B. Georgia Stanley should be seen second. *Rationale: Ms. Stanley is scheduled for x-rays and an MRI. She must be assessed before she leaves her room.*
   C. Andrew Hardy should be seen third. *Rationale: Mr. Hardy's blood glucose was 600 on admission and must be reevaluated do determine the effectiveness of treatment.*
   D. Gladys Harvey should be seen last. *Rationale: Ms. Harvey is experiencing routine post-op recovery and is stable.*

Health Promotion
1. Teach Ms. Stanley to avoid sudden head movements and position changes, to take prescribed medications, and to lie down in a quiet darkened room when feeling an impending attack. Discuss with her methods to maintain safety if an attack occurs when she is driving a car or using other mechanical equipment.
2. Teach Mr. Hardy to control his diabetes and make appropriate referrals for diabetic education. Teach him to take his prescribed antihypertensive medication, to be seen by an ophthalmologist annually, and to report black spots, floaters, cobwebs, or eye pain immediately.
3. D. *Rationale: Loud noises above 85 decibels may cause hearing loss.*

Nursing Process
1.

	Nursing Diagnosis	Rationale
Andrew Hardy	*Altered Nutrition: More than Body Requirements*	*Mr. Hardy had a blood glucose of 600. Lowering the blood glucose level is the highest priority for him.*

Gladys Harvey	*Sensory-Perceptual Alterations: Input Deficit* related to eye surgery	*Ms. Harvey's vision is decreased due to R eye patch from surgery.*
Georgia Stanley	*High Risk for Injury* related to vertigo	*Ms. Stanley has been experiencing vertigo that has resulted in falling.*
Kenneth Koch	*Pain* related to ear surgery	*Mr. Koch is experiencing pain at 9 on a scale of 1 to 10.*

2. D. *Rationale: Laser photocoagulation is the treatment for both forms of diabetic retinopathy. This treatment seals the leaking microaneurysms, and proliferating vessels are destroyed to reduce further damage.*

3. B. *Rationale: After eye surgery, place the patient in semi-Fowler's or Fowler's position on the unaffected side.*

4. C. *Rationale: Grilled chicken with lettuce and tomato are low in sodium. Ketchup, cheese, and potato chips are high in sodium.*

5. A, B, F. *Rationale: Diagnostic studies for Ménière's disease are caloric testing, Rinne and Weber tests, and glycerol test. These studies test impaired vestibular function and hearing.*

6. B. *Rationale: Coughing or sneezing increases intraocular pressure and may lead to postoperative complications. Avoid lifting more than 5 pounds. Lie on the unaffected side. Maintain eye patch to prevent injury to the eye.*

Communication

1. B, D, E, F. *Rationale: To improve communication with a patient with hearing loss, speak in a normal tone while facing the patient, and use short sentences and pauses to increase comprehension. Speak at a normal rate and avoid over articulating to make lip-reading easier. Reduce environmental noises to decrease distractions.*

Delegation

1.
   A. Andrew Hardy: The nursing assistant can obtain vital signs and blood glucose by finger stick, and assist with ambulating to maintain safety.
   B. Gladys Harvey: The nursing assistant can obtain vital signs and assist with ADLs as needed, including ambulation to maintain safety.
   C. Georgia Stanley: The nursing assistant can obtain vital signs, assist with ADLs, assist with ambulation to maintain safety, and prepare the room for the patient's return from radiology.
   D. Kenneth Koch: The nursing assistant can obtain vital signs and assist with ADLs as needed, including ambulation to maintain safety.

Content-Specific Questions

1. A. *Rationale: Hyphema is bleeding into the anterior chamber of the eye. Assessment of hyphema includes eye pain, decreased visual acuity, and seeing a reddish tint.*

2. A. *Rationale: Gentamicin may damage the eighth cranial nerve, resulting in hearing loss.*

3. C. *Rationale: The correct way to administer ear drops is to have the patient lie on the unaffected side, pull the pinna up and back, instill the ear drops, and have the patient remain on the side for approximately 5 minutes.*

Concept Map

Hint: Are there more detailed Independent Interventions that you can identify for this patient? Review Chapter 20 as you develop your second concept map addressing this patient's risk for visual impairment. How do your nursing diagnosis and planned interventions compare between the two concept maps?

Chapter 47: Assessing the Male and Female Reproductive Systems

1. **Answer: 3 Rationale:** The obese male may have enlarged breasts, called gynecomastia.

2. **Answer: 4 Rationale:** In the female, the clitoris is an erectile organ similar to the penis in the male.

3. **Answer: 2 Rationale:** The explanation should begin by explaining that the prostate gland surrounds the urethra.

4. **Answer: 1 Rationale:** PSA is the diagnostic test used to diagnose and monitor prostate cancer.

5. **Answer: 1 Rationale:** Testicular self-examination is one method of providing health management.

6. **Answer: 3 Rationale:** Following menopause the estrogen level drops and cholesterol increases, putting the woman at risk for cardiovascular disease.

7. **Answer: 1 Rationale:** When women of reproductive age become pregnant, menstruation normally stops until after delivery.

8. **Answer: 4 Rationale:** Pap smears are used to detect cervical cancers and precancerous lesions of the cervix.

9. **Answer: 3 Rationale:** Palpation is used to detect any lumps or changes in breast tissues.

10. **Answer: 2 Rationale:** Vaginal bleeding after menopause is not normal and should be reported to the healthcare provider.

Chapter 48: Nursing Care of Men with Reproductive System and Breast Disorders

1. **Answer: 4 Rationale:** This is stated in an appropriate way to allow the patient to feel free to ask any questions about his sexual concerns.

2. **Answer: 2 Rationale:** In a health teaching session with young men, the nurse should tell them about retracting the foreskin while showering, and cleaning regularly to decrease the presence of collection of secretions under the foreskin, which has been shown to increase the risk of penile cancer.

3. **Answer: 1 Rationale:** Sexually active men who have gonorrhea are especially susceptible to inflammation or infection of the epididymis.

4. **Answer: 2 Rationale:** Testicular cancer commonly occurs between the ages of 15 and 40.

5. **Answer: 3 Rationale:** Men with chronic prostatitis should increase their fluid intake to 3L/day and void often to decrease the irritation when voiding.

6. **Answer: 2, 4 Rationale:** In digital rectal examination for BPH, the prostate is asymmetrical and enlarged, while in prostate cancer the exam shows nodules and a fixed position. PSA is specific to the prostate and is released by both benign and malignant cells; however, in BPH the amounts of the free form of PSA and complex PSA would be different.

7. **Answer: 2 Rationale:** As the prostate enlarges around the urethra it begins to obstruct the outflow of urine from the bladder during urination, causing problems with urinary retention, frequency, and urgency.

8. **Answer: 3 Rationale:** The nurse needs to notify the surgeon because dark red fluid with obvious clots and painful bladder spasms could indicate that the patient may be hemorrhaging postoperatively.

9. **Answer: 1 Rationale:** Prostate cancer is the most common type of malignancy in American men.

10. **Answer: 4 Rationale:** Some studies have shown an increase in prostate cancer in men with diets high in red meats and fats. Informing the community of this relationship could help men change their dietary habits to decrease the risk of prostate cancer.

Chapter 49: Nursing Care of Women with Reproductive System and Breast Disorders

1. **Answer: 1 Rationale:** The nurse acknowledging the problem stated by the patient gives credence for the patient, but because the nurse is uncomfortable addressing the issue herself, she refers the patient to the physician.

2. **Answer: 2, 3, 4 Rationale:** Osteoporosis, cardiovascular disease, and fractures are all related to estrogen deprivation.

3. **Answer: 1200 Rationale:** This level can be achieved through diet and supplements if necessary.

4. **Answer: 1 Rationale:** Kegel exercises strengthen perineal muscle tone and minimize stress incontinence.

5. **Answer: 2 Rationale:** A health-promotion seminar for reducing the risk of cervical cancer should contain information about safe sex methods that reduce the incidence of genital infections from HPV, which is the most important risk factor.

6. **Answer: 4 Rationale:** For a woman with PMS, the nurse would recommend a decrease in sodium intake to help minimize the fluid retention due to the increased production of aldosterone, which results in sodium retention and edema.

7. **Answer: 2 Rationale:** Endometrial implantations tend to atrophy and disappear after menopause since ovarian hormones no longer stimulate them.

8. **Answer: 1, 3, 4 Rationale:** A teaching plan for home care of a woman following an abdominal hysterectomy should include no lifting to decrease chances of hemorrhage, reporting temperature > 100°F since this may be a sign of infection, and taking regular rest periods since she may be tired for several days postoperatively.

9. **Answer: 4 Rationale:** Risk factors for breast cancer are doubled for the 64-year-old with a positive family history.

10. **Answer: 3 Rationale:** *Grieving* is an appropriate nursing diagnosis since she is losing a portion of her body.

Chapter 50: Nursing Care of Patients with Sexually Transmitted Infections

1. **Answer: 2 Rationale:** Women and infants are disproportionately affected by STIs because women may not experience manifestations of the disease and pass the infection on to the infant through vaginal birth.

2. **Answer: 1 Rationale:** STIs must be treated by treating both partners to prevent reinfection from one to the other, since manifestations are not always demonstrated when the infection is present.

3. **Answer: 1, 4, 5 Rationale:** Topics of information when teaching a male to prevent an STI should include using a new condom with each sex act, careful handling to prevent damage to condom, and withdrawal from the vagina when the penis is erect, holding the condom against the base of the penis to prevent contamination of the penis.

4. **Answer: 4 Rationale:** Blisters and ulcers appear on the penis of a patient infected with genital herpes.

5. **Answer: 1 Rationale:** Genital warts are caused by a viral infection (not yeast).

6. **Answer: 4 Rationale:** Women with HPV genital infection should be advised to have a pelvic exam and Pap smear every year since this infection causes an increased risk in developing cervical cancer, and the annual exams would identify the cancer early.

7. **Answer: 2 Rationale:** Itching is the most common manifestation experienced by a woman with a vaginal infection.

8. **Answer: 3 Rationale:** When teaching a woman with an STI experiencing severe genital discomfort, a simple recommendation is to wear cotton underwear because it absorbs moisture and allows airflow better than other materials.

9. **Answer: 1 Rationale:** The male urethra and female cervix are initially affected by the gonorrheal organism.

10. **Answer: 3 Rationale:** Syphilis is a systemic infection that is caused by a spirochete that can affect a developing fetus.

Unit 13 Building Clinical Competence: Responses to Altered Reproductive Function
Functional Health Pattern: Sexuality-Reproductive Pattern

Functional Health Patterns
Hint: Think about your nonverbal communication techniques that can put the patient at ease and increase the patient's comfort.

Priority Setting
1. In what order would you visit these patients after report?
   A. Wendy Torrell should be seen first. *Rationale: Ms. Torrell has had major abdominal bleeding and is at risk for impaired tissue perfusion.*
   B. Tara Morris should be seen second. *Rationale: She has an elevated temperature and a significant infection that must be assessed. Her IV antibiotics need to be administered on time.*
   C. Barney Green should be seen third. *Rationale: Because Mr. Green is a postoperative patient, he is at risk for bleeding and infection. His output needs to be assessed because the Foley catheter was removed.*
   D. Regina Perkins should be seen last. *Rationale: Ms. Perkins is stable and is ready for discharge. By assessing her last, the nurse can provide discharge teaching at the same time.*

Health Promotion
1. Ms. Torrell should be encouraged to eat foods high in iron and folic acid, including dark green vegetables and deep yellow fruits and vegetables. She should take prescribed iron supplements and eat high-fiber foods to maintain normal bowel function.
2. Ms. Morris should be instructed to abstain from sexual intercourse until the infection has cleared. She should be instructed to use condoms unless she is in a monogamous relationship.

Nursing Process
1.

	Nursing Diagnosis	Rationale
Wendy Torrell	*Fluid Volume Deficit* related to blood loss	*Ms. Torrell lost enough blood to require replacement of 2 units of whole blood.*
Barney Green	*Altered Urinary Elimination Patterns* related to TURP	*Mr. Green is dribbling urine after the catheter is removed.*
Tara Morris	*Infection of Reproductive Organs* as evidenced by purulent vaginal drainage, pain, and fever	*Infection must be resolved to prevent damage to the reproductive organs.*
Regina Perkins	*Knowledge Deficit* related to postoperative care	*Ms. Perkins is recovering normally and is ready for discharge instruction.*

2. B. *Rationale: For Ms. Torrell the abdominal binder is used to control intra-abdominal bleeding. Abdominal binders can be used to support the abdominal muscles especially in obese patients, but there is no indication that these were the purpose in Ms. Torrell's case.*

3. C. *Rationale: Absorption of isotonic irrigating fluids during and after surgery may cause a hypervolemic and hyponatremic state.*

4. A. *Rationale: All are correct. The most important is to take all medications for the prescribed amount of doses to completely cure the infection.*

5. A. *Rationale: Beef and eggs are high in heme iron. Brown rice is high in nonheme iron. Heme iron foods promote absorption of nonheme iron foods when eaten together. Broccoli, asparagus, kidney beans, and green, leafy vegetables are high in folic acid.*

Communication

1. Some reproductive infections can cause scar tissue of the fallopian tubes. There would be a possibility of having difficulty becoming pregnant or developing a tubal pregnancy if that occurs. The doctor or healthcare provider can provide more information in her specific case.

2. Dribbling urine after the Foley catheter is removed following a TURP is common. Usually the dribbling stops once complete healing occurs. It is too early to determine if dribbling will be permanent.

Delegation

1.

A. Wendy Torrell: The nursing assistant can obtain vital signs, empty the Foley catheter every hour, and provide ADLs. He or she should be instructed not to get Ms. Torrell out of bed and to keep her NPO until it is determined surgery will not be necessary.

B. Barney Green: The nursing assistant can obtain vital signs and assist with ADLs. Mr. Green may need assistance with ambulation.

C. Tara Morris: The nursing assistant can obtain vital signs and assist with ADLs. He or she should be instructed to obtain a temperature every 2 hours until it is within normal limits for 24 hours.

D. Regina Perkins: The nursing assistant can obtain vital signs and offer breakfast prior to discharge. He or she can assist with packing belongings and can take Ms. Perkins to her car in a wheelchair once the discharge process is complete.

Content-Specific Questions

1. D. *Rationale: The priority nursing diagnosis with endometriosis is Anxiety related to risk for loss of reproductive function due to increased risk of infertility.*

2. B. *Rationale: Cialis is incompatible with many medications, such as nitrates, alpha blockers, antibiotics, and antifungals.*

3. A, C, F. *Rationale: VDRL and RPR blood tests measure syphilis antibody production. FTA-ABS is an antibody test used for symptomatic patients who test negative to VDRL.*

4. B. *Rationale: To prevent radiation damage to others, avoid close contact with pregnant women, infants, and children. Other factors related to radiation therapy are to sleep alone for the first week, eat less red meat, and use condoms for sexual contact.*

5. D. *Rationale: Vaginal bleeding after intercourse or between menstrual periods may be the first symptom of cervical cancer. Other answers are later symptoms of cervical cancer.*

6. C. *Rationale: Condoms provide the best protection of birth control when being treated for gonorrhea.*

Concept Map

Hint: As you prioritize identified nursing diagnoses and interventions, think about the other physical problems the patient has or might have and the psychological issues with which she must cope. Reviewing Chapter 14 will be helpful in developing your second concept map for this patient.

Evaluate Your Response: Cues for Critical Thinking Questions

Chapter 4: Nursing Care of Patients Having Surgery
A Patient Having Surgery

1. Safety concerns include ambulating and not tripping over scatter rugs or clutter. See the information in Chapter 3 on safety in the home.

2. Medications used to prevent an occurrence such as infection are called prophylactic medications. Her risks for infection are from the surgical wound and microvascular circulation in bone. Teach her to take the complete course of antibiotics prescribed and about the possible side effects of the antibiotic. Encourage her to notify the physician if side effects or adverse events occur.

3. When blood stops flowing, it clots. Her immobility is a concern and puts her at risk for thrombosis and emboli. She has a risk for bleeding secondary to the anticoagulant and should inform healthcare providers such as dentists that she is taking the anticoagulant.

4. Consider the risk for osteoporosis in addition to the degenerative changes Mrs. Overbeck experienced. She will need calcium sources and vitamin D.

Chapter 5: Nursing Care of Patients Experiencing Loss, Grief, and Death
A Patient Experiencing Loss and Grief

1. Review the physical manifestations of grief described in the chapter and compare and contrast those with the ones verbalized by Mrs. Rogers.

2. Consider the benefits of including Mrs. Rogers's daughter in a meeting of the staff. What type of questions would be most useful in making the daughter feel a part of the plan of care? Why would a statement such as "Why don't you do more for your mother" be inappropriate?

3. Consider the losses Mrs. Rogers has experienced. Review the material in the chapter on responses to loss. Think about the reasons you would not say, "Oh, you have a lot to live for." Think of two or three questions or statements that would help you assess the reason why Mrs. Rogers said this to you.

Chapter 6: Nursing Care of Patients with Problems of Substance Abuse
A Patient Having Withdrawal from Alcohol

1. Consider the interactions of prescribed or over-the-counter medications with alcohol. What if the patient has not taken prescribed medications because of chronic alcoholism?

2. Review the effects of Antabuse. Make a list of possible interactions and side effects.

3. *Imbalanced Nutrition: Less than Body Requirements* is an appropriate nursing diagnosis when a patient does not have sufficient nutritional intake to meet metabolic needs. What in Mr. Russell's history and physical assessment supports this diagnosis? What nutritional information should you provide?

Chapter 7: Nursing Care of Patients Experiencing Disasters
A Patient with Injuries from a Natural Disaster
1. Consider how Mr. Jones put himself at risk for infection (see Chapter 12). How could Mr. Jones have avoided exacerbating his skin lesions?
2. Since Mr. Jones has a history of elevated blood pressure that has not been consistently treated or monitored, cardiac status should be evaluated. Which tests are indicated? Also, could his decreased sensation and poor healing be related to cardiac impairment? Mr. Jones also has identifying data in his history and physical to suggest diabetes. Identify this data and tests that would be indicated.
3. Review risk factors for and causes and manifestations of infection in Chapter 12. Identify the factors that contributed to Mr. Jones's fever.
4. Consider Mr. Jones's environmental and personal situations. What information do you have about Mr. Jones that indicates a lack of interest in health maintenance? Are there signs of a change in outlook?

Chapter 9: Nursing Care of Patients in Pain
A Patient Experiencing Chronic Pain
1. Review the factors that affect an individual's response to pain. What have you observed in your own family and friends, as well as patients for whom you have cared?
2. Reflect on the benefits and disadvantages of each alternative. Make your decision based on knowledge about pain and about medications for pain.
3. What factors in Ms. Akers's illness and treatment increase her risk for constipation? What would you include in the plan specific to fluid intake and diet?

Chapter 10: Nursing Care of Patients with Altered Fluid, Electrolyte, and Acid–Base Balance
A Patient with Hypokalemia
1. Review the physiologic effects of potassium, especially its intracellular and neuromuscular effects.
2. Review the potential sites and causes of excess potassium loss.
3. Think about the effects of diuretics on potassium balance and the effects of hypokalemia on digitalis therapy. What is the primary indication for digitalis therapy and how does this contribute to the interaction of these three factors?
4. Review the section in Chapter 24 on the causes and management of constipation.

A Patient with Hyperkalemia
1. Review the causes and manifestations of hyperkalemia.
2. What are the potential effects of hyperkalemia on cardiac conduction? At what level of hyperkalemia are these likely to be seen?
3. Review collaborative treatment measures to rapidly reduce potassium levels. Why would these be used with a K1 of 8.5?
4. Think about the effects of anxiety on learning as you develop a plan to provide teaching to avoid future episodes of hyperkalemia. As you develop your plan, remember the potential long-term effects of chronic renal failure.

A Patient with Acute Respiratory Acidosis
1. Review normal gas exchange across the alveolar-capillary membrane and the processes that drive this exchange. Then review the role that carbon dioxide plays as a potential acid.
2. Describe the effect of acidosis on cerebral neurons. What manifestations of mental impairment may result?

3. Consider risk factors for choking such as alcohol consumption, taking large bites of food, or inadequate chewing.

Chapter 11: Nursing Care of Patients Experiencing Trauma and Shock
A Patient with Multiple Injuries
1. The definition of *Deficient Fluid Volume* is decreased intravascular, interstitial, and/or intracellular fluid. Which of Mrs. Souza's vital signs would support this definition? What other assessments could you make that would further support this diagnosis?
2. Consider the physiology of cellular metabolism. How long do brain cells live without oxygen? What happens if circulation is improved but the airway is blocked?
3. What can cause restlessness? Consider comfort, elimination, oxygenation, emotional status, and immobility.
4. List the multiple possibilities for entry of pathogens into the human body. Would age and physical condition increase the risk? What about transmission from healthcare personnel?

A Patient with Septic Shock
1. Review the pharmacologic effects of vasopressors. Consider the pathologic basis for septic shock and how these medications may be effective.
2. Review the content on respiratory acidosis in Chapter 10. What do these findings tell you? What is present in Ms. Huang's physical status that would cause these manifestations?
3. Review the content about colloidal intravenous solutions in this chapter. What would you expect these solutions to do when they are administered? How does this correlate to cardiac output? How do you assess increased circulatory volume?

Chapter 12: Nursing Care of Patients with Infections
A Patient with Acquired Immunity
1. Review the adult immunizations listed in this chapter. Consider the geographical area in which the patient lives. For example, patients living in areas at risk for Lyme disease should check with their physician about the new Lyme disease vaccine.
2. Review the concept of acquired immunity and the discussion of immunization in this chapter. What affect could nonimmunized persons have on their family and community?
3. Identify possible systemic and local reactions associated with immunizations. List manifestations that the patient should report to the primary caregiver.

Chapter 13: Nursing Care of Patients with Altered Immunity
A Patient with HIV Infection
1. Considering Ms. Lu's age, how effective is her immune system? How could lifestyle factors affect immune status?
2. At this stage of Ms. Lu's diagnosis, would you expect the physician to order a viral load test? Why or why not?
3. To what community resources could you refer Ms. Lu and her fiancé regarding their desire to have a child?

Chapter 14: Nursing Care of Patients with Cancer
A Patient with Cancer
1. Review content on altered nutrition in Chapter 22 and the content in this chapter on the nursing diagnosis *Imbalanced Nutrition: Less than Body Requirements*. Make a list of diagnostic tests for malnutrition with normal values.
2. Consider the type of cancers Mr. Casey has been diagnosed as having. Where in the body do these malignancies commonly metastasize? What would cause the pain?

3. Review a pharmacology book for medications that increase appetite and make a list of those appropriate to Mr. Casey.

4. Review the content in Chapter 11 on septic shock and outline manifestations. Develop a plan of care for Mr. Casey that is structured by priority of nursing diagnoses.

Chapter 16: Nursing Care of Patients with Integumentary Disorders

A Patient with Herpes Zoster

1. Consider environmental, economic, and language barriers. What agencies in your own city or state exist to provide help? What can you do other than make referrals? If you do make a referral, to whom would it be?

2. Review skin assessment guidelines in Chapter 15. How would you determine that the lesions had not improved? What manifestations would indicate secondary infection of the lesions? What would you do next if the lesions are still very painful and have not improved?

3. *Ineffective Role Performance* is defined as patterns of behavior and self-expression that do not match environmental context, norms, and expectations. Related factors include inadequate or inappropriate linkage with the healthcare system and poverty. Based on this information, what interventions would you use? How would you evaluate the effectiveness of your interventions?

A Patient with Malignant Melanoma

1. List reasons why people do not seek health care. Do you believe nurses can effect change? If so, what community activities would be most effective?

2. Consider attitudes toward the possibility of future illnesses. How would this affect your plan? What do you believe would be most effective in teaching this age group?

3. Think about what you know about taking prescribed antibiotics as well as the side effects of antibiotic therapy. What would you suggest that Mr. Sanders do?

4. *Powerlessness* is the perception that one's own actions will not significantly affect an outcome. Is this a common response to the diagnosis of cancer? Consider types of communications and interventions that would allow greater decision making for Mr. Sanders.

Chapter 17: Nursing Care of Patients with Burns

A Patient with a Major Burn

1. Review the effects of the major burn wound on the renal and gastrointestinal systems. What assessments would indicate effective fluid resuscitation?

2. What type of burns did Mr. Howard have on his arms? Consider the effect of compression on the peripheral vascular system. What assessments would you make to identify this complication?

3. Consider the type of pain the patient has. What do you think might happen if the narcotics were given by other routes, such as oral or intramuscular?

4. Review the effects of a major burn. Consider the damage to cell wall integrity and capillary beds. What effect does the shift of proteins and sodium have on intravascular volume?

Chapter 19: Nursing Care of Patients with Endocrine Disorders

A Patient with Graves' Disease

1. What effect does increased TH have on metabolism and cardiac rate and stroke volume? How does this effect compare to that of sympathetic stimulation?

2. Consider the effect of elevating any body part, such as elevating your leg above heart level for a sprained ankle. How does this affect venous return?

3. You will need to consider Mrs. Manuel from both a medical and a surgical perspective. How would you teach her to care for her incision? With removal of most of the thyroid gland, what manifestations would you be sure she knew about? What should she do if these occur?

A Patient with Hypothyroidism

1. Make a list of changes in body systems that occur with aging and with decreased TH levels. How would you determine what assessment findings were abnormal?

2. Consider the effects of the following factors: weakness, fatigue, problems with memory. What would you recommend she do in her home to increase her safety?

3. Prepare a list of manifestations of hyperthyroidism. Be sure they are in terms a patient would understand.

A Patient with Cushing's Syndrome

1. Review Ms. Domico's lab results and compare them to normal results. What altered the findings in her case?

2. How many ways can you think of to assess fluid balance? Consider weight, I&O, and skin. What other assessments provide information?

3. How does fatigue differ from "just being tired"? Would increasing hours of sleep be an intervention you would include? Why or why not?

A Patient with Addison's Disease

1. Review the functions of the hormones of the adrenal cortex in Chapter 18. Consider the effects of stress, and formulate your response with rationale.

2. Review content on fluid imbalance in Chapter 10. Make a list of assessments you might make that would indicate severe dehydration. What is the pathophysiology of fluid loss in the patient with Addison's disease?

3. Review content on sodium and potassium in Chapter 10 and make a list of foods you would suggest Mr. Sardoff eat.

Chapter 20: Nursing Care of Patients with Diabetes Mellitus

A Patient with Type 1 DM

1. How do the increased urinary output and increased osmolarity of the blood plasma affect the fluid status of the body? What is the response of the body to decreased intravascular volume?

2. Consider the effects of nicotine on blood vessels. How would these effects, when combined with the pathologic effects of long-standing hyperglycemia, affect blood vessel walls?

3. Review the information about chronic illness in Chapter 2. Powerlessness is a perceived lack of control over a situation and/or one's ability to significantly affect an outcome. What types of statements by a patient would help you make this nursing diagnosis?

4. Compare and contrast the developmental needs and tasks of the young adult and the older adult (see Chapter 2). Consider the teaching materials that might have to be adapted to physical changes in the older adult.

Chapter 22: Nursing Care of Patients with Nutritional Disorders

A Patient with Obesity

1. Review the physiology of cholesterol formation in the body and the factors that affect this process.

Appendix C

2. Consider developmental stages and teaching strategies for adult learners.
3. Think about individual factors, family and support group influences, and cultural factors that may affect recommended weight loss and exercise strategies.

A Patient with Malnutrition
1. Review the physiology of albumin and cholesterol formation in the body.
2. Review Mrs. Chow's diet and compare it to the food pyramid or recommendations for food intake to formulate your response.
3. Consider cultural influences and the patient's preferred foods as you plan a diet that is high in calories and protein.

Chapter 23: Nursing Care of Patients with Upper Gastrointestinal Disorders

A Patient with Oral Cancer
1. Review the major risk factors for oral cancer and identify the populations most likely to have these risk factors.
2. Work with your classmates to plan (and implement) an education program, considering the developmental/teaching needs of this group of young people.
3. Think about the possible causes for Mr. Chavez's refusal to talk (remember that assessment is the first step of the nursing process). How will you identify factors contributing to his behavior?

A Patient with Peptic Ulcer Disease
1. Review the physiology of the gastric mucosal barrier and the pathogenesis of peptic ulcer disease, and the effect of *H. pylori* infection on these processes.
2. Review physiologic responses to stress in your physiology or nursing fundamentals text; compare and apply this information with the physiology of the gastric mucosal barrier and the pathophysiology of ulcer development.
3. Consider Mr. O'Donnell's occupation and schedule, as well as the prescribed medications and when each should be taken.
4. Using journal and text resources as well as your classmates, identify as many stress reduction techniques as possible. Then sort your list into those that could be used while working, and identify ways to effectively teach each technique.

A Patient with Gastric Cancer
1. Review the healing process and the normal physiology of the stomach as you formulate your answer to this question.
2. Consider the surgery, immediate postoperative care, and what the patient and family should expect in developing your teaching plan.
3. Review Chapter 14 and nursing care related to chemotherapy.
4. Again, review Chapter 14 for nursing care measures for patients with cancer; also review Chapter 22 for strategies to prevent and manage malnutrition.

Chapter 24: Nursing Care of Patients with Bowel Disorders

A Patient with Acute Appendicitis
1. Review the acute inflammatory response to an infectious process and the role WBCs play in the immune response.
2. Review Chapter 4. Consider factors such as incision size, abdominal muscle disruption, and manipulation of the bowel in developing your response.
3. Consider points such as pain management, resumption of activities, incision care, and potential complications in developing your teaching plan. Consider the patient's education and developmental stage as well.

4. Review the effects of anxiety on recovery and learning. Identify nursing measures to reduce situational anxiety.

A Patient with Ulcerative Colitis
1. Review normal functions of the small and large intestine. Review the usual location of an ileostomy. Review fluid volume deficit in Chapter 10 for manifestations and assessment data.
2. Think about the effect of chronic blood loss and review the effect of malnutrition on the hemoglobin and hematocrit.
3. Review the home care section of inflammatory bowel disease for teaching points to include.
4. Review nursing care for the patient with diarrhea, as well as the procedure for ileostomy care.

A Patient with Colorectal Cancer
1. Review peripheral innervation and impulse transmission in your anatomy and physiology textbook; think about how nerves in the rectal region are disrupted in an abdominoperineal resection. Also review the phantom pain phenomenon in Chapter 9.
2. Compare elimination through a colostomy with "normal" bowel elimination through the anus. How do they differ in terms of the passage of flatus?
3. Review Procedure 24–1. Also review the procedure for administering an enema in your fundamentals or skills textbook.
4. Review this nursing diagnosis in your nursing diagnosis or nursing care planning handbook; be sure to individualize your plan to Mr. Cunningham's situation and needs.

Chapter 25: Nursing Care of Patients with Gallbladder, Liver, and Pancreatic Disorders

A Patient with Cholelithiasis
1. Review the composition of gallstones, as well as the physiology of gallbladder function and bile. Research and discuss dietary practices of the Chickasaw tribe (or of Native Americans).
2. Review Chapter 4 for care related to a laparotomy (incision into the abdomen).
3. As you develop your plan, consider Mrs. Red Wing's culture, job, and family obligations.

A Patient with Alcoholic Cirrhosis
1. Review the anatomy and physiology of the liver and its circulation, as well as the pathophysiology of cirrhosis and its complications.
2. Consult your nutrition textbook as needed for foods that are high in calories but low in protein and sodium. When planning for limited protein intake, be sure to include high-quality proteins and limit intake of lower-quality proteins such as legumes.
3. Review the pathophysiology of hepatic encephalopathy to develop your responses to this question.
4. Review therapeutic communication skills; consult your nursing diagnosis and care planning text book as you develop this care plan.

A Patient with Acute Pancreatitis
1. Review Chapter 6 for assessment data indicative of alcohol withdrawal.
2. Review both the pathophysiology of acute pancreatitis and the acute inflammatory process.
3. Consult your nutrition textbook or the American Dietetic Association website.
4. Consult your nursing care planning textbook to develop this care plan.

Chapter 27: Nursing Care of Patients with Urinary Tract Disorders

A Patient with Cystitis

1. Consider risk factors for UTI as well as factors affecting Mrs. Waisanen's immune function.
2. Consider the indications for short-course antibiotic therapy and the indications for conventional therapy. Think about factors such as cost, compliance, and the risk for adverse effects, as well as how antibiotics work to eradicate bacteria.
3. Identify why *Ineffective Health Maintenance* may be an appropriate nursing diagnosis for Mrs. Waisanen and the individual factors contributing to this diagnosis as you plan care.

A Patient with Urinary Calculi

1. Review the risk factors for urinary lithiasis.
2/3. Using the medications section of interdisciplinary care for the patient with urinary calculi in this chapter and your pharmacology textbook or drug handbook, review analgesia for the patient with renal colic and the intended and adverse effects of the drugs given to Mr. Leton.

A Patient with a Bladder Tumor

1. Review the risk factors for urinary tract tumors, looking for commonalities and considering the physiology of the bladder and urine formation and elimination.
2. Remembering that patients rarely present with one isolated health problem, review Mr. Hussain's health history for possible contributing factors to these manifestations. Then review Chapter 6 for nursing care of the patient with substance abuse. Why might Mr. Hussain experience alcohol withdrawal after 2 to 3 days of hospitalization?
3. Considering the surgery performed and its potential effects on physical function and body image, use your nursing care planning book or guide to identify possible interventions and outcomes for this nursing diagnosis.

A Patient with Urinary Incontinence

1. Consider the effects of menopause and estrogen deficiency on genital tissues, as well as the desired and possible adverse effects of Mrs. Giovanni's medications.
2. Consider not only Mrs. Giovanni's nursing diagnosis of *Impaired Skin Integrity*, but also her risk factors for urinary tract infection.
3. Identify factors that may contribute to situational low self-esteem in Mrs. Giovanni and nursing interventions to address this diagnosis.

Chapter 28: Nursing Care of Patients with Kidney Disorders

A Patient with Acute Glomerulonephritis

1. Review Chapter 12 and the use of antibiotics to treat infection.
2. Review Mr. Chang's history and the risk factors for acute glomerulonephritis.
3. Review the diagnostic tests used to differentiate different forms of glomerulonephritis.

A Patient with Acute Renal Failure

1. Of the categories of causative factors for acute renal failure (prerenal, intrarenal, postrenal), review the two most common and compare Ms. Devak's history and physical examination findings with these categories.
2. Consider the effects of renal failure and the stress response on other body systems. You may want to review peptic ulcer disease and stress gastritis in Chapter 23.
3. Consider both the phases of acute renal failure and their physiologic effects, as well as potential complications of a fractured femur.

4. When planning nursing care related to *Deficient Diversional Activity*, consider Ms. Devak's developmental stage, usual state of health, and mechanisms currently being used to maintain femur alignment.

A Patient with End-Stage Renal Disease

1. Review the usual onset, pathophysiology, and long-term effects of type 1 and type 2 diabetes (Chapter 20).
2. Consider the effects of urea and ammonia (both neurologic toxins) on brain function.
3. Consider the physiology of dialysis, the composition of dialysis solutions (dialysate), as well as potential planned and unplanned effects of peritoneal dialysis.
4. As you develop your response, think about not only the mechanism by which peritoneal dialysis is delivered, but also possible effects of the peritoneal dialysis cycle on body image.

Chapter 30: Nursing Care of Patients with Coronary Heart Disease

A Patient with Coronary Artery Bypass Surgery

1. Identify Mr. Clements's modifiable risk factors as you develop your plan. What barriers might need to be overcome to implement strategies to reduce his risk factors?
2. What strategies can you use to overcome denial without creating hostility or impairing the patient–nurse relationship?
3. Consider traditional family roles as well as those roles that are unique to these individuals. Identify measures you can use to enlist the spouse's support.
4. Think about therapeutic communications as you formulate your response. Will your age or gender potentially affect your ability to respond effectively to these concerns? Would referral to another healthcare provider be appropriate?

A Patient with Acute Myocardial Infarction

1. Review immediate treatment measures for MI. Are other means available for reestablishing coronary artery perfusion? If you are in a rural area without immediate access to a cardiac catheterization lab, how will this affect your response?
2. Review the section of this chapter on dysrhythmias and their treatment. Research protocols for treating frequent PVCs in the post-MI patient at your clinical facility.
3. Review the goals of cardiac rehabilitation and Mrs. Williams's individual risk factors as you develop your teaching plan.
4. Consider the value of using a therapeutic response to Mrs. Williams's statement concerning smoking. Also consider the risks associated with cigarette smoke. How can you respond without supporting Mrs. Williams's desire to smoke and without precipitating anger or resistance? Review Chapter 6.

A Patient with Supraventricular Tachycardia

1. Review the effects of sympathetic and parasympathetic nervous system stimulation on cardiac function.
2. Review the section on supraventricular tachycardias, as well as the antidysrhythmic medications for other treatment options.
3. Use your pharmacology textbook as you develop your teaching plan.

Chapter 31: Nursing Care of Patients with Cardiac Disorders

A Patient with Heart Failure

1. Review the prescribed medications and their interactions. Do not forget to consider Mr. Jackson's age in assessing his risk for toxicity and interactions.
2. Review therapeutic communications skills and the use of open-ended statements to evaluate the underlying message of Mr. Jackson's statement.

3. Review exercise recommendations for the patient with heart failure as well as cardiac rehabilitation principles (Chapter 30).
4. Review the rationale for aspirin therapy in the patient with CHD and its effects on platelets and clotting as you formulate your response.
5. Review Chapter 42 for causes of stroke and the section of Chapter 30 on atrial fibrillation.

A Patient with Mitral Valve Prolapse

1. Review the pathophysiology and manifestations of MVP, as well as the general treatment measures for valve disorders.
2. Think about the effects of progressive conditioning on cardiac function.
3. Consider the anxiety associated with heart conditions and with a potentially progressive disorder that could affect childbearing and other life activities, as well as ultimately necessitate surgery.
4. Review the manifestations of MVP and of mitral regurgitation.

Chapter 32: Nursing Care of Patients with Vascular and Lymphatic Disorders

A Patient with Hypertension

1. Review Mrs. Spezia's assessment data and the risk factors for primary hypertension.
2. Review the pathophysiology of primary hypertension and of obesity (Chapter 22), as well as the relationship between hypertension and coronary heart disease.
3. Think about resources that are available in your community for homeless people. Talk to community health and social service agencies to identify additional resources.
4. Correlate Mrs. Spezia's assessment data, the pathophysiology of hypertension, and the long-term effects of stress.
5. Use your nursing care planning and nursing diagnosis textbooks to help develop your care plan.

A Patient with Peripheral Vascular Disease

1. Review treatments for peripheral atherosclerosis, as well as lifestyle measures for preventing and treating atherosclerosis and coronary heart disease (Chapter 30).
2. Compare the pathophysiology of peripheral atherosclerosis, intermittent claudication, and coronary heart disease (Chapter 30) to identify similarities and differences.
3. Review the actions of beta blockers and their role in angina prophylaxis.
4. Use your nursing care planning and nutrition textbooks to help develop your care plan.

A Patient with Deep Vein Thrombosis

1. Review the pathophysiologic processes of venous thrombosis and inflammation.
2. Think about questions you could ask for further information as well as potential resources for Mrs. Hipps.
3. Consider assessment data to evaluate Mrs. Hipps's limitations and resources, as well as community resources to help meet her needs.
4. Use your nursing diagnosis and care planning textbooks to develop your plan of care.

Chapter 33: Nursing Care of Patients with Hematologic Disorders

A Patient with Folic Acid Deficiency Anemia

1. Consider the effects of Mrs. Matthews's rapid weight loss on fluid balance, as well as the effects of tissue hypoxia on cardiac output.

2. Refer to this chapter and your nutrition text. Be sure to consider Mrs. Matthews's age in designing your menu.
3. Consider factors such as Mrs. Matthews's recent dietary history, the folic acid content of foods, and other pertinent factors in the history and physical assessment.
4. In addition to general factors to consider for the older adult (don't forget transportation among other factors), also consider the possible effect of Mrs. Matthews's recent loss and the grieving process.

A Patient with Acute Myelocytic Leukemia

1. Review the physiology of white blood cells, and the immune and inflammatory responses.
2. Think about the risks created by hospitalization in terms of exposure to infection and invasive procedures.
3. Think about the effect of inability to perform self-care on self-esteem, self-confidence, and perception of power and control.
4. Use information provided in the nursing care and home care sections of this chapter as well as in Chapter 12.
5. Use your nursing care planning and fundamentals texts to develop your care plan.

A Patient with Hodgkin's Disease

1. Review Chapter 14 and the effects of chemotherapy and radiation on cancerous cells. Think about the advantages of combining these two therapies in terms of short- and long-term desired and adverse effects.
2. Consider the primary and potential risks for infection in community settings as you design your teaching plan. What teaching strategies will you use for a young adult with Mr. Quito's education and experience?
3. Review theories of development and the developmental tasks for the young adult.
4. Use your nursing fundamentals and nursing care planning texts for reference in developing your care plan.

A Patient with Hemophilia

1. Review the pathophysiology of hemophilia and its effect on the clotting process.
2. Consider both the ABCs and Maslow's hierarchy of needs as you respond to this question.
3. Think about the genetic transmission of hemophilia. How might Mr. Cruise's hemophilia affect any children that he has? Grandchildren?
4. Review your nursing fundamentals book, nursing skills book, and intravenous therapy text to develop your teaching plan. Also consider previous learning and developmental levels.
5. What evidence supports his as an appropriate nursing diagnosis for Mr. Cruise?

Chapter 35: Nursing Care of Patients with Upper Respiratory Disorders

A Patient with Peritonsillar Abscess

1/2. Review the manifestations of upper respiratory infections and management of these disorders.
3. Think about the primary uses of the nose, mouth, and pharynx as you consider nursing diagnoses related to upper respiratory disorders.

A Patient with Nasal Trauma

1. Consider other measures to restore the patient's sense of control over the situation. Consider the potentially traumatic effects of suction on the mucous membranes as well as possible infection control risks.

2. Review the implications and potential dangers of CSF leakage to help you develop your care plan.

3. Think about the benefits and drawbacks of immediate and delayed rhinoplasty.

A Patient with Total Laryngectomy

1. Review the options for speech rehabilitation. If available, practice using a speech generator. Practice esophageal speech.

2. Use your nursing care planning and nursing diagnoses handbook to develop your care plan. Consider Mr. Tom's age, occupation, and marital status in your plan of care.

3. Review Chapter 4 for surgical nursing care interventions, as well as your nursing fundamentals textbook for wound care strategies.

4. Consider measures to promote airway clearance and ventilation of all lung fields.

Chapter 36: Nursing Care of Patients with Ventilation Disorders

A Patient with Pneumonia

1. Review Mrs. O'Neal's assessment data and compare her history with identified risk factors for pneumonia.

2. Review normal immune and inflammatory responses and the role of white blood cells in these processes.

3. Review Chapter 11 and altered immune responses for the physiology and effects of anaphylactic shock.

4. Use your nursing care planning and nursing diagnosis textbooks to help develop your care plan.

A Patient with Tuberculosis

1. Consider available resources for mentally ill patients, as well as community and public health resources. Consider measures to ensure compliance with the prescribed treatment.

2. Contact your local public health department, the discharge planner for your unit, or the social services department in your clinical facility to help identify available resources.

3. Use the nursing care section under Pneumonia, and your nursing diagnosis or care planning handbook as you develop your care plan.

A Patient with Lung Cancer

1. Review Chapter 14 and use your pharmacology text to research the effects of these drugs and the rationale for combination chemotherapy.

2. Use Chapter 14 and your pharmacology text to identify probable side effects of this treatment regimen. Then use your nursing care planning book to identify appropriate nursing diagnoses and interventions.

3. Review the pathophysiology and collaborative care sections for lung cancer to develop your response to this question.

Chapter 37: Nursing Care of Patients with Gas Exchange Disorders

A Patient with COPD

1. Review the processes by which cigarette smoke inflicts damage on lung tissue. Use your pediatric and pathophysiology texts for additional information.

2. Review the physiology of the respiratory drive, as well as the effects of chronic elevated carbon dioxide levels in the blood.

3. Review the manifestations of COPD and its complications as well as the section of this chapter on respiratory failure.

4. Use your nursing diagnosis handbook to help identify appropriate goals and interventions for this nursing diagnosis.

A Patient with ARDS

1. As you respond to this question, consider additional treatment measures for ARDS and respiratory failure. Also consider the potential long-term consequences and complications of intubation and mechanical ventilation. Discuss strategies for communicating with Ms. Adamson's family and supporting coping and decision making by Ms. Adamson and her family in an instance such as this.

2. Think about the precipitating factors for ARDS and the factors that may precipitate respiratory failure in a patient with COPD. Consider the probable overall respiratory and general health status of the individual affected by each of these conditions.

3. Review the precipitating factors for ARDS and discuss strategies to prevent them.

4. Use your nursing care planning book to identify appropriate goals and nursing interventions for this nursing diagnosis.

Chapter 39: Nursing Care of Patients with Musculoskeletal Trauma

A Patient with a Hip Fracture

1. Consider Mrs. Carbolito's age and the fact that she is postmenopausal. What effect does estrogen have on bone health? What might have increased her risk for falls?

2. Review the principles of traction application. What purpose does it serve prior to surgery? What words could you use that she would understand? Think about the effects of trauma, pain, and suddenly finding oneself in a strange environment on listening and understanding verbal communications.

3. List how each of these manifestations would affect skin integrity, food intake, and bone healing.

A Patient with a Below-the-Knee Amputation

1. Design a sequential plan for Mr. Rocke's self-care of the stump. Consider his readiness to learn and the complexity of the care. Is there a risk in letting him assume total responsibility from the beginning? Why or why not?

2. List the factors used to describe Mr. Rocke. How do these affect his ability or willingness to follow up with medical care? What community agencies are available where you live or go to school that would be good sources of assistance and support for Mr. Rocke?

3. Review the information about exercise. How would Mr. Rocke's choice not to do exercises affect his ability to use a prosthesis to walk?

Chapter 40: Nursing Care of Patients with Musculoskeletal Disorders

A Patient with Osteoporosis

1. Review the effects of nicotine and caffeine on blood circulation to bones. What effect does alcohol play in bone loss?

2. Review foods that increase blood cholesterol levels. What is considered a normal cholesterol level? You may need to read content in Chapter 31. Knowing the patient needs calcium, what type of dairy products would you recommend?

3. List activities for the patient who is not able to be ambulatory. How many of the activities on your list would help prevent osteoporosis?

4. *Risk for Trauma* is defined as an increased risk for accidental tissue injury, such as a fracture. What interventions would you teach Mrs. Bauer to reduce this risk?

A Patient with Osteoarthritis

1. Review information about serum creatinine and BUN in a laboratory studies textbook or on the web. What medications are Mr. Cerulli taking that may be affecting these findings? Consider what teaching is necessary related to these findings.

2. What assessments are significant for confusion? If necessary, review content related to confusion. Review Mr. Cerulli's history in the case study and determine factors that may have contributed to his risk for confusion before, during, and after surgery.

3. *Acute Confusion* is defined as an abrupt onset of a cluster of global, transient changes and disturbances in attention, cognition, psychomotor activity, level of consciousness, and/or sleep–wake cycle. What assessments could you make to support this diagnosis for Mr. Cerulli? What interventions might you design for this diagnosis?

A Patient with Rheumatoid Arthritis

1. Think about the role differences in a 42-year-old woman and a 72-year-old woman. On the other hand, consider the effects of a chronic illness that may have been present for 30 years. Would your plan differ? Why or why not?

2. List the possible disabilities that may be caused by rheumatoid arthritis. How do you believe these would affect Mrs. James? What agencies in your community are available for support of people with this type of illness? Where would you go for literature to give Mrs. James?

3. *Ineffective Role Performance* is defined as behaviors and expressions that do not match norms or expectations. Do you believe this is an appropriate nursing diagnosis for Mrs. James? Why or why not? What interventions could be implemented for this diagnosis?

Chapter 42: Nursing Care of Patients with Intracranial Disorders

A Patient with a Seizure Disorder

1. List the teaching topics you would include for Ms. Carlson. Consider how her needs (e.g., for safety) would differ if she lived alone.

2. Describe statements you could use to help Ms. Carlson understand not only the dangers but also the legal issues involved. What if Ms. Carlson does not recognize these concerns?

3. What type of questions could you ask Ms. Carlson to determine why she feels this way? Would you personally find it embarrassing? How can you facilitate Ms. Carlson's understanding for this recommendation?

A Patient with a Stroke

1. What subjective manifestations does the patient with hypertension have? (Review content in Chapter 32.)

2. Consider referral to community resources as a volunteer tutor for adult literacy, gardening, and/or woodworking. Tutoring college students is another option.

3. Use statements that will encourage Mr. Boren to talk about his arm and how he feels about being unable to use it.

A Patient with a Subdural Hematoma

1. Review the manifestations of the types of intracranial hematomas. What assessments are specific to a subdural hematoma? Why is it important to know this?

2. What are some other interventions that might be used? How could family help? What if no family members are available?

3. *Acute Confusion* is a sudden onset of changes in attention, cognition, psychomotor activity, level of consciousness, and/or

sleep–wake cycle. What would you determine as priority nursing diagnoses and interventions for Mr. Lee?

A Patient with a Brain Tumor

1. Review content in the chapter on increased intracranial pressure and intracranial surgery. List collaborative and nursing interventions to decrease increased intracranial pressure.

2. What do these manifestations indicate? What would be your priority assessment? Who would you notify?

3. Practice the use of therapeutic communications and what response you would make.

4. Consider the reasons Ms. Lange feels powerless. What nursing interventions might decrease this feeling?

Chapter 43: Nursing Care of Patients with Spinal Cord Disorders and CNS Infections

A Patient with an SCI

1. What are the developmental tasks of a 19-year-old? How does the inability to meet these tasks affect emotional responses?

2. Think about questions that explore Mr. Valdez's fears in relation to sexuality. Practice questions and statements with friends until you are not embarrassed to ask them.

3. Consider how your own values and beliefs may differ from those of a patient.

4. What baseline assessments and information are necessary before developing a plan for urinary elimination needs? Why would self-catheterization be an option? What are the risks of long-term Foley catheterization?

A Patient with Bacterial Meningitis

1. List the environmental stimuli in the hospital setting. How could these be decreased? What effect do these stimuli have on cognition and behavior that is altered by an intracranial infection?

2. Think about how you would feel if Mr. Cook tried to hit you. How would you respond to him? To whom would you report this?

3. Why would Mr. Cook have pain? How would pain be manifested during the initial treatment period? Is it important to consider the respiratory effects of narcotics for him? Defend your answer.

Chapter 44: Nursing Care of Patients with Neurologic Disorders

A Patient with Alzheimer's Disease

1. Think about what information you would need and how you would collect it. Consider such factors as the age of family members, educational level of family members, and stage of the patient's AD. What else would you need to know?

2. Review the suggested activities in this section of the chapter. What others can you think of or have you seen used successfully? Osteoarthritis often results in joint stiffness and pain as well as problems with mobility. Would this affect your interventions? If so, how could they be adapted?

3. Consider the type of foods that might be prepared, the timing of meals, and interventions that might be used to decrease agitation before or during meals.

A Patient with Multiple Sclerosis

1. Outline a typical day's activities for Mr. McMurphy that would provide a balance between activity and rest. What assessments would you make to evaluate the effectiveness of this plan?

2. Consider how respiratory infections are spread. Why is Mr. McMurphy at increased risk?

3. The definition of *Risk for Injury* is that one is at risk as a result of environmental conditions interacting with the person's adaptive

and defensive resources. What factors in this patient's history and physical status would support this diagnosis? What interventions would you include in the care plan and why?

A Patient with Parkinson's Disease

1. Consider the adaptations that might be made to clothing and shoes. What adaptive devices might be useful?
2. What information would you need to know before you develop your interventions? Include that from Mr. Avneil and what might be available in the community and the long-term care facility.
3. *Chronic Sorrow* is a recurring pattern of sadness in response to continual loss. Consider the type of communications you would need to use with Mr. Avneil to identify his degree of sorrow. What other assessment might provide cues to support this diagnosis (think about eating and sleeping)? How might an activity such as reminiscence help?

Chapter 46: Nursing Care of Patients with Eye and Ear Disorders

A Patient with Glaucoma and Cataracts

1. What is the pathophysiology of glaucoma? How does a cataract affect glaucoma?
2. Consider the effects of corticosteroids on glaucoma. If Mrs. Rainey is to administer several medications at home, identify specific teaching guidelines for her.
3. Would you request a referral for home health visits? Why or why not? Think about the effect of transferring her for a brief admission to an assisted-living facility.

Chapter 48: Nursing Care of Men with Reproductive System and Breast Disorders

A Man with Prostate Cancer

1. Why would Mr. Turner be at risk for altered skin integrity? Outline the interventions you would include on his teaching plan that would promote skin integrity as he cares for himself at home.
2. Noncompliance is defined as behaviors that do not coincide with the therapeutic plan agreed upon by the person and the healthcare professional. Do you think Mr. Turner fully understood his treatment and agreed with his follow-up care? What could be done in the preoperative phase of Mr. Turner's care to better ensure his understanding and desire to have continued medical care?
3. What assessments indicate that Mr. Turner does or does not have bladder distention? Would you report this? If so, to whom?

Chapter 49: Nursing Care of Women with Reproductive System and Breast Disorders

A Woman with Endometriosis

1. What is the relationship between Mrs. Hall's manifestations and a decreased RBC count? Review the information in Chapter 32 and list assessments you would make to identify anemia.
2. List nonthreatening questions you would use to begin the discussion. How might it help to ask these questions at the beginning of the interview? Then list questions that you might use to collect

data about the couple's sexual history. Would you be embarrassed to ask them? If so, how might this in turn affect their responses?
3. *Situational Low Self-Esteem* is the state in which a person develops a negative perception of self-worth in response to a current situation. What information in Mrs. Hall's history might provide data to support this nursing diagnosis?

A Woman with Cervical Cancer

1. Consider developmental needs and how they differ by age.
2. Review the effects of radiation, discussed in Chapter 14.
3. Does fatigue differ from "feeling tired"? Can the fatigue from radiation be decreased? If so, how?

A Woman with Breast Cancer

1. Review the information in the chapter on the genetic factors that pose a risk for developing breast cancer. How could you explain this in terms understandable by Mrs. Clemments and her daughters?
2. List the different types of mastectomies. Consider the implications of the differences, and how this would affect your nursing care.
3. Review the information on chemotherapy in Chapter 14. List the types of chemotherapy and its common side effects. Consider the classifications of medications that are used to treat these side effects.
4. What factors in the treatment of Mrs. Clemments's treatment might disrupt the amount and quality of her sleep? What interventions might be used to improve her sleep pattern?

Chapter 50: Nursing Care of Patients with Sexually Transmitted Infections

A Patient with Gonorrhea

1. What manifestations does Ms. Cirit have that are typical of the disease? Would you make other assessments? If so, what are they?
2. Review the discussion of HIV in Chapter 13. Do you believe it is true that infection with gonorrhea may increase the risk of HIV? If so, how would you explain this to Ms. Cirit?
3. *Impaired Social Interaction* is a state of aloneness or rejection experienced by an individual that is perceived as negative. What assessments of Ms. Cirit might support this diagnosis? What interventions and expected outcomes would you develop?

A Patient with Syphilis

1. Describe the assessments you would expect to find in a man with early syphilis.
2. Consider topics such as number of sex partners, patterns of sexual activity, and use of safe sex practices. What other topics should be explored? How can you ask these questions without being embarrassed or embarrassing the patient?
3. List possible statements you might make. Do you believe this is a nursing responsibility? If you do not feel comfortable with this topic, what could you do?

GLOSSARY

Abrasion Partial-thickness denudation of an area of integument, generally resulting from falls or scrapes.

Absence seizure (petit mal seizure) A type of generalized seizure characterized by a sudden brief cessation of all motor activity accompanied by a blank stare and unresponsiveness.

Accommodation The ability of the eye to adjust to variations in distance.

Achalasia Absence of peristalsis of the esophagus and high gastro-esophageal sphincter pressure resulting in dilation and loss of tone in the esophagus.

Acidosis The condition in which the hydrogen ion concentration increases above normal (reflected in a pH below 7.35).

Acids A substance that releases hydrogen ions in solution.

Acne Disorder of the pilosebaceous (hair and sebaceous gland) structure, resulting in eruption of papules or pustules.

Acoustic neuroma or schwannoma Benign tumor of cranial nerve VIII.

Acquired immune deficiency syndrome (AIDS) A specific group of diseases or conditions that are indicative of severe immunosuppression related to infection with the human immunodeficiency virus.

Acquired immunity Immunity developed after exposure to a pathogen. See *Active immunity*.

Acromegaly Meaning literally "enlarged extremities," this is a condition resulting from excessive growth hormone secretion during adulthood.

Actinic keratosis Also called senile or solar keratosis, this is an epidermal skin lesion directly related to chronic sun exposure and photodamage.

Active immunity Production of antibodies or development of immune lymphocytes against specific antigens.

Active transport Movement of molecules across cell membranes and epithelial membranes against a concentration gradient; requires energy.

Acute coronary syndrome (ACS) A condition of unstable cardiac ischemia; includes unstable angina and acute myocardial ischemia with or without significant myocardial tissue injury.

Acute gastritis A benign, self-limiting disorder associated with ingestion of gastric irritants such as aspirin, alcohol, caffeine, or foods contaminated with certain bacteria.

Acute illness An illness that occurs rapidly, lasts for a relatively short time, and is self-limiting.

Acute lymphoblastic leukemia (ALL) Abnormal proliferation of lymphoblasts in the bone marrow, lymph nodes, and spleen; the most common type of leukemia in children and young adults.

Acute myeloblastic leukemia (AML) Uncontrolled proliferation of myeloblasts (granulocyte precursors) and hyperplasia of bone marrow and the spleen; the most common acute leukemia in adults.

Acute myocardial infarction (AMI) Necrosis (death) of myocardial cells.

Acute pain Pain of sudden onset that is usually self-limited and localized; it lasts for less than 6 months and has an identifiable cause, such as trauma, surgery, or inflammation.

Acute renal failure Abrupt onset of renal failure, often reversible.

Acute respiratory distress syndrome (ARDS) Noncardiac pulmonary edema and progressive refractory hypoxemia.

Acute tubular necrosis (ATN) A syndrome of abrupt and progressive decline in tubular and glomerular function.

Adaptive immune response A specific and systemic immune initiated by and directed against particular antigens.

Adaptive immunity Long-lasting and specific response of the lymphocytes to antigens.

Addiction A primary, chronic neurobiologic disease characterized by compulsive use of a substance despite negative consequences, such as health threats or legal problems.

Addisonian crisis A life-threatening response to acute adrenal insufficiency. Triggers include surgery, acute systemic illness, trauma, or abrupt withdrawal of long-term corticosteroid therapy.

Advance directive Also called a *living will*, this is a document in which a patient formally states preferences for health care in the event that he or she later becomes mentally incapacitated, and names a person who has durable power of attorney to serve as a substitute decision maker to implement the patient's stated preferences.

Aesthetic surgery See *Cosmetic surgery*.

Afterload The force the ventricles must overcome to eject their blood volume; the pressure in the arterial system ahead of the ventricles.

Agnosia The inability to recognize one or more subjects that were previously familiar; agnosia may be visual, tactile, or auditory.

Agranulocytosis Severe neutropenia, with less than 200 cells/μm.

Alcohol Alcohol and other CNS depressants act on other neurotransmitters in the brain such as gamma-aminobutyric acid (GABA). GABA is the most prevalent inhibitory neurotransmitter in the brain and has a major role in decreasing neuronal excitability. Alcohol creates an additive effect with GABA, further inhibiting arousal and depressing the autonomic nervous system.

Alcoholic cirrhosis (Laënnec's cirrhosis) The end result of alcoholic liver disease.

Alkalis Alkalis are bases that accept hydrogen ions in solution.

Alkalosis The condition where the hydrogen ion concentration decreases below normal (reflected in a pH above 7.45).

Alleles Different forms of a gene or DNA occupying the same place on a pair of chromosomes; an allele for each gene is inherited from each parent.

Allergy A hypersensitivity response to environmental or exogenous antigens.

Allografts Grafts between members of the same species but who have different genotypes and HLA antigens. See also *Homograft*.

Alopecia Loss of hair; baldness.

Alzheimer's disease (AD) A form of dementia characterized by progressive, irreversible deterioration of the general intellectual functioning.

Amenorrhea Absence of menstruation.

Amphetamine Central nervous system stimulant that causes arousal and an elevation of mood with a sense of increased strength, mental capacity, self-confidence, and a decreased need for food and sleep.

Amputation Partial or total removal of a body part.

Amyotrophic lateral sclerosis (ALS) Progressive, degenerative neurologic disease characterized by weakness and wasting of the involved muscles, without any accompanying sensory or cognitive changes; also called *Lou Gehrig's disease*.

Analgesic A medication that reduces or eliminates the perception of pain.

Anaphylactic shock Shock resulting from a widespread hypersensitivity reaction (called *anaphylaxis*). The pathophysiology in this type of shock includes vasodilation, pooling of blood in the periphery, and hypovolemia with altered cellular metabolism.

Anaphylaxis An acute systemic type I hypersensitivity reaction that occurs in response to an injected antigen.

Anaplasia The regression of a cell to an immature or undifferentiated cell type.

Anasarca Severe, generalized edema.

Androgens Hormones synthesized in the testes, ovaries, and adrenal cortex that promote expression of male sex characteristics.

Anemia An abnormally low number of circulating RBCs, hemoglobin concentration, or both.

Anergy Inability to react to specific antigens.

Anesthesia State produced by medications given intravenously, intraspinally, subcutaneously, or by inhalation to create temporary partial or total loss of sensation and consciousness in a patient for invasive procedures such as surgery or painful diagnostic tests.

Aneurysm Abnormal dilation of a blood vessel, commonly at a site of a weakness or tear in the vessel wall.

Angina pectoris (angina) Chest pain resulting from reduced coronary blood flow that causes a temporary imbalance between myocardial blood supply and demand.

Angioma (hemangioma) Benign vascular tumor.

Anion gap The difference between the sum of two measured anions, chloride and bicarbonate, and the principal measured cation, sodium.

Ankylosing spondylitis A chronic inflammatory arthritis that primarily affects the axial skeleton, leading to pain and progressive stiffening and fusion of the spine.

Anorexia Loss of appetite.

Anorexia nervosa An eating disorder characterized by a body weight less than 85% of expected for age and height, and an intense fear of gaining weight.

Anorgasmia Absence of orgasm.

Anosmia Inability to smell.

Anthropometric measurements Measurement of height, weight, triceps skin folds, and midarm circumference.

Antibodies Immunoglobulin molecules that bind with an antigen to inactivate it.

Antibody-mediated (humoral) immune response Activation of B cells to produce antibodies to respond to antigens such as bacteria, bacterial toxins, and free viruses.

Anticipatory grieving A combination of intellectual and emotional responses and behaviors by which people adjust their self-concept in the face of a potential loss.

Antigen A substance capable of evoking a specific immune response; usually a protein which the body recognizes as foreign, causing an immune response to be stimulated.

Antigenic substances Agents such as microorganisms, cells and tissues from other humans or animals, and some inorganic substances that stimulate an immune response.

Aortic valve The semilunar valve between the left ventricle of the heart and the aorta. It prevents blood from flowing backward into the ventricle.

Aortitis Inflammation of the aorta, usually the aortic arch.

Aphasia Defective or absent language function.

Apical impulse A normal, palpable pulsation (thrust) in the area of the midclavicular line in the left fifth intercostal space. It can be seen on inspection in about half of the adult population.

Aplastic anemia A condition manifested by failure of the bone marrow to produce all three types of blood cells.

Apnea Cessation of breathing lasting from a few seconds to a few minutes.

Appendectomy Surgical removal of the appendix.

Appendicitis Inflammation of the vermiform appendix.

Apraxia The inability to carry out a motor pattern (such as drawing a figure) even when strength and coordination are adequate.

Areflexia Lack of normal reflexes.

Arterial blood gas (ABG) A laboratory test used to evaluate acid–base balance and gas exchange.

Arteriovenous (AV) malformation A congenital intracranial lesion, formed by a tangled collection of dilated arteries and veins, that allows blood to flow directly from the arterial into the venous system, bypassing the normal capillary network.

Arthralgia Joint pain.

Arthritis Joint inflammation.

Arthroplasty The reconstruction or replacement of a joint.

Ascites Excess fluid in the peritoneal cavity.

Asphyxiation Oxygen deprivation.

Asthma Chronic inflammatory disorder of the airways that is characterized by recurrent episodes of wheezing, breathlessness, chest tightness, and coughing.

Astigmatism A condition that develops with abnormal curvature of the cornea or eyeball, causing the image to focus at multiple points on the retina.

Ataxia Uncoordinated, irregular gait and muscle movement; weakness.

Atelectasis Collapse of lung tissue following obstruction of the bronchus or bronchioles.

Atherosclerosis A form of arteriosclerosis in which deposits of fat and fibrin obstruct and harden the arteries.

Atopic dermatitis (eczema) Common inflammatory skin disorder of unknown cause.

Atrial kick Delivery of an additional bolus of blood to the ventricles resulting from atrial systole; occurs just prior to ventricular systole.

Atrial natriuretic peptide (ANP) A hormone released by atrial muscle cells in response to distention from fluid overload.

Aura Sensation preceding generalized seizure activity; may be a vague sense of uneasiness or an abnormal sensation.

Auscultatory gap A temporary disappearance of sound between the systolic and diastolic BP.

Autografting Transplanting of the patient's own tissue; the most successful type of tissue transplant.

Autoimmune disorder Failure of immune system to recognize itself, resulting in normal host tissue being targeted by immune defenses.

Autonomic dysreflexia Exaggerated sympathetic response that occurs in patients with spinal cord injuries at or above the T_6 level.

Autosome A single chromosome from any one of the 22 pairs of chromosomes not involved in sex determination (X or Y); humans have 22 pairs of autosomes.

Azotemia Increased blood levels of nitrogenous waste products.

B lymphocytes (B cells) Bursa-equivalent lymphocytes responsible for synthesizing antibodies in response to specific antigens.

Bacterial vaginosis Nonspecific vaginitis.

Bactericidal Capable of killing organisms without immune system intervention.

Bacteriostatic Inhibits growth of microorganisms, leaving the destruction to the host's immune system.

Bacteriuria Bacteria in the urine.

Balanced suspension traction Traction in which several forces of pull work in unison to raise and support the patient's injured extremity off the bed and maintain its alignment.

Balloon tamponade The application of pressure to stop esophageal bleeding using an inflatable balloon.

Bariatrics The healthcare science that focuses on patients who are extremely obese.

Basal cell carcinoma Epithelial tumor that is believed to originate either from the basal layer of the epidermis or from cells in the surrounding dermal structures. These tumors are characterized by an impaired ability of the basal cells of the epidermis to mature into keratinocytes, with mitotic division beyond the basal layer.

Basal metabolic rate (BMR) Test to measure the energy used when the body is at rest; rarely used due to the availability of more accurate thyroid tests.

Base excess (BE) A calculated value also known as buffer base capacity. Base excess reflects the degree of acid–base imbalance by indicating the status of the body's total buffering capacity.

Bases (or alkalis) Substances that accept hydrogen ions in solution.

Bell's palsy (facial paralysis) Disorder of the facial nerve (seventh cranial nerve), characterized by unilateral paralysis of the facial muscles.

Benign prostatic hyperplasia (BPH) Enlargement of the prostate gland.

Bereavement The time of mourning experienced after a loss.

Bile A greenish, watery solution containing bile salts, cholesterol, bilirubin, electrolytes, water, and phospholipids.

Biliary colic A severe, steady pain in the epigastric region or upper right quadrant of the abdomen caused by obstruction and increased pressure in the bile duct.

Binge-eating disorder A nutritional disorder characterized by recurrent episodes of binge eating—eating an excessive amount of food during a defined period of time and a sense of loss of control over eating during binge episodes.

Biofeedback An electronic method of measuring autonomic physiologic responses, such as brain waves, muscle contraction, and skin temperature, and then "feeding" this information back to the patient.

Biological markers Stable segments of DNA important for the construction of chromosome maps.

Bioterrorism Use of an etiologic agent (disease) to cause harm or kill a population, food, and/or livestock.

Biotherapy Treatment that modifies the biologic processes that result in malignant cells, primarily through enhancing the person's own immune responses.

Bivalving Process of splitting a cast down both sides to alleviate pressure on the injured extremity.

Blood clot See *Thrombus*.

Blood flow The volume of blood transported in a vessel, in an organ, or throughout the entire circulation over a given period of time.

Blood pressure The tension or pressure exerted by blood against arterial walls.

Blunt trauma The type of trauma that occurs when there is no communication from the damaged tissues to the outside environment.

Body mass index (BMI) Used to identify excess adipose tissue, BMI is calculated by dividing the weight (in kilograms) by the height (in meters squared, m^2).

Bone marrow transplant (BMT) Infusion of bone marrow cells to restore bone marrow function after chemotherapy or radiation. Allogeneic BMT uses donor bone marrow cells from a donor; autologous BMT uses the patient's own bone marrow.

Borborygmus The presence of excessive loud and hyperactive bowel sounds.

Botulism A severe, life-threatening form of food poisoning caused by *Clostridium botulinum*.

Brachytherapy A type of radiation therapy in which the source of radiation is placed directly into or adjacent to the tumor, a technique that delivers a high dose to the tumor and a lower dose to normal tissue.

Bradycardia A heart rate of less than 60 beats per minute.

Bradykinesia Slowed movements due to muscle rigidity.

Bradypnea Abnormally low respiratory rate.

Brain abscess Infection with a collection of purulent material within the brain tissue.

Brain death The cessation of cerebral blood flow with global brain infarction and permanent loss of all brain function.

Brain death criteria Clinical signs used to determine whether a comatose patient is brain dead.

Breakthrough pain Pain that exceeds baseline chronic or persistent pain, with or without baseline analgesia.

Bronchiectasis Permanent abnormal dilation of one or more large bronchi and destruction of bronchial walls, usually accompanied by infection.

Bronchitis Inflammation of the bronchi (airways).

Bruit An adventitious sound heard during auscultation; of venous or arterial origin.

Buffer A substance that prevents major changes in pH by removing or releasing hydrogen ions.

Bulimia nervosa An eating disorder characterized by recurring episodes of binge eating followed by purge behaviors such as self-induced vomiting, use of laxatives or diuretics, fasting, or excessive exercise.

Burn An injury resulting from exposure to heat, chemicals, radiation, or electric current.

Burn shock Hypovolemic shock resulting from the shift of a massive amount of fluid from the intracellular and intravascular compartments into the interstitium following burn injury.

Bursitis Inflammation of the bursa.

Cachexia The wasted physical appearance characteristic of cancer and other chronic illnesses. It is characterized by rapid depletion of the body's protein, particularly in skeletal muscle, with less rapid loss of fat.

Caffeine A methylxanthine stimulant that increases the heart rate and acts as a diuretic.

Calculi Presence of abnormal concentration or stones in the body occur in the gallbladder, kidneys, ureters, bladder, or urethra.

Cancer A family of complex diseases with manifestations that vary according to body system and type of tumor cells involved; marked by uncontrolled growth and the spread of abnormal cells.

Candidiasis Infection of mucous membranes caused by *Candida albicans*, a yeast-like fungus.

Cannabis sativa Cannabis sativa is the source of marijuana.

Carbuncle A group of infected hair follicles.

Carcinogen Cancer-causing agent.

Carcinogenesis The production or origin of cancer.

Carcinoma A tumor arising from epithelial tissue.

Cardiac arrest Sudden failure of the heart to pump.

Cardiac cycle The contraction and relaxation of the heart during one heartbeat.

Cardiac index (CI) Cardiac output adjusted for body size.

Cardiac output (CO) The amount of blood pumped by the ventricles into the pulmonary and systemic circulations in 1 minute.

Cardiac rehabilitation A long-term program of medical evaluation, exercise, risk factor modification, education, and counseling designed to limit the physical and psychologic effects of cardiac illness and improve the patient's quality of life.

Cardiac reserve The ability of the heart to respond to the body's changing need for cardiac output.

Cardiac tamponade Compression of the heart due to pericardial effusion, trauma, cardiac rupture, or hemorrhage.

Cardiogenic shock Shock that occurs when the heart's pumping ability is compromised to the point that it cannot maintain cardiac output and adequate tissue perfusion.

Cardiomegaly Enlargement of the heart.

Cardiomyopathy Primary abnormality of the heart muscle that affects its structural or functional characteristics.

Cardiovascular disease (CVD) Generic term for disorders of the heart and blood vessels.

Carpal spasm Decreased calcium levels cause the patient's hand and fingers to contract in response to occlusion of the blood supply by a blood pressure cuff (Trousseau's sign).

Carpal tunnel syndrome Compression of the median nerve as a result of inflammation and swelling of the synovial lining of the tendon sheaths.

Carrier Any individual who carries a single copy of an altered gene or mutation for a recessive condition on one chromosome of a chromosome pair and an unaltered form of that gene on the other chromosome. A carrier generally is not affected by the gene alteration; on the average, each person in the general population is a carrier of five or six gene mutations for recessive disorders.

Carriers (related to infections) Harbor the pathogen without showing evidence of clinical disease.

Catabolism Biochemical process involving the breakdown of complex structures into simpler forms.

Cataract Opacification (clouding) of the lens of the eye.

Celiac disease (celiac sprue, nontropical sprue) Chronic hereditary disorder characterized by sensitivity to the gliadin fraction of gluten, a cereal protein.

Cell cycle The four phases that occur during growth and development of a cell.

Cell-mediated (cellular) immune response Direct or indirect inactivation of antigen by lymphocytes.

Cellulitis A localized infection of the dermis and subcutaneous tissue.

Central pain Related to a lesion in the brain that may spontaneously produce high-frequency bursts of impulses that are perceived as pain.

Central nervous system depressants Central nervous system depressants, including barbiturates, benzodiazepines, paraldehyde, meprobamate, and chloral hydrate, are subject to abuse.

Central obesity See *Upper body obesity*.

Cerebral concussion Transient, temporary, neurogenic dysfunction caused by mechanical force to the brain.

Cerebral contusion Bruise on the surface of the brain.

Cerebral edema An increase in the volume of brain tissue due to abnormal accumulation of fluid in brain cells.

Cerumen Earwax.

Chalazion Granulomatous cyst or nodule of the lid.

Chancre Hard, syphilitic primary ulcer.

Cheilosis Cracks at corners of the mouth seen in vitamin B-complex deficiencies, especially riboflavin.

Chemotherapy Cancer treatment involving the use of cytotoxic medications to decrease tumor size, adjunctive to surgery or radiation therapy, or to prevent or treat suspected metastases.

Chlamydia A group of syndromes caused by *Chlamydia trachomatis*, a bacterium that behaves like a virus spreading within a host cell; spread by sexual contact and to the neonate by passage through the birth canal of an infected mother.

Cholecystectomy Removal of the gallbladder.

Cholecystitis Inflammation of the gallbladder, usually associated with stones in the cystic or common bile duct.

Cholelithiasis Formation of stones (calculi) within the gallbladder or biliary duct system.

Cholera Acute diarrheal illness caused by certain strains of *Vibrio cholerae*.

Chorea Jerky, rapid, involuntary movements.

Chromosome Genetic material carried by each cell; found in the cell nucleus.

Chronic bronchitis Excessive secretion of bronchial mucus characterized by a productive cough lasting 3 or more months in 2 consecutive years.

Chronic gastritis Disorders characterized by progressive and irreversible changes in the gastric mucosa.

Chronic illness A condition that requires continuing management over a long period—years or even decades.

Chronic hepatitis Chronic infection of the liver; the primary cause of liver damage leading to cirrhosis, liver cancer, and liver transplantation.

Chronic kidney disease (CKD) The presence of kidney damage for three or more months with loss of nephron units and decreased renal mass leading to progressive deterioration of glomerular filtration, tubular secretion, and reabsorption.

Chronic lymphocytic leukemia (CLL) Proliferation and accumulation of small, abnormal, mature lymphocytes in the bone marrow, peripheral blood, and body tissues; least common type of the major leukemias.

Chronic myelogenous leukemia (CML) Abnormal proliferation of all bone marrow elements, usually associated with a chromosome abnormality (the Philadelphia chromosome).

Chronic obstructive pulmonary disease (COPD) Chronic air flow obstruction due to chronic bronchitis and/or emphysema.

Chronic otitis media Condition involving permanent perforation of the tympanic membrane, with or without recurrent pus formation and often accompanied by changes in the mucosa and bony structures (ossicles) of the middle ear.

Chronic pain Prolonged pain, usually lasting longer than 6 months; pain that persists after the condition causing it has resolved; may be malignant or nonmalignant in origin

Chronic sorrow A cyclical, recurring, and potentially progressive pattern of pervasive sadness experienced in response to continual loss, throughout the trajectory of an illness or disability.

Chronic stump pain The result of neuroma formation, causing severe burning pain.

Chronic venous insufficiency A chronic disorder of inadequate venous return.

Chvostek's sign Contraction of the lateral facial muscles in response to tapping the face in front of the ear; caused by decreased blood calcium levels.

Chyme Thick, fluid mixture of food and gastric juices formed in the stomach during the digestive process.

Circulating nurse A registered nurse who coordinates and manages a wide range of activities before, during, and after surgical procedures.

Cirrhosis A progressive, irreversible disorder, eventually leading to liver failure; the end stage of chronic liver disease.

Closed fracture (simple fracture) Break in continuity of bone with skin still intact.

Clubbing Enlargement and blunting of the terminal portion of the fingers; associated with chronic hypoxemia.

Cluster headache A severe, unilateral vascular headache that occurs in groups, or clusters and is characterized by exacerbations and remissions; predominantly experienced by men ages 20 to 40.

Coagulation The process of creating a fibrin meshwork that cements blood components together to form an insoluble clot.

Cocaine A highly addictive stimulant/euphoric drug extracted from the leaves of the coca plant.

Code of ethics An established and agreed-on group of principles of conduct that provide a frame of reference for nursing behaviors that are congruent with professional values.

Cold sore See *Herpes simplex*.

Cold zone Considered the "safe zone" during a disaster, it is adjacent to the warm zone and is the area where a more in-depth triage of victims would occur; survivors may find shelter in this area, and command and control vehicles would be found here as well as the emergency transport vehicles.

Colectomy Surgical removal of the colon.

Collateral channels Connections between small arteries.

Collateral vessels Accessory pathways connected to the smaller arteries in the coronary system.

Colorectal cancer Malignant tumor arising from the epithelial tissues of the colon or rectum.

Colostomy Ostomy made in the colon.

Comedones Noninflammatory acne lesions.

Community-based care Centers on individual and family healthcare needs. The nurse practicing community-based care provides direct services to individuals to manage acute or chronic health problems and to promote self-care. The care is provided in the local community, is culturally competent, and is family centered.

Compartment A space enclosed by a fibrous membrane or fascia.

Compartment syndrome Condition in which excess pressure constricts the structures within a compartment and reduces circulation to muscles and nerves.

Complex regional pain syndrome Extremity pain that is severe, diffuse, and burning, and accompanied by vasomotor changes that affect skin color and temperature.

Concussion Brain injury resulting from a violent jar, shake, or impact with an object.

Conjunctivitis Inflammation of the conjunctiva.

Consanguinity Related by having a common ancestor; close blood relationship.

Conscious sedation Anesthesia that provides analgesia and amnesia, but in which the patient remains conscious. Patients are able to breathe independently and are cardiovascularly stable.

Consciousness A condition in which a person is aware of self and environment and is able to respond appropriately to stimuli; full consciousness requires both normal arousal and full cognition.

Constipation The infrequent (two or fewer bowel movements weekly) or difficult passage of stools.

Contact dermatitis Type of dermatitis caused by a hypersensitivity response or chemical irritation.

Continuous renal replacement therapy (CRRT) A form of hemodialysis in which blood is continuously circulated through a highly porous hemofilter from artery to vein or vein to vein.

Contractility The inherent capability of the cardiac muscle fibers to shorten.

Contracting The negotiation of a cooperative working agreement between the nurse and patient that is continuously renegotiated.

Contractures Permanent shortening of connective tissues.

Contralateral deficit Manifestations of a stroke on the side of the body opposite the side of the brain that is damaged.

Contusion Superficial tissue injury resulting from blunt trauma, such as a kick or blow from an object, that causes the breakage of small blood vessels and bleeding into the surrounding tissue.

Conventional weapons Weapons such as bombs and guns that are used more frequently than nonconventional terrorist weapons.

Convergence Moving the eyes inward toward the nose to see an object close to the face.

Co-occurring disorders Concurrent diagnosis of a substance-use disorder and a psychiatric disorder. One disorder can precede and cause the other, such as the relationship between alcoholism and depression.

Cor pulmonale Condition of right ventricular hypertrophy and failure that results from long-standing pulmonary hypertension.

Core competencies Standards that a profession agrees are essential for a person to be deemed competent in his or her field.

Corneal reflex Closure of eyelids (blinking) due to corneal irritation.

Corneal ulcer Local necrosis of the cornea, may be caused by infection, exposure trauma, or the misuse of contact lenses.

Coronary heart disease (CHD) Heart disease caused by impaired blood flow to the myocardium.

Coryza (rhinorrhea) Profuse nasal discharge.

Cosmetic surgery (aesthetic surgery) One of two fields within plastic surgery. Cosmetic surgery enhances the attractiveness of normal features.

Crackles Discontinuous lung sounds heard by auscultation; can be fine or coarse. Produced by air passing over airway secretions or the opening of collapsed airways.

Crepitation A grating sound heard on movement of a joint.

Creutzfeldt-Jakob disease (CJD, spongiform encephalopathy) Rare, progressive neurologic disease that causes brain degeneration without inflammation.

Critical pathway A healthcare plan designed to provide care with a multidisciplinary, managed action focus; developed for specific diagnoses, usually those that are high volume, high risk, and high cost.

Critical thinking Self-directed thinking that is focused on what to believe or do in a specific situation.

CRNA Certified registered nurse anesthetist; a nurse certified in anesthesia administration.

Crohn's disease (regional enteritis) Chronic, relapsing inflammatory disorder affecting the gastrointestinal tract.

Crossing over A process that occurs during meiosis in which homologous maternal and paternal chromosomes break and exchange corresponding sections of DNA and then rejoin; this process can cause an exchange of alleles between chromosomes and provides human diversity.

Cryosurgery The destruction of tissue by cold or freezing with agents such as fluorocarbon sprays, carbon dioxide snow, nitrous oxide, and liquid nitrogen.

Curettage The removal of lesions with a curette, a semisharp cutting instrument.

Curling's ulcers Acute ulcerations of the stomach or duodenum that form following a burn injury.

Cushing's ulcers Stress ulcers occurring as sequelae of head injury or central nervous system surgery.

Cutaneous melanoma See *Malignant melanoma*.

Cyanosis A bluish discoloration of the skin and mucous membranes due to oxygen deficiency.

Cystectomy Complete surgical removal of the urinary bladder and adjacent muscles and tissues.

Cystic fibrosis (CF) Inherited disorder of the exocrine glands that results in the secretion of abnormal amounts of mucus.

Cystitis Inflammation of the urinary bladder.

Cysts Benign closed sacs in or under the skin surface that are lined with epithelium and contain fluid or a semisolid material.

Cytokines Hormone-like polypeptides produced primarily by monocytes, macrophages, and T cells. Cytokines act as messengers of the immune system, facilitating communication between the cells to adjust or vary the inflammatory reaction or to initiate immune cell proliferation and differentiation.

Dawn phenomenon A rise in blood glucose between 4 AM and 8 AM that is not a response to hypoglycemia.

Death Irreversible cessation of circulatory and respiratory functions or irreversible cessation of all functions of the entire brain, including the brainstem.

Death anxiety Worry or fear related to death or dying.

Debridement Process of removing dead tissue from a wound.

Decerebrate posturing Abnormal posture with the neck extended; the jaw clenched; arms pronated, extended, and close to the sides; legs extended; and feet plantar flexed. Results from lesions of the midbrain, pons, or diencephalons.

Decorticate posturing Abnormal posture with the upper arms close to the sides; the elbows, wrists, and fingers flexed; the legs extended and internally rotated; and the feet plantar flexed. Results from lesions of the corticospinal tracts.

Deep venous thrombosis (DVT) Blood clot (thrombus) formation and inflammation within a deep vein, usually in the pelvis or lower extremities; a common complication of hospitalization, surgery, and immobilization.

Deformation Alteration of the spinal cord and soft tissues caused by abnormal movements from acceleration and deceleration forces.

Dehiscence An unintended separation of wound margins due to incomplete healing.

Dehydration Loss of water.

Delayed healing Healing that occurs at a slower rate than expected.

Delegation To effectively assign appropriate work activities to other members of the healthcare team. When the nurse delegates nursing care activities to another person, that person is authorized to act in the place of the nurse, while the nurse retains the accountability for the activities performed.

Delirium tremens (DT) A medical emergency usually occurring 3 to 5 days following alcohol withdrawal and lasting 2 to 3 days; characterized by paranoia, disorientation, delusions, visual hallucinations, elevated vital signs, vomiting, diarrhea, and diaphoresis.

Dementia A global impairment of cognitive function that usually is progressive and may be permanent; interferes with normal social and occupational activities.

Demyelination Destruction or removal of the myelin sheaths of nerves.

Depolarization The rapid inflow of sodium ions, causing an electrical change in which the inside of a cell becomes positive in relation to the outside.

Dermatitis Acute or chronic inflammation of the skin characterized by erythema and pain or pruritus.

Dermatome Area of skin innervated by cutaneous branches of a single spinal nerve.

Dermatophytes Fungi that cause superficial skin infections.

Dermatophytoses Superficial fungal infection of the skin; also called *ringworm*.

Diabetes insipidus A deficit of ADH causes excretion of large amounts of dilute urine, in some instances as much as 12 L/day. The patient has extreme thirst and drinks large volumes of water. If unable to replace the water loss, the patient becomes dehydrated and hypernatremic. Even though hyperosmolality is present, the urine is dilute and has a low specific gravity.

Diabetes mellitus (DM) Group of chronic disorders of the endocrine pancreas, all categorized under a broad diagnostic label. The condition is characterized by inappropriate hyperglycemia caused by a relative or absolute deficiency of insulin or by a cellular resistance to the action of insulin.

Diabetic ketoacidosis (DKA) A form of metabolic acidosis induced by stress in a person with type 1 diabetes.

Diabetic nephropathy A disease of the kidneys characterized by the presence of albumin in the urine, hypertension, edema, and progressive renal insufficiency.

Diabetic neuropathies Disorders of the peripheral nerves and the autonomic nervous system manifesting one or more of the following: sensory and motor impairment, muscle weakness and pain, cranial nerve disorders, impaired vasomotor function, impaired gastrointestinal function, and impaired genitourinary function.

Diabetic retinopathy The collective name for the changes in the retina that occur in the person with diabetes. The retinal capillary structure undergoes alterations in blood flow, leading to retinal ischemia and a breakdown in the blood retinal barrier.

Dialysate Dialysis solution.

Dialysis The diffusion of solute molecules across a semipermeable membrane from an area of higher concentration to one of lower concentration.

Diaphoresis Copious production of sweat.

Diarrhea An increase in the frequency, volume, and fluid content of the stool.

Diastolic blood pressure The minimum pressure maintained by elastic arterial walls during diastole (cardiac relaxation) to maintain blood flow through capillary beds; averages 80 mmHg in a healthy adult.

Differentiation A process occurring over many cell cycles that allows cells to specialize in certain tasks.

Diffuse brain injury (DBI) A brain injury from a high-speed acceleration–deceleration accident with widespread disruption of axons in the white matter.

Diffuse esophageal spasm Nonperistaltic contraction of esophageal smooth muscle.

Diffusion The process by which solute molecules move from an area of high solute concentration to an area of low solute concentration to become evenly distributed.

Dilemma A choice between two unpleasant, ethically troubling alternatives.

Diplopia Unilateral or bilateral double vision.

Disability The degree of observable and measurable impairment.

Disaster Event that requires extraordinary efforts beyond those needed to respond to everyday emergencies.

Disease Literally meaning "without ease," this term describes alterations in structure and function of the body or mind. Diseases may have mechanical, biologic, or normative causes.

Dislocation Separation of contact between two bones of a joint.

Dissection (aortic) A life-threatening emergency caused by a tear in the intima of the aorta with hemorrhage into the media.

Disseminated intravascular coagulation (DIC) A disruption of hemostasis characterized by widespread intravascular clotting and bleeding; a syndrome that develops as a complication of many other disorders.

Distributive shock Also called *vasogenic shock*, this includes several types of shock that result from widespread vasodilation and decreased peripheral resistance.

Diverticula Saclike projections of mucosa through the muscular layer of the colon.

Diverticulitis Inflammation in and around the diverticular sac; typically affects only one diverticulum, usually in the sigmoid colon.

Diverticulosis Indicates the presence of diverticula.

Dominant A characteristic or gene that is apparent even when the relevant gene is present in only one copy; a person with a dominant gene usually expresses that gene trait.

Do-not-resuscitate (DNR or "no-code") order Usually written by the physician for the patient who has a terminal illness or is near death, this order is usually based on the wishes of the patient and family that no cardiopulmonary resuscitation be performed for respiratory or cardiac arrest.

Dual diagnosis The coexistence of substance abuse/dependence and a psychiatric disorder in one individual (used interchangeably with *dual disorder* and *co-occurring disorders*).

Dual disorder See *Dual diagnosis*.

Dumping syndrome Complication of partial gastrectomy characterized by nausea, weakness, sweating, palpitation, syncope, sensation of warmth, and occasionally diarrhea.

Duodenal ulcers Peptic ulcer disease affecting the duodenum.

Durable power of attorney A document that can delegate the authority to make health, financial, and/or legal decisions on a person's behalf. It must be in writing and must state that the designated person is authorized to make healthcare decisions.

Dwarfism A condition characterized by short stature; insufficient pituitary growth hormone is one cause.

Dysarthria Difficulty speaking.

Dysfunctional uterine bleeding (DUB) Vaginal bleeding that is usually painless but abnormal in amount, duration, or time of occurrence.

Dysmenorrhea Pain associated with menstruation.

Dyspareunia Painful intercourse.

Dysphagia Difficulty swallowing.

Dysphonia Change in the tone of voice.

Dysplasia The loss of DNA control over differentiation occurring in response to adverse conditions.

Dyspnea Difficult or labored breathing.

Dysrhythmia Abnormal heart rate or rhythm.

Dysuria Painful urination.

Ecchymosis A flat, irregularly shaped lesion (bruise) of varying size with no pulsation; caused by blood collecting under skin.

Ectopic beats Impulses originating outside normal conduction pathways of the heart.

Edema Accumulation of fluid in the body's tissues; an excess accumulation of fluid in the interstitial space.

Ejection fraction (EF) The percentage of total blood remaining in the ventricle at the end of diastole (relaxation); normal is 50% to 70%.

Electrical bone stimulation Application of electrical current at the fracture site to treat fractures that are not healing appropriately. The electrical stress increases the migration of osteoblasts and osteoclasts to the fracture site. Mineral deposition increases, promoting bone healing.

Electrocardiography The graphic recording of the heart's electrical activity detected and recorded through electrodes placed on the surface of the body.

Electrolytes Substances that dissociate in solution to form charged particles called ions.

Electrosurgery The destruction or removal of tissue with high-frequency alternating current.

Embolic CVA Cerebrovascular accident occurring when a blood clot or clump of matter traveling through the cerebral blood vessels becomes lodged in a vessel too narrow to permit further movement.

Embolism Sudden obstruction of a blood vessel by a clot or debris.

Emergency Encompasses an unforeseen combination of circumstances calling for immediate action for a range of victims from one to many.

Emphysema Destruction of the walls of the alveoli, with resulting enlargement of abnormal air spaces.

Empyema Accumulation of purulent exudate in the pleural cavity.

Encephalitis An acute inflammation of the parenchyma of the brain or spinal cord.

End of life The final days or weeks of life when death is imminent.

Endocarditis Inflammation of the endocardium.

Endometriosis A condition in which multiple, small implants of endometrial tissue develop throughout the pelvic cavity.

Endoscopy Inspection of organs or cavities of the body using an endoscope.

Endotoxins Found in the cell wall of gram-negative bacteria, endotoxins are released only when the cell is disrupted. They act as activators of many human regulatory systems, producing fever, inflammation, and potentially clotting, bleeding, or hypotension when released in large quantities.

End-stage renal disease The final stage of chronic renal failure in which the kidneys are unable to excrete metabolic wastes and regulate fluid and electrolyte balance adequately; characterized by a glomerular filtration rate of less than 5% of normal.

Enophthalmos Sunken appearance of the eyes.

Enteral nutrition Administration of liquid nutritional formulas to meet calorie and protein needs in patients unable to consume adequate food; also called *tube feeding*.

Enucleation Surgical removal of an eye.

Epicondylitis (tennis elbow, golfer's elbow) Inflammation of the tendon at its point of origin into the bone.

Epididymitis Infection or inflammation of the epididymis.

Epidural hematoma (extradural hematoma) A collection of blood between the dura and the skull.

Epilepsy A disorder characterized by chronic seizure activity.

Epistaxis Nosebleed.

Equianalgesia/Equianalgesic Approximate equivalent doses of opioid analgesics as compared to morphine sulfate.

Erectile dysfunction Inability to attain and maintain an erection sufficient to permit satisfactory sexual intercourse.

Erosive gastritis See *Stress-induced (erosive gastritis)*.

Erysipelas Infection of the skin most often caused by group A *streptococci*.

Erythema A reddening of the skin.

Erythropoiesis Red blood cell production.

Eschar Hard, leathery crust that covers a burn wound and harbors necrotic tissue.

Escharotomy Surgical removal of eschar from the torso or extremity to prevent circumferential constriction.

Esophageal varices Enlarged, thin-walled veins that form in the submucosa of the esophagus.

Esophagojejunostomy Removal of the entire stomach with anastomosis of the distal esophagus to the jejunum.

Estrogen Hormone produced by the ovaries.

Ethics Principles of conduct. Ethical behavior is concerned with moral duty, values, obligations, and the distinction between right and wrong.

Euthanasia From the Greek for painless, easy, gentle, or good death, now commonly used to signify a killing prompted by a humanitarian motive.

Euthyroid Term describing normal thyroid hormone function.

Evisceration Protrusion of body contents through a surgical wound.

Exacerbation A period during chronic illness in which symptoms reappear.

Exfoliative dermatitis Inflammatory skin disorder characterized by excessive peeling or shedding of skin.

Exophthalmos Protrusion of the eyeballs.

Exotoxins Soluble proteins secreted into surrounding tissue by the microorganism. Exotoxins are highly poisonous, causing cell death or dysfunction.

External otitis Inflammation of the ear canal.

Extracapsular fractures Fractures of the trochanteric region.

Extracorporeal shock-wave lithotripsy (ESWL, transcutaneous shock-wave lithotripsy) Noninvasive technique for fragmenting kidney stones using shock waves generated outside the body.

Faith community nursing Also known as parish nursing, this is a nontraditional, community-based way of providing health promotion and health restoration nursing interventions to specific groups of people.

Family Two or more persons joined by emotional closeness and shared bonds and who identify themselves as being part of a family.

Fasciculations Involuntary twitching.

Fasciectomy (fascial excision) Process of excising the wound to the level of fascia.

Fat embolism syndrome (FES) Characterized by neurologic dysfunction, pulmonary insufficiency, and a petechial rash on the chest, axilla, and upper arms due to fat globules lodged in the pulmonary vascular bed or peripheral circulation.

Fecal impaction A rock-hard or putty-like mass of feces in the rectum.

Fecal incontinence Loss of voluntary control of defecation.

Fecalith A hard mass of feces.

Fibrocystic changes (FCC) Physiologic nodularity and breast tenderness that increases and decreases with the menstrual cycle.

Fibroid tumors (uterine leiomyoma) Solid benign tumors originating from smooth muscle of the uterus.

Fibromyalgia (fibrositis) A common rheumatic syndrome characterized by musculoskeletal pain, stiffness, and tenderness.

Filtration The process by which water and dissolved substances (solutes) move from an area of higher hydrostatic pressure to an area of lower hydrostatic pressure.

Fistula Abnormal opening or passage between two organs or spaces that are normally separated or an abnormal passage to the outside of the body.

Flaccidity Decreased muscle tone in disease or trauma of the lower motor neurons.

Flail chest Free-floating segment of the chest wall, resulting from two or more consecutive ribs fractured in multiple places.

Flap A piece of tissue whose free end is moved from a donor site to a recipient site while maintaining a continuous blood supply through its connection at the base or pedicle.

Flatus Gas in the digestive tract.

Fluid resuscitation Replacement of the extensive fluid and electrolyte losses associated with major burn injuries.

Fluid volume deficit (FVD) A decrease in intravascular, interstitial, and/or intracellular fluid in the body.

Fluid volume excess (FVE) Excess extracellular fluid resulting from retention of both water and sodium in the body.

Folic acid deficiency anemia An anemia resulting from folic acid deficiency, a necessary nutrient for DNA synthesis and RBC maturation.

Folliculitis Bacterial infection of the hair follicle, most commonly caused by *Staphylococcus aureus*.

Fracture A break in a bone usually due to trauma.

Freestanding outpatient surgical facilities Surgical units independent of a hospital with or without financial connections to a hospital or healthcare organization.

Friction rub The sound heard when two dry surfaces are rubbed together.

Frostbite An injury of the skin from freezing.

Full-thickness burn A burn that involves all layers of the skin, including the epidermis, dermis, and epidermal appendages.

Fulminant hepatitis Hepatitis with a rapid and severe onset and course.

Furuncle Often called a boil, but also an inflammation of the hair follicle.

Fusiform excision The removal of a full thickness of the epidermis and dermis, usually with a thin layer of subcutaneous tissue.

Galactorrhea Lactation not associated with pregnancy or nursing.

Gastric lavage Irrigation of the stomach with large quantities of normal saline.

Gastric mucosal barrier A protective barrier consisting of lipids, bicarbonate ions, and mucous gel that protects the stomach lining from the damaging effects of gastric juices.

Gastric outlet obstruction Obstruction of the pyloric region of the stomach and duodenum that impairs gastric outflow; a potential complication of peptic ulcer disease.

Gastric ulcers Ulcers of the stomach lining, usually in the lesser curvature and antrum; more common in older adults.

Gastritis Inflammation of the stomach lining.

Gastroduodenostomy (Billroth I) Excision of the pylorus of the stomach with the anastomosis of the upper stomach to the duodenum; commonly used partial gastrectomy procedure.

Gastroenteritis Inflammation of the gastrointestinal tract; not a specific disease, but a group of syndromes or a collection of related manifestations.

Gastroesophageal reflux Backward flow of gastric contents into the esophagus.

Gastroesophageal reflux disease (GERD) The reflux of acidic gastric contents into the lower esophagus.

Gastrojejunostomy (Billroth II) Subtotal excision of the stomach with closure of the duodenum and side-to-side anastomosis of the jejunum to the stomach; commonly used partial gastrectomy procedure.

Gastroparesis Slowed gastrointestinal motility, which causes early satiety.

Gene A sequence of DNA on a chromosome that represents a fundamental unit of heredity; occupies a specific spot on a chromosome (gene locus).

Gene expression When the protein product of a gene is visible (for example, through the presence of a body structure or identifiable through biochemical tests such as insulin or phenylalanine levels).

General anesthesia Deep sedation, which includes analgesia and muscle paralysis. This type of anesthesia requires respiratory maintenance without the aid of the patient's respiratory musculature.

Genital herpes (herpes simplex genitalis) An infection of the external genitalia caused by herpes simplex genitalis; transmitted by vaginal, anal, or oral–genital contact.

Genital warts (condyloma acuminatum, venereal warts) A sexually transmitted condition caused by the human papilloma virus.

Genotype The genes and the variations therein that a person inherits from his or her parents.

Germ cells Cells that give rise to a sperm or egg.

Gigantism Gigantism occurs when GH hypersecretion begins before puberty and the closure of the epiphyseal plates. The person becomes abnormally tall, often exceeding 7 ft (213 cm) in height, but body proportions are relatively normal.

Informed consent Disclosure of risks associated with the intended procedure or operation to the patient. The language of the document varies according to statutory and common law of each state.

Inhalants Inhaled solvents categorized into three types: anesthetics, volatile nitrites, and organic solvents.

Innate adaptive immunity Specific and nonspecific responses that prevent or limit the entry of invaders into the body, thereby limiting the extent of tissue damage and reducing the workload of the adaptive immune system.

Insulin A hormone that facilitates entry of glucose into fat and muscle cells for energy.

Insulin reaction Hypoglycemia in patients with type 1 diabetes mellitus.

Interdisciplinary care Care provided by members of the healthcare team in addition to medical professionals. Usually includes team members who address psychosocial and spiritual issues as well as physical care.

Intermittent claudication Cramping, aching ischemic pain in the calves, thighs, and buttocks that occurs with a predictable level of activity and is relieved by rest.

Intracerebral hematomas A collection of blood in the brain tissue, most often located in the frontal or temporal lobes.

Intracranial aneurysm Saccular outpouching of a cerebral artery that occurs at the site of a weakness in the vessel wall.

Intracranial hypertension See *Increased intracranial pressure.*

Intracranial pressure (ICP) The pressure within the cranial cavity, usually measured as the pressure within the lateral ventricles.

Intraductal papilloma A tiny wartlike growth on the inside of the peripheral mammary duct that causes discharge from the nipple.

Intraoperative phase The time during surgery, from beginning to end.

Iron deficiency anemia The most common type of anemia; results from inadequate iron for optimal RBC formation.

Irritable bowel syndrome (IBS) A motility disorder of the gastrointestinal tract characterized by alternating periods of constipation and diarrhea.

Ischemia Deficient blood flow to tissue resulting in reduced oxygen delivery.

Ischemic Deprived of oxygen.

Islets of Langerhans Hormone-producing cells (alpha cells, beta cells, and delta cells) scattered through the pancreas.

Isograft Tissue transplant where the donor and recipient are identical twins.

Jaundice Yellow-to-orange color visible in the skin and mucous membranes; most often the result of a hepatic disorder.

Joint arthroplasty Reconstruction or replacement of a joint.

Kaposi's sarcoma (KS) A vascular malignancy (a tumor of the endothelial cells lining small blood vessels) that presents as vascular macules, papules, or violet lesions affecting the skin and viscera. It is often the presenting symptom of AIDS.

Keloid Elevated, irregularly shaped, progressively enlarging scar arising from excessive amounts of collagen in the stratum corneum during scar formation in connective tissue repair.

Keratitis Inflammation of the cornea.

Keratin Keratin is a fibrous, water-repellent protein that gives the epidermis its tough, protective quality.

Keratosis Any skin condition in which there is a benign overgrowth and thickening of the cornified epithelium.

Ketoacidosis A condition of very high blood glucose and insufficient insulin that results in accumulation of ketones and fatty acids in the blood; a form of metabolic acidosis.

Ketonuria The presence of ketones in the urine.

Ketosis An accumulation of ketone bodies produced during the oxidation of fatty acids.

Kindling Long-term changes in brain neurotransmission that occur after repeated detoxifications.

Kinesthesia The ability to perceive movement and sense of position.

Korotkoff's sounds Sounds heard during auscultation of blood pressure.

Korsakoff's psychosis Secondary dementia caused by thiamine (B_1) deficiency that may be associated with chronic alcoholism; characterized by progressive cognitive deterioration, confabulation, peripheral neuropathy, and myopathy.

Kussmaul's respirations Deep, rapid respirations associated with compensatory mechanisms.

Kwashiorkor (protein energy malnutrition, PEM) Chronic protein deficiency with adequate calories to meet body needs.

Kyphosis Exaggerated thoracic curvature of the spine, common in older adults.

Labyrinthectomy Surgical removal of the labyrinth.

Labyrinthitis Inflammation of the inner ear.

Laceration Open wound that results from sharp cutting or tearing. Injuries to the integument are at risk for contamination from dirt, debris, or foreign objects.

Lacunar strokes Thrombotic stroke of smaller cerebral blood vessels in deeper parts of the brain or brain stem.

Laminectomy Removal of the lamina of the vertebrae.

Laparoscopic cholecystectomy Removal of the gallbladder using an endoscope.

Laryngectomy Removal of the larynx.

Laryngitis Inflammation of the larynx.

Leiomyoma See *Fibroid tumor.*

Leukemia A group of chronic malignant disorders of white blood cells and WBC precursors; characterized by replacement of bone marrow by malignant immature WBCs, abnormal immature circulating WBCs, and infiltration of malignant cells into other tissues.

Leukocytes Also called white blood cells, these are the primary cells involved in both nonspecific and specific immune system responses. These cells isolate the infecting organism or injury, destroy pathogens, and promote healing.

Leukocytosis An increase in the number of leukocytes in the blood (above $10,/mm^3$), usually caused by infection.

Leukopenia Abnormal decrease of circulating leukocytes, usually below $5/mm^3$; occurs when bone marrow activity is suppressed or when leukocyte destruction increases.

Leukoplakia Formation of white patches or spots on the mucous membranes or tongue; these lesions may become malignant.

Libido Sexual desire.

Lichen planus Benign inflammatory disorder of the mucous membranes and skin.

Lift A more sustained thrust than normal.

Lipoatrophy Atrophy of subcutaneous tissue.

Liposuction A method of changing the contours of the body by aspirating fat from the subcutaneous layer of tissue.

Lithiasis Stone formation.

Lithotripsy Crushing of renal calculi.

Living will A document that provides written directions about life-prolonging procedures to provide instructions when a person can no longer communicate in a life-threatening situation.

Lobectomy Surgical removal of a single lobe of lung.

Locked-in syndrome Patient is alert and fully aware of the environment, but is unable to communicate through speech or movement as a result of blocked efferent pathways to the brain.

Lordosis Increased lumbar curve.

Loss Loss may be defined as an actual or potential situation in which a valued object, person, body part, or emotion that was formerly present is lost or changed and can no longer be seen, felt, heard, known, or experienced. A loss may be temporary or permanent, complete or partial, objectively verifiable or perceived, physical or symbolic.

Lower body obesity (peripheral obesity) A waist-to-hip ratio of less than 0.8 in an obese individual.

Lung abscess Localized area of lung destruction or necrosis and pus formation.

Lung compliance Distensibility of the lungs.

Lyme disease An inflammatory disorder caused by a spirochete, *Borrelia burgdorferi*, which is transmitted primarily by ticks.

Lymphadenopathy The enlargement of lymph nodes (over 1 cm) with or without tenderness. It may be caused by inflammation, infection, or malignancy of the nodes or the regions drained by the nodes.

Lymphangitis Inflammation of a lymphatic vessel.

Lymphedema Edema of an extremity due to accumulated lymph; may be primary or secondary, resulting from inflammation, obstruction, or removal of lymphatic vessels.

Lymphocytes Lymphocytes account for 20% to 40% of circulating leukocytes. Lymphocytes are the principal effector and regulator cells of specific immune responses.

Lymphoid tissues Connective tissues containing lymphocytes; include tissues of the bone marrow, thymus, lymph nodes, and spleen.

Lymphoma Malignancy of lymphoid tissue.

Macrophages Monocytes mature into macrophages after settling into tissue. Macrophages are large phagocytes. They are important in the body's defense against chronic infections.

Macular degeneration Destructive changes in the macula due to injury or gradual failure of the outer pigmented layer of the retina (the retinal layer adjacent to the choroid), which removes cellular waste products and keeps the retina attached to the choroid.

Malabsorption A condition in which nutrients are ineffectively absorbed by the intestinal mucosa, resulting in their excretion in the stool.

Malignant hypertension A hypertensive emergency, marked by a diastolic pressure greater than 120 mmHg.

Malignant melanoma (cutaneous melanoma) Skin cancer that arises from melanocytes.

Malignant pain Pain associated with a life-threatening illness such as cancer but not limited to cancer pain.

Malnutrition Inadequate nutrient intake to meet body needs; may include deficiency of major nutrients (calories, carbohydrates, proteins, and fats) or micronutrients such as vitamins and minerals.

Manifestations Signs and symptoms of a disease or condition caused by alterations in structure or function.

Man-made disasters Either accidental or intentional, they are complex emergencies, technological disasters, material shortages, and other disasters not caused by natural hazards.

Marasmus (protein energy undernutrition) Insufficient protein and calorie intake to meet metabolic needs.

Mass casualty incidents Situations in which 100 or more casualties are involved, significantly overwhelming available emergency medical services, facilities, and resources.

Mastoidectomy Surgical removal of infected mastoid air cells.

Mastoiditis Bacterial infection of the mastoid process.

Maturity onset diabetes of the young (MODY) Diabetes in young obese adults.

Mean arterial pressure (MAP) The average pressure in the arterial circulation throughout the cardiac cycle; the product of cardiac output and systemic vascular resistance (SVR).

Medical-surgical nursing The health promotion, health care, and illness care of adults, based on knowledge derived from the arts and sciences and shaped by knowledge (the science) of nursing.

Meiosis The reduction of division of the cell occurring only in the sex cells of the testes and ovaries when the amount of genetic material is reduced in half (23 chromosomes).

Melanin Skin pigment that forms a protective shield to protect keratinocytes and nerve endings in the dermis from the damaging effects of ultraviolet light.

Melena Black, tarry stool that contains old, digested blood.

Ménière's disease Chronic disorder of unknown cause characterized by recurrent attacks of vertigo with tinnitus and a progressive unilateral hearing loss.

Meningitis Inflammation of the meninges of the brain and spinal cord.

Menopause Permanent cessation of menses.

Menorrhagia Excessive or prolonged menstruation.

Menstrual cycle Cyclic buildup of the uterine lining, ovulation, and sloughing of the lining occurring approximately every 28 days in nonpregnant females of childbearing age.

Menstruation Periodic shedding of the uterine lining in a woman of childbearing age who is not pregnant.

Metabolism Consisting of the breakdown of complex structures into simpler forms to produce energy (catabolism) and the combination of simpler molecules to produce and maintain more complex structures necessary to living organisms (anabolism).

Metaplasia A change in the normal pattern of differentiation such that dividing cells differentiate into cell types not normally found in that location in the body.

Metastasis Secondary tumor; the process by which spreading of malignant neoplasms occurs; the transfer of disease from one organ or part to another not directly connected with it.

Methcillin-resistant *Staphylococcus aureus* (MRSA) A strain of antibiotic-resistant *S. aureus* that colonizes the skin and nares.

Metrorrhagia Bleeding between menstrual periods; may be caused by hormonal imbalances, pelvic inflammatory disease, cervical or uterine polyps, uterine fibroids, or cervical or uterine cancer.

Microalbuminuria Protein in the urine.

Micturition Releasing urine from the urinary bladder (voiding).

Mild concussion Brain trauma resulting in a brief loss of consciousness that lasts from seconds to hours.

Minor trauma Injury to a single part or system of the body, usually treated in the hospital or emergency department.

Mitigation The action taken to prevent or reduce the harmful effects of a disaster on human health or property, it involves future-oriented activities to prevent subsequent disasters or to minimize their effects.

Mitosis The process of making new cells by cell division. Cell division through mitosis results in two cells called *daughter cells* that are genetically identical to the original cell, or *mother cell*, and to each other.

Mitral valve (bicuspid valve) Valve between the left atrium and ventricle in the heart; prevents blood from flowing backwards into the atrium.

Monosomic (monosomy) When one member of the chromosome pair is missing, for example, Turner syndrome (45, XO).

Morbid obesity Weight greater than 100% over ideal body weight.

Morton's neuroma A tumor-like mass formed within the neurovascular bundle of the intermetatarsal spaces.

Mosaicism A chromosome variation or abnormality that occurs after fertilization during mitosis at an early cell stage so not all cells are affected with the variation; for example, a child who is mosaic for Down syndrome will have some cells with two copies of chromosome 21 and some that have an extra chromosome 21.

Mourning The actions or expressions of the bereaved, including the symbols, clothing, and ceremonies that make up the outward manifestations of grief.

Multifactorial Health conditions determined by multiple factors, including genetic and environmental factors, each having an additive effect.

Multiple casualty incidents Incidents in which more than 2 but fewer than 100 persons are injured.

Multiple myeloma A malignancy in which plasma cells multiply uncontrollably and infiltrate the bone marrow, lymph nodes, spleen, and other tissues.

Multiple sclerosis (MS) A chronic demyelating autoimmune disease of the central nervous system.

Multiple trauma Most often the result of a motor vehicle crash, this type of trauma requires immediate intervention specifically focused on ensuring survival.

Murmur Sound made by turbulent blood flow through the heart.

Muscular dystrophy (MD) A group of inherited muscle diseases that cause progressive muscle degeneration and wasting.

Myasthenia gravis Chronic, progressive neuromuscular disorder characterized by fatigue and severe weakness of skeletal muscles.

Myelodysplastic syndrome A group of blood disorders characterized by abnormal-appearing bone marrow and cytopenia (low numbers of circulating blood cells). MDS is not a single disease; at least five variations of the disorder have been identified.

Myocarditis Inflammatory disorder of the heart muscle.

Myopia (nearsightedness) A condition in which the eyeball is elongated, causing the image to focus in front of the retina instead of on it.

Myringotomy Incision of the tympanic membrane.

Myxedema Systemic condition that develops from inadequate levels of thyroid hormone (hypothyroidism).

Myxedema coma A life-threatening complication of long-standing, untreated hypothyroidism, characterized by severe metabolic disorders (hyponatremia, hypoglycemia, lactic acidosis), hypothermia, cardiovascular collapse, impaired cognition, and coma.

Natural disasters Disasters caused by acts of nature or emerging diseases; some are unexpected and some are predictable through advanced meteorological technologies.

Natural killer cells (NK cells, null cells) Large, granular lymphocytes (found in the spleen, lymph nodes, bone marrow, and blood) that provide immune surveillance and resistance to infection, and play an important role in the destruction of early malignant cells.

Nausea An unpleasant sensation of sickness or queasiness; may or may not be followed by vomiting.

Necrosis Tissue cell death.

Neglect syndrome (unilateral neglect) A disorder of attention. In this syndrome, the person cannot integrate and use perceptions from the affected side of the body or from the environment on the affected side and, hence, ignores that part.

Neoplasm A mass of new tissue (a collection of cells) that grows independently of its surrounding structures and has no physiologic purpose.

Nephrectomy Removal of the kidney.

Nephrotic syndrome A condition marked by massive proteinuria, hypoalbuminemia, hyperlipidemia, and edema.

Neuralgia Nerve pain.

Neurogenic bladder Dysfunctional urinary bladder due to lesion of central or peripheral nervous system.

Neurogenic shock Shock resulting from an imbalance between parasympathetic and sympathetic stimulation of vascular smooth muscle. If parasympathetic overstimulation or sympathetic understimulation persists, sustained vasodilation occurs, and blood pools in the venous and capillary beds.

Neuropathic pain Pain resulting from abnormal impulse processing by the peripheral and central nervous systems following injury to the peripheral nerves.

Neuropathy Damage to peripheral nerves causing hyper- or hyposensation and leading to neuropathic pain and injury.

Neutropenia A decrease in circulating neutrophils.

Nevi (moles) Flat or raised macules or papules with rounded, well-defined borders.

Nicotine Nicotine, a stimulant, is found in tobacco and enters the system via the lungs (cigarettes and cigars) and oral mucous membranes (chewing tobacco as well as smoking).

Nociceptive pain Pain caused by stimulation of peripheral or visceral pain receptors.

Nociceptors Sensory nerve fibers that conduct pain impulses from the periphery to the central nervous system.

Nocturia Voiding two or more times at night.

Node Elements of the immune system connected by lymphatics. Upregulates immune function; does not synthesize hormones.

Nonconventional terrorist weapons Chemical, biological, and nuclear weapons of terrorism; used less frequently than conventional terrorist weapons.

Non-Hodgkin's lymphoma (NHL) Lymphoid tissue malignancies that do not contain Reed–Sternberg cells.

Nonunion A state that exists when the ends of a fracture fail to heal together.

Normal sinus rhythm (NSR) Normal heart rhythm, in which impulses originate in the sinus node and travel through normal conduction pathways without delay.

Nosocomial Pertaining to or occurring in a hospital.

Nosocomial infection Infection contracted during residence in a hospital or extended care facility.

Nuclear terrorism Use of a nuclear device to cause mass murder and devastation.

Nursing process The series of critical thinking activities nurses use as they provide care to patients; this logical approach to care ensures that patients receive comprehensive and effective care.

Nutrients Substances found in food that are used by the body to promote growth, maintenance, and repair.

Nutrition The process by which the body ingests, absorbs, transports, uses, and eliminates food.

Nystagmus Rapid involuntary eye movements.

Obesity An excess of body fat (adipose tissue).

Obstructive shock Shock caused by an obstruction in the heart or great vessels that either impedes venous return or prevents effective cardiac pumping action.

Occult blood/bleeding Blood or bleeding that is hidden or not readily apparent.

Office-based surgical suites A setting for many elective surgeries, although increasing malpractice insurance premiums have influenced their decline.

Oligomenorrhea Scant menses.

Oliguria Urine output of less than 400 mL in 24 hours.

Oncogene Gene capable of triggering cancerous characteristics.

Oncologic emergencies In caring for patients with cancer, nurses may encounter a number of emergency situations in which their role may be pivotal to the patient's survival. Most of these emergencies require astute observations, accurate judgments, and rapid action once the problem has been identified.

Oncology The study of cancer.

Onycholysis The separation of the distal nail plate from the nail bed.

Onychomycosis A fungal or dermatophyte infection of the nail plate.

Opiates Analgesics derived from the opium plant; produce analgesia by binding to opioid receptors within and outside the CNS; the most potent analgesics available, and the treatment of choice for acute moderate-to-severe pain. Examples include morphine, codeine, and fentanyl (Durgesic, Actiq). Also called narcotic analgesics.

Orchitis Infection or inflammation of the testicle.

Orthopnea Difficulty breathing when supine.

Orthostatic hypotension A decrease in systolic blood pressure of more than 10 to 15 mmHg and a drop in diastolic blood pressure on standing.

Osmosis The process by which water moves across a selectively permeable membrane from an area of lower solute concentration to an area of higher solute concentration.

Ossification The process of bone formation.

Osteitis deformans See *Paget's disease of bone*.

Osteoarthritis (OA) (degenerative joint disease) The most commonly occurring of all forms of arthritis. This disease is characterized by loss of articular cartilage in articulating joints and hypertrophy of the bones at the articular margins.

Osteomalacia (adult rickets) Metabolic bone disorder characterized by inadequate mineralization of bone matrix.

Osteomyelitis Infection within the bone that can lead to tissue death and necrosis.

Osteophytes Bony outgrowths often called "joint mice."

Osteoporosis Literally defined as "porous bones," a metabolic bone disorder characterized by loss of bone mass, increased bone fragility, and an increased risk of fractures.

Osteotomy An incision into or transection of the bone.

Ostomy General term for an operation in which an artificial opening is created.

Otitis media Inflammation or infection of the middle ear.

Otorrhea Leakage of cerebrospinal fluid through the ear.

Otosclerosis Abnormal bone formation in the osseous labyrinth of the temporal bone causing the footplate of the stapes to become fixed or immobile in the oval window. The result is a conductive hearing loss.

Ovarian cycle The female cycle that occurs from puberty until menopause in which the production of ova occur.

Oxyhemoglobin The combined form of hemoglobin and oxygen; found in arterial blood, it carries oxygen to body tissues.

Pacemaker A pulse generator used to provide an electrical stimulus to the heart when the heart fails to generate or conduct its own at a rate that maintains the cardiac output.

PaCO₂ Partial pressure of carbon dioxide in arterial blood.

Paget's disease of bone (osteitis deformans) A skeletal disorder that results from excessive osteoclastic activity. Paget's disease is characterized by bone deformity, especially of the long bones of the lower limbs, the pelvis, the lumbar vertebrae, and the skull.

Pain A subjective response to both physical and psychologic stressors.

Pain threshold The point at which a stimulus elicits a pain response.

Pain tolerance The amount of pain a person can endure before responding to it.

Palliative care An area of care that has evolved out of the hospice experience, but exists outside of hospice programs and is not restricted to the end of life. Palliative care is focused on the relief of physical, mental, and spiritual distress for individuals who have an incurable illness and is used earlier in the disease experience than hospice care. The goal of palliative care is to prevent and relieve suffering by early assessment and treatment of pain and other physical, psychosocial, and spiritual needs to improve the patient's quality of life.

Pallor Lack of color; paleness of skin.

Pancreatitis Inflammation of the pancreas.

Pannus Granulation tissue that forms in joints affected by rheumatoid arthritis and leads to the formation of scar tissue that immobilizes the joint.

PaO₂ Partial pressure of oxygen in arterial blood.

Papilledema Swelling of the optic nerve.

Paracentesis Aspiration of fluid from the peritoneal cavity.

Paralytic ileus Impaired propulsion or forward movement of bowel contents.

Paraplegia Paralysis of the lower portion of the body, sometimes involving the lower trunk.

Parasites Organisms that live within, on, or at the expense of the patient.

Parenteral nutrition (PN or TPN) Intravenous administration of carbohydrates (high concentrations of dextrose), protein (amino acids), electrolytes, vitamins, minerals, and fat emulsions.

Paresthesia An abnormal sensation of the skin, such as numbness, burning, or pricking.

Parish nursing A nontraditional, community-based way of providing health promotion and health restoration nursing interventions to a spiritual community.

Parkinson's disease (PD) Progressive, degenerative neurologic disease characterized by nonintentional tremor, bradykinesia, and muscle rigidity.

Paronychia An infection of the cuticle of the fingernails or toenails.

Paroxysmal Abrupt onset and termination.

Paroxysmal nocturnal dyspnea (PND) Attacks of acute shortness of breath that occur at night, waking up the patient.

Partial gastrectomy Removal of a portion of the stomach, usually the distal half to two-thirds.

Partial seizures Seizures that involve a restricted part of one cerebral hemisphere; may be simple partial (without loss of consciousness) or complex partial (with loss of consciousness).

Partial-thickness burn Burn that involves the entire dermis and the papillae of the dermis (superficial partial-thickness burn) or extends into the hair follicles (deep partial-thickness burn).

Passive immunity Temporary protection—provided by antibodies produced by other people or animals—against disease-producing antigens. Protection is gradually lost when these acquired antibodies are used up either by natural degradation or by combining with the antigen.

Pathogens Virulent organisms rarely found in the absence of disease.

Patient The person with whom and for whom nursing care is designed and implemented.

Patient-controlled analgesia (PCA) A pump with a control mechanism that allows the patient to self-manage pain.

Pediculosis capitis An infestation with head lice.

Pediculosis corporis An infestation with body lice.

Pediculosis pubis An infestation with pubic lice (often called "crabs").

Pelvic inflammatory disease (PID) A term used to describe infection of the pelvic organs.

Pemphigus vulgaris Chronic disorder of the skin and oral mucous membranes characterized by vesicle (blister) formation.

Penetrance The percentage or likelihood that an individual who has inherited a gene mutation will actually express the disease signs and symptoms in his or her lifetime.

Penicillin-resistant *Streptococcus pneumoniae* (PRSP) Infection transmitted by droplets from the respiratory tract; requires transmission-based droplet precautions.

Peptic ulcer/peptic ulcer disease (PUD) A break in the mucous lining of the gastrointestinal tract where it comes in contact with gastric juice; may affect any area of the gastrointestinal tract exposed to acid-pepsin secretions, including the esophagus, stomach, or duodenum.

Pericarditis Inflammation of the pericardium.

Perioperative nursing A specialized area of nursing practice that incorporates the three phases of the surgical experience: preoperative, intraoperative, and postoperative.

Peripheral vascular disease (PVD) Impaired blood supply to peripheral tissues, particularly the lower extremities.

Peripheral vascular resistance (PVR) The opposing forces or impedance to blood flow as the arterial channels become more and more distant from the heart.

Peristalsis Alternating waves of contraction and relaxation of involuntary muscles.

Peritoneal dialysis Procedure in which electrolytes, waste products, and excess water are removed from the body by diffusion using the peritoneum surrounding the abdominal cavity as the dialyzing membrane.

Peritonitis Inflammation of the peritoneum.

Pernicious anemia Anemia resulting from failure to absorb dietary vitamin B_{12} due to lack of intrinsic factor.

Persistent vegetative state (PVS) Condition of complete unawareness of self and the environment.

Personal protective equipment (PPE) Equipment used for the protection of personnel including gloves, masks, goggles, gowns, and biologic disposal bags (red bags); may also include hoods, helmets, head gear, and impermeable suits.

Pertussis (whooping cough) A highly contagious acute upper respiratory infection caused by the bacterium *Bordetella pertussis.*

Phagocytosis A process by which a foreign agent or target cell is engulfed, destroyed, and digested. Neutrophils and macrophages, known as phagocytes, are the primary cells involved in phagocytosis.

Phantom limb pain A confusing pain syndrome that occurs following surgical or traumatic amputation of a limb. The patient experiences pain in the missing body part even though there is complete mental awareness that the limb is gone.

Pharyngitis Acute inflammation of the pharynx.

Phenotype The expression of a person's entire physical, biochemical, and physiologic makeup, as determined by the individual's genotype and environmental factors.

Phimosis Constriction of the foreskin so that it cannot be retracted over the glans penis.

Plasmapheresis (plasma exchange) Removal of the plasma component from whole blood.

Plastic surgery The alteration, replacement, or restoration of visible portions of the body, performed to correct a structural or cosmetic defect.

Platelets (thrombocytes) Cell fragments that have no nucleus and cannot replicate.

Pleural effusion Collection of excess fluid in the pleural space.

Pleuritis Inflammation of the pleura.

Pneumonectomy Removal of an entire lung.

Pneumonia Inflammation of the lung parenchyma (the respiratory bronchioles and alveoli).

Pneumothorax Results when air enters the pleural space due to blunt and penetrating injuries to the chest.

Polycystic kidney disease A hereditary disease characterized by cyst formation and massive kidney enlargement.

Polycythemia (erythrocytosis) Excess RBCs characterized by a hematocrit higher than 55%.

Polydipsia Excessive thirst.

Polymorphisms The DNA sequences that are natural variations in a gene usually having no adverse effects on the individual.

Polymyositis A systemic connective-tissue disorder characterized by inflammation of connective tissue and muscle fibers leading to muscle weakness and atrophy.

Polyp Mass of tissue that arises from the bowel wall and protrudes into the lumen.

Polyphagia Excessive eating.

Polysubstance abuse The simultaneous use of many substances.

Polyuria Excessive output of urine.

Portal hypertension Elevated pressure in the portal venous system that causes rerouting of blood to adjoining lower pressure vessels.

Portal systemic (hepatic) encephalopathy Impaired consciousness and mental status due to the accumulation of toxic waste products in the blood (ammonia in particular) as blood bypasses the congested liver.

Postconcussion syndrome Persistent headache, dizziness, irritability, insomnia, impaired memory and concentration, and learning problems following a concussion; may last for several weeks or up to 1 year.

Postoperative phase Period when a procedure or surgery has been completed and the patient is recovering from the stress associated with the surgery.

Postpoliomyelitis syndrome A complication of a previous infection by the poliomyelitis virus.

Preload The amount of cardiac muscle fiber tension or stretch that exists at end diastole, just before ventricular contraction.

Premature ejaculation A common ejaculatory disorder in which semen is ejaculated before completion of sexual intercourse.

Premenstrual syndrome (PMS) Complex of symptoms characterized by irritability, depression, edema, and breast tenderness preceding the monthly menses.

Preoperative phase Time when preparation of the patient for surgery is conducted and completed.

Preparedness Actions that address preparations for and actions in dealing with the consequences of a disaster.

Presbycusis Age-related loss of the ability to hear high-frequency sounds, may occur because of cochlear hair cell degeneration or loss of auditory neurons in the organ of Corti.

Presbyopia Impaired near vision resulting from a loss of elasticity of the lens of the eye.

Pressure ulcer Ischemic lesion of the skin and underlying tissue caused by external pressure that impairs the flow of blood and lymph.

Priapism Sustained, painful erection that lasts at least 4 hours and is not associated with sexual arousal.

Primary hypertension (idiopathic, essential) A persistently elevated systemic blood pressure.

Primary polycythemia (polycythemia vera) A neoplastic stem cell disorder characterized by overproduction of red blood cells and, to a lesser extent, white blood cells and platelets.

Professional boundaries The borders between the vulnerability of the patient and the power of the nurse.

Progesterone Hormone produced by the ovary; works with estrogen to control the menstrual cycle.

Proptosis Forward displacement of the eye.

Prostatitis Inflammation of the prostate gland.

Protein-calorie malnutrition (PCM) Deficient protein and calories to meet metabolic needs.

Proteinuria Abnormal proteins in the urine.

Proto-oncogenes Normal genes that promote cell growth and repair.

Pruritus Subjective itching sensation producing an urge to scratch.

Psoriasis Chronic, noninfectious skin disorder that is characterized by raised, reddened, round circumscribed plaques covered by silvery white scales.

Psychogenic pain Pain that is experienced in the absence of any diagnosed physiologic cause or event.

Psychostimulants Psychostimulants such as cocaine and amphetamines have a high potential for abuse. Euphoria is the main subjective effect associated with cocaine and amphetamines, leading to addiction.

Ptosis Drooping of the eyelid.

Pulmonary edema An abnormal accumulation of fluid in the interstitial tissue and alveoli of the lung.

Pulmonary embolism Sudden occlusion of blood flow in a portion of the pulmonary vascular system, causing a ventilation-perfusion imbalance and impaired gas exchange.

Pulmonary hypertension Condition in which the pulmonary arterial pressure is elevated to an abnormal level.

Pulmonic valve The semilunar valve between the right ventricle and the pulmonary artery.

Pulse Rhythmic pressure wave that can be felt over an artery.

Pulse deficit Condition in which the radial pulse is less than the apical pulse, indicating weak, inefficient left ventricular contractions.

Pulse pressure The difference between the systolic and diastolic blood pressure.

Puncture wound Wound that occurs when a sharp or blunt object penetrates the integument.

Pupillary light reflex Reflex in which the pupil contracts in response to a bright light.

Pyelonephritis Upper urinary tract inflammation affecting the kidney and renal pelvis.

Pyoderma Purulent bacterial infection of skin.

Pyuria Pus in the urine.

Quadriplegia See *Tetraplegia*.

Quality assurance The process of ensuring quality control activities that evaluate, monitor, or regulate the standard of services provided to the consumer.

Rabies Viral (rhabdovirus) infection of the central nervous system transmitted by infected saliva that enters the human body through a bite or an open wound.

Radiation sickness One of the results of DNA mutation inside cells exposed to ionizing radiation.

Radiation therapy Therapy that uses radiation to kill a tumor, to reduce its size, to decrease pain, or to relieve obstruction.

Radiculopathy A condition in which one or more nerves, especially nerve roots, do not function normally

Radiological dispersion bomb Also called a "dirty bomb," it consists of a conventional explosive such as trinitrotoluene (TNT) packed with radioactive waste by-products from nuclear reactors that discharges deadly radioactive particles into the environment.

Raynaud's disease/phenomenon Disorders characterized by episodes of intense vasospasm in the small arteries and arterioles of the fingers and possibly the toes.

Reactive arthritis (Reiter's syndrome) An acute, nonpurulent inflammatory arthritis that complicates a bacterial infection of the genitourinary or gastrointestinal tracts.

Rebound tenderness Pain that occurs with withdrawal or release of pressure applied during abdominal palpation.

Recessive A characteristic that is apparent only when two copies of the gene encoding it are present, one from the mother and one from the father.

Reconstruction The recovery aspect of disaster response; during this period restoration, reconstitution, and mitigation take place.

Recovery The fifth of 5 stages of disaster. Activities include rebuilding and returning to some semblance of "normalcy" but also includes mitigation activities or planning to prevent subsequent disasters or to minimize the effects of future disasters.

Red blood cell (RBCs, erythrocytes) Blood cells shaped like a biconcave disk that contain hemoglobin required for oxygen transport to body tissues; the most common type of blood cell.

Referral source A person recommending home care services and supplying the agency with details about the patient's needs. The source may be a physician, nurse, social worker, therapist, or discharge planner.

Referred pain Pain that is perceived in an area distant from the site of the stimuli.

Reflex sympathetic dystrophy A group of poorly understood posttraumatic conditions involving persistent pain, hyperesthesias, swelling, changes in skin color and texture, changes in temperature, and decreased motion.

Reflux, urinary Backflow of urine toward the kidneys.

Refraction The bending of light rays as they pass from one medium to another medium of different optical density.

Refractory period A period in which myocardial cells are resistant to stimulation.

Regional anesthesia Anesthesia that desensitizes the area to be operated but does not involve the full central nervous system or cause sedation.

Regurgitation (valvular) Backflow of blood through an incompletely closed valve into the area it just left.

Rehabilitation The process of learning to live to one's maximum potential with a chronic impairment and its resultant functional disability.

Reiter's syndrome See *Reactive arthritis*.

Remission A period in which symptoms are not experienced even though the disease is still clinically present.

Renal artery stenosis Narrowing of the renal artery.

Renal colic Acute, severe, intermittent pain in the flank and upper outer abdominal quadrant generally associated with acute obstruction of a ureter and resulting ureteral spasm.

Renal failure A condition in which the kidneys are unable to remove accumulated metabolites from the blood, resulting in altered fluid, electrolyte, and acid–base balance.

Renal impairment (decreased renal reserve) A glomerular filtration rate of approximately 50% of normal with normal BUN and serum creatinine levels.

Renal insufficiency A glomerular filtration rate of 20% to 50% of normal with azotemia and some manifestations of renal failure.

Renal transplant The surgical insertion of a functioning kidney.

Renin–angiotensin mechanism An intrinsic system that responds to renal perfusion; a fall in renal blood flow (e.g. due to low BP or cardiac output) stimulates renin release, ultimately leading to vasoconstriction and sodium and water retention and increased BP and cardiac output.

Repolarization Restoration of the resting cell membrane potential following generation of an action potential.

Respiratory failure Inability of lungs to oxygenate the blood and remove carbon dioxide adequately to meet the body's needs, even at rest.

Respite care Short-term or intermittent home care, often using volunteers. These services exist to give the primary caregiver some relief from the burden of full-time care.

Response Occurs in the emergency stage of disaster response, after the impact of the disaster event has occurred, the community has been rapidly assessed for damage, and the types and extent of injuries suffered as well as the immediate needs of the community have been determined.

Reticular activating system (RAS) A system of reticular neurons within the reticular formation that passes steady streams of impulses through thalamic relays in order to stimulate the cerebral cortex into wakefulness.

Retinal detachment Separation of the retina or sensory portion of the eye from the choroid.

Retinitis pigmentosa Hereditary degenerative disease characterized by retinal atrophy and loss of retinal function progressing from the periphery to the central region of the retina.

Retractions A pulling in of the tissue of the precordium; a slight retraction just medial to the midclavicular line at the area of the apical impulse is normal and is more likely to be visible in thin patients.

Retrograde ejaculation Seminal fluid discharged into the bladder.

Reverse triage Working from the principle of the greatest good for the greatest number, reverse triage is an "upside-down triage" used in mass casualty events in which the victims who are most severely injured, requiring extensive resources with little chance of surviving, are treated last.

Rheumatic disorders Inflammatory diseases of connective tissues that affect joints, the muscles, and bones.

Rheumatic fever A systemic inflammatory disease caused by an abnormal immune response to pharyngeal infection by group A beta-hemolytic streptococci.

Rheumatic heart disease (RHD) Slowly progressive valvular deformity following acute or repeated attacks of rheumatic fever; characterized by rigid and deformed valve leaflets, fused valve commissures, and fibrosis of chordae tendineae.

Rheumatoid arthritis A chronic systemic autoimmune disease that causes inflammation of connective tissue, primarily in the joints.

Rhinitis Inflammation of the nasal cavities.

Rhinoplasty Surgical reconstruction of the nose.

Rhinorrhea Leakage of cerebrospinal fluid through the nose.

Ruptured disk See *Herniated intervertebral disk*.

Salmonellosis A form of food poisoning caused by ingestion of foods contaminated with one or more varieties of *Salmonella* bacteria.

Sarcoidosis Systemic disease characterized by granulomas in the lungs, lymph nodes, liver, eyes, skin, and other organs.

Sarcoma A tumor arising from supportive tissues.

Scabies Parasitic infestation caused by the mite *Sarcoptes scabiei*.

Sciatica Pain over the sciatic nerve.

Scleroderma (systemic sclerosis) Hardening of the skin, a chronic condition characterized by the formation of excess fibrous connective tissue and diffuse fibrosis of the skin and internal organs.

Sclerotherapy The removal of benign skin lesions with a sclerosing agent that causes inflammation with fibrosis of tissue.

Scoliosis A lateral curvature of the spine.

Scrub person Prepares the sterile field, surgical supplies, and equipment for surgical procedures; also assists surgeon and physician assistant by passing instruments, suctioning blood, and maintaining the sterile field.

Seborrheic dermatitis Common and chronic inflammatory disorder of the skin that involves the scalp, eyebrows, eyelids, ear canals, nasolabial folds, axillae, and trunk. The cause is unknown.

Sebum Sebaceous glands are found all over the body except on the palms and soles. These glands secrete an oily substance called sebum, which softens and lubricates the skin and hair and also decreases water loss from the skin in low humidity. Sebum also protects the body from infection by killing bacteria.

Secondary hypertension Elevated blood pressure resulting from an identifiable underlying process.

Seizure An episode of excessive and abnormal discharge of electrical activity within the central nervous system.

Semen Fluid containing sperm secreted by the male reproductive system glands.

Seminoma A tumor from seminal or germ tissue.

Septic arthritis The type of arthritis that develops when a joint space is invaded by a pathogen.

Septic shock One part of a progressive syndrome called systemic inflammatory response syndrome (SIRS). Beginning with an infection, SIRS progresses to bacteremia, then sepsis, then septic shock, and finally multiple organ failure syndrome.

Seroconversion Antibody response to a disease or vaccine.

Serum bicarbonate The serum bicarbonate (HCO_3^-) reflects the renal regulation of acid–base balance. It is often called the metabolic component of arterial blood gases. The normal HCO_3^- value is 22 to 26 mEq/L.

Severe acute respiratory syndrome (SARS) Lower respiratory illness of unknown etiology; spread by close person-to-person contact.

Sex chromosomes The chromosomes X or Y that indicate gender.

Sexually transmitted infection (STI, sexually transmitted disease, venereal disease) Any infection transmitted by sexual contact, including vaginal, oral, and anal intercourse.

Shigellosis (bacillary dysentery) An acute bowel infection caused by microorganisms of the *Shigella* genus.

Shingles See *Herpes zoster*.

Shock A clinical syndrome characterized by a systemic imbalance between oxygen supply and demand. This imbalance results in a state of inadequate blood flow to the peripheral tissues, causing life-threatening cellular dysfunction, hypotension, and oliguria.

Sickle cell anemia A hereditary, chronic hemolytic anemia characterized by episodes of sickling, during which RBCs become abnormally crescent shaped.

Sickle cell crisis Severe episodes of fever and intense pain that are the hallmark of sickle cell anemia.

Sinusitis Inflammation of the mucous membranes of one or more of the sinuses.

Sjögren's syndrome An autoimmune disorder that causes inflammation and dysfunction of exocrine glands throughout the body.

Skeletal traction Application of a pulling force through placement of pins into the bone.

Skin graft Surgical method of detaching skin from a donor site and placing it in a recipient site, where it develops a new blood supply from the base of the wound.

Skin tags Soft papules on a pedicle.

Skin traction Traction in which the cradle-like sleeve placed around the extremity exerts its pulling force through the patient's skin.

Sleep apnea Absence of airflow through the upper airways for 10 or more seconds.

Somatic cell Any cell in the body that is not a sex cell (ova and sperm).

Somatic pain Pain arising from nerve receptors originating in the skin or close to the surface of the body.

Somogyi phenomenon A morning rise in blood glucose to hyperglycemic levels following an episode of nocturnal hypoglycemia and a counterregulatory hormone response.

Spasticity Increased muscle tone in diseases involving the corticospinal motor tract.

Spermatocele A mobile, usually painless mass containing dead spermatozoa that forms in the epididymis.

Spinal cord injury (SCI) Injury to spinal cord, usually due to trauma.

Spinal cord tumors Benign or malignant, primary or metastatic tumor of the spinal cord.

Spinal shock Temporary loss of reflex function below the level of injury to the spinal cord.

Splenomegaly Enlargement of the spleen.

Sprain Tearing or stretching of a ligament that results from a twisting motion.

Sprue A chronic primary disorder of the small intestine in which the absorption of nutrients, particularly fats, is impaired.

Squamous cell carcinoma Malignant tumor of the squamous epithelium of the skin or mucous membranes.

Standard A statement or criterion that can be used by a profession and by the general public to measure quality of practice.

Starvation Inadequate dietary intake; the condition of being without food for long periods of time.

Status asthmaticus Severe, prolonged asthma that does not respond to routine treatment. Without aggressive therapy, status asthmaticus can lead to respiratory failure with hypoxemia, hypercapnia, and acidosis.

Status epilepticus Continuous seizure activity with only very short periods of calm occurring between intense and persistent seizures.

Steatorrhea Greasy, frothy, yellow stools resulting from excess fat in the feces.

Stem cell transplant (SCT) Infusion of donor stem cells to replace the recipient's blood cell lines (WBCs, RBCs, and platelets).

Stem cells (hemocytoblasts) Bone marrow precursor cells for all blood cells.

Stenosis Condition where valve leaflets fuse together and are unable to open or close fully.

Stoma Surface opening.

Stomatitis Inflammation of the oral mucosa.

Straight traction A pulling force applied in a straight line to the injured body part resting on the bed.

Strain Stretching or tearing of muscle fibers that results in bleeding into the tissues.

Stress incontinence Loss of usually less than 50 mL of urine occurring with increased abdominal pressure.

Stress-induced (erosive) gastritis Inflammation and superficial erosions of the gastric mucosa that may occur as a complication of other life-threatening conditions such as shock, severe trauma, major surgery, sepsis, burns, or head injury.

Striae A line above or below tissue that differs in color and texture from surrounding tissue.

Stridor High-pitched, harsh inspiratory sound indicative of upper airway obstruction.

Stroke (brain attack, cerebrovascular accident, CVA) A condition in which neurologic deficits occur as a result of decreased blood flow to a focal (localized) area of brain tissue from a blood clot, an embolus, or a cerebral vessel rupture.

Stroke volume (SV) The amount of blood pumped into the aorta with each contraction of the left ventricle.

Subdural hematoma A localized mass of blood that collects between the dura mater and the arachnoid mater.

Subluxation Partial separation (or dislocation) of the bones of a joint.

Substance abuse The use of any chemical in a fashion inconsistent with medical or culturally defined social norms despite physical, psychologic, or social adverse effects.

Substance dependence A severe condition occurring when the use of a chemical substance is no longer under an individual's control for at least 3 months. Continued use of the substance usually persists despite adverse effects on the person's physical condition, psychologic health, and interpersonal relationships (used interchangeably with addiction).

Sudden cardiac death (SCD) Unexpected death occurring within 1 hour of the onset of cardiovascular symptoms.

Sundowning A behavioral change in Alzheimer's disease characterized by increased agitation, time disorientation, and wandering during afternoon and evening hours.

Superficial burn Burn involving only the epidermal layer of the skin; most often results from damage from sunburn, ultraviolet light, minor flash injury (from a sudden ignition or explosion), or mild radiation burn associated with cancer treatment.

Surfactant A lipoprotein produced by the alveolar cells; interferes with adhesion of water molecules, reducing surface tension and helping to expand lungs.

Surge capacity The healthcare system's ability to rapidly expand beyond normal services to meet the increased demand for qualified personnel, medical care, and public health in the event of a large-scale disaster.

Surgery An invasive medical procedure performed to diagnose or treat illness, injury, or deformity. Although surgery is a medical treatment, the nurse assumes an active role in caring for the patient before, during, and after surgery.

Surgical debridement The process of excising a wound to the level of fascia (fascial excision) or sequentially removing thin slices of a burn wound to the level of viable tissue (sequential excision).

Surveillance Collecting and analyzing data to establish a baseline and determine a point at which there is a change or trend in the health of the population.